MW00359094

Autism Spectrum Disorders

Autism Spectrum Disorders

EDITED BY

David G. Amaral, PhD
Geraldine Dawson, PhD
Daniel H. Geschwind, MD, PhD

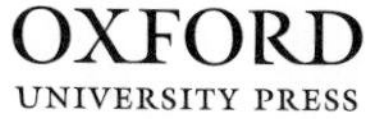

OXFORD
UNIVERSITY PRESS

Oxford University Press, Inc., publishes works that further
Oxford University's objective of excellence
in research, scholarship, and education.

Oxford New York
Auckland Cape Town Dar es Salaam Hong Kong Karachi
Kuala Lumpur Madrid Melbourne Mexico City Nairobi
New Delhi Shanghai Taipei Toronto

With offices in
Argentina Austria Brazil Chile Czech Republic France Greece
Guatemala Hungary Italy Japan Poland Portugal Singapore
South Korea Switzerland Thailand Turkey Ukraine Vietnam

Published by Oxford University Press, Inc.
198 Madison Avenue, New York, New York 10016
www.oup.com

Library of Congress Cataloging-in-Publication Data

Autism spectrum disorders / edited by David G. Amaral, Geraldine Dawson,
Daniel H. Geschwind.
p. ; cm.
Includes bibliographical references and index.
ISBN 978-0-19-537182-6 (hardcover : alk. paper)
1. Autism spectrum disorders. I. Amaral, David, 1950- II. Dawson, Geraldine.
III. Geschwind, Daniel H.
[DNLM: 1. Autistic Disorder. WS 350.6]
RC553.A88A8743 2011
616.85'882—dc22 2010030248

ISBN: 978-0-19-5371826

9 8 7 6 5 4 3 2 1

Printed in the United States of America
on acid-free paper

I dedicate this book,
To the founding families of the M.I.N.D. Institute,
who have inspired me with their courage and
their determination to help their own children and others like them.

To my parents, Ernie and Claire,
who have always supported my life as a scientist.

To my wonderful wife Tammy,
who has brought new meaning into my life.

and

To my children David Joseph, Jennie, Keith and Sarah
who remind me every day of what we are striving to accomplish.
D.G.A.

To my sister, Diana, for her constant love, support, and friendship, and to the many families of persons with autism spectrum disorders whose devotion and love for their children are the inspiration for my life's work.
G.D.

For their love, patience, support, and not least of all, their sense of humor, I am deeply grateful to my family, Sandy, Eli, Maya, and Jonah. I also thank my friends and colleagues, especially Portia Iversen and Jon Shestack, who first made me aware of the problems faced by individuals and families touched by autism and challenged me to do something about it.
D.H.G.

Preface

The disorder that we now know as autism was first formally described in 1943 by the Austrian born child psychiatrist, Leo Kanner, in his seminal paper "Autistic Disturbances of Affective Contact" (1943). For the next 20 years or more, "infantile autism" was considered to be a rare disorder affecting fewer than 5 in 10,000 individuals (Lotter, 1966). However, over the last 20 years, autism has come into the awareness of individuals from all walks of life and most of the world's countries. Kanner's autism has come to represent the classic form of a spectrum of disorders that are often conceived of as having core deficits in social functioning, communication, and repetitive behaviors; taken together these are now typically referred to as autism spectrum disorders (ASDs). Current estimates of the prevalence of autism spectrum disorders is on the order of 1 in 100 children (Rice, 2009), more frequent than many other childhood disorders that are often considered common, such as juvenile diabetes and childhood cancer.

One measure of the increased interest in autism research can be seen in the number of times Kanner's paper has been referenced in the peer reviewed scientific press. Overall, the paper has been cited nearly 2,300 times since its publication[1]. But, from 1945 until 1954, the paper was only cited 34 times. As illustrated in Figure 1, citations for the paper remained at a relatively low level until the 1990s, when there was a substantial increase in the rate at which this classic paper was referenced, paralleling an increase in biomedically based autism research.

There are many reasons for what could be considered a modern renaissance in autism research. Much of the credit for the increased research is due to the dedicated advocacy efforts of parents of children with autism throughout the world. One early example of this was Bernard Rimland, PhD, a psychologist and father of a son with autism. His influential book, *Infantile Autism: The Syndrome and Its Implications for a Neural Theory of Behavior* (which had a forward by Leo Kanner), published in 1964, dismissed the myth that early psychodynamic influences—the "refrigerator mother"—-caused autism. In short, Rimland reasoned that if many of the comorbid conditions of autism, such as epilepsy, were due to neural dysfunction, so should be the core features of autism. In retrospect, the chilling influence of psychoanalytic theory on biomedical research into autism's etiology could be considered remarkable, given that in his original paper, Kanner clearly saw autism as a biological, likely genetically mediated disorder in many cases.

Initially, advocacy groups such as the Autism Society of America were founded to advocate for research and more effective treatments of individuals with autism, but they did not focus their efforts on direct support of medical researchers. This organization shared a common mission with the National Autistic Society (a name adopted in 1975, when the original Autistic Children's Aid Society of North London, founded in 1962, was expanded to serve all of the United Kingdom). Autism first received widespread public attention through the Barry Levinson film *Rainman*. Dustin Hoffman, who portrayed a young man with autism and wanted his depiction of the disorder to be as accurate as possible, modeled his performance after an unusual autistic savant. The Oscar-winning best picture portrayed many of the social and communicative impairments of autism and particularly highlighted the circumscribed interests and the desire for routine and sameness in the environment.

Major impetus for the expansion of autism research was the founding in the mid-1990s of two parent advocacy organizations, the National Alliance for Autism Research (NAAR) and Cure Autism Now (CAN) that promoted not only the awareness of autism spectrum disorders, but also the need for research into the biological bases of autism. With the merger

1 These numbers are based on information from the Institute for Scientific Information (ISI) Web of Knowledge[sm]. Numbers reflect times the paper is cited in peer-reviewed journals and does not include references in books or the popular press.

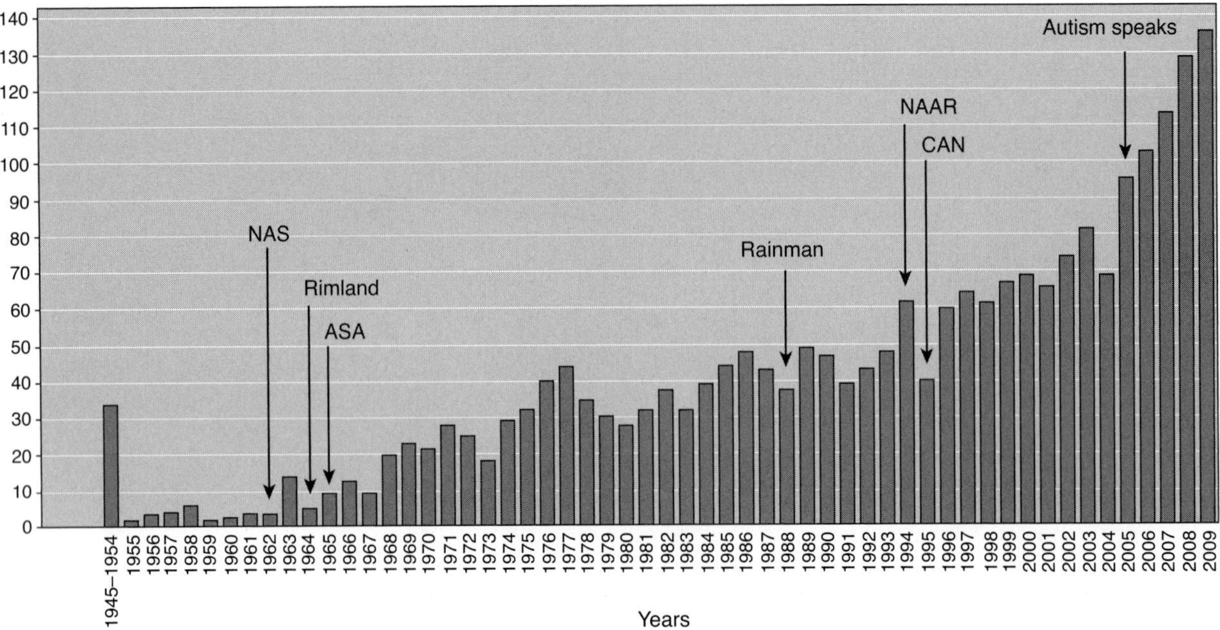

Figure 1 Citations of Kanner 1943. The graph displays the number of times the seminal paper by Kanner (1943) was referenced in the peer-reviewed scientific press from the time of publication to the end of 2009. Various events in the evolution of autism advocacy are indicated on the chart and are described in the text.

of these fund-raising and advocacy groups into Autism Speaks in 2005, a highly effective engine for worldwide autism research has been developed that has greatly expanded the scope and intensity of all levels of research concerning autism spectrum disorders. More recently, the Simons Foundation, which is focused primarily on genetic and neurobiological investigations, has also had a significant impact on funding of basic science research in autism. A 2009 study by Singh et al. found that the number of autism research grants funded in the U.S. from 1997 to 2006 increased 15% each year, with the majority of grants focused on genetics and neuroscience. This is a significant trend, but it must be acknowledged that it started from a very low baseline. At the beginning of this period, the total spending by the National Institutes of Health directed specifically at autism was estimated to be only about $6M dollars. Further, if one considers that estimates of disease costs indicate that the actual economic impact in the United States is $35 billion per year (Gantz, 2007), such an increase was clearly warranted. So, in many ways the rapid growth in funding for autism research is considered by many in the advocacy and research communities as necessary to make up for what could reasonably be framed as decades of neglect.

Fortunately, in addition to basic science funding, trends toward increased support in the areas of translational and clinical research have emerged in recent years, suggesting a transition from basic research to applied research that seeks to deliver real-world improvements for persons with autism. By 2008 the United States was spending over $222 million on autism research with 35% of the funding coming from private foundations. Given this brief history, it is not surprising that the field of autism research is moving rapidly forward and that knowledge about autism spectrum disorders is greatly increasing. In 2000, Medline listed 441 articles with the search terms "autism" or "autism spectrum disorders," whereas in 2009 the same terms identified 1,522 articles! Thus, from our perspective, the time was right to bring together summaries of as much of this new knowledge as possible into one volume—hence the genesis of this book. One now has the sense that this increase in research funding has finally created a critical mass of researchers from many different disciplines in the field, enabling true advances in understanding and treatment of autism. Here, the role of research advocacy groups in creating the proper permissive environment for the growth of the field via increasing governmental spending and by direct philanthropy cannot be overstated. Many of the advances described in this volume are a direct result of these efforts.

There are currently many excellent books that deal with various aspects of autism spectrum disorders. The guiding vision for this book was a core emphasis on ASD as a biological condition, so as to frame autism first and foremost from a biomedical perspective. We wished to provide a broad perspective on our current understanding of ASD, ranging from basic science to clinical symptomatology, to best clinical practices and social policy. We sought out leading authorities with diverse viewpoints and expertise, ranging from bench scientists to practitioners to parents and advocates. We encouraged authors to offer their own perspectives on the key themes guiding their field of study or interest, and provided commentary on the chapters from additional authors. Our goal was to paint the landscape of autism science and practice from a biomedical perspective, including what is currently known and where the field is heading.

Many books have provided detailed information and descriptions of the behavioral features and development of individuals with ASD. Although such information is also included in this book, we encouraged authors focusing primarily on behavior to consider biological constructs, such as how our current understanding of brain plasticity informs theories of behavioral development and intervention, and the role of pharmacological or other biological modulators of brain plasticity in facilitating conventional behavioral therapies in autism. Other authors considered how probes of brain function such as functional magnetic resonance imaging or magnetoencephalography may ultimately be sensitive readouts of the efficacy of behavior therapy.

Many of the most exciting recent advances have resulted from collaborative and interdisciplinary efforts at understanding autism. It is this realization that initially prompted the undertaking of this book project and provided a second guiding principle, namely that topics should be inclusive of all levels of research that will now or in the future affect research on ASD. Thus, every effort has been made to include topics that range from basic discovery of genetic and environmental risk factors to translational studies involving animal models to best practices in the fields of diagnosis, behavioral intervention, and medicine. Our hope is that those readers whose backgrounds are in the basic sciences will gain a better appreciation of challenges inherent in translating discoveries into clinical practice. Conversely, we hope that those readers whose primary interest is in clinical practice will learn how the basic sciences are pointing toward new directions for treatment and diagnosis that are derived from an increased understanding of the biology of ASD. Thus, this book is intended as much for the clinician, who is occupied primarily with diagnosis and treatment of individuals with autism, as for scientists who are studying selected biological features of autism spectrum disorders. Since the book is comprehensive in scope, we hope that it will be valuable to a wide audience, ranging from students who are entering the field of autism research, to advanced scientists who may be moving into the investigation of autism from some other area of research, to interested caregivers and educators. For most chapters, the authors have provided an introductory list of key points that summarize the most important ideas in their chapters, as well as future directions and challenges and suggested readings at the end, so as to provide a broad perspective on each topic.

A final guiding principle of the book is that the content will evolve over time. Currently, the book's 81 chapters are organized into several sections, with initial chapters discussing the history and phenomenology of autism spectrum disorders followed by deeper analyses of the core features of autism spectrum disorders. The book then moves to important comorbid psychiatric and medical conditions associated with autism and several chapters discussing different aspects of the broader autism phenotype. The next section delves into the neurobiological facets of autism spectrum disorders including what is known about brain chemistry, electrophysiology, imaging, and neuropathology, followed by a section on etiological factors. Here, recent findings in genetics and genomics based on many diverse approaches and models are presented; the emerging role of environmental factors is also covered. These etiological findings provide a solid foundation for translation into animal models, which we expect to play a rapidly expanding role in the biomedical research in ASD. Thus, this section is followed by a number of contributions on experimental animal models in species ranging from zebrafish to primates, as well as contributions on theoretical models of autism. These include primarily biologically based theories, those rooted in cognitive neuroscience, and those that bridge both areas. The penultimate section of the book is directed at treatment, which is the target that we all hope our research will influence. These chapters include several on a variety of behavioral and psychosocial interventions and summaries of current and future medical interventions including complementary and alternative medicine. We conclude with a number of chapters on "best practices" in diagnosis and treatment, as well as policy statements and perspectives related to the future of autism research and advocacy. Given the rapid pace of autism research, we fully expect that the content and complexion of the next edition of this book will be very different from the current one.

We thank the many contributors to this volume and the staff at Oxford University Press for their help in bringing it to fruition. We also want to express our gratitude to the parents and other family members, as well as many individuals with ASD themselves, who have fought hard for the resources that made much of the work discussed in this book possible. Their courage, tenacity, and dedication are an inspiration. We hope that this book adds impetus to continuing autism research efforts that ultimately improve the lives of persons with autism spectrum disorders and their families.

David G. Amaral,
The M.I.N.D. Institute, UC Davis

Geraldine Dawson,
Autism Speaks and University of
North Carolina at Chapel Hill

Daniel H. Geschwind,
The UCLA Center for Autism Research
and Treatment, UC Los Angeles

REFERENCES

Kanner, L. (1943). Autistic disturbances of affective contact. *Nervous Child, 2*, 217–250.

Ganz, M. L. (2007). The lifetime distribution of the incremental societal costs of autism, *Archives of Pediatrics and Adolescent Medicine, 161*, 343–349.

Lotter, V. (1966). Epidemiology of autistic conditions in young children I. Prevalence. *Social Psychiatry, 1*, 124–137.

Rice, C. (2009). Prevalence of autism spectrum disorders: Autism and Developmental Disabilities Monitoring Network, United States, 2006. *MMWR Surveillance Summaries, 58*, 1–20.

Singh, J., Illes, J., Lazzeroni, L., & Hallmayer, J. (2009). Trends in US autism research funding. *Journal of Autism and Developmental Disorders, 39*, 788–795.

Foreword

When our grandson Christian was diagnosed with autism in 2004 we were shocked. As a family involved with producing and developing some of our nation's most up-to-the-minute media, we were incredibly surprised and dismayed that we knew so little about the disorder. We were even more stunned to learn that the physicians and scientists to whom we reached out for help had very little information about autism. Like so many families around the United States we were left with more questions than answers. It was this quest for knowledge that became the catalyst in creating Autism Speaks.

Since the founding of Autism Speaks, we have moved closer to unlocking the mysteries of this often misunderstood disorder. The year 2010 marks the fifth anniversary of Autism Speaks, and we are proud that the past five years have seen accelerated scientific progress and a better understanding about autism. We have committed over $160 million dollars to autism scientific research, and we are aggressively examining a number of determinants, including genetic and environmental risk factors, biological systems and pathways, accompanying conditions, and most importantly, how to provide the best care possible for children and families.

Autism Spectrum Disorders provides a scholarly, yet accessible summary of the state of autism science, best practices, policy, legislation, and future directions. From language development, sleep disorders, and genetics to environmental toxicants, neuroscience, and early intensive interventions, this book delivers many of the answers that families like ours have been seeking. *Autism Spectrum Disorders* also exposes the knowledge gaps and unmet needs that our families continue to face every day.

What is clear now is that more has to be done for the autism community. Today, Autism Speaks is on the frontlines fighting for autism insurance reform. Until very recently, most families who received an autism diagnosis were denied insurance coverage for autism services—and for a disorder affecting one percent of children in the United States, this kind of treatment by insurance companies is not only negligent, it is outright discriminatory. Autism Speaks has been lobbying lawmakers around the clock, and at the time of this writing, 23 states have passed autism insurance laws, while an additional 25 have bills in progress. President Obama has made health care a priority. As part of this focus, he has allocated 85 million dollars in stimulus funds to autism research through the Recovery Act and is supporting language to end discrimination against autism in all insurance plans. Additionally, the Combating Autism Act, which was passed in 2006, authorizes nearly one billion dollars in expenditures over 5 years beginning in 2007, to combat autism spectrum disorders, Asperger's syndrome, Rett syndrome, childhood disintegrative disorder, and PDD-NOS through screening, education, early intervention, prompt referrals for treatment and services, and research.

On September 22, 2009, Autism Speaks hosted its second annual World Focus on Autism in New York City. There we announced our "Decade for Autism" challenge, a global call to action for international leaders and stakeholders to raise a combined $100 million dollars in their countries over the next 10 years for autism research, awareness, and service development. Our greatest wish is that 5 years from now—only halfway through the "Decade for Autism"—many of the questions raised here in this book will have been answered, and many of the pressing needs of the autism community will have been addressed. This book, hopefully, will inspire the scientific and professional community to continue with a sense of urgency in their efforts to find answers and use those answers to discover ways to effectively treat and prevent autism.

Suzanne and Bob Wright
Co-founders, Autism Speaks

Contents

Contributors

Ralph Adolphs, PhD
Division of Biology
California Institute of Technology
Pasadena, CA, USA

David G. Amaral, PhD
The M.I.N.D. Institute
University of California–Davis
Sacramento, CA, USA

Djesika Amendah, PhD
National Center on Birth Defects and Developmental Disabilities
Centers for Disease Control and Prevention
Atlanta, GA, USA

Evdokia Anagnostou, MD
Department of Pediatrics
Bloorview Research Institute
University of Toronto
Toronto, Ontario, Canada

Mary Catherine Aranda, MD
Maj, USAF, MC
Barksdale Air Force Base, LA, USA

Emma Ashwin, PhD
Autism Research Centre
Department of Psychiatry
University of Cambridge
Cambridge, UK

Paul Ashwood, PhD
The M.I.N.D. Institute
University of California–Davis
Sacramento, CA, USA

Bonnie Auyeung, PhD
Autism Research Centre
Department of Psychiatry
University of Cambridge
Cambridge, UK

Grace T. Baranek, PhD, OTR/L, FAOTA
Division of Occupational Science
Department of Allied Health Science
University of North Carolina at Chapel Hill
Chapel Hill, NC, USA

Simon Baron-Cohen
Autism Research Centre
Department of Psychiatry
University of Cambridge
Cambridge, UK

Margaret L. Bauman, MD
Harvard Medical School
Department of Pediatrics and Neurology
Massachusetts General Hospital
Lurie Center/LADDERS
Boston, MA, USA

Melissa D. Bauman, PhD
The M.I.N.D. Institute
University of California–Davis
Sacramento, CA, USA

Allison Bean
Department of Communication Sciences and Disorders
University of Iowa
Iowa City, IA, USA

Mark F. Bear, PhD
The Picower Institute for Learning and Memory
Howard Hughes Medical Institute
Department of Brain and Cognitive Sciences
Massachusetts Institute of Technology
Cambridge, MA, USA

Arthur L. Beaudet
Department of Molecular and Human Genetics
Baylor College of Medicine
Houston, TX, USA

Marlene Behrmann, PhD
Department of Psychology
Carnegie Mellon University
Pittsburgh, PA, USA

Peter H. Bell
Executive Vice President
Autism Speaks
Princeton, NJ, USA

Matthew K. Belmonte
Department of Human Development
Cornell University
Ithaca, NY, USA

Raphael Bernier
Department of Psychiatry and Behavioral Sciences
Autism Center
Center on Human Development and Disability
University of Washington
Seattle, WA, USA

Somer L. Bishop, PhD
Division of Developmental and Behavioral Pediatrics
Cincinnati Children's Hospital Medical Center
Cincinnati, OH, USA

Alicia Blaker-Lee, PhD
Whitehead Institute for Biomedical Research
Cambridge, MA, USA

Kelly Blankenship, DO
Department of Psychiatry
Indiana University School of Medicine
Christian Sarkine Autism Treatment Center
James Whitcomb Riley Hospital for Children
Indianapolis, IN, USA

James W. Bodfish, PhD
Departments of Psychiatry, Pediatrics, and Education
Carolina Institute for Developmental Disabilities
University of North Carolina at Chapel Hill
Chapel Hill, NC, USA

Patrick F. Bolton, PhD, FRCPsych
Social Genetic and Development Psychiatry Centre
Department of Child Psychiatry
The Institute of Psychiatry
Kings College
London, UK

Coleen Boyle, PhD
National Center on Birth Defects and Developmental Disabilities
Centers for Disease Control and Prevention
Atlanta, GA, USA

Catherine Bregere, PhD
Biology Division
California Institute of Technology
Pasadena, CA, USA

Timothy Buie, MD
Pediatric GI and Nutrition Associates
Massachusetts General Hospital for Children
Instructor in Pediatrics
Harvard Medical School
Boston, MA, USA

Jan K. Buitelaar, MD, PhD
Department of Cognitive Neuroscience
Donders Institute for Brain, Cognition and Behavior
Karakter Child and Adolescent Psychiatry University Centre
Radboud University Nijmegen Medical Centre
Nijmegen, The Netherlands

Karen Burner
Autism Center
Center on Human Development and Disability
Department of Psychology
University of Washington
Seattle, WA, USA

Rita M. Cantor, PhD
Department of Human Genetics
Center for Neurobehavioral Genetics
Department of Psychiatry and Biobehavioral Sciences
Semel Institute for Neuroscience and Human Behavior
David Geffen School of Medicine
University of California–Los Angeles
Los Angeles, CA, USA

Edward G. Carr†, PhD
Department of Psychology
Stony Brook University
Stony Brook, NY, USA

Kathryn K. Chadman
Department of Developmental Neurobiology
New York State Institute for Basic Research in Developmental Disabilities
Staten Island, NY, USA

Bhismadev Chakrabarti
University of Reading

Gina T. Chang, PhD
The Claremont Autism Center
Claremont Graduate University
Claremont, CA, USA

Marjorie H. Charlop, PhD
Department of Psychology
Claremont McKenna College
Claremont, CA, USA

Tony Charman
Behavioural & Brain Sciences Unit
University College London Institute of Child Health
London, UK

Diane C. Chugani, PhD
Wayne State University School of Medicine
Division of Clinical Pharmacology and Toxicology
Children's Hospital of Michigan
Detroit, MI, USA

John N. Constantino, MD
Departments of Psychiatry and Pediatrics
Washington University School of Medicine
St. Louis, MO, USA

Mark A. Corrales, MPP
U.S. Environmental Protection Agency
Washington, DC, USA

Neva M. Corrigan, PhD
Department of Radiology
University of Washington
Seattle, WA, USA

Eric Courchesne, PhD
Autism Center of Excellence
Department of Neurosciences
University of California–San Diego
San Diego, CA, USA

Daniel L. Coury, MD
Department of Pediatrics
The Ohio State University
Columbus, OH, USA

Jacqueline N. Crawley
Laboratory of Behavioral Neuroscience
Intramural Research Program
National Institute of Mental Health
National Institutes of Health
Bethesda, MD, USA

Stephen R. Dager, MD
Departments of Radiology and Bioengineering
University of Washington
Seattle, WA, USA

Susan A. Daniels, PhD
Office of Autism Research Coordination
National Institute of Mental Health
National Institutes of Health
Bethesda, MD, USA

Geraldine Dawson, PhD
Autism Speaks
University of North Carolina-Chapel Hill
Chapel Hill, NC, USA

Gianluca De Rienzo, PhD
Whitehead Institute for Biomedical Research
Cambridge, MA, USA

Elisabeth M. Dykens, PhD
Departments of Psychology and Human Development, Pediatrics, and Psychiatry
Vanderbilt Kennedy Center for Research on Human Development
Vanderbilt University
Nashville, TN, USA

Lisa R. Edelson, PhD
Department of Psychology
Boston University
Boston, MA, USA

Lauren M. Elder, PhD
Department of Psychology
University of Washington
Seattle, WA, USA

Craig A. Erickson, MD
Department of Psychiatry
Indiana University School of Medicine
Christian Sarkine Autism Treatment Center
James Whitcomb Riley Hospital for Children
Indianapolis, IN, USA

Anna J. Esbensen, PhD
Division of Developmental and Behavioral Pediatics
Cincinnati Children's Hospital Medical Center
Cincinnati, OH, USA

Annette Estes, PhD
Departments of Speech and Hearing Sciences and Psychology
University of Washington
Seattle, WA, USA

Eric Fombonne, MD
Department of Psychiatry
Montreal Children's Hospital
McGill University
Montreal, Quebec, Canada

Rosy M. Fredeen, PhD
University of California–Santa Barbara
Santa Barbara, CA, USA

Robin L. Gabriels, PsyD
Departments of Psychiatry and Pediatrics
University of Colorado at Denver and Health Sciences Center/The Children's Hospital Neuropsychiatric Special Care Program
Denver, CO, USA

Daniel Geschwind, MD, PhD
David Geffen School of Medicine
University of California–Los Angeles
Los Angeles, CA, USA

Christopher Gillberg, MD, PhD
Child and Adolescent Psychiatry
University of Gothenburg
Child Neuropsychiatry Clinic
Queen Silvia Children's Hospital
Sahlgrenska University Hospital
Gothenburg, Sweden

Daniel G. Glaze, MD
Department of Pediatrics and Neurology
Baylor College of Medicine
Houston, TX, USA

Paula Goines, BS
Department of Internal Medicine
University of California–Davis School of Medicine
Davis, CA, USA

Katherine Gotham, PhD
University of Michigan Autism and Communication Disorders Center
University of Michigan
Ann Arbor, MI, USA

Temple Grandin, PhD
Department of Animal Sciences
Colorado State University
Fort Collins, CO, USA

Alissa L. Greenberg, PhD
The Claremont Autism Center
Claremont Graduate University
Claremont, CA, USA

Jan S. Greenberg, PhD
University of Wisconsin–Madison
Madison, WI, USA

Stanley I. Greenspan†, MD
George Washington University Medical School
Washington, DC, USA

Roy Richard Grinker, PhD
Department of Anthropology
The George Washington University
Washington, DC, USA

Wouter B. Groen, MD, PhD
Department of Psychiatry
Donders Institute for Brain, Cognition and Behavior
Karakter Child and Adolescent Psychiatry University Centre
Radboud University Nijmegen Medical Centre
Nijmegen, The Netherlands

Scott D. Grosse, PhD
National Center on Birth Defects and Developmental Disabilities
Centers for Disease Control and Prevention
Atlanta, GA, USA

Arlene Hagen, PhD, MD
Montreal Children's Hospital
McGill University
Montreal, Quebec, Canada

Paul J. Hagerman, MD, PhD
Department of Biochemistry and Molecular Medicine
School of Medicine
University of California–Davis School of Medicine
Davis, CA, USA

Randi J. Hagerman, MD
Medical Director, M.I.N.D. Institute and Endowed Chair in Fragile X Research
Department of Pedaitrics
University of California–Davis School of Medicine
Davis, CA, USA

Francesca Happé
MRC SGDP Centre
Institute of Psychiatry
King's College London
London, UK

Martha R. Herbert, MD, PhD
Neurology and TRANSCEND Research Program
Massachusetts General Hospital
Harvard Medical School
Charlestown, MA, USA

Irva Hertz-Picciotto, PhD, MPH
Department of Public Health Sciences
School of Medicine
University of California–Davis
Davis, CA, USA

Kelly Heung, PhD
The M.I.N.D. Institute
University of California–Davis
Sacramento, CA, USA

Eric Hollander, MD
Department of Psychiatry and Behavioral Sciences
Albert Einstein College of Medicine and Montefiore Medical Center
Bronx, NY, USA

Jinkuk Hong, PhD
Waisman Center
University of Wisconsin–Madison
Madison, WI, USA

Elaine Hsiao
Biology Division
California Institute of Technology
Pasadena, CA, USA

Kara Hume, PhD
Frank Porter Graham Child Development Institute
University of North Carolina at Chapel Hill
Chapel Hill, NC, USA

Katherine Humphreys, PhD
Department of Clinical and Experimental Epilepsy
Institute of Neurology
University College
London, UK

Vanessa Hus, MSc
University of Michigan Autism and Communication Disorders Center
Department of Psychology
University of Michigan
Ann Arbor, MI, USA

Susan L. Hyman, MD
Golisano Children's Hospital at Strong
University of Rochester School of Medicine
Rochester, NY, USA

Marco Iacoboni, MD, PhD
Department of Psychiatry and Biobehavioral Sciences
Semel Institute for Neuroscience and Social Behavior
Brain Research Institute
David Geffen School of Medicine
University of California–Los Angeles
Los Angeles, CA, USA

Brooke Ingersoll, PhD
Department of Psychology
Michigan State University
East Lansing, MI, USA

Thomas R. Insel, MD
Office of the Director
National Institute of Mental Health
Bethesda, MD, USA

Suma Jacob, MD, PhD
Institute of Juvenile Research
Department of Psychiatry
University of Illinois–Chicago
Chicago, IL, USA

Marcel Adam Just
Department of Psychology
Carnegie Mellon University
Pittsburgh, PA, USA

Rajesh K. Kana, PhD
Department of Psychology
University of Alabama–Birmingham
Birmingham, AL, USA

Connie Kasari, PhD
Psychological Studies in Education
Center for Autism Research and Treatment
Department of Psychiatry
University of California–Los Angeles
Los Angeles, CA, USA

Hande Kaymakçalan, MD
Department of Genetics
Yale University School of Medicine
New Haven, CT, USA

Soeun Kim
Department of Molecular and Human Genetics
Baylor College of Medicine
Houston, TX, USA

Bryan H. King
Center for Child Health, Behavior and Development
Seattle Children's
Seattle, WA, USA

Ami Klin, PhD
Marcus Austim Center
Emory University School of Medicine
Center for Translational Social Neuroscience
Atlanta, GA, USA

Rebecca Knickmeyer, PhD
Department of Psychiatry
University of North Carolina School of Medicine
Chapel Hill, NC, USA

Lynn Kern Koegel, PhD
Koegel Autism Center
University of California–Santa Barbara
Santa Barbara, CA, USA

Robert L. Koegel, PhD
Department of Counseling, Clinical & School Psychology
Koegel Autism Center
University of California–Santa Barbara
Santa Barbara, CA, USA

Dilja D. Krueger, PhD
The Picower Institute for Learning and Memory
Massachusetts Institute of Technology
Cambridge, MA, USA

Janet E. Lainhart, MD
Departments of Psychiatry, Pediatrics and Psychology
Interdepartmental Neuroscience Program
The Brain Institute
University of Utah
Salt Lake City, UT, USA

Janine A. Lamb, PhD
Centre for Integrated Genomic Medical Research
University of Manchester
Manchester, UK

Rebecca J. Landa, PhD, CCC-SLP
The Kennedy Krieger Institute
The Johns Hopkins University School of Medicine
Baltimore, MD, USA

Angeli Landeros-Weisenberger, MD
Child Study Center
Yale University School of Medicine
New Haven, CT, USA

Nicholas Lange, ScD
Departments of Psychiatry and Biostatistics
Harvard University Schools of Medicine and Public Health
McLean Hospital
Belmont, MA, USA

James F. Leckman, MD
Child Study Center
Departments of Psychiatry, Psychology, and Pediatrics
Yale University School of Medicine
New Haven, CT, USA

Ann S. Le Couteur, BSc, MBBS
Institute of Health and Society
Newcastle University
Newcastle Upon Tyne, UK

Miriam Lense, MS
Departments of Psychology and Human Development
Vanderbilt Kennedy Center for Research on Human Development
Vanderbilt University
Nashville, TN, USA

Pat Levitt, PhD
Zilkha Neurogenetic Institute
Department of Cell and Neurobiology
Keck School of Medicine
University of Southern California
Los Angeles, CA, USA

Susan E. Levy, MD
Henry Cecil Professor of Pediatrics
The Children's Hospital of Philadelphia
University of Pennsylvania School of Medicine
Philadelphia, PA, USA

C. Enjey Lin, PhD
Department of Counseling, Clinical, and School Psychology
Koegel Autism Center
University of California–Santa Barbara
Santa Barbara, CA, USA

Jill Locke, PhD
University of Pennsylvania School of Medicine
The Children's Hospital of Philadelphia
Center for Autism Research
Philadelphia, PA, USA

Michael Lombardo
Autism Research Center
University of Cambridge
Cambridge, UK

Catherine Lord, PhD, ABPP
Urie Bronfenbrenner Collegiate Professor of Psychology, Pediatrics and Psychiatry
University of Michigan Autism and Communication Disorders Center
Ann Arbor, MI, USA

Molly Losh, PhD
Roxelyn and Richard Pepper Department of Communication Sciences and Disorders
Northwestern University
Evanston, IL, USA

Katherine A. Loveland, PhD
Departments of Psychiatry and Behavioral Sciences and Pediatrics
University of Texas Medical School
University of Texas Health Science Center at Houston
Houston, TX, USA

Rhiannon Luyster, PhD
Laboratories of Cognitive Neuroscience
Division of Developmental Medicine
Children's Hospital Boston
Harvard Medical School
Boston, MA, USA

Natalia Malkova, PhD
Biology Division
California Institute of Technology
Pasadena, CA, USA

David S. Mandell, ScD
Center for Mental Health Policy and Services Research
The Children's Hospital of Philadelphia
Center for Autism Research
University of Pennsylvania School of Medicine
Philadelphia, PA, USA

Beth McConnell, PhD
Offord Centre for Child Studies
Department of Psychiatry and Behavioural Neurosciences
McMaster University and McMaster Children's Hospital
Hamilton, ON, Canada

James T. McCracken, MD
Division of Child and Adolescent Psychiatry
Center for Autism Research and Treatment
UCLA Semel Institute
David Geffen School of Medicine
University of California–Los Angeles
Los Angeles, CA, USA

Christopher J. McDougle, MD
Department of Psychiatry
Indiana University School of Medicine
Christian Sarkine Autism Treatment Center
James Whitcomb Riley Hospital for Children
Indianapolis, IN, USA

Karla K. McGregor, PhD
Communication Sciences and Disorders
University of Iowa
Iowa City, IA, USA

Annie McLaughlin, PhD, BCBA-D
College of Education
University of Washington
Seattle, WA, USA

Judith H. Miles, MD, PhD
Department of Child Health, Division of Medical Genetics
Thompson Center for Autism & Neurodevelopmental Disorders
University of Missouri
Columbia, MO, USA

Nancy J. Minshew, MD
Departments of Psychiatry and Neurology
University of Pittsburgh School of Medicine
Pittsburgh, PA, USA

Meera E. Modi
Center for Translational Social Neuroscience
Department of Psychiatry and Behavioral Sciences
Yerkes National Primate Research Center
Atlanta, GA, USA

Eric M. Morrow, MD, PhD
Department of Molecular Biology, Cell Biology, and Biochemistry
Institute for Brain Science
Brown University
Department of Psychiatry
Brown University Medical School
Providence, RI, USA

Matthew W. Mosconi, PhD
Departments of Psychiatry and Pediatrics
University of Texas
Southwestern Medical Center
Dallas, TX, USA

Peter Mundy, PhD
Schools of Education and Medicine
Lisa Capps Chair in Neurodevelopmental Disorders and Education
School of Education and the M.I.N.D. Institute
University of California–Davis
Davis, CA, USA

Michael Murias, PhD
Department of Psychiatry and Behavioral Sciences
Autism Center
University of Washington
Seattle, WA, USA

Vivien Narcisa, BS
The M.I.N.D. Institute
University of California–Davis
Sacramento, CA, USA

Jeffrey L. Neul, MD, PhD
Blue Bird Circle Rett Center
Anthony and Cynthia Petrello Scholar
Jan and Dan Duncan Neurological Research Institute
Texas Children's Hospital
Department of Pediatrics
Baylor College of Medicine
Houston, TX, USA

Steven C. Noctor, PhD
Department of Psychiatry and Behavioral Sciences
The M.I.N.D. Institute
University of California–Davis
Sacramento, CA, USA

Samuel L. Odom, PhD
Director, FPG Child Development Institute
University of North Carolina at Chapel Hill
Chapel Hill, NC, USA

Gael I. Orsmond, PhD
Department of Occupational Therapy
Boston University
Boston, MA, USA

Sally Ozonoff, PhD
The M.I.N.D. Institute
University of California–Davis
Sacramento, CA, USA

Jeremy R. Parr, MBChB, MD, MRCPCH
Institute of Neuroscience
Newcastle University
Newcastle Upon Tyne, UK

Paul H. Patterson, PhD
Biology Division
California Institute of Technology
Pasadena, CA, USA

Georgina Peacock, MD, MPH
National Center on Birth Defects and Developmental Disabilities
Centers for Disease Control and Prevention
Atlanta, GA, USA

Leena Peltonen†, MD, PhD
Institute for Molecular Medicine Finland
University of Helsinki
Helsinki, Finland
Wellcome Trust Sanger Institute
Hinxton, Cambridge, UK
The Broad Institute
Cambridge, MA, USA

Richard Person, PhD
Department of Molecular and Human Genetics
Baylor College of Medicine
Houston, TX, USA

Joseph Piven, MD
Carolina Institute for Developmental Disabilities
University of North Carolina
Chapel Hill, NC, USA

Anne E. Porter
University of Texas Health Science Center at San Antonio
San Antonio, TX, USA

David J. Posey, MD
Department of Psychiatry
Indiana University School of Medicine
Christian Sarkine Autism Treatment Center
James Whitcomb Riley Hospital for Children
Indianapolis, IN, USA

Sara Quirke, BSc Psychology
Department of Psychiatry
Montreal Children's Hospital
McGill University
Montreal, Quebec, Canada

Isabelle Rapin, MD
Saul R. Korey Department of Neurology
Department of Pediatrics, and Rose F. Kennedy Center for Research on Intellectual and Developmental Disabilities
Albert Einstein College of Medicine
Bronx, NY, USA

Karola Rehnström, PhD
Institute for Molecular Medicine Finland
University of Helsinki
Helsinki, Finland
Wellcome Trust Sanger Institute
Hinxton, Cambridge, UK

Angela M. Reiersen, MD, MPE
Department of Psychiatry
Washington University School of Medicine
St. Louis, MO, USA

Todd Richards, PhD
Department of Radiology
University of Washington
Seattle, WA, USA

Patricia M. Rodier, PhD
University of Rochester
School of Medicine & Dentistry
Rochester, NY, USA

Sally J. Rogers, PhD
The M.I.N.D. Institute
University of California–Davis
Sacramento, CA, USA

John L. R. Rubenstein, MD, PhD
Department of Psychiatry
University of California–San Francisco
San Francisco, CA, USA

Michael Rutter, MD, FRS, FRCPsych, FBA, FMedSci
MRC Social, Genetic & Developmental Psychiatry Centre
Institute of Psychiatry
King's College London
London, UK

Maria L. Scattoni
Laboratory of Behavioral Neuroscience
Intramural Research Program
National Institute of Mental Health
National Institutes of Health
Bethesda, MD, USA

Suzanne Scherf, PhD
Department of Psychology
Carnegie Mellon University
Pittsburgh, PA, USA

Laura Schreibman, PhD
Autism Intervention Research Program
University of California–San Diego
San Diego, CA, USA

Cynthia M. Schumann, PhD
Department of Psychiatry and Behavioral Sciences
The M.I.N.D. Institute
University of California–Davis
Sacramento, CA, USA

Marsha Mailick Seltzer, PhD
Vaughan Bascom and Elizabeth M. Boggs Professor
Director, Waisman Center
University of Wisconsin-Madison
Madison, WI, USA

Dennis Shaw, MD
Department of Radiology
University of Washington
Seattle, WA, USA

Marwan Shinawi
Department of Molecular and Human Genetics
Baylor College of Medicine
Houston, TX, USA

Jill L. Silverman
Laboratory of Behavioral Neuroscience
Intramural Research Program
National Institute of Mental Health
Bethesda, MD, USA

Hazel Sive, PhD
Whitehead Institute for Biomedical Research
Massachusetts Institute of Technology
Cambridge, MA, USA

Leann Smith, PhD
Waisman Center
University of Wisconsin-Madison
Madison, WI, USA

Tristram Smith, PhD
School of Medicine and Dentistry
University of Rochester
Rochester, NY, USA

Craig Snyder
Ikon Public Affairs
Government Relations Chair
Autism Speaks
New York, NY, USA

Sarah J. Spence, MD, PhD
Department of Neurology
Children's Hospital Boston
Harvard Medical School
Boston, MA, USA

Matthew W. State, MD, PhD
Departments of Child Psychiatry, Psychiatry, and Genetics
Yale University School of Medicine
New Haven, CT, USA

Lindsey Sterling, PhD
Department of Psychiatry and Biobehavioral Sciences
UCLA Semel Institute
University of California–LA
Los Angeles, CA, USA

Kimberly A. Stigler, MD
Department of Psychiatry
Indiana University School of Medicine
Christian Sarkine Autism Treatment Center
James Whitcomb Riley Hospital for Children
Indianapolis, IN, USA

Wendy L. Stone, PhD
Director, UW Autism Center
Department of Psychology
University of Washington
Seattle, WA, USA

John A. Sweeney
Center for Cognitive Medicine
University of Illinois–Chicago
Chicago, IL, USA

Peter Szatmari, MD, MSc
Offord Centre for Child Studies
Department of Psychiatry and Behavioural Neurosciences
McMaster University and McMaster Children's Hospital
Hamilton, Ontario, Canada

Holly K. Tabor, PhD
Department of Pediatrics
University of Washington
Treuman Katz Center for Pediatric Bioethics
Seattle Children's Hospital
Seattle, WA, USA

Helen Tager-Flusberg, PhD
Department of Psychology
Boston University
Boston, MA, USA

Yukari Takarae, PhD
Center for Mind and Brain
University of California–Davis
Davis, CA, USA

Julie Lounds Taylor, PhD
Vanderbilt Kennedy Center
Department of Pediatrics and Special Education
Vanderbilt University
Nashville, TN, USA

Bonnie P. Taylor, PhD
Department of Psychiatry and Behavioral Sciences
Albert Einstein College of Medicine
Montefiore Medical Center
Bronx, NY, USA

Meagan Thompson, MA
Department of Psychology
Boston University
Boston, MA, USA

Richard D. Todd†, PhD, MD
Departments of Psychiatry and Genetics
Washington University School of Medicine
St. Louis, MO, USA

J. Bruce Tomblin, PhD
Department of Communication Sciences and Disorders
University of Iowa
Iowa City, IA, USA

Roberto Tuchman, MD
Miami Children's Hospital
Director, Autism and Neurodevelopment Program
Florida International University
College of Medicine
Miami, FL, USA

Judy Van de Water, PhD
Department of Internal Medicine
School of Medicine
University of California–Davis
Davis, CA, USA

Linn Wakeford, MS, OTR/L
Department of Allied Health Science
University of North Carolina at Chapel Hill
Chapel Hill, NC, USA

Katherine S. Wallace, MSW
The M.I.N.D. Institute
University of California–Davis
Sacramento, CA, USA

Christopher A. Walsh, MD, PhD
Manton Center for Orphan Disease Research
Children's Hospital Boston
Howard Hughes Medical Institute
Boston, MA, USA

Zachary Warren, PhD
Vanderbilt Kennedy Center for Research on Human Development
Departments of Pediatrics and Psychiatry
Vanderbilt University
Nashville, TN, USA

Sara Jane Webb, PhD
Department of Psychiatry and Behavioral Sciences
University of Washington
Seattle, WA, USA

Serena Wieder, PhD
Interdisciplinary Council for Developmental and Learning Disorders
Bethesda, MD, USA

Kerstin Wittemeyer, BSc, MSc, PhD
Autism Centre for Education and Research
School of Education
University of Birmingham
Birmingham, UK

Mu Yang
Laboratory of Behavioral Neuroscience
Intramural Research Program
National Institute of Mental Health
Bethesda, MD, USA

Marshalyn Yeargin-Allsopp, MD
National Center on Birth Defects and Developmental Disabilities
Centers for Disease Control and Prevention
Atlanta, GA, USA

Keith J. Yoder
Department of Psychology
University of Chicago
Chicago, IL, USA

Larry J. Young, PhD
Center for Translational Social Neuroscience
Department of Psychiatry and Behavioral Sciences
Yerkes National Primate Research Center
Atlanta, GA, USA

Xinna Zhang
Department of Molecular and Human Genetics
Baylor College of Medicine
Houston, TX, USA

Andrew Zimmerman, MD
Center for Autism and Related Disorders
Kennedy Krieger Institute
Baltimore, MD, USA

Lonnie Zwaigenbaum, MD
Autism Research Centre
Glenrose Rehabilitation Hospital
University of Alberta
Edmonton, AB, Canada

Autism Spectrum Disorders

Introduction

Isabelle Rapin

Autism Turns 65: A Neurologist's Bird's Eye View

Asking a neurologist to write the introduction to a book on the autism spectrum disorders (autism for short in this chapter) seems unexceptional in 2008 because it is now taken for granted that autism is the behavioral consequence of any one of a multitude of developmental disorders of the immature brain. Not so when I was in training in the 1950s. What has brought about such a profound change in perspective? This introduction highlights a few of the changes I have witnessed over a half-century, including ideas about causation, prevalence, language subtypes, epilepsy and language regression, sensorimotor symptoms, neuropathology/imaging, genetics, and intervention. Whereas this book provides in depth discussion of each of these issues and others, this limited bird's eye view makes no apology for the myopia of a single person's perspective.

Biology vs. Refrigerator Parents

As far as disorders of complex human behaviors are concerned, the first half of the twentieth century saw the ascendancy of the Freudian hypothesis that attributed to early psychic traumas even such a life-long disorder as schizophrenia, despite its fluctuating, deteriorating course. Kanner was an Austrian-born, Berlin-educated child psychiatrist who spent much of his professional life at the Harriet Lane Children's Hospital of Johns Hopkins Medical School in Baltimore. His astute and comprehensive 1943 description of autism in 11 children (Kanner, 1943) remains valid to this day. He characterized their disorder as "an inborn autistic disturbance of affective contact," yet emphasized their parents' lack of warmth. By 1954 he had compiled his observations on 100 children (Kanner, 1954) and expressed the view that highly educated mothers' (and fathers') parenting inadequacies were largely responsible for their children's autism. He must have swung back to the hypothesis of innateness because, according to his biographer Sanua (Sanua, 1990), at the 1969 national convention of parents of children with autism, Kanner said: "Herewith, I officially acquit you people as parents." His writings continued to reflect ambivalence, however, as in the 1979 edition of his textbook, *Child Psychiatry*, he still states, according to Sanua, that childhood schizophrenia—a term routinely used for autism until the 1970s, although allegedly not by Kanner—was more strongly correlated with parental attitudes than with genetic or metabolic factors. Predictably, the widely publicized views of this father of American child psychiatry and professor at a prestigious medical school were promptly disseminated and almost universally adopted in this country and abroad.

Because of the tenor of the times and lack of ostensible evidence for a neurologic basis for autism and other developmental disorders, 30 years were to go by before enough evidence had accumulated to refute the inadequate parenting theory of autism. The 1952 discovery of chlorpromazine's dramatic effectiveness in schizophrenia opened the door to an avalanche of new evidence regarding the role of neurotransmitters, neuromodulators, and neuropeptides in synaptic transmission. Their discrete distributions in the brain, together with progress in neuroendocrinology, ushered in the era of biologic psychiatry. The contemporaneous birth in the 1970s of neuroscience and expansion of the field of neuropsychology, coupled with the explosion of new technologies for studying the living brain, finally led to neurobiology's eclipsing Freudian psychiatry and theories of refrigerator mothers.

Two factors pushed the neurobiologic view of autism to the forefront and, perhaps prematurely, denied any causal relevance of deleterious early life experiences. The first factor was the 1964 congenital rubella epidemic which left in its wake a number of children with autism. Stella Chess, a child psychiatrist who worked at Bellevue Hospital in New York City, evaluated many of these children (Chess et al., 1971). They reinforced her long-standing opinion of autism as a disorder of the brain. The second factor was the realization that some third of the children with autism developed epilepsy (Deykin & MacMahon, 1979), to which I will come back later. Richard Schain, a child neurologist at the University of California in Los Angeles, had made the earlier seminal observation that about one-third of children with autism have elevated levels of serotonin in their platelets, but this report was overlooked until research on neurotransmitters progressed sufficiently (Schain & Freedman, 1961).

The late Bernard Rimland, a psychologist whose son has autism and is artistically gifted, wrote the first book defending the biologic basis of autism: *Infantile Autism: The Syndrome and Its Implications for a Neural Theory of Behavior* (Rimland, 1964). He was also the first and most influential parent advocate and achieved tremendous influence, which persists to this day. He collected thousands of questionnaires filled out by parents of children with autism from around the globe, a treasure trove of data waiting to be mined comprehensively. Rimland disseminated promptly and widely any new information with potential therapeutic implications, without waiting for empirical support. I assume he did so because of his burning desire to make sure parents had access to the newest potentially useful information, but this has resulted in the uncritical worldwide adoption of some unproven diets, other interventions, and theories about the causation of autism.

Mary Coleman, a child neurologist, atypically chose to limit her Washington DC practice to autism. Equally convinced that autism had a neurobiologic basis, she evaluated each child extensively for this possibility. Together with Christopher Gillberg, a child psychiatrist from Göteborg, Sweden, trained in pediatrics and epidemiology, she published *The Biology of the Autistic Syndromes* in 1985 (Coleman & Gillberg, 1985). Its 2000 third edition (Gillberg & Coleman, 2000) details not only clinical and epidemiologic evidence and management issues but also lists many of the rare genetic conditions occasionally associated with autism. The first 1987 edition of the encyclopedic *Autism and Other Developmental Disorders: A Handbook*, edited by the late Donald Cohen and colleagues (Cohen et al., 1987), is also in its third edition (Volkmar et al., 2005) and getting thicker with each iteration.

I particularly want to draw attention to the French child psychiatrist and electrophysiologist Gilbert LeLord of Tours, who started biologic studies of autism in the early 1970s (LeLord et al., 1973), because he and his colleagues have been bucking the mainstream of French psychiatry which, to this day, is strongly invested in psychoanalysis. LeLord eventually attracted a large cadre of collaborators whose many lines of quality research parallel autism studies in Anglo-Saxon, Scandinavian, and other countries. With the active help of parent-advocates, the Tours group organized a day school to educate children with autism, described in their 1995 book *Infantile Autism: Exchange and Development Therapy*, which particularly emphasizes social skills training (Barthélémy et al., 1995).

Controversies Regarding Prevalence and Classification

Information on the prevalence of autism has changed dramatically over the past half-century. At first only classic Kanner-type children, whom the DSM and ICD systems label Autistic Disorder, were counted, and their prevalence was quoted as ~1/2,500 children (e.g., Lotter, 1966; Ritvo et al., 1989). Lorna Wing, a London child psychiatrist, was among early clinicians to recognize the wide spectrum of severity of the social and other impairments of autism and the triad of behavioral domains affected (Wing & Gould, 1979). The psychologist Uta Frith's translation into English of Asperger's 1944 paper (Frith, 1991) contributed to awareness and acceptance of more mildly affected individuals as belonging on the autism spectrum, which helped swell the statistics. Wing (Wing & Potter, 2002) and others (e.g., Fombonne, 2003) attribute the recent so-called epidemic of autism, i.e., 1/110, largely to such changes in diagnostic criteria. I acknowledge up front that I have contributed to the "epidemic" in New York, as my threshold for an autism spectrum diagnosis dropped dramatically over the years. For example, I recently reviewed the chart of an 18-year-old musician about to enter college whose high functioning autism diagnosis was instantly obvious to me from his father's description over the phone. In the early nineties I had diagnosed this same child, then 4 years old, as having a "severe developmental language disorder with serious behavioral problems."

A factor strongly contributing to the increase in prevalence is availability, for the past 20 years or so, of standardized autism-focused diagnostic and screening instruments like the Childhood Autism Rating Scale (CARS) (Schopler et al., 1986); an autism-focused history, the Autistic Diagnostic Interview (ADI) (Le Couteur et al., 1989); the age-stratified Autistic Diagnostic Observation Schedule (ADOS) (Lord et al., 1989); and the Checklist for Autism in Toddlers (CHAT) (Baron-Cohen et al., 2000), to name some of the more widely applied tests. A consequence of their use in the clinic, not just for the selection of research subjects, is that a diagnosis of autism spectrum disorder became applicable to hitherto ignored individuals at both the very severe and mild ends of the spectrum. Still another factor is that many parents, at least in the United States, now push for an autism diagnosis because it brings with it access to more intensive services than a diagnosis of other developmental disorders. Their hope is that, through early intervention, their child may eventually be included in mainstream education. There is no exclusionary criterion for a diagnosis of autism. Use of standardized diagnostic instruments therefore resulted in many children with rare disorders who already carried a medical diagnosis being newly counted among those with autism, inasmuch as they fulfilled the behavioral diagnostic triad of autism, namely impaired sociability and communication, and a narrow perseverative behavioral repertoire. *Secondary autism* is the term widely used today for the minority—estimated at less than

20%—of children on the autism spectrum with an identifiable etiology (Rutter et al., 1994), be it genetic or unequivocally environmental, like congenital rubella.

Primary autism, the only group counted in early studies, encompasses the great majority of cases of autism without a known cause or associated somatic deficit, a fraction expected to shrink with advancing etiologic research. Individuals currently diagnosed with Asperger's syndrome and high functioning autistic disorder (HFA), and those with Pervasive Developmental Disorder Not-Otherwise-Specified (PDD-NOS), i.e., more mildly affected individuals, some without cognitive impairment, were not counted in early epidemiologic studies. The "autistic traits" of these individuals would not have made the diagnostic cut. It remains controversial how to classify persons with epilepsy or with other behavioral problems warranting an additional DSM/ICD psychiatric diagnosis. For example, should autism with attention deficit disorder with hyperactivity (ADHD) (Landgren et al., 1996) or bipolar disorder (Rzhetsky et al., 2007) be classified as primary autism with comorbidity or as secondary autism?

The bottom line is that because autism is a behaviorally, i.e., dimensionally defined, diagnosis, its classification is based on agreed-upon cut-off criteria along a behavioral continuum, not on dichotomous biologically based criteria. For all these reasons, prevalence figures are and will continue to remain approximate and disputed. Regardless of the reasons for its cause, the prevalence of autism spectrum diagnoses has risen dramatically over the past several decades.

Language Disorders, Language Regression, and Epilepsy in Autism

I will not attempt to cover here the vast neuropsychologic and electrophysiologic advances of recent decades, nor will I focus on the core deficits in sociability and joint attention. My colleagues and I did carry out exhaustive evaluations of anamnestic, neurologic, neuropsychologic, language, play, and behavioral dimensions in preschool children with autism compared to cognitively matched developmentally impaired controls who did not have autism (Rapin, 1996a). The child neuropsychologist Deborah Fein and her students have published a number of studies of these same children followed at school age, (e.g., Fein et al., 1999; Stevens et al., 2000). Here, I confine myself to studies of language to which I have personally contributed.

Language Disorder Subtypes in Autism

Delayed or absent language, together with impaired conversational use of language (pragmatics) constitute the second criterion for an autism diagnosis. Impoverished imaginative play is also a component of this criterion. I was fortunate to work with the late Doris A. Allen, a developmental psycholinguist with a background in education, psychology, and speech pathology. She directed the Therapeutic Nursery of the Einstein Division of Child Psychiatry, which, before she took it over in the mid-seventies, was still run by a psychoanalyst. Dr. Allen turned it around by addressing children's communication deficiencies, social and play deficits. A parent or other caretaker had to accompany the child to school every day because one of her focuses was to teach "in the trenches" more effective skills for managing the child's difficult behaviors (Allen & Mendelson, 2000).

Pooling our skills, Doris Allen and I developed an observational classification of developmental language disorders suitable for clinicians' use in their offices (Allen et al., 1988; Rapin, 1996b). We discovered that the subtypes of language disorders in unselected consecutive young children with autism evaluated clinically overlap those of children with developmental language disorders who do not have autism, except for major differences in subtype prevalence (Allen & Rapin, 1992; Tuchman et al., 1991a). Besides their signature pragmatic deficits, young children on the autism spectrum, verbal or not, all have comprehension deficits for conversational speech, whereas a sizable proportion of language disordered children without autism do not. We were struck that, in both groups, epilepsy is strongly linked to verbal auditory agnosia (VAA), the most severe subtype of receptive/expressive disorder for speech sound processing (phonology) (Tuchman et al., 1991b). VAA is characterized by dysfunction in auditory cortex, which jeopardizes the acquisition of verbal comprehension and expression at the language-learning age.

Until very recently (Kjelgaard & Tager-Flusberg, 2001; Tager-Flusberg & Joseph, 2003), studies of language in autism focused mainly on its impaired pragmatics (conversational use), a correlate of autism's social impairment, and on abnormal features like echolalia, pronominal reversal, perseverative questioning, and aberrant vocabulary and prosody. The accepted tenet was that phonology (speech sound production) and grammar (syntax and morphologic markers), although often delayed, were unaffected in autism. When children started to speak, often after a considerable delay, they did so competently and thus did not have "structural" language disorders. Our clinical observations in unselected preschoolers, together with a recent study at school age using formal tests, indicate that this is not true of some third of children (Rapin et al., 2009). It is the case that the intellectually deficient children on the autism spectrum are those who are most likely to have impaired expressive and receptive language. Yet, blaming global cognitive deficit for impaired expressive phonology and grammar and for an impoverished vocabulary begs the question of the neurologic basis of the deficient language. Having similar subtypes of language disorder in no way implies that autism and developmental language disorder are on a continuum or share a common etiology. It does suggest that they have in common dysfunction in a corresponding language network, although not necessarily in the same node of that network.

In more than three quarters of typically developing children and adults, even in the majority of those who are left-handed, it is well known that language depends strongly on the function of the left superior temporal (Wernicke's) and inferior frontal (Broca's) cortices and on the pathways that interconnect them (Galaburda et al., 1990). On average these areas are typically asymmetric, larger on the left than the right. Classically, lesions affecting Wernicke's area in adults compromise comprehension of the meaning of language (semantics) but not the production of phonology or syntax, and lesions affecting Broca's area interfere with language expression, specifically with phonology and syntax. Morphometric studies showed similarly reversed asymmetry, compared to normally developing controls, in a sample of children with autism and with developmental language disorders without autism (Herbert et al., 2002; Herbert et al., 2005), findings that support parallel involvement of language networks in both disorders. In an independent sample, De Fossé and colleagues (De Fossé et al., 2004) detected reversed asymmetry of frontal language cortex in children with developmental language disorders and among those with autism, only in those whose expressive phonology and grammar were impaired on formal testing; asymmetry was not reversed in those who did not fulfill criteria for this subtype of language disorder. The study provides further evidence for the existence of more than a single subtype of language disorder in autism.

Epilepsy and Language/Autistic Regression

We noted earlier that the occurrence of epilepsy (defined as at least two unprovoked seizures) in some one third of children with autism by adolescence provided critical evidence against the psychogenic etiology of autism (Deykin & MacMahon, 1979; Olsson et al., 1988; Tuchman et al., 1991b; Volkmar & Nelson, 1990). Earlier evidence indicated that infantile spasms (West syndrome), one of the malignant epileptic encephalopathies of infancy, may leave autism in its wake (Taft & Cohen, 1971); in other words, infantile spasms (or the encephalopathy responsible for the spasms) may damage permanently selective pathways required for sociability, communication, and behavioral flexibility. Despite recent intensive work, it remains controversial whether in these children autism and epilepsy arise from a common underlying molecular mechanism, or whether in some cases it is the seizures that, by damaging certain critical networks, are responsible for the autism and the intellectual impairment likely to accompany it (Tuchman et al., 2009). Parents' reports of regression of language and sociability around 15 to 30 months were greeted at first with skepticism. My doubting an identical story told to me by scores of mothers would have been foolish, especially when Japanese mothers gave identical reports (Kurita, 1985). The reality of regression finally received empirical corroboration when home videos documented language/autistic regression in some third of toddlers (Werner & Dawson, 2005). Its cause remains frustratingly elusive, however.

One possibility we and others explored was that covert epilepsy might be responsible for autistic regression. This hypothesis was based on awareness of the rare but dramatic language regression without autism well documented in older children in the context of epilepsy or of an epileptiform EEG without clinical seizures (acquired epileptic aphasia—Landau-Kleffner syndrome). A brief questionnaire brought out that language regression in children under age 3 is highly predictive of autism, whereas in older children it more often signals clinical or subclinical epilepsy (Shinnar et al., 2001). Overnight EEGs are more likely to reveal epileptiform activity, and seizures are more prevalent in older children with language regression than in the younger children, who are at much higher risk for autism (McVicar et al., 2005). Language regression per se is not a strong predictor of epilepsy in autism (Tuchman & Rapin, 1997). Thus, these studies indicate that the pathophysiologies of language regression in autism and in Landau-Kleffner syndrome differ and that epilepsy, be it overt or subclinical, seems to play a minor role in the language regression of autism.

Sensorimotor Deficits

As long as autism was considered a psychogenic disorder, sensorimotor symptoms were largely ignored, despite parents' concerns about them and despite articulate adults' descriptions of their own atypical sensory experiences (Grandin, 1995). Information regarding the sensory and motor symptoms of autism is sparse, yet they are targets of many expensive therapeutic attempts to influence them, with little empirical evidence of efficacy (Baranek, 2002).

Neurologic explanations are being sought for the frequent and puzzling co-occurrence in the same individual of hyper- and hyposensitivity to sound and visual, somatosensory, and other less well studied sensory inputs (Rapin, 2006). A notable change over the past decade is that researchers have started to think of the autistic brain as different rather than damaged and have started to investigate the brain basis of enhanced perception and talent of some individuals with autism (Mottron et al., 2006; Samson et al., 2006). This change was prompted, in part, by early studies of savants, most of whom had autism and all of whom had severe impairments outside their extraordinary talents (Obler & Fein, 1988; Treffert, 2005).

The main motor symptoms in autism are stereotypies, difficulty imitating and mastering complex motor tasks, persistent toe walking, and "hypotonia" (Akshoomoff et al., 2007). Parents view stereotypies, purposeless rhythmic, repetitive movements, as particularly troublesome because they are stigmatizing (Goldman et al., 2009). Stereotypies are widely regarded as enjoyable bad habits to be squashed, rather than as temporarily suppressible movement disorders in some ways akin to tics (Berthier et al., 2003; Rapin, 2001). Despite a large animal literature (Saka et al., 2004), little is known about the neurologic basis of stereotypies in humans.

Why is it that some individuals with autism do not imitate, are clumsy, and have trouble learning the sequence of movements required to tie their shoes or write (Fuentes et al., 2009)?

Rather than signaling lack of motivation, these inadequacies may signal inadequate procedural learning and inefficient cerebellar-basal ganglia-parietal circuitry (Mahone et al., 2006; Mostofsky et al., 2000). A characteristic of many children with autism is their impaired imitation of movements, for which lack of attention to the task does not seem to provide a convincing explanation (Vivanti et al., 2008). In a study of sensorimotor function comparing children with autism to children without autism but with either developmental language disorders or low IQ, we were unable to determine reliably whether failure to carry out motor tasks was due to inability to perform or impaired motivation (Mandelbaum et al., 2006). Functional neuroimaging suggests that poor imitation may reflect absent or dysfunctional mirror neurons, which play a crucial role in imitation (Iacoboni & Mazziotta, 2007; Rizzolatti & Craighero, 2004; Rogers, 2007).

A frequent motor characteristic of autism is toe-walking (Ming et al., 2007). No one knows why so many children with autism toe-walk in the absence of spasticity, bony or soft tissue structural abnormality.

Physical therapists regularly comment on "hypotonia," by which they mean increased joint mobility without weakness. Neurologists gave a score for hypotonia to a quarter of preschoolers with autism, but also, among those without autism, to a third of those with low IQ and 13% of those with language disorders (Rapin, 1996c). In the absence of a standardized metric for "hypotonia" in young children, the significance of these observations, their specificity and functional importance are undetermined. The literature is replete with reports of "hypotonia" in a large variety of children with chromosome anomalies and other developmental syndromes, but its basis is essentially never specified. It remains to be seen whether "hypotonia" in autism, when real, is a consequence of cerebellar or proprioceptive impairment, conceivably muscle mitochondrial dysfunction, or whether in some children cytogenetic or micro DNA rearrangements may have implicated a gene for collagen or elastin. In any case, in view of physical and occupational therapists' huge expenditures of effort to improve "hypotonia," this is a symptom that cries for much more rigorous definition and metric, longitudinal assessment of its functional significance, and specification of its almost certainly disparate causes.

Neuropathologic/Imaging Evidence

Autism had no known neuropathology until 20 years ago when Margaret Bauman, a child neurologist, and Thomas Kemper, a neuropathologist and anatomist, both from Boston, described subtle stunting of the soma and dendrites of some limbic neurons and, surprisingly, no neocortical pathology (Bauman & Kemper, 1985). Their report of a reduced number of Purkinje and granular cells in the cerebellum was a clap of thunder. This unexpected finding, amplified in subsequent papers (Bauman & Kemper, 2003), opened the door to a flood of morphometric studies of the cerebellum and to reconsideration of its role not only in autism but in other complex human behaviors like language, attention, and affect, to name but a few (Schmahmann, 2004). Kemper & Bauman also noted subtle differences in specific brain nuclei of children and adults (Kemper & Bauman, 2002), suggesting the possibility of an ongoing process in some individuals. The aberrant early growth curve of the brain in autism (Courchesne et al., 2007) bolsters this contention.

As technologies for neuroimaging advanced, a more detailed understanding of the anatomy and function of the autistic brain began to emerge. Recent computer-assisted morphologic studies of the neocortex revealed increased numbers of narrower neuronal minicolumns (Casanova, 2006). These may account for enlargement of the radiate white matter fibers that interconnect neocortical areas described in some of the children we had studied behaviorally (Herbert et al., 2004). Overconnectivity of some cortical circuitry, underconnectivity of others involving subcortical relays such as the basal ganglia, amygdala and other limbic areas, and the cerebellum are at the forefront of current investigations (Geschwind & Levitt, 2007; Minshew & Williams, 2007). Studies range from behavioral to morphometric and functional imaging, and from electrophysiology down to the level of the synapse (Zoghbi, 2003) and of neurotransmitters like dopamine, glutamate, and others (Yip et al., 2007).

Subtle neuronal migration defects were observed in a handful of severely affected individuals (Bailey et al., 1998), and an unsuspected variant of neuroaxonal dystrophy in two others (Weidenheim et al., 2001), not to mention the variety of other findings in individuals with defined etiologies like tuberous sclerosis (Asano et al., 2001), or fragile X, in which dendritic spines are thin and immature-looking (Hagerman et al., 2005). Signs suggesting inflammation (Vargas et al., 2005) point to neuroimmunologic abnormalities, long suspected but not demonstrated in children with a history of regression (Ashwood et al., 2006; Cabanlit et al., 2007; Wills et al., 2007). The National Alliance for Autism Research (NAAR), a parent-initiated group now part of Autism Speaks, supports the Autism Tissue Program (Pickett, 2001), which has raised awareness of the urgent need for continued tissue donation from affected individuals and nonaffected controls. Tissue enables investigators around the world to carry out studies of the cellular and molecular biology of autism that are impossible without this precious resource.

Genetics and Epigenetics

Awareness that genetics might be an important player in autism grew in the 1970s and'80s following early reports of strong concordance of autism in identical twins (Folstein & Rutter, 1977; Steffenburg et al., 1986). Genetic studies gained momentum in the mid-nineties after a parent advocacy group, Cure Autism Now (CAN), also currently part of Autism Speaks, sponsored the systematic collection of detailed family and personal histories and DNA from families with more than one rigorously diagnosed affected member. The resultant Autism Genetic Resource Exchange (AGRE) has enrolled many hundreds of families across the country and some abroad (Geschwind et al., 2001; Ylisaukko-oja et al., 2006). The NIH and Autism Speaks now support this extraordinarily valuable resource. I learned when I first came to Einstein 50 years ago the power of interdisciplinary coalitions of basic scientists working hand-in-hand with clinicians to elucidate the pathophysiology of obscure neurogenetic diseases, several of which generated novel biologic insights (Goldfischer et al., 1973; Purpura & Suzuki, 1976). This same multidisciplinary approach, yoked with spectacular technologic advances following the 2001 completion of the human genome project, has uncovered unexpected complexities of autism genetics (O'Roak & State, 2008). Single mutations with strong effects seem to be the exception in "primary" autism, judging from the small proportion of families with a typical Mendelian or mitochondrial pattern of inheritance. Multigenetic influence is likely in view of relatively weak linkages of the many newly discovered genes to "primary" autism and of the high prevalence of unaffected family members with lesser developmental deficits (Dawson et al., 2007). Stunningly rapid progress in genetics makes it a challenge to keep clinicians up-to-date; two Einstein medical students, whose knowledge of genetics was much fresher than mine, attempted to do so for pediatricians a few years ago (Muhle et al., 2004), and Roberto Tuchman and I more recently for neurologists (Rapin & Tuchman, 2008). The public needs to be reminded again and again that the brain, not genes, causes or explains behavior (Abrahams, B. S. and Geschwind, D. H., 2010). Any one gene is likely to accumulate many different mutations in different families, resulting in potentially different phenotypes. The role of genes in autism will not be understood until it becomes clear what protein each codes for and what roles the protein plays in the brain and its different cell types.

Hitherto unsuspected complexities in the inheritance of autism have important implications for genetic counseling. Prenatal diagnosis is not in the cards now and unlikely to become so, except for families with identified cytogenetic, Mendelian, or mitochondrial traits. Most cases of autism are sporadic, that is, neither parent carries a mutation identified in their child. An as yet unknown proportion of de novo mutations arise either in the gonad of one of the noncarrier parents or possibly in the early embryo. Such couples are at minimal risk of having another affected child, but that child's descendents, especially males, will be at high risk of inheriting the trait (Zhao et al., 2007). Some of these new traits are micro DNA deletions, duplications, or other rearrangements (Weiss et al., 2008), which may affect not only coding but also noncoding regulatory parts of one or more genes.

Postmitotic epigenetic effects, some of them environmentally mediated, may have direct biologic consequences or influence brain development indirectly. I witnessed an extreme example of a presumed epigenetic effect that caused a gross anatomic difference in a set of monozygotic twin girls with Joubert syndrome. One of the twins had autism and was very intellectually impaired, with a major motor handicap and much more severe cerebellar malformation than her sister (Raynes et al., 1999). Others have reported presumed epigenetic influences in phenotypically discordant monozygotic twins with tuberous sclerosis and autism (Humphrey et al., 2004). Epigenetic influences may be major or subtle. I cannot discount several parents who reported convincingly an abrupt autistic regression in their children following a stressful life event like a separation, a move, or a brief hospitalization that another child would have weathered without lasting consequence. Kurita and colleagues heard similar stories from several Japanese mothers (Kurita et al., 1992). These rare occurrences suggest the synergistic effect of a stressor in an individual vulnerable because of an inherent (genetic?) predisposition.

There is evidence to suggest that at least some autistic symptoms may reflect functional rather than structural changes in the brain. We (Rapin, 1996d) and others reported that children's behavior may improve when they have a fever, an effect that can persist for several days following defervescence (Curran et al., 2007). A provocative suggestion is that dysfunction of the locus coeruleus-noradrenergic system may account for these observations, with obvious potential implications for intervention (Mehler, 2008, Mehhler & Purpura, 2009).

A very recent realization is that the number of noncoding RNAs increases exponentially from lower organisms to man, in the face of fairly similar numbers of protein coding genes. These RNAs provide a plausible explanation for increasing brain complexity, as many are specific to the brain and especially active during its development (Mattick & Mehler, 2008; Mehler, 2008). Epigenetics, that is postmitotic control of gene expression, plays a crucial and very specific role in neuronal and neural network development and function. MicroRNAs can turn on and off messenger RNAs and noncoding RNAs, which control entire neural networks transiently or permanently. They are highly sensitive to environmental influences and therefore are potent epigenetic modulators of genetic developmental programs in response to random life events (Mehler & Mattick, 2007; Persico & Bourgeron, 2006). They may thus provide a partial explanation for the puzzling clinical observations of sudden language/autistic regression. By the same token they might play a role in the brain plasticity that underlies the behavioral amelioration that often results from intensive early education and competent parenting (Dawson, 2008; Helt et al., 2008).

Intervention: Psychopharmacology and Education

From my perspective, progress in the psychopharmacology of autism has been disappointing despite growing understanding of neurotransmitters and neuromodulators. Risperidone is the only FDA medication approved specifically for autism, and, at that, only for irritability and aggression (McCracken et al., 2002; Scahill et al., 2007). Yet it is prescribed extensively off-label in small doses in attempts to control stereotypies and other undesirable behaviors. It is known to affect both serotonin and dopamine receptors and has largely supplanted the dopamine blockers that were prescribed in the fifties and sixties. Stimulants, anticonvulsants, specific serotonin reuptake inhibitors, and many other psychotropic drugs are widely prescribed to help modify specific behaviors, but their very multiplicity indicates that none is a magic bullet (Mintz et al., 2006). I am impressed with potentially undesirable—especially long-term—side effects such as abnormal involuntary movements in susceptible children treated with dopamine reuptake inhibitors, and weight gain precipitated by risperidone. I believe that medications should be limited to specific behavioral indications, mostly in more severely affected children.

Without doubt the major revolution in the management of autism is early intervention and education. Ivar Lovaas's report (Lovaas, 1987) that intensive systematic operant conditioning had ameliorated the outcome of 9 of 19 preschoolers to the point of their becoming educable in regular classrooms was the second thunderclap in the field. The improvement was lasting, since 4 years after the training, 8 of the 9 were described as indistinguishable from their normally developing peers (McEachin et al., 1993). This impressive success was recently replicated in another small cohort (Sallows & Graupner, 2005) and no doubt in others. Up to the development of this strategy, prognosis for improvement in children with autistic disorder was dismal, professionals' attitudes defeatist, and intervention was viewed as largely futile. The news of an effective treatment that raised IQs and suppressed bad behaviors in some children spread like wildfire. The Lovaas Applied Behavior Analysis (ABA) approach has become dominant, at least for preschoolers, with the caveat that it works best in children with a reasonable intellect and that it is not a "cure" but can make some previously unreachable children available to less rigid educational approaches. The field of applied behavior analysis has developed dramatically over the years, spawning a number of less rigid early intervention curricula that incorporate naturalistic and developmental approaches to formal operant conditioning. Two of the most widely accepted are those of Eric Schopler (Schopler & Olley, 1982), which emphasizes structured teaching, and of Stanley Greenspan (Greenspan, 1992), based on child-centered play-based methods. Today's eclectic programs may borrow features from the three programs and others (Schreibman & Ingersoll, 2005). They tend to focus on pivotal social behaviors such as motivation, self-initiated interaction, responsiveness to cues, and others shown to enhance learning of language and other skills (Koegel et al., 2001). For example, adding to an ABA-based preschool program 30 minutes per day for 6 weeks of training in either joint attention or symbolic play yielded additional gains in language and sociability that were sustained for a year (Kasari et al., 2008).

The program I am most familiar with is a preschool for higher functioning children on the spectrum that focuses on teaching sociability and communication to the child and on training of parents to achieve control of their child's difficult behaviors (Mendelson et al., 2007). Most recently, two of my colleagues have published a curriculum (Dunn, 2005) and practical guidance for teachers of children able to be educated in regular classes (Fein & Dunn, 2007).

It is now clear that intervention is most likely to be effective in very early childhood, when development is fastest and the brain most plastic. Prospective study of the younger siblings of probands is currently providing the opportunity to compare affected and nonaffected infants from birth (Landa & Garrett-Mayer, 2006; Zwaigenbaum et al., 2005). The goal is to identify the earliest signs of autism so that intervention can start forthwith. Diagnosis of an autism spectrum disorder before age 3 years entitles children in the United States to intensive early intervention under the umbrella of federally mandated state-delivered agencies. After age 3 years children fall under the jurisdiction of local school districts, which may provide as much as full day, 11 months/year, specialized education and therapies. This educational revolution has turned around the management of children on the autism spectrum but is straining the resources of educators and parents. Many parents insist on every possible therapy in school and pay out of pocket for touted unconventional, unproven interventions they read about on the Internet (Levy & Hyman, 2005).

At this time in developed countries, many intensive interventions are recommended from toddlerhood to young adulthood. Desperate parents, anxious for their children not to miss out on any potentially helpful intervention, are often eager to try pharmacotherapy and, sadly, alternative and expensive treatments of dubious effectiveness. What is still glaringly missing is empirical evaluation of these disparate medical and educational approaches. Equally inadequate are programs for adults who may need ongoing more or less intensive support in their every day lives. Worse of all is the inequality of what can be provided for the rich and vocal and for the poor, especially in developing countries. It is urgent that effective interventions that parents can provide at home be devised, evaluated, and exported to needy children both here and abroad. There is no way teachers and therapists can do it all.

Summary and Conclusion

Autism has come full circle in a half-century, from an obscure "psychiatric disease" to the symptom of a partially understood deviance in brain development influenced by both genetics and the environment. I highlighted what I believe to be the main reasons for dramatic changes in its prevalence. I emphasized our complete lack of understanding of what triggers language/autistic regression and provided evidence against epilepsy as a major player in its occurrence. I presented my view of subtypes of language disorders in autism, pointing out that, besides their universally and persistently impaired use of language (pragmatics), some children have undisputable deficits at the level of receptive and expressive phonology and grammar. I did not discuss the potential role of inflammatory/immunologic factors in autism and, particularly, in regression. I only acknowledged major advances in electrophysiology, functional imaging, and neuropsychology. I mentioned anatomic and pathologic evidence suggesting that, at least in some individuals, autism might be an ongoing developmental process and stressed the dire need for more tissue for research. I pointed out that the study of sensorimotor deficits has been neglected for too long, a fertile area for neurologic study. I stressed that major progress in modern genetics applied to autism has yet to have a major impact on our understanding its cause or our ability to provide genetic counseling to most families. Finally, I stated that I considered advances in pharmacologic intervention disappointing, in contrast to my much more optimistic appraisal of progress in education, especially in toddlers who are being diagnosed at ever earlier ages. I hope that the detailed chapters of this book show my views to be overly pessimistic, but these do represent those of a clinician evaluating real children and attempting to inform their parents.

I choose to emphasize here the pressing need for empirical evidence to help weed out some of the many expensive and conflicting recommendations for evaluation and management. Providing all of these in the clinic and the school is breaking the bank, without proof of which are cost-effective. I did not spell out the many frankly exploitative panaceas touted to parents by word of mouth or on the Internet. I do not doubt the effectiveness of early, intensive, specialized education for many of the children, but there is a need for evidence-based research on the efficacy of the many expensive mainstream therapies they receive. Education, even though it does not "repair" the brain, can improve many symptoms and enable some high functioning adults to take an independent place in society. They demand, legitimately, to be considered somewhat different, but not "sick" (Chamak, 2008). In large part because of better education, even though some individuals will require long-term help, nowadays only the most severely affected will spend their days in idleness in institutions. That is real progress. And who would have predicted early on that autism would help advance basic neuroscience and education and that some individuals with autism would be recognized as able to make contributions to society that individuals without autism cannot make?

REFERENCES

Abrahams, B. S. and Geschwind, D. H. (2010) Connecting genes to brain in the autism spectrum disorders. *Archives of Neurology, 67*(4), 395–399.

Akshoomoff, N., Farid, N., Courchesne, E., & Haas, R. (2007). Abnormalities on the neurological examination and EEG in young children with pervasive developmental disorders. *Journal of Autism and Developmental Disorders, 37*(5), 887–893.

Allen, D. A., & Mendelson, L. (2000). Parent, child, and professional: Meeting the needs of young autistic children and their families in a multidisciplinary therapeutic nursery model. In S. Epstein, (Ed.), *Autistic spectrum disorders and psychoanalytic ideas: Reassessing the fit* (pp. 704–731). Analytic Press: Hillsdale, NJ.

Allen, D. A., & Rapin, I. (1992). Autistic children are also dysphasic. In H. Naruse & E. Ornitz (Eds.), Neurobiology of infantile autism (pp. 73–80). Amsterdam: Excerpta Medica.

Allen, D. A., Rapin, I., & Wiznitzer, M. (1988). Communication disorders of preschool children: The physician's responsibility. *Journal of Developmental and Behavioral Pediatrics, 9*, 164–170.

Asano, E., Chugani, D. C., Muzik, O., Behen, M., Janisse, J., Rothermel, R., et al. (2001). Autism in tuberous sclerosis complex is related to both cortical and subcortical dysfunction. *Neurology, 57*(7), 1269–1277.

Ashwood, P., Wills, S., & Van de Water, J. (2006). The immune response in autism: A new frontier for autism research. *Journal of Leukocyte Biology, 80*(1), 1–15.

Bailey, A., Luthert, P., Dean, A., Harding, B., Janota, I., Montgomery, M., et al. (1998). A clinicopathological study of autism. *Brain, 121*(5), 889–905.

Baranek, G. T. (2002). Efficacy of sensory and motor interventions for children with autism. *Journal of Autism and Developmental Disordorders, 32*(5), 397–422.

Baron-Cohen S., Wheelwright S., Cox A., Baird G., Charman T., Swettenham J., et al. (2000). Early identification of autism by the Checklist for Autism in Toddlers (CHAT). *Journal of the Royal Society of Medicine, 93*(10), 521–525.

Barthélémy C., Hameury, L., & LeLord G. (1995). *Infantile autism: Exchange and development theory*. Paris: Expansion Scientifique Publications.

Bauman, M. L., & Kemper, T. L. (1985). Histoanatomic observations of the brain in early infantile autism. *Neurology 35*, 866–874.

Bauman, M. L., & Kemper, T. L. (2003). The neuropathology of the autism spectrum disorders: What have we learned? *Novartis Foundation Symposium, 251*, 112–122.

Berthier, M. L., Kulisevsky, J., Asenjo, B., Aparicio, J., & Lara D. (2003). Comorbid Asperger and Tourette syndromes with localized mesencephalic, infrathalamic, thalamic, and striatal damage. *Developmental Medicine and Child Neurology, 45*(3), 207–212.

Cabanlit, M., Wills, S., Goines, P., Ashwood, P., & Van de Water, J. (2007). Brain-specific autoantibodies in the plasma of subjects with autistic spectrum disorder. *Annals of the New York Academy of Sciences, 1107*, 92–103.

Casanova, M. F. (2006). Neuropathological and genetic findings in autism: The significance of a putative minicolumnopathy. *Neuroscientist, 12*(5), 435–441.

Chamak, B. (2008). Autism and social movements: French parents' associations and international autistic individuals' organisations. *Sociology of Health and Illness, 30*, 76–96.

Chess, S., Korn, S. J., & Fernandez, P. B. (1971). Psychiatric disorders of children with congenital rubella. New York: Brunner/Mazel.

Cohen, D. J., Donnellan, A. M., & Paul R. (Eds.). (1987). *Handbook of autism and pervasive developmental disorders*. New York: Wiley.

Coleman. M., & Gillberg. C. (1985). The biology of the autistic syndromes. New York: Praeger.

Courchesne. E., Pierce K., Schumann, C. M., Redcay, E., Buckwalter, J. A., Kennedy, D. P., et al. (2007). Mapping early brain development in autism. *Neuron, 56*(2), 399–413.

Curran, L. K., Newschaffer, C. J., Lee, L. C., Crawford, S. O., Johnston, M. V., & Zimmerman, A. W. (2007). Behaviors associated with fever in children with autism spectrum disorders. *Pediatrics, 120*(6), e1386–e1392.

Dawson, G. (2008). Early behavioral intervention, brain plasticity, and the prevention of autism spectrum disorder. *Developmental Psychopathology, 20*(3), 775–803.

Dawson, G., Estes, A., Munson, J., Schellenberg, G., Bernier, R., & Abbott, R. (2007). Quantitative assessment of autism symptom-related traits in probands and parents: Broader Phenotype Autism Symptom Scale. *Journal of Autism and Developmental Disorders, 37*(3), 523–536.

DeFossé, L., Hodge, S. M., Makris, N., Kennedy, D. N., Caviness, V. S., Jr., McGrath, L., et al. (2004). Language-association cortex asymmetry in autism and specific language impairment. *Annals of Neurology, 56*(6), 757–766.

Deykin, E. Y., & MacMahon, B. (1979). The incidence of seizures among children with autistic symptoms. *American Journal of Psychiatry, 136*, 1310–1312.

Dun, M. (2005). *S.O.S.: Social Skills in Our Schools Program (A Social Skills program for children with Pervasive Developmental Disorders and their typical peers)*. Shawnee Mission KS: Autism and Asperger Publishing Co.

Fein, D., & Dunn, M. A. (2007). *Autism in your classroom: A general educator's guide to students with autism spectrum disorders.* Bethesda, MD: Woodbine House.

Fein, D., Stevens, M., Dunn, M., Waterhouse, L., Allen, D. A., Rapin, I., et al. (1999). Subtypes of pervasive developmental disorder: Clinical characteristics. *Child Neuropsychology*, 5(1), 1–23.

Folstein, S. E., & Rutter, M. (1977). Infantile autism: A genetic study of 21 twin pairs. *Journal of Child Psychology and Psychiatry, 18*, 297–321.

Fombonne, E. (2003). Epidemiological surveys of autism and other pervasive developmental disorders: An update. *Journal of Autism and Developmental Disorders, 33*(4), 365–382.

Frith U. (1991). *Autism and Asperger syndrome.* Cambridge,UK: Cambridge University Press.

Fuentes, C. T., Mostofsky, S. H., & Bastian, A. J. (2009). Children with autism show specific handwriting impairments. *Neurology, 73*(19), 1532–1537.

Galaburda, A. M., Rosen, G. D., & Sherman, G. F. (1990). Individual variability in cortical organization: Its relationship to brain laterality and implications to function. *Neuropsychologia, 28*(6), 529–546.

Geschwind, D. H., & Levitt, P. (2007). Autism spectrum disorders: Developmental disconnection syndromes. *Current Opinion in Neurobiology, 17*(1), 103–111.

Geschwind, D. H., Sowinski, J., Lord, C., Iversen, P., Shestack, J., Jones, P., et al. (2001). The autism genetic resource exchange: A resource for the study of autism and related neuropsychiatric conditions. *American Journal of Human Genetics, 69*(2), 463–466.

Gillberg, C., & Coleman, M. (2000). *The biology of the autistic syndromes*. London: MacKeith Press.

Goldman, S., Wang, C., Salgado, M. W., Greene, P. E., Kim, M., & Rapin, I. (2009). Motor stereotypies in children with autism and other developmental disorders. *Developmental Medicine and Child Neurology, 51*(1), 30–38.

Goldfischer, S., Moore, C. I., Johnson, A. B., Spiro, A. J., Valsamis, M. P., Wisniewski, H. E., Ritch, R. H., et al. (1973). Peroxisomal and mitochondrial defects in the cerebro-hepato-renal syndrome. *Science, 182*(107), 62–64.

Grandin, T. (1995). *Thinking in pictures and other reports from my life with autism.* New York: Doubleday.

Greenspan, S. I. (1992). *Infancy and early childhood: The practice of clinical assessment and intervention with emotional and developmental challenges.* Madison, CT: International Universities Press.

Hagerman, R. J., Ono, M. Y., & Hagerman, P. J. (2005). Recent advances in fragile X: A model for autism and neurodegeneration. *Current Opinion in Psychiatry, 18*(5), 490–496.

Helt, M., Kelley, E., Kinsbourne, M., Pandey, J., Boorstein, H., Herbert, M., et al. (2008). Can children with autism recover? If so, how? *Neuropsychology Review, 18*(4), 339–366.

Herbert, M. R., Harris, G. J., Adrien, K. T., Ziegler, D. A., Makris, N., Kennedy, D. N., et al. (2002). Abnormal asymmetry in language association cortex in autism. *Annals of Neurology, 52*(5), 588–596.

Herbert, M. R., Ziegler, D. A., Deutsch, C. K., O'Brien, L. M., Kennedy, D. N., Filipek, P. A., et al. (2005). Brain asymmetries in autism and developmental language disorder: A nested whole-brain analysis. *Brain, 128*, 213–226.

Herbert, M. R., Ziegler, D. A., Makris, N., Filipek, P. A., Kemper, T. L., Normandin, J. J., et al. (2004). Localization of white matter volume increase in autism and developmental language disorder. *Annals of Neurology, 55*(4), 530–540.

Humphrey, A., Higgins, J. N., Yates, J. R., & Bolton, P. F. (2004). Monozygotic twins with tuberous sclerosis discordant for the severity of developmental deficits. *Neurology, 62*(5), 795–798.

Iacoboni, M., & Mazziotta, J. C. (2007). Mirror neuron system: Basic findings and clinical applications. *Annals of Neurology, 62*(3), 213–218.

Kanner, L. (1943). Autistic disturbances of affective contact. *Nervous Child, 2*, 217–250.

Kanner, L. (1954). To what extent is early infantile autism determined by constitutional inadequacies? *Research Publications of the Association for Research in Nervous and Mental Diseases*, 33: 378–385.

Kasari, C., Paparella, T., Freeman, S., & Jahromi, L. B. (2008). Language outcome in autism: Randomized comparison of joint attention and play interventions. *Journal of Consulting and Clinical Psychology, 76*(1), 125–137.

Kemper, T. L. & Bauman, M. L. 2002. Neuropathology of infantile autism. *Molecular Psychiatry 7 (Supplement 2)*, S12–S13.

Kjelgaard, M. M., & Tager-Flusberg, H. (2001). An investigation of language impairment in autism: Implications for genetic subgroups. *Language and Cognitive Processes, 16*(2/3), 287–308.

Koegel, R. L., Koegel, L. K., & McNerney, E. K. (2001). Pivotal areas in intervention for autism. *Journal of Clinical Child Psychology, 30*(1), 19–32.

Kurita, H. (1985). Infantile autism with speech loss before the age of thirty months. *Journal of the American Academy of Child and Adolescent Psychiatry, 24*, 191–196.

Kurita, H., Kita, M., & Miyake, Y. (1992). A comparative study of development and symptoms among disintegrative psychosis and infantile autism with and without speech loss. *Journal of Autism and Developmental Disorders, 22*, 175–188.

Landa, R., & Garrett-Mayer, E. (2006). Development in infants with autism spectrum disorders: A prospective study. *Journal of Child Psychology and Psychiatry, 47*(6), 629–638.

Landgren, M., Pettersson, R., Kjellman, B., & Gillberg, C. (1996). ADHD, DAMP, and other neurodevelopmental/psychiatric disorders in 6-year-old children: Epidemiology and co-morbidity. *Developmental Medicine and Child Neurology, 38*, 891–906.

Le Couteur, A., Rutter, M., Lord, C., Rios, P., Robertson, S., Holdgrafer, M., et al. (1989). Autism Diagnostic Interview: A standardized observation of communication and social behavior. *Journal of Autism and Developmental Disorders, 19*(3), 363–387.

LeLord, G., Laffont, F., Jusseaume, P., & Stephant, J. L. (1973). Comparative study of conditioning of averaged evoked responses by coupling sound and light in normal and autistic children. *Psychophysiology, 10*(4), 415–425.

Levy, S. E., & Hyman, S. L. (2005). Novel treatments for autistic spectrum disorders. *Mental Retardation and Developmental Disabilities Research Reviews, 11*(2), 131–142.

Lord, C., Rutter, M., Goode, S., Heemsbergen, J., Jordan, H., Mawhood, L., et al. (1989). Autism Diagnostic Observation Schedule: A standardized observation of communicative and social behavior. *Journal of Autism and Developmental Disorders, 19*(2), 185–212.

Lotter, V. (1966). Epidemiology of autistic conditions in young children. *Social Psychiatry, 1*(3), 124–137.

Lovaas, O. I. (1987). Behavioral treatment and normal educational and intellectual functioning in young autistic children. *Journal of Consulting and Clinical Psychology, 55*(1), 3–9.

Mahone, E. M., Powell, S. K., Loftis, C. W., Goldberg, M. C., Denckla, M. B., & Mostofsky, S. H. (2006). Motor persistence and inhibition in autism and ADHD. *Journal of the International Neuropsychology Society, 12*(5), 622–631.

Mandelbaum, D. E., Stevens, M., Rosenberg, E., Wiznitzer, M., Steinschneider, M., Filipek, P., et al. (2006). Comparison of sensorimotor performance in school age children with autism, developmental language disorder, or low IQ. *Developmental Medicine and Child Neurology, 48*, 33–39.

Mattick, J. S., & Mehler, M. F. (2008). RNA editing, DNA recoding and the evolution of human cognition. *Trends in Neurosciences, 31*(5), 227–233.

McCracken, J. T., McGough, J., Shah, B., Cronin, P., Hong, D., Aman, M. G., et al. (2002). Risperidone in children with autism and serious behavioral problems. *New England Journal of Medicine, 347*(5), 314–321.

McEachin, J. J., Smith, T., & Lovaas, O. I. (1993). Long-term outcome for children with autism who received early intensive behavioral treatment. *American Journal of Mental Retardation, 97*(4), 359–372.

McVicar, K. A., Ballaban-Gil, K., Rapin, I., Moshé, S. L., & Shinnar, S. (2005). Epileptiform EEG abnormalities in children with language regression. *Neurology, 65*(1), 129–131.

Mehler, M. F. (2008). Epigenetics and the nervous system. *Annals of Neurology, 64*(6), 602–617.

Mehler, M. F., & Mattick, J. S. (2007). Noncoding RNAs and RNA editing in brain development, functional diversification, and neurological disease. *Physiological Review, 87*(3), 799–823.

Mehler, M. F. ,& Purpura, D. P. (2009). Autism, fever, epigenetics and the locus coeruleus. *Brain Research.Reviews. 59*(2), 388–392.

Mendelson, L., Dunn, M. A., & Miller, A. (2007). Let's get ready for social skills: A program for preschool children with pervasive developmental disorders. *Autism Spectrum Quarterly*, (Fall), 24–27.

Ming, X., Brimacombe, M., & Wagner, G. C. (2007). Prevalence of motor impairment in autism spectrum disorders. *Brain and Development, 29*(9), 565–570.

Minshew, N. J., & Williams, D. L. (2007). The new neurobiology of autism: Cortex, connectivity, and neuronal organization. *Archives of Neurology, 64*(7), 945–950.

Mintz, M., Alessandri, M., & Curatolo, P. (2006). Treatment approaches for the autism spectrum disorders. In R. Tuchman & I. Rapin (Eds.), *Autism: A neurological disorder of early brain development* (pp. 281–307). London: Mac Keith Press.

Mostofsky, S. H., Goldberg, M. C., Landa, R. J., & Denckla, M. B. (2000). Evidence for a deficit in procedural learning in children and adolescents with autism: Implications for cerebellar contribution. *Journal of the International Neuropsychology Society, 6*, 752–759.

Mottron, L., Dawson, M., Soulieres, I., Hubert, B., & Burack, J. (2006). Enhanced perceptual functioning in autism: An update, and eight principles of autistic perception. *Journal of Autism and Developmental Disorders, 36*(1), 27–43.

Muhle, R., Trentacoste, S. V., & Rapin, I. (2004). The genetics of autism. *Pediatrics, 113*(5), e472–e486.

Obler, L. K., & Fein, D. (1988). *The exceptional brain: Neuropsychology of talent and special abilities.* New York: Guilford 1Press.

Olsson, I., Steffenburg, S., & Gillberg, C. (1988). Epilepsy in autism and autisticlike conditions: A population- based study. *Archives of Neurology, 45*, 666–668.

O'Roak, B. J., & State, M. W. (2008). Autism genetics: Strategies, challenges, and opportunities. *Autism Research, 1*(1), 4–17.

Persico, A. M., & Bourgeron, T. (2006). Searching for ways out of the autism maze: Genetic, epigenetic, and environmental clues. *Trends in Neurosciences, 29*(7), 349–358.

Pickett, J. (2001). Current investigations in autism brain tissue research. *Journal of Autism and Developmental Disorders, 31*(6), 521–527.

Purpura, D. P., & Suzuki, K. (1976). Distortion of neuronal geometry and formation of aberrant synapses in neuronal storage disease. *Brain Research, 116*(1), 1–21.

Rapin, I. (Ed.). (1996a). *Preschool children with inadequate communication: Developmental language disorders, autism, low IQ.* London: Mac Keith Press.

Rapin, I. (1996b). Practitioner review: Developmental language disorders: A clinical update. *Journal of Child Psychology and Psychiatry, 37*(6), 643–655.

Rapin, I. (1996c). Neurological examination. In I. Rapin (Ed.), *Preschool children with inadequate communication: Developmental language disorders, autism, low IQ* (pp. 98–122). London: MacKeith Press.

Rapin, I. (1996d). Historical data. In I. Rapin (Ed.), *Preschool children with inadequate communication: Developmental language disorders, autism, low IQ* (pp. 58–97). London: Mac Keith Press.

Rapin, I. (2001). Autistic spectrum disorders: Relevance to Tourette syndrome. In D. J. Cohen, J. Jankovic & C. G. Goetz (Eds.), *Tourette syndrome* (pp. 89–101). Philadelphia: Lippincott Williams & Wilkins.

Rapin, I. (2006). Atypical sensory/perceptual responsiveness. In R. F. Tuchman & I. Rapin (Eds.), *Autism: A neurological disorder of early brain development.* London: Mac Keith Press.

Rapin, I., Dunn, M., Allen, D. A., Stevens, M., & Fein, D. (2009). Subtypes of language disorders in schoolage children with autism. *Developmental Neuropsychology, 34*(1), 1–9.

Rapin, I., & Tuchman, R. F. (2008). What is new in autism? *Current Opinion in Neurology, 21*(2), 143–149.

Raynes, H. R., Shanske, A., Goldberg, S., Burde, R., & Rapin, I. (1999). Joubert syndrome: Monozygotic twins with discordant phenotypes. *Journal of Child Neurology, 14*(10), 649–654.

Rimland, B. (1964). *Infantile autism: The syndrome and its implications for a neural theory of behavior.* New York: Appleton-Century-Crofts.

Ritvo, E. R., Freeman, B. J., Pingree, C., Mason-Brothers, A., Jorde, L., Jenson, W. R., et al. (1989). The UCLA-University of Utah epidemiologic survey of autism: Prevalence. *American Journal of Psychiatry, 146*, 194–199.

Rizzolatti, G., & Craighero, L. (2004). The mirror-neuron system. *Annual Review of Neuroscience, 27*, 169–192.

Rogers, S. (2007). Nature of motor imitation problems in school-aged males with autism. *Developmental Medicine and Child Neurology, 49*(1), 5.

Rutter, M., Bailey, A., Bolton, P., & Le Couteur, A. (1994). Autism and known medical conditions: Myth and substance. *Journal of Child Psychology and Psychiatry, 2*, 311–322.

Rzhetsky, A., Wajngurt, D., Park, N., & Zheng, T. (2007). Probing genetic overlap among complex human phenotypes. *Proceedings of the National Academy of Sciences of the United States of America, 104*(28), 11694–11699.

Saka, E., Goodrich, C., Harlan P., Madras, B. K., & Graybiel, A. M. (2004). Repetitive behaviors in monkeys are linked to specific striatal activation patterns. *Journal of Neuroscience, 24*(34), 7557–7565.

Sallows, G. O., & Graupner, T. D. (2005). Intensive behavioral treatment for children with autism: Four-year outcome and predictors. *American Journal of Mental Retardation, 110*(6), 417–438.

Samson, F., Mottron, L., Jemel, B., Belin, P., & Ciocca, V. (2006). Can spectro-temporal complexity explain the autistic pattern of performance on auditory tasks? *Journal of Autism and Developmental Disorders, 36*(1), 65–76.

Sanua, V. D. (1990). Leo Kanner (1894–1981): The man and the scientist. *Child Psychiatry and Human Development, 21*(1), 3–23.

Scahill, L., Koenig, K., Carroll, D. H., & Pachler, M. (2007). Risperidone approved for the treatment of serious behavioral problems in children with autism. *Journal of Child and Adolescent Psychiatry Nursing, 20*(3), 188–190.

Schain, R. J., & Freedman, D. X. (1961). Studies on 5-hydroxyindole metabolism in autistic and other mentally retarded children. *Journal of Pediatrics, 59*, 315–320.

Schmahmann, J. D. (2004). Disorders of the cerebellum: Ataxia, dysmetria of thought, and the cerebellar cognitive affective syndrome. *Journal of Neuropsychiatry and Clinical Neuroscience, 16*(3), 367–378.

Schopler, E., & Olley, J. G. (1982). Comprehensive educational services for autistic children: The TEACCH model. In C. R. Reynolds & T. R. Gutkin (Eds.), *The handbook of school psychology* (pp. 629–643). New York: Wiley.

Schopler, E., Reichler, R. J., & Renner, B. R. (1986). *The Childhood Autism Rating Scale (CARS) for diagnostic screening and classification in autism.* New York: Irvington.

Schreibman, L., & Ingersoll, B. (2005). Behavioral interventions to promote learning in individuals with autism. In F. R. Volkmar, R. Paul, A. Klin, & D. Cohen (Eds.), *Handbook of autism and pervasive developmental disorders* (pp. 882–896). New York: Wiley.

Shinnar, S., Rapin, I., Arnold, S., Tuchman, R. F., Shulman, L., Ballaban-Gil, K., et al. (2001). Language regression in childhood. *Pediatric Neurology, 24*(3), 185–191.

Steffenburg, S., Gillberg, C., & Holmgren, L. (1986). A twin study of autism in Denmark, Finland, Iceland, Norway, and Sweden. *Journal of Child Psychology and Psychiatry, 30*, 405–416.

Stevens, M. C., Fein, D. A., Dunn, M., Allen, D., Waterhouse, L. H., Feinstein, C., et al. (2000). Subgroups of children with autism by cluster analysis: A longitudinal examination. *Journal of the American Academy of Child and Adolescent Psychiatry, 39*(3), 346–352.

Taft, L. T., & Cohen, H. (1971). Hypsarrhythmia and infantile autism: A clinical report. *Journal of Autism and Childhood Schizophrenia, 1*, 327–336.

Tager-Flusberg, H., & Joseph, R. M. (2003). Identifying neurocognitive phenotypes in autism. *Philosophical Transactions of the Royal Society of London. Series B, Biological Sciences, 358*(1430), 303–314.

Treffert, D. A. (2005). The savant syndrome in autistic disorder. In M. F. Casanova (Ed.), *Recent developments in autism research* (pp. 27–55). New York: Nova Science.

Tuchman, R., Moshe, S. L., & Rapin, I. (2009). Convulsing toward the pathophysiology of autism. *Brain and Development, 31*(2), 95–103.

Tuchman, R. F., & Rapin, I. (1997). Regression in pervasive developmental disorders: Seizures and epileptiform EEG correlates. *Pediatrics, 99*(4), 560–566.

Tuchman, R. F., Rapin, I., & Shinnar, S. (1991a). Autistic and dysphasic children. I: Clinical characteristics. *Pediatrics, 88*(6), 1211–1218.

Tuchman, R. F., Rapin, I., & Shinnar, S. (1991b). Autistic and dysphasic children: II. Epilepsy. *Pediatrics, 88*(6), 1219–1225.

Vargas, D. L., Nascimbene, C., Krishnan, C., Zimmerman, A. W., & Pardo, C. A. (2005). Neuroglial activation and neuroinflammation in the brain of patients with autism. *Annals of Neurology, 57*, 67–81.

Venter, J. C., Adams, M. D., Myers, E. W., Li, P. W., Mural, R. J., Sutton, G. G., et al. (2001) The sequence of the human genome. *Science, 291*(5507), 1304–1351.

Vivanti, G., Nadig, A., Ozonoff, S., & Rogers, S. J. (2008). What do children with autism attend to during imitation tasks? *Journal of Experimental Child Psychology, 101*(3), 186–205.

Volkmar, F. R., & Nelson, D. S. (1990). Seizure disorders in autism. *Journal of the American Academy of Child and Adolescent Psychiatry, 29*, 127–129.

Volkmar, F. R., Paul, R., Klin, A., & Cohen, D. (Eds.). (2005). *Handbook of autism and pervasive developmental disorders.* New York: Wiley.

Weidenheim, K. M., Goodman, L., Dickson, D. W., Gillberg, C., Rastam, M., & Rapin, I. (2001). Etiology and pathophysiology of autistic behavior: Clues from two cases with an unusual variant of neuroaxonal dystrophy. *Journal of Child Neurology, 16*, 809–819.

Weiss, L. A., Shen, Y., Korn, J. M., Arking, D. E., Miller, D. T., Fossdal, R., et al. (2008). Association between microdeletion and microduplication at 16p11.2 and autism. *New England Journal of Medicine, 358*(7), 667–675.

Werner, E., & Dawson, G. (2005). Validation of the phenomenon of autistic regression using home videotapes. *Archives of General Psychiatry, 62*(8), 889–895.

Wills, S., Cabanlit, M., Bennett, J., Ashwood, P., Amaral, D., & Van de Water, J. (2007). Autoantibodies in autism spectrum disorders (ASD). *Annals of the New York Academy of Sciences, 1107*, 79–91.

Wing, L., & Gould, J. (1979). Severe impairments of social interaction and associated abnormalities in children: Epidemiology and classification. *Journal of Autism and Developmental Disorders, 9*, 11–29.

Wing, L., & Potter, D. (2002). The epidemiology of autistic spectrum disorders: Is the prevalence rising? *Mental Retardation and Developmental Disability Research Reviews*, *8*(3), 151–161.

Yip, J., Soghomonian, J. J., & Blatt, G. J. (2007). Decreased GAD67 mRNA levels in cerebellar Purkinje cells in autism: Pathophysiological implications. *Acta Neuropathologica (Berl)*, *113*(5), 559–568.

Ylisaukko-oja, T., Alarcon, M., Cantor, R. M., Auranen, M., Vanhala, R., Kempas, E., et al. (2006). Search for autism loci by combined analysis of Autism Genetic Resource Exchange and Finnish families. *Annals of Neurology*, *59*(1), 145–155.

Zhao, X., Leotta, A., Kustanovich, V., Lajonchere, C., Geschwind, D. H., Law, K., et al. (2007). A unified genetic theory for sporadic and inherited autism. *Proceedings of the National Academy of Sciences of the United States of America*, *104*(31), 12831–12836.

Zoghbi, H. Y. (2003). Postnatal neurodevelopmental disorders: meeting at the synapse? *Science*, *302*(5646), 826–830.

Zwaigenbaum, L., Bryson, S., Rogers, T., Roberts, W., Brian, J., & Szatmari, P. (2005). Behavioral manifestations of autism in the first year of life. *International Journal of Developmental Neuroscience*, *23*(2–3), 143–152.

Section I

Historical Perspective, Diagnosis and Classification, and Epidemiology

1 Michael Rutter

Autism Spectrum Disorders: Looking Backward and Looking Forward

Points of Interest

- Meaning of association with raised paternal age.
- Meaning of copy number variations.
- Nature of nongenetic causal influences.
- Nature of genetic liability at the molecular level.
- Transition from the broader phenotype to a handicapping disorder.

Introduction

It is now well over half a century since Kanner (1943) first postulated the syndrome of autism. He provided a remarkably incisive, detailed description and conceptual outline that has stood the test of time in almost all respects. Nevertheless, there have been huge changes in the understanding of autistic spectrum disorders (ASD), and research findings have clarified a range of crucial questions while, at the same time, presenting many further challenges. This chapter starts with a succinct summary of some of the main research accomplishments to date, then proceeds to outline a range of challenges that remain. Throughout, there is an emphasis on research findings and research challenges that have potentially important clinical implications.

Clinical Findings

The story starts with the validation of the differentiation between autism and a range of other child psychiatric disorders. This was shown by the distinctiveness of the clinical pattern, after matching groups for mental age, together with the finding that these differences persisted over time and were accompanied by a distinctive cognitive profile (Rutter, Greenfeld, & Lockyer, 1967; Lockyer & Rutter, 1969; Lockyer & Rutter, 1970). For a while, autism was regarded as an infantile psychosis, but numerous differences between autism and schizophrenia indicated that it was a mistake to see autism as an early manifestation of schizophrenia (Kolvin, 1971; Rimland, 1964; Rutter, 1972). Equally, although many individuals with autism also showed an intellectual disability, autism differed from general intellectual disability in numerous ways, including sex ratio, cognitive patterns, social class distribution, head circumference, and neuropathological findings (Rutter & Schopler, 1987).

Although Kanner had postulated that autism had a "constitutional" origin, he had not specified a neurodevelopmental origin as such. This was first demonstrated decisively by the finding that individuals with autism, who had shown no discernible neurological abnormality in early childhood, nevertheless showed a markedly increased rate of epileptic seizures in adolescence or early adult life (Rutter, 1970). More recent research (Bolton et al., in press) has shown that, in the majority of cases, seizures began after age 10 years. Epilepsy in the proband was not associated with an increased risk of epilepsy in relatives, but it was associated with the broader phenotype in other family members. Follow-up studies identified low IQ and a lack of language by age 5 as the key predictors of outcome (Eisenberg, 1956; Kanner, 1973; Howlin, Goode, Hutton, & Rutter, 2004).

Once the diagnostic criteria for autism became clarified, it became both possible and necessary to develop reliable and valid interview and observation measures. A range of assessment methods were developed but, over time, the autism diagnostic interview (Lord, Rutter, & Le Couteur, 1994; Rutter, Le Couteur, & Lord, 2003) and the autism diagnostic observation schedule (Lord et al., 1989; Lord, Rutter, DiLavore, & Le Couteur, 2001) came to be accepted as the best diagnostic methods available. Initially, most clinicians had assumed that children with autism were untestable by quantified psychometric approaches, and it was important that both the follow-up studies and detailed experimental studies showed that this was not the case (Lockyer & Rutter, 1969; Hermelin & O'Connor, 1970). To the contrary, given appropriate skilled testing, most individuals with autism are testable and moreover the psychometric findings proved stable over time.

As the concept of autism changed from a psychogenic variety of early-onset schizophrenia to an early-onset neurodevelopmental disorder, methods of treatment switched in parallel to developmentally oriented behavioral methods. It became clear from comparative studies that structure and focus in special education were the key features (Schopler, Brehm, Kinsbourne, & Reichler, 1971; Rutter & Bartak, 1973), and psychological methods of treatment that involved developmental and behavioral principles and partnership with parents were developed (Schopler & Reichler, 1971; Howlin et al., 1987; Marcus, Kunce, & Schopler, 2005). Moreover, systematic studies showed that these methods of intervention brought worthwhile benefits (National Research Council, 2001; Howlin, 1998).

As concepts of autism changed, attention turned to the possibility of genetic influences on the liability to autism. Initially, most commentators had dismissed the possibility on the grounds that the base-rate of autism in siblings was so low—estimated at ~2% in the 1960s. The key question, however, was whether the rate of autism in families exceeded the base rate in the general population. Expressed in this way, it became clear that there was a huge increase in relative risk of the order of 20- to 100-fold (Bolton et al., 1994). Moreover, twin studies showed that the familial loading was strongly genetically influenced (Bailey et al., 1995). Most psychiatric geneticists in the 1970s tended to think of genetic influences in relation to Mendelian transmission of an entirely determinative kind. The first systematic twin study (Folstein & Rutter, 1977a, 1977b) was important in demonstrating that the genetic liability extended beyond the traditional diagnosis to include a broader phenotype (Le Couteur et al., 1996). This provided a key indication of the necessity to broaden the concept of autism.

The altered concept of autism as a neurodevelopmental disorder meant that attention came to be paid to the possibility that some cases might arise on the basis of a medical condition of some kind. Gillberg (1992) claimed that this applied to as many as 37% of cases, but an overall review of the evidence suggested that the proportion was probably nearer 10% (Rutter, Bailey, Bolton, & Le Couteur, 1994). Nevertheless, 10% was sufficiently high to mean that the clinical assessment of individuals with autism had to include a proper assessment of possible associated medical conditions. The evidence was strongest in the case of the association with tuberous sclerosis (Smalley, 1998) and, to a lesser extent, the Fragile X anomaly (Bailey et al., 1993), but it included a mixed bag of other medical conditions and it was also found that the 5–10% rate of chromosome anomalies (albeit not diagnostically specific) seemed to be substantially increased above base population levels. The use of Wood's light to pick up cases of tuberous sclerosis became routine, as did the use of DNA methods to identify Fragile X. Although the meaning of chromosome anomalies was not clear, it also became standard practice to karyotype individuals. Interestingly, in his first report Kanner (an astute clinician) had noted the enlarged head size found in a substantial minority of individuals with autism. More recently, his findings have been amply confirmed initially by head circumference measurement (Fombonne, Rogé, Claverie, Courty, & Frémolle, 1999; Woodhouse et al., 1996), then later by structural brain imaging findings. During the last decade or so, systematic research has also been highly informative in showing that the enlarged brain size is not evident at birth but develops during the 1- to 3-year age period then tends to stabilize and not increase further (Courchesne, Carper, & Akshoomoff, 2003; Redcay & Courchesne, 2005). It seems highly likely that, although the mechanisms remain ill-understood, this is a neural feature that differentiates autism from other neurodevelopmental conditions.

A key breakthrough with respect to cognitive patterns came with Hermelin and O'Connor's (1970) demonstration of a basic mentalizing defect. This led the way to identification in the mid-1980s of an impaired Theory of Mind (ToM) associated with the majority of cases of autism (Baron-Cohen, Leslie, & Frith, 1985). Attention came to be focused on the possible role of specific cognitive deficits as the basis for the social abnormalities of autism (Rutter, 1983, 1987). The ToM finding has been amply confirmed as applying to the great majority of individuals with autism, although some 20% pass standard ToM tests (Frith, 2003a; Happé, 2003). One problem with the Theory of Mind notion, however, is that the social deficits repeatedly found in autism are evident long before ToM, at least as established in relation to standard tests, becomes apparent in normal children. This led the way to a study of key social cognitive deficits (especially joint attention) evident before the development of ToM (Mundy & Sigman, 1989; Sigman et al., 1999; Mundy & Burnette, 2005). In his initial case report, Kanner had argued that individuals with autism had a basically normal level of general intelligence. That has not proved to be the case, but what has become clearer is that savant skills (usually involving mathematics or memory, as evident in calendrical calculation or the ability to draw in detail from memory or similarly play a piece of music heard only once), or unusual specific cognitive skills (meaning skills—often on visuospatial or memory tests—that are both above the individual's own overall cognitive level and above general population norms) are common in autism—applying to some 1 in 4 autistic individuals (Howlin, Goode, Hutton, & Rutter, 2009). Moreover, systematic experimental studies have shown that these skills are real and not just peculiar tricks (Hermelin, 2001). Accordingly, explanations of autism need to account for both intellectual impairment and also marked intellectual skills (see also Happé & Frith, 2010).

About the same time as Kanner's first report, there was a report by Asperger (1944) of a somewhat similar syndrome. His account does not compare with Kanner's in terms of incisiveness, but it highlighted that autistic-like patterns could and did develop in individuals who lacked the global language delay that, at least up until that point, had been viewed as a necessary characteristic of autism. Although there were a number of reports of autistic psychopathy in the European literature in the years that followed (see van Krevelen, 1963), the diagnostic concept only became established after a key report by Lorna Wing (1981) and a publication of the English translation of Asperger's paper (Frith, 1991). Numerous epidemiological and clinical studies since then have amply confirmed the reality of this pattern, although views differ on the distinctiveness of the syndrome as different from autism in intellectually high functioning individuals (Klin, McPartland, & Volkmar, 2005; Szatmari et al., 2009). Nevertheless, whatever the answer to that query may prove to be, the descriptions played an important role in the acceptance of a broader spectrum of autism disorders. The extension upward into syndromes in the individuals of normal levels of overall intelligence was paralleled by the earlier demonstration by Wing and Gould (1979), of the extension downward to individuals with profound intellectual disability.

Numerous reports over the years had indicated that a substantial minority (25–33%) showed a pronounced developmental regression usually occurring at the end of the second year of life (Rutter, 2005a, 2008). Surprisingly, these reports gave rise to remarkably little in the way of systematic research, but home videos (Werner & Dawson, 2005) and, more recently, follow-up of siblings of individuals with autism (Bryson et al., 2007) have confirmed the reality of the pattern of regression. Moreover, it seems that this pattern may be particularly distinctive in autism, regression in other neurodevelopmental disorders being much less common (Baird et al., 2008; Pickles et al., 2009).

In 1966, there was a key discovery of a hitherto unrecognized syndrome involving characteristic loss of purposive hand movements—usually in the second year of life—and accompanied by a range of social and behavioral abnormalities (Rett, 1966). At first, it received little recognition, and its general acceptance was only established some years later by a key report by Hagberg, Aicardi, Dias, and Ramos (1983). Subsequently, it was found that in the great majority of cases, the disorder was due to a pathological mutation on the X chromosome (Amir et al., 1999). Although, for convenience, Rett syndrome was placed within ASD, it is clinically quite different with respect to diagnostic features, and particularly course and etiology (Rutter, 2005b). It occurs almost exclusively in females (contrasting with the male preponderance in ASD), there is deceleration of head growth in the early years (the opposite of the patterns in ASD), there is a loss of purposive hand movements (not found in ASD), and there is a later deterioration in motor function (Van Acker, Loncola, & Van Acker, 2005).

Although the claim that autism was a psychogenic disorder associated with poor parenting had long since become discredited (not because it was decisively disproven, but because of a lack of supporting evidence coupled with growing evidence for the importance of genetically influenced neurodevelopmental impairment), findings have shown that an autistic-like pattern develops in a substantial minority of individuals subjected to profound institutional deprivation (Rutter et al., 1999, 2007). It is similar to autism with respect to impaired social reciprocity and awareness of social context, as well as in the presence of abnormal preoccupations and circumscribed interests. It differs, however, in the greater presence of social approach and communicative flexibility, and especially in the marked diminution in autistic features as the individuals grow older (see also Rutter & Sonuga-Barke, 2010). The precise meaning of this pattern in relation to etiology remains unclear, but circumstantial evidence suggests that profound perceptual deprivation, arising from environmental conditions, may give rise to a similar pattern that is more ordinarily associated with autism. The same may apply to the autistic-like patterns found in some congenitally blind children (Hobson, Lee, & Brown, 1999).

Research Accomplishments Reflecting Technological Innovations

Dawson and her colleagues (Dawson, Finley, Phillips, & Galpert, 1985; Dawson, 1994) pioneered the EEG use of evoked event-related potentials to examine brain functioning in autism. The technique remains a useful one (Nelson & Luciana, 1998), especially as current studies focus on the earliest patterns of brain function in infants and toddlers at risk for autism. To date, however, the two technologies that have been most informative with respect to autism have been structural and functional brain imaging (Frith, 2003b) and molecular genetics (Bacchelli & Maestrini, 2006; Freitag, 2007). The former have been consistent in showing that autism is not due to a localized brain abnormality. The findings have also shown that the increased head size reflects an increased brain size (Redcay & Courchesne, 2005). Although the details are not yet entirely clear, it is generally accepted that the imaging data indicate that autism is associated with some form of abnormal neural connectivity. The functional imaging findings have also been instructive in showing that individuals with autism solve cognitive tasks using areas of the brain that differ from those used by typically developing individuals (Frith & Frith, 2008). Neurochemical findings have been, on the whole, rather uninformative, apart from the fact that it has been consistently found that blood serotonin levels are raised in a substantial minority of individuals with autism (although this does not show diagnostic specificity; Anderson & Hoshino, 2005). Molecular genetic evidence has pointed to several chromosomal regions likely to contain susceptibility genes. On the other hand, it has proved quite frustrating that specific genes underlying multifactorial autism have not, as yet, been identified. The most recent findings, bringing together several large-scale data sets, have shown the likely importance of copy number variations—meaning submicroscopic deletions and duplications (Persico & Bourgeron, 2006; Sebat et al., 2007; Autism Genome Project Consortium, 2007; Weiss et al., 2008).

Overview of Research Accomplishments

Looking back on the successful research strategies, it is evident that good use has been made of longitudinal studies with appropriate comparison groups, that the observation of the unexpected has been crucial, that the development of systematic standardized measures has greatly improved comparability across studies, and that knowledge on psychological processes associated with autism have greatly benefited from parallel studies in typically developing children. Quantitative genetics have been decisive in showing that the heritability of liability to autism is very high—probably in the region of 90%. Creative experimental strategies have been crucial in delineating the cognitive features associated with autism and structural and functional imaging has been invaluable in demonstrating the neural concomitants of these cognitive features. Molecular genetic strategies are likely to be highly informative, and there is replicated evidence of likely chromosomal regions that may be expected to contain susceptibility genes, but the identification of these genes remains a challenge for the future.

Some Inconclusive Research

There is no convincing evidence that the basic deficits associated with autism are regularly relieved by any form of psychotropic medication (Scahill & Martin, 2005). That is a striking negative finding because pharmacological interventions have proved of value in almost all other psychiatric disorders. Equally, there is no convincing evidence of any neurochemical abnormality specifically associated with autism (Anderson & Hoshino, 2005) and no convincing evidence of particular EEG patterns that are specifically associated with autism (Minshew, Sweeney, Baumann, & Webb, 2005). There are leads pointing to possible immune abnormalities associated with autism, but the evidence to date is inconclusive (Medical Research Council MRC, 2001; Pardo, Vargas, & Zimmerman, 2005). Finally, there is no convincing evidence that the benefits of psychological intervention are contingent on either very early or very intensive application. Authoritative reviews (National Research Council, 2001) have suggested that very early intensive intervention may be particularly effective, but it has to be said that the evidence in support is relatively scanty. On the other hand, there is growing evidence that comprehensive early behavioral treatments result in substantial worthwhile developmental gains (Rogers & Vismara, 2008). The uncertainties concern both the claims that these gains only occur with highly intensive, very early treatment, and the claims of full recovery.

Animal models have proved immensely informative in medicine because of their value in testing causal mechanisms (Hernandez & Blazer, 2005; Weatherall, 2006). They allow systematic study of the temporal sequence of events, and by the removal and add-back of hypothesized mediators (at the genetic, protein, physiological, behavioral, or social environment level), strong leverage on causal questions is possible. Of course, these are crucially dependent on the validity of the animal model—a particularly difficult challenge in the case of autism (Crawley, 2007). Mentalizing skills and language features cannot be assessed in rodents. Nevertheless, ingenious ways of measuring social interaction and communication in mice have been developed. Once one or more susceptibility genes have been identified, the possibilities could be transformed if a genetically modified mouse could be created, as was done in the case of Rett syndrome.

Two main varieties of model have been employed. First, there are those that focus on embryological origins—such as Rodier, Ingram, Tisdale, Nelson, and Romano's (1996) use of valproate to mimic the supposed prenatal effects of thalidomide on liability to autism. The thalidomide evidence is not very convincing (because it focuses on cranial nerve lesions that are not characteristic of autism), and the supposed validation through reproduction of cerebellar abnormalities (Ingram, Peckham, Tisdale, & Rodier, 2000) has the limitation of using a disputed human finding (see Bailey, Phillips, & Rutter, 1996). Second, targeted gene mutations may be used to examine gene effects—as has been done very successfully in the case of Rett syndrome (Guy, Hendrich, Holmes, Martin, & Bird, 2001; Shahbazian et al., 2002). Oxytocin knockout mice were found to display deficits in social recognition and social memory, but not in social approach (Crawley et al., 2007), leaving the parallel with autism somewhat uncertain. Cross-fostering can be used as an additional research tactic to check whether social differences between genetic strains might be an artifact of the rearing environment (Yang, Zhodzishsky, & Crawley, 2007). Because of the difficulties in the modeling of key features of autism in mice, the potential of mouse models is difficult to evaluate, but it would seem to be an avenue worth further exploration. Primates are closer to humans. Study of amygdala lesions in developing and mature macaque monkeys was informative in showing that it was unlikely that the amygdala has a fundamental role in the core social impairments found in autism, although it did play a role in fear responses that could be relevant (Prather et al., 2001; Bauman, Lavenex, Mason, Capitanio, & Amaral, 2004; Amaral & Corbett, 2003).

Some Misleading Research Claims

There have been many misleading therapeutic claims. These are too numerous to list but they include; fenfluramine (McDougle, 1997), secretin (Scahill & Martin, 2005), and holding therapy (Howlin, 1998). Of course, it is inevitable that some promising interventions may not prove their worth, but what is regrettable is that some of these claims have been in high-impact journals and accompanied by extremely uncritical statements from leading scientists. There is also the misleading claim that facilitated communication reveals normal functioning in autistic individuals. Early studies led to the claim that autism was caused by urinary polypeptide abnormalities, but when the research was undertaken with experimenters blinded to the diagnosis of the contributors of the samples it could not confirm the findings (Le Couteur, Trygstad, Evered, Gillberg, & Rutter, 1988). In recent times, there was the claim that MMR (Measles, Mumps, & Rubella vaccine) had led to a massive epidemic of autism. Although the claim was based on a very weak study, it too was published in a high-impact journal (Wakefield et al., 1998). Subsequent epidemiological research has been consistently negative with respect to the claim that MMR has led to a rise in the rate of autism (see Honda, Shimizu, & Rutter, 2005; Rutter, 2005) and well-conducted studies have also shown that the measles virus in tissues claims were mistaken (Baird et al., 2008; Hornig et al., 2008; D'Souza, Fombonne, & Ward, 2006; Afzal et al., 2006).

Earlier, there was a claim that at least one quarter of cases of autism were caused by the Fragile X anomaly (Gillberg & Wahlström, 1985), whereas better studies subsequently showed that the true proportion was probably below 5% (Bailey et al., 1993). Another early claim was that autism was due to perceptual inconstancy (Ornitz & Ritvo, 1968), or to vestibular dysfunction (Ornitz, 1978). This claim was based on comparisons that did not take account of mental age (see Yule, 1978, on the need to control for mental age), and the findings have not stood the test of rigorous testing. The same applies to claims regarding overselectivity (Lovaas & Schreibman, 1971), which proved to be a function of mental age (Schover & Newsom, 1976; Lovaas, Koegel, & Schreibman, 1979).

Looking Ahead: Remaining Puzzles and Challenges

Inevitably, as with any field of inquiry, numerous research challenges remain. Here, attention is primarily drawn to those that are likely to have important clinical implications. It is appropriate to start with three well-demonstrated clinical features that, nevertheless, remain very poorly understood. First, there is the question of what is the meaning of the regression that occurs in ASD (see Rutter, 2008). What brain mechanisms underlie its occurrence, and how often is it found in other developmental disorders of language? Recent evidence (Baird et al., 2008; Pickles et al., 2009) indicates that a developmental regression is particularly characteristic of autism and is much less frequent with other developmental language disorders. Finding from multiplex families suggest that there is no familial influence on regression other than that which concerns autism itself (Parr et al., in press). The likelihood is that it reflects a developmental change in the neural mechanisms underlying language related skills, rather than any extrinsic environmental influence, but what are those neural mechanisms?

What is the meaning of the savant skills in autism (Howlin et al., 2009), what brain mechanisms underlie their recurrence, and how often are they found in other neurodevelopmental disorders? With respect to both regression and savant skills, there is a need to question what leads to their occurrence and also to question whether it is a categorical feature or rather a dimensional characteristic that may be found in greater or lesser degrees. What is the meaning of epilepsy in autism? What brain mechanisms underlie its occurrence, and why is the peak age of onset in late adolescence (Minshew et al., 2005; Bolton et al., in press) rather than in early childhood, which is what is usually found in both the general population and in individuals with intellectual disability?

It is well established that there is a broader phenotype of autism, meaning a qualitatively similar pattern of social communicative and developmental impairments that is similar to that found in autism "proper," but that differs in not being associated with either intellectual disability or epilepsy (Bailey et al., 1995). Questions remain on how this is best identified and quantified (but see Dawson et al., 2007). What happens to individuals with a broader phenotype as they grow older? What mechanisms are involved in the transition of the broader phenotype to the more obviously handicapping disorder? Does this simply reflect a higher "dose" of the genetic liability or is there some kind of "two hit" mechanism, in which some other factor (either intrinsic or extrinsic) is implicated?

What are the origins of the intellectual disability found in so many individuals with autism? Some researchers who have focused on higher functioning individuals have tended to dismiss the issue on the grounds that it is simply some independent impairment having a different origin. This seems rather unlikely, given both the strength of the association and the fact that, within monozygotic twin pairs, one may show intellectual disability and the other not (Le Couteur et al., 1996). Moreover, experimental cognitive studies have shown substantial overlap in the pattern of impairments found in individuals with autism who are and who are not intellectually disabled.

Traditionally, autism has been conceptualized as a meaningful syndrome, but recently that concept has been challenged by claims that the individual components of autism may not only be more separate than appreciated, but also that they may reflect different genetic influences (Ronald, Happé, & Plomin, 2005). The question is a reasonable one, but it has to be said that the evidence in support of the claim is somewhat contradictory and inconclusive. What is needed (and not yet available) is evidence on the general prevalence of the different components of autism, individually measured in a way that does not necessitate the diagnostic concept. The key question then is to what extent the three main domains of impairment in autism co-occur.

A rather different question is why autism differs from most other psychiatric disorders in showing no substantial response to neuroleptics? There are minor benefits with respect to individual behavioral features, but the evidence to date is that there is no substantial effect on the basic features of autism. Does that mean that research has focused on the wrong neuroleptics or does it mean that the abnormalities should not be conceptualized in neurotransmitter terms but, rather, in terms of some other underlying mechanism, such as immunological abnormalities (Pardo, Vargas, & Zimmerman, 2005)? The supporting evidence on immune features is weak and inconclusive, but it constitutes a possibility worth investigating more thoroughly.

A recent well conducted study showed a quite strong association between high paternal age and an increased risk of ASD (Reichenberg et al., 2007). Two other studies (Cantor, Yoon, Furr, & Lajonchere, 2007; Croen, Najjar, Fireman, & Grether, 2007) have shown something similar, so it may be that this is a reasonably robust finding. Nonetheless, further replication is desirable and the question remains on what this association means. Why is the association mostly with paternal age rather than maternal age (although there is some evidence in support of both associations)? If confirmed, does the association mean that the nongenetic factor in autism should be conceptualized in terms of stochastic (random) developmental perturbations, rather than the influence of some specific environmental factor?

A somewhat similar question has to be posed with respect to the association with copy number variations (CNV) and with a high rate of chromosome abnormalities. The evidence to date suggests that it may not be the effect of a specific CNV (but see Eichler & Zimmerman, 2008; Weiss et al., 2008, with regard to CNVs on chromosome 16 and ASD unassociated with regression), or a specific chromosomal anomaly (apart from the association with interstitial duplications on chromosome 15 that are of maternal origin). Rather, the basic questions concern why individuals with ASD are much more likely than other people to have a chromosomal anomaly or microdeletions and microduplications, the nature of the biological consequences of CNV (Cook & Scherer, 2008), and the meaning of the indication that CNVs may be associated with schizophrenia as well as with autism (International Schizophrenia Consortium, 2008).

What mechanisms underlie the male preponderance in ASD? Baron-Cohen (2002) has argued that autism constitutes an extreme of "maleness," but that ignores the important finding that a male preponderance is common with most, but not all, early neurodevelopmental disorders (Rutter, Caspi, & Moffitt, 2003). Although there might be mechanisms that are specifically associated with each neurodevelopmental disorder, it seems likely that there will be some commonality underlying the male preponderance. What mechanism might this reflect? Might it reflect some influence on gene expression, for example?

It is already noted that major intellectual disability is a very important prognostic factor for poor outcome in autism, but what is surprising from the systematic long-term follow-up studies, is that a substantial proportion of individuals of normal intelligence nevertheless also have a poor adult outcome (Howlin et al., 2004). Why is this the case? Does it reflect some aspect of the underlying neural abnormality, or does it reflect inadequate interventions in childhood, or does it reflect inadequate services in adult life? Satisfactory answers to these questions have yet to be obtained.

The genetic evidence suggests that autism is usually a multifactorial disorder—meaning that multiple genetic influences and multiple environmental factors are likely to be implicated (Rutter, 2005b). But what are the nongenetic contributory causes of autism, and what mechanisms might be involved? Attention has rightly shifted from the unlikely hypothesis that poor parenting is responsible, to the more likely expectation that some prenatal or early postnatal factor might be implicated. Large-scale prospective studies beginning during pregnancy, and involving good biological measures, are clearly indicated (Magnus et al., 2006; Rønningen et al., 2006; Stotltenberg et al., 2010). Insofar as there are prenatal or early postnatal environmental causal effects, do they operate through toxicological, allergic, or immunological mechanisms? So far, it is unclear what the answers may be, but we must take seriously the possibility that there are important environmental features that play a role in the etiology of autism. Their elucidation is likely to be facilitated by gains in our understanding of genetic vulnerability (Geschwind & Levitt, 2007).

What is the neuropathology of autism (Amaral, Schumann, & Nordahl, 2008; Bailey et al., 1998; Bauman & Kemper, 2005)? There is abundant evidence that some form of neural underpinning is likely to be implicated in autism, but what is it? Evidence to date suggests that, ordinarily, prenatal abnormalities are likely to be responsible, but the evidence base is decidedly slim. Moreover, the postmortem studies are constrained by the fact that most deaths occur in individuals who have severe intellectual disability and epilepsy as well as autism. The question remains as to how far the neuropathological findings in this group generalize to the broader range of ASD. It is undoubtedly good that brain-banks are being established in the United States and Europe, but the findings so far are not providing definitive answers. On the other hand, the integration with imaging studies may constitute an important way forward (Munson et al., 2006; Schumann & Amaral, 2006; Courchesne et al., 2007; Kennedy & Courchesne, 2008).

What neural processes underlie the increase in brain size in the early preschool years? Prospective high-risk sibling studies with appropriate measures would help, but it is also essential that studies using animal models take on board the need to examine this key feature of the ASD phenotype. The experience with Rett syndrome, again, shows that this can be achieved (Guy et al., 2001). Moreover, the Rett example shows that, against expectation, the brain changes may be potentially reversible (Guy, Gan, Selfridge, Cobb, & Bird, 2007).

Claims have been made that dietary factors play a role in either the genesis of autism or the severity of impairments of autism. It has to be said that the evidence is, so far, rather unconvincing, but nevertheless it would be premature to rule out the possibility that dietary factors may play a role. For example, they seemed rather unlikely to be operative in ADHD, but good studies have indicated that they do play a role in a minority of cases (McCann et al., 2007). Although it seems unlikely that dietary factors play a primary role in the etiology of autism, they could constitute a contributory factor, and the possibility should be investigated. If they are shown to be operative, the further question arises as to what mechanisms might be involved.

A somewhat different question is what can be achieved through psychological interventions? There is good evidence in terms of their efficacy in reducing impairments and improving outcome. Nevertheless, it remains uncertain as to what extent efficacy depends on their early application at high intensity (Helt et al., 2008). Claims have been made that it does, but empirical evidence is thin. An important new randomized controlled trial of early intensive behavioral intervention (Dawson et al., 2009) showed there was a significant increase in IQ (albeit of modest size) in the treated group and not in controls. However, what this means is uncertain because there was no increase in social functioning as measured by the Vineland scale after 12 months. Also, the results showed there is no effect of the treatment on core features of autism assessed by the autism diagnostic observation schedule. Consequently, the study certainly does not support the Lovaas claims (Lovaas, 1987; McEachin, Smith, & Lovaas, 1993) about the huge benefits of early treatment leading to recovery.

What is also very new is the introduction of methods of treatment focussed on improving parental sensitivity and responsiveness. The randomized controlled trial undertaken by Green and his colleagues (2010) provides an excellent model of how RCTs should be undertaken. The findings were encouraging in showing substantial significant positive changes in parental sensitivity/responsivity, but disappointing in that there was only a very small improvement (relative to the control group) in the children's autistic features.

Moreover, we need to go on to ask what mechanisms mediate the observed efficacy. Also, do the children, apparently relieved of their major autistic handicaps, show a normalization of the social/cognitive deficits (Howlin, 2005)? The early reports from McEachin et al. (1993) reported that normalization was achieved in nearly half the cases, but subsequent studies have indicated that the benefits may be much more modest (Howard, Sparkman, Cohen, Green, & Stanislaw, 2005; Cohen, Amerine-Dickens, & Smith, 2006; Magiati, Charman, & Howlin, 2007). Also, follow-up studies of groups not receiving intensive interventions have shown that a few individuals with autism in the early preschool years, and a rather larger proportion with ASDs other than autism, cease to show autism by middle childhood. Do the findings indicate uncertainty over diagnosis at, say, 2 years, or has there been a true remission? Either way, the findings mean that caution should be exercised over therapeutic claims (Lord et al., 2006; Sutera et al., 2007).

What early psychological abnormalities precede the onset of the overt clinical manifestations? What is their meaning in terms of the abnormal psychology involved in autism and what is the meaning of the abnormal interconnectivity as found in imaging studies? How can the observations be translated into meaningful neural mechanisms? The empirical findings are persuasive, but it remains quite unclear what they mean in terms of what is going on in the brain. What are the brain mechanisms involved in compensatory processes? Up to now the greatest emphasis has been placed on impairments but, equally, it is clear that an important minority of individuals make remarkable progress. What is different about them and their experiences? We need to focus on protective mechanisms as well as on risk mechanisms. One of the interesting basic science findings concerns the identification of mirror neurons—meaning neurons that respond both to an individual's movements and to the observation of similar movements in another individual (Rizzolatti & Craighero, 2004). Clearly there is the potential that an abnormality in such mirror neurons might underly autism (see Dapretto, Lee, & Caplan, 2005), but do they actually underlie autism? How might that be tested in a rigorous systematic fashion? Fan, Decety, Yang, Liu, & Cheng (2010) used *mu* suppression on the EEG as an index of mirror neuron activity with findings casting doubt on the causal influence of mirror neurons in autism.? Also, if they are causal, the question remains as to why the psychological abnormalities are not manifest earlier than seems to be the case.

With respect to the genetic influences on liability to autism, a host of different questions arise. Are different genes involved in each of the key domains of autistic symptomatology? Will progress on identified genes require a focus on subgroups such as shown by language impairment (Alarcón, Yonan, Gilliam, Cantor, & Geshwind, 2005; Alarcón et al., 2008), insistence on sameness (Shao et al., 2003), or macrocephaly (Sacco et al., 2007)? Also, does the genetic liability vary between males and females? Will studies of gene expression help in establishing connections between genetic risk and specific brain structures (Alarcón et al., 2008; Nishimura et al., 2007)? Does the genetic liability operate dimensionally or categorically? What genetic factors and nongenetic factors operate in the transition from the broader phenotype to autism? What is the role of stochastic variation and developmental perturbations? Are these more relevant in sporadic cases of ASD than in familial cases (Sebat et al., 2007)? Also, are the relevant genes ones that code for proteins, or are they noncoding genes that influence genetic expression? To what extent is gene-environment interaction involved (see D'Amelio et al., 2005, for a suggestion of genetic vulnerability to organophosphates as used in pesticides)? To what extent is the genetic liability for autism shared with other neurodevelopmental disorders.

In recent years, evidence has emerged that a tiny minority of cases of autism are associated with single-gene pathological mutations (Persico & Bourgeron, 2006). The key question is whether the findings on these rare variants can be extrapolated to the broader range of multifactorial ASDs. On the one hand, it is clear that there are well-established examples in which rare Mendelian variants do seem to reflect the same pathophysiology as the much more common multifactorial disorders—as in the case of Alzheimer's disease. On the other hand, there are contrary examples (see below). In short, it would be wrong to dismiss the evidence derived from rare Mendelian variants but, equally, it would be wrong to assume that the findings extrapolate to the more frequent multifactorial varieties of ASD.

The problem is that many monogenic disorders can occasionally give rise to a clinical phenotype that is very much like ASD. The Fragile X anomaly, Down syndrome, and tuberous sclerosis all illustrate this point. In each case, the pathophysiology (insofar as it is known) seems not to mimic that seen in autism. The tubers of tuberous sclerosis are not found in ASD, and neither is the microcephaly of Down syndrome. Although it has been argued that the findings on correction of the Fragile X syndrome in mice has implications for autism (Dölen et al., 2007), that seems dubious. Why then should one suppose that the single-gene mutations (such as the X-linked neuroligins, SHANK-3 or neurexin) that are associated with ASD in a tiny handful of cases might involve mechanisms that could generalize more widely? The possible answer is that they affect neural processes (such as synaptic function and circadian rhythm or developmental disconnection) that might be applicable (Durand et al., 2007; Bourgeron, 2007; Geschwind & Levitt, 2007; Jamain et al., 2008). In addition, attention needs to be paid to the connection between neuronal activity and gene expression (Flavell & Greenberg, 2008). Research into the neural underpinnings of autism needs to be informed by an understanding of normal brain function. The fact that each of these genes seems to be associated with a wider range of phenotypes than just ASD is not necessarily an objection. Genes do not code for *DSM-IV* or *ICD-10* diagnostic categories! Nevertheless, unless the neural abnormalities can be shown to be specifically associated with ASD there must be doubts over the meaning of the finding.

Somewhat similar challenges arise with respect to CNV. Undoubtedly, they constitute an important new focus for genetic studies. On the other hand, for the most part, because the de novo mutations appear to apply to phenotypes that are quite varied (on the limited basis of the published data), it is unclear whether they will be informative on what may be specific for ASD. It remains uncertain what proportion of cases they account for, but it certainly seems to be a small proportion and, insofar as they are de novo mutations, they do not account for the familiality of ASD. What is clear is that such CNVs are much more common in a mixed range of neurodevelopmental disorders than they are in the general population. That raises the question about what it is that has brought about this increased proportion of CNV. Might this, for example, be a function of raised parental age in increasing the rate of developmental anomalies or perturbations—the parallel is the well-established association between maternal age and Down syndrome?

Some General Messages on Research Challenges

Clearly, there are a variety of specifics that warrant systematic attention, but here there is concentration only on general messages. First, it would appear that a greater focus is needed on neglected clinical issues. The examples of regression, savant skills, and epilepsy stand out in that connection.

Second, there is a need to use epidemiological methods in a more hypothesis-testing fashion. Two rather different examples may be provided. First, large-scale prospective epidemiological studies are required to look at the possibility that prenatal and early postnatal environmental risk factors are involved in etiology. Second, epidemiological research is needed to examine the possibility that autism does not constitute a meaningful, cohesive syndrome but rather three disparate domains of malfunction that happen to have been brought together as a result of prevailing diagnostic concepts.

Third, there is a need to increase the more searching creative use of the technologies such as imaging or molecular genetics. There is no doubt that these technologies provide powerful research tools, but progress will not come in throwing a technological bag of tricks at the problem. Rather, the technologies need to be used in hypothesis-testing fashion to examine competing alternative hypotheses.

Fourth, why is it taking so long to identify susceptibility genes for ASD? Larger and larger samples are unlikely to provide a sufficient solution, and it will be essential to use innovative strategies to focus on possibly meaningful subgroups, or possible interplay with stochastic variations, and on possible gene by environment interactions (see Dodge & Rutter, in press, for a fuller discussion). In addition, there may be value in focusing on the minority of cases of ASD born to children from consanguineous partnerships (Walsh et al., 2008).

Finally, funding agencies need to recognize that research advances usually derive from creative research that reflects often iconoclastic approaches born out of new ways of looking at old problems.

SUGGESTED READING

Bock, G., & Goode, J. (Eds.). (2003). *Autism: Neural basis and treatment possibilities*. Novartis Foundation Symposium 251. Chichester, UK: John Wiley.

Frith, U. (2003). *Autism: Explaining the enigma* (2nd ed.). Oxford: Blackwell.

Volkmar, F., Paul, R., Klin, A., & Cohen, D. (Eds). (2005). *Handbook of autism and pervasive developmental disorders* (3rd ed.). New York: John Wiley & Sons.

REFERENCES

Afzal, M. A., Ozoemena, L. C., O'Hare, A., Kidger, K. A., Bentley, M. L., & Minor, P. D. (2006). Absence of detectable measles virus genome sequence in blood of autistic children who have had their MMR vaccination during the routine Childhood Immunization Schedule of UK. *Journal of Medical Virology*, *78*, 623–630.

Alarcón, M., Abrahams, B. S., Stone, J. L., Duvall, J. A., Perederiy, J. V., Bomar, J. M., et al. (2008). Linkage association and gene-expression analyses identify *CNTNAP2* as an autism-susceptibility gene. *American Journal of Human Genetics*, *82*, 150–159.

Alarcón, M., Yonan, Y., Gilliam, T., Cantor, R., & Geschwind, D. (2005). Quantitative genome scan and ordered-subsets analysis of autism endophenotypes support language QTLs. *Molecular Psychiatry, 10*, 747–757.

Amaral, D. G., & Corbett, B. A. (2003). The amygdala, autism, and anxiety. In G. Bock & J. Goode (Eds.), *Autism: Neural basis and treatment possibilities*. Chichester, UK: John Wiley & Sons. 177–197.

Amaral, D. G., Schumann, C. M., & Nordahl, C. W. (2008). Neuroanatomy of autism. *Trends in Neurosciences, 31*, 137–144.

Amir, R. E., van den Veyver, I. B., Wan, M., Tran, C. Q., Francke, U., & Zoghbi, H. Y. (1999). Rett syndrome is caused by mutations in X-linked MECP2, encoding methyl-CpG-binding protein 2. *Nature Genetics, 23*, 185–188.

Anderson, G., & Hoshino, Y. (2005). Neurochemical studies of autism. In F. Volkmar, R. Paul, A. Klin, & D. Cohen (Eds.), *Handbook of autism and pervasive developmental disorders* (3rd ed., pp. 453–472). New York: John Wiley & Sons.

Asperger, H. (1944). Die "Autistischen Psychopathen" im Kindesalter. *Archiv fur Psychiatrie und Nervkrankheiten, 117*, 76–136. Translated in U. Frith (Ed.), *Autism and Asperger syndrome* (pp. 37–92). Cambridge, UK: Cambridge University Press.

Autism Genome Project Consortium, The. (2007). Mapping autism risk loci using genetic linkage and chromosomal rearrangements. *Nature Genetics, 39*, 319–328.

Bacchelli, E., & Maestrini, E. (2006). Autism spectrum disorders: Molecular genetic advances. *American Journal of Medical Genetics. Part C, Seminars in Medical Genetics, 142*, 13–23.

Bailey, A., Bolton, P., Butler, L., Le Couteur, A., Murphy, M., Scott, S., et al. (1993). Prevalence of the fragile X anomaly amongst autistic twins and singletons. *Journal of Child Psychology and Psychiatry, 34*, 673–688.

Bailey, A., Le Couteur, A., Gottesman, I., Bolton, P., Simonoff, E., Yuzda, E., et al. (1995). Autism as a strongly genetic disorder: Evidence from a British twin study. *Psychological Medicine, 25*, 63–77.

Bailey, A., Luthert, P., Dean, A., Harding, B., Janota, I., Montgomery, M., et al. (1998). A clinicopathological study of autism. *Brain, 121*, 889–905.

Bailey, A., Phillips, W., & Rutter, M. (1996). Autism: Towards an integration of clinical, genetic, neuropsychological, and neurobiological perspectives. *Journal of Child Psychology and Psychiatry, 37*, 89–126.

Baird, G., Charman, T., Pickles, A., Chandler, S., Loucas, T., Meldrum, D., et al. (2008). Regression, developmental trajectory, and associated problems in disorders in the autism spectrum: The SNAP Study. *Journal of Autism and Developmental Disorders, 38*, 1827–1836.

Baird, G., Pickles, A., Simonoff, E., Charman, T., Sullivan, P., Chandler, S., et al. (2008). Measles vaccination and antibody response in autism spectrum disorders. *Archives of Disease in Childhood, 93*, 832–837.

Baron-Cohen, S. (2002). The extreme male brain theory of autism. *Trends in Cognitive Sciences, 6*, 248–254.

Baron-Cohen, S., Leslie, A. M., & Frith, U. (1985). Does the autistic child have a "Theory of Mind"? *Cognition, 21*, 37–46.

Bauman, M. L., & Kemper, T. L. (2005). *The neurobiology of autism*. Baltimore, MD, Johns Hopkins University Press.

Bauman, M. D. M., Lavenex, P., Mason, W. A., Capitanio, J. P., & Amaral, D. G. (2004). The development of social behavior following neonatal amygdala lesions in Rhesus monkeys. *Journal of Cognitive Neuroscience, 16*, 1388–1411.

Bolton, P.F., Carcani-Rathwell, I., Hutton, J., Goode, S., Howlin, P., & Rutter, M. (In press). Features and correlates of epilepsy in autism. *British Journal of Psychiatry*.

Bolton, P., Macdonald, H., Pickles, A., Rios, P., Goode, S., Crowson, M., et al. (1994). A case-control family history study of autism. *Journal of Child Psychology and Psychiatry, 35*, 877–900.

Bourgeron, T. (2007). The possible interplay of synaptic and clock genes in autism spectrum disorders. In *Cold Spring Harbor Symposia on Quantitative Biology*. Cold Spring Harbor, NY: Cold Spring Laboratory Press.

Bryson, S. E., Zwaigenbaum, L., Brian, J., Roberts, W., Szatmari, P., Rombough, V., et al. (2007). A prospective case series of high-risk infants who developed autism. *Journal of Autism and Developmental Disorders, 37*, 12–24.

Cantor, R. M., Yoon, J., Furr, J., & Lajonchere, C. (2007). Paternal age and autism are associated in a family-based sample. *Molecular Psychiatry, 12*, 419–423.

Cohen, H., Amerine-Dickens, M., & Smith, T. (2006). Early intensive behavioral treatment: Replication of the UCLA model in a community setting. *Journal of Developmental and Behavioral Pediatrics, 27*, S145–155.

Cook, E. H. Jr., & Scherer, S. W. (2008). Copy-number variations associated with neuropsychiatric conditions. *Nature, 455*, 919–923.

Courchesne, E., Carper, R., & Akshoomoff, N. (2003). Evidence of brain overgrowth in the first year of life in autism. *Journal of the American Medical Association, 290*, 337–344.

Courchesne, E., Pierce, K., Schumann, C., Redcay, E., Buckwalter, J., Kennedy, D., et al.(2007). Mapping early brain development in autism. *Neuron, 56*, 399–413.

Crawley, J. N. (2007). Mouse behavioral assays relevant to the symptoms of autism. *Brain Pathology, 17*, 448–459.

Crawley, J. N., Chen, T., Puri, A., Washburn, R., Sullivan, T., Hill, J., et al. (2007). Social approach behaviors in oxytocin knockout mice: Comparison of two independent lines tested in different laboratory environments. *Neuropeptides, 41*, 145–163.

Croen, L. A., Najjar, D., Fireman, B., & Grether, J. (2007). Maternal and paternal age and risk of autism spectrum disorders? *Archives of Pediatrics and Adolescent Medicine, 161*, 334–340.

D'Amelio, M., Ricci, I., Sacco, R., Liu, X., D'Agruma, L., Muscarella, L., et al. (2005). Paraoxonase gene variants are associated with autism in North America, but not in Italy: Possible regional specificity in gene-environment interactions. *Molecular Psychiatry, 10*, 1006–1016.

Dapretto, M., Lee, S. S., & Caplan, R. (2005). A functional magnetic resonance imaging study of discourse coherence in typically developing children. *Neuroreport, 16*, 1661–1665.

Dawson, G. (1994). Frontal electroencephalographic correlates of individual differences in emotion expression in infants: A brain systems perspective on emotion. *Monographs of the Society for Research on Child Development, 59*, 135–151.

Dawson, G., Estes, A., Munson, J., Schellenberg, G., Bernier, R., & Abbott, R. (2007). Quantitative assessment of autism symptom-related traits in probands and parents: Broader phenotype autism symptom scale. *Journal of Autism and Developmental Disorders, 37*, 523–536.

Dawson, G., Finley, C., Phillips, S., & Galpert, L. (1985). Cognitive processing of verbal and musical stimuli in autistic children as indexed by P300 of the event-related potential. *Journal of Experimental and Clinical Neuropsychiatry, 7*, 626–636.

Dawson, G., Rogers, S., Munson, J., Smith, M., Winter, J., Greenson, J., et al. (2009). Randomized, controlled trial of an intervention for toddlers with autism: The early start Denver model. *Pediatrics, 125*, 17–23.

Dodge, K. A., & Rutter, M. (Eds.) (in press). *Gene-environment interactions in developmental psychopathology: So what?* New York: Guilford Press.

Dölen, G., Osterweil, E., Rao, B., Smith, G., Auerbach, B., Chattarji, S., et al. (2007). Correction of fragile X syndrome in mice. *Neuron, 56*, 955–962.

D'Souza, Y., Fombonne, E., & Ward, B.J. (2006). No evidence of persisting measles virus in peripheral blood mononuclear cells from children with autism spectrum disorder. *Pediatrics, 118*, 1664–2608.

Durand, C. M., Betancur, C., Boeckers, T. M., Bockmann, J., Chaste, P., Fauchereau, F., et al. (2007). Mutations in the gene encoding the synaptic scaffolding protein SHANK3 are associated with autism spectrum disorders. *Nature Genetics, 39*, 25–27.

Eichler, E., & Zimmerman, A. (2008). A hot spot of genetic instability in autism. *New England Journal of Medicine, 358*, 737–739.

Eisenberg, L. (1956). The autistic child in adolescence. *American Journal of Psychiatry, 112*, 607–612.

Fan, Y-T., Decety, J., Yang, C-Y., Liu, J-L., & Cheng, Y. (2010). Unbroken mirror neurons in autism spectrum disorders. *Journal of Child Psychology and Psychiatry, 51*, 981–988.

Flavell, S. W., & Greenberg, M. E. (2008). Signalling mechanisms linking neuronal activity to gene expression and human cognition. *Annual Review of Neuroscience, 31*, 563–590.

Folstein, S., & Rutter, M. (1977a). Infantile autism: A genetic study of 21 twin pairs. *Journal of Child Psychology and Psychiatry, 18*, 297–321.

Folstein, S., & Rutter, M. (1977b). Genetic influences and infantile autism. *Nature, 265*, 726–728.

Fombonne, E., Rogé, B., Claverie, J., Courty, S., & Frémolle, J. (1999). Microcephaly and macrocephaly in autism. *Journal of Autism and Developmental Disorders, 29*, 113–119.

Freitag, C. M. (2007). The genetics of autistic disorders and its clinical relevance: A review of the literature. *Molecular Psychiatry, 12*, 2–22.

Frith, U. (1991). *Autism and Asperger syndrome*. Cambridge: Cambridge University Press.

Frith, U. (2003a). *Autism: Explaining the enigma* (2nd ed.). Oxford: Blackwell.

Frith, C. (2003b). What do imaging studies tell us about the neural basis of autism? In: G. Bock & J. Goode (Eds), *Autism: Neural basis and treatment possibilities* (pp. 149–176). Chichester, UK: John Wiley & Sons.

Frith, C., & Frith, U. (2008). What can we learn from structural and functional brain imaging? In M. Rutter, D. Bishop, D. Pine, S. Scott, J. Stevenson, E. Taylor, et al. (Eds.), *Rutter's child and adolescent psychiatry* (5th ed., pp. 134–144). Oxford: Blackwell.

Geschwind, D. H., & Levitt, P. (2007). Autism spectrum disorders: Developmental disconnection syndromes. *Current Opinion in Neurobiology, 17*, 103–111.

Gillberg, C. (1992). Subgroups in autism: Are there behavioural phenotypes typical of underlying medical conditions? *Journal of Intellectual Disability Research, 36*, 201–214.

Gillberg, C., & Wahlström, J. (1985). Chromosome abnormalities in infantile autism and other childhood psychoses: A population study of 66 cases. *Developmental Medicine and Child Neurology, 27*, 293–304.

Green, J., Charman, T., McConachie, H., Aldred, C., Slonims, V., Howlin, P. et al. (2010). Parent-mediated communication-focused treatment in children with autism (PACT): a randomized controlled trial. *Lancet, 375*, 2152–2160.

Guy, J., Gan, J., Selfridge, J., Cobb, S., & Bird, A. (2007). Reversal of neurological defects in a mouse model of Rett syndrome. *Science, 315*, 1143–1147.

Guy, J., Hendrich, B., Holmes, M., Martin, J. E., & Bird, A. (2001). A mouse Mecp2-null mutation causes neurological symptoms that mimic Rett syndrome. *Nature Genetics, 27*, 322–326.

Hagberg, B., Aicardi, J., Dias, K., & Ramos, O. (1983). A progressive syndrome of autism, dementia, ataxia, and loss of purposeful hand use in girls: Rett's syndrome; report of 35 cases. *Annals of Neurology, 14*, 471–479.

Happé, F. (2003). Cognition and autism: One deficit too many? In G. Bock & J. Goode (Eds.), *Autism: Neural basis and treatment possibilities* (pp. 198–212). Chichester, UK: John Wiley & Sons.

Happé F., & Frith, U. (2010). Introduction: The beautiful otherness of the autistic mind. In: F. Happé & U. Frith (Eds.) *Autism and talent* (pp. 1–12). Oxford University Press, UK.

Helt, M., Kelley, E., Kinsbourne, M., Pandey, J., Boorstein, H., Herbert, M., et al. (2008). Can children with autism recover? If so, how? *Neuropsychology Review, 18*, 339–66.

Hermelin, B. (2001). *Bright splinters of the mind: A personal story of research with autistic artists*. London: Jessica Kingsley.

Hermelin, B., & O'Connor, N. (1970). *Psychological experiments with autistic children*. New York City: Pergamon Press.

Hernandez, L. M., & Blazer, D. G. (2005). *Genes, behavior, and the social environment: Moving beyond the nature/nurture debate*. Washington, DC: National Academies Press.

Hobson, R., Lee, A., & Brown, R. (1999). Autism and congenital blindness. *Journal of Autism and Developmental Disorders, 29*, 45–56.

Honda, H., Shimizu, Y., & Rutter, M. (2005). No effect of MMR withdrawal on the incidence of autism: A total population study. *Journal of Child Psychology and Psychiatry, 46*, 572–579.

Hornig, M., Brieses, T., Buie, T., Mauman, M. L., Lauwers, G., Siemetzki, U., et al. (2008). Lack of association between measles virus vaccine and autism with enteropathy: A case-control study. *PLoS ONE, 3*, e3140.

Howard, J. S., Sparkman, C. R., Cohen, H. G., Green, G., & Stanislaw, H. (2005). A comparison of intensive behavior analytic and eclectic treatments for young children with autism. *Research in Developmental Disabilities, 26*, 359–383.

Howlin, P. (1998). Practitioner review: psychological and educational treatments for autism. *Journal of Child Psychology and Psychiatry, 39*, 307–322.

Howlin, P. (2005). The effectiveness of interventions for children with autism. *Journal of Neural Transmission, Suppl. 69*, 101–119.

Howlin, P., Goode, S., Hutton, J., & Rutter, M. (2004). Adult outcome for children with autism. *Journal of Child Psychology and Psychiatry, 45*, 212–229.

Howlin, P., Goode, S., Hutton, J., & Rutter, M. (2009). Savant skills in autism: Psychometric approaches and parental reports *Philosophical Transactions of the Royal Society of London. Series B, Biological Sciences, 364*, 1359–1367.

Howlin, P., & Rutter, M. (with Berger, M., Hemsley, R., Hersov, L., & Yule, W.). (1987). *Treatment of autistic children*. Chichester, UK: Wiley.

Ingram, J. L., Peckham, S., Tisdale, B., & Rodier, P. (2000). Prenatal exposure of rats to valproic acid reproduces the cerebellar anomalies associated with autism. *Neurotoxicology and Teratology, 22*, 319–324.

International Schizophrenia Consortium. (2008). *Nature, 455*, 237–241.

Jamain, S., Radyushkin, K., Hammerschmidt, K., Granon, S., Boretius, S., Varoqueaux, F., et al. (2008). Reduced social interaction and ultrasonic communication in a mouse model of monogenic heritable autism. *Proceedings of the National Academy of Sciences of the United States of America, 5*, 1710–1715.

Kanner, L. (1943). Autistic disturbances of affective contact. *Nervous Child, 2*, 217–250.

Kanner, L. (1973). The birth of early infantile autism. *Journal of Autism and Childhood Schizophrenia, 3*, 93–95.

Kennedy, D. P., & Courchesne, E. (2008). The intrinsic functional organization of the brain is altered in autism. *NeuroImage, 39*, 1877–1885.

Klin, A., McPartland, J., & Volkmar, F. R. (2005). Chapter 4: Asperger syndrome. In F. R. Volkmar, R. Paul, A. Klin, & D. Cohen (Eds), *Handbook of autism and pervasive developmental disorders, volume 1.* (3rd ed., pp. 88–125). New York: John Wiley & Sons.

Kolvin, I. (1971). Psychoses in childhood: A comparative study. In M. Rutter (Ed.), *Infantile autism: Concepts, characteristics and treatment* (pp. 7–26). Edinburgh: Churchill Livingstone.

Le Couteur, A., Bailey, A., Goode, S., Pickles, A., Robertson, S., Gottesman, I., et al. (1996). A broader phenotype of autism: The clinical spectrum in twins. *Journal of Child Psychology and Psychiatry, 37*, 785–801.

Le Couteur, A., Trygstad, O., Evered, C., Gillberg, C., & Rutter, M. (1988). Infantile autism and urinary excretion of peptides and protein-associated peptide complexes. *Journal of Autism and Developmental Disorders, 18*, 181–190.

Lockyer, L., & Rutter, M. (1969). A five- to fifteen-year follow-up study of infantile psychosis. III. Psychological aspects. *British Journal of Psychiatry, 115*, 865–882.

Lockyer, L., & Rutter, M. (1970). A five- to fifteen-year follow-up study of infantile psychosis. IV: Patterns of cognitive ability. *British Journal of Social and Clinical Psychology, 9*, 152–163.

Lord, C., Pickles, A., McLennan, J., Rutter, M., Bregman, J., Folstein, S., et al. (1997). Diagnosing autism: Analyses of data from the Autism Diagnostic Interview. *Journal of Autism and Developmental Disorders, 27*, 501–517.

Lord, C., Risi, S., DiLavore, P., Shulman, C., Thurm, A., & Pickles, A. (2006). Autism from 2 to 9 years of age. *Archives of General Psychiatry, 63*, 694–701.

Lord, C., Rutter, M., DiLavore, P.C., & Le Couteur, A. (2001). *Autism Diagnostic Observation Schedule – Manual.* Los Angeles CA: Western Psychological Services.

Lord, C., Rutter, M., Goode, S., Heemsbergen, J., Jordan, H., Mawhood, L., et al. (1989). Autism diagnostic observation schedule: A standardized observation of communicative and social behavior. *Journal of Autism and Developmental Disorders, 19*, 185–212.

Lord, C., Rutter, M., & Le Couteur, A. (1994). Autism Diagnostic Interview-Revised: A revised version of a diagnostic interview for caregivers of individuals with possible pervasive developmental disorders. *Journal of Autism and Developmental Disorders, 24*, 659–685.

Lovaas, O. I. (1987). Behavioral treatment and normal educational and intellectual functioning in young autistic children. *Journal of Consulting and Clinical Psychology, 55*, 3–9.

Lovaas, O. I., Koegel, R., & Schreibman, L. (1979). Stimulus overselectivity in autism: A review of research. *Psychological Bulletin, 86*, 1236–1254.

Lovaas, O. I., & Schreibman, L. (1971). Stimulus overselectivity of autistic children in a two-stimulus situation. *Behaviour Research and Therapy, 9*, 305–310.

Magiati, I., Charman, T., & Howlin, P. (2007). A two-year prospective follow-up study of community-based early intensive behavioural intervention and specialist nursery provision for children with autism spectrum disorders. *Journal of Child Psychology and Psychiatry, 48*, 803–812.

Magnus, P., Irgens, L. M., Haug, K., Nystad, W., Skjaerven, R., & Stoltenberg, C.; MoBa Study Group. (2006). Cohort profile: The Norwegian Mother and Child Cohort Study (MoBa). *International Journal of Epidemiology, 35*, 1146–1150.

Marcus, L. M., Kunce, L. J., & Schopler, E. (2005). Chapter 42: Working with families. In F. R. Volkmar, R. Paul, A. Klin, & D. Cohen (Eds.), *Handbook of autism and pervasive developmental disorders, volume 2* (3rd ed., pp. 1055–1086). New York: John Wiley & Sons.

McCann, D., Barrett, A., Cooper, A., Crumpler, D., Dalen, L., Grimshaw, K., et al. (2007). Food additives and hyperactive behaviour in 3-year-old and 8/9-year-old children in the community: A randomised, double-blinded, placebo-controlled trial. *Lancet, 370*, 1560–1567.

McDougle, C. J. (1997). Psychopharmacology. In D. J. Cohen & F. R. Volkman (Eds.), *Handbook of autism and pervasive developmental disorders* (2nd ed., pp. 707–729). New York: John Wiley & Sons.

McEachin, J. J., Smith, T., & Lovaas, O. I. (1993). Long-term outcome for children with autism who received early intensive behavioral treatment. *American Journal of Mental Retardation, 97*, 359–372.

Medical Research Council. (2001). *MRC Review of Autism Research: Epidemiology and Causes.* London: Author.

Minshew, N. J., Sweeney, J. A., Baumann, M. L. & Webb, S. J. (2005). Chapter 18: Neurologic aspects of autism. In F. Volkmar, R. Paul, A. Klin, D. Cohen (Eds), *Handbook of autism and pervasive developmental disorders, volume 1* (3rd ed., pp. 473–514). New York: John Wiley & Sons.

Mundy, P., & Burnette, C. (2005). Chapter 25: Joint attention and neurodevelopmental models of autism. In F. R. Volkmar, R. Paul, A. Klin, & D. Cohen (Eds), *Handbook of autism and pervasive developmental disorders, volume 1* (3rd ed., pp. 650–681). New York: John Wiley & Sons.

Mundy, P., & Sigman, M. (1989). The theoretical implications of joint-attention deficits in autism. *Development and Psychopathology, 1*, 173–184.

Munson, J., Dawson, G., Abbott, R., Faja, S., Webb, S., Friedman, S., et al. (2006). Amygdalar volume and behavioral development in autism. *Archives of General Psychiatry, 63*, 686–693.

National Research Council (2001). *Educating children with autism.* (Committee on Educational Interventions for Children with Autism. Division of Behavioral and Social Sciences and Education). Washington, DC: National Academies Press.

Nelson, C. A., & Luciana, M. (1998). Electrophysiological studies II: Evoked potentials and event-related potentials. In C. E. Coffey & R. A. Brumback (Eds.), *Textbook of pediatric neuropsychiatry* (pp. 331–356). Washington, DC: American Psychiatric Press.

Nishimura, Y., Martin, C., Lopez, A., Spence, S., Alvarez-Retuerto, A., Sigman, M., et al. (2007). Genome-wide expression profiling of lymphoblastoid cell lines distinguishes different forms of autism and reveals shared pathways. *Human Molecular Genetics, 16*, 1682–1698.

Ornitz, E. M. (1978). Neurophysiologic studies. In M. Rutter & E. Schopler (Eds), *Autism: A reappraisal of concepts and treatment* (pp. 117–140). New York: Plenum Press.

Ornitz, E. M., & Ritvo, E. R. (1968). Perceptual inconstancy in early infantile autism: The syndrome of early infant autism and its variants including certain cases of childhood schizophrenia. *Archives of General Psychiatry, 18*, 76–98.

Pardo, C. A., Vargas, D., & Zimmerman, A. (2005). Immunity, neuroglia, and neuroinflammation in autism. *International Review of Psychiatry, 17*, 485–495.

Parr, J. R., Le Couteur, A., Baird, G., Rutter, M., Pickles, A., Fombonne, E., & The international Molecular Genetic Study of Autism Consortium (IMGSAC). (In press). Early developmental regression in autism spectrum disorder: Evidence from an International Multiplex Sample. *Journal of Autism and Developmental Disorders.*

Persico, A. M., & Bourgeron, T. (2006). Searching for ways out of the autism maze: Genetic, epigenetic, and environmental clues. *Trends in Neurosciences, 29*, 349–358.

Pickles, A., Simonoff, E., Conti-Ramsden, G., Falcaro, M., Simkin, Z., Charman, T., et al. (2009). Loss of language in early development of autism and specific language impairment. *Journal of Child Psychology and Psychiatry, 50*, 843–852.

Prather, M. D., Lavenex, P., Maudlin-Jourdan, M. L., Mason, W. A., Captianio, J. P., Mendoza, S. P., et al. (2001). Increased social fear and decreased fear of objects in monkeys with neonatal amygdala lesions. *Neuroscience, 106*, 653–658.

Redcay, E., & Courchesne, E. (2005). When is the brain enlarged in autism? A meta-analysis of all brain size reports. *Biological Psychiatry, 58*, 1–9.

Reichenberg, A., Gross, R., Weiser, M., Bresnahan, M., Silverman, J., Harlap, S., et al. (2007). Advancing paternal age and autism. *Archives of General Psychiatry, 63*, 1026–1032.

Rett, A. (1966). Über ein eigenartiges hirnatrophisches syndrom bei hyperamonaemie im kindesalter[Article in German]. *Wiener Medizinische Wochenschrift, 116*, 723–726.

Rimland, B. (1964). *Infantile autism: The syndrome and its implications for a neural theory of behaviour.* New York: Appleton-Century-Crofts.

Rizzolatti, G., & Craighero, L. (2004). The mirror-neuron system. *Annual Review of Neuroscience, 27*, 169–192.

Rodier, P. M., Ingram, J., Tisdale, B., Nelson, S., & Romano, J. (1996). Embryological origin for autism: Developmental anomalies of the cranial nerve motor nuclei. *Journal of Comparative Neurology, 370*, 247–261.

Rogers, S., & Vismara, L. (2008). Evidence-based comprehensive treatments for early autism. *Journal of Clinical Child and Adolescent Psychology, 37*, 8–38.

Ronald, A., Happé, F., & Plomin, R. (2005). The genetic relationship between individual differences in social and nonsocial behaviours characteristic of autism. *Developmental Science, 8*, 444–458.

Rønningen, K. S., Paltiel, L., Meltzer, H. M., Nordhagen, R., Lie, K. K., Hovengen, R., et al. (2006). The biobank of the Norwegian Mother and Child Cohort Study: A resource for the next 100 years. *European Journal of Epidemiology, 21*, 619–625.

Rutter, M. (1970). Autistic children: Infancy to adulthood. *Seminars in Psychiatry, 2*, 435–450.

Rutter, M. (1972). Childhood schizophrenia reconsidered. *Journal of Autism and Childhood Schizophrenia, 2*, 315–337.

Rutter, M. (1983). Cognitive deficits in the pathogenesis of autism. *Journal of Child Psychology and Psychiatry, 24*, 513–531.

Rutter, M. (1987). The role of cognition in child development and disorder. *British Journal of Medical Psychology, 60*, 1–16.

Rutter, M. (2005a). Incidence of autism spectrum disorders: Changes over time and their meaning. *Acta Paediatrica, 94*, 2–15.

Rutter, M. (2005b). Chapter 16: Genetic influences and autism. In F. R. Volkman, R. Paul, A. Klin, & D. Cohen (Eds.), *Handbook of autism and pervasive developmental disorders* (3rd ed., pp. 425–452). New York: John Wiley & Sons.

Rutter, M. (2008). *Thimerosal vaccine litigation.* Report to US vaccine court 2008.

Rutter, M., Andersen-Wood, L., Beckett, C., Bredenkamp, D., Castle, J., Groothues, C., et al. (1999). Quasi-autistic patterns following severe early global privation. English and Romanian Adoptees (ERA) Study Team. *Journal of Child Psychology and Psychiatry, 40*, 537–549.

Rutter, M., Bailey, A., Bolton, P., & Le Couteur, A. (1994). Autism and known medical conditions: Myth and substance. *Journal of Child Psychology and Psychiatry, 35*, 311–322.

Rutter, M., & Bartak, L. (1973). Special educational treatment of autistic children: A comparative study. II: Follow-up findings and implications for services. *Journal of Child Psychology and Psychiatry, 14*, 241–270.

Rutter, M., Greenfeld, D., & Lockyer, L. (1967). A five- to fifteen-year follow-up study of infantile psychosis. II: Social and behavioural outcome. *British Journal of Psychiatry, 113*, 1183–1199.

Rutter, M., Kreppner, J., Croft, C., Murin, M., Colvert, E., Beckett, C., et al. (2007). Early adolescent outcomes of institutionally deprived and non-deprived adoptees. III: Quasi-autism. *Journal of Child Psychology and Psychiatry, 48*, 1200–1207.

Rutter, M., Le Couteur, A., & Lord, C. (2003). *ADI-R Autism Diagnostic Interview –Revised: Manual.* Los Angeles: Western Psychological Services.

Rutter, M., & Schopler, E. (1987). Autism and pervasive developmental disorders: Concepts and diagnostic issues. *Journal of Autism and Developmental Disorders, 17*, 159–186.

Rutter, M., & Sonuga-Barke, E. (Eds.). (2010). Deprivation-specific psychological patterns: Effects of institutional deprivation. *Monographs of the Society for Research in Child Development, 75*(1), 1–252.

Sacco, R., Militerni, R., Frolli, A., Bravaccio, C., Gritti, A., Elia, M., et al. (2007). Clinical, morphological, and biochemical correlates of head circumference in autism. *Journal of Biological Psychiatry, 62*, 1038–1047.

Scahill, L., & Martin, A. (2005). Psychopharmacology. In F. Volkmar, R. Paul, A. Klin, & D. Cohen (Eds), *Handbook of autism and pervasive developmental disorders, volume 2* (3rd ed., pp. 425–452). New York: John Wiley & Sons.

Schopler, E., Brehm, S. S., Kinsbourne, M., & Reichler, R. J. (1971). Effect of treatment structure on development in autistic children. *Archives of General Psychiatry, 24*, 415–421.

Schopler, E., & Reichler, R. J. (1971). Parents as cotherapists in the treatment of psychotic children. *Journal of Autism and Childhood Schizophrenia, 1*, 87–102.

Schover, L. R., & Newsom, C. D. (1976). Overselectivity, developmental level, and overtraining in autistic and normal children. *Journal of Abnormal Psychology, 71*, 108–114.

Schumann, C. M., & Amaral, D. G. (2006). Stereological analysis of amygdala neuron number in autism. *Journal of Neuroscience, 26*, 7674–7679.

Sebat, J. Lakshmi, B., Malhotra, D., Troge, J., Lese-Martin, C., Walsh, T., et al. (2007). Strong association of de novo copy number mutations with autism. *Science, 316*, 445–449.

Shahbazian, M. D., Young, J. I., Yuva-Paylor, L. A., Spencer, C., Antalffy, B., Noebels, J., et al. (2002). Mice with truncated MeCP2 recapitulate many Rett syndrome features and display hyperacetylation of histone H3. *Neuron, 35*, 243–254.

Shao, Y., Cuccaro, M., Hauser, E., Raiford, K., Menold, M., Wolpert, C., et al. (2003). Fine mapping of autistic disorder to chromosome 15q11-q13 by use of phenotypic subtypes. *American Journal of Human Genetics, 72*, 539–548.

Sigman, M., Ruskin, E., Arbeile, S., Corona, R., Dissanayake, C., Espinosa, M., et al. (1999). Continuity and change in the social competence of children with autism, Down syndrome, and developmental delays. *Monographs of the Society for Research in Child Development, 64*, 1–114.

Smalley, S. L. (1998). Autism and tuberous sclerosis. *Journal of Autism and Developmental Disorders, 28*, 407–414.

Stoltenberg, C., Schjolberg, S., Bresnahan, M., Hornig, M., Hirtz, D., Dalh, C., et al. (2010) The Autism Birth Cohort: a paradigm for gene-environment–timing research. *Molecular Psychiatry, 15*, 676–680.

Szatmari, P., Bryson, S., Duku, E., Vaccarella, L., Zwaigenbaum, L., Bennett, T., et al. (2009). Similar developmental trajectories in autism and Asperger syndrome: from early childhood to adolescence. *Journal of Child Psychology and Psychiatry, 50*, 1459–1467.

Sutera, S., Pandey, J., Esser, E. L., Rosenthal, M. A., Wilson, L. B., Barton, M., et al. (2007). Predictors of optimal outcome in toddlers diagnosed with autism spectrum disorders. *Journal of Autism and Developmental Disorders, 37*, 98–107.

Van Acker, R., Loncola, J. A., & Van Acker, E. Y. (2005). Rett syndrome: A pervasive developmental disorder. In F. R. Volkmar, R. Paul, A. Klin, & D. Cohen (Eds.), *Handbook of autism and pervasive developmental disorders* (3rd ed., pp. 126–164). New York: John Wiley & Sons.

van Krevelen, D. (1963). On the relationship between early infantile autism and autistic psychopathy. *Acta Paedopsychiatrica, 30*, 303–323.

Wakefield, A. J., Murch, S. H., Anthony, A., Linnell, J., Casson, D. M., Malik, M., et al. (1998). Ileal-lymphoid-nodular hyperplasia, non-specific colitis, and pervasive developmental disorder in children. *Lancet, 351*, 637–641.

Walsh, T., McClellan, J. M., McCarthy, S. E., Addington, A. M., Pierce, S. B., Cooper, G. M., et al. (2008). Rare structural variants disrupt multiple genes in neurodevelopmental pathways in schizophrenia. *Science, 320*, 539–543.

Weatherall, D. (2006). *The use of non-human primates in research*. An independent working group report. London: The Academy of Medical Sciences, MRC, Royal Society and Wellcome Trust.

Weiss, L., Shen, Y., Korn, J., Arking, D., Miller, D., Fossdal, R., et al. (2008). Autism Consortium. Association between microdeletion and microduplication at 16p11.2 and autism. *New England Journal of Medicine, 358*, 667–675.

Werner, E., & Dawson, G. (2005). Validation of the phenomenon of autistic regression using home videotapes. *Archives of General Psychiatry, 62*, 889–895.

Wing, L. (1981). Asperger's syndrome: A clinical account. *Psychological Medicine, 11*, 115–129.

Wing, L., & Gould, J. (1979). Severe impairments of social interaction and associated abnormalities in children: Epidemiology and classification. *Journal of Autism and Developmental Disorders Schizophrenia, 9*, 11–29.

Woodhouse, W., Bailey, A., Rutter, M., Bolton, P., Baird, G., & Le Couteur, A. (1996). Head circumference in autism and other pervasive developmental disorders. *Journal of Child Psychology and Psychiatry, 37*, 665–671.

Yang, M., Zhodzishsky, V., & Crawley, J. N. (2007). Social deficits in BTBR *T + tf*/J mice are unchanged by cross-fostering with C57BL/6J mothers. *International Journal of Developmental Neuroscience, 25*, 515–521.

Yule, W. (1978). Chapter 10: Research methodology: What are the "correct controls"? In M. Rutter, & E. Schopler (Eds.), *Autism: A reappraisal of concepts and treatment* (pp. 155–162). New York: Plenum Press.

2 Diagnosis of Autism Spectrum Disorders

Katherine Gotham, Somer L. Bishop, Catherine Lord

Points of Interest

- History of autism and ASD classification.
- Current criteria for and presentation of pervasive developmental disorders.
- Potential revisions to ASD criteria and classification framework.
- Participant characteristics that affect diagnosis.
- Instruments and methods for assessing ASD.
- Diagnostic issues often overlooked in research.

Introduction

Since its original description by Leo Kanner in 1943, autism has come to be recognized as a neurodevelopmental disorder that manifests in infancy or early childhood and encompasses both delays and deviance in a "triad" of behavioral domains (Wing & Gould, 1979): reciprocal social interaction, communication, and restricted and repetitive behaviors and interests. Autism is thought to be the cornerstone of a spectrum of disorders, commonly referred to as autism spectrum disorders (ASD) or pervasive developmental disorders (PDD). This spectrum includes Asperger's syndrome (AS), and Pervasive Developmental Disorder-Not Otherwise Specified (PDD-NOS, or atypical autism), as well as two very rare disorders, Rett's disorder and Childhood Disintegrative Disorder (CDD).

Studies of monozygotic twin concordance for autism, and of families in which parents have multiple affected children, have established that risk for ASD is influenced by genetic factors (Morrow et al., 2008; Constantino & Todd, 2008). A "broader phenotype" of social impairments in family members of individuals with ASD continues to generate interest as a potential window into the genetic transmission of these disorders (Dawson et al., 2007). Though associations have been shown between increased rates of ASD and genetic, chromosomal, and/or brain abnormalities, no biological marker adequately accounts for a significant minority of cases with reasonable specificity. Therefore diagnosis is currently based on behavioral phenotype alone.

In this chapter, we provide an overview of the history of autism and ASD classification, including criteria for and presentation of each of the PDDs, participant characteristics that affect diagnosis, instruments and methods for assessing ASD, innovative uses for the diagnostic measures, and diagnostic issues often overlooked in research.

Epidemiology and Diagnosis

Whereas autism was previously thought to occur in approximately 4 children out of 10,000 based on epidemiological studies published in the 1960s, the autism spectrum currently is thought to have a combined prevalence rate of 50–60 out of 10,000 school-age children (Chakrabarti & Fombonne, 2005; CDC, 2007). Refinements to diagnostic criteria, addressed later in this chapter, surely have impacted these prevalence rates (D. Bishop, Whitehouse, Watt, & Line, 2008). Growing ASD prevalence and awareness of the disorders in turn demand greater research attention to the boundaries of and within this spectrum. Indeed, one of the primary issues in ASD diagnosis today is a debate about the clinical and biological validity of distinct categorical disorders within the spectrum (see below).

ASD is more prevalent among males, with an approximate gender ratio of 4:1. There seems to be a higher proportion of severe cognitive impairment in females with ASD than in males (Fombonne, 2005a). It is speculated that gender may be differently associated with various etiological subtypes in ASD (Miles et al., 2005). Though we may come to see subgroups with different ASD severity levels and cognitive ranges in which sex ratios differ from that in the overall population, at this point there is no specific profile of ASD impairments that distinguishes girls from boys (except for greater female prevalence in Rett's disorder).

Factors such as race, ethnicity, and socioeconomic class are not thought to influence presentation of ASD. We mention them here, however, because they have been associated with age of first diagnosis, and with over- or underdiagnosis of ASD, depending on the specific group. Kanner noted that the parents of his sample were well educated and high achieving, leading to a notion that autism was more prevalent among the higher socioeconomic classes. Later, more rigorous studies of SES and ASD found that autism crosses social class (Schopler, Andrews, & Strupp, 1980; Wing, 1980). However, early diagnosis of children with lower SES is often impeded by less sensitive referral sources, limited access to specialized clinics, and the cost of a diagnostic evaluation. Accurate diagnosis for a complicated case of ASD may span a couple of years and require thousands of dollars (Shattuck & Grosse, 2007). One study found that children from poor or near-poor families receive an initial diagnosis up to 11 months later than children from wealthier families (Mandell, Novak, & Zubritsky, 2005). Age of identification was significantly higher for African American and Latino children than for white children in another study in which the entire sample had low SES (Mandell, Listerud, & Levy, 2002), although this was not replicated in two more recent studies (Mandell et al., 2005; Wiggins, Baio, & Rice, 2006). In 2009 Mandell and his research team examined age of diagnosis by race and other factors in over 76,000 Medicaid-enrolled children with new diagnoses of an ASD. They found that African American children were diagnosed with an ASD at a mean age of 70.8 months, compared to the overall sample mean of 68.4, whereas Latino and Asian children tended to receive diagnoses at younger ages than did children in other ethnic groups, including Caucasian children (Mandell, Morales, et al., 2009). The author postulates that the findings might be due to the amelioration of ethnicity-related disparities in impoverished samples, or perhaps a phenomenon in which the most severely impaired children within some ethnic groups are the only ones to be identified in early childhood, decreasing the observed age of diagnosis for a particular group. Indeed, another study by the same team found that black and Hispanic children were less likely to have a documented ASD than were white children (Mandell, Wiggins, et al., 2009). Research is currently being done to determine the influence of cultural factors in observing and reporting autism behaviors, as well as differences in ASD prevalence across racial/ethnic groups (Mandell, Wiggins, et al., 2009; Bhasin & Schendel, 2007; Overton, Fielding, & Garcia de Alba, 2007; Schieve, Rice, & Boyle, 2006).

Diagnostic Classification

In 1943, Kanner used the term "infantile autism" to describe 11 children who exhibited limited interest in and impaired social response to others from infancy onward (Kanner, 1943). These children were either nonverbal or had impaired communication, as well as behavioral rigidity. Virtually simultaneously, Hans Asperger described a similar group of male children (Asperger, 1944), but the fact that Kanner published in English and Asperger in German barred the comparison of these findings. For decades, most mental health professionals continued to think of children with this behavioral profile as having "childhood schizophrenia" (Tidmarsh & Volkmar, 2003), until the work of Rutter and Kolvin in the 1970s distinguished the two conditions in terms of clinical characteristics and outcome (Rutter, 1970, 1972; Kolvin, 1971). Whereas childhood schizophrenia was characterized by disordered personality, thought, and mood and blunted affect, usually with normal intelligence and an onset after 11 years of age, "infantile autism" was noted from infancy or shortly after in children with a range of intellectual functioning, and was marked by speech delay, ritualistic behaviors, and deficits in social relationships and imaginative play.

In 1980, the *Diagnostic and Statistical Manual of Mental Disorders*, 3rd edition (DSM-III; APA, 1980), first included "infantile autism" under a new diagnostic category of Pervasive Developmental Disorder, partly in recognition of Wing's "triad of impairments" often associated with intellectual disabilities (Wing & Gould, 1979). With the 1987 revisions, DSM-III-R changed the diagnostic label to "autistic disorder." Also, "Not Otherwise Specified" categories were added to this version of the DSM, thereby creating PDD-NOS. The World Health Organization's *International Statistical Classification of Diseases and Related Health Problems*, 10th Revision (ICD-10; WHO, 1990), which included Rett's disorder and CDD in the Pervasive Developmental Disorder category, came into widespread use in 1994. The DSM-IV was published in the same year (APA, 1994), and had PDD criteria revised to correspond to ICD-10 criteria for these disorders.

The DSM-IV PDD classifications and a brief overview of their criteria are presented below (see also Tidmarsh & Volkmar, 2003). Because ICD-10 categories and criteria are so similar to DSM-IV classification, the former system will not be reviewed in depth here. ICD-10 includes more subtypes of PDD than does DSM-IV. Nonetheless, the similarity between these systems has already had a profound impact by enabling international merging of datasets and comparison of research findings (e.g. International Molecular Genetic Study of Autism, Gong et al., 2008; Autism Genome Project et al., 2007).

Autistic Disorder

In the DSM-IV, autistic disorder is diagnosed when six symptoms are present across the three domains of qualitative impairment in social interaction, communication, and restricted repetitive and stereotyped patterns of behavior, interests, and activities. At least two of the symptoms must be from the social domain, with at least one symptom present from each of the other two domains. Social, language, or play abnormalities or delays must be present before the age of 3, and Rett's disorder and CDD must first be ruled out before assigning a diagnosis of autistic disorder.

Impairment in social reciprocity is believed to be the central defining characteristic of autism (Williams White, Koenig, & Scahill, 2007; Carter, Davis, Klin, & Volkmar, 2005). Difficulties in social interaction present in various ways within and across individuals, such as a toddler who does not direct eye contact or a changed facial expression to her parent when something startles her, but looks up briefly in the direction of the noise and continues playing, an adolescent who interjects abruptly during a group conversation to bring up his own interest in videogames, or an adult who makes no response to another's comment about having a terrible day.

Delay, impairment in, or absence of communication strategies is also characteristic of autism. These difficulties are evident in both verbal (e.g., late onset of phrase speech, pronoun reversal, stereotyped speech) and nonverbal (e.g., minimal use of gestures) aspects of communication. Recent factor analyses of standardized diagnostic measures, the Autism Diagnostic Observation Schedule (ADOS; Lord et al., 2000) and the Autism Diagnostic Interview–Revised (ADI-R; Lord, Rutter, & LeCouteur, 1994), have shown that social and communication domain items from these measures load onto a single factor (Gotham et al., 2008; Georgiades et al., 2007; Lecavalier et al., 2006), and therefore it is possible that these two symptoms domains will be merged in DSM-V criteria for autistic disorder.

Restricted, repetitive behaviors and interests (RRBs) comprise the third domain of autism symptomatology. These include repetitive motor mannerisms (e.g., hand flapping), unusual sensory interests (e.g., squinting one's eyes to peer at a wind-up toy), and restricted or unusual topics of interest (e.g., collecting ticket stubs, learning and reciting everything there is to know about the Roman emperor Nero). Based on recent analyses of the factor structure and developmental course of behaviors in the RRB domain, some researchers have suggested that this third domain of behavior be split into two separate categories: "repetitive sensory motor behaviors," which include motor mannerisms, sensory interests, and repetitive use of objects, and "insistence on sameness behaviors," such as compulsions and rituals and overreliance on routines (Cuccaro et al., 2003; Bishop, Richler, & Lord, 2006; Richler, Bishop, Kleinke, & Lord, 2007).

Asperger's Syndrome (AS)

Like autism, AS is also marked by social impairment and restricted interests and behaviors. Development of speech is not delayed in AS, but communication abnormalities are often present, including flat intonation, pedantic speech (e.g., "Could I trouble you to answer some questions with regard to this new development?"), and diminished conversational reciprocity, often associated with restricted topics of interest. According to DSM-IV, autistic disorder must be ruled out before a diagnosis of AS can be made. When this rule is observed, the prevalence of AS is very low, making it difficult to gather samples large enough to study potential differences between this disorder and high functioning autism (HFA; or autism without intellectual disability) (see Szatmari, 2000). The DSM-IV rule-out criterion is therefore often ignored, with many clinical and research facilities each tending to use their own AS criteria.

Earlier studies suggested that children with AS differed from those with HFA with regard to impoverished motor skills (Gillberg, 1989) and profiles of discrepantly high verbal IQ (Volkmar et al., 1994). However, the lack of standardization of diagnosis has made these findings difficult to corroborate (Klin, Paul, Schultz, & Volkmar, 2005), and a number of more recent reviews have found little evidence of distinction between AS and HFA (Macintosh & Dissanayake, 2004; Frith, 2004; see also Howlin, 2003). For example, Bennett, Szatmari, and colleagues (2008) found that grouping 6- to 8-year-olds by the presence or absence of structural language impairment (deficits in grammar or syntax) explained more variance in outcome through ages 15–17 on an array of dimensions, including adaptive behavior and scores on the Autism Behavior Checklist (Krug, Arick, & Almond, 1980), than did grouping the sample by clinical diagnoses of AS and HFA. Similarly, Cuccaro and colleagues (2007) found no differences in repetitive behaviors between individuals with diagnoses of AS versus HFA. Based on widespread disagreement in the field about how to diagnose AS, as well as lack of evidence of differences between AS and HFA, there are likely to be significant changes in how AS is conceptualized in future DSM and ICD editions.

Pervasive Developmental Disorder, Not-Otherwise-Specified (PDD-NOS)

PDD-NOS diagnoses are assigned to children who do not meet onset criteria for autistic disorder or whose pattern of impairments falls short of the required number of symptoms in each domain. An individual with PDD-NOS may have symptoms meeting criteria in the social and one other domain, but exhibit no symptoms in the remaining domain, or alternatively, he/she may have a subthreshold number of symptoms in all three domains. Because this category does not have specific criteria of its own, it is often used as a "catch-all" diagnosis for individuals with a spectrum disorder difficult to specify, or for young children to whom professionals do not yet feel comfortable giving an autism diagnosis (Walker et al., 2004; Lord et al., 2006). In a study of interrater diagnostic reliability using three expert raters, the agreement for PDD-NOS (versus autism or AS) was not better than chance (Mahoney et al., 1998). Walker and colleagues (2004) suggested that the reliability and utility of the category may be improved by creating a separate designation for individuals with significant social and communication impairment without restricted, repetitive behaviors (RRBs). However, other studies have indicated that most individuals with PDD-NOS *do* have RRBs (Matson, Dempsey, LoVullo, & Wilkins, 2008; Bishop et al., 2006), so this revised definition would only account for a very small proportion of PDD-NOS cases.

PDD-NOS and AS may have dimensional differences from autism in some cases, but their utility as distinct, reliable categorical disorders will depend on evidence of their specific value in determining etiology and treatment (Volkmar & Lord, 2007). For future DSM and ICD versions, it will be important to examine whether PDD-NOS should remain a "catch-all" diagnosis or whether the population currently identified with this label could be divided into more definable subtypes, with the "NOS" label used less frequently for cases that fall short of meeting criteria for any PDD subtype.

Rett's Disorder

This rare disorder appears primarily in girls. Development in infancy is not obviously abnormal initially, but soon head growth slows and fine and gross motor skills may be lost. The loss may include language skills and social interest as well. Social interaction usually improves by late childhood or adolescence, though severe mental retardation and motor impairment are persistent. Rett's Disorder is characterized by stereotypical motor behaviors, most prominently hand-wringing, and breathing abnormalities, such as breathholding or hyperventilation; seizure activity is common. Mutations to X-linked gene MECP2 account for most cases (Amir et al., 1999).

Because Rett syndrome is associated with a identifiable genetic mutation, it has been argued that it should not be considered within the autism spectrum. However, more recently, as various genetic associations become apparent within this spectrum, the proposal has been made to give an ASD diagnosis on the basis of behavioral characteristics regardless of genetic findings, with genetic or chromosomal abnormalities coded on a separate axis. Thus, children with other identified disorders (e.g., genetic syndromes, fetal alcohol spectrum disorders) could receive an additional diagnosis of ASD if they meet behavioral criteria for social and communication impairments.

Childhood Disintegrative Disorder

Also rare, with prevalence estimated at 2 cases per 100,000 children (Fombonne, 2005b), CDD is differentiated from autism by a marked regression between 2 and 10 years of age following normal development in at least the first two years of life. In CDD, skills are lost in two or more of the following areas: language, social interaction, motor skills, play, or adaptive behavior. Though regression occurs in other ASDs as well (approximately 20–33% of children on the autism spectrum develop some single words in infancy and then lose them, usually between the ages of 18 and 24 months; even more children "lose" other social or communication skills; Luyster et al., 2005), in non-CDD regression, the developed speech is often very limited (i.e., 3–10 single words) and only present for a few weeks or months. Additionally, while loss of eye contact or other signs of social interest and engagement or play skills are often reported in children with autism, regressions in autism, unlike CDD regressions, are less frequently accompanied by losses in adaptive or motor skills.

It once seemed likely that CDD was etiologically distinct from autism. However researchers have recently questioned whether this disorder represents an arbitrary distinction from autism on the basis of the timing of the regression, the level of the child's skills before the regression, and the type of skills lost. Studies about the validity of CDD as a distinct disorder have suggested that CDD may be accompanied by higher rates of epilepsy, increased fearfulness, and lower intellectual functioning (or less discrepancy between verbal and nonverbal IQ) than is seen in autism (Kurita, Osada, & Miyake, 2004; Malhotra & Gupta, 2002; Volkmar & Rutter, 1995). At this time, it remains unclear whether CDD represents extremes on all three dimensions of autism-like regression (e.g., lateness of regression, strength of prior skills, and amount of skills affected by the regression) or a unique disorder.

Factors That Affect the Presentation of ASD

ASDs are heterogeneous disorders, and individuals with these diagnoses can look quite different from each other. A nonverbal 16-year-old who avoids eye contact and spins in circles might share a diagnosis of autism with a hyperactive, verbally fluent 4-year-old who seeks out others to talk at length about his interest in maps and state capitals. Because ASDs are developmental disorders, they both influence and are influenced by developmental levels of the individual (such as language level, "mental age," and chronological age). Thus, diagnosticians must be familiar with the range of factors that can affect the presentation of ASD across individuals. Furthermore, although autism spectrum disorders are considered some of the most reliably diagnosable psychiatric disorders of childhood (Volkmar & Lord, 2007), current classification systems may be most useful in the diagnosis of somewhat verbal, school-age children with mild-to-moderate intellectual disability. Special considerations must be taken, therefore, when assessing individuals on the "extremes" of the spectrum: very young children and adults; individuals with severe intellectual disability and those with average to above-average intelligence; and individuals with very limited or very strong verbal skills.

Chronological Age

As with any developmental disorder, chronological age has a significant impact on the way in which ASD symptoms manifest. Individuals behave differently at different phases in development, and these changes affect the presentation of their symptoms, as well as the contexts in which they should be evaluated. Most individuals with ASD continue to exhibit social and communication difficulties and restricted or repetitive behaviors across the lifespan, but the particular nature of these symptoms is likely to change dramatically with age.

In recent years, a great deal of attention has been given to identifying symptoms of ASD in very young children. Early identification of autism has been emphasized in clinical research and practice due to the reported benefits of early intervention. Current research suggests that autism can be diagnosed reliably by age 2 and nonautism ASD by age 3 (Turner, Stone, Pozdol, & Coonrod, 2006; Chawarska, Klin, Paul, & Volkmar, 2006). Some first signs in infants that are associated with later ASD diagnoses include failure to respond to one's name, poor eye contact, and an array of unusual reactions to sensory properties of objects (Dawson et al., 2004; Baranek, 1999). Although the field continues to make gains in the area of early assessment and diagnosis (see Chapter 5 in this volume), many professionals are still not well versed in the range of social and communication abilities exhibited by typically developing infants and toddlers. Knowledge of chronological age expectations in normal development is therefore essential for all professionals working with this population (see Bishop, Luyster, Richler, & Lord, 2008).

Unlike infants and toddlers, adolescents and adults with ASD have received relatively little attention in the recent literature, particularly with regard to assessment and diagnosis. Adolescents and adults with ASD often exhibit greater social interest than younger children, but have exaggerated, stilted, or otherwise abnormal means of interacting, including poor social reciprocity and difficulty sustaining interactions. Across many studies, the use of communicative speech increases from childhood to adulthood, but aspects of communication remain impaired in ASD into adulthood, particularly those related to social functioning, such as gestures, perseveration, or overly literal interpretation of language (Seltzer, Shattuck, & Abbeduto, 2004). Based on a more limited body of research, the presence of RRBs seems to be relatively stable into adulthood, though the particular manifestation of these behaviors may change, for example, shifting from a toddler who seeks out only toys that have buttons, to an adolescent conversing about her restricted interest in constellations (Seltzer et al., 2004).

As a result of rising prevalence estimates and increased public awareness of ASD, more and more adults are presenting for initial evaluations with concerns about ASD. However, because ASD is normally diagnosed during childhood, most empirically derived assessment tools were designed for and validated on samples of children with ASD. Future research will need to dedicate more attention to developing best practice guidelines for assessment and diagnosis of adults with suspected ASD.

Mental Retardation

Intellectual disability was once thought to be present in most autism cases, but findings from more recently recruited samples estimate that 29–60% of children with autism fall in the normal range of nonverbal IQ (Fombonne, 2005a; Tidmarsh & Volkmar, 2003). Although there is a great deal of variability in developmental trajectories and outcomes for children with ASD, nonverbal IQ has been found to be one of the best prognostic indicators (Thurm, Lord, & Lee, 2007; Venter, Lord, & Schopler, 1992). Consequently, information about a child's cognitive abilities is important in programming and planning for the future.

Because skill expectations are different for children at different developmental levels, knowledge about a child's cognitive abilities is necessary in order to accurately assess his/her social and communication skills. We would not expect, for example, the same level of social sophistication from a 14-year-old with mild intellectual disability as we would if his cognitive abilities were in the average range. Thus, as mentioned previously, it is essential that clinicians familiarize themselves with typical social behaviors for individuals at different developmental stages, taking into account both chronological and mental age. This is necessary in order to "separate" the behaviors related to ASD from those related to intellectual disability. Studies comparing children with ASD to children with nonspectrum developmental delays (e.g., Down syndrome, intellectual disability of unknown etiology), have provided essential information about behaviors that are more or less specific to ASD, and have shown that even children with significant delays (without ASD) exhibit social competencies, such as joint attention skills, that many children with ASD do not (Dawson et al., 2004; Bishop, Gahagan, & Lord, 2007).

It is more difficult to make diagnostic differentiations in children with profound levels of intellectual disability. These individuals are very likely to meet criteria for ASD because their general level of functioning falls below a preschool level. In these cases, it may not be possible to differentiate individuals with profound mental retardation in whom the ASD is "primary" from those in whom the intellectual disability is the central cause of their difficulties. Furthermore, as discussed below, diagnostic instruments for ASD do not have the same psychometric properties when applied to populations of individuals with very severe cognitive disabilities.

Language

As is the case with nonverbal skills, language abilities vary widely among children and adults with ASD. Whereas many or most children with autism were once expected to be nonverbal or minimally verbal, these rates have changed dramatically with the recognition of milder cases, as well as greater access to early language intervention. In one study of children with relatively severe ASD, about 40% of school-age children had complex fluent speech by age 9, and the proportion of completely nonverbal children was less than 15% (Lord et al., 2006), indicating that previous estimates of 50% of children with ASD being nonverbal are no longer valid.

Assessing social difficulties and communication impairments across a range of language levels from nonverbal to fluent requires expertise in various instruments (as discussed later) but also an understanding of the *range* of behaviors associated with the autism spectrum. It is important to recognize that individuals with more limited language abilities who do not have ASD still employ nonverbal forms of communication, such as gestures and eye contact, to initiate social interactions. Therefore, understanding the numerous ways in which humans communicate and what is expected for individuals at different developmental stages is required in order to be able to distinguish ASD from other disorders.

Comorbid Disorders

Comorbidity of ASD with other psychiatric disorders occurs frequently and may have great impact on the already heterogeneous presentation of these disorders. Some of the most common comorbid disorders include anxiety, depression, hyperactivity, attention problems, obsessive-compulsive features, oppositional-defiant disorder, tics, and epilepsy. Tuberous sclerosis and Fragile X account for a relatively small proportion of ASD cases (though conversely, a significant proportion of children with these disorders have autism or ASD) (Lord & Spence, 2006; see also Chapter 46, this volume). Schizophrenia has also been reported to co-occur with ASD, though infrequently. Adults with ASD may sometimes receive a schizophrenia diagnosis because of social isolation, flat affect, speaking their thoughts aloud, and/or endorsing the idea of "hearing voices" based on a literal interpretation, e.g., someone was speaking in the next room and could be heard despite not being immediately present (Fitzgerald, 1999).

Physical disabilities, such as blindness, deafness, or conditions that impair or prohibit motor coordination, also impact ASD presentation and diagnosis. These disabilities can affect social development; they also can render irrelevant certain behaviors that influence diagnosis, e.g., eye contact in blind children, or response to name in deaf children. These conditions may also prevent a referred individual's participation in standard forms of assessment (e.g., a child with cerebral palsy who cannot construct block designs for cognitive testing).

Many of these disorders have social implications, and some of them are associated with specific kinds of repetitive behaviors, especially motor mannerisms, which can make diagnosis of ASD and comorbid disorders challenging. Comorbidity is more the rule than the exception in assessment today, due to high rates of co-occurring conditions within individuals on the autism spectrum (Sterling, Dawson, & Estes, 2008; Matson & Nebel-Schwalm, 2007).

While ASDs are commonly thought to be life-long disorders, there has been a great deal of recent interest and research on "optimal outcome" children—those who come to function in the normal range of cognitive, adaptive, and social skills, and thus no longer qualify for an ASD diagnosis. Though the accuracy and standardization of assessment and diagnosis may play a role in the observation of this phenomenon, a subtype of children on the spectrum who "recover" would likely be associated with and influenced by many of the factors described in this section—such as strong initial language and cognitive abilities and younger chronological age at identification (Helt et al., 2008).

Assessment of ASD

Diagnostic assessment of ASD is carried out by a number of professionals, e.g., physicians, psychologists, and educators. The type of professional or service system making the diagnosis will often affect how that diagnosis will be used to obtain services: distinct labels from different professionals are usually needed for eligibility of insurance or governmental funding, educational placement, or treatment planning (Shattuck & Grosse, 2007). Regardless of the assessment venue or the qualifications of the evaluator, it is vital that all professionals undertaking ASD assessment have clinical experience, skill, and familiarity with individuals with ASD and related disorders. Diagnosticians should be aware of best practices in the field and utilize standardized instruments. At the same time, clinical judgment has been found to contribute to the stability of ASD diagnosis beyond the classification from common standardized measures (Lord et al., 2006). Thus, even when required training has been completed for use of a particular diagnostic measure, a background of clinical experience with individuals with ASD is integral to competent diagnostic practice. Frequent, active contact with individuals with ASD led to excellent interrater reliability for clinical diagnosis in DSM-IV field trials, compared to fair reliability in less experienced professionals (Volkmar et al., 1994). Beginning professionals must have access to adequate supervision, and "experts" must maintain a high rate of ongoing clinical involvement with the ASD population.

Components of a Diagnostic Assessment

Before proceeding with a behavioral assessment for ASD, appropriate steps should be taken to ensure that the referred individual is physically healthy. These may include a physical exam to take growth measurements and rule out medical disorders that might obscure the presentation of ASD, as well as hearing, speech, and language assessments. In some cases, additional neurological or genetic testing may be indicated (see the American Academy of Pediatrics Council on Children with Disabilities guidelines for autism evaluation, Johnson et al., 2007).

A multidisciplinary assessment for ASD should include a caregiver-based developmental history that addresses milestones and noted abnormalities in the individual's earliest years. A pregnancy and birth history should be taken, as well as an overview of the referred individual's general health, including sleeping and eating behaviors, and a family history documenting relatives with ASD, genetic conditions, and mental health issues. Teachers or daycare providers can also assist in providing additional information about the individual's behavior.

In addition to obtaining information from parents and teachers about an individual's behavior, a diagnostic assessment should always include a direct observation of the referred individual. The child or adult with ASD should be seen personally by the diagnostician, and ideally, the observation should include the administration of a semistructured observational measure to assess the presence of symptoms associated with ASD (see below). The direct assessment should also include cognitive and language testing, as verbal and nonverbal abilities directly affect how symptoms of ASD manifest. Furthermore, a home or school visit may be useful for directly observing behavior problems or peer relationships that occur outside of the clinic setting.

When evaluating adolescents and adults who have the cognitive and language abilities to report on their own symptoms, it may also be appropriate to incorporate self-report measures into the diagnostic assessment. Standardized self-report questionnaires such as the Autism Spectrum Quotient (AQ: Baron-Cohen, Wheelwright, Skinner, Martin, & Clubley, 2001—see below) have been developed to obtain symptom reports directly from the referred individual. These instruments hold promise as a means of gaining a better understanding about the perspectives and internal experiences of individuals with ASD. However, given that lack of insight is one of the features of ASD, further work is required to understand the extent to which adolescents and adults with ASD are capable of providing valid reports about their own strengths and difficulties (see Bishop & Seltzer, submitted).

Following the assessment, diagnostic feedback should be provided to the parents or referred adult both in person and in a written report. The family should be provided with information about ASD, and the clinician may wish to discuss coping skills and support resources with the family (Lord & McGee, 2001). If the primary clinician is not a psychiatrist, parents should have the option of requesting a psychiatric consult to discuss the patient's medication needs, if any.

Because of the time, expertise, number of professionals, waiting lists, and costs, multidisciplinary assessments may not be a reality for all families with children with ASD, nor is it necessary in all contexts (e.g., confirming a previous diagnosis for research inclusion). However, clinicians should attempt to review information from as many of the above-mentioned sources as possible when making a clinical diagnosis of ASD. Communication between professionals from various disciplines promotes accurate and efficient diagnosis.

Differential Diagnosis

Many psychiatric disorders impact social communication, thus differential diagnosis of ASD can be complicated. Some of the most common non-ASD diagnoses given to children referred for ASD evaluations are language disorders, such as receptive-expressive language disorder or pragmatic language impairment, attention-deficit/hyperactivity disorder (ADHD), and intellectual disability. In each case, social and communication impairments should be assessed relative to the individual's developmental level (Volkmar & Lord, 2007). Other diagnoses that referred children may have received in error include right hemisphere learning problems, hearing disabilities, obsessive compulsive disorder (OCD), schizoid personality disorder, attachment disorder, selective mutism, and Landau-Kleffner syndrome (characterized by language loss and seizure onset; Landau & Kleffner, 1998). While some differential diagnoses are more likely to be ruled out before an ASD diagnosis is made (e.g., schizoid personality disorder or selective mutism), others may warrant consideration as comorbid disorders (e.g., language disorders or intellectual disability).

Diagnostic Measures

Diagnosis of ASD has benefited from the development of standardized measures. This review will touch on the clinical utility and psychometric properties of a few questionnaires, interviews, and observational measures that have historical importance or current relevance in ASD diagnosis. See Lord and Corsello (2005) for a more detailed review of ASD diagnostic instruments.

Though measures vary in their purpose and convenience (thus clinical diagnosticians and research projects employ a range of the measures described below, as well as others), a number of instruments have come to be included in an internationally recognized "best practice" diagnostic assessment for ASD. These include the parent/caregiver interview, the Autism Diagnostic Interview-Revised (ADI-R; Lord et al., 1994), and the standardized clinical observation, the Autism Diagnostic Observation Schedule (ADOS; Lord et al., 2000), as well as the Social Communication Questionnaire (SCQ; Rutter, Bailey, & Lord, 2003) and the Social Responsiveness Scale (SRS; Constantino, 2002). The ADI-R and ADOS exist in 20 authorized translations worldwide, the SCQ in 17, and the SRS in 18. Due in part to the widespread use of these instruments, research findings can be more easily compared and samples collapsed across data collection sites.

Despite the strong predictive validity of some of the assessment tools described below, an individual's diagnosis of ASD should never depend on the diagnostic classification of a single measure or combination of measures. Be it for access to early intervention, educational services, or inclusion in a research sample, the ability of an experienced clinician is required to integrate information from standardized diagnostic instruments and other sources into a clinical diagnosis.

Questionnaires

Questionnaires offer the advantage of being able to collect a large amount of information in a relatively short amount of time. As part of a diagnostic assessment, questionnaires can also be useful for gathering information from multiple informants, such as teachers, daycare workers, or, in the case of adult clients, supervisors, siblings, or spouses. A number of questionnaires have been designed to assess behaviors characteristic of ASD. Whereas earlier questionnaires relied on general and vague descriptions of behavior, such as "social interest" or "emotional connection," more recently developed instruments inquire about specific, empirically identified symptoms of ASD that are intended to differentiate children with ASD from those who are typically developing or who have nonspectrum disorders. Nevertheless, even recently developed questionnaires have limitations, including reliance on the report of "lay observers" (e.g., parents), as well as inter-reporter differences in the way that questions are interpreted. Thus, whereas these tools can be useful for quickly gauging the types of behaviors that a child exhibits in different settings, questionnaires used as part of a diagnostic assessment should be combined with information from a parent interview and child observation.

Questionnaires developed to assist in the diagnosis of ASD include the Autism Behavior Checklist (ABC; Krug, Almond, & Arick, 1993), the Gilliam Autism Rating Scale (GARS; Gilliam, 1995), the Social Communication Questionnaire (SCQ; Rutter, Bailey, & Lord, 2003), and the Autism Spectrum Screening Questionnaire (ASSQ: Ehlers, Gillberg, & Wing, 1999). The ABC may be filled out by parents or teachers and inquires about behaviors related to sensory interests, body and object use, language and social interaction, and self-help. Based on findings that the instrument does not always adequately distinguish between individuals with autism and those with nonspectrum disorders (Volkmar et al., 1988, Eaves, Campbell, & Chambers, 2000), the ABC may be more appropriate for documenting change in response to treatment or education, rather than as a diagnostic measure (Lord & Corsello, 2005). Similarly, the GARS, which is also a parent-rated questionnaire intended to indicate autism likelihood, has been shown to underidentify children as having autism (sensitivity = .48) (South et al., 2002), suggesting that it should not be used as a primary diagnostic tool. The SCQ is a parent checklist based on questions from the Autism Diagnostic Interview (see below). Though the SCQ works relatively well for identifying children with ASD in certain populations (especially when used together with the Autism Diagnostic Observation Schedule—see below), cut-offs may need to be adjusted for younger children (see Corsello et al., 2007). The ASSQ is another brief symptom checklist for use in a clinical setting. It is specifically intended to identify characteristics of Asperger's syndrome and high functioning autism, and thus is not appropriate for use with the full range of individuals referred for ASD diagnostic assessment.

Questionnaires that have been designed as continuous measures of ASD symptoms or traits include the Social Responsiveness Scale (SRS; Constantino, 2002) and the Autism Spectrum Quotient (AQ: Baron-Cohen, Wheelwright, Skinner, Martin, & Clubley, 2001). The SRS is a parent- or teacher-rated questionnaire that consists of 65 items assessing communication, social interaction, and repetitive and stereotyped behaviors and interests. When parent and teacher ratings are combined, the measure has excellent specificity for indicating the presence of ASD (.96) versus other disorders, but sensitivity is relatively low (.75) (Constantino et al., 2007). When only a parent rating is used, specificity is still good (.84), though sensitivity is less clear (Constantino et al., 2007). In its current format, the SRS is only validated for children between the ages of 4 and 18 years, though an adult research version of the instrument is currently being developed (see Constantino & Todd, 2005). For adults with suspected ASD, the Autism Spectrum Quotient (AQ) is available as a continuous measure of ASD traits. The AQ is a self-report measure for adults with average or above average intelligence. Adapted versions of the instrument have been validated for use with adolescents (Baron-Cohen, Hoekstra, Knickmeyer, & Wheelwright, 2006) and children aged 4–11 (Auyeung, Baron-Cohen, Wheelwright, & Allison, 2008) with suspected ASD. Parent-report versions of the AQ are also available to supplement the self-report forms (see Baron-Cohen et al., 2001; Baron-Cohen et al., 2006).

Interviews

Like questionnaires, diagnostic interviews collect information from informants about an individual's behaviors. An advantage of the interview format is that the interviewer has some control over the way in which questions are interpreted, because clarification can be provided when necessary. Semistructured interviews that are scored by the interviewer are also advantageous, because, as opposed to more subjective interpretations of behavior (e.g., a parent rating a behavior as normal/abnormal, mild/severe), scores are derived from a trained interviewer's objective assessment of a behavioral description. On the other hand, interviews are often lengthy and thus time-consuming. Furthermore, unlike questionnaires, which can be mailed and completed anywhere, interviews require face-to-face contact between an informant and a trained examiner.

The Autism Diagnostic Interview-Revised (ADI-R; Lord et al., 1994) is a standardized, semistructured parent interview that is administered by a trained clinician in approximately 2–3 hours. Diagnostic algorithms, which yield a classification of "autism" or "nonspectrum," are overinclusive for individuals with nonverbal mental ages below 18 months and those with severe to profound intellectual disability (Lord, Storoschuk, Rutter, & Pickles, 1993; Nordin & Gillberg, 1998). However, the measure has good to excellent predictive validity for most other developmental groups, especially when used in combination with the Autism Diagnostic Observation Schedule (see Risi et al., 2006). Although some researchers have used ADI-R scores to measure severity of autism symptoms and improvement over time, the ADI-R was developed with the goal of distinguishing individuals with ASD from those without ASD. Thus, more research is required to determine the extent to which higher scores on the ADI-R correspond to "more severe" autism, as well as whether current scores can be used to track changes over time.

The Diagnostic Interview for Social and Communication Disorders (DISCO; Wing, Leekam, Libby, Gould, & Larcombe,

2002) is another semistructured, standardized interview used in ASD assessment. It is primarily intended to assist in clinical assessment of an individual rather than to yield a categorical diagnosis, although diagnostic algorithms for research use have been created (Leekam, Libby, Wing, Gould, & Taylor, 2002). Unlike the ADI-R, the DISCO assesses a number of non-ASD-specific behaviors, including maladaptive behaviors and those related to daily living skills.

Observational Measures

Observation by a trained clinician is a critical component of any ASD diagnostic evaluation, and a diagnosis should never be made without first directly observing and interacting with a referred individual. Use of a standardized observation instrument is also recommended, because the observational period can be structured to specifically elicit behaviors associated with an ASD diagnosis. For example, in the absence of any particular demands, an individual who is allowed to talk at length about a particular topic may appear socially skilled, but as soon as he is encouraged to talk about something outside of his interests, his difficulties with conversation and social reciprocity will become more apparent. Thus, employing some type of semistructured observation measure is preferable to simply watching an individual referred for ASD.

The Childhood Autism Rating Scale (CARS; Schopler, Reichler, & Renner, 1986) is one of the most widely used autism diagnostic scales. Originally designed to be scored based on an examiner's observations, the CARS is often used now as a general rating of all information available (e.g., scores may be derived from parent report, as well as from direct observation). Created before the current diagnostic classification systems, it is likely that the CARS overidentifies certain children (e.g., young nonspectrum children with intellectual disability) as having autism, while underestimating the difficulties of high-functioning children with ASD (see Lord & Corsello, 2005; Van Bourgondien, Marcus, & Schopler, 1992). Consequently, whereas it may be useful in some cases as a screening measure or a summary coding of all clinical information, care should be taken in using the CARS as the only observation measure in a diagnostic assessment.

The Autism Diagnostic Observation Schedule (ADOS; Lord et al., 2000) is a semistructured, standardized observation of children and adults referred for ASD. Like the ADI-R, its companion measure, the ADOS was created by operationalizing DSM-IV criteria for autism. Both original and revised diagnostic algorithms (see Gotham, Risi, Pickles, & Lord, 2007) show strong predictive validity, with the revised set of algorithms showing better specificity in lower-functioning populations. Because of its strong discriminant validity, the ADOS is widely used in international clinical and research efforts. It is useful in standardizing clinical observation, but must be considered in conjunction with a developmental history and clinical judgment of an experienced clinician.

With the recent interest in early diagnosis of ASD, several observational measures have been developed for use in very young children at risk for ASD and other communication disorders. The Communication and Symbolic Behavior Scales (CSBS; Wetherby & Prizant, 2002) evaluates communication and symbolic abilities in babies and toddlers and can be useful in identifying children who may require further evaluation. The Screening Tool for Autism in Toddlers (STAT: Stone, Coonrod, & Ousley, 2000) is an interactive screening measure for children between 24 and 35 months. The STAT has been shown to distinguish 2-year-old children with autism from those with nonspectrum developmental delays, but it is less good at picking up children with milder ASD symptoms (e.g., children with PDD-NOS). More recently, the Autism Observation Scale for Infants (AOSI: Bryson, Zwaigenbaum, McDermott, Rombough, & Brian, 2004) was developed to identify very young children (6 to 18 months) who may be at risk for ASD. Finally, the ADOS has been adapted for use with children aged 12 to 30 months; see Luyster et al., 2009, for description and psychometric analysis of this new toddler module.

Though direct observation is a crucial component of ASD diagnostic assessment, children and adults do not always behave as they normally would when they are "under the microscope," being observed by professionals in an unfamiliar setting. Furthermore, it is not always possible to observe an individual's full range of strengths and difficulties within a relatively short clinical observation period. Questionnaires and interviews provide information about behaviors that occur across various settings outside of a clinical context. As such, all three sources of information (questionnaires, interviews, and observations) are valuable components of a thorough ASD assessment.

Complementary Assessment Measures

In addition to ASD-specific diagnostic instruments, measures of cognitive, adaptive, and language abilities should be included in an ASD diagnostic evaluation. Individuals with ASD often have significantly discrepant verbal and performance IQ scores, so cognitive tests that yield separate verbal and nonverbal IQ scores should be selected. When working with individuals with less sophisticated language abilities, tests with lower language demands, such as the Mullen Scales of Early Learning (Mullen, 1995) and the Differential Ability Scales (DAS; Elliot, 1990), are sometimes preferable to tests that rely more on verbal instructions (e.g., the Wechsler Intelligence Scale for Children; Wechsler, 2003). Adaptive functioning is most commonly assessed with a parent interview, such as the Vineland Adaptive Behavior Scales, 2nd edition (Vineland-II; Sparrow, Cicchetti, & Balla, 2005), which yields separate normalized scores and age equivalents in the domains of communication, daily living skills, socialization, and motor skills. Language testing is also an important component of an ASD assessment. Tests should be selected such that receptive and expressive language skills are evaluated separately (see Paul, 2007).

Supplementary assessment tools may be indicated depending on the particular behavioral profile, or on the intervention, educational, or vocational needs of an individual referred for diagnostic assessment. Measures might be drawn from other areas of psychopathology to assess for comorbidities or to evaluate particular aspects of learning or achievement. For example, the Child Behavior Checklist (CBCL) is a parent/caregiver questionnaire that results in a total score, an Internalizing and Externalizing Scale score, and Syndrome and DSM Oriented Scales, one of which is a Pervasive Developmental Disorder Problems scale (Achenbach & Rescorla, 2000). The CBCL is not intended to be diagnostic, but can be used to identify a range of behavioral issues (ASD-specific and otherwise) to target for intervention. The Repetitive Behavior Scale–Revised (RBS-R; Bodfish, Symons, Parker, & Lewis, 2000) evaluates a range of repetitive behaviors seen in individuals with ASD and other developmental disorders and may be useful both for diagnostic purposes and for tracking changes in these behaviors over time. Other questionnaires that can be used to assess problematic behaviors in ASD include the Aberrant Behavior Checklist (Aman & Singh, 1994) and the Nisonger Child Behavior Rating Form (Tasse, Aman, Hammer, & Rojahn, 1996). The PDD Behavior Inventory (PDD-BI: Cohen, Schmidt-Lackner, Romanczyk, & Sudhalter, 2003) includes questions about adaptive and maladaptive behaviors, and is designed to evaluate responsiveness to intervention in children with ASD. For educational or vocational planning for individuals with ASD, the Psychoeducational Profile, 3rd edition (PEP-3; Schopler, Lansing, Reichler, & Marcus, 2004) and the Adolescent and Adult Psychoeducational Profile (AAPEP; Mesibov, Schopler, & Carson, 1989) may be used.

Though this list is far from exhaustive, we have attempted to review some of the more widely used instruments in ASD assessment. Evaluators should always keep in mind that certain accommodations may be necessary in order to obtain valid assessments of individuals with ASD, such as supplementing verbal directions with visual supports (e.g., schedules or reward systems), or using tests outside of the standard age range (e.g., administering a preschool language test to an older child with limited verbal abilities).

Looking Ahead

The field has made great strides in designing and validating instruments for use in ASD assessment and diagnosis, as well as in revising diagnostic criteria to be more inclusive of individuals across the full autism spectrum. However, there are many challenges that lie ahead in terms of further refining classification criteria and diagnostic instruments to meet current needs. As mentioned previously, more research is needed in the area of assessment methods for very young and/or very cognitively impaired individuals, and for adults across the range of abilities. It will be necessary to examine how well current diagnostic standards, which are largely based on observations of school-age children with ASD, apply to very young or older individuals. Do the same symptoms continue to be diagnostically relevant as individuals grow older, or should core symptoms of the disorder be defined relative to a person's developmental stage?

Some researchers have proposed shifting from a categorical approach in ASD diagnosis toward a more dimensional framework. Continuous measures of social and communication difficulties could be used to describe a child's level of social impairment/competence across different domains. Since many childhood disorders are characterized by social difficulties, this would aid in identifying areas of strength and difficulty in children with various disorders (including ASD), which could then be used to guide intervention efforts for these children.

Another advantage of thinking dimensionally about ASD symptoms rather than relying primarily on categorical distinctions is that we may be able to develop more meaningful measures of severity. There is currently no well-defined benchmark for "average autism," so it is difficult to classify children as mild or severe, especially since a child may have very severe symptoms in one domain of behavior and relatively mild symptoms in another. Quantitative approaches to measuring symptoms across domains could improve our ability to describe different developmental trajectories and responses to treatment, which would in turn further efforts to identify subgroups of children with ASD and to isolate endophenotypes that may map onto specific genetic or neurobiological findings.

Conclusions

Standardized diagnostic criteria and "best practice" assessment measures have been associated with more comparable research findings and the ability to reliably describe younger and milder cases of autism spectrum disorders. Current research is underway to explore the relationship between participant characteristics such as gender, ethnicity, cognitive and language abilities, and comorbid disorders with specific ASD symptoms and severity. Further advancements in ASD diagnostic practices are needed to identify subtypes for neurobiological, genetic, and treatment research, as well as to define boundaries or dimensional gradations within the spectrum for clinical and research use.

Challenges and Future Directions

- Achieving consistent early identification practices across geographic regions and within socioeconomic and ethnic groups
- Revising international classification criteria to reflect data on symptom specificity and presentation

- Identifying symptom profiles in historically overlooked populations, such as individuals with severe intellectual disability and adults with ASD
- Measuring autism severity as a means to subtype groups within the spectrum

SUGGESTED READINGS

Fombonne, E. (2005). The changing epidemiology of autism. *Journal of Applied Research in Intellectual Disabilities, 18*, 281–294.

Lord, C., Risi, S., DiLavore, P., Shulman, C., Thurm, A., & Pickles, A. (2006). Autism from 2 to 9 years of age. *Archives of General Psychiatry, 63*(6), 694–701.

Risi, S., Lord, C., Gotham, K., Corsello, C., Szatmari, P., Cook, E., et al. (2006). Combining information from multiple sources in the diagnosis of autism spectrum disorders. *Journal of the American Academy of Child and Adolescent Psychiatry, 45*, 1094–1103.

REFERENCES

Achenbach, T. M., & Rescorla, L. A. (2000). *Manual for ASEBA preschool forms and profiles.* Burlington: University of Vermont, Research Center for Children, Youth, & Families.

Aman, M. G., & Singh, N. N. (1994). *Aberrant Behavior Checklist—Community. Supplementary Manual.* East Aurora, NY: Slosson Educational Publications.

American Psychiatric Association (1980). *Diagnostic and statistical manual* (3rd ed.). Washington, DC: APA Press.

American Psychiatric Association (1994). *Diagnostic and Statistical Manual of Mental Disorders* (4th ed.). Washington, DC: APA Press.

Amir, R. E., Van den Veyver, I. B., Wan, M., Tran, C. Q., Francke, U., & Zoghbi, H. Y. (1999). Rett syndrome is caused by mutations in X-linked MeCP2, encoding methyl-CpG-binding protein 2. *Nature Genetics, 23*, 185–188.

Asperger, H. (1944/1991). Die "autistischen psychopathen" in kind esalter. Archive fur Psychiatrie und Nervenkrankheiten, 117, 76–136. Translated by U. Frith (Ed.), Autism and Asperger syndrome (1991, pp. 37–92). Cambridge: Cambridge University.

Autism Genome Project Consortium et al. (2007). Mapping autism risk loci using genetic linkage and chromosomal rearrangements. *Nature Genetics, 39*(3), 319–328.

Auyeung, B., Baron-Cohen, S., Wheelwright, S., & Allison, C. (2008). The Autism Spectrum Quotient: Children's version (AQ-Child). *Journal of Autism and Developmental Disorders, 38*(7), 1230–1240.

Baranek, G. (1999). Autism during infancy: A retrospective video analysis of sensory-motor and social behaviors at 9–12 months of age. *Journal of Autism and Developmental Disorders, 29*(3), 218–224.

Baron-Cohen, S., Hoekstra, R. A., Knickmeyer, R., & Wheelwright, S. (2006). The Autism-Spectrum Quotient (AQ)—Adolescent version. *Journal of Autism and Developmental Disorders, 36*, 343–350.

Baron-Cohen, S., Wheelwright, S., Skinner, R., Martin, J., & Clubley, E. (2001). The Autism-Spectrum Quotient (AQ): Evidence from Asperger syndrome/high-functioning autism, males and females, scientists and mathematicians. *Journal of Autism and Developmental Disorders, 31*, 5–17.

Bennett, T., Szatmari, P., Bryson, S., Volden, J., Zwaigenbaum, L., Vaccarella, L., et al. (2008). Differentiating autism and Asperger syndrome on the basis of language delay or impairment. *Journal of Autism and Developmental Disorders, 38*, 616–625.

Bhasin, T. K., & Schendel, D. (2007). Sociodemographic risk factors for autism in a US metropolitan area. *Journal of Autism and Developmental Disorders, 37*, 667–677.

Bishop, D. V. M., Whitehouse, A. J. O., Watt, H. T., & Line, E. A. (2008). Autism and diagnostic substitution: Evidence from a study of adults with a history of developmental language disorder. *Developmental Medicine and Child Neurology, 50*(5), 341–345.

Bishop, S. L., & Seltzer, M. M. (submitted). Self-reported symptoms in adults with autism spectrum disorders.

Bishop, S. L., Gahagan, S., & Lord, C. (2007). Re-examining the core features of autism: A comparison of autism spectrum disorder and fetal alcohol spectrum disorder. *Journal of Child Psychology and Psychiatry, 48*(11), 1111–1121.

Bishop, S. L., Luyster, R., Richler, J., & Lord, C. (2008). Diagnostic assessment. In K. Chawarska, A. Klin, & F. R. Volkmar (Eds.), *Autism spectrum disorders in infants and toddlers: Diagnosis, assessment, and treatment* (pp. 23–49). New York: Guilford.

Bishop, S. L., Richler, J., & Lord, C. (2006). Association between restrictive and repetitive behaviors and nonverbal IQ in children with autism spectrum disorders. *Child Neuropsychology, 12*, 247–267.

Bodfish, J. W., Symons, F. J., Parker, D. E., & Lewis, M. H. (2000). Varieties of repetitive behavior in autism: Comparisons to mental retardation. *Journal of Autism and Developmental Disorders, 30*(3), 237–243.

Bryson, S. E., Zwaigenbaum, L., McDermott, C., Rombough, V., & Brian, J. (2004). The Autism Observation Scale for Infants: Scale development and reliability data. *Journal of Autism and Developmental Disorder, 38*, 731–738.

Carter, A. S., Davis, N. O., Klin, A., & Volkmar, F. R. (2005). Social development in autism. In F. R. Volkmar, R. Paul, A. Klin, & D. Cohen (Eds.), *Handbook of autism and pervasive developmental disorders: Vol. 1. Diagnosis, development, neurobiology, and behavior* (pp. 312–334). Hoboken, NJ: Wiley.

Centers for Disease Control (2007). Prevalence of autism spectrum disorders—Autism and developmental disabilities monitoring network, six sites, United States, 2000. *CDC Morbidity and Mortality Weekly Report, 56*, 1–11.

Chakrabarti, S., & Fombonne, E. (2005). Pervasive developmental disorders in preschool children: confirmation of high prevalence. *American Journal of Psychiatry, 162*, 1133–1141.

Chawarska, K., Klin, A., Paul, R., & Volkmar, F. (2006). Autism spectrum disorder in the second year: Stability and change in syndrome expression. *Journal of Child Psychology and Psychiatry, 48*(2), 128–138.

Cohen, I. L., Schmidt-Lackner, S., Romanczyk, R., & Sudhalter, V. (2003). The PDD Behavior Inventory: A rating scale for assessing response to intervention in children with pervasive developmental disorder. *Journal of Autism and Developmental Disorders, 33*, 31–45.

Constantino, J. N. (2002). *The Social Responsiveness Scale.* Los Angeles: Western Psychological Services.

Constantino, J. N., LaVesser, P. D., Zhang, Y., Abbacchi, A. M., Gray, T., & Todd, R. D. (2007). Rapid quantitative assessment of autistic social impairment by classroom teachers. *Journal of the American Academy of Child and Adolescent Psychiatry, 46*, 1668–1676.

Constantino, J. N., & Todd, R. D. (2005). Intergenerational transmission of subthreshold autistic traits in the general population. *Biological Psychiatry, 57*, 655–660.

Constantino, J. N., & Todd, R. D. (2008). Genetic epidemiology of pervasive developmental disorders. In J. Hudziak (Ed.), *Developmental psychopathology and wellness: Genetic and environmental influences* (pp. 209–224). Arlington, VA: American Psychiatric Publishing.

Corsello, C., Hus, V., Pickles, A., Risi, S., Cook, E. H., Leventhal, B. N., et al. (2007). Between a ROC and a hard place: Decision making and making decisions about using the SCQ. *Journal of Child Psychology and Psychiatry, 48*, 932–940.

Cuccaro, M., Nations, L., Brinkley, J., Abramson, R., Wright, H., Hall, A., et al. (2007). A comparison of repetitive behaviors in Asperger's disorder and high functioning autism. *Child Psychiatry and Human Development, 37*, 347–360.

Cuccaro, M. L., Shao, Y., Grubber, J., Slifer, M., Wolpert, C. M., Donnelly, S. L., et al. (2003). Factor analysis of restricted and repetitive behaviors in autism using the Autism Diagnostic Interview-R. *Child Psychiatry and Human Development, 34*(1), 3–17.

Dawson, G., Estes, A., Munson, J., Schellenberg, G., Bernier, R., & Abbott, R. (2007). Quantitative assessment of autism symptom-related traits in probands and parents: Broader Phenotype Autism Symptom Scale. *Journal of Autism and Developmental Disorders, 37*, 523–536.

Dawson, G., Toth, K., Abbott, R., Osterling, J., Munson, J., Estes, A., et al. (2004). Early social attention impairments in autism: Social orienting, joint attention, and attention to distress. *Developmental Psychology, 40*(2), 271–283.

Eaves, R. C., Campbell, H. A., & Chambers, D. (2000). Criterion-related and construct validity of the Pervasive Developmental Disorders Rating Scale and the Autism Behavior Checklist. *Psychology in the Schools, 37*, 311–321.

Ehlers, S., Gillberg, C., & Wing, L. (1999). A screening questionnaire for Asperger syndrome and other high-functioning autism spectrum disorders in school age children. *Journal of Autism and Developmental Disorders, 29*, 129–141.

Elliot, C. D. (1990). *Differential abilities scale (DAS)*. San Antonio, TX: Psychological Corporation.

Fitzgerald, M. (1999). Differential diagnosis of adolescent and adult Pervasive Developmental Disorders/Autism Spectrum Disorders (PDD/ASD): A not uncommon diagnostic dilemma. *International Journal of Psychiatry in Medicine, 16*, 145–148.

Fombonne, E. (2005a). The changing epidemiology of autism. *Journal of Applied Research in Intellectual Disabilities, 18*, 281–294.

Fombonne, E. (2005b). Epidemiological studies of Pervasive Developmental Disorders. In: F. R. Volkmar, A. Klin, R. Paul, & D. J. Cohen (Eds.), *Handbook of autism and pervasive developmental disorders* (3rd ed., Vol. 1, pp. 42–69). New York: Wiley.

Frith, U. (2004). Emmanuel Miller lecture: Confusions and controversies about Asperger syndrome. *Journal of Child Psychology and Psychiatry, 45*, 672–686.

Georgiades, S., Szatmari, P., Zwaigenbaum, L., Duku, E., Bryson, S., Roberts, W., et al. (2007). Structure of the autism symptom phenotype: A proposed multidimensional model. *Journal of the American Academy of Child and Adolescent Psychiatry, 46*(2), 188–196.

Gillberg, C. (1989). Asperger syndrome in 23 Swedish children. *Developmental Medicine and Child Neurology, 31*, 520–531.

Gilliam, J. E. (1995). *Gilliam Autism Rating Scale*. Austin, TX: ProED.

Gong, X., Bacchelli, E., Blasi, F., Toma, C., Betancur, C., Chaste, P., et al. IMGSAC (2008). Analysis of X chromosome inactivation in autism spectrum disorders. *American Journal of Medical Genetics. Part B, Neurosychiatric Genetics, 147B*(6), 830–835.

Gotham, K., Risi, S., Dawson, G., Tager-Flusberg, H., Joseph, R., Carter, A., et al. (2008). A replication of the Autism Diagnostic Observation Schedule (ADOS) revised algorithms. *Journal of the American Academy of Child and Adolescent Psychiatry, 47*(6), 643–651.

Gotham, K., Risi, S., Pickles, A., & Lord, C. (2007). The Autism Diagnostic Observation Schedule (ADOS): Revised algorithms for improved diagnostic validity. *Journal of Autism and Developmental Disorders, 37*, 400–408.

Helt, M., Kelley, E., Kinsbourne, M., Pandey, J., Boorstein, H., Herbert, M., et al. (2008). Can children with autism recover? If so, how? *Neuropsychology Review, 18*, 339–366.

Howlin, P. (2003). Outcome in high-functioning adults with autism with and without early language delays: Implications for the differentiation between autism and Asperger syndrome. *Journal of Autism and Developmental Disorders, 33*, 3–13.

Johnson, C. P., Myers, S. M., & American Academy of Pediatrics Council on Children with Disabilities (2007). Identification and evaluation of children with autism spectrum disorders. *Pediatrics, 120*(5), 1183–1215.

Kanner, L. (1943). Autistic disturbances of affective contact. *Nervous Child, 2*, 217–250.

Klin, A., Pauls, R., Schultz, R., & Volkmar, F. (2005). Three diagnostic approaches to Asperger Syndrome: Implications for research. *Journal of Autism and Developmental Disorders, 35*, 221–234.

Kolvin, I. (1971). Studies in childhood psychoses. I. Diagnostic criteria and classification. *British Journal of Psychiatry, 118*, 381–384.

Krug, D. A., Arick, J. R., & Almond, P. J. (1980). *Autism screening instrument for educational planning*. Portland, OR: ASIEP Educational.

Krug, D. A., Arick, J. R., & Almond, P. J. (1993). *Autism screening instrument for educational planning* (2nd ed.). Austin, TX: ProEd.

Kurita, H., Osada, H., & Miyake, Y. (2004). External validity of Childhood Disintegrative Disorder in comparison with Autistic Disorder. *Journal of Autism and Developmental Disorders, 34*(3), 355–362.

Landau, W. M., & Kleffner, F. R. (1998). Syndrome of acquired aphasia with convulsive disorder in children. 1957. *Neurology, 51*(5), 1241.

Lecavalier, L., Aman, M., Scahill, L., McDougle, C., McCracken, J., Vitiello, B., et al. (2006). Validity of the Autism Diagnostic Interview-Revised. *American Journal of Mental Retardation, 111*(3), 199–215.

Leekam, S. R., Libby, S. J., Wing, L., Gould, J., & Taylor, C. (2002). The Diagnostic Interview for Social and Communication Disorders: Algorithms for ICD-10 childhood autism and Wing and Gould autistic spectrum disorder. *Journal of Child Psychology and Psychiatry and Allied Disciplines, 43*(3), 327–342.

Lord, C., & Corsello, C. (2005). Diagnostic Instruments in Autistic Spectrum Disorders. In F. R. Volkmar, R. Paul, A. Klin, &

D. J. Cohen (Eds.), *Handbook of autism and pervasive developmental disorders* (pp. 730–770). New York: Wiley.

Lord, C., & McGee, J. (2001). *Educating children with autism spectrum disorders: Report of the Committee on Early Intervention in Autism.* Washington, DC: National Academy of Sciences.

Lord, C., Risi, S., DiLavore, P., Shulman, C., Thurm, A., & Pickles, A. (2006). Autism from 2 to 9 years of age. *Archives of General Psychiatry, 63*(6), 694–701.

Lord, C., Risi, S., Lambrecht, L., Cook, E. H., Jr., Leventhal, B. L., DiLavore, P. C., et al. (2000). The Autism Diagnostic Observation Schedule-Generic: A standard measure of social and communication deficits associated with the spectrum of autism. *Journal of Autism and Developmental Disorders, 30,* 205–223.

Lord, C., Rutter, M. L., & LeCouteur, A. (1994). The Autism Diagnostic Interview-Revised: A revised version of a diagnostic interview for caregivers of individuals with possible pervasive developmental disorders. *Journal of Autism and Developmental Disorders, 24,* 659–685.

Lord, C., & Spence, S. (2006). Autism spectrum disorders: phenotype and diagnosis. In S. Moldin & J. Rubenstein (Eds). *Understanding autism: From basic neuroscience to treatment* (pp. 1–23). New York, NY: Taylor & Francis.

Lord, C., Storoschuk, S., Rutter, M., & Pickles, A. (1993). Using the ADI-R to diagnose autism in preschool children. *Infant Mental Health Journal, 14,* 1234–1252.

Luyster, R., Gotham, K., Guthrie, W., Coffing, M., Petrak, R., Pierce, K., et al. (2009). The Autism Diagnostic Observation Schedule—Toddler Module: A new module of a standardized diagnostic measure for ASD. *Journal of Autism and Developmental Disorders, 39*(9), 1305–1320.

Luyster, R., Richler, J., Risi, S., Hsu, W., Dawson, G., Bernier, R., et al. (2005). Early regression in social communication in autism spectrum disorders: A CPEA study. *Developmental Neuropsychology, 27*(3), 311–336.

Macintosh, K. E., & Dissanayake, C. (2004). Annotation: The similarities and differences between autistic disorder and Asperger's disorder: A review of the empirical evidence. *Journal of Child Psychology and Psychiatry, 45,* 421–434.

Mahoney, W. J., Szatmari, P., MacLean, J. E., Bryson, S., Bartolucci, G., Walter, S., et al. (1998). Reliability and accuracy of differentiating pervasive developmental disorder subtypes. *Journal of the American Academy of Child and Adolescent Psychiatry, 37,* 278–285.

Malhotra, S., & Gupta, N. (2002). Childhood Disintegrative Disorder: Re-examination of the current concept. *European Child and Adolescent Psychiatry, 11,* 108–114.

Mandell, D. S, Listerud, J., & Levy, S. E. (2002). Race differences in the age at diagnosis among Medicaid-eligible children with autism. *Journal of American Academy of Child and Adolescent Psychiatry, 41,* 1447–1453.

Mandell, D., Morales, K., Xie, M., Polsky, D., Stahmer, A., & Marcus, S. (2009). Factors associated with age of diagnosis among Medicaid-enrolled children with autism spectrum disorders in the United States. *International Meeting for Autism Research,* Chicago, Illinois, May 7, 2009.

Mandell, D., Novak, M., & Zubritsky, C. (2005). Factors associated with age of diagnosis among children with autism spectrum disorders. *Pediatrics, 116*(6), 1480–1487.

Mandell, D., Wiggins, L., Arnstein Carpenter, L., Daniels, J., DiGiuseppi, C., Durkin, M., et al. (2009). Racial/ethnic disparities in the identification of children with autism spectrum disorders. *American Journal of Public Health, 99*(3), 493–498.

Matson, J., Dempsey, T., LoVullo, S., & Wilkins, J. (2008). The effects of intellectual functioning on the range of core symptoms of autism spectrum disorders. *Research in Developmental Disabilities, 29,* 341–350.

Matson, J., & Nebel-Schwalm, M. (2007). Comorbid psychopathology with autism spectrum disorder in children: An overview. *Research in Developmental Disabilities, 28*(4), 341–352.

Mesibov, G., Schopler, E., & Caison, W. (1989). The Adolescent and Adult Psychoeducational Profile: Assessment of adolescents and adults with severe developmental handicaps. *Journal of Autism and Developmental Disorders, 19,* 33–40.

Miles, J., Takahashi, T. N., Bagby, S., Pahota, S. K, Vaslow, D. F., Wang, C. H., et al. (2005). Essential versus complex autism: Definition of fundamental prognostic subtypes. *American Journal of Medical Genetics, 135,* 171–180.

Morrow, E., Yoo, S., Flavell, S., Kim, T, Lin, Y. Hill, R., et al. (2008). Identifying autism loci and genes by tracing recent shared ancestry. *Science, 321*(5886), 218–223.

Mullen, E. (1995). *Mullen Scales of Early Learning* (AGS ed.). Circle Pines, MN: American Guidance Service.

Nordin, V., & Gillberg, C. (1998). The long-term course of autistic disorders: Update on follow-up studies. *Acta Psychiatrica Scandinavica, 97,* 99–108.

Overton, T., Fielding, C., & Garcia de Alba, R. (2007). Differential diagnosis of Hispanic children referred for Autism Spectrum Disorders: Complex issues. *Journal of Autism and Developmental Disorders, 37,* 1996–2007.

Paul, R. (2007). *Language disorders from infancy through adolescence: Assessment and intervention* (3rd ed.). St. Louis: Mosby-Year Book.

Richler, J., Bishop, S. L., Kleinke, J. R., & Lord, C. (2007). Restrictive and repetitive behaviors in young children with autism spectrum disorders. *Journal of Autism and Developmental Disorders, 37,* 73–85.

Risi, S., Lord, C., Gotham, K., Corsello, C., Szatmari, P., Cook, E., et al. (2006). Combining information from multiple sources in the diagnosis of autism spectrum disorders. *Journal of the American Academy of Child and Adolescent Psychiatry, 45,* 1094–1103.

Rutter, M. (1970). Autistic children: Infancy to adulthood. *Seminars in Psychiatry, 2,* 435–450.

Rutter, M. (1972). Childhood schizophrenia reconsidered. *Journal of Autism and Childhood Schizophrenia, 2*(4), 315–337.

Rutter, M., Bailey, A., & Lord, C. (2003). *Social Communication Questionnaire (SCQ).* Los Angeles: Western Psychological Services.

Schieve, L. A., Rice, C., & Boyle, C. (2006). Parental report of diagnosed autism in children aged 4–17 years—United States—2003–2004. *CDC Morbidity and Mortality Weekly Report, 55,* 481–486.

Schopler, E., Andrews, C. E., & Strupp, K. (1980). Do autistic children come from upper middle-class parents? *Journal of Autism and Developmental Disorders, 10,* 91–103.

Schopler, E., Lansing, M., Reichler, R., & Marcus, L. (2004). *Psychoeducational Profile, Third Edition (PEP-3).* Austin, TX: Pro-Ed, USA.

Schopler, E., Reichler, R., & Renner, B. (1986). The childhood autism rating scale (CARS) for diagnostic screening and classification of autism. Part of the series *Diagnosis and teaching curricula for autism and developmental disabilities*. New York: Irvington.

Seltzer, M., Shattuck, P., & Abbeduto, L. (2004). Trajectory of development in adolescents and adults with autism. *Mental Retardation and Developmental Disabilities Research Reviews, 10*(4), 2004, 234–247.

Shattuck, P. T., & Grosse, S. D. (2007). Issues related to the diagnosis and treatment of autism spectrum disorders. *Mental Retardation and Developmental Disabilities Research Reviews, 13*, 129–135.

South, M., Williams, B. J., McMahon, W. M., Owley, T., Filipek, P. A., Shernoff, E., et al. (2002). Utility of Gilliam Autism Rating Scale in research and clinical populations. *Journal of Autism and Developmental Disorders, 32*, 593–599.

Sparrow, S. S., Cicchetti, D. V., & Balla, D. A. (2005). *Vineland Adaptive Behavior Scales* (2nd ed.). Circle Pines, MN: American Guidance Service.

Sterling, L., Dawson, G., & Estes, A. (2008). Characteristics associated with presence of depressive symptoms in adults with autism spectrum disorder. *Journal of Autism and Developmental Disorders, 38*(6), 1011–1018.

Stone, W. L., Coonrod, E. E., & Ousley, O. Y. (2000). Screening tool for autism in two-year-olds (STAT): Development and preliminary data. *Journal of Autism and Developmental Disorders, 30*(6), 607–612.

Szatmari, P. (2000). The classification of autism, Asperger's syndrome, and pervasive developmental disorder. *Canadian Journal of Psychiatry, 45*(8), 731–738.

Tassé, M. J., Aman, M. G., Hammer, D., & Rojahn, J. (1996). The Nisonger Child Behavior Rating Form: Age and gender effects and norms. *Research in Developmental Disabilities, 17*, 59–75.

Thurm, A., Lord, C., & Lee, L. (2007). Predictors of language acquisition in preschool children with autism spectrum disorders. *Journal of Autism and Developmental Disorders, 37*(9), 1721–1734.

Tidmarsh, L., & Volkmar, F. R. (2003). Diagnosis and epidemiology of autism spectrum disorders. *Canadian Journal of Psychiatry, 48*(8), 517–525.

Turner, L., Stone, W., Pozdol, S., & Coonrod, E. (2006). Follow-up of children with autism spectrum disorders from age 2 to age 9. *Autism, 10*(3), 243–265.

Van Bourgondien, M., Marcus, L., & Schopler, E. (1992). Comparison of DSM-III-R and childhood autism rating scale diagnoses of autism. *Journal of Autism and Developmental Disorders, 22*(4), 493–506.

Venter, A., Lord, C., & Schopler, E. (1992). A follow-up study on high functioning autistic children. *Journal of Child Psychology and Psychiatry, 33*(3), 489–507.

Volkmar, F. R., Cicchetti, D. V., Dykens, E., Sparrow, S. S., Leckman, J. F., & Cohen, D.F. (1988). An evaluation of the Autism Behavior Checklist. *Journal of Autism and Developmental Disorders, 18*, 81–97.

Volkmar, F. R., Klin, A., Siegel, B., Szatmari, P., Lord, C., Campbell, M., et al. (1994). Field trial for autistic disorder in DSM-IV. *American Journal of Psychiatry, 151*, 1361–1367.

Volkmar, F. R., & Lord, C. (2007). Diagnosis and definition of autism and other pervasive developmental disorders. In F. R. Volkmar (Ed.), *Autism and pervasive developmental disorders* (2nd ed., pp. 1–31). Cambridge: Cambridge University Press.

Volkmar, F. R., & Rutter, M. (1995). Childhood Disintegrative Disorder: Results of the DSM-IV autism field trial. *Journal of the American Academy of Child and Adolescent Psychiatry, 34*, 1092–1095.

Walker, D., Thompson, A., Zwaigenbaum, L., Goldberg, J., Bryson, S., Mahoney, W., et al. (2004). Specifying PDD-NOS: A comparison of PDD-NOS, Asperger syndrome, and autism. *Journal of the American Academy of Child and Adolescent Psychiatry, 43*, 172–180.

Wechsler, D. (2003). *Wechsler Intelligence Scales for Children* (4th ed.). San Antonio, TX: Psychological Corporation.

Wetherby, A., & Prizant, B. (2002). *Communication and Symbolic Behavior Scales Developmental Profile—First Normed Edition.* Baltimore, MD: Paul H. Brookes.

Wiggins, L. D., Baio, J., & Rice, C. (2006). Examination of the time between first evaluation and first autism spectrum diagnosis in a population-based sample. *Journal of Developmental and Behavioral Pediatrics, 27*, 79–87.

Williams White, S., Koenig, K., & Scahill, L. (2007). Social skills development in children with autism spectrum disorders: A review of the intervention research. *Journal of Autism and Developmental Disorders, 37*, 1858–1868.

Wing, L. (1980). Childhood autism and social class: A question of selection? *British Journal of Psychiatry*, 137, 410–417.

Wing, L., & Gould, J. (1979). Severe impairments of social interaction and associated abnormalities in children: Epidemiology and classification. *Journal of Autism and Developmental Disorders, 9*(1), 11–29.

Wing, L., Leekam, S. R., Libby, S. J., Gould, J., & Larcombe, M. (2002). The Diagnostic Interview for Social and Communication Disorders: Background, inter-rater reliability and clinical use. *Journal of Child Psychology and Psychiatry and Allied Disciplines, 43*, 307–325.

World Health Organization (1990). *International Classification of Diseases* (10th ed.). Diagnostic Criteria for Research. Geneva: WHO.

3 Ami Klin

Asperger's Syndrome: From Asperger to Modern Day

Points of Interest

- The DSM-IV and ICD-10 definitions of Asperger's syndrome reflect an unhelpful compromise based on seminal, historical descriptions but limited evidence or operationalization, which collectively render these definitions virtually irrelevant.
- The lack of consensual definitions has given rise to a wide range of usages of the term that reflect popularity among investigators and in the community rather than replicable, empirical findings; this state of affairs renders the literature on external validity uninterpretable.
- Forthcoming updates of DSM-IV and ICD-10 will take place in suboptimal conditions of evidence, while the stakes for clinical practice and advocacy could not be higher given the increasingly larger numbers of individuals diagnosed and the proliferation of support agencies coalescing around the term to provide sorely needed services.
- Knowledge advancements of developmental factors mediating outcome, discovered through prospective and longitudinal studies, are likely to elucidate the utility of empirically derived categorical subtypes of the autism spectrum disorders.

Introduction

Asperger's syndrome (AS) is one of the pervasive developmental disorders (PDD)—a group of neurodevelopmental conditions of early onset characterized by impairments in social interaction and communication, and by restricted interest and behaviors. The prototypical PDD is autism. Unlike autism, however, AS is marked by a lack of any clinically significant delay in spoken or receptive language, cognitive development, self-help skills, or curiosity about the environment.

Over 60 years after its initial description, the nosologic validity of AS relative to autism without intellectual disabilities (or higher functioning autism; HFA) and relative to the residual PDD category or Pervasive Developmental Disorder Not-Otherwise-Specified (PDD-NOS), is still questionable. A large number of studies seeking to test its external validity on the basis of genetic, neurobiological, neurostructure and neurofunction, neuropsychological, treatment, and outcome research have yielded conflicted data (Klin, McPartland, et al., 2005). This research, however, is difficult to interpret because of fundamental ambiguities inherent in the formal definitions of the syndrome (i.e., definitions provided by the *Diagnostic and Statistical Manual* published by the American Psychiatric Association; DSM-IV-TR, APA, 2000; and by the *International Classification of Diseases* published by the World Health Organization; ICD-10, WHO, 1992). This state of affairs has meant assignment of the diagnosis to participants in clinical and experimental research cannot be easily standardized for compliance with a consensual approach. This, in turn, makes comparison of results across studies virtually impossible.

A failure in formal definitions to yield distinguishable diagnostic groups has led to a multitude of usages of the term AS in research, clinical practice, and advocacy. Some definitions single out one variable defined rather simplistically as delays in the acquisition of single words or phrase speech, dichotomizing diagnostic assignment into autism and AS on the basis of presence or absence of this criterion, respectively. Others consider all individuals with autism spectrum disorders (ASD) with preserved intellectual skills as having AS. Others consider AS a diagnosis encompassing individuals who have milder symptoms or whose social presentation is marked by some difficulties without necessarily leading to functional impairment. In the research literature, a "conservative" approach has been to list autism with preserved intellectual skills, or HFA, and AS as equivalent terms, in this way circumventing the need to define either one. This is typically done despite the rule in formal nosology—the "precedence rule," according to which if an individual meets criteria for autism he or she should not receive a diagnosis of AS.

While the validity status of AS has generated a controversial and not very productive debate, the clinical and real-life challenges faced by the vast majority of individuals with this condition are an incontrovertible reality regardless of which diagnostic construct is assigned to them. In fact, the formalization of AS in official diagnostic manuals in the 1990s has led to a great explosion in public awareness of "higher functioning" individuals with ASD. As a result, a large number of support and advocacy groups and organizations were formed around the world coalescing around the term AS. Thousands of individuals who were until then almost invisible to their surrounding communities—in many ways, struggling within the hidden environments of family and self-support only—were now "discovered" by the educational and mental health structures capable of fostering their growth. With this new awareness came also fascination by the media, with both good and detrimental results. The portrayal of individuals with AS as eccentric intellectuals—"the geek syndrome"—introduced stereotyped views that sensationalized intellectual prodigies while ignoring the majority's life struggles. Juxtaposed to this media portrayal came the advocacy for stopping the "medicalization" of the term "AS," defining it instead as a "style of learning," something to be contrasted to "neurotypical" learning, rather than a psychiatric diagnosis intended to entitle the person to comprehensive treatments, appropriate educational programs, and community supports. While achieving political correctness and a semblance of integration, this movement also diluted the term, making it even harder for advocates to secure sorely needed services without which these individuals are unlikely to fulfill the promise of independent, self-supporting, and productive adult lives.

Against this clinical, research, and cultural backdrop, the future nosologic status of AS continues to be discussed, now with greater urgency given the forthcoming update of formal classification systems (i.e., DSM-V), and the uncertainty as to whether or not the term will be included within the PDDs. This chapter provides an overview of the historical and research background of AS leading to current debates, the changing nature of this discussion given the transformative changes in autism research in general in the past decade, the unchanging nature of these individuals' needs whether or not the term survives new updates in psychiatric classification, and suggestions for a future more likely to clarify old questions while raising new and more scientifically helpful ones. This future should avoid past sterile debates and focus more intensively on the developmental nature of this and related disorders of social and communicative functioning. To anchor this discussion in clinical realities, an overview of clinical features, treatment, and support services is also provided.

History and Nosology of Asperger's Syndrome (AS)

Although AS was accorded formal diagnostic status only in the 1990s (in DSM-IV; APA, 1994; and in ICD-10; WHO, 1992), the original description appeared in 1944 (Asperger, 1944), only one year after Kanner's seminal account of autism (Kanner, 1943). The first influential description of Asperger's work appeared in English only in 1981 (Wing, 1981), the year after Hans Asperger's death. But it was only in the 1990s, and particularly after the publication of DSM-IV and ICD-10, that his work became better known. Since then, however, the clinical and research literature making use of the term AS has grown exponentially. To exemplify this growth, publications including AS in their title in PsychINFO grew from a handful before 1981, to maybe a few more than 10 between 1981 and 1990, to 140 between 1991 and 2000, to 452 in since 2001. The numbers since 1991 still represent only about 10% of the number of publications including the word "autism" in their title. Since 2001, the use of the term "autism spectrum disorder" (ASD) has also been growing exponentially. From fewer than 10 titles during the 1990s, there have been close to 260 titles since 2001. And the term is now commonly used in grant applications and large research meetings, particularly as more and more investigators in a whole range of disciplines from molecular genetics to social policy are baffled by the heterogeneity of autism related disorders. It is possible that the increasingly more popular term ASD will gradually replace the term AS in future clinical and research work.

Hans Asperger's Original Construct

In 1944 Hans Asperger, an Austrian pediatrician with interest in special education, described four children who had difficult integrating socially into groups (Asperger, 1944). These 4 children were 6 to 11 years of age, and all appeared to have intact if not gifted intellectual functioning. This text was translated in 1991 by Uta Frith, who also added some background on his professional training and clinical practice (Frith, 1991). Unaware of Kanner's publication (1943), Asperger termed the condition he described *Autistischen Psychopathen im Kindesalter*, or autistic psychopathy in childhood, echoing Bleuler's (1916) use of the term "autism" in schizophrenia to signify extreme egocentrism. He contrasted this condition from schizophrenia, however, by emphasizing the stable and enduring nature of the social impairments and by voicing the optimistic view that unlike in schizophrenia, his patients were able to eventually develop some relationships. His term is probably better translated into today's psychiatric nomenclature as a stable personality disorder marked by social isolation. His use of the term "autism" marked his belief that difficulties in socialization represented the defining feature of the condition.

The four children had come to Asperger's attention, to some extent, because of school failure and behavioral problems displayed in social situations, including aggression, noncompliance, and negativism. He did not consider these to be willful transgressions of social mores but reflections of a true inability to understand others, particularly their nonverbal signals and communications. He described a marked reduction in the quantity and diversity of facial expressions and in the use of gesture, and profound difficulties in understanding nonverbal cues conveyed by others. They were verbose, and their own spontaneous communications were marked by correct formal language structures but highly idiosyncratic form. There were frequent circumstantial utterances (e.g., failing to distinguish information about the world from their own autobiographical narration); speech typically involved long-winded and incoherent verbal sequences failing to convey a clear message or thought (e.g., tangential speech triggered by a series of nonmeaningful associations); and conversation was profoundly one-sided (e.g., failing to demarcate changes of topic or to introduce new materials, thus leading to other people's confusion). The children also displayed unusual and highly circumscribed interests which absorbed their attention and learning, often appeared to preclude the acquisition of practical and self-help skills, and dominated the content of their communications with others. Their emotional presentation was marked by poor empathy, the tendency to intellectualize feelings, and a profound lack of intuitive understanding of other people's affective experiences and intentions. They were also motorically clumsy, unable to participate in group sports, and often lagged in the acquisition of motor coordination skills such as riding a bike or producing good penmanship.

Other important features of Asperger's description included his belief that the condition could not be recognized in early childhood because speech, language and intellectual curiosity in the environment appeared intact in the first few years of life. Also, he thought that there was a clear familial nature to his syndrome, as similar traits in parents or close relatives could be found in almost every case. Almost always, both affected individuals and vulnerable family members were male.

With the exception of one brief communication that appeared in the year before his death (Asperger, 1979), Asperger's work was published in German, and remained largely unknown in the English-speaking world until Wing's publication in the 1981. In contrast, Leo Kanner's (1943) description of 11 children with "autistic disturbances of affective contact," whom he had begun to see in the 1930s, was published in English by someone who was the founding figure of child psychiatry in the United States, and became an instant classic. Although both men's native language was German, World War II and the lack of academic communication across languages signified that neither had knowledge of the other's work, at least not in the 1940s and 1950s. And yet, there were clear commonalities in the syndromes they described. Their patients had profound difficulties in social interaction, affect, and communication, and displayed unusual and idiosyncratic patterns of interest. The main differences related to Asperger's observation that his patients' speech and language acquisition as well as intellectual functioning were less commonly delayed, motor deficits were more likely, onset was later in childhood, and all of his initial cases occurred in boys. More importantly, however, there were significant differences in terms of aspects and severity of symptomatology in the areas of social-emotional functioning, communication and cognitive skills, motor mannerisms, and circumscribed interests. In retrospect, however, some of these differences appear to have been a function of the presentation of the specific children initially described by Kanner and Asperger rather than some fundamental markers denoting two fully independent syndromes. Kanner's patients included preschoolers, were less verbal, and some were considerably more cognitively disabled. Asperger's patients were primarily school-age children, and were highly verbal and cognitively intact if not gifted. Consequently, Kanner's initial description became associated with the "classically" cognitively impaired or "lower functioning" child with autism, whereas Asperger's initial description became associated with the more cognitively able and highly verbal older child with ASD.

That the nature of patients originally described by Kanner and Asperger was a more important factor in accounting for differences separating the two accounts is clear in some of the work appearing subsequently. For example, Robinson and Vitale (1954) described three cases of children aged 8 to 11 years who showed a pattern of circumscribed interests reminiscent of Asperger's patients. The children were interested in developmentally precocious topics such as chemistry, nuclear fission, transportation systems, astronomy, and electricity, among others. They talked about these topics incessantly in one-sided conversations with peers and adults. They were socially isolated, had little adherence to social niceties, and their play revolved almost exclusively around their interests. Kanner (1954) was the invited discussant of this paper. The descriptions reminded him of "infantile autism" (the term that had by then become the common clinical construct used to denote autism). But he felt that these children were less socially withdrawn and more affectively engaged with others than the children he had described in previous years. Still they lacked friends and did not participate in group activities. As the paper focused on circumscribed interests, Kanner suggested that the various topics dominated the lives of these children, monopolizing their learning and interfering with their ability to engage others in reciprocal relationships. And because these interests were so unusual, consisting of collections of facts rather than conceptual inquiries or hobbies; they could not be shared with others and could not easily become a springboard for vocational learning. It is of interest, therefore, that Kanner's incisive clinical observations greatly resembled those of Asperger when he was called to describe children similar to those Asperger encountered in his original case studies.

An equivalent example in Asperger's writings—the description of "lower functioning" children—cannot be found in the English literature, but it may be available in his considerable body of work from 1944 to the time of his death. But one important difference set Asperger's and Kanner's accounts apart, and to some extent influenced their power to generate research. While Asperger's frame of reference was special education on the one hand—his patients were not willful transgressors of rules but children who could not process social information—and the prevailing concept of schizophrenia on the other hand—his patients had a stable, longstanding personality structure marked by social disabilities—Kanner's frame of reference was deeply developmental. Influenced by the work of Arnold Gesell, a developmentalist at the Yale Child Study Center, Kanner described autism as a congenital disorder partially because of his appreciation of the fact that his children failed to display social communication, learning, and play skills that were effortlessly acquired by much younger, typically developing children. While Asperger's description was primarily clinical in nature, Kanner ventured into learning structures (e.g., difficulty in integrating information in learning) and other observations (e.g., macrocephaly) that generated a wide array of cognitive and other hypotheses that are still very much relevant to this day. It was probably not a coincidence that 2 years after Kanner's description of autism, Scheerer and colleagues (1945) published an exquisite set of neuropsychological experiments involving one of Kanner's patients, which foreshadowed much of cognitive research that began to appear only in the 1970s and 1980s.

Evolving Conceptualization of as in the 1980s

Although historically Kanner's and Asperger's clinical syndromes appeared more complementary than mutually exclusive, the introduction of Asperger's work to English-based psychiatry was inherently tied to the question of whether the diagnostic constructs they described were "the same or different." To some extent, this introduction was first made by Van Krevelen (1963), who made a deliberate attempt to distinguish the concept of "autistic psychopathy" from Kanner's autism (Van Krevelen, 1971) and concluded that they were sharply different. His discussion clearly separated onset patterns, social and communicative functions, and intellectual and language abilities that are characteristic of lower functioning children with ASD from those that are more characteristic of higher functioning children. Kanner never discussed this distinction, whereas Asperger appeared to support it later in life (Asperger, 1979; Hippler & Klicpera, 2003).

As noted, awareness of Asperger's syndrome did not increase until Lorna Wing's (1981) influential case series was published. She described 34 individuals, aged 5 to 35 years, of whom 19 had a clinical presentation similar to that described by Asperger, whereas the remaining sample had a current presentation similar to the syndrome but onset patterns and early history were different. Concerned that the term "psychopathy" might connote sociopathic behavior (rather than the intended personality disorder), and hoping to ground the condition in developmental terms (thus ensuring that no support to the position blaming autism on parents could be derived from this work), Wing chose the eponymous "Asperger's Syndrome" instead of "autistic psychopathy." She summarized Asperger's original text and proposed some modifications for the syndrome on the basis of her case studies. Although Asperger thought that the condition was unrecognizable prior to age 3 years, Wing suggested that several difficulties were present in the first 2 years of life, including problems in socialization, speech, and communication; pronounced narrow interests and restricted behaviors; and restrictive imaginative play. She also suggested that AS could be found in girls and in individuals with mild intellectual disabilities.

While Wing's publication set in motion a great surge of interest in AS, it also blurred the distinctions made by Van Krevelen, essentially bringing Asperger's construct within the triad of impairments involving social, communication, and imaginative symptoms (Wing, 1986). There was palpable progress made in fostering awareness of the challenges of higher functioning individuals, but also an unexpected consolidation of the "same or different" preoccupation in the field, which Wing subsequently thought of as a major and unjustified distraction (Wing, 2000). And yet the two decades that followed Wing's initial publication on AS were primarily characterized by such attempts at separating autism from AS. Several definitions were derived from her account on the basis of the experience of influential clinical investigators (Gillberg & Gillberg, 1989; Szatmari et al., 1989; Tantam, 1988), yielding results that fell on either side of the "same or different" question. The use of different definitions yielded, not surprisingly, different groups for comparison (Klin, Pauls, et al., 2005). This undermined any attempt to interpret this literature, and failed to shed light on developmental mechanisms of interest that might account for differential outcomes, and which could be proven diagnostically meaningful (Klin, McPartland, et al., 2005).

Formalization of AS as a Diagnostic Category in DSM-IV and ICD-10

As noted, AS was not officially recognized until the 10th edition of the *International Classification of Diseases* (ICD-10; WHO, 1992) and the 4th edition of the *Diagnostic and Statistical Manual* (DSM-IV; APA, 1994). The coordinated and simultaneous inclusion in both systems followed limited evidence provided by a large, joint field trial that revealed that AS could be differentiated from autism unaccompanied by intellectual disabilities or higher functioning autism (HFA) on the basis of some limited data (Volkmar et al., 1994). This work was prompted by the recognition that autism is a clinically heterogeneous disorder and that the characterization of subtypes of PDD or ASD might help behavioral and biological research by allowing the identification of clinically more homogeneous groups (Bailey et al., 1998; Rutter, 1999; Volkmar et al., 1997). An awareness of the large number of individuals with serious social disability who did not meet strict criteria for autism was a further concern. For some disorders like Rett's syndrome (Amir et al., 1999), this approach facilitated neurobiological research.

This hope, however, was not realized in the subtyping of the more commonly found PDDs, namely autism, AS, and PDD-NOS. To begin with, there was some ambivalence about the inclusion of AS as a "new" category, impacting on the final definition adopted in DSM-IV and ICD-10, which has proven highly problematic in many respects. Limitations of the adopted formal definition of AS were pointed out almost immediately (Miller & Ozonoff, 1997). It has since been criticized as overly narrow (Eisenmajer et al., 1996; Szatmari et al., 1995), rendering the diagnostic assignment of AS improbable or even "virtually impossible" (Mayes et al., 2001; Miller & Ozonoff, 2000). Equally concerning, criteria were modified by investigators for a given study, or were disregarded altogether in favor of the investigator's own criteria (see Klin, McPartland, et al., 2005 for a discussion). Studies attempting to compare different diagnostic schemes (e.g., Ghaziuddin et al., 1992; Leekam et al., 2000; Klin, Pauls, et al., 2005; Kopra et al., 2008; Woodbury-Smith et al., 2005) invariably revealed, not surprisingly, discordance in case assignment among the various schemes adopted.

The DSM-IV Definition of AS

The DSM-IV approach to the definition of AS was to adopt the triad of symptom clusters used for the definition of autism, namely qualitative impairments in social interaction and communication, and restricted repetitive and stereotyped patterns of behavior. And while the text accompanying the definition of AS in the text revision of DSM-IV (DSM-IV-TR; APA, 2000) was modified, the formal criteria for the diagnosis were not (as these cannot be changed but in a new edition of the manual). In DSM-IV, symptom requirements in the social and restrictive behaviors cluster are identical for AS and autism (or Autistic Disorder). In contrast to autism, there are no symptom requirements in the communication cluster, despite the fact that communication difficulties are universally reported in AS (Paul, in press). In essence, therefore, DSM-IV makes a distinction between autism and AS solely on the basis of the onset criteria. In autism, any concerns prior to the age of 3 years involving social interaction, social communication, or symbolic/imaginative play are sufficient for the criteria to be met. In contrast, any concern involving cognitive development (during childhood), self-help skills, or more broadly defined adaptive behavior (other than social interaction but including social communication) would rule out the diagnosis of AS. The overinclusive nature of onset criteria for autism and overexclusive nature of onset criteria for AS (and any ambiguities left in the definition, e.g., how to distinguish social interaction from social communication) are resolved in terms of the "precedence rule," according to which if an individual meets criteria for autism, he or she cannot be assigned the diagnosis of AS (Volkmar & Klin, 2000). Moreover, the clinical literature is replete with cases who defy this classification on the basis of a mixture of developmental features such as early language delays, or early cognitive delays (consistent with autism), and maybe adolescent presentation with no deficits in formal language skills or learning (more consistent with AS).

The impracticality of this scheme led to attempts at systematic modification, which, however, have not been followed up in subsequent research. They did, however, highlight pros and cons of possible alternatives for the current DSM-IV scheme. One influential approach has been to divide children with an early-emerging social disability but apparently normative cognitive development in terms of whether or not there were single words by age 2 years, and phrase speech (typically defined as non-echolalic 3-word combinations used meaningfully for communication) by the age of 3 years (i.e., AS is assigned if a child meets these criteria, and autism is assigned if the child does not (e.g., Gilchrist et al., 2001; Szatmari, 1995; 2000). Although this approach allows for important research on developmental paths and outcome, it greatly narrows the potential lines of distinction between autism and AS in that other aspects of onset as well as any unique features in the child's current presentation are disregarded (Volkmar & Klin, 2000). In essence, given that individuals with HFA may not present with speech delays as defined, there is a potential for the resultant samples (of individuals with HFA and AS) to overlap considerably in terms of other symptomatology, thus increasing the potential for type II errors (i.e., not finding differences) in such studies. Other practical concerns include the fact that many individuals with AS are not diagnosed as young children (McConachie et al., 2005; Mandell et al., 2005) and some are even diagnosed in adulthood (in fact, more frequently now than before), making the attainment of reliable and valid, as well as detailed developmental history quite challenging.

An additional factor contributing to the weakening of the AS construct is the fact that the benchmark diagnostic instruments in ASD—the *Autism Diagnostic Interview–Revised* or ADI-R; reference; and the *Autism Diagnostic Observation Schedule* or ADOS; reference—which are keyed in to DSM-IV criteria and are virtually universally required in research of ASD, do not include any of the PDD subtypes, limiting the resulting classification to Autism (or Autistic Disorder), ASD (often equated with PDD-NOS), and non-ASD. While it is clear that AS never achieved sufficient validity to be included in the instruments, the instruments were never adjusted by any investigators to attempt a better operationalization of the construct.

The result of these enduring nosologic quandaries has been a virtual abandonment of DSM-IV criteria and rules for the diagnostic assignment of AS. And yet, the construct survives nevertheless, having acquired what can be termed as "usage validity." As noted, the vast majority of clinical and research publications equate AS with autism without intellectual disabilities, or expand its meaning to encompass borderland expressions of ASD. Invariably, however, the term is used for school-age children, adolescents, and adults but not for young children, negating, therefore, its neurodevelopmental nature (and curiously perpetuating Asperger's original assertion that the condition cannot be identified in the first years of life).

Subtyping of the Autism Spectrum Disorders and the Diagnostic Status of AS

The need for subtyping of the autism spectrum disorders (ASD) is based on several different challenges in clinical practice and research. The ASDs are early-emerging neurodevelopmental disorders that impact on most domains of social and communicative functioning, with associated impact on cognitive and adaptive functioning. They are vastly heterogeneous in genotype and phenotype, which in turn likely reflects multiple etiologies and pathogenetic courses (Volkmar et al., 2004). These multiple levels of variability are often viewed as one of the greatest obstacles blocking the advancement of research on causes and treatments of these disorders. The advancement of meaningful clinical subtypes could yield more homogeneous samples, with the hope that these in turn could translate into advances in research on etiology, treatment specificity, and outcome optimization.

As noted, the separation between AS and autism was thought to provide a starting point for reducing heterogeneity, thus empowering research. However, the tentative inclusion of AS in DSM-IV and ICD-10 was not followed by research substantiating clear-cut distinctions in regard to traditional external validators such as etiology, developmental course, learning profiles, differential treatment response, or differential outcome (see Klin, McPartland, et al., 2005 for a review). Much of the validation work was thought to be confounded by the lack of a common nosologic framework and by circular reasoning, when validating factors were not clearly independent of the defining diagnostic criteria used to assign participants to different groups in the first place (Frith, 2004). This frustration intensified the use of the term "ASD," which blurs the categorical boundaries among the most common PDDs—autism, AS, and PDD-NOS—into a hypothesized continuum of affectedness (Wing, 1986; Wing & Gould, 1979). The term "spectrum" implies that a number of meaningful dimensions could generate the full range of syndrome expression (not unlike, for example, the spectrum of light) (Klin, 2009). These dimensions, if validated, could be considered as factors mediating the relationship between etiology(ies) and behavioral expressions. Several of such dimensions—also called "endophenotypes"—have been proposed at multiple levels of causation, from gene(s) and gene combinations, neuroanatomic abnormalities and disease processes, to onset patterns, neurocognitive abnormalities, combinations of symptom clusters, and levels of developmental skills such as language and intellectual endowment (e.g., Dawson et al., 2002; DiCicco-Bloom et al., 2006).

These endophenotypes, however, are still a work in progress, but collectively, this work further reinforces the need for subtyping research. And yet, discussions of subtyping of the PDDs typically focus primarily on the creation of categorical subdivisions of ASDs, their validation, and utility (Volkmar & Klin, 2005; Volkmar et al., 2009). There is a ubiquitous expectation that subtyping solutions in one domain of research or clinical practice should necessarily apply to other domains of clinical science (Klin, 2009). And yet, there is no reason to assume that factors underlying classification for one purpose should necessarily apply in the case of other purposes. For example, classification for clinical management and decisions on eligibility for educational services should be inclusive, reflecting the consensus that programming for persons with ASD should be determined on the basis of individualized profiles of strengths and deficits, and not on basis of the person's specific PDD diagnosis (NRC, 2001). In contrast, classification for the purpose of brain research should focus on the mechanism of interest in a given study. For example, several studies have suggested accelerated brain growth in the infancy period of children with ASD (e.g., Courschene et al., 2001). The full potential of this finding depends to some extent on quantified evaluation of the behavioral correlates of accelerated brain growth, including, for example, a specific timetable for onset and course of the atypical patterns of brain growth (Hazlett et al., 2005).

In this light, defining the purposes and expectations for diagnostic subtyping is critical (Klin, 2009; Volkmar et al., 2009). While current data available do not support validation of the PDD subcategory of AS (Frith, 2004; Klin et al., 2005b; Witwer & Lecavalier, 2008), they do not necessarily refute the premise that meaningful onset patterns may in fact delineate meaningful clinical entities. They only refute the simplistic notion that poorly defined and poorly operationalized behavioral statements are a sufficient basis to create distinguishable and meaningful diagnostic constructs, particularly if these are dependent on ascertainment of onset patterns carried out for individuals who are already adolescents or adults. While it is important not to perseverate on the seminal descriptions of 15 children made by two influential clinicians over 60 years ago (Kanner, 1943; Asperger, 1944) with the hope that research "by exegesis" might solve our current nosologic quandary, it is equally important not to prematurely foreclose the possibility that the vastly heterogeneous social disabilities encompassed by the term "ASD" cannot gain from better, developmental cognitive science research on mechanisms of socialization and their unfolding during the first years of a child's life (Johnson, 2001). For example, following from the experience-expectant model of child development (Johnson & Karmiloff-Smith, 2004) in which the genetically determined schedule of neural maturation matches the timing of adaptive tasks, disruptions of socialization processes occurring at different times are likely to result in different outcomes (Jones & Klin, 2009). Similarly, different outcomes are likely to result from a wide range of permutations of intact and impaired mechanisms of social cognition. What might be the consequences of these developmental processes to eventual outcomes, including any meaningful clusters of symptoms and abilities in individuals with ASD, is not known at present.

The potential contribution of developmental cognitive neuroscience is typically left unexplored in nosology research, which tends to go back to the classic clinical descriptions. For example, while Kanner emphasized the congenital nature of autism (Kanner, 1943), Asperger emphasized the later onset of the condition he described (1944). This incidental point of departure in the two accounts subsequently led to the hypothesis that presence or absence of speech delays could lead to meaningfully different clinical entities. This scenario should be considered hopelessly simplistic given current knowledge of developmental psychopathology and development cognitive science. The ASDs are quintessential neurodevelopmental disorders. By all accounts, diagnosis of vulnerabilities consistent with this diagnosis can be made within the first 2 or 3 years of life (Chawarska et al., 2007) if not earlier (e.g., Klin et al., 2004). It would be naïve to disregard the fact that variability in developmental profiles early in life might not have consequences for phenotypic variability later in life.

Two parallel sets of advancements bode well for this field: First, our knowledge of normative processes in child development has increased dramatically in the past 10 years, although autism research has been slow in fully assimilating new investigative paradigms, technologies, and concepts (Klin et al., 2008). Second, the advent of prospective studies of large cohorts of genetically at-risk infants, a proportion of whom will develop autism, carries the promise of shedding light on this critical period of pathogenesis hitherto confined to knowledge based on retrospective accounts or less-than-ideal methods of infancy research (Zwaigenbaum et al., 2007). As knowledge accrues from these efforts, it is very likely that a great deal of what we know about ASD will have to updated if not fully modified.

In this light, the future of nosologic research on AS needs to rely on these advancements if the field is to move forward beyond the sterile debates as to whether autism and AS represent "same or different" diagnostic entities. Clearly, several of the validation problems briefly described above could only be systematically tackled if there were some agreement as to a set of criteria, comprehensively detailed and uniformly utilized according to standardized ascertainment procedures. But at the root of this problem is the fact that the all-important onset criteria have been, universally, ascertained retrospectively, often many years after the person's early childhood. It is possible that the advent of prospective studies will answer some of these questions more productively. For example, meaningful differential patters of onset or developmental mechanisms can be used as independent variables, whereas diagnostic assignment later on in life can be analyzed as dependent variables, thus exploring the full range of meaningful diagnostic outcomes associated with clusters of well-quantified, early symptoms or developmental profiles (e.g., language, communication, social cognition). This effort might yield systematic mapping of developmental factors on trajectories and eventual outcomes, thus avoiding circular reification of definitions, and moving instead to a developmentally based and empirically derived nosology of the higher functioning ASDs (Klin, 2009). Such studies are underway, and there is some hope that they will be available prior to DSM-V, the next update of the formal diagnostic system used in the United States and several other countries. In their absence, a new round of arbitrary decisions impacting on the definition of AS is likely, maybe yielding to the concept of "usage validity" (i.e., the most popular patterns of use), or, more likely, removing the construct in favor of a more encompassing construct such as ASD.

Diagnosis and Clinical Features

The diagnosis of AS requires the demonstration of qualitative impairments in social interaction and restricted patterns of interest, criteria that are identical to autism. In contrast to autism, there are no criteria in the cluster of language and communication symptoms, and onset criteria differ in that there should be no clinically significant delay in language acquisition, cognitive, and self-help skills. These symptoms result in significant impairment in social and occupational functioning (APA, 2000).

Social and Communication Functioning

In some contrast to the social presentation in autism, individuals with AS find themselves socially isolated but are not usually withdrawn in the presence of other people, typically approaching others but in an inappropriate or eccentric fashion. For example, they may engage the interlocutor, usually an adult, but also same-age peers, in one-sided conversation characterized by long-winded, pedantic speech about a favorite and often unusual and narrow topic. They may express interest in friendships and in meeting people, but their wishes are invariably thwarted by their awkward approaches and insensitivity to the other person's feelings, intentions, and nonliteral and implied communications (e.g., signs of boredom, haste to leave, and need for privacy). They may also react inappropriately to or fail to interpret the valence of the context of the affective interaction, often conveying insensitivity, formality, or general disregard for the other person's emotional expressions. They may be able to describe correctly, in cognitive and often formalistic fashion, other people's emotions, expected intentions, and social conventions; however, they are unable to act on this knowledge in an intuitive and spontaneous fashion, thus losing the tempo of the interaction. Their poor intuition and lack of spontaneous adaptation are accompanied by marked reliance on formalistic rules of behavior and rigid social conventions. This presentation is largely responsible for the impression of social naïveté and behavioral rigidity that is so forcefully conveyed by these individuals.

Circumscribed Interests

Individuals with AS typically amass a large amount of factual information about a topic in an intense fashion (Klin,

Danovitch, et al., 2007). The actual topic may change from time to time, but often dominates the content of social exchange. Frequently the entire family may be immersed in the subject for long periods of time. This behavior is peculiar in the sense that oftentimes extraordinary amounts of information are learned about very circumscribed, and occasionally unusual topics (e.g., snakes, names of stars, TV guides, deep fat fryers, weather information, sports statistics, personal information on politicians or celebrities) without a genuine understanding of the broader phenomena involved. This symptom may not always be easily recognized in childhood because strong interests in certain topics, such as dinosaurs or fashionable fictional characters, are ubiquitous. In younger and older children with AS, however, special interests typically interfere with learning in general because they absorb so much of the person's attention and motivation, and also interfere with the person's ability to engage in more reciprocal forms of conversation with others.

Speech, Language, and Communication

Although significant abnormalities of speech and formal language skills are not typical of individuals with AS, there are at least three aspects of their communication patterns that are of clinical interest (Klin, McPartland, et al., 2005; Paul, in press). First, speech may be marked by poor prosody, although inflection and intonation may not be as rigid and monotonic as in autism. There is often a constricted range of intonation patterns that is used with little regard to the communicative function of the utterance (e.g., assertions of fact, humorous remarks). Rate of speech may be unusual (e.g., too fast) or may lack in fluency (e.g., jerky speech), and often there is poor modulation of volume (e.g., voice is too loud despite physical proximity to conversational partner). The latter feature may be particularly noticeable in the context of a lack of adjustment to the given social setting (e.g., social contact occurring in a library or at a funeral). These various oddities can be extremely stigmatizing given low tolerance for these oddities among members of the general community.

A second important communication pattern of interest relates to the fact that speech may often be tangential and circumstantial, conveying a sense of looseness of associations and incoherence. Even though in a very small number of cases this symptom may be an indicator of a possible thought disorder, the lack of contingency in speech is more typically a result of the one-sided, egocentric conversational style (e.g., unrelenting monologues about the names, codes, and attributes of innumerable TV stations in a country); failure to provide the background for comments and to clearly demarcate changes in topic of conversation; and failure to suppress vocal output accompanying internal thoughts.

A third noticeable symptom relates to a communication style that is often characterized by marked verbosity. The child or adult may talk incessantly, usually about a favorite subject, often in complete disregard to the listener's interest, engagement, or attempt to interject a comment or change the subject of conversation. Despite such forceful monologues, the individual with AS may never come to a point or conclusion. And attempts by the interlocutor to elaborate on issues of content or logic, or to shift the conversation to related topics, are often unsuccessful.

Motor Difficulties

Although Asperger noticed pronounced "motoric clumsiness" in his patients, attempts to use this symptom as a point of differentiation between the diagnosis of AS (where motoric dysfunction is contrasted with preserved intellectual skills) and the diagnosis of autism (where presumably motor skills are at a higher or at least commensurate level with intellectual skills) have yielded conflicted results. Comparisons of individuals with AS and autism at similar cognitive levels have generally suggested that motor deficits are displayed by individuals with both syndromes (Smith, 2000). Patterns of acquisition of motor skills, or potential developmental factors underlying possible differences in motoric functioning later in life have not been systematically studied.

Practically, however, individuals with AS may have a history of delayed acquisition of motor skills, such as pedaling a bike, catching a ball, opening jars, and climbing outdoor play equipment. They are often visibly awkward and poorly coordinated and may exhibit stilted or bouncy gait patterns and odd posture.

Comorbid Features

The most common disorders co-occurring with AS are depression and anxiety. Estimates of comorbid anxiety and/or depression in individuals with AS are as high as 65 percent, and some researchers have suggested that these elevated rates represent a distinction between AS and higher functioning autism (HFA) (Ellis et al., 1994; Fujikawa et al., 1987; Ghaziuddin, 2002; Ghaziuddin et al., 1998; Green et al., 2000; Howlin & Goode, 1998). Other data suggest, however, that individuals with AS and HFA are equally at increased risk for problems with anxiety and depression, with no differences between the groups (Kim et al., 2000). Anxiety in AS has been observed to stem from several sources. Concern about possible violations of rigid routines or rituals can be anxiety-provoking for individuals with AS. They frequently rely on particular schedule or methods of completing daily activities that, when violated, result in significant upset. Conversely, when placed in a context in which no clear schedule or set of expectations is known, anxiety may result. Also, devoid of an intuitive sense of other people's intentions and unspoken rules of social engagement, and yet often painfully aware of previous experiences of social failure, there may be great anticipatory anxiety relative to social encounters, the outcomes of which are perceived as situations these individuals have little control over.

Equally common to anxiety and typically appearing in early adolescence, depressive symptoms represent the result of the unique pairing of social desire in the absence of social intuition or skill. Chronically frustrated by their repeated experiences of failure to engage others and form friendships or romantic relationships, individuals with AS often become despondent, negativistic, and bitter, or even clinically depressed, which may require treatment, including psychopharmacological treatment.

Several other comorbid conditions have been reported. Hyperactivity and inattention are common among children with AS (Eisenmajer et al., 1996; Schatz et al., 2002), and many children with the disorder are often initially misdiagnosed with attention-deficit/hyperactivity disorder as mental health providers or educational professionals fail to appreciate the neurodevelopmental nature of their social and communication difficulties. Some studies have associated AS with Tourette's syndrome (Kerbeshian & Burd, 1986; Littlejohns et al., 1990; Marriage et al., 1993, obsessive-compulsive disorder (Thomsen, 1994), and psychotic conditions (Gillberg, 1985). Some studies have investigated the notion that the combination of preserved intellectual and linguistic capacities with limited empathy and social understanding might predispose individuals with AS to violent or criminal behavior (Everall & Le Couteur, 1990; Scragg & Shah, 1994), but this hypothesis is unsupported by other studies (Ghaziuddin et al., 1991). Nevertheless, these individuals' lack of "common sense," reduced intuition, and extreme "gullibility" at times leads to unintentional transgressions of rules that may have legal consequences which can be grave. For example, the combination of extreme social isolation and technical competencies in operating computers often result in unlimited, typically unsupervised Internet use with the attending perils that this medium poses to naïve users. Serious crimes can be committed through naïve, reckless, or otherwise unguided or unsupervised use of the Internet, including crimes for which there are mandatory sentences (e.g., downloading of illegal images).

Course and Prognosis

There are no systematic long-term follow-up studies of children with AS as of this writing, partially because of nosologic issues. Many children are able to attend regular education classes with additional support services, although these children are especially vulnerable to being seen as eccentric and being teased or victimized; others require special education services, usually not because of academic deficits but because of their social and behavioral difficulties. Asperger's initial description predicted a positive outcome for many of his patients, who were often able to use their special talents for the purpose of obtaining employment and leading self-supporting lives. His observation of similar traits in family members (e.g., fathers, grandfathers) may also have made him more optimistic about the ultimate outcome. Although his account was tempered somewhat over time, Asperger continued to believe that a more positive outcome was a central criterion differentiating individuals with his syndrome from those with Kanner's autism. Although some clinicians have informally concurred with this statement, particularly in regard to gainful employment, independence, and establishing a family, no studies using consensual definitions of the condition have to date addressed long-term outcome in longitudinal follow-ups. Clearly, since cognitive and language levels are probably the most important factors in predicting outcome (Howlin, 2005), the perception of differences between individuals with autism and those with AS relative to prognosis in adulthood might be confounded by perceptions of the definitions of these conditions (i.e., AS being associated with higher level of cognitive and language skills).

Medical and Neurobiological Factors

Several reports of medical abnormalities associated with AS have appeared, but, due to nosological issues and the preponderance of case reports and or small studies, no factors have been reliably associated with AS across studies. Wing (1981) reported high frequency of perinatal problems (nearly half of her original sample) among individuals with AS. Other reports have associated AS with medical conditions, including aminoaciduria (Miles & Capelle, 1987) and ligamentous laxity (Tantam et al., 1990). A case series by Gillberg (1989) reported high frequencies of medical anomalies common to both AS and autism, but these results have not been consistently replicated (Rutter et al., 1994). Epilepsy occurs more frequently in individuals with ASD than in the general population (Tuchman & Rapin, 2002), and this increased rate has been detected in case series investigating individuals with AS (Cederlund & Gillberg, 2004). Anomalies have also been detected in eye movements and visual scanning in individuals with ASDs (Sweeney et al., 2004), particularly in natural viewing of social scenes (Klin et al., 2002) but these findings have not yet been shown to distinguish AS from other ASDs. Neurochemical studies of autism spectrum disorders have produced inconsistent results. The most robust finding is elevated blood serotonin levels, but other studies have reported atypicalities in peptide excretion, neuroendocrine/HPA function, amino acid levels, uric acid excretion, and central cholinergic and gabaergic receptors. Some of these findings have been seriously challenged in more recent studies (Cass et al., 2008). At any rate, none of these findings seems to apply differentially to AS versus other ASDs (Anderson & Hoshino, 2005).

In recent years extensive neuroimaging research has been conducted to investigate structural anomalies in the brains of individuals with AS. However, no clear common pathology has emerged in individuals with AS, both with respect to typical individuals and in terms of differentiation among other ASDs. Berthier and colleagues (Berthier et al., 1990) reported MRI results indicating left frontal macrogyria and bilateral opercular polymicrogyria in patients with AS. Other studies have reported gray tissue anomalies (McAlonan et al., 2002), left temporal lobe damage (Jones & Kerwin, 1990), left occipital hypoperfusion (Ozbayrak et al., 1991), and dysmorphology superior to the ascending ramus of the Sylvian fissure proximal to the intersection of the middle frontal gyrus and the precentral sulcus (Volkmar et al., 1996). The most robust neuroanatomical findings (applying to ASDs in general) are of rapid brain growth in early childhood leading to increased brain volume that normalizes in mid-childhood, and reduced size of the corpus callosum (Minshew et al., 2005) although once again, there have been no claims that such findings differentiate AS from other ASD subtypes.

Functional imaging has also provided information about ASDs, though, as is the case for structural findings, minimal evidence exists to indicate reliable differences among AS and other ASDs. FMRI and event-related potential studies of hemodynamic and electrophysiological brain responses have detected abnormalities in brain activity associated with face-processing mechanisms in inferotemporal cortex (Dawson et al., 2005; Schultz, 2005), and some of these anomalies have been specifically replicated in adults (but not children) with AS (O'Connor et al., 2005). Single Photon Emission Computed Tomography (SPECT) imaging has suggested abnormal right-hemisphere functioning in AS (McKelvey et al., 1995), which is consistent with the hypothesis that neuropsychological profiles of individuals with AS, but not of those with autism, are marked by strengths and deficits consistent with a nonverbal learning disability (Klin et al., 1995; Rourke et al., 1989). Other research has found dysfunction in brain regions subserving social cognition (anterior cingulate cortex, prefrontal cortex, temporoparietal junction, amygdala, and periamygdaloid cortex; Schultz & Robins, 2005). An emerging body of research suggests problems with functional connectivity among separate brain regions in ASDs (Just et al., 2004) and, specifically, in AS (Welchew et al., 2005). Though brain imaging technologies have shed some light on the pathobiology of ASDs, current research fails to present a clear picture of the specific neurobiological underpinnings of AS or factors that distinguish it from other PDD subtypes.

Genetics

Asperger's (1944) original description of the disorder noted common symptoms in family members, especially fathers, and empirical research since that time has supported this observation. Overall, ASDs are among the most heritable of psychiatric conditions, although genetic etiology and pattern of heritability is still poorly understood (Rutter, 2005). Many case reports have reported AS, ASD, or autistic-like traits in family members, particularly among fathers (Bowman, 1988; DeLong & Dwyer, 1988; Ghaziuddin, 2005; Gillberg et al., 1992; Gillberg & Cederlund, 2005; Volkmar et al., 1996; Wolff & McGuire, 1995), and recurrence rate in siblings of children with an ASD is considerably higher than the population base rate (Rutter, 2005). Some family history studies have also indicated associations with other psychiatric disorders including depression, schizophrenia, and schizoid personality disorders (Ghaziuddin et al., 1993). Klin and colleagues (Klin, Pauls, et al., 2005) reported rates of ASDs or the broader autism phenotype in parents and grandparents of probands with AS that were triple the rate found for the same relatives of probands with HFA (17% vs. 5%). Though this finding suggests AS may have an even stronger genetic component than autism, the preponderance of research suggests shared genetic mechanisms common to all ASDs (Frith, 2004; Rutter, 2005). Though no clear genetic etiology has been established for the majority of ASDs in general, or AS in particular, a subgroup of individuals have identifiable genetic abnormalities (perhaps 10%) which include translocations, balanced translocations, and de novo translocations (chromosomes 1, 5, 11, 13, 14, 15, 17; Cederlund & Gillberg, 2004; Anneren et al., 1995; Tentler et al., 2001; 2003), autosomal fragile site (Saliba & Griffiths, 1990), Fragile X syndrome (Bartolucci & Szatmari, 1987), and 21p+ (Cederlund & Gillberg, 2004), among others. As in other areas of medical, neurobiological, and genetic research, however, none of these findings have been claimed to differentiate individuals with AS from those with other PDD subtypes.

Treatment

As in autism, treatment of AS is essentially supportive and symptomatic and, to a great extent, overlaps with the treatment guidelines applicable to individuals with autism unaccompanied by mental retardation, or higher functioning autism (HFA) (Attwood, 2006; Klin & Volkmar, 2000; Ozonoff et al., 2002; Powers & Poland, 2002). One initial difficulty encountered by families is proving eligibility for services. As these children are often very verbal and many of them do well academically, educational authorities might judge that the deficits—primarily social and communicative—are not within the scope of educational intervention. In fact, these two aspects should be the core of any educational intervention and curriculum for individuals with this condition.

In regard to learning strategies, skills, concepts, appropriate procedures, cognitive strategies, and behavioral norms may be more effectively taught in an explicit and rote fashion, using a parts-to-whole verbal instruction approach, in which the verbal steps are in the correct sequence for the behavior to be effective. Additional guidelines should be derived from the individual's neuropsychological profile of assets and deficits. Typically, however, individuals with AS have very poor organizational skills, which are more globally described as executive function deficits. They require specific and explicit help with planning ahead, breaking down problems into accomplishable components, executing them in a stepwise fashion while keeping in mind the overall goal of the activity, among many other challenges.

The acquisition of self-sufficiency skills in all areas of adaptive functioning should be a priority (Klin, Saulnier, et al., 2007; Saulnier & Klin, 2007). There should be a concerted effort to prepare children for independent, self-supporting life. Areas of proficiency in adulthood should include personal hygiene, grooming, and management of clothing; awareness of and capable management of health issues; an operationalized view of what is private and what can be displayed or otherwise be spoken in public; sexuality; home management, including budgeting, purchasing, cooking, cleaning, and disposing of unnecessary items; budgeting, paying bills, and complying with financial and personal duties such as maintaining financial records and paying taxes; knowledge of how to deal with authority, including police, how to behave in situations of emergency, how to manage telemarketers, how to avoid falling prey to offers that are "too good to be true," critical knowledge of perils associated with Internet use, management of "junk" electronic and paper mail, among many others critical aspects of real life.

The tendency of individuals with AS to rely on rigid rules and routines can be used to foster positive habits and enhance the person's quality of life and that of family members. Specific problem-solving strategies, usually following a verbal algorithm, may be taught for handling the requirements of frequently occurring, troublesome situations (e.g., involving novelty, intense social demands, or frustration). Training is usually necessary for recognizing situations as troublesome and for selecting the best available learned strategy to use in such situations. Social and communication skills are best taught by a communication specialist with an interest in pragmatics in speech in the context of both individual and small-group therapy. Communication skills training should include appropriate nonverbal behavior (e.g., the use of gaze for social interaction, monitoring and patterning of voice inflection, verbal decoding of nonverbal behaviors of others, social awareness, perspective taking skills, and correct interpretation of ambiguous communications such as nonliteral language.

Often adults with AS fail to meet entry requirements for jobs in their area of training (e.g., college degree) or fail to maintain a job because of their poor interview skills, social disabilities, eccentricities, or anxiety attacks. It is important, therefore, that they be trained for and placed in jobs for which they are not neuropsychologically impaired and in which they will enjoy a certain degree of support and shelter. Therefore, it is preferable that the job not involve intensive social demands, time pressure, or the need to quickly improvise or generate solutions to novel situations.

The available experience with self-support groups suggests that individuals with AS enjoy the opportunity to meet others with similar problems and may develop relationships around an activity or subject of shared interest. Special interests may be use as a way of creating social opportunities through hobby groups. Supportive psychotherapy, as well as pharmacological interventions, may be helpful in dealing with feelings of despondency, frustration, and anxiety, although a more direct, problem-solving focus is thought to be more beneficial than an insight-oriented approach. Recently, the use of especially adapted forms of cognitive behavioral therapy has been shown to be effective and beneficial, particularly in regard to, but not limited to, anxiety symptoms.

Conclusions

The inclusion of the term "Asperger's syndrome" (AS) as one of the pervasive developmental disorders in the DSM-IV and ICD-10 has decisively contributed to greater awareness of individuals with autism spectrum disorders with preserved cognitive and language functioning. This in turn has generally translated into greater availability of services and supports to persons who previously had to fend for themselves in their daily challenges with only the support of their families and often with the disservice of misconceptions of the origins of their behavioral difficulties. In this light, the term "Asperger's syndrome" has certainly had a beneficial impact on the community of individuals with autism spectrum disorders and their families (Wing, 2000).

In contrast to this positive outcome, research on the external validity of the construct relative to other PDD subtypes has been undermined by the lack of operationalized and consensual definitions of the condition, the virtual irrelevance of the DSM-IV and ICD-10 formal definitions, and the rather arbitrary way in which the term has been used in clinical investigations. As researched in the past, this issue is not likely to be clarified in the future without radical changes. The forthcoming update of formal nosology presents an opportunity for such changes, but there is little definitive evidence to base decisions on. The alternatives available are not appealing: (1) to maintain the tentative status of AS within formal PDD nosology and, in so doing, to possibly perpetuate for yet another decade the current situation; or (2) to remove the term from formal PDD nosology and, in so doing, to leave the community without a term previously used as a coalescing force for advocacy.

At present, an empirically based decision is rather difficult because while AS has not been shown to differ from other PDD subtypes on a whole array of important variables, it has not been shown to be the same either because research on this issue has been uninterpretable. While one can state that the onus should be on disproving the nil hypothesis (i.e., that AS is meaningfully different from related PDD subtypes), the construct of Asperger's syndrome has taken a life of its own with many real-life consequences as alluded to before. A possible solution for this quandary will not help nosology in the short term, but it can rephrase the question in a way that valuable insights may eventually follow. This solution involves deriving the more far-reaching implications of the fact that autism spectrum disorders (ASD) are the quintessential neurodevelopmental disorders, and that a great many aspects of interest in investigations and clinical practice should be conceptualized in light of developmental psychopathology processes (Klin et al., 2003). Thus fully quantifying key aspects of developmental skills and symptomatology in infants and toddlers with ASD and then following these children longitudinally while casting the search for meaningful categorical subtypes as dependent, outcome variables might free this debate from some sterile, past discussions. We still do not know what are important mediators of outcome beyond the obvious notion that IQ and language matter. In other words, we still do not know what are the dimensions that generate the spectrum of autism conditions beginning in early infancy.

Two parallel sets of advancements bode well for this field: first, our knowledge of normative processes in child development has increased dramatically since the early 1990s, although autism research has been slow in fully assimilating new investigative paradigms, technologies, and concepts (Volkmar et al., 2004). Second, the advent of prospective studies of large cohorts of genetically at-risk infants, a proportion of which will develop autism, carries the promise of shedding light on this critical period of pathogenesis. Until recently, our knowledge of this period of development was confined to retrospective accounts or less-than-ideal methods of infancy research (Zwaigenbaum et al., 2007). As knowledge accrues from these efforts, it is very likely that a great deal of what we know about ASD will have to be reappraised and updated, if not fully modified.

In regard to nosology and classification of ASD, prospective work singling out relevant patterns of onset and examining the range of associated symptomatic expressions over time is likely to systematize the search for empirically defined subtypes. This should allow for an examination of their utility in terms of response to treatment and outcomes. This process has begun with the identification of earlier- and later-onset autism (Landa et al., 2007), and possibly the existence of regressive subtypes (Lord et al., 2004; Siperstein & Volkmar, 2004; Werner & Dawson, 2005). It is possible, however, that these distinctions are still too crude, and are going to be remediated only by more detailed and quantified analyses of infancy data than those performed to date (Jones & Klin, 2009).

As new genes or genetic anomalies are found to be associated with ASD, some have argued for an etiology-based nosology as a viable approach to reduce the marked heterogeneity of phenotypic expressions of this family of conditions: there would be many "autisms," each corresponding to a "disease process." However, genotypic variability seems to be as baffling as phenotypic variability, if not more. For example, although more and more susceptibility loci are being identified, each is thought to account for only a small number of overall cases (e.g., Weiss et al., 2008). Likewise, de novo mutations may play a causal role in a relatively large percentage (~ 10%) of individuals with autism who do not have an affected first-degree family relative (e.g., Zhao et al., 2007). Other disorders, such as Rett syndrome, in which the genetic mutation has been identified nevertheless retain the clinical diagnosis based on clinical features, recognizing that not all cases that fit the clinical diagnosis have the underlying mutation and that the clinical diagnosis has utility in terms of describing clinical course and prognosis.

Given the multiplicity of possible causes, it is in fact surprising that ASD are identified, reliably, as a fairly unitary, though variable, syndrome (Jones & Klin, 2009). Beginning with Kanner's original description, consensus on core diagnostic features has remained relatively stable. Autism-specific diagnostic instruments have strong sensitivity and specificity by age 2 years, and among experienced clinicians, agreement in diagnostic assignment is typically high (Klin et al., 2000; Lord & Corsello, 2005). These factors highlight homogeneity of basic features despite the wide range of genomic causes and varying outcomes.

But the interclinician reliability for the assignment of an ASD diagnosis is high relative to the differentiation of children with ASD vs. non-ASD. This is not so for the differentiation of ASD subtypes (i.e., autism, AS, and PDD-NOS). Thus it seems that the balance is tilted toward the adoption of the all-encompassing ASD construct, a disregard of the other subtypes, with the addition of maybe a dimensional qualifier such as level of cognitive or language functioning. This might be a palatable, interim solution until the subtyping enterprise can be more solidly derived from prospective, longitudinal research of early-emerging developmental pathways leading to social communication disabilities.

Challenges and Future Directions

- Prospective, longitudinal studies of well-characterized infants and toddlers with ASD identifying meaningful and quantified outcomes as dependent variables is likely to yield empirically derived subtyping schemes for the pervasive developmental disorders;
- In the absence of well-operationalized and consensually accepted definitions of AS, research on its external validity in the future is likely to fail. This will perpetuate the current unsatisfactory situation, which includes a complete disregard of the DSM-IV definition and the adoption of a whole array of other definitions in clinical research. The decision of whether or not to include AS in the forthcoming DSM-V will be made under less than optimal conditions and yet it is likely to have a far-reaching impact on the community; and
- "AS" is a term around which many affected individuals, their families, and advocacy agencies coalesce to advance factors beneficial to this community. In case AS is excluded from DSM-V, it will be critically important to minimize the deleterious impact of this decision on the entitlements of the individuals with this condition, or on their advocates' power to increase public awareness of their needs and challenges.

SUGGESTED READINGS

Attwood, T. (2006). *The complete guide to Asperger's syndrome.* London: Kingsley.

Klin, A., Volkmar, F. R., & Sparrow, S. S. (2000). *Asperger syndrome.* New York: Guilford.

Ozonoff, S., Dawson, G., & McPartland, J. (2003). *A parent's guide to Asperger syndrome and high-functioning autism.* New York: Guilford.

REFERENCES

American Psychiatric Association (1994). *Diagnostic and statistical manual of mental disorders* (4th ed.; DSM-IV). Washington, DC: Author.

American Psychiatric Association (2000). *Diagnostic and statistical manual of mental disorders* (4th ed., text rev.; DSM-IV-TR). Washington, DC: Author.

Amir, R. E., Van den Veyver, I. B., Wan, M., Tran, C. Q., Francke, U., & Zoghbi, H. Y. (1999). Rett syndrome is caused by mutations in X-linked MECPw, encoding methyl-CpG-binding protein 2. *Nature Genetics, 23*(2), 185–188.

Anderson, G., & Hoshino, Y. (2005). Neurochemical studies of autism. In: F. R. Volkmar, R. Paul, A. Klin, & D. Cohen (Eds.), *Handbook of autism and pervasive developmental disorders* (3rd ed., Vol. 1, pp. 453–472). Hoboken, NJ: Wiley.

Anneren, G., Dahl, N., Uddenfeldt, U., & Janols, L. (1995). Asperger syndrome in a boy with a balanced de novo translocation. *American Journal of Medical Genetics, 56,* 330–331.

Asperger, H. (1944). Die "Autistischen Psychopathen" im kindesalter. *Archiv für Psychiatrie und Nervenkrankheiten, 117,* 76–136.

Asperger, H. (1979). Problems of infantile autism. *Communication, 13,* 45–52.

Attwood, T. (2006). *The complete guide to Asperger's syndrome.* London: Kingsley.

Bailey, A., Palferman, S., Heavey, L., & Le Couteur, A. (1998). Autism: The phenotype in relatives. *Journal of Autism and Developmental Disorders, 28,* 369–392.

Bartolucci, G., & Szatmari, P. (1987). Possible similarities between the fragile X and Asperger's syndrome. *American Journal of Diseases in Childhood, 141*(6), 601–602.

Berthier, M. L., Starkstein, S. E., & Leiguarda, R. (1990). Developmental cortical anomalies in Asperger's syndrome: Neuroradiological findings in two patients. *Journal of Neuropsychiatry and Clinical Neurosciences, 2*(2), 197–201.

Bleuler, E. (1916). *Lehrbuch der Psychiatrie.* Trans. A. A. Brill (1951), *Textbook of psychiatry.* New York: Dover.

Bowman, E. P. (1988). Asperger's syndrome and autism: The case for a connection. *British Journal of Psychiatry, 152,* 377–382.

Cass, H., Gringras, P., March, J., McKendrick, I., O'Hare, A. E., Owen, L., & Pollin, C. (2008). Absence of urinary opioid peptides in children with autism. *Archives of Diseases in Childhood, 93,* 745–750.

Cederlund, M., & Gillberg, C. (2004). One hundred males with Asperger syndrome: A clinical study of background and associated factors. *Developmental Medicine and Child Neurology, 46*(10), 652–660.

Chawarska, K., Klin, A., Paul, R., & Volkmar, F. R. (2007). Autism spectrum disorders in the second year: Stability and change in syndrome expression. *Journal of Child Psychology and Psychiatry, 48*(2), 128–138.

Courschene, E., Karns, C. M., Davis, H. R., Ziccardi, R., Carper, R. A., Tigue, Z. D., Chisum, H. J. et al. (2001). Unusual brain growth patterns in early life in patients with autism disorder: An MRI study. *Neurology, 57,* 245–254.

Dawson, G., Webb, S. J., & McPartland, J. (2005). Understanding the nature of face processing impairment in autism: Insights from behavioral and electrophysiological studies. *Developmental Neuropsychology, 27*(3), 403–424.

Dawson, G., Webb, S., Schellenberg, G. D., Dager, S., Friedman, S., Aylward, E., & Richards, T. (2002). Defining the broader phenotype of autism: Genetic, brain, and behavioral perspectives. *Development and Psychopathology, 14,* 581–611.

DeLong, G. R., & Dwyer, J. T. (1988). Correlation of family history with specific autistic subgroups: Asperger's syndrome and bipolar affective disease. *Journal of Autism and Developmental Disorders, 18*(4), 593–600.

DiCicco-Bloom, E., Lord, C., Zwaigenbaum, L., Courchesne, E., Dager, S. R., Schmitz, C., et al. (2006). The developmental neurobiology of autism spectrum disorder. *Journal of Neuroscience, 26*(26), 6897–6906.

Eisenmajer, R., Prior, M., Leekam, S., Wing, L., Gould, J., Welham, M., et al. (1996). Comparison of clinical symptoms in autism and Asperger's disorder. *Journal of the American Academy of Child and Adolescent Psychiatry, 35,* 1523–1531.

Ellis, H. D., Ellis, D. M., Fraser, W., & Deb, S. (1994). A preliminary study of right hemisphere cognitive deficits and impaired social judgments among young people with Asperger syndrome. *European Child & Adolescent Psychiatry, 3*(4), 255–266.

Everall, I. P., & Le Couteur, A. (1990). Firesetting in an adolescent with Asperger's syndrome. *British Journal of Psychiatry, 157,* 284–287.

Frith, U. (Ed.). (1991). *Autism and Asperger syndrome* (pp. 37–92). Cambridge, UK: Cambridge University Press.

Frith, U. (2004). Emanuel Miller lecture: Confusions and controversies about Asperger syndrome. *Journal of Child Psychology and Psychiatry, 45*(4), 672–686.

Fujikawa, H., Kobayashi, R., Koga, Y., & Murata, T. (1987). A case of Asperger's syndrome in a nineteen-year-old who showed psychotic breakdown with depressive state and attempted suicide after entering university. *Japanese Journal of Child and Adolescent Psychiatry, 28*(4), 217–225.

Ghaziuddin, M. (2002). Asperger syndrome: Associated psychiatric and medical conditions. *Focus on Autism and Other Developmental Disabilities, 17*(3), 138–144.

Ghaziuddin, M. (2005). A family history study of Asperger syndrome. *Journal of Autism and Developmental Disorders, 35*(2), 177–182.

Ghaziuddin, N., Metler, L., Ghaziuddin, M., Tsai, L., et al. (1993). Three siblings with Asperger syndrome: A family case study. *European Child and Adolescent Psychiatry, 2*(1), 44–49.

Ghaziuddin, M., Tsai, L. Y., & Ghaziuddin, N. (1991). Brief report: Violence in Asperger syndrome, a critique. *Journal of Autism and Developmental Disorders, 21*(3), 349–354.

Ghaziuddin, M., Tsai, L. Y., & Ghaziuddin, N. (1992). Brief report: A comparison of the diagnostic criteria for Asperger syndrome. *Journal of Autism and Developmental Disorders, 22*(4), 643–649.

Ghaziuddin, M., Weidmer-Mikhail, E., Ghaziuddin, N. (1998). Comorbidity of Asperger syndrome: A preliminary report. *Journal of Intellectual Disability Research, 42*(4), 279–283.

Gilchrist, A., Green, J., Cox, A., Burton, D., Rutter, M., & Le Couteur, A. (2001). Development and current functioning in adolescents with Asperger syndrome: A comparative study. *Journal of Child Psychology and Psychiatry, 42,* 227–240.

Gillberg, C. (1985). Asperger's syndrome and recurrent psychosis: A case study. *Journal of Autism and Developmental Disorders, 15*(4), 389–397.

Gillberg, C. (1989). Asperger syndrome in 23 Swedish children. *Developmental Medicine and Child Neurology, 31,* 520–531.

Gillberg, C., & Cederlund, M. (2005). Asperger syndrome: Familial and pre- and perinatal factors. *Journal of Autism and Developmental Disorders, 35*(2), 159–166.

Gillberg, I. C., & Gillberg, C. (1989). Asperger syndrome: Some epidemiological considerations. *Journal of Child Psychology and Psychiatry, 30,* 631–638.

Gillberg, C., Gillberg, I. C., & Steffenburg, S. (1992). Siblings and parents of children with autism: A controlled population-based study. *Developmental Medicine and Child Neurology, 34*(5), 389–398.

Green, J., Gilchrist, A., Burton, D., & Cox, A. (2000). Social and psychiatric functioning in adolescents with Asperger syndrome compared with conduct disorder. *Journal of Autism and Developmental Disorders, 30,* 279–293.

Hazlett, H. C., Poe, M. D., Gerig, G., Smith, R. G., Provenzale, J., Ross, A., et al. (2005). An MRI and head circumference study of brain size in autism: Birth through age two years. *Archives of General Psychiatry, 62,* 1366–1376.

Hippler, K., & Klicpera, C. (2003). A retrospective analysis of the clinical case records of "autistic psychopaths" diagnosed by Hans Asperger and his team at the University Children's Hospital, Vienna. *Philosophical Transactions of the Royal Society, Series B, Biological Sciences, 358,* 291–301.

Howlin, P. (2005). Outcomes in autism spectrum disorders. In F. R. Volkmar, R. Paul, A. Klin, & D. J. Cohen (Eds.), *Handbook of autism and pervasive developmental disorders* (3rd ed., pp. 201–221). New York: Wiley.

Howlin, P., & Goode, S. (1998). Outcome in adult life for people with autism and Asperger's syndrome. In F. R. Volkmar (Ed.), *Autism and pervasive developmental disorders* (pp. 209–241). Cambridge: Cambridge University Press.

Johnson, M. (2001). Functional brain development in humans. *Nature Reviews Neuroscience, 2,* 475–483.

Johnson, M. H., & Karmiloff-Smith, A. (2004). Neuroscience perspectives on infant development. In G. Bremner & A. Slater (Eds.), *Theories of infant development* (pp. 121–141). Malden: Blackwell.

Jones, P. B., & Kerwin, R. W. (1990). Left temporal lobe damage in Asperger's syndrome. *British Journal of Psychiatry, 156,* 570–572.

Jones, W., & Klin, A. (2009). Heterogeneity and homogeneity across the autism spectrum: The role of development. *Journal of the American Academy of Child and Adolescent Psychiatry, 48*(5), 1–3.

Just, M. A., Cherkassky, V. L., Keller, T. A., & Minshew, N. J. (2004). Cortical activation and synchronization during sentence comprehension in high-functioning autism: Evidence of underconnectivity. *Brain, 127*(8), 1811–1821.

Kanner, L. (1943). Autistic disturbances of affective contact. *Nervous Child, 2,* 217–253.

Kanner, L. (1954). Discussion of Robinson and Vitale's paper on "Children with circumscribed interests." *American Journal of Orthopsychiatry, 24,* 764–766.

Kerbeshian, J., & Burd, L. (1986). Asperger's syndrome and Tourette syndrome: The case of the pinball wizard. *British Journal of Psychiatry, 148,* 731–736.

Kim, J., Szatmari, P., Bryson, S., Streiner, D. L., & Wilson, F. J. (2000). The prevalence of anxiety and mood problems among children with autism and Asperger syndrome. *Autism, 4,* 117–132.

Klin, A. (2009). Subtyping the autism spectrum disorders: Theoretical, research, and clinical considerations. In S. Goldstein, J. Naglieri, & S. Ozonoff (Eds.), *Assessment of autism spectrum disorders* (pp. 91–116). New York: Guilford.

Klin, A., Chawarska, K., Paul, R., Rubin, E., Morgan, T., Wiesner, L., et al. (2004). Autism in a 15-month-old child. *American Journal of Psychiatry, 161*(11), 1981–1988.

Klin, A., Chawarska, K., Volkmar, F. R. (2008). Opportunities for research: Concepts and future directions. In K. Chawarska, A. Klin, & F. R. Volkmar (Eds.), *Autism spectrum disorders in infants and toddlers: Diagnosis, assessment and treatment* (pp. 327–336). New York: Guilford.

Klin, A., Danovitch, J. H., Merz, A. B., Dohrmann, E. H., & Volkmar, F. R. (2007). Circumscribed interests in higher-functioning individuals with autism spectrum disorders: An exploratory study. *Research and Practice for Persons with Severe Disabilities, 32*(2), 89–100.

Klin, A., Jones, W., Schultz, R. T., & Volkmar, F. R. (2003). The Enactive Mind—from actions to cognition: Lessons from autism. *Philosophical Transactions of the Royal Society of London. Series B, Biological Sciences, 358,* 345–360.

Klin, A., Jones, W., Schultz, R., Volkmar, F., & Cohen, D. (2002). Defining and quantifying the social phenotype in autism. *American Journal of Psychiatry, 159*(6), 895–908.

Klin, A., McPartland, J., & Volkmar, F. R. (2005). Asperger syndrome. In F. R. Volkmar, R. Paul, A. Klin, & D. J. Cohen (Eds.), *Handbook of autism and pervasive developmental disorders* (3rd ed. pp. 88–125). New York: Wiley.

Klin, A., Pauls, D., Schultz, R., & Volkmar, F. R. (2005). Three diagnostic approaches to Asperger syndrome: Implications for research. *Journal of Autism and Developmental Disorders, 35*(2), 221–234.

Klin, A., Saulnier, C. A., Sparrow, S. S., Cicchetti, D. V., Volkmar, F. R., & Lord, C. (2007). Social and communication abilities and disabilities in higher functioning individuals with autism spectrum disorders. *Journal of Autism and Developmental Disorders, 37*(4), 748–759.

Klin, A. & Volkmar, F. R. (2000). Treatment and intervention guidelines for individuals with Asperger syndrome. In A. Klin, F. R. Volkmar, & S. S. Sparrow (Eds.), *Asperger syndrome* (pp. 340–366). New York: Guilford.

Klin, A., Volkmar, F. R., & Sparrow, S. S. (Eds.) (2000). *Asperger syndrome.* New York: Guilford.

Klin, A., Volkmar, F. R., Sparrow, S. S., Cicchetti, D. V., & Rourke, B. P. (1995). Validity and neuropsychological characterization of Asperger syndrome. *Journal of Child Psychology and Psychiatry, 36*(7), 1127–1140.

Kopra, K., von Wendt, L., Nieminen-von, W., & Paavonen, E. J. (2008). Comparison of diagnostic methods for Asperger syndrome. *Journal of Autism and Developmental Disorders, 38*(8), 1567–1573.

Landa, R. J., Holman, K. C., & Garrett-Mayer, E. (2007). Social and communication development in toddlers with early and later diagnosis of autism spectrum disorders. *Archives of General Psychiatry, 64*(7), 853–864.

Leekam, S., Libby, S., Wing, L., Gould, J., & Gillberg, C. (2000). Comparison of ICD-10 and Gillberg's criteria for Asperger syndrome. *Autism, 4,* 11–28.

Littlejohns, C. S., Clarke, D. J., & Corbett, J. A. (1990). Tourette-like disorder in Asperger's syndrome. *British Journal of Psychiatry, 156*, 430–433.

Lord, C., & Corsello, C. (2005). Diagnostic instruments in autism spectrum disorders. In F. R. Volkmar, R. Paul, A. Klin, & D. Cohen (Eds.), *Handbook of autism and pervasive developmental disorders* (3rd ed., Vol. 1, pp. 730–771). Hoboken, NJ: Wiley.

Lord, C., Shulman, C., & DiLavore, P. (2004). Regression and word loss in autistic spectrum disorders. *Journal of Child Psychology and Psychiatry, 45*(5), 936–955.

Mandell, D. S., Walrath, C. M., Manteuffel, B., Sqro, G., & Pinto-Martin, J. (2005). Characteristics of children with autistic spectrum disorders served in comprehensive community-based mental health settings. *Journal of Autism and Developmental Disorders, 35*(3), 313–321.

Marriage, K., Miles, T., Stokes, D., & Davey, M. (1993). Clinical and research implications of the co-occurrence of Asperger's and Tourette syndrome. *Australian and New Zealand Journal of Psychiatry, 27*(4), 666–672.

Mayes, S. D., Calhoun, S. L., & Crites, D. L. (2001). Does DSM-IV Asperger's disorder exist? *Journal of Abnormal Child Psychology, 29*, 263–271.

McAlonan, G., Daly, E., Kumari, V., Critchley, H. D., van Amelsvoort, T., Suckling, J., et al. (2002). Brain anatomy and sensorimotor gating in Asperger's syndrome. *Brain, 125*(7), 1594–1606.

McConachie, H., Le Couteur, A., & Honey, E. (2005). Can a diagnosis of Asperger syndrome be made in very young children with suspected autism spectrum disorder? *Journal of Autism and Developmental Disorders, 42*(2), 227–240.

McKelvey, J. R., Lambert, R., Mottron, L., & Shevell, M. I. (1995). Right-hemisphere dysfunction in Asperger's syndrome. *Journal of Child Neurology, 10*(4), 310–314.

Miles, S. W., & Capelle, P. (1987). Asperger's syndrome and aminoaciduria: A case example. *British Journal of Psychiatry, 150*, 397–400.

Miller, J., & Ozonoff, S. (2000). The external validity of Asperger disorder: Lack of evidence from the domain of neuropsychology. *Journal of Abnormal Psychology, 109*, 227–238.

Miller, J. N., & Ozonoff, S. (1997). Did Asperger's cases have Asperger disorder? A research note. *Journal of Child Psychology and Psychiatry, 38*(2), 247–251.

Minshew, N., Sweeney, J., Bauman, M., & Webb, S. (2005). Neurologic aspects of autism. In F. R. Volkmar, R. Paul, A. Klin, & D. J. Cohen (Eds.), *Handbook of autism and pervasive developmental disorders* ((3rd ed., Vol. 1, pp. 473–514). Hoboken, NJ: Wiley.

National Research Council (2001). *Educating children with autism.* Washington, DC: National Academies Press.

O'Connor, K., Hamm, J. P., & Kirk, I. J. (2005). The neurophysiological correlates of face processing in adults and children with Asperger's syndrome. *Brain and Cognition, 59*(1), 82–95.

Ozbayrak, K. R., Kapucu, O., Erdem, E., & Aras, T. (1991). Left occipital hypoperfusion in a case with Asperger syndrome. *Brain and Development, 13*(6), 454–456.

Ozonoff, S., Dawson, G., & McPartland, J. (2002). *A parent's guide to Asperger syndrome and high-functioning autism.* New York: Guilford.

Paul, R. (in press). Social communication in Asperger syndrome and higher functioning autism. In A. Klin, J. McPartland, & F. R. Volkmar (Eds.), *Asperger syndrome* (2nd ed.). New York: Guilford.

Powers, M., & Poland, J. (2002). *Asperger syndrome and your child: A parent's guide.* New York: HarperCollins.

Robinson, J. F., & Vitale, L. J. (1954). Children with circumscribed interests. *American Journal of Orthopsychiatry, 24*, 755–764.

Rourke, B., Young, G. C., & Leenaars, A. A. (1989). A childhood learning disability that predisposes those afflicted to adolescent and adult depression and suicide risk. *Journal of Learning Disabilities, 22*, 169–185.

Rutter, M. (1999). The Emanuel Miller Memorial Lecture 1998. Autism: Two-way interplay between research and clinical work. *Journal of Child Psychology and Psychiatry, 40*(2), 169–188.

Rutter, M. (2005). Genetic influences and autism. In F. R. Volkmar, R. Paul, A. Klin, & D. J. Cohen (Eds.), *Handbook of autism and pervasive developmental disorders* (3rd ed., Vol. 1, pp. 425–452). Hoboken, NJ: Wiley.

Rutter, M., Bailey, A., Bolton, P., & Le Couteur, A. (1994). Autism and known medical conditions: Myth and substance. *Journal of Child Psychology and Psychiatry, 35*(2), 311–322.

Saliba, J. R., & Griffiths, M. (1990). Brief report: Autism of the Asperger type associated with an autosomal fragile site. *Journal of Autism and Developmental Disorders, 20*(4), 569–575.

Saulnier, C. A., & Klin, A. (2007). Social and communication abilities and disabilities in higher functioning individuals with autism and Asperger syndrome. *Journal of Autism and Developmental Disorders, 37*(4), 788–793.

Schatz, A. M., Weimer, A. K., & Trauner, D. A. (2002). Brief report: Attention differences in Asperger syndrome. *Journal of Autism and Developmental Disorders, 32*(4), 333–336.

Scheerer, M., Rothmann, E., & Goldstein, K. (1945). A case of "idiot savant": An experimental study of personality organization. *Psychological Monographs, 58*(4).

Schultz, R. T. (2005). Developmental deficits in social perception in autism: The role of the amygdala and fusiform face area. *International Journal of Developmental Neuroscience, 23*(2–3), 125–141.

Schultz, R., & Robins, D. (2005). Functional neuroimaging studies of autism spectrum disorders. In F. R. Volkmar, R. Paul, A. Klin & D. J. Cohen (Eds.), *Handbook of autism and pervasive developmental disorders* (3rd ed., Vol. 1, pp. 515–533). Hoboken, NJ: Wiley.

Scragg, P., & Shah, A. (1994). Prevalence of Asperger's syndrome in a secure hospital. *British Journal of Psychiatry, 165*(5), 679–682.

Siperstein, R., & Volkmar, F. (2004). Brief report: Parental reporting of regression in children with pervasive developmental disorders. *Journal of Autism and Developmental Disorders, 34*(6), 731–734.

Smith, I. M. (2000). Motor functioning in Asperger syndrome. In A. Klin, Volkmar, F. R. & S. S. Sparrow (Eds.), *Asperger syndrome* (pp. 97–124). New York: Guilford.

Sweeney, J. A., Takarae, Y., Macmillan, C., Luna, B., & Minshew, N. J. (2004). Eye movements in neurodevelopmental disorders. *Current Opinion in Neurology, 17*(1), 37–42.

Szatmari, P., Archer, L., Fisman, S., Streiner, D. L., & Wilson, F. (1995). Asperger's syndrome and autism: Differences in behavior, cognition, and adaptive functioning. *Journal of the American Academy of Child and Adolescent Psychiatry, 34*, 1662–1671.

Szatmari, P., Bartolucci, G., & Bremner, R. (1989). Asperger's syndrome and autism: Comparison of early history and outcome. *Developmental Medicine and Child Neurology, 31*(6), 709–720.

Szatmari, P., Bryson, S. E., Streiner, D. L., Wilson, F., Archer, L., & Ryerse, C. (2000). Two-year outcome of preschool children with autism or Asperger's syndrome. *American Journal of Psychiatry, 157*, 1980–1987.

Tantam, D. (1988). Annotation: Asperger's syndrome. *Journal of Child Psychology and Psychiatry, 29*(3), 245–255.

Tantam, D., Evered, C., & Hersov, L. (1990). Asperger's syndrome and ligamentous laxity. *Journal of the American Academy of Child and Adolescent Psychiatry, 29*(6), 892–896.

Tentler, D., Brandberg, G., Betancur, C., Gillberg, C., Anneren, G., Orsmark, C., et al. (2001). A balanced reciprocal translocation t(5;7)(q14;q32) associated with autistic disorder: Molecular analysis of the chromosome 7 breakpoint. *American Journal of Medical Genetics, 105*(8), 729–736.

Tentler, D., Johannesson, T., Johansson, M., Rastamm, M., Gillberg, C., Orsmark, C., et al. (2003). A candidate region for Asperger syndrome defined by two 17p breakpoints. *European Journal of Human Genetics: EJHG, 11*(2), 189–195.

Thomsen, P. H. (1994). Obsessive-compulsive disorder in children and adolescents: A 6–22-year follow-up study: Clinical descriptions of the course and continuity of obsessive-compulsive symptomatology. *European Child and Adolescent Psychiatry, 3*(2), 82–96.

Tuchman, R., & Rapin I. (2002). Epilepsy in autism. *Lancet Neurology, 1*(6), 352–358.

Van Krevelen, D. A. (1963). On the relationship between early infantile autism and autistic psychopathy. *Acta Paedopsychiatrica, 30*, 303–323.

Van Krevelen, D. A. (1971). Early infantile autism and autistic psychopathy. *Journal of Autism and Childhood Schizophrenia, 1*(1), 82–86.

Volkmar, F. R., & Klin, A. (2000). Diagnostic issues in Asperger syndrome. In A. Klin, F. R. Volkmar, & S. S. Sparrow (Eds.), *Asperger syndrome* (pp. 25–71). New York: Guilford.

Volkmar, F. R., & Klin, A. (2005). Issues in the classification of autism and related conditions. In F. R. Volkmar, R. Paul, A. Klin, & D. J. Cohen (Eds.), *Handbook of autism and pervasive developmental disorders* (3rd ed., Vol. 1, pp. 5–41). New York: Wiley.

Volkmar, F. R., Klin, A., & Cohen, D. J. (1997). Diagnosis and classification of autism and related conditions: Consensus and Issues. In D. J. Cohen & F. R. Volkmar (Eds.), *Handbook of autism and pervasive developmental disorders* (2nd ed., pp. 5–40). New York: Wiley.

Volkmar, F. R., Klin, A., Schultz, R. B., Bronen, R., Marans, W. D., Sparrow, S. S., & Cohen, D. J. (1996). Grand rounds in child psychiatry: Asperger syndrome. *Journal of the American Academy of Child and Adolescent Psychiatry, 35, 118–123.*

Volkmar, F. R., Klin, A., Siegel, B., Szatmari, P., Lord, C., Campbell, M., et al. (1994). DSM-IV autism/pervasive developmental disorder field trial. *American Journal of Psychiatry, 151*, 1361–1367.

Volkmar, F. R., Lord, C., Bailey, A., Schultz, R. T., & Klin, A. (2004). Autism and pervasive developmental disorders. *Journal of Child Psychology and Psychiatry, 45*(1), 1–36.

Volkmar, F. R., State, M., & Klin, A. (2009). Autism and autism spectrum disorders: Diagnostic issues for the coming decade. *Journal of Child Psychology and Psychiatry, 50*(1–2), 108–115.

Weiss, L. A., Shen, Y., Korn, J. M., et al. (2008). Association between microdeletion and microduplication of 16p11.2 and autism. *New England Journal of Medicine, 358*(7), 667–675.

Welchew, D. E., Ashwin, C., Berkouk, K., Salvador, R., Suckling, J., Baron-Cohen, S., et al. (2005). Functional disconnectivity of the medial temporal lobe in Asperger's syndrome. *Biological Psychiatry, 57*(9), 991–998.

Werner, E., & Dawson, G. (2005). Validation of the phenomenon of autistic regression using home videotapes. *Archives of General Psychiatry, 62*(8), 889–895.

Wing, L. (1981). Asperger's syndrome: A clinical account. *Psychological Medicine, 11*, 115–129.

Wing. L. (1986). Clarification on Asperger's syndrome. *Journal of Autism and Developmental Disorders, 16*(4), 513–515.

Wing, L. (2000). Past and future of research on Asperger syndrome. In A. Klin, F. R. Volkmar, & S. S. Sparrow (Eds.), *Asperger syndrome* (pp. 418–432). New York: Guilford.

Wing, L., & Gould, J. (1979). Severe impairments of social interaction and associated abnormalities in children: Epidemiology and classification. *Journal of Autism and Childhood Schizophrenia, 9*, 11–29.

Witwer, A. N., & Lecavalier, L. (2008). Examining the validity of autism spectrum disorder subtypes. *Journal of Autism and Developmental Disorders, 38*(9), 1611–1624.

Wolff, S., McGuire R. J. (1995). Schizoid personality in girls: A follow-up study: What are the links with Asperger's syndrome? *Journal of Child Psychology and Psychiatry, 36*(5), 793–817.

Woodbury-Smith, M., Klin, A., & Volkmar, F. R. (2005). Asperger's syndrome: A comparison of clinical diagnoses and those made according to the ICD-10 and DSM-IV. *Journal of Autism and Developmental Disorders, 35*(2), 235–240.

World Health Organization (1992). *The ICD-10 classification of mental and behavioural disorders: Clinical descriptions and diagnostic guidelines.* Geneva: World Health Organization.

Zhao, X., Leotta, A., Kustanovich, V., et al. (2007). A unified theory for sporadic and inherited autism. *Proceedings of the National Academy of Sciences of the United States of America, 104*, 12831–12836.

Zwaigenbaum, L., Thurm, A., Stone, W., Baranek, G., Bryson, S., Iverson, J., et al. (2007). Studying the emergence of autism spectrum disorders in high-risk infants: Methodological and practical issues. *Journal of Autism and Developmental Disorders, 37*(3), 466–480.

4 Sally Ozonoff, Kelly Heung, Meagan Thompson

Regression and Other Patterns of Onset

Points of Interest

- Dichotomous classification of onset (early onset, regression) is insufficient to describe the many ways that symptoms of autism emerge in early development.
- Parent report methods for measuring regression may not be reliable.
- Prospective investigations of high risk samples suggest that regression may be much more common in children with autism than previously thought.
- Symptoms of autism appear to emerge slowly during the first year of life. Behavioral signs of autism are not present at or shortly after birth in most children, as Kanner once suggested.

Introduction

The onset of autism is usually described as occurring in one of two patterns. In one onset prototype, children show abnormalities in social and communicative development in the first 12 months of life. The most common initial symptom recognized by parents is delayed speech development (De Giacomo & Fombonne, 1998), but a growing body of literature suggests that social and nonverbal communicative delays predate the language abnormalities that typically lead to diagnosis. Behaviors that discriminate between young children with autism, developmental delays, and typical development are orienting to name, looking at the faces of others, joint attention, affect sharing, and imitation (Baranek, 1999; Osterling & Dawson, 1994; Stone et al., 1994, 1999; Werner, Dawson, Osterling, & Dinno, 2000; Wetherby et al., 2004). A few studies suggest that symptoms can be detected before the first birthday in some children (Baranek, 1999; Werner et al., 2000), but these very early differences appear to be nonspecific (e.g., sleeping, eating, temperament patterns) and do not differentiate children with developmental delays from those with autism (Werner et al., 2005). Group differences are more reliably present and consistently found across studies in the second year of life (Palomo et al., 2006). This so-called early onset pattern is thought to occur in the majority of individuals with autism.

In the second pattern of onset, regressive autism, children appear to be developing typically for the first year or two of life. Between the first and second birthday, they lose skills that they had previously acquired, accompanied by the onset of autistic symptoms. The earliest literature on autism made no mention of this onset pattern. Kanner (1943), for example, did not report any loss of previously acquired skills in the 11 cases he described initially. The phenomenon was first reported in the 1970s by researchers in Japan (as cited in Kobayashi & Murata, 1998) and further described in the following decade (Hoshino et al., 1987; Kurita, 1985; Volkmar & Cohen, 1989).

Domains of Loss

The developmental areas most affected by regression are communication and social abilities. Much less frequently, adaptive and motor losses are reported (Davidovitch et al., 2000; Ozonoff et al., 2005; Siperstein & Volkmar, 2004). Several studies have found loss of language skills to be the most common type of regression reported by parents (Goldberg et al., 2003; Siperstein & Volkmar, 2004), possibly because speech is so eagerly awaited and salient to parents. Regression typically also involves loss of social interest and behaviors. As described by Rogers and DiLalla (1990), "the onset of their children's symptoms began with a change in or loss of the child's previous apparently normal social behavior. A loss of interest in others, the loss of eye contact, increasing isolation, the loss of interpersonal initiative including normal play were among the behaviors that the parents reported" (p. 866). Almost all parents who reported loss of words also described loss of social skills (Goldberg et al., 2003; Lord et al., 2004). Ozonoff and colleagues (2005) found loss of eye contact to be the most frequently reported change in social behavior, with 90% of parents of children with regression reporting such a loss. The second most frequently lost social behavior was a loss of social interest, which was reported in 61% of children with regressive autism (Ozonoff et al., 2005).

Timing of Loss

Regression is most often observed between the first and second birthday, with mean or median ages of regression reported across different samples between 16 and 20 months (Goldberg et al., 2003; Kurita, 1985; Ozonoff et al., 2005; Shinnar et al., 2001). In a large epidemiological sample, parents of children with regression first became concerned about development at a mean age of 19.8 months (Fombonne & Chakrabarti, 2001), which is consistent with the smaller studies.

Prevalence of Regression

Fombonne and Chakrabarti (2001) reviewed six early studies that reported regression rates in the range of 22% to 50%. Similar rates have been found in other studies. Rogers and DiLalla (1990) and Tuchman and Rapin (1997) reported approximately 30% of their samples displayed a loss of skills. Kurita (1985) reported that 37% of his sample showed speech loss. In these and other similar studies, which do not use epidemiological or community-based samples, sample sizes are typically small and cases may be ascertained in a manner that is biased toward greater severity (e.g., through clinics or hospitals). Samples from epidemiological studies provide better estimates of prevalence. In one such study, Taylor et al. (2002) reported a 25% rate of developmental regression in a large cohort of children with autism born between 1979 and 1998 in London. Another epidemiological study undertaken in California found that 34.7% of 277 children with autism had histories of regression (Byrd et al., 2002). Thus, both epidemiological and individual sample studies indicate that regression in autism occurs in a substantial minority of cases and is not a rare form of onset.

Later Outcomes

Several studies have compared the later outcomes of children with regression to those of their peers with early onset autism, with varying results. Hoshino et al. (1987) reported more severe speech and behavioral problems, as well as lower adaptive levels, in children with regression. Rogers and DiLalla (1990) found that children with regression had significantly lower IQs than those who did not lose speech. However, Short and Schopler (1988) found no statistically significant differences in IQ between early onset and regression cases, and one early study actually found a better prognosis for children who had experienced a regression (Harper & Williams, 1975). In most studies, the results have been mixed. Richler et al. (2006) reported on a large (n = 351) multisite sample (mean age 9 years) and found that children with regressive autism displayed significantly lower social reciprocity and verbal IQ than children with autism without regression, but found no differences on twelve other measures of intelligence, autism severity, and adaptive skills. Other studies (Brown & Prelock, 1995; Kobayashi & Murata, 1998; Meilleur & Fombonne, 2009; Wiggins, Rice, & Baio, 2009) have reported similarly mixed results, with some skills lower in children who regressed, but other skills no different from children with early onset autism. These studies assessed outcome at a variety of ages and many were based on small samples. A recent study examined two different cohorts of children with autism (ages 6–9 years and 16–19 years at data collection) from a large community-based sample, comparing functioning in children with and without regression. No differences were found between the onset groups in autism severity, intellectual function, or social, communicative, and adaptive outcomes. Similarly, no significant differences were found between the onset groups in any of the potential etiological factors examined, such as rate of seizures, MMR vaccination history, gastrointestinal symptoms, prenatal or neonatal risk factors, and family history (Heung, 2008). Similar findings of virtually no group differences between children with and without regression on a range of outcome measures have been reported by others (e.g., Hansen et al., 2008; Werner, Dawson, Munson, & Osterling, 2005). Hansen et al.'s investigation examined a large sample and had excellent statistical power to detect group differences, but nevertheless found very few. Thus, while some earlier studies suggested otherwise, large-scale investigations, some of which followed children for years after onset, indicate that regression histories are not necessarily associated with poorer developmental outcomes.

Potential Etiologies of Regression

The mechanisms underlying autistic regression (or for that matter, early onset autism) are unknown. Accelerated rates of head growth have been reported in several studies of young children with autism, suggesting that processes of synaptic growth and pruning may go awry and lead to autism. However, no differences in head circumference trajectories were found between children with signs of autism early in life and those with regression in one recent study (Webb et al., 2007); head growth was accelerated in both groups.

The possibility that seizures or other electrophysiological disruptions contribute to regression has also been suggested (Mantovani, 2000), in part due to the apparent reversibility of "autistic-like" features with anticonvulsant treatment found in a small subset of individuals with another regressive condition, Landau-Kleffner syndrome (Deonna, Ziegler, Maeder, Ansermet, & Roulet, 1995; Nass, Gross, Wisoff, & Devinsky, 1999; Neville et al., 1997). Kobayashi and Murata (1998) found epilepsy to be twice as frequent in children with a history of regression than in children without such a history

(31% versus 15%). Hoshino et al. (1987) also found a higher incidence of epileptic seizures and febrile convulsions in children who had experienced regression (23% versus 5%). However, this finding is not universal. Among their sample of children on the autism spectrum, Tuchman and Rapin (1997) found no difference in the frequency of reported epilepsy between children with autistic regression and those without (12% and 11%, respectively). Similarly, Shinnar et al. (2001) found that regression was actually more common in children with autism without seizures. Neither Hansen et al. (2008), Baird et al. (2008), or Heung (2008) found differences in rates of epilepsy between regression and no regression groups.

Past research has occasionally suggested that psychosocial stressors might trigger regression in a vulnerable child. Kurita (1985) found that events such as the birth of siblings, parental discord, and change of residence were occasionally reported just before the regression. Rutter (1985) noted, however, that the specific life events that have been associated with developmental regression are relatively minor and common to many children, questioning their causal association. Clearly, the majority of children who experience such stressors do not suffer from regression.

Immunizations

Wakefield et al. (1998) linked autism to MMR vaccination in their study of 12 autistic children with gastrointestinal (GI) symptoms such as chronic constipation, pain, bloating, and esophageal reflux. The GI symptoms reportedly began around the same time that the children's autistic symptoms appeared. Endoscopy revealed lymphonodular hyperplasia and macroscopic evidence of colitis. These findings led Wakefield and his colleagues to hypothesize that the children's regressive autism was induced by the MMR vaccinations through a series of events involving mucosal damage, increased permeability of the intestines, and gastrointestinal absorption of toxic neuropeptides, causing central nervous system dysfunction and behavioral regression (Hansen & Ozonoff, 2003).

Wakefield et al.'s (1998) paper was later retracted by 10 of the study's 13 authors (Murch et al., 2004), in part due to the paucity of epidemiological evidence supporting the theory (e.g., Dales, Hammer, & Smith, 2001; Farrington, Miller, & Taylor, 2001; Kaye, del Mar Melero-Montes, & Jick, 2001; Taylor et al., 2002; Uchiyama, Kurosawa, & Inaba, 2007). For example, Taylor et al. (1999) found no evidence of changes in incidence or age at diagnosis associated with the introduction of the MMR vaccine in the United Kingdom in 1988. A later study by this group (Taylor et al., 2002) compared three groups of children: (1) children who received the MMR vaccine before their parents became concerned about their development, (2) children who received the vaccine after such concern, and (3) children who had not received the vaccine at all. Findings showed no significant differences in incidence of regression between these three groups.

In addition to the lack of epidemiological evidence for MMR influence, there is also little support in the literature for a specific regressive phenotype of autism that Wakefield (1998) termed "autistic enterocolitis." One large study found more GI symptoms in children with regression than those without regression (Richler et al., 2006), but this has not been reported in several other empirical studies. Fombonne and Chakrabarti (2001) analyzed one epidemiological sample and two clinical samples of children (total N = 262) and found no association between developmental regression and GI symptoms; only 2.1% of the samples experienced both problems, and this rate did not exceed chance expectations. In addition, this study compared children who were exposed to the MMR immunization with those who were not exposed and found no difference in the reported rates of regression between the two groups. These authors also found no evidence that children with regressive autism have symptom or severity profiles that are different from children with early onset autism (Fombonne & Chakrabarti, 2001). Similar lack of association between GI problems and regression has been reported by several other groups (Baird et al., 2008; Hansen et al., 2008; Heung, 2008; Taylor et al., 2002).

Concerns about MMR extended to other combinations of vaccines, to the increasing number of vaccines, and then to potentially toxic components of vaccines. One such component that attracted much attention was thimerosal, a mercury-containing preservative found in vaccines. James and colleagues (2004) found that, compared to controls, some children with autism have a severe deficiency of glutathione, which is required for heavy metal detoxification and excretion. Contrary to this hypothesis, however, increases (rather than decreases) in the incidence of autism following discontinuation of thimerosal-containing vaccines have been reported in Denmark (Madsen et al., 2003) and California (Schechter & Grether, 2008). Andrews et al. (2004) found no relationship between vaccine doses (and thus, levels of thimerosal exposure) and subsequent neurodevelopmental disorders including autism. Some have suggested that symptoms of autism are similar to those of mercury poisoning (e.g., Bernard et al., 2001; Blaxill, Redwood, & Bernard, 2004), but this was refuted by Nelson and Bauman (2003) who found no link between either the clinical manifestations or the neuropathology of autism and mercury poisoning. Thus, there is no direct support for the hypothesis that immunizations contribute to autism and/or developmental regression. Recently, research is focusing on whether certain medical conditions that can be associated with autism, such as mitochondrial disorders, may increase vulnerability to adverse effects of vaccines (Poling, 2006; Weissman et al., 2008).

Genetics

It has been suggested that autism with regression may represent a different genetic subtype. One study (Xi et al., 2007) examined a group of 31 boys with autism and speech loss for mutations in MeCP2, the gene that causes Rett syndrome, another condition involving developmental regression. Only one sequence variant was found, leading the authors to conclude that mutations in the coding region of the MeCP2 gene are not common causes of regression in autism.

Both Schellenberg et al. (2006) and Molloy et al. (2005) conducted linkage analyses in large cohorts of siblings with autism and found different linkage signals for pairs with and without regression, suggesting a possible genetic susceptibility to the regressive form of onset. The association found by Molloy et al.'s group was not replicated in the International Molecular Genetic Study of Autism Consortium (IMGSAC) cohort of affected siblings (Parr et al., 2006), however. The methods of the two studies differed in that the Molloy et al. study examined only siblings concordant for regression (n = 34 pairs), while the IMGSAC study included all pairs in which at least one sibling had experienced language loss (n = 58), of which only 12 were concordant for regression. Therefore, these linkage findings require further investigation and replication. The low rate of concordance for regression (20.7%) in the IMGSAC sample is, in and of itself, an important finding, suggesting that the regression phenotype is likely to be etiologically heterogeneous and multifactorial.

The liability to autism includes not only the full autism syndrome but also qualitatively similar but milder deficits (e.g., shyness, intense interests, speech delays, or other communication difficulties). This subclinical set of social and language differences seen in nonautistic relatives of individuals with autism is called the broader autism phenotype (BAP) and is found in 12 to 50% of relatives of those with autism (Lainhart et al., 2002). The BAP is considered an index of genetic vulnerability to autism (Piven, 2001).

Lainhart et al. (2002) compared the BAP in relatives of children with early onset and regressive autism. In a sample of 88 children, they found that parents of children with and without regression showed similar rates of the BAP (27.8% versus 32.9%, $p = 0.33$). Both groups had significantly higher rates of the BAP when compared to parents of children without autism (3.6%; $p \leq 0.01$). The authors argued that these findings suggest that environmental factors are unlikely to be the sole cause of regressive autism. That is, if regressive autism were caused solely by nongenetic factors, such as immunizations, one would instead expect to find similar rates of the BAP in relatives of children with regressive autism and the general population, both of which would be significantly lower than relatives of children with early onset autism (Lainhart et al., 2002).

Case Studies of Onset Types

We end this section with two case studies that illustrate the traditionally defined patterns of onset described so far in this chapter. These case descriptions were reconstructed from both parent responses on the Autism Diagnostic Interview–Revised (ADI-R; Lord et al., 1994; Rutter et al., 2003) and family videos collected as part of an IRB-approved home movie study (Ozonoff et al., 2008). Unique to these case studies, family home movies were systematically analyzed by coders unaware of the child's diagnosis or the purposes of the study, trained to reliability on an objective coding system (Werner & Dawson, 2005). Coded data was divided into four developmental periods, each 4 months long. To account for differences in the amount of footage available in each period, raw duration and frequency scores were converted to proportion and rate scores, respectively. Means for each period were calculated and graphs of the developmental trajectories are presented in Figure 4-1. The rates of key social-communicative behaviors are thus objectively quantified during the window of development when autism symptoms emerge, illustrating the two prototypical patterns of onset described in this chapter. Informed consent was obtained from parents prior to participation in the research project, as well as prior to the writing of these descriptions (which use pseudonyms and disguise identifying characteristics).

Case 1: Isaac, Early Onset Autism

Isaac was the product of a full-term pregnancy with no reported complications. His medical history is unremarkable. He is the first child born to parents with no family history of autism. He has two younger sisters who are typically developing.

Birth to 5 months: On the ADI-R, Isaac's parents reported that they had concerns about his development "from birth, coming home from the hospital" and said that they had noticed "no eye contact around two weeks." Corroborating these reports, family home video taken at three months of age shows Isaac fixating on the ceiling fan while his grandfather attempts to engage him in a social game. Although his grandfather's face is animated and just a few inches away, Isaac never looks at him. By three months of age, his parents had already become concerned specifically about the possibility that their son had autism, although they had little experience or knowledge of the condition.

6 to 10 months: During this time, Isaac continued to ignore the social approaches of others and demonstrated multiple unusual visual and repetitive behaviors. At 10 months he is observed on video repetitively flipping and rolling a marker across the floor. Coding of home videos shows that Isaac rarely oriented to his name, vocalized, or smiled at others during this period. He also shows an elevated level of unusual visual behavior, such as prolonged staring at objects (see Figure 4-1).

11 to 15 months: In home video from this period, Isaac continues to be socially isolated. At 12 months, he can be observed on camera failing to respond to his mother's repeated attempts to engage him in a game of peek-a-boo. Instead, his attention remains focused on a large hairbrush that he is spinning on the tiled bathroom floor. At 11 months of age, his parents refer him to the first author for an autism diagnostic evaluation. He is diagnosed with Autistic Disorder at 13 months.

16 to 20 months: During this period, Isaac begins receiving intensive early behavioral intervention and speech therapy. Home video footage at this time shows Isaac repeatedly pushing a button on a musical toy and putting his face up close to the blinking lights that accompany the song. At 16 months, he fails to make eye contact or respond to his

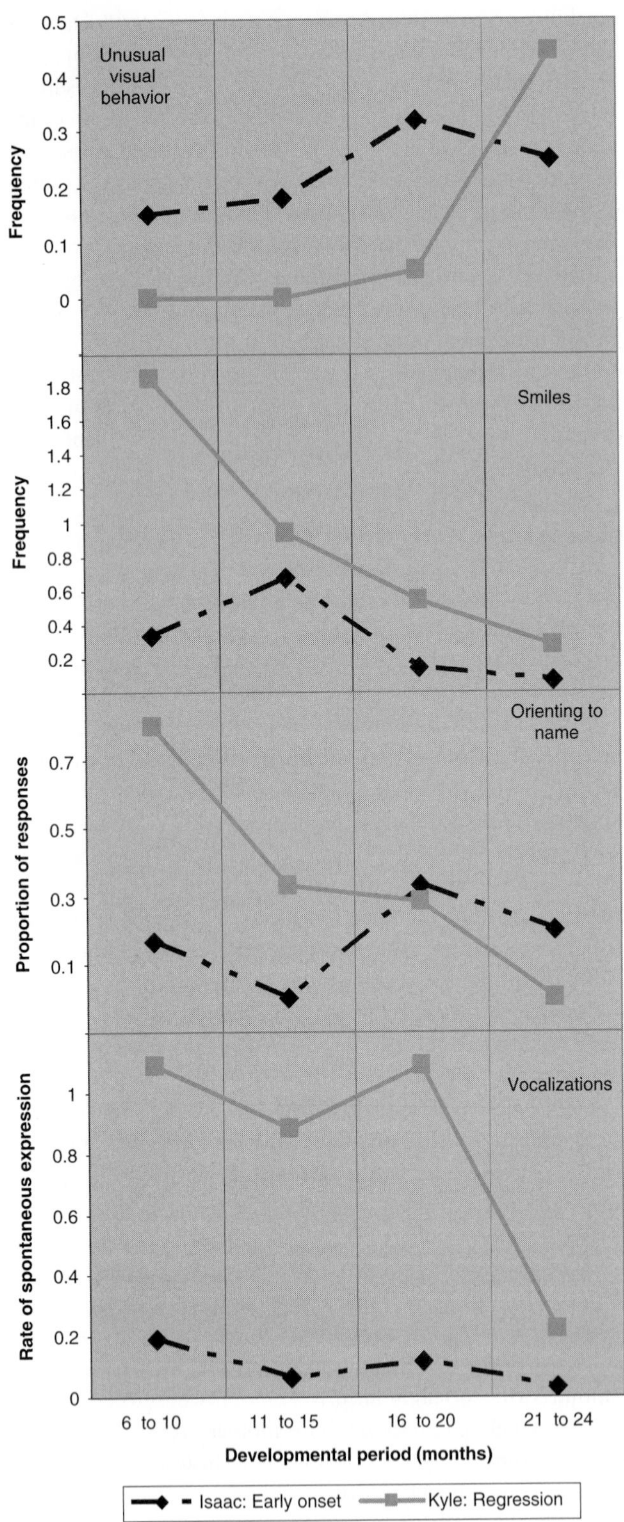

Figure 4–1. Developmental trajectories of key behaviors coded from home video.

father's verbal prompts when they are looking through a picture book together.

21 to 24 months: Footage from just prior to his second birthday shows Isaac repetitively waving a flashlight on the ceiling and examining it from the corner of his eyes. Coded data from this period show that he rarely responded to his name, smiled at others, or vocalized. He continued to meet full criteria for Autistic Disorder when retested as part of a research study at 24 months of age.

Case 2: Kyle, Autistic Regression

Kyle is the only child of parents with no family history of autism. He was born at full term; no complications were experienced during pregnancy, labor, or delivery. His medical history in the first year and a half of life revealed nothing significant. Onset of GI problems around 18 months of age was reported.

0 to 5 months: Parent report and observation of family home videos from this time period indicate that Kyle was socially well engaged, displaying frequent reciprocal smiles and babbling often. At 5 months, for example, he is seen on video playing peek-a-boo with his mother, laughing, and babbling reciprocally to continue the game.

6 to 10 months: Kyle continues to demonstrate high rates of warm positive affect, eye contact, and vocalizations throughout this period (see Figure 4-1). At 9 months he is observed on video imitating his mother blowing raspberries, laughing, and taking turns in this social game.

11 to 15 months: Both by parent report and as observed on home video, Kyle's behavior becomes more variable, particularly toward the end of this period. Home video at 11 months captures several word approximations ("nye-nye," "hi," "yeah"), bright smiles toward others, and immediate orientation when his name is called. Between 13 and 15 months he begins to appear more interested in objects than people, displays less positive affect, and demonstrates a few repetitive behaviors, but these concerning behaviors are interspersed with some typical social interactions, moments of excellent eye contact, and clearly directed smiles on home video. For example, at 13 months Kyle is filmed pushing plastic balls around the edge of a table as he circles it multiple times. Although his mother is sitting a few feet away, he does not approach her or look in her direction, even when accidentally backing into her, but later turns to his father, who is filming, and gives a broad smile. Similarly, at 15 months, Kyle is seen running back and forth across the living room, flapping his hands and sporadically squealing in a high-pitched manner as he approaches people and smiles. Kyle's parents reported on the ADI-R that they began to have concerns about Kyle's development at 15 months, when he "lost interaction and connectedness and began to withdraw socially."

16 to 20 months: During this period, Kyle's symptoms become much more pronounced on video and by parent report. At 20 months he is observed making repeated stereotyped vocalizations and failing to orient to his mother, who is just a few feet away. While playing outside, he is seen flapping his hands and sifting repetitively through a pile of rocks.

He ignores others when they call or approach him. No word-like vocalizations are coded on video.

21 to 24 months: Home movies taken just before his second birthday show Kyle playing with a string of beads, repeatedly setting them on the edge of a table and closely watching as they slide over the side. He does not respond to the social overtures of others in any video clips. Kyle was diagnosed with Autistic Disorder at 27 months of age.

Problems with Traditional Views of Onset

Despite the prototypicality of these two case descriptions, as well as the progress that has been made in the last half century in describing the regression phenotype, a number of difficulties with traditionally held views about onset have become evident with time. One problem is that definitions of regression and methods of describing onset differ across studies and newer research has shown that results can be quite influenced by these measurement differences. A second issue is that recent research has not always upheld previous views or clinical intuitions about the central features of and differences between onset types. Finally, prospective studies provide new data that do not fully support the findings of onset investigations that used retrospective methods (parent recall or home video analysis). Therefore, we may need to revise current conceptualizations of how the symptoms of autism emerge in the first years of life. It is to these topics that we move in the following sections.

Definition and Measurement Issues

Until relatively recently, when prospective studies that follow children from infancy through the window of autism susceptibility have been conducted, the only methodologies to investigate the early autism phenotype and onset patterns were retrospective. One method is the analysis of home movies of children later diagnosed with autism spectrum disorders. While this reduces potential reporting biases of parent interviews, home movie methodology suffers from several biases (Palomo et al., 2006). There is tremendous variability across families in the amount, content, and quality of footage of early development that is captured on video. Many families do not tape their children early in life, so home movie studies are not representative of all children with autism. Many families turn off video cameras when children are not behaving as expected or in a positive manner. Finally, home movie analysis is a very time-intensive method of collecting information about early development that is not practical for routine research use. Thus, most studies of the early autism phenotype (and clinical practice) have employed parent report, a more efficient method of collecting early history. However, parent report can be biased by knowledge of the child's eventual diagnosis, poor recall, or lack of sensitivity to developmental differences. Retrospective reports are subject to problems of memory and interpretation (Finney, 1981; Robbins, 1963) and need to be used with caution when examining hypotheses that demand precision in estimating event dates and frequencies (Henry, Moffitt, Caspi, Langley, & Silva, 1994). When people are asked to recall particular episodes, they often report them as having occurred more recently than they did, an error called "forward telescoping" (Loftus & Marburger, 1983). This phenomenon has been described specifically in investigations using parent report to study autism onset (Lord et al., 2004). Thus, it is critical to understand the degree of accuracy in parent reports of regression, particularly since other methods (e.g., video analysis) are labor intensive and require expert training.

One widely used instrument that collects detailed parent recollections of early development is the ADI-R, a "gold standard" research interview used in diagnosis (Lord et al., 1994; Rutter et al., 2003). This instrument has a section of 18 questions that collect detailed information about potential losses, including specific skills lost, duration of losses, and potential factors associated with the losses. It first asks about language losses (question 11, "Were you ever concerned that [your child] might have lost language skills during the first years of life?"). If the parent responds in the affirmative, the interviewer then probes for the number of words lost, how they were used prior to the loss, the duration of establishment of the skill, and the duration of loss of the skill. To meet ADI-R criteria for loss of language, at least five words must have been used spontaneously, meaningfully, and communicatively for at least three months before being lost for at least three months. If there are losses indicated by the parent that do not meet these criteria (e.g., words lost that fail to meet the quantity or duration criteria or other communicative losses, like loss of babbling or gesture use), they can be recorded on the form, but the child does not meet ADI-R criteria for word loss. There is no consensus in the field yet as to how to handle parent-reported losses that are subthreshold. Parents can give very convincing descriptions of 4 word losses or of losses of 5+ words that had not consistently been in the child's vocabulary for the three months required to meet ADI-R criteria. In most studies, these children would not be included in a language regression group.

A later ADI-R item asks parents about losses in other domains (question 20, "Has there ever been a period when [your child] seemed to get markedly worse or dropped further behind in his/her development?"). If the parent indicates yes, then possible losses in motor, self-help, play, and social abilities are probed, in that order. If the parent does not endorse other losses, no querying is done nor examples given. This may lead to underendorsement of losses, particularly in the social domain. In our experience, parents do not as readily regard social behaviors as acquired skills or specific developmental achievements that can be lost. However, when examples are provided, such as asking whether the child got markedly worse in their eye contact or lost interest in interacting with them, parents occasionally recognize this pattern and change their report.

The vast majority of children losing language also lose behaviors indicative of social interest and engagement, such as direct gaze and response to name (Goldberg et al., 2003; Lord, Shulman, & DiLavore, 2004; Ozonoff et al., 2005), but the converse is not always true. Some children show marked changes only in social development and do not lose spoken language. While it is very uncommon for children to retain acquired speech when experiencing a clear loss of social interest and engagement, many children have not acquired language at the time of the regression and therefore have no language to lose (Goldberg et al., 2003; Kurita, 1985; Ozonoff et al., 2005). Hansen et al. (2008) found that only 18% of a large (n = 138) sample of children with regression lost language skills alone, while 46% exhibited social losses alone, and 36% had losses in both language and social behaviors. Goldberg et al. (2003) found similar rates in a smaller sample, with language losses reported to occur about 2 months after losses of direct gaze, orientation to name, and social exchanges.

There is debate about whether definitions of regression should require loss of language and how children who only lose social milestones should be classified. Early studies tended to characterize regression as speech loss (Brown & Prelock, 1995; Kurita, 1985; Rogers & DiLalla, 1990) without including loss of social milestones as part of the criteria. Requiring the loss of language excludes from the regression group children who only experience social losses without substantial language loss. In many studies, such children were placed into the no-regression or early onset group (Kurita, 1985; Lainhart et al., 2002). However, recent studies suggest that there are very few differences between children who lose both words and social skills and those who experience losses in social milestones alone (Lord et al., 2004; Luyster et al., 2005). In a multisite study of children with ASD, Luyster et al. (2005) compared 125 children with word loss to 38 children with nonword loss (regression in areas other than language). They found no differences between the two regression groups. Children with word loss and nonword loss regression lost the same skills, including prespeech behaviors, games, and routines, and phrase comprehension, with almost exactly the same frequency (Luyster et al., 2005). Therefore, more recent studies have expanded definitions of regression to include losses in domains other than language (Davidovitch et al., 2000; Fombonne & Chakrabarti, 2001; Kobayashi & Murata, 1998).

Not surprisingly, the prevalence of regression is dependent on the definitions used. When a narrower definition that required language loss was used, only 15% of a large epidemiological sample of children with ASD met criteria for regression, whereas when losses in either language or social behaviors was used to classify onset patterns, 41% were found to have experienced losses (Hansen et al., 2008). Thus, requiring loss of language appears to significantly underestimate the frequency of developmental regression.

There is one published study that reports the test-retest reliability of parent report of regression. Richler et al. (2006) reported data from the multisite Collaborative Programs of Excellence in Autism (CPEA) sample (n = 351). The ADI-R was used initially to determine study eligibility and then later a detailed interview about regression was conducted by telephone. The time lag between administration of these two instruments was not specified in the study, but ranged from several months to several years. Conflicting information about word loss on the ADI-R and regression interview was apparent for 18.9% of the sample, with 12.3% reporting no loss on the ADI-R, but loss on the phone interview and 6.6% demonstrating the opposite pattern.

In unpublished data from our lab, we administered the same instrument (ADI-R) on two occasions, an average of 2 years apart. Four of 34 parents (11.8%) reported conflicting information on the ADI-R at times 1 and 2, with two feeling that their child had not regressed when asked at a mean age of 34.4 months but reporting a definite regression when asked again at a mean age of 57.4 months, and two displaying the opposite pattern (regression reported at time 1 but denied at time 2). This study also examined concurrent reliability of report of regression using two different parent report instruments. We used both the ADI-R and the Early Development Questionnaire (EDQ), a measure that asks 45 questions about social and communication development in the first 18 months of life, as well as 25 detailed questions about regression. We found that 7 of 40 parents of children with autism (17.5%) gave inconsistent information about regression across the two measures. In all cases, report on the ADI-R indicated no losses (either definite reports of no regression, 7.5%, or losses that fell short of the criteria, 10%), while report on the EDQ suggested some regression. Similarly, another investigation conducted at the M.I.N.D. Institute, the Childhood Autism Risk from Genetics and Environment (CHARGE) study (Hansen et al., 2008), found that 23 of 245 parents (9.4%) from a largely independent sample gave inconsistent information about regression on these two measures.

When reports of onset are inconsistent, it is quite difficult to determine which is accurate. Two home movie studies (Goldberg, Thorsen, Osann, & Spence, 2008; Werner & Dawson, 2005) have compared parent report with videotape footage and shown that parent report is generally valid, but poorer for reports of social than word loss and for reports of regression than no regression. Specifically, the Goldberg et al. study found 85% concordance between parental reports and independent video coders' ratings of loss or no loss of spoken language, but only 49% concordance between parent and home video coders' reports of social losses. Parents were more consistent when reporting no loss than when reporting loss across both language and social domains (Goldberg et al., 2008). Thus, neither parent report nor home video analysis can be considered a gold standard method of documenting whether a child displayed early signs of autism or experienced a regression in skills and the respective limitations of each method need to be recognized by researchers.

As we end this section, we provide a few recommendations that may improve the quality of future data acquisition using parent report, the more feasible of the retrospective methods currently in use. First, interviewers need to be well trained to ask questions fully (with appropriate probes) without being too leading. They should realize that parents not only may have difficulty recalling specific behaviors and their exact timing, but also may not define or conceptualize behaviors in the same way as interviewers. Examples and queries are permitted on the ADI-R, a semistructured interview that encourages examiners to ask additional questions until they are certain that the parents have understood the behavior being measured and have given a valid response. Parents often do not ask for clarification of questions and it is the interviewer's job to anticipate when this is necessary. Parents may misinterpret failures to progress as regression and this is an additional difficulty that examiners need to be aware of during their queries. It is not uncommon for an initial positive response to questions about regression to change to a negative report of losses after further probing, when it becomes clear that although the child failed to gain anticipated new skills, he did not experience any actual losses of acquired skills. This kind of querying needs to be balanced by the recognition that subtle losses of skills are indeed possible.

Evidence for Other Patterns of Loss

A second problem with current definitions of onset is that dichotomous categorical conceptualizations do not capture all the different ways that autism can emerge. The traditional view of regression has been that development is typical prior to the loss of skills. For example, Rogers and DiLalla (1990) reported that parents of children with later onset autism "were emphatic about the normalcy of their children's behavior in the first year of life. The onset of their children's symptoms began with a change in or a loss of the child's previous apparently normal social behavior" (p. 866). Data from recent studies, however, have raised doubt regarding the universality of typical development prior to regression. Ozonoff et al. (2005) identified a subset of children who presented abnormalities prior to regression. Of 31 children with regression, 45% were reported by parents to have displayed social and communication delays prior to the onset of the losses. This subset of children were reported by their parents to have never displayed several typical early-developing social behaviors, such as joint attention, showing, and social games (Ozonoff et al., 2005). Kurita (1985) also described a subset of children who showed signs of abnormalities prior to regression. Of the 97 autistic children with speech loss in his study, 78.3% showed some developmental abnormalities before the onset of the speech loss, including lack of stranger anxiety and limited social responsiveness (Kurita, 1985). Goldberg et al. (2003) reported that over two thirds of their sample with regression were already delayed in their language acquisition prior to the loss of skills. Similarly, Heung (2008) found that two thirds of subjects with regression had some indication of delayed language or social development prior to the onset of their regression. These studies and others (Meilleur & Fombonne, 2009; Richler et al., 2006; Wiggins et al., 2009) suggest that mixed onset features, with evidence of both early delays and later losses, are quite common.

Further evidence that traditional onset classifications are insufficient comes from the CHARGE study, a large epidemiological investigation of genetic and environmental risks for autism. Using an independent measure of regression, the EDQ (described above), Hansen and colleagues (2008) demonstrated that even children whose parents reported no evidence of regression on the ADI-R occasionally reported subtle losses of specific skills on the EDQ. Figure 4-2 displays the distribution of scores on the EDQ as a function of onset subtype. This finding is consistent with another report that some children whose parents reported no losses indicative of regression on the ADI-R nevertheless demonstrated subtle loss of skills on home video (Werner & Dawson, 2005).

Some parents report neither early signs of autism nor later regression. For example, in one sample, less than a third of parents of children who did not experience a regression reported concerns before the first birthday and, in fewer than half, were these concerns specifically social or autistic-like in nature (De Giacomo & Fombonne, 1998). In another sample, approximately one third of parents identified only nonspecific temperament or physiological patterns (e.g., irritability, passivity, eating or sleeping problems) before the first birthday "which evolved into typical autistic features like stereotypical behavior, aloneness, and a lack of eye contact in the second year of life" (Rogers & DiLalla, 1990, p. 866). In our own data, we have found that many parents who do not report a regression also report several intact early social behaviors. For example, 35% stated that their child often looked at others during social interactions in the first 18 months of life, 50% smiled back when others smiled at them, and 28% enjoyed interactive games such as peek-a-boo (Ozonoff et al., 2005).

Collectively, these findings suggest that there is an additional pattern of symptom emergence that is characterized by intact early social development and/or nonspecific abnormalities that are followed by a failure to progress and gain new skills as expected. It has been hypothesized that this pattern may be due to failures to use intact early dyadic social reciprocity skills to support the typical maturational processes of speech acquisition, intentional communication, and triadic

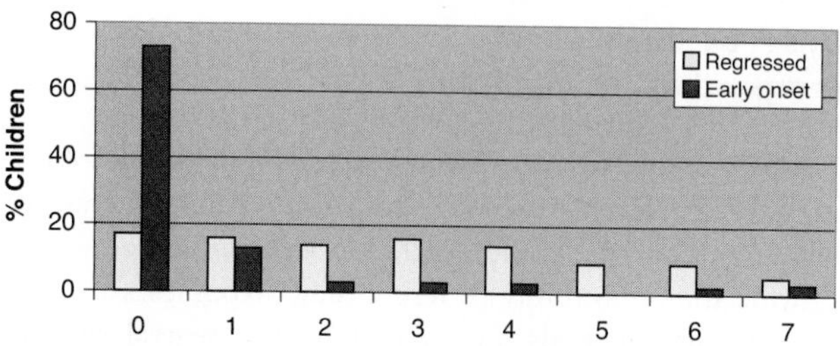

Figure 4–2. Number of skills lost in children with and without regression. Data from Hansen, R. L., Ozonoff, S., Krakowiak, P., Angkustsiri, K., Jones, C., Deprey, L. J., et al. (2008). Regression in autism: Prevalence and associated factors in the CHARGE study. *Ambulatory Pediatrics, 8*(1), 25–31.

social interactions (Chawarska et al., 2007). In such cases, the intact early behaviors fade away because they are not reinforced by the natural predisposition to seek and communicate with others. What might seem like a loss of skills is simply a failure to progress and transform the basic skills into their more developmentally advanced versions. Klin et al. (2004) used the term "pseudo-regression" to describe this pattern and it has also been referred to as "developmental stagnation" (Siperstein & Volkmar, 2004) and "developmental plateau" (Hansen et al., 2008; Kalb, Law, Landa, & Law, 2010). Little empirical research has been conducted on this pattern, and little is known about whether it differs from other onset patterns in phenotypic features unrelated to symptom emergence. A recent study suggests that the plateau onset pattern may be associated with better adaptive outcomes (Jones & Campbell, 2010).

Data from two large population-based studies at the M.I.N.D. Institute reinforce the notion of additional onset patterns beyond the traditionally defined categories. Byrd et al. (2002) recruited a random sample of children with autism from California's Regional Centers, which provide services for persons with developmental disabilities. Two cohorts were studied, one born in 1983–1985 and the other in 1993–1995. The CHARGE study, described above, is a large epidemiological sample also recruited from the Regional Center system, with the birth cohort extending from 1998 to 2004. The ADI-R was employed in both studies. Not only does it ask about regression, as described above, but also it asks about "onset as perceived with hindsight" (Question 4). Examining the intersection of these questions is informative to onset typology. Traditional definitions of onset suggest that most or all children without regression displayed symptoms early in life, while most or all with regression had typical early development. Thus, there should be very few, if any, subjects in the shaded diagonals of Tables 4-1 and 4-2. As is evident, however, almost half of both samples fell in these cells.

In summary, recent research suggests that there may be several different patterns of symptom emergence. Whether these are best characterized as additional onset types or conceptualized in some other way is not yet clear. We will return to this topic after finishing this section with insights from recent prospective studies of autism onset.

Table 4–1.
Data from Byrd et al., 2002

	Loss of Skills (ADI-R Q 11 or 25)	
	No	Yes
Symptoms before 1st birthday (ADI-R Q 4)	Early Onset N = 82 28.7%	Mixed N = 34 11.9%
Symptoms after 1st birthday (ADI-R Q 4)	Plateau N = 96 33.6%	Regression N = 74 25.9%

Notes: n = 286. Byrd, R., et al. (2002). *Report to the legislature on the principal findings from the epidemiology of autism in California: A comprehensive pilot study*. Davis: M.I.N.D. Institute, University of California, Davis.

Onset as Measured in Prospective Investigations

Prospective investigations are a very helpful method of studying onset, because they reduce errors due to parental recall and biases introduced by selective home videotaping, as well as provide the opportunity to test specific hypotheses through experimental methods. In the past decade, several research groups have instigated prospective investigations that study children at higher risk for autism because they have one or more siblings with the condition. Several infant sibling studies have now been published and thus far all have failed to find differences before the first birthday (at 4, 6, and 9 month visits of the respective studies) between children who are later diagnosed with autism and those who develop typically (Landa & Garrett-Mayer, 2006; Nadig et al., 2007; Zwaigenbaum et al., 2005; see also Yirmiya & Ozonoff, 2007 for a summary of this work). Bryson and colleagues (2007), in a consecutive case series of infant siblings followed prospectively from 6 months of age, describe several children whose symptoms are not present at their 6 and 12 month visits, but emerge slowly during the second year of life. Not a single child who developed autism (n = 9) displayed marked limitations in social reciprocity at 6 months. All nine infants were described as interested in social interactions, responsive to others, demonstrating sustained eye contact and social smiles. Most of the children did not experience an explicit loss of previously acquired skills that would meet established definitions of regression either. Two prospective case studies (Dawson et al., 2000; Klin et al., 2004) report on children who were noted to be symptomatic by the first birthday, but who presented with mostly intact social behavior at 6 months and did not experience a clear regression as symptoms began to emerge.

Table 4–2.
Data from Hansen et al., 2008

	Loss of Skills (ADI-R Q 11 or 25)	
	No	Yes
Symptoms before 1st birthday (ADI-R Q 4)	Early Onset N = 123 35%	Mixed N = 58 17%
Symptoms after 1st birthday (ADI-R Q 4)	Plateau N = 94 27%	Regression N = 76 22%

Notes: n = 351. Hansen, R. L., Ozonoff, S., Krakowiak, P., Angkustsiri, K., Jones, C., Deprey, L. J., et al. (2008). Regression in autism: Prevalence and associated factors in the CHARGE study. *Ambulatory Pediatrics, 8*(1), 25–31.

Data from the UC Davis Infant Sibling study (Ozonoff et al., 2010) are consistent with this published research. We followed 90 infants with older siblings with autism from birth through age 3. At each visit, they were administered the Mullen Scales of Early Learning, among other measures, and parents completed detailed questionnaires eliciting concerns about development and presence of autism symptoms. After each visit, the examiner made summary ratings of the infant's eye contact, social reciprocity, spontaneous engagement, initiatives, shared affect, and vocalizations. Interactions between the examiner and infant were also recorded and coded later by research staff unaware of the infant's group membership or outcome. The first 13 infants to be diagnosed with autism are included in Table 4-3, which depicts a reconstruction of the onset of developmental concerns and autism symptoms in these children.

Data used to rate onset of concerns included, at all ages, Mullen scores, parent concerns elicited at the end of each session, and examiner summary ratings of social engagement. At 18 months and up, scores on the Autism Diagnostic Observation Schedule (Lord et al., 2000), Social Communication Questionnaire (Rutter et al., 2003), and Modified-Checklist for Autism in Toddlers (Robins et al., 2001) were used as well. Table 4-3 demonstrates the rarity of children with developmental concerns at 6 months and the gradual emergence of concerns over time. Four of the five infants seen at 6 months were in the average range on all developmental tests, had no concerns raised by parents, and were rated as typical in social engagement by experienced examiners unaware of group status. The fifth infant (Child 5 in Table 4-3) scored low on motor testing, and both parents and examiners expressed concern about motor development, but social, communicative, and cognitive development were all in the average range. At 12 months, concerns had been raised about 5 of 11 children seen at this age, but over half the group continued to present relatively normally to both examiners and parents and to score in the average range on standardized testing. By 18 months, however, concerns had been raised about all children with eventual autism/ASD outcomes and 3 were formally diagnosed.

On the ADI-R, none of these 13 children was rated as having significant regression in development by their parents. Two parents noted loss of individual skills: loss of eye contact between 12 and 18 months in Child 6 and loss of gestures and language comprehension between 18 and 24 months in Child 11. Concerns had already been raised about the development of both children prior to these losses (see Table 4-3). No parents reported that their child had acquired and then lost language.

The scarcity of children with symptoms before 12 months, combined with the lack of parent-reported regression, was initially unexpected but is consistent with the results of retrospective studies reported in the previous section. To further examine the validity of this phenomenon, we used growth curve analyses to examine developmental trajectories of examiner summary ratings of social engagement. Analyses revealed a significant group by time effect (F 3, 49.38) = 9.71, $p < .001$). As seen in Figure 4-3, the interaction effect was due to a significant decline in social engagement over time in the autism/ASD group. Post hoc tests revealed no group differences at 6 months. At 12 months, the autism/ASD group scored significantly lower than a group with no family history of autism (Low-Risk Typical group; Beta = .604, t = 2.44, $p < .05$).

Table 4–3.
Onset of concerns and age of diagnosis in infants with autism/ASD outcomes

Child	6 Months	12 Months	18 Months	24 Months	36 Months
1	No concerns	No concerns	Concerns	Diagnosed	Diagnosed
2	No concerns	No concerns	Concerns	Diagnosed	Diagnosed
3	No concerns	Concerns	Concerns	Diagnosed	Diagnosed
4	No concerns	Concerns	Diagnosed	Diagnosed	Diagnosed
5	Concerns	Concerns	Diagnosed	Diagnosed	Diagnosed
6		Concerns	Concerns	Concerns	Diagnosed
7		Concerns	Diagnosed	Diagnosed	Diagnosed
8		No concerns	Concerns	Concerns	Diagnosed
9		No concerns	Concerns	Concerns	Diagnosed
10		No concerns	Concerns	Diagnosed	Diagnosed
11		No concerns	Concerns	Concerns	Diagnosed
12			Concerns	Diagnosed	Diagnosed
13			Concerns	Concerns	Diagnosed

Notes: Data from the UC Davis Infant Sibling Study (Ozonoff et al., 2010). Blank entries indicate the child was not seen at that visit.

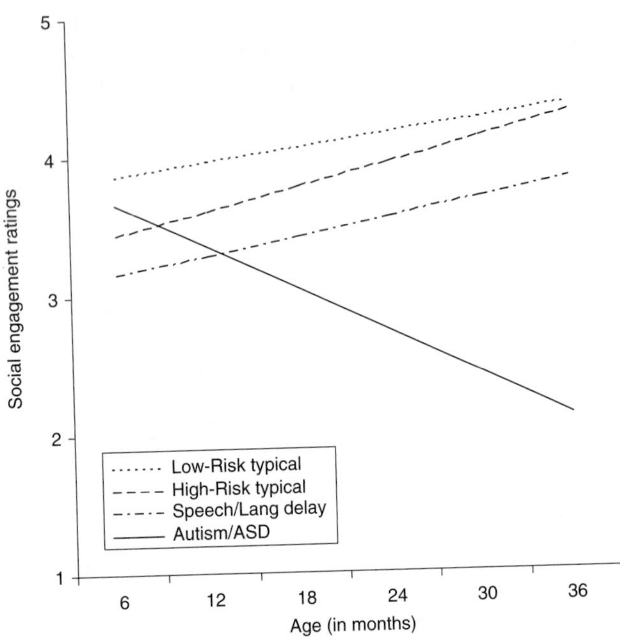

Figure 4–3. Developmental trajectories of social engagement ratings.

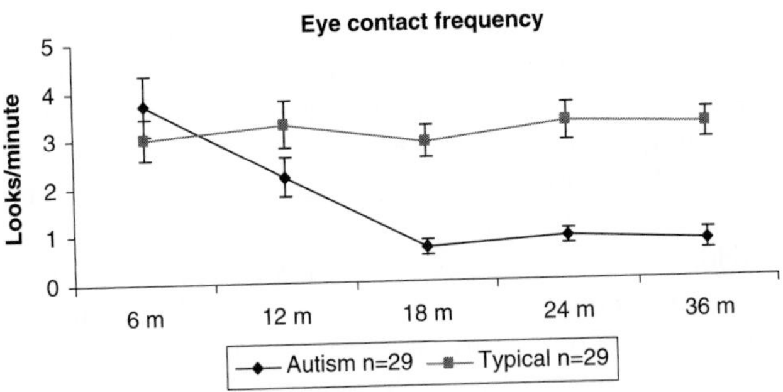

Figure 4–4. Frequency of eye contact with the examiner coded during the session.

By 24 months and later, the autism/ASD group had significantly lower scores than a Speech Delay group, a group with a positive family history of autism but who was developing typically (High Risk Typical group), and the Low Risk Typical group (Beta = .814, $t = 3.22$, $p < .01$). Coded data of the frequency of eye contact, vocalizations, and shared affect during the lab visit were highly consistent with the picture revealed by the examiner summary ratings, indicating again intact skills during the first year of life, followed by diminishing rates of social and communicative behaviors over time. See Figure 4-4. Similar declining trajectories in the onset of autism in infant siblings have also been reported by other research teams (Dawson, Munson, Webb, Nalty, Abbott, & Toth, 2007; Landa, Holman, & Garrett-Mayer, 2007).

Thus, infant sibling studies are consistent with retrospective studies in finding that for many, perhaps most, children with autism symptoms emerge gradually over the first 18 months or so of life.

Summary

The research literature reviewed in this chapter suggests that onset of autism is a gradual process that involves both diminishment of certain key social behaviors and failure to progress in other more advanced social-communicative processes over time. Autism appears to *emerge* over the first year and a half of life and is not present in most cases from shortly after birth, as once suggested by Kanner (1943).

Data from both retrospective and prospective studies are consistent in finding that two-category onset classification systems do not fit the empirical data well. There is evidence that the traditionally defined categories of early onset and regressive autism are overly narrow prototypes that may not in fact be very common. There is ample evidence of other ways in which symptoms emerge that are not captured by these prototypes. One possibility is that we need to expand the number of categories used to describe onset. For example, perhaps there are four rather than two categories of onset, adding a plateau and a mixed group. We suggest another possibility, however. We hypothesize that symptom emergence may better be considered as a continuum. The two extremes of this continuum are anchored by the traditionally defined, prototypical early onset and regressive cases, such as those of Isaac and Kyle described above, but many intermediate phenotypes containing mixed features and varying degrees of early deficits, subtle diminishments, failures to progress, and frank losses are also possible. We propose that variable combinations and timings of these processes across children lead to symptoms exceeding the threshold for diagnosis at different points in the first 24 months for different children, as also suggested by Landa et al. (2007).

A second insight from the body of research summarized in this chapter is that regression may be much more common than initially thought. If defined narrowly, in the traditional manner (requiring loss of language, as in the ADI-R criteria), regression is relatively rare. If defined more broadly, to include diminishment in social engagement, regression may be the rule rather than the exception. However, losses are subtle, are usually preceded by some early concerns, and are followed by failures to progress in other areas, rather than characterized by typical development followed by catastrophic losses, as traditionally defined. Others have suggested that many, even most, children with autism undergo some regression during the course of symptom onset (Dawson et al., 2007). Along these lines, we propose that symptom emergence may better be conceptualized as a continuum characterized by the amount and timing of regression. In this conceptualization, at one end of the continuum lie children who display loss of social interest so early that the regression is difficult to see and symptoms appear to have always been present. At the other end of the continuum lie children who experience losses of social interest and communication skills so late that the regression appears quite dramatic.

Conclusions

Thus, it is clear that existing definitions of onset patterns will need to undergo further development as new data emerges from future studies. Investigations using prospective samples may be especially fruitful because they will be less affected by potential videotaping, reporting, and recall biases inherent in retrospective studies. Further research clarifying whether onset is better conceptualized categorically (dichotomously) or dimensionally is urgently needed for etiologic studies, which have been hindered already by the tremendous heterogeneity of the autism phenotype. Finally, future research should strive to find early processing or biological markers that may predict who will develop autism prior to the onset of behavioral symptoms. It is possible that infants who are behaviorally asymptomatic at 6 and 12 months may show differences in lower-level underlying processes that can impact later development. For example, differences in visual attention, such as prolonged visual fixations (Landry & Bryson, 2004), might lead to joint attention deficits or behavioral rigidity a few months later. Deficits in the dorsal stream visual pathway, which is specialized for quick processing of global, low spatial-frequency information, could create a cascade of functional differences in brain regions downstream. Recently, McCleery et al. (2007) found high luminance contrast sensitivity in a subgroup of younger siblings of children with autism on a task measuring the integrity of the magnocellular visual pathway (part of the dorsal stream). Two of the infants developed autism, leading the authors to speculate that early abnormalities in the magnocellular pathway might be a risk marker for autism. Thus, research on lower level processes that may signal an affected child prior to the onset of behavioral signs could permit interventions to be applied that might significantly lessen disability or perhaps even prevent the disorder from developing.

Finally, this body of work has clinical implications for screening, diagnosis, and intervention. Universal screening has been recommended by the American Academy of Pediatrics at 18 and 24 months (Johnson et al., 2007), but many have hoped that identification even earlier than this might be possible. The research reviewed here suggests that identification of autism prior to the first birthday will be a major challenge and may not possible in many children. In fact, for the large group of infants whose autism emerges through diminishment in skills, they may be showing few or no behavioral signs of the disorder at the first birthday. Therefore, screening twice, at both 18 and 24 months, is essential, as many children will be missed at the earlier time point. Given the gradual and protracted course of symptom emergence, we urge professionals to consider referring children for intervention at the point that there is a suspicion of autism and not wait for a definitive diagnosis. Finally, development of treatments appropriate for infants and young toddlers is an urgent priority.

Challenges and Future Directions

- Studies of larger, community-ascertained samples at high risk for autism must be conducted, ideally with enrollment during pregnancy or shortly after birth, prior to the emergence of developmental concerns that may bias subject inclusion and study results
- Identification of risk markers prior to the onset of behavioral signs of autism
- Development of diagnostic criteria appropriate for infants and toddlers
- Development of screening guidelines that incorporate results of recent research on infants at risk for autism
- Development of treatments appropriate for infants and toddlers

SUGGESTED READINGS

Goldberg, W. A., Thorsen, K. L., Osann, K., & Spence, A. M. (2008). Use of home videotapes to confirm parental reports of regression in autism. *Journal of Autism and Developmental Disorders, 38*, 1136–1146.

Werner, E., Dawson, G., Munson, J., & Osterling, J. (2005). Variation in early developmental course in autism and its relation with behavioral outcome at 3–4 years of age. *Journal of Autism and Developmental Disorders, 35*, 337–350.

Zwaigenbaum, L., Bryson, S., Lord, C., Rogers, S., Carter, A., et al. (2009). Clinical assessment and management of toddlers with suspected ASD: Insights from studies of high-risk infants. *Pediatrics, 123*, 1383–1391.

REFERENCES

Andrews, N., Miller, E., Grant, A., Stowe, J., Osborne, V., & Taylor, B. (2004). Thimerosal exposure in infants and developmental disorders: A retrospective cohort study in the United Kingdom does not support a causal association. *Pediatrics, 114*(3), 584–591.

Baird, G., Charman, T., Pickles, A., Chandler, S., Loucas, T., Meldrum, D., et al. (2008). Regression, developmental trajectory, and associated problems in disorders in the autism spectrum: The SNAP study. *Journal of Autism and Developmental Disorders, 38*(10), 1827–1836.

Baranek, G. T. (1999). Autism during infancy: A retrospective video analysis of sensory-motor and social behaviors at 9–12 months of age. *Journal of Autism and Developmental Disorders, 29*(3), 213–224.

Bernard, S., Enayati, A., Redwood, L., Roger, H., & Binstock, T. (2001). Autism: A novel form of mercury poisoning? *Medical Hypotheses, 56*, 462–471.

Blaxill, M. F., Redwood, L., & Bernard, S. (2004). Thimerosal and autism? A plausible hypothesis that should not be dismissed. *Medical Hypotheses, 62*(5), 788–794.

Brown, J., & Prelock, P. A. (1995). The impact of regression on language development in autism. *Journal of Autism and Developmental Disorders, 25*(3), 305–309.

Byrd, R., et al. (2002). *Report to the legislature on the principal findings from the epidemiology of autism in California: A comprehensive pilot study*. Davis: M.I.N.D. Institute, University of California, Davis.

Bryson, S. E., Zwaigenbaum, L., Brian, J., Roberts, W., Szatmari, P., Rombough, V., et al. (2007). A prospective case series of high-risk infants who developed autism. *Journal of Autism and Developmental Disorders, 37*(1), 12–24.

Chawarska, K., Klin, A., Paul, R., & Volkmar, F. (2007). Autism spectrum disorder in the second year: Stability and change in syndrome expression. *Journal of Child Psychology and Psychiatry, 48*(2), 128–138.

Dales, L., Hammer, S. J., & Smith, N. J. (2001). Time trends in autism and in MMR immunization coverage in California. *Journal of the American Medical Association, 285*(9), 1183–1185.

Davidovitch, M., Glick, L., Holtzman, G., Tirosh, E., & Safir, M. P. (2000). Developmental regression in autism: Maternal perception. *Journal of Autism and Developmental Disorders, 30*(2), 113–119.

Dawson, G., Munson, J., Webb, S. J., Nalty, T., Abbott, R., & Toth, K. (2007). Rate of head growth decelerates and symptoms worsen in the second year of life in autism. *Biological Psychiatry, 61*, 458–464.

Dawson, G., Osterling, J., Meltzoff, A. N., & Kuhl, P. (2000). Case study of the development of an infant with autism from birth to 2 years of age. *Journal of Applied Developmental Psychology, 21*, 299–313.

De Giacomo, A., & Fombonne, E. (1998). Parental recognition of developmental abnormalities in autism. *European Child and Adolescent Psychiatry, 7*(3), 131–136.

Deonna, T., Ziegler, A.-L., Maeder, M.-I., Ansermet, F., & Roulet, E. (1995). Reversible behavioral autistic-like regression: A manifestation of a special (new?) epileptic syndrome in a 28-month-old child: A 2-year longitudinal study. *Neurocase, 1*(2), 91–99.

Farrington, C. P., Miller, E., & Taylor, B. (2001). MMR and autism: Further evidence against a causal association. *Vaccine, 19*(27), 3632–3635.

Finney, H. C. (1981). Improving the reliability of retrospective survey measures. *Evaluation Review, 5*, 207–229.

Fombonne, E., & Chakrabarti, S. (2001). No evidence for a new variant of measles-mumps-rubella-induced autism. *Pediatrics, 108*(4), E58.

Goldberg, W. A., Osann, K., Filipek, P. A., Laulhere, T., Jarvis, K., Modahl, C., et al. (2003). Language and other regression: Assessment and timing. *Journal of Autism and Developmental Disorders, 33*(6), 607–616.

Goldberg, W. A., Thorsen, K. L., Osann, K., & Spence, A. M. (2008). Use of home videotapes to confirm parental reports of regression in autism. *Journal of Autism and Developmental Disorders, 38*, 1136–1146.

Hansen, R. L., & Ozonoff, S. (2003). Alternative theories: Assessment and therapy options. In S. Ozonoff & S. J. Rogers (Eds.), *Autism spectrum disorders: A research review for practitioners* (pp. 187–207). Washington, DC: American Psychiatric Publishing.

Hansen, R. L., Ozonoff, S., Krakowiak, P., Angkustsiri, K., Jones, C., Deprey, L. J., et al. (2008). Regression in autism: Prevalence and associated factors in the CHARGE study. *Ambulatory Pediatrics, 8*(1), 25–31.

Harper, J., & Williams, S. (1975). Age and type of onset as critical variables in early infantile autism. *Journal of Autism and Childhood Schizophrenia, 5*(1), 25–36.

Henry, B., Moffitt, T. E., Caspi, A., Langley, J., & Silva, P. A. (1994). On the "remembrance of things past": A longitudinal evaluation of the retrospective method. *Psychological Assessment, 34*, 49–68.

Heung, K. (2008). Is autistic regression too narrowly defined? Doctoral dissertation, University of California, Davis. *University Microfilms International.*

Hoshino, Y., Kaneko, M., Yashima, Y., Kumashiro, H., Volkmar, F. R., & Cohen, D. J. (1987). Clinical features of autistic children with setback course in their infancy. *Japanese Journal of Psychiatry and Neurology, 41*(2), 237–245.

James, S. J., Cutler, P., Melnyk, S., Jernigan, S., Janak, L., Gaylor, D. W., et al. (2004). Metabolic biomarkers of increased oxidative stress and impaired methylation capacity in children with autism. *American Journal of Clinical Nutrition, 80*(6), 1611–1617.

Johnson, C. P., & Myers, S. M. (2007). Identification and evaluation of children with autism spectrum disorders. *Pediatrics, 120*(5): 1183–1215.

Jones, L. A., & Campbell, J. M. (2010). Clinical characteristics associated with language regression for children with autism spectrum disorders. *Journal of Autism and Developmental Disorders, 40*(1), 54–62.

Kalb, L. G., Law, J. K., Landa, R., & Law, P. A. (2010). Onset patterns prior to 36 months in autism spectrum disorders. *Journal of Autism and Developmental Disorders, 40*(11), 1389–1402.

Kanner, L. (1943). Autistic disturbances of affective contact. *Nervous Child, 2*, 217–250.

Kaye, J. A., del Mar Melero-Montes, M., & Jick, H. (2001). Mumps, measles, and rubella vaccine and the incidence of autism recorded by general practitioners: A time trend analysis. *British Medical Journal, 322*(7284), 460–463.

Klin, A., Chawarska, K., Paul, R., Rubin, E., Morgan, T., Wiesner, L., et al. (2004). Autism in a 15-month-old child. *American Journal of Psychiatry, 161*(11), 1981–1198.

Kobayashi, R., & Murata, T. (1998). Setback phenomenon in autism and long-term prognosis. *Acta Psychiatrica Scandinavica, 98*(4), 296–303.

Kurita, H. (1985). Infantile autism with speech loss before the age of thirty months. *Journal of the American Academy of Child Psychiatry, 24*(2), 191–196.

Lainhart, J. E., Ozonoff, S., Coon, H., Krasny, L., Dinh, E., Nice, J., et al. (2002). Autism, regression, and the broader autism phenotype. *American Journal of Medical Genetics, 113*(3), 231–237.

Landa, R., & Garrett-Mayer, E. (2006). Development in infants with autism spectrum disorders: A prospective study. *Journal of Child Psychology and Psychiatry, 47*(6), 629–638.

Landa, R., Holman, K. C., & Garrett-Mayer, E. (2007). Social and communication development in toddlers with early and later diagnosis of autism spectrum disorders. *Archives of General Psychiatry, 64*(7), 853–864.

Landry, R., & Bryson, S. E. (2004). Impaired disengagement of attention in young children with autism. *Journal of Child Psychology and Psychiatry, 45*(6), 1115–1122.

Loftus, E. F., & Marburger, W. (1983). Since the eruption of Mt. St. Helens, has anyone beaten you up? Improving the accuracy of retrospective reports with landmark events. *Memory and Cognition, 11*, 114–120.

Lord, C., Risi, S., Lambrecht, L., Cook, E. H., Leventhal, B. L., DiLavore, P. C., et al. (2000). The Autism Diagnostic Observation Schedule—Generic: A standard measure of social and communication deficits associated with the spectrum of autism. *Journal of Autism and Developmental Disorders, 30*(3), 205–223.

Lord, C., Rutter, M., & Le Couteur, A. (1994). Autism Diagnostic Interview-Revised: A revised version of a diagnostic interview for caregivers of individuals with possible pervasive developmental disorders. *Journal of Autism and Developmental Disorders, 24*(5), 659–685.

Lord, C., Shulman, C., & DiLavore, P. (2004). Regression and word loss in autistic spectrum disorders. *Journal of Child Psychology and Psychiatry and Allied Disciplines, 45*, 1–21.

Luyster, R., Richler, J., Risi, S., Hsu, W. L., Dawson, G., Bernier, R., et al. (2005). Early regression in social communication in autism spectrum disorders: A CPEA Study. *Developmental Neuropsychology, 27*(3), 311–336.

Madsen, K. M., Lauritsen, M. B., Pedersen, C. B., Thorsen, P., Plesner, A. M., Andersen, P. H., et al. (2003). Thimerosal and the occurrence of autism: Negative ecological evidence from Danish population-based data. *Pediatrics, 112*(3 Pt 1), 604–606.

Mantovani, J. F. (2000). Autistic regression and Landau-Kleffner syndrome: Progress or confusion? *Developmental Medicine and Child Neurology, 42*(5), 349–353.

McCleery, J., Allman, E., Carver, L., & Dobkins, K. (2007). Abnormal magnocellular pathway visual processing in infants at risk for autism. *Biological Psychiatry, 62*(9), 1007–1014.

Meilleur, A. S., & Fombonne, E. (2009). Regression of language and non-language skills in pervasive developmental disorders. *Journal of Intellectual Disability Research, 53*, 115–124.

Molloy, C. A., Keddache, M., & Martin, L. J. (2005). Evidence for linkage on 21q and 7q in a subtest of autism characterized by developmental regression. *Molecular Psychiatry, 10*, 741–746.

Murch, S. H., Anthony, A., Casson, D. H., Malik, M., Berelowitz, M., Dhillon, A. P., et al. (2004). Retraction of an interpretation. *Lancet, 363*(9411), 750.

Nadig, A. S., Ozonoff, S., Young, G. S., Rozga, A., Sigman, M., & Rogers, S. J. (2007). Failure to respond to name is indicator of possible autism spectrum disorder. *Archives of Pediatrics and Adolescent Medicine, 161*, 378–383.

Nass, R., Gross, A., Wisoff, J., & Devinsky, O. (1999). Outcome of multiple subpial transections for autistic epileptiform regression. *Pediatric Neurology, 21*(1), 464–470.

Nelson, K. B., & Bauman, M. L. (2003). Thimerosal and autism? *Pediatrics, 111*(3), 674–679.

Neville, B. G., Harkness, W. F., Cross, J. H., Cass, H. C., Burch, V. C., Lees, J. A., et al. (1997). Surgical treatment of severe autistic regression in childhood epilepsy. *Pediatric Neurology, 16*(2), 137–140.

Osterling, J., & Dawson, G. (1994). Early recognition of children with autism: A study of first birthday home videotapes. *Journal of Autism and Developmental Disorders, 24*(3), 247–257.

Ozonoff, S., Iosif, A. M., Baguio, F., Cook, I. C., Hill, M. M., Hutman, T., Rogers, S. J., Sangha, S., Sigman, M., Steinfeld, M.B., & Young, G. S. (2010). A prospective study of the emergence of early behavioral signs of autism. *Journal of the American Academy of Child and Adolescent Psychiatry, 49*(3), 256–266.

Ozonoff, S., Young, G. S., Goldring, S., Greiss-Hess, L., Herrera, A. M., Steele, J., et al. (2008). Gross motor development, movement abnormalities, and early identification of autism. *Journal of Autism and Developmental Disorders, 38*, 644–656.

Ozonoff, S., Williams, B. J., & Landa, R. (2005). Parental report of the early development of children with regressive autism: The delays-plus-regression phenotype. *Autism, 9*(5), 461–486.

Palomo, R., Belinchon, M., & Ozonoff, S. (2006). Autism and family home movies: A comprehensive review. *Journal of Developmental and Behavioral Pediatrics, 27*(2), S59–S68.

Parr, J. R., Lamb, J. A., Bailey, A. J., & Monaco, A. P. (2006). Response to paper by Molloy et al.: Linkage on 21q and 7q in autism subset with regression. *Molecular Psychiatry, 10*(8), 741–746.

Piven, J. (2001). The broad autism phenotype: A complementary strategy for molecular genetic studies of autism. *American Journal of Medical Genetics, 105*(1), 34–35.

Poling, J. S. (2006). Developmental regression and mitochondrial dysfunction in a child with autism. *Journal of Child Neurology, 21*, 170–172.

Richler, J., Luyster, R., Risi, S., Hsu, W. L., Dawson, G., Bernier, R., et al. (2006). Is there a "regressive phenotype" of Autism Spectrum Disorder associated with the measles-mumps-rubella vaccine? A CPEA study. *Journal of Autism and Developmental Disorders, 36*(3), 299–316.

Robins, D. L., Fein, D., Barton, M. L., & Green, J. A. (2001). The Modified Checklist for Autism in Toddlers: An initial study investigating the early detection of autism and pervasive developmental disorders. *Journal of Autism and Developmental Disorders, 31*, 131–144.

Robins, L. C. (1963). The accuracy of parental recall of aspects of child development and child rearing practices. *Journal of Abnormal Social Psychology, 66*, 261–270.

Rogers, S. J., & DiLalla, D. L. (1990). Age of symptom onset in young children with pervasive developmental disorders. *Journal of the American Academy of Child and Adolescent Psychiatry, 29*(6), 863–872.

Rutter, M. (1985). The treatment of autistic children. *Journal of Child Psychology and Psychiatry and Allied Disciplines, 26*(2), 193–214.

Rutter, M., Bailey, A., Lord, C., & Berument, S. K. (2003). *Social Communication Questionnaire.* Los Angeles, CA: Western Psychological Services.

Rutter, M., Le Couteur, A., & Lord, C. (2003). *Autism Diagnostic Interview-Revised (ADI-R).* Los Angeles, CA: Western Psychological Services.

Schechter, R., & Grether, J. K. (2008). Continuing increases in autism reported to California's developmental services system. *Archives of General Psychiatry, 65*, 19–24.

Schellenberg, G. D., Dawson, G., Sung, Y. J., Estes, A., Munson, J., et al. (2006). Evidence for multiple loci from a genome scan of autism kindreds. *Molecular Psychiatry, 11*, 1049–1060.

Shinnar, S., Rapin, I., Arnold, S., Tuchman, R. F., Shulman, L., Ballaban-Gil, K., et al. (2001). Language regression in childhood. *Pediatric Neurology, 24*(3), 183–189.

Short, A. B., & Schopler, E. (1988). Factors relating to age of onset in autism. *Journal of Autism and Developmental Disorders, 18*(2), 207–216.

Siperstein, R., & Volkmar, F. (2004). Parental reporting of regression in children with pervasive developmental disorders. *Journal of Autism and Developmental Disorders, 34*(6), 731–734.

Stone, W. L., Hoffman, E. L., Lewis, S. E., & Ousley, O. Y. (1994). Early recognition of autism. Parental reports vs. clinical observation. *Archives of Pediatric and Adolescent Medicine. 148*(2), 174–179.

Stone, W. L., Lee, E. B., Ashford, L., Brissie, J., Hepburn, S. L., et al. (1999). Can autism be diagnosed accurately in children under 3 years? *Journal of Child Psychology and Psychiatry, 40*(2), 219–226.

Taylor, B., Miller, E., Lingam, R., Andrews, N., Simmons, A., & Stowe, J. (2002). Measles, mumps, and rubella vaccination and bowel problems or developmental regression in children with autism: Population study. *British Medical Journal, 324*(7334), 393–396.

Taylor, B., Miller, E., Farrington, C. P., Petropoulos, M. C., Fayot-Mayaud, I., Li, J., et al. (1999). Autism and measles, mumps and rubella vaccine: No epidemiological evidence for a causal association. *Lancet, 353*, 2026–2029.

Tuchman, R. F., & Rapin, I. (1997). Regression in pervasive developmental disorders: Seizures and epileptiform electroencephalogram correlates. *Pediatrics, 99*(4), 560–566.

Uchiyama, T., Kurosawa, M., & Inaba, Y. (2007). MMR-vaccine and regression in autism spectrum disorders: Negative results presented from Japan. *Journal of Autism and Developmental Disorders, 37*, 210–217.

Volkmar, F. R., & Cohen, D. J. (1989). Disintegrative disorder or "late onset" autism. *Journal of Child Psychology and Psychiatry, 30*(5), 717–724.

Wakefield, A. J., Murch, S. H., Anthony, A., Linnell, J., Casson, D. M., Malik, M., et al. (1998). Ileal-lymphoid-nodular hyperplasia, non-specific colitis, and pervasive developmental disorder in children. *Lancet, 351*(9103), 637–641.

Webb, J., Nalty, T., Munson, J., Brock, C., Abbott, R., & Dawson, G. (2007). Rate of head circumference growth as a function of autism diagnosis and history of autistic regression. *Journal of Child Neurology, 22*(10), 1192–1190.

Weissman, J. R., Kelley, R. I., Bauman, M. L., Cohen, B. H., Murray, K. F., et al. (2008). Mitochondrial disease in autism spectrum disorder patients: A cohort analysis. *PLoS ONE, 3*, 1–6.

Werner, E., & Dawson, G. (2005). Validation of the phenomenon of autistic regression using home videotapes. *Archives of General Psychiatry, 62*, 889–895.

Werner, E., Dawson, G., Munson, J., & Osterling, J. (2005). Variation in early developmental course in autism and its relation with behavioral outcome at 3–4 years of age. *Journal of Autism and Developmental Disorders, 35*(3), 337–350.

Werner, E., Dawson, G., Osterling, J., & Dinno, N. (2000). Recognition of autism spectrum disorder before one year of age: A retrospective study based on home videotapes. *Journal of Autism and Developmental Disorders, 30*(2), 157–162.

Wetherby, A. M., Woods, J., Allen, L., Cleary, J., Dickinson, H., & Lord, C. (2004). Early indicators of autism spectrum disorders in the second year of life. *Journal of Autism and Developmental Disorders, 35*(5), 473–493.

Wiggins, L. D., Rice, C. E., & Baio, J. (2009). Developmental regression in children with an autism spectrum disorder identified by a population-based surveillance system. *Autism, 13*, 357–374.

Xi, C. Y., Ma, H. W., Lu, Y., Zhao, Y. J., Hua, T. Y., et al. (2007). MeCP2 gene mutation analysis in autistic boys with developmental regression. *Psychiatric Genetics, 17*(2), 113–116.

Yirmiya, N., & Ozonoff, S. (2007). The very early phenotype of autism. *Journal of Autism and Developmental Disorders, 37*, 1–11.

Zwaigenbaum, L., Bryson, S., Rogers, T., Roberts, W., Brian, J., & Szatmari, P. (2005). Behavioral manifestations of autism in the first year of life. *International Journal of Developmental Neuroscience, 23*, 143–152.

5 Lonnie Zwaigenbaum

Screening, Risk, and Early Identification of Autism Spectrum Disorders

Points of Interest

- Retrospective studies and prospective studies of high-risk infants indicate that ASD symptoms are often apparent by 12 months of age, and include atypicalities in social and communication development, play interests, and regulation of attention, emotions, and functions essential to physical well-being, such as eating and sleeping.
- Recent screening data suggest that both the Modified–Checklist for Autism in Toddlers (M-CHAT) and the Infant Toddler Checklist (ITC) have the potential to efficiently identify very young children with ASD, including some that may not be flagged by parental concerns or surveillance by community physicians.
- Future evaluation of ASD screening should adopt a broader health systems perspective in order to more fully gauge the potential impacts of screening, and to gain further support among health care providers and policy-makers.

Introduction

The clinical heterogeneity and varying patterns of onset of the autism spectrum disorders (ASD) as discussed by Lord, and by Ozonoff in this volume, highlight the complex challenges associated with developing a comprehensive early detection strategy. However, it is essential to develop effective approaches to identify and diagnose children with ASD early in life. ASD is one of the most prevalent forms of developmental disability, occurring in approximately 1 in 150 children (Bertrand et al., 2001; Chakrabarti & Fombonne, 2001; Yeargin-Allsopp et al., 2003; Fombonne, Zakarian, Bennett, Meng, & McLean-Heywood, 2006; Scott, Baron-Cohen, Bolton, & Brayne, 2002; see Fombonne in this volume for a detailed review). Earlier diagnosis creates opportunities for children with ASD to benefit more fully from intervention (e.g., Harris & Handleman, 2000). Gains through early intervention can reduce the burden-of-suffering and enhance the quality of life for affected children and their families, and may ultimately reduce the considerable family and societal costs related to ASD across the lifespan (Jacobson & Mulick, 2000; Jarbrink & Knapp, 2001). Earlier diagnosis also allows parents to be better informed about recurrence risk to later-born children, and better able to monitor for early signs of autism (Zwaigenbaum et al., 2005) and other related concerns (Bailey, Palferman, Heavey, & Le, 1998; Dawson et al., 2002). Overall, the frequency, burden of suffering, long-term cumulative costs, and efficacy of early intervention provide a strong rationale for efforts aimed at earlier identification and diagnosis of ASD.

There is considerable evidence to suggest that autism and other ASDs could be diagnosed at an earlier age than is the current norm. Although there are published reports of ASD diagnoses being established as early as 14–15 months (Chawarska, Klin, Paul, & Volkmar, 2007; Landa, Holman, & Garrett-Mayer, 2007), a recent report by the Centers for Disease Control and Prevention (Autism and Developmental Disabilities Monitoring Network, 2007) indicated that the median age of ASD diagnosis across 14 U.S. states ranged from 49 to 66 months. Howlin and Moore in their survey of 1300 families in the UK, found that these parents typically became concerned around 18 months of age, and sought out medical attention by age 2 (Howlin & Moore, 1997). Often parents were offered reassurances without recognition of the seriousness of their concerns, followed eventually by a referral for a more specialized assessment, and then, further delays: many children were seen by at least 3 different consultants before receiving a diagnosis of autism. The experience of parents in North America has been similar (Mandell, Novak, & Zubritsky, 2005; Siegel, Pliner, Eschler, & Elliott, 1988). Studies in both the UK and North America have suggested that the delays in diagnosis experienced by families of children with Asperger's syndrome are more extreme (Howlin & Asgharian, 1999; Mandell et al., 2005). Consistent with the survey by Howlin and Moore (Howlin & Moore, 1997), several studies have found that 80–90% of parents of children with ASD recall developmental concerns dating back to the first two years of life (De Giacomo A. & Fombonne, 1998; Ohta, Nagai, Hara, & Sasaki, 1987; Rogers & DiLalla, 1990; Gillberg et al., 1990). Analyses of home videos also demonstrate that many children with autism show signs of impairment long before they are diagnosed (Adrien et al., 1992; Osterling & Dawson, 1994; Osterling, Dawson, & Munson, 2002; Werner, Dawson, Osterling, & Dinno, 2000). Prospective studies of high-risk infants ascertained by a positive family history (older sibling with ASD; discussed in detail below) have also identified behavioral profiles specific to ASD as early as 12–18 months (Zwaigenbaum et al., 2005; Landa et al., 2007; Brian et al., 2008). Clearly, there are opportunities to accelerate the process that occurs between the initial emergence of ASD symptoms and confirmation of diagnosis. Fortunately, there have been advances in the development of measures and service models aimed at early detection of ASD that could facilitate earlier diagnosis, lessen the burden on families, and improve opportunities for children to benefit from intervention.

To highlight advances in early identification of ASD and priorities for future research, this chapter will focus on current knowledge about early signs, strengths and limitations of current screening options, and implications for early diagnosis.

Early Signs of ASD

ASD screening measures draw heavily from the literature on parents' retrospective descriptions of early concerns, as well as data from analyses of early home videos. Concerns involving delayed speech and language development (and/or lack of responsiveness, e.g., when the child's name is called) are among the most common (De Giacomo & Fombonne, 1998; Coonrod & Stone, 2004). Other recollections include atypical reactivity (from passive and underreactive to irritable and difficult to console, with features of both extremes in some children) and disruption in the social-communicative, play, sensory, and motor domains of development (Hoshino et al., 1987; Tuchman & Rapin, 1997). Concerns may also be expressed about medical or regulatory functions such as sleeping and eating (Young, Brewer, & Pattison, 2003). In 20–50% of children with ASD, parents retrospectively describe a pattern of regression involving loss of speech and/or social-emotional connectedness during the second year of life, most often around 18 months of age (see Chapter 4 in this volume for a detailed review) (Young et al., 2003; Baranek, 1999; Adrien et al., 1991; Dawson et al., 2004; Rutter & Lord, 1987). Analysis of early home videos also suggests that many children later diagnosed with ASD show signs of atypical development by their first birthday or shortly afterward (Gray & Tonge, 2001). Social-communicative findings from home videos include atypical patterns of social orienting, joint attention (i.e., sharing attention with others), imitation, and affect regulation, as well as reduced use of gestures (Osterling & Dawson, 1994; Maestro et al., 2001; Maestro et al., 2002; Volkmar, Chawarska, & Klin, 2005; Yirmiya, Gamliel, Shaked, & Sigman, 2007). Infants later diagnosed with ASD show decreased variety and appropriateness of object-oriented play compared to infants later diagnosed with mental retardation (Baranek et al., 2005).

Emerging data from prospective studies of infants with an older sibling with ASD also show that behavioral risk indicators can be identified early in life (Zwaigenbaum et al., 2007). These "infant siblings" have an increased risk of developing ASD, estimated at 5–8% (Ritvo et al., 1989; Sumi, Taniai, Miyachi, & Tanemura, 2006), or roughly 20-fold higher than the risk in the general population (Rice et al., 2007). Complementing this approach is research aimed at identifying features that differentiate ASDs from other developmental disorders and from typical development among 12- to 24-month-olds who have failed a screen for communication deficits (Wetherby et al., 2004; Wetherby, Watt, Morgan, & Shumway, 2007). In both types of studies, participants are assessed systematically early in development, and then evaluated for ASD at 24–36 months, when reliable diagnoses are more possible. To date, findings from prospective research are highly consistent with risk markers identified in retrospective studies. Impairments and/or delays associated with ASD are observed by 12–18 months in one or more of the following domains: (1) *Social-communication*: atypicalities in eye gaze, orienting to name, social smiling, and social interest and affect, with reduced expression of positive emotion (Zwaigenbaum et al., 2005; Landa et al., 2007; Bryson et al., 2007; Wetherby et al., 2004); (2) *Language*: delays in babbling (especially back-and-forth social babbling), verbal comprehension and expression, and in gesturing (Mitchell et al., 2006; Landa et al., 2007; Bryson et al., 2007; Wetherby et al., 2004; Brian et al., 2008); (3) *Play*: delays in the development of motor imitation (Zwaigenbaum et al., 2005) and functional use of toys (Landa et al., 2007; Wetherby et al., 2004), as well as unusually repetitive actions with toys and other objects (Zwaigenbaum et al., 2005; Bryson et al., 2007; Wetherby et al., 2004; Ozonoff et al., 2008); (4) *Visual*: atypicalities in visual tracking and fixation, and prolonged visual examination of toys and other objects (Zwaigenbaum et al., 2005; Bryson et al., 2007; Loh et al., 2007; Wetherby et al., 2004; Ozonoff et al., 2008); (5) *Motor*: delayed fine and gross motor skills (Landa et al., 2007; Iverson & Wozniak, 2007) and atypical motor mannerisms (Loh et al., 2007; Wetherby et al., 2004).

Overall, there is convergent evidence from both retrospective and prospective studies that ASD symptoms emerge, in the vast majority of cases, in the first two years of life, affecting multiple domains of development, including social, communication, and repetitive interests/behaviors (the so-called "autistic triad") as well as regulation of attention, behavioral reactivity, motor activity, and in some children, regulatory behavior such as eating and sleeping (for review, see Zwaigenbaum et al., 2009). However, the application of knowledge regarding behavioral signs of ASD toward the important goals of early detection and diagnosis is a complex process. Clearly, a systematic population health strategy is required to effectively identify children with these early signs, and then to ensure that these children receive specialized diagnostic assessments and intervention services in a timely manner. Continuing education efforts aimed at physicians and other health/developmental service providers working with young children have been an important part of this strategy (First Signs Inc., 2009; see www.firstsigns.org). However, there is growing consensus that formal ASD screening, integrated into a broader framework of developmental surveillance, is needed for meaningful progress toward lowering the average age of diagnosis (see Johnson & Myers, 2007; Greenspan et al., 2008 for detailed discussion). The next section outlines recommended practice models aimed at surveillance and screening for ASD, and describes currently available ASD screening tools in detail.

Surveillance and Screening for ASD

Surveillance and screening are different but complementary processes aimed at detecting individuals at increased risk of a disorder for further assessment, with the goal of reducing or preventing subsequent disability through earlier initiation of intervention. *Surveillance* consists of an ongoing and multifaceted evaluative process that includes inquiry about parents' concerns and observations of the child, and is aimed at obtaining an overall picture of the child's developmental health over time (Dworkin, 1989). Decisions regarding the need for further evaluation are made based on clinical judgment. *Screening* involves administering and scoring a specific instrument (i.e., parent questionnaire, observational tool, or a combination) to identify at-risk individuals in need of further assessment. Developmental surveillance can also include the administration of standardized tools, but with the aim of gathering additional information to help inform clinical decisions, rather than using scoring cut-points as a basis for referral.

The following terms are used to describe the measurement properties of screening tools; i.e., classification accuracy. "Sensitivity" refers to the proportion of children with ASD who are correctly identified as "high-risk" by a screen; a child with ASD who is not identified by the screen is considered to be a "false negative." "Specificity" is the proportion of children who do not have ASD who are correctly classified by the screen (a child who does not have ASD yet fails the screen is considered to be a "false positive"). Children with and without ASD who are correctly classified by the screen can be considered to be "true positives" and "true negatives," respectively. Thus, the "case positive rate" of a screen, relevant to allocating resource needed for follow-up assessments, is the total number of "true positives" and "false positives." Positive predictive value (PPV) is the likelihood of having the diagnosis, given a positive screen. Negative predictive value (NPV) is the likelihood of not having the diagnosis, given a negative screen. Notably PPV and NPV vary with the base rate of ASD in the group being screened. For a screening test of given sensitivity and specificity, the PPV will be higher when disorder is more prevalent within the population, and lower when the disorder is rarer. Sensitivity and specificity are often considered to be intrinsic properties of a screening test; however there is evidence that these parameters can vary, based on the severity of symptoms in the group being screened. For example, children with severe symptoms are more likely to be correctly identified than those with milder or more equivocal symptoms. In general, the properties of the screening instrument should be evaluated in populations similar to those in which they are to be implemented, and one should be cautious about extrapolating from one context to another, particularly if there are differences in base rates and/or symptom severity (for more detailed discussion, see Sackett, Haynes, Guyatt, & Tugwell, 1991).

Over the past decade, several professional groups, including the American Academy of Neurology (Filipek et al., 2000), the American Academy of Child and Adolescent Psychiatry (Volkmar, Cook, Jr., Pomeroy, Realmuto, & Tanguay, 1999), and the American Academy of Pediatrics (Johnson & Myers, 2007; AAP Committee on Children with Disabilities, 2001) have issued practice parameters focused on the early identification and diagnosis of children with ASD. The way in which screening is incorporated varies somewhat among these statements. The AAP and other groups initially recommended an approach that combines developmental surveillance with ASD-specific screening: screening is targeted to children who are flagged due to concerns regarding language development or other early signs of ASD, or due to a positive family history or other known biological risk factor. This approach is considered *second-stage* or targeted screening, in that the screen is targeted to children who have been identified as being at increased risk. In contrast, subsequent practice parameters from Johnson, Myers, and the AAP Counsel on Children with Disabilities (Johnson & Myers, 2007) recommend developmental surveillance and monitoring for ASD-related concerns as well as ASD screening for *all* children at ages 18 and 24 months regardless of concerns; that is, *first-stage*, or universal screening.

First-stage screening has the potential advantage of higher sensitivity but also potential disadvantages in terms of resource demands to support screening and necessary follow-up of children who are flagged by the screen, particularly those who do not truly have ASD (i.e., false positives). Second-stage screening also presents challenges. To be effective, general developmental surveillance must identify children with ASD for further assessment. However, there is evidence that general screeners miss some children flagged by ASD-specific screens (Pinto-Martin et al., 2008). Recent reports also indicate that first-level ASD screening identifies children with the diagnosis who are not detected by experienced clinicians through routine surveillance (Wetherby, Brosnan-Maddox, Peace, & Newton,

2008; Robins, 2008). To date, first- and second-level screening approaches have not been directly compared.

The next section will provide a review of instruments that have been evaluated as first- or second-level screens and have published psychometric information about the accuracy of detecting children with ASD in children younger than 36 months of age. Recognizing that decisions about implementing ASD screening requires more than a consideration of sensitivity and specificity, a more general evaluation framework focused on clinically meaningful endpoints and overall impacts on the health system will also be discussed.

Review of Available Screening Tools

Checklist for Autism in Toddlers (CHAT)

Much of the recent progress in ASD screening can be traced back to conceptual and methodological contributions from the Checklist for Autism in Toddlers by Baron-Cohen and colleagues (Baron-Cohen, Allen, & Gillberg, 1992; Baron-Cohen et al., 1996; Baron-Cohen et al., 2000). This work was the first to show that some children with ASD could be identified via a screening questionnaire as early as 18 months of age (Baron-Cohen et al., 1992). The CHAT is also the only ASD-screening tool that has been assessed in a true population sample with comprehensive follow-up to identify children who were initially misclassified.

Initially, 41 infant siblings of children with ASD and 50 low-risk control children were assessed with the CHAT at 18 months, and subsequently evaluated at age 3½ years, blind to group status and CHAT scoring. Four children, all in the sibling group, were diagnosed with autism, each of whom at 18 months had failed 3 key CHAT items: gaze monitoring, protodeclarative pointing (i.e., pointing to show), and pretend play (Baron-Cohen et al., 1992). The CHAT was then expanded to 5 key items: the original 3 based on direct observation, plus parents' reports for pointing to show and pretend play. The screen was then administered by home visitors (mainly nurses) to a population-based sample (N = 16,235) of 18-month-olds, and again at 20 months to children who had failed any item. Children with severe developmental delays (including motor impairments) were excluded at the discretion of the home visitor. Diagnostic assessments (including the Autism Diagnostic Interview–Revised; ADI-R) were completed within 2 months on the 12 children who failed all 5 key CHAT items, on 22 of 44 children who passed "gaze monitoring" but failed at least one other key item (termed "developmental delay" risk group), and on 16 of the remaining 16,179 children (termed "normal") who passed all key items. *Ten of 12 children failing all key items were diagnosed with autism, compared to none of the 38 children in the two contrast groups.* The authors did not calculate sensitivity and specificity from these data, and rightly so, given that these estimates would be biased by lack of diagnostic information on half of the "developmental delay" risk group and almost the entire "normal" group at this stage. Sensitivity would be overestimated, to the extent that some children in the untested group may have received a diagnosis of autism if they'd received the same follow-up evaluation as the screen-positive group. As well, specificity would be underestimated by excluding from the denominator the large number of children who passed the screen and truly did not have autism. However, sensitivity and specificity estimates have been reported for other measures (e.g., the M-CHAT; see below) despite lack of diagnostic assessment of toddlers who screen negative. For comparison, the sensitivity of the CHAT at 18 months would be calculated as 100% (all 10 children diagnosed with autism at 20 months had failed the screen) and the specificity as 95% (only 2 of 40 children who were not diagnosed at this stage failed the screen).

Cox et al. (1999) reported a 2-year follow-up of the sample of children assessed at 20 months. Of the 10 children initially diagnosed with autism, each had the diagnosis confirmed at age 42 months (although for one child, the diagnosis was changed to PDD). Of the 40 children who were not diagnosed at 20 months, 9 received a diagnosis at age 42 months (7 with PDD, and 2 with Asperger's syndrome, all from the "developmental delay" risk group). In other words, both the CHAT *and* a comprehensive assessment by an expert clinician failed to identify an autism spectrum disorder at 20 months in almost half of the children who were diagnosed at 42 months. The "developmental delay" criteria were redefined as "medium-risk criteria" for autism in the 6-year follow-up paper (Baird et al., 2000), with the original cutoff of all 5 key items failed redefined as "high-risk criteria."

Additional children with ASDs were identified by surveillance methods at 42 months. The original sample of 16,235 was rescreened using a "Checklist for Referral" by a health practitioner or by a questionnaire mailed to parents (Baird et al., 2000). Based on this checklist, 22 children in addition to those in the subsample reported by Cox et al. (1999) were identified as possibly having ASD (Baird et al., 2000); these children were each seen for a diagnostic assessment. In total, the research team identified 24 children with autism at 42 months out of the original sample screened at 18 months (Charman et al., 2001). Of these 24 children, only 10 were considered to have failed the CHAT at 18 months using the original ("high-risk") criteria (sensitivity = 41.7%), whereas 19 of 24 children with ASD at 42 months met threshold for "medium-" or "high-risk" criteria on the 18-month CHAT (sensitivity = 79.2%). Case ascertainment at 6-year follow-up was even more comprehensive. The investigators mailed a second screening questionnaire to parents of children in the original sample (of which 47.8% were completed and returned), and reviewed case records of children diagnosed with ASD at regional centers and special education needs registers to identify members of the original sample (Baird et al., 2000). Children identified by these procedures were assessed, with diagnoses confirmed by consensus best-estimate review of case records, cognitive and language testing, and the ADI-R. In all, 50 children with autism and 44 children with other

ASDs were identified, a total of 94 children with ASD. Sensitivity and specificity of the CHAT were estimated for autism and for "all PDDs" (equivalent to ASD) for both high- and medium-risk criteria. Based on the original criteria (i.e., all 5 key items failed on two occasions), sensitivity of the CHAT at 18 months for a later diagnosis of autism is only 18% (9 of 50), although the positive predictive value is high (75%). The sensitivity for other forms of PDD is only 2.3% (1 of 44), for an overall sensitivity for ASD of 11.7%. Using less stringent criteria (failing "medium-risk" criteria on a single occasion) increases sensitivity for autism to 38% (19 of 50), but positive predictive value drops to 4.7% (19 of 407). Similarly, the sensitivity of these less stringent criteria for ASD as a whole at 6-year follow-up is 35.1% (33 of 94 cases correctly identified), with a positive predictive value of 8.1% (33 of 407).

Baird and colleagues (2000) suggested that the low sensitivity of the CHAT may be due to dichotomous scoring of critical items (i.e., ever vs. never), which would miss children that rarely, as opposed to never, demonstrate targeted skills. Requiring that skills be absent based on both observation *and* parent report may also be overly stringent. The authors acknowledged that the low sensitivity of the CHAT limits its utility as a stand-alone screener.

Although the CHAT was developed for first-stage screening, a subsequent study assessed its sensitivity and specificity in a clinically referred sample. Scambler, Rogers, and Wehner (2001) evaluated the CHAT in 26 children with established diagnoses of autism and in 18 children with other developmental delays, including 6 with Down syndrome. Participants ranged in age from 2 to 3 years (mean = 33 months). The purpose of the study was to assess whether expanding the "medium-risk" CHAT screening criteria to include children who fail protodeclarative pointing *or* pretend play (rather than just those who fail protodeclarative pointing) would improve overall classification rate. The original "medium-risk" criteria correctly identified 17 of 26 children with autism (sensitivity = 65%), whereas the modified criteria identified 22 (sensitivity = 85%), without any change in false positive rate (no child with a diagnosis of developmental delay failed the CHAT by either criteria). Two-year follow-up of the sample indicated that improved classification by the modified criteria was maintained (Scambler, Hepburn, & Rogers, 2006). Although these data are encouraging, findings from a convenience sample of children with established diagnoses will not necessarily generalize to a community screening context. In particular, there may have been a selection bias toward children with more straightforward clinical presentations. Assessing agreement between screening and diagnostic measures in a cross-sectional study is very different from using a screening tool to predict future diagnoses in a longitudinal study. Ultimately, research with the CHAT (Baird et al., 2000; Baron-Cohen et al., 1996; Cox et al., 1999) illustrates how estimates of the sensitivity and specificity may be influenced by several factors other than characteristics of the test or criteria used to establish risk status, including sampling strategy, age at screening, duration of follow-up, and case detection methods.

Nevertheless, Scambler et al.'s (2001; 2006) findings suggest that using broader screening thresholds and targeting older toddlers (i.e., 2 years rather than 18 months) may yield higher sensitivity while retaining high levels of specificity.

Subsequent modifications to the CHAT have successfully used these strategies, most notably, the Modified Checklist for Autism in Toddlers (Robins, Fein, Barton, & Green, 2001), discussed below. In addition, Baron-Cohen and colleagues have developed the Quantitative–Checklist for Autism in Toddlers (Q-CHAT; Allison et al., 2008). In contrast to the CHAT, the Q-CHAT is limited to parent-report, items are scored on a 5-point Likert scale (rather than "ever" vs. "never"), and cover a broader range of ASD symptoms. Preliminary Q-CHAT data from 160 preschool children with ASD (including 41 younger than 36 months) and 2360 low-risk 18- to 24-month-olds indicate large group differences in total score, although no specific screening cutoffs have yet been established (Allison et al., 2008).

Modified Checklist for Autism in Toddlers (M-CHAT)

The M-CHAT, developed by Fein and colleagues (Robins et al., 2001), differs from the CHAT in two main ways. The M-CHAT covers a broader range of developmental domains, including sensory and motor abnormalities, imitation, and response to name, and is administered as a parent-completed questionnaire, with no observational component. It includes two questions covering critical CHAT items (pointing to show and pretending, but not gaze monitoring). The M-CHAT was initially assessed in 24 month-olds, although it has since been reported in toddlers aged 16 to 30 months.

Robins et al. (2001) evaluated the M-CHAT in toddlers being seen for routine checkups with their community physician (n = 1122 from 98 selected practices) and in toddlers referred to early intervention programs due to language delays or other developmental concerns (n = 171). Parents were contacted if: (1) at least 3 of 23 items were endorsed, (2) 2 of 6 critical items were endorsed (see below), or (3) the clinician noted concerns. Critical items were selected by a discriminant function analysis (DFA) of the first 600 participants, and included pointing to indicate interest, responding to name, showing interest in other children, bringing objects to show, looking where someone points, and imitating. In total, telephone interviews were conducted with parents of 132 toddlers, and 58 positive screens were confirmed. Subsequent ASD diagnoses were assigned by clinical judgment, using a semistructured DSM-IV-based interview and the Childhood Autism Rating Scale (CARS), as well as standardized assessments of language, cognitive, and adaptive skills. A total of 39 children were diagnosed with ASD, at a mean age of 27.6 months, including 3 of 1122 who were referred at well-child visits (i.e., first-level screening) and 36 of 171 from early intervention services (i.e., a second-level screening context). Children who did not meet M-CHAT criteria or who were "OK on phone interview" did not receive further assessment. The sensitivity and specificity of the M-CHAT for ASD, using 3 of 23 items as the screening cutoff, was initially estimated to be 97% and 95% respectively, and using the criteria of 2 of the 6 critical items, 95% and 98% respectively. However, *these estimates assume that there were no cases of ASD among the children who were not seen for clinical assessment*, i.e., no cases among the 1235 "screen negative" children, including 74 who were flagged by the questionnaire but whose risk status was not confirmed during the phone interview. A follow-up study by (Kleinman et al., 2008) included 1416 toddlers drawn from the original sample and a second replication sample, each recruited from both low- and high-risk settings (i.e., from community physicians and early intervention services). Participants were rescreened using the M-CHAT, 2 years after the initial screen (follow-up rate = 57%; mean age = 58 month), and were assessed for ASD if screen positive on the parent questionnaire and telephone interview. Seven children with ASD were identified either by rescreening or by clinical referral after the initial screen, although it was not reported whether these cases came from the original or replication samples.

Despite these follow-up data, the sensitivity and specificity of the M-CHAT *cannot* truly be estimated in the initial cohort (Robins et al., 2001) because toddlers below the screening cutoff received no further evaluation. With this constraint, the proportion of toddlers diagnosed with ASD who exceeded the M-CHAT cutoff simply reflects whether the procedures for selecting participants for clinical assessment were followed consistently. For example, there was one child who received a diagnosis but had 2 (rather than 3 or more) positive items; presumably this child was one of the first 600 participants assessed prior to the change in cutoff criteria, or else had 2 of the 6 critical items. Because the sampling frame for the M-CHAT was not geographically defined, even for the low-risk sample, surveillance for subsequent ASD diagnoses in screen negative toddlers depended on individual follow-up rather than review of community-wide medical and/or educational records.

However, the positive predictive value (PPV) of the M-CHAT *can* be accurately estimated, as this relies on diagnostic information from the screen positive group only. Both the case positive rate and PPV are relevant to resource planning, as these parameters describe the expected proportion of toddlers who will require further assessment, and within this group, the expected rate of ASD. In the M-CHAT replication study by Kleinman et al. (2008), 189 of 3309 of the low-risk sample were screen positive (case positive rate = 5.7%), of whom 19 were diagnosed with ASD (PPV = 0.11). It would be difficult to justify comprehensive, ASD-specific assessments for 5.7% of all toddlers in the community, particularly when only about 1 in 10 are expected to result in an ASD diagnosis. In contrast, when the questionnaire is followed up by the structured telephone (or in-person) interview clarifying parents' responses on endorsed items, the case positive rate drops to 31 of 3309 (<1%), and the PPV increases accordingly (19 of 31, or 0.65). This approach essentially combines first- and second-stage screening. First, at-risk toddlers are identified from the general community using the questionnaire, and then the number of potential referrals is reduced by further screening using the follow-up interview, reducing costs and potentially improving feasibility. With further recruitment to a total of 6776 screened toddlers, Fein and colleagues (Pandey et al., 2008) has reported the positive predictive value of the M-CHAT by age (16–23 months versus 24 months and older) and risk group: 0.28 for younger, low-risk infants; 0.61 for older, low-risk infants; 0.79 for younger, high-risk infants; and 0.74 for older, high-risk infants. As in Robins et al.'s (2001) original report, more cases of ASD were found among the high-risk group (155 of 726; 21.3%) than the low-risk group (29 of 6050; 0.5%), but the false positive rate even among the low-risk group was relatively low, particularly in toddlers 24 months or older. Moreover, over 90% of screen positive children in both the older and younger high-risk groups and the older low-risk group, and 72% of the younger low-risk group, had atypical development when other diagnoses (e.g., language delay, global developmental delay, as well as ASD) were considered. In an independent sample of 14- to 27-month-old low-risk toddlers assessed in community pediatricians' offices, Robins (2008) reported that 466 of 4797 (9.7%) met screening criteria on the M-CHAT questionnaire. Of 362 toddlers from the group whose parents participated, 61 (1.3% of the total sample) screened positive on the follow-up interview. Of 41 toddlers from this group who were subsequently seen for diagnostic evaluation, 21 were diagnosed with ASD, an additional 17 were diagnosed with other developmental delays/disorders, and 3 were typically developing. Thus, of the toddlers who were assessed, 57% were diagnosed with ASD (21 cases, or 0.4% of the total sample of screened toddlers), and of the nondiagnosed children 17 of 20 (85%) had other developmental delays. Only 4 of 21 toddlers with ASD were clinically flagged by their pediatricians, whereas no toddlers with ASD were identified by their pediatricians who weren't also identified by the M-CHAT questionnaire and interview (Robins, 2008).

Overall, the M-CHAT shows considerable promise as a combined first- and second-stage screen for ASD. Recent studies (Kleinman et al., 2008; Pandey et al., 2008; Robins, 2008) have addressed some of the limitations of the M-CHAT evaluation (Charman et al., 2001). First, a follow-up study consisting of rescreening the original screened cohort of toddlers has been initiated (Kleinman et al., 2008), although a more comprehensive follow-up of screen-negative toddlers is still needed. Second, whereas the screening properties of the M-CHAT were first described in a combined sample from low- and high-risk settings, both Pandey et al. (2008) and Robins (2008) have reported data specific to low-risk settings in a large number of toddlers (combined sample size over 10,000). Third, in these recent reports, the follow-up procedures are described more explicitly, and evidence is provided that the screen positive rate drops substantially when questionnaire responses are clarified by the interview (e.g., from 9.7% to 1.3% in Robins, 2008). Finally, recognizing that sensitivity and specificity estimates are uncertain without follow-up of screen negative toddlers, psychometric assessment of the M-CHAT has shifted to positive predictive value. Pandey et al. (2008) and Robins (2008) reported that over 50% of screen positive children seen for assessment were diagnosed with ASD, and in the latter study, most were not independently flagged by their community pediatrician as being at increased risk. With a case positive rate of around 1%, the M-CHAT appears to identify a substantial number of toddlers with ASD who might not otherwise be flagged at an early age, without generating excessive burden on diagnostic services.

Infant Toddler Checklist (ITC)

The Infant–Toddler Checklist (Wetherby et al., 2004) is a component of the Communication and Symbolic Behavior Scales Developmental Profile (CSBS DP), developed by Wetherby and Prizant (2002). In contrast to ASD-specific measures such as the CHAT and M-CHAT, the ITC is designed to be a broadband screener for communication delays. This parent-completed questionnaire includes 24 items focused on social communication milestones that are rated on a 3- to 5-point scale, and an open-ended question about current concerns regarding the child's development. A unique strength of the ITC is that it has been standardized in a normative sample of over 2000 children, and thus in addition to screening cutoffs, results can be reported as standard scores for infants and toddlers aged 6 to 24 months (Wetherby & Prizant, 2002).

Wetherby et al. (2004) reported a study of 3021 children aged 12–24 months recruited from selected childcare and health care agencies. An additional 5 children under 24 months with known developmental delay (DD) also participated. Children scoring below the 10th percentile on the ITC (n = 377), a random sample of children scoring above this cutoff (n = 230), and the 5 children with known delays were invited for further assessment using an observational component of the CSBS-DP, the "Behavioral Sample." Assessments were completed in 490 children, excluding 122 who were lost to follow-up. Children scoring below the 10th percentile on the Behavioral Sample, a random sample scoring above this cutoff (n's not reported separately), as well as the 5 children with known DD were invited for additional cognitive and language assessment, which was completed in 298 children (i.e., 147 were lost to follow-up). Finally, children with communication delays (based on the Behavioral Sample) were selected for further assessment, including 71 from the main sample and the 5 children with known DD. Based on parent-report from a related study, 10 of 71 were suspected of having ASD; these 10 children, as well as 21 other randomly selected children with "communication delay" and the 5 children with known DD formed a group of 36 children who were evaluated for clinical diagnoses. Overall, 18 children were diagnosed with ASD (9 with autism, 9 with PDD NOS), and 18 children with DD. Among the 5 children who were originally recruited due to known DD, 3 were ultimately diagnosed and included in the ASD group, and the other 2 (both with Down syndrome) were among the final DD group. A typically developing (TD) group was selected for comparison, including 18 nondelayed children who had completed the first three steps of the study. Seventeen of the 18 children in the ASD group (94.4%) had a positive screen on the ITC, as did 15 in the DD group (83.3%), and 2 in the TD group (11.1%). The sensitivity of the ITC was 88.9% for the combined ASD and DD groups (i.e., 32 of 36), although nonrandom selection and dropout may have inflated this estimate, given that screen negative children were underrepresented in the assessed sample relative to the original screened sample. Inclusion of participants with known DD at the outset also reduces the interpretability of the summary statistics. That being said, the study was one of the first to confirm that children with ASD could be identified using a broadband screener and thus referred for more specialized assessments. Additional insights were gained by comparison of toddlers in the ASD and DD groups using a videotape coding scheme developed by Wetherby and Woods (2004). The "Systematic Observation of Red Flags" (SORF) consists of 29 items derived from DSM-IV and studies of early signs of autism (e.g., home videotape studies; Osterling & Dawson, 1994), scored 0 (absent) to 2 (present at least 3 times), and is coded from videotapes of the Behavioral Sample. Significant differences between the ASD and DD groups were found for 9 items: (1) lack of appropriate gaze; (2) lack of warm, joyful expression with gaze; (3) lack of sharing enjoyment or interest; (4) lack of response to name; (5) lack of coordination of gaze, facial expression, gesture, and sound; (6) lack of showing; (7) unusual prosody; (8) repetitive movements or posturing of body, arms, hands, or fingers; and (9) repetitive movements with objects (Wetherby et al., 2004).

Wetherby, Brosnan-Madox, Peace, & Newton (Wetherby et al., 2008) conducted a more definitive evaluation of the ASD screening properties of the ITC in a cumulative community sample of 5385 6- to 24-month-olds recruited from health and childcare services (i.e., included the sample reported by Wetherby et al., 2004). Service providers were encouraged to administer the ITC each time the child was seen, thus, some children who entered the study at the early end of the age range were assessed on multiple occasions. Children were assessed using the Behavioral Sample of the CSBS DP if they met criteria for a positive screen on the ITC, or if parents reported concerns. Screening data were linked to an ongoing study of ASD prevalence in Florida, which identified potential ASD cases using 3 strategies: (1) SORF scoring from the Behavioral Sample; (2) responses to a questionnaire asking parents whether the child had received a clinical ASD diagnosis; and (3) information from state-funded ASD services. Identified children were invited for confirmatory diagnostic assessments by the research team. In total, 60 children were diagnosed with ASD, 56 of whom were screen positive on at least one ITC. Some ITCs were positive as early as 9–11 months, although in some cases, an initial screen was negative at 9–11 months, and did not become positive until a later administration. Some parents did not agree to have their child assessed until 2 or more ITC were failed, illustrating the potential added value of serial screening over time, as well as the challenges associated with evaluating screening outcomes, given that follow-up is voluntary. Parental concerns were assessed independent of ITC status over time. Most parents of children with ASD expressed concern by age 24 months, but relying on parental concerns alone would have led to later identification than the ITC screen. Although the ITC is not specific for ASD (i.e., does not differentiate ASD from other communication disorders), its estimated sensitivity was very high, at 93% (i.e., 56 of 60). Notably, the SORF as coded from the CSBS DP Behavioral Sample appears to differentiate well between ASD and other communication disorders, as reported by Wetherby et al. (2004). Hence, although additional research and replication by other groups is needed, these two components of the CSBS DP may constitute an effective combined first- and second-level screening strategy for ASD.

Early Screening of Autistic Traits Questionnaire (ESAT)

The ESAT (Swinkels et al., 2006) is a 14-item two-stage screening instrument designed for use at 14–15 months of age. Items were initially selected based on review of findings from parents' retrospective reports and home video analyses. A preliminary 19-item version of the ESAT was pretested with a community sample of parents and other caregivers of 8- to 20-month-olds to assess the frequency of item endorsement in a low-risk sample, and then with a sample of 478 parents of children aged 14–226 months previously diagnosed with ASD, who were asked to retrospectively report on their children based on behaviors recalled at age 14 months. A comparison group of parents of 76 children aged 34–201 months who were diagnosed with ADHD also completed the ESAT retrospectively, based on 14-month behaviors. Fourteen items were selected that best differentiated children with ASD from the ADHD and low-risk groups based on retrospective report, which constituted the long version of the ESAT, with a screening cutoff of 3 or more items. A shorter, prescreening version of the ESAT was also established, consisting of 4 items that identified 94% of the children with ASD but only 2% of the low-risk sample. Further pilot testing of the 14-item ESAT was conducted by parents of 34 preschool children with ASD (aged 14–48 months), who also completed the screen retrospectively based on the child's behavior at age 14 months. As in the first retrospective sample, most parents endorsed the 3 or more items on the ESAT necessary to screen positive.

The ESAT was then evaluated in a random population sample of 31,724 toddlers at a mean age of 14.9 months (Dietz, Swinkels, van Daalen, van Engeland, & Buitelaar, 2006). Screening was carried out in two stages. First, the entire sample was screened at well-child visits by their health providers using the 4-item prescreen. Second, parents endorsed at least 1 item on the prescreen were asked to complete further screening using the 14-item ESAT during a home visit by a study psychologist. A total of 370 children were positive on the prescreen (1.2% of the total sample), 255 of whom participated in the second stage. Of 100 who were screen positive on the 14-item ESAT, 73 were seen for a more comprehensive diagnostic assessment by a child psychiatrist on the study team, with 18 receiving an ASD diagnosis, consistent with a positive predictive value of 25% and an ASD rate of 0.57 per 1000, well below the expected prevalence rates. Of the remaining 55 screen-positive children who were seen for assessment, 13 were diagnosed with intellectual disability and 18 with language delay; the rest were considered to have other mental health or developmental problems, none were considered to be typically developing. Follow-up to age 42 months reclassified 2 children initially diagnosed with ASD with non-ASD developmental disorders, but 2 children from the delayed group (one with intellectual disability, one with language delay) were reclassified as ASD, so the total rate of ASD was unchanged (2 additional children diagnosed with ASD were lost to follow-up; (van Daalen et al., 2009).

Although the ESAT showed promise in differentiating ASD from typical development (as well as ADHD) in pilot work (Swinkels et al., 2006), the overall rate of 0.57 in 1000 is only about 10% of the expected population prevalence of ASD. Consistent with findings from the CHAT (Baird et al., 2000), screening children younger than 18 months (and perhaps limiting the prescreen to only 4 items) may have contributed to low sensitivity of the ESAT. Establishing screening cut-points based on retrospective data from older pilot samples may have also undermined the validity of the ESAT for prospective screening of younger children.

Screening Tool for Autism in Two-Year-Olds (STAT)

The STAT was developed by Stone and Ousley (Stone, Ousley, & Littleford, 1997) as a second-stage screen for autism for children between 24 and 35 months of age. Scoring is based on behavior observed during a structured interactive assessment of motor imitation, play skills, requesting, and directing attention. Cutoff criteria were established in a "development sample" of 7 children with autism and 33 children with other developmental disorders, and were then were evaluated in a "validation sample" of 12 children with autism and 21 children with other disorders. Both samples were recruited from consecutive referrals to a university-based clinic. Screening with the STAT and diagnostic assessment were completed independently at the same clinic visit, and clinical diagnoses were based on DSM-IV criteria, Childhood Autism Rating Scale (CARS) scores, and standard cognitive measures. Cutoff criteria were selected that best distinguished children with autism from clinical controls in the development sample. To pass each of the three domains (imitation, play, and directing attention) the child must receive credit on at least two items within that domain. These criteria were independently assessed in the validation sample: 10 of 12 children with autism failed at least 2 domains (sensitivity = 83%), compared to 3 of 21 in the nonautism group (specificity = 86%).

The STAT was further assessed in 26 children with autism (AUT) and 26 children with language impairment or other developmental delays (DD/LI; children with PDD-NOS were excluded) (Stone, Coonrod, Turner, & Pozdol, 2004) matched on age and mental age. As in the initial study, the sample was divided into development and validation samples. The revised STAT scoring weighted the 4 domains equally (maximum score of 1 for each domain), and was based on the total item score rather than the number of domains passed. ROC curves determined that a scoring cutoff of 2 was associated with maximal sensitivity (100%) and specificity = 81% in the developmental sample, and a sensitivity of 92% and specificity of 85% in the validation sample. The STAT was then evaluated in a sample of 50 children with autism, 39 with DD/LI, and 15 with PDD-NOS. There was excellent interobserver and test-retest reliability for the STAT classification of high-risk versus low-risk (kappas = 1.0 and .90, respectively) and excellent agreement between the STAT and ADOS (autism cutoff) when the sample was restricted to children with autism and DD/LI (only 2 of 52 children scoring in the STAT high-risk range failed to exceed ADOS threshold for autism). However, children with a clinical diagnosis of PDD-NOS were roughly equally divided into the "high-risk" and "low-risk" categories by the STAT (Stone et al., 2004).

Stone, McMahon and Henderson (2008) recently assessed the screening properties of the STAT in a group of high-risk 12- to 23-month-olds, including 59 younger siblings of children with ASD, and 12 toddlers referred for suspected ASD. A higher cutoff score than recommended for 2-year-olds was required for optimal classification of toddlers with and without ASD, as determined by follow-up diagnostic assessment after age 2. The STAT did not effectively discriminate 12- and 13-month-olds who later developed ASD from those do not; in contrast, a cutoff score of 2.75 was associated with a sensitivity of 0.93 and specificity of 0.83 for later diagnoses of ASD in 14- to 23-month-olds. These data should be considered preliminary, as validation in a second sample has not yet been completed, and the majority of ASD cases were identified from the referred sample.

The STAT has a number of strengths as a second-level screen. It can discriminate children with autism from those with DD/LI with a high degree of sensitivity and specificity, and there is excellent agreement between the STAT high-risk category and an ADOS classification of autism. Its interactive format also allows for greater standardization, assessment of relatively subtle differences between autism and DD/LI that may be difficult to ascertain in a questionnaire, and generates rich observational data. The potential limitations of the STAT are that it is less sensitive to PDD-NOS than to autism, and requires more training and expertise than parent questionnaires. Screening using the STAT is more resource intensive than a questionnaire such as the M-CHAT. However, in a clinical setting, the STAT provides an effective second-stage screen that is both sensitive and specific for autism, and may yield clinically informative data that can help guide both additional assessment, and initial intervention planning for toddlers as young as 14 months at increased risk of ASD.

Pervasive Developmental Disorders Screening Test - II (PDDST-II)

The PDDST-II is a parent-report questionnaire that includes components designed for first-stage and second-stage screening. Its psychometric properties are described in a published manual (Siegel, 2004), but have not been reported in peer-reviewed publications.

The PDDST-II - Stage 1 was designed to be used in primary care settings, and includes 23 items based on behaviors "emerging between 12 and 24 months." The standardization sample included 656 preschool children who had been referred due to suspected autism (not all of whom actually had an ASD, but all had "at least a few autistic symptoms"), and 256 ex-preterm infants who were expected to show a high rate of early atypical development (but not autism). Sensitivity and specificity estimates are based on agreement between item and group classification. For example, a true positive is recorded when a child in the suspected autism group scores positive on a PDDST-II item. Hence, although this instrument is intended to be used as a first-stage screen, its evaluation is based on classification into groups defined by clinical suspicion rather than by individual diagnoses.

The PDDST-II - Stage 2 was designed for use in developmental clinics where children are often first assessed for possible developmental disorders. The index population was patients with diagnoses of Autistic Disorder or PDD-NOS (N = 318). The comparison group was patients clinically referred for an autism evaluation but who eventually received non–autistic spectrum disorder diagnoses such as mental retardation or developmental language disorders (N = 62). Estimates of sensitivity and specificity for the PDDST-II are not yet available.

Social Communication Questionnaire (SCQ)

The SCQ (formerly, Autism Screening Questionnaire; Berument, Rutter, Lord, Pickles, & Bailey, 1999) is a 40-item parent questionnaire based on the Autism Diagnostic Interview–Revised (ADI-R) (Lord, Rutter, & Le Couteur, 1994). Because of its close relationship to the ADI-R, the SCQ was designed for use in individuals age 4 and older, although it has subsequently been evaluated in younger samples. Screening criteria for the SCQ were initially established in a sample of 200 individuals aged 4–40 years (160 with ASD, and 40 with other developmental disorders, such as language disorders and intellectual disability). A score of 15 was associated with a sensitivity of .85 and specificity of .75 in this sample. There are relatively little data on the screening properties of the SCQ in younger children, and research to date suggests that classification accuracy is poorer than in children 4 and older. Corsello et al. (2007) reported on a consecutive referral sample of 590 children aged 2–16 years, including 200 who were age 4 and younger

(157 with ASD, and 43 with nonspectrum disorders). The original cutoff of 15 was associated with sensitivity = .68 and specificity = .74 in this age group (data in children 36 months and younger are not reported separately). Lowering the screening cut-point to 11 increased sensitivity to .80, but reduced specificity to .60; similarly, raising the cut-point to 17 increased specificity to .80 but reduced sensitivity to .58 (Corsello et al., 2007). At least 3 other groups have evaluated in the SCQ in children younger than age 5 referred for a suspected diagnosis of ASD (Lee, David, Rusyniak, Landa, & Newschaffer, 2007; Allen, Silove, Williams, & Hutchins, 2007; Eaves, Wingert, Ho, & Mickelson, 2006), reporting sensitivity of .54–.71 using the original cutoff score of 15. Only two of these studies included children 36 months of age and younger (Lee et al., 2007; Allen et al., 2007), and neither of these reported data in this younger subgroup separate from older preschoolers. As well, the samples in all 4 studies that have evaluated the SCQ in children younger than 5 (Lee et al., 2007; Allen et al., 2007; Corsello et al., 2007; Eaves et al., 2006) are drawn from children referred for specialized assessments at tertiary care centers, the majority of whom were ultimately diagnosed with ASD. In other words, these were highly select samples that may not easily generalize to other level 2 screening contexts. Hence, there are insufficient data to assess or recommend the SCQ as an early screening tool for ASD.

Summary and Recommendations

There are now a number of empirically supported screening measures that differentiate ASD from typical development (and to a lesser extent, from other developmental delays) in children younger than 36 months. The CHAT remains the only screener that has been assessed in a general population sample, and with sufficiently comprehensive follow-up to identify children with ASD who were missed by the initial screen. Estimates of CHAT sensitivity are very low (18% for the originally proposed "high-risk" criteria, 38% for "moderate risk" criteria), although differences in sensitivity compared to newer tools are magnified by the follow-up duration. The ESAT has been assessed in a total population cohort of 14-month-olds but its low case detection rate (which may have arisen from the brief "prescreening" component) raises questions about potential sensitivity.

In contrast, both the M-CHAT and ITC have shown considerable promise as ASD screens in community samples, although not "population samples" in the strictest sense—only selected health and childcare agencies participated in evaluation studies. The ITC has excellent sensitivity for ASD (93%, based on multimethod ascertainment of ASD cases among the screened sample), although as a broadband screener is not specific to ASD and thus must be combined with additional levels of assessment to differentiate ASD from other communication disorders (Wetherby et al., 2008). Other broadband screeners such as the Pediatric Evaluation of Developmental Status have been less effective at identifying toddlers with early signs of ASD (Pinto-Martin et al., 2008), so there may be specific features of the ITC (e.g., a focus on communication development) that are critical. The sensitivity of the M-CHAT cannot be directly estimated from available data, as follow-up assessments have mainly been limited to screen-positive children. However, when the parent questionnaire was combined with a follow-up interview in two large community samples, the M-CHAT identified a high-risk group from which over 50% were diagnosed with ASD (i.e., PPV >50%) (Pandey et al., 2008; Robins, 2008). Both the ITC and M-CHAT identify toddlers at risk of autism who might not otherwise be detected through routine developmental surveillance using clinical judgment and/or parental concerns, yet do not appear to overidentify children who are typically developing (Robins, 2008; Wetherby et al., 2008). Hence, the ITC and M-CHAT could be effective first-stage screening options when part of a multistage early detection strategy for ASD. In contrast, the STAT is specifically designed to be used as a second-stage screener. In this context, the STAT has been reported to have excellent sensitivity and specificity for autism in 24- to 35-month-olds (Stone et al., 2004), and based on preliminary data in a high-risk sample, perhaps in children as young as 14–23 months (Stone et al., 2008).

Assessing the measurement properties of early detection tools is only the first step toward understanding the potential impacts of ASD screening programs. Evaluation of ASD screening should adopt a broader health systems perspective in order to more fully gauge its potential impacts, and to gain support among health care providers and policy-makers. Although ensuring that individual tools will accurately classify children with and without ASD is an essential prerequisite for implementing a screening program, there are other important considerations related to how screening ultimately impacts children, families, and society as a whole. The positive benefits of screening for children with ASD depend on timely access to specialized assessment and intervention services. Concerns about lengthy waiting lists and/or overreferral of children who meet screening criteria for reasons other than ASD (i.e., false positives) may contribute to low uptake of ASD screening into pediatric practice (Dosreis, Weiner, Johnson, & Newschaffer, 2006) and delays in referral of children with identified concerns (Kennedy, Regehr, Rosenfield, Roberts, & Lingard, 2004). Options for multistage screening that can take place in the community (e.g., the combined M-CHAT questionnaire and interview; the ITC followed by a second-stage screener such as the SORF or the STAT) could help limit the number of referrals for specialized assessment, without significantly sacrificing case detection rate. Screening programs also require clinicians with the expertise to make relevant differential diagnoses in children referred for assessment, as children with other disorders who are identified through the process of screening will have service needs as well. Specialized training may be needed to support clinicians faced with increasingly complex diagnostic questions as children are referred due to suspected ASD at younger ages: for example, differentiating

ASD from the broader range of impairments in emotional expression and referential communication that can be observed in infants with an older sibling with ASD, and assessing whether early joint attention behaviors are consistent with developmental level in toddlers with cognitive delays (see Zwaigenbaum et al., 2009 for detailed discussion). As well, screening is difficult to justify unless earlier initiation of treatment leads to improvements in long-term outcomes. Although children participating in ASD treatment research have generally been 3 years of age and older, consistent with the usual timing of diagnosis, recent studies suggest that substantial gains can be achieved by interventions initiated prior to 24 months (Vismara, Colombi, & Rogers, 2009; Dawson et al., 2010; see Chapter 61 in this volume for details). There are theoretical advantages to treating ASD earlier in development due to increased neural plasticity and less severe interfering behaviors than are observed in older children (Dawson, 2008). The degree to which child-related outcomes can be improved through earlier diagnosis and intervention is not yet known, but there may be added benefits to families including reduced parental stress and frustration associated with delays in diagnosis (Howlin & Asgharian, 1999) and increased sense of empowerment and efficacy related to active participation in intervention (Vismara et al., 2009).

The relative effects of implementing ASD screening, and enhancing the expertise and service capacity of specialized diagnostic and treatment programs remain to be assessed, but it seems likely that a comprehensive strategy that includes all of these components will better address the needs of children and families than screening alone. Evaluation of ASD screening should focus on meaningful end-points such as age of initial referral and diagnosis of ASD, treatment outcomes of children identified through positive screening, family experience related to screening misclassification, and health service costs/utilization related to additional referrals (both true and false positives). Screening uptake might be improved if stakeholders such as families, clinicians, and health and policy decision-makers are engaged from the earliest stages of implementation, in an effort to better understand community-specific challenges (e.g., access to diagnostic services), and to ensure outcomes of greatest interest to each group are targeted and measured.

Further research is clearly needed, but the availability of measures with adequate sensitivity and specificity lends important support to current pediatric practice guidelines recommending broader implementation of ASD screening (Johnson & Myers, 2007). As well, although community physicians have a critical role in identifying early signs of ASD, early intervention, daycare/preschool, and speech and language services are the "point-of-entry" to developmental services for many families. Providers in these settings are often the first to observe the at-risk child's development in sufficient depth to identify early markers of autism. The use of a standardized ASD screen may help ensure that children with ASD are detected earlier and more consistently, so that children can be referred for a specialized diagnostic assessment in a timely manner. Further research assessing the utility of ASD screening tools in a wide range of community-based therapeutic settings is warranted.

Conclusions

Detailed knowledge about early signs of ASD from retrospective and prospective research has helped guide the development of screening measures aimed at facilitating earlier diagnosis and entry into intervention programs. Although the evidence-base for ASD screening is not yet fully established, recent data suggest community-wide screening can effectively augment general surveillance efforts to identify appropriate children for referral. Future research evaluating ASD screening should adopt a broader health systems perspective and focus on outcomes meaningful to families, clinicians and health and policy decision-makers.

Challenges and Future Directions

- Future research aimed at improving early detection of ASD should consider whether biological differences such as accelerated head growth might add predictive power to current approaches based on early behavioral markers.
- Consistent with clinical heterogeneity in ASD, early developmental and behavioral trajectories can be variable, making early detection and diagnosis of children across the spectrum more difficult using a single strategy. Children with milder symptoms and/or more advanced intellectual development may be more difficult to identify using existing screening methods.
- Early detection and diagnosis of ASD must be accompanied by timely access to effective, developmentally appropriate interventions that lead to improved outcomes. However, the availability of specialized assessment and treatment services for ASD varies considerably across communities (both nationally and internationally), and there may be significant disparities related to factors influencing access to health care.
- Future research on early identification and screening of ASD should consider these "real-world" health systems challenges, and engage key stakeholders to ensure that findings lead to meaningful change in clinical practice and policy.

SUGGESTED READINGS

Ozonoff, S., Heung, K., Byrd, R., Hansen, R., & Hertz-Picciotto, I. (2008). The onset of autism: Patterns of symptom emergence in the first years of life. *Autism Research,1*, 320–328.

Pandey, J., Verbalis, A., Robins, D., Boorstein, H., Klin, A., Babitz, T., et al. (2008). Screening for autism in older and younger toddlers with the Modified Checklist for Autism in Toddlers. *Autism, 12*, 512–535.

Wetherby, A. M., Brosnan-Maddox, S., Peace, V., & Newton, L. (2008). Validation of the Infant-Toddler Checklist as a broadband screener for autism spectrum disorders from 9 to 24 months of age. *Autism,12*, 487–511.

Zwaigenbaum, L., Bryson, S., Rogers, T., Roberts, W., Rogers, T., Brian, J., et al. (2005, Apr.–May). Behavioral manifestations of autism in the first year of life. *International Journal of Developmental Neurosciences, 23*(2–3),143–152.

Zwaigenbaum, L., Thurm, A., Stone, W., Baranek, G., Bryson, S., Iverson, J., et al. (2007). Studying the emergence of autism spectrum disorders in high-risk infants: methodological and practical issues. *Journal of Autism and Developmental Disorders, 37*, 466–480.

REFERENCES

AAP Committee on Children with Disabilities (2001). Technical report: The pediatrician's role in the diagnosis and management of autistic spectrum disorder in children. *Pediatrics, 107*, 1221–1226.

Adrien, J. L., Faure, M., Perrot, A., Hameury, L., Garreau, B., Barthelemy, C., et al. (1991). Autism and family home movies: preliminary findings. *Journal of Autism and Developmental Disorders, 21*, 43–49.

Adrien, J. L., Perrot, A., Sauvage, D., Leddet, I., Larmande, C., Hameury, L., & Barthelemy, C. (1992). Early symptoms in autism from family home movies. Evaluation and comparison between 1st and 2nd year of life using I.B.S.E. scale. *Acta Paedopsychiatrica, 55*, 71–75.

Allen, C. W., Silove, N., Williams, K., & Hutchins, P. (2007). Validity of the Social Communication Questionnaire in Assessing Risk of Autism in Preschool Children with Developmental Problems. *Journal of Autism and Developmental Disorders, 37*, 1272–1278.

Allison, C., Baron-Cohen, S., Wheelwright, S., Charman, T., Richler, J., Pasco, G., et al. (2008). The Q-CHAT (Quantitative CHecklist for Autism in Toddlers): A normally distributed quantitative measure of autistic traits at 18-24 months of age: preliminary report. *Journal of Autism and Developmental Disorders, 38*, 1414–1425.

Autism and Developmental Disabilities Monitoring Network (2007). Prevalence of autism spectrum disorders—autism and developmental disabilities monitoring network, 14 sites, United States, 2002. *Morbidity and Mortality Weekly Report Surveillance Summaries, 56*, 12–28.

Bailey, A., Palferman, S., Heavey, L., & Le Couteur, A. (1998). Autism: the phenotype in relatives. *Journal of Autism and Developmental Disorders, 28*, 369–92.

Baird, G., Charman, T., Baron-Cohen, S., Cox, A., Swettenham, J., Wheelwright, S., et al. (2000). A screening instrument for autism at 18 months of age: a 6-year follow-up study. *Journal of the American Academy of Child and Adolescent Psychiatry, 39*, 694–702.

Baranek, G. T. (1999). Autism during infancy: a retrospective video analysis of sensory-motor and social behaviors at 9–12 months of age. *Journal of Autism and Developmental Disorders, 29*, 213–224.

Baranek, G. T., Barnett, C. R., Adams, E. M., Wolcott, N. A., Watson, L. R., & Crais, E. R. (2005). Object play in infants with autism: methodological issues in retrospective video analysis. *American Journal of Occupational Therapy, 59*, 20–30.

Baron-Cohen, S., Allen, J., & Gillberg, C. (1992). Can autism be detected at 18 months? The needle, the haystack, and the CHAT. *British Journal of Psychiatry, 161*, 839–843.

Baron-Cohen, S., Cox, A., Baird, G., Swettenham, J., Nightingale, N., Morgan, K., et al. (1996). Psychological markers in the detection of autism in infancy in a large population. *British Journal of Psychiatry, 168*, 158–163.

Baron-Cohen, S., Wheelwright, S., Cox, A., Baird, G., Charman, T., Swettenham, J., et al. (2000). Early identification of autism by the Checklist for Autism in Toddlers (CHAT). *Journal of the Royal Society of Medicine, 93*, 521–525.

Bertrand, J., Mars, A., Boyle, C., Bove, F., Yeargin-Allsopp, M., & Decoufle, P. (2001). Prevalence of autism in a United States population: the Brick Township, New Jersey, investigation. *Pediatrics, 108*, 1155–1161.

Berument, S. K., Rutter, M., Lord, C., Pickles, A., & Bailey, A. (1999). Autism screening questionnaire: Diagnostic validity. *British Journal of Psychiatry, 175*, 444–451.

Brian, J., Bryson, S. E., Garon, N., Roberts, W., Smith, I. M., Szatmari, P., et al. (2008). Clinical assessment of autism in high-risk 18-month-olds. *Autism, 12*, 433–456.

Bryson, S. E., Zwaigenbaum, L., Brian, J., Roberts, W., Szatmari, P., Rombough, V., et al. (2007). A prospective case series of high-risk infants who developed autism. *Journal of Autism and Developmental Disorders, 37*, 12–24.

Chakrabarti, S., & Fombonne, E. (2001). Pervasive developmental disorders in preschool children. *Journal of the American Medical Association, 285*, 3141–3142.

Charman, T., Baron-Cohen, I., Baird, G., Cox, A., Wheelwright, S., Swettenham, J., et al. (2001). Commentary: The Modified Checklist for Autism in Toddlers. *Journal of Autism and Developmental Disorders, 31*, 145–148.

Chawarska, K., Klin, A., Paul, R., & Volkmar, F. (2007). Autism spectrum disorder in the second year: stability and change in syndrome expression. *Journal of Child Psychology and Psychiatry, 48*, 128–138.

Coonrod, E. E., & Stone, W. (2004). Early concerns of parents of children with autistic and nonautistic disorders. *Infants and Young Children, 17*, 258–268.

Corsello, C., Hus, V., Pickles, A., Risi, S., Cook, E. H., Leventhal, B. L., et al. (2007). Between a ROC and a hard place: Decision making and making decisions about using the SCQ. *Journal of Child Psychology and Psychiatry, 48*, 932–940.

Cox, A., Klein, K., Charman, T., Baron-Cohen, S., Swettenham, J., Drew, A., et al. (1999). Autism spectrum disorders at 20 and 42 months of age: Stability of clinical and ADI-R diagnosis. *Journal of Child Psychology and Psychiatry, 40*, 719–732.

Dawson, G. (2008). Early behavioral intervention, brain plasticity, and the prevention of autism spectrum disorder. *Developmental Psychopathology, 20*, 775–803.

Dawson, G., Rogers, S., Munson, J., Smith, M., Winter, J., Greenson, J., et al. (2010). Randomized controlled trial of the Early Start Denver Model: a developmental behavioral intervention for toddlers with autism: Effects on IQ, adaptive behavior, and autism diagnosis. *Pediatrics, 125*, e17-23.

Dawson, G., Toth, K., Abbott, R., Osterling, J., Munson, J., Estes, A., et al. (2004). Early social attention impairments in autism: social orienting, joint attention, and attention to distress. *Developmental Psychology, 40*, 271–283.

Dawson, G., Webb, S., Schellenberg, G. D., Dager, S., Friedman, S., Aylward, E., & Richards, T. (2002). Defining the broader phenotype of autism: genetic, brain, and behavioral perspectives. *Development and Psychopathology, 14*, 581-611.

De Giacomo A., & Fombonne, E. (1998). Parental recognition of developmental abnormalities in autism. *European Child and Adolescent Psychiatry, 7*, 131–136.

Dietz, C., Swinkels, S., van Daalen, E., van Engeland, H., & Buitelaar, J. K. (2006). Screening for autistic spectrum disorder in children aged 14–15 months. II: population screening with the Early Screening of Autistic Traits Questionnaire (ESAT). Design and general findings. *Journal of Autism and Developmental Disorders, 36*, 713–722.

Dosreis, S., Weiner, C. L., Johnson, L., & Newschaffer, C. J. (2006). Autism spectrum disorder screening and management practices among general pediatric providers. *Journal of Developmental and Behavioral Pediatrics, 27*, S88–S94.

Dworkin, P. H. (1989). British and American recommendations for developmental monitoring: the role of surveillance. *Pediatrics, 84*, 1000–1010.

Eaves, L. C., Wingert, H. D., Ho, H. H., & Mickelson, E. C. R. (2006). Screening for autism spectrum disorders with the social communication questionnaire. *Journal of Developmental and Behavioral Pediatrics, 27*, S95–S103.

Filipek, P. A., Accardo, P. J., Ashwal, S., Baranek, G. T., Cook, E. H., Jr., Dawson, G., et al. (2000). Practice parameter: screening and diagnosis of autism: report of the Quality Standards Subcommittee of the American Academy of Neurology and the Child Neurology Society. *Neurology, 55*, 468–479.

First Signs Inc. (2009). Developmental disability, early intervention, developmental delays, autism screening and early intervention autism: First signs [Online]. Available at www.firstsigns.org

Fombonne, E., Zakarian, R., Bennett, A., Meng, L., & McLean-Heywood, D. (2006). Pervasive developmental disorders in Montreal, Quebec, Canada: prevalence and links with immunizations. *Pediatrics, 118*, e139–e150.

Gillberg, C., Ehlers, S., Schaumann, H., Jakobsson, G., Dahlgren S. O., & Lindblom, R. (1990). Autism under age 3 years: A clinical study of 28 cases referred for autistic symptoms in infancy. *Journal of Child Psychology and Psychiatry, 31*, 921–934.

Gray, K. M., & Tonge, B. J. (2001). Are there early features of autism in infants and preschool children? *Journal of Paediatrics and Child Health, 37*, 221–226.

Greenspan, S. I., Brazelton, T. B., Cordero, J., Solomon, R., Bauman, M. L., Robinson, R., et al. (2008). Guidelines for early identification, screening, and clinical management of children with autism spectrum disorders. *Pediatrics, 121*, 828–830.

Harris, S. L., & Handleman, J. S. (2000). Age and IQ at intake as predictors of placement for young children with autism: a four- to six-year follow-up. *Journal of Autism and Developmental Disorders, 30*, 137–142.

Hoshino, Y., Kaneko, M., Yashima, Y., Kumashiro, H., Volkmar, F. R., & Cohen, D. J. (1987). Clinical features of autistic children with setback course in their infancy. *Japanese Journal of Psychiatry and Neurology, 41*, 237–245.

Howlin, P., & Asgharian, A. (1999). The diagnosis of autism and Asperger syndrome: findings from a survey of 770 families. *Developmental Medicine and Child Neurology, 41*, 834–839.

Howlin, P., & Moore, A. (1997). Diagnosis of autism: A survey of over 1200 patients in the UK. *Autism, 1*, 135–162.

Iverson, J. M., & Wozniak, R. H. (2007). Variation in vocal-motor development in infant siblings of children with autism. *Journal of Autism and Developmental Disorders, 37*, 158–170.

Jacobson, J. W., & Mulick, J. A. (2000). System and cost research issues in treatments for people with autistic disorders. *Journal of Autism and Developmental Disorders, 30*, 585–593.

Jarbrink, K., & Knapp, M. (2001). The economic impact of autism in Britain. *Autism, 5*, 7–22.

Johnson, C. P., & Myers, S. M. (2007). Identification and evaluation of children with autism spectrum disorders. *Pediatrics, 120*, 1183–1215.

Kennedy, T., Regehr, G., Rosenfield, J., Roberts, S. W., & Lingard, L. (2004). Exploring the gap between knowledge and behavior: a qualitative study of clinician action following an educational intervention. *Academic Medicine, 79*, 386–393.

Kleinman, J. M., Robins, D. L., Ventola, P. E., Pandey, J., Boorstein, H. C., Esser, E. L., et al. (2008). The Modified Checklist for Autism in Toddlers: A follow-up study investigating the early detection of autism spectrum disorders. *Journal of Autism and Developmental Disorders, 38*, 827–839.

Landa, R. J., Holman, K. C., & Garrett-Mayer, E. (2007). Social and communication development in toddlers with early and later diagnosis of autism spectrum disorders. *Archives of General Psychiatry, 64*, 853–864.

Lee, L. C., David, A. B., Rusyniak, J., Landa, R., & Newschaffer, C. J. (2007). Performance of the Social Communication Questionnaire in children receiving preschool special education services. *Research in Autism Spectrum Disorders, 1*, 126–138.

Loh, A., Soman, T., Brian, J., Bryson, S. E., Roberts, W., Szatmari, P., et al. (2007). Stereotyped motor behaviors associated with autism in high-risk infants: a pilot videotape analysis of a sibling sample. *Journal of Autism and Developmental Disorders, 37*, 25–36.

Lord, C., Rutter, M., & Le Couteur, A. (1994). Autism Diagnostic Interview-Revised: a revised version of a diagnostic interview for caregivers of individuals with possible pervasive developmental disorders. *Journal of Autism and Developmental Disorders, 24*, 659–685.

Maestro, S., Muratori, F., Barbieri, F., Casella, C., Cattaneo, V., Cavallaro, M. C., et al. (2001). Early behavioral development in autistic children: the first 2 years of life through home movies. *Psychopathology, 34*, 147–152.

Maestro, S., Muratori, F., Cavallaro, M. C., Pei, F., Stern, D., Golse, B., et al. (2002). Attentional skills during the first 6 months of age in autism spectrum disorder. *Journal of the American Academy of Child and Adolescent Psychiatry, 41*, 1239–1245.

Mandell, D. S., Novak, M. M., & Zubritsky, C. D. (2005). Factors associated with age of diagnosis among children with autism spectrum disorders. *Pediatrics, 116*, 1480–1486.

Mitchell, S., Brian, J., Zwaigenbaum, L., Roberts, W., Szatmari, P., Smith, I., et al. (2006). Early language and communication development of infants later diagnosed with autism spectrum disorder. *Journal of Developmental and Behavioral Pediatrics, 27*, S69–S78.

Ohta, M., Nagai, Y., Hara, H., & Sasaki, M. (1987). Parental perception of behavioral symptoms in Japanese autistic children. *Journal of Autism and Developmental Disorders, 17*, 549–563.

Osterling, J., & Dawson, G. (1994). Early recognition of children with autism: a study of first birthday home videotapes. *Journal of Autism and Developmental Disorders, 24*, 247–257.

Osterling, J. A., Dawson, G., & Munson, J. A. (2002). Early recognition of 1-year-old infants with autism spectrum disorder versus mental retardation. *Development and Psychopathology, 14*, 239–251.

Ozonoff, S., Macari, S., Young, G. S., Goldring, S., Thompson, M., & Rogers, S. J. (2008). Atypical object exploration at 12 months of age is associated with autism in a prospective sample. *Autism, 12*, 457–472.

Pandey, J., Verbalis, A., Robins, D., Boorstein, H., Klin, A., Babitz, T., et al. (2008). Screening for autism in older and younger toddlers with the Modified Checklist for Autism in Toddlers. *Autism, 12*, 513–535.

Pinto-Martin, J. A., Young, L. M., Mandell, D. S., Poghosyan, L., Giarelli, E., & Levy, S. E. (2008). Screening strategies for autism spectrum disorders in pediatric primary care. *Journal of Developmental and Behavioral Pediatrics, 29*, 345–350.

Rice, C. E., Baio, J., Van Naarden, B. K., Doernberg, N., Meaney, F. J., & Kirby, R. S. (2007). A public health collaboration for the surveillance of autism spectrum disorders. *Pediatric and Perinatal Epidemiology, 21*, 179–190.

Ritvo, E. R., Jorde, L. B., Mason-Brothers, A., Freeman, B. J., Pingree, C., Jones, M. B., McMahon, W. M., Petersen, P. B., Jenson, W. R., & Mo, A. (1989). The UCLA-University of Utah epidemiologic survey of autism: recurrence risk estimates and genetic counseling. *American Journal of Psychiatry, 146*, 1032–1036.

Robins, D. L. (2008). Screening for autism spectrum disorders in primary care settings. *Autism, 12*, 537–556.

Robins, D. L., Fein, D., Barton, M. L., & Green, J. A. (2001). The Modified Checklist for Autism in Toddlers: an initial study investigating the early detection of autism and pervasive developmental disorders. *Journal of Autism and Developmental Disorders, 31*, 131–144.

Rogers, S. J., & DiLalla, D. L. (1990). Age of symptom onset in young children with pervasive developmental disorders. *Journal of the American Academy of Child and Adolescent Psychiatry, 29*, 863–872.

Rutter, M., & Lord, C. (1987). Language disorders associated with psychiatric disturbance. In W. Yule & M. Rutter (Eds.), *Language development and disorders* (pp. 206–233). Philadelphia: Lippincott.

Sackett, D. L., Haynes, R. B., Guyatt, G. H., & Tugwell, P. (1991). Helping patients follow the treatments you prescribe. In *Clinical epidemiology: A basic science for clinical medicine* (pp. 249–281). Toronto: Little, Brown and Company.

Scambler, D. J., Hepburn, S. L., & Rogers, S. J. (2006). A two-year follow-up on risk status identified by the checklist for autism in toddlers. *Journal of Developmental and Behavioral Pediatrics, 27*, S104–S110.

Scambler, D. J., Rogers S.J., & Wehner, E. A. (2001). Can the checklist for autism in toddlers differentiate young children with autism from those with developmental delays? *Journal of the American Academy of Child and Adolescent Psychiatry, 40*, 1457–1463.

Scott, F. J., Baron-Cohen, S., Bolton, P., & Brayne, C. (2002). Brief report: prevalence of autism spectrum conditions in children aged 5–11 years in Cambridgeshire, UK. *Autism, 6*, 231–237.

Siegel, B. (2004). *The Pervasive Developmental Disorders Screening Test II (PDDST-II)*. San Antonio, Texas: Psychological Corporation.

Siegel, B., Pliner, C., Eschler, J., & Elliott, G. R. (1988). How children with autism are diagnosed: difficulties in identification of children with multiple developmental delays. *Journal of Developmental and Behavioral Pediatrics, 9*, 199–204.

Stone, W. L., Coonrod, E. E., Turner, L. M., & Pozdol, S. L. (2004). Psychometric properties of the STAT for early autism screening. *Journal of Autism and Developmental Disorders, 34*, 691–701.

Stone, W. L., McMahon, C. R., & Henderson, L. M. (2008). Use of the Screening Tool for Autism in Two-Year-olds (STAT) for children under 24 Months: An exploratory study. *Autism, 12*, 557–573.

Stone, W. L., Ousley, O. Y., & Littleford, C. D. (1997). Motor imitation in young children with autism: what's the object? *Journal of Abnormal Child Psychology, 25*, 475–485.

Sumi, S., Taniai, H., Miyachi, T., & Tanemura, M. (2006). Sibling risk of pervasive developmental disorder estimated by means of an epidemiologic survey in Nagoya, Japan. *Journal of Human Genetics, 51*, 518–522

Swinkels, S. H., Dietz, C., van, D. E., Kerkhof, I. H., van, E. H., & Buitelaar, J. K. (2006). Screening for autistic spectrum in children aged 14 to 15 months. I: the development of the Early Screening of Autistic Traits Questionnaire (ESAT). *Journal of Autism and Developmental Disorders, 36*, 723–732.

Tuchman, R. F., & Rapin, I. (1997). Regression in pervasive developmental disorders: seizures and epileptiform electroencephalogram correlates. *Pediatrics, 99*, 560–566.

van Daalen, E., Kemner, C., Dietz, C., Swinkels, S. H., Buitelaar, J. K., & van Engeland, H. (2009). Inter-rater reliability and stability of diagnoses of autism spectrum disorder in children identified through screening at a very young age. *European Child and Adolescent Psychiatry, 18*, 663–674.

Vismara, L. A., Colombi, C., & Rogers, S. J. (2009). Can one hour per week of therapy lead to lasting changes in young children with autism? *Autism, 13*, 93–115.

Volkmar, F., Chawarska, K., & Klin, A. (2005). Autism in infancy and early childhood. *Annual Review of Psychology, 56*, 315–336.

Volkmar, F., Cook, E. H., Jr., Pomeroy, J., Realmuto, G., & Tanguay, P. (1999). Practice parameters for the assessment and treatment of children, adolescents, and adults with autism and other pervasive developmental disorders. *Journal of the American Academy of Child and Adolescent Psychiatry, 38(Suppl. 12)*, 32S–54S.

Wetherby, A., & Prizant, B. (2002). *Communication and symbolic behavior scales—Developmental profile*. Baltimore: Brookes.

Wetherby, A. M., Watt, N., Morgan, L., & Shumway, S. (2007). Social communication profiles of children with autism spectrum disorders late in the second year of life. *Journal of Autism and Developmental Disorders, 37*, 960–975.

Werner, E., Dawson, G., Osterling, J., & Dinno, N. (2000). Brief report: Recognition of autism spectrum disorder before one year of age: A retrospective study based on home videotapes. *Journal of Autism and Developmental Disorders, 30*, 157–162.

Wetherby, A. M., Brosnan-Maddox, S., Peace, V., & Newton, L. (2008). Validation of the Infant-Toddler Checklist as a broadband screener for autism spectrum disorders from 9 to 24 months of age. *Autism,12*, 487–511.

Wetherby, A. M., Woods, J., Allen, L., Cleary, J., Dickinson, H., & Lord, C. (2004). Early indicators of autism spectrum disorders in the second year of life. *Journal of Autism and Developmental Disorders, 34*, 473–493.

Wetherby, A., & Woods, J. (2004). *SORF: Systematic Observation of Red Flags for Autism Spectrum Disorders in Young Children*. Unpublished manual, Florida State University, Tallahassee, FL.

Yeargin-Allsopp, M., Rice, C., Karapurkar, T., Doernberg, N., Boyle, C., & Murphy, C. (2003). Prevalence of autism in a US metropolitan area. *Journal of the American Medical Association, 289*, 49–55.

Yirmiya, N., Gamliel, I., Shaked, M., & Sigman, M. (2007). Cognitive and verbal abilities of 24- to 36-month-old siblings of children with autism. *Journal of Autism and Developmental Disorders, 37*, 218–229.

Young, R. L., Brewer, N., & Pattison, C. (2003). Parental identification of early behavioural abnormalities in children with autistic disorder. *Autism*, *7*, 125–143.

Zwaigenbaum, L., Bryson, S., Lord, C., Rogers, S., Carter, A., Carver, L., et al. (2009). Clinical assessment and management of toddlers with suspected autism spectrum disorder: Insights from Studies of High-Risk Infants. *Pediatrics*, *123*, 1383–1391.

Zwaigenbaum, L., Bryson, S., Rogers, T., Roberts, W., Brian, J., & Szatmari, P. (2005). Behavioral manifestations of autism in the first year of life. *International Journal of Developmental Neurosciences*, *23*, 143–152.

Zwaigenbaum, L., Thurm, A., Stone, W., Baranek, G., Bryson, S., Iverson, J., et al. (2007). Studying the emergence of autism spectrum disorders in high-risk infants: methodological and practical issues. *Journal of Autism and Developmental Disorders*, *37*, 466–480.

6 Eric Fombonne, Sara Quirke, Arlene Hagen

Epidemiology of Pervasive Developmental Disorders

Points of Interest

- The best estimate of prevalence for all PDDs combined is 0.7% (1 in 143 children is affected), and several recent surveys even point at figures closer to 1%.
- The proportion of children with cognitive functioning within the normal range is 30% for autistic disorder and 55% for all PDDs.
- There is a consistent male overrepresentation for autistic disorder, childhood disintegrative disorder, and all PDDs.
- Regression, or loss of skills in the developmental course, occurs in about 1 in 4 children with PDD.
- Upward trends in rates of prevalence cannot be directly attributed to an increase in the incidence of the disorder as changes in referral patterns and availability of services, heightened public awareness, decreasing age at diagnosis, and changes over time in diagnostic concepts and practices confound the interpretation of data.
- Diagnostic substitution (the reclassification as PDD of a child who had previously received a different diagnosis) has been shown to contribute to the increase of prevalence in several studies.

The aims of this chapter are to provide an up-to-date review of the methodological features and substantive results of published epidemiological surveys of the prevalence of pervasive developmental disorders (PDD). This chapter updates previous reviews (Fombonne, 2003a; Fombonne, 2005) with the inclusion of new studies made available since then. The specific questions addressed in this chapter are: (1) what is the range of prevalence estimates for autism and related pervasive developmental disorders, and what are the correlates of PDD in epidemiological surveys?; and (2) what interpretation can be given to time trends observed in prevalence rates of PDDs?

Selection of Studies

The studies were identified through systematic searches from the major scientific literature databases (MEDLINE, PSYCINFO, EMBASE) and from prior reviews (Fombonne, 2003a, 2003b; Fombonne, 2005; Williams et al., 2006). Only studies published in the English language were included. Surveys that relied only on a questionnaire-based approach to define caseness (for example, Ghanizadeh, 2008) were also excluded, as the validity of the diagnosis is uncertain in these studies. Overall, 61 studies published between 1966 and 2009 were selected that surveyed PDDs in clearly demarcated, nonoverlapping samples. Of these, 48 studies provided information on rates of autistic disorder, 13 studies on Asperger's disorder (later referred to as Asperger's syndrome; AS), and 12 studies on childhood disintegrative disorder (CDD). A total of 27 studies provided estimates on all PDDs combined, of which 14 provided rates for specific PDD subtypes as well, and 13 only for the combined category of PDD.

Surveys were conducted in 18 countries, including 16 studies from the UK, 13 from the United States, and 7 from Japan. The results of over half of the studies (N = 33) have been published since 2001. The age range of the population included in the surveys is spread from birth to early adult life, but most studies have relied on school-age samples. Similarly, there was huge variation in the size of the population surveyed (range: 826 to 4.9 million; mean: 267,000; median: 44,900), with some recent studies conducted by the U.S. Centers for Disease Control (CDC, 2007b; 2009) relying on very large samples of several hundreds of thousands of individuals.

Study Designs

In designing a prevalence study, two major features are critical for the planning and logistics of the study, as well as for the interpretation of its results: case definition, and case ascertainment (or case identification methods) (Fombonne, 2007).

Case Definition

Over time, the definitions of autism have changed as illustrated by the numerous diagnostic criteria that were used in both epidemiological and clinical settings (see Figure 6-1). Starting with the narrowly defined Kanner's autism (1943), definitions progressively broadened in the criteria proposed by Rutter (1970), and then ICD-9 (1977), DSM-III (1980) and DSM-III-R (1987), and more recently in the 2 major nosographies used worldwide, ICD-10 (1992) and DSM-IV (American Psychiatric Association [APA], 1994). The early diagnostic criteria reflected the more qualitatively severe forms of the phenotype of autism, usually associated with severe delays in language and cognitive skills. It is only in the 1980s that less severe forms of autism were recognized, either as a qualifier for autism occurring without mental retardation (so-called "high-functioning" autism), or as separate diagnostic categories (Pervasive Developmental Disorders Not-Otherwise-Specified–PDD NOS) within a broader class of autism spectrum disorders (ASD) denominated "pervasive developmental disorders" (PDD, an equivalent to ASD) in current nosographies. While it had been described in the literature as early as 1944 (Asperger, 1944), one type of PDD, Asperger's disorder, appeared in official nosographies only in the 1990s, and then with unclear validity, especially with respect to its differentiation from "high-functioning" autism. Subtypes of PDD that existed in DSM-III subsequently disappeared (i.e., Autism–residual state). While there is generally high interrater reliability on the diagnosis of PDDs and commonality of concepts across experts, some differences persist between nomenclatures about the terminology and precise operationalized criteria of PDDs. For example, DSM-IV (1994) has a broad category of PDD NOS, sometimes referred to loosely as "atypical autism," whereas ICD-10 (1992) has several corresponding diagnoses for clinical presentations that fall short of autistic disorder, that include Atypical autism (F84.1, a diagnostic category that existed already in ICD-9), Other PDD (F84.8), and PDD-, unspecified (F84.9). As a result, studies that refer to "atypical autism" must be carefully interpreted, and no direct equivalence with the DSM-IV concept of PDD NOS should be assumed. In recent years, the definitions of syndromes falling on the autism spectrum have been expanded further with reference to the broader autism phenotype, and, with an increasing reliance on a dimensionalization of the autism phenotype. As no impairment or diagnostic criteria are available for these milder forms, the resulting boundaries with the spectrum of PDDs are left uncertain. Whether or not this plays a role in more recent epidemiological studies is difficult to know, but the possibility should be considered in assessing results for the new generation of surveys.

Broader autism phenotype: a pattern of mild developmental deficits similar to, but less severe than, symptoms of autism seen in relatives of subjects affected with a pervasive development disorder.

Case Identification

When an area or population have been identified for a survey, different strategies have been employed to find subjects matching the case definition retained for the study. Some studies have relied solely on existing service providers databases (Croen et al., 2002); on special educational databases (Gurney et al., 2003; Fombonne et al., 2006; Lazoff et al., 2010); or on national registers (Madsen et al., 2002) for case identification. These studies have the limitation in common of relying on a population group that happened to access the service provider or agencies rather than sampling from the population at large. As a result, subjects with the disorder who are not in contact with these services are yet unidentified and not included as cases, leading to a underestimation of the prevalence proportion.

Other investigations have relied on a multistage approach to identify cases in underlying populations. The aim of the first screening stage of these studies is to cast a wide net in order to identify subjects possibly affected with a PDD, with the final diagnostic status being determined at a next phase. The process utilized by the researchers often consists of sending letters or brief screening scales requesting school and health professionals and/or other data sources to identify possible cases of autism. Few of these investigations relied on systematic sampling techniques that would ensure a near complete coverage of the target population. Moreover, each investigation differed in several key aspects of this screening stage. First, the thoroughness of the coverage of all relevant data sources varied enormously from one study to another. In addition, the surveyed areas were not comparable in terms of service development, reflecting the specific educational or health care systems of each country and of the period of investigation. Second, the type of information sent out to professionals invited to identify children varied from simple letters, including a few clinical descriptors of autism-related symptoms or diagnostic checklists rephrased in nontechnical terms, to more systematic screening strategy based on questionnaires or rating scales of known reliability and validity. Third, variable participation rates in the first screening stages provide another source of variation in the screening efficiency of surveys, although refusal rates tended, on average, to be very low.

Few studies provided an estimate of the reliability of the screening procedure. The sensitivity of the screening methodology is also difficult to gauge in autism surveys and the proportion of children truly affected with the disorder but not identified in the screening stage (the "false negatives") remains generally unmeasured. The usual approach, which consists of sampling at random screened negative subjects in order to estimate the proportion of false negatives and adjusting the

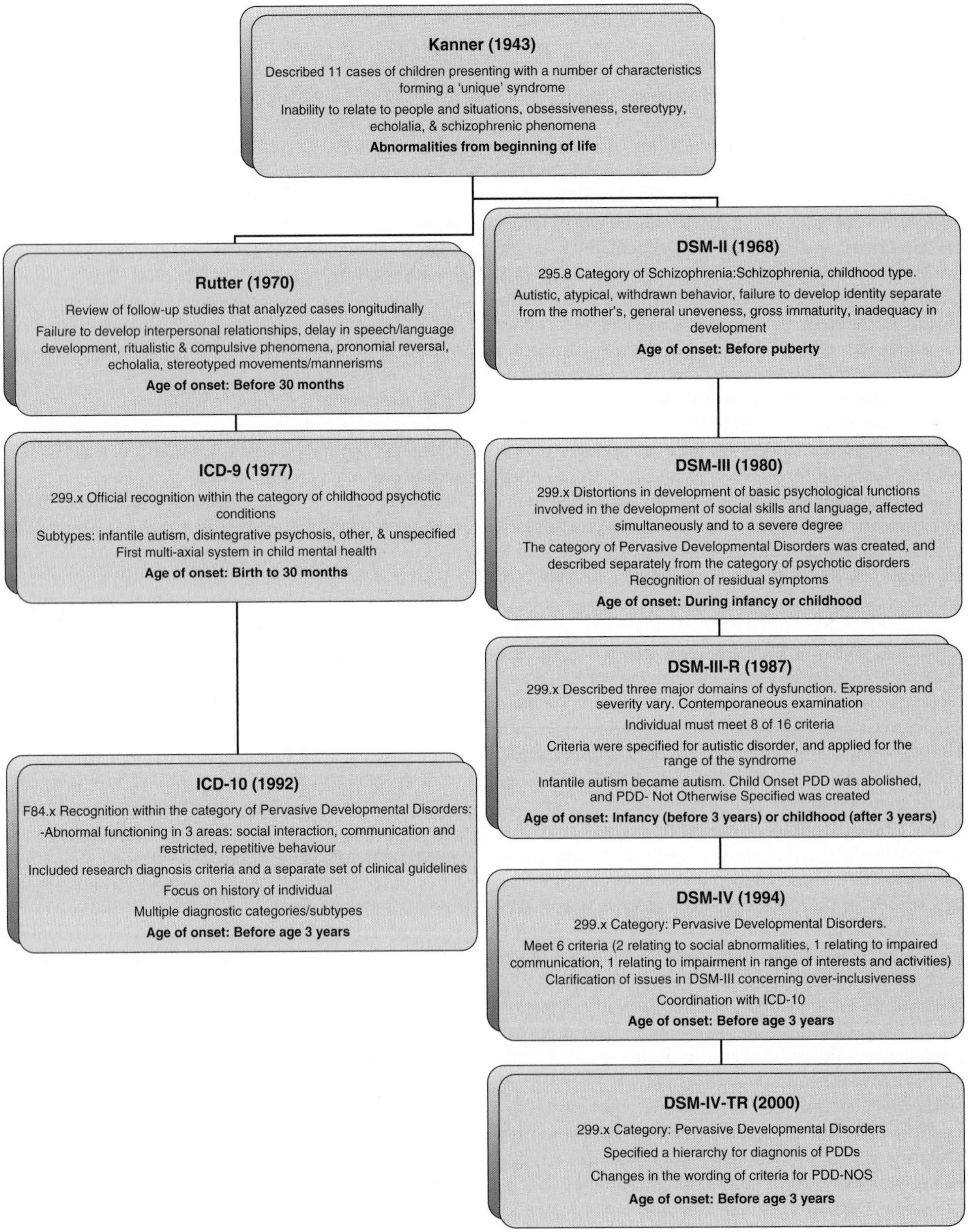

Kanner (1943)

Described 11 cases of children presenting with a number of characteristics forming a 'unique' syndrome

Inability to relate to people and situations, obsessiveness, stereotypy, echolalia, & schizophrenic phenomena

Abnormalities from beginning of life

Rutter (1970)

Review of follow-up studies that analyzed cases longitudinally

Failure to develop interpersonal relationships, delay in speech/language development, ritualistic & compulsive phenomena, pronomial reversal, echolalia, stereotyped movements/mannerisms

Age of onset: Before 30 months

ICD-9 (1977)

299.x Official recognition within the category of childhood psychotic conditions

Subtypes: infantile autism, disintegrative psychosis, other, & unspecified

First multi-axial system in child mental health

Age of onset: Birth to 30 months

ICD-10 (1992)

F84.x Recognition within the category of Pervasive Developmental Disorders:

-Abnormal functioning in 3 areas: social interaction, communication and restricted, repetitive behaviour

Included research diagnosis criteria and a separate set of clinical guidelines

Focus on history of individual

Multiple diagnostic categories/subtypes

Age of onset: Before age 3 years

DSM-II (1968)

295.8 Category of Schizophrenia:Schizophrenia, childhood type.

Autistic, atypical, withdrawn behavior, failure to develop identity separate from the mother's, general uneveness, gross immaturity, inadequacy in development

Age of onset: Before puberty

DSM-III (1980)

299.x Distortions in development of basic psychological functions involved in the development of social skills and language, affected simultaneously and to a severe degree

The category of Pervasive Developmental Disorders was created, and described separately from the category of psychotic disorders

Recognition of residual symptoms

Age of onset: During infancy or childhood

DSM-III-R (1987)

299.x Described three major domains of dysfunction. Expression and severity vary. Contemporaneous examination

Individual must meet 8 of 16 criteria

Criteria were specified for autistic disorder, and applied for the range of the syndrome

Infantile autism became autism. Child Onset PDD was abolished, and PDD- Not Otherwise Specified was created

Age of onset: Infancy (before 3 years) or childhood (after 3 years)

DSM-IV (1994)

299.x Category: Pervasive Developmental Disorders.

Meet 6 criteria (2 relating to social abnormalities, 1 relating to impaired communication, 1 relating to impairment in range of interests and activities)

Clarification of issues in DSM-III concerning over-inclusiveness

Coordination with ICD-10

Age of onset: Before age 3 years

DSM-IV-TR (2000)

299.x Category: Pervasive Developmental Disorders

Specified a hierarchy for diagnonis of PDDs

Changes in the wording of criteria for PDD-NOS

Age of onset: Before age 3 years

Figure 6–1. Historical changes in diagnostic concepts and criteria.

estimate accordingly, has not been used in these surveys for the obvious reason that, due to the low frequency of the disorder, it would be both imprecise and very costly to undertake such estimations. As a consequence, prevalence estimates must be understood as underestimates of "true" prevalence rates. The magnitude of this underestimation is unknown in each survey.

When the screening phase is completed, subjects identified as positive screens go through the next step involving a more in-depth diagnostic evaluation to confirm their case status. Similar considerations about the methodological variability across studies apply to these more intensive assessment phases. In the studies reviewed, participation rates in second-stage assessments were generally high. The source of information used to determine caseness usually involved a combination of data coming from different informants (parents, teachers, pediatricians, other health professionals, etc.) and data sources (medical records, educational sources), with an in-person assessment of the person with autism being offered in some but not all studies. Obviously, surveys of very large populations as those conducted in the United States by the CDC (2007a, 2007b, 2009) or in national registers (Madsen et al., 2002) did not include a direct diagnostic assessment of all subjects by the research team. However, these investigators could generally confirm the accuracy of their final caseness determination by undertaking, on a randomly selected subsample, a more complete diagnostic workup. The CDC surveys have established a methodology for surveys of large populations that relies on screening of population using multiple data sources, a systematic review and scoring system for the data gathered in the screening phase combined with, in the less obvious cases, input from experienced clinicians with known reliability and validity. This methodology is adequate for large samples, and is likely to be used in the future for surveillance efforts.

When subjects were directly examined, the assessments were conducted with various diagnostic instruments, ranging from a typical unstructured examination by a clinical expert (but without demonstrated psychometric properties), to the use of batteries of standardized measures by trained research staff. The Autism Diagnostic Interview (Le Couteur et al., 1989) and/or the Autism Diagnostic Observational Schedule (Lord et al., 2000) have been increasingly used in the most recent surveys.

Prevalence Estimations

We now present the results of the 61 studies in several tables that summarize results by type of PDD or for PDD as a spectrum of disorders. Characteristics of samples surveyed in these studies are briefly summarized.

Autistic Disorder

Prevalence estimates for autistic disorder are summarized in Table 6-1. There were 48 studies (including 13 in the UK, 6 in the United States, and 6 in Japan), half of them published since 1999. The sample size varied from 826 to 4.95 millions, with a median of 35,300 (mean: 212,500) subjects in the surveyed populations. The age ranged from 3 to 15 years, with a median age of 8.5 years. The number of subjects identified with autistic disorder ranged from 6 to 5,032 (median: 51). Males consistently outnumbered females in 40 studies where gender differences were reported, with a male/female ratio ranging from 1.33:1 to 16.0:1 in 39 studies (1 small study had no girls at all), leading to an average male/female ratio of 4.4:1. Prevalence rates varied from 0.7/10,000 to 72.6/10,000 with a median value of 12.9/10,000. Prevalence rates were negatively correlated with sample size (Spearman's r: -0.71; $p < .001$), with small-scale studies reporting higher prevalence rates. The correlation between prevalence rate and year of publication was significant (Spearman's r: 0.69; $p < .001$), indicative of higher rates in more recent surveys. Therefore, a current estimate for the prevalence of autistic disorder must be derived from more recent surveys with an adequate sample size. In 23 studies published since 2000, the median rate was 21.6/10,000 (mean rate: 21.9/10,000). After exclusion of the 2 studies with the smallest and largest sample sizes, the results were very similar (mean rate: 22.4/10,000). Thus, the best current estimate for autistic disorder is 22/10,000. In 25 studies where the proportion of subjects with IQ within the normal range was reported, the median value was 30% (interquartile range: 17.5%–50%). In these surveys, there was a significant correlation between a higher proportion of normal IQ subjects and a higher male/female ratio (Spearman's r: 0.53; $p = .007$), a result consistent with the known association between gender and IQ in autism. Over time, there were minor associations between the year of publication of the survey and the sample male/female ratio (Spearman's r: 0.36; $p = 0.024$) and the proportion of subjects without mental retardation (Spearman's r: 0.32; $p = 0.11$). Taken in conjunction with the much stronger increase over time in prevalence rates, these results suggest that the increase in prevalence rates is not entirely accounted for by the inclusion of milder forms (i.e., less cognitively impaired) of autistic disorder, albeit this might have contributed to it to some degree.

Asperger's Syndrome

Epidemiological studies of Asperger's syndrome (AS) are sparse, due to the fact that it was acknowledged as a separate diagnostic category only in the early 1990s, in both ICD-10 and DSM-IV. Two epidemiological surveys have been conducted which *specifically* investigated AS prevalence (Kadesjö et al., 1999; Ehlers & Gillberg, 1993). However, only a handful ($N < 5$) of cases were identified in these surveys, with the resulting estimates being unacceptably imprecise. In addition, since there was no separate report for children meeting criteria for autistic disorder, it remains unclear if these subjects would have also met criteria for autistic disorder and how prevalence rates would be affected if hierarchical rules were followed to diagnose both disorders. A recent

Table 6–1.
Prevalence surveys of autistic disorder

Year of Publication	Authors	Country	Area	Size of Target Population	Age	Number of Subjects with Autism	Diagnostic Criteria	% with normal IIQ	Gender ratio (M:F)	Prevalence Rate/10,000	95% CI
1966	Lotter	UK	Middlesex	78,000	8–10	32	Rating scale	15.6	2.6 (23/9)	4.1	2.7; 5.5
1970	Brask	Denmark	Aarhus County	46,500	2–14	20	Clinical	–	1.4 (12/7)	4.3	2.4; 6.2
1970	Treffert	USA	Wisconsin	899,750	3–12	69	Kanner	–	3.06 (52/17)	0.7	0.6; 0.9
1976	Wing et al.	UK	Camberwell	25,000	5–14	17[1]	24 items rating scale of Lotter	30	16 (16/1)	4.8[2]	2.1; 7.5
1982	Hoshino et al.	Japan	Fukushima-Ken	609,848	0–18	142	Kanner's criteria	—	9.9 (129/13)	2.33	1.9; 2.7
1983	Bohman et al.	Sweden	County of Västerbotten	69,000	0–20	39	Rutter criteria	20.5	1.6 (24/15)	5.6	3.9; 7.4
1984	McCarthy et al.	Ireland	East	65,000	8–10	28	Kanner	—	1.33 (16/12)	4.3	2.7; 5.9
1986	Steinhausen et al.	Germany	West Berlin	279,616	0–14	52	Rutter	55.8	2.25 (36/16)	1.9	1.4; 2.4
1987	Burd et al.	USA	North Dakota	180,986	2–18	59	DSM-III	—	2.7 (43/16)	3.26	2.4; 4.1
1987	Matsuishi et al.	Japan	Kurume City	32,834	4–12	51	DSM-III	—	4.7 (42/9)	15.5	11.3; 19.8
1988	Tanoue et al.	Japan	Southern Ibaraki	95,394	7	132	DSM-III	—	4.07 (106/26)	13.8	11.5; 16.2
1988	Bryson et al.	Canada	Part of Nova-Scotia	20,800	6–14	21	New RDC	23.8	2.5 (15/6)	10.1	5.8; 14.4
1989	Sugiyama & Abe	Japan	Nagoya	12,263	3	16	DSM-III	—	—	13.0	6.7; 19.4
1989	Cialdella & Mamelle	France	1 département (Rhône)	135,180	3–9	61	DSM-III like	—	2.3	4.5	3.4; 5.6
1989	Ritvo et al.	USA	Utah	769,620	3–27	241	DSM-III	34	3.73 (190/51)	2.47	2.1; 2.8
1991[4]	Gillberg et al.	Sweden	South-West Gothenburg + Bohuslän County	78,106	4–13	74	DSM-III-R	18	2.7 (54/20)	9.5	7.3; 11.6
1992	Fombonne & du Mazaubrun	France	4 régions 14 départements	274,816	9 & 13	154	Clinical-ICD-10 like	13.3	2.1 (105/49)	4.9	4.1; 5.7

1992	Wignyosumarto et al.	Indonesia	Yogyakarita (SE of Jakarta)	5,120	4–7	6	CARS	0	2.0 (4/2)	11.7	2.3; 21.1
1996	Honda et al.	Japan	Yokohama	8,537	5	18	ICD-10	50.0	2.6 (13.5)	21.08	11.4; 30.8
1997	Fombonne et al.	France	3 départements	325,347	8–16	174	Clinical ICD-10-like	12.1	1.81 (112/62)	5.35	4.6; 6.1
1997	Webb et al.	UK	South Glamorgan, Wales	73,301	3–15	53	DSM-III-R	—	6.57 (46/7)	7.2	5.3; 9.3
1997	Arvidsson et al.	Sweden (West coast)	Mölnlycke	1,941	3–6	9	ICD-10	22.2	3.5 (7/2)	46.4	16.1; 76.6
1998	Sponheim & Skjeldal	Norway	Akershus County	65,688	3–14	34	ICD-10	47.1[3]	2.09 (23/11)	5.2	3.4; 6.9
1999	Taylor et al.	UK	North Thames	490,000	0–16	427	ICD-10	—	—	8.7	7.9; 9.5
1999	Kadesjö et al.	Sweden (Central)	Karlstad	826	6.7–7.7	6	DSM-III-R/ ICD-10 Gillberg's criteria (Asperger's syndrome)	50.0	5.0 (5/1)	72.6	14.7; 130.6
2000	Baird et al.	UK	South-East Thames	16,235	7	50	ICD-10	60	15.7 (47/3)	30.8	22.9; 40.6
2000	Powell et al.	UK	West Midlands	25,377	1–5	62	Clinical/ ICD10/ DSM-IV	—	—	7.8	5.8; 10.5
2000	Kielinen et al.	Finland	North (Oulu et Lapland)	27,572	5–7	57	DSM-IV	49.8[7]	4.12[7] (156/50)	20.7	15.3; 26.0
2001	Bertrand et al.	USA	Brick Township, New Jersey	8,896	3–10	36	DSM-IV	36.7	2.2 (25/11)	40.5	28.0; 56.0
2001	Fombonne et al.	UK	Angleterre et Pays de Galles	10,438	5–15	27	DSM-IV/ ICD-10	55.5	8.0 (24/3)	26.1	16.2; 36.0
2001	Magnússon & Saemundsen	Iceland	Whole Island	43,153	5–14	57	Mostly ICD-10	15.8	4.2 (46/11)	13.2	9.8; 16.6
2001	Chakrabarti & Fombonne	UK (Midlands)	Staffordshire	15,500	2.5–6.5	26	ICD10/ DSM-IV	29.2	3.3 (20/6)	16.8	10.3; 23.2
2001	Davidovitch et al.	Israel	Haiffa	26,160	7–11	26	DSM-III-R/ DSM-IV	—	4.2 (21/5)	10.0	6.6;14.4
2002	Croen et al.	USA	California DDS	4,950,333	5–12	5,038	CDER "Full syndrome"	62.8[5]	4.47 (4116/921)	11.0	10.7;11.3
2002	Madsen et al.	Denmark	National Register	63,859	8	46	ICD-10	—	—	7.2	5.0–10.0

(*Continued*)

Table 6–1. *(Contd.)*

Year of Publication	Authors	Country	Area	Size of Target Population	Age	Number of Subjects with Autism	Diagnostic Criteria	% with Normal IQ	Gender Ratio (M:F)	Prevalence Rate/10,000	95% CI
2004	Tebruegge et al.	UK	Kent	2,536	8–9	6	ICD-10	—	0.0 (6/0)	23.7	9.6; 49.1
2005	Chakrabarti & Fombonne	UK (Midlands)	Staffordshire	10,903	4–7	24	ICD-10/DSM-IV	33.3	3.8 (19/5)	22.0	14.4; 32.2
2005	Barbaresi et al.	USA, Minnesota	Olmstead County	37,726	0–21	112	DSM-IV	—	—	29.7	24.0; 36.0
2005	Honda et al.[6]	Japan	Yokohama	32,791	5	123	ICD-10	25.3	2.5 (70/27)	37.5	31.0; 45.0
2006	Fombonne et al.	Canada (Quebec)	Montreal Island	27,749	5–17	60	DSM-IV	—	5.7 (51/9)	21.6	16.5; 27.8
2006	Gillberg et al.	Sweden	Göteborg	32,568	7–12	115	Gillberg's criteria	—	3.6 (90/25)	35.3	29.2; 42.2
2006	Baird et al.	UK	South Thames, London	56,946	9–10	81	ICD-10	47	8.3 (≈ 72/9)	38.9	29.9; 47.8
2007	Ellefsen et al.	Denmark	Faroe Islands	7,689	8–17	12	ICD-10 Gillberg criteria for AS		3.0 (9/3)	16.0	7.0; 25.0
2007	Oliveira et al.	Portugal	Mainland and Azores	67,795	6–9	115	DSM-IV	17	2.9	16.7	14.0; 20.0
2007	Latif & Williams	UK	Wales	39,220	0–17	50	Kanner	—	—	12.7	9.0;17.0
2008	Williams et al.	UK	South West (Avon)	14,062	11	30	ICD-10	86.7	5.0 (25/5)	21.6	13.9; 29.3
2009	van Balkom et al.	Netherlands	Aruba (Caribbean)	13,109	0–13	25	DSM-IV	36.0	7.3 (22/3)	19.1	12.3; 28.1
2010	Lazoff et al.	Canada	Montreal	23,635	5–17	60	DSM-IV	—	5.0 (50/10)	25.4	19.0; 31.8

[1] This number corresponds to the sample described in Wing & Gould (1979).
[2] This rate corresponds to the first published paper on this survey and is based on 12 subjects among children aged 5 to 14 years.
[3] In this study, mild mental retardation was combined with normal IQ, whereas moderate and severe mental retardation were grouped together.
[4] For the Goteborg surveys by Gillberg et al. (Gillberg, 1984; Steffenburg & Gillberg, 1986; Gillberg et al., 1991) a detailed examination showed that there was overlap between the samples included in the 3 surveys; consequently only the last survey has been included in this table.
[5] This proportion is likely to be overestimated and to reflect an underreporting of mental retardation in the CDER evaluations.
[6] This figure was calculated by the author and refers to prevalence data (not cumulative incidence) presented in the paper (the M:F ratio is based on a subsample).
[7] These figures apply to the whole study sample of 206 subjects with an ASD.

survey of high-functioning PDDs in Welsh mainstream primary schools has yielded a relatively high (uncorrected) prevalence estimate of 14.5/10,000, but no separate rate was available for AS, specifically (Webb et al., 2003).

Other recent surveys have examined samples with respect to the presence of both autistic disorder and Asperger's syndrome. Thirteen studies (already listed in Table 6-1), published since 1998, provided usable data (Table 6-2). The median population size was 16,200, and the median age 8.0 years. Numbers of children with AS varied from 6 to 427, with a median sample size of 32. There was a 160-fold variation in estimated rates of AS (range: 0.3 to 48.4/10,000) that demonstrates the lack of reliability of these estimates. The median value was 10.5/10,000. With the exception of one study (Latif & Williams, 2007), the number of children with autistic disorder was consistently higher than that of children with AS. The prevalence ratio (Table 6-2, right-hand column) exceeded 1, with a median value of 2.1, indicating that the rate of AS was consistently *lower* than that for autism (Table 6-2). The unusually high rate of AS relative to autistic disorder obtained in Latif and Williams's study (2007) appeared to be inflated due to the inclusion of high-functioning autism in the AS definition. The epidemiological data on AS are therefore of dubious quality, reflecting the difficult nosological issues that have surrounded the inclusion of AS in recent nosographies as well as the lack of proper measurement strategies that ensure a reliable difference between AS and autistic disorder.

Childhood Disintegrative Disorder

Twelve surveys provided data on childhood disintegrative disorder (CDD) (Table 6-3). In 5 of these, only 1 case was reported; no case of CDD was identified in 4 other studies. Prevalence estimates ranged from 0 to 9.2/100,000, with a median rate of 1.8/100,000. The pooled estimate, based on 11 identified cases and a surveyed population of about 560,000 children, was 1.9/100,000. Gender was reported in 10 of the 11 studies, and males appear to be overrepresented with a male/female ratio of 9:1. The upperbound limit of confidence interval associated to the pooled prevalence estimate (3.4/100,000) indicates that CDD is a quite rare condition, with about 1 case occurring for every 112 cases of autistic disorder.

Prevalence for Combined PDDs

A new objective of more recent epidemiological surveys was to estimate the prevalence of all disorders falling onto the autism spectrum, thereby prompting important changes in the conceptualization and design of surveys. However, before reviewing the findings of these studies mostly conducted since 2000, we examine to which extent findings of the first generation of epidemiological surveys of a narrow definition of autism also informed our understanding of the modern concept of autism spectrum disorders.

Unspecified Autism Spectrum Disorders in Earlier Surveys

In previous reviews, we documented that several studies performed in the 1960s and 1970s had provided useful information on rates of syndromes similar to autism but not meeting of the strict diagnostic criteria for autistic disorder then in use (Fombonne, 2003a, 2003b; Fombonne, 2005). At the time, different labels were used by authors to characterize these clinical pictures, such as the triad of impairments involving deficits in reciprocal social interaction, communication, and imagination (Wing & Gould 1979), autistic mental retardation (Hoshino et al., 1982), borderline childhood psychoses (Brask, 1970) or "autistic-like" syndromes (Burd et al., 1987). These syndromes would be falling within our currently defined autistic spectrum, probably with diagnostic labels such as atypical autism and/or PDD NOS. In 8 of 12 surveys providing separate estimates of the prevalence of these developmental disorders, higher rates for the atypical forms were actually found compared to those for more narrowly defined autistic disorder (see Fombonne, 2003a, Table 3, p. 172). However, this group received little attention in previous epidemiological studies, and these subjects were not defined as "cases" and therefore not included in the numerators of prevalence calculations, thereby underestimating systematically the prevalence of what would be defined today as the spectrum of autistic disorders. For example, in the first survey by Lotter (1966), the prevalence would rise from 4.1 to 7.8/10,000 if these atypical forms had been included in the case definition. Similarly, in Wing et al.'s study (1976), the prevalence was 4.9/10,000 for autistic disorder, but, adding the figure of 16.3/10,000 (Wing & Gould, 1979) corresponding to the triad of impairments, the prevalence for the whole PDD spectrum was in fact 21.1/10,000. For the purpose of historical comparison, it is important to be attentive to this earlier figure, bearing in mind that the study was conducted in the early 1970s for the field work and that autism occurring in subjects with an IQ within the normal range was not yet being investigated. Progressive recognition of the importance and relevance to autism of these less typical clinical presentations has led to changes in the design of more recent epidemiological surveys (see below), that are now using case definitions that incorporate upfront these milder phenotypes.

Newer Surveys of PDDs

The results of surveys that estimated the prevalence of the whole spectrum of PDDs are summarized in Table 6-4. Of the 27 studies listed, 14 also provided separate estimates for autistic disorder and other PDD subtypes; the other 13 studies provided only an estimate for the combined PDD rate. All these surveys were published since 2000, and the majority since 2006; the studies were performed in 8 countries (including 10 in the UK and 8 in the United States). Sample sizes ranged from 2,536 to 4,247,206 (median: 32,568; mean: 243,156).

Table 6–2.
Asperger's syndrome (AS) in recent autism surveys

			Assessment			Autism		Asperger Syndrome		
	Size of Population	Age Group	Informants	Instruments	Diagnostic Criteria	N	Rate/ 10,000	N	Rate/ 10,000	Autism/ AS Ratio
Sponheim & Skjeldal, 1998	65,688	3–14	Parent Child	Parental Interview + direct observation, CARS, ABC	ICD-10	32	4.9	2	0.3	16.0
Taylor et al., 1999	490,000	0–16	Record	Rating of all data available in child record	ICD-10	427	8.7	71	1.4	6.0
Kadesjö et al., 1999	826	6.7–7.7	Child Parent Professional	ADI-R, Griffiths Scale or WISC, Asperger Syndrome Screening Questionnaire	DSM-III-R/ICD-10 Gillberg's criteria (Asperger syndrome)	6	72.6	4	48.4	1.5
Powell et al., 2000	25,377	1–4.9	Records	ADI-R Available data	DSM-III-R DSM-IV ICD-10	54	—	16	—	3.4
Baird et al., 2000	16,235	7	Parents Child Other data	ADI-R Psychometry	ICD-10 DSM-IV	45	27.7	5	3.1	9.0
Chakrabarti & Fombonne, 2001	15,500	2.5–6.5	Child Parent Professional	ADI-R, 2 wks multidisciplinary assessment, Merrill-Palmer, WPPSI	ICD-10 DSM-IV	26	16.8	13	8.4	2.0
Chakrabarti & Fombonne, 2005	10,903	2.5–6.5	Child Parent Professional	ADI-R, 2 wks multidisciplinary assessment, Merrill-Palmer, WPPSI	ICD-10 DSM-IV	24	22.0	12	11.0	2.0
Fombonne et al., 2006	27,749	5–17	School registry	Clinical	DSM-IV	60	21.6	28	10.1	2.1
Ellefsen et al., 2007	7,689	8–17	Parent Child Professional	DISCO, WISC-R, ASSQ	ICD-10 Gillberg AS criteria	21	28.0	20	26.0	1.1
Latif & Williams, 2007	39,220	0–17	?	Clinical	Kanner, Gillberg AS criteria	50	12.7	139	35.4	0.36
William et al., 2008	14,062	11	Medical records and educational registry	Clinical	ICD-10	30	21.6	23	16.6	1.3
van Balkom et al., 2009	13,109	0–13	Clinic series	Review of medical records	DSM-IV	25	19.1	2	1.5	12.5
Lazoff et al., 2010	23,635	5–17	School registry	Review of educational records	DSM-IV	60	25.4	23	9.7	2.6

Table 6–3.
Surveys of childhood disintegrative disorder (CDD)

Study	Country (Region/State)	Size of Target Population	Age Group	Assessment	N	M/F	Prevalence Estimate (/100,000)	95% CI (/100,000)
Burd et al., 1987	USA (North Dakota)	180,986	2–18	Structured parental interview and review of all data available–DSM-III criteria	2	2/–	1.11	0.13–3.4
Sponheim & Skjeldal, 1998	Norway (Akershus County)	65,688	3–14	Parental interview and direct observation (CARS, ABC)	1	?	1.52	0.04–8.5
Magnusson et Saemundsen, 2001	Iceland (whole island)	85,556	5–14	ADI-R, CARS and psychological tests–mostly ICD-10	2	2/–	2.34	0.3–8.4
Chakrabarti & Fombonne, 2001	UK (Staffordshire, Midlands)	15,500	2.5–6.5	ADI-R, two weeks multidisciplinary assessment, Merrill-Palmer, WPPSI–ICD-10/DSM-IV	1	1/–	6.45	0.16–35.9
Chakrabarti & Fombonne, 2005	UK (Staffordshire, Midlands)	10,903	2.5–6.5	ADI-R, two weeks multidisciplinary assessment, Merrill-Palmer, WPPSI–ICD-10/DSM-IV	1	1/–	9.17	0–58.6
Fombonne et al., 2006	Montreal, Canada	27,749	5–17	DSM-IV, special needs school survey	1	1/–	3.60	0–20.0
Gillberg et al., 2006	Sweden, Götenborg	102,485	7–24	DSM-IV, review of medical records of local diagnostic center	2	1/1	2.0	0.2–7.1
Ellefsen et al., 2007	Faroe Islands, Denmark	7,689	8–17	DISCO, Vineland, WISC-R, ICD-10/DSM-IV	0	—	0	—
Kawamura et al., 2008	Japan, Toyota	12,589	5–8	DSM-IV, population based screening at 18 and 36 mths	0	—	0	—
Williams et al., 2008	UK, Avon	14,062	11	ICD-10, educational and medical record review	0	—	0	—
van Balkom et al., 2009	Netherlands, Aruba	13,109	0–13	Clinic medical record review	0	—	0	—
Lazoff et al., 2010	Canada, Montreal	23,635	5–17	DSM-IV, special needs school survey	1	1/0	4.23	0.0–24.0
Pooled Estimates		**559,951**			**11**	**9/1**	**1.96**	**1.1–3.4**

The median age of samples ranged from 5.0 to 12.5, with 8.0 years being both the modal and median age. The diagnostic criteria used in the 25 studies where they were specified reflect reliance on modern diagnostic schemes by all authors (10 studies used ICD-10, 17 the DSM-IV or DSM-IV-TR, both schemes being used simultaneously in 2 studies). In 14 studies where IQ data were reported, the proportion of subjects within the normal IQ range varied from 30% to 85.3% (median: 57.1%; mean: 56.1%), a proportion that is higher than that for autistic disorder and reflects the lesser degree of association, or lack thereof, between intellectual impairment and milder forms of PDDs. Overrepresentation of males was the rule, with male/female ratio ranging from 2.7:1 to 15.7:1 (mean: 5.5; median: 4.9). There was a 6-fold variation in prevalence proportions that ranged from a low 30.0/10,000 to a high of 181.1/10,000. However, some degree of consistency is found

Table 6–4.
Newer epidemiological surveys of pervasive developmental disorders

References	Country	Area	Size	Age	N	Diagnostic Criteria	% With Normal IQ	Gender Ratio (M:F)	Prevalence/ 10,000	95% CI
Baird et al., 2000	UK	South East Thames	16,235	7	94	ICD-10	60%	15.7 (83 : 11)	57.9	46.8–70.9
Bertrand et al., 2001	USA	New Jersey	8,896	3–10	60	DSM-IV	51%	2.7 (44 : 16)	67.4	51.5–86.7 *
Chakrabarti & Fombonne, 2001	UK	Stafford	15,500	4–7	96	ICD-10	74.2%	3.8 (77 : 20)	61.9	50.2–75.6
Madsen et al., 2002	Denmark	National register	—	8	738	ICD-10	—	—	30.0	—
Scott et al., 2002	UK	Cambridge	33,598	5–11	196	ICD-10	—	4.0 (—)	58.3 *	50 67 *
Yeargin-Allsopp et al., 2003	USA	Atlanta	289,456	3-10	987	DSM-IV	31.8%	4.0 (787 : 197)	34.0	32–36
Gurney et al., 2003	USA	Minnesota	—	8–10	—	—	—	—	52.0** 66.0	— —
Icasiano et al., 2004	Australia	Barwon	≈ 54,000	2–17	177	DSM-IV	53.4%	8.3 (158 : 19)	39.2	—
Tebruegge et al., 2004	UK	Kent	2,536	8–9	21	ICD-10	—	6.0 (18:3)	82.8	51.3–126.3
Chakrabarti & Fombonne, 2005	UK	Stafford	10,903	4–6	64	ICD-10	70.2%	6.1 (55 : 9)	58.7	45.2–74.9
Baird et al., 2006	UK	South Thames	56,946	9–10	158	ICD-10	45%	3.3 (121 : 37)	116.1	90.4–141.8
Fombonne et al., 2006	Canada	Montreal	27,749	5–17	180	DSM-IV	—	4.8 (149 : 31)	64.9	55.8–75.0
Harrison et al., 2006	UK	Scotland	134,661	0–15	443‡	ICD-10, DSMIV	—	7.0 (369 : 53)	44.2‡	39.5–48.9

Gillberg et al., 2006	Sweden	Göteborg	32,568	7 12	262	DSM-IV	—	3.6 (205:57)	80.4	71.3–90.3
CDC, 2007a	USA	6 states	187,761	8	1,252	DSM-IV-TR	38% to 60%[§]	2.8 to 5.5	67.0	—[§]
CDC, 2007b	USA	14 states	407,578	8	2,685	DSM-IV-TR	55.4%[†]	3.4 to 6.5	66.0	63–68
Ellefsen et al., 2007	Denmark	Faroe Islands	7,689	8–17	41	DSM-IV, Gillberg's criteria	68.3%	5.8 (35 : 6)	53.3	36–70
Latif & Williams, 2007	UK	South Wales	39,220	0–17	240	ICD-10, DSM-IV, Kanner's & Gillberg's criteria	—	6.8 —	61.2	54–69*
Wong et al., 2008	China	Hong Kong	4,247,206	0–14	682	DSM-IV	30%	6.6 (592 : 90)	16.1 (1986–2005) 30.0 (2005)	— —
Nicholas et al., 2008	USA	South Carolina[††]	47,726	8	295	DSM-IV-TR	39.6%	3.1 (224 : 71)	62.0	56–70
Kawamura et al., 2008	Japan	Toyota	12,589	5–8	228	DSM-IV	66.4%	2.8 (168 : 60)	181.1	158.5–205.9 *
Williams et al., 2008	UK	Avon	14,062	11	86	ICD-10	85.3%	6.8 (75:11)	61.9	48.8–74.9
Baron–Cohen et al., 2009	UK	Cambridgeshire	8,824	5–9	83	ICD-10	—	—	94[‡‡]	75 - 116
Kogan et al., 2009	USA	nationwide	77,911	3–17	913	—	—	4.5 (746:167)	110	94 - 128
Van Balkom et al., 2009	Netherlands	Aruba	13,109	0–13	69	DSM-IV	58.8%	6.7 (60:9)	52.6	41.0-66.6
CDC, 2009	USA	11 states	307,790	8	2,757	DSM-IV	59%	4.5 (–)	89.6	86 - 93
Lazoff et al., 2010	Canada	Montreal	23,635	5–17	187	DSM-IV	—	5.4 (158:29)	79.1	67.8–90.4

* calculated by the author.

§ specific values for % with normal IQ and confidence intervals are available for each state prevalence.

† average across 7 states.

‡ estimated using a capture-recapture analysis, the number of cases used to calculate prevalence was estimated to be 596.

** these are the highest prevalences reported in this study of time trends. The prevalence in 10-year-olds is for the 1991 birth cohort, and that for 8-year-olds for the 1993 birth cohort. Both prevalences were calculated in the 2001–2002 school year.

†† children aged 8, born either in 2000 and 2002, and included in the two CDC multisite reports.

‡‡ rate based on Special Education Needs register. A figure of 99/10,000 is provided from a parental and diagnostic survey. Other estimates in this study vary from 47 to 165/10,000 deriving from various assumptions made by the authors.

in the center of this distribution, with a median rate of 62.0/10,000 and a mean rate of 69.2/10,000 (interquartile range: 53.3–80.4/10,000). This mean rate coincides with the rate reported recently for PDDs in 14 sites (CDC, 2007b); the CDC value represents, however, an average, and that study conducted at 14 different sites utilizing the same methodology found a 3-fold variation of rate by state. Alabama had the lowest rate of 3.3/1,000 whereas New Jersey had the highest value with 10.6/1,000 (CDC, 2007b). As expected, a new CDC report on 307,000 U.S. children aged 8 and born 4 years later than children from the previous survey reported an average prevalence of 89.6/10,000 (CDC, 2009). Again, substantial variation across states was reported as prevalence ranged from 4.2/1,000 in Florida to 12.1/1,000 in Arizona and Missouri. One factor associated with the prevalence increase in the CDC monitoring survey was improved quality and quantity of information available through records, indicative of greater awareness about ASD among community professionals. As surveillance efforts continue, it is likely that awareness and services will develop in states that were lagging behind, resulting in a predictable increase in the average rate for the United States as time elapses. These CDC findings apply to other countries as well, and prevalence estimates from any study should always be regarded in the context of the imperfect sensitivity of case ascertainment that results in downward biases in prevalence proportions in most surveys.

As an illustration, the 4 surveys in Table 6-4 with the lowest rates probably underestimated the true population rates. In the Danish investigation (Madsen et al., 2002), case finding depended on notification to a National Registry, a method which is usually associated with lower sensitivity for case finding. The Hong Kong (Wong et al., 2008) and Australian (Icasiano et al., 2004) surveys have relied on less systematic ascertainment techniques. The Atlanta survey by the CDC (Yeargin-Allsopp et al., 2003) was based on a very large population and included younger age groups than subsequent CDC surveys, and age specific rates were in fact in the 40–45/10,000 range in some birth cohorts (Fombonne, 2003a, 2003b). Case finding techniques employed in the other surveys were more proactive, relying on multiple and repeated screening phases, involving both different informants at each phase and surveying the same cohorts at different ages, which certainly enhanced the sensitivity of case identification (Chakrabarti & Fombonne, 2005; Baird et al., 2006). Assessments were often performed with standardized diagnostic measures (i.e., ADI-R and ADOS) which match well the more dimensional approach retained for case definition.

Overall, results of recent surveys agree that an average figure of 70/10,000 can be used as the current estimate for the spectrum of PDDs.

> Regression: a loss of skills including language (the child stops using 5 to 30 words that he had gained) often associated with contemporaneous changes in social and play skills.

Regressive Autism in Population Surveys

The studies of regression or loss of skills in the developmental course of PDDs has gained much attention in recent years. As there is evidence that regression is associated with younger age at identification (Shattuck et al., 2009), and with slight increase in severity of autistic symptoms and cognitive deficits (Meilleur & Fombonne, 2009; Fombonne & Chakrabarti, 2001; Parr et al., submitted), we examined how often regression was reported and how it was measured in population based studies, and, when available, the age at regression and the outcome (Table 6-5). Ten studies reported the frequency of regression in the survey sample. Interestingly, Lotter (1966) documented in the first epidemiological survey of autism that a "set-back" had occurred in almost one third of the children. There has been no standardized way to evaluate regression, and the methods have relied on record abstraction or parents' retrospective recall. Regression has often focused on the loss of language skills, with or without the loss of other (social, play) skills. Regression ranged from 12.5% (Sugiyama & Abe, 1989) to 38.6% (Baird et al., 2008), with a median rate of 23%. In the majority of studies, the age at regression is the 6 months preceding the 2nd birthday or close to age 2, which differentiates this pattern of loss from that seen in CDD. Symptoms of CDD are typically observed at the end of the 3rd year of life and are characterized by marked developmental and behavioral changes and deterioration that result in profound, lasting, autistic and cognitive impairments. Two studies provided separate figures for a strict definition of autism compared to atypical or milder forms. In one study (Taylor et al., 2002), regression occurs at comparable frequency in typical and atypical autism, whereas in the other (Baird et al., 2008) there is a marked difference between the 38.6% figure of regression (including both definite and lower level) in autism as opposed to a much lower corresponding figure of 10.6% in the broadly defined ASD group. Finally, in 3 studies where some kind of outcome data were reported, all studies pointed at higher symptom severity in the regressive group. Overall, these results do not differ from studies of regression based on clinical samples and they confirm that a loss of skills in the development of PDD children is common, affecting about 1 in 4 children with ASD.

In conclusion, conducted in different regions and countries by different teams, the convergence of estimates around 70 per 10,000 for all PDDs combined is striking especially when derived from studies with improved methodology. This estimate is now the best estimate for the prevalence of PDDs currently available. However, this represents an average and conservative figure, and it is important to recognize the substantial variability that exists between studies, and within studies, across sites or areas. The prevalence figure of 70/10,000 (equivalent to 7/1,000 or 0.7%) translates into 1 child out of 143 suffering from a PDD. It should be noted, however, that some studies have reported rates that are even two to three times higher (Baird et al., 2006; Kawamura et al., 2008), and that the most recent and reliable estimates point at a 0.9% to 1% prevalence.

Table 6–5.
"Regressive" autism in population-based studies

Authors	Measurement of Regression	Proportion of Study Sample with Regression/Loss	Age at Regression	Skills Lost	Diagnosis	Outcome
Lotter, 1966	"set-back" in development	31.2%	18–27 months (N = 3) 27–36 months (N = 4) 3 to 4.5 years (N = 3)[2]	Loss of some ability (i.e., speech) or failure to progress after a satisfactory beginning	Kanner's autism	All but 2 of the children with a set-back (80%) had a low (< 55) IQ, compared to 63.4% in the group without set-back
Sugiyama & Abe, 1989	Developmental checkups from 18 months to age 3	12.5%	2 years	Loss of a few words or of one-word sentences	DSM-III autism	
Bertrand et al., 2001	Question to parents during clinical evaluation[1]	24%	12–18 months	Single words and social smiling	All had autistic disorder	
Fombonne & Chakrabarti, 2001	ADI-R items on regression before age 5	15.6%	19.8 months	Any language, social, play, or motor skill	—	Trend ($p = .08$) for children with regression to have lower IQ scores (IQ < 70) than nonregressive children (21.5%)
Taylor et al., 2002	Abstraction of medical records	25%	—	Deterioration in any aspect of a child's development or reported loss of skills	Typical autism (23%); atypical autism (27%)	
Icasiano et al., 2004	Parental interview	27.1%[3] 5.6%[3]		Previously acquired language skills Previously acquired motor skills	Autism spectrum disorders	
CDC, 2007a	Abstraction of all records by an ASD clinician reviewer	19.0%[4]	24 months (median age across 6 sites)	Loss of previously acquired skills in social, communication, play, or motor areas	Autism spectrum disorders	
CDC, 2007b	Abstraction of all records by an ASD clinician reviewer	19.7% [5]	24 months (median age across 14 sites)	Loss of previously acquired skills in social, communication, play, or motor areas	Autism spectrum disorders	
Baird et al., 2008	ADI-R items (11–15, and 20) on regression	30.2% (8%)[7] 8.4% (2.6%)[7]	25 months 25 months	Definite language regression[6] Lower level regression[6]	Narrow autism (broad ASD)	Increase in severity of autistic symptoms in both regression groups
CDC, 2009	Abstraction of all records by an ASD clinician reviewer	21.9%[8]	19 months (median age across 11 sites)	Loss of previously acquired skills in social, communication, play, or motor areas	Autism spectrum disorders	

[1] "Did your child experience any loss of previously acquired skills?"
[2] In the 3 children with an onset after age 3, the setback was "severe and fairly rapid" (Lotter, 1966, p. 130) (these cases would probably meet criteria for CDD).
[3] Potential overlap between these 2 groups was not reported.
[4] Weighted average computed by the authors (238 out of 1252; range: 12.5%–26.9%).
[5] Weighted average computed by the authors (530 out of 2685; range: 13.8%–31.6%).
[6] Definite regression: at least 5 words used before regression, and strict language regression with or without regression of other skills; Lower level regression: loss of fewer words than five words, or of babble, or regression of other skills than language. The rates for definite and lower level regression can be summed up to derive a frequency of "any" regression.
[7] The first rate is for narrow autism, the figure within brackets is for broad ASD.
[8] Weighted average computed by the authors (603 out of 2757; range: 13.3%–29.6%).

Time Trends in Prevalence and Their Interpretation

The debate on the hypothesis of a secular increase in rates of autism has been obscured by a lack of clarity in the measures of disease occurrence used by investigators, or rather in the interpretation of their meaning. In particular, it is crucial to differentiate prevalence from incidence. Prevalence is useful to estimate needs and plan services; however, only incidence rates can be used for causal research. Both prevalence and incidence estimates will increase when case definition is broadened and case ascertainment is improved. Time trends in rates can therefore only be gauged in investigations that hold these parameters under strict control over time. These methodological requirements must be borne in mind while reviewing the evidence for a secular increase in rates of PDDs, or testing for the "epidemic" hypothesis. The "epidemic" hypothesis emerged in the 1990s when, in most countries, increasing numbers were diagnosed with PDDs leading to an upward trend in children registered in service providers databases that was paralleled by higher prevalence rates in epidemiological surveys. These trends were interpreted by some observers as evidence that the actual population incidence of PDDs was going up (what the term "epidemic" means); however, alternative explanations to explain the rise in numbers of children diagnosed with PDDs had to be ruled out first before attaining this conclusion.

Prevalence: the proportion of individuals in a population who suffer from a defined disorder at any point in time.

Incidence: the number of new cases occurring in a population over a period of time.

Several approaches to assessing this question have been used in the literature and these fall into 5 broad categories.

1. Use of Inappropriate Referral Statistics

Increasing numbers of children referred to specialist services or known to special education registers have been taken as evidence for an increased incidence of autism-spectrum disorders. Upward trends in national registries, medical, and educational databases have been seen in many different countries (Taylor et al., 1999; Madsen et al., 2002; Shattuck, 2006; Gurney et al., 2003), all occurring in the late 1980s and early 1990s. However, trends over time in *referred* samples are confounded by many factors such as referral patterns, availability of services, heightened public awareness, decreasing age at diagnosis, and changes over time in diagnostic concepts and practices, to name only a few. Failure to control for these confounding factors was obvious in some recent reports (Fombonne, 2001), such as the widely quoted reports from California Developmental Database Services (CDDS, 1999; CDDS, 2003). First, these reports applied to numbers rather than rates, and failure to relate these numbers to meaningful denominators left the interpretation of an upward trend vulnerable to changes in the composition of the underlying population. For example, the population of California was 19,971,000 in 1970 and rose to 35,116,000 as of July 1, 2002, a change of +75.8%. Second, the focus on the year-to-year changes in absolute numbers of subjects known to California state-funded services detracts from more meaningful comparisons. For example, as of December 2007, the total number of subjects with a PDD diagnosis was 31,332 in the 3–21 age group (including all CDER autism codes) (California Department of Developmental Services, December 2007). The population of 3–21 year olds of California was 9,976,768 on July 1, 2007 (Census Bureau for the US, 2009). If one applies the 2007 average U.S. rate of 67/10,000 deriving from the CDC (2007b), one would expect to have 66,844 subjects with a PDD, within this age group, living in California. The expected number is twice as high as the number of subjects recorded in the public service at the same time. The discrepancy would be more pronounced if the latest CDC figures of 9/1,000 (Table 6-4; CDC, 2009) were used to estimate the expected number of Californian residents with a PDD. Certainly, these calculations do not support the "epidemic" interpretation of the California DDS data, and confirm the selective nature of the referred sample. Unfortunately, these data have been misused in many ways to infer population trends and causes for autism in California, for which they are simply not suited. The upward trends in the DDS database simply suggest that children identified in the California DDS database were only a subset of the population prevalence pool and that the increasing numbers reflect merely an increasing proportion of children receiving services. Third, with one exception (see below), no attempt was made to adjust the trends for changes in diagnostic concepts and definitions. However, major nosographical modifications were introduced during the corresponding years with a general tendency in most classifications to broaden the concept of autism (as embodied in the terms "autism spectrum" or "pervasive developmental disorder"). Fourth, age characteristics of the subjects recorded in official statistics were portrayed in a misleading manner where the preponderance of young subjects was presented as evidence of increasing rates in successive birth cohorts (Fombonne, 2001). The problems associated with disentangling age from period and cohort effects in such observational data are well known in the epidemiological literature and deserve better statistical handling. Fifth, the decreasing age at diagnosis leads in itself to increasing numbers of young children being identified in official statistics (Wazana et al., 2007) or referred to specialist medical and educational services. Earlier identification of children from the prevalence pool may therefore result in increased service activity that may lead to a misperception by professionals of an "epidemic"; however, an increase in referrals does not necessarily mean increased *incidence*. A more refined analysis of the effect of a younger age at diagnosis using cumulative incidence data by age 5 years showed that 12% of the increase in incidence from the 1990 to the 1996 birth cohort could be explained by this factor, and up to 24% with an extrapolation to the 2002 cohort (Hertz-Picciotto & Delwiche, 2009). Although younger age at diagnosis can explain only a small proportion of the increase in diagnoses in this analysis, it does play a role in several published reports though its effect would attenuate as the cohort becomes older. Hertz-Picciotto and Delwiche's analysis (2009) of the California DDS data is also limited by their reliance on the DDS database that reflected changes in regional referral patterns, especially during that period.

Another study of this dataset was subsequently launched to demonstrate the validity of the "epidemic" hypothesis (MIND, 2002). The authors relied on DDS data and aimed at ruling out changes in diagnostic practices and immigration into California as factors explaining the increased numbers. While immigration was reasonably ruled out, the study comparing diagnoses of autism and mental retardation over time was impossible to interpret in light of the extremely low (< 20%) response rates. Furthermore, a study only based on cases registered for services cannot rule out that the proportion of cases within the general population who registered with services has changed over time. For example, assuming a constant incidence and prevalence at 2 different time points (i.e., hypothesizing no epidemic), the number of cases known to a public agency delivering services could well increase by 200% if the proportion of cases from the community referred to services rises from 25% to 75% in the same interval. In order to eliminate this plausible (see above) explanation, data over time are needed *both* on referred subjects *and* on nonreferred (or referred to other services) subjects. Failure to address this phenomenon precludes any inference to be drawn from a study of the California DDS database population to the California population (Fombonne, 2003a). The conclusions of this report were therefore simply unfounded.

2. The Role of Diagnostic Substitution

One possible explanation for increased numbers of a diagnostic category is that children presenting with the same developmental disability may receive one particular diagnosis at one time, and another diagnosis later. Such diagnostic substitution (or switching) may occur when diagnostic categories become increasingly familiar to health professionals and/or when access to better services is ensured by using a new diagnostic category. The strongest evidence of "diagnostic switching" contributing to the prevalence increase was produced in all U.S. states in a complex analysis of Department of Education Data in 50 U.S. states (Shattuck, 2006), indicating that a relatively high proportion of children previously diagnosed as having mental retardation were subsequently identified as having a PDD diagnosis. Shattuck showed that the odds of being classified in autism category increased by 1.21 during 1994–2003. In the meantime, the odds decreased significantly of being classified in the learning disability (LD) (odds ratio: OR = 0.98) and the mental retardation (MR) categories (OR = 0.97). He further demonstrated that the growing prevalence of autism was directly associated with decreasing prevalence of LD and MR within states, and that a significant downward deflection in the historical trajectories of LD and MR occurred when autism became reported in the United States as an independent category in 1993–94. Finally, this author showed that, from 1994 to 2003, the mean increase for the combined category of *Autism + Other Health Impairments +Trauma Brain Injury + Developmental Delay* was 12/1000, whereas the mean decrease for MR and LD was 11/1000 during the same period. One exception to that was California, for which previous authors had debated the presence of diagnostic substitution between MR and autism (Croen et al., 2002; Eagle, 2004). The previous investigations have largely relied on ecological, aggregated data that have known limitations. Using individual level data, a new study has reexamined the hypothesis of diagnostic substitution in the California DDS dataset (King & Bearman, 2009) and has shown that 24% of the increase in caseload was attributable to such diagnostic substitution (from the mental retardation to the autism category). It is important to keep in mind that other types of diagnostic substitution are likely to have occurred as well for milder forms of the PDD phenotype, from various psychiatric disorders (including childhood schizoid "personality" disorders; Wolff & Barlow, 1979) that have not been studied yet (Fombonne, 2009). For example, children currently diagnosed with Asperger's disorder were previously diagnosed with other psychiatric diagnoses (i.e., obsessive-compulsive disorder, school "phobia," social anxiety, etc.) in clinical settings before the developmental nature of their condition was fully recognized.

Diagnostic substitution occurs when an individual presenting with a diagnosis at one point in time receives another diagnosis later and is "re-classified".

Evidence of diagnostic substitution within the class of developmental disorders has also been provided in UK studies. Using the General Practitioner Research Database, Jick and Kaye (2003) have shown that the incidence of specific developmental disorders (including language disorders) decreased by about the same amount that the incidence of diagnoses of autism increased in boys born from 1990 to 1997. A more recent UK study (Bishop et al., 2008) has shown that up to 66% of adults previously diagnosed as children with developmental language disorders would meet diagnostic criteria for a broad definition of PDD. This change was observed for children initially diagnosed with specific language impairments, but even more so for those with a pragmatic language impairment.

3. Comparison of Cross-Sectional Epidemiological Surveys

As shown earlier, epidemiological surveys of autism each possess unique design features that could account almost entirely for between-studies variation in rates; therefore, time trends in rates of autism are difficult to gauge from published prevalence rates. The significant correlation previously mentioned between prevalence rate and year of publication for autistic disorder could merely reflect increased efficiency over time in case identification methods used in surveys as well as changes in diagnostic concepts and practices (Kielinen et al., 2000; Webb et al., 1997; Magnusson et al., 2001; Shattuck, 2006; Bishop et al., 2008). In studies using capture-recapture methods, it is apparent that up to a third of prevalent cases may be missed by an ascertainment source, even in recently conducted studies (Harrison et al., 2006). Evidence that method factors could account for most of the variability in published prevalence estimates comes from a direct comparison of 8 recent surveys conducted in the UK and the United States (Fombonne, 2005). In each country, 4 surveys were conducted around the same year and with similar age groups. As there is no reason to expect huge between-area differences in rates, prevalence estimates should therefore be comparable within each country. However, there was a 6-fold variation in rates for UK surveys, and a 14-fold variation in U.S. rates. In each set of studies, high rates derived from surveys where intensive population-based screening techniques were employed whereas lower rates were obtained from studies relying on passive administrative methods for case finding. Since no passage of time was involved, the magnitude of these gradients in rates can only be attributed to differences in case identification methods across surveys. Even more convincing evidence comes from the large survey by the CDC on 408,000 U.S. children aged 8 and born in 1994 (CDC, 2007b) where an average prevalence of 66/10,000 was reported for 14 U.S. states. One striking finding of this report is that there was more than a 3-fold variation in state specific rates that ranged from a low 33/10,000 for Alabama to a high of 106/10,000 in New Jersey. It would be surprising if there were truly this much variance in the number of children with autism in different states in the United States. These substantial differences most certainly reflected ascertainment variability across sites in a study that was otherwise performed with the same methods and at the same time. In the more recent CDC 11 states study (CDC, 2009), the same variability is reported again. Prevalence was significantly lower (7.5/1,000) in states that had access to health sources only compared to that (10.2/1,000) of states where educational data was also available. The authors also reported that the quality and quantity of information available in abtracted records (the main method for case ascertainment) had increased between the 2002 and 2006. Together with a reported average decrease of 5 months for the age at diagnosis and a larger increase in the non–mentally retarded population, these factors suggest that improved sensitivity in case ascertainment in the CDC monitoring network has contributed substantially to the increase in prevalence. Thus, no inference on trends in the incidence of PDDs can be derived from a simple comparison of prevalence rates over time, since studies conducted at different periods are likely to differ even more with respect to their methodologies.

4. Repeat Surveys in Defined Geographical Areas

Repeated surveys, using the same methodology and conducted in the same geographical area at different points in time, can potentially yield useful information on time trends provided that methods are kept relatively constant. The Göteborg studies (Gillberg et al., 1991; Gillberg, 1984) provided three prevalence estimates that increased over a short period of time from 4.0 (1980) to 6.6 (1984) and 9.5/10,000 (1988), the gradient being even steeper if rates for the urban area alone are considered (4.0, 7.5, and 11.6/10,000, respectively) (Gillberg et al., 1991). However, comparison of these rates is not straightforward, as different age groups were included in each survey. Secondly, the increased prevalence in the second survey was explained by improved detection among the mentally retarded, and that of the third survey by cases born to immigrant parents. That the majority of the latter group was born abroad suggests that migration into the area could be a key explanation. Taken in conjunction with a change in local services and a progressive broadening of the definition of autism over time that was acknowledged by the authors (Gillberg et al., 1991), these findings do not provide evidence for an increased incidence in the rate of autism. Similarly, studies conducted in Japan at different points in time in Toyota (Kawamura et al., 2008) and Yokohama (Honda et al., 1996 and 2005) showed rises in prevalence rates that their authors interpreted as reflecting the effect of both improved population screening of preschoolers and of a broadening of diagnostic concepts and criteria.

Two separate surveys of children born 1992–1995 and 1996–1998 in Staffordshire in the UK (Chakrabarti & Fombonne, 2001, 2005) were performed with rigorously identical methods for case definition and case identification. The prevalence for combined PDDs was comparable and not statistically different in the 2 surveys (Chakrabarti & Fombonne, 2005), suggesting no upward trend in overall rates of PDDs, at least during the short time interval between studies. In two recent CDC surveys (2007a, 2007b), the prevalence at six sites included in the 2000 and 2002 surveys remained constant at 4 sites, and increased in 2 states (Georgia and West Virginia), most likely due to improved quality of survey methods at these sites. In the 2009 CDC report, an average increase of 57% in prevalence was reported in 10 sites with 2002 and 2006 data, with a smaller increase in Colorado. Increases of different magnitude and directions were reported in all subgroups, making it difficult to detect a particular explanation. The CDC researchers identified a number of factors associated with the change in prevalence but could not conclude on the hypothesis of a real change in the risk of ASD in the population.

5. Successive Birth Cohorts

In large surveys encompassing a wide age range, increasing prevalence rates among most recent birth cohorts could be interpreted as indicating a secular increase in the incidence of the disorder, provided that alternative explanations can confidently be eliminated. This analysis was used in two large French surveys (Fombonne & du Mazaubrun, 1992; Fombonne et al., 1997). The surveys included birth cohorts from 1972 to 1985 (735,000 children, 389 of whom had autism), and, pooling the data of both surveys, age-specific rates showed no upward trend (Fombonne et al., 1997).

An analysis of special educational disability from Minnesota showed a 16-fold increase in the number of children identified with a PDD from 1991–1992 to 2001–2002 (Gurney et al., 2003). The increase was not specific to autism since, during the same period, an increase of 50% was observed for all disability categories (except severe mental handicap), especially for the category including ADHD. The large sample size allowed the authors to assess age, period, and cohort effects. Prevalence increased regularly in successive birth cohorts; for example, among 7-year-olds, the prevalence rose from 18/10,000 in those born in 1989, to 29/10,000 in those born in 1991 and to 55/10,000 in those born in 1993, suggestive of birth cohort effects. Within the *same* birth cohorts, age effects were also apparent since for children born in 1989 the prevalence rose with age from 13/10,000 at age 6, to 21/10,000 at age 9, and 33/10,000 at age 11. As argued by the authors, this pattern is not consistent with what one would expect from a chronic nonfatal condition diagnosed in the first years of life. Their analysis also showed a marked period effect that identified the early 1990s as the period where rates started to increase in all ages and birth cohorts. Gurney et al. (2003) further argued that this phenomenon coincided closely with the inclusion of PDDs in the federal Individual with Disabilities Educational Act (IDEA) funding and reporting mechanism in the United States. A similar interpretation of upward trends had been put forward by Croen et al. (2002) in their analysis of the California DDS data, and by Shattuck (2006) in his well-executed analysis of trends in the Department of Education data in all U.S. states.

Conclusion on Time Trends

As it stands now, the recent upward trend in rates of *prevalence* cannot be directly attributed to an increase in the *incidence* of the disorder, or to an "epidemic" of autism. There is good evidence that changes in diagnostic criteria, diagnostic substitution, changes in the policies for special education, and the increasing availability of services are responsible for the higher prevalence figures. It is also noteworthy that the rise in number of children diagnosed occurred at the same time in many countries (in the early 1990s), when radical shifts occurred in the ideas, diagnostic approaches, and services for children with PDDs. Alternatively, this might, of course, reflect the effect of environmental influences operating simultaneously in different parts of the world. However, there has been no proposed and legitimate risk mechanism to account for this worldwide effect. Most of the existing epidemiological data are inadequate to properly test hypotheses on changes in the incidence of autism in human populations. Moreover, due to the relatively low frequency of autism and PDDs, power is seriously limited in most investigations, and variations of small magnitude in the incidence of the disorder are very likely to go undetected. Equally, the possibility that a true increase in the incidence of PDDs has also partially contributed to the upward trend in prevalence rates cannot, and should not, be eliminated based on available data.

Conclusion

Epidemiological surveys of autism and PDDs have now been conducted in many countries. Methodological differences in case definition and case finding procedures make between survey comparisons difficult to perform. However, from recent studies, a best estimate of 70/10,000 (equivalences = 7/1,000; or 0.7%; or 1 child in about 143 children) can be confidently derived for the prevalence of autism spectrum disorders. Current evidence does not strongly support the hypothesis of a secular increase in the incidence of autism, but power to detect time trends is seriously limited in existing datasets. While it is clear that prevalence estimates have increased over time, this increase most likely represents changes in the concepts, definitions, service availability, and awareness of autistic-spectrum disorders in both the lay and professional public. To assess whether or not the incidence has increased, methodological factors that account for an important proportion of the variability in rates must be tightly controlled. New survey methods have been developed to be used in multinational comparisons; ongoing surveillance programs are currently under way and will soon provide more meaningful data to evaluate this hypothesis. The possibility that a true change in the underlying incidence has contributed to higher prevalence figures remains to be adequately tested. Meanwhile, the available prevalence figures carry straightforward implications for current and future needs in services and early educational intervention programs.

Challenges and Future Directions

- The boundaries of the spectrum of PDDs with both severe developmental and neurogenetic disorders and mild forms of atypical development remain uncertain and unreliable. Measures of impairment will need to be added to symptom and developmental assessments in order to refine case definitions for epidemiological studies and other research endeavors.
- Future epidemiological surveys should estimate the proportion of "false negatives" in order to estimate the sensitivity of case ascertainment methods and obtain more

accurate rates. Current prevalence rates underestimate the "true" prevalence rates as they are not adjusted to compensate for missed cases.

- Monitoring trends in prevalence and incidence is needed. It will require methods that allow meaningful comparisons over time of cases defined and ascertained with stable approaches.

SUGGESTED READINGS

Centers for Disease Control. Prevalence of autism spectrum disorders—Autism and developmental disabilities monitoring network, United States, 2006. *Morbidity and Mortality Weekly Report Surveillance Summary 2009*, *58*, 1–14.

Chakrabarti, S., & Fombonne, E. (2001). Pervasive developmental disorders in preschool children. *Journal of the American Medical Association*, *285*(24), 3093–3099.

Fombonne, E. (2007) Epidemiology. In A. Martin & F. Volkmar (Eds.), *Lewis's child and adolescent psychiatry: A comprehensive textbook* (4th ed., pp. 150–171). Lippincott, Williams, and Wilkins.

Shattuck, P. T. (2006). The contribution of diagnostic substitution to the growing administrative prevalence of autism in US special education. *Pediatrics*, *117*(4), 1028–1037.

REFERENCES

American Psychiatric Association. (1980). *Diagnostic and statistical manual of mental disorders* (3rd ed.). Washington, DC: Author.

American Psychiatric Association. (1987). *Diagnostic and statistical manual of mental disorders* (3rd ed., rev.). Washington, DC: Author.

American Psychiatric Association. (1994). *Diagnostic and statistical manual of mental disorders*. (4th ed.). Washington, DC: Author.

American Psychiatric Association. (2000). *Diagnostic and statistical manual of mental disorders* (4th ed., text rev.; DSM-IV-TR). Washington, DC: Author.

Arvidsson, T., Danielsson, B., Forsberg, P., Gillberg, C., Johansson, M., & Kjellgren, G. (1997). Autism in 3–6 year-olds in a suburb of Goteborg, Sweden. *Autism*, *2*, 163–173.

Baird, G., Charman, T., Baron-Cohen, S., Cox, A., Swettenham, J., Wheelwright, S., et al. (2000). A screening instrument for autism at 18 months of age: A 6-year follow-up study. *Journal of the American Academy of Child and Adolescent Psychiatry*, *39*, 694–702.

Baird, G., Charman, T., Pickles, A., Chandler, S., Loucas, T., Meldrum, D., et al. (2008). Regression, developmental trajectory, and associated problems in disorders in the autism spectrum: The SNAP study. *Journal of Autism and Developmental Disorders*, *38*(*10*), 1827–1836.

Baird, G., Simonoff, E., Pickles, A., Chandler, S., Loucas, T., Meldrum, D., et al. (2006). Prevalence of disorders of the autism spectrum in a population cohort of children in South Thames: The special needs and autism project (SNAP). *Lancet*, *368*(9531), 210–215.

Barbaresi, W. J., Katusic, S. K., Colligan, R. C., Weaver, A. L., & Jacobsen, S. J. (2005). The incidence of autism in Olmsted County, Minnesota, 1976–1997: Results from a population-based study. *Archives of Pediatrics and Adolescent Medicine*, *159*(1), 37–44.

Baron-Cohen, S., Scott, F. J., Allison, C., Williams, J., Bolton, P., Matthews, F. E., et al. Prevalence of autism-spectrum conditions: UK school-based population study. *British Journal of Psychiatry*, *194*(6), 500–509.

Bertrand, J., Mars, A., Boyle, C., Bove, F., Yeargin-Allsopp, M., & Decoufle, P. (2001). Prevalence of autism in a United States population: The Brick Township, New Jersey, investigation. *Pediatrics*, *108*(5), 1155–1161.

Bishop, D. V., Whitehouse, A. J., Watt, H. J., & Line, E. A. (2008). Autism and diagnostic substitution: Evidence from a study of adults with a history of developmental language disorder. *Developmental Medicine and Child Neurology*, *50*(5), 341–345.

Bohman, M., Bohman, I., Bjorck, P., & Sjoholm, E. (1983). Childhood psychosis in a northern Swedish county: Some preliminary findings from an epidemiological survey. In M. Schmidt & H. Remschmidt (Eds.), *Epidemiological approaches in child psychiatry* (pp. 164–173). Stuttgart: Georg Thieme Verlag.

Brask, B. (1970). A prevalence investigation of childhood psychoses. Paper presented at the *Nordic Symposium on the Care of Psychotic Children*, Oslo.

Bryson, S. E., Clark, B. S., & Smith, I. M. (1988). First report of a Canadian epidemiological study of autistic syndromes. *Journal of Child Psychology and Psychiatry and Allied Disciplines*, *29*(4), 433–445.

Burd, L., Fisher, W., & Kerbeshan, J. (1987). A prevalance study of pervasive developmental disorders in North Dakota. *Journal of the American Academy of Child and Adolescent Psychiatry*, *26*, 700–703.

California Department of Developmental Services. (2003, April). *Autism spectrum disorders: Changes in the California caseload–An update 1999 through 2002*. Available at http://www.dds.ca.gov/Autism/pdf/AutismReport2003.pdf

California Department of Developmental Services. (1999, March 1). *Changes in the population of persons with autism and pervasive developmental disorders in California's Developmental Services System: 1987 through 1998*. Report to the Legislature March 1, 1999, 19 pages. Available at http://www.dds.ca.gov

California Department of Developmental Services (2007, December). Table 34. Retrieved January 28, 2009 from http://www.dds.ca.gov/FactsStats/docs/Dec07_QRTTBLS.pdf.

Census Bureau for the US. Accessed January 28, 2009. http://www.census.gov/popest/states/asrh/SC-EST2007-01.html.

Centers for Disease Control. (2007a). Prevalence of autism spectrum disorders—Autism and developmental disabilities monitoring network, six sites, United States, 2000. *Morbidity and Mortality Weekly Report Surveillance Summary*, *56*(1), 1–11.

Centers for Disease Control. (2007b) Prevalence of autism spectrum disorders—Autism and developmental disabilities monitoring network, 14 sites, United States, 2002. *Morbidity and Mortality Weekly Report Surveillance Summary*, *56*(1), 12–28.

Centers for Disease Control. (2009). Prevalence of autism spectrum disorders—Autism and developmental disabilities monitoring network, United States, 2006. *Morbidity and Mortality Weekly Report Surveillance Summary 2009*, *58*, 1–14.

Chakrabarti, S., & Fombonne, E. (2001). Pervasive developmental disorders in preschool children. *Journal of the American Medical Association*, *285*(24), 3093–3099.

Chakrabarti, S., & Fombonne, E. (2005). Pervasive developmental disorders in preschool children: Confirmation of high prevalence. *American Journal of Psychiatry*, *162*(6), 1133–1141.

Cialdella, P., & Mamelle, N. (1989). An epidemiological study of infantile autism in a French department (Rhone): A research note. *Journal of Child Psychology and Psychiatry and Allied Disciplines, 30*(1), 165–175.

Croen, L. A., Grether, J. K., Hoogstrate, J., & Selvin, S. (2002). The changing prevalence of autism in California. *Journal of Autism and Developmental Disorders, 32*(3), 207–215.

Davidovitch, M., Holtzman, G., & Tirosh, E. (2001, March). Autism in the Haifa area: An epidemiological perspective. *Israeli Medical Association Journal, 3*, 188–189.

Eagle, R. S. (2004). Commentary: Further commentary on the debate regarding increase in autism in California. *Journal of Autism and Developmental Disorders, 34*(1), 87–88.

Ehlers, S., & Gillberg, C. (1993). The epidemiology of Asperger syndrome: A total population study. *Journal of Child Psychology and Psychiatry and Allied Disciplines, 34*(8), 1327–1350.

Ellefsen, A., Kampmann, H., Billstedt, E., Gillberg, I. C., & Gillberg, C. (2007). Autism in the Faroe islands: An epidemiological study. *Journal of Autism and Developmental Disorders, 37*(3), 437–444.

Fombonne, E. (2001). Is there an epidemic of autism? *Pediatrics, 107*, 411–413.

Fombonne, E. (2003a). Epidemiological surveys of autism and other pervasive developmental disorders: An update. *Journal of Autism and Developmental Disorders, 33*(4), 365–382.

Fombonne, E. (2003b). The prevalence of autism. *Journal of the American Medical Association, 289*(1), 1–3.

Fombonne, E. (2005). Epidemiology of autistic disorder and other pervasive developmental disorders. *Journal of Clinical Psychiatry, 66* (Suppl. 10), 3–8.

Fombonne, E. (2007) Epidemiology. In A. Martin & F. Volkmar (Eds.), *Lewis's child and adolescent psychiatry: A comprehensive textbook* (4th ed., pp. 150–171). Lippincott, Williams, and Wilkins.

Fombonne, E. (2009). Commentary: On King and Bearman. *International Journal of Epidemiology, 38*(5), 1241–1242.

Fombonne, E., & Chakrabarti, S. (2001). No evidence for a new variant of measles-mumps-rubella-induced autism. *Pediatrics, 108*(4), E58.

Fombonne, E., & du Mazaubrun, C. (1992). Prevalence of infantile autism in four French regions. *Social Psychiatry and Psychiatric Epidemiology, 27*(4), 203–210.

Fombonne, E., du Mazaubrun, C., Cans, C., & Grandjean, H. (1997). Autism and associated medical disorders in a French epidemiological survey. *Journal of the American Academy of Child and Adolescent Psychiatry, 36*(11), 1561–1569.

Fombonne, E., Simmons, H., Ford, T., Meltzer, H., & Goodman, R. (2001). Prevalence of pervasive developmental disorders in the British nationwide survey of child mental health. *Journal of the American Academy of Child and Adolescent Psychiatry, 40*(7), 820–827.

Fombonne, E., Zakarian, R., Bennett, A., Meng, L., & McLean-Heywood, D. (2006). Pervasive developmental disorders in Montreal, Quebec, Canada: Prevalence and links with immunizations. *Pediatrics, 118*(1), e139–e150.

Ghanizadeh, A. (2008). A preliminary study on screening prevalence of pervasive developmental disorder in school children in Iran. *Journal of Autism and Developmental Disorders, 38*(4), 759–763.

Gillberg, C. (1984). Infantile autism and other childhood psychoses in a Swedish urban region: Epidemiological aspects. *Journal of Child Psychology and Psychiatry and Allied Disciplines, 25*(1), 35–43.

Gillberg, C., Steffenburg, S., & Schaumann, H. (1991). Is autism more common now than ten years ago? *British Journal of Psychiatry, 158*, 403–409.

Gillberg, C., Cederlund, M., Lamberg, K., & Zeijlon, L. (2006). Brief report: "The autism epidemic." The registered prevalence of autism in a Swedish urban area. *Journal of Autism and Developmental Disorders, 36*(3), 429–435.

Gurney, J. G., Fritz, M. S., Ness, K. K., Sievers, P., Newschaffer, C. J., & Shapiro, E. G. (2003). Analysis of prevalence trends of autism spectrum disorder in Minnesota. *Archives of Pediatrics and Adolescent Medicine, 157*(7), 622–627.

Harrison, M. J., O'Hare, A. E., Campbell, H., Adamson, A., & McNeillage, J. (2006). Prevalence of autistic spectrum disorders in Lothian, Scotland: An estimate using the "capture-recapture" technique. *Archives of Disease in Childhood, 91*(1), 16–19.

Hertz-Picciotto I., & Delwiche L. (2009). The rise in autism and the role of age at diagnosis. *Epidemiology 38*(5), 84-90.

Honda, H., Shimizu, Y., Misumi, K., Niimi, M., & Ohashi, Y. (1996). Cumulative incidence and prevalence of childhood autism in children in Japan. *British Journal of Psychiatry, 169*, 228–235.

Honda, H., Shimizu, Y., & Rutter, M. (2005). No effect of MMR withdrawal on the incidence of autism: A total population study. *Journal of Child Psychology and Psychiatry and Allied Disciplines, 46*(6), 572–579.

Hoshino, Y., Kumashiro, H., Yashima, Y., Tachibana, R., & Watanabe, M. (1982). The epidemiological study of autism in Fukushima-Ken. *Folia Psychiatrica et Neurologica Japonica, 36*, 115–124.

Icasiano, F., Hewson, P., Machet, P., Cooper, C., & Marshall, A. (2004). Childhood autism spectrum disorder in the Barwon region: A community based study. *Journal of Paediatrics and Child Health, 40*(12), 696–701.

ICD-9. (1977). *The ICD-9 classification of mental and behavioural disorders: Clinical descriptions and diagnostic guidelines*. Geneva, World Health Organization.

ICD-10. (1992). *The ICD-10 classification of mental and behavioural disorders: Clinical descriptions and diagnostic guidelines*. Geneva, World Health Organization.

Jick, H., Kaye, J. A., & Black, C. (2003). Epidemiology and possible causes of autism changes in risk of autism in the UK for birth cohorts 1990–1998. *Pharmacotherapy, 23*(12), 1524–1530.

Kadesjo, B., Gillberg, C., & Hagberg, B. (1999). Brief report: Autism and Asperger syndrome in seven-year-old children: A total population study. *Journal of Autism and Developmental Disorders, 29*(4), 327–331.

Kawamura, Y., Takahashi, O., & Ishii, T. (2008). Reevaluating the incidence of pervasive developmental disorders: Impact of elevated rates of detection through implementation of an integrated system of screening in Toyota, Japan. *Psychiatry and Clinical Neurosciences, 62*(2), 152–159.

Kielinen, M., Linna, S.-L., & Moilanen, I. (2000). Autism in northern Finland. *European Child and Adolescent Psychiatry, 9*, 162–167.

King, M., & Bearman, P. (2009). Diagnostic change and the increase in prevalence of autism. *International Journal of Epidemiology, 38*(5), 1224–1234.

Kogan, M. D., Blumberg, S. J., Schieve, L. A., Boyle, C. A., Perrin, J. M., Ghandour, R. M., et al. (2009). Prevalence of parent-reported diagnosis of autism spectrum disorder among children in the US, 2007. *Pediatrics, 124* (5), 1395–1403.

Latif, A. H., & Williams, W. R. (2007). Diagnostic trends in autistic spectrum disorders in the South Wales valleys. *Autism, 11*(6), 479–487.

Lazoff, T., Zhong L., Piperni, T., & Fombonne, E. (2010). Prevalence rates of PDD among children in a Montreal School Board. *Canadian Journal of Child Psychiatry, 55*(11), 715–720.

Le Couteur, A., Rutter, M., Lord, C., Rios, P., Robertson, S., Holdgrafer, M., et al. (1989). Autism diagnostic interview: A standardized investigator-based instrument. *Journal of Autism and Developmental Disorders, 19*, 363–387.

Lord, C., Risi, S., Lambrecht, L., Cook, E. H., Jr., Leventhal, B. L., DiLavore, P. C., et al. (2000). The Autism Diagnostic Observation Schedule-Generic: A standard measure of social and communication deficits associated with the spectrum of autism. *Journal of Autism and Developmental Disorders, 30*(3), 205–223.

Lotter, V. (1966). Epidemiology of autistic conditions in young children: I. Prevalence. *Social Psychiatry, 1*, 124–137.

Madsen, K. M., Hviid, A., Vestergaard, M., Schendel, D., Wohlfahrt, J., Thorsen, P., et al. (2002). A population-based study of measles, mumps, and rubella vaccination and autism. *New England Journal of Medicine, 347*(19), 1477–1482.

Magnusson, P., & Saemundsen, E. (2001). Prevalence of autism in Iceland. *Journal of Autism and Developmental Disorders, 31*(2), 153–163.

Matsuishi, T., Shiotsuki, M., Yoshimura, K., Shoji, H., Imuta, F., & Yamashita, F. (1987). High prevalence of infantile autism in Kurume city, Japan. *Journal of Child Neurology, 2*, 268–271.

McCarthy, P., Fitzgerald, M., & Smith, M. (1984). Prevalence of childhood autism in Ireland. *Irish Medical Journal, 77*, 129–130.

Meilleur, A. A., & Fombonne, E. (2009). Regression of language and non-language skills in pervasive developmental disorders. *Journal of Intellectual Disability Research, 53*(2), 115–124.

MIND Institute. (2002, October 17). *Report to the Legislature on the Principal Findings from the epidemiology of autism in California. A comprehensive pilot study*. University of California, Davis.

Nicholas, J. S., Charles, J. M., Carpenter, L. A., King, L. B., Jenner, W., & Spratt, E. G. (2008). Prevalence and characteristics of children with autism-spectrum disorders. *Annals of Epidemiology, 18*(2), 130–136.

Oliveira, G., Ataide, A., Marques, C., Miguel, T. S., Coutinho, A. M., Mota-Vieira, L., et al. (2007). Epidemiology of autism spectrum disorder in Portugal: Prevalence, clinical characterization, and medical conditions. *Developmental Medicine and Child Neurology, 49*(10), 726–733.

Parr, J. R., Le Couteur, A., Baird, G., Fombonne, E., Rutter, M., Bailey, A. J., & International Molecular Genetic Study of Autism Consortium (IMGSAC). (submitted). Early developmental regression in autism: Evidence from an International Multiplex Sample.

Powell, J., Edwards, A., Edwards, M., Pandit, B., Sungum-Paliwal, S., & Whitehouse, W. (2000). Changes in the incidence of childhood autism and other autistic spectrum disorders in preschool children from two areas of the West Midlands, UK. *Developmental Medicine and Child Neurology, 42*, 624–628.

Ritvo, E., Freeman, B., Pingree, C., Mason-Brothers, A., Jorde, L., Jenson, W., et al. (1989). The UCLA-University of Utah epidemiologic survey of autism: Prevalence. *American Journal of Psychiatry, 146*, 194–199.

Rutter, M. (1970). Autistic children: Infancy to adulthood. *Seminars in Psychiatry, 2*(4), 435–450.

Scott, F. J., Baron-Cohen, S., Bolton, P., & Brayne, C. (2002). Brief report: Prevalence of autism spectrum conditions in children aged 5–11 years in Cambridgeshire, UK. *Autism, 6*(3), 231–237.

Shattuck, P. T. (2006). The contribution of diagnostic substitution to the growing administrative prevalence of autism in US special education. *Pediatrics, 117*(4), 1028–1037.

Shattuck, P. T., Durkin, M., Maenner, M., Newschaffer, C., Mandell, D. S., Wiggins, L., et al. (2009). Timing of identification among children with an autism spectrum disorder: Findings from a population-based surveillance study. *Journal of the American Academy of Child and Adolescent Psychiatry, 48*(5), 474–483.

Sponheim, E., & Skjeldal, O. (1998). Autism and related disorders: Epidemiological findings in a Norwegian study using icd-10 diagnostic criteria. *Journal of Autism and Developmental Disorders, 28*, 217–227.

Steffenburg, S., & Gillberg, C. (1986). Autism and autistic-like conditions in Swedish rural and urban areas: a population study. *British Journal of Psychiatry, 149*(1), 81–87.

Steinhausen, H.-C., Gobel, D., Breinlinger, M., & Wohlloben, B. (1986). A community survey of infantile autism. *Journal of the American Academy of Child Psychiatry, 25*, 186–189.

Sugiyama, T., & Abe, T. (1989). The prevalence of autism in Nagoya, Japan: A total population study. *Journal of Autism and Developmental Disorders, 19*, 87–96.

Tanoue, Y., Oda, S., Asano, F., & Kawashima, K. (1988). Epidemiology of infantile autism in southern Ibaraki, Japan: Differences in prevalence in birth cohorts. *Journal of Autism and Developmental Disorders, 18*, 155–166.

Taylor, B., Miller, E., Farrington, C., Petropoulos, M.-C., Favot-Mayaud, I., Li, J., et al. (1999, June 12). Autism and measles, mumps, and rubella vaccine: No epidemiological evidence for a causal association. *Lancet, 353*, 2026–2029.

Taylor, B., Miller, E., Lingam, R., Andrews, N., Simmons, A., & Stowe, J. (2002). Measles, mumps, and rubella vaccination and bowel problems or developmental regression in children with autism: Population study. *British Medical Journal, 324*(7334), 393–396.

Tebruegge, M., Nandini, V., & Ritchie, J. (2004). Does routine child health surveillance contribute to the early detection of children with pervasive developmental disorders? An epidemiological study in Kent, UK. *BMC Pediatrics, 4*, 4.

Treffert, D. A. (1970). Epidemiology of infantile autism. *Archives of General Psychiatry, 22*, 431–438.

van Balkom, I. D. C., Bresnahan, M., Vogtländer, M. F., van Hoeken, D., Minderaa, R., Susser, E., et al. (2009). Prevalence of treated autism spectrum disorders in Aruba. *Journal of Neurodevelopmental Disorders, 1*, 197–204.

Wazana, A., Bresnahan, M., & Kline, J. (2007). The autism epidemic: Fact or artifact? *Journal of the American Academy of Child and Adolescent Psychiatry, 46*(6), 721–730.

Webb, E., Lobo, S., Hervas, A., Scourfield, J., & Fraser, W. (1997). The changing prevalence of autistic disorder in a Welsh health district. *Developmental Medicine and Child Neurology, 39*, 150–152.

Webb, E., Morey, J., Thompsen, W., Butler, C., Barber, M., & Fraser, W. I. (2003). Prevalence of autistic spectrum disorder in children attending mainstream schools in a Welsh education authority. *Developmental Medicine and Child Neurology, 45*(6), 377–384.

Wignyosumarto, S., Mukhlas, M., & Shirataki, S. (1992). Epidemiological and clinical study of autistic children in Yogyakarta, Indonesia. *Kobe Journal of Medical Sciences, 38*(1), 1–19.

Williams, J. G., Brayne, C. E., & Higgins, J. P. (2006). Systematic review of prevalence studies of autism spectrum disorders. *Archives of Disease in Childhood, 91*(1), 8–15.

Williams, E., Thomas, K., Sidebotham, H., & Emond, A. (2008). Prevalence and characteristics of autistic spectrum disorders in the ALSPAC cohort. *Developmental Medicine and Child Neurology*, *50*(9), 672–677.

Wing, L., & Gould, J. (1979). Severe impairments of social interaction and associated abnormalities in children: Epidemiology and classification. *Journal of Autism and Developmental Disorders*, *9*, 11–29.

Wing, L., Yeates, S., Brierly, L., & Gould, J. (1976). The prevalence of early childhood autism: Comparison of administrative and epidemiological studies. *Psychological Medicine*, *6*, 89–100.

Wolff, S., & Barlow, A. (1979). Schizoid personality in childhood: A comparative study of schizoid, autistic and normal children. *Journal of Child Psychology and Psychiatry*, *20* (1), 29–46.

Wong, V. C., & Hui, S. L. (2008). Epidemiological study of autism spectrum disorder in China. *Journal of Child Neurology*, *23*(1), 67–72.

Yeargin-Allsopp, M., Rice, C., Karapurkar, T., Doernberg, N., Boyle, C., & Murphy, C. (2003). Prevalence of autism in a US metropolitan area[comment]. *Journal of the American Medical Association*, *289*(1), 49–55.

7 Roy Richard Grinker, Marshalyn Yeargin-Allsopp, Coleen Boyle

Culture and Autism Spectrum Disorders: The Impact on Prevalence and Recognition

Points of Interest

- Autism exists throughout the world, even in societies that have no name for it.
- Understanding how culture influences the recognition, definition, and treatment of autism may lead to better prevalence estimates.
- Public and private funding agencies now support epidemiological research in low and middle-income countries to explore how autism varies internationally in terms of its clinical manifestation and the extent of disability associated with the disorder.
- Autism spectrum disorders and *explanations* of developmental disorders (scientific or otherwise) are products of the interplay between biological, psychological, and cultural phenomena.
- Local factors affecting "administrative" prevalence estimates include poverty, access to services, racial discrimination, stigma, cultural beliefs about what kinds of behavior are "normal" and "abnormal," and a nation's health and public health infrastructure.

Awareness of the prevalence and phenotypes of autism spectrum disorders (ASD) has increased significantly over the past decade, especially in North America and the United Kingdom. Knowledge about ASD has also begun to spread internationally to countries such as India, South Korea, and Kenya, where the fields of developmental psychology, developmental pediatrics, and child psychiatry are less robust and where clinicians and educators do not generally distinguish ASD from other neurodevelopmental disorders, such as intellectual disability or learning disorders.

A search of published ASD research activities across the globe, however, might suggest that there is little knowledge about ASD outside of North America and Western Europe. Indeed, there are insufficient data to estimate the prevalence of autism in the Caribbean, Central and South America, Eastern Europe, the Middle East, South and Southeast Asia, and the entire continent of Africa (see Table 7-1; Figures 7-1 and 7-2). Mapping the prevalence of autism, as seen in Figure 7-2, can be misleading, as it does not reflect the history of autism research or the recent growth around the world in awareness and expertise. For example, Hans Asperger, whose studies of ASD were foundational to the field today and whose descriptions are, for the most part, still relevant today, was Austrian. Leo Kanner, the psychiatrist who first described autism, was Austrian-American and was deeply influenced by an Italian scientist, de Sanctis, who in 1906 published case reports on early onset "dementia praecox" (probably autism) in a group of children with intellectual disability.

In addition, despite the absence of international epidemiological studies, awareness, advocacy, and opportunities for treatment and education of children and adults with ASD are advancing rapidly throughout the world. Today, national autism societies exist in more than 100 different countries, and scientific research on ASD is underway in eastern and southern Africa, India, several Middle Eastern countries, Mexico, Venezuela, and a host of other nations.

For a number of reasons, continued growth of international research on ASDs, and neurodevelopmental disorders in general, should be expected. First, the number of child mental health professionals in non-Western countries is rising. Second, recent large-scale collaborations between UNICEF, WHO, the World Bank, and university-based scientists, have led to improved recognition of developmental and intellectual disabilities among children living in poverty in the developing world, as evidenced by a high-profile series of articles on child development in *The Lancet* in 2007. In war-torn countries, some United Nations peacekeepers are now trained to provide services to individuals with autism.

Third, as low and middle-income countries advance economically, and infectious diseases and child mortality

Table 7–1.
Autism prevalence around the world (2000–2009)

Continent/Region	Country	Prevalence	Reference
North America	United States	~90/10,000 = 1/110	ADDM 2009
	Canada	~65/10,000 = 1/154	Fombonne et al. 2006
Caribbean	Dominican Republic, Aruba, other	**Insufficient Data**	
Central America	Mexico, Costa Rica, Panama, other	**Insufficient Data**	
South America	Venezuela, Brazil, Chile, other	**Insufficient Data**	
Europe	UK	~116/10,000 = 1/86	Baird et al., 2006
	Sweden	~53/10,000 = 1/188	Gillberg et al., 2006
	Finland	~12/10,000 = 1/833	Kielinen et al., 2000
	Denmark	~12/10,000 = 1/833	Lauritsen et al., 2004
	Iceland	~13/10,000 = 1/769	Magnusson & Saemundsen, 2001
	France, Spain, Italy, Greece, other	**Insufficient Data**	
Eastern Europe	Russia, Poland, others	**Insufficient Data**	
Middle East	Israel, Qatar, Saudi Arabia, other	**Insufficient Data**	
Africa	All regions	**Insufficient Data**	
South-central Asia	India, Bangladesh, others	**Insufficient Data**	
Eastern Asia	Japan	~89/10,000 = 1/112	Honda et al., 2005
	China	**Insufficient Data**	
	Korea	**Insufficient Data**	
Southeast Asia	Taiwan, Singapore, Thailand, other	**Insufficient Data**	
Oceania	Australia	~39/10,000 = 1/256	Icasiano et al., 2004
	New Zealand	**Insufficient Data**	

[1] Table based on data published 2000 or later.
[2] Some findings may not be comparable across sites due to differences in study design, case ascertainment techniques, and among sample populations.

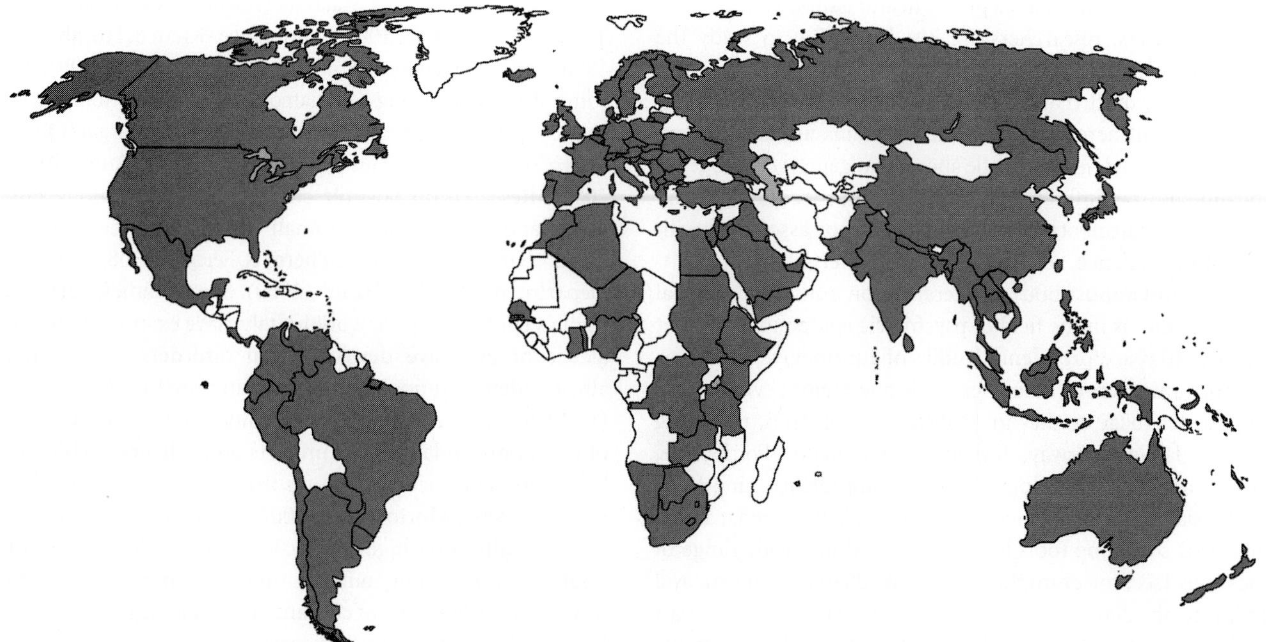

Figure 7–1. Map of autism societies around the world as of 2008 (Map courtesy of Tamara Daley).

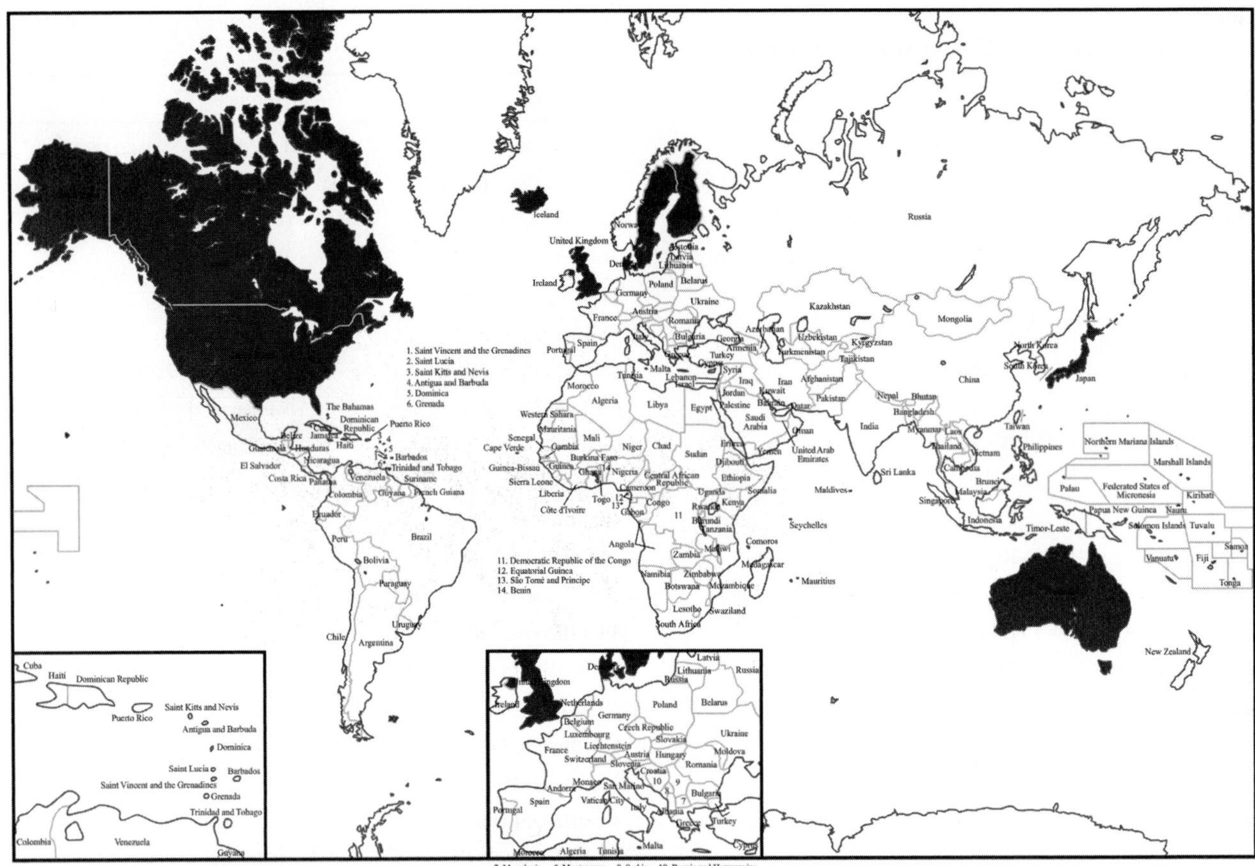

Figure 7–2. Map of autism prevalence studies around the world (2000–2008).

become less of a concern, disability and child development become more prominent as public health issues.

Nonetheless, researchers are just beginning to study the extent to which ASD varies across cultures. Although most researchers expect that the onset and core symptoms of ASD are consistent across cultures, this remains an assumption. ASD experts to date know little about how genetic heterogeneity and cultural differences interact to influence the kind and range of impairments that are essential to or associated with ASD, its prevalence, course, or familial patterns.

The most robust body of literature on autism as a global phenomenon is in the field of psychiatric epidemiology. Over the past 40 years, prevalence studies of autism have been conducted in numerous countries, with one major review citing English-language studies in 13 different countries, including France, Japan, Norway, Iceland, and Finland (Fombonne, 2003, 2009). Epidemiological findings are forthcoming from East Asia and South America (Montiel-Nava & Peña, 2008) and ASD screening tools have been tested in a wide range of locations (see, for example, Lung et al., 2010 on Taiwan, and Eldin et al., 2008 on the Middle East). However, the vast majority of prevalence studies have been conducted in the United Kingdom and North America.

A few case reports and screenings have been published for other countries, such as Malaysia (Kasmini & Zasmani, 1995), Taiwan (Chang et al., 2003), Zimbabwe (Khan & Hombarume, 1996), and the United Arab Emirates (Sartawi, 1999), with some studies reporting associated medical conditions such as mitochondrial respiratory chain disorders in Portugal (Oliveira et al., 2007) and Möbius sequence in Brazil (Bandim et al., 2002). Research on possible clusters of autism among Europeans and Americans of Somali origin is in the beginning stages (Barnevik-Olsson, Gillberg, & Fernell, 2008; Minnesota Department of Public Health, 2009). Some studies, such as La Malfa's epidemiological work in Italy, have examined the prevalence of pervasive developmental disorders (PDD) in an already identified pool of children with intellectual disabilities (La Malfa et al., 2004). Others examine ASD as one of a group of conditions in large-scale projects on challenging childhood behaviors or developmental disorders in general (Holden & Gitleson, 2006; Morton et al., 2002). At least one British study noted significantly higher prevalence of childhood cognitive disabilities, including autism, among citizens of Pakistani origin, whose high rate of consanguineous marriage is believed to be related to a rate of birth defects that is higher than the general population in the United Kingdom (Morton et al., 2002).

DSM criteria for ASD have been tested in multiple countries, and genetic research involves samples from populations throughout Western Europe. However, with the exception of Lotter's brief, anecdotal survey of autism prevalence in six African countries (1978) and Probst's exploratory survey of the stresses and demands of parents of children with autism in Brazil, Germany, Greece, and Italy (1998), there are, to our knowledge, no published cross-national studies that address the impact of culture on ASD. There is also very little information about how the genetics, biology, risk factors, treatment, and course of ASD differ across continents, countries, or ethnic groups. This chapter focuses on the international prevalence and diagnosis of autism because these are the areas in which international scientific publications exist. We consider the effect of culture on the conceptualization and identification of ASD, with special attention to the question of how studies of the sociocultural contexts of ASD, and neuropsychiatric disorders in general, can help us frame future international ASD research.

Given the fact that the majority of research on ASD has been carried out within the mental health field, we situate the research within the larger framework of psychiatric and psychological studies. However, we recognize that as research on ASD progresses, a greater number of studies will consider ASD from alternative, nonpsychiatric perspectives, such as within the context of a neurodevelopmental disorders framework.

Recognition and Epidemiology

Research to date has highlighted cross-national differences in the symptoms and course of psychiatric disorders. For example, although the age of onset and prevalence of both schizophrenia and obsessive-compulsive disorder are remarkably consistent across the globe, sex ratios, comorbid conditions, symptom expression, severity, and prognosis vary significantly (Hopper et al., 2007; Horwath & Weissman, 2000; Lemelson, 2003). Moreover, although researchers may use standardized assessments and criteria (at the very least, DSM and ICD criteria) to determine whether an individual constitutes a "case" of autism, clinicians who are not integrated into a research community—physicians and psychologists who see patients in private or clinic settings—may conform to folk categories of illness or rely on past training and personal clinical experience. Even with standardized criteria, considerable subjectivity and differences in clinical assessments exist, since the diagnosis depends on patient or caretaker narrative and behavioral observation rather than laboratory tests. Indeed, variations in diagnosis within and between societies can sometimes be explained in terms of the differences between research and clinical practice.

Cross-cultural variations in psychiatric diagnoses can be found, even between communities whose scientific traditions are often assumed to be similar, such as the United States and the United Kingdom. In a landmark study of the differences between British and American psychiatrists (whose scientific cultures are not dramatically different), R. E. Kendell (1971) and his colleagues showed a video of a socially awkward man, described as a 30-year-old bachelor, and asked British and American psychiatrists to give a diagnosis based only on the video. Sixty-nine percent of the American psychiatrists diagnosed the man with schizophrenia; only 2% of British psychiatrists gave that diagnosis (a large number of the British clinicians gave a diagnosis of manic-depressive illness). Shifts in classification occur for many reasons—such as the need to screen and treat soldiers in military conflicts, shifts in the way the insurance industry conceptualizes appropriate reimbursements, and public attitudes about the stigma of mental illness—that have little to do with advances in science and much to do with social and historical context (Grinker, 2010a). The classifications of the most empirically verifiable disorders, such as bacterial or viral infections, evolve and are formed by consensus. A disorder, even one with a clear cause or biomarker, is only a disorder when a society construes it as such. Thus, although Asperger's disorder is scheduled for elimination from the proposed DSM-5, this does not mean that Asperger's once existed as a real disease and now has disappeared. Asperger's was useful when a non-stigmatizing term was needed for people with the disorder, but clinicians now question it for both cultural and scientific reasons. From the perspective of culture, Asperger's is fast becoming obsolete as a scientific category as the stigma of autism declines. Societies throughout the world are beginning to appreciate the strengths and capabilities of people with autism, and people with autism increasingly feel less self-stigma and may advocate for their needs in public forums. From the perspective of science, clinicians recognize that almost everyone with Asperger's also fits the profile of the more classic autistic disorder. Indeed, in the current diagnostic manual, the DSM-IV, a child who has good language acquisition and intelligence qualifies as autistic if, in addition to having restricted interests and problems with social interactions, he has just one of the following symptoms, which are common among children with Asperger's: difficulty conversing, an inability to engage in make-believe play or repetitive or unusual use of language. Even the best available diagnostic instruments, such as the ADOS and ADI-R, cannot clearly identify distinct subtypes on the autism spectrum (Grinker, 2010b).

The social construction of psychiatric classification can be illustrated by the differences between ASD diagnostic classification and research in the United States and France. In the United States, the American Psychiatric Association removed autism from the category of "psychosis" in 1980, but the French child psychiatric establishment, which uses its own indigenous manual of mental disorders, the *Classification Française des Troubles Mentaux de l'Enfant et de l'Adolescent* (CFTMEA), classified autism as a psychosis until November 2004. French health professionals also conceptualize the etiology of autism in a manner that is different from other European countries and consider the American classification of PDDs to be a product of Anglo-American culture.

Since French health professionals generally view autism as a problem that lies within family social relationships and with the mother-child relationship in particular, there are only a few psychiatric or medical centers with expertise on autism as a genetic or brain disorder.

In recent years, a battle has erupted between French parents, armed with scientific studies and classifications from the United States and the United Kingdom, and French child psychiatrists. French health professionals generally retain a more restricted concept of autism and are openly hostile to behavioral interventions, such as the Treatment and Education of Autistic and Related Communication-Handicapped Children (TEACCH) program or Applied Behavioral Analysis, and to parent and parent association efforts to shift the locus of autism treatment from the hospital to the school (Chamak, 2008). Despite the efforts of parents, autism research and treatment in France continues to be guided largely by psychoanalytic thought, in particular the idea that autism is a disorder of object relations. Research on treatment emphasizes play therapy and interactive techniques to facilitate the growth of autonomy and a sense of self.

A clinical trial is underway in Lille, France, on the controversial therapy called "packing," in which a child is wrapped tightly in wet, refrigerated sheets, for approximately sixty minutes while clinicians attempt to talk with them about their feelings. The therapy is based on an argument that a child's ability to establish a proper relationship between his internal world and his external, social reality depends on his ability to merge his body and his body image (Spinney, 2007).

One reason for the absence of a large number of cross-national studies in mental health is that, in addition to being expensive and difficult to coordinate, the standardized assessments and classifications needed for such studies are of somewhat recent origin. American psychiatrists and psychologists have become keenly interested in diagnostic classification only in the last 3 decades. As one result, psychiatric epidemiological studies using comparable methods did not begin in earnest until the 1970s, and there were few cross-national studies conducted until the 1990s. The World Health Organization (WHO) international studies of schizophrenia began in 1968 and eventually included thirty research sites in nineteen countries and involved a 26-year follow-up period. These studies represent the most ambitious and lengthy cross-cultural explorations of the manifestations, course, and outcomes of a mental illness. Yet, as recently as 2004, only two prevalence studies of mental disorders among European adults had used comparable methods of ascertainment at the same time in more than one country (ESEMeD/MHEDEA, 2004). However, if we accept Cohen and Volkmar's assertion about autism, in relation to the DSM-IV and ICD-9 criteria that "There is no other developmental or psychiatric disorder of children (or perhaps of any age) for which such well-grounded and internationally accepted diagnostic criteria exist," cross-national studies should be feasible (Cohen & Volkmar, 1997).

Although there is a rapidly growing literature on international studies of neurodevelopmental disorders, and ASD in particular, there are few estimates of the prevalence of physical disabilities among children in low and middle-income countries and even fewer of behavioral disorders (Yeargin-Allsopp & Boyle, 2002). Researchers have made significant progress internationally, studying some disorders in childhood that have a neurodevelopmental component, such as cerebral palsy and epilepsy. Among psychiatric disorders, ADHD and conduct disorder have been studied extensively across the globe (Faraone et al., 2003; Polanczyk et al., 2007). However, epidemiological research on childhood onset disorders lags behind the epidemiology of such disorders in adults. Even within the area of the epidemiology of child mental disorders, more is known about psychiatric disorders in older children and adolescents than in younger children.

One area of progress in the diagnosis and epidemiology of autism across cultures has been at the level of screening, in particular the development of brief screening tools that can be validated in numerous languages and dialects and administered with minimal training. For example, the Childhood Autism Rating Scale (CARS) (Schopler et al., 1988), a 15-item, behavioral rating scale has been shown to be both sensitive and specific for ASD; the Autism Behavior Checklist (ABC) (Krug et al., 1980) includes 57 items but nonetheless takes less than 20 minutes to complete; and the Autism Spectrum Screening Questionnaire (ASSQ) (Ehlers et al., 1999), a 10-minute, 25-item rating scale appears to be particularly good at screening for high-functioning autism and Asperger's disorder. These scales have been used successfully in international research, have proved both reliable and specific, and are thus valuable in clinical and community-based settings. A broader approach, especially applicable in low and middle-income countries, is to screen children initially for an array of neurodevelopmental disabilities and then administer a condition-specific assessment for children who screen positive. This model was initially developed by Durkin et al. (1992) using a short questionnaire that includes only ten questions (known as the "ten questions screen"). More recently, the ten questions screen has been adapted by Indian researchers as part of the International Clinical Epidemiology Network (INCLEN) in India for a community-based screening study of autism and other developmental disorders among children ages 2–9 years.

In research settings in which scientists trained in the diagnosis of developmental disabilities are available, screenings are useful as a first-stage diagnostic tool. More lengthy and substantial diagnostic assessments are then performed with tools such as the Autism Diagnostic Observation Schedule (ADOS) (Lord et al., 1999) and the Autism Diagnostic Interview (ADI) (Rutter et al., 2003), both of which have been translated, validated, and are available for purchase in twelve European languages and Korean. Numerous other translations are underway, but more are needed. As one researcher in Thailand noted (where no translations of these tools have been validated), even when researchers and clinicians can characterize ASD as conforming to DSM-IV criteria, they cannot confirm the diagnoses in the absence of Thai-translated, standardized investigator-based instruments and structured observational schedules (Chuthapisith et al., 2007).

Conducting Prevalence Studies in International Settings

In the United States and United Kingdom, investigators now ideally use a two-stage approach to estimate autism prevalence, and this approach is capable of detecting more cases than ever before. In general, the approach involves a screening phase to identify a pool of children who may have an ASD, followed by a diagnostic confirmation stage. The methods for both phases vary widely, and their validity is dependent on the clinical and educational infrastructure in the country or setting. The screening stage can range from a general population screen in a primary care setting, as done by Honda et al. (2005), to a screening of children identified in high-risk settings, such as special education schools. High-risk screening can be based on canvassing records in schools or health care settings that target children with developmental delays or administering an autism screening instrument to a knowledgeable informant, such as a parent, guardian or teacher, or a combination of these two.

The targeted approach to case screening has become easier in many countries in recent years due to better awareness of autism and, presumably, a combination of more accurate clinical diagnosis and critical policy level changes that promote identification. For example, in the United States, beginning in the 1991–1992 school year, autism became a separate area of "exceptionality," meaning that children with autism could receive special education services specifically designated for children with autism. The U.S. Department of Education required schools to report, as part of an annual "child count," the number of children receiving these services under the autism classification. The child count made it significantly easier to locate potential case children from school records. To add even more cases, the CDC studies examined records of children with educational classifications beyond autism, such as behavior disorders and intellectual disabilities, since all children with autism are not necessarily classified by schools as autistic. In low and middle-income countries, a records-based screening approach may not be feasible, because of the absence of records or because the diagnosis of autism is either unknown or rarely used. In such situations, researchers will have to screen individuals rather than records.

In the best of circumstances, a researcher can combine a record review with individual screening. During the individual screening, parents and teachers fill out standardized third-party questionnaires such as the Autism Screening Questionnaire (ASQ) or the Autism Spectrum Syndrome Screening Questionnaire (ASSQ). These questionnaires, which have been studied extensively for their reliability—i.e., to make sure that independent researchers using them with the same case would come to the same conclusion—help epidemiologists identify potential cases, especially when two or more instruments with different sensitivities are used together. However, in some countries, it may be impractical to use parent self-administered screening tools for a variety of reasons. For example, many parents in low and middle income countries may have low literacy, especially mothers (since women often have more limited access to education then men), and may thus be unable to complete the surveys. Also, for political reasons, parents in some countries may be afraid of having their child's health condition codified in writing.

In the second stage—diagnostic confirmation—epidemiologists ideally use trained diagnosticians to confirm case status among those who screen positive. If the screening phase was based on a record review, a standardized review process is established to determine case status (for examples, see Barbaresi et al., 2005; Honda et al., 2005; Williams et al., 2005; Powell et al., 2000; Lauritsen et al., 2004; and Autism and Developmental Disabilities Monitoring Network [ADDM], 2009). Because the study population is much smaller at the confirmation stage, assessments can be done in person with each child, preferably with more than one structured, reliable diagnostic assessment, such as the combination of the ADOS (a *synchronic* observation schedule over one 2- to 3-hour period of time) and the ADI (an extended parent/guardian interview that provides a detailed history, or *diachronic* perspective, on the child). Ideally, for both methods (record-based and in-person assessments) the confirmatory diagnoses are then validated by outside consultants using a group of randomly selected cases (some with and some without an autism diagnosis). This second stage is especially important for validating the less clear-cut cases, such as the ones on the border between two different diagnoses or between a diagnosis and none at all.

We have entered a period in history in which autism awareness is at an all-time high and in which the diagnosis of autism has broadened to include a range of different people along a wide spectrum. This is largely due to the current use of the two-stage case-finding approach, which yields many more cases of autism than the older studies. In addition, researchers ideally employ quality control measures, such as blinded reviewers, to establish interrater reliability. However, it must be stressed that it is exceedingly difficult and expensive to use such thorough and rigorous methods. Implementation of the gold standard assessments for autism is particularly challenging in low-income countries. Extensive training is necessary to obtain test reliability. Considerable participant burden is associated with the length of time, often several hours, to administer the assessments. Furthermore, in countries in which little research has been conducted on child development, the validity of results from such protocols will be hampered by the absence of established, documented norms of child development for a given population. Epidemiological studies in the low and middle-income country setting will therefore benefit from the development of more efficient and affordable diagnostic assessments.

Challenges to ASD Surveillance

The epidemiology of ASD should be understood in the context of the many challenges inherent in applying diagnostic criteria to growing and developing children in different cultural contexts. It is not feasible to produce a list of criteria for a disability that will be relevant at all developmental levels, and what counts as normal or abnormal development will vary from culture to culture. There is the obvious problem that researchers who study school-age children face the difficult task of reliably defining cases on the basis of information presented in teacher reports (which can be heavily influenced by a multitude of factors, such as class size, teacher training, and the local, cultural attitudes toward discipline and about what kinds of behaviors are age appropriate) and parent reports (which are influenced by the particularities of the parent who completes the report). For some childhood onset psychiatric disorders, estimates may appear higher in a country with great awareness among parents, educators, and clinicians; access to services; or in which the national government mandates the use of "autism" as a diagnostic term. In contrast, estimates may be lower in a country with little awareness, few services, and lack of research studies, especially of administrative prevalence. For example, school and clinic records of "autism" and "traumatic brain injury" grew tremendously following the 1991–1992 school year, when the U.S. Department of Education first introduced these terms to the American public school system (Newschaffer et al., 2005).

Previous studies confirm significant variations among locations, even within the same country, as the Centers for Disease Control and Prevention showed from their multisite surveillance network. Recent prevalence estimates for Arizona and Missouri (12.1 per 1000) were higher than those from Florida (ADDM, 2009). Research in Australia has demonstrated considerable variability in diagnostic rates across states and between state and national records. In Queensland, the number of diagnoses of ASD exceeds that of other states, since Queensland requires a DSM-IV diagnosis for eligibility for services but other Australian states do not (Skellern et al., 2005).

Moreover, clinicians will not make or record a particular diagnosis, and parents will not seek it, unless the diagnostic term is meaningful and in current use. Thus, for example, the Navajo Indians of the American Southwest tend to classify autism as "perpetual childhood" (Conners & Donnellan, 1995), and throughout most of India, clinicians call autism *paagol*, the Hindi word for "madness" (Daley, 2002, 2003). School and clinic records for a child with ASD, if there are any records kept, will not list the word "autism." In rural South Korea, the catch-all "brain disorder" can be used for children with disorders including traumatic brain injury, autism, epilepsy, speech and language disorders, Down syndrome, and other clearly genetic disorders. In this setting, record reviews will yield few cases of autism.

Researchers should expect to encounter additional obstacles when attempting to do public health screening in general and ascertain and classify neurodevelopmental disorders in societies with low access to services. Illness categories are beneficial only if there is something one can do with them. Thus, for many American adults with ASD who require public assistance, it makes little sense to carry an autism diagnosis in states where services for adults with autism are provided only under the category of intellectual disability, or formerly "mental retardation." In urban India, where there are few autism-related services, a clinician is unlikely to give a diagnosis of autism since the clinician may believe that it would only confuse the family, the school system, and potential service providers (Daley & Sigman, 2002; Daley, 2003). Indian pediatricians interviewed by Daley (2003) and Grinker (2007) use a much more well-known category—mental retardation, popularly glossed as "madness"—even if it is sometimes inaccurate, and they will justify it by arguing that the treatments and educational services in India for someone with mental retardation are identical to those for someone with autism. For this reason, records-based approaches to the epidemiology of autism in societies where "autism" is uncommonly used as a diagnostic term are not feasible. Even in societies where the concept of autism does exist, people may not seek care from the experts who are familiar with the term. Indeed, epidemiologists should not assume that the population being studied shares the researchers' understanding about the relationship between the symptoms being studied and the name of the disease. In Korea, for example, despite dramatic changes in autism awareness, the word for autism (*chap'ae*) has quite negative connotations because many people mistakenly believe that all individuals with the diagnosis are profoundly intellectually disabled and nonverbal. The Korean research team in the first author's prevalence study of ASD worked hard to explain to teachers and parents the concept of an autism *spectrum* (Grinker, 2007). Toward this goal, researchers asked the child psychiatrists who led the information sessions at the "mainstream" elementary schools to remove from their presentations a film about autism because it depicted a quite impaired young man with autistic disorder.

Furthermore, in some developing countries there may be opposition to research on disorders that are not life threatening. It has been suggested that research on developmental disabilities in general is a low priority in many low-income countries where there are more pressing issues such as diseases that cause infant and child mortality (Durkin, 2002, p. 206). Consequently, in many countries, due to the lack of administrative records on child health, researchers need to be referred to potential cases by a wide range of individuals, such as priests and ministers, pediatricians, community leaders, and teachers. Researchers may need to conduct door-to-door household surveys and individual screenings of all children in a community (see, for example, Islam et al., 1993; Thorburn et al., 1992; Durkin, Hasan, & Hasan, 1998). Even then, parents and health officials may strongly oppose the introduction of a diagnostic category that is new and thus confusing.

Social stigma influences diagnosis. In South Korea, children that American clinicians might diagnose with autism are often diagnosed with reactive attachment disorder (RAD), pejoratively referred to as "lack of love" (*aejŏng kyŏlpip*), a term that parallels the older American concept of the "refrigerator mother." In Korea, RAD is thought to be a condition mimicking autism, caused by a mother's absence of attachment to her child (Shin et al., 1999). Many parents prefer a RAD diagnosis to autism.

First, unlike autism, RAD or lack of love can be ameliorated by giving love and thus is not a permanent condition. Koreans widely consider autism to be untreatable (Grinker, 2007). Second, RAD, unlike autism, is not a genetic condition. Thus, while RAD may stigmatize the mother, autism would stigmatize the whole family—past, present, and future. This fear of autism as a genetic disorder is found in many other countries as well, where parents fear that a child's diagnosis of autism will marginalize the family from the social networks to which they feel they are entitled, and harm other family members' marriage prospects (such as the autistic child's siblings). Third, and perhaps most importantly, the diagnosis makes sense. Korea has been undergoing dramatic social change for the last 50 years, emerging from the total devastation of the Korean War to becoming the twelfth largest economy in the world, ahead of countries like Australia, Switzerland, and Sweden. Noting the increase in working mothers and nuclear, as opposed to extended, households, Korean sociologists and child health experts argue that children left with nannies or in daycare cannot form appropriate or lasting attachments with their mothers, and that the failure of attachment leads to RAD.

Such attitudes are not unique to Korea. Hypotheses about the causative role of environmental factors, such as poor parenting and social stressors, in ASD, attachment disorders, and other childhood onset problems, have considerable traction in impoverished or rapidly changing societies. In South Africa, for example, child psychiatrists argue that the role of such stressors have been grossly underrepresented in research on child development: young children are exposed to many forms of violence, parental substance abuse is common, and many children are orphaned or raised by multiple caretakers and with little continuity of care (Hugo et al., 2003).

Despite such obstacles at the clinical level, improvements in diagnostic specification with screening tools and "gold standard" assessments have opened the possibility for rigorous and comparable studies of ASD across cultures. Regardless of whether a society has a word for autism or maintains that autism is a rare condition, epidemiologists can ascertain cases. Children with ASD in a range of different countries have been identified in prevalence studies and can thus form cohorts for studies of etiology and intervention (Vogel & Holford, 1999).

As more diagnoses are made and recorded in school and clinic records, there will be greater opportunities for records-based epidemiological studies. In addition, advances in disability legislation and the growth of advocacy organizations in a number of countries, such as Brazil, China, India, Malawi, South Africa, and Uganda (Braddock & Parish, 2001) as well as at the transnational level (for example, the United Nations, UNICEF, PAHO, WHO, and the World Bank) have made it possible for children with autism to obtain appropriate educational placements and have their diagnoses recorded in school records. As just one example, the well-known TEACCH program has been studied and subsequently adopted in numerous countries and is currently under development in China, India, Mexico, Morocco, Nigeria, and the Philippines, among other places.

Despite the progress in the epidemiology of ASD, there are only a handful of studies that examined the incidence of autism: the rate of occurrence of new cases in a population over a specified period of time (Fombonne, 2007; Rothman and Greenland, 1998; Kleinbaum et al., 1982). This absence is understandable due to the fact that the emergence of ASD in early childhood is insidious, and it is thus often difficult to determine disease onset, which is necessary to examine incidence. Of the studies that have examined incidence, the date of first diagnosis is usually used as a proxy for onset of the disorder. Incidence studies are particularly challenging in a low or middle-income country setting where autism is not routinely diagnosed and symptom onset is not well documented (Figure 7-3).

Despite all of these challenges, there are ongoing efforts to facilitate and standardize the epidemiologic approach to autism research from an international perspective. However, the approaches to autism epidemiology have to be based on local capacity and other attributes in a country. A large-scale initiative sponsored by the parent advocacy organization Autism Speaks distinguishes three separate approaches: one exclusively using records for those settings where most children with an ASD can be identified in schools and health care settings; another utilizing disease registry systems established in some countries as a mechanism to track the health of the population; and a third approach, for those countries with an undeveloped service system, which requires community canvassing or more generalized screening. The intent is to facilitate research within each of these settings and to explore how autism varies in terms of its clinical manifestation and the extent of disability associated with the disorder.

Effect of Social Organization, Culture, and Language on Prevalence Studies and Services

Social Organization and Culture

The WHO studies of schizophrenia constituted the first large-scale effort to explore the role of social organization and culture in influencing the prevalence and outcomes of a mental illness. However, the concept of "culture," broadly defined as the system of meanings through which people organize and make sense of their lives, has long been a central feature of psychiatric description and should not be used only in reference to non-Western societies. For example, researchers have considered how poverty, occupation, social class, and marriage systems affect mental illness in the United States. Epidemiological studies of schizophrenia as early as the 1930s (Faris & Dunham, 1939) noted differences in the prevalence of schizophrenia in urban and rural areas in the United States.

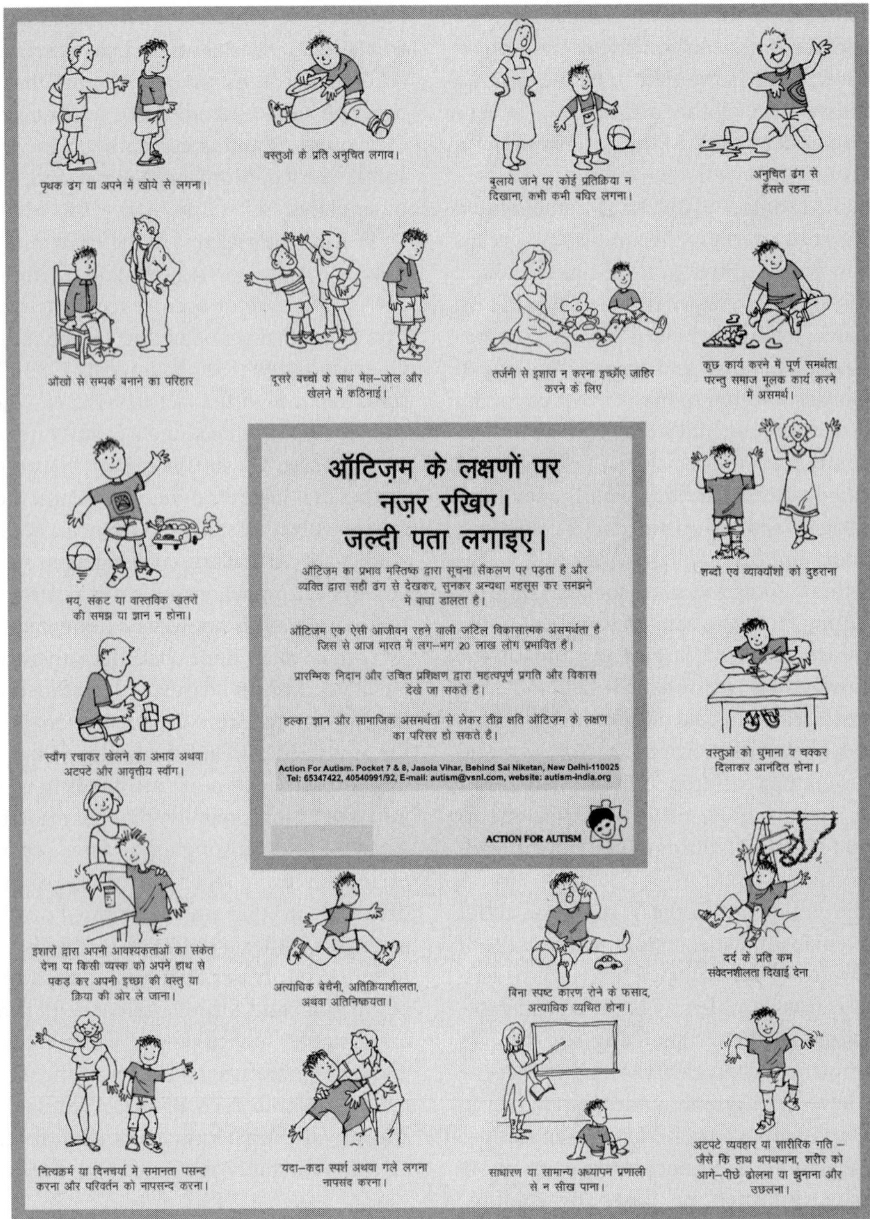
पृथक ढग या अपने मे खोये से लगना।
वस्तुओं के प्रति अनुचित लगाव।
बुलाये जाने पर कोई प्रतिक्रिया न दिखाना, कभी कभी बधिर लगना।
अनुचित ढग से हँसते रहना
आँखो से सम्पर्क बनाने का परिहार
दूसरे बच्चो के साथ मेल–जोल और खेलने मे कठिनाई।
तर्जनी से इशारा न करना इच्छाँए जाहिर करने के लिए
कुछ कार्य करने मे पूर्ण समर्थता परन्तु समाज मूलक कार्य करने मे असमर्थ।
ऑटिज़्म के लक्षणों पर नज़र रखिए।
जल्दी पता लगाइए।
ऑटिजम का प्रभाव मस्तिष्क द्वारा सूचना सँकलण पर पड़ता है और व्यक्ति द्वारा सही ढग से देखकर, सुनकर अन्यथा महसूस कर समझने मे बाधा डालता है।
ऑटिजम एक ऐसी आजीवन रहने वाली जटिल विकासात्मक असमर्थता है जिस से आज भारत मे लग–भग 20 लाख लोग प्रभावित है।
प्रारम्भिक निदान और उचित प्रशिक्षण द्वारा महत्वपूर्ण प्रगति और विकास देखे जा सकते है।
हल्का ज्ञान और सामाजिक असमर्थता से लेकर तीव्र क्षति ऑटिजम के लक्षण का परिसर हो सकते है।
Action For Autism. Pocket 7 & 8, Jasola Vihar, Behind Sai Niketan, New Delhi-110025
Tel: 65347422, 40540991/92, E-mail: autism@vsnl.com, website: autism-india.org
ACTION FOR AUTISM
भय, संकट या वास्तविक खतरो की समझ या ज्ञान न होना।
शब्दो एवं व्यावयाँशो को दुहराना
स्वाँग रचाकर खेलने का अभाव अथवा अटपटे और आवृत्तीय स्वाँग।
वस्तुओ को घुमाना व चक्कर दिलाकर आनदित होना।
इशारो द्वारा अपनी आवश्यकताओं का संकेत देना या किसी व्यस्क को अपने हाथ से पकड़ कर अपनी इच्छा की वस्तु या क्रिया की ओर ले जाना।
अत्याधिक बेचैनी, अतिक्रियाशीलता, अथवा अतिनिष्क्रयता।
बिना स्पष्ट कारण रोने के फसाद, अत्याधिक व्यथित होना।
दर्द के प्रति कम संवेदनशीलता दिखाई देना
नित्यक्रम या दिनचर्या मे समानता पसन्द करना और परिवर्तन को नापसन्द करना।
यदा–कदा स्पर्श अथवा गले लगना नापसंद करना।
साधारण या सामान्य अध्यापन प्रणाली से न सीख पाना।
अटपटे व्यवहार या शारीरिक गति – जैसे कि हाथ थपथपाना, शरीर को आगे–पीछे ढोलना या झुनाना और उछलना।

Figure 7–3. Hindi poster. Autism experts in India are promoting autism awareness through educational programs and posters, such as this one, in Hindi, that depict and describe a range of symptoms. For example, the poster describes the symptom at the top left as "Aloof in Manner"; the caption at the bottom right is "Unusual behavior of body movement such as flapping hands, rocking, or jumping." Courtesy of Merry Barua, Action for Autism (India).

Numerous studies highlight racial disparities in the diagnosis of schizophrenia (Mishler, 1965; Ruiz, 1982), with most researchers agreeing that the disparities are the result not of true differences in prevalence but rather racism, cultural misunderstandings, misdiagnosis, and mismanagement (Whaley, 2001). Among the mentally ill, poor people are also overrepresented, perhaps a legacy to the day when insane asylums also served as poorhouses.

As recently as 1984, Sanua, echoing Lotter (1978), argued that autism was not a universal phenomenon, but a culture-bound disorder, "an illness of Western Civilization" (Sanua, 1984). And for decades following Kanner's original description of the parents of children with autistic disorder as highly educated, upper-middle-class workers, researchers focused on social class as a possible risk factor for autism, one result of which was the concept of the refrigerator mother (usually the educated, working, professional mother). Even today, some scientists continue to argue that ASD occurs more often in the offspring of scientists, engineers, mathematicians, and computer experts, and those with a sociobiological perspective have hypothesized that the increase in the prevalence of higher-functioning autism and Asperger's disorder in the United States and the United Kingdom is the result of intermarriage between highly educated parents (Baron-Cohen, 2004). The development of computer technologies, they argue, makes it possible for autistic adults to find gainful employment, marry, and reproduce. The delay in finding a suitable mate may lead to an increase in parental age, which has been shown in some studies, but not all, to be a risk factor for ASD (Durkin et al., 2008; Croen et al., 2007; Shelton et al., 2010; Grether et al., 2009).

The hypothesis of an association between autism and high socioeconomic status (SES) stands in stark contrast to the large body of research consistently showing that low socioeconomic status is the strongest predictor of childhood disabilities (Durkin, 2002). It is important to point out that none of the claims associating autism or changing prevalence rates to computer technology or to higher SES has been proven. One research team (Cuccaro et al., 1996) did find that school-based clinicians, pediatricians, and psychiatrists were biased in favor of giving autism diagnoses to children of parents of high SES. In a survey of pediatricians, Stone (1987) found that a majority believed there was a true association between autism and SES. It is possible that such a bias explains, at least in part, the fact that African American children subsequently diagnosed with autism are at least 2.5 times less likely to receive a diagnosis at their first specialty visit than a white child with autism (Mandell et al., 2002). With respect to diagnosis, Bearman and colleagues (Liu, King and Bearman 2009; Fountain, King, and Bearman 2010) correlate lower age of diagnosis and increased diagnosis with higher socio-economic status, and social networks. All of these studies indicate that cultural attitudes about SES influence diagnostic practice, but SES does not appear to determine whether or not someone actually has autism.

Nevertheless, poverty, racial discrimination, and marginalization have real effects on outcomes among children with mental illnesses and disabilities (Brown & Rogers, 2003). Researchers have paid special attention to the differences in prevalence and course of mental illnesses between rural and urban environments. Rutter's comparison of the prevalence of psychiatric disorders among 10-year-olds showed significantly higher prevalence of disorders (25.4%) in London than in the Isle of Wight (12%). Rutter et al. (1975) concluded that higher rates of family conflicts, parental psychopathology, and poverty in London were positively associated with higher rates of psychiatric disorders in the children (Rutter et al., 1975). Similarly, in the Ontario Child Health Study, Offord et al. found higher rates of all psychiatric disorders in 4- to 16-year-olds in urban areas (Offord et al., 1987).

The World Health Organization studies on schizophrenia, conducted in the 1970s, showed that prevalence was consistent across rural and urban areas but that outcomes differed significantly depending on geographic location. Although schizophrenia occurs with similar frequency all over the world, people with schizophrenia in the sites in developing countries, such as Agra, India, do better over time than those in industrialized countries. They need less care, fewer medicines, and have fewer traumatic, psychotic episodes. For example, as Hopper (2003) documents, psychiatrists in Madras, India, note that individuals with schizophrenia have had surprising success finding spouses. Thara, Padmavati, and Srinivasan (2004) attribute this success to the importance of one aspect of *dharma*, the duty to marry for the sake of the extended family and the continuity of the lineage. The institution of marriage "adapts and endures, accommodating even those whose nuptial capital would seem to be seriously devalued, given the persistent stigma attached to mental illness in India" (Hopper, 2003, p. 78). Hopper associates marriage of disabled persons with a measure of "social recovery" (2007). We need similar information about ASD to know if certain cultural conditions help people with ASD improve their ability to learn, communicate, and participate in social and economic life. Comparisons to schizophrenia may be useful. For example, in comparison to ASD, is there less stigma attached to the person with schizophrenia in some cultures because the onset of the disorder is in late adolescence, after a family and a community have had nearly two decades to form an attachment to the person? Is there greater stigma attached to a person with autism because the onset is so early?

Both developmental disorders and *explanations* of developmental disorders (scientific or otherwise) are products of the interplay between biological, psychological, and cultural phenomena. In part, as the result of the WHO studies, public health officials increasingly see disabilities as simultaneously both neurologically and culturally constructed. By including culture as a variable in medical research, scientists understand that an illness motivates behaviors in multiple areas of social life. A diagnosis of autism, for example, mobilizes kin groups toward common action or conflict and influences financial planning, choices about residence, reproduction, and employment. In the research community, changes in epidemiological methods produce different rates that can directly influence government policies and educational practices. Changes in educational practices also influence scientific research. Thus, in Italy, mandatory inclusion of children with disabilities, following national inclusion legislation in the 1970s, facilitated lively scholarly work on the course of ASD among children who are educated alongside unimpaired peers, as well as research on early diagnosis of autism (Levi & Bernabei, 2005).

Health services research is one area in which mental health professionals have shown that cultural differences within a single population, like the United States, can lead to disparities in recognition, diagnosis, and care. Availability of clinical services, access to and utilization of services, and cultural appropriateness of services vary considerably among ethnic minorities in the United States. As a result of centuries of racism and discrimination, many African Americans, for example, do not trust government health care institutions and so may not seek care. (Indeed, there is a long history of psychiatric misdiagnosis in African American patients.) Native Americans, a largely rural population, not only live in areas with low access to services, but often utilize traditional healers rather than doctors in clinic settings; some do not see ASD as pathological and may not seek any care at all (Conners &

Donnellan, 1995). Asian Americans underutilize the mental health care system in the United States because of the shame and stigma associated with mental illness. Latinos underutilize the mental health care system because of language barriers (USDHHS, 1999), and Latino parents of autistic children are more likely than the general population to use "nontraditional" treatments (Levy & Hyman, 2003).

For ASD, David Mandell showed that, on average, white children in the United States receive an autism diagnosis approximately 18 months earlier than African American children (Mandell et al., 2002). In the United States, rural children with autism received a diagnosis approximately 5 months later than urban children, and near-poor children received a diagnosis approximately 1 year later than children whose families had an income >100% above the poverty level (Mandell, Novak, & Zubritsky, 2005). Mandell and Novak (2005) urge researchers to conduct research on "the complex relationship between culture and treatment, focusing on cultural differences in the behavioral phenotype of ASD, recognition of symptoms, interpretation of symptoms, families' decisions regarding medical and educational interventions, and interactions between families and the healthcare system" (2005, p. 114). One implication of this recommendation is that even as researchers begin to study autism in other cultures, Americans have not yet resolved the questions that exist in our own society about when and how race, ethnicity, and class, among other cultural factors, influence diagnosis.

In most low and middle-income countries, where there are few or no services for children with special needs, family management and treatment of children with developmental disabilities are influenced directly by socioeconomic and demographic changes. As societies rapidly urbanize (today, for example, one fourth of the population of South Korea lives in Seoul) nuclear families replace extended ones. Parents thus lose the primary source of social support for disabled persons and are compelled to seek help elsewhere, from charitable organizations and other associational communities (such as churches and newly formed autism societies) and from local and national governments. The demands become even greater in households with two working parents.

Taken together, the impact of sociocultural factors on autism recognition, epidemiology, and services reveals an additional and important aspect of our contemporary understandings of autism: the degree to which autism can be conceptualized as a disability as well as a disorder. Disability is fundamentally about a person's interaction with an environment of discrimination, exclusion, and barriers to functioning. The concept of "environment" comprises attitudes, natural or built physical barriers, and policies or systems that may limit an individual's potential. Toward the goal of providing a common language for defining and comparing disabilities across cultures, the WHO developed the International Classification of Functioning, Disability, and Health (ICF). The ICF (which classifies health status), together with the ICD (which classifies disease status), can help experts predict functional outcomes, the need for services, work potential, and possibilities for successful integration into community life (WHO, 2001).

Language

Researchers conducting international studies of developmental disabilities should remain vigilant about preconceived notions of culture. First, at a time of unprecedented population movements across national borders, "culture" is no longer synonymous with place. The rich person in India and the rich person in England may be more culturally similar in terms of values associated with health and disease than the rich and the poor person in either one of those countries (Gupta & Ferguson, 1992). Thus, "culture" should not necessarily be equated with race, class, ethnicity, or nationality only. Second, culture cannot be easily measured and perhaps should not be. Each location demands different methods and types of description. An ethnographic study of help-seeking for ASD in the United States would likely focus primarily on the relationship between parents and health care providers, while the same study in Kenya would likely focus on an extended-family disease management group and how the family negotiates a plurality of coexisting medical and religious systems. Recognizing the particularities of each location leads to a third point: autism may be universal, but the contexts in which it occurs are distinctive. This claim can be illustrated with reference to children's acquisition of language and use of language in social situations.

Language delay and the ability to use language for social interaction are central features of the diagnostic criteria for ASD, and the two are inextricably related. Indeed, though language acquisition is universal, the process and speed of language acquisition varies across cultures, in large part because of differences in socialization. Samoan children, for example, learn certain forms of language much later than one would expect them to, not because they are developmentally delayed but because they are restricted from doing so (Duranti & Ochs, 1996). In Samoa, some syntactic operations are restricted to highly formalized occasions in Samoan society from which children are excluded, and so they do not learn them until adulthood. However, Samoan children learn how to use emotion-marked particles (words, prefixes, or suffixes, that index internal states, such as "oops!" or "wow!") very early in childhood—earlier than American children do—because emotion-marked particles are considered part of "baby language." This Samoan example highlights the fact that language is not a single entity. Children learn different aspects of language at different times in different societies, depending on the way a society organizes its verbal resources and exposes children to them.

Another way of approaching the relationship between language and social behavior is to study how children are both socialized through language and socialized to use language

(Ochs & Schieffelin, 1984; Ochs, 1998). Caregivers not only communicate to their children about the kinds of social behaviors that are acceptable, but they give children explicit instructions about how and when to speak in different social situations. For example, the Kaluli of Papua New Guinea do not consider babbling or any form of vocalization other than speech to be a mode of communication, and a Kaluli child who does not use words is not expected to respond to the vocal communication of others (Schieffelin, 2005). In this area of Papua New Guinea, a parent or teacher report on communicative skills in early childhood would no doubt be influenced by these perspectives.

Similarly, to return to the Samoan example, Samoan children interact with caregivers in a way that restricts direct, dyadic exchanges of meaning. Samoan society is highly stratified, with social interaction organized according to rank. A child who wants something will make the request only of someone who is of higher rank, perhaps an adult. But this adult will not respond directly to the child. Instead he will pass on the request to a third person, someone of lower rank. It is not known what impact such triadic patterns of communication might have on screening for abnormalities in social behavior using measures of social responsiveness designed in the United States, but the mere existence of such variations suggests that researchers should pay close attention to how communication can be shaped by society and culture.

In developing screening tools for autism, for example, items can be tailored to language impairment in particular languages and cultures. It is well known, for example, that English speakers with autism exhibit features such as echolalia, delayed echolalia, and monotonic speech. In addition, a commonly reported impairment is pronominal reversal; in fact, it was one of the diagnostic criteria for autism in the DSM-III. But pronominal reversal would seldom be observed in Korea, since pronouns are rarely used. In Korea one would find other abnormalities. In Korea, as one example, people on the autism spectrum commonly exhibit a particular language impairment: they generally cannot use language to distinguish social rank. The Korean language employs suffixes as honorifics that denote levels of politeness and respect and which are used in nearly every sentence a person speaks. However, a young person with autism may, for example, thank an elderly man with the equivalent of "Thanks, Dude," and thank his younger sister as if she is an elderly woman, "Thank you, Madame." In Korea, and most likely in other societies that employ grammatical forms to convey respect or mark one's place in a hierarchy, abnormalities in language and communication suggestive of an ASD can be identified in a screening instrument that includes a question about the appropriate or inappropriate use of honorifics.

Apart from screening, researchers face the problem of validating assessments in the native language of the community being studied. Unfortunately, researchers all too often use an assessment in a non-native language, such as English in India, or a lingua franca in sub-Saharan Africa (e.g., Swahili in East Africa). There are other related issues. In communities that are ethnically and linguistically heterogeneous, what language does one use to conduct the research, and in particular, the assessments? When studying the role of culture, where does one draw the line between cultural groups? In India, for example, a single community or school system may consist of families from more than a dozen cultural and language groups. In that setting, what language should be chosen for the assessments?

Even when a translation has been validated, it is useful to do focus groups with parents and teachers prior to the beginning of the study to discuss language issues. For example, prior to beginning a prevalence study of elementary school-aged children in Korea, the first author conducted a focus group in which several mothers objected to some of the vocabulary used by the Korean child psychiatrists who translated and validated the protocols. The most objectionable word was *isanghan*, a word the Korean survey translators used to screen for odd behaviors because it means "unusual" but which parents interpreted to mean "bizarre" or "freakish." Thus, even native health care practitioners may not be able to anticipate problems with translation, since the meaning of a concept in the medical community may differ significantly from that in the general public (the classic American example being "hypertension," which Americans have long defined as excessive strain or nervousness, but which the medical community has defined as high blood pressure).

Interventions from a Global Perspective

Numerous interventions have been developed for the treatment of ASD in North America and Western Europe—behavioral/educational, medical, nutritional, and pharmacologic—although many are untested. However, there have been several reviews of the benefits of behavioral/educational interventions in children with ASD, and the results are encouraging (NRC, 2001; Dawson & Osterling, 1997; Evans et al., 2003; Rogers and Vismara, 1998, 2008). Although the specifics of these educational interventions vary, there is general consensus that the core components of a "successful" program include at least the following: entry into intervention as soon as an ASD diagnosis is seriously considered; active engagement of the child in intensive, daily instructional programs for a minimum of the equivalent of a full school day throughout the year; low, adequate student-to-teacher ratios; and promotion of opportunities for interaction with typically developing peers. A recent report of a randomized, controlled trial in the United States of an intervention with toddlers, the Early Start Denver Model, shows tremendous promise (Dawson, 2010). Nonetheless, some interventions in Western Europe, and South America, continue to focus on the treatment of maternal psychopathology, since the refrigerator mother hypothesis persists in those areas where psychoanalytic theory still dominates child psychology and psychiatry.

In the Netherlands and in several Scandinavian countries, there is extensive government support for both children and adults with ASD, providing both groups with behavioral treatment programs, even for mildly autistic individuals. In the Netherlands, the government provides a residence ("Work Home") for adults who are unable to live independently. Multidisciplinary teams located in the Regional Institutions for Outpatient Mental Health Care (RIAGG) provide diagnostic and treatment services, including in-home training, daycare programs, placement in special educational centers, and residential placement. However, despite these services, the waiting lists for assessment by the RIAGGs are long, and educational programs are lacking. Moreover, as in many countries, autism services in the Netherlands are technically available under the Dutch disability laws only for people with a diagnosis of autistic disorder and not the other PDDs (van Engeland, 2005). In Sweden, the government has focused largely on the establishment of treatment homes, in the tradition of Rudolph Steiner's concept of curative education (or Heilpedagogie) (Rydelius, 2005), some of them arranged into villages. A similar model has been adopted by organizations in other countries, such as the Camphill communities in the United Kingdom, Ireland, Scotland, the United States, and Canada.

However, while progress has been made in increasing the number and availability of treatments for ASD throughout the world, a search of the English language literature (Pub Med, 2000 to the present) yielded little information on interventions for neurodevelopmental disorders (including autism) in low-income countries. Three articles discussed behavioral modification, early intervention, and medication for children with autism in India (Daley, 2002, 2003; Kalra, 2005; Karande, 2006). Kalra (2005), in an evaluation of behavior modification and early intervention, found improvement in core symptoms of autism in some children. Karande (2006) recommended the use of psychotropic drugs and counseling for parents and teachers in the treatment of autism in India. Daley (2002) emphasized that the responsibility for interventions lies primarily with the parents since there are few special education services for autism and few psychologists and speech/language pathologists available for treating autism.

Because information on interventions for autism in non-Western countries is scarce, we can use other neurodevelopmental disorders as a model for how a successful intervention plan can be implemented. Olusanya (2007) described a program in Nigeria to detect hearing loss in infants. A pilot program for neonatal screening for hearing loss was developed with financial support from a local nongovernmental organization (NGO). In the first year, more than 3,000 children were screened and fitted with hearing aids at no cost to the parents. This public-private partnership for screening and intervention was noted as a model for other low and middle-income countries. While not focusing on autism per se, in South Africa there was an audit of referrals from primary care facilities (mostly managed by nurses) for a range of mental health services, many of which were for intellectual disability and scholastic problems in children under 19 years old. Following the audit, a recommendation was made that a professional "counselor" be responsible for providing psychological assessment and intervention services at the primary care level (Petersen, 2004). One would imagine that these "counselors" would be the first professionals to identify and diagnose children with autism as well as other developmental disabilities.

There are few estimates of the prevalence of autism in China, although one recent study in Hong Kong suggests a comparatively low rate of 16.1 per 10,000 among children less than 15 years old (Wong & Hui, 2008). Given the Chinese government's March 2009 census, showing 251,660,000 persons ages 0–14 (approximately 19% of the total population), even such a low rate would mean there are at least 402,656 children in that age group with autism in China (National Population and Family Planning Commission, 2009). Unfortunately, although the Ministry of Education in China has recently become concerned about services for children with disabilities overall, there are not enough programs and trained personnel to provide for children with disabilities, including autism.

There are few child psychiatrists in China, and these practice in the largest cities. Common diagnoses for Chinese children with autism include intellectual disability, hyperactive syndrome, childhood schizophrenia, and sporadic encephalitis (Tao & Yang, 2005). There is, nonetheless, a Chinese classification of mental disorders adopted from the ICD-9 but which uses the term "childhood autism" instead of autistic disorder.

Autism services in China, when available, include a mix of traditional treatments (i.e., herbs and acupuncture, which are increasingly popular as treatments for autism in China, although there are no studies of their effectiveness) and more contemporary treatments (i.e., sensory integration and Applied Behavioral Analysis/ABA) (Clark & Zhou, 2005). Part of the reason for the paucity of services for autism lies in the fact that it was not until the 1980s that special education of any type began in China, and when services are available, most of the resources have been put into services for children with physical disabilities. There is one exemplary private program, the "Stars and Rain" Education Institute for Children with Autism in Beijing. It is reported to have served nearly 500 children (ages 3–6) across China since 1993. The program uses an ABA approach to treatment along with a parent training model. However, at a cost of approximately $36 per week, it is not feasible for most Chinese families. There are also limited programs in psychiatric facilities and no public school programs designed specifically for children with autism. There may, however, be some children who receive special services because they have an accompanying intellectual disability in addition to autism.

Future Growth in Global Research

Greater global awareness of both the characteristic features and prevalence of ASD has led to a range of new research activities on ASD supported by public institutions in both the United States (i.e., the Centers for Disease Control and Prevention [CDC], the National Institute of Mental Health [NIMH], and the National Institute for Child Health and Development [NICHD]) and in other countries (i.e., the National Institute of Mental Health and Neurosciences in India [NIMHANS], the National Institute for Health and Medical Research [INSERM] in France, and the National Health Research Institutes [NHRI] in Taiwan). Biological and genetic research on autism is expanding in Europe. In France, for example, the Paris Autism Research International Sibpair genome study has been analyzing samples from Italy, Sweden, France, Norway, the United States, Austria, and Belgium (Phillipe et al., 1999).

As reported prevalence estimates increased, funding increased. Between 1997 and 2008, when government funding for most medical research was unchanged, annual funding for autism studies at the National Institutes of Health increased from $22 million to $118 million (http://www.iacc.hhs.gov/portfolio-analysis/2008/index.shtml). Progress has also been made through new laws: the Combating Autism Act (signed into law by President Bush in February 2007) was designed to support autism research, and the French Chossy Act (December 1996) reclassified autism as a handicap rather than solely a psychiatric illness and thus ensured disability rights for autistic individuals.

Even more noticeable than these forms of public participation, philanthropists and the families of autistic individuals have founded private foundations to support basic scientific research on ASD and improve the availability and quality of services. Donors are contributing millions of dollars to parent advocacy organizations, private schools, and foundations in the United States (e.g., for example, the Autism Science Foundation, Autism Speaks, and the Simons Foundation) and in the United Kingdom (e.g., the National Autistic Society or NAS). The NAS, founded in 1962, has grown considerably over the past decade to include more than 17,000 members. It has launched a telephone helpline that, according to their website, took 38,000 telephone calls in 2007. As a result, even scientists who never before had an interest in autism, but worked in a related area such as neuroscience or genetics, are joining an increasingly long parade of autism researchers who are able to secure funding through these private foundations. Between 2003 and 2004 the number of grant applications to the National Alliance for Autism Research, then the leading private foundation for autism research (before its merger with Autism Speaks), doubled. In 2009 alone, the Simons Foundation and Autism Speaks awarded $51,526,058 and $23,416,615 respectively for autism research projects (http://iacc.hhs.gov/events/2010/102210/materials.shtml). Much of the force behind the growth of research and advocacy has come from funding through the telecommunications or entertainment field: for example, Bob Wright, former president and CEO of NBC Universal, founder of Autism Speaks; the Fondation France Télécom in France, which supports Autisme France; and Carlos Slim, the magnate who controls the Mexican telecommunications company Teléfonos de México.

Conclusions

This chapter described a significant number of obstacles to conducting international research on ASD but also highlighted opportunities for advancing knowledge about how autism varies across different settings. Even a preliminary cross-cultural exploration of the epidemiology of autism and the role that culture plays in diagnosis and treatment shows that ASD exists throughout the world, even in societies that have no name for it. The study of the cultural variations in ASD is therefore not so much a matter of whether ASD exists, but rather the *contexts* in which it takes shape. The increased funding for research by private and public institutions constitutes just one important step to meet the challenges of epidemiological research on autism across cultures. This chapter also argued that ASD should be conceptualized as a cultural phenomenon and as a disability—not just as a phenomenon of Western civilization, and not just a disease. Understanding how culture influences the recognition and definition of autism spectrum disorders will facilitate cross-cultural adaptations of screening and diagnostic tools, and generate knowledge that can one day be translated into a better understanding of its etiology and improved treatments, services, education, and community integration of people on the autism spectrum.

Challenges and Future Directions

- Provide support to low and middle-income countries for community education and awareness.
- Develop more efficient and affordable diagnostic assessments that are reliable and valid in multiple languages and societies.
- In addition to ascertaining prevalence, epidemiological studies should develop low cost, appropriate services for children identified through screening, surveillance, and research efforts.
- In order to develop culturally appropriate services, including educational programs, future epidemiological studies should study the impact of autism on the child as well as his/her family.

SUGGESTED READINGS

Daley, T. (2002). The need for cross-cultural research on the pervasive developmental disorders. *Transcultural Psychiatry, 39*(4), 531–550.

Fombonne, E. (2009). Epidemiology of pervasive developmental disorders. *Pediatric Research, 65*(6): 591–598.

Grinker, R. R. (2007). *Unstrange minds: Remapping the world of autism.* New York: Basic Books.

Ochs, E., Kremer-Sadlik, T., Gainer Sirota, K., & Solomon, O. (2004). Autism and the social world: An anthropological perspective. *Discourse Studies, 6*(2), 147–183.

Trostle, J. A. (2005). *Epidemiology and culture.* Cambridge: Cambridge University Press.

APPENDIX

Table 7–2.
Appendix: Selected epidemiological studies

Europe					
Gillian Baird, F. R.C. Paed Guy's and St Thomas' Hospital London, UK Tony Charman, PhD Behavioural & Brain Sciences Unit Institute of Child Health University College London, UK	The South Thames Special Needs and Autism Project (SNAP)	UK (South Thames)	Birth cohort study of the prevalence of ASD from 12 districts in the South Thames area.	56,946 children (18 month birth cohort July 1990–Dec 1991) screened at age 9 years; in-depth assessment age 9 to 14 years.	ASD subgroup(s): All ASD subgroups Diagnostic criteria: ICD-10 Source of cases: ongoing assessments
Jean Golding, PhD Institute of Child Health University of Bristol, St Michael's Hill, BS2 8BJ Bristol, UK	Avon Longitudinal Study of Parents and Children (ALSPAC)	UK (Avon)	Prospective cohort starting in pregnancy to identify the environmental and genetic antecedents of the autistic spectrum disorders, and of the traits that make up the autistic spectrum.	Children born in 1991–1992	ASD subgroup(s): All ASDs Diagnostic criteria: ICD-10 Source of cases: Service provider records for ascertainment of ASD; traits identified from maternal completion of sets of questions completed at different ages
Eric Fombonne, MD, FRCPsych(UK) McGill University and Montreal Children's Hospital Montreal, Quebec	Staffordshire Surveys	UK (Staffordshire)	Successive prevalence studies of PDDs among preschoolers, to examine temporal trends and changes in risk factors overtime.	160 case children identified from children born from 1992 to 1998	ASD subgroup(s): All ASD subgroups Diagnostic criteria: DSM-IV, ICD-10 Source(s) of cases: repeated screening of the general population
Camilla Stoltenberg, MD, PhD, Norwegian Institute of Public Health (NIPH), Oslo, Norway Nydalen, 0403 Oslo, Norway	The ASD Healthcare and Registry Project	Norway	Pilot study to monitor the prevalence of ASD in Norway, and possibly providing the foundations for a permanent national ASD registry.	Children born in Norway 1999 or later who have been given an ASD diagnosis in the Norwegian health care system	ASD subgroup(s): All ASD subgroups Diagnostic criteria: All ICD-10; F84.0–F84.9 will be included. Expected sample size: 1000–2000 cases.

(Continued)

Table 7–2. *(Contd.)*

Christopher Gillberg, MD, PhD Gothenburg University Gothenburg, Sweden	**Bergen Child Study: the Autism Spectrum Study**	Norway (Bergen)	Cross-sectional study to determine prevalence rates of ASD, test the ASSQ as a screening device for ASD, assess ASD risk factors using screening devices and neuropsychological/ neuroimaging.	Case children identified from 7- to 9-year olds in 2003 in Bergen, Norway.	ASD subgroup(s): All ASD subgroups Diagnostic criteria: DSM-IV (plus Gillberg criteria for Asperger's syndrome) Source of cases: general population screen- and clinic-referred cases
W. Ian Lipkin, MD Center for Infection and Immunity Mailman School of Public Health Columbia University New York, NY 10032	**Gene-Environment Interactions in an Autism Birth Cohort (ABC)**	Norway	Nested case-control study focused on the role of gene-environment interactions in the etiology of ASD. The ABC study builds on the Norwegian Mother and Child Cohort Study (MoBa).	Children born in 1999 through May 2008 and screened at 36 months for ASD.	ASD subgroups: All ASD subgroups Diagnostic criteria: DSM-IV Source of cases; Screening of the MoBa cohort of children at 36 months; referrals (parents or provider-based); search of health registries
Christopher Gillberg, MD, PhD Gothenburg University Gothenburg, Sweden	**Göteborg Prevalence studies of Autism Spectrum Disorders.**	Sweden (Göteborg)	Cross-sectional prevalence study of ASD.	Case children identified from clinic and population screening of 7- to 9-year-olds in Goteborg, Sweden.	ASD subgroup(s): All ASD subgroups included Diagnostic criteria: DSM-IV criteria (plus Gillberg criteria for Asperger's syndrome) Source of cases: general population screen- and clinic-referred cases
Paul Lichtenstein, PhD Department of Medical Epidemiology, Karolinska Institute, Stockholm, Sweden	**Child and Adolescent Twin Study in Sweden (CATSS)**	Sweden	Cohort study of liveborn twins to examine genetic and environmental influences for ASD and comorbid conditions (e.g., ADHD).	All twins (n = 24,000) born in Sweden during 1994–2001. (Expected number of twin pairs with ASD = 800.)	ASD Subgroup(s): All ASD subgroups Diagnostic criteria: DSM-IV (plus Gillberg criteria for Asperger's syndrome). Source of cases: general population screening with A-TAC and clinical testing
Christopher Gillberg, MD, PhD Gothenburg University Gothenburg, Sweden	Faroe Islands ASD Genetic Epidemiology Study	Faroe Islands, Denmark	Cross-sectional prevalence study to estimate the prevalence of ASD and examine the genetic and environmental (mercury) risk factors for ASD in a genetically homogeneous population.	All children in the Faroe Islands, aged 7–15 years (n = 44 ASD cases).	ADS subgroup(s): All ASD subgroups included Diagnostic criteria: DSM-IV criteria (plus Gillberg criteria for Asperger's syndrome) Source of cases: school-based screening and clinic-referred cases

(Continued)

Table 7–2. *(Contd.)*

Paul Thorsen, MD, PhD, Institute of Public Health, NANEA at Department of Epidemiology, University of Aarhus Aarhus, Denmark	Danish national case-control study on infantile autism	Denmark	Case-control study to examine the association between genetic factors and the development of infantile autism, and to develop the methodological expertise for studying genetic markers for autism.	473 case children born in Denmark from 01/01/1990 to12/31/1999 and diagnosed before age 10 years.	ASD subgroup(s): Infantile autism diagnosed before age 10 years Diagnostic criteria: ICD-8 and ICD-10 Source(s) of cases: Danish Psychiatric Central Registry and Danish National Patient Registry
Marko Kielinen, PhD and Marja-Leena Mattila, MD Department of Paediatrics Clinic of Child Psychiatry University of Oulu Oulu, Finland	Autism in Northern Finland	Finland (Oulu and Lapland)	Retrospective cohort study to estimate the prevalence of autism in Oulu and Lapland, and to examine secular changes in incidence.	152, 732 children born between 1979–1994 and age 3–18 in 1996–1997 (time period for case ascertainment)	ADS subgroup(s): Autistic disorder and Asperger's disorder Diagnostic criteria: DSM-IV, ICD-10 (Gillberg & Szatmari, et al. criteria) Sources of Cases: Hospital records and the records of the central institutions of the intellectually disabled
Marko Kielinen, PhD and Marja-Leena Mattila, MD Department of Paediatrics Clinic of Child Psychiatry University of Oulu Oulu, Finland	An Epidemiological and Diagnostic Study of Asperger´s disorder	Finland (Oulu and Lapland)	Retrospective cohort study to evaluate the diagnostic process and prevalence rates of Asperger´s disorder.	5484 children born in year 1992 and screened in 2000–2001; 125 screened positive and 110 examined; 19 Asperger case children and 13 children with autistic disorder	ADS subgroup(s): Autistic disorder and Asperger's disorder Diagnostic criteria: DSM-IV, ICD-10 (Gillberg and Szatmari et al. criteria) Sources of Cases: Population screening followed by semistructured observation and testing
Evald Sæmundsen, PhD State Diagnostic and Counseling Center Kopavogur, Iceland	Prevalence of autism spectrum disorders in Iceland in children born in 1994–1998.	Iceland	Cross-sectional survey too examine the prevalence of ASD in Iceland and to identify risk factors associated with ASD.	Children born 1994–1998 identified through medical and other service system records through January 2008	ASD subgroup(s): All ASD subgroups listed in the ICD-10 Diagnostic Criteria: ICD-10 Source of cases: Service records of the referral center for autism and other developmental disabilities
Manuel Posada, PhD, MD, Research Institute for Rare Diseases, Health Institute Carlos III 28029. Madrid, Spain,	Spanish Autistic Spectrum Disorders Register (TEAR in Spanish and SASDR in English)	Spain (four regions)	Population-based registry and a nested case-control study to study the feasibility and costs of a population screening program using the M-CHAT and analyze risk factors for in incident cases.	Children 18–36 months of age in 2006	ASD subgroup(s): All ASD subgroups Diagnostic Criteria: DSM-IV-TR Source of cases: population-based screening in the following venues: Public Health Care System-Well Child Care visits (WCC) and Compulsory Vaccination Program Parent's organizations, ASD settlements and educational and social services

(*Continued*)

Table 7–2. *(Contd.)*

Astrid Moura Vicente, PhD Instituto Nacional de Saúde Av. Padre Cruz 1649-016 Lisboa, Portugal	Epidemiology of Autism in Portugal	Portugal	Cross-sectional study to estimate the prevalence of autism and to describe its clinical characterization and associated medical conditions.	Children born in 1990, 1991, and 1992, living in mainland Portugal or the Azores and attending elementary school in the school year of 1999/2000	ASD subgroup(s): Autistic disorder Diagnostic criteria: DSM-IV Source(s) of cases: School-based screening followed by clinical assessment
The Americas					
Eric Fombonne, MD, FRCPsych(UK) McGill University and Montreal Children's Hospital Montreal, Quebec	Prevalence of Pervasive Developmental Disorders in Montreal, Quebec	Canada (Quebec)	Retrospective cohort study to evaluate time trends in relation to use of thimerosal-containing vaccines and MMR.	180 case children identified from children born between 1997 and 1998 and ascertained in 2003	ASD subgroup(s): All ASDs Diagnostic criteria: DSM-IV Sources of Cases: special educational registers
CDC: Diana Schendel, PhD National Center on Birth Defects and Developmental Disabilities Centers for Disease Control and Prevention Atlanta, GA 30333 California: Lisa Croen, PhD Colorado: Lisa Miller, MD, MSPH Maryland: Craig Newschaffer, PhD North Carolina: Julie Daniels, PhD Pennsylvania: Jennifer Pinto-Martin, PhD, MPH,	The CADDRE Study: Child Development and Autism	USA (6 sites: California, Colorado, Georgia, Maryland, North Carolina, and Pennsylvania)	Population-based case-cohort study to investigate risk factors for ASD and phenotypic subgroups of ASD.	Children born from September 2003 through August 2005; Eligible children must be 30–60 months of age during data collection. Expected sample size is 650 children with ASD across 6 sites.	ASD subgroup(s): All ASDs subgroups Diagnostic criteria: DSM IV Source of cases: intensive screening and case finding in clinics and special programs for young children with developmental delays
Catherine Rice, PhD National Center on Birth Defects and Developmental Disabilities, Centers for Disease Control and Prevention 1600 Clifton Road, MS-E-86 Atlanta, GA 30333	Autism and Developmental Disabilities Monitoring Network (ADDM)	USA (Alabama, Arizona, Colorado, Florida, Georgia, Maryland, Missouri, North Carolina, Pennsylvania, South Carolina, Wisconsin)	Ongoing population-based surveillance of ASD in 8-year-old children in 11 sites in the United States to determine prevalence and trends.	Children who are 8 years old (selected states) beginning in 2000 and monitored biannually	ASD subgroups included: All ASDs Diagnostic criteria: Systematic review of service provider records—education (selected sites) and medical—by expert clinicians using DSM-IV criteria Sources of case: school, medical, and other service provider records
Lisa Croen, PhD Kaiser Permanente Northern California Division of Research Oakland, CA 94612	Childhood Autism Perinatal Study (CHAPS)	USA (Northern California)	Case-control study to investigate prenatal and perinatal risk factors for autism spectrum disorders.	Children born 1995–1999 in a Kaiser Permanente hospital in northern CA	ASD subgroup(s): All ASD subgroups Diagnostic criteria: DSM-IV Source of cases: Kaiser Permanente electronic medical records

(Continued)

Table 7–2. *(Contd.)*

Lisa Croen, PhD Kaiser Permanente Northern California Division of Research Oakland, CA 94612	Early Autism Risks Longitudinal Investigations (EARLI)	USA (multisite study—Northern California, Pennsylvania, and Maryland)	Prospective, longitudinal, cohort study to identify early autism risk factors and biomarkers based on an enriched-risk pregnancy cohort.	Women who have at least one ASD-affected child who have a subsequent pregnancy. Women will be followed through their pregnancies and the infants will be followed through age 3.	ASD subgroup(s): All ASD subgroups Diagnostic criteria: DSM-IV Source of cases (proband child) clinical care providers, service providers, educational system, self-referrals.
Lisa Croen, PhD Kaiser Permanente Northern California Division of Research Oakland, CA 94612	Early Markers for Autism Study (EMA)	USA (Northern California)	Case-control study to identify early (prenatal and neonatal) biomarkers for autism spectrum disorders.	Children born July 2000–Sept. 2001	ASD: All ASD subgroups Diagnostic criteria: DSM-IV Source of cases: Regional Center of Orange County (review of service provider records)
Michaeline Bresnahan, PhD Columbia University School of Public Health New York City	Aruba Autism Project	Aruba	Retrospective birth cohort study to examine prevalence and cumulative incidence of ASD in Aruba.	All children born in Aruba in 1990–1999 and followed through 2003.	ASD subgroup(s) included: Autistic Disorder, PDD-NOS, Asperger, Rett, disintegrative Diagnostic Criteria: DSM-IV Source of Cases: clinical/medical records
Cecilia Montiel-Nava, PhD School of Education La Universidad del Zulia. Maracaibo, Estado Zulia, Venezuela	Epidemiological Findings of Autism Spectrum Disorders in Maracaibo County	Venezuela (Maracaibo County)	Cross-sectional survey to estimate the prevalence of autism spectrum disorders (ASD) among children between 3 and 7 years of age in Maracaibo County.	Children aged 3 to 7 years, and children born in the 2003 (5 years old).	ASD subgroup(s): All ASDs Diagnostic criteria: DSM-IV criteria Source of cases: School-based screening and clinic-referred cases
Cristiane Silvestre de Paula Pervasive Developmental Disorders Program; Mackenzie Presbyterian University, Brazil São Paulo, Brazil.	Prevalence of pervasive developmental disorders in southeast Brazil: A pilot study	Brazil (Atibaia)	Cross-sectional survey to estimate the prevalence of pervasive developmental disorders in southeast Brazil.	7- to 12-year-old children	ASD subgroup(s): All ASDs combined Diagnostic Criteria: DSM IV criteria Source of cases: population based screening study
Middle East, Africa, Asia, and Australia					
Shlomo (Sol) Eaglstein, PhD Department of Research, Planning and Training State of Israel Ministry of Social Affairs Jerusalem 93,420 Israel.	The Israeli Ministry of Social Affairs (MOSA) Autism Registry.	Israel (Jerusalem)	Population-based registry to estimate the prevalence of autism/ASD in Israel, by means of detecting the number and age of people diagnosed who apply for services and to track placement (home, special education, assisted living, etc).	Expected sample size 4,000 case children (12/07)	ASD subgroup(s) included: Autism, Asperger's syndrome, and PDD-NOS. Diagnostic criteria: DSM-IV Source of cases: children applying for services.

(Continued)

Table 7–2. *(Contd.)*

Hideo Honda, M.D. Ph.D. Yokohama Rehabilitation Centre Yokohama, Japan	Cumulative incidence and prevalence of childhood autism in children in Japan Japan (Yokohama)	Japan (Yokohama City)	Cumulative incidence study of "childhood autism." Attempt to replicate earlier epidemiological study using identical methods in a large population with screening beginning at 18 months.	Cumulative incidence up to age 5 years was calculated for childhood autism among a birth cohort from four successive years (1988 to 1991).	"Childhood Autism:" (ICD-10) Source of cases: Yokohama City Routine Health Checkup (18 months).
MKC Nair, MD, PhD Professor of Pediatrics & Director, Child Development Centre, Medical College Campus, Thiruvananthapuram, Kerala, India 695,011 Dr. Narendra K. Arora Executive Director-INCLEN The INCLEN Trust International New Delhi, India 110,049	Neuro-developmental Disabilities among Children In India: An INCLEN Study	**India (5 regions)**	Cross-sectional study to examine the prevalence of 10 neurodevelopmental disabilities, including ASDs, in children aged 2–9 years in India and gather information on potentially modifiable risk factors.	9,000 children aged 2–9 years old will be screened with a neurodevelopmental disability screening tool. Children with autism will be determined based on a clinical examination applying agreed on study criteria for ASDs	ASD subgroup(s): All subgroups of ASD Diagnostic criteria: DSM-IV Source of cases: Community based household screening
Richard Grinker, PhD George Washington University, Washington, DC 20052 Young Shin Kim, MD, MS, MPH, PhD Yale Child Study Center New Haven, CT 06520	Study 1: The Prevalence of Autistic Spectrum Disorder (ASD) in Korean School-age Children Study 2: Prospective Examination of 6-year Cumulative Incidence of ASDs: A Total Population Study	South Korea (Ilsan)	Study 1: Birth cohort study to examine the prevalence of ASD; to establish a population-based cohort of children with ASD for future genetic and environmental studies, to investigate public attitudes about ASD; and to examine patterns of service utilization in Korean children with ASD. Study 2: Prospective birth cohort study to examine the incidence proportion of ASD in children followed from birth to age 6 years.	Study 1: 36, 592 cases screened 9/2005-8/2006, confirmative diagnoses completed 2/2006-7/2009, among children born 1995-2000. Study 2: 2001–2002 birth cohort; screened at age 6 years in 2007–2008	ASD subgroups: All ASD subtypes Diagnostic criteria DSM IV using ADOS and ADI-R Source of cases: Study: community based screening; family referrals; and disability registry

(Continued)

Table 7–2. *(Contd.)*

Craig J. Newschaffer, PhD Associate Professor of Epidemiology Center for Autism and Developmental Disabilities Epidemiology Department of Epidemiology	Epidemiologic Research on Autism in China	China (Shandong Province)	Pilot study to examine methods for population-based screening to estimate prevalence estimation toward capacity-building for conducting epidemiologic research on ASD in China.	3- to 5-year-old children residing in the Weicheng district of Weifang Prefecture of Shandong Province.	ASD subgroup(s) included: ADI-defined autism. Diagnostic criteria: ADI-R.
Joe Cubells, MD, PhD Department of Human Genetics Emory University School of Medicine Atlanta, GA 30322 USA	Genetic Epidemiology of Autism in China: Phase 1	China (Wuiiang County near Beijing)	Pilot study to develop, validate, and field test culturally appropriate screening methods for identifying potential ASD cases in the offspring of mothers who were enrolled prior to pregnancy in a large longitudinal cohort study assembled in 1994–1996.	Children born in 1994–1996 and assessed in late 2008–2009	ASD subgroup(s): All ASD subtypes Diagnostic criteria: DSM-IV Source of cases: Local health centers where original study participants receive their health care.
Virginia C. N. Wong, MD Division of Child Neurology, Developmental Paediatrics, and Neurohabilitation Department of Pediatrics & Adolescent Medicine, The University of Hong Kong, Hong Kong, China	Epidemiological Study of Autism Spectrum Disorder in Hong Kong	China (Hong Kong)	Retrospective cohort study to investigate the epidemiological pattern of ASD in Chinese children.	Children aged under 15 years who had a diagnosis of ASD in 1986 to 2005	ASD subgroup(s): All cases Diagnostic Criteria: DSM-III-R or DSM-IV Source of cases: Autism Spectrum Disorder Registry for Children in Hong Kong
Li-Ching Lee, PhD, ScM Department of Epidemiology Bloomberg School of Public Health Johns Hopkins University Baltimore MD 21205	Population-based prevalence study of autism spectrum disorders in Taiwan	Taiwan	Pilot activities to support development of epidemiology and clinical capacity for a population-based prevalence study.	Children in first and second grades, aged 6–7, to be ascertained in 2009.	ASD subgroup(s): All ASD subgroups Diagnostic Criteria: DSM-IV Source of cases: Screening of children in first and second grades.
Glenys Dixon, PhD Telethon Institute for Child Health Research Centre for Child Health Research University of Western Australia Perth, Australia	The West Australian Autism Register	Western Australia (WA)	Ongoing population-based registry of ASD for WA to describe the pattern of autism diagnoses and prevalence rates of ASD in WA.	1500 case children ongoing starting in 1999	ASD subgroup(s): All ASD subtypes Diagnostic criteria: DSM-IV Source of Cases: case reporting by diagnosing clinicians and WA service system records

REFERENCES

Autism and Developmental Disabilities Monitoring Network 2006 Principal Investigators (ADDM). (2009, December 18). Prevalence of autism spectrum disorders: Autism and Developmental Disabilities Monitoring Network, United States, (2006), Surveillance summaries. *Morbidity and Mortality Weekly Report, 58*(No. SS#10).

Baird, G., Simonoff, E., Pickles, A., Chandler, S., Loucas, T., Meldrum, D., & Charman, T. (2006). Prevalence of disorders of the autism spectrum in a population cohort of children in South Thames: The Special Needs and Autism Project (SNAP). *Lancet, 368,* 210–215.

Bandim, J. M., Ventura, L. O., Miller, M. T., Almeida, H. C., & Santos Costa, A. E. (2002). Autism and Möbius sequence: An exploratory study of children in Northeastern Brazil. *Arquivos de Neuro-Psiquiatrica, 61*(2-A), 181–185.

Barbaresi, W., Katusic, S., Colligan, R., Weaver, A., & Jacobsen, S. (2005). The incidence of autism in Olmsted County, Minnesota, 1976–1997: Results from a population-based study. *Archives of Pediatric and Adolescent Medicine, 159,* 37–44.

Barnevik-Olsson, M., Gillberg, C., & Fernell, E. (2008). Prevalence of autism in children born to Somali parents living in Sweden: A brief report. *Developmental Medicine and Child Neurology, 50*(8), 598–601.

Baron-Cohen, S. (2004). *The essential difference: Male and female brains and the truth about autism.* New York: Basic Books.

Braddock, D. L., & Parish, S. L. (2001). An institutional history of disability. In G. L. Albrecht, K. D. Seelman, & M. Bury (Eds.), *Handbook of disability studies* (pp. 11–68). Thousand Oaks, CA: Sage.

Brown, J. R., & Rogers, S. J. (2003). Cultural issues in autism. In S. Ozonoff, S. J. Rogers, & R. L. Hendren (Eds.), *Autism spectrum disorders: A research review for practitioners.* Washington, DC: American Psychiatric Publishing.

Chamak, B. (2008). Autism and social movements: French parents' associations and international autistic individuals' organizations. *Sociology of Health and Illness, 30*(1), 76–96.

Chang, H.-L., Juang, Y.-Y., Wang, W.-T., Huang, C.-I., Chen, C.-Y., & Hwang, Y.-S. (2003). Screening for autism spectrum disorder in adult psychiatric outpatients in a clinic in Taiwan. *General Hospital Psychiatry, 25,* 284–288.

Chuthapisth, J, Ruangdaraganon, N., Sombuntham, T., & Roongpraiwan, R. (2007). Language development among the siblings of children with autism spectrum disorder. *Autism, 11*(2), 153–164.

Clark, E. & Zhou, Z. (2005). Autism in China: From acupuncture to applied behavioral analysis. *Psychology in the Schools, 42*(3), 285–295.

Cohen, D. J., & Volkmar, F. R. (1997). Conceptualizations of autism and intervention practices: international perspectives. In D. J. Cohen & F.R. Volkmar, (Eds.), *Handbook of autism and pervasive developmental disorders* (2nd ed., pp. 947–950). New York: Wiley.

Connors, J. L., & Donnellan, A. M. (1995). Walk in beauty: Western perspectives on disability and Navajo family/cultural resilience. In H. McCubbin, E. Thomson., A. Thompson, & J. Fromer (Eds.), *Resiliency in ethnic minority families: Native and immigrant American families* (Vol. 1, pp. 159–182). New York: Sage.

Croen, L. A., Najjar, D. V., Fireman, B., & Grether, J. K. (2007). Maternal and paternal age and risk of autism spectrum disorders. *Archives of Pediatrics and Adolescent Medicine, 161*(4), 334–340.

Cuccaro, M. L., Wright, H. H., Rownd, C. V., & Abramson, R. K. (1996). Brief report: Professional perceptions of children with developmental difficulties: The influence of race and socioeconomic status. *Journal of Autism and Developmental Disorders, 26*(4), 461–469.

Daley, T. (2002). The need for cross-cultural research on the pervasive developmental disorders. *Transcultural Psychiatry, 39*(4), 531–550.

Daley, T. (2003). From symptom recognition to diagnosis: Children with autism in urban India. *Social Science and Medicine, 58,* 1323–1335.

Daley, T., & Sigman, M. (2002). Diagnostic conceptualization of autism among Indian psychiatrists, psychologists, and pediatricians. *Journal of Autism and Developmental Disorders, 32*(1), 13–23.

Dawson, G., Rigers, S., Munson, J., Smith, M., Winter, J., Greenson, J., & Varley, J. (2010). Randomized, controlled trial of an intervention for toddlers with autism: the Early Start Denver Model. *Pediatrics, 125*(1), e17–23.

Dawson, G. & Osterling, J. (1997). Early intervention in autism: Effectiveness and common elements of current approaches. In M. J. Guralnick (Ed.), *The effectiveness of early intervention: Second generation research* (pp. 307–326) Baltimore: Brookes.

Duranti, A., & Ochs, E. (1996). Use and acquisition of genitive constructions in Samoan. In D. Slobin, J. Gerhardt, A. Kyratzis, & G. Jiansheng (Eds.), *Social interaction, social context, and language: Essays in honor of Susan Ervin-Tripp* (pp. 175–190). Mahwah, NJ: Erlbaum.

Durkin, M. S. (2002). The epidemiology of developmental disabilities in low-income countries. *Mental Retardation and Developmental Disabilities Research Reviews, 8,* 206–211.

Durkin, M. S., Davidson, L. L., Hasan, Z. M., Hasan, Z., Hauser, W. A., Khan, N., et al. (1992). Estimates of the prevalence of childhood seizure disorders in communities where professional resources are scarce: Results from Bangladesh, Jamaica, and Pakistan. *Pediatric and Perinatal Epidemiology, 6,* 166–180.

Durkin, M. S., Hasan, Z. M., & Hasan, K. Z. (1998). Prevalence and correlates of mental retardation among children in Karachi, Pakistan. *American Journal of Epidemiology, 147,* 281–288.

Durkin, M. S., Maenner, M. J., Newschaffer, C. J., Lee, L.-C., Cunniff, C. M., Daniels, J. L., et al. (2008, October 21). Advanced paternal age and the risk of autism spectrum disorders. *American Journal of Epidemiology, 168*(11), 1268–1276. Epub.

Durkin, M. S., Maenner, MJ, Meaney, F. J., Levy, S.E., DiGuiseppi C., Nicholas, J. S., et al. (2010). Socioeconomic inequality in the prevalence of autism spectrum disorder: evidence from a US cross-sectional study. *PLoS One,* 5: e11551.

Ehlers, S., Gillberg, C., & Wing, L. (1999). A screening questionnaire for Asperger's syndrome and other high-functioning autism spectrum disorders in school age children. *Journal of Autism and Developmental Disorders, 29,* 129–140.

Eldin, A. S., Habib, D., Noufal, A., Farrag, S., Bazaid, K., Al-Sharbati, M., & Gaddour, N. (2008). Use of M-CHAT for a multinational screening of young children with autism in the Arab countries. *International Review of Psychiatry, 20*(3), 281–289.

ESEMeD/MHEDEA (2004). Prevalence of mental disorders in Europe: Results from the European Study of the Epidemiology of Mental Disorders (ESEMeD) project. *Acta Psychiatrica Scandinavica, 109*(suppl. 420), 21–27.

Evans, J., Harden, A., Thomas, J., & Benefield, P. (2003). *Support for pupils with emotional and behavioural difficulties (EBD) in mainstream primary school classrooms: A systematic review of the effectiveness of interventions* [online]. *NFER (National Foundation for Education Research).* eppi.ioe.ac.uk/EPPIWebContent/reel/**review.../EBD/EBD1**.pdf

Faraone, S. V., Sergeant, J., Gillberg, C., & Biederman, J. (2003). The worldwide prevalence of ADHD: Is it an American condition? *World Psychiatry, 2*(2), 104–113.

Faris, R. E. L., & Dunham, H. W. (1939). *Mental disorders in urban areas: An ecological study of schizophrenia and other psychoses.* New York: Hafner.

Fombonne, E. (2003). Epidemiological surveys of autism and other pervasive developmental disorders: an update. *Journal of Autism and Developmental Disorders, 33*(4), 365–382.

Fombonne, E., Zakarian, R., Bennet, A., Meng, L., & McLean-Heywood, D. (2006) . Pervasive developmental disorders in Montreal, Quebec, Canada: Prevalence and links with immunizations. *Pediatrics, 118*(1), 139–150.

Fombonne, E. (2007). Epidemiology and child psychiatry. In A. Martin, F. Volkmar, M. Lewis (Eds.), *Lewis's child and adolescent psychiatry: A comprehensive textbook* (pp. 149–170). Lippincott, Williams, & Wilkins.

Fombonne, E. (2009). Epidemiology of pervasive developmental disorders. *Pediatric Research, 65*(6), 591–598.

Fountain, C., King, M.D., & Bearman, P.S. (2010). Age of diagnosis for autism: individual and community factors among 10 birth cohorts. *Journal of Epidemiology and Community Health,* Epub, October 25.

Gillberg, C., Lamberg, K., & Zeijlon, L. (2006). The autism epidemic. the registered prevalence of autism in a Swedish urban area. *Journal of Autism and Development Disorders, 36*(3), 429–435.

Grinker, R. R. (2007). *Unstrange minds: Remapping the world of autism.* New York: Basic Books.

Grinker, R.R. (2010a). "In Retrospect: The Five Lives of the Psychiatry Manual." *Nature* (November 11), *468*: 168–170.

Grinker, R.R. (2010b). "Disorder Out of Chaos." *New York Times,* February 10, A23.

Grether, J. K, Anderson, M. C., Croen, L. A., Smith, D., Windham, G. C. (2009) Risk of autism and increasing maternal and paternal age in a large North American population. *American Journal of Epidemiology, 170*: 1118–1126.

Gupta, A., & Ferguson, J. (1992). Beyond culture: space, identity, and the politics of difference. *Cultural Anthropology, 7*(1), 6–23.

Holden, B., & Gitleson, J. P. (2006). A total population study of challenging behavior in the county of Hedmark, Norway: prevalence and risk markers. *Research in Developmental Disabilities, 27*(4), 456–465.

Honda, H., Yasuo Shimizu, Miho Imai, & Yukari Nitto. (2005). Cumulative incidence of childhood autism: a total population study of better accuracy and precision. *Developmental Medicine and Child Neurology, 47,* 10–18.

Hopper, K. (2003). Interrogating the meaning of culture in the WHO international studies of schizophrenia. In J. Jenkins (Ed.), *Schizophrenia, culture, and subjectivity: The edge of experience* (pp. 62–86). Cambridge: Cambridge University Press.

Hopper, K., Harrison, G., Janca, A., & Sartorius, N. (Eds.). (2007). *Recovery from schizophrenia: an international perspective: A report from the WHO collaborative project, the international study of schizophrenia.* Oxford: Oxford University Press.

Horwath, E., & Weissman, M. M. (2000). The epidemiology and cross-national presentation of obsessive–compulsive disorder. *Psychiatric Clinics of North America, 23*(3), 493–507.

Hugo, C. J., Boshoff, D. E. L., Traut, A., Zungu-Dirwayi, N., & Stein, D. J. (2003). Community attitudes toward and knowledge of mental illness in South Africa. *Social Psychiatry and Psychiatric Epidemiology, 38,* 715–719.

Icasiano, F., Hewson, P., Machet, P., Cooper, C., & Marshall, A. (2004). Childhood autism spectrum disorder in the Barwon region: a community based study. *Journal of Paediatrics and Child Health, 40*(12), 696–701.

Islam, S., Durkin, M. S., & Zaman, S. (1993). Socioeconomic status and the prevalence of mental retardation in Bangladesh. *Mental Retardation, 31,* 412–417.

Kalra, V., Seth, R., & Sapra, S. (2005). Autism: experiences in a tertiary hospital. *Indian Journal of Pediatrics, 72*(3), 227–230.

Karande, S. (2006). Autism: a review for family physicians. *Indian Journal of Medical Sciences (Practitioner's Section), 60*(5), 205–215.

Kasmini, K., & Zasmani, S. (1995). Asperger's syndrome: a report of two cases from Malaysia. *Singapore Medical Journal, 36,*641–643.

Kendell, R. E., Cooper, J. E., Gourlay, A. J., Copeland, J. R. M., Sharpe, L., & Gurland, B. J. (1971). Diagnostic criteria of American and British psychiatrists. *Archives of General Psychiatry, 25*(2), 123–130.

Khan, N., & Hombarume, J. (1996). Levels of autistic behavior among the mentally handicapped children in Zimbabwe. *Central African Journal of Medicine, 42*(2), 39.

Kielinen, M., Linna, S. L., & Moilanen, I. (2000). Autism in northern Finland. *European Child and Adolescent Psychiatry, 9*(3), 162–167.

King, M. & Bearman, P. (2010). Diagnostic change and the increased prevalence of autism. *International Journal of Epidemiology, 38,* 1224–1234.

Kleinbaum, D. G., Kupper, L. K., & Morgenstern, H. (1982). Measures of disease frequency: Incidence. *Epidemiology and research: Principles and quantitative measures* (pp. 97–115). New York: Wiley.

Krug, D. A., Arick, J. R., & Almond, P. J. (1980). Behavior checklist for identifying severely handicapped individuals with high levels of autism behavior. *Journal of Child Psychology and Psychiatry and Allied Disciplines, 21*(3), 221–229.

La Malfa, G., Lassi, S., Bertelli, M., Salvini, R., & Placidi, G. F. (2004). Autism and intellectual disability: a study of prevalence on a sample of the Italian population. *Journal of Intellectual Disability Research, 48*(3), 262–267.

Lauritsen, M. B., Pedersen, C. B., & Mortensen, P. B. (2004). The incidence and prevalence of pervasive developmental disorders: a Danish population-based study. *Psychological Medicine, 34,* 1339–1346.

Lemelson, R. (2003). Obsessive-compulsive disorder in Bali: the cultural shaping of a neuropsychiatric disorder. *Transcultural Psychiatry, 40*(3), 377–408.

Levi, G., & Bernadbei, P. (2005). Italy. In F. R. Volkmar, R. Paul, A. Klin, & D. Cohen (eds.), *Handbook of autism and pervasive developmental disorders* (3rd ed., pp. 1221–1223). New York: Wiley.

Levy, S., & Hyman, S. (2003). Use of complementary and alternative treatments for children with autistic spectrum disorders is increasing. *Pediatric Annals, 32*, 685–691.

Liu, K., King, M., & Bearman, P. (2009). Social influence and the autism epidemic. *American Journal of Sociology, 115*(5), 1387–1434.

Lord, C., Rutter, M. L., DiLavore, P. C., & Risi, S. (1999). *Autism Diagnostic Observation Schedule–WPS*. Los Angeles: Western Psychological Services.

Lotter, V. (1978). Childhood autism in Africa. *Journal of Child Psychology and Psychiatry, 19*, 231–244.

Lung, F., Shu, B., Chiang, T., & Lin, S. (2010). Parental concerns based general developmental screening tool and autism risk: the Taiwan national birth cohort study. *Pediatric Research, 67*(2), 226–231.

Maenner, M. J. & Durkin, M. S. (2010). Trends in the prevalence of autism on the basis of special education data. *Pediatrics*, 126(5): 1018–1025.

Magnusson, P., & Saemundsen, E. (2001). Prevalence of autism in Iceland. *Journal of Autism and Developmental Disorders, 31*(2), 153–163.

Mandell, D. S., Listerud, J., Levy, S. E., & Pinto-Martin, J. A. (2002). Race differences in the age at diagnosis among Medicaid-eligible children with autism. *Journal of the American Academy of Child and Adolescent Psychiatry, 41*(12), 1447–1453.

Mandell, D. S., & Novak, M. M. (2005). The role of culture in family's treatment decisions for children with autism spectrum disorders. *Mental Retardation and Developmental Disabilities Research Reviews, 11*(2), 110–115.

Mandell, D. S., Novak, M. M., & Zubritsky, C. D. (2005). Factors associated with age of diagnosis among children with autism spectrum disorders. *Pediatrics, 116*(6), 1480–1486.

Minnesota Department of Public Health. (2009). *Autism spectrum disorders among preschool children participating in the Minneapolis public schools early childhood special education programs*. St. Paul, MN. Available at www.health.state.mn.us/ommh/projects/autism/index.cfm.

Mishler, E. G., & Scotch, N. A. (1965, April). Sociocultural factors in the epidemiology of schizophrenia: a review. *International Journal of Psychiatry, 1*, 258–305.

Montiel-Nava, C., & Peña, J. A. (2008). Epidemiological findings of pervasive developmental disorders in a Venezuelan study. *Autism, 12*(2), 191–202.

Morton, R., Sharma, V., Nicholson, J., Broderick, M., & Poyser, J. (2002). Disability in children from different ethnic populations. *Child: Care, Health, and Development, 28*(1), 87–93.

National Population and Family Planning Commission of the People's Republic of China. (2009, March 9). Available at http://www.chinapop.gov.cn/wxzl/rkgk/200903/t20090309_166730.htm Accessed March 16, 2009 (In Chinese).

National Research Council (Committee on Educational Interventions for Children with Autism). (2001). *Educating children with autism*. Washington, DC: National Academies Press.

Newschaffer, C. J., Falb, M. D., & Gurney, J. G. (2005). National autism prevalence trends from United States special education data. *Pediatrics, 115*, 277–282.

Ochs, E. (1998). *Culture and language development: Language acquisition and language socialization in a Samoan village*. Cambridge: Cambridge University Press.

Ochs, E. & Schieffelin, B. (1984). Language acquisition and socialization: Three developmental stories. In R Shweder & R. LeVine, (Eds.), *Culture theory: Mind, self, and emotion* (pp. 263–301). Cambridge: Cambridge University Press.

Offord, D. R., Boyle, M. H., Szatmari, P., Rae-Grant, N. I., Links, P. S., Cadman, D. T., et al. (1987). Ontario Child Health Study: I. Six-month prevalence of disorder and rates of service utilization. *Archives of General Psychiatry, 44*, 832–836.

Olivera, G., Assunção, A., Marques, C., Miguel, T. S., Coutinho, A. M., Mota-Vieira, L., & Vicente, A. M. (2007). Epidemiology of autism spectrum disorder in Portugal: prevalence, clinical characterization, and medical conditions. *Developmental Medicine and Child Neurology, 49*(10), 726–733.

Olusanya, B. O. (2007). Promoting effective interventions for neglected health conditions in developing countries. *Disability and Rehabilitation, 29*(11–12), 973–976.

Petersen, I. (2004). Primary level psychological services in South Africa: can a new psychological professional fill the gap? *Health, Policy, and Planning, 19*(1), 33–40.

Philippe, A., Martinez, M., Guilloud-Bataille, M., Gillberg, C., Råstam, M., Sponheim, E., & Leboyer, M. (1999). Genome-wide scan for autism susceptibility genes. Paris Autism Research International Sibpair Study. *Human Molecular Genetics, 8*(5), 805–812.

Polanczyk, G., de Lima, M., Horta, B., Biederman, J. & Rohde, L. (2007). The worldwide prevalence of ADHD: a systematic review and metaregression analysis. *American Journal of Psychiatry, 16*(6), 942–948.

Powell, J. E., Edwards, A., Edwards, M., Pandit, B. S., Sungum-Paliwal, S. R., & Whitehouse, W. (2000). Changes in the incidence of childhood autism and other autism spectrum disorders in preschool children from two areas of the West Midlands, UK. *Developmental Medicine and Child Neurology, 42*, 624–628.

Probst, P. (1998). Child health-related cognitions of parents with autistic children: A cross-national exploratory study. In U. P. Gielen and A. L. Comunian (Eds.), *The family and family therapy in international perspective* (pp. 461–483). Trieste: Lint.

Rogers, S. J. (1998). Empirically supported comprehensive treatments for young children with autism. *Journal of Clinical Child and Adolescent Psychology, 27*, 167–178.

Rogers, S. J., & Vismara, L. A. (2008). Evidence-based comprehensive treatments for early autism. *Journal of Clinical Child and Adolescent Psychology, 37*(1), 8–38.

Rothman, K. J., & Greenland, S. (1998). Measures of disease frequency. In K. J. Rothman & S. Greenland (Eds.), *Modern epidemiology* (pp. 29–64). Philadelphia: Lippincott-Raven.

Ruiz, D. S. (1982). Epidemiology of schizophrenia: some diagnostic and sociocultural considerations. *Phylon, 43*(4), 315–326.

Rutter, M., Cox, A., Tupling, C., Berger, M., & Yule, M. (1975). Attainment and adjustment in two geographical areas: I. The prevalence of psychiatric disorder. *British Journal of Psychiatry, 126*, 493–509.

Rutter, M., Le Couteur, A., & Lord, C. (2003). *Manual for the ADI-WPS version*. Los Angeles: Western Psychological Services.

Rydelius, P.-A. (2005). Sweden and other Nordic nations. In F. R. Volkmar, R. Paul, A. Klin, & D. Cohen (Eds.), *Handbook of autism and pervasive developmental disorders* (3rd ed., pp. 1238–1243). New York: Wiley.

Sanua, V. D. (1984). Is infantile autism a universal phenomenon? An open question *International Journal of Social Psychiatry, 30*(3), 163–174.

Sartawi, A. M. (1999). Educational and behavioural characteristics of autistic children in the United Arab Emirates. *International Journal of Rehabilitation Research, 22*(1), 337–339.

Schieffelin, B. B. (2005). *The give and take of everyday life: Language socialization of Kaluli children*. Tucson: Fenestra.

Schopler, E., Reichler, R. J., & Brenner, B. R. (1988). *The Childhood Autism Rating Scale* (CARS). Los Angeles: Western Psychological Services.

Shelton, J. F., Tancredi, D. J., & Hertz-Picciotto, I. (2010). Independent and dependent contributions of advanced maternal and paternal ages to autism risk. *Autism Research*, 3, 30–39.

Shin, Y., Lee, K., Min, S., & Emde, R. N. (1999). A Korean syndrome of attachment disturbance mimicking symptoms of pervasive developmental disorder. *Infant Mental Health Journal*, *20*(1), 60–76.

Skellern, C. M., McDowell, M., & Schluter, P. (2005). Diagnosis of autism spectrum disorders in Queensland: variations in practice. *Journal of Pediatrics and Child Health*, *41*, 407–412.

Spinney, L. (2007). Therapy for autistic children causes outcry in France. *Nature*, *370*, 645–646.

Stone, W. L. (1987). Cross-disciplinary perspectives on autism. *Journal of Pediatric Psychology*, *12*, 615–630.

Tao, K., & Yang, X. (2005). China. In F. R. Volkmar, R. Paul, A. Klin, & D. Cohen (Eds.), *Handbook of autism and pervasive developmental disorders* (3rd ed., pp. 1203–1206). New York: Wiley.

Thara, R., Padmavati, R., & Srinivasan, T. N. (2004). Focus on psychiatry in India. *British Journal of Psychiatry*, *184*, 366–373.

Thorburn, M. J., Desai, P., Paul, T. J., Malcolm, L., Durkin, M., & Davidson, L. (1992). Identification of childhood disability in Jamaica: the ten question screen. *International Journal of Rehabilitation Research*, *15*, 115–127.

U.S. Department of Health and Human Services (USDHHS). (1999). *Mental health: A report of the Surgeon General.* Rockville, MD: U.S. Department of Health and Human Services, Substance Abuse and Mental Health Services Administration, Center for Mental Health Services, National Institutes of Health, National Institute of Mental Health.

van Engeland, H. (2005). The Netherlands. In F. R. Volkmar, R. Paul, A. Klin, & D. Cohen (Eds.), *Handbook of autism and pervasive developmental disorders* (3rd ed., pp. 1233–1235). New York: Wiley.

Vogel, W., & Holford, L. (1999). Child psychiatry in Johannesburg, South Africa: a descriptive account of cases presenting at two clinics in 1997. *European Child and Adolescent Psychiatry*, *8*, 181–188.

Whaley, A. L. (2001). Cultural mistrust and the clinical diagnosis of paranoid schizophrenia in African American patients.*Journal of Psychopathology and Behavioral Assessment*, *23*(2), 93–100.

Williams, K., Glasson, E. J., Wray, J., Tuck, M., Helmer, M., Bower, C. I., et al. (2005). Incidence of autism spectrum disorders in children in two Australian states. *Medical Journal of Australia*, *182*(3), 108–111.

Wong, V. C. N., & Hui, S. L. H. (2008). Epidemiological study of autism spectrum disorder in China. *Journal of Child Neurology*, *23*(1), 67–72.

World Health Organization. (2001). *International classification of functioning, disability, and health*. Geneva: WHO.

Yeargin-Allsopp, M., & Boyle, C. (2002). Overview: the epidemiology of neurodevelopmental disorders. *Mental Retardation and Developmental Disabilities Research Reviews*, *8*, 113–116.

Commentary

Patrick F. Bolton

Issues in the Classification of Pervasive Developmental Disorders

Introduction

The rationale for classifying childhood onset mental problems, including neurodevelopmental disorders such as autism, is that it aids in communication and the nosological entities predict aspects of the natural history of the condition, its response to treatment as well as the causes of the phenomena. By their nature, classification systems can never be complete and perfect, as they continually need to be revised and updated as knowledge accrues (Taylor & Rutter, 2002; Angold & Costello, 2009).

Approaches to the classification of mental problems have evolved over the years and have moved from a system based on psychoanalytic theory to more phenomenologically based approaches. Modern schemes really began with the introduction of DSM-III and ICD-9 in the 1970s, both of which are based largely on descriptions of patterns of symptomatology.

One of the key developments in the nosology of childhood psychopathology was the implementation of a multiaxial diagnostic scheme. The need for a multiaxial scheme stemmed from the recognition that psychopathology is often multifaceted in its presentation and that multiple factors, often occurring in combination, may be etiologically relevant. For example, both the presence of a specific medical condition and certain psychosocial stresses may be relevant in the development of a child's problems.

Although the advent of ICD-10 and DSM-IV represented a major step in nosological classification, several advances in knowledge have taken place over the last 15 years, and this has led to a realization of the need to revise our diagnostic scheme and work toward the publication of new editions of the main classificatory systems for psychopathology, ICD-11 and DSM-V.

Within this context it is timely, therefore, to consider the classification of the pervasive developmental disorders and the areas in which revisions might need to be made.

Unresolved Issues in ICD-10 and DSM-IV

The term Pervasive Developmental Disorder (PDD) was coined in order to reflect the fact that autism, the prototypical form of Pervasive Developmental Disorder, is characterized by problems in development that pervade both social, language/communication, play, and intellectual development. The need for an umbrella term that encompassed a number of different possible conditions falling under the generic heading PDD, reflected the fact that there was some uncertainty as to whether different subtypes or forms of presentation were meaningfully associated with different causes, natural history, and response to treatment. The conditions listed under the Pervasive Developmental Disorder category in DSM-IV and ICD-10 are summarized in Table C1-1. Although the two classificatory

Table C1–1.
ICD-10 and DSM 1V classification of pervasive developmental disorders

DSM 1V	ICD-10
Autism	Autism
Asperger's	Asperger's
	Atypical Autism
PDD NOS	PDD Other
	PDD Unspecified
Rett Syndrome	Rett Syndrome
	Childhood Disintegrative Disorder
Childhood Disintegrative Disorder	Overactive disorder associated with mental retardation and stereotyped movements

schemes were similar in many respects, there were some notable differences.

First, The World Health Organization (WHO) published two versions of ICD-10: a clinical diagnostic scheme as well as research diagnostic scheme (WHO, 1993). The clinical diagnostic scheme provided prototypical descriptions of the specific disorder (e.g., autism), and the onus was on the clinician to determine whether or not the child's presentation best fitted with one or other prototype. By contrast, the research diagnostic criteria followed a similar approach to that adopted in DSM-IV by specifying a list of symptoms that had to be present in different domains of function: to meet diagnostic criteria individuals had to manifest a specific number of symptoms within each domain. The rational for adopting these different approaches in ICD-10 was that it was considered that the approach of pattern matching to a "gestalt" that was exemplified in the clinical diagnostic scheme better reflected expert clinical practice, whereas the symptom count approach was better suited for research, as more detailed operationalization of the diagnostic criteria was likely to increase the reliability of diagnosis. The drawback of the symptom count approach was that the criteria were not externally validated and potentially led to premature conceptual closure, with critics pointing out that diagnosis is not simply an exercise in counting symptoms. Of course, the two approaches are not mutually exclusive and, in practice, it is possible to adopt a combined approach by specifying that a case meets clinical and research diagnostic criteria.

Second, ICD-10 and DSM-IV adopted different multiaxial schemes. Although both systems place PDD on axis 1, DSM 1V classifies personality disorders and the degree of intellectual disability on axis 2, the presence of medical conditions on axis 3, associated psychosocial and environmental problems on axis 4, and the overall level of function on axis 5. By contrast, in ICD-10, axis 2 is used to classify specific developmental disorders, axis 3 the intellectual level, axis 4 medical conditions, axis 5 psychosocial influences, and axis 6 the level of functioning. Personality disorders are classified on axis 1 in ICD-10.

At this stage there seems to be little reason to argue that PDD should be moved from axis 1 to another axis. However, clear guidance on how associated features of PDD such as language delays and impairments should be dealt with is necessary, as speech and language delay is currently one of the diagnostic criteria for autism, but is not a necessary feature. As language level is a key predictor of outcome, it would arguably make sense to separately classify the presence of language impairment on axis 2.

Third, when the two classificatory systems were being formulated, there was a good deal of uncertainty as to where the boundaries should be drawn between autism and other pervasive developmental disorders and what other possible subtypes of PDD should be delineated. The main dilemmas centered on the degree of possible heterogeneity and how to classify cases that did not meet all the criteria for a diagnosis of autism. At the time, the main questions focused on whether and how to separately classify cases of Asperger's syndrome and Rett's syndrome and what to do with atypical presentations in terms of atypical symptom profiles and atypical ages of onset. Asperger's paper and description of the eponymous syndrome had only recently been translated from German into English (Wing, 1981), and some differences from autism in the presenting and associated features raised the possibility that it might represent a different condition. The findings from studies of schizoid disorder of childhood (Wolff & Barlow, 1979; Wolff & Chick, 1980; Wolff, 1991), fueled the speculation that children presenting in these ways may constitute a separate subgroup. Accordingly, Asperger's syndrome was included as a separate category in both schemes. Similarly, Rett's syndrome had also only relatively recently been characterized on the basis of symptomatology, regression, and course (Rett, 1986), but as the cause was unknown at that time, it was classified as a PDD rather than a genetic disorder, despite the fact that it was strongly suspected to be a single gene disorder.

The two classificatory systems took quite different approaches to the classification of other atypical presentations. In DSM-IV they were all lumped together and classified as PDD Not-Otherwise-Specified (PDD-NOS). There were no operationalized criteria for PDD-NOS. By contrast, four additional diagnostic categories were created in ICD-10.

1. Atypical autism was used to classify cases that nearly met the full criteria for a diagnosis of autism, but there were insufficient symptoms in one domain to meet criteria for autism or the presentation was atypical in terms of age of onset.
2. PDD "other" was used to classify cases that were thought to have a PDD but did not meet criteria for autism or atypical autism. There were no operationalized criteria for this diagnosis.
3. The category of PDD unspecified was created for cases where findings were conflicting, inconsistent, or incomplete. For example, if findings from observational assessments did not agree with parental reports of the child's development, or if observational assessments suggested the diagnosis, but there was no informant available to provide details of the early developmental history.
4. ICD-10 also included a diagnostic category of uncertain nosological status termed "over active disorder with mental retardation and stereotyped movements."

The aim in ICD-10 was to attempt to split PDD into various different putative subtypes.

Fourth, the operational definition of Asperger's syndrome has given rise to some confusion over how to differentiate it from high functioning autism (i.e., cases where there was no significant speech/language delay and where the individual is of normal intelligence, yet speech and language development was deviant). The dilemma has been that these cases could meet criteria for both autism and Asperger's syndrome (Volkmar, Klin, et al., 1996; Volkmar, Klin, et al., 1998).

An additional concern was that PDD "other" and PDD unspecified in ICD-10 and PDD-NOS in DSM-IV were not operationally defined, so there was a good deal of uncertainty as to when these diagnoses should be made.

Clearly one of the issues to address in future revisions of the nosological scheme concerns the approach to subtyping and the number of subtypes to be included under the rubric of pervasive developmental disorders (see below).

Fifth, the two classificatory systems took rather different approaches to hierarchical rules within the schemes. In ICD-10 the diagnosis of one condition often precluded the diagnosis of other disorders, whereas in DSM-IV this was less frequently the case, although a hierarchical approach was sometimes adopted. As a consequence in DSM-IV it was more often possible to diagnose two conditions concurrently. The rationale for including hierarchical rules was that the significance of symptoms may be different when they occur in the presence of a major disorder (Matson & Nebel-Schwalm, 2007). For example, high levels of activity were thought to be common features in individuals with autism and not necessarily indicative of the presence of hyperkinesis/attention deficit/hyperactivity. Accordingly, the diagnosis of ADHD/hyperkinesis was precluded in individuals with a diagnosis of autism both in ICD-10 and DSM 1V. Here again, the findings over the last 15 years highlight the need to reconsider some of these hierarchical rules and the best approach to adopt for classifying complex presentations that are characterized by admixtures of symptomatology of various kinds (Matson & Nebel-Schwalm, 2007).

In addition to these extant issues, a number of new issues have emerged as methods have developed and the evidence base has advanced. These are outlined below.

Recent Advances and New Issues

The Concept of "Autism Spectrum Disorder"

One of the most significant conceptual shifts has been the adoption of the notion that autism is part of a "spectrum of disorder." Lorna Wing was the first to put forward the idea that autism is a spectrum disorder and proposed a typology based on the pattern of social impairment (Wing & Gould, 1979; Wing, 1997). Subsequent genetic epidemiological data has helped underpin the concept of autism as a spectrum disorder. For example, findings from family and twin studies have clearly shown that the liability to autism confers a risk not just for autism, but for a range of manifestations that can include several PDD variants such as Asperger's syndrome, atypical autism and PDD other/PDD-NOS (Bolton, Macdonald, et al., 1994; Bailey, Le Couteur, et al., 1995; Bailey, Palferman, et al., 1998). The findings provide unequivocal support for the concept of a spectrum of manifestations, but the spectrum typology proposed by Wing has not been widely adopted or extensively investigated.

The genetic epidemiological data also showed that the liability to autism confers a risk for social and communication difficulties and unusual patterns of interests and activities that extend well beyond the traditional concepts of a pervasive developmental disorder, to include impairments in just one domain of function (Bolton, Macdonald, et al., 1994; Bailey, Le Couteur et al., 1995; Bailey, Palferman et al., 1998).

These findings have led to uncertainty over where the line should be drawn between autism spectrum disorder and normal variation in personality, social behavior, and function. Indeed, the lack of any clear demarcation between the broader autism phenotype and normal variation in behavior has been used to argue that autism is the extreme of a normally distributed set of traits, in much the same way that obesity can be considered to be the extreme of normal variation in weight. Accordingly, researchers have developed and investigated dimensional models of the phenotype (Constantino & Todd, 2003; Constantino, Gruber, et al., 2004). The findings from these studies have provided interesting new insights, but it should nevertheless be emphasized that the absence of a clear discontinuity in the distribution of trait questionnaire scores does not unequivocally prove that autism is the extreme of normal variation in autistic traits for several reasons.

First, the distribution of scores in siblings of individuals with autism has a long upper tail, raising the possibility that there may be a discontinuity. Second, the autism phenotype is associated with features that are not commonly found in the general population, such as macrocephaly, epilepsy, and intellectual disability. The findings indicate that at some point there is a discontinuity or threshold at which point there is a qualitative change in manifestation. The findings are potentially consistent with the liability threshold model. Alternatively, they may reflect a second hit event or heterogeneity. For example, it may be that, as for intellectual disability, a mixed model applies, where individuals fall at the extreme of the distribution either because they have a specific genetic or medical problem or because the factors responsible for variation within the normal range have conspired together to place individuals at the extreme of the normal distribution.

As such, although the development and construction of a dimensional measure of the autistic traits has much to commend it, there are a number of methodological challenges to overcome in developing a suitable measure, conceptual issues to resolve, and uncertainties about when a dimensional or categorical model is most informative. Until these issues have been resolved, most effort has gone into the development of measures of the severity of autism spectrum disorder.

Measuring the Severity of Autism Spectrum Disorder

The reasons for developing a scale of the severity of autism spectrum disorder are in order to use the measure: (1) as an index of liability to the condition, (2) to predict outcome, (3) to assess response to treatment. The approach to constructing a measure will differ in each of these circumstances. For example, a measure to quantify response to treatment will need to be a measure of current severity and be sensitive to change. By contrast a measure for the purpose of predicting outcome will need to be designed to assess severity at a particular time point in development, when the scale is going to have good predictive properties and be of maximal clinical use for planning future service provision and advising families.

For the purpose of classification, the primary goals are to quantify liability and predict outcome. Typically severity is estimated on the basis of symptomatology and symptom severity can be quantified in a number of ways. These include (1) counting the total number of symptoms, (2) measuring the intrusiveness or contextual sensitivity of symptomatology, (3) determining the persistence and duration of symptoms over time.

Symptom Count

Up to now the majority of studies have chosen to examine the number of symptoms as a metric of severity. However, the approach is not as simple as it might at first seem. For example, the list of symptoms has to be delineated and a decision made as to how to score them and whether to give each symptom equal weight in computing the score. So far the choice of symptoms has been determined on the basis of the instrument used to evaluate them and in part, therefore, on the instruments' ability to discriminate between cases and controls. Obviously selecting symptoms in this way can affect the properties of the distribution observed. Moreover each symptom has typically been given equal weight, yet the rating scales tend to have more items covering some symptom domains than others, so again this has the potential to influence the distributional properties of the scale.

A related challenge in deriving a severity score is to develop a means of equating scores in individuals with no speech to scores in those with speech, where a higher score is potentially possible simply because individuals with speech can manifest phenomena such as neologism, pronominal reversal, and stereotypic and repetitive speech. The limited investigation of this issue so far conducted suggests that language impairments may not lead to long-lasting differences in severity (Loucas, Charman, et al., 2008). Similar considerations apply to the estimation of symptom severity in individuals with an associated intellectual disability, where again the repertoire of symptoms will be modified by the presence of the intellectual disability.

Developmental Changes

Another issue is that the type and number of symptoms will change and vary with age and over time. To some degree the problem can be circumvented by focusing on a particular age and stage of development and evaluating the symptomatology at that time point. This is the approach taken for example by the Autism Diagnostic Interview-Revised (Lord, Pickles, et al., 1997; Lord, Rutter, et al., 1994), which focuses in part on symptomatology that is exhibited between the ages of 4 to 5 years. Clearly, this approach leaves open the issue of what to do with children younger than 4 to 5, where the number and type of symptoms develops and unfolds considerably. Focusing on a specific age period also leads to inherent problems in accurately assessing symptom count in older individual or young adults, where recall bias is likely to be present.

Sources of Information

Reports on symptomatology can be obtained from various sources, including parents and teachers, but symptomatology can also be evaluated during observational assessments using instruments such as the Autism Diagnostic Observation Schedule-Generic (Lord, Rutter et al., 1989). The comparative validity of measures derived from an observational assessment lasting an hour compared with reports of behavior occurring over the course of months or a year is unknown. It may be that a combination of questionnaire, interview-based reports, and observational methods will be the most accurate way of quantifying symptom severity, but as yet the best approach to combining information from various sources is still unclear.

Dimensions of Severity

Another consideration concerns our conceptualization of autism spectrum disorder as a cohesive unitary phenomenon. Recent findings have challenged this view and have raised the possibility that autism spectrum disorder represents a "compound phenotype" comprising several interrelated dimensions relating to social, communication, and repetitive behaviors. These ideas have stemmed in part from twin study data that have suggested that there may be overlapping as well as distinct genetic and environmental determinants of each dimension (Ronald, Happe, et al., 2005; Ronald, Happe, et al., 2006; Happe & Ronald, 2008). If autism spectrum disorder were a compound phenotype, then this would have implications for assessing severity and indicate that it should be assessed on a number of different dimensions. Currently, the notion that autism spectrum disorder represents a compound phenotype has not been conclusively established (Constantino, Gruber, et al., 2004). For the time being therefore, it is best to focus on the development of a unitary measure of symptom severity.

Other Approaches to Measuring Severity

An alternative way of estimating the severity of a condition is to assess change in symptomatology over time, but although it is known that autistic symptomatology can wax or wane, the relationship to liability and outcome has not been systematically investigated. Similarly, the degree to which symptoms vary across situations (e.g., home or school) or intrude into other activities or disrupt family life can be used as a metric of severity. But here again, the approach has not been evaluated.

Yet another approach to measuring severity is to evaluate the level of social role impairment associated with the symptoms and quantifying this, for example by using the Childhood Global Assessment Scale (Bird, Yager, et al., 1990) or by measuring the level of adaptive function. Severity estimates using these approaches are likely to be influenced by intellectual level, as well as the presence of any comorbid disorders and other features associated with autism (e.g., speech and language impairment). Nevertheless, these approaches could potentially capture severity more comprehensively, but whether such measures relate more closely to liability or better predict outcome is uncertain, with variable findings with respect prognosis (Nordin & Gillberg, 1998; Szatmari, Bryson, et al., 2003; Howlin, Goode, et al., 2004; Baghdadli, Picot, et al., 2007).

The current published research on the utility of each of the approaches to quantifying severity is extremely limited. Most research has focused on estimating severity from symptom count. Even here, the data are inconsistent with some, but not all, studies suggesting that symptom count is associated with the familial liability to autism spectrum disorder (Bolton, Macdonald, et al., 1994; Szatmari, Jones, et al., 1996; Spiker, Lotspeich, et al., 2002; Szatmari, Merette, et al., 2008). The evidence from studies of identical twins (one of whom has an autism spectrum disorder) suggests however, that symptom severity is only weakly correlated with liability if at all (Le Couteur, Bailey, et al., 1996) or exhibits correlations in only some domains (Kolevzon, Smith, et al., 2004). It remains uncertain, therefore, how closely symptom severity indexes liability.

Similarly, it remains unclear how well symptom count predicts prognosis, after the presence of associated features such as speech/language and intellectual level has been taken into consideration. Findings from some studies suggest that symptom severity is associated with outcome, others do not (Nordin & Gillberg, 1998; Szatmari, Bryson, et al., 2003; Howlin, Goode, et al., 2004; Baghdadli, Picot, et al., 2007; Billstedt, Gillberg, et al., 2007).

In the absence of any data on the utility of other approaches, the simplest way forward is to quantify severity using symptom count anchored developmentally within a specific time period such as the 4- to 5-year period adopted by the ADI(R) Interview, perhaps supplemented with measures derived from observational assessments.

There still remains one important issue. This concerns the criteria to adopt for the diagnosis of autism spectrum disorder and how broadly to define the concept. The dilemma here is that very little is known about the development and outcome of individuals with the broader autism phenotype (BAP), so it is unclear to what extent social role impairment is associated with the broader phenotype. Also, as the criteria for diagnosing the BAP are not well developed, the sensitivity and specificity of the criteria for diagnosis are not known. For the time being it seems sensible, therefore to retain a category of PDD other for diagnosing individuals with the BAP, but operationalized criteria will have to be created.

Developmental Issues

Although autism spectrum has by definition an onset within the first 3 years of life, it is evident that in some individuals symptomatology emerges within the first year or two, before the full syndrome has become manifest (Rogers, 2004; Elsabbagh & Johnson, 2007; Stefanatos, 2008). This is evident for example from the studies of infant siblings of individuals with autism spectrum disorders which have revealed that early social and communication difficulties can be identified prior to the manifestation of the full syndrome. At this stage, the specificity of these early manifestations is under investigation, but the findings nevertheless highlight the need to develop a system for classifying these phenomena. In the diagnostic scheme for children aged 0 to 3 (DC 0–3) (Zero-Three, 2005), the only option at present is to diagnose a multisystem developmental disorder in children under the age of 2 and pervasive developmental disorder for children aged 2+. However, these diagnoses have not been fully operationalized. At present, we know too little about the specificity of the early signs to be able to classify them under the rubric of PDD. However, there is no reason to refrain from diagnosing PDD in children under the age of 2 years if they meet diagnostic criteria. Otherwise, until we have a better understanding of the precursors of ASD, it would seem best to specify the type of developmental problem using the DC 0–3 scheme.

In addition to the question of classification of precursor symptomatology there is also the issue as to whether or not the occurrence of regression in development is an important feature to record in the classification scheme. Here again the findings are inconsistent, with some reports suggesting that the presence of regression may be associated with different manifestations, course, and possibly etiology, but other studies failing to identify any significant differences in those with and without regression (Rogers, 2004; Stefanatos, 2008). The picture has been further complicated by the recent suggestion that regression may be an almost universal feature in autism spectrum disorder albeit unobservable or unmeasurable in the subset of cases where regression occurs very early in development (Baird, Charman, et al., 2008; Pickles, Simonoff, et al., 2009). It will also have to be decided whether to subclassify the type of regression and stipulate the areas in which regression is observed (e.g., language, social, motor, intelligence, etc).

Another consideration concerns the fact that autism symptomatology also changes later on in development either becoming significantly more or less marked with age. There has been a tendency to consider autism as a disorder that is lifelong in manifestations, and certainly this is the case in many individuals (Howlin, Goode, et al. 2004). However, there are also reports of individuals who largely if not completely outgrow their autism. These findings raise the question as to whether or not autism should be a permanent lifelong diagnosis. It is perhaps worth emphasizing here that in the current DSM classification scheme it is possible to stipulate that the condition is in partial or full remission or the diagnosis was based on prior history. It makes sense to retain this subspecification.

Presentations in adulthood also raise issues about the differentiation of autism spectrum disorder and PDD other from schizoid and schizotypal personality disorder. This question has been little studied, but potential differentiating features include the developmental history, pragmatics of communication, form of prosody, and pattern of interests and activities.

Associated Features

Quite apart from the challenge of estimating symptom severity, there is an additional need to provide a means for quantification of the level of function in key features associated with autism, including speech/language and intellectual level. That is because these associated features constitute some of the best indices of prognosis (Nordin & Gillberg 1998; Szatmari, Bryson, et al., 2003; Baghdadli, Picot, et al., 2007; Billstedt, Gillberg, et al., 2007). One way of achieving this would be to specify the level of speech and language attainment using some standardized measure of speech language skills and to record this on axis 2, rather than simply the presence of speech language impairment. Similarly, intellectual ability (e.g., full scale IQ) can be recorded on axis 3, rather than simply specifying the degree of intellectual disability.

With respect to the measurement of the degree of social role impairment, both DSM and ICD-10 record the overall level of social impairment on axis 6 in ICD-10 and axis 5 on DSM, but agreed methods for measuring the degree of impairment would be desirable.

Heterogeneity

It is well established that autism spectrum disorder is etiologically heterogeneous, with an identifiable, probably causal medical condition found in some 10% of cases (Rutter, Bailey, et al., 1994). For example individuals with tuberous sclerosis, Fragile X syndrome, and abnormalities of chromosome 15 are at increased risk for developing an autism spectrum disorder, although they are not necessarily destined to do so (Feinstein & Reiss, 1998; Bolton, Dennis, et al., 2001; Bolton, Park, et al., 2002; Milner, Craig, et al., 2005). With the recent discovery of the association between autism spectrum disorder and copy number variants it is likely that other genetic and other submicroscopic chromosomal abnormalities will soon be established as new causes of autism spectrum disorder (Sebat, Lakshmi, et al., 2007; Christian, Brune, et al., 2008; Geschwind, 2009; Kumar & Christian, 2009). There is some evidence to suggest that the manifestations of autism spectrum disorder in individual with these comorbid medical conditions may differ in certain respects. For example, individuals with Fragile x syndrome are said to be socially avoidant and anxious (Cohen, Fisch, et al., 1988; Cohen, Vietze, et al., 1989). In many circumstances, individuals with a comorbid genetic condition also have an associated intellectual disability and epilepsy. Accordingly, there is a need to make allowances for this within the classificatory scheme. At present, all medical disorders are recorded on axis 4 in ICD-10 and axis 3 in DSM-IV, but there is no way of indicating which of the medical disorders is probably causal. One solution is to include a subcategory on axis 1 for individuals with autism spectrum deriving from an associated, likely causal medical condition, recording the associated medical disorder on axis 4. The list of currently accepted medical cause of autism spectrum disorder includes Fragile x syndrome, tuberous sclerosis, and abnormalities of chromosome 15 involving 15q11-13, but the list is likely to grow in the near future.

In addition to genetic and medical causes, it is now also apparent that individuals who experienced severe early deprivation may exhibit quasi-autistic-like manifestations that tend to resolve with time and nurturance (Rutter, Andersen-Wood, et al., 1999). Again, consideration needs to be given as to how to differentiate between these presentations and autism spectrum disorder and whether to classify the disturbance in social and communication development observed after extreme deprivation as a PDD or a form of attachment disorder.

Childhood disintegrative disorder, which currently is separately characterized on the basis of the prior period of normal development up until at least 2 years of age followed by a regression and loss of skills and the emergence of an autistic-like syndrome (Volkmar & Rutter, 1995; Mashiko, 2003; Kurita, Koyama, et al. 2004; Rogers, 2004), should be retained as a subtype of PDD, but consideration should be given to renaming it, as the current label can give a rather misleading impression. The rational for subtyping this group of children stems from the fact that rare neurological disorders are more often identified in these individuals.

A further potential subtype includes the children who have early difficulties in peer and social relationships as well as some language and communication difficulties and unusual experiences, who are later prone to develop psychotic illness, such as schizophrenia (Buitelaar & van der Gaag, 1998; Remschmidt & Theisen, 2005; de Bruin, de Nijs, et al., 2007). Current research suggests that among the individuals with a diagnosis of pervasive developmental disorder not otherwise specified in DSM there are a subset of children who meet criteria for so called multiple complex developmental disorder, and that this subgroup seems to be particularly at risk for developing psychotic illnesses later in development. It remains unclear as to quite how best to distinguish these children from children with autism spectrum disorders, but the limited available evidence indicates that some means of classifying these individuals is needed. Whether they should be classified under the rubric of pervasive developmental disorder or as a subtype of schizophrenia clearly needs to be decided.

Comorbidity

Although the diagnosis of some comorbid disorders has been precluded in ICD and DSM, recent reports have suggested that there are individuals who seem to meet criteria for autism and ADHD/hyperkinesis and that, at least in some cases, the associated hyperkinesis or ADHD can be treated reasonably successfully with the same medications used for ADHD. However, in many children with PDD and concurrent overactivity, restlessness, and impulsivity, medication is ineffective or gives rise to very problematic side effects. This has led to increasing speculation over the extent and basis of co-occurrence between autistic spectrum disorder symptomatology and ADHD/hyperkinetic symptomatology. There is some evidence to suggest that there are shared genetic risk factors for this symptomatic overlap (Ronald, Simonoff, et al. 2008; Mulligan, Anney, et al. 2009) but equally other evidence to suggest that the risk factors for ADHD/hyperkinesis in individuals with autism spectrum disorder may be rather different from those that ordinarily underlie pure ADHD/hyperkinesis (Simonoff, Pickles, et al., 2008). The issue clearly requires further research to resolve; but it is evident the classificatory systems in the future need in some way to be able to accommodate the situation when two sets of problems are present. There are various approaches that could be adopted to achieve this. For example, one approach is to set aside a diagnostic category for autistic hyperkinesis, just as there is a category for hyperkinetic conduct disorder in ICD-10. The alternative approach is to abandon the hierarchical structure of the classificatory scheme so that dual diagnosis of autism spectrum disorder and ADHD/hyperkinesis can be made. At present it is not really clear which of these options is to be preferred. The potential drawback of the dual diagnosis approach is that the ADHD/hyperkinetic disorder may have different origins, prognosis, and response to treatment when in the presence of autism spectrum disorder. It is evident, however, that there has been no research to support the retention of the category "overactive disorder with mental retardation and stereotyped movements" in ICD-11.

A review of the hierarchical rules relating to dual diagnosis with other disorder will also be required.

Future Approaches to Diagnosis and Classification

Currently, diagnosis and classification is based entirely on behavioral criteria, and this will be so for some time yet. In the future, however, it may be possible to better parse heterogeneity and classify cases by incorporating information on associated features, such as cognitive profile, structural and functional brain imaging findings, gene expression profile (Nishimura, Martin, et al., 2007; Geschwind, 2008; Hu, Sarachana, et al., 2009), other biomarker findings, and genotype. The multiaxial classification system may need to be adapted to allow findings from investigations in these domains to be included, perhaps by broadening the scope of each axis or by creating new axes.

Conclusions

It is evident that there have been a considerable number of advances in our understanding of the pervasive developmental disorders, and it is time for revisions to the current classificatory schemes. Equally it is evident that much remains to be determined and, in some areas, it is still uncertain as to what the best approach to classification should be. This is inevitable, and classificatory schemes continually need to be developed and honed for their purpose. It is hoped that at least with respect to the pervasive developmental disorders there will be an opportunity for closer integration of the ICD-10 and DSM-IV approaches as a comprehensive and unified approach has much to offer.

REFERENCES

Angold, A., & Costello, E. J. (2009). Nosology and measurement in child and adolescent psychiatry. *Journal of Child Psychology and Psychiatry, and Allied Disciplines, 50*(1–2), 9–15.

Baghdadli, A., Picot, M. C., et al. (2007). What happens to children with PDD when they grow up? Prospective follow-up of 219 children from preschool age to mid-childhood. *Acta Psychiatrica Scandinavica, 115*(5), 403–412.

Bailey, A., Le Couteur, A., et al. (1995). Autism as a strongly genetic disorder: Evidence from a British twin study. *Psychological Medicine, 25*(1), 63–77 issn: 0033–2917.

Bailey, A., Palferman, S., et al. (1998). Autism: The phenotype in relatives. *Journal of Autism and Developmental Disorders,* 28(5), 369–392.

Baird, G., Charman, T., et al. (2008). Regression, developmental trajectory and associated problems in disorders in the autism spectrum: The SNAP study. *Journal of Autism and Developmental Disorders, 38*(10), 1827–1836.

Billstedt, E., Gillberg, I. C., et al. (2007). Autism in adults: Symptom patterns and early childhood predictors: Use of the DISCO in a community sample followed from childhood. *Journal of Child Psychology and Psychiatry, and Allied Disciplines, 48*(11), 1102–1110.

Bird, H. R., Yager, T. J., et al. (1990). Impairment in the epidemiological measurement of childhood psychopathology in the community. *Journal of the American Academy of Child and Adolescent Psychiatry, 29*(5), 796–803.

Bolton, P., Macdonald, H., et al. (1994). A case-control family history study of autism. *Journal of Child Psychology and Psychiatry, and Allied Disciplines, 35,* 877–900.

Bolton, P. F., Dennis, N. R., et al. (2001). The phenotypic manifestations of interstitial duplications of proximal 15q with special reference to the autistic spectrum disorders. *American Journal of Medical Genetics, 105*(8), 675–685.

Bolton, P. F., Park, R. J., et al. (2002). Neuro-epileptic determinants of autism spectrum disorders in tuberous sclerosis complex. *Brain, 125*(Pt 6), 1247–1255.

Buitelaar, J. K., & van der Gaag, R. J. (1998). Diagnostic rules for children with PDD-NOS and multiple complex developmental disorder. *Journal of Child Psychology and Psychiatry, and Allied Disciplines, 39*(6), 911–919.

Christian, S. L., Brune, C. W., et al. (2008). Novel submicroscopic chromosomal abnormalities detected in autism spectrum disorder. *Biological Psychiatry, 63*(12), 1111–1117.

Cohen, I. L., Fisch, G. S., et al. (1988). Social gaze, social avoidance, and repetitive behavior in fragile X males: A controlled study. *American Journal of Mental Retardation, 92*(5), 436–446 issn: 0895–8017.

Cohen, I. L., Vietze, P. M., et al. (1989). Parent-child dyadic gaze patterns in fragile X males and in non-fragile X males with *autistic disorder. *Journal of Child Psychology and Psychiatry, and Allied Disciplines, 30*, 845–856.

Constantino, J. N., Gruber, C. P., et al. (2004). The factor structure of autistic traits. *Journal of Child Psychology and Psychiatry, and Allied Disciplines, 45*(4), 719–726.

Constantino, J. N., & Todd, R. D. (2003). Autistic traits in the general population: A twin study. *Archives of General Psychiatry, 60*(5), 524–530.

de Bruin, E. I., de Nijs, P. F., et al. (2007). Multiple complex developmental disorder delineated from PDD-NOS. *Journal of Autism and Developmental Disorders, 37*(6), 1181–1191.

Elsabbagh, M., & Johnson, M. H. (2007). Infancy and autism: Progress, prospects, and challenges. *Progress in Brain Research, 164*, 355–383.

Feinstein, C., & Reiss, A. L. (1998). Autism: The point of view from fragile X studies. *Journal of Autism and Developmental Disorders, 28*(5), 393–405.

Geschwind, D. H. (2008). Autism: Many genes, common pathways? *Cell, 135*(3), 391–395.

Geschwind, D. H. (2009). Advances in autism. *Annual Review of Medicine, 60*, 367–380.

Happe, F., & Ronald, A. (2008). The "fractionable autism triad": A review of evidence from behavioural, genetic, cognitive and neural research. *Neuropsychology Review, 18*(4), 287–304.

Howlin, P., Goode, S., et al. (2004). Adult outcome for children with autism. *Journal of Child Psychology and Psychiatry, and Allied Disciplines, 45*(2), 212–229.

Hu, V. W., Sarachana, T., et al. (2009). Gene expression profiling differentiates autism case-controls and phenotypic variants of autism spectrum disorders: Evidence for circadian rhythm dysfunction in severe autism. *Autism Research, 2*(2), 78–97.

Kolevzon, A., Smith, C. J., et al. (2004). Familial symptom domains in monozygotic siblings with autism. *American Journal of Medical Genetics. Part B, Neuropsychiatric Genetics, 129B*(1), 76–81.

Kumar, R. A., & Christian, S. L. (2009). Genetics of autism spectrum disorders. *Current Neurology and Neuroscience Reports, 9*(3), 188–197.

Kurita, H., Koyama, T., et al. (2004). Validity of childhood disintegrative disorder apart from autistic disorder with speech loss. *European Child and Adolescent Psychiatry, 13*(4), 221–226.

Le Couteur, A., Bailey, A., et al. (1996). A broader phenotype of autism: The clinical spectrum in twins. *Journal of Child Psychology and Psychiatry, and Allied Disciplines, 37*(7), 785–801 issn: 0021–9630.

Lord, C., Pickles, A., et al. (1997). Diagnosing autism: Analyses of data from the Autism Diagnostic Interview [see comments]. *Journal of Autism and Developmental Disorders, 27*(5), 501–517.

Lord, C., Rutter, M., et al. (1989). Autism diagnostic observation schedule: A standardized observation of communicative and social behaviour. *Journal of Autism and Developmental Disorders, 19*, 185–212.

Lord, C., Rutter, M., et al. (1994). Autism Diagnostic Interview-Revised: A revised version of a diagnostic interview for caregivers of individuals with possible pervasive developmental disorders. *Journal of Autism and Developmental Disorders, 24*(5), 659–685.

Loucas, T., Charman, T., et al. (2008). Autistic symptomatology and language ability in autism spectrum disorder and specific language impairment. *Journal of Child Psychology and Psychiatry, and Allied Disciplines, 49*(11), 1184–1192.

Mashiko, H. (2003). Heller's syndrome (childhood disintegrative disorder) [in Japanese]. *Ryoikibetsu Shokogun Shirizu*, (39), 524–527.

Matson, J. L., & Nebel-Schwalm, M. S. (2007). Comorbid psychopathology with autism spectrum disorder in children: An overview. *Research in Developmental Disabilities, 28*(4), 341–352.

Milner, K. M., Craig, E. E., et al. (2005). Prader-Willi syndrome: Intellectual abilities and behavioural features by genetic subtype. *Journal of Child Psychology and Psychiatry, and Allied Disciplines, 46*(10), 1089–1096.

Mulligan, A., Anney, R. J., et al. (2009). Autism symptoms in attention-deficit/hyperactivity disorder: A familial trait which correlates with conduct, oppositional defiant, language and motor disorders. *Journal of Autism and Developmental Disorders, 39*(2), 197–209.

Nishimura, Y., Martin, C. L., et al. (2007). Genome-wide expression profiling of lymphoblastoid cell lines distinguishes different forms of autism and reveals shared pathways. *Human Molecular Genetics, 16*(14), 1682–1698.

Nordin, V., & Gillberg, C. (1998). The long-term course of autistic disorders: Update on follow-up studies. *Acta Psychiatrica Scandinavica, 97*(2), 99–108.

Pickles, A., Simonoff, E., et al. (2009). Loss of language in early development of autism and specific language impairment. *Journal of Child Psychology and Psychiatry, and Allied Disciplines, 50*(7), 843–852.

Remschmidt, H., & Theisen, F. M. (2005). Schizophrenia and related disorders in children and adolescents. *Journal of Neural Transmission. Supplementum*, (69), 121–141.

Rett, A. (1986). History and general overview. *American Journal of Medical Genetics, 24*, 21–25.

Rogers, S. J. (2004). Developmental regression in autism spectrum disorders. *Mental Retardation and Developmental Disabilities Research Reviews, 10*(2), 139–143.

Ronald, A., Happe, F., et al. (2006). Genetic heterogeneity between the three components of the autism spectrum: A twin study. *Journal of the American Academy of Child and Adolescent Psychiatry, 45*(6), 691–699.

Ronald, A., Happe, F., et al. (2005). The genetic relationship between individual differences in social and nonsocial behaviours characteristic of autism. *Developmental Science, 8*(5), 444–458.

Ronald, A., Simonoff, E., et al. (2008). Evidence for overlapping genetic influences on autistic and ADHD behaviours in a community twin sample. *Journal of Child Psychology and Psychiatry, and Allied Disciplines, 49*(5), 535–542.

Rutter, M., Andersen-Wood, L., et al. (1999). Quasi-autistic patterns following severe early global privation: English and Romanian Adoptees (ERA) study team. *Journal of Child Psychology and Psychiatry, and Allied Disciplines, 40*(4), 537–549.

Rutter, M., Bailey, A., et al. (1994). Autism and known medical conditions: Myth and substance. *Journal of Child Psychology and Psychiatry, and Allied Disciplines, 35*, 311–322.

Sebat, J., Lakshmi, B., et al. (2007). Strong association of de novo copy number mutations with autism. *Science, 316*(5823), 445–449.

Simonoff, E., Pickles, A., et al. (2008). Psychiatric disorders in children with autism spectrum disorders: Prevalence, comorbidity, and associated factors in a population-derived sample. *Journal of the American Academy of Child and Adolescent Psychiatry, 47*(8), 921–929.

Spiker, D., Lotspeich, L. J., et al. (2002). Behavioral phenotypic variation in autism multiplex families: Evidence for a continuous severity gradient. *American Journal of Medical Genetics, 114*(2), 129–136.

Stefanatos, G. A. (2008). Regression in autistic spectrum disorders. *Neuropsychology Review, 18*(4), 305–319.

Szatmari, P., Bryson, S. E., et al. (2003). Predictors of outcome among high functioning children with autism and Asperger syndrome. *Journal of Child Psychology and Psychiatry, and Allied Disciplines, 44*(4), 520–528.

Szatmari, P., Jones, M. B., et al. (1996). High phenotypic correlations among siblings with autism and pervasive developmental disorders. *American Journal of Medical Genetics, 67*(4), 354–360.

Szatmari, P., Merette, C., et al. (2008). Decomposing the autism phenotype into familial dimensions. *American Journal of Medical Genetics. Part B, Neuropsychiatric Genetics: The official publication of the International Society of Psychiatric Genetics, 147B*(1), 3–9.

Taylor, E., & Rutter, M. (2002). Classification: Conceptual issues and substantive findings. In M. Rutter and E. Taylor (Eds.), *Child and Adolescent Psychiatry* (pp. 3–17). Oxford: Blackwell Science.

Volkmar, F. R., Klin, A., et al. (1996). Asperger's syndrome. *Journal of the American Academy of Child and Adolescent Psychiatry, 35*(1), 118–123.

Volkmar, F. R., Klin, A., et al. (1998). Nosological and genetic aspects of Asperger syndrome. *Journal of Autism and Developmental Disorders, 28*(5), 457–463.

Volkmar, F. R., & Rutter, M. (1995). Childhood disintegrative disorder: Results of the DSM-IV autism field trial. *Journal of the American Academy of Child and Adolescent Psychiatry, 34*(8), 1092–1095.

WHO. (1993). *The ICD-10 classification of mental and behavioural disorders: Diagnostic criteria for research.* Geneva: World Health Organization.

Wing, L. (1981). Asperger's syndrome: A clinical account. *Psychological Medicine, 11,* 115–129.

Wing, L. (1997). The autistic spectrum. *Lancet, 350*(9093), 1761–1766.

Wing, L., & Gould, J. (1979). Severe impairments of social interaction and associated abnormalities in children: Epidemiology and classification. *Journal of Autism and Developmental Disorders, 9,* 11–29.

Wolff, S. (1991). "Schizoid" personality in childhood and adult life. III: The childhood picture. *British Journal of Psychiatry, 159,* 629–635.

Wolff, S., & Barlow, A. (1979). Schizoid personality in childhood: A comparative study of schizoid, autistic and normal children. *Journal of Child Psychology and Psychiatry, and Allied Disciplines, 20*(1), 29–46 issn: 0021–9630.

Wolff, S., & Chick, J. (1980). Schizoid personality in childhood: A controlled follow-up study. *Psychological Medicine, 10,* 85–100.

Zero–Three. (2005). *Diagnostic Classification: 0–3R: Diagnostic Classification of Mental Health and Developmental Disorders of Infancy and Early Childhood: Revised Edition.* Washington, DC, Zero to Three Press.

Section II

Core Features and Developmental Trajectories

8 Peter Mundy

The Social Behavior of Autism: A Parallel and Distributed Information Processing Perspective

Points of Interest

- Joint attention impairments are a first-year onset symptom of autism, and a pivotal domain of development for early intervention and diagnosis.
- Hypothetically, joint attention impairments in autism are cardinal early behavioral symptoms of developmental neural interconnectivity impairments.
- In infancy frequent practice with the social coordination of attention to external object or events is internalized and becomes the ability to socially coordinate mental attention with others to internal representations of object or events. Hence, reduced practice with joint attention among children with autism is a source of their subsequent social-cognitive, symbolic, and social learning impairments.
- Joint attention impairments in autism entail problems in constructive self-referenced, self-regulated, and self-motivated behaviors, as much they involve problems in perceiving and interpreting the social behaviors of others.

Translational research has changed the way we think about, diagnose, and treat the social impairments of autism. Application of basic science to autism has begun to encourage new ways of thinking about the phylogenetic and ontogenetic development of human social-cognition. In particular, human social-cognition may be viewed as the outgrowth a special form of human information processing that we call joint attention (Mundy & Newell, 2007). As this chapter will describe, joint attention requires the parallel processing of information about one's own attention and the attention of other people. This requires the activation and functions of a distributed system of frontal and posterior cortical networks in the brain. Recognizing and understanding the parallel and distributed nature of joint attention impairment contributes to new perspectives about the development of social cognition, the social brain in all people including those with autism (Mundy, 2003). This new framework has emerged from the interplay between cognitive neuroscience, developmental science, and the science of psychopathology in autism. As such it provides a seminal illustration of a school of translational research that began more than two decades ago when a farsighted group outlined the new discipline of *developmental psychopathology* (Cicchetti, 1984; Sroufe & Rutter, 1984).

The chapter begins with a brief description of the history of thought and research on autism. One message of that first section is that a lack of precise understanding of social behavioral development impeded the accurate diagnosis of autism until the early 1990s, which was fifty years after it was initially described by Asperger (1944) and Kanner (1943). The second section of the chapter illustrates how social developmental research continues to be a vital source of information about the nature of autism. Indeed, research on autism has led to insights about the precise nature of joint attention development in infants that have contributed to the framework for a new model of human social-cognition development. As previously noted this model adopts a parallel and distributed information processing perspective on joint attention and social cognition. An advantage of this model is that it explicitly attempts to link developmental behavioral research on social pathology to a range of recent observations from research on neural connectivity, genetics, intervention, and ocular motor control in autism.

A Brief History of Research on the Social Impairments of Autism

Autism is a biologically based disorder that is characterized by impaired social development, impaired language and/or pragmatic communication skill acquisition, and the presence of repetitive behaviors and thoughts (Asperger, 1944; Bailey, Philips, & Rutter, 1996; Dawson, Osterling, Rinaldi, Carver, & McPartland, 2001; Kanner, 1943). The symptoms of autism may be observable by 24 months of age or earlier (Stone, Coonrod, & Ousley, 1997; Zwaigenbaum et al., 2005), with children expressing at least four different paths of symptom onset (Ozonoff, Heung, Byrd, Hansen, & Hertz-Picciotto, 2008). Some children may display clear symptoms by the end of the first year, some may display more typical development through the early part of the second year but reach a plateau. Still others may express mixed pictures of early delays, gains, and losses of developmental milestones.

Leo Kanner (1943) displayed impressive clinical acumen when he was able to discern three common characteristics that distinguished children with autism from those in a larger, varied clinical sample of children. He noted that children with autism appeared to have: (1) a common biological impairment, (2) of affective relatedness to others, which (3) resulted in a developmental disorder that primarily impaired the capacity for typical social interactions. The recognition of the biological, affective, and social behavioral syndrome triumvirate of autism was a remarkable achievement, and is as valid today as it was in 1944. Unfortunately, Kanner's initial perspective did not fit well with the psychodynamic zeitgeist of the time. The psychodynamic perspective emphasized the primacy of environmental over biological factors in the etiology of all psychopathology. Sufficient challenges were brought to bear in this regard that Kanner (1949) recanted his initial biological view of autism.

In the ensuing thirty years the science of autism drifted from conceptual model to conceptual model. Autism was characterized as a disorder caused by an aloof parenting style in which the children grew up to be emotionless (Bettelheim, 1959). Convincing evidence against the parenting style hypothesis was quickly marshaled (Rimland, 1964). However, the prototype of people with autism as emotionless and aloof remained for a long time. Little data were available to critically appraise this view because the social and emotional development of children with autism was rarely a focus of empirical inquiry through the 1970s. Rather, theory at that time suggested that sensory, perceptual or language impairments were primary in the etiology of autism (Mundy & Sigman, 1989). Although this was a scientifically valid perspective at the time, it implicitly relegated the social-emotional impairments of autism to the status of epiphenomenon.

The relegation of social-emotional symptoms to secondary status constrained the theory and methods used to establish the initial diagnostic criteria for autism. So, in the first attempts to establish a systematic diagnostic definition of autism (e.g., American Psychiatric Association [APA], 1980) only five criteria were proposed: (1) onset before 30 months of age; (2) a pervasive lack of responsiveness to other people; (3) gross deficits in language development; if speech is present, peculiar speech patterns such as immediate and delayed echolalia, metaphorical language, and pronominal reversal; (4) bizarre responses to various aspects of the environment, e.g., resistance to change, peculiar interest in or attachments to animate or inanimate objects; and (5) absence of delusions, hallucinations, loosening of associations, and incoherence as in schizophrenia.

Note that *only one criterion* was specific to the social deficits of autism and this was the broad and vague descriptor of a *pervasive lack of responsiveness to other people.* There had been so little research on defining the nature of the social deficits of autism through 1980 that we simply had no idea what was involved in this domain of autism, even though Kanner had argued that it was central to nature of the syndrome. Pat Howlin (1978) made this limit to our knowledge clear in an early review of research on the social deficits of autism. Howlin was able to cogently summarize the field of social developmental research on autism with 7 pages of text and 39 citations. Only a handful of the latter involved peer reviewed empirical research publications. Fortunately, in the intervening decade there was a virtual explosion of research on the social deficits of autism. When Howlin published a second review of research on the social development of autism, eight years later, her review required 24 pages and 116 citations to adequately cover the field (Howlin, 1986).

This welcome increase in information on the social nature of autism occurred because of translational research. Several groups in the United States, the United Kingdom and throughout the world began to recognize that theory and methods from the study of human infant and primate social development could provide useful tools to examine and define the social deficits of autism (e.g., Dawson & McKissick, 1984; Rogers & Pennington, 1991; Sigman & Ungerer, 1984). This new wave involved the translation of basic science on infant imitation, social learning, social cognition, preverbal communication, attachment, and other domains of early social development to autism. One fairly immediate and vital impact of this surge of translational research was the dawning awareness that the description of the social impairments of autism singularly as a "pervasive lack of responsiveness to others" was at best limited and, at worst, misguided. It established a narrow categorical prototype that many individuals with autism did not resemble (Mundy & Sigman, 1989; Wing & Gould, 1979).

Studies began to show that children with autism displayed a significant phenotypic range of social styles and social behaviors. Some children, often also affected by severe or moderate levels of mental retardation appeared to be aloof, and came closest to the description of "a pervasive impairments in responsiveness to others." However, many other children with mild mental retardation, or normal IQs were not pervasively underresponsive. Instead, some were passive but socially responsive in structured situations, and others were even proactive in initiating interactions. However, these "active but odd" children were atypical and maladaptive in conducting their interactions with other people (Wing & Gould, 1979; Volkmar et al., 1989; Fein et al., 1999).

By the end of the 1980s research had also shown that many children with autism had social strengths as well as weaknesses, rather than a *pervasive lack of responsiveness to others.*

They responded when others imitated them, some could learn from social modeling, many increased their social output in structured situations, and they varied greatly in their use of gestures and eye contact to communicate (Curcio, 1978; Lewy & Dawson, 1992; Mundy & Sigman, 1989). Perhaps most remarkably children with autism often displayed levels of attachment behaviors that were commensurate with their mental development and *not atypical* relative to other groups of children with commensurate developmental delays (Shapiro, Sherman, Calamari, & Koch, 1987; Sigman & Ungerer, 1984; Sigman & Mundy, 1989).

Consequently, by the early 1990s translational developmental research indicated that key elements of the nosology of autism were incorrect. Children with autism, as a group, did not display a *pervasive* lack of responsiveness to others. Not only was this inaccurate, it promoted a constricted view of autism that excluded many children with the syndrome who frequently made eye contact, or displayed caregiver attachment, or any of a number of other social abilities. The perseverance of this inaccurate taxonomic prototype likely contributed to a historic underestimation of the prevalence of autism (Wing & Potter, 2002). Indeed, only with the publication of the most recent nosology (e.g., American Psychiatric Association [APA], 1994) have we had had sufficiently well defined guidelines to begin to capture something of the full range of phenotypic variability expressed across individuals with this syndrome. Prior to this we simply could not identify all the children with autism in the 1970s, 1980s, and early 1990s because we limited ourselves to those that just met a very limited and restrictive social criterion.

The empirically based revisions of social diagnostic criteria of autism culminated in the criteria now common to both the systems used in the United States, Europe, and the world (APA, 1994; 2000; World Health Organization, 1992). In both systems the qualitative impairment in social interaction in autism became defined as the expression of at least two of the following: (1) a marked impairment in the use of multiple nonverbal behaviors such as eye-to-eye gaze, facial expression, body postures, and gestures to regulate social interaction; (2) a failure to develop peer relationships appropriate to developmental level; (3) a lack of spontaneous seeking to share enjoyment, interests, or achievements with other people (e.g., by a lack of showing, bringing, or pointing out objects of interest); and (4) lack of social or emotional reciprocity.

The criterion of a lack of appropriate peer skills is extremely useful, but not until 3 or 4 years of age. As a result, the early identification and diagnosis of the social deficits of autism relies on observation of the other three social symptoms. This chapter attempts to provide a detailed consideration of why the third symptom, a *lack of spontaneous seeking to share experience, enjoyment, interests, or achievements with other people*, is central to the description of the social pathology of autism. In the research literature we study the early development of spontaneously seeking to share experience with others with measures of joint attention development. While other domains of social behavior such as imitation, face processing, empathy, and pragmatic communication skills are prominent in the literature (Travis & Sigman, 1998), none of these is as central to the current social nosology of autism. Moreover, intervention and behavioral research indicate that the degree of early joint attention impairment is pivotal to the nature of autism because it is predictive of collateral social symptom, language, and cognitive outcomes (e.g., Bruinsma et al., 2004; Dawson et al., 2004; Charman, 2004; Kasari et al., 2006; Mundy & Crowson, 1997; Sigman & Ruskin, 1999). The recognition of the centrality of this social deficit in autism followed from the translation of basic research on how infants develop the ability to share experience with other people (Bruner, 1975).

How Infants Share Experiences with Other People

Well before infants learn to use symbols and language they begin to spontaneously share information with other people. They do so by coordinating their attention with another person and by using eye contact and gestures to show objects to others, or request aid obtaining and manipulating objects.

In 1975 Scaife and Bruner reported in *Nature* that between 6 to 18 months of age infants increasingly displayed the ability to follow the direction of gaze of a social partner. When a tester turned their head to the left or right many infants tracked and followed the visual attention of the testers with their own line of regard. This observation was groundbreaking. It was inconsistent with the prevailing notion of egocentrism or the idea that infants could not adopt dual perspectives, such as the perspective of self and another person, until late in the second year (Piaget, 1952). Scaife and Bruner's (1975) observations suggested that infants begin to discriminate and adapt their own visual perspective relative to another person's perspective much earlier in life than that.

Bruner (1975) adopted the general term "joint attention" for this domain of infant development. He recognized that this ability allowed infants and caregivers to adopt co-reference to the same object or event. One of Bruner's goals was to understand how young children learn in order to improve early educational curriculums. Instead of studying only how knowledge was acquired (learning), he studied how the ability to share knowledge in "social learning" develops, because this is essential to all forms of pedagogy. His work suggested that the development of the ability to participate in joint attention marked a critical turning point in some unknown set of early cognitive processes that were foundational to human social learning and education. More specifically, Bruner understood that co-reference was elementary to our human ability to perceive shared meanings and necessary for the development of symbolic thinking and language development.

In the early days of empirical research it became apparent that infants did not just develop one type of joint attention behavior. Rather they developed multiple forms of joint attention. The previously referred to type that involves infants' ability follow the direction of another person's gaze (Scaife & Bruner, 1975) is often called Responding to Joint Attention (RJA; Seibert, Hogan, & Mundy, 1982). It can be reliably assessed beginning at about 3 to 6 months of life by determining if infants correctly turn their head and/or eyes to follow the visual line of regard of another person (see Figure 8-1). Another dimension called Initiating Joint Attention (IJA) arises sometime in the first year, but no later than 8 to 9 months. It involves the infant's use of alternating eye contact or gestures (i.e., pointing or showing) to spontaneously "declare" and direct and coordinate attention to share an experience with a social partner (Bates, Benigni, Bretherton, Camaioni, & Volterra, 1979; Mundy et al., 2007; Figure 8-1).

The declarative, social information sharing functions of IJA and RJA can be juxtaposed with other early nonverbal behaviors that involve attention coordination for more instrumental and imperative purposes. Young infants also learn to prelinguistically direct the attention of other people to request aid in obtaining object or actions (Initiating Behavioral Requests-IBR). In addition they learn to respond to the attention directing bids that adults use to request objects or actions from infants or Responding to Behavioral Requests (RBR; Figure 8-1).

As the theory and measurement concerning infant joint attention was developing in the 1970s, the important practical issue of identifying valid markers of *infant* cognition came to the fore. The types of sensory motor measures used to assess infant "intelligence" and cognitive "risk" at the time were not sufficiently reliable or valid (Lewis & McGurk, 1972). Without valid measures it was challenging to identify many infants who were at risk for developmental disorders. It was also difficult to know what constituted valid targets for early cognitive intervention. This impasse began to clear as applications of basic research indicated that measures of infant visual attention could be used as valid indicators of current and future cognitive development in infancy (Bornstein & Sigman, 1986).

One laboratory for the translation of research on infant attention to clinical applications was created by Jeff Seibert

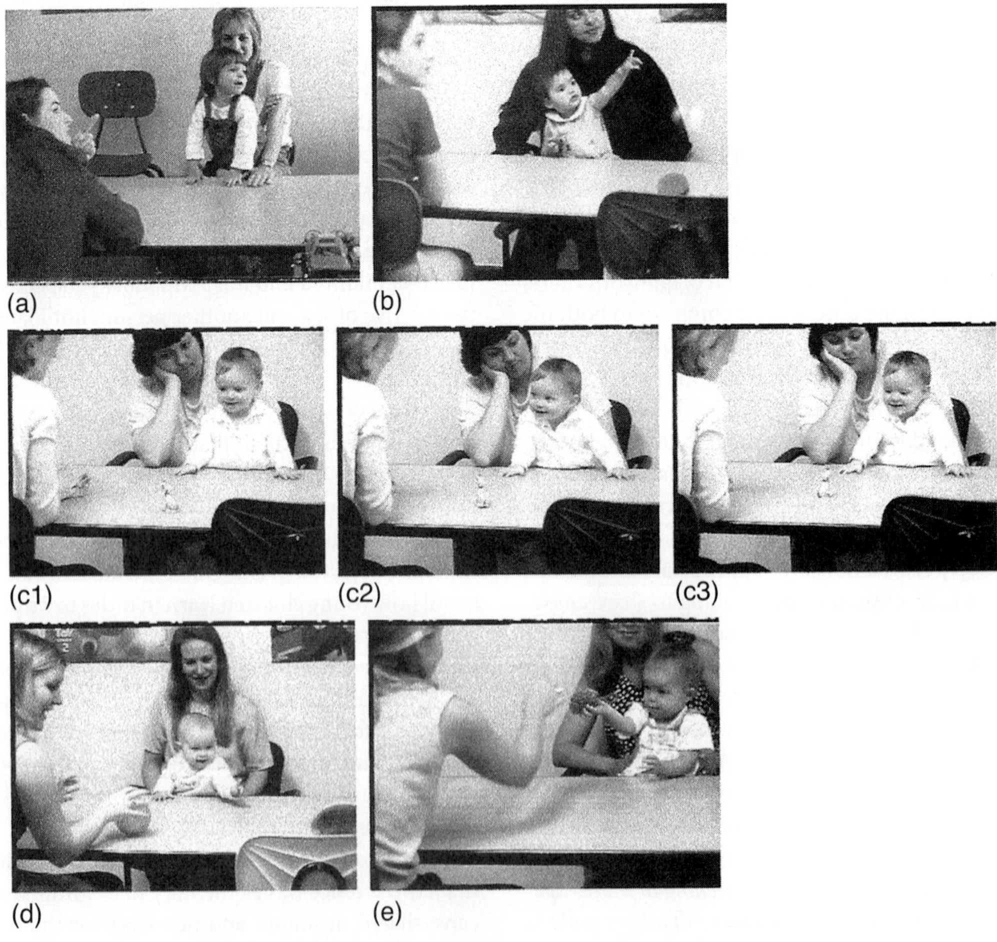

Figure 8–1. Illustrations of different types of infant social attention coordination behaviors: (a) Responding to Joint Attention-RJA, involving following an other person's gaze and pointing gesture; (b) Initiating Joint Attention-IJA, involving a conventional gesture "pointing" to share attention regarding a room poster; ($c_{1,2,3}$) IJA involving *alternating eye contact* to share attention with respect to a toy; (d) Initiating Behavior Request, involving pointing to elicit aid in obtaining an out-of-reach object; and (e) Responding to Behavior Requests, involving following an adult's open-palm "give it to me" gesture.

and Anne Hogan at the Debbie School of the University of Miami. The Debbie School served preschoolers who had moderate to severe motor and developmental impairments. Their motor impairments made the use of sensorimotor-based cognitive assessments and interventions extremely problematic. So Seibert, Hogan, and their graduate students began to develop an early assessment and intervention curriculum that focused on joint attention and preverbal communication skill development. This resulted in the Early Social Communication Scales (ESCS), which organized precise observations of joint attention and social attention coordination into a measurement instrument that could also be used to guide to early intervention (Seibert et al., 1982). A lasting contribution of the ESCS, along with related measures (see Stone, Coonrod & Ousley, 1997; Wetherby, Allen, Cleary, Kublin, & Goldstein, 2002) was that joint attention assessment turned out to be a powerful instrument for the study of the social pathology of autism.

Joint Attention and Defining The Social Deficits of Autism

To the best of my knowledge it was Frank Curcio (1978) who first noted that many children with autism capably initiated nonverbal requests but not joint attention bids in social interactions. Indeed, 50% of the elementary school–age children with autism he observed in classrooms systematically used eye contact and conventional gestures to express their requests. However, few if any children with autism displayed evidence of the use of eye contact or gestures to initiate nonverbal "declaratives" (i.e., display an IJA bid). Curcio concluded that impairments in the capacity to initiate declarative communicative functions, or what we now call initiating joint attention bids, could be central to the nature of the social impairments of autism. Numerous subsequent studies have indicated that Curcio was correct (e.g., Charman, 2004; Dawson et al., 2004; Loveland & Landry, 1986; Mundy et al., 1986; Sigman & Ruskin, 1999; Wetherby & Prutting, 1984).

In work with Marian Sigman at UCLA we compared mental age, chronological age, and IQ matched samples of 4- to 7-year-old children with autism or mental retardation as well as a mental-age matched sample of typically developing children. We found the children with autism displayed deficits in joint attention in interactions with unfamiliar testers as well as their familiar parents relative to both comparison groups (Mundy et al., 1986; Sigman et al., 1986). However, just as Curcio had observed, our sample of children with autism displayed levels of requesting that were comparable to those observed in the MR sample. Also similar to Curcio's data from older children, we observed that young children with autism did not display pervasive differences in eye contact relative to children with mental retardation on the ESCS, but rather strengths and weaknesses. They displayed comparable levels of eye contact in requesting and turn-taking social interactions. However, an eye contact disturbance specific to autism was clearly manifested in their diminished use of alternating gaze to spontaneously initiate sharing of their experience of a mechanical toy with the tester. This type of behavior is illustrated in Figure 8-1.

We cannot definitively know why a child does or does not engage in IJA during a social interaction. Nevertheless, during the administration of the ESCS adult testers often arrive at the impression that IJA behaviors, such as alternating eye contact, serve to share experience of an event or garner attention to the child's own experience of the event (Figure 8-1). Hence, it was not too surprising to find that higher or lower frequencies of alternating eye-contact in young children, with or without autism, were significantly related to parents' independent perceptions of their child's social relatedness (Mundy et al., 1994). Thus, it seemed reasonable to begin to consider to us the possibility that diminished IJA alternating eye-contact was crucial to what Kanner had characterized as impairments in relatedness and positive affective contact with others in autism (e.g., Mundy & Sigman, 1989).

The idea that IJA was related to a disturbance in positive social-affective contact in autism was subsequently supported by research that showed that about 60% of the IJA bids displayed by typical infants and children with mental retardation involved the conveyance of positive affect (Kasari, Sigman, Mundy, & Yirmiya, 1990; Mundy, Kasari, & Sigman, 1992). However, positive affect was much less frequently part of the IJA behaviors of children with autism (Kasari et al., 1990). It was not the case, though, that children with autism displayed significantly lower positive affect in requesting or turn-taking interactions. Hence, it was unlikely that the diminished positive affect in joint attention reflected a general aversion to social interactions. More recently we've come to suspect that the onset of the systematic conveyance of positive affect as part of IJA bids begins to develop early in life at about 8 to 10 months of age (Venezia, Messinger, Thorp, & Mundy, 2004). Thus, joint attention impairments reflect what are likely to be early arising deficits in the tendency of children with autism to socially share positive affect. This in turn may involve a disturbance in their early appreciation of the positive social *value* of shared attention. That is to say motivation factors or sensitivity to reward value of social gaze may play a role in joint attention disturbance in autism (Mundy, 1995).

Joint Attention Impairments and The Social-Cognitive Hypothesis

During the time that joint attention impairments in autism were first being described another kind of social developmental translational research was beginning to emerge. Premack and Woodruff (1978) began to describe observational methods that enabled them to evaluate whether primates were aware of the thoughts or intention of conspecifics. That is, they began to study if apes had a theory of mind (ToM). In the

United Kingdom Wimmer and Perner (1983) further operationalized the construct of theory of mind with the development of the false belief task. With this paradigm they began to study the course of development of ToM and social cognition in young preschool and elementary school–age children. Very quickly thereafter, other research groups in London began to translate Wimmer and Perner's basic "false belief" developmental paradigms to the study of autism. This led to another sequence of seminal observations regarding the defining features of social impairments in autism. Children with autism appeared to have more difficulty with the development of social cognition than other aspects of cognitive development (e.g., Baron-Cohen, Leslie, & Frith, 1985; Leslie & Happe, 1989; Frith, 1989).

Theory had previously linked the development of joint attention to the emergence of social cognition (Bretherton, 1991). However, the parallel observations of deficits in joint attention development and theory of mind development in autism during the mid-1980s provided the first empirical, albeit indirect, link between these two domains of development. Consequently, the social cognitive view of autism and typical social development became so compelling in the literature that joint attention disturbance began to be interpreted as a manifestation of social cognitive impairment in autism (Baron-Cohen, 1989; Leslie & Happe, 1989). This was also true for theory on typical development, where a prominent view remains that joint attention is not possible without social cognition (Tomasello & Call, 1997).

So, some have argued that social cognition, or the knowledge that other people's behavior is guided by mental, goal-directed intentions precedes and gives rise to joint attention (Tomasello, Carpenter, Call, Behne, & Moll, 2005). Therefore, impairments in social cognition may explain the cause of joint attention impairment in autism (Baron-Cohen, 1989). Alternatively, we have proposed that it may be inadvisable to use later arising knowledge base cognition (e.g., ToM) to explain what may be best viewed as a form of early developing social information processing that provides an essential foundation for subsequent social and cognitive development in people (Mundy, 2003; Mundy & Newell, 2007; Mundy & Sigman, 1989; Mundy, Sigman, & Kasari, 1993). This idea has emerged, in part, from considering the differences in IJA and RJA in autism and typical development.

The Dissociation of Joint Attention Impairment in Autism

To interpret the nature of IJA and RJA impairments in autism it is important to recognize that they dissociate in development. Both RJA and IJA are useful in the early identification and diagnosis of autism (e.g., Lord et al., 2000; Stone, Coonrod, & Ousley, 1997). However, RJA impairments are less evident for children with more advanced levels of cognitive development (Mundy et al., 1994, see Figure 8-2). Indeed, across studies of different age group of children there is at best inconsistent evidence of a robust syndrome-specific impairment in the ability to process the direction of gaze or respond to joint attention in people with autism (Nation & Penny, 2008). On the other hand, IJA deficits are observed in children with autism from preschool through adolescence, *and* IJA is a better discriminator of children with autism relative to children with other developmental disorders (e.g., Charman, 2004; Dawson et al., 2004; Hobson & Hobson, 2007; Mundy et al., 1986; Sigman & Ruskin, 1999). The correlates of IJA and RJA also diverge as much as they converge in studies of autism. Both IJA and RJA are related to executive inhibition and language development in autism (Bono et al., 2004; Dawson et al., 2002; Dawson et al., 2004; Griffith et al., 1999; Sigman & McGovern, 2005). However, to our knowledge, only IJA is significantly associated with individual differences in social and affective symptom presentation (Charman, 2004; Kasari et al., 1990; Kasari et al., 2007; Lord et al., 2003; Mundy et al., 1994; Naber et al., 2008; Sigman & Ruskin, 1999).

This literature emphasizes that joint attention deficits are neither absolute nor uniform in autism, and the impairment of IJA and RJA likely constitutes different developmental processes that are vital to symptom presentation in the syndrome. Moreover, of the two, deficits in initiating joint attention behavior appears be the more pathognomonic feature of autism (Mundy, 1995). Observations from intervention research also emphasize that autism is a disturbance of the spontaneous *generation* of social behaviors, as much as or more than a disturbance of perception and *response* to the social behaviors of others (Koegel et al., 2003). A similar interpretation is suggested by recent research with infant siblings of children with autism (Zwaigenbaum et al., 2005). Indeed, the centrality of initiating deficits, especially IJA, is highlighted in current nosology where it is "a lack of *spontaneous* seeking to share enjoyment, interests, or achievements with other people, (e.g., by a lack of showing, bringing, or pointing out objects of interest to other people)" that is described as one of the

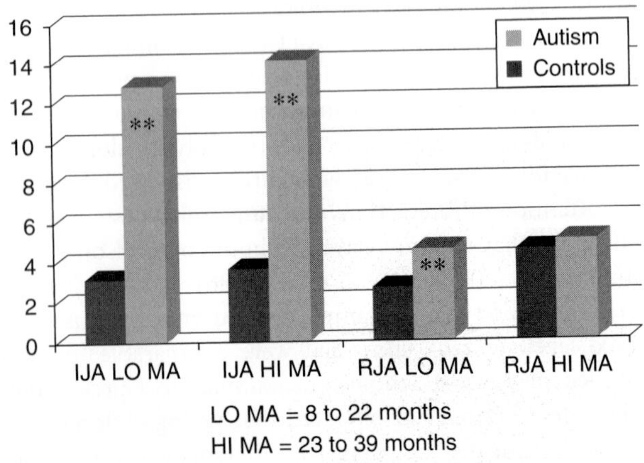

Figure 8–2. Illustration data on the moderating affect of mental age on diagnostic group differences on RJA versus IJA reported in Mundy et al. (1994).

primary social symptoms of autism (APA, 1994). Furthermore, the "gold standard" diagnostic observation instrument, the Autism Diagnostic Observation Schedule (ADOS), recognizes the primacy of IJA symptoms. Measures of both IJA and RJA are used in Module 1 diagnostic algorithms for the youngest children. However, Module 2 for older children only includes IJA measures in its diagnostic criteria (Lord et al., 2000).

Evidence of a developmental dissociation between IJA and RJA is also apparent in studies of typical infant development. Frequency measures of IJA and RJA are characterized by different growth patterns, and these domains display weak to nonsignificant correlations in infant development (e.g., Meltzoff & Brooks, 2008; Mundy et al., 2007; Sheinkopf et al., 2004; Slaughter & McDonald, 2003). They also have different patterns of correlations with childhood IQ (Ulvund & Smith, 1996), frontal brain activity (Caplan et al., 1993; Mundy et al., 2000); reward-based behavioral goal-inhibition and self-monitoring behaviors (Nichols et al., 2005), attention related self-regulation (Morales et al., 2005), and attachment (Claussen et al., 2002). These observations imply that the nature of the differences, as well as commonalities between IJA and RJA may be a key to conceptualizations of the joint attention impairments of autism.

Initiating Joint Attention Behaviors and Autism

It is essential to be precise about the nature of the behavioral expression of IJA impairments in autism, which are often equated with problems with pointing and showing gestures. However, diminished alternating gaze behavior (Figure 8-1) is a more powerful measure of IJA impairment in autism. This type of measure was superior to point and showing and correctly identified 94% of 54 preschool children with autism, mental retardation, and typical development (Mundy et al., 1986). Others have observed that IJA measured with the Early Social Communication Scales (ESCS; Seibert, Hogan, & Mundy, 1982) had a sensitivity of 83% to 97% and a specificity of 63% to 67% in discriminating fifty-three 3- to 4-year-olds with autism from controls (Dawson et al., 2004). Recent research indicates that most of the variance in ESCS-IJA scores is carried by alternating gaze behavior (Mundy et al., 2007). The IJA alternating gaze of 2-year-olds also predicts 4-year-old symptom outcomes in children with autism (Charman, 2004), as well as social cognition in typical 4-year-old children (Charman et al., 2000).

These developmental and measurement details are important for models of joint attention disturbance in autism. Often joint attention problems are viewed as growing out of developmental antecedent or successor processes that are considered to be more fundamental. A nonexhaustive list here includes affective processes, reward-sensitivity, executive attention control, social-orienting, identification, imitation and mirror neurons, intersubjectivity, and most prominently social cognition (e.g., Baron-Cohen, 1989; Charman, 2004; Dawson et al., 2004; Mundy et al., 1986; Williams, 2008). This reductionism has lead to a paradox where joint attention deficits are viewed as pivotal to autism, but also as an outgrowth of more basic processes. Charman (2004) recognized this paradox in noting that we often think of joint attention not as "a starting point [for autism], but merely a staging post in early social communicative development, and hence a 'postcursor' of earlier psychological and developmental processes... [which may] underlie the impaired development of joint attention skills in autism" (p. 321).

There are at least three problems with this perspective. First, stable individual differences in IJA alternating gaze are well established by 8 to 9 months in typical development (Mundy et al., 2007; Venezia et al., 2004), and the onset of cortical control of alternating gaze likely begins between 4 to 6 months (Mundy, 2003; Striano, Reid, & Hoel, 2006). Joint attention precursors would need to be present prior to this time. Second, there is little evidence that the association of joint attention with the etiology or outcomes of autism is mediated by more basic antecedent or successor processes. Dawson et al. (2004) observed that neither social-orienting measures nor empathy measures could account for relations between IJA and language development in a large sample of children with autism. Joint attention disturbance in autism also cannot be explained in terms of affect regulation or social relatedness measured with attachment measures (Capps, Sigman, & Mundy, 1994; Naber et al., 2008). Moreover, joint attention accounts for significant portions of variance in the language, symbolic play, and symptom development of children with autism above and beyond variance associated with executive functions, imitation, knowledge about others' intentions, or global measures of mental development (e.g., Charman 2004; Royers et al., 1998; Kasari et al., 2007; Naber et al., 2008; Rutherford et al., 2008; Sigman & Ruskin, 1999; Smith et al., 2007; Thurm et al., 2007; Toth et al., 2006).

A third issue is that precursor and successor process hypotheses rarely account for the dissociation of IJA and RJA (Mundy et al., 2007). Social-cognitive hypotheses suggest that RJA and IJA should be highly related because they are precursors of a common "mentalizing" ability involved in perceiving the intentions of others (e.g., Baron-Cohen, 1995; Tomasello, 1995). Executive attention or social-orienting hypotheses don't explicitly account for why IJA deficits are more pervasive than RJA deficits, even though both ostensively involve comparable attention inhibition and attention reorienting processes (e.g., Dawson et al., 1998; Mundy & Burnette, 2005). Imitation and mirror neuron theory emphasizes the role of deficits in processing and responding to the behavior of other people in the development of autism (e.g., Williams, 2008). Hypothetically, though, this should be more related to responsive joint attention than the spontaneous initiation of joint attention bids. Why then do IJA deficits appear to be the more robust form of joint attention disturbance in autism than RJA deficits? An answer may be perceived from a constructivists vantage point on joint attention and human social-learning (e.g., Bruner, 1975, 1995).

Learning and The Importance of Joint Attention

Early language learning often takes place in unstructured, incidental situations where parents spontaneously refer to a new object (Figure 8-3). How do infants know how to map their parents' vocal labels to the correct parts of the environment amid a myriad of potential referents? Baldwin (1995) suggested that they use RJA and use the direction of gaze of their parent's to guide them to the correct area of the environment, thereby reducing "referential" mapping errors. Infants' use of IJA also reduces the chance of referential mapping errors. IJA serves to denote something of immediate interest to the child. This assists parents to follow their child's attention to provide new information in a context when the child's interest and attention is optimal for learning (Tomasello & Farrar, 1986). Hence, joint attention may be conceived of as a self-organizing system that facilitates information processing in support of social learning (Mundy, 2003). This "learning function" is fundamental to joint attention (Bruner, 1975) and continues to operate throughout our lives (e.g., Bayliss et al., 2006; Nathan et al., 2007). Without the capacity for joint attention, success in many pedagogical contexts would be difficult. Imagine the school readiness problems of a 5-year-old who enters kindergarten but is not facile with coordinating attention with the teacher. Similarly, children, adolescents and adults who cannot follow, initiate, or join with the rapid-fire exchanges of shared attention in social interactions may be impaired in any social learning context, as well as in their very capacity for relatedness and relationships (Mundy & Sigman, 2006).

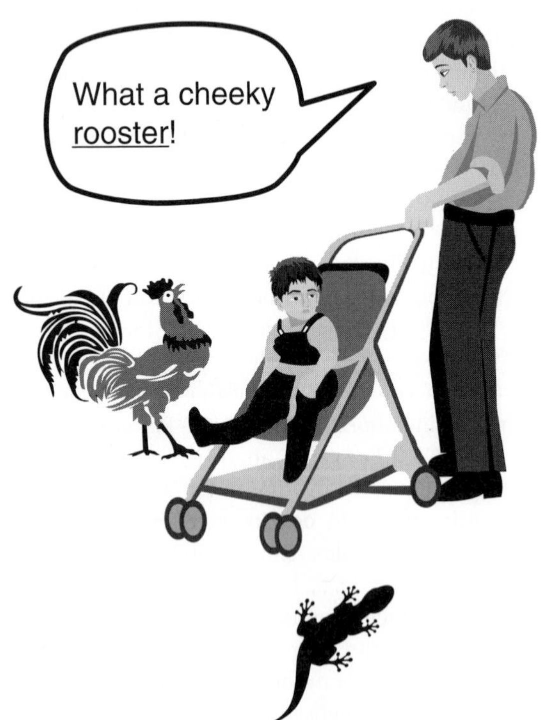

Figure 8–3. Illustration from Baldwin (1995) depicting the referential mapping problem encountered by infants in incidental social word learning situations. Source: Baldwin, D. (1995). Understanding the link between joint attention and language. In C. Moore & P. Dunham (Eds.), *Joint Attention: Its origins and role in development* (pp. 131–158). Hillsdale, NJ: Erlbaum.

If joint attention helps self-organize social learning, then the more that children engage in joint attention, the more optimal social-learning opportunities they help create for themselves. This may help to explain why the frequency with which infants engage in joint attention is positively related to their language acquisition and childhood IQ status (e.g., Mundy et al., 2007; Smith & Ulvund, 2003). More direct evidence of the links between joint attention and early learning is provided by the observation that coordinated social attention to pictures elicits electrophysiological evidence of enhanced neural activity (Striano, Reid, & Hoel, 2006) and recognition memory associated with greater depth of processing in 9-month-olds (Striano, Chen, Cleveland, & Bradshaw, 2006).

In light of the assumption that joint attention is basic to early learning, reconsider the observation that IJA and RJA dissociate in development. Theory and research suggest that this occurs because these forms of joint attention involve functions of two distinct neural networks (Mundy & Newell, 2007). In conjunction with this idea note that parallel and distributed cognitive theory suggests that learning occurs best in the context of the simultaneous activation of multiple neural networks during encoding (e.g., Munakata & McClelland, 2003; Otten et al., 2001). Taken together, these ideas raise two hypotheses. First, joint attention may involve the early development of a form of social information processing across multiple distributed neural networks. Second, impairments of joint attention may reflect deficits in the development of this parallel and distributed activation of cortical neural networks in autism.

Research has indicated that IJA is associated with frontal cortical activity (Caplan et al., 1993; Henderson et al., 2002; Mundy et al., 2000; Torkildsen et al., 2008), while RJA and related gaze-following behaviors are more closely tied to parietal and temporal cortical processes (e.g., Frieschen, Bayliss, & Tipper, 2007; Materna, Dicke, & Thern, 2008; Mundy et al., 2000). One interpretation of these data is that joint attention involves developments of functions of both the anterior and posterior cortical attention networks that have been described by Michael Posner and others (Posner & Rothbart, 2007), which is essential to typical human social learning. The basis for the first hypothesis is outlined in the next section.

The Two Neural Systems of Joint Attention and Social Cognition

The functions of the posterior network are common to many primates, but the anterior network is not well represented in primates other than humans (Astafiev et al., 2003; Emery, 2000; Gilbert & Burgess, 2008; Jellema, Baker, Wicker, &

Perrett, 2000). RJA appears to be most closely associated with the posterior system, which regulates relatively involuntary attention, begins to develop in the first 3 months of life, and prioritizes orienting to biologically meaningful stimuli. It is supported by neural networks of the parietal/precuneus and superior temporal cortices (Figure 8-4). These neural networks are active in the perception of the eye and head orientations of others, as well as the perception of spatial relations between self, other, and the environment. The posterior system is especially involved in control of orienting on a trial-by-trial basis, and the development of cognitive representations about the world built from information acquired through external senses (Dosenbach et al., 2007; Fuster, 2006; Cavanna & Trimble, 2006).

Initiating joint attention is supported by the later developing anterior attention network involved in the cognitive processing, representation, and regulation of self-initiated goal-directed action. This network includes the anterior cingulate, rostral medial superior frontal cortex, including the frontal eye fields, anterior prefrontal cortex, and orbital frontal cortex (e.g., Dosenbach et al., 2007; Fuster, 2006). The development of the intentional control of visual attention begins at about 3 to 4 months of age, when a pathway from the frontal eye fields (BA 8/9) that releases the superior colliculus from inhibition begins to be actively involved in the prospective control of saccades and visual attention (Canfield & Kirkham, 2001; Johnson, 1990). The function of this pathway may underlie 4-month-old infants' ability to suppress automatic visual saccades in order to respond to a second, more attractive stimulus (Johnson, 1995), and 6-month-olds' ability to respond to a peripheral target when central, competing stimuli are present (Atkinson, Hood, Wattam-Bell, & Braddick, 1992). We assume that the functions of this pathway also enable intentional gaze alternation between interesting events and social partners (Mundy, 2003). It is instructive to note at this juncture that research has long indicated that neonates and young infants at risk for cognitive delays, but not necessarily autism, display problems with visual disengagement from a visual stimulus (Sigman, Cohen, & Beckwith, 1997). So it is not clear if this early phase of the development of intentional control of visual attention should be considered to be a prime candidate in developmental models specific to joint attention disturbance in autism.

Differences in the functions and developmental timing of the anterior and posterior attention networks help to explain why IJA and RJA dissociate in development (Mundy et al., 2000; Mundy et al., 2007). However, although IJA and RJA follow distinct biobehavioral paths of development, it is also likely that they integrate in development. Indeed, EEG data indicates that activation of a distributed anterior and posterior cortical system predicts IJA development in infants (Henderson et al., 2002), and fMRI data indicate that activation of a distributed anterior-posterior cortical network is associated with the experience of joint attention in adults (Williams et al., 2005). These observations, among others, have motivated the description of a parallel and distribute information processing

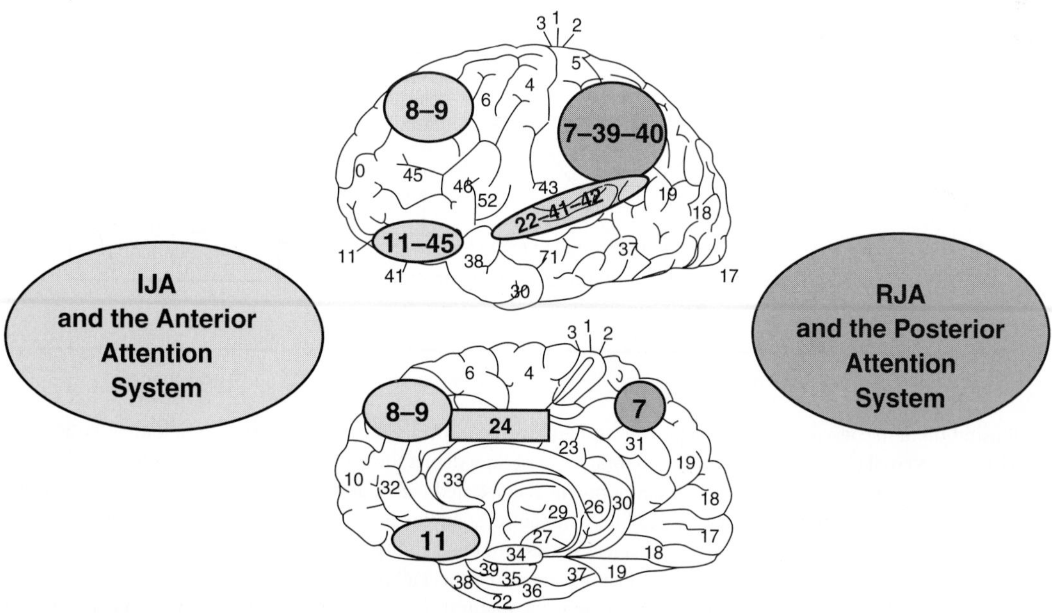

Figure 8–4. Illustration from Mundy & Newell (2007) depicting the lateral (top) and medial (bottom) illustrations of Brodmann's cytoarchitectonic areas of the cerebral cortex associated with Initiating Joint Attention and the anterior attention system, as well as RJA and the posterior attention systems. The former include areas 8 (frontal eye fields), 9 (prefrontal association cortex), 24 (anterior cingulate), and 11 and 47 (orbital prefrontal and insula association cortices—*not illustrated*). The latter include areas 7 (precuneus, posterior parietal association area), 22, 41, and 42 (superior temporal cortex), and 39 and 40 (parietal, temporal, occipital association cortex).
Source: Mundy, P., & Newell, L. (2007). Attention, joint attention, and social cognition. *Current Directions in Psychological Science, 16*, 269–274.

model (PDPM). In this model the integrative processing internal self-referenced information about one's own visual attention, with the processing of external information about the visual attention of other people is a defining feature of joint attention (Figure 8-5; Mundy & Newell, 2007; Mundy, Sullivan, & Mastergeorge, 2009). Indeed, neurocognitive theory has begun to claim that an emergent function of the human rostral medial frontal cortex is the capacity to switch attention between self-generated and perceptual information in support of social cognition (Gilbert & Burgess, 2008). The PDPM suggests that this utility is "allocated" to the rostral medial frontal cortex with development in large part as a function of the adequate biobehavioral exercise of joint attention in infancy.

According to the PDPM the joint attention, or the integration of information about self-attention and the attention of others, is a form of parallel processing that occurs across a distributed cortical network. It is first practiced in infancy and contributes to an information processing synthesis that plays a crucial role in human social cognition. The basic idea here is that human levels of self-awareness cannot develop without bidirectional interactive processing of information about self and others (e.g., Piaget, 1952). The potential role of parallel and distributed processing in synthesis in human social cognition has previously been recognized (Decety & Sommerville, 2003; Keysers & Perrett, 2006). However, the developmentally primary role of joint attention in this synthesis is less well recognized.

Social Cognition, Joint Attention, and The PDPM

Social-cognitive models often describe joint attention in terms of incremental stages of knowledge about the intentionality of other people. Baron-Cohen (1995) described a sequence of cognitive modules that included the *intentionality detector* (ID), a dedicated cognitive facility that attributes goal-directed behavior to objects or people; and the *eye direction detector* (EDD), which senses and processes information about eyes. These combine to form the *shared attention mechanism* (SAM), a cognitive module that represents self and other as attending to the same referent *and* attributes volitional states (intentionality) to direction of gaze of *other* people. As infancy ebbs the *theory of mind mechanism* replaces SAM and enables representation of the full range of mental states of others and enables us to make sense of others behaviors.

Tomasello et al. (2005) more explicitly described joint attention development in terms of three stages of what infants *know about other people.* In *understanding animate action*, 3- to 8-month-old infants can perceive contingencies between

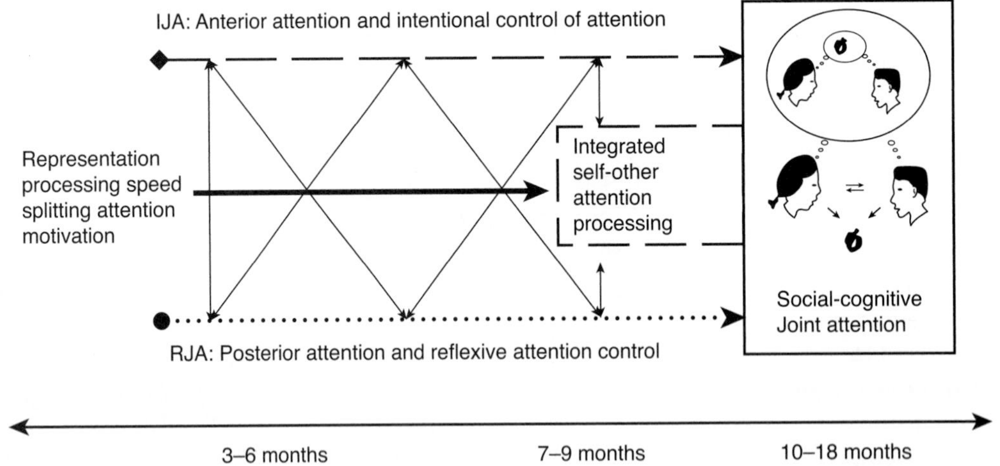

Figure 8–5. An illustration of the development of the parallel and distributed information processing system of joint attention and social cognition, from Mundy & Newell (2007). In this model, different types of lines depict the multiple paths of joint attention development. The posterior attention system path associated with RJA development is illustrated with a dotted line and the anterior attention system path associated with IJA development is illustrated with a dashed line. The central solid line in the figure depicts the developments of other processes during infancy that influence joint attention development such as representational ability, speed of processing, motivation, and the executive attention control, as well as each other during infancy. The diagonal arrows connect all paths throughout early development. This reflects the dynamic and coactive nature of joint attention development whereby the maturation of attention, cognitive, and affective systems interact in reciprocal cause-and-effect relations with experience, including the experiences children create for themselves through their own actions. Finally, the development of integrated self- and other-attention processing is considered to be a social attention executive function of the anterior system that emerges in the 4- to 9-months period. This is represented by the box. The capacity to integrate and share overt aspects of attention provides a foundation for the ability to share covert aspects of attention, such as representations, and social cognition.
Source: Mundy, P., & Newell, L. (2007). Attention, joint attention, and social cognition. *Current Directions in Psychological Science, 16*, 269–274.

their own animate actions and emotions relative to the animate actions and affect of others. However, they cannot represent the internal mental goals of others that are associated with these actions. In the next *understanding of pursuit of goals* stage, 9-month-olds become capable of shared action and attention on objects (e.g., building a block tower with parents).

Tomasello et al. (2005) suggest this stage involves *joint perception,* rather than *joint attention,* because the social-cognitive capacity to represent others' internal mental representations necessary for true joint attention is not yet available. However, this ability emerges between 12 and 15 months in the *understanding choice of plans* stage. This stage is heralded when infants become truly active in initiating episodes of joint engagement by alternating their eye-contact between interesting sights and caregivers (Tomasello et al., 2005). This shift to active alternating gaze indicates infants' appreciation that others make mental choices about alternative actions that affect their attention. Infants also now know themselves as agents that initiate collaborative activity based on their own goals. Hence, the development of "true" joint attention at this stage is revealed in the capacity to adopt two perspectives analogous to speaker-listener.

The capacity to adopt two perspectives is also assumed to be an intrinsic characteristic of symbolic representations. In this regard, Tomasello et al. (2005) raise a truly seminal hypothesis that symbolic thought is a *developmental transformation* of joint attention. They argue that symbols themselves serve to socially coordinate attention so that the intentions of the listener align with those of the speaker. In other words, *linguistic symbols both lead to and are dependent on the efficient social coordination of covert mental attention to common abstract representations among people.* This hypothesis fits well with the parallel and distributed information processing model (PDPM) of joint attention, but the PDPM places it in a substantially different developmental framework.

The PDPM does not emphasize functional segregation of cognitive systems implicit to modular perspectives, but instead emphasizes the cortically multidetermined nature of human cognition because of the "massively parallel nature of human brain networks and the fact that function also emerges from the flow of information between brain areas" (Ramnani et al., 2004, p. 613). Furthermore, cognitive development need not be construed only in terms of changes in discontinuous stages of knowledge. It can also be modeled as a continuous change in the speed, efficiency, and combinations of information processing that give rise to knowledge (Hunt, 1999). Specifically, the PDPM envisions joint attention development in terms of increased speed, efficiency, and complexity of processing of: (1) internal information about self-referenced visual attention, (2) external information about the visual attention of other people, and (3) the neural networks that integrate processing of self-generated visual attention information with processing of information about the visual attention behavior of other people (Mundy & Newell, 2007; Mundy et al., 2009).

Consequently, the notion that *true* joint attention does not emerge until requisite social-cognitive knowledge emerges at 12–15 months (Tomasello et al., 2005) is not germane to the PDPM. Rather, consistent with a growing empirical literature, the PDPM holds that the true joint processing of attention information begins to be practiced by infants by 3 to 4 months of age (D'Entremont, Hains, & Muir, 1997; Farroni, Massuccessi, & Francesca, 2002; Hood, Willen, & Driver, 1998, Morales et al., 1998, Striano Reed, & Hoel, 2006; Striano & Stahl, 2005). Indeed, even the types of active alternating gaze behaviors thought to mark the onset of true joint attention at 12–15 months (Tomasello et al., 2005) develop no later than at 8–9 months of life, and quite possibly earlier (Mundy et al., 2007; Venezia et al., 2004).

Equally important, the PDPM assumes that joint attention is not replaced by the subsequent development of social-cognitive processes. Instead, joint attention is thought to remain an active system of information processing that supports cognition through adulthood (Mundy & Newell, 2007; Mundy et al., 2009). As an example, recall the hypothesis that linguistic symbols enable the social coordination of covert attention to common mental representations across people (Tomasello et al., 2005). According to the PDPM symbolic thinking *involves* joint attention but does not *replace* joint attention. Just as 12-month-olds can shift eye contact or use pointing to establish a common visual point of reference with other people, 4-year-olds can use symbols to establish a common reference to covert mental representations with other people. Symbolic representations are often, if not always, initially encoded during the joint processing of information about the overt attention of self and of others directed toward some third object or event (Adamson et al., 2004; Baldwin, 1995; Werner & Kaplan, 1963). The PDPM combines that hypothesis with the connectionist notion that "representations can take the form of patterns of activity distributed across processing units" that occurred during encoding (Munakata & McClelland, 2003, p. 415). Together these two ideas lead to the assumption of the PDPM that *symbol acquisition incorporates the distributed activation of the joint self-attention and other-attention neural processing units, which were engaged during encoding, as part of their functional neural representational mappings.* Hence, the distributed joint attention processing system may always be activated as a network encoding that contributes to the intersubjectivity (i.e., shared attention and meaning) of symbolic thought.

In infancy the distributed joint attention processing system is initially effortful. However, thousands of episodes of practice allow the joint information processing of self-other attention to become efficient, less effortful, and even automatically activated in social engagement. As this occurs, joint attention becomes a social-executive "subroutine" that runs in support of symbolic thought, as well that capacity to maintain a shared focus in social interactions and in social-cognition (Mundy, 2003). The distributed neural activation patterns associated with joint attention are part of infants' sense of developing sense of relatedness to others (Mundy & Hogan, 1994; Mundy,

Kasari, & Sigman, 1993). Moreover, the distributed neural activation associated with joint attention can be thought of as an enduring stratum of a more *continuous spiral* of human social-neurocognitive development that supports, if not enables, later emerging human symbolic, linguistic, and social cognitive facilities (see Figure 8-6).

Inside-Out Processing and The PDPM

In addition to parallel and distributed processing, the PDPM may be distinguished from other models by its constructivist perspective on development. Rather than focusing on the development of knowledge *about others*, the PDPM gives equal footing to the significance of infants' development of their own intentional visual behavior in joint attention and social cognitive development (Mundy et al., 1993). The assumption here is that neonates and young infants receive greater quantities and fidelity of information about self-intended actions (e.g., active looking) through proprioception than they receive about other's intended actions through exteroceptive information processing. Thus, infants have the opportunity to learn as much *or more* about intentionality from their own actions as from observing the actions of others. A corollary of this assumption of the PDPM is that joint attention is an embodied form of cognition (Feldman & Narayanan, 2004). Its development is a constructivist process that involves self-perception as a foundation for the attribution of meaning to the perception of others behaviors.

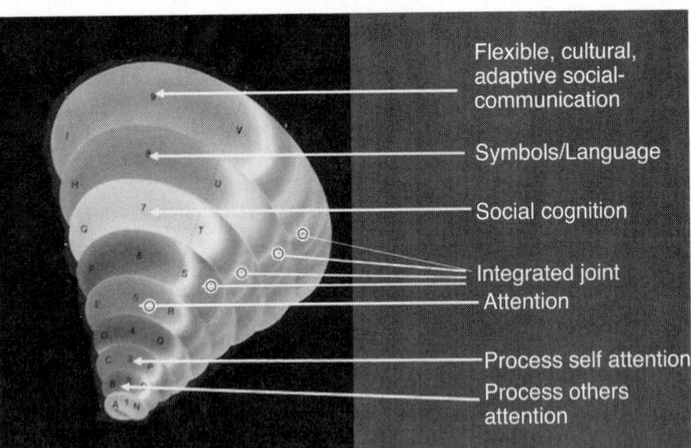

Figure 8-6. An illustration of the continuous nature of joint attention development. Development is modeled as a spiral in which the initial acquisition of the capacity for integrated processing of information about self and other attention (joint attention) remains an active but deeper layer of cognitive activity throughout life that supports symbolic thought, language, and cultural social exchange. Numbers of the spiral bands represent changing phases of development. The letters on each side of the spiral bands represent change and continuity in multiple developmental factors that may impact joint attention development, such as speed of information processing, representational development, and memory.

We have referred to this as the "inside-out" processing assumption of the PDPM (Mundy & Vaughan Van Hecke, 2008).

The general tenor of this constructivist assumption is nothing new. Bates et al. (1979) suggested that a sense of self-agency was basic to joint attention. More generally Piaget (1952) argued that infants do not learn through the passive perception of objects [or others] in the world. Rather, infants take action on objects and learn from their [causal] actions. They then modify their actions, observe changes in causal relations, and learn new things about the physical world. Thus, Piaget viewed the processing of self-initiated actions on objects as a singularly important fuel for the engines of cognitive development. The constructivist viewpoint is not only central to the PDPM, it is also a mainstay of contemporary connectionist biological principles of typical and atypical neurocognitive development (e.g., Blakemore & Frith, 2003; Elman, 2005; Mareschal et al., 2007; Meltzoff, 2007; Quartz, 1999).

The vast number of functional neural connections that are made in early postnatal brain development are thought to be too numerous to be specified by genes alone. Instead, genes specify relatively wide channels of potential neurodevelopmental architecture (e.g., Quartz, 1999). Within these prescribed channels the specifics of important functional connections in the developing nervous systems are sculpted by our experience. Since most of us experience relatively similar environments and experiences in early life developmental, brain organization displays significant similarities across most people (Mareschal et al., 2007). Greenough, Wallace, & Black (1987) refer to this gene-by-environment interaction in the ontogeny of neural connections as "experience expectant" neurodevelopment. Greenough et al. (1987) also explicitly noted the that infants' generation of actions, and observations of social reactions, likely play a role in experience expectant processes specific to neurodevelopmental basis of human social behavior. So, just as Piaget envisioned that infants learn about the physical world from their self-generated actions on objects, it is reasonable to think that a significant portion of what infants learn about the social world comes from their self-generated actions with people. One type of self-generated action that may be developmentally key in this regard is active vision.

Active Vision and The PDPM

One of the first and most vitally informative types of actions infants take involves the self-control of their looking behaviors, or active vision. The science of vision has moved away from the study of "seeing" or passive visual perception, to the study of "looking" or intentional, *active-vision* and attention deployment (Findlay & Gilchrist, 2003). Active vision in infancy begins to develop at 3–4 months (e.g., Canfield & Kirkham, 2001; Johnson, 1990, 1995). It involves the goal-directed selection of information to process, and can elicit contingent social behavior responses from other people, such as parental smiles, vocalizations, or gaze shifts. It also is one of the first types of volitional actions that infants use to control stimulation to order to self-regulate arousal and affect (Posner & Rothbart, 2007).

Vision and looking behavior have unique properties. Vision provides information regarding the relative spatial location of ourselves and other people. Moreover, direction of gaze conveys the distal and proximal spatial direction of our attention to others, and vice versa. Comparable information on the spatial direction of attention is not as clearly available from the other senses. This is especially true in the first 9 months of life, and for distal information. The importance of spatial visual information for the development of joint attention was emphasized by Butterworth and Jarrett (1991) in their influential article "What Minds Have in Common Is Space."

In some sense primate eyes are specialized for *social* spatial attention processing (e.g., Tomasello, Hare, Lehman, & Call, 2006). Frontal binocular eye positions allow for enhanced spatial processing and depth of perception through parallax perception. Intricate musculatures allow for rapid visual focus on objects that are far or near. Equally important, precise information about the spatial direction of attention is available from human eyes because of the highlighted contrast between the dark coloration of the pupil and iris versus the light to white coloration of the sclera. These observations have led to the suggestion that the ease of processing the direction of attention of *other peoples' eyes* contributed to the human phylogenetic and ontogenetic development of social cognition (e.g., Tomasello et al., 2006).

It is also the case, though, that these characteristics of the human eye allow the saccades of infants to be readily observed by other people. Consequently, infant saccades can effectively act as elicitors of contingent social feedback. When infants shift attention to an object, their parents may pick up and show them the object. When infants shift attention to their parents' eyes they may also receive a vocal, affective, or physical parental response. Thus, just as the characteristics of eyes make it easier for infants to perceive the attention of others, the signal value of eyes makes the active control of vision a likely nexus of infants' developing sense of agency. A corollary here is that a sense of visual self-agency may play a role in joint attention and social-cognitive development.

The notion that active vision has primacy in social development relates back to the time-honored observation that visual behavior is at least as important to human social development as physical contact (Rheingold, 1966; Robson, 1967). However, the contemporary literature on social-cognitive development emphasizes only the importance of the information infants gather from processing the visual attention of others (e.g., Johnson et al., 2005). It neglects the potential importance of the information infants' process about their own active vision, and socially contingent responses.

Alternatively, the active vision assumption of the PDPM offers one plausible explanation for why activation of the frontal eye fields (a cortical area involved in volitional saccadic control) is a consistent significant correlate of social cognition in imaging studies (Mundy, 2003). This is because the volitional control of active vision, via the frontal eye fields, may be central to developing an integrated sense of the relations between self-attention and other-attention, which is fundamental to joint attention and subsequent social cognition. This hypothesis leads to the testable prediction that the frontal eye fields should be less active in social-cognitive processing in older congenitally blind individuals than in sighted individuals (Mundy & Newell, 2007). If true, this hypothesis may also help to explain some of the developmental commonalities observed for children with autism and blind infants (Bigelow, 2003; Hobson, Lee, & Brown, 1999).

Dynamic Systems, Integrated Processing, and The PDPM

The PDPM emphasizes inside-out processing, constructivism, and the role of active vision in the development of joint attention. However, it *does not* maintain that the inside-out processing of self-attention is more important for social-cognitive development than outside-in processing of other's-attention. This is because the PDPM holds that social meaning, and even conscious self-awareness, cannot be derived from processing either self-attention or other's-attention in isolation (cf. Decety & Sommerville, 2003; Keysers & Perrett, 2006; Vygotsky, 1962). Ontogeny may be best viewed as a dynamic system that, through interactions of multiple factors over time and experience, coalesce into higher order integrations, structures, and skills (e.g., Smith & Thelen, 2003). The development of joint attention, or the joint processing of the attention of self and other, is such a dynamic system. Indeed, the pertinence of joint attention for human development derives in no small part from the unique synthesis that arises from of the rapid, parallel processing of self-attention and other-attention across distributed neural networks. Consequently, it is not possible to account for the role of joint attention in typical or atypical development with research or theory that focuses on only one of its elements in isolation.

The dynamic system of joint attention begins to synergize as frontal executive functions increasingly enable attending to multiple sources of information during infancy. According to one definition, executive functions involve the transmission of bias signals throughout the neural network to selectively inhibit comparatively automatic behavioral responses in favor of more volitional, planned, and goal-directed ideation and action in problem-solving contexts (Miller & Cohen, 2001). These bias signals act as regulators for the brain, affecting visual processes and attention as well as other sensory modalities and systems responsible for task-relevant response execution, memory retrieval, emotional evaluation, etc. *The aggregate effect of these bias signals is to guide the flow of neural activity along pathways that establish the proper mappings between inputs, internal states, and outputs needed to perform a given task* more efficiently (Miller & Cohen, 2001). According to this definition, joint attention development may be thought of as reflecting the emergence of frontal bias signals that establish the proper mappings across: (1) outside-in posterior cortical [temporal-precuneus] processing of inputs about the attention behaviors of other people and, (2) rostral medial frontal [BA 8-9, anterior cingulate] inside-out processing of internal states and outputs related to active vision. This mapping results in the integrated development of a distributed anterior and posterior cortical joint attention system.

It is conceivable that the early establishment of this mapping of the joint processing of attention is formative with respect to the shared neural network of representations self-other that Decety and Grezes (2006) suggest is essential to social cognition. It also may a play a role in what Keysers and Perrett (2006) have described as a Hebbian learning model of social cognition. Neural networks that are repeatedly active at the same time become associated, such that activity [e.g., representations] in one network triggers activity in the other (Hebb, 1949). Keysers and Perrett (2006)suggest that *common* activation of neural networks for processing self-generated information and information about conspecifics is fundamental to understanding the actions of others. This Hebbian learning process is fundamental to the hypothesized functions of simulation (Gordon, 1986) and mirror neurons (i.e., Decety & Summerville, 2003; Williams, 2008) that are commonly invoked in current models of social-cognitive development.

The PDPM is consistent with these interrelated ideas *and* suggests that Hebbian mapping in social cognition begins with integrated rostral medial frontal processing of information about self-produced visual attention and posterior processing of the attention of others. Moreover, the PDPM specifically operationalizes the study of development of this dynamic mapping system in terms of psychometrically sound measures of early joint attention development (Mundy et al., 2007). Indeed, IJA assessments may be relatively powerful in research on social cognitive development and autism, because they measure variance in the whole dynamic system, rather than any one of its parts alone.

Once well practiced the joint processing of attention information requires less mental effort. As the basic joint attention process is mastered and its "effort to engage" goes down it can become integrated as an executive function that contributes to the initial development and increasing efficiency of social-cognitive problem-solving. Thus, joint attention development may be envisioned as shifting from "learning to do joint attention" at 6 to 9 months to "learning from joint attention" in the second year of life (Mundy & Vaughan Van Hecke, 2008; Figure 8-7). In the learning-from phase the capacity to attend to multiple sources of information in "triadic attention" deployment becomes more common (Scaife & Bruner, 1975). Triadic attention contexts provide infants with rich opportunities to compare information gleaned through processing internal states associated with volitional visual attention deployment and the processing of the visual attention of others in reference to a common third object or event. Through simulation (Gordon, 1986) infants may begin to impute that others have intentional control over their looking behavior that is similar to their own.

The role of simulation in the learning-from phase of joint attention development is well illustrated by a recent sequence of elegant experimental studies. Twelve-month-olds often follow the "gaze direction" of testers, even if their eyes are closed. After 12 months, though, infants discriminate and follow the gaze of testers whose eyes are open but not closed. This suggests that infants' understanding of the meaning of the eye gaze of others may improve in this period leading older infants to inhibit looking in the "eyes closed" condition (Brooks & Meltzoff, 2002).

To examine this interpretation Meltzoff and Brooks (2008) conducted an experimental intervention. They provided 12-month-olds with the experience of blindfolds that occluded their own looking behavior. After gaining that experience, 12-month-olds did not follow the head-turn of blindfolded testers, but did follow the head-turn and gaze of non-blindfolded testers. Meltzoff and Brooks also provided 18-month-olds with experience with blindfolds that looked opaque but were transparent when worn. After this condition the 18-month-olds reverted to following the gaze of blindfolded social partners. These data strongly suggest that the infants demonstrated inside-out learning and constructed social-cognitive awareness about others' gaze based on the experience of effects of blindfolds on their own active vision.

The Distributed Information Processing Model and Autism

Assumptions of the PDPM bridge theory on the development of joint attention with phenomena observed in other disciplines of research with autism. Several of these will be briefly considered in this final section of the chapter. The first of these involves links with theory and research on neural connectivity impairments in autism.

Neural Connectivity and Activity Dependent Genes in Autism

Over the last 10 years several research groups have suggested that problems in functional connectivity between brain regions contribute to autism (e.g., Courchesne & Pierce, 2005; Geschwind & Levitt, 2007; Horowitz et al. 1998;Just et al., 2004; Lewis & Elman, 2008; Wickelgren, 2005). However, rather than specific to autism, impaired connectivity may be central to many forms of mental retardation and developmental disorders (Dierssen & Ramakers, 2006). So how do neurodevelopmental connectivity impairments lead to the specific social symptom impairments of autism, and how are these different from the connectivity impairments that characterize other developmental disorders?

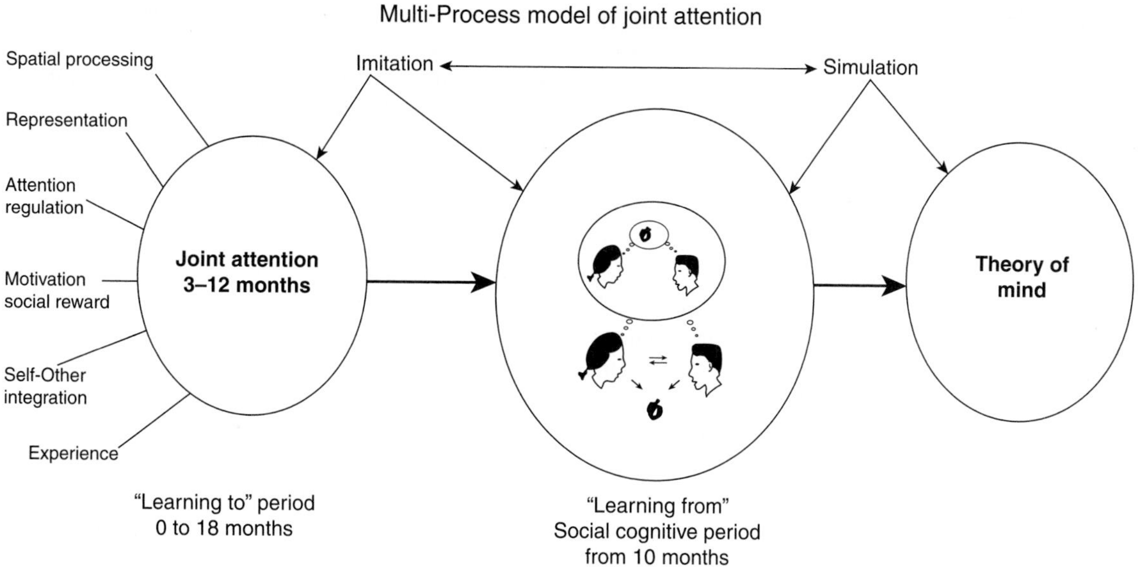

Multi-Process model of joint attention

Spatial processing
Representation
Attention regulation
Motivation social reward
Self-Other integration
Experience
Imitation ⟷ Simulation
Joint attention 3–12 months
Theory of mind
"Learning to" period 0 to 18 months
"Learning from" Social cognitive period from 10 months

Figure 8–7. In the first year the development of joint attention involves the "learning to" integration of executive, motivation, and imitation processes to support the routine, rapid, and efficient (error free) execution of patterns of behavior that enable infants to coordinate processing of *overt* aspects of visual self attention with processing of the social attention of other people. In the latter part of the first year and the second year infants can better monitor their own experiences and integrate it with information about the social partners during joint attention events. This provides a critical multimodal source of information to the infants about the convergence and divergence of self and others' experience and behavior during sharing information in social interactions. Theoretically, this provides the stage for the "learning from" phase of joint attention development. In this stage infants can control their attention to self-organize and optimize information processing in social learning opportunities. The integration of anterior and posterior self-other attention processing (Figure 8-5) provides a neural network that enriches encoding in social learning. The internalization of the overt joint processing of attention to the covert joint processing of attention to representations is part of an executive system that facilitates symbolic development and the social cognition. Indeed both symbolic thought and social cognition may be characterized by a transition from learning to *socially coordinate overt attention* to the capacity to *socially coordinate covert mental representations of the attention of self and others.*

One possibility is that mental retardation may be associated with connectivity impairments within proximal brain networks, but that autism may be characterized by more distal connectivity problems (Courchesne & Pierce, 2005; Lewis & Elman, 2008). Indeed, several studies suggest that distal connectivity problems between frontal and temporal parietal networks may be especially prominent in autism (Cherkassky, Kana, Keller, & Just, 2006; Courchesne & Pierce, 2005; Murias, Webb, Greenson, & Dawson, 2007; Wicker et al., 2008). The PDPM offers a moderately explicit developmental account of how the impairment of distal frontal-parietal pathways may have an early and robust effect specific to a disturbance of joint attention and related social symptom of autism, such as a lack of spontaneously sharing experiences with other people. The PDPM's focus on the fundamental relations between the joint processing of attention information, learning, and symbolic development also provide a means for understanding why variations in the strength of the disturbance of anterior-posterior connectivity could contribute to phenotypic variability in autism, such as the co-occurrence of mental retardation or specific language impairments.

The connectivity assumptions of PDPM also lead to the prediction that differences in the development of joint attention in typical and atypical children should be associated with measures of synchrony or coherence in cortical activity. There is some support for this, but currently available data are no more than suggestive in this regard (Mundy et al., 2000; Mundy et al., 2003). Nevertheless, the PDPM offers a conceptual framework that emphasizes the benefits of a multidisciplinary approach to neurodevelopment, attention, connectionist network models of development and autism. This emphasis is in line with the recent call for the multidisciplinary examination of relations between EEG or imaging coherence in developmental and intervention studies of autism (Dawson, 2008).

It also may be that mental retardation is associated with impairments of prenatal neural connectivity that are less activity dependent, but that autism involves a greater degree of postnatal connectivity impairments that are more activity dependent (Morrow, Yoo, Flavell, Kim, & Lin, 2008). Morrow et al. have recently observed several genome deletions in families of children with autism. The expression of three genes associated with the two largest deletions (*c3orf*58, NHE9, and PCDH10) is regulated by neuronal activity. From this observation Morrow et al. (2008) reasoned that defects in activity-dependent gene expression may be a cause of cognitive deficits in autism. They note that these genes likely have a defined temporal course of greater or lesser vulnerability to atypical expression depending on the timing and quality of the young child's postnatal activity and experience-dependent processes.

The PDPM proposes that problems with initiating joint attention activity may be especially key to understanding activity-dependent alterations of gene expression associated with autism. Some evidence consistent with this proposition stems from the observation that the activity of children with autism may affect and modify the attempts of caregivers to scaffold the development of joint attention in their children (Adamson et al., 2001). If the PDPM is correct in this regard, it will be important to build a better understanding of genetic influences on the typical range of expression individual differences in IJA in infant development. Little if any information currently exists on this topic. Fortunately, the recent observation of a surprising degree of longitudinal stability of individual differences in a sample of the 100 typical infants (Mundy et al., 2007) suggests that behavioral or metabolic genetic methods may be brought to bear in large-scale studies of the typical development of infant joint attention.

The PDPM, Visual Attention Control, and Autism

The work of several research groups indicates that basic mechanism of visual control may play a role in autism (Brenner, Turner, & Muller, 2007; Landry & Bryson, 2004; Johnson et al., 2005). Brenner et al. (2007) have noted that one of the essential issues for this line of research is to understand precisely, "how an ocular-motor system that is over-specialized for certain tasks and under-specialized for others early in life might affect later development in [social] domains such as joint attention" (p. 1302). The PDPM offers a guide in this regard. First, it encourages the research community to recognize the possibility that joint attention may not be a "later" development, but one that begins as part of the development of volitional visual attention control by the 4th month of life. In addition, the PDPM provides means for understanding how significantly altered early visual preferences could have a cascading effect on the development of intentional joint attention and autism (Mundy, 1995). In this regard, consider two recent studies.

McCleery et al. (2007) observed that magnocellular visual processing may be atypically enhanced in a sample of 6-month-old infant siblings of children with autism. Similarly Karmel et al. (2008) observed visual attention patterns that are consistent with a magnocellular bias in 6-month-olds in neonatal intensive care who later received the diagnosis of autism at 3 years of age. The magnocellular visual system contributes to orienting based on movement and contrast-sensitivity related to small achromatic differences in brightness. This system dominates early visual orienting. However, by 2- to 4-months visually orienting is increasingly influenced by the parvocellular system, which contributes to orienting based on high-resolution information about shape, or low-resolution information about color and shades of grey. The studies of Karmel et al. (2008) and McCleery et al. (2007) raise the possibility that a delay in the developmental shift from the magnocellular to parvocellular visual systems could alter what children with autism choose to attend to early in life.

Hypothetically, the maintenance of a magnocellular bias may lead to a relatively long-standing visual preference for stimuli or objects characterized by movement or achromatic contrasts, such as surface edges, power lines, spinning objects, the outlines of faces, or mouth movement. Reciprocally, the decreased influence of the parvocellular system could lead to developmental delays in the emergence of a visual attention bias to targets that are socially informative but involve differentiation based on high resolution of shape and color information, such as distal processing of eyes and facial expressions. Thus, the alteration of visual preferences during early critical periods of development could degrade the establishment of the dynamic system of internal information processing about active looking, relative to contingent social feedback, and information about the attention of other people (Mundy, 1995; Mundy & Burnette, 2005). Moreover, if magnocelluar guidance bias and connectivity impairments are orthogonal processes, combinations of varying levels of their effects could present as phenotypic differences in joint attention processing and social symptom expression in autism.

Early Intervention, Learning, Motivation, and the PDPM

The assumptions of the PDPM may also help to explain why joint attention is a pivotal skill in early intervention for children with autism (Bruinsma, Koegel, & Koegel, 2004; Charman, 2004; Mundy & Crowson, 1997). Improvements in pivotal skills, by definition, lead to positive changes in a broad array of *other* problematic behaviors. This appears to be the case with joint attention. It can be improved with early intervention (e.g., Kasari et al., 2006, 2007; Pierce & Schreibman, 1995; Rocha et al., 2007; Yoder & Stone, 2006), and joint attention improvement has collateral benefits on language, cognitive, and social development (Kasari et al., 2007; Jones, Carr, & Feely, 2006; Whalen & Schreibman, 2006). Joint attention also appears to mediate responsiveness to early intervention among children with autism (Bono et al., 2004; Yoder & Stone, 2006).

According to the PDPM, joint attention is a pivotal skill in autism because its improvement has multiple effects on social learning. Recall that joint attention facilitates the self-organization of information processing to optimize incidental as well as structured social learning opportunities (Baldwin, 1995). Hence, impairment in joint attention may be viewed as part of a broader social constructivist learning disturbance in autism. By the same token, effective intervention likely improves social constructivist learning in autism.

Second, the PDPM proposes that joint attention serves as a foundation for social cognitive development. Social cognitive development is defined in terms of advances in the processing of information about self and other, rather than singularly in terms of changes in knowledge about intentionality. Following connectionist cognitive theory (McClelland & Rogers, 2003; Otten et al., 2001), the PDPM assumes that information encoded during learning is stored as a distributed neural network activation pattern that involves parallel activation of networks of related semantic information. Additionally, whenever information is acquired during social learning and joint attention it is also encoded in parallel with the activation of a frontal-temporal-parietal neural network that maps relations between representations of information about self-directed attention and information about the attention of other people. Thus, every time we process information in social learning we encode it as an activation pattern in a distributed semantic network *in conjunction with* an activation pattern of the anterior-posterior cortical joint attention network (see Figures 8-4 & 8-5). Recall that deeper information processing and learning occurs best in the context of the simultaneous activation of multiple neural networks during encoding (Otten et al., 2001). If so, joint attention may lead to deeper processing because it adds activation of the distributed social attention network (a form of episodic encoding) to the network activation associated more directly with semantic information. This conjecture provides one interpretation of the observation that joint attention facilitates depth of processing in 9-month-olds (Striano, Chen, et al., 2006; Striano, Reid, et al., 2006). It also suggests that part of the learning disability of autism occurs because children with this disorder do not reap the full benefits of encoding semantic information in conjunction with episodic memory encoded within the integrated processing of self- and other-attention. This, in turn, may help to explain the attenuation of self-referenced memory effects in autism (Henderson et al., 2009).

Third, the PDPM argues that overt joint attention becomes increasingly internalized as a social executive function that supports the social coordination of covert mental attention to cognitive representations. The spontaneous coordination of mental attention cognitive representations is an essential element of symbolic thought (Tomasello et al., 2005). The PDPM assumes that months of practice of the social coordination of overt attention (i.e., joint attention) in the first years of life is required before this function can be internalized and transformed to an executive facility for the socially coordinated covert mental attention and symbolic thought. Thus, symbolic thought processes incorporate, but do not replace activation of the self-other joint attention system. Joint attention however does not necessarily involve symbolic process (Mundy et al., 1987).

These assumptions of the PDPM are consistent with two recent observations. Joint attention is a unique predictor of pretend play development in children with autism relative to measures of imitation or executive functions (Rutherford et al., 2008). Moreover, successful symbolic play intervention, which according to the PDPM must involve effects on joint attention, *is* associated with parallel collateral improvements in joint attention in autism. However, intervention with joint attention has less immediate impact on symbolic play behavior (Kasari et al., 2006).

Fourth, the joint processing of attention information also plays a fundamental role in social cognition defined in terms of the development of knowledge about intentions in self and other (Mundy & Newell, 2007). The assumption here is that when infants or primates practice monitoring others attention (RJA), statistical learning ultimately leads to the associative rule *where others' eyes go, their behavior follows* (Jellema, Baker, Wicker, & Perrett, D., 2000). Similarly, anterior monitoring or *self-awareness* of control of visual attention likely leads to awareness of the self-referenced associative rule that *where my eyes go, my intended behavior follows* (Mundy & Newell, 2007). An integration of the development of these "concepts" leads to the logical cognitive output *where others eyes go → their intended behavior follows,* which is a building block of social cognitive development (Mundy & Newell, 2007). Social cognition of this kind is thought to enable new and more efficient levels of social or cultural learning is atypical in autism.

Finally, the constructivist assumptions of the PDPM stress that motivation factors are part of a crucial fifth path of association between joint attention and social learning. Initiating joint attention requires "choosing" between behavior goals, such as fixated looking at an event, or alternating looking at the event and another person. Choosing among behavior goals is thought to involve frontal and medial cortical processing of the relative reward associated with different goals (Holroyd & Coles, 2002). Therefore, IJA impairment in autism may be expected to be related to deficits in biobehavioral processes associated with reward sensitivity and motivation (Dawson, 2008; Kasari et al., 1990; Mundy, 1995). Such a deficit, however, could take several forms.

Social stimuli could be aversive in some way for children with autism. However, the aversion hypothesis is complicated by observations of behaviors indicative of relatively intact caregiver-attachment in many children with autism and a willingness to engage in playful physical interactions with strangers (e.g., Mundy et al., 1986; Sigman & Ungerer, 1984). On the other hand, social stimuli may not be aversive. Rather, they may simply not be sufficiently positive to compel social-orienting and joint attention early in the life of children with autism (Dawson et al., 1998; Mundy, 1995). Finally, social stimuli could have a positive valence for children with autism, but be overshadowed by an atypically strong visual preference that make objects, rather that social elements of the world more "interesting" (Karmel et al., 2008; McCleery et al., 2006; Mundy & Crowson, 1997).

The construction of effective empirical approaches to address these alternatives is one of the outstanding challenges in the science of autism (Dawson, 2008; Koegel et al., 2003). Research on joint attention in relation to motivation and the perceived valence of objects in adults (Bayliss et al., 2006) offers one potential route for developmental and functional neurocognitive studies on this topic. For now, though, the literature on early intervention may be the best source of information in this regard. Early interventions studies offer some of the most systematic investigations to date of how to structure social engagements with young children with autism to modify and increase their motivation to initiate episodes of shared attention and shared experience with others (e.g., Kasari et al., 2006, 2007).

Conclusions

Only in its most expansive or grandiose interpretation can the PDPM be viewed as an explanatory model of joint attention, or autism. Nevertheless, the PDPM does serve a purpose. It presents a new perspective on joint attention that suggests its impairment in autism is more than an epiphenomenon associated with other fundamental precursor or successor processes. This alternative perspective can be summed up in terms of several general principles. First, autism is as much about impairments in self-generated activity as it is about problems in perceiving or responding to the behavior of others. Hence, we need to consider the neurodevelopmental processes and networks involved in initiating behavior and attention control, as well as those involved in perceiving and responding to the behaviors of others to understand this disorder (Mundy, 2003). Second, joint attention is a form of information processing that gives rise to social-cognitive knowledge. Third, joint attention is a form of *parallel and distributed processing* that involves the conjoint analysis of information from anterior cortical system for guidance of goal-directed attention and behavior, with posterior cortical processing external information about the attention related behavior of other people. Ultimately, joint attention becomes a social executive process that supports all subsequent cognition and learning that demands the rapid social coordination of mental attention to internal representations of object and events. Thus, neural network activation associated with joint attention is an enduring substrate that plays a role in the unique characteristics of human cognition throughout the lifespan (Mundy & Newell, 2007). Indeed, it may be one example of the type of "hot" executive functions that Zelazo, Qu, and Muller (2005) theorize are central to social cognition. Hot executive functions are those that entail motivation processes and affect-regulation specific to the support of successful goal-directed behavior in social engagements. It follows from this notion that individual differences in the operation of the social-executive function of joint attention, including the extreme variation displayed by people with autism, may be an expression of variance in motivation process.

Challenges and Future Directions

- To fully appreciate the significance of joint attention impairments in autism requires a deeper appreciation of the typical development of joint attention. This may necessitate a shift away from a singular emphasis on the stages of acquisition of social cognitive "knowledge" in the study of joint attention, to research on the development of joint attention as an information processing system associated with learning.
- Recent research suggests that the etiology of autism is associated with complex polygenetic processes. Studies also suggest that the early development joint attention is characterized by stable sources of individual differences by 9 months of age. One challenge for future research is to determine if the behavioral and metabolic genetic study of typical joint attention development in large samples of infants provides for identifying a subset of genetic contributions to autism.
- The constructivist hypothesis of the PDPM raises the challenge of creating paradigms for the study of neurocognitive systems involved in the generation and self-regulation of social behavior, as well as the perception and interpretation of the social behaviors of others. Without the former we will likely have a most incomplete picture of the development of the "social brain."
- Examination of parallel and distributed processing of joint attention requires measurement that is sensitive to temporal, parallel nature of information processing and well as localized-functional activation of distributed neural networks. Hence, future informative research on joint attention may be effectively joined with diffusion tensor imaging technology, as well as advances in EEG and MEG coherence analysis.
- The most direct tests of the PDPM of joint attention will likely require an integration of advances in biometric measurement (e.g., advances in EEG coherence methods) with advances in behavioral and pharmacological interventions that change the course of joint attention expression and development in children with autism. Fortunately, research on the latter has begun to emerge, and now studies of this kind await integration with the former.

SUGGESTED READINGS

Kasari, C., Paparella, T., Freeman, S., & Jahromi, L. (2008). Language outcomes in autism: Randomized comparison of joint attention and play interventions. *Journal of Consulting and Clinical Psychology*, *76*, 125–137.

Keysers, C., & Perrett, D. (2006). Demystifying social-cognition: A Hebbian perspective. *Trends in Cognitive Science*, *8*, 501–507.

Mundy, P., Block, J., Vaughan Van Hecke, A., Delgado, C., Venezia Parlade, M., & Pomares, Y. (2007). Individual differences and the development of infant joint attention. *Child Development*, *78*, 938–954.

ACKNOWLEDGMENT

The research and theory development reported in this paper were supported by NIH Grants HD 38052, and MH 071273, as well as the generous support of Marc Friedman and Marjorie Solomon for the Lisa Capps Endowment to the UC Davis Department of Psychiatry and M.I.N.D. Institute.

REFERENCES

Adamson, L., Bakeman, R., & Dekner, D. (2004). The development of symbol infused joint engagement. *Child Development, 75,* 1171–1187.

Adamson, L., McArthur, D., Markov, Y., Dunbar, B., & Bakeman, R. (2001). Autism and joint attention: Young children's responses to maternal bids. *Applied Developmental Psychology, 22,* 439–453.

American Psychiatric Association. (1980). *Diagnostic and statistical manual on mental disorders* (3rd ed.). Washington, DC: Author.

American Psychiatric Association. (1994). *Diagnostic and statistical manual on mental disorders* (4th ed.). Washington, DC: Author.

American Psychiatric Association. (2000). *Diagnostic and statistical manual on mental disorders* (4th ed., text revision). Washington, DC: Author.

Asperger, H. (1944). Die "Autistischen Psychopathen" im Kindesalter. *Archiv Für Psychiatrie und Nevenkrankheiten, 117,* 76–136.

Astafiev, S., Shulman, G., Stanley, C., Snyder, A., Essen, D., & Corbetta, M. (2003). Functional organization of human intraparietal and frontal cortex for attending, looking, and pointing. *Journal of Neuroscience, 23,* 4689–4699.

Atkinson, J., Hood, B., Wattam-Bell, J., & Braddick, O. (1992). Changes in infants' ability to switch attention in the first three months of life. *Perception, 21,* 643–653.

Bailey, A., Philips, W., & Rutter, M. (1996). Autism: Towards an integration of clinical, genetic, neuropsychological, and neurobiological perspectives. *Journal of Child Psychology and Psychiatry, 37,* 89–126.

Baldwin, D. (1995). Understanding the link between joint attention and language. In C. Moore & P. Dunham (Eds.), *Joint attentiozn: Its origins and role in development* (pp. 131–158). Hillsdale, NJ: Erlbaum.

Baron-Cohen, S. (1989). Joint attention deficits in autism: Towards a cognitive analysis. *Development and Psychopathology, 3,* 185–190.

Baron-Cohen, S., Leslie, A., & Frith, U. (1985). Does the autistic child have a theory of mind? *Cognition, 21,* 37–46.

Baron-Cohen, S. (1995). *Mindblindness.* Cambridge, MA: MIT Press.

Bates, E., Benigni, L., Bretherton, I., Camaioni, L., & Volterra, V. (1979). *The emergence of symbols: Cognition and communication in infancy.* New York: Academic Press.

Bayliss, A., Paul, M., Cannon, P., & Tipper, S. (2006). Gaze cuing and affective judgments of objects: I like what you look at. *Psychonomic Bulletin and Review, 13,* 1061–1066.

Bettelheim, B. (1959). Joey: A "mechanical boy." *Scientific American, 200,* 117–126.

Bigelow, A. (2003). The development of joint attention in blind infants. *Development and Psychopathology, 15,* 259–275.

Blakemore, S., & Frith, C. (2003). Self awareness and action. *Current Opinion in Neurobiology, 13, 219–224.*

Bono, M., Daley, T., & Sigman, M. (2004). Joint attention moderates the relation between intervention and language development in young children with autism. *Journal of Autism and Related Disorders, 34,* 495–505.

Bornstein, M., & Sigman, M. (1986). Continuity in mental development from infancy. *Child Development, 57,* 251–274.

Brenner, L., Turner, K., & Muller, R. (2007). Eye movement and visual search: Are there elementary abnormalities in autism? *Journal of Autism and Developmental Disorders, 37,* 1289–1309.

Bretherton, I. (1991). Intentional communication and the development of an understanding of mind. In D. Frye & C. Moore (Eds.), *Children's theories of mind: Mental states and social understanding* (pp. 49–75). Hillsdale, NJ: Erlbaum.

Brooks, R., & Meltzoff, A. (2002). The importance of eyes: How infants interpret adult looking behavior. *Developmental Psychology, 38,* 958–966.

Bruinsma, Y., Koegle, R., & Koegle, L. (2004). Joint attention and children with autism: A review of the literature. *Mental Retardation and Developmental Disabilities Research Reviews, 10,* 169–175.

Bruner, J. S. (1975). From communication to language: A psychological perspective. *Cognition, 3,* 255–287.

Bruner, J. S. (1995). From joint attention to the meeting of minds: An Introduction. In C. Moore & P. J. Dunham (Eds.). *Joint attention: Its origins and role in development* (pp. 1–14). Hillsdale, NJ: Erlbaum.

Butterworth, G., & Jarrett, N. (1991). What minds have in common is space: Spatial mechanisms in serving joint visual attention in infancy. *British Journal of Developmental Psychology, 9,* 55–72.

Canfield, R., & Kirkham, N. (2001). Infant cortical development and the prospective control of saccadic eye movements. *Infancy, 2,* 197–211.

Caplan, R., Chugani, H., Messa, C., Guthrie, D., Sigman, M., Traversay, J., et al. (1993). Hemispherectomy for early onset intractable seizures: Presurgical cerebral glucose metabolism and postsurgical nonverbal communication patterns. *Developmental Medicine and Child Neurology, 35,* 574–581.

Capps, L., Sigman, M., & Mundy, P. (1994). Attachment security in children with autism. *Development and Psychopathology, 6,* 249–262.

Cavanna, A., & Trimble, M. (2006). The precuneus: A review of its functional anatomy and behavioural correlates. *Brain, 10,* 1–20.

Charman, T. (2004). Why is joint attention a pivotal skill in autism? *Philosophical Transactions of the Royal Society of London, 358,* 315–324.

Charman, T., Baron-Cohen, S., Swettenham, J., Baird, G., Cox, A., & Drew, A. (2000). Testing joint attention, imitation, and play infancy precursors to language and theory of mind. *Cognitive Development, 15,* 481–498.

Cherkassky, V., Kana, R., Keller, T., & Just, M. (2006). Functional connectivity in the baseline resting state network in autism. *Neuroreport, 17,* 1687–1690.

Cicchetti, D. (1984). The emergence of developmental psychopathology. *Child Development, 55,* 1–7.

Claussen, A., Mundy, P., Malik, S., & Willoughby, J. (2002). Joint attention and disorganized attachment status in at risk infants. *Development and Psychopathology, 14,* 279–292.

Courchesne, E., & Pierce, K. (2005). Why the frontal cortex in autism might be talking only to itself: Local over-connectivity but long distance disconnection. *Current Opinion in Neurology, 15,* 225–230.

Curcio, F. (1978). Sensorimotor functioning and communication in mute autistic children. *Journal of Autism and Developmental Disorders, 8,* 281–292.

Dawson, G. (2008). Early behavioral intervention, brain plasticity, and the prevention of autism spectrum disorders. *Development and Psychopathology, 20,* 775–804.

Dawson, G., & McKissick, F. C. (1984). Self-recognition in autistic children. *Journal of Autism and Developmental Disorders, 14,* 383–394.

Dawson, G., Meltzoff, A., Osterling, J., Rinalidi, J., & Brown, E. (1998). Children with autism fail to orient to naturally occurring social stimuli. *Journal of Autism and Developmental Disorders, 28,* 479–485.

Dawson, G., Osterling, J., Rinaldi, J., Carver, L., & McPartland, J. (2001). Brief report: Recognition memory and stimulus-reward associations: Indirect support for the role of ventromedial prefrontal dysfunction in autism. *Journal of Autism and Developmental Disorders, 31,* 337–341.

Dawson, G., Toth, K., Abbott, R., Osterling, J., Munson, J., Estes, A. et al. (2004). Early social attention impairments in autism: Social orienting, joint attention, and attention in autism. *Developmental Psychology, 40,* 271–283.

Dawson, G., Webb, S., Schellenberg, G., Dager, S., Friedman, S., Ayland, E., et al. (2002). Defining the broader phenotype of autism: Genetic, brain, and behavioral perspectives. *Development and Psychopathology, 14,* 581–612.

Decety, J. & Grezes, J. (2006). The power of simulation: Imagining one's own and other's behavior. *Cognitive Brain Research, 1079,* 4–14.

Decety, J., & Sommerville, J. (2003). Shared representations between self and other: A social cognitive neuroscience view. *Trends in Cognitive Sciences, 7,* 527–533.

D'Entremont, B., Hains, S., & Muir, D. (1997). A demonstration of gaze following in 3- to 6- month-olds. *Infant Behavior and Development, 20,* 569–572.

Dierssen, M., & Ramakers, G. (2006). Dendritic pathology in mental retardation: From molecular genetics to neurobiology. *Genes, Brain, and Behavior, 5,* 48–60.

Dosenbach, N., Fair, D., Miezin, F., Cohen, A., Wenger, K., et al. (2007). Distinct brain networks for adaptive and stable task control in humans. *Proceedings of the National Academy of Sciences of the United States of America, 104,* 11073–11078.

Elman, J. (2005). Connectionist models of cognitive development: Where next? *Trends in Cognitive Science, 9,* 111–117.

Emery, N. (2000). The eyes have it: The neuroethology, function, and evolution of social gaze. *Neuroscience and Biobehavioral Reviews, 24,* 581–604.

Farroni, T. Massaccesi, S., & Francesca, S. (2002). Can the direction of gaze of another person shift the attention of a neonate? *Giornole-Italiano-di-Psicologia, 29,* 857–864.

Fein, D., Stevens, M., Dunn, M., Waterhouse, L., Allen, D., Rapin, I., & Feinstein, C. (1999). Subtypes of pervasive developmental disorders: Clinical characteristics. *Child Neuropsychology, 5,* 1–23.

Feldman, J., & Narayanan, S. (2004). Embodied meaning in a neural theory of language. *Brain and Language, 89,* 385–392.

Findlay, J., & Gilchrist, I. (2003). *Active vision: The psychology of looking and seeing.* New York: Oxford University Press.

Frieschen, A., Bayliss, A., & Tipper S., (2007). Gaze cueing of attention: Visual attention, social cognition, and individual differences. *Psychological Bulletin, 133,* 694–724.

Frith, U. (1989). *Autism: Explaining the enigma.* Oxford, UK: Basil Blackwell.

Fuster, J. (2006). The cognit: A network model of cortical representation. *International Journal of Psychophysiology, 60,* 125–132.

Geschwind, D., & Levitt, P. (2007). Autism spectrum disorders: developmental disconnection syndromes. *Current Opinion in Neurobiology, 17,* 103–111.

Gilbert, S., & Burgess, P. (2008). Social and nonsocial functions of rostral prefrontal cortex: Implications for education. *Mind, Brain, and Education, 2,* 148–156.

Gordon, R. (1986). Folk psychology as simulation. *Mind and Language, 1,* 158–171.

Greenough, W., Black, J., & Wallace, C. (1987). Experience and brain development. *Child Development, 58,* 539–559.

Griffith, E., Pennington, B., Wehner, E., & Rogers, S. (1999). Executive functions in young children with autism. *Child Development, 70,* 817–832.

Hebb, D. (1949). *The Organization of Behaviour.* New York: Wiley.

Henderson, H., Zahka, N., Kojkowski, N., Inge, A., Schwarz, C., Hileman, C., et al. (2009). Self referenced memory, social cognition, and symptom presentation in autism. *Journal of Child Psychology and Psychiatry, 50,* 853–861.

Henderson, L., Yoder, P., Yale, M., & McDuffie, A. (2002). Getting the point: Electrophysiological correlates of protodeclarative pointing. *International Journal of Developmental Neuroscience, 20,* 449–458.

Hobson, J., & Hobson, R. P. (2007). Identification: The missing link between joint attention and imitation. *Development and Psychopathology, 19,* 411–431.

Hobson, R. P., Lee, A., & Brown, R. (1999). Autism and congenital blindness. *Journal of Autism and Developmental Disorders, 12,* 45–66.

Holroyd, C., & Coles, M. (2002). The neural basis of human error processing: Reinforcement learning, dopamine, and the error related negativity. *Psychological Review, 109,* 679–709.

Hood, B., Willen, J., & Driver, J. (1998). Adult's eyes trigger shifts of visual attention in human infants. *Psychological Science, 9,* 131–134.

Horwitz, B., Rumsey, J., Grady, C., & Rapoport, S. (1998). The cerebral metabolic landscape in autism: Intercorrelations of regional glucose utilization. *Archives of Neurology, 45,* 749–755.

Howlin, P. (1978). The assessment of social behavior. In M. Rutter & E. Schopler (Eds.), *Autism: A reappraisal of concepts and treatment* (pp. 63–69). New York: Plenum.

Howlin, P. (1986). An overview of social behavior in autism. In E. Schopler & G. Mesibov (Eds.), *Social behavior in autism* (pp. 103–131). New York: Plenum.

Hunt, E. (1999). Intelligence and human resources: past, present and future. In P. Ackerman, P. Kyllonen, & R. Roberts (Eds) Learning and individual differences (pp. 3–30). Washington, D.C.: American Psychological Association.

Jellema, T., Baker, C., Wicker, B., & Perrett, D. (2000). Neural representation for the perception of intentionality of actions. *Brain and Cognition, 44,* 280–302.

Johnson, M. (1990). Cortical maturation and the development of visual attention in early infancy. *Journal of Cognitive Neuroscience, 2,* 81–95.

Johnson, M. (1995). The inhibition of automatic saccades in early infancy. *Developmental Psychobiology, 28,* 281–291.

Johnson, M., Griffin, R., Csibra, G., Halit, H., Farronni, T., et al. (2005). The emergence of the social brain network: Evidence from typical and atypical development. *Development and Psychopathology, 17,* 599–619.

Jones, E., Carr, E., & Feeley, K. (2006). Multiple effects of joint attention intervention for children with autism. *Behavior Modification, 30,* 782–834.

Just, M. A., Cherkassky, V., Keller, T., & Minshew, N. (2004). Cortical activation and synchronization during sentence comprehension in high functioning autism: evidence of underconnectivity. *Brain, 127*, 1811–1821.

Kanner, L. (1943). Autistic disorder of affective contact. *Nervous Child, 2*, 217–250.

Kanner, L. (1949). Problems of nosology and psychodynamics of early infantile autism. *American Journal of Orthopsychiatry, 19*, 416–426.

Karmel, B., Gardner, J., Swensen, L., Lennon, E., & London, E. (2008, March). Contrasts of medical and behavioral data from NICU infants suspect and non-suspect for autism spectrum disorder (ASD). Paper presented at the International Conference on Infant Studies, Vancouver.

Kasari, C., Freeman, S., & Paparella, T. (2006). Joint attention and symbolic play in young children with autism: a randomized controlled intervention study. *Journal of Child Psychology and Psychiatry, 47*, 611–620.

Kasari, C., Freeman, S., & Paparella, T. (2007, April). *The UCLA RCT on play and joint attention.* Paper presented at the Biennial Conference of the Society for Research on Child Development, Boston, MA.

Kasari, C., Sigman, M., Mundy, P., & Yirmiya, N. (1990). Affective sharing in the context of joint attention interactions of normal, autistic, and mentally retarded children. *Journal of Autism and Developmental Disorders, 20*, 87–100.

Keysers, C., & Perrett, D. (2006). Demystifying social-cognition: A Hebbian perspective. *Trends in Cognitive Science, 8*, 501–507.

Koegel, L., Carter, C., & Koegel, R. (2003). Teaching children with autism self-initiations as a pivotal response. *Topics in Language Disorders, 23*, 134–145.

Landry, R., & Bryson, S. (2004). Impaired disengagement of attention in young children with autism. *Journal of Child Psychology and Psychiatry, 45*, 115–1122.

Leslie, A., & Happe, F. (1989). Autism and ostensive communication: The relevance of meta-representation. *Development and Psychopathology, 1*, 205–212.

Lewis, J., & Elman, J. (2008). Growth-related neural organization and the autism phenotype: a test of the hypothesis that altered brain growth leads to altered connectivity. *Developmental Science, 11*, 135–155.

Lewis, M., & McGurk, H. (1972). Evaluation of intelligence in infants. *Science, 178*, 1174–1177.

Lewy, A., & Dawson, G. (1992). Social stimulation and joint attention in young autistic children. *Journal of Abnormal Child Psychology, 20*, 555–566.

Lord, C., Floody, H., Anderson, D., & Pickles, A. (2003, April). *Social engagement in very young children with autism: Differences across contexts.* The Society for Research in Child Development, Tampa, FL.

Lord, C., Lambrecht, L., Cook, E., Leventhal, B., DiLavore, P., et al. (2000). The Autism Diagnostic Observation Schedule-Generic: A standard measure of social communication deficits associated with the spectrum of autism. *Journal of Autism and Developmental Disorders, 30*, 205–223.

Loveland, K., & Landry, S. (1986). Joint attention and language in autism and developmental language delay. *Journal of Autism and Developmental Disorders, 16*, 335–349.

Mareschal, D., Johnson, M., Sirois, S., Spratling, S., Thomas, M., & Wasserman, G. (2007). *Neuroconstructivism I: How the brain constructs cognition.* New York: Oxford University Press.

Materna, S., Dicke, P., & Thern, P. (2008). Dissociable roles of the superior-temporal sulcus and the intraparietal sulcus in joint attention: A functional magnetic resonance imaging study. *Journal of Cognitive Neuroscience, 20*, 108–119.

McCleery, J. Allman, E., Carver, L., & Dobkins, K. (2007). Abnormal magnocellular pathway visual processing in infants at risk for autism. *Biological Psychiatry, 62*, 1007–1014.

McClelland, J., & Rogers, T. (2003). The parallel distributed processing approach to semantic cognition. *Nature Reviews: Neuroscience, 4*, 310–322.

Meltzoff, A., & Brooks, R. (2008). Self experiences a mechanism for learning about others: A training study in social cognition. *Developmental Psychology, 44*, 1–9.

Meltzoff, A. (2007). "Like me": a foundation for social cognition. *Developmental Science, 10*, 126–134.

Miller, E., & Cohen, J. (2001). An integrative theory of prefrontal cortex functioning. *Annual Review of Neurosciences, 24*, 167–2002.

Morales, M., Mundy, P., & Rojas, J. (1998). Following the direction of gaze and language development in 6-month olds. *Infant Behavior and Development, 21*, 373–377.

Morales, M., Mundy, P., Crowson, M., Neal, R., & Delgado, C. (2005). Individual differences in infant attention skills, joint attention, and emotion regulation behavior. *International Journal of Behavioral Development, 29*, 259–263.

Morrow, E., Yoo, S., Flavell, S., Kim, T., & Lin, Y. (2008). Identifying autism loci and genes by tracing recent shared ancestry. *Science, 32*, 218–225.

Munakata, Y., & McClelland, J. (2003). Connectionist models of development. *Developmental Science, 6*, 413–429.

Mundy, P. (1995). Joint attention and social-emotional approach behavior in children with autism. *Development and Psychopathology, 7*, 63–82.

Mundy, P. (2003). The neural basis of social impairments in autism: the role of the dorsal medial-frontal cortex and anterior cingulate system. *Journal of Child Psychology and Psychiatry and Allied Disciplines, 44*, 793–809.

Mundy, P. (in preparation). *Joint attention and our sharing minds.* New York: Guilford.

Mundy, P., Block, J., Vaughan Van Hecke, A., Delgado, C., Venezia Parlade, M., & Pomares, Y. (2007). Individual differences and the development of infant joint attention. *Child Development, 78*, 938–954.

Mundy, P., & Burnette, C. (2005). Joint attention and neurodevelopment. In F. Volkmar, A. Klin, & R. Paul (Eds.), *Handbook of autism and pervasive developmental disorders* (3rd ed., pp. 650–681). Hoboken, NJ: Wiley.

Mundy, P., Card, J., & Fox, N. (2000). EEG correlates of the development of infant joint attention skills. *Developmental Psychobiology, 36*, 325–338.

Mundy, P., & Crowson, M. (1997). Joint attention and early social communication: Implications for research on intervention with autism. *Journal of Autism and Developmental Disorders, 27*, 653–676.

Mundy, P., Fox, N., & Card, J. (2003). Joint attention, EEG coherence, and early vocabulary development. *Developmental Science, 6*, 48–54.

Mundy, P., & Hogan, A. (1994). Intersubjectivity, joint attention, and autistic developmental pathology. In D. Cicchetti & S. Toth (Eds.), *Rochester symposium of developmental psychopathology, Vol. 5*, A developmental perspective on the self and its disorders, (pp. 1–30). Hillsdale, NJ: Erlbaum.

Mundy, P., Kasari, C., & Sigman, M. (1992). Nonverbal communication, affective sharing, and intersubjectivity. *Infant Behavior and Development, 15*, 377–381.

Mundy, P., & Newell, L. (2007). Attention, joint attention, and social cognition. *Current Directions in Psychological Science, 16*, 269–274.

Mundy, P., & Sigman, M. (1989). Theoretical implications of joint attention deficits in autism. *Development and Psychopathology, 1*, 173–184.

Mundy, P., & Sigman, M. (2006). Joint attention, social competence, and developmental psychopathology. In D. Cicchetti and D. Cohen (Eds.), *Developmental psychopathology: Vol. 1. Theory and Methods* (2nd ed., pp. 293–332). Hoboken, NJ: Wiley.

Mundy, P., Sigman, M., & Kasari, C. (1993). The autistic person's theory of mind and early nonverbal joint attention deficits. In S. Baron-Cohen, H. Tager-Flusberg, D. Cohen, & F. Volkmar (Eds.), *Understanding other minds: Perspectives from autism* (pp. 181–201). Oxford, UK: Oxford University Press.

Mundy, P., Sigman, M., & Kasari, C. (1994). Joint attention, developmental level, and symptom presentation in children with autism. *Development and Psychopathology, 6*, 389–401.

Mundy, P., Sigman, M., Ungerer, J., & Sherman, T. (1986). Defining the social deficits of autism: The contribution of nonverbal communication measures. *Journal of Child Psychology and Psychiatry, 27*, 657–669.

Mundy, P., Sigman, M., Ungerer, J., & Sherman, T. (1987). Nonverbal communication and play correlates of language development in autistic children. *Journal of Autism and Developmental Disorders, 17*, 349–364.

Mundy, P., Sullivan, L., & Mastergeorge, A. (2009). A parallel and distributed processing model of joint attention and autism. *Autism Research, 2*, 2–21.

Mundy, P., & Vaughan Van Hecke, A. (2008). Neural Systems, Gaze Following, and the Development of Joint Attention. In C. Nelson & M. Luciana (Eds.), *Handbook of developmental cognitive neuroscience* (pp. 819–837). New York: Oxford University Press.

Murias, M., Webb, S., Greenson, J., & Dawson, G. (2007). Resting state cortical connectivity reflected in EEG coherence in individuals with autism. *Biological Psychiatry, 62*, 270–273.

Naber, F., Bakermans-Kranenburg, M., van Ijzendoorn, M., Dietz, C., Daalen E., et al., (2008). Joint attention development in toddlers with autism. *European Child and Adolescent Psychiatry, 17*, 143–152.

Nathan, M., Eilam, B., & Kim, S. (2007). To disagree we must all agree: How intersubjectivity structures and perpetuates discourse in a mathematics classroom. *Journal of Learning Sciences, 16*, 523–563.

Nation, K., & Penny, S. (2008). Sensitivity to eye gaze in autism: Is it normal? Is it automatic? Is it social? *Development and Psychopathology, 20*, 79–97.

Nichols, K. E., Fox, N., & Mundy, P. (2005). Joint attention, self-recognition, and neurocognitive functioning. *Infancy, 7*, 35–51.

Otten, L., Henson, R., Rugg, M. (2001). Depth of processing effects on neural correlates of memory encoding. *Brain, 125*, 399–412.

Ozonoff, S., Heung, K., Byrd, R., Hansen, R., & Hertz-Picciotto, I. (2008). The onset of Autism: Patterns of symptom emergence in the first years of life. *Autism Research, 1*, 320–328.

Piaget, J. (1952). *The origins of intelligence in children*. New York: Norton.

Pierce, K., & Schreibman, L. (1995). Increasing complex social behaviors in children with autism: Effects of peer implemented pivotal response training. *Journal of Applied Behavior Analysis, 28*, 285–295.

Posner, M., & Rothbart, M. (2007). Research on attention networks as a model for the integration of psychological science. *Annual Review of Psychology, 58*, 1–23.

Premack, D. & Woodruff, G. (1978) Does the chimpanzee have a theory of mind? *The Brain and Behavioral Sciences, 4*, 515–526.

Quartz, S. (1999). The Constructivist Brain. *Trends in Cognitive Science, 3*, 48–57.

Ramnani, N., Behrens, T., Penny, W., & Matthews, P. (2004). New approaches for exploring anatomical and functional connectivity in the human brain. *Biological Psychiatry, 56*, 613–619.

Rheingold, H. (1966). The development of social behavior in the human infant. *Monographs of the Society for Research in Child Development. 31*, 1–17.

Rimland, B. (1964). Infantile Autism: The Syndrome and Its Implications for a Neural Theory of Behavior. New York: Appleton-Century-Crofts.

Robson, K. (1967). The role of eye-to-eye contact in maternal infant attachment. *Journal of Child Psychology and Psychiatry, 8*, 13–25.

Rocha, M., Schriebman, L., & Stahmer, A. (2007). Effectiveness of training parents to teach joint attention with children with autism. *Journal of Early Intervention, 29*, 154–172.

Rogers, S. & Pennington, B. (1991). A theoretical approach to the deficits of infantile autism. *Development and Psychopathology, 3*, 137–162,

Royers, H., Van Oost, P., Bothutne, S. (1998). Immediate imitation and joint attention in young children with autism. *Development and Psychopathology, 10*, 441–450.

Rutherford, M., Young, G., Hepburn, S., & Rogers, S. (2008). A longitudinal study of pretend play in autism. *Journal of Autism and Developmental Disorders, 37*, 1024–1039.

Scaife, M., & Bruner, J. (1975). The capacity for joint visual attention in the infant. *Nature, 253*, 265–266.

Seibert, J. M., Hogan, A. E., & Mundy, P. C. (1982). Assessing interactional competencies: The Early Social-Communication Scales. *Infant Mental Health Journal, 3*, 244–258.

Shapiro, T., Sherman, M., Calamari, G., & Koch, D. (1987). Attachment in autism and other developmental disorders. *Journal of the American Academy of Child and Adolescent Psychiatry, 26*, 480–484.

Sheinkopf, S., Mundy, P., Claussen, A., & Willoughby, J. (2004). Infant joint attention skill and preschool behavioral outcomes in at-risk children. *Development and Psychopathology, 16*, 273–293.

Sigman, M., Cohen, S., & Bechwith, L. (1997). Why does infant attention predict intelligence? *Infant Behavior and Development, 20*, 133–140.

Sigman, M., & McGovern, C. (2005). Improvements in cognitive and language skills from preschool to adolescence in autism. *Journal of Autism and Developmental Disorders, 35*, 15–23.

Sigman, M., Mundy, P., Sherman, T., & Ungerer, J. (1986). Social interactions of autistic, mentally retarded, and normal children and their caregivers. *Journal of Child Psychology and Psychiatry, 27*, 647–656.

Sigman, M., & Ruskin, E. (1999). Continuity and change in the social competence of children with autism, Down syndrome, and developmental delays. *Monographs of the Society for Research in Child Development, 64* (1, Serial No. 256).

Sigman, M., & Ungerer, J. (1984). Attachment behaviors in autistic children. *Journal of Autism and Related Disabilities, 14*, 231–244.

Slaughter, V., & McConnell, D. (2003). Emergence of joint attention: Relationships between gaze following, social referencing, imitation, and naming in infancy. *Journal of Genetic Psychology, 164*, 54–71.

Smith, L., & Thelen, E. (2003). Development as a dynamic system. *Trends in Cognitive Science, 7*, 343–348.

Smith, L., & Ulvund, L. (2003). The role of joint attention in later development among preterm children: Linkages between early and middle childhood. *Social Development, 12*, 222–234.

Smith, V., Mirenda, P., & Zaidman-Zait, A. (2007). Predictors of expressive vocabulary growth in children with autism. *Journal of Speech, Language, and Hearing Research, 50*, 149–160.

Sroufe, A., & Rutter, M. (1984). The domain of developmental psychopathology. *Child Development, 55*, 17–29.

Stone, W., Coonrod, E., & Ousley, C. (1997). Brief report: Screening tool for autism in two year olds (STAT): Development and preliminary data. *Journal of Autism and Developmental Disorders, 30*, 607–612.

Striano, T., & Stahl, D. (2005). Sensitivity to triadic attention in early infancy. *Developmental Science, 8*, 333–343.

Striano, T., Chen, X., Cleveland, A., & Bradshaw, S. (2006). Joint attention social cues influence infant learning. *European Journal of Developmental Psychology, 3*, 289–299.

Striano, T., Reid, V., & Hoel, S. (2006). Neural mechanisms of joint attention in infancy. *European Journal of Neuroscience, 23*, 2819–2823.

Thurm, A., Lord, C., Lee, L., & Newschaffer, C. (2007). Predictors of language acquisition in preschool children with autism spectrum disorders. *Journal of Autism and Developmental Disorders, 37*, 1721–1734.

Tomasello, M. (1995). Joint attention as social-cognition. In C. Moore and P. Dunham (Eds.), *Joint attention: Its origins and role in development* (pp.103–130). Hillsdale, NJ: Lawrence Erlbaum.

Tomasello, M., & Farrar, M. J. (1986). Joint attention and early language. *Child Development, 57*, 1454–1463.

Tomasello, M., & Call, J. (1997). *Primate cognition*. New York: Oxford University Press.

Tomasello, M., Carpenter, M., Call, J., Behne, T., & Moll, H. (2005). Understanding sharing intentions: The origins of cultural cognition. *Brain and Behavior Sciences, 28*, 675–690.

Tomasello, M., Hare, B., Lehman, H., & Call, J. (2006). Reliance on head versus eyes in the gaze following of great apes and humans: the cooperative eyes hypothesis. *Journal of Human Evolution, 52*, 314–320.

Torkildsen, J., Thormodsen, R., Syvensen, G., Smith, L., & Lingren, M. (2008, March). *Brain correlates of nonverbal communicative comprehension in 20–24-month-olds*. Paper presented at the International Conference on Infant Studies, Vancouver, BC, Canada.

Toth, K., Munson, J., Meltzoff, A., & Dawson, G. (2006). Early predictors of communication development in young children with autism spectrum disorders: joint attention, imitation, and toy play. *Journal of Autism and Developmental Disorders, 36*, 993–1005.

Travis, L., & Sigman, M. (1998). Social deficits and interpersonal relationships in autism. *Mental Retardation and Developmental Disabilities Research Reviews, 4*, 65–72.

Ulvund, S., & Smith, L. (1996). The predictive validity of nonverbal communicative skills in infants with perinatal hazards. *Infant Behavior and Development, 19*, 441–449.

Venezia, M., Messinger, D., Thorp, D., & Mundy, P. (2004). Timing changes: The development of anticipatory smiling. *Infancy, 6*, 397–406.

Volkmar, F. R., Cohen, D. J., Bregman, J. D., Hooks, M. Y., & Stevenson, J. M. (1989). An examination of social typologies in autism. *Journal of the American Academy of Child and Adolescent Psychiatry, 28*, 82–86.

Vygotsky, L. (1962). *Thought and language*. Cambridge, MA: M.I.T. Press.

Werner, H., & Kaplan, B. (1963). *Symbol formation*. Oxford: Wiley.

Wetherby, A., Allen, L., Cleary, J., Kublin, K., & Goldstein, H. (2002). Validity and reliability of the communication and symbolic behavior scales developmental profile with very young children. *Journal of Speech, Language, and Hearing Research, 45*, 1202–1218.

Wetherby, A., & Prutting, C. (1984). Profiles of communicative and cognitive-social abilities in autistic children. *Journal of Speech and Hearing Research, 27*, 367–377.

Whalen, C., & Schreibman, L. (2006). The collateral effects of joint attention training on social initiations, positive affect, imitation, and spontaneous speech for young children with autism. *Journal of Autism and Developmental Disorders, 36*, 655–664.

Wickelgren, I. (2005). Autistic brains out of synch. *Science, 24*, 1856–1858.

Wicker, B., Fanlupt, P., Hubert, B., Tardif, C., Gepner, & Derulle, C. (2008). Abnormal cerebral effective connectivity during explicit emotional processing in adults with autism spectrum disorders. *Social-Cognitive Affective Neuroscience, 3*, 135–143.

Williams, J. (2008). Self-other relations in social development and autism: Multiple roles for mirror neurons and other brain bases. *Autism Research, 1*, 73–90.

Williams, J., Waiter, G., Perra, O., Perrett, D., Murray, A., & Whitten, A. (2005). An fMRI study of joint attention experience. *NeuroImage, 25*, 133–140.

Wimmer, H., & Perner, J. (1983). Beliefs about beliefs: Representation and constraint functions of wrong beliefs in young children. *Cognition, 13*, 102–128.

Wing, L., & Gould J. (1979). Severe impairments of social interaction and associated abnormalities in children: epidemiology and classification. *Journal of Autism and Developmental Disorders, 9*, 11–29.

Wing, L., & Potter, D. (2002). The epidemiology of autistic spectrum disorders: Is the prevalence rising? *Mental Retardation and Developmental Disabilities Research, 8*, 151–161.

World Health Organization (1992). *International statistical classification of diseases (ICD) and related health problems, Tenth Revision*. Geneva: World Health Organization.

Yoder, P., & Stone, W. (2006). Randomized comparison of two communication interventions for preschoolers with autism spectrum disorders. *Journal of Consulting and Clinical Psychology, 74*, 426–435.

Zelazo, P. D., Qu, L., Muller, U. (2005). Hot and cool aspects of executive function: Relations in early development. In W. Schneider, R. Schumann-Hegsteler & B. Sodian (eds.), *Young children's cognitive development: Interrelations among executive functioning, working memory, verbal ability and theory of mind* (pp. 71–93). Mahwah, NJ: Lawrence Erlbaum Associates.

Zwaigenbaum, L., Bryson, S., Rogers, T., Roberts, W., Brian, J., & Szatmari, P. (2005). Behavioral manifestations of autism in the first year of life. *International Journal of Neuroscience, 23*, 143152.

9 Language and Communication in Autism Spectrum Disorders

Helen Tager-Flusberg, Lisa Edelson, Rhiannon Luyster

Points of Interest

- Unique clinical features of language in ASD include stereotyped speech patterns, pronoun reversal, echolalia, and idiosyncratic words and phrases.
- There are universal impairments in pragmatic aspects of language: the use of language in social contexts, which are closely linked to deficits in theory of mind.
- Language skills, including articulation, vocabulary, and grammar, are quite heterogeneous. Different subtypes have been identified within the ASD population that may be associated with differences in etiology and neurobiological factors.
- Brain areas associated with language are often reduced in size in ASD. There are differences in brain organization, with less reliance on the left hemisphere for processing language and reduced connectivity between different brain regions that are critical for language perception and production.
- Atypical developmental trajectories within and across different domains of language are found. These may be grounded in infancy, and associated with impairments in prelinguistic developments in social engagement, gesture, imitation, and vocal productions.

When Leo Kanner (1943) first introduced his newly discovered syndrome, autistic disorder, impairments in language and communication were not listed among the core diagnostic features. The same held for Hans Asperger's (1944/1991) presentation of what is now referred to as Asperger's syndrome. Nevertheless, the detailed descriptions of the children by these pioneers included numerous examples of unusual speech and communication patterns that were evident in all their cases, and it is now recognized that, at least for autistic disorder, deficits in language and communication are defining criteria for diagnosis. Furthermore, most clinicians and researchers acknowledge the presence of aberrant communication among highly verbal people with Asperger's syndrome (Paul, Orlovski, Marcinko, & Volkmar, 2009; Tager-Flusberg, 2003).

By the end of the first year of life, most children are babbling, using gesture and vocalization to communicate with others, responding appropriately to words and simple phrases, and even speaking a few words that at least their parents understand. When these milestones are not met as expected, this can be an early warning sign that something may be awry. Indeed, surveys of parents whose children were later diagnosed with autism indicated that the most common causes for initial concern were delays in language and social-communicative abilities (Chawarska, Paul, Klin, Hannigen, Dichtel, & Volkmar, 2007; De Giacomo & Fombonne, 1998; Siklos & Kerns, 2007). Infants later diagnosed with autism spectrum disorder (ASD) show less joint attention behavior and produce fewer gestures and consonants (Landa, Holman, & Garrett-Mayer, 2007), all of which are key precursors to the acquisition of language (Luyster, Kadlec, Carter, & Tager-Flusberg, 2008). Given the critical role of language functioning in predicting outcomes in children with autism (Bennett et al., 2008; Billstedt, Gillberg, & Gillberg, 2007; Szatmari, Bryson, Boyle, Streiner, & Duku, 2003), there is now heightened interest in investigating this domain, with particular focus on targeting language and communication skills in early intervention programs (Dawson, 2008). In this chapter we provide an overview of the key features of atypical language and communication in ASD from a developmental perspective and then discuss some neurocognitive models that have been proposed as explanations for these impairments in ASD.

Defining the Language and Communication Impairment in ASD

Description of Language

Language is a multifaceted, hierarchically organized system that can be analyzed into specific components, each of which has expected patterns of development. The smallest linguistic unit is the *phoneme*, defined as a sound that can be discriminated from others within a language. For example, by changing a /b/ to a /p/, English has two words with different meanings, *bat* and *pat*. Phonology describes the way phonemes can be combined and used. It also encompasses nonspeech *suprasegmental* aspects, defined as those vocal patterns that are at a higher level than the phoneme, such as prosody, rhythm and melody that serve linguistic functions.

The smallest meaningful units of speech are called *morphemes*. These can be unbound, able to stand alone as lexical words (e.g., "walk"), or can be bound, requiring another morpheme for their usage, for example the past tense ending added to verbs -ed, or the negative morpheme un- that can be added to nouns, verbs, and other parts of speech. Morphemes can be combined to form words with new meanings, which in turn can be linked together to form sentences following predictable patterns of combinations, referred to as *syntax*. Within linguistics, morphology and syntax describe the rules governing each of these processes, and together form the *grammar* of a particular language. Sounds and rules cover the basic structure of a language, but these are all in service of expressing meaning, or *semantics*, in words and sentences. The semantic level of language connects most closely to world knowledge. For words, this includes both *intension*, the definition of a word, and *extension*, the range of exemplars to which that word refers. Sentential meaning is derived from the combination of words and grammatical rules.

Together, phonology, morphology, syntax, and semantics form our core linguistic knowledge. The domain of *pragmatics* refers to how context contributes to the interpretation of the meaning of language as it is used in social situations. It includes the functions served by utterances, also called *speech acts* (e.g., statements, requests), the rules of effective communication in discourse (e.g., conversation, narrative), and inferences about the intentions of the speaker, covering literal and nonliteral expressions (e.g., lies, sarcasm). Interpreting language in social contexts often goes beyond the spoken word, relying also on nonverbal cues such as gesture, facial and vocal expressions of affect, and body language.

Language is a highly complex system that is dependent on the interaction of multiple factors over the course of development. These include the input provided to the child that may vary in both quantitative and qualitative ways, and child-specific variables such as the motivation, cognitive, or neurological status of the individual. It is therefore not surprising that in ASD, core social and other neurocognitive impairments contribute significantly to the delays and deficits that are seen in the acquisition of language.

Deficits in Language and Communication

According to the *Diagnostic and Statistical Manual of Psychiatric Disorders* (DSM-IV-TR: American Psychiatric Association, 2000) autistic disorder is defined on the basis of at least one qualitative impairment in the domain of communicative abilities. These include: delay in, or total lack of, the development of spoken language; in individuals with adequate speech, marked impairment in the ability to initiate or sustain a conversation with others; stereotyped and repetitive use of language or idiosyncratic language; or lack of varied, spontaneous make-believe play or social imitative play appropriate to developmental level. These criteria are now viewed as reflecting distinct underlying mechanisms. Delays and deficits in language are associated with nonuniversal comorbid impairments in language processing (Bishop & Norbury, 2002; Rapin & Dunn, 2003, Tager-Flusberg, 2004); conversational problems reflect difficulties in theory of mind (Paul, Orlowski, Marcinko, & Volkmar, 2009; Tager-Flusberg, 2000); stereotyped language is an example of repetitive behavior (Bodfish, Symons, Parker, & Lewis, 2000; Gabriels, Cuccaro, Hill, Ivers, & Goldson, 2005); and the absence of play is a reflection of deficits in socialization and symbolic capacity (Naber et al., 2008).

Certain features of the language spoken by children with ASD are relatively unique and specific to this syndrome. One salient symptom of autism is the presence of odd or stereotyped speech patterns. Kanner (1943, 1946) noted several verbal rituals in his early observations of children with autism. Children with autism may quote scripts from favorite television shows or movies, engage in verbal rituals, or echo the speech of others (Rydell & Mirenda, 1994). Other children might use odd phrasing, perhaps incorporating vocabulary that is not age-appropriate (Ghaziuddin & Gerstein, 1996). Another striking feature of autistic children's use of language is their reversal of pronouns—referring to themselves as "you" and their conversational partner as "I." Although reversing personal pronouns is not unique to autism, it does occur more frequently in this group than in any other population (Lee, Hobson, & Chiat, 1994). Odd vocal patterns were noted in many early descriptions of autistic children's language both in echolalic and non-echolalic speech (Pronovost, Wakstein, & Wakstein, 1966). Kanner (1946) also commented on the autistic child's tendency to use words with special or unique meanings, not shared by others. The use of idiosyncratic lexical terms, or "neologisms," has been found even in higher functioning children and adults with autism (Volden & Lord, 1991).

Across the ASD population, including people with Asperger's syndrome, certain aspects of language are universally impaired. One example is the domain of pragmatics, as individuals with ASD have difficulty with the social aspects of language use, including turn-taking (Eales, 1993), conversational discourse (Paul et al., 2009; Tager-Flusberg & Anderson, 1991), processing contextually and socially appropriate comments (Eales, 1993; Loukusa et al., 2007), and understanding nonliteral language such as irony, sarcasm, and metaphor (Happé, 1995; MacKay & Shaw, 2004; Martin & McDonald, 2004). Another problem area is the appropriate use of prosody, or intonation patterns, when speaking. Individuals with ASD can produce grammatically correct sentences, but they may come across as sounding flat, robotic, or otherwise odd (Peppé, McCann, Gibbon, O'Hare, & Rutherford, 2007; Shriberg, Paul, McSweeny, Klin, Cohen, & Volkmar, 2001). They may also have trouble decoding the meaning of an utterance based on its stress patterns (Peppé et al., 2007) or miss affective content encoded in the voice (Korpilahti et al., 2007; Rutherford, Baron-Cohen, & Wheelwright, 2002).

In contrast to the universal nature of pragmatic deficits in autism spectrum disorders, other language skills vary on a broad continuum from intact linguistic abilities to failure to acquire any language (Diehl, Bennetto, Watson, Gunlogson, & McDonough, 2008; Kjelgaard & Tager-Flusberg, 2001; Lewis, Murdoch, & Woodyatt, 2007). One study of 9-year-old children found that, while a quarter of the children were able to speak fluently using complex sentences, another quarter were still effectively nonverbal (Anderson et al., 2007). Longitudinal studies suggest that variability in language skills increases with time, possibly due to mixed results of interventions (Charman, Taylor, Drew, Cockerill, Brown, & Baird, 2005).

Development of Language and Communication in ASD

Preverbal Period (0–12 Months)

From the moment they are born, infants come prepared to acquire language with a suite of mechanisms that include general learning systems, a bias toward attending to social stimuli in their environment including faces and voices, as well as domain-specific speech processing systems. Within a few short years they have mastered one of the most complex challenges they face, with seemingly little effort or explicit tuition. For children with ASD, the developmental pathway is affected, even before the acquisition of first words, and difficulties continue throughout childhood. Early in life most children communicate with their social partners. They begin to smile reciprocally, vocalize in response to other people, and engage in simple social routines. These early-appearing behaviors form an important foundation for the development of language. Children later diagnosed with ASD have been shown to have deficits in these reciprocal social communication skills within the first year of life. Early impairments have been noted in eye contact, imitation, social interest, shared positive affect, play skills, and joint engagement (Baranek, 1999; Bryson et al., 2007; Landa, Holman, & Garrett-Mayer, 2007; Zwaigenbaum et al., 2005).

Toward the end of the first year, infants typically exhibit a variety of communicative behaviors that are not usually seen in autism. These nonverbal communicative gestures express the same intentions for which words will be used in the coming months, such as requesting objects, rejecting offered actions, calling attention to objects or events, and commenting on their appearance. Gestural ability has been shown to be a strong predictor of later language in typically developing children (Rowe, Özçalişkan, & Goldin-Meadow, 2008; Watt et al., 2006) as well as children with developmental disabilities (Brady, Marquis, Fleming, & McLean, 2004) and ASD (Charman, Baron-Cohen, Swettenham, Baird, Drew, & Cox, 2003; Luyster, Kadlec, Carter, & Tager-Flusberg, 2008).

Parallel to these impairments in social communication during infancy, are early abnormalities in speech perception and preference. Typically developing children, when given a choice of listening to a nonspeech analog or infant-directed speech, consistently prefer to listen to the latter (Kuhl, 2004). This preference is viewed as instrumental in language development, in that the child is motivated to "tune in" to the sounds of their caregiver's speech. Infant-directed speech, moreover, is characterized by exaggerated phonetic and prosodic features that facilitate the emergence of early language. Young children identified with ASD do not show a preference for infant-directed speech, choosing instead to listen to the nonspeech analog (Kuhl, Coffey-Corina, Padden, & Dawson, 2005) or to other environmental sounds (Klin, 1991). There are important early language implications for these observations in ASD: A stronger preference for nonspeech sounds is associated with a greater degree of impairment in early expressive language (Kuhl et al., 2005).

By late infancy, these early disturbances in communication and speech development result in language differences for children later diagnosed with ASD. The majority show delays in the attainment of early milestones, in the production of babbling and first words, gestural communication, as well as in language comprehension (Colgan et al., 2006; Landa & Garrett-Mayer, 2006; Mitchell et al., 2006; Zwaigenbaum et al., 2005).

Early Language (12–30 Months)

The toddler years are characterized by language impairments for most children on the autism spectrum. Delays are evident in both receptive and expressive language. The receptive language deficits are quite striking and not usually seen in children with other language disorders, but these show up more on standardized testing than in parental reports of early language in ASD (Luyster et al., 2008), and are most likely related to the children's overall lack of social responsiveness.

Other atypical patterns may also be observed in the trajectory of language development. A significant minority (estimates usually ranging from about 15 to 40%) of children with ASD experience a loss (or *regression*) of verbal and nonverbal communication skills sometime in the second year of life (Goldberg et al., 2003; Hansen et al., 2008; Lord, Shulman, & DiLavore, 2004; Luyster et al., 2005). Several studies have found that these children show undetected symptoms of ASD within their first year of life, but they also often attain important early milestones in social and communication development. These early gains are followed by a loss of skill, usually some time between 16 and 21 months of age (Goldberg et al., 2003; Lord, Shulman et al., 2004; Luyster et al., 2005; Meilleur & Fombonne, 2009). Historically, these losses were defined strictly on the deterioration of language skills. Typically, children had mastered single words but not yet progressed to phrases, and then lost a substantial number of words during the regression. Recent conceptualizations of regression have included documentation of social-communication losses as well, particularly in the realm of social interest and reciprocity (Goldberg et al., 2003; Hansen et al., 2008; Luyster et al., 2005). Importantly, children who experience a regression generally do regain the lost skills, although the implications for later outcome remain unclear (Bernabei, Cerquiglini, Cortesi, & D'Ardia, 2007; Hansen et al., 2008; Ozonoff, Williams, & Landa, 2005; Richler et al., 2006; Werner, Dawson, Munson, & Osterling, 2005).

The close connection between language and social-communicative development is also evident when examining early predictors of language development in ASD. Just as the two domains are linked in the loss of skills, they are also linked in the mastery of skills. Language emergence is associated with a number of other symbolic and social-communicative skills. Joint attention (Adamson, Bakeman, Deckner, & Romski, 2009; Carpenter, Pennington, & Rogers, 2002; Charman et al., 2003; Dawson et al., 2004; Mundy, Sigman, & Kasari, 1990; Mundy, Sigman, Ungerer, & Sherman, 1987; Sigman & McGovern, 2005), imitation (Carpenter et al., 2002; Charman et al., 2003; Stone, Ousley, & Littleford 1997; Stone & Yoder 2001), gesture (Luyster et al., 2008), and play (Mundy et al., 1987; Sigman & McGovern, 2005) have all been found to be associated with language ability both concurrently and longitudinally. In addition to social-communicative factors, other child factors including general cognitive skills are highly correlated with language outcomes in children with ASD (Luyster et al., 2008; Thurm et al., 2007), and recent work by Sigman and her colleagues has highlighted the significance of parental responsiveness to the child's focus of attention and play as predictors of later language abilities, independent of the IQ or initial language skills of the child (Siller & Sigman, 2008).

During this period, children acquire a rich and varied vocabulary. By the age of 18 months, typically developing children show an exponential growth curve, learning several words each day. They do so by "fast-mapping" meaning to new words using a number of cues present in the environment. Several studies of children with ASD have found that they are able to exploit some, but not all, of these cues for learning the meanings of nouns, which may partially account for the slower growth and in certain cases, idiosyncratic meanings attached to some words. One cue that children with ASD are capable of using involves the inference that different objects are labeled with different words—the principle of "mutual exclusivity" (Preissler & Carey, 2005). In contrast, children with ASD are less able to use some social cues, such as the direction of a speaker's eye gaze (Baron-Cohen, Baldwin, & Crowson, 1997; Preissler & Carey, 2005), though if the objects are especially interesting and the speaker adds gestural or touch cues, children with ASD can rapidly learn the meanings of new words (McDuffie, Yoder, & Stone, 2006; Parish-Morris, Hennon, Hirsh-Pasek, Golinkoff, & Tager-Flusberg, 2007). At the heart of their difficulty is the use of combinations of social cues (eye gaze, facial expressions, etc.) that signal the speaker's intention, rather than simply a failure to attend to their social partner (Parish-Morris et al., 2007).

Caregivers also notice that their child's pragmatic uses of language are quite restricted. Whereas children with ASD may proficiently use language to meet their needs and wants (e.g., "More cookies"), they are less likely to use language in prosocial ways—directing someone's attention to an object or event of interest (e.g., "A doggie!"), or to use language to engage in a reciprocal exchange of thoughts or experiences (e.g., "Baby went night-night") (Loveland, Landry, Hughes, Hall, & McEvoy, 1988; Wetherby, Watt, Morgan, & Shumway, 2007). The speech acts missing among young children with ASD all involve social, rather than regulatory functions (Wetherby, 1986).

Later Language (30–48 Months)

During the preschool years, children acquire the morphosyntax of their language, continue to add new words to their vocabulary, and develop basic conversation skills. There are few longitudinal studies of grammatical development in ASD. Tager-Flusberg and her colleagues recruited a small group of preschoolers and found that they followed the same developmental path as typically developing children and children with Down syndrome (Tager-Flusberg et al., 1990). The children with autism and Down syndrome showed similar growth curves in the length of their utterances (MLU - Mean Length of Utterance), which is usually taken as a hallmark measure of grammatical development. In a follow-up study using the same language samples, Scarborough et al. (1991) compared the relationship between MLU and scores on a different index of grammatical development, which charts the emergence of a wide range of grammatical constructions: The IPSyn (Index of Productive Syntax). The main findings were that at higher MLU levels, MLU overestimated IPSyn scores for the children with ASD, because they used a narrower range of constructions and asked fewer questions, which accounts for a significant portion of the IPSyn score. These findings have been replicated in a cross-sectional study of preschoolers with ASD (Eigsti, Bennetto, & Dadlani, 2007).

Several studies of English-speaking children with ASD investigated the acquisition of grammatical morphology, using data from spontaneous speech samples. For example, Bartolucci, Pierce, & Streiner (1980) found that children with ASD were more likely to omit certain morphemes, particularly articles (*a, the*), auxiliary and copula verbs, past tense, third-person present tense, and present progressive. Tager-Flusberg (1989) also found that children with ASD were significantly less likely to mark past tense than were matched controls with Down syndrome. Similar findings were obtained on elicited production tasks of grammatical tense in children with lower overall levels of language (e.g., Bartolucci & Albers, 1974; Roberts, Rice, & Tager-Flusberg, 2004) as well as on grammaticality judgment tasks (Eigsti & Bennetto, 2009).

In comparison to grammatical development, lexical knowledge is an area of strength for children with ASD (Eigsti et al., 2007; Tager-Flusberg, Lord, & Paul, 2005). High-functioning children often score well on standardized vocabulary tests (Jarrold, Boucher, & Russell, 1997; Kjelgaard & Tager-Flusberg, 2001), they extend or generalize words they know to a broad range of exemplars, and their lexicons are organized in hierarchical semantic groups as in typically developing children (Boucher, 1988; Tager-Flusberg, 1985; Walenski, Mostofsky, Gidley-Larson, & Ullman, 2008). At the same time, certain classes of words may be underrepresented in the vocabularies of children with ASD. Tager-Flusberg (1992) found that children with ASD rarely used mental-state terms, particularly terms for cognitive states (e.g., *know, think, remember*) when conversing with their mothers. Other studies suggest that children with ASD have particular difficulties understanding social-emotional terms as measured on vocabulary tests such as the Peabody Picture Vocabulary Test (Eskes, Bryson, & McCormick, 1990; Hobson & Lee, 1989; van Lancker, Cornelius, & Needleman, 1991). Thus, while overall lexical knowledge is a relative strength in autism, acquiring words that map onto mental-state concepts may be specifically impaired.

In contrast to their typically developing peers who are successfully mastering early conversational skills, young children with ASD show difficulties in reciprocal and flexible dialogue. At a basic level, question-asking and question-answering may be diminished. More complex abilities such as introducing new topics of discussion, offering additional information, or providing clarification to ongoing discourse topics are also significantly affected (Capps, Kehres, & Sigman, 1998; Tager-Flusberg & Anderson, 1991). These difficulties emerge in early childhood (Hale & Tager-Flusberg, 2005a; Lord, Rutter, DiLavore, & Risi, 1999) and persist throughout the lifespan (de Villiers, Fine, Ginsberg, Vaccarella, & Szatmari, 2007; Dobbinson, Perkins, & Boucher, 1998; Volden, 2004).

Language in Older Children

For many children with ASD, the school years are characterized by continued growth of core language skills (Anderson et al., 2007). However, along with increased skills come new language difficulties that have particular impact on their social interactions with peers and to their academic success. Even for children who have optimal outcomes, losing their diagnosis of ASD and becoming fully integrated into academic settings, subtle impairments remain in the domains of semantics and pragmatics (Kelley, Paul, Fein, & Naigles, 2006).

Complex aspects of language prove to be particularly challenging for individuals with ASD. One example of this is language used in a nonliteral manner. Understanding irony (Kaland et al., 2005; Martin & McDonald, 2004), humor (Emerich, Creaghead, Grether, Murray, & Grasha, 2003; Lyons & Fitzgerald, 2004), idioms (Kerbel & Grunwell, 1998; Norbury, 2004), and metaphor (Happé, 1995) is often impaired in children with ASD, because they tend to interpret words or utterances in a literal or concrete way, rather than the intended meaning, which is often dependent on the context or delivery of the language through a combination of verbal and nonverbal signals.

This difficulty of interpreting intended meaning is especially salient in conversational discourse (Mitchell, Saltmarsh, & Russell, 1997) and reflects the fact that pragmatic deficits in language are more often found in unstructured social contexts than in structured tasks. These deficits, which are found in both Asperger's syndrome and high-functioning autism, take different forms including overly formal or pedantic speech, lack of reciprocal exchanges, problems with topic management, or handling breakdowns and repairs in conversation (Paul et al., 2009). But not all aspects of social language usage are impaired in ASD. For example, older children are quite able at judging and producing requests at different levels of politeness, depending on the status of their discourse partner (Volden & Sorenson, 2009). Sparing of these kinds of skills may be related to their intact knowledge of social stereotypes such as gender and race (Hirschfeld, Bartmess, White, & Frith, 2007).

Another area of deficit is in the production of narratives, which has implications for their ability to perform well in language arts and social studies classes in school. Children with ASD generally produce less coherent and complex stories (Diehl, Bennetto, & Young, 2006; Losh & Capps, 2003), they tend not to be able to flexibly use different referring expressions such as pronouns (Arnold, Bennetto, & Diehl, 2009), they are less likely to take the perspective of another person in a story (Garcia-Perez, Hobson, & Lee, 2008), and they often ignore the motivations of characters or causal connections in a plot line (Tager-Flusberg, 1995). Their personal narratives also tend to focus more on facts than in providing a meaningful interpretation of autobiographical events (Goldman, 2008).

Processing nonverbal aspects of communication continues to be an area of significant impairment for children and adults with ASD, which may partially explain their strong preference for communicating with others through the Internet. One example is in the use of prosody. Difficulties arise both in using prosody to clarify linguistic ambiguity (Diehl, Bennetto, Watson, Gunlogson, & McDonough, 2008) and in understanding its social significance (see McCann & Peppé, 2003,for a review; McCann, Peppé, Gibbon, O'Hare, & Rutherford, 2007), though these deficits in prosody are more apparent at the level of sentences rather than single words (Järvinen-Pasley, Peppé, King-Smith, & Heaton, 2008). Other nonlinguistic communicative cues, such as gestures, continue to show impairment through childhood into adolescence and beyond. For instance, individuals with ASD are less likely to use "beat gestures" while speaking (Lord et al., 1999), employ nonverbal cues of reciprocity such as nodding their head when a conversational partner is speaking (Garcia-Perez, Lee, & Hobson, 2007), respond to such cues in their conversational partner, or modulate eye contact (Paul et al., 2009). Thus, it is clear that even when structural aspects of language are acquired, people with ASD continue to experience significant problems in communicating effectively and appropriately in everyday social contexts.

Neurocognitive Models of Language and Communication in ASD

Variability in the Language Phenotypes

A hallmark feature of ASD is heterogeneity in etiology, neurobiological substrate, behavioral characteristics, developmental trajectory, and comorbidity. In an effort to distill some of the essential features that have both clinical and theoretical relevance, our review of the language characteristics and their development in ASD glosses over the fundamental variability that is seen in every study. Within language, heterogeneity takes on particular significance, in part because language itself is multifaceted, composed of intersecting systems of knowledge—sounds, words, morphosyntax, meaning—serving a full range of social-communicative functions. In ASD, any one or all of these systems can be affected. In recent years, considerable effort has been made to explore this heterogeneity to advance understanding about the mechanisms that may underlie the different phenotypes that are observed.

At a superficial level, three primary subtypes can be distinguished. At one end are the verbally fluent individuals who acquire a full and rich system of linguistic knowledge at the structural level (phonology, morphosyntax, vocabulary) that is indistinguishable from nonautistic individuals. For this group, language deficits are primarily limited to the domain of pragmatics. Interestingly, studies have shown that some proportion of older children who fit within this group experienced early delays in language, however once they reached initial milestones, the rate of acquisition was normal or even accelerated and by the end of the preschool period they were indistinguishable from children who experienced no delays in the early timing of language development (Bennett et al., 2008). At the other end are nonverbal individuals who fail to acquire the ability to speak (or communicate via other systems) beyond a rudimentary level of single words or short phrases. In general, the prognosis for acquiring useful speech is very poor for children who have not done so by age 5, however there are a number of cases in the literature of children who do achieve some success after this age if they continue to receive highly intensive behavioral treatment programs (Pickett, Pullara, O'Grady, & Gordon, 2009). The majority of children fall into a third group: They acquire language, albeit later, at a slower rate, and without fully catching up to age expectations. As more children with ASD receive early diagnoses and interventions, the proportion of children who acquire some degree of functional spoken language is increasing (Tager-Flusberg et al., 2005).

A diagnosis of ASD, even classic autism, does not require that a child has impaired language; conversational impairments are sufficient to meet criteria. Thus, the children who have linguistic deficits may be viewed as forming subtypes within the spectrum. Several researchers have proposed that children who are verbal but with impairments in phonology and morphosyntax (in addition to pragmatics) have a comorbid disorder of specific language impairment (SLI), because of the parallel deficits that are seen in these children (e.g., Bishop & Norbury, 2002; Tager-Flusberg, 2006). Clinical characteristics of SLI include lower overall language scores on standardized tests, impaired phonological processing as measured by repetition of nonsense words, and for English-speakers, morphosyntactic problems, particularly in the omission of tense markers and other grammatical features (Tager-Flusberg & Cooper, 1999). Like ASD, SLI is a heterogeneous disorder. For example, some children with SLI have articulation deficits, others do not; some have both receptive and expressive impairments, others only expressive; some have comorbid dyslexia, others do not (Tomblin & Zhang, 1999). A range of similar language deficits are seen in children with ASD (Rapin, Dunn, Allen, Stevens, & Fein, 2009; Tager-Flusberg, 2006; Tager-Flusberg et al. 2005; Whitehouse, Barry, & Bishop, 2008), though the added triad of autism-specific impairments contributes to how these are uniquely expressed in ASD on both structured tasks and in everyday language use. There is very little language research on the children at the nonverbal end of the continuum. These children are likely to have more severe autism-specific impairments, are more likely to be intellectually disabled (Luyster et al., 2008), and there is evidence that oral-motor impairments may explain why some children with ASD fail to acquire spoken language (Gernsbacher, Sauer, Geye, Schweigert, & Goldsmith, 2008). These children may have a comorbid dyspraxia, though this is a poorly understood developmental language disorder.

Given these different subtypes (or comorbidities), it is clear that no single etiology, neurological deficit, or theoretical framework can be developed to explain the language phenotypes associated with ASD. Instead, in recent years, researchers have attempted to exploit the variability in language to parse the population for genetic (e.g., Alarcon, Cantor, Liu, Gilliam, & Geschwind, 2002; Alarcon et al., 2008; Bradford et al., 2001), neurobiological (de Fossé et al., 2004), and cognitive (e.g., Norbury, Brock, Cragg, Einav, Griffiths, & Nation, 2009) studies with considerable success.

Neurobiology of Language in ASD

The classic language network is composed of Broca's area (regions in the inferior frontal gyrus) and Wernicke's area (regions in the posterior superior temporal gyrus and planum temporale). These areas are connected by a series of dorsal and ventral pathways, the most significant of which is the arcuate fasciculus, and they are supplemented by other cortical and subcortical regions, including the basal ganglia, thalamus, and cerebellum (for a recent review, see Friederici, 2009). Typically, portions of Broca's and Wernicke's areas (particularly in the pars triangularis and planum temporale) are asymmetric, larger in the left hemisphere; and functionally, the left hemisphere assumes a primary role in processing phonological, semantic, and grammatical aspects of language, although findings across studies using different methods are not consistent, and there is greater variability among females and non–right handed individuals (Keller, Crow, Foundas, Amunts, & Roberts, 2009; Wallentin, 2009). Developmental studies have found that with age, there is continued developmental growth in the structure and asymmetry of language-related cortices into early adulthood (Gogtay, et al., 2004; Sowell, Thompson, Leonard, Welcome, Kan, & Toga, 2004).

In children with developmental language disorders such as SLI and dyslexia, both structural and functional differences have been found in studies using magnetic resonance imaging. In general, these children have reduced volumes in the primary cortical language areas, reduced asymmetry in the frontal areas, and are functionally less left-lateralized (Tager-Flusberg, Lindgren, & Mody, 2008). In ASD, similar atypical structural patterns have been found, although findings across different studies vary, depending on the methods used (e.g., manual or automatic) and the age and characteristics of the participants. The majority of studies, which primarily have included only boys with ASD, report reduced volume of the pars triangularis and posterior language regions (e.g., McAlonan et al., 2005; Rojas, Camou, Reite, & Rogers, 2005; but see also, Knaus et al., 2009). Interestingly, a recent study suggested that reduced volumes in these regions may be associated with later onset of language (McAlonan et al., 2008). Reductions in left hemisphere asymmetry of frontal language regions has also been found in several studies and is associated with greater impairment in language abilities, or comorbid SLI (Herbert et al., 2002; Herbert et al., 2005; de Fossé et al., 2004). Several studies have found exaggerated left hemisphere asymmetry in the planum temporale, again associated with comorbid SLI (Herbert et al., 2002; de Fossé et al., 2004; but for different findings see Knaus et al., 2009; Rojas et al., 2005). Only one MRI study, conducted by Munson and his colleagues (Munson et al., 2006) included very young children with ASD to explore the relationship between brain structure and developmental trajectories in communication development, as measured by the Vineland Adaptive Behavior Scales (Sparrow, Balla, & Cicchetti, 1984). Interestingly, they found a significant inverse relationship between the size of the right amygdala and growth in communication scores, which may be taken as evidence for the role of atypical development of subcortical structures associated with social functioning in the acquisition of language use in young children with ASD.

Functional imaging studies of language have found atypical patterns of activation in children and adults with ASD. Several studies have found reduced activation in frontal areas in adults with ASD, but increased activation in posterior regions, on both syntactic (Just et al., 2004) and semantic processing tasks (Harris et al., 2006). However, this pattern was not found in adolescents with ASD, who demonstrated increased activation, relative to controls in both frontal and posterior language areas (Knaus et al., 2008). The most consistent findings across studies is reduced asymmetry of language processing, especially in Broca's area, and reduced correlations in activation patterns across language regions (Just et al., 2004; Harris et al., 2006; Kleinhans et al., 2008; Knaus et al., 2008; Muller et al., 1999), which is consistent with other work suggesting impaired connectivity in the brains of people with ASD (e.g., Courchesne & Pierce, 2005). A recent study found atypical activation to speech in toddlers with ASD (Redcay & Courchesne, 2008). In contrast to the control children, who activated the left hemisphere language network, toddlers with ASD primarily activated corresponding regions in the right hemisphere, confirming that these atypical patterns begin early in development. It is not known, however, the extent to which these differences in functional organization of language in ASD are related to fundamental differences in neuroanatomy that are present at birth, to behavioral language skills, or to compensatory mechanisms. Finally, it is surprising to note that, to date, there are no published studies of the neural processing of pragmatic aspects of language in individuals with ASD.

Mechanisms Associated with Language and Communication Impairments in ASD

Most researchers argue that more than one set of mechanisms is needed to explain the full range of language impairments that is seen across the different language phenotypes in ASD. Given the complexity of the language system itself, as well as its interactions with perceptual (visual, auditory), motor (articulation), memory, social, executive, and general cognitive capacities we are still many years from having anything close to a complete theoretical account that is grounded in a dynamic, developmental framework. Still, some progress has been made in specifying the neurocognitive mechanisms associated with the universal pragmatic impairments as well as with the linguistic deficits that characterize some portion of the population.

Pragmatic aspects of language typically entail an appreciation of the intentions, knowledge, and other mental states of a discourse partner (Sperber & Wilson, 1986). Such mental state understanding, or "theory of mind" skills, are important for the interpretation of intended meaning, nonliteral language, and conversational and narrative skills, all of which are impaired in individuals with ASD. According to this view, the pragmatic deficits in ASD are explained on the basis of deficits in theory of mind, and thus, are closely linked to aspects of the core social symptoms (Baron-Cohen, Tager-Flusberg, & Cohen, 2000). Studies have found significant relationships between performance on theory of mind tasks and conversational impairments (Hale & Tager-Flusberg, 2005b) as well as in understanding nonliteral meaning (Happé, 1993, 1994) that are independent of general cognitive and language skills. Thus, according to this model, impairments in theory of mind mechanisms underlie the pragmatic language problems that are found across most individuals with ASD (Paul et al., 2009; Tager-Flusberg, 2000).

There is less agreement on what might underlie the deficits in other language skills. At a neurobiological level, the evidence suggests that these deficits are associated with altered asymmetry, structural and functional impairments in inferior frontal regions in the left hemisphere, and reduced connectivity between frontal and temporal language regions.

These atypical neuroanatomical and functional patterns are also found in individuals with other developmental and acquired language disorders, and one theory that has been proposed as a unifying explanation for phonological and grammatical impairments across a range of disorders, including ASD, is the procedural deficit hypothesis, which claims that these impairments are related to neurocognitive abnormalities in the procedural memory system (Ullman, 2001; Walenski, Tager-Flusberg, & Ullman, 2006). The procedural memory system is involved in the learning and maintenance of cognitive and motor skills, particularly those that involve sequences, such as rule-governed combinations in phonology and grammar. This system is based on networks of interconnected brain regions, particularly in the left hemisphere, including frontal-basal ganglia, and frontal-cerebellar circuits (Ullman, 2001). The procedural deficit hypothesis proposes that the language impairments in ASD (and related disorders such as SLI; Ullman & Pierpont, 2005) are rooted in this neurocognitive system, and are thus associated with impairments in other functions (e.g., temporal processing, motor skills) that also depend on this network of structures. Because of the complexity of the neural bases of the procedural memory system, it is predicted that there will be significant individual variation in the specific nature and extent of the language (and other) impairments, that reflect the specific structures and connections that have been affected, as well as the compensatory systems that may be activated, such as the declarative memory system (Walenski et al., 2006). The nature of the deficits found among language-impaired individuals with ASD is consistent with this theoretical model, however, no studies have yet related language deficits to structural or functional abnormalities in the basal ganglia or cerebellum, both of which are central components of the procedural memory system.

Conclusions

Considerable progress has been made in advancing knowledge about the development and neurobiological bases of language and communication in ASD. For the majority of children with ASD, impairments in this domain involve fundamental alterations in the onset and rate of acquisition of major language milestones (Tager-Flusberg et al., 2005). Hallmark characteristics of the profile of language development involve dissociations in the developmental trajectory for different components of language. One example is the dissociation seen between form and function—or between structural and pragmatic aspects of language development (Tager-Flusberg, 1994). Other examples include relative dissociations between expressive and receptive processing systems and between lexical and phonological development (see Paul, Chawarska, Cicchetti, & Volkmar, 2008). These dissociations reveal differences in developmental timing that influence the interactions among language components, and between these components and other aspects of cognition.

Atypical developmental trajectories within and across domains of language and social cognition are grounded in atypical patterns of brain organization for language and associated functions, particularly hemispheric specializations that are typically present early in development (Flagg, Cardy, Roberts, & Roberts, 2005; Kuhl et al., 2005; Redcay & Courchesne, 2008). Infants are born biased to attend to human speech. Toward the end of the first year, infants' speech processing skills are rapidly changing as they are molded to their native language, resulting in an increase in cortical specialization for language (Kuhl, 2007). All experience is now deeply embedded in a social and cultural environment; infants no longer discriminate speech sounds that are not part of their everyday world. These developmental changes, which reflect advances in linguistic development, are crucially dependent on socially grounded experience (Kuhl, 2007). Indeed, change in speech perception and early language development are dependent on interactions with people, referred to as the "social gating" model (Kuhl, 2007). One possibility is that these early stages of development, between 6 and 12 months, mark the beginning of the atypical developmental pathways that can lead to ASD, including core language and communicative impairments. Failures to attend fully to socially mediated learning opportunities for language acquisition may have profound developmental consequences (Meltzoff, Kuhl, Movellan, & Sejnowski, 2009). This view is consistent with the developmental timing of changes in head size in some infants with ASD as reported in retrospective studies (e.g., Redcay & Courchesne, 2005) as well as in the genetic mechanisms relating to synaptic plasticity that have been implicated in recent studies (cf. Morrow et al., 2008). Even during this early period, there is likely to be heterogeneity, both in the mechanisms crucial for responding to the social environment, and in the mechanisms crucial for linguistic development (including perceptual, motor, and learning systems). Future research will investigate these very early developmental patterns using prospective longitudinal approaches (cf. Zwaigenbaum et al., 2007). In turn, these studies may shed light on the mechanisms that underlie the profound impairments seen in some children with ASD who fail to acquire any spoken language.

This review of the research on language and communicative impairments in ASD has a number of important clinical implications. First, it is now clear based on several studies that a history of delay in early language is not nearly as important from a diagnostic perspective as is a comprehensive evaluation of current language skills (e.g., Bennett et al., 2008). Second, we know that early intervention can jumpstart and significantly accelerate the rate of language acquisition in young children with ASD (Dawson, 2008). Finally, we should also be optimistic that since language skills continue to develop in older children (e.g., vocabulary, discourse and narrative abilities) and the neural substrates for language do not reach full maturity until the end of adolescence, ongoing treatment may also lead to continued growth in children with ASD throughout this period.

Challenges and Future Directions

- Little is known about the neurocognitive mechanisms associated with the failure to acquire language in some children with ASD. Methodological challenges of obtaining valid behavioral data and in acquiring measures of brain structure and function have slowed research into these important issues.
- Given the pervasive and lifelong impairments in pragmatic aspects of language that are universally found in individuals with ASD, an important priority for future research will be advancing our understanding of the neurobiology of these deficits.
- Evidence-based treatments for older children and adults with ASD, including interventions for pragmatic aspects of language and nonverbal communication skills need to be developed and implemented in the community.

SUGGESTED READINGS

Bishop, D. V. M. (2009). Genes, cognition, and communication: Insights from neurodevelopmental disorders. *Annals of the New York Academy of Sciences, 1156*, 1–18.

Kuhl, P. (2004). Early language acquisition: Cracking the speech code. *Nature Reviews Neuroscience, 5*, 831–843.

Tager-Flusberg, H. (2000). Language and understanding minds: Connections in autism. In S. Baron-Cohen, H. Tager-Flusberg, & D. J. Cohen (Eds.), *Understanding other minds: Perspectives from developmental cognitive neuroscience* (2nd ed., pp. 124–149). Oxford: Oxford University Press.

ACKNOWLEDGMENTS

Preparation of this chapter was supported by grants from Autism Speaks and the National Institute on Deafness and Other Communication Disorders (R21 DC 08637; RO1 DC 10290).

REFERENCES

Adamson, L., Bakeman, R., Deckner, D., & Romski, M. (2009). Joint engagement and the emergence of language in children with autism and Down syndrome. *Journal of Autism and Developmental Disorders, 39*, 84–96.

Alarcon, M., Abrahams, B. S., Stone, J. L., Duvall, J. A., Perederiy, J. V., Bomar, J. M., et al. (2008). Linkage, association, and gene-expression analyses identify CNTNAP2 as an autism-susceptibility gene. *American Journal of Human Genetics, 82*, 150–159.

Alarcon, M., Cantor, R. M., Liu, J., Gilliam, T. C., & Geschwind, D. H. (2002). Evidence for a language quantitative trait locus on chromosome 7q in multiplex autism families. *American Journal of Human Genetics, 70*, 60–71.

American Psychiatric Association. (2000). *Diagnostic and statistical manual of mental disorders* (4th ed., text rev.; DSM-IV-TR). Washington, DC: Author.

Anderson, D. K., Lord, C., Risi, S., Shulman, C., Welch, K., DiLavore, P. S., et al. (2007). Patterns of growth in verbal abilities among children with autism spectrum disorder. *Journal of Consulting and Clinical Psychology, 75*, 594–604.

Arnold, J., Bennetto, L., & Diehl, J. (2009). Reference production in young speakers with and without autism: Effects of discourse status and processing constraints. *Cognition, 110*, 131–146.

Asperger, H. (1944/1991). "Autistic psychopathy" in childhood. In U. Frith (Ed.), *Autism and Asperger syndrome* (pp. 37–91). Cambridge: Cambridge University Press.

Baranek, G. T. (1999). Autism during infancy: A retrospective video analysis of sensory-motor and social behaviors at 9–12 months of age. *Journal of Autism and Developmental Disorders, 29*, 213–224.

Baron-Cohen, S., Baldwin, D., & Crowson, M. (1997). Do children with autism use the speaker's direction of gaze strategy to crack the code of language? *Child Development, 68*, 48–57.

Baron-Cohen, S., Tager-Flusberg, H., & Cohen, D. J. (2000). *Understanding other minds: Perspectives from developmental cognitive neuroscience* (2nd ed.). Oxford: Oxford University Press.

Bartolucci, G., & Albers, R. J. (1974). Deictic categories in the language of autistic children. *Journal of Autism and Childhood Schizophrenia, 4*, 131–141.

Bartolucci, G., Pierce, S. J., & Streiner, D. (1980). Cross-sectional studies of grammatical morphemes in autistic and mentally retarded children. *Journal of Autism and Developmental Disorders, 10*, 39–50.

Bennett, T., Szatmari, P., Bryson, S., Volden, J., Zwaigenbaum, L., Vaccarella, L., et al. (2008). Differentiating autism and Asperger syndrome on the basis of language delay or impairment. *Journal of Autism and Developmental Disorders, 38*, 616–625.

Bernabei, P., Cerquiglini, A., Cortesi, F., & D'Ardia, C. (2007). Regression versus no regression in the autistic disorder: Developmental trajectories. *Journal of Autism and Developmental Disorders, 37*, 580–588.

Billstedt, E., Gillberg, I. C., & Gillberg, C. (2007). Autism in adults: symptom patterns and early childhood predictors; Use of the DISCO in a community sample followed from childhood. *Journal of Child Psychology and Psychiatry, 48*, 1102–1110.

Bishop, D. V. M., & Norbury, C. (2002). Exploring the borderlands of autistic disorder and specific language impairment: A study using standardized diagnostic instruments. *Journal of Child Psychology and Psychiatry, 43*, 917–929.

Bodfish, J., Symons, F., Parker, D., & Lewis, M. (2000). Varieties of repetitive behavior in autism: Comparisons to mental retardation. *Journal of Autism and Developmental Disorders, 30*, 237–243.

Boucher, J. (1988). Word fluency in high-functioning autistic children. *Journal of Autism and Developmental Disorders, 18*, 637–645.

Bradford, Y., Haines, J., Hutcheson, H., Gardiner, M., Braun, T., Sheffield, V., et al. (2001). Incorporating language phenotypes strengthens evidence of linkage to autism. *American Journal of Medical Genetics*, *105*, 539–547.

Brady, N. C., Marquis, J., Fleming, K., & McLean, L. (2004). Prelinguistic predictors of language growth in children with developmental disabilities. *Journal of Speech, Language, and Hearing Research*, *47*, 663–677.

Bryson, S. E., Zwaigenbaum, L., Brian, J., Roberts, W., Szatmari, P., Rombough, V., et al. (2007). A prospective case series of high-risk infants who developed autism. *Journal of Autism and Developmental Disorders*, *37*, 12–24.

Capps, L., Kehres, J., & Sigman, M. (1998). Conversational abilities among children with autism and children with developmental delays. *Autism*, *2*, 325–344.

Carpenter, M., Pennington, B., & Rogers, S. (2002). Interrelations among social-cognitive skills in young children with autism. *Journal of Autism and Developmental Disorders*, *32*, 91–106.

Charman, T., Baron-Cohen, S., Swettenham, J., Baird, G., Drew, A., & Cox, A. (2003). Predicting language outcome in infants with autism and pervasive developmental disorder. *International Journal of Language and Communication Disorders*, *38*, 265–285.

Charman, T., Taylor, E., Drew, A., Cockerill, H., Brown, J., & Baird, G. (2005). Outcome at 7 years of children diagnosed with autism at age 2: predictive validity of assessments conducted at 2 and 3 years of age and patterns of symptom change over time. *Journal of Child Psychology and Psychiatry*, *46*, 500–513.

Chawarska, K., Paul, R., Klin, A., Hannigen, S., Dichtel, L. E., & Volkmar, F. (2007). Parental recognition of developmental problems in toddlers with autism spectrum disorders. *Journal of Autism and Developmental Disorders*, *37*, 62–72.

Colgan, S. E., Lanter, E., McComish, C., Watson, L. R., Crais, E. R., & Baranek, G. T. (2006). Analysis of social interaction gestures in infants with autism. *Child Neuropsychology*, *12*, 307–319.

Courchesne, E., & Pierce, K. (2005). Why the frontal cortex in autism might be talking only to itself: local over-connectivity but long-distance disconnection. *Current Opinion in Neurobiology*, *15*, 225–230.

Dawson, G. (2008). Early behavioral intervention, brain plasticity, and the prevention of autism spectrum disorder. *Development and Psychopathology*, *20*, 775–803.

Dawson, G., Toth, K., Abbott, R., Osterling, J., Munson, J., Estes, A., et al. (2004). Early social attention impairments in autism: Social orienting, joint attention, and attention to distress. *Developmental Psychology*, *40*, 271–283.

de Fossé, L., Hodge, S. M., Makris, N., Kennedy, D. N., Caviness, V. S., Jr., McGrath, L., et al. (2004). Language-association cortex asymmetry in autism and specific language impairment. *Annals of Neurology*, *56*, 757–766.

de Giacomo, A., & Fombonne, E. (1998). Parental recognition of developmental abnormalities in autism. *European Child and Adolescent Psychiatry*, *7*, 131–136.

de Villiers, J., Fine, J., Ginsberg, G., Vaccarella, L., & Szatmari, P. (2007). Brief report: A scale for rating conversational impairment in autism spectrum disorder. *Journal of Autism and Developmental Disorders*, *37*, 1375–1380.

Diehl, J. J., Bennetto, L., Watson, D., Gunlogson, C., & McDonough, J. (2008). Resolving ambiguity: a psycholinguistic approach to understanding prosody processing in high-functioning autism. *Brain and Language*, *106*, 144–152.

Diehl, J. J., Bennetto, L., & Young, E. C. (2006). Story recall and narrative coherence of high-functioning children with autism spectrum disorders. *Journal of Abnormal Child Psychology*, *34*, 87–102.

Dobbinson, S., Perkins, M. R., & Boucher, J. (1998). Structural patterns in conversations with a woman who has autism. *Journal of Communication Disorders*, *31*, 113–134.

Eales, M. J. (1993). Pragmatic impairments in adults with childhood diagnoses of autism or developmental receptive language disorder. *Journal of Autism and Developmental Disorders*, *23*, 593–617.

Eigsti, I.-M., & Bennetto, L. (2009). Grammaticality judgements in autism: Deviance or delay? *Journal of Child Language*, *36*, 999–1201.

Eigsti, I.-M., Bennetto, L., & Dadlani, M. (2007). Beyond pragmatics: Morphosyntactic development in autism. *Journal of Autism and Developmental Disorders*, *37*, 1007–1023.

Emerich, D. M., Creaghead, N. A., Grether, S. M., Murray, D., & Grasha, C. (2003). The comprehension of humorous materials by adolescents with high-functioning autism and Asperger's syndrome. *Journal of Autism and Developmental Disorders*, *33*, 253–257.

Eskes, G. A., Bryson, S. E., & McCormick, T. A. (1990). Comprehension of concrete and abstract words in autistic children. *Journal of Autism and Developmental Disorders*, *20*, 61–73.

Flagg, E. J., Cardy, J. E., Roberts, W., & Roberts, T. P. (2005). Language lateralization development in children with autism: insights from the late field magnetoencephalogram. *Neuroscience Letters*, *386*, 82–87.

Friederici, A. (2009). Pathways to language: Fiber tracts in the human brain. *Trends in Cognitive Sciences*, *13*, 175–181.

Gabriels, R., Cuccaro, M., Hill, D., Ivers, B., & Goldson, E. (2005). Repetitive behaviors in autism: Relationships with associated clinical features. *Research in Developmental Disabilities*, *26*, 169–181.

Garcia-Perez, R. M., Hobson, R. P., & Lee, A. (2008). Narrative role-taking in autism. *Journal of Autism and Developmental Disorders*, *38*, 156–168.

Garcia-Perez, R. M., Lee, A., & Hobson, R. P. (2007). On intersubjective engagement in autism: A controlled study of nonverbal aspects of conversation. *Journal of Autism and Developmental Disorders*, *37*, 1310–1322.

Gernsbacher, M., Sauer, E., Geye, H., Schweigert, E., & Goldsmith, H. (2008). Infant and toddler oral- and manual-motor skills predict later speech fluency in autism. *Journal of Child Psychology and Psychiatry*, *49*, 43–50.

Ghaziuddin, M., & Gerstein, L. (1996). Pedantic speaking style differentiates Asperger syndrome from high-functioning autism. *Journal of Autism and Developmental Disorders*, *26*, 585–595.

Gogtay, N., Giedd, J. N., Lusk, L., Hayashi, K. M., Greenstein, D., Vaituzis, A. C., et al. (2004). Dynamic mapping of human cortical development during childhood through early adulthood. *Proceedings of the National Academy of Sciences of the United States of America*, *101*, 8174–8179.

Goldberg, W. A., Osann, K., Filipek, P. A., Laulhere, T., Jarvis, K., Modahl, C., et al. (2003). Language and other regression: Assessment and timing. *Journal of Autism and Developmental Disorders*, *33*, 607–616.

Goldman, S. (2008). Narratives of personal events in children with autism and developmental language disorders: Unshared memories. *Journal of Autism and Developmental Disorders*, *38*, 1982–1988.

Hale, C. M., & Tager-Flusberg, H. (2005a). The relationship between discourse deficits and autism symptomatology. *Journal of Autism and Developmental Disorders, 35*, 519–524.

Hale, C. M., & Tager-Flusberg, H. (2005b). Social communication in children with autism: The relationship between theory of mind in discourse development. *Autism, 9*, 157–178.

Hansen, R. L., Ozonoff, S., Krakowiak, P., Angkustsiri, K., Jones, C., Deprey, L. J., et al. (2008). Regression in autism: Prevalence and associated factors in the CHARGE study. *Ambulatory Pediatrics, 8*, 25–31.

Happé, F. (1993). Communicative competence and theory of mind in autism: A test of relevance theory. *Cognition, 48*, 101–119.

Happé, F. (1994). An advanced test of theory of mind: Understanding of story characters' thoughts and feelings by able autistic, mentally handicapped, and normal children and adults. *Journal of Autism and Developmental Disorders, 24*, 129–154.

Happé, F. G. E. (1995). Understanding minds and metaphors: insights from the study of figurative language in autism. *Metaphor and Symbolic Activity, 10*, 275–295.

Harris, G. J., Chabris, C. F., Clark, J., Urban, T., Aharon, I., Steele, S., et al. (2006). Brain activation during semantic processing in autism spectrum disorders via functional magnetic resonance imaging. *Brain and Cognition, 61*, 54–68.

Herbert, M. R., Harris, G. J., Adrien, K. T., Ziegler, D. A., Makris, N., Kennedy, D. N., et al. (2002). Abnormal asymmetry in language association cortex in autism. *Annals of Neurology, 52*, 588–596.

Herbert, M. R., Ziegler, D. A., Deutsch, C. K., O'Brien, L. M., Kennedy, D. N., Filipek, P. A., et al. (2005). Brain asymmetries in autism and developmental language disorder: a nested whole-brain analysis. *Brain, 128*, 213–226.

Hirschfeld, L., Bartmess, E., White, S., & Frith, U. (2007). Can autistic children predict behavior by social stereotypes? *Current Biology, 17*, R641–R642.

Hobson, R. P., & Lee, A. (1989). Emotion-related and abstract concepts in autistic people: Evidence from the British Picture Vocabulary Scale. *Journal of Autism and Developmental Disorders, 19*, 601–623.

Jarrold, C., Boucher, J., & Russell, J. (1997). Language profiles in children with autism: Theoretical and methodological implications. *Autism, 1*, 57–76.

Järvinen-Pasley, A., Peppé, S., King-Smith, G., & Heaton, P. (2008). The relationship between form and function level receptive prosodic abilities in autism. *Journal of Autism and Developmental Disorders, 38*, 1328–1340.

Just, M. A., Cherkassky, V. L., Keller, T. A., & Minshew, N. J. (2004). Cortical activation and synchronization during sentence comprehension in high-functioning autism: evidence of underconnectivity. *Brain, 127*, 1811–1821.

Kaland, N., Moller-Nielsen, A., Smith, L., Mortensen, E. L., Callesen, K., & Gottlieb, D. (2005). The Strange Stories test: A replication study of children and adolescents with Asperger syndrome. *European Child and Adolescent Psychiatry, 14*, 73–82.

Kanner, L. (1943). Autistic disturbance of affective contact. *Nervous Child, 2*, 217–250.

Kanner, L. (1946). Irrelevant and metaphorical language. *American Journal of Psychiatry, 103*, 242–246.

Keller, S. S., Crow, T., Foundas, A., Amunts, K., & Roberts, N. (2009). Broca's area: nomenclature, anatomy, typology, and asymmetry. *Brain and Language, 109*, 29–48.

Kelley, E., Paul, R., Fein, D., & Naigles, L. (2006). Residual language deficits in optimal outcome children with a history of autism. *Journal of Autism and Developmental Disorders, 36*, 807–828.

Kerbel, D., & Grunwell, P. (1998). A study of idiom comprehension in children with semantic-pragmatic difficulties. Part II: Between-groups results and discussion. *International Journal of Language and Communication Disorders, 33*, 23–44.

Kjelgaard, M. M., & Tager-Flusberg, H. (2001). An investigation of language impairment in autism: Implications for genetic subgroups. *Language and Cognitive Processes, 16*, 287–308.

Kleinhans, N. M., Muller, R. A., Cohen, D. N., & Courchesne, E. (2008). Atypical functional lateralization of language in autism spectrum disorders. *Brain Research, 1221*, 115–125.

Klin, A. (1991). Young autistic children's listening preferences in regard to speech: A possible characterization of the symptom of social withdrawal. *Journal of Autism and Developmental Disorders, 21*, 29–42.

Knaus, T. A., Silver, A. M., Lindgren, K. A., Hadjikhani, N., & Tager-Flusberg, H. (2008). fMRI activation during a language task in adolescents with ASD. *Journal of the International Neuropsychological Society, 14*, 967–979.

Knaus, T. A., Silver, A. M., Dominick, K. C., Schuring, M. D., Shaffer, N., Lindgren, K. A., et al. (2009). Age-related changes in the anatomy of language regions in autism spectrum disorder. *Brain Imaging and Behavior, 3*, 51–63.

Korpilahti, P., Jansson-Verkasalo, E., Mattila, M., Kuusikko, S., Sumoinen, K., Rytky, S., et al. (2007). Processing of affective speech prosody is impaired in Asperger syndrome. *Journal of Autism and Developmental Disorders, 37*, 1539–1549.

Kuhl, P. (2004). Early language acquisition: Cracking the speech code. *Nature Reviews Neuroscience, 5*, 831–843.

Kuhl, P. (2007). Is speech learning "gated" by the social brain? *Developmental Science, 10*, 110–120.

Kuhl, P. K., Coffey-Corina, S., Padden, D., & Dawson, G. (2005). Links between social and linguistic processing of speech in preschool children with autism: behavioral and electrophysiological measures. *Developmental Science, 8*, F1–F12.

Landa, R., & Garrett-Mayer, E. (2006). Development in infants with autism spectrum disorders: a prospective study. *Journal of Child Psychology and Psychiatry, 47*, 629–638.

Landa, R., Holman, K., & Garrett-Mayer, E. (2007). Social and communication development in toddlers with early and later diagnosis of autism spectrum disorders. *Archives of General Psychiatry, 64*, 853–864.

Lee, A., Hobson, R. P., & Chiat, S. (1994). I, you, me, and autism: An experimental study. *Journal of Autism and Developmental Disorders, 24*, 155–176.

Lewis, F. M., Murdoch, B. E., & Woodyatt, G. C. (2007). Communicative competence and metalinguistic ability: Performance by children and adults with autism spectrum disorder. *Journal of Autism and Developmental Disorders, 37*, 1525–1538.

Lord, C., Risi, S., & Pickles, A. (2004). Trajectory of language development in autistic spectrum disorders. In M. Rice & S. Warren (Eds.), *Developmental language disorders: From phenotypes to etiologies* (pp. 7–29). Mahwah, NJ: Erlbaum.

Lord, C., Rutter, M., DiLavore, P., & Risi, S. (1999). *Autism Diagnostic Observation Schedule (ADOS)*. Los Angeles: Western Psychological Services.

Lord, C., Shulman, C., & DiLavore, P. (2004). Regression and word loss in autistic spectrum disorders. *Journal of Child Psychology and Psychiatry, 4*, 936–955.

Losh, M., & Capps, L. (2003). Narrative ability in high-functioning children with autism or Asperger's syndrome. *Journal of Autism and Developmental Disorders, 33*, 239–251.

Loukusa, S., Leinonen, E., Kuusikko, S., Jussila, K., Mattila, M., Ryder, N., et al. (2007). Use of context in pragmatic language comprehension by children with Asperger syndrome or high-functioning autism. *Journal of Autism and Developmental Disorders, 37*, 1049–1059.

Loveland, K., Landry, S., Hughes, S., Hall, S., & McEvoy, R. (1988). Speech acts and the pragmatic deficits of autism. *Journal of Speech and Hearing Research, 31*, 593–604.

Luyster, R., Richler, J., Risi, S., Hsu, W. L., Dawson, G., Bernier, R., et al. (2005). Early regression in social communication in autism spectrum disorders: A CPEA study. *Developmental Neuropsychology, 27*, 311–336.

Luyster, R. J., Kadlec, M. B., Carter, A., & Tager-Flusberg, H. (2008). Language assessment and development in toddlers with autism spectrum disorders. *Journal of Autism and Developmental Disorders, 38*, 1426–1438.

Lyons, V., & Fitzgerald, M. (2004). Humor in autism and Asperger syndrome. *Journal of Autism and Developmental Disorders, 34*, 521–531.

MacKay, G., & Shaw, A. (2004). A comparative study of figurative language in children with autism spectrum disorders. *Child Language Teaching and Therapy, 20*, 13–32.

Martin, I., & McDonald, S. (2004). An exploration of causes of non-literal language problems in individuals with Asperger Syndrome. *Journal of Autism and Developmental Disorders, 34*, 311–328.

McAlonan, G. M., Cheung, V., Cheung, C., Suckling, J., Lam, G. Y., Tai, K. S., et al. (2005). Mapping the brain in autism. A voxel-based MRI study of volumetric differences and intercorrelations in autism. *Brain, 128*, 268–276.

McAlonan, G. M., Suckling, J., Wong, N., Cheung, V., Lienenkaemper, N., Cheung, C., et al. (2008). Distinct patterns of grey matter abnormality in high-functioning autism and Asperger's syndrome. *Journal of Child Psychology and Psychiatry, 49*, 1287–1295.

McCann, J., & Peppé, S. (2003). Prosody in autism spectrum disorders: a critical review. *International Journal of Language and Communication Disorders, 38*, 325–350.

McCann, J., Peppé, S., Gibbon, F. E., O'Hare, A., & Rutherford, M. (2007). Prosody and its relationship to language in school-aged children with high-functioning autism. *International Journal of Language and Communication Disorders, 42*, 682–702.

McDuffie, A., Yoder, P., & Stone, W. (2006). Labels increase attention to novel objects in children with autism and comprehension-matched children with typical development. *Autism, 10*, 288–301.

Meilleur, A., & Fombonne, E. (2009). Regression of language and non-language skills in pervasive developmental disorders. *Journal of Intellectual Disability Research, 53*, 115–124.

Meltzoff, A., Kuhl, P., Movellan, J., & Sejnowski, T. (2009). Foundations for a new science of learning. *Science, 325*, 284–288.

Mitchell, P., Saltmarsh, R., & Russell, H. (1997). Overly literal interpretations of speech in autism: Apprehending the mind behind the message. *Journal of Child Psychology and Psychiatry, 38*, 685–692.

Mitchell, S., Brian, J., Zwaigenbaum, L., Roberts, W., Szatmari, P., Smith, I., et al. (2006). Early language and communication development of infants later diagnosed with autism spectrum disorder. *Journal of Developmental and Behavioral Pediatrics, 27*, S69–S78.

Morrow, E., Yoo, S-Y, Flavell, S, Kim, T-K, Lin, Y, Hill, R. (2008). Identifying autism loci and genes by tracing recent shared ancestry. *Science, 321*, 218–223.

Muller, R. A., Behen, M. E., Rothermel, R. D., Chugani, D. C., Muzik, O., Mangner, T. J., et al. (1999). Brain mapping of language and auditory perception in high-functioning autistic adults: a PET study. *Journal of Autism and Developmental Disorders, 29*(1), 19–31.

Mundy, P., Sigman, M., & Kasari, C. (1990). A longitudinal study of joint attention and language development in autistic children. *Journal of Autism and Developmental Disorders, 20*, 115–128.

Mundy, P., Sigman, M., Ungerer, J., & Sherman, T. (1987). Nonverbal communication and play correlates of language development in autistic children. *Journal of Autism and Developmental Disorders, 17*, 349–364.

Munson, J., Dawson, G., Abbott, R., Faja, S., Webb, S., Friedman, S., et al. (2006). Amygdalar volume and behavioral development in autism. *Archives of General Psychiatry, 63*, 686–693.

Naber, F., Bakermans-Kranenburg, M., van Ijzendorn, M. Swinkels, S. Buitelaar, J., Dietz, C., et al. (2008). Play behavior and attachment in toddlers with autism. *Journal of Autism and Developmental Disorders, 38*, 857–866.

Norbury, C. F. (2004). Factors supporting idiom comprehension in children with communication disorders. *Journal of Speech Language and Hearing Research, 47*, 1179–1193.

Norbury, C., Brock, J., Cragg, L., Einav, S., Griffiths, H., & Nation, K. (2009). Eye-movement patterns are associated with communicative competence in autistic spectrum disorders. *Journal of Child Psychology and Psychiatry, 50*, 834–842.

Ozonoff, S., Williams, B. J., & Landa, R. (2005). Parental report of the early development of children with regressive autism: The delays-plus-regression phenotype. *Autism, 9*, 461–486.

Parish-Morris, J., Hennon, E., Hirsh-Pasek, K., Golinkoff, R., & Tager-Flusberg, H. (2007). Children with autism illuminate the role of social intention in word learning. *Child Development, 78*, 1265–1287.

Paul, R., Chawarska, K., Cicchetti, D., & Volkmar, F. (2008). Language outcomes of toddlers with autism spectrum disorders: A two year follow-up. *Autism Research, 1*, 97–107.

Paul, R., Orlovski, S., Marcinko, H., & Volkmar, F. (2009). Conversational behaviors in youth with high-functioning ASD and Asperger syndrome. *Journal of Autism and Developmental Disorders, 39*, 115–125.

Peppé, S., McCann, J., Gibbon, F., O'Hare, A., & Rutherford, M. (2007). Receptive and expressive prosodic ability in children with high functioning autism. *Journal of Speech, Hearing, and Language Research, 50*, 1015–1028.

Pickett, E., Pullara, O., O'Grady, J, & Gordon, B. (2009). Speech acquisition in older nonverbal individuals with autism: A review of features, methods, and prognosis. *Cognitive and Behavioral Neurology, 22*, 1–21.

Preissler, M., & Carey, S. (2005). The role of inferences about referential intent in word learning: Evidence from autism. *Cognition, 97*, B13–B23.

Pronovost, W., Wakstein, M., & Wakstein, D. (1966). A longitudinal study of speech behavior and language comprehension in fourteen children diagnosed as atypical or autistic. *Exceptional Children, 33*, 19–26.

Richler, J., Luyster, R., Risi, S., Hsu, W. L., Dawson, G., Bernier, R., et al. (2006). Is there a "regressive phenotype" of autism spectrum disorder associated with the measles-mumps-rubella vaccine? A CPEA study. *Journal of Autism and Developmental Disorders, 36*, 299–316.

Rapin, I., & Dunn, M. (2003). Update on the language disorders of individuals on the autistic spectrum. *Brain and Development, 25*, 166–172.

Rapin, I., Dunn, M., Allen, D., Stevens, M., & Fein, D. (2009). Subtypes of language disorders in school-age children with autism. *Developmental Neuropsychology, 34,* 66–84.

Redcay, E., & Courchesne, E. (2005). When is the brain enlarged in autism? A meta-analysis of all brain size reports. *Biological Psychiatry, 58,* 1–9.

Redcay, E., & Courchesne, E. (2008). Deviant functional magnetic resonance imaging patterns of brain activity to speech in 2–3-year-old children with autism spectrum disorder. *Biological Psychiatry, 64,* 589–598.

Roberts, J., Rice, M., & Tager-Flusberg, H. (2004). Tense marking in children with autism. *Applied Psycholinguistics, 25,* 429–448.

Rojas, D. C., Camou, S. L., Reite, M. L., & Rogers, S. J. (2005). Planum temporale volume in children and adolescents with autism. *Journal of Autism and Developmental Disorders, 35,* 479–486.

Rowe, M. L., Özçalişkan, Ş., & Goldin-Meadow, S. (2008). Learning words by hand: Gesture's role in predicting vocabulary development. *First Language, 28,* 182–199.

Rutherford, M. D., Baron-Cohen, S., & Wheelwright, S. (2002). Reading the mind in the voice: a study with normal adults and adults with Asperger syndrome and high functioning autism. *Journal of Autism and Developmental Disorders, 32,* 189–194.

Rydell, P. J., & Mirenda, P. (1994). Effects of high and low constraint utterances on the production of immediate and delayed echolalia in young children with autism. *Journal of Autism and Developmental Disorders, 24,* 719–735.

Scarborough, H. S., Rescorla, L., Tager-Flusberg, H., Fowler, A. E., & Sudhalter, V. (1991). The relation of utterance length to grammatical complexity in normal and language-disordered groups. *Applied Psycholinguistics, 12,* 23–45.

Shriberg, L. D., Paul, R., McSweeny, J. L., Klin, A., Cohen, D. J., & Volkmar, F. R. (2001). Speech and prosody characteristics of adolescents and adults with high-functioning autism and Asperger syndrome. *Journal of Speech, Language, and Hearing Research, 44,* 1097–1115.

Sigman, M., & McGovern, C. (2005). Improvement in cognitive and language skills from preschool to adolescence in autism. *Journal of Autism and Developmental Disorders, 35,* 15–23.

Siller, M., & Sigman, M. (2008). Modeling longitudinal change in the language abilities of children with autism: Parent behaviors and child characteristics as predictors of change. *Developmental Psychology, 44,* 1691–1704.

Siklos, S., & Kerns, K. A. (2007). Assessing the diagnostic experiences of a small sample of parents of children with autism spectrum disorders. *Research in Developmental Disabilities, 28,* 9–22.

Sowell, E. R., Thompson, P. M., Leonard, C. M., Welcome, S. E., Kan, E., & Toga, A. W. (2004). Longitudinal mapping of cortical thickness and brain growth in normal children. *Journal of Neuroscience, 24,* 8223–8231.

Sparrow, S., Balla, D., & Cicchetti, D. (1984). *Vineland Adaptive Behavior Scales.* American Guidance Service: Circle Pines, MN.

Sperber, D., & Wilson, D. (1986). *Relevance: Communication and cognition.* Cambridge, MA: Harvard University Press.

Stone, W., Ousley, O. Y., & Littleford, C. (1997). Motor imitation in young children with autism: What's the object? *Journal of Abnormal Child Psychology, 25,* 475–485.

Stone, W., & Yoder, P. J. (2001). Predicting spoken language level in children with autism spectrum disorders. *Autism, 5,* 341–361.

Szatmari, P., Bryson, S. E., Boyle, M. H., Streiner, D. L., & Duku, E. (2003). Predictors of outcome among high functioning children with autism and Asperger syndrome. *Journal of Child Psychology and Psychiatry, 44,* 520–528.

Tager–Flusberg, H. (1985). The conceptual basis for referential word meaning in children with autism. *Child Development, 56,* 1167–1178.

Tager–Flusberg, H. (1989). A psycholinguistic perspective on language development in the autistic child. In G. Dawson (Ed.), *Autism: New directions in diagnosis, nature, and treatment,* (pp. 92–115). New York: Guilford.

Tager-Flusberg, H. (1992). Autistic children's talk about psychological states: Deficits in the early acquisition of a theory of mind. *Child Development, 63,* 161–172.

Tager-Flusberg, H. (1994). Dissociations in form and function in the acquisition of language by autistic children. In H. Tager-Flusberg (Ed.), *Constraints on language acquisition: Studies of atypical children* (pp. 175–194). Hillsdale, NJ: Erlbaum.

Tager-Flusberg, H. (1995). "Once upon a ribbit": Stories narrated by autistic children. *British Journal of Developmental Psychology, 13,* 45–59.

Tager-Flusberg, H. (2000). Language and understanding minds: Connections in autism. In S. Baron-Cohen, H. Tager-Flusberg, & D. J. Cohen (Eds.), *Understanding other minds: Perspectives from developmental cognitive neuroscience* (2nd ed., pp. 124–149). Oxford: Oxford University Press.

Tager-Flusberg, H. (2003). Language and communicative deficits and their effects on learning and behavior. In M. Prior (Ed.), *Asperger syndrome: Behavioral and educational aspects,* (pp. 85–103). New York: Guilford.

Tager-Flusberg, H. (2004). Do autism and specific language impairment represent overlapping language disorders? In M. L. Rice & S. Warren (Eds.), *Developmental language disorders: From phenotypes to etiologies* (pp. 31–52). Mahwah, NJ: Erlbaum.

Tager-Flusberg, H. (2006). Defining language phenotypes in autism. *Clinical Neuroscience Research, 6,* 219–224.

Tager-Flusberg, H., & Anderson, M. (1991). The development of contingent discourse ability in autistic children. *Journal of Child Psychology and Psychiatry, 32,* 1123–1134.

Tager-Flusberg, H., Calkins, S., Noin, I., Baumberger, T., Anderson, M., & Chadwick-Denis, A. (1990). A longitudinal study of language acquisition in autistic and Down syndrome children. *Journal of Autism and Developmental Disorders, 20,* 1–22.

Tager-Flusberg, H., & Cooper, J. (1999). Present and future possibilities for defining a phenotype for specific language impairment. *Journal of Speech, Language, and Hearing Research, 42,* 1275–1278.

Tager-Flusberg, H., Lindgren, K. A., & Mody, M. (2008). Structural and functional imaging research on language disorders: Specific language impairment and autism spectrum disorders. In L. Wolf, H. Schreiber, & J. Wasserstein (Eds.), *Adult learning disorders: Contemporary issues* (pp. 127–157). Neuropsychology Handbook Series. New York: Psychology Press.

Tager-Flusberg, H., Paul, R., & Lord, C. (2005). Language and communication in autism. In F. Volkmar, R. Paul, A. Klin, & D. J. Cohen (Eds.), *Handbook of autism and pervasive developmental disorder* (3rd ed., Vol. 1, pp. 335–364). New York: Wiley.

Thurm, A., Lord, C., Lee, L.-C., & Newschaffer, C. (2007). Predictors of language acquisition in preschool children with autism spectrum disorders. *Journal of Autism and Developmental Disorders, 37,* 1721–1734.

Tomblin, J. B., & Zhang, X. (1999). Language patterns and etiology in children with specific language impairment.

In H. Tager-Flusberg (Ed.), *Neurodevelopmental disorders* (pp. 361–382). Cambridge, MA: MIT Press.

Ullman, M. (2001). A neurocognitive perspective on language: The declarative/procedural model. *Nature Reviews Neuroscience, 2*, 717–726.

Ullman, M., & Pierpont, E. I. (2005). Specific language impairment is not specific to language: The procedural deficits hypotheses. *Cortex, 41*, 399–433.

Van Lancker, D., Cornelius, C., & Needleman, R. (1991). Comprehension of verbal terms for emotions in normal, autistic, and schizophrenic children. *Developmental Neuropsychology, 7*, 1–18.

Volden, J. (2004). Conversational repair in speakers with autism spectrum disorder. *International Journal of Language and Communication Disorders, 39*, 171–189.

Volden, J., Coolican, J., Garon, N., White, J., & Bryson, S. (2009). Pragmatic language in autism spectrum disorder: Relationships to measures of ability and disability. *Journal of Autism and Developmental Disorders, 39*, 388–393.

Volden, J., & Lord, C. (1991). Neologisms and idiosyncratic language in autistic speakers. *Journal of Autism and Developmental Disorders, 21*, 109–130.

Volden, J., & Sorenson, A. (2009). Bossy and nice requests: Varying language register in speakers with autism spectrum disorder. *Journal of Communication Disorders, 42*, 58–73.

Walenski, M., Mostofsky, S., Gidley-Larson, J., & Ullman, M. (2008). Enhanced picture naming in autism. *Journal of Autism and Developmental Disorders, 38*, 1395–1399.

Walenski, M., Tager-Flusberg, H., & Ullman, M. (2006). Language in autism. In S. Moldin & J. Rubenstein (Eds.), *Understanding autism: From basic neuroscience to treatment.* New York: CRC Press/Taylor & Francis.

Wallentin, M. (2009). Putative sex differences in verbal abilities and language cortex: A critical review. *Brain and Language, 108*, 175–183.

Watt, N., Wetherby, A., & Shumway, S. (2006). Prelinguistic predictors of language outcome at 3 years of age. *Journal of Speech, Language, and Hearing Research, 49*, 1224–1237.

Werner, E., Dawson, G., Munson, J., & Osterling, J. (2005). Variation in early developmental course in autism and its relation with behavioral outcome at 3-4 years of age. *Journal of Autism and Developmental Disorders, 35*, 337–350.

Wetherby, A. (1986). Ontogeny of communication functions in autism. *Journal of Autism and Developmental Disorders, 16*, 295–316.

Wetherby, A. M., Watt, N., Morgan, L., & Shumway, S. (2007). Social communication profiles of children with autism spectrum disorders late in the second year of life. *Journal of Autism and Developmental Disorders, 3*, 960–975.

Whitehouse, A. J., Barry, J. G., & Bishop, D. V. (2008). Further defining the language impairment of autism: is there a specific language impairment subtype? *Journal of Communication Disorders, 41*, 319–336.

Zwaigenbaum, L., Bryson, S., Rogers, T., Roberts, W., Brian, J., & Szatmari, P. (2005). Behavioral manifestations of autism in the first year of life. *International Journal of Developmental Neuroscience, 23*, 143–152.

Zwaigenbaum, L., Thurm, A., Stone, W., Baranek, G., Bryson, S., Iverson, J. et al. (2007). Studying the emergence of autism spectrum disorders in high-risk infants: Methodological and practical issues. *Journal of Autism and Developmental Disorders, 37*, 466–480.

10 Wouter B. Groen, Jan K. Buitelaar

Cognitive and Neural Correlates of Language in Autism

Points of Interest

- The language impairments in autism are much more extensive than captured by the current diagnostic criteria, and even in relatively able subjects with autism, include phonological, semantic, syntactic, and pragmatic deficits.
- The language impairments in autism are linked to the neural architecture in autism.
- There is not only symptomatic overlap between autism and specific language impairment (SLI) but likely also shared neural substrates and shared genes.
- Future research into language impairments in autism should integrate studies in emotion understanding and in manipulating emotional context with that of language issues.
- Future research into language impairments in autism should combine a neural systems and a neurogenetic approach and integrate the still mostly separate research fields of autism and SLI.

To communicate with other people and to describe our thoughts and feelings, we use the faculty of language. This faculty relies on a complex set of cognitive processes and representations carried out by an intricate network of neural regions distributed across cortical and subcortical structures (Hillis, 2007). Since autism is a disorder in which the development of cortical (Courchesne & Pierce, 2005) and subcortical (Herbert et al., 2003) structures is affected, it is not surprising that the faculty of language is affected in autism as well. There is not only an impairment in verbal and nonverbal communication as described by formal DSM-IV and ICD-10 diagnostic criteria, the ability to use and understand language is affected as well. The linguistic deficits are, however, much more variable than the universal deficits in communication (Kjelgaard & Tager-Flusberg, 2001), and their neural correlates are therefore difficult to investigate. Nevertheless, there have been converging efforts from different disciplines to document the neural correlates underlying language in autism. In this chapter we aim to discuss recent evidence from structural, electrophysiological, and functional studies on the neural correlates of linguistic abnormalities in autism. We will argue that the linguistic features in autism cover a wider range of impairments than described in the DSM-IV criteria for autistic disorder and are more linked to the neural architecture in autism than earlier behavioral studies have suggested. Functional brain-imaging data show aberrant neural activation in semantic, syntactic, and pragmatic tasks of higher-order language functions, as well as in low-level sensory processes. Furthermore, we will argue that the abnormalities of low-level sensory processing of linguistic stimuli can be interpreted in the light of connectivity models in autism. Finally, we will discuss the relationship between language impairments and the other functional impairments in autism (social interaction and stereotyped and rigid behavior patterns), as well as the relationship between autism and specific language impairment (SLI). First of all, however, some background will be given on the current views of the typical cognitive architecture underlying language production and comprehension and discuss the anatomy of language. We will also briefly discuss the development of language in typically developing children.

Neural Architecture of Language

Linguists commonly describe language and language disorders in terms of phonology, semantics, syntax, and pragmatics. Whereas phonology deals with the perception and production of sound units whose concatenation produces words, semantics deals with the meaning of lexical items, syntax with the structure of words in sentences, and pragmatics with the conventions and rules governing the use of language for communication. From a neuroscientific perspective, however, there is no clear-cut relation between linguistic categories and cortical function.

Recent functional imaging studies have furthered the idea that the language system is organized in a large number of small but tightly clustered modules in both the left and right hemispheres with unique contributions to language processing. There is also increasing evidence that cortical language regions are not specific to language, but involve more reductionist processes that give rise to language as well as nonlinguistic functions (Bookheimer, 2002). The areas involved in language processing include the dorsolateral prefrontal cortex, premotor cortex, middle and inferior temporal cortices, anterior cingulate gyrus, supplementary motor area, supramarginal, and angular gyri in the posterior-inferior parietal cortex. The cerebellum and the thalamus also play a role (Price et al., 1999).

Among the regions already recognized in the nineteenth century are the left inferior frontal gyrus (Broca's area), which includes Brodmann area 44 and 45, and the posterior auditory association cortex (Wernicke's area) on the superior temporal gyrus (Brodmann area 22). Broca's area and Wernicke's area, along with the arcuate fasciculus that connects the two, play a key role in the traditional language model. This model essentially states that Wernicke's area controls language comprehension, and Broca's area language production (Dronkers, 2000). The model was mainly derived from lesion studies, in which damage to Wernicke's area typically results in impaired comprehension with less impairment in producing fluent, well-articulated speech. Damage to Broca's area results in relatively intact comprehension but poor speech fluency, which makes speakers with such lesions unable to create grammatically complex sentences. Yet, with the onset of neuroimaging techniques, researchers consistently found that not all patients with Broca's aphasia (relatively intact comprehension but poor speech fluency) have lesions in Broca's area and vice versa. The same applies to Wernicke's aphasia. Thus, speech perception is not always normal in patients with Broca's aphasia, and articulation of speech sounds is not always normal in patients with Wernicke's aphasia (Dronkers, 2000).

Growing insight in the cognitive processes underlying language has led to a refinement of the traditional twentieth-century language model. Current cognitive language models assume that language tasks are decomposable into discrete representations and, furthermore, assume that these representations are composites of features distributed across regions of the brain (Hillis, 2007). For example, the semantic representation of "train" includes features on how it moves, represented in cortical areas such as the middle temporal visual area dedicated to motion recognition. Features on how people get on trains may be represented closer to motor systems, so that semantic representations might be distributed across the temporal, parietal, and frontal cortex. So, for naming a picture of a train, a number of processing steps must be performed. These include abstracting the features that allow recognition of something familiar, access to its semantic representation, access to its syntactic role, access to its phonologic representation, and finally motor planning for articulating the word. However, overlapping networks of brain regions are essential for these tasks. Damage to the same regions, for example, can disrupt naming, written word, and spoken word comprehension. Yet, some areas are more likely to disrupt each of these tasks. In this model, Wernicke's area might be critical for linking the widespread representations to specific words. Broca's area might be critical for selecting certain types of semantic information to accomplish specific tasks (Hillis, 2007).

Development of Language in Typical Populations

Typically, infants show communicative behaviors such as eye gaze, facial expression, and vocal turn-taking from the first months of life. At 12 to 15 months of age, infants are able to understand and express a number of words. Combined with nonverbal communication, infants use their vocabulary to produce 1-word sentences with which they request objects, reject offered actions, or call attention to objects or events (Bates, 1976). In the second year of life, there is a gradual increase in receptive and expressive vocabulary, until at an average age of 18 months, children combine words into 2-word sentences with basic semantic relations. It is in that time that the word "explosion" begins, as children begin to understand the referential nature of words (Nazzi & Bertoncini, 2003). At the age of 2, children understand around 900 words and actively use around 300 words in 2-word sentences. At the age of 3, the average mean length of utterance is 3 (Tager-Flusberg et al., 2005). Using nonverbal clues such as eye gaze, children are then able to make fine distinctions between an object that an adult is naming and other objects. At the age of 4, almost all sounds are produced correctly. At the age of 6, children understand and use thousands of words, and are able to use them in complex syntactic forms.

Language and Cognitive Theories in Autism

Several psychological theories, such as the Weak Central Coherence (WCC) theory (Frith, 1996) and the impaired theory of mind (ToM) (Baron-Cohen et al., 1985), have attempted to explain the high-order language deficits in autism. The weak central coherence theory predicts that, since people with autism are biased toward local versus global processing, their ability to integrate contextual information into a composite whole is diminished. The high-order core deficit in central processing supposedly results in altered low-level processing. Several studies have indeed demonstrated a reduced ability to infer word-meaning from sentence context (Happe, 1997) or to infer global meaning from sentences

(Jolliffe & Baron-Cohen, 2000), yielding empirical evidence for the WCC account for at least the semantic and pragmatic language deficits in autism. However, WCC would also predict a superior performance on single-word tasks, as is the case in hyperlexia. Yet, hyperlexia is only rarely seen in autism. The majority of people with autism have difficulties with the meaning of isolated words as well as whole sentences.

ToM refers to the specific cognitive ability to infer other people's mental states and to understand that others have beliefs, desires, and intentions that are different from our own. It has been argued that early stages of ToM are necessary for the ability to use symbols such as words (Tager-Flusberg, 2000), and that impairment in ToM in autism therefore causes an inability to comprehend the meaning of words. Furthermore, acquisition of language may be mediated by shared or joined attention, which, in case of an impaired ToM, would be impaired as well (Kuhl et al., 2003). Semantic ability and false belief have indeed been found to correlate in children with autism (Tager-Flusberg, 2000).

The psychological framework provided by these top-down theories assumes that an impaired high-level cognitive function is causing the impairments in autism. This assumption has been criticized for several reasons. First, converging evidence suggests that abnormalities of the processing of low-level sensory information may lead to impairments in higher-order cognitive functions, rather than the other way around (Happe & Frith, 2006; Bertone et al., 2005). That is to say, altered low-level perceptual processing in autism should not be considered a by-product of weak central coherence. Quite on the contrary, perceptual abnormalities may give rise to weak central coherence. Second, these neuropsychological top-down theories are descriptive rather than explanatory, and finding the neural correlates of these theories has proven difficult, since their predictions of cortical functioning are too general to be falsifiable.

The Phenotype of Language Disorders in Autism

Impaired language function is frequently observed in people with autism, often in combination with mental retardation. Language dysfunction in autism is, however, much more variable than the universal deficits in communication (Kjelgaard & Tager-Flusberg, 2001). At one end of the autism spectrum there are children whose verbal abilities are within the normal range of functioning, and at the other there are some who never start to speak (Lord & Paul, 1997). In those with sufficient language and cognitive abilities, i.e., people with high functioning autism (HFA) and Asperger's syndrome, social communicative abilities remain impaired. Language tends to be used one-sidedly, nonreciprocally, and instrumentally rather than for social purposes (Fine et al., 1994). In their original descriptions of ASD, Kanner and Asperger both gave account of the typical language anomalies encountered in autism such as echolalia, pronoun reversal, utterances not related to the conversational context, and a lack of drive to engage in communication (Asperger, 1991; Kanner, 1943).

Articulation

It has been a widely held belief that the development of phonology progresses at a slower rate, but is not impaired in autism since phonologically correct echolalia is commonly found in low-functioning autism, suggesting that phonological perception and production is intact even in severely affected individuals (Tager-Flusberg, 1996). However, there is converging evidence for an articulation deficit in a subgroup of autistic children. A delayed developmental trajectory of phonology has been reported (Bartolucci et al., 1976), as well as a greater number of articulation distortion errors in people with HFA and the Asperger group than in typically developing speakers (Shriberg et al., 2001). Recently, Kjelgaard and colleagues found phonological processing deficits (as measured by repeating nonsense words) in autistic children, although only in those with concurrent impaired vocabulary and higher-order semantic and syntax deficits (Kjelgaard & Tager-Flusberg, 2001). This language profile was also found by another group in half of the children with poor communicative abilities (Rapin & Dunn, 2003). It thus seems that, in a subgroup of autistic children, phonology is impaired along with language comprehension and production. This clustering of symptoms may suggest that common causes underlie phonology and syntactic abilities in autism and also in other disorders such as specific language impairment.

Word Use

Difficulties in both understanding and expressing lexicon are the most widely recognized linguistic impairments in autism. Semantic impairments are most severe in people with low-functioning autism (LFA) and least severe in those with HFA and AS (Boucher, 2003). Delay in speech acquisition is one of the primary diagnostic characteristics, and the degree of language impairment is a key prognostic factor (Lord & Paul, 1997; Venter et al., 1992). Yet, the course and development of semantic difficulties is an underresearched area in autism. One comprehensive study revealed marked difficulties in lexical comprehension and expressive vocabulary in the majority of children with autism (Kjelgaard & Tager-Flusberg, 2001). Furthermore, a strong correlation was found between full-scale IQ and performance on tests for comprehension (Peabody Picture Vocabulary Test) and expression (Expressive Vocabulary Test) (Dunn & Dunn, 1997; Williams, 1997). This correlation suggests that semantic comprehension and expression are unimpaired in the most able people with autism, and especially in those with Asperger syndrome. Subtle semantic impairments are however also present in HFA and AS. Howlin and colleagues found a poor performance on tests for productive (British Picture Vocabulary Scale) and receptive (Expressive One Word Picture Vocabulary Test) semantic abilities for both AS and HFA (Gardner, 1982; Howlin, 2003; Dunn et al., 1997). While there was no significant difference for language comprehension between HFA and AS, ratings for language expression revealed a small but significant difference favoring the AS group. Thus, in accordance with clinical experience and anecdotal evidence, language abilities in people with HFA and AS differ mainly with respect to expressive abilities.

It has been suggested that the semantic difficulties in autism are a consequence of deficits in advanced conceptualization, since simple concepts referred to by lexical items are not affected in autism (Tager-Flusberg, 1981) and comprehension of terms referring to emotional states (Tager-Flusberg & Sullivan, 1995; Hobson & Lee, 1989) or abstract terms (Frith & Snowling, 1983) is more affected than comprehension of concrete words. Other studies, however, do not support this finding. Interference during a reading task was not different for concrete and abstract words (Eskes et al., 1990), and abstract terms that exist through human agency such as "war" and "peace" were not found to be used anomalously in autism (Perkins et al., 2006). Thus, the exact nature of the semantic deficits in autism remains to be established.

Syntax

As with the phonological properties of language in autism, syntactic impairments have not been well researched. Recent findings, however, do provide evidence for distinct and specific syntactic deficits in autistic children who acquire spoken language, and more noteworthy, they also show that, in those who do not acquire speech, the ability to acquire the grammar (and vocabulary) of signed language is impaired as well (Boucher, 2003). The distinct syntactic deficits in autism entail reduced expressive and receptive syntactic abilities, which have been found using the Clinical Evaluation of Language Fundamentals (CELF) (Kjelgaard & Tager-Flusberg, 2001) and mean utterance length in free play sessions (Eigsti et al., 2007). Contrary to the consistent findings on the length of syntactically complex utterances, the findings on grammatical morphemes such as verb tense markers and articles are inconsistent. Whereas earlier studies found more grammatical errors (Bartolucci & Albers, 1974; Bartolucci et al., 1980), a more recent well-matched study found no such errors in spontaneous autistic speech (Eigsti et al., 2007). Yet, Roberts and colleagues did find high rates of omissions of tense marking in a subgroup of children who were language impaired (Roberts et al., 2004). The inconsistency of findings on grammatical morphemes probably reflects the fact that subgroups are affected rather than all autistic people, so that sufficiently large subject groups are needed.

It has been a long-held belief that people with autism are better at language production than at language comprehension. The main reason for this assumption was a series of studies conducted in the seventies that compared autistic children with children with severe receptive language disorder. These studies revealed significant differences in comprehension of vocabulary and the production of syntactically complex utterances, favoring the children with receptive language disorder (Bartak et al., 1975; Cox et al., 1975; Cantwell et al., 1978). It was therefore argued that syntactic comprehension was more affected than production. However, in contrast with the above finding for syntax, a more recent study did not replicate a difference between *semantic* comprehension and expression (Kjelgaard & Tager-Flusberg, 2001). A language profile in autism with better production than comprehension could thus not be replicated. Nevertheless, evidence was found for two distinct language profiles in autism. The language profile in one subgroup entailed worse performance on tests of grammatical ability than vocabulary (Kjelgaard & Tager-Flusberg, 2001), possibly clustering with phonological impairments (Rapin & Dunn, 2003) (see also the "Phonology" section). The language profile in the other subgroup entailed impaired semantics and pragmatics (Rapin & Dunn, 2003). These subtypes suggest that syntactic and phonological deficits have a common cause, as have semantic and pragmatic deficits in autism. However, the distinction of subtypes was based on a number of studies with an autistic sample that was preselected for the presence of difficulties in language comprehension, so the extent to which these findings can be generalized to the broad autism spectrum remains to be established.

In summary, syntactic abilities in autism are characterized by sparse expressive language with immature syntax in a majority of children. There is some evidence for a clustering of syntactic/phonological deficits in a subgroup of children and a clustering of semantic/pragmatic deficits in a subgroup, but this will require confirmation in an unselected autistic population.

Pragmatics and Prosody

Pragmatics entails both the linguistic and nonlinguistic items that are covered by the defining criteria of autism. Linguistic pragmatics implies difficulties in the ability to disambiguate meaning, to structure coherent discourse, and to understand irony and implied meaning. The ability to understand other people's intentions, social rules of conduct, and nonverbal communication gestures is regarded as nonlinguistic pragmatics. Deficits in pragmatic functioning are evident at all developmental stages, even in highly verbal adults with autism (Lord & Paul, 1997; Tantam et al., 1993; Happe, 1993; Martin & McDonald, 2004; Baron-Cohen, 1997).

It should be noted that most research in autism on nonlinguistic pragmatic abilities, such as the ability to understand other people's intentions, as measured by ToM tests, involve language. Data on whether the deficit in ToM extends to people with autism with little or no language is sparse, making it difficult to disentangle the relative contributions of linguistic and nonlinguistic deficits in the sociocommunicative deficits in autism. Moreover, it has been argued that the syntactic ability to build subordinate clauses allows children to reason about mental states that are at odds with reality (e.g., "Jane *thinks* the cookies are in the cabinet") (De Villiers & De Villiers, 1995). Syntax mastery has indeed been found to correlate with performance on ToM tasks. However, using a nonverbal ToM test, Colle et al. found that children with autism selectively failed false-belief tasks, whereas children with SLI or typically developing children did not (Colle et al., 2007), indicating dissociation between verbal and pragmatic abilities.

A pragmatic ability closely related to language comprehension is the ability to perceive and use intonation, rhythm, tone of voice, and stress, referred to as prosody. The use of aberrant prosody is mentioned in the DSM-IV description of autism, and the perception of prosody in autism has been investigated by several authors. Rutherford and colleagues, for example, compared the ability of adults with ASD to attribute emotions to sentences spoken with an emotional tone of voice, and found that individuals with HFA or Asperger's syndrome have difficulties extracting mental-state information from vocalizations (Rutherford et al., 2002). Researchers found deficits in the perception and production of stress, intonation, and phrasing (Paul et al., 2005), as well as a preference for nonverbal sounds and an indifference to the mother's voice in children with autism (Dawson et al., 1998; Klin, 1991). The latter finding seems to indicate that deficits in the perception of prosody do not reflect an innate inability, but arise as a consequence of nonsocial orientation. However, the direction of causality may also be the other way around, or even be bidirectional. Finally, the relation between prosodic and verbal abilities in autism is not clear. Although using a relatively small study sample, Heaton et al. did not find a relation between the ability to perceive pitch in speech and nonspeech sounds and verbal ability (Heaton et al., 2008). This suggests that the WCC account does not adequately explain the relation between local auditory processing and global language ability.

In summary, linguistic and nonlinguistic pragmatic deficits and prosodic deficits are part of the most commonly affected domains of functioning measured across the spectrum of autism disorders. It appears that linguistic abilities facilitate pragmatic abilities, although they are not necessary per se for pragmatic competence.

The Neural Correlates of Language Disorders in Autism

Although autism is a heterogeneous disorder that includes many contradictory neurophysiological findings, several neural correlates underlying the linguistic deficits of autism have been reproduced in different investigative modalities. Some researchers focused on structural abnormalities (Herbert et al., 2002), while others addressed the perception of simple linguistic stimuli (Boddaert et al., 2003; Ceponiene et al., 2003) and higher-level linguistic functions (Harris et al., 2006; Kana et al., 2006). The results indicate that individuals with autism activate alternative and possibly less flexible networks during phonetic, semantic, syntactic, and pragmatic language processing. Abnormalities at an early level of information processing contribute to the hypothesis of a bottom-up etiology in which, for example, an alteration of auditory cortical processing leads to abnormal language development in early childhood.

Structural Abnormalities

After a long period of inconsistent findings in structural neuroimaging studies, data of recent studies converge to elucidate the underlying abnormalities in autism (see Palmen & van Engeland, 2004, for a review, as well as the chapters on Neurobiology of Autism in this book). The cortical areas that are most consistently affected in autism (the frontal, temporal, and cerebellar structures) all subserve language functions, although the cerebellum is only considered to play a facilitating role (Allen et al., 2004). Consequently, morphometric findings on the frontal and temporal language areas have been associated with language impairments in autism. Asymmetry reversal of the frontal language-related cortex was found (DeFosse et al., 2004; Herbert et al., 2002; Abell et al., 1999), as well as anterior and superior shifting of the left inferior frontal sulcus and superior temporal sulcus bilaterally (Levitt et al., 2003) and decreases of grey matter concentration bilaterally in the superior temporal sulcus (Boddaert, Chabane, Gervais, et al., 2004). Although cognitive functions are difficult to relate to morphometric findings in a one-to-one manner, the main conclusion of these studies is that the cortical development of language-related areas follows a different trajectory in autism, possibly in the context of a reduced left-lateralized hemispheric dominance. Whether these findings of aberrant development and collaboration between cortical areas are specific for autism is, however, not clear. As a consequence, there is a need to directly compare the neurobiological development and functioning in autism with other disorders of language such as SLI and dyslexia (see also Herbert et al., 2007 and the chapters on Neurobiology of Autism in this book).

Auditory Perception and Lower-Level Language Paradigms

Several authors have focused on clarifying two main questions in the field of language in autism: whether or not early sensory processes are deficient in autism and whether or not these early sensory processes are speech-specific. These questions are highly relevant to better understand the nature of language deficits in autism, since they allow inferences on the contribution of top-down versus bottom-up processes in the functional impairments in autism. Basically, bottom-up theories assume that early sensory deficits give rise to deficient high-level operations such as language and social behavior (e.g., the inability to speak in deaf people). Alternatively, top-down theories assume that the ability to perceive stimuli is not impaired. Yet, deficits in high-level processes such as social behavior could give rise to undirected attention, or attention directed to non–socially relevant clues, so that word-object associations do not develop efficiently in autistic children. In healthy children, joint attention has indeed been shown to be a prerequisite for acquiring language (Kuhl et al., 2003), suggesting a role for top-down influences in autism. Yet, it is still possible that sensory deficits give rise to deficits in joint attention. To shed light on this chicken-and-egg problem, much data has been collected using neurophysiological experiments that measure neural responses to stimuli at a millisecond scale.

Čeponienė et al. used an ERP oddball paradigm to examine the sensory and early attentional processing of speech and nonspeech sounds in children with HFA (Ceponiene et al., 2003). They found no differences in mismatch negativity (MMN, an index of automatic sound change detection, situated in time after the N1c wave and before the P3a wave), which suggests intact early perceptual abilities in autism. However, involuntary orienting (P3a) was different for speech sounds but not for nonspeech sounds in the HFA group. This finding supports the hypothesis of a speech-specific *post*sensory auditory impairment, suggesting that people with autism may perceive but not attend to linguistic stimuli. Contrary to Čeponienė's findings, Kasai et al. did find a delayed magnetic mismatch field for vowels (but not for tones) by using magnetoencephalography (Kasai et al., 2005). Thus, early perceptual processing in autism appeared to be deficient and speech-specific.

Others studies have confirmed the early perceptual processing deficits, but the speech specificity was not replicated: They reported smaller N1c waves in children with autism in an event-related paradigm with simple tones (Bruneau et al., 1999) and delayed MMN for both speech and nonspeech sounds (Oram Cardy et al., 2005). Whether or not cortical sound processing impairments are speech-specific, sound processing impairments may be fundamentally associated with language impairments. In a behavioral study, Groen et al. found no differences between children with and without autism in the ability to distinguish the parametrically morphed gender of speakers, but the response times differed between the groups (Groen et al., 2008). The authors argued that focus on different features in the voices, as a consequence of a difference in salience, caused the differences in response time. The results suggest that focus on different features in auditory objects may lead to a different development of higher-order cognitive systems such as language or pragmatics.

In an fMRI study that contrasted voices with environmental sounds, no differential activation between the two conditions was found in the autism group, suggesting that speech was not processed by a speech-specific cortical region (Gervais et al., 2004). The control group, on the other hand, showed greater activation for voices along the upper bank of the superior temporal sulcus bilaterally. The abnormal pattern of cortical activation in the autism group might reflect a bottom-up sensory impairment, or alternatively, it may be caused by an attention bias toward nonvocal sounds, which in turn may lead to the development of linguistic deficits in autistic children. This problem was tackled by a positron emission tomography (PET) study that investigated the auditory cortical processing of prelinguistic speech-like sounds that have an acoustic structure similar to speech (Boddaert et al., 2003; Boddaert, Chabane, Belin, et al., 2004). The study reported a reversed hemispheric dominance in the autism group and, compared with controls, less left-temporal activation and greater right middle frontal gyrus activation. The elegance of the study design was that top-down processing of language was less likely because the sounds were not perceived as language but rather as strange electronic tones. The acoustic structure was made to resemble speech sounds, such that any cortical processing differences reflected bottom-up linguistic abnormalities. The authors therefore speculated that the observed abnormal auditory processing led to an abnormal early stage of language development rather than that it reflects the consequences of abnormal language development.

The above-mentioned studies converge to the idea that impairments of information processing may lead to an abnormal developmental trajectory of language in autism. Studies of the maturational path of cortical language processing do indeed indicate an abnormal developmental trajectory in the form of reversed hemispheric dominance. Dawson et al. reported a strong relationship between language ability and hemispheric asymmetry in ERP, on the one hand, and vowel stimuli in autism, on the other (Dawson et al., 1989). Furthermore, in a MEG study using simple vowel stimuli, Flagg et al. found rightward instead of typical leftward hemispheric lateralization (Flagg et al., 2005). Reduced leftward hemispheric activation was also found in nonlinguistic neuroimaging studies (Gendry-Meresse et al., 2005; Chiron et al., 1995). Yet, the association of cortical processing impairments and impaired language in autism does not per se imply causality. That is, cortical sound processing impairments may cause language deficits, but language deficits may also cause cortical sound processing impairments. Alternatively, another factor such as a genetically programmed maldevelopment of neuroarchitecture in autism may give rise to both cortical sound processing impairments and language deficits.

In short, impaired cortical sound processing is reproduced reliably in autism. Whether or not the auditory processing abnormalities are speech-specific is still unclear, but early sensory impairments and their interplay with the maturational path of the cerebral cortex are likely to play a part in the abnormal language acquisition in autism.

Higher-Level Language Paradigms

Given the neuroimaging data found so far, it is unlikely that a deficit in a single cortical area can account for the phenotypic language deficits in autism, as is the case in poststroke aphasia. In the autistic brain, cortical regions seem to collaborate in a different fashion, and cortical areas that show hypoactivation or hyperactivation for one task may show normal activation for another task.

The first functional imaging study of higher-level language perception and generation in autism was a small exploratory PET study conducted in 1999 (Muller et al., 1999). In five autistic participants, sentence perception was associated with the reversal of normal left-hemisphere dominance, while sentence generation showed normal left inferior frontal activation. In a re-analysis of the data on the same subjects, which focused on three regions of interest, participants with autism had a reduced Broca's area (Broca's area is situated in the opercular and triangular sections of the inferior frontal gyrus) activation during language perception and production (Muller et al., 1998). A more recent fMRI study, using a reading paradigm that required the attribution of complex mental states contrasted with rest states, demonstrated more right frontal activation in the autism group, also indicating a reversal of hemisphere dominance (Takeuchi et al., 2004). These studies should, however, be considered exploratory because of their small sample sizes and multiple comparisons.

In an fMRI study by Harris et al., the semantic and perceptual processing of single words was assessed (Harris et al., 2006). Semantic processing (evaluating words as positive or negative) and perceptual processing (evaluating words as lower or UPPER case) were contrasted as well as processing of concrete and abstract words. The participants with autism had weaker left and right frontal activation, but greater temporal activation for semantic processing, relative to perceptual task conditions. More importantly, compared with the control group, there was little differential activation between semantic and perceptual processing in the autism group. The concrete versus abstract contrast also demonstrated less activation differences between the two conditions in the autism group.

Groen et al. investigated pragmatic and semantic language in adolescents with autism using fMRI. They hypothesized that the left inferior frontal gyrus (Broca's area), which has an integrating role, would be less activated during tasks that demand integration of social-pragmatic information such as speaker's age or gender with the content of the speaker's utterance. In the semantic-knowledge condition, activation of the LIF region did not differ between groups. In sentences that required integration of speaker information, the autism group showed abnormally reduced activation of the LIF region. The results suggest that people with autism may recruit the LIF region in a different manner in tasks that demand integration of social information.

In another fMRI study, abnormal Broca's and Wernicke's area (Wernicke's area is situated in the posterior section of the superior temporal gyrus and the Sylvian fissure) activation in autism was also demonstrated using a sentence comprehension task with syntactically demanding probes (Just et al., 2004). The autism group had less activation of Broca's area and adjacent areas and more Wernicke's area activation. Furthermore, the study showed a reduced synchronization of neural activation across the large-scale cortical network for language processing. The greater Wernicke's area activation was interpreted as a tendency for more extensive processing of the meanings of the individual words that make up a sentence in autism. The authors hypothesized that the reduced Broca's area activation may reflect a reduced ability to integrate the meaning of individual words into a coherent conceptual and syntactic structure. This may still hold, but Harris's study showed that Broca's area and Wernicke's area are also abnormally activated during the processing of single words when no syntactic demands are made (Harris et al., 2006).

The findings on underconnectivity were elaborated in an fMRI study in which autistic participants processed sentences with a high-imagery or low-imagery content (Kana et al., 2006). Measures of functional connectivity showed a reduced functional synchronization between the frontal and parietal areas. Again, the controls had greater Broca's area and adjacent area activation. In contrast to the control group, there were little activation differences between the two conditions in the autism group: The autism group seemed to process high- and low-imagery sentences similarly.

Thus, the neuroimaging data give rise to four main conclusions. First, the data indicate that people with autism tend to rely more on Wernicke's area (temporal region) and less on Broca's area (frontal region) for processing sentences and single words. Since Broca's area subserves integration processes (Hagoort et al., 2004) and Wernicke's area is more associated with semantic retrieval, the neuroimaging data present an intriguing parallel between the WCC's piecemeal processing style and the greater reliance on Wernicke's area neurally. It might thus well be that early sensory processes that highlight individual components in a composite whole give rise to the greater Wernicke's area activation rather than that Wernicke's area itself is malfunctioning.

Second, the neuroimaging data suggest that, during high-level processing in autism, cortical areas are used in a different manner and in reaction to other stimuli rather than that certain cortical areas are malfunctioning per se. An elegant example of this are two studies by the same group that assessed the neural basis of irony comprehension in autism. One study found hypoactivation of prefrontal and temporal regions during judgment of scenarios that involved irony (Wang et al., 2007). However, the other study, in which also scenarios that involved irony were presented, used a paradigm that demanded explicit attention to socially relevant clues, and found greater activation of the prefrontal and temporal regions (Wang et al., 2006).

Third, the task indifferent pattern of activation during language tasks in autism supports the idea that the neural networks that are temporarily recruited for a cognitive task cannot be reset as easily as in controls when the task is changed. There is theoretical evidence that suggests that less flexible network regrouping could be the result of abnormalities in low-level sensory processing (Gustafsson, 1997) in the sense that high-level processes are flooded with irrelevant information from low-level centers and the extra processing demand impedes the flexibility required for neural assemblies to form (Belmonte, Cook, et al., 2004). As such, less flexible network regrouping has been associated with models of aberrant connectivity in autism. This matter will be further discussed below. Interestingly, less flexible network regrouping might also be involved in the part of the triad of symptoms that involves rigidness and repetitive/restricted behavior. The correspondence between the triad of symptoms in relation to their putative causes will be also addressed below.

Fourth, autism is a heterogeneous disorder, and the same can be said about the neuroimaging results on language in autism. Some of the conflicting findings can be explained by the wide range of phenotypic variation with different intellectual levels and age groups studied. As a consequence of the difficulty to obtain large enough sample sizes, only a minority of the neuroimaging studies have evaluated the results at a search volume correct p-value and have used a random effects analysis and a direct group comparison.

Neural Architecture, Cortical Connectivity, and Language

Over two decades of research have shown that linguistic deficits are present in the majority of individuals with autism. Neurophysiological studies that sought the neural basis of these deficits have shown abnormalities at a basic, early level of sensory information processing in autism (Boddaert et al., 2003; Ceponiene et al., 2003). Quite likely, these findings reflect developmental abnormalities, and as such, they are in accordance with hypotheses on impaired integration of cortical information in autism. Basically, these theories state that cortical regions do not operate in synchrony, but show disorganized and inadequately selective development of connectivity (Rippon et al., 2007; Just et al., 2004; Belmonte, Allen, et al., 2004). Especially impaired connectivity between the frontal lobe and other systems has been implicated in autism (Courchesne, & Pierce, 2005). A growing body of evidence lends support for aberrant connectivity in autism, including deficits in physical connectivity, such as histopathology findings of neuroinflammatory microglial activation (Vargas et al., 2005), the abnormal developmental trajectory of brain size (Redcay & Courchesne, 2005), decreases in white matter structure integrity measured with DTI (Keller et al., 2007; Barnea-Goraly et al., 2004; Alexander et al., 2007), and deficits in computative connectivity measured as the synchrony of time series of activation of cortical regions (Kana et al., 2006; Wilson et al., 2006). Although it is tempting to ascribe a unidirectional causal relation to deficits in connectivity and impairments in autism such as abnormal language development, a bidirectional relation between connectivity and functional impairments in autism is more likely. In healthy adults, white matter integrity changes over time (Snook et al., 2005), suggesting that experiences influence neural connectivity. The sociocommunicative deficits in autism could likewise give rise to abnormal connectivity.

Yet, it has been argued that, in autism, genetic factors in interaction with environmental influences lead to an abnormal neural architecture that causes either increased or reduced neural connectivity, or both (Belmonte, Cook, et al., 2004). Both conditions could cause an abnormally low signal-to-noise ratio in developing neural assemblies, given the fact that there is excess noise in hyperconnected systems and the signal gets lost in the noise in hypoconnected systems. This may result in a failure to delimit activation in perceptual processing centers, forcing higher processing mechanisms to actively suppress irrelevant sensory information at a later, less efficient stage. These compensatory mechanisms can presumably not be reset as quickly as the normal mechanisms of selective attention. Empirically, the allocation of neural resources during higher-order language tasks does indeed seem to be more task-indifferent in autistic individuals than in controls. The observation of less flexible network regrouping in autism during different language task conditions (see also "Higher-Level Language Paradigms," above) can possibly be explained by the high neural demands that active filtering of relevant stimuli imposes (Belmonte, Cook, et al., 2004).

More direct evidence suggesting reduced cortico-cortico connectivity during language tasks in collaborating cortical areas has been provided as well (Just et al., 2004; Kana et al., 2006). Intraregional underconnectivity during a simple auditory task has also been reported (Wilson et al., 2006). The high-level processing deficits of linguistic stimuli might arise when an unfiltered flood of linguistic information reaches higher information processing units that have to evaluate and actively suppress irrelevant sensory inputs. The greater reliance on Wernicke's area for linguistic processing in autism (Just et al., 2004) might thus result from compensatory developmental processes that lead to a more self-reliant Wernicke's area. In a MEG study on contextual integration, semantic violations induced greater gamma-oscillations in the autism group (Braeutigam et al., 2008). Gamma oscillations reflect an increase in local collaboration, or local binding (Tallon-Baudry & Bertrand, 2006). Thus, this finding may reflect a failure to delimit activation in perceptual processing centers. There is a certain charm to this model of local over- and interregional underconnectivity in autism, since it elegantly explains behavioral findings of reduced integration of information in autism. Smith et al. found that individuals with autism benefited less from the addition of visual information (lipreading) in audiovisual speech perception (Smith & Bennetto, 2007). The integration of the two information streams was uniquely affected in the autism group. Data by Groen et al. demonstrated that children with autism were less able to integrate speech fragments so that they could be perceived as words (Groen et al., 2009). However, interpreting these behavioral data as evidence for impaired cortical synchronization in autism would be circular reasoning. More direct evidence of abnormal cortical synchrony in autism is needed to add strength to this model.

The Relationship Between Linguistic Impairments and Social and Restricted/ Repetitive Impairments in Autism

It should be noted that linguistic and communicative impairments comprise only one third of the triad of impairments in autism. Whether or not abnormal connectivity and the genetic constellation associated with communicative abilities contribute to the other behavioral domains in autism (social interaction and restricted and repetitive behaviors and interests) is unclear. This issue will be further discussed below.

The core deficits in autism are traditionally viewed as inherently intertwined, i.e., communicative, social and restricted/repetitive difficulties influence each other and are highly interdependent. Indeed, the acquisition of language is one of the strongest predictors of long-term positive academic and social outcome in children with autism (Gillberg, 1991). Conversely, joint attention and immediate imitation predict language ability at ages 3–4, and toy play and deferred imitation predict communication development at ages 4–6 (Toth et al., 2006). However, recent behavioral-genetic data from a large general population-based twin-pair study indicate that phenotypic correlations between traits usually associated with autism (social interaction, repetitive-restrictive behaviors, and communication) are low (Ronald et al., 2006). Even social interaction and communicative abilities were only modestly clustered with correlations of 0.2 to 0.4 (Happe et al., 2006). Furthermore, although each aspect of the triad of impairments was found to be highly heritable, cross-trait, cross-twin correlations were low, suggesting that most genetic effects are specific to one of the core symptoms. One might argue that these behavioral-genetic findings suggest that the neural underpinning of the separate parts of the triad of symptoms is trait-specific as well. However, a different pattern of genetic and environmental causal factors for each of the symptom domains of autism does not preclude the possibility of a common neural deficit. In fact, each of these causal patterns may lead to a common neural deficit that further compromises other neural functions and give rise to the triad of symptoms in various degrees.

Genetic, Endophenotypical, and Behavioral Correspondence Between Autism and Language Impairments

In the DSM-IV, there is an explicit contrast between autism and specific language impairment. Children with SLI have a specific disability to acquire age-appropriate language, while development in all other domains is normal (American Psychiatric Association, 1994). Children with autism, by contrast, may not only have a delay in language development, other developmental domains are affected as well, and there are also linguistic deviations that are not normal for any stage of development (Bishop, 2002). Nevertheless, the linguistic deficits observed in specific language impairment resemble the language impairment in autism. Children with SLI usually have limited vocabularies, produce immature speech sounds, and use basic grammatical structures (Newbury et al., 2005). The profile of language performance among a subgroup of children with autism mirrors the profile of SLI: Poorer performance on tests of grammatical ability than vocabulary, and difficulties with nonword repetition (Tomblin & Zhang, 1999; Dollaghan & Campbell, 1998; Kjelgaard & Tager-Flusberg, 2001). The overlap in both disorders suggests that autism and SLI involve a shared neural substrate and one or more shared genes (Kjelgaard & Tager-Flusberg, 2001). Family members of probands with autism have a higher than chance rate of language impairments, and family members of probands with SLI are at risk for autism (Piven & Palmer, 1997; Tomblin et al., 2003). However, parents of children with autism and parents of typically developing children did not differ in their language abilities, while parents of children with SLI performed less well on language tasks (Whitehouse et al., 2007). This may indicate that there are additional genes involved in SLI that are not present in families with autism. Interestingly, phenotypic similarity at a neural level has been found between language impaired boys with autism and boys with SLI (DeFosse et al., 2004). Segmented MRI scans showed larger right than left frontal language association cortexes in both groups. Since the inversed asymmetry was not present in the autism group that was linguistically unimpaired, these results also suggest that there is a common underlying (genetic) cause for the language impairments in autism and SLI. The CNTNAP2 gene on 7q32, involved in nerve cell communication, is associated with autism and SLI (Alarcon et al., 2008), which suggests that this genetic pathway could bridge the common elements of both disorders.

Conclusion

Parents often start being concerned about the development of their child when they notice delays in the development of speech, and a delay or lack of speech is one of the defining criteria in autism. Yet, linguistic functioning is highly variable among people with this disorder. At one end of the autism spectrum there are children whose verbal abilities are within the normal range of functioning, and at the other there are some who never start to speak. In those with sufficient language and cognitive abilities, social communicative abilities remain impaired. Language tends to be used one-sidedly, nonreciprocally, and instrumentally rather than for social purposes. When examined systematically, semantic, syntactic, and pragmatic deficits can be seen in most people with autism. A smaller number are known to have deficits in articulation.

Autism is a neurodevelopmental disorder with a complex, probably polygenic origin (Fisch, 2008), and the development of the brain is a dynamic process that is constantly evolving and changing in concert with the environment. It is therefore not surprising that research on the neural correlates of language deficits in autism has produced many different results that are hard to cover under one umbrella-model. However, a growing number of findings converge to the idea that early sensory impairments and atypical neural connectivity are likely to play a part in abnormal language acquisition in autism. That is, abnormal processing of low-level linguistic information points to perceptual difficulties, and impairments of information processing may lead to an abnormal developmental trajectory of language in autism. Abnormal high-level

Table 10–1.
Phenotype, brain structure, brain function, and genetics in autism and specific language impairment

	Autism Spectrum Disorders	Specific Language Impairment
Phenotype	• School age: Deficits in higher order language skills (comprehension and production of discourse and pragmatic language skills) are more severe than deficits in and syntax and semantics. Phonology is least affected. • Preschool age: All levels of language, both in expressive and receptive language. In the majority of children the phonologic and most of the syntactic impairments resolve over time. • Note: Some authors report subtypes with affected syntax-phonology and affected semantics pragmatics. • Echolalic and idiosyncratic utterances and pronoun reversal are common. • Language function is highly variable. Some individuals have superior language skills, sometimes present at a very young age.	• School age: Deficits in phonology and syntax are more severe than deficits in higher order lexical or pragmatic language skills, both in expressive and receptive language. • Preschool age: All levels of language, both in expressive and receptive language. The phonologic and syntactic typically do not resolve. • Note: Different subtypes are reported: Expressive phonological impairment, mixed receptive phonologic and syntactic impairment, lexical syntactic impairment, semantic-pragmatic impairment. • Echolalic and idiosyncratic utterances and pronoun reversal are rare.
Brain structure	• Larger head size in majority of children. • Reduced left-right hemispheric asymmetry.	• Larger head size in fraction of children. • Reduced left-right hemispheric asymmetry.
Brain function	• Increased activation of Wernicke's area and decreased activation of Broca's area. • Reduced left-right hemispheric asymmetry. • Task indifferent pattern of activation during language tasks (possibly reflecting less flexible network regrouping).	• Decreased activation of both Wernicke's and Broca's area. (not replicated, as a sufficient number of studies on this subject is lacking)
Genetics	• Linkage to 13q21 is involved in (language impairments in) autism. • Linkage to 7q is related to autism, but FOXP2 on 7q31 was found to be unrelated to autism (despite previous reports). • CNTNAP2 on 7q35 is associated with autism and is thought to be involved in nerve cell communication.	• 13q21 involved in literacy impairment but not in SLI. • The FOXP2 gene on 7q31 is related to a language disorder with orofacial dyspraxia, but it is not related to common forms of SLI. • CNTNAP2 is associated with SLI.

linguistic processing of the frontal and temporal language association cortices suggests that neural subsystems may be more self-reliant and less connected. In addition to these processes, the development of the brain in autism also relies on the environment that children with autism create for themselves. The double handicap of linguistic and pragmatic-social impairments prevents individuals with autism to fall back on adequate compensation strategies. Future interventions and investigations will need to carefully consider how the biological, environmental, and developmental features of language in autism are intertwined, and perhaps differently so for different individuals.

Challenges and Future Directions

- Future research should attempt to increase our understanding of the language problems in autism at various levels. Issues that ask for further exploration are:
  - the context-dependency of semantic, syntactic, and pragmatic language skills in autism, and the influence of implicit versus explicit learning processes to extract meaningful information from ongoing verbal discourse and communication.
  - It is unclear how the emotional context impacts linguistic understanding and production of subjects with autism. So far, research in emotion understanding and responding in autism has been focused almost exclusively on processing of visual stimuli, such as facial expressions of emotions. Much psycholinguistic research has been done on processing emotion words. An important finding is that valence and arousal of emotion words are processed separately by different brain areas. The amygdala, dorsomedial prefrontal cortex (PFC), and ventromedial PFC have been found to be associated with the arousal value of stimuli (Lewis et al., 2007; Kensinger et al., 2006), while valence is correlated with differential activity in the orbitofrontal cortex (Lewis et al., 2006) and the lateral regions

of prefrontal cortex (Kensinger et al.2006), although some studies have found amygdala response to valence as well (Anders et al., 2008). These two separate strings of research, i.e., research in emotion understanding and research in language abnormalities, should be brought more closely together.

- Another challenge is to integrate research in autism with that in SLI. This would include not only aggregating molecular-genetic data of samples with autism and SLI and testing for shared genetic risk factors, but also developing standardized neural system approaches to produce structural and functional maps of key language functions. For example, activations to the inferior frontal cortical areas in speaker identity paradigms (Groen et al., 2009) and functional connectivity between Broca and Wernicke's language areas may serve as intermediate phenotypes to define more homogeneous samples for molecular genetic studies. This will all converge in significant advances in our understanding of the molecular base of autism and the neural pathways to language impairments as one of the key symptom domains of autism.

SUGGESTED READINGS

Herbert, M. R., & Kenet, T. (2007). Brain abnormalities in language disorders and in autism. *Pediatric Clinics of North America, 54,* 563–583.

Williams, D., Botting, N., & Boucher, J. (2008). Language in autism and specific language impairment: Where are the links? *Psychological Bulletin, 134,* 944–963.

ACKNOWLEDGMENT

This chapter is based on Groen, W. B., Zwiers, M. P., van der Gaag, R. J., and Buitelaar, J. K. (2008). The phenotype and neural correlates of language in autism: An integrative review. *Neuroscience and Biobehavioral Reviews, 32*(8), 1416–1425.

REFERENCES

Abell, F., Krams, M., Ashburner, J., Passingham, R., Friston, K., Frackowiak, R., et al. (1999). The neuroanatomy of autism: A voxel-based whole brain analysis of structural scans. *Neuroreport, 10,* 1647–1651.

Alarcón, M., Abrahams, B. S., Stone J. L., Duvall J. A., Perederiy J. V., Bomar J. M., Sebat, J., Wigler, M., Martin C. L., Ledbetter D. H., Nelson S. F., Cantor R. M., & Geschwind D. H. (2008). Linkage, association, and gene-expression analyses identify CNTNAP2 as an autism-susceptibility gene. *American Journal of Human Genetics, 82*(1), 150–159.

Alexander, A. L., Lee, J. E., Lazar, M., Boudos, R., Dubray, M. B., Oakes, T. R., et al. (2007). Diffusion tensor imaging of the corpus callosum in Autism. *NeuroImage, 34,* 61–73.

Allen, G., Muller, R. A., & Courchesne, E. (2004). Cerebellar function in autism: Functional magnetic resonance image activation during a simple motor task. *Biological Psychiatry, 56,* 269–278.

American Psychiatric Association. (1994). *Diagnostic and statistical manual of mental disorders.* Washington, DC: Author.

Anders, S., Eippert, F., Weiskopf, N., & Veit R. (2008). The human amygdala is sensitive to the valence of pictures and sounds irrespective of arousal: An fMRI study. *Social Cognitive and Affective Neuroscience, 3,* 233–243.

Asperger, H. (1991). Autistic psychopathy (translation of the original paper by U. Frith). In U. Frith (Ed.), *Autism and Asperger syndrome.* Cambridge: Cambridge University Press.

Barnea-Goraly, N., Kwon, H., Menon, V., Eliez, S., Lotspeich, L., & Reiss, A. L. (2004). White matter structure in autism: Preliminary evidence from diffusion tensor imaging. *Biological Psychiatry, 55,* 323–326.

Baron-Cohen, S., Leslie, A. M., & Frith, U. (1985). Does the autistic child have a "theory of mind"? *Cognition, 21,* 37–46.

Baron-Cohen, S. (1997). Hey! It was just a joke! Understanding propositions and propositional attitudes by normally developing children and children with autism. *Israel Journal of Psychiatry and Related Sciences, 34,* 174–178.

Bartak, L., Rutter, M., & Cox, A. (1975). A comparative study of infantile autism and specific development receptive language disorder. I. The children. *British Journal of Psychiatry, 126,* 127–145.

Bartolucci, G., & Albers, R. J. (1974). Deictic categories in the language of autistic children. *Journal of Autism and Childhood Schizophrenia,* 131–141.

Bartolucci, G., Pierce, S. J., & Streiner, D. (1980). Cross-sectional studies of grammatical morphemes in autistic and mentally retarded children. *Journal of Autism and Developmental Disorders, 10,* 39–50.

Bartolucci, G., Pierce, S., Streiner, D., & Eppel, P. T. (1976). Phonological investigation of verbal autistic and mentally retarded subjects. *Journal of Autism and Childhood Schizophrenia,* 303–316.

Bates, E. (1976). *Language in context.* New York: Academic.

Belmonte, M. K., Allen, G., Beckel-Mitchener, A., Boulanger, L. M., Carper, R. A., & Webb, S. J. (2004). Autism and abnormal development of brain connectivity. *Journal of Neuroscience, 24,* 9228–9231.

Belmonte, M. K., Cook, E. H., Jr., Anderson, G. M., Rubenstein, J. L., Greenough, W. T., Beckel-Mitchener, A., et al. (2004). Autism as a disorder of neural information processing: Directions for research and targets for therapy. *Molecular Psychiatry,* 646–663.

Bertone, A., Mottron, L., Jelenic, P., & Faubert, J. (2005). Enhanced and diminished visuo-spatial information processing in autism depends on stimulus complexity. *Brain, 128,* 2430–2441.

Bishop, D. V. (2002) Speech and language difficulties. In M. Rutter & E. Taylor (Eds.), *Child and adolescent psychiatry.* Malden, MA: Blackwell.

Boddaert, N., Belin, P., Chabane, N., Poline, J. B., Barthelemy, C., Mouren-Simeoni, M. C., et al. (2003). Perception of complex sounds: Abnormal pattern of cortical activation in autism. *American Journal of Psychiatry, 160,* 2057–2060.

Boddaert, N., Chabane, N., Belin, P., Bourgeois, M., Royer, V., Barthelemy, C., et al. (2004). Perception of complex sounds in autism: Abnormal auditory cortical processing in children. *American Journal of Psychiatry, 161,* 2117–2120.

Boddaert, N., Chabane, N., Gervais, H., Good, C. D., Bourgeois, M., Plumet, M. H., et al. (2004). Superior temporal sulcus anatomical abnormalities in childhood autism: A voxel-based morphometry MRI study. *NeuroImage, 23*, 364–369.

Bookheimer, S. (2002). Functional MRI of language: New approaches to understanding the cortical organization of semantic processing. *Annual Review of Neuroscience, 25*, 151–188.

Boucher, J. (2003). Language development in autism. *International Journal of Pediatric Otorhinolaryngology, 67*(Suppl 1), S159–S163.

Braeutigam, S., Swithenby, S. J., & Bailey, A. J. (2008). Contextual integration the unusual way: A magnetoencephalographic study of responses to semantic violation in individuals with autism spectrum disorders. *European Journal of Neuroscience, 27*, 1026–1036.

Bruneau, N., Roux, S., Adrien, Jean L., & Barthelemy, C. (1999). Auditory associative cortex dysfunction in children with autism: Evidence from late auditory evoked potentials (N1 wave-T complex). *Clinical Neurophysiology, 110*, 1927–1934.

Cantwell, D., Baker, L., & Rutter, M. (1978). A comparative study of infantile autism and specific developmental receptive language disorder—IV. Analysis of syntax and language function. *Journal of Child Psychology and Psychiatry, 19*, 351–362.

Carper, R. A., Moses, P., Tigue, Z. D., & Courchesne, E. (2002). Cerebral lobes in autism: Early hyperplasia and abnormal age effects. *NeuroImage, 16*, 1038–1051.

Ceponiene, R., Lepisto, T., Shestakova, A., Vanhala, R., Alku, P., Naatanen, R., et al. (2003). Speech-sound-selective auditory impairment in children with autism: They can perceive but do not attend. *Proceedings of the National Academy of Sciences of the United States of America, 100*, 5567–5572.

Chiron, C., Leboyer, M., Leon, F., Jambaque, I., Nuttin, C., & Syrota, A. (1995). SPECT of the brain in childhood autism: Evidence for a lack of normal hemispheric asymmetry. *Developmental Medicine and Child Neurology, 37*, 849–860.

Colle, L., Baron-Cohen, S., & Hill, J. (2007). Do children with autism have a theory of mind? A non-verbal test of autism vs. specific language impairment. *Journal of Autism and Developmental Disorders, 37*, 716–723.

Courchesne, E., Karns, C. M., Davis, H. R., Ziccardi, R., Carper, R. A., Tigue, Z. D., et al. (2001). Unusual brain growth patterns in early life in patients with autistic disorder: An MRI study. *Neurology, 57*, 245–254.

Courchesne, E., & Pierce, K. (2005). Why the frontal cortex in autism might be talking only to itself: Local over-connectivity but long-distance disconnection. *Current Opinion in Neurobiology, 15*, 225–230.

Courchesne, E., Redcay, E., Morgan, J. T., & Kennedy, D. P. (2005). Autism at the beginning: Microstructural and growth abnormalities underlying the cognitive and behavioral phenotype of autism. *Development and Psychopathology, 17*, 577–597.

Cox, A., Rutter, M., Newman, S., & Bartak, L. (1975). A comparative study of infantile autism and specific developmental receptive language disorder. II. Parental characteristics. *British Journal of Psychiatry, 126*, 146–159.

Dawson, G., Finley, C., Phillips, S., & Lewy, A. (1989). A comparison of hemispheric asymmetries in speech-related brain potentials of autistic and dysphasic children. *Brain and Language, 37*, 26–41.

Dawson, G., Meltzoff, A. N., Osterling, J., Rinaldi, J., & Brown, E. (1998). Children with autism fail to orient to naturally occurring social stimuli. *Journal of Autism and Developmental Disorders, 28*, 479–485.

De Villiers, J., & De Villiers, P. (1995). Steps in the mastery of sentence complements. Paper presented at the biennial meeting of the Society for Research in Child Development. Indianapolis.

DeFosse, L., Hodge, S. M., Makris, N., Kennedy, D. N., Caviness, V. Jr, McGrath, L., et al. (2004). Language-association cortex asymmetry in autism and specific language impairment. *Annals of Neurology, 56*, 757–766.

Dollaghan, C., & Campbell, T. F. (1998). Nonword repetition and child language impairment. *Journal of Speech, Language, and Hearing Research, 41*, 1136–1146.

Dronkers, N. F. (2000). The pursuit of brain-language relationships. *Brain and Language, 71*, 59–61.

Dunn, L., Dunn, L., Whetton, C., & Burley, J. (1997). *British Picture Vocabulary Scale: revised.* Slough, Bucks: NFER Nelson.

Dunn, L. M., & Dunn, M. (1997). *Peabody picture vocabulary test.* Circle Pines, MN: American Guidance Service.

Eigsti, I. M., Bennetto, L., & Dadlani, M. B. (2007). Beyond pragmatics: Morphosyntactic development in autism. *Journal of Autism and Developmental Disorders, 37*, 1007–1023.

Eskes, G. A., Bryson, S. E., & McCormick, T. A. (1990). Comprehension of concrete and abstract words in autistic children. *Journal of Autism and Developmental Disorders, 20*, 61–73.

Fine, J., Bartolucci, G., Szatmari, P., & Ginsberg, G. (1994). Cohesive discourse in pervasive developmental disorders. *Journal of Autism and Developmental Disorders, 24*, 315–329.

Fisch, G. S. (2008). Syndromes and epistemology II: Is autism a polygenic disorder? *American Journal of Medical Genetics. Part A, 146A*, 2203–2212.

Flagg, E. J., Cardy, J. E., Roberts, W., & Roberts, T. P. (2005). Language lateralization development in children with autism: Insights from the late field magnetoencephalogram. *Neuroscience Letters, 386*, 82–87.

Frith, U. (1996). Cognitive explanations of autism. *Acta Paediatrica Supplement, 416*, 63–68.

Frith, U., & Snowling, M. (1983). Reading for meaning and reading for sound in autistic and dyslexic children. *British Journal of Developmental Psychology, 1*, 329–342.

Gardner, M. (1982). *Expressive one word vocabulary test.* Los Angeles: Western Psychological Services.

Gendry-Meresse, I., Zilbovicius, M., Boddaert, N., Robel, L., Philippe, A., Sfaello, I., et al. (2005). Autism severity and temporal lobe functional abnormalities. *Annals of Neurology, 58*, 466–469.

Gervais, H., Belin, P., Boddaert, N., Leboyer, M., Coez, A., Sfaello, I., et al. (2004). Abnormal cortical voice processing in autism. *Nature Neuroscience*, 801–802.

Gillberg, C. (1991). Outcome in autism and autistic-like conditions. *Journal of the American Academy of Child and Adolescent Psychiatry, 30*, 375–382.

Groen, W. B., Tesink, C., Petersson, K. M., Van Berkum, J., Van der Gaag, R. J., Hagoort, P., et al. (2009). Semantic, factual, and social language comprehension in adolescents with autism: An FMRI study. *Cerebral Cortex Epub, 20*, 1937–1945.

Groen, W. B., van Orsouw, L., Zwiers, M., Swinkels, S., van der Gaag, R. J., & Buitelaar, J. K. (2008). Gender in voice perception in autism. *Journal of Autism and Developmental Disorders 38*, 1819–1826.

Groen, W. B., van Orsouw, L., Huurne, N., Swinkels, S., van der Gaag, R. J., Buitelaar, J. K., et al. (2009). Intact spectral but abnormal temporal processing of auditory stimuli in autism. *Journal of Autism and Developmental Disorders, 39*, 742–750.

Gustafsson, L. (1997). Inadequate cortical feature maps: A neural circuit theory of autism. *Biological Psychiatry, 42*, 1138–1147.

Hagoort, P., Hald, L., Bastiaansen, M., & Petersson, K. M. (2004). Integration of word meaning and world knowledge in language comprehension. *Science, 304*, 438–441.

Happe, F. G. (1993). Communicative competence and theory of mind in autism: A test of relevance theory. *Cognition, 48*, 101–119.

Happe, F. G. (1997). Central coherence and theory of mind in autism: Reading homographs in context. *British Journal of Developmental Psychology, 15*, 1–12.

Happe, F., & Frith, U. (2006). The weak coherence account: Detail-focused cognitive style in autism spectrum disorders. *Journal of Autism and Development Disorders, 36*, 5–25.

Happe, F., Ronald, A., & Plomin, R. (2006). Time to give up on a single explanation for autism. *Nature Neuroscience*, 1218–1220.

Harris, G. J., Chabris, C. F., Clark, J., Urban, T., Aharon, I., Steele, S., et al. (2006). Brain activation during semantic processing in autism spectrum disorders via functional magnetic resonance imaging. *Brain and Cognition, 61*, 54–68.

Heaton, P., Hudry, K., Ludlow, A., & Hill, E. (2008). Superior discrimination of speech pitch and its relationship to verbal ability in autism spectrum disorders. *Cognitive Neuropsychology, 25*, 771–782.

Herbert, M. R., Harris, G. J., Adrien, K. T., Ziegler, D. A., Makris, N., Kennedy, D. N., et al. (2002). Abnormal asymmetry in language association cortex in autism. *Annals of Neurology, 52*, 588–596.

Herbert, M. R., & Kenet, T. (2007). Brain abnormalities in language disorders and in autism. *Pediatric Clinics of North America, 54*, 563–583.

Herbert, M. R., Ziegler, D. A., Deutsch, C. K., O'Brien, L. M., Lange, N., Bakardjiev, A., et al. (2003). Dissociations of cerebral cortex, subcortical, and cerebral white matter volumes in autistic boys. *Brain, 126*, 1182–1192.

Hillis, A. E. (2007). Aphasia: Progress in the last quarter of a century. *Neurology, 69*, 200–213.

Hobson, R. P., & Lee, A. (1989). Emotion-related and abstract concepts in autistic people: Evidence from the British Picture Vocabulary Scale. *Journal of Autism and Developmental Disorders, 19*, 601–623.

Howlin, P. (2003). Outcome in high-functioning adults with autism with and without early language delays: Implications for the differentiation between autism and Asperger syndrome. *Journal of Autism and Developmental Disorders, 33*, 3–13.

Jolliffe, T., & Baron-Cohen, S. (2000). Linguistic processing in high-functioning adults with autism or Asperger's syndrome. Is global coherence impaired? *Psychological Medicine, 30*, 1169–1187.

Just, M. A., Cherkassky, V. L., Keller, T. A., & Minshew, N. J. (2004). Cortical activation and synchronization during sentence comprehension in high-functioning autism: Evidence of underconnectivity. *Brain, 127*, 1811–1821.

Kana, R. K., Keller, T. A., Cherkassky, V. L., Minshew, N. J., & Just, M. A. (2006). Sentence comprehension in autism: Thinking in pictures with decreased functional connectivity. *Brain, 129*, 2484–2493.

Kanner, L. (1943). Autistic disturbances of affective contact. *Nervous Child, 2*, 217–250.

Kasai, K., Hashimoto, O., Kawakubo, Y., Yumoto, M., Kamio, S., Itoh, K., et al. (2005). Delayed automatic detection of change in speech sounds in adults with autism: A magnetoencephalographic study. *Clinical Neurophysiology, 116*, 1655–1664.

Keller, T. A., Kana, R. K., & Just, M. A. (2007). A developmental study of the structural integrity of white matter in autism. *Neuroreport, 18*, 23–27.

Kensinger, E. A., & Schacter, D. L. (2006). Processing emotional pictures and words: Effects of valence and arousal. *Cognitive, Affective, and Behavioral Neuroscience*, 110–126.

Kjelgaard, M. M., & Tager-Flusberg, H. (2001). An investigation of language impairment in autism: Implications for genetic subgroups. *Language and Cognitive Processes, 16*, 287–308.

Klin, A. (1991). Young autistic children's listening preferences in regard to speech: A possible characterization of the symptom of social withdrawal. *Journal of Autism and Developmental Disorders, 21*, 29–42.

Kuhl, P. K., Tsao, F. M., & Liu, H. M. (2003). Foreign-language experience in infancy: Effects of short-term exposure and social interaction on phonetic learning. *Proceedings of the National Academy of Sciences of the United States of America, 100*, 9096–9101.

Levitt, J. G., Blanton, R. E., Smalley, S., Thompson, P. M., Guthrie, D., McCracken, J. T., et al. (2003). Cortical sulcal maps in autism. *Cerebral Cortex, 13*, 728–735.

Lewis, P. A., Critchley, H. D., Rotshtein, P., & Dolan, R. J. (2007). Neural correlates of processing valence and arousal in affective words. *Cerebral Cortex, 17*, 742–748.

Lord, C., & Paul, R. (1997) Language and communication in autism. In D. Cohen & F. R. Volkmar (Eds.), *Handbook of autism and pervasive developmental disorders.* New York: Wiley.

Martin, I., & McDonald, S. (2004). An exploration of causes of non-literal language problems in individuals with Asperger syndrome. *Journal of Autism and Developmental Disorders, 34*, 311–328.

Muller, R. A., Behen, M. E., Rothermel, R. D., Chugani, D. C., Muzik, O., Mangner, T. J., et al. (1999). Brain mapping of language and auditory perception in high-functioning autistic adults: A PET study. *Journal of Autism and Developmental Disorders, 29*, 19–31.

Muller, R. A., Chugani, D. C., Behen, M. E., Rothermel, R. D., Muzik, O., Chakraborty, P. K., et al. (1998). Impairment of dentato-thalamo-cortical pathway in autistic men: Language activation data from positron emission tomography. *Neuroscience Letters, 245*, 1–4.

Nazzi, T., & Bertoncini, J. (2003). Before and after the vocabulary spurt: Two modes of word acquisition? *Developmental Science*, 136–142.

Newbury, D. F., Bishop, D. V., & Monaco, A. P. (2005). Genetic influences on language impairment and phonological short-term memory. *Trends in Cognitive Sciences*, 528–534.

Oram Cardy, J. E., Flagg, E. J., Roberts, W., & Roberts, T. P. (2005). Delayed mismatch field for speech and non-speech sounds in children with autism. *Neuroreport, 16*, 521–525.

Palmen, S. J., & van Engeland, H. (2004). Review on structural neuroimaging findings in autism. *Journal of Neural Transmission, 111*, 903–929.

Paul, R., Augustyn, A., Klin, A., & Volkmar, F. R. (2005). Perception and production of prosody by speakers with autism spectrum disorders. *Journal of Autism and Development Disorders, 35*, 205–220.

Perkins, M. R., Dobbinson, S., Boucher, J., Bol, S., & Bloom, P. (2006). Lexical knowledge and lexical use in autism. *Journal of Autism and Developmental Disorders, 36*, 795–805.

Piven, J., & Palmer, P. (1997). Cognitive deficits in parents from multiple-incidence autism families. *Journal of Child Psychology and Psychiatry, 38*, 1011–1021.

Price, C., Indefrey, P., & Turenhout, M. (1999)The neural architecture underlying the processing of written and spoken word forms. In C. M. Brown & P. Hagoort (Eds.), *The neurocognition of language.* New York: Oxford University Press.

Rapin, I., & Dunn, M. (2003). Update on the language disorders of individuals on the autistic spectrum. *Brain and Development, 25*, 166–172.

Redcay, E., & Courchesne, E. (2005). When is the brain enlarged in autism? A meta-analysis of all brain size reports. *Biological Psychiatry, 58*, 1–9.

Rippon, G., Brock, J., Brown, C., & Boucher, J. (2007). Disordered connectivity in the autistic brain: Challenges for the "new psychophysiology." *International Journal of Psychophysiology, 63*, 164–172.

Roberts, J. A., Rice, M. L., & Tager-Flusberg, H. (2004). Tense marking in children with autism. *Applied Psycholinguistics, 25*, 429–448.

Ronald, A., Happe, F., Price, T. S., Baron-Cohen, S., & Plomin, R. (2006). Phenotypic and genetic overlap between autistic traits at the extremes of the general population. *Journal of the American Academy of Child and Adolescent Psychiatry, 45*, 1206–1214.

Rutherford, M. D., Baron Cohen, S., & Wheelwright, S. (2002). Reading the mind in the voice: A study with normal adults and adults with Asperger syndrome and high functioning autism. *Journal of Autism and Developmental Disorders, 32*, 189–194.

Shriberg, L. D., Paul, R., McSweeny, J. L., Klin, A. M., Cohen, D. J., & Volkmar, F. R. (2001). Speech and prosody characteristics of adolescents and adults with high-functioning autism and Asperger syndrome. *Journal of Speech, Language, and Hearing Research, 44*, 1097–1115.

Smith, E. G., & Bennetto, L. (2007). Audiovisual speech integration and lipreading in autism. *Journal of Child Psychology and Psychiatry, 48*, 813–821.

Smitz, C. (2005). New aspects in the neuropathology of the forebrain in autism. Paper presented at Integrating the Clinical and Basic Sciences of Autism: A Developmental Biology Workshop.

Snook, L., Paulson, L. A., Roy, D., Phillips, L., & Beaulieu, C. (2005). Diffusion tensor imaging of neurodevelopment in children and young adults. *NeuroImage, 26*, 1164–1173.

Tager-Flusberg, H. (1981). On the nature of linguistic functioning in early infantile autism. *Journal of Autism and Developmeental Disorders, 11*, 45–56.

Tager-Flusberg, H. (1996). Brief report: Current theory and research on language and communication in autism. *Journal of Autism and Developmental Disorders, 26*, 169–172.

Tager-Flusberg H. (2000). *Language and understanding minds: Connections in autism.* In S. Baron-Cohen, H. Tager-Flusberg, & D. Cohen (Eds.), Oxford, Oxford University Press.

Tager-Flusberg H., Paul, R., & Lord, C. (2005) Language and communication in autism. In F. Volkmar, R.Paul, A. Klin, D. Cohen. (Eds), *Handbook of autism and pervasive developmental disorders.* New York: Wiley.

Tager-Flusberg, H., & Sullivan, K. (1995). Attributing mental states to story characters: A comparison of narratives produced by autistic and mentally retarded individuals. *Applied Psycholinguist, 16*, 241–256.

Takeuchi, M., Harada, M., Matsuzaki, K., Nishitani, H., & Mori, K. (2004). Difference of signal change by a language task on autistic patients using functional MRI. *Journal of Medical Investigation, 51*, 59–62.

Tallon-Baudry, C., & Bertrand, O. (2006). Gamma oscillations in humans. *Encyclopedia of Cognitive Science*, 1–6.

Tantam, D., Holmes, D., & Cordess, C. (1993). Nonverbal expression in autism of Asperger type. *Journal of Autism and Developmental Disorders, 23*, 111–133.

Tomblin, J. B., Hafeman, L. L., & O'Brien, M. (2003). Autism and autism risk in siblings of children with specific language impairment. *International Journal of Language and Communication Disorders, 38*, 235–250.

Tomblin, J. B., & Zhang, X. (1999) Language patterns and etiology in children with specific language impairment. In H. Tager-Flusberg (Ed.), *Neurodevelopmental disorders.* Cambridge, MA: MIT Press/Bradford Books.

Toth, K., Munson, J., Meltzoff, A. N., & Dawson, G. (2006). Early predictors of communication development in young children with autism spectrum disorder: Joint attention, imitation, and toy play. *Journal of Autism and Developmental Disorders, 36*, 993–1005.

Vargas, D. L., Nascimbene, C., Krishnan, C., Zimmerman, A. W., & Pardo, C. A. (2005). Neuroglial activation and neuroinflammation in the brain of patients with autism. *Annals of Neurology, 57*, 67–81.

Venter, A., Lord, C., & Schopler, E. (1992). A follow-up study of high-functioning autistic children. *Journal of Child Psychology and Psychiatry, 33*, 489–507.

Wang, A. T., Lee, S. S., Sigman, M., & Dapretto, M. (2006). Neural basis of irony comprehension in children with autism: The role of prosody and context. *Brain, 129*, 932–943.

Wang, A. T., Lee, S. S., Sigman, M., & Dapretto, M. (2007). Reading affect in the face and voice: Neural correlates of interpreting communicative intent in children and adolescents with autism spectrum disorders. *Archives of General Psychiatry, 64*, 698–708.

Whitehouse, A. J. O., Barry, J. G., & Bishop, D. V. M. (2007). The broader language phenotype of autism: A comparison with specific language impairment. *Journal of Child Psychology and Psychiatry, 48*, 822–830.

Williams, K. T. (1997). *Expressive vocabulary test.* Circle Pines, MN: American Guidance Service.

Wilson, T. W., Rojas, D. C., Reite, M. L., Teale, P. D., & Rogers, S. J. (2006). Children and adolescents with autism exhibit reduced MEG steady-state gamma responses. *Biological Psychiatry, 62*, 192–196.

11 James W. Bodfish

Repetitive Behaviors in Individuals with Autism Spectrum Disorders

Points of Interest

- A wide variety of discrete types of repetitive behaviors occurs in persons with autism spectrum disorders, including stereotyped movements, rituals and elaborate routines, insistence on sameness, and circumscribed interests, preoccupations, and attachments.
- Repetitive behaviors can be among the earliest recognized signs of autism in infants who go on to receive an ASD diagnosis and they tend to persist into adulthood in individuals with ASD.
- Repetitive behaviors can be associated with significant functional impairments; in at least a subset of cases repetitive behaviors and interests can significantly interfere with learning and socialization, and can be associated with mood and behavior problems that drive the need for intervention.

Repetitive behavior is one of three core features of autism (ICD-10, World Health Organization, 1990; DSM-IV, American Psychiatric Association, 1994). Repetitive behaviors frequently dominate the daily activity of children with autism, can significantly interfere with opportunities to develop functional behaviors, and are frequently the target of intervention and treatment. This is a rapidly growing area of research in autism, and much is now known about the clinical phenomenology, developmental course, neurobiology, and treatment of repetitive behaviors. Further, gaps in the current knowledge base on repetitive behaviors represent critical new areas for research in the pathogenesis and treatment of autism.

A central theme in the recent research findings in repetitive behavior is that while all cases by definition have expressed repetitive behaviors, several distinct subtypes of repetitive behavior appear to exist across persons with autism spectrum disorders. These subtypes may represent a viable strategy for uncovering at least some of the multiple pathogenic factors responsible for the clear heterogeneity of phenotypic expression in autism. In addition, isolation and understanding of specific discrete subtypes may help direct the development of novel forms of intervention.

Phenomenology

Varieties of Repetitive Behavior in Autism

The term "repetitive behavior" is an umbrella term used to refer to a broad class of actions linked by repetition, rigidity, and inappropriateness. In the *Diagnostic and Statistical Manual of Mental Disorders–4th Edition* (DSM-IV; APA, 1994), criteria for repetitive behavior can be met by a person exhibiting at least one of the following: "(a) encompassing preoccupation with one or more stereotyped and restricted patterns of interest that is abnormal either in intensity or focus; (b) apparently inflexible adherence to specific, nonfunctional routines or rituals; (c) stereotyped and repetitive motor mannerisms (e.g., hand or finger flapping or twisting or complex whole-body movements); or (d) persistent preoccupation with parts of objects." What becomes clear on examination of these criteria is that they are very broad, ranging from repetitive movements of the body to more cognitively mediated symptoms such as intense interests or hobbies. Although no single type of repetitive behavior may be specific to autism, previous studies have found that it is a pattern of multiple types of repetitive behavior that can best distinguish autism from other disorders (Bodfish et al., 2000; Bartak & Rutter, 1976).

Stereotyped Movements

Repetitive motor movements (e.g., hand flapping, body rocking, arm waving, hand and finger movements, repetitive postures) are commonly observed in normally developing infants and young children (e.g., Evans et al., 1997; Thelen, 1979), and are also commonly observed in other developmental and psychiatric conditions such as Tourette's syndrome, Fragile X syndrome, Rett syndrome, Parkinson's disease, and schizophrenia (Frith & Done, 1990; Turner, 1996). Although few studies have sought to compare the nature of repetitive motor behavior across clinical groups, there is evidence to suggest that there are important differences in the display of at least some forms of this behavior in autistic and nonautistic populations. In persons with mental retardation, the occurrence of stereotyped movements appears to be related to mental age (Smith & Van Houten, 1996). In contrast, individuals with autism engage in more frequent, severe, and longer bouts of stereotyped movements compared to age and ability matched controls (Freeman et al., 1981; Hermelin & O'Connor, 1963; Lord, 1995; Lord & Pickles, 1996; Szatmari, Bartolucci, & Bremner, 1989). Szatmari et al. (1989) showed that motor stereotypies were significantly more common in high-functioning adults with autism than in age and ability matched control subjects referred to outpatient psychiatry services for problems with social relationships (86% vs. 14%). Lord (1995), in her 12-month follow-up study of 2-year-olds referred for possible autism, reported that those who met diagnostic criteria for autism at age 3 showed significantly higher rates of stereotyped movements at ages 2 and 3 than those children failing to meet diagnostic criteria, despite the fact there was no difference between the groups in age of ability.

Repetitive Self-Injurious Behavior

There is evidence that certain forms of lower-order repetitive behavior such as repetitive self-injurious behavior (e.g., head hitting or banging, hand or arm biting) are not unique to autism. The self-injurious behavior described in autism is similar in prevalence to those described for individuals with nonspecific mental retardation (Freeman et al., 1981; McKenna, Thornton, & Turner, 1998). Furthermore, in autism, as in mental retardation, self-injury is negatively associated with IQ and positively correlated with severity of illness (Bartak & Rutter, 1976; Campbell et al., 1990; Freeman et al., 1981). Thus, it appears that repetitive self-injurious behavior in persons with autism is related to more nonspecific factors such as level of intellectual ability, or other associated developmental impairments.

Rituals and Routines

It can be difficult to distinguish the rigid and invariant routines that are described in autism (e.g., ordering, arranging, touching/tapping, hoarding), and the routines and rituals that are commonplace in individuals with obsessive compulsive disorder (e.g., de Silva, 1994), mental retardation (Lewis, Bodfish, Powell, & Golden, 1994), Tourette's syndrome (Swedo, Rapoport, Leonard, Lenane, & Cheslow, 1989), and many normal individuals. There has been little systematic comparison of the routines and rituals of autistic and nonautistic individuals. However, the limited evidence available indicates that these behaviors are significantly more prevalent and marked in individuals with autism relative to age and ability matched control subjects (Bartak & Rutter, 1976; Lord & Pickles, 1996). The extreme distress and catastrophic reaction shown by many autistic people in response to changes in routine is rarely described in nonautistic individuals. Similarly, rituals in autism are likely to be highly elaborate and extend to many areas of daily living (e.g., routines around self-care and dressing, eating routines, travel routines), whereas rituals in nonautistic individuals are largely restricted to personal activity (Turner, 1996). In support of these differences, Wing and Gould (1979) reported that the presence of elaborate routines differentiated those children and adolescents with a history of autism from those without (94% vs. 2%). To date, two studies have directly compared repetitive behavior presentation in autism and OCD (McDougle et al., 1995; Zandt, Prior, & Kyrios, 2006). Both studies found evidence for significant differences in repetitive behavior phenomenology; however, both focused primarily on compulsive/ritualistic kinds of repetitive behavior and consequently neither included a specific examination of the types of discrete repetitive behaviors frequently seen in autism (e.g., stereotyped movements, insistence on sameness, circumscribed interests).

Sameness and Resistance to Change

Although "insistence on sameness" is often considered to be specific to autism, only one study has explored the relative frequency of this class of behavior. Szatmari et al. (1989) reported such behavior to be significantly more common in high-functioning individuals with autism and Asperger's syndrome than in socially odd psychiatric control subjects, although specific prevalence rates were not given. The results of a study by Evans et al. (1997) indicate that this type of behavior is also characteristic of normally developing children between 2 and 4 years of age.

Interests, Preoccupations, and Attachments

Circumscribed interests in autism were originally described by Leo Kanner in his seminal paper in 1943 (Kanner, 1943). One case, Alfred L., was described in the following way:

> He has gradually shown a marked tendency toward developing one special interest which will completely dominate his day's activities. He talks of little else while the interest exists, he frets when he is not able to indulge in it (by seeing it, coming in contact with it, drawing pictures of it), and it is difficult to get his attention because of his preoccupation.

Circumscribed interests (also known as restricted behavior) range from preoccupations with highly unusual aspects of the environment (such as the serial numbers of electrical appliances) to intense and all-absorbing interests in more common hobbies (such as trains or computers). Szatmari et al. (1989) reported that 86% of a normally intelligent sample of individuals with autism had circumscribed interests in comparison to 37% of individuals diagnosed with Asperger's syndrome and 9% of outpatient control subjects. In contrast, Kerbeshian, Burd, and Fisher (1990) noted rates of 31% for high-functioning individuals with autism and 92% for individuals with Asperger's syndrome. It is sometimes assumed that circumscribed interests are more common in high-functioning individuals because they demand a higher level of ability. Although it is true that certain sophisticated circumscribed interests may be beyond the ability of some autistic individuals, it is likely for even severely disabled individuals with autism to demonstrate insistence on sameness or show very restricted patterns of interest and activity. The only study to compare levels of repetitive behavior in high and low ability individuals with autism reported that insistence on sameness was more commonly observed in mentally retarded, relative to normally intelligent, individuals with autism (82% vs. 42%), and both groups showed similar levels of circumscribed interests (71% vs. 84%) (Bartak & Rutter, 1976). DeLoache, Simcock, and Macari (2007) examined circumscribed interests in typically developing children and found that "extremely intense interests" (e.g., interest in tea sets, interest in brushes, interest in pouring liquids) occurred in 29% of their sample of 1 to 6 year olds. However, no clinical comparison group was included, and no screening or assessment of potential autism features/diagnoses was reported. Thus, while it is clear that focused interests and even perhaps unusual or circumscribed interests can occur in typically developing children, it is not clear if these persist in the same way that they do in autism or if they are associated with the same degree of functional impairment as appears to be the case in at least a subset of children and adults with autism.

While circumscribed interests (CI) per se are not indicative of autism, the results of previous studies of such interests in ASD provide information about the ways that interests in autism differ from interests seen in the course of typical development. Baron-Cohen and Wheelwright (1999) reported that persons with ASD were more likely to have interests that could be characterized within the knowledge domain of "folk physics," which involved knowledge about mechanical aspects of the world, as opposed to the domain of "folk psychology," which involves knowledge about social aspects of the world. Consistent with this finding, South et al. (2005) reported some common forms of circumscribed interests that were manifested by persons with ASD including an interest in vehicles, electronics, dinosaurs, particular animals, schedules, or numbers (South et al., 2005). Sasson et al. (2008) reported that images representing the types of objects commonly involved in circumscribed interests elicited a unique pattern of visual attention in children with ASD that was characterized by a more perseverative and repetitive attentional style relative to noncircumscribed interest images. Further, for children with ASD but not typically developing children the presence of CI images reduced overall visual exploration and especially exploration of social images. This latter finding suggests one way in which circumscribed interests could be associated with functional impairment in ASD: the presence of strong *non-social* interests could potentially diminish the types of social experiences that are important for experience-dependent brain and behavioral development.

Subtypes of Repetitive Behavior in Autism

As commonly conceptualized in autism, repetitive behaviors are assumed to represent a unitary domain of behavioral expression (e.g., DSM IV category 3 criteria for autism; ADI-R and ADOS repetitive behavior subdomain). However, there is growing evidence that there is considerable structure within the overall domain of repetitive behavior.

Several research groups have taken the concept of repetitive behavior variety an important step further by exploring whether the various discrete forms of repetitive behavior can be reliably and validly grouped into discrete subtypes. More than a psychometric exercise, a subtyping approach may have heuristic value in genetic, neurobiologic, and treatment response studies. For example, neuroimaging studies of OCD have demonstrated that distinct OC symptom subtypes are associated with dysregulation of separate but partially overlapping neural systems (Mataix-Cols, Rosario-Campos, & Leckman, 2005). To date, several studies have examined subtyping of repetitive behaviors (Cuccaro et al., 2003; Shao et al., 2003; Szatmari et al., 2006; Hus et al., 2007). These studies have typically identified two factors: a "lower-order" category called "Repetitive Sensory and Motor Behaviors" (RSMB), and a "higher-order" category labeled "Insistence on Sameness" (IS). Based on the findings of these studies, the 2-factor (lower-order, higher-order) has become the assumed model for the structure of repetitive behaviors. However, it is important to recognize that other subtyping studies of repetitive behaviors in autism have yielded more than 2 factors (Lam & Aman, 2007). In a study by Honey et al. (2006) of 2–4 year old children with autism, a third factor that included circumscribed interests was isolated, suggesting that circumscribed interest may be an independent subtype of repetitive behavior. In addition, closer examination of the items excluded in the earlier 2-factor studies suggests that there may be more structure present. In particular, in the solutions provided by Cuccaro et al. (2003) and Szatmari et al. (2006), the ADI-R items "Unusual Preoccupations," "Unusual Attachments," and "Circumscribed Interests" do not load on either factor and were therefore excluded. These types of repetitive behavior may be of particular interest in autism, because unlike motor stereotypies and compulsions (which are found in other disorders such as OCD, Tourette's syndrome, and mental retardation), these behaviors may be particularly characteristic of autistic disorder. In addition, the 2-factor solutions have accounted for a small amount of variance in each study (between 32 and 36%), suggesting the presence of other factors.

Lam, Bodfish, and Piven (2008) completed a large scale (n = 316) study of the structure of repetitive behaviors in autism in an attempt to systematically extend previous 2-factor studies by specifically including analysis of circumscribed interest items. They found evidence for a distinct interest/preoccupation/attachment factor and were able to account for significantly more variance in phenotypic expression than previous 2-factor models (Lam, Bodfish, & Piven, 2008). Also, 88% of the sample exhibited circumscribed interests as defined by this third factor, and, in contrast to the RSMB and the IS factors, only the circumscribed interest factor was unrelated to either IQ or severity of social-communication symptoms. These findings suggest that circumscribed interests are prevalent in autism, and their independence from co-occurring autism features indicates that circumscribed interests may be associated with unique pathogenic factors relative to the other symptoms of autism.

Factors That Moderate the Type and Severity of Expressed Repetitive Behaviors

Existing research findings suggest that several factors can influence the severity of repetitive behavior expression. Chronological age is likely to be one such moderating factor for the expression and severity of repetitive behaviors. It is now clear that both lower- and higher-order forms of repetitive behavior are present in many cases of autism by 2 to 3 years of age (Bishop, Richler, & Lord, 2006; Mooney, Gray, & Tonge, 2006; Militerni et al., 2002; Honey et al., 2006) and manifest with sufficient severity to warrant intervention (Bishop et al., 2006). Further, lifespan studies have indicated that repetitive behavior symptoms and associated impairment (behavioral rigidity) persists into adolescence and adulthood in most cases (Rumsey, Rappoport, & Sceery, 1985; Piven, Harper, Palmer, & Arndt, 1996). In the largest study of moderator variables to date (Bishop, Richler, & Lord, 2006; N = 830), nonverbal IQ was found to be more related to the presence of repetitive behavior in older (6–11 years) than younger (2–5 years) children with autism. Family factors, including parent/family accommodation of repetitive behaviors can also moderate the expression of repetitive behaviors (Lenane et al., 1990; Reaven & Hepburn, 2003; Boyd, Woodard, Storch, & Bodfish, 2007). Parents and siblings often become involved in a child's repetitive behaviors in efforts to reduce associated impairment such as the behavior problems or "meltdowns" that can occur when rituals, sameness behaviors, or circumscribed interests are not accommodated. Although such efforts are often well intentioned, they typically result in greater impairment and symptom severity by virtue of impacting family life and reinforcing symptom engagement. Thus, indirectly, mood and behavior problems (e.g., irritability, agitation, aggression, self-injury, screaming, disruptive behavior) may also moderate the expression of repetitive behaviors in children with autism (Bodfish et al., 2000; Gabriels et al., 2005). There is evidence that unique profiles of repetitive behaviors occur in specific genetic disorders associated with autism such as Fragile X syndrome, Williams syndrome, and Angelman syndrome (Moss, Oliver, Arron, Burbridge, & Berg, 2009), indicating that specific genetic factors in persons with autism may moderate the expression of specific subtypes of repetitive behavior. These various factors (e.g., age, cognitive ability, family factors, genetic factors) most likely interact in ways that are poorly understood at present to influence the specific pattern of repetitive behaviors seen clinically in persons with autism.

Developmental Course

The findings of early research in autism suggested that repetitive behaviors may not be clinically significant primarily because they did not appear to be early features of the disorder and they were presumed to be related to comorbid mental retardation and, thus, not an autism-specific core feature. Recent research findings call these early assumptions into question and more clearly establish the clinical significance of repetitive behaviors in autism. Recent developmental studies of autism have now shown that repetitive behaviors are among the earliest signs of the disorder during infancy (Landa, Holman, & Garrett-Mayer, 2007; Ozonoff et al., 2008; Watt, Wetherby, Barber, & Morgan, 2008), and the degree of severity of early repetitive behaviors (RBs) uniquely predicts the overall severity of autism in adolescence (Lord et al., 2006). Recent research has demonstrated that RBs can be identified as early as 12–18 months in infants who go on to develop autism (Morgan, Wetherby, & Barber, 2008; Ozonoff et al., 2008; Watt et al., 2008).

Retrospective developmental studies have found that there is some improvement in repetitive behavior severity with age but that age-related improvements are less pronounced on average than that seen for other core features of autism (Piven et al., 1996; Fecteau et al., 2003). In the longitudinal cohort study described by Rutter et al. (1967), some improvements in repetitive behavior severity were noted; however, all subjects with RBs in childhood continued to report difficulties in this domain 10 years later, and there was a tendency for increase in the frequency and complexity of these behaviors with age. Approximately 90% of adolescents and adults with autism report difficulties with repetitive behaviors (Seltzer et al., 2003; Howlin et al., 2004).

In support of the concept that repetitive behaviors in autism may not be a unitary phenomenon, there appear to be different developmental trajectories for discrete subtypes of repetitive behavior. For example, in a large scale (N = 320) study of children and adults with autism spectrum disorders (3–48 years of age) stereotyped movements were less frequent among older individuals, self-injurious behaviors and compulsive behaviors were comparable across age groups, and ritualistic/sameness were found to be more frequent among older individuals (Lam & Aman, 2007). In a comparison of younger and older children with ASD, younger children were more likely to exhibit motor and sensory repetitive behaviors, and older children were more likely to exhibit more complex repetitive behaviors (Militerni, Bravaccio, Falco, Fico, & Palermo, 2002). In another study of children with ASD who ranged in age from toddlers to 12-year-olds, most RBs, including self-injury, desire for sameness, restricted interests, and compulsions, were more frequent among the older than the younger children (Bishop, Richler, & Lord, 2006). However, when taking into account nonverbal IQ, the pattern of findings changed. Some repetitive behaviors did not show age-related patterns (such as restricted interests), whereas others (such as self-injury, desire for sameness, and compulsions) were less frequent among older children. Although there are discrepancies, there is some convergence in the findings relating to age and repetitive behaviors. A trend is observed of specific subtypes appearing to become less frequent with age (e.g., stereotyped movements), while other subtypes appear to increase in prevalence during middle and late childhood and often persist into adulthood (e.g., circumscribed interests). While the pattern of findings across studies is not strong enough to define the age-related pattern of this aspect of the behavioral phenotype of ASD, and there is a need to examine in more detail the age-related patterns across the lifespan, the results of these developmental studies do clearly support the concept that repetitive behaviors are a heterogeneous group of behaviors and that discrete subtypes likely exist.

Functional Significance

Disorders such as Tourette's syndrome and obsessive compulsive disorder (OCD) are characterized by repetitive behaviors, however the need to perform them is aversive and distressing. In part due to the communication deficits that are diagnostic of autism, it is not known whether repetitive behaviors in autism are aversive and distressing, or, whether repetitive behaviors represent an appetitive motivation to approach certain stimuli. Many functions have been hypothesized for repetitive behaviors in autism, including stress reduction, sensory stimulation, and reward (Lewis & Bodfish, 1998). For example the persistence of repetitive behaviors even in the face of aversive consequences has been taken by some as evidence of the rewarding nature of the behaviors. Several theorists have emphasized the apparently "self-stimulatory" nature of stereotyped movements and behaviors (Berkson & Davenport, 1962). This sensation/perception perspective has taken two theoretical forms. The perceptual reinforcement hypothesis (Lovaas et al., 1987) holds that repetitive behaviors are learned, operant self-stimulatory behavior for which the reinforcers are the perceptual stimuli automatically produced by the behavior. The sensorimotor integration hypothesis (Ornitz, 1971) holds that sensory deficits leave the individual reliant on kinesthetic (sensorimotor) feedback derived from the behavior. A functional analysis perspective (Iwata et al., 1982) emphasizes social consequences (e.g., social attention, escape from instruction/demands/interaction, tangible reinforcement), but also invokes "automatic" reinforcement which is similar to both the notion of sensory/perceptual reinforcement and also internal (biological) reward. Such internal factors could include increases in arousal (Hutt & Hutt, 1970) or reductions in stress. The functional consequences and maintaining factors of RB are far from firmly established however.

Given the evidence in support of the existence of discrete subtypes of repetitive behavior in autism, it is plausible that distinct subtypes may be associated with distinct psychological/motivational factors and thus distinct underlying psychobiology. If this is true, then heterogeneity in the expression of these underlying factors may contribute to the marked heterogeneity in both clinical expression and treatment response seen in autism. OCD can be conceptualized as an avoidance phenomenon (compulsions serve to neutralize or avoid obsessive or fearful thoughts). Further, OCD is presumed to be ego-dystonic with affected persons actively wanting to *not* engage in either compulsions or obsessions. These functional features do not seem to apply as easily to all forms of repetitive behavior in autism. While comorbid autism and OCD (i.e., an OCD overlay on top of autism) has been reported in the literature (Cath et al., 2008; Storch et al., 2007) this is not the typical presentation of repetitive behaviors in autism. A larger question is how much of the repetitive behavior symptomatology in autism is mediated by underlying anxiety, as is the case in OCD. Often in the case of autism, behaviors like stereotyped movements (e.g., hand-flapping) seem to be motivationally neutral or affectively linked to excitement/pleasure as much as anxiety or fear (Schultz & Berkson, 1995). This also seems true for behaviors like circumscribed or restricted interests (e.g., intense interest in trains) in persons with autism (Sasson et al., 2008). In these situations the distress/anxiety appears to come as a *consequence* of not having access to the behavior or interest (Powell et al., 1996) much like the case of frustrative nonreward. Thus repetitive behaviors in autism may involve functional manifestations similar to OCD (e.g., avoidance phenomenon like compulsions, rituals, or insistence on sameness) as well as those dissimilar to OCD (e.g., approach phenomenon like preoccupations, attachments, and circumscribed interests) (Lam, Bodfish, & Piven, 2008). One potential overarching commonality however is that in both OCD and autism, repetitive behavior can be mediated by its reward properties—presumably negative reinforcement in the case of OCD and some forms of repetitive behaviors in autism, and presumably positive reinforcement in the case of other forms of repetitive behavior in autism. If so, then the anticipatory-reward nature of the circumscribed interest subtype of repetitive behavior in autism may distinguish autism from other psychiatric disorders characterized by repetitive behaviors (e.g., OCD or OC spectrum disorders) that involve purely anxiety-reduction.

Repetitive Behaviors and Cognitive or Attentional Style in Autism

Part of the functional significance of repetitive behaviors may relate to the way in which repetitive behaviors are associated with particular cognitive features in autism. Baron-Cohen (1989) proposed that repetitive behavior develops in autism to combat a specific cognitive impairment, and that this behavior may develop as a coping strategy that allows the autistic individual to reduce the high level of anxiety resulting from a primary impairment in this ability to understand and infer the mental states of others. Similarly, Carruthers (1996) suggests that repetitive behavior functions to withdraw persons with autism from social contexts that are unpredictable and perhaps frightening. These cognitive accounts predict that levels of repetitive behavior will be highest when in novel and unpredictable social contexts. However, a number of studies have compared the frequency of repetitive behaviors during periods of social interaction and periods in which limited or no interpersonal demands are made, and have shown that rates of repetitive behavior are lowest during periods of social interaction and highest during periods devoid of interaction (Charlop, Schreibman, Mason, & Vesey, 1983; Clark & Rutter, 1981; Dadds, Schwartz, Adams, & Rose, 1988; Donnellan, Anderson & Mesaros 1984; Runco, Charlop, & Schreibman, 1986). In addition, studies that have examined the correlation of the severity of the repetitive behavior and social-communicative aspects of autism have found that these domains vary largely independent of one another (Bodfish et al., 2000; Happe, Ronald, & Plomin, 2006; Lam, Bodfish, & Piven, 2008) Thus, the model of repetitive behaviors occurring as a secondary consequence of core social-cognitive deficits in autism does not seem to be a viable model of repetitive behaviors in autism.

The executive dysfunction account of autism conceptualizes symptoms of restricted and repetitive behaviors to reflect the impaired ability to adapt flexibly to changing environmental contingencies (Russell, 1997; Turner, 1999). Executive functions refer to a range of abilities, including behavioral inhibition, planning, working memory, and mental flexibility (Lezak, 1995). These abilities require the integration of a variety of basic abilities (e.g., language and working memory) to achieve the higher-order processing of information, goal attainment, and appropriate emotional responses (Christ, Holt, White, & Green, 2007). Difficulties with cognitive flexibility are consistent with the clinical phenomenon of the repetitiveness and rigidity that characterizes autism: cognitive inflexibility is manifest as repetitive motor behaviors, perseverative responding, and difficulty with modulating ongoing cognitive and motor behavior (Lopez, Lincoln, Ozonoff, & Lai, 2005). Numerous studies have documented impaired executive function abilities in autism spectrum disorders (Ozonoff et al., 2004; Pennington & Ozonoff, 1996; Sergeant, Geurts, & Oosterlaan, 2002), and some have found that executive function deficits correlate with clinical ratings of repetitive behavior severity (Lopez, Lincoln, Ozonoff, & Lai, 2005). However, clearly not all studies of executive functioning indicate deficits in autism (e.g., Minshew, Goldstein, Muenz, & Payton, 1992). These seemingly contradictory results may reflect the fact that executive function is not a unitary construct, but may be subdivided into more elemental components (see Kenworthy, Black, Wallace, Ahluvalia, Wagner, & Sirian, 2005, for a review). Conceptually, this may map onto the notion of repetitive behavior subtypes such that specific executive functions may map onto specific types of repetitive behavior.

In line with the notion of separable executive subprocesses, Turner (1997) proposed two distinct and dissociable hypotheses: (1) an impaired capacity to regulate behavior via the inhibition of ongoing but inappropriate behavior may lead to repetition as the individual, unable to control attention and action in the usual manner, becomes "locked into" one line of thought or behavior; and (2) an inability spontaneously to generate novel behavior without prompting may lead to a lack of variety in responding, manifest as the repeated display of a restricted set of behaviors. In support of this model, performance on tasks designed to tap each of these key abilities has been shown to be related to the display of specific classes of repetitive behavior (Turner, 1996, 1997). However, results in this area are not entirely consistent. Barnard and colleagues (2008) examined word and design fluency and found no differences in the autism group relative to learning disabled controls. Additionally, phonological fluency has been found to be both intact (Minshew, Goldstein, & Siegel, 1997; Kleinhans, Akshoomoff, & Delis, 2005) and impaired (Rumsey & Hamburger, 1988, 1990) in high-functioning autism relative to both adult controls and adults with severe dyslexia. Further, two studies that attempted to replicate the association between repetitive behavior and generativity both failed to find such a relationship and instead both found generative ability to be correlated with severity of communication impairment in autism (Bishop & Norbury, 2005; Dichter et al., 2009).

Frith and Happe (1994) have suggested that the expression of repetitive behavior may be explained by the notion that individuals with autism do not show the drive for "central coherence" that characterizes normal information processing. The cognitive style of individuals with autism is characterized by preferential processing of local rather than global features of the environment and this may lead to a focus on seemingly insignificant details. This theory is particularly intriguing in light of certain subtypes of repetitive behavior such as insistence on sameness and circumscribed interests. To date, evidence in support of weak central coherence in autism has been mixed, and significant associations with specific forms of repetitive behavior have not been examined.

Atypical attentional processing has also been posited to be a mechanism associated with both downstream cognitive and behavioral deficits in autism (Burack, 1994; Casey et al., 1993; Courchesne et al., 1994; Dawson et al., 1998; Sasson et al., 2008; Wainwright-Sharp & Bryson, 1993). Perseverative attention, or an inability to disengage could also account for variance within the rigid and repetitive behaviors domain associated with the autism phenotype, especially higher order repetitive behaviors (Lewis & Bodfish, 1998; Turner, 1999). Recent evidence has linked circumscribed patterns of attentional orienting to specific aspects of clinical behavior in children and adolescents with autism (Sasson et al., 2008). Of particular relevance, significant correlations between perseverative attention (average duration of fixation during a passive viewing visual exploration task) and composite scores from the Repetitive Behavior Scales-Revised (RBS-R) in a sample of children and adolescents with autism. Circumscribed attentional patterns also have been shown to differentiate 12- to 24-month-olds who go on to receive a diagnosis of autism, reflected through the repetitive and stereotyped manipulation of objects (Morgan et al., 2008; Ozonoff et al., 2008; Watt et al., 2008).

Functional Impairment Associated with Repetitive Behaviors

Repetitive behaviors can cause significant impairment in individuals with autism and their families. In more severe cases these behaviors may consume the majority of waking hours of an individual and interfere with daily family activities. Moreover, children and adults with autism tend to become agitated, disruptive, or even aggressive when repetitive behaviors are interrupted. The presence of circumscribed interests, preoccupations, or unusual attachments may be particularly clinically significant because the presence of strong unusual interests or preoccupations may diminish the saliency of and response to more natural or typical rewards and sources of information and experience. As a result, experience-dependent learning and development may be constrained in a more direct way by persistent circumscribed interests as compared to other forms of repetitive behavior (e.g., stereotyped movements) which may not alter the saliency or reward value of ambient environmental events.

Despite clear indicators of functional impairment associated with repetitive behaviors, parents and clinicians sometimes debate whether or not to make repetitive behaviors the target of intervention. Some parents are struck by how "proficient" their child is in certain areas (e.g., memorizing facts, reciting movie scripts) and how this stands in contrast with all the other things their child is not able to do (e.g., socialize with peers, communicate clearly, adapt to preschool, etc.). In these situations parents sometimes express a fear to tread on these "islands of ability" (Mercier, Mottron, & Belleville, 2000). Another common scenario involves parents who have seen the "meltdowns" and negative side effects on their child's behavior that are related to preventing these repetitive behaviors and interests (Gabriel et al., 2005; Mercier et al., 2000). From a clinical perspective it is apparent that in at least a subset of cases repetitive behaviors and interests can significantly interfere with learning and socialization, and can become a motivating factor underneath the development of mood and behavior problems.

Phenomenologic and behavioral studies of autism have shown that repetitive behaviors persist into adulthood and can be the "residual symptom" of autism once social-communicative deficits improve (Shattuck et al., 2007; Piven et al., 1996). Thus, treatment directed at reducing the severity of repetitive behaviors carries the potential to increase the child's overall degree of flexibility and adaptability and thereby improve the overall trajectory of adaptive behavior development and functioning. In support of this clinical perspective, recent large-scale studies of family and parent functioning in the context of a child with autism have reported that repetitive and related problem behaviors are associated with elevated parent stress (Orsmond, Lin, & Seltzer, 2007), engender negative parenting styles (Smith et al., 2007; Orsmond & Seltzer, 2007; Lounds et al., 2007), and are among the most difficult aspects of autism that parents must deal with on a daily basis (South et al., 2005; Mercier et al., 2000). Thus repetitive behaviors and interests have the potential for interfering with experience-dependent brain and behavioral development and family well-being, and treatment can be seen as necessary when viewed as an approach to expand the child's behavioral repertoire rather than simply thwarting or punishing the child's repetitive behaviors and interests.

Pathogenesis

Deficits and Disorders Associated with Basal Ganglia Pathology

There is a confluence of evidence that implicates altered basal ganglia function in the mediation of repetitive behavior disorders. Historically, examinations of the functions of the basal ganglia have been limited to its role in motor control and movement disorders. Currently, the functions of the basal ganglia are grouped into circuits that include motor, cognitive, and behavioral/personality divisions (Visser, Bar, & Jinnah, 2000; Alexander, Delong, & Strick, 1986). Of interest is the fact that animal lesion studies and human neuropsychological studies of neurosurgery patients with well-defined lesions have demonstrated that abnormality of these basal ganglia circuits produces both the types of restricted repetitive behaviors seen in autism and the types of cognitive flexibility deficits presumed to be related to the expression of repetitive behaviors (Cummings, 1993; Masterman & Cummings, 1997).

A large number of studies using chemical lesioning and site-specific drug administration support the importance of basal ganglia structures in the mediation of drug-induced stereotypies (Lewis et al., 1994). In addition, there is growing evidence that OCD is associated with perturbations in basal ganglia function. For example, there is a significant degree of comorbid OCD in a variety of diseases of the basal ganglia, including Sydenham's Chorea, postencephalitic Parkinson's, toxic lesions of the striatum, and Tourette's syndrome (Rapoport, 1988). The ritualistic-repetitive behaviors that are a defining feature of autism are also observed in (OCD) and Tourette's syndrome (TS) (APA, 1994). Individuals with autism and OCD both exhibit compulsive rituals and rigidity while individuals with autism and TS share repetitive stereotyped motor behaviors (Eapen et al., 1997). Further, abnormalities in the basal ganglia have been implicated in all three of these disorders on the basis of multiple converging findings from structural and functional neuroimaging studies

(Rosenberg et al., 1998; Peterson & Kline, 1997; Peterson et al., 1993; Swedo et al., 1989; Scarone et al., 1992).

MRI Studies of Basal Ganglia in Autism

To date, seven studies have used MRI to investigate the neurobiology of repetitive behavior in autism. Two of these have reported enlarged basal ganglia volumes proportional to an increase in total brain volume (Herbert et al., 2003; study 1 in Sears et al., 1999), and five reported a disproportional increase in caudate nucleus volume (study 2 in Sears et al., 1999; Hollander et al., 2005; Langen et al., 2007; Rojas et al., 2006; Langen et al., 2009). McAlonan et al. (2002) reported no differences in caudate size between autism and typical control groups but did report that autism subjects had significantly decreased gray matter density in striatal areas. In several of these studies a correlation between repetitive behavior severity and caudate size was found (Langen et al., 2007; Rojas et al., 2006; Langen et al., 2009), however in some the magnitude of the correlation differed as a function of discrete type of RB (Sears et al., 1999; Hollander et al., 2005).

fMRI Studies of Fronto-Striatal Circuitry in Autism

The "frontostriatal hypothesis" of autism implicates the basal ganglia and its afferents to the frontal cortex (Robbins, 1997) and is supported by both neuropsychological and animal studies (Visser, Bar, & Jinnah, 2000; Masterman & Cummings, 1997; Lewis, Gluck, Beauchamp, Keresztury, & Mailman, 1990; Robbins, Mittleman, O'Brien, & Winn, 1990; Insel, 1992). There is a host of neuroimaging evidence indicating anomalous activation of prefrontal brain areas in individuals with autism during so-called cognitive control or executive tasks. The specific prefrontal regions affected and the direction of changes are heterogeneous across studies and related to the specific cognitive tasks utilized, supporting the widely held view that executive functions include a number of distinct cognitive processes. Hyperactivation in the left middle and inferior frontal gyri and orbitofrontal cortex has been reported during a go/no-go (i.e., motor inhibition) task, whereas hyperactivation of the left insula was observed in the same participants during a spatial Stroop (i.e., interference inhibition) task (Schmitz et al., 2006). Hyperactivation in the right superior, middle and inferior prefrontal cortex and the left inferior parietal cortex has been reported during an auditory novelty detection task (Gomot et al., 2008). Rostral anterior cingulate cortex hyperactivation during an antisaccade that predicted the magnitude of repetitive behaviors was reported by Thakkar and colleagues (2008). Finally, hypoactivation bilaterally in middle frontal, right superior frontal, and left inferior frontal regions has been reported during a Tower of London (i.e., problem solving) task (Just, Cherkassky, Keller, Kana, & Minshew, 2007).

Shafritz et al. (2008) reported hypoactivation in the striatum, as well as in the middle and inferior frontal gyri and anterior cingulate cortex (ACC) in autism during a standard visual target detection (i.e., oddball) task. Furthermore, the magnitude of ACC activation inversely correlated with repetitive behaviors in the autism sample. The anterior cingulate circuit is one of five parallel circuits that link the frontal lobes with subcortical structures. The anterior cingulate circuit projects to the ventral striatum, then to the ventral and rostrolateral globus pallidus and rostrodorsal substantia nigra, which, in turn, project to the medial dorsal nucleus of the thalamus, and then the circuit is completed via projections to the anterior cingulate (for a review, see Cummings, 1993). Injury to this circuit produces deficits on response inhibition tasks (Drewe, 1975), and other repetitive behavior disorders, such as Tourette's syndrome and obsessive compulsive disorder, are characterized by dysfunction within this circuit (Singer, Hahn, & Moran, 1991; Baxter, Phelps, Mazziotta, Guze, Schwartz, & Selin, 1987). To date, no fMRI studies have examined potential links between specific neurocognitive functions and discrete subtypes of repetitive behavior, and thus critical extensions of the neurobiologic study of specific types of repetitive behavior in autism remain to be explored.

Intervention

Behavioral and Psychosocial Intervention

An important distinction that can be made in the autism intervention literature is the differentiation of comprehensive treatment models (CTMs) from focused intervention practices (FIPs) (Odom, Boyd, Hall, & Hume, 2009). CTMs (e.g., Denver Model, LEAP, Lovaas Institute, TEACCH) are conceptually organized treatment packages to address a broad array of skills for children with autism. FIPs (e.g., prompting, reinforcement, PEC, visual supports, response interruption/redirection) are individual instructional practices that are used to address specific targeted skills or presenting symptoms. Seminal work by Odom, Rogers, and colleagues has involved the examination of both CTMs (Odom et al., 2009; Rogers & Vismara, 2008) and FIPs (Odom, Klingenberg, & Rogers, in press) in relation to accepted evidentiary criteria. As a result of this work, subsets of both CTMs and FIPs can be designated as "evidenced-based practices" for autism intervention. In this context, an important question is: what is the evidence base for CTMs and FIPs with respect to the treatment of repetitive behaviors in autism?

Although definitive evidence (e.g., multiple, independent, methodologically sound RCTs) for the efficacy of both CTMs and FIPs in autism is lacking, it is now clear that (1) specific evidenced-based practices for autism intervention can be identified, and (2) the development of young children with autism can be significantly improved by the delivery of these evidenced based CTMs and FIPs. While the bulk of this evidence for efficacy for specific CTMs and FIPs is in the area of specific targeted instruction in the areas of communication, social skills, play, cognition, and independence, there is evidence that specific FIPs (e.g., behavioral teaching strategies such as prompting, differential reinforcement, interruption/redirection; functional analysis based strategies such as the Positive Behavior Supports approach) can effectively reduce the occurrence of some types of repetitive behavior and the types of problem behaviors that can be associated with repetitive behaviors in autism such as aggression, noncompliance, and self-injury (Odom, et al., in press; Horner, Carr, Strain, Todd, & Reed, 2002).

Two gaps do exist however in this literature on evidenced-based behavioral and psychosocial intervention practices for repetitive behaviors in autism. First, given that there are a variety of discrete types of repetitive behaviors, virtually all of the behavioral/psychosocial intervention research has focused on the lower-order forms of repetitive behavior (stereotyped movements, self-injury) and as a result there are no established evidenced-based practices for treating the quintessential autistic repetitive behaviors like rituals, insistence on sameness/difficulty with change, and intense preoccupations, attachments, and interests (Bodfish, 2004). Second, existing studies and their resultant intervention practices have focused entirely on the frequency of occurrence of repetitive behaviors as outcomes and as a result fail to address the underlying aspect of behavioral inflexibility that is so characteristic of autism. This trait is evident perhaps most clearly in the "higher-order" or cognitive aspects of repetitive behaviors such as sameness behaviors, and restricted interests, which as noted have not been the focus of intervention research to date.

Evidenced-based forms of treatment for other neuropsychiatric disorders characterized by repetitive behaviors may be worthy of consideration in the search for novel forms of intervention to treat the higher-order types of repetitive behaviors and overarching behavioral inflexibility in autism. There is a consensus that cognitive behavioral therapy (CBT) is an effective treatment for child, adolescent, and adult neuropsychiatric disorders characterized by prominent repetitive behavior symptoms such as OCD (Abramowitz et al., 2005; March et al., 1997; Piacentini et al., 2002; POTS, 2004), Tourette's syndrome (Piacentini & Chang, 2005; Carr & Chong, 2005), stereotyped movement disorder (Miller, Singer, Bridges, & Waranch, 2006; Teng, Woods, & Twohig, 2006), and a variety of other repetitive behavior disorders (Woods & Miltenberger, 2001; Deckersbasch, Wilhelm, Keuthen, Baer, & Jenike, 2002; Byrd, Richards, Hove, & Friman, 2002; Wilner, 2006; Wilner & Goodey, 2006). Although a variety of CBT protocols exist (e.g., Exposure Response-Prevention, Habit Reversal Therapy [HRT]), each consists of three similar components: exposure (placing the patient in situations that elicit repetitive behavior symptoms); response prevention (deterring the stereotyped, ritualistic, or compulsive behaviors); and cognitive or behavioral therapy (training the patient or his family to identify and redirect to an alternative/competing response). In two previously reported case studies of an ERP-based intervention for children with autism (Lehmkuhl, Storch, Bodfish, & Geffen, in press; Reaven & Hepburn, 2003), the intervention was used to treat comorbid OCD symptoms (e.g., contamination thoughts or hand-washing rituals). To date, no studies have addressed the modification of ERP for the treatment of more autism-typical subtypes of repetitive behavior (e.g., insistence on sameness, complex rituals/routines, unusual and intense interests and preoccupations).

Medication Intervention

For persons with autism, symptoms of repetitive behaviors are common, and frequently form a source of significant interference in adapting to educational and social settings. These repetitive behaviors are commonly associated with emotional distress, tension, or dysphoria. While such behaviors can be responsive to behavioral treatments, in their severe forms of expression they are often difficult to manage by psychosocial efforts alone, and lead clinicians to attempt trials of treatment with medications.

Given the evidence linking dopamine functioning and the expression of repetitive behaviors, dopamine-blockade medications have been used for a long time clinically to target interfering repetitive behaviors and their associated mood and behavior problems. The older, high-potency neuroleptic haloperidol was studied extensively in autism in the 1970s and 1980s, and several controlled studies showed evidence of efficacy over placebo among young children treated with relatively low doses (e.g., 1–2 mg/day) (Campbell et al., 1978; Perry et al., 1989). However, the frequent emergence of harmful extrapyramidal symptoms (e.g., dyskinesia, akathisia) significantly limited the use of haloperidol. Older neuroleptics have now been replaced with atypical antipsychotics that combine dopamine and serotonin receptor antagonism. Considerable evidence now exists for the efficacy of these atypical neuroleptics in the treatment of mood and behavior problems in autism (Bryson, Rogers, & Fombonne, 2003), including a large multicenter randomized controlled trial comparing risperidone to placebo in 1010 children with autism aged 5–17 years presenting with clinically significant levels of irritability, tantrums, aggression, and self-injury (McCracken et al., 2002). In this trial, improvements were also found for stereotyped and ritualistic behaviors. While atypical neuroleptics are now established as viable interventions for at least some of the repetitive behaviors associated with autism and their clinical sequelae, they produce adverse effects such as tachycardia, sedation, and weight gain with metabolic symptoms in a significant minority of patients treated.

Because of the success of drug treatment for the management of repetitive behaviors in obsessive compulsive disorder (OCD), and evidence supporting abnormalities in the serotonin system in autism, there has been considerable interest in exploring the possible benefits of serotonergic-acting medications for the control of these repetitive movements associated with autism and other PDDs. Interest in serotonergic mechanisms in the manifestation of symptoms in autism has led to several prior clinical drug trials, with mixed results. Extant data suggest that adolescents and adults with autism may experience improvements in repetitive behaviors, anxiety, and other related symptoms (Bryson, Rogers, & Fombonne, 2003; Lewis & Bodfish, 2000; McDougle et al., 1997). A large-scale, multisite double-blind randomized controlled trial (n = 149) of children with autism spectrum disorders (age range 5 to 17 years) with clinical levels of repetitive behaviors found that the serotonergic antidepressant citalopram did not differ from placebo in terms of efficacy for repetitive behaviors but did produce significantly more adverse events (e.g., activation, impulsiveness) (King et al., 2009). Thus, while serotonergic antidepressants may be effective in adults with autism, in spite of their widespread use in children with autism, the existing evidence base on the efficacy and safety of serotonergic medications for children with autism is poor.

Conclusion

Understanding autism requires an appreciation of the various types of repetitive behaviors displayed by children and adults with autism, understanding how this variety of repetitive behaviors can affect the course of the disorder, and understanding how the putative neurobiology of repetitive behaviors can be conceptualized in a way that can inform treatment decisions. Although repetitive behaviors in autism are frequently conceptualized as being a single, unitary symptom domain in autism, it is now clear that this aspect of the autism phenotype involves multiple, distinct subtypes of repetitive behavior. This conceptualization of repetitive behavior subtypes is consistent with the reigning notion that autism is not a unitary entity in itself and that efforts to disaggregate the autism phenotype are needed to help identify the multiple pathogenic factors involved in the etiology and development of the disorder. While our understanding of the phenomenology, course, and pathophysiology of repetitive behaviors in autism is growing, evidence on safe, effective, and practical forms of intervention to manage the sequelae of repetitive behaviors still lags far behind what we know about treating other aspects of autism. Closing this gap will involve translating newly emerging evidence on repetitive behavior subtypes and potential subtype-specific pathogenesis into efforts to develop focused forms of behavioral, developmental, and pharmacologic forms of intervention for specific repetitive behavior subtypes.

Challenges and Future Directions

- The emerging discrete subtypes of repetitive behavior seen in ASD offer promise for helping parse the considerable clinical heterogeneity of ASD. It will be important to validate these subtypes by determining if discrete subtypes are associated with differences in developmental course, pathogenesis, and response to established treatments.
- The functional significance of the different forms of repetitive behavior in autism has not been established and this is an important step for guiding treatment decisions in other neurodevelopmental disorders characterized by repetitive behaviors (e.g., OCD, TS). Comparative studies of repetitive behaviors across conditions (ASD, OCD, TS, etc.) are needed to begin to determine the functional significance of the variety of repetitive behaviors in ASD.
- There are currently no evidenced-based focused treatments for repetitive behaviors in ASD despite the fact that in at least a significant subset of cases repetitive behaviors are associated with considerable functional impairment. Research is overdue on both psychosocial and psychopharmacological treatment development focusing on clinically significant repetitive behaviors in ASD.

SUGGESTED READINGS

Graybiel, A. M. (2008). Habits, rituals, and the evaluative brain. *Annual Review of Neuroscience, 31*, 359–387.

Lam, K. S., Bodfish, J. W., & Piven, J. (2008). Evidence for three subtypes of repetitive behaviors in autism that differ in familiarity and association with other symptoms. *Journal of Child Psychology and Psychiatry, and Allied Disciplines, 49*, 1193–1200.

Lord, C., Risi, S., DiLavore, P. S., Shulman, C., Thurm, A., & Pickles, A. (2006). Autism from 2 to 9 years of age. *Archives of General Psychiatry, 63*(6), 694–701.

Morgan, L., Wetherby, A. M., & Barber, A. (2008). Repetitive and stereotyped movements in children with autism disorders late in the second year of life. *Journal of Child Psychology and Psychiatry, 49*, 826–837.

REFERENCES

American Psychiatric Association. (1994). *Diagnostic and Statistical Manual of Mental Disorders, Fourth Edition, Text Revision.* (4th ed.) Washington, DC: Author.

Anderson, G. M., Freedman, D. X., Cohen, D. J., Volkmar, F. R., Hoder, E. L., McPhedran, P., et al. (1987). Whole blood serotonin in autistic and normal subjects. *Journal of Child Psychology and Psychiatry, and Allied Disciplines, 28*(6), 885–900.

Awad, G. A. (1996). The use of selective serotonin reuptake inhibitors in young children with pervasive developmental disorders: some clinical observations. *Canadian Journal of Psychiatry–Revue Canadienne de Psychiatrie, 41*(6), 361–366.

Barnard, L., Muldoon, K., Hasan, R., O'Brien, G., & Stewart, M. (2008). Profiling executive dysfunction in adults with autism and comorbid learning disability. *Autism, 12*(2), 125–141.

Baron-Cohen, S. (1989). Do autistic children have obsessions and compulsions? *British Journal of Clinical Psychology, 28*, 193–200.

Baron-Cohen, S. (1997). Are children with autism superior at folk physics? *New Directions for Child Development, 75*, 45–54.

Bartak, L., & Rutter, M. (1973). Special education treatment of autistic children: A comparative study. I: Design of study and characteristic of units. *Journal of Child Psychology and Psychiatry, and Allied Disciplines, 14*, 161–179.

Bartak, L., & Rutter, M. (1976). Differences between mentally retarded and normally intelligent autistic children. *Journal of Autism and Childhood Schizophrenia*, *6*, 109–120.

Berkson, G., & Davenport, R. K. (1962). Stereotyped movements of mental defectives. *American Journal of Mental Deficiency*, *66*, 849–852.

Bishop, S. L., Richler, J., & Lord, C. (2006). Association between restricted and repetitive behaviors and nonverbal IQ in children with autism spectrum disorders. *Child Neuropsychology*, *12*(4), 247–267.

Bodfish, J. W., Crawford, T. W., Powell, S. B., et al. (1995). Compulsions in adults with mental retardation: prevalence, phenomenology, and comorbidity with stereotypy and self injury. *American Journal of Mental Retardation*, *100*(2), 183–192.

Bodfish, J. W., Symons, F. J., Parker, D. E., & Lewis, M. H. (2000). Varieties of repetitive behavior in autism: comparisons to mental retardation. *Journal of Autism and Developmental Disorders*, *30*(3), 237–243.

Bryson, S. E., Rogers, S. J., Fombonne, E. (2003, September). Autism spectrum disorders: Early detection, intervention, education, and psychopharmacological management. *Canadian Journal of Psychiatry. Revue canadienne de psychiatrie*, *48*(8), 506–516.

Campbell, M., Anderson, L. T., Meier, M., Cohen, I. L., Small, A. M., Samit C., et al. (1978). A comparison of haloperidol and behavior therapy and their interaction in autistic children. *Journal of the American Academy of Child Psychiatry*, *17*, 640–655.

Campbell, M., Locascio, J. J., Choroco, M. C., Spencer, E. K., Malone, R. P., Kafantaris, V., et al. (1990). Stereotypies and tardive dyskinesia: Abnormal movements in autistic children. *Psychopharmacology Bulletin*, *26*, 260–266.

Carcani-Rathwell, I., Rabe-Hasketh, S., & Santosh, P. J. Repetitive and stereotyped behaviors in pervasive developmental disorders. *Journal of Child Psychology and Psychiatry*, *47*(6), 573–581.

Chugani, D. C., Muzik, O., Behen, M., Rothermel, R., Janisse, J. J., Lee, J., et al. (1999). Developmental changes in brain serotonin synthesis capacity in autistic and nonautistic children. *Annals of Neurology*, *45*(3), 287–295.

Clark, P., & Rutter, M. (1981). Autistic children's response to structure and to interpersonal demands. *Journal of Autism and Developmental Disorders*, *11*, 201–217.

Cook, E. H., Jr., Rowlett, R., Jaselskis, C., & Leventhal, B. L. (1992). Fluoxetine treatment of children and adults with autistic disorder and mental retardation. *Journal of the American Academy of Child and Adolescent Psychiatry*, *31*(4), 739–745.

Cuccaro, M. L., Shao, Y., Grubber, J., Slifer, M., Wolpert, C. M., Donnelly, S. L., et al. (2003). Factor analysis of restricted and repetitive behaviors in autism using the Autism Diagnostic Interview-R. *Child Psychiatry and Human Development*, *34*(1), 3–17.

Dawson, G., Meltzoff, A. N., Osterling, J., & Rinaldi, J. (1998). Neuropsychological correlates of early symptoms of autism. *Child Development*, *69*, 1276–1285.

Dawson, G., Munson, J., Estes, A., Osterling, J., McPartland, J., Toth, K., et al. (2002). Neurocognitive function and joint attention ability in young children with autism spectrum disorder versus developmental delay. *Child Development*, *73*(2), 345–358.

DeLoache, J. S., Simcock, G., & Macari, S. (2007). Planes, trains, automobiles—and tea sets: extremely intense interests in very young children. *Developmental Psychology*, *43*(6), 1579–1586.

de Silva, P. (1994). Obsession and compulsions: Investigation. In S. J. E. Lindsay & G. E. Powell (Eds.), *The handbook of clinical adult psychology* (2nd ed., pp. 51–70). London: Routledge.

Dichter, G., Felder, J., & Bodfish, J. (submitted). The neural correlates of social target detection in autism.

Dichter, G., Felder, J., Bodfish, J., Sikich, L., & Belger, A. (in press). Mapping social target detection with fMRI. *Social Cognitive and Affective Neuroscience*.

Donnellan, A. M., Anderson, J. L., & Mesaros, R. A. (1984). An observation of stereotypic behavior and proximity related to the occurrence of autistic child-gamily member interactions. *Journal of Autism and Developmental Disorders*, *14*, 205–210.

Eason, L. J., White, M. J., & Newsom, C. (1982). Generalized reduction of self-stimulatory behavior: An effect of teaching appropriate toy play to autistic children. *Analysis and Intervention in Developmental Disabilities*, *2*, 157–169.

Epstein, L. J., Taubman, M. T., & Lovaas, O. I. (1985). Changes in self-stimulatory behaviors with treatment. *Journal of Abnormal Child Psychology*, *13*, 281–294.

Esbensen, A. J., Seltzer, M. M., Lam, K. S., & Bodfish, J. W. (2008). Age-related differences in restricted repetitive behaviors in autism spectrum disorders. *Journal of Autism and Developmental Disorders*, *39*, *57–66*.

Evans, D. W., Leckman, J. F., Carter, A., Reznick, J. S., Henshaw, D., King, R. A., et al. (1997). Ritual, habit, and perfectionism: The prevalence and development of compulsive-like behavior in normal young children. *Child Development*, *68*, 58–68.

Freeman, B. J., Ritvo, E. R., Schroth, P. C., Tonick, I., Gurhrie, D., & Wake, L. (1981). Behavioral characteristics of high-and-low-IQ autistic children. *American Journal of Psychiatry*, *138*, 25–29.

Frith, D. D., & Done, D. J. (1990). Stereotyped behavior in madness and in health. In S. J. Cooper & C. T. Dourish (Eds.), *Neurobiology of stereotyped behaviour* (pp. 232–259). Oxford: Clarendon.

Frith, U. (1989). Autism: *Explaining the enigma*. Oxford: Blackwell.

Gabriels, R. L., Cuccaro, M. L., Hill, D. E., Ivers, B. J., & Goldson, E. (2005). Repetitive behaviors in autism: Relationships with associated clinical features. *Research in Developmental Disabilities*, *26*, 169–181.

Gordon, C. T., State, R. C., Nelson, J. E., Hamburger, S. D., & Rapoport, J. L. (1993). A double-blind comparison of clomipramine, desipramine, and placebo in the treatment of autistic disorder. *Archives of General Psychiatry*, *50*(6), 441–447.

Graybiel, A. M. (2008). Habits, rituals, and the evaluative brain. *Annual Review of Neuroscience*, *31*, 359–387.

Hanley, H. G., Stahl, S. M., & Freedman, D. X. (1977). Hyperserotonemia and amine metabolites in autistic and retarded children. *Archives of General Psychiatry*, *34*(5), 521–531.

Happe, F., Booth, R., Charlton, R., & Hughes, C. (2006). Executive function deficits in autism spectrum disorders and attention-deficit/hyperactivity disorder: examining profiles across domains and ages. *Brain and Cognition*, *61*(1), 25–39.

Happe, F., Ronald, A., & Plomin, R. (2006, October). Time to give up on a single explanation for autism. *Nature Neuroscience*, *9*(10).

Hermelin, B., & O'Connor, N. (1963). The response of self-generated behavior of severely disturbed children and severely subnormal controls. *British Journal of Social and Clinical Psychology*, *2*, 37–43.

Hollander, E., Anagnostou, E., Chaplin, W, Esposito, K., Haznedar, M. M., Licalzi, E., et al. (2005). Striatal volume on magnetic resonance imaging and repetitive behaviors in autism. *Biological Psychiatry*, *58*, 226–232.

Hughes, C., Russell, J., & Robbins, T. W. (1993). Evidence for executive dysfunction in autism. *Neuropsychologia, 32*, 477–492.

Hus, V., Pickles, A., Cook, E. H., Jr., Risi, S., & Lord, C. (2007). Using the Autism Diagnostic Interview—Revised to increase phenotypic homogeneity in genetic studies of autism. *Biological Psychiatry, 61*(4), 438–448.

Hutt, C., & Hutt, S. (1970). Stereotypies and their relation to arousal: A study of autism children. In S. Hutt & C. Hutt(Eds.), Behavior studies in psychiatry (pp 175–204). Oxford: Pergamon.

Iwata, B., Dorsey, M., Slifer, K., et al. Toward a functional analysis of self-injury. *Analysis and Intervention in Developmental Disabilities, 2*, 3–20.

Kanner, L. (1943). Autistic disturbances of affective contact. *Nervous Child, 2*, 217–250.

Kerbeshian, J., Burd, L., & Fisher, W. (1990). Asperger's syndrome: To be or not to be? *British Journal of Psychiatry, 156*, 721–725.

King, B. H., Hollander, E., Sikich, L., McCracken, J. T., Scahill, L., Bregman, J. D., et al. (2009, June). Lack of efficacy of citalopram in children with autism spectrum disorders and high levels of repetitive behavior: citalopram ineffective in children with autism. *Archives of General Psychiatry, 66*(6), 583–590.

Klin, A., Danovitch, J. H., Merz, A. B., & Volkmar, F. R. (2007). Circumscribed interests in higher functioning individuals with autism spectrum disorders: an exploratory study. *Research and Practice for Persons with Severe Disabilities, 32*(2), 89–100.

Koegel, R. L., & Covert, A. (1972). The relationship of self-stimulation to learning in autistic children. *Journal of Applied Behavior Analysis, 5*(4), 381–387.

Koegel, R. L., Firestone, P. B., Kramme, K. W., & Dunlap, G. (1974). Increasing spontaneous play by suppressing self-stimulation in autistic children. *Journal of Applied Behavior Analysis, 7*(4), 521–528.

Lam, K. S. L., & Aman, M. G. (2007). The Repetitive Behavior Scale-Revised: Independent validation in individuals with autism spectrum disorders. *Journal of Autism and Developmental Disorders.* Epub ahead of print.

Lam, K. S., Bodfish, J. W., & Piven, J. (2008). Evidence for three subtypes of repetitive behaviors in autism that differ in familiarity and association with other symptoms. *Journal of Child Psychology and Psychiatry, and Allied Disciplines, 49*, 1193–1200.

Langen, M., Durston, S., Staal, W. G., Palmen, S. J., & van Engeland, H. (2007, August). Caudate nucleus is enlarged in high-functioning medication-naïve subjects with autism. *Biological Psychiatry, 2007, 62*(3), 262–266.

Langen, M., Schnack, H. G., Nederveen, H., Bos, D., Lahuis, B. E., de Jonge, M. V., et al. (2009, August 15). Changes in the development trajectories of striatum in autism. *Biological Psychiatry, 66*(4), 327–333.

Lewis, M. H., & Bodfish, J. W. (1998). Repetitive behavior disorders in autism. *Mental Retardation and Developmental Disabilities Research Reviews, 4*, 80–89.

Lewis, M. H., Bodfish, J. W., Powell, S. B., & Golden, R. N. (1994). Compulsive and stereotyped behavior disorders in mentally retarded patients (Abstract). *Biological Psychiatry, 35*, 643–644.

Lopez, B. R., Lincoln, A. J., Ozonoff, S., et al. (2005). Examining the relationship between executive functions and restricted, repetitive symptoms of autistic disorder. *Journal of Autism and Developmental Disorders, 35*(4), 445–460.

Lord, C. (1995). Follow-up of 2-year-olds referred for possible autism. *Journal of Child Psychology and Psychiatry, and Allied Disciplines, 36*, 1365–1382.

Lord, C., Risi, S., DiLavore, P. S., Shulman, C., Thurm, A., & Pickles, A. (2006). Autism from 2 to 9 years of age. *Archives of General Psychiatry, 63*(6), 694–701.

Lovaas, O. I., Litrownik, A., & Mann, R. (1971). Response latencies to auditory stimuli in autistic children engaged in self-stimulatory behavior. *Behaviour Research and Therapy, 9*(1), 39–49.

Lovaas, I., Newsom, C., Hickman, C. (1987). Self-stimulatory behavior and perceptual reinforcement. *Journal of Applied Behavior Analysis, 20*, 45–68.

Mataix-Cols, D., Rosario-Campos, M. C., & Leckman, J. F. (2005). A multidimensional model of obsessive-compulsive disorder. *American Journal of Psychiatry, 162*(2), 228–238.

McCracken, J. T., McGough, J., Shah, B., Cronin P., Hong D., Aman M. D., et al. (2002). Risperidone in children with autism and serious behavioral problems. *New England Journal of Medicine, 347*, 314–321.

McDougle, C. J., Holmes, J. P., Carlson, D. C., Pelton, G. H., Cohen, D. J., Price, L. H. (1997). A double-blind, placebo-controlled study of risperidone in adults with autistic disorder and other pervasive developmental disorders. *Archives of General Psychiatry, 55*(7), 633–641.

McDougle, C. J., Kresch, L. E., Goodman, W. K., Naylor, S. T., Volkmar, F. R., Cohen, D. J., et al. (1995). A case-controlled study of repetitive thoughts and behavior in adults with autistic disorder and obsessive-compulsive disorder. *American Journal of Psychiatry, 152*(5), 772–777.

McDougle, C. J., Naylor, S. T., Cohen, D. J., Aghajanian, G. K., Heninger, G. R., & Price, L. H. (1996). Effects of tryptophan depletion in drug-free adults with autistic disorder. *Archives of General Psychiatry, 53*(11), 993–1000.

McDougle, C. J., Naylor, S. T., Cohen, D. J., Volkmar, F. R., Heninger, G. R., & Price, L. H. (1996). A double-blind, placebo-controlled study of fluvoxamine in adults with autistic disorder. *Archives of General Psychiatry, 53*(11), 1001–1008.

Mercier, C., Mottron, L., & Belleville, S. (2000). A psychosocial study on restricted interests in high functioning persons with pervasive developmental disorders. *Autism, 4*(4), 406–425.

Militerni, R., Bravaccio, C., Falco, C., Fico, C., & Palermo, M. T. (2002). Repetitive behaviors in autistic disorders. *European Child and Adolescent Psychiatry, 11*, 210–218.

Mooney, E. L., Gray, K. M., & Tonge, B. J. (2006). Early features of autism: Repetitive behaviors in young children. *European Child and Adolescent Psychiatry, 15*(1), 12–18.

Morgan, L., Wetherby, A. M., & Barber, A. (2008). Repetitive and stereotyped movements in children with autism disorders late in the second year of life. *Journal of Child Psychology and Psychiatry, and Allied Disciplines, 49*, 826–837.

Moss, J., Oliver, C., Arron, K., Burbridge, C., & Berg, K. (2009). The prevalance and phenomenology of repetitive behavior in genetic syndromes. *Journal of Autism and Developmental Disorders, 39*, 572–588.

Ornitz, E. M. (1971). Childhood autism: A disorder of sensorimotor integration. In M. Rutter (Ed.), Infantile autism: Concepts, characteristics, and treatment. London Churchill Livingstone.

Ozonoff, S., Cook, I., Coon, H., Dawson, G., Joseph, R. M., Klin, A., et al. (2004). Performance on Cambridge Neuropsychological Test Automated Battery subtests sensitive to frontal lobe function in people with autistic disorder: evidence from the Collaborative Programs of Excellence in Autism network. *Journal of Autism and Developmental Disorders, 34*(2), 139–150.

Ozonoff, S., & Jensen, J. (1999). Brief report: specific executive function profiles in three neurodevelopmental disorders. *Journal of Autism and Developmental Disorders, 29*(2), 171–177.

Ozonoff, S., Macari, S., Young, G. S., Goldring, S., Thompson, M., & Rogers, S. J. (2008). Atypical object exploration at 12 months of age is associated with autism in a prospective sample. *Autism, 12*(5), 457–472.

Ozonoff, S., Pennington, B. F., & Rogers, S. J. (1991). Executive function deficits in high-functioning autistic individuals: Relationship to theory of mind. *Journal of Child Psychology and Psychiatry, 32*, 1081–1105.

Perry, R., Campbell, M., Adams, P., Lynch, N., Spencer, E. K., Curren, E. L., et al. (1989). Long-term efficacy of haloperidol in autistic children: continuous versus discontinuous drug administration. *Journal of the American Academy of Child and Adolescent Psychiatry, 28*, 87–92.

Pierce, K., & Courchesne, E. (2001). Evidence for a cerebellar role in reduced exploration and stereotyped behavior in autism. *Biological Psychiatry, 49*, 655–664.

Piven, J., Harper, J., Palmer, P., & Arndt, S. (1996). Course of behavioral change in autism: A retrospective study of high-IQ adolescents and adults. *Journal of the American Academy of Child and Adolescent Psychiatry, 35*, 523–529.

Prior, M., & Macmillan, M. B. (1973). Maintenance of sameness in children with Kanner's syndrome. *Journal of Autism and Childhood Schizophrenia*, 154–167.

Ridley, R. M. (1994). The psychology of perseverative and stereotyped behavior. *Progress in Neurobiology, 44*, 221–231.

Runco, M. A., Charlop, A. H., & Schreibman, L. (1986). The occurrence of autistic children's self-stimulation as a function of familiar versus unfamiliar stimulus conditions. *Journal of Autism and Developmental Disorders, 16*, 31–44.

Sasson, N. J., Turner-Brown, L. M., Holtzclaw, T. N., Lam, K. S. L., & Bodfish, J. W. (2008). Children with autism demonstrate circumscribed attention during passive viewing of complex social and nonsocial picture arrays. *Autism Research, 1*, 31–42.

Schopler, E., Brehm, S., Kinsbourne, M., & Reichler, R. J. (1971). Effect of treatment structure on development in autism. *Archives of General Psychiatry, 24*, 415–421.

Sears, L. L., Vest, C., Mohamed, S., Bailey, J., Ranson, B. J., & Piven, J. (1999). An MRI study of the basal ganglia in autism. *Progress in Neuro-Psychopharmacology and Etiological Psychiatry, 23*, 613–624.

Seltzer, M. M., Krauss, M. W., Shattuck, P. T., Orsmond, G., Swe, A., & Lord, C. (2003). The symptoms of autism spectrum disorders in adolescence and adulthood. *Journal of Autism and Developmental Disorders, 33*, 565–581.

Seltzer, M. M., Shattuck, P., Abbeduto, L., & Greenberg, J. S. (2004). Trajectory of development in adolescents and adults with autism. *Mental Retardation and Developmental Disabilities Research Reviews, 10*, 234–247.

Shafritz, K., Dichter, G. S., Baranek, G., & Belger, A. (in press). The neural circuitry mediating cognitive flexibility deficits in autism. *Biological Psychiatry*.

Shao, Y., Cuccaro, M. L., Hauser, E. R., Raiford, K. L., Menold, M. M., Wolpert, C. M., et al. (2003). Fine mapping of autistic disorder to chromosome 15q11-q13 by use of phenotypic subtypes. *American Journal of Human Genetics, 72*(3), 539–548.

Shattuck, P. T., Seltzer, M. M., Greenberg, J. S., Orsmond, G. I., Bolt, D., Kring, S., et al. (2007). Change in autism symptoms and maladaptive behaviors in adolescents and adults with an autism spectrum disorder. *Journal of Autism and Developmental Disorders, 37*, 1735–1747.

Smith, E. A., & Van Houten, R. (1996). A comparison of the characteristics of self-stimulatory behaviors in "normal" children and children with developmental delays. *Research in Developmental Disabilities, 17*, 253–268.

South, M., Ozonoff, S., & McMahon, W. (2005). Repetitive behavior profiles in Asperger syndrome and high-functioning autism. *Journal of Autism and Developmental Disorders, 35*(2), 145–158.

Stone, W. L., Lee, E. B., Ashford, L., Brissie, J., Hepburn, S. L., Coonrod, E. E., et al. (1999). Can autism be diagnosed accurately in children under 3 years? *Journal of Child Psychology and Psychiatry, 40*(2), 219–226.

Swedo, S. E., Rapoport, J. L., Leonard, H., Lenane, M., & Cheslow, D. (1989). Obsessive-compulsive disorder in children and adolescents: Clinical phenomenology of 70 consecutive cases. *Archives of General Psychiatry, 46*(4), 335–341.

Szatmari, P., Bartolucci, G., & Bremmer, R. (1989). Asperger's syndrome and autism: Comparison of early history and outcome. *Developmental Medicine and Child Neurology, 31*, 709–720.

Szatmari, P., Georgiades, S., Bryson, S., Zwaigenbaum, L., Roberts, W., Mahoney, W., et al. (2006). Investigating the structure of the restricted, repetitive behaviors and interests domain of autism. *Journal of Child Psychology and Psychiatry, 47*(6), 582–590.

Tadevosyan-Leyfer, O., Dowd, M., Mankoski, R., Winklosky, B., Putnam, S., McGrath, L., et al. (2003). A principal components analysis of the Autism Diagnostic Interview-Revised. *Journal of the American Academy of Child and Adolescent Psychiatry, 42*(7), 864–872.

Taylor, S. F., & Liberzon, I. (2007). Neural correlates of emotion regulation in psychopathology. *Trends in Cognitive Sciences, 11*(10), 413–418.

Thelen, E. (1979).Rhythmical stereotypies in normal human infants. *Animal Behaviour, 27*(Pt3), 699–715.

Turner, M. A. (1996). Repetitive behavior and cognitive functioning in autism. Unpublished PhD thesis. University of Cambridge.

Turner, M. A. (1997). Towards an executive dysfunction account of repetitive behavior in autism. In J. Russell (Ed.), *Autism as an executive disorder* (pp. 57–100). Oxford: Oxford University Press.

Turner, M. A. (1999). Generating novel ideas: Fluency performance in high-functioning and learning disabled individuals with autism. *Journal of Child Psychology and Psychiatry, and Allied Disciplines, 40*(2), 189–201.

Varni, J. W., Lovaas, O. I., Koegel, R. L., et al. (1979). An analysis of observational learning in autistic and normal children. *Journal of Abnormal Child Psychology, 7*(1), 31–43.

Watt, N., Wetherby, A. M., Barber, A., & Morgan, L. (2008). Repetitive and stereotyped behaviors in children with autism spectrum disorders in the second year of life. *Journal of Autism and Developmental Disorders, 38*(8), 1518–1533.

Wheelwright, S., & Baron-Cohen, S. (2001). The link between autism and skills such as engineering, math, physics, and computing: a reply to Jarrold and Routh. *Autism, 5*(2), 223–227.

Wing, L., & Gould, J. (1979). Severe impairments of social interaction and associated abnormalities in children: Epidemiology and classification. *Journal of Autism and Developmental Disorders*, 11–29.

Zandt, F., Prior, M., & Kyrios, M. (2006). Repetitive behavior in children with high functioning autism and obsessive compulsive disorder. *Journal of Autism and Developmental Disorders, 37*, 251–259.

12 Rebecca J. Landa

Developmental Features and Trajectories Associated with Autism Spectrum Disorders in Infants and Toddlers

Points of Interest

- Developmental trajectory in the first 2 years of life may vary across different children with ASD, and across different aspects of development.
- The earlier that a parent becomes concerned about a child with autism, the more likely that the child will have more severe autism symptoms later.
- By the time children with autism reach the second birthday, 80% of parents have become concerned about the child's development.
- Some children with autism exhibit developmental regression, usually affecting social and/or language development, in the first two years of life.
- Early diagnosis of autism is quite stable, especially when made by a professional with expertise in early diagnosis of this disorder.

Over the course of the last decade, there has been a major emphasis on earlier detection of autism spectrum disorders (ASD) by researchers (e.g., Landa, 2008; Zwaigenbaum et al., 2007), public health agencies (Centers for Disease Control and Prevention; 2008), professional health care organizations (American Academy of Pediatrics [AAP]; Johnson et al., 2007), advocacy groups (Autism Speaks, 2007), and clinical providers. The primary reason for this emphasis on earlier detection is to permit earlier access to intervention, which is expected to improve outcomes for children with ASD (Harris & Handleman, 2000; Howard, Sparkman, Cohen, Green, & Stanislaw, 2005; Sallows & Graupner, 2005). Another reason for earlier detection is parents' need for accurate information about their children. Parents of children with ASD often recognize disruptions in their child's behavior or development well before the diagnosis of ASD is given. Recent studies have indicated that parents wish to be informed as early as possible about the presence of ASD in their young child (Johnson, Myers, & the Council on Children with Disabilities, 2007; Glascoe, 2005). All too often, parents are given inaccurate information about their child's well-being early in the child's life, which may lead to frustration and long-lasting mistrust of professionals. The reduction in familial stress (Goin & Meyers, 2004) and improved child outcomes that result from earlier detection of ASD lead to improved quality of life within families, and quite possibly reduced educational and long-term-care costs. Thus, efforts to detect ASD earlier in life have inestimable benefit for children with ASD, their families, and the community at large.

In the absence of a medical test for autism, research aimed at early detection of ASD has focused on behavioral signs of ASD. Both retrospective and prospective research approaches have been employed. Retrospective approaches involve obtaining past data about a child who has been diagnosed with ASD. Such data may come from medical records, interviewing or surveying parents about their memories of the child's earlier development (often many years in the past), and/or coding (e.g., counting frequency of occurrence and number of different types) behaviors exhibited by a child from home videos recorded earlier in the child's life. Prospective research may involve studies of community-based samples of children who received early developmental screening, studies of infants or toddlers who received assessment within a clinical setting, or studies of infants at high risk for ASD, as is the case for infants who have an older sibling with ASD (Landa, Holman, & Garrett-Mayer, 2007).

Both retrospective and prospective studies have provided insights into the earliest signs of ASD and about the process of early development in infants and toddlers who will later obtain a diagnosis of ASD. For example, studies employing both types of research strategies have indicated that development may be disrupted during the first year of life in some infants later diagnosed with ASD, and that the nature of the earliest signs of developmental disruption may be subtle or nonspecific to ASD. However, by the time of the first birthday, the social and communication characteristics that define autism in older children are observable in some children with ASD and differentiate those children from age peers with non-ASD developmental delay and typical development. The specific nature of the symptoms and the timing of their onset may differ from child to child. Longitudinal prospective studies indicate that trajectory of development over the first years of life may differ across children having an ASD diagnosis. These issues will be addressed within this chapter as the literature is reviewed on developmental features, diagnosis, and developmental trajectory associated with ASD in the first 3 years of life.

Parents' Early Concerns About Children Diagnosed with ASD

Parents of children with ASD are often the first to observe the signs of developmental disruption. These concerns may arise early, even in the first year of a child's life (Howlin & Asgharian, 1999). When concerns do arise so early, the later diagnosis is more likely to be autism than Pervasive Developmental Disorder Not-Otherwise-Specified (Chawarska et al., 2007a). Similarly, when parents recognized developmental disruption prior to 18 months of age, the child with autism was more likely to have more severe autism symptoms and greater speech delay, lower level of developmental functioning, lower adaptive skills, and a specific neurological disorder (e.g., epilepsy, cerebral palsy, meningitis) (Baghdadli, Picot, Pascal, Pry, & Aussilloux, 2003).

Parents of children later diagnosed with ASD first become concerned about their child at mean age 18 months (Howlin & Asgharian, 1999), with increasing numbers of parents expressing concerns as children approach their second birthday (Wetherby, Bronson-Maddox, Peace, & Newton, 2008). Less than half of the parents of children with ASD younger than 15 months of age expressed concerns about communication development on a communication checklist (Wetherby, Bronson-Maddox, Peace, & Newton, 2008). By the time of the second birthday, 80% of parents of children later diagnosed with ASD recall having been concerned about their child's development (De Giacomo & Fombonne, 1998). Parents' concerns most often focus on speech and language delays (De Giacomo & Fombonne, 1998; Hess & Landa, in press), and less often, concerns involved social, play, sensory, motor (Charman et al., 2000; Hess & Landa, in press) or medical or regulatory problems related to sleep, eating, and attention (De Giacomo & Fombonne, 1998). Parent concerns, as elicited by a structured questionnaire, have not been found to distinguish infants and toddlers later diagnosed with ASD from those later diagnosed with other developmental delay (Wetherby et al., 2008). These concerns are typically reported to a professional when the child is between 18 and 24 months of age (Rogers & DiLalla, 1990; Young, Brewer, & Pattison, 2003). Yet a diagnosis of ASD occurs considerably later, usually not until 4 years of age. The age at first diagnosis tends to be even later for urban, low SES (socioeconomic status) children (Fombonne, Simmons, Ford, Meltzer, & Goodman, 2001; Gray, Tonge & Brereton, 2006; Howlin & Asgharian, 1999; Mandell et al., 2002; Shattuck, Durkin, Maenner, Newschaffer, Mandell, Wiggins, et al., 2009; Wiggins, Baio, & Rice, 2006; Williams & Brayne, 2006).

What is Known about Signs of ASD in the First Year of Life?

Very little is known about ASD in the first year of life. Most information about developmental features of infants with ASD comes from retrospective studies. Prospective studies have provided only preliminary insights into the developmental features of infants later diagnosed with autism. This is because most studies have not yet followed these infants through the third birthday, the time when diagnosis becomes reliable (Ventola et al., 2006). Information about differences in infants (under 12 months of age) later diagnosed with ASD is reviewed below, with reference made to retrospective and prospective findings.

Attention

Evidence is accumulating that the attention system may be disrupted by 6–12 months of age in infants later diagnosed with ASD. In infants between the ages of 6 and 12 months, the literature describes two types of disruption in attention: difficulty with attention disengagement (Adrien et al., 1992; Maestro et al., 2002; Zwaigenbaum et al., 2005) and diminished attention to faces relative to objects (Baranek, 1999; Maestro et al., 2002; Osterling et al., 2002; Chawarska, Volkmar, & Klin, 2010; Pierce, Conant, Hazin, Stoner, & Desmond, 2011). The latter feature was noted to distinguish infants later diagnosed with ASD from those with non-ASD developmental delay as well as from those with typical development (Baranek, 1999; Maestro et al., 2002). The ability to direct attention to objects or to sustain the focus of attention on objects does not appear to be impaired in infants later diagnosed with ASD (Maestro et al., 2002).

Sensory and Motor Systems

Evidence for disruption in the sensory and motor systems in infants with ASD has emerged from retrospective and prospective studies. Sensory features may include hyposensitivity or hypersensitivity to sound and touch (Adrien et al., 1992; Baranek 1999) and excessive mouthing (Baranek, 1999; Maestro et al., 2002), which, in combination with other variables, distinguished infants with ASD from those with non-ASD developmental delay and those with typical development. Some of the motor abnormalities observed in this author's study of infant siblings of children with autism, such as head lag in older infants, may be related to an abnormality within the sensory system, including proprioception and feed-forward systems (Flanagan & Landa, 2007). Motor system disruption may involve gross or fine motor delays (Flanagan & Landa, 2007; Ozonoff et al., 2008a), atypical movements (including tremulousness, posturing, or persistent repetition of an age-appropriate behavior such as raspberries; Flanagan & Landa, 2007; Sparling, 1991), or hypotonicity or rigidity of limbs (Flanagan & Landa, 2007; Sparling, 1991). Diminished range of facial expressions and abnormalities related to vocalization or babbling (Maestro et al., 2002) could also be related to disruption in the motor system. It should be noted that motor system abnormalities are not likely to be specific to ASD (Ozonoff et al., 2008a), but may be predictive of social and communication impairments, including autism (Flanagan & Landa, 2007).

Social and Communication Systems

The two most frequently reported aspects of developmental disruption involving the social and/or communication systems involve decreased attention to faces (in infants as young as 6 months of age) and diminished response to name (beginning at 8 months of age; Baranek, 1999; Werner et al., 2000). In Baranek's (1999) study of 9- to 12-month-olds, response to name reliably distinguished infants with autism from those with mental retardation or typical development. Diminished affective responsiveness has also been reported in a retrospective study involving analysis of videotapes of infants (6 months and younger) who had outcomes of ASD versus typical development (Maestro et al., 2002). Social and communication initiation may also be diminished in infants with ASD (Adrien et al., 1993; Flanagan & Landa, 2007; Maestro et al., 2005; Maestro et al., 2002). There is conflicting evidence regarding abnormality of eye contact in infants with ASD (not different from typically developing age peers in a study of 8- to 10-month-olds; versus limited eye contact in case reports by Dawson, Osterling, Meltzoff, & Kuhl, 2000; Klin et al., 2004, and Sparling, 1991). Further evidence for social abnormalities in the first year of life comes from parents' report that their preschoolers with autism had never performed certain social behaviors that typically emerge in the first year of life, including showing anticipation of being lifted, showing affection toward others, showing interest in children other than siblings, reaching for a familiar person, and playing simple interaction games with others (Klin, Volkmar, & Sparrow, 1992).

What is Known about Signs of ASD in the Second Year of Life?

The literature provides more substantial information about predictors of ASD for children in the 1- to 2-year age range. The developmental features associated with ASD become increasingly clear with increasing chronological age (Landa, Holman, & Garrett-Mayer, 2007). Even the passage of a few months may permit recognition of an ASD clinical picture that was previously unclear. The nature of the developmental disruptions in 1-year-olds with ASD will vary from child to child in number, severity, and nature, as well as in the timing of onset and pattern of developmental trajectory. Nevertheless, the guiding principle that social impairment must be present for a diagnosis of ASD holds true even for children at this young age.

Retrospective Studies: 12 to 24 Months of Age

Retrospective studies indicate that at around the time of the first birthday, some children later diagnosed with ASD can be distinguished from their typically developing peers as well as from age peers with other types of developmental delays. In a retrospective study involving analysis of first birthday videotapes, Osterling and colleagues (2002) reported that 12-month-olds later diagnosed with ASD differed from those with intellectual disability and typical development in the frequency and duration of orienting to name and looking at people. There were other behaviors that failed to distinguish children with ASD from those with intellectual disability, but that distinguished both groups of impaired children from typically developing age peers. Such behaviors involved the use of gestures, looking at objects held by others, and the presence of repetitive actions. This supported findings from Osterling and Dawson's (1994) earlier retrospective study that children with ASD differed from 1-year-olds with typical development in the frequency with which they looked at others, showed or pointed to objects, and responded to their name. In addition to the social, communication, and play abnormalities, atypical patterns of sensory responsivity have also been identified in retrospective studies that reviewed home videos taken at about the time of the first birthday (Adrien et al., 1993; Baranek, 1999). Disruption in self-regulation has also been identified in 1-year-olds with ASD (Gomez & Baird, 2005). This finding emerged from a study in which parents completed a standardized temperament questionnaire (the Temperament and Atypical Behavior Scale (TABS) (Bagnato, Neisworth, Salvia, & Hunt, 1999). Based on TABS norms, parents' responses would have resulted in 86% of the children meeting criteria for regulatory disorder (Gomez & Baird, 2005).

In the latter half of the first year of life, multiple retrospective studies indicate that development of children with ASD diverges to a greater degree from typical patterns of development, qualitatively and/or quantitatively. For example, in a small longitudinal, retrospective study, Losche (1990) examined play behavior of children with ASD and typical development using videotapes taken between 4 and 42 months of age. No differences in presymbolic play behavior were noted between the groups until 22 months of age. At that age, however, the children with ASD exhibited a plateau in the frequency of goal-oriented object exploration. In contrast, children with typical development at that age displayed growth in play development, exhibiting greater diversity of play acts with objects and an increase in the frequency of those acts.

This timing of the plateau in children with ASD parallels the mean age at which parents become concerned about their children with ASD (Howlin & Asgharian, 1999), the mean age at which regression occurs (Luyster et al., 2005), and the timing of developmental slowing identified in prospective, longitudinal studies (Landa & Garrett-Mayer, 2006; Landa et al., 2007). Prior to this time (18 to 22 months of age), symptoms of ASD may be absent or too subtle to raise parents' concern. Support for this notion comes from Baird and colleagues' (2000) study of parents' responses on an autism screening questionnaire. Parents of 18-month-olds later diagnosed with ASD did not report that their children showed abnormality in protodeclarative pointing or gaze monitoring (Baird et al., 2000).

Prospective Studies: 12 to 18 Months of Age

Like retrospective studies, prospective studies suggest that, at around the time of the first birthday, some behavioral features are predictive of later developmental disruption, including a later diagnosis of ASD. The behavioral features represent all three of the diagnostic symptom domains for pervasive developmental disorders as defined in the *Diagnostic and Statistical Manual-IV* (American Psychiatric Association [APA], 1994): qualitative impairment in social behavior, qualitative impairment in communication behavior, and repetitive and stereotyped patterns of behavior and interest. Qualitative and quantitative differences in social development are characterized by decreased social responsivity, social initiation, and affective expression. Examples of disruption in social responsivity include poor response to name (Nadig et al., 2007), poor monitoring of others' gaze (Landa et al., 2007), and poor response to others' bids for joint attention (Sullivan et al., 2007). Difficulty with social initiation involves infrequent initiation of joint attention through pointing or showing (Landa et al., 2007), infrequent directing of play acts toward others (Landa et al., 2007), and infrequent initiation of social communication bids (Landa et al., 2007). Response to others' joint attention cues (shifts in gaze, head turn, pointing gesture) occurs less frequently and has a longer period of instability in 1-year-olds with ASD than in age peers without ASD (Sullivan et al., 2007). Young children with ASD also share positive affect with others less often than their non-ASD age peers (Landa et al., 2007). Qualitative and quantitative differences in communication are represented by receptive and expressive language delay (Landa & Garrett-Mayer, 2006) and decreased frequency of communicative bids directed toward others. Communication is characterized by a restricted repertoire of communicative forms, affecting gesture use and production of consonants compared to age peers with typical development or language delays (Landa et al., 2007). Play behavior in children with an early diagnosis of ASD was distinguished from children with typical development and language or social delays; action schema on toys was less diverse and fewer sequences of play acts on toys were exhibited (Landa et al., 2007). In addition, repetitive and stereotyped patterns of behavior and interests are also represented. Repetitive behavior and sensory preoccupation were reported in some 12-month-olds later diagnosed with ASD (Loh et al., 2007; Ozonoff et al., 2008b), especially involving the use of the arms compared to children with other developmental delays and typical development (Loh et al., 2007).

Prospective Studies: 18–24 Months of Age

The studies reviewed below focused on 18- to 24-month-olds with ASD and included a comparison group involving children with non-ASD delays.

An increased number of studies are available to shed light on behavioral abnormalities associated with ASD in 18- to 24-month-olds with ASD. As discussed in the review of retrospective studies above, ASD symptoms become more prominent or persistent in this timeframe, and thus become clearer indicators for concern about the presence of ASD. One illustration of this comes from Cox and colleagues' (1999) follow-up of children with ASD who were originally assessed at 20 months of age. At both the original assessment at 20 months and the follow-up assessment at 42 months of age, the Autism Diagnostic Interview-Revised (ADI-R; Lord, Rutter, & Le Couteur, 1994) was conducted to systematically elicit parents' memories and report of past and current autism-related behavior. Two ADI-R items, "Point for Interest" and "Use of Conventional Gestures" differentiated the ASD group at 20 and 42 months of age from children with language delay and typical development. But with increasing age, an increased number of ADI-R items differentiated children with ASD from other children. At 42 months of age, the items newly endorsed by parents of children with ASD included: "Seeking to Share Enjoyment," "Offering Comfort," "Nodding and Imaginative Play." As with Losche's (1990) report about play development, children with ASD are failing to exhibit the more complex and sophisticated social and play behavior that is expected at more advanced chronological ages. Cox and colleagues (1999) did not find any variables from the Repetitive Behaviors and Stereotyped Interests section of the ADI-R to differentiate the groups at either age. However, the ADI-R is based on parent report. Studies involving direct measurement of children's repetitive behaviors have yielded different results (see references to Wetherby's work below).

Studies involving direct assessment of 18- to 24-month-olds contribute additional insights into the early characteristics of ASD. One of the first such studies focused on children who had failed an autism screening (CHAT; Baron-Cohen, Allen, & Gillberg, 1992) at 18 months of age, and were thus considered at high risk for autism or other developmental delay. This sample of children was assessed extensively at 20 months of age (reviewed below). The children who were later diagnosed with ASD differed in multiple ways from those later diagnosed with a language delay. The children with ASD looked less at adults during play (Swettenham et al., 1998), exhibited decreased frequency of gaze shifts between objects and people (Charman et al., 1997; Swettenham et al., 1998), were less likely to look at the face of an adult expressing distress (Charman et al., 1997), and imitated less often (Charman et al., 1997). As noted above, Cox and colleagues (1999) found that, per concurrent parent report, 20-month-olds with ASD less often used conventional gestures, including the use of pointing for sharing interest, compared to language delayed and typically developing age peers. Thus, prior to the second birthday, children with ASD displayed abnormality in interpersonal synchrony. They provided few cues to their interaction partner to indicate their interest in being engaged.

Using a similar screening strategy to identify children at high risk for ASD, Wetherby and colleagues (2004) compared 50 children with ASD to 25 children with non-ASD developmental delay and 50 children with typical development at age 18 to 24 months. The children with ASD differed from the non-ASD group in that they less frequently displayed eye contact, coordinated gaze with nonverbal communicative behaviors (e.g., gestures), initiated joint attention, and responded to their name. In addition, the children with ASD exhibited unusual prosody, and more repetitive body movements and repetitive use of objects. The authors then rated videotaped lab-based behavior samples of the children using the Systematic Observation of Red Flags (SORF) for ASD (Wetherby & Woods, 2002). The ASD group differed from the Developmental Delay and Typically Developing groups on nine items, representing impaired social interaction, impaired communication, and repetitive behavior and restricted interests. These included lack of appropriate gaze; lack of warm, joyful expressions; lack of sharing interest or enjoyment; lack of response to name; lack of showing; lack of coordination of nonverbal communication; unusual prosody; repetitive movements with objects; and repetitive movements or posturing of body. Four behaviors differentiated the ASD and developmentally delayed (DD) groups from the typically developing (TD) group, but did not differentiate the ASD and DD groups from each other. These behaviors fall within the domain of communication, and could be considered early signs of nonspecific delay. They include: lack of pointing; lack of playing with a variety of toys; lack of response to contextual cues; and lack of communicative vocalizations with consonants. In later work, Wetherby and colleagues reported finding higher rates and a larger inventory of repetitive and stereotyped body movements and movements with objects in children with ASD than in age peers with developmental delay or typical development (Morgan, Wetherby, & Barber, 2008; Watt, Wetherby, Barber, & Morgan, 2008).

Wetherby, Watt, Morgan, and Shumway (2007) examined children who were first assessed between the ages of 18 and 24 months, and at 30 months of age received an "outcome" diagnosis of ASD, Developmental Delay, or Typically Developing. Based on data obtained via the Communication and Symbolic Behavior Scales Developmental Profile (Wetherby & Prizant, 2002) at the first assessment, the ASD and TD groups were found to differ on all social, communication, and play variables. The ASD and DD groups differed on frequency of gaze shifts between objects and people, response to pointing gestures, rate of communicating, frequency of initiation of joint attention, and variety of conventional gestures used communicatively. This parallels Landa and colleague's finding in early diagnosed 14-month-olds with ASD, but does not entirely parallel the findings involving later diagnosed 24-month-olds with ASD. In Landa and colleagues' (2007) study, the later diagnosed group of children with ASD did not differ from the language and/or social delayed group on the communication or play variables, nor on frequency of triadic gaze. Likewise, they did not differ from nondelayed controls in play behavior.

Early predictors of later ASD severity were examined by Wetherby and colleagues (2007). The following behaviors were predictive of later severity: frequency of behavior regulatory acts and rate of communicating; variety of conventional gestures and consonants; and variety of conventional actions on objects during play as well as variety of pretend play acts. Interestingly, frequency of shared positive affect and gaze shifts did not differentiate the DD and ASD groups, nor did these variables predict ASD severity. One explanation for this may be the coding protocol used by Wetherby's group. For shared positive affect and gaze shifts, the coding protocol required scorers to indicate whether or not the child exhibited that particular behavior within each of the six sampling conditions rather than coding frequency of occurrence of these behaviors. Since young children with ASD do produce some such behaviors (Landa et al., 2007; Charman et al., 1998), a more continuous variable involving frequency of occurrence of such events may be necessary to capture differences between toddlers with ASD and those with other types of developmental delays.

Another important finding emerged from Wetherby and colleagues' (2007) report: response to others' pointing gestures (response to joint attention cues) and initiation of joint attention were highly correlated with language comprehension. Wetherby and colleagues (2007) suggested that joint attention behavior in 18- to 24-month-olds may reflect representational skills rather than just social cognition. This is an interesting notion. Although one prospective, longitudinal study reported that the developmental trajectory of joint attention in the second year of life does not parallel that of word inventory, word combinations, or representational play (Landa et al., 2007; Sullivan et al., 2007), there appears to be a relationship between the developmental trajectories of initiation of joint attention and diversity of gestures produced between 14 and 24 months of age. Landa and colleagues (2007) reported that frequency of initiating joint attention through the use of showing or pointing gesture declines or plateaus between 14 and 24 months of age, much like that of gesture inventory. More research is needed to reveal the relationships between different types of communicative intents, responses to others' communicative bids, gestures, and other forms of communication. Understanding such relationships would have implications for intervention, where treatment focused on some of these aspects of development may result in collateral changes in other aspects.

Implications of the Presence of Early Signs of ASD

The retrospective and prospective literatures indicate that there are a number of different systems in which developmental processes may be disrupted in some younger siblings of children with ASD, even if they are not ultimately diagnosed with ASD. The same is true for children later diagnosed with ASD, whether or not they have a known family history of ASD. Affected aspects of development may involve motor (including muscle tone), attention, motivation and initiative, arousal and self-regulation, expression of emotion, social reciprocity, patterns of social orienting, and coordination and integration of movement/affect/vocalization/gaze. In some infants and toddlers, repetitive body movements and actions on objects are also observed. The behavioral features described above in infants and toddlers with ASD culminate in an abnormal ability to engage in flexible, adaptive, appropriate and well-synchronized social and communicative engagement with others. Although early disruption in these aspects of development does not always predict ASD, they signal the need for monitoring development, at least through the preschool years. Each of the systems mentioned above (attention, motor, affective, self-regulatory, social orienting, etc.) contribute substantially to children's ability to detect relevant saliency, orient to and anticipate social and communicative events, respond contingently and synchronously to the dynamic changes in others' facial and vocal behaviors, and initiate engagement with others in "readable" and predictable ways. For these children, adaptations to environmental input, particularly social input, may be beneficial. Such adaptations in input may include, for example, simplifying the movements required to successfully grasp toys, providing toys that provide rewarding sensory input to the child and that can be easily grasped and held, making social stimuli more salient and consistent in form, introducing highly predictable routines that are presented slowly and with the amount of sensory input that is satisfying to the child, and so forth. The next section of this chapter focuses on guidelines that may facilitate the early identification of children who may be in need of such adapted input, or who may be at high risk for a developmental disorder such as ASD.

Implications for Detecting ASD Prior to the First Birthday

As indicated above, the literature is populated with few studies, all involving small numbers of children, on which to base guidance for clinicians and parents in their efforts to identify infants who will later manifest the full complex of autism symptoms. The early signs of developmental disruption in infants with ASD are subtle, and may not involve the expected social impairments that are so clear in older children with ASD. Furthermore, standardized test scores may fall well within normal limits (Landa & Garrett-Mayer, 2006). Despite such quantitative scores, qualitative behavioral abnormalities or extremes may be present (Landa & Garrett-Mayer, 2006). During infancy, behavioral signs of disrupted development vary in number, nature, and severity (or intensity) from child to child. In addition, identifying infants who will later receive a diagnosis of developmental delay is complicated by the variation that characterizes typical development. Thus, there is a "gray zone" in which the boundaries between "typical" and "atypical" development are unclear. To address this challenge guidelines have been published for primary health providers (Johnson, Myers, & the Council on Children with Disabilities, 2007) for use beginning at age 9 months. These guidelines call for developmental surveillance at well visits conducted at 9, 18, and 24 months of age. During these visits, health care professionals are advised to: (1) elicit and attend to parents' concerns about their child's development; (2) document and maintain a developmental history; (3) make accurate observations of the child; (4) identify risk and protective factors; and (5) maintain an accurate record of documenting the process and findings. Since parents of children with developmental delays may not have initial concerns about their child (Hess & Landa, in press; King et al., 2005; Wetherby, Brosnan-Maddox, Peace, & Newton, 2008), the role of the health care provider is considerable in the early detection of developmental disorders, including ASD. Alternatively, parents' concerns may be more sensitive than developmental measures in some cases (Hess & Landa, in press).

Since guidelines for primary health care providers do not address infants younger than 9 months of age, providers may feel poorly equipped to recognize the earliest signs of developmental disruption or to know when to refer infants for developmental assessment. Since early signs of developmental disruption may be subtle, and there are no clear predictors of ASD from infancy, a prudent guideline for referring younger infants for a developmental assessment may be as follows: (1) refer if there is mild concern (expressed by parent or professional) and one or more risk factors exist (e.g., family history of language impairment or ASD, preterm birth, low birth weight); or (2) refer if there is at least moderate concern, regardless of presence of risk factors. Of course, regardless of risk factors, parents must always make the final decision about seeking a nonmedical developmental assessment. A developmental checklist is provided below (Table 12-1) to assist health care providers and other clinicians to systematically consider aspects of development that may be disrupted in infants at risk for ASD. When possible indicators of risk for ASD are observed or reported, the professional should inquire about the frequency, duration, and intensity of the display of the concerning behaviors. Determining the age at which the concerning behavior began to be exhibited is also important. Referral to an expert in infant development will clarify level of risk, and yield recommendations about how parents may stimulate, regulate, and engage their infants in ways that optimize the infant's development. Obtaining a medical evaluation

Table 12–1.
Developmental features to consider in infant developmental screening for 6- to 9-month-olds

Developmental Domain	Features to Observe or About Which to Query the Parent	Indicators of Possible Risk for ASD
Communication	__ Babbling (frequency, variety of sounds) __Infant watches the face of the person talking to him/her __Vocal turn-taking during engagement with parent __Quality of vocal tone	• Absent or rare occurrence of babbling • Reduced variety of sounds in babbling • No attention to face of speaker • Absence of vocal response to caregiver vocalization • Unusual high pitched squeals
Social Responsivity, Duration of Engagement, and Active Participation During Engagement	__Eye contact __Reciprocal smiling __Orients to name being called __Exhibits a range of facial expressions __Sustains attention to social input __ Initiative with toys and people __Social anticipation	• Gaze aversion, infrequent or brief duration eye contact • Absence of reciprocal smiling, or smiling occurs only when infant is touched, or a robust stimulus is needed to elicit a smile; infrequent social smiles • No response to name being called • Neutral affect • Brief duration of gaze during caregiver engagement with infant • Passivity, rarely reaches for objects without extra assistance from caregiver • Poor anticipation of being picked up or of social games (as in peek-a-boo)
Motor and Sensory	__Muscle tone __Coordinated movements __Motor milestones (sitting, crawling, rolling, supporting self on arms when prone) __Response to touch or other sensory experience __Feeding __Quality of body movements	• Hypotonicity • Poor coordination of hands together • Delay in milestone acquisition; head lag when pulled to sit from supine position • Hyper- or hyposensitive to touch or other sensory experience • Feeding difficulties (e.g., refusing categories of foods) • Unusual posturing or excessive repetition of movements
Play	__Variety of ways of exploring toys __ Variety of toys explored __Nature of object exploration	• Atypically intense focus on specific objects or parts of objects (e.g., wheels on a car) • Repetitive action on a particular object or class of objects (e.g., trying to make lids wobble) • Absence of object exploration or atypical patterns or intensity of exploration (e.g., holding toy close to eyes or in peripheral vision, excessive mouthing)
Self-regulatory	__Temperament __Soothe-ability	• Extreme temperament (including passivity, high reactivity, underresponsive) • Not easily soothed when upset; may be inconsolable

also may be appropriate to rule out known etiologies for the behavioral indicators of developmental disruption (Filipek et al., 1999).

Stability of Early Diagnosis of ASD

The age at which a diagnosis of ASD is made will depend on a variety of factors. There is consensus among autism clinical researchers that by the age of 3 years, a diagnosis of ASD can be made reliably, and that the stability of the diagnosis after this age is high. Two studies have focused on stability of ASD diagnosis in children younger than 2 years of age (Chawarska et al., 2007b; Cox et al., 1999). Chawarska and colleagues (2007b) studied short-term stability (from just under 24 months of age to 3 years of age) of the diagnosis of autism and Pervasive Developmental Disorder Not-Otherwise-Specified (PDD-NOS) in 31 children referred to a clinic for evaluation to rule out ASD. All children initially diagnosed with ASD remained on the spectrum, however two children shifted diagnosis from autism to PDD-NOS. In another study, Cox and colleagues (1999) reported high levels of stability of ASD diagnosis from 20 months of age to 42–46 months of age in children who had screened positive at 18 months of age an autism screening instrument (CHAT, Baron-Cohen, Allen, & Gillberg, 1992).

Several studies have examined stability of diagnosis of ASD in 2-year-olds. In studies where 2-year-olds diagnosed with autism or PDD-NOS were followed for at least 5 years, the stability of diagnosis ranged from 85 to 89% (Charman et al., 2005; Lord et al., 2006; Turner, Stone, Pozdol, & Coonrod, 2006). However, one study examining short-term stability of ASD diagnosis in 2-year-olds suggests that, under certain circumstances, early diagnosis of ASD may be unstable (Turner & Stone, 2007). One factor related to diagnostic instability was being younger than 30 months at the time of diagnosis. Stability of ASD diagnosis was 52% in children younger than 30 months of age compared to 87% in children 30 months or older. Two other factors related to diagnostic instability involved milder symptoms, especially social functioning, and higher cognitive test scores (Turner & Stone, 2007). These factors are similar to the predictors of improvement in 2-year-olds with ASD as reported by others (Charman et al., 2003; Lord, 1995). In general, stability of diagnosis in 2-year-olds is associated with experience of the diagnostician (Stone et al., 1999) and severity or pervasiveness of symptoms (Eaves & Ho, 2004; Lord et al., 2006; Moore & Goodson, 2003; Stone et al., 1999; Turner et al., 2006). Stability of diagnosis is greatest when the diagnostic "gold standard" is clinical judgment as opposed to diagnostic classification based on the scores of an autism diagnostic measure, such as the ADI-R (Chawarska et al., 2007b; Kleinman et al., 2008). For children whose diagnostic status shifts from ASD to non-ASD, lingering developmental delays often persist (Fein, Dixon, Paul, & Levin, 2005; Kleinman et al., 2008; Landa, Holman, & Garrett-Mayer, 2007; Turner & Stone, 2007). At present, predicting the children who will improve substantially and, thus, lose the ASD diagnosis is quite difficult. Sutera and colleagues (2007) found only one variable, motor functioning at age 2 years, was associated with optimal outcome (defined as losing the ASD diagnosis). With increasing age, diagnosis becomes more stable (Charman et al., 2005). The findings summarized above have implications for clinical practice. First, diagnosis of children younger than 3 years of age should be made only by clinicians with expertise in autism and in early child development. Second, when a diagnosis of ASD is made, parents should be informed that their child's diagnostic status or severity of symptoms could possibly change when assessed at an older age. Third, follow-up assessments are advised when risk for ASD is considered high, or when an ASD diagnosis is made, in a child younger than 3 years of age.

A word about false negatives is worthwhile. With the extensive media coverage about early signs of ASD, some parents begin to suspect that their child is showing signs of ASD and seek expert advice. Many times the expert who sees the child is a physician. If the physician conducts a screening (e.g., using the M-CHAT, a brief behavioral screening questionnaire, or some combination of formal or informal screening questionnaire and observation) and does not see clear signs of ASD, parents may be informed that their child is "normal." This is probably an accurate conclusion for many children. However, studies (Cox et al., 1999; Landa et al., 2007; Werner & Dawson, 2005) are showing that some children with ASD may exhibit few signs of early developmental disruption, with subsequent change in developmental trajectory (e.g., slowing, plateauing, or regression in development; see "Progression of ASD," below). Indeed, 9 children evaluated at 42 months of age had been judged to have typical development or language delay at 20 months of age (Cox et al., 1999), but were later diagnosed with ASD. In a prospective study of infant siblings of children with autism, Landa and colleagues (2007) reported that nearly half of the children diagnosed with ASD at 3 years of age had not been judged by an expert clinician to have ASD at 14 months of age, though all had been noted to have disruptions in one or more aspects of development. The possibility of "false negatives" may be heightened for toddlers having a positive family history of ASD, or in other high risk populations (e.g., preterm infants), but this author advises professionals to monitor development of toddlers when parents have early developmental concerns, regardless of the medical risk status of the child. The 8-step surveillance guidelines proposed by members of the American Academy of Pediatrics' Council on Children with Disabilities (Johnson et al., 2007) for early detection of ASD within pediatric offices, and the associated decision tree are supported by prospective and retrospective studies. As children approach their third birthday, the likelihood of false negatives diminishes and becomes less of a concern. The likely exception here is children with ASD who have no cognitive or language delays. These children tend to be identified once they are in school and begin to show difficulty in peer interactions.

Issues Related to Threshold for Diagnosing ASD in Children Younger Than 30 Months of Age

Determining the degree to which a young child must vary from typical development, qualitatively and quantitatively, in order to qualify for a diagnosis of ASD is a complex matter. It involves defining the boundaries between "typical" and disordered development, particularly in communication and social behavior. For children younger than 3 years of age, defining these boundaries can be quite difficult. In this author's longitudinal study of infant siblings of children with ASD, where children are tested at 6, 14, 18, 24, 30, and 36 months of age, expert clinicians indicate, at each assessment from 14 to 36 months of age, whether a child displays the signs of ASD, and if so, whether a clinical impression of ASD is warranted. For some children, this is quite difficult because the younger siblings of children with ASD present with a continuum of "typical" to abnormal or delayed functioning in one or more aspects of development, and positive symptoms may not be present or robust in early development (e.g., there can be no echolalia before spoken language begins to emerge). Thus, the research setting mimics community-based health centers, where professionals are faced with difficult decisions about whether to refer a child for developmental assessment, or for children who have received such assessment, whether to diagnose the child with ASD. In this author's lab, the concept of a continuum of risk for ASD is integrated into the process of establishing clinical impressions. We think of this continuum as beginning with typical development, where expected language, social, motor, cognitive, and behavioral milestones are met and displayed in contextually appropriate ways, with appropriate levels of flexibility and consistency. At the other end of the continuum is clear delay or impairment, where children fail to meet expected milestones, score abnormally on multiple standardized measures of different domains of development, and where clinical judgment of experts from different professional disciplines agree on the diagnosis of ASD. In Figure 12-1 below, this continuum is illustrated.

A behavior sampling guide is provided in Table 12-2. With little extra time or effort, this sample may be collected in a primary health care setting, as well as in a developmental screening center. It is entirely possible that a young child with ASD may perform "normally" in assessment contexts that involve familiar routines and tasks, especially if these do not require the child to integrate multiple aspects of development, as in a peek-a-boo task. Thus, parent report of behavior in different contexts and their sense of the level of "impairment" caused by their child's behavior or responsivity is important to elicit.

Progression of ASD

New insights into developmental trajectories associated with autism are emerging from the prospective, longitudinal studies of infant siblings of children with autism. As discussed above, most such studies are revealing that infants later diagnosed with ASD show only subtle, if any, signs of developmental disruption (Zwaigenbaum et al., 2005; Landa & Garrett-Mayer, 2006). The aspects of development that are disrupted may involve non-ASD specific domains, such as motor development (Bryson et al., 2007; Flanagan & Landa, 2007; Ozonoff et al., 2008a). Near the time of the first birthday, some children with ASD manifest sufficiently robust signs of impairment that ASD can be diagnosed by an expert (Landa, Holman, & Garrett-Mayer, 2007). Other children with ASD, however, do not exhibit clear symptomatology until sometime closer to the third birthday (Landa et al., 2007). This suggests that ASD has a progressive nature during the first few years of life in some, perhaps many, children affected with this disorder. Progression is conceptualized here as a "worsening," involving a shift from rather typical to atypical quality of behavior, a slowing of developmental trajectory or even a plateau in development, or intensification of behaviors that previously were considered subclinical (e.g., increase in repetitive behavior, poor eye contact), and/or there is a loss or attenuation in frequency of occurrence or diversity of previously exhibited behaviors or skills. Using this definition, toddlers with early diagnosis (as in the Landa et al., 2007, paper) may "worsen," as do toddlers with later onset ASD.

In the past, the nuances of trajectory in children with ASD were not easily defined because of the necessary reliance on retrospective research designs. Retrospective studies, primarily involving parents' recall of their now older child's early

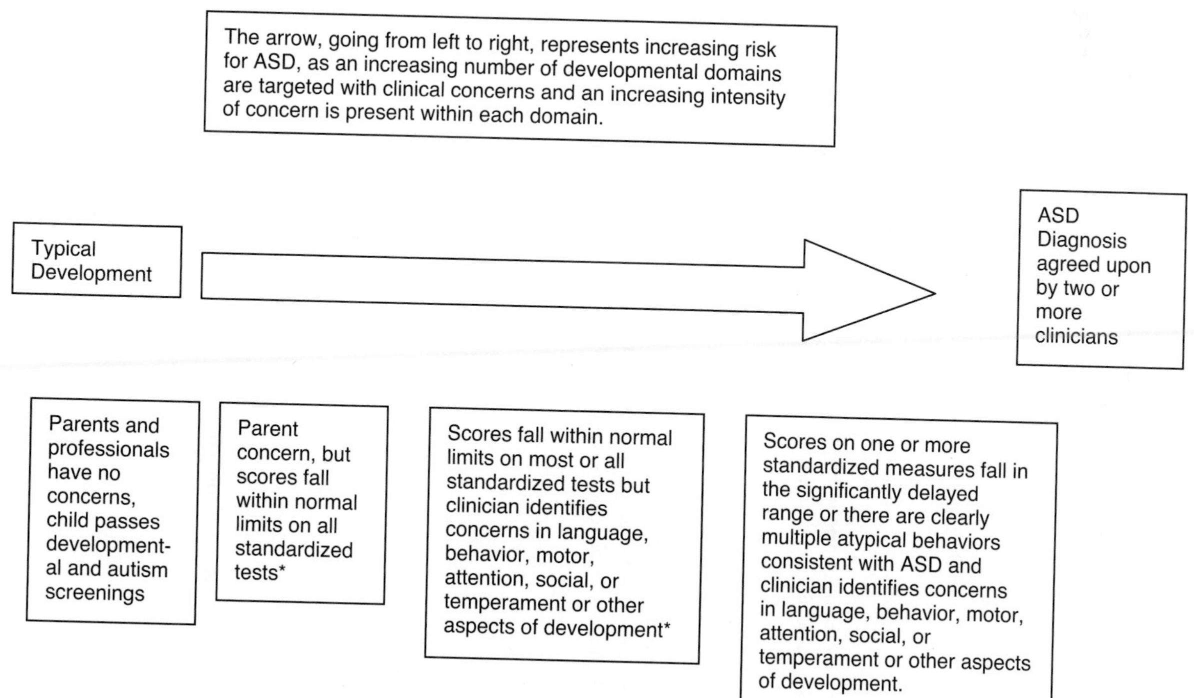

Figure 12–1. ASD risk continuum based on developmental features and parent concern for young children. * Increased weighting is given if the child is "at risk" based on medical or environmental factors (e.g., family history, preterm birth, low birth weight, health history, history of neglect, etc.).

Table 12–2.
Brief procedure for sampling ASD symptoms for children aged 9 to 30 months

Behavior to be Sampled*	Brief Sampling Procedure	Red Flag for ASD
Shared positive affect (looking at a person and smiling)	After playing with the child with some toys for a few minutes as a "warm up," comment on the child's activity or something else about the child and smile. Ask the parents how they elicit a smile from the child at home.	• The child does not smile back at you, and the parent reports that the child does not do so at home except within familiar routines or when anticipating a "tickle" or other physical contact.
Eye contact (looking directly into the eyes of another person)	Throughout the time you are with the child, note whether the child exhibits eye contact with you or their parent.	• The child rarely or never gives eye contact to the parent or to you when you speak to him or her, and the parent confirms that this pattern of behavior is characteristic of the child at home.
Initiation of joint attention (pointing something out for the purpose of sharing, not to ask for something)	Have a remote control toy set up in the room. Without drawing the child's attention to the toy, activate the toy. Remain quiet for a moment or so, watching to see whether the child will look back and forth from the toy to the parent or you, and whether the child will point the toy out to his or her parent.	• The child does not attempt to direct others' attention to the toy by pointing to it and the parents report that the child does not (or rarely will) point to show objects or events of interest to him or her.
Sustained engagement (at an early developmental level, this would involve remaining attentive to the other person, but taking a passive role; at a more mature developmental level, it would involve taking an active role in the interaction)	Ask the parent to engage the child in a familiar routine. Observe the child's reaction. Ask the parent if the child's engagement may also be sustained during less familiar activities or in activities that are not "favorites" of the child.	• The child is difficult to engage, shows only brief or no interest in the routine and the parents report that they are only successful at getting brief moments of engagement with their child. • The parent reports that the child only responds and stays engaged during favorite or familiar routines or activities, or in high affect activities.
Spontaneous imitation of others' actions	Present the parent with two sets of toys. For example, you may have two plastic toy drumsticks, two plastic plates, two forks, and a baby doll. Give one set to the parent and the other set to the child. Ask the parent to tap on the plate gently with the drumstick and to smile at their child as they do it, without telling their child what to do. They should pause, smiling at their child, and then repeat the action. Do this several times.	• The child does not attempt to imitate the parent's action and the parent reports that the child does not imitate without being asked to (or at all) at home.
Response to others' joint attention bids	Place a colorful appliqué on the wall at the child's eye level, 90° to the child's right or left. Place yourself directly opposite the child and point to the appliqué, keeping your finger close to your body (otherwise the child will simply track the movement of your arm movement and look in the direction of the appliqué). As you do this, say "Look *child's name.*"	• The child does not look in the direction of your pointing gesture and the parents report that the child does not look where others point, unless they are pointing to an object immediately in front of the child.

Behavior to be Sampled*	Brief Sampling Procedure	Red Flag for ASD
Response to name	Standing 45° to 90° from the child's midline, call the child's name in normal tone of voice. If the child does not respond immediately, pause briefly and repeat two more times. If the child does not respond, ask the parent if this is typical for the child and, if so, what the parents do at home to get the child's attention.	• The child does not respond to their name by looking directly at you when you call the child, and the parents confirm that the child inconsistently responds to their name (or does not respond to their name at all) at home.
Variety of consonants used communicatively	Create a situation in which the child is likely to be highly motivated to communicate. For example, show the child a bottle of bubbles and then blow a few bubbles. Wait and watch to see whether the child requests more bubbles by vocalizing (and what consonants are produced). Throughout the time spent with the child, observe whether the child attempts to communicate, and note number of different consonants used during these communicative bids (e.g., b, p, t, d, m, n, k).	• The child produces fewer than 5 consonants and the parent reports that the child's consonant repertoire (when communicating) is limited to five or fewer consonants at home. (This criterion is applied only to children age 12 months and older.)
A typical behaviors **		
Posturing of hand, arm, or mouth	Throughout the time spent with the child, note the child's body movements.	• The child holds arm, hand, fingers, mouth, or head in an unusual position. If there is tension in the muscles of the body part being positioned oddly, this is additional basis for concern. If the parent reports that the child shows such behaviors in the home, there is more evidence for concern.
Repetitive or unusual play with toys	Give the child the following toys and allow him or her to play with each one for a brief period: • Toy car • Doll with eyes that open and close, plate, fork, cup • Tin can and lid with wooden alphabet blocks (be sure the child is placed on a hard surface).	• Intense focus on the wheels of the car, flicking the doll's eyes for more than 5 seconds, attempting to make the lid wobble or roll, visual inspection of the letters on the blocks, lining up the blocks.
Motor	Throughout the time spent with the child, note the child's body movements.	• Low muscle tone, poor motor coordination, motor delays.
Unusual squealing	Observe the tonal quality of the child's vocalizations.	• Unusual tonal quality or squealing.
Echoing	Observe the child's verbalizations.	• Repeating segments of movies or television programs, echoing back part of all of what is said to him or her.

* *Absence of these behaviors may be red flags for ASD;* ** *Presence of these behaviors are red flags for ASD.*

development, revealed an important phenomenon involving "worsening" in children with ASD, which was conceptualized as regression. The precise definition of regression has been difficult to bring to consensus among experts beyond the general agreement that the loss of skills occurs mainly in the domains of language and/or social development. Definitions of language regression have focused mainly on the loss of spoken words, since regression usually occurs before children progress to more complex levels of language development (Kurita, 1996; Kurita, Kita, & Miyake, 1992; Kurita, 1985). Regression of social skills has been more difficult to quantify, especially when relying on parent memory of behavior that occurred many years ago.

The challenge of coming to consensus on the definition of regression in ASD is complicated by the variation in the nature of regression as reported by parents. Regression may occur in children whose parents reported previously typical development (constituting 49% of regression cases, per Wilson et al., [2003]). Alternatively, regression may occur in children whose development was previously recognized as delayed. In contrast to Wilson and colleagues (2003), a large collaborative database involving children with parental report of regression indicated that this is the more common phenomenon (Luyster et al., 2005). Some children lost only language skills, some lost only social skills, and others lost skills across multiple aspects of development (Luyster et al., 2005). Most children with regression (77%), however, reportedly lost skills in multiple aspects of development (Luyster et al., 2005). Age of regression varies from child to child, occurring at the mean age of 19 months (Luyster et al., 2005). Regardless of the nuances, however, regression of language and/or social skills rarely occurs in children with typical development or in children with non-ASD developmental delays (Burack & Volkmar, 1992; Lord, Shulman, & DiLavore, 2004; Luyster et al., 2005). Regression is estimated to occur in 20 to 33 percent of children with ASD (Goldberg et al., 2003; Rapin & Katzman, 1998; Rutter & Lord, 1987). Regression appears to occur with similar likelihood in children with or without a history of epilepsy (Luyster et al., 2005).

Prospective, longitudinal studies indicate that the onset of ASD symptoms may occur gradually, often without an accompanying parental report of regression. Our group (Landa, Holman, & Garrett-Mayer, 2007) identified this developmental pattern in about half of the children with ASD. These children were classified as "not ASD" at 14 months of age, with gradual emergence of autism symptoms culminating in a diagnosis of ASD at age 3 years. This group of children with "later ASD onset" had subtle developmental disruption, noted by an expert clinician at 14 months of age, but their social, communication, and play behavior at 14 months of age did not differ significantly from children without ASD. By 24 months of age, their social, communication, and play behavior paralleled that of the children with early onset ASD, and they were clearly distinguishable from the non-ASD groups. In some of the children with early ASD onset, and in all the children with later ASD onset, progressive worsening could be observed. Since the children diagnosed with ASD in this study (Landa et al., 2007) had an older sibling with autism, they were by definition from multiplex families. It is possible that the nature of regression in children from multiplex families is different from that observed within children from families having only one member with autism, where the genetic mechanism may be different (Sebat, Lakshmi, Malhotra, Troge, Lese-Martin, Walsh, Yamrom, et al., 2007). Despite this possibility, the phenomenon of progressive worsening was illustrated in Cox et al.'s (1999) prospective study of ASD as described above (see "False Negatives," above). Additional evidence for an increase in severity of ASD symptoms is provided by Stone and colleagues' (1999) study of diagnostic stability of ASD. In that study, 37 children diagnosed with ASD were assessed at mean age 31.4 months and again at mean age 45 months. Half of the 12 children initially diagnosed with PDD-NOS were judged by a secondary clinician to have a diagnosis of autism at the follow-up assessment. One longitudinal retrospective study involving videotape analysis of children with ASD at three age periods (10–12 months, 16–18 months, 24–26 months) highlighted what the prospective studies are showing: deficits in interaction and imitation become more prominent with increasing age (Receveur et al., 2005). Outcomes, as measured using standardized tests of verbal and nonverbal IQ and observational measures of severity of autism, were not significantly different for children with ASD whose parents did and did not report a history of regression (Werner, Dawson, Munson, & Osterling, 2005).

Conclusions

This chapter reviewed the literature on developmental features observed in children with ASD in the first 2 years of life. The matter of recognizing early signs of developmental disruption is a critical one, as it opens the door to early intervention. Parents and professionals contribute important insights to the early detection process. Early detection of ASD is usually a process, involving suspicion that something is amiss with the child's development, obtaining validation about concern, and discerning whether the diagnosis of ASD is appropriate. Given that the trajectory of development, such as slowing, plateau, or regression, may be a key factor in determining whether development is truly divergent from the typical path, a single point-in-time assessment for a very young child may not conclusively determine whether a diagnosis of ASD is appropriate. For some children, development will be sufficiently divergent from typical, and the signs of ASD may be clearly present at an early age. In such cases, a diagnosis of ASD may be made with some degree of confidence some time after the first birthday. Professionals are encouraged to become familiar with the early signs of ASD as well as common trajectories associated with this set of developmental disorders. In addition, they are encouraged to seek a clear understanding of parents' concerns and insights into their children throughout childhood, and especially during the first 3 years of life. Screening for developmental disorders, including an autism-specific screening, is a critical component of well-child visits to pediatricians. Once a diagnosis has been made, the early intervention community of professionals may join together with families to develop an individualized intervention program that draws from the empirical literature of instructional strategies and addresses developmentally appropriate goals, strategically targeting core deficits of ASD within the comprehensive program.

Challenges and Future Directions

- Research is needed to define biomarkers of autism that may help with preclinical identification of autism.
- Assessment protocols and tools for identifying subtle developmental disruption early in life are needed to aid in the design of efficacious early intervention or enrichment programs for infants and toddlers at risk for autism.
- A system is needed to ensure that all children are screened for autism in the first and second years of life.

SUGGESTED READINGS

Johnson, C. P., Myers, S. M., and the Council on Children With Disabilities. (2007). Identification and evaluation of children with autism spectrum disorders. *Pediatrics, 120*(5), 1183–1215.

Landa, R. (2008). Autism spectrum disorders in the first 3 years of life. In B. K. Shapiro & P. J. Accardo (Eds.) *Autism frontiers: Clinical issues and innovations* (pp. 97–123). Baltimore, MD: H. Brookes.

Landa, R. (2008). Diagnosis of autism spectrum disorder in the first three years of life. *Nature Clinical Practice Neurology, 4*, 138–147.

Zwaigenbaum, L., Bryson, S., Lord, C., Rogers, S., Chawarska, K., Constantino, J., et al. (2009). Clinical assessment and management of toddlers with suspected ASD: Insights from studies of high-risk infants. *Pediatrics, 123*(5), 1383–1391.

ACKNOWLEDGMENTS

Support for the preparation of this chapter was provided through by grants R01 MH 59630-06A2 and U54MH066417 (Studies to Advance Autism Research and Treatment) from the National Institute of Mental Health, and Autism Speaks, awarded to Rebecca Landa (PI).

REFERENCES

Adrien, J. L., Barthelemy, C., Perrot, A., & Roux, S. (1992). Validity and reliability of the Infant Behavioral Summarized Evaluation (IBSE): A rating scale for the assessment of young children with autism and developmental disorders. *Journal of Autism and Developmental Disorders, 22*(3), 375–394.

Adrien, J. L., Lenoir, P., Martineau, J., & Perrot, A. (1993). Blind ratings of early symptoms of autism based upon family home movies. *Journal of the American Academy of Child and Adolescent Psychiatry, 32*(3), 617–626.

American Psychiatric Association. (1994). *Diagnostic and statistical manual of mental disorders* (4th ed.; DSM-IV). Washington, DC: APA.

Autism Speaks. (2007). *ASD video glossary*. Retrieved December 17, 2008, from http://www.autismspeaks.org/video/glossary.php.

Baghdadli, A., Picot, M. C., Pascal, C., Pry, R., & Aussilloux, C. (2003). Relationship between age of recognition of first disturbances and severity in young children with autism. *European Child and Adolescent Psychiatry, 12*(3), 122–127.

Baird, G., Charman, T., Baron-Cohen, S., Cox, A., Swettenham, J., Wheelwright, S., et al. (2000). A screening instrument for autism at 18 months of age: A 6-year follow-up study. *Journal of the American Academy of Child and Adolescent Psychiatry, 39*(6), 694–702.

Baird, S., & Gomez, C. R. (2005). Identifying early indicators for autism in self-regulation difficulties. *Focus on Autism and Other Developmental Disabilities, 20*(2), 106–116.

Bagnato, S. J., Neisworth, J. T., Salvia, J. J., & Hunt, F. M. (1999). *Temperament and atypical behavior scale (TABS): Early childhood indicators of developmental dysfunction*. Baltimore, MD: Brookes.

Baranek, G. T. (1999). Autism during infancy: A retrospective video analysis of sensory-motor and social behaviors at 9–12 months of age. *Journal of Autism and Developmental Disorders, 29*(3), 213–224.

Baron-Cohen, S., Allen, J., & Gillberg, C. (1992). Can autism be detected at 18 months? The needle, the haystack, and the CHAT. *British Journal of Psychiatry, 161*(6), 839–843.

Bryson, S. E., Zwaigenbaum, L., Brian, J., Roberts, W., Szatmari, P., Rombough, V., et al. (2007). A prospective case series of high-risk infants who developed autism. *Journal of Autism and Developmental Disorders, 37*(1), 12–24.

Burack, J. A., & Volkmar, F. R. (1992). Development of low- and high-functioning autistic children. *Journal of Child Psychology and Psychiatry, 33*(3), 607–616.

Centers for Disease Control and Prevention. (2004). *Learn the signs: Act early*. Retrieved December 17, 2008, from http://www.cdc.gov/ncbddd/autism/actearly/.

Charman, T., Baron-Cohen, S., Swettenham, J., Baird, G., Cox, A., & Drew, A. (2000). Testing joint attention, imitation, and play as infancy precursors to language and theory of mind. *Cognitive Development, 15*(4), 481–498.

Charman, T., Baron-Cohen, S., Swettenham, J., Baird, G., Drew, A., & Cox, A. (2003). Predicting language outcome in infants with autism and pervasive developmental disorder. *International Journal of Language and Communication Disorders, 38*(3), 265–285.

Charman, T., Swettenham, J., Baron-Cohen, S., Cox, A., Baird, G., & Drew, A. (1997). Infants with autism: An investigation of empathy, pretend play, joint attention, and imitation. *Developmental Psychology, 33*(5), 781–789.

Charman, T., Swettenham, J., Baron-Cohen, S., Cox, A., Baird, G., & Drew, A. (1998). An experimental investigation of social-cognitive abilities in infants with autism: Clinical implications. *Infant Mental Health Review Special Issue: 6th World Congress, World Association of Infant Mental Health, 19*(2), 260–275.

Charman, T., Taylor, E., Drew, A., Cockerill, H., Brown, J., & Baird, G. (2005). Outcome at 7 years of children diagnosed with autism at age 2: Predictive validity of assessments conducted at 2 and 3 years of age and pattern of symptom change over time. *Journal of Child Psychology and Psychiatry, 46*(5), 500–513.

Chawarska, K., Paul, R., Klin, A., Hannigen, S., Dichtel, L. E., & Volkmar, F. (2007a). Parental recognition of developmental problems in toddlers with autism spectrum disorders. *Journal of Autism and Developmental Disorders, 37*(1), 62–72.

Chawarska, K., Klin, A., Paul, R., & Volkmar, F. (2007b). Autism spectrum disorder in the second year of life: Stability and change in syndrome expression. *Journal of Child Psychology and Psychiatry, 48*(2), 128–138.

Chawarska, K., Volkmar, F., & Klin, A. (2010). Limited attentional bias for faces in toddlers with autism spectrum disorders. *Archives of General Psychiatry, 67*(2), 178–185.

Cox, A., Klein, K., Charman, T., Baird, G., Baron-Cohen, S., Swettenham, J., et al. (1999). Autism spectrum disorders at 20 and 42 months of age: Stability of clinical and ADI-R diagnosis. *Journal of Child Psychology and Psychiatry, 40*(5), 719–732.

Dawson, G., Osterling, J., Meltzoff, A. N., & Kuhl, P. (2000). Case study of the development of an infant with autism from birth to two years of age. *Journal of Applied Developmental Psychology, 21*(3), 299–313.

De Giacomo, A. & Fombonne, E. (1998). Parental recognition of developmental abnormalities in autism. *European Child and Adolescent Psychiatry, 7*(3), 131–136.

Eaves, L. C., & Ho, H. H. (2004). The very early identification of autism: Outcome to age 4½–5. *Journal of Autism and Developmental Disorders, 34*(4), 267–378.

Fein, D., Dixon, P., Paul, J., & Levin, H. (2005). Brief report: Pervasive developmental disorder can evolve into ADHD: Case illustrations. *Journal of Autism and Developmental Disorders, 35*(4), 525–534.

Fenson, L., Dale, P. S., Reznick, J. S., Thal, D., Bates, E., Hartung, J. P., et al. (1993). *The MacArthur Communicative Development Inventories: User's guide and technical manual.* San Diego, CA: Singular.

Filipek, P. A., Accardo, P. J., Baranek, G. T., Cook, E. H., Dawson, G., Gordon, B., et al. (1999). The screening and diagnosis of autistic spectrum disorders. *Journal of Autism and Developmental Disorders, 29*(6), 439–484.

Flanagan, J., & Landa, R. (2007, November). *Earlier indicators of autism may promote healthier outcomes in high risk infants.* Presented at the National Prevention and Health Promotion Summit, Washington, DC.

Fombonne, E., Simmons, H., Ford, T., Meltzer, H., & Goodman, R. (2001). Prevalence of pervasive developmental disorders in the British Nationwide Survey of Child Mental Health. *Journal of the American Academy of Child and Adolescent Psychiatry, 40*(7), 820–827.

Glascoe, F. P. (2005). Screening for developmental and behavioral problems. *Mental Retardation and Developmental Disabilities Research Reviews, 11*(3), 173–179.

Goin, R. P., & Myers, B. J. (2004). Characteristics of infantile autism: Moving toward earlier detection. *Focus on Autism and Other Developmental Disabilities, 19*(1), 5–12.

Goldberg, W. A., Osann, K., Filipek, P. A., Laulhere, T., Jarvis, K., Modahl, C., et al. (2003). Language and other regression: Assessment and timing. *Journal of Autism and Developmental Disorders, 33*(6), 607–616.

Gomez, C. R., & Baird, S. (2005). Identifying indicators for autism in self-regulation difficulties. *Focus on Autism and Other Developmental Disabilities, 20*(2), 106–116.

Gray, K. M., Tonge, B. J., & Brereton, A. V. (2006). Screening for autism in infants, children, and adolescents. *International Review of Research in Mental Retardation, 32*, 197–227.

Harris, S. L., & Handleman, J. S. (2000). Age and IQ at intake as predictors of placement for young children with autism: A four- to six-year follow-up. *Journal of Autism and Developmental Disorders, 30*(2), 137–142.

Hess, C. R., & Landa, R. J. (in press). Predictive and concurrent validity of parent concern about young children at risk for autism.

Howard, J. S., Sparkman, C. R., Cohen, H. G., Green, G., & Stanislaw, H. (2005). A comparison of intensive behavior analytic and eclectic treatments for young children with autism. *Research in Developmental Disabilities, 26*(4), 359–383.

Howlin, P., & Asgharian, A. (1999). The diagnosis of autism and Asperger syndrome: Findings from a survey of 770 families. *Developmental Medicine and Child Neurology, 41*(12), 834–839.

Johnson, C. P., Myers, S. M., & Council on Children with Disabilities. (2007). Identification and evaluation of children with autism spectrum disorders. *Pediatrics, 120*(5), 1183–1215.

King, T. M., Rosenberg L. A., Fuddy, L., McFarlane, E., Sia, C., & Duggan, A. K. (2005). Prevalence and early identification of language delays among at-risk three-year-olds. *Journal of Developmental and Behavioral Pediatrics, 26*(4), 293–303.

Kleinman, J. M., Ventola, P. E., Pandey, J., Verbalis, A. D., Barton, M., Hodgson, S., et al. (2008). Diagnostic stability in very young children with autism spectrum disorders. *Journal of Autism and Developmental Disorders, 38*(4), 606–615.

Klin, A., Chawarska, K., Paul, R., Rubin, E., Morgan, T., Wiesner, L., et al. (2004). Autism in a 15-month-old child. *American Journal of Psychiatry, 161*(11), 1981–1988.

Klin, A., Volkmar, F. R., & Sparrow, S. S. (1992). Autistic social dysfunction: Some limitations of the theory of mind hypothesis. *Journal of Child Psychology and Psychiatry, 33*(5), 861–876.

Kurita, H. (1985). Infantile autism with speech loss before the age of thirty months. *Journal of the American Academy of Child Psychiatry, 24*(2), 191–196.

Kurita, H. (1996). Specificity and developmental consequences of speech loss in children with pervasive developmental disorders. *Psychiatry and Clinical Neurosciences, 50*, 181–184.

Kurita, H., Kita, M., & Miyake, Y. (1992). A comparative study of development and symptoms among disintegrative psychosis and infantile autism with and without speech loss. *Journal of Autism and Developmental Disorders, 22*(2), 175–188.

Landa, R. (2008). Neurobiological origins and innovative treatment of autism. NIH STAART annual meeting, Washington, DC.

Landa, R., & Garrett-Mayer, E. (2006). Development in infants with autism spectrum disorders: A prospective study. *Journal of Child Psychology and Psychiatry, 47*(6), 629–638.

Landa, R. J., Holman, K. C., & Garrett-Mayer, E. (2007). Social and communication development in toddlers with early and later diagnosis of autism spectrum disorders. *Archives of General Psychiatry, 64*(7), 853–864.

Lord, C., Rutter, M., & Le Couteur, A. (1994). Autism Diagnostic Interview—Revised: A revised version of a diagnostic interview for caregivers of individuals with possible pervasive developmental disorders. *Journal of Autism and Developmental Disorders, 24*(5), 659–685.

Loh, A., Soman, T., Brian, J., Bryson, S. E., Roberts, W., Szatmari, P., et al. (2007). Stereotyped motor behaviors associated with autism in high risk infants: A pilot videotape analysis of a sibling sample. *Journal of Autism and Developmental Disorders, 37*(1), 25–36.

Lord, C. (1995). Follow-up of two-year-olds referred for possible autism. *Journal of Child Psychology and Psychiatry, 36*(8), 1365–1382.

Lord, C., Risi, S., DiLavore, P. S., Shulman, C., Thurm, A., & Pickles, A. (2006). Autism from 2 to 9 years of age. *Archives of General Psychiatry, 63*(6), 694–701.

Lord, C., Shulman, C., & DiLavore, P. (2004). Regression and word loss in autistic spectrum disorders. *Journal of Child Psychology and Psychiatry, 45*(5), 936–955.

Losche, G. (1990). Sensorimotor and action development in autistic children from infancy to early childhood. *Journal of Child Psychology and Psychiatry, 35*(5), 749–761.

Luyster, R., Richler, J., Risi, S., Hsu, W., Dawson, G., Bernier, R., et al. (2005). Early regression in social communication in autism spectrum disorders: A CPEA study. *Developmental Neuropsychology, 27*(3), 311–336.

Maestro, S., Muratori, F., Cavallaro, M. C., Pei, F., Stern, D., Golse, B., et al. (2002). Attentional skills during the first 6 months of age in autism spectrum disorder. *Journal of the American Academy of Child and Adolescent Psychiatry, 41*(10), 1239–1245.

Maestro, S., Muratori, F., Cesari, A., Cavallaro, M. C., Paziente, A., Pecini, C., et al. (2005). Course of autism signs in the first year of life. *Psychopathology, 38*(1), 26–31.

Mandell, D. S., Listerud, J., Levy, S. E., & Pinto-Martin, J. A. (2002). Race differences in the age at diagnosis among Medicaid-eligible children with autism. *Journal of the American Academy of Child and Adolescent Psychiatry, 41*(12), 1447–1453.

Moore, V., & Goodson, S. (2003). How well does early diagnosis of autism stand the test of time? Follow-up study of children assessed for autism at age 2 and development of an early diagnostic service. *Autism, 7*(1), 47–63.

Morgan, L., Wetherby, A. M., & Barber, A. (2008). Repetitive and stereotyped movements in children with autism spectrum disorders late in the second year of life. *Journal of Child Psychology and Psychiatry, 49*(8), 826–837.

Mullen E. (1995). *Mullen Scales of Early Learning* (AGS ed.). Circle Pines, MN: American Guidance Service.

Nadig, A. S., Ozonoff, S., Young, G. S., Rozga, A., Sigman, M., & Rogers, S. J. (2007). A prospective study of response to name in infants at risk for autism. *Archives of Pediatric and Adolescent Medicine, 161*(4), 378–383.

Osterling, J. A., & Dawson, G. (1994). Early recognition of children with autism: A study of first birthday home videotapes. *Journal of Autism and Developmental Disorders, 24*(3), 247–257.

Osterling, J. A., Dawson, G., & Munson, J. (2002). Early recognition of 1-year-old infants with autism spectrum disorder versus mental retardation. *Development and Psychopathology, 14*(2), 239–251.

Ozonoff, S., Young, G. S., Goldring, S., Greiss-Hess, L., Herrera, A.M., Steele, J., et al. (2008a). Gross motor development, movement abnormalities, and early identification of autism. *Journal of Autism and Developmental Disorders, 38*(4), 644–656.

Ozonoff, S., Macari, G. S., Young, S., Goldring, M., Thompson, M., & Rogers, S. J. (2008b). Atypical object exploration at 12 months of age is associated with autism in a prospective sample. *Autism, 12*(5), 457–472.

Pierce, K., Conant, D., Hazin, R., Stoner, R., & Desmond, J. (2011). A preference for geometric patterns early in life is a risk factor for autism. *Archives of General Psychiatry, 68*(1), 101–109.

Rapin, I., & Katzman, R. (1998). Neurobiology of autism. *Annals of Neurology, 43*(1), 7–14.

Receveur, C., Lenoir, P., Desombre, H., Roux, S., Barthelemy, C., & Malvy, J. (2005). Interaction and imitation from infancy to 4 years of age in children with autism. *Autism, 9*(1), 69–82.

Rogers, S., & DiLalla, D. L. (1990). Age of symptom onset in young children with pervasive developmental disorders. *Journal of the American Academy of Child and Adolescent Psychiatry, 29*(6), 863–872.

Rutter, M., & Lord, C. (1987). Language disorders associated with psychiatric disturbance. In W. Yale & M. Rutter (Eds.), *Language development and disorders* (pp. 206–233). Philadelphia, PA: Lippincott.

Sallows, G. O., & Graupner, T. D. (2005). Intensive behavioral treatment for children with autism: Four-year outcome and predictors. *American Journal of Mental Retardation, 110*(6), 417–438.

Sebat, J., Lakshmi, B., Malhotra, D., Troge, J., Lese-Martin, C., Walsh, T., et al. (2007). Strong association of de novo copy number mutations with autism. *Science, 316*(5823), 445–449.

Shattuck, P. T., Durkin, M., Maenner, M., Newschaffer, C., Mandell, D. S., Wiggins, L., Lee, et al. (2009). Timing of identification among children with an Autism Spectrum Disorder: Findings from a population-based surveillance study. *American Journal of Epidemiology, 48*(5), 474–483.

Sparling, J. W. (1991). A prospective case report of infantile autism from pregnancy to four years. *Journal of Autism and Developmental Disorders, 21*(2), 229–236.

Stone, W. L., Lee, E. B., Ashford, L., Brissie, J., Hepburn, S. L., Coonrod, E. E., et al. (1999). Can autism be diagnosed accurately in children under 3 years of age? *Journal of Child Psychology and Psychiatry, 40*(2), 219–226.

Sullivan, M., Finelli, J., Marvin, A., Garret-Mayer, E., Bauman, M., & Landa, R. (2007). Response to joint attention in toddlers at risk for autism spectrum disorder: A prospective study. *Journal of Autism and Developmental Disorders, 37*(1), 37–48.

Sutera, S., Pandey, J., Esser, E. L., Rosenthal, M. A., Wilson, L.B., Barton, M., et al. (2007). Predictors of optimal outcome in toddlers diagnosed with autism spectrum disorders. *Journal of Autism and Developmental Disorders, 37*(1), 98–107.

Swettenham, J., Baron-Cohen, S., Charman, T., Cox, A., Baird, G., & Drew, A. (1998). The frequency and distribution of spontaneous attention shifts between social and nonsocial stimuli in autistic, typically developing, and nonautistic developmentally delayed infants. *Journal of Child Psychology and Psychiatry, 39*(5), 747–753.

Turner, L. M., & Stone, W. L. (2007). Variability in outcome for children with an ASD diagnosis at age 2. *Journal of Child Psychology and Psychiatry, 48*(8), 793–802.

Turner, L. M., Stone, W. L., Pozdol, S. L., & Coonrod, E. E. (2006). Follow-up of children with autism spectrum disorders from age 2 to age 9. *Autism, 10*(3), 243–265.

Ventola, P. E., Kleinman, J., Pandey, J., Barton, M., Allen, S., Green, J., et al., (2006). Agreement among four diagnostic instruments for autism spectrum disorders in toddlers. *Journal of Autism and Developmental Disorders, 36*(7), 839–847.

Watt, N., Wetherby, A. M., Barber, A., & Morgan, L. (2008). Repetitive and stereotyped behaviors in children with autism spectrum disorders in the second year of life. *Journal of Autism and Developmental Disorders, 38*(8), 1518–1533.

Werner, E., & Dawson, G. (2005). Validation of the phenomenon of autistic regression using home videotapes. *Archives of General Psychiatry, 62*(8), 889–895.

Werner, E., Dawson, G, Munson, J., & Osterling, J. (2005). Variation in early developmental course in autism and its relation with behavioral outcome at 3–4 years of age. *Journal of Autism and Developmental Disorders, 35*(3), 337–350.

Werner, E., Dawson, G., Osterling, J., & Dinno, N. (2000). Brief report: Recognition of autism spectrum disorder before one year of age: A retrospective study based on home videotapes. *Journal of Autism and Developmental Disorders, 30*(2), 157–162.

Wetherby, A. M., Brosnan-Maddox, S., Peace, V., & Newton, L. (2008). Validation of the Infant-Toddler Checklist as a broadband screener for autism spectrum disorders from 9 to 24 months of age. *Autism, 12*(5), 487–511.

Wetherby, A. M., & Prizant, B. M. (2002). *Communication and symbolic behavior scales: Developmental profile, 1st normed ed.* Baltimore, MD: Brookes.

Wetherby, A. M., Watt, N., Morgan, L., & Shumway, S. (2007). Social communication profiles of children with autism spectrum disorders late in the second year of life. *Journal of Autism and Developmental Disorders, 37*(5), 960–975.

Wetherby, A. M., & Woods, J. (2002). Early indicators of autism spectrum disorders in the second year of life. Retrieved December 17, 2008, from http://firstwords.fsu.edu/pdf/ASD.pdf.

Wetherby, A. M., Woods, J., Allen, L., Cleary, J., Dickinson, H., & Lord, C. (2004). Early indicators of autism spectrum disorders in the second year of life. *Journal of Autism and Developmental Disorders, 34*(5), 473–493.

Wiggins, L. D., Baio, J., & Rice, C. (2006). Examination of the time between first evaluation and first autism spectrum diagnosis in a population-based sample. *Journal of Developmental and Behavioral Pediatrics, 27*(Suppl2), S79–S87.

Williams, J., & Brayne, C. (2006). Screening for autism spectrum disorders: What is the evidence? *Autism, 10*(1), 11–35.

Wilson, S., Djukic, A., Shinnar, S., Dharmani, C., & Rapin, I. (2003). Clinical characteristics of language regression in children. *Developmental Medicine and Child Neurology, 45*(8), 508–514.

Young, R. L., Brewer, N., & Pattison, C. (2003). Parental identification of early behavioural abnormalities in children with autistic disorder. *Autism, 7*(2), 125–143.

Zwaigenbaum, L., Bryson, S., Rogers, T., Roberts, W., Brian, J., & Szatmari, P. (2005). Behavioral manifestations of autism in the first year of life. *International Journal of Developmental Neuroscience, 23*(2–3), 143–152.

Zwaigenbaum, L., Thurm, A., Stone, W., Baranek, G., Bryson, S., Iverson, J., et al. (2007). Studying the emergence of autism spectrum disorders in high-risk infants: Methodological and practical issues. *Journal of Autism and Developmental Disorders, 37*(3), 466–480.

13 Tony Charman

Development from Preschool Through School Age

Points of Interest

- Do we know if diagnosis from age 2 is reliable and stable?
- What features are associated with better social and communication outcomes?
- When do associated features such as mental health problems begin to emerge?

Over the past decade there has been remarkable progress in our understanding of the early development of children with autism spectrum disorders. Until the 1990s it was rare for children to receive a diagnosis of autism until the age of 3 or 4 years. Therefore, much of the historical literature in both the clinical and research fields starts with descriptions of children with autism at age 4 to 5 years or older. Several factors have driven this change, including efforts to improve earlier identification with the recognition that earlier-delivered intervention may improve outcomes and prevent "secondary" neurodevelopmental disturbances (Dawson, 2008; Mundy, 2003), the development of prospective screening instruments to indentify possible cases of autism from the first few years of life (Charman & Baron-Cohen, 2006; Zwaigenbaum & Stone, 2006), and the use of the genetic high-risk research design of prospectively studying younger siblings of children with a diagnosis of autism from the first year of life (Yirmiya & Ozonoff, 2007). This decade of work has uncovered important evidence regarding the developmental trajectory of autism spectrum disorder from toddlerhood, through the preschool years into school age and beyond. An even more recent development has been the application of modern neuroimaging and neuroscientific experimental approaches to infants, toddlers, and young preschool children with autism spectrum disorders (Courchesne et al., 2007). While many of the insights gained from these clinical and experimental studies have proved clinically useful—in particular with respect to questions about when autism can be diagnosed reliably and how stable the diagnosis is over the course of the preschool years as well as the ability to predict (at least at a group level) outcomes many years later—they have also raised considerable challenges. Among the most notable challenges are the substantial variability in early development trajectory in children with autism and our difficulty in disentangling the extent to which these variable trajectories for individual children are due to intrinsic versus extrinsic factors. This chapter will summarize the state of our current knowledge of these issues and identify challenges for future research and clinical studies.

Diagnosis and Developmental Trajectory Through the Preschool Years

There is a degree of irony that while both psychiatric classification systems are clear that, at least to meet criteria for the core disorder of childhood autism (ICD-10; World Health Organization, 1993) or autistic disorder (DSM-IV-TR; American Psychiatric Association, 2000), symptoms of autism are usually present in the first 3 years of life as evidenced by abnormalities in social interaction, language as used in social communication, and early play skills, until the 1990s few studies had been conducted with samples under the age of 3 years. This is not to challenge the notion that in many if not most cases of autism spectrum disorder, excepting perhaps those with very high IQ or those who meet criteria for Asperger's syndrome, there is some developmental anomaly within the first 3 years. Some recent evidence suggests that, at least in the case of childhood autism, early developmental perturbation that in some but not all cases meets recognized criteria for regression might occur for the majority as opposed to the minority of cases (Landa et al., 2007; Pickles et al., 2009). It may well be that parents do not always notice or pick up on more subtle changes in their children's social and communicative development from infancy to toddlerhood unless there is frank regression, most typically evidenced in a loss of expressive language skills. Rather, it is to point out that apart from rare exceptions (Gillberg et al., 1990) until the mid-1990s the majority of information about development from toddlerhood through the preschool years came from retrospectively reported information from parents. The growth in our knowledge base regarding the presentation of autism in the preschool years over the past decade is demonstrated by a simple experiment. In August 2008 entering the search terms "autism" and "toddlers" into PudMed identified 88 articles. Seventy-seven of these were published *after* 2000, 57 of which were dated from 2005.

One of the most significant challenges and concerns of this new era of prospectively studying children with autism spectrum disorders from the age of 2 and 3 years concerned diagnosis. Given the relative lack of experience of applying the diagnostic criteria to children of this age, even among the relatively expert clinical teams conducting such studies, one critical question quickly arose: Was the diagnosis accurate and stable when applied at this age? Fortunately, many research teams were studying cohorts of toddlers by the mid-1990s, and evidence regarding the issues of diagnostic accuracy and stability began to emerge as the cohorts were followed into preschool and in the mid-2000s into the school-age years. What emerged from these programs of work were some clear messages (autism *can* be accurately diagnosed in 2-year-olds) but also some areas of uncertainty that will take continued study to resolve (in some cases diagnosis appears less stable). This research will be reviewed next.

Table 13-1 summarizes the diagnostic outcome studies that have followed cohorts of children from initial diagnostic assessments around the age of 2 years into the preschool years and, in several of the more recent studies (Charman et al., 2005; Lord et al., 2006; Turner et al., 2006), into the school-age years. The first series of studies (Cox et al., 1999; Lord, 1995; Moore & Goodson, 2003; Stone et al., 1999) all showed high stability of diagnosis in particular for "core" autism, with somewhat lower stability for broader autism spectrum disorder (ASD) and Pervasive Developmental Disorder Not-Otherwise-Specified (PDD-NOS). The movement across the ASD/PDD-NOS diagnostic category boundary was somewhat different in the different studies, with Stone et al. (1999) finding that 4 out of 12 children who met broader ASD criteria at the initial assessment did not meet criteria for an autism spectrum disorder at follow-up, whereas Cox et al. (1999) found that 7 from 31 children who did not receive an autism spectrum diagnosis at the initial assessment met criteria for broader ASD at follow-up. Several of the studies (Cox et al., 1999; Lord, 1995; Stone et al., 1999) concluded that, for 2-year-olds, expert clinical judgment is more reliable than the standard diagnostic instruments—the Autism Diagnostic Interview-Revised (ADI-R; Lord et al., 1994) and the Autism Diagnostic Observation Schedule-Generic (ADOS-G; Lord et al., 2000). Several studies also found that behaviors from the third symptom cluster that defines autism—restricted and repetitive behaviors and activities—were less evident at 2 years of age than at 3 to 5 years of age (Cox et al., 1999; Moore & Goodson, 2003; Stone et al., 1999). The samples in these early studies differ in a number of characteristics, including how and for what purposes they were ascertained (for example, prospectively using the CHAT screening instrument in the Cox et al. study vs. following clinical referral for possible autism in the Lord, Moore and Goodson, and Stone et al. studies), IQ, language ability, and the different use and implementation both of standard diagnostic instruments but also of DSM-IV and ICD-10 diagnostic criteria, and these differences might account for the differences found.

The more recent studies differ from the earlier ones in a number of features, most notably considerably larger sample sizes (N = 172, Lord et al., 2006; N = 77, Kleinman et al., 2008) and follow-up periods that extend to age 7 years in the Charman et al. (2005) study and age 9 years in the Lord et al. (2006) and Turner et al. (2006) studies. Broadly, the lessons learned are the same—that the diagnosis of autism is highly stable in these samples but that of broader ASD is less so. Lord et al. (2006) found that age 2 scores on measures of repetitive and restricted behaviors and activities predicted an autism diagnosis at age 9 years. In some of these more recent studies there was greater movement from having an ASD diagnosis at age 2 years to a nonspectrum diagnosis at age 4 (Kleinman et al., 2008; Turner & Stone, 2007). While the authors report the factors associated with these "good outcomes"—mainly higher IQ and better language competency—it is important to remain cautious regarding predictors of poorer or better outcomes. However, the general pattern is of high stability of diagnosis for autism, replicating the earlier pioneering longitudinal work of Sigman and colleagues, who found high stability of diagnosis of children from 4 years of age through to mid-childhood (13 years) and young adulthood (19 years) (McGovern & Sigman, 2005; Sigman & Ruskin, 1999).

For clinicians the lesson is to accept that autism is a *developmental* disorder and at a very young age there may be less certainty regarding the pattern of behavior that a child is showing and the likelihood of their continuing to meet diagnostic criteria into the future. Charman and Baird (2002) discuss the importance of understanding the diagnostic process as an iterative process to be worked out between clinician teams and parents over time and that concepts such as a "working diagnosis" can be helpful. However, at the same time, clinical teams need to be aware of the need to provide sufficient certainty regarding the child's condition that they are not refused appropriate services following assessment. One other important clinical reminder is that while the trajectory of early emerging impairments in social and communication development accompanied by rigid and repetitive behaviors and interests characterizes many children on the autism spectrum, there is a subgroup of particularly verbal and able children who go onto to receive a diagnosis of autism (sometimes called "high functioning autism") or Asperger's syndrome who may not receive a diagnosis in the preschool years. There is also another group who might meet diagnostic criteria for an autism spectrum disorder who do

Table 13–1.
Studies of diagnostic stability from preschool into the school-age years

Reference	Age Time 1	Age Time 2	Diagnoses at Time 1	Findings
Lord (1995)	31 months	50 months	16 CA, 14 NS	Diagnosis largely stable; Clinical judgment more reliable than ADI-R
Stone et al. (1999)	31 months	45 months	25 CA, 12 ASD, 8 NS	CA diagnosis largely stable; ASD less so (4 out of 12 moved to NS at Time 2); Fewer repetitive symptoms at Time 1
Cox et al. (1999)	21 months	45 months	9 CA, 3 ASD, 31 NS	CA diagnosis largely stable; NS less so (7 out of 31 moved to ASD at Time 2); Fewer repetitive symptoms at Time 1; Clinical judgment more reliable than ADI-R
Moore & Goodwin (2003)	34 months	53 months	16 CA, 3 ASD, 1 NS	Diagnosis stable (slight movement between CA and ASD only)
Charman et al. (2005)	25 months	85 months	26 CA	Diagnosis largely stable (3 moved to ASD and 1 to NS at Time 2)
Turner et al. (2006)	31 months	109 months	18 CA, 7 ASD	Diagnosis largely stable (2 CA moved to NS and 1 ASD moved to NS at Time 2)
Lord et al. (2006)	29 months	112 months	84 CA, 46 ASD, 42 NS	Diagnosis of CA largely stable (12 from 84 moved to ASD and 1 to NS at Time 2); ASD less so (27 of 46 moved to CA and 5 to NS at Time 2); NS less so (2 from 42 moved to CA and 9 to ASD at Time 2)
Chawarska et al. (2007)	22 months	36 months	19 CA, 9 ASD	Diagnosis of ASD stable (2 of 19 CA cases moved to ASD at Time 2); Clinical judgment more reliable than ADI-R and ADOS-G
Turner & Stone (2007)	29 months	53 months	38 CA, 10 ASD	Diagnosis stability moderate only (6 of 38 CA cases moved to ASD and 13 moved to NS at Time 2; 6 of 10 cases of ASD moved to NS at Time 2)
Kleinman et al. (2008)	27 months	53 months	46 CA, 15 ASD, 16 NS	Diagnosis stability moderate only (15 of 61 ASD cases moved to NS at Time 2)

CA = ICD-10 childhood autism/DSM-IV autistic disorder; ASD = PDD-NOS, atypical autism; NS = nonspectrum.

not receive an explicit diagnosis—those individuals with moderate to severe intellectual disability or those with an already identified preexisting associated medical condition, such as Fragile X or Down syndrome. In a recent epidemiological study Baird et al. (2006) found that, for cases meeting research diagnostic criteria for an autism spectrum disorder following in-depth assessment, low IQ predicted those who had not received a clinical diagnosis by local clinical services by age 10 years. One final caveat is that the studies summarized in Table 13-1 largely come from expert research clinical centers specifically studying young cohorts of children. In community settings in many countries there is evidence including from recent studies that for many children and their families a diagnosis is not confirmed until children are well into the school-age years (Howlin & Asgharian, 1999; Wiggins et al., 2006).

One final feature that emerges from these longitudinal studies is that, aside from the issue of diagnostic or categorical stability, the developmental trajectory of symptoms measured using a continuous or dimensional (as opposed to a categorical) metric changes over time (see also Honey et al., 2008). For example, Charman et al. (2005) described how the trajectories of the social, communication, and repetitive domain scores on the ADI-R had different developmental trajectories over time, consistent with the notion that the various aspects that make up the autism phenotype might not be tied together as closely as suggested by the current classification systems. This notion has also received support from a twin study demonstrating that, while each component of the autism phenotype is highly heritable, there is only very modest commonality in the heritability of the three components (Ronald et al., 2006). The recognition that autism is a complex neurodevelopmental condition and that the presentation changes (in different ways in different individuals) over time presents considerable challenges to genetic and neuroscientific investigations (Happé et al., 2006). Longitudinal studies tracing the behavioral autism phenotype will therefore be important not only for informing clinicians regarding diagnostic practice but also for answering basic science questions regarding influences on the etiology and course of the disorder.

Language and Communication Development from Toddlerhood to the School-Age Years

Delayed language milestones are common in many preschool children with autism spectrum disorders, and the diagnostic criteria include both a delay in the emergence of language and the atypical use of nonverbal social-communication abilities including joint attention behaviors, social imitation, and pretend play abilities. However, while it is not uncommon for 2- and 3-year-olds with core autism (as opposed to those with Asperger's syndrome) to be nonverbal, language and nonverbal communication abilities typically do begin to develop throughout the preschool period as children enter kindergarten and school (Charman, Drew, et al., 2003; Luyster et al., 2007). Previously, the prognosis in terms of the proportion of children with autism who go on to develop functional language was considered poor, with papers from the 1970s and 1980s suggesting that perhaps only 50% of children develop functional speech (DeMyer et al., 1973; Freeman et al., 1985)—a reflection of the severely autistic and intellectually delayed cohorts who were first studied longitudinally. However, more recently it has become clear that language onset and outcomes are very variable, but generally more positive, for children with the spectrum of autism disorders. For example, in the large clinical cohort recently described by Hus and colleagues (N = 983; mean age 8 years, SD 5 years, range 4 to 52 years; Hus et al., 2007) only 9.8% had no single words (using the ADI-R criteria of 5 or more words used on a daily basis excluding "mama," "papa," etc.), 41.0% had delay in single word onset (> 24 months) but had single words when assessed, and half were not delayed in single word onset (49.2%; data from Hus et al., 2007, Table 5, p. 443). For phrase speech, the comparable figures were 24.0% of individuals with no phrase speech when assessed, 51.3% with delayed phrase speech onset (>33 months) but with phrased speech when assessed, and one quarter were not delayed in phrase speech (24.7%; data from Hus et al., 2007, Table 5, p. 443). A longitudinal study with a subgroup (N = 206) of the same cohort measured language ability at age 2, 3, 5, and 9 years (Anderson et al., 2007). This allowed sophisticated statistical modeling using growth curves to plot the trajectory of language development through the preschool years into school age. At a group level, the trajectory of growth in language abilities was slower for the children with a diagnosis of autism than for the children with PDD-NOS or a nonspectrum developmental disorder. However, within each diagnostic group language growth and outcomes were very variable—and this variability increased over time—with some children in each group making such good progress that their language abilities were at the expected level at age 9 years, whereas other children in each group, in particular a subset of the children with "core" autism, made very little progress at all (see Figure 13-1). Age 2 symptom severity, nonverbal cognitive abilities, and joint attention skills were significant predictors of language outcomes at age 9 years. Anderson et al. (2007) conclude that their study "offers messages of both hope and realism" (p. 602) regarding the language outcomes of children receiving an early diagnosis of autism spectrum disorder.

There is also increasing recognition that while expressive language competencies might be the most evident delay for some preschool children with autism spectrum disorders, receptive abilities can be relatively more delayed (Charman, Drew, et al., 2003; Hudry et al., 2008; Luyster et al., 2007). This is clinically important but requires sensitive handling to explain that what parents sometimes take as "understanding" is often understanding of familiar routines and contextual cues rather than language comprehension per se. However, this finding is important as it is related to the appropriate focus of development, psycholinguistic approaches to communication intervention for preschool children with autism (see below).

Over the past 20 years there has been increasing interest in delineating the emergence of language competencies in children with autism spectrum disorder from toddlerhood through the preschool years. In part, this is to aid the clinical ability to determine likely prognosis—clinicians will recognize how parents understandably desire to be told if their child will talk and when. However, it has also helped develop our theoretical understanding of how (albeit sometimes delayed) language develops in autism. This is important both to understand if the mechanisms underpinning (delayed) language development are the same as or different from those in typically developing infants—about which a great deal is known (Bloom, 2000)—and to inform communication-based approaches to early intervention (see below).

Many studies over the past 20 years have demonstrated the perhaps unsurprising fact that over time individual variability is relatively stable in cohorts of preschoolers with autism—that is, early language competence predicts later language competence—including in some studies that followed children into the school-age period (e.g. Charman et al., 2005; Lord & Schopler, 1989; Mundy et al., 1990; Sigman & Ruskin, 1999; Venter et al., 1992). However, theoretically more interesting has been the question of whether earlier-emerging social communication abilities predict later language development. A strong psycholinguistic tradition from the study of normative language development has shown that this is the case for typically developing infants and toddlers (Bates et al., 1989; Carpenter et al., 1998; Morales et al., 2000; Mundy & Gomes, 1998). Given that many preschoolers with autism spectrum

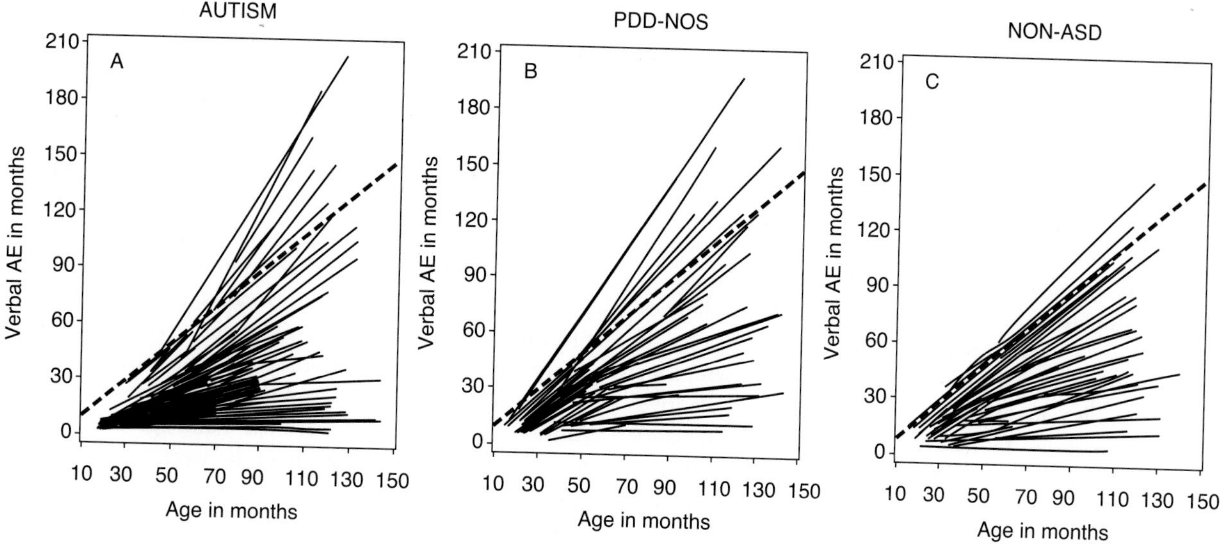

Figure 13–1. Language growth curves from 2 to 9 years. Copyright © 2007 by the American Psychological Association. Reproduced with permission from Anderson, D. K., Lord, C., Risi, S., Shulman, C., Welch, K., DiLavore, P. S., et al. (2007). Patterns of growth in verbal abilities among children with autism spectrum disorder. *Journal of Consulting and Clinical Psychology, 75*, 594–604.

disorders are impaired in their development of language ability *and* of early social communication abilities, the question of whether such associations also hold for toddlers and preschoolers with autism is both of clinical but also of theoretical interest. Demonstrating that the same association holds between early social communication abilities and later language development might suggest that similar developmental mechanisms are operating—albeit at a slower rate than in the typical case. Mundy et al. (1990) were the first to provide evidence to support this position, finding that joint attention behaviors (alternating gaze, pointing, showing, and gaze following) measured at 45 months were associated with language outcomes 13 months later. Sigman and Ruskin (1999) extended this finding by demonstrating associations from the preschool years to later language ability at 12 years of age. Stone and colleagues have also demonstrated longitudinal associations between various aspects of imitation and play as well as joint attention abilities at 2 years of age and language abilities measured at 4 years of age. This pattern has now been replicated in several other studies (e.g. Toth et al., 2006), including one that followed children with autism spectrum disorders from toddlerhood (20 months) into the preschool years (42 months; Charman, Baron-Cohen, et al., 2003).

These findings are both of theoretical and practical importance. Theoretically they suggest that since some of the associations seen in preschoolers with autism spectrum disorders are similar to that seen in typical development it might be the case that the mechanisms that operate are similar too. This is relevant to informing approaches to communication-based approaches to intervention. Although individual stability of skills (language to language) or of one "precursor" skill to another later emerging skill (joint attention to language; Charman et al., 2000) may tell us something about intrinsic characteristics of the child, they may also suggest routes to intervention. Evidence consistent with this proposition was provided by Siller and Sigman (2002), who demonstrated that individual differences in maternal synchronicity (sometimes called "sensitivity") measured in joint play interactions was associated with later language outcomes even over many years. The circle is squared, so to speak, by several recent randomized controlled intervention trials. These have used a variety of social-communication strategies, including the promotion of joint attention, imitation, and joint social engagement skills both directly delivered by therapists (Kasari et al., 2006, 2008; Yoder & Stone, 2006) and delivered by training parents in these methods (Aldred et al., 2004; Drew et al., 2002), and found that language outcomes (and in the case of the Aldred et al. study social outcomes) can be improved. For developmentalists, this convergence of evidence that for preschool children with autism spectrum disorders there are both naturalistic associations over time between early social communication skills and later language outcomes and that these can be altered by targeted intervention in controlled studies is as close to evidence for a development mechanism as it is possible to get (Bradley & Bryant, 1983).

Social Development and Adaptive Behavior Development into the School-Age Years

While the development of language and communication abilities has understandably been the focus of much research interest in delineating the developmental trajectory of children with autism spectrum disorders from preschool to the school-age years, it is also of considerable importance to measure and understand the influences on social development. This reflects not only the central place that social development—both the characteristic social impairments that are the primary feature of the diagnostic criteria but also the continuing emergence of positive social interests and competencies—has in our understanding of autism but also the changing social environment that children encounter as they emerge from the preschool period. When children enter kindergarten or preschool and then school their social milieu and the challenges they face in terms of forming friendships and social relationships changes considerably. Several studies have looked at the trajectory of social development in autism—both in terms of symptom measures but also in terms of everyday socially adaptive behavior, as measured by instrument such as the Vineland Adaptive Behavior Scales (VABS; Sparrow et al., 1984, 2006).

Initial studies used retrospective designs to document the changes in autism symptoms, including social behaviors, comparing current to past symptoms by parent report on the ADI-R. Piven et al. (1996) studied 38 adolescents and adults and found reductions on all 3 symptom domains compared to retrospective report at age 4 to 5 years. Fecteau et al. (2003) compared parent current report of symptoms at a mean age of 13 years with retrospective report at age 4 to 5 years in a sample of 28 children and adolescents and found significant reduction in symptoms on each of the 3 ADI-R domain scores, with most improvement shown in social symptoms. Interestingly, both studies reported fewest improvements in the repetitive behaviors and restricted interests domains. Piven et al. (1996) caution against the reliability of retrospective parental report that can be subject to biases in both directions (remembering things as "much worse" than they were in the light more recent improved behaviors and skills; and underreporting current symptoms as they are an improvement on the past) and also that the particular items included in the ADI-R algorithm that was developed to capture a lifetime diagnosis with age 4 to 5 years being considered the prototypical age at which autism symptoms are fully emerged and the presence at any point in a child's past (ADI-R "ever" ratings) might underestimate current social and communication difficulties in school-age children, adolescents, and adults.

A prospective longitudinal study by Szatmari and colleagues (Starr et al., 2003; Szatmari et al., 2003) has followed a group of high-IQ children and adolescents with autism (N = 41) and Asperger's syndrome (N = 17) from their initial diagnostic assessment at age 4 to 6 years over two years to age 6 to 8 years (Starr et al., 2003) and then to young adolescence (10 to 13 years; Szatmari et al., 2003). They found somewhat different patterns for the diagnostic groups with slight increases in social and communication symptoms on the ADI-R for the Asperger's group but reductions in social symptoms, but not communication symptoms, for the "high functioning" autism group (Starr et al., 2003). For neither group did scores on the repetitive and rigid behaviors change over time. The Szatmari et al. (2003) report focused on predictors of later outcomes and found that early language and nonverbal abilities were the strongest predictors but also reported lower adaptive behavior on the VABS in adolescence compared to childhood. As summarized above, in their diagnostic outcome study Charman et al. (2005) also reported ADI-R symptom domain scores and found that from 2 to 7 years of age social and communication symptoms diminished (while those in the repetitive behavior domain initially increased and then decreased. One striking finding from this study was the increasing variability of the level of social symptoms over time and also among the general trends to diminished social impairment different children made progress across different timepoints as measured at age 2, 3, 4, to 5 (this timepoint only was retrospective) and 7 years. What this study does not answer is the underlying explanation for why some children, for example, make considerable progress between age 3 and age 4–5 years, while for others the most gains are made between 5 and 7 years. This pattern of individual variability is illustrated in Figure 13-2. While longitudinal studies are valuable, only randomized trials have the power to indicate likely causative effects of extrinsic factors, and only larger cohort studies (such as the Anderson et al. (2007) language study described above) the power to model different subgroup trajectories. Moss et al. (2008) reported ADI-R scores in a cohort of 35 children assessed at age 4 years and again at age 11 years and found that social and nonverbal communication domain scores were significantly reduced over time but repetitive behavior domain scores did not change. Lord et al. (2006) also presented ADI-R and ADOS scores at age 2 and age 9 years but found a somewhat different pattern. On the ADI-R, scores increased in each of the 3 domains (Lord et al., 2006, Table 2). On the ADOS-G the pattern was somewhat different, with a reduction in social domain scores and repetitive behavior domain scores for both children with an age-2 diagnosis of autism and PDD-NOS but little change in communication domain scores. Comparing findings across these different studies is not possible due to differences in the child characteristics, measures used and timepoints of the assessments, as well as extrinsic factors (such as interventions; likely differing etiologies) that were not controlled and often not measured. However, in line with our current conception of autism spectrum disorders as developmental disorders there is change in social symptoms as children enter the school-age years, and at a group level the most consistent finding is that social symptoms diminish. However, what is notable in line with the data presented on language above is that variability increases over time. At a clinical level this can be frustrating for clinicians and for parents alike—what parents want to know is what the future holds for their own child. From the clinician's perspective extrapolating from group data to an individual child is not possible. This high-lights the need for continuing longitudinal and controlled intervention trials in order to better inform prognosis and also to identify those individuals most in need of the most intensive interventions.

The above studies examined the trajectories of social impairments as measured by the diagnostic instruments the ADI-R and ADOS, but there are other facets of social development that are not always well captured by such instruments, in particular everyday social, communication, and daily living

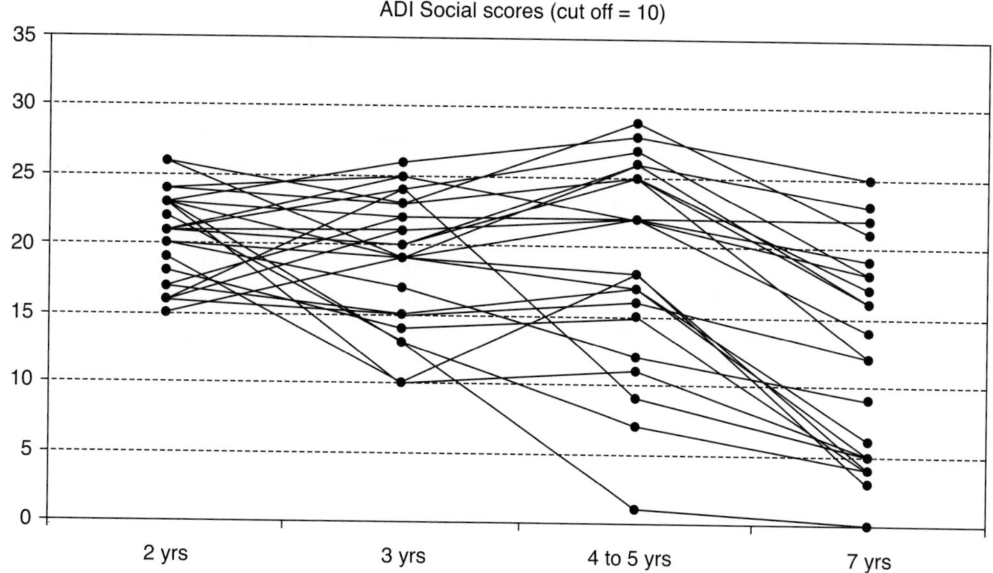

Figure 13–2. ADI-R Reciprocal Social Interaction Domain scores from Charman, T., Taylor, E., Drew, A., Cockerill, H., Brown, J. A., & Baird, G. (2005). Outcome at 7 years of children diagnosed with autism at age 2: Predictive validity of assessments conducted at 2 and 3 years of age and pattern of symptom change over time. *Journal of Child Psychology and Psychiatry, 46,* 500–513.

adaptive skills. Several studies have shown that early social communication behaviors such as joint attention, imitation, and play are predictive of later language and social outcomes (Charman et al., 2003; Toth et al., 2006). Recent, more experimental studies have indicated that individual differences in key brain regions such as the amygdala are also associated with behavioral outcomes, reflecting the fact that autism is a neurobiobehavioral disorder (Munson et al., 2006; Mosconi et al., 2009).

Several cross-sectional studies have used the VABS (Sparrow et al., 1984) with samples of school-age children with an autism spectrum disorder. At least 2 findings have a high degree of consistency across samples. The first is that overall adaptive outcome is significantly lower than IQ, and the second is that, perhaps unsurprisingly, socialization skills are most delayed in comparison to communication and especially daily living skills (Carpentieri & Morgan, 1996; Freeman et al., 1999; Klin et al., 2007; Liss et al., 2001; Saulnier & Klin, 2007; although see Klin et al, 2007, Figure 1, for a example in the Michigan sample where daily livings skills are as depressed compared to IQ as socialization skills).

These findings are clinically important for several reasons. First, even for individuals who perform at or above age expectations within the adult-directed and relatively contained and predictable psychometric test situation their everyday "street smarts" (Klin et al., 2007) coping behavior can be significantly impaired. Indeed, the discrepancy between IQ scores and adaptive functioning is often most notable in individuals with high IQs, and Klin and colleagues found that socialization and daily living skills standard scores were 2 to 3 standard deviations below Full Scale IQ scores in 2 independent samples. This study also found that adaptive skills (in terms of standard scores) decreased with age, suggesting that the "lag" between measured intelligence and everyday coping widened between the early school years and late adolescence (see Szatmari et al, 2003; summarized above). Note however, that other studies have found no association between age and adaptive ability (e.g. Schatz & Hamden-Allen, 1995), and one study even found a positive association (Freeman et al., 1999). Further longitudinal studies are required to understand which developmental pattern is most representative. Both Klin et al. and Szatmari et al. found only marginal associations between autistic social and communication impairments and adaptive skills, suggesting that everyday adaptive behavior needs to be the target of intervention studies, alongside social understanding and skills and language and communication skills.

Alongside the discrepancy between a child's intellectual ability and his/her adaptive functioning, many children with autism spectrum disorders, including those with average or above average IQ, have significant difficulties with self-help and self-organization. This is related to their problems with the components of executive function, including set-shifting, generating ideas, and planning (Russo et al., 2007). Instruments such as the Behavioural Assessment of Dysexecutive Syndrome for Children (BADS-C; Emslie et al., 2003) can be helpful when used in conjunction with a structured parents and teacher rating scale, (e.g. the Adaptive Behaviour Assessment System-Second Edition [ABAS-II; Harrison & Oakland, 2003] or the Vineland Adaptive Behaviour Scale-II [Sparrow et al., 2006]) for determining whether executive functioning difficulties are affecting daily functioning (Bolte & Poustka, 2002). Gilotty et al. (2002) found negative associations between executive dysfunctions, including the ability to initiate behaviors and working memory, as measured by the Behavior Rating

Inventory of Executive Function (BRIEF; Gioia et al., 2000) and adaptive skills as measured by the VABS. One clinical lesson from these findings is that in particular as the social and organizational challenges of the school environment increase as children enter high school and teaching moves from a one-teacher, one-classroom environment to a many-teachers, many-classrooms environment, children with autism may need support to manage this more challenging environment (see Ozonoff, 1998; for examples of everyday strategies to overcome executive difficulties). Executive difficulties also impact on a child's ability to learn in the classroom environment, and a detailed psychometric assessment can identify specific executive difficulties that can inform approaches to remediation (see Box 13-1).

Box 13–1
Case description of a girl with specific executive difficulties.

Reprinted with permission from Charman, et al. (2008).

Case description
Lucy is an 8-year-old girl. Observed behavior in class: Lucy is distractible, daydreams, misunderstands the teacher's instructions, loses her possessions, and is always in the wrong place; her math and literacy skills are very weak. Her teacher believes she has poor attention and that her behavior is attention-seeking as, when an adult works with her, she is able to perform much better. Initial observations, using time-sampling, indicate that Lucy is off-task 70% of the time. An age matched peer is only off-task 22% of the time in the same lesson.

Assessment results
Assessments show that Lucy has average intellectual ability (Full Scale IQ: 90) but very poor executive skills (e.g. D-KEFS Colour-Word Interference, Scaled score: 3, Tower, Scaled Score: 3. BADS-C, Standard Score: 55). She finds it hard to plan her work although she can follow individually given instructions well; she does nothing when given open-ended tasks; cannot organize herself unless following a repetitive and learned routine; cannot hold instructions in her head or generate an understanding of what the instructions mean in practical terms, and does not know when to apply rules.

Intervention
Interventions need to focus on providing a model or framework within which Lucy can operate. At the beginning of every task she should be shown each step that she will need to take; she should be shown the end-point of what she is trying to achieve, and she should be taken through the steps needed to achieve this goal. By following this process and achieving success on several occasions, she will be able to learn how to apply the same series of steps to similar situations—i.e., she will develop a template to use in the future. When faced with changes to the task, she will need support to adapt her learned system. She should be provided with a visual timetable of the day's events and the things she needs for each session so that she can begin to learn to organize herself and see the sequence of events ahead of her.

A number of recently developed standardized instruments exist that test a range of cognitive abilities that make up the executive system (Delis-Kaplan Executive Function System [D–KEFS]; Delis et al., 2001; NEPSY; Korkman et al., 1997). Alongside routine psychometric assessment of IQ and language and communication skills, psychometric assessment of executive abilities, as well as attention and memory abilities (e.g. Working Memory Test Battery for Children (WMTB-C; Pickering & Gathercole, 2001); Test of Everyday Attention in Children (TEA-Ch; Manly et al., 1998)) can be helpful in identifying why a seemingly bright child is struggling either with learning or with managing the complex school environment. Based on a detailed psychometric assessment of executive, memory and attention difficulties bespoke approaches to intervention to bootstrap executive or memory difficulties can then be implemented to help a child fulfill their learning potential within the school environment and at home.

The Emergence of Comorbid Psychiatric Disorders in the School Age-Years

It is common for preschool children with an autism spectrum disorder to manifest behavior problems, and advice on management should form part of the postdiagnostic support provided by clinical services (Herring et al., 2006). However, several recent studies using questionnaire measures have reported high rates of psychiatric problems in school-age children and adolescents with autism spectrum disorders (Steinhausen & Metzke, 2004; Sukhodolsky et al., 2008). Two recent studies have used structured parental interviews that assess psychiatric disorder "caseness" and also found high rates. Leyfer et al. (2006) described rates of lifetime psychiatric disorder in 5- to 17-year-old children with autism, using a new interview, the Autism Comorbidity Interview-Parent and Lifetime Version (ACI-PL), modified from the KSADS (Chambers et al., 1985). Just less than three quarters met criteria for one or more DSM-IV disorders, with the most commonly reported disorders being specific phobia (44%), obsessive compulsive disorder (36%), and ADHD (30%). Studying a population-derived sample of 10- to 14-year-olds with autism or a broader autism spectrum disorder, Simonoff et al. (2008) found that 70% of participants had at least one comorbid disorder and 41% had 2 or more. The most common diagnoses were social anxiety disorder (29%), attention-deficit/hyperactivity disorder (28%) and oppositional-defiant disorder (28%). Simonoff and colleagues systematically examined whether the presence of psychiatric disorders was systematically associated with child (e.g., low IQ), parental (e.g., parent mental health difficulties), or contextual (e.g., deprivation) factors, but found few associations. Simonoff et al. (2008) suggest that the presence of an autism spectrum disorder "trumps" other risk factors that are commonly associated with childhood psychiatric disorders. They conclude that "Psychiatric disorders are common and frequently multiple in children with autism spectrum disorders. They may provide targets for intervention and should be routinely evaluated in the clinical assessment of this group" (Simonoff et al., 2008, p. 921). There are issues regarding the extent to which these disorders should be considered truly "comorbid"—an independently occurring disorder unrelated to the primary symptoms of autism itself—or whether psychiatric symptom scales are endorsed by parents on the basis of autistic symptoms (see also Pine et al., 2008). While further research including direct assessments of mental state in school-age children is warranted to help determine the answer to this conundrum, the challenges of interviewing children with low IQ and the veracity and representativeness of self-report in children (and indeed adults) with autism spectrum disorders are considerable. It might be that in the future advances in genetics or neuroimaging experimental methods will help disentangle these issues, although for now clinicians, educators, and parents need to be aware that cognitive and behavioral manifestations that resemble those seen in children and adolescents without autism but with psychiatric disorders are common in autism spectrum disorders.

Conclusions

It is now widely recognized that there is very large heterogeneity in the children for whom a clinical diagnosis of "autism spectrum disorder" is clinically appropriate and that etiology will differ from case to case, moving some researchers from the biological fields of science to coin the term "the autisms" (Geschwind & Levitt, 2007). However, autism remains quintessentially a *developmental* disorder and heterogeneity in many, if not most, domains of functioning increases with age. Thus, predicting outcomes into the school years for children seen as toddlers and preschoolers can be very difficult. Determining the influence of intrinsic and extrinsic factors—and the interplay between the two (see Dawson, 2008)—remains a significant challenge but one in which the pace of research is at last beginning to catch up with the questions that parents understandably ask of clinicians ("How will my child do in school?"; "Will they go to college and be able to live independently?") (see Howlin et al., 2009; Rogers & Visnara, 2008; for reviews). The evidence base for interventions for preschool and school-age children has, until recent years, been woefully inadequate (see chapters by Green; Kasari; Rogers; Schreibman and Smith; for reviews). However, there are an increasing number of published studies including randomized controlled trials that provide evidence for the benefit of interventions, including those that focus on areas of core deficit such as communication (Aldred et al., 2004; Howlin et al., 2007; Kasari et al., 2008; Yoder & Stone, 2006).

The findings of the longitudinal studies summarized earlier and those of intervention trials offer both hope but also caution. Hope because some children with autism make significant progress as they enter the school-age years. Caution because in all cohort and intervention studies some children make little progress and because development can bring with it new challenges and problems such as mental health difficulties. Over the past decade there has understandably been a great focus on toddlers and preschoolers with autism spectrum disorders, with great advances in knowledge and clinical practice about early risk signs and early detection and diagnosis. The challenges faced by school-age children with autism spectrum disorders differ from those of the toddler, whose parents or caregivers structure much of their everyday world. An increasing emphasis on social group activities, self-organized behavior, and formal learning as children enter school can be a very challenging change for many children with autism spectrum disorders and much work remains to be done for us to understand how to help children with autism, their families, and educators to meet these challenges.

Challenges and Future Directions

- We need to integrate information on behavioral developmental trajectories with emerging developmental neurobiological accounts.
- The developmental trajectory of individual children differs significantly, and we do not know how much individual trajectories are influenced by intrinsic versus extrinsic factors.
- Better-controlled studies on the effects of intervention and schooling are needed.

SUGGESTED READINGS

Anderson, D. K., Lord, C., Risi, S., Shulman, C., Welch, K., DiLavore, P. S., et al. (2007). Patterns of growth in verbal abilities among children with autism spectrum disorder. *Journal of Consulting and Clinical Psychology, 75*, 594–604.

Charman, T., Taylor, E., Drew, A., Cockerill, H., Brown, J. A., & Baird, G. (2005). Outcome at 7 years of children diagnosed with autism at age 2: Predictive validity of assessments conducted at 2 and 3 years of age and pattern of symptom change over time. *Journal of Child Psychology and Psychiatry, 46*, 500–513.

Charman, T., & Baird, G. (2002). Practitioner review: Diagnosis of autism spectrum disorder in 2-and 3-year-old children. *Journal of Child Psychology and Psychiatry and Allied Disciplines, 43*, 289–305.

Lord, C., Risi, S., DiLavore, P. S., Shulman, C., Thurm, A., & Pickles, A. (2006). Autism from 2 to 9 years of age. *Archives of General Psychiatry, 63*, 694–701.

REFERENCES

Aldred, C., Green, J., & Adams, C. (2004). A new social communication intervention for children with autism: pilot randomised controlled treatment study suggesting effectiveness. *Journal of Child Psychology and Psychiatry, 45*, 1420–1430.

American Psychiatric Association. (2000). *Diagnostic and Statistical Manual of Mental Disorders* (4th ed., text rev.; DSM-IV-TR). Washington, DC: Author.

Anderson, D. K., Lord, C., Risi, S., Shulman, C., Welch, K., DiLavore, P. S., et al. (2007). Patterns of growth in verbal abilities among children with autism spectrum disorder. *Journal of Consulting and Clinical Psychology, 75,* 594–604.

Baird, G., Simonoff, E., Pickles, A., Chandler, S., Loucas, T., Meldrum, D., et al. (2006). Prevalence of disorders of the autism spectrum in a population cohort of children in South Thames: the Special Needs and Autism Project (SNAP). *Lancet, 368,* 210–215.

Bates, E., Thal, D., Fenson, L., Whitesell, K., & Oakes, L. (1989). Integrating language and gesture in infancy. *Developmental Psychology, 25,* 1004–1019.

Bloom, P. (2000). *How children learn the meaning of words.* Cambridge, MA: MIT Press.

Bolte, S., & Poustka, F. (2002). The relation between general cognitive level and adaptive behavior domains in individuals with autism with and without co-morbid mental retardation. *Child Psychiatry and Human Development, 33,* 165–172.

Bradley, L., & Bryant, P. E. (1983). Categorizing sounds and learning to read: A causal connection. *Nature, 301,* 419–421.

Carpenter, M., Nagell, K., & Tomasello, M. (1998). Social cognition, joint attention, and communicative competence from 9 to 15 months of age. *Monographs of the Society for Research in Child Development, 63,* 1–143.

Carpentieri, S., & Morgan, S. B. (1996). Adaptive and intellectual functioning in autistic and nonautistic retarded children. *Journal of Autism and Developmental Disorders, 26,* 611–620.

Chambers, W. J., Puig-Antich, J., Hirsch, M., Paez, P., Ambrosini, P. J., Tabrizi, M. A., et al. (1985). The assessment of affective disorders in children and adolescents by semistructured interview: Test-retest reliability of the schedule for affective disorders and schizophrenia for school-age children. *Archives of General Psychiatry, 42,* 696–702.

Charman, T., & Baird, G. (2002). Practitioner review: Diagnosis of autism spectrum disorder in 2-and 3-year-old children. *Journal of Child Psychology and Psychiatry and Allied Disciplines, 43,* 289–305.

Charman, T., Baird, G., Simonoff, E., Loucas, T., Chandler, S., Meldrum, D., et al. (2008). Cross-cultural validation of the Social Communication Questionnaire (SCQ) as a screener for autism spectrum disorders: Practical considerations. *Journal of the American Academy of Child and Adolescent Psychiatry, 47,* 720.

Charman, T., & Baron-Cohen, S. (2006). Screening for autism spectrum disorders in populations: Progress, challenges, and questions for future research and practice. In T. Charman & W. Stone (Eds.), *Social and communication development in autism spectrum disorders: Early identification, diagnosis, and intervention* (pp. 61–87). New York: Guilford.

Charman, T., Baron-Cohen, S., Swettenham, J., Baird, G., Cox, A., & Drew, A. (2000). Testing joint attention, imitation, and play as infancy precursors to language and theory of mind. *Cognitive Development, 15,* 481–498.

Charman, T., Baron-Cohen, S., Swettenham, J., Baird, G., Drew, A., & Cox, A. (2003). Predicting language outcome in infants with autism and pervasive developmental disorder. *International Journal of Language and Communication Disorders, 38,* 265–285.

Charman, T., Drew, A., Baird, C., & Baird, G. (2003). Measuring early language development in pre-school children with autism spectrum disorder using the MacArthur Communicative Development Inventory (Infant Form). *Journal of Child Language, 30,* 213–236.

Charman, T., Howlin, P., Berry, B., & Prince, E. (2004). Measuring developmental progress of children with autism spectrum disorder on school entry using parent report. *Autism, 8,* 89–100.

Charman, T., Taylor, E., Drew, A., Cockerill, H., Brown, J. A., & Baird, G. (2005). Outcome at 7 years of children diagnosed with autism at age 2: predictive validity of assessments conducted at 2 and 3 years of age and pattern of symptom change over time. *Journal of Child Psychology and Psychiatry, 46,* 500–513.

Courchesne, E., Pierce, K., Schumann, C. M., Redcay, E., Buckwalter, J. A., Kennedy, D. P., et al. (2007). Mapping early brain development in autism. *Neuron, 56,* 399–413.

Cox, A., Klein, K., Charman, T., Baird, G., Baron-Cohen, S., Swettenham, J., et al. (1999). Autism spectrum disorders at 20 and 42 months of age: Stability of clinical and ADI-R diagnosis. *Journal of Child Psychology and Psychiatry, 40,* 719–732.

Dawson, G. (2008). Early behavioral intervention, brain plasticity, and the prevention of autism spectrum disorder. *Development and Psychopathology, 20,* 775–803.

Delis, D. C., Kaplan, E., & Kramer, J. H. (2001). *Delis-Kaplan Executive Function System (D–KEFS).* San Antonio, TX: Harcourt.

DeMyer, M. K., Barton, S., DeMyer, W. E., Norton, J. A., Allen, J., & Steele, R. (1973). Prognosis in autism: a follow-up study. *Journal of Autism and Childhood Schizophrenia, 3,* 199–246.

Drew, A., Baird, G., Baron-Cohen, S., Cox, A., Slonims, V., Wheelwright, S., et al. (2002). A pilot randomised control trial of a parent training intervention for pre-school children with autism - Preliminary findings and methodological challenges. *European Child and Adolescent Psychiatry, 11,* 266–272.

Emslie, H., Wilson, C., Burden, V., Nimmo-Smith, I., & Wilson, B. A. (2003). *Behavioural Assessment of the Dysexecutive Syndrome for Children (BADS-C).* Lutz, FL: Psychological Assessment Resources.

Fecteau, S., Mottron, L., Berthiaume, C., & Burack, J. A. (2003). Developmental changes of autistic symptoms. *Autism, 7,* 255–268.

Freeman, B. J., Del'Homme, M., Guthrie, D., & Zhang, F. (1999). Vineland adaptive behavior scale scores as a function of age and initial IQ in 210 autistic children. *Journal of Autism and Developmental Disorders, 29,* 379–384.

Freeman, B. J., Ritvo, E. R., Needleman, R., & Yokota, A. (1985). The stability of cognitive and linguistic parameters in autism: a five-year prospective study. *Journal of the American Academy of Child and Adolescent Psychiatry, 24,* 459–464.

Geschwind, D. H., & Levitt, P. (2007). Autism spectrum disorders: developmental disconnection syndromes. *Current Opinion in Neurobiology, 17,* 103–111.

Gillberg, C., Ehlers, S., Schaumann, H., Jakobsson, G., Dahlgren, S. O., Lindblom, R., et al. (1990). Autism under age 3 years: A clinical-study of 28 cases referred for autistic symptoms in infancy. *Journal of Child Psychology and Psychiatry and Allied Disciplines, 31,* 921–934.

Gilotty, L., Kenworthy, L., Sirian, L., Black, D. O., & Wagner, A. E. (2002). Adaptive skills and executive function in autism spectrum disorders. *Child Neuropsychology, 8,* 241–248.

Gioia, G., Isquith, P., Guy, S., & Kenworthy, L. (2000). *BRIEF: Behavior Rating Inventory of Executive Function.* Odessa, FL: Psychological Assessment Resources.

Happe, F., Ronald, A., & Plomin, R. (2006). Time to give up on a single explanation for autism. *Nature Neuroscience, 9,* 1218–1220.

Harrison, P., & Oakland, T. (2003). *Adaptive Behavior Assessment System—Second Edition (ABAS—II).* San Antonio, TX: Harcourt.

Herring, S., Gray, K., Taffe, J., Tonge, B., Sweeney, D., & Einfeld, S. (2006). Behaviour and emotional problems in toddlers with pervasive developmental disorders and developmental delay: associations with parental mental health and family functioning. *Journal of Intellectual Disability Research, 50*, 874–882.

Honey, E., McConachie, H., Randle, V., Shearer, H., & Le Couteur, A. S. (2008). One-year change in repetitive behaviours in young children with communication disorders including autism. *Journal of Autism and Developmental Disorders, 38*, 1439–1450.

Howlin, P., & Asgharian, A. (1999). The diagnosis of autism and Asperger syndrome: findings from a survey of 770 families. *Developmental Medicine and Child Neurology, 41*, 834–839.

Howlin, P., Gordon, R. K., Pasco, G., Wade, A., & Charman, T. (2007). The effectiveness of Picture Exchange Communication System (PECS) training for teachers of children with autism: a pragmatic, group randomised, controlled trial. *Journal of Child Psychology and Psychiatry, 48*, 473–481.

Howlin, P., Magiati, I., & Charman, T. (2009). A systematic review of early intensive behavioural interventions (EIBI) for children with autism. *American Journal on Intellectual and Developmental Disabilities, 114*, 23–41.

Hudry, K., Leadbitter, K., Temple, K., Clifford, S., Slonims, V., McConachie, H., Aldred, C., Charman, T., & the PACT Consortium. (2008, May). Agreement across measures of language and communication in preschoolers with core autistic disorder. *Presentation at the 7th International Meeting for Autism Research.* London.

Hus, V., Pickles, A., Cook, E. H., Risi, S., & Lord, C. (2007). Using the Autism Diagnostic Interview-Revised to increase phenotypic homogeneity in genetic studies of autism. *Biological Psychiatry, 61*, 438–448.

Kasari, C., Paparella, T., Freeman, S., & Jahromi, L. B. (2008). Language outcome in autism: Randomized comparison of joint attention and play interventions. *Journal of Consulting and Clinical Psychology, 76*, 125–137.

Kasari, C., Freeman, S., & Paparella, T. (2006). Joint attention and symbolic play in young children with autism: a randomized controlled intervention study. *Journal of Child Psychology and Psychiatry, 47*, 611–620.

Kleinman, J. M., Ventola, P. E., Pandey, J., Verbalis, A. D., Barton, M., Hodgson, S., et al. (2008). Diagnostic stability in very young children with autism spectrum disorders. *Journal of Autism and Developmental Disorders, 38*, 606–615.

Klin, A., Saulnier, C. A., Sparrow, S. S., Cicchetti, D. V., Volkmar, F. R., & Lord, C. (2007). Social and communication abilities and disabilities in higher functioning individuals with autism spectrum disorders: The Vineland and the ADOS. *Journal of Autism and Developmental Disorders, 37*, 748–759.

Korkman, M., Kirk, U., & Kemp, S. (1997). *NEPSY.* San Antonio, TX: Harcourt.

Landa, R. J., Holman, K. C., & Garrett-Mayer, E. (2007). Social and communication development in toddlers with early and later diagnosis of autism spectrum disorders. *Archives of General Psychiatry, 64*, 853–864.

Leyfer, O. T., Folstein, S. E., Bacalman, S., Davis, N. O., Dinh, E., Morgan, J., et al. (2006). Comorbid psychiatric disorders in children with autism: Interview development and rates of disorders. *Journal of Autism and Developmental Disorders, 36*, 849–861.

Liss, M., Harel, B., Fein, D., Allen, D., Dunn, M., Feinstein, C., et al. (2001). Predictors and correlates of adaptive functioning in children with developmental disorders. *Journal of Autism and Developmental Disorders, 31*, 219–230.

Lord, C. (1995). Follow-up of two-year-olds referred for possible autism. *Journal of Child Psychology and Psychiatry and Allied Disciplines, 36*, 1365–1382.

Lord, C., Risi, S., DiLavore, P. S., Shulman, C., Thurm, A., & Pickles, A. (2006). Autism from 2 to 9 years of age. *Archives of General Psychiatry, 63*, 694–701.

Lord, C., Risi, S., Lambrecht, L., Cook, E. H., Leventhal, B. L., DiLavore, P. C., et al. (2000). The Autism Diagnostic Observation Schedule-Generic: A standard measure of social and communication deficits associated with the spectrum of autism. *Journal of Autism and Developmental Disorders, 30*, 205–223.

Lord, C., & Schopler, E. (1989). Stability of assessment results of autistic and non-autistic language impaired children from preschool years to early school age. *Journal of Child Psychology and Psychiatry, 30*, 575–590.

Luyster, R., Lopez, K., & Lord, C. (2007). Characterizing communicative development in children referred for Autism Spectrum Disorders using the MacArthur-Bates Communicative Development Inventory (CDI). *Journal of Child Language, 34*, 623–654.

Manly, T., Robertson, I. H., Anderson, V., & Nimmo-Smith, I. (1998). *Test of Everyday Attention for Children (TEA-Ch).* London: Harcourt.

Moore, V., & Goodson, S. (2003). How well does early diagnosis of autism stand the test of time? Follow-up study of children assessed for autism at age 2 and development of an early diagnostic service. *Autism, 7*, 47–63.

Morales, M., Mundy, P., Delgado, C. E. F., Yale, M., Neal, R., & Schwartz, H. K. (2000). Gaze following, temperament, and language development in 6-month-olds: A replication and extension. *Infant Behavior and Development, 23*, 231–236.

Mosconi, M. W., Cody-Hazlett, H., Poe, M. D., Gerig, G., Gimpel-Smith, R., & Piven, J. (2009). Longitudinal study of amygdala volume and joint attention in 2- to 4-year-old children with autism. *Archives of General Psychiatry, 66*, 509–516.

Moss, J., Magiati, I., Charman, T., & Howlin, P. (2008). Stability of the autism diagnostic interview-revised from pre-school to elementary school age in children with autism spectrum disorders. *Journal of Autism and Developmental Disorders, 38*, 1081–1091.

Mundy, P. (2003). Annotation: The neural basis of social impairments in autism: the role of the dorsal medial-frontal cortex and anterior cingulate system. *Journal of Child Psychology and Psychiatry and Allied Disciplines, 44*, 793–809.

Mundy, P., & Gomes, A. (1998). Individual differences in joint attention skill development in the second year. *Infant Behavior and Development, 21*, 469–482.

Mundy, P., Sigman, M., & Kasari, C., (1990). A longitudinal study of joint attention and language development in autistic children. *Journal of Autism and Developmental Disorders, 20*, 115–128.

Munson, J., Dawson, G., Abbott, R., Faja, S., Webb, S. J., Friedman, S.D., Shaw, D., Artru, A., & Dager, S. R, (2006). Amygdalar volume and behavioral development in autism. *Archives of General Psychiatry, 63*, 686–693.

Ozonoff, S. (1998). Assessment and remediation of executive dysfunction in autism and Asperger syndrome. In E. Schopler,

G. B. Mesibov, & L. J. Kunce (Eds.), *Asperger syndrome or high-functioning autism?* (pp. 263–289). New York: Plenum.

Pickering, S., & Gathercole, S. (2001). *Working Memory Test Battery for Children (WMTB-C)*. London: Harcourt.

Pickles, A., Simonoff, E., Conti-Ramsden, G., Falcaro, M., Simkin, Z., Charman, T., et al. (2009). Loss of language in early development of autism and specific language impairment. *Journal of Child Psychology and Psychiatry, 50*, 843–852.

Pine, D. S., Guyer, A. E., Goldwin, M., Towbin, K. A., & Leibenluft, E. (2008). Autism spectrum disorder scale scores in pediatric mood and anxiety disorders. *Journal of the American Academy of Child and Adolescent Psychiatry, 47*, 652–661.

Piven, J., Harper, J., Palmer, P., & Arndt, S. (1996). Course of behavioral change in autism: A retrospective study of high-IQ adolescents and adults. *Journal of the American Academy of Child and Adolescent Psychiatry, 35*, 523–529.

Rogers, S. J., & Vismara, L. A. (2008). Evidence-based comprehensive treatments for early autism. *Journal of Clinical Child and Adolescent Psychology, 37*, 8–38.

Ronald, A., Happe, F., Bolton, P., Butcher, L. M., Price, T. S., Wheelwright, S., et al. (2006). Genetic heterogeneity between the three components of the autism spectrum: A twin study. *Journal of the American Academy of Child and Adolescent Psychiatry, 45*, 691–699.

Russo, N., Flanagan, T., Iarocci, G., Berringer, D., Zelazo, P. D., & Burack, J. A. (2007). Deconstructing executive deficits among persons with autism: Implications for cognitive neuroscience. *Brain and Cognition, 65*, 77–86.

Saulnier, C. A., & Klin, A. (2007). Brief report: Social and communication abilities and disabilities in higher functioning individuals with autism and Asperger syndrome. *Journal of Autism and Developmental Disorders, 37*, 788–793.

Schatz, J., & Hamdanallen, G. (1995). Effects of Age and IQ on adaptive-behavior domains for children with autism. *Journal of Autism and Developmental Disorders, 25*, 51–60.

Sigman, M., & McGovern, C. W. (2005). Improvement in cognitive and language skills from preschool to adolescence in autism. *Journal of Autism and Developmental Disorders, 35*, 15–23.

Sigman, M., & Ruskin, E. (1999). Continuity and change in the social competence of children with autism, Down syndrome, and developmental delays. *Monographs of the Society for Research in Child Development, 64*, 1–114.

Siller, M., & Sigman, M. (2002). The behaviors of parents of children with autism predict the subsequent development of their children's communication. *Journal of Autism and Developmental Disorders, 32*, 77–89.

Simonoff, E., Pickles, A., Charman, T., Chandler, S., Loucas, T., & Baird, G. (2008). Psychiatric disorders in children with autism spectrum disorders: Prevalence, comorbidity, and associated factors in a population-derived sample. *Journal of the American Academy of Child and Adolescent Psychiatry, 47*, 921–929.

Sparrow, S. S., Balla, D. A., & Cicchetti D. (1984). *Vineland Adaptive Behavior Scales*. Circle Pines, MN: American Guidance Service.

Sparrow, S. S., Balla, D. A., & Cicchetti D. (2006). *Vineland Adaptive Behavior Scales–II*. Circle Pines, MN: American Guidance Service.

Starr, E., Szatmari, P., Bryson, S., & Zwaigenbaum, L. (2003). Stability and change among high-functioning children with pervasive developmental disorders: A 2-year outcome study. *Journal of Autism and Developmental Disorders, 33*, 15–22.

Steinhausen, H. C., & Metzke, C. W. (2004). Differentiating the behavioural profile in autism and mental retardation and testing of a screener. *European Child and Adolescent Psychiatry, 13*, 214–220.

Stone, W. L., Lee, E. B., Ashford, L., Brissie, J., Hepburn, S. L., Coonrod, E. E., et al. (1999). Can autism be diagnosed accurately in children under 3 years? *Journal of Child Psychology and Psychiatry and Allied Disciplines, 40*, 219–226.

Sukhodolsky, D. G., Scahill, L., Gadow, K. D., Arnold, L. E., Aman, M. G., McDougle, C. J., et al. (2008). Parent-rated anxiety symptoms in children with pervasive developmental disorders: Frequency and association with core autism symptoms and cognitive functioning. *Journal of Abnormal Child Psychology, 36*, 117–128.

Szatmari, P., Bryson, S. E., Boyle, M. H., Streiner, D. L., & Duku, E. (2003). Predictors of outcome among high functioning children with autism and Asperger syndrome. *Journal of Child Psychology and Psychiatry and Allied Disciplines, 44*, 520–528.

Toth, K., Munson, J., Meltzoff, A. N., & Dawson, G. (2006). Early predictors of communication development in young children with autism spectrum disorder: Joint attention, imitation, and toy play. *Journal of Autism and Developmental Disorders, 36*, 993–1005.

Turner, L. M., & Stone, W. L. (2007). Variability in outcome for children with an ASD diagnosis at age 2. *Journal of Child Psychology and Psychiatry, 48*, 793–802.

Turner, L. M., Stone, W. L., Pozdol, S. L., & Coonard, E. E. (2006). Follow-up of children with autism spectrum disorders from age 2 to age 9. *Autism, 10*, 243–265.

Venter, A., Lord, C., & Schopler, E. (1992). A follow-up-study of high-functioning autistic-children. *Journal of Child Psychology and Psychiatry and Allied Disciplines, 33*, 489–507.

Wiggins, L. D., Baio, J., & Rice, C. (2006). Examination of the time between first evaluation and first autism spectrum diagnosis in a population-based sample. *Journal of Developmental and Behavioral Pediatrics, 27*, S79–S87.

World Health Organization. (1993). *Mental disorders: A glossary and guide to their classification in accordance with the 10th Revision of the International Classification of Diseases: Research Diagnostic Criteria (ICD-10)*. Geneva: WHO.

Yirmiya, N., & Ozonoff, S. (2007). The very early autism phenotype. *Journal of Autism and Developmental Disorders, 37*, 1–11.

Yoder, P., & Stone, W. L. (2006). Randomized comparison of two communication interventions for preschoolers with autism spectrum disorders. *Journal of Consulting and Clinical Psychology, 74*, 426–435.

Zwaigenbaum, L., & Stone, W. (2006). Early screening for autism spectrum disorders in clinical practice. In T. Charman & W. Stone (Eds.), *Social and communication development in autism spectrum disorders: Early identification, diagnosis, and intervention* (pp. 88–113). New York: Guilford.

14

Marsha Mailick Seltzer, Jan S. Greenberg, Julie Lounds Taylor, Leann Smith, Gael I. Orsmond, Anna Esbensen, Jinkuk Hong

Adolescents and Adults with Autism Spectrum Disorders

Points of Interest

- Improvement in autism symptoms and behavior problems is evident during adolescence and adulthood, although the majority of individuals with ASD remain significantly affected and dependent at least partially on the support of others.
- Comorbid psychiatric disorders affect approximately half of adolescents and adults with ASD. The majority is prescribed psychotropic medications; and once beginning medications the probability of discontinuing such medications is very low.
- Almost one quarter of adults continue in some type of postsecondary education once leaving high school, and about 20% achieve competitive or supported employment in the community. However, nearly half of adults attend day activity centers or sheltered workshops, and fewer than 10% have no structured day activity.
- Relationships between adolescents and adults with ASD and their parents and siblings are largely positive, although behavior problems interfere with close family relationships at these stages of life.
- High levels of maternal warmth and low levels of maternal criticism are longitudinally predictive of reduced behavior problems and autism symptoms in adolescents and adults, suggesting possible avenues for intervention.

Autism Spectrum Disorders (ASDs) are often conceptualized as disorders of childhood. However, for most affected individuals, autism lasts throughout the life course, although the severity of symptoms often declines with advancing age (for a review, see Seltzer, Shattuck, Abbeduto, & Greenberg, 2004). As most individuals with ASD live a full lifespan, many more years are spent in adolescence and adulthood than in childhood. Nevertheless, the bulk of research and clinical knowledge is focused on early identification of ASD, the early years after the diagnosis, and the response to early intervention.

In this chapter, we focus on autism during adolescence and adulthood. We summarize the available research and provide an in-depth report of the findings from our ongoing longitudinal study, "Adolescents and Adults with Autism (AAA)." Our focus in this chapter is on (1) the developmental course of autism symptoms and behavior problems during adolescence and adulthood, (2) physical and psychiatric comorbidities during these life stages, (3) the transition from school to adult life, and (4) family relations. Our goal is to present a multidimensional description of ASD during adolescence and adulthood.

Overview of the AAA Study

Our longitudinal study began in 1998 and it will extend through 2012, encompassing 12 years in the lives of each participating family during the 14-year study period. The inclusion criteria were as follows: the son or daughter was age 10 or older when the study began, had received an ASD diagnosis (autistic disorder, Asperger's disorder, or PDD-NOS) from an independent health or educational professional, and had a research-administered Autism Diagnostic Interview-Revised (ADI-R, Lord et al., 1994) profile consistent with the specific ASD diagnosis. Nearly all (94.6%) of the 406 sample members met ADI-R lifetime criteria for a diagnosis of autistic disorder. Case-by-case review of the other sample members (5.4%) determined that their ADI-R profile was consistent with their autism spectrum diagnosis (either Asperger's or PDD-NOS). Many sample members (44.2%) had been given multiple diagnoses on the autism spectrum; 37.2% have received two diagnoses (most commonly autistic disorder and PDD-NOS in 28.3% of the sample), and 5.3% received all three diagnoses on the autism spectrum. For this reason, we refer to our sample members as having ASD, even though nearly all qualify for a diagnosis of autistic disorder.

Half of the families were from Wisconsin (n = 202), and half from Massachusetts (n = 204). We used identical recruitment (distributing information through service agencies, schools, clinics) and data collection methods in both states. When the study began, two thirds of the probands (65.1%) were living in the parental home. Currently (in 2009), the proportion who are coresiding is lower (41.6%), reflecting out-of-home placement during the past decade. Additionally, some sample members made educational transitions into (n = 61) and out of (n = 92) high school during the study period.

At Time 1, the probands ranged in age from 10 to 52 (mean = 21.91, SD = 9.41). Two thirds (63.8%) were under age 22. Their characteristics are consistent with what we would expect based on epidemiological studies of autism (Fombonne, 2003). Three fourths (73.2%) were male. One quarter (24.4%) had a seizure disorder, and a similar number (25.6%) were nonverbal or only spoke in single words. The majority (70.2%) had intellectual disability (ID).

We chose to include a wide age range of individuals with ASD for two reasons. First, the behavioral manifestations of developmental disabilities often change with age (Hodapp, 2004). Age-related change in the behavioral phenotype has been examined in adults with Down syndrome, Fragile X syndrome, Williams syndrome, and Prader-Willi syndrome (Dykens, 2004; Hodapp & Ricci, 2002; Jerrold et al., 2001; Wright-Talamante et al., 1996), but less is known about the life course trajectory of ASD. By examining behavioral change longitudinally across a broad range of ages, it is possible to describe the life course trajectory of autism symptoms and related behavior problems.

Our second rationale for including a broad age range is to be able to examine a number of age-related transitions. As noted above, our study includes adolescents and adults who transitioned into and out of high school, and moved out of the family home (and sometimes back). Once our study is completed, we will have collected pre- and posttransition measures on individuals who experience each of these transitions, and we will thus be able to examine their impacts on the unfolding lives of individuals with ASD in adolescence and adulthood.

We collect data from the families every 18 months. Thus far (between 1998 and 2009), we have conducted six repeated in-depth interviews with mothers, conducted a Daily Diary Study with the mothers, collected saliva from mothers to measure cortisol as a biomarker of daily stress, administered questionnaires to fathers and both adolescent and adult siblings, and administered cognitive assessments and interviews with the adolescents and adults with ASD.

More detailed descriptions of our methodology and findings can be found in publications from our research group (e.g., Greenberg, Seltzer, Hong, & Orsmond, 2006; Lounds, Greenberg, Seltzer, & Shattuck, 2007; Orsmond & Seltzer, 2009; Shattuck et al., 2007; and Seltzer et al., 2003).

Developmental Course of Autism Symptoms and Behavior Problems

Only a few studies have examined the developmental course of autism during adolescence and adulthood, and these studies agree that although there is a gradual pattern of improvement, residual levels of impairment remain clinically significant and continue to limit quality of life (Billstedt et al., 2005; Fombonne, 2003; Howlin et al., 2000, 2004; Kobayashi & Murata, 1998; Mawhood et al., 2000; Nordin & Gillberg, 1998; Piven et al., 1996; Rutter et al., 1967). Furthermore, development may be "splintered," with improvement evident in only some of behaviors and symptoms and with different timing of improvements across behaviors (Seltzer et al., 2003). Additionally, there can be plateaus, and for some individuals, symptoms may even worsen (Gillberg & Steffenberg, 1987). Behavior problems are often exhibited by people with ASD (Aman et al., 2003; Hollander et al., 2003; Lecavalier, 2005; Shea et al., 2004; Tonge & Enfield, 2003). However, our research (Shattuck et al., 2007) was the first prospective study to have examined change in behavior problems among adolescents and adults with ASD.

Our retrospective and prospective analyses indicated that improvement in symptoms and behavior problems is evident during adolescence and adulthood. Although 95% of our sample qualified for a diagnosis of autistic disorder during childhood (using the ADI-R), by the time our study began, only about half (54.8%) currently showed symptoms severe enough to qualify for this diagnosis (Seltzer et al., 2003). Building on this pattern of improvement, our prospective analyses (Shattuck et al., 2007) indicated that between Times 1 and 4 of our study (spanning a 4.5-year period), the sample members improved significantly on 57% of the ADI-R algorithm items that rated current functioning, most prominently in the domain of restricted, repetitive behaviors and interests.[1] No item assessing current functioning worsened significantly, on average, over this 4.5-year period. These prospective analyses also revealed that internalizing, externalizing, and asocial behavior problems were significantly less frequent at Time 4 than Time 1. The subgroup who did not have ID and who had better language ability at Time 1 improved the most (Shattuck et al., 2007).

A similar pattern of improvement was evident in a life course analysis of restricted repetitive behaviors (RRBs) in individuals with ASD ranging from 2 to 62 years of age, combining data from seven studies including ours (Esbensen, Seltzer, Lam, & Bodfish, 2009). Over 700 individuals with ASD were rated on the Repetitive Behavior Scale-Revised (Bodfish, Symons, Parker & Lewis, 2000; Lam & Aman, 2007). In cross-sectional cohort comparisons, RRBs were found to be less frequent and less severe among older than younger individuals, corroborating that autism symptoms abate with age. Further, we found that discrete types of RRBs had unique age-related patterns. For example, restricted interests were the most prevalent RRB across most ages, although they were markedly less prevalent among older individuals with ASD than younger individuals in these cohort comparisons and showed the steepest slope of age-related differences. Self-injurious repetitive behaviors were the least prevalent RRB across all ages. Stereotyped movements were common among young children with ASD, more so than rituals and compulsions, but became less prevalent than these other RRBs in adulthood. These unique patterns of age-related differences suggest that RRBs are a heterogeneous group of behaviors, and further confirm the findings reported in Lam and Aman (2007) that RRBs are not uniform in their age-related patterns.

On a less optimistic note, our sample members with ASD continued to struggle with social isolation in adolescence and adulthood. Overall, we found that fewer than 10% had reciprocal friendships with age peers, and nearly half had no peer relationships (Orsmond, Krauss, & Seltzer, 2004). Those who had peer relationships were more likely to be adolescents than adults, and had less impairment in reciprocal social interaction, as measured by current ratings on the ADI-R, than those who did not have friends. Although friendships were rare, the sample members more frequently engaged in recreational activities, including exercise (74.5% exercised at least once a week), working on a hobby (41.3% at least weekly), participating in group recreational activities (35.3% at least weekly), attending religious services (30.6% at least weekly), and socializing with relatives, neighbors, or people they knew from school or work (22.6%, 20.9%, and 13.2%, respectively, at least once a week).

In summary, past research suggests, and our findings confirm that, unlike some other developmental disabilities (e.g., Down syndrome, Fragile X syndrome) that evidence flat or declining patterns of functioning during adulthood, ASD shows a gradually improving pattern with respect to autism symptoms and behavior problems, on average. Nevertheless, the majority of the adolescents and adults in our sample remain significantly impaired and, as described below, at least partially dependent on the assistance of others.

Physical and Psychiatric Comorbidities

Fully 25–50% of individuals with ASD have comorbid health problems (Billstedt et al., 2005; Bryson & Smith, 1998). Up to 12% have disorders of known or suspected genetic origin (Kielinen et al., 2004). Lifetime rates of epilepsy are high (up to 40%), especially among those with ID, with seizures often developing during adolescence (Billstedt et al., 2005; Fombonne, 2003). Disrupted sleep is reported in 40–80% of children with ASD (Richdale, 1999).

In our sample of adolescents and adults, health problems were common. Only 29% were rated by their mothers as being in excellent health. According to maternal report, disrupted sleep was frequent (70% of adolescents and adults had disrupted sleep, with 35% having disrupted sleep once a week or more often). Also, many reported that their son or daughter had gastrointestinal (GI) problems (58%, with 22% having GI problems once a week or more often). One quarter (25%) had seizures. Of those who had seizures, most reported tonic-clonic (63%), absence (31%), or complex partial (26%) seizures, and some had multiple types of seizures. Fully 12% of the sample had at least one emergency room visit in the past year, with some reporting more than 50 visits.

Studies of children with ASD find consistently high rates of comorbid psychiatric disorders. Studies have shown that approximately three fourths of children with autism, PDD, and Asperger's syndrome met symptom criteria for at least one other comorbid psychiatric disorder (de Bruin, 2007; Ghaziuddin et al., 1998, Leyfer et al., 2006). Other studies report that children with ASD have higher rates of a variety of psychiatric disorders than typically developing children, including mood disorders, anxiety disorders, and oppositional defiant disorder (Gadow, Devincent, Pomeroy & Azizian, 2004, 2005; Kim et al., 2000).

Rates of comorbid psychiatric disorders remain high as individuals with ASD enter adolescence and adulthood. Ghaziuddin et al. (1998) reported that about 50% of adolescents and adults with Asperger's syndrome met diagnostic criteria for a comorbid psychiatric disorder. Bradley et al. (2004) found that 67% of adolescents and adults diagnosed with both autism and severe intellectual disability met at least one clinical cutoff for a psychiatric disorder. Tsakanikos and colleagues (2006) reported somewhat lower rates in their large community-based study of adults who had both autism and intellectual disability, with 36% of the sample having a psychiatric disorder.

We examined this issue in our sample of adolescents and adults with ASD (Kring, Greenberg, & Seltzer, 2008) and found that approximately half (52%) of the sample members had at least one comorbid psychiatric diagnosis, according to maternal report. Anxiety disorders were the most prevalent, with over 40% of the individuals with ASD in our sample having received an anxiety disorder diagnosis, of which a large subgroup had obsessive-compulsive disorder. Depression also was quite prevalent among these adolescents and adults (23.9%). We do not have data about whether the probability of receiving diagnoses of anxiety and depression increases for children with ASD during adolescence, whether anxiety and depressive symptoms increase in severity, or whether these comorbid conditions increase in individuals with ASD at any greater rate than in the general population during adolescence. These all remain important questions for future research.

There remains considerable debate about the prevalence of psychotic disorders among individuals with ASD. Some reports indicate higher rates of schizophrenia and bipolar disorder in individuals with ASD (e.g., Billstedt et al., 2005), but other investigations have shown rates comparable to individuals with other types of DDs (Tsakinikos et al., 2006) and to the general population (Kobayashi & Murata, 1998; Lainhart &

Folstein, 1994; Morgan et al., 2003). In our study, 5.9% of the adolescents and adults with ASD had a diagnosis of bipolar disorder and 2.6% had a diagnosis of schizophrenia (Kring et al., 2008), which is substantially higher than in the general population (estimated at 0.4%–1.6% for bipolar disorder and 0.5%–1.5% for schizophrenia; APA, 2000).

Relatively little is known about the extent to which individuals with ASD and comorbid psychiatric disorders have more severe symptoms of autism, elevated behavior problems, and more physical health problems than those with autism and no comorbid psychiatric disorders. Kim et al. (2000) found evidence that children with ASD who also had anxiety or depression had elevated levels of behavior problems (Kim et al., 2000). In our study of adolescents and adults, those with ASD and a comorbid psychiatric diagnosis had significantly more repetitive behaviors, higher levels of asocial behaviors, poorer overall health, more frequent GI problems, and more difficulty sleeping than those with ASD only (Kring et al., 2008).

Adolescents and adults with ASD are frequently prescribed medications for psychiatric and health problems. There is some evidence supporting the efficacy of psychotropic medications in reducing behavior problems (Anderson et al., 1989; Gordon et al., 1993; Hellings et al., 2006; McDougle et al., 1996; Research Units on Pediatric Psychopharmacology Autism Network, 2002). However, these medications carry the risk of side effects (Aman, Lam & Von Bourgondien, 2005; Tsai, 1999), which may adversely affect health (Law, 2007).

We conducted a longitudinal analysis of medications taken by the adolescents and adults with ASD in our sample, spanning the 4.5 years between Times 1 and Time 4 of our study (Esbensen, Greenberg, Seltzer & Aman, 2009). We found that a total of 57% of our sample members were taking at least one prescription psychotropic medication, and 37% were taking at least one prescription nonpsychotropic medication at the beginning of the study (with 70% taking at least one prescription medication of either type at Time 1). The proportion of individuals taking these medications increased significantly over time, with 81% taking at least one medication 4.5 years later (64% taking at least one psychotropic medication and 50% taking at least one nonpsychotropic medication at Time 4). We calculated the conditional probabilities of continuing or altering medication status over the 4.5-year study period, and the findings were highly informative about medication practices over time. Our data showed that once adolescents and adults with ASD are prescribed medications, they are highly likely to stay medicated. This pattern was more pronounced for psychotropic medications (approximately 11 times more likely to remain on psychotropic medications than to *stop* taking them) than for nonpsychotropic medications (nearly five times more likely to stay on nonpsychotropic medications than to stop during the 4.5 year study period). Thus, a considerable number of individuals with ASD are being prescribed psychotropic medications, and once prescribed it is likely that they will remain on these medications for many years.

To summarize, our data confirm past research that adolescents and adults with ASD have a high rate of comorbidities at these stages of life, particularly psychiatric diagnoses. Not surprisingly, this is a highly medicated population. Juxtaposed against this pattern of multiple diagnoses and high rates of psychotropic medications is the pattern of improvement in autism symptoms and behavior problems, reported above. An unanswered question is whether the increasing use of psychotropic medication may account for some of the behavioral and symptomatic improvements evident in our sample members, or whether the trajectory of improvement reflects the natural course of ASD in adolescence and adulthood.

The Transition from School to Adult Life

Change is often extremely stressful for individuals with ASD, but they must face many age-related transitions. The transition out of high school signifies the end of the entitlement to educational services mandated by federal law. Moving to one's own home is a daunting challenge for many individuals with ASD, and lack of independence results in continued family caregiving. Residence in a group home or supported living also continues to challenge parents who must provide oversight in a service system marked by very high staff turnover and questionable quality of services. Over time, there is an increasing risk of parental marital disruption, health decline, and death, which in turn may have consequences for the timing of other transitions for individuals with ASD. Each transition has its own ecology, but the timing, antecedents, and consequences are poorly understood.

In 2006, there were nearly 224,000 children and adolescents in the primary and secondary school systems with an ASD diagnosis; the number of students served with an ASD diagnosis increased 650% between 1996 and 2006, and 34% between 2004 and 2006 (IDEA, 2008). The number of children diagnosed with ASD began rising rapidly in the early 1990s (Gurney et al., 2003), and children from that generation are now exiting the school system, putting an extreme burden on an already overtaxed adult service system (Howlin, Alcock, & Burkin, 2005). Although this increase in the prevalence of ASD may be due in part to diagnostic substitution (Shattuck, 2006), nevertheless many of these adolescents and young adults are in need of formal and informal supports during and after transition.

There is considerable variability in the age when individuals with ASD exit the educational system. Some higher-functioning individuals graduate from high school with their similarly aged peers. Others take advantage of IDEA and continue in school until age 22. Once they leave school and lose entitlement to services, there is an increase in parental responsibility. Leaving high school does not necessarily imply the receipt of a diploma. Howlin et al. (2004) reported that 78% of their sample left high school without a formal diploma, fewer than one third were working, and the majority of jobs did not require a skill and were poorly paid (Howlin et al., 2005), all of which are stressful for the individual and the family.

We conducted preliminary analyses examining the postsecondary educational and employment activities in which individuals with ASD participated during their first 18 months after exiting the secondary school system. Nearly one quarter of our sample members (23%) went on to some type of postsecondary education; the majority of these (70%) were in school more than 10 hours a week. Another 22% did not pursue postsecondary education, but obtained a competitive or supported job in the community. However, the most prevalent activity for our sample members after exiting high school was participation in day activity centers or sheltered workshops (46%). The remaining 9% had no employment activities. Although the proportion of adults with ASD who had no regular daytime activities is cause for concern, our data suggest that most are able to find some type of regular day activity after leaving high school. Nevertheless, the fact that approximately half of the sample members were in segregated day programs or workshops for individuals with developmental disabilities points to the challenge of finding community employment for these adults.

An increasing number of adults with ASD live apart from their parents. Rumsey et al. (1985) reported that 36% of the adults in their sample lived away from their parents. Gillberg and Steffenberg (1987), reporting on the birth cohort with autism born in Goteburg, Sweden, between 1961 and 1968, found an even split between those who lived with their parents and those in nonfamily settings. In other studies, the proportion of adults living away from parents was about two thirds (Howlin et al., 2004; Wolf & Goldberg, 1986). Therefore, although some adults with ASD continue to live with their parents, a substantial number move into nonfamily settings. No recent study has described the living arrangements of adults with ASD, with the exception of Howlin et al. (2004), which reported on a British sample.

We examined the percentage of adults with ASD who were living with their families at our most recent wave of data collection. Results were similar to what was found by Gillberg and Steffenberg (1987); fewer than half of the individuals with ASD were living with parents or other relatives (41.6%). Of those who were not living with family, 62% were living in a community residence or foster home, and 34% were living in semi-independent or independent housing. Narrowing the sample to those who were between the ages of 10 and 22 years at the start of the study, we found that over 82% were residing with parents at the first time point (in 1998). At the most recent time point, 10 years later, the percentage living with family dropped to 61%. Just over one half of those who moved out of the family home went to live in semi-independent or independent settings, while the other half lived in community residences, foster homes, or institutionalized settings. In sum, the percentage of adolescents and adults with ASD living with family in our sample was slightly higher than Howlin et al.'s (2004) British sample, with younger adults more likely to live with family than older adults.

In another analysis, we profiled adult lives of individuals with ASD and contrasted them with another well-defined group of adults with ID, namely adults with Down syndrome (DS; Esbensen, Bishop, Seltzer, Greenberg, & Taylor, 2010). Using data from a linked longitudinal study of adults with DS (Krauss & Seltzer, 1999), analyses included 70 adults with ASD, and 70 adults with DS who were matched on age and ID (all had ID). Dependent variables included residential arrangements, social contact with friends, vocational activities, and an overall composite of adult success that combined these three domains.

Our analyses revealed significant differences between the adults with ASD and the adults with DS in residential independence and social contact with friends. On average, adults with ASD lived in less independent residential settings than did adults with DS. Furthermore, only 8% of these adults with ASD visited with friends several times a week, compared to 25% of adults with DS. Given these differences, it was not surprising that adults with ASD scored lower on the composite measure of adult success than did adults with DS. Our findings suggest that the difficulties in attaining adult independence that have been reported in other studies of individuals with ASD (Ballaban-Gil, Rapin, Tuchman, & Shinnar, 1996; Eaves & Ho, 2008; Howlin et al., 2004; Kobayashi, Murata, & Yoshinaga, 1992) cannot be accounted for only by impairments in cognitive abilities, as ID was controlled in our study. Instead, there are characteristics or behaviors associated with the ASD phenotype that place adults with ASD at an elevated risk for poorer adult outcomes.

We also examined the role of adult services (occupational therapy, psychiatric services, or transportation services) in promoting adult success, and found that the number of services received was related to greater adult success for adults with DS, but was unrelated to adult success for those who had ASD (Esbensen et al., 2010). This finding points to the need to develop new, more effective methods of service delivery targeted specifically to meet the needs of adults with ASD.

In summary, the transition from adolescence to adulthood brings many changes to the lives of individuals with ASD. About one quarter pursue some type of postsecondary education after leaving high school, and about one fifth had obtained supported or independent jobs in the community. However, nearly half were in segregated vocational settings and a few had no day activity, which is cause for concern. Regarding residential transitions, it is common for individuals to move out of the family home once they reach adulthood, and about half of those who move away from home live either independently or in semi-independent settings. Their lifestyles are considerably more restricted than counterparts with Down syndrome. Finally, the receipt of formal services is associated with greater adult success for those with DS but not for those with ASD, suggesting a need for the development of more effective services for persons with ASD in adulthood.

Family Relationships

Although adulthood signifies a time of increasing independence from the family, for individuals with disabilities, the role of the family remains predominant throughout the life course and critical to maintaining a high quality of life (Seltzer, Krauss, Orsmond, & Vestal, 2000). Our study provided the opportunity to assess parent-child relationships during adolescence and adulthood and also the relationships between the individual with ASD and his or her unaffected siblings. These are reported in this section, along with findings about how the family environment is associated with changes in the symptoms of autism and behavior problems during these stages of life.

Parent-Child Relationships in Adolescence and Adulthood

Research on young children with ASD has shown that, despite the communication and social challenges associated with this disorder, strong bonds of attachment are formed, and interactions between parents and the child are positive (see Rutgers, Bakermans-Kranenburg, van Ijendoorn, & van Berckelaer-Onnes, 2004, for a review). Nevertheless, mothers may experience the relationship as quite different from their relationships with their other (unaffected) children.

These patterns characterizing the mother-child relationship tend to persist into adolescence and adulthood. In our study, we assessed the degree of positive affect felt by mothers toward their son or daughter with ASD and the mother's perception of reciprocated positive affect from the adult child to her (Orsmond, Seltzer, Greenberg, & Krauss, 2006). The Positive Affect Index (Bengtson & Roberts, 1991) assessed the dimensions of affection, respect, fairness, understanding, and trust in the parent-child relationship, each rated on a 6-point scale, with scores of 5 or 6 signifying a high degree of positive affect with respect to the particular dimension. We found a strong pattern of positive affect felt by the mother for the son or daughter. Fully 90.1% of the mothers gave ratings of either a 5 or a 6 for the degree of affection she felt toward her son or daughter with ASD and more than three fourths of the mothers (78.2%) gave rates of either 5 or 6 with respect to the degree to which she respects her son or daughter with ASD. About half of the mothers rated their feelings of fairness toward (57.9%) and understanding of (53.0%) their son or daughter with ASD at the high end of the scale (i.e., a rating of 5 or 6), but only about one third (38.1%) of the mothers felt that they trusted their adolescent or adult child to this degree.

There were lower ratings of reciprocated positive affect from the adolescent or adult with ASD, as perceived by the mother. Just under two thirds of the mothers perceived the highest levels (i.e., a rating of 5 or 6) of affection from their son or daughter, and about two fifths (39.6%) felt that their adolescent or adult child had the highest levels of respect for them. Only about one quarter of the mothers perceived a high level of reciprocated feelings of fairness (27.7%) and understanding (29.2%) from their son or daughter. However, three fourths (74.3%) felt that their adolescent or adult child with ASD trusted them at the highest levels.

We also rated mothers' expression of warmth toward their adolescent or adult son or daughter with ASD, using standardized and independent ratings of the Five Minute Speech Sample (Magana, Goldstein, Karno, Miklowitz, Jenkins, & Falloon, 1986). Consistent with the data on positive affect, over one third (35.6%) of mothers were rated as expressing moderately high to high degrees of warmth when describing their child with ASD, half (50.5%) expressed some to moderate degrees of warmth, and only 10.4% were rated as expressing no or very little warmth in the relationship (Orsmond et al., 2006).

Thus, the descriptive data suggest that relationships between mothers and their adolescent or adult child with ASD are positive during these stages of life, with the most positive aspects being the exchange of affection between the mother and her adolescent or adult child. Contrary to historical characterizations of mothers of individuals with autism (Bettelheim, 1967), the majority of mothers in our sample had warm and positive relationships with their adolescent son or daughter.

Sibling Relationships in Adolescence and Adulthood

The sibling relationship is one of the most important family relationships, as it typically lasts the longest. Siblings of individuals with an ASD often become the guardians when their parents are no longer able to provide care, due to illness or death. Thus, maintaining a positive sibling relationship and sibling psychological well-being is crucial to the long-term quality of life of individuals with an ASD. Moreover, sibling well-being has the potential to impact maternal well-being. We have found that mothers who have a child with an ASD and another child with a diagnosed disability report higher levels of depressive symptoms and anxiety and lower levels of family adaptability and cohesion, compared to mothers whose only child with a disability has an ASD (Orsmond, Lin, & Seltzer, 2007). These differences were observed when the children were adolescents and adults, suggesting that the effects of such caregiving experiences continue beyond childhood.

Our research has been among the first to examine sibling well-being and sibling relationships specifically during the life stages of adolescence and adulthood. Prior research has focused on childhood (e.g., Knott et al., 1995; Rivers & Stoneman, 2003) or included siblings in broad age ranges that span childhood through adolescence and young adulthood (e.g. Bägenholm & Gillberg, 1991; Kaminsky & Dewey, 2001; Ross & Cuskelly, 2006). Taking a developmental perspective will help us understand the unique challenges to siblings and the family at different life stages (Orsmond & Seltzer, 2007).

As siblings during adulthood are establishing their independent lives, we observed fewer shared activities between adult siblings than was reported for adolescent siblings (Orsmond, Kuo, & Seltzer, 2009). However, feelings of closeness in the sibling relationship did not differ between the samples of adolescent and adult siblings, suggesting fewer changes in the quality of sibling relationships across these life stages. For both age groups, behavior problems manifested by the brother or sister with an ASD were associated with fewer shared sibling activities and a more distant sibling relationship. Interestingly, support from parents was particularly important to adult siblings, wherein adult siblings who reported greater support from their parents reported a closer sibling relationship (Orsmond et al., 2009).

We also examined the extent to which sibling relationships in adulthood, when one sibling has an ASD, are distinct from sibling relationships in adulthood when one sibling has Down syndrome (Orsmond & Seltzer, 2007). Using data from the same linked longitudinal study on adults with DS as mentioned above (Krauss & Seltzer, 1999), we found that siblings of adults with an ASD have less contact with their brother or sister, and report lower levels of closeness in the sibling relationship and more pessimism about their brother or sister's future, than do siblings of adults with DS (Orsmond & Seltzer, 2007).

Comparing sibling well-being among adolescent and adult siblings of individuals with ASD, we did not find a significant age-related difference in their report of depressive symptoms (Orsmond et al., 2009), suggesting stability in the risk of depression among siblings of individuals with ASD from adolescence to adulthood. Focusing on the adolescent sample, we found that one third reported depressive symptoms on the Center for Epidemiological Studies Depression Scale (CES-D) above the clinical cutoff score of 16. Compared to community samples of adolescents, this rate is not elevated, but there was considerable variability within our sample, and sisters reported significantly higher rates of depressive and anxiety symptoms than brothers (Orsmond & Seltzer, 2009). Realizing that siblings are at risk of negative outcomes both because of family stress (such as maternal distress or behavior problems manifested by the brother or sister with an ASD) and because of genetic vulnerabilities, we have examined the variability in depressive symptoms in these siblings from a diathesis-stress perspective (e.g., Bauminger & Yirmiya, 2001). We found support for this model, in that the siblings with the highest level of depressive symptoms were those who experienced a greater number of stressful life events in the past year and also were rated by their mothers as showing more subclinical symptoms of the autism phenotype (Orsmond & Seltzer, 2009).

Taken together, our research findings on siblings suggest an altered path of sibling relationships that may put individuals with an ASD at risk of limited support after their parents are deceased. At the same time, we have identified some factors that might put siblings themselves at risk of adverse outcomes (e.g., the experience of stressful life events), and these could serve as screening factors to identify siblings who might need additional individual supports to help promote their well-being into adulthood. Nevertheless, the majority of siblings remain involved with their adult brother or sister with ASD and function in the nonclinical range psychologically.

The Family Environment and Expressed Emotion

One aspect of the family environment that has been receiving increasing attention for families of individuals with disabilities is *expressed emotion* (EE). EE is a measure of emotional intensity in the family and specifically refers to criticism or emotional overinvolvement of one family member toward another. In individuals with mental health problems such as schizophrenia and bipolar disorder, EE has been a strong predictor of outcomes including relapse (Butzlaff & Hooley, 1998; Lopez et al., 2004). Concomitantly, in studies of families of individuals with developmental disabilities, EE, particularly criticism, has consistently be related to elevated behavior problems in both children and adults (Chadwick, Kusel, & Cuddy, 2008; Hastings, Daley, Burns, & Beck, 2006; Hastings & Lloyd, 2007). When considering the association between EE and the behavioral functioning of individuals with developmental disabilities, it is important to consider that these relationships are likely bidirectional. Behavior problems have been repeatedly documented as a significant source of stress for parents (Hastings et al., 2005; Herring et al., 2006; Lounds et al., 2007), which may in turn relate to elevated levels of EE in the home. Conversely, high levels of EE may serve to maintain or even exacerbate children's behavior problems (Hastings & Lloyd, 2007).

Expressed Emotion is a qualitative measure of the amount or degree of emotion displayed. The measure is usually applied to caretakers or to family members in a home setting.

In our research, we have examined the bidirectional associations between aspects of the family environment and the behavior problems and autism symptoms in adolescents and adults with ASD. Before discussing our findings, it is particularly important to note that although the family environment may have an impact on the behavioral functioning of the individuals with ASD, this does not imply that the child's ASD is *caused* by the family. In the past, mothers of children with ASD were wrongly accused of causing their child's autism by being emotionally cold and distant. In contrast with this inaccurate and stigmatizing early belief, research subsequently has shown that parents of children with ASD interact with their children in ways that are just as sensitive and responsive as parents of children with other developmental disabilities and parents of typically developing children (Siller & Sigman, 2002; van IJzendoorn et al., 2007). Furthermore, there is clear consensus that ASD is a complex neurodevelopmental disorder that is strongly genetic in origin (Folstein & Rosen-Sheidley, 2001). Despite the genetic etiology of ASD, however, it is still possible to explore ways in which the phenotypic expression of ASD may be influenced by family factors. This has been our focus in several studies.

In one set of analyses, we explored the bidirectional effects of maternal EE, specifically criticism and emotional overinvolvement, on the behavior problems and autism symptoms of adolescents and adults with ASD. Using a subsample of coresiding mothers and children at Time 2 and Time 3 of our study, cross-lagged panel analyses revealed that high levels of EE were associated with increases in internalizing, externalizing, and asocial behavior in the adolescents and adults with ASD over an 18-month period. A high level of EE was also related to increasingly severe autism symptoms (Greenberg et al., 2006). Of note, most families in our study did not have abnormally elevated levels of EE, perhaps reflecting successful coping and adaptation by these families (Greenberg et al., 2006). These findings also underscore that, even in the absence of extreme levels of EE, the family environment is still an important influence on development in adolescents and adults with ASD.

In a separate set of analyses (Smith, Greenberg, Seltzer, & Hong, 2008), we examined the bidirectional impact of prosocial family processes such as warmth, praise, and relationship quality on behavior problems and autism symptoms, using the same longitudinal design. We found that high levels of warmth and praise were associated with the abatement of repetitive behaviors over time. Additionally, a positive mother-child relationship quality was associated with reductions in internalizing and externalizing problems, repetitive behaviors, and impairments in social reciprocity 18 months later in our sample of adolescents and adults with ASD.

Interestingly, in these analyses, the majority of effects flowed from parent to child, although we did find some evidence of reciprocal child-to-mother effects in a few instances. Overall, we found that the majority of mothers in our sample expressed low levels of criticism and high levels of warmth toward their son or daughter with ASD and that positive aspects of the family emotional climate were associated with improvements in behavior problems and autism symptoms during adolescence and adulthood. These findings highlight how a positive family environment can act as a mechanism for improving the quality of life for individuals with ASD.

Taken together, the findings from our investigations of EE and warmth in families of adolescents and adults with ASD suggest that some aspects of the family environment may be useful targets for future interventions. Specifically, reducing criticism and increasing warmth, praise, and relationship quality may serve not only to improve the family emotional climate but also to reduce behavior problems and alleviate autism symptoms during adolescence and adulthood. In families of individuals with mental health problems, family psychoeducation programs have been shown to be very effective for reducing levels of EE, leading to reductions in family burden and better outcomes for the individuals with a mental health condition (Hogarty et al., 1991; Klaus & Fristad, 2005; Lopez, Toprac, Crismon, Boemer, & Baumgartner, 2005; Miklowitz et al., 2004). These interventions typically involve weekly group sessions wherein multiple family members are provided with education on the nature, course, and management of the condition as well as activities to practice problem-solving. Although the challenges associated with parenting an adolescent or adult with ASD are distinct from those faced by families coping with psychiatric conditions, some aspects are similar, such as managing difficult behaviors and navigating the service system. As such, a family psychoeducation intervention may be one potentially promising model that could be effectively adapted for families of individuals with ASD during adolescence and adulthood.

Conclusion

Much remains to be learned about individuals with ASD during adolescence and adulthood. Studies of those who become symptom-free and who lead normative adult lives will have great importance for informing our understanding of ASD across the life course. In addition, it will be profitable to examine the cohort of individuals with ASD who remain supported by their families or by the formal service system in order to identify the constellation of services, employment opportunities, and living arrangements that promote a high quality of life. In particular, the identification of factors that ease the transition out of high school will be valuable.

Challenges and Future Directions

- Other research is needed to reveal more about the health of individuals with ASD, especially as they reach midlife and old age. The many comorbid physical and psychiatric conditions that characterize this population, and their heavy prescription medication use, make it important to determine the long-range consequences of health problems and medication practices that often begin in childhood.
- Behavior problems continue during adolescence and adulthood in individuals with ASD and remain major risk factors for disrupted family relationships and a limited quality of life. Therefore, more research is needed to develop and evaluate interventions aimed at reducing behavior problems during adolescence and adulthood, as they represent risk factors throughout the life course.
- The young children who receive an ASD diagnosis today may have a very different life course than the cohort that has been followed in the AAA study. Changing diagnostic patterns, improved early detection and diagnosis, more widespread early intervention, and more supportive societal attitudes might signal a more promising life course for those who reach adolescence and adulthood in the future. Yet it is only by studying this population longitudinally, extending into the adolescent and adult years, that we will be able to disentangle cohort differences from the true developmental course of the behavioral phenotype of autism and related disorders.

SUGGESTED READINGS

Esbensen, A. J., Seltzer, M. M., Lam, K. S., & Bodfish, J. W. (2009). Age-related differences in restricted repetitive behaviors in the autism spectrum disorder over the lifespan. *Journal of Autism and Developmental Disorders, 39*, 57–66.

Greenberg, J. S., Seltzer, M. M., Hong, J., & Orsmond, G. I. (2006). Bidirectional effects of expressed emotion and behavior problems and symptoms in adolescents and adults with autism. *American Journal of Mental Retardation, 111*, 229–249.

Seltzer, M. M., Krauss, M. W., Shattuck, P. T., Orsmond, G., Swe, A., & Lord, C. (2003). The symptoms of autism spectrum disorders in adolescence and adulthood. *Journal Autism and Developmental Disorders, 33*, 565–581.

Shattuck, P. T., Seltzer, M. M., Greenberg, J. S., Orsmond, G. I., Bolt, D., Kring, S., et al. (2007). Change in autism symptoms and maladaptive behaviors in adolescents and adults with an autism spectrum disorder. *Journal of Autism and Developmental Disorders, 37*, 1735–1747.

Smith, L. E., Greenberg, J. S., Seltzer, M. M., & Hong, J. (2008). Symptoms and behavior problems of adolescents and adults with autism: Effects of mother-child relationship quality, warmth, and praise. *American Journal of Mental Retardation, 113*, 378–393.

ACKNOWLEDGMENTS

This chapter was prepared with the support of grants from the National Institute on Aging (R01 AG08768 to M.M. Seltzer), and the National Institute of Child Health and Human Development (T32 HD07489 to L. Abbeduto, and P30 HD03352 to M. M. Seltzer).

NOTES

1 Statistically significant improvement was found for the following symptoms: neologisms, friendships, range of facial expression, direct gaze, social smiling, seeking to share enjoyment with others, inappropriate facial expression, use of others' body to communicate, compulsions and rituals, circumscribed interests, unusual sensory interests, hand and finger mannerisms, unusual preoccupations, repetitive use of objects or interest in parts of objects, and other complex mannerisms and body movements.

REFERENCES

Aman, M. G., Lam, K. S., & Von Bourgondien, M. E. (2005). Medication patterns in patients with autism: Temporal, regional, and demographic influences. *Journal of Child and Adolescent Psychopharmacology, 15*, 116–126.

Aman, M. G., Lam, K. S. L., & Collier-Crespin, A. (2003). Prevalence and patterns of use of psychoactive medicines among individuals with autism in the Autism Society of Ohio. *Journal of Autism and Developmental Disorders, 33*, 527–534.

Anderson, L. T., Campbell, M., Adams, P., Small, A. M., Perry R., & Shell, J. (1989). The effects of haloperidol on discrimination learning and behavioral symptoms in autistic children. *Journal of Autism and Developmental Disorders, 19*, 227–239.

American Psychiatric Association (2000). Diagnostic and statistical manual of mental disorders (4th ed., text rev.; DSM-IV-TR). Washington, DC: Author.

Bägenholm, A., & Gillberg, C. (1991). Psychosocial effects on siblings of children with autism and mental retardation: A population-based study. *Journal of Mental Deficiency Research, 35*, 291–307.

Ballaban-Gil, K., Rapin, I., Tuchman, R., & Shinnar, S. (1996). Longitudinal examination of the behavioral, language, and social changes in a population of adolescents and young adults with autistic disorders. *Pediatric Neurology, 15*, 217–233.

Bauminger, N., & Yirmiya, N., (2001). The functioning and well-being of siblings of children with autism: Behavioral-genetic and familial contributions. In J. A. Burack, T. Charman, N. Yirmiya, & P. R. Zelazo (Eds.), *The development of autism: Perspectives from theory and research* (pp. 61–80): Maywah, NJ: Erlbaum.

Bengtson, V. L., & Roberts, R. E. L. (1991). Intergenerational solidarity in aging families: An example of formal theory construction. *Journal of Marriage and the Family, 53*, 856–870.

Bettelheim, B. (1967). *The empty fortress: Infantile autism and the birth of the self.* New York: Free Press.

Billstedt, E., Gillberg, C., & Gillberg, C. (2005). Autism after adolescence: Population-based 13- to 22-year follow-up study of 120 individuals with autism diagnosed in childhood. *Journal of Autism and Developmental Disorders, 35*, 351–360.

Bodfish, J., Symons, F., Parker., D, & Lewis, M. (2000). Varieties of repetitive behavior in autism: Comparisons to mental retardation. *Journal of Autism and Developmental Disorders, 30*, 237–243.

Bradley, E. A., Summers, J. A., Wood, H. L., & Bryson, S. E. (2004). Comparing rates of psychiatric and behavior disorders in adolescents and young adults with severe intellectual disability with and without autism. *Journal of Autism and Developmental Disorders, 34*, 151–161.

Bryson, S. E., & Smith, I. M. (1998). Epidemiology of autism: Prevalence, associated characteristics, and implications for research and service delivery. *Mental Retardation and Developmental Disabilities Research Reviews, 4*, 97–103.

Butzlaff, R. L., & Hooley, J. M. (1998). Expressed emotion and psychiatric relapse: A meta-analysis. *Archives of General Psychiatry, 55*, 547–552.

Chadwick, O., Kusel, Y., & Cuddy, M. (2008). Factors associated with the risk of behavior problems in adolescents with severe intellectual disabilities. *Journal of Intellectual Disability Research, 52*, 864–876.

de Bruin, E. L., Ferdinand, R. F., Meester, S., de Nijs, P. F. A., & Verheij, F. (2007). High rates of psychiatric co-morbidity in PDD-NOS. *Journal of Autism and Developmental Disorders, 37*, 877–886.

Dykens, E. M. (2004). Maladaptive and compulsive behavior in Prader-Willi syndrome: New insights from older adults. *American Journal of Mental Retardation, 109*, 142–153.

Eaves, L. C., & Ho, H. H. (2008). Young adult outcomes of autism spectrum disorders. *Journal of Autism and Developmental Disorders, 38*, 739–747.

Esbensen, A. J., Bishop, S. L., Seltzer, M. M., Greenberg, J. S., & Taylor, J. L. (2010). Comparisons between individuals with autism spectrum disorders and individuals with Down syndrome in adulthood. *American Journal of Intellectual and Developmental Disabilities*, 115, 277–290.

Esbensen, A. J., Greenberg, J. S., Seltzer, M. M., & Aman, M. G. (2009). A longitudinal investigation of psychotropic and non-psychotropic medication use among adolescents and adults with autism spectrum disorders. *Journal of Autism and Developmental Disorders, 39*, 1339–1349.

Esbensen, A. J., Seltzer, M. M., Lam, K. S., & Bodfish, J. W. (2009). Age-related differences in restricted repetitive behaviors in the autism spectrum disorder over the lifespan. *Journal of Autism and Developmental Disorders, 39*, 57–66.

Folstein, S. E., & Rosen-Sheidley, B. (2001). Genetics of autism: Complex aetiology for a heterogeneous disorder. *Nature Reviews Genetics, 2*, 943–955.

Fombonne, E. (2003). Epidemiological surveys of autism and other pervasive developmental disorders: An update. *Journal of Autism and Developmental Disorders, 33*, 365–382.

Gadow, K. D., DeVincent, C. J., Pomeroy, J., & Azizian, A. (2004). Psychiatric symptoms in preschool children with PDD and clinic and comparison samples. *Journal of Autism and Developmental Disorders, 34*, 379–393.

Gadow, K. D., DeVincent, C. J., Pomeroy, J., & Azizian, A. (2005). Comparison of DSM-IV symptoms in elementary school-age children with PDD versus clinic and community samples. *Autism, 9*, 392–415.

Ghaziuddin, M., Weidmer-Mikhail, E., & Ghaziuddin, N. (1998). Comorbidity of Asperger syndrome: A preliminary report. *Journal of Intellectual Disability Research, 42*, 279–283.

Gillberg, C., & Steffenburg, S. (1987). Outcome and prognostic factors in infantile autism and similar conditions: A population-based study of 46 cases followed through puberty. *Journal of Autism and Developmental Disorders, 17*, 273–287.

Gordon, C. T., State, R. C., Nelson, J. E., Hamburger, S. D., & Rapoport, J. L. (1993). A double-blind comparison of clomipramine, desipramine, and placebo in the treatment of autistic disorder. *Archives of General Psychiatry, 50*, 441–447.

Greenberg, J. S., Seltzer, M. M., Hong, J., & Orsmond, G. I. (2006). Bidirectional effects of expressed emotion and behavior problems and symptoms in adolescents and adults with autism. *American Journal of Mental Retardation, 111*, 229–249.

Gurney, J., Fritz, M., Ness, K., Sievers, P., Newschaffer, C., & Shapiro, E. (2003). Analysis of prevalence trends of autism spectrum disorder in Minnesota. *Archives of Pediatrics and Adolescent Medicine, 157*, 622–627.

Hastings, R. P., Daley, D., Burns, C., & Beck, A. (2006). Maternal distress and expressed emotion: Cross-sectional and longitudinal relationships with behavior problems of children with intellectual disabilities. *American Journal of Mental Retardation, 111*, 48–61.

Hastings, R. P., Kovshoff, H., Ward, N. J., degli Espinosa, F., Brown, T., & Remington, B. (2005). Systems analysis of stress and positive perceptions in mothers and fathers of pre-school children with autism. *Journal of Autism and Developmental Disorders, 35*, 635–644.

Hastings, R. P., & Lloyd, T. (2007). Expressed emotion in families of children and adults with intellectual disabilities. *Mental Retardation and Developmental Disabilities Research Reviews, 13*, 339–345.

Hellings, J. A., Zarcone, J. R., Reese, R. M., Valdivinos, M. G., Marquis, J. G., Fleming, K. K., et al. (2006). A crossover study of risperidone in children, adolescents, and adults with mental retardation. *Journal of Autism and Developmental Disorders, 36*, 401–411.

Herring, S., Gray, K., Taffe, J., Tonge, B., Sweeney, D., & Einfeld, S. (2006). Behavior and emotional problems in toddlers with pervasive developmental disorders and developmental delay: Associations with parental mental health and family functioning. *Journal of Intellectual Disability Research, 50*, 874–882.

Hodapp, R. M. (2004). Studying interactions, reactions, and perceptions: Can genetic disorders serve as behavioral proxies? *Journal of Autism and Developmental Disabilities, 34*, 29–34.

Hodapp, R. M., & Ricci, L. A. (2002). Behavioral phenotypes and educational practice: The unrealized connection. In G. O'Brien & O. Udwin (Eds.), *Behavioral phenotypes in clinical practice* (pp. 137–151). London: MacKeith.

Hogarty, G. E., Anderson, C. M., Reiss, D. J., Kornblith, S. J., Greenwald, D. P., Ulrich, R. F., et al. (1991). Family psychoeducation, social skills training, and maintenance chemotherapy in aftercare treatment of schizophrenia. *Archives of General Psychiatry, 48*, 340–347.

Hollander, E., Phillips, A. T., & Yeh, C. C. (2003). Targeted treatments for symptom domains in child and adolescent autism. *Lancet, 362*, 732–734.

Howlin, P., Alcock, J., & Burkin, C. (2005). An 8 year follow-up of a specialist supported employment service for high-ability adults with autism or Asperger syndrome. *Autism, 9*, 533–549.

Howlin, P., Goode, S., Hutton, J., & Rutter, M. (2004). Adult outcome for children with autism. *Journal of Child Psychology and Psychiatry, 45*, 212–229.

Howlin, P., Mawhood, L., & Rutter, M. (2000). Autism and developmental receptive language disorder-A follow-up comparison in early adult. II: Social, behavioural, and psychiatric outcomes. *Journal of Child Psychology and Psychiatry and Allied Disciplines, 41*, 561–578.

IDEAdata.org. (2008). Annual report tables. Available at www.ideadata.org/PartBdata.asp. Accessed July 15, 2008.

Jerrold, C., Baddeley, A. D., Hewes, A. K., & Phillips, C. (2001). A longitudinal assessment of diverging verbal and non-verbal abilities in the Williams syndrome phenotype. *Cortex, 27*, 423–431.

Kaminsky, L., & Dewey, D. (2001). Sibling relationships of children with autism. *Journal of Autism and Developmental Disorders, 31*, 399–410.

Kielinen, M., Rantala, H., Timonen, E., Linna, S. L., & Moilanen, I. (2004). Associated medical disorders and disabilities in children with autistic disorder: A population-based study. *Autism, 8*, 49–60.

Kim, J. A., Szatmari, P., Bryson, S. E., Streiner, D. L., & Wilson, F. J. (2000). The prevalence of anxiety and mood problems among children with autism and Asperger syndrome. *Autism, 4*, 117–132.

Klaus, N., & Fristad, M. A. (2005). Family psychoeducation as a valuable adjunctive intervention for children with bipolar disorder. *Directions in Psychiatry, 25*, 217–229.

Knott, F., Lewis, C., & Williams, T. (1995). Sibling interactions of children with learning disabilities: A comparison of autism and Down's syndrome. *Journal of Child Psychology and Psychiatry, 56*, 965–976.

Kobayashi, R., & Murata, T. (1998). Behavioral characteristics of 187 young adults with autism. *Psychiatry and Clinical Neurosciences, 52*, 383–390.

Kobayashi, R. Murata, T., & Yoshinaga, T. (1992). A follow-up study of 201 children with autism in Hyushu and Yamaguchi Areas, Japan. *Journal of Autism and Developmental Disorders, 22*, 395–422.

Krauss, M. W., & Seltzer, M. M. (1999). An unanticipated life: The impact of lifelong caregiving. In H. Bersani (Ed.), *Responding to the challenge: International trends and current issues in developmental disabilities.* Brookline, MA: Brookline.

Kring, S. R., Greenberg, J. S., & Seltzer, M. M. (2008). Adolescents and adults with autism with and without co-morbid psychiatric disorders: Differences in maternal well-being. *Journal of Mental Health Research in Intellectual Disabilities, 1*, 53–74.

Lainhart, J. E., & Folstein, S. E. (1994). Affective disorders in people with autism: A review of published cases. *Journal of Autism and Developmental Disorders, 24,* 587–601.

Lam, K. S. L., & Aman, M. G. (2007). The Repetitive Behavior Scale–Revised: Independent validation in individuals with autism spectrum disorders. *Journal of Autism and Developmental Disorders, 37,* 855–866.

Law, D. (2007). Physical health: How to minimise the risks faced by patients with schizophrenia. *Mental Health Practice, 10,* 26–28.

Lecavalier, L. (2005). An evaluation of the Gilliam Autism Rating Scale. *Journal of Autism and Developmental Disorders, 35,* 795–805.

Leyfer, O. T., Folstein, S. E., Bacalman, S., Davis, N. O., Dinh, E., Morgan, J., et al. (2006). Co-morbid psychiatric disorders in children with autism: Interview development and rates of disorders. *Journal of Autism and Developmental Disorders, 36,* 849–861.

Lord, C., Rutter, M., & Le Couteur, A. (1994). Autism Diagnostic Interview-Revised: A revised version of a diagnostic interview for caregivers of individuals with possible pervasive developmental disorders. *Journal of Autism and Developmental Disorders, 24,* 659–685.

Lopez, S. R., Hipke, K. N., Polo, A. J., Jenkins, J. H., Karno, M., Vaughn, C., Snyder, K. S. (2004). Ethnicity, expressed emotion, attributions, and course of schizophrenia: Family warmth matters. *Journal of Abnormal Psychology, 113,* 428–439.

Lopez, M. A., Toprac, M. G., Crismon, M. L., Boemer, C., & Baumgartner, J. (2005). A psychoeducational program for children with ADHD or depression and their families: Results from the CMAP feasibility study. *Community Mental Health Journal, 41,* 51–66.

Lounds, J. J., Seltzer, M. M., Greenberg, J. S., & Shattuck, P. (2007). Transition and change in adolescents and young adults with autism: Longitudinal effects on maternal well-being. *American Journal of Mental Retardation, 112,* 401–417.

Magana, A. B., Goldstein, J. M., Karno, M., Miklowitz, D. J., Jenkins, J., & Falloon, I. R. (1986). A brief method for assessing expressed emotion in relatives of psychiatric patients. *Psychiatry Research, 17,* 203–212.

Mawhood, L., Howlin, P., & Rutter, M. (2000). Autism and developmental receptive language disorder: A comparative follow-up in early adult life. I: Cognitive and language outcomes. *Journal of Child Psychology and Psychiatry and Allied Disciplines, 41,* 547–559.

McDougle, C. J., Naylor, S. T., Cohen, D. J., Volkmar, F. R., Heninger, G. R., & Price, L. (1996). A double blind, placebo-controlled study of fluvoxamine in adults with autistic disorder. *Archives of General Psychiatry, 53,* 1001–1008.

Miklowitz, D. J., George, E. L., Axelson, D. A., Kim, E. Y., Birmaher, B. Schneck, C., et al. (2004). Family-focused treatment for adolescents with bipolar disorder. *Journal of Affective Disorders, 82,* 113–128.

Morgan, C. N., Roy, M., & Chance, P. (2003). Psychiatric comorbidity and medication use in autism: A community survey. *Psychiatric Bulletin, 27,* 378–381.

Nordin, V., & Gillberg, C. (1998). The long-term course of autistic disorders: Update on follow-up studies. *Acta Psychiatrica Scandinavica, 97,* 99–108.

Orsmond, G., Krauss, M. W., & Seltzer, M. M. (2004). Peer relationships and social and recreational activities among adolescents and adults with autism. *Journal of Autism and Developmental Disorders, 34,* 245–256.

Orsmond, G. I., Kuo, H., & Seltzer, M. M. (2009). Siblings of individuals with autism spectrum disorder: Sibling relationships and well-being in adolescence and adulthood. *Autism, 13,* 59–80.

Orsmond, G. I., Lin, L.-Y., & Seltzer, M. M. (2007). Mothers of adolescents and adults with autism: Parenting multiple children with disabilities. *Intellectual and Developmental Disabilities, 45,* 257–270.

Orsmond, G. I., & Seltzer, M. M. (2007). Siblings of individuals with autism spectrum disorders across the life course. *Mental Retardation Developmental Disabilities Research Reviews, 13,* 313–320.

Orsmond, G. I., & Seltzer, M. M. (2009). Adolescent siblings of individuals with an autism spectrum disorder: Testing a diathesis-stress model of sibling well-being. *Journal of Autism and Developmental Disorders, 39,* 1053–1065.

Orsmond, G. I., Seltzer, M. M., Greenberg, J. S., & Krauss, M. W. (2006). Mother-child relationship quality among adolescents and adults with autism. *American Journal of Mental Retardation, 111,* 121–137.

Piven, J., Harper, J., Palmer, P., & Arndt, S. (1996). Course of behavioral change in autism: A retrospective study of high-IQ adolescents and adults. *Journal of the Academy of Child and Adolescent Psychiatry, 35,* 523–529.

Research Units on Pediatric Psychopharmacology (RUPP) Autism Network. (2002). Double-blind placebo-controlled trial of risperidone in children with autism. *New England Journal of Medicine, 347,* 314–321.

Richdale, A. (1999). Sleep problems in autism: Prevalence, cause, and intervention. *Developmental Medicine and Child Neurology, 41,* 60–66.

Rivers, J. W., & Stoneman, Z. (2003). Sibling relationships when a child has autism: Marital stress and support coping. *Journal of Autism and Developmental Disorders, 33,* 383–394.

Ross, P., & Cuskelly, M. (2006). Adjustment, sibling problems, and coping strategies of brothers and sisters of children with autistic spectrum disorder. *Journal of Intellectual and Developmental Disability, 31*(2), 77–86.

Rumsey, J. M., Rapoport, J. L., & Sceery, W. R. (1985). Autistic children as adults: Psychiatric, social, and behavioral outcomes. *Journal of the American Academy of Child and Adolescent Psychiatry, 24,* 465–473.

Rutgers, A. H., Bakermans-Kranenburg, M. J., van Ijzendoorn, M. H., & van Berckelaer-Onnes, I. A. (2004). Autism and attachment: A meta-analytic review. *Journal of Child Psychology and Psychiatry, 45,* 1123–1134.

Rutter, M., Greenfeld, D., & Lockyer, L. (1967). A five to fifteen year follow-up study of infantile psychosis. II. Social and behavioural outcome. *British Journal of Psychiatry, 113,* 1183–1199.

Seltzer, M. M., Shattuck, P., Abbeduto, L., & Greenberg, J. S. (2004). The trajectory of development in adolescents and adults with autism. *Mental Retardation and Developmental Disabilities Research Reviews, 10,* 234–247.

Seltzer, M. M., Krauss, M. W., Orsmond, G. I., & Vestal, C. (2000). Families of adolescents and adults with autism: Uncharted territory. In L. M. Glidden (Ed.), *International review of research on mental retardation* (Vol. 23). San Diego: Academic.

Seltzer, M. M., Krauss, M. W., Shattuck, P. T., Orsmond, G., Swe, A., & Lord, C. (2003). The symptoms of autism spectrum disorders in adolescence and adulthood. *Journal Autism and Developmental Disorders, 33,* 565–581.

Shattuck, P. T. (2006). The contribution of diagnostic substitution to the growing administrative prevalence of autism in US special education. *Pediatrics, 117,* 1028–1037.

Shattuck, P. T., Seltzer, M. M., Greenberg, J. S., Orsmond, G. I., Bolt, D., Kring, S., et al. (2007). Change in autism symptoms and maladaptive behaviors in adolescents and adults with an autism spectrum disorder. *Journal of Autism and Developmental Disorders, 37,* 1735–1747.

Shea, S., Turgay, A., Carroll, A., Schulz, M., Orlik, H., Smith, I., et al. (2004). Risperidone in the treatment of disruptive behavioral symptoms in children with autistic and other pervasive developmental disorders. *Pediatrics, 114,* 634–641.

Siller, M., & Sigman, M. (2002). The behaviors of parents of children with autism predict the subsequent development of their children's communication. *Journal of Autism and Developmental Disorders, 32,* 77–89.

Smith, L. E., Greenberg, J. S., Seltzer, M. M., & Hong, J. (2008). Symptoms and behavior problems of adolescents and adults with autism: Effects of mother-child relationship quality, warmth, and praise. *American Journal of Mental Retardation, 113,* 378–393.

Tonge, B. J., & Einfeld, S. (2003). Psychopathology and intellectual disability: The Australian Child to Adult Longitudinal Study. *International Review of Research in Mental Retardation, 26,* 61–91.

Tsai, L. Y. (1999). Psychopharmacology in autism. *Psychosomatic Medicine, 61,* 651–665.

Tsakanikos, E., Costello, H., Holt, G., Bouras, N., Sturmey, P., & Newton, T. (2006). Psychopathology in adults with autism and intellectual disability. *Journal of Autism and Developmental Disorders, 36,* 1123–1129.

Van Ijzendoorn, M. H., Rutgers, A. H., Bakermans-Kranenburg, M. J., Swinkels, S. H. N., van Daalen, E., Dietz, C., et al., (2007). Parental sensitivity and attachment in children with autism spectrum disorder: Comparison with children with mental retardation, with language delays, and with typical development. *Child Development, 78,* 597–608.

Wolf, L. C., & Goldberg, B. (1986). Autistic children grow up: An eight to twenty-four year follow-up study. *Canadian Journal of Psychiatry, 31,* 550–556.

Wright-Talamante, C., Cheema, A., Riddle, J. E., Luckey, D. W., Taylor, A. K., & Hagerman, R. J. (1996). A controlled study of longitudinal IQ changes in females and males with fragile X syndrome. *American Journal of Medical Genetics, 64,* 350–355.

Commentary

Katherine A. Loveland

Issues in Defining the Core Features of Autism Through the Lifespan

The quest to define autism in terms of its central characteristics has evolved greatly over the past fifty years, as evidenced both by changing descriptions of the syndrome in the Diagnostic and Statistical Manual (DSM) of the American Psychiatric Association, and by changes in the topics most researched by investigators in the field. In this commentary I discuss some of the outstanding issues that must be confronted if we are to attain a better understanding and definition of autism (hereafter referred to as Autism Spectrum Disorder or ASD, for simplicity) and move beyond the limitations of present diagnostic models.

Since the syndrome was first identified, the core characteristics of ASD have been a source of controversy (see Mundy, chapter 8, this volume). Much ink has been expended in the battle to secure the high ground in this controversy, with adherents to various positions claiming to have identified the "real" underlying deficit in ASD, from which all else proceeds. As in the ancient Indian parable of the blind men and the elephant, however, scholars have naturally tended to interpret ASD according to the conceptual and methodological lenses through which they have viewed it. Thus, for example, over the decades psychodynamic models gave way to those involving language, perception and cognition, emotion, social cognition, or neuropsychological differences, reflecting the models and approaches current in the behavioral and medical sciences at the time. Why should ASD pose such problems to our attempts to define its essential characteristics?

Clinicians and researchers have long recognized that difficulties and disagreements in specifying the core characteristics of ASD stem in part from the wide heterogeneity among individuals with this type of disorder. Individuals vary not only in the severity of autistic behaviors, but also in other characteristics such as intellectual ability, level of language development, motor skills and behaviors, sensory differences, early social communication as well as emotional behavior and responsivity (see Loveland & Tunali, 2005, for review). This wide range of presentations has led to the currently accepted practice of referring to "Autism Spectrum Disorders," a term that embraces all forms of the disorder and suggests the image of a vector along which individuals can be located according to their severity.

Although the concept of the spectrum is in many ways an improvement over a model that does not recognize degrees of severity, it too is incomplete as a characterization of a developmental disorder such as ASD, since the spectrum concept does not necessarily encompass the idea of change with development. The task of specifying the core characteristics of ASD is further complicated when we consider the implications of a lifespan perspective. For example, Lord et al. (2006) and others have found that a consequence of the move to greater inclusiveness in the definition of ASD is that children on the margins of the definition, i.e., those with less classical presentations, are less likely to exhibit stability of diagnosis with increasing age. Charman (chapter 13, this volume) also emphasizes that heterogeneity among individuals with ASD actually increases as they become older, with various "core characteristics" progressing and skills developing at different rates. Thus, the fact that ASD is developmental in nature becomes critical to our consideration of the autism spectrum and the question of core characteristics: ASD must be conceptualized not as a discrete and static disorder presenting at a particular point in time, but as a *complex developmental process or pathway* that differs from the typical and that extends across the lifespan of the individual. An implication of this view is that over the life of the individual, ASD will present differently at different chronological ages, as a function of a complex combination of influences both within and outside the person. Among these are the genotype of the individual, maturational stage, family resources and functioning, social experiences with peers, the individual's own actions, changing social expectations of the individual as he or she matures, and many others. Current efforts to specify the earliest observable behavioral markers for high risk of ASD in infants (e.g., Brian et al., 2008; see also chapter 12, this volume) demonstrate that many of the characteristics we regard as essential to the syndrome of ASD emerge over time rather than being fully manifested when development first departs from a typical pathway. Thus, we can expect that ASD, far from being a discrete constellation of clinical signs that once it arrives remains fixed in its manifestations over time, is instead a moving target—a target moreover that moves with the child, developing as she or he develops, being constantly shaped by factors both within the individual and originating in the environment.

It is no wonder then, that there remains controversy about what unifies this disorder, with its changing manifestations over the lifespan of the individual. In the face of such frustrating complexity one might reasonably look for a way to characterize ASD that does not depend on behavioral characteristics of the phenotype to unify our concept of ASD across the lifespan. The tremendous growth in basic biomedical research on ASD that has occurred in the past 15 years represents in part a search for a way to find order amid chaos.

At the present time scientific and methodological advances in the biomedical sciences, particularly in imaging and genetics, have led to a widely accepted goal of characterizing ASD according to its basis in biological differences. This goal has been adopted in part because of the overwhelming evidence that biological differences from the typical population are present, and also because their discovery has the potential to lead to medical treatments or even prevention. Therefore, the search for the essentials of the syndrome has moved conceptually from the behavioral to the biological level. In recent years the study of the autism phenotype has become less a focus of the attempt to pin down the true nature of the syndrome, and more an adjunct to studies of genetics, neurobiology, and other biomedical approaches that fit within the reductionist program and that have the potential to lead to specific medical treatments. Although a detailed discussion of such research efforts is beyond the scope of this chapter, it is safe to say that as interesting and promising as such studies are, they have as yet not resulted in an improved specification of the core characteristics of autism. Numerous genetic discoveries have pointed to the involvement of a variety of genes, but it has become clear that the phenotype of ASD is multiply determined and that the genetic picture is likely to remain complex (see for review Geschwind, 2009; also see Section VI, this chapter). Similarly, some exciting findings resulting from neuroimaging of children and adults with ASD, for example evidence of differences in functional connectivity among brain regions (e.g., Just, Cherkassky, Keller, Kana, & Minshew, 2007), have opened new vistas in the ways we think about the brain and how it develops in ASD. However, rather than pointing to clear and specific markers that could simplify the early diagnosis of autism, the findings of biomedical studies have continued instead to reveal the great complexity of the disorder. As a consequence of this inherent complexity, a model of ASD across the lifespan of the individual that is both comprehensive and realistic will by necessity include the effects of many influences beyond those of genotype and brain maturation and will suggest mechanisms by means of which these influences lead to particular outcomes.

We can illustrate in a simplified way, using the metaphor of a snowball that grows larger as it rolls downhill, how secondary psychopathologies comorbid with ASD might arise, and worsen, over the life of an individual. If ASD is considered as a developmental pathway, then factors affecting development either supportively or adversely have their effects not only at a single time point but continuously and cumulatively over time. Just as the snowball grows larger as it rolls downhill accumulating more snow, an individual's developmental pathway will tend to depart from the typical to a greater and greater degree over time if the supportive influences are not sufficient to mitigate the effects of those that are adverse. A key feature of this model is that influences are not one-way, but transactional, such that a child's actions on the environment help to determine the feedback that the child receives, shaping not only future behaviors but ultimately the child him- or herself. If unusual or maladaptive behaviors are met with negative feedback from the child's environment (chiefly, the social environment), the child with ASD will be very likely to experience stress and anxiety. The result is that the child with ASD is exposed to frequent episodes of negative, highly stressful experiences.

The cumulative effects of negative experiences throughout life can have a profound effect on the well-being of the individual with ASD. These experiences, whether minor (e.g., frustration at being made to change activities) or major in nature (e.g., a lengthy and very upsetting experience with a large crowd of noisy people; being socially rejected for acting differently) might arguably affect individuals with ASD more severely than would be typical, in part because of the difficulty in emotional self-regulation associated with ASD, which renders them less able to regain equilibrium after an upset (see Loveland, 2005, for further discussion), and because of underlying genetic susceptibilities. Consequently, as families, educators, and clinicians well know, periods of emotional upset may be lengthy and exhausting for both the individual and others. Such episodes may constitute repeated stressors to the developing brain that have as their longer-term outcome psychiatric comorbidities such as anxiety disorders, depression, and other mood disorders, as well as other behavioral problems. A number of studies have documented the developmental pathway toward anxiety disorders in children who are by temperament highly reactive, showing that such a mechanism is not limited to ASD but is generally applicable to human neurodevelopment (see Bradley, 2000, for an excellent discussion of this topic; see also Schore, 1996, 1997). Given that verbal persons with ASD frequently struggle painfully with social relationships and learning to behave appropriately, it is not surprising that in adulthood many of them are more troubled by accumulated psychiatric disorders than by the symptoms of ASD itself.

Even if we accept the complexity that comes with a truly developmental way of viewing ASD, we are still left with the question of heterogeneity among individuals on the spectrum, and the consequent difficulties in both clinical diagnosis and research. If the heterogeneity of phenotype in the autism spectrum is as great as research suggests; if the neurobiological and biomedical correlates of ASD, including genetics, are not only exceedingly complex but also highly variable among individuals; if the characteristics of individuals with ASD become more, not less, heterogeneous with development; if linking genotypes to the categorical phenotype of ASD has proven increasingly complex; then can we in fact expect to define core characteristics that are common to all persons with ASD regardless of age, sex, developmental level, severity, genotype, etc.?

Perhaps we have been asking the wrong question.

Perhaps it is time to move away from the traditional scheme of psychiatric classification that depends on identifying a number of specific symptoms in order to determine whether an individual does or does not meet the criteria for a particular diagnostic category. The dichotomous (yes or no) approach to clinical classification has utility from a practical standpoint, of course, in that it is easier to determine a patient's eligibility for treatments, services, insurance coverage, educational programs, etc., if he or she can be said to fall within a particular category. On the other hand, for reasons discussed above, the dichotomous, categorical approach is a poor model to use as a basis for understanding a developmental disorder such as ASD. In the clinical realm, it encourages the clinician, the educator, and the family to think of ASD as a distinct and reified entity, that one either has or does not have. In the realm of research, the dichotomous classification scheme encourages investigators to classify together under the same diagnostic umbrella, as it were, individuals who though technically meeting the same diagnostic criteria, are nonetheless widely different in numerous ways.

A number of authors have in the past few years argued in favor of adopting a new approach to psychiatric classification, not only of ASD but of other psychiatric disorders as well (e.g., Craddock, O'Donovan, & Owen, 2009; Geschwind, 2009; O'Donovan, Craddock, & Owen, 2009). In addition to the increasingly obvious shortcomings of the dichotomous classification scheme as noted above, there are other reasons to revise the approach we use to guide our clinical practice and research. We now know that psychopathologies long conceptualized as separate and discrete are in fact overlapping in both behavioral and biological characteristics. For example, Craddock et al. (2009) in their recent discussion of relationships among schizophrenia, bipolar disorder, and mixed psychoses argued that current genetic findings are not compatible with dichotomous methods of classification. They further suggested that we must use methods of classification that capture phenotypic variability within and among individuals of the same diagnostic category and must link this variability to its biological substrates.

An approach that holds much promise for overcoming some of the limitations of the current diagnostic scheme grows out of the search for genotype/phenotype relationships in behavioral genetics. The concept of the *endophenotype* refers to quantifiable component characteristics that lie between a complex genotype and phenotype (see DeGeus & Boomsma, 2001; Gottesman & Gould, 2003; and Viding & Blakemore, 2007, for reviews and discussion of this topic). Endophenotypes may be behavioral or biological in nature. Ideally, a behavioral or biological marker should meet the following criteria to be selected as an endophenotype (Viding & Blakemore, 2007): (1) It should be reliably measurable; (2) It should be to some extent heritable; (3) Some association between the behavioral or cognitive phenotype and the proposed endophenotype should be demonstrated; (4) There should be evidence that the proposed endophenotype and the behavioral or cognitive phenotype have some shared genetic basis; (5) There should be evidence of a causal relationship such that the phenotype would not be realized without the presence of the endophenotype. Some possible behavioral/cognitive endophenotypes relevant to developmental psychopathology are self-regulation of emotions, behaviors, and choices; inhibition; ability to sustain attention; ability to manage attention flexibly and appropriately (e.g., to switch attention as needed, to selectively attend, etc.); motivational differences (e.g., readiness to initiate, response to rewards); temperament of the individual; motor skills; executive functions (e.g., planning and organizing), and others. Endophenotypes may also be biological, as in specific neuroanatomical or neurofunctional, physiological or biochemical characteristics of the individual. Because they are simpler components of complex disorders, endophenotypes presumably have much greater potential for being linked to a specific genetic or neurobiological basis. Because they do not constitute in themselves whole syndromes, but rather elements, it is also possible to imagine that different complex syndromes may share certain endophenotypes. If so, comparative studies of disorders that apparently share certain endophenotypes (e.g., Craddock et al., 2009) may shed light on the processes that lead to expression of these endophenotypes as well as of broad phenotypes such as ASD.

In fact, there is growing evidence from both clinical observation and scientific investigations that ASD has many overlaps with other disorders, not only in behavioral symptoms but in definable brain abnormalities and in its genetic basis. Increasingly, investigators have begun to identify these areas of overlap, and to consider possible relationships among the syndromes as they are currently defined. Clinical experience as well as a growing literature suggests that there is an unusually high prevalence of comorbid psychiatric disorders with ASD (although cf. Melville et al., 2008, who found that the rate of such disorders was not greater than that in a general sample of comparable persons with intellectual disability). For example it is very common for individuals with ASD, particularly those with greater intellectual ability and language skills, to show prominent symptoms of anxiety (Groden, Cautela, Prince, & Berryman, 1994; Kim, Szatmari, Bryson, Streiner, & Wilson, 2000; Leyfer et al., 2006; Loveland, 2005; Mazefsky, Folstein, & Lainhart, 2008; Russell & Sofronoff, 2005) as well as major mood disorders including depression and bipolar disorder (Ghaziuddin & Zafar, 2008). Also commonly found in individuals with ASD are symptoms of attention-deficit/hyperactivity disorder (ADHD; Pearson et al., 2006; Ryden & Bejerot, 2008) and obsessive-compulsive disorder (OCD; Rossi, 2006). Some investigators have also found evidence that these psychopathologies are more common among parents of individuals with ASD than in the typical population (e.g., Mazefsky, Folstein & Lainhart, 2008), suggesting that there may be a heritable risk factor involved. These findings support the idea that the relationship between ASD and other psychopathologies is a fertile ground in which to seek potential endophenotypes.

As an example, the possible overlap of obsessive-compulsive disorder (OCD) and ASD has been explored in a number of recent studies. The question of overlap between OCD and ASD has long been the subject of controversy, since both disorders involve repetitive behaviors (see chapter 17, this volume). Although there are qualitative differences between the compulsive behaviors and obsessive thoughts that typically occur in OCD and repetitive, stereotyped behaviors typically observed in ASD, it is nonetheless possible that there is underlying commonality. Russell, Mataix-Cols, Anson, and Murphy (2005), studying adults with a primary diagnosis of OCD and those with a diagnosis of ASD, concluded that up to 50% of their sample with ASD had obsessions and compulsions that were similar to those of the patients with OCD and were not accounted for by stereotyped and repetitive behaviors characteristic of ASD. Bejerot and Mortberg (2009) found that adults with OCD were much more likely (50% of the sample) to have been bullied at school as children than were those with social phobia (20%) or a reference group (27%). The investigators argued that this finding was due to overlap between the characteristics of OCD and ASD, since their sample with OCD also had more signs of low social skills. Obsessive-compulsive symptoms in parents have also been found to be positively associated with measures of restricted interests and repetitive behavior in their child with ASD (Abramson et al., 2005; Hollander, King, Delaney, Smith, & Silverman, 2003; Kano, Ohta, Nagai, Pauls, & Leckman, 2004), suggesting that an endophenotype for repetitive behaviors may exist as a heritable trait that could be linked to a genetic basis. In fact, a number of studies have identified genes that are associated with the risk of both OCD and ASD (e.g., McDougle, Epperson, Price, & Gelernter, 1998; Wendland et al., 2008). Executive dysfunction has also been found in the first-degree relatives of individuals with OCD as well as the relatives of individuals with ASD (Delorme et al., 2007) and has been suggested as an endophenotype common to both disorders.

Behavioral or biological evidence of possible endophenotypes has been gathered from comparisons of ASD with other disorders as well. Recent evidence that schizophrenia, like ASD, is a disorder of neurodevelopment has led to reopening the question of overlap between the two disorders (Nylander, Lugnegard, & Hallerback, 2008). Genetic studies of schizophrenia and bipolar disorder (BPD) indicate that some loci confer risk of both disorders and risk of ASD as well (see Craddock et al., 2009, for review). Genes in the chromosomal 8p region may confer risk of disorders including schizophrenia, BPD, ASD, and depression, as well as some nonpsychiatric diseases (Tabarés-Seisdedos & Rubenstein, 2009). Deletion of 15q13.3 has been found to be associated with risks of both ASD and BPD (Ben-Shachar et al., 2009). Findings such as these lend weight to the argument that ASD shares endophenotypes with other disorders, and that further research to specify these endophenotypes will lead to a better understanding of how such disorders develop, and how development leads to expression of different clinical outcomes in different individuals.

A wide variety of possible endophenotypes relevant to ASD and related disorders have been proposed. If borne out by subsequent research, these candidate endophenotypes may be used to reduce the heterogeneity that results from using clinical classifications to form study samples. Among these are response monitoring (linked to abnormalities of anterior cingulate cortex) (Thakkar et al., 2008); inattention and hyperactivity (Tani et al., 2006); problems in executive functioning and motor skills (Rommelse et al., 2009); style of face-processing (Adolphs, Spezio, Parlier, & Piven, 2008); response variability (shared with ADHD and Tourette's syndrome; Geurts et al., 2008); a local bias in visual information processing (Wang, Mottron, Peng, Berthiaume, & Dawson, 2007); diminishment of a cingulate cortex "self" response when deciding what to do next or imagining oneself doing so (Chiu et al., 2008); a quantitative measure of ASD symptomatology particularly social relatedness (Social Responsiveness Scale) linked to loci on chromosomes 11 and 17 (Duvall et al., 2007); a metabolic endophenotype related to oxidative stress and linked to a genetic basis (James et al., 2006); and language delay (Spence et al., 2006). In addition some studies have begun to rule out potential endophenotypes for ASD, such as visual motor reconstruction (Block Design task) (de Jonge, Kemner, Naber, & van Engeland, 2009); and TPH2 alleles and haplotypes and GLO1 alleles (Sacco et al., 2007). Thus, the tools are beginning to be available to develop a way of classifying the characteristics of individuals with ASD (and other disorders) according to endophenotypes, which are measurable, linked to both genotype and phenotype, and can be assorted differently for different individuals. Such an approach would not dispel the heterogeneity present in ASD; rather, it would acknowledge variation among individuals while providing a more potentially useful way to characterize them.

The Core Characteristics of ASD Reconsidered

I have argued that despite many years of productive research on ASD, we have continued to try to classify individuals using a method that does not reflect what we have learned about this complex disorder. Neither the developmental nature of ASD nor the heterogeneity of expression it finds in different individuals is captured by the current categorical classification system. Not surprisingly, the current system has proven to be a poor basis for forming samples for research, particularly genetic research, and it has failed to shed much light on the ways individuals with ASD change over the course of their lives. The question of core characteristics reflects the current diagnostic system, and thus it too may need to be reconsidered.

Devising a way to characterize ASD that will address the issues I have discussed is neither simple nor straightforward. At this time we have few established endophenotypes for ASD that meet the criteria mentioned above (see Viding & Blakemore, 2007). Moreover there is much we do not know about development in ASD, particularly in those individuals who may be described as within the "Broader Autism Phenotype." With this in mind, I offer the following suggested directions for future investigation.

Researchers should embrace the study of individual differences in the ASD phenotype. The great majority of studies on ASD have been nomothetic in approach, seeking to find commonalities among persons with ASD in order to determine standards for diagnosis, education, treatment, neural basis, etc. However, variations among individuals may be informative in ways that cannot be achieved using a nomothetic approach, in which variations are typically regarded as "noise" to be controlled or eliminated through matching. Towgood, Meuwese, Gilbert, Turner, and Burgess (2009) recommended that investigators consider using the multiple case series approach often used in neuropsychology, because it permits the investigator to identify variability that may be lost in a typical group comparisons approach and that may be important to understanding the disorder(s) under study. Such studies may add to our ability to isolate relationships between genotype and phenotypes in ASD and establish whether they do or do not meet the criteria for an endophenotype.

More research should be focused on adults with ASD, including the ways the manifestations of the disorder have changed over time. At present we know much less about adults with ASD than we do about children. In particular the factors that lead to more- and less-desirable outcomes is deserving of study. Fortunately in Western countries many individuals with ASD do receive services and supports that lead to improvements in their functioning over time, at least in some areas. As the large prospective study by Seltzer et al. (chapter 14, this volume) demonstrates, development continues in adulthood in persons with ASD, just as it does in typical persons. Overt symptoms of ASD tend to become less pronounced as the individual reaches adulthood, particularly in those with higher intellectual functioning and those who have received remediation. One can speculate, as do Seltzer et al. in their chapter, that thanks to better identification and more available early intervention, those who are children now can look forward to a still better outcome in adulthood than those of the earlier cohorts who are now adults. However there remain major gaps in our knowledge. For example, we are only beginning to observe the lives of persons with ASD over 50 years of age; how their behavioral and cognitive symptoms change with aging remains largely unexplored.

Researchers should continue to identify endophenotypes that contribute to the larger ASD phenotype and its variations as well as commonalities between ASD and other disorders. The constellation of endophenotypes we call ASD is not so distinct from other disorders as was once thought (ADHD, OCD, schizophrenia, BPD, etc.). Not only do such disorders seem to co-occur frequently, but there is evidence that they overlap in both phenotypes and genotypes. It should be possible, then, to use comparisons among these disorders to help clarify the relationship of genotype to endophenotype, and endophenotype to phenotype. Indeed studies of this nature are already taking place at an accelerating rate, and it seems likely that this type of research will play a very important role in advancing our knowledge of how and why ASD occurs.

Researchers should work toward creating a "lexicon" of endophenotypes that is not applicable only to a single disorder, but to multiple disorders, and that may become the basis for a new clinical classification system. Under such a system the emphasis might be on specifying the endophenotypes expressed in that individual, their severity, and their implications for treatment, rather than classifying the individual as a whole. Ultimately, a more fine-grained and precise description of an individual with ASD might resemble not a point along a single spectrum (vector) for ASD severity, but a cloud of points in an n-dimensional space where n represents the number of relevant quantifiable endophenotypes considered. Such a hypothetical system of classification would offer the advantage of avoiding the necessity of using categories labeled "Not Otherwise Specified," which as currently used are by nature heterogeneous and vague. It would also provide more specific and quantifiable ways of dealing with the heterogeneity of the "Broader Autism Phenotype" (BAP) in research.

Finally, the approach I have sketched in this commentary, though as yet far from being realized, offers both the researcher and the clinician one further advantage over the present categorical method. By removing the necessity of dichotomous classification for psychopathologies, it serves to emphasize that in the human population there is no clear, sharp line between the normal and the abnormal but instead, the concept of the spectrum applies to everyone.

REFERENCES

Abramson, R. K., Ravan, S. A., Wright, H. H., Wieduwilt, K., Wolpert, C. M., Donnelly, S. A., et al. (2005). The relationship between restrictive and repetitive behaviors in individuals with autism and obsessive compulsive symptoms in parents. *Child Psychiatry and Human Development, 36*(2), 155–165.

Adolphs, R., Spezio, M. L., Parlier, M., & Piven, J. (2008). Distinct face-processing strategies in parents of autistic children. *Current Biology, 18*(14), 1090–1093.

Bachevalier, J., & Loveland, K. (2006). The orbitofrontal–amygdala circuit and self-regulation of socio-emotional behavior in autism. *Neuroscience and Biobehavioral Reviews, 30*, 97–117.

Barnhill, J. & Horrigan, J. P. (2002). Tourette's syndrome and autism: A search for common ground. *Mental Health Aspects of Developmental Disabilities, 5*(1), 7–15.

Baron-Cohen, S. (1989). Do autistic children have obsessions and compulsions? *British Journal of Child Psychology, 28*, 193–200.

Bartz, J. A. & Hollander, E. (2006). Is obsessive-compulsive disorder an anxiety disorder? *Progress in Neuropsychopharmacology and Biological Psychiatry, 30*(3), 338–352.

Bejerot, S., & Mortberg, E. (2009). Do autistic traits play a role in the bullying of obsessive-compulsive disorder and social phobia sufferers? *Psychopathology, 42*(3), 170–176.

Ben-Shachar, S., Lanpher, B., German, J. R., Qasaymeh, M., Potocki, L., Nagamani, S. C., et al. (2009). Microdeletion 15q13.3: A locus with incomplete penetrance for autism, mental retardation, and psychiatric disorders. *Journal of Medical Genetics, 46*(6), 382–388.

Billstedt, E., Gillberg, I. C., & Gillberg, C. (2007). Autism in adults: Symptom patterns and early childhood predictors; Use of the DISCO in a community sample followed from childhood, *Journal of Child Psychology and Psychiatry, 48*(11), 1102–1110.

Bradley, S. J. (2000). *Affect regulation and the development of psychopathology*. New York: Guilford.

Brian, J., Bryson, S. E., Garon, N., Roberts, W., Smith, I. M., Szatmari, P., et al. (2008). Clinical assessment of autism in high-risk 18-month-olds. *Autism, 12*(5), 433–456.

Chiu, P. H., Kayali, M. A., Kishida, K. T., Tomlin, D., Klinger, L. G., Klinger, M. R., et al. (2008). Self responses along cingulate cortex reveal quantitative neural phenotype for high-functioning autism. *Neuron*, 57(3), 463–473.

Craddock, N., O'Donovan, M. C., & Owen, M. J. (2009). Psychosis genetics: Modeling the relationship between schizophrenia, bipolar disorder, and mixed (or "schizoaffective") psychoses. *Schizophrenia Bulletin, 35* (3), 482–490.

DeGeus, E. J. C., & Boomsma, D. I. (2001). A genetic neuroscience approach to human cognition. *European Psychologist, 6*, 241–253.

de Jonge, M., Kemner, C., Naber, F., & van Engeland, H. (2009). Block design reconstruction skills: Not a good candidate for an endophenotypic marker in autism research. *European Child and Adolescent Psychiatry, 18*(4), 197–205.

Delong, R. (2007). GABA(A) receptor alpha5 subunit as a candidate gene for autism and bipolar disorder: A proposed endophenotype with parent-of-origin and gain-of-function features, with or without oculocutaneous albinism. *Autism, 11*(2), 135–147.

Delorme, R., Gousse, V., Roy, I., Trandafir, A., Mathieu, F., Mouren-Simeoni, M., et al. (2007). Shared executive dysfunctions in unaffected relatives of patients with autism and obsessive-compulsive disorder. *European Psychiatry, 22*(1), 32–38.

Duvall, J. A., Lu, A., Cantor, R. M., Todd, R. D., Constantino, J. N., Geschwind, D. H. (2007). A quantitative trait locus analysis of social responsiveness in multiplex autism families. *American Journal of Psychiatry, 164*(4), 656–662.

Eaves, L. C., & Ho, H. H. (2008). Young adult outcome of autism spectrum disorders. *Journal of Autism and Developmental Disorders, 38*(4), 739–747.

Fair, D. A., Dosenbach, N. U. F., Church, J. A., Cohen, A. L., Brahmbhatt, S., Miezin, F. M., et al. (2007). Development of distinct control networks through segregation and integration. *Proceedings of the National Academy of Sciences of the United States of America, 104*(33), 13507–13512.

Geschwind, D. H. (2009). Advances in autism. *Annual Review of Medicine, 60*, 367–380.

Geurts, H. M., Grasman, R. P., Verté, S., Oosterlaan, J., Roeyers, H., van Kammen, S. M., et al. (2008). Intra-individual variability in ADHD, autism spectrum disorders and Tourette's syndrome. *Neuropsychologia, 46*(13), 3030–3041.

Ghaziuddin, M., & Zafar, S. (2008). Psychiatric comorbidity of adults with autism spectrum disorders. *Clinical Neuropsychiatry: Journal of Treatment Evaluation, 5*(1), 9–12.

Golubchik, P., & Weizman, A. (2008). The role of neurosteroids in development of pediatric psychopathology. In M. S. Ritsner & A. Weizman (Eds.), *Neuroactive steroids in brain function, behavior and neuropsychiatric disorders: Novel strategies for research and treatment* (pp. 539–553). New York: Springer Science.

Gottesman, I. I. & Gould, T. D. (2003). The endophenotype concept in psychiatry: Etymology and strategic intentions. *American Journal of Psychiatry, 160*(4), 636–645.

Hofvander, B., Delorme, R., Chaste, P., Nyden, A., Wentz, E., Stahlberg, O., et al. (2009). Psychiatric and psychosocial problems in adults with normal-intelligence autism spectrum disorders. *BMC Psychiatry, 9*, 35.

Hollander, E., Anagnostou, E., Chaplin, W., Esposito, K., Haznedar, M. M., Licalzi, E., et al. (2005). Striatal volume on magnetic resonance imaging and repetitive behaviors in autism. *Biological Psychiatry, 58*(3), 226–232.

Hollander, E., King, A., Delaney, K., Smith, C. J., & Silverman, J. M. (2003). Obsessive-compulsive behaviors in parents of multiplex autism families. *Psychiatry Research, 117*(1), 11–16.

Hranilovic, D., Bujas-Petkovic, Z., Vragovic, R., Vuk, T., Hock, K., & Jernej, B. (2007). Hyperserotonemia in adults with autistic disorder. *Journal of Autism and Developmental Disorders, 37*(10), 1934–1940.

James, S. J., Melnyk, S., Jernigan, S., Cleves, M. A., Halsted, C. H., Wong, D. H., et al. (2006). Metabolic endophenotype and related genotypes are associated with oxidative stress in children with autism. *American Journal of Medical Genetics. Part B, Neuropsychiatric Genetics, 141B*(8), 947–956.

Just, M. A., Cherkassky, V. L., Keller, T. A., Kana, R. K., &Minshew, N. J. (2007). Functional and anatomical cortical underconnectivity in autism: Evidence from an FMRI study of an executive function task and corpus callosum morphometry. *Cerebral Cortex, 17*(4), 951–961.

Kano, Y., Ohta, M., Nagai, Y., Pauls, D. L., & Leckman, J. F. (2004). Obsessive-compulsive symptoms in parents of Tourette syndrome probands and autism spectrum disorder probands. *Psychiatry and Clinical Neurosciences, 58*(4), 348–352.

Kim, J. H. A., Szatmari, P., Bryson, S. E., Streiner, D. L., & Wilson, F. J. (2000). The prevalence of anxiety and mood problems among children with autism and Asperger syndrome. *Autism, 4*(2), 117–132.

Leckman, J. F., & Kim, Y.-S. (2006). A primary candidate gene for obsessive-compulsive disorder. *Archives of General Psychiatry, 63*(7), 717–720.

Levallois, S., Beraud, J., & Jalenques, I. (2007). Les patients souffrant d'une maladie du spectre autistique presentent-ils des stereotypies ou des troubles obsessionnels compulsifs (TOCs)? [Are repetitive behaviors of patients with autistic disorders, stereotypies or obsessive-compulsive disorders?]. *Annales Medico-Psychologiques, 165*(2), 117–121.

Leyfer, O. T., Folstein, S. E., Bacalman, S., Davis, N. O., Dinh, E., Morgan, J., et al. (2006). Comorbid psychiatric disorders in children with Autism: Interview development and rates of disorders. *Journal of Autism and Developmental Disorders, 36*(7), 849–861.

Lord, C., Risi, S., DiLavore, P. S., Shulman, C., Thurm, A., & Pickles, A. (2006). Autism from 2 to 9 years of age. *Archives of General Psychiatry, 63*, 694–701.

Loveland, K. A. (2001). Toward an ecological theory of Autism. In J. A. Burack, T. Charman, N. Yirmiya, & P. R. Zelazo (Eds.), *The development of autism: Perspectives from theory and research*. New Jersey: Erlbaum Press.

Loveland, K. (2005). Social-emotional impairment and self-regulation in Autism spectrum disorders. In J. Nadel and D. Muir (Eds.), *Emotional development: Recent research advances* (pp. 365–382). New York: Oxford University Press.

Mazefsky, C. A., Folstein, S. E., & Lainhart, J. E. (2008). Overrepresentation of mood and anxiety disorders in adults with autism and their first-degree relatives: What does it mean? *Autism Research*, 1(3), 193–197.

McDougle, C. J., Epperson, C. N., Price, L. H. & Gelernter, J. (1998). Evidence for linkage disequilibrium between serotonin transporter protein gene (SLC6A4) and obsessive compulsive disorder. *Molecular Psychiatry*, *3*(3), 270–273.

Melville, C. A., Cooper, S., Morrison, J., Smiley, E., Allan, L., Jackson, A., et al. (2008). The prevalence and incidence of mental ill-health in adults with autism and intellectual disabilities. *Journal of Autism and Developmental Disorders*, *38*(9), 1676–1688.

Nylander, L., Lugnegard, T., & Hallerback, M. U. (2008). Autism spectrum disorders and schizophrenia spectrum disorders in adults: Is there a connection? A literature review and some suggestions for future clinical research. *Clinical Neuropsychiatry: Journal of Treatment Evaluation*, *5*(1), 43–54.

O'Donovan, M. C., Craddock, N. J., & Owen, M. J. (2009). Genetics of psychosis: Insights from views across the genome. *Human Genetics*, *126* (1), 3–12.

Pearson, D. A., Loveland, K. A., Lachar, D., Lane, D. M., Reddoch, S. L., Mansour, R., & Cleveland, L. A. (2006). A comparison of behavioral and emotional functioning in children and adolescents with Autistic Disorder and PDD-NOS. *Child Neuropsychology*, *12*(4–5), 321–333.

Rommelse, N. N., Altink, M. E., Fliers, E. A., Martin, N. C., Buschgens, C. J., Hartman, C. A., et al. (2009). Comorbid problems in ADHD: Degree of association, shared endophenotypes, and formation of distinct subtypes; Implications for a future DSM. *Journal of Abnormal Child Psychology*, *37*(6), 793–804.

Ronald, A., Happé, F., & Plomin, R. (2005). The genetic relationship between individual differences in social and nonsocial behaviours characteristic of autism. *Developmental Science*, *8*(5), 444–458.

Rossi, L. (2006). Obsessive-compulsive disorder and related conditions. *Psychiatric Annals*, *36*(7), 514–517.

Rubin, K. H., & Mills, R. S. (1991). Conceptualizing developmental pathways to internalizing disorders in childhood. *Canadian Journal of Behavioural Science/Revue Canadienne des Sciences du Comportement*, *23*(3), 300–317.

Rump, K., Giovannelli, J. L., Minshew, N. J., & Strauss, M. S. (2009). The development of emotion recognition in individuals with autism. *Child Development*, *80*(5), 1434–1447.

Russell, A. J., Mataix-Cols, D., Anson, M., & Murphy, D. G. M. (2005). Obsessions and compulsions in Asperger syndrome and high-functioning autism. *British Journal of Psychiatry*, *186*(6), 525–528.

Russell, E., & Sofronoff, K. (2005). Anxiety and social worries in children with Asperger syndrome. *Australian and New Zealand Journal of Psychiatry*, *39*(7), 633–638.

Ryden, E., & Bejerot, S. (2008). Autism spectrum disorders in an adult psychiatric population: A naturalistic cross-sectional controlled study. *Clinical Neuropsychiatry: Journal of Treatment Evaluation*, *5*(1), 13–21.

Sacco, R., Papaleo, V., Hager, J., Rousseau, F., Moessner, R., Militerni, R., et al. (2007). Case-control and family-based association studies of candidate genes in autistic disorder and its endophenotypes: TPH2 and GLO1. *BMC Medical Genetics*, *8*, 11.

Sakurai, T., Ramoz, N., Reichert, J. G., Corwin, T. E., Kryzak, L., Smith, C. J., et al. (2006). Association analysis of the NrCAM gene in autism and in subsets of families with severe obsessive-compulsive or self-stimulatory behaviors. *Psychiatric Genetics*, *16*(6), 251–257.

Scahill, L., McDougle, C. J., Williams, S. K., Dimitropoulos, A., Aman, M. G., McCracken, J. T., et al. (2006). Children's Yale-Brown Obsessive Compulsive Scale Modified for Pervasive Developmental Disorders. *Journal of the American Academy of Child and Adolescent Psychiatry*, *45*(9), 1114–1123.

Schore, A. N. (1996). The experience-dependent maturation of a regulatory system in the orbital prefrontal cortex and the origin of developmental psychopathology. *Development and Psychopathology*, *8*, 59–87.

Schore, A. N. (1997). Early organization of the nonlinear right brain and development of a predisposition to psychiatric disorders. *Development and Psychopathology*, *9*(4), 595–631.

Spence, S. J., Cantor, R. M., Chung, L., Kim, S., Geschwind, D. H., & Alarcón, M. (2006). Stratification based on language-related endophenotypes in autism: attempt to replicate reported linkage. *American Journal of Medical Genetics. Part B, Neuropsychiatric Genetics*, *141B*(6), 591–598.

Tabarés-Seisdedos, R., & Rubenstein, J. L. (2009). Chromosome 8p as a potential hub for developmental neuropsychiatric disorders: Implications for schizophrenia, autism and cancer. *Molecular Psychiatry*, *14*(6), 563–589.

Tani, P., Lindberg, N., Appelberg, B., Nieminen-Von Wendt, T., von Wendt, L., & Porkka-Heiskanen, T. (2006). Childhood inattention and hyperactivity symptoms self-reported by adults with Asperger syndrome. *Psychopathology*, *39*(1), 49–54.

Taylor, E. (2009). Managing bipolar disorders in children and adolescents. *Nature Reviews Neurology*, *5*(9), 484–491.

Thakkar, K. N., Polli, F. E., Joseph, R. M., Tuch, D. S., Hadjikhani, N., Barton, J. J. S., et al. (2008). Response monitoring, repetitive behaviour and anterior cingulate abnormalities in autism spectrum disorders (ASD). *Brain*, *131*(9), 2464–2478.

Toichi, M. (2006). Obsessive and compulsive traits in pervasive developmental disorder [in Japanese]. *Japanese Journal of Child and Adolescent Psychiatry*, *47*(2), 127–134.

Towgood, K. J., Meuwese, J. D. I., Gilbert, S. J., Turner, M. S., & Burgess, P. W. (2009). Advantages of the multiple case series approach to the study of cognitive deficits in autism spectrum disorder. *Neuropsychologia*, *47*(13), 2981–2988.

Viding, E., & Blakemore, S. (2007). Endophenotype approach to developmental psychopathology: Implications for autism research. *Behavioral Genetics*, *37*, 51–60.

Wang, L., Mottron, L., Peng, D., Berthiaume, C., & Dawson, M. (2007). Local bias and local-to-global interference without global deficit: A robust finding in autism under various conditions of attention, exposure time, and visual angle. *Cognitive Neuropsychology*, *24*(5), 550–574.

Wendland, J. R., DeGuzman, T. B., McMahon, F., Rudnick, G., Detera-Wadleigh, S. D., & Murphy, D. L. (2008). SERT Ileu425Val in autism, Asperger syndrome and obsessive-compulsive disorder. *Psychiatric Genetics*, *18*(1), 31–39.

Section III

Psychiatric and Medical Comorbidities

15 Elisabeth M. Dykens, Miriam Lense

Intellectual Disabilities and Autism Spectrum Disorder: A Cautionary Note

Points of Interest

- Approximately two thirds of children with autism spectrum disorders have co-occurring intellectual disabilities, and autism is also associated with several genetic syndromes that involve intellectual disabilities.
- Persons with intellectual disabilities, including those with specific genetic etiologies, are underrepresented in autism research, often due to specific exclusionary criteria.
- Research findings from studies of individuals with autism and high IQ may not necessarily extend to lower functioning individuals with autism spectrum disorders.
- Researchers must more explicitly justify their reasoning for excluding individuals with low IQ from their research programs.
- Many research designs could be adapted to also include people with intellectual disabilities, as exemplified in phenotypic studies of persons with genetic syndromes with or without intellectual disabilities.
- Individuals with autism and low IQ or with specific genetic syndromes need to be included in research to further our understanding of the causes and mechanisms associated with autism.

This chapter presents a cautionary tale about the impact of the broader definition of autism on how investigators are conducting their research. Diagnostically, the autism spectrum has expanded to include milder types of autism that are not necessarily associated with intellectual disabilities. At the same time, the inclusionary criteria for autism studies have narrowed to primarily include persons with high IQs, to the exclusion of those with autism and low IQs or with co-occurring syndromes or neurological disorders.

In considering this broader diagnostic scope and more narrow focus on higher IQ individuals, it is important to note that intellectual disabilities (previously termed mental retardation) have long been associated with autism spectrum disorders. The DSM-IV-TR (APA, 2000) notes that up to 75% of children with ASD have co-occurring intellectual disabilities, but for many reasons, this estimate may no longer be accurate. This chapter provides a brief review of the prevalence of intellectual disabilities in ASD, and although not exhaustive, the review highlights the co-occurrence of ASD and intellectual disabilities, and factors that complicate these prevalence studies.

Beyond intellectual disabilities per se, autism is also associated with specific genetic etiologies, and many of these syndromes also involve intellectual disabilities. A growing body of literature now describes how autism spectrum disorder (ASD) is manifest in people with such diagnoses as tuberous sclerosis, Fragile X, Prader-Willi, Angelman, and other syndromes. Syndromes that involve both ASD and intellectual disabilities provide unique windows into genetic and neurobiological factors associated with autism (Dykens, Sutcliffe, & Levitt, 2004). Even so, having a known etiology is typically an exclusionary criterion for most autism studies.

Indeed, despite the robust associations between intellectual disabilities and ASD, persons with low IQ or with genetic syndromes are increasingly excluded from research in ASD. We provide data in support of this disquieting research trend, as reflected in a review we conducted of published, peer-reviewed studies. Why are children or adults with ASD and intellectual disabilities, with or without a co-occurring genetic syndrome, increasingly excluded from published ASD research?

Decades ago, studies in autism relied primarily on those with intellectual disabilities, as this reflected the conceptual framework of autism at that time. The pendulum now appears to have swung in the opposite direction, whereby persons with intellectual disabilities are routinely excluded from study protocols. The chapter discusses several possible reasons for this trend, including arguments both for and against including those with low IQs in autism research. The chapter concludes with recommendations that facilitate the inclusion of those with intellectual disabilities into future research in ASD.

Prevalence of Intellectual Disabilities in ASD

Intellectual disabilities affects from 1.5% to 3% of the population, and although the term "mental retardation" was previously used in the United States, a name change to "intellectual disabilities" occurred across the major disability research and service organizations approximately 3 years ago. Beyond a change in terms, there is general agreement across several diagnostic systems that intellectual disabilities consist of: (1) an IQ score of 70 or less as determined on standardized testing; (2) co-occurring deficits in adaptive functioning (in 3 or more areas); and (3) an onset that begins in the developmental years, before age 18 (APA, 2000).

Beyond these general similarities, the major diagnostic schemas differ somewhat in their approaches. The DSM-IV-TR and ICD-10 require standardized IQ and adaptive behavior testing in order to classify persons into traditional levels of delay (mild, moderate, severe, profound). The American Association of Intellectual and Developmental Disabilities (AAIDD) rejects these classifications, as they suggest inherent deficits within people. Instead, the AAIDD adopts an approach based on the intensity of environmental supports that people need to function their best (Luckasson et al., 2002). While there is considerable merit to this perspective, the AAIDD system has not been widely adopted, and the majority of researchers continue to use traditional diagnostic systems.

Given such definitions of intellectual disabilities, how often do intellectual disabilities occur in ASDs? Based on findings to date, no one knows for certain, and estimates vary widely. Table 15-1 summarizes selected prevalence studies on ASD that included IQ data. These epidemiological studies were international in scope, based in the UK, United States, China, Australia, Japan, Portugal, Finland, and Iceland.

As Table 15-1 reveals, the prevalence estimates of intellectual disabilities in ASD range from a low of 34% to a high of 84%, with a median of 65% across the 14 studies. This estimate of intellectual disabilities in ASD is lower than the 75% noted in DSM-IV-TR, but remains impressively high. Indeed, based on these studies, the majority of children with ASD have co-occurring intellectual disabilities.

Even so, several caveats are in order, as the same challenges for epidemiological studies of ASD in general hold true for studies that report intellectual disabilities as a co-occurring or secondary condition of ASD. These methodological concerns include: variable sample sizes and age ranges of participants across studies, with low sample sizes having less reliable estimates; and different diagnostic criteria for ASD across studies and over time.

Diagnostic criteria for autism ranges from rating scales or checklists, typically seen in earlier work, to more rigorous and contemporary diagnoses based on DSM or ICD criteria, or such diagnostic interviews as the ADOS and ADI-R. Comparing rates over time is also complicated by the broadening of the autism diagnostic criteria to include milder forms of ASD, as reflected in the DSM-IV-TR (APA, 2000). An additional source of variance relates to different methods used to identify mental retardation or intellectual disabilities across studies. For these reasons, Table 15-1 only includes studies that: were published after 2000; used well-accepted diagnostic criteria for autism; and included participants' IQ scores as opposed to their levels of delay (e.g., mild intellectual disabilities).

IQ levels do, however, differ substantially across diagnoses included under the umbrella of autism spectrum disorders. By definition, those with Asperger's disorder do not have clinically significant delays in language or cognitive development, but share the qualitative impairments in social interaction and restricted stereotypes or repetitive interests and activities that characterize autism in general. In pervasive developmental disorder not-otherwise-specified (PDD-NOS), intellectual disabilities may or may not be present, as this term is used to describe children with social impairments along with the presence of either restricted interests or impairment in cognitive or communicative skills. PDD-NOS is often a default diagnosis used to describe children who have mild or absent symptoms in one of the three core domains of autism. Children with autistic disorder have impairments in all three core domains of autism, and are more likely to have co-occurring intellectual disabilities. Even so, the term "high-functioning autism" is often used to describe persons with relatively high IQs, or those in the average range or higher.

Table 15–1.
ASD prevalence studies from 2000 to 2008 that included DSM-IV or ICD-10 ASD diagnostic criteria and IQ data

Lead Author	Dx Criteria	Study N	N with ASD	% ASD with ID
Baird et al., 2000	ICD-10	16,235	50	40%
Baird et al., 2006	ICD-10	56,946	81	53%
Bertrand, 2001	DSM-IV	8,896	36	63%
Chakrabarti & Fombonne, 2001	ICD-10, DSM-IV	15,500	26	71%
Chakrabarti & Fombonne, 2005	ICD-10, DSM-IV	10,903	24	67%
Fombonne, 2001	DSM-IV, ICD-10	10,438	27	44%
Honda, 2005	ICD-10	32,791	123	75%
Icasiano, 2004	DSM-IV	54,000	177	47%
Kawamura, 2008	DSM-IV	12,589	288	34%
Kielinen et al., 2000	ICD-10	152,732	187	50%
Magnússon et al., 2001	ICD-10	43,153	57	84%
Oliveira, 2007	DSM-IV	67,795	115	83%
Wong, 2008	DSM-IV	4,247,206	682	70%
Yeargin-Allsopp, 2003	DSM-IV	289,456	987	68%

Note: ID = Intellectual disabilities (formerly mental retardation).

Examining subtypes of ASD, Witwer and Lecavalier (2008) reviewed 22 studies that compared clinical differences between two of more groups of children with reliably-established diagnoses of autism, Asperger's disorder, or PDD-NOS. For studies in this review that reported IQ scores, we calculated the mean IQ for each subtype of ASD. As expected, the average IQ of persons with Asperger's disorder was 103.1, based on 12 studies that included a group with this disorder. Eleven studies in the Witwer and LeCavalier (2008) review included a group with PDD-NOS, and their average IQ was 86.1. Surprisingly, however, the average IQ of children with autistic disorder was 82.3, with just two of the 13 studies that included a group with autism reporting an average IQ of less than 70. Many of the studies stipulated low IQ as an exclusionary criteria, and we return to this trend later in the chapter.

Genetic Syndromes Associated with ASD and Intellectual Disabilities

A second, related issue concerns genetic syndromes. Recent estimates suggest that approximately 10% or less of the population of persons with ASD have a known co-occurring genetic syndrome (Herman et al., 2007; Muhle, Trentascoste, & Rapin, 2004; see also the chapters by State, Lamb, and Geschwind in this book). So called "syndromic autism" varies in prevalence and core autism features across different syndromes, but collectively are not believed to represent a major proportion of the population of persons with ASD. Table 15-2 summarizes the estimated occurrence rates of ASD in selected genetic syndromes. While this review is not exhaustive, it aptly demonstrates that autism is reasonably prevalent in certain genetic syndromes.

Table 15–2.
Selected genetic intellectual disability syndromes associated with ASD

Lead Author	Syndrome	% Estimate ASD
Chahrour, 2007	Rett, MCEP2 mutations	80–100%
Cook, 2001	15q11-q13 duplications	80–100%
Moss, 2008	Cornelia de Lange syndrome	62%
Peters, 2004	Angelman syndrome	42% (primarily class I deletions)
Rogers, 2001	Fragile X syndrome	30%
Sikora, 2006	Smith-Lemi-Opitz	75%
Smalley, 1998	Tuberous sclerosis	25%
Veltman, 2005	Prader-Willi syndrome	25% (38% UPD; 18% deletions)
Vorstman, 2006	22q11.2 deletion (VCFS)	50%

Note: UPD = uniparental disomy; VCFS = Velocardiofacial syndrome.

Given the heterogeneity of ASD, these genetic syndromes provide important perspectives that can fast-track candidate gene discoveries in ASD (see Muhle et al., 2004 for a thoughtful review). Examining two syndromes with high rates of co-occurring ASD, for example, Nishimura et al. (2007) identified several common genes that were dysregulated in subjects with autism and Fragile X syndrome, and autism due to 15q11-q13 duplications. Beyond their promising findings of shared molecular pathways in ASD, this study demonstrates the utility of syndromic-based research in autism.

Our purpose here is not to justify the scientific merit of examining "syndromic autism," but to highlight a research practice that may not serve the field well. On the one hand, for researchers who examine behavior in people with syndromes, the syndrome is the focus of study, and phenotypic studies may or may not include assessments of ASD along with other syndrome characteristics. Thus, one might assess autism in Prader-Willi syndrome (Veltman et al., 2005), along with other salient characteristics of this syndrome such as hyperphagia (Dykens et al., 2007), jigsaw puzzle skills (Verdine et al., 2008), or associations between the behavioral phenotype and genetic subtypes and age (Dykens et al., 2008). Phenotypic studies are not rooted in the autism field, but will include ASD assessments to the extent needed to accurately depict the syndrome's phenotypic expression.

In contrast, researchers rooted in the autism field, who focus exclusively on ASD, generally exclude participants with known etiologies or intellectual disabilities. Instead, these researchers examine individuals with what some refer to as "pure autism," or idiopathic, primary, or nonsyndromic autism. While these studies are essential, such syndromic versus nonsyndromic research practices have led to a growing separation of research and disability communities. Such separation is reflected in different professional conferences and journals that cater to each of these groups, as well as in separate, national efforts to develop ASD versus syndrome-based databanks, biobanks, or patient registries. Thus, persons with Fragile X, Down, Prader-Willi, or other syndromes are either excluded from or not well represented in databases connected to the Autism Treatment Network or Simons Simplex or Sibling Studies. Though the Autism Genetic Resource Exchange (AGRE) includes representative proportions of individuals with genetic syndromes and autism, the overall numbers of these individuals are too low for meaningful analyses.

At the same time, many syndrome-specific advocacy or parent groups are now developing their own data repositories, biobanks, or research registries. On the one hand, this separation seems logical, as not all parents or researchers who study syndromes need be concerned with autism, especially in syndromes where autism is relatively infrequent. But to the extent that persons with genetic syndromes also have ASD or brush up against issues related to ASD, then sharing data, registries, and resources would accelerate the pace of discoveries and of more effective treatments for persons with (or without) syndromic autism.

A Year in the Life of an Autism Journal

What are the current practices regarding intellectual disabilities for researchers who publish studies pertaining to ASD? Are the IQs of participants routinely reported? How many studies include or exclude those with low IQs? To address these questions, we selected a long-standing and highly regarded autism journal, the *Journal of Autism and Developmental Disorders* (*JADD*), and reviewed all studies published in 2008. Although not an exhaustive review of ASD work, we reasoned that studies published in 2008 would likely be representative of other recent years, and that a leading journal in autism would pull for quality submissions that included such methodological details as IQ scores. For the journal review we identified how IQ was reported (as an average, range, or not at all) in child versus adult participants, and when possible, we tallied or extracted mean IQ scores from each study.

As shown in Table 15-3, the vast majority of publications for both children and adults with ASD included participants with high IQs. Regarding children, 60 studies used either high IQ *or* low IQ children, with 77% of articles including children with high IQs only. Typically these studies had a required IQ score of greater than 75, 80, or 90 as an inclusionary criterion. In contrast, 23% of articles included children with low IQs only. Examining the actual numbers of participants enrolled in these 60 articles, 83% of research subjects had high IQs, and 17% low IQs.

Some studies of children with ASD included those with both low *and* high IQs: 19 studies included children with IQs less than 70 along with children with higher IQs. Of the 16 studies using low and high IQ children that reported actual IQ data, 10 reported a mean IQ greater than 70, and the mean IQ across these 10 studies was 77.80. Six studies reported mean IQs less than 70, with an overall average IQ of 66. Thus, while these 16 studies included some low IQ participants, on average most had IQs greater than 70, suggesting that the majority of participants were relatively high functioning.

Our review of 2008 *JADD* articles also indicates that adults are less often studied than children, and that the vast majority of adult studies only include high-functioning individuals. Of the 30 studies on adults with ASD, just 3 included persons with low IQs, and 27 with high IQs—the average IQ of these adults was 106.4. Thus, 9 times as many studies were published on high IQ adults than low IQ adults with ASD.

Examining the actual numbers of adult participants, 73% had high IQs, and surprisingly, the three studies of lower IQ adults represented over one quarter (27%) of adult subjects. This relatively high percentage is due to the fact that 2 of the 3 studies were based in large institutions for persons with intellectual disabilities. While such settings offer increased numbers of participants, they may not be representative of persons with ASD growing into adulthood today.

A final observation stemming from our 2008 *JADD* review is that the majority of studies (70%) included IQ data of some sort. Of the 47 articles that did not do so, 28% were parent surveys; 21% were case studies or single-subject interventions that may or may not have included formal developmental testing; 19% were genetic, medical, or physiological studies; 17% used large-scale or population-based datasets; and 15% sampled teachers or educators about their students with ASD. While there is room for improvement, the majority of articles that focused on children or adults with ASD included some index of intellectual functioning.

In summary, this "year in the life of an autism journal" confirms that published studies in ASD primarily include children and adults with relatively high IQs. While one could argue that 2008 may not be representative, there are no glaring or obvious cohort differences to suggest that 2008 differs dramatically from 2007 or 2009. As well, relative to other journals focused on autism, there is no reason to suspect that *JADD* is more or less likely to pull for submissions on high versus low functioning autism.

Table 15–3.
Data on low versus high IQ in children and adults with ASD as published in the 2008 volume of *JADD*

	Number of Studies	Number of Participants	Mean IQ, other IQ data
Low-IQ Children	14	380	*M* IQ = 58.21 (based on 9 studies) 2 studies noted "profound or severe" ID 3 studies stipulated IQ < 70
High-IQ Children	46	1,861	*M* IQ = 102.10 (based on 35 studies) 6 studies stipulated IQ > 70 or 75 4 studies stipulated IQ > 80 or 90 1 study noted IQ range (85–115)
Low- & High-IQ Children	19	690	*M* IQ = 72.73 (based on 16 studies) 2 studies noted IQ range (53–124; 52–85) 1 study noted % no ID, mild, moderate, severe ID
Low-IQ Adults	3	210	% noted for mild, moderate, severe, profound ID
High-IQ Adults	27	572	*M* IQ = 106.4 (based on 22 studies) 4 studies stipulated IQ > 70, 80, or 90 1 study noted IQ range (73 to 129)

Based on studies summarized in Table 15-1, approximately 65% of persons with ASD also have an intellectual disability. Yet our journal review suggests that only 10% to 23% of published articles are focused on persons with ASD and intellectual disabilities. In contrast, from 77% to 90% of studies we sampled in 2008 were restricted to persons with high IQs. Assuming that studies on all persons on the autism spectrum are critically important steps toward discovery, why are those with lower IQs not well represented in today's research landscape?

Reasons for Excluding Those with Intellectual Disabilities from ASD Research

Researchers present several explanations about why those with intellectual disabilities are often excluded from contemporary autism work. Some suggest that with the broadening of the autism diagnostic criteria, the field is now "catching up" or balancing out work based on a previous conceptual model of autism that primarily included lower functioning individuals. If this is indeed the case, we would expect to see an eventual shift toward a middle ground, with approximately equal numbers of studies that focus on low or high IQ participants, or that include a wider range of IQ in the same study.

A common explanation for excluding those with intellectual disabilities is that the demands of a particular research task or protocol are too difficult for those with low IQ. Tasks that require, for example, a high cognitive load, higher-order or abstract reasoning, or insight into one's thoughts or emotions are all better suited for those with higher IQs. In addition, some methodologies, such as functional neuroimaging, require that participants comply, remain still, and respond to various button presses or stimuli while in the scanner, and these are more challenging for those with lower IQs. By virtue of their better-developed cognitive and communicative skills, higher-functioning persons with ASD have provided novel insights into the phenomenology of ASD, as well as on neural functioning and basic mechanisms associated with the wider autism spectrum.

Even so, generations of biobehavioral scientists have specialized in the field of intellectual disabilities, and used a variety of methodologies that assess cognitive, neural, social, emotional, and adaptive functioning. Further, functional and structural neuroimaging studies have now been conducted in persons with intellectual disabilities and with Fragile X, Prader-Willi, Williams, and other syndromes. Techniques to enhance valid imaging data from persons with intellectual disabilities include behavioral interventions to decrease movement in the scanner and increase compliance, the use of mock scanners, and new methods of acquiring imaging data. These approaches hold much promise for imaging work in persons with intellectual disabilities and ASD.

Some experimental tasks can also be adapted to those with low IQ, while other experimental tasks can simply be used "as is" in persons with intellectual disabilities. Examples of specific methodologies or tasks gleaned from the 2008 *JADD* review that were limited to high-functioning persons but could easily be used across the IQ spectrum include: wearing actigraphy watches; playing cards with a peer; deciding if a speaker was male or female; taking a hearing test; providing saliva samples for cortisol assays; and identifying moods on feeling thermometers. The inclusion of those with low IQs may not necessarily be methodologically challenging for these or other ASD studies.

A second issue, however, is that some researchers are understandably striving to recruit a homogeneous sample of high-functioning persons with ASD. Presumably, their hypotheses and research questions demand that they focus exclusively on this high-IQ subgroup. Surprisingly few investigators, however, specify why their questions pertain only to high-functioning individuals, nor do their publications necessarily explain the scientific rationale for excluding those with lower IQs. Without a well-articulated rationale for using IQ cutoffs, excluding those with intellectual disabilities seems arbitrary; over the long term, this practice may not reflect well on the broader ASD field.

A third point is that because autism is a spectrum disorder, some investigators assume that findings from high IQ individuals will automatically apply to those with lower IQs. By definition, findings from ASD in its more "pure" form must apply to those with ASD and intellectual disabilities. Given the heterogeneity of ASDs, however, it seems shaky at best to assume that processes in high IQ individuals will simply extend to those with ASD and intellectual disabilities. Actually, this is an empirical question, and data are needed from both low- and high-IQ persons with ASD to determine if findings from individuals with high IQ are applicable to those with intellectual disabilities. Of concern, however, is that most researchers do not seem to be tackling this question, and are increasingly shying away from studies that include individuals with both low and high IQ.

Ideas for ASD Research That Includes Intellectual Disabilities

Table 15-1 suggests that approximately 65% or more of persons with ASD also have an intellectual disability, yet these individuals are not well represented in national ASD research networks, data repositories, or in published articles on ASD. Although far from comprehensive, our journal review suggests that a minority of published articles (from 10% to 23%) focus on persons with ASD and intellectual disabilities. A further concern applies to IQ across autism spectrum diagnoses. Calculating means IQs from Witwer and Lecavalier's (2008) review of ASD diagnoses, we found the expected high IQ in those with Asperger's disorder (M = 103.1), a lower IQ in those with PDD-NOS (M = 86.1), and a surprisingly high average IQ in participants with autistic disorder (M = 82.3). Although autistic disorder often includes those with intellectual disabilities, the reliably diagnosed participants in this review were relatively high functioning. Although further work is needed to explore these trends, it appears that those with lower IQs are not well represented in published research. As this imbalance may impede new insights into ASD, how can we increase the inclusion of those with intellectual disabilities into current ASD research?

A first step is for investigators to ask if their study hypotheses only apply to those with ASD and high IQs. Do investigators know for certain that their data will be compromised by adding those with intellectual disabilities to their study? Or are preliminary data needed on how those with low IQs might perform on a given task in order to make an informed decision about IQ inclusionary criteria and data integrity?

Perhaps intellectual disabilities should be a human subject characteristic that investigators are required to address in IRB and grant applications. Just as investigators must specify their rationale for the inclusion or exclusion of children, women, and ethnic/minority participants, maybe they should also specify the scientific rationale for excluding those with low IQs. Although this idea is not likely to be formally adopted, being asked to justify the exclusion of those with intellectual disabilities could sharpen investigators thinking about the role of IQ in their design.

Assuming that study hypotheses could be extended to those with low IQs, a second step is for investigators to think creatively about their methodology. How could tasks or experimental manipulations be adapted in order to glean meaningful data from participants with ASD and intellectual disabilities? Are extra supports, costs, or accommodations needed in order to include those with intellectual disabilities? Specific ways of examining persons with a broad range of IQs may be extracted from research on the behavioral phenotypes of persons with genetic etiologies of intellectual disabilities. In this work, IQ is rarely used to truncate samples, and all persons with a given genetic syndrome are included in research, regardless of their IQ. IQ effects are assessed in phenotypic data, which then inform links between underlying molecular genetics of syndromes, neurological functioning, and behavioral phenotypes.

Recent recommendations for dimensional assessments of cognitive, linguistic, adaptive, and social functioning in ASDs (Volkmar, State, & Klin, 2009) are similar to approaches taken in most phenotypic studies, and hint at the idea of moving away from low IQ as an exclusionary criterion in ASD research. Instead, IQ could be cast as a continuous variable that informs the broad autism phenotype.

Conclusion

Intellectual disabilities remain a highly prevalent co-occurrence with ASD. Our review of recent, well-conducted ASD epidemiology studies suggests that approximately 65% of those with an ASD have intellectual disabilities. As well, certain genetic intellectual disability syndromes are characterized by relatively high rates of ASD. Even so, persons with ASD and intellectual disabilities or with specific genetic etiologies, are not well represented in today's ASD research landscape. The exclusion, or relatively poor representation, of those with low IQs or genetic syndromes is reflected in large-scale databases, biobanks, and participant registries, as well as in published, peer-reviewed articles. Our admittedly limited sampling of "a year in the life of an autism journal" revealed that only 23% of articles on children, and 10% on adults, included persons with intellectual disabilities. Examining the numbers of children enrolled in these studies, 83% were high functioning, and 17% had intellectual disabilities.

The current research practice of truncating IQ and focusing primarily on those with high IQs does not represent the full scope of autism as a spectrum disorder, limits generalizability of findings, and does not represent the majority of persons who have autism spectrum disorder. This chapter describes several ideas for increasing the representation of those with intellectual disabilities into future ASD research.

This chapter sounds a strong cautionary note about research practices. It does not aim to detract from the critical importance of studies of "pure" autism, or those with high IQs, idiopathic autism, or no known genetic etiology. These samples are essential for ongoing, multisite efforts aimed at candidate gene discovery, or linking ASD candidate genes to specific aspects of the ASD phenotype. Similarly, the cautionary note does not aim to promote research focused exclusively on those with low IQs or with syndromic autism. Rather, a more equitable or balanced inclusion of individuals with low and high IQs is essential for future discoveries about the etiologies, mechanisms, and treatments of ASD.

Future Directions and Challenges

- Researchers should aim to increase numbers of individuals with lower IQ or syndromic autism in autism research programs and large-scale databases and biobanks. Studies of individuals with differing types of syndromic autism may provide information on common genetic or molecular pathways.
- Instead of setting IQ cutpoints, researchers should examine IQ as a continuous variable that can affect other areas of the phenotype.
- If researchers choose to exclude individuals with intellectual disability or syndromic autism, they should provide rationalizations for why these exclusions are necessary for their research question and should address whether or not their findings would extend to the broader phenotype.
- Researchers will need to think creatively about how to adapt research paradigms (if necessary) to include lower functioning individuals, which may include specific supports, accommodations, or additional costs. Researchers in the field of autism can look to the field of behavioral phenotypes in genetic syndromes for how these adaptations have been put into practice to successfully include lower functioning individuals in research.

ACKNOWLEDGMENTS

This chapter was supported in part by NICHD Grants P30HD15052NICHD, and R01 R01HD135681. The authors thank Robert Hodapp for his helpful comments on an earlier draft of this manuscript.

REFERENCES

American Psychiatric Association. (2000). *Diagnostic and statistical manual of mental disorders* (4th ed., text rev.; DSM-IV-TR). Washington, DC: Author.

Baird, G., Charman, T., Baron-Cohen, S., Cox, A., Swettenham, J., Wheelwright, S., et al. (2000). A screening instrument for autism at 18 months of age: A six-year follow-up study. *Journal of the American Academy of Child and Adolescent Psychiatry, 389*, 694–702.

Bertrand, J., Mars, A., Boyle, C., Bove, F., Yeargin-Allsopp. M., & Decoufle, P. (2001). Prevalence of autism in a United States population: The Brick Township, New Jersey investigation. *Pediatrics, 108*, 1155–1161.

Chahrour, M., & Zoghbi, H. Y. (2007). The story of Rett syndrome: From clinic to neurobiology. *Neuron, 56*, 422–437.

Chakrabarti, S., & Fombonne, E. (2001). Pervasive developmental disorders in preschool children. *Journal of the American Medical Association, 285*, 3093–3099.

Chakrabarti, S., & Fombonne, E. (2005). Pervasive developmental disorders in preschool of children: Conformation of high prevalence. *American Journal of Psychiatry, 162*, 1133–1141.

Cook, E. H. (2001). Genetics of autism. *Child and Adolescent Clinics of North America, 10*, 33–350.

Dykens, E. M., Maxwell, M, Patino, E., Kossler, R., & Roof, E. (2007). Assessment of hyperphagia in Prader-Willi syndrome. *Obesity, 15*, 1816–1826.

Dykens, E. M., & Roof, E. (2008). Behavior in Prader-Willi syndrome: Relationship to genetic subtypes and age. *Journal of Child Psychology and Psychiatry, 49*, 1001–1008.

Dykens, E. M., Sutcliffe, J. S., & Levitt, P. (2004). Contrasting autism and 15q11-q13 disorders: Behavioral, genetic, and pathophysiological issues. *Mental Retardation and Developmental Disability Research Reviews, 10*, 284–291.

Fombonne, E., Simmons, H., Ford, T., Meltzer, H., & Goodman, R. (2001). Prevalence of pervasive developmental disorders in the British nationwide survey of child mental health. *Journal of the American Academy of Child and Adolescent Psychiatry, 40*, 820–827.

Herman, G. E., Henninger, N., Ratliff-Schaub, K., Pastore, M., Fitzgerald, S., & McBride, K. L. (2007). Genetic testing in autism: How much is enough? *Genetics in Medicine, 9*(5), 268–274.

Honda, H., Shimizu, Y., & Rutter, M. (2005). No effects of MMR withdrawal on the incidence of autism: A total population study. *Journal of Child Psychology and Psychiatry, 46*(6), 572–579.

Icasiano, F., Hewson, P., Macher, P., Cooper, C., & Marshall, A. (2004). Childhood autism spectrum disorder in the Barwon region: A community based study. *Journal of Paediatrics and Child Health, 40*, 696–701.

Kawamura, Y., Takahashi, O., & Ishii, T., (2008). Reevaluating the incidence of pervasive developmental disorders: Impact of elevated rates of detection through implementation of an integrated system of screening in Toyota, Japan. *Psychiatry and Clinical of Neurosciences, 62*, 152–159.

Kielinen, M., Linna, S. L., & Moilanen, I. (2000). Autism in Northern Finland. *European Child and Adolescent Psychiatry, 9*(3), 162–167.

Luckasson, R., Schclock, R. L., Spitalnik, D., Spreast, S., Tasse, M., Snell, M. E., et al. (2002). *Mental retardation: Definition, classification, and systems of supports.* Washington, DC: American Association on Intellectual and Developmental Disabilities.

Magnússon, P., & Saemundsen, E. (2001). Prevalence of autism in Iceland. *Journal of Autism and Developmental Disorders, 31*(2), 153–163.

Moss, J. F., Oliver, C., Berg, K., Kaur, G., Jephcott, L., & Cornish, K. (2008). Prevalence of autism spectrum phenomenology in Cornelia de Lange and Cri du Chat syndromes. *American Journal of Mental Retardation, 113*, 278–291.

Muhle, R., Trentacoste, S. V., & Rapin, I. (2004). The genetics of autism. *Pediatrics, 113*, 472–486.

Nishimura, Y., Martin, C. L., Lopez, A. V., Spence, S. J., Alvarez-Retuerto, A., et al. (2007). Genome-wide expression profiling of lymphoblastoid cell lines distinguishes different forms of autism and reveals shared pathways. *Human Molecular Genetics, 16*, 1682–1698.

Oliveira, G., Ataide, A., Marques, C., Miguel, T. S., Coutinho, A. M., Mota-Vieira, L., et al. (2007). Epidemiology of autism spectrum disorders in Portugal: Prevalence, clinical characterization, and medical conditions. *Developmental Medicine and Child Neurology, 49*, 726–733.

Peters, S. U., Beaudet, A. L., Madduri, N., & Bacino, C. A. (2004). Autism in Angelman syndrome: Implications for autism research. *Clinical Genetics Journal, 128*, 110–113.

Rogers, S. J., Wehmer, D. E., & Hagerman R. (2001). The behavioral phenotype in fragile X syndrome: Symptoms of autism in very young children with fragile X syndrome, idiopathic autism, and other developmental disorders. *Journal of Developmental and Behavioral Pediatrics, 22*, 409–417.

Sikora, D. M., Petti-Kekel, K., Penfield, J., Merkens, L. S., & Steiner, R. D. (2006). The near universal presence of autism spectrum disorders in children with Smith-Lemi-Opitz syndrome. *American Journal of Medical Genetics. Part A, 140A*, 1511–1518. doi: 10.1002/ajmg.a.31294.

Smalley, S. (1998). Autism and tuberous sclerosis. *Journal of Autism and Developmental Disorders, 28*, 407–414.

Veltman, W. M., Craig, E. E., & Bolton, P. F. (2005). Autism spectrum disorders in Prader-Willi and Angelman syndromes: A systematic review. *Psychiatric Genetics, 15*, 243–254.

Verdine, B. M., Troseth, G., Hodapp, R. M., & Dykens, E. M. (2008). Strategies and correlates of jigsaw puzzle performance by persons with Prader-Willi syndrome. *American Journal of Mental Retardation, 113*, 343–355.

Volkmar, F. R., State, M., & Klin, A. (2009). Autism and autism spectrum disorders: Diagnostic issues for the coming decade. *Journal of Child Psychology and Psychiatry. 50*, 108–115.

Vorstman, J. A., Morcus, M. E., Duijiff, S. N., et al. (2006). The 22q11.2 deletion in children: High rate if autistic disorders and early inset psychotic symptoms. *Journal of the American Academy of Child and Adolescent Psychiatry, 45*, 1104–1113.

Witwer, A. N., & Lecavalier, L. (2008). Examining the validity of autism spectrum disorder subtypes. *Journal of Autism and Developmental Disorders, 38*, 1611–1624.

Wong, V. C., & Hui, S. L., (2008). Epidemiological study of autism disorder in China. *Journal of Child Neurology, 23*, 67–72.

Yeargin-Allsopp, M., Rice, C., Karapurkar, T., Doernberg, N., Boyle, C., Murphy, C., et al. (2003). Prevalence of autism in a US metropolitan area. *Journal of the American Medical Association, 289*(1), 49–55.

16 Bonnie P. Taylor, Eric Hollander

Comorbid Obsessive-Compulsive Disorders

Points of Interest

- Converging research suggests substantial overlap in phenomenology, comorbidity, course, family and genetic findings, neurobiology, cognitive functioning, and treatment response, across ASD and putative OCSDs. These data support the existence of a valid repetitive behavior domain that cuts across traditional diagnostic boundaries.
- The overlap in repetitive behaviors across nosological categories can also be conceptualized as a symptom-based dimension, or continuum, that encompasses "normal" behavior and extends beyond in degree and/or severity.
- Grouping the diverse repetitive behaviors into homogeneous, independent subfactors (i.e., dimensions) will allow future research to reveal unique neurobiological underpinnings associated with each, which will provide insight into the development of new treatment approaches.
- Accumulating empirical research across academic disciplines is supporting the conceptualization of higher-and lower-order dimensions of repetitive behaviors across OCD spectrum diagnostic categories.
- Recent findings are emerging that suggest a familial link and genetic vulnerability for the higher-order repetitive behaviors in autism and OCD, which may represent an underlying endophenotype. Neuroimaging data supports these findings.

Restricted and repetitive behavior is a core symptom domain of autism spectrum disorder (ASD). Behaviors categorized within this symptom domain range, however, both in form and severity. Moreover, repetitive behaviors are not unique to ASD, and in fact, they are recognized across various DSM-IV diagnostic categories. This overlap of repetitive behaviors across various disorders was studied by the Research Planning Agenda for the DSM-V Work Group on Obsessive-Compulsive Disorders and Related Disorders (OCDRD), which proposed a putative Obsessive-Compulsive Spectrum Disorders (OCSDs) grouping.

A variety of disparate disorders have been conceptualized as being a part of the OCSDs category (Hollander, Kim, Braun, Simeon, & Zohar, 2009; Hollander, Wang, Braun, & Marsh, 2009). While autism might fit into such a category, given the importance of childhood specialists (e.g., pediatricians, pediatric neurologists) and childhood history in the diagnosis and ongoing treatment of ASD, it is unlikely that autism will be a part of the final consideration (Hollander, Kim, Braun, Simeon, & Zohar, 2009). The other disorders being considered as part of the OCSDs span across various traditional DSM-IV diagnostic categories, potentially including anxiety disorders (e.g., obsessive-compulsive disorder [OCD]), impulse control disorders (e.g., trichotillomania [TTM]), personality disorders (e.g., obsessive-compulsive personality disorder [OCPD]), somatoform disorders (e.g., body dysmorphic disorder [BDD]), Tourette's and other tic disorders, stereotyped movement disorders, and Sydenham's and other Pediatric Autoimmune Neuropsychiatric Disorders Associated with Streptococcal Infections (PANDAS) (Hollander, Kim, et al., 2009). Converging data is emerging that suggests that, in addition to sharing the core symptom of repetitive thoughts and behaviors, these seemingly distinct disorders may also exhibit a similar course, comorbidity, familial and genetic features, brain circuitry, and treatment response profile (Hollander, Kim, et al., 2009; Hollander, Wang, Braun, & Marsh, 2009).

An alternative way to conceptualize repetitive behaviors across disorders is to identify and examine "symptom dimensions" that are empirically derived from factor analytic studies. These dimensions encompass "normal behavior" and extend beyond in degree and/or severity. As will be discussed later in the chapter, such factors may each be related to a distinct genetic contribution, neurobiological underpinnings, comorbidity, treatment response profile, and course of illness.

Regardless of whether this overlap is conceptualized from a "spectrum" or "dimensional" standpoint, the relevance is of interest both heuristically and clinically. Heuristically, these commonalities may suggest a common underlying neuropathological mechanism for this core symptom domain across autism and other putative OCD spectrum disorders. This knowledge, in turn, can provide insight into the development of new treatment approaches.

Chapter 11 of this book details more fully the types and the range of repetitive behaviors that are specific to ASD. The relationship between ASD and other OCSDs, including autoimmune disorders, stereotyped movement disorders, and Tourette's and other tic disorders will be detailed elsewhere in this book. This chapter will therefore focus primarily on the overlap of repetitive, restricted, and/or stereotyped patterns of behavior, interests, and/or activities that characterize both ASD and related OCD spectrum disorders including OCD, OCPD, BDD, and TTM. This chapter will be organized into the following sections: First, the symptomatic commonalities in repetitive behaviors between ASD and other OCSDs will be outlined. Next, research findings related to the frequent comorbidity, similar course, and potentially overlapping genetic, neurobiological, and neuropsychological correlates across these disorders will be summarized. Finally, different approaches to subtyping the diverse symptoms that comprise the repetitive behavior domain will be presented. This is important because the identification of homogeneous subgroups will arm investigators with more power to uncover the unique pathogenesis that underlies each repetitive phenotype.

Commonalities in Repetitive Behaviors in Autism and Other OCSDs

Autism

The term "repetitive behavior" in autism encompasses a wide range of heterogeneous symptoms and activities, each characterized by nonfunctional repetition, rigidity, and/or inflexibility. The DSM-IV describes repetitive behaviors in autistic disorders as an abnormally circumscribed interest or preoccupation (e.g., focus on subway maps), an unreasonable insistence on sameness, inflexible persistence in following nonfunctional routines or rituals (e.g., eating the same food for lunch, everyday, at exactly 12:00 noon), and/or stereotyped and repetitive motor mannerisms (e.g., hand flapping and body rocking). Individuals with ASD may also engage in repetitive behaviors such as lining up objects, ensuring symmetry, ritualistic behavior, and repetitive language. Clinically, other repetitive behaviors are commonly observed in individuals with ASD, but are either not mentioned in the DSM-IV, or are referred to as "associated symptoms." These include repetitive self-injurious behaviors (e.g., head banging and wrist biting), pathological repetitive grooming (e.g., hair pulling, skin-picking, nail biting), hoarding, Pica, dyskinesias, and unusual sensory interests such as repetitive sniffing and/or mouthing objects.

Traditionally, the repetitive behaviors in autism have been conceptualized as a single, unitary symptom domain. More recently, however, research findings are supporting the existence of multiple, distinct subtypes of repetitive behavior, which have been subcategorized into higher- and lower-order behaviors (Hollander et al., 1998). Briefly, higher-order behaviors, which are cognitively mediated, include complex behaviors such as circumscribed interests, repetitive language, and object attachments. Lower-order behaviors are thought to involve the more primitive brain, and include repetitive sensory and motor behaviors such as stereotyped movements, repetitive manipulations of objects, body rocking, finger flicking, and repetitive touching. As will be discusses later in this chapter, growing empirical research supports the existence of higher- and lower-order subtypes of repetitive behaviors not only in ASD, but also across diagnostic categories within the putative OCSDs.

Obsessive Compulsive Disorder (OCD)

OCD is classified in the DSM-IV as an anxiety disorder; however, it is primarily characterized by repetitive thoughts and behaviors, and irresistible impulses and urges, not by anxiety per se. In fact, the *International Statistical Classification of Diseases and Related Health Problems-10th Revision* (ICD-10; World Health Organization, 2003), which is the classification of diseases by the World Health Organization, does not classify OCD as an anxiety disorder. Rather, the ICD-10 categorizes OCD under the umbrella "Neurotic, stress-related and somatoform disorders." Although anxiety is mentioned as regularly being present, it is not the defining feature of OCD in the ICD-10. Along these lines, a redefining of the OCSDs as being a separate chapter within the anxiety disorders, or a separate category altogether, is currently being discussed for DSM-V (Bartz & Hollander, 2006).

Repetitive behaviors in OCD are manifested as obsessions and compulsions. The DSM-IV describes an obsession as a repetitive thought or impulse that is subjectively experienced as intrusive and/or inappropriate, and thereby causes anxiety and distress. A compulsion is characterized as the engagement in a repetitive action, aimed at avoiding or relieving the anxiety that is caused by the obsession. These symptoms parallel the complex higher-order repetitive behaviors displayed in ASD, such as ritualistic behaviors, preoccupations, and a desire to maintain sameness.

Obsessive-Compulsive Personality Disorder (OCPD)

Since its conception, the distinction between OCPD and OCD has been controversial. Adding to the confusion, the symptomatic profile of OCPD has changed over the past few decades. For example, DSM-II characterized "obsessive-compulsive personality" as an inflexible adherence to standards, severe introversion, and rigidity. DSM-III (American Psychiatric Association [APA], 1980) added affective constriction, perfectionism, and a lack of awareness of how one's behavior affects others. In 1987, the DSM-III-R (APA, 1987) minimized focus on affective restriction and added excessive preoccupation and hoarding. Today, OCPD is classified in DSM-IV (APA, 2000) as a Cluster C Personality Disorder, and is characterized by a pervasive preoccupation with organization (e.g., details, rules, lists, order, schedules), perfectionism, excessive devotion to work, inflexible morality, insistence that other's follow their rules, hoarding, miserly spending, and/or rigidity and stubbornness.

It is at once apparent that many of these symptoms substantially overlap with both the obsessions and compulsions in OCD, and the repetitive behaviors exhibited in ASD. Furthermore, written descriptions of OCPD in the DSM-IV, including language such as "prone to repetition," "inflexible," "rigid," and "difficulty acknowledging the viewpoints of others," further highlight the observable commonalities between OCPD, ASD and OCD.

Importantly, *hoarding*, a compulsion to excessively collect things without discarding, traverses ASD, OCD, and OCPD. For example, hoarding is included as part of the diagnostic criteria of OCPD; it is considered a compulsion in OCD; and it not uncommonly co-occurs with ASD (McDougle, Kresch, et al., 1995; Russell, Mataix-Cols, Anson, & Murphy, 2005).

Trichotillomania (TTM)

Trichotillomania (TTM) is characterized by the recurrent pulling out of one's hair in the scalp, eyelashes, face, nose, pubic area, eyebrow, etc., often resulting in noticeable bald patches. In the DSM-IV, TTM is classified as an impulse disorder, although, it has an indisputable compulsive quality to it. Moreover, similar to the function of compulsions in OCD, hair pulling is thought to reduce anxiety in individuals with TTM (Woods et al., 2006). A preoccupation with symmetry, which is also exhibited in autism and OCD, has also been suggested to trigger TTM.

Body Dysmorphic Disorder (BDD)

Body dysmorphic disorder (BDD) is classified as a somatoform disorder in the DSM-IV, and is characterized by a recurrent and intense preoccupation with imagined ugliness and/or a physical defect. In order to mitigate these obsessions, individuals with BDD engage in repetitive mirror-checking, camouflaging, frequent requests for reassurance, and/or skin-picking (Frare, Perugi, Ruffolo, & Toni, 2004; Hollander, Neville, Frenkel, Josephson, & Liebowitz, 1992; Phillips, 1996). These repetitive behaviors clearly resemble compulsions in OCD. The focus of the obsession, however, may differ between BDD and OCD: in BDD the preoccupation is centered on a perceived physical defect, whereas in OCD, the preoccupation may encompass a broad range of content.

It is readily apparent from the descriptions above that there is substantial overlap in the repetitive thoughts and behaviors that manifest in ASD, OCD, and other OCD spectrum disorders such as OCPD, TTM, and BDD. Additional support for the existence of a valid repetitive behavior domain, which cuts across traditional diagnostic boundaries, is rapidly accumulating from diverse disciplines. These findings will be discussed below, highlighting similarities in the comorbidity, course, family and genetic research, neurobiology, neuropsychology, and treatment response profile across OCSDs.

Comorbidity

The co-occurrence of two disorders, referred to as comorbidity, is one piece of evidence that suggests a common underlying pathophysiology between the co-existing diseases. Several obstacles hamper investigations of disorders that may be comorbid with ASD. First, to date, there are no standard, reliable measures of assessing comorbidity in ASD (Ghaziuddin, Ghaziuddin, & Greden, 2002; Matson, Smiroldo, & Hastings, 1998). Further, individuals with ASD frequently present with intellectual disability (Matson et al., 1998), which in itself is associated with the stereotypies and other repetitive behaviors displayed in idiopathic autism (Matson et al., 1997). As such, it is sometimes difficult to disentangle the origin of these repetitive behaviors.

In spite of the aforementioned assessment difficulties, recent studies have attempted to estimate comorbidity with ASD. For example, a 2.7% lifetime prevalence of Asperger's syndrome was found in individuals diagnosed with OCD (LaSalle et al., 2004). This is well above current estimates of Asperger's disorder in the general population (Fombonne & Tidmarsh, 2003). Conversely, approximately 25% of adults with Asperger's syndrome were found to have comorbid OCD (Russell et al., 2005).

The occurrence of other OCD spectrum disorders with each other has frequently been reported. For example, patients with BDD have a 30% lifetime prevalence of OCD (Gunstad & Phillips, 2003). Further, a high incidence of OCD has been reported in patients with TTM (Ferrao, Miguel, & Stein, 2009) and OCPD (Gunderson et al., 2000; Skodol et al., 1995) Similarly, patients with a current diagnosis of OCD have a higher lifetime prevalence rate for BDD and pathological grooming conditions compared to controls (i.e., 16% vs. 3%, and 41% vs. 17%, respectively) (Bienvenu et al., 2000).

Recent studies have estimated that hoarding and saving compulsions occur in 15–40% of OCD patients (Hanna, 1995; Mataix-Cols, Nakatani, Micali, & Heyman, 2008; Rasmussen & Eisen, 1992). Hoarding has also been reported in up to 30% of individuals with autism (McDougle, Kresch, et al., 1995; Russell et al., 2005). Hoarding, in turn, has been associated with other OCSDs, including pathological repetitive grooming such as TTM (9%), skin picking (39%), and nail biting (39%) (Samuels et al., 2002).

In summary, comorbidity has been reported among OCD, ASD, and hoarding, as well as between TTM, BDD, and OCD. This co-occurrence is one piece of evidence in favor of a common etiology across the disorders.

Course

In addition to the similarities in symptoms and comorbidity discussed above, autism and OCD spectrum disorders have parallels relating to the course of illness (see Figure 16-1). With regard to the course of ASD, abnormalities are thought to be present from birth, but must be present prior to the age of three to meet formal DSM-IV criteria. Autism is a chronic and lifelong illness, though some improvement may be seen in symptom domains over time (Fecteau, Mottron, Berthiaume, & Burack, 2003; Piven, Harper, Palmer, & Arndt, 1996). In terms of gender, males are affected with autism significantly more often than females, as evidenced by the approximately 4 to 1 male to female ratio (Fombonne, 2005).

OCD, in contrast, has a bimodal age of onset, with peaks during puberty, and then again during early adulthood (Zohar, 1999). It has been suggested that early-onset OCD is most similar to the course of autism, as it is also more prevalent in males than females (Tukel et al., 2005), and follows a chronic course (Fontenelle, Mendlowicz, Marques, & Versiani, 2003; Sobin, Blundell, & Karayiorgou, 2000). When hoarding is accompanied with symptoms of OCD, the hoarding symptoms appear to have an earlier age of onset (Pertusa et al., 2008).

Less is known regarding the course of BDD, TTM, and OCDPD. Demographic data, and illness duration of BDD appears to be similar to that of OCD (Phillips et al., 2007). TTM has a mean age of onset between 9 and 13 years of age, and is widely viewed to have a persistent course. Males may have a later age of onset than females. (Lochner, Seedat, & Stein, 2009). According to the DSM-IV (APA, 2000), OCPD is typically diagnosed in late adolescence or young adulthood, and it occurs almost twice as frequently in males than females.

With specific regard to the developmental course of repetitive behaviors, recent findings suggest that they are one of the earliest signs to appear in autism, occurring during the first and second year of life (Ozonoff et al., 2008; Watt, Wetherby, Barber, & Morgan, 2008). Significant repetitive behaviors continue to be reported by adolescents and adults with ASD (Esbensen, Seltzer, Lam, & Bodfish, 2009; Fecteau et al., 2003). Some studies suggest that the developmental trajectory differs for different repetitive behaviors in ASD. For example, motor and sensory repetitive behaviors have been found to occur more frequently in younger children (aged 2–4), with the repetitive behaviors becoming more complex by age 7–11 (Bishop, Richler, & Lord, 2006; Militerni, Bravaccio, Falco, Fico, & Palermo, 2002). Similarly, a recent study by Esbensen et al. (2009) found that stereotyped movements were more frequent in young children than in adults. Some studies have reported that whereas restricted interests, unusual preoccupations, and complex stereotypy may decrease with age (Esbensen et al., 2009; Seltzer et al., 2003), ritualistic behavior and a need for sameness appear to be frequent in older individuals with autism (Esbensen et al., 2009). Retrospective data have also suggested some improvement in repetitive behavior with age, but not as pronounced as improvements in the social and language domains (Fecteau et al., 2003; Piven et al., 1996) that together define autism.

In terms of the course of repetitive behaviors across the OCD spectrum, Hollander theorized that over time, the lower-order symptom dimension of repetitive behaviors, which serve to mediate arousal, progress into higher order, cognitively mediated repetitive behaviors (Hollander, personal communication). For example, as previously mentioned, young children with autism often engage in perseverative, self-stimulatory behaviors including hand flapping, rocking, lining objects up, and opening and closing doors. Similarly, young children with other OCD spectrum disorders may engage in comorbid, self-stimulatory trichotillomania. In older children with autism, these lower-order behaviors may be supplemented and/or substituted by higher order OCD spectrum behaviors such as checking, washing, counting, repetitive requesting, and repetitive asking for reassurance. Comorbid OCD spectrum

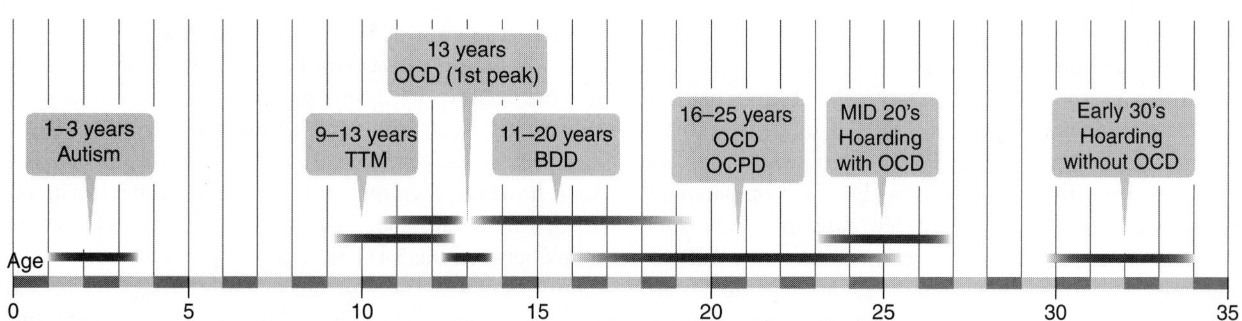

Figure 16–1. Timeline of average age of onset of disorders with a core repetitive behavior domain. Horizontal gray bands represent the approximate age range of onset for each corresponding disorder, with the bolder, middle color signifying the average. Vertical gray lines each represent one year.

disorders at this age might include BDD, as well as grooming and checking rituals.

Taken together, there is some overlap in the course of ASD and OCD spectrum disorders. Most notably, there is a greater male to female ratio in ASD, OCD, OCDPD, and hoarding, and the course is similar as well. Developmental research is beginning to depict a possible age-related trend for repetitive behaviors, with the earlier years being characterized by motor and sensory-related repetitive behaviors (e.g., stereotypy, TTM) that are later accompanied and/or replaced with higher-order repetitive thoughts and behaviors (e.g., obsessions, rituals). This is interesting given the earlier average age of onset for disorders characterized by motor-sensory related repetitive behaviors (e.g., autism and TTM) compared to the later onset for the more cognitively mediated repetitive behaviors (see Figure 16-1.) Clearly, more research is needed to determine the validity of this age-related trajectory.

Family Studies

Family studies, which demonstrate a high occurrence of OCD spectrum disorders in relatives of probands with OCD spectrum disorders, suggest a possible genetic link across them. For example, OCD has been found to be more prevalent in relatives of autistic probands compared to relatives of Down syndrome probands (Bolton, Pickles, Murphy, & Rutter, 1998) and control probands (Micali, Chakrabarti, & Fombonne, 2004).

In terms of other OCSDs, compared to first-degree relatives of control probands, first-degree relatives of probands with OCD have been reported to have a greater frequency of OCPD (5.8% vs.11.5%, respectively) and pathological grooming symptoms (10% vs.17%, respectively) (Samuels et al., 2000). Relatives of probands with early-onset OCD have a particularly high prevalence of OCD compared to control relatives (22.7% vs. 0.9%) (do Rosario-Campos et al., 2005), which is of particular interest given the observation that early-onset OCD is similar in course and gender ratio to that of autism. A familial link has similarly been reported in TTM, with relatives of probands with TTM approximately 20% more likely to exhibit OCD and TTM compared to control probands (Christenson, Mackenzie, & Reeve, 1992; Lenane et al., 1992).

With regard to a family history related to repetitive behaviors per se, Hollander et al. (2003) found that autistic probands who engaged in high levels of repetitive behaviors were more likely to have parents with OCD compared to autistic probands who exhibited few repetitive behaviors (15% vs. 4%, respectively). More recent studies have utilized quantitative symptoms dimensions to examine familial linkage. For example, Abramson et al. (2005) reported a positive correlation between the "Insistence on Sameness" factor on the Autism Diagnostic Interview-Revised (ADI-R) in subjects with autism and obsessive-compulsive behaviors in parents. Studies that examined sibling-pair correlations similarly found a significant familial relationship for the "Insistence on Sameness," as well as for the "Circumscribed Interest" factor, on the ADI (Lam, Bodfish, & Piven, 2008; Szatmari et al., 2006). Interestingly, neither of these studies found a familial relationship for the lower-order "Repetitive Sensory and Motor" factor. Along these lines, a multiplex family study also reported a familial pattern for higher-, but not lower-, order repetitive behaviors in first-degree relatives of individuals with ASD (Silverman et al., 2002). Higher-order repetitive behavior in idiopathic OCD has also been linked to a family history of OCD spectrum disorders. More specifically, OCD probands whose obsessions and compulsions included ordering and symmetry were more likely to have a relative with OCD (Alsobrook, Leckman, Goodman, Rasmussen, & Pauls, 1999; Hanna, Fischer, Chadha, Himle, & Van Etten, 2005).

In summary, family studies typically show that relatives of probands with OCD spectrum disorders have an increased risk of also having an OCD spectrum disorder. Further, research is emerging that is making a strong case for a familial link for higher-order repetitive behaviors in autism and OCD, which may represent an underlying endophenotype.

Genetics

Genetic linkage and association studies have reported genetic relationships between OCD and some OCD spectrum disorders. For example, linkage analysis has revealed that individuals with more severe OCD displayed an autism susceptibility gene on chromosomes 1, 6, and 19 (Buxbaum et al., 2004). The chromosome 15q11-q13, in particular, has been implicated in repetitive behaviors in autism. Moreover, families sharing high scores on the "Insistence on Sameness" factor of the ADI showed increased linkage at the GABRB3 locus in 15q11- q13 (Shao et al., 2003).

As with OCD, the serotonin transporter (5-HTT) is considered to be a candidate gene for autism. Investigations have isolated a genetic linkage of autism to the chromosome 17q11.2 region that harbors the serotonin transporter gene (SLC6A4) (Cantor et al., 2005; McCauley et al., 2004; Risch et al., 1999). Moreover, Brune, et al. (2006) reported an association between 5HTTLPR long/long genotype of the SLC6A4 and repetitive sensory-motor behaviors. Similarly, a link has been reported between novel variants at the serotonin transporter locus and rigid compulsive behavior (Sutcliffe et al., 2005). Associations with the 5-HTTLPR polymorphism, have, however, been mixed (Conroy et al., 2004; Devlin et al., 2005; Kim et al., 2002; Yirmiya et al., 2001). Nevertheless, a link between the 5-HT transporter and repetitive behaviors is consistent with the abundance of 5-HT receptors housed in the basal ganglia, which, as will be discussed in the following section, has been implicated in the expression of repetitive behaviors (Di Giovanni, Di Matteo, Pierucci, Benigno, & Esposito, 2006).

Other genes have also been implicated in repetitive behaviors. More specifically, studies show that dopamine transporter knockout mice exhibit a greater insistence on fixed patterns of action (Berridge, Aldridge, Houchard, & Zhuang, 2005). Other studies have found that a mitochondrial aspartate/glutamate carrier polymorphism on chromosome 2 was associated with routines and rituals in individuals with autism (Silverman et al., 2006). In addition, a significant allele sharing for hoarding phenotypes has been found for markers at 4q34–35, 5q35.2–35.3, and 17q2 (Zhang et al., 2002).

Neuroimaging

Current neuroimaging and cognitive findings across OCD spectrum disorders provides further evidence of a common underlying pathophysiology. More specifically, neuroimaging research has tended to show dysfunction in the cortico-striatal-thalamo-cortical circuit (sometimes referred to as the "OCD circuit"), which includes the basal ganglia, anterior cingulate, dorsolateral and orbitofrontal cortex, and the thalamus. As will be discussed in the next section, abnormalities in this pathway are supported by reduced performance on cognitive tasks that are mediated by these brain regions.

In terms of aberrant functioning within structures of the basal ganglia, recent MRI studies have revealed enlarged bilateral (Herbert et al., 2003; Sears et al., 1999) and right (Hollander, Anagnostou, et al., 2005) caudate volume in patients with autism compared to controls. The variability in findings may be a result of the positive correlation between right caudate volumes and higher order repetitive behaviors (Hollander, Anagnostou, et al., 2005). This hypothesis is consistent with increased right caudate volume reported in patients with OCD (Scarone et al., 1992), who also exhibit higher order repetitive behaviors. These data suggest a possible common underlying neural pathway associated with the higher order, cognitive mediated repetitive behaviors across both ASD and OCD.

In subjects with trichotillomania, smaller left putamen volume and increased grey matter density in the left stratum has been reported relative to normal controls (Chamberlain et al., 2008; O'Sullivan et al., 1997). Furthermore, a negative correlation has found between TTM severity and striatal activity, in that, more severe hair pulling was associated with a greater reduction in striatal activity (Stein et al., 2002).

Abnormalities in the anterior cingulate cortex have also been frequently reported across OCD-related disorders. For example, reduced metabolism and volume in the anterior cingulate have been observed in individuals with ASD relative to healthy controls (Haznedar et al., 1997; Haznedar et al., 2000; Ohnishi et al., 2000). Further, white matter disruption in the anterior cingulate has been reported in autism (Barnea-Goraly et al., 2004), as well as in OCD (Szeszko et al., 2005).

A differential pattern of cingulate activity has been shown for OCD patients with and without hoarding symptoms (Saxena et al., 2004). More specifically, OCD patients who also exhibit hoarding symptoms displayed reduced metabolism in the posterior cingulate gyrus compared to controls, and in the dorsal anterior cingulate compared to nonhoarding OCD patients. These data, together with findings of an earlier age of onset for hoarding with OCD versus hoarding without OCD, distinct susceptibility genes for hoarding, as well as, as will be discussed later in the chapter, an empirically derived hoarding factor in OCD, suggest that compulsive hoarding may be an independent subtype of repetitive behaviors.

Few studies have specifically investigated the neural structures involved in repetitive behaviors. Hollander et al. (2005) found a positive correlation between the severity of repetitive behaviors and right caudate and putamen volumes in patients with autism. This association was particularly strong for the higher-order OCD spectrum repetitive behaviors, such as insistence on sameness/resistance to change. Sears et al. (1999) similarly reported that enlarged caudate volume in autism was correlated with difficulties with minor change in routine, compulsions and rituals, and complex motor mannerisms.

Taken together, replicated neuroimaging findings have revealed a link between higher-order repetitive behaviors and structures in the basal ganglia, and the anterior cingulate cortex. This finding suggests that dysfunction in this circuitry may lead to the expression of higher-order repetitive behaviors across OCD spectrum disorders. Alternatively, subtle structural and/or functional alterations along the corticostriatal pathway may be associated with different symptom presentations of repetitive behavior. More research is needed linking brain imaging findings to distinct repetitive behaviors.

Neuropsychology

Structures within the corticostriatal neural pathway, which as discussed above, have been found abnormal in neuroimaging studies of OCSDs, play a prominent role in the mediation of executive functions. As such, one would expect executive dysfunction to be significant in the neuropsychological literature of OCD spectrum disorders.

Executive function is an umbrella term used to describe cognitive functions involved in planning and executing complex behavior such as organization, inhibition, initiation of action, self-monitoring, cognitive flexibility and set-shifting. Many of these functions are characteristic of ASD and OCD spectrum disorders. For example, in autism, difficulty inhibiting behavior may lead to repetitive verbalizations and/or actions, and in OCSDs, it may manifest as difficulty repressing unwanted obsessions, and/or controlling compulsions such as hair pulling.

Neuropsychological studies have in fact demonstrated deficits in response inhibition in individuals with OCSDs, albeit with variable results. Bohne et al. (2008) reported poor motor inhibition in patients with TTM, but not in patients with OCD. In contrast, Chamberlain et al. (2006) found that both patients with TTM and patients with OCD showed impaired motor inhibition, though the impairment was more significant in patients with TTM. Variable findings have also been reported regarding inhibition in autistic samples (Ozonoff, Strayer, McMahon, & Filloux, 1994; Shafritz, Dichter, Baranek, & Belger, 2008). However, it is of considerable interest that during a response inhibition task, functional brain imaging studies have correlated reduced inhibitory control with hypometabolism in the anterior cingulate in individuals with ASD (Anagnostou, 2006; Kana, Keller, Minshew, & Just, 2007). This is consistent with dysfunction in the anterior cingulate, which, as previously discussed, has frequently been reported across OCD spectrum disorders.

Another executive function that is often impaired in individuals with OCDRS is cognitive flexibility. Poor flexibility can manifest in preservative, stereotyped behavior, rigidity, and inflexibility. A recent study compared cognitive set shifting between subjects with TTM, OCD, and controls. Deficits in cognitive flexibility were demonstrated only in patients with OCD relative to controls (Chamberlain et al., 2006). In contrast other studies have found impaired cognitive set-shifting in subjects with TTM compared to controls (Stanley, Hannay, & Breckenridge, 1997). In samples of autistic individuals, executive deficits have been found in set-shifting (Ozonoff et al., 2004) as well as in an increased rate of perseverative responding compared to controls (Turner, 1999).

Few studies have explored the relationship between performance on tests of executive functioning and repetitive behavior. Turner (1999) reported that poorer performance on tasks that measure initiation and inhibition of response were associated with higher levels of repetitive behavior, in both high- and low-functioning patients with autism. In contrast, Ozonoff et al. (2004) reported no relationship between performance on tasks of executive functioning and repetitive behavior. More recently, Lopez et al. (2005) found that repetitive behaviors are associated with some, but not other executive functions. More specifically, in adults with autistic disorder, repetitive behavior was correlated with cognitive flexibility, response inhibition, and working memory, but not with planning or fluency.

In summary, executive dysfunction in response inhibition, cognitive flexibility, and perseveration has been demonstrated in OCSDs, albeit with some inconsistency. Variable findings in studies of executive function are not surprising, however, as these functions each comprise of a range of independent processes, and different research measures tap into different functional components. It is interesting, however, that an fMRI study that examined neural activity during an executive task demonstrated a relationship between executive function impairment, repetitive behavior, and frontostriatal circuitry. Similar interdisciplinary research will help to relate executive functioning to the expression of repetitive behaviors and the integrity of brain structures in OCD related disorders.

Pharmacology/Treatment Response

Common neurotransmitter systems, and a similar response profile to psychopharmacological treatments, have been found across some OCD spectrum disorders. For example, treatment with clomipramine has been reported to be more effective than desipramine for patients with OCD (Hollander & Kahn, 2003; Leonard et al., 1989), ASD (Gordon, State, Nelson, Hamburger, & Rapoport, 1993), BDD (Hollander et al., 1999), and TTM (Swedo et al., 1989). In addition, selective serotonin reuptake inhibitors (SSRIs) are the first-line treatment for OCD and BDD.

Treatment with SSRIs has similarly been efficacious in reducing repetitive behaviors in ASD in some but not all studies. For example, in randomized controlled clinical trials of children, adolescents, and adults treated with fluoxetine (Buchsbaum et al., 2001; Hollander, Phillips, et al., 2005) and fluvoxamine (McDougle, et al., 1996), significant improvements in repetitive symptoms were demonstrated compared to placebo. A recent study, however, that compared citalopram to placebo, found no difference in outcome between the treatment conditions (King et al., 2009). The discrepancy in findings may be the result of differences in methodology between studies (e.g., dosing, age of sample, etc.), as well as individual variability. Alternatively, since SSRIs effectively reduce anxiety in samples with autism (Buchsbaum et al., 2001; Hollander, Phillips, et al., 2005) (Steingard, Zimnitzky, DeMaso, Bauman, & Bucci, 1997), which is likely to be associated with reduced rigidity in adherence to routines and rituals (Soorya, Kiarashi, & Hollander, 2008), SSRIs may exert their effect on the higher-order repetitive behaviors. Future outcome studies with SSRIs may benefit by examining the relationship between treatment response, higher- vs. lower-order repetitive behaviors, and anxiety.

Nevertheless, there is strong evidence that implicates serotonin in playing a role in the expression of repetitive symptoms. For example, Hollander et al. (2000) found that the sensitivity of the 5HT1d receptor was associated with the severity of repetitive behaviors in adults with autism. Further, as previously reported, the serotonin transporter (5-HTT) has been studied as a possible candidate gene for autism.

Dopaminergic abnormalities have also been implicated in both ASD and OCD (Denys, Zohar, & Westenberg, 2004; Hollander, Baldini Rossi, Sood, & Pallanti, 2003; McCracken et al., 2002). For instance, children treated with the antipsychotic risperidone showed reductions in stereotypy, hyperactivity, and aggressive symptoms compared to those on placebo. Significant improvement in repetitive behaviors in children with ASD has also been associated with divalproex treatment (Hollander et al., 2006). Other support for dopamine's role in OCD spectrum disorders is the common use of dopamine blockers as augmentative treatment in individuals with treatment-resistant OCD (Pallanti, Bernardi, Antonini, Singh, & Hollander, 2009). Moreover, dopaminergic neurotransmission plays a significant role in mediating the function of structures in the basal ganglia, which as previously discussed are associated with the expression of repetitive behaviors, and are aberrant in many OCD spectrum disorders.

Phenotypes of ASD and OCSDs

As discussed throughout this chapter, the repetitive behaviors that are displayed in ASD and other OCD spectrum disorders lie across a broad spectrum that ranges from repetitive body movements to more cognitively mediated symptoms, such as circumscribed interests and obsessions. Several approaches have attempted to reduce the heterogeneity of repetitive behaviors into meaningful categories. The traditional method has been to consider whether or not the symptoms are *egodystonic*, that is, whether the individual perceives them as irrational and/or unreasonable. Importantly, when symptoms are egodystonic, they provoke significant mental distress (e.g., anxiety). In attempt to diminish that stress and anxiety, compulsions and rituals are performed, for example in OCD and BDD. With regard to TTM, tension is thought to mount immediately before, or during, attempts to avoid hair-pulling, followed by a sense of relief and pleasure during hair-pulling.

In contrast, repetitive behaviors exhibited in ASD and OCPD are not subjectively recognized as excessive or senseless, and do not provoke anxiety. Thus, they are *egosyntonic*. For example, many individuals with Asperger's disorder derive satisfaction and comfort from their preoccupations. Assessment of perceived rationality in ASD, however, is difficult due to impaired introspection that is inherent in the disorder. For patients with OCPD, obsessions and compulsions are also viewed as enjoyable, and, in fact, these patients will readily explain why their behaviors are rational.

One drawback of the egodystonic, egosyntonic classification of repetitive behaviors is that the same behavior may be subjectively experienced differently. As such, it becomes unclear as to whether the behavior is functioning as an anxiolytic in one individual relative to another. For example, one patient may engage in excessive list-making to reduce the significant subjective distress created by an egodystonic obsession. Alternatively, list making may be related to a preoccupation with detail, as in OCPD, and in this case, it is likely to be enjoyable, not resisted, and therefore, egosyntonic. Another shortcoming of this distinction stems from the discovery that there is a continuum of insight (i.e., degree of understanding of the problematic or irrational nature of the symptoms) into a patient's OCD-like symptoms. For example, Foa et al. (1995) conducted a field study for the DSM-IV and found that of 432 individuals with OCD, only 8% currently lacked insight, and 5% reported that they never had insight. This study propelled the DSM-IV to replace the egodystonic attribute of repetitive behaviors in OCD, and add a "poor insight" specifier. Poor insight is characterized as not realizing that obsessions and actions are excessive and unreasonable, and significantly interfere with daily life.

In contrast to egodystonicity, poor insight in OCD has been associated with treatment outcome, as well as with specific types of obsessions. For example, Tolin, Abramowitz, Kozak, and Foa (2001) found that poor insight was associated with religious obsessions, fears of making mistakes, and unwanted obsessional impulses to act aggressively. Other studies have found that poor insight was found more often in individuals with somatic obsessions (e.g., physical appearance, fears of illness), compared to other OCD symptoms (Abramowitz, Franklin, Schwartz, & Furr, 2003; McKay, Neziroglu, & Yaryura-Tobias, 1997; Neziroglu, Pinto, Yaryura-Tobias, & McKay, 2004). This is consistent with a finding in BDD, which also involves somatic symptoms, which reported a negative correlation between insight and symptoms severity (Eisen, Phillips, Coles, & Rasmussen, 2004). Poor insight in OCD has also been associated with poor psychopharmacological and behavioral treatment outcome (Raffin, Guimaraes Fachel, Ferrao, Pasquoto de Souza, & Cordioli, 2009; Shetti et al., 2005) and an earlier age of onset (Catapano et al., 2009).

With advances in theory and research, greater specificity of the structure of the repetitive behavior domain of OCD spectrum disorders has been conceptualized. In particular, various research groups have utilized factor analytic methods to mathematically derive independent underlying dimensions (also called factors or subtypes) of repetitive symptoms. Importantly, each of these homogeneous subtypes may be associated with a unique etiology and treatment response profile.

Using this technique, the most established factors that have emerged in the autism literature are the "lower order" and the "higher order" subtypes of repetitive behaviors. More recently, however, the structure of the repetitive behaviors has become even more specific, as additional distinct factors have been identified. In the earlier research (Cuccaro et al., 2003; Szatmari et al., 2006) factor analyses were performed on the symptoms items of the Autism Diagnostic Interview-Revised (ADI-R), a clinical assessment that focuses on the three main autism symptom domains (i.e., reciprocal social interaction; communication and language; and restricted and repetitive, stereotyped interests and behaviors). The results of these factor analyses yielded "lower-" and "higher-" order factors, in both children and adults. As previously mentioned, the lower-order factor, also referred to as "Repetitive Sensory and Motor Behaviors," includes symptoms such as hand and finger mannerisms, repetitive use of objects or parts of objects, unusual sensory interests, stereotyped body movements, and rocking. These repetitive behaviors are thought to be self-stimulatory and serve to modulate the level of arousal. The higher-order repetitive domain, called "Insistence on Sameness," comprises symptoms such as resistance to trivial changes in routine and environment, compulsions, and rituals. These repetitive thoughts and behaviors are thought to be mediated by higher cognitive processes.

Several groups have, in fact, demonstrated that the higher- and lower-order repetitive domains are correlated with level of cognitive functioning. More specifically, whereas higher-order repetitive symptoms have been associated with higher intellectual functioning (Militerni et al., 2002), lower-order repetitive behaviors have been linked with intellectual disability (Bishop et al., 2006; Militerni et al., 2002). Consistent with this, symptoms that comprise the lower-order domain, such as stereotyped motor movements, have also been linked to neurological dysfunction (Peterson et al., 2003; Sears et al., 1999), and as such, are also manifested in neurological-based OCSDs such as Tourette's syndrome (TS), Sydenham's chorea, as well as ASD.

More recently, a distinct third repetitive behavior factor in autism has been identified, also derived from the items on the ADI-R (Lam et al., 2008). This factor materialized because, in contrast to the earlier research, ADI-R items that did not load on either the "Repetitive Sensory and Motor Behaviors" or "Insistence on Sameness" factor were not excluded from the analysis. This third factor, described as "Circumscribed Interests" includes circumscribed interests, unusual preoccupations, and unusual attachment to objects.

In attempt to provide even more definition and structure to the repetitive domain, recent investigations have utilized instruments that more explicitly delineate repetitive behaviors. For example, a factor analysis using the items on the Repetitive Behavior Scale-Revised (RBS-R), conducted by Lam and Anon (2007), derived 5 subscales in children and adults with ASD. They included "Ritualistic/Sameness Behavior" (repetitive performance of activities of daily living, resistance to change, need for sameness), "Stereotypic Behavior" (repeated, purposeless body movements), "Self-injurious Behavior," "Compulsive Behavior" (repetitive behavior performed according to a rule, or until its "just right"), and "Restricted Interests" (limited range of interest, focus or activity). In contrast, Anagnostou et al. investigated the structure of the Yale-Brown Obsessive Compulsive Scale (Y-BOCS) in individuals with autism (unpublished data). Results yielded four empirically derived distinct factors, which comprised higher-order repetitive behaviors (e.g., ordering, washing, repeating, checking, ritualistic eating and rituals), lower-order repetitive behaviors (self-injurious behaviors, touching, rubbing), hoarding, and obsessions.

If the overlap of symptoms between ASD and other OCD spectrum disorders is meaningful, then repetitive symptoms within disorders should share a similar underlying factor structure, or should overlap with one or more established repetitive factor domains. Bloch et al. (2008) recently conducted a large-scale meta-analysis to validate the factor structure of the Y-BOCS in OCD. This study yielded 4 factors, including "Forbidden Thoughts" (obsessions involving aggression, sexual, religious, and somatic content, as well as checking compulsions), "Symmetry" (symmetry obsessions, and repeating, ordering, and counting compulsions), "Cleaning" (cleaning and contamination), and "Hoarding" (hoarding obsessions and compulsions).

Examination of the factor structure of repetitive behaviors on the Y-BOCS between ASD and OCD samples is notable for interesting similarities and differences (see Figure 16-2). For example, the repetitive symptoms intrinsic to each disorder

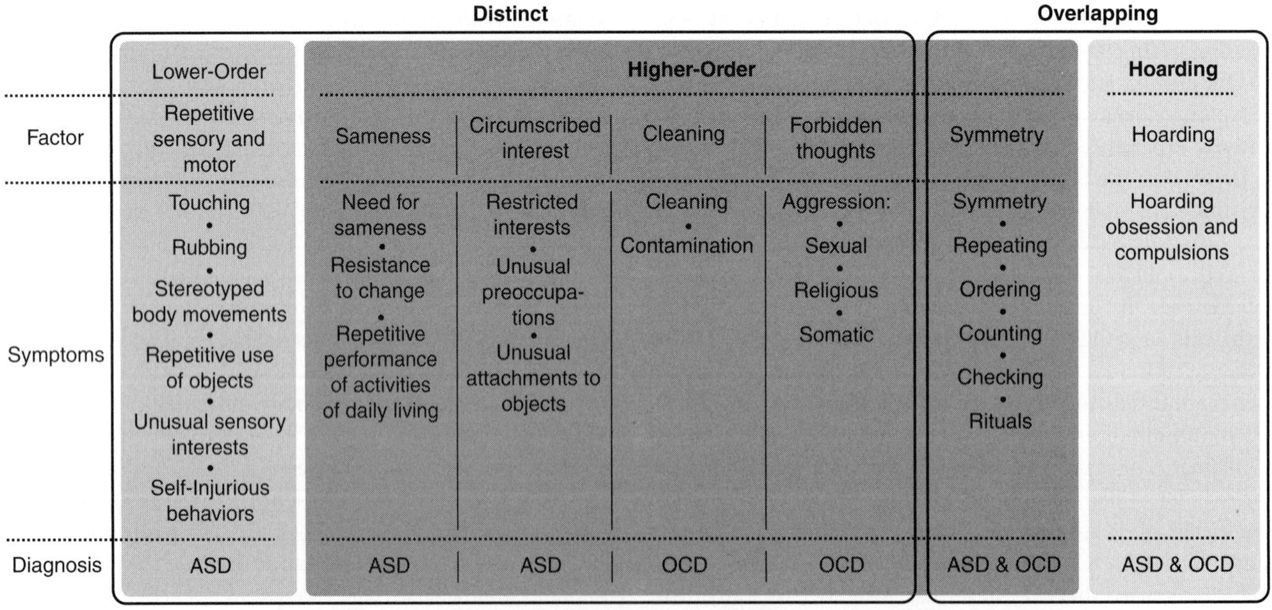

	Distinct					Overlapping	
	Lower-Order	Higher-Order					Hoarding
Factor	Repetitive sensory and motor	Sameness	Circumscribed interest	Cleaning	Forbidden thoughts	Symmetry	Hoarding
Symptoms	Touching • Rubbing • Stereotyped body movements • Repetitive use of objects • Unusual sensory interests • Self-Injurious behaviors	Need for sameness • Resistance to change • Repetitive performance of activities of daily living	Restricted interests • Unusual preoccupations • Unusual attachments to objects	Cleaning • Contamination	Aggression: • Sexual • Religious • Somatic	Symmetry • Repeating • Ordering • Counting • Checking • Rituals	Hoarding obsession and compulsions
Diagnosis	ASD	ASD	ASD	OCD	OCD	ASD & OCD	ASD & OCD

Figure 16–2. Summary of distinct and overlapping repetitive factors in autism spectrum disorder (ASD) and obsessive-compulsive disorder (OCD). Distinct repetitive factors found only in ASD include the lower order "Repetitive Sensory and Motor" factor and the higher order "Sameness" and "Circumscribed Interest" factors. Distinct factors found in OCD include the higher order repetitive factors of "Cleaning" and "Forbidden Thoughts." Overlapping factors, which have been derived in both samples of ASD and OCD, include the higher order "Symmetry" factor, and a "Hoarding" factor.

loaded similarly to yield 2 analogous factors. The first, characterized as a distinct hoarding subtype, was derived in both the ASD and OCD samples. The validity of hoarding as a discrete subtype is supported by previous research, which suggests that hoarding is associated with a distinct biological and genetic profile, poor insight, and resistance to psychological and pharmacological treatments (Abramowitz et al., 2003; Lochner et al., 2005).

The second repetitive dimension uncovered in both samples involves repeating, ordering, symmetry, counting, and rituals. This is referred to as the "Symmetry" factor in OCD, and the "Higher-order" repetitive factor in ASD. Strong support for a distinct higher-order, cognitively mediated repetitive factor comes from family and genetic studies. As previously discussed, family studies have demonstrated a familial link for the "Insistence on Sameness" and "Circumscribed Interests" factors of the RRBS, as well as the "Insistence on Sameness" factor of ADI-R (Abramson et al., 2005; Lam et al., 2008; Silverman et al., 2002; Szatmari et al., 2006). Furthermore families sharing high scores on the "Insistence on Sameness" factor of the ADI showed increased linkage at the GABRB3 locus in 15q11-q13 (Shao et al., 2003). In contrast, no familial or genetic link has been reported for the lower-order sensory motor repetitive behaviors. Neuroimaging findings, which suggest a positive correlation between higher-order repetitive behaviors and caudate and putamen volumes (Hollander, Anagnostou, et al., 2005; Sears et al., 1999), also point in the direction of a unique etiology for this repetitive domain.

A distinction in the underling factor structure of repetitive behaviors between the ASD and OCD sample is that the lower-order repetitive factor, which is consistently yielded in studies of ASD, was not reported in the OCD sample. This lack of finding supports previous research that suggests lower-order repetitive behavior is in fact a homogeneous neurologically based factor (Peterson et al., 2003; Sears et al., 1999), associated with intellectual disability (Bishop et al., 2006; Militerni et al., 2002) but not common in OCD (McDougle, Kresch, et al., 1995). In contrast, a subtype of "Forbidden Thoughts" was identified in OCD, but not ASD, samples. This concurs with a study that directly compared the Y-BOCS in adults with OCD and ASD, and found that patients with OCD were significantly more likely to experience aggressive, sexual, religious, and somatic obsessions compared to patients with ASD (McDougle, Krystal, Price, Heninger, & Charney, 1995). It is also of interest to note that aggressive, religious, and somatic obsessions have been associated with an unfavorable treatment response (Erzegovesi et al., 2001; Ferrao et al., 2006; Mataix-Cols, Marks, Greist, Kobak, & Baer, 2002) and with poor insight (Catapano et al., 2009; Erzegovesi et al., 2001; Raffin et al., 2009), thus mounting further support to the validity of this subtype.

To the authors' knowledge, no studies have been performed looking at the structure of repetitive symptoms in BDD, OCPD, or TTM. Within the framework of the empirically validated repetitive symptom dimensions described above, however, it is not difficult to conceptualize where they may fit in. For example, as the content of obsessions in BDD are somatic in nature, they would seemingly load with the "Forbidden Thoughts" factor that also includes somatic preoccupations. Similarly, the repetitive behaviors exhibited in TTM, stereotypic movement disorder, skin picking, and Tourette's syndrome should effectively superimpose on the lower-order repetitive cluster found in ASD.

As can be seen, the heterogeneous repetitive behaviors across OCD spectrum disorders can be reduced and more specifically categorized into discrete repetitive domains. Individuals with these disorders, in turn, could be subgrouped accordingly. For example, one individual diagnosed with ASD may predominately engage in self-stimulatory behavior whereas another may primarily experience extreme resistance to trivial changes. The former patient in this example could be reclassified into the lower-order repetitive behaviors subtype, and the latter could be categorized within the higher-order domain. Alternatively, another individual with autism may display symptoms within both dimensions, or may even have a combination of symptoms across dimensions. This is also the case for individuals with other OCD spectrum disorders, who would be classified within the same repetitive clusters. Grouping the diverse repetitive behaviors into homogeneous domains will provide future research with more statistical power to reveal the unique neurobiological underpinnings associated with each dimension. This will, in turn, inform the development of new treatment approaches, with the ultimate goal of offering patients personalized treatment that will match their unique pattern of symptom dimensions to specific and targeted treatments.

Conclusions

Evidence is converging across multiple disciplines to support the conceptualization of discrete dimensions of repetitive behaviors across OCD spectrum disorders. Importantly, this subtyping appears to reduce heterogeneity in research studies to allow for the identification of OCD spectrum endophenotypes. For example, recent findings have demonstrated that higher-order repetitive behaviors across disorders have familial and genetic linkage, as well as similar neurobiological findings. In contrast, lower-order repetitive behaviors appear not to be influenced by genetics, but rather by neurological insult, including intellectual disability. Hoarding has also manifested as a distinct repetitive dimension across OCD spectrum disorders, with a unique underlying neuropathophysiology.

Challenges and Future Directions

- Future studies that examine repetitive behaviors in OCD spectrum disorders would benefit by using measures that assess the full range of thoughts, actions, and behaviors within this domain. This would allow for a more the precise identification of homogeneous dimensions within the core repetitive behavior domain.

- More interdisciplinary studies are needed to delineate the unique neurobiological underpinnings associated with each repetitive symptom dimension.
- Studies are needed to examine the possibility of a differential treatment response between patients with symptoms that load primarily on one repetitive symptom dimension versus another.

SUGGESTED READINGS

Hollander, E., Kim, S., Braun, A., Simeon, D., & Zohar, J. (2009). Cross-cutting issues and future directions for the OCD spectrum. *Psychiatry Research, 170*(1), 3–6.

Hollander, E., Cartwright, C., & Wong, C. M. (1998). A dimensional approach to the autism spectrum. *CNS Spectrums, 3*(3), 22–39.

Stein, D. J., Denys, D., Gloster, A. T., Hollander, E., Leckman, J. F., Rauch, S. L., et al. (2009). Obsessive-compulsive disorder: Diagnostic and treatment issues. *Psychiatric Clinics of North America, 32*(3), 665–685.

REFERENCES

Abramowitz, J. S., Franklin, M. E., Schwartz, S. A., & Furr, J. M. (2003). Symptom presentation and outcome of cognitive-behavioral therapy for obsessive-compulsive disorder. *Journal of Consulting and Clinical Psychology, 71*(6), 1049–1057.

Abramson, R., Ravan, S., Wright, H., Wieduwilt, K., Wolpert, C., Donnelly, S., et al. (2005). The relationship between restrictive and repetitive behaviors in individuals with autism and obsessive compulsive symptoms in parents. *Child Psychiatry and Human Development, 36*(2), 155–165.

Alsobrook, I. J., Leckman, J. F., Goodman, W. K., Rasmussen, S. A., & Pauls, D. L. (1999). Segregation analysis of obsessive-compulsive disorder using symptom-based factor scores. *American Journal of Medical Genetics, 88*(6), 669–675.

American Psychiatric Association (APA). (1980). *Diagnostic and statistical manual of mental disorders* (3rd ed.). Washington, DC: Author.

American Psychiatric Association. (1987). *Diagnostic and statistical manual of mental disorders* (3rd ed., rev.). Washington, DC: Author.

American Psychiatric Association. (2000). *Diagnostic and statistical manual of mental disorders* (4th ed., text rev.; DSM-IV-TR). Washington, DC: Author.

Anagnostou, E. (2006). fMRI of response inhibition in ASD. *International Meeting for Autism Research.* Montreal, CA.

Barnea-Goraly, N., Kwon, H., Menon, V., Eliez, S., Lotspeich, L., & Reiss, A. L. (2004). White matter structure in autism: preliminary evidence from diffusion tensor imaging. *Biological Psychiatry, 55*(3), 323–326.

Bartz, J. A., & Hollander, E. (2006). Is obsessive-compulsive disorder an anxiety disorder? *Progress in Neuropsychopharmacology and Biological Psychiatry, 30*(3), 338–352.

Berridge, K. C., Aldridge, J. W., Houchard, K. R., & Zhuang, X. (2005). Sequential super-stereotypy of an instinctive fixed action pattern in hyper-dopaminergic mutant mice: a model of obsessive compulsive disorder and Tourette's. *BMC Biology, 3*, 4.

Bienvenu, O. J., Samuels, J. F., Riddle, M. A., Hoehn-Saric, R., Liang, K. Y., Cullen, B. A., et al. (2000). The relationship of obsessive-compulsive disorder to possible spectrum disorders: results from a family study. *Biological Psychiatry, 48*(4), 287–293.

Bishop, S. L., Richler, J., & Lord, C. (2006). Association between restricted and repetitive behaviors and nonverbal IQ in children with autism spectrum disorders. *Child Neuropsychology, 12*(4–5), 247–267.

Bloch, M. H., Landeros-Weisenberger, A., Rosario, M. C., Pittenger, C., & Leckman, J. F. (2008). Meta-analysis of the symptom structure of obsessive-compulsive disorder. *American Journal of Psychiatry, 165*(12), 1532–1542.

Bohne, A., Savage, C. R., Deckersbach, T., Keuthen, N. J., & Wilhelm, S. (2008). Motor inhibition in trichotillomania and obsessive-compulsive disorder. *Journal of Psychiatric Research, 42*(2), 141–150.

Bolton, P. F., Pickles, A., Murphy, M., & Rutter, M. (1998). Autism, affective, and other psychiatric disorders: patterns of familial aggregation. *Psychological Medicine, 28*(2), 385–395.

Brune, C. W., Kim, S. J., Salt, J., Leventhal, B. L., Lord, C., & Cook, E. H., Jr. (2006). 5-HTTLPR genotype-specific phenotype in children and adolescents with autism. *American Journal of Psychiatry, 163*(12), 2148–2156.

Buchsbaum, M. S., Hollander, E., Haznedar, M. M., Tang, C., Spiegel-Cohen, J., Wei, T. C., et al. (2001). Effect of fluoxetine on regional cerebral metabolism in autistic spectrum disorders: a pilot study. *International Journal of Neuropsychopharmacology, 4*(2), 119–125.

Buxbaum, J. D., Silverman, J., Keddache, M., Smith, C. J., Hollander, E., Ramoz, N., et al. (2004). Linkage analysis for autism in a subset families with obsessive-compulsive behaviors: evidence for an autism susceptibility gene on chromosome 1 and further support for susceptibility genes on chromosome 6 and 19. *Molecular Psychiatry, 9*(2), 144–150.

Cantor, R. M., Kono, N., Duvall, J. A., Alvarez-Retuerto, A., Stone, J. L., Alarcon, M., et al. (2005). Replication of autism linkage: fine-mapping peak at 17q21. *American Journal of Human Genetics, 76*(6), 1050–1056.

Catapano, F., Perris, F., Fabrazzo, M., Cioffi, V., Giacco, D., De Santis, V., et al. (2010). Obsessive-compulsive disorder with poor insight: A three-year prospective study. *Progress in Neuropsychopharmacology and Biological Psychiatry, 34(2)*, 323–330.

Chamberlain, S. R., Fineberg, N. A., Blackwell, A. D., Robbins, T. W., & Sahakian, B. J. (2006). Motor inhibition and cognitive flexibility in obsessive-compulsive disorder and trichotillomania. *American Journal of Psychiatry, 163*(7), 1282–1284.

Chamberlain, S. R., Menzies, L. A., Fineberg, N. A., Del Campo, N., Suckling, J., Craig, K., et al. (2008). Grey matter abnormalities in trichotillomania: morphometric magnetic resonance imaging study. *British Journal of Psychiatry, 193*(3), 216–221.

Christenson, G. A., Mackenzie, T. B., & Reeve, E. A. (1992). Familial trichotillomania. *American Journal of Psychiatry, 149*(2), 283.

Conroy, J., Meally, E., Kearney, G., Fitzgerald, M., Gill, M., & Gallagher, L. (2004). Serotonin transporter gene and autism: a haplotype analysis in an Irish autistic population. *Molecular Psychiatry, 9*(6), 587–593.

Cuccaro, M. L., Shao, Y., Grubber, J., Slifer, M., Wolpert, C. M., Donnelly, S. L., et al. (2003). Factor analysis of restricted and repetitive behaviors in autism using the Autism Diagnostic Interview-R. *Child Psychiatry and Human Development, 34*(1), 3–17.

Denys, D., Zohar, J., & Westenberg, H. G. (2004). The role of dopamine in obsessive-compulsive disorder: preclinical and clinical evidence. *Journal of Clinical Psychiatry, 65*(Suppl 14), 11–17.

Devlin, B., Cook, E. H., Jr., Coon, H., Dawson, G., Grigorenko, E. L., McMahon, W., et al. (2005). Autism and the serotonin transporter: the long and short of it. *Molecular Psychiatry, 10*(12), 1110–1116.

Di Giovanni, G., Di Matteo, V., Pierucci, M., Benigno, A., & Esposito, E. (2006). Serotonin involvement in the basal ganglia pathophysiology: could the 5-HT2C receptor be a new target for therapeutic strategies? *Current Medicinal Chemistry, 13*(25), 3069–3081.

do Rosario-Campos, M. C., Leckman, J. F., Curi, M., Quatrano, S., Katsovitch, L., Miguel, E. C., et al. (2005). A family study of early-onset obsessive-compulsive disorder. *American Journal of Medical Genetics. Part B, Neuropsychiatric Genetics, 136B*(1), 92–97.

Eisen, J. L., Phillips, K. A., Coles, M. E., & Rasmussen, S. A. (2004). Insight in obsessive compulsive disorder and body dysmorphic disorder. *Comprehensive Psychiatry, 45*(1), 10–15.

Erzegovesi, S., Cavallini, M. C., Cavedini, P., Diaferia, G., Locatelli, M., & Bellodi, L. (2001). Clinical predictors of drug response in obsessive-compulsive disorder. *Journal of Clinical Psychopharmacology, 21*(5), 488–492.

Esbensen, A. J., Seltzer, M. M., Lam, K. S., & Bodfish, J. W. (2009). Age-related differences in restricted repetitive behaviors in autism spectrum disorders. *Journal of Autism and Developmental Disorders, 39*(1), 57–66.

Fecteau, S., Mottron, L., Berthiaume, C., & Burack, J. A. (2003). Developmental changes of autistic symptoms. *Autism, 7*(3), 255–268.

Ferrao, Y. A., Miguel, E., & Stein, D. J. (2009). Tourette's syndrome, trichotillomania, and obsessive-compulsive disorder: how closely are they related? *Psychiatry Research, 170*(1), 32–42.

Ferrao, Y. A., Shavitt, R. G., Bedin, N. R., de Mathis, M. E., Carlos Lopes, A., Fontenelle, L. F., et al. (2006). Clinical features associated to refractory obsessive-compulsive disorder. *Journal of Affective Disorders, 94*(1–3), 199–209.

Foa, E. B., Kozak, M. J., Goodman, W. K., Hollander, E., Jenike, M. A., & Rasmussen, S. A. (1995). DSM-IV field trial: obsessive-compulsive disorder. *American Journal of Psychiatry, 152*(1), 90–96.

Fombonne, E. (2005). Epidemiology of autistic disorder and other pervasive developmental disorders. *Journal of Clinical Psychiatry, 66*(Suppl 10), 3–8.

Fombonne, E., & Tidmarsh, L. (2003). Epidemiologic data on Asperger disorder. *Child and Adolescent Psychiatric Clinics of North America, 12*(1), 15–21, v–vi.

Fontenelle, L. F., Mendlowicz, M. V., Marques, C., & Versiani, M. (2003). Early- and late-onset obsessive-compulsive disorder in adult patients: an exploratory clinical and therapeutic study. *Journal of Psychiatric Research, 37*(2), 127–133.

Frare, F., Perugi, G., Ruffolo, G., & Toni, C. (2004). Obsessive-compulsive disorder and body dysmorphic disorder: a comparison of clinical features. *European Psychiatry, 19*(5), 292–298.

Ghaziuddin, M., Ghaziuddin, N., & Greden, J. (2002). Depression in persons with autism: implications for research and clinical care. *Journal of Autism and Developmental Disorders, 32*(4), 299–306.

Gordon, C. T., State, R. C., Nelson, J. E., Hamburger, S. D., & Rapoport, J. L. (1993). A double-blind comparison of clomipramine, desipramine, and placebo in the treatment of autistic disorder. *Archives of General Psychiatry, 50*(6), 441–447.

Gunderson, J. G., Shea, M. T., Skodol, A. E., McGlashan, T. H., Morey, L. C., Stout, R. L., et al. (2000). The Collaborative Longitudinal Personality Disorders Study: development, aims, design, and sample characteristics. *Journal of Personality Disorders, 14*(4), 300–315.

Gunstad, J., & Phillips, K. A. (2003). Axis I comorbidity in body dysmorphic disorder. *Comprehensive Psychiatry, 44*(4), 270–276.

Hanna, G. L. (1995). Demographic and clinical features of obsessive-compulsive disorder in children and adolescents. *Journal of the American Academy of Child and Adolescent Psychiatry, 34*(1), 19–27.

Hanna, G. L., Fischer, D. J., Chadha, K. R., Himle, J. A., & Van Etten, M. (2005). Familial and sporadic subtypes of early-onset obsessive-compulsive disorder. *Biological Psychiatry, 57*(8), 895–900.

Haznedar, M. M., Buchsbaum, M. S., Metzger, M., Solimando, A., Spiegel-Cohen, J., & Hollander, E. (1997). Anterior cingulate gyrus volume and glucose metabolism in autistic disorder. *American Journal of Psychiatry, 154*(8), 1047–1050.

Haznedar, M. M., Buchsbaum, M. S., Wei, T. C., Hof, P. R., Cartwright, C., Bienstock, C. A., et al. (2000). Limbic circuitry in patients with autism spectrum disorders studied with positron emission tomography and magnetic resonance imaging. *American Journal of Psychiatry, 157*(12), 1994–2001.

Herbert, M. R., Ziegler, D. A., Deutsch, C. K., O'Brien, L. M., Lange, N., Bakardjiev, A., et al. (2003). Dissociations of cerebral cortex, subcortical and cerebral white matter volumes in autistic boys. *Brain, 126*(Pt 5), 1182–1192.

Hollander, E., Allen, A., Kwon, J., Aronowitz, B., Schmeidler, J., Wong, C., et al. (1999). Clomipramine vs desipramine crossover trial in body dysmorphic disorder: selective efficacy of a serotonin reuptake inhibitor in imagined ugliness. *Archives of General Psychiatry, 56*(11), 1033–1039.

Hollander, E., Anagnostou, E., Chaplin, W., Esposito, K., Haznedar, M. M., Licalzi, E., et al. (2005). Striatal volume on magnetic resonance imaging and repetitive behaviors in autism. *Biological Psychiatry, 58*(3), 226–232.

Hollander, E., Baldini Rossi, N., Sood, E., & Pallanti, S. (2003). Risperidone augmentation in treatment-resistant obsessive-compulsive disorder: a double-blind, placebo-controlled study. *International Journal of Neuropsychopharmacology, 6*(4), 397–401.

Hollander, E., Cartwright, C., Wong, C., DeCaria, C., DelGiudice-Asch, G., Buchsbaum, M., et al. (1998). A dimensional approach to the autism spectrum. *CNS Spectrums, 3*(3), 22–39.

Hollander, E., & Kahn, J. (2003). Review: In obsessive-compulsive disorder, clomipramine may be more effective than selective serotonin reuptake inhibitors after controlling for other factors. *Evidence-Based Mental Health, 6*(1), 23.

Hollander, E., Kim, S., Braun, A., Simeon, D., & Zohar, J. (2009). Cross-cutting issues and future directions for the OCD spectrum. *Psychiatry Research, 170*(1), 3–6.

Hollander, E., King, A., Delaney, K., Smith, C. J., & Silverman, J. M. (2003). Obsessive-compulsive behaviors in parents of multiplex autism families. *Psychiatry Research, 117*(1), 11–16.

Hollander, E., Neville, D., Frenkel, M., Josephson, S., & Liebowitz, M. R. (1992). Body dysmorphic disorder. Diagnostic issues and related disorders. *Psychosomatics, 33*(2), 156–165.

Hollander, E., Novotny, S., Allen, A., Aronowitz, B., Cartwright, C., & DeCaria, C. (2000). The relationship between repetitive behaviors and growth hormone response to sumatriptan challenge in adult autistic disorder. *Neuropsychopharmacology, 22*(2), 163–167.

Hollander, E., Phillips, A., Chaplin, W., Zagursky, K., Novotny, S., Wasserman, S., et al. (2005). A placebo controlled crossover trial of liquid fluoxetine on repetitive behaviors in childhood and adolescent autism. *Neuropsychopharmacology, 30*(3), 582–589.

Hollander, E., Soorya, L., Wasserman, S., Esposito, K., Chaplin, W., & Anagnostou, E. (2006). Divalproex sodium vs. placebo in the treatment of repetitive behaviours in autism spectrum disorder. *International Journal of Neuropsychopharmacology, 9*(2), 209–213.

Hollander, E., Wang, A. T., Braun, A., & Marsh, L. (2009). Neurological considerations: autism and Parkinson's disease. *Psychiatry Research, 170*(1), 43–51.

Kana, R. K., Keller, T. A., Minshew, N. J., & Just, M. A. (2007). Inhibitory control in high-functioning autism: decreased activation and underconnectivity in inhibition networks. *Biological Psychiatry, 62*(3), 198–206.

Kim, S. J., Cox, N., Courchesne, R., Lord, C., Corsello, C., Akshoomoff, N., et al. (2002). Transmission disequilibrium mapping at the serotonin transporter gene (SLC6A4) region in autistic disorder. *Molecular Psychiatry, 7*(3), 278–288.

King, B. H., Hollander, E., Sikich, L., McCracken, J. T., Scahill, L., Bregman, J. D., et al. (2009). Lack of efficacy of citalopram in children with autism spectrum disorders and high levels of repetitive behavior: citalopram ineffective in children with autism. *Archives of General Psychiatry, 66*(6), 583–590.

Lam, K. S., & Aman, M. G. (2007). The Repetitive Behavior Scale-Revised: independent validation in individuals with autism spectrum disorders. *Journal of Autism and Developmental Disorders, 37*(5), 855–866.

Lam, K. S., Bodfish, J. W., & Piven, J. (2008). Evidence for three subtypes of repetitive behavior in autism that differ in familiality and association with other symptoms. *Journal of Child Psychology and Psychiatry, 49*(11), 1193–1200.

LaSalle, V. H., Cromer, K. R., Nelson, K. N., Kazuba, D., Justement, L., & Murphy, D. L. (2004). Diagnostic interview assessed neuropsychiatric disorder comorbidity in 334 individuals with obsessive-compulsive disorder. *Depression and Anxiety, 19*(3), 163–173.

Guroff, J. J. (1992). Rates of Obsessive Compulsive Disorder in first degree relatives of patients with trichotillomania: a research note. *Journal of Child Psychology and Psychiatry, 33*(5), 925–933.

Leonard, H. L., Swedo, S. E., Rapoport, J. L., Koby, E. V., Lenane, M. C., Cheslow, D. L., et al. (1989). Treatment of obsessive-compulsive disorder with clomipramine and desipramine in children and adolescents. A double-blind crossover comparison. *Archives of General Psychiatry, 46*(12), 1088–1092.

Lochner, C., Kinnear, C. J., Hemmings, S. M., Seller, C., Niehaus, D. J., Knowles, J. A., et al. (2005). Hoarding in obsessive-compulsive disorder: clinical and genetic correlates. *Journal of Clinical Psychiatry, 66*(9), 1155–1160.

Lochner, C., Seedat, S., & Stein, D. J. (2009). Chronic hair-pulling: Phenomenology-based subtypes. *Journal of Anxiety Disorders, 24*(2), 196–202

Lopez, B. R., Lincoln, A. J., Ozonoff, S., & Lai, Z. (2005). Examining the relationship between executive functions and restricted, repetitive symptoms of autistic disorder. *Journal of Autism and Developmental Disorders, 35*(4), 445–460.

Mataix-Cols, D., Marks, I. M., Greist, J. H., Kobak, K. A., & Baer, L. (2002). Obsessive-compulsive symptom dimensions as predictors of compliance with and response to behaviour therapy: results from a controlled trial. *Psychotherapy and Psychosomatics, 71*(5), 255–262.

Mataix-Cols, D., Nakatani, E., Micali, N., & Heyman, I. (2008). Structure of obsessive-compulsive symptoms in pediatric OCD. *Journal of the American Academy of Child and Adolescent Psychiatry, 47*(7), 773–778.

Matson, J. L., Hamilton, M., Duncan, D., Bamburg, J., Smiroldo, B., Anderson, S., et al. (1997). Characteristics of stereotypic movement disorder and self-injurious behavior assessed with the Diagnostic Assessment for the Severely Handicapped (DASH-II). *Research in Developmental Disabilities, 18*(6), 457–469.

Matson, J. L., Smiroldo, B. B., & Hastings, T. L. (1998). Validity of the Autism/Pervasive Developmental Disorder subscale of the Diagnostic Assessment for the Severely Handicapped-II. *Journal of Autism and Developmental Disorders, 28*(1), 77–81.

McCauley, J. L., Olson, L. M., Dowd, M., Amin, T., Steele, A., Blakely, R. D., et al. (2004). Linkage and association analysis at the serotonin transporter (SLC6A4) locus in a rigid-compulsive subset of autism. *American Journal of Medical Genetics. Part B, Neuropsychiatric Genetics, 127*(1), 104–112.

McCracken J. T., McGough, J., Shah, B., et al, for Research Units on Pediatric Psychopharmacology Autism Network (2002). Risperidone in children with autism and serious behavioral problems. *New England Journal of Medicine, 347*, 314–332.

McDougle, C. J., Kresch, L. E., Goodman, W. K., Naylor, S. T., Volkmar, F. R., Cohen, D. J., et al. (1995). A case-controlled study of repetitive thoughts and behavior in adults with autistic disorder and obsessive-compulsive disorder. *American Journal of Psychiatry, 152*(5), 772–777.

McDougle, C. J., Krystal, J. H., Price, L. H., Heninger, G. R., & Charney, D. S. (1995). Noradrenergic response to acute ethanol administration in healthy subjects: comparison with intravenous yohimbine. *Psychopharmacology (Berl), 118*(2), 127–135.

McDougle, C. J., Naylor, S. T., Cohen, D. J., Volkmar, F. R., Heninger, G. R., & Price, L. H. (1996). A double-blind, placebo-controlled study of fluvoxamine in adults with autistic disorder. *Archives of General Psychiatry, 53*(11), 1001–1008.

McKay, D., Neziroglu, F., & Yaryura-Tobias, J. A. (1997). Comparison of clinical characteristics in obsessive-compulsive disorder and body dysmorphic disorder. *Journal of Anxiety Disorders, 11*(4), 447–454.

Micali, N., Chakrabarti, S., & Fombonne, E. (2004). The broad autism phenotype: findings from an epidemiological survey. *Autism, 8*(1), 21–37.

Militerni, R., Bravaccio, C., Falco, C., Fico, C., & Palermo, M. T. (2002). Repetitive behaviors in autistic disorder. *European Child and Adolescent Psychiatry, 11*(5), 210–218.

Neziroglu, F., Pinto, A., Yaryura-Tobias, J. A., & McKay, D. (2004). Overvalued ideation as a predictor of fluvoxamine response in patients with obsessive-compulsive disorder. *Psychiatry Research, 125*(1), 53–60.

O'Sullivan, R. L., Rauch, S. L., Breiter, H. C., Grachev, I. D., Baer, L., Kennedy, D. N., et al. (1997). Reduced basal ganglia volumes in trichotillomania measured via morphometric magnetic resonance imaging. *Biological Psychiatry, 42*(1), 39–45.

Ohnishi, T., Matsuda, H., Hashimoto, T., Kunihiro, T., Nishikawa, M., Uema, T., et al. (2000). Abnormal regional cerebral blood flow in childhood autism. *Brain, 123*(Pt 9), 1838–1844.

Ozonoff, S., Cook, I., Coon, H., Dawson, G., Joseph, R. M., Klin, A., et al. (2004). Performance on Cambridge Neuropsychological Test Automated Battery subtests sensitive to frontal lobe function in people with autistic disorder: evidence from the Collaborative Programs of Excellence in Autism network. *Journal of Autism and Developmental Disorders, 34*(2), 139–150.

Ozonoff, S., Macari, S., Young, G. S., Goldring, S., Thompson, M., & Rogers, S. J. (2008). Atypical object exploration at 12 months of age is associated with autism in a prospective sample. *Autism, 12*(5), 457–472.

Ozonoff, S., Strayer, D. L., McMahon, W. M., & Filloux, F. (1994). Executive function abilities in autism and Tourette syndrome: an information processing approach. *Journal of Child Psychology and Psychiatry, 35*(6), 1015–1032.

Pallanti, S., Bernardi, S., Antonini, S., Singh, N., & Hollander, E. (2009). Ondansetron augmentation in treatment-resistant obsessive-compulsive disorder: a preliminary, single-blind, prospective study. *CNS Drugs, 23*(12), 1047–1055.

Pertusa, A., Fullana, M. A., Singh, S., Alonso, P., Menchon, J. M., & Mataix-Cols, D. (2008). Compulsive hoarding: OCD symptom, distinct clinical syndrome, or both? *American Journal of Psychiatry, 165*(10), 1289–1298.

Peterson, B. S., Thomas, P., Kane, M. J., Scahill, L., Zhang, H., Bronen, R., et al. (2003). Basal ganglia volumes in patients with Gilles de la Tourette syndrome. *Archives of General Psychiatry, 60*(4), 415–424.

Phillips, K. A. (1996). Body dysmorphic disorder: diagnosis and treatment of imagined ugliness. *Journal of Clinical Psychiatry, 57*(Suppl 8), 61–64; discussion 65.

Phillips, K. A., Pinto, A., Menard, W., Eisen, J. L., Mancebo, M., & Rasmussen, S. A. (2007). Obsessive-compulsive disorder versus body dysmorphic disorder: a comparison study of two possibly related disorders. *Depression and Anxiety, 24*(6), 399–409.

Piven, J., Harper, J., Palmer, P., & Arndt, S. (1996). Course of behavioral change in autism: a retrospective study of high-IQ adolescents and adults. *Journal of the American Academy of Child and Adolescent Psychiatry, 35*(4), 523–529.

Raffin, A. L., Guimaraes Fachel, J. M., Ferrao, Y. A., Pasquoto de Souza, F., & Cordioli, A. V. (2009). Predictors of response to group cognitive-behavioral therapy in the treatment of obsessive-compulsive disorder. *European Psychiatry, 24*(5), 297–306.

Rasmussen, S. A., & Eisen, J. L. (1992). The epidemiology and clinical features of obsessive compulsive disorder. *Psychiatric Clinics of North America, 15*(4), 743–758.

Risch, N., Spiker, D., Lotspeich, L., Nouri, N., Hinds, D., Hallmayer, J., et al. (1999). A genomic screen of autism: evidence for a multilocus etiology. *American Journal of Human Genetics, 65*(2), 493–507.

Russell, A. J., Mataix-Cols, D., Anson, M., & Murphy, D. G. (2005). Obsessions and compulsions in Asperger syndrome and high-functioning autism. *British Journal of Psychiatry, 186*, 525–528.

Samuels, J., Bienvenu, O. J., III, Riddle, M. A., Cullen, B. A., Grados, M. A., Liang, K. Y., et al. (2002). Hoarding in obsessive compulsive disorder: results from a case-control study. *Behaviour Research and Therapy, 40*(5), 517–528.

Samuels, J., Nestadt, G., Bienvenu, O. J., Costa, P. T., Jr., Riddle, M. A., Liang, K. Y., et al. (2000). Personality disorders and normal personality dimensions in obsessive-compulsive disorder. *British Journal of Psychiatry, 177*, 457–462.

Saxena, S., Brody, A. L., Maidment, K. M., Smith, E. C., Zohrabi, N., Katz, E., et al. (2004). Cerebral glucose metabolism in obsessive-compulsive hoarding. *American Journal of Psychiatry, 161*(6), 1038–1048.

Scarone, S., Colombo, C., Livian, S., Abbruzzese, M., Ronchi, P., Locatelli, M., et al. (1992). Increased right caudate nucleus size in obsessive-compulsive disorder: detection with magnetic resonance imaging. *Psychiatry Research, 45*(2), 115–121.

Sears, L. L., Vest, C., Mohamed, S., Bailey, J., Ranson, B. J., & Piven, J. (1999). An MRI study of the basal ganglia in autism. *Progress in Neuropsychopharmacology and Biological Psychiatry, 23*(4), 613–624.

Seltzer, M. M., Krauss, M. W., Shattuck, P. T., Orsmond, G., Swe, A., & Lord, C. (2003). The symptoms of autism spectrum disorders in adolescence and adulthood. *Journal of Autism and Developmental Disorders, 33*(6), 565–581.

Shafritz, K. M., Dichter, G. S., Baranek, G. T., & Belger, A. (2008). The neural circuitry mediating shifts in behavioral response and cognitive set in autism. *Biological Psychiatry, 63*(10), 974–980.

Shao, Y., Cuccaro, M. L., Hauser, E. R., Raiford, K. L., Menold, M. M., Wolpert, C. M., et al. (2003). Fine mapping of autistic disorder to chromosome 15q11-q13 by use of phenotypic subtypes. *American Journal of Human Genetics, 72*(3), 539–548.

Shetti, C. N., Reddy, Y. C., Kandavel, T., Kashyap, K., Singisetti, S., Hiremath, A. S., et al. (2005). Clinical predictors of drug nonresponse in obsessive-compulsive disorder. *Journal of Clinical Psychiatry, 66*(12), 1517–1523.

Silverman, J. M., Buxbaum, J. D., Ramoz, N., Reichenberg, A., Hollander, E., Schmeidler, J., et al. (2008). Autism related routines and rituals associated with a mitochondrial aspartate/glutamate carrier polymorphism. *American Journal of Medical Genetics. Part B, Neuropsychiatric Genetics, 147*(3), 408–410.

Silverman, J. M., Smith, C. J., Schmeidler, J., Hollander, E., Lawlor, B. A., Fitzgerald, M., et al. (2002). Symptom domains in autism and related conditions: evidence for familiality. *American Journal of Medical Genetics, 114*(1), 64–73.

Skodol, A. E., Oldham, J. M., Hyler, S. E., Stein, D. J., Hollander, E., Gallaher, P. E., et al. (1995). Patterns of anxiety and personality disorder comorbidity. *Journal of Psychiatric Research, 29*(5), 361–374.

Sobin, C., Blundell, M. L., & Karayiorgou, M. (2000). Phenotypic differences in early- and late-onset obsessive-compulsive disorder. *Comprehensive Psychiatry, 41*(5), 373–379.

Soorya, L., Kiarashi, J., & Hollander, E. (2008). Psychopharmacologic interventions for repetitive behaviors in autism spectrum disorders. *Child and Adolescent Psychiatric Clinics of North America, 17*(4), 753–771, viii.

Stanley, M. A., Hannay, H. J., & Breckenridge, J. K. (1997). The neuropsychology of trichotillomania. *Journal of Anxiety Disorders, 11*(5), 473–488.

Stein, D. J., van Heerden, B., Hugo, C., van Kradenburg, J., Warwick, J., Zungu-Dirwayi, N., et al. (2002). Functional brain imaging and pharmacotherapy in trichotillomania. Single photon emission computed tomography before and after treatment with the selective serotonin reuptake inhibitor citalopram. *Progress in Neuropsychopharmacology and Biological Psychiatry, 26*(5), 885–890.

Steingard, R. J., Zimnitzky, B., DeMaso, D. R., Bauman, M. L., & Bucci, J. P. (1997). Sertraline treatment of transition-associated anxiety and agitation in children with autistic disorder. *Journal of Child and Adolescent Psychopharmacology, 7*(1), 9–15.

Sutcliffe, J. S., Delahanty, R. J., Prasad, H. C., McCauley, J. L., Han, Q., Jiang, L., et al. (2005). Allelic heterogeneity at the serotonin transporter locus (SLC6A4) confers susceptibility to autism and rigid-compulsive behaviors. *American Journal of Human Genetics, 77*(2), 265–279.

Swedo, S. E., Leonard, H. L., Rapoport, J. L., Lenane, M. C., Goldberger, E. L., & Cheslow, D. L. (1989). A double-blind comparison of clomipramine and desipramine in the treatment of trichotillomania (hair pulling). *New England Journal of Medicine, 321*(8), 497–501.

Szatmari, P., Georgiades, S., Bryson, S., Zwaigenbaum, L., Roberts, W., Mahoney, W., et al. (2006). Investigating the structure of the restricted, repetitive behaviours and interests domain of autism. *Journal of Child Psychology and Psychiatry, 47*(6), 582–590.

Szeszko, P. R., Ardekani, B. A., Ashtari, M., Malhotra, A. K., Robinson, D. G., Bilder, R. M., et al. (2005). White matter abnormalities in obsessive-compulsive disorder: a diffusion tensor imaging study. *Archives of General Psychiatry, 62*(7), 782–790.

Tolin, D. F., Abramowitz, J. S., Kozak, M. J., & Foa, E. B. (2001). Fixity of belief, perceptual aberration, and magical ideation in obsessive-compulsive disorder. *Journal of Anxiety Disorders, 15*(6), 501–510.

Tukel, R., Ertekin, E., Batmaz, S., Alyanak, F., Sozen, A., Aslantas, B., et al. (2005). Influence of age of onset on clinical features in obsessive-compulsive disorder. *Depression and Anxiety, 21*(3), 112–117.

Turner, M. A. (1999). Generating novel ideas: fluency performance in high-functioning and learning disabled individuals with autism. *Journal of Child Psychology and Psychiatry, 40*(2), 189–201.

Watt, N., Wetherby, A. M., Barber, A., & Morgan, L. (2008). Repetitive and stereotyped behaviors in children with autism spectrum disorders in the second year of life. *Journal of Autism and Developmental Disorders, 38*(8), 1518–1533.

Woods, D. W., Flessner, C. A., Franklin, M. E., Keuthen, N. J., Goodwin, R. D., Stein, D. J., et al. (2006). The Trichotillomania Impact Project (TIP): exploring phenomenology, functional impairment, and treatment utilization. *Journal of Clinical Psychiatry, 67*(12), 1877–1888.

World Health Organization. (2003). *International statistical classification of diseases and related health problems, 10th Revision.* Retrieved from http://www.who.int/classifications/icd/en/ on February 5, 2006.

Yirmiya, N., Pilowsky, T., Nemanov, L., Arbelle, S., Feinsilver, T., Fried, I., et al. (2001). Evidence for an association with the serotonin transporter promoter region polymorphism and autism. *American Journal of Medical Genetics, 105*(4), 381–386.

Zhang, H., Leckman, J. F., Pauls, D. L., Tsai, C. P., Kidd, K. K., & Campos, M. R. (2002). Genomewide scan of hoarding in sib pairs in which both sibs have Gilles de la Tourette syndrome. *American Journal of Human Genetics, 70*(4), 896–904.

Zohar, A. H. (1999). The epidemiology of obsessive-compulsive disorder in children and adolescents. *Child and Adolescent Psychiatric Clinics of North America, 8*(3), 445–460.

17

Suma Jacob, Angeli Landeros-Weisenberger, James F. Leckman

Interface Between Autism Spectrum Disorders and Obsessive-Compulsive Behaviors: A Genetic and Developmental Perspective

Points of Interest

- Autism Spectrum Disorders (ASD) include obsessive-compulsive behaviors (OCB) that partially overlap with obsessive-compulsive disorder (OCD).
- The symptoms that most closely resemble the repetitive behaviors seen in ASD include:
  - Ordering and arranging, counting, doing and redoing often prompted by sensory phenomena urges, or a need to have things feel, look, or sound "just right";
  - Rituals associated with sleep-wake transitions, separation from attachment figures, as well as habits associated with dressing and grooming; and
  - Collecting or hoarding.
- OCB associated with ASD are partially independent of genetic associations with the social disabilities of ASD, suggesting that a different set of genes influence OCB versus social behavioral deficits.
- Several family-genetic studies have indicated that OCD itself may be part of a broader autism disorder phenotype, because there is increased risk of OCD or traits in close family relatives of individuals with autism.
- Many typically developing children display OCB as toddlers and in the preschool age range. These behaviors are also frequently persistent in individuals with genetically determined intellectual disabilities including Fragile X syndrome, Prader-Willi syndrome, and Smith-Magenis syndrome.
- Specific vulnerability genes associated with OCB in ASD have not been identified. Like ASD, OCB are likely to prove to be multidimensional and polygenic. Some of the vulnerability genes may prove to be generalist genes influencing the phenotypic expression of both ASD and OCD, while others will be specific to subcomponents of the ASD phenotype.

Autism Spectrum Disorders (ASD) are severe neurodevelopmental disorders characterized by impairments in reciprocal communication and social interactions, accompanied by restricted interests and/or stereotyped patterns of behaviors (Lord, Cook, et al., 2000; Lord, Leventhal, et al., 2001). The prevalence of ASD is currently estimated to be at least 6 per 1000 children (Yeargin-Allsopp, Rice, et al., 2003; Fombonne, 2005). Family and twin studies indicate that ASD have a strong genetic component (Folstein & Rutter, 1977; Bailey, Le Couteur, et al., 1995; Folstein & Rosen-Sheidley, 2001; Veenstra-VanderWeele & Cook, 2004; Gupta & State, 2007). It is also clear that ASD are etiologically heterogeneous. This heterogeneity can markedly reduce the power of gene-localization methods, including linkage analysis (Zhang & Risch, 1996; Gu, Province, et al., 1998; Alcais & Abel, 1999). Some of the core features of ASD (e.g. phrase speech delay and repetitive behaviors) may themselves be familial traits (Silverman, Smith, et al., 2002; Kolevzon, Smith, et al., 2004; Ronald, Happe, et al., 2006a; Ronald, Viding, et al., 2006b; Freitag, 2007; Yrigollen, Han, et al., 2008) and may thus be useful phenotypes for identifying ASD-related genes.

Obsessive-compulsive behaviors (OCB) are one of the behavioral phenotypes that have shown the greatest promise for identifying different ASD-related phenotypes based on cross-sectional and family-genetic, linkage, and association studies (Bolton, Pickles, et al., 1998; Bejerot, Nylander, et al., 2001; Buxbaum, Silverman, et al., 2004; Bejerot, 2007; Cath, Ran, et al., 2008; Cullen, Samuels, et al., 2008; Ivarsson & Melin, 2008). At the surface, this would naturally lead to questions concerning the heritability of obsessive-compulsive disorder (OCD) and the possibility that some of these behaviors might be shared in common across OCD and ASD. It is clear that twin and family-genetic studies suggest that genetic factors play a role in the transmission and expression of OCD (Pauls, 2008). Although earlier studies have indicated that the vertical transmission of OCD in families is consistent with the effects of a single major autosomal gene (Cavallini, Pasquale, et al., 1999), it is likely that there are a number of vulnerability genes involved. Similar to ASD, etiologic heterogeneity may be reflected in phenotypic variability, making it highly desirable to dissect the OCD, at the level of the phenotype, into valid quantitative heritable components.

Questions are increasingly being raised concerning the degree to which the OCB seen in many individuals with ASD are related to their social difficulties (Mandy & Skuse, 2008). Nevertheless major questions remain concerning the precise nature of the OCB seen in ASD and whether and how closely these behaviors resemble those seen in OCD. We undertake this review with the firm belief that identifying genetic risk factors for ASD, OCB, and related phenotypes and characterizing their role in early brain development will be important in understanding the molecular pathogenesis of ASD, as well as for defining methods for better diagnostics, and developing therapeutic approaches (Abrahams & Geschwind, 2008). In order to achieve this goal, common phenotypic measurements are needed. Consequently, the question of "what phenotype is being evaluated" will be a key focus as we review the available data concerning the broader autism phenotype (Piven, Palmer, et al., 1997; Bolton, Pickles, et al., 1998; Cath, Ran, et al., 2008).

Clinical Phenotypes

A major issue in considering the phenotypic overlap between ASD and OCD concerns the degree to which the behaviors and mental states described as "compulsive" or "obsessional" are really the same across the two sets of disorders. Terms used to describe the OCB seen in ASD include repetitive interests, behaviors, and activities (RIBAs) (Bodfish, Symons, et al., 2000; Charman & Swettenham, 2001; Mandy & Skuse, 2008). Questionnaire, interview, and direct observation data all point to the presence of a range of OCB in ASD that, to some extent, are dependent on the individual's mental age (Table 17-1; Esbensen, Seltzer, et al., 2009). While there are a few overlapping items such as ordering/arranging, collecting, and the need for things to be "just right," it is also clear that the range of repetitive behaviors include some seen in young typically developing children that may persist for a longer period of time in individuals with ASD and OCD.

From the ASD perspective, information collected during formal evaluations using the Autism Diagnostic Interview, Revised (ADI-R), (Lord, Rutter, et al., 1994) provides a sense of what behaviors are typical of some individuals with ASD. For example, Frazier and colleagues (Frazier, Youngstrom, et al., 2008) recently reported the results of both exploratory and confirmatory factor analysis of the ADI-R and confirmed the existence of a Stereotyped Behavior and Restricted Interests factor that includes each of the ratings on the repetitive behavior domain of the ADI-R (R1: circumscribed interests; R2: compulsive routines; R3: stereotyped motor mannerisms; and R4 preoccupation with objects; Table 17-1). A number of other questionnaires and direct observation measures contain similar constructs (Berument, Rutter, et al., 1999; Bodfish, Symons, et al., 2000; Wetherby, Watt, et al., 2007). At present, the most detailed of these scales is the Repetitive Behavior Scale-Revised, which includes 43 items divided into 5 domains (Table 17-1). Of interest, scores in each of these domains are sensitive to both chronological and mental age. The scores in each domain decrease with advancing chronological age and are higher in the presence of intellectual disability (Esbensen, Seltzer, et al., 2009). The slope of the decline with chronological age was steepest for the stereotyped repetitive behaviors and the ritualistic/sameness repetitive behaviors domains.

However, typically developing young children beginning around the second year of life develop a variety of rituals, habits, routines, and preferences, some of which resemble the behaviors associated with ASD and OCD (Evans, Leckman, et al., 1997; Zohar & Felz, 2001). The idea that compulsive ritualistic behaviors may be normative in young children is not new. Gesell and his colleagues (Gesell, 1928; Gesell & Llg, 1943) were among the first to recognize that young children—particularly those around the age of two and a half—begin to establish rigid routines that Gesell termed the "ritualisms of the ritualist." Rather than addressing emotional needs, Gesell believed children engage in rituals to master the tasks of a specific developmental epoch, for instance, matters of feeding, toileting, and dressing. More than 80% of parents report the presence of a bedtime ritual for children by the age of three years. It is less well known that these compulsive ritualistic behaviors manifest in most typically developing children in a regular sequence. After the emergence of a bedtime ritual, the need to arrange things "just right" or in a symmetrical pattern appears, followed by the child's being very concerned with dirt and germs, and finally, the need to collect and store objects. With the exception of hoarding, each of these behaviors peaks at the age of three years. (Evans, Leckman, et al., 1997) Hoarding, in contrast, shows a monotonic increase, at least until the age of six years, when more than 60% of normal children display this trait (Evans, Leckman, et al., 1997; Zohar & Felz, 2001). The earlier the age at which these compulsive behaviors appear, the more advanced the child's developmental level. It is also striking that children with severe intellectual disabilities, including many children with ASD whose mental age remains in the low range, show a persistence of many of these obsessive-compulsive behaviors (Evans & Gray, 2000; Greaves, Prince, et al., 2006). From this perspective, one could ask whether the repetitive behaviors seen in some children with ASD are little more than the persistence or increase in severity or frequency of these "normal" repetitive behaviors.

The complex clinical presentation of OCD can be summarized using a few consistent and temporally stable symptom dimensions (Mataix-Cols, Rosario-Campos, et al., 2005). These can be understood as a spectrum of potentially overlapping features that are likely to be continuous with "normal" worries and extend beyond the traditional nosological boundaries of OCD. Although the understanding of the dimensional structure of obsessive-compulsive (OC) symptoms is still imperfect, recent large-scale meta-analysis of data from more than 5,000 individuals provides the clearest picture of the

Table 17–1.
Overlapping phenotypes and assessment tools

Class	Description	Measurement
DSM-IV-TR criteria #3 for Autistic Disorder	Restricted repetitive and stereotyped patterns of behavior, interests, and activities, as manifested by at least one of the following: - Encompassing preoccupation with one or more stereotyped and restricted patterns of interest that is abnormal either in intensity or focus - Apparently inflexible adherence to specific, nonfunctional routines or rituals - Stereotyped and repetitive motor manners (e.g., hand or finger flapping or twisting, or complex whole-body movements) Persistent preoccupation with parts of objects	*Autism Diagnostic Interview-Revised* (Lord et al., 1994) R1. Encompassing preoccupation or circumscribed pattern of interest: circumscribed interests and unusual preoccupations R2. Apparently compulsive adherences to nonfunctional routines or rituals including verbal rituals and compulsions/rituals R3: Stereotyped and repetitive motor mannerisms including hand and finger mannerisms as well as other complex mannerisms R4: Preoccupations with part-objects or nonfunctional elements of materials including the repetitive use of objects and unusual sensory interests *Autism Screening Questionnaire* (Berument et al., 1999): Eight items loaded on a single factor: Repetitive used objects; Unusual sensory interests; Compulsions and rituals; Unusual preoccupations; Use of other's body to communicate; Complex body mannerisms; Unusual attachment to objects; and Circumscribed interests. *Repetitive and Stereotyped Movement (RSM) Scales* (Wetherby & Morgan, 2007) Direct observation: RSM with Body: Flaps; Rubs body; Pats body; and/or Stiffens body parts and postures; RSM with Objects; Restricted preoccupation in intensity or focus with restricted interest; Swipes; Rubs/Squeezes; Rolls/Knocks Over; Rocks/Flips; Spins/Wobbles; insists on sameness or difficulty with change in activity; Collects; Moves/Places; Lines up/Stacks and/or Clutches *Repetitive Behavior Scale-Revised* (RBS-R, Bodfish et al., 2000) Questionnaire completed by parent, teacher, or caregiver, five empirical derived subscales: Stereotyped behavior; Self-injurious behavior; Compulsive "just-right" behavior; Ritualistic/sameness; and Restricted interests
Obsessive-Compulsive Behaviors Within Pervasive Developmental Disorders	Beginning from an obsessive-compulsive symptom perspective, investigators have adapted the "compulsions" portion of the Y-BOCS symptom checklist. The symptoms that most closely resemble the repetitive behaviors seen in ASD include ordering and arranging, counting, doing and redoing often prompted by sensory phenomena urges, and rituals associated with sleep-wake transitions, separation from attachment figures, as well as habits associated with dressing and grooming, ordering and arranging, and collecting	*Children's Yale-Brown Obsessive Compulsive Scale for Pervasive Developmental Disorders* (CY-BOCS-PDD, Scahill et al., 2006) 9 classes of compulsions are included in the CY-BOCS-PDD checklist. The same nine categories are present in the CY-BOCS symptom checklist: Washing/cleaning; Checking; Repeating rituals; Counting compulsions; Ordering/arranging; Hoarding/saving compulsions; Excessive games/superstitious behaviors; Rituals involving other persons; and Miscellaneous compulsions. The content of only two of the CY-BOCS categories were modified for this scale: repeating rituals for the CY-BOCS-PDD includes: "touching in patterns; rocking; Spinning, twirling, pacing; spinning objects; and Echolalia." Likewise, the Miscellaneous Compulsions category for the CY-BOCS-PDD includes: "Repetitive sexual behavior (masturbation, grabbing at crotch)."

(*Continued*)

Table 17–1. (*Contd.*)

Class	Description	Measurement
Classic Obsessive-Compulsive Disorder Behaviors	Obsessive-compulsive disorder is clinically heterogeneous. There are a variety of obsessive-compulsive dimensions that are usually prompted by anxious intrusive thoughts or images or sensory phenomena.	*Children's Yale-Brown Obsessive Compulsive Scale for Pervasive Developmental Disorders* (CY-BOCS-PDD, Scahill1 et al., 1997): This scale is modeled on the original Yale-Brown Obsessive Compulsive Scale (Y-BOCS, Goodman et al., 1989) with 8 categories of obsessions (Contamination obsessions; Aggressive obsessions; Sexual obsessions; Hoarding/saving obsessions; Magical thoughts/superstitious obsessions; Somatic obsessions; Religious obsessions; and Miscellaneous obsessions) and 9 categories of compulsions (see above). *Dimensional Yale-Brown Obsessive Compulsive Scale* (DY-BOCS, Rosario-Campos et al., 2006): This scale specifically rates the severity of obsessive-compulsive (OC) symptoms within multiple symptom dimensions. Although the understanding of the dimensional structure of (OC) symptoms is still imperfect, recent large-scale meta-analysis of data from more than 5,000 individuals provides the clearest picture of data of the interrelationship of these symptom dimensions (Bloch3 et al., in press). The four factors validated by this meta-analysis are included in the DY-BOCS: (Factor I) FORBIDDEN THOUGHTS—Aggressive, sexual, religious, and somatic obsessions and checking compulsions; (Factor II) SYMMETRY—Symmetry obsessions and repeating, ordering, and counting compulsions; (Factor III) CLEANING—Cleaning and contamination; and (Factor IV); HOARDING—Hoarding obsessions and compulsions. The Miscellaneous obsessions and compulsions were not included in these analyses.
Normative Repetitive Behaviors	Mental age–dependent multidimensional rituals associated with sleep-wake transitions, separation from attachment figures, as well as habits associated with dressing and grooming,; ordering and arranging, and collecting. The content of many of these items resembles the symptom dimensions that are commonplace in pediatric-onset as well as adult-onset OCD: worries about harm and separation; ordering and arranging; contamination worries and collecting.	*Childhood Routine Inventory*: (CRI, Evans et al., 1997): 19 items, parental report: Prefer to have things done in a particular order or in a certain way (i.e., is he/she a "perfectionist"?); Very attached to one favorite object? Very concerned with dirt, cleanliness, or nearness? Arrange objects, or perform certain behaviors until they seem "just right" to him/her? Have persistent habits? Line up objects in straight lines or symmetrical patterns? Prefer the same household schedule or routine every day? Act out the same thing over and over in pretend play? Insist on having certain belongings around the house "in their place"? Repeat certain actions over and over? Have strong preferences for certain foods? Like to eat food in a particular way? Seem very aware of, or sensitive to how certain clothes feel? Has a strong preference for wearing (or not wearing) certain articles of clothing? Collect or store objects? Seem very aware of certain details at home (such as flecks of dirt on the floor, imperfections in toys and clothes)? Strongly prefer to stick to one game or activity rather than change to a new one? Make requests or excuses that would enable him/her to postpone going to bed? Prepare for bedtime by engaging in a special activity or routine, or by doing or saying things in a certain order or certain way?

interrelationship of these symptom dimensions (Bloch, Landeros-Weisenberger, Rosario, et al., 2008). The four factors that emerged from this systematic analysis were: (Factor I) Forbidden thoughts—Aggression, sexual, religious, and somatic obsessions and checking compulsions; (Factor II) Symmetry—Symmetry obsessions and repeating, ordering, and counting compulsions; (Factor III) Cleaning—Cleaning and contamination; and (Factor IV) Hoarding—Hoarding obsessions and compulsions. While any of these may be present in individuals with ASD, Factor II is particularly common. This symptom dimension is also one where various sensory phenomena are commonplace. These sensory elements often occur prior to the repetitive movement and include localized tactile and muscle-skeletal sensations that are associated with an urge to perform certain repetitive behaviors; "just-right" perceptions associated with sensory stimuli such as visual, tactile, or auditory; as well as a feeling of incompleteness, which refers to an inner sense of discomfort that can only be relieved by performing the repetitive behaviors (Prado, Rosario, et al., 2008).

Efforts to use the Yale-Brown Obsessive Compulsive Scale (Y-BOCS) in assessing the OCB in ASD began with the work of McDougle and colleagues (McDougle, Kresch, et al., 1995). They recruited 50 ASD subjects (with or without significant intellectual disability) and compared them to 50 age- and sex-matched individuals with OCD. They reported that compared to the OCD group, the ASD patients were significantly less likely to experience thoughts with aggressive, contamination, sexual, religious, or somatic content. With regard to compulsions, cleaning behaviors were less common in the ASD group. However, other compulsions including repetitive ordering; hoarding; touching, tapping, or rubbing; as well as self-damaging or self-mutilating behavior occurred significantly more frequently in the ASD patients.

More recently, Russell and colleagues (Russell, Mataix-Cols, et al., 2005) studied 40 individuals with high-functioning ASD and compared them to a matched group of individuals with OCD. Although the OCD group had higher OC symptom severity ratings, up to 50% of the ASD group reported at least moderate levels of interference with daily functioning from their OC symptoms. Some of the most frequent OC symptoms reported from the Y-BOCS symptom checklist in the high-functioning ASD group included: obsessions of contamination (60%), symmetry (55%), aggressive content (50%), and hoarding (43%); as well as compulsions of checking (60%), cleaning (55%), and repeating (43%). In addition, Cath and colleagues (Cath, Ran, et al., 2008) also used the Y-BOCS to compare a group of individuals with high-functioning ASD with either comorbid OCD or comorbid social anxiety disorder (SAD) to individuals with either OCD or SAD alone and to a group of normal controls. Twelve subjects were in each of the four groups of comorbid ASD, OCD, SAD or control. The factor scores for the four OC symptom dimensions were then compared across the four groups. Although few significant differences were observed, the mean values for all of the OC symptom dimensions were higher in the OCD group and in the ASD comorbid group compared to the SAD and the normal control groups. While this study needs to be replicated with a larger number of subjects in each group and with the addition of a pure ASD contrast group, these findings bring to mind a recent report by Pine and colleagues (Pine, Guyer, et al., 2008) that found that pediatric patients with mood disorders exhibit higher scores on ASD symptom scales than healthy children or children with non-OCD anxiety disorders.

There has also been an effort to adjust the available OCD severity rating scales such as the Children's Yale-Brown Obsessive Compulsive Scale (CY-BOCS) for use in children with ASD (Scahill, McDougle, et al., 2006). This has led to the creation of CY-BOCS modified for pervasive developmental disorders (CY-BOCS-PDD; Table 17-1). Scores on the CYBOCS-PDD only modestly correlated with the repetitive behavior domain of the ADI-R and they also failed to discriminate between measures of repetitive behavior and maladaptive behavior (Scahill, McDougle, et al., 2006). This suggests that these two scales may be measuring partially distinctive traits. Another approach would be to use the Dimensional Yale-Brown Obsessive Compulsive Scale (DY-BOCS; Rosario-Campos, Miguel, et al., 2006). The DY-BOCS separately assesses the clinical severity associated with each OC symptom dimension. The use of this scale in family-genetic, twin, linkage, and association studies would allow investigators to better characterize the nature of the OC traits seen in the relatives of ASD probands.

Neuropsychological Endophenotypes

Yet another approach is to identify potentially informative endophenotypes based on neuropsychological test performance or on brain imaging findings. Ideally, traits identified in this manner would be evident in unaffected family members as well as the probands. One example of this approach is reported by Delorme and his colleagues (Delorme, Gousse, et al., 2007). They administered five tests assessing executive functions (Tower of London, verbal fluency, design fluency, trail making, and association fluency) to 58 unaffected first-degree relatives (parents and siblings) of probands with ASD and 64 unaffected first-degree relatives of individuals with OCD. Only the Tower of London results showed similarities between the ASD relatives and the OCD relatives, suggesting shared executive dysfunction in this domain. There are several endophenotypes of this sort that have recently emerged in OCD. For example, Chamberlain and colleagues (Chamberlain, Menzies, et al., 2008) identified reduced activation of several cortical regions, including the lateral orbitofrontal cortex, in both OCD patients and a matched group of unaffected first-degree relatives, during a reversal learning task. It would be useful to know if a similar result would be seen in the first-degree relatives of ASD probands.

Recently, Bloch and colleagues (Bloch, Landeros-Weisenbergerm, et al., 2008) discovered that as many as half of the pediatric OCD cases have a marked discrepancy between verbal and performance IQ scores. This association of verbal-performance IQ discrepancy and OCD was still significant after adjusting for full-scale IQ, age, and gender and excluding OCD subjects with comorbid ADHD or a tic disorder. This finding is of potential interest given that Williams, Goldstein, et al. (2008) also found a similar profile of lower performance IQ scores relative to verbal IQ scores in 18% to 32% of children with high-functioning ASD.

Evidence for a Familial Relationship Between Autism Spectrum Disorders and Obsessive-Compulsive Behaviors

The advantages and disadvantages to specific approaches to studying the role of genetic factors in ASD are presented in Table 17-2. Figure 17-1 presents the range of genetic and environmental factors that interact over the course of brain development that lead to the emergence of autistic disorder and related OCB phenotypes.

Twin and Family Studies

In 1977, Folstein and Rutter found that while many of the nonautistic co-twins in their ASD twin study did not meet the criteria for autism, they showed ASD traits which in turn sparked a renewed interest in identifying heritable "lesser variants." This finding led, in part, to the initiation of two large studies done more or less in parallel (Bolton, Macdonald, et al., 1994; Piven, Palmer, et al., 1997). The results taken together indicate that the first-degree relatives of individuals with ASD have an increased tendency to show social reticence and communication difficulties as well as an insistence on sameness.

Subsequently, there have been at least three family-genetic studies that have indicated that OCD itself may be part of the "broader autism phenotype." There are data to suggest that the association between ASD and OCD may be strongest in families of individuals on the more severe end of the autism spectrum disorder (i.e., those with autistic disorder), especially those with prominent repetitive behaviors (Bolton, Pickles, et al., 1998; Hollander, King, et al., 2003; Wilcox,

Table 17–2.
Overview of approaches in studying genetics of obsessive-compulsive behaviors and autism spectrum disorders

Study Design & Methods	Advantages	Disadvantages
Family-Twin	Study role of genetic effects (concordance of identical vs. fraternal twin pairs) as well as the shared vs. unique environmental effects	**Rare disorders are harder because more efforts to access large sample sizes**
Family-Trio	Reduces genotyping errors because parents of probands are included, so that maternal vs. paternal transmission can be studied	More laborious for ascertainment; difficult to obtain specimens from parents, especially for later onset disorders
Case-Control	Easy and less expensive to perform with access to larger sample sizes	Matching for many variables is challenging, especially ethnic variation in large or combined samples
Quantitative	May be used for polygenetic disorders and to estimate heritability or strength of genetic influences on particular traits	Limited by assumptions underlying specific modes of inheritance and analytic methods for evaluating multiple genes with small effect sizes
Linkage	Linkage recombination maps allow researchers to locate novel regions or genes by testing for genetic linkage of the already known markers	For complex traits, poor reproducibility (improves with larger samples and a larger number of studies); often there are broad peaks with low resolution (never improves)
Candidate Gene	Testing direct hypotheses for specific genes; focused, less expensive	Limited by known pathophysiologic differences or candidates based on treatment responses. Difficult to find novel genes (given many unknown genes in multigenetic disorders)
Array technology	Can provide information on thousands of targets in a single experiment (e.g., genes, mRNA, CNV, etc.) The possibility of inducing neural pluripotent stem cells from individuals with ASD is particularly exciting	Large numbers of targets relate to computational and statistical challenges
Epigenetic	May provide insight into heritable traits with limited or unclear evidence for DNA sequence variation	Many nongenetic factors may cause the organism's genes to behave differently; limited by studying one of many mechanisms at a time (e.g., methylation)

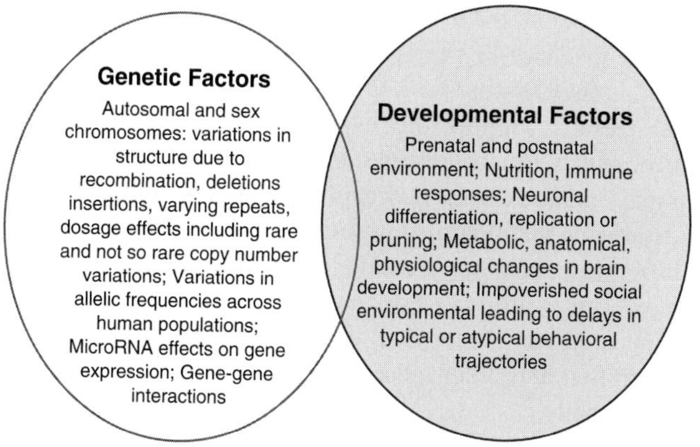

Genetic Factors
Autosomal and sex chromosomes: variations in structure due to recombination, deletions insertions, varying repeats, dosage effects including rare and not so rare copy number variations; Variations in allelic frequencies across human populations; MicroRNA effects on gene expression; Gene-gene interactions

Developmental Factors
Prenatal and postnatal environment; Nutrition, Immune responses; Neuronal differentiation, replication or pruning; Metabolic, anatomical, physiological changes in brain development; Impoverished social environmental leading to delays in typical or atypical behavioral trajectories

Figure 17–1. Developmental and genetic variables and their interaction influence the emergence of obsessive-compulsive behaviors in individuals with autism spectrum disorders. Both genes and events affecting the course of brain development can influence the emergence of autism spectrum disorders (ASD) and obsessive-compulsive behaviors (OCB). Some genes may also influence an individual's exposure to risk (and protective) environments. There is also a growing body of evidence on the importance of gene–environment interactions (G × E) in relation to ASD and obsessive-compulsive disorder such that even adverse experiences might have a negligible effect in the absence of relevant susceptibility genes and yet have a very large effect in the presence of such genes.

Tsuang, et al., 2003). Specifically, Bolton and colleagues (Bolton, Pickles, et al., 1998) studied the pattern of familial aggregation of psychiatric disorders in relatives of 99 autistic and 36 Down syndrome probands and found that motor tics, OCD, and affective disorders were significantly more common in relatives of autistic probands. Those relatives with OCD were also more likely to exhibit autistic-like social and communication impairments. Subsequently, Wilcox, Tsuang, et al. (2003) interviewed 300 family members of autistic probands (120 first-degree, 150 second-degree, and 30 third-degree relatives). In addition, they interviewed 290 family members of probands with more broadly defined pervasive developmental disorders (PDD; 121 first-degree, 139 second-degree, and 30 third-degree relatives) and 310 family members of a healthy control group (123 first-degree, 149 second-degree, and 38 third-degree relatives). They found a significant concentration of psychiatric disorders, primarily OCD and other anxiety disorders, in just the relatives of the autistic probands. The degree of mental illness in the families of autistic probands was more than five times higher than in either the PDD contrast group ($x^2 = 8.45$, $p < 0.001$) or the healthy control group ($x^2 = 9.58$, $p < 0.001$).

The finding that OCD was largely seen in the families of probands with autistic disorder is striking and requires replication, particularly in light of the following findings reported by Hollander and colleagues (Hollander, King, et al., 2003). They evaluated the parents of autistic disorder probands with high vs. low rates of repetitive behaviors as measured by scores on R1 and R2 subscales of the ADI-R (Table 17-1). They found that children who had high total scores on the repetitive behavior domain of the ADI-R were significantly more likely, by a factor greater than 3, to have one or both parents with OC traits or OCD compared with children who had low total scores in this domain ($x^2 = 4.70$, $p = 0.03$). This was especially true of the fathers, 27% of whom met criteria for OCD as opposed to just 7% of the mothers. In future studies, it will be of interest to examine the OC symptom dimensions that are the most prominent in these fathers. Our prediction is that OC symptoms associated with ordering, symmetry, counting, doing and redoing, and the need for things to be "just right" would be particularly common. It will also be important to determine if this association was more common among the fathers of children with autism compared to the fathers of children with a development disorder that is not autism.

Quantitative Genetics

Quantitative genetic studies are designed to evaluate the relative strength of genetic and environmental influences on variations of particular traits within a population. In human research, this is most commonly studied using twin and adoptee designs. They are highly dependent on the assumptions underlying the models being used to evaluate the available data and as such, cannot "prove" that a particular model is true. The most that can be said is that a particular model is "consistent with the available data." Another challenge for quantitative genetic studies in autism is that analytic methods for evaluating multiple genes of small effect size, as found in autism, are still in their early stages of development.

In relation to ASD, several quantitative genetic studies have sought to estimate the heritability of ASD-related OCB. Using items from the ADI-R, in a large sample (N = 457) of individuals within 212 multiple affected sibships, Silverman and colleagues (Silverman, Smith, et al., 2002) found evidence that the severity of an autistic person's ASD-related OCB were largely unrelated to their level of social-communication impairment. This finding was supported by a subsequent study from the same group (Kolevzon, Smith, et al., 2004), which compared intrafamilial to interfamilial trait variability to estimate familiality. In a sample of 15 pairs of identical twins and one set of quadruplets, they found no evidence supporting the view that ASD-related OCB were related to their level of social-communication impairment.

Subsequently, investigators (Ronald, Happe, et al., 2005; Ronald, Happe, et al., 2006a) completed two twin studies that yielded a similar conclusion. First, they gave a questionnaire to parents and teachers of over 3,000 twins, who were part of the Twins Early Development Study, a cohort of twins born in the UK between 1994 and 1996. This questionnaire had 10 items designed to measure possible "social impairments" (social and communication deficits typical of ASD) and six items addressing "nonsocial behaviors relevant to autism."

Only modest correlations between these two scales were found using either the parent data or the teacher data (n = 3,090). In the formal twin analyses looking at additive genetic variance vs. shared and unshared environmental factors, they reported that both traits were highly heritable (62% to 76%), but that the genetic correlation between social impairments and nonsocial behaviors relevant to autism was quite low. This led the authors to predict that "over half of the genes found to be associated with quantitative variation in social behaviors will not be found to be associated with nonsocial behaviors associated with autism." In sum, the available quantitative genetic literature is consistent with the view that the OCB associated with ASD are partially genetically independent of those associated with the social disabilities of ASD.

Linkage Analyses

Although there is considerable evidence for a strong genetic component to the intergenerational vulnerability to develop ASD, several genome-wide screens for susceptibility genes have been carried out with limited success in consistently identifying specific loci. This is likely to reflect the presence of a multiplicity of genes of modest effect as well as phenotypic, genetic, and population diversity. Among the available genome-wide studies, Alarcon and colleagues (2002) were the first to explore the OCB subphenotype. In addition to finding strong quantitative trait locus evidence for age-of-first-word on chromosome 7q, they also reported a smaller broad peak on 7q for restrictive-repetitive behavior phenotype that is considered a distinct locus.

Subsequently, Buxbaum and colleagues (Buxbaum, Silverman, et al., 2004) systematically assessed the value of severe OCB in order to define a more homogeneous subset of individuals with autism. OCB were assessed using the ADI-R (Table 17-1). In the sample with more severe OCB, the strongest evidence for linkage was at the marker D1S1656 (Chromosome 1: 245.1cM) where the multipoint nonparametric linkage (NPL) score was just above 3.00. The authors concluded that their data supported the presence of an ASD susceptibility gene associated with OCB on chromosome 1 and provided modest support for the presence of OCB-related ASD susceptibility genes on chromosomes 6 and 19.

Another study that explicitly sought to identify genetic loci associated with the OCB of ASD was reported by Shao and colleagues (Shao, Cuccaro, et al., 2003). They limited their focus to a specific region on chromosome 15q11-13 and utilized a novel technique called ordered subset analysis (OSA) to ensure a greater degree of sample homogeneity with regard to the OCB associated with ASD ("insistence on sameness" = IS). Individual IS scores were computed by summing a subset of the total items in the "restricted, repetitive, and stereotyped behaviors and interests" domain of the ADI-R items designed to measure this type of OCB. Their analysis of families sharing high scores on the IS factor increased the probability for linkage evidence in the 15q11-q13 region from a logarithm of odds (LOD) score of 1.45 to a LOD score of 4.71. While their results support the hypothesis that the analysis of phenotypicly homogeneous subtypes may be a powerful tool in mapping the disease-susceptibility genes of complex traits, it is notable that this chromosomal region was not one of the chromosomal regions identified in the Buxbaum et al. (2004) study. This is probably explained by the fact that Buxbaum's group used very severe OCB to define a homogeneous subset of families; and Shao focused on subjects with IS to create homogeneity.

Several autism linkage studies have pointed to the 17q region near the serotonin transporter gene (SERT; Stone et al., 2004; Sutcliffe et al., 2005). The highest LOD score for a linkage peak in the 17q11.2 region (where SERT is located) was found when all male affected sibling pairs were considered (Stone et al., 2004), but no similar peak in this region was present when sibling pairs had at least one affected female (Sutcliffe et al., 2005). This suggests that sex differences also need to be considered in studying genetic risk for OCB-related subphenotype.

Candidate Gene Studies

Serotonin Genes

Serotonergic pathways have been consistently implicated in the pathobiology of both ASD and OCD (Pardo & Eberhart, 2007; Goddard, Shekhar, et al., 2008). Several serotonergic genes have been evaluated as candidate genes in both ASD and OCD including SERT (*SLC6A4*), tryphophan hydroxylase (TH2), and *SLC6A4*, the serotonin 5-HT(2B) receptor gene.

SERT, *SLC6A4*

The SERT gene is located on 17q11.1–q12 and is called *SLC6A4* because it belongs to the monoamine transporter family. SERT has 13-14 exons with alternate splicing of exon 1B. It also has a well-characterized functional polymorphism upstream of the coding sequence. The promoter region of SERT contains a polymorphism with "short" and "long" repeats that leads to variation in the levels of gene transcription (McDougle, Epperson, et al., 1998). The long (L) allele consists of 16 copies of a 20-23 base pair repeat unit and the short (S) allele contains 14 copies. In addition to these length variants, there is a single nucleotide polymorphism (SNP) (rs25531, A→G) that changes the functional status of the L allele (Hu, Frank, et al., 2006). Another SNP (rs25532, C→T) also affects gene expression suggesting further categorization of functional variants (Wendland, DeGuzman, et al., 2008). Unrecognized SNP variability related to functional expression may explain some of the contradictory results with combined subgroups when examining disorder association.

Initially, OCD studies reported a family-based association with the L allele in European-American families (McDougle et al., 1998) and that OCD probands were more likely to carry two copies of the long allele or L/L (48% vs. 32%; Bengel, Greenberg, et al., 1999). However, L allele associations were not found with OCD patients of Afrikaner, Mexican, Jewish, German, French, or other descent (Frisch, Michaelovsky, et al., 2000; Camarena, Rinetti, et al., 2001; Di Bella, Erzegovesi, et al., 2002; Chabane, Millet, et al., 2004; Walitza, Wewetzer, et al., 2004; Bloch, Landeros-Weisenberger, Sen, et al., 2008). There was no overall association in a Korean sample, but there was a very low percentage of L/L genotypes, and the L/L group combined with the S/L group had higher scores for religious/somatic-related symptoms on the Y-BOCS (Kim, Lee, et al., 2005). Population differences of polymorphism frequencies, SNP variability, how polymorphisms are grouped or combined, and sample ascertainment or phenotype variability contribute to the complexity of the possible association of SERT polymorphisms and OCD.

SERT polymorphism studies in ASD have also yielded complex and mixed results that are likely due to phenotypic and ethnic heterogeneity. There have been reports of increased occurrence of the S allele variant in an American ASD sample (Cook, Courchesne, et al., 1997) and the tendency for the L variant in a German sample (Klauck, Poustka, et al., 1997). Although there are some population specific replications (Devlin et al., 2005), the range of mixed results reported in the literature likely reflects methodological and sample differences.

A few studies have focused on subphenotypes of ASD that include OCB. For example, a Dutch group found that the 12/12 long allele genotype of Intron 2 VNTR had the highest severity of OCB (Mulder, Anderson, et al., 2005). They did not find significant differences between L or S SERT polymorphisms. In an independent American sample (Brune, Kim, et al., 2006), there were no significant subphenotype relationships with the Intron 2 VNTR genotypes but there was an L/L genotype association with the stereotyped and repetitive motor mannerisms subdomain of the ADI-R. Sutcliffe and collaborators reported that the presence of novel SERT variants, including Gly56Ala, Ile425Leu, and Leu550Val, was correlated with high scores on OCB items of the ADI-R scale (Sutcliffe, Delahanty, et al., 2005). This study illustrates the importance of looking for rare versus common variants.

Indeed, it has been suggested that rare gene variants associated with OCD phenotypes may be found in up to 2% of OCD cases (Wendland, DeGuzman, et al., 2008) and as many as 10% of cases of ASD (Freitag, 2007). Examining rare variants is an alternative method to the broader scale genome-wide evaluations which seek to find common variants accounting for common diseases. In both ASD and OCD it seems possible that uncommon, relatively highly penetrant functional variants may more directly contribute to these relatively common diseases.

For example, the SERT Ileu425Val was originally found in six individuals with OCD (two of whom also had Asperger's disorder) within two unrelated families among 112 OCD probands (Ozaki, Goldman, et al., 2003; Wendland, DeGuzman, et al., 2008). The total frequency of SERT Ileu425Val in all populations that have been genotyped (3155 individuals) is 0.61%. It is a hypermorphic mutation, which produces a gain of SERT function (Prasad, Zhu, et al., 2005). SERT Ileu425Val was reported in a male sibling pair, both of whom had ASD (Sutcliffe, Delahanty, et al., 2005). Because it was also present in the probands' unaffected mother and three sisters but not their unaffected brother, Sutcliffe and colleagues suggested that this might be due to a male-biased genetic risk for ASD. This group also reported 19 other SERT variants (four coding, and 15 in 50 and intronic regions) and examined their association with rigid-compulsive traits in their ASD sample (Sutcliffe et al., 2005). Wendland and colleagues summarized that Ileu425Val has been identified in 15 clinically evaluated individuals, including nine with OCD and one with obsessive compulsive personality disorder from five families out of a total OCD sample of 530 probands/families (Wendland, DeGuzman, et al., 2008). Of the 14 cases where SERT was also genotyped, it is important to note that Ileu425Val occurred together with the L allele or LL (or L_AL_A) genotype. Looking over all diagnoses in this rare variant sample, social dysfunction disorders such as ASD and social phobia were present in 5/8 men but only 1/6 women, suggesting sex differences of clinical phenotype.

Tryptophan Hydroxylase *(TPH2)*

The *TPH2* gene has been studied in ASD and OCD because it is the rate-limiting enzyme responsible for 5-HT synthesis in the brain. Coon and colleagues reported a possible association between the *TPH2* gene and two SNP variants (rs4341581 in intron 1 and rs11179000 in intron 4) in ASD, especially in patients reported to have more severe repetitive and stereotyped behaviors (Coon, Dunn, et al., 2005). Similarly, Mössner and colleagues studied *TPH2* and found two common SNPs in a different region of the gene (rs4570625 and rs4565946 in intron 2) to be associated with childhood onset OCD in a family-based sample of 71 trios (Mossner, Walitza, et al., 2006). More recent studies have failed to replicate these initial studies of *TPH2* and OCD association. When rs4341581, rs11179000, and a different set of eight SNPs were selected to cover the 95 kb region of the *TPH2* gene and tested in a large cohort of 352 families with ASD, no significant associations in the overall group or in any clinically defined subsets of families with either severe OCB or self-stimulatory behaviors were found (Ramoz, Cai, et al., 2006). On a larger, independent sample of Italian and American probands with ASD, *TPH2* alleles and haplotypes were not significantly associated with the overall sample, with repetitive and stereotyped behavior measures, and with endophenotypic analyses for 5-HT blood levels, cranial circumference, and urinary peptide excretion rates (Sacco, Papaleo, et al., 2007).

5-HT(2B) Receptor Gene

Given that atypical antipsychotics are sometimes successful in augmenting OCD treatment with SSRIs, the 5HT(2B) receptor is a potential candidate for involvement in the neurobiology of OCD. 5HT(2B) is located on chromosome 2q36-37.1, and the 2q region was implicated in a genome scan with 56 individuals from seven families with multiplex pediatric probands (Hanna, Veenstra-VanderWeele, et al., 2002). DNA from probands from these seven families, along with 10 unrelated control subjects and 10 unrelated ASD probands, were studied, but no evidence for a functional mutation was found.

Glutamate Genes

The glutamatergic system has been implicated in the neurobiology of both ASD and OCD (Bhattacharyya & Chakraborty, 2007; Pardo & Eberhart, 2007; Pittenger, Kelmendi, et al., 2008). A majority of studies have examined the role of a high affinity glutamate transporter and several of the glutamate receptors.

SLC1A1

The *SLC1A1* gene is located on chromosome 9p24 and belongs to the monoamine transporter family as a neuronal glutamate transporter expressed in the brain. Similar to SERT, the glutamate transporter is important for the excitatory actions of glutamate and for maintaining extracellular concentrations within a normal range. The chromosomal region of *SLC1A1* showed suggestive linkage in a genome-wide scan of seven, large extended pedigrees of probands with early onset OCD (Hanna, Veenstra-VanderWeele, et al., 2002) and linkage in 42 pedigrees with early onset OCD (Willour, Yao Shugart, et al., 2004). In addition, three studies have reported an association between markers at *SLC1A1* and independent OCD samples (Arnold, Sicard, et al., 2006; Dickel, Veenstra-VanderWeele, et al., 2007; Stewart, Fagerness, et al., 2007). In a collaborative autism genome-wide linkage project, *SLC1A1* was identified as a candidate gene because it fell close to the linkage peak at 9p24.1 that occurred in families with female probands with ASD (Szatmari, Paterson, et al., 2007). Brune and colleagues tested three SNPS (rs301430, rs301979, rs301434) previously associated with OCD and looked for haplotype associations in 86 strictly defined trios with ASD (Brune, Kim, et al., 2006). In males only, Family-Based Association Tests showed nominally significant associations between ASD and rs301979 as well as the rs301430–rs301979 haplotype under a recessive model.

Glutamate Receptor Genes

The glutamate receptor 6 gene (*GRIK2* or *GLUR6*) plays a role in synaptic transmission related to learning a memory. It became a candidate gene after studies indicated chromosome 6q21 as a region linked to ASD (Philippe, Martinez, et al., 1999; Jamain, Betancur, et al., 2002). *GRIK2* is a member of the ionotropic kainate receptor family that is expressed during brain development. Although some studies have reported that markers within *GRIK2* are associated with ASD (Jamain, Betancur, et al., 2002; Shuang, Liu, et al., 2004; Kim, Kim, et al., 2007), these same markers do not replicate in all ethnic populations (Dutta, Das, et al., 2007). In a study of *GRIK2* with 156 OCD probands of European descent, the I867 allele on exon 16 was transmitted less often than expected (Delorme, Krebs, et al., 2004). Future research needs to examine subgroups of ASD with more severe OCB as well as to examine the genetics of other genes within the glutaminergic pathway. For example, mRNA levels of several genes in the glutamate system (including *SLC1A3*, glutamate receptor AMPA1, and glutamate receptor binding proteins) were abnormal in brain samples of 10 individuals with ASD as compared with 23 matched controls (Purcell, Jeon, et al., 2001).

GABA Receptor Genes

GABA is the main inhibitory neurotransmitter in the human brain and it binds to two distinct receptor types: the ionotrophic $GABA_A$ and $GABA_C$ receptors with Cl^- channels and fast synaptic transmission, or the metabotrophic GABA type B ($GABA_B$) G-coupled protein for prolonged inhibitory signals. Three $GABA_A$ receptor genes (*GABRB3*, *GABRA5*, and *GABRG3*) are located in the 15q11-q13 chromosomal region. Several studies have shown linkage to markers near or within *GABRB3* to be associated ASD (Cook, Courchesne, et al., 1997; Philippe, Martinez, et al., 1999; Martin, Menold, et al., 2000; Buxbaum, Silverman, et al., 2002; Shao, Cuccaro, et al., 2003; McCauley, Olson, et al., 2004; Curran, Roberts, et al., 2005; Kim, Kim, et al., 2007), although other studies have failed to replicate this association (Maestrini, Lai, et al., 1999; Salmon, Hallmayer, et al., 1999; Tochigi, Kato, et al., 2007). Recently, Kim and colleagues examined SNPs within the 15q11-q13 for association with specific restrictive-repetitive behavior phenotypes measured on the ADI-R and ADOS (Kim, Kim, et al., 2007). Among 93 SNPs, 5 SNPs showed nominally significant association, three of five were close in proximity to $GABA_A$, and two of the five near $GABA_A$ showed genotype-phenotype interactions with an ADI-R subdomain related to inflexible language behavior. Only one study has examined $GABA_A$ receptor genes in individuals with OCD (Zai, Arnold, et al., 2005). They reported nominally significant trends toward biased transmission of the -7265A allele and associations with elevated Y-BOCS severity.

Chromosomal Abnormalities Associated with Both ASD and OCB

Prevalence of chromosomal abnormalities in individuals with ASD is estimated between 5% to 10% (Zhao, Leotta, et al., 2007). Here we focus on those chromosomal alterations that have been associated with the presence of OCB.

Fragile X and Other X-linked Syndromes

The most prevalent chromosomal abnormality associated with ASD is Fragile X syndrome (FXS). Molecular testing for the FMR-1 gene is recommended in individuals diagnosed with ASD and probands identified with FXS are excluded from most genetics studies of ASD. The behavioral phenotype of FXS includes OC behaviors as well as stereotypic behavior, gaze aversion, inattention, impulsivity, hyperactivity, hyperarousal, social anxiety, withdrawal, social deficits with peers, abnormalities in communication, and unusual responses to sensory stimuli. The full mutation is described as having more than 200 CGG repeats in the 5' untranslated region of the FMR1 located at Xq27.3 and typically involves an altered pattern of methylation. There is transcriptional silencing of the FMR1 gene and lack of the FMR1 protein called FMRP. Recent studies suggest that some males with the premutation also have social, emotional, and cognitive deficits, although sample sizes are small or clinically referred (Dorn, Mazzocco, et al., 1994; Tassone, Hagerman, et al., 2000; Hagerman & Hagerman, 2002; Aziz, Stathopulu, et al., 2003; Goodlin-Jones, Tassone, et al., 2004; Moore, Daly, et al., 2004).

A study of men and women with the premutation, but without age-related Fragile X–associated tremor/ataxia syndrome (FXTAS), reported higher levels of OC symptoms on the Symptom Checklist-90-R (Hessl, Tassone et al., 2005). In men only, elevated FMR1 mRNA, rather than CGG repeat size or percent of FMRP expression (peripheral lymphocyte immunocytochemistry), was significantly associated with increased OC symptoms and psychotic episodes with and without FXTAS symptoms. An association with elevated FMR1 mRNA and anxiety in women, but only in women with skewed X activation ratio toward active premutation alleles, was also found. Previous studies have shown elevated levels of anxiety and OCB in some females with FXS (Lachiewicz, 1992).

In a recent cytogenetic analysis of 26 patients with OCD, 21% of the peripheral cells of one male patient with OCD were found to have a fragile site at Xq27-q28 (Wang & Kuo, 2003). This was determined to be in the region of FRAXE mutation, a hyperexpansion of the CCG repeat in the 5' untranslated region of the FMR2 gene (Wang & Kuo, 2003). Typically FRAXE is associated with mild or borderline mental retardation ($50 < IQ < 85$; Gecz, 2000). In this patient's family, expansion of FRAXE CCG repeats and methylation cosegregated with OCD in the proband and a speech impairment in a maternal uncle. Unfortunately, the specific OCD symptom presentation in this individual was not reported.

Hendriksen and Vles (2008) also recently reported on the results of a questionnaire study of 351 males with Duchenne muscular dystrophy (DMD). DMD is characterized by progressive proximal muscular dystrophy and is the result of mutations in a very large gene that encodes dystrophin and is located at Xp21.2. In this study, 11 of the subjects were reported to have ASD and of this number three (27%) also had OCD. Unfortunately, no details were provided concerning either the nature of the ASD or OCD symptomatology.

Finally, several other studies involving individuals with other X-chromosome abnormalities have suggested a link between ASD and OCB. For example, El Abd and colleagues (1999) identified five women with deteriorating social skills as well as attentional problems, impulsive and aggressive behaviors, and prominent OCB. All of these women had a subphenotype of Turner's syndrome with a small, active, early replicating, ring X chromosome and inactive specific transcript (XIST) locus confirmed by fluorescent in situ hybridization. There have been at least eight other cases with similar karyotypes and behavioral-cognitive phenotypes that included intellectual disabilities and developmental delays (El Abd, Patton, et al., 1999). In another case report, a patient with Asperger's syndrome, OCD, and major depression was discovered to have 45X/46XY mosaicism (Fontenelle, Mendlowicz, et al., 2004). An earlier study (Telvi, Lebbar, et al., 1999) reported that two (7%) patients were diagnosed with ASD in a sample of 27 patients with 45X/46XY mosaicism, but the nature and severity of OCB was not assessed.

Prader-Willi Syndrome and Other Disorders Associated with Chromosomal Alterations in the 15q11–q13 Region

Duplications and deletions of genes within this chromosomal region have been associated with both ASD and OCB. Inherited duplications of 15q11-q13 (mostly maternal) have been observed in 1% to 3% of cases of ASD, either as interstitial duplications or supernumerary isodicentric marker chromosomes containing one or two extra copies of this region (Veenstra-VanderWeele & Cook, 2004). If the paternal copy of this region is deleted, Prader-Willi syndrome (PWS) occurs. In contrast, the loss of the maternal copy of this region is associated with Angelman's syndrome. PWS is of interest because the clinical presentation of these individuals frequently includes mild to moderate intellectual disability and social deficits as well as OCB. The OCB include: hoarding of non-food items; ordering/arranging things; requiring symmetry and exactness; preference for daily routines; verbal perseveration or talking too much; the need to know, ask, tell, or rewrite; and repeating rituals with grooming, toileting, or showering (Dykens & Cohen, 1996; Dykens & Roof, 2008). The majority of individuals with PWS have a paternally derived interstitial deletion of 15q11-13, but 25% have maternal uniparental disomy 15 (UPD), and 2% to 5% have imprinting defects (Dykens & Roof, 2008). Recent studies suggest that those with maternal UPD are at greater risk for ASD symptomatology than those with paternal deletions of 15q11-q13 (Milner, Craig, et al., 2005; Dimitropoulos & Schultz, 2007). Although Milner et al. (2005) found no clear differences in OC symptom severity comparing PWS cases due to paternal deletions vs. maternal UPD, Zarcone, Napolitano, et al. (2007) more recently reported that PWS individuals with the long type TI deletion had more compulsions regarding personal cleanliness (i.e., excessive bathing/grooming) while those with the short type TII deletion were more likely to have OC symptoms in the symmetry and ordering domain.

Smith-Magenis Syndrome and Alterations in the Region of 17p11.2

Behavioral issues with patients with duplications of 17(p11.2p11.2) are notable for variable symptoms including expressive language delay, attention problems, hyperactivity, and intellectual disability. A subset of these patients also displays OCB (Potocki, Chen, et al., 2000; Nakamine, Ouchanov, et al., 2008). For example, Nakamine, Ouchanov, et al. (2008) recently described an individual who inherited a 17p(11.2p11.2) duplication de novo on a paternal chromosome and whose clinical presentation included an expressive language delay, ASD, and OCB, whereas another patient inherited the duplication on a maternal chromosome and presented with hyperactivity and OCB (Potocki, Chen, et al., 2000).

Future Directions for OCB and the Broader Phenotype of ASD

In this final section, we point to the need for greater specification of component ASD and OCB phenotypes over the course of development, and then briefly consider a few of the emerging areas of research including the expanded use of genome-wide association studies, the availability of DNA microarrays, the importance of noncoding RNAs, copy number variation, and epigenetic programming.

Greater Specification of Relevant Phenotypes Over the Course of Development

Currently available data suggest that, with rare exceptions, ASD is typically a multidimensional, polygenic disorder in which the effects of individual genes are much smaller than previously thought. It is likely that certain genes will differentially influence the emergence of specific domains of ASD-related behaviors. At the moment, a number of scales have been developed to measure restricted repetitive and stereotyped patterns of behavior. One additional scale, the DY-BOCS, has been developed for use in studies of individuals with OCD. The value of this scale for ASD has not been evaluated. Rating the severity of each of the OC or symptom categories, including the symmetry dimension, in ASD family-genetic, twin, linkage, and association studies would allow investigators to determine whether or not this set of OC symptoms predominates in ASD probands and their relatives.

In any case, additional research is needed to sort out which of the available scales provides the best coverage and how these behaviors correlate, or not, with (1) the social and communicative deficits seen in ASD and/or (2) repetitive behaviors seen in other disorders such as OCD as well as with the repetitive behaviors that are normally seen in typically developing children; as well as to what extent these phenotypes change with advancing chronological age and are influenced by the individual's mental age. When examining subgroupings of OCB in ASD, it has recently been reported that circumscribed interests or insistence on sameness may have a stronger familial relationship whereas stereotypies/repetitive motor behaviors may be related to severity or intellectual disability (Lam et al., 2008). It is important to note that that there were no significant differences in OCB overall and in subgroupings except for repetitive sensory behaviors when 33 pairs of sex-, IQ-, and age-matched children with Asperger's or high-functioning autism were compared (Cuccaro et al., 2007). In addition to questionnaire and interview data, future studies need to collect data acquired by direct observation. Performance on standardized neuropsychological tasks (and perhaps on the associated patterns of brain activation) may also provide valuable endophenotypes for future studies, but this will require testing unaffected (or less affected) family members (Chamberlain, Menzies, et al., 2008).

Gene Array Studies

Given the sequencing of the human genome, it is now possible to monitor expression levels of thousands of genes simultaneously using DNA microarrays. Gene expression profiling of peripheral blood of a small number of ASD patients has led to the preliminary identification of a subset of genes relating to glutamatergic neurotransmission (Purcell, Jeon, et al., 2001). Nishimura and colleagues used microarray analyses to study males with autism with known Fragile X mutation (FMR1-FM) or duplication of 15q11-13 (dup-15q) (Nishimura, Martin, et al., 2007). By comparing mRNA expression profiles in lympoblastoid cells, they identified 68 genes dysregulated in both groups with genetically known causes related to autism phenotype. In search of common molecular pathways, they discovered that the cytoplasmic FMR1 interacting protein 1 (CYFIP1) was upregulated in dup-15q individuals. Using animal neural tissue models, they also showed common regulation of downstream genes JAKMIP1 and GRP155. In addition, they demonstrated that lympoblastoid expression in humans can mirror these animal neural expressions by showing differential expression of JAKMIP1 and GRP155 in male sibling pairs discordant for idiopathic ASD. Thus far, only one of these gene expression studies (Hu, Sarachana, et al., 2009) has incorporated the OCB associated with ASD as a subtype to study (Baron, Tepper, et al., 2006; Hu, Frank, et al., 2006; Gregg, Frank, et al., 2008; Hu, Sarachana, et al., 2009).

Work using DNA microarrays in ASD has begun, but in the future it will permit investigators to use hundreds, or perhaps thousands of genes to assess an individual's genetic vulnerability and to use these sets of genes in research that explores developmental change and continuity, comorbidity with other disorders, as well as gene-gene and gene-environment interactions. We also anticipate that the use of gene expression data will increase as sample sizes grow, and that gene expression information will be better integrated with a greater specification of the relevant phenotypes including OCB associated with ASD.

Perhaps the most exciting development is the capacity to induce pluripotent "stem" cells by reprogramming somatic cells from patients with ASD. This will permit investigators to recapitulate neuronal development in vitro by differentiating neuronal progenitors of various CNS lineages and compare patterns of expression in ASD cell lines vs. those seen in typically developing individuals as well as OCD patients (Gurdon & Melton, 2008).

Noncoding RNAs

Another discovery with far-reaching implications for future genetic research is the importance of noncoding RNAs. MicroRNAs (miRNAs) are short, 20-22 bases, noncoding RNAs that typically suppress translation and destabilize messenger RNAs that bear complementary target sequences. Many miRNAs are expressed in a tissue-specific manner and may contribute to the maintenance of cellular identity. Remarkably, recent studies suggest that tissue-specific miRNAs may function at multiple hierarchical stages within gene regulatory networks, from targeting hundreds of effector genes to controlling the levels of key transcription factors (Makeyev & Maniatis, 2008). This multilevel regulation may permit individual miRNAs to profoundly affect the gene expression program of differentiated cells. It is also possible that specific miRNAs could alter cellular identities.

Copy Number Variation

Genomic microduplications and microdeletions, also known as copy number variants (CNVs) refer to differences in the number of copies of a particular region of DNA within the genome of an individual. Recent reports have suggested the possibility that CNVs play a role in the development of complex disorders including ASD and schizophrenia (Sebat, Lakshmi, et al., 2007). Genomic structural variation is not entirely new to the field of ASD genetics, as chromosomal disorders were among the earliest identified genetic abnormalities associated with ASD phenotypes. The increased resolution of array-based approaches suggests that the proportion of cases attributable to structural variants will be considerably higher than the 6% to 7% identified by standard cytogenetic techniques. CNVs with a potentially large impact on ASD susceptibility include maternal duplication(15)q11-q13, deletion(22)q13-SHANK3, deletion(16)p.11.2, deletion(X)p22-NLGN4, deletion(X)q13-NLGN3, homodeletion(4)q28.3, and PCDH10, and there are more than a dozen CNVs with moderate or mild effects that probably require other genetic (or nongenetic) factors to take the phenotype across the ASD threshold (Cook & Scherer, 2008). Again, it will be critical for investigators to consider the relevant ASD subphenotypes including OCBs as they analyze these formidable data sets.

Epigenetic Programming

Epigenetics is another emerging field of potential promise for understanding the origins of ASD. Epigenetics is a fundamental part of eukaryotic biology. Epigenetic programming involves the modification of DNA and the chromatin proteins that associate with it during key periods of development. Frequently these modifications have enduring effects on gene expression in key brain regions. In addition, some epigenetic alterations can be passed from one generation to the next. For example, there is now compelling data for the presence of developmental windows during which the genetically determined microcircuitry of key limbic–hypothalamic–midbrain structures are susceptible to early environmental influences and that these influences powerfully shape an individual's responsivity to psychosocial stressors and their capacity to parent the next generation (Kaffman & Meaney, 2007). These early environmental influences have been shown to alter the pattern of methylation of the promoter region of the glucocortoid receptor gene in the hippocampus. This epigenetic change stably alters the level of glucocortoid receptor gene expression and hypothalamic-pituitary-adrenal responses to stress. Imprinted genes expressed in the brain are numerous, and it is clear that they play an important role in nervous system development and function. Epigenetic modulations, mediated in part by DNA methylation, RNA-associated silencing, and histone modification, can transform dynamic environmental experiences into altered genomic function and the emergence of stable alterations in phenotypic outcome. Behavioral analyses of rare imprinted disorders, such as Rett syndrome, FXS, PWS, and Angelman's syndrome, will continue to provide insight regarding the phenotypic impact of imprinted genes in the brain, and can be used to guide the study of normal behavior as well as more common, but genetically complex, disorders such as ASD (Zhao, Pak, et al., 2007; Goos & Ragsdale, 2008).

Conclusion

The last three decades of research have demonstrated that ASD is more genetically heterogeneous than initially thought. Important progress toward the understanding of genetic influences in ASD has been made by the combination of family and twin studies, segregation analyses, parametric and nonparametric linkage analyses, and association studies, as well as the study of rare genetic variants. The currently available data suggest that, with few exceptions, ASD is typically a multidimensional, polygenic disorder in which the effects of individual genes are much smaller than previously thought. This implies that in a majority of cases, ASD vulnerability is determined by a multiplicity of genes interacting with specific environmental risk factors over the course of development. One of the relevant phenotypes within the broader ASD phenotype is OCB. Like ASD itself, the etiologies of OCB are likely to prove to be multidimensional and polygenic, and significant progress is being made in assessing the relevant symptom domains (and neuropsychological endophenotypes) and their interrelationship with the family of vulnerability genes that underlie OCD and related disorders.

Challenges and Future Directions

- Challenges include the marked clinical heterogeneity of the autism spectrum disorders (ASD) and the frequent occurrence of obsessive compulsive behaviors (OCB) in very young (2–6 years) typically developing individuals.
- OCB may be an important clinical phenotype within the broader ASD nosological categorization. Like ASD, OCB

may be related to a broad set of disorders and have its own polygenic liability. This highlights the challenge of identifying multiple etiologies across the spectrum of a diagnostic category.

- Methodological challenges of imprecise or varying phenotypic definitions, insufficient power, varying designs, genotyping inconsistencies, and different modes of analyses contribute as well.
- In order to discover molecular and genetic mechanisms, collaborative approaches need to generate shared samples, resources, and novel genomic technologies, as well as more refined phenotypes and innovative statistical approaches.
- At present the most promising area is the induction of pluripotent "stem" cells by reprogramming somatic cells from patients with ASD. This will permit investigators to recapitulate neuronal development in vitro by differentiating neuronal progenitors of various CNS lineages and comparing patterns of expression in ASD cell lines, stratified by the presence and degree of OCB, versus those seen in typically developing individuals.
- There is a growing need to identify the range of molecular pathways involved in OCB related to ASD in order to develop novel treatment interventions. Recent advances in treatment trials with known genetic disorders like Fragile X illustrate the promise of such translational research.

SUGGESTED READINGS

Matson, J. L., & Dempsey, T. (2009). The nature and treatment of compulsions, obsessions, and rituals in people with developmental disabilities. *Research in Developmental Disabilities, 30*(3), 603–611.

Losh, M., Sullivan, P. F., Trembath, D., & Piven, J. (2008). Current developments in the genetics of autism: from phenome to genome. *Journal of Neuropathology and Experimental Neurology, 67*(9), 829–837.

Pauls, D. L. (2008). The genetics of obsessive compulsive disorder: A review of the evidence. *American Journal of Medical Genetics. Part C, Seminars in Medical Genetics, 148C*(2), 133–139.

ACKNOWLEDGMENTS

Portions of the research described in this review were supported by grants from the National Institutes of Health: K23MH082121 (SJ), T32 MH 19126 (AL-W), and K05MH076273 (JFL) and a NARSAD Young Investigator Award (SJ). The authors also gratefully acknowledge Edwin H. Cook Jr.'s, comments on an earlier version of this chapter.

REFERENCES

Abrahams, B. S., & Geschwind, D. H. (2008). Advances in autism genetics: on the threshold of a new neurobiology. *Nature Reviews Genetics, 9*(5), 341–355.

Alarcon, M., Cantor, R. M., Lui, J., Gilliam, T. C., Geschwind, D. H., & Autism Genetic Research Exchange Consortium. (2002). "Evidence for a language quantitative trait locus on chromosome 7q in multiplex autism families." *American Journal of Human Genetics, 70*(1), 60–71.

Alcais, A., & Abel, L. (1999). Maximum-Likelihood-Binomial method for genetic model-free linkage analysis of quantitative traits in sibships. *Genetic Epidemiology, 17*(2), 102–117.

Arnold, P. D., Sicard, T., Burroughs, E., Richter, M. A., & Kennedy, J. L. (2006). Glutamate transporter gene SLC1A1 associated with obsessive-compulsive disorder. *Archives of General Psychiatry, 63*(7), 769–776.

Aziz, M., Stathopulu, E., Callias, M., Taylor, C., Turk, J., Oostra, B., et al. (2003). Clinical features of boys with fragile X premutations and intermediate alleles. *American Journal of Medical Genetics. Part B, Neuropsychiatric Genetics, 121B*(1), 119–127.

Bailey, A., Le Couteur, A., Gottesman, I., Bolton, P., Simonoff, E., Yuzda, E., et al. (1995). Autism as a strongly genetic disorder: evidence from a British twin study. *Psychological Medicine, 25*(1), 63–77.

Baron, C. A., Tepper, C. G., Liu, S. Y., Davis, R. R., Wang, N. J., Schanen, N. C., et al. (2006). Genomic and functional profiling of duplicated chromosome 15 cell lines reveal regulatory alterations in UBE3A-associated ubiquitin-proteasome pathway processes. *Human Molecular Genetics, 15*(6), 853–869.

Bejerot, S. (2007). An autistic dimension: a proposed subtype of obsessive-compulsive disorder. *Autism, 11*(2), 101–110.

Bejerot, S., Nylander, L., & Lindström, E. (2001). Autistic traits in obsessive-compulsive disorder. *Nordic Journal of Psychiatry, 55*(3), 169–176.

Bengel, D., Greenberg, B. D., Corá-Locatelli, G., Altemus, M., Heils, A.,Li, Q., et al. (1999). Association of the serotonin transporter promoter regulatory region polymorphism and obsessive-compulsive disorder. *Molecular Psychiatry, 4*(5), 463–466.

Berument, S. K., Rutter, M., Lord, C., Pickles, A., & Bailey, A. (1999). Autism screening questionnaire: diagnostic validity. *British Journal of Psychiatry: The Journal of Mental Science, 175*, 444–451.

Bhattacharyya, S., & Chakraborty, K. (2007). Glutamatergic dysfunction: Newer targets for anti-obsessional drugs. *Recent Patents on CNS Drug Discovery, 2*(1), 47–55.

Bloch, M. H., Landeros-Weisenberger, A., Rosario, M. C., Pittenger, C., & Leckman, J. F. (2008). Meta-Analysis of the symptom structure of obsessive-compulsive disorder. *American Journal of Psychiatry, 165*(12), 1532–1542.

Bloch, M. H., Landeros-Weisenberger, A., Sen, S., Dombrowski, P., Kelmendi, B., Coric, V., et al. (2008). Association of the serotonin transporter polymorphism and obsessive-compulsive disorder: systematic review. *American Journal of Medical Genetics. Part B, Neuropsychiatric Genetics, 147B*(6), 850–858.

Bodfish, J. W., Symons, F. J., Parker, D. E., & Lewis, M. H. (2000). Varieties of repetitive behavior in autism: comparisons to mental retardation. *Journal of Autism and Developmental Disorders, 30*(3), 237–243.

Bolton, P., Macdonald, H., Pickles, A., Rios, P., Goode, S., Crowson, M., et al. (1994). A case-control family history study of autism. *Journal of Child Psychology and Psychiatry, 35*(5), 877–900.

Bolton, P. F., Pickles, A., Murphy, M., & Rutter, M. (1998). Autism, affective, and other psychiatric disorders: patterns of familial aggregation. *Psychological Medicine, 28*(2), 385–395.

Brune, C. W., Kim, S. J., Salt, J., Leventhal, B. L., Lord, C., & Cook, E. H., Jr. (2006). 5-HTTLPR genotype-specific phenotype in children and adolescents with autism. *American Journal of Psychiatry, 163*(12), 2148–2156.

Buxbaum, J. D., Silverman, J., Keddache, M., Smith, C. J., Hollander, E., Ramoz, N., et al. (2004). Linkage analysis for autism in a subset families with obsessive-compulsive behaviors: evidence for an autism susceptibility gene on chromosome 1 and further support for susceptibility genes on chromosome 6 and 19. *Molecular Psychiatry, 9*(2), 144–150.

Buxbaum, J. D., Silverman, J. M., Smith, C. J, Greenberg, D. A., Kilifarski, M., Reichert, J., et al. (2002). Association between a GABRB3 polymorphism and autism. *Molecular Psychiatry, 7*(3), 311–316.

Camarena, B., Rinetti, G., Cruz, C., Hernández, S., de la Fuente, J. R., & Nicolini, H. (2001). Association study of the serotonin transporter gene polymorphism in obsessive-compulsive disorder. *International Journal of Neuropsychopharmacology, 4*(3), 269–272.

Cath, D. C., Ran, N., Smit, J. H., van Balkom, A. J., & Comijs, H. C. (2008). Symptom overlap between autism spectrum disorder, generalized social anxiety disorder, and obsessive-compulsive disorder in adults: a preliminary case-controlled study. *Psychopathology, 41*(2), 101–110.

Cavallini, M. C., Pasquale, L., Bellodi, L., & Smeraldi, E. (1999). Complex segregation analysis for obsessive compulsive disorder and related disorders. *American Journal of Medical Genetics, 88*(1), 38–43.

Chabane, N., Millet, B., Delorme, R., Lichtermann, D., Mathieu, F., Laplanche, J. L., et al. (2004). Lack of evidence for association between serotonin transporter gene (5-HTTLPR) and obsessive-compulsive disorder by case control and family association study in humans. *Neuroscience Letters, 363*(2), 154–156.

Chamberlain, S. R., Menzies, L., Hampshire, A., Suckling, J., Fineberg, N. A., del Campo, N., et al. (2008). Orbitofrontal dysfunction in patients with obsessive-compulsive disorder and their unaffected relatives. *Science, 321*(5887), 421–422.

Charman, T., & J. Swettenham (2001). The relationship between repetitive behaviours and social impairments in pre-school children with autism: Implications for developmental theory. In: J. Barack, T. Charman, N. Yirmiya, & P. Zelazo (Eds.), *The development of autism: Perspectives from theory and research* (pp. 325–345). Mahwah, NJ: Erlbaum.

Cook, E. H., Jr., Courchesne, R., Lord, C., Cox, N. J., Yan, S., Lincoln, A., et al. (1997). Evidence of linkage between the serotonin transporter and autistic disorder. *Molecular Psychiatry, 2*(3), 247–250.

Cook, E. H., Jr., & Scherer, S.W. (2008). Copy-number variations associated with neuropsychiatric conditions. *Nature, 455*(7215), 919–923.

Coon, H., Dunn, D., Lainhart, J., Miller, J., Hamil, C., Battaglia, A., et al. (2005). Possible association between autism and variants in the brain-expressed tryptophan hydroxylase gene (TPH2). *American Journal of Medical Genetics. Part B, Neuropsychiatric Genetics, 135B*(1), 42–46.

Cullen, B., Samuels, J., Grados, M., Landa, R., Bienvenu, O. J., Liang, K. Y., et al. (2008). Social and communication difficulties and obsessive-compulsive disorder. *Psychopathology, 41*(3), 194–200.

Cuccaro, M. L., Nations, L., Brinkley, J., Abramson, R. K., Wright, H. H., Hall, A., et al. (2007). A comparison of repetitive behaviors in Asperger's disorder and high functioning autism. *Child Psychiatry and Human Development, 37*(4), 347–360.

Curran, S., Roberts, S., Thomas, S., Veltman, M., Browne, J., Medda, E., et al. (2005). An association analysis of microsatellite markers across the Prader-Willi/Angelman critical region on chromosome 15 (q11-13) and autism spectrum disorder. *American Journal of Medical Genetics. Part B, Neuropsychiatric Genetics, 137B*(1), 25–28.

Delorme, R., Gousse, V., Roy, I., Trandafir, A., Mathieu, F., Mouren-Siméoni, M. C., et al. (2007). Shared executive dysfunctions in unaffected relatives of patients with autism and obsessive-compulsive disorder. *European Psychiatry, 22*(1), 32–38.

Delorme, R., Krebs, M. O., Chabane, N., Roy, I., Millet, B., Mouren-Simeoni, M. C., et al. (2004). Frequency and transmission of glutamate receptors GRIK2 and GRIK3 polymorphisms in patients with obsessive compulsive disorder. *Neuroreport, 15*(4), 699–702.

Devlin, B., Cook, E. H., Jr., Coon, H., Dawson, G., Grigorenko, E. L., McMahon, W., et al. (2005). Autism and the serotonin transporter: the long and short of it. *Molecular Psychiatry, 10*(12), 1110–1116.

Di Bella, D., Erzegovesi, S., Cavallini, M. C., & Bellodi, L. (2002). Obsessive-compulsive disorder, 5-HTTLPR polymorphism, and treatment response. *Pharmacogenomics Journal, 2*(3), 176–181.

Dickel, D. E., Veenstra-VanderWeele, J., Bivens, N. C., Wu, X., Fischer, D. J., Van Etten-Lee, M., et al. (2007). Association studies of serotonin system candidate genes in early-onset obsessive-compulsive disorder. *Biological Psychiatry, 61*(3), 322–329.

Dimitropoulos, A., & Schultz, R. T. (2007). Autistic-like symptomatology in Prader-Willi syndrome: a review of recent findings. *Current Psychiatry Reports, 9*(2), 159–164.

Dorn, M. B., Mazzocco, M. M., & Hagerman, R. J. (1994). Behavioral and psychiatric disorders in adult male carriers of fragile X. *Journal of the American Academy of Child and Adolescent Psychiatry, 33*(2), 256–264.

Dutta, S., Das, S., Guhathakurta, S., Sen, B., Sinha, S., Chatterjee, A., et al. (2007). Glutamate receptor 6 gene (GluR6 or GRIK2) polymorphisms in the Indian population: a genetic association study on autism spectrum disorder. *Cellular and Molecular Neurobiology, 27*(8), 1035–1047.

Dykens, E. M., & Cohen, D. J. (1996). Effects of Special Olympics International on social competence in persons with mental retardation. *Journal of the American Academy of Child and Adolescent Psychiatry, 35*(2), 223–229.

Dykens, E. M., & Roof, E. (2008). Behavior in Prader-Willi syndrome: relationship to genetic subtypes and age. *Journal of Child Psychology and Psychiatry, 49*(9), 1001–1008.

El Abd, S., Patton, M. A., Turk, J., Hoe, H., & Howlin, P. (1999). Social, communicational, and behavioral deficits associated with ring X Turner syndrome. *American Journal of Medical Genetics, 88*(5), 510–516.

Esbensen, A. J., Seltzer, M. M., Lam, K. S., Bodfish, J. W. (2009). Age-related differences in restricted repetitive behaviors in autism spectrum disorders. *Journal of Autism and Developmental Disorders* 39(1), 57–66.

Evans, D. W., & Gray, F. L. (2000). Compulsive-like behavior in individuals with Down syndrome: its relation to mental age level, adaptive and maladaptive behavior. *Child Development, 71*(2), 288–300.

Evans, D. W., Leckman, J. F., Carter, A., Reznick, J. S., Henshaw, D., King, R. A., et al. (1997). Ritual, habit, and perfectionism: the prevalence and development of compulsive-like behavior in normal young children. *Child Development, 68*(1), 58–68.

Folstein, S., & Rutter, M. (1977). Infantile autism: a genetic study of 21 twin pairs. *Journal of Child Psychology and Psychiatry, 18*(4), 297–321.

Folstein, S. E., & Rosen-Sheidley, B. (2001). Genetics of autism: complex aetiology for a heterogeneous disorder. *Nature Reviews Genetics, 2*(12), 943–955.

Fombonne, E. (2005). Epidemiology of autistic disorder and other pervasive developmental disorders. *Journal of Clinical Psychiatry, 66*(Suppl 10), 3–8.

Fontenelle, L. F., Mendlowicz, M. V., Bezerra de Menezes, G., dos Santos Martins, R. R., & Versiani, M. (2004). Asperger syndrome, obsessive-compulsive disorder, and major depression in a patient with 45,X/46,XY mosaicism. *Psychopathology, 37*(3), 105–109.

Frazier, T. W., Youngstrom, E. A., Kubu, C. S., Sinclair, L., & Rezai, A. (2008). Exploratory and confirmatory factor analysis of the autism diagnostic interview-revised. *Journal of Autism and Developmental Disorders, 38*(3), 474–480.

Freitag, C. M. (2007). The genetics of autistic disorders and its clinical relevance: a review of the literature. *Molecular Psychiatry, 12*(1), 2–22.

Frisch, A., Michaelovsky, E., Rockah, R., Amir, I., Hermesh, H., Laor, N., et al. (2000). Association between obsessive-compulsive disorder and polymorphisms of genes encoding components of the serotonergic and dopaminergic pathways. *European Neuropsychopharmacology, 10*(3), 205–209.

Gecz, J. (2000). The FMR2 gene, FRAXE, and non-specific X-linked mental retardation: clinical and molecular aspects. *Annals of Human Genetics, 64*(Pt 2), 95–106.

Gesell, A. (1928). *Infancy and human growth.* New York: Macmillan.

Gesell, A., & Llg, F. L. (1943). *Infant and child in the culture of today.* New York: Harper & Row.

Goddard, A. W., Shekhar, A., Whiteman, A. F., & McDougle, C. J. (2008). Serotoninergic mechanisms in the treatment of obsessive-compulsive disorder. *Drug Discovery Today, 13*(7–8), 325–332.

Goodlin-Jones, B. L., Tassone, F., Gane, L. W., & Hagerman, R. J. (2004). Autistic spectrum disorder and the fragile X premutation. *Journal of Developmental and Behavioral Pediatrics, 25*(6), 392–398.

Goos, L. M., & Ragsdale, G. (2008). Genomic imprinting and human psychology: cognition, behavior, and pathology. *Advances in Experimental Medicine and Biology, 626*, 71–88.

Greaves, N., Prince, E., Evans, D. W., & Charman, T. (2006). Repetitive and ritualistic behaviour in children with Prader-Willi syndrome and children with autism. *Journal of Intellectual Disability Research, 50*(Pt 2), 92–100.

Gregg, J. P., Lit, L., Baron, C. A., Hertz-Picciotto, I., Walker, W., Davis, R. A., et al. (2008). Gene expression changes in children with autism. *Genomics, 91*(1), 22–29.

Gu, C., Province, M., Todorov, A., & Rao, D. C. (1998). Meta-analysis methodology for combining non-parametric sibpair linkage results: genetic homogeneity and identical markers. *Genetic Epidemiology, 15*(6), 609–626.

Gupta, A. R., & State, M. W. (2007). Recent advances in the genetics of autism. *Biological Psychiatry, 61*(4), 429–437.

Gurdon, J. B., & Melton, D. A. (2008). Nuclear reprogramming in cells. *Science, 322*(5909), 1811–1815.

Hagerman, R. J., & Hagerman, P. J. (2002). The fragile X premutation: into the phenotypic fold. *Current Opinion in Genetics and Development, 12*(3), 278–283.

Hanna, G. L., Veenstra-VanderWeele, J., Cox, N. J., Boehnke, M., Himle, J. A., Curtis, G. C., et al. (2002). Genome-wide linkage analysis of families with obsessive-compulsive disorder ascertained through pediatric probands. *American Journal of Medical Genetics, 114*(5), 541–552.

Hendriksen, J. G., & Vles J. S. (2008). Neuropsychiatric disorders in males with duchenne muscular dystrophy: frequency rate of attention-deficit hyperactivity disorder (ADHD), autism spectrum disorder, and obsessive–compulsive disorder. *Journal of Child Neurology, 23*(5), 477–481.

Hessl, D., Tassone, F., Loesch, D. Z., Berry-Kravis, E., Leehey, M. A., Gane, L. W., et al. (2005 Nov 5). Abnormal elevation of FMR1 mRNA is associated with psychological symptoms in individuals with the fragile X premutation. *American Journal of Medical Genetics. Part B, Neuropsychiatric Genetics, 139B*(1), 115–121.

Hollander, E., King, A., Delaney, K., Smith, C. J., & Silverman, J. M. (2003). Obsessive-compulsive behaviors in parents of multiplex autism families. *Psychiatry Research, 117*(1), 11–16.

Hu, V. W., Frank, B. C., Heine, S., Lee, N. H., & Quackenbush, J. (2006). Gene expression profiling of lymphoblastoid cell lines from monozygotic twins discordant in severity of autism reveals differential regulation of neurologically relevant genes. *BMC Genomics, 7*, 118.

Hu, V. W., Sarachana, T., Kim, K. S., Nguyen, A., Kulkarni, S., Steinberg, M. E., et al. (2009). Gene expression profiling differentiates autism case-controls and phenotypic variants of autism spectrum disorders: evidence for circadian rhythm dysfunction in severe autism. *Autism Research, 2*(2), 78–97.

Ivarsson, T., & Melin, K. (2008). Autism spectrum traits in children and adolescents with obsessive-compulsive disorder (OCD). *Journal of Anxiety Disorders, 22*(6), 969–978.

Jamain, S., Betancur, C., Quach, H., Philippe, A., Fellous, M., Giros, B., & Paris Autism Research International Sibpair (PARIS) Study. (2002). Linkage and association of the glutamate receptor 6 gene with autism. *Molecular Psychiatry, 7*(3), 302–310.

Kaffman, A., & Meaney, M. J. (2007). Neurodevelopmental sequelae of postnatal maternal care in rodents: clinical and research implications of molecular insights. *Journal of Child Psychology and Psychiatry, 48*(3–4), 224–244.

Kim, S. A., Kim, J. H., Park, M., Cho, I. H., & Yoo, H. J. (2007). Family-based association study between GRIK2 polymorphisms and autism spectrum disorders in the Korean trios. *Neuroscience Research, 58*(3), 332–335.

Kim, S. J., Lee, H. S., & Kim, C. H. (2005). Obsessive-compulsive disorder, factor-analyzed symptom dimensions, and serotonin transporter polymorphism. *Neuropsychobiology, 52*(4), 176–182.

Klauck, S. M., Poustka, F., Benner, A., Lesch, K. P., & Poustka, A. (1997). Serotonin transporter (5-HTT) gene variants associated with autism? *Human Molecular Genetics*, 6(13), 2233–2238.

Kolevzon, A., Smith, C. J., Schmeidler, J., Buxbaum, J. D., & Silverman, J. M. (2004). Familial symptom domains in monozygotic siblings with autism. *American Journal of Medical Genetics. Part B, Neuropsychiatric Genetics, 129B*(1), 76–81.

Lachiewicz, A. M. (1992). Abnormal behaviors of young girls with fragile X syndrome. *American Journal of Medical Genetics, 43*(1–2), 72–77.

Lam, K. S., Bodfish, J. W., & Piven, J. (2008). Evidence for three subtypes of repetitive behavior in autism that differ in familiality and association with other symptoms. *Journal of Child Psychology and Psychiatry, 49*(11), 1193–1200.

Lord, C., Cook, E. H., Jr., Leventhal, B. L., & Amaral, D. G. (2000). Autism spectrum disorders. *Neuron, 28*(2), 355–363.

Lord, C., Leventhal, B. L., & Cook, E. H., Jr. (2001). Quantifying the phenotype in autism spectrum disorders. *American Journal of Medical Genetics, 105*(1), 36–38.

Lord, C., Rutter, M., & Le Couteur, A. (1994). Autism Diagnostic Interview-Revised: a revised version of a diagnostic interview for caregivers of individuals with possible pervasive developmental disorders. *Journal of Autism and Developmental Disorders, 24*(5), 659–685.

Maestrini, E., Lai, C., Marlow, A., Matthews, N., Wallace, S., Bailey, A., et al. (1999). Serotonin transporter (5-HTT) and gamma-aminobutyric acid receptor subunit beta3 (GABRB3) gene polymorphisms are not associated with autism in the IMGSA families. The International Molecular Genetic Study of Autism Consortium. *American Journal of Medical Genetics, 88*(5), 492–496.

Makeyev, E. V., & Maniatis, T. (2008). Multilevel regulation of gene expression by microRNAs. *Science, 319*(5871), 1789–1790.

Mandy, W. P., & Skuse, D. H. (2008). What is the association between the social-communication element of autism and repetitive interests, behaviours, and activities? *Journal of Child Psychology and Psychiatry, 49*(8), 795–808.

Martin, E. R., Menold, M. M., Wolpert, C. M., Bass, M. P., Donnelly, S. L., Ravan, S. A., et al. (2000). Analysis of linkage disequilibrium in gamma-aminobutyric acid receptor subunit genes in autistic disorder. *American Journal of Medical Genetics, 96*(1), 43–48.

Mataix-Cols, D., Rosario-Campos, M. C., & Leckman, J. F. (2005). A multidimensional model of obsessive-compulsive disorder. *American Journal of Psychiatry, 162*(2), 228–238.

McCauley, J. L., Olson, L. M., Delahanty, R., Amin, T., Nurmi, E. L., Organ, E. L., et al. (2004). A linkage disequilibrium map of the 1-Mb 15q12 GABA(A) receptor subunit cluster and association to autism. *American Journal of Medical Genetics. Part B, Neuropsychiatric Genetics, 131B*(1), 51–59.

McDougle, C. J., Epperson, C. N., Price, L. H., & Gelernter, J. (1998). Evidence for linkage disequilibrium between serotonin transporter protein gene (SLC6A4) and obsessive compulsive disorder. *Molecular Psychiatry, 3*(3), 270–273.

McDougle, C. J., Kresch, L. E., Goodman, W. K., Naylor, S. T., Volkmar, F. R., Cohen, D. J., et al. (1995). A case-controlled study of repetitive thoughts and behavior in adults with autistic disorder and obsessive-compulsive disorder. *American Journal of Psychiatry, 152*(5), 772–777.

Milner, K. M., Craig, E. E., Thompson, R. J., Veltman, M. W., Thomas, N. S., Roberts, S., et al. (2005). Prader-Willi syndrome: intellectual abilities and behavioural features by genetic subtype. *Journal of Child Psychology and Psychiatry, 46*(10), 1089–1096.

Moore, C. J., Daly, E. M., Schmitz, N., Tassone, F., Tysoe, C., Hagerman, R. J., et al. (2004). A neuropsychological investigation of male premutation carriers of fragile X syndrome. *Neuropsychologia, 42*(14), 1934–1947.

Mossner, R., Walitza, S., Geller, F., Scherag, A., Gutknecht, L., Jacob, C., et al. (2006). Transmission disequilibrium of polymorphic variants in the tryptophan hydroxylase-2 gene in children and adolescents with obsessive-compulsive disorder. *International Journal of Neuropsychopharmacology, 9*(4), 437–442.

Mulder, E. J., Anderson, G. M., Kema, I. P., Brugman, A. M., Ketelaars, C. E., de Bildt, A., et al. (2005). Serotonin transporter intron 2 polymorphism associated with rigid-compulsive behaviors in Dutch individuals with pervasive developmental disorder. *American Journal of Medical Genetics. Part B, Neuropsychiatric Genetics, 133B*(1), 93–96.

Nakamine, A., Ouchanov, L., Jiménez, P., Manghi, E. R., Esquivel, M., Monge, S., et al. (2008). Duplication of 17(p11.2p11.2) in a male child with autism and severe language delay. *American Journal of Medical Genetics. Part A, 146A*(5), 636–643.

Nishimura, Y., Martin, C. L., Vazquez-Lopez, A., Spence, S. J., Alvarez-Retuerto, A. I., Sigman, M., et al. (2007). Genome-wide expression profiling of lymphoblastoid cell lines distinguishes different forms of autism and reveals shared pathways. *Human Molecular Genetics, 16*(14), 1682–1698.

Gregg, J. P., Lit, L., Baron, C. A., Hertz-Picciotto, I., Walker, W., Davis, R. A., et al. (2008). Gene expression changes in children with autism. *Genomics, 91*, 22–29.

Ozaki, N., Goldman, D., Kaye, W. H., Plotnicov, K., Greenberg, B. D., Lappalainen, J., et al. (2003). Serotonin transporter missense mutation associated with a complex neuropsychiatric phenotype. *Molecular Psychiatry, 8*(11), 933–936.

Pardo, C. A., & Eberhart, C. G. (2007). The neurobiology of autism. *Brain Pathology, 17*(4), 434–447.

Pauls, D. L. (2008). The genetics of obsessive compulsive disorder: a review of the evidence. *American Journal of Medical Genetics. Part C, Seminars in Medical Genetics, 148*(2), 133–139.

Philippe, A., Martinez, M., Guilloud-Bataille, M., Gillberg, C., Rastam, M., Sponheim, E., et al. (1999). Genome-wide scan for autism susceptibility genes. Paris Autism Research International Sibpair Study. *Human Molecular Genetics, 8*(5), 805–812.

Pine, D. S., Guyer, A. E., Goldwin, M., Towbin, K. A., & Leibenluft, E. (2008). Autism spectrum disorder scale scores in pediatric mood and anxiety disorders. *Journal of the American Academy of Child and Adolescent Psychiatry, 47*(6), 652–661.

Pittenger, C., Kelmendi, B., Wasylink, S., Bloch, M. H., & Coric, V. (2008). Riluzole augmentation in treatment-refractory obsessive-compulsive disorder: a series of 13 cases, with long-term follow-up. *Journal of Clinical Psychopharmacology, 28*(3), 363–367.

Piven, J., Palmer, P., Jacobi, D., Childress, D., & Arndt, S. (1997). Broader autism phenotype: evidence from a family history study of multiple-incidence autism families. *American Journal of Psychiatry, 154*(2), 185–190.

Potocki, L., Chen, K. S., Park, S. S., Osterholm, D. E., Withers, M. A., Kimonis, V., et al. (2000). Molecular mechanism for duplication 17p11.2- the homologous recombination reciprocal of the Smith-Magenis microdeletion. *Nature Genetics, 24*(1), 84–87.

Prado, H. S., Rosario, M. C., Lee, J., Hounie, A. G., Shavitt, R. G., & Miguel, E. C. (2008). Sensory phenomena in obsessive-compulsive disorder and tic disorders: a review of the literature. *CNS Spectrums, 13*(5), 425–432.

Prasad, H. C., Zhu, C. B., McCauley, J. L., Samuvel, D. J., Ramamoorthy, S., Shelton, R. C., et al. (2005). Human serotonin transporter variants display altered sensitivity to protein kinase G and p38 mitogen-activated protein kinase. *Proceedings of the National Academy of Sciences of the United States of America, 102*(32), 11545–11550.

Purcell, A. E., Jeon, O. H., Zimmerman, A. W., Blue, M. E., & Pevsner, J. (2001). Postmortem brain abnormalities of the glutamate neurotransmitter system in autism. *Neurology, 57*(9), 1618–1628.

Ramoz, N., Cai, G., Reichert, J. G., Corwin, T. E., Kryzak, L. A., Smith, C. J., et al. (2006). Family-based association study of TPH1 and TPH2 polymorphisms in autism. *American Journal of Medical Genetics. Part B, Neuropsychiatric Genetics, 141B*(8), 861–867.

Ronald, A., Happe, F., Bolton, P., Butcher, L. M., Price, T. S., Wheelwright, S., et al. (2006a). Genetic heterogeneity between the three components of the autism spectrum: a twin study. *Journal of the American Academy of Child and Adolescent Psychiatry, 45*(6), 691–699.

Ronald, A., Happe, F., & Plomin, R. (2005). The genetic relationship between individual differences in social and nonsocial behaviours characteristic of autism. *Developmental Science, 8*(5), 444–458.

Ronald, A., Viding, E., Happé, F., & Plomin, R. (2006b). Individual differences in theory of mind ability in middle childhood and links with verbal ability and autistic traits: a twin study. *Social Neuroscience, 1*(3–4), 412–425.

Rosario-Campos, M. C., Miguel, E. C., Quatrano, S., Chacon, P., Ferrao, Y., Findley, D., et al. (2006). The Dimensional Yale-Brown Obsessive-Compulsive Scale (DY-BOCS), an instrument for assessing obsessive-compulsive symptom dimensions. *Molecular Psychiatry, 11*(5), 495–504.

Russell, A. J., Mataix- Cols, D., Anson, M., & Murphy, D. G. (2005). Obsessions and compulsions in Asperger syndrome and high-functioning autism. *British Journal of Psychiatry: The Journal of Mental Science, 186*, 525–528.

Sacco, R., Papaleo, V., Hager, J., Rousseau, F., Moessner, R., Militerni, R., et al. (2007). Case-control and family-based association studies of candidate genes in autistic disorder and its endophenotypes: TPH2 and GLO1. *BMC Medical Genetics, 8*, 11.

Salmon, B., Hallmayer, J., Rogers, T., Kalaydjieva, L., Petersen, P. B., Nicholas, P., et al. (1999). Absence of linkage and linkage disequilibrium to chromosome 15q11-q13 markers in 139 multiplex families with autism. *American Journal of Medical Genetics, 88*(5), 551–556.

Scahill, L., McDougle, C. J., Williams, S. K., Dimitropoulos, A., Aman, M. G., McCracken, J. T., & Research Units on Pediatric Psychopharmacology Autism Network. (2006). Children's Yale-Brown Obsessive Compulsive Scale modified for pervasive developmental disorders. *Journal of the American Academy of Child and Adolescent Psychiatry, 45*(9), 1114–1123.

Scahill, L., Riddle, M. A., McSwiggin-Hardin, M., Ort, S. I., King R. A., Goodman W. K., et al. (1997). "Children's Yale-Brown Obsessive Compulsive Scale: reliability and validity." *Journal of the American Academy of Child and Adolescent Psychiatry, 36*(6), 844–852.

Sebat, J., Lakshmi, B., Malhotra, D., Troge, J., Lese-Martin, C., Walsh, T., et al. (2007). Strong association of de novo copy number mutations with autism. *Science, 316*(5823), 445–449.

Shao, Y., Cuccaro, M. L., Hauser, E. R., Raiford, K. L., Menold, M. M., Wolpert, C. M., et al. (2003). Fine mapping of autistic disorder to chromosome 15q11-q13 by use of phenotypic subtypes. *American Journal of Human Genetics, 72*(3), 539–548.

Shuang, M., Liu, J., Jia, M. X., Yang, J. Z., Wu, S. P., Gong, X. H., et al. (2004). Family-based association study between autism and glutamate receptor 6 gene in Chinese Han trios. *American Journal of Medical Genetics. Part B, Neuropsychiatric Genetics, 131B*(1), 48–50.

Silverman, J. M., Smith, C. J., Schmeidler, J., Hollander, E., Lawlor, B. A., Fitzgerald, M., & Autism Genetic Research Exchange Consortium. (2002). Symptom domains in autism and related conditions: evidence for familiality. *American Journal of Medical Genetics, 114*(1), 64–73.

Stewart, S. E., Fagerness, J. A., Platko, J., Smoller, J. W., Scharf, J. M., Illmann, C., et al. (2007). Association of the SLC1A1 glutamate transporter gene and obsessive-compulsive disorder. *American Journal of Medical Genetics. Part B, Neuropsychiatric Genetics, 144B*(8), 1027–1033.

Stone, J. L., Merriman, B., Cantor, R. M., Yonan, A. L., Gilliam, T. C., Geschwind, D. H., et al. (2004). Evidence for sex-specific risk alleles in autism spectrum disorder. *American Journal of Human Genetics, 75*(6), 1117–1123.

Sutcliffe, J. S., Delahanty, R. J., Prasad, H. C., McCauley, J. L., Han, Q., Jiang, L., et al. (2005). Allelic heterogeneity at the serotonin transporter locus (SLC6A4) confers susceptibility to autism and rigid-compulsive behaviors. *American Journal of Human Genetics, 77*(2), 265–279.

Szatmari, P., Paterson, A. D., Zwaigenbaum, L., Roberts, W., Brian, J., Liu, X. Q., et al. for The Autism Genome Project Consortium. (2007). Mapping autism risk loci using genetic linkage and chromosomal rearrangements. *Nature Genetics, 39*(3), 319–328.

Tassone, F., Hagerman, R. J., Chamberlain, W. D., & Hagerman, P. J. (2000). Transcription of the FMR1 gene in individuals with fragile X syndrome. *American Journal of Medical Genetics, 97*(3), 195–203.

Telvi, L., Lebbar, A., Del Pino, O., Barbet, J. P., & Chaussain, J. L. (1999). 45,X/46,XY mosaicism: report of 27 cases. *Pediatrics, 104*(2 Pt 1), 304–308.

Tochigi, M., Kato, C., Koishi, S., Kawakubo, Y., Yamamoto, K., Matsumoto, H., et al. (2007). No evidence for significant association between GABA receptor genes in chromosome 15q11-q13 and autism in a Japanese population. *Journal of Human Genetics, 52*(12), 985–989.

Veenstra-VanderWeele, J., & Cook, E. H., Jr. (2004). Molecular genetics of autism spectrum disorder. *Molecular Psychiatry, 9*(9), 819–832.

Walitza, S., Wewetzer, C., Gerlach, M., Klampfl, K., Geller, F., Barth, N., et al. (2004). Transmission disequilibrium studies in children and adolescents with obsessive-compulsive disorders pertaining to polymorphisms of genes of the serotonergic pathway. *Journal of Neural Transmission, 111*(7), 817–825.

Wang, H. S., & Kuo, M. F. (2003). Tourette's syndrome in Taiwan: an epidemiological study of tic disorders in an elementary school at Taipei County. *Brain and Development, 25*(Suppl 1), S29–31.

Wendland, J. R., DeGuzman, T. B., McMahon, F., Rudnick, G., Detera-Wadleigh, S. D., & Murphy, D. L. (2008). SERT Ileu425Val in autism, Asperger syndrome and obsessive-compulsive disorder. *Psychiatric Genetics, 18*(1), 31–39.

Wetherby, A. M., Watt, N., Morgan, L., & Shumway, S. (2007). Social communication profiles of children with autism spectrum disorders late in the second year of life. *Journal of Autism and Developmental Disorders, 37*(5), 960–975.

Wilcox, J. A., Tsuang, M. T., Schnurr, T., & Baida-Fragoso, N. (2003). Case-control family study of lesser variant traits in autism. *Neuropsychobiology, 47*(4), 171–177.

Williams, D. L., Goldstein, G., Kojkowski, N., & Minshew, N. J. (2008). Do individuals with high functioning autism have the IQ profile associated with nonverbal learning disability? *Research in Autism Spectrum Disorders, 2*(2), 353–361.

Willour, V. L., Yao Shugart, Y., Samuels, J., Grados, M., Cullen, B., Bienvenu, O. J., 3rd, et al. (2004). Replication study supports evidence for linkage to 9p24 in obsessive-compulsive disorder. *American Journal of Human Genetics, 75*(3), 508–513.

Yeargin-Allsopp, M., Rice, C., Karapurkar, T., Doernberg, N., Boyle, C., & Murphy, C. (2003). Prevalence of autism in a US metropolitan area. *Journal of the American Medical Association, 289*(1), 49–55.

Yrigollen, C. M., Han, S. S., Kochetkova, A., Babitz, T., Chang, J. T., Volkmar, F. R., et al. (2008). Genes controlling affiliative behavior as candidate genes for autism. *Biological Psychiatry, 63*(10), 911–916.

Zai, G., Arnold, P., Burroughs, E., Barr, C. L., Richter, M. A., & Kennedy, J. L. (2005). Evidence for the gamma-amino-butyric acid type B receptor 1 (GABBR1) gene as a susceptibility factor in obsessive-compulsive disorder. *American Journal of Medical Genetics. Part B, Neuropsychiatric Genetics, 134B*(1), 25–29.

Zarcone, J., Napolitano, D., Peterson, C., Breidbord, J., Ferraioli, S., Caruso-Anderson, M., et al. (2007). The relationship between compulsive behaviour and academic achievement across the three genetic subtypes of Prader-Willi syndrome. *Journal of Intellectual Disability Research, 51*(Pt 6), 478–487.

Zhang, H., & Risch, N. (1996). Mapping quantitative-trait loci in humans by use of extreme concordant sib pairs: selected sampling by parental phenotypes. *American Journal of Human Genetics, 59*(4), 951–957.

Zhao, X., Leotta, A., Kustanovich, V., Lajonchere, C., Geschwind, D. H., Law, K., et al. (2007). A unified genetic theory for sporadic and inherited autism. *Proceedings of the National Academy of Sciences of the United States of America, 104*(31), 12831–12836.

Zhao, X., Pak, C., Smrt, R. D., & Jin, P. (2007). Epigenetics and Neural developmental disorders: Washington DC, September 18 and 19, 2006. *Epigenetics, 2*(2), 126–134.

Zohar, A. H., & Felz, L. (2001). Ritualistic behavior in young children. *Journal of Abnormal Child Psychology, 29*(2), 121–128.

18 Angela M. Reiersen, Richard D. Todd†

Attention-Deficit/Hyperactivity Disorder (ADHD)

This chapter is dedicated to Dr. Richard Todd, who died prior to the publication of this book (for further comment, see acknowledgment at end of chapter).

Points of Interest

- ADHD symptoms are common in ASD, yet DSM-IV-TR does not allow codiagnosis of ADHD and ASD.
- Among individuals with ASD, the presence of ADHD is associated with more severe impairment and higher likelihood of additional comorbid psychopathology.
- Recent evidence suggests some of the same genetic influences affect the development of both ASD and ADHD.
- ADHD symptoms in ASD often respond to standard ADHD medications such as stimulants, atomoxetine, and alpha adrenergic agents. Neuroleptics can also reduce ADHD symptoms in ASD.
- Distinguishing between ASD-related and ADHD-related social impairments may be helpful when planning nonpharmacologic interventions such as social skills training.
- Revision of diagnostic criteria to allow a diagnosis of ADHD for individuals with ASD may facilitate identification and treatment of ADHD symptoms.

Introduction

Attention-deficit/hyperactivity disorder (ADHD) is one of the most common childhood-onset neurodevelopmental disorders. The DSM-IV ADHD symptom criterion lists nine inattentive and nine hyperactive-impulsive symptoms. ADHD subtypes are defined as predominantly inattentive, predominantly hyperactive-impulsive, or combined type, depending on whether there are at least six symptoms in one or both of the two symptom categories. Some of the symptoms and behaviors commonly seen in autism spectrum disorders (ASD) could fit the description of ADHD symptoms, but may have an entirely different underlying mechanism when they occur in ASD. For example, an individual with autism may exhibit the DSM-IV ADHD inattentive symptom of not listening, but this may be due to specific deficits in the areas of communication and joint attention rather than general difficulty in paying attention. Also, some individuals with autism may have excessive motor activity due to frequent repetitive/stereotyped movements, but this may have a different quality than the restlessness and excessive movement that is typical of hyperactivity in ADHD. Social anxiety may lead to fidgeting in social situations, which could also be misinterpreted as a hyperactive symptom of ADHD. If one considers DSM diagnoses in terms of a diagnostic hierarchy, then it can be argued that ADHD-like symptoms (particularly those that could be explained by decreased social attention) are always present in severe forms of ASD, and an additional diagnosis of ADHD may seem redundant. However, if ADHD symptoms in ASD are associated with more severe impairment or altered response to treatment, then it may be important to diagnose and treat ADHD when it co-occurs with an ASD. This chapter reviews the existing literature on co-occurrence of ASD and ADHD in clinical and epidemiological samples, discusses genetic and other biological mechanisms that may contribute to the co-occurrence of these symptoms, briefly discusses the treatment of ADHD symptoms in ASD, and provides some general comments on diagnostic nosology and areas in need of further research.

ADHD in ASD: Prevalence and Clinical Significance

DSM-IV-TR prohibits the diagnosis of both ADHD and ASD in the same individual (APA, 2000). In part due to this exclusion criterion, many studies of ASD or ADHD exclude individuals who show signs of the other diagnosis. However,

ADHD symptoms are very common in ASD, and in some cases these ADHD symptoms may be of very high clinical and etiological relevance.

Several studies have investigated the prevalence of ADHD symptoms and diagnoses among individuals with ASD (DeVincent, Gadow, Delosh, & Geller, 2007; Gadow & DeVincent, 2005; Gadow, DeVincent, & Pomeroy, 2006; Gadow, DeVincent, Pomeroy, & Azizian, 2004, 2005; Goldstein & Schwebach, 2004; Hattori et al., 2006; Lecavalier, Gadow, Devincent, & Edwards, 2009; Ogino et al., 2005; Sturm, Fernell, & Gillberg, 2004; Yoshida & Uchiyama, 2004). Results of clinic-based studies are described in Table 18-1. In summary, these studies indicate that if the DSM exclusion criterion prohibiting co-diagnosis of ASD and ADHD is ignored, about 40–80% of clinically ascertained individuals with ASD meet criteria for an ADHD diagnosis. Some investigators of the relationship between ADHD and ASD suggest these two disorders may actually belong in the same diagnostic spectrum (Hattori et al., 2006). Others describe evidence that the presence of ADHD symptoms in a subset of children with ASD represents a co-occurring psychiatric syndrome that presents very similarly in children with ASD as it does in those without ASD (Gadow et al., 2006; Lecavalier et al., 2009).

Through a small retrospective chart review of 27 children with autism or Pervasive Developmental Disorder Not-Otherwise-Specified (PDD-NOS), Goldstein and Schwebach found that 26% of these children met symptom criteria for combined type ADHD, 33% met criteria for the inattentive

Table 18–1.
Studies of attention-deficit/hyperactivity disorder in patients with autism spectrum disorders

Study Authors, Year	Number of Subjects, Diagnoses	Percent of ASD Subjects Meeting Criteria for ADHD	Other Key Findings
Goldstein & Schwebach, 2004	N = 27, autism or PDD-NOS	59% of all ASD subjects	26% had combined type ADHD 33% had inattentive ADHD
Yoshida & Uchiyama, 2004	N = 53, high functioning ASD	68% of all ASD subjects	23% had combined type ADHD 38% had inattentive ADHD 8% had hyperactive-impulsive ADHD
Sturm, Fernell, & Gillberg, 2004	N = 101, 90% Asperger's, 9% PDD-NOS, 1% high-functioning autism	75% of all ASD subjects	95% had attention problems 56% had hyperactivity 50% had impulsivity
Hattori et al., 2006	N = 15 ASD subjects N = 20 ADHD subjects N = 40 controls	Following the DSM-IV exclusion criterion, Subjects with PDD were excluded from the ADHD group in this study.	ASD and ADHD groups both had higher ASD and ADHD symptom ratings than controls. ADHD symptom ratings were similar between ASD and ADHD groups. The authors questioned whether ASD and ADHD are distinct disorders.
Gadow et al., 2006	N = 449 with parent ADHD ratings, N = 441 with teacher ADHD ratings. 35% Autism, 22% Asperger's, 43% PDD-NOS	53% of all 3–12 year old ASD subjects had ADHD (same overall percentage whether by parent or teacher rating).	ASD subjects with combined type ADHD had more oppositional, aggressive, and autistic symptoms than those with inattentive ADHD. Inattentive subtype was the most common. ADHD subtypes and associated comorbidity patterns were similar in ASD subjects and non-ASD control subjects. Some analyses were first reported separately for preschool and elementary school age groups (Gadow et al., 2004, 2005).
Lee & Ousley, 2006	N = 58 autistic disorder, N = 12 Asperger's, N = 13 PDD-NOS	78% of all ASD subjects 83% of autism subjects 58% of Asperger's disorder subjects 77% of PDD-NOS subjects	Combined type ADHD was the most common subtype in autistic disorder, but inattentive type was the most common in Asperger's disorder and PDD-NOS.
Holtmann, Bolte, & Poustka, 2007	N = 182 ASD subjects, split into high and low ADHD groups for comparison on CBCL measures.		ASD subjects with ADHD had higher internalizing and externalizing symptoms. They also had higher impairment on the social interaction subscale of the ADI-R.

type, and 41% did not meet symptom criteria for ADHD (Goldstein & Schwebach, 2004). Sturm, Fernell, and Gillberg performed a larger chart review of 101 Swedish children with pervasive developmental disorders (90% Asperger's disorder, 9% PDD-NOS, 1% high-functioning autism), and found that 95% had "attentional problems," 56% had "hyperactivity," and 50% had "impulsiveness." They also reported that 75% had symptoms consistent with an ADHD diagnosis (Sturm et al., 2004). Yoshida and Uchiyama evaluated 53 Japanese children with high-functioning pervasive developmental disorders, and found that 68% met criteria for ADHD: 38% had the inattentive type, 23% had combined type, and about 8% had the hyperactive-impulsive type (Yoshida & Uchiyama, 2004). Hattori and colleagues compared ratings of ADHD and ASD symptoms in 20 children with ADHD, 15 children with ASD, and 40 normal controls. They found that the ASD and ADHD groups both had higher ratings of ASD and ADHD symptoms than controls. Based on their findings, they questioned whether ADHD and autism spectrum disorders are truly distinct (Hattori et al., 2006).

Lee and Ousley also investigated ADHD symptoms in a clinical sample of 83 children and adolescents with ASD, and found that 78% had symptoms consistent with an ADHD diagnosis (Lee & Ousley, 2006). They found that while the combined subtype was most common in autistic disorder, the inattentive subtype was the most common subtype in Asperger's disorder and PDD-NOS.

Kenneth Gadow and colleagues have published a number of studies investigating the validity of ADHD diagnoses in ASD (DeVincent et al., 2007; Gadow, Devincent, & Schneider, 2008; Gadow & DeVincent, 2005; Gadow, Devincent, & Drabick, 2008; Gadow et al., 2006; Gadow et al., 2004, 2005; Lecavalier et al., 2009). In a group of 6- to 12-year-old clinic-referred patients with ASD (38% with autism), they found that 59% of ASD males and 67% of ASD females had ADHD. In this study, the inattentive subtype was the most common form of ADHD among children with ASD, just as it was among non-ASD clinical and nonreferred community comparison groups (Gadow et al., 2005). Findings were similar in a study of preschoolers (Gadow et al., 2004). The same research group reported that children with the combination of ASD and combined type ADHD had more oppositional, aggressive, and autistic symptoms than those with the combination of ASD plus inattentive type ADHD (Gadow et al., 2006). Another analysis found that children with ASD who have the combination of ADHD and tics have particularly high levels of psychopathology, suggesting that the combination of ADHD and tics may be an indicator of a more complex psychiatric disorder (Gadow & DeVincent, 2005). This group also reported an association between sleep problems and increased ADHD symptoms among children with ASD (DeVincent et al., 2007). Another study found that ADHD symptom severity was associated with higher rates of medication treatment and current use of special education services among children with ASD (Gadow, Devincent, & Schneider, 2008). In ASD children, the combination of oppositional-defiant disorder (ODD) plus ADHD was associated with particularly high rates of medication use, co-occurring psychiatric symptoms, and adverse environmental factors indicative of disadvantage (Gadow, Devincent, & Drabick, 2008). In one of their most recent papers, this group of investigators concludes that ADHD and several other DSM psychiatric diagnoses are valid constructs in children with ASD (Lecavalier et al., 2009).

Holtmann, Bolte, and Poustka also explored the association of ADHD symptoms with autistic behavior domains and co-occurring psychopathology. In children with ASD, they found that ADHD symptoms were associated with more impairment on the social interaction subscale of the Autism Diagnostic Interview-Revised (ADI-R) as well as higher levels of internalizing and externalizing symptoms measured using the Child Behavior Checklist (Holtmann, Bolte, & Poustka, 2007).

Population-based studies are also important in determining the prevalence of ADHD among individuals with ASD. Simonoff and colleagues have reported the presence of ADHD in 28% of 112 10- to 14-year-old children with ASD from a population-derived cohort. They also found that those with ADHD had very high rates of additional comorbidity, with a second comorbid psychiatric diagnosis in 84% of ASD subjects who had ADHD (Simonoff et al., 2008). Of note, the prevalence of ADHD among ASD subjects from this population-based sample is somewhat lower than reported in the clinic-based studies shown in Table 18-1, and this difference may be due to referral bias. Since individuals with the combination of ASD plus ADHD have higher rates of additional comorbidity and impairment, the ASD subjects with ADHD (and higher comorbidity) may be more likely to present to clinics for treatment.

Social Impairment in ADHD

There are also a few studies of autistic symptoms in children and adolescents whose primary diagnosis is ADHD. In order to distinguish this from social impairment that may be due to ADHD itself, it is helpful to have an awareness of the typical social deficits that are very common in ADHD. It has long been recognized that children with ADHD are often socially impaired, and many published papers have described the phenomenology and treatment of social difficulties that are frequently present in ADHD (de Boo & Prins, 2007; Reiersen & Todd, 2008). Sociometric studies requiring children within a group to comment on their relationships with specific peers indicate that children with ADHD are often rejected by their peers (Blachman & Hinshaw, 2002; Hoza, Gerdes, et al., 2005; Hoza, Mrug, et al., 2005). Some of the social impairment can be attributed to the direct effects of ADHD symptoms on social behaviors. For example, impulsive and intrusive behaviors may lead to difficulties in making and keeping friends if peers are annoyed by such behaviors. Co-occurring psychopathology such as social anxiety and oppositional behaviors (Jensen et al., 2001), and cognitive impairments such as working memory and executive deficits (Diamantopoulou, Rydell, Thorell, & Bohlin, 2007) may also contribute to the social deficits seen in ADHD. A conceptual framework for social deficits in ADHD is presented in Table 18-2. The extent of overlap between mechanisms of social impairment in ADHD and autism remains unclear.

In addition to some of the social difficulties that have been classically described in ADHD, several recent clinic- and population-based studies indicate that children with a primary diagnosis of ADHD often have additional deficits in the areas of social reciprocity, communication impairment, and repetitive/stereotyped behaviors that suggest the presence of mild ASD symptoms or diagnoses (Clark, Feehan, Tinline, & Vostanis, 1999; Hattori et al., 2006; Reiersen, Constantino, & Todd, 2008; Reiersen, Constantino, Volk, & Todd, 2007; Santosh & Mijovic, 2004; Mulligan et al., 2009; Nijmeijer et al., 2009; Grzadzinski et al., 2010).

Clark and colleagues studied autistic symptoms using the Autism Criteria Checklist in a clinical sample of 49 children with ADHD and estimated that 65–85% had difficulties in social interaction and communication (Clark et al., 1999).

Santosh and Mijovic examined evidence of autistic-like symptoms through a chart review of 309 child and adolescent patients with ICD-10 Hyperkinetic Disorder (HKD),

Table 18–2.
A conceptual framework for social deficits in ADHD

Social Deficit Category	Specific Behaviors/Problems/Perceptions that may Lead to Social Impairment/ Relationship Difficulties/Rejection by Peers
Social Deficits Directly Resulting from ADHD Symptoms:	
1. Inattention	-Fails to notice/attend to social cues. -Forgets social plans/promises. -Loses others' things. -Appears disorganized. -Fails to focus on conversations. -Unable to persist in prolonged games. -Unable to attend to and learn appropriate social protocols.
2. Hyperactivity	-Moves quickly between peer activities. -Has increased energy that tires others out. -Talks too much/monopolizes the conversation. -Unable to sit still for a game or conversation with peers.
3. Impulsivity	-Rapidly/unexpectedly changes plans based on impulses. -Shows impulsive aggressive behaviors. -Impulsively makes comments that offend others. -Impulsively intrudes on others' space. -Insists on being first. -Poor at taking turns.
Social Deficits Resulting from Co-Occurring Problems:	
1. Poor emotional regulation	-Has emotional outbursts that disrupt activities and annoy others. -Unpleasant mood makes social interactions unpleasant for peers. -Social anxiety leads to social avoidance.
2. Oppositional Behavior	-Unwilling to go with others' plans or consider others' opinions. -Argumentative with peers.
3. Autistic symptoms	-Decreased desire for close friendships leads to social avoidance. -Decreased ability to read/understand social cues. -Decreased empathy with failure to respond appropriately to peer emotions. -Odd/repetitive behaviors that annoy peers. -Poor reciprocal communication/conversation skills. -Insistence on playing games related to own unusual or hyperfocused interests. -Rigid/stereotyped play behaviors. -Few shared interests with peers.
Social Deficits Resulting from Specific Cognitive or Language Deficits:	
1. Low overall IQ	-Perceived by others as "not smart." -Unable to logically solve social problems. -Failure to notice when being taken advantage of by peers. -Difficulty learning social skills

(Continued)

Table 18–2. *(Contd.)*

Social Deficit Category	Specific Behaviors/Problems/Perceptions that may Lead to Social Impairment/ Relationship Difficulties/Rejection by Peers
2. Poor executive function	-Difficulty planning social responses. -Difficulty adjusting behavior appropriately for social context. -Difficulty distinguishing between appropriate vs. inappropriate social behaviors. -Difficulty deciding when to use specific social skills.
3. Poor working memory	-Unable to process complex social situations. -Difficulty holding in mind social context information. -Trouble keeping in mind topic of game/conversation. -Difficulty remembering steps necessary to play a game. -Difficulty remembering promises to peers. -Difficulty interacting/conversing with more than one peer at a time.
4. Language impairment	-Has odd speech patterns that peers find strange or difficult to understand. -Difficulty communicating leads to decreased ability to confide in peers, converse, or develop meaningful friendships.

a diagnosis similar to DSM-IV combined type ADHD. Compared to 2048 psychiatric controls without HKD, ASD, or obsessive-compulsive disorder diagnoses, the patients with HKD were more likely to exhibit the "autistic symptom triad" of impaired social interaction, impaired communication, and repetitive/stereotyped behaviors. Santosh and Mijovic found evidence of two types of social impairment in their HKD subjects, which they named relationship difficulty and social communication difficulty. Those with evidence of social communication difficulty had more developmental delays and autistic-like symptoms such as repetitive/stereotyped behaviors and language problems. On the other hand, those with relationship difficulty had more conduct problems, mood symptoms, and environmental stressors. The authors suggested children with relationship difficulty may benefit from more family interventions, while those with social communication difficulty may require more social skills training (Santosh & Mijovic, 2004).

Grzadzinski and colleagues (2010) recently found evidence of autistic traits in a clinical sample of 75 children with DSM-IV-TR ADHD who did not have any history of an ASD diagnosis. They found that 32% of these children had elevated autistic traits based on a Social Responsiveness Scale (SRS) T-score ≥ 60. Those with elevated SRS scores showed evidence of non-structural language abnormalities on the Children's Communication Checklist-2 and greater oppositional behaviors, but did not show greater anxiety or ADHD symptoms.

Because clinic-based studies are prone to referral bias, it is also important to examine the relationship between ADHD and autistic symptoms in subjects ascertained through population-based samples. In our own population-based studies of ADHD, we have used the Social Responsiveness Scale (SRS) as a measure of autistic traits. This 65-item parent- or teacher-rated scale focuses on deficits in reciprocal social behavior, but also includes items assessing the other two autism symptom domains of communication impairment and stereotyped/repetitive behaviors (Constantino & Gruber, 2005; Constantino, Przybeck, Friesen, & Todd, 2000). Elevated SRS scores correlate highly with Autism Diagnostic Interview-Revised (ADI-R) algorithm scores (Constantino et al., 2003). In a population-based sample of Missouri twins, we found statistically significant SRS score elevations in children and adolescents with DSM-IV ADHD. SRS scores were highest in children with DSM-IV combined type ADHD or a severe combined subtype of ADHD defined using latent class analysis of DSM-IV ADHD symptoms (Reiersen et al., 2007). We also found that among children with ADHD, those with parent-reported motor coordination problems on the Child Behavior Checklist (CBCL) were more likely to have elevated autistic symptoms than those without parent-reported motor problems (Reiersen, Constantino, et al., 2008). This is consistent with a Scandinavian concept of Deficits in Attention, Motor Control, and Perception (DAMP), a syndrome that has recently been redefined as a combination of ADHD plus Developmental Coordination Disorder (DCD). Children with DAMP frequently show evidence of ASD in addition to their ADHD and DCD symptoms (Gillberg, 2003).

Examination of the ADHD-enriched International Multicenter ADHD Genetics (IMAGE) study sample has also revealed evidence of elevated ASD symptoms in subjects with ADHD. The Social Communication Questionnaire (SCQ) and Children's Social Behavior Questionnaire (CSBQ) were used as measures of autistic traits in this study. Analyses using the SCQ suggested autistic symptoms in ADHD are familial and associated with neurodevelopmental and oppositional-defiant disorders (Mulligan et al., 2009). Additional analyses using the CSBQ in Dutch participants within the IMAGE sample also showed elevated levels of autistic traits in ADHD probands and their siblings compared to controls, but weak and nonsignificant cross-sibling cross-trait correlations suggested the familiality of ASD symptoms may be largely independent from ADHD familiality (Nijmeijer et al., 2009).

Underlying Biology and Genetics

Evidence for Genetic Overlap

Based on studies described above, it is apparent that ASD and ADHD symptoms frequently co-occur. The biological mechanisms underlying the co-occurrence of these two types of symptoms remains to be elucidated. Some recent studies suggest that some of the same genetic influences may affect both ASD and ADHD symptoms. Smalley and colleagues found statistically significant overlap between genetic linkage peaks on review of autism and ADHD linkage studies (Smalley, Loo, Yang, & Cantor, 2005). Nijmeijer, Arias-Vasquez, and colleagues (2010) performed a QTL linkage analysis of autistic symptoms in the ADHD-enriched IMAGE sample, and hypothesized that one of their suggestive linkage peaks (at 15q24) may be pleiotropic for ADHD and ASD since the height of this peak was reduced when a measure of ADHD symptoms was included as a covariate. In a recent study of 12,206 8-year-old twins, Ronald and colleagues found evidence for substantial overlap of genetic influences on autistic and ADHD symptoms (Ronald, Simonoff, Kuntsi, Asherson, & Plomin, 2008). They estimated genetic correlation (r_g) for ASD and ADHD traits in the range of 0.54–0.57 and non-shared environmental correlation (r_e) in the range of 0.15–0.35, depending on rater (parent vs. teacher) and sex. Similarly, a study of 674 young adult Australian twins suggested overlapping genetic influences on self-reported autistic and ADHD symptoms (Reiersen et al., 2008), with r_g estimated at 0.72 and r_e estimated at 0.26. While there is evidence of substantial genetic overlap from the above twin studies, both studies estimated that only a small proportion of environmental influences were shared between the two disorders. So, while common genetic factors may underlie both ADHD and ASD, environmental influences may predispose individuals to one disorder or the other. The degree of overlap of genetic and environmental influences on the two disorders may vary depending upon the age of ADHD and ASD symptom assessment. Ronald, Edelson, Asherson, and Saudino (2010) recently reported a study of autistic-like traits and ADHD behaviors in 2-year-old twins which suggested a smaller degree of genetic overlap (r_g = 0.26), complete overlap of common environmental influences (r_c = 1.00), and the possibility that non-shared environmental influences tend to increase one of the two symptom domains while decreasing the other (r_e = −0.17). Additional types of neurodevelopmental disorders may also show genetic overlap with ASD and ADHD. For example, another twin study by Lichtenstein, Carlstrom, Rastrom, Gillberg, and Ankarsater (2010) suggested that ADHD, tic disorders, and developmental coordination disorders are all influenced by genetic and environmental factors that also contribute to ASD. Perhaps even where the same genetic predispositions toward psychopathology are present, the timing or type of environmental insults may result in different forms of psychopathology. Gene-gene interactions may also influence the specific type of symptoms that develop.

So far, there are few reported examples of specific genetic variations associated with both ADHD and autistic symptoms. In our own Missouri twin sample, we found that among children with severe combined type ADHD, those with the DRD4 7-repeat allele were more likely to have clinically elevated autistic traits as measured by the SRS (Reiersen, Neuman, et al., 2008). Although there was evidence of an interaction between prenatal nicotine exposure and the DRD4 7-repeat allele in producing risk for severe combined type ADHD (Neuman et al., 2007), no main or interaction effects of smoking were found for SRS score (Reiersen, Neuman, et al., 2008). This may be one example where a gene can influence both ADHD and autism symptoms, but environmental interactions with this gene may be different for autism and ADHD symptoms. Another recent study found an association between a Monoamine Oxidase A gene promoter polymorphism and ADHD symptoms in children with ASD (Roohi, DeVincent, Hatchwell, & Gadow, 2009). Children with the 4-repeat allele had higher parent-rated ADHD symptoms than those with the 3-repeat allele. The same research group found lower levels of ADHD symptoms and language deficits but higher levels of tics and social anxiety in ASD subjects homozygous for the DAT1 10-repeat allele (Gadow, Roohi, DeVincent, & Hatchwell, 2008). Using the IMAGE and Tracking Adolescents' Individual Lives (TRAILS) samples, Nijmeijer, Hartman, and colleagues (2010) found evidence that interaction of perinatal risk factors with catechol O-methyltransferase gene (COMT) and the serotonin transporter gene (SLC6A4) may influence ASD symptoms in children with ADHD. These association studies should be considered preliminary, and require replication.

There are also some well-known complex genetic syndromes that can produce both ASD and ADHD. Two examples are 22q11 deletion syndrome (also known as velocardiofacial syndrome or DiGeorge syndrome) (Antshel et al., 2007; Fine et al., 2005; Gothelf et al., 2004; Niklasson, Rasmussen, Oskarsdottir, & Gillberg, 2002; Ousley, Rockers, Dell, Coleman, & Cubells, 2007; Vorstman et al., 2006) and Fragile X premutation (Farzin et al., 2006). In the case of 22q11 deletion syndrome, the proportion of these individuals having ADHD and ASD diagnoses varies by study, and appears affected by whether formal evaluation for ASD was done and whether the researchers adhered to the DSM-IV exclusion prohibiting codiagnosis of ADHD and ASD (Reiersen, 2007). The 22q11 deletion is also associated with increased risk of psychotic disorders such as schizophrenia (Murphy, 2005; Ousley et al., 2007). In addition to the above example, copy number variation (insertions/deletions) in other gene regions have shown evidence of association with autism (Glessner et al., 2009; Hogart, Wu, Lasalle, & Schanen, 2010; Kakinuma & Sato, 2008; Kusenda & Sebat, 2008) and/or

ADHD (Elia et al., 2009), and frequently the regions of duplication/deletion include genes that are thought to be involved in neurodevelopment. As in the example of 22q11 deletion syndrome, some of the same copy number variants that increase risk for ADHD and/or autism may also increase the risk for other psychiatric disorders such as schizophrenia (Cook & Scherer, 2008; Williams, Owen, & O'Donovan, 2009). In a recent review of the shared heritability of ADHD and ASD, Rommelse, Franke, Geurts, Hartman, and Buitelaar (2010) suggest future studies should include family-based designs which obtain data on ADHD symptoms, ASD symptoms, endophenotypic measures, and environmental measures from all family members. They also discuss several potential candidate pleiotropic genes based on existing studies of both disorders.

Potential Biological Mechanisms

A vast number of genes involved in neurodevelopment and/or neurotransmission might theoretically affect both ASD and ADHD symptoms, but genes relevant to the brain's dopaminergic system may be of particular relevance. Stimulant medications used to treat ADHD increase dopaminergic neurotransmission, and many ADHD candidate genes are related to the dopamine system (Faraone et al., 2005; McGough, 2005; Neuman et al., 2007; Todd et al., 2005; Todd & Neuman, 2007). Dopaminergic neurons innervate both the frontal cortical attention regions and midbrain motor control regions (Todd & Botteron, 2001), and dysfunction of the dopaminergic system has been implicated in motor dysfunction, ADHD, and autism (Nieoullon, 2002). Also of note, motor abnormalities have been described in both ADHD and ASD (Mahone et al., 2006; Mostofsky, Burgess, & Gidley Larson, 2007), and the syndrome described as Deficits in Attention, Motor Control, and Perception (DAMP) typically includes autistic features along with ADHD and motor coordination deficits (Gillberg, 2003). Certain aberrant cognitive processes may be relevant to both ASD and ADHD, and these may also be affected by dysfunction in the dopaminergic system. For example, executive function deficits have been found in ADHD, ASD, and in motor coordination disorders (Geurts, Verte, Oosterlaan, Roeyers, & Sergeant, 2004; Goldberg et al., 2005; Livesey, Keen, Rouse, & White, 2006; Pennington & Ozonoff, 1996; Piek, Dyck, Francis, & Conwell, 2007; Piek et al., 2004; Sergeant, Geurts, & Oosterlaan, 2002). Our own research group has proposed a dopaminergic synapse-based model in which interaction between dopamine system gene polymorphisms and prenatal nicotine exposure influences the development of ADHD and/or autistic symptoms (Reiersen, Constantino, et al., 2008; Reiersen, Neuman, et al., 2008; Todd & Neuman, 2007). If individuals with a combination of ASD and ADHD respond to typical stimulant treatments, this would support the hypothesis that the mechanism of ADHD symptoms is similar, whether or not ASD is present. And in fact, individuals with ASD often do respond to typical ADHD treatments as described below. However, different effects of prenatal exposure to nicotine on ADHD versus ASD suggests some differences in the underlying mechanisms that produce ADHD versus ASD.

Treatment of ADHD Symptoms in ASD

A number of studies have evaluated the effects of medication treatment on ADHD-like symptoms in autistic disorder (Hazell, 2007). In his review of this treatment literature, Hazell concluded that methylphenidate, atomoxetine, some anticonvulsants, guanfacine, and donepezil showed evidence of moderate benefit. Atypical neuroleptics such as risperidone and quetiapine also improved ADHD symptoms in autism, but commonly had side effects of weight gain and sedation. Often medication studies for treatment of autism have included outcome measures related to ADHD symptoms, but only a few studies have specifically targeted individuals with the combination of ASD and ADHD symptoms. The use of methylphenidate for treatment of ADHD symptoms in ASD is supported by two placebo-controlled trials and a retrospective and prospective effectiveness study (Handen, Johnson, & Lubetsky, 2000; RUPP, 2005; Santosh, Baird, Pityaratstian, Tavare, & Gringras, 2006). The effectiveness of guanfacine is supported by a chart review, a small open-label trial, and a small double-blind, placebo-controlled, cross-over trial (Handen, Sahl, & Hardan, 2008; Posey, Puntney, Sasher, Kem, & McDougle, 2004; Scahill et al., 2006). The use of atomoxetine is supported by small open-label and placebo-controlled trials (Arnold et al., 2006; Posey et al., 2006; Troost et al., 2006).

One retrospective and prospective effectiveness study by Santosh and colleagues compared treatment responses of children with ADHD only to those with comorbid ADHD and ASD (Santosh et al., 2006). They concluded that stimulants were as effective in children with ASD plus ADHD as they were in children with ADHD alone, but also acknowledged that randomized, controlled trials are needed to further investigate the efficacy of stimulants for treating ADHD symptoms in ASD. They did not find a significant difference in side effects between groups, but they noted a trend toward increased dysphoria and obsessionality in the ASD group (Santosh et al., 2006), so they recommended caution with stimulant dosing and close monitoring for side effects in patients with ASD. Double-blind, randomized trials directly comparing stimulant response between a pure ADHD group and a group presenting with the combination of ASD and ADHD symptoms are needed to further investigate any difference in response rates and side effects.

As mentioned earlier, 22q11 deletion syndrome is a special case of a genetic disorder associated with both ADHD and ASD. Though some experts have been concerned about use of stimulants in these individuals due to their risk for psychotic symptoms, results of an open-label study suggested that stimulants are safe and effective for treating ADHD in 22q11 deletion syndrome (Gothelf et al., 2003).

Nonpharmacological treatments may also be very important in reducing ADHD symptoms in ASD. Educational accommodations for individuals with ASD should take into account the presence of any ADHD-like symptoms. For example, children who have ADHD symptoms may need more help organizing tasks and assignments, may pay attention better if sitting near the front of the classroom, may require instructions to be repeated more than once or written down for the student, and may benefit from extended time for completion of examinations.

Social skills therapies may be helpful for children with ASD and for children with ADHD. However, the type of therapy may be different depending on the nature of the social deficits that are present. Children who mainly have social reciprocity deficits typical of autism spectrum disorders may need more training in the areas of appropriate social communication (pragmatics, etc.) as well as education regarding situationally appropriate behaviors in various contexts. They may also need encouragement to initiate and maintain social interactions. Children with high levels of ADHD symptoms may benefit more from social skills therapies geared toward reducing inappropriate social behaviors that result directly from ADHD symptoms (for example, difficulty waiting turn, intrusiveness, and poor self-control due to impulsivity).

Box 18–1
Optimizing diagnostic nosologies

- Co-occurrence of multiple neurodevelopmental disorders is common, but current diagnostic criteria do not fully take this into account.
- Revision of DSM to allow diagnosis of ASD and ADHD in the same individual may encourage clinicians to assess and treat ADHD symptoms when they occur along with ASD.
- Future studies aimed at disentangling ASD from ADHD symptoms may lead to improved tailoring of treatment according to the symptom variations, strengths, and weaknesses of individual patients.

Conclusions

Given the studies showing frequent co-occurrence of ADHD and autistic symptoms and the evidence that ADHD symptoms in ASD are associated with higher levels of co-occurring psychopathology and impairment, it appears important to assess for ADHD symptoms in ASD. Individuals with the combination of ASD and ADHD may have a more complex neurodevelopmental disorder than those with ASD alone. They may have different comorbidity profiles and a different long-term prognosis. Also, individuals with the combination of ASD and ADHD may benefit from specific treatment of ADHD symptoms (for example, standard ADHD medications plus social skills interventions that target classic ADHD-type social impairment in addition to ASD-type social impairment). Revision of DSM diagnostic criteria to allow codiagnosis of ASD and ADHD may encourage clinicians to assess and treat ADHD symptoms in patients with ASD. Future studies may address the issues of disentangling ASD from ADHD symptoms and tailoring treatment according to symptom variations, strengths, and weaknesses of individual patients.

Challenges and Future Directions

- Detailed phenotypic studies aimed at disentangling the measurement of ADHD and ASD symptoms may contribute to better diagnostic classification as well as the development of new treatments to specifically target different types of social impairment that are present in ASD and/or ADHD.
- Studies including neurocognitive testing and functional neuroimaging may help to clarify similarities and differences in brain function between ASD and ADHD.
- Further genetic studies considering gene-gene interaction, gene-environment interaction, and timing of environmental insults may further elucidate the mechanisms of abnormal brain development that can lead to ASD, ADHD, or both.
- Future treatment studies should include randomized, double-blind clinical trials directly comparing treatment response between ASD+ADHD and ADHD-only groups.

SUGGESTED READINGS

de Boo, G. M., & Prins, P. J. (2007). Social incompetence in children with ADHD: possible moderators and mediators in social-skills training. *Clinical Psychology Review, 27*(1), 78–97.

Gillberg, C. (2003). Deficits in attention, motor control, and perception: a brief review. *Archives of Disease in Childhood, 88*(10), 904–910.

Hazell, P. (2007). Drug therapy for attention-deficit/hyperactivity disorder-like symptoms in autistic disorder. *Journal of Paediatrics and Child Health, 43*(1–2), 19–24.

Reiersen, A. M., & Todd, R. D. (2008). Co-occurrence of ADHD and autism spectrum disorders: phenomenology and treatment. *Expert Review of Neurotherapeutics, 8*(4), 657–669.

Rommelse, N. N. J., Franke, B., Geurts, H. M., Hartman, C. A., & Buitelaar, J. K (2010). Shared heritability of attention-deficit/hyperactivity disorder and autism spectrum disorder. *European Child and Adolescent Psychiatry, 19*(3), 281–295.

ACKNOWLEDGMENT

Dr. Todd was involved in the early planning of this work, but died due to complications of leukemia on August 22, 2008, prior to completion of this chapter. Much of his recent research focused on the genetic epidemiology of childhood onset psychiatric disorders, including ADHD and autism. He was a caring physician with a special talent for working with patients affected by autism spectrum disorders and their families. He was also an excellent mentor and a valued colleague. This chapter is dedicated to his memory.

REFERENCES

American Psychiatric Association. (2000). *Diagnostic and statistical manual of mental disorders* (4th ed., text rev.; DSM-IV-TR). Washington, DC: Author.

Antshel, K. M., Aneja, A., Strunge, L., Peebles, J., Fremont, W. P., Stallone, K., et al. (2007). Autistic spectrum disorders in velocardio facial syndrome (22q11.2 deletion). *Journal of Autism and Developmental Disorders, 37*(9), 1776–1786.

Arnold, L. E., Aman, M. G., Cook, A. M., Witwer, A. N., Hall, K. L., Thompson, S., et al. (2006). Atomoxetine for hyperactivity in autism spectrum disorders: placebo-controlled crossover pilot trial. *Journal of the American Academy of Child and Adolescent Psychiatry, 45*(10), 1196–1205.

Blachman, D. R., & Hinshaw, S. P. (2002). Patterns of friendship among girls with and without attention-deficit/hyperactivity disorder. *Journal of Abnormal Child Psychology, 30*(6), 625–640.

Clark, T., Feehan, C., Tinline, C., & Vostanis, P. (1999). Autistic symptoms in children with attention deficit-hyperactivity disorder. *European Child and Adolescent Psychiatry, 8*(1), 50–55.

Constantino, J. N., Davis, S. A., Todd, R. D., Schindler, M. K., Gross, M. M., Brophy, S. L., et al. (2003). Validation of a brief quantitative measure of autistic traits: comparison of the social responsiveness scale with the Autism Diagnostic Interview-Revised. *Journal of Autism and Developmental Disorders, 33*(4), 427–433.

Constantino, J. N., & Gruber, C. P. (2005). *Social Responsiveness Scale (SRS) manual.* Los Angeles: Western Psychological Services.

Constantino, J. N., Przybeck, T., Friesen, D., & Todd, R. D. (2000). Reciprocal social behavior in children with and without pervasive developmental disorders. *Journal of Developmental and Behavioral Pediatrics, 21*(1), 2–11.

Cook, E. H., Jr., & Scherer, S. W. (2008). Copy-number variations associated with neuropsychiatric conditions. *Nature, 455*(7215), 919–923.

de Boo, G. M., & Prins, P. J. (2007). Social incompetence in children with ADHD: possible moderators and mediators in social-skills training. *Clinical Psychology Review, 27*(1), 78–97.

DeVincent, C. J., Gadow, K. D., Delosh, D., & Geller, L. (2007). Sleep disturbance and its relation to DSM-IV psychiatric symptoms in preschool-age children with pervasive developmental disorder and community controls. *Journal of Child Neurology, 22*(2), 161–169.

Diamantopoulou, S., Rydell, A. M., Thorell, L. B., & Bohlin, G. (2007). Impact of executive functioning and symptoms of attention deficit hyperactivity disorder on children's peer relations and school performance. *Developmental Neuropsychology, 32*(1), 521–542.

Elia, J., Gai, X., Xie, H. M., Perin, J. C., Geiger, E., Glessner, J. T., et al. (2009, June 23). Rare structural variants found in attention-deficit hyperactivity disorder are preferentially associated with neurodevelopmental genes. *Molecular Psychiatry.* Electronically published June 23.

Faraone, S. V., Perlis, R. H., Doyle, A. E., Smoller, J. W., Goralnick, J. J., Holmgren, M. A., et al. (2005). Molecular genetics of attention-deficit/hyperactivity disorder. *Biological Psychiatry, 57*(11), 1313–1323.

Farzin, F., Perry, H., Hessl, D., Loesch, D., Cohen, J., Bacalman, S., et al. (2006). Autism spectrum disorders and attention-deficit/hyperactivity disorder in boys with the fragile X premutation. *Journal of Developmental and Behavioral Pediatrics, 27*(2 Suppl), S137–144.

Fine, S. E., Weissman, A., Gerdes, M., Pinto-Martin, J., Zackai, E. H., McDonald-McGinn, D. M., et al. (2005). Autism spectrum disorders and symptoms in children with molecularly confirmed 22q11.2 deletion syndrome. *Journal of Autism and Developmental Disorders, 35*(4), 461–470.

Gadow, K. D., Devincent, C., & Schneider, J. (2008). Predictors of psychiatric symptoms in children with an autism spectrum disorder. *Journal of Autism and Developmental Disorders, 38*(9), 1710–1720.

Gadow, K. D., & DeVincent, C. J. (2005). Clinical significance of tics and attention-deficit hyperactivity disorder (ADHD) in children with pervasive developmental disorder. *Journal of Child Neurology, 20*(6), 481–488.

Gadow, K. D., Devincent, C. J., & Drabick, D. A. (2008). Oppositional defiant disorder as a clinical phenotype in children with autism spectrum disorder. *Journal of Autism and Developmental Disorders, 38*(7), 1302–1310.

Gadow, K. D., DeVincent, C. J., & Pomeroy, J. (2006). ADHD symptom subtypes in children with pervasive developmental disorder. *Journal of Autism and Developmental Disorders, 36*(2), 271–283.

Gadow, K. D., DeVincent, C. J., Pomeroy, J., & Azizian, A. (2004). Psychiatric symptoms in preschool children with PDD and clinic and comparison samples. *Journal of Autism and Developmental Disorders, 34*(4), 379–393.

Gadow, K. D., Devincent, C. J., Pomeroy, J., & Azizian, A. (2005). Comparison of DSM-IV symptoms in elementary school-age children with PDD versus clinic and community samples. *Autism, 9*(4), 392–415.

Gadow, K. D., Roohi, J., DeVincent, C. J., & Hatchwell, E. (2008). Association of ADHD, tics, and anxiety with dopamine transporter (DAT1) genotype in autism spectrum disorder. *Journal of Child Psychology and Psychiatry, 49*(12), 1331–1338.

Geurts, H. M., Verte, S., Oosterlaan, J., Roeyers, H., & Sergeant, J. A. (2004). How specific are executive functioning deficits in attention deficit hyperactivity disorder and autism? *Journal of Child Psychology and Psychiatry, 45*(4), 836–854.

Gillberg, C. (2003). Deficits in attention, motor control, and perception: a brief review. *Archives of Disease in Childhood, 88*(10), 904–910.

Glessner, J. T., Wang, K., Cai, G., Korvatska, O., Kim, C. E., Wood, S., et al. (2009). Autism genome-wide copy number variation reveals ubiquitin and neuronal genes. *Nature, 459*(7246), 569–573.

Goldberg, M. C., Mostofsky, S. H., Cutting, L. E., Mahone, E. M., Astor, B. C., Denckla, M. B., et al. (2005). Subtle executive impairment in children with autism and children with ADHD. *Journal of Autism and Developmental Disorders, 35*(3), 279–293.

Goldstein, S., & Schwebach, A. J. (2004). The comorbidity of pervasive developmental disorder and attention deficit hyperactivity disorder: results of a retrospective chart review. *Journal of Autism and Developmental Disorders, 34*(3), 329–339.

Gothelf, D., Gruber, R., Presburger, G., Dotan, I., Brand-Gothelf, A., Burg, M., et al. (2003). Methylphenidate treatment for attention-deficit/hyperactivity disorder in children and adolescents with velocardiofacial syndrome: an open-label study. *Journal of Clinical Psychiatry, 64*(10), 1163–1169.

Gothelf, D., Presburger, G., Levy, D., Nahmani, A., Burg, M., Berant, M., et al. (2004). Genetic, developmental, and physical factors associated with attention deficit hyperactivity disorder in patients with velocardiofacial syndrome. *American Journal of Medical Genetics. Part B, Neuropsychiatric Genetics, 126*(1), 116–121.

Grzadzinski, R., Di Martino, A., Brady, E., Mairena, M. A., O'Neale, M., Petkova, E., et al. (2010, November 25). Examining autistic traits in children with ADHD: Does the autism spectrum extend to ADHD? *Journal of Autism and Developmental Disorders*, electronically published.

Handen, B. L., Johnson, C. R., & Lubetsky, M. (2000). Efficacy of methylphenidate among children with autism and symptoms of attention-deficit hyperactivity disorder. *Journal of Autism and Developmental Disorders, 30*(3), 245–255.

Handen, B. L., Sahl, R., & Hardan, A. Y. (2008). Guanfacine in children with autism and/or intellectual disabilities. *Journal of Developmental and Behavioral Pediatrics, 29*(4), 303–308.

Hattori, J., Ogino, T., Abiru, K., Nakano, K., Oka, M., & Ohtsuka, Y. (2006). Are pervasive developmental disorders and attention-deficit/hyperactivity disorder distinct disorders? *Brain and Development, 28*(6), 371–374.

Hazell, P. (2007). Drug therapy for attention-deficit/hyperactivity disorder-like symptoms in autistic disorder. *Journal of Paediatrics and Child Health, 43*(1–2), 19–24.

Hogart, A., Wu, D., Lasalle, J. M., & Schanen, N. C. (2010). The comorbidity of autism with the genomic disorders of chromosome 15q11.2-q13. *Neurobiology of Disease, 38*(2), 181–191.

Holtmann, M., Bolte, S., & Poustka, F. (2007). Attention deficit hyperactivity disorder symptoms in pervasive developmental disorders: association with autistic behavior domains and coexisting psychopathology. *Psychopathology, 40*(3), 172–177.

Hoza, B., Gerdes, A. C., Mrug, S., Hinshaw, S. P., Bukowski, W. M., Gold, J. A., et al. (2005). Peer-assessed outcomes in the multimodal treatment study of children with attention deficit hyperactivity disorder. *Journal of Clinical Child and Adolescent Psychology, 34*(1), 74–86.

Hoza, B., Mrug, S., Gerdes, A. C., Hinshaw, S. P., Bukowski, W. M., Gold, J. A., et al. (2005). What aspects of peer relationships are impaired in children with attention-deficit/hyperactivity disorder? *Journal of Consulting and Clinical Psychology, 73*(3), 411–423.

Jensen, P. S., Hinshaw, S. P., Kraemer, H. C., Lenora, N., Newcorn, J. H., Abikoff, H. B., et al. (2001). ADHD comorbidity findings from the MTA study: comparing comorbid subgroups. *Journal of the American Academy of Child and Adolescent Psychiatry, 40*(2), 147–158.

Kakinuma, H., & Sato, H. (2008). Copy-number variations associated with autism spectrum disorder. *Pharmacogenomics, 9*(8), 1143–1154.

Kusenda, M., & Sebat, J. (2008). The role of rare structural variants in the genetics of autism spectrum disorders. *Cytogenetic and Genome Research, 123*(1–4), 36–43.

Lecavalier, L., Gadow, K. D., Devincent, C. J., & Edwards, M. C. (2009). Validation of DSM-IV model of psychiatric syndromes in children with autism spectrum disorders. *Journal of Autism and Developmental Disorders, 39*(2), 278–289.

Lee, D. O., & Ousley, O. Y. (2006). Attention-deficit hyperactivity disorder symptoms in a clinic sample of children and adolescents with pervasive developmental disorders. *Journal of Child and Adolescent Psychopharmacology, 16*(6), 737–746.

Lichtenstein, P., Carlstrom, E., Rastam, M., Gillberg, C., & Anckarsater, H. (2010). The genetics of autism spectrum disorders and related neuropsychiatric disorders in childhood. *American Journal of Psychiatry, 167*(11), 1357–1363.

Livesey, D., Keen, J., Rouse, J., & White, F. (2006). The relationship between measures of executive function, motor performance, and externalising behaviour in 5- and 6-year-old children. *Human Movement Science, 25*(1), 50–64.

Mahone, E. M., Powell, S. K., Loftis, C. W., Goldberg, M. C., Denckla, M. B., & Mostofsky, S. H. (2006). Motor persistence and inhibition in autism and ADHD. *Journal of the International Neuropsychological Society, 12*(5), 622–631.

McGough, J. J. (2005). Attention-deficit/hyperactivity disorder pharmacogenomics. *Biological Psychiatry, 57*(11), 1367–1373.

Mostofsky, S. H., Burgess, M. P., & Gidley Larson, J. C. (2007). Increased motor cortex white matter volume predicts motor impairment in autism. *Brain, 130*(Pt 8), 2117–2122.

Mulligan, A., Anney, R. J., O'Regan, M., Chen, W., Butler, L., Fitzgerald, M., et al. (2009). Autism symptoms in Attention-Deficit/Hyperactivity Disorder: a familial trait which correlates with conduct, oppositional defiant, language, and motor disorders. *Journal of Autism and Developmental Disorders, 39*(2), 197–209.

Murphy, K. C. (2005). Annotation: velo-cardio-facial syndrome. *Journal of Child Psychology and Psychiatry, 46*(6), 563–571.

Neuman, R. J., Lobos, E., Reich, W., Henderson, C. A., Sun, L. W., & Todd, R. D. (2007). Prenatal smoking exposure and dopaminergic genotypes interact to cause a severe ADHD subtype. *Biological Psychiatry, 61*(12), 1320–1328.

Nieoullon, A. (2002). Dopamine and the regulation of cognition and attention. *Progress in Neurobiology, 67*(1), 53–83.

Nijmeijer, J. S., Arias-Vasquez, A., Rommelse, N. N., Altink, M. E., Anney, R. J., Asherson, P., et al. (2010). Identifying loci for the overlap between attention-deficit/hyperactivity disorder and autism spectrum disorder using a genome-wide QTL linkage approach. *Journal of the American Academy of Child and Adolescent Psychiatry, 49*(7), 675–685.

Nijmeijer, J. S., Hartman, C. A., Rommelse, N. N., Altink, M. E., Buschgens, C. J., Fliers, E. A., et al. (2010). Perinatal risk factors interacting with catechol O-methyltransferase and the serotonin transporter gene predict ASD symptoms in children with ADHD. *Journal of Child Psychology and Psychiatry, 51*(11), 1242–1250.

Nijmeijer, J. S., Hoekstra, P. J., Minderaa, R. B., Buitelaar, J. K., Altink, M. E., Buschgens, C. J., et al. (2009). PDD symptoms in ADHD, an independent familial trait? *Journal of Abnormal Child Psychology, 37*(3), 443–453.

Niklasson, L., Rasmussen, P., Oskarsdottir, S., & Gillberg, C. (2002). Chromosome 22q11 deletion syndrome (CATCH 22): neuropsychiatric and neuropsychological aspects. *Developmental Medicine and Child Neurology, 44*(1), 44–50.

Ogino, T., Hattori, J., Abiru, K., Nakano, K., Oka, E., & Ohtsuka, Y. (2005). Symptoms related to ADHD observed in patients with pervasive developmental disorder. *Brain and Development, 27*(5), 345–348.

Ousley, O., Rockers, K., Dell, M. L., Coleman, K., & Cubells, J. F. (2007). A review of neurocognitive and behavioral profiles associated with 22q11 deletion syndrome: implications for clinical evaluation and treatment. *Current Psychiatry Reports, 9*(2), 148–158.

Pennington, B. F., & Ozonoff, S. (1996). Executive functions and developmental psychopathology. *Journal of Child Psychology and Psychiatry, 37*(1), 51–87.

Piek, J. P., Dyck, M. J., Francis, M., & Conwell, A. (2007). Working memory, processing speed, and set-shifting in children with developmental coordination disorder and attention-deficit-hyperactivity disorder. *Developmental Medicine and Child Neurology, 49*(9), 678–683.

Piek, J. P., Dyck, M. J., Nieman, A., Anderson, M., Hay, D., Smith, L. M., et al. (2004). The relationship between motor coordination, executive functioning, and attention in school aged children. *Archives of Clinical Neuropsychology, 19*(8), 1063–1076.

Posey, D. J., Puntney, J. I., Sasher, T. M., Kem, D. L., & McDougle, C. J. (2004). Guanfacine treatment of hyperactivity and inattention in pervasive developmental disorders: a retrospective analysis of 80 cases. *Journal of Child and Adolescent Psychopharmacology, 14*(2), 233–241.

Posey, D. J., Wiegand, R. E., Wilkerson, J., Maynard, M., Stigler, K. A., & McDougle, C. J. (2006). Open-label atomoxetine for attention-deficit/hyperactivity disorder symptoms associated with high-functioning pervasive developmental disorders. *Journal of Child and Adolescent Psychopharmacology, 16*(5), 599–610.

Reiersen, A. M. (2007). Psychopathology in 22q11 deletion syndrome. *Journal of the American Academy of Child and Adolescent Psychiatry, 46*(8), 942; author reply 942–944.

Reiersen, A. M., Constantino, J. N., & Todd, R. D. (2008). Co-occurrence of motor problems and autistic symptoms in attention-deficit/hyperactivity disorder. *Journal of the American Academy of Child and Adolescent Psychiatry, 47*(6), 662–672.

Reiersen, A. M., Constantino, J. N., Volk, H. E., & Todd, R. D. (2007). Autistic traits in a population-based ADHD twin sample. *Journal of Child Psychology and Psychiatry, 48*(5), 464–472.

Reiersen, A. M., Neuman, R. J., Reich, W., Constantino, J. N., Volk, H. E., & Todd, R. D. (2008). Intersection of autism and ADHD: Evidence for a distinct syndrome influenced by genes and by gene-environment interactions. In J. J. Hudziak (Ed.), *Developmental psychopathology and wellness: Genetic and environmental influences* (pp. 191–208). Arlington, VA: American Psychiatric Publishing.

Reiersen, A. M., & Todd, R. D. (2008). Co-occurrence of ADHD and autism spectrum disorders: phenomenology and treatment. *Expert Review of Neurotherapeutics, 8*(4), 657–669.

Rommelse, N. N. J., Franke, B., Geurts, H. M., Hartman, C. A., & Buitelaar, J. K. (2010). Shared heritability of attention-deficit/hyperactivity disorder and autism spectrum disorder. *European Child and Adolescent Psychiatry, 19*(3), 281–295.

Ronald A., Edelson, L. R., Asherson, P., Saudino, K. J. (2010). Exploring the relationship between autistic-like traits and ADHD behaviors in early childhood: findings from a community twin study of 2-year-olds. *Journal of Abnormal Child Psychology, 38*(2), 185–196.

Ronald, A., Simonoff, E., Kuntsi, J., Asherson, P., & Plomin, R. (2008). Evidence for overlapping genetic influences on autistic and ADHD behaviours in a community twin sample. *Journal of Child Psychology and Psychiatry, 49*(5), 535–542.

Roohi, J., DeVincent, C. J., Hatchwell, E., & Gadow, K. D. (2009). Association of a monoamine oxidase-a gene promoter polymorphism with ADHD and anxiety in boys with autism spectrum disorder. *Journal of Autism and Developmental Disorders, 39*(1), 67–74.

RUPP. (2005). Randomized, controlled, crossover trial of methylphenidate in pervasive developmental disorders with hyperactivity. *Archives of General Psychiatry, 62*(11), 1266–1274.

Santosh, P. J., Baird, G., Pityaratstian, N., Tavare, E., & Gringras, P. (2006). Impact of comorbid autism spectrum disorders on stimulant response in children with attention deficit hyperactivity disorder: a retrospective and prospective effectiveness study. *Child: Care, Health, and Development, 32*(5), 575–583.

Santosh, P. J., & Mijovic, A. (2004). Social impairment in Hyperkinetic Disorder: Relationship to psychopathology and environmental stressors. *European Child and Adolescent Psychiatry, 13*(3), 141–150.

Scahill, L., Aman, M. G., McDougle, C. J., McCracken, J. T., Tierney, E., Dziura, J., et al. (2006). A prospective open trial of guanfacine in children with pervasive developmental disorders. *Journal of Child and Adolescent Psychopharmacology, 16*(5), 589–598.

Sergeant, J. A., Geurts, H., & Oosterlaan, J. (2002). How specific is a deficit of executive functioning for attention-deficit/hyperactivity disorder? *Behavioural Brain Research, 130*(1–2), 3–28.

Simonoff, E., Pickles, A., Charman, T., Chandler, S., Loucas, T., & Baird, G. (2008). Psychiatric disorders in children with autism spectrum disorders: prevalence, comorbidity, and associated factors in a population-derived sample. *Journal of the American Academy of Child and Adolescent Psychiatry, 47*(8), 921–929.

Smalley, S. L., Loo, S. K., Yang, M. H., & Cantor, R. M. (2005). Toward localizing genes underlying cerebral asymmetry and mental health. *American Journal of Medical Genetics. Part B, Neuropsychiatric Genetics, 135*(1), 79–84.

Sturm, H., Fernell, E., & Gillberg, C. (2004). Autism spectrum disorders in children with normal intellectual levels: associated impairments and subgroups. *Developmental Medicine and Child Neurology, 46*(7), 444–447.

Todd, R. D., & Botteron, K. N. (2001). Is attention-deficit/hyperactivity disorder an energy deficiency syndrome? *Biological Psychiatry, 50*(3), 151–158.

Todd, R. D., Huang, H., Smalley, S. L., Nelson, S. F., Willcutt, E. G., Pennington, B. F., et al. (2005). Collaborative analysis of DRD4 and DAT genotypes in population-defined ADHD subtypes. *Journal of Child Psychology and Psychiatry, 46*(10), 1067–1073.

Todd, R. D., & Neuman, R. J. (2007). Gene-environment interactions in the development of combined type ADHD: evidence for a synapse-based model. *American Journal of Medical Genetics. Part B, Neuropsychiatric Genetics, 144B*(8), 971–975.

Troost, P. W., Steenhuis, M. P., Tuynman-Qua, H. G., Kalverdijk, L. J., Buitelaar, J. K., Minderaa, R. B., et al. (2006). Atomoxetine for attention-deficit/hyperactivity disorder symptoms in children with pervasive developmental disorders: a pilot study. *Journal of Child and Adolescent Psychopharmacology, 16*(5), 611–619.

Vorstman, J. A., Morcus, M. E., Duijff, S. N., Klaassen, P. W., Heineman-de Boer, J. A., Beemer, F. A., et al. (2006). The 22q11.2 deletion in children: high rate of autistic disorders and early onset of psychotic symptoms. *Journal of the American Academy of Child and Adolescent Psychiatry, 45*(9), 1104–1113.

Williams, H. J., Owen, M. J., & O'Donovan, M. C. (2009). Schizophrenia genetics: new insights from new approaches. *British Medical Bulletin, 91*, 61–74.

Yoshida, Y., & Uchiyama, T. (2004). The clinical necessity for assessing attention deficit/hyperactivity disorder (AD/HD) symptoms in children with high-functioning pervasive developmental disorder (PDD). *European Child and Adolescent Psychiatry, 13*(5), 307–314.

19

J. Bruce Tomblin, Karla McGregor, Allison Bean

Specific Language Impairment

Points of Interest

- The deficits in specific language impairment (SLI) extend beyond language.
- The language deficits that are common in SLI involve the meaning (semantics) system and the structural (grammatical) system. Speech sound disorders (phonology) and disorders of language use (pragmatics) are less common.
- The range of severity of language deficits in children with SLI is more limited than that found in children with ASD.
- The nature of the overlap of SLI and ASD within affected children, as well as near family members remains a topic of debate.
- *CNTNAP2* appears to be a liability gene for ASD and SLI.

SLI, also called developmental aphasia, dysphasia, developmental language disorder, or language delay, is a developmental disorder characterized by limitations in language learning. Children with SLI are less capable than their unaffected same-age peers at understanding or expressing language. Any or all domains of language—syntax, morphology, phonology, semantics, and pragmatics—may be affected and, in any given child, one domain of language may be more severely affected than another. The extent to which they are behind their peers varies from mild to severe. The hallmarks of SLI vary with age: toddlers with SLI typically present with late onset of first words (Trauner, Wulfeck, Tallal, & Hesselink, 2000); preschoolers are often late to acquire grammatical inflections and function words (Leonard, 1998; Rice & Wexler, 1996); school children frequently have difficulty with sentence repetition (Conti-Ramsden, Botting, & Faragher, 2001), word finding (Lahey & Edwards, 1999; McGregor, Newman, Reilly, & Capone, 2002), and narrative formulation (Johnston, 2008; Liles, 1985). Learning to read and write is often problematic as well (Catts, 1993). Some children do seem to "outgrow" SLI early in life, but once children enter school, the severity of their deficits remains relatively stable (Tomblin, Zhang, Buckwalter, & O'Brien, 2003). Older children and young adults present with a broad range of academic difficulties (Young et al., 2002). Follow-ups beyond the late teens are rare, but one study of seventeen 30-year-olds who had severe receptive and expressive SLI as children revealed persistent problems with spoken and written language as well as deficits in phonological processing, verbal short-term memory, and theory of mind (Clegg, Hollis, Mawhood, & Rutter, 2005). Even among adults who seem to have compensated for their SLI, weaknesses emerge in formal assessments that stress the linguistic system (Tomblin, Freese, & Records, 1992).

As the name implies, the clinical manifestations of SLI are limited to language. By definition, there are no broader, clinically significant deficits in cognition or delays in motor, social, or emotional development (American Psychiatric Association, 1994, *Diagnostic and statistical manual of mental disorders*). Nevertheless, it is common for children with SLI to struggle in academic and social settings and to have difficulty with peer relationships (Young et al., 2002; Clegg et al., 2005).

This chapter will summarize the status of research on the nature and etiology of SLI. Because late emergence of language and, in many cases, subsequent limitations in language learning also characterize children with autism spectrum disorders (ASD), we will pay particular attention to similarities and differences that may exist between SLI and autism with regard to symptoms and etiology. At the end of the chapter we will examine models of the relationships between ASD and SLI.

Prevalence

SLI is a common developmental disorder. In the United States, prevalence is estimated at 7.4% (Tomblin, Records,

Buckwalter, et al., 1997). Of course, prevalence estimates are a rather direct function of the test cutoffs used for identification. In the study conducted by Tomblin and colleagues (1997), children randomly sampled from the states of Iowa and Illinois were identified as having SLI if they scored at least 1.25 standard deviations below the mean on at least two of six measures of language. If the distributions of these scores had matched perfectly the distribution of the scores collected from children nationwide during the norming of these tests, one would expect 10% of the children to fall at or below 1.25 standard deviations of the mean (a score of -1.25 standard deviations is equivalent to the 10th percentile). Therefore, it is quite sensible that the prevalence estimate obtained by Tomblin and colleagues was close to 10%. A cutoff of -1 would have yielded a higher estimate of prevalence; -2 a lower one. The logical relationship between rather arbitrary test cutoffs and prevalence does not diminish the validity of the diagnosis. In societies that place high value on articulate language, being among the least articulate 3%, 10%, or even 15%, of the society is nearly certain to limit success and well-being.

Diagnosis

The diagnosis of SLI is based solely on certain patterns of strength and weakness rather than etiology. In this respect, it is similar to many developmental disorders such as autism. A clinician may diagnose SLI in children who have poor language achievement and yet the common causes of slow language development such as mental retardation, autism, or limitations in motor control and hearing acuity can be excluded (Stark & Tallal, 1981). Frank neurological problems are also excluded in cases of SLI; however as we will note later, subtle differences in brain structure are likely. SLI is typically diagnosed in the preschool or early school years (Stanton-Chapman, Chapman, Bainbridge, & Scott, 2002), although diagnoses are possible at both earlier and later points in development. The clinician commonly documents poor performance on a battery of standardized language tests as well as some detriment to the function of the child in familial, social, academic, or professional settings. For example, interviews with the teacher, observations of the child in classroom situations, and curriculum-based assessments may reveal the functional impact on academics (Westby, 2006). Clinicians may also supplement standardized tests and functional assessments with dynamic assessments, tasks that measure the ability to learn aspects of language over time rather than extant knowledge of the language at a single point in time (Pena, Iglesias, & Lidz, 2001).

There is no universally agreed on test battery nor a particular test score that defines SLI. In recent years, tasks that involve repetition of nonwords (1996), sentence repetition (Conti-Ramsden et al., 2001), and marking of tense and agreement in English speakers (Rice & Wexler, 1996) have been proposed as sensitive indicators of SLI; however these markers have not been shown to be specific to SLI, as poor performance on these is also found in other populations of children with developmental disorders (see, for instance, Eadie et al., 2002; Grant et al., 1997). Tests that are well standardized and appropriately normed for the test-taker and that include measures of comprehension and production in all language domains would be considered best practice (Bishop, 1997). Depending on the age of the test-taker, tests that measure written as well as spoken language may be included. Guidelines set forth in the International Classification of Diseases (World Health Organization, 1993) specify that children diagnosed with SLI score at least 2 standard deviations below age level on standardized measures of language. Bishop and Edmundson (1987) associated severe SLI with scores of at least 2 standard deviations below the mean on any measure and moderate SLI with scores of at least 1.5 standard deviations below the mean on two or more measures. Specific cutoffs vary from lab to lab, clinic to clinic, and school to school (Aram, Morris, & Hall, 1993).

Diagnosis of SLI and ASD Compared

Current standards for the diagnosis of autism require a delay in the development of language and persistent qualitative abnormalities in the social use of language. Subsequent to the delay in language onset, a substantial variation in the use of language form (syntax, morphology, and phonology) and content can been seen among children with ASD. SLI is primarily characterized by deficits in the development of the form and content of language. Thus, whereas children with ASD may or may not have form and content deficits, all children with SLI will have such deficits and these are likely to be persistent through much if not all of childhood. Children with ASD are also required to have impairments in social interactions and the presence of repetitive stereotyped behaviors for diagnosis. In contrast, children with such social and behavioral deficits would be excluded from a diagnosis of SLI (Leonard, 1998). As such, SLI and autism by definition are exclusive of each other because of this exclusionary condition within the construct of SLI. This exclusionary requirement was established to highlight the fact that often language impairment can be found in the absence of other conditions; however, the requirement that SLI be independent of autism must be recognized for what it is—a diagnostic criterion established purely by fiat. We therefore acknowledge that there is certainly a reasonable chance that the developmental conditions that contribute to SLI could also contribute to autism. Therefore, overlap in behavioral characteristics and etiology should be considered as viable and requires empirical consideration.

One way that SLI and ASD might overlap is that SLI could developmentally progress into autism. Two studies recently reported data showing that some children initially diagnosed as language impaired and perhaps SLI as young children were later found to meet diagnostic qualifications for ASD. Conti-Ramsden et al. (2006) reported that approximately 4 percent of adolescents with a history of SLI demonstrated characteristics necessary for a diagnosis of ASD, as considered by the ADOS and ADI-R; a rate nearly 10 times what would be expected for the general population. These authors concluded that this was due to the developmental progression of SLI into ASD. Bishop et al. (2008) also reported that 21% of adults who had earlier been identified as having specific speech and language impairments in early childhood met criteria for ASD using the ADOS-G and ADI-R. These authors interpreted their data and those of Conti-Ramsden et al. (2006) as indicative of diagnostic substitution in childhood. This substitution of language impairment for autism was considered to be the result of narrower criteria for autism at the time of the initial diagnosis. With changes in diagnostic criteria over time, children who earlier were not viewed as presenting ASD came to meet the criteria for ASD as the criteria shifted.

Behavioral Profile

An early sign of SLI is the late emergence of spoken words during the second year of life (Trauner et al., 1995). (Charman, Drew, Baird, & Baird, 2003; Ellis Weismer, et al., 2008; Luyster, Lopez, & Lord, 2007) Even after the child with SLI has begun to use words, subsequent word learning remains slow relative to same-age peers. For example, preschoolers with SLI require twice the numbers of exposures to new words before they can learn them (Gray, 2003). Once a word has been learned, semantic representation of the word is typically fragile as characterized by word-finding problems in preschoolers and school-age children with SLI, as well as sparse lexical semantic representations and semantic category knowledge (Kail & Leonard, 1986; McGregor et al., 2002). As compared to expression, comprehension of words is an area of relative strength (Thal & Tobias, 1992).

In general, the grammatical development of children with SLI is even more limited than their word learning. In the preschool years, they tend to produce short sentences that lack nonobligatory arguments and grammatical inflections (van der Lely, 1998). Inflections that mark finite tense and agreement on verbs (e.g, he play*s*, he play*ed*) are particularly prone to omission (Rice & Wexler, 1996). Children with SLI continue to lag behind their same-age peers in grammatical development once they have entered school. For example, they rarely use sentences that involve noncanonical word order (e.g., *the dog was kissed by the cat*), auxiliary inversion (e.g., *is he going to the store?*), conjoined clauses (e.g., *he is happy but she is sad*), or embedded clauses (e.g, *we knew he could swim*) (Johnston & Kamhi, 1984; Leonard, 1995). Careful testing reveals that comprehension of these advanced sentence structures is often problematic as well (Bishop, 1997; van der Lely, 1994). Though no longer frequent in their spoken language, omissions of grammatical inflections characterize their written language (Scott & Windsor, 2000).

For many children with SLI, speech sound production is an area of relative strength (Kjelgaard & Tager-Flusberg, 2001; Shriberg, Tomblin, & McSweeny, 1999). Shriberg and colleagues (1999) reported the comorbidity of speech sound deficits and SLI to be less than 2%. Despite this sparing of speech sound production abilities, children with SLI have often been shown to be poorer than typically developing age mates in tasks that place demands on phonological skills such as those requiring repetition of lengthy unfamiliar phonological sequences (nonword repetition) (Bishop et al., 1996; Conti-Ramsden & Botting, 2000), the conscious identification and manipulation of sound units of words (deletion or blending of syllables or phonemes) (Kamhi et al., 1988), and perceptual discriminations of synthetic speech or syllabic words (Coady et al., 2007; Montgomery, 2003).

Pragmatics and the social use of language is generally considered a relative strength for children with SLI: 85% score higher on measures of pragmatic communication than semantics and syntax (Tomblin, Zhang, Weiss, Catts, & Ellis Weismer, 2004). That said, children with SLI present with a variety of pragmatic difficulties including attributing emotions to others and understanding utterances that are not literally true (Botting & Conti-Ramsden, 2008; Farmer, 2000), even after controlling for overall language ability (Botting & Conti-Ramsden, 2008). These children also demonstrate difficulty with basic social tasks. They interact differently than their normally developing peers in classroom contexts, are less preferred by their peers, and experience significantly fewer peer contacts (Bishop & Baird, 2001; Botting & Conti-Ramsden, 2008; Craig, 1993; Fujiki, Brinton, & Todd, 1996). These difficulties may, in part, be attributed to the difficulty that children with SLI demonstrate in their conversational exchanges. Because they have difficulty taking the perspective of their conversational partner (Farrant, Fletcher, & Mayberry, 2006), children with SLI tend to contribute too little or too much information, make irrelevant comments, and/or ask inappropriate questions (Adams & Bishop, 1989; Marton, Abramoff, & Rosenzweig, 2005). These are long-term problems that increase with age, leading to an increased risk of victimization by 11 years of age (Conti-Ramsden & Botting, 2004). Thus, although pragmatics is not a prominent area of difficulty for them, children with SLI are not unscathed in social communication.

A subgroup of children with SLI with pragmatic difficulties that overshadow their grammatical deficits but do not meet the criteria for a diagnosis of ASD have been described (Bishop & Norbury, 2002; Botting & Conti-Ramsden, 1999). This profile has been referred to as semantic-pragmatic language impairment or more recently pragmatic language impairment (PLI; Bishop, 2000; Brook & Bowler, 1992). These children do not represent misdiagnosed cases of ASD, but rather are a group of children who have some features of both autism and SLI. Children with PLI have been described as sociable, talkative children who produce stereotyped language with abnormal prosody, focusing conversation on topics of their own particular interest. However, these same children have good reciprocal interactions and do not show nonverbal repetitive behaviors that are characteristic of ASD (Bishop & Norbury, 2002).

Behavioral Profiles of SLI and ASD Compared

To summarize, children with SLI have widespread deficits in communication development, but with particular difficulties with grammar and phonological working memory along with relative strengths in speech sound production and pragmatics. The language and communication profiles of children with ASD are more completely described in Chapters 9 and 27 in this volume. In those chapters we find that the skills of children with ASD with regard to form and content can vary widely. With regard to those aspects of language most often viewed as "markers of SLI," there are data that show that some, but not all, of the children with ASD show poor grammatical skills (Botting & Conti-Ramsden, 2003; Kjelgaard & Tager-Flusberg, 2001; Roberts et al., 2004) and also poorer phonological short-term memory as shown in their nonword repetition (Botting & Conti-Ramsden, 2003; Kjelgaard & Tager-Flusberg, 2001; Whitehouse et al., 2007). These data have provided the basis for an active debate over the presence or nature of an overlap of SLI and ASD, as will be discuss further at the end of this chapter.

As noted earlier in the diagnostic contrast of SLI and ASD, impaired reciprocal social interactions are grounds for ruling out SLI, whereas such impairments are required of children with ASD. Additionally, the use of language for socially adapted appropriate communication has been well documented to be a prominent feature of ASD. Therefore, an overlap in the full range of pragmatics deficits between SLI and ASD has been essentially prohibited by this exclusionary condition. Also as noted above, children with SLI have been shown to have difficulties with pragmatics, but these deficits are generally less prominent than those seen in ASD. Furthermore, there is some question as to whether the pragmatic difficulties in SLI are a primary part of the communication problems of children with SLI or secondary to the form and content difficulties they experience (Redmond & Rice, 1998). Thus, pragmatics and social communication skills are clearly the developmental domain where there is little overlap between SLI and ASD. It remains unclear, however, as to whether this is evidence that these are naturally different developmental disorders or whether a naturally occurring relationship has been severed by the imposition of exclusionary standards for SLI. Studies concerned with underlying neurological function could shed light on this.

Neurological Findings and SLI

Questions concerning brain function among children with SLI have been informed by theory but limited by the technology that is available. Thus, in concert with research concerned with other developmental disorders such as autism and dyslexia, most of the search for neural anatomical bases of SLI has focused on whether there are differences in relative brain volumes across different brain regions. In particular, interest has focused on the cortical regions of the inferior frontal cortex including Broca's area and the temporal parietal region often defined as the perisylvian region including Wernicke's area. Within individuals with typical language development these regions are usually larger in the left hemisphere (leftward asymmetry) than the right. Likewise, measures of functional brain activity using fMRI or an intracarodid amobarbitol (Wada) test during language tasks have shown a common left hemispheric dominance for language tasks. This convergence of anatomical and functional asymmetry has supported the viewpoint that anatomical differences in these language areas could contribute to functional outcomes (for a cautionary viewpoint, see Eckert et al., 2006).

Early autopsy findings by Galaburda et al. (1985) suggested that developmental dyslexia and other developmental language disorders such as SLI might be associated with the absence of expected asymmetry of the perisylvian region. Soon after this, a neuropathological study of a deceased child with a diagnosis of developmental dysphasia was reported to have abnormal symmetry of the perisylvian region (Cohen et al., 1989). These findings generated considerable interest in this region as MRI imaging became available. Jernigan et al. (1991) reported that children with SLI had smaller-than-expected left perisylvian volumes, and at the same time Plante and colleagues (Plante et al., 1989; Plante et al., 1991) reported reduced left asymmetry of the perisylvian region. Similar results regarding reduced rates of leftward asymmetry of the perisylvian region in children with SLI were reported by Gauger et al. (1997). Preis et al. however, did not find abnormal symmetry in the perisylvian region (Preis et al., 1998). Gauger et al. also extended the regions of interest for SLI to the inferior frontal cortex, where they also found the volume of the left pars triangularis to be smaller in children with SLI than controls. Evidence that abnormal asymmetries in the perisylvian region were further supported by Leonard and colleagues who found reduced asymmetry in this region differentiated children with SLI from children with dyslexia and normal readers (Leonard et al., 2002). More recently De Fosse et al. (2004) also found a rightward asymmetry in the inferior frontal cortex of children with SLI. Surprisingly, the planum temporale was found to have more leftward asymmetry in the children with SLI than among typically developing children in this study. Herbert et al. (2005) performed a nested hierarchical analysis ranging from whole brain through major anatomical lobes to smaller regions defined as parcellation units with images from children with SLI. Similar to De Fosse et al., they found more rightward asymmetry in the frontal language areas and more leftward asymmetry in the perisylvian language areas.

Most of the research concerning brain structure and SLI has concentrated on the study of brain regions that have long been associated with language functions. Such an approach assumes that there are language-specific brain regions and that language can be viewed as a special cognitive faculty. Under the alternate view that language arises from a widely distributed nonmodular neural system, Herbert and colleagues (Herbert et al., 2003; Herbert et al., 2005) examined larger-scale brain regions including subcortical structures. From this larger perspective they found little evidence of abnormal asymmetry at these whole brain–level analyses, despite having found such asymmetries at the more local parcellation units. At this larger-scale analysis they did find that children with SLI (and children with ASD) presented larger cortical volume due to greater amounts of white matter, in other words, greater amounts of connectivity via myelinated fiber tracts. Although connectivity is generally considered important for neural networks, excessive connectivity could result in inefficient and noisy processing.

These findings are beginning to reveal replicable differences between brain structure of typically developing children and those with SLI. Those studies concerned with patterns of asymmetry in the two principal language regions support the notion that variations in basic neurodevelopmental processes involving these language regions contribute to the liability for SLI. It seems that this vulnerability is more consistently found in the inferior frontal region than in the perisylvian region, and some evidence of more general abnormalities involving general brain size can be found. Of course these conclusions assume that these differences in asymmetry and volume are laid down during early development and are not themselves the product of poor language learning (Locke, 1994). Furthermore, it is clear that although there appear to be anatomical effects that are robust enough for group differences, there are often cases of either abnormal asymmetry accompanied by normal language or normal patterns of asymmetry accompanied by abnormal language. Thus, as Herbert et al. (2003) note, these anatomic findings do not point to a simple deterministic relationship with language development.

Neurological Findings in SLI and ASD Compared

There have been substantially more structural imaging studies of individuals with autism (see Section II of this book) than SLI. Far more brain regions and brain features have been examined in autism than in SLI, where the focus has largely been on language regions. Among these is a small set of studies that has directly contrasted children with SLI and children with ASD. In addition to reporting on findings concerned with SLI, the De Fosse et al. (2004) study described earlier compared children with SLI with children with ASD who either presented with poor language or had normal language abilities. Patterns of abnormal asymmetry in the inferior frontal cortex were found for the children with SLI and the children with ASD who were also language impaired. Likewise both the SLI and children with ASD and language impairment showed the unexpected exaggerated L > R asymmetry described earlier. The children with normal language but with ASD did not show these abnormal asymmetric relationships. Herbert et al. (2005) used children with ASD who were described as being high functioning and therefore would be likely to have had normal structural language abilities and may have been similar to De Fosse's normal language ASD group. Despite this, they also found patterns of asymmetry similar to those of the De Fosse study for both anterior and posterior parcellation units involved with language. Thus, they also found the unexpected abnormal exaggerated L > R in both groups. Also, as we noted earlier, this study found larger overall cortical size in both groups. Herbert and Kenet (2007) have concluded from these findings that autism and SLI share many, although not all, neurological features and thus could be viewed as overlapping conditions.

Familial Aggregation of SLI

If SLI and ASD are overlapping conditions, we would expect that they share, in part, etiological origins. One clue to the origins of SLI is that it tends to aggregate in families (Beitchman et al., 1992; Neils & Aram, 1986; Tallal et al., 1989; Tomblin, 1989). Familial aggregation is one piece of evidence in support of a genetic contribution to the etiology of SLI. Of course, as in all cases of complex developmental disorders, the behavioral manifestations of SLI are multidetermined: both genes and the environment participate. Certainly, genes are not the whole story. Three well-documented environmental risks for SLI are low maternal education (Stanton-Chapman et al., 2002; Tomblin, Smith, & Zhang, 1997), higher birth order (Hoff-Ginsberg, 1998; Stanton-Chapman et al., 2002; Tomblin, 1990), and single-parent homes (Stanton-Chapman et al., 2002). These risks pertain to the care-giving environment. Mothers with limited formal education are less knowledgeable about childcare and development than more educated mothers (Furstenberg, Brooks-Gunn, & Chase-Lansdale, 1989). If these mothers are the sole head of household or have many children, the time they can devote to any one child is limited. More siblings and fewer parents obviously make for less opportunity for dyadic interactions between child and adult, interactions known to facilitate language development (Tomasello & Farrar, 1986). Whereas none of these factors alone would cause SLI, a child with a vulnerable genotype faced with these environmental factors is at greater risk.

In any study of familial aggregation, results will vary depending on the phenotype, or behavioral profile, examined. Some studies of familial aggregation of SLI employ a broader phenotype; they include speech, language, and reading problems; whereas others employ a narrower phenotype. In the Tomblin (1989) study the phenotype was limited to specific language and speech sound disorders. Tomblin and Buckwalter (1994) have also found that SLI diagnosed on the basis of direct assessment occurs in 21% of the first-degree relatives of SLI probands and at a rate of 28% in the male relatives of these probands. Rice and colleagues (1998) reported very similar rates of speech/language impairment in the nuclear family members of probands who were identified by their failure to mark tense in obligatory contexts. More recently, Tallal and colleagues (Tallal et al., 2001) also tested family members of SLI probands and probands with normal language status. They reported a rate of 31% SLI in the families of the SLI probands and 7.1% in the control families. Thus, across a large number of studies using a range of methods of ascertainment and measurement of the language phenotype, support for the familiality of SLI can be found.

Twin studies of specific language impairment have provided evidence that this familial feature to SLI is at least partially genetically influenced. Lewis and Thompson (1992) reported concordance rates of 86% for monozygotic (MZ) and 48% for dizygotic (DZ) twins with speech and language problems. Bishop, North, and Donlan (1995) reported a concordance of .46 and .70 for the DZ and MZ twins, respectively, for twins ascertained for specific speech and language impairments. Later, Tomblin and Buckwalter (1998) looked at twins with a language-impaired proband and found a concordance for the MZ pairs of .96 and .69 for the DZ pairs and obtained a group difference heritability of .45. Dale and colleagues (1998) also have reported group differences heritability in a large-scale twin study. Using delays in vocabulary development of 2-year-olds as a phenotype, these investigators found heritability rates of .73. In the study by Dale and colleagues (1998) heritability was lower, as the cutoff score for language delay was shifted from the 5th percentile upward toward the 16th percentile, suggesting that there may be unique genetic contributions to particularly low language abilities. This research group (Spinath et al., 2004) has reported similar results for a phenotype that included grammar as well as vocabulary. In this study, group differences heritability for children with low language was higher than individual differences heritability (h^2) for a sample of children that included typically developing children. Thus heritability increased with severity; however variation in severity involved both verbal and nonverbal abilities.

In most of the studies up to this point, the phenotype was often one that allowed language, nonverbal IQ, and speech sound status to covary. During the last few years, research has come to focus on the question of which of these aspects of the phenotype are most likely to be genetically influenced. Initially the question focused on the covariance of language and nonverbal IQ. Hayiou-Thomas and colleagues (2005) reported that heritability of poor language accompanied by low nonverbal IQ (nonspecific language impairment; NLI) was much higher than was found for children who had discrepancies between language and nonverbal IQ (SLI). These findings suggested that the heritability of poor language was only found when it occurred with poor nonverbal skills, suggesting that the genetic influence was not limited to language, but perhaps "generalist" genes. DeThorne and colleagues (DeThorne et al., 2005) pointed out that the children with SLI in the Hayiou-Thomas et al. study had less severe language impairment as well as better nonverbal IQ, and the NLI children had more severe language impairment. Thus language severity and nonverbal IQ were confounded. DeThorne and colleagues examined this question further by controlling for this confound and demonstrated that heritability of language impairment was independent of the child's nonverbal IQ. Consequently, these findings support the contention that poor language is genetically influenced regardless of nonverbal IQ. Collectively, these studies would also seem to be in agreement with Bishop, North, and Donlan (1995), who had earlier concluded that the genetic studies of SLI should dispense with a nonverbal IQ criterion as a part of the phenotype.

In most of the twin studies on SLI, phonological deficits in the form of speech sound disorders were considered as a part of the general specific speech and language disorder phenotype. Bishop and Hayiou-Thomas (2008) reexamined the Hayiou-Thomas et al. (2005) data and reported low heritability of SLI in children with nonverbal IQs above 85, but high heritabilities of speech sound ability in children with similar nonverbal IQs. Likewise, heritability of clinically identified SLI was higher than SLI identified via population sampling. This latter difference was attributed to greater rates of children with SLI and comorbid speech sound disorder in the clinically identified group. These authors argue that the prior reports of substantial heritability of SLI may be due to the confounding of speech sound disorder in several of these studies. This conjecture is given further support by studies showing substantial heritability estimates for speech sound disorder (Bishop et al., 1995; DeThorne et al., 2006; Lewis & Thompson, 1992) and phonological memory (Bishop et al., 1996). These results would suggest that phonological abilities including speech sounds production skills may be, in their own right heritable, and that characterization of these aspects of the broader language phenotype should be employed in genetic studies of children with SLI. Whether all of the heritability of SLI can be attributed to speech sound abilities will require additional research.

Familial Aggregation of SLI and ASD

Earlier we reviewed evidence suggesting that SLI may be comorbid with autism and this comorbid condition may account for a substantial subgroup of individuals with autism. Alternatively, SLI has also been considered to be a milder variant of autism. Each of these accounts implies that autism spectrum disorders and SLI may share a common liability factor. This sharing could be either in a subgroup of children with ASD or it could span all individuals and differ with respect to the strength of the effect. The later view allows the traits that comprise autism and SLI to be dimensional, and thus the familial liability may be expressed in subclinical behavioral levels of some or all of these behavioral dimensions in the near relatives of children with autism or SLI. Thus, a very reasonable place to look for this shared liability is within families. If autism and SLI are related due to a common familial etiology, we should expect to see a co-occurrence of SLI and autism features among near relatives of children with SLI or autism.

The first investigation of this sort can be seen in Folstein and Rutter (1977), who found increased rates of language problems in nonautistic co-twins of autistic probands. More recently, Le Couteur and colleagues (1996) reported additional support for these results in a follow-up of the Folstein and Rutter twin study with a new sample of twins. Similar findings of familial loading of communication deficits in nonautistic family members of probands with autism have been found in studies of the Broader Autism Phenotype (BAP) hypothesis (Bishop et al., 2006; Plumet et al., 1995; Cox et al., 1975; Boutin et al., 1997; Bolton et al., 1994; Le Couteur et al., 1996; Landa et al., 1992; Folstein et al., 1999; Szatmari et al., 2000). In all these studies, near relatives of probands with ASD were evaluated with respect to language related disorders. One study (Tomblin et al., 2003) examined this relationship between ASD and SLI by obtaining evidence for ASD in siblings of probands with SLI. A comparison of the sibling scores from SLI and the ASD probands on the Autism Behavior Checklist (ABC; Krug et al., 1980) did not show a significant difference, however all siblings with scores on the ABC indicative of risk were sibs of probands with low language. Furthermore the rate of diagnosed autism in the siblings of probands with SLI was significantly higher than population estimates for the prevalence of autism at that time. Thus, these data provided partial support for a reciprocal familial relationship between ASD and SLI. Although the studies above found that near relatives of probands with autism were liable for communication deficits, it should be recognized that several studies have not found such evidence (Szatmari et al., 1993; Fombonne & Du Mazaubrun, 1992; Gillberg et al., 1992; Fombonne et al., 1997; Pilowsky et al., 2003; Bishop et al., 2004). Bishop et al. (2006) observed that many of the studies showing a relationship used measures based on history or report from family members regarding communication status, whereas those that did not find an elevated rate of language impairment in family members of probands with autism employed language tests. These language tests were typically focused on language form and meaning rather than communication function; whereas the historical reports could reflect poor communication function. Bishop et al. (2006) predicted that if both communication function and structure were systematically measured in the siblings of children with ASD, it would be likely that the excess deficits would be concentrated in social communication. Bishop et al. (2006) explored this using a structured questionnaire that spanned communication function and structure. Elevated rates of poor communication were found in the relatives of the autism probands; however, this elevated rate was not concentrated in the domain of communication function. These results provided support for a more generalized language impairment to be a part of the BAP, and thus could be considered to suggest that SLI may overlap with ASD. More recently however, Whitehouse, Barry, and Bishop (Whitehouse et al., 2007) tested the language structure and social communication abilities among parents of children with ASD and parents of children with SLI. It is noteworthy in this study that the parents of the two groups were similar in nonverbal IQ and education. In fact, the parents in this study were well above average on nonverbal IQ. Despite this matching, the parents of the SLI probands were found to have poorer phonological and language skills than the parents of ASD probands. In contrast, the parents of ASD probands had poorer social communication skills than the parents of SLI probands. These data support the view that SLI and ASD do not share common liability factors so long as a distinction is made between the structural aspects of language and the social functional aspects of communication. Thus, currently, the extent to which there is a shared etiology or liability between ASD and SLI remains unclear.

Molecular Genetic Evidence

Linkage Studies

In the past 9 years there have been reports of two genome-wide scans for developmental language disorders. Bartlett and colleagues (Bartlett et al., 2002) reported suggestive linkage of phenotype of receptive language impairment to a locus on 2p in family members from 5 families originally ascertained for schizophrenia. A linkage of reading to 13q (*SLI3*) was also reported in this study. The SLI consortium in England (Newbury, Ishikawa-Brush, et al., 2002) performed a sib-pair genome-wide scan with SLI probands that resulted in linkage to loci at chromosomes 16q (*SLI1*) and 19q. The language trait linked to chromosome 19q (*SLI2*) was one that represented the children's ability to express words and sentences. The chromosome 16q locus was linked to a measure of phonological working memory (PM) requiring remembering and repeating nonsense words. A subsequent study by this same research group was able to replicate the linkage of PM to *SLI1* and *SLI2* in a new sample, but when the samples were combined PM was only linked to *SLI1* (Newbury et al., 2004). Two additional analyses of these data provided further support for the linkage of PM to the SLI1 locus and sentence usage including grammar and vocabulary for *SLI2* (Monaco, 2007; Falcaro et al., 2008). Previous work has shown that phonological memory is a sensitive indicator of SLI and may be an important cognitive skill for language development (Dollaghan & Campbell, 1998; Ellis Weismer et al., 1999; Conti-Ramsden & Hesketh, 2003). To date, no fine mapping results have been published pointing to the possible causal locus for *SLI1*, and it will be important to further replicate these findings in independent samples.

Candidate Gene Studies

To date one gene (FOXP2) has been found to be strongly implicated in language development (Lai et al., 2001). These results came from the study of one family with a point mutation of FOXP2 and high rates of speech and language impairment. However, several studies have not found evidence of this gene contributing to SLI in the general population (Newbury, Bonora, et al., 2002; Meaburn et al., 2002; O'Brien et al., 2003). Thus, although FOXP2 appears to affect neural systems important for normal speech and language development, it does not appear to be a very common basis for language impairment. This failure to find association or linkage of language impairment to FOXP2 in population samples is consistent with other studies (Bartlett et al., 2002; SLI Consortium, 2004). Our group (O'Brien et al., 2003) did find an association of language impairment to two markers flanking FOXP2 in the region of WNT2, suggesting that a language-related locus other than FOXP2 may reside nearby. One significant association was to a marker within the CFTR gene, and these findings have been replicated by Bartlett (2004). Recently, Tyson and colleagues (2004) reported a microdeletion at 7q31.3 in a child with a complex balanced translocation involving chromosomes 5, 6, and 7. This child presented with language impairment and also cleft palate. These authors concluded that their results supported the O'Brien et al. (2003) results that suggest that a gene concerned with language disorders lies in the 7q31.2-31.3 region.

Bartlett et al. (2004) reported candidate region studies for two additional regions that had been found promising on an initial genome linkage study (Bartlett et al., 2002). In this study significant linkage was again found for a reading phenotype at chromosome 13q (*SLI3*).

Overlaps in Genetic Bases of SLI and ASD

If ASD and SLI co-occur in families, a reasonable hypothesis might be that there is a shared genetic liability for SLI and ASD. Previously, we reviewed the current molecular genetics research on SLI. Far more research has been conducted on the genetics of ASD. There have been at least 18 reported genome-wide linkage scans and now two genome-wide association scans (see, for instance, Freitag, 2007). Strikingly, none of these studies have reported linkage or association to the *SLI1* or *SLI2* regions. The most widely replicated linkage findings have involved a region on chromosome 7q and 2q. The studies concerning the 7q locus in autism has been particularly interesting to those studying the genetics of SLI, because in many cases, these linkage signals have been improved when the phenotype was narrowed to focus on language (Alarcon et al., 2005; Alarcon et al., 2002; Wassink et al., 2001; Alarcon et al., 2005). One gene in this region is *FOXP2*, which as we noted earlier has been implicated in speech and language. The fact that *FOXP2* was in the region where these linkages were found led some research groups to examine *FOXP2* in ASD samples to determine if *FOXP2* might be the source of the linkage. In the majority of these studies no association was found between *FOXP2* and ASD (Newbury, Bonora, et al., 2002; Gauthier et al., 2003; Wassink et al., 2002); however, Gong and colleagues have reported an association of markers within *FOXP2* to autism in a sample of Chinese individuals of Han descent (Gong et al., 2004).

Thus, so far, common genetic variation within *FOXP2* has not been shown to be associated with either SLI or ASD. Recently however, the 7q region has yielded rather robust findings with regard to another gene, *CNTNAP2*. This gene is in the 7q35 region and also lies under the linkage peak found in the earlier linkage studies on autism cited above. The CNTNAP2 protein is a member of the neurexin superfamily that is concerned with cell adhesion and is expressed in brain. Bakkalouglu et al. (2008), Alarcon et al. (2008), and Arking et al. (2008) simultaneously published papers showing that common and rare genetic polymorphisms within *CNTNAP2* were associated with autism. Bakkalouglu et al. reported a case with mental retardation and ASD who had a chromosomal inversion that disrupted *CNTNAP2*. Furthermore, these authors resequenced *CNTNAP2* in 635 individuals with autism and 942 controls and found an elevated but nonsignificant rate of rare variants that yielded changes in the amino acid sequence of CNTNAP2. In both the Bakkalouglu et al. and the Arking et al. studies the phenotype was based on autism diagnosis. In the Alarcon et al. study, the phenotype most strongly associated with *CNTNAP2* was a quantitative trait concerned with the age at which the parents reported the child with ASD acquiring the first word, and therefore these findings implicated CNTNAP2 as a possible genetic cause of language problems with or without autism. Soon after these reports of *CNTNAP2* association, Vernes et al. (2008) reported that *CNTNAP2* was a downstream regulatory target of *FOXP2* and that the same genetic polymorphism reported to be associated with autism by Alarcon et al. (2008) was also associated with phonological short-term memory in a sample of children with SLI. These findings have provided the first strong evidence supporting a shared etiology between autism and SLI.

Two other regions that have been reported to be linked to SLI lie at 13q and 2q. Both these regions were found to be linked to phenotypes associated with SLI by Bartlett and colleagues (Bartlett et al., 2002, Bartlett et al., 2004). The region of linkage on chromosome 13q has also been linked to autism in two studies (Barrett et al., 2001; Bradford et al., 2001). Likewise the region on 2q linked to SLI was found to be linked to autism in one study also by Barrett and colleagues (Barrett et al., 2001).

Thus, out of the 5 regions (*SLI1*, *SLI2*, *SLI3*, 2q, and 7q35), three of these fall into regions that have also been implicated in autism. Thus, although the molecular genetics findings are by no means conclusive that there is genetic overlap, these molecular data are consistent with the quantitative genetic findings showing some evidence of shared familial/genetic liability between autism and SLI.

Hypotheses on the Relationship of SLI and Autism

Throughout this chapter we have described the behavioral and etiologic findings concerning SLI and have provided comparisons and contrasts of these features with ASD. As noted earlier, there has been a long-standing interest in possible ties between autism and SLI. This has resulted in several different hypotheses being proposed.

The first account associating SLI and autism was that of Bartak, Rutter, and Cox (Bartak et al., 1975; Bartak et al., 1977), where it was hypothesized that these conditions represented different points on a single dimension of severity of language impairment (Figure 19-1). At this time, these authors considered the possibility that the social and behavioral features of autism resulted from the language impairment. Therefore this model assumed that ASD and SLI would have common etiologies and the difference was in the severity of expression and the development of secondary abnormal social responses to communication difficulties. Their research, however, provided evidence that clear qualitative differences existed between these two conditions, and thus the model of SLI and autism lying on a single continuum was rejected. Soon, Rutter (1978) introduced a model of autism wherein ASD was formed from deficits in three domains of development (language, social interest, rigidity). Within this conceptualization, ASD was a mixture of these three domains. As a part of this model, some researchers began to report that the nonautistic relatives of autistic individuals were likely to demonstrate milder forms of one or more of the particular components of the full syndrome of autism, and this led to the notion of a broader autism phenotype (BAP: Piven, 1999). This provided a means for SLI to overlap with autism with regard to the language dimension while contrasting with autism on the other two dimensions, as depicted in Figure 19-2.

A feature of the mixture model would be that all children with ASD would present with SLI-like language problems. As we noted earlier, children with SLI often have particular difficulties with the development of grammatical morphology and with the accurate repetition of novel words. Tager-Flusberg (Tager-Flusberg, 2004; Kjelgaard & Tager-Flusberg, 2001) found that indeed a subgroup of children with autism presented a similar profile of deficits. Additionally, they found some children with autism who had normal language ability albeit poor social communication. Thus, Tager-Flusberg proposed that many but not all children with autism presented with comorbid SLI (see Figure 19-3). Thus, like the mixture model, SLI and autism overlap, but unlike the mixture model, they are considered as distinct, since children could present with ASD and not SLI and obviously SLI but not ASD. As such, SLI and ASD would be viewed as comorbid and therefore likely to have related if not shared etiologies.

Recently, Whitehouse and colleagues (Whitehouse et al., 2007; Whitehouse et al., 2008) have argued against this notion of an overlap between SLI and ASD, claiming that SLI and ASD, although similar in some surface manifestations of language deficits, differ with regard to the underlying bases of these deficits. They suggest that the apparent signs of SLI among children with ASD do not hold on closer inspection and that the overlap in familial risk is likewise weak and not well founded. These authors have concluded that there is no basis for claiming that SLI and ASD are related at the behavioral symptom or etiologic level. They concluded that children with SLI present with a disorder that involves deficits in phonological working memory and grammatical development whereas children with autism have impairments in language use and social interactions as well as restricted interests and behaviors. Even in cases where there appears to be symptom overlap, such as with nonword repetition, the underlying reasons for poor repetition differs between the two groups. Thus, within this viewpoint we should expect that these are independent

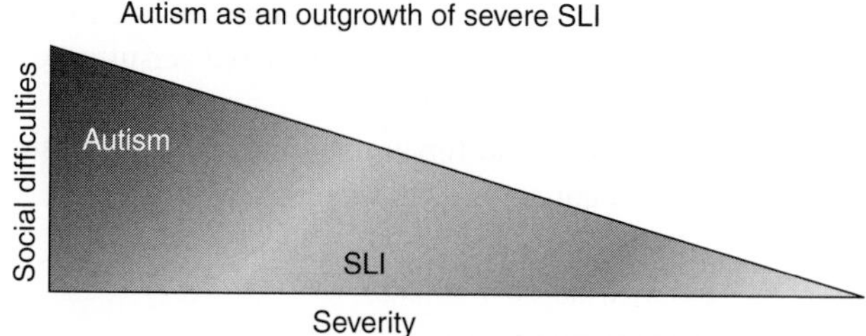

Figure 19–1. Autism as a result of severe specific language impairment. As the severity of SLI increases, the odds of social difficulties increase.

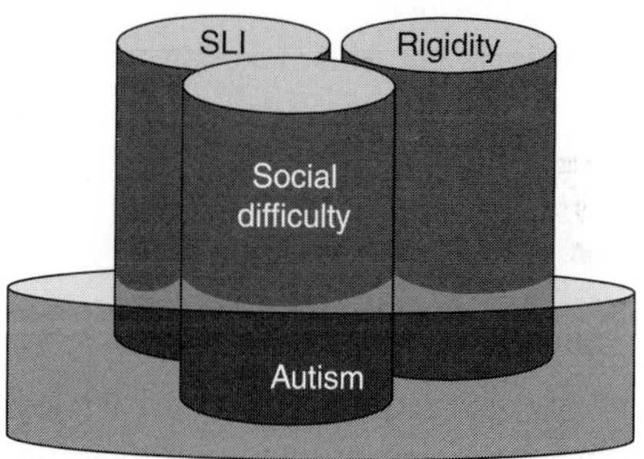

Figure 19–2. Autism as a composite disorder containing SLI.

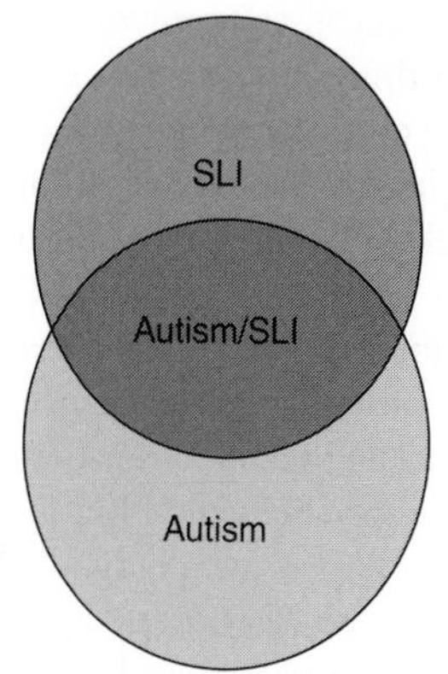

Figure 19–3. SLI and autism as comorbid conditions.

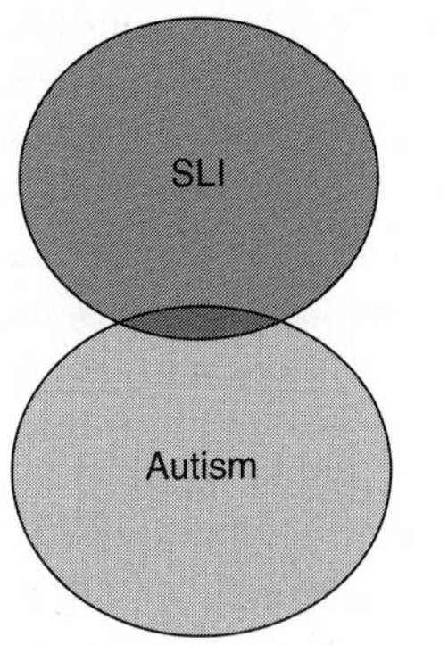

Figure 19–4. SLI and autism as independent conditions where overlap is no greater than expected by chance.

disorders and that would only co-occur at levels expected by chance (see Figure 19-4).

It should be noted that these conclusions by Whitehouse and Bishop were reached prior to the publication of the data on *CNTNAP2.* As noted earlier, allelic variation in *CNTNAP2* is associated with autism and in particular age of first-word production in these children and it is also associated with phonological memory measured by nonword repetition in children with SLI. If *CNTNAP2* does confer liability for both autism and SLI, it would provide for quite strong support for these two conditions being comorbid. What remains unclear is whether *CNTNAP2* is a gene that influences a wide range of neural developmental phenotypes, or whether it impacts on brain systems that are particularly important for language.

Conclusion

For nearly three decades SLI has served as a model of developmental language disorder that can be examined without the influence of other developmental disorders. As researchers have approached SLI, we can find that some seem to make the assumption that SLI represents a unique form of poor language and thus the etiologic systems that underlie SLI are also unique to SLI and distinct from those that cause poor language development in children with other developmental disorders. Within this vein of thinking a full account of SLI will consist of a set of unique language features (markers) that map onto a unique etiologic system. Plomin once described this type of model for developmental disorders when applied to genetics as One Gene One Disorder (OGOD). In such a case we would also not expect overlap between SLI and other developmental disorders to exceed chance levels. If it does, we would need to consider that this is due to something analogous to phenocopy. The specificity of SLI in this model would also extend to its distinctiveness from individual differences within the normal population. The recent findings of an etiologic overlap in the form of similar risk alleles being shared between autism and SLI challenges this model of SLI.

These findings of overlap between SLI and autism suggest that we need to rethink our basic assumptions about SLI, and this rethinking may also have an impact on views of the language impairments in autism. An alternative perspective may be that that cutting across ability levels (poor, average, or high) and across various disability groups will be a common set of causal factors that account for an important fraction of the individual differences in children's development of language content and structure. This viewpoint was voiced by Leonard (1987), when he concluded that SLI is likely to represent the tail end of the normal distribution of language ability and is fully consistent with the quantitative trait locus model that Plomin (1994) described as an alternative. In this regard, it is quite possible to expect that etiologic factors such as risk variants of *CNTNAP2* will be found in excess in other populations with developmental language problems and indeed even will be found in typically developing children. These etiologies alone are most likely probabilistic rather than deterministic and it is only as they work in concert with other risk factors that different symptom complexes emerge.

Karmiloff-Smith (1992) has emphasized that development is complex and dynamic. Within this view developmental processes are clearly shared across children who are then growing up in diverse circumstances (biologically and culturally), thus there are likely to be shared and unique features across all children, and these may vary over development. It may be more important to focus on understanding these developmental processes as they generate differences and similarities across children throughout development. Such reconceptualization will hopefully lead to deeper insights into autism and SLI.

Challenges and Future Directions

- In order to directly test whether there is a subgroup of children with autism who also have SLI, research methods that have been developed to test for continuities or discontinuities in individual differences should be applied to this problem (see, for instance, Lenzenweger, 2004; Markon & Krueger, 2006; Ruscio et al., 2006).
- Parallel genetic studies of children with autism and children with SLI using high density SNP platforms for GWAS or nextgen sequencing for rare variants and carefully selected language phenotype and endophenotypes should provide a means to test for shared versus unique risk genetic variants.
- Parallel structural and functional imaging studies using children with autism and children with SLI.

SUGGESTED READINGS

Leonard, L. (1998). *Children with specific language impairment.* Cambridge, MA: MIT Press.

Bavin, E. (2009). *The Cambridge handbook of child language.* Cambridge, UK: Cambridge University Press.

Bishop, D. (2006). What causes Specific Language Impairment? *Current Directions in Psychological Science, 15,* 217–221.

REFERENCES

Alarcon, M., Abrahams, B. S., Stone, J. L., Duvall, J. A., Perederiy, J. V., Bomar, J. M., et al. (2008). Linkage, association, and gene-expression analyses identify CNTNAP2 as an autism-susceptibility gene. *American Journal of Human Genetics, 82*(1), 150–159. Retrieved from PM:18179893.

Alarcon, M., Cantor, R. M., Liu, J., Gilliam, T. C., & Geschwind, D. H. (2002). Evidence for a language quantitative trait locus on chromosome 7q in multiplex autism families. *American Journal of Human Genetics, 70,* 60–71.

Alarcon, M., Yonan, A. L., Gilliam, T. C., Cantor, R. M., & Geschwind, D. H. (2005). Quantitative genome scan and ordered-subsets analysis of autism endophenotypes support language QTLs. *Molecular Psychiatry, 10*(8), 747–757. Retrieved from ISI:000230827800006

American Psychiatric Association (1994). *Diagnostic and statistical manual of mental disorder* (4th ed.). Washington, DC: Author.

Aram, D. M., Morris, R., & Hall, N. E. (1993). Clinical and research congruence in identifying children with specific language impairment. *Journal of Speech and Hearing Research, 36,* 580–591.

Arking, D. E., Cutler, D. J., Brune, C. W., Teslovich, T. M., West, K., Ikeda, M., et al. (2008). A common genetic variant in the neurexin superfamily member CNTNAP2 increases familial risk of autism. *American Journal of Human Genetics, 82*(1), 160–164. Retrieved from PM:18179894.

Bakkaloglu, B., O'Roak, B. J., Louvi, A., Gupta, A. R., Abelson, J. F., Morgan, T. M., et al. (2008). Molecular cytogenetic analysis and resequencing of contactin associated protein-like 2 in autism spectrum disorders. *American Journal of Human Genetics, 82*(1), 165–173. Retrieved from PM:18179895.

Barrett, S., Beck, J. C., Bernier, R., Bisson, E., Braun, T. A., Casavant, T. L., et al. (2001). An autosomal genomic screen for autism (Vol. 88, pp. 609, 1999). *American Journal of Medical Genetics, 105*(8), 609–615.

Bartak, L., Rutter, M., & Cox, A. (1975). A comparative study of infantile autism and specific developmental receptive language disorder: I. The children. *International Journal of Psychiatry, 126,* 127–145.

Bartak, L., Rutter, M., & Cox, A. (1977). A comparative study of infantile autism and specific developmental receptive language disorders. III. Discriminant function analysis. *Journal of Autism and Childhood Schizophrenia, 7*(4), 383–396.

Bartlett, C. W., Flax, J. F., Logue, M. W., Smith, B. J., Vieland, V. J., Tallal, P., et al. (2004). Examination of potential overlap in autism and language loci on chromosomes 2, 7, and 13 in two independent samples ascertained for specific language impairment. *Human Heredity, 57*(1), 10–20.

Bartlett, C. W., Flax, J. F., Logue, M. W., Vieland, V. J., Bassett, A. S., Tallal, P., et al. (2002). A major susceptibility locus for specific language impairment is located on 13q21. *American Journal of Human Genetics,* 71, 45–55.

Beitchman, J. H., Hood, J., & Inglis, A. (1992, Apr). Familial transmission of speech and language impairment: a preliminary investigation. *Canadian Journal of Psychiatry–Revue Canadienne de Psychiatrie, 37*(3), 151–156.

Bishop, D. V. M. (1997) *Uncommon understanding: Development and disorders of language comprehension in children.* United Kingdom: Psychology Press.

Bishop, D. V. M. (2000). Pragmatic language impairment: A correlate of SLI, a distinct subgroup, or part of the autistic continuum? In D.V.M. Bishop & L.B. Leonard (Eds.), *Speech and language impairments in children: Causes, characteristics, intervention and outcome* (pp. 99–113). Hove, UK: Psychology Press.

Bishop, D. V. M., & Adams, C. (1989). Conversational characteristics of children with semantic-pragmatic disorder: II. What features lead to a judgment of inappropriacy? *British Journal of Disorders of Communication, 24,* 241–263.

Bishop, D. V. M., & Baird, G. (2001). Parent and teacher report of pragmatic aspects of communication: Use of the Children's Communication Checklist in a clinical setting. *Developmental Medicine and Child Neurology, 43*(12), 809–818.

Bishop, D. V. M., & Edmundson, A. (1987). Language impaired 4-year-olds: Distinguishing transient from persistent impairment. *Journal of Speech and Hearing Disorders, 52,* 156–173.

Bishop, D. V., Maybery, M., Wong, D., Maley, A., & Hallmayer, J. (2006). Characteristics of the broader phenotype in autism: a study of siblings using the Children's Communication Checklist-2. *American Journal of Medical Genetics. Part B, Neuropsychiatric Genetics, 141B*(2), 117–122.

Bishop, D. V., Maybery, M., Wong, D., Maley, A., Hill, W., & Hallmayer, J. (2004). Are phonological processing deficits part of the broad autism phenotype? *American Journal of Medical Genetics. Part B, Neuropsychiatric Genetics, 128B*(1), 54–60. Retrieved from PM:15211632.

Bishop, D. V. M., & Hayiou-Thomas, M. E. (2008). Heritability of specific language impairment depends on diagnostic criteria. *Genes, Brain, and Behavior, 7*(3), 365–372. Retrieved from ISI:000254611500012.

Bishop, D. V. M., & Norbury, C. F. (2002). Exploring the borderlands of autistic disorder and specific language impairment: A study using standardised diagnostic instruments. *Journal of Child Psychology and Psychiatry, 43*(7), 917–929.

Bishop, D. V. M., North, T., & Donlan, C. (1995). Genetic basis of specific language impairment: Evidence from a twin study. *Developmental Medicine and Child Neurology, 37*(1), 56–71.

Bishop, D. V. M., North, T., & Donlan, C. (1996). Nonword repetition as a behavioral marker of inherited language impairment: Evidence from a twin study. *Journal of Child Psychology and Psychiatry and Allied Disciplines, 37*(4), 391–403.

Bishop, D. V. M., Whitehouse, A. J. O., Watt, H. J., & Line, E. A. (2008). Autism and diagnostic substitution: evidence from a study of adults with a history of developmental language disorder. *Developmental Medicine and Child Neurology, 50*(5), 341–345.

Bolton, P., Macdonald, H., Pickles, A., Rios, P., Goode, S., Crowson, M., et al. (1994). A case-control family history study of autism. *Journal of Child Psychology and Psychiatry, 35*(5), 877–900.

Botting, N., & Conti-Ramsden, G. (2003). Autism, primary pragmatic difficulties, and specific language impairment: can we distinguish them using psycholinguistic markers? *Developmental Medicine and Child Neurology, 45*(8), 515–524. Retrieved from ISI:000184341700003.

Botting, N., & Conti-Ramsden, G. (2008). The role of language, social cognition and social skill in the functional social outcomes of young adolescents with and without a history of SLI. *British Journal of Developmental Psychology, 26*(2), 281–300.

Boutin, P., Maziade, M., Merette, C., Mondor, M., Bedard, C., & Thivierge, J. (1997). Family history of cognitive disabilities in first-degree relatives of autistic and mentally retarded children. *Journal of Autism and Developmental Disorders, 27*(2), 165–176. Retrieved from PM:9105967.

Bradford, Y., Haines, J., Hutcheson, H., Gardiner, M., Braun, T., Sheffield, V., et al. (2001). Incorporating language phenotypes strengthens evidence of linkage to autism. *American Journal of Medical Genetics, 105*(6), 539–547. Retrieved from ISI:000170244500011.

Brook, S., & Bowler, D., 1992, Autism by another name? Semantic and pragmatic impairments in children. *Journal of Autism and Developmental Disorders, 22*(1), 61–81.

Catts, H. W. (1993). The relationship between speech-language impairments and reading disabilities. *Journal of Speech and Hearing Research, 36*, 948–958.

Charman, T., Drew, A., Baird, C., & Baird, G. (2003). Measuring early language development in preschool children with autism spectrum disorder using the MacArthur Communicative Development Inventory (Infant Form). *Journal of Child Language, 30*(1), 213–236.

Clegg, J., Hollis, C., Mahwood, L., & Rutter, M. (2005). Developmental language disorders–a follow-up in later adult life. Cognitive, language and psychosocial outcomes. *Journal of Child Psychology and Psychiatry, 46*, 128–149.

Coady, J. A., Evans, J. L., Mainela-Arnold, E., & Kluender, K. R. (2007). Children with specific language impairments perceive speech most categorically when tokens are natural and meaningful. *Journal of Speech, Language, and Hearing Research, 50*(1), 41–57.

Cohen, M., Campbell, R., & Yaghmai, F. (1989). Neuropathological abnormalities in developmental dysphasia. *Annals of Neurology, 25*(6), 567–570. Retrieved from PM:2472772.

Conti-Ramsden, G., & Botting, N. (1999). Classification of children with specific language impairment: Longitudinal considerations. *Journal of Speech, Language, and Hearing Research, 42*, 1195–1204.

Conti-Ramsden, G., & Botting, N. (2000). Non-word repetition and tense marking tasks as behavioural markers for SLI: The relationship between measures and with different sub-groups of children. Poster shown at the 21st Annual Symposium on Research in Child Language Disorders. Madison, WI.

Conti-Ramsden G. & Botting N. (2004). Social difficulties and victimization in children with SLI at 11 years of age. *Journal of Speech, Language, and Hearing Research, 47*,145–161.

Conti-Ramsden, G., Botting, N., & Faragher, B. (2001). Psycho linguistic markers for specific language impairment (SLI). *Journal of Child Psychology and Psychiatry and Allied Disciplines, 42*(6), 741–748.

Conti-Ramsden, G., & Hesketh, A. (2003). Risk markers for SLI: a study of young language-learning children. *International Journal of Language and Communication Disorders, 38*(3), 251–263. Retrieved from ISI:000183673500003.

Conti-Ramsden, G., Simkin, Z., & Botting, N. (2006). The prevalence of autistic spectrum disorders in adolescents with a history of specific language impairment (SLI). *Journal of Child Psychology and Psychiatry, 47*(6), 621–628.

Cox, A., Rutter, M., Newman, S., & Bartak, L. (1975). A comparative study of infantile autism and specific developmental receptive language disorder. II. Parental characteristics. *British Journal of Psychiatry, 126*, 146–159.

Craig, H. (1993). Social skills of children with specific language impairment: Peer relationships. *Language, Speech and Hearing Services in Schools, 24*, 206–215.

Dale, P. S., Simonoff, E., Bishop, D. V. M., Eley, T. C., Oliver, B., Price, T. S., et al. (1998). Genetic influence on language delay in two-year-old children. *Nature Neuroscience, 1*(4), 324–328.

De Fosse, L., Hodge, S. M., Makris, N., Kennedy, D. N., Caviness, V. S., McGrath, L., et al. (2004). Language-association cortex asymmetry in autism and specific language impairment. *Annals of Neurology, 56*(6), 757–766.

DeThorne, L. S., Hart, S. A., Petrill, S. A., Deater-Deckard, K., Thompson, L. A., Schatschneider, C., et al. (2006). Children's history of speech-language difficulties: Genetic influences and associations with reading-related measures. *Journal of Speech, Language, and Hearing Research, 49*(6), 1280–1293.

DeThorne, L. S., Petrill, S. A., Hayiou-Thomas, M. E., & Plomin, R. (2005). Low expressive vocabulary: Higher heritability as a function of more severe cases. *Journal of Speech, Language, and Hearing Research, 48*(4), 792–804. Retrieved from ISI:000233974900007.

Dollaghan, C., & Campbell, T. F. (1998). Nonword repetition and child language impairment. *Journal of Speech, Language, and Hearing Research, 41*(5), 1136–1146.

Eadie, P. A., Fey, M. E., Douglas, J. M., & Parsons, C. L. (2002). Profiles of grammatical morphology and sentence imitation in children with specific language impairment and Down syndrome. *Journal of Speech, Language, and Hearing Research, 45*(4), 720–732.

Eckert, M. A., Leonard, C. M., Possing, E. T., & Binder, J. R. (2006). Uncoupled leftward asymmetries for planum morphology and functional language processing. *Brain and Language, 98*(1), 102–111.

Ellis Weismer, S., Tomblin, J. B., Zhang, X., Gaura, J., Buckwalter, P., & Jones, M. (1999). Nonword repetition performance in second graders with and without language impairment. Vol. Poster presented at the 20th Annual Symposium on Research in Child Language Disorders. Madison, WI.

Ellis Weismer, S., Gernsbacher, M., Roos, E., Karasinski, C., Hollar, C., Esler, A., & Stronach, S. (2008, June). Understanding comprehension in toddlers on the autism spectrum. Poster presented at the Symposium for Research in Child Language Disorders.

Falcaro, M., Pickles, A., Newbury, D. F., Addis, L., Banfield, E., Fisher, S. E., et al. (2008). Genetic and phenotypic effects of phonological short-term memory and grammatical morphology in specific language impairment. *Genes, Brain, and Behavior, 7*(4), 393–402.

Farrant, B., Fletcher, J., & Mayberry, M. (2006). Specific language impairment, theory of mind, and visual perspective taking: Evidence for simulation theory and the developmental role of language. *Child Development, 77*, 1842–1853.

Farmer, M. (2000). Language and social cognition in children with specific language impairment. *Journal of Child Psychology and Psychiatry and Allied Disciplines, 41*, 627–636.

Folstein, S. E., & Rutter, M. (1977). Infantile autism: a genetic study of 21 twin pairs. *Journal of Child Psychology and Psychiatry, 18*(4), 297–321. Retrieved from PM:0000562353.

Folstein, S. E., Santangelo, S. L., Gilman, S. E., Piven, J., Landa, R., Lainhart, J., et al. (1999). Predictors of cognitive test patterns in autism families. *Journal of Child Psychology and Psychiatry, 40*(7), 1117–1128.

Fombonne, E., Bolton, P., Prior, J., Jordan, H., & Rutter, M. (1997). A family study of autism: cognitive patterns and levels in parents and siblings. *Journal of Child Psychology and Psychiatry, 38*(6), 667–683.

Fombonne, E., & Du Mazaubrun, C. (1992). Prevalence of infantile autism in four French regions. *Social Psychiatry and Psychiatric Epidemiology, 27*(4), 203–210. Retrieved from PM:0001411750.

Freitag, C. M. (2007). The genetics of autistic disorders and its clinical relevance: a review of the literature. *Molecular Psychiatry, 12*(1), 2–22.

Fujiki, M., Brinton, B., & Todd, C. M. (1996). Social skills of children with specific language impairment. *Language, Speech, and Hearing Services in Schools, 27*, 195–202.

Furstenberg, F. F., Brooks-Gunn, J., & Chase-Lansdale, P. L. (1989). Teenaged pregnancy and childbearing. *American Psychologist, 44*, 313–320.

Galaburda, A. M., Sherman, G. F., Rosen, G. D., Aboitiz, F., & Geschwind, N. (1985). Developmental dyslexia: Four consecutive patients with cortical anomalies. *Annals of Neurology, 18*, 222–233.

Gauger, L. M., Lombardino, L. J., & Leonard, C. M. (1997). Brain morphology in children with specific language impairment. *Journal of Speech, Language, and Hearing Research, 40*(6), 1272–1284.

Gauthier, J., Joober, R., Mottron, L., Laurent, S., Fuchs, M., De Kimpe, V., et al. (2003). Mutation screening of FOXP2 in individuals diagnosed with autistic disorder. *American Journal of Medical Genetics. Part A, 118A*(2), 172–175.

Gillberg, C., Gillberg, I. C., & Steffenburg, S. (1992). Siblings and parents of children with autism: a controlled population-based study. *Developmental Medicine and Child Neurology, 34*(5), 389–398.

Gong, X. H., Jia, M. X., Ruan, Y., Shuang, M., Liu, J., Wu, S. P., et al. (2004). Association between the FOXP2 gene and autistic disorder in Chinese population. *American Journal of Medical Genetics. Part B, Neuropsychiatric Genetics, 127B*(1), 113–116. Retrieved from ISI:000221136100022.

Grant, J., Karmiloff-Smith, A., Gathercole, S. A., Paterson, S., Howlin, P., Davies, M., et al. (1997). Phonological short-term memory and its relationship to language in Williams syndrome. *Cognitive Neuropsychiatry, 2*(2), 81–99.

Gray, S. (2003). Word learning by preschoolers with specific language impairment: What predicts success? *Journal of Speech, Language, and Hearing Research, 46*, 56–67.

Hayiou-Thomas, M. E., Oliver, B., & Plomin, R. (2005). Genetic influences on specific versus nonspecific language impairment in 4-year-old twins. *Journal of Learning Disabilities, 38*(3), 222–232.

Herbert, M. R., & Kenet, T. (2007). Brain abnormalities in language disorders and in autism. *Pediatric Clinics of North America, 54*(3), 563–583.

Herbert, M. R., Ziegler, D. A., Deutsch, C. K., O'Brien, L. M., Kennedy, D. N., Filipek, P. A., et al. (2005). Brain asymmetries in autism and developmental language disorder: a nested whole-brain analysis. *Brain, 128*, 213–226.

Herbert, M. R., Ziegler, D. A., Makris, N., Bakardjiev, A., Hodgson, J., Adrien, K. T., et al. (2003). Larger brain and white matter volumes in children with developmental language disorder. *Developmental Science, 6*(4), F11–F22.

Hoff-Ginsberg, E. (1998). The relation of birth order and socioeconomic status to children's language experience and language development. *Applied Psycholinguistics, 19*(4), 603–629.

Jernigan, T. L., Hesselink, J. R., Sowell, E., & Tallal, P. A. (1991). Cerebral structure on magnetic resonance imaging in language- and learning-impaired children. *Archives of Neurology, 48*(5), 539–545.

Johnston, J. (2008) Narratives: Twenty-five years later. *Topics in Language Disorders, 28*(2), 93–98.

Johnston, J., & Kahmi, A. (1984). The same can be less: Syntactic and semantic aspects of the utterances of language impaired children. *Merrill-Palmer Quarterly, 30*, 65–86.

Kail, R., & Leonard, L. B. (1986). Word-finding abilities in children with specific language impairment. *Monographs of the American Speech-Language-Hearing Association*, no. 25.

Kamhi, A. G., Catts, H. W., Mauer, D., Apel, K., & Gentry, B. F. (1988). Phonological and spatial processing abilities in language- and reading-impaired children. *Journal of Speech and Hearing Disorders, 53*(3), 316–327.

Karmiloff-Smith, A. (1992). *Beyond modularity: A developmental perspective on cognitive science.* Cambridge, MA: MIT Press.

Kjelgaard, M., & Tager-Flusberg, H. (2001). An investigation of language impairment in autism: Implications for genetic subgroups. *Language and Cognitive Processes, 16*, 287–308.

Krug, D., Arick, J., & Almond, P. (1980). Behavior checklist for identifying severely handicapped individuals with high levels of autism behavior. *Journal of Child Psychology and Psychiatry and Allied Disciplines, 21*, 221–229.

Lahey, M., & Edwards, J. (1999). Naming errors of children with specific language impairment. *Journal of Speech, Language, and Hearing Research, 42*, 195–205.

Lai, C. S., Fisher, S., Hurst, J. A., Vargha-Khadem, F., & Monaco, A. (2001). A forkhead-domain gene is mutated in a severe speech and language disorder. *Nature, 413*, 519–523.

Landa, R., Piven, J., Wzorek, M. M., Gayle, J. O., Chase, G. A., & Folstein, S. E. (1992). Social language use in parents of autistic individuals. *Psychological Medicine, 22*(1), 245–254.

Le Couteur, A., Bailey, A., Goode, S., Pickles, A., Robertson, S., Gottesman, I., et al. (1996). A broader phenotype of autism: The clinical spectrum in twins. *Journal of Child Psychology and Child Psychiatry, 37*, 785–801.

Lenzenweger, M. F. (2004). Consideration of the challenges, complications, and pitfalls of taxometric analysis. *Journal of Abnormal Psychology, 113*(1), 10–23. doi:doi:10.1037/0021-843X.113.1.10. Retrieved from US: American Psychological Association.

Leonard, L. B. (1995). Functional categories in the grammars of children with specific language impairment. *Journal of Speech and Hearing Research, 38*, 1270–1283.

Leonard, L. (1998). *Children with specific language impairment.* Cambridge, MA: MIT Press.

Leonard, C. M., Lombardino, L. J., Walsh, K., Eckert, M. A., Mockler, J. L., Rowe, L. A., et al. (2002). Anatomical risk factors that distinguish dyslexia from SLI predict reading skill in normal children. *Journal of Communication Disorders, 35*(6), 501–531.

Leonard, L. B. (1987). Is specific language impairment a useful construct? In S. Rosenberg (Ed.), *Advances in applied psycholinguistics, Vol. 1: Disorders of first-language development; Vol. 2: Reading, writing, and language learning* (pp. 1–39). Cambridge monographs and texts in applied psycholinguistics. New York: Cambridge University Press.

Lewis, B. A., & Thompson, L. A. (1992). A study of developmental speech and language disorders in twins. *Journal of Speech and Hearing Research, 35*(5), 1086–1094.

Locke, J. L. (1994). Gradual emergence of developmental language disorders. *Journal of Speech and Hearing Research, 37*(3), 608–616.

Luyster, R., Lopez, K., & Lord, C. (2007). Characterizing communicative development in children referred for autism spectrum disorder using the MacArthur–Bates Communicative Development Inventory (CDI). *Journal of Child Language, 34*(3), 623–654.

Markon, K. E., & Krueger, R. F. (2006). Information-theoretic latent distribution modeling: distinguishing discrete and continuous latent variable models. *Psychological Methods, 11*(3), 228–243.

Marton, K., Abramoff, B., & Rosenzweig, S. (2005). Social cognition and language in children with specific language impairment (SLI). *Journal of Communication Disorders, 38*, 143–162.

McGregor, K. K., Newman, R. M., Reilly, R. M., & Capone, N. C. (2002). Semantic representation and naming in children with specific language impairment. *Journal of Speech, Language, and Hearing Research, 45*, 998–1014.

Meaburn, E., Dale, P. S., Craig, I. W., & Plomin, R. (2002). Language-impaired children: No sign of the FOXP2 mutation. *Neuroreport, 13*(8), 1075–1077. Retrieved from ISI:000176823600027.

Monaco, A. P. (2007). Multivariate linkage analysis of specific language impairment (SLI). *Annals of Human Genetics, 71*, 660–673.

Montgomery, J. W. (2003) Working memory and comprehension in children with specific language impairment: What we know so far. *Journal of Communication Disorders, 36*(3), 221–231.

Neils, J., & Aram, D. M. (1986). Family history of children with developmental language disorders. *Perceptual and Motor Skills, 63*, 655–658.

Newbury, D. F., Bonora, E., Lamb, J. A., Fisher, S. E., Lai, C. S. L., Baird, G., et al. (2002). FOXP2 is not a major susceptibility gene for autism or specific language impairment. *American Journal of Human Genetics, 70*(5), 1318–1327.

Newbury, D. F., Cleak, J. D., Banfield, E., Marlow, A. J., Fisher, S. E., Monaco, A. P., et al. (2004). Highly significant linkage to the SLI1 locus in an expanded sample of individuals affected by specific language impairment. *American Journal of Human Genetics, 74*(6), 1225–1238.

Newbury, D. F., Ishikawa-Brush, Y., Marlow, A. J., Fisher, S. E., Monaco, A. P., Stott, C. M., et al. (2002). A genomewide scan identifies two novel loci involved in specific language impairment. *American Journal of Human Genetics, 70*(2), 384–398. Retrieved from ISI:000173254300011.

O'Brien, E. K., Zhang, X. Y., Nishimura, C., Tomblin, J. B., & Murray, J. C. (2003). Association of specific language impairment (SLI) to the region of 7q31. *American Journal of Human Genetics, 72*(6), 1536–1543.

Pena, E. D., Iglesia, A., & Lidz, C. S. (2001). Reducing test bias through dynamic assessment of children's word learning ability. *American Journal of Speech Language Pathology, 10*, 138–154.

Pilowsky, T., Yirmiya, N., Shalev, R. S., & Gross-Tsur, V. (2003). Language abilities of siblings of children with autism. *Journal of Child Psychology and Psychiatry and Allied Disciplines, 44*(6), 914–925. Retrieved from ISI:000184996200012.

Piven, J. (1999). Genetic liability for autism: the behavioural expression in relatives. *International Review of Psychiatry, 11*(4), 299–308.

Plante, E., Swisher, L., & Vance, R. (1989). Anatomical correlates of normal and impaired language in a set of dizygotic twins. *Brain and Language, 37*(4), 643–655.

Plante, E., Swisher, L., Vance, R., & Rapcsak, S. (1991). MRI findings in boys with specific language impairment. *Brain and Language, 41*(1), 52–66.

Plomin, R. (1994). The genetic basis of complex behavior. *Science, 264*, 1733–1739.

Plumet, M. H., Goldblum, M. C., & Leboyer, M. (1995). Verbal skills in relatives of autistic females. *Cortex, 31*(4), 723–733. Retrieved from ISI:A1995TN06300009.

Preis, S., Jancke, L., Schittler, P., Huang, Y., & Steinmetz, H. (1998). Normal intrasylvian anatomical asymmetry in children with developmental language disorder. *Neuropsychologia, 36*(9), 849–855.

Redmond, S. M., & Rice, M. L. (1998). The socioemotional behaviors of children with SLI: Social Adaptation or Social Deviance? *Journal of Speech, Language, and Hearing Research, 41*(3), 688–700. Retrieved from PM:9638932.

Rice, M. L., Haney, K. R., & Wexler, K. (1998). Family histories of children with SLI who show extended optional infinitives. *Journal of Speech, Language, and Hearing Research, 41*(2), 419–432.

Rice, M. L., & Wexler, K. (1996). Toward tense as a clinical marker of specific language impairment in English-speaking children. *Journal of Speech and Hearing Research, 39*(6), 1239–1257.

Roberts, J. A., Rice, M. L., & Tager-Flusberg, H. (2004). Tense marking in children with autism. *Applied Psycholinguistics, 25*(3), 429–448. Retrieved from ISI:000222466200006.

Ruscio, J., Haslam, N., & Ruscio, A. (2006). *Taxometric method: A practical guide.* Mahwah, NJ: Erlbaum.

Rutter, M. (1978). Diagnosis and Definition. In M. Rutter & E. Schopler (Eds.), *Autism* (pp. 1–26). New York: Plenum.

Scott, C. M., & Windsor, J. (2000). General language performance measures in spoken and written narrative and expository discourse of school-age children with language learning disabilities. *Journal of Speech, Language, and Hearing Research, 43*, 324–339.

Shriberg, L., Tomblin, J., & McSweeny, J. (1999). Prevalence of speech delay in 6-year-old children and comorbidity with language impairment. *Journal of Speech, Language, and Hearing Research, 42*, 1461–1481.

SLI Consortium. (2004). A genomewide scan identifies two novel loci involved in specific language impairment. *American Journal of Human Genetics, 70*, 384–398.

Spinath, F. M., Price, T. S., Dale, P. S., & Plomin, R. (2004). The genetic and environmental origins of language disability and ability. *Child Development, 75*(2), 445–454.

Stanton-Chapman, T. L., Chapman, D. A., Bainbridge, N. L., & Scott, K. G. (2002). Identification of early risk factors for language impairment. *Research in Developmental Disabilities, 23*(6), 390–405.

Stark, R. E., & Tallal, P. (1981). Selection of children with specific language deficits. *Journal of Speech and Hearing Disorders, 46*, 114–122.

Szatmari, P., Jones, M. B., Tuff, L., Bartolucci, G., Fisman, S., & Mahoney, W. (1993). Lack of cognitive impairment in first-degree relatives of children with pervasive developmental disorders. *Journal of the American Academy of Child and Adolescent Psychiatry, 32*(6), 1264–1273.

Szatmari, P., MacLean, J. E., Jones, M. B., Bryson, S. E., Zwaigenbaum, L., Bartolucci, G., et al. (2000). The familial aggregation of the lesser variant in biological and nonbiological relatives of PDD probands: a family history study. *Journal of Child Psychology and Psychiatry, 41*(5), 579–586. Retrieved from PM:10946750.

Tager-Flusberg, H. (2004). Do autism and specific language impairment represent overlapping language disorders? In M. Rice & S. Warren (Eds.), *Developmental language disorders: From phenotypes to etiologies* (pp. 31–52). Mahwah, NJ: Erlbaum.

Tallal, P., Hirsch, L. S., Realpe-Bonilla, T., Miller, S., Brzustowicz, L. M., Bartlett, C., et al. (2001). Familial aggregation in specific language impairment. *Journal of Speech, Language, and Hearing Research, 44*(5), 1172–1182.

Tallal, P., Ross, R., & Curtiss, S. (1989). Familial aggregation in specific language impairment. *Journal of Speech and Hearing Research, 54*, 167–173.

Thal, D., & Tobias, S. (1992). Communicative gestures in children with delayed onset of expressive vocabulary. *Journal of Speech and Hearing Research, 35*, 1281–1289.

Tomasello, M., & Farrar, J. (1986). Joint attention and early language. *Child Development, 57*,1454–1463.

Tomblin, J. B. (1989). Familial concentration of developmental language impairment. *Journal of Speech and Hearing Disorders, 54*(2), 287–295.

Tomblin, J. B. (1990). The effect of birth order on the occurrence of developmental language impairment. *British Journal of Disorders of Communication, 25*(1), 77–84.

Tomblin, J. B., & Buckwalter, P. R. (1994). Studies of genetics of specific language impairment. In R.V. Watkins & M. L. Rice (Eds.), *Specific language impairments in children* (pp. 17–34). Communication and language intervention series. Baltimore; MD, US: Paul H. Brookes Publishing Co.

Tomblin, J. B., & Buckwalter, P. R. (1998). The heritability of poor language achievement among twins. *Journal of Speech and Hearing Research, 41*, 188–199.

Tomblin, J. B., Freese, P. R., & Records, N. L. (1992). Diagnosing specific language impairment in adults for the purpose of pedigree analysis. *Journal of Speech and Hearing Research, 35*, 832–843.

Tomblin, J. B., Hafeman, L. L., & O'Brien, M. (2003). Autism and autism risk in siblings of children with specific language impairment. *International Journal of Language and Communication Disorders, 38*(3), 235–250.

Tomblin, J. B., Smith, E., & Zhang, X. (1997). Epidemiology of specific language impairment: Parental and perinatal risk factors. *Journal of Communication Disorders, 30*, 325–344.

Tomblin, J. B., Records, N. L., Buckwalter, P., Zhang, X., Smith, E., & O'Brien, M. (1997). Prevalence of specific language impairment in kindergarten children. *Journal of Speech and Hearing Research, 40*, 1245–1260.

Tomblin, J. B., Zhang, X., Weiss, A., Catts, H., & Ellis Weismer, S. (2004). Dimensions of individual differences in communication skills among primary grade children. In: Rice, M. L., Warren, S. F., editors. *Developmental language disorders: From phenotypes to etiologies.* Mahwah, NJ: Erlbaum.

Trauner, D., Wulfeck, B., Tallal, P., & Hesselink, J. (1995). Neurologic and MRI profiles of language impaired children. (Technical Report, Publication No. CND-9513). San Diego, CA: Center for Research in Language, UCSD.

Tyson, C., McGillivray, B., Chijiwa, C., & Rjcan-Separovic, E. (2004). Elucidation of acryptic interstitial 7q331.3 deletion in a patient with a language disorder and mild mental retardation by array-CGH. *American Journal of Medical Genetics, 129A*, 254–260.

van der Lely, H. K. J. (1998). G-SLI in children: Movement, economy and deficits in the computational syntactic system. *Language Acquisition, 7*, 161–193.

van der Lely, H. K. J. (1994). Canonical linking rules: Forward vs. reverse linking in normally developing and specifically language impaired children. *Cognition, 51*(1), 29–72.

Vernes, S. C., Nicod, J., Elahi, F. M., Coventry, J. A., Kenny, N., Coupe, A. M., Bird, L. E., Davies, K. E., & Fisher, S. E. (2006). Functional genetic analysis of mutations implicated in a human speech and language disorder. *Human Molecular Genetics, 15*, 3154–3167.

Wassink, T. H., Piven, J., Vieland, V. J., Huang, J., Swiderski, R. E., Pietila, J., et al. (2001). Evidence supporting WNT2 as an autism susceptibility gene. *American Journal of Medical Genetics, 105*(5), 406–413. Retrieved from PM:11449391.

Wassink, T. H., Piven, J., Vieland, V. J., Pietila, J., Goedken, R. J., Folstein, S. E., et al. (2002). Evaluation of FOXP2 as an autism susceptibility gene. *American Journal of Medical Genetics, 114*(5), 566–569.

Westby, C. (2006). There's more to passing than knowing the answers: Learning to do school. In T. A. Ukrainetz (Ed.), *Contextualized language intervention: Scaffolding PreK-12 literacy achievement* (pp. 319–387). Eau Claire, WI: Thinking Publications.

Whitehouse, A. J. O., Barry, J. G., & Bishop, D. V. M. (2007). The broader language phenotype of autism: a comparison with specific language impairment. *Journal of Child Psychology and Psychiatry, 48*(8), 822–830.

Whitehouse, A. J. O., Barry, J. G., & Bishop, D. V. M. (2008). Further defining the language impairment of autism: Is there a specific language impairment subtype? *Journal of Communication Disorders, 41*(4), 319–336.

World Health Organization. (1993). *The ICD-10 classification for mental and behavioural disorders: Diagnostic criteria for research.* Geneva: World Health Organization.

Young, A. R., Beitchman, J. H., Johnson, C., Douglas, L., Atkinson, L, Escobar, M., & Wilson, B. (2002). Young adult academic outcomes in a longitudinal sample of early identified language impaired and control children. *Journal of Child Psychology and Psychiatry, 43*(5), 635–645.

20 Anxiety and Mood Disorders in Individuals with Autism Spectrum Disorder

Peter Szatmari, Beth McConnell

Points of Interest

- To establish comorbidity, assessment measures must establish that anxiety/mood symptoms are independent of the core symptoms of ASD and are causing additional distress or impairment.
- Anxiety and mood disorders are more common in individuals with ASD than in the general population.
- Prevalence estimates for anxiety disorders range from 10 to 50%.
- Prevalence estimates for mood disorders range from 25 to 50%.
- When an individual with ASD presents with a significant change in behavior (e.g., increase in aggressive behavior; intensification of restricted interests), clinicians should be aware that anxiety and/or mood symptoms may be a contributing factor.
- Cognitive behavior therapy can be used successfully with individuals with ASD for the treatment of anxiety.

The social and communication deficits and restricted behavior that characterize autism spectrum disorders (ASD) make it challenging for affected individuals to navigate a complex social world. Too often individuals with ASD have the added stress of managing anxiety and mood problems. Considering how anxiety and depression can affect behavior in a typically developing person, it is easy to appreciate how the added burden of an internalizing disorder can impact the day to day functioning of individuals with ASD.

The study of anxiety and mood disorders is a relatively new area in the field of ASDs. For many years, it was thought that people with ASD could not express anxious or depressive symptoms, given that early estimates suggested more than 50% were nonverbal. More recently, DSM-IV has stipulated that comorbid anxiety and mood disorders could not be diagnosed in individuals with ASD. Such disorders were thought to be part of the ASD phenotype or could not be assessed properly in individuals with ASD. This has had the unfortunate effect of not recognizing this type of comorbidity and the attendant impairment that it entails. Since treatment of anxiety and mood disorders has progressed remarkably in the last 10 years with now good evidence of effective treatments, it would be important to screen for and diagnose these conditions. Fortunately, many clinicians and researchers now recognize that comorbid psychiatric symptoms are a significant and often disabling issue for this population. The present chapter highlights a number of issues and questions that research is beginning to address:

1. How common are anxiety and affective disorders in the ASD population?
2. How do we assess and treat psychiatric comorbidity in this group?
3. What are the causes and correlates of anxiety and mood disorders for individuals with ASD?
4. What should clinicians and researchers do next to further our understanding of these issues?
5. What are the clinical implications of comorbidity for this population?

What Does Comorbidity Mean?

Before beginning a review of the literature, it is worth considering what comorbidity actually means. The term was originally coined by Feinstein (1970) to describe the co-occurrence of two diseases either by chance, by shared vulnerability, or by some common etiologic mechanism. There are two types of comorbidity: sequential and simultaneous. Simultaneous comorbidity refers to the co-occurrence of two disorders that arise at the same time. Sequential comorbidity refers to the situation when one disorder precedes another disorder. In this circumstance, it is possible that one disorder is a true risk factor for the other disorder. However, it is also possible that the two disorders share a third, common, risk factor that gives rise to both. The distinction between simultaneous and sequential comorbidity is an important one, since the meaning of the comorbidity and its mechanism may be different in these two circumstances.

The determination of comorbidity can be confusing when this involves two psychiatric disorders. For example, individuals with autism often have symptoms of "sensory defensiveness"; that is, they put their hands over their ears, or get upset at the feel of certain clothes, or smells. These are not part of the diagnostic criteria for ASD or of any other disorder yet they may occur in other conditions as well. These might be considered associated symptoms or behaviors, but are not an example of comorbidity. Similarly, an individual with ASD may present with sadness, poor sleep, lack of motivation, and being a picky eater. The assessment of comorbidity must make a determination as to which of these symptoms is part of ASD, and which is part of a possible comorbid mood disorder. Poor sleep, lack of motivation, and being a picky eater are behaviors seen in both ASD and depression. How does one decide? The key is to determine whether there was a change over time in symptom presentation. If depression were a true diagnosis, then the symptoms of sadness, poor sleep, etc., would have to occur in a constellation, represent a change in behavior, and not be present from early in development.

In addition to observing a change in adaptive functioning, it is important to determine whether the symptoms are associated with added impairment over and above the primary diagnosis. An individual with ASD may develop new symptoms of depression and poor sleep, but unless those symptoms cause, or are associated with, extra impairment it is not possible to make another, comorbid diagnosis. ASD itself is associated with considerable impairment in terms of adaptive functioning and performance in certain roles. While a child with an ASD might have comorbid anxiety or mood symptoms, it can be difficult to establish whether or not the impairment associated with those symptoms is over and above the impairment due to autism itself. To meet criteria for a comorbid disorder, it is important that there be impairment specifically due to that comorbidity. Again, there must be a deterioration in adaptive functioning if a comorbid disorder occurs. This can often be hard to demonstrate if a person with ASD is already profoundly impaired due to his or her autism or intellectual disability.

Measurement

Quantitative research using questionnaire data has repeatedly shown that anxiety symptoms are more common in individuals with ASD than in the general population or controls with other developmental disabilities. When compared to the general population, anxiety symptoms are 3 to 4 times more common among high-functioning children with ASD than their age- and sex-matched counterparts (Kim, Szatmari, Bryson, Streiner, & Wilson, 2000). Several studies have shown that anxiety symptoms are also more common among the ASD population than other clinical groups (e.g., non-ASD clinical controls, language impaired controls, IQ- and age-matched controls; Bradley et al., 2004; Gillott, Furniss, & Walter, 2001; Gillot & Standen, 2007; Weisbrot, Gadow, DeVincent, & Pomeroy, 2005).

The most reliable prevalence estimates of anxiety and affective *disorders* (as opposed to symptoms) are from studies using semistructured diagnostic interviews. Unlike self-report questionnaires, diagnostic interviews allow clinicians to probe for additional details to determine whether endorsed symptoms are sufficiently impairing and persistent to warrant a clinical diagnosis of a mood or anxiety disorder. The problem is that it is unclear whether the instruments that have been traditionally used to measure psychiatric disorder in typically developing children are appropriate for those with ASD. To date, two measures have been developed to assess psychiatric comorbidity specifically in the ASD population: The Schedule for the Assessment of Psychiatric Problems with Autism (and Other Developmental Disorders) (SAPPA; Bolton & Rutter, 1988) and the Autism Comorbidity Interview-Present and Lifetime Versions (ACI-PL; Leyfer, 2006).

The SAPPA is a semistructured interview used to assess psychiatric disturbances in individuals with an ASD. The SAPPA corresponds to the Research Diagnostic Criteria (RDC; Spitzer, Endicott, & Robins, 1978) with respect to major psychiatric disorders. The SAPPA is still under development but has been used in three follow-up studies (Bradley & Bolton, 2006; Hutton, 1998; McConnell et al., 2011). The primary purpose of the SAPPA is to identify an episode of *new* behaviors and/or symptoms that are independent of ASD-related symptoms exhibited since early development. The interviewer must first establish a baseline of behaviors to which any change in behavior or symptoms (an "episode" of change) is compared. In order for an "episode" of a psychiatric disorder to be deemed clinically significant, it must meet one of the following criteria: psychiatric symptoms (anxiety, mood, delusions, hallucinations, catatonia, etc.) that are present for at least 3 days, OR a change in behavior that is outside the range of normal variation for an individual, present for at least 1 week AND definite decline in level of social functioning as indicated by at least two of the following: loss of interest in "play," loss of self-care, loss of social participation, loss of initiative, need for change in supervision/placement.

The ACI-PL is a modified version of the Kiddie Schedule for Affective Disorders and Schizophrenia (KSADS; Chambers et al., 1985), an instrument used to assess for the presence of psychiatric disorders in typically developing children and adolescents. The ACI-PL has been piloted in one study (Leyfer et al., 2006). The major modifications made to the KSADS to develop the ACI-PL include an introductory section to ascertain a baseline of emotional and behavioral functioning against which to evaluate psychiatric symptomatology. The administration of this instrument also includes descriptions of how specific disorders typically present in children with ASD. The ACI-PL also attempts to assess whether certain symptoms are applicable to a particular child. For instance, if a child has not demonstrated an understanding of guilt in the past then asking questions about feelings of guilt in the context of depression is not appropriate (Leyfer et al., 2006).

Both the SAPPA and ACI-PL highlight the need to assess whether or not psychiatric symptoms are a departure from an individual's baseline level of functioning. There is also an emphasis on ensuring that the symptoms are causing significant and persistent impairment in functioning beyond the impairment caused by the ASD alone. Both can elicit information from the parent (or guardian) and the individual with ASD. A common problem is that many people with ASD are nonverbal and cannot be interviewed. In that situation, a reliance on behavioral manifestations of anxiety and depression as observed by a parent is warranted (Matson & Nebel-Schwalm, 2007; Matson et al., 1997). The approach used by the SAPPA and ACI-PL is theoretically appropriate and represents a movement toward establishing a gold standard for the assessment of comorbidity in the ASD population.

Prevalence

We carried out a systematic review to identify all the studies that reported on the comorbidity of anxiety and mood disorders in ASD (also see Wood et al., 2009, for a useful review). We specifically focused on papers that used diagnostic interviews to assess comorbidity. We also wished to provide a systematic review of studies discussing potential causes and correlates of comorbidity and treatment studies of the accompanying disorder. We were able to identify 8 studies that used a structured or semistructured approach to making a diagnosis. The prevalence estimates from these studies for specific disorders are summarized in Table 20-1 and described in more detail below.

Specific Phobias

In a sample of 44 children and adolescents with ASD, Muris et al. (1998) identified specific phobias in 63% of the sample, the highest estimate to date for any anxiety disorder. Other studies report prevalence estimates ranging from less than 10% to as high as 43% (Rumsey et al., 1985; Green et al., 2000; Klin et al., 2005).

It has been argued that fears and phobias are part of the ASD phenotype (Evans, Canavera, Kleinpeter, Maccubbin, & Taga, 2005). Using mental age–matched children, chronologically age-matched children, and children with Down syndrome as comparisons, Evans et al. (2005) explored what types of fears children with ASD exhibit and whether these fears are normative given their developmental level. They found that ASD children had more situational fears and more fears of medical situations. They also found that externalizing problems (e.g., impulsivity, hyperactivity) were associated with these fears, whereas fears were "less symptomatic" in the other groups. Leyfer et al. (2006) also found discord between the types of fears endorsed by typically developing children and those with ASD. Such data suggest that certain fears may be part of the syndrome of ASD and not simply a developmental phase that the children will outgrow.

OCD

Estimates for OCD range from less than 10% to as high as 37% (Klin et al., 2005; Leyfer et al., 2006; McConnell et al., 2011). When assessing for the presence of obsessions and compulsions in individuals with ASD it can be difficult to ascertain if the symptoms have the required ego-dystonic quality. One must also be certain that obsessions do not merely reflect intense interests. Adherence to routines and rituals are also characteristic of ASD and needs to be distinguished from the anxiety-reducing compulsive behaviors seen in OCD. See Chapter 16 for a comprehensive discussion of OCD in the ASD population.

Social Phobia

Fear and avoidance of social situations and social awkwardness are extremely common in ASD. Prevalence estimates for social phobia range from 7 to 23% (Klin et al., 2005; Leyfer et al., 2006). Determining whether anxiety is attributable to the social (e.g., fear of negative evaluation or looking stupid) versus nonsocial (e.g., unfamiliar people, noise, change in routine) aspects of a situation is a critical distinction when making a diagnosis of social anxiety. On the other hand, it has been argued that poor social skills and increased awareness of social deficits in high-functioning individuals with ASD make them especially vulnerable to social anxiety (Meyer, Mundy, Van Hecke, & Durocher, 2006; Wing, 1981). Understanding the source of anxiety in social situations is, therefore, critical to making an appropriate diagnosis.

Generalized Anxiety Disorder (GAD)

In the first study of comorbidity in autism, Rumsey et al. (1985) reported symptoms of chronic generalized worry in half of an adult sample of men with autism. However, the worry symptoms were judged to be part of the autism symptomatology, and an additional diagnosis of GAD was not assigned. While subsequent studies report prevalence rates between 20 and 35% for GAD, a recent study reported GAD in only 2.4% of the study sample (Leyfer et al., 2006; see Table 20-1). Leyfer et al. described the anxiety exhibited by children in their sample as being more trait-like and less variable in content than one would expect from GAD. McConnell et al. reported much higher rates of GAD in a population of adolescents and young adults with high-functioning autism and Asperger's syndrome (AS). Further clinical research is needed to clarify the nature, chronicity, and variability of worry symptoms and how they manifest in the ASD population.

Table 20–1.
Summary of prevalence data on comorbid psychiatric disorders among individuals with autism spectrum disorders

Study	Sample Size	Age	Measure	Disorders	Percent
McConnell, Vaccarella, Tuff, Bryson, & Szatmari	n = 70	13–22 x = 19	KSADS & SAPPA	GAD	25.7
				OCD	7.1
				Panic Disorder	7.1
				Separation Anxiety	N/A
				Social Phobia	8.6
				Specific Phobia	N/A
				Major Depressive Disorder	31
				Dysthymia	0
				Bipolar Disorder	
Leyfer, Folstein, Bacalman, Davis, Dinh, & Morgan	n = 109	5–17 x = 9.2	ACI-PL	GAD	2.4
				OCD	37.2
				Panic Disorder	0
				Separation Anxiety	11.9
				Social Phobia	7.5
				Specific Phobia	44.3
				Major Depressive Disorder	10.1
				Bipolar 1 Disorder	1.9
				Bipolar 2 Disorder Cyclothymia	0.9
					0.94
Bradley & Bolton (2006)	n = 36	14–20 x = 16.5	SAPPA	Depressive disorder	22.2
				Bipolar Disorders	5.5
Klin, Pauls, Schultz, & Volkmar (2005)	n = 47	8–32 x = 16.8	KSADS or SCID	GAD	19.1
				OCD	23.4
				Panic Disorder	23.4
				Separation Anxiety	29.8
				Social Phobia	
				Specific Phobia	
				Major Depressive Disorder	
				Bipolar 1 Disorder	
				Bipolar 2 Disorder	
				Cyclothymia	
Green, Gilchrist, Burton, & Cox (2000) (diagnoses based on ICD-10 criteria)	n = 20	11–19 x = 13.8	IOW(1) and IOW(S)*	GAD	35
				OCD	25
				Panic Disorder	10
				Separation Anxiety	5
				Social Phobia	25
				Phobia Anxiety Disorder	
				Major Depression	
				Dysthymia	
Muris & Steerneman (1998)	n = 44	2–18 x = 9.7	DISC (anxiety section)	Agoraphobia	45.5
				Avoidant Disorder	18.2
				GAD	11.4
				OCD	22.7
				Overanxious Disorder	9.1
				Panic Disorder	27.3
				Separation Anxiety	20.5
				Social Phobia	63.6
				Specific Phobia	
Szatmari, Bartoucci, & Bremner (1989) Asperger's syndrome group High-functioning autism group	n = 28 n = 25	8–18 x = 14.3 7–32 x = 23.3	DICA DICA	OCD	29
				Overanxious disorder	32
				Separation Anxiety	4
				OCD	17
				Overanxious Disorder	17
				Separation Anxiety	0
Rumsey, Rapoport, & Sceery (1985)	n = 14	18–39 x = 28	DIS & DICA	Chronic Generalized Anxiety	50
				Separation Anxiety	14
				Simple Phobia	7

* IOW: Isle of Wight Semistructured Informant and Subject Interviews

Panic Disorder

Reported rates for panic disorder are consistently below 10% (Leyfer et al., 2006; McConnell et al., 2011; Muris & Steerneman, 1998; Rumsey et al., 1985). Although some studies report discrete episodes of panic attacks among individuals with ASD, it appears that few evolve into full-blown panic disorder. A relatively high rate of agoraphobia (45%) was reported in the Muris and Steerneman sample, but no details regarding the nature of the anxiety were provided. Individuals with ASD may feel anxious in a variety of situations for a variety of reasons. Establishing whether anxiety is related to having panic symptoms is critical for establishing a diagnosis of agoraphobia. Clinically, a diagnosis of specific phobia may be more appropriate if the avoidance occurs in response to only a few specific situations.

Post Traumatic Stress Disorder (PTSD)

Few studies have looked at the rates of PTSD in the ASD population. Our study identified a single case triggered by severe bullying at school (McConnell et al., 2011).

Mood Disorders

The rates for mood disorders are also high in the ASD population. In a sample of adolescents with Asperger's syndrome, 25% were found to have chronically low mood or dysthymia (Green et al., 2000). Klin et al. (2005) diagnosed depression in 34% of a sample of adolescents and young adults with ASD. In a population-based study comparing the rate of psychiatric disturbances between individuals with mental retardation with and without autism, 50% of the autism group was diagnosed with depression (Bradley, Summers, Wood, & Bryson, 2004). The rate of mood disorders in the McConnell sample was 31% (n = 22/70). Depression was the most common mood disorder diagnosed in the sample (n = 20), but dysthymia was also reported (n = 6). No episodes of mania or hypomania were identified.

Summary

As seen in Table 20-1, there is significant variability in prevalence estimates for anxiety and affective disorders in the ASD population. Depending on the specific disorder, estimates range from approximately 10% to 63% (Bradley & Bolton, 2006; Green, Gilchrist, Burton, & Cox, 2000; Klin, Pauls, Schultz, & Volkmar, 2005; Leyfer, et al, 2006; Muris & Steerneman, 1998; Szatmari, Bartolucci, & Bremner, 1989). The range in prevalence estimates is due, in part, to variability in the criteria for judging whether or not a symptom is independent of the ASD diagnosis. In addition, the lack of a truly valid and reliable instrument to assess for psychiatric disorders in the ASD population makes the data difficult to summarize and interpret in a meaningful way, even when diagnostic interviews are used by experienced clinicians.

Among the ASD population with a diagnosed Axis-I disorder, rates of multiple disorders are not uncommon. For example, in the McConnell et al. study (2011), 41% had more than one such diagnosis. Anxiety and mood disorders had the highest rate of co-occurrence, with 21% of the sample meeting criteria for both. In addition, nearly half the cases with comorbid anxiety and mood disorders had an additional diagnosis of an externalizing disorder (i.e., ADHD, conduct disorder, or oppositional disorder). By comparison, only one third of the cases diagnosed with an externalizing disorder did not have a comorbid diagnosis of an anxiety and/or mood disorder. Thus, behavioral problems occurred predominantly in the presence of clinically significant persistent anxiety and/or affective symptoms.

Research with typically developing teens presenting with depression has also shown a high rate of comorbidity between depression and aggressive behavior (Knox, King, Hanna, Logan, & Ghaziuddin, 2000). Given the frequency with which children and adolescents with ASDs are treated for behavioral problems, it is important to consider that anxiety and/or mood symptoms may be important factors in the development of aggressive behavior in adolescence and young adulthood. Otherwise, interventions may be misguided by failing to also target the underlying internalizing disorders.

This pattern of comorbidity is commonly seen in psychiatric clinics among adolescents without ASDs. But it is interesting to speculate on how the clinical manifestations of anxiety and mood disorders are modified by the ASD. It is unfortunate that few studies have reported on the manifestations of anxiety and mood disorders in the ASD population and how the ASD phenotype is modified by the comorbid disorder. Anecdotally, McConnell et al. (2011) saw that children with anxiety and mood disorders tended to demonstrate an increase in their restricted interests and preoccupations. This led to more social withdrawal and apparent apathy. Anxiety was also associated with more repetitive questioning and ruminating over worries, concerns, and past events. Both the anxiety and mood disorders were frequently associated with pacing, inappropriate laughter and sleep disturbance. Aggressive behavior of a reactive nature, often in response to teasing and bullying at school or to limitations imposed at home, were frequent in those who had anxiety and depression.

Causes and Correlates

Finally, it is not known whether risk factors for anxiety and mood disorders are specific to ASD or similar to those reported in other adolescents with similar disorders. Very little is known about the correlates of mood disorders in ASD children, and only a few studies report on correlates for comorbid anxiety disorder. It has been reported that adolescents with ASDs who are depressed have a higher frequency of a family history of depression and more negative life events than ASD adolescents without mood disorder (Ghaziuddin, Alessi, &

Greden, 1995; Ghaziuddin & Greden, 1998). While it may be true that a family history of depression and negative life events might be associated with depression in this population, these correlates do not explain why such comorbid disorders are more common in this group than in the general population (unless the mood problems are indeed more common in their parents and are genetically transmitted). To understand specifically why such comorbid disorders might be particularly prevalent one needs to think of characteristics of ASD children that could be associated with increased risk.

IQ

Several studies have found that higher IQ is associated with greater levels of anxiety and depressive symptoms in children and adults with ASD (Gadow et al., 2008; Lecavalier et al., 2006; Sterling, Dawson, Estes, & Greenson, 2007; Sukhodolsky et al., 2008; Weisbrot et al., 2005). This does not imply that lower functioning individuals are unaffected but does suggest a degree of heterogeneity within the ASD population. Such heterogeneity may be mediated by a number of additional factors. For example, Sukhodolsky et al. (2008) found that anxiety was not only associated with higher IQ but with the presence of functional language and more stereotyped behavior. The same study also found that higher IQ *combined* with greater impairment in social reciprocity led to more severe anxiety. Interestingly, social phobia and specific phobia occurred with equal frequency in the lower and higher IQ groups. One implication of this finding, as suggested by Sukhodolsky et al., is that these two disorders are more a part of the core phenotype of ASD compared to other disorders.

Stressors

Gillot and Standen (2007) found high levels of anxiety to be associated with certain types of stressors, including sensory stimuli, anticipation, coping with change, and unpleasant events. Individuals with higher levels of anxiety were less capable of coping with these stressors. During the diagnostic interview, McConnell et al. (2011) made notes regarding precipitating events, if any, of depressive episodes. Participants reported a variety of events, including moving, death of a family member, loss of significant relationships, and bullying. Their findings are consistent with previous research indicating that life stressors contribute to the onset of depression in individuals with ASD (Ghaziuddin, Alessi, & Greden, 1995), just as they do in typically developing individuals (Kendler, Karkowski, & Prescott, 1999). Anecdotal evidence suggests that teasing and bullying experienced at school were particularly important background factors in the precipitation of the anxiety and mood disorders.

Social Information Processing

Although social impairments are characteristic of ASD, that does not mean that affected individuals lack awareness of social situations or their own limitations. On the contrary, research suggests that many children with ASD are capable of self-reporting social difficulties and are sensitive to the reactions of others (Meyer et al., 2006; Wing, 1981). Furthermore, it may be that increased social awareness in high functioning individuals with ASD makes such individuals especially vulnerable to anxiety and mood problems (Sterling, Dawson, Estes, & Greenson, 2007; Wing, 1981). An emerging area of research attempts to identify the types of social information processing deficits that may contribute to this vulnerability (Hedley & Young, 2006; Meyer, Mundy, Van Heckem, & Durocher, 2006). Hedley and Young (2006) found an association between depressive symptoms and a measure of social comparison. Specifically, adolescents with AS who rated themselves as "more different" than others also reported greater depressive symptomatology. Other research suggests an association between the social information processing patterns of adolescents with AS and anxiety and mood symptoms (Meyer et al., 2006). For example, a tendency toward social encoding errors and hostile intent attributions was associated with greater comorbidity.

Treatment

Psychological Intervention

Cognitive behavior therapy (CBT) is recognized as an effective treatment for anxiety and mood disorders in both adults and children without ASD. Adapting CBT for use with the ASD population has been attempted in several case studies with positive results (Cardaciotto & Herbert, 2004; Hare, 1997; Reaven & Hepburn, 2003).

Using a CBT protocol developed for use with adults with social phobia, Cardaciotto and Herbert (2004) describe only minor modifications to the treatment plan for a 23-year-old male with Asperger's syndrome. In addition to exposure exercises and cognitive therapy, the social skill deficits of the participant were identified and targeted in treatment. Appropriate verbal and nonverbal social skills were explained and rehearsed in session. Following treatment, the participant continued to report fear in social situations but experienced a reduction in anxiety symptoms. The participant also reported less impairment and avoidance in response to his fears.

Reaven and Hepburn (2003) reported successfully treating a 7-year-old female with AS for OCD. A comprehensive assessment distinguished obsessions and compulsions (e.g., contamination obsessions, "need to know") from the child's intense interests and preoccupations. The CBT protocol was adapted principally from March and Mulle (1998) and is outlined in the article. Reaven and Hepburn (2003) also discuss the types of modifications that may be necessary when undertaking CBT with children with ASD. These include the liberal use of visual supports to reinforce intervention strategies and the involvement of parents to maximize the generalization of strategies learned in treatment.

While case reports are useful preliminary steps toward identifying potentially effective treatment for anxiety and mood difficulties in individuals with ASD, more rigorous methods are required to assess efficacy. To date, the literature includes two randomized controlled trials of CBT in a group of children with Asperger's syndrome or ASD (Sofronoff, Attwood, & Hinton, 2005; Wood et al., 2009). Children in the first study were identified with anxiety through questionnaires and assigned to one of two treatment groups (Sofronoff et al., 2005); a child-only treatment group and a child and parent treatment group in which the parent was trained as a cotherapist. A waitlist control group was also included in the study. The treatment protocol included a variety of CBT techniques that have shown effectiveness with typically developing children with anxiety. Relative to a waitlist control group, both intervention groups showed significant reductions in anxiety levels. In the study by Wood et al. (2009), 47 children with ASD were randomized to receive a modified form of CBT or waitlist control condition. The experimental group received 16 sessions consisting of behavioral experimentation, parent training, and school consultation. At the end of treatment, 78.5% of the experimental group had made a clinically significant improvement compared to 8.7% in the control group (number needed to treat = 2). These results are consistent with research evaluating interventions with typically developing children, which has shown that including both the child and parent in the treatment process leads to greater improvements.

Pharmacological Intervention

The issue of medication efficacy is complex. There is now reasonably good evidence that antidepressants such as selective serotonin reuptake inhibitors are effective among typical children and youth with anxiety disorders and major depression (Hetrick, Merry, McKenzie, Sindahl, & Proctor, 2007). There is a concern about increased suicidal *thinking* (Olfson & Shaffer, 2007) but no evidence of more suicide *attempts* on SSRIs than placebos. Whether or not medications are more effective than CBT is somewhat unclear. There are no controlled clinical trials of SSRIs to treat depression or anxiety when it is comorbid with ASD. Kolevzon et al. (2006) recently published a comprehensive systematic review of SSRIs in ASD and concluded that although the quality of the evidence is poor and more rigorous studies are required, there is some evidence that SSRIs can reduce significant anxiety symptoms in ASD.

Conclusions

The prevalence data presented in this review highlight the importance of doing a systematic assessment for comorbid anxiety and mood disorders in children and adolescents with ASD who present with a change in behavior. Clinicians must be alert for episodes of depression, especially in those who present with significant anxiety symptoms, increased aggressive behavior, and/or intensifying restricted interests and preoccupations. Anecdotal evidence suggests the importance of ensuring that the social context for these adolescents and young adults remains supportive and encouraging. To prevent the development of a comorbid disorder, it may now be time to focus on *changing* the social context of the adolescent with ASD rather than attempting to "treat" the ASD, as service providers did during childhood. If a comorbid anxiety or mood disorder does occur, there is now some evidence for the usefulness of medication as well as cognitive behavior therapy (Sofronoff et al.; Cardaciotto & Herbert, 2004; Wood et al., 2009). Health care professionals working in the field of developmental disabilities will need to develop skills in this form of treatment. In addition, mental health professionals can no longer justify excluding ASD youth and adults from the benefits of their services. Finally, perhaps it is ironic to point out that while those with good language and nonverbal problem-solving skills have a better outcome when it comes to autistic symptoms and overall adaptation they appear to be at higher risk for often debilitating anxiety and mood disorder. It's as if this particularly vulnerable population of high-functioning adolescents with ASD cannot win in their developmental struggles!

Challenges and Future Directions

- Ensuring that we have reliable ways to assess for psychiatric comorbidity in this vulnerable population should be a primary goal for future research. Both the SAPPA and ACI-PL are promising measures but the development of consensus guidelines detailing how anxiety and mood disorders present in the ASD population are essential and outstanding.
- We also need consensus guidelines to address two questions paramount to making a valid and reliable clinical diagnosis: (1) Is the anxiety/mood symptom independent of the core symptoms of ASD? (2) Is the anxiety/mood symptom causing significant distress or impairment above and beyond that caused by the ASD diagnosis? The majority of studies have relied on measures validated on the typically developing population. The problem with relying exclusively on such measures is the lack of consideration for how anxiety presents in individuals with ASD and how some core features of ASD can be mistakenly attributed to other disorders (e.g., distinguishing between preoccupations and obsessions). Only once guidelines are established and reliable measures become available can we compare studies in a meaningful manner.
- As seen in Table 20-1, there is great variability in prevalence estimates and only eight studies from which to draw conclusions. There is clearly a need for more clinical research using diagnostic interviews and comparison groups.

As much as possible, researchers need to provide clinical details to convey how critical distinctions are made in the diagnostic process (e.g., distinguishing obsessions from preoccupations; judging whether symptoms cause significant distress/impairment). As assessment methods and measures are refined, consistency between prevalence estimates will no doubt emerge.

- Another important area of research is studying the development of comorbid anxiety and mood symptoms over time. We were not able to identify any longitudinal studies that investigate the developmental trajectories of these symptoms from early childhood to adolescence. This is critical in understanding the earliest manifestations of the comorbidity and in developing early interventions to reduce further morbidity.

SUGGESTED READING

White, S. W., Oswald, D., Ollendick, T., & Scahill, L. (2009). Anxiety in children and adolescents with autism spectrum disorders. *Clinical Psychology Review, 29*, 216–229.

Wood, J. J., Drahota, A., Sze, K., Har, K., Chiu, A., & Langer, D. A. (2009). Cognitive behavioral therapy for anxiety in children with autism spectrum disorders: a randomized, controlled trial. *Journal of Child Psychology and Psychiatry, 50*, 224–234.

Kolevzon, A., Mathewson, K. A., & Hollander, E. (2006). Selective serotonin reuptake inhibitors in autism: a review of efficacy and tolerability. *Journal of Clinical Psychiatry, 67*(3), 407–414.

REFERENCES

Bolton, P., & Rutter, M. (1988). *Schedule for assessment of psychiatric problems associated with autism (and other developmental disorders).* (Available from the Department of Child Psychiatry, Institute of Psychiatry, London, England).

Bradley, E. A., & Bolton, P. (2006). Episodic psychiatric disorders in teenagers with learning disabilities with and without autism. *British Journal of Psychiatry, 189*, 361–366.

Bradley, E. A., Summers, J. A., Wood, H. L., & Bryson, S. E. (2004). Comparing rates of psychiatric and behavior disorders in adolescents and young adults with severe intellectual disability with and without autism. *Journal of Autism and Developmental Disorders, 34*, 151–161.

Cardaciotto, L., & Herbert, J. D. (2004). Cognitive behavior therapy for social anxiety disorder in the context of Asperger's syndrome: A single-subject report. *Cognitive and Behavioral Practice, 11*, 75–81.

Chambers, W. J., Puig-Antich, J., Hirsch, M., Paez, P., Ambrosini, P. J., Tabrizi, M. A., et al. (1985). The assessment of affective disorders in children and adolescents by semistructured interview. *Test-retest reliability of the schedule for affective disorders and schizophrenia for school-age children*, present episode version. *Archives of General Psychiatry, 42*, 696–702.

Evans, D. W., Canavera, K., Kleinpeter, F. L., Maccubbin, E., & Taga, K. (2005). The fears, phobias and anxieties of children with autism spectrum disorders and down syndrome: Comparisons with developmentally and chronologically age matched children. *Child Psychiatry and Human Development, 36*, 3–26.

Feinstein, A. R. (1970). The pre-therapeutic classification of co-morbidity in chronic disease. *Journal of Chronic Disease, 23*, 455–468.

Gadow, K. D., DeVincent, C., & Schneider, J. (2008). Predictors of psychiatric symptoms in children with an autism spectrum disorder. *Journal of Autism and Developmental Disorders.*

Ghaziuddin, M., Alessi, N., & Greden, J. F. (1995). Life events and depression in children with pervasive developmental disorders. *Journal of Autism and Developmental Disorders, 25*, 495–502.

Ghaziuddin, M., & Greden, J. (1998). Depression in children with autism/pervasive developmental disorders: A case-control family history study. *Journal of Autism and Developmental Disorders, 28*, 111–115.

Gillot, A., Furniss, F., & Walter, A. (2001). Anxiety in high-functioning children with autism. *Autism, 5*, 277–286.

Gillott, A., & Standen, P. J. (2007). Levels of anxiety and sources of stress in adults with autism. *Journal of Intellectual Disabilities, 11*, 359–370.

Green, J., Gilchrist, A., Burton, D., & Cox, A. (2000). Social and psychiatric functioning in adolescents with Asperger syndrome compared with conduct disorder. *Journal of Autism and Developmental Disorders, 30*, 279–293.

Hare, D. J. (1997). The use of cognitive-behavior therapy with people with Asperger syndrome. *Autism, 1*, 215–225.

Hedley, D., & Young, R. (2006). Social comparison processes and depressive symptoms in children and adolescents with Asperger syndrome. *Autism, 10*, 139–153.

Hetrick, S., Merry, S., McKenzie, J., Sindahl, P., & Proctor, M. (2007). Selective serotonin reuptake inhibitors (SSRIs) for depressive disorders in children and adolescents. *Cochrane Database Systematic Review, 18*, CD004852.

Hutton, J. (1998). *Cognitive decline and new problems arising in association with autism.* Doctor of Clinical Psychology Thesis, Institute of Psychiatry, University of London.

Kendler, K. S., Karkowski, L. M., & Prescott, C. A. (1999). Causal relationship between stressful life events and the onset of major depression. *American Journal of Psychiatry, 156*, 837–841.

Kim, J. A., Szatmari, P., Bryson, S. E., Streiner, D. L., & Wilson, F. J. (2000). The prevalence of anxiety and mood problems among children with autism and Asperger syndrome. *Autism, 4*, 117–132.

Klin, A., Pauls, D., Schultz, R., & Volkmar, F. (2005). Three diagnostic approaches to Asperger syndrome: Implications for research. *Journal of Autism and Developmental Disorders, 35*, 221–234.

Knox, M., King, C., Hanna, G. L., Logan, D., & Ghaziuddin, N. (2000). Aggressive behaviour in clinically depressed adolescents. *Journal of the American Academy of Child and Adolescent Psychiatry, 39*(5), 611–618.

Kolevzon, A., Mathewson, K. A., & Hollander, E. (2006). Selective serotonin reuptake inhibitors in autism: a review of efficacy and tolerability. *Journal of Clinical Psychiatry, 67*(3), 407–414.

Lainhart, J. E., & Folstein, S. E. (1994). Affective disorders in people with autism: A review of published cases. *Journal of Autism and Developmental Disorders, 24*, 587–601.

Lecavalier, L. (2006). Behavioral and emotional problems in young people with pervasive developmental disorders: Relative prevalence, effects of subject characteristics, and empirical classification. *Journal of Autism and Developmental Disorders, 36*, 1101–1114.

Leyfer, O. T., Folstein, S. E., Bacalman, S., Davis, N. O., Dinh, E., Morgan, J., et al. (2006). Comorbid psychiatric disorders in children with autism: Interview development and rates of disorders. *Journal of Autism and Developmental Disorders, 36*, 849–861.

March, J., & Mulle, K. (1998). *OCD in children and adolescents: A cognitive-behavioral treatment manual.* New York: Guilford.

Matson, J. L., & Nebel-Schwalm, M. S. (2007). Comorbid psychopathology with autism spectrum disorder in children: An overview. *Research in Developmental Disabilities, 28*, 341–352.

Matson, J. L., Smiroldo, B. B., Hamilton, M., & Baglio, C. S. (1997). Do anxiety disorders exist in persons with severe and profound mental retardation? *Research in Developmental Disabilities, 18*, 39–44.

McConnell, B. A., Vaccarella, L., Tuff, L., Bryson, S. E., & Szatmari, P. (2011, submitted). Anxiety and mood disorders in adolescents with autistic spectrum disorders.

Meyer, J. A., Mundy, P. C., Van Hecke, A., & Durocher, J. S. (2006). Social attribution processes and comorbid psychiatric symptoms in children with Asperger syndrome. *Autism, 10*, 383–402.

Muris, P., Steerneman, P., Merckelbach, H., Holdrinet, I., & Meesters, C. (1998). Comorbid anxiety symptoms in children with pervasive developmental disorders. *Journal of Anxiety Disorders, 12*, 387–393.

Olfson, M., & Shaffer, D. (2007). SSRI prescriptions and the rate of suicide. *American Journal of Psychiatry, 164*(12), 1907–1908.

Reaven, J., & Hepburn, S. (2003). Cognitive-behavioral treatment of obsessive-compulsive disorder in a child with Asperger syndrome. *Autism, 7*, 145–164.

Rumsey, J. M., Rapoport, J. L., & Sceery, W. R. (1985). Autistic children as adults: Psychiatric, social, and behavioral outcomes. *Journal of the American Academy of Child Psychiatry, 24*, 465–473.

Sofronoff, K., Attwood, T., & Hilton, S. (2005). A randomized controlled trial of a CBT intervention for anxiety in children with Asperger syndrome. *Journal of Child Psychology and Psychiatry, 46*, 1152–1160.

Spitzer, R. L., Endicott, J., & Robins, E. (1978). Research diagnostic criteria: Rationale and reliability. *Archives of General Psychiatry, 35*, 773–782.

Sterling, L., Dawson, G., Estes, A., & Greenson, J. (2007). Characteristics associated with presence of depressive symptoms in adults with autism spectrum disorder. *Journal of Autism and Developmental Disorders, 38*(6), 1011–1018.

Sukhodolsky, D. G., Scahill, L., Gadow, K. D., Arnold, L. E., Aman, M. G., McDougle, C. J., et al. (2008). Parent-rated anxiety symptoms in children with pervasive developmental disorders: Frequency and association with core autism symptoms and cognitive functioning. *Journal of Abnormal Child Psychology, 36*(1), 117–128.

Szatmari, P., Bartolucci, G., & Bremmer, R. (1989). Asperger's syndrome and autism: Comparison of early history and outcome. *Developmental Medicine and Child Neurology, 31*, 709–720.

Weisbrot, D. M., Gadow, K. D., DeVincent, C. J., & Pomeroy, J. (2005). The presentation of anxiety in children with pervasive developmental disorders. *Journal of Child and Adolescent Psychopharmacology, 15*, 477–496.

White, S. W., Oswald, D., Ollendick, T., & Scahill, L. (2009). Anxiety in children and adolescents with autism spectrum disorders. *Clinical Psychology Review, 29*, 216–229.

Wood, J. J., Drahota, A., Sze, K., Har, K., Chiu, A., & Langer, D. A. (2009). Cognitive behavioral therapy for anxiety in children with autism spectrum disorders: a randomized, controlled trial. *Journal of Child Psychology and Psychiatry, 50*, 224–234.

Wing, L. (1981). Asperger's syndrome: A clinical account. *Psychological Medicine, 11*, 115–129.

21 Stereotypy and Self-Injury

Lindsey Sterling, Annie McLaughlin, Bryan H. King

Points of Interest

- Stereotypy and self-injury are behaviors commonly associated with a number of developmental disorders, including autism spectrum disorders.
- A variety of neurological systems have been implicated in the expression of stereotypy and self-injury, particularly the dopaminergic, opioidergic, and glutamatergic systems.
- Animal models provide insight into putative neurological mechanisms and social/emotional factors that may contribute to the development and maintenance of stereotypy and self-injury.
- It has been demonstrated that impoverished environments and sensory deprivation can impact the development of stereotypy and self-injury in a variety of animal species, including humans.
- Pharmacological and behavioral treatments have been somewhat efficacious in ameliorating stereotypy and self-injury, though much work still needs to be done to successfully target these symptoms.

Stereotypy is a core feature of autistic disorder and refers to behavior(s) that are typically repetitive and nonfunctional or non–goal directed (Berkson, 1967). A child might cock her head and look out of the corner of her eyes at her hand while she waves it side to side in front of a ceiling light. Another may hold a string between his thumb and index finger and appear to become lost in its dance as he wiggles it rapidly up and down or from side to side. He may turn a toy car upside down and incessantly spin its wheels rather than play with it as intended.

"A low grade… child [with profound intellectual disability who] would rush about, leaping over or knocking against articles of furniture, or dashing her head against the walls or floor, so that, if left alone for a minute or two her face and hands would be hurt and bruised. Along with motor restlessness there was often a strange indifference to pain." From Ireland, 1898.

Some stereotyped behaviors are associated with tissue damage; for example, repetitive licking can cause dry, cracked skin. Other behaviors appear to be quite specifically designed to cause injury—like head banging and face slapping and have been described in case reports dating back over a century (e.g., Ireland, 1898). These behaviors pose a serious risk of bodily tissue damage and increase the risk of hospitalization. They can also lead to intensive and possibly restrictive special education programming, reduced opportunities for social interactions, and physical restraint. Significant medical problems can also arise as a result of self-injurious behaviors such as cataracts, retinal detachment, permanent scars, contusions, soft tissue lacerations, and even death. Among families affected by autism, higher repetitive behaviors increase perceived stress on families (Bishop et al., 2007). The effect of self-injurious behaviors on families and care providers can be absolutely overwhelming.

For all of these behaviors, the fact that they are repetitive and seem so compelling perhaps begs the question of how they can be truly "non–goal directed." Indeed, stereotyped behaviors are typically discriminated from involuntary movements like tics because they are more rhythmic and under some measure of voluntary control (e.g., Crosland et al., 2005).

Additional confusion about the nonfunctional nature of these behaviors might also derive from the fact that stereotypy exists on a continuum and within a context. The child who incessantly bounces a ball on the pavement despite the complaints of neighbors may be internally motivated to hone his basketball skills, or reinforced by the sight or sound or feel of the activity, or even by the psychological impact he is having on the neighborhood. It is thus perhaps more accurate to suggest for stereotypy that the goals of the behavior are not always immediately apparent or that they are atypical or uniquely held. However, it is also the case that certain environmental and physiological factors are likely to increase the probability for expression of stereotypy that is regarded as pathological because of its intensity and interference. In this chapter we will review the biology and treatment of stereotypy with a focus on stereotyped self-injury as an extreme manifestation of this behavior.

Definitions of Stereotypy and SIB

As noted earlier, over the past several decades, definitions of stereotypy have incorporated both a description of the behavior—as repetitive, topographically invariant, and often rhythmical—as well as purposeless (Baumeister & Rollings, 1976; LaGrow & Repp, 1984).

Stereotypy: behavior that is repetitive, topographically invariant, often rhythmical, and seemingly without purpose.

This latter qualifier allows one to discriminate stereotyped basketball bouncing from basketball practice; to discriminate stereotyped hair twirling from grooming; string wiggling from untangling; pacing from ambulating. The *Diagnostic and Statistical Manual of Mental Disorders-4th Edition-Text Revision* (DSM-IV-TR; APA, 2000) highlights hand or finger flapping and complex whole-body movements in the diagnostic criteria for autism as well as a variety of other examples in the criteria for stereotypic movement disorder (Table 21-1). Although some behaviors, for instance, amphetamine-induced stereotypies in the rat (Fowler et al., 2003), and body rocking in humans (Ross, Yu, & Kropla, 1998) are highly rhythmic, not all stereotyped acts are consistently so. Repetitive hitting may occur at different rates and even involve different targets. Although a potentially helpful discrimination between perseveration and stereotypy has been suggested as a function of whether the behavior involves excessive activity (Ridley, 1994), this distinction is complicated. In practice, stereotypy invariably reduces other, typically more adaptive behaviors because of their mutual incompatibility. Thus, stereotypy is virtually always perseverative, but a perseveration may not be stereotyped.

Table 21–1.
DSM-IV-TR Diagnostic criteria for stereotypic movement disorder

A. Repetitive, seemingly driven, and nonfunctional motor behavior (e.g., hand shaking or waving, body rocking, head banging, mouthing of objects, self-biting, picking at skin or bodily orifices, hitting own body).

B. The behavior markedly interferes with normal activities or results in self-inflicted bodily injury that requires medical treatment (or would result in an injury if preventive measures were not used).

C. If mental retardation is present, the stereotypic or self-injurious behavior is of sufficient severity to become a focus of treatment.

D. The behavior is not better accounted for by a compulsion (as in obsessive-compulsive disorder), a tic (as in tic disorder), a stereotypy that is part of a pervasive developmental disorder, or hair pulling (as in trichotillomania).

E. The behavior is not due to the direct physiological effects of a substance or a general medical condition.

F. The behavior persists for 4 weeks or longer.

Specify if:

With self-injurious behavior: if the behavior results in bodily damage that requires specific treatment (or that would result in bodily damage if protective measures were not used).

DSM-IV-TR incorporates all of the above features in the diagnostic criteria for stereotypic movement disorder (Table 21-1). In this definition, the fact that stereotyped movements can occur in the context of intellectual disability, or in conditions other than an autism spectrum disorder, is highlighted by exclusions. For example, criterion C allows for concurrent diagnoses of mental retardation and stereotypic movement disorder only when the latter behavior becomes a focus of treatment. And criterion D essentially allows for the diagnosis of a pervasive developmental disorder to absorb the presence of stereotypic movement disorder. However, because self-injurious behavior, and even intense stereotypy that may be a focus of treatment, is not necessarily clear from the diagnosis of autism alone, it is best to utilize this diagnosis in autism when all other criteria are met (e.g., "stereotypic movement disorder with self-injurious behavior" should be included as a diagnosis in addition to an ASD if the stereotypic behavior is a focus of treatment).

Relationship Between Stereotypy and SIB

Self-injurious behavior (SIB) has long been viewed as occurring on a continuum of other stereotyped behaviors. Some early stereotypy scoring conventions in animal models place self-injurious behavior at the extreme end of the scale. In humans, stereotypy is regarded as a precursor of SIB (Schroeder et al., 1990; Richman & Lindauer, 2005), and SIB is viewed as an extreme manifestation of stereotypy (Gal, Dyck, & Passmore, 2009).

Prevalence of Stereotypy and SIB

Studies that have examined the prevalence of stereotypy are influenced by sampling strategies, but rates can be upward of 30% in institutional settings (Dura, Mulick, & Rasnake, 1987). The prevalence of self-injury in people with intellectual disabilities also varies, and estimates between 4%

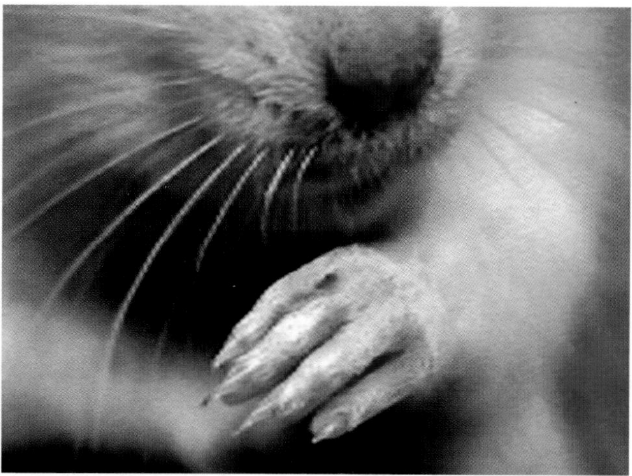

Figure 21–2. Lesion on the dorsum of the paw from self-biting in a rat treated with pemoline.

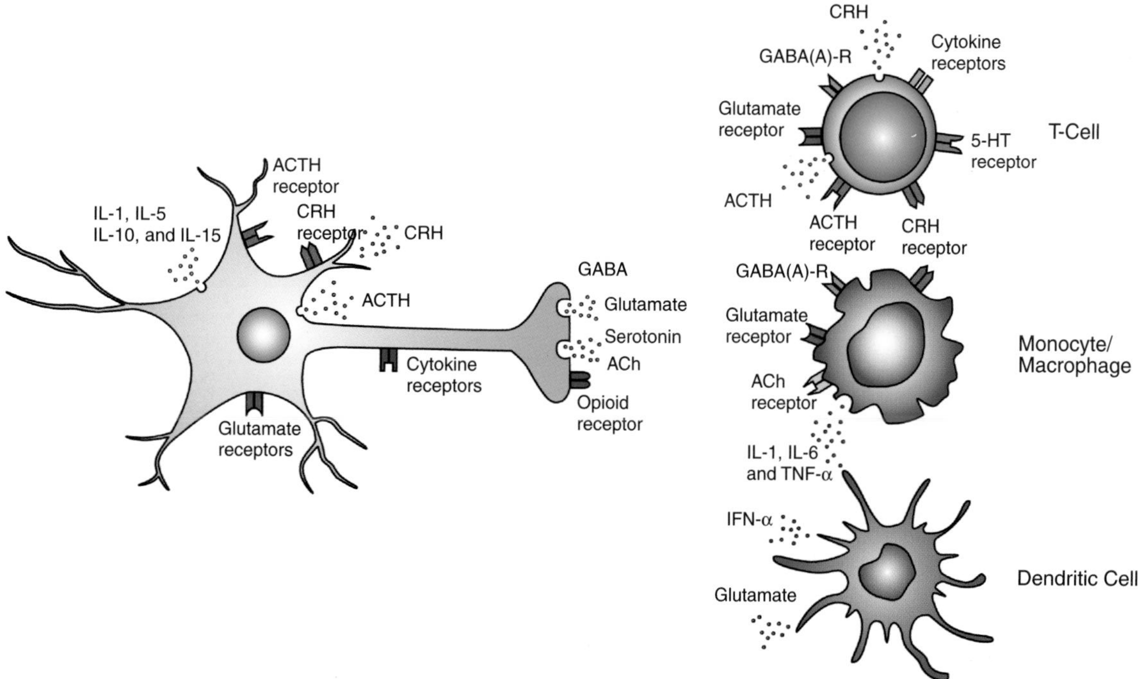

Figure 24–2. Cross-talk between the immune and central nervous systems. Intercommunication between the cells of the immune and nervous systems is possible on several levels. Neurons, microglia, and astrocytes can produce various cytokines and express cytokine receptors. This enables them to direct immune cells as well as respond to various immunological stimuli. In turn, cells of the immune system are able to secrete various neurotransmitters, such as glutamate, and express receptors for many of these molecules. This allows immune cells to impact neural processes and respond to neural stimuli. These mechanisms permit extensive cross-talk between the immune system and neural systems. Illustration by Milo Careaga.

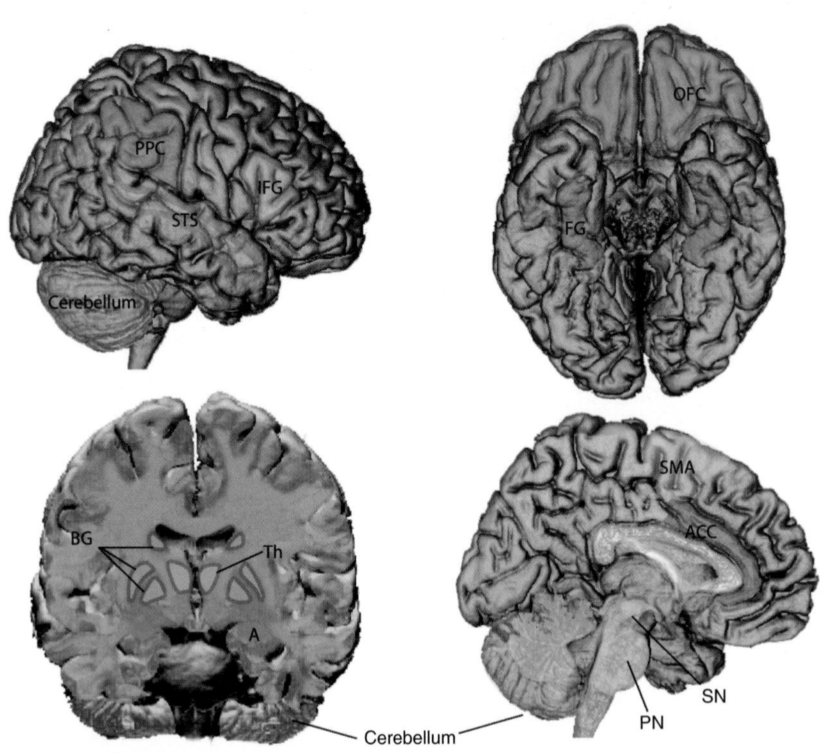

Social Impairment	Communication Deficits	Repetitive Behaviors
OFC - Orbitofrontal Cortex ACC - Anterior Cingulate Cortex FG - Fusiform Gyrus STS - Superior Temporal Sulcus A - Amygdala Mirror Neuron Regions IFG - inferior frontal gyrus PPC - posterior parietal cortex	IFG - Inferior frontal gyrus (Broca's Area) STS - Superior Temporal Sulcus SMA - Supplementary Motro Area BG - Basal Ganglia SN - Substantia Nigra Th - Thalamus PN - Pontine Nuclei Cerebellum	OFC - Orbitofrontal Cortex ACC - Anterior Cingulate Cortex BG - Basal Ganglia Th - Thalamus

Figure 31–1. Brain areas that have been implicated in the mediation of the three core behaviors that are impaired in autism: social behavior, language and communication, and repetitive and stereotyped behaviors. *Adapted from* Amaral, D. G., Schumann, C. M., & Nordahl, C. W. (2008). Neuroanatomy of autism. *Trends in Neuroscience, 31*, 137–145, *with permission from Trends in Neurosciences.*

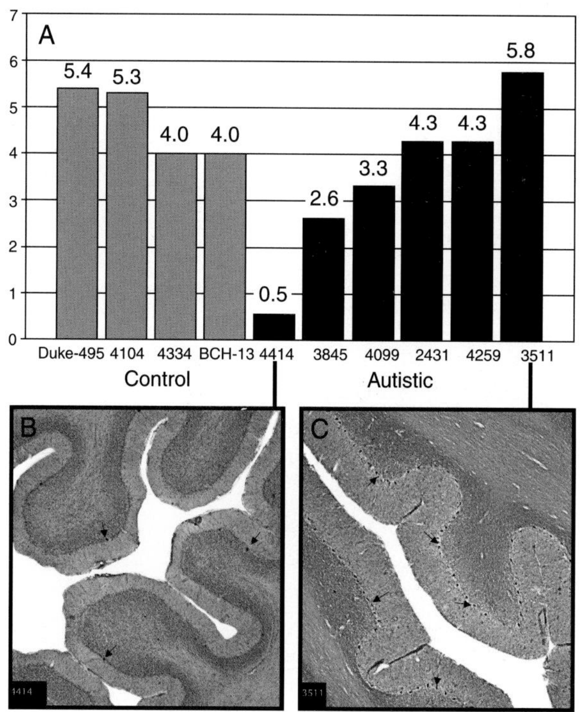

Figure 31–3. (A) Number of Purkinje neurons per millimeter in control (light gray bars) and autistic (black bars) cases from calbindin-D28k-immunostained series. Photographs illustrate the variability in Purkinje cell density within autism group in (B) 4414 with reduced Purkinje cell density and (C) 3611 with Purkinje cell density in the normal range. Adapted from Whitney et al., 2008, with kind permission from Springer Science+Business Media.

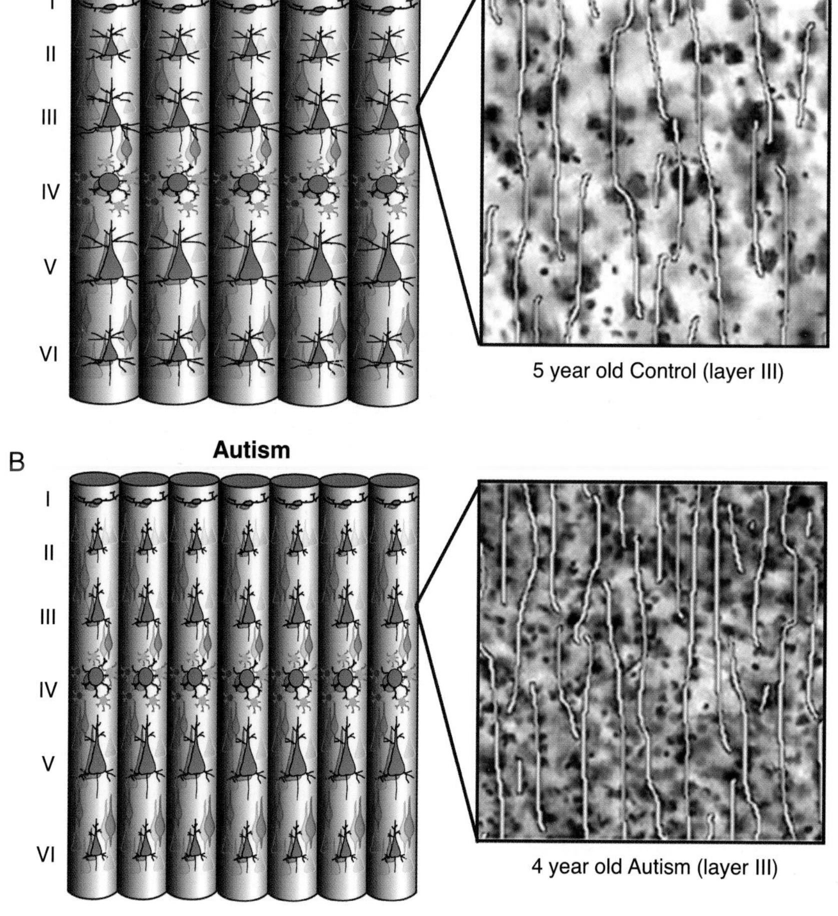

Figure 31–5. Model of the minicolumnar hypothesis proposed by Casanova et al. (2002, 2006) that there are an abnormal number and width of minicolumns in the cortex of individuals with autism. Each so-called minicolumn contains approximately 80–100 neurons (see schematic of minicolumn formation in Figure 31.8). (A) Model depicts a decreased intercolumnar width in the autism case relative to controls. (B) Nissl images were adapted with permission from Casanova et al. (2006), in which the distance between cell-body defined minicolumns was found to be reduced in layer III of dorsolateral prefrontal cortex (BA 9) in a 4-year-old autism case relative to a 5-year-old control. Given the narrower neuropil area between columns, one would also predict a decrease in the dendritic arborization of BA 9 neurons (as depicted in the model, A).

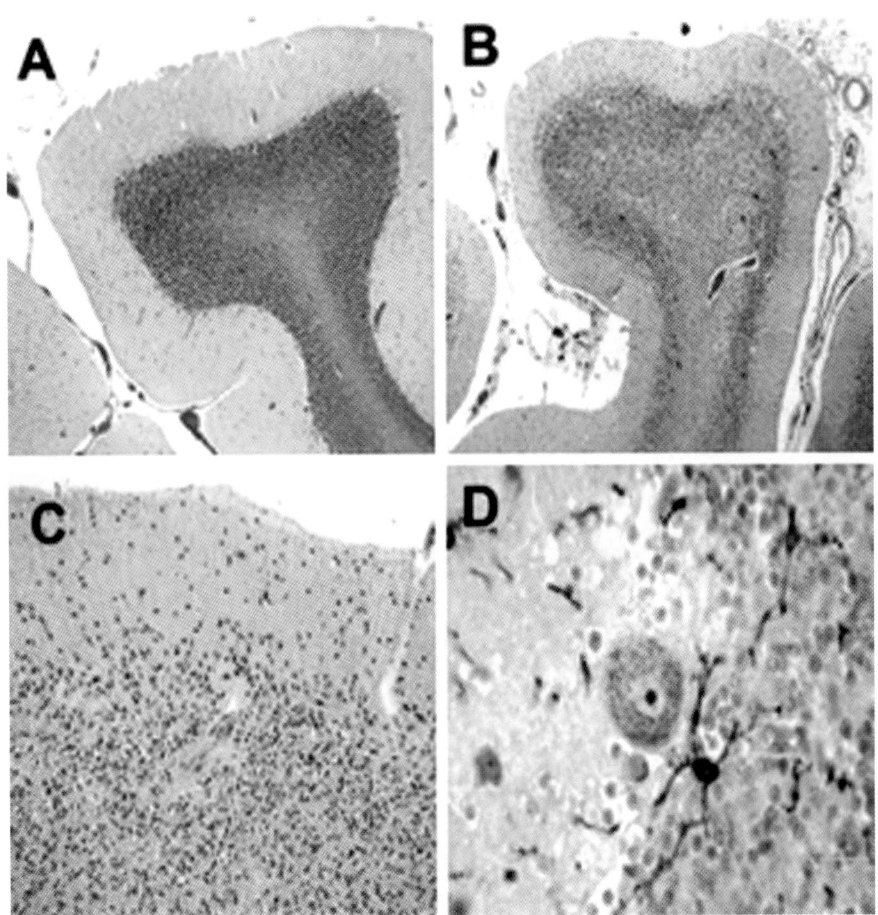

Figure 31–6. (A) Normal appearance of the cerebellum in a control patient; (B–C) atrophic folia and marked loss of Purkinje and granular cells in the cerebellum of an autistic patient (H&E stain); (D) microglia activation seen with anti-MHC class II immunostaining. Adapted with permission from Vargas et al., 2005.

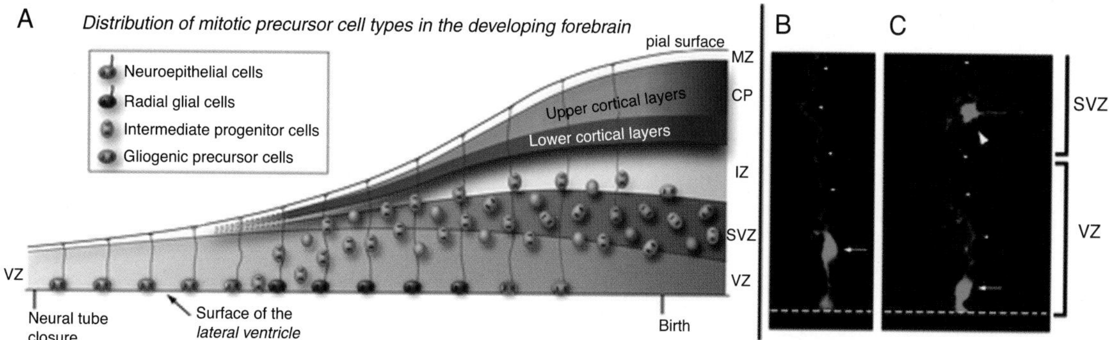

Figure 31–7. (A) Scheme depicting precursor cell types in the embryonic brain. After neural tube closure, the embryonic proliferative zone is composed of a single population of neuroepithelial cells (red) which transition into radial glial cells (dark blue) at the onset of neurogenesis in the ventricular zone (VZ). They undergo division at the surface of the lateral ventricle and possess a long thin pial fiber that reaches the pial surface. Radial glial cell divisions produce neurons and intermediate progenitor cells (light blue). Intermediate progenitor cell bodies are primarily located in the subventricular zone (SVZ); divisions occur away from the surface of the lateral ventricle and produce multiple neurons. At the conclusion of neurogenesis radial glial cells begin producing astrocytes (green), and translocate to the SVZ, where gliogenesis continues after birth. (B) Micrograph showing an example of a radial glial cell labeled with fluorescent reporter gene. Radial glia are bipolar cells with a single process that contacts the ventricular surface (dotted line) and a single pial process that ascends toward the pial surface (small arrowheads). The cell body (arrow) is located in the VZ. (C) Micrograph showing a radial glial cell (arrow) and a daughter intermediate progenitor cell (large arrowhead) labeled with fluorescent reporter gene. The intermediate progenitor cell maintains contact with the radial glial cell pial fiber (small arrowheads).

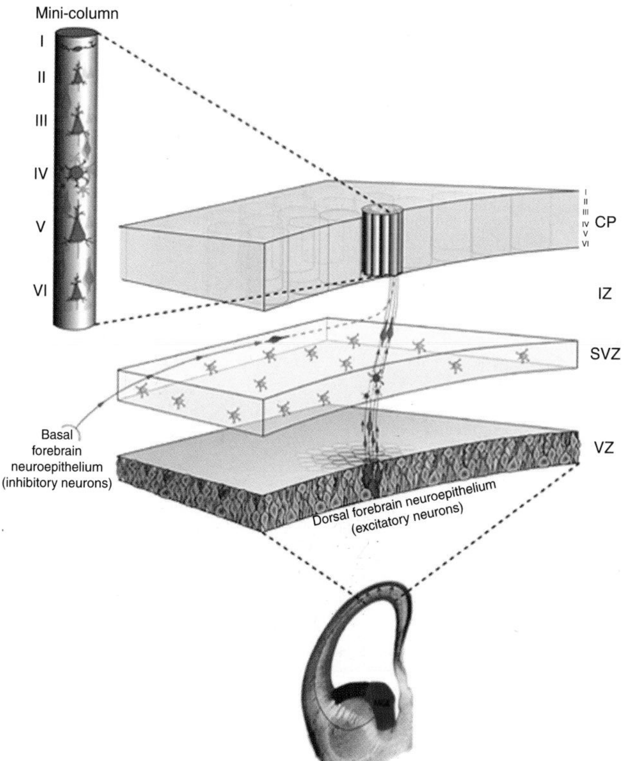

Figure 31–8. Scheme depicting the formation of minicolumn and cortical column functional units in the cerebral cortex. Each minicolumn contains approximately 80–100 neurons. Multiple minicolumns together form a single cortical column. As proposed by Rakic (1988), proliferative units in the ventricular zone (VZ) of the dorsal forebrain produce neurons that are destined for a single minicolumn functional unit (dark blue column) in the cortical plate (CP). Each proliferative unit in the VZ may comprise 5–10 radial glial cells. Each radial glial cell possesses a single pial fiber that stretches across the cortical wall to the pial surface of the brain. The pial fiber guides the migration of newborn neurons from the proliferative zones to their respective minicolumn functional units in the CP. Neighboring proliferative units in the VZ produce neurons that are destined for different minicolumns in the CP (grey columns). Radial glial cells produce both neurons and intermediate progenitor cells, which migrate away from the ventricle along their parental pial fiber. Recent work shows that intermediate progenitor cells undergo additional rounds of division in the subventricular zone (SVZ) to produce multiple neurons. Excitatory projection neurons are derived from the VZ of the dorsal forebrain, and migrate radially along radial glial cell fibers. Inhibitory interneurons are derived from the VZ of the medial ganglionic eminence (MGE, red) in the basal forebrain, and migrate tangentially into the overlying cerebral cortex. Mechanisms that guide migrating interneurons to specific minicolumns remain to be determined.

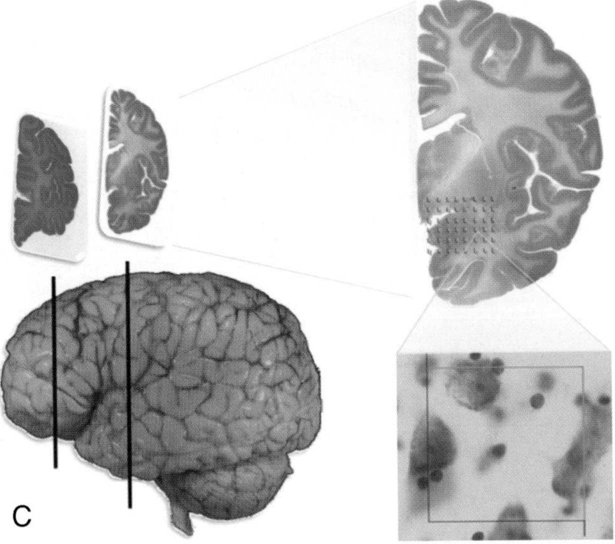

Box Figure 31–C

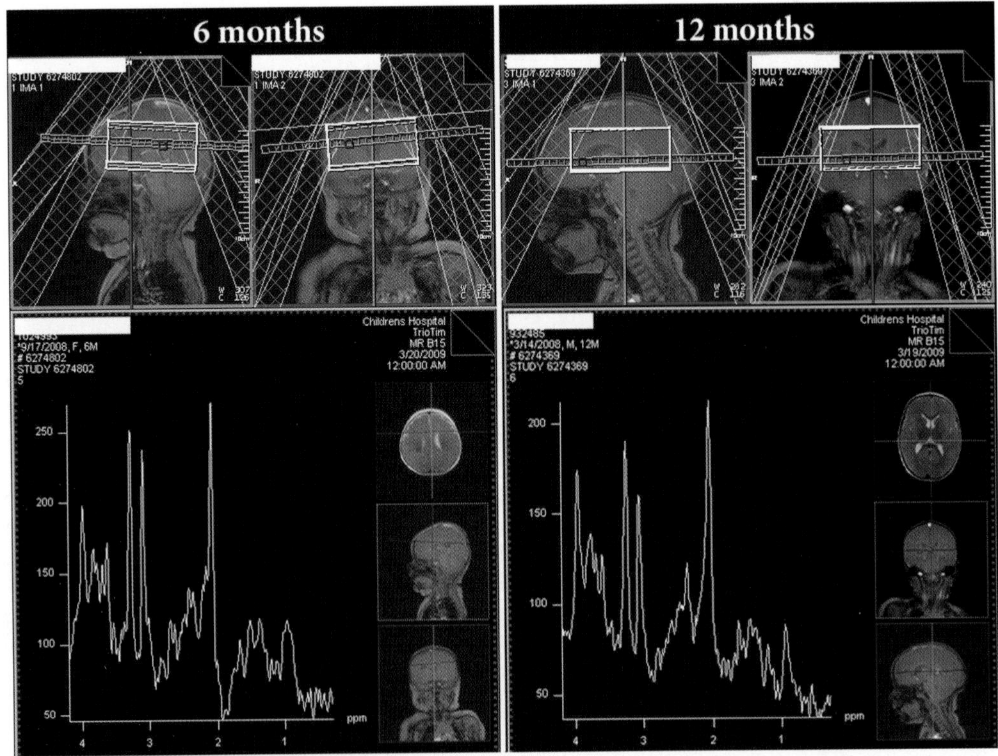

Figure 33–3. Example 3-D PEPSI spectra, acquired over 4.5 minutes on a clinical 3 Tesla scanner, showing the 3-D anatomical volume, individual voxel placement (blue box) and outer volume sat band positioning for a 6m infant without a family history of ASD and for a 12m infant at high risk for an ASD due to an older affected sibling. Each example shows one 0.3 cc voxel out of the 8,192 collected concurrently.

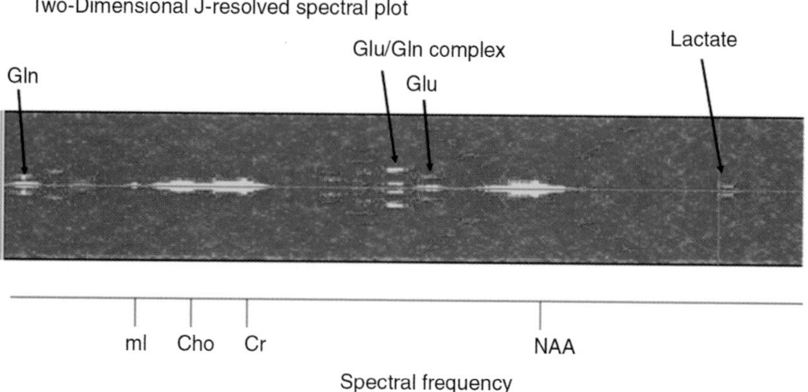

Figure 33–4. A 2-D J-resolved spectral image acquired over 20 minutes from a 64 cc volume at 3 Tesla. Spectral resonances for glutamine, glutamate, Glu/Gln complex, lactate, as well as myoinositol, choline, creatine, and NAA are shown. Data were acquired as a function of echo time, using progressively increasing echo times to record signal change that can differentiate between chemicals.

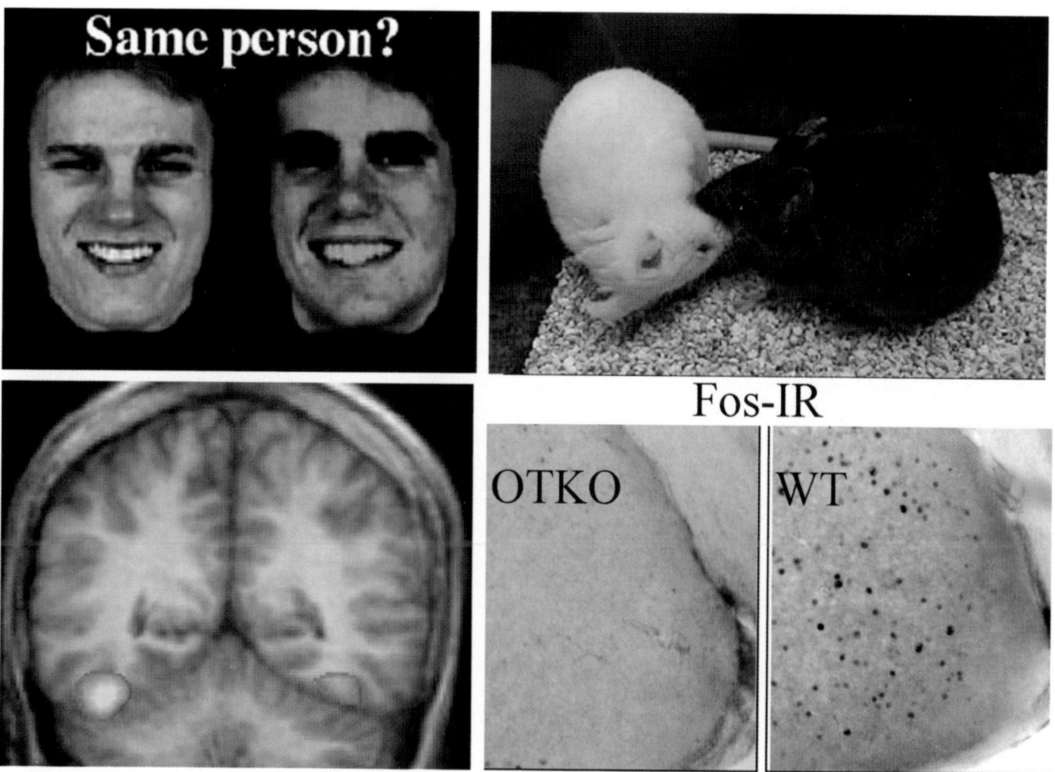

Figure 34–7. Social Information Processing in Humans and Rodents. Individuals with autism show reductions in the activation of the fusiform face area, a structure regulated by amygdala activation, as measured by fMRI, when viewing human faces compared to controls (Left Panel). Analogously, OTKO mice show reduced activity of the medial amygdala in response to olfactory investigation, as evidenced by the expression of c-Fos (a neuronal marker of activity), compared with wild-type mice (Right Panel). Adapted with permission from Schultz, R. T. (2005). Developmental deficits in social perception in autism: The role of the amygdala and the fusiform face area. *International Journal of Developmental Neuroscience, 23*(2–3), 125–141, and Ferguson, J. N., Aldagm, J. M., Insel, T. R., & Young, L. J. (2001). Oxytocin in the medial amygdala is essential for social recognition in the mouse. *Journal of Neuroscience*, *21*, 8278–8285.

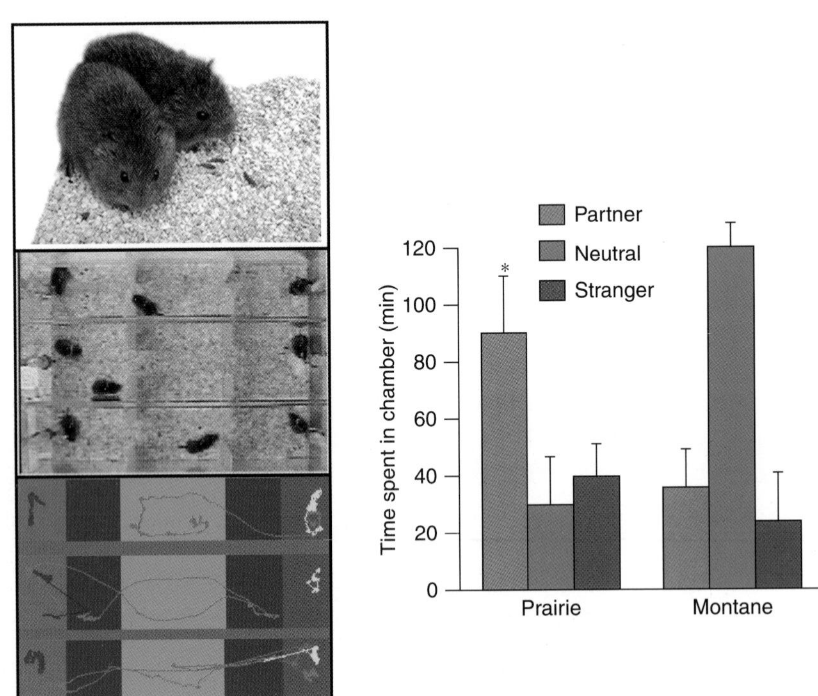

Figure 34–8. Partner Preference Test. Social attachment in prairie voles is measured using the partner preference test. In this behavioral test a male is paired with an unfamiliar female vole and allowed to cohabitate for a period of time (Upper Panel). The pair is then separated, and the partner female is tethered in the partner preference apparatus along with a stranger female. The male is then placed in the apparatus and allowed to wander freely for 3 hours (Middle Panel). The amount of time the male spends with either the partner female or the stranger female is recorded and analyzed using behavior analysis software (Lower Panel). If the male is shown to have spent twice as much time with the partner female than with the stranger female, he is said to have formed a partner preference. Partner preference is a marker of social attachment. Prairie voles easily form a partner preference after about 24 hours of cohabitation. Montane voles, however, fail to show a preference for their partner after as much as 2 weeks of cohabitation.

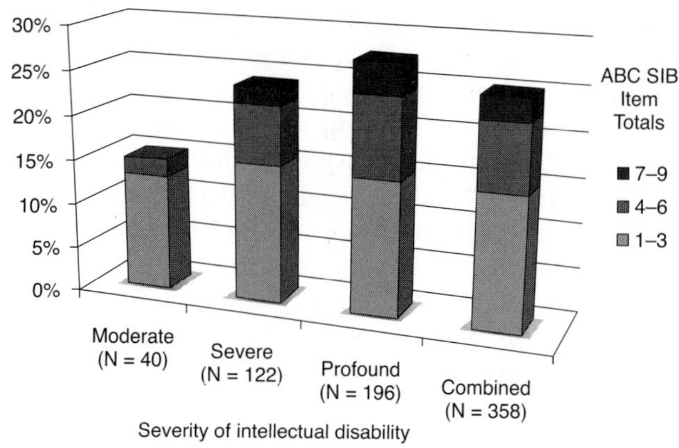

Figure 21–1. Relationship between severity of intellectual disability and severity of self-injurious behavior (SIB) as assessed by total score on the SIB items of the Aberrant Behavior Scale in an institutional setting.

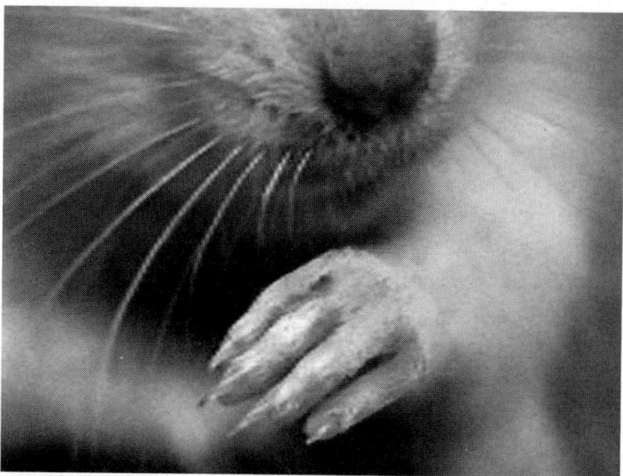

Figure 21–2. Lesion on the dorsum of the paw from self-biting in a rat treated with pemoline. (See Color Plate Section for a color version of this figure.)

(Oliver, Hall, Hales, Murphy, & Watts, 1998) and 16% (Schroeder, Rojahn, & Oldenquist, 1991) have been reported. Several years ago, King and colleagues surveyed a large institutional setting of adults with mostly severe to profound intellectual disability in the context of a study looking at the relationship between whole blood serotonin and behavior. Caretakers completed the Aberrant Behavior Checklist (ABC) on 358 residents. The total scores on the three items of the ABC provide a sense of the distribution of SIB as it relates to severity of intellectual disability.

Thelen's (1981) seminal work demonstrated that stereotyped behaviors are part of typical development, and may help infants to gain motor mastery. Students taking exams commonly exhibit stereotyped mannerisms presumed to reflect or to allay anxiety (Rafaeli-Mor, Foster, & Berkson, 1999).

In genetic syndromes such as Lesch-Nyhan, Prader-Willi, Cornelia de Lange, Cri du Chat, and Smith-Magenis, self-injury is common (and in some cases so frequent as to be considered part of the clinical manifestations of the disorder itself), while in people with other disabilities such as Down syndrome, SIB appears to be more associated with severity of intellectual disability than with trisomy 21 per se. Both visual and auditory sensory impairment increase the likelihood of stereotypy and self-injury (Troster, Brambring, & Beelman, 1991; Bachara & Phelan, 1980; Murdoch, 1996; McHugh & Pyfer, 1999; Gal, Dyck, & Passmore, 2009), as discussed in more detail below.

Predisposing Factors and Biology of SIB

As suggested above, many conditions have been associated with stereotyped SIB, including specific genetic disorders, intellectual disability more broadly, sensory impairment, and severe deprivation and neglect. There are also more purely psychological constructs for repetitive self-injury, but all invoke a failure of self-regulation with attendant neurophysiological underpinnings. Experience from the use of pharmacological agents, animal models, and patients in clinical settings exhibiting stereotypy and self-injurious behavior (SIB) advances our understanding of potential underlying neurobiological processes involved in its expression.

Neuropharmacology of Stereotypy and SIB

In the 1960s, stereotypic behaviors were reported in people abusing amphetamine (e.g., Ellinwood, 1967), prompting researchers to explore the role of agents that stimulate the central nervous system (CNS) in the expression of repetitive motor behavior (Lewis, Gluck, Bodfish, Beauchamp, & Mailman, 1996). Because amphetamines increase the concentration of dopamine at the synapse, understanding dopamine function in the production of stereotypy became a logical focus of research. As reviewed by King (2002), a number of such dopaminergic manipulations have been explored. Experimenter-induced dopaminergic lesions, for example, through administration of neurotoxins such as 6-hydroxydopamine (6-OHDA), have been conducted in attempts to isolate brain regions or systems related to the etiology or expression of stereotypy and self-injury.

In one of the earliest such studies, 6-OHDA was injected bilaterally into the substantia nigra of young adult male rats (Ungerstedt, 1968). Subsequent injection of a single dose of the dopamine agonist apormorphine 3 days later resulted in stereotypy and SIB—including violent self-biting and compulsive gnawing. Similar behaviors, then characterized as *self-aggressiveness,* were observed in mice and rats administered high doses of the stimulant 5-phenyl-2-imino-4oxo-oxazolidine, or pemoline (Genovese, Napoli, & Bolego-Zonta, 1969). Pemoline has subsequently been used in a number of studies to investigate drug-induced repetitive behavior in animal models (King, 2002; Muehlmann, Brown, & Devine, 2008).

These behavioral effects were first described in detail in rats by Mueller and Hsiao (1980). Injection of high doses of pemoline resulted in persistent self-biting (primarily of the medial foreleg) and stereotypy, as well as other behaviors including hyperactivity, abnormal social and sensorimotor behavior, and unresponsiveness or avoidance of moderate levels of sensory stimuli. These behaviors appeared in as few as 3 hours or as many as 2 days, and persisted despite a variety of efforts to interrupt the behavior including prodding with a cotton swab, presentation of highly palatable food, the introduction of a nondrugged cagemate, banging on the cage with a metal can, or even dousing with water. Mueller and Hsiao (1980) noted that the pemoline-induced biting response was similar to certain aspects of the normal grooming sequence exhibited by rodents. Specifically, areas groomed initially in a typical sequence were the areas of most likely injury. Therefore, the authors posited that the pemoline-induced self-biting behavior was a fragmented grooming response. Because pemoline-induced behaviors, including hyperactivity, stereotypy, abnormal social behavior, avoidance of physical contact, and grooming-associated self-mutilation, are similar to those observed in the de Lange (Mueller & Hsiao, 1980) or Lesch-Nyhan syndromes (Mueller & Nyhan, 1982), pemoline was an early rodent model utilized to elucidate self-injury in individuals with mental retardation.

In a more recent study examining the relation between stereotypy and the dopaminergic system in humans, Bodfish and colleagues (1995) measured blink rates in individuals with intellectual disability and repetitive behavior disorders versus control subjects. Previous evidence has implicated the dopamine system in the regulation of spontaneous eye blinks in humans, as documented in individuals with dopamine-related pathologies. For example, persons with Parkinsonism have decreased dopamine levels, and have lower blink rates (Karson, 1983; Karson et al., 1984), while patients with schizophrenia, and presumably increased dopamine levels, demonstrate higher blink rates (Mackert et al., 1991). Using eye blink rate as a dependent variable of dopaminergic function, Bodfish and colleagues (1995) found that individuals with stereotypy exhibited lower blink rates than the control group, providing further evidence for the role of the dopaminergic system in stereotypic behavior in humans.

Taken together, the directionality of impaired dopaminergic function (e.g., enhanced or diminished), and its relationship to stereotypy, is perplexing. Stereotypy appears to be associated both with increased synaptic concentrations of dopamine (e.g., amphetamine abuse) and also decreased synaptic concentrations of dopamine and consequent increased sensitivity of dopamine receptors. Thus, dopamine-induced stereotypy can be attenuated using dopamine antagonists, such as haloperidol, in primates (Ridley, Baker, & Scraggs, 1979). Many clinical reports demonstrate successes with the use of dopamine antagonists for stereotyped behavior and/or self-injurious behaviors (King, 2000). Largely as a result of the Research Units on Pediatric Pharmacology (RUPP) trial (RUPP, 2002), the atypical antipsychotic and dopamine antagonist risperidone has an FDA approved indication for the treatment of behaviors including self-injury in autism.

At the same time, pharmacologically induced stereotyped behavior also responds to manipulations of other neurotransmitters, calling into question the specificity of the role of dopamine. In both the pemoline and 6-OHDA models of self-biting behavior, glutamatergic antagonists have been shown to exert important effects to prevent the emergence of self-injury (King et al., 1998; Muehlmann & Devine, 2008). Evidence suggests dopaminergic and glutamatergic interactions in the neostriatum play a role in the development and expression of self-biting in the pemoline model (King et al., 1998). The potential utility of glutamate antagonists in treating SIB and related behaviors remains a focus of research, but while clinical case reports of successes with drugs like dextromethorphan and lamotrigine (Welch & Sovner, 1992; Davanzo & King, 1996) have been described, no controlled trials with these or related agents have been undertaken.

The opiate system has long been implicated in the expression of stereotypy with early observations of morphine-induced behavior (Ayhan & Randrup, 1972; Charness, Amit, & Taylor, 1975). Subsequent studies linked opiate-induced stereotypy with both dopaminergic and glutamatergic effects (Feigenbaum & Yanai, 1984; Capone et al., 2008). However, given the role of the endogenous opioid system in pain responsivity and brain reward mechanisms (reviewed in Harris, 1992), it has been posited that repeated SIB could be associated with increased release of endogenous opioid peptides that inhibit pain, leading to opioid-mediated reward (e.g., Sandman, 1988). Self-injurious behavior might thus be a means of self-administering opioid peptides. In clinical observations made over a century ago (Ireland, 1898) and subsequently (Symons, 2002) it has also been suggested that individuals with developmental disabilities such as autism have altered pain sensitivity or responsivity that may be related to the opioid system (Gillberg, 1995). However, reports are inconsistent, with some findings indicating normal response to pain in individuals with autism (e.g., Nader, Oberlander, Chambers, & Craig, 2004). Further, the ability to discriminate atypical pain perception from an atypical pain response (including an atypical affective response) is a significant challenge in autism.

If endogenous opioid release reinforces or maintains SIB, then blocking the effects of opioids with antagonists could interrupt this cycle. Many clinical studies have examined naltrexone in this regard. A literature review of 27 research articles (Symons, Thompson, & Rodriguez, 2004) revealed that treatment with naltrexone improved symptoms relative to baseline in 80 percent of subjects. Fifty-three percent of subjects showing improvement in SIB had a diagnosis of autism. An additional review of 3 case reports, 8 case series, and 14 clinical studies suggests naltrexone treatment is generally efficacious in treating SIB in autism (Elchaar, Maisch, Augusto, & Wehring, 2006). Other reviews (e.g., King, 2000) have indicated mixed results for the efficacy of naltrexone in treating SIB, including the results of larger controlled trials;

heterogeneous findings may reflect inconsistencies in study design and symptoms measured.

Self-injurious behavior and stereotypy have also been associated with serotonin function in human and nonhuman primates. As reviewed by King and colleagues (1998), hypotheses regarding the role of serotonin in SIB developed in the 1970s were based on animal studies demonstrating that the administration of serotonin agonists attenuate aggressive behavior. More recently, it has been shown that in small rodents called bank voles, administration of citalopram, a selective serotonin reuptake inhibitor (SSRI), prevents the increase of stereotypy after stress (Schoenecker & Heller, 2001). However, reports have failed to show evidence of altered serotonin system function in rhesus monkeys with SIB (Tiefenbacher, Davenport, Novak, Pouliot, & Meyer, 2003; Weld et al., 1998). A number of studies have reported reduced serotonin function in human patients with psychiatric illness (e.g., personality disorder, depression, bulimia nervosa) and with history of self-injurious behavior (New et al., 1997; Herpertz, Steinmeyer, Marx, Oidtmann, & Sass, 1995; Rinne, Westenberg, den Boer, & van den Brink, 2000; Steiger et al., 2001). Case reports and open label trials of treatment with the SSRIs, including sertraline (Hellings, Kelley, Gabrielli, Kilgore, & Shah, 1996) and fluoxetine (Cook, Rowlett, Jaselskis, & Leventhal, 1992; King, 1991; Markowitz, 1992) have been moderately effective in improving self-injury in adults with autism and mental retardation. Notably, dysregulation of the serotonin system has long been reported in autism (see Chapter 32, this volume, for review). A review of the literature, including 2 controlled trials and 10 open-label trials or chart reviews revealed SSRIs have been somewhat efficacious in improving global functioning in individuals with autism (Kolevzon, Mathewson, & Hollander, 2006), but a recent large study was negative (King et al., 2009). Interestingly, it has been proposed that serotonin levels are more specifically related to SIB and aggression, which are common features of autism, rather than to the core features comprising the full syndrome of autism (Schroeder et al., 2001).

Impoverished Environments and Social/Sensory Deprivation on the Development of Stereotypy and SIB

A variety of animal species demonstrate stereotypic or self-injurious behavior when housed in confined environments, including zoo enclosures and standard laboratory cages (e.g., Harris, 1992; Hosey & Skyner, 2007; Marriner & Drickamer, 1994; Wolfer et al., 2004; Würbel, 2001), perhaps because captivity hinders ability to appropriately adjust to the environment by engaging in species-specific behaviors. For example, a variety of rodents caged as research models engage in bar-mouthing (Cooper, Odberg, & Nicol, 1996; Garner & Mason, 2002; Nevison, Hurst, & Barnard, 1999; Powell, et al., 1999); parrots demonstrate oral and locomotor stereotypies when housed in impoverished conditions (Meehan, Garner, & Mench, 2004); horses housed in a confined stable or barn exhibit stereotypic behavior, including crib-biting, weaving, and box walking (Bachmann, Audigé, & Stauffacher, 2003; Waters, Nicol, & French, 2002); nonhuman primates demonstrate stereotypic and self-injurious behavior when housed in captivity (Lutz, Well, & Novak, 2003; Tarou, Bloomsmith, & Maple, 2005). Self-injury in nonhuman primates usually consists of self-biting, where rips and slashes of the skin or muscle may occur (Novak et al., 1998).

Nonhuman primates also exhibit stereotyped and self-injurious behaviors as a consequence of social deprivation (e.g., Harlow, Dodsworth, & Harlow, 1965). In his classic early experiments, Harlow and his colleagues (1965) described the emergence of "autistic self-clutching and rocking" behavior when monkeys were housed in total social isolation. Others have observed similar phenomena. For example, increased amount of time spent in individual cages was associated with self-injury, self-biting, hair-pulling, body-flipping, and swinging in rhesus monkeys (Lutz et al., 2003); greater amount of time spent singly housed (separate from their mothers) during infant and juvenile periods was significantly related to development of abnormal behaviors, including locomotor stereotypies and self-injury (Bellanca & Crockett, 2002). Similarly, rhesus monkeys reared by artificial surrogates were significantly more likely to self-bite than monkeys reared by peers or mothers (Lutz, Davis, Ruggiero, & Suomi, 2007).

Evidence suggests that humans are also susceptible to the development of stereotypy as a result of social deprivation. Children reared in orphanages with a paucity of caregiver social-emotional interactions and limited opportunity to develop relationships with their caregiver exhibit a variety of developmental delays. Drawing on theories of infant-mother attachment (e.g., Ainsworth, 1979), it has been proposed that early experience devoid of warm, nurturing, and socially-emotionally responsive adults is related to problem behavior and delayed development of appropriate social-emotional behavior. As summarized by the St. Petersburg-USA Orphanage Research Team (2008), research compiled over six decades across a number of countries has demonstrated that children reared in severely deficient institutional environments demonstrate delays in physical growth and general behavior development, and engage in atypical behavior, including stereotyped self-stimulation. While conditions vary across orphanages, according to Rutter (1999), the institutionalized children typically "remained in cots all day, had few if any toys or playthings, and were fed gruel through bottles with large teats (often left propped up for self-feeding); there was no personalised caregiving and very little talk or interaction with caregivers" (p. 538). A number of reports have suggested that a subset of children reared in such conditions display behaviors consistent with an autism spectrum disorder, including difficulty establishing friendships, developing empathy, using eye contact and gestures appropriately, and lack of proper language development and ability to engage in reciprocal conversation (e.g., Hoksbergen, ter Laak, Rijk, van Dijkum, & Stoutjesdijk, 2005;

Rutter et al., 1999). Rutter (1999) termed this constellation of behaviors, observed in 6% of a sample of 111 children adopted from Romanian orphanages, "quasi-autistic patterns." Though children described in Rutter's sample demonstrated circumscribed interests, they did not engage in stereotypic behavior such as rocking. However, Hoksbergen and colleagues (2005) reported that 13 of 80 (16%) Romanian adoptees showed symptoms of autism; eleven of the children exhibiting symptoms of autism engaged in stereotypic behavior, including rocking, and four of the children engaged in other stereotypic behavior.

A number of reports have indicated that sensory deprivation produces similar "autistic-like" behaviors in children, specifically as a result of congenital blindness (Brown, Hobson, Lee, & Stevenson, 1997). Sensory deprivation may limit the capacity to explore one's surroundings, as well as impede the ability to communicate effectively and develop the skills necessary to engage reciprocally and socially with others. In 1969, Wing compared children aged 4 to 16 years with perceptual impairments (e.g., congenital receptive aphasia, congenital executive aphasia, congenital partial blindness combined with partial deafness) to groups of children with autism, Down syndrome, and typical development with respect to behaviors characteristic of autism. In addition to exhibiting social difficulties, the group with partial blindness/deafness showed similar patterns of abnormal body movements, defined as jumping, spinning, toe-walking, and flapping arms or legs, as the group with autism. Since that time, a number of studies have reported similar behaviors in children with sensory impairments. Brown and colleagues (1997) compared congenitally blind children to age- and IQ-matched children using measures of autism-related behaviors. The blind group demonstrated significantly more communication difficulties than the sighted children, as well as more postural oddities and motor stereotypies. In a sample of 25 congenitally blind children, 19 (73%) demonstrated stereotyped behaviors, including body rocking, repetitive handling of objects, hand and finger mannerisms, eye pressing and eye poking, and jumping (Fazzi et al., 1999). Fazzi and colleagues suggested that repetitive body movements (hand mannerisms, jumping) might be interpreted as self-comforting behaviors, performed as a means of controlling anxiety or reducing tension in stressful situations; conversely, eye pressing, typically observed when the child was alone or bored, may increase levels of stimulation. These observations are consistent with previous reports of young blind infants and preschoolers who demonstrate stereotypies such as rocking and hand and finger mannerisms when aroused, and eye poking during more monotonous situations (e.g., Tröster, Brambring, & Beelmann, 1991). Taken together, these findings suggest stereotypies may represent a process of achieving an optimal state of arousal (Fazzi et al., 1999).

Inasmuch as sensory impairments may also compromise important social interactions, it is noteworthy that a number of studies have shown that reduced social contact may be a significant contributor to the development of stereotypy. Lewis and colleagues (1996) followed a group of rhesus monkeys deprived of social contact with their mother or peers for the first 6–9 months of life. Socially isolated monkeys exhibiting stereotyped behavior failed to exhibit a component of associative conditioned learning that requires inattention to irrelevant or redundant information, which is mediated in part by central dopamine function. Further, deprived monkeys showed potentiated response (i.e., increased stereotyped behaviors) to apomorphine, compared to control monkeys, suggesting long-term or permanent alterations in dopamine receptor sensitivity (Lewis et al., 1996). Examination of brain tissue in the group of socially isolated monkeys confirmed alterations in dopamine function, characterized by reduced dopamine innervation of the corpus striatum. These findings suggest a disrupted dopaminergic system is a consequence of social deprivation and directly related to the expression of stereotypic behaviors.

Thus, stereotypy appears to emerge as a result of being reared in environments lacking certain features essential for proper development. Impoverished environments and perceptual/sensory impairments inhibit one's ability to explore his or her surroundings, observe social behavior, interact with others, and at times, develop the social-emotional relationships necessary to facilitate a safe and secure attachment. A subset of young animals and children who are reared in such conditions appear to develop social and communication deficits, as well as repetitive behavior and stereotypy, which are common features of autism spectrum disorders. Given observations of analogous behavioral patterns exhibited by children as a result of these distinct conditions (impoverished environments, perceptual/sensory deprivation, and autism), one might consider the common elements inherent in each. Children in each condition experience barriers to developing social communication, rendering it difficult to achieve connections and establish relationships with other people. The impedances to developing these skills may differ in each situation; for example, an impoverished environment would limit opportunities to interact with a caregiver during a crucial period in the formation of attachment relationships, perceptual/sensory deprivation might pose challenges to interpreting social cues and responses such as facial expression, and a child with ASD may have diminished attention to faces and limited perspective taking. In each case, social-communication deficits and stereotypy emerge. These commonalities may have implications for possible shared mechanisms of intervention. For example, the St. Petersburg-USA Orphanage Research Team (2008) employed interventions that successfully altered the social-emotional-relationship experience of children from impoverished environments by providing training to caregivers to increase social-emotional responsiveness and support, and changing structural organization of orphanages in St. Petersburg, Russian Federation. Results of the intervention indicated substantial improvements in typically developing children and children with disabilities, in terms of physical growth, general behavioral development, social-emotional-relationship behaviors, and various measures of attachment. These findings provide support for the potential utility of behavioral interventions and environmental enrichment in treating children with atypical behavior, regardless of its etiology.

In sum, impoverished environments and social deprivation appear to impact the development and maintenance of stereotyped behaviors and SIB in primates and other species. Dopamine function is clearly altered as a result of stressful environments in some cases. While environmental enrichment may enhance brain development and attenuate atypical behavior in mice (Lewis, 2004) and rats (see Sackett, Novak, & Kroeker, 1999, for a review), little work has been done to examine effects of enrichment on primate brain morphology. The neurological and behavioral changes resulting from environmental enrichment reported using rodent models support the notion that the behavioral treatment (e.g., enhanced socialization) can impact brain plasticity in addition to modifying behavior. This is particularly relevant given recent advances in the use of behavioral interventions to treat humans exhibiting stereotypy and SIB.

Animal Models Pertinent to Autism

It has been hypothesized that early risk factors for the development of autism are those that may alter a child's responses to and perception of his or her environmental surroundings (Dawson, Sterling, & Faja, 2008). Distorted interactions between child and environment may disturb critical input supporting proper brain development. As such, the study of animals experiencing environmental challenges, including impoverished housing conditions or deprivation, provide models of experience-dependent changes in behavior and associated neuropathology.

Lewis, Tanimura, Lee, and Bodfish (2007) reviewed and expanded on studies of deer mice exhibiting repetitive behaviors associated with environmental restriction. Findings suggest that repetitive behaviors are the most common consequence of physical confinement, and enriching environmental conditions reduces the presence of these behaviors. Moreover, stereotypy was associated with alterations in cortical-basal ganglia circuitry, elucidating possible etiology and underlying neuropathology in individuals with autism exhibiting such behavior (see also Cromwell & King, 2004).

In a study of Orange-Wing Amazon parrots, Garner, Meehan, and Mench (2003) demonstrated that increased stereotypy was associated with poor performance (i.e., perseveration) on a gambling task measuring executive function. Deficits in executive function are consistently reported in autism (e.g., Hill & Frith, 2003; Pennington & Ozonoff, 1996). Based on previous evidence (Norman & Shallice, 1986), the authors suggested that repetition of responses made by parrots during the gambling task is indicative of disinhibition of the behavioral control mechanisms of the dorsal basal ganglia, which parallels neural circuitry of stereotypy in humans.

Animal models of stereotypy developing as a consequence of social deprivation (e.g., Lutz et al., 2003) are also of particular relevance to understanding autism. It has been proposed that initial damage to anatomical structures and systems supporting social function in autism (e.g., the amygdala), results in failure to assign social stimuli as salient, reducing inherent reward value of social stimuli, thereby hindering experience with such stimuli and specialization of cortical brain regions involved in social perception (Dawson et al., 2005; Schultz, 2005). Recent experiments by Bauman and colleagues (2008) are particularly salient in this regard. Juvenile rhesus monkeys received bilateral amygdala or hippocampal lesions and were assessed for later development of repetitive and stereotyped behaviors. Interestingly, these neonatal lesions resulted in distinctly different stereotypies depending on the brain structure involved, and did not develop until fully a year after the initial brain lesions. While a direct connection between nonhuman and human primates is a conceptual leap, these studies are consistent with the suggestion that a child's lack of social experience may contribute to and exacerbate more complex social perceptual deficits later in life. As such, animal models of social deprivation (including lesions that interfere with social communication) and consequential behavioral abnormalities may shed light on developmental processes associated with the emergence of symptoms associated with autism.

Using animal models to understand physiological responses to *changes* in the environment can also inform our understanding of the physiological aspects of SIB in humans. Many individuals with autism are characterized by insistence on sameness and experience difficulty with changes in routine. In a study of adult rhesus monkeys with SIB, exposure to the stress of housing relocation was associated with increase in self-biting behavior, sleep disturbance, and elevated levels of cortisol (Davenport, Lutz, Tiefenbacher, Novak, & Meyer, 2008). These findings lend support to the notion that life stresses, particularly change in environment, may exacerbate SIB in individuals with autism.

Evaluation and Treatment of Stereotypy and Self-Injury

Perhaps the best way to treat stereotypy and self-injury is to prevent it. Specific attention should be paid to those with autism who are at particularly increased risk for the development of the behavior such as those with sensory impairments or severe intellectual disability. The effectiveness of functional communication training is well established as a means to impact maladaptive self-injurious and other behaviors (see Carr & Durand, 1985).

Based on consensus development (AAMR, 2000) the first line of assessment methods for psychiatric and behavior problems in the context of intellectual disability include an interview with family/caregiver, direct observation of behavior, medical history and physical examination, functional behavior assessment, medication and side-effects evaluation, and unstructured psychiatric diagnostic interview. From a behavioral intervention standpoint, first line treatments for challenging behaviors, and SIB in particular, include client and family education, functional behavior assessment, and managing the environment. Educating the family and the client about behavior problems and how to manage them can decrease stress and address situations that predispose to the expression of the behavior. A comprehensive assessment of stereotypy and/or self-injury will include a variety of assessments and examine the whole person. For a review of positive behavior support strategies, see Chapter 65 (this volume).

Current best practices in the field of applied behavior analysis for the assessment of stereotypy and self-injury focus on a function based model (Rapp & Vollmer, 2005a). Applied behavior analysis determines the functional relationships between the environment and behavior (Skinner, 1953). Procedures using these principles have been used to assess and treat a variety of behaviors including stereotypy and self-injury. Indeed, some 400 papers have been written since 1964 that specifically described behavioral intervention for SIB (Kahng, Iwata, & Lewin, 2002).

The standard of care for the treatment of stereotypy and self-injury has developed significantly over the past three decades primarily due to advances in behavior analysis. Research has consistently focused on decreasing the stereotypy and/or self-injury while increasing adaptive behaviors. However, early attempts at reducing stereotypy and self-injury were based on punishment. Current approaches have developed with advances in an assessment methodology that incorporates reinforcers that are specifically linked to the putative function of the challenging behavior. While these strategies have brought about significant change to the methodology of assessment and treatment, the use of restraint, seclusion, and even punishment may still be necessary to prevent immediate harm to some individuals with self-injury (Brown, Genel, & Riggs, 2000). Clinicians who employ restraint in the management of self-injury, do so in the context of a comprehensive behavior plan with specific procedures to decrease the use of restraint (Fisher, Piazza, Bowman, Hanley, & Adelinis, 1997).

With the behavioral approach, it is believed that stereotypy is an operant behavior that is maintained or reinforced by its consequences (Rapp & Vollmer, 2005). When determining the function of the behavior, information is gathered to identify the challenging behavior and possible replacement behaviors. There are two basic approaches to determining the function of the behavior: a functional assessment and/or a functional analysis. A functional assessment usually is based on observations that are conducted in the natural environment and do not require environmental manipulation during the initial data collection. Indirect assessments include rating scales that can be filled out by teachers, parents, and occasionally even the affected individual. The indirect assessments require no direct observations but can help determine the function of the challenging behavior. A functional analysis involves more systematic manipulation of environments to isolate potential variables that impact the behavior (Iwata et al., 1982/1994).

During a functional analysis, potential antecedents and consequences are systematically manipulated so that their effects on the problem behavior can be observed and measured. Such functional analyses usually consist of three test conditions: (1) contingent attention, (2) contingent escape, (3) alone. A control condition (sometimes called the play condition) where there are no demands on the individual and reinforcement is continuously available is also assessed. Each of the conditions is repeated over multiple sessions in order to determine if the behavior occurs more often under particular circumstances.

When analyzing the data from a functional analysis, the problem behavior is expected to be elevated in the conditions that maintain the behavior. For example, if the frequency of the problem behavior is high in the contingent attention condition, it suggests that the behavior is maintained by social positive reinforcement. If the problem behavior is high during the contingent escape condition, the behavior is maintained by negative reinforcement. If the problem behavior is high in the alone condition, the behavior is maintained by automatic or sensory reinforcement. It is of course possible for the problem behavior to serve multiple functions.

Due to the potential harm that could be caused, particular precautions during a functional analysis need to be addressed. In order to assess self-injury, the behavior needs to occur and thus there is the potential to cause harm. However, allowing the behavior to occur during specific functional analysis conditions with the appropriate professional supervision could lead to an intervention that could potentially lower the behavior in the future. Another risk of conducting a functional analysis is the potential that the challenging behavior could come under control of contingencies that previously did not control the behavior. Because of the risks, it is extremely important that whoever conducts the functional analysis has specific training in the methodology.

A number of tools are routinely used in the service of assessing or monitoring treatment response in persons with SIB and stereotypy. The Aberrant Behavior Checklist (ABC; Aman, Singh, Stewart, & Field, 1985) and the Repetitive Behavior Scale-Revised (RBS-R; Bodfish et al., 2000; Lam & Aman, 2007) are each used widely as general assessment tools for problem behavior and for self-injury in particular. These scales may be sensitive to pharmacological or other interventions and are being utilized as outcome measures in clinical trials (RUPP, 2002; Aman, 2003; King et al., 2009). The Challenging Behavior Interview (Oliver, McClintock, Hall, Smith, Dagnan, & Stenfert-Kroese, 2003) can be used to capture problem behaviors including self-injury as well as its severity. The Motivation Assessment Scale (MAS; Durand & Crimmins, 1988) can be helpful in suggesting the possible function of the behavior. Joosten and colleagues recently modified this scale and administered it to a population of children with intellectual disability and stereotyped and repetitive behaviors. They observed that both intrinsic and extrinsic motivators are commonly associated with these behaviors. The Self-Injurious Behavior Trauma Scale (SIT; Iwata, Pace, Kissel, Nau, & Farber, 1990) has also been used in some studies to classify the type of injury, number of wounds, severity of wounds, and injuries based on location.

Interventions for stereotypy and self-injury need to be matched with the function of the behavior so that the problem behavior becomes ineffective and irrelevant. Interventions can be based on positive reinforcement (extinction, differential reinforcement of other behavior, differential reinforcement of alternative behavior, differential reinforcement of incompatible behavior, and noncontingent reinforcement), negative reinforcement (extinction, noncontingent negative reinforcement, differential negative reinforcement, and response chain interruption), and/or automatic reinforcement (noncontingent competing reinforcers, sensory extinction, and differential reinforcement).

Treatment of non–socially mediated (automatically reinforced) stereotypy or self-injurious behavior is difficult, since the exact mechanism that maintains the behavior is difficult to identify. King (1995) has suggested that some forms of stereotypy associated with self-restraining behavior may be compulsive or driven, and might be more likely to yield to treatments that are commonly utilized for obsessive-compulsive disorder.

While the use of punishment is controversial, it is important to discuss the behavioral aspects and ethical considerations for its use. "Punishment" is a behavioral term that describes a response that immediately follows a stimulus that decreases the future frequency of a similar response (Azrin & Holz, 1966). For example, the use of a disapproving look to decrease whining, a stern "no" to stop a child from hitting, a manual restraint to stop a person from self-injury are all classified as punishment simply because they decrease the likelihood that the similar behavior will occur again. Ethical considerations include that the least restrictive alternative interventions have been tried and found unsuccessful, the type of punishment is consistent with local laws, the appropriate training has been conducted for all involved prior to the use of punishment, and a risk-benefit analysis confirms a greater risk without the use of punishment. For a comprehensive review of ethical guidelines of punishment see Bailey and Burch (2005).

It is common that challenging behavior serves more than one function. When this happens it is important to develop multicomponent treatments. As noted above, medications are commonly utilized in the treatment of stereotypy and SIB, and optimal approaches will address medical issues and behavioral issues concurrently.

Beyond behavior change, the measurement of quality of life and social validity are receiving increasing attention. Quality of life captures the broad range of social issues relating to the person's sense of self and patterns of daily living with respect to family, community, and society (Schalock, 1990). Social validity assessments are designed to gather the perspective of a given treatment's social acceptability in a particular setting (Schwartz & Baer, 1991). Symons, Koppekin, & Wehby (1999) have reviewed studies that assessed social validity and quality of life following the treatment of people with self-injurious behaviors. They observed that reducing self-injury is a necessary component to an intervention, but it may not be enough to result in important life changes. Of the 138 studies they reviewed, only about a third included a quality of life measurement, and most of these were anecdotal with poorly defined terms. Objective and reliable quality of life measurements should be considered among the outcomes for interventions with this population.

Indeed, whether the interventions focus on behavioral or medical strategies, it is critical that a variety of outcomes be monitored. Typically data collected as a plan unfolds will inform appropriate fine-tuning, or the exploration of new directions in search of the best outcomes.

Conclusions

Between 4% and 16% of individuals with intellectual disabilities engage in stereotypy and self-injurious behavior. Stereotypy and self-injury are commonly observed in individuals with autism spectrum disorders, and/or significant intellectual disability, and can have a substantial impact on level of functioning. Research examining underlying biological factors and neurological processes has facilitated the development of improved pharmacological and behavioral treatments for individuals struggling with these behaviors. Animal models have also provided insight into putative mechanisms contributing to stereotypy and self-injury in humans. Studies examining the detrimental impact of impoverished environments and social/emotional deprivation underscore the role of one's surroundings and the importance of social interaction in development. Understanding the interaction between neurological processes and social/emotional functioning may facilitate development of more effective treatment strategies.

Much progress has been made in recent years concerning the conceptualization and measurement of stereotypy and SIB. However, much work remains to better understand the factors that lead to the development and maintenance of these behaviors. That these behaviors form part of the core autism phenotoype highlights the potential for greater exploration of the links between stereotypy and developmental and social function.

The field has yet to produce a definition that fully encompasses the essence of stereotypy. In particular, the assertion that such behaviors are produced with a lack of goal or purpose contradicts much of our understanding regarding the nature of stereotypy. Given that stereotypic behavior arises as a result of impoverished environments, sensory deprivation, increased stress or discomfort, and other circumstances, it has been suggested that such behaviors are expressed to self-calm, self-regulate, experience sensations, or even explore oneself and one's surroundings. Stereotypy occurs as part of the normal developmental process, suggesting there is a purpose to the behaviors in infancy; the fact that they persist in individuals with a variety of developmental disabilities might indicate the continued need or reliance on the behaviors in persons with altered developmental trajectories.

In moving toward a better understanding of stereotypy, more work needs to be done in a number of areas. Various neurotransmitter and brain systems have been implicated in the development and maintenance of stereotypy, particularly dopamine. However, the directionality of disrupted neurotransmitter function remains unclear. Further, given that pharmacologically induced stereotyped behavior responds to manipulations of a number of neurotransmitters, the specificity for the role of any particular neurotransmitter system is still under debate. Elucidating the pathways of these systems will in turn lead to more targeted pharmacological treatment options.

Research has indicated that children who have been reared in impoverished environments, children with perceptual impairments, and children with autism engage in stereotypy, suggesting commonalities across these conditions. Perhaps consistent among them are barriers to developing appropriate communication skills, and lack of opportunity to form social-emotional connections and relationships with others. Animal models exist in which similar behaviors emerge spontaneously after early developmental or environmental manipulations and may significantly advance our understanding of effective interventions. Thus, environmental enrichment can impact brain development in rats and mice, and enhancement of social-emotional relationships has been shown to improve development generally and stereotypy more specifically in children reared in orphanages. Future research will no doubt examine pre- and posttreatment brain morphology in humans who benefit from such intervention, to better elucidate underlying neurological mechanisms involved in the expression of stereotypy. In the meantime, continued elaboration of animal models of stereotypy, perhaps in the context of other social-communication deficits, will facilitate our understanding of these behaviors in individuals with ASD.

Challenges and Future Directions

- Examine the factors that lead to the development and maintenance of stereotypy and self-injury.
- Continued development and refinement of the definition of stereotypy to include and better understand the role of possible underlying motivating factors.
- Examine pre- and post-treatment brain morphology in humans to better elucidate underlying neurological mechanisms involved in the expression of stereotypy.
- Continued elaboration of animal models of stereotypy to facilitate our understanding of these behaviors in individuals with ASD and/or intellectual disability.

SUGGESTED READINGS

Iwata, B. A., Dorsey, M. R., Slifer, K. J., Bauman, K. E., & Richman, G. S. (1994). Toward a functional analysis of self-injury. *Journal of Applied Behavior Analysis, 27,* 197–209. (Reprinted from *Analysis and Intervention in Developmental Disabilities, 2,* 3–20, 1982.)

King, B. H. (2002). Pemoline and other dopamine models of self-biting behavior. In S. R. Schroeder, M. L. Oster-Granite, & T. Thompson (Eds.), *Self-injurious behavior* (pp. 181–189). Washington, DC: American Psychological Association.

Lewis, M. H., Gluck, J. P., Bodfish, J. W., Beauchamp, A. J., & Mailman, R. B. (1996). Neurological basis of stereotyped movement disorder. In R. L. Sprague & K. M. Newell (Eds.), *Stereotypy: Brain behavior relationships* (pp. 37–67).

ACKNOWLEDGMENTS

This work was supported in part by grant no. NICHD P50 HD055782 to B.H.K.

REFERENCES

Ainsworth, M. D. (1979). Infant–mother attachment. *American Psychologist, 34,* 932–937.

Alborz, A., Bromley, J., Emerson, E., Kiernan, C., & Qureshi, H. (1994). *Challenging behavior survey: Individual schedule.* Manchester, UK: Hester Adrian Research Centre, University of Manchester.

Aman, M. G. (2003). *Annotated bibliography on the aberrant behavior checklist (June 2003 update).* Columbus: Ohio State University.

Aman, M. G., Singh, N. N., Stewart, A. W., & Field, C. J. (1985). The Aberrant Behavior Checklist: A behavior rating scale for the assessment of treatment effects. *American Journal of Mental Deficiency, 89,* 485–491.

Aman, M. G., Tassé, M. J., Rojahn, J., & Hammer, D. (1996). The Nisonger CBRF: A child behavior rating form for children with developmental disabilities. *Research in Developmental Disabilities, 17,* 41–57.

American Psychiatric Association. (2000). *Diagnostic and statistical manual of mental disorders* (4th ed., text rev.; DSM-IV-TR). Washington, DC: Author.

Ayhan I. H., & Randrup A. (1972). Role of brain noradrenaline in morphine-induced stereotyped behaviour. *Psychopharmacologia, 27*(3), 203–212.

Azrin, N. H., & Holz, W. C. (1966). Punishment. In W. K. Honig (Ed.), *Operant behavior: Areas of research and application* (pp. 380–447). New York: Appleton-Century-Crofts.

Bachara, G. H., & Phelan, W. J. (1980). Rhythmic movement in deaf children. *Perceptual and Motor Skills, 50,* 933–934.

Bachmann, I., Audigé, L., & Stauffacher, M. (2003). Risk factors associated with behavioural disorders of crib-biting, weaving, and box-walking in Swiss horses. *Equine Veterinary Journal, 35,* 158–163.

Bailey, J. S., & Burch, M. R. (2005). *Ethics for behavior analysts.* Mahwah, NJ: Erlbaum.

Baroff, G. S., & Tate, B. G. (1968). The use of aversive stimulation in the treatment of chronic self-injurious behavior. *Journal of the American Academy of Child Psychiatry, 7,* 454–470.

Bauman, M. D., Toscano, J. E., Babineau, B. A., Mason, W. A., & Amaral, D. G. (2008). Emergence of stereotypies in juvenile monkeys (Macaca mulatta) with neonatal amygdala or hippocampus lesions. *Behavioral Neuroscience, 122,* 1005–1015.

Baumeister, A. A., & Rollings, J. P. (1976). Self-injurious behavior. In N. Ellis (Ed.), *International Review of Research in Mental Retardation,* 8. New York: Academic Press.

Bellanca, R. U., & Crockett, C. M. (2002). Factors predicting increased incidence of abnormal behavior in male pigtailed macaques. *American Journal of Primatology, 58,* 57–69.

Berkson, G. (1967). Abnormal stereotyped motor acts. In J. Zubin, & H. Hunt (Eds.), *Comparative psychology* (pp. 76–94). New York: Grune and Stratton.

Berkson, G., & Tupa, M. (2000). Early development of stereotyped and self-injurious behaviors. *Journal of Early Intervention, 23,* 1–19.

Berkson, G., Tupa, M., & Sherman, L. (2001). Early development of stereotyped and self-injurious behaviors: I. Incidence. *American Journal of Mental Retardation, 106,* 539–547.

Bishop, S. L., Richler, J., Cain, A. C., & Lord, C. (2007) Predictors of perceived negative impact in mothers of children with autism spectrum disorder. *American Journal of Mental Retardation, 112,* 450–461.

Bodfish, J. W., Powell, S. B., Golden, R. N., & Lewis, M. H. (1995). Blink rates as an index of dopamine function in adults with mental retardation and repetitive behavior disorders. *American Journal of Mental Retardation, 99,* 335–344.

Bodfish, J. W., Symons, F. J., & Lewis, M. H. (1999). *Repetitive behavior scales.* Western Carolina Center Research Reports.

Bodfish, J. W., Symons, F. J., Parker, D. E., & Lewis, M. H. (2000) Varieties of repetitive behavior in autism: Comparisons to mental retardation. *Journal of Autism and Developmental Disorders, 30,* 237–243.

Borthwick-Duffy, S. A., Eyman, R. K., & White, J. F. (1987). Client characteristics and residential placement patterns. *American Journal of Mental Deficiency, 92,* 24–30.

Briere, J., & Gil, E. (1998). Self-mutilation in clinical and general population samples: Prevalence, correlates, and functions. *American Journal of Orthopsychiatry, 68,* 609–620.

Brown, R. L., Genel, M., & Riggs, J. A. (2000). Use of seclusion and restraint in children and adolescents. *Archives of Pediatrics and Adolescent Medicine, 154,* 653–656.

Brown, R., Hobson, R. P., Lee. A., & Stevenson, J. (1997). Are there "autistic-like" features in congenitally blind children? *Journal of Child Psychology and Psychiatry, 39,* 693–703.

Bruhl, H. H., Fielding, L. H., Joyce, M., Peters, W., & Wiesler, N. (1982). Thirty month demonstration project for the treatment of self-injurious behavior in severely retarded individuals. In J. H. Hollis & C. E. Meyers (Eds.), *Life-threatening behavior: analysis and intervention* (pp. 191–275). Washington, DC: American Association on Mental Deficiency.

Bruininks, R. H., Woodcock, R. W., Weatherman, R. F., & Hill, B. K. (1996). *Scales of independent behavior–revised.* Chicago, IL: Riverside.

Burgess, J. W., & Villablanca, J. R. (2007). Ontogenesis of morphine-induced behavior in the cat. *Brain Research, 1134*(1), 53–61.

Capone, F., Adriani, W., Shumilina, M., Izykenova, G., Granstrem, O., Dambinova, S., et al. (2008). Autoantibodies against opioid or glutamate receptors are associated with changes in morphine reward and physical dependence in mice. *Psychopharmacology (Berl), 197*(4), 535–548.

Carr, E. D., & Durand, V. M. (1985). Reducing behavior problems through functional communication training. *Journal of Applied Behavior Analysis, 18,* 111–126.

Charness, M. E., Amit, Z., & Taylor, M. (1975). Morphine induced stereotypic behavior in rat. *Behavioral Biology, 13*(1), 71–80.

Cohen, I. L. (2003). Criterion-related validity of the PDD Behavior Inventory. *Journal of Autism and Developmental Disorders, 33,* 47–53.

Collins, M. S., & Cornish, K. (2002). A survey of the prevalence of stereotypy, self-injury, and aggression in children and young adults with Cri du Chat syndrome. *Journal of Intellectual Disability Research, 46,* 133–140.

Cook, E. H., Jr., Rowlett, R., Jaselskis, C., & Leventhal, B. L. (1992). Fluoxetine treatment of children and adults with autistic disorder and mental retardation. *Journal of the American Academy of Child and Adolescent Psychiatry, 31,* 739–745.

Cooper, J. J., Odberg, F., & Nicol, C. J. (1996). Limitations on the effectiveness of environmental improvement in reducing stereotypic behaviour in bank voles *(Clethrionomys glareolus). Applied Animal Behaviour Science, 48,* 237–248.

Cromwell, H. C., & King, B. H. (2004). The role of the basal ganglia in the expression of stereotyped, self-injurious behaviors in developmental disorders. *International Review of Research in Mental Retardation, 29,* 120–158.

Crosland, K. A., Zarcone, J. R., Schroeder, S., Zarcone, T., & Fowler, S. (2005). Use of an antecedent analysis and a force sensitive platform to compare stereotyped movements and motor tics. *American Journal of Mental Retardation, 110,* 181–192.

Davanzo, P. A., & King, B. H. (1996). Open trial lamotrigine in the treatment of self-injurious behavior in an adolescent with profound mental retardation. *Journal of Child and Adolescent Psychopharmacology, 6*(4), 273–279.

Davenport, M. D., Lutz, C. K., Tiefenbacher, S., Novak, M. A., & Meyer, J. S. (2008). A rhesus monkey model of self-injury: effects of relocation stress on behavior and neuroendocrine function. *Biological Psychiatry, 63,* 990–996.

Dawson, G., Sterling, L., & Faja, S. (2008). Autism: Risk factors, risk processes, and outcome. In M. deHaan & M. R. Gunnar (Eds.), *Handbook of developmental neuroscience.* New York: Guilford.

Dawson, G., Webb, S. J., Wijsman, E., Schellenberg, G., Estes, A., Munson, J., et al. (2005). Neurocognitive and electrophysiological evidence of altered face processing in parents of children with autism: Implications for a model of abnormal development of social brain circuitry in autism. *Development and Psychopathology, 17,* 679–697.

De Lissavoy, V. (1961). Head-banging in early childhood. *Journal of Pediatrics, 58,* 109–114.

Derby, K. M., Fisher, W. W., & Piazza, C. C. (1996). The effects of contingent and noncontingent attention on self-injury and self-restraint. *Journal of Applied Behavior Analysis, 29,* 107–110.

Durand, V. M., & Crimmins, D. B. (1988). Identifying variables maintaining self-injurious behavior. *Journal of Autism and Developmental Disorders, 18,* 99–117.

Einfeld, S. L., & Tonge, B. J. (1992). *Manual for the Developmental Behaviour Checklist.* Clayton, Melbourne, and Sydney: Monash University Center for Developmental Psychiatry and School of Psychiatry, University of New South Wales.

Elchaar, G. M., Maisch, N. M., Augusto, L. M., & Wehring, H. J. (2006). Efficacy and safety of naltrexone use in pediatric patients with autistic disorder. *Annals of Pharmacotherapy, 40,* 1086–1095.

Ellinwood, E. J., Jr. (1967). Amphetamine psychosis: I. Description of the individuals and process. *Journal of Mental and Nervous Disease, 144*, 273–282.

Expert Consensus Guideline Series. Treatment of psychiatric and behavioral problems in mental retardation. (2000). *American Journal of Mental Retardation, 105*, 159–226.

Favell, J. E., Azrin, N. H., Baumeister, A. A., Carr, E. G., Dorsey, M. F., Forehand, R., et al. (1982). The treatment of self-injurious behavior. *Behavior Therapy, 13*, 529–554.

Fazzi, E., Lanners, J., Danova, S., Ferrarri-Ginevra, O., Gheza, C., Luparia, A., et al. (1999). Stereotpyed behaviours in blind children. *Brain and Development, 21*, 522–528.

Feigenbaum, J., & Yanai, J. (1984). The role of dopaminergic mechanisms in mediating the central behavioral effects of morphine in rodents. *Neuropsychobiology. 11*, 98–105.

Fisher, W. W., Grace, N. C., & Murphy, C. (1996). Further analysis of the relationship between self-injury and self-restraint. *Journal of Applied Behavior Analysis, 29*, 103–106.

Fisher, W. W., Piazza, C. C., Bowman, L. G., Hagopian, L. P., Owen, J. C., & Slevin, I. (1992). A comparison of two approaches for identifying reinforcers for persons with severe to profound disabilities. *Journal of Applied Behavior Analysis, 25*, 491–498.

Fisher, W. W., Piazza, C. C., Bowman, L. G., Hanley, G. P., & Adelinish, J. D. (1997). Direct and collateral effects of restraints and restraint fading. *Journal of Applied Behavior Analysis, 30*, 105–120.

Fowler, S. C., Birkestrand, B., Chen, R., Vorontsova, E., & Zarcone, T. (2003). Behavioral sensitization to amphetamine in rats: changes in the rhythm of head movements during focused stereotypies. *Psychopharmacology (Berl), 170*, 167–177.

Gal, E., Dyck, M. J., & Passmore, A. (2009). The relationship between stereotyped movements and self-injurious behavior in children with developmental or sensory disabilities. *Research in Developmental Disabilities, 30*, 342–352.

Garner, J. P. (2005). Stereotypies and other abnormal repetitive behaviors: potential impact on validity, reliability, and replicability of scientific outcomes. *Institute for Laboratory Animal Research Journal, 46*(2), 106–117.

Garner, J. P., & Mason, G. J. (2002). Evidence between the relationship of cage stereotypies and behavioural disinhibition in laboratory rodents. *Behavioural Brain Research, 136*, 83–92.

Garner, J. P., Meehan, C. L., & Mench, J. A. (2003). Stereotypies in caged parrots, schizophrenia, and autism: evidence for a common mechanism. *Behavioural Brain Research, 145*, 125–134.

Genovese, E., Napoli, P. A., & Bolego-Zonta, N. (1969). Self-aggressiveness: a new type of change induced by pemoline. *Life Sciences, 8*, 513–515.

Gillberg, C. (1995). Endogenous opioids and opiate antagonists in autism: brief review of empirical findings and implications for clinicians. *Developmental Medicine and Child Neurology, 37*, 239–245.

Griengl, H., Sendera, A., & Dantendorfer, K. (2001). Naltrexone as a treatment of self-injurious behavior: A case report. *Acta Psychiatrica Scandinavica, 103*, 234–136.

Gualtieri, C. T., & Schroeder, S. R. (1989). Pharmacotherapy of self-injurious behavior: Preliminary tests of the D-1 hypothesis. *Psychopharmacology Bulletin, 25*, 364–371.

Hall, S., Oliver, C., & Murphy, G. (2001). Early development of self-injurious behavior: An empirical study. *American Journal of Mental Retardation, 106*, 113–122.

Harlow, H. F., Dodsworth, R. O., & Harlow, M. K. (1965). Total social isolation in monkeys. *Proceedings of the National Academy of Sciences of the United States of America, 54*, 90–97.

Harris, J. C. (1992). Neurobiological factors in self-injurious behavior. In J. K. Luiselli, J. L. Matson., & N. N. Singh (Eds.), *Self-injurious behavior: Analysis, assessment, and treatment* (pp. 59–92). New York: Springer-Verlag.

Hellings, J. A., Kelley, L. A., Gabrielli, W. F., Kilgore, E., & Shah, P. (1996). Sertraline response in adults with mental retardation and autistic disorder. *Journal of Clinical Psychiatry, 57*, 333–336.

Herpertz, S., Steinmeyer, S. M., Marx, D., Oidtmann, A., & Sass, H. (1995). The significance of aggression and impulsivity for self-mutilative behavior. *Pharmacopsychiatry, 28S*, 64–72.

Hill, E. L., & Frith, U. (2003). Understanding autism: insights from mind and brain. *Philosophical Transactions of the Royal Society of London. Series B, Biological Sciences, 358*, 281–289.

Hoksbergen, R., ter Laak, J., Rijk, K., van Dijkum, C., & Stoutjesdijk, F. (2005). Post-institutional autistic syndrome in Romanian adoptees. *Journal of Autism and Developmental Disorders, 35*, 615–623.

Hosey, G. R., & Skyner, L. J. (2007). Self-injurious behavior in zoo primates. *International Journal of Primatology, 28*, 1431–1437.

Hyman, P., Oliver, C., & Hall, S. (2002). Self-injurious behavior, self-restraint, and compulsive behaviors in Cornelia de Lange Syndrome. *American Journal of Mental Retardation, 107*, 146–154.

Ireland, W. W. (1898). *Mental affections of children, idiocy, imbecility and insanity.* Oxford: Churchill.

Isley, E. M., Kartsonis, C., McCurley, C. M., Weisz, K. E., & Roberts, M. S. (1991). Self-restraint: A review of etiology and applications in mentally retarded adults with self-injury. *Research in Developmental Disabilities, 12*, 87–95.

Iwata, B. A., Dorsey, M. F., Slifer, K. J., Bauman, K. E., & Richman, G. S. (1982). Towards a functional analysis of self-injury. *Analysis and Intervention in Developmental Disabilities, 2*, 3–20.

Iwata, B. A., Dorsey, M. R., Slifer, K. J., Bauman, K. E., & Richman, G. S. (1994). Toward a functional analysis of self-injury. *Journal of Applied Behavior Analysis, 27*, 197–209. (Reprinted from *Analysis and Intervention in Developmental Disabilities, 2*, 3–20, 1982.)

Iwata, B. A., Pace, G. M., Dorsey, M. F., Zarcone, J. R., Vollmer, T. R., Smith, R. G., et al. (1994). The functions of self-injurious behavior: An experimental-epidemiological analysis. *Journal of Applied Behavior Analysis, 27*, 215–240.

Iwata, B. A., Pace, G. M., Kissel, R. C., Nau, P. A., & Farber, J. M. (1990). The self-injury trauma (SIT) scale: A method for quantifying surface tissue damage caused by self-injurious behavior. *Journal of Applied Behavior Analysis, 23*, 99–110.

Iwata, B. A., Wallace, M. D., Kahng, S., Lindberg, J. S., Roscoe, E. M., Conners, J., et al. (2000). Skill acquisition in the implementation of functional analysis methodology. *Journal of Applied Behavior Analysis, 33*, 181–194.

Jones, R. S. P., Wint, D., Ellis, N. C. (1990). The social effects of stereotyped behavior. *Journal of Mental Deficiency Research, 34*, 261–268.

Joosten, A. V., Bundy, A. C., & Einfeld, S. L. (2009) Intrinsic and extrinsic motivation for stereotypic and repetitive behavior. *Journal of Autism and Developmental Disorders, 39*, 521–531.

Kahng, S., Iwata, B. A., & Lewin, A. B. (2002). Behavioral treatment of self-injury. *American Journal of Mental Retardation, 107*, 212–221.

Kanner, L. (1943). Autistic disturbances of affective contact. *Nervous Child, 2,* 217–250.

Karson, C. N. (1983). Spontaneous eye-blink rates and dopaminergic systems. *Brain, 106,* 643–653.

Karson, C. N., Burns, R. S., LeWitt, P. A., Foster, N. L., & Newman, R. P. (1984). Blink rates and disorders of movement. *Neurology, 34,* 677–678.

Kelley, A. E. (2001, May). Measurement of rodent stereotyped behavior. *Current protocols in neuroscience.* Chapter 8: Unit 8.8.

Kennedy, C. H., Meyer, K. A., Knowles, T., & Shukla, S. (2000). Analyzing the multiple functions of stereotypical behavior for students with autism: Implications for assessment and treatment. *Journal of Applied Behavior Analysis, 33,* 559–571.

King, B. H. (1991). Fluoxetine reduced self-injurious behavior in an adolescent with mental retardation. *Journal of Child and Adolescent Psychopharmacology, 1,* 321–329.

King, B. H. (1993). Self-injury by people with mental retardation: A compulsive behavior hypothesis. *American Journal of Mental Retardation, 100,* 654–665.

King, B. H. (2000). Pharmacological treatment of mood disturbances, aggression, and self-injury in persons with pervasive developmental disorders. *Journal of Autism and Developmental Disorders, 30,* 439–445.

King, B. H. (2002). Pemoline and other dopamine models of self-biting behavior. In S. R. Schroeder, M. L. Oster-Granite, & T. Thompson (Eds.), *Self-injurious behavior* (pp. 181–189). Washington, DC: American Psychological Association.

King, B. H., Cromwell, H. C., Ly, H. T., Behrstock, S. P., Schmanke, T., & Maidment, N. T. (1998). Dopaminergic and glutamatergic interactions in the expression of self-injurious behavior. *Developmental Neuroscience, 20,* 180–187.

King, B. H., Hollander, E., Sikich, L., McCracken, J. T., Scahill, L., Bregman, J. D., et al. STAART Psychopharmacology Network. (2009). Lack of efficacy of Citalopram in children with autism spectrum disorders and high levels of repetitive behavior. *Archives of General Psychiatry, 6,* 583–590.

Kolevzon, A., Mathewson, K. A., & Hollander, E. (2006). Selective serotonin reuptake inhibitors in autism: a review of efficacy and tolerability. *Journal of Clinical Psychiatry, 67,* 407–414.

Korsgaard, S., Povlsen, U. J., & Randrup, A. (1985). Effects of apomorphine and haloperidol on "spontaneous" stereotyped licking behaviour in the Cebus monkey. *Psychopharmacology, 85,* 240–243.

Kurtz, P. F., Chin, M. D., Huete, J. M., Tarbox, R. S. F., O'Connor, J. T., Paclawskyj, T. R., et al. (2003). Functional analysis and treatment of self-injurious behavior in young children: A summary of 30 cases. *Journal of Applied Behavior Analysis, 36,* 205–219.

LaGrow, S. J., & Repp, A. C. (1984). Stereotypic responding: A review of intervention research. *American Journal of Mental Deficiency, 89,* 595–609.

Lam, K. S., & Aman, M. G. (2007). The Repetitive Behavior Scale-Revised: Independent validation in individuals with autism spectrum disorders. *Journal of Autism and Developmental Disorders, 37,* 855–866.

Lambert, N., Nihira, K., & Leland, H. (1993). AAMR Adaptive Behavior Scales-School (ABS-S:2). Pro-Ed, Inc., Austin, TX.

Lerman, D. C., Iwata, B. A., Smith, R. G., & Vollmer, T. R. (1994). Restraint fading and the development of alternative behaviour in the treatment of self-restraint and self-injury. *Journal of Intellectual Disability Research, 38,* 135–148.

Lerman, D. C., & Vorndran, C. M. (2002). On the status of knowledge for using punishment: Implications for treating behavior disorders. *Journal of Applied Behavior Analysis, 35,* 431–464.

Lewis, M. H. (2004). Environmental complexity and central nervous system development and function. *Mental Retardation and Developmental Disabilities Research Reviews, 10,* 91–95.

Lewis, M. H., & Baumeister, A. A. (1982). Stereotyped mannerisms in mentally retarded persons: Animal models and theoretical analyses. In N. R. Ellis (Ed.), *International review of research in mental retardation* (pp. 123–161). New York: Academic.

Lewis, M. H., Gluck, J. P., Bodfish, J. W., Beauchamp, A. J., & Mailman, R. B. (1996). Neurological basis of stereotyped movement disorder. In R. L. Sprague & K. M. Newell (Eds.), *Stereotypy: Brain behavior relationships* (pp. 37–67). Washington, DC: American Psychological Association.

Lewis, M. H., Tanimura, Y., Lee, L. W., & Bodfish, J. W. (2007). Animal models of restricted repetitive behavior in autism. *Behavioural Brain Research, 176,* 66–74.

Lutz, C. K., Davis, E. B., Ruggiero, A. M., & Suomi, S. J. (2007). Brief report: Early predictors of self-biting in socially-housed rhesus macaques (Macaca mulatta). *American Journal of Primatology, 69,* 584–590.

Lutz, C., Well, A., & Novak, M. (2003). Stereotypic and self-injurious behavior in rhesus macaques: a survey and retrospective analysis of environment and early experience. *American Journal Primatology, 60,* 1–15.

MacDonald, R., Green, G., Mansfield, R., Geckeler, A., Gardenier, N., Anderson, J., et al. (2007). Stereotypy in young children with autism and typically developing children. *Research in Developmental Disabilities, 28,* 266–277.

Mace, F. C., & Mauk, J. E. (1995). Bio-behavioral diagnosis and treatment of self-injury. *Mental Retardation and Developmental Disabilities Research Reviews, 1,* 104–110.

Mackert, A., Flechtner, K. M., Woyth, C., & Frick, K. (1991). Increased blink rates in schizophrenics: Influences of neuroleptics and psychopathology. *Schizophrenia Research, 4,* 41–47.

Markowitz, P. I. (1992). Effect of fluoxetine on self injurious behavior in the developmentally disabled: A preliminary study. *Journal of Clinical Psychopharmacology, 12,* 27–31.

Marriner, L. M., & Drickamer, L. C. (1994). Factors influencing stereotypic behavior of primates in a zoo. *Zoo Biology, 13,* 267–275.

Matson, J. L. (1995). *Manual for the Diagnostic Assessment for the Severely Handicapped-II.* Baton Rouge: Louisiana State University.

Matson, J. L. (1997). *Manual for the assessment of dual diagnosis.* Baton Rouge: Louisiana State University.

Matson, J. L., & LoVullo, S. V. (2008). A review of behavioral treatments for self-injurious behaviors of persons with autism spectrum disorders. *Behavior Modification, 32,* 61–76.

McClintock, K., Hall, S., & Oliver, C. (2003). Risk markers associated with challenging behaviours in people with intellectual disabilities: A meta-analytic study. *Journal of Intellectual Disability Research, 47,* 405–416.

McHugh, E., & Pyfer, J. (1999). The development of rocking among children who are blind. *Journal of Visual Impairment and Blindness, 93,* 82–95.

Meehan, C. L., Garner, J. P., & Mench, J. A. (2004). Environmental enrichment and development of cage stereotypy in orange-winged Amazon parrots (Amazona amazonica). *Developmental Psychobiology, 44,* 209–218.

Moore, J. W., Edwards, R. P., Sterling-Turner, H. E., Riley, J., DuBard, M., & McGeorge, A. (2002). *Journal of Applied Behavior Analysis, 35*, 73–77.

Morrison, K., & Rosales-Ruis, J. (1997). The effect of object preferences on task performance and stereotypy in a child with autism. *Research in Developmental Disabilities, 18*, 127–137.

Muehlmann, A. M., Brown, B. D., & Devine, D. P. (2008). Pemoline (2-amino-5-phenyl-1,3-oxazol-4-one)-induced self-injurious behavior: a rodent model of pharmacotherapeutic efficacy. *Journal of Pharmacology and Experimental Therapeutics, 324*, 214–223.

Muehlmann, A. M., & Devine, D. P. (2008). Glutamate-mediated neuroplasticity in an animal model of self-injurious behaviour. *Behavioural Brain Research, 189*, 32–40.

Mueller, K., & Hsiao, S. (1980). Pemoline-induced self-biting in rats and self-mutilation in the de Lange syndrome. *Pharmacology, Biochemistry, and Behavior, 13*, 627–631.

Mueller, K., & Nyhan, W. L. (1982). Pharmacologic control of pemoline-induced self-injurious behavior in rats. *Pharmacology, Biochemistry, and Behavior, 18*, 891–894.

Murdoch, H. (1996). Stereotyped behaviours in deaf and hard of hearing children. *American Annals of the Deaf, 141*, 379–386. *Journal of Autism and Developmental Disorders, 15*, 149–161.

Murphy, G., Hall, S., Oliver, C., & Kissi-Debra, R. (1999). Identification of early self-injurious behaviour in young children with intellectual disability. *Journal of Intellectual Disability Research, 43*, 149–163.

Nader, R., Oberlander, T. F., Chambers, C. T., & Craig, K. D. (2004). Expression of pain in children with autism. *Clinical Journal of Pain, 20*, 88–97.

Nevison, C. M., Hurst, J. L., & Barnard, C. J. (1999). Strain-specific effects of cage enrichment in male laboratory mice (Mus musculus). *Animal Welfare, 8*, 361–389.

New, A. S., Trestman, R. L., Mitropoulou, V., Benishay, D. S., Coccaro, E., Silverman, J., et al. (1997). Serotonergic function and self-injurious behavior in personality disorder patients. *Psychiatry Research, 69*, 17–26.

Nihira, K., Foster, R., Shellhaas, M., & Leland, H. (1974). *AAMD Adaptive Behavior Scale.* Washington, DC: American Association on Mental Deficiency.

Norman, D. A., & Shallice, T. (1986). Attention to action: willed and automatic control of behavior. In: R. J. Davidson, G. E. Schwartz, & D. Shapiro (Eds.), *Consciousness and self-regulation: advances in research and theory* (pp. 1–18). New York: Plenum.

Novak, M. A., Kinsey, J. H., Jorgensen, M. J., & Hazen, T. J. (1998). Effects of puzzle feeders on pathological behavior in individually housed rhesus monkeys. *American Journal of Primatology, 46*, 213–227.

Oliver, C., Hall, S., Hales, J., Murphy, G., & Watts, D. (1998). The treatment of severe self-injurious behavior by the systematic fading of restraints: Effects on self-injury, self-restraint, adaptive behavior, and behavioral correlates of affect. *Research in Developmental Disabilities, 19*, 143–165.

Oliver, C., McClintock, K., Hall, S., Smith, M., Dagnan, D., & Stenfert-Kroese, B. (2003). Assessing the severity of challenging behavior: Psychometric properties of the challenging behavior interview. *Journal of Applied Research in Intellectual Disabilities, 16*, 53–61.

Pace, G. M., Iwata, B. A., Edwards, G. L., & McCosh, K. C. (1986). Stimulus fading and transfer in the treatment of self-restraint and self-injurious behavior. *Journal of Applied Behavior Analysis, 19*, 381–389.

Pennington, B. F., & Ozonoff, S. (1996). Executive functions and developmental psychopathology. *Journal of Child Psychology and Psychiatry, 37*, 51–87.

Peterson, R. F., & Peterson, L. R. (1968). The use of positive reinforcement in the control of self-destructive behavior in a retarded boy. *Journal of Experimental Child Psychology, 6*, 351–360.

Piazza, C. C., Adelinis, J. D., Hanley, G. P., Goh, H., & Delia, M. D. (2000). An evaluation of the effects of matched stimuli on behaviors maintained by automatic reinforcement. *Journal of Applied Behavior Analysis, 33*, 13–27.

Pollock J., & Kornetsky C. (1996). Reexpression of morphine-induced oral stereotypy six months after last morphine sensitizing dose. *Pharmacology, Biochemistry, and Behavior, 53*, 67–71.

Powell, S. B., Newman, H. A., Pendergast, J. F., & Lewis, M. (1999). A rodent model of spontaneous stereotypy: Initial characterization of developmental, environmental, and neurobiological factors. *Physiology and Behavior, 66*, 355–363.

Powers, K. V., Roane, H. S., & Kelley, M. E. (2007). Treatment of self-restraint associated with the application of protective equipment. *Journal of Applied Behavior Analysis, 40*, 577–581.

Rafaeli-Mor, N., Foster, L., & Berkson, G. (1999). Self-reported body-rocking and other habits in college students. *American Journal of Mental Retardation, 104*, 1–10.

Rapp, J. T., & Miltenberger, R. G. (2000). Self-restraint and self-injury: A demonstration of separate functions and response classes. *Behavioral Interventions, 15*, 37–51.

Rapp, J. T., & Vollmer, T. R. (2005a). Stereotypy I: A review of behavioral assessment and treatment. *Research in Developmental Disabilities, 26*, 527–547.

Rapp, J. T., & Vollmer, T. R. (2005b). Stereotypy II: A review of neurological interpretations and suggestions for an integration with behavioral methods. *Research in Developmental Disabilities, 26*, 548–564.

Reiss, S. (1988). *Test manual for the Reiss Screen for maladaptive behavior.* Orland Park, IL: International Diagnostic Systems.

Research Units on Pediatric Psychopharmacology Autism Network (RUPP). (2002). Risperidone in children with autism and serious behavioral problems. *New England Journal of Medicine, 347*, 314–321.

Richman, D. M., & Lindauer, S. E. (2005). Longitudinal assessment of stereotypic, proto-injurious, and self-injurious behavior exhibited by young children with developmental delays. *American Journal of Mental Retardation, 110*, 439–450.

Ridley, R. M. (1994). The psychology of perseverative and stereotyped behavior. *Progress in Neurobiology, 44*, 221–231.

Ridley, R. F., Baker, H. F., & Scraggs, P. R. (1979). The time course of the behavioral effects of amphetamine and their reversal by haloperidol in primate species. *Biological Psychiatry, 14*, 753–765.

Rinne, T., Westenberg, H. G., den Boer, J. A., & van den Brink, W. (2000). Serotonergic blunting to meta-chlorophenylpiperazine (m-CPP) highly correlates with sustained childhood abuse in impulsive and autoaggressive female borderline patients. *Biological Psychiatry, 47*, 548–556.

Rojahn, J., Matlock, S. T., & Tassé, M. J. (2000). The stereotyped behavior scale: psychometric properties and norms. *Research in Developmental Disabilities, 21*, 437–454.

Rojahn, J., Mulick, J. A., McCoy, D., & Schroeder, S. R. (1978). Setting effects, adaptive clothing, and the modification of head-banging and self-restraint in two profoundly retarded adults. *Behavior Analysis and Modification, 2,* 185–196.

Rojahn, J., Schroeder, S. R., & Hoch, T. A. (2008). *Self-injurious behavior in intellectual disabilities.* The Netherlands: Elsevier.

Rooker, G. W., & Roscoe, E. M. (2005). Functional analysis of self-injurious behavior and its relation to self-restraint. *Journal of Applied Behavior Analysis, 38,* 537–542.

Ross, L. L., Yu, D., & Kropla, W. C. (1998). Stereotyped behavior in developmentally delayed or autistic populations: Rhythmic or nonrhythmic? *Behavior Modification, 22,* 321–234.

Rutter, M., Andersen-Wood, L., Beckett, C., Bredenkamp, D., Castle, J., Groothues, C., et al. (1999). Quasi-autistic patterns following severe early global privation. *Journal of Child Psychology and Psychiatry, 40,* 537–549.

Sackett, G. P., Novak, M. F. S. X., & Kroeker, R. (1999). Early experience effects on adaptive behavior: theory revisited. *Mental Retardation and Developmental Disabilities Research Reviews, 5,* 30–40.

Saloviita, T. (2000). The structure and correlates of self-injurious behavior in an institutional setting. *Research in Developmental Disabilities, 21,* 501–511.

Sandman, C. A. (1988). Beta-endorphin disregulation in autistic and self-injurious behavior: a neurodevelopmental hypothesis. *Synapse, 2,* 193–199.

Schalock, R. L. (1990). *Quality of life: Perspectives and issues.* Washington, DC: American Association on Mental Retardation.

Schoenecker, B., & Heller, K. E. (2001). The involvement of dopamine (DA) and serotonin (5-HT) in stress induced stereotypies in bank voles (Clethrionomys glareolus). *Applied Animal Behaviour Science, 73,* 311–319.

Schroeder, S. R., Mulick, J., & Rojahn, J. (1980). The definition, taxonomy, epidemiology, and ecology of self-injurious behavior. *Journal of Autism and Developmental Disorders, 10,* 417–432.

Schroeder, S. R., Oster-Granite, M. L., Berkson, G., Bodfish, J. W., Breese, G. R., Cataldo, M. F., et al. (2001). Self-injurious behavior: gene-brain-behavior relationships. *Mental Retardation and Developmental Disabilities Research Reviews, 7,* 3–12.

Schroeder, S. R., Rojahn, J., Mulick, J. A., & Schroeder, C. S. (1990). Self-injurious behavior. In J. L. Matson (Ed.), *Handbook of behavior modification with the mentally retarded* (2nd ed., pp. 141–180). New York: Plenum.

Schroeder, S., Rojahn, J., & Oldenquist, A. (1991). Treatment of destructive behaviors among people with mental retardation and developmental disabilities: Overview of the problem. In *Treatment of destructive behaviors in persons with developmental disabilities* (NIH Publication No. 91–2410, pp. 173–220). Washington, DC: U. S. Department of Health and Human Services.

Schultz, R. (2005). Developmental deficits in social perception in autism: the role of the amygdala and fusiform face area. *International Journal of Developmental Neuroscience, 23,* 125–141.

Schwartz, I. S., & Baer, D. M. (1991). Social validity assessments: Is current practice state of the art? *Journal of Applied Behavior Analysis, 24,* 189–204.

Sher, L., & Stanley, B. H. (2008). The role of endogenous opioids in the pathophysiology of self-injurious and suicidal behavior. *Archives of Suicide Research, 12,* 299–308.

Silverman, K. J., Watanabe, K., Marshall, A. M., & Baer, D. M. (1984). Reducing self-injury and corresponding self-restraint through the strategic use of protective clothing. *Journal of Applied Behavior Analysis, 17,* 545–552.

Skinner, B. F. (1953). *Science and human behavior.* New York: Macmillan.

Smith, R. G., Iwata, B. A., Vollmer, T. R., & Pace, G. M. (1992). On the relationship between self-injurious behavior and self-restraint. *Journal of Applied Behavior Analysis, 25,* 433–445.

Smith, R. G., Lerman, D. C., & Iwata, B. A. (1996). Self-restraint as a positive reinforcement for self-injurious behavior. *Journal of Applied Behavior Analysis, 29,* 99–102.

Sparrow, S. S., Cicchetti, D. V., & Balla, D. A. (2005). *Vineland II–Vineland Adaptive Behavior Scales (2nd ed.) teacher rating form manual.* Circle Pines, MN: AGS.

St. Petersburg-USA Orphanage Research Team. (2008). The effects of early social-emotional and relationship experience on the development of young orphanage children. *Monographs of the Society for Research in Child Development, 73,* 1–15.

Steiger, H., Koerner, N., Engelberg, M. J., Israel, M., Ng Ying Kin N. M., & Young, S. N. (2001). Self-destructiveness and serotonin function in bulimia nervosa. *Psychiatry Research, 103,* 15–26.

Symons, F. J. (2002). Pain and self-injury: mechanisms and models. In S. Schroeder, T. Thompson, & M. L. Oster-Granite (Eds.), *Self-injurious behavior: genes, brain, and behavior* (pp. 223–234). Washington, DC: American Psychological Association.

Symons, F. J., Koppekin, A., & Wehby, J. H. (1999). Treatment of self-injurious behavior and quality of life for persons with mental retardation. *Mental Retardation, 37,* 297–307.

Symons, F. J., Sperry, L. A., Dropik, P. L., & Bodfish, J. W. (2005). The early development of stereotypy and self-injury: A review of research methods. *Journal of Intellectual Disability Research, 49,* 144–158.

Symons, F. J., Thompson, A., & Rodriguez, M. C. (2004). Self-injurious behavior and the efficacy of naltrexone treatment: a quantitative synthesis. *Mental Retardation and Developmental Research Reviews, 10,* 193–200.

Szatmari, P., Georgiades, S., Bryson, S., Zwaigenbaum, L., Roberts, W., Mahoney, W., et al. (2006). Investigating the structure of the restricted, repetitive behaviours and interests domain of autism. *Journal of Child Psychology and Psychiatry and Allied Disciplines, 47,* 582–590.

Tarou, L. R., Bloomsmith, M. A., & Maple, T. L. (2005). Survey of stereotypic behavior in prosimians. *American Journal of Primatology, 65,* 181–196.

Tate, B. G., & Baroff, G. S. (1966). Aversive control of self-injurious behavior in a psychotic boy. *Behaviour Research and Therapy, 4,* 281–287.

Thelen, E. (1981). Rhythmical behavior in infancy: An ethological perspective. *Developmental Psychology, 17,* 237–257.

Thompson, T., & Caruso, M. (2002). Self-injury: Knowing what we're looking for. In S. Schroeder, M. L. Oster-Granite, & T. Thompson (Eds.), *Self-injurious behavior: Gene-brain-behavior relationships* (pp. 3–21). Washington, DC: APA.

Tiefenbacher, S., Davenport, M. D., Novak, M. A., Pouliot, A. L., & Meyer, J. S. (2003). Fenfluramine challenge, self-injurious behavior, and aggression in rhesus monkeys. *Physiology and Behavior, 80,* 327–331.

Tröster, H., Brambring, M., & Beelmann, A. (1991). Prevalence and situational causes of stereotyped behaviors in blind infants and preschoolers. *Journal of Abnormal Child Psychology, 19,* 569–590.

Ungerstedt, U. (1968). 6-Hydroxydopamine induced degeneration of central monoamine neurons. *European Journal of Pharmacology, 5,* 107–110.

Vandebroek, I., Berchmoes, V., & Odberg, F. O. (1998). Dissociation between MK-801- and captivity-induced stereotypies in bank voles. *Psychopharmacology (Berl)*, *137*, 205–214.

Vollmer, T. R., & Vorndran, C. M. (1998). Assessment of self-injurious behavior maintained by access to self-restraint materials. *Journal of Applied Behavior Analysis*, *31*, 647–650.

Wallace, M. D., Doney, J. K., Mintz-Resudek, C. M., and Tarbox, R. S. F. (2004). Training educators to implement functional analyses. *Journal of Applied Behavior Analysis*, *37*, 89–92.

Waters, A. J., Nicol, C. J., & French, N. P. (2002). Factors influencing the development of stereotypic and redirected behaviours in young horses: findings of a four year prospective epidemiological study. *Equine Veterinary Journal*, *34*, 572–579.

Weld, K. P., Mench, J. A., Woodward, R. A., Bolesta, M. S., Suomi, S. J., & Higley, J. D. (1998). Effect of tryptophan treatment on self-biting and central nervous system serotonin metabolism in rhesus monkeys (Macaca mulatta). *Neuropsychopharmacology*, *19*, 314–321.

White, T., & Schultz, S. K. (2000). Naltrexone treatment for a 3-year-old boy with self-injurious behavior. *American Journal of Psychiatry*, *157*, 1574–1582.

Wing, L. (1969). The handicaps of autistic children: A comparative study. *Journal of Child Psychology and Psychiatry*, *10*, 1–40.

Wolery, M., Kirk, K., & Gast, D. L. (1985). Stereotypic behavior as a reinforcer: Effects and side effects. *Journal of Autism and Developmental Disorders*, *15*, 149–161.

Wolfer, D. P., Litvin, O., Morf, S., Nitsch, R. M., Lipp, H. P., & Würbel, H. (2004). Laboratory animal welfare: cage enrichment and mouse behaviour. *Nature*, *432*, 821–822.

Würbel, H. (2001). Ideal homes? Housing effects on rodent brain and behaviour. *Trends in Neurosciences*, *24*, 207–211.

22 Matthew W. Mosconi, Yukari Takarae, John A. Sweeney

Motor Functioning and Dyspraxia in Autism Spectrum Disorders

Points of Interest

- Motor impairments are present in the majority of individuals with ASD and may include deficits in vestibular functions, fine and gross motor abilities, eye movements, motor learning, and complex motor sequencing.
- Motor systems lend themselves to translational studies in ASD because their neurophysiological substrates are well defined via animal and human lesion studies, they have quantifiable spatial and temporal characteristics, and they can be administered to individuals across the autism spectrum with a range of cognitive disability.
- Neurophysiological, neuroimaging, and histological studies have identified alterations in ASD in multiple brain regions involved in motor functions, including sensorimotor cortices, basal ganglia, cerebellum, and brainstem nuclei.
- Motor disturbances appear to be among the first manifestations of developmental abnormalities in ASD and thus could serve as biomarkers of disease detectable in the first years of life.
- New family data on eye movement impairments suggests similar profiles in unaffected first-degree relatives and probands, indicating that these deficits may be familial and could serve as viable intermediate phenotypes for family-genetic research.

Investigation of neurobehavioral aspects of autism spectrum disorders (ASD; including autism, Asperger's syndrome, and Pervasive Developmental Disorder-NOS) primarily has focused on an analysis of abnormalities in complex cognitive operations including social cognition, communication, and executive functioning, which represent the defining clinical characteristics of the disorder. However, recent behavioral, neurophysiological, neuroimaging, and histological evidence suggests that motor system development is also abnormal in ASD. These observations highlight the need for systematic investigation of the developmental trajectory and causes of atypical motor function and dyspraxia (i.e., difficulty in planning and executing sequences of movements) in these disorders.

Histology: The study of microscopic anatomy of brain cells performed by examining slices of tissue under a light microscope or electron microscope.

Dyspraxia: The partial loss of the ability to coordinate and perform purposeful movements and gestures that is not accounted for by other primary motor or sensory impairments.

Neurobehavioral studies of ASD have more recently devoted increased attention to dyspraxia, postulating that impairments in learning complex motor sequences may relate to social communication deficits such as impaired imitation (Dapretto et al., 2006; Martineau, Cochin, Magne, & Barthelemy, 2008; Williams et al., 2006b). While there is evidence for impairment in learning complex motor behaviors in the context of social interaction, these impairments also include more basic motor functions that are not specific to social learning. Converging evidence from behavioral and neurophysiological research (see below) indicate that individuals with ASD demonstrate deficits in vestibular control, gross and fine motor movements, and eye movements, and they are dyspraxic when performing both social and nonsocial behaviors.

Kanner (1943) and Asperger (1944, as translated by Frith, 1991) each noted a diverse set of motor atypicalities in their original case studies, including hand and finger stereotypies, lack of appropriate posturing in response to being held among young children, awkward motility, slow reflexes, delays in walking and an absence of crawling, and overall clumsiness. Motor abnormalities consistent with these observations have since been documented in more systematic analyses. These studies have identified impairments in vestibular functions (Baranek, 1999; Bryson et al., 2007; Gepner, Mestre, Masson, &

de Schonen, 1995; Kohen-Raz, Volkmar, & Cohen, 1992; Minshew, Sung, Jones, & Furman, 2004; Molloy, Dietrich, & Bhattacharya, 2003; Teitelbaum, Teitelbaum, Nye, Fryman, & Maurer, 1998), gross (e.g., Jansiewicz et al., 2006; Rinehart, Tonge, Bradshaw, Iansek, Enticott, & McGinley, 2006b; Vernazza-Martin et al., 2005) and fine motor skills (e.g., Freitag, Kleser, Schneider, & von Gontard, 2007; Green et al., 2002; Williams, Goldstein, & Minshew, 2006a), eye movements (e.g., Takarae, Minshew, Luna, Krisky, & Sweeney, 2004a; Takarae, Minshew, Luna, & Sweeney, 2004b; Thakkar et al., 2008), complex motor sequences (e.g., Dziuk et al., 2007; Rogers, Bennetto, McEvoy, & Pennington, 1996), and motor learning (e.g., Haswell, Izawa, Dowell, Mostofsky, & Shadmehr, 2009; D'Cruz et al., 2009). Still, current classification systems devote minimal attention to this area of impairment. The *Diagnostic and Statistical Manual–Fourth Edition* includes motor stereotypies within the restricted, repetitive behavior domain. It also notes that nonspecific neurological symptoms may be present, including primitive reflexes and delayed development of hand dominance (American Psychiatric Association [APA], 2000). Further, abnormalities of posture are noted to be characteristic of autism, and "motor clumsiness" is described as a feature of Asperger's disorder. The potential utility of disturbances of motor systems and dyspraxia to diagnostic practice remains largely unexplored, however, as does the potential of investigations of disturbances in these domains to clarify ASD pathophysiology.

Stereotypies: Nonpurposeful repetitive, ritualistic movements, postures, or utterances.

Motor system dysfunction affects a myriad of behaviors and thus may have critical implications for the development of core social and cognitive deficits in ASD. For example, early emerging dyspraxia and motor imitation deficits reported in children with ASD (see Williams, Whiten, & Singh, 2004, for a review) are known to affect oromotor skill development and concomitant maturation of language ability (Mandelbaum et al., 2006; Rogers, Hepburn, Stackhouse, & Wehner, 2003). Similarly, impaired visual pursuit ability, as demonstrated previously in ASD (Takarae et al., 2004a), may limit children's ability to visually follow shifts in eye gaze and attention that are inherent in social referencing and joint attention. Delays in basic motor operations and vestibular control also have been noted in individuals with ASD, including abnormal postural stability (Minshew et al., 2004). Similarly, gross and fine motor deficits are observed clinically and consistently have been identified in comprehensive neuropsychological investigations of children (Williams et al., 2006a) and adolescents and adults with ASD (Freitag et al., 2007; Ming, Brimacombe, & Wagner, 2007; Minshew, Goldstein, & Siegel, 1997). Hypotonia and dyspraxia are common in ASD, with estimated prevalence rates of 25% to 51% and 34% to 75% respectively (Ming et al., 2007; Rapin, 1996). Motor deficits also are observed in approximately 80% of genetic syndromes currently known to be associated with ASD, suggesting clear advantages in studying motor disturbances in ASD for understanding etiological pathways (Abrahams & Geschwind, 2010). Taken together, these observations indicate that motor impairments are related to alterations in widely distributed neural networks, including those involved in vestibular control, gross motor movements such as walking, fine motor skill movements, oculomotor processes, and motor praxis.

Hypotonia: Disorder that causes low muscle tone (the amount of tension or resistance to movement in a muscle), often involving reduced muscle strength.

Multiple factors unique to motor impairments make them ideally suited for studies of atypical brain maturation in ASD (see Table 22-1). First, neural system correlates of motor

Table 22–1.
Factors supporting increased research focus on motor development in ASD

- Current neurobehavioral studies suggest that motor impairments are present in the majority of individuals with ASD. These deficits affect multiple motor systems, including those involved in vestibular functions, fine and gross motor abilities, eye movements, motor learning, and motor sequencing.
- Neural systems underlying motor behavior are well mapped via animal and human studies, making studies of motor development directly translational.
- Neurophysiological, neuroimaging, and histological studies implicate brain regions involved in motor functions, including sensorimotor cortices, basal ganglia, cerebellum, and brain stem nuclei.
- Motor disturbances appear to be among the first manifestations of developmental abnormalities in ASD and thus could serve as biomarkers of this disorder detectable in the first years of life. These deficits also may contribute to a cascade of social-communication and cognitive deficits.
- Approximately 80% of genetic syndromes currently known to be associated with ASD are characterized by motor impairments, suggesting several candidate genetic mechanisms.
- Family studies of motor deficits suggest similar profiles in unaffected first-degree relatives and probands. These findings indicate that motor impairments may be familial and could serve as viable intermediate phenotypes for genetic studies.
- Minimal task demands relative to higher-order cognitive/behavioral paradigms make motor tasks more suitable for young children and individuals with cognitive impairment.
- Practice effects for motor tasks are relatively modest compared to cognitive paradigms, making motor tasks more suitable for longitudinal studies.
- Precise quantitative measurements of temporal and spatial components of motor behaviors are available, enabling detailed models of neural system dysfunction.

behavior are well understood via studies of neurological conditions involving focal brain lesions, unit recording studies with behaving nonhuman primates, and functional neuroimaging studies. These studies have laid a foundation for translational research to develop better models of the links between brain and behavioral abnormalities in ASD. As an example, studies of patients with cerebellar damage including the vermis reveal failures to modulate the amplitude of eye movements when fatigued or during adaptation paradigms (Golla et al., 2008; Xu-Wilson, Chen-Harris, Zee, & Shadmehr, 2009). In contrast, patients with cerebellar lesions that do not extend to the vermis do not show deficits on these paradigms. These findings are compelling in the context of studies documenting Purkinje cellular abnormalities within the vermis in ASD (Bailey et al., 1998; Kemper & Bauman, 2002) and hypoplasia of oculomotor vermal lobules VI–VII (see Stanfield et al., 2008, for a meta-analysis). Second, in contrast to studies of higher-order cognition that rely on tasks that cannot be readily applied to animal models, motor system studies are directly translational, since identical behaviors can be studied in human and animal models under identical task conditions. Third, the understanding of complex task instructions that is required for many higher cognitive tasks is not relevant for motor system studies, so motor system studies using identical task conditions can be conducted across a wide range of age and general cognitive abilities. Fourth, practice effects are relatively modest with motor system studies compared to higher-order cognitive tasks (Kida, Oda, & Matsumura, 2005), so that they are particularly suitable for longitudinal studies of developmental processes. Fifth, precise quantitative measurements of motor behaviors are available, making it possible to study temporal and spatial dynamics of relevant neural operations in detail. Sixth, motor impairments are among the first manifestations of developmental abnormalities in ASD. They are present in infants later diagnosed with ASD (Teitelbaum et al., 1998) and predict the severity of clinical symptoms that emerge later in life (Dziuk et al., 2007; Gernsbacher, Sauer, Geye, Schweigert, & Hill, 2008). Additionally, although motor impairments alone are not sufficient for early identification of ASD (Provost, Lopez, & Heimerl, 2007), distinct patterns of motor impairments might be associated with unique patterns of development in ASD, such as early emergent or regressive courses (Ozonoff et al., 2008). Hence, assessment of motor skills might be useful for predicting developmental pathways for particular individuals and thus applying more individualized treatments and interventions. Finally, motor impairments might provide viable quantitative familial phenotypes associated with particular subtypes within ASD. For instance, unaffected parents of children with ASD have oculomotor impairments that are similar to those in affected individuals (Koczat, Rogers, Pennington, & Ross, 2002; Mosconi, Kay, D'Cruz, Guter, Kapur, et al., 2010) suggesting that certain eye movement impairments and associated neurophysiological alterations might be useful phenotypes for genetic research.

Cerebellar vermis: Narrow central structure within the cerebellum between the two hemispheres.

Purkinje cells: GABAergic neurons located in the cerebellar cortex and vermis that are the sole output of the cerebellar cortex to deep cerebellar nuclei.

Phenotype: Observable characteristics or traits of an organism, including morphology, development, or physiological properties, that result from the expression of an organism's genes as well as the influence of environmental factors.

Despite the multiple advantages of motor system research for resolving important questions about the pathophysiology of ASD, progress in understanding these disturbances has been modest. The generalizability of many studies of motor impairments in ASD has been limited by small sample sizes that cannot adequately account for biological and behavioral heterogeneity, reliance on clinical ratings rather than objective measurements of motor system function, a lack of longitudinal data that is necessary for understanding changes in motor deficits over the course of development, and failures to compare patients to suitable control samples (e.g., IQ-matched controls).

Motor System Neurophysiology and Its Dysfunction in ASD

Several distinct but highly interacting sensorimotor systems exist within the human central nervous system, reflecting the diversity of our motor capabilities. Cortico-cortical, cortico-striatal, and cortico-thalamo-cerebellar loops each innervate lower motor neurons indirectly through the brain stem (Dum & Strick, 1992; He, Dum, & Strick, 1993, 1995). Histological and single-cell recording studies of nonhuman primates indicate that efferent cortical pathways related to motor control predominantly derive from frontal cortex (Dum & Strick, 1991), including the primary motor cortex (Brodmann's area 4) and the lateral and medial zones of premotor cortex (Brodmann's area 6), as well as from the intraparietal sulcus and inferior parietal lobule (Brodmann's areas 5 and 7; Leichnetz, 2001; Cavada & Goldman-Rakic, 1989). While the primary motor and premotor areas of the frontal lobe are essential for the execution of basic and complex motor acts, supplementary motor areas, prefrontal cortex (PFC) and parietal cortex have been shown to be involved in the planning of complex motor sequences (Catalan, Honda, Weeks, Cohen, & Hallett, 1998; Grafton, Hazeltine, & Ivry, 2002; Honda et al., 1998). Frontoparietal integrity is therefore critical for efficiently executing everyday motor sequences and gestures, likely because integrating motor planning with spatial perceptual processes is necessary in order to optimize motor plans and actions. Disturbances in frontoparietal function are associated with dyspraxia, and thus are implicated by demonstrations of dyspraxia and imitation impairments in individuals with ASD (Dowell, Mahone, & Mostofsky, 2009; Dziuk et al., 2007; Jansiewicz et al., 2006; Rogers et al., 1996).

In addition to frontoparietal systems, frontostriatal loops contribute to the execution and inhibition of motor output (DeLong & Strick, 1974). The basal ganglia is a network of subcortical gray matter structures, including the caudate nucleus, putamen, globus pallidus, and substantia nigra, that are involved in the planning, initiation, and inhibition of motor commands (DeLong, 1990; Kaji, 2001). Frontal cortical inputs into the basal ganglia are excitatory and involve glutamatergic innervations that synapse with neurons in the caudate nucleus and putamen (Pollack, 2001), two structures collectively referred to as the "corpus striatum." Dopaminergic neurons in the substantia nigra also provide input to the striatum (Khan et al., 2000; Yung et al., 1995). Direct and indirect pathways project to the globus pallidus and modulate ventral thalamic nuclei output to primary motor and premotor cortices, thus completing frontostriatal loops that are crucial for initiating and inhibiting goal-directed movements (Alexander, Crutcher, & DeLong, 1990; Rolls, 1994). Dysfunction within the basal ganglia can cause failures in motor inhibition, manifesting as repetitive motor movements or stereotypies similar to those observed in people with ASD (Ames, Cummings, Wirshing, Quinn, & Mahler, 1994; Canales & Graybiel, 2000). Additionally, some individuals with ASD show slowed walking patterns similar to patients with Parkinson's disease (Damasio & Maurer, 1978; Mari, Castiello, Marks, Marraffa, & Prior, 2003; Vernazza-Martin et al., 2005; Vilensky, Damasio, & Maurer, 1981), a disorder involving reduced dopaminergic input to the striatum (Dauer & Przedborski, 2003).

Motor commands generated through frontoparietal and frontostriatal loops are subsequently adjusted by the cerebellum (Houk & Wise, 1995; Ito, 1984; Stein & Glickstein, 1992). The cerebellum detects deviations between an intended movement and actual movement to correct motor output in real time. Through its projections to primary and premotor cortices, the cerebellum reduces these deviations in future planned action (Ohyama, Nores, Murphy, & Mauk, 2003). The cerebellum thus acts to continuously modulate motor behavior on line and enable more precise performance. These functions primarily are performed via the coordination of signals from motor cortices relayed to the cerebellum via pontine nuclei, where motor intentions and consequences of motor acts are compared (Brodal, 1978). Efferent pathways exiting deep cerebellar nuclei, including the dentate nuclei, interpositus nuclei, and fastigial nuclei, through the superior cerebellar peduncle, continuously modulate motor output via thalamic and brain stem projections (Middleton & Strick, 1997; 2001). Disturbances to cortico-cerebellar systems thus lead to ataxia or failures to accurately coordinate planned motor behavior (Timmann et al., 2008). In addition, the cerebellar vermis is involved in motor learning and adaptation. The vermis mediates implicit motor learning and oculomotor control in nonhuman and human primates (Catz & Thier, 2007; Soetedjo, Kojima, & Fuchs, 2008; Takagi, Tamargo, & Zee, 2003; Takagi, Zee, & Tamargo, 1998; 2000; Thier, Dicke, Haas, Thielert, & Catz, 2002). Gait abnormalities (Damasio et al., 1978; Esposito & Venuti, 2008; Hallett et al., 1993; Rinehart et al., 2006b; Rinehart, Tonge, Iansek, et al., 2006c; Teitelbaum et al., 1998; Vernazza-Martin et al., 2005) and alterations in oculomotor control (Takarae et al., 2004a; Takarae et al., 2004b) in individuals with ASD have parallels with movement abnormalities of patients with cerebellar lesions implicating cerebellar dysfunction in ASD.

Ataxia: Gross lack of coordination of muscle movements often implicating cerebellar dysfunction.

Vestibular Modulation of Motor Control in ASD

Both the vestibular nuclei and the reticular formation help control posture in response to perturbations of the body in space (Keshner & Cohen, 1989). The vestibular nuclei make adjustments according to information from the inner ear, while the reticular formation controls postural stability based on an integration of inputs from motor centers in the cortex, basal ganglia, and brain stem (Drew, Prentice, & Schepens, 2004; Fitzpatrick & Day, 2004). These movements often are anticipatory, such as the excitation of lower limb muscles prior to lifting a heavy object. The reticular formation, therefore, is part of a feedforward motor planning process that initially stabilizes the body by altering posture and then, via its connections with the cerebellum, readjusts body position to maintain stability during the performance of motor actions (Kennedy, Ross, & Brooks, 1982).

Abnormalities in postural control have been reported in individuals with ASD, but these abnormalities have not been observed consistently when individuals were compared with IQ-matched control subjects, or beyond the first years of life. Baranek (1999) observed abnormal postural behaviors in 9- to 12-month-old children later diagnosed with ASD relative to typically developing children, but the children later diagnosed with ASD did not differ in their rate of abnormal posturing relative to age- and IQ-matched infants. Bryson and colleagues (2007) reported poor motor stability at age 6 months in three out of nine infants later diagnosed with ASD. Teitelbaum and colleagues (1998) reported that a small (3/3) subset of infants later diagnosed with ASD demonstrated abnormalities in early postural control, including sitting upright and righting from supine to prone position. These results are difficult to interpret because quantitative data regarding either behavior are not provided, and because only three children were observed. In contrast, more consistent deficits were observed for behaviors involving the coordination of complex motor movements of the arms, such as crawling. Kanner (1943) observed inconsistent postural control disturbances among his patients with ASD. He noted that multiple children did not demonstrate changes in their posture in response to being held. Failures to alter posture in response to being held could reflect disturbances in vestibular control or could be attributable to poor social awareness in developing infants with ASD. Follow-up examination of the constituent components underlying abnormal postural responses in young infants identified with ASD now may be more clearly teased apart with the advent of infant sibling studies and retrospective videotape analyses that allow children later diagnosed with ASD to have their behavior within the first year of life retrospectively reviewed.

Studies of postural control in children beyond the first years of life and adults with ASD have been inconsistent, possibly due to differences in patient and control sample characteristics. The first quantitative study of postural control in ASD examined a large sample (N = 91) of cognitively impaired children and adults with ASD who were not age-matched with their non-ASD cognitively impaired subjects (Kohen-Raz et al., 1992). The ASD and non-ASD cognitively impaired subjects had underdeveloped postural stability relative to the typically developing controls, but only the subjects with ASD showed paradoxically superior stability when vision was occluded or somatosensory input was obstructed. These observations have not been replicated by subsequent studies that have noted decreased postural stability in children with ASD, but increased postural stability with visually perceptible external motion and more profound deficits when vision was occluded (Gepner & Mestre, 2002; Molloy et al., 2003). It is not clear why the original Kohen-Raz et al. paradoxical vision occlusion findings for postural stability have not been replicated, but these results may point to significant heterogeneity along the autism spectrum in motor dysfunction that may be unique to individuals with cognitive impairment. A more recent dynamic posturography study of a large sample of children and adults with ASD (N = 79) indicated that non–mentally retarded individuals with ASD have underdeveloped postural stability that is disproportionate under conditions in which somatosensory input is disrupted (Minshew et al., 2004). Examining cross-sectional data, the authors also suggested that the development of postural stability was delayed in children with ASD and that it does not achieve healthy adult levels in adulthood. The deficits observed across these studies suggest that postural instability is evident in at least a subset of individuals with ASD and not unique to those individuals with cognitive impairment.

Currently, several questions remain unanswered regarding postural stability mechanisms in ASD: (1) Do observed deficits in postural control affect only a minor subset of individuals with ASD (e.g., those with cognitive impairment) and under specific conditions (e.g., when sensory input is eliminated), or do a greater proportion of affected individuals show subtle alterations when laboratory-based analyses of behavior are performed? (2) Are these abnormalities more prominent within the first year of life? (3) Are abnormalities in the development of postural stability evident exclusively in social contexts as suggested by observations that infants with ASD do not conform to physical gestures of caregivers? and (4) Is postural dyscontrol, if present, stable over time or does it reflect delayed maturation of brain stem circuitries that eventually "catch up" to normative trajectories? Further research is needed to address these questions.

Gross Motor Impairments in Individuals with ASD

Gross motor deficits observed in individuals with ASD suggest that both corticostriatal and corticocerebellar circuits are affected. Kanner (1943) originally reported that some children with autism walk late, walk clumsily, and/or never crawl prior to walking. Similarly, Asperger (1944, as translated by Frith, 1991) noted consistent clumsiness among the patients that he studied, suggesting that a broad range of motor abilities are impacted and that these disturbances persist throughout development. Disentangling the role of frontostriatal and corticocerebellar systems in the gross motor disturbances characteristic of autism and Asperger's disorder has been difficult. Some researchers have suggested that the "autistic gait" is similar to that of individuals with Parkinson's disease, characterized by bradykinesia, longer movement duration and deceleration, and lower peak velocity (Damasio et al., 1978; Mari et al., 2003; Vernazza-Martin et al., 2005; Vilensky et al., 1981), indicating that patterns of impaired motor preparation and inhibition evidenced in ASD may reflect frontostriatal pathology. Still, findings from several studies of early gait characteristics have been more consistent with patterns of cerebellar, rather than basal ganglia dysfunction. Rinehart and colleagues (Rinehart et al., 2006b) reported that, subsequent to learning to walk, children with ASD show persistent atypical gait with increased variation in overall stride length similar to patients with cerebellar ataxia. Their qualitative ratings of gait parameters revealed that both individuals with autism and individuals with Asperger's disorder were less coordinated, smooth, and consistent. Individuals with autism showed abnormal arm postures likely reflecting poor balance, and individuals with Asperger's disorder evidenced head and trunk postural atypicalities that may reflect interference of the frontostriatal motor preparation network. Esposito and Venuti (Esposito et al., 2008) found that, relative to developmentally delayed children without ASD and typically developing children, children diagnosed with ASD who were within their first six months of walking had problems performing typical heel-to-toe transfers of weight while walking, showed asymmetric postures of their arms while walking, and exhibited increased rates of a "waddling" walking style, again similar to patterns evidenced by some patients with cerebellar abnormalities. The picture is not entirely clear, however, as these same individuals further showed stereotyped movements while walking, implicating frontostriatal systems. Gait disturbances thus are documented in both individuals with autism and individuals with Asperger's disorder, and each subgroup demonstrates early emerging atypicalities that include poor balance and postural stability. While these behavioral disturbances reflect, at least in part, basal ganglia dysfunction, they are not identical to the pronounced bradykinesia and motor initiation/inhibition deficits characteristic of Parkinson's disease patients. Similarly, overlap with patients experiencing cerebellar ataxia is considerable but not complete.

Bradykinesia: Slowness of movement due to dysfunction of the basal ganglia and related structures.

Disturbances in these circuits emerge early and thus may be useful as screening indices early in development. In a study of parents' first concerns regarding their developing children with ASD, Chawarska and colleagues (2007) indicated that, next to reduced rates of sharing enjoyment, the primary indicator was delay in walking. Teitelbaum and colleagues also observed gross motor and sequential motor movement abnormalities by age 3 to 6 months in infants later diagnosed with autism (1998) and those later diagnosed with Asperger's disorder (2004). The most consistent abnormalities observed were lateralized asymmetries in crawling and walking as well as poor sequencing of component behaviors implicating corticostriatal circuitry and cerebellar feedback loops. Gross motor disturbances have been reported for children with ASD beyond the first years of life as well. Ahsgren and colleagues (2005) reported that 31/32 children and adolescents with ASD demonstrated some form of ataxia consistent with cerebellar pathology. Williams and colleagues (2006a) indicated that 8-year-old children with ASD without cognitive impairments show deficits in manual motor strength relative to age- and IQ- matched healthy controls. Hallett and colleagues (1993) reported that 4/5 adults with autism showed mild clumsiness and upper limb posturing during gait. Finally, Vernazza-Martin and colleagues (2005) reported that children with ASD walk with smaller steps and more irregular oscillation of upper limbs, head, and trunk than age-matched non-ASD children. Taken together, these findings indicate that the sequential processing of complex motor movements involving corticostriatal circuitry as well as the calibration of these movements modulated by corticocerebellar circuits are disrupted in ASD, and that these deficits present as delays within the first year of life and continue to manifest throughout childhood and later years as subtle deviations in gross motor coordination.

Neuroimaging studies aiming to define the neural pathways associated with motor disturbances in ASD have yielded inconsistent results likely due to limitations in early MRI capabilities (e.g., reduced resolution), small sample sizes in the context of biological and behavioral heterogeneity, and failures to assess widely distributed networks involving long-distance connective white matter fiber tracts and their terminal fields. The ability to investigate grey and white matter volumes with standard MR sequences, white matter tracts through diffusion tensor imaging (DTI) and functional activation and connectivity with fMRI, ERP, and PET, now make it possible to simultaneously study the anatomic and neurophysiological substrates of motor dysfunction.

MRI studies of the basal ganglia in ASD have suggested that the caudate nucleus is enlarged (Haznedar et al., 2006; Hollander et al., 2005; Langen, Durston, Staal, Palmen, & van Engeland, 2007; Langen et al., 2009; Rojas et al., 2006; Sears et al., 1999; Stanfield et al., 2008, but see Hardan, Kilpatrick, Keshavan, & Minshew, 2003; McAlonan et al., 2008, for discrepant results), although it is unclear whether this enlargement is disproportionate to overall brain enlargement (Herbert et al., 2003), consistent across affected individuals (Hardan et al., 2003; McAlonan et al., 2008), and/or specific to the caudate nuclei as opposed to other striatal gray matter (McAlonan et al., 2008). Still, an association between caudate volume and repetitive motor behaviors in ASD has been reported (Hazlett, Poe, Smith, Gerig, & Piven, 2005; Hollander et al., 2005; Rojas et al., 2006; Sears et al., 1999) suggesting that the caudate nucleus is involved in some motor abnormalities in ASD.

Studies of the cerebellum in ASD also have yielded inconsistent findings. Studies of selective hypoplasia of vermal lobules VI–VII (Courchesne, Yeung-Courchesne, Press, Hesselink, & Jernigan, 1988; Hashimoto et al., 1995; Kaufmann et al., 2003; Schaefer et al., 1996) have not always been replicated (Holttum, Minshew, Sanders, & Phillips, 1992; Kleiman, Neff, & Rosman, 1992; Manes et al., 1999; Piven, Saliba, Bailey, & Arndt, 1997), owing perhaps to the fact that confounding factors (i.e., comparability of IQ in cases and controls) are not consistently taken into account. In contrast, histopathological studies provide strong and consistent evidence for cerebellar pathology in ASD. Reduced density of GABAergic Purkinje cells of the cerebellar vermis (50% to 60% cell loss) and hemispheres (42% cell loss) along with reduced granule cell number are the most consistent and frequently reported neuropathological findings in ASD (Bailey et al., 1998; Bauman, 1991; Bauman & Kemper, 1985, 2005; Ritvo et al., 1986). In one study, reduced Purkinje cell number and size in vermian lobules VI–VII and VIII–X was noted in all ASD cases examined (Arin, Bauman, & Kemper, 1991). This pathology may be related to comorbid seizure disorders (Crooks, Mitchell, & Thom, 2000) as subsequent analyses have indicated that only about half of postmortem cases show reduced Purkinje cell density (Whitney, Kemper, Bauman, Rosene, & Blatt, 2008). Further evidence for cerebellar pathology is found in studies of glutamate decarboxylase (GAD) 65 and 67, isoform tracers that catalyze glutamate to GABA within the cerebellum. Studies of GAD 65 and 67 reveal reduced isoforms in Purkinje cells (Yip, Soghomonian, & Blatt, 2007, 2009), and increased GAD67 production within basket and stellate cells (Yip, Soghomonian, & Blatt, 2008). More recent investigations of white matter integrity within the cerebellum indicate that intrahemispheric and efferent white matter tracts show decreased fractional anisotropy (an index of white matter integrity) in individuals with Asperger's disorder (Catani et al., 2008). Although the precise mechanisms contributing to reduced fractional anisotropy within the cerebellum are not known, these findings suggest that connective pathways within the cerebellum and pathways projecting from the cerebellum to brain stem and thalamus are abnormal in ASD. The functional significance of cerebellar pathology remains unclear, and likely is diverse. However, the consistency of cerebellar pathology findings in ASD, the central role for the cerebellum in motor control, and the consistency of findings of disrupted motor control in ASD together highlight the importance of corticocerebellar circuitry in motor control dysfunction in patients with ASD.

Hypoplasia: Underdevelopment of an organ reflecting a decreased number of cells.

Granule cells: Tiny cells found within the innermost granular layer of the cerebellum and other brain regions, including the hippocampus and olfactory bulbs.

Basket and stellate cells: GABAergic interneurons that synapse with Purkinje cells within the molecular layer of the cerebellum.

Fractional anisotropy: A scalar value between 0 and 1 used to describe the degree of anisotropy of a diffusion process. This value is often extracted from diffusion tensor images (DTI) to index the integrity of white matter within the brain because water typically diffuses parallel to white matter tracts.

Fine Motor Impairments in Individuals with ASD

The neural control of fine motor manipulations involves neural systems that overlap considerably with those underlying gross motor movements, but these systems also require greater precision and rely on axons to more distal limbs. Premotor areas of the frontal lobe play a major role in the planning and control of complex and sequential voluntary movements (Kornhuber, 1978; Petrides, 2005). Distal and local motor pathways are dissociated at their origin, within the somatotopically organized motor cortex, and again diverge within the spinal cord (Dawnay & Glees, 1986).

Somatotopy: The correspondence of receptors in regions of the body via respective nerve fibers to specific functional areas of the cerebral cortex.

Although some early findings suggested that individuals with ASD show relatively superior (Jones & Prior, 1985) or intact (Ozonoff, Pennington, & Rogers, 1991; Rumsey & Hamburger, 1988) dexterity, subsequent studies utilizing increasingly sensitive assessment tools have documented consistent patterns of deficit in children and adolescents with ASD (Freitag et al., 2007; Ghaziuddin, 2008; Green et al., 2002; Mostofsky, Burgess, & Gidley Larson, 2007; Vanvuchelen, Roeyers, & De Weerdt, 2007). Comprehensive neuropsychological studies of large samples of children (N = 56, Williams et al., 2006a) and adults (N = 33, Minshew et al., 1997) have indicated that performance on measures of motor strength, fine motor planning and motor speed is impaired in patients with ASD. These results suggest that both simple and complex motor behaviors are impacted, and that deficits are detectable with standardized neuropsychological measures across a large proportion of affected children and adults.

Consistent with large-scale neuropsychological studies, assessments of smaller samples of individuals with ASD have revealed fine motor abnormalities. Green and colleagues (2002) reported that 9 of 11 children with Asperger's syndrome ages 6.5 to 11.5 showed fine motor dexterity scores within the 5th percentile or lower relative to other children their age. Fourteen of 16 adolescent males with high-functioning autism or Asperger's syndrome studied by Freitag and colleagues (2007) demonstrated slowed alternation between prone and supine hand positions, as well as poor dynamic balance (i.e., jumping forward or side-to-side), each of which were associated with level of autistic symptomatology. Studies of graphomotor skills also suggest fine motor abnormalities, including demonstrations of macrographia (Beversdorf et al., 2001) and poor fine motor control (Mayes & Calhoun, 2003) in large samples of average-IQ and cognitively impaired children with ASD.

Impaired performance across gross and fine motor skills suggests that disturbances likely involve abnormalities of the upper motor neuron systems above the brain stem. Tracts involved in gross and fine motor skills diverge below the brain stem (Dawnay et al., 1986), so evidence that each set of abilities is affected in ASD to a relatively similar degree suggests a common supratentorial origin of motor impairments. Freitag and colleagues' (2007) finding that both gross and fine motor impairments are associated with the severity of autistic symptoms suggests that motor disturbances may contribute to the core traits of the disorder, or have pathophysiological mechanisms that relate to the causes of those traits.

Functional MRI studies of fine motor behavior in individuals with ASD directly implicate the basal ganglia and cerebellum. Mostofsky and colleagues (2009) reported that children with ASD ages 8 to 12 years demonstrated reduced ipsilateral anterior cerebellar activation and increased supplementary motor area activation relative to age- and IQ-matched controls during a finger tapping task. The authors also documented reduced coherence of activation between cortical and cerebellar regions of interest in ASD. Allen and Courchesne (2003) observed more diffuse cerebellar activation across lobules VI–VII among average-IQ patients with ASD performing a finger tapping task in which they received verbal cues to press a button as many times as possible within a fixed duration. Using an identical paradigm, Muller and colleagues (Muller,

Pierce, Ambrose, Allen, & Courchesne, 2001) identified decreased frontostriatal activation within eight participants with ASD suggesting that, despite the relative simplicity of these motor tasks and individuals' ability to perform the motor behaviors comparable to age-matched controls, robust alterations in frontostriatal and frontocerebellar networks in individuals with ASD are evident. Interestingly, Muller et al.'s results also highlighted increased activation in patients with ASD within areas typically not recruited for simple motor behaviors. These areas included precuneus, inferior parietal lobule, superior temporal gyrus, and PFC. Allen, Muller, and Courchesne (2004) suggest that disturbances of motor systems in ASD may show characteristics consistent with the "crowding effect" in which spared tissue performs the function of typically specialized brain regions that are dysfunctional (Teuber, 1974). It has been proposed that the functions normally subserved by more primitive systems, such as motor skills mediated by the paleocerebellum, are disrupted by aberrant Purkinje cell development, and that functions are subsequently carried out by more recently evolved systems within the neocerebellum and neocortex (Allen et al., 2004). The higher level neural system's ongoing need to compensate for disturbances in lower level systems in ASD may result in their being limited in their capacity to support the ontogenesis of higher-order cognitive operations such as executive functions and language. Evidence that areas not typically involved in fine motor manipulations are recruited for simple finger tapping tasks in ASD suggest that motor impairments could contribute to a cascade of effects disrupting developments in higher level systems that typically support complex cognitive operations.

Paleocerebellum: The anterior lobe of the cerebellum, which was one of the phylogenetically earliest parts of the hindbrain to develop in mammals.

Neocerebellum: The phylogenetically youngest part of the cerebellum comprising most of the cerebellar cortex and vermis.

Oculomotor Impairments in ASD

Oculomotor paradigms, which typically require sensory analysis, sensorimotor transformation, and motor control with varying levels of cognitive planning, are heavily dependent on effective integration of multiple neural systems. Brain regions that are involved in the control of eye movements include the PFC; frontal, parietal, and supplementary eye fields; basal ganglia; thalamus; superior colliculus; cerebellum; and brain stem. Structural magnetic resonance imaging and histological studies have documented that many of these brain areas are affected in ASD (Carper & Courchesne, 2005; Cody, Pelphrey, & Piven, 2002; Courchesne et al., 1988; Courchesne, Press, & Yeung-Courchesne, 1993; Sears et al., 1999; Tsatsanis et al., 2003). Consistent with these findings, several studies suggest that conjugate eye movements are abnormal in ASD (see below), including both saccades and smooth pursuit, and that these deficits may be familial (Koczat et al., 2002; Mosconi et al., 2010).

Saccade Impairments in Individuals with ASD

Saccades are rapid ballistic eye movements that are typically made to focus gaze on objects of interest. Studies of saccadic eye movements provide opportunities to examine relevant motor circuitry as well as higher-level cognitive processes that modulate the use of saccades in a context appropriate manner. Peak velocity of saccades is determined primarily by the brain stem, while accuracy of saccades heavily depends on the cerebellum, especially the cerebellar vermis. Latency of saccades is primarily determined by a balance between input from cortical eye fields and basal ganglia to the superior colliculus. The PFC provides top-down modulation of saccade planning and execution using context-relevant information and behavioral plans that continue over time (see Figure 22-1).

Exogenous Saccades

Findings from early studies suggested that brain circuitry supporting the planning and execution of saccades is intact in individuals with ASD when saccades are guided by exogenous

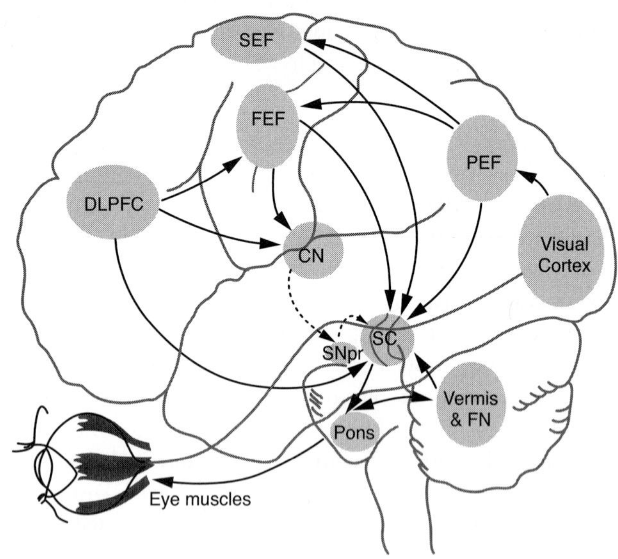

Figure 22-1. Lateral view of human cerebral cortex and projections to superior colliculus (SC) involved in saccade generation. Cortical and subcortical areas involved in oculomotor control, with excitatory and inhibitory pathways depicted in solid and broken lines, respectively. Direct excitatory pathways to the SC shown are from the dorsolateral prefrontal cortex (DLPFC), frontal eye fields (FEF), parietal eye fields (PEF), and supplementary eye fields (SEF). Indirect cortical input from the DLPFC and FEF are through the caudate nucleus (CN), which inhibits the SC. Cerebellar connections (vermis and fastigial nuclei [FN]) and pontine connections to the SC are also shown.

sensory information, such as the sudden appearance of visual targets (these saccades are often called prosaccades or visually guided saccades). Minshew, Luna, and Sweeney (1999) observed no abnormalities in average peak velocity, duration, latency, or accuracy of exogenous saccades in 26 adolescents and adults with ASD when they were compared to age-and IQ-matched typically developing subjects, suggesting brain circuitry supporting basic saccade planning and execution is intact. A more recent study that used higher resolution measures (Takarae et al., 2004b), however, reported greater trial-to-trial variability in saccade accuracy in a larger sample (n = 46) of individuals with ASD compared to age- and IQ-matched typically developing individuals. Increased trial-to-trial variations in saccade accuracy with lack of consistent alteration in average saccade accuracy in subjects with ASD is a pattern similar to effects seen after chronic lesions in lobules VI and VII in the cerebellar vermis, which are critical for achieving saccade accuracy (Thier, Dicke, Haas, & Barash, 2000). A potential link to the cerebellar vermis is also suggested by histological and MRI studies documenting abnormalities of the cerebellar vermis in ASD (Bailey et al., 1998; Cody et al., 2002; Courchesne et al., 1988; Kemper & Bauman, 1998; Ritvo et al., 1986).

Takarae and colleagues (2004b) compared the accuracy of exogenous saccades of subjects with ASD who had delays in early language acquisition with those who did not. While both ASD groups had increased trial-to-trial variability in saccade accuracy, the group who did not have early language delays also had saccadic hypometria (tendency to undershoot saccades relative to target locations). Thus, it is possible that some individuals with ASD without language delays have a different pattern of neural system dysfunction that involves more severe cerebellar impairments. Perhaps more importantly, these findings suggest that development of basic motor circuitry supporting exogenous saccades may be associated with a specific pattern of early cognitive development. A cross-sectional study by Luna and colleagues (2007) has shown that reduced average saccade accuracy is present in children with ASD, but not in adolescents or adults. Thus, reductions in saccade accuracy might be resolved by adolescence, possibly by compensatory mechanisms or delayed brain maturation.

A functional MRI study by Takarae and colleagues (2007) reported altered patterns of brain activation in individuals with ASD during execution of exogenous or visually guided saccades. They examined brain activation in 13 individuals with ASD and 14 age- and IQ-matched typically developing controls during performance of a visually guided saccade task. The ASD group had reduced activation relative to the control group in brain areas that are typically involved in executing exogenous saccades, including the frontal, supplementary, and parietal eye fields, and cerebellar hemispheres. This is consistent with the observed behavioral deficits, since these regions receive and utilize experience related to error in previous saccades from the cerebellum to reduce error in future saccades. More strikingly, the ASD group also demonstrated increased activation in the dorsolateral PFC, caudate, thalamus, and dentate nucleus, all of which are more typically involved in endogenous or cognitive control of saccadic eye movements and much less so during exogenous saccades in typically developing individuals. These observations parallel findings of compensatory neurocircuitry alterations in manual motor control studies discussed above (Mostofsky et al., 2009; Muller et al., 2001), and indicate that frontostriatal systems might be providing compensatory input to the sensorimotor circuitry during exogenous saccadic eye movements in individuals with ASD. This would suggest that PFC is called on to perform computational functions other than those for which it is specialized, which over the course of development might reduce its ability to perform its typical functions.

Some studies of exogenous saccades in ASD have used a temporal gap or an overlap between offset of central cue and presentation of peripheral targets to vary the level of attentional investment in the central cue location at the time a new peripheral target elicits a saccade. There have been reports, though inconsistent, of abnormal saccade latencies using exogenous saccade tasks with this type of manipulation. Van der Geest and colleagues (2001) reported no abnormalities of saccade latency in gap and overlap trials in 16 children with ASD and 15 age- and IQ-matched typically developing subjects. However, they did report a reduced difference between latencies in gap and overlap conditions that primarily resulted from shorter latencies among individuals with ASD in the overlap condition. Kawakubo and colleagues (2007) examined saccade latencies using a gap-overlap paradigm in 7 adults with PDD with mental retardation and 9 typically developing control subjects. They found shorter saccade latencies and increased rates of express saccades in overlap trials in subjects with ASD compared to controls. In contrast, Goldberg and colleagues (2002) reported longer saccade latencies in gap and overlap trials as well as trials with synchronous central cue offset and peripheral target onset in a sample of 11 adolescents with ASD compared to 11 age- and IQ-matched control subjects. Kawakubo and colleagues (2007) showed significantly longer saccade latencies during overlap trials in 17 adults with ASD and cognitive impairment when they were compared to chronological age–matched typically developing adults.

These studies, though not all using IQ- and age-matched comparison groups, demonstrated abnormalities in saccade latency in individuals with ASD when the task had higher demand for attention disengagement, suggesting dysregulation of visual spatial attention in ASD. Kawakubo and colleagues (2007) examined presaccadic event related potentials during a gap-overlap task in 17 adults with ASD and cognitive impairment. They found that presaccadic positive potentials that are related to disengagement of attention (Csibra, Johnson, & Tucker, 1997) were greater in participants with ASD compared to the IQ-matched control group with mental retardation or chronological age–matched control groups. These results suggest that deficits in attentional disengagement in ASD and underlying physiological abnormalities are specific to ASD and are not exclusively a generalized manifestation of cognitive impairment.

Endogenous Saccades

In contrast to findings regarding exogenous saccades, deficits during tasks that evaluate the intentional or endogenous control of saccades have been consistently reported in individuals with ASD. Endogenous control of saccades involves making saccades based on a cognitive plan rather than as a relatively automatic response to sensory input. These have been examined to evaluate capacities for voluntary response inhibition and working memory that are primarily supported by PFC, anterior cingulate cortex (ACC), and striatal systems. The ability to execute endogenous goal-directed saccades develops throughout adolescence into early adulthood, and thus has a prolonged period for neural plasticity (Luna, Garver, Urban, Lazar, & Sweeney, 2004). Endogenous saccades have been examined using antisaccade paradigms where subjects are required to voluntarily inhibit a saccade toward a target and instead make a saccade away from the new target, and using oculomotor delayed response (or memory-guided saccade) tasks, where subjects are required to make saccades to remembered target locations. In both paradigms, subjects are required to make saccades based on an internal plan rather than to the locations of unpredictably appearing sensory stimuli.

Increased rates of saccade inhibition errors during antisaccade tasks have been reported in ASD when compared to age- and IQ-matched typically developing control subjects, reflecting a reduced ability to voluntarily suppress the natural response tendency to look toward suddenly appearing targets (Luna et al., 2007; Goldberg et al., 2002; Minshew, Luna, & Sweeney, 1999). A cross-sectional study by Luna and colleagues (2007) examined developmental changes in endogenous saccades in 19 children (8–12 years of age), 21 adolescents (13–17 years), and 21 adults (18–33 years) with ASD and age- and IQ-matched typically developing control groups. They reported that saccade inhibition errors during an antisaccade task decreased with age in both ASD and control groups, but error rates in the ASD group were higher overall and did not reach the error rates observed in the control group even in adulthood. Latencies of antisaccades, the time needed to initiate a volitional saccade away from a target, gradually reduced with age in the control group but not in the ASD group. Mosconi, Kay, D'Cruz, Seidenfeld, et al. (2009) also found increased antisaccade error rates, and reported that error rates were associated with higher-order repetitive behaviors in ASD. The implications of these findings point to frontostriatal system disturbances as a cause of repetitive behaviors in ASD.

Studies of oculomotor delayed-response tasks have also documented poor performance in subjects with ASD. Minshew and colleagues (1999) demonstrated that adolescents and young adults with ASD had difficulty shifting their eyes accurately to remembered locations. This finding was not replicated by Goldberg and colleagues (2002), who reported no abnormalities in the accuracy of memory-guided saccades in subjects with ASD, although they did report a prolonged latency of saccades to remembered targets. In the previously mentioned developmental study, Luna and colleagues (2007) also reported that latencies of memory-guided saccades were longer in subjects with ASD than typically developing controls. Further, the ASD group's age-related improvements were limited to childhood and adolescence, while no improvement was observed from adolescence to adulthood. In contrast, the control group showed progressive reductions in response latency through childhood to adulthood. As with antisaccades, the accuracy of memory-guided saccades improved with age only in the control group, and no age-related improvement was observed in the ASD group. This suggests an alteration in maturational processes that leads to a persistent reduction in the ability to quickly make and initiate behavioral plans.

Goldberg and colleagues (2002) examined a different type of endogenous saccades, predictive saccades, using a task where targets alternated between two positions at a fixed time interval. Because of the predictability of the target sequence, subjects typically begin to make anticipatory saccades to the expected target appearance after only a few target presentations. Switching to use learned target timing to execute saccades depends on function of the frontostriato-thalamocortical loop (Simo, Krisky, & Sweeney, 2005). High-functioning individuals with ASD had fewer anticipatory saccades and more variable response latencies than age- and IQ-matched control individuals, suggesting that individuals with ASD are less able to take advantage of the predictable timing and location of targets. Using a similar paradigm, D'Cruz and colleagues (2009) reported that individuals with ASD show abnormalities in the timing of predictive rightward, but not leftward saccades. These findings suggest abnormalities in response timing systems within the left basal ganglia.

To investigate neural substrates of impairments in endogenous saccades, Luna and colleagues (2002) conducted an fMRI study of individuals with ASD performing an oculomotor delayed-response task. Eleven individuals with ASD demonstrated reduced activation in the dorsolateral PFC and the posterior cingulate cortex when performing the task. Other circuitry involved in performing the task, including cortical eye fields, ACC, basal ganglia, thalamus, and lateral cerebellum, had similar levels of activation in ASD and age- and IQ-matched control groups. Thakkar and colleagues (Thakkar et al., 2008) used fMRI to investigate the neural substrates of antisaccade performance in 12 subjects with ASD. During the study, rostral ACC (rACC) activation during incorrect trials was greater than that for correct trials in healthy controls but not for subjects with ASD. Individuals with ASD showed increased rACC activation during correct trials compared to controls and reduced fractional anisotropy within white matter tracts underlying ACC. Both increased rACC activation on correct trials and decreased fractional anisotropy in rACC white matter were associated with more severe repetitive behavior. Taken together, these fMRI findings of endogenous saccade performance in ASD are consistent with the idea that dysfunction in the PFC and ACC may not only contribute to deficits in the generation of endogenous saccades, but be a marker for alterations in prefrontal systems that cause higher-order cognitive deficits that are widely observed in individuals with ASD (Hill, 2004).

Smooth Pursuit

Whereas saccades are used to acquire target objects that are located in the visual periphery, smooth pursuit is used to follow an object in motion that is already foveated. Neural systems that support smooth pursuit largely overlap with those that support saccades, though there are dissociable subdivisions in each relevant brain area for saccades and smooth pursuit and, thus, each type of eye movement could be selectively impaired (Rosano et al., 2002). Relevant brain circuitry includes extrastriate areas of visual cortex such as Area MT (also called V5), which is devoted to the processing of visual motion information; cortical eye fields and cerebellum, which are involved in translating sensory information to motor commands; and the basal ganglia, which are involved in initiating motor commands and perhaps predictive aspects of pursuit (Lencer & Trillenberg, 2008; Sharpe, 2008). Visual pursuit requires rapid, temporally precise integration of activity within these brain areas in order to visually track moving targets through space. Visual pursuit is typically described using a two-stage model. During the initiation or "open-loop" stage (first 100 ms after pursuit onset), control of pursuit is almost exclusively dependent on sensory analysis of visual motion that is performed primarily by contralateral area MT (Carl & Gellman, 1987; Lisberger & Movshon, 1999; Newsome, Wurtz, Dursteler, & Mikami, 1985). Analysis of visual motion information is passed from MT to the parietal and frontal eye fields, each of which project through the pons and the cerebellum to deep brainstem oculomotor areas to generate smooth pursuit eye movements (Yamada, Suzuki, & Yee, 1996). After the initial open-loop period of pursuit, the subsequent "closed-loop" stage of sustained pursuit relies primarily on memory for target velocity, predictions about target movement, and feedback about performance rather than an analysis of actual visual motion. The cortical eye fields, prefrontal cortex, striatum, and cerebellum play a crucial role during closed-loop pursuit to drive predictive pursuit using extraretinal information (Lencer et al., 2008; O'Driscoll et al., 2000).

Several studies have reported visual pursuit impairments in ASD. Scharre and Creedon (1992) and Rosenhall, Johansson, and Gillberg (1988) each noted difficulty eliciting pursuit responses in ASD. However, the latter study reported that pursuit accuracy was in the normal range in a small subset of participants with ASD who were able to initiate pursuit. It is important to note, however, that the time that these studies were conducted did not allow for the use of current criteria for diagnosing ASD. Perhaps more importantly, age- and IQ-matched control groups were not included in either study. A more recent report by Kemner, van der Geest, Verbaten, and van Engeland (2004) compared visual pursuit in subjects with PDD and age- and IQ-matched control subjects and reported an approximate 10% reduction in pursuit accuracy.

A study with a large sample performed by Takarae and colleagues (2004a) used three different pursuit tasks to characterize both open- and closed-loop pursuit in 60 high-functioning subjects with ASD and 94 age- and IQ-matched typically developing control subjects. They reported reduced pursuit accuracy in 3 different tasks during the closed-loop stage. This group difference in closed-loop pursuit was specific to older subjects with ASD, suggesting age-related improvement in visual pursuit performance in controls that was reduced in ASD. Closed-loop pursuit depends on internal representations of target movement and feedback about performance, and this pattern of developmental curtailment of closed-loop pursuit is similar to maturational failures for endogenous saccades that also depend on memory about targets and internally set goals. Takarae and colleagues also found lateralized reduction in accuracy of smooth pursuit and primary catch-up saccades in the ASD group during rightward open-loop pursuit. This hemifield-specific impairment could be related to disturbances in the left extrastriate areas that extract visual motion information, or in the feedforward projections from the left extrastriate areas to oculomotor areas that transform visual information into appropriate motor commands. In a follow-up study with an independent sample, Takarae, Luna, Minshew, and Sweeney (2008) observed significant associations between visual motion perception in psychophysical studies with pursuit latency in individuals with ASD, suggesting contributions of visual motion processing disturbances to problems in pursuit initiation in this population. Of note, slower pursuit initiation was only observed in participants with ASD who did not have early language delays. In contrast, pursuit latency and open-loop pursuit gain were correlated with manual motor skills only in the ASD group with language delays. Thus, the observed impairment of open-loop pursuit is likely part of more general sensorimotor alterations in individuals with language delays as well as being related to alteration in visual input or functional connectivity between extrastriate and sensorimotor areas.

In order to examine the neural substrates of pursuit impairments in ASD, Takarae and colleagues (2007) examined brain activation during visual pursuit of predictable target movement in 13 participants with ASD and 14 age- and IQ-matched typically developing control participants. They reported reduced activation in brain areas that mediate sensorimotor transformations, including cortical eye fields, and areas that are involved in acquisition of skilled motor responses, such as dorsolateral PFC, cingulate motor areas, and the presupplementary motor area. These findings suggest that abnormalities in brain circuitry that are involved in motor learning might be a contributing factor for pursuit impairments in ASD.

Visual Fixation and Vestibulo-Ocular Reflexes

Several studies have demonstrated, albeit inconsistently, that individuals with ASD have unusual visual scanning patterns when they examine human faces and social scenes (Klin, Jones,

Schultz, Volkmar, & Cohen, 2002; Pelphrey et al., 2002; van der Geest, Kemner, Verbaten, & van Engeland, 2002; van der Geest, Kemner, Camfferman, Verbaten, & van Engeland, 2002) and make fewer visual fixations during visual search (Kemner, van Ewijk, van Engeland, & Hooge, 2008). While these studies are designed to evaluate how individuals with ASD extract visual information from their social environments, few studies have investigated brain systems supporting sustained visual fixation. Stability of visual fixation depends on the integrity of cerebellar–brain stem systems, more specifically a balance between activity of burst neurons in the paramedian pontine reticular formation that drive eye movements and omnipause neurons in the raphe interpositus nucleus that inhibit burst neurons and receive input from the cerebellar vermis (Fuchs, Kaneko, & Scudder, 1985).

Nowinski, Minshew, Luna, Takarae, and Sweeney (2005) examined rates of square-wave jerks during central and eccentric fixation and ocular drift during eccentric fixation in 52 individuals with ASD and 52 age- and IQ-matched typically developing control subjects. Square-wave jerks are intrusive eye movements that consist of two saccades: the first saccade, which results from reduced inhibitory input to the brain stem, takes the eyes off the target object and is followed by a second saccade that corrects eye position to return to the target. Rates and size of square-wave jerks increase when inhibitory input is disrupted (Dell'Osso, Abel, & Daroff, 1977; Zee, Yee, Cogan, Robinson, & Engel, 1976). Speed of ocular drift during eccentric gaze increases after lesions in the flocculus and paraflocculus of the cerebellum (Zee, Leigh, & Mathieu-Millaire, 1980), and thus depends on cerebellar integrity. Nowinski and colleagues (2005) found no alterations in rates of square wave jerks and speed of ocular drift in ASD suggesting that this system is largely preserved in ASD. They did find that the amplitude of square-wave jerks was larger in individuals with ASD while fixating peripheral targets and when the participant was asked to maintain central fixation without a visual target. Further, the second corrective saccade to refoveate the target (the second saccade of square wave jerks) was executed more quickly in individuals with ASD when they were asked to maintain central fixation without visual stimuli. These findings suggest a subtle imbalance between excitatory and inhibitory processes in the brain stem, which was sufficient to alter amplitude and timing of square-wave jerks. The cerebellar vermis is considered critical in using proprioceptive information about extraocular muscles to maintain fixation with the absence of visual stimuli and sends input to the brain stem (Zee et al., 1980). Because the metrics of square-wave jerks were most affected in the condition without visual stimuli, it is possible that disturbances in vermal input are the source of reduced inhibitory control of relevant brain stem neurons. This is consistent with the previously described observation of saccadic dysmetria in ASD (Takarae et al., 2004b) that also suggests abnormalities of the cerebellar vermis.

While the study of visual fixation indicates subtle abnormalities in the cerebellar–brain stem system, studies of the vestibulo-ocular reflex (VOR) have not indicated reduced cerebellar oculomotor system integrity in ASD. VOR stabilizes visual images of stationary objects on the retina during transient head rotation by compensating for the movement of orbits with eye rotation. The VOR system is particularly sensitive to effects of cerebellar nodulus and uvula lesions (Waespe, Cohen, & Raphan, 1985; Wiest, Deecke, Trattnig, & Mueller, 1999). Early studies comparing children with ASD and typically developing children reported similar duration (Ritvo et al., 1969) but a statistically longer time constant for VOR in darkness (Ornitz, 1985; Ornitz, Atwell, Kaplan, & Westlake, 1985) and shorter duration in lighted conditions for children with ASD (Ornitz, 1985; Ornitz et al., 1985; Ornitz, Brown, Mason, & Putnam, 1974; Ritvo et al., 1969). These studies, however, did not match patient and control groups by IQ, and examinations of individual data suggest that the group differences might have been driven by a few subjects with extreme performance abnormalities while the majority of children with ASD performed at levels similar to the control group. A more recent study by Goldberg and colleagues (2000) examined VOR in darkness in 13 children with ASD and 10 age- and IQ-matched typically developing children and found no differences in time constant of VOR between groups. Findings from studies of VOR thus suggest that cerebellar–brain stem systems supporting these oculomotor processes are largely preserved in ASD.

In summary, eye movement studies indicate that subcortical circuitry supporting visual fixation, VOR, and exogenous saccades are largely preserved in ASD, although modest disturbances in sensorimotor transformations implicating cerebellar dysfunction are present when subjects make visually guided saccades to sensory targets and when they fixate remembered target locations in darkness. When tasks place greater demands on higher cognitive processes of behavioral inhibition, planning, working memory, and motor learning, deficits in individuals with ASD are more consistently observed. This pattern of findings has been observed in impairments in antisaccade and oculomotor delayed response tasks, closed-loop pursuit, and predictive saccade tasks. Developmental trajectories that are observed in these tasks suggest that maturation in brain systems that support endogenous eye movements may reach a developmental plateau earlier in ASD and not reach the same level of ability/performance as typically developing individuals.

Eye Movement Abnormalities in Unaffected Family Members of Individuals with ASD

Recent data indicate that unaffected parents and siblings of individuals with ASD show saccade and smooth pursuit abnormalities that are similar to those observed in individuals with ASD (Mosconi et al., 2010). Studying 57 first-degree relatives (42 parents and 15 siblings) of individuals with autistic disorder, Mosconi and colleagues found that family members demonstrated saccade hypometria, reduced closed-loop pursuit gain, reduced rightward open-loop pursuit gain, impaired response timing mechanisms for rightward predictive saccades, and increased rates of response suppression errors on an antisaccade task. These findings indicate that pontocerebellar circuitry alterations implicated in ASD by studies of saccade inaccuracy, increased trial-wise saccade amplitude variability, and reduced closed-loop pursuit gain may be familial. Similarly, rightward lateralized deficits in open-loop smooth pursuit and predictive saccade timing suggest left-hemisphere dysfunction affecting temporoparietal and basal ganglia systems, respectively. Last, impaired antisaccade performance is consistent with PFC abnormalities that also were implicated in the one previous study of eye movements in unaffected family members that identified inhibitory control deficits on a memory guided saccade task (Koczat et al., 2002). This profile of impairments has direct implications for shared neurocircuitry dysfunction in individuals with ASD and their first-degree relatives. Future studies are needed to examine relationships between eye movement performance in probands and family members (these studies did not examine family trios), identify whether these impairments are heritable, and investigate gene variants in ASD that are associated with neurophysiological developments underlying saccade and smooth pursuit abnormalities. Still, these recent data indicating parallel eye movement alterations in independent sets of probands and family members support the viability of eye movement alterations as intermediate phenotypes for future genetic and neurobiological studies of ASD.

Coordination of Complex Motor Sequences: Evidence of Dsypraxia in ASD

The neurophysiology of planning and executing motor sequences is less well understood than that regulating the initiation and precision of motor acts. Single-cell recording studies of behaving primates and human functional neuroimaging studies indicate that performing response sequences engages premotor cortex and basal ganglia to a significantly greater degree than the performance of single responses (Chan, Rao, Chen, Ye, & Zhang, 2006; Lecas, Requin, Anger, & Vitton, 1986; Requin, Riehle, & Seal, 1988; Rosenbaum, 1980; Tanji & Kurata, 1985; Wise, 1985), while also integrating unique connections with PFC, presupplementary motor area and parietal cortex (Grafton & Hamilton, 2007; Hamilton & Grafton, 2008; Seal & Commenges, 1985). Sequence learning and voluntary execution of motor sequences are organized at the neocortical level within the supplementary (SMA) and presupplementary motor areas and the inferior parietal lobule (Bapi, Miyapuram, Graydon, & Doya, 2006; Bischoff-Grethe, Goedert, Willingham, & Grafton, 2004; Grafton et al., 2002). Premotor and posterior parietal cortex are engaged during the planning phase of complex action sequences (Johnson-Frey, Newman-Norlund, & Grafton, 2005; Kawashima et al., 1996; Tunik, Rice, Hamilton, & Grafton, 2007) while the SMA is a vital node for the final assembly of action elements into a sequential motor plan (Gentilucci et al., 2000). Grafton and Hamilton (2007) noted that the anterior intraparietal sulcus also is involved in goal representation for motor actions, while activity in the inferior frontal gyrus is sensitive to the local kinematic features of how an object is acted upon. In addition, these frontoparietal systems engage dorsolateral PFC that is known to store previously learned information in short-term or working memory and to organize complex behavioral plans. Utilizing this widely distributed neural system, frontoparietal motor planning and execution systems rely on previously learned motor behaviors to initiate sequences of actions that together allow rapid and adaptive management of complex environmental demands.

Numerous neurobiological and behavioral studies suggest that at least a portion of individuals with ASD are dyspraxic, demonstrating a reduced ability to organize or initiate motor sequences despite intact performance of constituent movements (Hughes, 1996; Jones et al., 1985; Leary & Hill, 1996; Minshew et al., 1997; Rogers et al., 1996). Dyspraxia is typically considered as a deficit that occurs in the context of spared basic motor skills, so that considering behavioral manifestations of dyspraxia in ASD is complicated, requiring demonstration that the dyspraxia is either more severe than can be accounted for by basic motor system deficits or occurs in contexts where basic motor deficits do not influence behavioral performance. Available evidence indicates that a subset of individuals with ASD show impairments in complex purposeful behavior that are disproportionate to their deficits in basic motor skills. Dziuk and colleagues (2007) reported that, although basic motor skills predicted a significant proportion of variance in overall praxis scores, differences in praxis performance exceeded deficits expected based on impairment in basic motor abilities. Additional research is needed to clarify the extent to which deficits in complex motor sequences are attributable to more fundamental motor impairments, but current evidence indicates that individuals with ASD show impairments in planning and implementing sequential motor responses that can not be explained fully by deficits in basic motor abilities.

Evidence of dyspraxia in ASD suggests that alterations in frontoparietal circuitry involving premotor cortex, SMA, pre-SMA, posterior parietal cortices, and the inferior parietal lobule negatively impact motor behavior in ASD. Frontoparietal connections have not been adequately investigated with functional neuroimaging during tasks evaluating motor praxis, but enlargement of inter-cortical white matter (indexed by MRI segmentation of cerebral white matter; Herbert et al., 2003; Herbert et al., 2004) and minicolumnar abnormalities in ASD (including increased minicolumnar width and number, smaller neurons and nucleolar cross sections, and increased neuron density; Casanova, 2004; Casanova, Buxhoeveden, Switala, & Roy, 2002; Casanova, van Kooten, Switala, van Engeland, Heinsen, et al., 2006) suggest that corticocortical pathways necessary for complex cognitive processing (e.g., coordinated motor movements) are altered during development. Mostofsky, Burgess, and Gidley Larson (2007) indicated that increased left motor and premotor cortical white matter volume was related to soft neurological signs (including incoordination, immature reflexes, and poor perceptual or sensorimotor integration) in patients with ASD. Schmitz, Daly, and Murphy (2007) reported reduced prefrontal parenchymal volumes associated with increased motor reaction time in patients with ASD. Examining neural circuits involved in praxis in individuals with ASD with functional neuroimaging is one critical next step for understanding neurophysiological mechanisms of dyspraxia in this population.

Minicolumn: A vertical column through the cortex comprising 80–120 neurons (except in visual cortex) that is the most basic organizational structure of neocortex.

Considerable variability in praxis ability exists among individuals with ASD, both between individuals and within individuals over time. Rinehart and colleagues (Rinehart, Tonge, Bradshaw, Iansek, Enticott, & Johnson, 2006a) reported that individuals with autism show greater variability in reaction time on a motor planning task relative to both an Asperger's group and a group of age-matched typically developing controls. The authors further demonstrated that movement related potentials (MRP) thought to be associated with SMA and motor cortical activity were less robust for patients with autism relative to healthy controls during premovement phases. Individuals with Asperger's disorder showed less robust peak activity during movement planning, but none of the comparisons between the Asperger's group and controls reached statistical significance. In a related study, Rinehart and colleagues (Rinehart, Bradshaw, Brereton, & Tonge, 2002) observed protracted motor preparation times for individuals with autism as well as a failure to benefit from the predictability of stimulus sequences as reflected by an absence of differences between their reaction time to predictable versus unpredictable cues. These patterns of abnormality were not observed for individuals with Asperger's disorder (although it should be noted that the Asperger's disorder group did show increased movement times that did not reach statistical significance). These studies highlight two major insights: First, significant variability both among individuals with autism and between individuals with autism and Asperger's disorder can be large with some measures, and this may explain some of the inconsistencies in the literature on motor impairments in autism (e.g., Rogers et al., 2003 reported oromotor and action on object imitation impairments, but no differences between children with autism and typically developing controls on manual gesture imitation tasks). Also, if the variability reducing functions of corticocerebellar networks fail to effectively regulate motor output in ASD, it too may explain some differences within subjects in terms of the consistency of deficits observed on motor tasks. Second, evidence of dyspraxia in a subset of individuals with autism likely reflects motor planning dysfunction that typically relies on SMA connections with PFC and the striatum. Individuals with Asperger's disorder also showed reduced peak amplitude of movement related potentials during the motor preparation phase, but this difference is not as robust as found for individuals with autism. Postmovement cortical activity was largely intact for both groups in this study. Hypotheses regarding a similarity between patients with Parkinson's disease (who show characteristic pre- and postmovement cortical abnormalities; Cunnington, Iansek, Bradshaw, & Phillips, 1995) and ASD (Damasio et al., 1978; Vilensky et al., 1981) are thus informative but also limiting in that the pattern of frontostriatal dysfunction has both similarities and differences in these disorders.

Movement related potentials: Electrophysiological changes in cortex leading up to voluntary muscle movement that reflect the cortical contribution to the premotor planning of movement.

Studies of motor planning also indicate that dyspraxia is linked to core features of ASD. Dziuk and colleagues (2007) found that the level of dyspraxia in children with ASD was associated with their overall level of impairment in social, communication, and repetitive behavior domains measured with the Autism Diagnostic Observation Scale (ADOS; Lord et al., 2000). Similarly, Rogers and colleagues (2003) reported that children with ASD who were "weak imitators" (defined as those performing below the mean level for age- and IQ-matched developmentally delayed children on tasks of imitation of sequential motor actions) had greater overall symptomatology, poorer social responsiveness, and weaknesses in fine motor skill relative to "strong imitators" with ASD. These studies suggest that either the core features of ASD result from a shared neurological basis with dyspraxia (e.g., similar neural alterations across different brain systems), or that impaired coordination of motor actions may contribute to the social and communicative deficits observed in ASD as well as patterns of repetitive behavior. Clearly dyspraxia is not a stand-alone cause of core features of ASD, as the majority of children with dyspraxia do not develop an ASD. However, evidence that dyspraxia contributes to delayed development in oromotor and imitation skills integral to language and social development (Crary, Landess, & Towne, 1984; Dewey, Roy, Square-Storer, & Hayden, 1988; Stone, Ousley, & Littleford, 1997) and that motor impairments precede or at least coincide with the emergence of core social and communication impairments in ASD (Baranek, 1999; Bryson et al., 2007; Teitelbaum et al., 1998) together suggest that dyspraxia may be one contributing factor to impairments that are core to the disorder (DeMyer, Hingtgen, & Jackson, 1981). Considerable development of the neurobiological systems associated with motor coordination and complex motor behavior precede the development of social and communication systems (Lawrence & Hopkins, 1976; Simonds & Scheibel, 1989), consistent with the hypothesis that early motor system dysfunction may have downstream effects for developing social and communication systems in ASD. Nonmotor brain systems have been shown to take on motor functions during childhood and adolescence in individuals with ASD (Muller et al., 2001; Takarae et al., 2007), indicating that these regions may be developmentally compromised in part because they are called on to provide ongoing compensation for deficits in motor skill and sequencing.

This is a novel and exciting hypothesis that may be important for understanding the sequential pattern of brain development in individuals with ASD.

Recent data on motor learning suggest that alternative mechanisms may be used to adapt motor behavior to consistent changes in external demands. Assessment of motor adaptation provides a useful clinical approach for evaluating the functional integrity of the cerebellum (Werner, Bock, Gizewski, Schoch, & Timmann, 2009; Xu-Wilson et al., 2009) and thus has been investigated in several studies of ASD. Gidley-Larson and colleagues (2008) and Mostofsky and colleagues (2004) each reported intact motor adaptation in ASD when either visual (Gidley-Larson study only) or proprioceptive feedback (both studies) was altered. In contrast, D'Cruz and colleagues (2008) administered an intrasaccadic target displacement task known to elicit saccade adaptation and found that individuals with ASD demonstrated reduced adaptation relative to controls for rightward saccades, and increased adaptation for leftward saccades compared to controls. Haswell and colleagues (2009) also reported disrupted motor generalization when subjects with ASD were required to rely on visual, as opposed to proprioceptive feedback. The authors examined the trajectories of reaching movements while children with ASD and age-matched healthy controls moved a robotic arm toward a visual target. During task trials, a perpendicular force was applied to the robotic arm causing subjects to modify the trajectories of their responses. Working in the left workspace, both groups of subjects learned to make more direct paths toward the visual target over trials. Two generalization conditions then were administered in the right workspace: (1) subjects made identical joint rotations as compared to the learning trials; and (2) subjects made identical hand motions as the learning trials. Therefore, condition 1 examined the generalization of learned proprioceptive feedback in a different workspace, and condition 2 examined the generalization of learned visual feedback in a different workspace. Children with ASD generalized learning to the proprioceptive feedback condition, but not to the visual feedback condition. Children with ASD therefore may show intact abilities to apply proprioceptive feedback during motor learning, but they appear to be impaired when having to rely on visual feedback to guide learned motor responses. Interestingly, performance during the generalization of visual feedback was associated with social dysfunction in ASD, suggesting that reduced skill in integrating visual feedback regarding motor performance may impact social development in ASD.

Are Mirror Neurons Involved in Dyspraxia in ASD?

Additional insights into complex motor learning and planning can be gained by examining "mirror neuron systems," the consideration of which recently has been popular in the ASD literature. Mirror neurons—neurons responsive during the observation as well as the performance of motor acts—were first identified in studies of nonhuman primates (Di Pellegrino, Fadiga, Fogassi, Gallese, & Rizzolatti, 1992; Gallese, Fadiga, Fogassi, & Rizzolatti, 1996; Rizzolatti et al., 1988). Subsequent human functional neuroimaging studies have indicated that rostroventral motor cortex (Area F5) activation increases both during the execution as well as the observation of hand and mouth movements (Arbib, Billard, Iacoboni, & Oztop, 2000; Fogassi et al., 2005; Grezes, Armony, Rowe, & Passingham, 2003; Kaplan & Iacoboni, 2006; Molnar-Szakacs, Kaplan, Greenfield, & Iacoboni, 2006). Discrete clusters of mirror neurons within the dorsal convexity and adjacent posterior bank of the arcuate sulcus in the macaque monkey have been found to selectively respond during the voluntary production of meaningful hand gestures as well as when these gestures are observed while being performed by others (Fogassi et al., 2005). However, the mirror quality of these neurons was evident only for meaningful movements with objects and not for meaningful social or communicative gestures (Arbib et al., 2000; Buccino et al., 2004), suggesting that it is the observation of intentional action related to manipulating objects rather than the intentions or communicative meaning of the actor's movements that is tied to the engagement of these neurons.

Mirror neuron characteristics also are observed within cell clusters located in the lateral bank of the inferior parietal lobule and in the superior temporal sulcus (Fogassi et al., 2005; Sakata, Taira, Murata, & Mine, 1995). Visual systems within the inferior parietal lobule and superior temporal sulcus show increased neuronal firing rates in the presence of an object even when an individual is instructed or cued not to act on the object (Grafton et al., 2007). This mirror neuron system activates in response to others' meaningful actions on objects, putatively reflecting the learning and storage of motor actions that guide response planning and execution regarding that class of objects (Jeannerod, Arbib, Rizzolatti, & Sakata, 1995; Jeannerod & Decety, 1995). This system allows an individual to understand that an action sequence is taking place, differentiate this action sequence from other actions, and use this information to guide subsequent motor behavior. Mirror neurons thus may contribute to complex motor learning, planning, and execution. Because of their social features, interest in this neuron population has been intense in the ASD community.

Deficits in the performance of overlearned motor sequences have been observed in ASD (Dziuk et al., 2007; Mostofsky et al., 2006; Rogers et al., 1996; Vernazza-Martin et al., 2005), and hypoactivation in brain regions believed to have some cells with mirror neuron properties has been documented in functional MRI studies of individuals with ASD (Dapretto et al., 2006; Martineau et al., 2008; Williams et al., 2006b). Findings from these studies suggest that imitation impairments in ASD may be related to alterations of mirror neuron systems, and that mirror neuron disturbances may contribute to social interaction deficits and dyspraxia in ASD (Williams et al., 2004). However, research on skilled motor gestures indicates that the errors made by individuals with ASD are not confined to social imitation but also are evident in response to explicit instructions and with tool-use (Mostofsky et al., 2006). Thus, despite the intuitive appeal of the idea, there is significant risk of overinterpreting available evidence to infer a direct and pivotal role of mirror neuron disturbances in the social features of ASD.

Motor Development in Infants and Young Children with ASD

Examining the early development of motor systems in ASD may facilitate not only an earlier diagnosis, but also an understanding of behavioral and neurobiological phenotypes that will be useful in genetic research. Studies of the infant siblings of children with ASD are providing exciting new clues into the early development of these disorders. Results suggest that, overall, motor impairments are robust and prevalent across the majority of infants who go on to develop an ASD. Further, evidence indicates that not only do motor symptoms appear early, but they precede the onset of social and communication features of ASD.

Retrospective parent reports (Chawarska et al., 2007) and histological findings of pathology likely originating within the second trimester (Bauman et al., 1985) each have indicated that ASDs typically have a prenatal or early postnatal onset. Still, ASDs seldom are diagnosed prior to age three years (Mandell, Novak, & Zubritsky, 2005) suggesting that the emergence of symptoms often is not discernible until ages at which children typically achieve social and communication milestones and actively are engaged in peer interactions. The discrepancy between presumed onset and identification of ASD is likely related to multiple factors, not the least of which is an absence of knowledge regarding infantile developmental trajectories of affected individuals. There is an overarching assumption that symptoms of ASD are present early in ontogeny and that delays in obtaining formal diagnoses reflect a failure to recognize behavioral indicators or a failure to obtain adequate resources to aid in the detection of these indicators. However, this assumption has only inconsistently been supported by empirical evidence, and there may be variability in the onset of the pathophysiological and clinical presentation that will prove informative.

Recent studies of infant siblings later identified with ASD challenge the assumption that behavioral indicators are present within the first 6 months of life. Studies of ASD infants' development within the first year of life have failed to detect behavioral features of ASD prior to age 9–12 months (Landa, Holman, & Garrett-Mayer, 2007; Osterling & Dawson, 1994; Zwaigenbaum et al., 2005) suggesting that: (1) the core symptoms are not present early in ontogeny, (2) current methodology is not sensitive enough to reliably measure core features, or (3) the early behavioral development of infants with ASD does not map cleanly onto the behavioral phenotype evident after the first year of life. In contrast to the absence of consistent evidence for social and nonverbal communication deficits prior to age 12 months in children later diagnosed with ASD, an emerging and consistent literature regarding motor abnormalities within the first year of life suggests that this domain of impairment may be detectable earlier. In two independent studies of early development of infants later diagnosed with ASD, Teitelbaum and colleagues (1998) and Bryson and colleagues (2007) collectively identified motor dysfunction prior to age 12 months in 24/26 infants studied. Teitelbaum and colleagues (2004) reported similar findings for a sample of infants later diagnosed with Asperger's syndrome. While Teitelbaum's studies did not examine social or communication behaviors, Bryson and colleagues (2007) reported that hallmark characteristics of ASD, including deficits in social reciprocity, eye contact, and social referencing, were largely absent at age 6 months despite motor impairment in 7 out of 9 infants studied. Motor impairments included poor visual tracking, limited motor control when grasping or reaching for objects, and difficulty sitting independently. Additional motor disturbances were observed at 12 and 18 months, including abnormal, repetitive motor behaviors and odd posturing. Interestingly, the two infants identified with ASD at age 3 years who did not show motor abnormalities by age 6 months did, in fact, demonstrate motor impairments by age 12 months. These infants also were the only two observed that were identified as having ASD but who did not meet criteria on both the Autism Diagnostic Inventory (Lord, Rutter, & Le Couteur, 1994) and ADOS. Although these studies collectively examined only a small sample of children with ASD, results do suggest that motor impairments are associated with ASD and may precede aberrant development in more complex cognitive functions, including executive impairment, deficits in socialization, and atypical communication development.

These reports have significant implications for the early identification of infants with ASD and for understanding pathophysiological mechanisms. In addition, this research points to the importance of future studies examining the relationship between early emerging motor impairments and the altered development of complex cognitive processes involving both social and communication skills in children with ASD. Elucidating the neurobiological basis of motor control deficits may help resolve several controversies about the timing of alteration and specific pathophysiological mechanisms associated with the earliest manifestations of ASD.

Factors Associated with Motor Deficits in ASD

Initial reports of motor abnormalities in ASD relied largely on retrospective accounts of major developmental milestones, and suggested that motor impairments in ASD were confined to early childhood gross motor abilities. Deviations in vestibular control, gross and fine motor skill, oculomotor processes, and complex motor learning and adaptation across development are not yet well understood. The severity of disturbances among individuals with ASD in gross motor and fine motor systems may diminish over the lifespan, but oculomotor impairment and dyspraxia appear to persist throughout development (Freitag et al., 2007). Further, developmental failures may cause some abnormalities of motor control, such as the neocortical/cognitive control of planned actions, to deviate from normative trajectories so that greater differences can be seen later rather than earlier in life. These observations have critical implications for understanding the developmental pathophysiology of ASD.

Currently available evidence suggests that dysfunction in basic motor and sensorimotor circuits may be compensated for by the recruitment of alternative neural networks as demonstrated in functional imaging studies of manual (Muller et al., 2001) and oculomotor (Takarae et al., 2007) systems in patients with ASD. These compensations may mitigate basic motor impairments, but consequently adversely affect developments in more complex processes that rely on the "borrowed" higher-order systems. Elucidating the developmental neurobiology of ASD thus will require a mechanistic approach in which the neural system characteristics of component motor processes are investigated with longitudinal functional and anatomical imaging studies.

While there appear to be high rates of motor system dysfunction in ASD, alterations of motor systems are of course not specific to ASD and therefore are not specific diagnostic indicators. Thus, many of the motor problems in ASD may be sensitive but not specific markers for ASD—similar to other domains of deficit associated with the disorder when considered in isolation. For example, Provost, Lopez, and Heimerl (2007) reported gross and fine motor delays in children with ASD ages 21–41 months but also indicated that these deficits were not disproportionate in children with ASD relative to children with specific motor delays. Studies of oculomotor and praxis performance comparing individuals with ASD and cognitive impairment with age- and IQ-matched individuals have not been performed, but are necessary for clarifying the specificity of motor impairments to ASD phenotypes relative to the cognitive delays often associated with these disorders. Impairments that are specific to the disorder are of especial interest, especially those that have not been reported for other developmental or neuropsychiatric disorders studied. In this regard, the observation of left-lateralized abnormalities on eye movement testing, for example reduced rightward open-loop pursuit gain (Takarae et al., 2004a), has not been identified in other neuropsychiatric disorders with smooth pursuit impairments, and this is a potentially important observation. Overreliance on proprioceptive relative to visual feedback during motor adaptation also may be specific to ASD (Haswell et al., 2009). Further, most neuroimaging studies of motor functions performed to date have not typically included cognitively impaired individuals with ASD, making it difficult to generalize findings regarding the integrity of motor systems to a broader population of affected individuals. While the requirements of functional imaging studies often preclude the inclusion of severely cognitively impaired individuals, novel strategies for acquiring anatomical data, including morphometric and diffusion weighted imaging, may provide a basis for useful studies of brain-behavior linkages across the autism spectrum and spectrum of cognitive ability. Additionally, studies of familial motor phenotypes may provide insights into pathophysiological mechanisms relevant to severely impaired and less impaired individuals.

Demarcation of ASD subgroups has been attempted with analysis of motor performance patterns. Initial reports provided inconsistent evidence for disproportionate motor impairments in individuals with Asperger's syndrome relative to individuals with autism (Gillberg, 1989; Manjiviona & Prior, 1995; Szatmari, Tuff, Finlayson, & Bartolucci, 1990). Motor impairments in individuals with Asperger's syndrome have been documented for a range of motor skills (Lopata, Hamm, Volker, & Sowinski, 2007; Sahlander, Mattsson, & Bejerot, 2008), but few studies have found evidence for a dissociation between Asperger's syndrome and autism on the basis of motor functioning. Rinehart and colleagues (2002) reported that individuals with autism show lateralized delays in performing motor responses to visual-spatial cues presented to the right visual field consistent with left hemisphere underdevelopment. In contrast, individuals with Asperger's syndrome did not show this pattern of motor delay but did show impaired motor preparation abilities as demonstrated by increased response latencies to predictable targets. Studies have rarely compared Asperger's syndrome and autism directly, but a few have found significant group differences (Ghaziuddin, Butler, Tsai, & Ghaziuddin, 1994; Manjiviona et al., 1995; Miller & Ozonoff, 2000) or disproportionate impairment in individuals with autism (Gepner et al., 2002; Ghaziuddin & Butler, 1998). Gepner and Mestre (2002) reported poor postural stability and postural adaptation to environmental motion in individuals with autism relative to individuals with Asperger's syndrome. Comparisons between these groups are difficult owing to the inconsistency of Asperger's syndrome diagnostic criteria applied across studies (Volkmar, 1999) and the tendency of many studies to include small samples of each diagnostic group and consequently combine these samples. Studies directly comparing these subpopulations will need to utilize consistent diagnostic classification criteria along with comprehensive and more sensitive motor measures to thoroughly parse neurobehavioral profiles.

Summary and Conclusions

The analysis of motor system deficits presents a unique opportunity to study alterations in brain systems that cause neurodevelopmental disorders such as ASD. Motor abnormalities in ASD have their onset early in ontogeny and involve multiple widely distributed neurophysiological systems. Several features unique to motor systems make them ideally suited for the translational studies needed to link genetic mechanisms to neurophysiological and cognitive substrates of ASD. Motor systems can be more reliably assessed than many complex cognitive operations, and can be examined from the first moments of postnatal life. This aspect allows researchers to reliably detect early emerging motor impairments in infants with ASD and track these impairments over time using quantitative objective laboratory procedures. Studies of infants later diagnosed with ASD indicate that motor impairments may be among the earliest indicators of behavioral pathology, and thus they may be useful for identifying high risk individuals for early intervention. Motor disturbances also can be assessed across wide levels of cognitive ability enabling the examination both of higher-functioning individuals with ASD and individuals with ASD whose cognitive abilities are in the impaired range. Finally, recent evidence

Table 22–2.
Motor system deficits and brain regions most directly implicated in neuroimaging and neurobehavioral studies of ASD*

	Frontal Lobe	Temporoparietal Lobes	Basal Ganglia	Cerebellum	Brain Stem Nuclei
Vestibular functions Poor balance Poor postural control	—	**Somatosensory cortex**	—	**Spinocerebellum; interposed nuclei**	**Reticular formation**
Walking movements Bradykinesia Variable stride rates Poor balance	**Primary motor cortex**	—	**Substantia nigra; striatum**	**Spinocerebellum; interposed nuclei**	—
Writing and finger movements Dysgraphia Impaired grooved pegboard performance	**Dorsal premotor, supplementary motor and primary motor cortex**	**Superior temporal gyrus; precuneus; inferior parietal lobule**	**Striatum**	**Anterior cerebellum (lobules V–VI); lateral cerebellum; inferior vermis (lobule VIII); dentate nuclei**	—
Saccades Dysmetria Increased amplitude variability Increased latencies Increased response inhibition error rate Memory guided saccade inaccuracy	**Frontal eye field; supplementary eye field; DLPFC; anterior cingulate cortex**	**Parietal eye field; inferior parietal lobule**	**Caudate nucleus Substantia nigra pars reticulata**	**Vermis (lobules VI–VII); fastigial nuclei**	**PPRF; superior colliculus**
Smooth pursuit Reduced rightward open-loop gain Reduced closed-loop gain	**Frontal, supplementary and parietal eye fields**	**MT/V5**	—	**Vermis (lobules VI–VII); fastigial nuclei**	**PPRF**
Fixation Large amplitude square-wave jerks Reduced latency of corrective saccades	—	—	—	**Vestibulocerebellum; vestibular nuclei Vermis (lobules VI-VII)**	**Superior colliculus**
Motor sequences/learning Dyspraxia Impaired saccadic adaptation Impaired manual adaptation with visual feedback	**Inferior frontal gyrus; DLPFC; premotor, presupplementary motor, supplementary motor and primary motor cortices**	**Inferior parietal lobule; intraparietal sulcus; superior temporal sulcus**	**Striatum**	**Lateral hemispheres; dentate nuclei; vermis (lobules VI–VII); fastigial nuclei**	—

* This is not an exhaustive list of brain regions involved in each aspect of motor behavior. Brain regions were included if they were identified in previous neuroimaging studies of ASD or are directly implicated by neurobehavioral findings.
MT/V5: middle temporal area/visual cortical area 5; DLPFC: dorsolateral prefrontal cortex; PPRF: paramedian pontine reticular formation.

indicates that motor disturbances are evident in the majority of individuals with ASD and that these disturbances involve multiple neurophysiological systems. Impairments in gross motor, fine motor, oculomotor, and coordinated motor sequencing skills implicating corticocortical, frontostriatal, and corticocerebellar circuitry dysfunction in individuals with ASD all have been observed and they parallel findings of neuroanatomical and neurofunctional abnormalities. The extent to which these neural systems are affected in parallel, or differentially in different individuals, remains to be fully clarified (Table 22-2).

Higher level cognitive functioning impairments are often emphasized in the examination of ASD development, including language skills, executive functions, and social processes, but these are particularly difficult to characterize with the mechanistic, neurobiologically informed approaches that are provided by motor and sensorimotor studies. For example, although deficits in imitating observed gestures are robust and consistently noted in individuals with ASD (see Williams et al., 2004, for a review), the neural systems that enable individuals to implicitly learn, integrate, and execute the complex motor sequences inherent in motor praxis seldom have been systematically assessed in studies of ASD. However, by studying discrete motor processes and their underlying neurobiology, a clearer picture of the developmental neurophysiology of ASD may be drawn and insights into brain-behavior mechanisms that can be more closely linked to candidate genes are possible. A potential contributory role of motor system disturbances to the later emergence of social, language, and cognitive deficits also can be evaluated.

ASDs are characterized by complex and diverse sets of impairments. It is now recognized that single-factor models focusing on only one cognitive/behavioral process or brain region can not sufficiently account for the full constellation of clinical disturbances in ASD that involve pathology across multiple levels of the neuroaxis. Motor disturbances traditionally have not been included in these unitary frameworks because they are much less disabling features of the disorder than communication and social deficits. However, motor system research lends itself to translational studies, some of which have been initiated and offer preliminary evidence converging around gene-brain-behavior associations that provide a suitable model for investigating the neurobiology of motor impairments in ASD. Evidence also exists suggesting that motor profiles may distinguish individuals with Asperger's syndrome and individuals with autism, and individuals with autism with and without language delay, and thus may offer a focus for studies aimed at teasing apart subgroups of individuals with ASD in a neurobiologically informed manner that will be useful as quantitative phenotypes for genetic research. Motor disturbances in ASD, therefore, require increased behavioral, neurobiological, and genetic research attention, and should be included in models characterizing the pervasive and complex behavioral impairments that characterize ASD and related neurodevelopmental disorders.

Challenges and Future Directions

- Integrating converging findings on the profound and diverse motor deficits and dyspraxia in ASD into the definitions of the disorder(s) that currently are under revision will be important for fully elucidating these disorders and parsing heterogeneity.
- Longitudinal neurobehavioral and imaging studies of the development of motor skills are needed. Existing evidence suggests that motor impairments are among the earliest abnormalities to emerge in ASD development. Further, neuroimaging studies indicate that higher order neural systems may compensate for motor neurocircuitry dysfunction in a way that may alter the maturation of those systems and contribute to higher-level cognitive and social communication deficits.
- Motor profiles may distinguish individuals with Asperger's syndrome and individuals with autism, and individuals with autism with and without language delay, and thus may offer a focus for studies aimed at teasing apart subgroups of individuals with ASD in a neurobiologically informed manner.
- Identifying shared motor impairments in individuals with ASD and their unaffected first-degree relatives could offer clues to pathophysiological mechanisms, indicate disrupted neural systems that cosegregate within families, and provide direction for future genetic research.
- Cerebellar pathology has been consistently reported in ASD, but the functional impairments associated with these abnormalities are poorly understood. In addition, the extent to which this pathology is attributed to a history of seizures has been questioned (Crooks, Mitchell, & Thom, 2000; Whitney et al., 2008), suggesting that examination of motor skills in individuals with ASD with a history of seizures should be investigated relative to those without a history of seizures.

SUGGESTED READINGS

Blatt, G. J. (2005). GABAergic cerebellar system in autism: a neuropathological and developmental perspective. *International Review of Neurobiology, 71*, 167–178.

Grafton, S. T., Hamilton, A. F., Gowen, E., & Miall, R. C. (2007). Evidence for a distributed hierarchy of action representation in the brain. *Human Movement Science, 26*, 590–616.

Nayate, A., Bradshaw, J. L., & Rinehart, N. J. (2005). Autism and Asperger's disorder: are they movement disorders involving the cerebellum and/or basal ganglia? *Brain Research Bulletin, 67*, 327–334.

Sweeney, J. A., Takarae, Y., Macmillan, C., Luna, B., & Minshew, N. J. (2004). Eye movements in neurodevelopmental disorders. *Current Opinion in Neurology, 17*, 37–42.

REFERENCES

Abrahams, B. S., & Geschwind, D. H. (2010). Connecting genes to brain in the autism spectrum disorders. *Archives of Neurology, 67*, 395–399.

Ahsgren, I., Baldwin, I., Goetzinger-Falk, C., Erikson, A., Flodmark, O., & Gillberg, C. (2005). Ataxia, autism, and the cerebellum: a clinical study of 32 individuals with congenital ataxia. *Developmental Medicine and Child Neurology, 47*, 193–198.

Alexander, G. E., Crutcher, M. D., & DeLong, M. R. (1990). Basal ganglia-thalamocortical circuits: parallel substrates for motor, oculomotor, "prefrontal" and "limbic" functions. *Progress in Brain Research, 85*, 119–146.

Allen, G., & Courchesne, E. (2003). Differential effects of developmental cerebellar abnormality on cognitive and motor functions in the cerebellum: an fMRI study of autism. *American Journal of Psychiatry, 160*, 262–273.

Allen, G., Muller, R. A., & Courchesne, E. (2004). Cerebellar function in autism: functional magnetic resonance image activation during a simple motor task. *Biological Psychiatry, 56*, 269–278.

American Psychiatric Association (2000). *Diagnostic and statistical manual* (4th ed., text rev.; DSM-IV-TR). Washington, DC: Author.

Ames, D., Cummings, J. L., Wirshing, W. C., Quinn, B., & Mahler, M. (1994). Repetitive and compulsive behavior in frontal lobe degenerations. *Journal of Neuropsychiatry and Clinical Neurosciences, 6*, 100–113.

Arbib, M. A., Billard, A., Iacoboni, M., & Oztop, E. (2000). Synthetic brain imaging: grasping, mirror neurons and imitation. *Neural Networks, 13*, 975–997.

Arin, D. M., Bauman, M., & Kemper, T. L. (1991). The distribution of Purkinje cell loss in the cerebellum in autism. *Neurology, 41*, 301.

Asperger, H. (1944/1991). "Autistic psychopathy" in childhood. In U. Frith (Ed., & Trans.), *Autism and Asperger syndrome* (pp. 37–92). New York: Cambridge University Press.

Bailey, A., Luthert, P., Dean, A., Harding, B., Janota, I., Montgomery, M., et al. (1998). A clinicopathological study of autism. *Brain, 121*(Pt 5), 889–905.

Bapi, R. S., Miyapuram, K. P., Graydon, F. X., & Doya, K. (2006). fMRI investigation of cortical and subcortical networks in the learning of abstract and effector-specific representations of motor sequences. *NeuroImage, 32*, 714–727.

Baranek, G. T. (1999). Autism during infancy: a retrospective video analysis of sensory-motor and social behaviors at 9–12 months of age. *Journal of Autism and Developmental Disorders, 29*, 213–224.

Bauman, M. L. (1991). Microscopic neuroanatomic abnormalities in autism. *Pediatrics, 87*, 791–796.

Bauman, M., & Kemper, T. L. (1985). Histoanatomic observations of the brain in early infantile autism. *Neurology, 35*, 866–874.

Bauman, M. L., & Kemper, T. L. (2005). Neuroanatomic observations of the brain in autism: a review and future directions. *International Journal of Developmental Neuroscience, 23*, 183–187.

Beversdorf, D. Q., Anderson, J. M., Manning, S. E., Anderson, S. L., Nordgren, R. E., Felopulos, G. J., et al. (2001). Brief report: macrographia in high-functioning adults with autism spectrum disorder. *Journal of Autism and Developmental Disorders, 31*, 97–101.

Bischoff-Grethe, A., Goedert, K. M., Willingham, D. T., & Grafton, S. T. (2004). Neural substrates of response-based sequence learning using fMRI. *Journal of Cognitive Neuroscience, 16*, 127–138.

Brodal, P. (1978). Principles of organization of the monkey corticopontine projection. *Brain Research, 148*, 214–218.

Bryson, S. E., Zwaigenbaum, L., Brian, J., Roberts, W., Szatmari, P., Rombough, V., et al. (2007). A prospective case series of high-risk infants who developed autism. *Journal of Autism and Developmental Disorders, 37*, 12–24.

Buccino, G., Vogt, S., Ritzl, A., Fink, G. R., Zilles, K., Freund, H. J., et al. (2004). Neural circuits underlying imitation learning of hand actions: an event-related fMRI study. *Neuron, 42*, 323–334.

Canales, J. J., & Graybiel, A. M. (2000). A measure of striatal function predicts motor stereotypy. *Nature Neuroscience, 3*, 377–383.

Carl, J. R., & Gellman, R. S. (1987). Human smooth pursuit: stimulus-dependent responses. *Journal of Neurophysiology, 57*, 1446–1463.

Carper, R. A., & Courchesne, E. (2005). Localized enlargement of the frontal cortex in early autism. *Biological Psychiatry, 57*, 126–133.

Casanova, M. F. (2004). White matter volume increase and minicolumns in autism. *Annals of Neurology, 56*, 453.

Casanova, M. F., Buxhoeveden, D. P., Switala, A. E., & Roy, E. (2002). Minicolumnar pathology in autism. *Neurology, 58*, 428–432.

Casanova, M. F., van Kooten, I. A., Switala, A. E., van Engeland, H., Heinsen, H., Steinbusch, H. W., et al. (2006). Minicolumnar abnormalities in autism. *Acta Neuropathologica, 112*, 287–303.

Catalan, M. J., Honda, M., Weeks, R. A., Cohen, L. G., & Hallett, M. (1998). The functional neuroanatomy of simple and complex sequential finger movements: a PET study. *Brain, 121*(Pt 2), 253–264.

Catani, M., Jones, D. K., Daly, E., Embiricos, N., Deeley, Q., Pugliese, L., et al. (2008). Altered cerebellar feedback projections in Asperger syndrome. *NeuroImage, 41*, 1184–1191.

Catz, N., & Thier, P. (2007). Neural control of saccadic eye movements. *Developments in Ophthalmology, 40*, 52–75.

Cavada, C., & Goldman-Rakic, P. S. (1989). Posterior parietal cortex in rhesus monkey: I. Parcellation of are as based on distinctive limbicand sensorycorticocortical connections. *Journal of Comparative Neurology, 287*, 393–421.

Chan, R. C., Rao, H., Chen, E. E., Ye, B., & Zhang, C. (2006). The neural basis of motor sequencing: an fMRI study of healthy subjects. *Neuroscience Letters, 398*, 189–194.

Chawarska, K., Paul, R., Klin, A., Hannigen, S., Dichtel, L. E., & Volkmar, F. (2007). Parental recognition of developmental problems in toddlers with autism spectrum disorders. *Journal of Autism and Developmental Disorders, 37*, 62–72.

Cody, H., Pelphrey, K., & Piven, J. (2002). Structural and functional magnetic resonance imaging of autism. *International Journal of Developmental Neuroscience, 20*, 421–438.

Courchesne, E., Press, G. A., & Yeung-Courchesne, R. (1993). Parietal lobe abnormalities detected with MR in patients with infantile autism. *American Journal of Roentgenology, 160*, 387–393.

Courchesne, E., Yeung-Courchesne, R., Press, G. A., Hesselink, J. R., & Jernigan, T. L. (1988). Hypoplasia of cerebellar vermal lobules VI and VII in autism. *New England Journal of Medicine, 318*, 1349–1354.

Crary, M. A., Landess, S., & Towne, R. (1984). Phonological error patterns in developmental verbal dyspraxia. *Journal of Clinical Neuropsychology, 6*, 157–170.

Crooks, R., Mitchell, T., & Thom, M. (2000). Patterns of cerebellar atrophy in patients with chronic epilepsy: a quantitative neuropathological study. *Epilepsy Research, 41*, 63–73.

Csibra, G., Johnson, M. H., & Tucker, L. A. (1997). Attention and oculomotor control: a high-density ERP study of the gap effect. *Neuropsychologia, 35*, 855–865.

Cunnington, R., Iansek, R., Bradshaw, J. L., & Phillips, J. G. (1995). Movement-related potentials in Parkinson's disease: Presence and predictability of temporal and spatial cues. *Brain, 118*(Pt 4), 935–950.

D'Cruz, A.-M., Mosconi, M. W., Nowinski, C. V., Kay, M., Seidenfeld, A., Rubin, L. H., et al. (2008). Saccadic adaptation in autism. Presented at the International Meeting for Autism Research. London.

D'Cruz, A. M., Mosconi, M. W., Steele, S., Rubin, L. H., Luna, B., Minshew, N., et al. (2009). Lateralized response timing deficits in autism. *Biological Psychiatry, 66*, 393–397.

Damasio, A. R., & Maurer, R. G. (1978). A neurological model for childhood autism. *Archives of Neurology, 35*, 777–786.

Dapretto, M., Davies, M. S., Pfeifer, J. H., Scott, A. A., Sigman, M., Bookheimer, S. Y., et al. (2006). Understanding emotions in others: mirror neuron dysfunction in children with autism spectrum disorders. *Nature Neuroscience, 9*, 28–30.

Dauer, W., & Przedborski, S. (2003). Parkinson's disease: mechanisms and models. *Neuron, 39*, 889–909.

Dawnay, N. A., & Glees, P. (1986). Somatotopic analysis of fibre and terminal distribution in the primate corticospinal pathway. *Brain Research, 391*, 115–123.

Dell'Osso, L. F., Abel, L. A., & Daroff, R. B. (1977). "Inverse latent" macro square-wave jerks and macro saccadic oscillations. *Annals of Neurology, 2*, 57–60.

DeLong, M. R. (1990). Primate models of movement disorders of basal ganglia origin. *Trends in Neurosciences, 13*, 281–285.

DeLong, M. R., & Strick, P. L. (1974). Relation of basal ganglia, cerebellum, and motor cortex units to ramp and ballistic limb movements. *Brain Research, 71*, 327–335.

DeMyer, M. K., Hingtgen, J. N., & Jackson, R. K. (1981). Infantile autism reviewed: a decade of research. *Schizophrenia Bulletin, 7*, 388–451.

Dewey, D., Roy, E. A., Square-Storer, P. A., & Hayden, D. (1988). Limb and oral praxic abilities of children with verbal sequencing deficits. *Developmental Medicine and Child Neurology, 30*, 743–751.

Di Pellegrino, G., Fadiga, L., Fogassi, L., Gallese, V., & Rizzolatti, G. (1992). Understanding motor events: a neurophysiological study. *Experimental Brain Research, 91*, 176–180.

Dowell, L. R., Mahone, E. M., & Mostofsky, S. H. (2009). Associations of postural knowledge and basic motor skill with dyspraxia in autism: implication for abnormalities in distributed connectivity and motor learning. *Neuropsychology, 23*, 563–570.

Drew, T., Prentice, S., & Schepens, B. (2004). Cortical and brainstem control of locomotion. *Progress in Brain Research, 143*, 251–261.

Dum, R. P., & Strick, P. L. (1991). The origin of corticospinal projections from the premotor areas in the frontal lobe. *Journal of Neuroscience, 11*, 667–689.

Dum, R. P., & Strick, P. L. (1992). Medial wall motor areas and skeletomotor control. *Current Opinion in Neurobiology, 2*, 836–839.

Dziuk, M. A., Gidley Larson, J. C., Apostu, A., Mahone, E. M., Denckla, M. B., & Mostofsky, S. H. (2007). Dyspraxia in autism: association with motor, social, and communicative deficits. *Developmental Medicine and Child Neurology, 49*, 734–739.

Esposito, G., & Venuti, P. (2008). Analysis of toddlers' gait after six months of independent walking to identify autism: a preliminary study. *Perceptual and Motor Skills, 106*, 259–269.

Fitzpatrick, R. C., & Day, B. L. (2004). Probing the human vestibular system with galvanic stimulation. *Journal of Applied Physiology, 96*, 2301–2316.

Fogassi, L., Ferrari, P. F., Gesierich, B., Rozzi, S., Chersi, F., & Rizzolatti, G. (2005). Parietal lobe: from action organization to intention understanding. *Science, 308*, 662–667.

Freitag, C. M., Kleser, C., Schneider, M., & von Gontard, A. (2007). Quantitative assessment of neuromotor function in adolescents with high functioning autism and Asperger syndrome. *Journal of Autism and Developmental Disorders, 37*, 948–959.

Fuchs, A. F., Kaneko, C. R., & Scudder, C. A. (1985). Brainstem control of saccadic eye movements. *Annual Review of Neuroscience, 8*, 307–337.

Gallese, V., Fadiga, L., Fogassi, L., & Rizzolatti, G. (1996). Action recognition in the premotor cortex. *Brain, 119*(Pt 2), 593–609.

Gentilucci, M., Bertolani, L., Benuzzi, F., Negrotti, A., Pavesi, G., & Gangitano, M. (2000). Impaired control of an action after supplementary motor area lesion: a case study. *Neuropsychologia, 38*, 1398–1404.

Gepner, B., Mestre, D., Masson, G., & de Schonen, S. (1995). Postural effects of motion vision in young autistic children. *Neuroreport, 6*, 1211–1214.

Gepner, B., & Mestre, D. R. (2002). Brief report: postural reactivity to fast visual motion differentiates autistic from children with Asperger syndrome. *Journal of Autism and Developmental Disorders, 32*, 231–238.

Gernsbacher, M. A., Sauer, E. A., Geye, H. M., Schweigert, E. K., & Hill, G. H. (2008). Infant and toddler oral- and manual-motor skills predict later speech fluency in autism. *Journal of Psychology and Psychiatry and Allied Disciplines, 49*, 43–50.

Ghaziuddin, M. (2008). Defining the behavioral phenotype of Asperger syndrome. *Journal of Autism and Developmental Disorders, 38*, 138–142.

Ghaziuddin, M., & Butler, E. (1998). Clumsiness in autism and Asperger syndrome: a further report. *Journal of Intellectual Disability Research, 42*(Pt 1), 43–48.

Ghaziuddin, M., Butler, E., Tsai, L., & Ghaziuddin, N. (1994). Is clumsiness a marker for Asperger syndrome? *Journal of Intellectual Disability Research, 38*(Pt 5), 519–527.

Gidley Larson, J. C., Bastian, A. J., Donchin, O., Shadmehr, R., & Mostofsky, S. H. (2008). Acquisition of internal models of motor tasks in children with autism. *Brain, 131*, 2894–2903.

Gillberg, C. (1989). Asperger syndrome in 23 Swedish children. *Developmental Medicine and Child Neurology, 31*, 520–531.

Goldberg, M. C., Landa, R., Lasker, A., Cooper, L., & Zee, D. S. (2000). Evidence of normal cerebellar control of the vestibulo-ocular reflex (VOR) in children with high-functioning autism. *Journal of Autism and Developmental Disorders, 30*, 519–524.

Goldberg, M. C., Lasker, A. G., Zee, D. S., Garth, E., Tien, A., & Landa, R. J. (2002). Deficits in the initiation of eye movements in the absence of a visual target in adolescents with high functioning autism. *Neuropsychologia, 40*, 2039–2049.

Golla, H., Tziridis, K., Haarmeier, T., Catz, N., Barash, S., & Thier, P. (2008). Reduced saccadic resilience and impaired saccadic adaptation due to cerebellar disease. *European Journal of Neuroscience, 27*, 132–144.

Grafton, S. T., & Hamilton, A. F. (2007). Evidence for a distributed hierarchy of action representation in the brain. *Human Movement Science, 26*, 590–616.

Grafton, S. T., Hazeltine, E., & Ivry, R. B. (2002). Motor sequence learning with the nondominant left hand: A PET functional imaging study. *Experimental Brain Research, 146*, 369–378.

Green, D., Baird, G., Barnett, A. L., Henderson, L., Huber, J., & Henderson, S. E. (2002). The severity and nature of motor impairment in Asperger's syndrome: a comparison with specific developmental disorder of motor function. *Journal of Child Psychology and Psychiatry and Allied Disciplines, 43*, 655–668.

Grezes, J., Armony, J. L., Rowe, J., & Passingham, R. E. (2003). Activations related to "mirror" and "canonical" neurones in the human brain: an fMRI study. *NeuroImage, 18*, 928–937.

Hallett, M., Lebiedowska, M. K., Thomas, S. L., Stanhope, S. J., Denckla, M. B., & Rumsey, J. (1993). Locomotion of autistic adults. *Archives of Neurology, 50*, 1304–1308.

Hamilton, A. F., & Grafton, S. T. (2008). Action outcomes are represented in human inferior frontoparietal cortex. *Cerebral Cortex, 18*, 1160–1168.

Hardan, A. Y., Kilpatrick, M., Keshavan, M. S., & Minshew, N. J. (2003). Motor performance and anatomic magnetic resonance imaging (MRI) of the basal ganglia in autism. *Journal of Child Neurology, 18*, 317–324.

Hashimoto,T.,Tayama,M.,Murakawa,K.,Yoshimoto,T.,Miyazaki,M., Harada, M., et al. (1995). Development of the brainstem and cerebellum in autistic patients. *Journal of Autism and Developmental Disorders, 25*, 1–18.

Haswell, C. C., Izawa, J., Dowell, L. R., Mostofsky, S. H., & Shadmehr, R. (2009). Representation of internal models of action in the autistic brain. *Nature Neuroscience, 12*, 970–972.

Hazlett, H., Poe, M., Smith, R., Gerig, G., & Piven, J. (2005). Update on a longitudinal MRI study of young children with autism. Presented at the International Meeting for Autism Research. Boston, MA.

Haznedar, M. M., Buchsbaum, M. S., Hazlett, E. A., LiCalzi, E. M., Cartwright, C., & Hollander, E. (2006). Volumetric analysis and three-dimensional glucose metabolic mapping of the striatum and thalamus in patients with autism spectrum disorders. *The American Journal of Psychiatry, 163*, 1252–1263.

He, S. Q., Dum, R. P., & Strick, P. L. (1993). Topographic organization of corticospinal projections from the frontal lobe: motor areas on the lateral surface of the hemisphere. *Journal of Neuroscience, 13*, 952–980.

He, S. Q., Dum, R. P., & Strick, P. L. (1995). Topographic organization of corticospinal projections from the frontal lobe: motor areas on the medial surface of the hemisphere. *Journal of Neuroscience, 15*, 3284–3306.

Herbert, M. R., Ziegler, D. A., Deutsch, C. K., O'Brien, L. M., Lange, N., Bakardjiev, A., et al. (2003). Dissociations of cerebral cortex, subcortical and cerebral white matter volumes in autistic boys. *Brain, 126*, 1182–1192.

Herbert, M. R., Ziegler, D. A., Makris, N., Filipek, P. A., Kemper, T. L., Normandin, J. J., et al. (2004). Localization of white matter volume increase in autism and developmental language disorder. *Annals of Neurology, 55*, 530–540.

Hill, E. L. (2004). Executive dysfunction in autism. *Trends in Cognitive Sciences, 8*, 26–32.

Hollander, E., Anagnostou, E., Chaplin, W., Esposito, K., Haznedar, M. M., Licalzi, E., et al. (2005). Striatal volume on magnetic resonance imaging and repetitive behaviors in autism. *Biological Psychiatry, 58*, 226–232.

Holttum, J. R., Minshew, N. J., Sanders, R. S., & Phillips, N. E. (1992). Magnetic resonance imaging of the posterior fossa in autism. *Biological Psychiatry, 32*, 1091–1101.

Honda, M., Deiber, M. P., Ibanez, V., Pascual-Leone, A., Zhuang, P., & Hallett, M. (1998). Dynamic cortical involvement in implicit and explicit motor sequence learning: A PET study. *Brain, 121*(Pt 11), 2159–2173.

Houk, J. C., & Wise, S. P. (1995). Distributed modular architectures linking basal ganglia, cerebellum, and cerebral cortex: their role in planning and controlling action. *Cerebral Cortex, 5*, 95–110.

Hughes, C. (1996). Brief report: planning problems in autism at the level of motor control. *Journal of Autism and Developmental Disorders, 26*, 99–107.

Ito, M. (1984). The modifiable neuronal network of the cerebellum. *Japanese Journal of Physiology, 34*, 781–792.

Jansiewicz, E. M., Goldberg, M. C., Newschaffer, C. J., Denckla, M. B., Landa, R., & Mostofsky, S. H. (2006). Motor signs distinguish children with high functioning autism and Asperger's syndrome from controls. *Journal of Autism and Developmental Disorders, 36*, 613–621.

Jeannerod, M., Arbib, M. A., Rizzolatti, G., & Sakata, H. (1995). Grasping objects: the cortical mechanisms of visuomotor transformation. *Trends in Neurosciences, 18*, 314–320.

Jeannerod, M., & Decety, J. (1995). Mental motor imagery: a window into the representational stages of action. *Current Opinion in Neurobiology, 5*, 727–732.

Johnson-Frey, S. H., Newman-Norlund, R., & Grafton, S. T. (2005). A distributed left hemisphere network active during planning of everyday tool use skills. *Cerebral Cortex, 15*, 681–695.

Jones, V., & Prior, M. (1985). Motor imitation abilities and neurological signs in autistic children. *Journal of Autism and Developmental Disorders, 15*, 37–46.

Kaji, R. (2001). Sensory-motor disintegration in the basal ganglia disorders. *Clinical Neurology, 41*, 1076–1078.

Kanner, L. (1943). Autistic disturbances of affective contact. *Nervous Child, 2*, 217–250.

Kaplan, J. T., & Iacoboni, M. (2006). Getting a grip on other minds: mirror neurons, intention understanding, and cognitive empathy. *Social Neuroscience, 1*, 175–183.

Kaufmann, W. E., Cooper, K. L., Mostofsky, S. H., Capone, G. T., Kates, W. R., Newschaffer, C. J., et al. (2003). Specificity of cerebellar vermian abnormalities in autism: a quantitative magnetic resonance imaging study. *Journal of Child Neurology, 18*, 463–470.

Kawakubo, Y., Kasai, K., Okazaki, S., Hosokawa-Kakurai, M., Watanabe, K., Kuwabara, H., et al. (2007). Electrophysiological abnormalities of spatial attention in adults with autism during the gap overlap task. *Clinical Neurophysiology, 118*, 1464–1471.

Kawashima, R., Itoh, H., Ono, S., Satoh, K., Furumoto, S., Gotoh, R., et al. (1996). Changes in regional cerebral blood flow during self-paced arm and finger movements: A PET study. *Brain Research, 716*, 141–148.

Kemner, C., van der Geest, J. N., Verbaten, M. N., & van Engeland, H. (2004). In search of neurophysiological markers of pervasive developmental disorders: smooth pursuit eye movements? *Journal of Neural Transmission, 111*, 1617–1626.

Kemner, C., van Ewijk, L., van Engeland, H., & Hooge, I. (2008). Brief report: eye movements during visual search tasks indicate enhanced stimulus discriminability in subjects with PDD. *Journal of Autism and Developmental Disorders, 38*, 553–557.

Kemper, T. L., & Bauman, M. (1998). Neuropathology of infantile autism. *Journal of Neuropathology and Experimental Neurology, 57*, 645–652.

Kemper, T. L., & Bauman, M. L. (2002). Neuropathology of infantile autism. *Molecular Psychiatry, 7*(Suppl 2), S12–S13.

Kennedy, P. R., Ross, H. G., & Brooks, V. B. (1982). Participation of the principal olivary nucleus in neocerebellar motor control. *Experimental Brain Research, 47*, 95–104.

Keshner, E. A., & Cohen, H. (1989). Current concepts of the vestibular system reviewed: 1. The role of the vestibulospinal system in postural control. *American Journal of Occupational Therapy, 43,* 320–330.

Khan, Z. U., Gutierrez, A., Martin, R., Penafiel, A., Rivera, A., & de la Calle, A. (2000). Dopamine D5 receptors of rat and human brain. *Neuroscience, 100,* 689–699.

Kida, N., Oda, S., & Matsumura, M. (2005). Intensive baseball practice improves the go/nogo reaction time, but not the simple reaction time. *Brain Research. Cognitive Brain Research, 22,* 257–264.

Kleiman, M. D., Neff, S., & Rosman, N. P. (1992). The brain in infantile autism: are posterior fossa structures abnormal? *Neurology, 42,* 753–760.

Klin, A., Jones, W., Schultz, R., Volkmar, F., & Cohen, D. (2002). Visual fixation patterns during viewing of naturalistic social situations as predictors of social competence in individuals with autism. *Archives of General Psychiatry, 59,* 809–816.

Koczat, D. L., Rogers, S. J., Pennington, B. F., & Ross, R. G. (2002). Eye movement abnormality suggestive of a spatial working memory deficit is present in parents of autistic probands. *Journal of Autism and Developmental Disorders, 32,* 513–518.

Kohen-Raz, R., Volkmar, F. R., & Cohen, D. J. (1992). Postural control in children with autism. *Journal of Autism and Developmental Disorders, 22,* 419–432.

Kornhuber, H. H. (1978). Cortex, basal ganglia, and cerebellum in motor control. *Electroencephalography and Clinical Neurophysiology, Supplement,* 449–455.

Landa, R. J., Holman, K. C., & Garrett-Mayer, E. (2007). Social and communication development in toddlers with early and later diagnosis of autism spectrum disorders. *Archives of General Psychiatry, 64,* 853–864.

Langen, M., Durston, S., Staal, W. G., Palmen, S. J., & van Engeland, H. (2007). Caudate nucleus is enlarged in high-functioning medication-naive subjects with autism. *Biological Psychiatry, 62,* 262–266.

Langen, M., Schnack, H. G., Nederveen, H., Bos, D., Lahuis, B. E., de Jonge, M. V., et al. (2009). Changes in the developmental trajectories of striatum in autism. *Biological Psychiatry, 66,* 327–333.

Lawrence, D. G., & Hopkins, D. A. (1976). The development of motor control in the rhesus monkey: evidence concerning the role of corticomotoneuronal connections. *Brain, 99,* 235–254.

Leary, M. R., & Hill, D. A. (1996). Moving on: autism and movement disturbance. *Mental Retardation, 34,* 39–53.

Lecas, J. C., Requin, J., Anger, C., & Vitton, N. (1986). Changes in neuronal activity of the monkey precentral cortex during preparation for movement. *Journal of Neurophysiology, 56,* 1680–1702.

Leichnetz, G. R. (2001). Connections of the medial posterior parietal cortex (area 7m) in the monkey. *Anatomical Record, 263,* 215–236.

Lencer, R., & Trillenberg, P. (2008). Neurophysiology and neuroanatomy of smooth pursuit in humans. *Brain and Cognition, 68,* 219–228.

Lisberger, S. G., & Movshon, J. A. (1999). Visual motion analysis for pursuit eye movements in area MT of macaque monkeys. *Journal of Neuroscience, 19,* 2224–2246.

Lopata, C., Hamm, E. M., Volker, M. A., & Sowinski, J. E. (2007). Motor and visuomotor skills of children with Asperger's disorder: preliminary findings. *Perceptual and Motor Skills, 104,* 1183–1192.

Lord, C., Risi, S., Lambrecht, L., Cook, E. H., Jr., Leventhal, B. L., DiLavore, P. C., et al. (2000). The autism diagnostic observation schedule-generic: a standard measure of social and communication deficits associated with the spectrum of autism. *Journal of Autism and Developmental Disorders, 30,* 205–223.

Lord, C., Rutter, M., & Le Couteur, A. (1994). Autism Diagnostic Interview-Revised: a revised version of a diagnostic interview for caregivers of individuals with possible pervasive developmental disorders. *Journal of Autism and Developmental Disorders, 24,* 659–685.

Luna, B., Doll, S. K., Hegedus, S. J., Minshew, N. J., & Sweeney, J. A. (2007). Maturation of executive function in autism. *Biological Psychiatry, 61,* 474–481.

Luna, B., Garver, K. E., Urban, T. A., Lazar, N. A., & Sweeney, J. A. (2004). Maturation of cognitive processes from late childhood to adulthood. *Child Development, 75,* 1357–1372.

Luna, B., Minshew, N. J., Garver, K. E., Lazar, N. A., Thulborn, K. R., Eddy, W. F., et al. (2002). Neocortical system abnormalities in autism: an fMRI study of spatial working memory. *Neurology, 59,* 834–840.

Mandelbaum, D. E., Stevens, M., Rosenberg, E., Wiznitzer, M., Steinschneider, M., Filipek, P., et al. (2006). Sensorimotor performance in school-age children with autism, developmental language disorder, or low IQ. *Developmental Medicine and Child Neurology, 48,* 33–39.

Mandell, D. S., Novak, M. M., & Zubritsky, C. D. (2005). Factors associated with age of diagnosis among children with autism spectrum disorders. *Pediatrics, 116,* 1480–1486.

Manes, F., Piven, J., Vrancic, D., Nanclares, V., Plebst, C., & Starkstein, S. E. (1999). An MRI study of the corpus callosum and cerebellum in mentally retarded autistic individuals. *The Journal of Neuropsychiatry and Clinical Neurosciences, 11,* 470–474.

Manjiviona, J., & Prior, M. (1995). Comparison of Asperger syndrome and high-functioning autistic children on a test of motor impairment. *Journal of Autism and Developmental Disorders, 25,* 23–39.

Mari, M., Castiello, U., Marks, D., Marraffa, C., & Prior, M. (2003). The reach-to-grasp movement in children with autism spectrum disorder. *Philosophical Transactions of the Royal Society of London. Series B, Biological Sciences, 358,* 393–403.

Martineau, J., Cochin, S., Magne, R., & Barthelemy, C. (2008). Impaired cortical activation in autistic children: is the mirror neuron system involved?. *International Journal of Psychophysiology, 68,* 35–40.

Mayes, S. D., & Calhoun, S. L. (2003). Analysis of WISC-III, Stanford-Binet:IV, and academic achievement test scores in children with autism. *Journal of Autism and Developmental Disorders, 33,* 329–341.

McAlonan, G. M., Suckling, J., Wong, N., Cheung, V., Lienenkaemper, N., Cheung, C., et al. (2008). Distinct patterns of grey matter abnormality in high-functioning autism and Asperger's syndrome. *Journal of Child Psychology and Psychiatry and Allied Disciplines, 49,* 1287–1295.

Middleton, F. A., & Strick, P. L. (1997). Cerebellar output channels. *International Review of Neurobiology, 41,* 61–82.

Middleton, F. A., & Strick, P. L. (2001). Cerebellar projections to the prefrontal cortex of the primate. *Journal of Neuroscience, 21,* 700–712.

Miller, J. N., & Ozonoff, S. (2000). The external validity of Asperger disorder: lack of evidence from the domain of neuropsychology. *Journal of Abnormal Psychology, 109,* 227–238.

Ming, X., Brimacombe, M., & Wagner, G. C. (2007). Prevalence of motor impairment in autism spectrum disorders. *Brain Development, 29,* 565–570.

Minshew, N. J., Goldstein, G., & Siegel, D. J. (1997). Neuropsychologic functioning in autism: profile of a complex information processing disorder. *Journal of the International Neuropsychological Society, 3*, 303–316.

Minshew, N. J., Luna, B., & Sweeney, J. A. (1999). Oculomotor evidence for neocortical systems but not cerebellar dysfunction in autism. *Neurology, 52*, 917–922.

Minshew, N. J., Sung, K., Jones, B. L., & Furman, J. M. (2004). Underdevelopment of the postural control system in autism. *Neurology, 63*, 2056–2061.

Molloy, C. A., Dietrich, K. N., & Bhattacharya, A. (2003). Postural stability in children with autism spectrum disorder. *Journal of Autism and Developmental Disorders, 33*, 643–652.

Molnar-Szakacs, I., Kaplan, J., Greenfield, P. M., & Iacoboni, M. (2006). Observing complex action sequences: The role of the fronto-parietal mirror neuron system. *NeuroImage, 33*, 923–935.

Mosconi, M. W., Kay, M., D'Cruz, A. M., Guter, S., Kapur, K., et al. (2010). Neurobehavioral abnormalities in first-degree relatives of individuals with autism. *Archives of General Psychiatry, 67*, 830–840.

Mosconi, M. W., Kay, M., D'Cruz, A. M., Seidenfeld, A., Guter, S., Stanford, L. D., et al. (2009). Impaired inhibitory control is associated with higher-order repetitive behaviors in autism spectrum disorders. *Psychological Medicine, 39*, 1559–1566.

Mostofsky, S. H., Bunoski, R., Morton, S. M., Goldberg, M. C., & Bastian, A. J. (2004). Children with autism adapt normally during a catching task requiring the cerebellum. *Neurocase, 10*, 60–64.

Mostofsky, S. H., Burgess, M. P., & Gidley Larson, J. C. (2007). Increased motor cortex white matter volume predicts motor impairment in autism. *Brain, 130*, 2117–2122.

Mostofsky, S. H., Dubey, P., Jerath, V. K., Jansiewicz, E. M., Goldberg, M. C., & Denckla, M. B. (2006). Developmental dyspraxia is not limited to imitation in children with autism spectrum disorders. *Journal of the International Neuropsychological Society, 12*, 314–326.

Mostofsky, S. H., Powell, S. K., Simmonds, D. J., Goldberg, M. C., Caffo, B., & Pekar, J. J. (2009). Decreased connectivity and cerebellar activity in autism during motor task performance. *Brain, 132*, 2413–2425.

Muller, R. A., Pierce, K., Ambrose, J. B., Allen, G., & Courchesne, E. (2001). Atypical patterns of cerebral motor activation in autism: a functional magnetic resonance study. *Biological Psychiatry, 49*, 665–676.

Newsome, W. T., Wurtz, R. H., Dursteler, M. R., & Mikami, A. (1985). Deficits in visual motion processing following ibotenic acid lesions of the middle temporal visual area of the macaque monkey. *Journal of Neuroscience, 5*, 825–840.

Nowinski, C. V., Minshew, N. J., Luna, B., Takarae, Y., & Sweeney, J. A. (2005). Oculomotor studies of cerebellar function in autism. *Psychiatry Research, 137*, 11–19.

O'Driscoll, G. A., Wolff, A. L., Benkelfat, C., Florencio, P. S., Lal, S., & Evans, A. C. (2000). Functional neuroanatomy of smooth pursuit and predictive saccades. *Neuroreport, 11*, 1335–1340.

Ohyama, T., Nores, W. L., Murphy, M., & Mauk, M. D. (2003). What the cerebellum computes. *Trends in Neurosciences, 26*, 222–227.

Ornitz, E. M. (1985). Neurophysiology of infantile autism. *Journal of the American Academy of Child Psychiatry, 24*, 251–262.

Ornitz, E. M., Atwell, C. W., Kaplan, A. R., & Westlake, J. R. (1985). Brain-stem dysfunction in autism. *Archives of General Psychiatry, 42*, 1018–1025.

Ornitz, E. M., Brown, M. B., Mason, A., & Putnam, N. H. (1974). Effect of visual input on vestibular nystagmus in autistic children. *Archives of General Psychiatry, 31*, 369–375.

Osterling, J., & Dawson, G. (1994). Early recognition of children with autism: a study of first birthday home videotapes. *Journal of Autism and Developmental Disorders, 24*, 247–257.

Ozonoff, S., Pennington, B. F., & Rogers, S. J. (1991). Executive function deficits in high-functioning autistic individuals: relationship to theory of mind. *Journal of Child Psychology and Psychiatry and Allied Disciplines, 32*, 1081–1105.

Ozonoff, S., Young, G. S., Goldring, S., Greiss-Hess, L., Herrera, A. M., Steele, J., et al. (2008). Gross motor development, movement abnormalities, and early identification of autism. *Journal of Autism and Developmental Disorders, 38*, 644–656.

Pelphrey, K. A., Sasson, N. J., Reznick, J. S., Paul, G., Goldman, B. D., & Piven, J. (2002). Visual scanning of faces in autism. *Journal of Autism and Developmental Disorders, 32*, 249–261.

Petrides, M. (2005). Lateral prefrontal cortex: architectonic and functional organization. *Philosophical Transactions of the Royal Society of London. Series B, Biological Sciences, 360*, 781–795.

Piven, J., Saliba, K., Bailey, J., & Arndt, S. (1997). An MRI study of autism: the cerebellum revisited. *Neurology, 49*, 546–551.

Pollack, A. E. (2001). Anatomy, physiology, and pharmacology of the basal ganglia. *Neurologic Clinics, 19*, 523–34, v.

Provost, B., Lopez, B. R., & Heimerl, S. (2007). A comparison of motor delays in young children: autism spectrum disorder, developmental delay, and developmental concerns. *Journal of Autism and Developmental Disorders, 37*, 321–328.

Rapin, I. (1996). Practitioner review: developmental language disorders: a clinical update. *Journal of Child Psychology and Psychiatry and Allied Disciplines, 37*, 643–655.

Requin, J., Riehle, A., & Seal, J. (1988). Neuronal activity and information processing in motor control: from stages to continuous flow. *Biological Psychology, 26*, 179–198.

Rinehart, N. J., Bradshaw, J. L., Brereton, A. V., & Tonge, B. J. (2002). Lateralization in individuals with high-functioning autism and Asperger's disorder: a frontostriatal model. *Journal of Autism and Developmental Disorders, 32*, 321–331.

Rinehart, N. J., Tonge, B. J., Bradshaw, J. L., Iansek, R., Enticott, P. G., & Johnson, K. A. (2006a). Movement-related potentials in high-functioning autism and Asperger's disorder. *Developmental Medicine and Child Neurology, 48*, 272–277.

Rinehart, N. J., Tonge, B. J., Bradshaw, J. L., Iansek, R., Enticott, P. G., & McGinley, J. (2006b). Gait function in high-functioning autism and Asperger's disorder: evidence for basal-ganglia and cerebellar involvement? *European Child and Adolescent Psychiatry, 15*, 256–264.

Rinehart, N. J., Tonge, B. J., Iansek, R., McGinley, J., Brereton, A. V., Enticott, P. G., et al. (2006c). Gait function in newly diagnosed children with autism: Cerebellar and basal ganglia related motor disorder. *Developmental Medicine and Child Neurology, 48*, 819–824.

Ritvo, E. R., Freeman, B. J., Scheibel, A. B., Duong, T., Robinson, H., Guthrie, D., et al. (1986). Lower Purkinje cell counts in the cerebella of four autistic subjects: Initial findings of the UCLA-NSAC autopsy research report. *American Journal of Psychiatry, 143*, 862–866.

Ritvo, E. R., Ornitz, E. M., Eviatar, A., Markham, C. H., Brown, M. B., & Mason, A. (1969). Decreased postrotatory nystagmus in early infantile autism. *Neurology, 19*, 653–658.

Rizzolatti, G., Camarda, R., Fogassi, L., Gentilucci, M., Luppino, G., & Matelli, M. (1988). Functional organization of inferior area 6 in the macaque monkey. *Experimental Brain Research, 71,* 491–507.

Rogers, S. J., Bennetto, L., McEvoy, R., & Pennington, B. F. (1996). Imitation and pantomime in high-functioning adolescents with autism spectrum disorders. *Child Development, 67,* 2060–2073.

Rogers, S. J., Hepburn, S. L., Stackhouse, T., & Wehner, E. (2003). Imitation performance in toddlers with autism and those with other developmental disorders. *Journal of Child Psychology and Psychiatry and Allied Disciplines, 44,* 763–781.

Rojas, D. C., Peterson, E., Winterrowd, E., Reite, M. L., Rogers, S. J., & Tregellas, J. R. (2006). Regional gray matter volumetric changes in autism associated with social and repetitive behavior symptoms. *BMC Psychiatry, 6,* 56.

Rolls, E. T. (1994). Neurophysiology and cognitive functions of the striatum. *Revue Neurologique, 150,* 648–660.

Rosano, C., Krisky, C. M., Welling, J. S., Eddy, W. F., Luna, B., Thulborn, K. R., et al. (2002). Pursuit and saccadic eye movement subregions in human frontal eye field: a high-resolution fMRI investigation. *Cerebral Cortex, 12,* 107–115.

Rosenbaum, D. A. (1980). Human movement initiation: specification of arm, direction, and extent. *Journal of Experimental Psychology. Generic, 109,* 444–474.

Rosenhall, U., Johansson, E., & Gillberg, C. (1988). Oculomotor findings in autistic children. *Journal of Laryngology and Otology, 102,* 435–439.

Rumsey, J. M., & Hamburger, S. D. (1988). Neuropsychological findings in high-functioning men with infantile autism, residual state. *Journal of Clinical and Experimental Neuropsychology, 10,* 201–221.

Sahlander, C., Mattsson, M., & Bejerot, S. (2008). Motor function in adults with Asperger's disorder: a comparative study. *Physiotherapy Theory and Practice, 24,* 73–81.

Sakata, H., Taira, M., Murata, A., & Mine, S. (1995). Neural mechanisms of visual guidance of hand action in the parietal cortex of the monkey. *Cerebral Cortex, 5,* 429–438.

Schaefer, G. B., Thompson, J. N., Bodensteiner, J. B., McConnell, J. M., Kimberling, W. J., Gay, C. T., et al. (1996). Hypoplasia of the cerebellar vermis in neurogenetic syndromes. *Annals of Neurology, 39,* 382–385.

Scharre, J. E., & Creedon, M. P. (1992). Assessment of visual function in autistic children. *Optometry and Vision Science, 69,* 433–439.

Schmitz, N., Daly, E., & Murphy, D. (2007). Frontal anatomy and reaction time in autism. *Neuroscience Letters, 412,* 12–17.

Seal, J., & Commenges, D. (1985). A quantitative analysis of stimulus- and movement-related responses in the posterior parietal cortex of the monkey. *Experimental Brain Research, 58,* 144–153.

Sears, L. L., Vest, C., Mohamed, S., Bailey, J., Ranson, B. J., & Piven, J. (1999). An MRI study of the basal ganglia in autism. *Progress in Neuropsychopharmacology and Biological Psychiatry, 23,* 613–624.

Sharpe, J. A. (2008). Neurophysiology and neuroanatomy of smooth pursuit: lesion studies. *Brain and Cognition, 68,* 241–254.

Simo, L. S., Krisky, C. M., & Sweeney, J. A. (2005). Functional neuroanatomy of anticipatory behavior: dissociation between sensory-driven and memory-driven systems. *Cerebral Cortex, 15,* 1982–1991.

Simonds, R. J., & Scheibel, A. B. (1989). The postnatal development of the motor speech area: a preliminary study. *Brain and Language, 37,* 42–58.

Soetedjo, R., Kojima, Y., & Fuchs, A. F. (2008). Complex spike activity in the oculomotor vermis of the cerebellum: a vectorial error signal for saccade motor learning? *Journal of Neurophysiology, 171,* 153–159.

Stanfield, A. C., McIntosh, A. M., Spencer, M. D., Philip, R., Gaur, S., & Lawrie, S. M. (2008). Towards a neuroanatomy of autism: a systematic review and meta-analysis of structural magnetic resonance imaging studies. *European Psychiatry, 23,* 289–299.

Stein, J. F., & Glickstein, M. (1992). Role of the cerebellum in visual guidance of movement. *Physiological Reviews, 72,* 967–1017.

Stone, W. L., Ousley, O. Y., & Littleford, C. D. (1997). Motor imitation in young children with autism: what's the object? *Journal of Abnormal Child Psychology, 25,* 475–485.

Szatmari, P., Tuff, L., Finlayson, M. A., & Bartolucci, G. (1990). Asperger's syndrome and autism: neurocognitive aspects. *Journal of the American Academy of Child and Adolescent Psychiatry, 29,* 130–136.

Takagi, M., Tamargo, R., & Zee, D. S. (2003). Effects of lesions of the cerebellar oculomotor vermis on eye movements in primate: binocular control. *Progress in Brain Research, 142,* 19–33.

Takagi, M., Zee, D. S., & Tamargo, R. J. (1998). Effects of lesions of the oculomotor vermis on eye movements in primate: saccades. *Journal of Neurophysiology, 80,* 1911–1931.

Takagi, M., Zee, D. S., & Tamargo, R. J. (2000). Effects of lesions of the oculomotor cerebellar vermis on eye movements in primate: smooth pursuit. *Journal of Neurophysiology, 83,* 2047–2062.

Takarae, Y., Luna, B., Minshew, N. J., & Sweeney, J. A. (2008). Patterns of visual sensory and sensorimotor abnormalities in autism vary in relation to history of early language delay. *Journal of the International Neuropsychological Society, 14,* 980–989.

Takarae, Y., Minshew, N. J., Luna, B., Krisky, C. M., & Sweeney, J. A. (2004a). Pursuit eye movement deficits in autism. *Brain, 127,* 2584–2594.

Takarae, Y., Minshew, N. J., Luna, B., & Sweeney, J. A. (2004b). Oculomotor abnormalities parallel cerebellar histopathology in autism. *Journal of Neurology, Neurosurgery, and Psychiatry, 75,* 1359–1361.

Takarae, Y., Minshew, N. J., Luna, B., & Sweeney, J. A. (2007). Atypical involvement of frontostriatal systems during sensorimotor control in autism. *Psychiatry Research, 156,* 117–127.

Tanji, J., & Kurata, K. (1985). Contrasting neuronal activity in supplementary and precentral motor cortex of monkeys. I. Responses to instructions determining motor responses to forthcoming signals of different modalities. *Journal of Neurophysiology, 53,* 129–141.

Teitelbaum, O., Benton, T., Shah, P. K., Prince, A., Kelly, J. L., & Teitelbaum, P. (2004). Eshkol-Wachman movement notation in diagnosis: the early detection of Asperger's syndrome. *Proceedings of the National Academy of the Sciences of the United States of America, 101,* 11909–11914.

Teitelbaum, P., Teitelbaum, O., Nye, J., Fryman, J., & Maurer, R. G. (1998). Movement analysis in infancy may be useful for early diagnosis of autism. *Proceedings of the National Academy of the Sciences of the United States of America, 95,* 13982–13987.

Teuber, H. L. (1974). Functional recovery after lesions of the nervous system. II. Recovery of function after lesions of the central nervous system: history and prospects. *Neurosciences Research Program Bulletin, 12,* 197–211.

Thakkar, K. N., Polli, F. E., Joseph, R. M., Tuch, D. S., Hadjikhani, N., Barton, J. J., et al. (2008). Response monitoring, repetitive behaviour and anterior cingulate abnormalities in autism spectrum disorders (ASD). *Brain, 131*, 2464–2478.

Thier, P., Dicke, P. W., Haas, R., & Barash, S. (2000). Encoding of movement time by populations of cerebellar Purkinje cells. *Nature, 405*, 72–76.

Thier, P., Dicke, P. W., Haas, R., Thielert, C. D., & Catz, N. (2002). The role of the oculomotor vermis in the control of saccadic eye movements. *Annals of the New York Academy of Sciences, 978*, 50–62.

Timmann, D., Brandauer, B., Hermsdorfer, J., Ilg, W., Konczak, J., Gerwig, M., et al. (2008). Lesion-symptom mapping of the human cerebellum. *Cerebellum, 7*, 602–606.

Tsatsanis, K. D., Rourke, B. P., Klin, A., Volkmar, F. R., Cicchetti, D., & Schultz, R. T. (2003). Reduced thalamic volume in high-functioning individuals with autism. *Biological Psychiatry, 53*, 121–129.

Tunik, E., Rice, N. J., Hamilton, A., & Grafton, S. T. (2007). Beyond grasping: representation of action in human anterior intraparietal sulcus. *NeuroImage, 36*(Suppl 2), T77–T86.

van der Geest, J. N., Kemner, C., Camfferman, G., Verbaten, M. N., & van Engeland, H. (2001). Eye movements, visual attention, and autism: a saccadic reaction time study using the gap and overlap paradigm. *Biological Psychiatry, 50*, 614–619.

van der Geest, J. N., Kemner, C., Camfferman, G., Verbaten, M. N., & van Engeland, H. (2002). Looking at images with human figures: comparison between autistic and normal children. *Journal of Autism and Developmental Disorders, 32*, 69–75.

van der Geest, J. N., Kemner, C., Verbaten, M. N., & van Engeland, H. (2002). Gaze behavior of children with pervasive developmental disorder toward human faces: a fixation time study. *Journal of Child Psychology and Psychiatry and Allied Disciplines, 43*, 669–678.

Vanvuchelen, M., Roeyers, H., & De Weerdt, W. (2007). Nature of motor imitation problems in school-aged boys with autism: a motor or a cognitive problem? *Autism, 11*, 225–240.

Vernazza-Martin, S., Martin, N., Vernazza, A., Lepellec-Muller, A., Rufo, M., Massion, J., et al. (2005). Goal directed locomotion and balance control in autistic children. *Journal of Autism and Developmental Disorders, 35*, 91–102.

Vilensky, J. A., Damasio, A. R., & Maurer, R. G. (1981). Gait disturbances in patients with autistic behavior: a preliminary study. *Archives of Neurology, 38*, 646–649.

Volkmar, F. (1999). Can you explain the difference between autism and Asperger syndrome. *Journal of Autism and Developmental Disorders, 29*, 185–186.

Waespe, W., Cohen, B., & Raphan, T. (1985). Dynamic modification of the vestibulo-ocular reflex by the nodulus and uvula. *Science, 228*, 199–202.

Werner, S., Bock, O., Gizewski, E. R., Schoch, B., & Timmann, D. (2009). Visuomotor adaptive improvement and aftereffects are impaired differentially following cerebellar lesions in SCA and PICA territory. *Experimental Brain Research, 201*, 429–439.

Whitney, E. R., Kemper, T. L., Bauman, M. L., Rosene, D. L., & Blatt, G. J. (2008). Cerebellar Purkinje cells are reduced in a subpopulation of autistic brains: a stereological experiment using calbindin-D28k. *Cerebellum, 7*, 406–416.

Wiest, G., Deecke, L., Trattnig, S., & Mueller, C. (1999). Abolished tilt suppression of the vestibulo-ocular reflex caused by a selective uvulo-nodular lesion. *Neurology, 52*, 417–419.

Williams, D. L., Goldstein, G., & Minshew, N. J. (2006a). Neuropsychologic functioning in children with autism: further evidence for disordered complex information-processing. *Child Neuropsychology, 12*, 279–298.

Williams, J. H., Waiter, G. D., Gilchrist, A., Perrett, D. I., Murray, A. D., & Whiten, A. (2006b). Neural mechanisms of imitation and "mirror neuron" functioning in autistic spectrum disorder. *Neuropsychologia, 44*, 610–621.

Williams, J. H., Whiten, A., & Singh, T. (2004). A systematic review of action imitation in autistic spectrum disorder. *Journal of Autism and Developmental Disorders, 34*, 285–299.

Wise, S. P. (1985). The primate premotor cortex: past, present, and preparatory. *Annual Review of Neuroscience, 8*, 1–19.

Xu-Wilson, M., Chen-Harris, H., Zee, D. S., & Shadmehr, R. (2009). Cerebellar contributions to adaptive control of saccades in humans. *Journal of Neuroscience, 29*, 12930–12939.

Yamada, T., Suzuki, D. A., & Yee, R. D. (1996). Smooth pursuit-like eye movements evoked by microstimulation in macaque nucleus reticularis tegmenti pontis. *Journal of Neurophysiology, 76*, 3313–3324.

Yip, J., Soghomonian, J. J., & Blatt, G. J. (2007). Decreased GAD67 mRNA levels in cerebellar Purkinje cells in autism: pathophysiological implications. *Acta Neuropathologica, 113*, 559–568.

Yip, J., Soghomonian, J. J., & Blatt, G. J. (2008). Increased GAD67 mRNA expression in cerebellar interneurons in autism: implications for Purkinje cell dysfunction. *Journal of Neuroscience Research, 86*, 525–530.

Yip, J., Soghomonian, J. J., & Blatt, G. J. (2009). Decreased GAD65 mRNA levels in select subpopulations of neurons in the cerebellar dentate nuclei in autism: an in situ hybridization study. *Autism Research, 2*, 50–59.

Yung, K. K., Bolam, J. P., Smith, A. D., Hersch, S. M., Ciliax, B. J., & Levey, A. I. (1995). Immunocytochemical localization of D1 and D2 dopamine receptors in the basal ganglia of the rat: light and electron microscopy. *Neuroscience, 65*, 709–730.

Zee, D. S., Leigh, R. J., & Mathieu-Millaire, F. (1980). Cerebellar control of ocular gaze stability. *Annals of Neurolgy, 7*, 37–40.

Zee, D. S., Yee, R. D., Cogan, D. G., Robinson, D. A., & Engel, W. K. (1976). Ocular motor abnormalities in hereditary cerebellar ataxia. *Brain, 99*, 207–234.

Zwaigenbaum, L., Bryson, S., Rogers, T., Roberts, W., Brian, J., & Szatmari, P. (2005). Behavioral manifestations of autism in the first year of life. *International Journal of Developmental Neuroscience, 23*, 143–152.

23 Roberto Tuchman

Epilepsy and Electroencephalography in Autism Spectrum Disorders

Points of Interest

- Epilepsy is approximately 10 to 30 times more prevalent in individuals with ASD than in the general population.
- The prevalence of seizures and epileptiform activity is highest in children with ASD with moderate to severe intellectual disability.
- Frequent seizures and epileptiform activity in the first 3 years of life are a risk factor for developing ASD with intellectual disability.
- Children with both ASD and epilepsy have poor developmental outcomes, and epilepsy is a risk factor for early mortality in ASD.
- ASD and epilepsy do not reflect singular entities with uniform etiologies; there is no one single treatment or treatment protocol for children with ASD and epilepsy; rational pharmacotherapy requires an understanding of the shared neuronal networks, genetic and molecular biological mechanisms that account for both ASD and the epilepsies.
- The best hope for improving developmental outcomes in children with ASD and epilepsy is early recognition and comprehensive treatment of both the ASD and epilepsy.

Autism Spectrum Disorders—Epilepsy: Definitions

Standardized classification systems for autism and epilepsy are essential, as both autism and epilepsy are heterogeneous disorders with multiple etiologies (Tuchman, Cuccaro, & Alessandri, 2010a). An understanding of the terminology for both autism and epilepsy is crucial in the interpretation of research studies on the relationship of what are now conceived of as the autisms (Geschwind & Levitt, 2007) and the epilepsies (Reynolds & Rodin, 2009).

Throughout this chapter the term "autism spectrum disorders" (ASD) is used to include children with autistic disorder, Pervasive Developmental Disorders Not-Otherwise-Specified (PDD-NOS) and Asperger's syndrome. In this chapter children with disintegrative disorder (DD) or Rett syndrome (RS) are discussed separately from those with autism. In DD and RS rates of seizures are significantly higher than in autism, and both are associated with regression of skills.

> Seizures are clinical events characterized by paroxysmal, stereotyped, relatively brief interruptions of ongoing behavior, associated with electrographic seizure patterns, and epilepsy is operationally defined as two unprovoked seizures of any type (ILAE, 1981). Seizures are the most dramatic aspect of epilepsy, although recent definitions of epilepsy have emphasized the neurologic, cognitive, psychological, and social consequences of this group of disorders (Fisher et al., 2005).

The term "subclinical" or "nonconvulsive" seizure is used to refer to electrographic patterns, without clinically recognizable cognitive, behavioral, or motor functions or apparent impairment of consciousness, and requires a concurrent EEG, with behavioral testing for identification; however there is significant controversy to what constitutes a seizure or an interictal event, and this differentiation becomes increasingly challenging in a child with complex behavioral manifestations as occurs in ASD (Besag, 1995). "Interictal epileptiform discharges" and "epileptiform activity" (both terms are used interchangeably) describe abnormal electroencephalogram (EEG) activity, specifically referring to spikes alone or accompanied by a slow wave, occurring either singly or in bursts, and lasting at most 1 or 2 seconds (Chatrian et al., 1974). This term is used to describe interictal paroxysmal activity, is not used to refer to seizure patterns, and the association of epileptiform activity with an epileptic disorder is variable (Worrell, Lagerlund, & Buchhalter, 2002). The terminology and standards used to determine epileptic activity, seizures, or epileptiform activity, in children with ASD has varied widely among studies (Kelley & Moshe, 2006).

Historical Perspective

Epilepsy has been associated with ASD since the initial description of the disorder by Leo Kanner in 1943 (Kanner, 1971). In the 1960s the first studies on the relationship of ASD to epilepsy and to EEG abnormalities emerged (Creak & Pampiglione, 1969; Hutt, Hutt, Lee, & Ounsted, 1965; Schain & Yannet, 1960; White, Demyer, & Demyer, 1964). These studies were among the first neurobiological studies to suggest that the behaviors of children with ASD were secondary to a disorder of brain function.

In the early1970s a relationship between infantile spasms, hypsarrhythmia, and ASD (Taft & Cohen, 1971) was first described. A Finnish study in 1981 (Riikonen & Amnell, 1981) confirmed the relationship between infantile spasms and ASD. Recent studies have found that up to 35% of children diagnosed with infantile spasms in the first year of life go on to develop the ASD phenotype with associated intellectual disability (ID) (Saemundsen, Ludvigsson, & Rafnsson, 2007). At the present time we are just beginning to appreciate the high number of children with epileptic encephalopathies who later go on to develop the ASD phenotype and how often ASD coexists in children with epilepsy (Clarke et al., 2005).

In the late 1970s and early 1980s there was an interest in specific aspects of the relationship of ASD to epilepsy and of epilepsy and EEG abnormalities to language disorders. During this period the increased risk of seizures in autism at puberty was highlighted (Deykin & MacMahon, 1979), the relationship of autism to tuberous sclerosis was recognized (Mansheim, 1979), and clinical researchers began to investigate the relationship of epilepsy and the EEG to language disorders (Deonna, Beaumanoir, Gaillard, & Assal, 1977; Holmes, McKeever, & Saunders, 1981). At the present time, the neurobiological basis of the secondary peak of seizures during adolescence in ASD is still not clear, tuberous sclerosis has become an important model to explore the neurobiological underpinnings of the association between ASD and epilepsy, and the relationship of language regression, epilepsy, and EEG abnormalities to ASD remains controversial.

In the 1980s studies on autism-epilepsy investigated the differences in rates of epilepsy in different groups of children with ASD (Olsson, Steffenburg, & Gillberg, 1988). During this time standardized criteria for ASD (Lord et al., 1989) and advances in the classification of the epilepsies (ILAE, 1981) emerged; both of these advances had a positive scientific impact on the study of ASD-epilepsy. By the 1990s the relationship between ASD and epilepsy had been established (Volkmar & Nelson, 1990). During the 1990s studies focused on the specific risk factors for development of epilepsy in children with ASD (Tuchman, Rapin, & Shinnar, 1991) and explored the relationship of epilepsy and EEG findings to autistic regression (Tuchman & Rapin, 1997).

Recently studies have found that individuals with ASD and epilepsy have poorer cognitive (lower IQ), adaptive, behavioral, and social outcomes than those with ASD without epilepsy (Hara, 2007; Turk et al., 2009). There is emerging evidence that the mortality in ASD may be twice as high as in the general population with a significant percentage of the deaths being associated or secondary to coexisting epilepsy (Billstedt & Gillberg, 2005; Gillberg, Billstedt, Sundh, & Gillberg, 2010; Mouridsen, Bronnum-Hansen, Rich, & Isager, 2008). There has also been recent interest in the effects of chronic seizure disorders such as mesial temporal lobe epilepsy on deficits in higher-order social cognitive tasks in adults (Schacher et al., 2006; Walpole, Isaac, & Reynders, 2008). One study suggested that epilepsy is not part of the broader autism phenotype (Mouridsen, Rich, & Isager, 2008), but how often ASD is part of the broader epilepsy phenotype is not known. There is a renewed interest in the relationship of ASD to epilepsy with a shift in focus to the molecular biology mechanisms common to both ASD (Bourgeron, 2009) and the epilepsies (Rakhade & Jensen, 2009).

Epidemiology

Neither ASD nor epilepsy is a singular entity with uniform etiologies (Guerrini, 2006; Happe, Ronald, & Plomin, 2006). In children with ASD, cognitive and motor impairments, age of epilepsy onset, severity of receptive language deficits, and genetic and molecular abnormalities are associated with an increased prevalence of epilepsy (Tuchman, Moshe, & Rapin, 2009). In children with epilepsy, younger age at seizure onset, cognitive impairment, temporal or frontal lobe onset of seizures, and intractable epilepsy are associated with an increased likelihood of coexisting social-communication and behavioral disorders (Hamiwka & Wirrell, 2009).

The recognition of clinical seizures and the classification of seizure type are difficult in the general population (Camfield & Camfield, 2003), and in children with ASD the challenge of diagnosing and classifying seizures is even greater, secondary to their diverse behavioral manifestations (Tuchman & Rapin, 2002). Studies on individuals with ASD have reported that all seizure types may be associated with autism (Tuchman & Rapin, 2002). In a group of 98 children with ASD, ages 6 to 13 years, all with intellectual disability, the predominant seizure types in order of frequency were generalized tonic-clonic, myoclonic, atypical absences, and partial complex seizures (Steffenburg, Hagberg, & Kyllerman, 1996). In addition this found that children who only had partial complex seizure types were less likely to have other evidence of brain damage such as severe intellectual disability, cerebral palsy, or visual impairments as contrasted to those with generalized epilepsies.

Epilepsy

The prevalence of epilepsy in ASD is highly variable and depends on the cohort studied, with rates ranging from 5% to 46% (Spence & Schneider, 2009). The reported rates of epilepsy in ASD are several-fold higher than the 0.5% to 1% prevalence of epilepsy in the general population (Hauser, Annegers, & Kurland, 1993). However, the prevalence of epilepsy in ASD is similar to prevalence of epilepsy in a population of children with intellectual disability, with the highest rates of seizures in those with severe cognitive impairments (Goulden, Shinnar, Koller, Katz, & Richardson, 1991; Murphy, Trevathan, & Yeargin-Allsopp, 1995; Steffenburg et al., 1996; Steffenburg, Hagberg, Viggedal, & Kyllerman, 1995). There is a paucity of information on how often ASD is found in children with epilepsy, although in a study conducted in a tertiary epilepsy clinic, approximately 30% of children with epilepsy screened positive for ASD (Clarke et al., 2005) and approximately 7% of children with seizures in the first year of life develop ASD (Saemundsen, Ludvigsson, Hilmarsdottir, & Rafnsson, 2007).

Studies suggest that there are two peaks of seizure onset in autism—one in early childhood and one in adolescence (Volkmar & Nelson, 1990). Studies that include younger children with autism, that is, prior to adolescence, have in general a prevalence rate of less than 10% (Fattal-Valevski et al., 1999; Hoshino et al., 1987; Voigt et al., 2000). In studies that include a high number of adolescents and adults with autism, the rates of seizures reported are higher than 30% (Giovanardi Rossi, Posar, & Parmeggiani, 2000; Kawasaki, Yokota, Shinomiya, Shimizu, & Niwa, 1997). In those that include a mixture of infants, children, adolescents, and adults the prevalence of epilepsy is 10% to 20% (Kobayashi & Murata, 1998; Tuchman & Rapin, 1997; Tuchman et al., 1991).

It is not uncommon for children who go on to develop ASD to have seizures in the first year of life, with one study of 246 children with ASD ages 4 to 15 years reporting that 80% had their seizure onset in the first year of life (Wong, 1993). Studies suggest that the prevalence of autism is highest among children whose seizures started around age 2 years or earlier and those with low cognitive level (Clarke et al., 2005) and that approximately 7% of children with epilepsy whose seizure onset is in the first year of life go on to develop ASD with intellectual disability (Saemundsen, Ludvigsson, Hilmarsdottir, et al., 2007). Children with autism who have a history of epilepsy at an early age likely reflect a subgroup that is associated with more significant insults to the developing brain. Seizures in the first year of life are a risk factor for ASD, and may reflect the role of early insults to the developing brain, genetic or environmental.

The secondary peak in seizure onset during adolescence and adulthood, although possibly unique to children with ASD as compared to other developmental disabilities, is not well understood. In a prospective population-based study of adolescents and adults with epilepsy and ASD ages 18 to 38 years, all with moderate to severe mental retardation, almost 50% of those with severe intellectual disability had epilepsy by early adult life as compared to 20% of those with moderate intellectual disability (Danielsson, Gillberg, Billstedt, Gillberg, & Olsson, 2005). This latter study did not find the secondary peak of epilepsy and found the highest risk of epilepsy in the first year of life. They did find that greater than 10% of individuals in their study developed epilepsy after age 18 years. They also pointed out that in their study they included individuals with ASD and epilepsy with congenital or acquired disorders, such as individuals with tuberous sclerosis and Rett syndrome. This would bias their study to finding a younger age of seizures, as this is a different population than that in other studies that have found a secondary peak (Giovanardi Rossi et al., 2000). The suggestion here is that the secondary peak is found among those with ASD and intellectual disability without a known etiology.

One intriguing study has found that during the decades of adulthood the prevalence of epilepsy in mental retardation and in cerebral palsy declines, while the prevalence of epilepsy in individuals with Down syndrome and ASD increases during this same period of time (McDermott et al., 2005). In contrast, in Rett syndrome the severity of epilepsy tends to decrease with age with lower seizure frequency and less severe seizures as these girls approach adulthood (Steffenburg, Hagberg, & Hagberg, 2001). These findings suggest that the observed second peak of seizure onset in adolescence and increasing prevalence of epilepsy into adulthood is secondary to an ongoing pathological process in individuals with ASD (Deykin & MacMahon, 1979; Hara, 2007), although clearly more research in this area is needed.

One of the most consistent findings on the coexistence of ASD and epilepsy is that intellectual disability is a significant risk factor for the development of epilepsy in ASD (Amiet et al., 2008) and that the highest rates of seizures are observed in those with the most severe intellectual disability (Pavone et al., 2004). The role of intellectual disability as a primary risk factor for the development of epilepsy in children with ASD was highlighted in the early 1990s in a study of a cohort of 314 children with ASD and 237 children with language disorder without ASD, evaluated over a 30-year period (Tuchman et al., 1991). The major risk factor for epilepsy identified in this study was severe intellectual disability, and this risk was heightened in the presence of severe intellectual disability with a motor deficit. In contrast, epilepsy occurred in 6% of children in the ASD group that was negative for severe intellectual disability, motor deficit, associated perinatal or medical disorder, or a positive family history of epilepsy. The prevalence of epilepsy in this group was similar to the 8% of language-impaired non-ASD children with the highest risk of epilepsy, regardless of whether they had ASD, or language impairment without ASD in those with the most severe receptive language disorder (Tuchman, et al., 1991). This study also found a statistically significant higher percentage of epilepsy in girls with ASD (24%) compared to boys with ASD (11%), which was attributed to the increased prevalence of cognitive and motor deficit in girls. In addition, this found a high risk for developing seizures in the first 5 years of life and that infantile spasms were overrepresented in ASD. A follow-up of this cohort of children into adulthood confirmed previous finding of a secondary peak of seizure onset during adolescence (Ballaban-Gil, Rapin, Tuchman, Freeman, & Shinnar, 1991).

In summary, best estimate of the prevalence on epilepsy in ASD is 8% in ASD without intellectual disability and 20% in ASD with intellectual disability (Amiet et al., 2008). Sample ascertainment and associated medical disorders contribute to the wide range of prevalence rates found in studies on epilepsy in ASD (Spence & Schneider, 2009; Tuchman et al., 2009). Variables such as early brain pathology and degree of intellectual disability are strong contributors to the risk of developing epilepsy in ASD. There are two peaks of seizure onset one occurring prior to age 5 years and one occurring into adolescence and adulthood. Studies on the prevalence of epilepsy in ASD clearly indicate that the highest prevalence of epilepsy, regardless of age or gender, is in individuals with ASD and ID (Elia, Musumeci, Ferri, & Bergonzi, 1995; Mouridsen, Rich, & Isager, 2000; Rossi, Parmeggiani, Bach, Santucci, & Visconti, 1995).

EEG Abnormalities

Studies on the prevalence of epileptiform activity in individuals with ASD and no clinical history of seizures range from 6% to 31% (Kagan-Kushnir, Roberts, & Snead, 2005), although rates as high as 60% have been reported (Chez et al., 2006). Despite documentation of the higher prevalence of epileptiform activity in ASD compared to the 1.5 to 4% rate of epileptiform activity in the general population (Capdevila, Dayyat, Kheirandish-Gozal, & Gozal, 2008; Cavazzuti, Cappella, & Nalin, 1980), there is significant controversy regarding the specificity of these findings to the ASD phenotype. For example in ADHD without epilepsy, epileptiform activity occurs in 6% to 30% of children (Hughes, DeLeo, & Melyn, 2000; Kaufmann, Goldberg-Stern, & Shuper, 2009; Richer, Shevell, & Rosenblatt, 2002), which is remarkably similar to the prevalence of epileptiform activity in children with ASD without seizures. The suggestion is that the high prevalence of epileptiform activity is secondary to the neuropathological processes common to neurodevelopmental disorders. However, there is emerging evidence that epileptiform activity can, independently of seizures or the underlying brain pathology, contribute to specific cognitive dysfunction (Sengoku, Kanazawa, Kawai, & Yamaguchi, 1990; Shewmon & Erwin, 1988) and, when it occurs early in brain development, can cause acute and long-lasting impairment of brain function and neurodevelopment (Galanopoulou & Moshe, 2009; Holmes & Lenck-Santini, 2006).

The term "transient cognitive impairment" is used to describe individuals with epileptiform EEG discharges in association with a momentary disruption of adaptive cerebral function (Aarts, Binnie, Smit, & Wilkins, 1984; Binnie, 2003). The controversy is whether treating this group of children in the absence of seizures is justifiable (Binnie, 2003; Pressler, Robinson, Wilson, & Binnie, 2005). Despite the higher prevalence of epileptic activity in ASD, there is a lack of evidence that treatment of the interictal epileptiform discharges has a positive impact on language, social, cognitive, or behavioral outcomes (Tharp, 2004; Tuchman, 2004).

All of the reports on EEG findings in children with ASD are retrospective reviews of clinical populations and are flawed secondary to selection bias. The studies with the highest rates of epileptiform activity are those from child neurologists who are being referred children with ASD for the evaluation of seizures. In addition, the technology used, such as ambulatory EEG, may be prone to artifacts that may be falsely interpreted as epileptiform (Jayakar, Patrick, Sill, Shwedyk, & Seshia, 1985). Furthermore an overnight sleep EEG study of healthy adults found that 13% had epileptiform activity (Beun, van Emde Boas, & Dekker, 1998), and how often epileptiform activity is present in overnight sleep EEG of infants, children, and adolescents is not known. Therefore the practical impact and relative value of epileptiform activity in children with ASD both from a prognostic and treatment perspective is not known (Baird, Robinson, Boyd, & Charman, 2006).

In summary, the prevalence of epileptiform activity in ASD without seizures is dependent on the type of EEG study done, the length of the EEG recording, methodology specific to collecting and interpretation of EEGs, and the specific population of children with ASD being studied. The significance of epileptiform activity in children with ASD without epilepsy and with or without regression is not known. There is much to be learned regarding the relationship of epilepsy and epileptiform activity to ASD. There is emerging evidence that seizures and frequent epileptiform activity can negatively impact the developmental trajectory and life of individuals with ASD. In addition, in rare instances an epileptic process could be causally related to communication deficits or sociocognitive dysfunction manifesting as behaviors that overlap with the ASD phenotype (Deonna & Roulet, 2006).

Autistic Regression and Epileptic Encephalopathy

Autistic Regression

Regression associated with ASD is usually related to the loss of only a few words but is accompanied by the loss of nonverbal communication skills and occurs in approximately 30% of children with autism (Goldberg et al., 2003; Lord, Shulman, & DiLavore, 2004; Luyster et al., 2005; Werner & Dawson, 2005). The language and social regression that occurs in a subgroup of children with ASD has been termed "autistic regression." Autistic regression may be superimposed on prior abnormal development and occurs prior to age 3 years and in most instances prior to age 2 years (Baird et al., 2008).

Children with ASD and late-onset autistic and cognitive regression that can include motor regression and loss of bowel and bladder use, usually occurring after age 3, are classified under the subgroup of childhood disintegrative disorder (Burd, Fisher, & Kerbeshian, 1989; Mouridsen, Rich, & Isager, 1999; Rapin, 1995; Rogers, 2004; Volkmar, 1992). The prevalence of epilepsy in childhood disintegrative disorder has been reported to be as high as 77% (Mouridsen et al., 2000), and EEG abnormalities are significantly more common in the histories of those with disintegrative disorder than those with infantile autism (Kurita, Kita, & Miyake, 1992). Children with childhood disintegrative disorder regress at a later age than children with ASD, have loss of more than just language and social skills, have significant cognitive impairment, and have a higher rate of seizures than children with ASD, including those with mental retardation and regression.

The other disorder under the ASD umbrella with a rate of seizures compatible with disintegrative disorder is Rett syndrome (Steffenburg et al., 2001). Rett and disintegrative disorder are both associated with regression and severe mental retardation. To what extent the high rate of seizures in this group is secondary to the severe degree of cognitive impairment present in both Rett and disintegrative disorder or what influence other specific variables such as metabolic or molecular factors, i.e., the role of MECP2, have in the development of seizures, remains unknown.

Since the early descriptions of regression in ASD, there has been a suggestion that the subgroup of children with autistic regression have a higher rate of epilepsy (Hoshino et al., 1987; Kurita, 1985). Some studies have found no differences in history of autistic regression in ASD children with epileptiform EEGs and epilepsy versus ASD children with a normal EEG and no epilepsy (Canitano, Luchetti, & Zappella, 2005; Hara, 2007). Contrary to results showing no relationship of regression to epilepsy in autism, one study found that autistic regression was more frequent in children with ASD and epilepsy versus those with ASD and no epilepsy (Hrdlicka et al., 2004). Giannotti et al. (2008) also found that epilepsy was more likely to occur in children with autistic regression. This latter study also found that children with autistic regression had more disrupted sleep than those with ASD without regression.

Epileptic Encephalopathy

The relationship of regression of language and epileptiform EEG abnormalities that occurs in a subgroup of children with ASD has been compared to children who have an epileptic encephalopathy.

> "Epileptic encephalopathy" is a conceptual term that captures the emerging evidence that epileptic activity, seizures, or interictal epileptiform discharges, can lead to cognitive and behavioral impairment above and beyond what might be expected from the underlying pathology (Berg et al., 2009).

Approximately 40% of all epilepsies that start in the first 3 years of life are characterized as epileptic encephalopathies (Guerrini, 2006), and the most common and recognized epilepsy syndromes associated with developmental stagnation or regression in cognitive and behavioral skills include: severe myoclonic epilepsy of infancy (Dravet syndrome, see Box 23-1), infantile spasms (West syndrome), Lennox-Gastaut syndrome, and Landau-Kleffner syndrome–continuous spike-waves during slow-wave sleep (Engel, 2001).

As a group the epileptic encephalopathies are commonly associated with poor developmental outcomes and many of the children affected develop an ASD phenotype (Tuchman et al., 2009). A common epileptic encephalopathy that has been associated with ASD is infantile spasms, an age-specific epilepsy syndrome with a peak age of presentation between 4 to 8 months of age (Zupanc, 2009). The prevalence of autism spectrum disorders is as high as 35% depending on the severity of intellectual disability (Saemundsen, Ludvigsson, & Rafnsson, 2007), with a heightened risk of ASD in the presence of identifiable structural lesions of the brain (Saemundsen, Ludvigsson, & Rafnsson, 2008).

A controversial example of an epileptic encephalopathy that can overlap and sometimes be confused with other conditions, as in children with language regression and an epileptiform EEG, is Landau-Kleffner syndrome, an acquired aphasia in association with an epileptiform EEG with spikes, sharp waves, or spike and wave discharges that are usually bilateral and occur predominantly over the temporal regions (Landau & Kleffner, 1998). On a continuum with Landau- Kleffner syndrome is continuous spike-waves during slow-wave sleep, an epileptic encephalopathy associated with the EEG pattern of electrical status epileptics during slow-wave sleep, various seizure types, and with cognitive, motor, and behavioral disturbances (Tassinari, Cantalupo, Rios-Pohl, Giustina, & Rubboli, 2009). Continuous spike-waves during slow-wave sleep and Landau-Kleffner syndrome are sleep-related epileptic encephalopathies with common clinical features including seizures,

Box 23–1

Dravet syndrome is a genetically determined infantile epileptic encephalopathy mainly caused by de novo mutations in the SCN1A gene (Scheffer, Zhang, Jansen, & Dibbens, 2009). Progressive decline or plateau in development occurs by 1 to 4 years of age, with intellectual disability and an autism phenotype commonly present especially in those with greater than five seizures per month (Wolff, Casse-Perrot, & Dravet, 2006). There is emerging evidence that vaccine encephalopathy, characterized by the appearance of seizures and regression in infants following vaccination, may be secondary to SCNA1 gene mutations, suggesting that vaccine encephalopathy could in fact be a genetically determined epileptic encephalopathy (Berkovic et al., 2006). Whether these findings have relevance to the controversy of vaccine encephalopathy and ASD (Berg, 2007), especially in those children with autistic regression and seizures or an epileptiform EEG, is not known. A susceptibility locus for ASD has been reported on chromosome 2 in the vicinity of the epilepsy-involved genes SCN1A and SCN2A (Weiss et al., 2003); how often SCNA1 mutations are present in children with autistic regression and epilepsy may be an instructive research question with implications to the larger vaccine and ASD debate.

regression, and epileptiform abnormalities that are activated by sleep (Nickels & Wirrell, 2008). In continuous spike-waves during slow-wave sleep there is a regression in global skills, while in Landau-Kleffner syndrome the primary clinical manifestation is a regression of language.

Landau-Kleffner syndrome can be differentiated from children with autistic regression and an epileptiform EEG or seizures based on variables such as age of onset of regression (age less than 3 years for autistic regression versus greater that 3 years of age for Landau-Kleffner syndrome), type of regression (primarily language in Landau-Kleffner syndrome), and sleep-related EEG findings, with more frequent epileptiform activity on the EEG, activated in sleep in Landau-Kleffner (McVicar, Ballaban-Gil, Rapin, Moshe, & Shinnar, 2005; Shinnar et al., 2001; Tuchman, 2009). The clinical differences between Landau-Kleffner syndrome and autistic regression with epilepsy or an epileptiform EEG suggests that they are overlapping but distinct phenotypes with potentially different etiologies and pathophysiology, as well as developmental outcomes.

In summary, there are many unanswered questions regarding autistic regression and its relationship to epilepsy and epileptiform activity on the EEG. Clinical reports suggest that children with epileptic encephalopathies are at high risk for developing ASD (Tuchman, 2006). There are also reports of children with early-onset seizures and autistic regression (Deonna, Roulet-Perez, Chappuis, & Ziegler, 2007; Deonna, Ziegler, Moura-Serra, & Innocenti, 1993; Humphrey, Neville, Clarke, & Bolton, 2006; Neville et al., 1997), however the contribution that epileptiform activity has in the development of autistic regression is not presently understood. Nevertheless, the epileptic encephalopathy model suggests that in the absence of seizures, an EEG needs to be considered when there is clinically significant loss of social and communicative functions and there is a clinical suspicion that epilepsy or that epileptiform activity may be contributing to the regression (Filipek et al., 2000). If abnormal electrical activity is found in a child with ASD with or without seizures, the interpretation and potential treatment needs to be based on the type, location, and frequency of the epileptiform activity within the clinical context of that individual child (Trevathan, 2005). There will be rare children with ASD and markedly abnormal sleep EEG suggestive of a sleep-related epileptic encephalopathy (Scheffer, Parry-Fielder, Mullen, & Saunders, 2006). However there is a lack of clinical signs and biomarkers that can presently guide a clinician to provide evidence-based guidelines for performing an EEG in children with ASD with or without regression (Kagan-Kushnir, Roberts, & Snead, 2005). Finally, in the child with autistic regression with epilepsy or frequent epileptiform activity, a work-up for metabolic and mitochondrial disorders should be strongly considered (Shoffner et al., 2009).

Treatments of Epilepsy and the EEG in ASD

ASD and epilepsy do not reflect singular entities with uniform etiologies (Guerrini, 2006; Happe et al., 2006), and it follows that there is no one single treatment or treatment protocol for children with ASD or epilepsy. An understanding of the shared neuronal networks, genetic and molecular biological mechanisms that account for both ASD and the epilepsies is emerging and essential to rational pharmacotherapy, but our knowledge is far from complete (Tuchman et al., 2009). The heterogeneity of clinical symptoms in children with ASD highlights the importance of a comprehensive assessment that includes investigation of underlying biological etiologies as well assessment of cognitive, language, affective, social, and behavioral function prior to initiating treatment and throughout the intervention process.

Conditions common to both epilepsy and ASD as separate disorders challenge both diagnostic and therapeutic strategies, when both disorders co-occur in the same child. Of importance is not missing treatable causes such as metabolic disorders, which may account for both the epilepsy and ASD (Zecavati & Spence, 2009). In addition, disorders of mitochondrial function, which may be more common than appreciated among children with childhood epilepsies, including a number of the epileptic syndromes associated with ASD, should be considered as potential etiologies (Lee et al., 2008).

The view of pharmacotherapy in epilepsy has evolved from the treatment of seizures to include targeting improvement in cognitive symptoms, mood, and psychiatric disorders (Devinsky, 2003). The psychotropic mechanism of action of several antiepileptic drugs is now well established, and there are several reviews that attempt to place this within the context of treating children with ASD and epilepsy (Di Martino & Tuchman, 2001; Ettinger, 2006; Ettinger & Argoff, 2007). Nevertheless, at the present time there are no randomized controlled trials or large clinical studies that have looked closely at the effects of these anticonvulsants in well-defined populations of children with ASD and epilepsy to guide a clinician in the treatment of a child with ASD and epilepsy. As such, the standard of care in children with both ASD and epilepsy is no different from treatment of seizures in other children with epilepsy without autism (Gillberg, 1991; Tuchman & Rapin, 2002).

Antiepileptic drugs are administered widely to children with ASD with and without epilepsy (Aman, Lam, & Collier-Crespin, 2003), and one of the most commonly reported medications used in the treatment of ASD and epilepsy is valproic acid. Several clinical reports of the use of valproic acid in children with ASD with or without clinical seizures but with epileptiform abnormalities on the EEG report overall behavioral improvement (Childs & Blair, 1997; Nass & Petrucha, 1990; Plioplys, 1994). An open trial in 14 individuals using divalproex sodium found improvement in core symptoms of ASD and the associated affective instability, impulsivity, and aggression, only in those children with autism and an abnormal EEG or seizure history (Hollander, Dolgoff-Kaspar, Cartwright, Rawitt, & Novotny, 2001). Hollander and colleagues reported the use of valproic acid in repetitive behaviors in repetitive compulsive behaviors and found improvement (Hollander et al., 2006), suggesting that valproic acid has a wide effect on numerous behaviors, as do other anticonvulsants, and highlighting the limitations on our knowledge of the mechanisms and specificity of this group of medications.

A study of 50 children with intractable epilepsy measured the effects of lamotrigine, an antiepileptic drug with a beneficial psychotropic profile, on 13 children with autism. Eight of these children showed a decrease in "autism symptoms" without a concomitant decrease in seizures, suggesting a specific benefit of lamotrigine in ASD (Uvebrant & Bauziene, 1994). In a subsequent double-blind placebo control trial of lamotrigine in 28 children with autism without seizures, no significant benefit was found on the Autism Behavior Checklist, the Aberrant Behavior Checklist, the Vineland Adaptive Behavior scales, the PL-ADOS, or the CARS; nevertheless, parents reported a beneficial effect of lamotrigine (Belsito, Law, Kirk, Landa, & Zimmerman, 2001). Clinical experience suggests that picking anticonvulsants with favorable psychotropic effects in children with autism and epilepsy is important. The problem is that generally small numbers of children limit the power of the studies, and these samples cannot be considered representative of all children with ASD and epilepsy (Garcia-Penas, 2005; Pellock, 2004). The findings of whether antiepileptic drugs have positive psychotropic effects on children with ASD with or without epilepsy are equivocal. For example, in an open-label study of levetiracetam in 10 children with ASD without epilepsy, positive effects were noted on measures of hyperactivity, impulsivity, mood instability, and aggression (Rugino & Samsock, 2002). However, a second study of levetiracetam in 20 children with ASD and no seizures found no positive effects on behavior (Wasserman et al., 2006).

Some clinicians have used the strategies recommended for the management of children with Landau-Kleffner syndrome in children with autistic regression and an epileptiform EEG with or without clinical seizures. Therapy in Landau-Kleffner syndrome has been the subject of numerous case reports or short series that have reported poorly documented improvements in language in response to anticonvulsants, especially valproate, ethosuximide, and the benzodiazepines (Marescaux et al., 1990). There are other positive reports of improvement with ACTH, steroids, or immunoglobulins (Lagae, Silberstein, Gillis, & Casaer, 1998; Mikati, Lepejian, & Holmes, 2002; Prasad, Stafstrom, & Holmes, 1996, Tsuru, 2000). Despite these reports, and because of the limited data documenting the specifics of language improvement, the role that these therapies have in autistic regression with an epileptiform EEG but without frequent seizures is controversial. In addition, as emphasized earlier, the clinical phenotype of autistic regression is not the same as that of Landau-Kleffner syndrome, and recommendations for treatments in children with autistic regression and epileptiform EEGs without epilepsy should not be extrapolated from treatments used in an epileptic encephalopathy. Furthermore in children with ASD it is rare to find the same frequency of epileptiform activity or intractability of epilepsy as is found in children with an epileptic encephalopathy.

Other potential interventions that have been used in epilepsy, such as vagal nerve stimulation and the ketogenic diet, have been tried in children with both epilepsy and ASD with mixed results (Danielsson, Viggedal, Gillberg, & Olsson, 2008; Evangeliou et al., 2003; Mantis, Fritz, Marsh, Heinrichs, & Seyfried, 2009; Park, 2003; Warwick, Griffith, Reyes, Legesse, & Evans, 2007). In children with ASD with and without intractable seizures that have undergone epilepsy surgery, there are reports of transient behavioral improvements; however core deficits in social communication functioning remain, as do other affective and social emotional issues, despite improvement in seizure control (Lewine et al., 1999; Nass, Gross, Wisoff, & Devinsky, 1999; Neville et al., 1997; Szabo et al., 1999; Taylor, Neville, & Cross, 1999). In addition, intellectual capacity influences response to intervention in children with ASD and epilepsy, and current medical and surgical interventions do not appear to dramatically alter intellectual ability (Danielsson et al., 2009).

At present we are just beginning to understand the mechanisms of epileptogenesis (Rakhade & Jensen, 2009) and the risks, risk processes, symptom emergence, and adaptation leading to impairments in the normal trajectory of sociocommunicative development and to ASD (Dawson, 2008). There is some emerging evidence that early and successful treatment of seizures and interictal epileptiform activity may be crucial to positive neurodevelopmental outcomes in children with epileptic encephalopathies (Arts & Geerts, 2009; Bombardieri, Pinci, Moavero, Cerminara, & Curatolo, 2010; Freitag & Tuxhorn, 2005; Jonas et al., 2005; Lux et al., 2005) and that early treatment of children at risk for ASD may prevent the full-blown syndrome from developing (Dawson, 2008). However there is still significant controversy and uncertainty regarding treatment approaches for children with ASD and epilepsy or those with autistic regression and an epileptiform EEG (Deonna & Roulet, 2006).

An emerging approach to the development of therapeutic agents specific to the ASD-epilepsy phenotype is based on our understanding of common mechanisms for ASD and epilepsy such as abnormalities of synaptic structure in ASD (Garber, 2007) and epilepsy (Caleo, 2009; Lado & Moshe, 2008). For example, in Rett syndrome abnormalities in synapse formation and modulation contribute to a higher rate of seizures, epileptiform activity, and to the ASD phenotype (Glaze, 2004; Zoghbi, 2003). Other mechanisms that can lead to both ASD and epilepsy are abnormalities in the genetic calcium channel signals, which are also involved in regulatory pathways and in energy metabolism (Gargus, 2009). In addition, genetic disorders such as Angelman's syndrome, where epilepsy and ASD commonly coexist (Dan, 2009), and animal models such as Pten mouse, where conditional deletion of Pten is associated with abnormalities in circadian rhythms, seizures, and social interaction deficits (Ogawa et al., 2007; Zhou et al., 2009), allow for the investigation of common mechanisms and potential targets for therapeutic drugs for individuals with ASD and epilepsy. A prototype clinical disorder that allows for investigation of the complex interrelationship between genetics, seizures, brain pathology, and the development of cognitive impairments and ASD is the tuberous sclerosis complex (Box 23-2).

In summary, the clinical heterogeneity, numerous coexisting conditions found in both ASD and epilepsy, and our limited understanding of the pathophysiology of the ASD-epilepsy

Box 23–2
Tuberous sclerosis complex and ASD-epilepsy phenotypes: common mechanisms and treatment

Tuberous sclerosis complex is a neurological disorder commonly associated with ASD, epilepsy, and cognitive impairments (Napolioni, Moavero, & Curatolo, 2009). Tuberous sclerosis, which occurs in about 1 in 6000 live births, is an autosomal dominant disorder, although up to 60% of affected children carry spontaneous mutations of one of two different genes causing the disorder, TSC2 and TSC1 (Curatolo, 2003). In tuberous sclerosis temporal lobe epileptiform discharges, a history of infantile spasms, and onset of seizures in the first 3 years of life appear to be risk factors for development of ASD (Bolton, 2004). There is also a suggestion that the proportion of the total brain volume occupied by tubers and age at seizure onset are the best predictors of cognitive function in individuals with tuberous sclerosis (Jansen et al., 2008), and that prolonged duration of infantile spasms, longer delays prior to initiation of treatment of the infantile spasms, and poor seizure control after cessation of infantile spasms are risk factors for development of intellectual disability in tuberous sclerosis complex (Goh, Kwiatkowski, Dorer, & Thiele, 2005). In addition, seizures unresponsive to treatment and tuberous sclerosis complex 2 mutations are associated with poor cognitive outcomes (Winterkorn, Pulsifer, & Thiele, 2007). Tuberous sclerosis complex has become an informative model to investigate molecular mechanisms and potential treatments for the ASD-epilepsy phenotype (Crino, 2008). In the mouse model of tuberous sclerosis, treatment with the mTor inhibitor rapamycin has been reported to prevent epilepsy and reverse learning deficits (Ehninger et al., 2008; Meikle et al., 2008; Zeng, Xu, Gutmann, & Wong, 2008). A recent report of rapamycin reducing seizures in a child with tuberous sclerosis complex raises the intriguing question of the clinical use of rapamycin for epilepsy, especially in children with an epileptic encephalopathy that are at high risk of developing ASD (Muncy, Butler, & Koenig, 2009).

phenotypes have challenged our ability to find effective treatments for individuals with epilepsy and ASD. In addition, a lack of clear clinical and biological markers to measure effectiveness, particularly developmental outcomes, hinders study design. The few studies that have been conducted have included small numbers of children, are based on short periods of observation, rely on incomplete diagnostic measures of either ASD or epilepsy, and measure efficacy in a limited fashion.

The importance of a comprehensive approach to treatment, especially in the early-onset epilepsies, is that if the epileptic activity interfering with the normal trajectory of development is eliminated, then intensive, frequent, and structured intervention may allow for the plasticity of the brain, now unburdened of the epileptic activity, to overcome the language, social, and cognitive deficits associated with ASD. There are no studies in individuals with ASD and epilepsy that use a comprehensive approach to treatment, incorporating behavioral, educational, medical, and surgical interventions (Tuchman, Cuccaro, & Alessandri, 2010b). Treatment of the seizures follows the standards of epilepsy management and is clearly indicated in all children with ASD with epilepsy, but when and how to treat epileptiform activity in the absence of seizures is not known.

Conclusion

The wide range of co-occurrence of seizures and epileptic activity is dependent on multiple variables that include age, presence of genetic syndrome or underlying brain pathology, and degree of intellectual disability. The best estimate of the prevalence on epilepsy in ASD is 8% in ASD without significant intellectual disability and 20% in ASD with intellectual disability. The prevalence of epileptiform activity in individuals with ASD and no clinical history of seizures is approximately 6% to 30% and is dependent on the type of EEG study done, the length of the EEG recording, methodology specific to collecting and interpretation of EEGs, and the specific population of children with ASD being studied. The prevalence of epilepsy and of epileptiform activity is significantly higher, greater than 50%, in those with severe intellectual disability, genetic syndromes, and other associated brain pathology.

An emerging consensus is that shared genetic and molecular mechanisms account for the common co-occurrence of ASD and epilepsy. In the overwhelming majority of children with ASD neither the epilepsy nor the epileptiform activity is frequent or intractable. ASD is a common developmental outcome of the early-onset epilepsies, such as the epileptic encephalopathies. The contribution of epileptic activity to brain development, and specifically to the language and sociocognitive dysfunction characteristic of ASD, remains inadequately studied and poorly understood. In children with epileptic encephalopathies the contribution of the seizures and epileptiform activity to brain development may in and of itself account for lower intellectual ability, adaptive function, and an ASD phenotype. This has important implications for treatment, as early and successful treatment of seizures and epileptiform activity is more likely to be associated with good neurodevelopmental outcomes.

Challenges and Future Directions

- Defining the clinical and biological determinants that account for the phenotypic convergence of ASD and epilepsy with lowered cognitive profiles, motor impairments, attention difficulties, hyperactivity, and mood problems.
- Identification of ASD-epilepsy phenotypes, defined by common clinical and biological criteria, such as those

with early- versus late-onset seizures, facilitating the search for common developmental genes for epilepsy and ASD.

- Determining in a population of children with epilepsy those at high risk for development outcomes associated with the ASD phenotype by characterizing subgroups based on etiology and brain pathology, as well as by seizure type, frequency, and EEG characteristics.
- Investigating the biological significance of interictal epileptiform discharges, the effect they have on neural networks critical for development of early social and communicative skills, and their usefulness as biomarkers defining subgroups of children with ASD.
- Development of biologically informative animal models with shared clinical features of ASD-epilepsy phenotypes, allowing for identification of common molecular mechanisms for ASD and epilepsy and identification of therapeutic targets for pharmacological intervention.

SUGGESTED READINGS

Tuchman, R., Moshe, S. L., & Rapin, I. (2009). Convulsing toward the pathophysiology of autism. *Brain and Development, 31*(2), 95–103.

Spence, S. J., & Schneider, M. T. (2009). The role of epilepsy and epileptiform EEGs in autism spectrum disorders. *Pediatric Research, 65*(6), 599–606.

Tuchman, R., Cuccaro, M., & Alessandri, M. (2010). Autism spectrum disorders and epilepsy: Moving towards a comprehensive approach to treatment. *Brain and Development, 32*(9), 719–730.

REFERENCES

Aarts, J. H., Binnie, C. D., Smit, A. M., & Wilkins, A. J. (1984). Selective cognitive impairment during focal and generalized epileptiform EEG activity. *Brain, 107*(Pt 1), 293–308.

Aman, M. G., Lam, K. S., & Collier-Crespin, A. (2003). Prevalence and patterns of use of psychoactive medicines among individuals with autism in the Autism Society of Ohio. *Journal of Autism and Developmental Disorders, 33*(5), 527–534.

Amiet, C., Gourfinkel-An, I., Bouzamondo, A., Tordjman, S., Baulac, M., Lechat, P., et al. (2008). Epilepsy in autism is associated with intellectual disability and gender: evidence from a meta-analysis. *Biological Psychiatry, 64*(7), 577–582.

Arts, W. F., & Geerts, A. T. (2009). When to start drug treatment for childhood epilepsy: the clinical-epidemiological evidence. *European Journal of Paediatric Neurology, 13*(2), 93–101.

Baird, G., Charman, T., Pickles, A., Chandler, S., Loucas, T., Meldrum, D., et al. (2008). Regression, developmental trajectory, and associated problems in disorders in the autism spectrum: the SNAP study. *Journal of Autism and Developmental Disorders, 38*(10), 1827–1836.

Baird, G., Robinson, R. O., Boyd, S., & Charman, T. (2006). Sleep electroencephalograms in young children with autism with and without regression. *Developmental Medicine and Child Neurology, 48*(7), 604–608.

Ballaban-Gil, K., Rapin, I., Tuchman, R., Freeman, K., & Shinnar, S. (1991). The risk of seizures in autistic individuals: Occurrence of a secondary peak in adolescence. *Epilepsia, 32*(S3), S84.

Belsito, K. M., Law, P. A., Kirk, K. S., Landa, R. J., & Zimmerman, A. W. (2001). Lamotrigine therapy for autistic disorder: a randomized, double-blind, placebo-controlled trial. *Journal of Autism and Developmental Disorders, 31*(2), 175–181.

Berg, A. (2007). Vaccines, encephalopathies, and mutations. *Epilepsy Currents, 7*(2), 40–42.

Berg, A., Berkovic, S., Brodie, M. J., Buchhalter, J. R., Cross, H., Boas, W., et al. (2009). Revised terminology and concepts for organization of the epilepsies: Report of the Commission on Classification and Terminology. Retrieved from http://www.ilae-epilepsy.org in August 2009.

Berkovic, S. F., Harkin, L., McMahon, J. M., Pelekanos, J. T., Zuberi, S. M., Wirrell, E. C., et al. (2006). De-novo mutations of the sodium channel gene SCN1A in alleged vaccine encephalopathy: a retrospective study. *Lancet Neurology, 5*(6), 488–492.

Besag, F. M. (1995). The therapeutic dilemma: treating subtle seizures or indulging in electroencephalogram cosmetics? *Seminars in Pediatric Neurology, 2*(4), 261–268.

Beun, A. M., van Emde Boas, W., & Dekker, E. (1998). Sharp transients in the sleep EEG of healthy adults: a possible pitfall in the diagnostic assessment of seizure disorders. *Electroencephalography and Clinical Neurophysiology, 106*(1), 44–51.

Billstedt, E., & Gillberg, C. (2005). Autism after adolescence: population-based 13- to 22-year follow-up study of 120 individuals with autism diagnosed in childhood. *Journal of Autism and Developmental Disorders, 35*(3), 351–360.

Binnie, C. D. (2003). Cognitive impairment during epileptiform discharges: is it ever justifiable to treat the EEG? *Lancet Neurology, 2*(12), 725–730.

Bolton, P. F. (2004). Neuroepileptic correlates of autistic symptomatology in tuberous sclerosis. *Mental Retardation and Developmental Disabilities Research Reviews, 10*(2), 126–131.

Bombardieri, R., Pinci, M., Moavero, R., Cerminara, C., & Curatolo, P. (2010). Early control of seizures improves long-term outcome in children with tuberous sclerosis complex. *European Journal of Paediatric Neurology, 14*(2), 146–149.

Bourgeron, T. (2009). A synaptic trek to autism. *Current Opinion in Neurobiology, 19*(2), 231–234.

Burd, L., Fisher, W., & Kerbeshian, J. (1989). Pervasive disintegrative disorder: are Rett syndrome and Heller dementia infantilis subtypes? *Developmental Medicine and Child Neurology, 31*(5), 609–616.

Caleo, M. (2009). Epilepsy: synapses stuck in childhood. *Nature Medicine, 15*(10), 1126–1127.

Camfield, P., & Camfield, C. (2003). Childhood epilepsy: what is the evidence for what we think and what we do? *Journal of Child Neurology, 18*(4), 272–287.

Canitano, R., Luchetti, A., & Zappella, M. (2005). Epilepsy, electroencephalographic abnormalities, and regression in children with autism. *Journal of Child Neurology, 20*(1), 27–31.

Capdevila, O. S., Dayyat, E., Kheirandish-Gozal, L., & Gozal, D. (2008). Prevalence of epileptiform activity in healthy children during sleep. *Sleep Medicine, 9*(3), 303–309.

Cavazzuti, G. B., Cappella, L., & Nalin, A. (1980). Longitudinal study of epileptiform EEG patterns in normal children. *Epilepsia, 21*(1), 43–55.

Chatrian, G. E., Bergamini, L., Dondey, M., Klass, D. W., Lennox-Buchthal, M., & PetersÈn, I. (1974). A glossary of terms most commonly used by clinical electroencephalographers. *Electroencephalography and Clinical Neurophysiology, 37*(5), 538–548. [doi: DOI: 10.1016/0013-4694(74)90099-6].

Chez, M. G., Chang, M., et al. (2006). Frequency of epileptiform EEG abnormalities in a sequential screening of autistic patients with no known clinical epilepsy from 1996 to 2005. *Epilepsy and Behavior, 8*(1), 267–271.

Childs, J. A., & Blair, J. L. (1997). Valproic acid treatment of epilepsy in autistic twins. *Journal of Neuroscience Nursing, 29*(4), 244–248.

Clarke, D. F., Roberts, W., Daraksan, M., Dupuis, A., McCabe, J., Wood, H., et al. (2005). The prevalence of autistic spectrum disorder in children surveyed in a tertiary care epilepsy clinic. *Epilepsia, 46*(12), 1970–1977.

Creak, M., & Pampiglione, G. (1969). Clinical and EEG studies on a group of 35 psychotic children. *Developmental Medicine and Child Neurology, 11*(2), 218–227.

Crino, P. B. (2008). Do we have a cure for tuberous sclerosis complex? *Epilepsy Currents, 8*(6), 159–162.

Curatolo, P. (Ed.). (2003). *Tuberous Sclerosis Complex: From basic science to clinical phenotypes*. London, United Kingdom: Mac Keith Press.

Dan, B. (2009). Angelman syndrome: current understanding and research prospects. *Epilepsia, 50*(11), 2331–2339.

Danielsson, S., Gillberg, I. C., Billstedt, E., Gillberg, C., & Olsson, I. (2005). Epilepsy in young adults with autism: a prospective population-based follow-up study of 120 individuals diagnosed in childhood. *Epilepsia, 46*(6), 918–923.

Danielsson, S., Viggedal, G., Gillberg, C., & Olsson, I. (2008). Lack of effects of vagus nerve stimulation on drug-resistant epilepsy in eight pediatric patients with autism spectrum disorders: a prospective 2-year follow-up study. *Epilepsy and Behavior, 12*(2), 298–304.

Danielsson, S., Viggedal, G., Steffenburg, S., Rydenhag, B., Gillberg, C., & Olsson, I. (2009). Psychopathology, psychosocial functioning, and IQ before and after epilepsy surgery in children with drug-resistant epilepsy. *Epilepsy and Behavior, 14*(2), 330–337.

Dawson, G. (2008). Early behavioral intervention, brain plasticity, and the prevention of autism spectrum disorder. *Development and Psychopathology, 20*(3), 775–803.

Deonna, T., Beaumanoir, A., Gaillard, F., & Assal, G. (1977). Acquired aphasia in childhood with seizure disorder: a heterogeneous syndrome. *Neuropediatrie, 8*(3), 263–273.

Deonna, T., & Roulet, E. (2006). Autistic spectrum disorder: evaluating a possible contributing or causal role of epilepsy. *Epilepsia, 47*(Suppl 2), 79–82.

Deonna, T., Roulet-Perez, E., Chappuis, H., & Ziegler, A. L. (2007). Autistic regression associated with seizure onset in an infant with tuberous sclerosis. *Developmental Medicine and Child Neurology, 49*(4), 320.

Deonna, T., Ziegler, A. L., Moura-Serra, J., & Innocenti, G. (1993). Autistic regression in relation to limbic pathology and epilepsy: report of two cases. *Developmental Medicine and Child Neurology, 35*(2), 166–176.

Devinsky, O. (2003). Psychiatric comorbidity in patients with epilepsy: implications for diagnosis and treatment. *Epilepsy and Behavior, 4*(Suppl 4), S2–10.

Deykin, E. Y., & MacMahon, B. (1979). The incidence of seizures among children with autistic symptoms. *American Journal of Psychiatry, 136*(10), 1310–1312.

Di Martino, A., & Tuchman, R. (2001). Antiepileptic drugs: affective use in autism spectrum disorders. *Pediatric Neurology, 25*(3), 199–207.

Ehninger, D., Han, S., Shilyansky, C., Zhou, Y., Li, W., Kwiatkowski, D. J., et al. (2008). Reversal of learning deficits in a Tsc2+/- mouse model of tuberous sclerosis. *Nature Medicine, 14*(8), 843–848.

Elia, M., Musumeci, S. A., Ferri, R., & Bergonzi, P. (1995). Clinical and neurophysiological aspects of epilepsy in subjects with autism and mental retardation. *American Journal of Mental Retardation, 100*(1), 6–16.

Engel, J., Jr. (2001). A proposed diagnostic scheme for people with epileptic seizures and with epilepsy: report of the ILAE Task Force on Classification and Terminology. *Epilepsia, 42*(6), 796–803.

Ettinger, A. B. (2006). Psychotropic effects of antiepileptic drugs. *Neurology, 67*(11), 1916–1925.

Ettinger, A. B., & Argoff, C. E. (2007). Use of antiepileptic drugs for nonepileptic conditions: psychiatric disorders and chronic pain. *Neurotherapeutics, 4*(1), 75–83.

Evangeliou, A., Vlachonikolis, I., Mihailidou, H., Spilioti, M., Skarpalezou, A., Makaronas, N., et al. (2003). Application of a ketogenic diet in children with autistic behavior: pilot study. *Journal of Child Neurology, 18*(2), 113–118.

Fattal-Valevski, A., Kramer, U., Leitner, Y., Nevo, Y., Greenstein, Y., & Harel, S. (1999). Characterization and comparison of autistic subgroups: 10 years' experience with autistic children. *Developmental Medicine and Child Neurology, 41*(1), 21–25.

Filipek, P. A., Accardo, P. J., Ashwal, S., Baranek, G. T., Cook, E. H., Jr., Dawson, G., et al. (2000). Practice parameter: screening and diagnosis of autism: report of the Quality Standards Subcommittee of the American Academy of Neurology and the Child Neurology Society. *Neurology, 55*(4), 468–479.

Fisher, R. S., van Emde Boas, W., Blume, W., Elger, C., Genton, P., Lee, P., et al. (2005). Epileptic seizures and epilepsy: definitions proposed by the International League Against Epilepsy (ILAE) and the International Bureau for Epilepsy (IBE). *Epilepsia, 46*(4), 470–472.

Freitag, H., & Tuxhorn, I. (2005). Cognitive function in preschool children after epilepsy surgery: rationale for early intervention. *Epilepsia, 46*(4), 561–567.

Galanopoulou, A. S., & Moshe, S. L. (2009). The epileptic hypothesis: developmentally related arguments based on animal models. *Epilepsia, 50*(Suppl 7), 37–42.

Garber, K. (2007). Neuroscience. Autism's cause may reside in abnormalities at the synapse. *Science, 317*(5835), 190–191.

Garcia-Penas, J. J. (2005). Tratamiento con fármacos antiepilépticos en los sindromes de regresión autista [Antiepileptic drugs in the treatment of autistic regression syndromes.]. *Revista de Neurologia, 40*(Suppl 1), S173–176.

Gargus, J. J. (2009). Genetic calcium signaling abnormalities in the central nervous system: seizures, migraine, and autism. *Annals of the New York Academy Sciences, 1151*, 133–156.

Geschwind, D. H., & Levitt, P. (2007). Autism spectrum disorders: developmental disconnection syndromes. *Current Opinion in Neurobiology, 17*(1), 103–111.

Giannotti, F., Cortesi, F., Cerquiglini, A., Miraglia, D., Vagnoni, C., Sebastiani, T., et al. (2008). An investigation of sleep characteristics, EEG abnormalities and epilepsy in developmentally regressed and non-regressed children with autism. *Journal of Autism and Developmental Disorders, 38*(10), 1888–1897.

Gillberg, C. (1991). The treatment of epilepsy in autism. *Journal of Autism and Developmental Disorders, 21*(1), 61–77.

Gillberg, C., Billstedt, E., Sundh, V., & Gillberg, I. C. (2010). Mortality in autism: A prospective longitudinal community-based study. *Journal of Autism and Developmental Disorders, 40*(3), 352–357.

Giovanardi Rossi, P., Posar, A., & Parmeggiani, A. (2000). Epilepsy in adolescents and young adults with autistic disorder. *Brain and Development, 22*(2), 102–106.

Glaze, D. G. (2004). Rett syndrome: of girls and mice—lessons for regression in autism. *Mental Retardation and Developmental Disabilities Research Reviews, 10*(2), 154–158.

Goh, S., Kwiatkowski, D. J., Dorer, D. J., & Thiele, E. A. (2005). Infantile spasms and intellectual outcomes in children with tuberous sclerosis complex. *Neurology, 65*(2), 235–238.

Goldberg, W. A., Osann, K., Filipek, P. A., Laulhere, T., Jarvis, K., Modahl, C., et al. (2003). Language and other regression: assessment and timing. *Journal of Autism and Developmental Disorders, 33*(6), 607–616.

Goulden, K. J., Shinnar, S., Koller, H., Katz, M., & Richardson, S. A. (1991). Epilepsy in children with mental retardation: a cohort study. *Epilepsia, 32*(5), 690–697.

Guerrini, R. (2006). Epilepsy in children. *Lancet, 367*(9509), 499–524.

Hamiwka, L. D., & Wirrell, E. C. (2009). Comorbidities in pediatric epilepsy: beyond "just" treating the seizures. *Journal of Child Neurology, 24*(6), 734–742.

Happe, F., Ronald, A., & Plomin, R. (2006). Time to give up on a single explanation for autism. *Nature Neuroscience, 9*(10), 1218–1220.

Hara, H. (2007). Autism and epilepsy: a retrospective follow-up study. *Brain and Development, 29*(8), 486–490.

Hauser, W. A., Annegers, J. F., & Kurland, L. T. (1993). Incidence of epilepsy and unprovoked seizures in Rochester, Minnesota: 1935–1984. *Epilepsia, 34*(3), 453–468.

Hollander, E., Dolgoff-Kaspar, R., Cartwright, C., Rawitt, R., & Novotny, S. (2001). An open trial of divalproex sodium in autism spectrum disorders. *Journal of Clinical Psychiatry, 62*(7), 530–534.

Hollander, E., Soorya, L., Wasserman, S., Esposito, K., Chaplin, W., & Anagnostou, E. (2006). Divalproex sodium vs. placebo in the treatment of repetitive behaviours in autism spectrum disorder. *International Journal of Neuropsychopharmacology, 9*(2), 209–213.

Holmes, G. L., & Lenck-Santini, P. P. (2006). Role of interictal epileptiform abnormalities in cognitive impairment. *Epilepsy and Behavior, 8*(3), 504–515.

Holmes, G. L., McKeever, M., & Saunders, Z. (1981). Epileptiform activity in aphasia of childhood: an epiphenomenon? *Epilepsia, 22*(6), 631–639.

Hoshino, Y., Kaneko, M., Yashima, Y., Kumashiro, H., Volkmar, F. R., & Cohen, D. J. (1987). Clinical features of autistic children with setback course in their infancy. *Japanese Journal of Psychiatry and Neurology, 41*(2), 237–245.

Hrdlicka, M., Komarek, V., Propper, L., Kulisek, R., Zumrova, A., Faladova, L., et al. (2004). Not EEG abnormalities but epilepsy is associated with autistic regression and mental functioning in childhood autism. *European Child and Adolescent Psychiatry, 13*(4), 209–213.

Hughes, J. R., DeLeo, A. J., & Melyn, M. A. (2000). The electroencephalogram in attention deficit-hyperactivity disorder: Emphasis on epileptiform discharges. *Epilepsy and Behavior, 1*(4), 271–277.

Humphrey, A., Neville, B. G., Clarke, A., & Bolton, P. F. (2006). Autistic regression associated with seizure onset in an infant with tuberous sclerosis. *Developmental Medicine and Child Neurology, 48*(7), 609–611.

Hutt, S. J., Hutt, C., Lee, D., & Ounsted, C. (1965). A behavioural and electroencephalographic study of autistic children. *Journal of Psychiatric Research, 3*(3), 181–197.

ILAE. (1981). ILAE Commission on Classification and Terminology of the International League Against Epilepsy: Proposal for revised clinical and electroencephalographic classification of epileptic seizures. *Epilepsia, 22,* 489–501.

Jansen, F. E., Vincken, K. L., Algra, A., Anbeek, P., Braams, O., Nellist, M., et al. (2008). Cognitive impairment in tuberous sclerosis complex is a multifactorial condition. *Neurology, 70*(12), 916–923.

Jayakar, P. B., Patrick, J. P., Sill, J., Shwedyk, E., & Seshia, S. S. (1985). Artifacts in ambulatory cassette electroencephalograms. *Electroencephalography and Clinical Neurophysiology, 61*(5), 440–443.

Jonas, R., Asarnow, R. F., LoPresti, C., Yudovin, S., Koh, S., Wu, J. Y., et al. (2005). Surgery for symptomatic infant-onset epileptic encephalopathy with and without infantile spasms. *Neurology, 64*(4), 746–750.

Kagan-Kushnir, T., Roberts, S. W., & Snead, O. C., 3rd. (2005). Screening electroencephalograms in autism spectrum disorders: evidence-based guideline. *Journal of Child Neurology, 20*(3), 197–206.

Kanner, L. (1971). Follow-up study of eleven autistic children originally reported in 1943. *Journal of Autism and Childhood Schizophrenia, 1*(2), 119–145.

Kaufmann, R., Goldberg-Stern, H., & Shuper, A. (2009). Attention-deficit disorders and epilepsy in childhood: incidence, causative relations, and treatment possibilities. *Journal of Child Neurology, 24*(6), 727–733.

Kawasaki, Y., Yokota, K., Shinomiya, M., Shimizu, Y., & Niwa, S. (1997). Brief report: electroencephalographic paroxysmal activities in the frontal area emerged in middle childhood and during adolescence in a follow-up study of autism. *Journal of Autism and Developmental Disorders, 27*(5), 605–620.

Kelley, R. K., & Moshe, S. L. (2006). Electrophysiology and epilepsy in autism. In R. Tuchman & I. Rapin (Eds.), *Autism: A neurological disorder of early brain development* (pp. 160–173). London: MacKeith Press.

Kobayashi, R., & Murata, T. (1998). Setback phenomenon in autism and long-term prognosis. *Acta Psychiatrica Scandinavica, 98*(4), 296–303.

Kurita, H. (1985). Infantile autism with speech loss before the age of thirty months. *Journal of the American Academy of Child Psychiatry, 24*(2), 191–196.

Kurita, H., Kita, M., & Miyake, Y. (1992). A comparative study of development and symptoms among disintegrative psychosis and infantile autism with and without speech loss. *Journal of Autism and Developmental Disorders, 22*(2), 175–188.

Lado, F. A., & Moshe, S. L. (2008). How do seizures stop? *Epilepsia, 49*(10), 1651–1664.

Lagae, L. G., Silberstein, J., Gillis, P. L., & Casaer, P. J. (1998). Successful use of intravenous immunoglobulins in Landau-Kleffner syndrome. *Pediatric Neurology, 18*(2), 165–168.

Landau, W. M., & Kleffner, F. R. (1957, 1998). Syndrome of acquired aphasia with convulsive disorder in children. *Neurology, 51*(5), 1241. (Also available at http://www.neurology.org/content/51/5/1241.2.full.html last accessed on 28 November 2010).

Lee, Y. M., Kang, H. C., Lee, J. S., Kim, S. H., Kim, E. Y., Lee, S. K., et al. (2008). Mitochondrial respiratory chain defects: underlying etiology in various epileptic conditions. *Epilepsia, 49*(4), 685–690.

Lewine, J. D., Andrews, R., Chez, M., Patil, A. A., Devinsky, O., Smith, M., et al. (1999). Magnetoencephalographic patterns of epileptiform activity in children with regressive autism spectrum disorders. *Pediatrics, 104*(3 Pt 1), 405–418.

Lord, C., Rutter, M., Goode, S., Heemsbergen, J., Jordan, H., Mawhood, L., et al. (1989). Autism Diagnostic Observation Schedule: a standardized observation of communicative and social behavior. *Journal of Autism and Developmental Disorders, 19*(2), 185–212.

Lord, C., Shulman, C., & DiLavore, P. (2004). Regression and word loss in autistic spectrum disorders. *Journal of Child Psychology and Psychiatry and Allied Disciplines, 45*(5), 936–955.

Lux, A. L., Edwards, S. W., Hancock, E., Johnson, A. L., Kennedy, C. R., Newton, R. W., et al. (2005). The United Kingdom Infantile Spasms Study (UKISS) comparing hormone treatment with vigabatrin on developmental and epilepsy outcomes to age 14 months: a multicentre randomised trial. *Lancet Neurology, 4*(11), 712–717.

Luyster, R., Richler, J., Risi, S., Hsu, W. L., Dawson, G., Bernier, R., et al. (2005). Early regression in social communication in autism spectrum disorders: a CPEA Study. *Developmental Neuropsychology, 27*(3), 311–336.

Mansheim, P. (1979). Tuberous sclerosis and autistic behavior. *Journal of Clinical Psychiatry, 40*(2), 97–98.

Mantis, J. G., Fritz, C. L., Marsh, J., Heinrichs, S. C., & Seyfried, T. N. (2009). Improvement of motor and exploratory behavior in Rett syndrome mice with restricted ketogenic and standard diets. *Epilepsy and Behavior, 15*(2), 133–141.

Marescaux, C., Hirsch, E., Finck, S., Maquet, P., Schlumberger, E., Sellal, F., et al. (1990). Landau-Kleffner syndrome: a pharmacologic study of five cases. *Epilepsia, 31*(6), 768–777.

McDermott, S., Moran, R., Platt, T., Wood, H., Isaac, T., & Dasari, S. (2005). Prevalence of epilepsy in adults with mental retardation and related disabilities in primary care. *American Journal of Mental Retardation, 110*(1), 48–56.

McVicar, K. A., Ballaban-Gil, K., Rapin, I., Moshe, S. L., & Shinnar, S. (2005). Epileptiform EEG abnormalities in children with language regression. *Neurology, 65*(1), 129–131.

Meikle, L., Pollizzi, K., Egnor, A., Kramvis, I., Lane, H., Sahin, M., et al. (2008). Response of a neuronal model of tuberous sclerosis to mammalian target of rapamycin (mTOR) inhibitors: effects on mTORC1 and Akt signaling lead to improved survival and function. *Journal of Neuroscience, 28*(21), 5422–5432.

Mikati, M. A., Lepejian, G. A., & Holmes, G. L. (2002). Medical treatment of patients with infantile spasms. *Clinical Neuropharmacology, 25*(2), 61–70.

Mouridsen, S. E., Bronnum-Hansen, H., Rich, B., & Isager, T. (2008). Mortality and causes of death in autism spectrum disorders: an update. *Autism, 12*(4), 403–414.

Mouridsen, S. E., Rich, B., & Isager, T. (1999). Epilepsy in disintegrative psychosis and infantile autism: a long-term validation study. *Developmental Medicine and Child Neurology, 41*(2), 110–114.

Mouridsen, S. E., Rich, B., & Isager, T. (2000). A comparative study of genetic and neurobiological findings in disintegrative psychosis and infantile autism. *Psychiatry and Clinical Neurosciences, 54*(4), 441–446.

Mouridsen, S. E., Rich, B., & Isager, T. (2008). Epilepsy and other neurological diseases in the parents of children with infantile autism. A case control study. *Child Psychiatry and Human Development, 39*(1), 1–8.

Muncy, J., Butler, I. J., & Koenig, M. K. (2009). Rapamycin reduces seizure frequency in tuberous sclerosis complex. *Journal of Child Neurology, 24*(4), 477.

Murphy, C. C., Trevathan, E., & Yeargin-Allsopp, M. (1995). Prevalence of epilepsy and epileptic seizures in 10-year-old children: results from the Metropolitan Atlanta Developmental Disabilities Study. *Epilepsia, 36*(9), 866–872.

Napolioni, V., Moavero, R., & Curatolo, P. (2009). Recent advances in neurobiology of tuberous sclerosis complex. *Brain and Development, 31*(2), 104–113.

Nass, R., Gross, A., Wisoff, J., & Devinsky, O. (1999). Outcome of multiple subpial transections for autistic epileptiform regression. *Pediatric Neurology, 21*(1), 464–470.

Nass, R., & Petrucha, D. (1990). Acquired aphasia with convulsive disorder: a pervasive developmental disorder variant. *Journal of Child Neurology, 5*(4), 327–328.

Neville, B. G., Harkness, W. F., Cross, J. H., Cass, H. C., Burch, V. C., Lees, J. A., et al. (1997). Surgical treatment of severe autistic regression in childhood epilepsy. *Pediatric Neurology, 16*(2), 137–140.

Nickels, K., & Wirrell, E. (2008). Electrical status epilepticus in sleep. *Seminars in Pediatric Neurology, 15*(2), 50–60.

Ogawa, S., Kwon, C. H., Zhou, J., Koovakkattu, D., Parada, L. F., & Sinton, C. M. (2007). A seizure-prone phenotype is associated with altered free-running rhythm in Pten mutant mice. *Brain Research, 1168*, 112–123.

Olsson, I., Steffenburg, S., & Gillberg, C. (1988). Epilepsy in autism and autisticlike conditions. A population-based study. *Archives of Neurology, 45*(6), 666–668.

Park, Y. D. (2003). The effects of vagus nerve stimulation therapy on patients with intractable seizures and either Landau-Kleffner syndrome or autism. *Epilepsy and Behavior, 4*(3), 286–290.

Pavone, P., Incorpora, G., Fiumara, A., Parano, E., Trifiletti, R. R., & Ruggieri, M. (2004). Epilepsy is not a prominent feature of primary autism. *Neuropediatrics, 35*(4), 207–210.

Pellock, J. M. (2004). Managing behavioral and cognitive problems in children with epilepsy. *Journal of Child Neurology, 19*(Suppl 1), S73–74.

Plioplys, A. V. (1994). Autism: electroencephalogram abnormalities and clinical improvement with valproic acid. *Archives of Pediatrics and Adolescent Medicines, 148*(2), 220–222.

Prasad, A. N., Stafstrom, C. F., & Holmes, G. L. (1996). Alternative epilepsy therapies: the ketogenic diet, immunoglobulins, and steroids. *Epilepsia, 37*(Suppl 1), S81–95.

Pressler, R. M., Robinson, R. O., Wilson, G. A., & Binnie, C. D. (2005). Treatment of interictal epileptiform discharges can improve behavior in children with behavioral problems and epilepsy. *Journal of Pediatrics, 146*(1), 112–117.

Rakhade, S. N., & Jensen, F. E. (2009). Epileptogenesis in the immature brain: emerging mechanisms. *Nature Reviews Neurology, 5*(7), 380–391.

Rapin, I. (1995). Autistic regression and disintegrative disorder: how important the role of epilepsy? *Seminars in Pediatric Neurology, 2*(4), 278–285.

Reynolds, E. H., & Rodin, E. (2009). The clinical concept of epilepsy. *Epilepsia, 50*(Suppl 3), 2–7.

Richer, L. P., Shevell, M. I., & Rosenblatt, B. R. (2002). Epileptiform abnormalities in children with attention-deficit-hyperactivity disorder. *Pediatric Neurology, 26*(2), 125–129.

Riikonen, R., & Amnell, G. (1981). Psychiatric disorders in children with earlier infantile spasms. *Developmental Medicine and Child Neurology, 23*(6), 747–760.

Rogers, S. J. (2004). Developmental regression in autism spectrum disorders. *Mental Retardation and Developmental Disabilities Research Reviews, 10*(2), 139–143.

Rossi, P. G., Parmeggiani, A., Bach, V., Santucci, M., & Visconti, P. (1995). EEG features and epilepsy in patients with autism. *Brain and Development, 17*(3), 169–174.

Rugino, T. A., & Samsock, T. C. (2002). Levetiracetam in autistic children: an open-label study. *Journal of Developmental and Behavioral Pediatrics, 23*(4), 225–230.

Saemundsen, E., Ludvigsson, P., Hilmarsdottir, I., & Rafnsson, V. (2007). Autism spectrum disorders in children with seizures in the first year of life: A population-based study. *Epilepsia, 48*(9), 1724–1730.

Saemundsen, E., Ludvigsson, P., & Rafnsson, V. (2007). Autism spectrum disorders in children with a history of infantile spasms: a population-based study. *Journal of Child Neurology, 22*(9), 1102–1107.

Saemundsen, E., Ludvigsson, P., & Rafnsson, V. (2008). Risk of autism spectrum disorders after infantile spasms: A population-based study nested in a cohort with seizures in the first year of life. *Epilepsia, 49*(11), 1865–1870.

Schacher, M., Winkler, R., Grunwald, T., Kraemer, G., Kurthen, M., Reed, V., et al. (2006). Mesial temporal lobe epilepsy impairs advanced social cognition. *Epilepsia, 47*(12), 2141–2146.

Schain, R. J., & Yannet, H. (1960). Infantile autism. An analysis of 50 cases and a consideration of certain relevant neurophysiologic concepts. *Journal of Pediatrics, 57*, 560–567.

Scheffer, I. E., Parry-Fielder, B., Mullen, S. A., & Saunders, K. (2006). Epileptiform EEG abnormalities in children with language regression. *Neurology, 67*(8), 1527.

Scheffer, I. E., Zhang, Y. H., Jansen, F. E., & Dibbens, L. (2009). Dravet syndrome or genetic (generalized) epilepsy with febrile seizures plus? *Brain and Development, 31*(5), 394–400.

Sengoku, A., Kanazawa, O., Kawai, I., & Yamaguchi, T. (1990). Visual cognitive disturbance during spike-wave discharges. *Epilepsia, 31*(1), 47–50.

Shewmon, D. A., & Erwin, R. J. (1988). The effect of focal interictal spikes on perception and reaction time. II. Neuroanatomic specificity. *Electroencephalography and Clinical Neurophysiology, 69*(4), 338–352.

Shinnar, S., Rapin, I., Arnold, S., Tuchman, R., Shulman, L., Ballaban-Gil, K., et al. (2001). Language regression in childhood. *Pediatric Neurology, 24*(3), 183–189.

Shoffner, J., Hyams, L., et al. (2010). Fever plus mitochondrial disease could be risk factors for autistic regression. *Journal of Child Neurology, 25*(4), 429–434.

Spence, S. J., & Schneider, M. T. (2009). The role of epilepsy and epileptiform EEGs in autism spectrum disorders. *Pediatric Research, 65*(6), 599–606.

Steffenburg, U., Hagberg, G., & Hagberg, B. (2001). Epilepsy in a representative series of Rett syndrome. *Acta Paediatrica, 90*(1), 34–39.

Steffenburg, U., Hagberg, G., & Kyllerman, M. (1996). Characteristics of seizures in a population-based series of mentally retarded children with active epilepsy. *Epilepsia, 37*(9), 850–856.

Steffenburg, U., Hagberg, G., Viggedal, G., & Kyllerman, M. (1995). Active epilepsy in mentally retarded children. I. Prevalence and additional neuro-impairments. *Acta Paediatrica, 84*(10), 1147–1152.

Szabo, C. A., Wyllie, E., Dolske, M., Stanford, L. D., Kotagal, P., & Comair, Y. G. (1999). Epilepsy surgery in children with pervasive developmental disorder. *Pediatric Neurology, 20*(5), 349–353.

Taft, L. T., & Cohen, H. J. (1971). Hypsarrhythmia and infantile autism: a clinical report. *Journal of Autism and Childhood Schizophrenia, 1*(3), 327–336.

Tassinari, C. A., Cantalupo, G., Rios-Pohl, L., Giustina, E. D., & Rubboli, G. (2009). Encephalopathy with status epilepticus during slow sleep: "The Penelope syndrome." *Epilepsia, 50*(Suppl 7), 4–8.

Taylor, D. C., Neville, B. G., & Cross, J. H. (1999). Autistic spectrum disorders in childhood epilepsy surgery candidates. *European Child and Adolescent Psychiatry, 8*(3), 189–192.

Tharp, B. R. (2004). Epileptic encephalopathies and their relationship to developmental disorders: do spikes cause autism? *Mental Retardation and Developmental Disabilities Research Reviews, 10*(2), 132–134.

Trevathan, E. (2005). To sleep, perchance to speak: the search for epileptic language regression. *Neurology, 65*(1), 11–12.

Tsuru, T., Mori, M., et al. (2000). Effects of high-dose intravenous corticosteroid therapy in Landau-Kleffner syndrome. *Pediatric Neurology, 22*(2), 145–147.

Tuchman, R. (2004). AEDs and psychotropic drugs in children with autism and epilepsy. *Mental Retardation and Developmental Disabilities Research Reviews, 10*(2), 135–138.

Tuchman, R. (2006). Autism and epilepsy: what has regression got to do with it? *Epilepsy Currents, 6*(4), 107–111.

Tuchman, R. (2009). CSWS-related autistic regression versus autistic regression without CSWS. *Epilepsia, 50*(Suppl 7), 18–20.

Tuchman, R., Cuccaro, M., & Alessandri, M. (2010a). Autism and epilepsy: Historical perspective. *Brain and Development, 32*(9), 709–718.

Tuchman, R., Cuccaro, M., & Alessandri, M. (2010b). Autism spectrum disorders and epilepsy: Moving towards a comprehensive approach to treatment. *Brain and Development, 32*(9), 719–730.

Tuchman, R., Moshe, S. L., & Rapin, I. (2009). Convulsing toward the pathophysiology of autism. *Brain and Development, 31*(2), 95–103.

Tuchman, R., & Rapin, I. (1997). Regression in pervasive developmental disorders: seizures and epileptiform electroencephalogram correlates. *Pediatrics, 99*(4), 560–566.

Tuchman, R., & Rapin, I. (2002). Epilepsy in autism. *Lancet Neurology, 1*(6), 352–358.

Tuchman, R., Rapin, I., & Shinnar, S. (1991). Autistic and dysphasic children. II: Epilepsy. *Pediatrics, 88*(6), 1219–1225.

Turk, J., Bax, M., Williams, C., Amin, P., Eriksson, M., & Gillberg, C. (2009). Autism spectrum disorder in children with and without epilepsy: impact on social functioning and communication. *Acta Paediatrica, 98*(4), 675–681.

Uvebrant, P., & Bauziene, R. (1994). Intractable epilepsy in children. The efficacy of lamotrigine treatment, including non-seizure-related benefits. *Neuropediatrics, 25*(6), 284–289.

Voigt, R. G., Dickerson, C. L., Reynolds, A. M., Childers, D. O., Rodriguez, D. L., & Brown, F. R. (2000). Laboratory evaluation of children with autistic spectrum disorders: a guide for primary care pediatricians. *Clinical Pediatrics (Phila), 39*(11), 669–671.

Volkmar, F. R. (1992). Childhood disintegrative disorder: issues for DSM-IV. *Journal of Autism and Developmental Disorders, 22*(4), 625–642.

Volkmar, F. R., & Nelson, D. S. (1990). Seizure disorders in autism. *Journal of the American Academy of Child and Adolescent Psychiatry, 29*(1), 127–129.

Walpole, P., Isaac, C. L., & Reynders, H. J. (2008). A comparison of emotional and cognitive intelligence in people with and without temporal lobe epilepsy. *Epilepsia, 49*(8), 1470–1474.

Warwick, T. C., Griffith, J., Reyes, B., Legesse, B., & Evans, M. (2007). Effects of vagus nerve stimulation in a patient with temporal lobe epilepsy and Asperger syndrome: case report and review of the literature. *Epilepsy and Behavior, 10*(2), 344–347.

Wasserman, S., Iyengar, R., Chaplin, W. F., Watner, D., Waldoks, S. E., Anagnostou, E., et al. (2006). Levetiracetam versus placebo in childhood and adolescent autism: a double-blind placebo-controlled study. *International Clinical Psychopharmacology, 21*(6), 363–367.

Weiss, L. A., Escayg, A., Kearney, J. A., Trudeau, M., MacDonald, B. T., Mori, M., et al. (2003). Sodium channels SCN1A, SCN2A, and SCN3A in familial autism. *Molecular Psychiatry, 8*(2), 186–194.

Werner, E., & Dawson, G. (2005). Validation of the phenomenon of autistic regression using home videotapes. *Archives of General Psychiatry, 62*(8), 889–895.

White, P. T., Demyer, W., & Demyer, M. (1964). EEG abnormalities in early childhood schizophrenia: A double-blind study of psychiatrically disturbed and normal children during promazine sedation. *American Journal of Psychiatry, 120*, 950–958.

Winterkorn, E. B., Pulsifer, M. B., & Thiele, E. A. (2007). Cognitive prognosis of patients with tuberous sclerosis complex. *Neurology, 68*(1), 62–64.

Wolff, M., Casse-Perrot, C., & Dravet, C. (2006). Severe myoclonic epilepsy of infants (Dravet syndrome): natural history and neuropsychological findings. *Epilepsia, 47*(Suppl 2), 45–48.

Wong, V. (1993). Epilepsy in children with autistic spectrum disorder. *Journal of Child Neurology, 8*(4), 316–322.

Worrell, G. A., Lagerlund, T. D., & Buchhalter, J. R. (2002). Role and limitations of routine and ambulatory scalp electroencephalography in diagnosing and managing seizures. *Mayo Clinic Proceedings, 77*(9), 991–998.

Zecavati, N., & Spence, S. J. (2009). Neurometabolic disorders and dysfunction in autism spectrum disorders. *Current Neurology and Neuroscience Reports, 9*(2), 129–136.

Zeng, L. H., Xu, L., Gutmann, D. H., & Wong, M. (2008). Rapamycin prevents epilepsy in a mouse model of tuberous sclerosis complex. *Annals of Neurology, 63*(4), 444–453.

Zhou, J., Blundell, J., Ogawa, S., Kwon, C. H., Zhang, W., Sinton, C., et al. (2009). Pharmacological inhibition of mTORC1 suppresses anatomical, cellular, and behavioral abnormalities in neural-specific Pten knock-out mice. *Journal of Neuroscience, 29*(6), 1773–1783.

Zoghbi, H. Y. (2003). Postnatal neurodevelopmental disorders: meeting at the synapse? *Science, 302*(5646), 826–830.

Zupanc, M. L. (2009). Clinical evaluation and diagnosis of severe epilepsy syndromes of early childhood. *Journal of Child Neurology, 24*(8 Suppl), 6S–14S.

24 Paula Goines, Andrew Zimmerman, Paul Ashwood, Judy Van de Water

The Immune System, Autoimmunity, Allergy, and Autism Spectrum Disorders

Points of Interest

- The immune system is complex and dynamic. It balances between defending the body from invaders and minimizing harmful overreactions to self-tissues and innocuous agents.
- Extensive reciprocal interactions exist between the immune and nervous systems. Activity in one system is capable of modifying the activity of the other.
- Several genes that have been linked to autism spectrum disorders have immunological significance.
- Individuals with autism and their family members have an increased incidence of immune system anomalies compared to the general population.
- Gestational exposure to brain-directed antibodies or various immune stimulants may be involved in some cases of autism.
- The exact mechanisms underlying the immunological observations in autism remain ambiguous, and are an active area of investigation.

Introduction

For three decades, immune anomalies have been described in subjects with autism spectrum disorders (ASD) and their family members. Examples include signs of inflammation in the brain and cerebrospinal fluid (Vargas, Nascimbene, et al., 2005) and gastrointestinal tract (Ashwood, Anthony, et al., 2004), as well as differences in both the humoral and cellular immune systems, (reviewed in Pardo, Vargas, et al., 2005; Ashwood, Wills, et al., 2006). In addition, autoimmune and allergy-associated disorders appear more frequently in ASD subjects and their families compared to "neurotypical" control populations (Ashwood & Van de Water, 2004; Silva, Correia, et al., 2004; Croen, Grether, et al., 2005; Ashwood, Wills, et al., 2006; Cabanlit, Wills, et al., 2007). The nature of the connection between behavior and the immune system in autism is the current focus of several exciting new studies. While the clinical significance of immune related findings in autism is unclear, it provides a valuable opportunity to understand the underlying biology of the disorder, and may lead to future therapies. The following is a discussion of the complex relationship between immune dysfunction and ASD. An overview of this relationship is depicted in Figure 24-1.

Immunity, Autoimmunity, and Allergy

Immune System 101

The immune system is intricately linked to every organ system in the body, where it demonstrates great versatility and specialization in different locations. For example, immune activity in the bacteria-filled gastrointestinal tract is very different from that found in the sterile blood stream. The lymphatic system is the major conduit for immune components. Reminiscent of the circulatory system, the lymphatics consist of a clear fluid called "lymph" mixed with an array of immune cells. Lymph and cells drain from tissues throughout the body, and filter through local lymph nodes, where more selective immune responses are initiated.

The immune system is made up of "innate" and "adaptive" branches. The innate branch is the first line of bodily defense. It responds rapidly and nonspecifically to injury or infection by recognizing the telltale signs of danger. Cells such as neutrophils and macrophages engulf pathogens, and secrete immune-stimulating species like cytokines, chemokines, and reactive oxygen species. Dendritic cells are antigen-presenting cells (APCs) that serve as the link between the innate and adaptive systems by

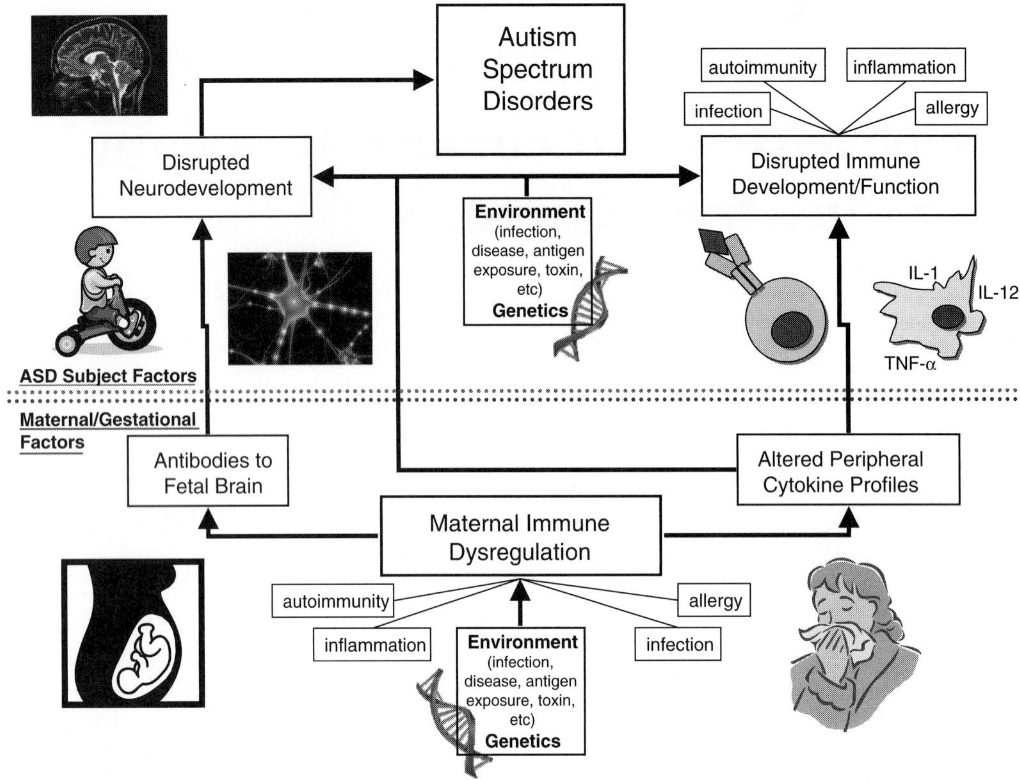

Figure 24–1. An overview of the relationship between immune dysfunction and autism spectrum disorders.

stimulating B and T cells under specific conditions. Natural killer (NK) cells are specialized members of the innate immune system that respond rapidly to viral infections and tumors by secreting cytokines and cytolytic molecules. These cells have additional importance in stimulating the adaptive immune system, maintaining pregnancy, and regulating autoimmune reactions (Perricone, Perricone, et al., 2008). Additional innate immune cells include mast cells, eosinophils, and basophils. Under normal conditions, such cells are important in defense against parasites, though they are more often associated with allergy/asthma in developed countries.

When the innate branch of the immune system cannot resolve the threat, the adaptive branch is called into action. The adaptive immune system is dominated by highly specialized B and T cells that focus the response on specific components of the invading agents, known as "antigens." When activated, B cells make targeted, antigen-specific antibodies, while T cells carry out antigen-specific helper and cytotoxic functions. With the continuing aid of the innate immune system, B and T cells orchestrate the elimination of the foreign antigens.

Autoimmunity and Allergy-Misfiring of Adaptive Immunity

A healthy immune system must be poised for attack against harmful pathogens. Simultaneously, it must be tolerant of harmless agents, since unnecessary immune responses can be destructive and energy depleting. Immune tolerance is

Autoimmunity

In order for the immune system to identify and destroy unwanted assailants, it must be able to distinguish between self-tissues and foreign invaders. The innate immune system achieves this by targeting features that are common among various pathogens, but are absent in host tissues. The adaptive immune system recognizes more specific features, and depends on a complex signaling network to discriminate between appropriate targets, self-tissues, and innocuous agents. Under normal circumstances, adaptive immune cells directed toward self-tissues are eliminated or regulated to prevent harmful immune reactions. However, if these cells persist and the identification or regulatory systems break down, the adaptive immune system may become activated to target the body's own tissues. This phenomenon is called "autoimmunity," and is observed in diseases like systemic lupus erythematosus, rheumatoid arthritis, and multiple sclerosis.

A major weapon used by the immune system to protect the body is a group of proteins called "antibodies." Produced by highly specialized "B cells," antibodies protect the body by flagging unwanted invaders for destruction and removal. In autoimmune disorders, antibodies are directed toward the body itself. Self-directed antibodies are called "autoantibodies." T cells are additional members of the adaptive immune system that become involved in autoimmunity. They help to facilitate immune reactions by activating B cells and directing various innate cells to carry out specific immune-related tasks. Autoreactive T cells encourage destructive immune reactions against self-tissues, and are key players in autoimmune processes.

Allergy

Each day the body is exposed to far more harmless agents than pathogens. The immune system is therefore poised to distinguish between innocuous and harmful environmental entities that are inhaled or ingested. Occasionally, the immune system mistakenly targets harmless environmental species, which are known as allergens. Some common allergens include dust mite antigen, pet dander, pollen, and peanuts. Adaptive immune cells can become activated to respond when the body encounters these allergens, and mount increasingly exuberant responses upon subsequent exposures. Symptoms of allergic reactions vary, ranging from mild irritation to severe anaphylactic shock and death.

Allergic responses usually include a specific subset of antibodies known as Immunoglobulin E, or IgE. Levels of IgE are often elevated among highly allergic individuals. IgE molecules target specific allergens, and help stimulate effector cells including mast cells, basophils, and eosinophils. Upon activation, these cells rapidly secrete immune stimulating factors, including histamine, which increase vasodilation and a rapid propagation of the immune response.

enabled by deletion and/or suppression of B and T cells that target self-tissues or innocuous environmental antigens. *Autoimmune disease* occurs when *self-antigen specific* B and T cells are activated to attack host tissues. For example, multiple sclerosis (MS) is an autoimmune condition where specific B and T cells destroy the myelin sheaths that insulate nerve axons. In contrast, *allergy* describes the activation of B and T cells that target *harmless environmental agents* like pollen, peanuts, or pet dander. The resulting hypersensitivity ranges from annoying, as is the case of allergic rhinitis, to potentially fatal in the case of severe asthma or anaphylaxis. Autoimmune and allergic diseases are each examples of a misdirected immune response with potentially severe pathological consequences for the host.

Immunity, Behavior, and the Central Nervous System

Central Nervous System (CNS) Immune Privilege

Historically, the central nervous system (CNS, brain and spinal cord) was thought to be sequestered from the body's peripheral immune system (Bailey, Carpentier, et al., 2006; Carson, Doose, et al., 2006). This was accepted for several reasons. First, the CNS lacks obvious lymphatic drainage. It was therefore thought that immune cells did not come into contact with components from the brain or spinal cord. Second, neurons have extremely low regenerative capacity, so damaging immune reactions within the CNS can destroy vital neural networks. Third, the bony cranium limits space for expansion of the brain due to the edema (swelling) that accompanies inflammation. Finally, neurons (nerve cells) were thought to lack expression of major histocompatibility complex (MHC) molecules, which are required for recognition by T cells. Despite these issues, it has become clear that the immune system does in fact interface with the CNS in many ways (Carson, Doose, et al., 2006). Overly exuberant systemic immune responses are restricted from the CNS through a combination of limited access and local immune suppression. The former is accomplished through an intact "blood-brain barrier," which under normal circumstances prevents the passage of most immune components. Local immune suppression and activation are achieved through the actions of local CNS cells such as astrocytes and microglia. These cells have immune functions including phagocytosis, cytokine secretion, and T cell activating capacity (Nelson, Soma, et al., 2002; Raivich, 2005; Bailey, Carpentier, et al., 2006). They are additionally far more immunosuppressive than their counterparts in the body periphery (Nelson, Soma, et al., 2002).

Neuroimmune Networks

The old dogma of CNS immune privilege has faded further as growing evidence suggests that the immune and nervous systems are actually highly interconnected. Complex interactions between the CNS and immune system begin early in development and continue throughout life (Haddad, Saade, et al., 2002; Steinman, 2004; Wrona, 2006; Bauer, Kerr, et al., 2007). Immune system factors such as MHC I, cytokines, and chemokines are important during several stages of neurodevelopment. Additionally, they are involved in CNS plasticity, functioning, and maintenance. Likewise, several proteins associated with the nervous system, such as neuropeptides, have a broad range of suppressive and activating effects on the development and function of the immune system, including the innervation of immune organs such as the lymph nodes and spleen (Rothwell, Luheshi, et al., 1996; Mehler & Kessler, 1998; Huh, Boulanger, et al., 2000; Biber, Zuurman, et al., 2002; Mignini, Streccioni, et al., 2003; Marques-Deak, Cizza, et al., 2005). A carefully established equilibrium and timing of immune and neural parameters is vital for normal development and functioning of each system. An insult to either system during a critical developmental stage may have life-long effects, such as changes in receptor distribution and/or number, as well as modifications in neuropeptide, cytokine, hormone, and neurotransmitter release (Merlot, Couret, et al., 2008) (Figure 24-2).

The adaptive immune system also has an important role in several CNS processes. T cell trafficking into the CNS is well characterized (Engelhardt & Ransohoff, 2005). Once in the brain, T cells aid in the repair of CNS injuries, (Hammarberg, Lidman, et al., 2000; Kipnis, Yoles, et al., 2001; Kerschensteiner, Stadelmann, et al., 2003), and are required for neurogenesis in the adult brain (Kipnis, Cohen, et al., 2004; Ziv, Ron, et al., 2006). Studies using immunodeficient mice have demonstrated the importance of adaptive immunity in learning

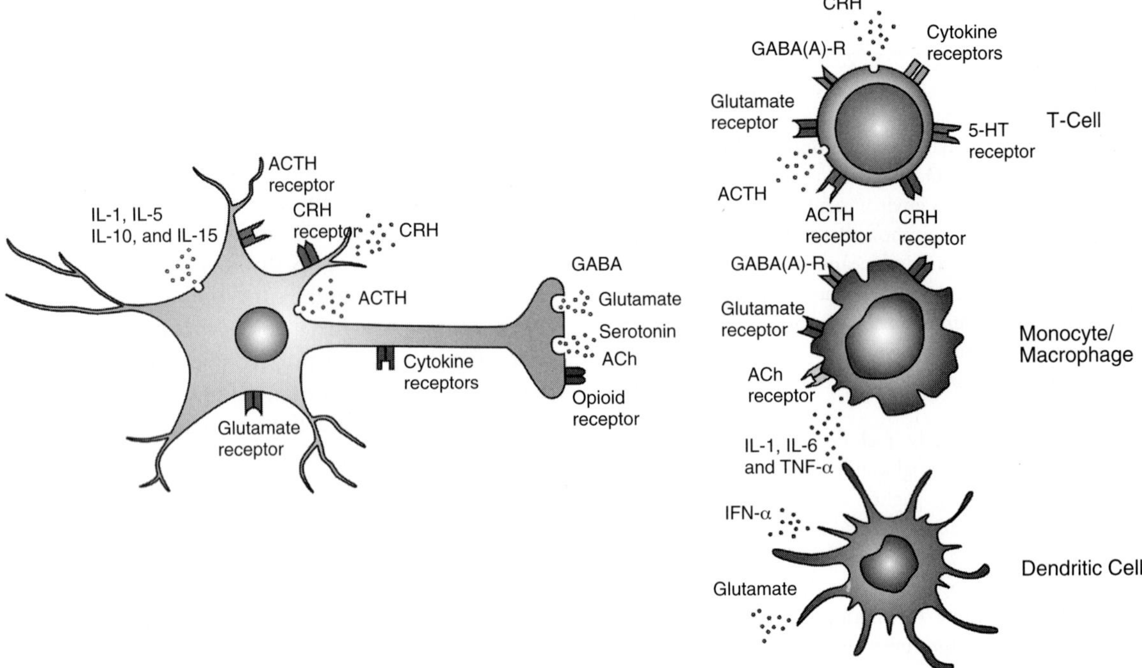

Figure 24–2. Cross-talk between the immune and central nervous systems. Intercommunication between the cells of the immune and nervous systems is possible on several levels. Neurons, microglia, and astrocytes can produce various cytokines and express cytokine receptors. This enables them to direct immune cells as well as respond to various immunological stimuli. In turn, cells of the immune system are able to secrete various neurotransmitters, such as glutamate, and express receptors for many of these molecules. This allows immune cells to impact neural processes and respond to neural stimuli. These mechanisms permit extensive cross-talk between the immune system and neural systems. Illustration by Milo Careaga. (See Color Plate Section for a color version of this figure.)

(Kipnis, Cohen, et al., 2004; Brynskikh, Warren, et al., 2008). SCID mice (*s*evere *c*ombined *i*mmuno *d*eficient, having no B or T cells) have reduced cognitive function compared to immunocompetent controls. Immunodeficient mice have difficulties with learning a new task, and take longer than control mice to adjust to changes in previously acquired tasks. It is currently unclear whether T cells interact with neurons directly or indirectly through soluble immune mediators called cytokines, or whether similar phenomena occur in humans.

Autoimmunity, Allergy, and Behavior

There is evidence that certain autoimmune disorders can have behavioral and psychological consequences. This has been explored in recent studies of patients with systemic lupus erythematosus (SLE) accompanied by neuropsychiatric symptoms (Diamond, Kowal, et al., 2006). Antibodies toward double stranded DNA isolated from the serum of neuropsychiatric SLE patients were found to cross-react with the NMDA receptor for the neurotransmitter glutamate (Diamond, Kowal, et al., 2006; Huerta, Kowal, et al., 2006). The neuropathogenic significance of these autoantibodies was established in a murine model. Following lipopolysaccharide (LPS) administration (to breach the integrity of the blood-brain barrier) and passive transfer of serum from patients with SLE, recipient mice demonstrated cognitive impairments. Further, brain histopathology revealed that the transferred human antibodies caused apoptotic neuronal death in the hippocampus (Kowal, DeGiorgio, et al., 2004). Elevated levels of circulating autoantibodies to nervous system components have been reported in a number of psychiatric disorders including ASD (discussed in detail below), schizophrenia, obsessive-compulsive disorder, pediatric autoimmune neuropsychiatric disorders associated with streptococcal infection (PANDAS), and Gilles de la Tourette's syndrome (TS) (Pandey, Gupta, et al., 1981; Kiessling, Marcotte, et al., 1994; Rothermundt, Arolt, et al., 2001; Perrin, Murphy, et al., 2004; Jones, Mowry, et al., 2005; Huerta, Kowal, et al., 2006; Yeh, Wu, et al., 2006). While brain-directed antibodies are clearly observed in many CNS disorders, their clinical relevance is uncertain because they are also found in some unaffected control subjects.

In addition to the capability of the immune system to affect brain function through autoimmune mechanisms, there is evidence that the CNS directly affects the inflammatory response. This has been observed in the autoimmune disorder rheumatoid arthritis. For example, Boyle et al. demonstrated that selective inhibition of spinal cord p38 MAP kinase in rats with adjuvant arthritis markedly decreased paw swelling, synovial inflammation, and joint destruction (Boyle, Jones, et al.,

2006). The data from this study suggest that peripheral inflammation is "sensed" by the CNS, which subsequently activates stress-induced kinases in the spinal cord via a mechanism involving the inflammatory cytokine TNFα. Intracellular p38 MAP kinase signaling processes this information and profoundly modulates the somatic inflammatory response.

While the pathophysiology of allergic and immune mediated–disorders such as asthma is fairly well understood, little is known about the influence of such disorders on brain activity and behavior. Costa-Pinto et al. (2005) described the neurobehavioral correlates of food allergy using an experimental murine model with high levels of IgE. They demonstrated that mice allergic to ovalbumin (OVA) have increased activity in the paraventricular nucleus of the hypothalamus (PVN) and the central nucleus of the amygdala (CeA). Both of these CNS areas are commonly associated with emotionality-related behavioral responses following a single intra-nasal challenge with OVA. Further, using a classical passive avoidance test, with OVA aerosol as the aversive stimulus, the authors noted that allergic mice avoided entering the dark compartment of the apparatus that had been previously associated with an aerosol spray of the allergen, in contrast to the nonallergic controls (Costa-Pinto, Basso, et al., 2005). These data suggest that through activation of specific brain regions, there is a modification of behavior after only one challenge with an allergen in a highly sensitized mouse model.

Autism Spectrum Disorders and Immunity

Immune Dysregulation in Subjects with ASD

Emerging evidence suggests that the immune system may play a role in the etiology of behavioral disorders like autism (reviewed in Ashwood, Wills, et al., 2006). Subjects with ASD demonstrate skewed immune activity compared to neurotypical populations. Some irregularities include decreased numbers of B and T cells, reduced lymphocyte responses to stimulation (Stubbs & Crawford, 1977; Warren, Cole, et al., 1990; Plioplys, Greaves, et al., 1994), increased numbers of monocytes (Sweeten, Posey, et al., 2003), skewed cytokine profiles (Sweeten, Posey, et al., 2003; Molloy, Morrow, et al., 2006), and abnormal immunoglobulin levels (Croonenberghs, Wauters, et al., 2002; Trajkovski, Ajdinski, et al., 2004; Heuer, 2008; Table 24-1; Figure 24-3).

Vargas et al. reported findings of an ongoing immune response in the postmortem brain of patients with ASD (Vargas, Nascimbene, et al., 2005). Brain regions especially affected included the cerebral cortex and cerebellum. Microglial and astroglial cells were found to be immunologically activated based on cell appearance and morphology. Additionally, altered glial fibrillary acidic protein (GFAP) staining and cytokine profiles were found in brain tissue and cerebrospinal fluid (CSF) from subjects with ASD.

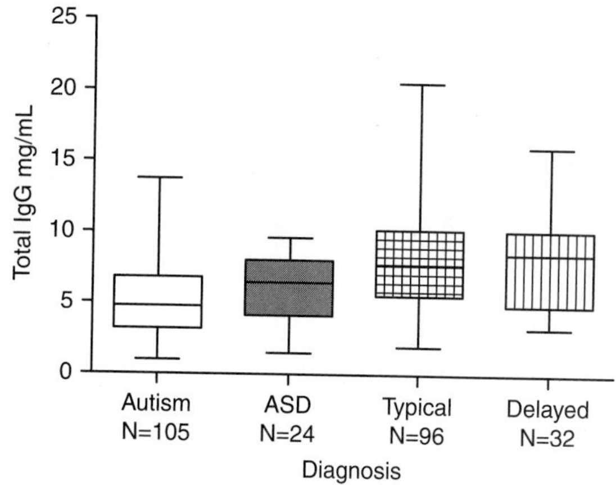

Figure 24–3. Relationship between ASD diagnosis and immunoglobulin levels.

Lymphocytes and antibody (IgG) were absent from the brain tissue, and accumulation of perivascular macrophages and monocytes was noted, which may be indicative of innate (as opposed to adaptive) immune activation. The sample size (n = 11) in this study was limited by the availability of postmortem tissue and may not be representative of the entire ASD spectrum, but did include patients over a wide range of ages and clinical symptoms. The studies by Vargas et al. (2005) have not yet been replicated, and additional CNS immunopathologies may exist. Two animal models have demonstrated similar immune activation ("neuroinflammation") in brain, along with behavioral changes in the offspring, following: (1) administration of terbutaline (a beta-2 adrenergic agonist) to neonatal rat pups (Zerrate, Pletnikov, et al., 2007); and (2) gestational administration in mice of antibodies to fetal brain from mothers of children with ASD (Singer et al., 2008).

Cytokines and ASD

Recent evidence suggests a correlation between the pluripotent cytokine TGF-β and ASD (Okada, Hashimoto, et al., 2007; Ashwood, Enstrom, et al., 2008). TGF-β has diverse roles in development, cell migration, apoptosis, and immune regulation (Letterio & Roberts, 1998). Additionally, this cytokine may play a role in CNS development, protection, and function (Gomes, Sousa Vde, et al., 2005). Two independent studies demonstrated low serum levels of TGF-β in individuals with ASD. Okada et al. reported their findings using ELISA among a group of adults with ASD compared to age-matched controls (Okada, Hashimoto, et al., 2007). Similar data were reported by Ashwood et al. in an extensively characterized group of 143 2- to 4-year-old children with ASD. Decreased TGF-β was found in ASD subjects compared to both neurotypical and non-ASD developmentally delayed controls (Ashwood, Enstrom, et al., 2008). Further, TGF-β

Table 24–1.
Evidence of altered immune function in subjects with autism

		Study Description	Reference
Altered Immunoglobulin Levels in Autism Subjects		**Serum IgG, IgG2, and IgG4** levels were **higher in autism** subjects than in normal controls. There was a correlation found between behavioral problems, total serum protein, and serum gamma globulin.	**(Croonenberghs, Wauters, et al., 2002)**
		Increased plasma IgG1, IgG4, and IgM in 35 **autistic subjects** compared to their siblings. No unrelated healthy controls were included.	**(Trajkovski, Ajdinski, et al., 2004)**
		Decreased total **plasma IgG and IgM** in a large group of **ASD subjects** compared to age matched developmentally delayed and healthy controls. Ig levels correlated with behavior, such that subjects with the most severe behavioral scores had the lowest Ig levels.	**(Heuer, 2008)**
		Young children with **autism** were found to have **significantly higher levels of IgG4** compared with age-matched typically developing and developmentally delayed control subjects.	**(Enstrom, Krakowiak, et al., 2008)**
Altered Cytokine and Inflammatory Profiles in Autism Subjects	**Circulatory Cytokine Profiles**	Plasma levels of several cytokines were measured in small group of autistic patients and age-matched normal controls ranging in age. The levels **of IL-12 and IFN-gamma** were significantly higher in autism subjects.	**(Singh, 1996)**
		Increased neopterin in peripheral blood of autism subjects compared to age and gender matched controls.	**(Sweeten, Posey, et al., 2003)**
		Decreased serum TGF-B in small groups of ASD subjects compared to matched healthy controls.	**(Okada, Hashimoto, et al., 2007)**
		Decreased plasma TGF-B in large group of ASD children compared to matched typically developing controls.	**(Ashwood, Enstrom, et al., 2008)**
		Increased plasma **Macrophage Migration Inhibitory Factor** (MIF) in large group of ASD subjects compared to controls. Lower MIF correlated with worse behavior, MIF gene polymorphisms also associated with ASD.	**(Grigorenko, Han, et al., 2008)**
		Large group of ASD subjects, especially those with the regressive version of the disorder had **increased** levels of plasma **leptin** compared to age-matched typically developing, mentally retarded, and sibling controls	**(Ashwood, Kwong, et al., 2008)**
	Tissue/Cellular Cytokine Expression	**Intracellular cytokines w**ere measured by FACS in blood from ASD subjects compared to healthy controls. Proportions **Th1 and IFN-g$^+$ cytotoxic cells** were lower in autistic children, while **Th2 and IL-4$^+$ cytotoxic T cells** were increased in autism compared to healthy controls.	**(Gupta, Aggarwal, et al., 1998)**
		Mucosal lymphocyte cytokine phenotypes in ASD subjects and neurotypical controls with and without gastrointestinal symptoms. ASD subjects had more lymphocyte infiltration and pro-inflammatory T cells (**IFN-g$^+$ or TNF-a$^+$**), and fewer regulatory (**IL-10$^+$**) T cells than controls.	**(Ashwood, Anthony, et al., 2004)**
		Postmortem **brain inflammation** in ASD subjects demonstrated by increased **MCP-1, TGF-B**, and **activated microglia/astroglia**. Increased MCP-1 in cerebrospinal fluid from live ASD subjects compared to controls.	**(Vargas, Nascimbene, et al., 2005)**
	Cytokine Expression in Cell Culture	Peripheral blood mononuclear cells from a large group of ASD subjects produced **more TNF-a, IL-1B,** and **IL-6** in the absence of stimulation, and after stimulation with LPS, PHA, tetanus, IL-12, and IL-18 compared to cells from normal siblings and healthy controls.	**(Jyonouchi, Sun, et al., 2001)**
		Unstimulated whole blood cultures from a small group of ASD subjects showed increased production of **IFN-g** and **IL-1RA** compared to healthy controls. A trend towards higher **IL-6** and **TNF-a** was also observed.	**(Croonenberghs, Bosmans, et al., 2002)**
		Cytokine production by PBMCs stimulated with LPS or dietary proteins in a group of ASD subjects compared to siblings and healthy controls. ASD cells produced high levels of **IFN-g** and **TNF-a** compared to controls.	**(Jyonouchi, Sun, et al., 2002)**
		Cytokine production by PBMCs stimulated with dietary proteins was compared between a large group of ASD subjects with and without GI symptoms and healthy controls. ASD subjects with GI symptoms made more **TNF-a** and **IL-12** after stimulation with milk proteins.	**(Jyonouchi, Geng, et al., 2005)**
		Increased production **of both Th1 and Th2** cytokines by PBMCs from 20 ASD children compared to matched controls.	**(Molloy, Morrow, et al., 2006)**

Altered Cellular Immunity in Autism Subjects	**Functional Differences**	**NK cell Activity**	Peripheral blood mononuclear cells from 31 autism subjects and no controls were tested for **cytotoxic potential**. Cells from 12 subjects had reduced cytotoxicity, which was not due to lower NK cell numbers.	**(Warren, Foster, et al., 1987)**
			NK cells from a large group of ASD subjects and healthy controls were compared. **RNA expression** of NK cell receptors and effector molecules was increased in ASD, as was **production of perforin, granzyme B,** and **IFN-gamma** under resting conditions. Functional characterization showed **reduced** NK cell **cytotoxicity,** and **production of perforin, granzyme B,** and **IFN-gamma** after stimulation compared to controls.	**(Enstrom, Lit, et al., 2008)**
			NK cell activity in peripheral blood was compared between a large group of ASD subjects and healthy controls. ASD subjects demonstrated **reduced NK cell activity** compared to controls. Authors suggest that low intracellular glutathione levels may be in part responsible.	**(Vojdani, Mumper, et al., 2008)**
		PBMC Activity	Decreased **lymphocyte proliferation** with PHA stimulation in 12 ASD children compared to normal controls.	**(Stubbs and Crawford, 1977)**
			Cellular response to human myelin basic protein in blood from a small group of autistic subjects and mentally disabled controls was analyzed using a macrophage migration inhibition factor test. Several autism subjects and no controls had **a cell-mediated immune response to brain tissue**.	**(Weizman, Weizman, et al., 1982)**
	Phenotypic or Quantitative Differences	**Monocytes**	Increased numbers of **monocytes** in peripheral blood of ASD subjects compared to age- and sex-matched controls.	**(Sweeten, Posey, et al., 2003)**
		Peripheral Blood Lymphocytes	36 autism subjects were shown to have **reduced** numbers of peripheral blood lymphocytes, **CD2$^+$ T** cells, **CD4$^+$** T cells, and **CD4$^+$CD45RA$^+$** lymphocytes in circulation compared to healthy age-matched subjects.	**(Warren, Yonk, et al., 1990)**
			Peripheral blood lymphocytes from 25 autistic subjects were characterized by FACS. Autistic subjects had **fewer total lymphocytes, CD4$^+$, and CD20$^+$** cells compared to siblings and healthy control subjects.	**(Yonk, Warren, et al., 1990)**
			Characterization of peripheral blood lymphocytes from 17 autism subjects, 8 Rett syndrome subjects, and no healthy controls. All had normal B and T cell numbers. Some autism subjects had **abnormal CD4:CD8 ratios,** and more incompletely activated T cells (**IL-2R negative non-naïve cells**). Results were not seen in the Rett syndrome subjects.	**(Plioplys, Greaves, et al., 1994)**
			Peripheral blood lymphocytes were characterized in 10 autistic subjects and 10 age- and sex-matched healthy controls. Autism subjects had **a lower percentage of helper-inducer cells**, a **lower ratio of helper: suppressor cells**, and a **lower** percentage of **interleukin-2receptor$^+$ lymphocytes** following stimulation. All findings correlated with behavioral severity.	**(Denney, Frei, et al., 1996)**
		Mucosal Immune Populations	Mucosal biopsies were compared using immunohistochemistry and histology between autism subjects and developmentally normal subjects with inflammatory bowel diseases (IBD). Autism subjects had **inflammation** that was less severe than IBD controls, though **basement membrane thickness, gamma-delta T cell, CD8$^+$ cell,** and **intraepithelial lymphocyte density** was **increased in autism** compared to IBD controls.	**(Furlano, Anthony, et al., 2001)**
			FACS and histological analysis of cell infiltrate in mucosal biopsies from a large group of autism children and normal controls with and without gut inflammation. ASD subjects had more **intraepithelial and lamina propria lymphocytes** compared to healthy noninflamed controls, which neared levels in inflamed healthy controls. **Eosinophil infiltration** was seen in ASD subjects, and was less severe in those on elimination diets.	**(Ashwood, Anthony, et al., 2003)**

levels correlated with behavioral measures, such that lower levels predicted worse behavior. In contrast, increased levels of TGF-β were found in brain tissue from postmortem brain, and CSF from living ASD subjects (Vargas, Nascimbene, et al., 2005). In addition, these authors described increased levels of the inflammatory chemokine MCP-1. It is unclear how these findings within the CNS relate to peripheral cytokine levels, specifically TGF-β. Collectively, these studies suggest that aberrant levels of TGF-β and other cytokines may have a lifelong role in various aspects of ASD. It is unknown whether the immune activation present is harmful or beneficial, or if immune treatments will be indicated for patients with ASD. Another point of view is that this immune activation may reflect persistence or reactivation of a fetal pattern, since similar phenomena occur normally in brain development with the appearance of MHC II on microglia during midgestation (Wierzba-Bobrowicz, Kosno-Kruszewska, et al., 2000).

The innate immune regulator macrophage inhibitory factor (MIF) has also been linked to ASD (Grigorenko, Han, et al., 2008). MIF is a unique proinflammatory regulator of many acute and chronic inflammatory diseases through activation of the innate immune system (Calandra & Roger, 2003). Furthermore, certain genetic polymorphisms in the MIF locus have been associated with autoimmune and inflammatory conditions (Gregersen & Bucala, 2003). Genotyping of two large populations found 2 polymorphisms in the promoter region of MIF that were associated with ASD. Additionally, plasma levels of MIF were higher in subjects with ASD, suggesting the possibility that the polymorphisms have functional significance (Grigorenko, Han, et al., 2008). Finally, it was found that higher levels of MIF correlated with more severe behavior (Grigorenko, Han, et al., 2008). The neurological significance of MIF is currently unknown, though this correlative evidence may represent another link between genetics and the immune system in neurologic disorders such as ASD.

An additional cytokine/hormone that has recently been linked to ASD is leptin (Ashwood, Kwong, et al., 2008), which is produced primarily by adipocytes, though it is also produced by lymphocytes (Sanna, Di Giacomo, et al., 2003). Leptin shares functional similarities with inflammatory cytokines such as IL-6 and IL-12 (Zhang, Proenca, et al., 1994) and has been implicated in various autoimmune diseases (Sanna, Di Giacomo, et al., 2003). Leptin is also capable of crossing the blood-brain barrier (Banks, 2001) to regulate food intake, and promotes the formation of CNS lesions in an animal model of multiple sclerosis (Matarese, Procaccini, et al., 2008). Ashwood et al. recently demonstrated that plasma leptin levels were elevated in a population of children with ASD compared to typically developing controls (Ashwood, Kwong, et al., 2008). This was especially dramatic among children with early-onset autism as opposed to those with clinical regression. Increased levels of leptin were also noted by Vargas et al to be present in postmortem brain tissue of persons with autism (Vargas, Nascimbene, et al., 2005).

Immunogenetics of ASD

Interestingly, several genes associated with autism are relevant to both the nervous and immune systems. Immunogenetic associations include PTEN (a negative regulator of the PI3K/AKT pathway) (Goffin, Hoefsloot, et al., 2001; Butler, Dasouki, et al., 2005; Boccone, Dessi, et al., 2006; Kwon, Luikart, et al., 2006), MET (a receptor tyrosine kinase; Campbell, Sutcliffe, et al., 2006; Campbell, D'Oronzio, et al., 2007), and Ca(V)1.2 (an L-type calcium channel; Splawski, Timothy, et al., 2004). Each of these genes is involved in regulation of the innate immune system, and alterations in these genes have the potential to affect development and function in both the immune and neural systems. Thus, it is highly possible that the genetic associations of these genes to ASD also contribute to both neural and immune dysfunction in ASD subjects.

In addition to genetic polymorphisms and protein levels, differential gene expression may also play a role in ASD. Local expression levels of several immunologically relevant genes have been characterized in ASD. There are increased transcript levels of many immune system–related genes in neocortical regions of ASD postmortem brain tissue (Garbett, Ebert, et al., 2008). Using microarray analysis, Garbett et al. demonstrated differential gene expression in the superior temporal gyrus between ASD and control tissues (Garbett, Ebert, et al., 2008). Several of the differentially expressed genes were immunologically relevant, and included heat shock proteins, chemokines, costimulatory molecules, and leptin receptors. Differences were also detected within immune pathways including NF-κB, TOLL, TNFR, P38MAPK, 4-1BB, IL-6, MET, and IL-2R, among others. Altered expression of many of the aforementioned genes can result in a susceptibility toward the development of autoimmune and immune-mediated sequelae.

In addition to cortical brain tissue, several other tissues have been used for gene expression analysis relating to ASD. This includes analysis of NK cells (Enstrom, Lit, et al., 2008; Gregg, Lit, et al., 2008), peripheral blood (Nishimura, Martin, et al., 2007), and cerebellar tissue (Fatemi, Halt, et al., 2001; Fatemi, Stary, et al., 2001; Yip, Soghomonian, et al., 2007). Many of these studies reported differences in genes associated with immune activity. In a recent study, gene expression profiles of peripheral blood were compared between well-characterized groups of ASD children and typically developing controls. This study revealed differential expression of several genes related to natural killer (NK) and cytotoxic (CD8+) T cell function (Gregg, Lit, et al., 2008). Further analyses uncovered several differences in NK cells derived from the ASD group when compared to the typically developing controls (Enstrom, Lit, et al., 2008). Increased expression of various NK cell receptors and effector molecules was found in resting cells from ASD children. Functional analysis also demonstrated that NK cells from ASD subjects had diminished cytotoxic ability, suggesting dysregulation on several levels among ASD children. Similar expression profiles were observed in a study of NK cells stimulated with IL-2 (Dybkaer, Iqbal, et al., 2007). The link between NK cells and ASD is not yet clear, however, NK cells produce cytokines and cytotoxic substances that could impact the CNS (Lambertsen, Gregersen, et al., 2004; Czlonkowska, Ciesielska, et al., 2005; Gilmore, Jarskog, et al., 2005). Interestingly, NK cells have various roles in both controlling and exacerbating autoimmunity (Perricone, Perricone, et al., 2008). As discussed below, autoimmune conditions have also been linked to ASD in several studies.

The major histocompatibility complex (MHC, types I and II) is a group of highly polymorphic genes on chromosome 6p known as human lymphocyte antigens (HLA). These genes are well known for their central role in the adaptive immune system, as they encode proteins that present self- and non-self-peptides to T cells for immune surveillance. They also have specific associations with autoimmune disorders, such as rheumatoid arthritis. Genes coding for TNF-α and complement are also located within the MHC and have been implicated in autism (Warren, Burger, et al., 1994; Jyonouchi, Geng, et al., 2005). In addition, MHC I is essential for cellular development of the visual system, demonstrating that immune factors are important for CNS plasticity during early brain development (Huh, Boulanger, et al., 2000; Boulanger, 2004). Association of particular HLA types, especially DR4, has been reported in children with autism (Warren, Odell, et al., 1996; Torres, Maciulis, et al., 2002; Lee, Zachary, et al., 2006), while another study showed no such link (Rogers, Kalaydjieva, et al., 1999). Lee et al. found a significant association with HLA DR4 in families with autism in East Tennessee and suggested that geographical factors may play a role in immune susceptibility (Lee, Zachary, et al., 2006). These same families also reported high rates of rheumatoid arthritis in first-degree relatives, a disorder that is typically associated with DR4. Recently Johnson et al. have demonstrated linkage disequilibrium for HLA DR4 from the maternal grandparents to the mothers of children with autism, thereby supporting a theory of prenatal immunogenetic susceptibility to autism (Johnson et al., 2009).

Autoimmunity in ASD

Various autoimmune phenomena have been described in subjects with ASD, although clinical autoimmune disorders are uncommon (Table 24-2). Exploration of autoimmunity in ASD began with several studies that demonstrated increased rates of autoimmune disorders among family members (especially mothers), including rheumatoid arthritis, psoriasis, type I diabetes, thyroid disease, and asthma (Comi, Zimmerman, et al., 1999; Sweeten, Bowyer, et al., 2003; Croen, Grether, et al., 2005; Molloy, Morrow, et al., 2006; Mouridsen, Rich, et al., 2007). In contrast, a study based on medical record review showed no increased rates of autoimmune diseases (Micali, Chakrabarti, et al., 2004). Differences in the occurrence of autoimmune disorders in families from different geographical areas may reflect local environmental factors and represent sampling biases (Lee, Zachary, et al., 2006). Another complicating factor may be that the onset of autoimmune disorders in family members may arise after the time of inquiry. The largest study to date, from the Danish National Registry, found increased rates of ulcerative colitis in mothers and type 1 diabetes in fathers of children with autism (Mouridsen, Rich, et al., 2007). Additional studies are needed to determine the nature and relevance of autoimmune disorders in families with autism.

Many independent studies have described circulating antibodies that are specific to various components in the central nervous system (CNS) in persons with autism (Wills, Cabanlit, et al., 2007). As early as 1982, Weizman et al. demonstrated that 13 of 17 patients with ASD had a cell-mediated response to brain tissues using a macrophage migration inhibition factor test (Weizman, Weizman, et al., 1982). Other putative CNS targets include myelin basic protein (Singh, Warren, et al., 1993), brain serotonin receptors (Todd & Ciaranello, 1985; Singh, Singh, et al., 1997), neurofilament proteins (Singh, Warren, et al., 1997), brain endothelial cell proteins (Connolly, Chez, et al., 1999), brain derived neurotrophic factor (Connolly, Chez, et al., 2005), heat shock protein (Evers, Cunningham-Rundles, et al., 2002), and caudate nucleus (Singh & Rivas, 2004). A recent study by Singer et al. identified a variety of brain-specific autoantibodies in the serum of subjects with autism spectrum disorders (Singer, Morris, et al., 2006). Interestingly, both subjects with autism and their nonautistic siblings had antibody reactivity to the cerebellum and cingulate gyrus that was different in intensity from controls (Singer, Morris, et al., 2006). A 2004 study suggested an increased prevalence of antibodies to cerebellar proteins found in Purkinje cells. These antibodies were also thought to cross react with the dietary protein gliadin (Vojdani, O'Bryan, et al., 2004). More recently, Zimmerman and colleagues reported antibody reactivity to fetal rat brain in plasma from subjects with autism and their mothers (Zimmerman, Connors, et al., 2007). It was further demonstrated that children with ASD had a different pattern than their siblings and typically developing control children. However, there was no clear delineation of patterns between children with ASD and children with other neurodevelopmental disorders.

Autoantibodies to proteins in human hypothalamus and thalamus, which appear to be specific for a subpopulation of children with ASD, were recently described by Cabanlit et al. (Cabanlit, Wills, et al., 2007). To further explore the possibility of autoantibodies directed toward proteins in their native state, or toward a protein of low abundance in the brain, immunohistochemical studies were performed using brain sections from the nonhuman primate macaque monkey (*Macca fascicularis*). Observations thus far have been restricted to the cerebellum and demonstrate that 21% of patients with ASD have intense staining of cerebellar Golgi cells, compared with 0% of controls (Wills, Cabanlit, et al., 2008). Moreover, there appeared to be a correlation between the cerebellar staining and the presence of an approximately 52 kDa band in cerebellum using Western blot analysis.

Autoantibodies such as those described herein have the potential to exert their effects through several different mechanisms. For example, some may act as ligands for a target

Table 24–2.
Autoantibodies and allergy in subjects with autism

		Study Description	Reference
Circulating Autoantibodies and ASD Subjects	**Myelin Basic Protein and Other Identified antigens**	Serum antibodies to Myelin Basic Protein more prevalent in ASD subjects compared to control groups (typically developing children, children with mental retardation or Down syndrome, normal adults)	(Singh, Warren, et al., 1993)
		Serum antibodies to Myelin Basic protein and *neuron axon filament protein* found more often in ASD children than in non-age-matched controls.	(Singh, Lin, et al., 1998)
		Serum antibodies to Myelin Basic Protein, *endothelial cells, BDNF* more prevalent in ASD subjects than healthy controls and controls without neurological illness.	(Connolly, Chez, et al., 2005)
		Subjects with ASD (wide age range) had serum antibodies against dietary antigens like *gliadin* more often than healthy age- and sex-matched controls. These antibodies cross-reacted with *cerebellar peptides,* myelin basic protein, *myelin-associated glycoprotein, gandlioside, sulfatide,* and other neural antigens.	(Vojdani, Campbell, et al., 2002), (Vojdani, O'Bryan, et al., 2004)
	Nonneural Antigen	Occurrence of serum antibodies against Heat shock protein 90 higher in autism group compared to normal controls and a group with autoimmune diseases	(Evers, Cunningham-Rundles, et al., 2002)
	Identified Neural Antigens	ASD subjects have serum antibodies to glial fibrillary acidic protein and neuron-axon filament protein more often than mentally retarded and healthy controls. Subjects vary greatly in age.	(Singh, Warren, et al., 1997)
		ASD subjects have serum antibodies to human serotonin receptors. ASD serum blocks serotonin receptor binding more heavily than healthy control serum.	(Todd & Ciaranello, 1985), (Singh, Singh, et al., 1997)
	Antibodies Directed toward Unidentified Neural Antigen(s)	Increased incidence/staining density of serum IgG specific to brain protein homogenate in ASD subjects compared to their parents and healthy control subjects. Antibodies not specific to MBP as determined by inhibition assay.	(Silva, Correia, et al., 2004)
		ASD subjects had antibodies to temporal cortex endothelial cells and nuclei more frequently than healthy controls and controls with nonneurological illness	(Connolly, Chez, et al., 1999)
		ASD subjects had serum antibodies to rat caudate nucleus, cerebral cortex, cerebellum more frequently than healthy controls.	(Singh & Rivas, 2004)
		ASD subjects had serum antibodies to human caudate nucleus, putamen, and prefrontal cortex more frequently than siblings and non-age-matched healthy controls.	(Singer, Morris, et al., 2006)
		Increased serum antibodies against protein homogenates from fetal rat brain (gestational day 18) in small group of ASD subjects, their mothers, and subjects with other neurological illnesses compared to healthy controls.	(Zimmerman, Connors, et al., 2007)
		IgG reactive to human hypothalamus and thalamus homogenates was found in plasma from ASD subjects more frequently than age-matched controls.	(Cabanlit, Wills, et al., 2007)
		Immunohistochemistry showed a higher prevalence of plasma IgG antibodies to rat cerebellum golgi cells in ASD subjects compared to plasma from age-matched healthy and mentally retarded control subjects.	(Wills, Cabanlit, et al., 2008)

Allergy and ASD Subjects	**Peripheral Allergic Sensitization**	**No Allergy Link Found**	Small group of ASD subjects had serum IgE levels within the normal range for their ages. No control group was included.	(Menage, Thibault, et al., 1992)
			ASD subjects showed no difference in serum IgE, frequency of allergic disorders, or positive skin prick tests compared to an age-matched healthy control group.	(Bakkaloglu, Anlar, et al., 2008)
			No diff in plasma IgE between ASD subjects and age-matched controls, even when considering location and season of birth.	(Heuer, 2008)
		Possible Allergy Link Found	ASD subjects had more blood eosinophils than a group of sex and age matched mentally retarded controls, but there was *no difference* in serum total and allergen-specific IgE levels.	(Renzoni, Beltrami, et al., 1995)
			Increased blood basophil sensitization and positive skin prick tests in a small group ASD subjects compared to small groups of healthy and neurological illness controls.	(Bidet, Leboyer, et al., 1993)
	Allergy and Diet		36 ASD subjects were given specific allergen–free diets (allergen for which they had a positive skin prick test). Subjects demonstrated improved behavior after 8 weeks, though no control group was present.	(Lucarelli, Frediani, et al., 1995)
			Comparison of cytokine production by PBMCs in response to stimulation by various dietary proteins (cows milk protein, Gliadin, and soy) in a group of ASD subjects, siblings, and healthy controls. ASD PBMCs were found to produce more IFN-gamma and TNF-alpha with stimulation at a higher rate than controls.	(Jyonouchi, Sun, et al., 2002)
			Increased cytokine production by blood mononuclear cells in response to dietary antigens in ASD subjects (especially those with gastrointestinal symptoms) compared to healthy controls.	(Jyonouchi, Geng, et al., 2005)
			As mentioned above, antibodies were found in serum of ASD subjects that were specific to dietary many antigens. These antibodies also cross-reacted with many neural antigens.	(Vojdani, Campbell, et al., 2002), (Vojdani, O'Bryan, et al., 2004)
		No Allergy Link	This study of current evidence shows that the link between elimination diets, autism, and improved behavior is weak. It calls for future well-controlled clinical studies to further explore any association.	(Millward, Ferriter, et al., 2008)

receptor. Such autoantibody-receptor interactions have the potential to induce excitotoxic death through excessive signaling (Portales-Perez, Alarcon-Segovia, et al., 1998; Sisto, Lisi, et al., 2006). Alternatively, autoantibodies to neural antigens can act antagonistically, and block an essential pathway. Such interference may lead to abnormal neural development and/or function. Finally, autoantibodies can mediate tissue destruction through complement fixation and cell-mediated cytotoxicity. If any of the above scenarios were to occur during a critical developmental window, consequences might include impaired neuronal function, altered receptor density and/or distribution, or improper release of neurotransmitters and/or cytokines. However, it is currently premature to speculate whether antibodies found in ASD subjects are pathogenically significant or merely an epiphenomenon. Thus, additional studies are under way to characterize any possible deleterious effects in animal models.

Allergy in Subjects with ASD

Some researchers have postulated that allergic disease may be associated with ASD, despite a number of studies suggesting no relationship. In 1992, six children with ASD were found to be within normal ranges for levels of total IgE and histamine (Menage, Thibault, et al., 1992). However, the small sample size and lack of control group require that these results be interpreted with caution (Menage, Thibault, et al., 1992). A larger study, including 43 ASD patients and age-/sex-matched, developmentally disabled non-ASD controls, showed no differences in total or allergen-specific IgE, though eosinophilia was more prevalent in the ASD group (Renzoni, Beltrami, et al., 1995). A neurotypical control group was not included in this study. A more recent study of over 116 subjects with autism and 96 neurotypical controls demonstrated that there was no difference in plasma IgE levels when the subjects were controlled for age, season, and geographic location (Heuer, 2008). There are additional reports of increased basophil sensitization and positive skin prick tests among ASD subjects compared to controls (Bidet, Leboyer, et al., 1993), though independent studies have contradicted these findings (Bakkaloglu, Anlar, et al., 2008).

The relationship between food allergy and ASD is highly controversial (Cormier & Elder, 2007). Over a decade ago, a study of 36 ASD patients suggested that a specific allergen-free diet was associated with improved behavior (Lucarelli, Frediani, et al., 1995). Whether these behavioral improvements were due to neurological phenomena, or simply increased comfort and disposition in the absence of allergic activity is unclear. There is little additional nonanecdotal evidence supporting any behavioral benefits of allergen-free diets (Cormier & Elder, 2007). Furthermore, several subsequent studies have reported negligible behavioral changes after elimination diets (Millward, Ferriter, et al., 2008).

Vojdani et al. have published a series of studies linking food hypersensitivity and CNS-specific autoantibodies. ASD subjects were observed to have an increased incidence of neural-protein-specific autoantibodies that cross-reacted with dietary antigens like milk butyrophilin (Vojdani, Campbell, et al., 2002) and gliadin (Vojdani, O'Bryan, et al., 2004). However, these studies have not been confirmed. A large 2005 study explored the cellular response to various food allergens in ASD subjects versus controls (Jyonouchi, Geng, et al., 2005). This study found an association between cytokine production against dietary proteins and GI symptoms in ASD. A large proportion of ASD subjects with GI symptoms were included in the study (75 out of 109), so it is possible that food allergy is most relevant among this subset of ASD subjects. One should also note that there is a difference between food allergy that is IgE mediated, and a food sensitivity that is not directly mediated by the immune system, such as lactose intolerance due to an enzyme deficiency.

In comparison to the literature linking autoimmunity and other immune dysfunctions to ASD, there is a dearth of evidence concerning associations of allergic diseases. Future studies that utilize large, well-described patient groups and well-matched controls will help to resolve lingering ambiguity.

Infections, Immunizations and Responses to Fever in Subjects with ASD

Although anecdotal evidence suggests that children with ASD appear to have frequent infections, available data show the overall infection rate to be similar to controls (Comi, Zimmerman, et al., 1999; Rosen, Yoshida, et al., 2007). Children with ASD have been shown to have fewer upper respiratory infections, more frequent genitourinary infections, and more total infections during the first 30 days of life when compared to neurotypical controls (Rosen, Yoshida, et al., 2007).

Childhood immunizations frequently have been perceived by families as causing autism due to the temporal relationship with regression, or loss of skills, and the emergence of autistic symptoms (Woo, Ball, et al., 2007). However, multiple epidemiological studies have negated a causative relationship (Taylor, Miller, et al., 1999; DeStefano & Chen, 2000). With respect to measles vaccine, a recent study found no evidence of RNA measles virus transcripts in bowel tissue from autism subjects (Hornig, Briese, et al., 2008). Furthermore, antibody responses to measles vaccine are similar in children with autism and controls (Baird, Pickles, et al., 2008). This is in contrast to previous studies (Singh & Jensen, 2003). Despite many reassuring studies, individual cases of regression following immunizations may occur due to underlying mitochondrial dysfunction on a genetic and cellular basis, which may also be exacerbated by the stress of fever and infection (Poling, Frye, et al., 2006). Further, one cannot rule out the possibility that a subset of children with autism react differentially to immunization due to underlying immune dysfunction. However, systematic evaluation of the immune response immediately following vaccination needs to be performed to examine this hypothesis.

Behaviors in children with autism frequently improve rapidly during fever, including reduced stereotypy, hyperactivity, irritability, and inappropriate speech (Curran, Newschaffer, et al., 2007). Although this "fever effect" can be difficult to separate from sickness behavior, up to 80% of families observe some degree of improvement, and anecdotal reports of marked changes occur frequently. There are many hypothetical reasons for these changes, including immune-mediated effects from cytokines, changes in synaptic membrane properties, and intracellular signaling. Further studies are needed to verify this intriguing, and potentially enlightening phenomenon.

Maternal Immunity and Autism Spectrum Disorders

Mothers of children with ASD have been shown to have various immune system abnormalities compared to mothers of neurotypical children (Ashwood, Wills, et al., 2006; Wills, Cabanlit, et al., 2007). This might be explained by genetic factors that relate to both ASD susceptibility and immune function. Given that several genes are linked to both ASD and the immune system (discussed above), it is likely that mothers of ASD children may possess similar genetic and immune profiles. Additionally, aberrant maternal immune activation during pregnancy can have a profound impact on fetal brain development.

Maternal Immunity and the Gestational Environment

Maternal immune responses (including infection, autoimmunity, and allergy) generate factors that have a direct impact on the gestational environment. Factors like cytokines, chemokines, and antibodies produced during pregnancy may carry various developmental consequences for the fetus. Increased rates of infection and other environmental factors may account for increased autism rates among children born in the spring months (Lee, Newschaffer, et al., 2008). This is consistent with early observations that autism can be associated with congenital rubella (Chess, 1977) as well cytomegalovirus (Stubbs, 1978; Markowitz, 1983), which were some of the earliest indicators of the neurobiological basis of autism.

Maternal Inflammation and Cytokines

Under normal conditions, the maternal immune system is uniquely regulated during pregnancy to maintain a pathogen-free yet noninflammatory environment for the developing fetus (Wegmann, Lin, et al., 1993; Chaouat, 2007). Robust maternal immune activation is associated with obstetrical, developmental, and/or behavioral complications (Jenkins, Roberts, et al., 2000; Shi, Fatemi, et al., 2003; Samuelsson, Jennische, et al., 2006; Smith, Li, et al., 2007; Raghupathy & Kalinka, 2008). During pregnancy, maternal cytokines may cross the placenta (in the case of IL-6; Zaretsky, Alexander, et al., 2004; Aaltonen, Heikkinen, et al., 2005; Ashdown, Dumont, et al., 2006; Samuelsson, Jennische, et al., 2006), or act on placental cells to stimulate the downstream production of mediators in the fetal compartment (Hauguel-de Mouzon & Guerre-Millo, 2006). Cytokines are involved in many diverse aspects of normal brain development including proliferation and differentiation of neural and glial cells (Mehler & Kessler, 1998). Fluctuations in levels of these molecules may alter neurodevelopment. Therefore, changes in maternal immune homeostasis can impact the fetus in many ways.

The effect of maternal immunity on the developing immune and central nervous systems has been studied extensively using both epidemiological studies and animal models (Holladay & Smialowicz, 2000; Meyer, Yee, et al., 2007) (Table 24-3). Findings from these studies may be relevant to psychiatric disorders such as autism and schizophrenia. Independent studies carried out in mice have shown that pregnant dams injected with immune-stimulating agents, including IL-6, IL-2, influenza, LPS, Poly I:C, and turpentine, gave birth to pups with behavioral differences, some of which are thought to be reminiscent of autism (Shi, Fatemi, et al., 2003; Samuelsson, Jennische, et al., 2006; Ponzio, Servatius, et al., 2007; Smith, Li, et al., 2007). A study by Meyer et al. showed that immune challenges during two critical periods of fetal development resulted in differential effects on future behavioral modifications, neuropathology, and fetal brain cytokine responses (Meyer, Yee, et al., 2007). These experiments suggest that the gestational environment may contribute to abnormalities in offspring born to mothers with excessive immune activation. The effects of such agents on the developing immune and nervous systems are likely dependent on the period of exposure and genetic susceptibility (Holladay & Smialowicz, 2000). This research supports the hypothesis that early immune/nervous system disturbances are capable of permanently altering either or both systems.

Maternal Autoantibodies

Cytokines are not the only link between maternal immune activity and fetal development. Maternal antibodies (IgG) are passed to the fetus to provide passive immunity throughout pregnancy (Simister, 2003). These antibodies serve this protective role until the child's immune system matures, and can be found in a child's circulation up to 6 months after birth (Heininger, Desgrandchamps, et al., 2006). Maternal antibodies are passed without regard to their specificity, meaning that both protective and autoantibodies have equal access. Therefore, maternal autoantibodies produced during pregnancy can target tissues in the developing fetus. In the case of autoimmune conditions like myasthenia gravis, the neonate may display transient signs of the disorder, which usually resolve soon after birth (Djelmis, Sostarko, et al., 2002). Alternatively, with systemic lupus erythematosus (SLE), maternal autoantibodies can cause long-term irreparable harm to developing organ systems (Motta, Rodriguez-Perez, et al., 2007).

Table 24–3.
Gestational exposure and offspring behavior

	Prenatal Exposure		
	LPS	Poly IC	Cytokines
Demonstration of behavioral phenotypes among offspring exposed in utero	Disrupted sensorimotor gating (Prepulse inhibition, PPI), reversed by antipsychotics (Borrell, Vela, et al., 2002)	Disrupted PPI w/acoustic startle, deficient open field exploration, novel object test and social interaction (Shi, Fatemi, et al., 2003) (Smith, Li, et al., 2007)	Macrophage IL-10 overexpression REDUCES behavioral problems in mice exposed in utero to Poly I:C (exploratory behavior, PPI, LI (Meyer, Murray, et al., 2008)
	Lower locomotive activity in elevated plus maze and more skips on beam walking (Bakos, Duncko, et al., 2004)	Decreased exploratory behavior, PPI, selective associative learning (LI, US-pre-exposure effect), spatial working memory, enhanced locomotor response to amphetamine, reversal learning. (Meyer, Feldon, et al., 2005), (Meyer, Feldon, et al., 2006).	Pups exposed prenatally to IL-2 had increased open-field activity, grooming and rearing behavior, abnormal motor learning (acquisition of classically conditioned eyeblink response) (Ponzio, Servatius, et al., 2007)
	Altered object recognition, passive avoidance, social interaction lower locomotive activity in elevated plus maze, water maze, and open field exploration (Golan, Lev, et al., 2005; Golan, Stilman, et al., 2006)	Deficient reversal learning, disrupted latent inhibition, both alleviated w/antipsychotics, enhanced locomotor response to amphetamine (Zuckerman, Rehavi, et al., 2003) (Zuckerman & Weiner, 2005)	Adults exposed prenatally to IL-6: impaired working memory (Morris water maze: increased escape latency and time spent near the pool wall) (Samuelsson, Jennische, et al., 2006)
	enhanced amphetamine-induced locomotor response and startle reflex (Fortier, Joober, et al., 2004)	disrupted sensorimotor gating (PPI) (Wolff & Bilkey, 2008), (Meyer, Nyffeler, et al., 2008) Disrupted PPI, open field, amphetamine-induced locomotion, cognitive impairment (Ozawa, Hashimoto, et al., 2006)	IL-6 deficient mice, or mice coadministered anti-IL-6 lack behavioral problems of WT mice exposed prenatally to Poly I:C alone (Smith, Li, et al., 2007)
Demonstrations of Neurobiological Differences among Offspring exposed in utero	Increased tyrosine hydroxylase in bed nucleus of the stria terminalis and shell nucleus acumbens, activated microglia and astroglia (increased MHCII), increased GFAP-in adult offspring (Borrell, Vela, et al., 2002)	Increased responses to antipsychotic (clozapine and chlorpromazine) and psychomimetic (ketamine) drugs (Shi, 2003)	Adult rats exposed prenatally to IL-6 had -neuronal loss and astrogliosis, with some sex differences. -Increased expression of GABA (Aalpha5), NR1, and GFAP mRNA. -Increased levels of the apoptosis marker caspase-3 (Samuelsson, Jennische, et al., 2006)
	Less myelin basic protein (MBP), more GFAP, altered microglial staining (Cai, Pan, et al., 2000) Decreased dopamine in nucleus accumbens (Bakos, Duncko, et al., 2004) Less tyrosine hydroxylase in mesencephalon, reduced striatal dopamine, increased microglia (Ling, Chang, et al., 2004)	Cerebellar pathology: Purkinje cell deficit, delayed granule cell migration (Shi, Smith, et al., 2009) GABAA receptor increase (Meyer, Feldon, et al., 2005), (Nyffeler, Meyer, et al., 2006), (Meyer, Feldon, et al., 2006)	

	Less oligodendrocyte-protein staining (Proteolipo Protein (PLP), MBP, 2', 3'-cyclic nucleotide phosphodiesterase (CNP)) (Bell & Hallenbeck, 2002), (Poggi, Park, et al., 2005, (Paintlia, 2004)		Large adult brain, Purkinje cell deficit (Fatemi, Earle, et al., 2002), (Smith, Li, et al., 2007)	
	Increased numbers and packing density of hippocampal pyramidal neurons and granular cells-(Golan, Lev, et al., 2005; Golan, Stilman, et al., 2006)		Increased dopamine turnover, decreased receptor binding (Ozawa, Hashimoto, et al., 2006)	
	Cell death in striatum, white matter, ventricular zone, increase GFAP, decreased MBP, astrogliosis, enlarged ventricles, gray matter lesions (Rousset, Chalon, et al., 2006), (Wang, Hagberg, et al., 2007)		Hippocampal necrosis, altered hippocampal morphology, increased dopamine release (Zuckerman, Rehavi, et al., 2003), (Zuckerman & Weiner, 2005)	
	Increased GFAP, fewer oligodendrocytes, increased cell death in fetal brain (Elovitz, Mrinalini, et al., 2006) Increased microglial activation and axonal injury, fewer oligodendrocytes (Nitsos, Rees, et al., 2006)		Delayed myelination, less MBP, smaller axon diameters (Makinodan, Tatsumi, et al., 2008)	
Demonstrations of Immunological Differences in Offspring exposed in utero (measured in stated compartments)	Amniotic fluid	Increased IL-1a (Fidel, Romero, et al., 1994)	**TNF-a** (Gilmore, Jarskog, et al., 2005)	Radio labeled **IL-2** administered to pregnant dam was found in amniotic fluid (Ponzio, Servatius, et al., 2007)
		Increased IL-8 (Nitsos, Rees, et al., 2006),(Kramer, Moss, et al., 2001)		
		Increased IL-1B (Gayle, Beloosesky, et al., 2004) Increased IL-6 (Fidel, Romero, et al., 1994), (Urakubo, Jarskog, et al., 2001), (Nitsos, Rees, et al., 2006),(Kramer, Moss, et al., 2001), (Gayle, Beloosesky, et al., 2004) Increased TNF-a (Urakubo, Jarskog, et al., 2001), (Gayle, Beloosesky, et al., 2004), (Xu, Chen, et al., 2006)		
	Fetal Brain	Increased IL-1B (Cai, 2000), (Paintlia, Paintlia, et al., 2004), (Elovitz, Mrinalini, et al., 2006), (Liverman, Kaftan, et al., 2006)	Increased IL-1B (Meyer, Nyffeler, et al., 2006), (Meyer, Feldon, et al., 2005)	Overexpression of **IL-10** reduces expression of inflammatory cytokines in animals exposed to Poly I:C (Meyer, Murray, et al., 2008)
		Increased TNF-a (Cai, Pan, et al., 2000), (Bell & Hallenbeck, 2002), (Paintlia, 2004), (Elovitz, Mrinalini, et al., 2006)	Increased TNF-a (Meyer, Nyffeler, et al., 2006)	
		Increased IFN-g (Bell and Hallenbeck 2002), (Elovitz, 2006)	Altered IL-10 (Meyer, Nyffeler, et al., 2006)	Pups prenatally exposed to **IL-6** had increased IL-6 levels in the hippocampus (Samuelsson, Jennische, et al., 2006)
		BDNF (Golan, Lev, et al., 2005)		

(Continued)

Table 24–3. (*Contd.*)

	Prenatal Exposure		
	LPS	Poly IC	Cytokines
	Increased IL-6 (Elovitz, Mrinalini, et al., 2006), (Liverman, Kaftan, et al., 2006), (Golan, Lev, et al., 2005)	Increased IL-6 (Meyer, Nyffeler, et al., 2006)	
Placenta	Increased **IL-1a** (Rounioja, Rasanen, et al., 2003), (Urakubo, Jarskog, et al., 2001),(Gayle, Beloosesky, et al., 2004) Increased **IL-1B** (Rounioja, Rasanen, et al., 2003),(Nitsos, Rees, et al., 2006), (Kramer, Moss, et al., 2001), (Ashdown, Dumont, et al., 2006), (Elovitz, Mrinalini, et al., 2006) **IL-6** (Urakubo, Jarskog, et al., 2001), (Gayle, Beloosesky, et al., 2004), (Nitsos, Rees, et al., 2006), (Kramer, Moss, et al., 2001), (Bell & Hallenbeck, 2002), (Ashdown, Dumont, et al., 2006), (Elovitz, Mrinalini, et al., 2006), (Xu, Chen, et al., 2006), (Beloosesky, Gayle, et al., 2006) **TNF-a** (Urakubo, Jarskog, et al., 2001), (Gayle, Beloosesky, et al., 2004), (Nitsos, Rees, et al., 2006), (Kramer, Moss, et al., 2001), (Bell & Hallenbeck, 2002), (Ashdown, Dumont, et al., 2006), (Elovitz, Mrinalini, et al., 2006), (Xu, Chen, et al., 2006), (Beloosesky, Gayle, et al., 2006) **IL-8** (Nitsos, Rees, et al., 2006), (Kramer, Moss, et al., 2001) **IL-10** (Bell & Hallenbeck, 2002) **IFN-g** (Elovitz, Mrinalini, et al., 2006)	Increased TNF-a (Gilmore, Jarskog, et al., 2005)	
Nonneural Fetal/Offspring Samples	**IL-1a** (Rounioja, Rasanen, et al., 2003)		Radio labeled IL-2 administered to pregnant dams was found in embryonic tissue (Ponzio, Servatius, et al., 2007)
	IL-6 (Rounioja, Rasanen, et al., 2003), (Beloosesky, Gayle, et al., 2006) serum **IL-6** (Borrell, Vela, et al., 2002) **IL-1B**, (Rounioja, Rasanen, et al., 2003), (Ashdown, Dumont, et al., 2006)		Pups prenatally exposed to IL-6 had increased IL-6 serum levels (Samuelsson, Jennische, et al., 2006)
	TNF-a (Rounioja, Rasanen, et al., 2003) increased serum **IL-2** (Borrell, Vela, et al., 2002) Reduction in offspring body weight (Bakos, Duncko, et al., 2004)		Pups exposed prenatally to IL-2 had accelerated T cell development, TH1 skewed differentiation, increased proliferative and cytotoxic responses to syngeneic B lymphoma cells or allogeneic splenocytes. (Ponzio, Servatius, et al., 2007)

Interesting murine models have demonstrated a link between the gestational immune environment and offspring behavior. NZB and BSXB are mouse strains that spontaneously develop autoimmune diseases, and often demonstrate behavioral abnormalities that are linked to cortical ectopias (Sakic, Szechtman, et al., 1997). It is unclear whether the ectopias are related to the autoimmune disease, or if they are the consequence of an unfavorable gestational environment due to maternal autoimmune disease. Denenberg et al. designed an elegant embryo transfer study to delineate the relationship between maternal autoimmunity, fetal brain development, and cortical ectopias. They demonstrated that mouse strains transferred to the uterus of an autoimmune mother demonstrate deficits in learning and increased autoimmune activity (Denenberg, Mobraaten, et al., 1991; Denenberg, Sherman, et al., 1996). The reverse situation, in which an autoimmune-prone strain was transferred to a nonautoimmune mother, resulted in offspring with improved learning and decreased autoimmunity compared to those that developed in a syngeneic autoimmune uterus (Denenberg, Mobraaten, et al., 1991; Denenberg, Sherman, et al., 1996).

Autoimmunity in Mothers of ASD Subjects

Autoimmune factors have been demonstrated in both subjects with ASD and their family members (Wills, Cabanlit, et al., 2007) (Table 24-4). As discussed above, primary relatives of subjects with ASD have a higher incidence of autoimmune disease than those of typically developing children (Money, Bobrow, et al., 1971; Sweeten, Bowyer, et al., 2003; Croen, Grether, et al., 2005). In 1990, Warren et al. observed that 6 of 11 mothers of children with autism had antibodies that were reactive to lymphocytes of their autistic child (Warren, Cole, et al., 1990). Additionally, a growing body of evidence suggests that some mothers of ASD children produce antibodies that target brain proteins. Recently, it was noted by Braunschweig et al. that a subset of mothers whose children have autism demonstrate antibodies that recognized human fetal brain proteins in a disease-specific pattern of reactivity when compared to mothers of typically developing controls (Braunschweig, Ashwood, et al., 2007). Similarly, Zimmerman and colleagues observed specific patterns of plasma reactivity to fetal rat brain protein by immunoblotting in mothers of ASD children. These antibodies differentially recognized fetal rat brain proteins when compared with plasma from mothers of typically developing children (Zimmerman, Connors, et al., 2007). Similar fetal brain–specific reactivity was also noted in samples taken during the second trimester of pregnancy (Croen, Braunschweig, et al., 2008). Subsequent studies by another group have confirmed that a subset of mothers with ASD children produce circulating antibodies reactive to human fetal brain proteins (Singer, Morris, et al., 2008).

While the role of these antibodies in ASD is currently unknown, in an early model, Dalton et al. utilized a murine model to test the pathogenicity of maternal serum to the fetus during pregnancy. Serum from a mother of three children (a typically developing child, a child with autism, and a child with severe language impairment) was introduced by intraperitoneal injection into gestating mice (Dalton, Deacon, et al., 2003). The offspring of the injected mice demonstrated behavioral changes and antibody deposition on Purkinje cells and other neurons. This was in contrast to the offspring of gestating mice injected with sera from mothers of typically developing children. This study suggested that a factor(s) present in the sera of mothers of children with ASD, possibly immunoglobulin, led to altered neurodevelopment behavioral changes in the offspring.

More recently, a primate model was used to assess behavioral consequences of prenatal exposure to the maternal antibodies described by Braunschweig et al. (Braunschweig, Ashwood, et al., 2007); (Martin, Ashwood, et al., 2008). IgG was isolated from mothers of children with ASD and typically developing controls, and injected into pregnant rhesus monkeys. The resulting offspring were assessed from birth until 15 months of age by trained observers. Significant increases in stereotypic behavior were observed in 3 of 4 offspring who received IgG from mothers of children with autism. In contrast, behavioral anomalies were not observed in the monkeys from control IgG-treated pregnancies. The stereotypic behaviors surfaced after weaning, and were more prevalent in unfamiliar situations. Stereotypic behaviors are one characteristic of ASD, suggesting a potential link between maternal anti–fetal brain IgG and changes in offspring behavior. An analogous study by Singer et al. demonstrated the transfer of serum antibodies from mothers of children with autism to gestating mice, led to behavioral changes in the offspring, including hyperactivity and decreased sociability (Singer et al., 2008). Immunohistochemical studies in this model showed immune activation of astrocytes and microglia in the offspring, similar to that observed in humans with autism by Vargas et al. (Vargas, Nascimbene, et al., 2005).

Maternal Allergy and ASD

There is very limited evidence linking the presence of maternal allergies to ASD. However a recent study suggested that midgestational allergic/asthmatic immune profiles may relate to the development of ASD. Croen et al. reported that mothers diagnosed during their second trimester with asthma or allergy are twice as likely to have a child with ASD than mothers without asthma or allergy (Croen, Grether, et al., 2005). A retrospective analysis of blood collected during the second trimester is currently underway to confirm these epidemiological findings with clinical evidence. It is possible that a subset of ASD may involve exposure to allergic/asthmatic immune activation during gestation. The development of ASD is likely dependent on the duration of the exposure, and whether it occurred during a critical neurodevelopmental window. Future, well-controlled epidemiological studies and animal modeling will be necessary to lend further credence to these findings.

Table 24–4.
Familial autoimmune and other noninfectious pathology related to autism

		Study Description	Reference(s)
Epidemiological Associations for Familial Non Infectious Diseases		Case study describing a family of ASD subject with high incidence of autoimmune disorders.	(Money, Bobrow, et al., 1971)
		More autoimmune disorders among primary family members of ASD subjects than typical controls.	(Comi, Zimmerman, et al., 1999)
		Increased familial autoimmunity among primary family members of ASD subjects.	(Sweeten, Bowyer, et al., 2003)
		Familial familial anxiety and obsessive compulsive disorder among ASD subjects, no autoimmune connection	(Micali, Chakrabarti, et al., 2004)
		Greater risk of ASD with maternal diagnosis of allergy/asthma during second trimester. No strong autoimmune association during pregnancy, however, there was a trend toward increased Type I diabetes and psoriasis.	(Croen, Grether, et al., 2005)
		Regressive ASD associated w/familial autoimmunity.	(Molloy, Morrow, et al., 2006)
		Increased Type 1 diabetes in fathers of ASD subjects, and ulcerative colitis among mothers of ASD subjects.	(Mouridsen, Rich, et al., 2007)
Antibodies to fetal tissue in mothers of ASD Subjects	**PBMC antigen**	Mothers of ASD subjects demonstrated increased antibody reactivity against the lymphocytes of their ASD children.	(Warren, Cole, et al., 1990)
	Rat Brain Antigen	Mothers of ASD subjects were shown to have IgG reactivity to rat fetal brain proteins.	(Zimmerman, Connors, et al., 2007)
	Human Brain Antigen	Plasma from mothers of ASD subjects showed IgG reactivity to human fetal brain proteins at 37 and 73kd unlike mothers of controls	(Braunschweig, Ashwood, et al., 2007)
		Mothers of ASD subjects were confirmed to have IgG reactivity to human fetal brain proteins.	(Singer, Morris, et al., 2008)
		Serum collected during the second trimester from mothers of ASD subjects showed increased IgG reactivity to human fetal brain proteins compared to serum from control pregnancies.	(Croen, Braunschweig, et al., 2008)
Animal Models: gestational exposure to maternal antibodies and offspring behavior		Conventionally reared mice from autoimmune-prone/behaviorally impaired strain of mice were compared to same strain transferred as embryos into mothers of alternative, non–autoimmune/behaviorally impaired strain. Behavioral improvements were observed in transferred offspring based on several measures.	(Denenberg, Sherman, et al., 1996)
		Serum from mother of ASD subject injected into pregnant rats. Offspring had altered exploration, motor coordination, and cerebellar magnetic resonance spectroscopy. Ig deposition was observed on offspring purkinje cells. Results not observed in rats exposed in utero to serum from control mothers.	(Dalton, Deacon, et al., 2003)
		Stereotypic behavior observed in monkeys exposed prenatally to IgG from mothers of ASD subjects who had previously demonstrated IgG reactivity to fetal brain. This was not observed in monkeys exposed to IgG from control mothers.	(Martin, Ashwood, et al., 2008) building on (Braunschweig, Ashwood, et al., 2007)
		Offspring from pregnant SLE mice producing DNA-specific, NMDAR-specific autoantibodies throughout gestation were observed. Histological abnormalities were observed in the fetal brain of exposed offspring, and adult offspring demonstrated cognitive impairments.	(Lee, Huerta, et al., 2009)

Conclusions

At this time, an overarching question with respect to the immune system in autism is whether it contributes to the pathogenesis of the disorder. Evidence of significant "immune anomalies" in autism has accumulated over the past 30 years, raising serious questions as to their origin and role in the development of the disorder. Many findings regarding the immune system in ASD have been inconsistent due to numerous methodologic factors, the most notable of which are the use of inappropriate and non–age matched control groups, as well as heterogeneous, ill-defined subject populations. However, more recent studies are gaining credibility through the use of age-matched controls and well-characterized subject populations. Additionally, promising animal models are under development that mirror characteristics of ASD (Crawley, 2007; Tordjman, Drapier, et al., 2007). Such models will expand our understanding of the disorder, and pave the way for more focused clinical studies. They will be especially useful for determining the effects of human antibodies from children with ASD, their mothers and other family members, on brain development and behavior.

The presence of autoantibodies in subjects with ASD and their mothers is intriguing, and suggests a previous exposure of CNS antigens to the immune system. This may be the result of injury or abnormal development that led to an immune response to brain antigens in some subjects with ASD. However, it must be emphasized that these autoantibodies have not as yet been firmly associated with pathology. In some cases, similar antibodies are found in diseases other than ASD, and they are not present in all subjects with ASD. It is not abnormal to detect autoantibodies in normal healthy controls, although elevated titers have usually been associated with CNS disorders. Increased prevalence of such antibodies among ASD subjects is possibly representative of ongoing immune activation. It is also possible that subjects with ASD are more prone to form these and other antibodies, even if they do not cause or maintain the disorder.

To date, there is extensive data suggesting that some mothers of ASD children have immune-related abnormalities. Maternal immune activity can influence the gestational environment, and impact fetal neurodevelopment. Accordingly, behavioral issues have been noted in offspring from pregnancies exposed to various insults that affect immune function. Currently, the majority of data correlating maternal immunity to ASD in human populations comes from analysis of a single blood sample collected years after the birth of an ASD child. This approach is only partially revealing for several reasons. First, cross-sectional retrospective analysis does not account for the dynamic nature of immune activity and fetal neurodevelopment, and fails to identify critical windows of susceptibility to exposure. Second, immune profiles in maternal plasma do not necessarily reflect the immune activity at the maternal-fetal interface. In order to lend strength to the mid- and postpregnancy findings, prospective longitudinal studies of maternal immune function measured in various biological specimens collected throughout relevant windows of development would be ideal. Current studies are attempting this study design by following the subsequent pregnancies of mothers who have an existing child with autism. Younger siblings of ASD children have an increased chance of developing the disorder compared to the general population (Ritvo, Jorde, et al., 1989), and are thus ideal subjects for a well-targeted prospective study. Clinically relevant immune profiles could then be obtained during pregnancy and postnatally, and analyzed for a link between early immunity and the manifestation of ASD (Landa & Garrett-Mayer, 2006). Given the importance of the intrauterine milieu and the possibility that ASD results from an early insult, prospective maternal-fetal immune studies hold considerable promise.

Finally, one must ask the question: Do these immune anomalies occur as epiphenomena with the varied genotypes and phenotypes of autism, or are they in fact responsible for initiating, maintaining, or exacerbating the disorder, at least in some patients? An attractive hypothesis is that in some children with ASD, immune dysregulation is indicative of disturbances in cellular or signaling pathways that are common to both the immune and neural systems. As evidence of detectable immune differences in autism subjects accumulates, the possibility of identifying biological markers of the disorder nears. Continued research may eventually allow for further clinical differentiation of the disorder with concomitant development of meaningful medical treatments, and an overall better understanding of pathogenic mechanisms in ASD.

Challenges and Future Directions

There remain many additional unexplored questions with respect to the immune system in autism. Among others, these include:

- The basic correlation of laboratory immune profiles to varying phenotypes of autism.
- A detailed analysis of the responses to immunization in children with and without autism.
- The characterization of antigenic proteins that are targeted by autoantibodies in both mothers and children with autism.
- Analysis of the cellular mechanisms of the "fever effect."
- The relationship between immune anomalies observed in mothers of ASD children and those observed in the ASD subjects themselves.

SUGGESTED READINGS

Ashwood, P., Wills, S., et al. (2006). The immune response in autism: a new frontier for autism research. *Journal of Leukocyte Biology, 80*(1), 1–15.

Pardo, C. A., & Eberhart, C. G. (2007, October). The neurobiology of autism. *Brain Pathology, 17*(4), 434–447.

Pardo, C. A., Vargas, D. L., & Zimmerman, A. W. (2005, December). Immunity, neuroglia, and neuroinflammation in autism. *International Review of Psychiatry (Abingdon, England), 17*(6), 485–495.

Wills, S., Cabanlit, M., Ashwood, P., Amaral, D., & Van de Water, J. (2007, June). Autoantibodies in autism spectrum disorders (ASD). *Annals of the New York Academy of Sciences, 1107*, 79–91.

REFERENCES

Aaltonen, R., Heikkinen, T., et al. (2005). Transfer of proinflammatory cytokines across term placenta. *Obstetrics and Gynecology, 106*(4), 802–807.

Ashdown, H., Dumont, Y., et al. (2006). The role of cytokines in mediating effects of prenatal infection on the fetus: implications for schizophrenia. *Molecular Psychiatry, 11*(1), 47–55.

Ashwood, P., Anthony, A., et al. (2003). Intestinal lymphocyte populations in children with regressive autism: evidence for extensive mucosal immunopathology. *Journal of Clinical Immunology, 23*(6), 504–517.

Ashwood, P., Anthony, A., et al. (2004). Spontaneous mucosal lymphocyte cytokine profiles in children with autism and gastrointestinal symptoms: mucosal immune activation and reduced counter regulatory interleukin-10. *Journal of Clinical Immunology, 24*(6), 664–673.

Ashwood, P., Enstrom, A., et al. (2008). Decreased transforming growth factor beta1 in autism: A potential link between immune dysregulation and impairment in clinical behavioral outcomes. *Journal of Neuroimmunology, 204*(1–2), 149–153.

Ashwood, P., Kwong, C., et al. (2008). Brief report: plasma leptin levels are elevated in autism: association with early onset phenotype? *Journal of Autism and Developmental Disorders, 38*(1), 169–175.

Ashwood, P., & Van de Water, J. (2004). Is autism an autoimmune disease? *Autoimmunity Reviews, 3*(7–8), 557–562.

Ashwood, P., Wills, S., et al. (2006). The immune response in autism: a new frontier for autism research. *Journal of Leukocyte Biology, 80*(1), 1–15.

Bailey, S. L., Carpentier, P. A., et al. (2006). Innate and adaptive immune responses of the central nervous system. *Critical Reviews in Immunology, 26*(2), 149–188.

Baird, G., Pickles, A., et al. (2008). Measles vaccination and antibody response in autism spectrum disorders. *Archives of Disease in Childhood, 93*(10), 832–837.

Bakkaloglu, B., Anlar, B., et al. (2008). Atopic features in early childhood autism. *European Journal of Paediatric Neurology, 12*(6), 476–479.

Bakos, J., Duncko, R., et al. (2004). Prenatal immune challenge affects growth, behavior, and brain dopamine in offspring. *Annals of the New York Academy of Sciences, 1018*, 281–287.

Banks, W. A. (2001). Leptin transport across the blood-brain barrier: implications for the cause and treatment of obesity. *Current Pharmaceutical Design, 7*(2), 125–133.

Bauer, S., Kerr, B. J., et al. (2007). The neuropoietic cytokine family in development, plasticity, disease and injury. *Nature Reviews Neuroscience, 8*(3), 221–232.

Bell, M. J., & Hallenbeck, J. M. (2002). Effects of intrauterine inflammation on developing rat brain. *Journal of Neuroscience Research, 70*(4), 570–579.

Beloosesky, R., Gayle, D. A., et al. (2006). N-acetyl-cysteine suppresses amniotic fluid and placenta inflammatory cytokine responses to lipopolysaccharide in rats. *American Journal of Obstetrics and Gynecology, 194*(1), 268–273.

Biber, K., Zuurman, M. W., et al. (2002). Chemokines in the brain: neuroimmunology and beyond. *Current Opinion in Pharmacology, 2*(1), 63–68.

Bidet, B., Leboyer, M., et al. (1993). Allergic sensitization in infantile autism. *Journal of Autism and Developmental Disorders, 23*(2), 419–420.

Boccone, L., Dessi, V., et al. (2006). Bannayan-Riley-Ruvalcaba syndrome with reactive nodular lymphoid hyperplasia and autism and a PTEN mutation. *American Journal of Medical Genetics. Part A, 140*(18), 1965–1969.

Borrell, J., Vela, J. M., et al. (2002). Prenatal immune challenge disrupts sensorimotor gating in adult rats. Implications for the etiopathogenesis of schizophrenia. *Neuropsychopharmacology, 26*(2), 204–215.

Boulanger, L. M. (2004). MHC class I in activity-dependent structural and functional plasticity. *Neuron Glia Biology, 1*(3), 283–289.

Boyle, D. L., Jones, T. L., et al. (2006). Regulation of peripheral inflammation by spinal p38 MAP kinase in rats. *PLoS Medicine, 3*(9), e338.

Braunschweig, D., Ashwood, P., et al. (2008). Autism: Maternally derived antibodies specific for fetal brain proteins. *Neurotoxicology, 29*(2), 226–231.

Brynskikh, A., Warren, T., et al. (2008). Adaptive immunity affects learning behavior in mice. *Brain, Behavior, and Immunity, 22*(6), 861–869.

Butler, M. G., Dasouki, M. J., et al. (2005). Subset of individuals with autism spectrum disorders and extreme macrocephaly associated with germline PTEN tumour suppressor gene mutations. *Journal of Medical Genetics, 42*(4), 318–321.

Cabanlit, M., Wills, S., et al. (2007). Brain-specific autoantibodies in the plasma of subjects with autistic spectrum disorder. *Annals of the New York Academy of Sciences, 1107*, 92–103.

Cai, Z., Pan, Z. L., et al. (2000). Cytokine induction in fetal rat brains and brain injury in neonatal rats after maternal lipopolysaccharide administration. *Pediatric Research, 47*(1), 64–72.

Calandra, T., & Roger, T. (2003). Macrophage migration inhibitory factor: a regulator of innate immunity. *Nature Reviews Immunology, 3*(10), 791–800.

Campbell, D. B., D'Oronzio, R., et al. (2007). Disruption of cerebral cortex MET signaling in autism spectrum disorder. *Annals of Neurology, 62*(3), 243–250.

Campbell, D. B., Sutcliffe, J. S., et al. (2006). A genetic variant that disrupts MET transcription is associated with autism. *Proceedings of the National Academy of Sciences of the United States of America, 103*(45), 16834–16839.

Carson, M. J., Doose, J. M., et al. (2006). CNS immune privilege: hiding in plain sight. *Immunological Reviews, 213*, 48–65.

Chaouat, G. (2007). The Th1/Th2 paradigm: still important in pregnancy? *Seminars in Immunopathology, 29*(2), 95–113.

Chess, S. (1977). Follow-up report on autism in congenital rubella. *Journal of Autism and Childhood Schizophrenia, 7*(1), 69–81.

Comi, A. M., Zimmerman, A. W., et al. (1999). Familial clustering of autoimmune disorders and evaluation of medical risk factors in autism. *Journal of Child Neurology, 14*(6), 388–394.

Connolly, A. M., Chez, M., et al. (2006). Brain-derived neurotrophic factor and autoantibodies to neural antigens in sera of children with autistic spectrum disorders, Landau-Kleffner syndrome, and epilepsy. *Biological Psychiatry, 59*(4), 354–363.

Connolly, A. M., Chez, M. G., et al. (1999). Serum autoantibodies to brain in Landau-Kleffner variant, autism, and other neurologic disorders. *Journal of Pediatrics, 134*(5), 607–613.

Cormier, E., & Elder, J. H. (2007). Diet and child behavior problems: fact or fiction? *Pediatric Nursing, 33*(2), 138–143.

Costa-Pinto, F. A., Basso, A. S., et al. (2005). Avoidance behavior and neural correlates of allergen exposure in a murine model of asthma. *Brain, Behavior, and Immunity, 19*(1), 52–60.

Crawley, J. N. (2007). Mouse behavioral assays relevant to the symptoms of autism. *Brain Pathology (Zurich, Switzerland), 17*(4), 448–459.

Croen, L. A., Braunschweig, D., et al. (2008). Maternal mid-pregnancy autoantibodies to fetal brain protein: the early markers for autism study. *Biological Psychiatry, 64*(7), 583–588.

Croen, L. A., Grether, J. K., et al. (2005). Maternal autoimmune diseases, asthma and allergies, and childhood autism spectrum disorders: a case-control study. *Archives of Pediatrics and Adolescent Medicine, 159*(2), 151–157.

Croonenberghs, J., Bosmans, E., et al. (2002). Activation of the inflammatory response system in autism. *Neuropsychobiology, 45*(1), 1–6.

Croonenberghs, J., Wauters, A., et al. (2002). Increased serum albumin, gamma globulin, immunoglobulin IgG, and IgG2 and IgG4 in autism. *Psychological Medicine, 32*(8), 1457–1463.

Curran, L. K., Newschaffer, C. J., et al. (2007). Behaviors associated with fever in children with autism spectrum disorders. *Pediatrics, 120*(6), e1386–1392.

Czlonkowska, A., Ciesielska, A., et al. (2005). Estrogen and cytokines production: The possible cause of gender differences in neurological diseases. *Current Pharmaceutical Design, 11*(8), 1017–1030.

Dalton, P., Deacon, R., et al. (2003). Maternal neuronal antibodies associated with autism and a language disorder. *Annals of Neurology, 53*(4), 533–537.

Denenberg, V. H., Mobraaten, L. E., et al. (1991). Effects of the autoimmune uterine/maternal environment upon cortical ectopias, behavior, and autoimmunity. *Brain Research, 563*(1–2), 114–122.

Denenberg, V. H., Sherman, G., et al. (1996). Effects of embryo transfer and cortical ectopias upon the behavior of BXSB-Yaa and BXSB-Yaa + mice. *Brain Research. Developmental Brain Research, 93*(1–2), 100–108.

Denney, D. R., Frei, B. W., et al. (1996). Lymphocyte subsets and interleukin-2 receptors in autistic children. *Journal of Autism and Developmental Disorders, 26*(1), 87–97.

DeStefano, F., & Chen, R. T. (2000). Autism and measles, mumps, and rubella vaccine: No epidemiological evidence for a causal association. *Journal of Pediatrics, 136*(1), 125–126.

Diamond, B., Kowal, C., et al. (2006). Immunity and acquired alterations in cognition and emotion: lessons from SLE. *Advances in Immunology, 89*, 289–320.

Djelmis, J., Sostarko, M., et al. (2002). Myasthenia gravis in pregnancy: report on 69 cases. *European Journal of Obstetrics, Gynecology, and Reproductive Biology, 104*(1), 21–25.

Dybkaer, K., Iqbal, J., et al. (2007). Genome wide transcriptional analysis of resting and IL2 activated human natural killer cells: gene expression signatures indicative of novel molecular signaling pathways. *BMC Genomics, 8*, 230.

Elovitz, M. A., Mrinalini, C., et al. (2006). Elucidating the early signal transduction pathways leading to fetal brain injury in preterm birth. *Pediatric Research, 59*(1), 50–55.

Engelhardt, B., & Ransohoff, R. M. (2005). The ins and outs of T-lymphocyte trafficking to the CNS: anatomical sites and molecular mechanisms. *Trends in Immunology, 26*(9), 485–495.

Enstrom, A., Krakowiak, P., et al. (2009). Increased IgG4 levels in children with autism disorder. *Brain, Behavior, and Immunity, 23*(3), 389–395.

Enstrom, A. M., Lit, L., et al. (2009). Altered gene expression and function of peripheral blood natural killer cells in children with autism. *Brain, Behavior, and Immunity, 23*(1), 124–133.

Evers, M., Cunningham-Rundles, C., et al. (2002). Heat shock protein 90 antibodies in autism. *Molecular Psychiatry, 7*(Suppl 2), S26–28.

Fatemi, S. H., Earle, J., et al. (2002). Prenatal viral infection leads to pyramidal cell atrophy and macrocephaly in adulthood: implications for genesis of autism and schizophrenia. *Cellular and Molecular Neurobiology, 22*(1), 25–33.

Fatemi, S. H., Halt, A. R., et al. (2001). Reduction in anti-apoptotic protein Bcl-2 in autistic cerebellum. *Neuroreport, 12*(5), 929–933.

Fatemi, S. H., Stary, J. M., et al. (2001). Dysregulation of reelin and Bcl-2 proteins in autistic cerebellum. *Journal of Autism and Developmental Disorders, 31*(6), 529–535.

Fidel, P. L., Jr., Romero, R., et al. (1994). Interleukin-1 receptor antagonist (IL-1ra) production by human amnion, chorion, and decidua. *American Journal of Reproductive Immunology (New York, N.Y.: 1989), 32*(1), 1–7.

Fortier, M. E., Joober, R., et al. (2004). Maternal exposure to bacterial endotoxin during pregnancy enhances amphetamine-induced locomotion and startle responses in adult rat offspring. *Journal of Psychiatric Research, 38*(3), 335–345.

Furlano, R. I., Anthony, A., et al. (2001). Colonic CD8 and gamma delta T-cell infiltration with epithelial damage in children with autism. *Journal of Pediatrics, 138*(3), 366–372.

Garbett, K., Ebert, P. J., et al. (2008). Immune transcriptome alterations in the temporal cortex of subjects with autism. *Neurobiology of Disease, 30*(3), 303–311.

Gayle, D. A., Beloosesky, R., et al. (2004). Maternal LPS induces cytokines in the amniotic fluid and corticotropin releasing hormone in the fetal rat brain. *American Journal of Physiology. Regulatory, Integrative, and Comparative Physiology, 286*(6), R1024–1029.

Gilmore, J. H., Jarskog, L. F., et al. (2005). Maternal poly I:C exposure during pregnancy regulates TNF alpha, BDNF, and NGF expression in neonatal brain and the maternal-fetal unit of the rat. *Journal of Neuroimmunology, 159*(1–2), 106–112.

Goffin, A., Hoefsloot, L. H., et al. (2001). PTEN mutation in a family with Cowden syndrome and autism. *American Journal of Medical Genetics, 105*(6), 521–524.

Golan, H., Stilman, M., et al. (2006). Normal aging of offspring mice of mothers with induced inflammation during pregnancy. *Neuroscience, 141*(4), 1909–1918.

Golan, H. M., Lev, V., et al. (2005). Specific neurodevelopmental damage in mice offspring following maternal inflammation during pregnancy. *Neuropharmacology, 48*(6), 903–917.

Gomes, F. C., Sousa Vde, O., et al. (2005). Emerging roles for TGF-beta1 in nervous system development. *International Journal of Developmental Neuroscience, 23*(5), 413–424.

Gregersen, P. K., & Bucala, R. (2003). Macrophage migration inhibitory factor, MIF alleles, and the genetics of inflammatory disorders: incorporating disease outcome into the definition of phenotype. *Arthritis and Rheumatism, 48*(5), 1171–1176.

Gregg, J. P., Lit, L., et al. (2008). Gene expression changes in children with autism. *Genomics, 91*(1), 22–29.

Grigorenko, E. L., Han, S. S., et al. (2008). Macrophage migration inhibitory factor and autism spectrum disorders. *Pediatrics, 122*(2), e438–445.

Gupta, S., Aggarwal, S., et al. (1998). Th1- and Th2-like cytokines in CD4+ and CD8+ T cells in autism. *Journal of Neuroimmunology, 85*(1), 106–109.

Haddad, J. J., Saade, N. E., et al. (2002). Cytokines and neuro-immune-endocrine interactions: a role for the hypothalamic-pituitary-adrenal revolving axis. *Journal of Neuroimmunology, 133*(1–2), 1–19.

Hammarberg, H., Lidman, O., et al. (2000). Neuroprotection by encephalomyelitis: rescue of mechanically injured neurons and neurotrophin production by CNS-infiltrating T and natural killer cells. *Journal of Neuroscience, 20*(14), 5283–5291.

Hauguel-de Mouzon, S., & Guerre-Millo, M. (2006). The placenta cytokine network and inflammatory signals. *Placenta, 27*(8), 794–798.

Heininger, U., Desgrandchamps, D., et al. (2006). Seroprevalence of Varicella-Zoster virus IgG antibodies in Swiss children during the first 16 months of age. *Vaccine, 24*(16), 3258–3260.

Heuer, L., Ashwood, P., Schauer, J., Goines, P., Krakowiak, P., Hertz-Picciotto, I., et al. (2008). Reduced levels of immunoglobulin in children with autism correlates with behavioral symptoms. *Autism Research, 1*(5), 275–283.

Holladay, S. D., & Smialowicz, R. J. (2000). Development of the murine and human immune system: differential effects of immunotoxicants depend on time of exposure. *Environmental Health Perspectives, 108*(Suppl 3), 463–473.

Hornig, M., Briese, T., et al. (2008). Lack of association between measles virus vaccine and autism with enteropathy: a case-control study. *PLoS ONE, 3*(9), e3140.

Huerta, P. T., Kowal, C., et al. (2006). Immunity and behavior: antibodies alter emotion. *Proceedings of the National Academy of Sciences of the United States of America, 103*(3), 678–683.

Huh, G. S., Boulanger, L. M., et al. (2000). Functional requirement for class I MHC in CNS development and plasticity. *Science (New York, N.Y.), 290*(5499), 2155–2159.

Jenkins, C., Roberts, J., et al. (2000). Evidence of a T(H) 1 type response associated with recurrent miscarriage. *Fertility and Sterility, 73*(6), 1206–1208.

Johnson, W. G., Buyske, S., Mars, A. E., Sreenath, M., Stenroos, E. S., Williams, T. A., et al. (2009). HLA-DR4 as a risk allele for autism acting in mothers of probands possibly during pregnancy. *Archives of Pediatrics and Adolescent Medicine, 163*, 542–546.

Jones, A. L., Mowry, B. J., et al. (2005). Immune dysregulation and self-reactivity in schizophrenia: do some cases of schizophrenia have an autoimmune basis? *Immunology and Cell Biology, 83*(1), 9–17.

Jyonouchi, H., Geng, L., et al. (2005). Evaluation of an association between gastrointestinal symptoms and cytokine production against common dietary proteins in children with autism spectrum disorders. *Journal of Pediatrics, 146*(5), 605–610.

Jyonouchi, H., Sun, S., et al. (2002). Innate immunity associated with inflammatory responses and cytokine production against common dietary proteins in patients with autism spectrum disorder. *Neuropsychobiology, 46*(2), 76–84.

Jyonouchi, H., Sun, S., et al. (2001). Proinflammatory and regulatory cytokine production associated with innate and adaptive immune responses in children with autism spectrum disorders and developmental regression. *Journal of Neuroimmunology, 120*(1–2), 170–179.

Kerschensteiner, M., Stadelmann, C., et al. (2003). Neurotrophic cross-talk between the nervous and immune systems: implications for neurological diseases. *Annals of Neurology, 53*(3), 292–304.

Kiessling, L. S., Marcotte, A. C., et al. (1994). Antineuronal antibodies: tics and obsessive-compulsive symptoms. *Journal of Developmental and Behavioral Pediatrics, 15*(6), 421–425.

Kipnis, J., Cohen, H., et al. (2004). T cell deficiency leads to cognitive dysfunction: implications for therapeutic vaccination for schizophrenia and other psychiatric conditions. *Proceedings of the National Academy of Sciences of the United States of America, 101*(21), 8180–8185.

Kipnis, J., Yoles, E., et al. (2001). Neuronal survival after CNS insult is determined by a genetically encoded autoimmune response. *Journal of Neuroscience, 21*(13), 4564–4571.

Kowal, C., DeGiorgio, L. A., et al. (2004). Cognition and immunity; antibody impairs memory. *Immunity, 21*(2), 179–188.

Kramer, B. W., Moss, T. J., et al. (2001). Dose and time response after intraamniotic endotoxin in preterm lambs. *American Journal of Respiratory and Critical Care Medicine, 164*(6), 982–988.

Kwon, C. H., Luikart, B. W., et al. (2006). Pten regulates neuronal arborization and social interaction in mice. *Neuron, 50*(3), 377–388.

Lambertsen, K. L., Gregersen, R., et al. (2004). A role for interferon-gamma in focal cerebral ischemia in mice. *Journal of Neuropathology and Experimental Neurology, 63*(9), 942–955.

Landa, R., & Garrett-Mayer, E. (2006). Development in infants with autism spectrum disorders: a prospective study. *Journal of Child Psychology and Psychiatry and Allied Disciplines, 47*(6), 629–638.

Lee, J. Y., Huerta, P. T., et al. (2009). Neurotoxic autoantibodies mediate congenital cortical impairment of offspring in maternal lupus. *Nature Medicine, 15*(1), 91–96.

Lee, L. C., Newschaffer, C. J., et al. (2008). Variation in season of birth in singleton and multiple births concordant for autism spectrum disorders. *Paediatric and Perinatal Epidemiology, 22*(2), 172–179.

Lee, L. C., Zachary, A. A., et al. (2006). HLA-DR4 in families with autism. *Pediatric Neurology, 35*(5), 303–307.

Letterio, J. J., & Roberts, A. B. (1998). Regulation of immune responses by TGF-beta. *Annual Review of Immunology, 16*, 137–161.

Ling, Z., Chang, Q. A., et al. (2004). Rotenone potentiates dopamine neuron loss in animals exposed to lipopolysaccharide prenatally. *Experimental Neurology, 190*(2), 373–383.

Liverman, C. S., Kaftan, H. A., et al. (2006). Altered expression of pro-inflammatory and developmental genes in the fetal brain in a mouse model of maternal infection. *Neuroscience Letters, 399*(3), 220–225.

Lucarelli, S., Frediani, T., et al. (1995). Food allergy and infantile autism. *Panminerva Medica, 37*(3), 137–141.

Makinodan, M., Tatsumi, K., et al. (2008). Maternal immune activation in mice delays myelination and axonal development in the hippocampus of the offspring. *Journal of Neuroscience Research, 86*(10), 2190–2200.

Markowitz, P. I. (1983). Autism in a child with congenital cytomegalovirus infection. *Journal of Autism and Developmental Disorders, 13*(3), 249–253.

Marques-Deak, A., Cizza, G., et al. (2005). Brain-immune interactions and disease susceptibility. *Molecular Psychiatry, 10*(3), 239–250.

Martin, L. A., Ashwood, P., et al. (2008). Stereotypies and hyperactivity in rhesus monkeys exposed to IgG from mothers of children with autism. *Brain, Behavior, and Immunity, 22*(6), 806–816.

Matarese, G., Procaccini, C., et al. (2008). The intricate interface between immune and metabolic regulation: a role for leptin in the pathogenesis of multiple sclerosis? *Journal of Leukocyte Biology, 84*(4), 893–899.

Mehler, M. F., & Kessler, J. A. (1998). Cytokines in brain development and function. *Advances in Protein Chemistry, 52*, 223–251.

Menage, P., Thibault, G., et al. (1992). An IgE mechanism in autistic hypersensitivity? *Biological Psychiatry, 31*(2), 210–212.

Merlot, E., Couret, D., et al. (2008). Prenatal stress, fetal imprinting, and immunity. *Brain, Behavior, and Immunity, 22*(1), 42–51.

Meyer, U., Feldon, J., et al. (2005). Towards an immuno-precipitated neurodevelopmental animal model of schizophrenia. *Neuroscience and Biobehavioral Reviews, 29*(6), 913–947.

Meyer, U., Feldon, J., et al. (2006). Immunological stress at the maternal-foetal interface: a link between neurodevelopment and adult psychopathology. *Brain, Behavior, and Immunity, 20*(4), 378–388.

Meyer, U., Murray, P. J., et al. (2008). Adult behavioral and pharmacological dysfunctions following disruption of the fetal brain balance between pro-inflammatory and IL-10-mediated anti-inflammatory signaling. *Molecular Psychiatry, 13*(2), 208–221.

Meyer, U., Nyffeler, M., et al. (2006). The time of prenatal immune challenge determines the specificity of inflammation-mediated brain and behavioral pathology. *Journal of Neuroscience, 26*(18), 4752–4762.

Meyer, U., Nyffeler, M., et al. (2008). Adult brain and behavioral pathological markers of prenatal immune challenge during early/middle and late fetal development in mice. *Brain, Behavior, and Immunity, 22*(4), 469–486.

Meyer, U., Yee, B. K., et al. (2007). The neurodevelopmental impact of prenatal infections at different times of pregnancy: the earlier the worse? *Neuroscientist, 13*(3), 241–256.

Micali, N., Chakrabarti, S., et al. (2004). The broad autism phenotype: findings from an epidemiological survey. *Autism, 8*(1), 21–37.

Mignini, F., Streccioni, V., et al. (2003). Autonomic innervation of immune organs and neuroimmune modulation. *Autonomic and Autacoid Pharmacology, 23*(1), 1–25.

Millward, C., Ferriter, M., et al. (2008). Gluten- and casein-free diets for autistic spectrum disorder. *Cochrane Database of Systematic Reviews (Online)*(2), CD003498.

Molloy, C. A., Morrow, A. L., et al. (2006). Familial autoimmune thyroid disease as a risk factor for regression in children with autism spectrum disorder: a CPEA study. *Journal of Autism and Developmental Disorders, 36*(3), 317–324.

Molloy, C. A., Morrow, A. L., et al. (2006). Elevated cytokine levels in children with autism spectrum disorder. *Journal of Neuroimmunology, 172*(1–2), 198–205.

Money, J., Bobrow, N. A., et al. (1971). Autism and autoimmune disease: a family study. *Journal of Autism and Childhood Schizophrenia, 1*(2), 146–160.

Motta, M., Rodriguez-C., Perez, et al. (2007). Outcome of infants from mothers with anti-SSA/Ro antibodies. *Journal of Perinatology, 27*(5), 278–283.

Mouridsen, S. E., Rich, B., et al. (2007). Autoimmune diseases in parents of children with infantile autism: a case-control study. *Developmental Medicine and Child Neurology, 49*(6), 429–432.

Nelson, P. T., Soma, L. A., et al. (2002). Microglia in diseases of the central nervous system. *Annals of Medicine, 34*(7–8), 491–500.

Nishimura, Y., Martin, C. L., et al. (2007). Genome-wide expression profiling of lymphoblastoid cell lines distinguishes different forms of autism and reveals shared pathways. *Human Molecular Genetics, 16*(14), 1682–1698.

Nitsos, I., Rees, S. M., et al. (2006). Chronic exposure to intra-amniotic lipopolysaccharide affects the ovine fetal brain. *Journal of the Society for Gynecologic Investigation, 13*(4), 239–247.

Nyffeler, M., Meyer, U., et al. (2006). Maternal immune activation during pregnancy increases limbic GABAA receptor immunoreactivity in the adult offspring: implications for schizophrenia. *Neuroscience, 143*(1), 51–62.

Okada, K., Hashimoto, K., et al. (2007). Decreased serum levels of transforming growth factor-beta1 in patients with autism. *Progress in Neuropsychopharmacology and Biological Psychiatry, 31*(1), 187–190.

Ozawa, K., Hashimoto, K., et al. (2006). Immune activation during pregnancy in mice leads to dopaminergic hyperfunction and cognitive impairment in the offspring: a neurodevelopmental animal model of schizophrenia. *Biological Psychiatry, 59*(6), 546–554.

Paintlia, M. K., Paintlia, A. S., et al. (2004). N-acetylcysteine prevents endotoxin-induced degeneration of oligodendrocyte progenitors and hypomyelination in developing rat brain. *Journal of Neuroscience Research, 78*(3), 347–361.

Pandey, R. S., Gupta, A. K., et al. (1981). Autoimmune model of schizophrenia with special reference to antibrain antibodies. *Biological Psychiatry, 16*(12), 1123–1136.

Pardo, C. A., Vargas, D. L., et al. (2005). Immunity, neuroglia, and neuroinflammation in autism. *International Review of Psychiatry (Abingdon, England), 17*(6), 485–495.

Perricone, R., Perricone, C., et al. (2008). NK cells in autoimmunity: a two-edg'd weapon of the immune system. *Autoimmunity Reviews, 7*(5), 384–390.

Perrin, E. M., Murphy, M. L., et al. (2004). Does group A beta-hemolytic streptococcal infection increase risk for behavioral and neuropsychiatric symptoms in children? *Archives of Pediatrics and Adolescent Medicine, 158*(9), 848–856.

Plioplys, A. V., Greaves, A., et al. (1994). Lymphocyte function in autism and Rett syndrome. *Neuropsychobiology, 29*(1), 12–16.

Poggi, S. H., Park, J., et al. (2005). No phenotype associated with established lipopolysaccharide model for cerebral palsy. *American Journal of Obstetrics and Gynecology, 192*(3), 727–733.

Poling, J. S., Frye, R. E., et al. (2006). Developmental regression and mitochondrial dysfunction in a child with autism. *Journal of Child Neurology, 21*(2), 170–172.

Ponzio, N. M., Servatius, R., et al. (2007). Cytokine levels during pregnancy influence immunological profiles and neurobehavioral patterns of the offspring. *Annals of the New York Academy of Sciences, 1107*, 118–128.

Portales-Perez, D., Alarcon-Segovia, D., et al. (1998). Penetrating anti-DNA monoclonal antibodies induce activation of human peripheral blood mononuclear cells. *Journal of Autoimmunity, 11*(5), 563–571.

Raghupathy, R., & Kalinka, J. (2008). Cytokine imbalance in pregnancy complications and its modulation. *Frontiers in Bioscience, 13*, 985–994.

Raivich, G. (2005). Like cops on the beat: the active role of resting microglia. *Trends in Neurosciences, 28*(11), 571–573.

Renzoni, E., Beltrami, V., et al. (1995). Brief report: allergological evaluation of children with autism. *Journal of Autism and Developmental Disorders, 25*(3), 327–333.

Ritvo, E. R., Jorde, L. B., et al. (1989). The UCLA-University of Utah epidemiologic survey of autism: recurrence risk estimates and genetic counseling. *American Journal of Psychiatry, 146*(8), 1032–1036.

Rogers, T., Kalaydjieva, L., et al. (1999). Exclusion of linkage to the HLA region in ninety multiplex sibships with autism. *Journal of Autism and Developmental Disorders, 29*(3), 195–201.

Rosen, N. J., Yoshida, C. K., et al. (2007). Infection in the first 2 years of life and autism spectrum disorders. *Pediatrics, 119*(1), e61–69.

Rothermundt, M., Arolt, V., et al. (2001). Review of immunological and immunopathological findings in schizophrenia. *Brain, Behavior, and Immunity, 15*(4), 319–339.

Rothwell, N. J., Luheshi, G., et al. (1996). Cytokines and their receptors in the central nervous system: physiology, pharmacology, and pathology. *Pharmacology and Therapeutics, 69*(2), 85–95.

Rounioja, S., Rasanen, J., et al. (2003). Intra-amniotic lipopolysaccharide leads to fetal cardiac dysfunction. A mouse model for fetal inflammatory response. *Cardiovascular Research, 60*(1), 156–164.

Rousset, C. I., Chalon, S., et al. (2006). Maternal exposure to LPS induces hypomyelination in the internal capsule and programmed cell death in the deep gray matter in newborn rats. *Pediatric Research, 59*(3), 428–433.

Sakic, B., Szechtman, H., et al. (1997). Neurobehavioral alterations in autoimmune mice. *Neuroscience and Biobehavioral Reviews, 21*(3), 327–340.

Samuelsson, A. M., Jennische, E., et al. (2006). Prenatal exposure to interleukin-6 results in inflammatory neurodegeneration in hippocampus with NMDA/GABA(A) dysregulation and impaired spatial learning. *American Journal of Physiology. Regulatory, Integrative, and Comparative Physiology, 290*(5), R1345–1356.

Sanna, V., Di Giacomo, A., et al. (2003). Leptin surge precedes onset of autoimmune encephalomyelitis and correlates with development of pathogenic T cell responses. *Journal of Clinical Investigation, 111*(2), 241–250.

Shi, L., Fatemi, S. H., et al. (2003). Maternal influenza infection causes marked behavioral and pharmacological changes in the offspring. *Journal of Neuroscience, 23*(1), 297–302.

Shi, L., Smith, S. E., et al. (2009). Activation of the maternal immune system alters cerebellar development in the offspring. *Brain, Behavior, and Immunity, 23*(1), 116–123.

Silva, S. C., Correia, C., et al. (2004). Autoantibody repertoires to brain tissue in autism nuclear families. *Journal of Neuroimmunology, 152*(1–2), 176–182.

Simister, N. E. (2003). Placental transport of immunoglobulin G. *Vaccine, 21*(24), 3365–3369.

Singer, H. S., Morris, C. M., et al. (2008). Antibodies against fetal brain in sera of mothers with autistic children. *Journal of Neuroimmunology, 194*(1–2), 165–172.

Singer, H. S., Morris, C. M., et al. (2006). Antibrain antibodies in children with autism and their unaffected siblings. *Journal of Neuroimmunology, 178*(1–2), 149–155.

Singh, V. K. (1996). Plasma increase of interleukin-12 and interferon-gamma. Pathological significance in autism. *Journal of Neuroimmunology, 66*(1–2), 143–145.

Singh, V. K., & Jensen, R. L. (2003). Elevated levels of measles antibodies in children with autism. *Pediatric Neurology, 28*(4), 292–294.

Singh, V. K., Lin, S. X., et al. (1998). Serological association of measles virus and human herpesvirus-6 with brain autoantibodies in autism. *Clinical Immunology and Immunopathology, 89*(1), 105–108.

Singh, V. K., & Rivas, W. H. (2004). Prevalence of serum antibodies to caudate nucleus in autistic children. *Neuroscience Letters, 355*(1–2), 53–56.

Singh, V. K., Singh, E. A., et al. (1997). Hyperserotoninemia and serotonin receptor antibodies in children with autism but not mental retardation. *Biological Psychiatry, 41*(6), 753–755.

Singh, V. K., Warren, R., et al. (1997). Circulating autoantibodies to neuronal and glial filament proteins in autism. *Pediatric Neurology, 17*(1), 88–90.

Singh, V. K., Warren, R. P., et al. (1993). Antibodies to myelin basic protein in children with autistic behavior. *Brain, Behavior, and Immunity, 7*(1), 97–103.

Sisto, M., Lisi, S., et al. (2006). Autoantibodies from Sjogren's syndrome induce activation of both the intrinsic and extrinsic apoptotic pathways in human salivary gland cell line A-253. *Journal of Autoimmunity, 27*(1), 38–49.

Smith, S. E., Li, J., et al. (2007). Maternal immune activation alters fetal brain development through interleukin-6. *The Journal of Neuroscience, 27*(40), 10695–10702.

Splawski, I., Timothy, K. W., et al. (2004). Ca(V)1.2 calcium channel dysfunction causes a multisystem disorder including arrhythmia and autism. *Cell, 119*(1), 19–31.

Steinman, L. (2004). Elaborate interactions between the immune and nervous systems. *Nature Immunology, 5*(6), 575–581.

Stubbs, E. G. (1978). Autistic symptoms in a child with congenital cytomegalovirus infection. *Journal of Autism and Childhood Schizophrenia, 8*(1), 37–43.

Stubbs, E. G., & Crawford, M. L. (1977). Depressed lymphocyte responsiveness in autistic children. *Journal of Autism and Childhood Schizophrenia, 7*(1), 49–55.

Sweeten, T. L., Bowyer, S. L., et al. (2003). Increased prevalence of familial autoimmunity in probands with pervasive developmental disorders. *Pediatrics, 112*(5), e420.

Sweeten, T. L., Posey, D. J., et al. (2003). High blood monocyte counts and neopterin levels in children with autistic disorder. *American Journal of Psychiatry, 160*(9), 1691–1693.

Taylor, B., Miller, E., et al. (1999). Autism and measles, mumps, and rubella vaccine: no epidemiological evidence for a causal association [see comments]. *Lancet, 353*(9169), 2026–2029.

Todd, R. D., & Ciaranello, R. D. (1985). Demonstration of inter-and intraspecies differences in serotonin binding sites by antibodies from an autistic child. *Proceedings of the National Academy of Sciences of the United States of America, 82*(2), 612–616.

Tordjman, S., Drapier, D., et al. (2007). Animal models relevant to schizophrenia and autism: validity and limitations. *Behavior Genetics, 37*(1), 61–78.

Torres, A. R., Maciulis, A., et al. (2002). The transmission disequilibrium test suggests that HLA-DR4 and DR13 are linked to autism spectrum disorder. *Human Immunology, 63*(4), 311–316.

Trajkovski, V., Ajdinski, L., et al. (2004). Plasma concentration of immunoglobulin classes and subclasses in children with autism in the Republic of Macedonia: retrospective study. *Croatian Medical Journal, 45*(6), 746–749.

Urakubo, A., Jarskog, L. F., et al. (2001). Prenatal exposure to maternal infection alters cytokine expression in the placenta, amniotic fluid, and fetal brain. *Schizophrenia Research, 47*(1), 27–36.

Vargas, D. L., Nascimbene, C., et al. (2005). Neuroglial activation and neuroinflammation in the brain of patients with autism. *Annals of Neurology, 57*(1), 67–81.

Vojdani, A., Campbell, A. W., et al. (2002). Antibodies to neuron-specific antigens in children with autism: possible cross-reaction with encephalitogenic proteins from milk, Chlamydia pneumoniae, and Streptococcus group A. *Journal of Neuroimmunology, 129*(1–2), 168–177.

Vojdani, A., Mumper, E., et al. (2008). Low natural killer cell cytotoxic activity in autism: The role of glutathione, IL-2 and IL-15. *Journal of Neuroimmunology, 205*(1–2), 148–154.

Vojdani, A., O'Bryan, T., et al. (2004). Immune response to dietary proteins, gliadin, and cerebellar peptides in children with autism. *Nutritional Neuroscience, 7*(3), 151–161.

Wang, X., Hagberg, H., et al. (2007). Effects of intrauterine inflammation on the developing mouse brain. *Brain Research, 1144*, 180–185.

Warren, R. P., Burger, R. A., et al. (1994). Decreased plasma concentrations of the C4B complement protein in autism. *Archives of Pediatrics and Adolescent Medicine, 148*(2), 180–183.

Warren, R. P., Cole, P., et al. (1990). Detection of maternal antibodies in infantile autism. *Journal of the American Academy of Child and Adolescent Psychiatry, 29*(6), 873–877.

Warren, R. P., Foster, A., et al. (1987). Reduced natural killer cell activity in autism. *Journal of the American Academy of Child and Adolescent Psychiatry, 26*(3), 333–335.

Warren, R. P., Odell, J. D., et al. (1996). Strong association of the third hypervariable region of HLA-DR beta 1 with autism. *Journal of Neuroimmunology, 67*(2), 97–102.

Warren, R. P., Yonk, L. J., et al. (1990). Deficiency of suppressor-inducer (CD4+CD45RA+) T cells in autism. *Immunological Investigations, 19*(3), 245–251.

Wegmann, T. G., Lin, H., et al. (1993). Bidirectional cytokine interactions in the maternal-fetal relationship: is successful pregnancy a TH2 phenomenon? *Immunology Today, 14*(7), 353–356.

Weizman, A., Weizman, R., et al. (1982). Abnormal immune response to brain tissue antigen in the syndrome of autism. *American Journal of Psychiatry, 139*(11), 1462–1465.

Wierzba-Bobrowicz, T., Kosno-Kruszewska, E., et al. (2000). Major histocompatibility complex class II (MHC II) expression during the development of human fetal cerebral occipital lobe, cerebellum, and hematopoietic organs. *Folia neuropathological/ Association of Polish Neuropathologists and Medical Research Centre, Polish Academy of Sciences, 38*(3), 111–118.

Wills, S., Cabanlit, M., et al. (2007). Autoantibodies in autism spectrum disorders (ASD). *Annals of the New York Academy of Sciences, 1107*, 79–91.

Wills, S., Cabanlit, M., et al. (2008). Detection of autoantibodies to neural cells of the cerebellum in the plasma of subjects with autism spectrum disorders. *Brain, Behavior, and Immunity, 1107*, 79–91.

Wolff, A. R., & Bilkey, D. K. (2008). Immune activation during mid-gestation disrupts sensorimotor gating in rat offspring. *Behavioural Brain Research, 190*(1), 156–159.

Woo, E. J., Ball, R., et al. (2007). Developmental regression and autism reported to the Vaccine Adverse Event Reporting System. *Autism, 11*(4), 301–310.

Wrona, D. (2006). Neural-immune interactions: an integrative view of the bidirectional relationship between the brain and immune systems. *Journal of Neuroimmunology, 172*(1–2), 38–58.

Xu, D. X., Chen, Y. H., et al. (2006). Tumor necrosis factor alpha partially contributes to lipopolysaccharide-induced intra-uterine fetal growth restriction and skeletal development retardation in mice. *Toxicology Letters, 163*(1), 20–29.

Yeh, C. B., Wu, C. H., et al. (2006). Antineural antibody in patients with Tourette's syndrome and their family members. *Journal of Biomedical Science, 13*(1), 101–112.

Yip, J., Soghomonian, J. J., et al. (2007). Decreased GAD67 mRNA levels in cerebellar Purkinje cells in autism: pathophysiological implications. *Acta Neuropathologica, 113*(5), 559–568.

Yonk, L. J., Warren, R. P., et al. (1990). CD4+ helper T cell depression in autism. *Immunology Letters, 25*(4), 341–345.

Zaretsky, M. V., Alexander, J. M., et al. (2004). Transfer of inflammatory cytokines across the placenta. *Obstetrics and Gynecology, 103*(3), 546–550.

Zerrate, M. C., Pletnikov, M., et al. (2007). Neuroinflammation and behavioral abnormalities after neonatal terbutaline treatment in rats: implications for autism. *Journal of Pharmacology and Experimental Therapeutics, 322*(1), 16–22.

Zhang, Y., Proenca, R., et al. (1994). Positional cloning of the mouse obese gene and its human homologue. *Nature, 372*(6505), 425–432.

Zimmerman, A. W., Connors, S. L., et al. (2007). Maternal antibrain antibodies in autism. *Brain, Behavior, and Immunity, 21*(3), 351–357.

Ziv, Y., Ron, N., et al. (2006). Immune cells contribute to the maintenance of neurogenesis and spatial learning abilities in adulthood. *Nature Neuroscience, 9*(2), 268–275.

Zuckerman, L., Rehavi, M., et al. (2003). Immune activation during pregnancy in rats leads to a postpubertal emergence of disrupted latent inhibition, dopaminergic hyperfunction, and altered limbic morphology in the offspring: a novel neurodevelopmental model of schizophrenia. *Neuropsychopharmacology, 28*(10), 1778–1789.

Zuckerman, L., & Weiner, I. (2005). Maternal immune activation leads to behavioral and pharmacological changes in the adult offspring. *Journal of Psychiatric Research, 39*(3), 311–323.

25 Timothy Buie

Gastrointestinal Problems in Individuals with Autism Spectrum Disorders

Points of Interest

- Gastrointestinal problems appear to be relatively common in children with autism.
- Speculation on a gastrointestinal cause of autism has not been supported by findings.
- The clinical presentation of gastrointestinal symptoms in children with autism may include behavioral problems including self-injury, aggression, and sleep disorder.
- Dietary restriction trials have not shown a benefit for the treatment of autism.
- The use of nutritional supplementation such as vitamin therapy is discussed.
- Inflammation in the GI tract and the potential neurological impact is reviewed.

Leo Kanner (1943) coined the term "autism." In his seminal paper, 11 children were described as having unusual neurobehavioral presentations but were otherwise reported to be healthy. Interestingly, eating disorders were identified in 6 of these children. Kanner believed these symptoms to be behavioral in nature rather than having a medical etiology. One child required a gastrostomy for nutrition support, and eventually the GI issues were reported to have resolved spontaneously.

We currently understand autism to be a condition with manifold presentations, complex genetic and potential environmental associations, and likely therefore no single cause or pathway. When training medical professionals, we point to conditions like Down's syndrome or William's syndrome with well-characterized medical presentations. These conditions have, through consistency of outcomes, taught us to be aware of a variety of medical complications seen as a result of the genetic condition. In autism, we lack this characteristic or phenotypical pattern.

Medical providers often hear from families that some children improve with dietary alterations or vitamin supplements, yet when these interventions are applied under study conditions, the response is often not seen. Perhaps an unrecognized subset of individuals with autism would respond to such treatments, but the research has provided no evidence of this.

Discussion of gastrointestinal issues in individuals with autism is important for several reasons:

1. A variety of studies support a high frequency of gastrointestinal complaints in this patient population.
2. Although the gastrointestinal complaints may or may not be related to the cause of autism, underlying gastrointestinal problems may exacerbate behaviors in children with autism.
3. There may become evident a phenotypical subgroup of individuals with autism who have characteristic gastrointestinal problems.
4. Ongoing genetic and environment studies may help to explain linkage of gastrointestinal problems and the neurobehavioral problems in autism.

This chapter will discuss the prevalence of gastrointestinal symptoms in individuals with autism. Some of the unusual clinical presentations of pain will be characterized. Speculated dietary and nutritional issues in children will be addressed. Inflammation in the GI tract will be discussed. Finally, some reflection on research pathways involving the GI problems in children with autism will be offered.

Overview of GI Problems in Children with ASD

Gastrointestinal function is profoundly complex, involving the gut (esophagus, stomach, the small and large intestines) and the central nervous system, which are impacted by exterior factors such as food intake, psychological influences, and the environment. In his book *The Second Brain* (1998), Gershon discusses the concept "neuro-gastroenterology." He describes the interaction between the big brain in the head and the nervous system of the GI tract (the second brain). We know little about the messages the gut sends to the brain and how that information is processed.

Prevalence

The prevalence of GI problems in individuals with autism must be understood relative to the prevalence of GI problems in the general population. Gastroesophageal reflux disease may be experience by 1 in 4 children at some time during childhood (Rudolph et al., 2001). Constipation accounts for 2% of all visits to the pediatrician (North American Society for Pediatric Gastroenterology, Hepatology, and Nutrition [NASPGHAN], 2006). Food allergy has been reported to be on the rise in the last few decades. All food allergies are currently reported at a prevalence of 5–8% (Sampson, 1999a) in pediatric patients. Peanut and nut allergy reports have doubled in the last 20 years to a prevalence of 2% of the population (Skripak, 2008). At a minimum, comorbidity of these GI conditions should be expected with similar frequency in individuals with autism.

Earlier papers evaluating gastrointestinal symptoms or problems in individuals with autism suggested a relatively low frequency. In a retrospective study presented by Fombonne & Chakrabarti (2001), a medical record review of 261 autistic children found a history of gastrointestinal symptoms in 18.8%. Taylor (2002) reported that 17% of individuals with autism had associated bowel problems, including 9% with constipation, 1.4% with constipation and diarrhea, 4% with diarrhea, 1.5% with food allergy, and 0.04% reporting nonspecific colitis with ileal lymphoid hyperplasia. Constipation and food allergy actually have a higher reported frequency in the general pediatric population (Bernheisel-Broadbent, 2001; Yong, 1998), which might suggest that the medical data were not complete in this study or that ascertainment of GI symptoms in these groups were difficult.

More recent papers show a wide range of prevalence of GI problems in individuals with autism. Malloy et al. (2003) reported a prevalence of GI problems in 24% of a general autism population, based on medical history intake information. Horvath and Perman (2002) reported a prevalence of GI disturbance in 76% of children in a survey study of a general autism population in the Baltimore area. This broad prevalence discrepancy could be due to differences in the groups evaluated or differences in the interpretation of GI problems assessed.

Perhaps the most compelling study that suggests a high prevalence of GI problems among individuals with autism was conducted by Valicenti-McDermott (2006). In this study, three groups of children were evaluated: children with autism, children with other neurological conditions (e.g., cerebral palsy or mental retardation), and children without neurological problems. Seventy percent of the children with autism had GI complaints, compared with 42% of the children with other neurological conditions and 28% of the nonneurologically impaired children. This not only suggests a higher frequency of GI issues in individuals with neurodevelopmental disorders but also suggests the problem is not simply related to nonspecific neurological dysfunction. The consistent pattern in most studies showing a higher-than-"baseline" frequency of GI issues continues to fuel discussion about possible autism/GI etiological relationships. Might we find reasons for a higher frequency of GI disease in this community of individuals?

Clinical Presentation

Children with autism have impaired or at least atypical communication. Because of this, families report difficulty recognizing when their child is sick. Certainly some children have obvious GI symptoms. Horvath (2002) described diarrhea (3 or more loose, watery stools per day) in 27% of 112 children with autism compared to 44 unaffected siblings who had no chronic diarrhea. This survey also reported constipation in 9.5% of children with autism (no greater frequency than unaffected comparisons), and that gaseousness, bloating, abdominal pain, and GE reflux were more frequent in children with autism than comparison. Afzal (2003) studied children with autism and unaffected children presenting to the gastroenterologist with abdominal pain; 36% of the children with autism had evidence of constipation by radiograph compared to 10% of the unaffected children. Both groups showed a higher frequency of constipation than reported in the general pediatric population. This study suggested that an abdominal x-ray may be useful in evaluating for constipation in children with autism. This may be valuable for two reasons: history of stool frequency may not be easily obtained from communication-impaired children, and even if regular stools are seen, it is not possible to assess for incomplete evacuation symptoms in many children with autism.

The Horvath study also described many non-GI presentations of GI pain or distress including sleep disturbance: "Children with ASD and GI symptoms had a higher prevalence of sleep disturbances (55%) compared with those who did not have GI symptoms (14%)." In this study of 36 children with autistic spectrum disorder, 61% of those with ASD and reflux esophagitis had nighttime wakings compared with 13% of those without reflux esophagitis. It is well known that sleep disturbance occurs frequently in this population (Honomichl et al., 2002). Many studies speak of difficulties with sleep induction as well as night awakening and early awakening (Patzold, 1998). GE reflux may be one of several potential factors in sleep disturbance, but should be considered. A trial of treatment for reflux may be warranted if this symptom is present.

The Horvath study also describes sudden irritability, unexplained crying, or aggressiveness as manifestations of pain. We have observed tapping or rubbing areas of the body where pain has occurred. Self-injurious behavior such as head-banging or self-biting may be a way of communicating distress in nonverbal individuals. Posturing behaviors as seen in Sandifer's syndrome have occurred in our practice. One nonverbal child went to the freezer and put an ice cube on her chest. She responded well to antiacid therapy for GE reflux. Another clinical observation suggested by several GI professionals is that children with autism and abdominal distress will seek pressure on the abdomen. This may include asking a parent to rub or press the abdomen or leaning over furniture to exert pressure.

The idea that children with autism merit consideration of medical treatment for GI disturbance seems to be common sense. However, because of communication impairment, many of the presentations are behaviors such as sleep disorder, aggression, and sudden irritability among others. Caregivers are taught to take a behavioral approach, prompting the child to calm down, have quiet hands or redirect the behaviors. In verbal children who may be able to explain their behaviors, we would ask What's wrong? or Why did you do that? It seems important to ask the same from children who are not able to explain. We should consider the possibility that some children acting out may have pain or distress in addition to other reasons for acting out.

Burd (1995) describes children with ASD who exhibit food selectivity or textural selectivity. Feeding difficulties are common (>30%) in children with developmental delays (Gouge, 1975), but reports of mealtime or feeding problems in unaffected children are common as well (18). Ahearn (2001) evaluated 30 ASD children with difficult eating behaviors and found food type or texture selectivity in 17 of 30 children. Palmer (1975) used applied behavioral analysis to broaden food acceptance in a child with food selectivity. Using a behavioral treatment plan, acceptance of a normal variety was achieved and maintained. Palmer makes the point that medical reasons should be considered when there is prolonged subsistence on pureed foods, delay or difficulty in sucking, swallowing, or chewing, and delay in self-feeding.

Toilet training is often delayed in ASD as in other developmental disorders. Dalrymple (1992) described problems of toilet training in autism. Of his surveyed patients with a mean age of 19.5 years, 22% did not have full success with toileting. Underlying medical issues such as constipation may present a barrier to successful toilet training.

Dietary and Nutritional Factors That May Be Seen in Children with ASD

Perhaps the greatest interest among researchers and families alike considering GI issues in autism focuses on the possibility that diet and nutrition play a role in autism causation and management.

When considering this relationship, several food-related factors need to be considered:

1. Allergy.
2. Food intolerance, as might be seen with inadequate digestion (e.g., lactose intolerance), which could be a cause of symptoms (abdominal pain, gas, and diarrhea).
3. Deficiency of vitamins or building block substances affecting normal neurotransmission.

Food Allergy and Celiac Disease

Food allergy and inflammation of the gut for other reasons could account for problems and symptoms in children with autism by several mechanisms. The GI symptoms of allergy could include pain, constipation, diarrhea, rash, and sleep disturbance. Determining food allergy is difficult, and various types of testing for allergy have pitfalls. Food elimination trials are fairly reliable at defining food intolerance, but do not lead to an exact diagnosis of food allergy, which by definition is an immune-mediated response (Sampson et al., 1999). Allergy can be evaluated by skin testing such as IgE RAST testing or IgG RAST testing among others. All tests risk identifying a clinically nonrelevant result and probably best serve as a guide to consider certain foods that could be an allergy culprit.

Studies concluding that children with ASD have a dietary allergy are often debated. Lucarelli (1995) evaluated 36 children with autism. These patients were evaluated by allergy skin testing for IgE levels, along with serum levels of IgG, IgA, and IgM specific antibodies for cow milk and egg proteins. The findings included: positive skin testing in 36% of children with autism compared to 5% in a control group of unaffected children. IgE level elevation was noted in 33% of the children with autism. In a separate study, Reichelt (1990) found IgA specific antibodies for gluten, gliadin, B-lactoglobulin, and casein in individuals with autism. Gluten proteins, which are present in wheat, rye, barley, and malt, have been suggested to contribute to autism and behavioral problems. In addition to the possibility of specific allergy to these foods, celiac disease or gluten enteropathy may occur. Celiac disease is an immune sensitivity to gluten proteins, which requires lifelong elimination of these foods.

Pursuing the question of the gut permeability and the potential for food sensitivity, D'Eufemia et al. (1996) evaluated 21 children with autism and 42 unaffected control children. The purpose of the study was to determine if increased passage of larger molecular sized substances across the gut barrier was present in children with autism, as increased permeability of larger molecular substances from the gut into the bloodstream might explain the potential for an increased sensitivity to certain peptides or proteins. The study found that 43% of the children with autism had increased permeability compared to unaffected control children, who showed no increased permeability, and suggested that with increased permeability, food-based or like-sized peptides that enter the bloodstream might induce allergic sensitization or cause "pharmacological" effects. This study attempted to address a theory known as opioid-excess theory (Panksepp, 1981).

Endogenous opioids may control developmental processes (Zagon, 1978). Self-stimulatory and self-injurious behavior has been linked to B-endorphin levels (Barron, 1983). Altered pain sensitivity has also been reported, and opioid antagonists such as naloxone and naltrexone have been used extensively in children with autism in attempts to modulate opioid associated symptoms (Panksepp, 1981). Sandyk (1986) briefly focuses on specific symptoms of autism that can be caused by abnormal endogenous opioid regulation. Sahley and Panksepp (1987) delineated the idea that abnormal brain opioid activity could play a role in the genesis of many autistic symptoms.

Maldigestion of dietary peptides forms the basis of the opioid peptide theory of autism. Several investigators have proposed that maldigestion of dietary proteins, particularly foods containing casein and gluten, produces small peptide molecules that may function as exogenous opioids. Peptides described as casomorphin (derived from milk) and gliadomorphin (derived from gluten foods) were identified in the urine of patients with schizophrenia and autism by Reichelt (1991). These peptides were shown, in vitro, to bind to opioid receptors and therefore are speculated to cause CNS effects by modulating opioid levels in the brain. Shattock (1990) supported this theory. Opioid peptide theory could provide a possible explanation for reports of clinical improvement when some autistic children are placed on restrictive diets without proof of allergic sensitivity. One criticism of the theory is the observation that these urinary peptides are also present in asymptomatic children and therefore may not exhibit a physiological effect.

Knivsberg (1990) placed a selected group of autistic children in a residential school on a gluten-free diet and reported improvement. He had screened these children prior to the diet and found evidence of the peptide gliadomorphin in their urine. He suggested this finding identified children who may have a problem with gluten. The gluten-free diet prescribed in this study would have potentially been helpful for children with celiac disease, food allergy to gluten products, or maldigestion of these food products. The conclusions may support the notion that at least a subgroup of patients could benefit from dietary change. Sponheim (1991) offered a limited study evaluating autistic children placed on a gluten-free diet and observed no behavioral improvement. He did not qualify the participants by identifying a gluten sensitivity marker. Several studies attempting to evaluate dietary reductions have been put forward since (Lucarelli, 1995; Whiteley 1999; Cade, 1999). These studies suggest that some participants do show behavioral response to dietary restriction.

A more recent trial by Knivsberg (2002), which addressed earlier limitations to tracking progress, suggested developmental progress was seen in individuals who had elevated urinary peptides to milk and gluten. Patients were divided into 2 groups, a casein-free, gluten-free group and a group that continued on milk and gluten. Ten children per group were monitored for a year by a blinded tester, and the dietary restricted group showed beneficial progress over unrestricted comparisons. This may represent a clear subset of proper candidates for dietary withdrawal.

Elder (2006) evaluated 15 children who were placed on a 12-week treatment cycle of a casein-free and gluten-free diet. This study was a blinded study, where the children received a diet that was free of casein and gluten for 12 weeks or a diet spiked with casein and gluten, and then the children were crossed over for 12 weeks to the alternative diet. Caregivers and observers were not aware what the child was receiving. No differences in developmental markers or behaviors were seen. This was a group of children with autism, unselected by any markers suggesting food intolerance. Interestingly, urinary peptides were evaluated for milk and gluten peptides during the diets and no differences were identified in children's urinary peptides while on or off milk or gluten.

At this time, the studies attempting to treat autistic symptoms with diet have not been sufficient to support the general institution of a diet for autism. Symptoms suggesting food allergy or dietary intolerance may prompt institution of a diet for these symptoms.

As we move forward, we need to consider the heterogeneity of the autism population. It seems unlikely that any diet, supplement, medicine, or even educational modality will work for every individual. Especially for dietary interventions, identifying a subgroup with characteristic presentation may allow a better prediction of response.

Celiac Disease

There is research that argues against a link between celiac disease and autism. Pavone (1997) evaluated a limited number of autistic children (11) for markers of celiac disease and found no correlation. He also conducted evaluations on 120 children documented with identifiable celiac disease for any indication of behavioral abnormalities. He found that none of the children exhibited autistic-like behaviors, concluding there was no connection between celiac disease and autism. This study is too small to conclude that celiac disease is no more frequent in autism, however with the high prevalence of both conditions in the general population (ASD seen in 1/166 individuals or even greater; Yeargin-Allsopp, 2003; and celiac disease seen in 1/133 individuals; Fasano, 2003), there will be an expected coincidence of these conditions. With such a common prevalence of celiac disease in the general population, celiac screening may be prudent in children with autism and any issues with GI disturbance or growth issues.

There is often disagreement between parent and professional (Ho, 1994) on the management of children with autism and what constitutes therapeutic benefit. Many parents institute dietary restrictions and report anecdotally that various benefits have occurred. Validated tracking tools are lacking to assess progress from therapeutic or nutritional trials. In her paper, Elder et al. (2006) reported that although measurable changes were not identified in children on a casein-free, gluten-free diet, some parents did notice subtle differences in their children when the diet was restricted. Perhaps alternate assays will allow recognition of currently subtle changes with intervention.

Dietary Intolerance

Beyond allergy or immune-mediated food problems that may account for dietary contribution to behavioral problems, food intolerance or nonimmune reaction to foods could result from inadequate digestion of food (e.g. lactose intolerance). Horvath (1999) described diminished lactase activity, measured via intestinal biopsy of autistic children with diarrhea who underwent endoscopies, 58% of the time. The reported prevalence of lactose intolerance in the general pediatric population falls well below the frequency reported in the Horvath study (Kretchmer, 1981). Possible reasons for lactase enzyme deficiency might include intestinal injury or diminished genetic expression of these enzymes. In the same study, Horvath measured pancreatic enzyme activity by performing secretin stimulation studies during endoscopy. He did not identify pancreatic enzyme deficiency when a limited number of children were evaluated.

Alberti (1999) suggests that poor breakdown of some food products could allow them to have a neurotransmitter effect, potentially accounting for altered behavior. He tested sulfation by dosing Paracetamol (acetaminophen) in children with autism and measuring metabolites in the urine compared to an age-matched unaffected control group. The sulfated metabolite of acetaminophen was lower in autistic children, raising the question whether consumption of certain foods requiring sulfation processing might exacerbate a metabolic dysfunction. Murch et al. (1993) discussed disruption of sulfation in intestinal inflammation (colitis). McFadden (1996) suggests that impaired sulfation has been found with increased frequency in individuals with several degenerative neurological and immunological conditions and might account for chemical and diet sensitivities in some children with autism.

Nutritional Deficiency

Model research regarding vitamin supplementation and neurological functioning is seen with the condition tryptophan deficiency. Young (1991) looked at the effects of dietary components including amino acids, carbohydrates, and folic acid supplementation on behavior. He reported that tryptophan depletion decreased serotonin levels and affected mood. Other studies suggest that tryptophan depletion alters pain perception. Some types of pain may improve with supplementation of tryptophan; others, including postoperative pain, actually worsened when supplemented with tryptophan. McDougle et al. (1996) found that autism symptoms worsened with tryptophan depletion.

Considering the model of tryptophan deficiency, debate has ensued regarding the use of specific vitamin supplementation as a potential treatment for autistic symptoms. Researchers have reported that various supplements may bring clinical improvement, including Vitamin B-6, Vitamin B-12, folic acid, calcium, magnesium, and zinc.

One theoretical reason that folate, B-6, and B-12 may have value is that they are necessary for serotonin production. It is also possible that these agents may alter metabolic pathways or modulate gene expression. Folic acid deficiency has been identified in patients with depression (Young, 1989), schizophrenia (Godfrey, 1990), and affective disorders (Coppen, 1986). Vitamin B-12 deficiency has been considered a potential factor contributing to neurological dysfunction perhaps because it aids protein synthesis and myelination (Herbert, 1975). Lowe (1981) could not identify deficiency of either folic acid or vitamin B-12 in autistic patients. More recent discussion of vitamin B-12 supplementation, particularly methyl B-12, focuses on the potential of methylation processing defects (James, 2009).

Vitamin B-6 (pyridoxine) supplementation was noted to improve behavior in autism (Rimland, 1974). A subsequent double blind, placebo-controlled trial supported the earlier report (Rimland, 1978). Discussing the metabolic approaches to the treatment of autism spectrum disorders, Page (2000) suggests that several well-designed studies including Coleman (1989), Kleijnen and Knipschild (1991), and Lelord (1988) support the idea that pyridoxine improves some symptoms of autism. Although the potential value is discussed, a Cochrane review (2005) of 14 studies evaluating B-6 supplementation did not find adequate data to support supplementation.

Several studies looking for nutritional deficiencies raise preliminary red flags. Hediger et al. (2008) reported decreased cortical bone thickness in a group of 75 children with ASD. This finding was present despite normal growth and unrestricted diet. Of the children studied, 12% had been in a milk-free diet, and this group had a significantly greater loss of cortical thickness. The long-term implications are not clear, but those children on calcium supplementation in their study were not spared. More work investigating malabsorption or required supplementation may be needed. Arnold et al. (2003) reported that children with autism had plasma amino acid profiles showing more essential amino acid deficiencies than age-matched controls and a trend for children on restricted diets to show greater deficiency. These studies do suggest there may be potential negative outcomes from restrictive diets and the need to continue a diet should be supported.

Many children with autism spectrum disorders receive vitamin and mineral supplements and other products every day on the basis of limited data. This limited information underscores the need for well-constructed clinical trials to evaluate these nutrients and better clarify if supplementation is a value and for whom it provides a benefit.

Mucosal Inflammatory Conditions Described in ASD

There are a number of reports discussing the findings of inflammation at endoscopy in children with autism. It is important to begin by saying that inflammation is going to be identified only in children who have presented with symptoms justifying an endoscopic procedure. This is true for all of the reports. Therefore discussion of GI findings cannot imply any known prevalence in the autism population, and at best describes abnormalities in a subset of individuals.

In his study of 36 children with GI symptoms and ASD brought to endoscopy, Horvath (1999) described esophagitis in 69.4%, gastritis in 42%, and duodenitis in 67% of these children. The high frequency of esophagitis was especially noteworthy because the children were primarily under evaluation for diarrhea.

Wakefield (1998) was the first to discuss inflammation in the lower GI tract among children with developmental disorders. This study evaluated 12 children with "regressive developmental disorder." Eleven of the patients were reported to have colitis by histology, and all had the endoscopic finding of prominent lymphoid nodules in the ileum (lymphoid nodular hyperplasia or LNH), colon, or both. He suggested that measles virus from vaccine potentially caused these intestinal changes, which led to GI symptoms and increased intestinal permeability and the subsequent development of autistic regression. In a larger study (Wakefield, 2000), he evaluated a group of 60 children with "regressive" autism. This study also evaluated a control group of unaffected children undergoing colonoscopy. In the affected group, 93% had ileal LNH; 14.3% of the unaffected children had these changes. Histologic colitis was seen in 88% of the affected but only 4.5% of the unaffected children.

Several contentious questions were raised by these reports:

1. The frequency of inflammation found was quite high. This may have reflected the severity of the patients being evaluated. As was seen in Horvath's study, there was a notable frequency of inflammation in endoscopy testing.
2. The finding of lymphoid nodular hyperplasia (LNH) was interpreted as an abnormality. Pediatric gastroenterologists have reported this finding as a developmentally normal or prominent following allergy or constipation (Turunen, 2004; MacDonald, 2007).The finding of lymphoid nodular hyperplasia has been noted in other conditions (Sabra, 1998). Allergy has been associated with LNH. Kokkonen (2002) reported that LNH was seen in the colon in 46 of 140 children undergoing colonoscopy for persistent and severe gastrointestinal symptoms. These children were not noted to have autism or other developmental issues. In this same study, ileal LNH was seen in 53 of 74 children tested, suggesting that LNH is common in children and not specific to the ASD population. He suggests LNH may be an expression of immune response. Wakefield et al. (2005) supports the contention that LNH is more prominent in autism and seems independent of allergy or constipation. This topic is one of ongoing discussion in the literature.
3. Wakefield suggested that the potential reason for colitis and LNH was measles virus infection from the measles, mumps, and rubella vaccination (MMR) accounting for the lesion. Alarge number of papers refute the idea that MMR administration is associated with the development of autism (Chen, 2004; Dales, 2001; DeStefano, 2004; Fombonne & Chakrabarti, 2001; Honda, 2005; Madsen, 2002; Afzal, 2006; D'Souza, 2006; among others). Taylor (2002) saw no change in the frequency of regression before and after the institution of MMR vaccination in England. He did note a possible association between nonspecific bowel problems and regression, but did not find that this related to MMR vaccination. Fombonne and Chakrabarti (2001) evaluated patient groups before and after the institution of MMR vaccination. He found no difference in the age of parent concern, the rate of developmental regression did not differ before and after MMR vaccine, and the intervals from MMR vaccine to parental recognition of autistic symptoms were comparable in autistic children with or without regression.

In 2008, Hornig et al. reported that in 25 children with autism and 13 unaffected controls, measles RNA was identified in only one affected and one unaffected child on intestinal biopsy. Although the presenting perception of most parents of children with autism was that they regressed following vaccination with MMR (regression was identified in 88% of the children with autism), the sequence of symptoms that would support Wakefield's theory was not present. Eighty percent of the children with autism did not present with a sequence of vaccination -> onset of GI symptoms -> autistic regression.

The discussion about vaccination as a cause of autism profoundly overshadowed the GI findings. If the children studied had significant GI pathology, regardless of suspected etiology, symptoms of pain, GI dysfunction, and perhaps behavioral issues would benefit from treatment of these noted GI disturbances.

Furlano (2001) reported that, although the histologic findings of colitis described in the autistic children were less severe than classical inflammatory bowel disease (IBD), immunohistochemical testing showed increased basement membrane thickness and mucosal gamma delta cell density compared to IBD. The significance of these findings is unclear.

Torrente (2002) described duodenal biopsy findings in 25 children with "regressive" autism. The biopsy findings were compared to 11 celiac patients, 5 patients with cerebral palsy and mental retardation, and 18 control patients with normal histology. Twenty-three of 25 autistic children had normal histology or nonspecific increased cellularity. Immunohistochemical studies showed an overall marked increase in mucosal lymphocyte density in autistic children compared to controls and MR-CP patients. The density of CD8 T-cells was also greater in the autistic patients than controls and MR-CP patients. IgG deposition in the basolateral enterocyte membrane and subepithelial basement membrane was seen in 23 of 25 autistic children but was not seen in the control or MR-CP patients. The significance of these findings remains unclear, as this specialized testing is not usually done on all patients undergoing intestinal biopsy. Evaluating the group of children Wakefield studied, Ashwood (2006) reported, "There is a unique pattern of peripheral blood and mucosal CD3+ lymphocytes intracellular cytokines, which is consistent with significant immune dysregulation, in this ASD cohort."

We may need to reconsider what we consider normal biopsies. We also need to consider the significance of microscopic inflammation. It may be that these findings are important in children with autism because these are a source of inflammation. Because children with autism have sensory processing abnormalities, perhaps low-grade inflammation can cause significant dysfunction in this population. It may be that the findings are not always clinically relevant. This is a primary focus of ongoing research.

Other considerations of impaired bowel health include an unhealthy bowel flora. Sandler et al. (2000) suggests that disruption of indigenous gut flora might promote colonization with bacteria that produce neurotoxins. He treated autistic children with oral Vancomycin, and 8 of 10 showed transient behavioral improvements. Brudnak (2002) and Linday (2001) describe the potential use of probiotic (nonpathogenic bacteria and yeast) agents such as Lactobacillus species and Saccharomyces Boulardii. The value of these organisms may be to normalize intestinal flora, provide digestive enzymes aiding nutrient absorption, minimizing allergen exposure, and to stimulate local immune responses in the intestine.

Evaluating children with ASD and GI symptoms, Horvath (1998) performed endoscopy and pancreatic function testing by administering secretin. Secretin is a neurotransmitter produced in the duodenum and stimulates the washout of pancreatic enzymes into the intestine. Following the procedure, he reported improvements in social behaviors including better eye contact, increased social awareness, and improved expressive language in 3 children. A flurry of studies followed, in effort to assess if secretin had a therapeutic benefit to treat the greater community of autistic children. Sandler (1999), Lightdale (2001), Roberts (2001) and others reported no sustained gastrointestinal or neurological benefit of secretin over placebo.

Functional GI issues include gastroesophageal reflux, recurrent abdominal pain, and irritable bowel syndrome. Population-based survey studies remain sorely lacking to fully determine how often children with ASD have gastrointestinal function problems. We cannot speculate on how frequently this will be seen in ASD, but should not assume that these conditions happen less frequently in the nonverbal child than in the verbal child.

Conditions such as recurrent abdominal pain, abdominal migraine, and irritable bowel syndrome (IBS) have no defining test to clarify the diagnosis. Symptom history is the best current method to identify these disorders and therefore may be difficult to ascertain in this population. Many children with ASD exhibit significant sensory processing dysfunction. Symptoms seen in sensory integration disorder such as altered pain perception are a primary component of IBS as well and may be a reason to consider this diagnosis in children with GI issues and ASD.

Speculations and Conclusions

In 2009, Campbell described the results of an exploratory, retrospective study indicating a genetic association of a functional variant of the MET gene (chromosome 7) in ASD patients in families with affected individuals who are reported to have co-occurring gastrointestinal conditions. A functional variant in the promoter of the gene encoding the MET receptor tyrosine kinase is associated with autism spectrum disorder, and MET protein expression is decreased in the temporal cortex of subjects with autism spectrum disorder. MET is a pleiotropic receptor that functions in both brain development and gastrointestinal repair. On the basis of these functions, the authors hypothesized that association of the autism spectrum disorder–associated MET promoter variant may be enriched in a subset of individuals with co-occurring autism spectrum disorder and gastrointestinal conditions. The sample consisted of 992 individuals from 214 families. Because the *C* allele disrupts transcription of the MET gene, the biological translation of these genetic findings is consistent with a hypothesis that reduced MET signaling may contribute to a syndrome that includes ASD with co-occurring gastrointestinal conditions. This finding may be one "biomarker" that if present may suggest a subgroup of individuals vulnerable to autism and comorbid gastrointestinal issues.

Another topic that may be relevant to GI issues and autism is the description of a higher frequency of children with mitochondrial dysfunction exhibiting autism (Oliviera et al., 2007). Children with mitochondrial dysfunction often have generalized motor dysfunction of the GI tract causing GER or constipation symptoms (Chitkara, 2003). The subgroup of children with autism and GI issues may suggest a subgroup of children meriting additional work-up for mitochondrial dysfunction.

Berney (2000) stated, "In the absence of a cure, the implementation of ideas will continue to outstrip factual evidence." Medical providers need to recognize that families of children with autism are not only looking for a cause or cure for autism, they are trying to assure that their child is as healthy as possible to prevent barriers to progress. As part of this, many children will be on diets or supplements. The use of complementary approaches to care is common in this population. Families have reported that 31.7% to 52% of children with autism have been treated with complementary approaches (Levy, 2003; Wong, 2006). Diets and complementary treatments are not unique to autism. Pediatric patients with chronic diseases often receive supplements to traditional treatments. Forty percent of pediatric patients with chronic disease report using CAM as part of their management (McCann, 2006). As we provide more definitive data about pathology and expectations in this population, one may expect speculative care to be reduced.

As a result of research to date, GI practitioners are now being asked to participate in the evaluation of children with ASD and GI symptoms. Pediatricians, family physicians, and gastroenterologists, first and foremost, need to be willing to consider that children with autism have a right to comorbid GI issues. The conditions of reflux, food sensitivity or allergy, constipation, diarrhea, and inflammatory bowel conditions are common in general pediatrics and should be expected to be identified in children with autism. As more prevalence data are available, we may find that some of these issues are more common in children with autism and may even be related to the phenotype of a subgroup. Until then, thoughtful care and evaluation should be offered to children with autism presenting for evaluation is needed.

Conclusions

Gastrointestinal conditions are common in children with autism. They may represent a comorbidity, but their presence may well exacerbate behaviors of autism. There remains debate about whether an underlying inflammatory condition of the bowel or environmental, dietary triggers might account for a contribution to causation of autism.

Challenges and Future Directions

- Broader understanding of the impact of medical comorbidity (including gastrointestinal illness and functional GI disorders such as constipation, acid reflux, and food allergy) on the well-being and behavior in children with autism is imperative.
- Evaluation of intestinal microflora in the setting of food allergy, inflammation, and functional GI motility conditions in children with autism may be valuable in explaining immune variation or autoimmune response in some individuals.
- Prospective tracking of GI conditions in children at risk for developing autism may help in characterizing GI phenomena versus outcomes that have resulted from intervention such as dietary selectivity, diet therapies, or other treatments.

SUGGESTED READING

Buie, T., Campbell, D. B., Fuchs, G. J., Furuta, G. T., Levy, J., Van de Water, J., et al. (2010). Evaluation, diagnosis, and treatment of gastrointestinal disorders in individuals with ASDs: A consensus report. *Pediatrics, 125*, S1–S18.

Carr, E. G., & Owen-Deschryver, J. S. (2007). Physical illness, pain, and problem behavior in minimally verbal people with developmental disabilities. *Journal of Autism and Developmental Disorders, 37*(3), 413–424.

Horvath, K., & Perman, J. A. (2002). Autistic disorder and gastrointestinal disease. *Current Opinion in Pediatrics, 14*, 583–587.

REFERENCES

Afzal, N., Murch, S., Thirrupathy, K., Berger, L., Fagbemi, A., & Heuschkel, R. (2003). Constipation with acquired megarectum in children with autism. *Pediatrics, 112*, 939–939.

Afzal, M. A., Ozoemena, L. C., O'Hare, A., Kidger, K. A., & Bentley, M. L. (2006). Absence of detectable measles virus genome sequence in blood of autistic children who have had their MMR vaccination during the routine childhood immunization schedule of UK. *Journal of Medical Virology, 78*, 623–630.

Ahearn, W. H., Castine, T., & Green, G. (2001). An assessment of food acceptance in children with autism or pervasive developmental disorder-not otherwise specified. *Journal of Autism and Developmental Disorders, 31*(5), 505–511.

Alberti, A., Pirrone, P., Elia, M., Waring, R., & Romano, C. (1999). Sulphation deficit in low-functioning autistic children: A pilot study. *Biological Psychiatry, 46*(3), 420–424.

Arnold, G. L., Hyman, S. L., Mooney, R. A., & Kirby, R. S. (2003). Plasma amino acids profiles in children with autism: Potential risk of nutritional deficiency. *Journal of Autism and Developmental Disorders, 33*(4), 449–454.

Ashwood, P., & Wakefield, A. J. (2006, April). Immune activation of peripheral blood and mucosal CD3+ lymphocyte cytokine profiles in children with autism and gastrointestinal symptoms. *Journal of Neuroimmunology, 173*(1–2), 126–134.

Barron, J., & Sandman, C. A. (1983). Relationship of sedative-hypnotic response to self-injurious behavior and stereotypy by mentally retarded clients. *American Journal of Mental Deficiency, 88*(2), 177–186.

Bentovim, A. (1970). The clinical approach to feeding disorders of childhood. *Journal of Psychosomatic Research, 14*, 267–276.

Berney, T. P. (2000). Autism: An evolving concept. *British Journal of Psychiatry, 176*, 20–25.

Bernhisel-Broadbent, J. (2001). Diagnosis and management of food allergy. *Current Allergy Reports, 1*(1), 67–75.

Brudnak, M. A. (2002). Probiotics as an adjuvant to detoxification protocols. *Medical Hypotheses, 58*(5), 382–385.

Burd, D., Shantz, J., Swearingen, W. S., Ahearn, W. H., & Kerwin, M. L. (1995). The treatment of food selectivity [poster, Assn for Behavioral Analysis].

Cade, R., Privette, M., Fregley, M., Rowland, N., Sun, Z., Zele, V., et al. (1999). Autism and schizophrenia: Intestinal disorders. *Nutritional Neuroscience, 3*, 57–72.

Campbell, D. B., Buie, T. M., Winter, H., Bauman, M., Sutcliffe, J. S., Perrin, J. M., et al. (2009, March). Distinct genetic risk based on association of MET in families with co-occurring autism and gastrointestinal conditions. *Pediatrics, 123*(3), 1018–1024.

Chen, W., Landau, S., Sham, P., & Fombonne, E. (2004). No evidence for links between autism, MMR, and measles virus. *Psychologie Medicale, 34*, 543–553.

Chitkara, D. K., Nurko, S., Shoffner, J. M., Buie, T., & Flores, A. (2003, April). Abnormalities in gastrointestinal motility are associated with diseases of oxidative phosphorylation in children. *American Journal of Gastroenterology, 98*(4), 871–877.

Coleman, N. (1989). Autism: Non-drug biological treatments. In C. Gilberg (Ed.), *Diagnosis and treatment of autism* (pp. 219–235). New York: Plenum.

Coppen, A., Chaudhry, S., & Swade, C. (1986). Folic acid enhances lithium prophylaxis. *Journal of Affective Disorders, 10*, 9–13.

D'Eufemia, P., Celli, M., Finocchiaro, R., Viozzi, L., Zaccagnini, M., Cardi, E., et al. (1996). Abnormal intestinal permeability in children with autism. *Acta Paediatrica, 85*, 1076–1079.

D'Souza, Y., Fombonne, E., & Ward, B. J. (2006). No evidence of persisting measles virus in peripheral blood mononuclear cells from children with autism spectrum disorder. *Pediatrics, 118*, 1664–1675.

Dales, L., Hammer, S. J., & Smith, N. J. (2001). Time trends in autism and in MMR immunization coverage in California. *JAMA: The journal of the American Medical Association, 285*, 1183–1185.

Dalrymple, N. J., & Ruble, L. A. (1992). Toilet training and behaviors of people with autism: Parent views. *Journal of Autism and Developmental Disorders, 22*(2), 265–275.

DeStefano, F., Bhasin, T. K., Thompson, W. W., Yeargin-Allsopp, M., & Boyle, C. (2004). Age at first measles-mumps-rubella vaccination in children with autism and school-matched control subjects: A population-based study in metropolitan Atlanta. *Pediatrics, 113*, 259–266.

Elder, J., Shankar, M., Shuster, J., Theriaque, D., Burns, S., & Sherrill, L. (2006). The gluten-free, casein-free diet in autism: Results of a preliminary double blind clinical trial. *Journal of Autism and Developmental Disorders, 36*(3), 413–420.

Fasano, A., Berti, I., Gerarduzzi, T., et al. (2003). Prevalence of celiac disease in at-risk and not-at-risk groups in the United States. *Archives of Internal Medicine, 163*(3), 268–292.

Fombonne, E., & Chakrabarti, S. (2001). No evidence for a new variant of measles-mumps-rubella-induced autism. *Pediatrics, 108*(4), E58, 368–373.

Furlano, R. I., Anthony, A., Day, R., Brown, A., McGarvey, L., Thomson, M. A., et al. (2001). Colonic CD-8 and gamma delta T-cell infiltration with epithelial damage in children with autism. *Journal of Pediatrics, 138*(3), 366–372.

Gershon, M. D. (1998). *The second brain.* New York: HarperCollins.

Godfrey, P. S., Toone, B. K., Carney, M. W. P., Flynn, T. G., Bottiglieri, T., Laundy, M., et al. (1990). Enhancement of recovery from psychiatric illness by methylfolate. *Lancet, 336*, 392–395.

Gouge, A. L., & Ekvall S. W. (1975). Diets of handicapped children: Physical, psychological, and socioeconomic correlations. *American Journal of Mental Deficiency, 80*, 149–157.

Hediger, M. L., England, L. J., Molloy, C. A., Yu, K., Manning-Courtney, P., & Mills, J. L. (2008). Reduced bone cortical thickness in boys with autism or autism spectrum disorder. *Journal of Autism and Developmental Disorders, 38*(5), 848–856.

Herbert, V. (1975). Drugs effective in megaloblastic anemias. In L. Goodman, & A. Gillman (Eds.), *Pharmacological basis of therapeutics* (5th ed.). New York: Macmillan.

Ho, H. H., Miller, A., & Armstrong, R. W. (1994). Parent-professional agreement on diagnosis and recommendations for children with developmental disorders. *Children's Health Care, 23*(2), 137–148.

Honda, H., Shimizu, Y., & Rutter, M. (2005). No effect of MMR withdrawal on the incidence of autism: A total population study. *Journal of Child Psychology and Psychiatry, and Allied Disciplines, 46*, 572–579.

Hornig, M., Briese, T., Buie, T., Bauman, M. L., Lauwers, G., et al. (2008). Lack of association between measles virus vaccine and autism with enteropathy: A case-control study. *PLoS ONE, 3*(9), e3140.

Horvath, K., Stefanatos, G., Sokolski, K. N., Wachtel, R., Nabors, L., & Tildon, T. (1998). Improved social and language skills after secretin administration in patients with autistic spectrum disorders. *Journal of the Association for Academic Minority Physicians, 9*(1), 9–15.

Horvath, K., Papadimitriou, J. C., Rabsztyn, A., et al. (1999). Gastrointestinal abnormalities in children with autistic disorder. *Journal of Pediatrics, 135*, 559–563.

Horvath, K., & Perman, J. A. (2002). Autistic disorder and gastrointestinal disease. *Current Opinion in Pediatrics, 14*, 583–587.

James, S. J., Melnyk, S., Fuchs, G., Reid, T., Jernigan, S., Pavliv, O., et al. (2009). Efficacy of methylcobalamin and folinic acid treatment on glutathione redox status in children with autism. *American Journal of Clinical Nutrition, 89*(1), 425–430.

Kanner, L. (1943). Autistic disturbances of affective contact. *Nervous Child, 12*, 217–250.

Kleijnen, J., & Knipchild, P. (1991). Niacin and vitamin B-6 in mental functioning: A review of controlled trials in humans. *Biological Psychiatry, 29*, 931–941.

Knivsberg, A. M., Wiig, K., Lind, G., Nogland, M., & Reichelt, K. L. (1990). Dietary intervention in autistic syndromes. *Developmental Brain Dysfunction, 3*, 315–327.

Knivsberg, A. M., Reichelt, K. L., Hoien, T., & Nodland, M. (2002). A randomized, controlled study of dietary intervention in autistic syndromes. *Nutritional Neuroscience, 5*(4), 251–261.

Kokkonen, J., & Karttunen, T. J. (2002) Lymphonodular hyperplasia on the mucosa of the lower gastrointestinal tract in children: An indication of enhanced immune response? *Journal of Pediatric Gastroenterology and Nutrition, 34*(1), 42–46.

Kretchmer, N. (1981). In R. M. Suskind (Ed.), Textbook of pediatric nutrition (pp. 189–215). New York: Raven.

Lelord, G., Barthelemy, C., & Martineau, N. (1988). Clinical and biological effects of vitamin B-6 plus magnesium in autistic subjects. In J. Laklam & R. Reynolds (Eds.), *Vitamin B-6 responsive disorders in humans* (pp. 329–356). New York: Liss.

Levy, S., Mandell, D., Merhar, S., Ittenbach, R. & Pinto-Martin, J. (2003, December). Use of complementary and alternative medicine among children recently diagnosed with autistic spectrum disorder. *Journal of Developmental and Behavioral Pediatrics, 24*(6), 418–423.

Lightdale, J. R., Hayer, C., Duer, A., Lind-White, C., Jenkins, S., Siegel, B., et al. (2001). Effects of intravenous secretin on language and behavior of children with autism and gastrointestinal symptoms: A single-blinded, open-label pilot study. *Pediatrics, 108*(5), E90.

Linday, L. A. (2001). Saccharomyces Boulardii: Potential adjunctive treatment for children with autism and diarrhea. *Journal of Child Neurology, 16*(5), 387.

Lowe, T. L., Cohen, D. J., Miller, S., & Young, J. G. (1981). Folic acid and B-12 in autism and neuropsychiatric disturbances of childhood. *Journal of the American Academy of Child Psychiatry, 20*, 104–111.

Lucarelli, S., Frediani,T., Zingoni, A. M., Ferruzzi, F., Giardini, O., Quintieri, F., et al. (1995). Food allergy and infantile autism. *Panminerva Medica, 37*(3), 137–141.

Madsen, K. M., Hviid, A., Vestergaard, M., Schendel, D., & Wohlfahrt, J., et al. (2002). A population-based study of measles, mumps, and rubella vaccination and autism. *New England Journal of Medicine, 347*, 1477–1482.

MacDonald, T. T., & Domizio, P. (2007). Autistic enterocolitis is it a histopathological entity? *Histopathology, 50*(3), 371–379.

McCann, L. J., & Newell, S. J. (2006). Survey of paediatric complementary and alternative medicine use in health and chronic illness, *Archives of Disease in Childhood, 91*, 173–174.

McDougle, C. J., Naylor, S. T., Cohen, D. J., Aghajanian, G. K., Heninger, G. R., & Price, L. H. (1996). Effects of tryptophan depletion in drug-free adults with autistic disorder. *Archives of General Psychiatry, 53*(11), 993–1000.

McFadden, S. A. (1996). Phenotypic variation in xenobiotic metabolism and adverse environmental response: Focus on sulfur-dependent detoxification pathways. *Toxicology, 111*(1–3), 43–65.

Molloy, C. A., & Manning-Courtney, P. (2003). Prevalence of chronic gastrointestinal symptoms in children with autism and autistic spectrum disorders. *Autism, 7*, 165–171.

Murch, S. H., MacDonald, T. T., Walker-Smith, J. A., Levin, M., Lionetti P., & Klein, N. J. (1993). Disruption of sulphated glycoaminoglycans in intestinal inflammation. *Lancet, 341*, 711–731.

North American Society for Pediatric Gastroenterology, Hepatology, and Nutrition. (2006, September). Evaluation and treatment of constipation in infants and children: Recommendations of the North American Society for Pediatric Gastroenterology, Hepatology, and Nutrition. *Journal of Pediatric Gastroenterology and Nutrition, 43*(3), e1–13.

Nye, C., & Brice, A. (2005, October 19). Combined vitamin B6-magnesium treatment in autism spectrum disorder. *Cochrane Database of Systematic Reviews (Online)*, (4), CD003497.

Oliveira, G., Ataíde, A., Marques, C., Miguel, T. S., Coutinho, A. M., & Mota-Vieira, L. (2007, October). Epidemiology of autism spectrum disorder in Portugal: Prevalence, clinical characterization, and medical conditions. *Developmental Medicine and Child Neurology, 49*(10), 726–733.

Page, T. (2000). Metabolic approaches to the treatment of autism spectrum disorders. *Journal of Autism and Developmental Disorders, 30*(5), 463–469.

Palmer, S., Thompson, R. J., & Linscheid, T. R. (1975). Applied behavioral analysis in the treatment of childhood feeding problems. *Developmental Medicine and Child Neurology, 17*, 333–339.

Panksepp, J. (1981). Brain opioids: A neurochemical substrate for narcotic and social dependence. In S. J. Cooper (Ed.), *Theory in psychopharmacology* (Vol. 1). London: Academic.

Patzold, L. M., Richdale, A. L., & Tonge, B. J. (1998). An investigation into sleep characteristics of children with autism and Asperger's disorder. *Journal of Paediatrics and Child Health, 34*(6), 528–533.

Pavone, L., Fiumara, A., Bottaro, G., Mazzone, D., & Coleman, M. (1997). Autism and celiac disease: Failure to validate the hypothesis that a link might exist. *Biological Psychiatry, 42*(1), 72–75.

Reichelt, K. L., Ekrem, J., & Scott, H. (1990). Gluten, milk proteins, and autism: The results of dietary intervention on behavior and peptide secretion. *Journal of Applied Nutrition, 42*, 1–11.

Reichelt, W. H., Ekrem, J., Stensrud, M., & Reichelt, K. L. (1998). Peptide excretion in celiac disease. *Journal of Pediatric Gastroenterology and Nutrition, 26*, 305–309.

Reichelt, K. L., Knivsberg, A. M., Lind, G., & Nodland, M. (1991). Probable etiology and possible treatment of childhood autism. *Brain Dysfunction, 4*, 308–319.

Rimland, B. (1974). An orthomolecular study of psychotic children. *Journal of Orthomolecular Psychiatry, 3*, 371–377.

Rimland, B., Callaway, E., & Dreyfus, P. (1978). The effect of high doses of vitamin B-6 on autistic children: A double-blind crossover study. *American Journal of Psychiatry, 135*(4), 472–475.

Roberts, W., Weaver, L., Brian, J., Bryson, S., Emelianova, S., Griffiths, A. M., et al. (2001). Repeated doses of porcine secretin in the treatment of autism: A randomized placebo-controlled trial. *Pediatrics, 107*(5), E71.

Rudolph, C. D., Mazur, L. J., Liptak, G. S., Baker, R. D., Boyle, J. T., Colletti, R. B., et al. (2001). North American Society for Pediatric Gastroenterology and Nutrition. Guidelines for evaluation and treatment of gastroesophageal reflux in infants and children: Recommendations of the North American Society for Pediatric Gastroenterology and Nutrition. *Journal of Pediatric Gastroenterology and Nutrition, 32*(suppl 2), S1–S31.

Ryan, D., Honomichl, B. L., Goodlin-Jones, M. B., Gaylor, E., & Anders, T. F. (2002). Sleep patterns of children with pervasive developmental disorders. *Journal of Autism and Developmental Disorders, 32*(6), 553–561.

Sabra, S., Bellanti, J. A., & Colon, A. R. (1998). Ileal lymphoid nodular hyperplasia, non-specific colitis, and pervasive developmental disorder in children. *Lancet, 352*, 234–235.

Sahley, T. L., & Panksepp, J. (1987). Brain opioids and autism: An updated analysis of possible linkages. *Journal of Autism and Developmental Disorders, 17*(2), 201–216.

Sampson, H. A. (1999a). Food Allergy. Part 1: Immunopathogenesis and clinical disorders. *Journal of Allergy and Clinical Immunology, 103*(5 pt 1), 717–728.

Sampson, H. A. (1999b). Food Allergy. Part 2: Diagnosis and management. *Journal of Allergy and Clinical Immunology, 103*(6), 981–998.

Sandler, A. D., Sutton, K. A., DeWeese, B. S., Girardi, M. A., Sheppard, V., & Bodfish, J. W. (1999). Lack of benefit of a single dose of synthetic human secretin in the treatment of autism and pervasive developmental disorder. *New England Journal of Medicine, 341*(24), 1801–1806.

Sandler, R. H., Finegold, S. M., Bolte, E. R., Buchanan, C.P., Maxwell, A. P., Vaisanen, M. L., et al. (2000). Short term benefit from oral vancomycin treatment of regressive-onset autism. *Journal of Child Neurology, 16*(5), 429–435.

Sandyk, R., & Gillman, M. A. (1986). Infantile autism: A dysfunction of the opioids? *Medical Hypotheses, 19*(1), 41–45.

Shattock, P., Kennedy, A., Rowell, F., & Berney, T. (1990). Role of neuropeptides in autism and their relationships with classical neurotransmitters. *Brain Dysfunction, 3*, 328–345.

Skripak, J. M., & Wood, R. A. (2008, June). Peanut and tree nut allergy in childhood. *Pediatric Allergy and Immunology, 19*(4), 368–373.

Sponheim, E. (1991). Gluten-free diet in infantile autism. A therapeutic trial. *Tidsskrift for den Norske laegeforening: Tidsskrift for praktisk medicin, ny raekke, 111*(6), 704–707.

Taylor, B., Miller, E., Lingam, R., Andrews, N., Simmons, A., et al. (2002). Measles, mumps, and rubella vaccination and bowel problems or developmental regression in children with autism: Population study. *BMJ (Clinical research ed.), 324*, 393–396.

Torrente, F., Ashwood, P., Day, R., Machado, N., Furlano, R. I., Anthony, A., et al. (2002). Small intestinal enteropathy with epithelial IgG and complement deposition in children with regressive autism. *Molecular Psychiatry, 7*(2), 375–382.

Turunen, S., Karttunen, T. J., & Kokkonen, J. (2004). Lymphoid nodular hyperplasia and cow's milk hypersensitivity in children with chronic constipation. *Journal of Pediatrics, 145*, 606–611.

Valicenti-McDermott, M., McVicar, K., Rapin, I., Wershil, B. K., Cohen, H., et al. (2006). Frequency of gastrointestinal symptoms in children with autistic spectrum disorders and association with family history of autoimmune disease. *Journal of Developmental and Behavioral Pediatrics, 27*, S128–136.

Wakefield, A. J., Anthony, A., Murch, S. H., Thomson, M., Montgomery, S. M., Davies, S., et al. (2000). Enterocolitis in children with developmental disorders. *American Journal of Gastroenterology, 95*(9), 2285–2295.

Wakefield, A. J., Ashwood, P., Limb, K., & Anthony, A. (2005, August). The significance of ileo-colonic lymphoid nodular hyperplasia in children with autistic spectrum disorder. *European Journal of Gastroenterology and Hepatology, 17*(8), 827–836.

Wakefield, A. J., Murch, S. H., Anthony, A., Linnell, J., Casson D. M., Malik, M., et al. (1998). Ileal-lymphoid-nodular hyperplasia, non-specific colitis, and pervasive developmental disorder in children. *Lancet, 351*(9103), 637–641 (Note: Lancet has subsequently withdrawn this paper from it's journal).

Whiteley, P., Rodgers, J., Savery, D., & Shattock, P. (1999). A gluten-free diet as an intervention for autism and associated spectrum disorder. *Autism, 3*(1), 45–65.

Wong, H. L., & Smith, R. G. (2006). Patterns of complementary and alternative medical therapy use in children diagnosed with autism spectrum disorders. *Journal of Autism and Developmental Disorders, 36*, 901–909.

Yeargin-Allsopp, M., Rice, C., Karapurkar, T., Doernberg, N., Boyle, C., & Murphy, C. (2003). Prevalence of autism in a US metropolitan area. *Journal of the American Medical Association, 289*, 49–55.

Yong, D., & Beattie, R. M. (1998). Normal bowel habits and prevalence of constipation in primary school children. *Ambulatory Child Health, 4*, 277–282.

Young, S. N., & Ghadirian, A. M. (1989). Folic acid and psychopathology. *Progress in Neuro-Psychopharmacology and Biological Psychiatry, 13*, 841–863.

Young, S. (1991). The (1989) Borden award lecture: Some effects of dietary components (amino acids, carbohydrate, folic acid) on brain serotonin synthesis, mood, and behavior. *Canadian Journal of Physiology and Pharmacology, 69*, 893–903.

Zagon, I. S., & McLaughlin, P. J. (1978). Perinatal methadone exposure and its influence on the behavioral ontogeny of rats. *Pharmacology, Biochemistry, and Behavior, 9*, 665–672.

26

Anne E. Porter, Daniel G. Glaze

Sleep Problems

Points of Interest

- Sleep disorders affect approximately 20 to 30% of the general pediatric population. In the ASD population the prevalence is much higher and is estimated at between 44 and 86%. The most commonly reported problem is insomnia, which can include inability to initiate sleep and difficulty maintaining sleep.
- Children with ASD are at risk for other medical problems and frequently receive psychotropic medications, both of which can impact sleep. The etiology of sleep problems in children with ASD is likely multifactorial, including genetic and environmental factors as well as medical and behavioral issues.
- The most common parasomnia reported in children with ASD is bruxism (18%). Other reported parasomnias include sleepwalking and night wakings associated with either inconsolable screaming or a frightening dream.
- Sleep problems experienced by children are frequently associated with disturbances in neurocognition and behavior. In children, common consequences of poor sleep include difficulty with mood regulation and impulse control, hyperactivity or daytime sleepiness, poor concentration and impaired memory. The impact of impaired sleep on daytime functioning may be even more severe in children with poor self-regulation, a deficit common in children with ASD. Poor sleep may exacerbate existing behavioral problems.
- Parent report measures are a quick and easy way for clinicians to screen for sleep problems. The two most commonly used measures in the pediatric population are the Children's Sleep Habits Questionnaire (CSHQ) and the BEARS. Objective measures of disturbed sleep include at home use of a physical activity monitor, or actigraph, and clinical polysomnography.
- Sleep problems should be treated first with behavioral therapy. If problems persist, consideration can be give to use of pharmacologic sleep aids.

Introduction

Sleep problems in children with autism spectrum disorders (ASD) are a significant issue and warrant a place in routine clinical evaluation. Evidence consistently indicates that children with an autism spectrum disorder are more likely to have a sleep disorder than typically developing children. A wide range of sleep disorders are reported in this population, with the most common being insomnia, including difficulty falling asleep and staying asleep. Furthermore, sleep disorders negatively impact the daytime functioning of both the child and family members, as well as exacerbate coexisting medical, psychiatric, psychosocial, and developmental problems. Progress has been made in understanding pediatric sleep disorders that will contribute to better care for children with ASD and sleep problems. Reliable and valid methods for identifying and characterizing sleep problems in children exist, including short screening questionnaires that can be easily administered at any point of contact. When sleep problems are identified, effective treatments are available. In this chapter we will consider an overview for the clinician of the clinical presentations of sleep disorders in children with autism spectrum disorders, as well as discuss the evaluation and treatment of these disorders.

Epidemiology

Prevalence and Correlates

Sleep disorders affect approximately 20 to 30% of the general pediatric population (Owens, Spirito, et al., 2000b; Sadeh, Raviv, et al., 2000). In the ASD population the prevalence is much higher and is estimated at between 44 and 86% (Richdale & Prior 1995; Wiggs & Stores, 1996; Patzold, Richdale, et al., 1998; Allik, Larsson, et al., 2006). This high prevalence cannot be explained by level of cognitive functioning alone. A study of parent-reported sleep problems in children with pervasive developmental disorder (PDD) and normal intelligence found that 78% of parents reported sleep problems in these children, compared to 26% of parents of an age- and gender-matched group of typically developing children (Couturier, Speechley, et al., 2005). Further, a large study comparing children with ASD (n = 303; ADI and ADOS confirmed) to children with developmental delays, but no ASD (n = 63) and typically developing children (n = 163) found that children with ASD had a higher prevalence of parent-reported sleep problems than either of the two comparison groups. Fifty-three percent of children in the ASD group had at least one frequent sleep problem, compared to 46% and 32%, respectively, of the developmentally delayed and typically developing groups (Schreck, Mulick, et al., 2004). It appears ASD may be a risk factor for sleep problems independent of level of cognitive functioning.

The most commonly reported problems include inability to initiate sleep and difficulty maintaining sleep (Table 26-1). Parents have reported that their children with ASD have trouble going to bed on time, wake frequently during the night, and wake early (Richdale & Prior, 1995; Johnson et al., 2008; Krakowiak et al., 2008; Richdale et al., 2009). Also reported are irregular sleep-wake patterns and poor sleep routines (Hoshino, Watanabe, et al., 1984; Clements, Wing, et al., 1986; Quine 1991; Patzold, Richdale, et al., 1998; Owens, Spirito, et al., 2000b; Schreck & Mulick, 2000; Honomichl, Goodlin-Jones, et al., 2002; Meltzer, 2008). During objective evaluations using actigraphy, children with ASD exhibited less total sleep time in 24 hours than children with developmental delay without ASD and typically developing children (Goodlin-Jones et al., 2008). The children with developmental delay exhibited more and longer awakenings after sleep onset than the ASD or typically developing children. The presentation of sleep problems in children with ASD is discussed in more detail later in this chapter.

As with other aspects of the ASD phenotype, sleep problems are a complex and variable phenomenon in this group. The high number of children who experience at least one sleep problem warrants screening for sleep problems in all children with ASD. There are some subgroups that are at increased risk. A 2008 study using the Children's Sleep Habits Questionnaire found that children with developmental regression were significantly more likely to experience sleep problems than children who did not have a regressive-onset of autism (Giannotti, Cortesi, et al., 2008). Similarly to typically developing children, sleep problems are more likely to be reported in children younger than 5 years and are more severe in children with intellectual disability (Richdale & Prior, 1995).

Table 26–1.
Commonly reported sleep problems in autism spectrum disorders

Sleep Problem	Reported Prevalence
Insomnia	40–80%; General Pediatric Population 10–30%
Circadian Rhythm Disorder	4–35%; General Pediatric Population 1%
Delayed Sleep Phase	
Irregular Sleep Schedule	
Parasomnias	Not known; in a small case report study RBD occurred in 45%
Bruxism	
NREM Parasomnias (Sleep walking; Night Terrors)	
REM Sleep Behavior Disorder	

Note: Sleep Disordered Breathing (Obstructive sleep apnea) and Sleep Related Movement Disorders not listed; prevalence not known, but may be similar to the general pediatric population.

Typical Sleep Architecture

Children with autism are subject to the same general sleep expectations as typically developing children, and deviation from these norms is significant even when the child "doesn't seem to need much sleep." It is therefore important to understand the sleep patterns that typically developing children manifest at different ages.

Toddler: Ages 0 to 2 Years

Just after birth, infants lack a circadian rhythm, and their sleep/wake cycle varies without regard to dark and light cycles. During the first few months of life they develop a diurnal sleep cycle and by 9 months 70% of infants are sleeping primarily in the evening with one to two naps during the day. By age 1 year, toddlers typically require 10 to 12 hours of sleep per night and may take one or two naps of 2 to 3 hours duration during the day (Meltzer & Mindell, 2006). The most common problems at this age are night wakings, which may be as common as 42% of toddlers, and bedtime resistance (Glaze, 2004). Behavioral patterns that are established at this time can impact the child later in life, including cosleeping and developing a bedtime ritual (Glaze, 2004).

Preschool: Age 3 to 5 Years

During this period children's sleep needs typically decrease from 13 hours to 11 hours by 5 years of age (Glaze, 2004).

Napping also decreases, and children may take only one nap and for a shorter time. Night wakings become less common, with somewhere between 15 to 30% affected (Mindell & Owens, 2003). Further reinforcement of a bedtime routine is important at this age, as some children will continue to demonstrate their increasing independence through bedtime resistance. Cosleeping is a common cause of sleep disturbance at this age (Mindell & Owens, 2003).

School-age: Age 6 to 12 Years

Children of this age require approximately 10 to 11 hours of sleep and no longer require a nap. Daytime sleep may be present, although it may be a symptom of abnormal sleep patterns (Mindell & Owens, 2003; Glaze, 2004). Common issues at this age include sleepwalking, nightmares, bruxism, and sleep disordered breathing. This period is also associated with changes in circadian rhythm, and children may shift from an externally enforced sleep schedule to intrinsic preferences, e.g., morning versus evening alertness (Mindell & Owens, 2003). Children should be allowed to direct their own bedtime to some degree in order to establish a routine that fits the child's circadian rhythm and maintains a full night of sleep (i.e., staying up later by 30 minutes is only appropriate if the child is able to alter his or her morning routine.

Adolescents: Age 12 to 18 Years

Sleep requirements drop further in this period. Most teens require approximately 9 hours of sleep per night, although the average teen gets 7 hours of sleep per night. Approximately 11 to 30% of adolescents and teenagers experience a sleep disorder at this age (Glaze, 2004). The increasing independence during these years, as well as increased responsibility at home and at school can contributed to compromised sleep. Environmental factors, such as caffeine, nicotine, alcohol, or drugs may reduce the quantity or quality of a child's sleep, while resulting daytime sleepiness may increase the use of these substances. Further, the onset of puberty may cause changes in circadian rhythm, shifting sleep phase later by approximately 2 hours. Children in this age group in the United States are frequently getting less sleep than is needed, and insufficient sleep is a primary problem in this group.

Sleep Problems in ASD

The term "sleep problems" encompasses a variety of phenotypes, including several well-characterized sleep disorders. Although there is no official system for classifying pediatric sleep disorders, common systems have developed around the adult literature and clinical practice.

The most widely used system is the International Classification of Sleep Disorders: Diagnostic and Coding Manual (American Academy of Sleep Medicine, 2005), which defines the following classes of sleep disorders: insomnia, sleep related breathing disorders, hypersomnias, circadian rhythm disorders, parasomnias, sleep related movement disorders, isolated symptoms, and other sleep disorders. Each of these classes is further subdivided based on etiology or presentation. Children with ASD most commonly present with a subset of these sleep disorders, and this chapter will focus on this subset.

Insomnia

The most common sleep problem experienced by children with ASD is insomnia. Over half of 167 parents surveyed with a modified Children's Sleep Habits Questionnaire (see section on screening) reported that their child with ASD experienced insomnia 5 to 7 nights per week (Liu, Hubbard, et al., 2006). In practice, insomnia is an umbrella term that includes problems that contribute to difficulty initiating sleep or difficulty maintaining sleep. Diagnostically, the American Academy of Sleep Medicine defines insomnia as persistent difficulty with sleep initiation, maintenance, or quality that occurs despite opportunities for sufficient sleep and that results in daytime impairment (The American Academy of Sleep Medicine). In many cases the diagnosis may come from parent report rather than directly from the child. A child with insomnia may present with difficult behavior surrounding bedtime routines, impaired daytime functioning, or daytime sleepiness.

Two major contributors to insomnia are difficulty falling asleep once in bed and waking during the night. This same previously mentioned study found that the average sleep latency, or the time that it takes for a child to fall asleep once in bed, was 33 minutes, although it was reported to be as long as 150 minutes in some cases (Liu, Hubbard, et al., 2006). This large variation is supported by another study that compared parent assessment of sleep problems to objective laboratory assessment (Malow, Marzec, et al., 2006). Children who were assessed by their parents as having moderate or severe sleep problems were found to have an average sleep latency of 97 minutes. This was significantly longer than the average 30-minute sleep latency in children with ASD but mild or no sleep problems. This suggests that when sleep problems are present, difficulty initiating sleep is a common occurrence. Difficulty falling asleep is also reported as a primary concern among parents (Malow, Marzec, et al., 2006). Bedtime resistance may be a behavioral issue, related to hypersensitivity, or other problem behaviors, or it may indicate an underlying abnormality in circadian rhythm.

Another symptom of insomnia is awakening during the night. Night wakings are normal and benign in children less than six months of age, but persist in approximately 25 to 50% of children after this age (Mindell & Owens, 2003). Waking during the night is frequently a result of negative sleep associations. Children who share a bed, or who require a specific stimulus to fall asleep are more likely to wake during the night. If the stimulus, such as parent's presence, is not available during the might then returning to sleep can be difficult. Parents may not be aware that their child wakes during the night if the child stays in his or her own room. Actigraphy can be used to assess sleep/wake patterns. A 1995 study of 39 children with autism found that night wakings were common, occurring as often as 3.2 nights per 2-week period.

In nearly half of these cases the child was awake for longer than 30 minutes (Richdale & Prior, 1995).

Insomnia can be caused by a variety of different factors. The ICSD-2 divides insomnias by causative factor including adjustment insomnia, psychophysiological insomnia, paradoxical insomnia, idiopathic insomnia, insomnia due to mental disorder, inadequate sleep hygiene, behavioral insomnia of childhood, insomnia due to drug or substance, insomnia due to medical condition, and insomnia not otherwise specified (American Academy of Sleep Medicine, 2005). While insomnia is usually considered to be a disorder experienced by adults, many of these factors may be relevant to children with ASD and will be discussed.

Adjustment Insomnia

Adjustment insomnia is marked by the occurrence of a specific stressor and is transient. The stressor may be a new environment but may also be a recent change in the child's life that is not clearly associated with bedtime. Children with ASD may be predisposed to adjustment insomnia due to difficulties in transitions that are inherent to the disorder. Parents who mention a recent onset of insomnia should be queried about the duration and about any changes that may have taken place in the child's life at that time. In many cases this type of insomnia will resolve on its own once the child has adjusted to a new environment.

Inadequate Sleep Hygiene

Sleep hygiene refers to the physical and behavioral environment surrounding sleep. Good sleep hygiene, or positive sleep habits, promote healthy sleep and eliminate factors that might disturb sleep. Good sleep hygiene practices include: maintaining regular and developmentally appropriate bedtimes and out-of-bedtimes; making the bedroom a media-free zone (no television, computers, video games, etc.); establishing a regular bedtime routine that is conducive to sleep (e.g., nightly bath, story, etc.); avoidance of caffeine and stimulation activity in close proximity to bedtime, and appropriate parent/caretaker expectations. Poor sleep hygiene may contribute or exacerbate sleep problems.

Behavioral Insomnia of Childhood, Limit-Setting Type

Limit-setting sleep disorder is an inability to go to sleep due to insufficient enforcement of good bedtime behaviors by parents (Mindell & Owens, 2003). In some cases parents are inconsistent with bedtime. In the absence of consistent structure, children are more likely to resist or completely refuse bedtime on any given night. This results in delayed sleep onset and shorter total sleep time, although sleep quality after onset is usual normal (Meltzer & Mindell, 2006). Children may also experience symptoms of insomnia if parents do not teach them good sleep hygiene. Allowing children to fall asleep with the television on, have access to video games after bedtime, or fall asleep in the parents bed are all examples of behaviors that will impair sleep by failing to set appropriate limits. Data published in 2006 from a survey of parents regarding their children with ASD reported that over half of the 167 participating children expressed resistance to bedtime and 16% shared a bed with parents (Liu, Hubbard, et al., 2006). This rate of cosleeping in a study with an average participant age of 8.8 years is considerably higher than a typically developing population at the same age. Limit-setting insomnia should be ruled out or identified and addressed through behavioral means in any investigation of pediatric insomnia. Particularly with cosleeping, parents may feel that falling asleep in mom or dad's bed is acceptable if it helps a child who will not fall asleep alone. However, accommodating a child's difficulty with bedtime either masks a potentially treatable intrinsic insomnia or causes primary insomnia. Parents should be queried about their bedtime routine with the child.

Behavioral Insomnia of Childhood, Sleep-Onset Association Type

Sleep-onset association type insomnia refers to a situation in which a child cannot fall asleep without a particular stimulus present (Meltzer & Mindell, 2006). Commonly reported negative stimuli include needing a parent present to fall asleep or needing to be driven around in the car. These behavioral accommodations are typically not sustainable and negatively impact parents' lives to a significant degree. When the required stimulus is not present, bedtime resistance and insomnia develops. As with limit-setting insomnia, the stimulus becomes either a mask for other etiology, or it becomes an obstacle to consistent healthy sleep patterns. This behavioral disorder typically occurs in toddlers or young children, but may be present at older ages in children with developmental disorders. When identified in parent-interview, sleep-onset association disorder can be addressed with behavioral changes called extinction that will gradually wean the child off the stimulus.

Insomnia Due to Other Medical Problems

Children with ASD are at risk for other medical problems and frequently receive psychotropic medications, both of which can impact sleep. Medical problems can include gastrointestinal problems such as gastroesophageal reflux and be particularly bothersome in relation to sleep. Epilepsy, which is resent in approximately one third of children with ASD (Giovanardi Rossi, Posar, et al., 2000), may also impact sleep. Partial seizures of temporal lobe origin have been found to reduce REM sleep in adults, even when the seizures occur during the day (Bazil, Castro, et al., 2000). REM sleep has been implicated in memory consolidation and learning. The possibility that sleep problems may be secondary to an existing medical condition, as well as a review of the medications a child is receiving, deserve consideration when children with ASD are experiencing sleep problems.

Sleep Related Breathing Disorders

Sleep disordered breathing (SDB) is a respiratory sleep disorder that involves some degree of obstruction to upper airways. SDB ranges from primary snoring to severe obstructive sleep apnea (OSA). Primary snoring does occur and can be benign, but snoring is more often a sign that OSA is present. OSA is a severe form of SDB and occurs when airflow ceases completely due to upper-airway obstruction. Signs of OSA include a repeated sequence of a snore, silence (breathing stops), and a gasp or snort as breathing resumes (Mindell & Owens, 2003). This sequence can cause small disruptions in sleep. These disruptions may be imperceptible to the patient but nonetheless fragment sleep and may result in daytime sleepiness and daytime cognitive/behavior problems including inattention and hyperactivity. Risk factors for OSA include tonsilar hypertrophy, obesity, hypotonia, family history, and ethnicity (higher in African American children; Mindell & Owens, 2003). OSA can be treated with weight-loss (when obesity is present), tonsillectomy and/or adenoidectomy, or continuous airway pressure (CPAP) when not otherwise resolved (Meltzer & Mindell, 2006). Children with ASD may have difficulty tolerating CPAP and may need a period of desensitization. Sleep disordered breathing has been reported by parents to occur in nearly 25% of surveyed children with ASD, although more data regarding the exact prevalence is needed (Liu, Hubbard, et al., 2006).

Circadian Rhythm Abnormalities

Circadian rhythm abnormalities include disruptions in the sleep-wake cycle that prohibit normal sleep. The most common type of circadian rhythm abnormality is delayed sleep phase syndrome (DSPS). This is an abnormality in circadian rhythm that results in sleep onset more than 2 hours after normal sleep time (Meltzer & Mindell, 2006). As the name implies, the child's internal circadian rhythm is active but latent. Children with DSPS do not respond to typical cues for sleep onset, such as low light or regular bedtime, but do experience appropriate sleep duration and quality after sleep onset at a later time. The two signs of DSPS are (1) a child who falls asleep easily and consistently at a delayed hour, or (2) a child who is predictably difficult to wake the next morning, but who will wake on their own if allowed to sleep in (Meltzer & Mindell, 2006). DSPS is most often addressed with behavioral changes to the sleep-wake schedule. Specifically, the child is slowly (over a period of several weeks or months) retrained to a more appropriate sleep cycle by using the natural sleep time as a starting point and gradually moving bedtime forward.

It is unclear exactly how common DSPS is in children with ASD but it appears to occur with at an elevated prevalence from the general pediatric population. A 2008 study of regression and disturbed sleep in children with autism found that 16% of children with nonregressive autism and 35% of children with regressive onset autism had DSPS (Giannotti, Cortesi, et al., 2008). Both of these rates were significantly different from the reported 1% of typically developing controls with DSPS. Diagnosis was based on parent report questionnaire and sleep diary. Other studies support the presence and significance of this problem in children with autism. Wiggs and Stores collected sleep data from parent report, sleep diary, and actigraphy on 69 families with an ASD child (Wiggs & Stores, 1996). Of the 44 children who reported disturbed sleep, 4 experienced symptoms of DSPS. This same study found that a second circadian rhythm abnormality, irregular sleep phase syndrome, was reported in 2 of the 44 children. Additional objective studies are needed to accurately assess the prevalence of DSPS in children with ASD, but it does appear to be a prevalent complaint.

Parasomnias

Parasomnias refer to problems that disturb sleep after it has been initiated. These include bruxism, nightmares, night terrors, sleepwalking, and REM sleep behavior disorder. Bruxism is the term used for repetitive teeth grinding during sleep. Approximately 14 to 20% of children in the general pediatric population grind their teeth during sleep, but this prevalence is likely higher in children with developmental or cognitive delays. Children are rarely aware of the condition, and parents who hear the grinding most often identify it. Bruxism can cause dental damage and may also cause muscle pain and headaches. Nightmares or frightening dreams may affect as many as 50% of young children, with decreasing prevalence as children age (Mindell & Owens, 2003). Removing negative or overstimulating images from the bedroom or practicing relaxation techniques prior to bedtime may help alleviate nightmares. Night terrors are episodes of waking during the night and expressing symptoms of intense fear. Night terrors differ from nightmares in that they occur during slow-wave sleep rather then REM sleep, generally occur earlier in the evening, and are rarely recalled by children.

Sleepwalking occurs in as many as 40% of children, and 3 to 4% experience episodes either monthly or weekly (Mindell & Owens, 2003). Sleepwalking has a strong genetic component, and a family history may be present in as many as 90% of cases. Although sleepwalking is benign, parents are able to protect the child from secondary injury by locking doors and windows, gating stairs, and removing obstructions or dangerous objects from the child's environment. If episodes occur at predictable times, scheduled awakenings can be planned to avoid the episode. Waking the child every night 15 to 20 minutes prior to the episode for 1 to 2 weeks may resolve the problem.

REM sleep behavior disorder (RBD) is a less commonly observed parasomnia, but may be more common in children with ASD than typically developing children. During healthy REM sleep there is muscular paralysis. RBD is characterized by loss of this atonia, resulting in patients acting out dreams. Patients may kick or punch the air, run from bed, or demonstrate other complex muscle movements (American Academy of Sleep Medicine, 2005). Daytime sleepiness may be observed if sleep is fragmented as a result of RBD. In the general population RBD most often occurs in adult males and is associated with neurodegenerative disease such as Parkinson's, Alzheimer's dementia, and multiple sclerosis. Evidence suggests that RBD may also occur at an increased incidence in children with ASD. A polysomnographic study of 11 children with a DSM-IV diagnosis of autism, ages 3 to 9 years, found that 5 met criteria for RBD (Thirumalai, Shubin, et al., 2002). RBD should be diagnosed by polysomnography, but is suggested if parents report observing any of the symptoms above. RBD may occur in combination with other sleep disorders.

As a group, parasomnias are reported to occur in approximately 53% of children with ASD. The most common parasomnia reported in this group is bruxism (18%). A reported 4% of children with ASD sleepwalk, 5% awaken during the night with inconsolable screaming, and 4% awaken from a frightening dream. Questions that may trigger identification of parasomnias are available in the CSHQ (see section on evaluation below).

Sleep Related Movement Disorders

Restless leg syndrome (RLS) is characterized by unpleasant sensations that are associated with a desire to move, and relief with such movement. These sensations occur more frequently at rest or lying down and during the evening (ICSD-2). RLS is usually considered in adults, but can have its onset in childhood. RLS is often, although not always, associated with periodic leg movement disorder (PLMD). PLMD is characterized by brief (second) jerks during non-REM sleep. These rapid movements may be accompanied by short arousals. Although the etiology of these disorders is unknown, RLS may include a history of iron-deficient anemia. Further, there appears to be a genetic component, and a family history of RLS is associated with increased risk. RLS is also associated with a diagnosis of ADHD (Mindell & Owens, 2003). RLS may be difficult to diagnosis in children with autism without polysomnography due to core deficits in communication. RLS may present as difficulty falling asleep or difficulty staying in bed at bedtime. While the diagnosis of RLS is based on clinical criteria, the diagnosis of PLMD is based on the findings of overnight polysomnography ("sleep study"), which may suggest or support the diagnosis of RLS in those children unable to provide sufficient clinical information.

Etiology

The etiology of sleep problems in children with ASD is likely multifactorial, including genetic and environmental factors as well as medical and behavioral issues. Disturbances in the sleep-wake cycle may contribute to the occurrence of sleep problems in these children. The sleep-wake cycle is regulated by many factors but the primary driving force is the circadian rhythm, which is the cycle of sleep-related hormones and internal signals. Disorders of the circadian rhythm can produce sleep problems, most commonly difficulty initiating and maintaining sleep. The circadian clock is located in the suprachiasmatic nucleus of the hypothalamus and, among other things, determines the release of sleep-related hormones such as melatonin. The circadian clock, in combination with changes in light, determines the production of melatonin from the pineal gland. Bright light suppresses melatonin production, but in dim-light conditions the level of endogenous melatonin can be measured using saliva, and the time of melatonin increase, referred to as dim-light melatonin onset (DMLO), can be used as a marker for circadian rhythm. Typically the DMLO should occur just prior to average time of sleep onset. Studies indicate that melatonin regulation in children with ASD may be abnormal compared to controls. Specifically, children with ASD may have elevated melatonin levels during the day and decreased levels of melatonin at night (Ritvo, Ritvo, et al., 1993; Nir, Meir, et al., 1995; Kulman, Lissoni, et al., 2000). This pattern is the opposite from that seen in typically developing children. A 2005 study assessed 6-sulphatoxymelatonin, a primary melatonin metabolite that is excreted in urine, and found that children with ASD showed significantly lower concentrations of 6-SM relative to age- and gender-matched controls (Tordjman, Anderson, et al., 2005). These studies together suggest that circadian rhythm abnormalities may more common in children with ASD and likely contribute to disturbed sleep in children with ASD.

Impact

Daytime Functioning

Sleep problems experienced by children are frequently associated with disturbances in neurocognition and behavior. In children, common consequences of poor sleep include difficulty with mood regulation and impulse control, hyperactivity or daytime sleepiness, poor concentration, and impaired memory. The impact of impaired sleep on daytime functioning may be even more severe in children with poor self-regulation, a deficit common in children with ASD. Poor sleep may exacerbate existing behavioral problems.

Data collected by the Autism Treatment Network (ATN) in 2006 found quantitative impairments in daytime functioning in children with ASD and sleep problems. Participants were 54 parents of children with a diagnosis on the autism spectrum, confirmed by ADI and ADOS. Parents reported their child's sleep using the Children's Sleep Habits Questionnaire (CSHQ) and completed behavioral questionnaires, including the Aberrant Behavior Checklist (ABC), the Child Behavior Checklist (CBCL), the Pervasive Developmental Disorder Behavior Index (PDDBI), and the Behavior Rating Inventory for Executive Functioning (BRIEF). Parents who reported sleep problems on the CSHQ also reported significantly increased scores in several behavioral subdomains.

Children were reported to have increased irritability, stereotypy, and hyperactivity, as well as deficits in executive function, including planning and organization.

These observations are consistent with reports from other studies indicating that poor nighttime sleep negatively impacts daytime functioning. In a study of children with an ADOS confirmed diagnosis of ASD and who underwent polysomnography, children with poor sleep were scored significantly higher by their caregivers on the affective problems scale of the Child's Behavior Checklist (CBCL) than children with good sleep (Malow, Marzec, et al., 2006). A study of questionnaire data from 55 parents who self-identified as having a child with ASD (ages 5–12 years) found that children with sleep problems also had more severe autism symptoms, as assessed using the Gilliam Autism Rating Scale (Schreck, Mulick, et al., 2004). Parent-report data from a study of 32 children with Asperger's syndrome (AS) or high functioning autism (HFA) indicates that children with AS/HFA and insomnia have more severe autism behaviors, as measured by the Autism Spectrum Screening Questionnaire, and worsened social behaviors, as assessed by the Strengths and Difficulties Questionnaire (Allik, Larsson, et al., 2006).

The majority of studies of sleep and behavior have found a statistical association, but do not provide support for a clear causal relationship, However, there is evidence that improving sleep problems improves behavior. A case study a 5-year-old female with pervasive developmental disorder not-otherwise-specified, and sleep disordered breathing found improved socialization and reduced stereotypy (Malow, McGrew, et al., 2006). Studies in typically developing children have also found improved behavior with successful treatment of sleep problems, although these results have not yet been replicated in large number in children with ASD. A study of children ages five to 13 years who underwent adenenotonsillectomy as treatment for sleep-disordered breathing found that hyperactivity was reduced in these children, and that attention improved (Chervin, Ruzicka, et al., 2006).

Sleep problems in children can also impact parents' sleep and cause significant stress for the family. Parents of children with sleep problems are more likely to have difficulty sleeping themselves, in part due to demands placed on them by the child's nighttime arousal. A study of 32 children with ASD and their parents found that not only did children have poorer sleep quality than a control group of 25 typically developing children, but parents of the ASD group reported significantly earlier wake times, shorter time in bed, and shorter actual sleep time than parents of the typically developing group (Meltzer, 2008). Parents of children with ASD also report higher levels of daytime stress, particularly if the child's daytime behavior was worsened due to poor sleep. It is not clear whether there is a causal relationship between poor sleep and parental daytime stress. However, a 2001 study found that when the child's sleep problems were successfully treated, the level of maternal stress was reduced. Paternal stress was not affected by improved sleep in the child, although father's satisfaction with their own sleep was improved in the treatment group (Wiggs & Stores, 2001). It is possible that the relationship between child's sleep problems and parental stress is bidirectional.

Screening and Identification

Parent Report

Parent report measures are a quick and easy way for clinicians to screen for sleep problems. The two most commonly used measures in the pediatric population are the Children's Sleep Habits Questionnaire (CSHQ)(Owens, Spirito, et al., 2000a) and the BEARS. However, other instruments are available, including screening guidelines for obstructive sleep apnea (American Academy of Pediatrics, 2002). Due to the overwhelming evidence that sleep problems occur frequently in children with autism, significantly impact cognition and behavior, contribute to family stress, and may be treatable, it is imperative that all children with a diagnosis of autism spectrum disorder be assessed for the presence of comorbid sleep problems, either at the time of first diagnosis or during follow-up care.

The BEARS is a clinician-administered questionnaire that consists of five items and allows parents to report the presence of bedtime issues. These include problems with bedtime and initiating sleep, excessive daytime sleepiness, night awakenings, regularity and duration of sleep, and snoring. See below for a list of BEARS items and sample questions. These questions may be modified to best query for the child's age and developmental level.

BEARS (Owens & Dalzell, 2005)

1. Bedtime: Does your child have any problems going to **B**ed or any problems falling asleep?
2. Excessive daytime sleepiness: Does your child seem **E**xcessively sleepy during the day and/or have difficulty waking up in the morning?
3. Awakenings: Does your child **A**waken during the night or have any unusual behaviors during the night?
4. Regularity and Duration of Sleep: Does your child have a **R**egular sleep schedule and get enough sleep each night?
5. Snoring: Does your child **S**nore or have any problems breathing during the night?

If parents answer yes to any of the five questions then the clinician is prompted to ask about the specifics of the problem. This instrument allows clinicians to inquire about sleep problems during a routine clinic visit, and, without being overly burdensome, will provide the clinician with some indication of need for further evaluation or for referral for formal sleep evaluation. The BEARS was developed by Judith Owens and has been used clinically since 2005 (Owens & Dalzell, 2005).

The Children's Sleep Habits Questionnaire (CSHQ) is a parent-report questionnaire developed by Judith Owens for use in children ages 4–12 years (Owens, Spirito, et al., 2000a). Parents are asked to rate each of 33 sleep-disturbance items based on their frequency during a "typical" recent week. Behaviors are rated on a 3-point scale: "usually" if the behavior occurred 5 to 7 times per week; "sometimes" for 2 to 4 times per week; and "rarely" for 1 or fewer times per week. The CSHQ asks parents to report how often their child has experienced each of a list of specific sleep behaviors during the past 7 days, e.g., snoring. Parents are also asked to separately report whether or not the behavior was a problem. Parent responses are numerically coded and classified into eight domain scores: (1) Bedtime Resistance; (2) Sleep Onset Delay; (3) Sleep Duration; (4) Sleep Anxiety; (5) Nightwakings; (6) Parasomnias; (7) Sleep Disordered Breathing; and (8) Daytime Sleepiness. All items contribute to a composite score, which has been shown to be clinically significant. Children who have a composite sleep score greater than 41 are considered to have sleep problems and should be considered for further evaluation. The CSHQ is designed based on common clinical presentations of the sleep disorders most often seen in children, and specific answers will provide some characterization of problems that are present.

Information about the child's sleep-wake cycle over a period of days can be collected using a sleep diary. The clinician can choose the duration of a sleep diary, but a typical period is 1 to 2 weeks. An informative sleep diary should allow parents to complete a continuous measure of their child's sleep over the period, clearly delineating sleep and wake periods. Each 24-hour period should be recorded as fully as possible, including naps and nighttime waking (if observed by parents). Parents should also be asked to provide a daily log of their child's routine and diet, including bedtime, consumption of caffeinated beverages, medications that might affect sleep, or any deviation from the typical routine. An example of a sleep diary is included in Figure 26-1. The sleep diary differs from other parent-report measures in that it is a structured free report rather than guided response, and because it provides more comprehensive child's sleep over a period of days. If parents are encouraged to complete the diary diligently, it may be possible to identify variation in sleep patterns from night to night as well as provide a better understanding of the home environment and some assessment of sleep latency (if the child is put to bed at 8:00 PM but sleep does not begin until 9:00 PM).

Objective Assessment

Nighttime sleep can be assessed objectively at home by using a physical activity monitor called an actigraph. Children can wear the watch-sized actigraph on their wrist or, if necessary, on their ankle. The actigraph contains a motion sensor that records activity over a period of time, often 1 or more weeks. Data from actigraphy provides a measure of all waking and sleep time, including exact times that the child went to sleep and all naps. When combined with information regarding bedtime and out-of-bed time, this data can be used to calculate sleep latency, total sleep time, and sleep efficiency (the percent of time in bed that is spent asleep). Caregivers should be asked to complete a concurrent daily sleep diary to provide a context for the data and aid in interpretation. The most informative actigraphy data relies on compliance from both the parents and the child. Children with sensory issues may have difficulty wearing a novel object, although undergoing a period of desensitization prior to beginning data collection may help address this difficulty.

Polysomnography (PSG) is the "gold standard" for assessing sleep (Meltzer & Mindell, 2006) and provides information regarding sleep architecture and disruption. PSG combines electroencephalogram (EEG), electromyogram (EMG), and electro-oculogram (EOG), with additional assessment of respiratory activity to quantitatively describe all aspects of the child's sleep over the course of a given night. Although PSG is widely acknowledged as the best tool for diagnosing and characterizing the sleep, and specifically sleep disorders such as PLMD and sleep disordered breathing, it has several drawbacks. Chiefly, PSG only provides data from a single or short series of nights rather than an assessment over a larger time period. The children are evaluated in the unfamiliar environment of a clinical sleep laboratory. Many children with ASD may experience difficulty tolerating the placement of the sensors and the novel environment of the sleep laboratory. Careful planning and preparation of the child and the parents are necessary for the successful completion of the polysomnographic study (Mindell, Emslie, et al., 2006).

Treatment

It is critical that sleep problems be reliably identified because there are interventions available that can alleviate or cure the problems and possibly improve the consequent adverse behavioral and cognitive effects. Parents are frequently under the misconception that the sleep problems are "part of the autism" and that they cannot be treated. Both behavioral and pharmacological treatments exist and can be used in this population. Figure 26-2 presents an algorithm for screening children for sleep problems and referral for sleep evaluation or other subspecialty evaluation.

Treatment of sleep problems in children with ASD can be complicated by the many other medications and therapies that are used to treat these children. However, it is import to first manage medical and behavior problems that may contribute or exacerbate sleep problems. Specific sleep disorders such as obstructive sleep apnea should be appropriately evaluated and managed. In general, guidelines published by the American Academy of Pediatrics mandate that sleep problems should be treated first with behavioral therapy (Mindell, Emslie, et al., 2006). If problems persist, consideration can be given to use of pharmacologic sleep aids.

CONTINUOUS SLEEP DIARY

Please shade times during which the child was asleep. If the child is wearing an activity monitor, please indicate time when the watch was taken off and put back on with two vertical bars connected by a line.

Date	12:00 PM	1:00 PM	2:00 PM	3:00 PM	4:00 PM	5:00 PM	6:00 PM	7:00 PM	8:00 PM	9:00 PM	10:00 PM	11:00 PM	12:00 AM	1:00 AM	2:00 AM	3:00 AM	4:00 PM	5:00 AM	6:00 AM	7:00 AM	8:00 AM	9:00 AM	10:00 AM	11:00 AM
Ex.																								
__-__																								
__-__																								
__-__																								
__-__																								
__-__																								
__-__																								
__-__																								

DAILY SLEEP DIARY

1. Who completed this diary? (e.g., Mother, Father, caregiver, etc.)

   ____

2. What time did your child go to bed last night? __ __:__ __AM/AM

3. What time did your child get up this morning? __ __:__ __AM/AM

4. Did your child go to school yesterday? Yes or No (circle one)

5. Was your child sick yesterday? Yes or No (circle one)

6. Did your child start any new medications yesterday? (circle one)

   Yes or No

   If so, list medications: ______________________________

7. Did your child stop any old medications yesterday? Yes or No (circle one)
   If so, list medications:

8. How many 8 oz. beverages containing caffeine did your child drink yesterday? ______

9. How would rate your child's sleep last night overall? (circle one)

   Very good   Good   Fair   Poor   Very Poor

8. Please add any comments you think may be relevant to your child's sleep, e.g. travel, specials events, etc: ______________________________

____

Figure 26–1. Sleep diary.

Behavioral Therapy

Sleep hygiene refers to bedtime practices, and particularly those that promote sleep onset and healthy sleep. Good sleep hygiene habits include setting a consistent and developmentally appropriate bedtime, removing electronics from the bedroom, avoiding caffeine, developing a step-down routine for bedtime and an appropriate bedtime ritual, and adjusting the environmental conditions to help entrain the circadian rhythm cycle. Low light and cool temperatures in the evening will help promote sleep onset, and bright light and warmer temperatures will help promote wakefulness. Exposure to early morning bright light helps advance the sleep phase, while evening bright light may delay sleep onset. An appropriate sleep hygiene plan should be developed in discussion with the family to meet their needs and ensure appropriate expectations. Sleep hygiene may not resolve sleep problems completely, but can contribute to improvement of the child's sleep and may be used in concert with other behavioral and pharmacological therapies.

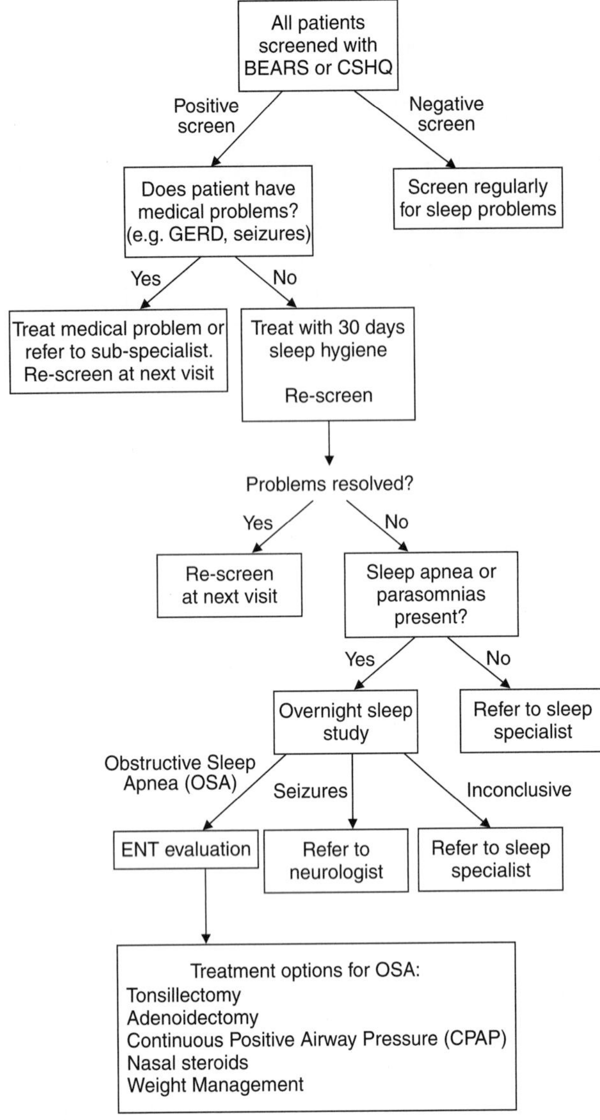

Figure 26–2. Decision tree for screening and assessment of sleep problems in children with autism spectrum disorder.

Specific behavioral interventions can be developed to address sleep-onset association and limit-setting type insomnia. Extinction involves putting the child to bed at a particular bedtime and then ignoring the child's inappropriate behaviors until the following morning. This technique forces children to resolve their need for a particular stimulus on their own, although it may be unpalatable to parents. Graduated extinction allows parents to check on the child, but with increasing delay over a period of 1 to 2 weeks. As with extinction, the goal is to wean children off sleep associations that are unsustainable and teach children to "self-soothe"(Mindell & Owens, 2003). Other step-down rituals can be devised based on the child's ability to tolerate bedtime changes and the parents desire to institute good bedtime habits. High-functioning children may respond to incentive-based interventions. In this case it is important to select incentives that are desired and that can be immediately awarded.

Pharmacotherapies

If behavioral therapy fails to address the child's sleep problems, treatment with a pharmacologic agent may be indicated. Many parents treat the symptoms of their child's sleep problem with secondary pharmacologic agents, often without a physician's oversight. Regardless of whether the treatment is prescription or over-the-counter, a physician should work with parents to develop and oversee a good plan for pharmacologic management. However, the lack of evidence supporting most pharmacological treatments has left parents and physicians without a reliable roadmap.

The lack of attention to pharmacologic management of sleep problems in children with autism may be due to the lack of treatment studies children in general. In response to this dearth of published evidence, the AAP has identified children with ASD as a high priority population for clinical trials of pharmacologic sleep therapies (Mindell, Emslie, et al., 2006). However, several studies have been released that build on existing literature to provide evidence for several different pharmacologic treatments of sleep problems in these children. Additionally, a consensus paper was published in 2005 that reviewed commonly used pharmacologic treatments for insomnia (Owens, Babcock, et al., 2005). This statement sets forth recommendations for treatment and dosing that are based primarily on clinical experience rather than evidence based on well-designed and controlled clinical trials.

This consensus statement and other published reviews discuss prescription and nonprescription medications that are commonly used to treat insomnia. Typically these are in the class of sedatives or hypnotics, although some psychotropic medications provide secondary benefits to sleep. As yet there are no pediatric guidelines for pharmacologic management of sleep problems, and the FDA has not approved any medications labeled for treatment of pediatric sleep problems. We present here a summary of the most frequently used medications. In particular, more evidence is needed to fully assess the use of these medications in children with ASD (Mindell, Emslie, et al., 2006). Pharmacologic intervention should be initiated after a thorough sleep evaluation and should be paired with behavioral interventions.

Melatonin

Melatonin is an endogenous neuropetide that is secreted by the pineal gland in response to signals from the circadian clock. Typically, endogenous melatonin levels are low during the day and peak prior to nighttime sleep onset, although evidence (discussed previously in this chapter) indicates that this rhythm may be disrupted in some children with ASD. This explanation of sleep problems in this population theoretically supports treatment with exogenous melatonin, although as yet the literature has not connected a response to treatment with melatonin to an underlying melatonin abnormality. Regardless, exogenous melatonin is a commonly used over-the-counter sleep aid. Melatonin has been studied in children with ASD and found to be a safe and effective treatment for insomnia.

A 2006 double-blinded, placebo-controlled cross-over trial in 11 children found that 5 mg of melatonin daily for 4 weeks significantly reduced both sleep latency and number of night wakings (Garstang & Wallis, 2006). These results have been supported by two open-label trials in children with ASD. An open-label study of the long-term safety and efficacy of melatonin was conducted in a group of 25 children with autism. Children were given 3 mg of controlled release melatonin at the start of the study, but were titrated up to as much as 6 mg per day if necessary. The study found that after 24 weeks patients had improved sleep, as evidenced by sleep diary and CSHQ. Further, children who discontinued melatonin at 16 weeks returned to disturbed sleep patterns but showed improvement after treatment resumed (Giannotti, Cortesi, et al., 2006). A large-scale clinical trial of melatonin in 107 children ages 2–18 showed that melatonin effectively resolved sleep problems in 25% of patients at doses of melatonin starting at 0.75 mg per day and titrated up to 6 mg as necessary. An additional 60% of patients reported improved sleep, although sleep problems were still present. Only three patients in this study reported experiencing side effects including morning sleepiness and increased enuresis, which resolved when the dose was lowered (Andersen, Kaczmarska, et al., 2008). Other studies have found that patients did not experience any side effects as a result of the melatonin. These studies support the use of melatonin to treat insomnia in children with ASD. Possible side effects of melatonin include hypotension, bradycardia, nausea, and headache. Melatonin may also exacerbate comorbid autoimmune diseases (Owens, Babcock, et al., 2005).

Clonidine

Catapres, known by the trade name of Clonidine, is an alpha-adrenergic receptor agonist that was originally developed as a nasal decongestant for adults. During initial clinical trials investigators observed that Clonidine had bradycardic and hypotensive effects, and it has since become a treatment for hypertension (Reed & Findling, 2002). Although Clonidine may cause insomnia in adults, it is soporific in children and is commonly prescribed to treat sleep problems in children with neurological disorders as well as ADHD (Reed & Findling, 2002). Clonidine may also be used to treat problems with impulsivity, inattention, and hyperactivity. Clonidine is not labeled to treat pediatric sleep problems, although studies have shown that it can improve insomnia in some children. A 1996 study found that Clonidine improved sleep problems in 85% of 62 children with ADHD, ages 4 to 17 years (Prince, Wilens, et al., 1996). Data from a 2008 open-label study of Clonidine in 19 children with ASD showed that parent report of sleep initiation improved, and that side effects were tolerable. Reported side effects from this study included lethargy, tachycardia, daytime sedation, and hypotension (Ming, Gordon, et al., 2008). These side effects were rare, and in only one case was the child withdrawn from the study due to side effects. Bradycardia, dry mouth, and depressed consciousness have also been reported (Reed & Findling, 2002).

Benzodiazapines

Benzodiazepines have historically been used to treat adult anxiety disorders and as sedatives and anticonvulsants in pediatric patients. Medications in this class function as gamma-aminobutyric acid (GABA) agonists to decrease neuronal excitability across the central nervous system. A variety of structurally variant benzodiazepines are now used to help children fall asleep and stay asleep for the course of the night. In particular these medications may be used to suppress night terrors or other partial-arousal parasomnias, as well as to treat circadian rhythm disorders (Reed & Findling, 2002; Mindell & Owens, 2003). The most commonly used of this class are clonazepam (Klonopin), lorazepam (Ativan), flurazeam (Dalmane), quazepam (Doral), temazepam (Restoril), estazolam (ProSam), and triazolam (Halcion) (Reed & Findling, 2002). These medications differ primarily on time of onset, which ranges from 15 minutes to an hour, and half life, which can be 3 to 120 hours (Reed & Findling, 2002). Side effects of benzodiazepines include daytime drowsiness, a worsening of insomnia with withdrawal of the drug (rebound insomnia), other withdrawal symptoms such as phonophobia, photophobia, and seizures, as well as anterograde amnesia (Reed & Findling, 2002). Short-acting benzodiazapines are generally associated with the withdrawal effects and amnesia, while longer-acting variants are more likely to produce daytime residual effects. Clinical trials have been limited to adults and no studies exist in an ASD population. No medications in this class are FDA approved for treatment of pediatric sleep problems, and guidelines for pediatric dosing do not exist.

Zolipidem (Ambien) and Zaleplon (Sonata)

Both Zolipidem and Zaleplon are both used clinically to treat adults and adolescents with primary insomnia (Mindell & Owens, 2003). Similar to benzodiazepines, these medicines act as GABA-agonists to inhibit the central nervous system. Unlike the previous class of medications, zolipidem and zaleplon are associated with limited daytime effects and reduced tolerance. Side effects do include daytime sleepiness, confusion, anterograde amnesia, and rebound insomnia (Mindell & Owens, 2003). Results from studies in children in general are lacking, and no studies have been conducted in children with ASD.

Chloral Hydrate

Chloral hydrate is one of the oldest treatments for sleep problems, although its use has declined since it was introduced in the 1870s (Reed & Findling, 2002). Today chloral hydrate is used to treat sleep-onset delay and circadian rhythm abnormalities, particularly in children with neurologic abnormalities or blindness. Adult studies have not shown chloral hydrate to have a benefit over placebo in treating insomnia. Side effects include gastrointestinal distress, nausea, vomiting, liver toxicity, dizziness, light-headedness, and respirator depression (Mindell & Owens, 2003). Discontinuation after prolonged use can cause withdrawal, including seizures and delirium. Use of chloral hydrate has also been associated with adverse events, including cardiac arrhythmias and central nervous system depression in children (Reed & Findling, 2002).

Antidepressants

Tricyclic and newer serotonergic antidepressants have been used with increasing frequency to treat partial arousals and nocturnal enuresis (Reed & Findling, 2002). Trazadone, nefazodone, and aroxetine are commonly used to treat the former, while imipramine hydrochloride is the most common antidepressant to treat the latter. These medications work by suppressing deep sleep and decreasing arousals during sleep-stage transitions. Side effects of antidepressants include daytime sleepiness and dry mouth. There is also concern for cardiac arrhythmias (Reed & Findling, 2002).

Antihistamines

Antihistamines are the most commonly recommended nonprescription medication for sleep problems. Data published from a survey of community based pediatricians found that 68% of physicians who have recommended a nonprescription medication recommended antihistamine at least once (Owens, Rosen, et al., 2003). Nonprescription antihistamines are also commonly chosen by parents of children with sleep problems without a physician's recommendation. H_1 receptor agonists such as diphenhydramine, hydroxyzine, and chlorpheniramine act by crossing the blood-brain barrier to depress the central nervous system. Decreased alertness and slowed reaction are typically achieved 2 to 3 hours after administration, and half-life ranges from 3 to 9 hours. Side effects include impaired daytime functioning and poor sleep quality (Reed & Findling, 2002). Second- and third-generation antihistamines, such as terfenadine and loraditine, may have fewer residual daytime effects (Mindell & Owens, 2003).

Prognosis (for the Field)

Sleep problems are a frequent and serious concern in children with ASD. Numerous studies have been conducted on the prevalence of sleep problems, and the percent of children with ASD who experience difficulty sleeping ranges from between 44 and 86% (Richdale & Prior, 1995; Wiggs & Stores, 1996; Patzold, Richdale, et al., 1998; Allik, Larsson, et al., 2006). Sleep problems in this group have been consistently found to be more common than in either typically developing or developmentally delayed children. This increased risk and, even at the lowest prevalence estimates, high comorbid occurrence, put sleep problems near the top of the list of medical conditions affecting children with ASD.

Although evidence that children with autism are much more likely than typically developing children to experience disturbed sleep has accumulated over the past decade, the prevailing understanding at one time was that poor sleep was "part of the autism" and did not warrant further clinical attention. In fact, children with ASD and sleep problems may have more impaired neurocognitive functioning and worse behavior than children with ASD and normal sleep (Schreck, Mulick, et al., 2004; Malow, Marzec, et al., 2006).

In response to the high prevalence and clinical severity, sleep problems are diagnosable, often in the pediatrician's office. Expedient screening questionnaires are available, and these can be both administered and assessed by most physicians who see children with ASD (Owens, Spirito, et al., 2000a; Owens & Dalzell, 2005). Referral to a sleep specialist may be necessary, but even in this case screening questionnaires are an efficient and effective way to identify children for further evaluation. Assessment for sleep problems should be a routine part of clinical care for children with ASD.

Available and effective treatments further justify attention to sleep problems in this population. A 2005 consensus statement provides guidelines the use of behavioral and pharmacotherapy by community-based pediatricians (Owens, Babcock, et al., 2005). Behavioral therapy should be tried first, followed by pharmacotherapy if necessary and supervised by a pediatric sleep specialist when possible. Future advancements in this field require data from well-designed clinical trials of sleep medications in children with ASD.

Conclusion

This review supports the opinion that sleep problems in children with ASD are a significant issue that should be part of the routine clinical evaluation of these children. Sleep problems occur frequently in ASD and negatively impact on the child's sleep, as well as the sleep of parents and caretakers. Additionally, sleep problems negatively impact on daytime cognition and behavior of these children, and the quality of life of their families. There is a need for further characterization of specific sleep problems in ASD and comparison of differences and prevalences to children with other developmental problems and typically developing children. Effective treatment has the potential to reverse the nighttime and daytime impact of sleep problems in these children. We are challenged to develop reliable screening paradigms for the primary care physician and the ASD specialists. To develop effective treatment protocols for the sleep problems of children with ASD we need to better understand the pathophysiology and the relationship of other medical problems and medications. Well-designed clinical trials of behavioral and pharmacological therapies are necessary to establish an evidence basis for the management of sleep problems.

Challenges and Future Directions

- Sleep problems should be part of the routine clinical evaluation of children with an autism spectrum disorder.

- Reliable screening paradigms are needed to aid primary care physicians and specialists in evaluating children with ASD.
- Well-designed clinical trials of behavioral and pharmacological therapies are needed to establish an evidence base for management of sleep problems.
- Effective management requires better understanding of the pathophysiology of sleep problems in children with ASD, including relationship to other medical problems and treatments.
- Better understanding of the epidemiology of sleep problems in children with ASD will aid identification and treatment.

REFERENCES

Allik, H., Larsson, J. O., et al. (2006). Insomnia in school-age children with Asperger syndrome or high-functioning autism. *BMC Psychiatry, 6*, 18.

American Academy of Pediatrics. (2002). Clinical practice guideline: Diagnosis and management of childhood obstructive sleep apnea syndrome. *Pediatrics, 109*(4), 704–712.

American Academy of Sleep Medicine. (2005). *International classification of sleep disorders, 2nd ed.: Diagnostic and coding manual.* Westchester, IL: American Academy of Sleep Medicine.

Andersen, I. M., Kaczmarska, J., et al. (2008). Melatonin for insomnia in children with autism spectrum disorders. *Journal of Child Neurology, 23*(5), 482–485.

Bazil, C. W., Castro, L. H., et al. (2000). Reduction of rapid eye movement sleep by diurnal and nocturnal seizures in temporal lobe epilepsy. *Archives of Neurology, 57*(3), 363–368.

Chervin, R. D., Ruzicka, D. L., et al. (2006). Sleep-disordered breathing, behavior, and cognition in children before and after adenotonsillectomy. *Pediatrics, 117*(4), e769–778.

Clements, J., Wing, L., et al. (1986). Sleep problems in handicapped children: A preliminary study. *Journal of Child Psychology and Psychiatry, 27*(3), 399–407.

Couturier, J. L., Speechley, K. N., et al. (2005). Parental perception of sleep problems in children of normal intelligence with pervasive developmental disorders: Prevalence, severity, and pattern. *Journal of the American Academy of Child and Adolescent Psychiatry, 44*(8), 815–822.

Garstang, J., & Wallis, M. (2006). Randomized controlled trial of melatonin for children with autistic spectrum disorders and sleep problems. *Child: Care, Health, and Development, 32*(5), 585–589.

Giannotti, F., Cortesi, F., et al. (2006). An open-label study of controlled-release melatonin in treatment of sleep disorders in children with autism. *Journal of Autism and Developmental Disorders, 36*(6), 741–752.

Giannotti, F., Cortesi, F., et al. (2008). An investigation of sleep characteristics, EEG abnormalities and epilepsy in developmentally regressed and non-regressed children with autism. *Journal of Autism and Developmental Disorders, 38(10), 1888–1897.*

Giovanardi Rossi, P., Posar, A., et al. (2000). Epilepsy in adolescents and young adults with autistic disorder. *Brain and Development, 22*(2), 102–106.

Glaze, D. G. (2004). Childhood insomnia: Why Chris can't sleep. *Pediatric Clinics of North America, 51*(1), 33–50, vi.

Goodlin-Jones, B. L., Tang, K., et al. (2008). Sleep patterns in preschool-age children with autism, developmental delay, and typical development. *Journal of the American Academy of Child and Adolescent Psychiatry, 47*, 930–938.

Honomichl, R. D., Goodlin-B. L., Jones, et al. (2002). Sleep patterns of children with pervasive developmental disorders. *Journal of Autism and Developmental Disorders, 32*(6), 553–561.

Hoshino, Y., Watanabe, H., et al. (1984). An investigation on sleep disturbance of autistic children. *Folia Psychiatrica et Neurologica Japonica, 38*(1), 45–51.

Johnson, K. P., Malow, B. A. (2008). Assessment and pharmacologic treatment of sleep disturbance in autism. *Child and Adolescent Psychiatric Clinics of North America, 17*, 773–785.

Krakowiak, P., Goodlin-Jones, B., et al. (2008). Sleep problems in children with autism spectrum disorders, developmental delays, and typical development: A population-based study. *Journal of Sleep Research, 17*, 197–206.

Kulman, G., Lissoni, P., et al. (2000). Evidence of pineal endocrine hypofunction in autistic children. *Neuroendocrinology Letters, 21*(1), 31–34.

Liu, X., Hubbard, J. A., et al. (2006). Sleep disturbances and correlates of children with autism spectrum disorders. *Child Psychiatry and Human Development, 37*(2), 179–191.

Malow, B. A., Marzec, M. L., et al. (2006). Characterizing sleep in children with autism spectrum disorders: A multidimensional approach. *Sleep, 29*(12), 1563–1571.

Malow, B. A., McGrew, S. G., et al. (2006). Impact of treating sleep apnea in a child with autism spectrum disorder. *Pediatric Neurology, 34*(4), 325–328.

Meltzer, L. J. (2008). Brief report: Sleep in parents of children with autism spectrum disorders. *Journal of Pediatric Psychology, 33*(4), 380–386.

Meltzer, L. J., & Mindell, J. A. (2006). Sleep and sleep disorders in children and adolescents. *Psychiatric Clinics of North America, 29*(4), 1059–1076; abstract x.

Mindell, J. A., Emslie, G., et al. (2006). Pharmacologic management of insomnia in children and adolescents: Consensus statement. *Pediatrics, 117*(6), e1223–1232.

Mindell, J. A., & Owens, J. A. (2003). *A clinical guide to pediatric sleep: Diagnosis and management of sleep problems.* Philadelphia: Lippincott Williams & Wilkins.

Ming, X., Gordon, E., et al. (2008). Use of clonidine in children with autism spectrum disorders. *Brain and Development,* 30(7), 454–460.

Nir, I., Meir, D., et al. (1995). Brief report: Circadian melatonin, thyroid-stimulating hormone, prolactin, and cortisol levels in serum of young adults with autism. *Journal of Autism and Developmental Disorders, 25*(6), 641–654.

Owens, J. A., Babcock, D., et al. (2005). The use of pharmacotherapy in the treatment of pediatric insomnia in primary care: Rational approaches. A consensus meeting summary. *Journal of Clinical Sleep Medicine, 1*(1), 49–59.

Owens, J. A., & Dalzell, V. (2005). Use of the BEARS sleep screening tool in a pediatric residents' continuity clinic: A pilot study. *Sleep Medicine, 6*(1), 63–69.

Owens, J. A., Rosen, C. L., et al. (2003). Medication use in the treatment of pediatric insomnia: Results of a survey of community-based pediatricians. *Pediatrics, 111*(5 Pt 1), e628–635.

Owens, J. A., Spirito, A., et al. (2000a). The Children's Sleep Habits Questionnaire (CSHQ): Psychometric properties of a survey instrument for school-aged children. *Sleep, 23*(8), 1043–1051.

Owens, J. A., Spirito, A., et al. (2000b). Sleep habits and sleep disturbance in elementary school-aged children. *Journal of Developmental and Behavioral Pediatrics, 21*(1), 27–36.

Patzold, L. M., Richdale, A. L., et al. (1998). An investigation into sleep characteristics of children with autism and Asperger's Disorder. *Journal of Paediatrics and Child Health, 34*(6), 528–533.

Prince, J. B., Wilens, T. E., et al. (1996). Clonidine for sleep disturbances associated with attention-deficit hyperactivity disorder: A systematic chart review of 62 cases. *Journal of the American Academy of Child and Adolescent Psychiatry, 35*(5), 599–605.

Quine, L. (1991). Sleep problems in children with mental handicap. *Journal of Mental Deficiency Research, 35*(Pt 4), 269–290.

Reed, M. D., & Findling, R. L. (2002). Overview of current management of sleep disturbances in children: I-Pharmacotherapy. *Current Therapeutic Research, 63*(Suppl B), B18–37.

Richdale, A. L., & Prior, M. R. (1995). The sleep/wake rhythm in children with autism. *European Child and Adolescent Psychiatry, 4*(3), 175–186.

Richdale, A. L., Schreck, K. A. (2009). Sleep problems in autism spectrum disorders: Prevalence, natured, and biopsychosocial aetiologies. *Sleep Medicine Review*, doi: 10.1016/j.smrv.2009.02.003

Ritvo, E. R., Ritvo, R., et al. (1993). Elevated daytime melatonin concentrations in autism: A pilot study. *European Child and Adolescent Psychiatry, 2*(2), 75–78.

Sadeh, A., Raviv, A., et al. (2000). Sleep patterns and sleep disruptions in school-age children. *Developmental Psychology, 36*(3), 291–301.

Schreck, K. A., & Mulick, J. A. (2000). Parental report of sleep problems in children with autism. *Journal of Autism and Developmental Disorders, 30*(2), 127–135.

Schreck, K. A., Mulick, J. A., et al. (2004). Sleep problems as possible predictors of intensified symptoms of autism. *Research in Developmental Disabilities, 25*(1), 57–66.

Thirumalai, S. S., Shubin, R. A., et al. (2002). Rapid eye movement sleep behavior disorder in children with autism. *Journal of Child Neurology, 17*(3), 173–178.

Tordjman, S., Anderson, G. M., et al. (2005). Nocturnal excretion of 6-sulphatoxymelatonin in children and adolescents with autistic disorder. *Biological Psychiatry, 57*(2), 134–138.

Wiggs, L., & Stores, G. (1996). Severe sleep disturbance and daytime challenging behaviour in children with severe learning disabilities. *Journal of Intellectual Disability Research, 40*(Pt 6), 518–528.

Wiggs, L., & Stores, G. (2001). Behavioural treatment for sleep problems in children with severe intellectual disabilities and daytime challenging behaviour: Effect on mothers and fathers. *British Journal of Health and Psychology, 6*(Pt 3), 257–269.

Perspective Article

Christopher Gillberg

Autism as a Medical Disorder

Autism spectrum disorders (ASDs)—including autistic disorder, atypical autism (also referred to as autistic-like condition and pervasive developmental disorder not-otherwise-specified/PDD-NOS), Asperger's disorder, and childhood disintegrative disorder—are often lifelong conditions that are, rightly, considered to be the territory of psychiatrists, psychologists, special education teachers, speech and language pathology therapists (SLPs), geneticists, neurophysiologists, neuroradiologists, and neurochemists. In everyday practice, special education teachers, psychologists, and SLPs are probably the specialists who interact the most with children, adolescents, and adults with ASD and their families. Almost by tradition, ASD has come to be regarded as a set of functional disabilities that are best contained within the realm of "psychoeducation." Only rarely, if at all, is autism looked at from the point of view of general clinical medicine, which is quite surprising, given the great amount of data that exist to suggest that autism is a collection of medical disorders rather than a specific disorder in its own right (Gillberg & Coleman, 2000, 2009).

In population-based studies, children with autistic disorder have an identifiable medical disorder—such as tuberous sclerosis or the Fragile X syndrome—in about 25% of all cases (Gillberg & Coleman, 1996). In males with Asperger's disorder, a similar medical condition may currently be identified in about 15% of all cases (Cederlund & Gillberg, 2005). These figures do not include epilepsy—which occurs in 5% to 40% of individuals with ASD, depending on age, gender, and ASD diagnostic subgroup (highest in autistic disorder, lowest in Asperger's disorder)—as a "medical disorder." In children with autistic disorder seen in specialized clinics, these rates of medical disorders can be either higher or lower, depending on the "niche" of the clinic. In child psychiatric clinics, the rate is likely to be low as a consequence of diagnostic overshadowing. For instance, when tuberous sclerosis is diagnosed in a pediatric or neurologic clinic, there is a high risk that the autistic disorder diagnosis will not be made (because of the stance on the part of the pediatrician or neurologist that *the* diagnosis—tuberous sclerosis—has already been made) and referral to the child psychiatric clinic will not happen, leading to underrepresentation of autism with tuberous sclerosis in the latter setting. On the other hand, in the specialized epilepsy clinic, where the child neurologist may be well aware of the very common co-occurrence of autism, epilepsy, and intellectual disability, the diagnosis of autistic disorder may be made in more than half of the clientele, depending on the number of severely mentally retarded individuals seen in that clinic. This subgroup of children with autism, epilepsy, and severe intellectual disability is likely to have a very high rate of "underlying" or otherwise associated medical disorders.

Conversely, there are a number of conditions, be they "neurological," "neurodevelopmental," or "medical" syndromes, that have a high rate (more than expected by chance, i.e., more than a few percent) or a very high rate (more than twenty percent) of several autism symptoms associated with them, and for which the diagnosis of autistic disorder or ASD is very often appropriate (Gillberg & Coleman, 2000). In the diagnostic category of autistic disorder, each one of these conditions contributes only a small fraction (up to a few percent) of the variance, but, taken together, they account for a very large minority of all cases with autistic disorder.

Conditions that have a More than Coincidental Chance of being Associated with ASD

Several of the "conditions associated with autism" (CAA) are listed in Table PA-1. Some of them, including Down syndrome, have a very much lower rate of autism symptoms than the remainder of these syndromes, but, nonetheless, much higher than expected in the general population. Every medical doctor working with individuals with ASD needs to be aware of the existence of these conditions so that a correct diagnosis can be made as early as possible. The list is not exhaustive, and "new" autism-associated disorders will be discovered over the next several years, illustrating the need for autism doctors to keep abreast of progress in the field of so called behavioral phenotype syndromes, including genetic and toxic disorders.

Some of the CAA have a rather specific link with autism (e.g., tuberous sclerosis, Moebius syndrome, thalidomide embryopathy, and Smith-Lemli-Opitz syndrome), some increase the risk for a whole host of neurodevelopmental problems, including autism, and others probably co-occur with autism, not because they themselves contribute to the risk of

Table PA–1.
Conditions associated with autism spectrum disorders (i.e., conditions with a high rate of associated autistic symptomatology)

Condition	Reference(s)
*Genetic/neurodevelopmental/neurocutaneous syndromes/disorders**	
Angelman	Steffenburg et al., 1996
CHARGE association	Johansson et al., 2006
Cohen	Howlin, 2001
Cornelia De Lange	Bhuyian et al., 2006
Di George (22q11del)	Niklasson, 2009
Down	Howlin et al., 1995
Fragile X	Gillberg, 1983
Fragile X premutation	Aziz et al., 2003
Hypomelanosis of Ito	Akefeldt & Gillberg 1991
Joubert	Holroyd et al., 1991
Klinefelter	Kielinen et al., 2004
	Kleine Levin Berthier et al., 1992
Landau Kleffner	Neville et al., 1997
Lujan-Fryns	Stathopulu et al., 2003
Moebius sequence	Johansson et al., 2001
Neurofibromatosis	Gillberg & Forsell 1984
Noonan	Ghaziuddin et al., 1994
Oculoauriculovertebral spectrum (including Goldenhar)	Johansson et al., 2007
Smith Magenis	Hicks et al., 2008
Smith Lemli Opitz	Tierney et al., 2001
Sotos	Zappella et al., 1992
Tuberous sclerosis	Hunt & Dennis 1987
Williams	Gillberg & Rasmussen 1994
Psychiatric disorders	
ADHD	Gillberg, 1983a
Anorexia nervosa	Gillberg, 1983b
Selective mutism	Kopp & Gillberg, 1997
Tourette syndrome	Kadesjö & Gillberg, 2000
Personality disorders	Anckarsäter et al., 2006
Metabolic disorders	
Ehlers Danlos syndrome	Fehlow et al., 1993
Galactosemia	
Marfan syndrome	Tantam et al., 1990
Mucopolysaccharidosis, including Sanfilippo	Colville & Bax, 1996
Smith-Lemli-Opitz syndrome	Tierney et al., 2000
Movement disorders/neuromuscular disorders	
Cerebral palsy	Goodman, 2002
Developmental coordination disorder (DCD)	Kadesjö & Gillberg, 1999
Catatonia	Wing & Shah, 2000
Duchenne muscular dystrophy	Komoto et al., 1984
Steinert myotrophic dystrophy†	Ekström et al., 2008
Peroxisomal disorders	
Leber congenital amaurosis	Curless et al., 1991
Mitochondrial disorders	
HEADD (Hypotonia, epilepsy, autism, developmental delay)	Fillano et al., 2002
Other mitochondrial disorders	Oliveira et al., 2005
Amino acid disorders	
PKU	separate chapter
Cystathionine beta-symthetase deficiency	separate chapter
Homocysteine	separate chapter
Urea cycle disorders	Görker & Tüzün 2005
Endocrine disorders	
Hypothyroidism	separate chapter
Congenital/perinatal infections	
Rubella	Chess, 1977
Herpes	Gillberg 1986
CMV	Stubbs et al., 1984
Toxoplasmosis	
Teratogenic syndromes/toxins	
Fetal alcohol spectrum disorder†	Aronson et al., 1997
Fetal cocaine syndrome	Davis et al., 1992
Thalidomide syndrome	Strömland et al., 1994
Valproic syndrome	Williams et al., 2001
Disorders affecting the visual system	
Retinopathy of Prematurity/ ROP)	Ek et al., 1998
Other conditions	
Consequences of being born prematurely	Limperopoulos et al., 2005
Effects of perinatal asphyxia and Hypoxic Ischemic Encephalopathyy (HIE)	Badawi et al., 2006

autism, but, just like autism, reflect underlying brain problems that may have identifiable or nonidentifiable underlying causes (e.g., ADHD, DCD, prematurity, and HIE).

Genetic Aspects

Autistic features are highly heritable. The heritability of autistic disorder in cases where there is no diagnosed CAA is on the order of 90%. However, there is no evidence, as yet, that any small number of genes account for most of the variance of this heritability. Instead, a number of different genes have been identified (so far mostly neurodevelopmental, including neuroligin and SHANK-3 genes) that each account for a small proportion of all cases (Lamb, chapter 38, this volume), and it does not seem unreasonable that when they are all taken together, they will explain more than half of the total variance.

Pre-, peri-, neo-, and Postnatal Brain Damage

A number of potentially pre- and perinatal brain damaging factors—including extreme prematurity, postmaturity, and perinatal asphyxia—are known to be statistically associated with a risk of being diagnosed with ASD (Badawi et al., 2006; Limperopolus, 2009; Gillberg & Cederlund, 2005).

What Is the Appropriate Level of Work-up in Individuals Presenting with Autistic Symptomatology?

There is now often animated discussion concerning the need for a "full" medical work-up in ASD. Mental retardation, or learning disability, is present in a large minority of all individuals with ASD, and in the majority of those with autistic disorder (Fernell & Gillberg, 2010). Most clinicians would not question the need for an in-depth medical appraisal of all children diagnosed as suffering from a learning disability. To see colleagues who advocate for a "full" medical work-up for children with mental retardation, regardless of presumed cause, but then argue against the need to go into some depth when it comes to trying to unravel the pathogenetic chain of events in autistic disorder, is conceptually pathetic and scientifically unsound. Children with autistic disorder are more—not less—in need of a full medical evaluation than children with mental retardation without autistic symptomatology. The medical work-up of children with ASD needs to be considered at various levels, including screening, behavioral diagnosis, physical and neuromotor examination, and laboratory investigations of varying kinds.

Screening

Screening for autism can, theoretically, be done in well-baby clinics, schools, and in connection with health checks in adults. These settings represent general population screens, and have been used in a number of epidemiological studies. However, it is still debatable whether general screening for autism should be universally recommended. Screening for autism among 18-month-old babies is successful in identifying severe cases and very few false positives (if false positive is defined as being "normal"). However, a majority of the moderately and mildly affected children with ASD are often missed in such screening efforts (Fernell & Gillberg, 2010). If screening for ASD of young children is done, it appears that 30 months could be a much better age, at which time the majority of cases with autistic disorder and some degree of intellectual disability would probably be picked up (Pandey et al., 2008, Fernell et al., 2010). Nevertheless, it would be important to continue to be on the look-out for ASD at older ages even if thorough screening of 2- to 3-year-olds has been performed. Cases of Asperger's syndrome and atypical autism will continue to cause diagnostic problems well into school age, and it is still common for children with these ASDs to be correctly diagnosed only around age ten years or later.

Screening in clinics is an altogether different issue and is, in the author's opinion, to be recommended. ASD screening would be particularly important in highly specialized clinics (such as learning disability, ADHD, and Tourette clinics) where many children have ASD "comorbidity."

There are several useful screening instruments, including the Checklist for Autism in Toddlers (CHAT; Baron-Cohen et al., 1992), the Modified CHAT (M-CHAT; Robin et al., 2001), and the Social Communication Questionnaire (SCQ; Berument et al., 1999) for 2- to 4-year-olds; the Five to Fifteen Questionnaire (FTF; Kadesjö et al., 2004) for school-age children; Autism, Tics, ADHD, and other comorbidities (A-TAC; Hansson et al., 2005), which can also be used as a telephone interview, and the Autism Spectrum Screening Questionnaire (ASSQ; Ehlers & Gillberg, 1993) for school age children and adolescents; and the Autism Quotient (AQ; Baron-Cohen, 2001) for adults. All these instruments have proven good psychometric properties. The ASSQ has been used in studies of altogether more than ten thousand children and has good to excellent validity for ASD, at least in preadolescent school children.

Diagnosis

For the diagnosis of ASD, a baseline of five different types of instruments should be used in all cases: (1) a parent/caregiver diagnostic interview for ASD, which—depending on age of the individual assessed, need for in-depth overall assessment, and type of ASD diagnosis suspected—could be the Diagnosis of Social and Communication Disorders (DISCO; Wing et al., 2002), the Autism Diagnostic Interview-Revised (ADI-R; Lord et al., 1994), the 3-di (Skuse et al., 2004), the Autism Spectrum or Asperger Syndrome Diagnostic Interview (ASDI; Gillberg et al., 2001), or another investigator-based interview that the clinician is well acquainted with; (2) questionnaires to parents and teachers, such as the FTF (see above) for coexisting problems, an extremely important part of the diagnostic process given the extremely high rate of coexisting problems, such as learning problems, ADHD, and tics (almost 100%) in ASD (the DISCO, unlike the other investigator-based diagnostic interviews has quite a large portion on such coexisting problems); (3) an ASD observation of the child, which could be the Autism Diagnostic Observation Schedule (ADOS; DiLavore et al., 1995) or another structured observation scheme; (4) a neuropsychological assessment, which must include a measure to cover overall intellectual and adaptive level—if possible, one of the Wechsler scales, portions of the Vineland (Sparrow et al., 1984), and the Global Assessment of Functioning (GAF) scale (APA, 2000); and last, but not least, (5) a thorough medical assessment by a physician well educated in child neuropsychiatry or child neurology, or both.

The Basic Medical Examination of a Child with ASD

All children with a diagnosis of an ASD—regardless of diagnostic subgroup within that category—should have all of the following: thorough physical examination (including specifically for minor physical anomalies and skin lesions), a brief motor screening test, tests of hearing and vision, a chromosomal analysis now including array CGH and a test for the FMR-1 (Fragile X) gene. In addition, the physician must survey the child's medical and developmental history, family history, and pre-, peri-, and postnatal events in interview with the parent/caregiver. If the DISCO is used, much of this part of the medical assessment will already have been covered. This is the minimum level of medical work-up. Most children with ASD will need further tests, as detailed below.

Apart from blood pressure, heart rate, height, and weight (which may all be important from the perspective of possible medication and need for physical training), and head circumference (which can suggest micro- or macrocephalus, both of which are overrepresented in ASD), the physical examination should focus on finding any signs of CAA. For instance, skin lesions could provide important indications that the child might be suffering from tuberous sclerosis (chagrin patches, ash-leaf and confetti hypopigmentations, perinasal rash), hypomelanosis of Ito (hypopigmented loops, whirls), or NF1 (café au lait spots, fibromas, axillar freckles). Some such lesions are best observed under a Wood's lamp (which should be available in the specialist autism clinic). Hypogonadism (especially if combined with obesity) could suggest Prader-Willi syndrome, whereas hypertrophy of the testicles could be a sign of Fragile X syndrome. A characteristic facial morphology is seen in Williams syndrome, 22q11 deletion syndrome, CHARGE association, Moebius sequence, and many other rare disorders. Submucous cleft soft palate and (operated) cardiac abnormalities are encountered in 22q11 deletion syndrome. Scoliosis is often present in variants of the Rett syndrome complex. Pitting of the nails is typical of tuberous sclerosis. Unexpected tallness could be a sign of XXY, XYY, or XXX syndrome. Minor physical anomalies are overrepresented in ASD and could be either a sign of a specific well-established genetic disorder or an indication that it might be appropriate to consult with a clinical geneticist. Many of these disorders above will now be picked up using modern molecular genetic screening. Low-seated ears are particularly common in autism. This physical anomaly could contribute to the variance of increased rates of otitis media found in ASD (Rosenhall et al., 2003, Skuse et al., 2009). Hypertelorism (increased distance between the eyes) is another common anomaly found in ASD. Occasionally this sign may signal underlying callosal dysgenesis.

The neuromotor examination should have a focus on functional capacity in the fields of gross and fine motor skills (often moderately impaired in Asperger's syndrome, sometimes in other ASD variants), and coordination skills including diadochokinesis (one of the more consistent areas of motor dysfunctions in ASD, sometimes indicating underlying cerebellar pathology; Teitelbaum et al., 1998, Rogers, 2009, Gillberg & Kadesjo, 2003). It is interesting to note that 90%+ of syndromes associated with ASD have significant motor problems associated. Many children with ASD meet full criteria for developmental coordination disorder (DCD), and the motor problems may need targeted interventions in their own right. The medical motor examination suggested by Kadesjö and Gillberg (1999), or the very brief six-item screen published by Gillberg et al. (1983), is usually sufficient when it comes to establishing this type of problem. Muscle tone is important to assess; many children with ASD have moderate to marked hypotonia, and this may seriously affect their daily life skills. If unrecognized, this problem might lead to reduced quality of life throughout the life span in ASD. Conversely, hypertonus, which could be a sign of mild cerebral palsy, is also often missed. Loss of hand skills or "refusal" to use hands for purposeful activities may be an indicator of Rett syndrome.

Actually, in the United States, the actual data is < 1/500 for chromosomal karyotype abnormalities, but 10% to 20% with The chromosomal analysis should include an array CGH (because 10% of all individuals with ASD have chromosomal abnormalities that can be demonstrated by this technique), and, possibly, depending on developments in the field over the next few years, assessment for presence of unusual copy number variants (CNVs), which are more common in ASD compared to other populations.

The FMR-1 gene should be screened for in all individuals with a diagnosis in the autism spectrum. This is both because the Fragile X syndrome is a disorder in the CAA group (in which it accounts, relatively speaking, for a large proportion of cases, and because the clinical examination findings and family history, although quite often very typical and almost diagnostic, may sometimes be very uncharacteristic of the syndrome.

More In-Depth Medical Investigation for Some Children with ASD

All preadolescent children with ASD and concomitant moderate, severe, or profound intellectual disability; all children with ASD and epilepsy or a clinical history suggestive of seizures; and all children with ASD and clear-cut regression (including those diagnosed as having childhood disintegrative disorder) are in need of more extensive medical investigations. Boys and girls with any of the characteristics described should be screened for the Angelman syndrome gene, and for other abnormalities (monosomy, trisomy, or partial tetrasomy) at chromosome 15q11-13. All girls in any of these groups should be screened for the MecP2 gene abnormality, even when the clinical picture is not consistent with classic Rett syndrome. Again, when in doubt, the physician should refer for evaluation by a clinical geneticist. EEGs should be performed and include registration during slow sleep. Depending on the clinical history and presentation, an MRI (sometimes SPECT) should be performed. The possibility of neurometabolic disorders, amino-acidopathies, and mitochondrial disease should be carefully considered on an individual basis.

Children with ASD and a suggested X-linked pattern of inheritance—regardless of IQ—should have testing for neuroligin mutations (Toro et al., 2010). If there is any indication of tuberous sclerosis in the family (poliosis or "white lock syndrome," confetti pigmentations, enamel or nail pitting), a full evaluation for this syndrome may be called for.

The Medical Examination of an Adult with ASD

If a person is diagnosed with ASD for the first time as an adult, the need for an extensive medical investigation may or may not be different from that outlined for children. On the one hand, it is unlikely that a severe disorder such as tuberous sclerosis could have been completely missed (not least because of the severity of the signs and symptoms of tuberous sclerosis in cases associated with autism) for 20 years or more (but there are always exceptions, and the present author has seen a few cases with autism where the tuberous sclerosis diagnosed was missed for 10, 13, and 25 years in spite of glaring clinical signs). Generally speaking, the need for a full medical work-up in adults with ASD is probably somewhat less acute than in children. On the other hand, some of the risk factors for ASD that were relatively common in the past (e.g., rubella embryopathy), and which are not considered likely causes of ASD in young children in the Western world today, need to be looked for specifically. It is perhaps important to mention that thalidomide embryopathy, although very rare, produced a very high proportion of autistic syndromes in affected individuals.

Adults with a diagnosis of ASD, whether given in childhood or later, who develop clear psychotic symptoms in early adult age, should be considered from the point of view of possible 22q11deletion syndrome, even when the physical phenotype is not characteristic of that syndrome.

Follow-up, Reappraisal, and Coexisting Problems

The making of the diagnosis of ASD can never be seen as an end point in itself. Follow-up and reappraisal are always needed. Also, ASD is virtually always an indicator that the individual affected has other problems that need diagnosis and intervention. For instance, intellectual disability, nonverbal learning disability, epilepsy, hearing and visual problems, DCD, ADHD, tics, anxiety, and depression are all very commonly encountered in ASD, not to mention the already discussed very high rate of CAA. Also, it is not uncommon for a toddler to present with extreme degrees of hyperactivity, to be diagnosed with ADHD and put on stimulant medication, only to reveal an "underlying" ASD (sometimes erroneously attributed to the medication). Some children with a core ASD problem presenting with extreme hyperactivity will actually calm down in a structured education setting to the extent that a stimulant is never considered. Conversely, the diagnosis of ASD may overshadow the diagnosis of ADHD (and the current diagnostic manuals actually support not making dual diagnoses of ASD and ADHD, which will hopefully be rectified in upcoming versions of the DSM and ICD), which may lead to a situation in which appropriate ADHD interventions for the child may be withheld for many years.

ASDs are often part of a spectrum of difficulties that involve social, communication, activity, attentional, language, and overall developmental problems. Quite a number of children actually meet criteria for ASD, ADHD, speech-language impairment, learning disability, and disability. Many of these have been diagnosed in Scandinavia as suffering from DAMP (Deficits in Attention, Motor Control, and Perception) with autistic features. When they first come to specialist attention (be it to a pediatrician, child psychiatrist, child psychologist, audiologist, speech language therapist, or a physiotherapist) at the age of 2–4 years, it may be impossible to say exactly which of the neurodevelopmental diagnoses mentioned apply. It is clear that the child has an Early Symptomatic Syndrome Eliciting Neurodevelopmental Clinical Examination ("ESSENCE"; Gillberg, 2009), and equally clear that there will very likely be persistent problems over many years, but unclear whether the most appropriate diagnosis in the longer term is ASD, ADHD, DCD, tic disorder, learning disability, speech-language impairment, or a combination of some or all of these. This means that preschool children presenting with ASD symptomatology need to be followed up and reappraised over a long period of time, usually many years to come. The clinician is faced with a child with a neurodevelopmental disorder presenting at varying ages with slightly or markedly different symptomatology. In the author's practice, it is quite common for a 3-year-old to be diagnosed with autistic disorder, followed by ADHD at age 6 years, and Tourette syndrome at 9 years. At about 10 years, the clinical presentation of the ASD is no longer that of autistic disorder, but, strikingly, of Asperger's syndrome. At age 20 years, the severe ADHD problems are at the clinical forefront of the ESSENCE syndrome, precluding academic and vocational success.

Epilepsy can develop at any time in the life of the child, adolescent, or young adult with an ASD (Danielsson et al., 2005). Signs of an underlying CAA can arise throughout childhood. Minor to moderate motor coordination, hearing, and visual problems may not present in a sufficiently clear manner leading to diagnoses of DCD, hearing loss or impairment and severe refractory errors being missed at the time of original diagnosis. Again, careful medical follow-up is required.

Medicines/Pharmacological Interventions

The majority of children with ASD should currently not be given any medication, at least not medication for their ASD. It is very important for the physician to keep abreast of developments in the field of biomedical therapies—including psychopharmacotherapy—so that he/she can provide well-founded guidance in the almost nightmarish jungle of suggested biomedical cures for autism that exist and which parents and others will grasp for, sometimes in desperation because psychoeducation and developmental interventions do not always lead to significant improvement.

Even though there is good evidence (see Canitano & Candurra, 2008) that risperidone is moderately effective for treating behavior problems associated with autism, the risk of substantial or even dramatic weight gain is very considerable, and no studies have demonstrated any really overwhelmingly positive results over a longer period of time. There is also good evidence that haloperidol has similar positive effects, including over a period of 6 months (Perry et al., 1989). One study has suggested that risperidone might be a bit more effective than haloperidol (Miral et al., 2008) in reducing behavioral abnormalities in autistic disorder. These classes of drugs (atypical and typical neuroleptics) are the only pharmacotherapies for ASD than can be said to have a relatively stable scientific foundation. They should be seriously considered in cases with the combination of violent behaviors, self-injury, hyperactivity, impulsivity, and sleep problems (see below for treatment of sleep disorder).

Two of the most commonly associated conditions in ASD, epilepsy and ADHD, are very often, if not always, treated with various kinds of medications. When they are present in ASD, they should be treated along similar guidelines as those that are employed for children without ASD. However, there are some caveats. In the case of epilepsy, there is particular concern that the antiepileptic drugs used not lead to further negative behavioral effects.

In the experience of the present author, the two antiepileptic drugs that have the least behavioral toxicity in a majority of ASD cases are lamotrigine and valproic acid. If possible, these drugs should be preferred in the initial stages of medical treatment for epilepsy in ASD. Both appear to have some positive effects on mood, and may contribute toward stabilizing mood in the—not infrequent—cases where there are bipolar swings both as regards mood and autistic features. Equally, however, it is understood that epilepsy is often difficult to treat in ASD, and several other drugs may have to enter into the equation. Generally speaking, benzodiazepines, especially clonazepam, can have very negative behavioral effects in ASD, and the author has seen many cases who have deteriorated in their autistic symptomatology during treatment with this type of drug (and prompt amelioration when the drug was withdrawn or changed to another class of antiepileptic medication). Also, even though carbamazepine is probably *the* drug with the most clinical "experience" in this field, it can have some rather negative effects, including increase in repetitive behaviors, obsessive questioning, and compulsive rituals of various kinds.

In the case of ADHD, both stimulants and atomoxetine can have some very beneficial effects on hyperactivity, attention deficit, and impulsivity in ASD. However, in the group with moderate or severe levels of intellectual disability, one must not expect dramatic improvements, even though, occasionally, even in this extremely severely disabled group with autism, severe learning disability and autism, unexpected major positive development is produced. It is a possibility that when ASD, ADHD, and tics occur together in the same individual, atomoxetine may be the preferred first-line drug for the treatment of inattention and hyperactivity, given the indications that it usually has no negative effects on tics. However, in the experience of the author, stimulants do not generally increase tic severity in individuals with this combination of symptoms.

It is not rare for a child to have autism, ADHD, and epilepsy. In such cases, stimulants and atomoxetine can be combined with antiepileptic drug treatment, usually with no adverse effects on seizure activity.

Children with ASD very often react in unexpected ways to "normal" doses of commonly used medications. This ranges from overreaction to very small doses all the way through to only minor effects of doses that are considered well above the recommended dose range. One has to strike a balance here, start with very low doses and then increase over a period of several weeks, sometimes even months in order to be able to arrive at the best possible dosage.

Sleep problems are important quality-of-life reducers both for many people with ASD, and, not least, for their caregivers. Before any drug treatment is considered for such problems, there is a need to establish whether or not the child (or adult) actually suffers from a "real" sleep problem or whether diurnal rhythms and other people's needs have produced the experienced need for help. However, sleep problems in ASD are very often severe, and need to be addressed not just with psychoeducation but also with other interventions, including pharmacological treatment. Melatonin appears to be a very effective and safe medication at least in relatively low-functioning individuals with autism and sleep onset problems. Such therapy will be effective only if adequate sleep hygiene measures (including sleeping in a dark, not semi-lit or well-lit, room) are taken in combination with the medication. Physical exercise to the limit of exhaustion during the daytime will also alleviate sleep problems (and sometimes hyperactivity, violent behaviors, and self-injury as well), as will listening to favorite music (earphones), in some cases.

Fish oils (specifically Omega-3) have become almost a panacea treatment for just about everything during the last several years. Although there is, as yet, no evidence that such treatment has any effects on autism, studies are currently underway looking at the effect of Omega-3 in ASD. There is preliminary evidence that ADHD symptoms, particularly when present in the context of autistic symptoms, could be ameliorated by Omega-3-therapy in a small, but not negligible, proportion of cases (Jonsson et al., 2008).

Medical Information

Parents, siblings, and children with ASD themselves, need oral and written information about the diagnosis, and about specific medical aspects of the disorder (Nydén et al., 2008). It is essential to have available such written information (booklets or brochures) at autism clinics and in neuropsychiatric, general psychiatric, or developmental/neurologic clinics catering to the needs of families affected by ASD.

REFERENCES

Åkefeldt, A., Gillberg, C., & Larsson, C. (1991). Prader-Willi syndrome in a Swedish rural county: Epidemiological aspects. *Developmental Medicine and Child Neurology, 33*, 715–721.

American Psychiatric Association. (2000). *Diagnostic and statistical manual of mental disorders. Fourth edition. Text revision.* Washington, DC: American Psychiatric Association.

Anckarsäter, H., Ståhlberg, O., Håkansson, C., Niklasson, L., Nydén, A., Jutblad S-B., et al. (2006). The impact of ADHD and autism spectrum disorders on temperament, character and personality development. *American Journal of Psychiatry, 163*, 1239–1244.

Aronson, M., Hagberg, B., & Gillberg, C. (1997). Attention deficits and autistic spectrum problems in children exposed to alcohol during gestation: a follow-up study. *Developmental Medicine and Child Neurology, 39*, 583–587.

Aziz, M., Stathopulu, E., Callias, M., Taylor, C., Turk, J., Oostra, B., et al. (2003). Clinical features of boy with fragile X premutations and intermediate alleles. *American Journal of Medical Genetics B Neuropsychiatric Genetics, 121B*:119–127.

Badawi, N., Dixon, G., Felix, J. F., Keogh, J. M., Petterson, B., Stanley, F. J., Kurinczuk, J. J. (2006). Autism following a history of newborn encephalopathy: more than a coincidence?. *Developmental Medicine and Child Neurology, 48*, 85–89.

Baron-Cohen, S., Allen, J., & Gillberg, C. (1992). Can autism be detected at 18 months? The needle, the haystack and the CHAT. *British Journal of Psychiatry, 161*, 839–843.

Baron-Cohen, S., Wheelwright, S., Skinner, R., Martin, J., & Clubley, E. (2001). The autism-spectrum quotient (AQ): evidence from Asperger syndrome/high functioning autism, males and females, scientists and mathematicians. *Journal of Autism Developmental Disorders, 31*, 5–17.

Berthier, M. L., Santamaria, J., Encabo, H., & Tolosa ES. (1992). Recurrent hypersomnia in two adolescent males with Asperger's syndrome. *J Am Acad Child Adolesc Psychiatry, 31*, 735–738.

Berument, S. K., Rutter, M., Lord, C., Pickles, A., & Bailey, A. (1999). Autism screening questionnaire: diagnostic validity. *British Journal of Psychiatry, 75*, 444–451.

Bhuiyan, Z. A., Kein, M., Hammond, P., van Haeringen, A., Mannens, M. M., van Berckelaer, I., et al. (2006). Genotype-phenotype correlations of 39 patients with Cornelia De Lange syndrome: the Dutch experience. *Journal of Medical Genetics, 43*, 568–575.

Canitano, R., & Scandurra, V. (2008). Risperidone in the treatment of behavioral disorders associated with autism in children and adolescents. *Neuropsychiatric Disease and Treatment, 4*, 723–730.

Chess, S. (1977). Follow-up report on autism in congenital rubella. *Journal of Autism and Childhood Schizophrenia, 7*, 69–81.

Coleman, M., & Gillberg, C. (2009). *The biology of the autistic syndromes* (4th ed.). Oxford: Oxford University Press.

Colville, G. A., & Bax, M. A. (1996). Early presentation in the mucopolysaccharide disorders. *Child Care Health Development, 22*, 31–36.

Curless, R. G., Flynn, J. T., Olsen, K. R., & Post MJ. (1991). Leber congenital amaurosis in siblings with diffuse dysmyelination. *Pediatric Neurology, 7*, 223–225.

Danielsson, S., Gillberg, I. C., Billstedt, E., Gillberg, C., & Olsson, I. (2005). Epilepsy in young adults with autism: a prospective population-based follow-up study of 120 individuals diagnosed in childhood. *Epilepsia, 46*, 918–923.

Davis, E., Fennoy, I., Laraque, D., Kanem, N., Brown, G., & Mitchell, J. (1992). Autism and developmental abnormalities in children with perinatal cocaine exposure. *Journal of the National Medical Association, 84*, 315–319.

DiLavore, P. C., Lord, C., & Rutter, M. (1995). The pre-linguistic autism diagnostic observation schedule. *Journal of Autism and Developmental Disorders, 25*, 355–379.

Ehlers, S., & Gillberg, C. (1993). The epidemiology of Asperger syndrome: A total population study. *Journal of Child Psychology and Psychiatry, 34*, 1327–1350.

Ek, U., Fernell, E., Jacobsson, L., & Gillberg, C. (1998). Relation between blindness due to retinopathy of prematurity and autistic spectrum disorders: a population-based study. *Developmental Medicine and Child Neurology, 140*, 297–301.

Ekstrom, R. A., Osborn, R. W., & Hauer PL. (2008). Surface electromyographic analysis of the low back muscles during rehabilitation exercises. *Journal of Orthopaedic and Sports Physical Therapy, 38*, 736–745.

Fehlow, P., Bernstein, K., Tennstedt, A., & Walther, F. (2003). Early infantile autism and excessive aerophagy with symptomatic megacolon and ileus in a case of Ehlers-Danlos syndrome. *Pädiatrie und Grenzgebiete, 31*, 259–267.

Fernell, E., & Gillberg, C. (2010). Autism spectrum disorder diagnoses in Stockholm preschoolers: Research in developmental disabilities. [Epub ahead of print]

Fernell, E., Norrelgren, F., Eriksson, M., Höglund-Carlsson, L., Hedvall, Å., Svensson, L., et al. (2009). Autism in preschool children: A study of 200 representative Stockholm children with autism spectrum disorders coming for intervention before age 4.5 years. Submitted.

Fillano, J. J., Goldenthal, M. J., Rhodes, C. H., & Marín-García, J. (2002). Mitochondrial dysfunction in patients with hypotonia, epilepsy, autism, and developmental delay: HEADD syndrome. *Journal and Child Neurology, 17*, 435–439.

Ghaziuddin, M., Bolyard, B., & Alessi, N. (1994). Autistic disorder in Noonan syndrome. *Journal of Intellectual Disability Research, 38*, 67–72.

Gillberg, C. (1983a). Are autism and anorexia nervosa related? letter. *British Journal of Psychiatry, 142*, 428.

Gillberg, C. (1983b). Identical triplets with infantile autism and the fragile-X syndrome. *British Journal of Psychiatry, 143*, 256–260.

Gillberg, C. (1983c). Perceptual, motor and attentional deficits in Swedish primary school children: Some child psychiatric aspects. *Journal of Child Psychology and Psychiatry, 24*, 377–403.

Gillberg, C. (1986). Brief report: Onset at age 14 of atypical autistic syndrome; A case report of a girl with herpes simplex encephalitis. *Journal of Autism and Developmental Disorders, 16*, 369–375.

Gillberg, C., Carlström, G., Rasmussen, P. (1983). Hyperkinetic disorders in seven-year-old children with perceptual, motor and attentional deficits. *Journal of Child Psychology and Psychiatry, 24*, 233–246.

Gillberg, C., & Cederlund, M. (2005). Asperger syndrome: familial and pre- and perinatal factors. *Journal of Autism Developmental Disorders, 35*, 159–166.

Gillberg, C., & Coleman, M. (1996). Autism and medical disorders: A review of the literature. *Developmental Medicine and Child Neurology, 38*,191–202.

Gillberg, C., & Coleman, M. (2000). *The biology of the autistic syndromes* (3d ed.). Cambridge: Cambridge University Press.

Gillberg, C., Gillberg, I. C., Råstam, M., & Wentz, N. (2001). The Asperger Syndrome Diagnostic Interview (ASDI): a preliminary study of a new structured clinical interview. *Autism, 5*, 57–66.

Gillberg, C., & Forsell, C. (1984). Childhood psychosis and neurofibromatosis—More than a coincidence? *Journal of Autism and Developmental Disorders, 14*, 1–8.

Gillberg, C., & Kadesjö, B. (2003). Why bother about clumsiness? The implications of having developmental coordination disorder (DCD). *Neural plasticity, 10*, 59–68.

Gillberg, C., & Rasmussen, P. (1994). Brief report: Four case histories and a literature review of Williams syndrome and autistic behavior. *Journal of Autism and Developmental Disorders, 24*, 381–393.

Goodman, D. M., Mendez, E., Throop, C., & Ogata, E. S. (2002). Adult survivors of pediatric illness: the impact on pediatric hospitals. *Pediatrics, 110*, 583–589.

Görker, I., & Tüzün, U. (2005). Autistic-like findings associated with a urea cycle disorder in a 4-year-old girl. *Journal of Psychiatry Neuroscience, 30*, 133–135.

Hansson, S.-L., Svanström, A., Råstam, M., Gillberg, I. C., Gillberg, C., & Söderström, H. (2005). Psychiatric telephone interview with parents for screening of childhood autism-tics, attention-deficit hyperactivity disorder and other comorbidities (A-TAC): Preliminary reliability and validity. *British Journal of Psychiatry, 187*, 262–267.

Hicks, M., Ferguson, S., Bernier, F., & Lemay, J. F. (2008). A case report of monozygotic twins with Smith-Magenis syndrome. *Journal of Developmental and Behavioral Pediatrics, 29*, 42–46.

Holroyd, S., Reiss, A. L., & Bryan, R. N. (1991). Autistic features in Joubert syndrome: a genetic disorder with agenesis of the cerebellar vermis. *Biological Psychiatry, 33*, 854–855.

Howlin, P. (2001). Autistic features in Cohen syndrome: a preliminary report. *Developmental Medicine and Child Neurology, 43*, 692–696.

Howlin, P., Wing, L., & Gould, J. (1995). The recognition of autism in children with Down syndrome—Implications for intervention and some speculations about pathology. *Dev Med Child Neurol, 37*, 406–414. Erratum in: *Developmental Medicine and Child Neurology, 37*, 672.

Hunt, A., & Dennis, J. (1987). Psychiatric disorder among children with tuberous sclerosis. *Developmental Medicine and Child Neurology, 29*, 190–198.

Johansson, M., Billstedt, E., Danielsson, S., Strömland, K., Miller, M., Granström, G., et al. (2007). Autism spectrum disorders and underlying brain mechanism in the oculoauriculovertebral spectrum. *Developmental Medicine and Child Neurology, 49*, 280–288.

Johansson, M., Råstam, M., Billstedt, E., Danielsson, S., Strömland, K., Miller, M., et al. (2006). Autistic spectrum disorders and underlying brain pathology in CHARGE association. *Developmental Medicine and Child Neurology, 48*, 40–50.

Johansson, M., Wentz, E., Fernell, E., Strömland, K., Miller, M. T., & Gillberg, C. (2001). Autistic spectrum disorders in Möbius sequence: a comprehensive study of 25 individuals. *Developmental Medicine and Child Neurology, 43*, 338–345.

Johnson, M., Östlund, S., Fransson, G., Kadesjö, B., & Gillberg, C. (2009). Omega-3/Omega-6 fatty acids for attention-deficit/hyperactivity disorder: A randomized placebo-controlled trial in children and adolescents. *Journal of Attention Disorders, 12*, 394–401.

Kadesjö, B., & Gillberg, C. (1999). Developmental coordination disorder in Swedish 7-year-old children. *Journal of the American Academy of Child and Adolescent Psychiatry, 38*, 820–828.

Kadesjö, B., & Gillberg, C. (2000). Tourette's disorder: Epidemiology and comorbidity in primary school children. *Journal of the American Academy of Child and Adolescent Psychiatry, 39*, 548–555.

Kadesjö, B., Gillberg, C., & Hagberg, B. (1999). Brief report: Autism and Asperger syndrome in seven-year-old children: A total population study. *Journal of Autism and Developmental Disorders, 29*, 327–331.

Kadesjö, B., Janols, L. O., Korkman, M., Michelson, K., Strand, G., Trillingsgaard, A., et al. (2004). The FTF (Five to Fifteen): The development of a parent questionnaire for the assessment of ADHD and comorbid conditions. *European Child and Adolescent Psychiatry, 13*(Suppl 3), 3–13.

Kielinen, M., Rantala, H., Timonen, E., Linna, S. L., & Moilanen, I. (2004). Associated medical disorders and disabilities in children with autistic disorder: a population-based study. *Autism, 8*, 49–60.

Komoto, J., Usui, S., Otsuki, S., & Terao, A. (1984). Infantile autism and Duchenne muscular dystrophy. *Journal of Autism and Developmental Disorders, 14*, 191–195.

Kopp, S., & Gillberg, C. (1997). Selective mutism: A population-based study: Research note. *Journal of Child Psychology and Psychiatry, 38*, 257–262.

Limperopoulos, C. (2009). Autism spectrum disorders in survivors of extreme prematurity. *Clinics in Perinatology, 36*, 791–805.

Limperopoulos, C., Soul, J. S., Gauvreau, K., Huppi, P. S., Warfield, S. K., Bassan, H., et al. (2005). Late gestation cerebellar growth is rapid and impeded by premature birth. *Pediatrics, 115*, 688–695.

Lord, C., Rutter, M., & Le Couteur, A. (1994). Autism Diagnostic Interview-Revised: a revised version of a diagnostic interview for caregivers of individuals with possible pervasive developmental disorders. *Journal of Autism and Developmental Disorders, 24*, 659–685.

Miral, S., Gencer, O., Inal-Emiroglu, F. N., Baykara, B., Baykara, A., & Dirik, E. (2008). Risperidone versus haloperidol in children and adolescents with AD: a randomized, controlled, double-blind trial. *European and Child Adolescent Psychiatry, 17*, 1–8.

Neville, B. G., Harkness, W. F., Cross, J. H., Cass, H. C., Burch, V. C., Lees, J. A., et al. (1997). Surgical treatment of severe autistic regression in childhood epilepsy. *Pediatric Neurology, 16*, 137–140.

Niklasson, L., Rasmussen, P., Óskardòttir, S., & Gillberg, C. (2009). Autism, ADHD, mental retardation and behavior problems in 100 individuals with 22q11 deletion syndrome. *Research in Developmental Disabilities, 30*, 763–773.

Nydén, A., Myrén, K. J., & Gillberg, C. (2008). Long-term psychosocial and health economy consequences of ADHD, autism, and reading-writing disorder: A prospective service evaluation project. *Journal of Attention Disorders, 12*, 141–148.

Oliveira, G., Diogo, L., Grazina, M., Garcia, P., Ataíde, A., Marques, C., et al. (2005). Mitochondrial dysfunction in autism spectrum disorders: a population-based study. *Developmental and Medicine Child Neurology, 47*, 185–189.

Pandey, J., Verbalis, A., Robins, D. L., Boorstein, H., Klin, A. M., Babitz, T., et al. (2008). Screening for autism in older and younger toddlers with the Modified Checklist for Autism in Toddlers. *Autism, 12*, 513–535.

Perry, R., Campbell, M., Adams, P., Lynch, N., Spencer, E. K., Curren, E. L., et al. (1989). Long-term efficacy of haloperidol in autistic children: continuous versus discontinuous drug administration. *Journal of the American Academy of Child and Adolescent Psychiatry, 28*, 87–92.

Robins, D. L., Fein, D., Barton, M. L., & Green J. A. (2001). The Modified Checklist for Autism in Toddlers: an initial study investigating the early detection of autism and pervasive developmental disorders. *Journal of Autism and Developmental Disorders, 31*, 131–144.

Rogers, S. J. (2009). What are infant siblings teaching us about autism in infancy? *Autism Research, 2*, 125–137.

Rosenhall, U., Nordin, V., Brantberg, K., & Gillberg, C. (2003). Autism and auditory brain stem responses. *Ear and Hearing, 24*, 206–214.

Skuse, D., Mandy, W., Steer, C., Miller, L., Goodman, R., Lawrence, K., et al. (2008). Social communication competence and functional adaptation in a general population of children: Preliminary evidence for sex-by-verbal IQ differential risk. *Journal of the American Academy of Child and Adolescent Psychiatry, 48*, 128.

Skuse, D., Warrington, R., Bishop, D., Chowdhury, U., Lau, J., Mandy, W., et al. (2004). The developmental, dimensional and diagnostic interview (3di): a novel computerized assessment for autism spectrum disorders. *Journal of the American Academy of Child and Adolescent Psychiatry, 43*, 548–558.

Sparrow, S., Balla, D., & Cicchetti, D. (1984). *Vineland Adaptive Behaviour Scales.* Circle Pines, MN: American Guidance Service.

Stathopulu, E., Ogilvie, C. M., & Flinter, F. A. (2003). Terminal deletion of chromosome 5p in a patient with phenotypical features of Lujan-Fryns syndrome. *American Journal of Medical Genetics, Part A, 119A*, 363–366.

Steffenburg, S., Gillberg, C. L., Steffenburg, U., & Kyllerman, M. (1996). Autism in Angelman syndrome: a population-based study. *Pediatric Neurology, 14*, 131–136.

Strömland, K., Nordin, V., Miller, M., Åkerström, B., & Gillberg, C. (1994). Autism in thalidomide embryopathy: A population study. *Developmental Medicine and Child Neurology, 36*, 351–356.

Stubbs, E. G., Ash, E., & Williams, C. P. (1984). Autism and congenital cytomegalovirus. *Journal of Autism and Developmental Disorders, 14*, 183–189.

Tantam, D., Evered, C., & Hersov, L. (1990). Asperger's syndrome and ligamentous laxity. *Journal of the American Academy of Child and Adolescent Psychiatry, 29*, 892–896.

Teitelbaum, P., Teitelbaum, O., Nye, J., Fryman, J., & Maurer, R. G. (1998). Movement analysis in infancy may be useful for early diagnosis of autism. *Proceedings of the National Academy of Sciences of the United States of America, 95*, 13982–13987.

Tierney, E., Nwokoro, N. A., & Kelley, R. I. (2000). Behavioral phenotype of RSH/Smith-Lemli-Opitz syndrome. *Mental Retardation and Developmental Disabilities Research Reviews, 6*, 131–134.

Tierney, E., Bukelis, I., Thompson, R. P., et al. (2001). Abnormalities of cholesterol metabolism in autism spectrum disorders. *American Journal and Medicine Genetics B Neuropsychiatry Genetics, 141*, 666–668.

Williams, G., King, J., Cunningham, M., Stephan, M., Kerr, B., & Hersh, J. H. (2001). Fetal valproate syndrome and autism: additional evidence of an association. *Developmental and Medicine Child Neurology, 43*, 202–206.

Wing, L., Leekam, S. R., Libby, S. J., Gould, J., & Larcombe, M. (2002). The Diagnostic Interview for Social and Communication Disorders: background, inter-rater reliability and clinical use. *Journal of Child and Psychology and Psychiatry, 43*, 307–325.

Wing, L., & Shah, A. (2000). Catatonia in autistic spectrum disorders. *British Journal of Psychiatry, 176*, 357–356.

Zappella, M. (1992). Hypomelanosis of Ito is common in autistic syndromes. *European Child and Adolescent Psychiatry, 1*, 170–177.

Section IV

Broader Autism Phenotype

27 Molly Losh, Ralph Adolphs, Joseph Piven

The Broad Autism Phenotype

Points of Interest

- The broad autism phenotype (BAP) represents a constellation of subtle personality and language characteristics that may reflect genetic liability to autism.
- The BAP is not typically associated with any functional impairment.
- The BAP may be associated with specific neurocognitive features also implicated in autism.
- Studying features of the BAP could aid genetic and biological studies of the etiologic basis of autism, by targeting features that are more amenable to genetic and neurobiological investigation than the full clinical syndrome of autism.

The BAP: Historical Perspective and Overview

More than 60 years have passed since Leo Kanner published his detailed clinical descriptions of 11 children sharing what he described as an "extreme autistic aloneness." That landmark study served as the first formal documentation of autism. Less well recognized, however, is that Kanner's insightful case studies also described a potential *forme fruste* of autism that he observed among relatives. Kanner documented among some parents and relatives of his patients mild characteristics that mirrored in quality many of the core features of autism, noting a preoccupation with "abstractions of a scientific, literary, or artistic nature, and limited in genuine interest in people." (1943, p. 250). A decade later, Leon Eisenberg further described relatives, and fathers in particular as "perfectionistic to an extreme ... pre-occupied with detailed minutiae to the exclusion of concern for over-all meanings" (1957, p. 721).

These insightful clinical observations would portend empirical evidence that autism is largely genetic in etiology, and importantly, that genetic liability to autism can be expressed through subtle behavioral and language features among relatives. Initially however, these early observations were misinterpreted in the context of psychodynamic theory, prominent at the time, in which parents were typically branded responsible for the development of children's psychopathology (Freud, 1923; Jung, 1921). Central in propagating the myth that parental behavior was causal in the etiology of autism was Bruno Bettelheim's *Empty Fortress* (1967), which developed the notion of "refrigerator mothers" and helped to launch a harmful legacy of doubt, blame, and misunderstanding of autism and its etiology. Although Kanner's observations of parental characteristics were oft recruited to bolster evidence for this damaging concept, careful review of Kanner's early writings makes clear his strong conviction that the root cause of autism was biological (see excerpt from Kanner's original observations of autism, Box 27-1). It was not for several decades, though, that empirical evidence would demonstrate definitively the biological basis of autism, first through observations that autism frequently co-occurred with epilepsy (Rutter, 1970), and then in the twin study of Folstein and Rutter (1977). This landmark study would also serve to ignite interest in and study of the broad autism phenotype, or BAP. Indeed, this study not only detected markedly higher concordance rates of autism among monozygotic (MZ) than dizygotic twins (evidence for a genetic etiology), but also found even higher MZ concordance for a more broadly defined phenotype including subclinical language and cognitive features that would propel a series of family-genetic studies aimed at studying and characterizing features that could index genetic liability to autism among unaffected relatives.

This broad autism phenotype now figures prominently in contemporary research as a promising avenue for identifying genetically meaningful features and neurobiological substrates involved in autism. To date, however, the BAP remains a poorly understood construct. There currently exists no consensus regarding those key features that comprise the BAP, and measurement tools vary widely across studies and

Box 27–1

The children's aloneness from the beginning of life makes it difficult to attribute the whole picture exclusively to ... early parental relations with our patients. We must, then, assume that these children have come into the world with innate inability to form the usual, biologically provided affective contact with people, just as other children come into the world with innate physical or intellectual handicaps. If this assumption is correct, a further study of our children may help to furnish concrete criteria regarding the still diffuse notions about the constitutional components of emotional reactivity. For here we seem to have pure-culture examples of *inborn autistic disturbances of affective contact.* Leo Kanner. Autistic Disturbances of Affective Contact *The Nervous Child.*, Vol II, No. 3, 1943

research groups. These factors have contributed in no small measure to difficulties implementing BAP features in genetic and neurobiological studies.

The goal of this chapter is to consider in depth the clinical phenomenon of the BAP, as well as to synthesize existing findings and recent developments in the study of the BAP in order to produce a consistent definition of the BAP, and to identify gaps in knowledge and methodological challenges currently inhibiting effective implementation of characteristics of the BAP in gene-finding and neurobiological studies. To this end, we begin by describing methodological considerations in assessment of the BAP and then delve into research describing the clinical picture of the BAP and principal domains of functioning that comprise this phenomenon, as well as the cognitive and neuropsychological features associated with the BAP. Discussion of clinical and empirical significance of the BAP concludes the chapter.

Assessment of the BAP

Since Folstein and Rutter's (1977) twin study findings cast explanatory light on Kanner's original observations of personality styles among parents of autistic individuals, the BAP has been studied using a wide array of measurement tools, ranging from informant questionnaires to direct clinical interview assessments with both subjects and informants. Additionally, studies have differed greatly in subject ascertainment and matching strategies, resulting in a methodological din that complicates synthesis of findings across studies. Therefore, before describing the components of the BAP, we first review the various tools employed for measuring the BAP, and discuss methodological inconsistencies across studies.

Methodological Differences

Measurement Tools

Unlike autism, where standard diagnostic instruments such as the Autism Diagnostic Interview and Autism Diagnostic Observational Schedule are now widely used, there exists no gold standard measure of the BAP that is applied consistently across groups. Among the earliest developed and most commonly used is the clinically structured family history interview, and the Autism Family History Interview (AFHI) in particular (Bolton et al., 1994). In the AFHI, an informant is asked detailed questions concerning their own behavior and dispositions as well as those of their first- and second-degree relatives across domains that parallel the defining features of autism (i.e., social, communication, and rigid/repetitive interests and behaviors). Both child and adult functioning are queried, and features are typically rated as absent, probably/mildly present, or definitely present, based either on ratings of interviews or blinded interview vignettes (Bolton et al., 1994; Piven et al., 1997; Szatmari et al., 1993). Using a related approach, the Broad Phenotype Autism Symptom Scale (BPASS; Dawson et al., 2007) assesses similar domains, but measures each trait on a continuous 5-point scale aimed at capturing behaviors ranging from impairment to above average skill in each domain. Like the AFHI, the BPASS includes probes about early development as well as current functioning and was developed specifically to assess features of the BAP among relatives. These informant-based methods have the advantage of efficiently assessing multiple family members. Yet, because they are based on an informant's impression, they may lack the sensitivity and specificity of direct clinical assessment.

Structured subject and informant personality interviews have also been applied to the study of the BAP. Piven et al. (1994) used the Modified Personality Assessment Schedule (MPAS; Tyrer, 1988) to examine traits conceptually related to autism (Piven et al., 1997; Murphy et al., 2000; Losh et al., 2008). In this method, interviewers begin by soliciting autobiographical accounts of dispositions throughout development (e.g., questions about childhood friendships, experiences in school, jobs, spousal relationships). Subjects are then guided through a number of questions to probe personality characteristics relevant to autism and the BAP, namely, *rigid* or *perfectionistic* personality, and *socially aloof* disposition/behavior. These traits correspond to the ritualistic/repetitive and social symptom domains of autism, respectively. Informants are then separately interviewed and asked these same questions. Concrete behavioral examples are solicited through interviews to substantiate trait endorsement. Ratings are assigned by combining both subject and informant interviews. As an extension of a clinical interview and based on a "life story" of an individual as seen through the eyes of both the subject and informant, the MPAS has face validity, but is time intensive and requires considerable training for reliable administration and rating.

Other direct assessment measures have focused on more specific characteristics of the BAP, namely, the Pragmatic Rating Scale (PRS; Landa et al., 1992) and the Friendship Interview (FI; Santangelo & Folstein, 1995). The PRS is a scale for rating conversational ability that taps pragmatic skills that correspond roughly to Gricean Maxims of conversation (i.e., quantity, relation/relevance, and manner). Ratings are based on a conversational sample, and rated by coders blind to group status. The Friendship Interview was developed to provide a reliable and relatively easy-to-administer measure of one aspect of social behavior—the quality and number of an individual's friendships. It involves a series of questions aimed at measuring the degree to which an individual possesses emotionally reciprocal friendships.

Adequate reliability has been shown for the MPAS (Tyrer et al., 1984), the PRS and FI (Landa et al., 1992; Piven et al., 1997), as well as the family history method and the BPASS (Bolton et al., 1994; Dawson et al., 2007), and these instruments provide a face valid index of features that have been hypothesized to comprise the BAP. However, the interviews involved can be lengthy and require considerable training for reliable administration and rating. As such, several groups have used questionnaires to study the BAP.

Several questionnaire measures used in studies of the BAP were originally developed to study or screen for autism. The Autism Spectrum Quotient (ASQ; Baron-Cohen, Wheelwright, Skinner et al., 2001) is a self-administered questionnaire that was developed initially to identify individuals with high-functioning autism, and has since been applied in studies of relatives at risk for displaying the BAP as well as the general population. Another tool initially used with autistic individuals, but applied to studies of the BAP among siblings, is the Children's Communication Checklist (Bishop, 1998), a parent/care-giver questionnaire designed to assess language and communication deficits in children. This instrument has been shown to discriminate relatives (siblings) of individuals with autism from controls on specific language features (Bishop et al., 2006).

The Social Responsiveness Scale (SRS) is a brief instrument completed by parents or teachers that assesses autism features, and social reciprocity in particular, on a single dimension, ranging from typical functioning to autistic. Twin studies have shown high heritability for SRS scores (Constantino et al., 2003), and an adult version has been developed to study mild traits among parents (Constantino et al., 2005). Because the SRS is measured on a quantitative scale, it is ideal for genetic studies, where quantitative measures typically wield greater power to detect linkage and association in complex disorders such as autism (e.g., van den Oord, 1999). Duvall et al. (2007) have in fact employed this tool in a genomewide linkage study including individuals with autism and their relatives, finding several suggestive linkage signals. The development and implementation of such quantitative measures certainly represents a promising avenue for genetic research. This issue is considered later in greater depth.

One questionnaire instrument specifically developed to study the BAP is the Broad Autism Phenotype Questionnaire (BAPQ; Hurley et al., 2007). This measure was designed to efficiently, validly, and reliably measure particular personality and language characteristics that have been hypothesized to define the BAP, including social personality, rigid personality, and pragmatic language deficits (Piven et al., 1997), in nonautistic parents of autistic individuals. The BAPQ was derived from prior work with the direct assessment measures of personality and pragmatic language, the MPAS and PRS, and yields three subscales providing quantitative indices relevant to the three DSM-IV domains of autism (American Psychiatric Association, 1994): social deficits, stereotyped-repetitive behaviors and pragmatic language impairments. While originally developed as a tool to screen for the BAP, the BAPQ appears to identify features of the BAP with adequate sensitivity and specificity when compared to ratings derived from gold standard clinical interviews (Hurley et al., 2007). Case-control differences in a large sample of parents of autistic individuals (~ N = 750) compared to a large population sample of parents unrelated to an autistic individual (~ N = 750; Piven, personal communication), have continued to support the validity of this instrument.

Study Design Considerations

A variety of methods exist for studying the BAP, and interpretation of findings across these varying approaches can be fettered by such methodological differences. Other complicating factors important to consider include differences across studies in diagnostic criteria, and ascertainment and matching procedures. For instance, not all studies have been limited to individuals with idiopathic autism (e.g., many did not screen for fragile X syndrome or other monogenic conditions related to autism), and different diagnostic definitions have been employed over time with various iterations of the DSM, thereby introducing sample heterogeneity that could influence findings. Studies have also varied in the inclusion and definition of control groups. Some have included no controls, others have examined relatives of individuals with Down syndrome to control for the stress of parenting a child with a disability, and still others have included relatives of individuals with genetically based conditions that could also result in subtle phenotypic manifestations among family members (e.g., schizophrenia, specific language impairment).

Each of these approaches has its advantages and disadvantages, but when considered together, studies using various control groups have offered complementary perspectives and methods for understanding the BAP. For instance, early studies without control groups provided detailed case study descriptions that highlighted phenotypes for subsequent investigation in systematic case-control studies. The inclusion of control groups is of course necessary for determining whether observed features occur at elevated rates in autism families and for teasing out effects of environmental stressors related to parenting a child with a disability. Studies using comparison groups have therefore been critical in defining the BAP. Important to consider from this work is how best to interpret findings from studies including different control groups, such as those including relatives of individuals with developmental delay caused by noninherited conditions (e.g., nondisjunction Down syndrome) versus those investigations including disorders conferring genetic risk among unaffected relatives.

Examining other inherited conditions can offer a means of examining autism-specific features that aggregate in families.

However, this strategy could also obscure detection of meaningful phenotypes associated with liability to autism and other disorders. That is, given evidence of phenotypic, neurobiological, and genetic overlap of autism with disorders such as specific language impairment and fragile X syndrome (e.g., Kjelgaard & Tager-Flusberg, 2001; deFosse et al., 2004; Belmonte & Bourgeron, 2006), it would follow that relatives of individuals who are carriers of the genes involved in these conditions may show phenotypes overlapping with the broad autism phenotype. In this case, associated phenotypes could be missed unless a control group without genetic liability is studied as well. Recent research is bearing out this scenario, showing, for example, that whereas parents of individuals with autism show elevated rates of pragmatic language violations when compared to parents of individuals with Down syndrome, their pragmatic language use is highly similar to parents of individuals with specific language impairment (Ruser et al., 2008). This in no way diminishes the validity of the concept of the BAP, but rather, adds important information about the continuum of liability to autism and its overlap with other conditions, and highlights an important methodological consideration for studies of the BAP.

An additional factor affecting family-study findings concerns the ascertainment strategies employed, as these have varied in important ways over time. Epidemiological sampling has been employed in a few studies (e.g., Ritvo et al., 1989; Piven et al., 1997), but more commonly cases have been recruited from existing clinical samples, through advocacy organizations, or other means that could introduce selection biases. The types of relatives examined have also varied—parents and siblings are commonly studied, but larger-scale family studies have also examined other collaterals (e.g., grandparents, aunts, uncles). Again, these different approaches all add valuable information that in aggregate provides compelling evidence for the existence of a BAP, but which may also introduce variation that could affect findings (e.g., traits of the BAP might be expected to express more profoundly among first-degree relatives than among more distant collaterals). Brief mention here of these important concerns serves to highlight these issues in interpreting the discussion of features believed to comprise the BAP, to follow.

Domains of the BAP

As touched on already, Kanner's original observations of autism included descriptions of socially reserved and single-minded personality characteristics among parents. With evidence in hand of a biological basis for autism from Folstein and Rutter's (1977) twin study, and encouraged by the potential of studying these fundamental, genetically meaningful traits, a series of family studies were launched in the 1980s and 1990s in an effort to further define the features that comprise the BAP (e.g., Bolton et al., 1994; Bailey et al., 1995; Le Couteur et al., 1996; Piven et al., 1994; Piven Palmer, Jacobi, et al., 1997). Based on family history informant interviews, as well as direct assessments, this carefully conducted work documented a constellation of personality, language, and cognitive features that while very subtly expressed, mirrored in quality the core features of autism. Below are those chief domains that have been described as comprising the BAP.

Personality Features of the BAP

In an early study by Wolff et al. (1988) and follow-up work with the same sample (Narayan et al., 1990), personality features were assessed among parents of individuals with autism and control parents of individuals with intellectual disabilities using a structured clinical interview for evaluating personality disorders. This pair of studies found that autism parents, and fathers in particular, were more often rated as "schizoid" (16/35 parents rated as such vs. 0/39 control parents of individuals with intellectual disability of unspecified etiology). In these studies schizoid personality was defined by limited empathic responsiveness, emotional detachment, and rigidity and restricted interests, features which were characterized by the authors as real and observable, but at the same time "quite subtle."

Subsequent research with the Autism Family History Interview indicated the presence of similar social features among family members and nonautistic co-twins (Bolton et al., 1994; Bailey et al., 1995; Le Couteur et al., 1996). In the first large-scale systematic study of relatives, Bolton et al. (1994) described among parents and siblings social characteristics including lack of affection, limited friendships, and lack of typical social play among children. Repetitive behaviors and traits akin to the "rigid" personality features observed by Narayan et al. (1990) were also observed among unaffected relatives (Bolton et al., 1994), but were found to be less common than social characteristics. It was in this initial family history study that such traits (along with language characteristics, to be discussed shortly) were first formally described as constituting a broad autism phenotype.

After Bolton's important work, which was confirmed in an expanded twin sample studied by Bailey et al. (1995), several studies followed that were aimed at further investigating and refining measurement of the BAP (see Table 27-1). Employing direct assessment interviews of personality features using the MPAS, described previously, Piven et al. (1994) studied 87 parents of autistic individuals and 38 parents of Down syndrome probands. Comparisons of blind ratings derived from subject and informant interviews indicated that parents of autistic individuals displayed significantly higher rates of three social characteristics—aloof, untactful, and undemonstrative. In a later study of parents from multiplex families using the MPAS, Piven, Palmer, Landa, et al. (1997) confirmed these patterns, finding that relatives of individuals with autism more commonly displayed social reticence or aloofness, and in the Friendship Interview reported fewer reciprocal friendships than controls. Additionally, the autism parent group was more likely than controls to display "rigid" or inflexible and perfectionistic personalities, showing relatively

Table 27–1.
Family studies of relatives of individuals with autism

Study	Sample	*n*	Method	Findings
August et al., 1981	Siblings	71	Informant and direct	Elevated rates of MR or language delays
Baird & August, 1985	Siblings	51	Informant	Elevated rates of MR
DeLong & Dwyer, 1988	1st- and 2nd-degree relatives	929	Informant	Elevated rates of depression
Piven et al., 1990	Siblings	67	Informant	High rates of social dysfunction and cognitive disorder
Minton et al., 1982	Siblings	50	Direct assessment	Elevated rates of MR
Wolff et al., 1988	Parents	35	Direct assessment	High rates of "schizoid" personality (defined by limited empathy, emotional detachment, rigidity and restricted interests, and "unusual" communication)
Freeman et al., 1989	Parents and sibs	280	Direct assessment	No group differences in cognitive or language ability
Narayan et al., 1990	Parents and sibs	53 (including 35 parents studied in Wolff et al., 1988)	Direct assessment and educational records	Higher vocabulary scores in fathers. No educational differences in siblings
Smalley & Asarnow, 1990	Parents and sibs	25	Direct assessment	No differences in cognition or language
Landa et al., 1991	Parents	41	Direct assessment	Less coherent narratives
Gillberg et al., 1992	Parents and sibs	101		No differences in learning disorders or language problems
Piven et al., 1990	Siblings	67	Informant	Elevated rates of psychiatric disorders
Landa et al., 1992	Parents	43	Direct assessment	Increased rates of pragmatic language violations
Ozonoff et al., 1993	Parents and sibs	118	Neuropsych	No significant differences in executive function
Szatmari et al., 1993	Parents and sibs	181	Informant and direct	No significant differences in cognition or social adaptation
Piven et al., 1994	Parents	87	Direct Assessment	Higher rates of social features (aloof, untactful, undemonstrative)
Bolton et al., 1994	Parents and sibs	332	Informant	Social, communication, and repetitive features more common
DeLong & Nohria, 1994	1st- and 2nd-degree relatives	420	Informant	Higher rates of affective disorder
Szatmari et al., 1995	Parents	103	Informant	Social isolation more common
Smalley et al., 1995	Parents and sibs	96	Direct assessment	Elevated rates of depression and social phobia
Plumet et al., 1995	Parents and sibs	47	Direct assessment	No differences in language skills of parents, difference in sibs
Leboyer et al., 1995	Parents and sibs	48	Direct assessment	No difference in verbal or visuospatial skills in parents. Lower verbal in sibs
Boutin et al., 1997	Parents and sibs	156	Informant and direct	Higher rates of cognitive delays
Hughes et al., 1997	Parents and sibs	97	Neuropsych	Impaired executive functioning
Baron-Cohen & Hammer, 1997	Siblings	30	Neuropsych	Bias toward local processing and impaired theory of mind
Piven, Palmer, Landa, et al., 1997	1st- and 2nd-degree relatives	133	Informant	Higher rates of social, communication, and repetitive features

(Continued)

Table 27–1. *(Contd.)*

Study	Sample	*n*	Method	Findings
Piven, Palmer, Landa, et al., 1997	Parents	48	Direct assessment, questionnaire, NEO-PI	Higher rates of aloof, rigid, hypersensitivity, pragmatic language violations, and less reciprocal friendships
Piven & Palmer, 1997	Parents	48	Direct assessment	Lower performance on executive function, performance IQ, and reading measures
Bolton et al., 1998	1st-, 2nd-, and 3rd-degree relatives	1238	Informant and direct	Higher rates of depression and OCD
Piven & Palmer, 1999	Parents and 2nd-degree relatives	48	Informant and direct	Higher rates of depression and social phobia
Folstein et al., 1999	Parents and sibs	253	Informant and direct	Higher rates of language related difficulties in parents
Hollander et al., 2003	Parents	114	Informant and direct	Higher rates of OCD in parents whose children showed more severe repetitive behaviors
Micali et al., 2004	Parents	152	Informant	Higher rates of depression and anxiety in mothers
Bishop et al., 2004	Parents and sibs	233	Direct assessment	No significant differences in phonological processing
Bishop et al., 2004	Parents	69	Informant	Social and communication features more common
Kano et al., 2004	Parents	28	Direct assessment	OCD symptoms higher in fathers
Bishop et al., 2006	Siblings	42	Informant	Delays in language related skills
Shaked et al., 2006	Siblings	24	Neuropsych	No significant differences on theory of mind
Wong et al., 2006	Parents and sibs	211	Neuropsych	No differences in executive skill of planning or cognitive flexibility. Weaknesses in generativity
Bolte et al., 2006	Parents	125	Informant	Higher rates of reserved and depressive characteristics
Dalton et al., 2007	Siblings	12	Neuropsych	Decreased gaze fixation, diminished fusiform gyrus activation, and reduced amygdala volume
Schmidt et al., 2008	Parents	22	Informant and direct	Lower PIQ and phonological processing. No differences in receptive/expressive language or family history of language difficulty
Hurley et al., 2007	Parents	86	Informant	Higher rates of aloof, rigid, and pragmatic language violations
Losh & Piven, 2007	Parents	48	Neuropsych	Impairments on theory of mind task
Losh et al., 2008	Parents	65	Direct	Elevated rates of social, communication, and rigid features
Daniels et al., 2008	Parents	1,227	Medical records	Higher rates of schizophrenia, depression, and personality disorder among mothers
Adolphs et al., 2008	Parents	42	Neuropsych	Atypical face processing

little interest in seeking novelty or change in their environment and activities and increased attention to detail. Finally, this study found higher rates of anxiety-related traits of hypersensitivity and anxious/worrying personality. To validate these clinical observations, the NEO Personality Inventory (NEO-PI) was administered to parents (Costa & McCrae, 1985). The NEO-PI is a standardized questionnaire based on the Five-Factor model of personality, and was developed to assess quantitative dimensions of normal personality traits. In nearly all cases, features assessed through the MPAS were found to correlate significantly with conceptually related domains on the NEO-PI. Social features (e.g., aloof) correlated negatively with components of the Extraversion factor (warmth and gregariousness) measured by the NEO-PI, and the "Rigid" personality feature measured by the MPAS was negatively correlated with the Openness dimension and agreeableness. The former identifies individuals with a preference for routine and familiar experiences, an unwillingness to try new activities and avoidance of novelty. The combination describes individuals (negative openness and negative agreeableness) who are more than just closed to changes in experience but in addition display what has been referred to as "interpersonal rigidity" (Paul Costa, personal communication; Costa & McCrae, 1985), and thus suggests an additional social aspect of this characteristic that is consistent with an overall conceptualization of the BAP as involving both social deficits and rigidity. Further, the MPAS-measured anxiety features (Anxious/worrying and Hypersensitivity) were significantly correlated with several facets of neuroticism on the NEO-PI. Such associations between clinically derived personality ratings and objective standardized instruments supported the validity of the personality traits measured by the MPAS and which were hypothesized to constitute features of the BAP.

The MPAS was subsequently employed in two additional studies, both yielding similar findings. Murphy et al. (2000) used an informant-only version of the MPAS and the AFHI with parents and adult siblings of 99 families of autistic individuals originally studied by Bolton and colleagues (Bolton et al., 1994; Bolton et al., 1998) as well as 36 families of individuals with Down syndrome. They again found among parents of individuals with autism a higher incidence of aloof or shy dispositions, as well as elevated rates of hypersensitivity and anxious/worrying personality style. Factor analysis of MPAS traits indicated three broad factors. Two factors were described as social in nature ("withdrawn" and "difficult"), and the third factor, dubbed "tense," appeared to capture anxiety-related traits. In a later investigation Losh et al. (2008) examined features assessed in the MPAS among parents from families differing in genetic liability to autism—multiple-incidence families (MIAF) with two or more children with autism, single-incidence autism families (SIAF), and control families of individuals with Down syndrome (DWNS). Because families with multiple incidences of autism are likely to represent cases of higher genetic loading than single-incidence cases (Piven & Folstein, 1994), it was hypothesized that "dosage" effects would be observed for the principal characteristics conferring genetic susceptibility to autism, in which such features would express most profoundly among MIAF parents, less strongly among SIAF parents, and least of all among comparison parents from DWNS families, who should display population base rates.

Results confirmed this prediction for both the social (aloof) and rigid features of the BAP. Aloof was present among 29% of MIAF parents, 17% of SIAF parents, and 3% of the DWNS parent group. This finding was bolstered by

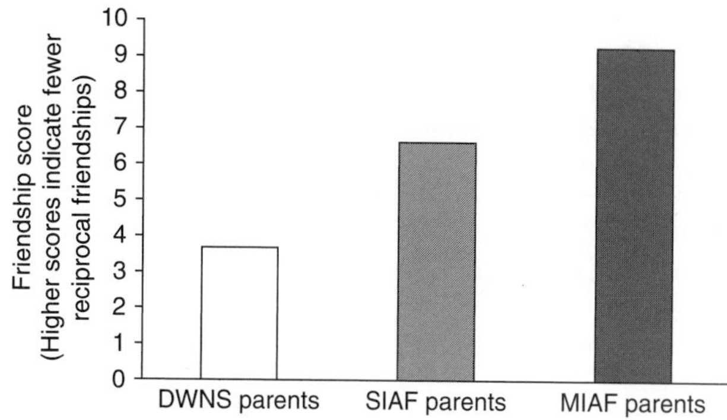

Figure 27–1. Quality of friendships across family types varying in genetic liability to autism. Higher scores represent fewer and/or less emotionally reciprocal friendships.

results from the Friendship Interview, also administered to parents, where an identical pattern was observed with multiplex parents reporting the fewest friendships, DWNS the most, and simplex parents falling intermediate between the two groups. Figure 27-1 depicts these findings, showing the mean quality of friendships, with higher scores corresponding to fewer and lower quality (i.e., less emotionally reciprocal) friendships. Similarly, the rigid feature was present in 48% of MIAF parents, 23% of SIAF parents, and 10% of parents in the DWNS groups.

Szatmari et al. (2000) previously found a similar "dosage" effect in BAP expression across families differing in genetic liability to autism. Szatmari's findings were particularly compelling in that they included not only multiple- and single-incidence families, but also nonbiological relatives of adopted individuals with autism. As predicted, adoptive parents showed no evidence of the BAP, whereas single- and multiple-incidence families showed increasing expression.

Together, these converging findings suggest that particular personality features are sensitive markers of genetic liability to autism. Important to note, however, is that the traits of the BAP were not observed among all parents. Furthermore, evidence suggests that when present, such traits were expressed quite subtly (as noted early on by Wolff et al., 1988; and Narayan et al., 1990). To illustrate, we present a vignette of a parent participating in this study, who was rated as BAP (+) for displaying both traits of rigid and aloof (Box 27-2). As is apparent from this brief account, this individual's preference for routine is relatively subtle, with the only hint that this trait may interfere with daily life coming from his spouse. And socially, this individual displays no evidence of autistic impairment, but instead simply a more reticent social disposition. As such, it may be that the features of the BAP are most aptly described as personality styles, rather than functional impairment within any particular domain. Studies of psychiatric disorders among relatives of individuals with autism have addressed this question, and are described below.

Box 27–2
Parent of an autistic individual rated as having the broad autism phenotype (rigid and aloof personality)

Mr A., a 41 year old college professor, describes himself as very organized and a planner. He gives as an example the fact that he always writes out his lectures verbatim before class. He is most comfortable in life with routine and says he is happiest with no surprises. He requests that all his courses be scheduled at the same time each semester and feels out of sorts when his routine is interrupted. His wife notes that he protests when asked to drop off a letter on the way to work because it disrupts his routine.

He has always been uncomfortable socially and describes himself as a loner with no interest in having friends. As a child he spent more time with books than people. He doesn't see the point of "chit chat". He prefers there be a purpose to conversations and avoids unstructured social gatherings (e.g., having coffee with colleagues at work).

Psychiatric Disorder and the BAP

A number of studies have observed elevated rates of axis I psychiatric disorders in first-degree relatives of autistic individuals, including affective disorder in adult siblings (Piven et al., 1991), and major affective disorder, and anxiety disorder in parents (including social phobia and generalized anxiety disorders; Bolton et al., 1998; Daniels et al., 2008; Hollander et al., 2003; Micali et al., 2004; Piven & Palmer, 1999; Smalley et al., 1995). Elevated rates of obsessive-compulsive disorder in relatives have been reported in some studies (Bolton et al., 1998; Hollander et al., 2003; Micali et al., 2004) but not in others (Piven et al., 1991; Piven & Palmer, 1999).

Given the familiality of these conditions, it is possible that these behavioral manifestations may be expressions of the underlying genetic liability for autism. The overlap in the phenomenology of generalized anxiety, social phobia, and obsessive-compulsive symptoms could be construed as reflecting aspects of the autistic phenotype, while the phenomenology of major affective disorder is qualitatively distinct from the defining features of autism. Bolton et al. (1998) using the family history method, and Piven and Palmer (1999) using direct assessment of both the BAP and psychiatric disorder, explored whether high rates of psychiatric disorder were occurring in parents with the BAP. Neither study found elevated rates of affective disorder occurring disproportionately in those individuals with the BAP. The number of parents with anxiety disorder was insufficient to examine this relationship in the study by Piven and Palmer. However, Bolton et al. (1998) reported that a high rate of OCD in parents occurred in association with social and communication manifestations of the BAP, suggesting that it may be a variable manifestation of the same genetic liability leading to the BAP. Piven and Palmer (1999) found suggestive evidence that affective disorders may occur at higher rates in those parents who do *not* display the BAP and who have a spouse with the BAP, suggesting that high rates of affective disorder in parents of autistic individuals may result from assortative mating of an individual with major affective disorder to an individual with the BAP.

Finally, the observation that particular personality characteristics are common in relatives of autistic individuals raises the question of whether these characteristics are associated with impairment and warrant diagnosis as a personality disorder. Piven (2002) examined the parents from 25 multiple-incidence autism families and 30 Down syndrome (DS) families using the Structured Interview for DSM-III-R Personality Disorder (SIDP-R) (Pfohl, 1989). While four autism and none of the control parents were found to have an avoidant personality disorder (Fischer's Exact, $p = .045$) for the most part, the majority of autism parents did not have evidence of personality disorder or impairment related to the presence of particular personality characteristics such as aloof or rigid personality. On the whole, then, while psychiatric disorders may occur more commonly in parents of individuals with autism, whether or not they are to be considered a component of the BAP is still unclear.

Language and Academic Profiles Associated with the BAP

Severe language impairment is a defining feature of autism (APA, 1994) and among the most debilitating among the constellation of features that characterize this serious disorder. Twin and family studies have repeatedly documented qualitatively similar, but generally more subtly expressed language profiles among relatives, in the key domains that most robustly define the autism language phenotype—delayed language acquisition and pragmatic language abilities (Table 27-2).

A growing body of literature has documented delays in early language milestones among siblings of individuals with autism, including delayed lexical (i.e., word acquisition) and morphosyntactic (i.e., grammatical) development (Gamliel et al., 2007; Shaked et al., 2006; Yirmiya et al., 2001, Yirmiya et al., 2006, Yirmiya et al., 2007). Additionally, elevated rates of delayed first words and phrase speech have been reported retrospectively

Table 27–2.
Key language phenotypes associated with autism and the BAP

Key Language Phenotypes in Autism and the BAP	Autism/PDD	Relatives
Language Delays	+	+
• lexicon	+	+
• morphosyntax	+	+
Pragmatic impairments	+	+
• Prosody	+	+
• Conversation	+	+
• Narrative	+	+

among parents of individuals with autism (Bolton et al., 1994; Folstein et al., 1999; Murphy et al., 2000; Pickles et al., 2000; Piven, Palmer, Jacobi, et al., 1997). Indeed, delayed language was among the characteristics observed among nonautistic co-twins in Folstein and Rutter's twin study (1977). Using the AFHI, subsequent studies noted delayed language milestones, articulation problems, and delays in reading and spelling among relatives (Bolton et al., 1994; Bailey et al., 1995; Piven et al., 1990).

The most consistently observed language feature among relatives was pragmatic language use. Pragmatic language skills include connected speech in specific social-communicative contexts (conversation, narrative, etc.) and is the facet of language most closely tied to interpersonal interaction (Tager-Flusberg, 2000). Impaired pragmatic language use is universally observed across the autistic spectrum (Capps et al., 1998; Capps et al., 2000; Losh & Capps, 2003, 2006; Loveland & Tunali, 1993; Tager-Flusberg, 1995, 2000), even in those very high functioning individuals who do not show delayed language acquisition. Evidence of impaired pragmatic language skills among parents appeared in Leo Kanner's original clinical descriptions, in which he noted among parents a disdain for conversational interaction and a pedantic communicative style (1943). Wolff and colleagues (Wolff & Morris, 1971; Wolff et al., 1988) further described both over- and under communicativeness and verbal disinhibition among parents.

More systematic characterization of such pragmatic language styles was reported in two influential studies conducted by Landa and colleagues (Landa et al., 1991; Landa et al., 1992). In the first, parents were provided with story stems and asked to produce a complete narrative based on the initial prompt. Analyses revealed among autism parents a tendency to produce more tangential, fragmented accounts (i.e., noncontingent discourse), and stories that were rated on a global scale (by raters blind to group status) as significantly lower in quality than those from controls. In a second investigation, focusing on pragmatic language abilities of parents, Landa et al. (1992) employed the Pragmatic Rating Scale (PRS, described earlier). Applying the PRS to language samples from a semistructured conversation with parents of individuals with autism and controls, Landa et al. found the language samples from autism parents to be most notably characterized by topic preoccupation, overly talkativeness, detailed and confusing accounts marked by multiple tangents and abrupt topic changes with insufficient causal links and background information. Importantly, such features are qualitatively similar to the pragmatic language profiles noted among autistic individuals (Capps et al., 1998; Tager-Flusberg, 1991).

These findings were replicated in a later study of multiple-incidence families (Piven, Palmer, Landa, et al., 1997). Ruser et al. (2008) also confirmed this pattern in a study comparing parents of individuals with autism, parents of individuals with specific language impairment (SLI), and parents of individuals with Down syndrome. Some evidence exists to suggest that SLI and autism may overlap in etiology and phenotypes (e.g., Kjelgaard & Tager-Flusberg, 2001), and this study aimed to determine whether shared pragmatic language profiles may exist in relatives at increased liability to autism and SLI. Using a modified version of the PRS, in which several items were combined and emotional expression and grammatical errors were also assessed, both parents of individuals with autism and parents of individuals with SLI scored higher on the modified PRS (i.e., committed more pragmatic language violations) than parents of individuals with Down syndrome. These results provide intriguing evidence that pragmatic language use may provide a marker of the genes involved in autism, and potentially in a related language disorder (SLI).

Findings from the Losh et al. (2008) study of multiple- and single-incidence autism families further suggest that pragmatic language profiles provide a sensitive marker of genetic liability to autism. Using the PRS to compare multiple- and single-incidence families, investigators found that as with the personality features, rigid and aloof, pragmatic language violations were most common among MIAF parents, who averaged ~4 pragmatic language violations during semistructured conversation, less so among SIAF parents, averaging ~2.5 errors, and the least frequent among DWNS parents, who committed on average fewer than one pragmatic language violation during conversation (Figure 27-2).

In addition to language delays and particular pragmatic language styles, early twin studies and family studies using family history methods reported cognitive delays, intellectual disability, and difficulties with early reading and spelling among siblings and family members (Folstein & Rutter, 1977; August et al., 1981; Baird & August, 1985; Folstein et al., 1999; Minton et al., 1982; Piven, Palmer, Jacobi, et al., 1997), raising the possibility that genetic liability to autism could manifest as a pervasive cognitive deficit, rather than more specific and subtle personality and language features. Later studies did not find evidence for intellectual disability among relatives that was not associated with autism (Fombonne et al., 1997; Piven & Palmer, 1997; Szatmari et al., 1993; Bailey et al., 1995), although developmental problems in reading and spelling have been reported repeatedly (Folstein et al., 1999; Piven & Palmer, 1997).

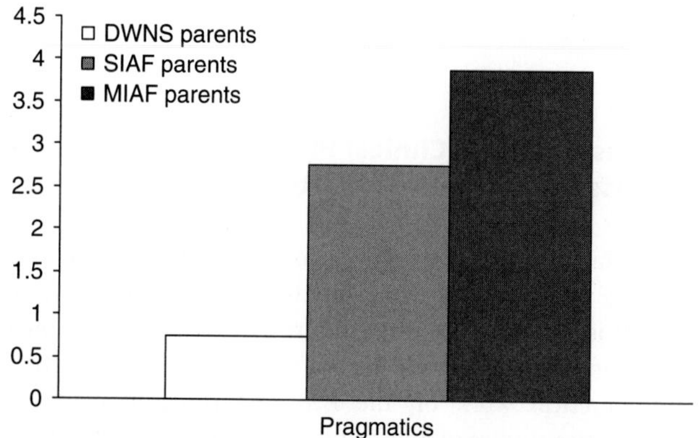

Figure 27–2. Mean number of pragmatic language violations measured by the PRS, across families differing in genetic liability to autism.

To further investigate whether cognitive and language disability may comprise part of the manifestation of genetic liability to autism, relatives' performance on standardized cognitive and language tests has been examined. This body of work has yielded equivocal results. On standardized intelligence tests, a discrepancy in verbal and performance abilities has been described in several separate case-control studies. Minton et al. (1982) found lower verbal IQ than performance IQ among siblings of individuals with autism. LeBoyer et al. (1995) also found a verbal-performance split, with performance IQ significantly higher among siblings, but this was specific to brothers of female autistic individuals. Investigating, parents' IQ profiles, several groups have reported lower performance IQs than controls (Folstein, Santangelo, Gilman, Piven, et al., 1999; Piven & Palmer, 1997; Schmidt, Kimel, Winterrowd, et al., 2008), and higher verbal IQs were observed in another study of parents and siblings (Fombonne et al., 1997). Other studies, however, have failed to detect differences in IQ (e.g., Bishop, et al., 2004; Pilowsky, et al., 2003; Szatmari et al., 1993; Szatmari et al., 1995).

Not unlike the picture in autism, conflicting findings present a somewhat muddled picture of the cognitive profiles of relatives, and studies employing standardized language tests of language have yielded similarly inconsistent results. Examining parents' performance on standardized tests of language, and phonological processing, Folstein et al. (1999) and Piven and Palmer (1997) reported deficits among the autism parent group on nonsense word reading, which taps phonological awareness. A later study also reported problems in nonword repetition among parents (Schmidt et al., 2008), a deficit that has also been observed in autism (Kjelgaard & Tager-Flusberg, 2001). These findings bolstered arguments favoring a shared etiology of autism and specific language impairment, where such phonological processing deficits are a hallmark (see Williams et al., 2008 for review), and could indicate overlapping pathophysiology and potential shared targets for intervention particular to specific symptom domains in autism. Yet studies have failed to replicate these findings consistently (e.g., Bishop et al., 2004), and therefore the findings require further study before their relevance to autism and the BAP can be evaluated.

What is the BAP? Clinical Phenotype and Associated Endophenotypes

Evaluating the array of findings across personality, psychiatric, language, and cognitive domains, the key question is, What actually is the BAP? To begin to address this question, and offer a nomenclature that may assist in structuring theoretical and empirical work on the BAP, returning to Kanner's original case studies of autism may be instructive. Among his original 11 patients, Kanner described clinical features and functional impairment in three key domains. These children displayed functional impairments in their ability "to relate themselves in the ordinary way to people and situations from the beginning of life," along with impaired social communicative behaviors marked by "monotonously repetitious" language, and restricted and repetitive interests and behaviors accompanied by "an anxiously obsessive desire for the maintenance of sameness." These clinical observations focused foremost on functional impairment associated with the features Kanner observed.

Applying this paradigm to findings from studies of the relatives of individuals with autism, the picture emerging is one of a subtle constellation of personality and language features among nonautistic relatives that parallel the defining features of autism, and which are distinct from a pervasive developmental disorder or autism spectrum disorder by virtue of a *lack* of functional impairment—i.e., particular social dispositions (social reticence or aloof personalities), particular profiles of communication that are similar in quality to those observed in autism [literal language, some problems with the social use of language (pragmatics)], and rigid or perfectionistic personality style. (Further study will determine whether language and cognitive delays reported retrospectively, and now being observed in the infant-sibling literature, may be developmental precursors to such features.) Thus, whereas the BAP has at times been characterized broadly as an autism spectrum disorder or pervasive developmental disorder (and often captured by cutoff scores on scales also intended to assess autism, e.g., Bishop et al., 2004), most family-study research has described a much more subtle phenotype that would not qualify as an autism spectrum disorder by virtue of a lack of associated functional impairment (this issue is considered in greater depth in a later section). And whereas psychiatric disorders and cognitive measures (e.g., IQ profiles or intellectual disability) have in some studies shown familial aggregation or heritability among families of individuals with autism, findings are somewhat inconsistent, and these features are not qualitatively similar to the core characteristics of autism. They may therefore be most fruitfully considered as associated but not constitutional features of the BAP.

How then should we conceptualize other associated features that do not correspond to the clinical features of autism, and yet show robust segregation within families of individuals with autism, such as the neurocognitive abilities described in the section to follow (e.g., social cognition)? Are they part of the BAP? Defined in this way, such features are not part of the BAP per se, but instead, associated characteristics that may throw into sharper relief understanding of the pathogenesis of the BAP (and autism). This important distinction may also help to clarify the often fuzzy boundary separating subthreshold clinical variant from endophenotype (or intermediate phenotype) which may or may not be present in affected individuals. The endophenotype concept was originally introduced by John and Lewis (1966), who in their studies of insect biology argued the merits of an empirical approach focused not on "obvious and external" *exo*phenotypes, but instead on *endo*phenotypes, which are "microscopic and internal" (p. 152). Later applied to psychiatry by Gottesman and Shields (1967, 1972), the endophenotype concept has since been used to decompose complex psychiatric disorders into more fundamental components that are more proximal to underlying biology, are assessed by experimentally based methods rather than clinical observation, and which hold the possibility of more direct genotype-phenotype associations than the complex clinical phenomena that comprise clinical diagnoses (Allen et al., 2009). In the case of autism and related disorders, then, the "microscopic and internal" endophenotype can therefore offer a foothold between complex clinical phenotype and genetic mechanisms. Presented below are findings from a handful of studies that point toward specific neurocognitive features associated with the BAP, which may serve as promising endophenotype candidates.

The Neurocognitive Underpinnings of the BAP: Identifying Endophenotypes

The validity of the BAP as a clinical phenomenon is apparent from the numerous case-control studies that have documented repeatedly a constellation of personality and language features among relatives, paralleling in quality the core features of autism. However, like autism, this construct is still considerably removed from underlying mechanisms that could give rise to these profiles, and which are mediated by those genes and neural circuits underlying autism. The BAP is also difficult to measure in a way that can be efficiently and reliably applied to genetic studies, where phenotypes reflecting specific biological substrates are ideal.

Language Processing

Whereas profiles from omnibus tests of cognition and language have produced inconsistent results, more specific tests of language processing have shown some promise in the way of defining particular cognitive-linguistic systems related to the BAP. In particular, robust patterns of difference have been documented on tests of rapid automatized naming (RAN). RAN is a sensitive index of reading ability (Wolf & Bowers, 2000), and is known to tap such fundamental language skills as phonological processing and memory, articulation, and linguistic processing speed (Denckla & Cutting, 1999; Denckla & Rudel, 1972, 1974, 1976; Holland, McIntosh, & Huffman, 2004). The rapid automatized naming (RAN) task first appeared in *The Mental Examiner's Handbook* as a bedside measure of recovery from brain injury in the mid-1900s. Patients were shown a series of randomly repeating squares printed in primary colors and instructed to name the colors as quickly as possible, with speed and accuracy serving as measures of recovery. The RAN was soon used experimentally in patients with focal brain lesions to study brain-behavior relationships (Geschwind & Fusillo, 1966). These early studies revealed that the RAN taps a number of important language processing skills that could be localized to specific regions of the brain, and which reflected stages of brain development (Denckla, 1972). In particular, subsequent research has shown that response speed measured by the RAN is linked to myelin deposition over the course of development, and resulting advances in language related skills (Mabbott et al., 2006). Deficits in rapid naming have also been associated with decreased connectivity (Deutsch et al., 2005), establishing further a link to neurocognitive underpinnings of this language related skill.

Piven and Palmer (1997) first reported slower RAN among parents of children with autism in contrast to controls, and in an expanded study involving over 300 parents of children with autism Losh et al. (2010) again found slower times and more errors among parents, as well as among a smaller group (n = 38) of high-functioning individuals with autism (see Figure 27-3). Further, significant parent-child correlations were detected for time and number of errors, supporting a genetic influence. Associations were also detected with features of the BAP. Both aloof personality style and language features of the BAP were associated with longer times to complete the task, a finding that could implicate limited verbal fluency in the language and associated social features of the BAP. Results further indicated that parents who were rated positive for the rigid personality trait were more likely to commit errors, or to become momentarily "stuck" on a prior color. This latter finding could reflect underlying difficulties in cognitive flexibility among parents showing the rigid trait of the BAP, as limitations therein could conceivably relate to this personality style. Because this task has been linked with particular neural circuitry, the RAN and similar tasks may provide neurocognitive markers of genetic liability to autism. Such links have begun to be addressed more directly through studies of neuropsychological abilities among relatives, as well as more direct research into brain activity, described below.

Social Cognition, Executive Function, and Central Coherence

In an effort to understand the underpinnings of the personality features of the BAP, Losh et al. (2009) conducted a neuropsychological assessment of high-functioning individuals with autism

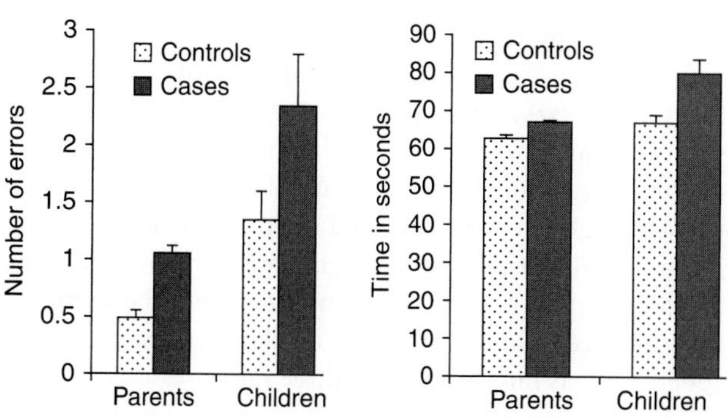

Figure 27–3. RAN performance in individuals with autism and parents.

and parents of autistic individuals (both with and without the BAP, defined by personality characteristics of aloof and rigid), across the three principal neurocognitive domains that have each been proposed as key cognitive abilities in which impairments may explain the autistic phenotype—social cognition, central coherence, and executive function. The study's aims were threefold: (1) to provide an in-depth characterization of the neuropsychological profile of the BAP; (2) to identify patterns of performance within and across neuropsychological domains that were common to both autistic individuals and parents with and without the BAP; and (3) to identify cosegregation between clinical phenotype (aloof, rigid, pragmatic language) and neuropsychological functioning that might serve to carve out specific phenotypic subtypes and that could form the basis for stronger genotype-phenotype associations.

The study assessed performance using a battery of tasks selected to assess processing comprehensively within a given domain and which could provide links to studies of subjects with circumscribed neurological lesions and fMRI studies that could shed light on specific neural structures that are involved in autism, and potentially the BAP. In particular, measures of social cognition, executive function, and central coherence were selected based on (1) their ties to the neuropsychological domains of interest, both theoretically and from their usage in prior neuropsychological investigations; (2) psychometric properties, including reliability and indication that each was appropriate for administration to all participants (i.e., suitable for both individuals with autism, parents, and controls) without danger of floor or ceiling effects; and (3) additional empirical evidence from fMRI and/or lesion studies suggesting associations with particular structures or regions of the brain thought to be important for the three domains and putatively implicated also in autism.

In brief, measures of social cognition tapped the ability to infer social-emotional information from various channels—the eye region of the face (via the Reading the Mind from the Eyes Task (Baron-Cohen, Wheelwright, Hill et al., 2001), facial information in general (through the Movie Stills and Trustworthiness of Faces tasks, Adolphs et al., 1998), and biological motion (through pointlight stimuli in which an actor was adorned with light emitting diodes and instructed to move across a stage in ways that conveyed different emotions—e.g., trudging slowly, dancing, lively strutting, etc.). Images were presented with only the points of light visible, such that no facial or contextual information was available. Measures of executive function included the commonly used Tower of Hanoi, which involves planning a sequence of moves that transfer an initial configuration of rings onto a particular peg, abiding by certain rules; and the trail making test, which is a measure of set shifting and cognitive control of interference in which sequences of numbers and letters must be alternately used to trace to an end point as quickly as possible. Central coherence was tapped through three measures used in prior work—(1) the embedded figures test, which involves detection of simple geometric figures obscured within a more complex design; (2) sentence completion, in which subjects must complete sentence stems and responses are rated as local or global based on their interpretation within the context of the whole sentence [e.g., the sea tastes of salt and *pepper* (local) vs. *water* (global)]; and finally (3) a block design task that taps the relative salience of parts over wholes through presentation of unsegmented designs followed by segmented designs in which the participant's task is to construct a design using blocks based on a model that is either presented complete or presegmented. The latter condition (segmented) breaks the gestalt for typically developing subjects and renders processing of figure-parts easier.

Findings revealed that individuals with autism displayed impairment on all of the social cognitive measures, but performed comparably to controls on measures of executive function, and 2/3 measures of central coherence (showing a tendency to complete sentences with local responses). Findings within the parent groups indicated that those autism parents who did not display features of the BAP performed comparably to controls on all measures, yet parents with the social features of the BAP (aloof) showed marked differences from controls on measures of social cognition (see Figure 27-4 for examples of tasks). As illustrated in Table 27-3, in all social cognitive measures, differences were observed in *both* individuals with autism and parents with the social BAP. By contrast, parents (with and without the BAP) performed similarly to controls on tasks of executive function and central coherence.

Others have reported differences between autism relatives and controls on social cognitive measures (e.g., Baron-Cohen & Hammer, 1997; Baron-Cohen, Wheelwright, Hill, et al., 2001; Gokcen et al., 2009), yet the present findings suggest that such differences may cosegregate specifically with the clinically expressed social features of the BAP. Further, these data suggest that specific social cognitive profiles shared by individuals with autism and a subgroup of parents (i.e., those with the BAP) may involve a number of different social cognitive skills—making complex social judgments of trustworthiness from facial information (trustworthiness of faces), interpreting the emotional content of complex scenes with and without affective facial information (movie stills), inferring emotions from very subtle variations in facial expression (morphed faces), and interpreting complex emotional content from biological motion (point light).

Importantly, patterns of performance were in some instances qualitatively different in the autistic and parent groups, perhaps suggesting a pathoplasticity in these features, where common underlying mechanisms manifest variably in autism and the BAP. In the trustworthiness of faces task, for instance, individuals with autism judged negative faces as significantly "more positive" than controls (i.e., they were overly trusting), whereas BAP (+) parents judged positively valenced faces as "more negative" than controls and BAP (-) parents (illustrated in Figure 27-5). Such a divergence in performance demonstrates how the underlying *forme fruste* of the disorder (trouble characterizing social stimuli) may manifest variably based on experience, and level of functioning (i.e., autism vs. clinically unaffected parents). The BAP may therefore provide a mechanism for investigating the role of experience in autism

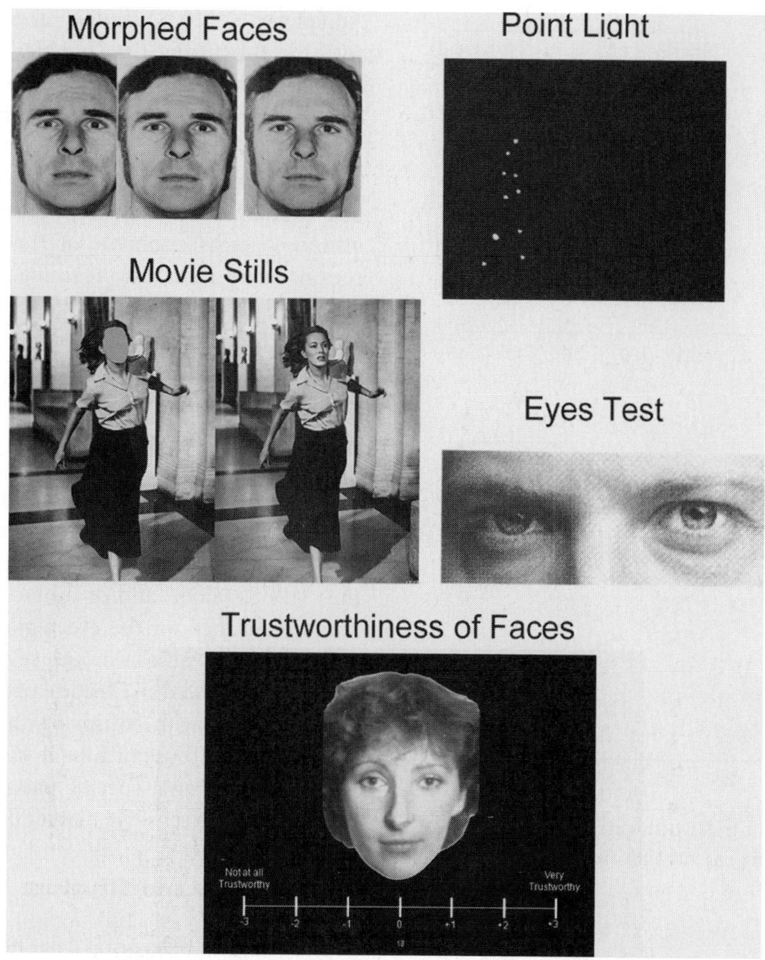

Figure 27–4. Measures of social cognition defining autism and the broad autism phenotype. Morphed Faces involve interpretation of faintly expressed emotions. Point Light stimuli tap the ability to read emotions from biological motion. The Movie Stills task indexes reliance on facial expressions when making emotional judgments. The Eyes Test requires interpretation of complex thoughts and emotions from only the eye region of the face. Finally, the Trustworthiness of Faces task measures complex social judgments based on facial stimuli varying gender, facial expression, and positioning.

Table 27–3.
Summary of findings (* denotes predicted difference detected at p < .05)

	Autism	BAP+ Parents
Social Cognition		
Eyes Task	*	*
Morphed Faces	*	*
Trustworthiness of Faces	*	*
Movie Stills	*	*
Point Light	*	*
Executive Function		
Tower of Hanoi	-	-
Trailmaking Test	-	-
Central Coherence		
Embedded Figures	-	-
Sentence Completion	*	-
Block Design	-	-

(as will the emergent literature on infant siblings of individuals with autism).

Executive function and central coherence measures did not discriminate parents with or without the BAP in this study. Several prior studies have demonstrated among relatives executive control deficits and a local processing bias as well as limited drive for central coherence (Jolliffe & Baron-Cohen, 1997; Bolte & Poustka, 2006; Happe et al., 2001; Hughes, Leboyer, & Bouvard, 1997; Hughes, Plumet, & Leboyer, 1999; Piven & Palmer, 1997). However, some other studies have also failed to detect differences in these domains (Szatmari et al., 1993; Ozonoff et al., 1993; de Jonge et al., 2009), raising the possibility that effects within these domains are more subtle and/or heterogeneous. Also, the net cast by the executive function task battery in the study by Losh et al. (2009) was not as broad as some other studies' and this may have reduced the ability to capture group differences. A related issue concerns the neurocognitive correlates of the rigid/perfectionistic features of the BAP. It is possible that this feature may not constitute as valid a construct as the social features of the BAP, or alternatively,

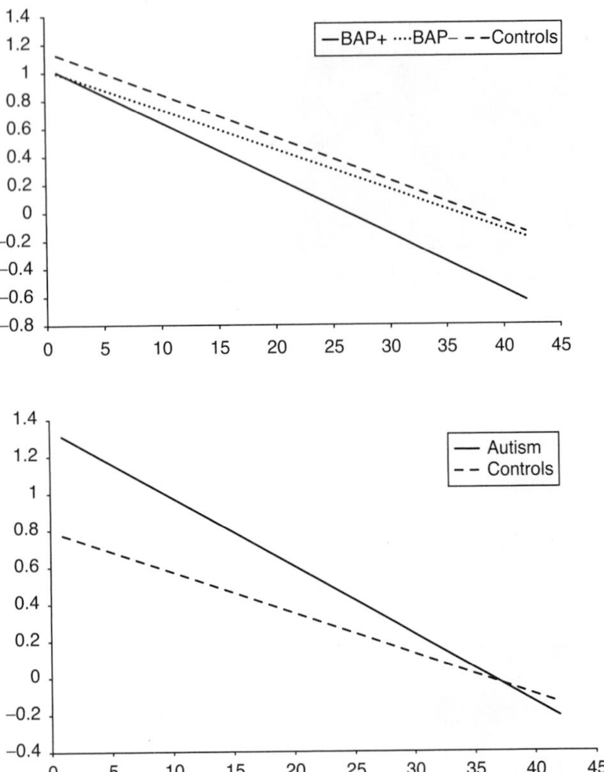

Figure 27–5. Judgments of the trustworthiness of faces by high functioning adults with autism, parents with and without the BAP, and respective control groups.

may relate to additional cognitive mechanisms not considered in this study (e.g., sensorimotor processing, which has been associated with repetitive behaviors in autism, Perry, Minassian, Lopez, et al., 2007). Nevertheless, the consistency of differences in social cognition, detected both in autism and parents with social features of the BAP point toward this domain as an important focus for future work teasing out the brain, and ultimately gene basis of autism and the BAP.

Further evidence that social cognition may be important to study in the BAP comes from an eye tracking study of face processing in parents of individuals with autism. Adolphs et al. (2008) studied face processing among parents with the BAP using the "bubbles" method (Gosselin et al., 2001). In this procedure, subjects were presented with obscured facial expressions containing randomly revealed "bubbles" of clarity of an underlying whole face and asked to determine whether each stimulus represented happiness or anger. That is, in some trials portions of the eye region were visible, whereas segments of the mouth, nose, and other regions were randomly revealed on other trials. Analyses examined those regions of the face that were present when accurate judgments were made, thereby providing a direct measure of perceptual processing strategies while judging emotional information. The number of bubbles (i.e., size of the region revealed) was adjusted on a trial-by-trial basis in order to maintain a relatively stable performance accuracy of ~80%. Whereas neurotypical control parents were found to rely heavily on the eye region, parents of individuals with autism who displayed social personality features measured by the MPAS (aloof and/or untactful) showed significantly reduced reliance on the eye regions (see Figure 27-6), and enhanced focus on the mouth region. Prior work by Spezio et al. (2007) showed an identical pattern among high-functioning individuals with autism on this task. These findings are consistent with those of Klin et al. (2002) and Pelphrey et al. (2002), suggesting a specific pattern of face processing that may constitute a sensitive marker of genetic liability to autism.

Brain Activity and Structure

Moving beyond behavioral data, neurocognitive features have been studied among relatives using more direct indices of brain activity. Using ERP, Dawson et al. (2005) showed that when viewing faces and nonsocial stimuli, parents of individuals with autism exhibited atypical neural responses. As has been observed in autism, parents of children with autism failed to show the typical shorter latency N170 to faces than nonface stimuli. Furthermore, they did not exhibit the typical right hemisphere lateralization when viewing faces. Abnormal brain activation has also been noted among siblings of individuals with autism. In a study of face processing ability in unaffected siblings, Dalton et al. (2007) found that siblings showed

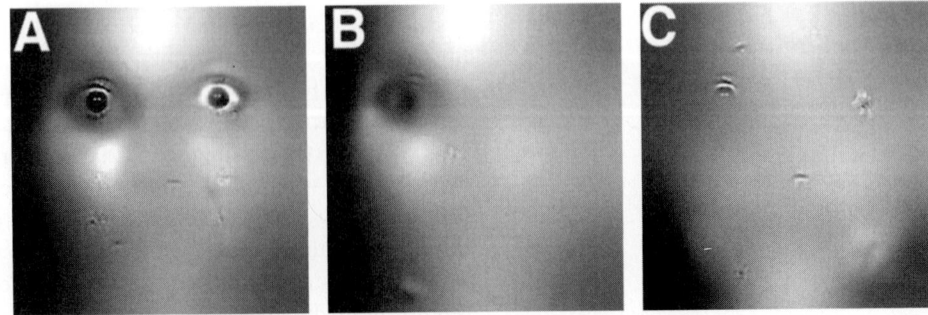

Figure 27–6. (A) shows facial regions used by controls when making accurate judgments; (B) depicts those regions used more often by control parents than BAP (+); and (C) depicts the difference between controls vs. BAP (–) parents.

reduced gaze fixation to eye regions of still faces, and fMRI conducted during the face viewing task revealed reduced activation in the fusiform gyrus, a brain structure largely devoted to face processing. Taken together, these findings are notable in their similarity to what has been observed in autism, suggesting they may serve as neural trait markers of genetic liability.

Just as studies of the BAP have trailed behind those of autism, cognitive neuroscience studies of the BAP have emerged only relatively recently. To date these studies have reported similarities between what has been found in prior studies with autism. Established findings on the neurobiological basis of autism may therefore provide a logical guide for pursuing this investigation—i.e., given what is known from neurobiological studies of autism, one can formulate hypotheses about what one might expect to find in the BAP. These first-order hypotheses would include the amygdala and visual cortices in the temporal lobe as key brain structures that mediate abnormal processing of faces and eye gaze (Pelphrey et al., 2005). They would include structural connectivity, specifically the idea that there may be altered white matter and reduced long-range connectivity in the brain. And they would include functional connectivity, such as the prediction that the "default network" of the brain would not be normally activated during rest. Evidence briefly reviewed here supports these hypotheses. Further work using magnetic resonance imaging (structural, BOLD-based, and diffusion-imaging) as well as complementary careful postmortem studies of brains will be required to delineate the neurocognitive basis of the BAP.

It will also be critical eventually to test hypotheses about how the brains of people with the BAP might *differ* from those with autism. Rather than assuming that, like the full syndrome, all biological measures in the BAP will look qualitatively similar to those in autism, only milder, it may be that there are other patterns. For instance, it might be that only certain brain regions in the BAP share features with autism. Alternatively, it may be that the endophenotype that mediates between genetic liability and phenotype looks rather different in the BAP and in autism (as observed in findings of differing patterns of trustworthiness judgments among parents with the BAP and high-functioning individuals with autism; Losh et al., 2009). Attention to such complexities will be important for establishing not only the biological basis of autism, but also the range of phenotypic expression arising from such biological substrates.

Summary: The Significance of the Concept of a BAP

Defining Boundaries Between Autism, the BAP, and Typical Development

The BAP can provide a useful tool for defining the varied clinical expressions of genetic liability to autism, and demarcating the clinical boundaries of autism in particular. Autism has been conceptualized as both a categorical entity (DSM-IV) and as constituting one end of a continuum of continuously distributed traits in the population (e.g., Constantino, 2009). The former characterization makes sense in the clinical arena, where autism is a syndrome associated with functional impairment and warranting treatment. The latter conceptualization has had increasing relevance in research studies aimed at understanding underlying pathogenesis. Clinical and research fields have wrestled with the interface of these overlapping domains in developing a nomenclature applicable to their purpose. This issue is evident in the gradual evolution from the terms "autism" and "pervasive developmental disorder" to the increasingly common use of the term "autism spectrum disorders" for identifying this group of related clinical conditions.

A question then arises about the boundary between the BAP and "autism spectrum disorders" and the usefulness of making this distinction. As reviewed earlier, Piven and Palmer (1999) examined parents with the BAP using a structured interview for personality disorder and for the most part found that these individuals did not have evidence of a personality disorder (i.e., they had no evidence of significant clinical impairment). While understanding the characteristics of the BAP may be useful in understanding families, and parents in particular, of individuals with autism and in providing optimal care, the BAP does not appear to be an indication for treatment. Therefore conceptualizing the BAP as part of an underlying continuum of distributed traits in the population that are genetically related to but not equivalent to autism or an autism spectrum disorder may be a useful distinction to make in the clinical arena. Given the increasing demands on the health care system for services for autism spectrum disorders, defining this upper boundary of autism (as opposed to a lower boundary between individuals with so-called low-functioning autism and those with mental retardation without autism) between individuals with an autism spectrum disorder (i.e., high-functioning autism and Asperger's syndrome) and those with the BAP may be an important distinction for clinicians to keep in mind when they see characteristics in family members that are qualitatively similar to autism, and that may have a determining role in lifestyle preferences, but are not associated with significant functional impairment.

In a related vein, studies of the BAP may also inform studies of the underlying nature of personality traits in the general population. For instance, do features of the BAP actually differ in etiology from these personality and language traits that can occur (though at much lower rates) in the general population? In other words, is social reticence in one who has no family history of autism etiologically distinct from the aloof dispositions described as comprising the BAP among relatives of individuals with autism? And how do environmental factors contribute, potentially differentially, in these different cases? Implicit in Kanner's original writings, and generally explicit in current empirical treatment of the BAP is the notion that features of the BAP are due to shared genetic variance associated with autism and thus distinct in etiology from personality traits observed in the general population.

A definitive answer to this question will require systematic studies of neurobiology and genetic variation related to such traits in populations varying in genetic liability to autism.

Genetic Significance of the BAP

Progress in understanding the etiology of autism may be hastened by parallel studies of the BAP. Whereas autism by definition involves all three symptom domains, in the BAP, features disaggregate and may occur independently, consistent with twin studies indicating that although the component features of autism all have strong genetic effects, they seem largely independent in patterns of transmission, with relatively little phenotypic or genetic overlap (Ronald et al., 2005, 2006). As a distilled expression of latent liability, the BAP can therefore provide a glimpse at the *forme fruste* of the disorder of autism, and its often complex and variable phenotypic manifestation. For example, in findings discussed earlier, Losh et al. (2009) identified impairments among individuals with autism and parents with the BAP, who shared differences in reading social cues across various social cognition tasks relative to controls. However, they were at times expressed in different ways (e.g., varying profiles judging trustworthiness). In this way, the BAP may prove critical in focusing on core behavioral and neuropsychological features and helping to narrow the empirical target from an otherwise highly complex and heterogeneous phenotype (i.e., a diagnosis of autism), to more specific component features that are likely to be more amenable to genetic and neurobiological study.

Whereas the clinically observable features of the BAP (aloof and rigid personality, pragmatic language profiles) are hypothesized to arise from a smaller constellation of genes (and/or gene-environment interactions) than autism, they do not seem to constitute endophenotypes in the strict sense of this term, at least in the same way as associated neurocognitive features, given the latter category's greater proximity to underlying biology (e.g., social cognition, brain activation, shorter N170 latency to facial stimuli; Allen et al., 2009). However, the BAP may prove critical in the detection of such endophenotypes. Because not all parents show the clinical features of the BAP, endophenotypes would be hypothesized to be present among the subgroup of parents who do. Support for this hypothesis comes from studies previously reviewed showing that language processing (RAN) and social cognitive profiles segregate with features of the clinically defined BAP (Adolphs et al., 2008; Losh & Piven, 2007; Losh et al., 2009; Losh et al., 2010). Thus, while the distinction between clinical phenotype (e.g., the BAP) and endophenotype (e.g., brain structure) is important to consider, these constructs are likely to be studied most profitably when considered jointly.

The BAP may therefore help to guide genetic studies by offering, as an alternative to the search for "autism genes," a more focused detection effort involving specific endophenotypes underlying components of the BAP, and that are linked in a more straightforward way to underlying susceptibility genes. The promise of the BAP for guiding genetic studies is supported by recent molecular genetic studies implementing phenotypic subgrouping in affected individuals and their parents (e.g., Alarcon et al., 2005; Duvall et al., 2007; Buxbaum et al., 2004; Autism Genome Project Consortium, 2008). Though still in its incipience, this approach of more precise phenotyping using features of the BAP and, eventually, endophenotypes, has already proven to be a method that strengthens power to detect linkage and association. When implemented into the large-scale collaborative efforts currently underway, such techniques may afford increased power and sensitivity for defining different etiologic pathways and, ultimately, leading to important new knowledge of the pathogenetics of autism.

Conclusions

As reviewed in this chapter, considerable evidence now exists to suggest that genetic liability to autism may be expressed through subtle behavioral and language features among relatives. Such features are similar in quality to the defining features of autism, but much milder in expression and do not appear to be associated with any functional impairment. Furthermore, the features of the BAP appear more common among relatives from families with multiple incidences of autism, providing further support for the idea that such features index genetic liability. Research is beginning to document the neuropsychological basis of the BAP, and such findings will be critical in moving forward in defining the brain and gene basis of autism.

Challenges and Future Directions

- Findings reviewed in this chapter support further study of the component features of the BAP and the neuropsychological characteristics that underlie the components of this construct.
- Evidence suggests that as a distilled expression of genetic liability, the BAP may offer a useful guide in studies of the brain and gene basis of autism.
- An important direction for future work will be to identify and/or develop efficient and standardized methods for measurement of the BAP that may be helpful for large-scale population and genetic studies.

Suggested Readings

Eisenberg, L. (1957). The fathers of autistic children. *American Journal of Orthopsychiatry, 27*, 715–724.

Folstein, S., & Rutter, M. (1977). Infantile autism: A genetic study of 21 twin pairs. *Journal of Child Psychology and Psychiatry, 18*, 297–321.

Losh, M., Adolphs, R., Poe, M., Penn, D., Couture, S., Baranek, G., et al. (2009). The Neuropsychological profile of autism and the broad autism phenotype. *Archives of General Psychiatry, 66*, 518–526.

ACKNOWLEDGMENT

The authors wish to thank Morgan Parlier for her important contributions to many of the studies reviewed in this chapter.

REFERENCES

Adolphs, R., Tranel, D., & Damasio, A. R. (1998). The human amygdala in social judgment. *Nature, 393*, 470–474.

Adolphs, R., Spezio, M., Parlier, M., & Piven, J. (2008). Distinct face-processing strategies in parents of autistic children. *Current Biology,18*(14), 1090–1093.

Alarcon, M., Yonan, A. L., Gilliam, T. C., Cantor, R. M., & Geschwind, D. H. (2005). Quantitative genome scan and Ordered-Subsets Analysis of autism endophenotypes support language QTLs. *Molecular Psychiatry, 10*, 747–757.

Allen, A., Griss, M., Folley, B., Hawkins, K., & Pearlson, G. (2009). Endophenotypes in schizophrenia: A selective review. *Schizophrenia Research, 109*, 24–37.

American Psychiatric Association. (1994). *Diagnostic and statistical manual of mental disorders* (4th ed.). Washington, DC: Author.

August, G. J., Stewart, M. A., & Tsai, L. (1981). The incidence of cognitive disabilities in the siblings of autistic children. *British Journal of Psychiatry, 138*, 416–422.

Bailey, A., Le Couteur, A., Gottesman, I., Bolton, P., Simonoff, E., Yuzda, E., et al. (1995). Autism as a strongly genetic disorder: Evidence from a British twin study. *Psychological Medicine, 25*, 63–77.

Baird, T. D., & August, G. J. (1985). Familial heterogeneity in infantile autism. *Journal of Autism and Developmental Disorders, 15*, 315–321.

Baron-Cohen, S., & Hammer, J. (1997). Parents of children with Asperger syndrome: What is the cognitive phenotype? *Journal of Cognitive Neuroscience, 9*, 548–554.

Baron-Cohen, S., Wheelwright, S., Hill, J., Raste, Y., Plumb, I. (2001). The Reading the Mind in the Eyes Test Revised Version: A study with normal adults, and adults with Asperger syndrome or high-functioning autism. *Journal of Child Psychology and Psychiatry, 42*, 241–251.

Baron-Cohen, S., Wheelwright, S., Skinner, R., Martin, J., & Clubley, E. (2001). The autism-spectrum quotient (AQ): Evidence from Asperger syndrome/high-functioning autism, males and females, scientists and mathematicians. *Journal of Autism and Developmental Disorders, 31*, 5–17.

Belmonte, M. K., & Bourgeron, T. (2006). Fragile X syndrome and autism at the intersection of genetic and neural networks. *Nature Neuroscience, 9*, 1221–1225.

Bettelheim, B. (1967). *The empty fortress: Infantile autism and the birth of the self.* New York: Free Press.

Bishop, D. V. (1998). Development of the Children's Communication Checklist (CCC): A method for assessing qualitative aspects of communicative impairment in children. *Journal of Child Psychology and Psychiatry, 39*, 879–891.

Bishop, D. V., Maybery, M., Maley, A., Wong, D., Hill, W., & Hallmayer J. (2004). Using self-report to identify the broad phenotype in parents of children with autistic spectrum disorders: A study using the Autism-Spectrum Quotient. *Journal of Child Psychology and Psychiatry, 45*, 1431–1436.

Bishop, D. V., Maybery, M., Wong, D., Maley, A., & Hallmayer, J. (2006). Characteristics of the broader phenotype in autism: A study of siblings using the children's communication checklist-2. *American Journal of Medical Genetics, 141*, 117–122.

Bolte, S., & Poustka, F. (2006). The broader cognitive phenotype of autism in parents: How specific is the tendency for local processing and executive dysfunction? *Journal of Child Psychology and Psychiatry and Allied Disciplines, 47*, 639–645.

Bolton, P., MacDonald, H., Pickles, A., Rios, P., Goode, S., Crowson, et al. (1994). A case-control family history study of autism. *Journal of Child Psychology and Psychiatry, 35*, 877–900.

Bolton, P. F., Pickles, A., Murphy, M., & Rutter, M. (1998). Autism, affective, and other psychiatric disorders: Patterns of familial aggregation. *Psychological Medicine, 28*, 385–395.

Boutin, P., Maziade, M., Mérette, C., Mondor, M., Bédard, C., & Thivierge, J. (1997). Family history of cognitive disabilities in first-degree relatives of autistic and mentally retarded children. *Journal of Autism and Developmental Disorders, 27*, 165–176.

Buxbaum, J. D., Silverman, J., Keddache, M., Smith, C. J., Hollander, E., Ramoz, N., et al. (2004). Linkage analysis for autism in a subset of families with obsessive-compulsive behaviors: Evidence for an autism susceptibility gene on chromosome 1 and further support for susceptibility genes on chromosome 6 and 19. *Molecular Psychiatry, 9*, 144–150.

Capps, L., Kehres, J., & Sigman, M. (1998). Conversational abilities among children with autism and developmental delay. *Autism, 2*, 325–344.

Capps, L., Losh, M., & Thurber, C. (2000). The frog ate a bug and made his mouth sad: Narrative competence in children with autism. *Journal of Abnormal Child Psychology, 28*, 193–204.

Constantino, J. N., Hudziak, J. J., & Todd, R. D. (2003). Deficits in reciprocal social behavior in male twins: Evidence for a genetically independent domain of psychopathology. *Journal of the American Academy of Child and Adolescent Psychiatry, 42*, 458–467.

Constantino, J. N., & Todd, R. D. (2005). Intergenerational transmission of subthreshold autistic traits in the general population. *Biological Psychiatry, 57*(6), 655–660.

Constantino, J. N. (2009). How continua converge in nature: Cognition, social competence, and autistic syndromes. *Journal of the American Academy of Child and Adolescent Psychiatry, 48*, 97–98.

Costa, P. T. J., & McCrae, R. R. (1985). *The NEO Personality Inventory Manual.* Odessa, FL: Psychological Assessment Resources.

Dalton, K. M., Nacewicz, B. M., Alexander, A. L., & Davidson, R. J. (2007). Gaze-fixation, brain activation, and amygdala volume in unaffected siblings of individuals with autism. *Biological Psychiatry, 61*(4), 512–520.

Daniels, J. L., Forssen, U., Hultman, C. M., Cnattingius, S., Savitz, D. A., Feychting, M., et al. (2008). Parental psychiatric disorders associated with autism spectrum disorders in the offspring. *Pediatrics, 121*, e1357–e1362.

Dawson, G., Estes, A., Munson J., Schellenberg, G., Bernier, R., & Abbott, R. (2007). Quantitative assessment of autism symptom-related traits in probands and parents: Broader phenotype autism symptom scale. *Journal of Autism and Developmental Disorders, 37*(3), 523–536.

Dawson, G., Webb, S. J., Wijsman, E., Shellenberg, G., Estes, A., Munson, J., et al. (2005). Neurocognitive and electrophysiological evidence of altered face processing in parents of children with autism: Implications for a model of abnormal development of social brain circuitry in autism. *Development and Psychopathology, 17*(3), 679–697.

De Fosse, L., Hodge, S. M., Makris, N., Kennedy, D. N., Caviness, V. S., Jr., McGrath, L., et al. (2004). Language-association cortex asymmetry in autism and specific language impairment. *Annals of Neurology, 56*, 757–766.

de Jonge, M., Kemner, C., Naber, F., & van Engeland, H. (2009). Block design reconstruction skills: Not a good candidate for an endophenotypic marker in autism research. *European Child and Adolescent Psychiatry, 18*, 197–205.

DeLong, G. R., & Dwyer, J. T. (1988). Correlation of family history with specific autistic subgroups: Asperger's syndrome and bipolar affective disease. *Journal of Autism and Developmental Disorders, 18*, 593–600.

DeLong, R., & Nohria, C. (1994). Psychiatric family history and neurological disease in autistic spectrum disorders. *Developmental Medicine and Child Neurology, 36*, 441–448.

Denckla, M. B. (1972). Color-naming defects in dyslexia boys. *Cortex, 10*, 186–202.

Denckla, M. B., & Cutting, L. E. (1999). History and significance of rapid automatized naming. *Annals of Dyslexia, 49*, 29–42.

Denckla, M. B., & Rudel, R. G. (1972). Color-naming in dyslexia boys. *Cortex, 8*, 164–176.

Denckla, M. B., & Rudel, R. G. (1974). Rapid "'automatized'" naming of pictured objects, colors, letters and numbers by normal children. *Cortex, 10*, 186–202.

Denckla, M. B., & Rudel, R. G. (1976). Rapid "automatized" naming (R.A.N), dyslexia differentiated from other learning disabilities. *Neuropsychologia, 14*(4), 471–479.

Deutsch, G. K., Dougherty, R. F., Bammer, R., Siok, W. T., Gabrieli, J. D., & Wandell, B. (2005). Children's reading performance is correlated with white matter structure measured by diffusion tensor imaging. *Cortex, 41*(3), 354–363.

Duvall, J. A., Lu, A., Cantor, R. M., Todd, R. D., Constantino, J. N., & Geschwind, D. H. (2007). A Quantitative trait locus analysis of social responsiveness in multiplex autism families. *American Journal of Psychiatry, 164*, 656–662.

Eisenberg, L. (1957), The fathers of autistic children. *American Journal of Orthopsychiatry, 27*, 715–724.

Falconer, D. S. (1965). The inheritance of liability to certain diseases estimated from incidences among relatives. *Annals of Human Genetics, 29*, 51–71.

Fombonne, E., Bolton, P., Prior, J., Jordan, H., & Rutter, M. (1997). A family study of autism: Cognitive patterns and levels in parents and siblings. *Journal of Child Psychology and Psychiatry, 38*, 667–683.

Folstein, S., & Rutter, M. (1977). Infantile autism: A genetic study of 21 twin pairs. *Journal of Child Psychology and Psychiatry, 18*, 297–321.

Folstein, S. E., Santangelo, S. L., Gilman, S. E., Piven, J., Landa, R., Lainhart, J., et al. (1999). Predictors of cognitive test patterns in autism families. *Journal of Child Psychology and Psychiatry, 40*(7), 1117–1128.

Freeman, B., Ritvo, E., Mason-Brothers, A., Pingree, C., Yokota, A., Jenson, W., et al. (1989). Psychometric assessment of first-degree relatives of 62 probands in Utah. *American Journal of Psychiatry, 146*, 361–364.

Freud, S. (1923). *The interpretation of dreams*. New York: Macmillan.

Gamliel, I., Yirmiya, M., & Sigman, M. (2007). The development of young siblings of children with autism from 4 to 54 months. *Journal of Autism and Developmental Disorders, 37*, 171–183.

Geschwind, N., & Fusillo, M. (1966). Color-naming defects in association with alexia. *Archives of Neurology, 15*, 137–143.

Gillberg, C., Gillberg, I. C., & Steffenburg, S. (1992). Siblings and parents of children with autism: A controlled population-based study. *Developmental Medicine and Child Neurology, 34*, 389–398.

Gokcen, S., Bora, S., Eremis, S., Kesikci, H., & Aydin, C. (2009). Theory of mind and verbal working memory deficits in parents of autistic children. *Psychiatry Research, 166*, 46–53.

Gosselin, F., & Schyns, P. G. (2001). Bubbles: A technique to reveal the use of information in recognition tasks. *Vision Research, 41*, 2261–2271.

Gottesman, I. I., & Shields, J. (1967). A polygenic theory of schizophrenia. *Proceedings of the National Academy of Sciences of the United States of America, 58*, 199–205.

Gottesman, I. I., & Shields, J. (1972). *Schizophrenia and genetics: A twin vantage point*. New York: Academic.

Happe, F., Briskman, J., & Frith, U. (2001). Exploring the cognitive phenotype of autism: Weak central coherence in parents and siblings of children with autism: I. Experimental tests. *Journal of Child Psychology and Psychiatry and Allied Disciplines, 42*, 299–307.

Holland, J., McIntosh, D., & Huffman, L. (2004). The role of phonological awareness, rapid automatized naming, and orthographic processing in word reading. *Journal of Psychoeducational Assessment, 22*, 233–260.

Hollander, E., King, A., Delaney, K., Smith, C. J., & Silverman, J. M. (2003). Obsessive-compulsive behaviors in parents of multiplex autism families. *Psychiatry Research, 117*, 11–16.

Hughes, C., Leboyer, M., & Bouvard, M. (1997). Executive function in parents of children with autism. *Psychological Medicine, 27*, 209–220.

Hughes, C., Plumet, M., & Leboyer, M. (1999). Towards a cognitive phenotype for autism: Increased prevalence of executive dysfunction and superior spatial span amongst siblings of children with autism. *Journal of Child Psychology and Psychiatry, 40*, 705–718.

Hurley, R., Losh, M., Childress, D., & Piven, J. (2007). The Broad Autism Phenotype Questionnaire. *Journal of Autism and Developmental Disorders, 37*(9), 1679–1690.

John, B., & Lewis, K. R. (1966). Chromosome variability and geographic distribution in insects. *Science, 152*(3723), 711–721.

Jolliffe, T., & Baron-Cohen, S. (1997). 'Are People with Autism and Asperger Syndrome Faster than Normal on the Embedded Figures Test?' *Journal of Child Psychology and Psychiatry and Allied Disciplines, 38*, 527–534

Jung, C. G. (1921). *Psychologische Typen*. Zurich: Rascher.

Kanner, L. (1943). Autistic disturbances of affective contact. *Nervous Child, 2*, 217–250.

Kano, Y., Ohta, M., Nagai, Y., Pauls, D. L., & Leckman, J. F. (2004). Obsessive-compulsive symptoms in parents of Tourette syndrome probands and autism spectrum disorder probands. *Psychiatry and Clinical Neurosciences, 58*, 348–352.

Kjelgaard, M. M., & Tager-Flusberg, H. (2001). An investigation of language impairment in autism: Implications for genetic subgroups. *Language and Cognitive Processes, 169*(2–3), 287–308.

Klin, A., Jones, W., Schultz, R., Volkmar, F., & Cohen, D. (2002). Visual fixation patterns during viewing of naturalistic social situations as predictors of social competence in individuals with autism. *Archives of General Psychiatry, 59*, 809–816.

Landa, R., Piven, J., Wzorek, M. M., Gayle, J. O., Chase, G. A., & Folstein, S. E. (1992). Social language use in parents of autistic individuals. *Psychological Medicine, 22*, 245–254.

Landa, R., Wzorek, M., Piven, J., Folstein, S., & Isaacs, C. (1991). Spontaneous narrative discourse characteristics of parents of autistic individuals. *Journal of Speech and Hearing Research, 34*, 1339–1345.

Leboyer, M., Plumet, M. H., Goldblum, M. C., Perez-Diaz, F., & Marchaland, C. (1995). Verbal versus visuospatial abilities in relatives of autistic females. *Developmental Neuropsychology, 11*, 139–155.

Le Couteur, A., Bailey, A., Goode, S., Pickles, A., Robertson, S., Gottesman, I. I., et al. (1996). A broader phenotype of autism: The clinical spectrum in twins. *Journal of Child Psychology and Psychiatry, 37*, 785–801.

Liu, X. Q., Paterson, A. D., Szatmari, P., & Autism Genome Project Consortium. (2008). Genome-wide linkage analyses of quantitative and categorical autism subphenotypes. *Biological Psychiatry, 64*, 561–570.

Losh, M., Adolphs, R., Poe, M., Penn, D., Couture, S., Baranek, G., et al. (2009). The Neuropsychological profile of autism and the broad autism phenotype. *Archives of General Psychiatry, 66*, 518–526.

Losh, M., & Capps, L. (2003). Narrative ability in high-functioning children with autism or Asperger's syndrome. *Journal of Autism and Developmental Disorders, 33*(3), 239–251.

Losh, M., & Capps, L. (2006). Understanding of emotional experience in autism: Insights from the personal accounts of high-functioning children with autism. *Developmental Psychology, 42*(5), 809–818.

Losh, M., Childress, D., Lam, K., & Piven, J. (2008). Defining key features of the broad autism phenotype: A comparison across parents of multiple- and single-incidence autism families. *American Journal of Medical Genetics. Part B, Neuropsychiatric Genetics, 147B*, 424–433.

Losh, M., Esserman, D., & Piven, J. (2010). Rapid Automatized Naming as an index of genetic liability to autism. *Journal of Neurodevelopmental Disorders, 2*, 109–116.

Losh, M., & Piven, J. (2007). Social-cognition and the broad autism phenotype: Identifying genetically meaningful phenotypes. *Journal of Child Psychology and Psychiatry, 48*(1), 105–112.

Loveland, K., & Tunali, B. (1993). Narrative language in autism and the theory of mind hypothesis: A wider perspective. In S. Baron-Cohen, H. Tager-Flusberg, & D. J. Cohen (Eds.), *Understanding other minds: Perspectives from autism*. Oxford, UK: Oxford University Press.

Mabbott, D. J., Noseworthy, M., Bouffet, E., Laughlin, S., & Rockel, C. (2006). White matter growth as a mechanism of cognitive development in children. *NeuroImage, 33*(3), 936–946.

Micali, N., Chakrabarti, S., & Fombonne, E. (2004). The broad autism phenotype: Findings from an epidemiological survey. *Autism, 8*(1), 21–37.

Minton, J., Campbell, M., Green, W. H., Jennings, S., & Samit, C. (1982). Cognitive assessment of siblings of autistic children. *Journal of the American Academy of Child Psychiatry, 21*, 256–261.

Murphy, M., Bolton, P., Pickles, A., Fombonne, E., Piven, J., & Rutter, M. (2000). Personality traits of the relatives of autistic probands. *Psychological Medicine, 30*, 1411–1424.

Narayan, S., Moyes, B., & Wolff, S. (1990). Family characteristics of autistic children: A further report. *Journal of Autism and Developmental Disorders, 20*, 523–535.

Ozonoff, S., Rogers, S. J., Farnham, J. M., & Pennington, B. F. (1993). Can standard measures identify subclinical markers of autism? *Journal of Autism and Developmental Disorders, 23*, 429–441.

Pelphrey, K. A., Morris, J. P., & McCarthy, G. (2005). Neural basis of eye gaze processing deficits in autism. *Brain, 128*, 1038–1048.

Pelphrey, K., Sasson, N., Reznick, J., Paul, G., Goldman, B., & Piven, J. (2002). Visual scanning of faces in autism. *Journal of Autism and Developmental Disorders, 32*, 249–261.

Perry, W., Minassian, A., Lopez, B., Maron, L., & Lincoln, A. (2007). Sensorimotor gating deficits in adults with autism. *Biological Psychiatry, 61*(4), 482–486.

Pfohl, B., Blum, N., Zimermann, M., & Stangel, D. (1989). *Structured Interview for DSM-III-R Personality Disorders (SIDP-R)*. Department of Psychiatry, University of Iowa, Iowa City, IA.

Pickles, A, Starr, E., Kazak, S., Bolton, P., Papanikolaou, K., Bailey, A., et al. (2000). Variable expression of the autism broader phenotype: Findings from extended pedigrees. *Journal of Child Psychology and Psychiatry, 41*, 491–502.

Pilowsky, T., Yirmiya, N., Shalev, R. S., & Gross-Tsur, V. (2003). Language abilities of siblings of children with autism. *Journal of Child Psychology and Psychiatry, 44*, 914–925.

Piven, J. (2002). The genetics of personality: The example of the broad autism phenotype. In J. Benjamin, R. P. Ebstein, & R. H. Belmaker (Eds.), *Molecular genetics and the human personality* (pp. 43–62). Washington, DC: American Psychiatric Publishing.

Piven, J., & Folstein, S. (1994). The genetics of autism. In M. Bauman & T. Kemper (Eds.), *The neurobiology of autism* (pp. 18–44). Baltimore: Johns Hopkins University Press.

Piven, J., Gayle, J., Chase, J., Fink, B., Landa, R., Wrozek, M., et al. (1990). A family history study of neuropsychiatric disorders in the adult siblings of autistic individuals. *Journal of the American Academy of Child and Adolescent Psychiatry, 29*, 177–183.

Piven, J., Landa, R., Gayle, J., Cloud, D., Chase, G., & Folstein, S. (1991). Psychiatric disorders in the parents of autistic individuals. *Journal of the American Academy of Child and Adolescent Psychiatry, 30*, 471–478.

Piven, J., & Palmer, P. (1997). Cognitive deficits in parents from multiple-incidence autism families. *Journal of Child Psychology and Psychiatry, 38*, 1011–1022.

Piven, J., & Palmer, P. (1999). Psychiatric disorder and the broad autism phenotype: Evidence from a family study of multiple-incidence autism families. *American Journal of Psychiatry, 156*(4), 557–563.

Piven, J., Palmer, P., Jacobi, D., Childress, D., & Arndt, S. (1997). Broader autism phenotype: Evidence from a family history study of multiple-incidence autism families. *American Journal of Psychiatry, 154*(2), 185–190.

Piven, J., Palmer, P., Landa, R., Santangelo, S., Jacobi, D., & Childress, D. (1997). Personality and language characteristics in parents from multiple-incidence autism families. *American Journal of Medical Genetics. Part B, Neuropsychiatric Genetics, 74*, 398–411.

Piven, J., Wzorek, M., Landa, R., Lainhart, J., Bolton, P., Chase, G. A., et al. (1994). Personality characteristics of the parents of autistic individuals. *Psychological Medicine, 24*, 783–795.

Plumet, M. H., Goldblum, M. C., & Leboyer, M. (1995). Verbal skills in relatives of autistic females. *Cortex, 31*, 723–733.

Ritvo, E., Freeman, B., Pingree, C., Mason-Brothers, A., Jorde, L., Jenson, W., et al. (1989). The UCLA-University of Utah epidemiologic survey of autism: Prevalence. *American Journal of Psychiatry, 146*, 194–199.

Ronald, A., Happe, F., & Plomin, R. (2005). The genetic relationship between individual differences in social and non-social behaviours characteristic of autism. *Developmental Science, 8*, 444–458.

Ronald, A., Happe, F., Thomas, P., Baron-Cohen, S., & Plomin, R. (2006). Phenotypic and genetic overlap between autistic traits at the extremes of the general population. *Journal of the American Academy of Child and Adolescent Psychiatry, 45*, 1206–1214.

Rudel, R. G., & Denckla, M. B. (1974). Relation of forward and backward digit repetition to neurological impairment in children with learning disabilities. *Neuropsychologia, 12*(1), 109–118.

Ruser, T. F., Arin, D., Dowd, M., Putnam, S., Winklosky, B., Rosen-Sheidley, B., et al. (2008). Communicative competence in parents of children with autism and parents of children with specific language impairment. *Journal of Autism and Developmental Disorders, 37*, 1323–1336.

Rutter, M. (1970). Autistic children: Infancy to adulthood. *Seminars in Psychiatry, 2*, 435–450.

Santangelo, S. L., & Folstein, S. E. (1995). Social deficits in the families of autistic probands. *American Journal of Human Genetics, 57*, 89.

Schmidt, G., Kimel, L. Winterrowd, E., Pennington, B., Hepburn, S., & Rojas, D. (2008). Impairments in phonological processing and nonverbal intellectual function in parents of children with autism. *Journal of Clinical and Experimental Neuropsychology, 30*(5), 557–567.

Shaked, M., Gamliel, I., & Yirmiya, N. (2006). Theory of mind abilities in young siblings of children with autism. *Autism, 10*, 173–187.

Smalley, S. L., & Asarnow, R. F. (1990). Brief report: Cognitive subclinical markers in autism. *Journal of Autism and Developmental Disorders, 20*, 271–278.

Smalley, S. L., McCracken, K., & Tanguay, P. (1995). Autism, affective disorders, and social phobia. *American Journal of Medical Genetics. Part B, Neuropsychiatric Genetics, 60*, 19–26.

Spezio, M. L., Adolphs, R., Hurley, R. S., & Piven, J. (2007). Abnormal use of facial information in high-functioning autism. *Journal of Autism and Developmental Disorders, 37*, 929–939.

Szatmari, P., Jones, M. B., Fisman, S., Tuff, L., Bartolucci, G., Mahoney, W. J., et al. (1995). Parents and collateral relatives of children with pervasive developmental disorders: A family history study. *American Journal of Medical Genetics. Part B, Neuropsychiatric Genetics, 60*, 282–289.

Szatmari, P., Jones, M. B., Tuff, L., Bartolucci, G., Fisman, S., & Mahoney, W. (1993). Lack of cognitive impairment in first-degree relatives of children with pervasive development disorders. *Journal of the American Academy of Child and Adolescent Psychiatry, 32*, 1264–1273.

Szatmari, P., MacLean, J. E., Jones, M. B., Bryson, S. E., Zwaigenbaum, L., Bartolucci, G., et al. (2000). The familial aggregation of the lesser variant in biological and nonbiological relatives of PDD probands: A family history study. *Journal of Child Psychology and Psychiatry, 41*, 579–586.

Tager-Flusberg, H. (1995). Once upon a ribbit: Stories narrated by autistic children. *British Journal of Developmental Psychology, 13*, 45–59.

Tager-Flusberg, H. (2000). Language and understanding minds: Connections in autism. In S. Baron-Cohen, H. Tager-Flusberg, & D. J. Cohen (Eds.). *Understanding other minds: Perspectives from autism*. Oxford, UK: Oxford University Press.

Tager-Flusberg, H., & Anderson, M. (1991). The development of contingent discourse ability in autistic children. *Journal of Child Psychology and Psychiatry, 32*(7), 1123–1134.

Tyrer, P. (1988). Personality Assessment Schedule. In P. Tyrer (Ed.), *Personality disorders: Diagnosis, management and course* (pp. 140–167). London: Butterworth.

Tyrer, P., Owen, R. T., & Cicchetti, D. V. (1984). The brief scale for anxiety: A subdivision of the Comprehensive Psychopathological Rating Scale. *Journal of Neurology, Neurosurgery, and Psychiatry, 47*, 970–975.

van den Oord, E. (1999). A comparison between different designs and tests to detect QTLs in association studies. *Behavior Genetics, 29*, 245–256.

Williams, D., Botting, N., & Boucher, J. (2008). Language in autism and specific language impairment: Where are the links? *Psychological Bulletin, 134*, 944–963.

Wolf, M., & Bowers, P. G. (2000). Naming-speed processes and developmental reading disabilities: An introduction to the special issue on the double-deficit hypothesis. *Journal of Learning Disabilities, 33*, 322–324.

Wolff, W. M., & Morris, L. A. (1971). Intellectual and personality characteristics of parents of autistic children. *Journal of Abnormal Psychology, 77*(2), 155–161.

Wolff, S., Narayan, S., & Moyes, B. (1988). Personality characteristics of parents of autistic children: A controlled study. *Journal of Child Psychology and Psychiatry, 29*(2), 143–153.

Wong, D., Mayberry, M., Bishop, D. V. M., Maley, A., & Jallmayer, J. (2006). Profiles of executive function in parents and siblings of individuals with autism spectrum disorders. *Genes, Brain, and Behavior, 5*, 561–576.

Yirmiya, N., Gamliel, I., Pilowsky, T., Baron-Cohen, S., Feldman, R., & Sigman, M. (2006). The development of siblings of children with autism at 4 and 14 months: Social engagement, communication, and cognition. *Journal of Child Psychology and Psychiatry, 47*, 511–523.

Yirmiya, N., Gamliel, I., Shaked, M., & Sigman, M. (2007). Cognitive and verbal abilities of 24- to 36-month-old siblings of children with autism. *Journal of Autism and Developmental Disorders, 37*, 218–229.

Yirmiya, N., Shaked, M., & Erel, O. (2001). Comparing siblings of individuals with autism and siblings of individuals with other diagnoses: An empirical summary. In E. Schopler, N. Yirmiya, C. Shulman, & L. Marcus (Eds.). *The research basis for autism intervention* (pp. 59–73). New York: Plenum.

28 Janet E. Lainhart, Nicholas Lange

The Biological Broader Autism Phenotype

Points of Interest

- To be a member of the Biological Broader Autism Phenotype, the rates of a biological alteration must be elevated above that of the general population in individuals with autism, in unaffected relatives generally, and in autism families specifically.
- No biological feature is currently required for the diagnosis of autism. Macrocephaly and increased rate of head and brain growth during early childhood are not included in the diagnostic criteria for autism. The absence of any biological feature does not exclude a diagnosis of autism at present.
- Hyperserotonemia is the only biological feature that has been shown to meet all criteria for inclusion in the Broader Autism Phenotype.
- Most intermediate phenotypes of the Biological Broader Autism Phenotype have yet to be discovered.

Introduction

At present, the Broader Autism Phenotype (BAP) is comprised of milder and partial cognitive, behavioral, and biological characteristics that are qualitatively the same as or conceptually similar in nature to the individual characteristics associated with autism. The biological subset of the present-day BAP is its smallest and most vital subdivision. The Biological Broader Autism Phenotype (BBAP) is the group of alterations in the development, structure, or function of the brain, other bodily systems, and their components that are inherited with autism in families. The key candidate members of the BBAP are the primary foci of this chapter.

Phenotype: an observable physical, biological, or behavioral characteristic influenced by genetic factors and the interaction between genes and environment.

Box 28–1

Intermediate phenotype (IP, in autism): a behavioral, cognitive, or biological trait found more commonly in affected and unaffected autism family members than in the general population. In the causal chain of developmental events, these phenotypes are in an intermediate position between the cause and the full diagnosis. As a result, the strength of the statistical association may be significantly stronger between a cause and an intermediate phenotype than between a cause and the full diagnosis. Components of the BAP are sometimes referred to as intermediate phenotypes. Gottesman and Shields (1972) introduced the term "endophenotype" during the course of their twin study in schizophrenia. As originally described by these pioneers, intermediate phenotypes and endophenotypes are conceptually identical (Gottesman & Gould, 2003; Szatmari et al., 2007). The first twin study of the genetic influences in autism suggested an inherited clinical phenotype broader than autism itself (Folstein & Rutter, 1972). The notion that a measurable trait, present in individuals with severe disorders such as schizophrenia or autism, could be present in some unaffected family members revolutionized thinking in neuropsychiatry.

It has been nearly 70 years since the clinical evidence that characteristics broader than autism may be inherited in families first emerged. Dr. Leo Kanner, in his eloquent clinical description of 11 children with autism, described particular traits and tendencies in unaffected family members, many of whom were gifted and outstanding individuals

(Kanner, 1943). Research evidence for an inherited phenotype broader than autism was derived over 30 years ago from the first twin study of autism (Folstein & Rutter, 1977). In this landmark study, co-twins of their sibling with autism were found to have increased rates of the disorder. Equally important, co-twins who did not have autism were found to have increased rates of cognitive difficulties, especially those involving language acquisition and socioemotional difficulties. These results led Folstein and Rutter to hypothesize the BAP, namely that autism is linked genetically to a range of difficulties broader than the disorder itself, with autism as the most severe form. Subsequent twin and family studies have confirmed that an inherited phenotype broader than autism exists (Bailey et al., 1995; Bolton et al., 1994; Folstein et al., 1999; Le Couteur et al., 1996; Piven et al., 1997). Nonautistic family members were found to have increased rates of delayed onset of spoken language, articulation problems, reading and spelling difficulties, specific social difficulties, occasionally repetitive interests and behaviors, and other features, alone or in combination. Twenty percent (20%) of members of families having one child with idiopathic autism have communication or social, cognitive, or behavioral features of the BAP (Bolton et al., 1994). The prevalence rate of the BAP has been estimated to be 30% or higher in families that have two or more children with idiopathic autism (Piven et al., 1997). These studies also confirmed that intellectual subnormality (mental retardation) found in many children with autism was not present in unaffected family members any more than in the general population.

Familial resemblance: a phenotype or phenotypes that show greater similarity in family members than in unrelated pairs of individuals (Rice, 2008). Exchangeable terms for familial resemblance are "familiality" and "familial aggregation." Familial resemblance provides essential evidence that a phenotype may be inherited in families, but resemblance within families can also be due to shared environments.

Idiopathic autism: autism without a known and specific medical cause. Roughly 90% of all known cases of autism are idiopathic; the remaining 10% arise from medical causes. Current evidence suggests that multiple genes and gene-environment interactions are involved in idiopathic autism but the majority of these are not yet known. Medical causes of autism include Fragile X syndrome, a genetic disorder in which there are long and abnormally repeated copies of DNA on the X chromosome, and tuberous sclerosis, a genetic disorder of the nervous system and the skin. Congenital rubella, an in utero rubella virus infection, is now known to be a rare medical cause of a form of autism.

If social, communication, and behavioral aspects of the BAP are known, and related neuropsychological aspects are being clarified (Losh et al., 2009), why is it important that research also focus on biological aspects of the BAP, the BBAP? It is self-evident that biological phenotypes are more proximal to the genetic mechanisms and the causal chain of events leading to autism than are cognitive and behavioral phenotypes. The biological and neurobiological determinants of autism and their potential genetic liabilities, however, remain in large part unknown. The present thinness of biological knowledge is somewhat surprising since autism has long been known to have the highest heritability of any neuropsychiatric disorder, of 0.7 for the narrow phenotype restricted to autism, and as high as 0.9 for the combined narrow and broader autism phenotypes (Geschwind, 2009). In addition, most features of the cognitive-behavioral BAP, as currently understood, are too variable and nonspecific to aid effective identification of the genes and neurobiological mechanisms involved in autism. Features of the cognitive-behavioral BAP, such as impairments in language, reading, and social functioning, can be due to many different genetic, biological, and nonbiological causes. The history of medicine has shown recurrently that the most pivotal advances in the differentiation of disorders with overlapping signs and symptoms and the discovery of different disease subtypes of clinical syndromes such as autism, have been biological. The biology of a disorder can be measured objectively, accurately, and reliably and include specific alterations in development, structure, and function of systems of the body such as the central nervous system and its most important component, the brain.

Biological dimensions of autism and the BAP bring autism research into twenty-first century medicine. Further insights in the biology of autism during development will increase understanding of pathological mechanisms and risk genes involved across the lifespan; identify nongenetic risk and protective factors, gene-environment interactions, and the earliest possible signs of the disorder; hasten development of effective and safe biology-based medical treatments of the disorder at all stages of life; and quantify the risk of recurrence specific to individual families. More detailed biological knowledge of unaffected carriers of autism liability will help answer major questions and concerns of scientist-clinicians and family members, such as why some children in families have autism while some of their siblings and other relatives have only the milder and more isolated difficulties of the BAP. A critical need in autism research today is to understand the alterations in development, structure, and function of the brain and other biological systems in the human body that are linked to the disorder.

Figure 28-1 is a description of the causal chain leading to autism. Genes that increase autism risk are believed to interact with each other and with environmental factors to alter the normal course of brain development and result in pathological processes and mechanisms. Abnormal brain development results in pathological alterations of brain structure, microstructure, function, and chemistry that have yet to be described comprehensively. According to current theory, all such pathologies result in autism when, as a whole, they reach a critical but unknown severity threshold. It is likely that the variable phenotypic expression within the BAP seen clinically results from isolated or combined subthreshold deviations of brain structure, microstructure, and function. Although the recognition and description of autism as a distinct clinical syndrome was a major advance in child psychiatry and medicine, it is evident from Figure 28-1 that present-day research falls far short of the required understanding of its biological basis.

Box 28–2

The present-day Broader Autism Phenotype

At present, the working BAP is a set of observable behaviors and cognitive tendencies that occur at increased rates in family members of children and adults with autism. These appear to be inherited in families in addition to the "narrow phenotype," the phenotype restricted to autism (and also Asperger's syndrome and PDD-NOS). The behaviors appear identical or conceptually similar to some of the behaviors observed in autism but occur in more isolated form and tend to be milder. New characteristics of the BAP are being discovered in infant siblings of autism probands (Elsabbagh et al. 2009a; Elsabbagh et al., 2009b). In an example family, the many behaviors of the child with autism may include lack of interest in and response to other children, no spoken language, hand-flapping, and intellectual subnormality. Family members without autism (or PDD-NOS) are all of average or above average intelligence but some have single or multiple isolated tendencies conceptually similar to some of the behaviors seen in the affected child. For instance, the child's father may be an expert in computer programming and have difficulty conversing with others and behaviors indicative of a tendency toward social aloofness. The child's mother, a physician, may have a history of reading and spelling problems as a child. One sibling may have had articulation problems, delayed onset of spoken language during early childhood, and mild impairments in eye contact. Three other siblings may exhibit typical development in these and other areas. In this example family, the father, mother and one sibling have had manifestations of the BAP.

Three key questions drive BBAP research, and these three questions must be answered precisely to determine if a biological feature is a member of the BAP. First, is the rate of the biological characteristic increased in individuals with autism when compared to that of the general population? Second, is this rate also increased in nonautistic family members: monozygotic co-twins, siblings, or parents? Third, and very important, does the biological feature show resemblance within families? When familial resemblance is present, family members of an individual with autism who has the biological feature are, by definition, more likely to have the feature themselves when compared to family members of individuals with autism in whom it is not present.

Example

The general strategy for answering the three key questions when identifying new intermediate phenotype (IP) members of the BBAP, and some of the complexities involved, are described using the volume of amygdala as an example. Biostatistical terms have been included in the following description; their definitions and further examples in the BBAP can be found in Appendix A. References for the studies mentioned below are cited in the amygdala and hippocampus part of Section 2.

First, there must be sufficient evidence that a particular alteration of amygdalar volume is associated with autism. Case-control studies provide this evidence and suggest that mean amygdala volume is increased in young children with autism and decreased in older children and adolescents with autism relative to that of healthy control subjects. Some studies report no case-control differences. When the findings across studies are not consistent, meta-analysis is often performed to determine the standardized overall effect size of all of the studies combined. In a meta-analysis, the overall effect size of the autism-control difference in amygdala volume was insignificant, as indicated by its 95% confidence interval.

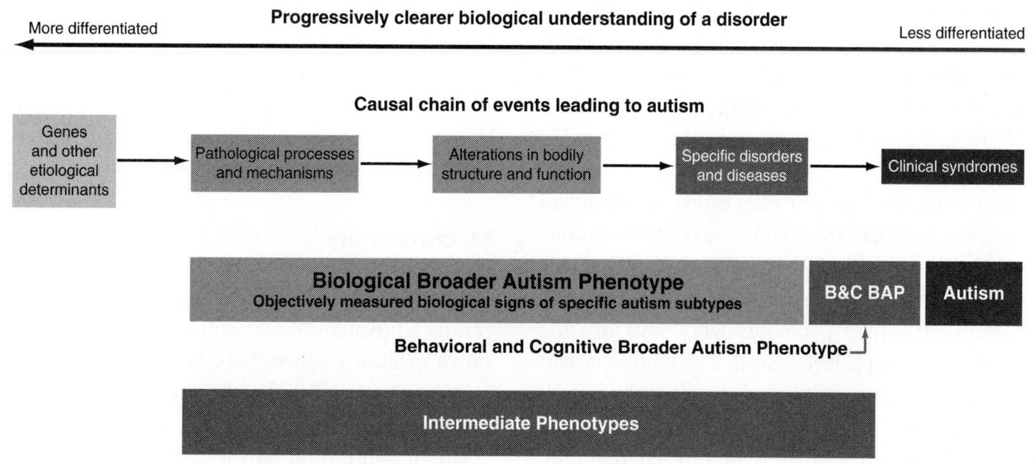

Figure 28–1. Description of the causal chain leading to autism.

In the case of amygdala volume, high variation was found between reported group differences in mean volume and their standard errors. When the heterogeneity of study results does not arise from the disorder itself, it can limit the statistical power to detect true volumetric differences and in some cases annul the meta-analytic findings altogether. Controlling the false discovery rate is an alternative way to assess the veracity of multistudy findings, especially when the number of studies is large.

An initial, small, and insignificant overall effect size may suggest that amygdala volume is not associated with autism. Amygdala volume appeared, however, to decrease with age in the autism but not the control groups, a significant age by group interaction. This finding raises the possibility that amygdala volume, as a potential IP, may vary with age, or that a pattern of age-related changes in amygdala volume, as could be ascertained by a longitudinal study, may be more significantly associated with autism than a single volume measurement at any age. If additional studies of volumetric changes in the amygdala in older children replicate the association with autism, and relationships between amygdala volume and specific symptoms of autism continue to be found, such would suggest that amygdala volume may mediate the effect of causative mechanisms on some signs of the disorder.

Proband: the first individual in a family who comes to clinical attention and is diagnosed with a particular disease or disorder. In this chapter, proband refers to the index case of autism in a family.

The next step in identifying the potential IP examines amygdala volume in unaffected family members: members of twin pairs without autism, and unaffected parents and siblings. Two exploratory studies found decreased mean volumes in unaffected older siblings but not in parents. Due to their small sample sizes, these studies are not sufficient to rigorously test amygdala volume as a potential IP. Sample size is an important consideration since autism is a heterogeneous disorder clinically and genetically. In addition, mutations in autism risk genes identified to date are sometimes inherited but often occur de novo (spontaneously, not inherited) in affected individuals. There may be inherited and noninherited (sporadic) forms of idiopathic autism (Zhao et al., 2007). Large sample sizes and elegant statistical modeling are needed to account for these factors properly. Additional replication studies may confirm that overall mean amygdala volume is decreased in unaffected older siblings and parents.

The third step is to determine if alterations in amygdala volume in autism are familial. Are unaffected relatives of children with autism who have alterations of amygdala volume more likely to have decreased amygdala volume compared to unaffected relatives of autism probands who have normal amygdala volumes? At a simple level, familial resemblance can be tested quantitatively with correlation statistics and categorically using the odds ratio. The participants for analysis need to be probands with autism and their unaffected relatives. Familial resemblance is tested more rigorously with multilevel mixed effects models. A simple mixed-effects model combines and separates odds ratios by treating them as repeated measures of a common association. If amygdala volumes in affected individuals and their unaffected relatives remain significantly correlated, then these volumetric deviations would meet the three necessary criteria for a potentially genetically informative member of the BBAP.

The fourth step is to determine how useful the IP is in identifying individuals with autism and unaffected family members. This step requires a shift from the comparison of case-control means to phenotypic classifications of individuals. The classification ability of a variety of amygdala size alterations is tested by balancing sensitivity and specificity depending on the purpose of the classification. For family genetic studies, specificity is often maximized to minimize false positives. In addition, the classification strategy must have high predictive values for the presence and absence of autism family membership and be highly reliable. To be a useful IP, the relative risk and the odds ratio should be high; the phenotype of decreased amygdala volume should occur in probands and their unaffected relatives at a much higher rate than in the general population. Because autism is a heterogeneous disorder, it is possible that a particular IP may be helpful in only a subgroup of autism families.

The final step is to further refine the amygdala volume phenotype for use in molecular genetic studies. This refinement requires additional research to describe in the finest detail possible the alteration in amygdala development that is most specific to affected and unaffected autism family members. Such refinement will increase the sensitivity (more power), specificity (fewer false positives) and predictive value of the phenotype to help identify new autism risk genes and biological mechanisms involved in the disorder.

As autism research moves into the era of personalized and genomic medicine in the twenty-first century, the preceding example raises another important issue: reliability. Proper assessment of the reliability and validity of imaging measurements, for instance the reliability of measurement of amygdala volume in vivo across time and across different sites, is more complex than many clinicians and researchers currently realize (Lange et al., 2010; Brain Development Cooperative Group, corresponding author: Nicholas Lange, 2011).

Section 1. Craniofacial Features

Macrocephaly

Macrocephaly, a head circumference greater than the 97th percentile equivalent to 1.88 standard deviations (SDs) above the mean specific to age and sex, is one of the most common physical features associated with autism. Macrocephaly in autism is usually due to megalencephaly, abnormal enlargement of the brain, at some time during development (Bailey et al., 1993; Courchesne et al., 1999; Kemper & Bauman, 2002).

Affected Individuals

On average, macrocephaly is present in 20% of affected individuals (Fombonne et al., 1999). There is an increased rate of macrocephaly in twins with autism (Bailey et al., 1995), an intriguing finding because head circumference tends to be smaller in typically developing twins than in singletons (Buckler & Green, 2008). The significant association between autism and macrocephaly has been replicated in multiple independent samples, in singletons and twins, simplex and multiplex families, children and adults, cognitively high- and low-functioning affected individuals, and in epidemiological and clinical samples (Lainhart et al., 2006). Published rates of macrocephaly range from 14% to 42% of cases (Bailey et al., 1995; Bolton et al., 1994; Courchesne et al., 2003; Davidovitch et al., 1996; Dementieva et al., 2005; Deutsch & Joseph, 2003; Fidler et al., 2000; Fombonne et al., 1999; Gillberg & de Souza, 2002; Lainhart et al., 1997; Lainhart et al., 2006; Miles et al., 2000; Sacco et al., 2007; Stevenson et al., 1997; Woodhouse et al., 1996).

Simplex, multiplex: the type of family as determined by number of its members with an autism spectrum disorder (ASD). If only one individual in a family is affected with an ASD, it is a simplex family. Families are termed multiplex if two or more of its members are so affected.

Box 28–3

Associated Features. Biological features that occur at higher rates in individuals with autism are termed "associated features" at present, as they are found in some but not all children and adults with the disorder. For example, some infants and young children who develop autism have an increased rate of head and brain growth during early childhood but some do not. Some older individuals with autism have macrocephaly but most do not. Because associated features occur in some but not all children with autism, they are not required for a diagnosis of autism. Similarly, the absence of any associated feature does not exclude a diagnosis of autism. For example, a normal rate of head and brain growth during infancy or early childhood does not mean that a child does not have autism. The diagnosis of autism is currently based on clusters of significantly impairing characteristic behaviors in the three areas of development in every affected child (reciprocal social interaction, communication, and range and flexibility of interests, behaviors, and tendencies) and clinical onset before three years of age. Biological features that occur in unaffected individuals with the BAP are also associated features. They occur at higher rates in unaffected family members but are not all present in every family member who carries risk genes for autism. Research efforts are underway to discover biological features that are present in all children with autism or at least all children with a biological subtype of autism. As such biological features are discovered, validated and found reliable, it will become increasingly likely that medical tests will be developed to diagnose autism.

Macrocephaly and megalencephaly develop in some but not all children with autism during the first few years of life, the period in which postnatal brain growth is the most rapid and when signs and symptoms of autism become apparent (Courchesne et al., 2003; Hazlett et al., 2005; Lainhart et al., 1997; Sparks et al., 2002). During the final, slower period of brain growth, from roughly 5–12 years of age, rates of macrocephaly remain increased (Lainhart et al., 2006) but brain growth may be less in children with autism compared to that in typical development although the head continues to grow at a normal rate (Aylward et al., 2002). By late adolescence and early adulthood, mean brain volume is no different from that of typical controls even though the rate of macrocephaly is still elevated. Evidence supporting the latter hypothesis, however, comes solely from combining the results of cross-sectional studies of head circumference and brain volume performed at different stages of late development (Lainhart et al., 2005). The trajectory of brain growth during late neurodevelopment in autism is only now being studied longitudinally in the same individuals over time (Bigler et al., 2010; Lange et al., 2010). Megalencephaly is found occasionally in postmortem examination of older individuals with autism, indicating that brain enlargement is still present in some people with autism later in life (Bailey et al., 1998).

Macrocephaly appears to be a component of a more general tendency toward larger head size in autism. The distribution of standardized head circumferences in autism appears unimodal with larger mean and greater variance when compared to that found in typical development (Lainhart et al., 2006). Taller children and adults with autism tend to have larger heads (Lainhart et al., 2006; Sacco et al., 2007) as in typical development. Increased height, however, does not explain all cases of macrocephaly in twins or singletons with autism (Bailey et al., 1995; Lainhart et al., 1997; Lainhart et al., 2006; Miles et al., 2000). Differences between standardized head circumference and height in autism also appear unimodal and symmetric with larger mean and greater variance relative to typical individuals, as in standardized head circumference (Lainhart et al., 2006). Rates of macrocephaly are also increased in other ASDs, such as PDD-NOS (Woodhouse et al., 1996).

Macrocephaly may identify unique subgroups of individuals with autism who have clinical features and risk genes that are different from the majority of individuals with autism who are normocephalic (i.e., have normal sized heads). There are no significant differences between macrocephalic and normocephalic autism with respect to sex ratio, age at onset, history of early regression, verbal and performance IQ and their discrepancy, total ADI-R algorithm score, verbal versus nonverbal language, incidence of seizures, minor/major congenital anomalies, sibling recurrence risk, maternal education, or parental socioeconomic status (SES; Lainhart et al., 2006; Miles et al., 2000). Evidence suggests that macrocephaly in autism is associated with an increased rate of delay in the onset of spoken words (Lainhart et al., 2006), a positive history of allergic/immune disorders in the affected child and first-degree relatives (Sacco et al., 2007), and greater cognitive processing difficulty when switching from local contextual detail to global processing (White et al., 2009). The latter neuropsychological finding appears to be specific to macrocephaly in autism; it is not found in healthy children with benign macrocephaly or in children with autism who are not macrocephalic. Recent genetic findings, described in the next section, indicate that macrocephaly, particularly extreme macrocephaly, appears to be a genetically informative covariate in autism.

Extreme Macrocephaly

Some children with autism have extreme macrocephaly, a head circumference that is three or more standard deviations above the mean for their age and sex. It is well known in medicine that distributional extremes may arise from developmental mechanisms separate from those affecting central distributional tendencies (Szatmari et al., 2007). Extreme macrocephaly is sometimes associated with a mutation in the PTEN gene on chromosome 10q23.3 (Buxbaum et al., 2007). The mutation may be inherited from a parent or it may occur de novo. When the PTEN mutation is inherited, the transmitting parent often has extreme macrocephaly, and siblings without autism may have macrocephaly and developmental delays. The rate of a mutation in the PTEN gene in children with autism accompanied by extreme macrocephaly is not yet known. When children with autism and any degree of macrocephaly (extreme or not extreme) are examined, the mutation is present in about one in 88 cases (1.2%) (Buxbaum et al., 2007). The rate in epidemiological samples of macrocephalic children with nonautistic idiopathic developmental is not yet known. A mutation in the PTEN gene is found more frequently in clinical samples of referred individuals. In children with macrocephaly whose families were referred for genetic counseling, a PTEN mutation was found in 10.5% of 19 children with ASD and 5% of 20 children with idiopathic nonautistic developmental delay (Orrico et al., 2008). A mutation in the PTEN gene was found in 18.6% of 59 macrocephalic individuals who had a neurodevelopmental disorder and had been referred for mutation testing; about half of the individuals with a PTEN mutation had an ASD and half had nonspecific developmental delay (Varga et al., 2009). The rate of a PTEN mutation increased with increasing head circumference: 11.6% of referred individuals whose head circumferences ranged from two to 3.9 standard deviations above the mean and 23.1% in individuals whose head circumferences were four or more standard deviations above the mean for age and sex (Varga et al., 2009).

PTEN gene: the phosphatase and tensin homolog gene. PTEN encodes a protein involved in tumor suppression and in brain development and brain function, including neuronal survival and growth, synaptic plasticity, memory, and learning (Butler et al., 2005; Buxbaum et al., 2007; Delatycki et al., 2003; Goffin et al., 2001; Greer & Wynshaw-Boris, 2006; Herman et al., 2007; Kwon et al., 2006; Parisi et al., 2001; Zori et al., 1998). A mutation in the PTEN gene may be inherited from a parent or may occur de novo (i.e., occurring spontaneously in the child). When inherited, the recurrence risk for PTEN-related hamartoma tumor syndromes, a spectrum of disorders in which multiple benign tumor-like malformations termed hamartomas that occur in the skin and other parts of the body may be as high as 50% and possibly associated with autism.

Microcephaly

Microcephaly, a head circumference roughly two standard deviations below average for an individual of a particular age and height, occurs in 3–7% of individuals with autism (Fombonne et al., 1999; Lainhart et al., 1997; Lainhart et al., 2006; Miles et al., 2000). In most studies, the microcephaly rate is identical to that of the general population.

Unaffected Family Members

In a twin study of autism, macrocephaly was only found in twins and co-twins who had autism (Bailey et al., 1995). No monozygotic (MZ, identical) or dizygotic (DZ, nonidentical) co-twins who did not have autism, including nonautistic co-twins who had signs of the cognitive-behavioral BAP, were macrocephalic (Bailey et al., 1995). When unaffected parents and siblings are compared to the general population, the rate of macrocephaly appears to be increased significantly in parents but not siblings (Fidler et al., 2000; Lainhart et al., 2006; Miles et al., 2000; Stevenson et al., 1997).

Familial Resemblance

For singletons with autism, resemblance between head circumference in parents and their children with autism is similar to parent-child resemblance in the general population (Fidler et al., 2000; Lainhart et al., 2006). In MZ twins concordant for autism, the within-twin pair variance for head circumference is no less than the between-twin variance (Le Couteur et al., 1996), indicating that head size is equally similar in members of identical twin pairs and in twins from different families. Macrocephaly, in general, does not appear to cluster in child-parent pairs within families; recall, however, the previous exception for extreme macrocephaly. The rate of macrocephaly in at least one parent appears to be identical for macrocephalic and nonmacrocephalic individuals with autism (Lainhart et al., 2006; Miles et al., 2000).

Increased Rate of Head Growth During Infancy

Affected Individuals

An atypical rate of head and brain growth during infancy is found in some but not all children with autism. The percent of children with autism who have an abnormal rate of head and brain growth during infancy varies widely from study to study, from almost 0 to over 70% (Courchesne et al., 2003; Dawson et al., 2007; Dementieva et al., 2005; Hazlett et al., 2005; Mraz et al., 2007; Torrey et al., 2004; van Daalen et al., 2007). Some studies suggest that the increased rate of growth occurs in early childhood but only after the first year (Dissanayake et al., 2006). One study, which analyzed growth curves for individual children with autism, suggests that an abnormally increased rate of head growth during the first year is followed by a deceleration to a more normal rate of growth from 12 to 36 months of age (Dawson et al., 2007). If the findings are replicated, they would suggest that, for individuals with autism, abnormally increased rate of head and brain growth occurs during the appearance of subtle subclinical manifestations of autism and that a normative deceleration of growth commences as severity of clinical symptoms increase and the full disorder unfolds. Similar to decreases in brain volume with age during later neurodevelopment in autism, an atypical normalization of head and brain growth rates during early childhood may be pathologic.

Unaffected Family Members

Rate of head growth during infancy appears to be increased in some very young siblings of children with autism. Increased head and brain growth have been found both in infant siblings who have high symptom levels and are therefore at highest risk of a future autism diagnosis, and in young siblings who have few symptoms and are most likely to be unaffected (Elder et al., 2008). A dose-response effect may exist, in which "dose" refers to the level of autistic symptoms observed by parents. Young siblings who showed the highest level of autistic symptoms on the Modified Checklist for Autism in Toddlers and the Early Developmental Interview (Werner et al., 2005) had the largest head circumferences at 12 months of age. Children who had the largest head circumferences at 12 months of age had the greatest observed deceleration in rate of head growth thereafter.

Facial Features

Facial features are of interest in autism as potential intermediate phenotypes or covariates that may identify genetic and other etiological subtypes of the disorder (Miles et al., 2005). Prenatal craniofacial development is related to prenatal brain development, and many risk genes involved in abnormal craniofacial development have been discovered (Kjaer, 1995; Wilkie & Morriss-Kay, 2001).

Affected Individuals

Craniofacial anomalies, usually minor but sometimes major, are known to occur in about one third of individuals with idiopathic autism (Miles et al., 2000), and a recent meta-analysis showed a high overall effect size for an increased minor anomaly score (Cohen's D = 0.84; Ozgen et al., 2010). Significant facial asymmetry has been found using modern methods of objective measurement in a large sample of boys with multiplex autism, with case-control differences in facial depth in the supra- and periorbital region overlying the right hemisphere frontal pole of the brain (Hammond et al., 2008).

Unaffected Family Members

Right-dominant facial asymmetry, similar to that found in the boys with autism described above, has also been found in unaffected mothers but not fathers in multiplex autism families (Hammond et al., 2008). The pattern of facial asymmetry correctly classified two thirds of the unaffected siblings (sight unseen) in the multiplex families as having facial features closer in similarity to the average facial features of the autism group than those of the typically developing control group.

Summary of Potential Craniofacial Features of the Biological BAP

Table 28B-1 is a summary of present-day research findings on head circumference, macrocephaly, and early childhood head growth rate in relatives of individuals with idiopathic autism (see Appendix B).

Lack of familial resemblance between affected individuals and unaffected co-twins, parents, and siblings nullifies the hypothesis that macrocephaly is usually inherited with autism in families. In MZ twins and nuclear families, macrocephaly associated with idiopathic autism is increased in affected individuals but not in unaffected twins or siblings. Macrocephaly does not appear to cluster in families. Findings to date suggest that affected macrocephalic individuals are no more likely to have a parent with macrocephaly than are affected normocephalic individuals. The biological underpinnings of these phenomena are yet to be understood. Extreme macrocephaly may provide an important exception and a reliable, genetically informative covariate in autism that may identify a subgroup of affected individuals and families with a distinct set of risk genes. Macrocephaly may be genetically linked to autism in these uncommon families.

Current findings also suggest that an atypical pattern of head and brain growth during very early childhood and possibly into adolescence may prove to have a stronger association with autism in general than macrocephaly itself. A more refined understanding of macrocephaly associated with autism is needed, including associated neuropsychological features and changes in brain structure, white matter microstructure, and functional connectivity. In addition, segregation of specific atypical patterns of head growth during early and later childhood within autism families needs to be tested.

A pattern of rightward facial asymmetry has been identified as a potential intermediate phenotype in at least a subgroup of multiplex autism families. Craniofacial features can now be easily, objectively, and reliably measured using 3D digital photogrammetry (Wong et al., 2008) and other developing technologies.

Section 2. Brain Structure, Function, and Connectivity

Total and Regional Brain Volume, Gray Matter Volume, and White Matter Volume

Although there is a multitude of structural neuroimaging studies of children and adults with autism, there are very few corresponding studies of unaffected twins, parents, and siblings. This section describes only the strongest replicated results to date in affected individuals and on regions of the brain that have been examined in unaffected relatives. For twin studies, data are not yet available on brain structure alteration frequencies in nonautistic co-twins compared to the co-twins in the general population; only comparisons to singletons and familial resemblance within twin pairs have been reported.

Affected Individuals

According to the combined findings of cross-sectional imaging studies, total brain volume (TBV) in singletons is statistically increased in young children but not older individuals with autism (reviewed in Lainhart et al., 2005; Rojas et al., 2004). Nevertheless, a meta-analysis of imaging studies published between 1984 and 2006 (Stanfield et al., 2008) showed significantly larger brain volumes in autism without any significant age-related effect (mean age of 3.9 to 30.3 years across studies) or IQ, with overall effect sizes of 0.32 for TBV, 0.51 for total intracranial volume (TICV) and 0.62 for the cerebrum. Generalized increases in total gray matter (GM) and white matter (WM) volumes have been found in very young children with autism (Hazlett et. al., 2005). Volumetric differences in older affected individuals vary greatly from study to study but appear to be more striking in GM than in WM (Lainhart et al., 2006), appearing as complex patterns of localized increases and decreases in left temporal lobe GM, parietal lobe GM bilaterally, and, in some studies, the occipital and frontal lobe GM (Brun et al., 2009; Hardan et al., 2006; Hyde et al., 2009). A cross-sectional study of cortical thickness suggests an age by group interaction; cortical thickness decreased between 10 and 60 years of age in typically developing but not in ASD groups (Raznahan et al., 2009). Cortical thickness was decreased in children and increased in adults with ASD in most but not all studies (Raznahan et al., 2009; Jiao et al., 2009, Hyde et al., 2009; Hadjikhani et al., 2006, Hardan et al., 2006).

Unaffected Family Members

A voxel-based analysis comparing parents of children with autism and control parents found widespread local increases in GM volume in frontal, occipital, parietal, and temporal lobes (Peterson et al., 2006). Increased GM volume in the parents of children with autism included areas involved in "mentalizing," i.e., considering the mental state of others, important in empathy, which is known to be impaired in many individuals with autism. Large increases in GM volume have also been seen in the mirror neuron system, regions important in the development of social cognition and implicated in autism. Decreased GM volume has been observed in vermal lobules XIII and IX of the left cerebellum (Peterson et al., 2006). Cortical thickness has not yet been examined in unaffected family members.

No differences between unaffected parents and controls have been found for TBV, TICV, total GM volume, total WM volume, lobar volumes, or the lateral and third ventricles (Rojas et al., 2004; Palmen et al., 2005b; Peterson et al., 2006). The absence of increased TICV in parents differs from the results of head circumference studies that report increased macrocephaly rates in parents of children with autism. This discrepancy does not appear to be due to changes in skull thickness that could increase head circumference but not TICV (Tate et al., 2007) but may be due in part to a detection problem caused by the generally smaller sample sizes of parents in imaging studies compared to those in head circumference studies.

Familial Resemblance

Familial resemblance of TBV in autism has not yet been examined in parent-affected child or unaffected-affected sibling pairs. A brain volume study of MZ twin pairs with autism and twins discordant for autism (most of the discordant twins have PDD-NOS or cognitive/behavioral characteristics of the BAP) shows twin resemblance on TICV, TBV, and cerebral and lobar WM volumes (Kates et al., 2004). The intraclass correlation coefficients for pairs concordant and discordant for autism do not significantly differ, and the correlations are similar to those reported in typically developing twins (Wallace et al., 2006). Patterns of cerebral cortical folding, assessed with a gyrification index, are highly discordant across MZ twin pairs that included twins concordant and discordant for autism (Kates et al., 2009).

Amygdala and Hippocampus

Affected Individuals

Replicated recent findings in volumetric studies of the amygdala show increased mean volume in preschool-age children with autism (Mosconi et al., 2009; Schumann et al., 2009) and decreased volume in older individuals (Nacewicz et al., 2006; Rojas et al., 2004; Salmond et al., 2003). Potential functional implications of abnormal volumetric development of the amygdala are found in a study of preschool-age children with autism, where increased size of the amygdala was correlated with severity of social-communication impairment at 5–6 years of age (Munson et al., 2006; Schumann et al., 2009). Some studies of children and young adults with autism have found no differences from typically developing controls (Corbett, 2009; Palmen et al., 2006; Zeegers et al., 2009). The recent meta-analysis of very heterogeneous studies of amygdala volume in autism published up to the year 2006 found no significant group effect and an age-related decrease in autism relative to controls (Stanfield et al., 2008).

A significant degree of heterogeneity is also present in studies of hippocampal volume in autism. Although hippocampal volume appears stable with age and unaffected in autism in a recent meta-analysis (Stanfield et al., 2008), several other studies have reported increased volume of the left hippocampus in older children and adults with autism (Rojas et al., 2004; Rojas et al., 2006; Salmond et al., 2005). Subtle shape differences have also been observed (Dager et al., 2007; Nicolson et al., 2006).

Unaffected Family Members

Mean amygdala volume appears to be decreased in unaffected siblings (Dalton et al., 2007), while parents of children with autism appear unaffected (Rojas et al., 2004). Mean left hippocampal volume, by manual tracing, was larger in parents of simplex children with autism compared with control adults (Rojas et al., 2004) but this finding was not replicated in a voxel-based comparison of parents (Peterson et al., 2006).

Familial Resemblance

In MZ autism twins pairs (five co-twins with autism, four with PDD-NOS, and five with no diagnosis), the intra-twin correlation coefficients for amygdala and hippocampal volumes were 0.66 and 0.91 respectively (Mitchell et al., 2009). Resemblance has not yet been examined within families.

Corpus Callosum and Caudate Nucleus

Affected Individuals

Decreased size of the corpus callosum in autism is a highly replicated finding (reviewed in Lainhart et al., 2005), including a small yet significant effect size (-0.28) found in a recent meta-analysis (Stanfield et al., 2008). Increased caudate volume has also been observed, with a moderate effect size (0.41) in studies published before 2007 (Stanfield et al., 2008). More recent studies are in agreement and show that caudate volume is associated with repetitive behaviors in autism (Langen et al., 2007; Langen et al., 2009; Rojas et al., 2006). Cross-sectional data suggest aberrant volumetric changes in the caudate between childhood and young adulthood (Langen et al., 2009). The corpus callosum and caudate have not yet been examined in unaffected family members.

Cerebellum

Affected Individuals

Increased cerebellar volume (effect size 0.72) and small to moderate effect sizes for reduced volumes of vermal lobules VI–VII and VIII–X (-0.27 and -0.43, respectively) have been reported (Stanfield et al., 2008). Studies of vermal lobules VI–VII produced heterogeneous results affected by age and IQ; increasing age and IQ were associated with smaller vermal area (Peterson et al., 2006; Stanfield et al., 2008).

Unaffected Family Members

The small number of parents of children with autism studied to date show no differences in total cerebellar volume relative to control adults (Palmen et al., 2005b), but increased GM volume in the left cerebellum and decreased GM volume in verbal lobules XIII and IX has been suggested (Peterson et al., 2006).

Brain Stem

Affected Individuals

Reduced midbrain volume has been observed in autism (effect size, -0.77), while the medulla and pons appear unaffected (Stanfield et al., 2008). The reliability of these findings, however, is compromised by large observed between-study heterogeneity. The brain stem has not been examined in unaffected relatives of autism probands.

Brain Function and Brain Connectivity

In other neuropsychiatric disorders, neurophysiological measures of brain function are among the strongest candidates for genetically informative IPs. In autism, these measures include eye movements ("eye-tracking"), neural activity measured on the scalp with electroencephalography (EEG) and magnetoencephalography (MEG), and in vivo neuroimaging of neural activity using positron emission tomography (PET), single-photon computed tomography (SPECT), and functional magnetic resonance imaging (fMRI). PET and SPECT studies of the serotonin system in the brain are reviewed in Section 3.

Affected Individuals

Though not yet reported in unaffected family members, several MEG findings in individuals with autism are particularly noteworthy as potential intermediate phenotypes (reviewed in Roberts et al., 2008). In typically developing children and adults, peak magnetic responses evoked by auditory stimuli presented at 50 and 100 milliseconds earlier (M50, M100) measured in time windows of short duration (roughly 40 milliseconds) indicate very early rapid temporal signal processing in the auditory cortex. In addition, the expected M100 in the right hemisphere is greater than that in the left hemisphere of the brain (termed "rightward asymmetry"). Children with autism, however, exhibit M100s that are equal on the right and left (hemispheric symmetry). This lack of typical asymmetry may be related to language impairment in the disorder (Schmidt et al., 2009). The delay ("latency") of right-hemisphere M50 in childhood appears to account for a substantial amount of variance in overall language ability in specific language impairments and in autism. A delay time of 84.6 milliseconds between stimulus presentation and the initial evoked response ("latency cutoff") has been found to indicate receptive language impairment in children with 70% sensitivity and 92% specificity (Oram Cardy et al., 2008).

A variety of neurophysiological measures have shown significant case-control differences in samples of individuals with autism and have been used to test family members. Differences in individuals with autism include abnormalities of eye-gaze fixation, evoked response, local oscillatory activity, localization of brain areas activated and rapid temporal aspects of brain activation in response to a variety of stimuli.

A preliminary family study using SPECT reports a variety of patterns of hypoperfusion in frontal, parietal, and temporal cortex as well as the caudate nucleus in 8 affected children (Degirmenci et al., 2008).

Unaffected Family Members

Parents and unaffected siblings have shown decreased perfusion in frontal and parietal regions, and siblings have shown additional hypoperfusion in the caudate nucleus (Degirmenci et al., 2008). Eye-tracking studies have indicated that unaffected siblings of children with autism have decreased fixation on eyes when looking at faces, similar to the decreased fixation found in individuals with autism (Dalton et al., 2007). This study also found that in individuals with autism, unaffected siblings, and typically developing controls (to a lesser extent), variation in the duration of eye fixation is strongly related to variation in the extent of right and left fusiform gyri activation measured by fMRI. No significant association was found between eye fixation duration and amygdala activation in individuals with autism in unaffected siblings or controls (Dalton et al., 2007). Parents of children with autism have exhibited atypical evoked responses when looking at faces (Dawson et al., 2005), atypical patterns of fMRI brain activation during visual search and empathy tasks (Baron-Cohen et al., 2006), and decreased synchronization of oscillatory brain activity as recorded by MEG (Rojas et al., 2008). Taken together, these atypical responses may indicate deficits in the binding of perceptual stimuli and abnormalities in neuronal connectivity and function in specific cortical areas.

Summary of Brain Structure, Function, and Connectivity in the Biological BAP

Table 28B-2 is a summary of structural brain imaging studies of unaffected twins, parents, and siblings to date. Table 28B-3 is a summary of brain function and brain connectivity studies to date. (See Appendix B for both tables.)

Structural imaging data contributed by unaffected relatives of children with autism are far too limited to draw any preliminary conclusions about whether or not particular alterations in brain volume may be part of the BBAP. Regional increases in GM volume in localized areas in all lobes of the brain and in the cerebellum in parents and decreased amygdala volume in unaffected siblings have yet to be replicated. Inconsistent differences in the left hippocampal volumes of parents may be due to heterogeneity of the BBAP, but the small sample sizes and the variety of image analysis methods used to date contribute to this ambiguity.

Structural imaging studies of unaffected family members are severely lacking, and testing for familiality nonexistent. Decreased size of the corpus callosum and midbrain, increased caudate volume, and emergent findings of regional alterations in cortical thickness have been found and replicated in children and adults with autism, but have yet to be evaluated in unaffected relatives. Twin studies have the potential to help understand how variations in brain structure and function mediate genetic and environmental effects on cognitive, behavioral, and emotional characteristics of autism and the BAP. Imaging studies comparing autistic and nonautistic members of twin pairs are in very early stages of development (Belmonte & Carper, 2006; Kates et al., 1998; Kates et al., 2004; Mitchell et al., 2009), have extremely small sample sizes, and thus have very limited statistical power to detect any differences if they exist. Also, it is not clear if these preliminary findings are due to autism or confounding factors related to twinning. To date, neuroimaging studies of twins with autism have not considered the prenatal, perinatal, and postnatal factors known to differ in twins and singletons or perinatal factors such as birth order effects in twinning that may also differ and influence brain development. Carefully designed studies that enable the direct comparison of MZ and DZ twins with autism and control twins are needed to evaluate these potentially separable effects.

The many mixed, inconsistent, and negative volumetric findings in children and adults with autism may suggest that the future yield of studies examining alterations in regional brain volumes as possible components of the BBAP is low except in a few brain regions. Recent studies showing complex patterns of increased and decreased GM volume within brain structures suggest that newer methods allowing more detailed examination of anatomy may be much more powerful than older methods that yielded only volumetric measures of whole structures. Almost all volumetric brain imaging studies in autism have been cross-sectional in design, and many age-related changes that have driven research in the field are based on cross-sectional data combined across studies. Limited conclusions about developmental processes can be drawn from cross-sectional data, and more longitudinal studies are needed (Kraemer et al., 2002). Longitudinal growth trajectories may be more informative phenotypic measures in affected and unaffected individuals than cross-sectional volumes at any given age. Many neuropathological changes due to autism may be detectable only at higher resolutions than usually used. Methods that bridge the gap between in vivo (during life) imaging studies of children and adults with autism at currently available resolutions and in vivo nonhuman studies at the very high resolutions provided by bright field, immunofluoresence, and electron microscopy are critically needed.

The identification of specific measures of neural function as potential IPs in autism research is severely lacking when compared, for instance, to corresponding research in schizophrenia and bipolar disorder (Ivleva et al., 2009; Jeste & Nelson, 2009). Structural and functional brain connectivity studies of unaffected relatives are lacking, as are tests of connectivity pattern aggregation within families. Normal short-range and intra- and interhemispheric long-range connectivity is essential between cortical areas whose functions must be tightly synchronized within very brief and rapidly evolving temporal windows to enable efficient and effective information processing. The paucity of studies of long-range underconnectivity between cortical areas in autism seems at odds with this major, replicated finding that is currently driving much interdisciplinary research in the field.

Section 3. Other Biomedical Features

Serotonin

In children with autism, elevated levels of serotonin in the blood, a measurable biological trait, was first reported in 1961. This finding remains one of the oldest and most robust biological findings in autism research (Anderson, 2002).

Box 28–4

Serotonin. Serotonin is a neurotransmitter that plays an essential role in sleep, appetite, mood, anxiety, social affiliation, impulsivity, arousal, aggression, and reaction to stress (Anderson, 2002). Brain serotonin was discovered in 1953. Serotonin, often abbreviated as 5-HT (5-hydroxytryptamine), is synthesized from the dietary amino acid precursor tryptophan and found in the brain, intestines, blood platelets (regulating blood clotting), blood vessels, and in the muscle of some organs. Serotonin plays critical roles in both fetal brain development and postnatal brain function throughout life, is present in the oocyte (egg cell), and is involved in very early embryonic patterning (Levin et al., 2006), in embryonic thalamocortical axonal guidance, in the formation of cortical sensory maps (Bonnin et al., 2007), and in craniofacial development (Moiseiwitsch, 2000).

Affected Individuals

Hyperserotonemia has been found repeatedly in individuals with autism. Mean levels of blood serotonin are 25–50% higher in autism than in typical control samples. A recent study shows a bimodal distribution with roughly 50% of affected children and young adults having blood serotonin levels greater than one standard deviation above that of typically developing controls; 20% have levels greater that two standard deviations above this normal level compared to 0% typically developing controls (Mulder et al., 2004). The same study showed that although a small proportion of the nonautistic comparison children with mental retardation have hyperserotonemia, they do not have increased mean levels of serotonin, suggesting some specificity to autism. Hyperserotonemia has also been found in children with PDD-NOS (Mulder et al., 2004).

Hyperserotonemia: elevated levels of serotonin in whole blood or platelet-rich plasma—a measurable biological trait possibly linked genetically to autism.

Several abnormalities of the serotonin system in the brain in autism are noteworthy. There is evidence of autism-related altered functioning of serotonin receptors in the brain from at least the late 1980s (McBride et al., 1989). A number of PET studies show alteration of brain serotonin synthesis and atypical neurodevelopmental trajectories in children with autism (Chugani et al., 1997; Chugani et al., 1999). In children with autism 2–4 years of age, increases in total and frontal lobe cortical GM volume of 10% and 16% respectively are reported to be associated with a particular form (allele) of one of the serotonin transporter genes (the 5HTTLRP short polymorphism of the SLC6A4 gene), a relationship that is absent in adults with the disorder (Raznahan et al., 2009; Wassink et al., 2007). The association between brain anatomy and serotonin transporter genotype in children but not adults with autism suggests that the effects of serotonin transporter genes on brain morphometry may be age-dependent.

By employing SPECT, a preliminary but important study of adults with Asperger's syndrome has provided evidence of decreased cortical density of 5-HT2_A serotonin receptors, as indexed by decreased receptor binding, relative to that of typical control adults (Murphy et al., 2006). Decreased binding is found in the anterior and posterior cingulate, bilateral frontal, and superior temporal lobes and in the left parietal lobe. Decreased receptor binding in the cingulate and frontal cortices is related to increased severity of impairment in reciprocal social interaction as measured by the Autism Diagnostic Interview-Revised (ADI-R). Decreased serotonin transporter binding is also found in individuals with autism. Adults with autism show highly significant decreases in serotonin transporter binding in widespread areas throughout the brain, including in all four lobes, limbic and subcortical regions, and the cerebellum (Nakamura et al., 2010). Children and adolescents with autism appear to have a decrease in cortical serotonin transporter binding, particularly in the medial frontal cortex, which is more pronounced with increasing age (Makkonen et al., 2008).

Unaffected Family Members

The observation that hyperserotonemia is also present in a sizable proportion of unaffected relatives is an important and complex finding that is not yet fully understood. A recent PET study of unaffected parents of children with autism and control adults has shown that mean cortical serotonin receptor binding potential in unaffected parents is decreased in all four lobes of the brain (effect sizes ~0.9), its standard deviation is reduced by 50%, and it is negatively correlated with blood platelet serotonin levels but not in controls (Goldberg et al., 2009).

Familial Resemblance

Hyperserotonemia in autism is familial and appears to be related to the degree of genetic liability to autism and recurrence risk (Abramson et al., 1989; Cook et al., 1990; Leboyer et al., 1999; Leventhal et al., 1990). Serotonin levels are elevated in multiplex individuals compared to simplex individuals with autism (Abramson et al., 1989; Cook & Leventhal, 1996; Piven et al., 1991). Serotonin levels are also elevated in children with autism compared to their first-degree relatives and are correlated positively with those of their unaffected parents and siblings (Leventhal et al., 1990). First-degree relatives are 2.4 times more likely to be hyperserotonemic if the child with autism is hyperserotonemic. Further research on molecular genetic differences in the serotonin system of unaffected relatives who are hyperserotonemic compared to relatives who are not is underway (Cross et al., 2008).

Summary of Serotonin Components of the Biological BAP

Table 28B-4 is an up-to-date summary of brain and blood serotonin system studies in autism and unaffected relatives and siblings (see Appendix B).

Hyperserotonemia meets criteria for a potential genetically informative IP, thus a possible component of the BBAP. It is increased in affected individuals and in unaffected parents and siblings and also tends to cluster in the families of hyperserotonemic individuals with autism. Although hyperserotonemia in autism has been known for many years, its genetic and molecular mechanisms remain unknown. Emerging biostatistical evidence of associations between brain and blood platelet levels of serotonin and brain structure and function may provide further clues. To our knowledge, serotonin transporter and serotonin receptor densities have not yet been studied in the same individuals to help discern their functional relationship in autism. Further integrative research advances in molecular genetics, animal models, neuroimaging, and biostatistics are needed for a thorough understanding of this oldest candidate biomarker in autism.

Immune Factors

Normal functioning of the immune system requires finely balanced, complex interactions of its many components, including a wide variety of immune cell types, proteins, and other biochemicals, tissues, and organs of the body. A number of studies have investigated the potential dysfunction of the immune system in individuals with autism and their relatives. The work of the late Dr. Reed Warren in Utah during the 1980s and early 1990s first brought the potential role of immunologic factors and the genes that control them to the forefront of autism research (Warren et al., 1986). The plausibility of immune system differences in unaffected family members was soon introduced. Dr. Warren was very careful in his earliest autism research to focus his immune hypotheses and their specificity on some but not all children with autism and their families, positing the existence and identifiability of familial subgroups in which immune factors were somehow linked to the disorder. He also acknowledged that if immune system abnormalities were involved in some cases of autism, then they may be related directly or indirectly to its pathogenesis, and hence that their presence may contribute to autism risk or be a consequence of the risk or atypical brain development. Recent studies employing advanced immunologic and molecular genetic technology have provided convergent evidence supporting Dr. Warren's original hypotheses.

Box 28–5

Biological marker (biomarker): a characteristic that is measured objectively and evaluated as an indicator of normal biological processes, pathogenic processes, or pharmacologic responses to a therapeutic intervention (Biomarker Definitions Working Group, 2001). One may refer to a characteristic or phenotype as a biomarker if it is minimally affected by the will, behavior, and attitudes of subjects or the evaluator or by transient environmental influences (Kraemer et al., 2002). If such a characteristic or phenotype is a statistic derived from an image, it must also be shown to be on a causal pathway of a clinical endpoint to fulfill the additional requirement for an imaging biomarker. The potential to identify useful biomarkers of autism will be greatly expanded by the further understanding of its pathogenesis. At present, however, without useful theory or models of its pathogenic underpinnings, biomarker research in autism is and needs to be conducted in the opposite direction.

Affected Individuals

In autism, studies have found abnormalities of cell-mediated and antibody-mediated components of the adaptive immune system that responds to new health threats throughout the lifespan. A preliminary comprehensive examination of immune components in individuals with autism and their unaffected siblings suggests subtle but important impairment of the cell-mediated part of the immune system in some children with autism (Saresella et al., 2009). Alterations are found in the levels of a number of different types of cells in different stages of immune function maturation and in levels of the substances they secrete (cytokines) that are important in cellular communication. Decreases in mean levels of fully differentiated cell subtypes that direct other immune cells (CD4+ T lymphocytes, also known as "helper" cells) have been observed. Mean levels of subtypes of "killer cells" (CD8+ T lymphocytes) that kill cells dangerous to the body, such as cells infected with viruses, are altered. Levels of "naive killer cells" (cells that have not yet been exposed to antigens such as viruses) are increased and levels of "effector memory cells" (cells that remember and quickly recognize infectious agents long after the original infection) are decreased (Saresella et al., 2009). A decrease in mean levels of immunoglobulins, specifically IgG and IgM, has been observed recently in a sample of individuals with autism compared to typically developing controls (Heuer et al., 2008). A minority of children with autism appear to have antibodies to fetal and adult brain proteins and to brain proteins from the basal ganglia, frontal lobe, cingulate gyrus, and cerebellum (Silva et al., 2004; Singer et al., 2006; Zimmerman et al., 2007; Wills et al., 2009). Finally, an association of a functional variant of the gene for the macrophage inhibitory factor (MIF) with autism and increased mean levels of plasma MIF indicates abnormality of the innate immune system that provides natural defenses against invading microorganisms (Grigorenko et al., 2008). The variant of the MIF gene appears to be associated with stereotyped repetitive behaviors in autism.

Macrophage migration inhibitory factor (MIF): a cytokine protein encoded by a gene on chromosome 22q11.2. MIF is part of the innate immune system, the body's first-line defense system against infection, and is produced by a wide variety of immune cells including macrophages and by cells and tissues of the body that are in direct contact with the natural environment such as the lungs, the skin, and the gastrointestinal and genitourinary tracts. MIF is also produced by endocrine tissues involved in the body's response to stress: the hypothalamus, pituitary, and adrenal glands (Calandra & Roger, 2003). MIF activates macrophages and T cells, promoting the function of both innate and adaptive immune responses. Although it is an important general defense against pathogens that cause infections, abnormally high levels during infections or at the wrong time could potentially affect early brain development.

Unaffected Family Members

The finding that antibodies to brain proteins are found in some children with autism led to studies that tested the hypothesis that in some cases of autism maternal antibodies to brain tissue may cross the placenta during pregnancy and affect the brain of the developing child. These studies yielded tantalizing preliminary evidence in mice and rhesus monkeys showing that offspring had behavioral deficits including hyperactivity and stereotypic behaviors (Dalton et al., 2003; Martin et al., 2008). A number of human studies find antibodies to brain tissue in unaffected mothers of children with autism and increased rates of autoimmune diseases in mothers and other relatives (Braunschweig et al., 2008; Comi et al., 1999; Croen 2005; Croen et al., 2008; Molloy et al., 2006; Singer et al., 2008; Sweeten et al., 2003). Several studies have measured the rates of autoimmune diseases in relatives of individuals with autism but not yet in these individuals themselves. A very large epidemiological study of autoimmune disorders in parents and siblings of children with autism, using the Denmark Medical Registry, found that of the 3325 children studied who had ASD, including 1089 with autism, 6.8% had a parent or sibling with a diagnosed autoimmune disease prior to their diagnosis of autism. This study confirmed an increased risk of autism in children born to parents who have type-1 diabetes and an increased risk of an ASD when mothers have rheumatoid arthritis or celiac disease (Atladóttir et al., 2009). It is important to note, however, that the majority of children with autism are born to parents who do not have these autoimmune disorders. Unaffected children in autism families show signs of immune dysregulation similar to the affected children with autism in a preliminary study (Saresella et al., 2009). If confirmed by replication and familial resemblance is demonstrated, the findings described here would indicate that a particular pattern of immune dysregulation is an IP of an immune-related subtype of autism.

Familial Resemblance

It appears that only one study to date has investigated the intrafamilial resemblance of immune findings, specifically those protein bands reactive to human brain tissue, in children with autism and their parents (Silva et al., 2004). No significant correlations were found.

Summary of Potential Immune Factors of the Biological BAP

Table 28B-5 is an up-to-date summary of studies of the immune system in children and adults with autism and their affected and unaffected siblings and first-degree relatives (see Appendix B).

Preliminary studies point to candidate intermediate phenotypes that may be found in patterns of immune system imbalance in some autism families. The association between autism and specific types of autoimmune diseases in fathers and mothers suggests the involvement of various a number of complex mechanisms. There appear to be at least two potentially separable mechanisms operating independently or in tandem: (1) a common genetic background may increase risk of autoimmune disease in a parent and autism in an offspring, and (2) the effects of maternal autoimmune disease during pregnancy may alter the intrauterine environment of the developing child in a way that increases autism risk. It appears certain that parental history of specific autoimmune diseases identifies a potential and very important etiological and clinical subtype of autism. Twin studies and carefully designed family studies are needed to further clarify what immunological characteristics are genetically informative biological phenotypes, which are not, and how immunological factors are related to alterations in brain development.

Section 4. Classification Research

The utility of any modern scientific method can be measured in large part by its context-specific predictive performance.

One important goal of scientific research of the BBAP is to employ routine medical tests, such as blood tests, eye-tracking measures, and brain scans, to phenotype individuals with autism or identify those at risk for autism objectively. Biological phenotypes are needed to correctly identify babies who carry autism risk genes and are therefore at increased risk of developing the disorder. If they become available, such biological phenotypes could be used to diagnose individuals with specific subtypes of autism, to identify unaffected family members who carry risk genes for autism, to help predict long-term outcome, and to determine what interventions are most likely to be effective for individuals at different stages of the disorder. Biological phenotypes have the potential to bring the practice of personalized medicine to autism, to make preventive interventions tailored specifically to the needs of individuals across the lifespan and improve the lives of people with autism or at risk for autism.

Classification research in autism seeks to discover biological methods that identify individuals with the disorder and discriminate them from individuals who are typically developing and individuals who have other developmental and neuropsychiatric disorders. Classification methods must have very high sensitivity, specificity, reliability, and predictive performance to be clinically useful. Table 28B-6 is a summary of current published findings (see Appendix B). Intensive research is currently underway to develop and test additional novel classification methods not summarized in Table 28B-6 in autism and their extensions to the BAP. Diffusion tensor imaging (DTI) technology is being developed to identify valid, accurate, and reliable autism versus control differences in white matter microstructure in key regions of the brain (Lange et al., 2010 and to locate differences in the shape and diffusion properties of white matter fiber bundles (Chung et al., 2010; Fletcher et al., 2009). Functional MRI is being used to measure functional brain connectivity in the default mode network and during performance of specific tasks (Anderson et al., 2010). If biological phenotypes with high classification ability for autism are discovered, it will be important to determine if they can correctly classify a large proportion of unaffected individuals who are related to persons with autism (BAP sensitivity), and individuals who do not have any relatives with ASDs (BAP specificity). Only one study that objectively measured right-dominant facial asymmetry (Hammond et al., 2008) tested the sensitivity of this measure in unaffected family members (67% in siblings) and none, to our knowledge, have tested specificity or replicated these findings in independent samples.

Summary of Classification Research in the Biological BAP

Table B6 is a summary of autism classification methods published to date, providing the proportion of individuals with autism who were identified correctly by the method as indeed having autism (sensitivity) and the proportion of nonautistic individuals who were identified correctly by the method as unaffected (specificity). Also included is a biological measure that may identify children with receptive language impairment associated with autism and other disorders.

Classification research in autism is producing many exciting preliminary results. Brain imaging analysis, electrophysiological methods, and 3D measures of craniofacial features now provide some ways to find patterns of alteration that are associated with autism and that perform well in discriminating individuals with autism from typically developing individuals. Among these are alterations in brain structure sizes, gyral morphometry, regional cortical thicknesses, spatial distributions of GM and WM density, white matter microstructure, reconstructed WM tract shapes, ocular function, and facial asymmetry. Studies are now needed that determine if the findings can be replicated in independent samples. To our knowledge, none have been replicated to date, except for Lange et al. (2010). Also required are performance-based comparisons of classification methods, testing discriminating ability for autism subgroups, including group comparisons of individuals with other developmental and neuropsychiatric disorders, and extensions to unaffected relatives.

Conclusion

How far has autism research progressed in identifying alterations in development, structure, and function of the brain and other body systems that indicate liability to autism in families, not only in individuals with the disorder but also in unaffected relatives? This chapter concludes with a critical appraisal of progress in identifying components of the biological BAP and suggested guidelines for future research.

Most biological alterations hypothesized to be members of the BAP do not meet genetic epidemiology criteria for potential genetically informative intermediate phenotypes. Biological findings associated with autism result from small-sample and very heterogeneous case-control studies lacking probative power. Many relevant published reports include only significant differences between group means. Typically, individuals in these groups are not phenotyped on the trait or characteristic of interest. The ability of the biological finding to classify individuals is rarely tested. Even when a biological feature is used to phenotype individuals, the performance of the classification method has yet to be tested in an independent sample, a major omission which can in some cases yield misleading and spurious results perhaps due to circular analysis (Kriegeskorte et al., 2009) and other analytic traps. In addition, most of the biological findings associated with autism have yet to be investigated in unaffected relatives. Some biological features studied in unaffected parents or siblings have not yet been measured in individuals with autism. When affected and unaffected relatives have been examined, they are usually not related, and thus familial aggregation cannot be determined. Finally, the relative performance of biological features that are increased in affected and unaffected relatives have yet to be compared to that of ASDs per se in identifying individuals who are likely to carry autism risk genes. In order to be more useful than ASDs per se, the intermediate biological phenotype should be at least 50 to 100 times more common in members of autism families than in general population (Szatmari et al., 2007). Biological alterations will be most helpful in identifying unaffected relatives who may have liability to autism when the alterations have high sensitivity and high specificity.

Biological Broader Autism Phenotype findings to date are consistent with biological subtypes of autism and risk genes being inherited or occurring de novo. Although macrocephaly does not appear to show familiality, extreme macrocephaly may cluster in a subset of autism families. Approximately 4.8% of individuals with autism have extreme macrocephaly (Lainhart et al., 2006), and these individuals appear to be at increased risk of having inherited or de novo mutations in the PTEN gene. Case series studies suggest that when the mutation is inherited, macrocephaly and developmental delay may be inherited along with autism in these families. Similarly, hyperserotonemia, which occurs in approximately 20% of individuals with autism, may identify a biological subtype of autism and autism families. Present-day findings suggest that the biological broader phenotype of autism is heterogeneous, as is autism itself (Geschwind, 2009). Alterations of bodily structure and function that are linked genetically to autism may not be identical in all families.

Major advances in Biological Broader Autism Phenotype research require innovative cross-disciplinary combinations of the scientific methods of autism clinical research, neuroscience, genetic epidemiology, neurostatistics, immunology, and other areas of medicine, in addition to novel ideas concerning developmental neuropsychiatric phenotypes. Recent genotype-phenotype relation discoveries in neuropsychiatry have shown strikingly complex and heterogeneous phenotypes associated with specific genetic loci (see Suggested Reading). Neuroimaging and neurophysiologic research are being rapidly transformed by powerful new ways of examining brain developmental, microstructure, function, local and global neural networks, connectivity, and biochemistry. As described in the Classification Research section of this chapter, autism research is on the brink of an explosion of individual biological characteristics as potential biomarkers and intermediate phenotypes of autism and the broader autism phenotype. Which of these will meet the criteria for a potentially informative intermediate phenotype, if any? Which combinations of biological phenotypes suggested by classification methods have the best diagnostic and subtyping ability for affected individuals and for identifying unaffected relatives who may have autism risk genes? How are the various phenotypes related within and across affected individuals and their families? What is the molecular biological and microstructural basis of the phenotypes? How do these phenotypes develop in autism families, and why? Do the phenotypes only discriminate individuals with autism and their relatives from typically developing individuals and their relatives, or are they also able to separate individuals with other developmental and neuropsychiatric disorders? Over three decades since the Broader Phenotype of Autism was first described, autism research now has the collaborative methods and technology to determine exactly what is inherited with autism in families.

Challenges and Future Directions

- Biological autism research needs to progress from a predominant focus on case-control mean differences to examination of distributions, classification and phenotyping of individuals, and testing for sensitivity, specificity, accuracy, and positive and negative predictive value.
- Large-scale biological studies of individuals with autism, their families, and control families, with replication in independent samples, are needed. The most effective studies will combine epidemiological and advanced statistical methods with reliable neuroimaging and other sophisticated biological phenotyping.
- Etiological heterogeneity, de novo as well as inherited mutations, phenotypic complexity, and individual heterogeneity are major research challenges in the search for the Biological Broader Autism Phenotype.

RECOMMENDED READING

Allen, A. J., Griss, M. E., Folley, B. S., Hawkins, K. A., & Pearlson, G.D. (2009). Endophenotypes in schizophrenia: A selective review. *Schizophrenia Research, 109*, 24–37.

Carroll, L. S., & Owen, M. J. (2009). Genetic overlap between autism, schizophrenia, and bipolar disorder. *Genome Medicine, 1*(10), 102.

Fernandez, B. A., Roberts, W., Chung, B., Weksberg, R., Meyn, S., Szatmari, P., et al. (2010). Phenotypic spectrum associated with de novo and inherited deletions and duplications at 16p11.2 in individuals ascertained for diagnosis of autism spectrum disorder. *Journal of Medical Genetics, 47*(3), 195–203.

Szatmari. P., Maziade, M., Zwaigenbaum, L., Merette, C., Roy, M.-A., Joober, R., et al. (2007). Informative phenotypes for genetic studies of psychiatric disorders. *American Journal of Medical Genetics Part B (Neuropsychiatric Genetics), 144B*, 581–588.

ACKNOWLEDGMENTS

We most gratefully acknowledge the help of Molly DuBray, MA, Alyson Froehlich, PhD, Anna Cariello, and Jason Cooperrider in the preparation of this chapter. Our autism research is supported by Grant Numbers RO1 MH080826 (JEL, NL), RO1 MH084795 (JEL, NL), and P50 MH060450 (J. Coyle, NL) from the National Institute of Mental Health. The content of this chapter is solely the responsibility of the authors and does not necessarily represent the official views of the National Institute of Mental Health or the National Institutes of Health.

APPENDIX A. DEFINITIONS AND DESCRIPTIONS OF BIOSTATISTICAL TERMS AND CONCEPTS

Accuracy: the percentage of correct test results, whether positive or negative, if the test is unbiased. For example, suppose that in a population of N = 100 individuals, 9 have autism and 91 do not. If the entire population is tested and it is found that 7 individuals with autism were identified as such (true positives, TP = 7) and 76 of those without autism were also identified correctly (true negatives, TN = 76), then the accuracy of the test for autism is (7 + 76)/100 or 83%. Formula: Accuracy = (TP + TN)/N. See *Bias, Precision.*

Bias: the amount by which a measurement, test or any statistic misses its "bulls-eye," its expected accurate value. See *Accuracy, Precision.*

Case-control study: a study of a select number of participants with autism (cases) and selected typically developing or nonautistic subjects, perhaps with dyslexia, OCD or ADHD (healthy or psychiatric controls) with respect to one more characteristics. If the cases and controls have similar characteristics other than the characteristic of primary interest, either by group or in case-control pairs, then the study is a **matched case-control study**. Case-control studies can be *retrospective* (looking back in time after the cases are already known) and *prospective* (looking forward in time when the cases are not yet known).

Coefficient of variation: the standard deviation expressed as a percentage of the mean; see *Mean, Standard deviation*. The coefficient of variation is preferred to standard deviation as a measure of variability when comparing an ensemble of measurements having different means and standard deviations and when mean and standard deviation are correlated (van Belle et al., 2004). Since the coefficient of variation normalizes standard deviation with respect to the mean, standard deviations can be compared on the same scale across brain regions or other measurements in health and in autism (Caviness et al., 1999; Kennedy et al. 1998; Lange et al., 1997). Formula: Coefficient of variation = Standard deviation/Mean.

Correlation (linear, Pearson): a number between -1 and 1 (inclusive) that represents the strength of the linear association between two sets of measurements. An association is linear if it can be characterized completely by a straight line on a plot of one set of measurements against the other; see *Regression (linear)*. Any association that appears curved or otherwise nonlinear is not accounted for in this definition of correlation. Other definitions of correlation exist to acknowledge these types of association, such as those based on the ranks of the observations (Kendall and Spearman correlations) and not the observations themselves.

Covariate: a characteristic, such as extreme macrocephaly, that is able to subtype autism families, given the characteristic's presence or absence. When present, the characteristic may show familial aggregation and be more strongly linked to potential risk genes.

Cross-sectional: a study or set of data that contain information on a subject or subjects collected at only one point in time, space, or space-time for all subjects. For instance, a study of fractional anisotropy in the genu of the corpus callosum in autism in which each subject has been scanned only once is a cross-sectional study, and the data collected constitute a cross-sectional data set. Also see *Mean, Standard Deviation, Longitudinal.*

Effect size: a research result that has been standardized for use in meta-analysis or hypothesized during the design of a research study or experiment; see *Meta-analysis*. For example, a standardized difference between the average brain size in a sample of subjects with autism and that of a comparison group, such as a two-sample t statistic, is an effect size. When effect sizes differ significantly across autism studies having the same goal, in an attempted meta-analysis for instance, then researchers not only have an opportunity to design and conduct better studies and meta-analyses but also to identify possible biological sources of autism heterogeneity. Effect size is best not used, however, as the sole criterion to formulate study objectives because it is but a single-number summary of several other useful results from a study, such as the mean, standard deviation, and correlation, that are useful in their own right (van Belle, 2002).

False discovery rate (FDR, its realized value): the percentage of incorrect positive test results ("false positives," FP) among a large number of positive test results that is designed to properly interpret the multitude of results. Examples of its use include crosswalks through genome-wide association studies (GWAS) for differentially expressed genes and in vivo imaging studies that involve a large number of images or image elements. For example, suppose that the test described in the previous examples for sensitivity and specificity has been replaced by a genetic test that has much greater specificity but identically poor sensitivity, and further that it has been administered to an entire high-risk population of 100,000 in which 9000 individuals have autism (see *Sensitivity, Specificity*). Suppose that the number of individuals identified incorrectly as having autism is 1 (FP = 1) and that the number of individuals identified correctly as having autism is 7000 (TP = 7000). (The test indeed has poor sensitivity, missing 2,000 autism cases in this hypothetical example.) The realized FDR of the test is 1/(1 + 7000) or 0.00014, a possibly acceptable low rate for this test. Controlling the false discovery rate is a wiser although less stringent approach to assessing the veracity of a scientific discovery than is the p-value concept and its variations for interpreting a multiplicity of research findings and their comparisons; see *P-value*. Principled control of the FDR requires the choice of an acceptable rate akin to the a priori significance level of 5% below which a single p-value is interpreted by convention as significant. The FDR method yields a value that is in between the potentially overconservative Bonferroni correction for multiple comparisons and an uncorrected p-value.

Intraclass correlation coefficient: See *Reliability.*

Longitudinal: a study or set of data that contains measurements of a subject or subjects at one or more points in time, space, or space-time for one or more subjects. For instance, a study of fractional anisotropy in the genu of the corpus callosum in autism in which one or more subjects have been scanned two or more times is a longitudinal study and the data collected constitute a longitudinal data set. Some but not all subjects may have only one data point or a varying number of repeated measurements. Autism studies with repeated measures per subject are often more powerful than those having only one measurement per subject to detect group differences when they exist (Lange, 2003). Also see *Mean, Standard Deviation, Cross-sectional.*

Mean (arithmétic mean): the simple average, the sum of measurements divided by their number. For instance, in autism research, a comparison of mean fractional anisotropy (FA), one measure of local directional flow coherence along axons showed that FA is lower in the autism group in the genu of the corpus callosum (Alexander et al., 2007) when only one measurement per subject was available; these are cross-sectional means; see *Cross-sectional*. If more than one measurement is available for some or all subjects, over time for example, then there are two sets of means, one for each individual and one for each of the groups; these are longitudinal means; see *Longitudinal*. Although the group means remain equal to the average in each group, the standard deviation of the group means and of their difference are often significantly lower because standard deviations of the individual means can be taken into account. See *Standard deviation.*

Meta-analysis: a systematic method for analyzing and synthesizing results from independent autism research studies, taking into account all pertinent information (van Belle et al., 2004). Meta-analyses attempt to mimic multicenter studies (such as multicenter controlled clinical trials) to increase statistical power; see *Sensitivity*. The aggregation of many small and heterogeneous autism studies, however, does not guarantee an increase in power; in fact, power can decrease. The validity of an increase in meta-analysis depends strongly on decisions of experts in autism research on which data or study results to combine and how to combine them, and depends on two conditions applied impartially: the quality of each study must be ascertained prior to combination, and the studies to be combined must be homogeneous. The first condition is met by expert review, and there are methods to assess the magnitude of possible inhomogeneity across studies of autism (DerSimonian & Laird, 1986). Also see *Effect size.*

Odds ratio: the ratio of the odds of having autism when a (biological) factor associated with the disorder is either present or absent. The odds of an event (having autism) is defined as the chance that the event occurs divided by the chance it does not occur. Case-control studies are most often best analyzed using the odds ratio rather than the relative risk; see *Case-control study, Relative risk.* The odds ratio and relative risk are nearly equal when the estimated prevalence of autism barely differs when the factor is present or absent. The odds ratio can be very different from the relative risk, which considers the effect of the factor on the chances of having the disorder and not on the chances of *not* having the disorder. The difference between the odds ratio and relative risk is important when, for instance, the rates of the disorder with and without the factor may be small but differ greatly. For example, autism spectrum disorder (ASD), including Asperger's syndrome and PDD-NOS, was estimated by the CDC in 2010 to affect as many as 1 out of 150 individuals in the United States. This rate may be much higher when a high-risk gene for autism (currently unidentified) is either present or absent, and the odds ratio will be greater than the relative risk. The odds ratio is always greater than the relative risk when autism is more prevalent (as can be determined from cross-sectional or longitudinal data) or incident (as can be determined from longitudinal data) when the factor is present (Holland, 1989; Schmidt & Kohlman, 2008). Although an individual may be rightfully concerned about the risk of autism when the gene is present, another and perhaps more relevant concern may be knowing the chances of autism with or without the gene compared to those of *not* having autism when the gene is either present or absent. The first type of odds, in the numerator of the odds ratio, is defined as the chance of having the disorder divided by the chance of not having the disorder when the gene is present. The second type of odds, in the denominator of the odds ratio, is defined again as the chance of having the disorder divided by the chance of not having the disorder, but when the gene is absent.

Precision: the reciprocal of the variance of a measurement, test, or any statistic. For example, if the variance of measurements of the volume of Heschl's gyrus, a small brain region important in language development, obtained by manual tracing performed on each of 100 MR images from different individuals is 11, then the precision of these measurements is 1/11 = 0.091. It is important to note that greater precision does not necessarily imply greater accuracy; it is possible that some or all measurements taken in a study of autism are precise yet inaccurate . See *Bias.*

Predictive value, negative: the percentage of correct negative test results among all negative test results, whether correct or not. For example, if 9 individuals in a high-risk population of 100 have autism, the number of individuals the test correctly identifies as not having autism is 76 (true negatives, TN = 76), and the number of individuals the test incorrectly identifies as not having autism is 5 (false negatives, FN = 2), then the negative predictive value of the test is 76/(76 + 2) or 97%. The test to predict if an individual does not have autism is valuable. Formula: Negative predictive value = TN/(TN + FN).

Predictive value, positive: the percentage of correct positive test results among all positive test results, whether correct or not. For example, if 9 individuals in a high-risk population of 100 have autism, the number of times the test correctly identifies the individuals with autism is 7 (TP = 7), and the number of individuals the test incorrectly identifies as having autism is 15 (FP = 15), then the positive predictive value of the test is 7/(7 + 15) or 58%, slightly greater than a chance coin flip. The test to predict if an individual has autism is not valuable. Formula: Positive predictive value = TP/(TP + FP).

P-value: the probability of observing an event at least as extreme as an event that could be observed under a null hypothesis. The p-value will be small if an alternative hypothesis provides a better description of the observed event, as in courtroom logic: innocent (the null hypothesis) until proven guilty (an alternative hypothesis) beyond a reasonable doubt (the p-value). A well-designed research study defines and applies a careful procedure to collect evidence (data) in an attempt to demonstrate that an alternate state of nature may be more likely than the default state. Accepted statistical principles are then applied to the data to yield a p-value. If small enough, for instance less than 5%, the p-value is then an indication that the study has yielded a statistically significant finding suggesting that the actual state of nature is different from the state presumed by the null hypothesis. For instance, suppose a researcher believes that there are less than 10 individuals with autism spectrum disorder (ASD), including Asperger's syndrome and PDD-NOS, in a specific population of 1500 individuals. The null hypothesis is that there are exactly 10 individuals with autism in this population according to the 2010 CDC estimate. A test for autism is applied to this population and identifies 2 individuals with autism, an extreme finding according to the null hypothesis. The p-value associated with this finding is 0.0103, the probability that the event would be observed in this population when 10 are present (under the null hypothesis). This p-value may be is an acceptably low value to reject the null hypothesis since it is less than the conventional **significance level** of 0.05 adopted for a single hypothesis test. In general, a study finding becomes more significant statistically, but not necessarily scientifically, as its p-value decreases. Also see *False Discovery Rate.*

Regression (linear): a principle or method that quantifies the association of an uncertain measurement with one or more measurements that are considered to be certain. For instance, when the ages of subjects with autism are known (that is, considered to be certain) the hemispheric asymmetry of diffusivity along localized regional brain circuitry in all directions (mean diffusivity, an uncertain measurement) has been shown by an application of linear regression to increase with age. This regression effect of age on mean diffusivity is not equivalent to the correlation between mean diffusivity and age, which is obtained by treating both measurements, symmetrically, as uncertain; see *Correlation (linear).* The magnitude of age-related increases in mean diffusivity can, however be easily obtained from this correlation by multiplying it by the standard deviations of age and dividing it by the standard deviation of mean diffusivity; see *Standard deviation.* Whereas a correlation treats both measurements as uncertain, regression methods break this symmetry and treat one set of measurements as being certain. Analysis of variance (ANOVA), analysis of covariance (ANCOVA) and many other statistical methods are special cases of linear regression. As a historical note, the term "regression" in this context was used by the inventor of this approach,

Sir Francis Galton, first cousin of Charles Darwin, who studied how the heights of sons "regressed" toward the heights of their fathers and coined the term "regression toward the mean" which is a central idea behind the technique.

Relative risk: the chance that an individual having a certain (biological) characteristic has autism divided by the chance that a similar individual without this characteristic has autism. Suppose, for instance, that a hypothetical study has found a significant and positive correlation between autism and hyperserotonemia (see Section 3. Serotonin) and estimates that the chance an individual with an elevated blood serotonin level (hyperserotonemia) greater than two standard deviations above the normal level has a 4.7% chance of having autism. The hypothetical study has also found that an individual with hyperserotonemia that is only 0.2 standard deviations above the normal level has a 1.3% chance of having autism. The hypothetical relative risk of autism for the individual with extreme hyperserotonemia is 4.7%/1.3% = 0.047/0.013 = 3.6. In this hypothetical example, the individual with extreme hyperserotonemia is 3.6 times more likely to have autism than is the individual having a blood serotonin level that is only slightly elevated. Obtaining the relative risk is feasible only when autism prevalence (from cross-sectional or longitudinal data) or incidence (from longitudinal data) is available. A benefit of using the relative risk to quantify autism risk is that it is a single-number summary that is easy to calculate and begin to understand, a benefit that may also be its major detriment. A considerable disadvantage of using the relative risk in autism research is that many different autism-biology relationships can give rise to the same relative risk because information about serotonin levels and potentially important autism features is missing, making it difficult to generalize a relative risk finding to heterogeneous populations (van Belle, 2002; Schmidt & Kohlman, 2008). Also see *Odds Ratio.*

Reliability: the ratio of measurement variance between individuals to the total variance of the measurements. Total variance includes measurement variance between individuals and the variance of repeated measurements for each individual. For instance, suppose one needs to know the reliability of volume measurements of Heschl's gyrus, and a researcher has measured the volume of Heschl's gyrus manually three times for each subject in a sample of subjects with autism. If the volumetric variance between subjects in this sample is 11 and the average variance of repeated measurements for each subject is three, then the reliability of the manual tracing method (performed by this researcher) is 11/(11 + 3) or 79%, an acceptably high fraction for research and some clinical purposes. This definition of reliability is equivalent to the definition of the **intraclass correlation coefficient**, which is in turn equivalent to Cohen's κ (Fleiss & Cohen, 1973).

Sensitivity: the percentage of correct positive test results ("true positives," TP) for the presence of a condition among all test results from a population having the condition, both correct (TP) and incorrect ("false negatives," FN). For example, if nine individuals in a population of 100 have autism and the number of correct results for a test of autism is 7 (TP = 7 and FN = 2), then the sensitivity of the test is 7/(7 + 2) or 78%, an unacceptably low fraction. The sensitivity of a test is equivalent to its statistical **power**, which by current scientific convention should be at least 80%. Formula: Sensitivity = TP/(TP + FN).

Specificity: the percentage of correct negative test results ("true negatives," TN) for the presence of a condition among all test results over a population not having the condition, both correct (TN) and incorrect ("false positives," FP). For example, if 91 individuals in a population of 100 do not have autism, and the number of correct results of a test for autism is 76 (TN = 76 and FP = 15), then the specificity of the test is 76/(76 + 15) or 84%, an unacceptably low fraction. The **significance level** of a test is equal to one minus its specificity, which by current scientific convention should be no greater than 5%. Formula: Specificity = TN/(TN + FP).

Standard Deviation (SD): a measure of spread around a mean of measurements; see *Mean*. The SD is the square root of the variance; see *Variance*. It is in the same units (for instance cm^3) as the measurements themselves and of their mean. It is often true that roughly 68% of the measurements lie within 1 SD of their mean and 95% within two SDs when most the data are spread symmetrically on either side of the mean. The SD is a measure of uncertainty in the value of a single measurement and not of the uncertainty in the value of their mean. The standard deviation of the mean is termed the *standard error* (SE) or *standard error of the mean* (SEM) to make the distinction clear. The standard error of the mean is equal to the SD divided by the square root of the number of measurements. Formula: SEM = $SD/\sqrt{n}$. For instance, research suggests that fractional anisotropy (FA), one measure of local directional flow along brain circuits, is low for individuals with autism in the genu of the corpus callosum, a major "information superhighway" between the brain hemispheres (Alexander et al., 2007). The SD of an FA measurement for each of the 43 individuals in the study with autism was 0.042, and the mean FA in the autism group was 0.663. The SD and mean FA for the 34 healthy control individuals were 0.037 and 0.692 when taking performance IQ into account for all subjects. Is FA in the genu of a subject with autism different from that of a healthy individual, on average, or are the observed differences due only to chance fluctuations? Critical in answering this question are the SEs of the mean in the autism and control groups and, more importantly, of their difference. The SEM in the autism group was 0.0010 (= 0.042/43) and that of the control group was 0.0011 (= 0.037/34), not significantly different from each other. The SE of the mean group difference was roughly 0.0046 when taking performance IQ into account since it is correlated with a diagnosis of autism. (This SEM was obtained from the published data by a common albeit seemingly complex formula found in many textbooks.) The standardized difference in FA means was -2.97 = (0.663 - 0.692)/0.00976, a difference that is unlikely if FA is identical in the two groups, having a p-value of 0.002, which is significant statistically; see *P-value*.

Variance: the sum of squared differences between a group of measurements and their mean, divided by their number less 1 (for an unbiased measure if the mean is unknown prior to data collection); see *Mean, Standard Deviation*.

APPENDIX B. TABULAR SUMMARY OF LITERATURE REVIEW

Table 28B–1. Macrocephaly

Family Study Design: Twin Study
Measurement: Head circumference was compared.
Autism sample: An epidemiological sample of N = 25 same-sex pairs of monozygotic (MZ) and N = 20 same-sex pairs of dizygotic (DZ) twins were examined.
Control sample: Typical twins reference data were used.

(*Continued*)

Table 28B–1. *(Contd.)*

Association in autism: For male twins less than 16 years of age, macrocephaly was present in 38.9% of twins with autism versus 9% of typically developing (TD) twins.

Association with nonautistic relative: There was no increased rate of macrocephaly in nonautistic co-twins.

Familial resemblance: The within-twin pair variance for head circumference was not significantly less than the between-twin variance in MZ twins concordant for autism.

Reference: Bailey et al., 1995; Le Couteur et al., 1996

Family Study Design: Autism Probands and their Parents

Measurement: Head circumference was compared.

Autism sample: N = 100 autism probands were examined. The number of parents included in the study is not reported.

Control sample: Reference data were used.

Association in autism: Twenty-four percent (24%) of autism probands were macrocephalic.

Association with nonautistic relative: The rate of macrocephaly for parents is not provided.

Familial resemblance: The resemblance was uncertain. Sixty-two percent (62%) of autism macrocephalic probands had at least one parent with macrocephaly. Data for parents of nonmacrocephalic probands were not provided.

Reference: Stevenson et al., 1997

Family Study Design: Autism Probands, Parents, and Unaffected Siblings

Measurement: Head circumference was compared.

Autism sample: N = 41 autism probands, N = 23 fathers, N = 30 mothers, and N = 44 unaffected siblings were examined.

Control sample: N = 21 children with nonautistic tuberous sclerosis or seizure disorder, N = 5 fathers, N = 12 mothers, and N = 19 siblings were examined.

Association in autism: Macrocephaly was present in 12.2% of autism probands versus 9.5% of comparison children, a statistically negligible difference.

Association with nonautistic relative: Macrocephaly was not specific to autism families. It was present in 18.9% of parents and 11.4% of siblings in autism families versus 17.6% of parents and 0% siblings in comparison families, again a statistically negligible difference.

Familial resemblance: A father-proband correlation of 0.52 was observed ($p < 0.001$), and the mother-proband correlation of 0.38 was also significant ($p < 0.02$). The estimated heritability in autism families was 47%, indistinguishable from that observed in the control families.

Reference: Fidler et al., 2000

Family Study Design: Autism Probands and their Parents

Measurement: Head circumference was compared.

Autism sample: N = 137 autism probands and N = 121 parents were examined.

Control sample: Existing reference data were used.

Association in autism: Macrocephaly was present in 23.3% of autism probands.

Association with non-autistic relative: Macrocephaly was present in 39% of parents of the combined sample of macrocephalic and normocephalic probands.

Familial resemblance: None was observed. Forty-five percent (45%) of 20 macrocephalic autism probands and 37% of 59 normocephalic autism probands had at least one parent with macrocephaly ($p > 0.6$, binomial proportions test).

Reference: Miles et al., 2000

Family Study Design: Autism Probands, Parents, and Siblings

Measurement: Head circumference was compared.

Autism sample: Collaborative Programs of Excellence in Autism (CPEA) Network Study data were used. N = 208 autism probands and N = 71 affected siblings were examined. Unaffected relatives examined included N = 76 mothers, N = 71 fathers, and N = 78 siblings.

Control sample: Typical controls and reference data were used.

Association in autism: Macrocephaly was present in 17.3% of autism probands versus 4.3% of controls. Macrocephaly was also present in 20.8% of autism probands having parental data and in 14.1% of their affected siblings.

Association with nonautistic relative: Macrocephaly was present for parents but not unaffected siblings. Macrocephaly was present in 19.7% of mothers, 16.9% of fathers, 2.9% of both parents, 33.3% of either parent, and 5.1% of unaffected siblings.

Familial resemblance: Thirty-five point seven percent (35.7%) of macrocephalic autism probands had at least one parent with macrocephaly, and 32.7% of autism probands without macrocephaly had at least one parent with macrocephaly. For head circumference, parent-proband child resemblance was similar to the resemblance between the parents and their TD children in the general population.

Reference: Lainhart et al., 2006

Family Study Design: ASD Probands and Younger Siblings

Measurement: Head circumference was compared.

Autism sample: N = 28 male children with autism or PDD-NOS were examined. In a separate study, N = 77 infant siblings, male and female, of children with ASD were examined.

Control sample: CDC reference data were used.

Association in autism: For the ASD children, mean rate of head growth during the first year of life and mean head circumference at 1 year of age were greater than those of the reference data. Individual growth curves had been estimated.

Association with nonautistic relative: An abnormal rate of head circumference growth during the first year of life was also observed. Quantitatively similar findings to those observed in the ASD children were observed in their infant siblings, including infants who had high levels of signs indicating risk for autism and siblings who had low levels of the signs.

References: Dawson et al., 2007; Elder et al., 2008

Table 28B–2.
Total brain volume and regional brain volume

Family Study Design: Twin Study

Measurement: Total and regional brain volumes were compared.

Autism sample: N = 1 pair of MZ male twins discordant for autism (7.5 years of age) was examined. The twin with autism also had ADHD (verbal IQ (VIQ) 73, performance IQ (PIQ) 91) and the non-autistic twin was had signs of the BAP and also mild ADHD (VIQ 97, PIQ 95).

Control sample: N = 5 age-matched male TD singletons (mean full-scale IQ (FSIQ 119) were examined.

Association in autism: Compared to the nonautistic MZ twin, the autism twin had smaller total intracranial volume (TICV), and when adjusting for TICV the following were smaller in autism: caudate, amygdala, hippocampus (by 34–55%), cerebellar lobules VI–VII (by 26%). Compared to the singleton controls, the autism twin had smaller TICV (z score difference: -2.35). The following regional volumes were disproportionately smaller than TICV (z-score difference): frontal lobe (Lt -5.78, Rt -3.13), superior temporal gyrus (STG) (Lt -3.22, Rt -2.12), amygdala (Lt -4.22, Rt -3.19), hippocampus (Lt -4.09, Rt -5.20).

Association with nonautistic relative: Compared to the singleton controls, the nonautistic twin had smaller TICV (z score difference: -1.02) and disproportionately smaller frontal lobe than TICV (z score difference: Lt -3.48, Rt -1.97).

Familial resemblance: The frontal lobe was disproportionately smaller than expected for TICV in the twin with autism and the co-twin with the BAP.

Reference: Kates et al., 1998

Family Study Design: Twin Study

Measurement: Total and regional brain volume were compared.

Autism sample: N = 16 pairs of MZ twins (N = 7 concordant for autism; N = 9 discordant for autism) were examined.

Control sample: N = 16 age- and gender-matched unrelated singletons were examined.

Association in autism: Compared to the nonautistic MZ twin, the autism twin had decreased cerebral white matter (WM) volume (due to frontal, temporal, and occipital regions) and increased ventricular total volume. No differences were found in TICV, cerebral gray matter (GM) volume, and cerebellar GM or WM volume.

Association with nonautistic relative: Compared to the singleton controls, the nonautistic twin had decreased cerebral WM volume (due to frontal, temporal, and occipital regions). No differences were found in TICV, cerebral GM volume, cerebellar WM or GM volume, and ventricular volume.

Familial resemblance: The MZ twins concordant for autism had high intraclass correlation coefficients (ICCs) for volumes of cerebral GM and WM, cerebellar GM and WM, and ventricles. The MZ twins discordant for autism also had high ICCs for cerebral GM and WM and ventricular volumes but had significantly decreased ICC for volumes of cerebellar GM and WM.

Reference: Kates et al., 2004

Family Study Design: Twin Study

Measurement: Total and regional brain volumes were compared.

Autism sample: N = 1 pair of MZ male twins discordant for autism (13 yrs old) was examined. The twin with autism had a VIQ= 106 and PIQ= 88, the nonautistic twin was a BAP and had a VIQ= 108 and PIQ= 96. N = 13 age-matched singletons were also examined.

Control sample: N = 25 age-matched TD controls were examined. Association in autism: Smaller total brain volume (TBV) was found in the autism twin compared to the singleton autism and typical controls. Regional brain volume differences (as percent of TBV) as well as greater left frontal lobe and smaller right cerebellum were also found. No cerebrum differences were found.

Association with nonautistic relative: Smaller TBV was found in the BAP twin compared to the singleton autism and typical controls. No regional brain volume differences were found.

Familial resemblance: TBV was smaller in autism and BAP twins.

Reference: Belmonte & Carper, 2006

Family Study Design: Twin Study

Measurement: Total and regional brain volumes were studied.

Autism sample: N = 14 pair of MZ twins (ages 5–14 yrs old) with at least one twin with an autism diagnosis were examined (36% concordant for autism, 28% co-twin PDD-NOS, 36% co-twin no diagnosis).

Control sample: N = 14 singleton age- and gender-matched TD comparison subjects were examined.

Association in autism: ICC for TBV was 0.93 in MZ twins. Right (but not left) dorsolateral prefrontal cortical volumes for autism were significantly larger than those of comparison subjects but not co-twins. The genu and anterior of the corpus callosum were smaller for children with autism relative to comparison subjects but not to co-twins. Relative to comparison subjects cerebellar lobules VI and VII were significantly smaller in co-twins and tended to be smaller in children with autism.

Association with nonautistic relative: Differences in those concordant for autism versus not concordant for autism were not tested.

Reference: Mitchell et al., 2009

Family Study Design: Nuclear Families (Parents)

Measurement: Total and regional brain volumes were compared.

Autism sample: N = 19 parent couples of autistic probands were examined.

Control sample: N = 20 matched healthy control parent couples were examined.

Association in autism: From the researchers' prior work, TBV was increased above the control mean in 17 of the 19 autism probands (Palmen et al., 2004; Palmen et al., 2005a).

Association with nonautistic relative: No significant differences were found in TICV, TBV, or regional brain volumes between the autistic proband parents and the control parents.

Reference: Palmen et al., 2005b

(*Continued*)

Table 28B–2. *(Contd.)*

Family Study Design: Nuclear Families (Parents and Unrelated Adults with Autism)

Measurement: TBV, hippocampus, and amygdala volumes were compared.

Autism sample: N = 17 parents of autism proband children and N = 15 adults with autism were examined.

Control sample: N = 17 control adults were examined. Association in autism: In the autism adults, left hippocampal volume was increased and left amygdala volume was decreased.

Association with nonautistic relative: Left hippocampal volume was increased in parents. No amygdala differences in parents were found.

Reference: Rojas et al., 2004

Family Study Design: Nuclear Families (Parents)

Measurement: Regional GM volumes were compared.

Autism sample: N = 23 parents of autistic probands (N = 18 families, N = 15 mothers, N = 8 fathers) were examined.

Control sample: N = 23 control participants (8 males) were examined. Association in autism: Not tested.

Association with nonautistic relative: GM was altered in ASD parents compared to controls. No TBV or hippocampal differences were found.

Reference: Peterson et al., 2006

Table 28B–3.
Brain function and brain connectivity

Family Study Design: Nuclear Family (Twin)

Measurement: Functional magnetic resonance (fMRI) activation in response to a frequent congruent visual condition versus a rare incongruent condition was examined. The functionally demanding task required simultaneous attending to location, color, and orientation.

Autism sample: One pair of MZ male twins discordant for autism, age 13 years (Twin L autism: VIQ 106, PIQ 88; Twin M BAP: VIQ 108, PIQ 96), was examined.

Association in autism: In the autistic twin, there was a significant differential activation only in the left superior temporal gyrus (STG) (Broadmann Area [BA] 22) and similar network activated in the two conditions.

Association with nonautistic relative: In the BAP twin there was activation in two separate networks for the two different conditions where easy and accurate performance of the cognitively high-demand task occurred.

Familial resemblance: No resemblance.

Reference: Belmonte & Carper, 2006

Family Study Design: Nuclear Family (Siblings)

Measurement: Eye movements, facial recognition and emotion discrimination, and fMRI brain activation were examined.

Autism sample: The following participants were examined: Study I: N = 14 males with autism (11 verbally fluent); Study II: N = 16 males with autism (14 verbally fluent); Study III: N = 12 children with autism, N = 10 unaffected siblings (ages 8–25yr old).

Control sample: The following control participants were studied: Study I: N = 12 TD males; Study II: N = 16 typical males; Study III: N = 12 matched typical children.

Association in autism: In Studies I & II, the autism group spent less time fixating on eyes, but there was marked variability within the group. In the autism but not control group, brain activation in the amygdala and right anterior fusiform gyrus was strongly positively related to the amount of time spent fixating on eyes.

Association with nonautistic relative: Similar to the children with autism, unaffected siblings spent less time fixating on eyes than controls (Study III). There was no significant difference between the autism group and the unaffected sibling group on time spent fixating on eyes. The eye fixation time was strongly positively related to right and left fusiform gyrus but not amygdala activation in unaffected siblings.

Reference: Dalton et al., 2005; Dalton et al., 2007

Family Study Design: Nuclear Family (Parents)

Measurement: event-related potential (ERP) response to face and nonface stimuli was compared.

Autism sample: N = 21 parents of autistic children were examined.

Control sample: N = 21 parents of TD children were examined.

Association in autism: Previous studies had shown that children and adults with autism have atypical ERPs to faces. These studies had failed to show a negative component (N170) latency advantage to face compared to nonface stimuli, and a bilateral, rather than the normal right-lateralized, pattern of N170 distribution.

Association with nonautistic relative: Parents of children with autism had atypical ERP response to faces that mirrored the response seen in affected individuals.

Reference: Dawson et al., 2005

Family Study Design: Nuclear Family (Parents)

Measurement: fMRI brain activation was recorded during a visual search task (Embedded Figures Task) and an empathy task (Reading the Mind in the Eyes Task).

Autism sample: N = 12 parents of children with Asperger's syndrome were examined.

Control sample: N = 12 matched parents of TD controls were examined.

Association in autism: Not reported.

Association with nonautistic relative: Both mothers and fathers of children with Asperger's syndrome showed atypical brain functioning compared to control parents on both tasks—they had less activation in visual cortex bilaterally (BA 19) and more activation in left medial temporal gyrus and dorsolateral prefrontal cortex (PFC).

Reference: Baron-Cohen et al., 2006

(Continued)

Table 28B–3. *(Contd.)*

Family Study Design: Nuclear Family (Parents)

Measurement: Magnetoencephalography (MEG) transient evoked and induced gamma-band power and inter-trial phase-locking consistency were recorded.

Autism sample: N = 11 adults with autism and N = 16 parents of children with autism, not related to the adults with autism, were examined.

Control sample: N = 16 control adults were examined.

Association in autism: In adults with autism, higher induced and lower evoked gamma-band power (40 Hz) and lower phase-locking factor measure of phase consistency of neuronal response to external stimuli was found. The potential endophenotypes in autism are MEG gamma-band phase consistency and changes in evoked verse induced power.

Association with nonautistic relative: The parents of children with autism had the same results as the adults with autism.

Familial resemblance: The adults with autism and the parents were not related.

Reference: Rojas et al., 2008; Wilson et al., 2007

Table 28B–4.
Serotonin

Family Study Design: Nuclear Family (Parents)

Measurement: Serotonin ($5\text{-}HT_2$) receptor cortical binding potential (BP) density was measured by positron emission tomography (PET, [^{18}F]setoperone PET in this case) with 12 cortical regions of interest and cortex-to-cerebellum ratio. Left and right cortical areas examined: frontal, inferior frontal, parietal, inferior parietal, lateral temporal, occipital.

Autism sample: N = 19 parents (8 females, 11 males) from 11 autism multiplex families, with no neurological or psychiatric disorders during 6 months prior to study and no medicine or substance use, were examined.

Control sample: N = 17 typical control adults (9 females, 8 males) were examined. Age and sex were covariates in all analyses.

Association in autism: There are no data concerning the affected children.

Association with nonautistic relative: Mean whole blood platelet serotonin showed no difference. The mean composite cortical $5\text{-}HT_2$ receptor BP was significantly lower in parents (effect size 0.9). The mean $5\text{-}HT_2$ BP was significantly lower in parents in every left and right cortical area examined (range: means 77–88% lower in parents versus controls). Also, variance of 5-HT BP was less in parents. There was significant negative correlation of mean platelet 5-HT with cortical $5\text{-}HT_2$ BP in parents but not in the controls (composite BP r = -0.59; 8 of 12 cortical regions of interest (ROIs), r = -0.52 to -0.65).

Familial resemblance: Not examined.

Reference: Goldberg et al., 2009

Family Study Design: Nuclear Family (Children with Autism, Parents and Siblings)

Measurement: Plasma serotonin levels were compared.

Autism sample: N = 17 children with autism and their mothers (N = 17) and fathers (N = 12) were examined. All parents were nonautistic.

Control sample: Control mothers were examined.

Association in autism: No comparison sample was examined.

Association with nonautistic relative: Plasma serotonin levels in autism mothers were significantly different than in mothers of TD children (P = 0.002).

Familial resemblance: Plasma serotonin levels correlated between autism mothers and their children, but differed between autistic children and their fathers and siblings.

Reference: Anderson, 2007; Connors et al., 2006

Family Study Design: Nuclear Family (First-Degree Relatives)

Measurement: Whole blood serotonin was compared.

Autism sample: N = 62 autism subjects and N = 122 of their first-degree relatives were examined.

Control sample: Age- and sex-matched controls were examined.

Association in autism: Increased rate of hyperserotonemia was found.

Association with nonautistic relative: Hyperserotonemia was found in 51% of mothers, 45% of fathers, 87% of siblings of autism probands.

Reference: Leboyer et al., 1999

Family Study Design: Nuclear Family (Parents and Siblings)

Measurement: Quantity of platelet $5\text{-}HT_2$ serotonin binding sites was compared.

Autism sample: N = 12 autism probands, N = 6 of their siblings, and N = 22 of their parents were examined.

Control sample: Adult and child controls were examined.

Association in autism: No case-control differences in platelet serotonin receptor binding sites, whole blood serotonin, or plasma norepinephrine (noradrenaline) were found.

Association with nonautistic relative: No autism relative-controls differences were found.

Familial resemblance: Significant correlation of total number of platelet serotonin binding sites in 11 autism probands and their fathers was found.

Reference: Perry et al., 1991

Family Study Design: Nuclear Family (Parents and Siblings)

Measurement: Levels of whole blood serotonin and plasma norepinephrine (noradrenaline) were compared.

Autism sample: N = 47 autism probands and their siblings, mothers, and fathers were examined.

Control sample: Not reported.

Association in autism: The mean whole blood 5-HT level was higher in autistic probands than parents and siblings.

(Continued)

Table 28B–4. *(Contd.)*

Association with nonautistic relative: Twenty-three of 47 families had at least one member with hyperserotonemia and 10 had two or more members with hyperserotonemia; in five families every member had hyperserotonemia.

Familial resemblance: Familiality of hyperserotonemia. If the autistic child of a family was hyperserotonemic, the first-degree relatives were 2.4 times more likely to be hyperserotonemic than if the autistic child was not hyperserotonemic.

Reference: Leventhal et al., 1990

Family Study Design: Nuclear Family (Parents and Siblings)

Measurement: Whole blood serotonin and plasma norepinephrine (noradrenaline) were compared.

Autism sample: N = 16 children with autism, N = 21 of their siblings, and N = 53 of their parents were examined.

Control sample: Not reported.

Association in autism: Not reported.

Association with nonautistic relative: Rate of hyperserotonemia increased.

Familial resemblance: Seven of 10 families with one hyperserotonemic member had two or more hyperserotonemic members.

Reference: Cook et al., 1990

Table 28B–5.
Immune factors

Family Study Design: Nuclear Family (Siblings)

Measurement: Antibodies reactive to human adult cerebellar extract, adult monkey cerebellar extract, and adult monkey brain sections.

Autism sample: N = 63 children with ASD and N = 25 of their unaffected siblings were examined.

Control sample: N = 63 age-matched healthy control children and N = 21 children with nonspecific developmental delay were examined.

Association in autism: 21% of the children with ASD had antibody to a 52kDa band protein from human adult cerebellum, compared to 2% of healthy control children and 5% of children with nonspecific developmental delay. Only antibodies from the ASD children reacted with a 52kDa protein band from adult monkey cerebellum. Antibodies from children with ASD showed specific immunohistochemical staining of slices of adult monkey brain cerebellum. Staining of cerebellar white matter was infrequently observed in the ASD children but was more common than in controls. Twenty-one percent of the ASD children, but none of the healthy children or developmentally delayed children, showed intense staining of cerebellar Golgi cells, large granule cell layer interneurons. The correlation between immunoreactivity to the Golgi cells and reactivity to the 52kDa band was strong in the ASD children ($r = 0.76$, $p = 0.0001$). There was no significant correlation in control children. No immunoreactivity to cerebellar Purkinje cells was observed.

Association with nonautistic relatives: None of the unaffected siblings had antibody to human or monkey cerebellar proteins. Intense immunoreactivity to cerebellar Golgi cells was found in 1 (4%) of the siblings.

Familial Resemblance: Not reported.

Reference: Wills et al., 2009

Family Study Design: Nuclear Family (Siblings)

Measurement: Multiple immune parameters were compared.

Autism sample: N = 20 children with autism ages 5–17 years and N = 15 of their unaffected siblings age 3–16 years were examined.

Control sample: N = 20 healthy control children ages 3–15 years were examined.

Association in autism: Mean numbers of subpopulations of CD4+ and CD8+ T lymphocytes, including naive and post-thymic differentiated cells, and mean levels of some cytokines were found to be altered in autistic children, suggesting dysregulation of the cell-mediated immune system.

Association with nonautistic relative: There was a similar pattern of immune dysregulation in healthy unaffected siblings as found in the children with autism.

Familial Resemblance: Not reported.

Reference: Saresella et al., 2009

Family Study Design: Nuclear Family (Mothers)

Measurement: Tissue protein medleys from human fetal and adult brain, duodenum (small intestine), and kidney were examined in mothers of children with autism.

Autism sample: N = 61 mothers of autism probands (AU) (36 regressive onset, 25 early onset) were examined.

Control sample: N = 62 mothers of TD children and N = 40 mothers of non-ASD children with developmental disabilities (DD) were examined. The case-control mothers were matched on maternal age, parity, and age of offspring (average age 3.5 years, range 2–5 years).

Association with nonautistic relative: Rate of plasma antibodies tested against human fetal (but not human adult) brain proteins was increased in some of the autism mothers. No association was found between maternal reactivity to human fetal proteins and history of current maternal autoimmune disorder. Reactivity to 37kDa and 73kDa protein bands from human fetal brain was significantly more common in the autism mothers including: a) reactivity to 37kDa fetal brain protein (found in 25–26% of Au mothers; 2–5% of DD mothers; 8.1% of TD mothers; odds ratio (OR) = 5.96 AP versus TD mothers; b) reactivity to both 37kDa and 73dDa fetal brain proteins: 11.5% (7 of 61) AP mothers; 0% of DD and TD mothers. The autism children of six of these seven mothers (86%) had a regressive onset.

Reference: Braunschweig et al., 2008

Family Study Design: Nuclear Family (Mother)

Measurement: Maternal blood drawn at midpregnancy was tested for maternal autoantibody to fetal brain protein.

Autism sample: N = 84 mothers of children with autism, where 19% of the autism offspring had a regressive onset, were examined.

(Continued)

Table 28B–5. *(Contd.)*

Control sample: N = 49 mothers (TD) of children with mental retardation (MR) or DD and N = 160 mothers of children not requiring DD services were examined.

Association with nonautistic relative: Reactivity to fetal brain 39kDa protein band was found in 7% of Au mothers versus 0% of MR mothers and 2% of TD mothers (p = 0.09 and 0.07); 1.2% (1 of 84) of autism mothers versus 0% of MR mothers and 2.6% of TD mothers had autoantibody reactivity to both 37kDa and 73kDa.

Reference: Croen et al., 2008

Family Study Design: Mothers Only

Measurement: The antibody source was serum. The tissue source was homogenated rodent fetal and adult brain and human fetal and adult brain of the following regions: BA9, caudate, cerebellum, and cingulate gyrus.

Autism sample: N = 100 mothers of children with autism, where 48 of the autism children had a history of social and language regression, were examined. (Some analyses had N = 20–25 autism mothers.)

Control sample: N = 100 age-matched control mothers (TD) were examined. Some analyses had n = 20–25 TDs.

Association in autism: Children with autism were not tested for the antibodies; only their mothers were tested.

Association with nonautistic relative: A personal history of autoimmune disease was present in 24 of 100 autism mothers and 12 of 100 TD mothers (OR = 2.32, p = 0.028).

There was little overlap in the antibodies autism mothers had to fetal and adult tissue in both rodent and human brain. Autism and TD mothers did not differ in antibodies to glial fibrillary acidic protein (GFAP) or myelin basic protein (MBP). No autism versus TD mother difference was found in serum levels of a brain-derived neurotrophic factor (BDNF). Mean serum immunoglobulin G (IgG) concentration was not different in Au and TD mothers. Sera from autism mothers contained antibodies that differed from TD mothers against prenatally expressed brain proteins. Antibodies to human fetal brain proteins were found in 10% of Au mothers (36kDa band) and 2% of TD mothers. Mean levels of human adult brain antibodies, against the caudate (155kDa) and frontal lobe (BA9, 63kDa), were significantly different in the mothers. It is not known if the antibodies in Au mothers have pathological consequences.

Reference: Singer et al., 2008

Family Study Design: Nuclear Family (Children with Autism and Siblings)

Measurement: IgG antibody source was plasma. Tissue source was protein extracts from thalamus and hypothalamus of the adult human brain.

Autism sample: N = 63 children with autism were examined.

Control sample: N = 25 unaffected siblings, N = 63 TD children and N = 21 children with other DD controls were examined.

Association in autism: Multiple bands of autoreactivity were observed: 52kDa band for the thalamus and 46 and 42kDa bands for thalamus and hypothalamus. Autoreactivity for the thalamus in plasma from children with autism was significantly greater than TD children, unaffected siblings, and DD controls. Circulating autoantibodies against thalamus and hypothalamus in children with autism but not their unaffected siblings suggest potential autoimmune sequelae specific to the disorder. The autoantibodies could be pathogenic or an epiphenomenon suggesting damage/injury to these areas of the brain.

Association with nonautistic relative: Autoreactivity for thalamus or hypothalamus was not increased in plasma from unaffected siblings; their levels were similar to TD and DD children.

Reference: Cabanlit et al., 2007

Family Study Design: Nuclear Family (Mothers and their Children with Autism; Unrelated Unaffected Siblings)

Measurement: The antibody source was serum. The tissue sources were fresh rat brain protein homogenates (fetal, postnatal, and adult rats) and tissue slices, and human GFAP and MBP.

Autism sample: N = 11 mothers of autism children (Au) 2–18 years after the birth of the autism proband and N = 12 male children with autism (7 regressive onset; 2 seizures) were examined.

Control sample: N = 10 mothers of TD children, 14 male children with other neurodevelopmental disorders (DD), 10 TD siblings (5 female, 5 male) of autism children (unrelated to probands and mothers in the study) and 4 TD children (2 female, 2 male) were examined.

Association in autism: Multiple varied reactive bands to postnatal and adult rat brain protein homogenates did not differentiate the groups. The pattern of reactivity to fetal rat brain proteins did differentiate Au mothers, their autism children, and DD children, from TD mothers, TD children, and TD siblings of autism probands unrelated to ones in the study. Reactivity to human GFAP and MBP did not differentiate Au verses TD mothers. No correlation of reactivity to regression, epilepsy, birth order in autism children, or to age, history of autoimmune disease, or parity in Au mothers was found. Antibodies from children with autism also recognized/reacted against different fetal rat brain proteins than TD controls and unrelated autism siblings; DD children reacted similarly to autism children (therefore, no specificity to autism).

Association with nonautistic relative: Autism mothers had different patterns of serum immunoreactivity to fetal rat brain protein, but not postnatal or adult rat brain proteins, than control mothers. Maternal reactivity persisted up to 18 years postdelivery.

Familial resemblance: Not reported.

Reference: Zimmerman et al., 2007

Family Study Design: Nuclear Family (ASD Children and Some of their Unaffected Siblings)

Measurement: The antibody source was serum. The tissue source was fresh human brain of the following regions: PFC (BA10), caudate, putamen, cerebellum, deep cerebellar nuclei, and cingulate gyrus.

(Continued)

Table 28B–5. *(Contd.)*

Autism sample: N = 29 children with ASD (3–12 yrs old) were examined: 22 low-functioning autism and 2 high-functioning autism, 1 Asperger's, 3 syndromal autism, 1 childhood disintegrative disorder. N = 9 nonautistic siblings (4–8 yrs old) of 8 of the children with autism.

Control sample: N = 13 unrelated typical controls (9–17 yrs old) were examined.

Association in autism: More autism and ASD children had 100 kDa bands than TD children (caudate: autism 100%, ASD 97%, TD 77% [p = 0.017]; putamen: autism 100%, ASD 100%, TD 69%; [p < 0.0001]; PFC [BA 10]: autism 95%, ASD 97%, TD 69% [p = .012]). Band density was measured as peak height and/or area under the curve. The autism children had increased density in the 73 kDa band in cerebellum and cingulate, the 160 kDa band in PFC (BA10), and the 36 kDa band in cerebellum. To date, the precise structural proteins involved are not known. Antibody repertoires may be pathological factors or secondary immune responses to previously damaged tissue. More autism than TD children had autoimmune complexes in the basal ganglia and frontal lobe and greater intensity of antigen-antibody complexes in the cingulate gyrus and cerebellum. Autism children had higher 73kDa density bands in cerebellum and cingulum.

Association with nonautistic relative: As mentioned above, mean levels of antibrain antibodies against cingulated gyrus and cerebellum were increased in a small number of unaffected siblings (N = 9), similar to their siblings with autism (N = 8), in comparison to TD children (N = 13). It is not clear if the latter represents an inherited tendency for a genetically determined defect or if it is an irrelevant trait.

Reference: Singer et al., 2006

Family Study Design: Nuclear Family (Children with Autism and their Parents)

Measurement: The tissue source was frozen human brain tissue. Reactivity to adult human brain extracted from a male 39 years of age, containing many different protein antigens, was measured.

Autism sample: N = 171 autism children 2–14 years of age and N = 171 parents of the autism children were examined.

Control Sample: N = 54 otherwise healthy children who were surgical patients were examined. Parent controls were the parents of 100 nonautistic patients.

Association in autism: The presence of numerous bands on immunoblot against human tissue was found in both autism and controls. Reactivity to protein 20kDa occurred in affected children but not their parents. The protein was not MBP.

Association with nonautistic relative: No reactivity to protein 20kDa in autism parents was observed.

Familial resemblance: No parent-autism child correlations for Section 32 (the 20kDa protein) were observed, and very low heritability estimates were found.

Reference: Silva et al., 2004

Family Study Design: Nuclear Family (Mother)

Measurement: Maternal serum antibodies to rodent Purkinje cells and neurons were used.

Autism sample: One mother had three children: a 9-year-old unaffected boy, a high-functioning girl 8 years of age with autism without a history of regression, and a boy 6 years of age with severe specific language disorder with onset after a regression at 18 months. Only the mother was examined.

Control Sample: N = 4 control mothers who each had one to four children.

Association with nonautistic relative: The autism mother had IgG that reacted to adult rat brain, specifically to the cytoplasm of cerebellar Purkinje cells, some large brain stem neurons, and to the Purkinje cell layer in developing mouse cerebellum. When serum from the mother was injected into a pregnant mouse, the mice offspring pups had behavioral deficits (less exploratory behavior and impaired performance on rods, but no impairment in memory acquisition). Immune staining and metabolism (studied with magnetic resonance spectroscopy) of the mice offspring cerebella was altered. There was no reaction from control mothers' serum.

Reference: Dalton et al., 2003

Family Study Design: Children with Autism, their Parents, and Unaffected Siblings

---

Measurement: Presence of plasma antibodies to serotonin receptors in human hippocampal membranes was measured.

Autism sample: N = 15 children with autism, N = 42 of their parents, and N = 17 of autistic unaffected siblings were examined.

Control sample: N = 12 unrelated TD controls were examined.

Association in autism: No evidence was found of plasma antibodies from children with autism binding to serotonin receptors $5HT_{1A}$ or $5H_{T2}$. There was no evidence of autoantibodies to serotonin receptors in autism probands or their relatives.

Association with nonautistic relative: There was no evidence of plasma antibodies from parents or unaffected siblings of autism probands binding to serotonin receptors.

Reference: Cook et al., 1993

Family Study Design: Nuclear Family (Mothers)

Measurement: Frequency of maternal immunologic disorders was compared.

Autism sample: Mothers of N = 407 children with autism were examined.

Control sample: Mothers of N = 2095 control children were examined.

Association with nonautistic relative: Mothers of autism probands showed no increased rate of autoimmune diseases in the 4–year period surrounding the pregnancy with the child who developed autism.

Reference: Croen et al., 2005

Family Study Design: Nuclear Family

Measurement: Frequency of autoimmune disorders.

Autism sample: Parents of N = 101 autism probands were examined.

Control sample: Parents of N = 101 children with an autoimmune disorder and N = 101 control children were examined.

(Continued)

Table 28B–5. *(Contd.)*

Association with nonautistic relative: There was an increased rate of autoimmune disorders in families of PDD-NOS children, especially in parents. Hypothyroid disease and rheumatic fever were more common in autism families.

Reference: Sweeten et al., 2003

Family Study Design: Nuclear Family

Measurement: Frequency of autoimmune disorders was compared.

Autism sample: N = 61 families of patients with autism were examined.

Control sample: N = 46 healthy controls were examined.

Association with nonautistic relative: There was an increased rate of autoimmune disorders in mothers and first-degree relatives in general.

Familial resemblance: As the number of family members with autoimmune disorders increased, the risk of autism in the family was greater.

Reference: Comi et al., 1999

Family Study Design: Nuclear Family

Measurement: Frequencies of null alleles at the C4A and C4B loci was compared.

Autism sample: N = 19 individuals with autism and unaffected family members were examined.

Control sample: TD controls were examined.

Association in autism: The rate of the C4A null allele was increased.

Association with nonautistic relative: Mothers of autism probands had significantly increased frequencies of C4A null allele (58% in mothers, 27% controls). Unaffected siblings also had increased C4A null alleles, although it was nonsignificant from controls.

Reference: Warren et al., 1991

Family Study Design: Nuclear Family (First-Degree Relatives of Children with ASD)

Measurement: Frequency of familial autoimmune disorders was measured.

Autism sample: Medical records of children born in Denmark from 1993 to 2004 with an ASD diagnosis (N = 3325, of which 1089 had an infantile autism diagnosis) were examined.

Control sample: Unaffected family members (siblings and parents) of children with autism and families of children born during the same time without an autism diagnosis (N = 685,871) were included in the study.

Association with nonautistic relative: Maternal history of celiac disease and rheumatoid arthritis were associated with increased risk of ASD. Type-1 diabetes in fathers and mothers was associated with an increased risk for autism. Maternal and familial thyrotoxicosis was related to lower risk for ASD.

Reference: Atladottir et al., 2009

Table 28B–6.
Classification

Method: Shape Representations of WM Fibers Passing Through the Splenium of the Corpus Callosum Extracted from Diffusion Tensor Images (DTI).

Sample: N = 41 males with high-functioning autism and N = 32 TD controls, matched for age, handedness, IQ, and head size, were examined.

Autism sensitivity: 72%

Autism specificity: 72%

Reference: Adluru et al., 2009

Method: A Combination of Cerebellar and Cerebral WM and GM Volumes, and Areas of Anterior Vermis and Posterior Vermis in the Medial Lobe of the Cerebellum.

Sample: N = 30 low-functioning autism, N = 12 high-functioning autism, and N = 13 normal controls (all boys, 1.7–5.2yrs of age) were examined.

Autism sensitivity: 94.7%

Autism specificity: 92.3%

Reference: Akshoomoff et al., 2004

Method: White Matter Cumulative Distribution Related to Size of Gyral Window.

Sample: N = 14 males with autism (8–38yrs of age, IQs 65–107) and N = 28 TD control males, matched for age and handedness, were examined.

Autism sensitivity: 67%

Autism specificity: 89%

Reference: Casanova et al., 2009

Method: A Whole-Brain Structural MRI Pattern Classification Approach in a Spatially Distributed Neural Network (Limbic, Frontal-Striatal, Frontotemporal, Frontoparietal, and Cerebellar Systems).

Sample: N = 22 ASD and N = 22 healthy controls (all adult males, matched for age, IQ, and GM, WM, and TBV) were examined.

Autism sensitivity: 77% for GM images (predictive power 81%); 73% for WM images (predictive power 68%).

Autism specificity: 86% for GM images; 64% for WM images.

Reference: Ecker et al., 2009

Method: Computerized Binocular Infrared Pupillography, with Transient Papillary Light Reflex Latency and Constriction Amplitude.

Sample: N = 24 males with ASD and N = 43 TD males (6–16 yrs of age) were examined.

Autism sensitivity: 91.7%

Autism specificity: 93%

Reference: Fan et al., 2009

(Continued)

Table 28B–6. *(Contd.)*

Method: Cortical Thickness and Cortical Volume of 33 Cortical Regions in Each Hemisphere were Used. Classification Methods Identified Seven Key Regions. Decreased Areas Included Bilateral Pars Triangularis, Left Medial Orbitofrontal and Parahippocampal Gyri, and Left Frontal Pole. Increased Areas Included Left Caudal Anterior Cingulate and Left Precuneus.
Sample: N = 22 children with ASD (mean age 9.2 +/- 2.1 years) and N = 16 age-matched community volunteer children were examined. Autism sensitivity: Cortical thickness: 95%; Cortical volume: 77% Autism specificity: Cortical thickness: 75%; Cortical volume: 69% Reference: Jiao et al., 2009
Method: A Combination of Left Fusiform Gyrus GM, Right Temporal Stem WM, and Right Inferior Temporal Gyrus GM Volumes.
Sample: N = 33 males with high-functioning autism and N = 24 control males were examined. Autism sensitivity: 85% Autism specificity: 83% Reference: Neeley et al., 2007
Method: Voxelwise Cortical Thickness Based on 40,000 Points, by Measuring the Goodness of Each Point as a Classifier and the Discriminative Characteristics of Regions.
Sample: N = 16 high-functioning males with autism and N = 11 TD males (mean age 14.5 years, SD 4.6) were examined. Autism sensitivity: Classification accuracy: 89% Reference: Singh et al., 2008
Method: Automated Vocalization Analysis of 12-hour Audio-Recordings from the Natural Home Environment.
Sample: Young children, N = 34 autism, N = 30 nonautistic language delay, and N = 76 TD, were examined. Autism sensitivity: Classification accuracy: 77 to 90% Reference: Xu et al., 2009
Method: MEG Latency of Right-Hemisphere M50.
Sample: N = 14 autism, N = 10 Asperger's syndrome, N = 5 nonautistic specific language impairment, and N = 6 TD controls (all children 7–18 yrs old) were examined. Impaired language sensitivity: 70% Impaired language specificity: 92% Reference: Oram Cardy et al., 2008
Method: MEG Latency of Right-Hemisphere 500 Hz M100.
Sample: N = 25 autism spectrum disorder (9 with language impairment, 16 without language impairment) and N = 17 TD controls (all children, ASD mean age 10.20 years, sd 2.15) were examined. Sensitivity for ASD: 75% Specificity: 81% Reference: Roberts et al., 2010

REFERENCES

Abramson, R. K., Wright, H. H., Carpenter, R., Brennan, W., Lumpuy, O., Cole, E., et al. (1989). Elevated blood serotonin in autistic probands and their first-degree relatives. *Journal of Autism and Developmental Disorders, 19*(3), 397–407.

Adluru, N., Hinrichs, C., Chung, M. K., Lee, J. E., Singh, V., Bigler, E. D., et al. (2009). Classification in DTI using shapes of white matter tracts. *IEEE Engineering in Medicine and Biology Society, 1*, 2719–2722.

Akshoomoff, N., Lord, C., Lincoln, A. J., Courchesne, R. Y., Carper, R. A., Townsend, J., et al. (2004). Outcome classification of preschool children with autism spectrum disorders using MRI brain measures. *Journal of the American Academy of Child and Adolescent Psychiatry, 43*(3), 349–357.

Allen, A. J., Griss, M. E., Folley, B. S., Hawkins, K. A., & Pearlson, G. D. (2009). Endophenotypes in schizophrenia: A selective review. *Schizophrenia Research, 109*, 24–37.

Alexander, A. L., Lee, J. E., Lazar, M., Boudos, R., DuBray, M. B., Oakes, T. R., et al. (2007). Diffusion tensor imaging of the corpus callosum in autism. *NeuroImage, 34*(1), 61–73.

Anderson, G. M. (2002). Genetics of childhood disorders: XLV. Autism, Part 4: Serotonin in autism. *Journal of the American Academy of Child and Adolescent Psychiatry, 41*(12), 1513–1516.

Anderson, G. (2007). Measurement of plasma serotonin in autism. *Pediatric Neurology, 36*(2), 138.

Anderson, J. S., Druzgal, T. J., Froehlich, A., DuBray, M. B., Lange, N., Alexander, A. L., et al. (2010). Decreased interhemispheric functional connectivity in autism. *Cerebral Cortex*, Epub date: October 12, doi:10.1093/cercor/bhq190.

Anderson, J. S., Lange, N., Froehlich, A., DuBray, M. B., Druzgal, T. J., Froimowitz, M. P., et al. (2010). Decreased left posterior insular activity during auditory language processing in autism. *American Journal of Neuroradiology, 31*, 131–139.

Akshoomoff, N., Lord, C., Lincoln, A. J., Courchesne, R. Y., Carper, R. A., Townsend, J., et al. (2004). Outcome classification of preschool children with autism spectrum disorders using MRI brain measures. *Journal of the American Academy of Child and Adolescent Psychiatry, 43*(3), 349–357.

Atladóttir, H. O., Pedersen, M. G., Thorsen, P., Mortensen, P. B., Deleuran, B., Eaton, W. W., et al. (2009). Association of family history of autoimmune diseases and autism spectrum disorders. *Pediatrics, 124*(2), 687–694.

Aylward, E. H., Minshew, N. J., Field, K., Sparks, B. F., & Singh, N. (2002). Effects of age on brain volume and head circumference in autism. *Neurology, 59*(2), 175–183.

Bailey, A., Le Couteur, A., Gottesman, I., Bolton, P., Simonoff, E., Yuzda, E., et al. (1995). Autism as a strongly genetic disorder: Evidence from a British twin study. *Psychological Medicine, 25*(1), 63–77.

Bailey, A., Luthert, P., Bolton, P., Le Couteur, A., Rutter, M., & Harding, B. (1993). Autism and megalencephaly. *Lancet, 341*, 1225–1226.

Bailey, A., Luthert, P., Dean, A., Harding, B., Janota, I., Montgomery, M., et al. (1998). A clinicopathological study of autism. *Brain, 121*(Pt 5), 889–905.

Baron-Cohen, S., Ring, H., Chitnis, X., Wheelwright, S., Gregory, L., Williams, S., et al. (2006). FMRI of parents of children with Asperger Syndrome: A pilot study. *Brain and Cognition, 61*(1), 122–130.

Belmonte, M. K., & Carper, R. A. (2006). Monozygotic twins with Asperger syndrome: Differences in behaviour reflect variations in brain structure and function. *Brain and Cognition, 61*(1), 110–121.

Bigler, E. D., Abildskov, T., DuBray, M. B., Froehlich, A., Alexander, A. L., Lange, N., et al. (2010, February). *Stability of brain volume from mid-childhood through adolescence and early adulthood in autism.* Accepted for presentation, 2010 International Neuropsychological Society Meeting, Acapulco, Mexico.

Biomarkers Definitions Working Group. (2001). Biomarkers and surrogate endpoints: Preferred definitions and conceptual framework. *Clinical Pharmacology and Therapeutics, 69*, 89–95.

Bolton, P., Macdonald, H., Pickles, A., Rios, P., Goode, S., Crowson, M., et al. (1994). A case-control family history study of autism. *Journal of Child Psychology and Psychiatry, 35*, 877–900.

Bonnin, A., Torii, M., Wang, L., Rakic, P., & Levitt, P. (2007). Serotonin modulates the response of embryonic thalamocortical axons to netrin-1. *Nature Neuroscience, 10*(5), 588–597.

Brain Development Cooperative Group (corresponding author: Nicholas Lange. (2011). Total and regional brain volumes in a population-based normative sample: The NIH study of normal brain development. In revision for *Cerebral Cortex*.

Braunschweig, D., Ashwood, P., Krakowiak, P., Hertz-Picciotto, I., Hansen, R., Croen, L.A., et al. (2008). Autism: Maternally derived antibodies specific for fetal brain proteins. *Neurotoxicology, 29*(2), 226–231.

Brun, C. C., Nicolson, R., Lepore, N., Chou, Y. Y., Vidal, C. N., DeVito, T. J., et al. (2009). Mapping brain abnormalities in boys with autism. *Human Brain Mapping, 30*, 3887–3900.

Buckler, J. M., & Green, M. (2008). The growth of twins between the ages of 2 and 9 years. *Annals of Human Biology, 35*(1), 75–92.

Butler, M. G., Dasouki, M. J., Zhou, X. P., Talebizadeh, Z., Brown, M., Takahashi, T. N., et al. (2005). Subset of individuals with autism spectrum disorders and extreme macrocephaly associated with germline PTEN tumour suppressor gene mutations. *Journal of Medical Genetics, 42*(4), 318–321.

Buxbaum, J. D., Cai, G., Chaste, P., Nygren, G., Goldsmith, J., Reichert, J., et al. (2007). Mutation screening of the PTEN gene in patients with autism spectrum disorders and macrocephaly. *American Journal of Medical Genetics. Part B, Neuropsychiatric Genetics, 144B*(4), 484–491.

Cabanlit, M., Wills, S., Goines, P., Ashwood, P., & Van de Water, J. (2007). Brain-specific autoantibodies in the plasma of subjects with autistic spectrum disorder. *Annals of the New York Academy of Sciences, 1107*, 92–103.

Calandra, T., & Roger, T. (2003). Macrophage migration inhibitory factor: a regulator of innate immunity. *Nature Reviews Immunology, 3*, 791–800.

Carroll, L. S., & Owen, M. J. (2009). Genetic overlap between autism, schizophrenia, and bipolar disorder. *Genome Medicine, 1*(10), 102.

Casanova, M. F., El-Baz, A., Mott, M., Mannheim, G., Hassan, H., Fahmi, R., et al. (2009). Reduced gyral window and corpus callosum size in autism: Possible macroscopic correlates of a minicolumnopathy. *Journal of Autism and Developmental Disorders, 39*, 751–764.

Caviness, V. S., Jr., Lange, N. T., Makris, N., Herbert, M. R., & Kennedy, D. N. (1999). MRI-based brain volumetrics: emergence of a developmental brain science. *Brain and Development, 21*(5), 289–295.

Chung, M. K., Adluru, N., Lee, J. E., Lazar, M., Lainhart, J. E., & Alexander, A. L. (2010). Cosine series representation of 3D curves and its application to white matter fiber bundles in diffusion tensor imaging. *Statistics and Its Interface, 3*(1), 69–80.

Chugani, D. C., Muzik, O., Behen, M., Rothermel, R., Janisse, J. J., Lee, J., et al. (1999). Developmental changes in brain serotonin synthesis capacity in autistic and nonautistic children. *Annals of Neurology, 45*(3), 287–295.

Chugani, D. C., Muzik, O., Rothermel, R., Behen, M., Chakraborty, P., Mangner, T., et al. (1997). Altered serotonin synthesis in the dentatothalamocortical pathway in autistic boys. *Annals of Neurology, 42*(4), 666–669.

Comi, A. M., Zimmerman, A. W., Frye, V. H., Law, P. A., & Peeden, J. N. (1999). Familial clustering of autoimmune disorders and evaluation of medical risk factors in autism. *Journal of Child Neurology, 14*(6), 388–394.

Connors, S. L., Matteson, K. J., Sega, G. A., Lozzio, C. B., Carroll, R. C., & Zimmerman, A. W. (2006). Plasma serotonin in autism. *Pediatric Neurology, 35*(3), 182–186.

Cook, E. H., & Leventhal, B. L. (1996). The serotonin system in autism. *Current Opinion in Pediatrics, 8*(4), 348–354.

Cook, E. H., Jr., Leventhal, B. L., Heller, W., Metz, J., Wainwright, M., & Freedman, D. X. (1990). Autistic children and their first-degree relatives: Relationships between serotonin and norepinephrine levels and intelligence. *Journal of Neuropsychiatry and Clinical Neurosciences, 2*(3), 268–274.

Cook, E. H., Jr., Perry, B. D., Dawson, G., Wainwright, M. S., & Leventhal B. L. (1993). Receptor inhibition by immunoglobulins: Specific inhibition by autistic children, their relatives, and control subjects. *Journal of Autism and Developmental Disorders, 23*(1), 67–78.

Corbett, B. A., Carmean, V., Ravizza, S., Wendelken, C., Henry, M. L., Carter, C., et al. (2009). A functional and structural study of emotion and face processing in children with autism. *Psychiatry Research, 173*(3), 196–205.

Courchesne, E., Carper, R., & Akshoomoff, N. (2003). Evidence of brain overgrowth in the first year of life in autism. *Journal of the American Medical Association, 290*(3), 337–344.

Courchesne, E., Muller, R. A., Saitoh, O. (1999). Brain weight in autism: Normal in the majority of cases, megalencephalic in rare cases. *Neurology, 52*, 1057–1059.

Croen, L. A., Braunschweig, D., Haapanen, L., Yoshida, C. K., Fireman, B., Grether, J. K., et al. (2008). Maternal mid-pregnancy autoantibodies to fetal brain protein: The early markers for autism study. *Biological Psychiatry, 64*(7), 583–588.

Croen, L. A., Grether, J. K., Yoshida, C. K., Odouli, R., & Van de Water, J. (2005). Maternal autoimmune diseases, asthma and allergies, and childhood autism spectrum disorders: A case-control study. *Archives of Pediatrics and Adolescent Medicine, 159*(2), 151–157.

Cross, S., Kim, S. J., Weiss, L. A., Delahanty, R. J., Sutcliffe, J. S., Leventhal, B. L., et al. (2008). Molecular genetics of the platelet serotonin system in first-degree relatives of patients with autism. *Neuropsychopharmacology, 33*(2), 353–560.

Dager, S. R., Wang, L., Friedman, S. D., Shaw, D. W., Constantino, J. N., Artru, A. A., et al. (2007). Shape mapping of the hippocampus in young children with autism spectrum disorder. *American Journal of Neuroradiology, 28*(4), 672–677.

Dalton, P., Deacon, R., Blamire, A., Pike, M., McKinlay, I., Stein, J., et al. (2003). Maternal neuronal antibodies associated with autism and a language disorder. *Annals of Neurology, 53*(4), 533–537.

Dalton, K. M., Nacewicz, B. M., Alexander, A. L., & Davidson, R. J. (2007). Gaze-fixation, brain activation, and amygdala volume in unaffected siblings of individuals with autism. *Biological Psychiatry, 61*(4), 512–520.

Dalton, K. M., Nacewicz, B. M., Johnstone, T., Schaefer, H. S., Gernsbacher, M. A., Goldsmith, H. H., et al. (2005). Gaze fixation and the neural circuitry of face processing in autism. *Nature Neuroscience, 8*(4), 519–526.

Dawson, G., Munson, J., Webb, S. J., Nalty, T., Abbott, R., & Toth, K. (2007). Rate of head growth decelerates and symptoms worsen in the second year of life in autism. *Biological Psychiatry, 61*(4), 458–464.

Dawson, G., Webb, S. J., Wijsman, E., Schellenberg, G., Estes, A., Munson, J., et al. (2005). Neurocognitive and electrophysiological evidence of altered face processing in parents of children with autism: Implications for a model of abnormal development of social brain circuitry in autism. *Development and Psychopathology, 17*(3), 679–697.

Davidovitch, M., Patterson, B., & Gartside, P. (1996). Head circumference measurements in children with autism. *Journal of Child Neurology, 11*(5), 389–393.

Degirmenci, B., Miral, S., Kaya, G. C., Iyilikçi, L., Arslan, G., Baykara, A., et al. (2008). Technetium-99m HMPAO brain SPECT in autistic children and their families. *Psychiatry Research, 162*(3), 236–243.

Delatycki, M. B., Danks, A., Churchyard, A., Zhou, X. P., & Eng, C. (2003). De novo germline PTEN mutation in a man with Lhermitte-Duclos disease which arose on the paternal chromosome and was transmitted to his child with polydactyly and Wormian bones. *Journal of Medical Genetics, 40*(8), e92.

Dementieva, Y. A., Vance, D. D., Donnelly, S. L., Elston, L. A., Wolpert, C. M., Ravan, S. A., et al. (2005). Accelerated head growth in early development of individuals with autism. *Pediatric Neurology, 32*(2), 102–108.

DerSimonian, R., & Laird, N. (1986). Meta-analysis in clinical trials. *Controlled Clinical Trials, 7*, 177–188.

Deutsch, C. K., & Joseph, R. M. (2003). Brief report: Cognitive correlates of enlarged head circumference in children with autism. *Journal of Autism and Developmental Disorders, 33*(2), 209–215.

Dissanayake, C., Bui, Q. M., Huggins, R., & Loesch, D. Z. (2006). Growth in stature and head circumference in high-functioning autism and Asperger disorder during the first 3 years of life. *Development and Psychopathology, 18*(2), 381–393.

Ecker, C., Rocha-Rego, V., Johnston, P., Mourao-Miranda, J., Marquand, A., Daly, E. M., et al. (2010). Investigating the predictive value of whole-brain structural MR scans in autism: A pattern classification approach. *NeuroImage, 49*(1), 44–56.

Efron, B., & Morris, C. (1977). Steins' paradox in statistics. *Scientific American, 236*, 119–127.

Elder, L. M., Dawson, G., Toth, K., Fein, D., & Munson, J. (2008). Head circumference as an early predictor of autism symptoms in younger siblings of children with autism spectrum disorder. *Journal of Autism and Developmental Disorders, 38*(6), 1104–1111.

Elsabbagh, M., Volein, A., Csibra, G., Holmboe, K., Garwood, H., Tucker, L., et al. (2009). Neural correlates of eye gaze processing in the infant broader autism phenotype. *Biological Psychiatry, 65*(1), 31–38.

Elsabbagh, M., Volein, A., Holmboe, K., Tucker, L., Csibra, G., Baron-Cohen, S., et al. (2009). Visual orienting in the early broader autism phenotype: Disengagement and facilitation. *Journal of Child Psychology and Psychiatry and Allied Disciplines, 50*(5), 637–642.

Fan, X., Miles, J. H., Takahashi, N., & Yao, G. (2009). Abnormal transient pupillary light reflex in individuals with autism spectrum disorders. *Journal of Autism and Developmental Disorders, 39*(11), 1499–1508.

Fernandez, B. A., Roberts, W., Chung, B., Weksberg, R., Meyn, S., Szatmari, P., et al. (2009, September 24). Phenotypic spectrum associated with de novo and inherited deletions and duplications at 16p11.2 in individuals ascertained for diagnosis of autism spectrum disorder. *Journal of Medical Genetics.* [Epub ahead of print].

Fidler, D. J., Bailey, J. N., & Smalley, S. L. (2000). Macrocephaly in autism and other pervasive developmental disorders. *Developmental Medicine and Child Neurology, 42*(11), 737–740.

Fleiss, J. L., & Cohen, J. (1973). The equivalence of weighted kappa and the intraclass correlation coefficient as measures of reliability. *Educational and Psychological Measurement, 33*, 613–619.

Fletcher, P. T., Whitaker, R. T., Tao, R., DuBray, M. B., Froehlich, A., Ravichandran, C., et al. (2010). Microstructural connectivity of the arcuate fasciculus in adolescents with high-functioning autism. *NeuroImage, 51*(3), 1117–1125.

Folstein, S., & Rutter, M. (1977). Infantile autism: A genetic study of 21 twin pairs. *Journal of Child Psychology and Psychiatry and Allied Disciplines, 18*(4), 297–321.

Folstein, S. E., Santangelo, S. L., Gilman, S. E., Piven, J., Landa, R., Lainhart, J., et al. (1999). Predictors of cognitive test patterns in autism families. *Journal of Child Psychology and Psychiatry, 40*(7), 1117–1128.

Fombonne, E., Roge, B., Claverie, J., Courty, S., & Fremolle, J. (1999). Microcephaly and macrocephaly in autism. *Journal of Autism and Developmental Disorders, 29*(2), 113–119.

Geschwind, D. H. (2009). Advances in autism. *Annual Review of Medicine, 60*, 367–380.

Gillberg, C., & de Souza, L. (2002). Head circumference in autism, Asperger syndrome, and ADHD: A comparative study. *Developmental Medicine and Child Neurology, 44*(5), 296–300.

Goffin, A., Hoefsloot, L. H., Bosgoed, E., Swillen, A., & Fryns, J. P. (2001). PTEN mutation in a family with Cowden syndrome and autism. *American Journal of Medical Genetics, 105*(6), 521–524.

Goldberg, J., Anderson, G. M., Zwaigenbaum, L., Hall, G. B., Nahmias, C., Thompson, A., et al. (2009). Cortical serotonin type-2 receptor density in parents of children with autism spectrum disorders. *Journal of Autism and Developmental Disorders, 39*(1), 97–104.

Gottesman, I. I., & Gould, T. D. (2003). The endophenotype concept in psychiatry: etymology and strategic intentions. *American Journal of Psychiatry, 160*(4), 636–645.

Gottesman, I. I., & Shields, J. (1972). *Schizophrenia and genetics: A twin study vantage point.* New York: Academic.

Greer, J. M., & Wynshaw-Boris, A. (2006). Pten and the brain: Sizing up social interaction. *Neuron, 50*(3), 343–345.

Grigorenko, E. L., Han, S. S., Yrigollen, C. M., Leng, L., Mizue, Y., Anderson, G. M., et al. (2008). Macrophage migration inhibitory factor and autism spectrum disorders. *Pediatrics, 122*(2), e438–445.

Hadjikhani, N., Joseph R. M., Snyder J., & Tager-Flusberg H. (2006). Anatomical differences in the mirror neuron system and social cognition network in autism. *Cerebral Cortex*, 16(9), 1276–1282.

Hammond, P., Forster-Gibson, C., Chudley, A. E., Allanson, J. E., Hutton, T. J., Farrell, S. A., et al. (2008). Face-brain asymmetry in autism spectrum disorders. *Molecular Psychiatry, 13*(6), 614–623.

Hardan, A. Y., Muddasani, S., Vemulapalli, M., Keshavan, M. S., & Minshew, N. J. (2006). An MRI study of increased cortical thickness in autism. *American Journal of Psychiatry, 163*, 1290–1292.

Hazlett, H. C., Poe, M., Gerig, G., Smith, R. G., Provenzale, J., Ross, A., et al. (2005). Magnetic resonance imaging and head circumference study of brain size in autism: Birth through age 2 years. *Archives of General Psychiatry, 62*(12), 1366–1376.

Herman, G. E., Butter, E., Enrile, B., Pastore, M., Prior, T. W., & Sommer, A. (2007). Increasing knowledge of PTEN germline mutations: Two additional patients with autism and macrocephaly. *American Journal of Medical Genetics. Part A, 143*(6), 589–593.

Heuer, L., Ashwood, P., Schauer, J., Goines, P., Krakowiak, P., Hertz-Picciotto, I., et al. (2008). Reduced levels of immunoglobulin in children with autism correlates with behavioral symptoms. *Autism Research, 1*(5), 275–283.

Holland, P. (1989). A note on the Mantel-Haenszel log-odds-ratio estimator and the sample marginal rates. *Biometrics, 45*, 1009–1016.

Huang, C. H., & Santangelo, S. L. (2008). Autism and serotonin transporter gene polymorphisms: A systematic review and meta-analysis. *American Journal of Medical Genetics. Part B, Neuropsychiatric Genetics, 147B*(6), 903–913.

Hyde, K. L., Samson, F., Evans, A. C., & Mottron, L. (2009, September 29). Neuroanatomical differences in brain areas implicated in perceptual and other core features of autism revealed by cortical thickness analysis and voxel-based morphometry. *Human Brain Mapping* [Epub ahead of print]. doi:10.1002/hbm.20887

Im, K., Lee, J. M., Lyttelton, O., Kim, S. H., Evans, A. C., & Kim, S. I. (2008). Brain size and cortical structure in the adult human brain. *Cerebral Cortex, 18*(9), 2181–2191.

Ivleva, E. I., Morris, D. W., Moates, A. F., Suppes, T., Thaker, G. K., & Tamminga, C. A. (2009, November 30). Genetics and intermediate phenotypes of the schizophrenia-bipolar disorder boundary. *Neuroscience and Biobehavioral Reviews* [Epub ahead of print]. doi:10.1016/j.neubiorev.2009.11.022

Jeste, S. S., & Nelson, C. A., 3rd (2009). Event related potentials in the understanding of autism spectrum disorders: An analytical review. *Journal of Autism and Developmental Disorders, 39*(3), 495–510.

Jiao, Y., Chen, R., Ke, X., Chu, K., Lu, Z., & Herskovits, E. H. (2009, December 21). Predictive models of autism spectrum disorder based on brain regional cortical thickness. *NeuroImage* [Epub ahead of print]. doi:10.1016/j.neuroimage.2009.12.047

Kanner, L. (1943). Autistic disturbances of affective contact. *Nervous Child, 2*, 217–250.

Kates, W. R., Burnette, C. P., Eliez, S., Strunge, L. A., Kaplan, D., Landa, R., et al. (2004). Neuroanatomic variation in monozygotic twin pairs discordant for the narrow phenotype for autism. *American Journal of Psychiatry, 161*(3), 539–546.

Kates W. R., Ikuta I., & Burnette C. P. (2009). Gyrification patterns in monozygotic twin pairs varying in discordance for autism. *Autism Research, 2*(5), 267–278.

Kates, W. R., Mostofsky, S. H., Zimmerman, A. W., Mazzocco, M. M., Landa, R., Warsofsky, I. S., et al. (1998). Neuroanatomical and neurocognitive differences in a pair of monozygous twins discordant for strictly defined autism. *Annals of Neurology, 43*(6), 782–791.

Kemper, T. L., & Bauman, M. L. (2002). Neuropathology of infantile autism. *Molecular Psychiatry, 7*(Suppl 2), S12–13.

Kennedy, D. N., Lange, N., Makris, N., Bates, J., Meyer, J., & Caviness, V. S., Jr. (1998). Gyri of the human neocortex: an MRI-based analysis of volume and variance. *Cerebral Cortex, 8*(4), 372–384.

Kjaer, I. (1995). Human prenatal craniofacial development related to brain development under normal and pathologic conditions. *Acta Odontologica Scandinavica, 53*(3), 135–143.

Kraemer, H. C., Schultz, S. K., & Arndt, S. (2002). Biomarkers in psychiatry: Methodological issues. *American Journal of Geriatric Psychiatry, 10*(6), 653–659.

Kriegeskorte, N., Simmons, W. K., Bellgowan, P. S., & Baker, C. I. (2009). Circular analysis in systems neuroscience: the dangers of double dipping. *Nature Neuroscience, 12*(5), 535–540.

Kwon, C. H., Luikart, B. W., Powell, C. M., Zhou, J., Matheny, S. A., Zhang, W., et al. (2006). Pten regulates neuronal arborization and social interaction in mice. *Neuron, 50*(3), 377–388.

Lainhart, J. E., Bigler, E. D., Bocian, M., Coon, H., Dinh, E., Dawson, G., et al. (2006). Head circumference and height in autism: A study by the Collaborative Program of Excellence in Autism. *American Journal of Medical Genetics. Part A, 140*(21), 2257–2274.

Lainhart, J. E., Lazar, M., Bigler, E. D., & Alexander, A. L. (2005). The brain during life in autism: Advances in neuroimaging research. In M. F. Casanova (Ed.), *Recent developments in autism research* (pp. 57–108). Hauppauge, NY: Nova Science Publishers.

Lainhart, J. E., Piven, J., Wzorek, M., Landa, R., Santangelo, S. L., Coon, H., et al. (1997). Macrocephaly in children and adults with autism. *Journal of the American Academy of Child and Adolescent Psychiatry, 36*(2), 282–290.

Lainhart, J. E., Ravichandran, C., Froehlich, A., DuBray, M. B., Abildskov, T., Bigler, E. D., Lange, N. (2010). Growth curves for longitudinal regional brain volumes in autism vs. typical development. Accepted for presentation at IMFAR 2010, Philadelphia.

Lange, N. (2003). What can modern statistics offer imaging neuroscience? *Statistical Methods in Medical Research, 12*(5), 447–469.

Lange, N., DuBray, M. B., Lee, J. E., Froimowitz, M. P., Froehlich, A., Adluru, N., et al. (2010). Atypical asymmetry of superior temporal gyrus and temporal stem white matter microstructure in autism. *Autism Research, 3*, 350–358.

Lange, N., Froimowitz, M. P., Lainhart, J. E., & The Brain Development Cooperative Group. (2010). Effects of brain development and demography on IQ in a large representative sample of healthy children and adolescents. *Developmental Neuropsychology*, accepted.

Lange, N., Giedd, J. N., Castellanos, F. X., Vaituzis, A. C., & Rapoport, J. L. (1997). Variability of human brain structure size: ages 4–20 years. *Psychiatry Research, 74*(1), 1–12.

Langen, M., Durston, S., Staal, W. G., Palmen, S. J., & van Engeland, H. (2007). Caudate nucleus is enlarged in high-functioning medication-naive subjects with autism. *Biological Psychiatry, 62*(3), 262–266.

Langen, M., Schnack, H. G., Nederveen, H., Bos, D., Lahuis, B. E., de Jonge, M. V., et al. (2009). Changes in the developmental trajectories of striatum in autism. *Biological Psychiatry, 66*(4), 327–333.

Leboyer, M., Philippe, A., Bouvard, M., Guilloud-Bataille, M., Bondoux, D., Tabuteau, F., et al. (1999). Whole blood serotonin and plasma beta-endorphin in autistic probands and their first-degree relatives. *Biological Psychiatry, 45*(2), 158–163.

Le Couteur, A., Bailey, A., Goode, S., Pickles, A., Robertson, S., Gottesman, I., et al. (1996). A broader phenotype of autism: The clinical spectrum in twins. *Journal of Child Psychology and Psychiatry, 37*(7), 785–801.

Leventhal, B. L., Cook, E. H., Jr., Morford, M., Ravitz, A., & Freedman, D. X. (1990). Relationships of whole blood serotonin and plasma norepinephrine within families. *Journal of Autism and Developmental Disorders, 20*(4), 499–511.

Levin, M., Buznikov, G. A., & Lauder, J. M. (2006). Of minds and embryos: Left-right asymmetry and the serotonergic controls of pre-neural morphogenesis. *Developmental Neuroscience, 28*(3), 171–185.

Losh, M., Adolphs, R., Poe, M., Couture, S., Penn, D., Baranek, G., et al. (2009). The neuropsychological profile of autism and the broad autism phenotype. *Archives of General Psychiatry, 66*, 518–526.

Makkonen, I., Riikonen, R., Kokki, H, Airaksinen, M. M., & Kuikka, J. T. (2008). Serotonin and dopamine transporter binding in children with autism determined by SPECT. *Developmental Medicine and Child Neurology, 50*(8), 593–597.

Martin, L. A., Ashwood, P., Braunschweig, D., Cabanlit, M., Van de Water, J., & Amaral, D. G. (2008). Stereotypies and hyperactivity in rhesus monkeys exposed to IgG from mothers of children with autism. *Brain, Behavior, and Immunity, 22*(6), 806–816.

McBride, P. A., Anderson, G. M., Hertzig, M. E., Sweeney, J. A., Kream, J., Cohen, D. J., et al. (1989). Serotonergic responsivity in male young adults with autistic disorder. Results of a pilot study. *Archives of General Psychiatry, 46*(3), 213–221.

McNamara, I. M., Borella, A. W., Bialowas, L. A., & Whitaker-Azmitia, P. M. (2008). Further studies in the developmental hyperserotonemia model (DHS) of autism: Social, behavioral, and peptide changes. *Brain Research, 1189*, 203–214.

Miles, J. H., Hadden, L. L., Takahashi, T. N., & Hillman, R. E. (2000). Head circumference is an independent clinical finding associated with autism. *American Journal of Medical Genetics, 95*(4), 339–350.

Miles, J. H., Takahashi, T. N., Bagby, S., Sahota, P. K., Vaslow, D. F., Wang, C. H., et al. (2005). Essential versus complex autism: Definition of fundamental prognostic subtypes. *American Journal of Medical Genetics. Part A, 135*(2), 171–180.

Mitchell, S. R., Reiss, A. L., Tatusko, D. H., Ikuta, I., Kazmerski, D. B., Botti, J. A., et al. (2009). Neuroanatomic alterations and social and communication deficits in monozygotic twins discordant for autism disorder. *American Journal of Psychiatry, 166*(8), 917–925.

Moiseiwitsch, J. R. (2000). The role of serotonin and neurotransmitters during craniofacial development. *Critical Reviews in Oral Biology and Medicine, 11*(2), 230–239.

Molloy, C. A., Morrow, A. L., Meinzen-Derr, J., Dawson, G., Bernier, R., Dunn, M. et al. (2006). Familial autoimmune thyroid disease as a risk factor for regression in children with Autism Spectrum Disorder: A CPEA Study. *Journal of Autism and Developmental Disorders, 36*(3), 317–324.

Mosconi, M. W., Cody-Hazlett, H., Poe, M. D., Gerig, G., Gimpel-Smith, R., & Piven, J. (2009). Longitudinal study of amygdala volume and joint attention in 2- to 4-year-old children with autism. *Archives of General Psychiatry, 66*(5), 509–516.

Mraz, K. D., Green, J., Dumont-Mathieu, T., Makin, S., & Fein, D. (2007). Correlates of head circumference growth in infants later diagnosed with autism spectrum disorders. *Journal of Child Neurology, 22*(6), 700–713.

Mulder, E. J., Anderson, G. M., Kema, I. P., de Bildt, A., van Lang, N. D., den Boer, J. A., et al. (2004). Platelet serotonin levels in pervasive developmental disorders and mental retardation: Diagnostic group differences, within-group distribution, and behavioral correlates. *Journal of the American Academy of Child and Adolescent Psychiatry, 43*(4), 491–499.

Munson, J., Dawson, G., Abbott, R., Faja, S., Webb, S. J., Friedman, S. D., et al. (2006). Amygdala volume and behavioral development in autism. *Archives of General Psychiatry, 63*(6), 686–693.

Murphy, D. G., Daly, E., Schmitz, N., Toal, F., Murphy, K., Curran, S., et al. (2006). Cortical serotonin 5-HT2A receptor binding and social communication in adults with Asperger's syndrome: An in vivo SPECT study. *American Journal of Psychiatry, 163*(5), 934–936.

Nacewicz, B. M., Dalton, K. M., Johnstone, T., Long, M. T., McAuliff, M. T., Oakes, T. R., et al. (2006). Amygdala volume and nonverbal social impairment in adolescent and adult males with autism. *Archives of General Psychiatry, 63*, 1417–1428.

Nakamura K., Sekine Y., Ouchi S., Tsujii M., Yoshikawa E., Futatsubashi M., et al. (2010). Brain serotonin and dopamine transporter binding in adults with high-functioning autism. *Archives of General Psychiatry, 67*(1), 59–68.

Neeley, E. S., Bigler, E. D., Krasny, L., Ozonoff, S., McMahon, W., & Lainhart, J. E. (2007). Quantitative temporal lobe differences: Autism distinguished from controls using classification and regression tree analysis. *Brain and Development, 29*(7), 389–399.

Nicolson, R., DeVito, T. J., Vidal, C. N., Sui, Y., Hayashi, K. M., Drost, D. J., et al. (2006). Detection and mapping of hippocampal abnormalities in autism. *Psychiatry Research, 148*(1), 11–21.

Oram Cardy, J. E., Flagg, E. J., Roberts, W., & Roberts, T. P. (2008). Auditory evoked fields predict language ability and impairment in children. *International Journal of Psychophysiology, 68*(2), 170–175.

Orrico, A., Galli, L., Buoni, S., Orsi, A., Vonella, G., Sorrentino, V. (2008). Novel PTEN mutations in neurodevelopmental disorders and macrocephaly. *Clinical Genetics, 75*, 195–198.

Ozgen, H. M., Hop, J. W., Hox, J. J., Beemer, F. A., & van Engeland, H. (2010). Minor physical anomalies in autism: A meta-analysis. *Molecular Psychiatry, 15*(3), 300–307.

Palmen, S. J., Durston, S., Nederveen, H., & van Engeland, H. (2006). No evidence for preferential involvement of medial temporal lobe structures in high-functioning autism. *Psychological Medicine, 36*(6), 827–834.

Palmen, S. J., Hulshoff Pol, H. E., Kemner, C., Schnack, H. G., Durston, S., Lahuis, B. E., et al. (2005a). Increased gray-matter volume in medication-naive high-functioning children with autism spectrum disorder. *Psychological Medicine, 35*(4), 561–570.

Palmen, S. J., Hulshoff Pol, H. E., Kemner, C., Schnack, H. G., Janssen, J., Kahn, R. S., et al. (2004). Larger brains in medication naïve high-functioning subjects with pervasive developmental disorder. *Journal of Autism and Developmental Disorders, 34*(6), 603–613.

Palmen, S. J., Hulshoff Pol, H. E., Kemner, C., Schnack, H. G., Sitskoorn, M. M., Appels, M. C., et al. (2005b). Brain anatomy in non-affected parents of autistic probands: A MRI study. *Psychological Medicine, 35*(10), 1411–1420.

Parisi, M. A., Dinulos, M. B., Leppig, K. A., Sybert, V. P., Eng, C., & Hudgins, L. (2001). The spectrum and evolution of phenotypic findings in PTEN mutation positive cases of Bannayan-Riley-Ruvalcaba syndrome. *Journal of Medical Genetics, 38*(1), 52–58.

Perry, B. D., Cook, E. H., Jr., Leventhal, B. L., Wainwright, M. S., & Freedman, D. X. (1991). Platelet 5-HT2 serotonin receptor binding sites in autistic children and their first-degree relatives. *Biological Psychiatry, 30*(2), 121–130.

Peterson, E., Schmidt, G. L., Tregellas, J. R., Winterrowd, E., Kopelioff, L., Hepburn, S., et al. (2006). A voxel-based morphometry study of gray matter in parents of children with autism. *Neuroreport, 17*(12), 1289–1292.

Piven, J., Palmer, P., Jacobi, D., Childress, D., & Arndt, S. (1997). Broader autism phenotype: Evidence from a family history study of multiple-incidence autism families. *The American Journal of Psychiatry, 154*(2), 185–190.

Piven, J., Tsai, G. C., Nehme, E., Coyle, J. T., Chase, G. A., & Folstein, S. E. (1991). Platelet serotonin, a possible marker for familial autism. *Journal of Autism and Developmental Disorders, 21*(1), 51–59.

Raznahan, A., Pugliese, L., Barker, G. J., Daly, E., Powell, J., Bolton, P. F., et al. (2009). Serotonin transporter genotype and neuroanatomy in autism spectrum disorders. *Psychiatric Genetics, 19*(3), 147–150.

Rice, T. K. (2008). Familial resemblance and heritability. *Advances in Genetics, 60*, 35–49.

Roberts, T. P. L., Khan S. Y., Rey M., Monroe J. F., Cannon K., Blaskey L., et al. (2010). MEG detection of delayed auditory evoked responses in autism spectrum disorders: Toward an imaging biomarker for autism. *Autism Research, 3*(1), 8–18.

Roberts, T. P., Schmidt, G. L., Egeth, M., Blaskey, L., Rey, M. M., Edgar, J. C., et al. (2008). Electrophysiological signatures: Magnetoencephalographic studies of the neural correlates of language impairment in autism spectrum disorders. *International Journal of Psychophysiology, 68*(2), 149–160.

Rojas, D. C., Maharajh, K., Teale, P., & Rogers, S. J. (2008). Reduced neural synchronization of gamma-band MEG oscillations in first-degree relatives of children with autism. *BMC Psychiatry, 8*, 66.

Rojas, D. C., Peterson, E., Winterrowd, E., Reite, M. L., Rogers, S. J., & Tregellas, J. R. (2006). Regional gray matter volumetric changes in autism associated with social and repetitive behavior symptoms. *BMC Psychiatry, 13*(6), 56.

Rojas, D. C., Smith, J. A., Benkers, T. L., Camou, S. L., Reite, M. L., & Rogers, S. J. (2004). Hippocampus and amygdala volumes in parents of children with autistic disorder. *American Journal of Psychiatry, 161*(11), 2038–2044.

Sacco, R., Militerni, R., Frolli, A., Bravaccio, C., Gritti, A., Elia, M., et al. (2007). Clinical, morphological, and biochemical correlates of head circumference in autism. *Biological Psychiatry, 62*(9), 1038–1047.

Salmond, C. H., Ashburner, J., Connelly, A., Friston, K. J., Gadian, D. G., & Vargha-Khadem, F. (2005). The role of the medial temporal lobe in autistic spectrum disorders. *The European Journal of Neuroscience, 22*(3), 764–772.

Salmond, C. H., de Haan, M., Friston, K. J., Gadian, D. G., & Vargha-Khadem, F. (2003). Investigating individual differences in brain abnormalities in autism. *Philosophical Transactions of the Royal Society of London. Series B, Biological Sciences, 358*(1430), 405–413.

Saresella, M., Marventano, I., Guerini, F. R., Mancuso, R., Ceresa, L., Zanzottera, M., et al. (2009). An autistic endophenotype results in complex immune dysfunction in healthy siblings of autistic children. *Biological Psychiatry, 66*(10), 978–984.

Schmidt, C. O., & Kohlmann, T. (2008). When to use the odds ratio or the relative risk. *International Journal of Public Health, 53*, 165–167.

Schmidt, G. L., Rey, M. M., Oram Cardy, J. E., & Roberts, T. P. (2009). Absence of M100 source asymmetry in autism associated with language functioning. *Neuroreport, 20*(11), 1037–1041.

Schumann, C. M., Barnes, C. C., Lord, C., & Courchesne, E. (2009). Amygdala enlargement in toddlers with autism related to severity of social and communication impairments. *Biological Psychiatry, 66*(10), 942–949.

Silva, S. C., Correia, C., Fesel, C., Barreto, M., Coutinho, A. M., Marques, C., et al. (2004). Autoantibody repertoires to brain tissue in autism nuclear families. *Journal of Neuroimmunology, 152*(1–2), 176–182.

Singer, H. S., Morris, C. M., Gause, C. D., Gillin, P. K., Crawford, S., & Zimmerman, A. W. (2008). Antibodies against fetal brain in sera of mothers with autistic children. *Journal of Neuroimmunology, 194*(1–2), 165–172.

Singer, H. S., Morris, C. M., Williams, P. N., Yoon, D. Y., Hong, J. J., & Zimmerman, A. W. (2006). Antibrain antibodies in children with autism and their unaffected siblings. *Journal of Neuroimmunology, 178*(1–2), 149–155.

Singh, V., Mukherjee, L., & Chung, M. K. (2008). Cortical surface thickness as a classifier: Boosting for autism classification. *Medical Image Computing and Computer-Assisted Intervention, 11*, 999–1007.

Sparks, B. F., Friedman, S. D., Shaw, D. W., Aylward, E. H., Echelard, D., Artru, A. A., et al. (2002). Brain structural abnormalities in young children with autism spectrum disorder. *Neurology, 59*(2), 184–192.

Stanfield, A. C., McIntosh, A. M., Spencer, M. D., Philip, R., Gaur, S., & Lawrie, S. M. (2008). Towards a neuroanatomy of autism: A systematic review and meta-analysis of structural magnetic resonance imaging studies. *European Psychiatry, 23*(4), 289–299.

Stevenson, R. E., Schroer, R. J., Skinner, C., Fender, D., & Simensen, R. J. (1997). Autism and macrocephaly. *Lancet, 349*(9067), 1744–1745.

Sweeten, T. L., Bowyer, S. L., Posey, D. J., Halberstadt, G. M., & McDougle, C. J. (2003). Increased prevalence of familial autoimmunity in probands with pervasive developmental disorders. *Pediatrics, 112*(5), e420.

Szatmari, P., Maziade, M., Zwaigenbaum, L., Merette, C., Roy, M. A., Joober, R., et al. (2007). Informative phenotypes for genetic studies of psychiatric disorders. *American Journal of Medical Genetics. Part B, Neuropsychiatric Genetics, 144B*(5), 581–588.

Tate, D. F., Bigler, E. D., McMahon, W., & Lainhart, J. (2007). The relative contributions of brain, cerebrospinal fluid-filled structures, and non-neural tissue volumes to occipital-frontal head circumference in subjects with autism. *Neuropediatrics, 38*, 18–24.

Torrey, E. F., Dhavale, D., Lawlor, J. P., & Yolken, R. H. (2004). Autism and head circumference in the first year of life. *Biological Psychiatry, 56*(11), 892–894.

van Belle, G. (2002). *Statistical rules of thumb* (2nd ed.). New York: Wiley.

van Belle, G., Fisher, L. D., Heagerty, P. J., & Lumley, T. S. (2004). *Biostatistics: A methodology for the health sciences* (2nd ed.). New York: Wiley.

van Daalen, E., Swinkels, S. H., Dietz, C., van Engeland, H., & Buitelaar, J. K. (2007). Body length and head growth in the first year of life in autism. *Pediatric Neurology, 37*(5), 324–330.

Varga, E. A., Pastore, M., Prior, T., Herman, G. E., & McBride, K. L. (2009). The prevalence of PTEN mutations in a clinical pediatric cohort with autism spectrum disorders, developmental delay, and macrocephaly. *Genetics in Medicine, 11*(2), 111–117.

Wallace, G. L., Schmitt, J. E., Lenroot, R., Viding, E., Ordaz, S., Rosenthal, M. A., et al. (2006). A pediatric twin study of brain morphometry. *Journal of Child Psychology and Psychiatry, 47*(10), 987–993.

Warren, R. P., Margaretten, N. C., Pace, N. C., & Foster, A. (1986). Immune abnormalities in patients with autism. *Journal of Autism and Developmental Disorders, 16*(2), 189–197.

Warren, R. P., Singh, V. K., Cole, P., Odell, J. D., Pingree, C. B., Warren, W. L., & White, E. (1991). Increased frequency of the null allele at the complement C4b locus in autism. *Clinical and Experimental Immunology, 83*(3), 438–440.

Wassink, T. H., Hazlett, H. C., Epping, E. A., Arndt, S., Dager, S. R., Schellenberg, G. D., et al. (2007). Cerebral cortical gray matter overgrowth and functional variation of the serotonin transporter gene in autism. *Archives of General Psychiatry, 64*(6), 709–717.

Werner, E., Dawson, G., Munson, J., & Osterling, J. (2005). Variation in early developmental course in autism and its relation with behavioral outcome at 3–4 years of age. *Journal of Autism and Developmental Disorders, 35*(3), 337–350.

White, S., O'Reilly, H., & Frith, U. (2009). Big heads, small details, and autism. *Neuropsychologia, 47*(5), 1274–1281.

Wilkie, A. O., & Morriss-Kay, G. M. (2001). Genetics of craniofacial development and malformation. *Nature Reviews Genetics, 2*(6), 458–468.

Wills, S., Cabanlit, M., Bennett, J., Ashwood, P., Amaral, D. G., & Van de Water, J. (2009). Detection of autoantibodies to neural cells of the cerebellum in the plasma of subjects with autism spectrum disorders. *Brain, Behavior, and Immunity, 23*(1), 64–74.

Wilson, T. W., Rojas, D. C., Reite, M. L., Teale, P. D., & Rogers, S. J. (2007). Children and adolescents with autism exhibit reduced MEG steady-state gamma responses. *Biological Psychiatry, 62*(3), 192–197.

Wong, J. Y., Oh, A. K., Ohta, E., Hunt, A. T., Rogers, G. F., Mulliken, J. B., et al. (2008). Validity and reliability of craniofacial anthropometric measurement of 3D digital photogrammetric images. *Cleft Palate-Craniofacial Journal, 45*(3), 232–239.

Woodhouse, W., Bailey, A., Rutter, M., Bolton, P., Baird, G., & Le Couteur, A. (1996). Head circumference in autism and other pervasive developmental disorders. *Journal of Child Psychology and Psychiatry, 37*(6), 665–671.

Xu, D., Gilkerson, J., Richards, J., Yapanel, U., & Gray, S. (2009). Child vocalization composition as discriminant information for automatic autism detection. *Annual International Conference of the IEEE Engineering in Medicine and Biology Society, 1*, 2518–2522.

Zeegers, M., Pol, H. H., Durston, S., Nederveen, H., Schnack, H., van Daalen, E., et al. (2009). No differences in MR-based volumetry between 2- and 7-year-old children with autism spectrum disorder and developmental delay. *Brain and Development, 31*(10), 725–730.

Zhao, X., Leotta A., Kustanovich V., Lajonchere C., Geschwind D. H., Law K., et al. (2007). A unified genetic theory for sporadic and inherited autism. *Proceedings of the National Academy of Sciences of the United States of America, 104*(31), 12831–12836.

Zimmerman, A. W., Connors, S. L., Matteson, K. J., Lee, L. C., Singer, H. S., Castaneda, J. A., et al. (2007). Maternal antibrain antibodies in autism. *Brain, Behavior, and Immunity, 21*(3), 351–357.

Zori, R. T., Marsh, D. J., Graham, G. E., Marliss, E. B., & Eng, C. (1998). Germline PTEN mutation in a family with Cowden syndrome and Bannayan-Riley-Ruvalcaba syndrome. *American Journal of Medical Genetics, 80*(4), 399–402.

29 Autism as a Quantitative Trait

John N. Constantino

Points of Interest

- Across several different measurement methods, the symptoms and traits that uniquely characterize autism spectrum conditions have been found to be continuously distributed in the general population. Thus, it may be arbitrary where cutoffs are drawn for the categorical designation of affected versus unaffected status, when those designations are made exclusively on the basis of behavioral symptoms.
- Variation in subclinical autistic traits is highly heritable, and subclinical autistic traits aggregate in the first-degree male relatives of individuals with familial autistic syndromes.
- Quantitative characterization of autistic severity can be conducted rapidly and feasibly, such that clinical course and response to intervention can be reliably ascertained by repeated measures over time.
- Quantitative autistic symptomatology may constitute an autism endophenotype in multiple-incidence autism families.

Research in child development over the past several decades has revealed that clinical neuropsychiatric syndromes often represent the severe ends of continuous distributions of core competencies and/or deficiencies that occur in nature. This concept was seminally applied to child psychopathology by Achenbach and colleagues (see Achenbach & Ruffle, 2000), who developed and validated an empirically based dimensional system of measurement; the implementation of that system in studies involving hundreds of thousands of children has revolutionized the way in which disorders of behavior and development are understood. Although on the surface, the difference between categorical ("all-or-nothing") and dimensional classification systems may appear trivial, a paradigm shift between the two can have profound implications for the exploration of neural mechanisms underlying behavior, the enhancement of statistical power in molecular genetic studies, the monitoring of effects of intervention, and helping parents understand (and accept) the nature of a psychiatric condition in a child. In recent years, the conceptualization of autistic syndromes as the severe end of a quantitative distribution of social impairment in nature has garnered considerable attention in science.

Genetic Mechanisms Underlying Quantitative Traits

The fact that a variety of rare single-gene disorders now account for some 10–15% of autistic syndromes (at the time of this writing) might seem to reinforce a categorical concept of autism; that the "autisms" actually represent a collection of such discrete disorders of social cognition. It is indeed possible that quantitative variation in autistic severity might be accounted for by variation in the severity of each rare-but-discrete disorder, or by variable penetrance within each condition. There are now documented examples of both phenomena occurring in autism, however it is still not known whether rare, as-yet-undiscovered causes comprise the bulk of the remaining 85% of autism cases, or whether multigenic mechanisms, strongly suspected in familial cases of autism, are predominantly at play. Multigenic mechanisms of causation have been identified for other complex conditions (diabetes, obesity, hypertension) and specific diseases (see below), in which common susceptibility alleles of relatively minor effect exert joint or interactive effects on the condition of interest. It is furthermore possible that some autistic syndromes arise from deleterious epistatic interactions involving both common and rare genetic factors.

When considering the manner in which disparate genetic mechanisms map to autistic syndromes, it is helpful to consider whether genetic variations are rare or common, operate singly or in combination with other genes, whether they are inherited or arise "de novo" in a given generation and whether they produce autism alone or autism accompanied by other major developmental disorders or anomalies. These factors have known associations with the likelihood of recurrence in families, such that approaches to gene-finding may be optimized by hypothesizing specific mechanisms of transmission within specific subsets of families in which autistic syndromes arise. For example, common inherited susceptibility alleles may be more likely to be identifiable in families in which multiple members are affected to varying degrees, whereas rare de novo (germline) mutations of large effect are more likely to be responsible for sporadic cases of ASD.

Advances in the elucidation of the genetic structure of other complex diseases have revealed ways in which specific genetic mechanisms can result in quantitative distributions that bear striking similarities to those observed in autism spectrum conditions. For example, in the short-segment variety of Hirschsprung's disease—a disorder of neuronal migration to the large intestine affecting boys 5 times more commonly than girls—the length of the gut that is affected (a straightforward quantitative index measured in centimeters) is associated with the number of recessive susceptibility alleles possessed by the patient, and is predictive of sibling recurrence risk (Amiel et al., 2008). This multifactorial genetic mechanism contrasts with the rarer and more severe long-segment Hirschsprung's disease, which follows a dominant pattern of autosomal transmission of single gene mutations of major effect. In schizophrenia, a neurodevelopmental disorder in which the normal process of synaptic pruning in adolescence is believed to be dramatically accelerated (in contrast to the disruption in synapse formation that is believed to occur in autism), sporadic cases have been associated with an elevated occurrence of de novo copy number variations (CNVs), some of which are the same as those observed in excess among sporadic cases of autism. Understanding how specific inherited susceptibilities affect the time course of the development of functional connections in the brain will no doubt bring us closer to understanding how phenotypic overlap in mental disorders such as autism, ADHD, schizophrenia, and bipolar disorder might occur.

Whatever the cause, what is observed in nature is a very wide, and in essence, continuous distribution of autistic symptoms and traits (Constantino & Todd, 2003; Ronald, Happe, Price, Baron-Cohen & Plomin, 2006; Skuse et al. 2009) comprising the so-called autism spectrum. Existing taxonomies attempt to subdivide this spectrum into discrete clinical syndromes (Asperger's syndrome, PDD-NOS, autistic disorder) but to date there is no evidence that these conditions breed true in families or are caused by their own specific genetic or neural mechanisms. It is possible that such syndromes represent the phenotypic result of interactions between specific quantitative abilities (e.g., intelligence) and disabilities (e.g., autistic social impairment), in which there are threshold effects for the phenotypic expression of such parameters as language and stereotypic motor behavior (see below). In addition to its implications for understanding causal mechanisms in the development of autistic syndromes, the conceptualization of autism as a quantitative trait has potentially far-reaching implications for understanding how autistic syndromes change in severity over the course of development or in response to intervention.

Quantitative Variation in Autistic Symptomatology in Affected Families

Numerous studies, using various methods of measurement, have documented the aggregation of autistic syndromes, symptoms, or traits in the close relatives of children with autism. Such observations of familial aggregation have ranged from a full diagnosis of autistic disorder (for which siblings of children with autism have a relative risk of 20 or higher; see Lauritsen, Pedersen, & Mortensen, 2005), to milder autistic syndromes (Asperger's syndrome, Pervasive Developmental Disorder Not-Otherwise-Specified; see Pickles et al., 2000), to subclinical behavioral features of the autistic syndrome (Constantino et al., 2006; Sung et al., 2005; Szatmari et al., 2000; Virkud Todd, Abbacchi, Zhang, & Constantino, 2009; Constantino et al., 2010b), to personality traits that are akin to autistic symptoms (Piven, Palmer, Jacobi, Childress, & Arndt, 1997). Lauritsen and colleagues (Lauritsen et al., 2005) additionally observed that the siblings of children with Asperger's syndrome in the Danish National Register had a 13 times higher-than-general-population risk for the development of full-blown autism, which constitutes some of the strongest evidence to date that the two disorders share common underlying genetic susceptibility factors. In addition to this aggregation of behavioral traits in family members, it has recently been suggested that electrophysiologic abnormalities (Dawson et al., 2005) and functional magnetic resonance imaging (fMRI) variations (Dalton, Nacewicz, Alexander, & Davidson, 2007) similar to those associated with autism are appreciable in the unaffected first-degree relatives of some children with autism.

Most recently, studies that have carefully differentiated simplex autism (single family member affected, also referred to as sporadic autism) from multiplex autism (two or more family members affected, also referred to as familial autism) have suggested that familial aggregation of subclinical autistic traits may occur only in multiplex autism (Losh, Childress, Lam, & Piven, 2008; Virkud et al., 2009; Constantino et al., 2010b), providing further evidence for differentiation of mechanisms of genetic transmission for sporadic versus familial forms of the disorder. Furthermore, differences in patterns of aggregation of quantitative autistic traits between male and female family members of multiplex autism families—as depicted below (Virkud et al., 2009)—suggest that the gender disparities that have been observed for nearly all familial autistic syndromes are reflected also in raw scores for subclinical traits among unaffected first-degree relatives (Constantino & Todd, 2003; Skuse et al., 2009), see Figure 29-1.

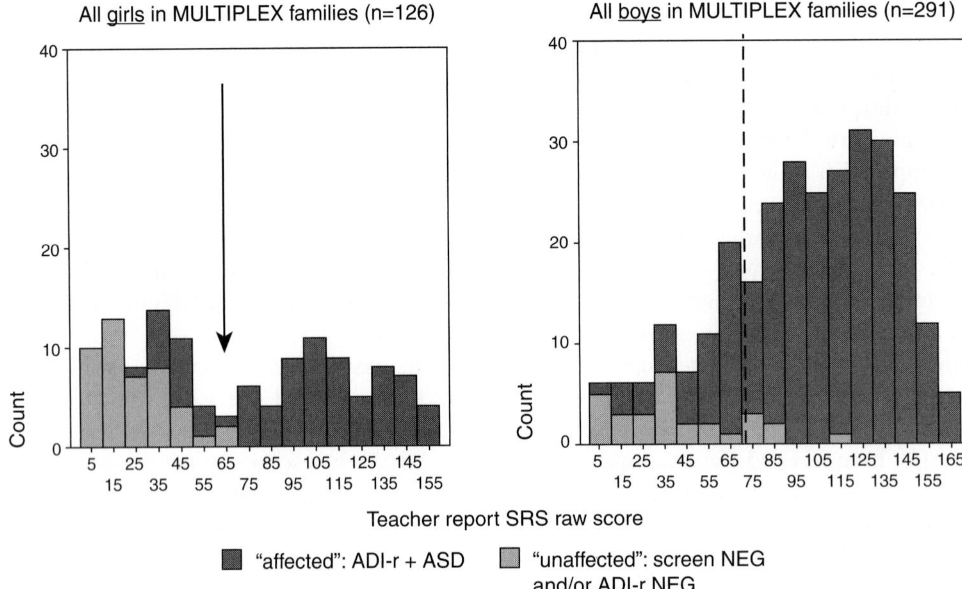

Figure 29–1. Distribution of RAW teacher-report Social Responsiveness Scale (SRS) scores for ALL assessed children in each family type (all of the boys in the simplex families, all of the boys in the multiplex families, all of the girls in the same set of multiplex families). A teacher-report SRS T-score of 60, the quantitative threshold used for comparison of less-affected/unaffected male siblings in multiplex versus simplex families (see text) is denoted by the hatched line in the right hand panel. Each bin is shaded to depict the respective numbers of children categorically-designated as affected or unaffected.

The Factoral Structure of Quantitative Autistic Traits

A key aspect of quantitative variation in autistic symptomatology involves the extent to which the three components of the autistic syndrome (social deficits, communicative deficits, and stereotypic behavior/restricted interests) covary. Although some methodologic approaches have yielded data suggesting that symptoms comprising the three respective criterion sets for a DSM-IV diagnosis of autism might arise independently of one another (Happe & Ronald, 2008), factor, cluster, and latent class analyses of autistic symptomatology in large samples of clinically affected families have revealed substantial overlap in these symptom sets. For example, Spiker and colleagues (Spiker, Lotspeich, Dimiceli, Myers, & Risch, 2002) studied affected sibling pairs with autism, and found that empirically derived clusters of symptoms within families differed not by specific symptom sets, but by the degree of impairment that existed (mild, moderate, or severe) across all three DSM-IV criterion domains for autism. Their findings were most consistent with a model of autistic symptomatology arising from a single, heritable, continuously distributed deficit that might influence dysfunction in all three symptom domains.

Similarly, Sung and colleagues (Sung et al., 2005) examined features of the broader autism phenotype in the relatives of autistic probands and found evidence for the primary aggregation of highly heritable social deficits that explained variation in symptomatology across other domains of the autistic syndrome. Constantino and colleagues (Constantino et al., 2004; Constantino et al., 2007; Constantino & Todd, 2000) applied factor, cluster, and latent class analysis to diagnostic interview and quantitative trait data from families affected by autism and consistently observed a unitary factor structure across data sources and methods of analysis, reinforcing a unitary, syndromic structure for autistic impairment (whether clinical or subclinical in severity) in families affected by autism. A recent principal components factor analysis of an accumulated Washington University sample of 1,799 boys from 1,799 separate families, representing the full range of variation in autistic severity from unaffected to severely affected (by full-blown autistic disorder), yielded the factor structure depicted in the Scree Plot below (Figure 29-2), indicating that a primary factor accounted for over one third of the variance with all other possible factors contributing only minor components of variance (Constantino et al., manuscript in preparation). It is noteworthy that in this observation and in previous studies, the symptoms that loaded most strongly onto the principal factor represented all three of the DSM-IV criterion domains for autism. Subsequent to the original reports summarized above, Gotham, Lord, and colleagues (Gotham, Risi, Pickles, & Lord, 2007; Lord et al., 2006) factor analyzed data from thousands of structured diagnostic observations of children with autism and concluded that the symptoms comprising social deficiency and the communicative deficiency loaded onto a single factor.

Even at face value, a review of typical autistic traits reveals aspects of overlap across symptom domains that provide insight into key unifying constructs. The tendency for the

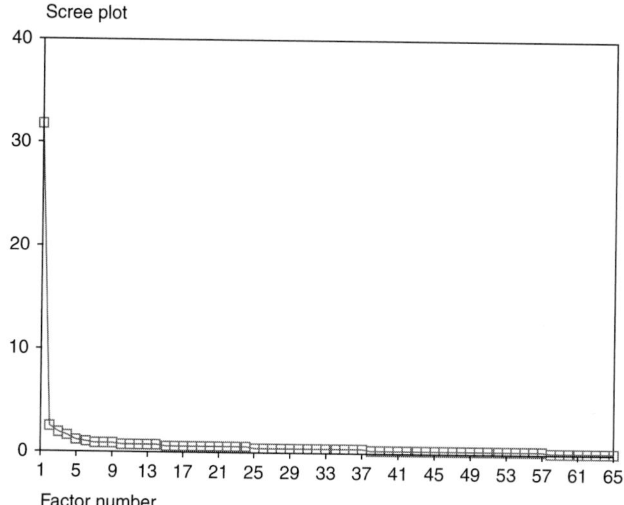

Figure 29–2. Scree plot of principal components analysis of SRS sample of 1,799 boys from 1,799 separate families, representing the full range of variation in autistic severity from unaffected to severely affected by clinical autistic syndromes.

social ability of individuals with ASD to be compromised by an over focus on the details of a social context ("missing the forest for the trees") is highly reminiscent of the over focus on details that characterizes young affected children's unusual (stereotypic) play with toys and older children's restricted range of interests. Thus, it is conceivable that an underlying deficit in the assignment of salience (Klin, Jones, Schultz, Volkmar, & Cohen, 2002) and the consequent absorption with details could underlie the social, stereotypic/behavioral, and even the communicative deficits (e.g., sentence comprehension compromised in the context of preserved decoding of individual words) that characterize autistic syndromes. Such unifying neuropsychological deficits in autism are beginning to be supported by neuroimaging studies that suggest an overabundance of short-range rather than long-range functional neural connections (reviewed elsewhere in this volume).

These observations provide a new framework for understanding quantitative variation in autistic symptomatology and challenge the 3-criterion taxonomy for differentiating specific pervasive developmental disorders (PDDs) in DSM-IV, by raising the possibility that each of the common disorders (autistic disorder, Asperger's syndrome, Pervasive Developmental Disorder Not-Otherwise-Specified) lie along a continuous distribution of impairment with a more parsimonious underlying factor structure. In such a reconceptualization, variation in autistic severity interacts with variation in other domains of development (general cognition, temperament, proneness to anxiety) to produce specific profiles of individual adaptation. For example, Asperger's syndrome, which is described in DSM-IV as a separate disorder (defined as autistic impairment without substantive language delay, and generally characterized by average to above average intellectual functioning), can be viewed as an autistic syndrome that is compensated by a level of intellectual functioning that is adequate to sustain normal language development, even in the presence of a level of social impairment that is otherwise typically associated with language impairment. In that sense it may be the preservation of a relatively high level of general cognition—not the existence of a separate pervasive developmental disorder entity—that uncouples the usual association between social and communicative impairment observed in autistic syndromes.

Molecular genetic studies are now just beginning to add to our knowledge of the factoral structure of autistic syndromes. While many disparate mutations have been associated with the same triad of symptoms observed in autism, quantitative trail loci (QTL) analyses have indicated that common autism susceptibility alleles may preferentially confer risk for joint phenotypes comprised of subclinical symptoms in all 3 criterion domains for autism (St. Pourcain et al., 2010) or among specific subsets of autistic patients, for example those with versus without severe language delays (Alarcon, Yonan, Gilliam, Cantor, & Geschwind, 2005) or those with versus without gastrointestinal symptoms (Campbell et al., 2010). It has also been observed that a given large chromosomal rearrangement or allelic variation associated with autism (i.e., occurring more commonly in ASD than in the general population) might have highly variable phenotypic expression, as observed for 16p11 deletions that are found in patients with autism, patients with mental retardation without autism, and in normal individuals within autism-affected families (Bijlsma et al., 2009). Finally, it is well recognized that syndromes of specific language impairment (SLI) can be inherited independently from autism, however a number of studies have observed that language disorders with distinct autistic qualities (pronoun reversal, socially inappropriate phrases) and/or accompanied by very mild levels of social deficiency aggregate in the unaffected siblings of autistic probands (Constantino et al., 2010b). Ultimately molecular genetic studies are poised to make major contributions to our understanding of how (and in what combinations) the various clinical manifestations of autism arise, and this in turn will inform strategies for intervention for specific subgroups. It is highly conceivable that the severity distribution that constitutes familial autism is fully continuous with the distribution of subclinical autistic symptomatology that is appreciable in the general population (described below). It has recently been demonstrated for other complex diseases such as hypertension that variation within the normal phenotypic range can be caused by variation in the same genes that are responsible for clinical disease states (Ji et al., 2008) and this has been preliminarily observed for autism (St. Pourcain et al., 2010). From an evolutionary standpoint, it is possible that inherited factors that are actually adaptive when phenotypic expression is mild may be highly preserved in the population and may result in clinical disease states only when severely expressed or in interaction with other genetic or environmental factors.

Quantitative Variation in Autistic Symptomatology in the General Population

Several large general population studies involving symptom counts (Ronald et al., 2006; Skuse et al., 2009), or quantitative measurements of the severity of autistic social impairment (Constantino & Todd, 2003) have revealed that the distribution of autistic symptoms is continuous in nature; this is shown for a general population twin sample in the histogram below (Figure 29-3). Thus it may be highly arbitrary where distinctions are drawn between the designation of affected versus unaffected status as suggested above, ASD can be viewed as the extreme end of a normative distribution for reciprocal social behavior (and its associated traits) that occurs in nature. The average male with a current designation of PDD-NOS scores at about the 1st percentile of this distribution for severity of autistic social impairment. Females who score at the 1st percentile of the distribution for girls are less than half as likely to be clinically diagnosed as boys at this percentile cutoff (Constantino et al., 2010b) which may in part explain the gender ratio reported for clinical autistic syndromes as they are currently defined (see below).

It is important to note that variation in the general population is highly heritable, at the same level of genetic influence that autism itself is believed to be inherited (Constantino & Todd, 2003; 2005; Ronald, Happe, Price, Baron-Cohen, & Plomin, 2006).This appears to be true throughout the distribution, i.e., both for social competency and social deficiency. This does not necessarily imply that social competency and social deficiency are controlled by the same genetic factors, but that possibility exists, and is being actively explored. What is known about genetic influences on "subthreshold" autistic traits is that they overlap at least partially with those that influence some forms of autism, because, as discussed above, they preferentially aggregate in the unaffected family members of many children with ASD (Constantino et al., 2006; Virkud et al., 2009), particularly those for whom other members of the family are also fully affected by ASD (so-called multiple-incidence or "multiplex" ASD; see Table 29-1).

A consistent feature of autistic traits throughout the general population distribution is sexual dimorphism; raw severity scores for boys are slightly but significantly shifted toward the pathological end, in comparison to scores for girls. In order to ascertain whether gender-specific genetic effects account for this shift, Constantino & Todd (2003) studied opposite sex dizygotic twins. Opposite-sex twin pairs represent a gender-comparison condition in which common environmental influences can be modeled and controlled for. The results of structural equation modeling applied to these data indicated that the genes influencing autistic traits appeared to be the same for males and females in the general population. Lower prevalence (and severity) of autistic traits in females was found not to be a function of sex-linked genetic influences, but rather the possible result of increased sensitivity to early environmental influences (in females), which operate to reduce the phenotypic expression of genetic susceptibility factors and promote social competency (Constantino & Todd, 2003). If the same genetic structure holds true for autistic traits in the clinical range of severity, it would indicate that given similar levels of genetic susceptibility, girls are relatively protected (compared to boys) from phenotypic expression of this liability.

The question also arises whether inherited influences or quantitative autistic traits are the same as or different from those influences involved in other dimensional domains of psychopathology. Twin designs are capable of answering such questions about genetic overlap, as long as the various traits of interest are all measured in the subjects in a given genetically informative sample. A series of studies in the general population have indicated that (1) scores for internalizing behavior

Table 29-1.
Mean Social Responsiveness Scale (SRS) scores as a function of gender, ASD-affectation status, and family type

	Simplex Autism Families	Multiplex Autism Families	*p Student's t-test*
Affected Boys *(raw teacher-report SRS)*	87.8 (SD = 28.3) n = 80	104.7 (SD = 33.8) n = 262	.0001
Unaffected Boys *(raw teacher-report SRS)*	30.7 (SD = 23.5) n = 89	40.3 (SD = 28.8) n = 29	.035*
Affected Girls *(raw teacher-report SRS)*		97.5 (SD = 36.0) n = 81	
Unaffected Girls *(raw teacher-report SRS)*		23.0 (SD = 16.3) n = 45	
Fathers *(spouse-report SRS)*	23.8 (SD = 17.5) n = 41	34.3 (SD = 23.3) n = 58	.01
Mothers *(spouse-report SRS)*	23.9 (SD = 20.1) n = 41	27.0 (SD = 17.8) n = 58	*ns*

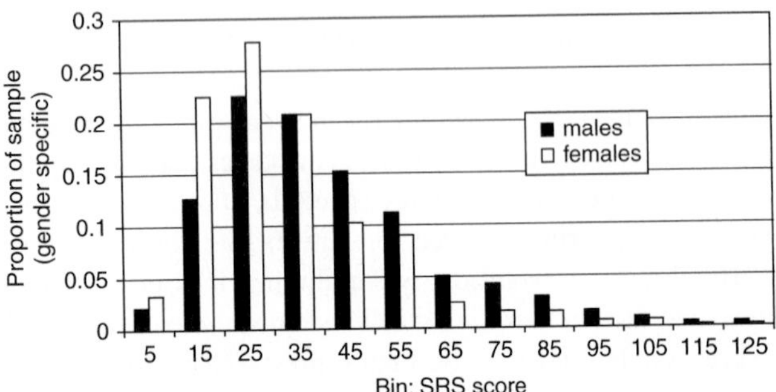

Figure 29-3. Distribution of Social Responsiveness Scale (SRS) scores as a function of sex (n = 1576) in a general population twin sample.

and externalizing behavior explained only a minority of the variance in quantitative autistic trait scores (Constantino & Todd, 2003); (2) there is moderate phenotypic and/or genetic overlap between attention problem syndromes and quantitative autistic traits (Constantino & Todd, 2003; Lichtenstein et al., 2010); (3) elevation in quantitative autistic trait scores may exacerbate co-occurring psychopathologic syndromes (Constantino & Todd, 2000); and (4) youths with severe mood or anxiety disorders exhibit substantially higher autistic trait scores than healthy controls (Pine, Guyer, Goldwin, Towbin, & Leibenluft, 2008) and the level of impairment incurred by these and other variations in personality and behavior may be predicted in part by co-occurrence of subclinical autistic symptomatology (Kanne, Christ, & Reiersen, 2009). Recently Lichtenstein et al., (2010) analyzed data from one of the largest twin studies (n= 10,895 – twin pairs) ever to ascertain data on symptoms of neurodevelopmental disorders in children. It revealed that while about 80% of the variation in liability for autism spectrum disorders was due to genetic effects, bivariate analyses suggested that a substantial share of the genetic variance was shared respectively with ADHD, developmental coordination disorder, tic disorders and learning disorder. Taken together, these results indicate that autistic traits represent an inherited component of developmental abnormality that is largely independent of some domains of child psychopathology, but overlapping with a number of other neurodevelopmental syndromes. When subclinical autistic traits co-occur with other (nonautistic) child psychiatric syndromes, they operate to exacerbate the latter, and can compound functional impairment.

Intergenerational Transmission of Quantitative Autistic Traits

As would be expected for any inherited trait, general populations studies have revealed that correlations for quantitative indices of social impairment are moderate between first-degree relatives (intraclass correlations on the order of 0.30–0.40)—this is true within and across generations, i.e., for correlations between siblings, and for correlations between parents and their children (Constantino & Todd, 2005). There is also substantial correlation for quantitative autistic traits between spouses in both the general population (Constantino & Todd, 2005) and in clinically affected families (Virkud et al., 2009), consistent with the phenomenon of preferential mating. In the general population, when both parents score in the upper quartile for quantitative autistic trait characteristics, mean trait scores of their offspring are significantly shifted toward the pathologic end of the distribution (effect size 1.5). In clinically affected multiplex families enrolled in research studies, however, it has not yet been apparent (at the time of this writing) that there exists gross overrepresentation of such concordantly elevated couples among autism-affected families, in comparison to what would be expected by chance (Virkud et al., 2009).

The Clinical Ascertainment of Autistic Severity

A variety of established and emerging rating scales for social impairment in autism are capable of reliably quantifying its severity—these include checklists or questionnaires of current functioning completed by adult informants (usually parents, teachers, or both) who have observed a child routinely in his/her naturalistic social contexts, assessments of developmental history as provided by parents, or direct observations of social behavior in response to structured or semistructured social prompts. Each domain of observation can provide a unique and valuable vantage point for assessing the severity of autistic social impairment (as well as its relationship to other domains of development and psychopathology) in a given child. There are many ways in which multi-informant characterization of a developing child can help avoid misclassification that would otherwise arise from single-informant or single-context assessment (Kanne, Abbacchi, & Constantino, 2009). Young children with milder forms of ASD who might be rapidly identified by an experienced day-care teacher could go unrecognized if observed exclusively at home, since young parents are often inexperienced with respect to normative trajectories of social development. Moreover, such children can be reasonably competent in one-on-one social interactions with caring adults who can support and scaffold their interpersonal behavior, but have a great deal of difficulty in less structured social contexts in the company of larger numbers of close-aged peers. This extends into childhood and adolescence as well—there are many children who respond reasonably appropriately to a clinician-examiner in the context of a structured diagnostic assessment, but may be observed by teachers to display floridly inappropriate social behavior when in an unstructured context at school (lunch, gym, recess, bathroom breaks between classes). For these reasons it is useful to acquire information from multiple sources (ideally direct clinical observation, parent-report, and teacher-report, see Constantino et al. (2007)) in the clinical evaluation of social impairment in a child suspected of having an ASD.

Other Implications of a Quantitative Structure for Autism

The quantitative distributions depicted in this chapter suggest that it may be arbitrary where a line is drawn between the condition of being affected versus unaffected by autism; the place where that line is drawn (a percentile cutoff versus a cutoff that correlates with clinical or other psychometric designations) has serious implications for epidemiologic, genetic, and neurobiologic studies that might be confounded by misclassification. For example the seemingly straightforward calculation of recurrence risk becomes complicated by the possibility that subtle degrees of affectedness may be appropriate to include as episodes of recurrence (Constantino et al., 2010b). A new generation of clinical epidemiologic research will need to explore the extent to which quantitative "recurrence" relates to patterns of aggregation in families and extended pedigrees as potential moderating variables such as twin versus singleton gestation.

Recognizing that a wide range of quantitative autistic traits may be present in the siblings of children with autism, it is possible to explore whether the association between phenotype and underlying genetic or neurobiologic mechanisms might be more appreciable when considering quantitative autistic trait information from all siblings in affected families rather than restricting analysis to the transmission of categorical disease states. A quantitative molecular genetic analysis utilizing quantitative trait information from all children of participating families (not just the fully affected subjects) has indicated that linkage signals in a multiplex family registry were substantially enhanced when adopting this approach as depicted below in Figure 29-4 (Duvall et al., 2007). The principal linkage signal derived from this approach has now been replicated in an independent sample (Coon et al., 2010) and overlaps with a strong linkage signal declined from the autism genome project (Autism Genome Project Consortium et al., 2007).

Quantitative Autistic Traits and Endophenotypes

In addition, a quantitative conceptualization of autism motivates the search for endophenotypes, which are inherited, quantitative phenotypic components of a syndrome. Endophenotypes, if they exist for autism, should be appreciable in some or many of the unaffected family members of clinically affected individuals, and might more closely map to specific genetic, neurobiologic, or psychologic factors that contribute to (but are not by themselves sufficient to cause) the phenotypic expression of the syndrome itself. Endophenotypes are not the same as associated symptoms of a condition (e.g., self-injurious behavior in Lesch-Nyan syndrome), but rather core components of the syndrome that appear in subclinical forms in unaffected relatives. Subclinical autistic traits exhibiting a unitary factor structure (as described earlier in this chapter) appear to constitute a social endophenotype for males in multiple-incidence (multiplex) autistic families (Virkud et al., 2009; Constantino et al., 2010b), and the search for more precise endophenotypic components of the autistic syndrome is under way. The findings from sibling and family studies that explore candidate endophenotypes can generally be interpreted on the basis of the matrix of possible results depicted in Table 29-2.

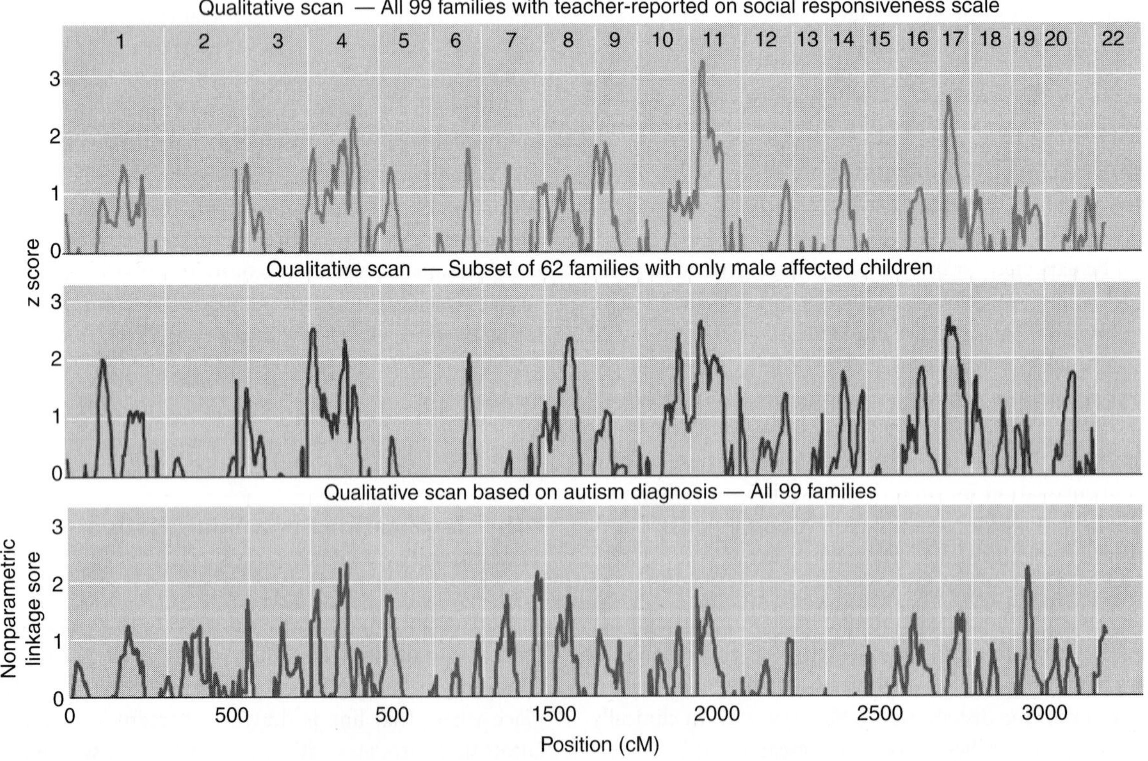

Figure 29–4. Linkage analysis of 99 AGRE families comparing results from Quantitative Trait Locus (QTL) analysis (top and middle) incorporating unchanged analysis of 99 AGRE families, showing contrasting results of a quantitative approach in which phenotypic information and genotypes of all siblings in each family were incorporated (top and middle panels, illustrating accentuation of a number of linkage scan across the genome) versus a qualitative scales in which only the information from affected sibling pairs was incorporated.

Table 29–2.
Matrix of interpretation of results from family studies of candidate autism endophenotypes

	Autistic Proband	ASD-Affected Degree Relatives	Unaffected 1st Degree Relatives in multiplex Families	Unaffected 1st Degree Relatives in Simplex Families	Unrelated Controls	Interpretation
Test Result	+	-	-	-	-	Poss. Severity Index
Test Result	+	+	-	-	-	ASD Phenotype
Test Result	+	+	+		-	ASD Endophenotype
Test Result	+	+	+	+	-	Inherited Trait*

**Possibly not Specific to autism, OR an endophenotype associated with genes shared by simplex and multiplex ASD.*

As an example of the way in which two candidate endophenotypes might interact to confer susceptibility to autistic social impairment, Reiersen, Constantino, and Todd (2008) analyzed data on inattention and motor coordination deficits (separately inherited domains of quantitative neurodevelopmental deficiency) in over 800 children in the general population and showed how their co-occurrence is associated with the development of autistic social impairment, as shown below. These associations are reminiscent of a syndrome of Deficits in Attention, Motor Coordination, and Perception (DAMP) that has been observed and described in the child psychiatric literature in Figure 29-5 (Landgren, Pettersson, Kjellman, & Gillberg, 1996).

The current list of proposed candidate endophenotypes for autism is long, but the series of investigations required to establish them as true endophenotypes (through studies confirming heritability, patterns of familial aggregation, trait-like stability, and specific association with autism) is long as well. Some of the more promising endophenotypic candidates (in addition to subclinical behavioral autistic traits, see above) include head circumference trajectory in infancy (Constantino et al., 2010a), laterality (handedness), electrophysiologic and brain activation responses to socially-relevant auditory and visual stimuli, sensory dysfunction, EEG/ERP abnormality, neuroimaging phenotypes (Di Martino et al., 2009; Scott-Van Zeeland et al., 2010; Kaiser et al., 2011), an array of neuropsychologic deficits (theory of mind, self-other representation, social motivation, capacity for shared intentionality, abnormalities in gaze cueing and/or joint attention), a variety of language endophenotypes (prosodic deficits, sentence comprehension abnormalities, timing of developmental milestones such as age of first word or first phrase), motor coordination problems, involuntary/repetitive motor movements, obsessionality, and inattention. Each of these might be uniquely influenced by specific brain networks that could become targets of preventive or therapeutic interventions.

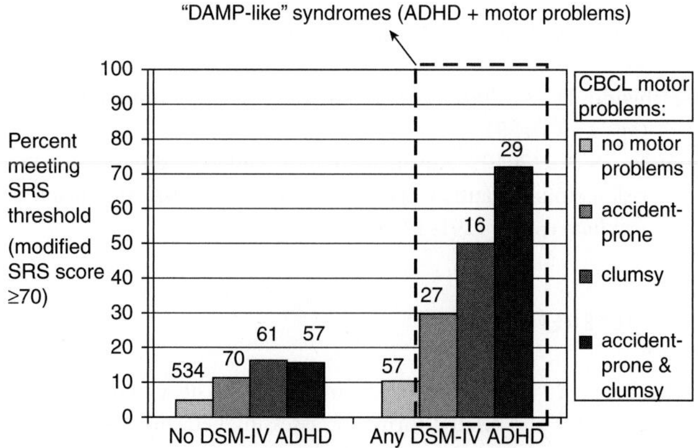

Figure 29–5. Percentage of subjects with clinically significant autistic traits, stratified by presence or absence of DSM-IV attention-deficit/hyperactivity disorder (ADHD) and by endorsement of Child Behavior Checklist (CBCL) motor problem items. N = 851. Number of subjects in each group is shown above each bar. DAMP = deficits in attention, motor control, and perception.

The Interface Between Social Impairment and General Cognition

Finally, it is important to consider the implications of the interaction between quantitative distributions of social deficiency (accompanied by relative deficiency in communication and the presence of stereotypic behaviors and/or restricted interests as occurs in the autistic syndrome) and quantitative variation in general cognition, which are orthogonal developmental constructs that can be differentiated from one another within the normal distribution of IQ in the population. Autism can occur in the context of low IQ (narrowly-defined, severe autistic disorders were once believed to be accompanied by intellectual disability in some 70 per cent of cases), high IQ, or anything in between, and it is often difficult to know whether syndromes of combined social and cognitive impairment represent a cognitive disorder with secondary social impairment, the reverse, or some combination of two independent conditions. And even if largely uncorrelated within the general population, clinical syndromes of severe deficiency in any developmental domain can exert expectable consequences on other developmental domains.

Co-occurrence of deficiencies across multiple domains can make it difficult (but crucial) to disentangle the relative contributions of impairments in each respective domain to the clinical syndrome of an individual child. A common example is the clinical scenario of a toddler who presents with language delay; it is perplexing (yet potentially relevant to the choice of intervention strategy) to determine whether that delay is most attributable to a primary cognitive deficit, an autistic syndrome, a specific language impairment, or some combination of dimensional variants of these conditions. If each domain is fundamentally quantitative in nature, it will ultimately require established maps of the expectable relations between the variables (analogous to the height versus weight norms used in pediatric practice) to accurately ascertain their relative contributions in a given case of developmental delay. We eagerly await a next generation of developmental-epidemiologic studies (some of which are currently under way) that will map the ways in which quantitative variations in such fundamental domains of development (especially cognition, capacity for reciprocal social behavior, language, emotional regulation, sensorimotor function and interpersonal experience) interact with one another over the course of development from infancy to adulthood. It is possible that such studies will pave the way for a new system of characterizing *all* syndromes of developmental delay, along measurable quantitative axes, each of which might allow more precise associations with contributing neural mechanisms (Constantino, 2009).

Conclusion

The deficits that characterize autistic syndromes–including those in the current diagnostic criterion domains of reciprocal social behavior, social communication and repetitive behavior/restricted interests–are continuously distributed in nature and may share common underlying genetic and neural mechanisms. Integrating quantitative approaches to characterization of neurodevelopmental syndromes will help advance the search for genetic, psychologic neurobiologic and endophenotypic components of their underlying cause(s), and provides a basis for repeated-measurement strategies that can track developmental course and response to intervention. Given what is currently known, the designation of autism affectation status (in a categorical sense) for any given individual a) should be contextualized with respect to published distributions in clinical and non-clinical populations; and b) is best informed by data from multiple social contexts.

Challenges and Future Directions

- The fundamental factor structure of quantitative autistic traits is a subject of ongoing controversy and some of the findings have varied as a function of different measurement methods. Clarification of the factor structure—specifically whether autism is truly syndromic or rather a function of the convergence of separable components of dysfunction—will have significant implications for studies of the causes and early development of ASD, as well as for approaches to intervention.
- The question of whether a high degree of social competence represents simply the absence of deficiency in reciprocal social behavior, or subsumes other abilities and developmental competencies remains unanswered. Future research on the roots of social competence may reveal key characteristics inherent in resiliency as well as contribute to better understanding of the genetic architecture of social development.
- It is hoped that a next generation of genetic-epidemiologic studies will map the ways in which quantitative variations in various developmental competencies interact with each other over time (see chapter by Cantor). Thus, rather than characterizing children on the basis of presence or absence of deficiency of one kind or another, a more comprehensive approach to assessment that simultaneously assimilates the contributions of quantitative variation in all major developmental domains (e.g. cognition, language, reciprocal social behavior, attention, affect regulation, life events) will allow for a more precise understanding of the contributing factors (and therefore potential targets of intervention) in children with syndromes of developmental delay. Such assessment will also help clarify the boundaries and interactions between such conditions as autism, specific language impairment, and intellectual disability.

SUGGESTED READINGS

Constantino, J. N. (2009). How continua converge in nature: cognition, social competence, and autistic syndromes. *Journal of the American Academy of Child and Adolescent Psychiatry*, *48*(2), 97–98.

Geschwind, D. H. (2008). Autism: many genes, common pathways? *Cell*, *135*(3), 391–395.

Kendler, S. K. (2010). Advances in our understanding of genetic risk factors for autism spectrum disorders. *American Journal of Psychiatry*, *167*, 1291–1293

REFERENCES

Achenbach, T. M., & Ruffle, T. M. (2000). The Child Behavior Checklist and related forms for assessing behavioral/emotional problems and competencies. *Pediatric Review*, *21*(8), 265–271.

Alarcon, M., Yonan, A. L., Gilliam, T. C., Cantor, R. M., & Geschwind, D. H. (2005). Quantitative genome scan and ordered-subsets analysis of autism endophenotypes support language QTLs. *Molecular Psychiatry*, *10*(8), 747–757.

Amiel, J., Sproat-Emison, E., Garcia-Barcelo, M., Lantieri, F., Burzynski, G., Borrego, S., et al. (2008). Hirschsprung disease, associated syndromes, and genetics: a review. *Journal of Medical Genetics, 45*(1), 1–14.

Autism Genome Project Consortium, Szatmari, P., Paterson, A.D., Zwaignebaum, L., Roberts, W., Brian, J. et al. (2007). Mapping autism risk loci using genetic linkage and chromosomal rearrangements. *Nature Genetics, 39*(3), 319–328.

Bijlsma, E. K., Gijsbers, A. C., Schuurs-Hoeijmakers, J. H., van Haeringen, A., Fransen van de Putte, D. E., Anderlid, B. M., et al. (2009). Extending the phenotype of recurrent rearrangements of 16p11.2: deletions in mentally retarded patients without autism and in normal individuals. *European Journal of Medical Genetics, 52*(2–3), 77–87.

Campbell, D. B., Warren, D., Sutcliffe, J. S., Lee, E. B., & Levitt, P. (2010). Association of MET with social and communication phenotypes in individuals with autism spectrum disorder. *American Journal of Medical Genetics. Part B, Neuropsychiatric Genetics, 153B*(2), 438–446.

Constantino, J. N. (2009). How continua converge in nature: Cognition, social competence, and autistic syndromes. *Journal of the American Academy of Child and Adolescent Psychiatry, 48*(2), 97–98.

Constantino, J. N., Gruber, C. P., Davis, S., Hayes, S., Passanante, N., & Przybeck, T. (2004). The factor structure of autistic traits. *Journal of Child Psychology and Psychiatry, 45*(4), 719–726.

Constantino, J. N., Lajonchere, C., Lutz, M., Gray, T., Abbacchi, A., McKenna, K., et al. (2006). Autistic social impairment in the siblings of children with pervasive developmental disorders. *American Journal of Psychiatry, 163*(2), 294–296.

Constantino, J. N., Lavesser, P. D., Zhang, Y., Abbacchi, A. M., Gray, T., & Todd, R. D. (2007). Rapid quantitative assessment of autistic social impairment by classroom teachers. *Journal of the American Academy of Child and Adolescent Psychiatry, 46*(12), 1668–1676.

Constantino JN, Majmudar P, Bottini A, Arvin M, Virkud Y, Simons P, Spitznagel E. (2010a). Infant head growth in male siblings of children with and without autism spectrum disorders. *Journal of Neurodevelopmental Disorders, 2*, 39–46.

Constantino J.N., Zhang Y., Abbacchi A., Frazier T.W., & Law P. (2010b). Sibling recurrence and the genetic epidemiology of autism. *American Journal of Psychiatry, 167*(11), 1349–56.

Constantino, J. N., & Todd, R. D. (2000). Genetic structure of reciprocal social behavior. *American Journal of Psychiatry, 157*(12), 2043–2045.

Constantino, J. N., & Todd, R. D. (2003). Autistic traits in the general population: A twin study. *Archives of General Psychiatry, 60*(5), 524–530.

Constantino, J. N., & Todd, R. D. (2005). Intergenerational transmission of subthreshold autistic traits in the general population. *Biological Psychiatry, 57*(6), 655–660.

Coon, H., Villalobos, M.E., Robison, F.J., Camp, N.J., Cannon, D.S., Allen-Brady, K., et al. (2010). Genome-wide linkage using the Social Responsiveness Scale in Utah autism pedigrees. *Molecular Autism, 8*(1), 8.

Dalton, K. M., Nacewicz, B. M., Alexander, A. L., & Davidson, R. J. (2007). Gaze-fixation, brain activation, and amygdala volume in unaffected siblings of individuals with autism. *Biological Psychiatry, 61*(4), 512–520.

Dawson, G., Webb, S. J., Wijsman, E., Schellenberg, G., Estes, A., Munson, J., et al. (2005). Neurocognitive and electrophysiological evidence of altered face processing in parents of children with autism: Implications for a model of abnormal development of social brain circuitry in autism. *Developmental Psychopathology, 17*(3), 679–697.

Di Martino, A., Shehzad, Z., Kelly, C., Krain, R., Dylan, G., Uddin, L., et al. (2009). Relationship between cingulo-insular functional connectivity and autistic traits in neurotypical adults. *American Journal of Psychiatry, 166*(8), 891–899.

Duvall, J. A., Lu, A., Cantor, R. M., Todd, R. D., Constantino, J. N., & Geschwind, D. H. (2007). A quantitative trait locus analysis of social responsiveness in multiplex autism families. *American Journal of Psychiatry, 164*(4), 656–662.

Gotham, K., Risi, S., Pickles, A., & Lord, C. (2007). The Autism Diagnostic Observation Schedule: Revised algorithms for improved diagnostic validity. *Journal of Autism and Developmental Disorders, 37*(4), 613–627.

Happe, F., & Ronald, A. (2008). The "fractionable autism triad": A review of evidence from behavioural, genetic, cognitive, and neural research. *Neuropsychology Review, 18*(4), 287–304.

Ji, W., Foo, J. N., O'Roak, B. J., Zhao, H., Larson, M. G., Simon, D. B., et al. (2008). Rare independent mutations in renal salt handling genes contribute to blood pressure variation. *Nature Genetics, 40*(5), 592–599.

Kaiser, M. D., Hudac, C. M., Shultz, S., Lee, S. M., Cheung, C., Berken, A. M., et al. (2010). Neural signatures of autism. *Proceedings of the National Academy of Sciences of the United States of America, 107*(49), 21223–21228.

Kanne, S. M., Abbacchi, A. M., & Constantino, J. N. (2009). Multi-informant ratings of psychiatric symptom severity in children with autism spectrum disorders: The importance of environmental context. *Journal of Autism and Developmental Disorders, 39*(6), 856–864.

Kanne, S. M., Christ, S. E., & Reiersen, A. M. (2009). Psychiatric symptoms and psychosocial difficulties in young adults with autistic traits. *Journal of Autism and Developmental Disorders, 39*(6), 827–833.

Klin, A., Jones, W., Schultz, R., Volkmar, F., & Cohen, D. (2002). Visual fixation patterns during viewing of naturalistic social situations as predictors of social competence in individuals with autism. *Archives of General Psychiatry, 59*(9), 809–816.

Landgren, M., Pettersson, R., Kjellman, B., & Gillberg, C. (1996). ADHD, DAMP, and other neurodevelopmental/psychiatric disorders in 6-year-old children: Epidemiology and co-morbidity. *Developmental Medicine and Child Neurology, 38*(10), 891–906.

Lauritsen, M. B., Pedersen, C. B., & Mortensen, P. B. (2005). Effects of familial risk factors and place of birth on the risk of autism: A nationwide register-based study. *Journal of Child Psychology and Psychiatry, 46*(9), 963–971.

Lichtenstein P., Carlstrom E., Rastam M., Gillberg C., Anckarsater H. (2010). The genetics of autism spectrum disorders and related neuropsychiatric disorders in childhood. *American Journal of Psychiatry, 167*(11), 1291–1293.

Lord, C., Risi, S., DiLavore, P. S., Shulman, C., Thurm, A., & Pickles, A. (2006). Autism from 2 to 9 years of age. *Archives of General Psychiatry, 63*(6), 694–701.

Losh, M., Childress, D., Lam, K., & Piven, J. (2008). Defining key features of the broad autism phenotype: A comparison across parents of multiple- and single-incidence autism families. *American Journal of Medicine Genetics. Part B, Neuropsychiatric Genetics, 147B*(4), 424–433.

Pickles, A., Starr, E., Kazak, S., Bolton, P., Papanikolaou, K., Bailey, A., et al. (2000). Variable expression of the autism broader phenotype: Findings from extended pedigrees. *Journal of Child Psychology and Psychiatry, 41*(4), 491–502.

Pine, D. S., Guyer, A. E., Goldwin, M., Towbin, K. A., & Leibenluft, E. (2008). Autism spectrum disorder scale scores in pediatric mood and anxiety disorders. *Journal of the American Academy of Child and Adolescent Psychiatry, 47*(6), 652–661.

Piven, J., Palmer, P., Jacobi, D., Childress, D., & Arndt, S. (1997). Broader autism phenotype: Evidence from a family history study of multiple-incidence autism families. *American Journal of Psychiatry, 154*(2), 185–190.

Reiersen, A. M., Constantino, J. N., & Todd, R. D. (2008). Co-occurrence of motor problems and autistic symptoms in attention-deficit/hyperactivity disorder. *Journal of the American Academy of Child and Adolescent Psychiatry, 47*(6), 662–672.

Ronald, A., Happe, F., Price, T. S., Baron-Cohen, S., & Plomin, R. (2006). Phenotypic and genetic overlap between autistic traits at the extremes of the general population. *Journal of the American Academy of Child and Adolescent Psychiatry, 45*(10), 1206–1214.

Scott-Van Zeeland, A. A., Abrahams, B. S., Alvarez-Retuerto, A. I., Sonnenblick, L. I., Rudie, J. D., Ghahremani, D., et al. (2010). Altered functional connectivity in frontal lobe circuits is associated with variation in the autism risk gene CNTNAP2. *Science Translational Medicine, 2*(56), p. 56ra80.

St. Pourcain B., Wang K., Glessner J. T., Golding J., Steer C., Ring S. M., et al. (2010). Association between a high-risk autism locus on 5p14 and social communication spectrum phenotypes in the general population. *American Journal of Psychiatry. 167*(10), 1283.

Skuse, D., Mandy, W., Steer, C., Miller, L., Goodman, R., Lawrence, K., et al. (2009). Social communication competence and functional adaptation in a general population of children: Preliminary evidence for sex-by-verbal IQ differential risk. *Journal of the American Academy of Child and Adolescent Psychiatry, 48*(2), 12–137

Spiker, D., Lotspeich, L. J., Dimiceli, S., Myers, R. M., & Risch, N. (2002). Behavioral phenotypic variation in autism multiplex families: Evidence for a continuous severity gradient. *American Journal of Medical Genetics, 114*(2), 129–136.

Sung, Y. J., Dawson, G., Munson, J., Estes, A., Schellenberg, G. D., & Wijsman, E. M. (2005). Genetic investigation of quantitative traits related to autism: Use of multivariate polygenic models with ascertainment adjustment. *American Journal of Human Genetics, 76*(1), 68–81.

Szatmari, P., Bryson, S. E., Streiner, D. L., Wilson, F., Archer, L., & Ryerse, C. (2000). Two-year outcome of preschool children with autism or Asperger's syndrome. *American Journal of Psychiatry, 157*(12), 1980–1987.

Virkud, Y. V., Todd, R. D., Abbacchi, A. M., Zhang, Y., & Constantino, J. N. (2009). Familial aggregation of quantitative autistic traits in multiplex versus simplex autism. *American Journal of Medicine Genetics. Part B, Neuropsychiatric Genetics, 150B*(3), 328–334.

Commentary

Jeremy R. Parr, Kerstin Wittemeyer,
Ann S. Le Couteur

The Broader Autism Phenotype: Implications for Research and Clinical Practice

Over the last two decades, the broader autism phenotype (BAP) has become a focus for researchers and clinicians alike; this is in part due to its central role in the conceptualization of autistic spectrum disorders (ASD) and its importance for identifying ASD susceptibility genes. Studies of very young children with ASD, and prospective studies of siblings of children with ASD (at-risk, or high risk sibling studies) have provided important insights about "typical" development, our understanding of early ASD characteristics and subsequent developmental trajectories, and the range of possible outcomes for affected individuals (which includes BAP). For clinicians and researchers, who await the publication of the DSM-V and ICD-11 clinical conceptualizations of ASD phenotypes, the need to have a better understanding of what constitutes the BAP is a priority. Using the context of the findings reported in this series of chapters, this commentary will summarize some of the important challenges and opportunities for BAP research and the implications for clinicians who diagnose and provide services for children with ASD, and their families.

Research Aspects

In Chapter 27, Losh et al. provide a welcome overview of the historical context of BAP research. The parental phenotype was once considered an etiological factor in the development of ASD in their children (see Bettelheim, 1967); during this period joint working between parents (who were understandably distressed by these erroneous theories) and researchers was a challenge. Perhaps inevitably, research then focused on core autism to identify the biological underpinning of this severe organic neurodevelopmental disorder (Rutter, 1970). As discussed in several of the Chapters in this section, the 1990s saw a surge in interest in the BAP. Following twin and family studies published in the mid-late 1990s and more recent research over the last decade (reviewed by Losh et al., Chapter 27), we now have a better understanding of the behaviors and traits associated with BAP. Core characteristics include social communication difficulties and behavioral rigidity (see Chapter 27, and Parr et al. and the International Molecular Genetic Study of Autism Consortium [IMGSAC] (in preparation)). A broad range of social (see Chapters 27 and 29), and communication impairments (in particular reciprocal communication impairments, and pragmatic difficulties) (reviewed by Groen & Buitelaar, Chapter 10) are frequently reported. In common with ASD, qualitatively similar elements of rigidity, perfectionism, and obsessive-compulsive disorder are also present (see Jacob et al., Chapter 17). Delineation of these repetitive BAP traits has been particularly difficult (Bailey et al., 1998). Furthermore, disentangling these repetitive traits from other psychiatric disorders (for example obsessive-compulsive disorder per se) remains challenging, and progress has been slow (Jacob et al., Chapter 17). Finally, as discussed by Losh et al. (Chapter 27), the relationship between mood disorders (particularly affective disorder) and the BAP remains poorly understood. Depression and/or anxiety may be related to the BAP itself, rather than a consequence of having a child (or children) with ASD (see Losh et al., Chapter 27). For both BAP and ASD, further research is needed to ascertain whether affective disorder is integral to the phenotypes, or present as a consequence of the impact of their behavioral characteristics.

Historically, in contrast with other areas of ASD research, a small number of groups have investigated the BAP, and overall research capacity has been limited. However, understanding the BAP has become of critical importance to our conceptualization of ASD, and its etiology. As a consequence, the BAP will continue to receive increased attention during the next decade. As with other complex neurodevelopmental disorders (for example attention-deficit/hyperactivity disorder [ADHD] and schizophrenia), careful characterization of the whole phenotypic spectrum, rather than a focus on the more severe phenotypes is necessary in order to fully investigate their neurobiological basis (Bailey & Parr, 2003).

In ASD research, the BAP was first identified in families with twins, or affected relative pairs ("multiplex families") with ASD (see Losh et al., Chapter 27). More recently, researchers have described BAP characteristics in the context of normative trait variation in general population samples (reviewed by Constantino, Chapter 29, and Losh et al., Chapter 27). This approach investigates common social communication difficulties and rigidity traits in the population and proposes that these lie on a dimension with ASD itself (see Constantino, Chapter 29). As discussed by Losh et al. in Chapter 27, different approaches to investigating the BAP have resulted in the development of different methods of BAP assessment (for example structured interviews and observation measures vs. parent and self-report questionnaires), undertaken on different populations (ASD families vs. the general population; see Losh et al., Chapter 27). Similar variability exists in the approaches taken in biological BAP research (Lainhart & Lange, Chapter 28). Losh et al. also highlight that few studies have controlled for the effect of having a child with a neurodevelopmental disorder (although see De Jonge et al. & IMGSAC, in preparation). There has been little opportunity to compare the validity of these different methodologies and potentially contrasting or complementary approaches.

The lack of comparative data from studies using different methods in the same population severely limits our conceptual understanding of the BAP (see Lainhart & Lange, Chapter 28; and Losh, Chapter 27). In the future, investigating general population samples, and samples of relatives from ASD families using the same BAP measures, for example the revised Family History Interviews (Parr et al. & IMGSAC, in preparation) and questionnaires such as the Social Responsiveness Scale (Constantino et al., 2003) will assist us in refining our behavioral measures and methods, and identifying how best to conceptualize ASD/BAP. It is possible that a combination of questionnaire screening, more in-depth interviewing, and hypothesis driven neurocognitive and functional imaging/ biological investigations of individuals across the behavioral spectrum might advance our understanding of the extent and impact of the phenotype (Losh et al., Chapter 27; Lainhart & Lange, Chapter 28).

Despite progress in better characterizing the BAP and utilizing relatives' data, many aspects remain poorly understood: More is known about the BAP in relatives from multiplex ASD families than singleton families. The relationship between the quality and severity of ASD in affected individuals, and BAP traits in their parents or other relatives requires further study; as discussed by Losh et al. (Chapter 27), understanding familiality (the extent to which traits in parents relate to their children's ASD) has methodological implications for researchers attempting to reduce genetic heterogeneity, by utilizing phenotypic information in the search for autism susceptibility genes (Bailey & Parr, 2003). In molecular genetic studies, relatives' BAP data could be used dimensionally or categorically (for example QTL methods, or haplotype, or parent of origin analysis). Dimensionalization of the BAP has been relatively straightforward (see Constantino, Chapter 29), but when to classify relatives of individuals with ASD as being "affected" with the BAP remains uncertain. The extent to which BAP status can confidently be assigned according to behavioral thresholds based on an interview or questionnaire scale is not yet known. Considering the utility of relatives' BAP status for genetic studies, as genetic influences may be different in singleton and multiplex families, as highlighted by our recent appreciation of the etiological role of de novo copy number variants (CNVs) in ASD, including parents in genetic studies is not likely to be a useful strategy in all families. This is further complicated by stoppage effects on reproduction, which results in families who might have had multiple children with a disability, deciding not to have further children following the diagnosis of one child (see Jones et al., 1988).

Considering the genetic and phenotypic heterogeneity of ASD, how best can relatives' BAP data be utilized in the search for susceptibility genes? While biological testing in individuals with ASD and those with the BAP is at an early stage, having a better understanding of brain structure, function, and neuronal connectivity, and potentially biological markers will help us understand the phenotypic spectrum (Bailey & Parr, 2003, and Lainhart & Lange, Chapter 28). Lainhart and Lange highlight the limited evidence supporting biological aspects of the BAP; the amount of research in this area is in stark contrast to that undertaken of the core ASD phenotypes. However, both fields suffer from a lack of replicated neurobiological findings. However, as the genetic liability to autism is likely to be expressed at a brain level, psychological (social cognition, executive functioning, face processing), neuroimaging (for example functional MRI or magnetoencephalography), and neurophysiological testing in combination may help us understand differences and similarities between the BAP and ASD, their genetics, and eventually the extent of environmental influences. Relatives (with and without the BAP) should be encouraged to donate brain tissue to repositories (such as the Autism Tissue Program) so that neuropathological studies can explore the cellular and molecular differences in the brains of individuals from across the behavioral spectrum.

Finally, translational research using BAP data has not been a priority to date, partly because the focus has been on characterization and methods. Researchers are starting to think about how relatives' BAP status might directly influence clinical practice, and here, we cite two examples: First, researchers could explore the use of parents' and other relatives' BAP data in genetic counseling for families who request information about the recurrence risk of ASD in their family. If parents with BAP were found to be at greater risk of having a second child with ASD, parental BAP status would allow us to give a revised (if still generic) recurrence risk of having another child with ASD. Such data could be used by parents to make better informed family planning decisions. Second, there are also nonmedical translational uses of BAP status. Parents are increasingly encouraged to deliver social communication and play-based intervention for their children; however, researchers are starting to explore whether parental BAP could potentially affect the delivery of parent-mediated intervention.

One hypothesis is that parents with BAP, who may find it difficult to vary their own social communication style, may find delivering effective intervention more challenging than parents without the BAP. Research evaluating the quality of intervention delivery will be necessary to ensure equal access to potentially effective intervention for all children.

Clinical Aspects

Clinicians in the 1980s and 1990s learned to diagnose autism; in the last decade, diagnosing children with Asperger's syndrome and Pervasive Developmental Disorder Not-Otherwise-Specified (PDD-NOS), has been a challenge. During the next decade, deciding who reaches ASD threshold according to DSM-V and ICD-11 will further challenge pediatricians, child psychiatrists, and their multidisciplinary teams. The majority of clinicians come across the BAP in the context of diagnostic assessments for children, adolescents, and adults. Since Kanner's first description of autism, there has been a shift in clinicians' and researchers' judgment about the threshold of the ASD behavioral phenotype, where that ends, and where the BAP begins. Over recent decades the use of diagnostic terminology has changed from an emphasis on a narrow definition of "core" autism to an acceptance of a broader concept of autism spectrum disorders. The increased awareness among families and professionals of autism, and a preparedness to accept a broader spectrum has contributed to the increase in the detected prevalence of ASD (see Chapter 6 by Fombonne et al.). Correspondingly, what we understand to be "BAP" is likely to change as research and clinical practice evolves further. For example, parents of children with ASD give descriptions of behavior from their own childhood that are compatible with a diagnosis of ASD using current classification. Some of these parents continue to have significant difficulties in adult life and may have developed adaptive strategies to manage some of their difficulties. In some circumstances, it may be appropriate to discuss the merits of referral to adult diagnostic services.

The revisions that result in the DSM-V and ICD-11 classifications may lead to a further widening of the autism spectrum; the implications for clinical and research practice are considerable. In that context, assessment tools such as ADI-R and ADOS were originally constructed for studies of children with autism. They can be used to evaluate clinical presentations across the differential diagnosis of PDD/ASD for individuals whose difficulties impair their functioning. However ADI-R and ADOS were not designed to evaluate individuals with qualitatively similar behavioral traits, but not ASD; such individuals who may have the BAP, are unlikely to reach threshold on either "gold standard" diagnostic measure. The challenge for clinicians and researchers alike is how best to identify and characterize this broader spectrum. Existing BAP measures have been developed to capture those qualitatively similar characteristics not identified by existing diagnostic tools (see Losh et al., Chapter 27, and Constantino, Chapter 29). For instance the Family History Interview was revised with the structure and scoring system of the ADI-R in mind, in order to allow true dimensionalization of the full ASD continuum (Parr et al. & the IMGSAC, in preparation). Whether these measures (or their subsequent revisions) are useful in clinical practice remains to be seen.

One striking aspect of the BAP chapters is the lack of research evidence about the clinical impact of the BAP across the lifespan. In our experience, BAP behaviors and traits may be associated with a certain set of relative strengths, but can also lead to significant functional impairments, including difficulties with social and marital relationships, and problems in the school or workplace. If ASD is indeed a continuum, functional impairment must be associated with the BAP, otherwise, by inference, all individuals with BAP characteristics and functional impairments would be classified as having ASD itself. For clinicians using future classification systems, the critical question will be whether individuals who present with subthreshold behaviors (BAP) and functional impairment should receive an ASD diagnosis. In our current clinical practice, using DSM-IV criteria, this is not the case, and when a clinical diagnosis is not possible due to subthreshold characteristics, clinicians are left to find a "form of words" to summarize the individual's ASD related impairment and potential support that might be beneficial (Parr & Le Couteur, clinical observations). One form of words used in our practice is: "John has social communication difficulties and behavioural rigidity, which are similar to, but less severe than those seen in children with ASD. Nevertheless, support would be beneficial in various settings, such as (to be specified by clinician)." For children who have a sibling with ASD, this wording is more acceptable to parents and service providers, as it can be placed in the context of ASD within the family. A greater challenge is faced by families in which there is no family history of ASD. The term "BAP" is mostly used in relation to families in which there is an index ASD case, is rarely understood outside clinical services, and is not useful to families who need to access support from education or social care services. We suggest also using the above descriptive wording and terminology when there is no ASD family history; however, in our experience accessing appropriate support is likely to be even more difficult in this context.

Evidence about whether we should provide "intervention" (for example support with social skills) to children and adults with BAP traits in order to ameliorate difficulties in their daily life is very limited. For very young children, intervention studies would be possible through identification of children with the BAP from at-risk study cohorts; such studies will increase our knowledge of whether the developmental trajectories of children with BAP can be altered by early intervention. Effective early intervention might reduce the risk of children developing additional behavior problems and comorbidities such as anxiety and mood disorder. Such evidence could be used to make a compelling case for intervention for young individuals with the BAP; however, as capacity to provide intervention to children with full-blown ASD remains limited in some countries this might not be prioritized. For older siblings of children with ASD, increased developmental surveillance may be appropriate, and intervention commenced when necessary; however, such a strategy would have considerable resource implications for families and local services. For adults with the BAP, social support in the workplace, including mentorship about effectively managing colleagues, may be helpful for some individuals (Parr & Le Couteur, clinical experience). Systematic evaluations of such workplace-based support are currently underway for adults with Asperger's syndrome (Howlin et al., 2005); whether such data are applicable to adults with BAP will require further evaluation. For young people and adults with ASD, bullying is encountered frequently, and is associated with low self-esteem and impacts on patient well-being. Individuals with the BAP may also be at increased risk of being bullied, thus awareness programs within educational settings should focus on a broader spectrum of children, rather than ASD alone.

Conclusions

Further understanding the BAP will have benefits to all. Clinicians, researchers, and families of individuals with ASD keenly await the findings of BAP research studies described in the chapters from this section during the next few years. As BAP research capacity continues to build, critical questions about genetics, developmental trajectories for infant siblings, and the impact of the BAP will become known. Whether the BAP holds the key to understanding the complex spectrum of ASD phenotypes remains to be seen.

REFERENCES

Bailey, A., Palferman, S., Heavey, L., & Le Couteur, A. (1998). Autism: The phenotype in relatives. *Journal of Child Psychology and Psychiatry and Allied Disciplines, 28*, 369–392.

Bailey A., & Parr J. (2003). Implications of the broader phenotype for concepts of autism. *Novartis Foundation Symposium, 251*, 26–35.

Bettelheim, B. (1967). *The empty fortress: Infantile autism and the birth of the self.* New York: Free Press.

Constantino, J. N., & Todd, R. D. (2003). Autistic traits in the general population: A twin study. *Archives of General Psychiatry, 60*, 524–530.

Howlin, P., Alcock, J., & Burkin, C. (2005). An 8-year follow-up of a specialist supported employment service for high-ability adults with autism or Asperger syndrome. *Autism, 9*, 533–549.

Jones, M. B., & Szatmari, P. (1988). Stoppage rules and genetic studies of autism. *Journal of Autism and Developmental Disorders, 18*, 31–40.

Rutter, M. (1970). Autistic children: infancy to adulthood. *Seminars in Psychiatry, 2*, 435–450.

Section V

Neurobiology

30 John L. R. Rubenstein

Developmental Neurobiology of Autism Spectrum Disorders

Points of Interest

- Many ASD susceptibility genes encode proteins that regulate synapse development and activity-dependent neural responses.
- Postulation of three additional mechanisms that may contribute to ASD:
  - Evolutionary-driven expansion of cerebrum and cerebellar size through signaling systems such as those activated by fibroblast growth factors.
  - Imbalance in the excitatory/inhibitory ratio in local and extended circuits.
  - The hormonal effects of the male genotype.

Autism Spectrum Disorders are extremely heterogeneous. While genetic etiologies are unquestionably involved (see below), one can't ignore epigenetic and environmental mechanisms, although the magnitude of their roles is uncertain. Since ASD have their onset in early childhood, all etiologies must interfere with brain development. In this perspective, I have addressed some of the neurodevelopmental mechanisms whose derailment may lead to ASD. In the introduction, I briefly review the neuroanatomical and genetic features of ASD, because they provide a context for the developmental models that I discuss later.

Neuroanatomical Landscape of ASD

ASD show no simple or single neuroanatomical phenotype that points to obvious neurodevelopment mechanisms. However, structural neuroimaging and histological studies (reviewed in Amaral et al., 2008; Bauman, et al., 2006; Carper et al., 2006) provide evidence for anatomical defects, at least in some individuals. These defects are the subject of another chapter in this volume; here I highlight a few points based on the reviews listed above.

1. Brain volume measurements show evidence for a modest increase in cerebrum growth (~10%; affecting both the white and grey matter) during early childhood (years 1–3), with the largest effect in the frontal lobes (dorsolateral and medial, but not orbital); the growth rate then decreases.
2. Cerebellar defects: cerebellar size increases (~7%) in children under age 5, but decreases in older patients; there are reduced numbers (~30% decrease) of Purkinje neurons in patients age 4–67 years.
3. Reduced cell size and increased density in the "limbic" areas (amygdala, hippocampus, entorhinal cortex, medial septal nucleus, mammillary body, and anterior cingulated; the increased density in the amygdala was not replicated by Amaral et al., 2008). There appears to be decreased dendrite complexity in the hippocampus. The dorsolateral prefrontal cortex also shows increased cell density, because of reduced space between cortical "minicolumns" in layer III (Casanova, 2006). There are decreased numbers of neurons in the amygdala and in the fusiform gyrus based on unbiased stereological studies in subjects without epilepsy. The earlier density findings were based on anatomical techniques open to bias and in brains of subjects most of whom also had epilepsy.
4. Increased amygdala size (15%) in 8- to 12-year-old ASD boys, followed by reduced postadolescent neuronal number (Amaral et al., 2008).

Genetic Landscape of Autism Spectrum Disorders (ASD)

The genetic landscape of Autism Spectrum Disorders (ASD) has several salient features that provide the boundary conditions for considering the breadth of its etiological mechanisms (Abrahams & Geschwind, 2008; Bonora et al., 2006; Sutcliffe, 2008; Walsh, Morrow, & Rubenstein, 2008):

1. ASD are heritable—concordance rates in monozygotic twins (~60–90%) are roughly 10-fold higher than in dizygotic twins and siblings, and first-degree relatives show a ~50-fold increased risk for autism compared to the population prevalence (1/150) (Bailey et al., 1995; Smalley et al., 1988).
2. ASD affect four times as many boys as girls. The mechanism(s) for this remains elusive; its elucidation could be fundamental to understanding the factors that predispose to ASD.
3. ASD are genetically heterogeneous. Defined mutations, genetic syndromes, and de novo copy number variation probably account for about 10–20% of cases; none of these causes individually accounts for more than 1–2% (Walsh, Morrow, & Rubenstein, 2008).
4. The genes currently linked to the ASD do not appear to selectively cause ASD. For instance, mutations of many genes cause mental retardation without ASD, and alleles of Neurexin1 and AHI1 are associated with ASD and schizophrenia (Ingason et al., 2007; Walsh et al., 2008).
5. Many cases of ASD may result from more complex genetic mechanisms, including co-inheritance of multiple alleles and/or epigenetic modifications (Freitag, 2007; Gupta & State, 2007).
6. Approximately 10% of sporadic cases of ASD are associated with de novo copy number variations in either single genes or sets of genes (Sebat et al., 2007).
7. Analysis of families of shared ancestry has identified recessive alleles of several genes that previously were unknown to cause ASD (Morrow et al., 2008).

Therefore, ASD, or at least risk for ASD, may be caused by a very large number of genes and alleles of those genes; the magnitude of that number is unknown. Gene variants that weaken the development and/or function of critical components of cognitive and emotional processing can alone, or in combination with other genes or environmental variables, increase the probability of ASD. While this poses a huge problem for understanding and treating ASD, it does suggest a paradigm for their conceptualization. The paradigm is to elucidate the developmental and neural pathways (anatomical, cellular and molecular) which tie together the known molecular/genetic defects causing ASD, and that cause neural systems defects that are postulated to contribute to ASD. Herein, I attempt to lay a foundation for this paradigm, by examining some of the pathways that appear to be disrupted by known causes of ASD.

Neural System Dysfunction: Localized Versus Distributed Developmental Defects

ASD are probably caused by alterations in the structural organization and/or function of neural systems that process social information, language, and sensorimotor integration. Neural system lesions can be localized or distributed (Rubenstein, 2006). A localized lesion that weakens or disables one component of a circuit can impede the function of the entire circuit, generating a behavioral phenotype. This phenotype can likewise be generated by defects in another component of the same circuit. Thus, related behavioral syndromes can be generated by a variety of anatomical defects.

Distributed lesions can be caused by defects that are common to many regions of a given neural system, or to multiple neural systems. For instance, mutation of genes that are broadly expressed, such as those that cause Fragile X mental retardation (FRAXA; FMR1), Rett syndrome (MeCP2), or tuberous sclerosis (TSC1 & 2), will disrupt neural function throughout the nervous system.

Developmental defects can alter the connectivity between brain regions; these can be distributed or localized. Distributed defects include general abnormalities in axon or dendrite growth, synaptogenesis, action potential initiation/propagation, or myelination. It is not known whether these types of abnormalities are found in autism, although there is evidence for connectivity defects from functional imaging studies (Kana et al., 2006; Geschwind & Levitt, 2007) and from mutations in or near genes that encode proteins implicated in the development of axon tracts: PCDH10 (protocadherin 10; Morrow et al., 2008), neurexins/neuroligins (Jamain et al., 2003; The Autism Genome Project Consortium, 2007), and Ig superfamily contactin proteins (Alarcón et al., 2008; Fernandez et al., 2008; Morrow et al., 2008; Roohi et al., 2008).

Currently, it is unclear whether or not there are localized connectivity defects in ASD. However, based on analyses of mouse mutants, there are many examples for genetic lesions that selectively alter development of specific brain connections, such as the corpus callosum (Paul et al., 2007), or connectivity of axons that comprise the internal capsule (Garel & Rubenstein, 2004; Molyneaux et al., 2007; Price et al., 2006; Uemura et al., 2007).

Localized lesions are exemplified by mutation of genes that are expressed in neurons that share common features, such as the Dlx1&2 homeobox transcription factors, which regulate the development of most forebrain GABAergic neurons, or TBR1, a T-box transcription factor that regulates the development of most early-born cortical glutamatergic neurons (Hevner et al., 2001). Likewise, localized lesions can be generated by mutations of genes that regulate the development of particular parts of the brain, such as Fgf17, which controls the size and character of the frontal cortex and cerebellum (Cholfin & Rubenstein, 2007), or Emx2, which controls the size and character of the occipital cortex (O'Leary et al., 2007). I will discuss some of these examples below, and speculate as to their relevance to some forms of ASD.

FGF Genes–Core Regulators That Pattern the Growth and Nature of the Frontal Cortex and Cerebellum

During evolution of the mammalian brain, perhaps the most salient morphological change has been the increased surface area of the neocortex with the concomitant increased laminar complexity of the late-born superficial layers (layers II, III, and IV) (Hill & Walsh, 2005; Bystron et al., 2008). The human brain is roughly three times larger than chimpanzee brain. In addition, the prefrontal cortex of humans and greater apes is disproportionately large compared to the rest of the neocortex of lesser apes, monkeys, and less complex mammals (Ongür & Price, 2000; Semendeferi et al., 2002). The prefrontal cortex is the center of cognition and decision-making.

Evolutionarily advantageous innovations can also come with liabilities, particularly if selective pressures have not reduced the frequency of design flaws. Thus, perhaps the benefits of the prefrontal cortex enlargement in humans have come with imperfections that underlie some of the etiologies of neuropsychiatric disorders including ASD. Therefore, insights into some forms of ASD may come from understanding the mechanisms that underlie prefrontal cortex development, including mechanisms that control the size, nature, and connections of its subdivisions.

The brain of ASD patients shows a trend for increased brain volume (and head circumference) apparently due to precocious growth during early postnatal life, followed by a deceleration at later stages (Piven et al., 1995; Carper et al., 2006; Amaral et al., 2008). Enlargements are greatest in the frontal lobes, although increases are also found in the temporal and parietal lobes. Within the frontal lobe, increases are seen in the dorsolateral and medial regions, but not the orbitofrontal cortex. Currently, prenatal and neonatal retrospective studies of ASD head circumference do not report enlargement (Hobbs et al., 2007).

The mechanisms for the postnatal brain enlargement are unknown, although insights may come from understanding the basic mechanisms that regulate cortical growth and patterning.

Over the last decade, fibroblast growth factor (FGF)–signaling has been shown to play a central role in regulating cortical regional properties and growth (Grove & Fukuchi-Shimogori, 2003; Sur & Rubenstein, 2005), and in particular promoting development of the frontal cortex (Garel et al., 2003; Storm et al, 2006; Cholfin & Rubenstein, 2007, 2008). These secreted proteins are produced by patterning centers embedded within the embryonic brain, including at the rostral end of the neural tube (Storm et al., 2006; Cholfin & Rubenstein, 2007, 2008). While Fgf8 has the major role in this process (Garel et al., 2003; Storm et al., 2006), other Fgf genes have smaller but perhaps more interesting roles. For instance Fgf17$^{-/-}$ null mutant mice are viable, but have a subtle reduction in their prefrontal cortex. The defect is selective to the dorsomedial prefrontal cortex, including the anterior cingulate cortex, while apparently not affecting the orbitofrontal cortex (Cholfin & Rubenstein, 2007; Cholfin & Rubenstein, 2008). Like Fgf8, Fgf17 also patterns the regions flanking the midbrain/hindbrain patterning center—including the tectum and the cerebellum (Xu et al., 2000). Thus, Fgf17$^{-/-}$ mice have defects in the prefrontal cortex, inferior colliculus, and cerebellum. In this regard, it is noteworthy that alterations in cerebellar vermis size are seen in ASD (Amaral et al., 2008; Bauman et al., 2006). While there is little understanding of the mechanism(s) for this, the En2 transcription factor, which lies downstream of FGF-signaling, may contribute to some forms of ASD (Benayed et al., 2005).

The behavior of Fgf17$^{-/-}$ mice shed light on the phenotype of individuals with prefrontal cortex, tectal, and cerebellar defects. They show deficiencies in assays of social recognition and interaction, as well as reductions in neonatal vocalizations (Scearce-Levie et al., 2008). At this point, we can't directly ascribe these phenotypes to specific neuroanatomical lesions, although is seems very likely that the dorsomedial prefrontal hypoplasia strongly contributes to the social deficits. However, given prefrontal-thalamic-cerebellar connectivity (Dum & Strick, 2006), one can not dismiss the behavioral importance of the cerebellar deficit. Furthermore, the hypoplasia of the inferior colliculus could contribute to the vocalization deficits. In any case, the key point is that lesion of a signal gene (Fgf17) disrupts functions of neural systems required for behaviors that are similar to those that are abnormal in ASD.

The analysis of mutations that reduce expression from Fgf8 and Fgf17 show that these genes promote growth of the cortex, and particularly of the dorsomedial frontal cortex—the region that shows the largest increase in size in ASD (Amaral et al., 2008). Thus, perhaps, there is overactivity of the FGF-signaling pathway in some forms of ASD. This could be due to several mechanisms, including increased expression of FGF ligands and/or increased signaling through the receptors and downstream transduction pathway. In this regard, mutation of several components that repress this pathway, including the PTEN phosphatase and TSC1/TSC2, are linked to ASD (see below). Of note, PTEN and TSC1/TSC2 regulate many steps in neural development and function, including synaptic signaling.

Dlx Genes—Gateway to Forebrain Inhibitory Neuron Development and Function

The Dlx homeobox transcription factors are broadly expressed prenatally in progenitors of forebrain GABAergic neurons, as well as postnatally in subsets of mature GABAergic neurons, such as in cortical interneurons (Cobos, Calcagnotto et al., 2005; Cobos et al., 2006). Mutations that simultaneously block the function of pairs of mouse Dlx genes disrupt development (particularly migration and differentiation) of most forebrain GABAergic neurons (including cortical interneurons, and projection neurons of the striatum, pallidum, central nucleus of the amygdala, and the reticular nucleus of the thalamus; Anderson, Eisenstat, Shi, & Rubenstein, 1997; Anderson, Qiu, et al., 1997; Long et al., 2008). Such mutations have the potential to disrupt function within these regions in addition to the communication between the neocortex, basal ganglia, and thalamus with obvious detrimental affects on cognitive and emotional functions (Fanselow & Poulos, 2005; Yin & Knowlton, 2006; LeDoux, 2007).

Whereas mice lacking pairs of Dlx genes die neonatally, mice lacking Dlx1 are viable. However, after ~1 month, there is a selective degeneration of a subset of cortical interneurons that results in epilepsy (Cobos, Calcagnotto et al., 2005). Thus, $Dlx1^{-/-}$ mutants have an age-dependent onset of seizures analogous to a subset of ASD patients who have late onset of epilepsy (Levisohn, 2007). Furthermore, Dlx genes regulate craniofacial morphogenesis, including the ossicles (Qiu et al., 1995; Jeong et al., 2008). As a result, Dlx1 mutants have reduced hearing acuity (Polley et al., 2006), which has obvious implications for auditory comprehension, but also suggests that analysis of craniofacial morphology may provide important insights into the etiologies of ASD.

While mutations in the Dlx2 and Dlx5 genes have been detected in some autistic individuals, it is unknown whether these contribute to the development of ASD (Hamilton et al., 2005), or comorbid symptoms such as epilepsy. Despite the lack of firm evidence implicating Dlx mutations genes in ASD susceptibility, I suggest that examining the function of the Dlx genes is illustrative of a genetic pathway whose dysfunction could predispose to ASD through defects in forebrain inhibitory neurons (Rubenstein & Merzenich, 2003). This could be through Dlx function in the neocortex and/or basal ganglia (including the amygdala). For instance, in the cortex, reduced Dlx dosage (function) would weaken inhibitory tone in the cortex, thereby increasing the ratio of excitation/inhibition, which would decrease the signal-to-noise ratio, altering neural processing and predisposing to epilepsy. In the basal ganglia, Dlx mutations could alter development of the striatum and pallidum—key components of the cortico–basal ganglia–thalamic circuit that is important in controlling Pavlovian (appetitve) learning, habit learning, and goal directed behaviors (Yin & Knowlton, 2006). Thus, understanding the genetic circuits downstream of the Dlx genes will identify genes required for forebrain inhibitory neuronal function—perhaps many of these, alone or in combination with other genes—are susceptibility factors for ASD.

Currently, the Dlx genes are known to (directly or indirectly) regulate the expression of large numbers of genes that are implicated in GABAergic neuronal development. For example, there is evidence that the Arx transcription factor is downstream of Dlx (Cobos, Broccoli, & Rubenstein, 2005b; Colasante et al., 2008; Long et al., 2009). Mutation of human Arx can cause epilepsy and autism, and in mice results in defects in cortical interneuron development (Colombo et al., 2007). Dlx genes also promote the expression of glutamic acid decarboxylase and vesicular GABA transporter (Stuhmer et al., 2002; Long et al., in press), and thereby will have profound functions in regulating inhibitory tone. Indeed, reduced Dlx dosage is associated with reduced synapse formation and reduced expression of neurexin3, a neuroligin ligand (Cobos, Long, & Rubenstein, unpublished). Dlx repression of the Pak3 kinase is implicated in regulating neurite growth (Cobos et al., 2007); and human Pak3 mutants have mental retardation (van Galen & Ramakers, 2005). Finally, Dlx genes promote the balance of neuronal vs. oligodendrocyte production, and thereby reduced Dlx function can reduce the number of GABAergic neurons, while perhaps altering the extent of myelination (Petryniak et al., 2007).

In sum, the Dlx genes can regulate the development and function of a single generic class of neurons: forebrain inhibitory neurons (e.g., interneurons in the cortex, and projection neurons in the basal ganglia). As such, alterations in the function of the Dlx genes, or of genes downstream of them, can weaken forebrain inhibitory tone, and thereby impact neural systems that underlie cognition. The future will determine to what extent alterations in the Dlx-regulated genetic network contribute to ASD susceptibility.

Detection of Salient Synaptic Information: Signal/Noise Processing

Molecular lesions that alter the development and/or function of excitatory, inhibitory, and neuromodulatory synapses can disrupt neural systems that process cognition and social behaviors. For instance, mutations that alter the balance of excitatory and inhibitory synaptic function may impede the ability to detect salient sensory signals above ambient noise, affect maturation of cortical regions (Hensch, 2005), and have been postulated to contribute to some forms of ASD (Rubenstein & Merzenich, 2003). For instance, selective interneuron apoptosis leads to epilepsy in $Dlx1^{-/-}$ mutants (Cobos, Calcagnotto et al., 2005).

The high prevalence of epilepsy in ASD (compared with its general-population prevalence) suggests an increase in the excitatory/inhibitory balance in ASD. However, current evidence from some mouse models of ASD provides evidence for decreased excitatory/inhibitory balance. For instance, female mice lacking one copy of MeCP2 (the gene responsible for Rett syndrome) show reduced synaptic excitation (Dani et al., 2005). Likewise, mice expressing a human allele of neuroligin3 found in an autistic individual, showed increased synaptic inhibition (Tabuchi et al., 2007). Nevertheless, one would expect a decreased signal-to-noise ratio (reduced signal salience) in the cortical/hippocampal circuits of these mutants. Therefore, there is good reason to continue exploring the model that disruption of excitatory/inhibitory balance, through multiple molecular/cellular mechanisms, contributes to ASD. Whether or not reduced synaptic excitation can evolve into epilepsy remains to be seen.

Male/Female Ratio

One of the great mysteries of ASD, and other neuropsychiatric disorders of childhood, such as attention deficit disorder, is the roughly 4:1 ratio of affected boys to girls. This could arise because maleness may bias cognitive style, emotional response, and instinctual behavior (Baron-Cohen et al., 2005; see Chapter 18 this book). It is this author's unsubstantiated opinion that some males are more likely to have a highly focused cognitive style that is less subject to emotional influences, and that males are less interested in verbal communication. This idea is akin to the Extreme Male Brain Model of Autism (Baron-Cohen et al., 2005). This bias may sensitize the male brain toward ASD, to the effects of certain alleles, or to environmental factors.

If this conception were correct, how would this male cognitive and behavioral style arise? While there are several ASD-susceptibility genes on the X chromosome (e.g., Arx, Fmr1, MeCP2, Neuroligin3 and 4), this far from accounts for the increased male prevalence of ASD. Thus, other models should be considered. Perhaps the simplest model is that male:female hormonal differences, such as brain concentrations of androgens and estrogens, account for bias (androgens are converted to estrogens in the brain via aromatase; males have higher estrogen concentrations). These hormones are potent regulators of behavior. Furthermore, exposure to them during various stages of brain development has multiple effects, including regulating cell survival (which modulates the number of neurons in particular nuclei: sexually dimorphic nucleus of the preoptic area, and the anteroventral periventricular nucleus), and regulating neuronal connectivity and function (McCarthy, 2008). For instance, estrogens can regulate synapse numbers through controlling the numbers of dendritic spines in some hypothalamic nuclei (ventromedial nucleus and the arcuate nucleus). In addition, estrogens appear to regulate the expression of glutamic acid decarboxylase in the arcuate nucleus of the hypothalamus, and thus can modulate GABA signaling (McCarthy, 2008). Estrogens also can modulate whether GABA is excitatory or inhibitory, via expression of the potassium-chloride cotransporter KCC2 (Galanopoulou, 2005). Finally, androgens can predispose males to GABA-mediated excitoxicity (Nunez & McCarthy, 2008). Therefore, sex steroids could modulate excitatory/inhibitory balance, which could sensitive the male brain to ASD. Perhaps one should consider attempting to devise a therapy for ASD that modulates sex-steroid signaling in males.

Genetic Susceptibility Factors

In the following sections I discuss specific genetic lesions that predispose to ASD, and consider, when feasible, how their functions fit within the developmental models of ASD discussed above. Many of these lesions alter synaptic function and signaling (Zoghbi, 2003; Hong et al., 2005; Walsh, Morrow, & Rubenstein, 2008).

Molecular Pathways Linking Synaptic and Nonsynaptic Signals with Changes in Gene Expression and Protein Synthesis

Tuberous Sclerosis (TSC1&2) and PTEN

Children with TSC (autosomal dominant) have greatly increased rates of autism (25–50%), epilepsy, and mental retardation (Wiznitzer, 2004). TSC1 (hamartin, 9q34) and TSC2 (tuberin, 16p13) encode GTPase-activating proteins that inhibit the activity of the small G-protein Rheb. TSC1/TSC2 are tumor suppressors, because they repress growth responses through reducing activity of mTOR kinase (Inoki et al., 2005). mTOR promotes protein synthesis and other processes that increase cell growth.

TSC1/TSC2 are integral regulators of signal-transduction cascades downstream of signaling pathways for signals that activate receptor tyrosine kinases such as EGFs, FGFs, IGFs, and neurotrophins (Inoki et al., 2005). These signals activate a family of phosphatidylinositol lipid kinases (phosphatidylinositol-3 kinases, PI3K) that in turn activate the serine-threonine kinase AKT, which then represses TSC1/TSC2 (Inoki et al., 2005). TSC1/TSC2 are also regulated by intracellular amino acid concentration and by the ATP/AMP ratio—the end product of this regulation is to promote appropriate levels of protein synthesis and cell size (Inoki et al., 2005).

While TSC patients develop focal CNS lesions (tubers), it is likely that the general function of TSC1&2 in most/all neurons underlies the ASD symptoms. For example, reduced TSC dosage in hippocampal pyramidal neurons results in increased size of the cell body and dendritic spines (Tavazoie et al., 2005)—this is intriguing given the increased size of the brain in some children with autism.

Further clues that implicate this signaling cascade in ASD come from the observation that some patients with mutations in the phosphatidylinositol phosphatase (PTEN; 10q23.31) have ASD with macrocephaly (Butler et al., 2005). PTEN reduces activity of the PI3K pathway through dephosphorylation of phosphatidylinositol-tris-phosphate. Mice lacking CNS function of PTEN have increased signaling through the AKT, TSC, and mTOR pathway (Kwon et al., 2006). These mutants have enlarged brains that are associated with increased dendritic and axonal arbors and increased dendritic spines and synapses. PTEN mutant mice also exhibit abnormal social behavior, further implicating this signaling pathway in autism (Kwon et al., 2006).

Neurofibromatosis Type I (NF1)

Neurofibromin, encoded by the Neurofibromatosis type I (NF1) gene (chr17: 26470278–26670503), regulates many signaling pathways, including those downstream of adenylate cyclase, AKT-mTOR, and Ras-GTPase. As a result, patients can have learning deficits and ASD (Marui et al., 2004). Mouse mutants recapitulate many of these features, and have developmental defects including abnormal patterning of the somatosensory cortex (Lush et al., 2008).

MET

MET encodes a receptor tyrosine kinase (7q31), which is an oncogene that mediates hepatocyte growth factor (HGF)/scatter factor signaling. MET has an important role in neuronal migration in the forebrain and cerebellum, as well as immune and gastrointestinal function. Mouse mutants have reduced cortical interneurons and a hypoplastic cerebellum. Campbell et al. (2006) identified a common functional allele in the promoter region of the MET gene that is associated with ASD.

Control of Translation and Protein Stability

Fragile X (FRAXA; FMR1)

Mutations that reduce expression (usually through CGG triplet-expansion) of this X-linked gene (Xq27.3) cause mental retardation, and these boys often have ASD (Belmonte & Bourgeron, 2006). Dendrites in FMR1 mutant humans and mice have an immature morphology (too long and thin). This phenotype may result from the observation that FMR1 encodes an RNA-binding protein whose functions includes translation regulation in dendrites. There is evidence that activation of metabotropic glutamate receptors leads to FMR1-regulated protein synthesis in dendrites—including production of proteins, such as PSD-95, that participate in excitatory synaptic transmission (Todd et al., 2003; Bear et al., 2004). Thus, FMR1 may function in part through transducing excitatory synaptic signals into changes in the protein constituents that modify synaptic function and structure. Indeed, reducing mGluR5 dosage partially rescues the phenotype of FMR1 mouse mutants (Dölen et al., 2007).

UBE3A

UBE3A (chr15: 23133489–23204888) is an imprinted gene that encodes an E6-associated protein (E6-AP) that contains an E3 ubiquitin ligase possessing two independent functions: a transcriptional coactivation and an ubiquitin-protein ligase activity, that can regulate the degradation of the transcriptional complexes (Ramamoorthy & Nawaz, 2008). Loss of UBE3A function causes Angelman's syndrome, often characterized by autistic features (Peters et al., 2004). UBE3A is also found at synapses, and maternal deficiency results in abnormal dendritic morphology (Dindot et al., 2008).

Axon and Synapse Formation/Function

Neuroligins (NLGN3 and NLGN4)

Neuroligins encode plasma membrane proteins that are implicated in regulating synapse development through binding neurexin proteins (Varoqueaux et al., 2006). There is evidence that specific combinations and splice forms of neuroligin/neurexin proteins can specify whether an excitatory or an inhibitory synapse will form (Chih et al., 2006). Mutations in two X-linked neuroligins (NLGN3 and NLGN4; Xq13 and Xp22.33, respectively) have been found in rare cases of autism (Jamain et al., 2003). Furthermore, a de novo deletion in neurexin1 (NRX1) has been identified in a pair of affected siblings (Autism Genome Project Consortium, 2007).

Mice with a loss-of-function mutation in the murine NLGN4 ortholog Nlgn4, exhibit deficits in reciprocal social interactions and communication (Jamain et al., 2008). Furthermore, mice engineered to express a neuroligin-3 mutation implicated in ASD have increased inhibitory synaptic transmission (Tabuchi et al., 2007).

Protocadherin 10 (PCDH10)

Protocadherin 10 (OL-Protocadherin) (4q28) encodes a cadherin superfamily protein that is essential for pathfinding of striatal, thalamocortical, and corticothalamic axons through the ventral telencephalon (Uemura et al., 2007). There is a >300 kb deletion near PCDH10 in an individual with ASD from a consanguinous family—the deletion is postulated to alter its expression (Morrow et al., 2008).

Ig-Superfamily Cell Adhesion Proteins: Contactin 3 & 4 (CNTN3 & 4) and CNTNAP2

Genetic variations, including deletions, have been mapped near to the CNTN members of the Immunoglobulin superfamily: CNTN3 (BIG-1; chr3: 74394412–74653033), CNTN4 (chr3: 2908921–3073040), and CNTNAP2 (chr7: 147667553–147745775) (Alarcón et al., 2008; Fernandez et al., 2008; Morrow et al., 2008; Roohi et al., 2008). The encoded axonal plasma membrane proteins are part of a family known to engage in cell adhesion (Yoshihara et al., 1995), and are implicated in axon pathfinding (Kaneko-Goto et al., 2008).

SHANK3 (ProSAP2)

SHANK3 (22q13.3) encodes a protein associated with the postsynaptic density of excitatory synapses, and can promote dendritic spine maturation. Rare mis-sense mutations in SHANK3 have been identified in autistic individuals (Moessner et al., 2007). Furthermore this region of chromosome 22 is a site of recurrent deletions in ASD (Sebat et al., 2007). Bourgeron and colleagues propose that a protein complex that includes SHANK3 and Neuroligins3&4 participates in the assembly of postsynaptic structures.

Neurotransmitters/Neuromodulators

Oxytocin and Vasopressin Receptors (OXTR; AVPR1a)

Oxytocin and vasopressin peptides are neuromodulators expressed by neurons in the hypothalamus and the amygdala. Axons from these neurons selectively ramify within circuits that are implicated in regulating social behaviors; these neuropeptides have demonstrated functions in mediating social behaviors (Young et al., 2005). There is growing evidence that the receptors for oxytocin (OXTR; 3p25–p26) and arginine vasopressin 1a (AVPR1a; 12q14–15) are associated with ASD (Wu et al., 2005; Yirmiya et al., 2006).

Serotonin Transporter (SLC6A4)

Serotonin has potent effects on multiple behavioral dimensions and developmental processes. Serum serotonin levels are increased in a subset of autistic individuals. Although this is not a specific diagnostic finding, it increases the potential importance that some alleles of the serotonin transporter gene (SLC6A4, SERT; 17q11.2) are associated with ASD (Sutcliffe et al., 2005; Brune et al., 2007).

Ion Channels

Calcium Channels (CACNA1C; CACNA1H; SCN1A; SCN2A)

Mis-sense mutations in the L-type (CACNA1C, Cav1.2; 12p13.3) and the T-type (CACNA1H, Cav3.2) calcium channels have been identified in rare cases of ASD (Splawski et al., 2004, 2006).

Sodium Channels (SCN1A; SCN2A)

Rare mis-sense mutations have been identified in two voltage-gated sodium channel genes (SCN1A: 2q24;SCN2A; 2q23–q24.3) (Weiss et al., 2003). A deletion near SCN7A (chr2: 166969785–167051724) has also been identified in a recessive form of ASD (Morrow et al., 2008).

Sodium/Hydrogen Exchanger (NHE9)

NHE9 (also known as SLC9A9; chr3: 144466754–145049979) encodes a (Na^+, K^+)/H^+ exchanger disrupted in a pedigree with a developmental neuropsychiatric disorder and mild mental retardation (de Silva et al., 2003). Likewise, a deletion near NHE9 has been identified in a recessive form of ASD (Morrow et al., 2008). Of note, mutations of NHE6, a related transporter, cause X-linked mental retardation and a phenotype mimicking Angelman's syndrome (Gilfillan et al., 2008).

Metabolic Genes

Phenylalanine Hydroxylase (PAH)

Historically, the elucidation that autism can be caused by phenylketonuria (hyperphenylalaninemia), was one of the turning points in establishing the biological etiology of autism (Cohen et al., 2005). There are several hundred alleles of phenylalanine hydroxylase (12q23.2) (www.pahdb.mcgill.ca), many of which, in the homozygous phenotype, can cause phenylketonuria. The rarity of ASD caused by phenylketonuria, may be attributed to the fact that neonatal screening and dietary treatment are now commonplace.

D7-Dehydrocholesterol Reductase Smith-Lemli-Opitz (SLO)

The SLO gene encodes D7-dehydrocholesterol reductase (DHCR7; 11q12–q13); loss-of-function mutations cause accumulation of D7-dehydrocholesterol. This recessive disorder has broad developmental affects, including ASD in a high proportion of patients (Sikora et al., 2006). While SLO is a rare cause of autism, it demonstrates that disruption of cholesterol metabolism, and related pathways, need to be considered as etiologic mechanisms.

Regulation of Gene Expression

Rett Syndrome (MeCP2)

Girls with Rett syndrome commonly exhibit ASD symptoms; males generally die prenatally. This syndrome is due to loss-of-function mutations of the methyl-CpG-binding protein 2 (MeCP2; Xq28) (Moretti & Zoghbi, 2006). Some mutations result in milder symptoms that include ASD in both boys and girls. MeCP2 is a nuclear protein that binds to methylated CpG dinucleotides. It recruits a corepressor complex that is implicated in transcriptional repression. The brain of mouse MeCP2 mutants shows subtle increases and decreases in the expression of large numbers of genes; there is now evidence that MeCP2 is both a transcriptional activator and repressor (Chahrour et al., 2008). Among the genes that show altered expression include ubiquitin protein ligase E3A (UBE3A) and b3 GABA A receptor (Gabrb3) (LaSalle, 2007); these are imprinted genes in the Angelman's disease locus—inheritance of a maternal duplication of this region (15q11.2–q13) is the most commonly associated chromosomal abnormality found in ASD (Schanen, 2006). There is evidence that MeCP2 mutants also showed increased Dlx5 expression (Horike et al., 2005; Miyano et al., 2008); however, this finding was not replicated by Schüle et al. (2007).

MeCP2's association with ASD alludes to the possibility that epigenetic modifications of chromatin (e.g., cytosine methylation and histone methylation/acetylation) and parent of origin effects (imprinting) may have broader roles in contributing to ASD (Schanen, 2006).

Arx

Arx encodes a homeobox transcription factor (chrX: 24931732–24943986); it is expressed in cortical progenitors and subcortical differentiating GABAergic neurons, including those that become cortical interneurons. Mice lacking this gene have defects in several aspects of telencephalic development, including differentiation of cortical interneurons (Kitamura et al., 2002; Colombo et al., 2007). The Dlx genes promote their expression (Cobos et al., 2005). Affected children often have severe epilepsy (infantile spasms) and severe mental retardation, but mild cases have been identified with ASD (Wallerstein et al., 2008), although Arx mutations are very rare in ASD (Chaste et al., 2007).

RNF8, Encoding a RING Finger Protein

RNF8 (chr6: 37429726–37470492) encodes a RING finger ubiquitin ligase and transcriptional coactivator of RXR-alpha (Takano et al., 2004). Thus, like UBE3A, it can regulate the activity of nuclear steroid receptors (see above). Furthermore, RNF8 can transduce DNA-damage signals via histone ubiquitylation and checkpoint protein assembly (Huen et al., 2007). Morrow et al. (2008) discovered a deletion near RNF8 in a recessive form of ASD.

Engrailed2 (EN2)

Alleles of the En2 homeobox transcription factor (7q36), which regulates cerebellum development, has been associated with ASD (Benayed et al., 2005). Mouse mutants exhibit social deficits (Cheh et al., 2006). EN2 is downstream of FGF-signaling from the midbrain/hindbrain patterning center (Liu & Joyner, 2001).

Distal-less 2 and 5 (Dlx2 and Dlx5)

Mis-sense mutations of the Dlx2 (2q31.1) and Dlx5 (7q21.3) homeobox transcription factors have been identified in individuals with ASD (Hamilton et al., 2005). As discussed above, these genes regulate development of forebrain GABAergic neurons and may be dysregulated in Rett syndrome (see above).

Genes of Unknown Function

Joubert Syndrome: Abelson's Helper Integration 1 Gene (AHI1)

Joubert syndrome is characterized by partial or complete agenesis of the cerebellar vermis; ~25% of these patients have autistic disorder. In a subset of Joubert patients, mutations have been found in the Abelson's helper integration 1 gene (AHI1; chr6: 135646805–135860596), encoding a protein of unknown function (Alvarez-Retuerto et al., 2008). These patients may also show deficits in axon pathfinding, based on defects in the decussation of the pyramidal tract (Ferland et al., 2004). Of note, AHI1 is also implicated in schizophrenia (Ingason et al., 2007).

Conclusion

The rapidly growing list of genes and alleles that contribute to ASD susceptibility suggests that many more genes will be discovered that are involved in this set of disorders. While this complexity is unsettling in terms of understanding and treating autism spectrum disorders, I hope that this review has been useful in suggesting some of the emerging themes of molecular and neural pathways/systems that underlie ASD.

Challenges and Future Directions

- Identify the mechanisms that promote growth, regional pattern formation, and connectivity of the cerebral cortex, and particularly of the prefrontal cortex, including those mechanisms that underlie the evolution of the human prefrontal cortex.
- Identify the mechanisms that regulate excitatory/inhibitory balance within local cortical circuits, as well as within extended circuited such as the cortical-striatal-thalamic loop.
- Identify mechanisms that underlie the increased ASD susceptibility of males.

SUGGESTED READINGS

Cholfin, J. A., & Rubenstein, J. L. (2007). Patterning of frontal cortex subdivisions by Fgf17. *Proceedings of the National Academy of Sciences of the United States of America, 104*(18), 7652–7657.

Rubenstein, J. L. R., & Merzenich, M. M. (2003). Model of autism: Increased ratio of excitation/inhibition in key neural systems. *Genes, Brain, and Behavior, 2,* 255–267.

Walsh C. A., Morrow E. M., & Rubenstein J. L. R. (2008). Autism and brain development. *Cell, 135*(3), 396–400.

REFERENCES

Abrahams, B. S., & Geschwind, D. H. (2008). Advances in autism genetics: On the threshold of a new neurobiology. *Nature Reviews Genetics, 9*(5), 341–355.

Alarcón, M., Abrahams, B. S., Stone, J. L., Duvall, J. A., Perederiy, J. V., Bomar, J. M., et al. (2008). Linkage, association, and gene-expression analyses identify CNTNAP2 as an autism-susceptibility gene. *American Journal of Human Genetics, 82*(1), 150–159.

Alvarez Retuerto, A. I., Cantor, R. M., Gleeson, J. G., Ustaszewska, A., Schackwitz, W. S., Pennacchio, L. A., et al. (2008). Association of common variants in the Joubert syndrome gene (AHI1) with autism. *Human Molecular Genetics, 17*(24), 3887–3896.

Amaral, D. G., Schumann, C. M., & Nordahl, C. W. (2008). Neuroanatomy of autism. *Trends in Neurosciences, 31*(3), 137–145.

Anderson, S. A., Eisenstat, D. D., Shi, L., & Rubenstein, J. L. (1997). Interneuron migration from basal forebrain to neocortex: Dependence on Dlx genes. *Science (New York, N.Y.), 278*(5337), 474–476.

Anderson, S. A., Qiu, M., Bulfone, A., Eisenstat, D. D., Meneses, J., Pedersen, R., et al. (1997). Mutations of the homeobox genes Dlx-1 and Dlx-2 disrupt the striatal subventricular zone and differentiation of late born striatal neurons. *Neuron, 19*(1), 27–37.

Autism Genome Project Consortium. (2007). Mapping autism risk loci using genetic linkage and chromosomal rearrangements. *Nature Genetics, 39*(3), 319–328.

Bauman, M. L., Anderson, G., Perry, E., & Ray, M. (2006). Neuroanatomical and neurochemical studies of the autistic brain: current thought and future directions. In S. O. Moldin & J. L. R. Rubenstein (Eds.), *Understanding autism: From basic neuroscience to treatment* (pp. 303–322). New York: CRC.

Baron-Cohen, S., Knickmeyer, R. C., & Belmonte, M. K. (2005). Sex differences in the brain: Implications for explaining autism. *Science (New York, N.Y.), 310*(5749), 819–823.

Bailey, A., Le Couteur, A., Gottesman, I., Bolton, P., Simonoff, E., Yuzda, E., et al. (1995). Autism as a strongly genetic disorder: Evidence from a British twin study. *Psychological Medicine, 25*(1), 63–77.

Bear, M. F., Huber, K. M., & Warren, S. T. (2004). The mGluR theory of fragile X mental retardation. *Trends in Neurosciences, 27*(7), 370–377.

Belmonte, M. K., & Bourgeron, T. (2006). Fragile X syndrome and autism at the intersection of genetic and neural networks. *Nature Neuroscience, 9*(10), 1221–1225.

Benayed, R., Gharani, N., Rossman, I., Mancuso, V., Lazar, G., Kamdar, S., et al. (2005). Support for the homeobox transcription factor gene ENGRAILED 2 as an autism spectrum disorder susceptibility locus. *American Journal of Human Genetics, 77*(5), 851–868.

Boccone, L., Dessi, V., Zappu, A., Piga, S., Piludu, M. B., Rais, M., et al. (2006). Bannayan-Riley-Ruvalcaba syndrome with reactive nodular lymphoid hyperplasia and autism and a PTEN mutation. *American Journal of Medical Genetics. Part A, 140*(18), 1965–1969.

Bonora, E., Lamb, J. A., Barnby, G., Bailey, A. J., & Monoco, A. P. (2006). Genetic basis of autism. In S. O. Moldin & J. L. R. Rubenstein (Eds.), *Understanding autism: From basic neuroscience to treatment* (pp. 49–74). New York: CRC.

Brune, C. W., Kim, S. J., Salt, J., Leventhal, B. L., Lord, C., & Cook, E. H., Jr. (2007). 5-HTTLPR genotype-specific phenotype in children and adolescents with autism. *American Journal of Psychiatry, 163*(12), 2148–2156.

Buxhoeveden, D. P., Semendeferi, K., Buckwalter, J., Schenker, N., Switzer, R., & Courchesne, E. (2006). Reduced minicolumns in the frontal cortex of patients with autism. *Neuropathology and Applied Neurobiology, 32*(5), 483–491.

Butler, M. G., Dasouki, M. J., Zhou, X. P., Talebizadeh, Z., Brown, M, Takahashi T. N., et al. (2005). Subset of individuals with autism spectrum disorders and extreme macrocephaly associated with germline PTEN tumour suppressor gene mutations. *Journal of Medical Genetics, 42*(4), 318–321.

Bystron, I., Bzlakemore, C., & Rakic, P. (2008). Development of the human cerebral cortex: Boulder Committee revisited. *Nature Reviews Neuroscience, 9*(2), 110–122.

Campbell, D. B., Sutcliffe, J. S., Ebert, P. J., Militerni, R., Bravaccio, C., Trillo, S., et al. (2006). A genetic variant that disrupts MET transcription is associated with autism. *Proceedings of the National Academy of Sciences of the United States of America, 103*(45), 16834–16839.

Carper, R. A., Wideman, G. M., & Courchesne, E. (2006). Structural neuroimaging. In S. O. Moldin & J. L. R. Rubenstein (Eds.), *Understanding autism: From basic neuroscience to treatment* (pp. 349–377). New York: CRC.

Casanova, M. F. (2006). Neuropathological and genetic findings in autism: The significance of a putative minicolumnopathy. *Neuroscientist, 12*(5), 435–441.

Chahrour, M., Jung, S. Y., Shaw, C., Zhou, X., Wong, S. T., Qin, J., et al. (2008). MeCP2, a key contributor to neurological disease, activates and represses transcription. *Science (New York, N.Y.), 320*(5880), 1224–1229.

Chaste, P., Nygren, G., Anckarsäter, H., Råstam, M., Coleman, M., Leboyer, M., et al. (2007). Mutation screening of the ARX gene in patients with autism. *American Journal of Medical Genetics. Part B, Neuropsychiatric Genetics, 144B*(2), 228–230.

Cheh, M. A., Millonig, J. H., Roselli, L. M., Ming, X., Jacobsen, E., Kamdar, S., et al. (2006). En2 knockout mice display neurobehavioral and neurochemical alterations relevant to autism spectrum disorder. *Brain Research, 1116*(1), 166–176.

Chez, M. G., Chang, M., Krasne, V., Coughlan, C., Kominsky, M., & Schwartz, A. (2006). Frequency of epileptiform EEG abnormalities in a sequential screening of autistic patients with no known clinical epilepsy from 1996 to 2005. *Epilepsy and Behavior: E&B, 8*(1), 267–271.

Chih, B., Gollan, L., & Scheiffele, P. (2006). Alternative splicing controls selective trans-synaptic interactions of the neuroligin-neurexin complex. *Neuron, 51*(2), 171–178.

Cholfin, J. A., & Rubenstein, J. L. (2007). Patterning of frontal cortex subdivisions by Fgf17. *Proceedings of the National Academy of Sciences of the United States of America, 104*(18), 7652–7657.

Cholfin, J. A., & Rubenstein, J. L. (2008). Frontal cortex subdivision patterning is coordinately regulated by Fgf8, Fgf17, and Emx2. *Journal of Comparative Neurology, 509*(2), 144–155.

Cobos, I., Borello, U., & Rubenstein, J. L. (2007). Dlx transcription factors promote migration through repression of axon and dendrite growth. *Neuron, 54*(6), 873–888.

Cobos, I., Broccoli, V., & Rubenstein, J. L. R. (2005). The vertebrate ortholog of *Aristaless* is regulated by *Dlx* genes in the developing forebrain. *Journal of Comparative Neurology, 483*(3), 292–303.

Cobos, I., Calcagnotto, M. E., Vilaythong, A. J., Thwin, M. T., Noebels, J. L., Baraban, S. C., et al. (2005). Mice lacking Dlx1 show subtype-specific loss of interneurons, reduced inhibition, and epilepsy. *Nature Neuroscience, 8*(8), 1059–1068.

Cobos, I., Long, J. E., Thwin, M. T., & Rubenstein, J. L. (2006). Cellular patterns of transcription factor expression in developing cortical interneurons. *Cerebral Cortex, 16*(Suppl 1), i82–i88.

Cohen, D., Pichard, N., Tordjman, S., Baumann, C., Burglen, L., Excoffier, E., et al. (2005). Specific genetic disorders and autism: Clinical contribution towards their identification. *Journal of Autism and Developmental Disorders, 35*(1), 103–116.

Colasante, G, Collombat, P., Raimondi, V., Bonanomi, D., Ferrai, C., Maira, M., et al. (2008). Arx is a direct target of Dlx2 and thereby contributes to the tangential migration of GABAergic interneurons. *Journal of Neuroscience, 28*(42), 10674–10686.

Colombo, E., Collombat, P., Colasante, G., Bianchi, M., Long, J., Mansouri, A., et al. (2007). Inactivation of Arx, the murine ortholog of the X-linked lissencephaly with ambiguous genitalia gene, leads to severe disorganization of the ventral telencephalon with impaired neuronal migration and differentiation. *Journal of Neuroscience, 27*(17), 4786–4798.

Courchesne, E., Carper, R., & Akshoomoff, N. (2003). Evidence of brain overgrowth in the first year of life in autism. *JAMA: The journal of the American Medical Association, 290*(3), 337–344.

Dani, V. S., Chang, Q., Maffei, A., Turrigiano, G. G., Jaenisch, R., & Nelson, S. B. (2005). Reduced cortical activity due to a shift in the balance between excitation and inhibition in a mouse model of Rett syndrome. *Proceedings of the National Academy of Sciences of the United States of America, 102*(35), 12560–12565.

de Silva, M. G., Elliott, K., Dahl, H. H., Fitzpatrick, E., Wilcox, S., Delatycki, M., et al. (2003). Disruption of a novel member of a sodium/hydrogen exchanger family and DOCK3 is associated with an attention deficit hyperactivity disorder-like phenotype. *Journal of Medical Genetics, 40*(10), 733–740.

Dindot, S. V., Antalffy, B. A., Bhattacharjee, M. B., & Beaudet, A. L. (2008). The Angelman syndrome ubiquitin ligase localizes to the synapse and nucleus, and maternal deficiency results in abnormal dendritic spine morphology. *Human Molecular Genetics, 17*(1), 111–118.

Dölen, G, Osterweil, E., Rao, B. S., Smith, G. B., Auerbach, B. D., Chattarji, S., et al. (2007). Correction of fragile X syndrome in mice. *Neuron, 56*(6), 955–962.

Dum, R. P., & Strick, P. L. (2006). Cerebellar networks and autism. In S. O. Moldin & J. L. R. Rubenstein (Eds.), *Understanding autism: From basic neuroscience to treatment* (pp. 155–174). New York: CRC.

Fanselow, M. S., & Poulos, A. M. (2005). The neuroscience of mammalian associative learning. *Annual Review of Psychology, 56*, 207–234.

Ferland, R. J., Eyaid, W., Collura, R. V., Tully, L. D., Hill, R. S., Al-Nouri, D., et al. (2004). Abnormal cerebellar development and axonal decussation due to mutations in AHI1 in Joubert syndrome. *Nature Genetics, 36*(9), 1008–1013.

Fernandez, T., Morgan, T., Davis, N., Klin, A., Morris, A., Farhi, A., et al. (2008). Disruption of Contactin 4 (CNTN4) results in developmental delay and other features of 3p deletion syndrome. *American Journal of Human Genetics, 82*(6), 1385.

Freitag, C. M. (2007). The genetics of autistic disorders and its clinical relevance: A review of the literature. *Molecular Psychiatry, 12*(1), 2–22.

Galanopoulou, A. S. (2005). GABA receptors as broadcasters of sexually differentiating signals in the brain. *Epilepsia, 46* (Suppl 5), 107–112.

Garel, S., Huffman, K. J., & Rubenstein, J. L. R. (2003). A caudal shift in neocortical patterning in a *Fgf8* hypomorphic mouse mutant. *Development (Cambridge, England), 130*, 1903–1914.

Garel, S., & Rubenstein, J. L. (2004). Intermediate targets in formation of topographic projections: Inputs from the thalamocortical system. *Trends in Neurosciences, 27*(9), 533–539.

Geschwind, D. H., & Levitt, P. (2007). Autism spectrum disorders: Developmental disconnection syndromes. *Current Opinion in Neurobiology, 17*(1), 103–111.

Gilfillan, G. D., Selmer, K. K., Roxrud, I., Smith, R., Kyllerman, M., Eiklid, K., et al. (2008). SLC9A6 mutations cause X-linked mental retardation, microcephaly, epilepsy, and ataxia, a phenotype mimicking Angelman syndrome. *American Journal of Human Genetics, 82*(4), 1003–1010.

Grove, E. A., & Fukuchi-Shimogori, T. (2003). Generating the cerebral cortical area map. *Annual Review of Neuroscience, 26*, 355–380.

Gupta, A. R., & State, M. W. (2007). Recent advances in the genetics of autism. *Biological Psychiatry, 61*(4), 429–437.

Hamilton, S. P., Woo, M., Carlson, E. J., Ghanem, N., Ekker, M., & Rubenstein, J. L. R. (2005). Analysis of four DLX homeobox genes in autistic probands. *BMC Genetics*, 6, 52.

Happe, F., Ronald, A., & Plomin, R. (2007). Time to give up on a single explanation for autism. *Nature Neuroscience, 9*(10), 1218–1220.

Hardan, A. Y., Muddasani, S., Vemulapalli, M., Keshavan, M. S., & Minshew, N. J. (2006). An MRI study of increased cortical thickness in autism. *American Journal of Psychiatry, 163*(7), 1290–1292.

Hazlett, H. C., Poe, M., Gerig, G., Smith, R. G., Provenzale, J., Ross, A., et al. (2005). Magnetic resonance imaging and head circumference study of brain size in autism: Birth through age 2 years. *Archives of General Psychiatry, 62*(12), 1366–1376.

Hensch, T. K. (2005). Critical period plasticity in local cortical circuits. *Nature Reviews Neuroscience, 6*(11), 877–888.

Hevner, R. F., Shi, L., Justice, N., Hsueh, Y., Sheng, M., Smiga, S., et al. (2001). Tbr1 regulates differentiation of the preplate and layer 6. *Neuron, 29*(2), 353–366.

Hill, R. S., & Walsh, C. A. (2005). Molecular insights into human brain evolution. *Nature, 437*(7055), 64–67.

Hobbs, K., Kennedy, A., Dubray, M., Bigler, E. D., Petersen, P. B., McMahon, W, et al. (2007). A retrospective fetal ultrasound study of brain size in autism. *Biological Psychiatry, 62*(9), 1048–1055.

Hong, E. J., West, A. E., & Greenberg, M. E. (2005). Transcriptional control of cognitive development. *Current Opinion in Neurobiology, 15*(1), 21–28.

Horike, S., Cai, S., Miyano, M., Cheng, J. F., & Kohwi-Shigematsu, T. (2005). Loss of silent-chromatin looping and impaired imprinting of DLX5 in Rett syndrome. *Nature Genetics, 37*(1), 31–40.

Huen, M. S., Grant, R., Manke, I., Minn, K., Yu, X., Yaffe, M. B., et al. (2007). RNF8 transduces the DNA-damage signal via histone ubiquitylation and checkpoint protein assembly. *Cell, 131*(5), 901–914.

Ingason, A., Sigmundsson, T., Steinberg, S., Sigurdsson, E., Haraldsson, M., Magnusdottir, B. B., et al. (2007). Support for involvement of the AHI1 locus in schizophrenia. *European Journal of Human Genetics: EJHG, 15*(9), 988–991.

Inoki, K., Corradetti, M. N., & Guan, K. L. (2005). Dysregulation of the TSC-mTOR pathway in human disease. *Nature Genetics, 37*(1), 19–24.

Jamain, S., Quach, H., Betancur, C., Rastam, M., Colineaux, C., Gillberg, I. C., et al. (2003). Paris Autism Research International Sibpair Study. Mutations of the X-linked genes encoding neuroligins NLGN3 and NLGN4 are associated with autism. *Nature Genetics, 34*(1), 27–29.

Jamain, S., Radyushkin, K., Hammerschmidt, K., Granon, S., Boretius, S., Varoqueaux, F., et al. (2008). Reduced social interaction and ultrasonic communication in a mouse model of monogenic heritable autism. *Proceedings of the National Academy of Sciences of the United States of America, 105*(5), 1710–1715.

Jeong, J., Li, X., McEvilly, R., Rosenfeld, M., Lufkin, T., & Rubenstein, J. (2008). Dlx genes pattern mammalian jaw primordium by regulating both lower jaw- and upper jaw-specific genetic programs. *Development, 135*, 2905–2916.

Juranek, J., Filipek, P. A., Berenji, G. R., Modahl, C., Osann, K., & Spence, M. A. (2006). Association between amygdala volume and anxiety level: Magnetic resonance imaging (MRI) study in autistic children. *Journal of Child Neurology, 21*(12), 1051–1058.

Kana, R. K., Keller, T. A., Cherkassky, V. L., Minshew, N. J., & Just, M. A. (2006). Sentence comprehension in autism: Thinking in pictures with decreased functional connectivity. *Brain, 129*, 2484–2493.

Kaneko-Goto, T., Yoshihara, S., Miyazaki, H., & Yoshihara, Y. (2008). BIG-2 mediates olfactory axon convergence to target glomeruli. *Neuron, 57*(6), 834–846.

Kitamura, K., Yanazawa, M., Sugiyama, N., Miura, H., Iizuka-Kogo, A., Kusaka, M., et al. (2002). Mutation of ARX causes abnormal development of forebrain and testes in mice and X-linked lissencephaly with abnormal genitalia in humans. *Nature Genetics, 32*(3), 359–369.

Kwon, C. H., Luikart, B. W., Powell, C. M., Zhou, J., Matheny, S. A., Zhang, W., et al. (2006). Pten regulates neuronal arborization and social interaction in mice. *Neuron, 50*(3), 377–388.

LaSalle, J. M. (2007). The odyssey of MeCP2 and parental imprinting. *Epigenetics, 2*(1), 5–10.

LeDoux, J. (2007). The amygdala. *Curr Biol, 17*(20), R868–R874.

Levisohn, P. M. (2007). The autism-epilepsy connection. *Epilepsia, 48*(Suppl 9), 33–35.

Levitt, P., Eagleson, K. L., & Powell, E. M. (2004). Regulation of neocortical interneuron development and the implications for neurodevelopmental disorders. *Trends in Neurosciences, 27*(7), 400–406.

Lisman, J. E., & Grace, A. A. (2005). The hippocampal-VTA loop: Controlling the entry of information into long-term memory. *Neuron, 46*(5), 703–713.

Liu, A., & Joyner, A. L. (2001). Early anterior/posterior patterning of the midbrain and cerebellum. *Annual Review of Neuroscience, 24*, 869–896.

Long, J. E., Swan, C., Liang, W. S., Cobos, I., Potter, G. B., & Rubenstein, J. L. R. (2009). Dlx1 & 2 and Mash1 transcription factors control striatal patterning and differentiation through parallel and overlapping pathways. *Journal of Comparative Neurology, 512*, 556–572.

Lush, M. E., Li, Y., Kwon, C. H., Chen, J., & Parada, L. F. (2008). Neurofibromin is required for barrel formation in the mouse somatosensory cortex. *Journal of Neuroscience, 28*(7), 1580–1587.

Marui, T., Hashimoto, O., Nanba, E., Kato, C., Tochigi, M., Umekage, T., et al. (2004). Association between the neurofibromatosis-1 (NF1) locus and autism in the Japanese population. *American Journal of Medical Genetics. Part B, Neuropsychiatric Genetics, 131B*(1), 43–47.

McCarthy, M. M. (2008). Estradiol and the developing brain. *Physiological Reviews, 88*(1), 91–124.

Miyano, M., Horike, S. I., Cai, S., Oshimura, M., & Kohwi-Shigematsu, T. (2008). DLX5 expression is monoallelic and Dlx5 is upregulated in the Mecp2-null frontal cortex. *Journal of Cellular and Molecular Medicine, 12*(4), 1188–1191.

Moessner, R., Marshall, C. R., Sutcliffe, J. S., Skaug, J., Pinto, D., Vincent, J., Zwaigenbaum, L., Fernandez, B., Roberts, W., Szatmari, P., & Scherer, S. W. (2007). Contribution of SHANK3 mutations to autism spectrum disorder. *American Journal of Human Genetics, 81*(6), 1289–1297.

Moldin, S. O., & Rubenstein, J. L. R. (2006). *Understanding autism: From basic neuroscience to treatment.* New York: CRC.

Moldin, S. O., Rubenstein, J. L. R., & Hyman, S. E. (2006). Autism speaks to neuroscience [Commentary]. *Journal of Neuroscience, 26*(26), 6893–6896.

Molyneaux, B. J., Arlotta, P., Menezes, J. R., & Macklis, J. D. (2007). Neuronal subtype specification in the cerebral cortex. *Nature Reviews Neuroscience, 8*(6), 427–437.

Moretti, P., & Zoghbi, H. Y. (2006). MeCP2 dysfunction in Rett syndrome and related disorders. *Current Opinion in Genetics and Development, 16*(3), 276–281.

Morrow, E. M., Yoo, S. Y., Flavell, S. W., Kim, T. K., Lin, Y., Hill, R. S., et al. (2008). Identifying autism loci and genes by tracing recent shared ancestry. *Science (New York, N.Y.), 321*(5886), 218–223.

Nuñez, J. L., & McCarthy, M. M. (2008). Androgens predispose males to GABAA-mediated excitotoxicity in the developing hippocampus. *Experimental Neurology, 210*(2), 699–708.

O'Leary, D. D., Chou, S. J., & Sahara, S. (2007). Area patterning of the mammalian cortex. *Neuron, 56*(2), 252–269.

Ongür, D., & Price, J. L. (2000). The organization of networks within the orbital and medial prefrontal cortex of rats, monkeys, and humans. *Cerebral Cortex, 10*(3), 206–219.

Paul, L. K., Brown, W. S., Adolphs, R., Tyszka, J. M., Richards, L. J., Mukherjee, P., et al. (2007). Agenesis of the corpus callosum: Genetic, developmental, and functional aspects of connectivity. *Nature Reviews Neuroscience, 8*(4), 287–299.

Persico, A. M., & Bourgeron, T. (2006). Searching for ways out of the autism maze: Genetic, epigenetic, and environmental clues. *Trends in Neurosciences, 29*(7), 349–358.

Peters, S. U., Beaudet, A. L., Madduri, N., & Bacino, C. A. (2004). Autism in Angelman syndrome: Implications for autism research. *Clinical Genetics, 66*(6), 530–536.

Petryniak, M. A., Potter, G. B., Rowitch, D. H., & Rubenstein, J. L. (2007). Dlx1 and Dlx2 control neuronal versus oligodendroglial cell fate acquisition in the developing forebrain. *Neuron, 55*(3), 417–433.

Piven, J., Arndt, S., Bailey, J., Havercamp, S., Andreasen, N. C., & Palmer, P. (1995). An MRI study of brain size in autism. *American Journal of Psychiatry, 152*, 1145–1149.

Polley, D. B., Cobos, I., Merzenich, M. M., & Rubenstein, J. L. (2006). Severe hearing loss in Dlxl mutant mice. *Hearing Research, 214*(1–2), 84–88.

Price, D. J., Kennedy, H., Dehay, C., Zhou, L., Mercier, M., Jossin, Y., et al. (2006). The development of cortical connections. *European Journal of Neuroscience, 23*(4), 910–920.

Qiu, M., Bulfone, A., Martinez, S., Meneses, J. J., Shimamura, K., Pedersen, R. A., et al. (1995). Role of Dlx-2 in head development and evolution: Null mutation of Dlx-2 results in abnormal morphogenesis of proximal first and second branchial arch derivatives and abnormal differentiation in the forebrain. *Genes and Development, 9*, 2523–2538.

Ramamoorthy, S., & Nawaz, Z. (2008). E6-associated protein (E6-AP) is a dual function coactivator of steroid hormone receptors. *Nuclear Receptor Signaling, 6*, e006.

Reichenberg, A., Gross, R., Weiser, M., Bresnahan, M., Silverman, J., Harlap, S., et al. (2006). Advancing paternal age and autism. *Archives of General Psychiatry, 63*(9), 1026–1032.

Roohi, J., Montagna, C., Tegay, D. H., Palmer, L. E., Devincent, C., Pomeroy, J. C., et al. (2008). Disruption of contactin 4 in 3 subjects with autism spectrum disorder. *Journal of Medical Genetics, 46*(3), 176–178.

Rubenstein, J. L. R. (2006). Comments on the genetic control of forebrain development. *Clinical Neuroscience Research, 6*, 169–177.

Rubenstein, J. L. R. & Merzenich, M. M. (2003). Model of autism: Increased ratio of excitation/inhibition in key neural systems. *Genes, Brain, and Behavior, 2*, 255–267.

Scearce-Levie, K., Roberson, E. D., Gerstein, H., Cholfin, J. A., Mandiyan, V. S., Shah, N. M., et al. (2008). Abnormal social behaviors in mice lacking Fgf17. *Genes, Brain, and Behavior, 7*(3), 344–354.

Schanen, N. C. (2006). Epigenetics of autism spectrum disorders. <http://www.ncbi.nlm.nih.gov/pubmed/16987877> *Human Molecular Genetics, 15*(Spec No 2), R138–R150.

Schüle, B., Li, H. H., Fisch-Kohl, C., Purmann, C., & Francke, U. (2007). DLX5 and DLX6 expression is biallelic and not modulated by MeCP2 deficiency. *American Journal of Human Genetics, 81*(3), 492–506.

Schwarz, J. M., & McCarthy, M. M. (2008). Steroid-induced sexual differentiation of the developing brain: Multiple pathways, one goal. *Journal of Neurochemistry, 105*(5), 1561–1572.

Sebat, J., Lakshmi, B., Malhotra, D., Troge, J., Lese-Martin, C., Walsh, T., et al. (2007). Strong association of de novo copy number mutations with autism. *Science (New York, N.Y.)* [Epub ahead of print].

Semendeferi, K., Lu, A., Schenker, N., & Damasio, H. (2002). Humans and great apes share a large frontal cortex. *Nature Neuroscience, 5*(3), 272–276.

Sikora, D. M., Pettit-Kekel, K., Penfield, J., Merkens, L. S., & Steiner, R. D. (2006). The near universal presence of autism spectrum disorders in children with Smith-Lemli-Opitz syndrome. *American Journal of Medical Genetics. Part A, 140*(14), 1511–1518.

Smalley, S. L., Asarnow, R. F., & Spence, M. A. (1988). Autism and genetics: A decade of research. *Archives of General Psychiatry, 45*, 953–961.

Splawski, I., Yoo, D. S., Stotz, S. C., Cherry, A., Clapham, D. E., Keating, M. T. (2006). CACNA1H mutations in autism spectrum disorders. <http://www.ncbi.nlm.nih.gov/pubmed/16754686> *Journal of Biological Chemistry, 281*(31), 22085–22091.

Storm, E., Garel, S., Borello, U., Hebert, J. M., Martinez, S., McConnell, S., et al. (2006). Dose-dependent functions of Fgf8 in regulating telencephalic patterning centers. *Development (Cambridge, England), 133*(9), 1831–1844.

Stühmer, T., Anderson, S. A., Ekker, M., & Rubenstein, J. L. R. (2002). Ectopic expression of the *Dlx* genes induces glutamic acid decarboxylase and *Dlx* expression. *Development (Cambridge, England), 129*, 245–252.

Sur, M., & Rubenstein, J. L. (2005). Patterning and plasticity of the cerebral cortex. *Science (New York, N.Y.), 310*(5749), 805–810.

Sutcliffe, J. S., Delahanty, R. J., Prasad, H. C., McCauley, J. L., Han, Q., Jiang, L., et al. (2005). Allelic heterogeneity at the serotonin transporter locus (SLC6A4) confers susceptibility to autism and rigid-compulsive behaviors. *American Journal of Human Genetics, 77*(2), 265–279.

Sutcliffe, J. S. (2008). Genetics: Insights into the pathogenesis of autism. *Science (New York, N.Y.), 321*(5886), 208–209.

Tabuchi, K., Blundell, J., Etherton, M. R., Hammer, R. E., Liu, X., Powell, C. M., et al. (2007). A neuroligin-3 mutation implicated in autism increases inhibitory synaptic transmission in mice. *Science (New York, N.Y.), 318*(5847), 71–76.

Takano, Y., Adachi, S., Okuno, M., Muto, Y., Yoshioka, T., Matsushima-Nishiwaki, R., et al. (2004). The RING finger protein, RNF8, interacts with retinoid X receptor alpha and enhances its transcription-stimulating activity. *Journal of Biological Chemistry, 279*(18), 18926–18934.

Tavazoie, S. F., Alvarez, V. A., Ridenour, D. A., Kwiatkowski, D. J, & Sabatini, B. L. (2005). Regulation of neuronal morphology and function by the tumor suppressors Tsc1 and Tsc2. *Nature Neuroscience, 8*(12), 1727–1734.

Todd, P. K., Mack, K. J., & Malter, J. S. (2003). The fragile X mental retardation protein is required for type-I metabotropic glutamate receptor-dependent translation of PSD-95. *Proceedings of the National Academy of Sciences of the United States of America, 100*(24), 14374–14378.

Uemura, M., Nakao, S., Suzuki, S. T., Takeichi, M., & Hirano, S. (2007). OL-Protocadherin is essential for growth of striatal axons and thalamocortical projections. *Nature Neuroscience, 10*(9), 1151–1159.

van Galen, E. J., & Ramakers, G. J. (2005). Rho proteins, mental retardation, and the neurobiological basis of intelligence. *Progress in Brain Research, 147*, 295–317.

Varoqueaux, F., Aramuni, G., Rawson, R. L., Mohrmann, R., Missler, M., Gottmann, K., et al. (2006). Neuroligins determine synapse maturation and function. *Neuron, 51*(6), 741–754.

Wallerstein, R., Sugalski, R., Cohn, L., Jawetz, R., & Friez, M. (2008). Expansion of the ARX spectrum. *Clinical Neurology and Neurosurgery, 110*(6), 631–634.

Walsh, C. A., Morrow E. M., & Rubenstein J. L. R. (2008). Autism and brain development. *Cell, 135*(3), 396–400.

Walsh, T., McClellan, J. M., McCarthy, S. E., Addington, A. M., Pierce, S. B., Cooper. G. M., et al. (2008). Rare structural variants disrupt multiple genes in neurodevelopmental pathways in schizophrenia. *Science (New York, N.Y.), 320*(5875), 539–543.

Weiss, L. A., Escayg, A., Kearney, J. A., Trudeau, M., MacDonald, B. T., Mori, M., et al. (2003). Sodium channels SCN1A, SCN2A, and SCN3A in familial autism. *Molecular Psychiatry, 8*(2), 186–194.

Wiznitzer, M. (2004). Autism and tuberous sclerosis. *Journal of Child Neurology, 19*(9), 675–679.

Wu, S., Jia, M., Ruan, Y., Liu, J., Guo, Y., Shuang, M., et al. (2005). Positive association of the oxytocin receptor gene (OXTR) with autism in the Chinese Han population. *Biological Psychiatry, 58*(1), 74–77.

Xu, J., Liu, Z., & Ornitz, D. M. (2000). Temporal and spatial gradients of Fgf8 and Fgf17 regulate proliferation and differentiation of midline cerebellar structures. *Development (Cambridge, England), 127*(9), 1833–1843.

Yin, H. H., & Knowlton, B. J. (2006). The role of the basal ganglia in habit formation. *Nature Reviews Neuroscience, 7*(6), 464–476.

Yirmiya, N., Rosenberg, C., Levi, S., Salomon, S., Shulman, C., Nemanov, L., et al. (2006). Association between the arginine vasopressin 1a receptor (AVPR1a) gene and autism in a family-based study: Mediation by socialization skills. *Molecular Psychiatry, 11*(5), 488–494.

Yoshihara, Y., Kawasaki, M., Tamada, A., Nagata, S., Kagamiyama, H., & Mori, K. (1995). Overlapping and differential expression of BIG-2, BIG-1, TAG-1, and F3: Four members of an axon-associated cell adhesion molecule subgroup of the immunoglobulin superfamily. *Journal of Neurobiology, 28*(1), 51–69.

Young, L. J., Murphy Young, A. Z., & Hammock, E. A. (2005). Anatomy and neurochemistry of the pair bond. *Journal of Comparative Neurology, 493*(1), 51–57.

Zhao, Y., Marín, O., Hermesz, E., Powell, A., Flames, N., Palkovits, M., et al. (2003). The LIM-homeobox gene Lhx8 is required for the development of many cholinergic neurons in the mouse forebrain. *Proceedings of the National Academy of Sciences of the United States of America, 100*(15), 9005–9010.

Zoghbi, H. Y. (2003). Postnatal neurodevelopmental disorders: Meeting at the synapse? *Science (New York, N.Y.), 302*(5646), 826–830.

31 Cynthia M. Schumann, Steven C. Noctor, David G. Amaral

Neuropathology of Autism Spectrum Disorders: Postmortem Studies

Points of Interest

- Compared to disorders such as Alzheimer's disease, relatively few autistic brains have been neuropathologically investigated, and even fewer have been subjected to quantitative analysis.
- Lower numbers of neurons have been reported in the amygdala, the fusiform gyrus of the temporal lobe, and the cerebellum.
- One current line of research emphasizes alterations in the basic columnar organization of the neocortex.
- Provocative data signs of ongoing inflammation are observed in the autistic brain.

Considerable progress in understanding the behavioral impairments of autism has been made over the last 65 years since Kanner (1943) first described a group of children with autistic-like disturbances, though the underlying neuropathology of the disorder remains elusive. Autism is a *clinically defined* disorder marked by impairments in reciprocal social interaction, abnormal development and use of language, and repetitive and ritualized behaviors, and a narrow range of interests that manifest by 3 years of age. These behavioral disturbances suggest that certain parts of the brain may be more pathological than others. Regions that constitute the "social brain" for example, might be preferentially impacted by autism. We recently compiled a list of neural systems involved in the functions that could be most affected by the core behavioral features of autism (Figure 31-1) to suggest where one might expect to find neuropathology (Amaral et al., 2008). Several brain regions have been implicated in social behavior through experimental animal studies, lesion studies in human patients, or functional imaging studies (Adolphs, 2001). These include regions of the frontal lobe, the cingulate cortex, the superior temporal cortex, the parietal cortex, and the amygdala. Language function is distributed throughout several cortical and subcortical regions. Foremost for expressive language function is Broca's area in the inferior frontal gyrus and portions of the supplementary motor cortex. Wernicke's area is essential for receptive language function, and the superior temporal sulcus plays a role in both language processing and social attention (Redcay, 2008). Finally, the repetitive or stereotyped behaviors of autism share many similarities with the abnormal of obsessive-compulsive disorder that implicate regions such as the orbitofrontal cortex and caudate nucleus.

Autism is increasingly considered to be a *heterogeneous* disorder with multiple causes and courses. Because there is a great range in the severity of symptoms associated with autism, it is described as a spectrum disorder. Mental retardation is a common correlate of autism representing the "low" end of the spectrum, and there are a number of comorbid symptoms, such as epilepsy, that have neurological underpinnings and affect some, but not all, individuals with autism. The comorbid symptoms of autism must be taken into consideration for the interpretation of the neuropathology of autism. Epilepsy, for example, is associated with pathology of the cerebral cortex, amygdala, cerebellum, and hippocampal formation, all of which have also been implicated in autism. Thus, if one analyzes the brain of an individual who has autism as well as epilepsy, it is not clear whether the observed pathology is related to the core features of autism, to the cause, effects or treatment of epilepsy, or perhaps to some peculiar convergence of the two disorders. Unfortunately, the majority of cases evaluated in earlier postmortem studies of the autistic brain (Table 31-1) involved brains from individuals who had comorbid seizure disorders and mental retardation.

There is also substantial heterogeneity in the onset of autism. Some children have signs of developmental delays within the first 18 months of life. However, 25–40% of children with autism initially demonstrate near-normal development until 18–24 months, when they regress into an autism that is generally indistinguishable from early onset autism (Werner & Dawson, 2005; Hansen et al., 2008; Ozonoff et al., 2008). The possibility that there is early-onset versus regressive phenotypes of autism might have important implications

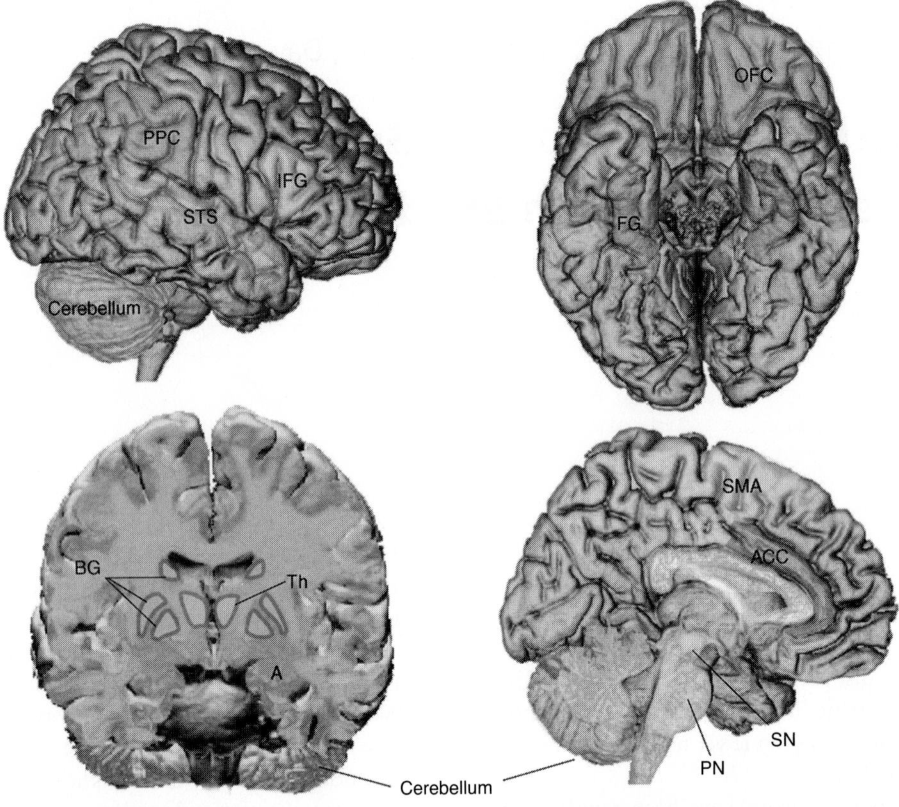

Social impairment	Communication deficits	Repetitive behaviors
OFC – Orbitofrontal cortex ACC – Anterior cingulate cortex FG – Fusiform gyrus STS – Superior temporal sulcus A – Amygdala IFG – Inferior frontal gyrus PPC – Posterior parietal cortex	IFG – Inferior frontal gyrus (Broca's area) STS – Superior temporal sulcus SMA – Supplementary motor area BG – Basal ganglia SN – Substantia nigra Th – Thalamus PN – Pontine nuclei	OFC – Orbitofrontal cortex ACC – Anterior cingulate cortex BG – Basal ganglia Th – Thalamus

Figure 31–1. Brain areas that have been implicated in the mediation of the three core behaviors that are impaired in autism: social behavior, language and communication, and repetitive and stereotyped behaviors. *Adapted from* Amaral, D. G., Schumann, C. M., & Nordahl, C. W. (2008). Neuroanatomy of autism. *Trends in Neuroscience, 31*, 137–145, *with permission from Trends in Neurosciences.* (See Color Plate Section for a color version of this figure.)

Table 31–1.
Neuropathological studies of autism using postmortem brain from 1980–2010

Author	Year	Sample Size and Characteristics	Approach and Region of Interest	Major Findings
Williams et al.	1980	4A (3M, 1F; ages 4, 14, 27, 33; 2S; 4MR); no C	qualitative observation—whole brain	Nerve cell loss and replacement gliosis in atrophic orbitofrontal and temporal regions in 2 cases; smaller neurons in CA4; ↓ Purkinje cell density in 1 case
Bauman & Kemper	1985	1A (1M; age 29; no S; 1MR); 1C (1M; age 25)	qualitative observation—whole brain	↑ cell density and ↓ cell size in hippocampus, subiculum, entorhinal cortex, septal nuclei, mammillary body and amygdala. ↓ density of Purkinje cells, neurons small and pale
Coleman et al.	1985	1A (1F; age 21; no S; 1MR); 2C (2F; ages 18, 25)	2D cell counts auditory cortex and Broca's area	No differences, except for ↓ glia in left auditory cortex and ↓ density of pyramidal neurons in right auditory association cortex

(*Continued*)

Table 31–1. *(Contd.)*

Author	Year	Sample Size and Characteristics	Approach and Region of Interest	Major Findings
Ritvo et al.	1986	4A (4M; ages 10, 19, 19, 22; no S; 3MR); 3C (3M; ages 3, 10, 13)	2D cell counts in cerebellum	↓ Purkinje cell density in cerebellar hemisphere and vermis
Bauman & Kemper	1987	1A (1F; age 11; no S; ?MR); 2C (?M; ?F; age-matched)	qualitative observation—amygdala & hippocampus	↑ cell density in amygdala & hippocampus
Bauman & Kemper	1990	1A (1M; age 12; no S; no MR); 2C (2M; age-matched)	qualitative observation—amygdala, hippocampus & cerebellum	↑ cell density of smaller neurons in limbic system; ↓ density of Purkinje cells; enlarged neurons in deep cerebellar nuclei and inferior olive
Bauman	1991	5A (4M, 1F; ages 9–29; 4S; 4MR)	review of earlier findings	↑ cell density in limbic system (4/5) and ↓ Purkinje cell density in cerebellum (5/5)
Hof et al.	1991	1A (1F; age 24; no S; 1MR)	qualitative observation—cerebral cortex and limbic system	Microcephaly (773 g); neurofibrillary tangles, especially in layer II and III of temporal cortex, probably due to severe head banging
Kemper & Bauman	1993	6A (5M, 1F; ages 9–29; 4S; 5MR); 6C (6M; age- and sex-matched)	qualitative/density measures—limbic system and cerebellum	Small and densely packed neurons in limbic system (6/6); anterior cingulate coarse and poorly laminated in 5/6; ↓ Purkinje cell #s in cerebellum (6/6)
Guerin et al.	1996	1A (1F; age 16; 1S 1MR)	qualitative observations—whole brain	Microcephaly, ↑ ventricular dilation, thin corpus callosum
Raymond et al.	1996	2A (1M; ages 7, 9; no S; 2MR); 2C (?M, ?F; ages 8, 13)	Golgi analysis in hippocampus	Smaller neurons in CA4; less dendritic branching in CA1 and CA4
Rodier et al.	1996	1A (1F; age 21; 1S; 1MR); 1C (1M; age 80)	qualitative observation—pons, medulla and cerebellum	Near-complete absence of facial nucleus and superior olive and shortening of the brainstem
Bailey et al.	1998	6A (6M; ages 4, 20–27 years; 3S; 6MR); 7C (5M, 2F; age-matched)	qualitative/density measures—whole brain	Megalencephaly (4/6); abnormalities in inferior olives (4/6); ↓ Purkinje cells in all adults; cortical dysgenesis in at least 50%
Blatt et al.	2001	4A (4M; ages 19–22; 2S; 4MR); 3C (3M; ages 16, 19, 24)	GABAergic, serotonergic, cholinergic, glutamatergic autoradiography in hippocampus	↓ GABA(A) receptor binding
Perry et al.	2001	7A (6M, 1F; ages ~24; ~4S; ~7MR); 10C (8M, 2F; ages ~32); 9MR (5M, 4F; ages ~32)	cholinergic immunohistochemistry in frontal and parietal cortex and basal forebrain	30% ↓ M1 receptor binding in parietal cortex; 65–73% ↓ α4 nicotinic receptor binding in frontal and parietal cortex; ↑ BDNF in forebrain
Casanova et al.	2002	2AS (2M; ages 22 and 79 years; ?S; no MR); 18C (18M; ages 9–98)	minicolumn analyses Layer III of prefrontal and temporal cortex	Cell columns were more numerous, smaller, and less compact in prefrontal layer III
Casanova et al.	2002	9A (7M, 1F; ages ~12; 5S; 7MR); 9C (?M, ?F; ages ~15)	minicolumn analyses Layer III of prefrontal and temporal cortex	Cell columns more numerous, smaller and less compact in prefrontal layer III
Fatemi et al.	2002	5A (5M; ages ~25; ?S; ?MR); 5C (≥ 4M; ages ~24)	density and size measure of Purkinje cells in cerebellum	24% smaller Purkinje cells in cerebellum; no differences in density

(Continued)

Table 31–1. *(Contd.)*

Author	Year	Sample Size and Characteristics	Approach and Region of Interest	Major Findings
Mukaetova-Ladinska et al.	2004	2A (2M; ages 29, 31; ?S; ?MR); 2C (1M, 1F; ages 19, 34)	MAP2 immunohistochemistry & Nissl in dorsolateral prefrontal cortex	"Ill defined neurocortical layers" & ↓ MAP2 immunoreactive neurons
Ray et al.	2005	3A (3M; ages 29, 31, 32; ?S; ?MR); 3C (2M, 1F; ages 12, 29, 72)	nAchR immunohistochemistry in thalamus	↓ α7 and β2 immunoreactive neurons in paraventricular nucleus & nucleus reuniens
Vargas et al.	2005	15A (12M, 3F; ages 5–44; 6S; 12MR); 12C (9M, 3F; ages 5–46)	neuroinflammation in cerebellum, mid frontal, & cingulate (immunostained for HLA-DR, etc.)	↑ activated microglia and astroglia and qualitative loss of Purkinje cells in cerebellum
Buxhoeveden	2006	2A (2M; ages 3, 41; ≥1S, ≥MR); 5C (5M; ages 2, 21, 34, 44, 75)	minicolumnar width in layer III in frontal cortex	↓ minicolumnar width in dorsal and orbital frontal cortex
Casanova	2006	6A (4M, 2F; ages 4–24; 2S; ?MR); 6C (4M, 2F; ages 4–25)	minicolumnar width in layer III of S1, BA4,9, 17	↓ minicolumnar width; smaller neurons; 23% ↑ in neuron density in layer III of BA9
Hutsler et al.	2006	8A (8M; ages 15–45, no S; ?MR); 8C (8M; ages 14–45)	cortical thickness on postmortem MRI	no difference in cortical thickness
Martchek et al.	2006	5A (?M, ?F; ages 19–54; ≥ 1S; ?MR); 4C (?M, ?F; ages 25–55)	stereological neuron # in locus coeruleus	no difference in neuron # in locus coeruleus
Schumann & Amaral	2006	9A (9M; ages 11–44; no S; ?MR); 10C (10M; ages 10–44)	stereological neuron # and size in amygdala	↓ neuron # in whole amygdala and lateral nucleus
Kennedy	2007	4A (4M; ages 3, 15, 34, 41; 1S; 3MR); 5C (5M; ages 2, 16, 21, 44, 75)	stereological spindle neuron # in frontal insula	no difference in spindle neuron #
Guptill et al.	2007	4A (4M; ages 19–22; 3S; 3MR); 3C (3M; ages 16–24)	multiple-concentration GABAergic autoradiography in the hipppocampus	Non-significant 20% ↓ in # of benzodiazepine binding sites
Yip et al.	2007	8A (6M, 2F; ages 16–30); 8C (8M; ages 16–30)	in situ GAD67 mRNA in cerebellum	40% reduction in GAD67 mRNA in Purkinje cells
Kulesza & Mangunay	2008	5A (5M; ages 8–32); 2C (2M; ages 26, 29)	morphology of neurons in the medial superior olive	↓ cell body size; abnormal shape and orientation
Van Kooten et al.	2008	7A(4M, 3F; ages 4–23; 4S; ?MR); 10C (8M, 2F; ages 4–65)	stereological neuron # in fusiform gyrus, V1 & cortical gray	↓ neuron densities in layer III, total neuron # in layers III,V, and VI, and mean perikaryal volumes in layers V/VI in fusiform. No differences in V1 or total cortical gray
Whitney et al.	2008	6A (5M, 1F; ages 13–54; ≥1S; ?MR); 4C (3M, 1F; ages 17–53)	calbindin-D28k immunohistochemistry in cerebellum	No difference in density of Purkinje cells

(Continued)

Table 31–1. *(Contd.)*

Author	Year	Sample Size and Characteristics	Approach and Region of Interest	Major Findings
Yip et al.	2008	same as Yip et al., 2007	in situ hybridization for GAD67 mRNA in cerebellum	28% upregulated GAD67 in basket cells of cerebellum
Yip et al.	2009	same as Yip et al., 2007	in situ hybridization for GAD65 mRNA in cerebellum	↓ GAD65 mRNA levels in cerebellar dentate nuclei
Whitney et al.	2009	same as Whitney et al., 2008	parvalbumin immunohistochemistry in cerebellum	No difference in basket or stellate cells
Simms et al.	2009	9A (9M; ages 15–54; ≥5S; ≥4MR); 4C (4M; ages 20–53)	density and size of neurons in anterior cingulate	↓ cell size in layers I–III and layers V–VI of area 24b and cell packing density in layers V–VI of area 24c
Oblak et al.	2009	7A (6M, 1F; ages 19–30; 4S; 9MR); 9C (9M; ages 19–43)	multiple-concentration ligand-binding study of GABA(A) in anterior cingulate	↓ GABA(A) receptors and benzodiazepine binding sites in anterior cingulate cortex
Lawrence et al.	2010	5A (5M; ages 13–54; ≥2S; ?MR); 5C (5M; ages 14–63)	density of GABAergic interneurons immunostained with Ca+ binding proteins in hippocampus	↑ immunoreactive interneuron density for calbindin in dentate gyrus, ↑ calretinin in CA1, ↑ parvalbumin in CA1 and CA3
Avino et al.	2010	8A (8M; ages 10–45; ≥2S; ≥7MR); 8C (8M; ages 11–51)	Spatial extent of gray-white transition in BA 7, 9, 21	"indistinct" boundary of layer VI and underlying white matter
Casanova et al.	2010	7A (5M, 2F; ages 4–67; ?S; ?MR); 7C (5M; 2F; ages 4–65)	minicolumnar width in BA 4, 9, 10, 11, 17, 24, 43, 44	↓ minicolumnar width in supra- and infragranular layers, most notable in BA 44.
Hutsler & Zhang	2010	10A (10M; ages 10–44; 4S; ≥6MR); 15C (15M; ages 11–15)	Golgi analysis of spine density of pyramidal neurons in BA 7, 9, 21	↑ apical dendrite spine density in layer II of BA 7, 9, 21 and Layer V of BA 21
Kulesza et al	2010	9A (8M, 1F; ages 2–36; ≥1S; ?MR); 4C (1M, 3F; ages 4–32)	neuronal morphology and density in superior olivary complex	↓ neuron density in superior olive; ↓ cell size in medial superior olive
Morgan et al.	2010	13A (13M; ages 3–41; ≥6S; ≥2MR); 9C (13M; ages 2–44)	microglia activation in BA 9/46 (immunostained for iba-1)	↑ microglial density in BA 9/46 and ↑ cell size in underlying white matter
Oblak et al.	2010a	*16A (15M, 1F; ages 3–30; 7S; ?MR); 19C (18M, 1F; ages 16–43)	density of GABA(A) receptors in anterior and posterior cingulate and fusiform gyrus	↓ GABA(B) receptor density
Oblak et al.	2010b	*15A (13M, 2F; ages 14–37; 7S; ?MR); 17C (16M, 1F; ages 16–43)	ligand-binding autoradiography of GABA(B) posterior cingulate and fusiform	↓ GABA(A) receptors and benzodiazepine binding sites and ↑ binding affinity
Santos et al.	2010	4A (2M, 2F; ages 4–11; ≥1S; ?MR); 3C (2M, 1F; ages 4–14)	stereological von Economo and pyramidal neuron # in frontal insula layer V	↑ ratio of von Economo to pyramidal neurons

(*Continued*)

Table 31-1. *(Contd.)*

Author	Year	Sample Size and Characteristics	Approach and Region of Interest	Major Findings
Wegiel et al.	2010	13A (9M, 4F; ages 4–62; ≥6S; ≥8MR); 14C (9M, 5F; ages 4–64)	qualitative neuropathological exam	multiregional heteropias (4/13) and flocculonodular, subependymal, or multifocal cerebral dysplasia (12/13)
Zikopoulos & Barbas	2010	5A (4M, 1F; ages 30–44; ≥1S; ?MR); 4C (2M, 2F; ages 36–42)	Light and electron microscopy of myelinated axons in frontal white matter	↓ # large axons, ↑ GAP-43 expression, ↑ # of thin axons below BA 32; ↓ myelin thickness below BA 11.

*regions analyzed varied by case (mean n = 8 per group per region)
A, autism spectrum disorder; C, control; M, male; F, female; S, seizure disorder; MR, mental retardation.

for the types and time courses of neuropathology that one might expect to encounter. Increasingly, researchers refer to "the autisms" rather than a single autism phenotype (Geschwind & Levitt, 2007; Amaral et al., 2008). There is no consistent genetic etiology of autism even though estimates of heritability are as high as 90% (Levitt & Campbell, 2009). The autism spectrum disorders are likely to involve multiple genes and complex interactions between genetic risk and environmental factors. When one takes all of these into consideration, it would be surprising if the neuropathology of autism were identical across all affected individuals. Whether there is a core neuropathology that is common to all, or at least most, individuals with autism remains to be determined.

Magnetic resonance imaging (MRI) studies have provided the greatest contribution to our understanding of how the brains in people with autism deviate from typical development and function. As discussed elsewhere in this book, there is substantial evidence indicating that the brain is undergoing an abnormal developmental time course that appears to include a period of early overgrowth in some individuals with autism, particularly noted in the frontal, temporal, and cingulate cortices and the amygdala (Courchesne et al., 2007; Amaral et al., 2008). Structural MRI is well equipped to deal with the *phenotypically diverse* nature of autism spectrum disorders by providing a reliable method for studying brain growth and function in large numbers of subjects over time. However, if brain size is an indication of aberrant neurological development, what does this really tell us about the neuropathology of autism? If the brain is larger in young children with autism, are there too many neurons, glia, synapses, and so forth? Does the underlying neuropathology differ between brain regions and tissue types? If the difference in brain size does not persist into adulthood, what neuropathological underpinnings account for this phenomenon of an abnormal growth trajectory?

Studies analyzing postmortem brain tissue acquired from individuals with autism provide an approach for understanding the underlying neuropathology. But, due to the limited number of cases and documentation available, these studies are currently not well positioned to deal with the heterogeneity of autism spectrum disorders. It may be obvious, but critical to point out, that postmortem studies are limited to observing the end result of each case's neuropathology due to their particular type of autism, comorbid symptoms, and individualized exposure to environmental factors. Well-designed postmortem studies must control for confounding factors such as age and gender, and excluding or segregating comorbid conditions such as epilepsy. The use of postmortem techniques as a tool for studying the neuropathology of autism is still very much in its infancy. Efforts have historically been hindered by poor tissue quality and small sample sizes, with fewer than *100* autism cases studied to date and a mean sample size of 6 autism cases per study (Table 31-1). In addition, nearly all of the brains studied have been from adults with autism, which is well after the time of peak aberrant neurological growth highlighted by MRI studies. Despite these limitations, with the availability of more abundant, high-quality postmortem tissue and by employing modern neuroanatomical techniques such as stereological methods for counting neurons and in situ hybridization for evaluating expression levels of genes, providing a more complete picture of the neuropathology of the autism spectrum disorders may be possible in the near future.

In this chapter, we first review the studies of the last 30 years that have utilized postmortem tissue and contributed to our current understanding of the neuropathology of autism (Table 31-1). Since autism, at its core, is a disorder of early development, we then review the pre- and postnatal stages of brain development. During this brief review of ontogenesis we speculate about how disruptions in the progressive and regressive events of brain development might result in the known pathology of autism. We next review data indicating that autism may involve ongoing inflammatory processes in the central nervous system. Finally, we discuss our ideas about the future direction of postmortem neuropathological studies, the need for better preparation of brain tissue to maximize the use of each precious case, and how best to serve the needs of multiple research specialties that must accommodate both classical histology and modern molecular approaches.

Historical Perspective

Margaret Bauman and Tom Kemper carried out the initial groundbreaking studies during the mid-1980s to early 1990s to systematically describe pathology in a sample of postmortem brains from people with autism during life. Before that time, most reports were case studies in which autism was not clearly identified, and in most cases, comorbid pathology such as seizure disorder, environmental insult (e.g., thalidomide exposure), severe mental retardation, self-injurious behavior, or another known neurodevelopmental disorder (e.g., phenylketonuria) was also present (Williams et al., 1980; Bauman & Kemper, 1985, 1990; Coleman et al., 1985; Hof et al., 1991; Guerin et al., 1996; Raymond et al., 1996; Rodier et al., 1996). Concurrently, during the early 1990s, a more consistent clinical definition of autism was beginning to emerge (DSM-IV, American Psychiatric Association, 1994) which enabled Kemper and Bauman (Kemper & Bauman, 1993) to collect and describe six cases of idiopathic autism, five of which had mental retardation and four of which had epilepsy. In a side-by-side comparison of each autism case with an age- and sex-matched control (see Box 31-1), the most consistent finding Kemper and Bauman reported was in the cerebellum. In all six autism cases they examined, there were fewer Purkinje cells in the cerebellar hemispheres. This observation had also been reported by Ritvo and colleagues (Ritvo et al., 1986) in a study in which they examined the brains from four males with autism, three of whom also had mental retardation, compared to three male controls; they found a lower Purkinje cell density in the cerebellar hemispheres and vermis in the autism group. In all six of the cases they studied, Kemper and Bauman (1993) also observed that olivary neurons tended to cluster at the periphery of the nuclear complex. In three of the young autism cases, the neurons in the inferior olive were large, whereas the neurons were small and pale in the adult autism cases. A near absence of the facial nucleus and superior olive was also reported in a female autism case study (Rodier et al., 1996). In addition to the cerebellum, Kemper and Bauman (1993) also observed that neurons in the amygdala and hippocampus of most autism cases appeared unusually small and more densely packed than in age-matched controls. The only area of consistent abnormality in the cerebral cortex of their cases was the anterior cingulate cortex, which appeared unusually coarse and poorly laminated.

In the late 1990s, Anthony Bailey and colleagues (1998) carried out a similar comprehensive qualitative and semi-quantitative study of six cases of autism with mental retardation, four of which had seizures, compared to seven controls. In four of the six autism brains, the brain weights were approximately 20% greater than normal for their age; two of the cases also had indications of macrocephaly in childhood clinical records. Cortical dysgenesis, which is a general term to describe malformation of cortical development, was observed in four of the six autism cases, particularly in the cerebellum and frontal cortex. These observations included increased cortical thickness in the frontal, cingulate, temporal, and parietal cortices; high neuronal density in the hippocampus and frontal and cingulate cortices; neurons present in the molecular layer of the frontal cortex; irregular laminar patterns in the superior frontal gyrus; and poor gray-white matter boundaries in the frontal cortex. Ectopic (misplaced) gray matter and an increased number of neurons were observed in the white matter of the inferior cerebellar peduncle and/or frontal cortex in three of the autism cases. Olivary dysplasia was present in three autism cases, as well as olivary ectopic neurons in two other cases. As described by both Kemper and Bauman (1993) and Ritvo (1986), Bailey et al. (1998) also reported lower numbers of Purkinje cells in the cerebellum in all five of the adult cases with autism, but not in the 4-year-old child with autism and mental retardation.

At the turn of the century, three major factors changed the way postmortem studies of autism were conducted. The first was the widespread adoption of the Autism Diagnostic Interview-Revised (ADI-R; Lord et al., 1994) as a tool to confirm autism in a postmortem case by interviewing the parents or caregivers. Autism became more clearly defined as a clinical disorder in which cases were categorized as autistic disorder or autism spectrum disorder, which includes Pervasive Developmental Disorder Not-Otherwise-Specified (PDD-NOS) and the more loosely defined diagnosis of Asperger's syndrome. Another important change was the establishment of the Autism Tissue Program (ATP) by the National Alliance for Autism Research (NAAR) (now under the direction of Autism Speaks), which supports the collection and distribution of autism brain tissue. The ATP has defined cases of autism by the ADI-R diagnosis thus facilitating modern studies utilizing postmortem autism brain tissue.

The second factor that altered the course of neuropathological studies of autism was that analytic tools, such as modern three-dimensional stereological quantitative techniques, replaced the use of density measures to become the standard for evaluating cellular pathology in postmortem brain tissue. Prior to 2006, reports on the neuropathology of autism (Table 31-1, Box 31-1) were based on two-dimensional observations to describe alterations in neuronal density, or neurons per unit volume, in a given region of brain tissue. However, it had become abundantly clear that density measurements were prone to a number of methodological artifacts, leading to interpretive problems. Haug et al. (1984), for example, found that the process of tissue fixation results in differential shrinkage of brains at different ages; shrinkage was found to be inversely proportional to age. The implication of this finding is that differences in the density of neurons may reflect changes in the volume of the tissue rather than changes in total cell number. Many investigators concluded that the only way to unambiguously interpret pathological changes in neuron number was to actually count a representative sample of neurons in a defined volume (West et al., 1991). This led to the genesis of modern "unbiased" stereological techniques that have now become standard practice for studies to describe cytoarchitectural abnormalities in human brain tissue (Box 31-1). These techniques require larger samples of brain tissue to obtain reliable measures and consequently, with better clinical definition, the sample sizes reported by postmortem autism studies are beginning to increase.

The third major factor influencing the course of neuropathological studies of autism over the last ten years was the dramatic increase in MRI studies reported in the literature that helped to guide postmortem studies on where and when

Box 31–1
Quantitative neuropathological methods then and now

The cellular alterations underlying aberrant brain growth and function in autism have been a focus of study for more than 25 years. However, over time the experimental approaches employed have changed dramatically. Bauman and Kemper (1985; Kemper & Bauman, 1993) carried out the first, groundbreaking systematic postmortem studies of autism, in which histological sections from age-matched autism and control brains, stained for cell bodies, were viewed side-by-side under a dual-headed microscope (Figure 31-A). Increases in neuronal density were observed in the subjects with autism, primarily in the amygdala and hippocampus. However, several studies have raised methodological concerns about the interpretation of density measurements as an accurate representation of neuron number. Concerns have focused on the observation of differential tissue shrinkage during postmortem processing in subjects of different ages (Haug et al., 1984). The potential impact of these confounds on observed cellular density has led many investigators to conclude that the only way to unambiguously interpret pathological changes in neuron number is to actually count a representative sample of neurons in a defined volume (West et al., 1991). Such "unbiased" stereological techniques have therefore increasingly become standard practice in postmortem cytoarchitectural studies. Stereological studies are often carried out on a microscope fitted with a camera and motorized stage controlled via software on a computer (Figure 31-B with permission from MBF Bioscience). In this approach, a representative number of evenly spaced histological sections covering the entirety of the brain region of interest are selected (Figure 31-C, See Color Plate Section for a color version of this figure), the appropriate cellular staining is applied and the region of interest is manually defined on each section. The cell population of interest is then three-dimensionally sampled across the region. An observer, blinded to the condition of the subject from which the tissue was obtained, counts cells at each location in an evenly-spaced grid of "disector counting frames" randomly oriented on each section to produce an estimate of the total number of cells for that brain region. A few experiments employing stereological methodology have now been carried out in subjects with autism, including those by Schumann and Amaral (2006) and Van Kooten et al. (2008), which found decreased neuron numbers in the amygdala and fusiform gyrus, respectively.

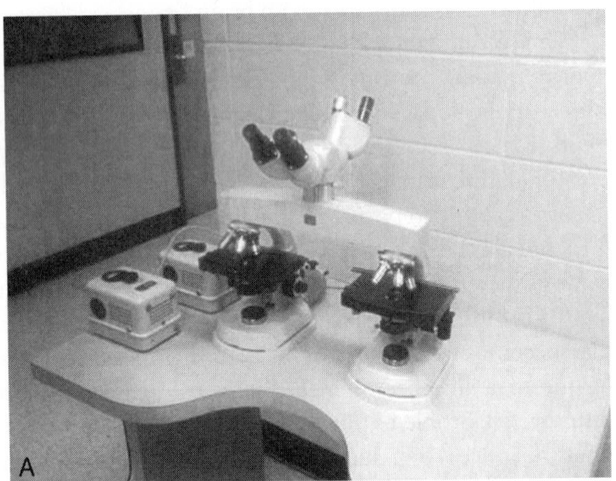
A

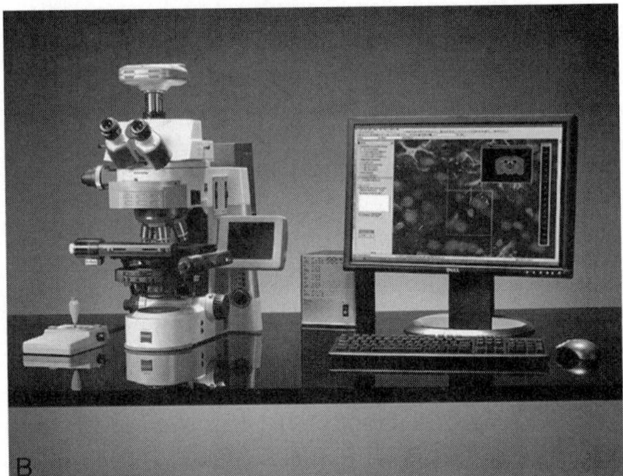
B

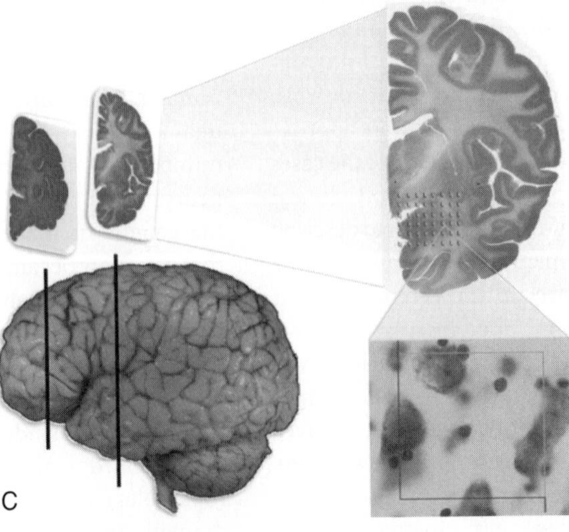
C

in the brain pathology might be present. MRI studies have consistently found increases in brain size in younger children with autism, particularly in frontal and temporal cortices as well as the amygdala and cerebellum, followed by an abnormal growth pattern through adolescence and adulthood (Courchesne et al., 2007; Amaral et al., 2008). Below we discuss the postmortem quantitative studies of the last ten years by the major areas of interest: amygdala, cerebellum, and the frontal, cingulate, and temporal cortices.

Amygdala

Schumann and Amaral (2006) were the first to carry out a neuropathology study of the brain in individuals with autism using unbiased stereological methods. They measured the number and size of neurons in the entire amygdaloid complex and in individual nuclei in nine male postmortem cases of autism, without seizure disorder, compared to ten typically developing age-matched male controls ranging in age from 10 to 44 years at death. They found that the autism group had significantly fewer neurons in the total amygdala and in the lateral nucleus than the controls (Figure 31-2). Whereas the average number of neurons in the control amygdala was about 12.2 million, the average in the amygdala in the autistic brains was about 10.8 million or about 85% of the total in the control brains. They did not find increased neuronal density or decreased size of neurons as Kemper and Bauman (1993) had initially reported. These findings have yet to be replicated

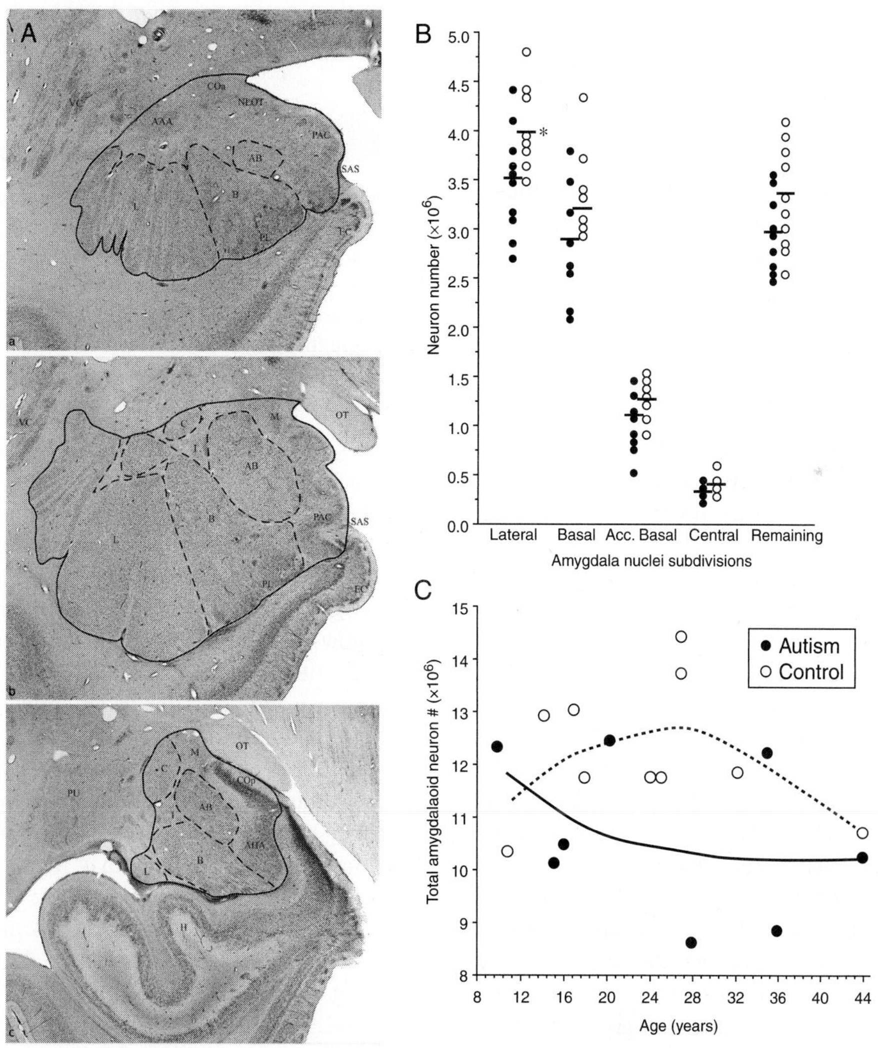

Figure 31–2. (A) Brightfield photomicrograph of Nissl-stained coronal sections through rostral (*a*), midrostrocaudal (*b*), and caudal (*c*) levels of the amygdala. AAA, Anterior amygdaloid area; AB, accessory basal nucleus; AHA, amygdalohippocampal area; B, basal nucleus; C, central nucleus; COa, anterior cortical nucleus; COp, posterior cortical nucleus; EC, entorhinal cortex; H, hippocampus; I, intercalated nuclei; L, lateral nucleus; M, medial nucleus; NLOT, nucleus of the lateral olfactory tract; OT, optic tract; PAC, periamygdaloid cortex; PL, paralaminar nucleus; PU, putamen; SAS, semiannular sulcus; VC, ventral claustrum. Scale bar, 2 mm. (B) Number of neurons in five subdivisions of the amygdala of autism (filled circle) and control (open circle) brains. The asterisk indicates significant difference ($p < 0.03$) in neuron number between autism and control lateral nuclei. (C) Bivariate scattergram of the number of neurons in the total amygdala of autism (solid black line) and control (dotted black line) brains by age. Adapted from Schumann & Amaral (2006), with permission from *Journal of Neuroscience*.

in an independent sample of brains, which is an important step in confirming decreased neuron numbers in the amygdala as a characteristic feature of autism. It is important to emphasize that this is a population difference with both the control brains and the autistic brains demonstrating a wide range of neuronal numbers.

Taken together with the findings from previous magnetic resonance imaging studies, the autistic amygdala shows multiple signs of pathology. It appears to undergo an abnormal pattern of postnatal development that includes precocious enlargement and ultimately a lower number of neurons. It will be important to determine in future studies whether decreased neuronal numbers in the amygdala is a unique characteristic of autism or whether cell loss occurs in other brain regions as well. If the lower number of neurons in the amygdala is found to be a reliable characteristic of autism, what might account for this finding? Two possible hypotheses are: (1) fewer neurons were generated during early development, or (2) a normal or even excessive number of neurons was generated initially, which would be consistent with MRI findings of a larger amygdala in early childhood (Schumann et al., 2004; Schumann, Barnes, Lord, & Courchesne, 2009), but some of these neurons have subsequently been eliminated during adulthood. Unfortunately, there is currently no evidence to support or reject either of these possibilities, and systematic stereological studies on younger autism and control cases are needed.

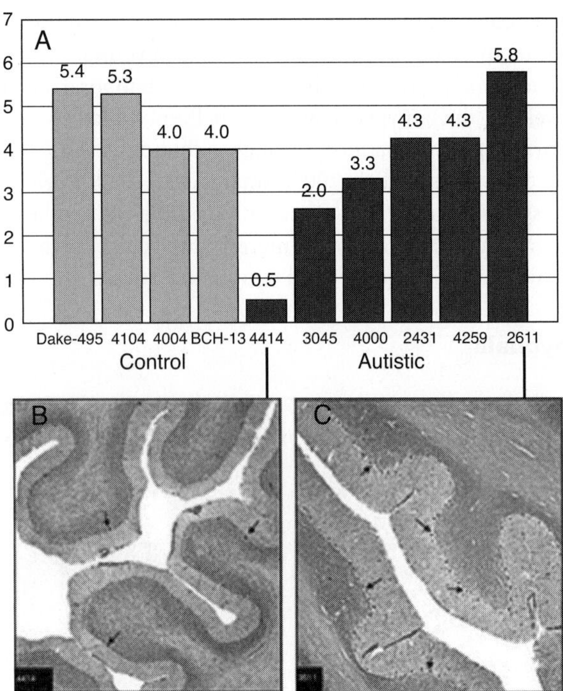

Figure 31–3. (A) Number of Purkinje neurons per millimeter in control (light gray bars) and autistic (black bars) cases from calbindin-D28k-immunostained series. Photographs illustrate the variability in Purkinje cell density within autism group in (B) 4414 with reduced Purkinje cell density and (C) 3611 with Purkinje cell density in the normal range. Adapted from Whitney et al., 2008, with kind permission from Springer Science+Business Media. (See Color Plate Section for a color version of this figure.)

Cerebellum

Of the 32 postmortem cases of autism reported in the literature in which the cerebellum was studied, 21 (or 66%) showed lower density of Purkinje cells, particularly in the more lateral parts or hemispheres of the structure (Ritvo et al., 1986; Kemper & Bauman, 1993; Bailey et al., 1998, Palmen et al., 2004; Whitney et al., 2008). Even though this is one of the most striking and consistent descriptive findings in neuropathological analyses in the autistic brain, a comprehensive stereological study of the actual number of Purkinje neurons in the whole cerebellum has yet to be carried out.

Recent studies from Blatt and colleagues have found that some, but not all, cases of autism show a reduction in the *density* of Purkinje neurons (using immunostaining for calbindin-D28k rather than standard Nissl staining), as well as a decrease in basket and stellate cell densities (Whitney et al., 2008; Whitney et al., 2009) (Figure 31-3). Fatemi and colleagues (2002) reported no differences in the density of Purkinje cells in the cerebellum in five adult cases of autism compared to five adult controls, but found a 24% decrease in the size of Purkinje neurons in the autism group. Blatt and colleagues have also reported substantial alterations in the GABAergic system of the cerebellum, including a 40% reduction in GAD67 mRNA in Purkinje cells, 28% upregulation of GAD67 in basket cells, and decreased levels of GAD65 mRNA in cerebellar dentate nuclei of eight individuals with autism compared to eight controls (Yip, Soghomonian, & Blatt, 2007, 2008, 2009).

The observation of decreased Purkinje cell density appears to be in stark contrast to some reports from MRI studies of an enlarged cerebellum in autism (Courchesne et al., 2007) implying potentially a higher number of neurons. Several factors, however, make it impossible to compare findings from the two methods. At least 20 of the 32 brains examined in postmortem studies came from individuals who also had mental retardation (Ritvo et al., 1986; Kemper & Bauman, 1993; Bailey et al., 1998; Palmen et al., 2004; Whitney et al., 2008). Almost half of the brains were from individuals with epilepsy, and some were from individuals who were taking anticonvulsive medications that might themselves damage Purkinje cells. By contrast, most of the MRI studies were conducted with high-functioning autistic individuals and typically excluded subjects with seizure disorders. So, two very different cohorts of subjects are being studied with these different techniques.

Whether the observations of lower Purkinje cell density actually reflect fewer Purkinje cell numbers in the autistic brain awaits confirmation with unbiased stereological neuron-counting methods. As discussed in detail later in this chapter, an interesting hypothesis has emerged that neuroinflammation in the brain of individuals with autism, indicated by the presence of an increased number of activated microglia, may be associated with the loss of Purkinje cells in the cerebellum (Vargas et al., 2005).

Frontal Cortex

Although the frontal cortex is one of the most prominent areas of study in the search for potential neuropathology in autism, very little work has been conducted with postmortem brain tissue in this region. Structural MRI studies suggest that the frontal lobe, and in particular, the prefrontal cortex, may show the greatest degree of aberrant development in the brains of children with autism (Carper et al., 2002; Carper & Courchesne, 2005). Yet, no systematic postmortem study to date has explored the underlying neurobiology of the identified aberrant growth in the frontal cortex. Seven recent studies (Table 31-1) have utilized frontocortical tissue; findings include an increased spine density on the apical dendrite of pyramidal neurons in layer II (Hutsler & Zhang, 2010), the presence of ill-defined cortical layers (Mukaetova-Ladinska et al., 2004), and an indistinct boundary between gray and white matter (Avino & Hutsler, 2010) in the dorsolateral prefrontal region. An electron microscopy study of the white matter underlying the orbitofrontal cortex found decreased myelin thickness in 5 autism cases relative to 4 controls (Zikopoulos & Barbas, 2010).

Von Economo (a.k.a. spindle) neurons have been recent focus of interest in autism, although clear evidence of pathology has yet to be found. Von Economo neurons are unique, large cells localized to the anterior cingulate and frontal insular region of great apes and man, and are suspected to play a role in higher order cognitive function and emotional behavior (Allman et al., 2001; Allman et al., 2005). Two recent studies with small sample sizes have failed to find a difference in the number of von Economo neurons in the frontal insular region in autism cases relative to controls (Kennedy et al., 2007; Santos et al., 2010) However, a recent stereological study found a higher ratio of von Economo neurons to pyramidal neurons in layer V of the frontal insula in four autism cases relative to three controls (Santos et al., 2010), suggesting that von Economo neuron pathology may become evident in autism with larger sample sizes.

The frontal cortex has also been the focus of studies of minicolumnar organization of neurons, finding reduced intercolumnar width and increased cell density in dorsolateral prefrontal cortex (Casanova et al., 2002; Buxhoeveden et al., 2006; Casanova et al., 2006; Casanova et al., 2010). These findings are discussed in greater detail later in this chapter.

Anterior Cingulate Cortex

As described above, the anterior cingulate cortex (ACC) was the only region of neocortex noted by Kemper and Bauman (1993) to show abnormalities; they observed the cortex of autism cases to be unusually coarse and poorly laminated compared to controls. Abnormalities in the ACC have since been reported by Blatt and colleagues, including decreases in cell size in layers I–III and layers V–VI of area 24b and in cell packing density in layers V–VI of area 24c (Simms et al., 2009). The authors also observed irregular lamination in three of nine autism brains and increased density of neurons in the subcortical white matter in the remaining cases. A preliminary study of von Economo (a.k.a. spindle) neuron density was also carried out, but no significant differences in the autism cases were detected (Simms et al., 2009). Instead, the study appeared to uncover two subsets of autism cases, one that displayed an increase in von Economo neuron density and another with reduced density compared to controls. In another study by the same group, decreases in the mean density of GABA(A) and GABA(B) receptors and benzodiazepine binding sites were found in the ACC (Oblak et al., 2009; 2010), suggesting an alteration in GABAergic innervation of the ACC; this could potentially lead to a disturbance of the delicate balance between excitation and inhibition in this cortical area.

Another prominent theory, postulated by Herbert et al. (2004) and Courchesne & Pierce (2005), suggests excessive short-range and diminished long-range connectivity in the white matter underlying the frontal and anterior cingulate cortices. Herbert et al. (2004) reported that increased white matter volume in children with autism is restricted to superficial radiate white matter (i.e., corona radiata and "U" fibers), with no difference reported in deep and bridging white matter (e.g., corpus callosum, internal capsule, etc.). A recent postmortem study of single axons in white matter underlying the anterior cingulate cortex of autism cases found an excessive number of thin axons, which link neighboring areas together, and a decreased number of large axons, that communicate over long distances (Zikopoulos & Barbas, 2010). Interestingly, this study also found an over expression of growth-associated protein (GAP-43 kDa), which is expressed at high levels during rapid axon growth (Benowitz & Routtenberg, 1997), in the white matter underlying the ACC in the autism cases relative to controls. Although this study was carried out in a small sample and included cases with other neurological conditions (i.e. schizophrenia, epilepsy, depression), the findings have important implications for understanding the underlying neurobiology of aberrant connectivity in autism as reported by structural MRI and diffusion tensor imaging (DTI) studies.

Temporal Cortex

In a recent longitudinal MRI study of young children, the temporal cortex was found to undergo an abnormal growth trajectory in children with autism as well as display the greatest degree of aberrant enlargement among the cortical lobes (Schumann et al., 2010). Postmortem studies designed to examine the underlying pathology of this abnormal growth have yet to be carried out. The only study of temporal cortex, and the only other study of stereological neuron number in the autism brain (besides Schumann & Amaral, 2006, on the amygdala) was carried out by Van Kooten, Schmitz, and colleagues (2008) on the fusiform gyrus, a visual area implicated in processing faces and located midrostrocaudal on the inferior surface of the temporal lobe. In seven postmortem brains from patients with autism compared to ten controls, they found that the autism group showed significantly lower neuronal densities within layer III; lower total neuron numbers in layers III, V, and VI; and smaller mean perikaryal volumes of neurons in layers V and VI (Figure 31-4). Although the findings of this study were based on a relatively small sample size, and require replication, the results have implications for the cellular basis of abnormalities of face perception in people with autism. Pathology may originate from events in the fusiform directly, or from pathology in other brain regions with which the fusiform connects, such as the amygdala, which has also been shown to have a reduction in neuron number in autism patients (Schumann & Amaral, 2006). It will be important to determine in future studies whether decreased neuronal numbers in both the fusiform gyrus and amygdala result in the functional impairments associated with autism or, alternatively, are caused by hypoactivation or underuse during early development.

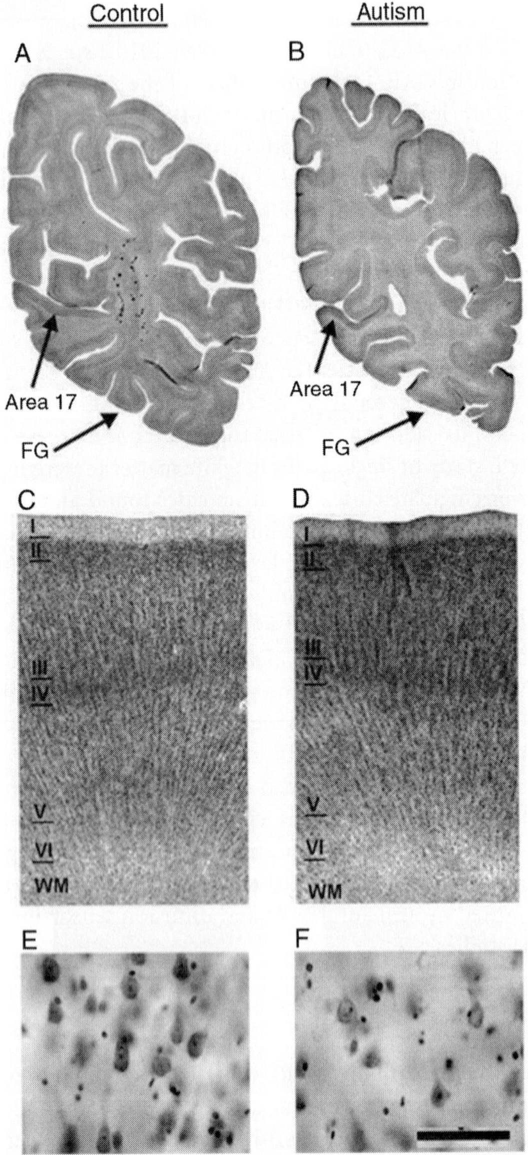

Figure 31–4. Photomicrographs of 200 μm thick coronal sections of the brain hemispheres through the level of the fusiform gyrus from a control (A, C, E) and a patient with autism (B, D, F), a cross-section of cortex from the fusiform gyrus (C, D; scale bar = 400μm), and layer III of the fusiform gyrus from each subject at high magnification (E, F; scale bar = 50 μm). Adapted with permission from van Kooten et al., 2008.

Blatt and colleagues have proposed widespread abnormalities in the GABAergic system of the brain in individuals with autism, including the fusiform gyrus and hippocampus. Reductions in the mean density of GABA(A) and GABA(B) receptors and benzodiazepine binding sites were recently reported in the fusiform gyrus (Oblak et al., 2010a; 2010b). Decreased GABA(A) receptor binding has also been reported in the hippocampus (Blatt et al., 2001); the decreased binding is likely due to a decrease in the density of binding sites rather than an altered affinity (Guptill et al., 2007). In a recent study, a subpopulation of GABAergic interneurons immunoreactive to calcium binding proteins were found to be decreased in the hippocampus of autism cases relative to controls (Lawrence et al., 2010). However, alterations in the GABAergic system in autism are not specific to the temporal cortex, as Blatt and colleagues have reported similar pathology in the cerebellum and cingulate cortices (Oblak et al., 2009, 2010a, 2010b; Yip et al., 2007, 2008, 2009), but instead appear to be a common feature that may disrupt global inhibitory control in the autistic brain.

Alterations of the Columnar Structure of the Neocortex: The Minicolumn Hypothesis

Increasing interest has been placed on the notion, advanced by Casanova and colleagues (Casanova et al., 2002; Buxhoeveden et al., 2006; Casanova et al., 2006; Casanova et al., 2010), that there are an abnormal number and width of minicolumns (Figure 31-5) in the cortex of individuals with autism. As described in further detail below, minicolumn formation has been associated with early stages of cortical development when postmitotic neurons ascend in linear arrays along a radial glial scaffolding (Rakic, 1988). Within the first year of life, there is a dramatic increase in dendritic growth. By 2 years of age, the minicolumns are spaced further apart with a lower cell density in a given region of cortex. Dendritic bundles and axonal fascicles that extend throughout several layers of the cortex occupy the space between minicolumns (Jones, 2000; Rockland & Ichinohe, 2004). Casanova and colleagues (Casanova et al., 2002; Buxhoeveden et al., 2006; Casanova et al., 2006) have posed the reasonable question of whether there is perturbation in the fundamental organization of minicolumns in the autistic brain.

Sixteen cases of autism (at least 9 with seizures and at least 10 with mental retardation) have been examined for

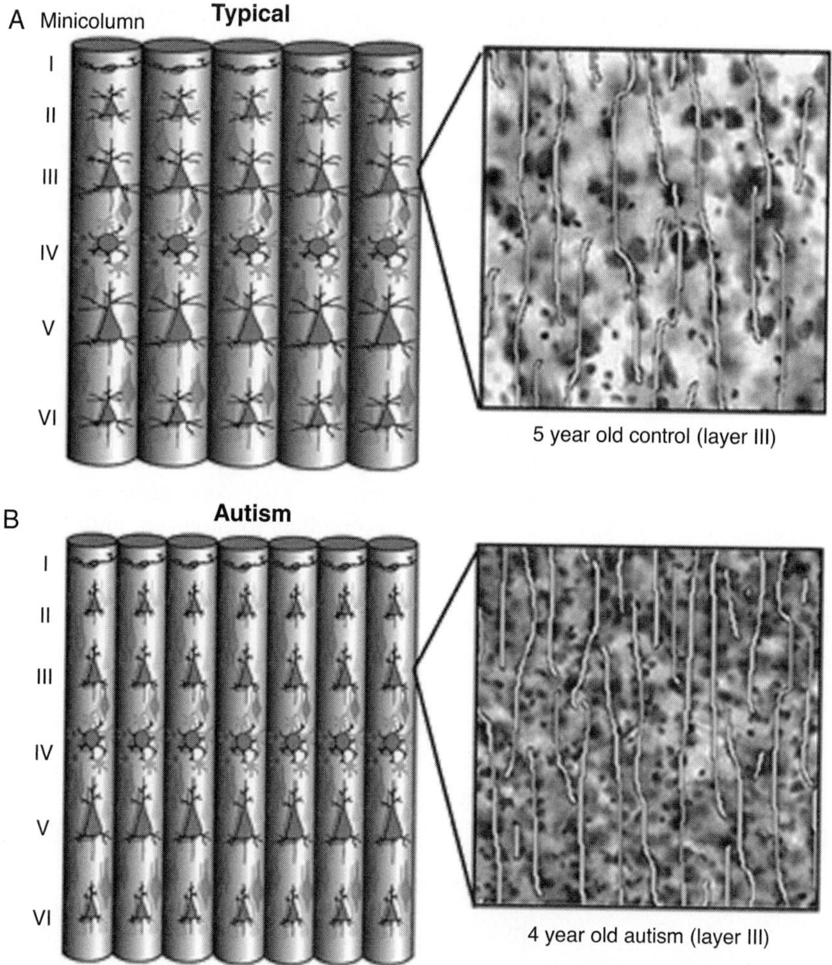

Figure 31–5. Model of the minicolumnar hypothesis proposed by Casanova et al. (2002, 2006) that there are an abnormal number and width of minicolumns in the cortex of individuals with autism. Each so-called minicolumn contains approximately 80–100 neurons (see schematic of minicolumn formation in Figure 31-8). (A) Model depicts a decreased intercolumnar width in the autism case relative to controls. (B) Nissl images were adapted with permission from Casanova et al. (2006), in which the distance between cell-body defined minicolumns was found to be reduced in layer III of dorsolateral prefrontal cortex (BA 9) in a 4-year-old autism case relative to a 5-year-old control. Given the narrower neuropil area between columns, one would also predict a decrease in the dendritic arborization of BA 9 Neurons (as depicted in the model, A). (See Color Plate Section for a color version of this figure.)

minicolumnar pathology in cortical layer III in three independent studies using varying techniques (Casanova et al., 2002; Buxhoeveden et al., 2006; Casanova et al., 2006). The most consistent finding in these studies is reduced intercolumnar width of the minicolumns in dorsolateral prefrontal cortex (BA 9/46). In a recent follow-up study, Casanova and colleagues (2010) determined that diminished minicolumnar width is not limited to layer III, but instead is present across supra- and infragranular cell layers, most notably in BA 44 (pars opercularis) in the frontal cortex of autism cases. These findings, coupled with increases in neuronal density on the order of 23% noted by Casanova et al. (2006), imply that there should be a greater number of neurons in BA 9 of the autistic cortex. Given the narrower neuropil area between columns, one would also predict a decrease in the dendritic arborization of dorsolateral prefrontal cortical neurons. These neuropathological questions are ripe for analysis using systematic stereological methods. One would predict an increased number of neurons in the prefrontal cortex in autism cases, given evidence of increased volume at young ages and reduction of minicolumnar spacing; however such a study has yet to be carried out.

Neuroinflammation in Autism

There is emerging evidence that an anomalous immune response during vulnerable periods of brain development could contribute to the neuropathology associated with autism (Ashwood & Van de Water, 2004; Pardo et al., 2005; Ashwood et al., 2006). Interactions between the immune and nervous systems begin early in embryogenesis and persist throughout an individual's lifetime, with successful neurodevelopment contingent on a normal and balanced immune response (Boulanger & Shatz, 2004; Wrona, 2006). Two cell populations act as directors and effectors of the immune response. Microglia primarily act as the resident phagocytes, constantly eliminating damaged neurons, accumulated debris, and infectious agents. Astroglia, meanwhile, are classically considered to act as directors of the immune response via detection and release of a wide array of cytokines and chemokines. Both microglia and astroglia participate in several additional functions during development, including histogenesis, synaptogenesis, neuronal dendritic arborization, and regulation of neuron numbers (Marin-Teva et al., 2004; Schmitz & Rezaie, 2008). In adulthood, microglia play a dual role; in addition to cytotoxic, phagocytic, and antigen-presenting capabilities, they also demonstrate cytoprotective and neurotrophic functions (for review see Pardo et al., 2005).

Microglia undergo morphological changes based on the current state of the immune response. "Resting" ramified microglia (Figure 31-6), with small cell bodies and long thin processes, are commonly found throughout the typically developing brain across life span for constant surveillance of the local environment to detect inflammatory signals (Nimmerjahn et al., 2005). When infection is presented, microglia may be "activated" by a variety of factors, including pro-inflammatory cytokines, necrotic factors, glutamate receptor agonists, and changes in extracellular potassium concentration. Once the microglial cell is activated, the processes thicken and retract to move rapidly to the site of the insult. The cell body has the appearance of swelling with the uptake of MHC class II proteins and secretes cytotoxic and pro-inflammatory signaling molecules including cytokines and chemokines. These *activated* microglia interact with neurons to fight off infection, typically with minimal damage to healthy brain cells. "Ameboid" microglia in the activated state are commonly observed in the typically developing brain in high concentrations during the prenatal period responding to large amounts of extracellular debris and apoptotic cells that is a consequence of programmed death (Rezaie & Male, 1999).

Although microglial and astroglial activation is often a beneficial response, dysfunction of the immune system

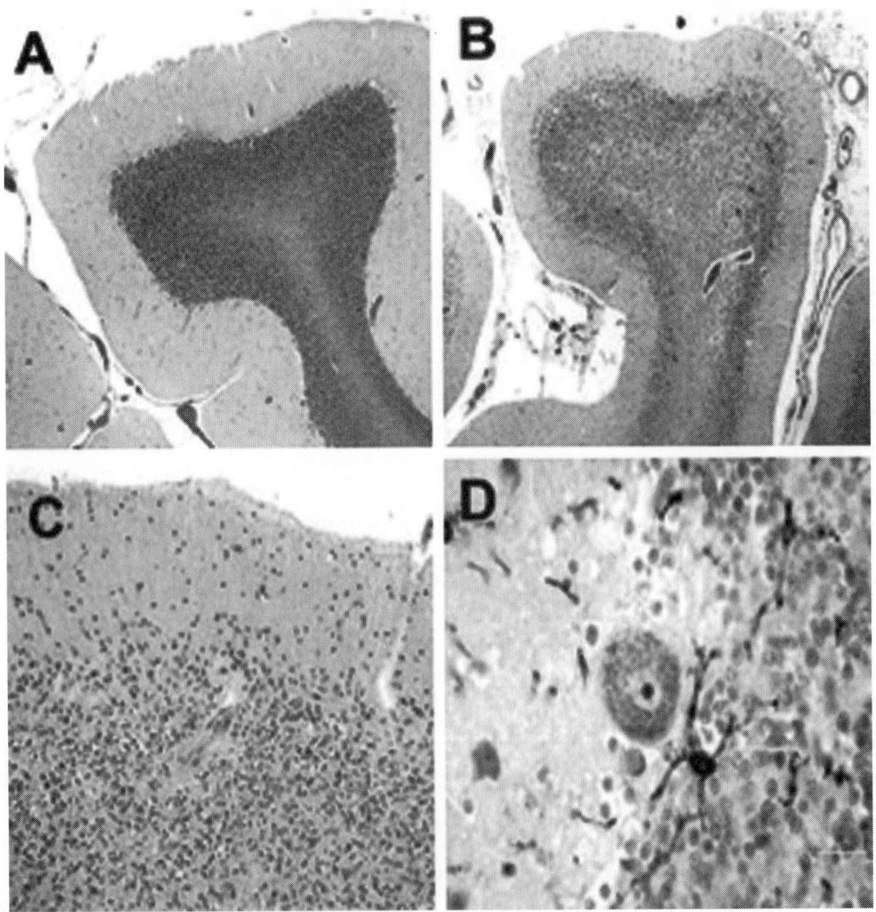

Figure 31–6. (A) Normal appearance of the cerebellum in a control patient; (B–C) Atrophic folia and marked loss of Purkinje and granular cells in the cerebellum of an autistic patient (H&E Stain); (D) Microglia activation seen with anti-MHC class II immunostaining. Adapted with permission from Vargas et al., 2005. (See Color Plate Section for a color version of this figure.)

resulting in a chronic state of neuroinflammation could have detrimental effects on the developing brain and potentially lead to neuronal cell death and alterations in neuronal connectivity (Streit et al., 2005). Ongoing neuroinflammatory processes, as evidenced by the presence of activated microglia and astroglia in cases of autism, was first described by Vargas et al. (2005). They observed excessive microglial activation in the cerebellum and frontal cortex in postmortem brain tissue in a subset of 11 autistic patients (age range 5–44 years) using immunocytochemical staining for MHC class II markers (HLA-DR). The excessive microglial activation was particularly prominent in the granular cell layer of the cerebellum. Vargas and colleagues speculated that the presence of activated microglia near Purkinje neurons in the cerebellum may be related to the commonly noted reduction of Purkinje cells in autism patients, given the regulatory role that microglia play in normal Purkinje neuron death (Marin-Teva et al., 2004) (Figure 31-6). Recently, Morgan and colleagues reported increases in activated microglia number and size in some, but not all, cases of autism in dorsolateral prefrontal cortex and amygdala using an antibody to ionized calcium binding adaptor molecule-1 (Iba-1); a marker that visualizes both resting and activated microglia (Morgan et al., 2010; Morgan et al., personal communication).

At present, the role of microglial activation in autism remains unclear. It is possible that aberrant microglial activity directly contributes to abnormal neurodevelopment, with activation triggered by genetic or environmental factors that otherwise would not be significantly disruptive. Alternately, it may be a largely healthy response to an exogenous insult such as viral infection, or a genetic alteration that, for example, produces an excessively large population of neurons that must be reduced. Interestingly, elevations in pro-inflammatory cytokine and chemokine levels have also been reported in the brain tissue and cerebrospinal fluid of patients with autism (Vargas et al., 2005, Li et al., 2009). An emerging hypothesis is that cytokine levels may be impacted by prenatal maternal infection (see Patterson, 2009, for review). Further evaluation is necessary to define the precise role of the immune response and microglial activation in the pathogenesis of autism. If glial activation in autism is demonstrated to be deleterious, anti-inflammatory agents represent a highly promising future avenue for biotheraputic research.

Future Perspective

Autism is clearly a pathological disorder of neural development, but when and how the pathology occurs remains elusive. Typical brain development is comprised of several stages, including the proliferation and migration of neurons, synaptic growth, and eventually cell death and dendritic pruning. Any deviation at one or more of these stages could produce catastrophic downstream effects. As evident from the previous section, the field of postmortem human brain research in autism is still young and we have few clues to point to a particular stage in which development goes awry. We therefore now ask the reverse question, if a particular stage of development did go awry, what would the resulting pathology look like? Below we describe the normal stages of brain development and speculate, based on the current findings of autistic neuropathology, about the particular stage at which brain development may deviate from normal, leading to autism. However, we would like to reiterate that it is unlikely that a single neuropathological event will account for all autism; future studies will need to be powered and designed to detect various patterns that underlie the "autisms."

Fundamentals of Brain Development

The human central nervous system (CNS) is the most complex organ system in vertebrates and contains a greater variety of cell types than is found in any other organ system. The mature brain is comprised of approximately 100 billion neurons, and perhaps 10 times as many glial cells. Remarkably, the generation of nearly one trillion diverse, complex cell types is accomplished during a brief span of intense proliferation that encompasses approximately 3 months during gestation. Not surprisingly, this period of development is sensitive to genetic abnormalities and/or environmental interference. In fact, it is not surprising that there are occasionally errors of development leading to disorders such as autism; what is surprising given the complexity of the enterprise, is that neurodevelopment is generally successful and results in an individual that is "typically developing."

CNS cells are generated in two proliferative zones that line the ventricular system of the developing brain. Each proliferative zone is home to a distinct class of precursor cell. The primary proliferative zone, the ventricular zone (VZ) is directly adjacent to the lumen of the ventricle. Radial glial cells are the principle precursor cell type in the VZ. The secondary proliferative zone, the subventricular zone (SVZ), appears at the onset of neurogenesis in many CNS regions (Boulder Committee, 1970). SVZ precursor cells are generated by radial glial cells in the VZ, and then migrate radially to establish the SVZ compartment superficial to the VZ (see Figure 31-7). Both VZ and SVZ precursor cells produce neurons in the embryonic forebrain (Noctor et al., 2007). The VZ proliferative zone becomes depleted during development and is not present in the adult brain, but the SVZ remains as a neurogenic compartment in the mature and a similar structure is present in the adult dentate gyrus (Ihrie & Alvarez-Buylla, 2008).

Proliferation in the Developing Brain

Advances in the field of molecular biology have provided exciting new tools that can be applied to investigations of the developing CNS. New molecular tools allow researchers to control the expression of specific genes both regionally and temporally in the CNS. For example, the gene sequence for

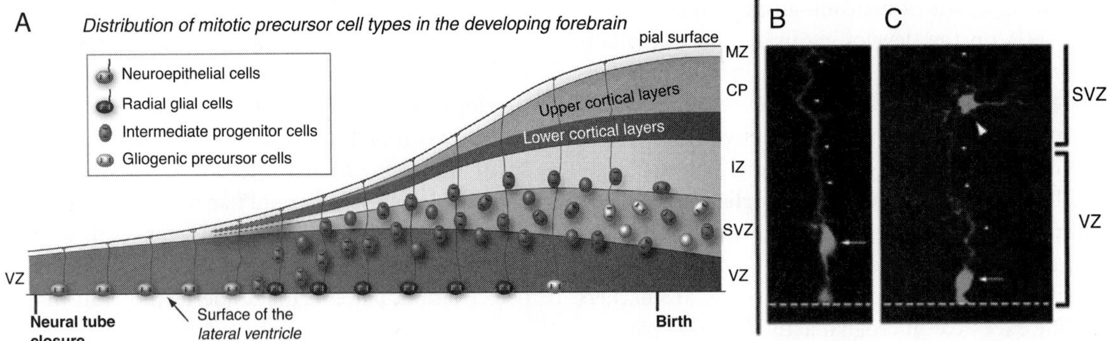

Figure 31–7. (A) Scheme depicting precursor cell types in the embryonic brain. After neural tube closure, the embryonic proliferative zone is composed of a single population of neuroepithelial cells which transition into radial glial cells at the onset of neurogenesis in the ventricular zone (VZ). They undergo division at the surface of the lateral ventricle and possess a long thin pial fiber that reaches the pial surface. Radial glial cell divisions produce neurons and intermediate progenitor cells. Intermediate progenitor cell bodies are primarily located in the subventricular zone (SVZ); Divisions occur away from the surface of the lateral ventricle and produce multiple neurons. At the conclusion of neurogenesis radial glial cells begin producing astrocytes, and Translocate to the SVZ, where gliogenesis continues after birth. (B) Micrograph showing an example of a radial glial cell labeled with fluorescent reporter gene. Radial glia are bipolar cells with a single process that contacts the ventricular surface (dotted line) and a single pial process that ascends toward the pial surface (small arrowheads). The cell body (arrow) is located in the VZ. (C) Micrograph showing a radial glial cell (arrow) and a daughter intermediate progenitor cell (large arrowhead) labeled with fluorescent reporter gene. The intermediate progenitor cell maintains contact with the radial glial cell pial fiber (small arrowheads). (See Color Plate Section for a color version of this figure.)

fluorescent reporter proteins has proven invaluable for detailed characterization of specific cell types, such as neural precursor cells in the developing brain. Fluorescent reporter proteins have allowed researchers to visualize neural precursor cells in living tissue. This capability has been used to identify neuronal and glial precursor cells in the developing brain, to characterize their patterns of cell division, cell production potential, and finally to characterize the daughter cells produced by precursor cells.

Glial cells and neurons had long been considered distinct cell types that were produced by separate precursor cell types in the developing brain. However, recent studies have demonstrated that glial functions are much broader, and that astrocytes in particular have much closer functional and lineal relationships with neurons than previously realized. Not only are astrocytes crucial partners with neurons in synaptic communication in the mature brain (Stevens, 2008), but they also generate neurons in several regions of the adult brain including the cortical SVZ (Doetsch et al., 1999), and the dentate gyrus (Seri et al., 2001). Astrocytes are lineally descended from embryonic radial glial cells (Noctor et al., 2004); the two cell types can be considered as representing different generations in the same immediate family. Radial glia are a specialized astroglial cell that is transiently present in the developing brain (Misson et al., 1988). Radial glia are bipolar cells that have a soma in the proliferative ventricular zone, a short descending process that contacts the ventricular lumen, and an ascending process that spans the wall of the developing brain to contact the pial membrane (Figure 31-7). Radial glial pial processes radiate outward from the ventricle to the surface of the brain, a pattern that dominates the appearance of the brain during early stages of development, and to a degree dictates organization of the mature CNS. Radial glial cells are the principle neuronal precursor cell type in the embryonic CNS (Malatesta et al., 2000; Miyata et al., 2001; Noctor et al., 2001; Noctor et al., 2002; Anthony et al., 2004). Radial glia generate neurons through one of two mechanisms: directly through an asymmetric division that produces a single neuron, or indirectly through a division that produces an SVZ intermediate progenitor cell that subsequently divides symmetrically to produce two neurons (Martínez-Cerdeño et al., 2006b). Most SVZ intermediate progenitor cells appear to undergo a single symmetric division to produce two neurons. But, in some cases they undergo multiple divisions that produce four or more neurons (Haubensak et al., 2004; Miyata et al., 2004; Noctor et al., 2004). A given radial glial cell division can therefore produce either a single neuron or multiple neurons. The exact number of radial glial cells in the embryonic brain has not been determined, nor has the total number of radial glial or intermediate progenitor divisions, but it is likely that billions of cell divisions are required to produce the 20 billion cortical neurons that populate the human cerebral cortex.

Most regions of the adult CNS are organized into discrete functional units. The cerebral cortex is a laminated sheet of tissue that is 2 to 4 mm thick, and organized into six horizontally arranged layers. This elaborate organization is further broken down into functional units that are arranged as radial columns, or cortical columns, that span across the six cortical layers (Mountcastle, 1997) (Figure 31-8). Each cortical column comprises multiple "minicolumns" in which a narrow column of approximately 80–100 radially arranged neurons span the cortical layers (Mountcastle, 1997). Neurons in each cortical

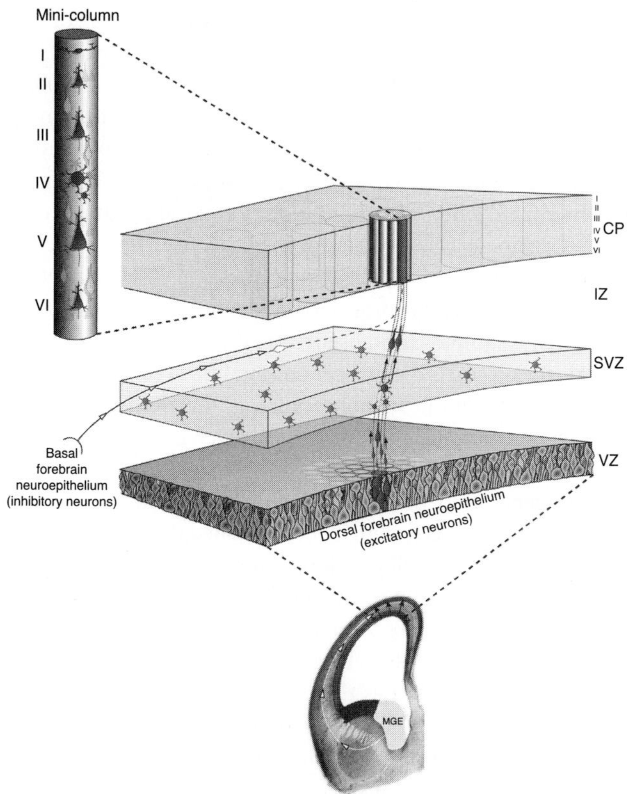

Figure 31–8. Scheme depicting the formation of minicolumn and cortical column functional units in the cerebral cortex. Each minicolumn contains approximately 80–100 neurons. Multiple minicolumns together form a single cortical column. As proposed by Rakic (1988), proliferative units in the ventricular zone (VZ) of the dorsal forebrain produce neurons that are destined for a single mini-column functional unit (dark column) in the cortical plate (CP). Each proliferative unit in the VZ may comprise 5–10 radial glial cells. Each radial glial cell possesses a single pial fiber that stretches across the cortical wall to the pial surface of the brain. The pial fiber guides the migration of newborn neurons from the proliferative zones to their respective minicolumn functional units in the CP. Neighboring proliferative units in the VZ produce neurons that are destined for different minicolumns in the CP (grey columns). Radial glial cells produce both neurons and intermediate progenitor cells, which migrate away from the ventricle along their parental pial fiber. recent work shows that intermediate progenitor cells undergo additional rounds of division in the subventricular zone (SVZ) to produce multiple neurons. Excitatory projection neurons are derived from the VZ of the dorsal forebrain, and migrate radially along radial glial cell fibers. Inhibitory interneurons are derived from the VZ of the medial ganglionic eminence (MGE) in the basal forebrain, and migrate tangentially into the overlying cerebral cortex. Mechanisms that guide migrating interneurons to specific minicolumns remain to be determined. (See Color Plate Section for a color version of this figure.)

column respond to similar stimuli and perform similar functions. The columnar, or radial organization of the cerebral cortex, is thought to derive from the organization of precursor cells in the embryonic ventricular zone. Rakic's Radial Unit Hypothesis proposes that precursor cells in the VZ (radial glia) are organized into discrete proliferative units that provide a proto-map of cortical columns in the adult cerebral cortex (Rakic, 1988). The Radial Unit Hypothesis predicts that each proliferative unit in the VZ produces the cortical neurons that populate a cortical column; each proliferative radial glial cell produces the cortical neurons that populate a single minicolumn (Figure 31-8). More recent data that shows substantial neurogenesis in the embryonic SVZ (Haubensak et al., 2004; Miyata et al., 2004; Noctor et al., 2004), has lead to modifications of the Radial Unit Hypothesis to account for the contribution of additional proliferative precursor cells in the SVZ (Kriegstein et al., 2006; see Figure 31-8). Subtle changes in the pattern of radial glial division and/or SVZ precursor cell division could produce measurable changes in the total number of neurons in the adult brain. Thus, aberrant regulation of cell proliferation within the VZ or SVZ may contribute to changes in cell number (Schumann et al., 2006; van Kooten et al., 2008), cell density and minicolumnar width (Casanova et al., 2002; Buxhoeveden et al., 2006; Casanova et al., 2006) (Figure 31-5), and ultimately increased brain size (Courchesne et al., 2007; Schumann et al., 2010) as reported in some cases of autism.

Regulation of Precursor Cell Proliferation

Proliferation is tightly regulated during brain development. Precursor cells follow a specific program that generates the proper number of neurons and glia. A wide variety of factors, including neurotransmitter substances, growth factors, and hormones, bind with receptors expressed by embryonic precursor cells and regulate cell division in the developing brain. For example, the classical neurotransmitters GABA and glutamate differentially regulate proliferation in the ventricular and subventricular zones during neocortical development (LoTurco et al., 1995; Haydar et al., 2000). Neurosteroids, such as estradiol, are also present in the embryonic proliferative zones and induce proliferation of precursor cells in the embryonic and adult brain (Martínez-Cerdeño et al., 2006a). Radial glial cells are coupled to one another through connexin gap junction channels that transmit electrical signals (LoTurco & Kriegstein, 1991). New evidence indicates that waves of calcium activity are also transmitted through gap junction channels and regulate radial glial cell proliferation (Weissman et al., 2004). Proteins such as beta-catenin promote proliferation versus differentiation of progenitor cells during cortical development (Chenn & Walsh, 2002). Blood vessels also appear to play an important role in proliferation. Precursor cells are often located in niches along the border of blood vessels in neurogenic regions of the adult brain (Palmer et al., 2000; Seri et al., 2004), as well as in the embryonic brain (Javaherian & Kriegstein, 2009; Stubbs et al., 2009). Furthermore, Temple and colleagues have found that endothelial cells release soluble factors that stimulate self-renewal of embryonic and adult precursor cells (Shen et al., 2004).

These findings indicate that endothelial cells, and perhaps factors circulating in the blood, regulate cell genesis during brain development.

Mutations in specific genes that regulate precursor cell behavior have been identified in Autism Spectrum Disorders. The genes *MCPH1* and *ASPM* are required for proper levels of proliferation during brain growth, and mutations in these genes produce microcephalic brains (Shen et al., 2005). Gene mutations that produce macrocephalic brains have also been identified. For example, mutations in the phosphatase and tensin homologue deleted on the chromosome 10 (PTEN) gene have been associated with large head size and autism (Zori et al., 1998; Goffin et al., 2001). PTEN is a tumor suppressor gene that controls cell size and number (Kwon et al., 2006). PTEN instructs cells to stop dividing, prevents cells from growing too rapidly, and in some cases instructs cells to undergo programmed cell death (Chu & Tarnawski, 2004). Together these functions prevent the formation of tumors and regulate the size of organs during development. Mice in which the PTEN gene has been deleted present with larger brains and hypertrophied neurons with abnormal cellular processes (Kwon et al., 2006). As described above, larger brain size has been reported in autism (Amaral et al., 2008). A recent study identified PTEN mutations in autism spectrum disorders, mentral retardation and developmental delays (Varga et al., 2009; McBride et al., 2010). Additional studies have reported that PTEN mutations are associated with some cases of autism spectrum disorders (Abrahams & Geschwind, 2008; see Chapters by State and colleagues, Lamb, and Morrow & Walsh in this volume). The cause of larger brain size observed in individuals with PTEN mutations has not been determined but may result from dysregulated precursor cell proliferation during development, hypertrophied neurons, decreased cell death, or a combination of the three.

Determination of Cell Fate

The determination of cell fate occurs at regional, local, and cellular levels. The regional expression patterns of different transcription factors along the rostrocaudal axis of the developing nervous system reveals one mechanism by which cortical cells acquire specific identities (Schuurmans & Guillemot, 2002). While all radial glial cells share characteristic morphological features, they nonetheless constitute a heterogeneous population based on protein expression patterns (Kriegstein & Gotz, 2003). This may explain how different regions of the developing telencephalon generate different classes of cortical cells. For example, excitatory pyramidal cells and astrocytes are generated by Pax6 expressing cells in the dorsal telencephalon, while inhibitory interneurons are generated by Dlx-1/2 expressing cells in the ganglionic eminences of the embryonic ventral telencephalon (Anderson et al., 1997; Figure 31-8). The expression of transcription factors such as Dlx-1/2 is likely an early step in the commitment of telencephalic cells to a specific fate. The expression of these factors may even correlate with the phenotype of specific neuronal subtypes. Indeed, new evidence indicates that subregions of the ganglionic eminences express different transcription factors and give rise to interneuron subtypes (Nery et al., 2002). Local environmental factors also play a role in determining the fate of neurons in the developing cortex. Transplantation studies demonstrate that the laminar fate of cortical neurons can be altered when transplantation of cortical precursor cells occurs during specific phases of the cell cycle (McConnell & Kaznowski, 1991). Furthermore, expression of transcription factors is crucial for the normal differentiation of cortical neurons. For example, the absence of the transcription factor Foxg1 during cortical neurogenesis induces deep layer cortical neurons to adopt the phenotype of Cajal-Retzius neurons that are normally found in the superficial layer 1 of the neocortex (Hanashima et al., 2004).

The generation of sufficient numbers of the diverse cell types in the nervous system is accomplished through two basic types of progenitor cell divisions, symmetric and asymmetric (Gotz & Huttner, 2005). Symmetric divisions generate two daughter cells that are similar, while asymmetric divisions generate two daughter cells that differ from one another. Recent evidence indicates that these types of divisions might occur in different proliferative zones, asymmetric divisions occur more frequently at the surface of the ventricular lumen, while symmetric divisions occur more frequently in the SVZ (Noctor et al., 2004). Radial glial cells divide asymmetrically at the ventricular lumen to generate either a single neuron, or a subventricular zone progenitor cell that subsequently generates two neurons. Therefore, each radial glial cell division can generate either one neuron directly, or two neurons indirectly. Thus, determination of daughter cell fate after radial glial divisions impacts the total number of neurons generated at a given time during development. A shift toward production of single neurons would decrease the total numbers of neurons being generated, while a shift toward the production of SVZ progenitor cells would double the neuronal output at a given time. Therefore, regulation of daughter cell fate during neurogenesis impacts the neuronal density for a given neocortical layer or structure. Invertebrate studies have revealed a number of molecules that are differentially segregated in nascent daughter cells during progenitor cell divisions. Some of these fate-determining molecules, such as Notch and Numb, are also expressed in mammalian proliferative zones and research into their role in determining daughter cell fate continues (Pearson & Doe, 2004; Bultje et al., 2009).

Migration in the Developing Brain

Neurons in the adult brain are organized into complex, intricately interconnected groups of nuclei and laminae. One of the remarkable aspects of brain development is that neurons are not born in their adult location, but instead must migrate distances of 7000 μm or more, from the proliferative zones to reach their final destination (Rakic, 1988). To put this into perspective, this is comparable to a person scaling a wall greater in height than Yosemite's 3,000 foot high El Capitan.

Despite the complexity of the task, this feat is achieved with such regularity and precision that there is little variation in the architectonic pattern of brain structures from one person to the next. In the developing neocortex, excitatory cortical neurons are generated in an inside-out sequence such that the deepest layers of the cerebral cortex are generated and migrate into the cortical mantle before the superficial layers. Thus, as development proceeds neurons must migrate progressively longer distances and through an increasing number of cortical cells. The radial glial cells that generate neurons play an important role in the migration of newborn cortical neurons. Radial glia are bipolar cells that have a long pial process that ascends from the cell body in the proliferative VZ, to the pial surface of the developing brain. Newborn excitatory neurons attach themselves to the pial process and migrate toward the cortical plate using the pial process as a directional guide (Rakic, 1971). In fact, many neurons piggy-back along the pial process of their parental radial glial cell (Noctor et al., 2001; Noctor et al., 2004; Noctor et al., 2008), demonstrating the importance of lineage relationships in the developing brain. Newborn cortical neurons extend a leading process toward the overlying cortical plate and migrate radially along the pial fiber of the parent radial glial cell until they reach their destination in the cortical plate, at which point they detach from the pial fiber. This form of migration relies on cell-cell adhesion molecules that interact between radial glial fibers and migrating neurons (Hatten, 1990). Recent data demonstrates that gap junctions play an important role in mediating the adhesion between migrating neurons and radial glial processes (Elias et al., 2007). Neuronal migration is also regulated by a number of extracellular signaling molecules such as neurotransmitter substances acting through the NMDA receptor (Komuro & Rakic, 1993). Migrating neurons depend on additional signaling molecules to reach the correct location in the developing brain. For example, the reelin protein acts through its constituent receptor molecules to guide migrating neurons to the cortical plate, and arrest migration once the neurons have reached their proper location (Tissir & Goffinet, 2003). Reelin may play a distinct role in neuronal functioning in the mature brain. Reductions in reelin protein have been reported in a few select regions of the cerebral cortex and in the cerebellum (Fatemi et al., 2005). Given current understanding of reelin function in the developing mammalian brain, a reduction in reelin protein could be predicted to alter the trajectory of migratory neurons, resulting in the ectopic location of neurons in the forebrain. Examination of the reelin gene (RELN) has detected missense mutations in some cases of autism, but at a very low frequency, leading some to suggest that reelin may not play a major role in the etiology of autism (Bonora et al., 2003). Future studies on the regulation of reelin protein expression may shed light on the role that reelin protein plays in the autistic brain.

Recent experiments employing time-lapse imaging of fluorescently labeled cells in cultured brain tissue have revealed that the patterns of neuronal migration in the neocortex are more complex than originally thought. Experiments in the 1990s discovered that inhibitory cortical neurons are generated in the ventral forebrain and migrate tangentially into the overlying dorsal neocortex (De Carlos et al., 1996; Anderson et al., 1997; Tamamaki et al., 1997; Wichterle et al., 1999). Interneurons do not appear to migrate along radial glial fibers during their journey from the ventral into the dorsal cortex. In fact, they appear to travel perpendicular to the radial glial matrix. It has yet to be determined whether they rely on cellular guides such as developing axonal pathways, or rather are guided solely along gradients of chemoattractive and repulsive factors (Marin & Rubenstein, 2003). Some syndromic forms of autism, for example mutations of CNTNAP2 in an Amish family with epilepsy, MR, and autism, appear to involve disruption of neuronal migration (Strauss et al., 2006), which likely occurs focally in the anterior frontal and temporal lobes (Alarcon et al., 2008). Thus, regional specificity may arise from either differences in protomap related genes, or regional cell adhesion molecules involved in migration.

Recent work in rodents shows that excitatory neurons undergo four distinct stages of migration that can be identified based on the morphology and position of the neurons. After being generated, cortical neurons enter stage one of migration, leaving the ventricular surface and rapidly ascending to the SVZ. During stage two, cortical neurons acquire a multipolar morphology and remain stationary in the SVZ for one day or longer. After sojourning in the SVZ (Bayer & Altman, 1991), many cortical neurons enter stage three, and make a retrograde movement back toward the ventricular lumen. Finally neurons enter stage four, during which they reverse polarity back toward the cortical plate and commence radial migration along the pial fiber (Noctor et al., 2004). Similar ventricular directed movements have been reported for GABAergic interneurons after they have migrated into the dorsal cortex (Nadarajah & Parnavelas, 2002). The ventricle directed movements exhibited by these distinct cell types suggests that both excitatory and inhibitory neurons can respond to some of the same cues during their cortical migrations, and also hints at a potential source of important migration guidance molecules located near the ventricular lumen of the developing brain. Yet another form of migration, termed chain migration, has been identified for olfactory bulb interneurons as they migrate from their birthplace in the cortical subventricular zone along the rostral migratory stream into the olfactory bulb (Lois et al., 1996). Despite differences in the identified forms of migration, all neurons appear to rely on a shared set of intracellular molecules that are involved in extension of the leading process and transport of cellular structures such as the nucleus (Feng & Walsh, 2001; Schaar et al., 2004).

Abnormal Cell Migration

Neuronal migration is thus a complex interplay between the migrating cell and its environment that relies on intracellular machinery as well as extrinsic signaling factors. Given the complexity of this task, it is not surprising that a number of nervous system malformations have been identified that result from defects in neuronal migration (Feng & Walsh, 2001). Neurons depend on different molecules for the successful progression from one stage of migration to the next. For example, deletion or mutation in the doublecortin gene prevents neurons from transitioning from stage two to stage three. Doublecortin is an X-linked gene, and males with a deletion or mutation in this gene are affected with lissencephaly, i.e., a greatly reduced and smooth cortical surface. Heterozygous females present with a milder form of neuropathology called "double cortex." In this condition, a second band of grey matter is located below the normal location of the cortical laminae (des Portes et al., 1998; Gleeson et al., 1998). This secondary band of tissue consists of neurons that did not progress beyond stage two of migration (LoTurco, 2004). These neurons can fire action potentials, but they do not appear to elaborate the initial axonal process that precedes stage three of migration in the embryonic neocortex (Bai et al., 2003). Another molecule that has been associated with migration failure, Filamin A, is required for leading process extension that precedes transition to stage four of migration. Individuals with a mutation in this gene present with a form of neuropathology termed "periventricular nodular heterotopia," in which large clusters or nodules of cortical neurons are found along the surface of the lateral ventricles. Periventricular nodular heterotopias have also been identified in subjects with fragile X syndrome (Moro et al., 2006), which results from CGG repeat expansion in the *FMR1* gene. The range of neuropathology associated with migration failure varies from severe brain malformations found in lissencephaly, to small ectopic clusters of neurons. In each case, varying proportions of neurons fail to migrate to their proper destination. Afflicted individuals present with mental retardation in severe cases, but even mild malformations are often associated with epilepsy. It is of interest that Bailey and colleagues reported a number of instances of ectopic cortical neuronal clusters in their survey of neuropathology in the autistic brain (Bailey et al., 1998). Recent work identifying alterations in cortical column structure in some autistic brains may also be related (Casanova et al., 2002; Buxhoeveden et al., 2006; Casanova et al., 2006). The etiology of altered minicolumn structure has not been determined, but may result from altered dendritic arborization, increased numbers of proliferative units in the VZ.

Axonal Outgrowth

Neurons are polarized cells that possess a single axon and, typically, multiple dendrites. The proper development of axons and dendrites is crucial for normal functioning, since a single neuron in the adult brain can make thousands of connections with neighboring and distant cells. Neurons begin elaborating processes immediately after being generated. During migration neurons extend and retract multiple leading processes as they migrate through the developing brain tissue toward their destination. These temporary processes serve specific purposes during development but are not retained by the neurons as they differentiate to assume their adult morphology. However, neurons do elaborate some processes during development that are retained as the cells mature, and these processes can determine with which cells a given neuron will communicate. Work in the embryonic cortex shows that sister neurons develop and maintain multiple contacts with one another during migration (Noctor et al., 2001; Noctor et al., 2004; Noctor et al., 2008), and that these contacts presage adults patterns of connectivity (Yu et al., 2009). In the cerebral cortex, most excitatory neurons elaborate an axonal process before initiating radial migration to the cortical plate (Noctor et al., 2004), and these processes can grow substantial distances across the cerebral hemispheres during gestation (Schwartz & Goldman-Rakic, 1991). While migrating cells express and rely on functional neurotransmitter receptors (Komuro & Rakic, 1993; Flint et al., 1998; Komuro & Rakic, 1998), they do not appear to form synaptic connections until after they have reached their destination. Migrating neurons do not have synapses, which precludes the synaptic release of neurotransmitter on these cells, but nonsynaptic release of transmitters before synapse development has been described in the developing brain, including the hippocampus (Demarque et al., 2002). Axon outgrowth can be summarized as occurring in four distinct stages: initial axonal outgrowth, axon pathfinding, pruning, and stabilization (Hedin-Pereira et al., 1999). Numerous molecules that regulate these processes have been identified and are well characterized, including those that guide axon pathfinding such as slit/robo (Dickson & Gilestro, 2006).

A number of MRI studies suggest that there are alterations in connectivity in the autistic brain. Herbert et al. (2003) postulated that the abnormal brain enlargement observed in children with autism is disproportionately accounted for by increased white matter based on their findings of large increases in white matter, but no difference in gray matter, in 7- to 11-year-old boys. Of six studies investigating cerebral gray and white matter volumes in autism, three in very young children (1.5–4 years) have reported findings that are consistent with Herbert's suggestion (Courchesne et al., 2001; Hazlett et al., 2005; Schumann et al., 2010). However, studies carried out with subjects who are in later childhood and adolescence are less consistent with Herbert's hypothesis. Two studies found no difference in white matter in later childhood and adolescence (7–18 years; Lotspeich et al., 2004; Palmen et al., 2005), and one found no difference in adolescence and early adulthood (13–29 years; Hazlett et al., 2006). Herbert et al. examined a narrower age range restricted to preadolescent children (7–11 years) and reported a 13% increase in white matter (Herbert et al., 2003), which is restricted to superficial radiate white matter, with no difference reported in deep and bridging white matter Herbert et al. (2004). As discussed earlier, a recent study of post-mortem human tissue found a decreased number of large axons that project long distances beneath the anterior cingulate cortex, an increased number of thin local projection axons, and increased expression of

GAP-43 (Zikopoulos & Barbas, 2010). While provocative, these observations should be confirmed and extended in studies that include a larger sample size.

Synaptogenesis is initiated at points of axodendritic contact between neurons. Functional synapses can form relatively quickly, in some cases within minutes after required pre- and postsynaptic proteins and material have been transported to the site (McAllister, 2007). Synapse development requires the presence of postsynaptic density, receptors, active zone proteins, synaptic vesicles, and transsynaptic adhesion molecules. Transsynaptic molecules in particular are thought to regulate early stages of synapse formation. Two classes of transsynaptic proteins, neuroligins and β-neurexins, have received considerable attention after the discovery that mutated forms of these proteins are found in some autistic patients (Jamain et al., 2003; Comoletti et al., 2004; Szatmari et al., 2007). Neuroligins are postsynaptic proteins that bind with high affinity to members of the presynaptic β-neurexin family of proteins. The formation of the neuroligin–β-neurexin complex is thought to be sufficient and necessary for synapse formation (McAllister, 2007). Multiple isoforms of neuroligin and neurexin have been identified, and each is associated with different types of synapses. The neuroligin-3 and neuroligin-4 isoforms garnered attention after the discovery that mutations in the genes that code these proteins were identified in some patients with autism (Jamain et al., 2003; Comoletti et al., 2004). The mutated forms of the protein can still induce synapse formation, but bind with their transsynaptic partners at a lower affinity (Jamain et al., 2003), which suggests the possibility that some synapses may be altered in these autistic patients. Mutated genes that code for proteins in the β-neuroexin family have also been identified and are linked to some cases of autism (Szatmari et al., 2007). Furthermore, mutated genes that code for additional proteins required for synaptogenesis, such as shank3 (Durand et al., 2007), and protocadherin 10 (Morrow et al., 2008), have been identified in families with autistic children. These data highlight the importance of proper synaptic formation and point toward the potential etiology of some types of autism.

The Role of Cell Death

Some reports indicate that as many as 50% of all neurons that are generated during the development of the CNS die soon after the formation of synapses. The discovery that neuron–target cell interactions are crucial for cell survival suggested that young neurons receive trophic support from their target cells with which they connect (Levi-Montalcini & Booker, 1960a, 1960b). The subsequent isolation and characterization of nerve growth factor led to the discovery of a large family of survival factors, called neurotrophins, which are secreted by target tissues. Most immature neurons depend on access to neurotrophins for survival; neurons that fail to make proper synaptic connections do not receive sufficient trophic support and do not survive. In addition, some neurons also depend on trophic support from cells that innervate them (Raff et al., 1993). The neurotrophic theory predicts that the developing nervous system can "correct" for some errors in proliferation or migration by eliminating those cells that do not succeed in making proper connections. Furthermore, the embryonic proliferative zones produce a greater number of cells than is generally required to ensure a higher degree of success during formation of CNS structures. Newborn neurons must therefore compete with one another for access to trophic support from target tissues in much the same way that neighboring trees compete with one another for access to sunlight. Additional signaling pathways also play a role in the programmed cell death of young neurons, such as the caspase family of cysteine proteases (Kuan et al., 2000).

As mentioned above and described in further detail elsewhere in this book, MRI studies have reported increased brain volume in some regions of the frontal lobes in young autistic children, but decreased brain volume in the same areas later in adolescence (for review see Courchesne et al., 2007). Additional groups have weighed in on this issue and generally concur that there is an enlargement of cortical brain volume in young autistic children, but it is not yet clear whether these changes are retained beyond childhood (Amaral et al., 2008). Although the etiology underlying these changes in cortical neuroanatomy has not been determined, the early overgrowth of brain tissue followed by possible degeneration is reminiscent of the neurotrophic theory. This suggests that an alteration in two distinct developmental processes could be associated with some forms of autism. An initial phase of increased proliferation in the ventricular and/or subventricular zone would increase cell numbers and could explain increased volume of grey cortical matter. Failure of these cells to form proper synaptic connections, and thus failure to receive sufficient trophic support, would then reduce cell numbers in affected structures and could explain the reduced brain volume reported for older children and adolescents. Furthermore, some cells in the brain appear to undergo programmed cell death, or apoptosis. Factors that promote and inhibit apoptosis have been identified. Interestingly, expression of the anti-apoptotic factor bcl2 is reduced in some cortical regions of individuals with autism, while the pro-apoptotic factor p53 may be overexpressed in the autistic brain (Fatemi & Halt, 2001). These patterns of expression would both lead to an increase in cell death, which could explain the smaller brain volumes that have been reported in some studies. Neurotrophins can regulate the activity of apoptotic factors such as p53, pointing to specific intracellular signaling pathways that might be activated in the autistic brain.

Establishment and Maintenance of Dendritic and Axonal Arbors

Just as the developing brain produces a greater number of cells than is needed, many neurons initially make an excessive number of synaptic connections (Scheiffele, 2003).

The changes in grey matter volume reported in autistic children discussed above could also result from an exuberant production of neuronal processes and cell-cell interactions, followed by excessive pruning of these processes and synapse retraction. The assembly of mature neural networks relies on tightly controlled cell-cell interactions, and candidate molecules that play crucial roles in these processes have been identified. For example, the α1-chimaerin family of proteins, which are expressed in neurons during differentiation and synaptogenesis (Lim et al., 1992), regulate process growth and pruning along dendritic arbors during brain development (Buttery et al., 2006; Beg et al., 2007). These molecules are crucial for normal development. Neurons, in which expression of α1-chimaerin protein has been decreased, sprout overabundant dendritic processes (Buttery et al., 2006). In contrast neurons in which α1-chimaerin protein is overexpressed have longer dendrites with a greater number of processes. Genes that code for proteins such as α1-chimaerin are candidates for consideration in neurodevelopmental disorders, such as autism, that may result from abnormal patterns of connectivity in the CNS. Indeed, a genomewide screen for linkage with autism conducted in 2001 identified α1-chimaerin as a potential gene of interest (IMGSAC, 2001), which, although speculative, may contribute to diminished long-range connectivity (Courchesne & Pierce, 2005; Geschwind & Levitt, 2007).

Conclusions

Research into the neuropathology of autism is still in its infancy. Progress has been hindered, in part, by the lack of availability of a large number of postmortem brains, particularly from early postnatal periods. Given the inherent heterogeneity in the etiologies and trajectories of the autisms, it is likely that various patterns of neuropathology will be observed if an adequate number of brains become available for analyses. It is fair to say that the technology for sophisticated neuropathological analyses is available once the brains have been obtained. Indications that there are fewer neurons in the fusiform gyrus and amygdala beg the question of whether there were always fewer neurons or whether a neurodegenerative process occurs in autism. While the minicolumn hypothesis is important in focusing future neuropathological efforts, it will be critical to combine this research with estimates of cell number, size, and complexity. Similarly, studies indicating persistent inflammation of the autistic brain are provocative, but must be replicated across multiple brain regions and in larger samples of autistic brains. In the end, the relatively subtle neuropathology observed thus far in the autistic brain provides some hope that the behavioral impairments associated with the syndrome are not due to massive neural alteration, but rather to a more subtle, although pervasive, modulation of brain activity. If so, intervention leading to normalized behavior may be more feasible.

Challenges and Future Directions

- Progress into the neuropathology of autism will require an international collaborative effort to acquire an adequate number of brain specimens for analysis.
- Fundamental studies of neuronal organization using modern quantitative, stereological techniques as well as classical methods (e.g., Golgi) will need to be carried out to understand whether the autistic brain is characterized by abnormal cell proliferation and/or cell loss and if there are fundamental differences in the structure of neurons in the autism brain.
- Sophisticated clinical phenotyping of donors will be essential to account for neuropathology associated with comorbid syndromes and the heterogeneity of the autisms in the neuropathological findings that are obtained from postmortem studies.

SUGGESTED READINGS

Amaral, D. G., Schumann, C. M., & Nordahl, C. W. (2008) Neuroanatomy of autism. *Trends in Neurosciences, 31*, 137–145.

American Psychiatric Association. (1994). Diagnostic and statistical manual of mental disorders (4th ed.). Washington, DC: Author.

Bailey, A. (2008). Postmortem studies of autism. *Autism Research, 1*(5), 265.

Schmitz, C., & Rezaie, P. (2008). The neuropathology of autism: Where do we stand? *Neuropathology and Applied Neurobiology, 34*(1), 4–11.

ACKNOWLEDGMENTS

Original research described in this chapter by the authors was supported by grants from the National Institute of Mental Health (R01 MH41479-18) and by the M.I.N.D. Institute. As always, we are grateful to the individuals and their families who contribute autism research.

REFERENCES

Abrahams, B. S., & Geschwind, D. H. (2008). Advances in autism genetics: on the threshold of a new neurobiology. *Nature Reviews Genetics, 9*, 341–355.

Adolphs, R. (2001). The neurobiology of social cognition. *Current Opinion in Neurobiology, 11*, 231–239.

Alarcón, M., Abrahams, B. S., Stone, J. L., Duvall, J. A., Perederiy, J. V., Bomar, J. M., et al. (2008). Linkage, association, and gene-expression analyses indentify CNTNAP2 as an autism-susceptibility gene. *American Journal of Human Genetics, 82*, 150–159.

Allman, J. M., Hakeem, A., Erwin, J. M., Nimchinsky, E., & Hof, P. (2001). The anterior cingulate cortex: The evolution of an interface between emotion and cognition. *Annals of the New York Academy Sciences, 935*, 107–117.

Allman, J. M., Watson, K. K., Tetreault, N. A., & Hakeem, A. Y. (2005). Intuition and autism: a possible role for Von Economo neurons. *Trends in Cognitive Sciences, 9*, 367–373.

Amaral, D. G., Schumann, C. M., & Nordahl, C. W. (2008). Neuroanatomy of autism. *Trends in Neurosciences, 31*, 137–145.

Anderson, S. A., Eisenstat, D. D., Shi, L., & Rubenstein, J. (1997). Interneuron migration from basal forebrain to neocortex: dependence on dlx genes. *Science, 278*, 474–476.

Anthony, T. E., Klein, C., Fishell, G., & Heintz, N. (2004). Radial glia serve as neuronal progenitors in all regions of the central nervous system. *Neuron, 41*, 881–890.

Ashwood, P., & Van de Water, J. (2004). Is autism an autoimmune disease? *Autoimmunity Reviews, 3*, 557–562.

Ashwood, P., Wills, S., & Van de Water, J. (2006). The immune response in autism: a new frontier for autism research. *Journal of Leukocyte Biology, 80*, 1–15.

Avino T. A., & Hutsler J. J. (2010). Abnormal cell patterning at the cortical gray-white matter boundary in autism spectrum disorders. *Brain Research, 1360*, 138–46.

Bai, J., Ramos, R. L., Ackman, J. B., Thomas, A. M., Lee, R. V., & LoTurco, J. J. (2003). RNAi reveals doublecortin is required for radial migration in rat neocortex. *Nature Neuroscience, 6*, 1277–1283.

Bailey, A., Luthert, P., Dean, A., Harding, B., Janota, I., Montgomery, M., Rutter, M., & Lantos, P. (1998). A clinicopathological study of autism. *Brain, 121*, 889–905.

Bauman, M. L. (1991). Microscopic neuroanatomic abnormalities in autism. *Pediatrics, 87*, 791–795.

Bauman, M. L., & Kemper, T. L. (1985). Histoanatomic observations of the brain in early infantile autism. *Neurology, 35*, 866–874.

Bauman, M. L., & Kemper, T. L. (1987). Limbic involvement in a second case of early infantile autism. *Neurology, 37*, 147.

Bauman, M. L., & Kemper, T. L. (1990). Limbic and cerebellar abnormalities are also present in an autistic child of normal intelligence. *Neurology, 40*(suppl. 1), 359.

Bayer, S. A., & Altman, J. (1991) *Neocortical development.* New York: Raven.

Beg, A. A., Sommer, J. E., Martin, J. H., & Scheiffele, P. (2007). Alpha2-Chimaerin is an essential EphA4 effector in the assembly of neuronal locomotor circuits. *Neuron, 55*, 768–778.

Benowitz, L. I., & Routtenberg, A. (1997). GAP-43: an intrinsic determinant of neuronal development and plasticity. *Trends in Neurosciences, 20*(2), 84–91.

Bonora, E., Beyer, K. S., Lamb, J. A., Parr, J. R., Klauck, S. M., et al. (2003). Analysis of reelin as a candidate gene for autism. *Molecular Psychiatry, 8*, 885–892.

Boulanger, L. M., & Shatz, C. J. (2004). Immune signalling in neural development, synaptic plasticity, and disease. *Nature Reviews Neuroscience, 5*, 521–531.

Boulder Committee (1970). Embryonic vertebrate central nervous system: revised terminology. *Anatomical Record, 166*, 257–261.

Bultje, R. S., Castaneda-Castellanos, D. R., Jan, L. Y., Jan, Y. N., Kriegstein, A. R., & Shi, S. H. (2009). Mammalian Par3 regulates progenitor cell asymmetric division via notch signaling in the developing neocortex. *Neuron, 63*, 189–202.

Buttery, P., Beg, A. A., Chih, B., Broder, A., Mason, C. A., & Scheiffele, P. (2006). The diacylglycerol-binding protein alpha1-chimaerin regulates dendritic morphology. *Proceedings of the National Academy of Sciences of the United States of America, 103*, 1924–1929.

Buxhoeveden, D. P., Semendeferi, K., Buckwalter, J., Schenker, N., Switzer, R., & Courchesne, E. (2006). Reduced minicolumns in the frontal cortex of patients with autism. *Neuropathology and Applied Neurobiology, 32*, 483–491.

Carper, R., & Courchesne, E. (2005). Localized enlargement of the frontal lobe in autism. *Biological Psychiatry, 57*, 126–133.

Carper, R. A., Moses, P., Tigue, Z. D., & Courchesne, E. (2002). Cerebral lobes in autism: early hyperplasia and abnormal age effects. *NeuroImage, 16*, 1038–1051.

Casanova, M. F., Buxhoeveden, D. P., Switala, A. E., & Roy, E. (2002). Minicolumnar pathology in autism. *Neurology, 58*, 428–432.

Casanova M. F., El-Baz A., Vanbogaert E, Narahari P, Switala A. (2010). A topographic study of minicolumnar core width by lamina comparison between autistic subjects and controls: possible minicolumnar disruption due to an anatomical element in-common to multiple laminae. *Brain Pathology, 20*(2), 451–458.

Casanova, M. F., van Kooten, I. A., Switala, A. E., van Engeland, H, Heinsen, H., Steinbusch, H. W., et al. (2006). Minicolumnar abnormalities in autism. *Acta Neuropathologica, 112*, 287–303.

Chenn, A., & Walsh, C. A. (2002). Regulation of cerebral cortical size by control of cell cycle exit in neural precursors. *Science, 297*, 365–369.

Chu, E. C., & Tarnawski, A. S. (2004). PTEN regulatory functions in tumor suppression and cell biology. *Medical Science Monitor, 10*, RA235–241.

Coleman, P. D., Romano, J., Lapham, L., & Simon, W. (1985). Cell counts in cerebral cortex of an autistic patient. *Journal of Autism and Developmental Disorders, 15*, 245–255.

Comoletti, D., De Jaco, A., Jennings, L. L., Flynn, R. E., Gaietta, G., Tsigelny, I., et al. (2004). The Arg451Cys-neuroligin-3 mutation associated with autism reveals a defect in protein processing. *Journal of Neuroscience, 24*, 4889–4893.

Courchesne, E., Karns, C., Davis, H. R., Ziccardi, R., Carper, R., Tigue, Z., et al. (2001). Unusual brain growth patterns in early life in patients with autistic disorder: An MRI study. *Neurology, 57*, 245–254.

Courchesne, E., & Pierce, K. (2005). Why the frontal cortex is autism might be talking only to itself: local over-connectivity but long-distance disconnection. *Current Opinion in Neurobiology, 15*, 225–230.

Courchesne, E., Pierce, K., Schumann, C. M., Redcay, E., Buckwalter, J. A., Kennedy, D. P., et al. (2007). Mapping early brain development in autism. *Neuron, 56*, 399–413.

De Carlos, J. A., Lopez-Mascaraque, L., & Valverde, F. (1996). Dynamics of cell migration from the lateral ganglionic eminence in the rat. *Journal of Neuroscience, 16*, 6146–6156.

des Portes, V., Pinard, J. M., Billuart, P., Vinet, M. C., Koulakoff, A., Carrie, A., et al. (1998). A novel CNS gene required for neuronal migration and involved in X-linked subcortical laminar heterotopia and lissencephaly syndrome. *Cell, 92*, 51–61.

Dickson, B. J., & Gilestro, G. F. (2006). Regulation of commissural axon pathfinding by slit and its Robo receptors. *Annual Review of Cell and Developmental Biology, 22*, 651–675.

Doetsch, F., Caillé, I., Lim, D. A., García-Verdugo, J. M., & Alvarez-Buylla, A. (1999). Subventricular zone astrocytes are neural stem cells in the adult mammalian brain. *Cell, 97*, 703–716.

Durand, C. M., Betancur, C., Boeckers, T. M., Bockmann, J., Chaste, P., Fauchereau, F., et al. (2007). Mutations in the gene encoding the synaptic scaffolding protein SHANK3 are associated with autism spectrum disorders. *Nature Genetics, 39*, 25–27.

Elias, L. A., Wang, D. D., & Kriegstein, A. R. (2007). Gap junction adhesion is necessary for radial migration in the neocortex. *Nature, 448*, 901–907.

Fatemi, S. H., & Halt, A. R. (2001). Altered levels of Bcl2 and p53 proteins in parietal cortex reflect deranged apoptotic regulation in autism. *Synapse, 42*, 281–284.

Fatemi, S. H., Halt, A. R., Realmuto, G., Earle, J., Kist, D. A., Thuras, P., et al. (2002). Purkinje cell size is reduced in cerebellum of patients with autism. *Cellular and Molecular Neurobiology, 22*, 171–175.

Fatemi, S. H., Snow, A. V., Stary, J. M., Araghi-Niknam, M., Reutiman, T. J., Lee, S., et al. (2005). Reelin signaling is impaired in autism. *Biological Psychiatry, 57*, 777–787.

Feng, Y., & Walsh, C. A. (2001). Protein-protein interactions, cytoskeletal regulation, and neuronal migration. *Nature Reviews Neuroscience, 2*, 408–416.

Flint, A. C., Liu, X., & Kriegstein, A. R. (1998). Nonsynaptic glycine receptor activation during early neocortical development. *Neuron, 20*, 43–53.

Geschwind, D. H., & Levitt, P. (2007). Autism spectrum disorders: developmental disconnection syndromes. *Current Opinion in Neurobiology, 17*, 103–111.

Gleeson, J. G., Allen, K. M., Fox, J. W., Lamperti, E. D., Berkovic, S., Scheffer, I., et al. (1998). Doublecortin, a brain-specific gene mutated in human X-linked lissencephaly and double cortex syndrome, encodes a putative signaling protein. *Cell, 92*, 63–72.

Goffin, A., Hoefsloot, L. H., Bosgoed, E., Swillen, A., & Fryns, J. P. (2001). PTEN mutation in a family with Cowden syndrome and autism. *American Journal of Medical Genetics, 105*, 521–524.

Gotz, M., & Huttner, W. B. (2005). The cell biology of neurogenesis. *Nature Reviews Molecular Cell Biology*, 6(10), 777–88,

Guerin, P., Lyon, G., Barthelemy, C., et al. (1996). Neuropathological study of a case of autistic syndrome with severe mental retardation. *Developmental Medicine and Child Neurology, 38*, 203–211.

Guptill, J. T., Booker, A. B., Gibbs, T. T., Kemper, T. L., Bauman, M. L. and Blatt, G. J. (2007). [3H]-flunitrazepam-labeled benzodiazepine binding sites in the hippocampal formation in autism: a multiple concentration autoradiographic study. *Journal of Autism and Developmental Disorders*, 37(5), 911–920.

Hanashima, C., Li, S. C., Shen, L., Lai, E., & Fishell, G. (2004). Foxg1 suppresses early cortical cell fate. *Science, 303*, 56–59.

Hansen, R. L., Ozonoff, S., Krakowiak, P., Angkustsiri, K., Jones, C., Deprey, L. J., et al. (2008). Regression in autism: prevalence and associated factors in the CHARGE Study. *Ambulatory Pediatrics, 8*, 25–31.

Hatten, M. E. (1990). Riding the glial monorail: a common mechanism for glial-guided neuronal migration in different regions of the developing mammalian brain. *Trends in Neurosciences, 13*, 179–184.

Haubensak, W., Attardo, A., Denk, W., & Huttner, W. B. (2004). Neurons arise in the basal neuroepithelium of the early mammalian telencephalon: a major site of neurogenesis. *Proceedings of the National Academy of Sciences of the United States of America, 101*, 3196–3201.

Haug, H., Kuhl, S., Mecke, E., Sass, N. L., & Wasner, K. (1984). The significance of morphometric procedures in the investigation of age changes in cytoarchitectonic structures of human brain. *Journal für Hirnforsch, 25*, 353–374.

Haydar, T. F., Wang, F., Schwartz, M. L., & Rakic, P. (2000). Differential modulation of proliferation in the neocortical ventricular and subventricular zones. *Journal of Neuroscience, 20*, 5764–5774.

Hazlett, H. C., Poe, M., Gerig, G., Smith, R. G., Provenzale, J., Ross, A., et al. (2005). Magnetic resonance imaging and head circumference study of brain size in autism: birth through age 2 years. *Archives of General Psychiatry, 62*, 1366–1376.

Hazlett, H. C., Poe, M. D., Gerig, G., Smith, R. G., & Piven, J. (2006). Cortical gray and white brain tissue volume in adolescents and adults with autism. *Biological Psychiatry, 59*, 1–6.

Hedin-Pereira, C., Lent, R., & Jhaveri, S. (1999). Morphogenesis of callosal arbors in the parietal cortex of hamsters. *Cerebral Cortex, 9*, 50–64.

Herbert, M. R., Ziegler, D. A., Deutsch, C. K., O'Brien, L. M., Lange, N., Bakardjiev, A., et al. (2003). Dissociations of cerebral cortex, subcortical, and cerebral white matter volumes in autistic boys. *Brain, 126*, 1182–1192.

Herbert, M. R., Ziegler, D. A., Makris, N., Filipek, P. A., Kemper, T. L., Normandin, J. J., et al. (2004). Localization of white matter volume increase in autism and developmental language disorder. *Annals of Neurology, 55*, 530–540.

Hof, P. R., Knabe, R., Bovier, P., & Bouras, C. (1991). Neuropathological observations in a case of autism presenting with self-injury behavior. *Acta Neuropathologica, 82*, 321–326.

Hutsler, J. J., & Zhang, H. (2010) Increased dendritic spine densities on cortical projection neurons in autism spectrum disorders. *Brain Research, 1309*, 83–94.

Ihrie, R. A., & Alvarez-Buylla, A. (2008). Cells in the astroglial lineage are neural stem cells. *Cell and Tissue Research, 331*, 179–191.

IMGSAC IMGSoAC. (2001). A genomewide screen for autism: strong evidence for linkage to chromosomes 2q, 7q, and 16p. *American Journal of Human Genetics, 69*, 570–581.

Jamain, S., Quach, H., Betancur, C., Rastam, M., Colineaux, C., Gillberg, I. C., et al. (2003). Mutations of the X-linked genes encoding neuroligins NLGN3 and NLGN4 are associated with autism. *Nature Genetics, 34*, 27–29.

Javaherian, A., & Kriegstein, A. (2009). A stem cell niche for intermediate progenitor cells of the embryonic cortex. *Cerebral Cortex, 1*, i70–77.

Jones, E. (2000). Microcolumns in the cerebral cortex. *Proceedings of the National Academy of Sciences of the United States of America, 97*, 5019–5021.

Kanner, L. (1943). Autistic disturbances of affective contact. *Nervous Child, 2*, 217–250.

Kemper, T. L., & Bauman, M. L. (1993). The contribution of neuropathologic studies to the understanding of autism. *Neurologic Clinics, 11*, 175–187.

Kennedy, D. P., Semendeferi, K., & Courchesne, E. (2007). No reduction of spindle neuron number in frontoinsular cortex in autism. *Brain and Cognition, 64*, 124–129.

Komuro, H., & Rakic, P. (1993). Modulation of neuronal migration by NMDA receptors. *Science, 260*, 95–97.

Komuro, H., & Rakic, P. (1998). Orchestration of neuronal migration by activity of ion channels, neurotransmitter receptors, and intracellular Ca2+ fluctuations. *Journal of Neurobiology, 37*, 110–130.

Kriegstein, A. R., & Gotz, M. (2003). Radial glia diversity: a matter of cell fate. *Glia, 43*, 37–43.

Kriegstein, A. R., Noctor, S., & Martínez-Cerdeño, V. (2006). Patterns of neural stem and progenitor cell division may underlie evolutionary cortical expansion. *Nature Reviews Neuroscience, 7*, 883–890.

Kuan, C. Y., Roth, K. A., Flavell, R. A., & Rakic, P. (2000). Mechanisms of programmed cell death in the developing brain. *Trends in Neuroscience, 23*, 291–297.

Kulesza, R. J. Jr, Lukose, R., Stevens, L.V. (2010). Malformation of the human superior olive in autistic spectrum disorders. *Brain Research, 1367*, 360–371.

Kwon, C. H., Luikart, B. W., Powell, C. M., Zhou, J., Matheny, S. A., Zhang, W., et al. (2006). Pten regulates neuronal arborization and social interaction in mice. *Neuron, 50*, 377–388.

Lawrence, Y. A., Kemper, T. L., Bauman, M. L., & Blatt, G. J. (2010). Parvalbumin-, calbindin-, and calretinin-immunoreactive hippocampal interneuron density in autism. *Acta Neurologica Scandinavica, 121*(2), 99–108.

Levi-Montalcini, R., & Booker, B. (1960a). Destruction of the sympathetic ganglia in mammals by an antiserum to a nerve-growth protein. *Proceedings of the National Academy of Sciences of the United States of America, 46*, 384–391.

Levi-Montalcini, R., & Booker, B. (1960b). Excessive growth of the sympathetic ganglia evoked by a protein isolated from mouse salivary glands. *Proceedings of the National Academy of Sciences, 46*, 373–384.

Levitt, P., & Campbell, D. B. (2009). The genetic and neurobiologic compass points toward common signaling dysfunctions in autism spectrum disorders. *Journal of Clinical Investigation, 119*, 747–754.

Li, X., Chauhan, A., Sheikh, A. M., Patil, S., Chauhan, V., Li, X. M., et al. (2009). Elevated immune response in the brain of autistic patients. *Journal of Neuroimmunology, 207*, 111–116.

Lim, H. H., Michael, G. J., Smith, P., Lim, L., & Hall, C. (1992). Developmental regulation and neuronal expression of the mRNA of rat n-chimaerin, a p21rac GAP:cDNA sequence. *Biochemical Journal, 287*(Pt 2), 415–422.

Lois, C., García-Verdugo, J. M., & Alvarez-Buylla, A. (1996). Chain migration of neuronal precursors. *Science, 271*, 978–981.

Lord, C., Rutter, M., & Le Couteur, A. (1994). Autism Diagnostic Interview-Revised: a revised version of a diagnostic interview for caregivers of individuals with possible pervasive developmental disorders. *Journal of Autism and Developmental Disorders, 24*, 659–685.

Lotspeich, L. J., Kwon, H., Schumann, C. M., Fryer, S. L., Goodlin-Jones, B. L., Buonocore, M. H., et al. (2004). Investigation of neuroanatomical differences between autism and Asperger syndrome. *Archives of General Psychiatry, 61*, 291–298.

LoTurco, J. (2004). Doublecortin and a tale of two serines. *Neuron, 41*, 175–177.

LoTurco, J. J., & Kriegstein, A. R. (1991).Clusters of coupled neuroblasts in embryonic neocortex. *Science, 252*, 563–566.

LoTurco, J. J., Owens, D. F., Heath, M. J. S., Davis, M. B. E., & Kriegstein, A. R. (1995). GABA and glutamate depolarize cortical progenitor cells and inhibit DNA synthesis. *Neuron, 15*, 1287–1298.

Malatesta, P., Hartfuss, E., & Gotz, M. (2000). Isolation of radial glial cells by fluorescent-activated cell sorting reveals a neuronal lineage. *Development, 127*, 5253–5263.

Marin-Teva, J. L., Dusart, I., Colin, C., Gervais, A., van Rooijen, N., & Mallat, M. (2004). Microglia promote the death of developing Purkinje cells. *Neuron, 41*, 535–547.

Marin, O., & Rubenstein, J. L. (2003). Cell migration in the forebrain. *Annual Review of Neuroscience, 26*, 441–483.

Martínez-Cerdeño, V., Noctor, S. C., & Kriegstein, A. R. (2006a). Estradiol stimulates progenitor cell division in the ventricular and subventricular zones of the embryonic neocortex. *European Journal of Neuroscience, 24*, 3475–3488.

Martínez-Cerdeño, V., Noctor, S. C., & Kriegstein, A. R. (2006b). The role of intermediate progenitor cells in the evolutionary expansion of the cerebral cortex. *Cerebral Cortex, 16*, 152–161.

McAllister, A. K. (2007). Dynamic aspects of CNS synapse formation. *Annual Review of Neuroscience, 30*, 425–450.

McConnell, S. K., & Kaznowski, C. E. (1991). Cell cycle dependence of laminar determination in developing neocortex. *Science, 254*, 282–285.

McBride, K. L., Varga, E. A., Pastore, M. L., Prior, T. W., Manickam, K., Atkin, J. F., & Herman, G. E. (2010) Confirmation study of PTEN mutations among individuals with autism or developmental delays/mental retardation and macrocephaly. *Autism Research, 3(3)*, 137–141.

Misson, J. P., Edwards, M. A., Yamamoto, M., & Caviness, V. S., Jr., (1988). Identification of radial glial cells within the developing murine central nervous system: studies based upon a new immunohistochemical marker. *Brain Research. Developmental Brain Research, 44*, 95–108.

Miyata, T., Kawaguchi, A., Okano, H., & Ogawa, M. (2001). Asymmetric inheritance of radial glial fibers by cortical neurons. *Neuron, 31*, 727–741.

Miyata, T., Kawaguchi, A., Saito, K., Kawano, M., Muto, T., & Ogawa, M. (2004). Asymmetric production of surface-dividing and non-surface-dividing cortical progenitor cells. *Development, 131*, 3133–3145.

Morgan, J. T., Chana, G., Pardo, C. A., Achim, C., Semendeferi, K., Buckwalter, J., Courchesne, E., & Everall, I. P. (2010). Microglial activation and increased microglial density observed in the dorsolateral prefrontal cortex in autism. *Biological Psychiatry, 15*;68(4), 368–376.

Moro, F., Pisano, T., Bernadina, B. D., Polli, R., Murgia, A., Zoccante, L., et al. Periventricular heterotopia in fragile X syndrome. *Neurology, 67(4)*, 713–715.

Morrow, E. M., Yoo, S. Y., Flavell, S. W., Kim, T. K., Lin, Y., Hill, R. S., et al. (2008). Identifying autism loci and genes by tracing recent shared ancestry. *Science, 321*, 218–223.

Mountcastle, V. B. (1997). The columnar organization of the neocortex. *Brain, 120*, 701–722.

Mukaetova-Ladinska, E. B., Arnold, H., Jaros, E., Perry, R., & Perry, E. (2004). Depletion of MAP2 expression and laminar cytoarchitectonic changes in dorsolateral prefrontal cortex in adult autistic individuals. *Neuropathology and Applied Neurobiology, 30*, 615–623.

Nadarajah, B., & Parnavelas, J. G. (2002). Modes of neuronal migration in the developing cerebral cortex. *Nature Reviews Neuroscience, 3*, 423–432.

Nery, S., Fishell, G., & Corbin, J. G. (2002). The caudal ganglionic eminence is a source of distinct cortical and subcortical cell populations. *Nature Neuroscience, 5*, 1279–1287.

Nimmerjahn, A., Kirchhoff, F., & Helmchen, F. (2005). Resting microglial cells are highly dynamic surveillants of brain parenchyma in vivo. *Science, 308*, 1314–1318.

Noctor, S. C., Flint, A. C., Weissman, T. A., Dammerman, R. S., & Kriegstein, A. R. (2001). Neurons derived from radial glial cells establish radial units in neocortex. *Nature, 409*, 714–720.

Noctor, S. C., Flint, A. C., Weissman, T. A., Wong, W. S., Clinton, B. K., & Kriegstein, A. R. (2002). Dividing precursor cells of the embryonic cortical ventricular zone have morphological and molecular characteristics of radial glia. *Journal of Neuroscience, 22*, 3161–3173.

Noctor, S. C., Martínez-Cerdeño, V., Ivic, L., & Kriegstein, A. R. (2004). Cortical neurons arise in symmetric and asymmetric division zones and migrate through specific phases. *Nature Neuroscience, 7*, 136–144.

Noctor, S. C., Martínez-Cerdeño, V., & Kriegstein, A. R. (2007). Contribution of intermediate progenitor cells to cortical histogenesis. *Archives of Neurology, 64*, 639–642.

Noctor, S. C., Martinez-Cerdeño, V., & Kriegstein, A. R. (2008). Distinct behaviors of neural stem and progenitor cells underlie cortical neurogenesis. *Journal of Comparative Neurology, 508*, 28–44.

Oblak, A., Gibbs, T. T., & Blatt, G. J. (2009). Decreased GABA(A) receptors and benzodiazepine binding sites in the anterior cingulate cortex in autism. *Autism Research, 2*, 205–219.

Oblak, A., Gibbs, T. T., & Blatt, G. J. (2010a). Reduced GABA(A) receptors and benzodiazepine binding sites in the posterior cingulate cortex and fusiform gyrus in autism. *Brain Research*, Sept 19, *Epub ahead of print*.

Oblak, A., Gibbs, T. T., & Blatt, G. J. (2010b). Decreased GABA(B) receptors in the cingulate cortex and fusiform gyrus in autism. *Journal of Neurochemistry, 114*(5), 1414–1423.

Ozonoff, S., Heung, K., Byrd, R., Hansen, R., & Hertz-Picciotto, I. (2008). The onset of autism: patterns of symptom emergence in the first years of life. *Autism Research, 1*, 320–328.

Palmen, S. J., Hulshoff, Pol, H. E., Kemner, C., Schnack, H. G., Durston, S., Lahuis, B. E., et al. (2005). Increased gray-matter volume in medication-naive high-functioning children with autism spectrum disorder. *Psychological Medicine, 35*, 561–570.

Palmen, S. J., van Engeland, H., Hof, P. R., & Schmitz, C. (2004). Neuropathological findings in autism. *Brain, 127*, 2572–2583.

Palmer, T. D., Willhoite, A. R., & Gage, F. H. (2000). Vascular niche for adult hippocampal neurogenesis. *Journal of Comparative Neurology, 425*, 479–494.

Pardo, C. A., Vargas, D. L., & Zimmerman, A. W. (2005). Immunity, neuroglia, and neuroinflammation in autism. *International Review of Psychiatry, 17*, 485–495.

Patterson, P. H. (2009). Immune involvement in schizophrenia and autism: etiology, pathology, and animal models. *Behavioural Brain Research, 204*, 313–321.

Pearson, B. J., & Doe, C. Q. (2004). Specification of temporal identity in the developing nervous system. *Annual Review of Cell and Developmental Biology, 20*, 619–647.

Raff, M. C., Barres, B. A., Burne, J. F., Coles, H. S., Ishizaki, Y., & Jacobson, M. D. (1993). Programmed cell death and the control of cell survival: lessons from the nervous system. [Review]. *Science, 262*, 695–700.

Rakic, P. (1971). Guidance of neurons migrating to the fetal monkey neocortex. *Brain Research, 33*, 471–476.

Rakic, P. (1988). Specification of cerebral cortical areas. *Science, 241*, 170–176.

Raymond, G. V., Bauman, M. L., & Kemper, T. L. (1996). Hippocampus in autism: a golgi analysis. *Acta Neuropathologica, 91*, 117–119.

Redcay, E. (2008). The superior temporal sulcus performs a common function for social and speech perception: implications for the emergence of autism. *Neuroscience and Biobehavioral Reviews, 32*, 123–142.

Rezaie, P., & Male, D. (1999). Colonisation of the developing human brain and spinal cord by microglia: a review. *Microscopy Research and Technique, 45*, 359–382.

Ritvo, E. R., Freeman, B. J., Scheibel, A. B., Duong, T., Robinson, H., Guthrie, D., et al. (1986). Lower Purkinje cell counts in the cerebella of four autistic subjects: initial findings of the UCLA-NSAC autopsy research report. *American Journal of Psychiatry, 143*, 862–866.

Rockland, K. S., & Ichinohe, N. (2004). Some thoughts on cortical minicolumns. *Experimental Brain Research, 158*, 265–277.

Rodier, P. M., Ingram, J. L., Tisdale, B., Nelson, S., & Romano, J. (1996). Embryological origin for autism: developmental anomalies of the cranial nerve motor nuclei. *Journal of Comparative Neurology, 370*, 247–261.

Santos, M., Uppal, N., Butti, C., Wicinski, B., Schmeidler, J., Giannakopoulos, P., Heinsen, H., Schmitz, C., & Hof, P. R. (2010). von Economo neurons in autism: A stereologic study of the frontoinsular cortex in children. *Brain Research*, Aug 27, *Epub ahead of print.*

Schaar, B. T., Kinoshita, K., & McConnell, S. K. (2004). Doublecortin microtubule affinity is regulated by a balance of kinase and phosphatase activity at the leading edge of migrating neurons. *Neuron, 41*, 203–213.

Scheiffele, P. (2003). Cell-cell signaling during synapse formation in the CNS. *Annual Review of Neuroscience, 26*, 485–508.

Schmitz, C., & Rezaie, P. (2008). The neuropathology of autism: where do we stand? *Neuropathology and Applied Neurobiology, 34*, 4–11.

Schumann, C. M., & Amaral, D. G. (2006). Stereological analysis of amygdala neuron number in autism. *Journal of Neuroscience, 26*, 7674–7679.

Schumann, C. M., Barnes, C. C., Lord, C., & Courchesne, E. (2009). Amygdala enlargement in toddlers with autism related to severity of social and communication impairments. *Biological Psychiatry, 15;66*(10), 942–949.

Schumann, C. M., Bloss, C., Barnes, C. C., Wideman, G. M., Carper, R., Akshoomoff, N., et al. (2010). Longitudinal magnetic resonance imaging study of cortical development through early childhood in autism. *Journal of Neuroscience, 24*;30(12), 4419–4427.

Schumann, C. M., Hamstra, J., Goodlin-Jones, B. L., Lotspeich, L. J., Kwon, H., Buonocore, M. H., et al. (2004). The amygdala is enlarged in children but not adolescents with autism; the hippocampus is enlarged at all ages. *Journal of Neuroscience, 24*, 6392–6401.

Schuurmans, C., & Guillemot, F. (2002). Molecular mechanisms underlying cell fate specification in the developing telencephalon. *Current Opinion in Neurobiology, 12*, 26–34.

Schwartz, M. L., & Goldman-Rakic, P. S. (1991). Prenatal specification of callosal connections in rhesus monkey. *Journal of Comparative Neurology, 307*, 144–162.

Seri, B., Garcia-Verdugo, J. M., Collado-Morente, L., McEwen, B. S., & Alvarez-Buylla, A. (2004). Cell types, lineage, and architecture of the germinal zone in the adult dentate gyrus. *Journal of Comparative Neurology, 478*, 359–378.

Seri, B., García-Verdugo, J. M., McEwen, B. S., & Alvarez-Buylla, A. (2001). Astrocytes give rise to new neurons in the adult mammalian hippocampus. *Journal of Neuroscience, 21*, 7153–7160.

Shen, J., Eyaid, W., Mochida, G. H., Al-Moayyad, F., Bodell, A., Woods, C. G., & Walsh, C. A. (2005). ASPM mutations identified in patients with primary microcephaly and seizures. *Journal of Medical Genetics, 42*, 725–729.

Shen, Q., Goderie, S. K., Jin, L., Karanth, N., Sun, Y., Abramova, N., et al. (2004). Endothelial cells stimulate self-renewal and expand neurogenesis of neural stem cells. *Science, 304*, 1338–1340.

Simms, M. L., Kemper, T. L., Timbie, C. M., Bauman, M. L., & Blatt, G. J. (2009). The anterior cingulate cortex in autism: heterogeneity of qualitative and quantitative cytoarchitectonic features suggests possible subgroups. *Acta Neuropathologica. 118*(5), 673–684.

Stevens, B. (2008). Neuron-astrocyte signaling in the development and plasticity of neural circuits. *Neurosignals, 16*, 278–288.

Strauss, K. A., Puffenberger, E. G., Huentelman, M. J., Gottlieb, S., Dobrin, S. E., Parod, J. M., et al. (2006). Recessive symptomatic focal epilepsy and mutant contactin-associated protein-like 2. *New England Journal of Medicine, 354*, 1370–1377.

Streit, W. J., Conde, J. R., Fendrick, S. E., Flanary, B. E., & Mariani, C. L. (2005). Role of microglia in the central nervous system's immune response. *Neurological Research, 27*, 685–691.

Stubbs, D., DeProto, J., Nie, K., Englund, C., Mahmud, I., Hevner, R., et al. (2009). Neurovascular congruence during cerebral cortical development. *Cerebral Cortex, 19*(Suppl1), i32–41.

Szatmari, P., Paterson, A. D., Zwaigenbaum, L., Roberts, W., Brian, J., Liu, X. Q., et al. (2007). Mapping autism risk loci using genetic linkage and chromosomal rearrangements. *Nature Genetics, 39*, 319–328.

Tamamaki, N., Fujimori, K. E., & Takauji, R. (1997). Origin and route of tangentially migrating neurons in the developing neocortical intermediate zone. *Journal of Neuroscience, 17*, 8313–8323.

Tissir, F., & Goffinet, A. M. (2003). Reelin and brain development. *Nature Reviews Neuroscience, 4*, 496–505.

van Kooten, I. A., Palmen, S. J., von Cappeln, P., Steinbusch, H. W., Korr, H., Heinsen, H., et al. (2008). Neurons in the fusiform gyrus are fewer and smaller in autism. *Brain, 131*, 987–999.

Varga, E. A., Pastore, M., Prior, T., Herman, G. E., & McBride, K. L. (2009). The prevalence of PTEN mutations in a clinical pediatric cohort with autism spectrum disorders, developmental delay, and macrocephaly. *Genetics in Medicine, 11*, 111–117.

Vargas, D. L., Nascimbene, C., Krishnan, C., Zimmerman, A. W., & Pardo, C. A. (2005). Neuroglial activation and neuroinflammation in the brain of patients with autism. *Annals of Neurology, 57*, 67–81.

Wegiel, J., Kuchna, I., Nowicki, K., Imaki, H., Wegiel, J., Marchi, E., Ma, S.Y., Chauhan, A., Chauhan, V., Bobrowicz, T.W., de Leon, M., Louis, L.A., Cohen, I.L., London, E., Brown, W.T., Wisniewski, T. (2010). The neuropathology of autism: defects of neurogenesis and neuronal migration, and dysplastic changes. Acta Neuropathologica, *119*(6), 755–770.

Weissman, T. A., Riquelme, P. A., Ivic, L., Flint, A. C., & Kriegstein, A. R. (2004). Calcium waves propagate through radial glial cells and modulate proliferation in the developing neocortex. *Neuron, 43*, 647–661.

Werner, E., & Dawson, G. (2005). Validation of the phenomenon of autistic regression using home videotapes. *Archives of General Psychiatry, 62*, 889–895.

West, M. J., Slomianka, L., & Gundersen, H. J. (1991). Unbiased stereological estimation of the total number of neurons in the subdivisions of the rat hippocampus using the optical fractionator. *Anatomical Record, 231*, 482–497.

Whitney, E. R., Kemper, T. L., Bauman, M. L., Rosene, D. L., & Blatt, G. J. (2008). Cerebellar Purkinje cells are reduced in a subpopulation of autistic brains: a stereological experiment using calbindin-D28k. *Cerebellum, 7*, 406–416.

Whitney, E. R., Kemper, T. L., Rosene, D. L., Bauman, M. L., & Blatt, G. J. (2009). Density of cerebellar basket and stellate cells in autism: evidence for a late developmental loss of Purkinje cells. *Journal of Neuroscience Research, 87*, 2245–2254.

Wichterle, H., García-Verdugo, J. M., Herrera, D. G., & Alvarez-Buylla, A. (1999). Young neurons from medial ganglionic eminence disperse in adult and embryonic brain. *Nature Reviews Neuroscience, 2*, 461–466.

Williams, R. S., Hauser, S. L., Purpura, D. P., DeLong, G. R., & Swisher, C. N. (1980). Autism and mental retardation: neuropathologic studies performed in four retarded persons with autistic behavior. *Archives of Neurology, 37*, 749–753.

Wrona, D. (2006). Neural-immune interactions: an integrative view of the bidirectional relationship between the brain and immune systems. *Journal of Neuroimmunology, 172*, 38–58.

Yip, J., Soghomonian, J. J., & Blatt, G. J. (2007). Decreased GAD67 mRNA levels in cerebellar Purkinje cells in autism: pathophysiological implications. *Acta Neuropathologica, 113*, 559–568.

Yip, J., Soghomonian, J. J., & Blatt, G. J. (2008). Increased GAD67 mRNA expression in cerebellar interneurons in autism: implications for Purkinje cell dysfunction. *Journal of Neuroscience Research, 86*, 525–530.

Yip, J., Soghomonian, J. J., & Blatt, G. J. (2009). Decreased GAD65 mRNA levels in select subpopulations of neurons in the cerebellar dentate nuclei in autism: an in situ hybridization study. *Autism Research, 2*, 50–59.

Yu, Y. C., Bultje, R. S, Wang, X., & Shi, S. H. (2009). Specific synapses develop preferentially among sister excitatory neurons in the neocortex. *Nature, 458*, 501–504.

Zikopoulos B., & Barbas H. (2010). Changes in prefrontal axons may disrupt the network in autism. *Journal of Neuroscience*, 3;30(44), 14595–609.

Zori, R. T., Marsh, D. J., Graham, G. E., Marliss, E. B., & Eng, C. (2008). Germline PTEN mutation in a family with Cowden syndrome and Bannayan-Riley-Ruvalcaba syndrome. *American Journal of Medical Genetics, 80*, 399–402.

32 Diane C. Chugani

Neurotransmitters

Points of Interest

- There is evidence for alterations in many neurotransmitters in autism; the most compelling evidence at this time is for alterations in serotonin and GABA neurotransmission.
- The relationship between neurotransmitters measured in blood and the levels of the transmitter in the central nervous system is not well understood.
- Neurotransmitter changes occur in genetic disorders associated with autism in which the gene mutation does not directly affect a neurotransmitter-related gene (synthetic or degradative enzymes, receptor, transporter, etc.).
- Altered neurotransmitter function during brain development may play a role in altered brain development in autism and provide a mechanism for pharmacological intervention.

Neurotransmitters have been the focus of numerous studies aimed at understanding autism, beginning nearly 50 years ago when Schain and Freedman (1961) first reported elevated serotonin in the blood of autistic subjects. Serotonin still remains the neurotransmitter that has been most studied in autism. There is some evidence for alterations in many transmitters, including GABA, glutamate, dopamine, norepinephrine, acetylcholine, and opioid peptides. This literature has been summarized in great detail recently (Lam et al., 2006). This review will focus on the evidence for two neurotransmitters for which there is the strongest link to autism, serotonin and GABA. For each of these neurotransmitters, the evidence for alterations in autism and the significance for altered neurotransmission on brain development and behavior are discussed.

Serotonin

Serotonin Synthesis and Degradation

Serotonin content in different parts of the body is determined by a vast number of factors. Serotonin is synthesized from the precursor tryptophan (Hamon et al., 1981). Tryptophan is an essential amino acid that must be derived from the diet, and constitutes only 1% of the total amino acid pool. In the blood, the majority of tryptophan is bound to plasma protein. It is the free plasma tryptophan that is available to be transported into the brain. Tryptophan is transported into the brain via the large neutral amino acid carrier (LAT1), where it competes for transport with the other large neutral amino acids (Pardridge et al., 1977; Smith et al., 1987). The first, and rate limiting step, of serotonin synthesis is the formation of 5-hydroxytryptophan catalyzed by the enzyme tryptophan hydroxylase (TPH) (Figure 32-1). Tryptophan hydroxylase is only 50% saturated with tryptophan, resulting in the dependence of brain serotonin levels on the plasma concentration of free tryptophan as well as the plasma levels of the other large neutral amino acids (Fernstrom & Wurtman, 1971).

There are 2 genes encoding tryptophan hydroxylase, TPH1 and TPH2 (Sakowski et al., 2006). TPH1 is localized to the pineal gland and throughout the periphery. TPH2 is found in the brain and in the gastrointestinal nervous system (Zhang et al., 2004). The current dogma is that the majority of the serotonin synthesized in the body is generated by the enterochromaffin cells in the gastrointestinal tract (Gershon & Tack, 2007). However, tryptophan hydroxylase is located at many peripheral sites, and the assertion that the majority of serotonin in the body is synthesized in the gastrointestinal tract is not well documented. There is much evidence that serotonin synthetic enzymes are ubiquitously distributed and that serotonin is involved in many different functions throughout the body. Many of these functions might be related to aspects of autism, and its causes. In addition to the gastrointestinal tract and the central nervous system, serotonin is synthesized in bronchial epithelium, taste papillae, thyroid parafollicular cells, ovaries, thymus, pancreas, breast, skin, and arteries (Eddahibi et al., 2006; Ortiz-Alvarado et al, 2006; Matsuda et al., 2004; Stull et al., 2007; Slominski et al., 2002; Ni et al., 2008). TPH and aromatic amino acid decarboxylase (AADC) mRNAs are expressed in the heart, and serotonin is produced and released in cardiomyocytes (Ikeda et al., 2005). TPH-1 mRNA and TPH protein is expressed in trigeminal neurons and is regulated during the estrous cycle (Berman et al., 2006). Serotonin plays an important role in

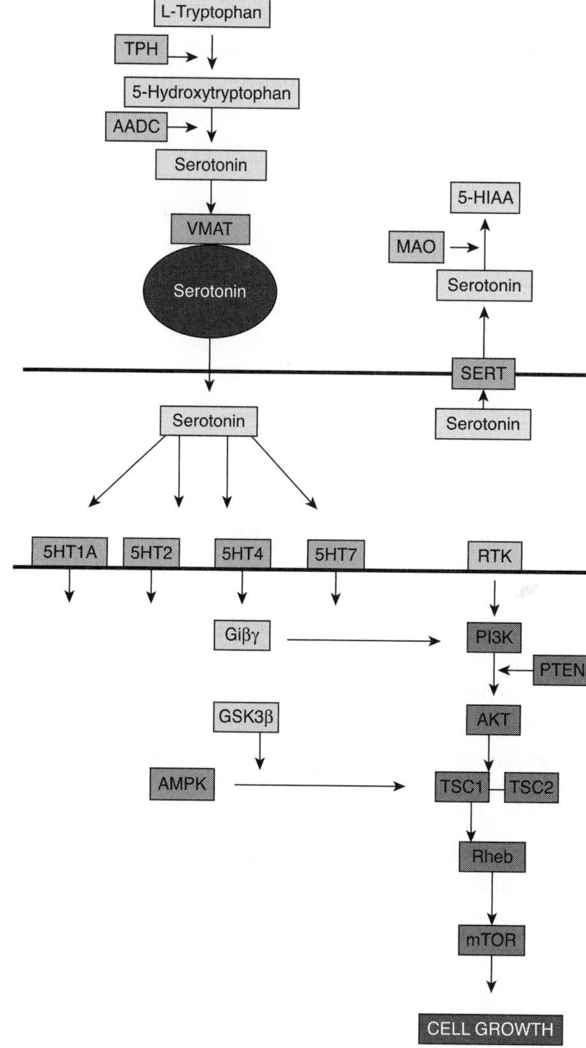

Figure 32–1. Model demonstrating interaction of serotonergic pathway with the receptor tyrosine kinase (RTK) mediated phosphatidyl inositol 3-kinase/Akt (PI3K) pathway. The synthesis of serotonin from tryptophan catalyzed by tryptophan hydroxylase (TPH) and aromatic amino acid decarboxylase (AADC). Serotonin is stored in synaptic vesicles mediated by the vesicular monoamine transporter (VMAT). Following release from the terminal, serotonin diffuses to both synaptic and extrasynaptic serotonin receptors. Several classes of serotonin receptors have been linked to modulation of the PI3K pathway, including 5HT1A, 5HT2, 5HT4, and 5HT7. Serotonin is taken back up into the terminal by the serotonin transporter (SERT) and metabolized by monamine oxidase (MAO) to 5-hydroxyindole acetic acid (5HIAA). Growth factors such as brain-derived growth factor (BDNF) and insulin-like growth factor (IGF) stimulate cell growth by binding to the receptor tyrosine kinase (RTK) which results in changing the activity of enzymes, causing activation of subsequent components of the pathway. Components of the pathway include phosphatidyl inositol 3-kinase (PI3K), Akt (also known as protein kinase B), tuberous sclerosis complex 1 (TSC1), tuberous sclerosis complex 2 (TSC2), Ras homologue enriched in brain (Rheb), mammalian target of rapamycin complex 1 (mTOR), and PTEN (phosphatase and tensin homologue deleted on chromosome 10). There is evidence that activation of serotonin receptors can change the activity of component of this pathway in part mediated by the G-protein Giβγ and glycogen synthase kinase 3β (GSK3β).

mammary gland function. TPH mRNA is elevated during pregnancy and lactation, and serotonin is present in mammary epithelium and in milk (Matsuda et al., 2004). Elevated plasma serotonin in autism might also be affected by changes in storage and degradation. Plasma serotonin is taken up by platelets through serotonin transporters (Ni & Watts, 2006), and is cleared by liver and lung endothelium (Nocito et al., 2007). Serotonin is metabolized by the enzyme monoamine oxidase to produce its major metabolite 5-hydroxyindoleacetic acid (5HIAA) (for review see Bortolato et al., 2008).

Serotonin Transporter and Receptors

The serotonin transporter (SERT or 5HTT) mediates uptake of serotonin following release at the synapse and at other sites such as the platelet. The gene for the serotonin transporter has two forms, the short and the long form, that are common in the general population. The short variant of the SERT gene has 30–40% lower mRNA expression leading to 50% lower serotonin uptake than transporters produced by the long form (Lesch et al., 1996). To date, 15 receptors for serotonin have been identified, and these are expressed in the brain and throughout the body where they regulate numerous processes (for review see Berger et al., 2009).

Altered Blood Serotonin in Autism

Current evidence now suggests that autism is likely to be caused by dysfunction of many genes (Zhao et al., 2007). Given that many different genes can cause autism, it is striking that 30–50% of autistic individuals show elevated serotonin in the blood (Schain & Freedman, 1961). This result has been replicated by several groups (Hoshino et al., 1984; Anderson et al., 1987; Cook et al., 1990), and extended with the recognition that blood serotonin is also elevated in the first-degree relatives of autistic individuals (Leventhal et al., 1990; Piven et al., 1999; Cook et al., 1994; Leboyer et al., 1999).

Altered Brain Serotonin in Autism

In light of the robust changes observed in blood serotonin, a number of investigators asked whether serotonin in brain was altered by measuring the serotonin metabolite 5HIAA in cerebrospinal fluid. Several studies spanning 20 years of investigation found no difference between autistic and nonautistic control groups in cerebrospinal fluid levels of 5HIAA (for details, see Lam et al., 2006). We used a molecular imaging approach with the tracer alpha[^{11}C]methyl-tryptophan (AMT) imaged with positron emission tomography (PET) (Chugani et al., 1997; Chugani et al., 1999, Chandana et al., 2005). Two fundamentally different types of serotonergic abnormality were found in children with autism. The first is a difference in whole brain serotonin synthesis capacity in autistic children compared to age-matched nonautistic children. Serotonin synthesis capacity was greater than 200% of adult values until the age of 5 years and then declined toward adult values in nonautistic children. In contrast, serotonin synthesis capacity in autistic children increased gradually between the ages of 2 years and 15 years to values 1.5 times the adult normal values (Chugani et al., 1999). These data suggested that humans undergo a period of high brain serotonin synthesis capacity during early childhood, and that this developmental process is disrupted in autistic children. We also found focal abnormalities in brain serotonin synthesis. Asymmetries of AMT uptake in frontal cortex, thalamus, and cerebellum were visualized in children with autism (Chugani et al., 1997). These results lead to the hypothesis that the dentate-thalamo-cortical pathway may be disrupted in some children with autism. Subsequently, we measured brain serotonin synthesis in a large group of autistic children with AMT PET and related these data to handedness and language function (Chandana et al., 2005). Autistic children demonstrated several patterns of abnormal cortical involvement, including right cortical, left cortical, and absence of abnormal asymmetry. Groups of autistic children defined by presence or absence and side of cortical asymmetry, differed on a measure of language as well as handedness. Autistic children with left cortical AMT decreases showed a higher prevalence of severe language impairment, whereas those with right cortical decreases showed a higher prevalence of left and mixed handedness.

There are several possible explanations for the asymmetries of cortical serotonin synthesis observed in children with autism. First, cortical asymmetry of serotonin synthesis may be normal during early brain development. The presence of abnormal cortical asymmetry in serotonin synthesis observed in approximately one half of the autistic children might represent another manifestation of the abnormality in the developmental regulation of serotonin synthesis. Second, early damage to the dominant left hemisphere leads to compensatory changes in the right hemisphere to support language based on the recognition that damage to the dominant left hemisphere leads to compensatory changes to the right hemisphere to support language (Rasmussen & Milner, 1977; Muller et al., 1999; Curtiss & de Bode, 2003). Evidence for a compensatory change to facilitate language function on the right in autism comes from a study using structural imaging by Herbert et al. (2002), which showed abnormal structural asymmetry in language association cortex in autistic boys. They reported that language-related inferior frontal cortex was 27% larger on the right in the autistic group compared to 17% larger on the left in control subjects.

Genetic Evidence Linking Serotonin to Autism

Blood serotonin levels have been linked to an interaction of the serotonin transporter gene (SLC6A4) and integrin beta3 (ITGB3) (Weiss et al., 2006a,b). This finding was recently replicated and additional interactions between these 2 genes were found, including an additive effect of the HTR5A gene, an interaction of TPH1 and SLC6A4, and an interaction between HTR1D and SLC6A4 for blood serotonin level (Coutinho et al., 2007). As mentioned above, the serotonin transporter has 2 forms. There have been conflicting reports regarding the relative roles of the short and long form in autism (reviewed in Devlin et al., 2005). More recently, the short allele of the 5HTT receptor was associated with higher gray matter volume in young boys with autism (Wassink et al., 2007). Furthermore, cortical enlargement in autism was reported to be associated with the "low activity" allele of the monamine oxidase A gene (Davis et al., 2008).

Single nucleotide polymorphisms in intron 1 and 4 of TPH2, the brain-specific form of tryptophan hydroxylase, showed an association with autism (Coon et al., 2005). Several recent studies report association of genes that may impact serotonin metabolism in autism. One such study reports the presence of a susceptibility mutation in a promoter variant of the tryptophan 2,3-dioxygenase gene (Nabi et al., 2004). Tryptophan 2,3-dioxygenase is a rate-limiting enzyme in the metabolism of tryptophan (by the kynurenine pathway), the precursor of serotonin. A mutation that results in decreased activity of this enzyme could decrease the metabolism of tryptophan by this pathway and increase the level of whole body serotonin content. Furthermore, tryptophan 2,3-dioxygenase, as well as indoleamine 2,3-dioxygenase (which also catalyses tryptophan metabolism by the kynurenine pathway), are expressed in the placenta and have a role in the prevention of allogeneic rejection of the fetus (Munn et al., 1998; Suzuki et al., 2001). Another recent study investigated the effect of maternal genotypes for monoamine oxidase-A (MAO-A) on the risk of autism in their offspring. Jones et al. (2004) reported that maternal genotypes containing specific polymorphisms at the MAO-A locus show significant negative effects on the intelligence quotient (IQ) in children with autism. These results are consistent with those of a study which found that a low activity MAO-A allele, due to an upstream variable-number tandem repeat region, is associated with both lower IQ and more severe autistic behavior in children, as compared to the high-activity allele (Cohen et al., 2003). The serotonin transporter is highly expressed in the brush border membrane of the human placenta and may mediate transport of serotonin from the maternal circulation to the developing fetus (Balkovetz et al., 1989). Given that there is expression of the serotonin transporter in the placenta, a maternal modifier effect of the serotonin transporter might be a risk factor for autism.

Altered Serotonin in Autism Caused by Genes Not Related to Serotonin

There are several studies showing alterations in serotonergic neurotransmission in Rett syndrome, as well as in the MECP2-null mouse model of Rett syndrome. Decreased levels of the serotonin metabolite 5HIAA were reported in the CSF from 32 patients with Rett syndrome compared to age matched control subjects (Zoghbi et al., 1989). Serotonin concentrations in whole brain from MECP2-null mice showed no difference at birth, but were significantly lower at 42 days of age compared to wild-type mice (Ide et al., 2005). However, these changes were not specific to serotonin, and changes in other transmitters were also reported. Further evidence that the serotonergic system is involved in MECP2, is the report that the selective serotonin uptake inhibitor fluoxetine induced upregulation of MECP2_e1 and MECP2_e2 transcripts in adult rat brain (Cassel et al., 2005). Conversely, significantly increased brain serotonin content has been reported in a Drosophila FraX model (Zhang et al., 2005). Finally, there is evidence for interaction of the 5HT2C receptor with PTEN (Ji et al., 2006; Muller & Carey, 2006).

Serotonin as a Neurotrophin

Serotonin displays both fast actions as a neurotransmitter and longer-term actions as a neurotrophin. This neurotrophic action may be in part through serotonin regulation of growth factors. For example, serotonin has been reported to stimulate the release of IGF1 and S100b (Lauder, 1993; Lambert & Lauder, 1999). S100b is a trophic factor released from astrocytes by a 5HT1A-mediated mechanism (Whitaker-Azmitia et al., 1996; Azmitia et al., 1996; Ahlemeyer et al., 2000; Eriksen & Druse, 2001). Treatment with selective serotonin reuptake inhibitors has been shown to increase mRNA for BDNF and its receptor trkB (Nibuya et al., 1996; Chen et al., 2001), levels of IGF1 (Khawaja et al., 2004), and FGF2 (Maragnoli et al., 2004) in hippocampus.

Many of these trophic factors are receptor tyrosine kinases that signal through the phosphatidyl inositol 3-kinase/Akt (PI3K) pathway (Figure 32-1). The phosphinositide products of the PI3K recruit Akt and PDK to the membrane resulting in phosphorylation of Akt. There is evidence that serotonin may directly couple to the PI3K pathway. For example, 5HT1A agonists lead to activation of Akt in cultured hippocampal neurons, an action blocked by the 5HT1A antagonist WAY100635 (Cowen et al., 2005; Hsuing et al., 2005). In vivo treatment with agents that increase serotonin resulted in an increase in phosphorylation of GSK-3β, a substrate for Akt (Li et al., 2004). The same results were obtained with the 5HT agonist 8-OH-DPAT and the phosphorylation was inhibited by WAY100635. Alterations in brain growth have long been recognized in autism. Macrocephaly was early recognized in a subset of persons with autism. Recently, mutations in PTEN, a regulator of the PI3K pathway, were shown in cases of autism with extreme macrocephaly (Butler et al., 2005; Varga et al., 2009). Both Akt1 and Akt3 are involved in the attainment of normal brain size (Easton et al., 2005). Thus, serotonin might play a role in brain growth and brain size through PI3K signaling.

Role of Serotonin in Brain Development

Evidence from both pharmacological and gene knockout experiments demonstrates that serotonin plays a role in modulation of synaptogenesis. Immunocytochemistry for serotonin and [^{3}H]citalopram binding to serotonin uptake sites both have demonstrated a transient serotonergic innervation of primary sensory cortex between postnatal days 2 and 14 during the period of synaptogenesis in rat cortex (D'Amato et al., 1987, Cases et al., 1995). Two early studies (Bennett-Clarke et al., 1996, Lebrand et al., 1996) reported that this transient innervation actually represented transient expression of the high-affinity serotonin transporter and vesicular monoamine transporter by glutamatergic thalamocortical neurons. The serotonin transporter is transiently expressed by glutamatergic thalamocortical afferents (Bennett-Clarke et al., 1996, Lebrand et al., 1996) during the first 2 postnatal weeks in rats. During this period, these thalamocortical neurons take up and store serotonin, although they do not synthesize serotonin. While the role of serotonin in glutamatergic neurons whose cell bodies are located in sensory nuclei of the thalamus is not yet known, there is evidence that the serotonin concentration must be neither too high nor too low during this period. Thus, depletion of serotonin delays the development of the barrel fields of the rat somatosensory cortex (Blue et al., 1991; Osterheld-Haas & Hornung, 1996) and decreases the size of the barrel fields (Bennett-Clarke et al., 1994). Conve-rsely, increased serotonin during this critical period, as in the MAO-A knockout mouse, results in increased tangential arborization of these axons, resulting in blurring of the boundaries of the cortical barrels (Cases et al., 1996). Decreased or increased brain serotonin during this period of development results in disruption of synaptic connectivity in sensory cortices (Cases et al., 1995; Bennett-Clarke et al., 1994; Cases et al., 1996). Furthermore, disruption of serotonin transporter functions impairs the cerebral glucose metabolism response to whisker stimulation (Esaki et al., 2005). The effect of serotonin on synaptogenesis and synaptic function is not limited to the sensory cortices. For example, Yan et al. (1997)have reported that depletion of serotonin with PCA or5,7-dihydroxytryptamine in neonatal rat pups resulted in large decreases in the numbers of dendritic spines in hippocampus. Finally, alterations of serotonergic function during development have lasting functional changes into adulthood (Ansorge et al., 2004; Gross et al., 2002).

Gamma-Aminobutyric Acid (GABA)

Gamma-aminobutyric acid (GABA) is synthesized from glutamate catalyzed by the enzyme glutamic acid decarboxylase (GAD), of which there are two forms identified: GAD_{65} and GAD_{67} (Kaufman et al., 1991). There are three types of GABA receptors, $GABA_A$ and $GABA_C$ are ligand-gated ion channels, and $GABA_B$ is a G protein coupled receptor (Bowery, 1993). Gamma-aminobutyric acid (GABA) induces fast inhibition by acting on $GABA_A$ receptors in the mature brain, while activation of $GABA_A$ receptors in neonatal brain produces depolarization due to the high intracellular chloride concentration in immature neurons (Yuste & Katz, 1991; Owens et al., 1996; Rivera et al., 1999). The $GABA_A$ receptor complex is composed of 5 polypeptide subunits to form a chloride channel (Nayeem et al., 1994). These polypeptide subunits have been classified based on sequence, and subunit classes have been designated $\alpha, \beta, \gamma, \delta, \varepsilon, \pi, \rho$ (Barnard et al., 1998), and θ (Whiting, 1999). The $GABA_A$ receptor complex incorporates binding sites not only for GABA, but also for benzodiazepines, barbiturates, steroid anesthetics (Olsen et al., 1991; MacDonald & Olsen, 1994; Olsen & Sapp, 1995), volatile general anesthetics (Olsen et al., 1991; Harrison et al., 1993), and possibly alcohols (Mahmoudi et al., 1997).

Pathological Evidence for Altered GABA Neurotransmission in Autism

A number of studies have addressed GAD and GABA receptors in postmortem autism brain and body fluids, by biochemical, receptor binding, western blotting, and mRNA expression methods. Abnormalities of GABA have been detected in blood and platelets of subjects with autism (Rolf et al., 1993). Fatemi et al. (2002) reported reduced GAD_{65} and GAD_{67} protein expression using western blotting in parietal and cerebellar cortices in 9 specimens from autistic adults aged 19–30 years compared to 7 age-matched controls. Blatt and colleagues have studied expression of GAD_{65} and GAD_{67} expression in different cerebellar cell groups. This group has reported decreased GAD_{67} mRNA levels in cerebellar Purkinje cells in autistic subjects (Yip et al., 2007), whereas GAD_{67} was increased in cerebellar interneurons (Yip et al., 2008). Finally, Yip et al. (2009) found decreased GAD_{65} mRNA levels in a subpopulation of cells in cerebellar dentate nuclei. Oblak et al. (2009) measured GABA receptor binding with [^{3}H]muscimol and benzodiazepine binding site with [^{3}H]flunitrazepam in anterior cingulate cortex in specimens from 7 autism subjects aged 19–30 years, compared with control subjects aged 16–43. They found large decreases in the maximum number of binding sites in both ligands in supragranular and infragranular layers of the anterior cingulate cortex. Fatemi, Reutiman, Folsom, and Thuras (2009) examined expression of four $GABA_A$ receptor subunits in using western blotting and found significantly decreased GABRA1, GABRA2, GABRA3, and GABAB3 subunit expression in parietal cortex, GABRA1 and GABRB3 in cerebellum and GABRA1 in superior frontal cortex in specimens from autistic subjects compared to controls. The same group also found decreased GABAB subunit expression in the same three brain regions (Fatemi, Folsom, Reutiman, and Thuras, 2009). These studies suggest widespread decreases in expression of the GABA synthetic enzymes as well as $GABA_A$ and $GABA_B$ receptors.

Genetic and Imaging Evidence for a Role of GABA in Autism

Cytogenetic studies have reported abnormalities in chromosome 15 in autism, specifically 15q11-13, the region that encodes several $GABA_A$ receptor subunit genes (GABRB3, GABRA5, and GABRG3; Silva et al., 2002; Menold et al., 2001; Buxbaum et al., 2002). Menold et al. (2001) reported two single nucleotide polymorphisms located within the GABRB3 gene in autism. Moreover, symptoms of autism can be associated with both Prader-Willi and Angelman's syndromes, both of which involve alterations in the chromosome 15q11-13 region (for a review, Nicholls & Knepper, 2001). Although autism and Angelman's syndrome are distinct disorders, there is considerable overlap among them, with both conditions characterized by language deficit, seizures, mental impairment, behavioral abnormalities, and sleep disturbances. The region 15q11-13 contains the disease loci for Angelman's syndrome (UBE3A) resulting from deletion or mutation within maternal chromosome 15q11-13 (Kishino et al., 1997). Based on investigations of a GABRB3 gene knockout mouse (Homanics, 1997; DeLorey, 1998), it was suggested that the lack of GABRB3 gene could contribute to most of the clinical symptoms in Angelman's syndrome. Interestingly, Angelman's patients with a maternal deletion of 15q11-13 leading to the loss of β3 subunit of GABA receptor showed significantly decreased binding of [^{11}C]flumazenil in frontal, parietal, hippocampal, and cerebellar regions in a PET study (Holopainen et al., 2001). Lucignani et al. (2004) studied 6 adults with Prader-Willi syndrome and found decreased [^{11}C]flumazenil binding in insula and cingulate, frontal, and temporal neocortices compared to normal control subjects. These studies demonstrate the utility of PET in elucidating the functional consequence of specific genetic abnormalities. Similarly, $GABA_A$ receptor binding, measured with $GABA_A$ receptor channel ligand ([(35)S]t-butylbicyclophosphorothionate) and benzodiazepine ligand ([(3)H]Ro 15-4513), was decreased in a GABAB3 knockout mouse but not in a UBE3A knockout mouse (Sinkkonen et al., 2003). The same 15q11-13 region has been implicated in autism based on several observations showing chromosomal duplications in autistic individuals and evidence of linkage disequilibrium in autistic families (Cook, 1997; Bass, 2000). Specifically, linkage disequilibrium was identified in GABRB3 and GABRA5, as well as at the Angelman's syndrome gene UBE3A in autism families (Cook, 1998; Martin, 2000; Nurmi, 2001). Expression of nonimprinted 15q11-13 GABA receptor subunit genes was significantly reduced specifically in the female 15q11-13 duplication (Hogart et al., 2008).

Role of GABA in Brain Development

It is well demonstrated that GABA mechanisms are involved in the refinement of ocular dominance columns. Treatment with GABAergic drugs during a critical period alters the time course of this development (Hensch et al., 1998). There is abundant evidence that developmental changes in GABA neurotransmission are related to critical periods of activity-dependent synaptic plasticity in response to sensory experience in animals (Wolf et al., 1986; Ramoa et al., 1988, Reiter & Stryker, 1988). Furthermore, there are dramatic changes in $GABA_A$ receptor subunit composition in developing brain, for example in visual cortex (Huntsman et al., 1994; Huang et al., 1999), somatosensory cortex (Golshani et al., 1997; Huntsman et al., 1995), and cerebellum (Carlson et al., 1998). A specific role for benzodiazepine-sensitive $GABA_A$ receptors in the critical period for establishing ocular dominance has been suggested by investigators, who have demonstrated that infusion of diazepam can restore visual cortex plasticity in mice with gene-targeted disruption of the 65-kD isoform of the GABA synthetic enzyme glutamic acid decarboxylase (GAD_{65}) (Hensch et al., 1998). GAD_{65} knockout mice showed no shift in ocular dominance with eye closure during the critical period. However, ocular dominance shift in response to eye closure did occur in these mice if diazepam was infused in the visual cortex during the critical period.

Conclusion

There is abundant evidence for changes in neurotransmitters in autism. These changes in some cases might be directly caused by changes in genes directly relevant to the transmitter, such as enzymes involved in syntheses and degradation, transporters, or receptors. In other cases, the changes in the neurotransmitter might result from altered brain development due to mutation in a trophic factor or signaling pathway, infection, or other environmental event. As illustrated for both serotonin and GABA, neurotransmitters themselves affect brain development, and alterations in neurotransmitters at critical periods of brain development can lead to long-lasting changes in brain connectivity, affecting behavior. Although human pathology studies can provide distinct anatomical detail for localization of neurotransmitters and proteins relevant to their function, postmortem measures are limited to a snapshot in time at the age and condition of death. Such studies will not be able to provide a definition of neurotransmitter changes through development for the many different causes of autism. Animal studies based on particular genes or environmental factors leading to autism can be used to understand the effects of these factors on brain development and be used for preclinical testing of therapeutic agents. Ultimately, however, longitudinal molecular imaging studies aimed at relevant neurotransmitters would be needed to define development changes in a particular neurotransmitter in cases in which the cause of autism is known.

Challenges and Future Directions

Although neurotransmitters in autism has been a subject of study for nearly 50 years, knowledge of the role of the multitude of transmitters and their associated signaling partners in autism is limited. New tools are now available to allow a greater depth of understanding of how neurotransmitters might be altered by different causes of autism at different stages of development over the lifespan.

- Use of animal genetic models of human genetic or environmental causes of autism with microarray techniques to determine the expression of mRNAs for all neurotransmitter related genes, including enzymes mediating synthesis and degradation, transporters, receptors, signaling pathways.
- Use of molecular imaging techniques in humans with known genetic or environmental causes of autism to follow up on discoveries from animal models.
- Employ pharmacological treatment strategies aimed at correcting neurotransmitter abnormalities during development to correct developmental errors.

SUGGESTED READINGS

Berger, M., Gray, J. A., & Roth, B. L. (2009). The expanded biology of serotonin. *Annual Review of Medicine, 60*, 355–366.

Chugani, D. C. (2005). Pharmacological intervention in autism: Targeting critical periods of brain development. *Clinical Neuropsychiatry, 2*(6), 346–353.

Gaspar, P., Cases, O., & Maroteaux, L. (2003). The developmental role of serotonin: news from mouse molecular genetics. *Nature Reviews Neuroscience, 4*, 1002–1012.

Lam, K. S. L., Aman, M. G., & Arnold, L. E. (2006). Neurochemical correlates of autistic disorder: A review of the literature. *Research in Developmental Disabilities, 27*, 254–289.

Pardo, C. A., & Eberhart, C. G. (2007). The neurobiology of autism. *Brain Pathology (Zurich, Switzerland), 17*, 434–447.

REFERENCES

Ahlemeyer, B., Beier, H., Semkova, I., Schaper, C., & Krieglstein, J. (2000). S-100beta protects cultured neurons against glutamate- and staurosporine-induced damage and is involved in the anti-apoptotic action of the 5 HT(1A)-receptor agonist, Bay x 3702. *Brain Research, 858*(1), 121–128.

Anderson, G. M., Freedman, D. X., Cohen, D. J., Volkmar, F. R., Hoder, E. L., McPhedran, P., et al. (1987). Whole blood serotonin in autistic and normal subjects. *Journal of Child Psychology and Psychiatry and Allied Disciplines, 28*(6), 885–900.

Ansorge, M. S., Zhou, M., Lira, A., Hen, R., & Gingrich, J. A. (2004). Early-life blockage of the 5-HT transporter alters emotion behavior in adult mice. *Science, 29*, 879–881.

Azmitia, E. C., Gannon, P. J., Kheck, N. M., & Whitaker-Azmitia, P. M. (1996). Cellular localization of the 5-HT1A receptor in primate brain neurons and glial cells. *Neuropsychopharmacology, 14*(1), 35–46.

Balkovetz, D. F., Tiruppathi, C., Leibach, F. H., Mahesh, V. B., & Ganapathy, V. (1989). Evidence for an imipramine-sensitive serotonin transporter in human placental brush-border membranes. *Journal of Biological Chemistry, 264*(4), 2195–2198.

Beaulieu, J-M., Zhang, X., Rodriguiz, R. M., Sotnikova, T. D., Cools, M. J., Wetsel, W. C., et al. (2008). Role of GSK3β in behavioral abnormalities induced by serotonin deficiency. *Proceedings of the National Academy of Sciences of the United States of America, 105*(4), 1333–1338.

Barnard, E. A., Skolnick, P., Olsen, R. W., Mohler, H., Sieghart, W., Biggio, G., et al. (1998). International Union of Pharmacology: XV. Subtypes of g-aminobutyric acidA receptors: Classification on the basis of subunit structure and receptor function. *Pharmacology, 50*, 291–313.

Bass, M. P., Menold, M. M., Wolpert, C. M., Donelly, S. L., Ravan, S. A., Hauser, E. R., et al. (2000). Genetic studies in autistic disorder and chromosome 15. *Neurogenetics, 2*, 219–226.

Bennett-Clarke, C. A., Chiaia, N. L., & Rhoades, R. W. (1996). Thalamocortical afferents in rat transiently express high-affinity serotonin uptake sites. *Brain Research, 733*, 301–306.

Bennett-Clarke, C. A., Leslie, M. J., Lane, R. D., & Rhoades, R. W. (1994). Effect of serotonin depletion on vibrissae-related patterns in the rat's somatosensory cortex. *Journal of Neuroscience, 14*, 7594–7607.

Berman, N. E. J., Puri, V., Chandrala, S., Puri, S., Macgregor, R., Liverman, C. S., et al. (2006). Serotonin in trigeminal ganglia of female rodents: relevance to menstrual migraine. *Headache, 46*, 1230–1245.

Berger, M., Gray, J. A., & Roth, B. L. (2009). The expanded biology of serotonin. *Annual Review of Medicine, 60*, 355–366.

Blue, M. E., Erzurumlu, R. S., & Jhaveri, S. (1991). A comparison of pattern formation by thalamocortical and serotonergic afferents in the rat barrel field cortex. *Cerebral Cortex, 1*, 380–389.

Bortolato, M., Chen, K., & Shih, J. C. (2008). Monoamine oxidase inactivation: from pathophysiology to therapeutics. *Advanced Drug Delivery Reviews, 60*(13–14), 1527–1533.

Bowery, N. (1993). GABAB receptor pharmacology. *Annual Review of Pharmacology and Toxicology, 33*, 109–147.

Butler, M. G., Dasouki, M. J., Zhou, X. P., Talebizadeh, Z., Brown, M., Takahashi, T. N., et al. (2005). Subset of individuals with autism spectrum disorders and extreme macrocephaly associated with germline PTEN tumour suppressor gene mutations. *Journal of Medical Genetics, 42*(4), 318–321.

Buxbaum, J. D., Silverman, J. M., Smith, C. J., Greenberg, D. A., Kilifarski, M., Reichert, J., et al. (2002). Association between a GABRB3 polymorphism and autism. *Molecular Psychiatry, 7*(3), 311–316.

Carlson, B. X., Elster, L., & Schousboe, A. (1998). Pharmacological and functional implications of developmentally-regulated changes in GABA(A) receptor subunit expression in the cerebellum. *European Journal of Pharmacology, 352*, 1–14.

Cases, O., Seif, I., Grimsby, J., Gaspar, P., Chen, K., Pournin, S., et al. (1995). Aggressive behavior and altered amounts of brain serotonin and norepinephrine in mice lacking MAOA. *Science, 268*, 1763–1766.

Cases, O., Vitalis, T., Seif, I., De Maeyer, E., Sotelo. C., & Gaspar, P. (1996). Lack of barrels in the somatosensory cortex of monoamine oxidase A-deficient mice, role of a serotonin excess during the critical period. *Neuron, 16*, 297–307.

Cassel, S., Carouge, D., Gensburger, C., Anglard, P. Burgun, C., Dietrich, J. B., et al. (2006). Fluoxetine and cocaine induce the epigenetic factors MeCP2 and MBD1 in adult rat brain. *Molecular Pharmacology, 70*(2), 487–492.

Chandana, S. R., Behen, M. E., Juhasz, C., Muzik, O., Rothermel, R. D., Mangner, T. J., et al. (2005). Significance of abnormalities in developmental trajectory and asymmetry of cortical serotonin synthesis in autism. *International Journal of Developmental Neuroscience, 23*, 171–182.

Chen, B., Dowlatshahi, D., MacQueen, G. M., Wang, J., & Young L. T. (2001). Increased hippocampal BDNF immunoreactivity in subjects treated with antidepressant medication. *Biological Psychiatry, 50*, 260–265.

Chugani, D. C., Muzik, O., Behen, M. E., Rothermel, R. D., Lee, J., & Chugani, H. T. (1999). Developmental changes in brain serotonin synthesis capacity in autistic and non-autistic children. *Annals of Neurology, 45*, 287–295.

Chugani, D. C., Muzik, O., Rothermel, R., Behen, M., Chakraborty, P. K., Mangner, T. J., et al. (1997). Altered serotonin synthesis in the dentatothalamo-cortical pathway in autistic boys. *Annals of Neurology, 14*, 666–669.

Cohen, I. L., Liu, X., Schutz, C., White, B. N., Jenkins, E. C., Brown, W. T., et al. (2003). Association of autism severity with a monoamine oxidase a functional polymorphism. *Clinical Genetics, 64*, 190–197.

Cook, E. H., Jr., Charak, D. A., Arida, J., Spohn, J. A., Roizen, N. J., & Leventhal, B. L., (1994). Depressive and obsessive-compulsive symptoms in hyperserotonemic parents of children with autistic disorder. *Psychiatry Research, 52*(1), 25–33.

Cook, E. H., Jr., Courchesne, R. Y., Cox, N. J., Lord, C., Gonen, D., Guter, S. J., et al. (1998). Linkage-disequilibrium mapping of autistic disorder, with 15q11-13 markers. *American Journal of Human Genetics, 62*, 1077–1083.

Cook, E. H., Jr., Leventhal, B. L., Heller, W., Metz, J., Wainwright, M., & Freedman, D. X., (1990). Autistic children and theirfirst-degree relatives: relationships between serotonin and norepinephrine levels and intelligence. *Journal of Neuropsychiatry and Clinical Neurosciences, 2*(3), 268–274.

Cook, E. H., Jr., Lindgren, V., Leventhal, B. L., Courchesne, R., Lincoln, A., Shulman, C., et al. (1997). Autism or atypical autism in maternally but not paternally derived proximal 15q duplication. *American Journal of Human Genetics, 4*, 928–934.

Coon, H., Dunn, D., Lainhart, J., Miller, J., Hamil, C., Battaglia, A., et al. (2005). Possible association between autism and variants in the brain-expressed tryptophan hydroxylase gene (TPH2). *American Journal of Medical Genetics. Part B, Neuropsychiatric Genetics, 135B*, 42–46.

Coutinho, A. M., Sousa, I., Martins, M., Correia, C., Morgadinho, T., Bento, C., et al. (2007). Evidence for epistasis between SLC6A4 and ITGB3 in autism etiology and in the determination of platelet serotonin levels. *Human Genetics, 121*(2), 243–256.

Cowen, D. S., Johnson-Farley, N. N., & Travkina, T. (2005). 5-HT1A Receptors couple to activation of Akt, but not extracellular-regulated kinase (ERK) in cultured hippocampal neurons. *Journal of Neurochemistry, 93*, 910–917.

Curtiss, S., & de Bode, S. (2003). How normal is grammatical development in the right hemisphere following hemispherectomy? The root infinite stage and beyond. *Brain and Language, 86*, 193–206.

D'Amato, R. J., Blue, M. E., Largent, B. L., Lynch, D. R., Ledbetter, D. J., Molliver, M. E., et al. (1987). Ontogeny of the serotonergic projection to rat neocortex, transient expression of a dense innervation to primary sensory areas. *Proceedings of the National Academy of Sciences of the United States of America, 84*, 4322–4326.

Davis, L. K., Hazlett, H. C., Librant, A. L., Nopoulos, P., Sheffield V. C., Piven, J., et al. (2008). Cortical enlargement in autism is associated with a functional VNTR in the monoamine oxidase a gene. *American Journal of Medical Genetics. Part B, Neuropsychiatric Genetics, 147B*, 1145–1151.

DeLorey, T. M., Handforth, A., Anagnostaras, S. G., Homanics, G. E., Minassian, B. A., Asatourian, A., et al. (1998). Mice lacking the β3 subunit of the GABAA receptor have the epilepsy phenotype and many of the behavioral characteristics of Angelman syndrome. *Journal of Neuroscience, 18*, 8505–8514.

Devlin, B., Cook, E. H., Jr., Coon, H., Dawson, G., Grigorenko, E. L., McMahon, W., et al. (2005). CPEA Genetics Network: Autism and the serotonin transporter, the long and short of it. *Molecular Psychiatry*, 10(12), 1110–1116.

Easton, R. M., Cho, H., Roovers, K., Shineman, D. W., Mizrahi, M., Forman, M. S., et al. (2005). Role for Akt3/protein kinase Bgamma in attainment of normal brain size. *Molecular and Cellular Biology, 25*(5), 1869–1878.

Eddahibi, S., Guignabert, C., Barlier-Mur, A-M., Dewachter, L., Fadel, E., Dartevelle, P., et al. (2006). Cross talk between endothelial and smooth muscle cells in pulmonary hypertension. *Circulation, 113*, 1857–1864.

Eriksen, J. L., & Druse, M. J. (2001). Astrocyte-mediated trophic support of developing serotonin neurons: effects of ethanol, buspirone, and S100B. *Brain Research. Developmental Brain Research, 131*(1–2), 9–15.

Esaki, T., Cook, M., Shimoji, K., Murphy, D. L., Sokoloff, L., & Holmes, A. (2005). Developmental disruption of serotonin transporter function impairs cerebral responses to whisker stimulation in mice. *Proceedings of the National Academy of Sciences of the United States of America, 102*(15), 5582–5587.

Fatemi, S. H., Folsom, T. D., Reutiman, T. J., & Thuras, P. D. (2009). Expression of GABB receptors is altered in brains of subjects with autism. *Cerebellum, 8*(1), 64–69.

Fatemi, S. H., Halt, A. R., Stary, J. M., Kanodia, R., Schulz, S. C., & Realmuto, G. R. (2002). Glutamic acid decarboxylase 65 and 67 kDa proteins are reduced in autistic parietal and cerebellar cortices. *Biological Psychiatry, 52,* 805–810.

Fatemi, S. H., Reutiman, T. J., Folsom, T. D., & Thuras, P. D. (2009). GABAA receptor downregulation in brains of subject with autism. *Journal of Autism and Developmental Disorders, 39*(2), 223–230.

Fernstrom, J. D., & Wurtman, R. J. (1971). Brain serotonin content: Physiological dependence on plasma tryptophan levels. *Science, 173,* 149–151.

Gaspar, P., Cases, O., & Maroteaux, L. (2003). The developmental role of serotonin: news from mouse molecular genetics. *Nature Reviews Neuroscience, 4,* 1002–1012.

Gershon, M. D., & Tack, J. (2007). The serotonin signaling system: from basic understanding to drug development for functional GI disorders. *Gastroenterology, 132,* 397–414.

Golshani, P., Truong, H., & Jones, E. G. (1997). Developmental expression of GABAA receptor subunit and GAD genes in mouse somatosensory barrel cortex. *Journal of Comparative Neurology, 383,* 199–219.

Gross, C., Zhuang, X., Stark, K., Ramboz, S., Oosting, R., Kirby, L., et al. (2002). Serotonin1A receptor acts during development to establish normal anxiety-like behavior in the adult. *Nature, 416,* 396–400.

Hamon, M., Bourgoin, S., Artaud, F. E., & Mestikawy, S. (1981). The respective roles of tryptophan uptake and tryptophan hydroxylase in the regulation of serotonin synthesis in the central nervous system. *Journal of Physiology, 77,* 269–279.

Harrison, N. L., Kugler, J. L., Jones, M. V., Greenblatt, E. P., & Pritchett, D. B. (1993). Positive modulation of human g-aminobutyric acid type A and glycine receptor by the inhalation anesthetic isoflurane. *Molecular Pharmacology, 44,* 628–632.

Hensch, T. K., Fagiolini, M., Mataga, N., Stryker, M. P., Baekkeskov, S., & Kash, S. F. (1998). Local GABA circuit control of experience-dependent plasticity in developing visual cortex. *Science, 282,* 1504–1508.

Herbert, M. R., Harris, G. J., Adrien, K. T., Ziegler, D. A., Makris, N., Kennedy, D. N., et al. (2002). Abnormal asymmetry in language association cortex in autism. *Annals of Neurology, 52,* 589–596.

Hogart, A., Wu, D., Lasalle, J. M., & Schanen, N. C. (2008, September 20). The comorbidity of autism with the genomic disorders of chromosome 15q11.2-q13. *Neurobiology of Disease, 18* [Epub ahead of print].

Holopainen, I. E., Metsähonkala, E. L., Kokkonen, H., Parkkola, R. K., Manner, T. E., Någren, K., et al.(2001). Decreased binding of [11C]flumazenil in Angelman syndrome patients with GABAA receptor β3 subunit deletions. *Annals of Neurology, 49,* 110–113.

Homanics, G. E., DeLorey, T. M. Firestone, L. L., Quinlan, J. J., Handforth A., Harrison, N. L., et al. (1997). Mice devoid of -aminobutyrate type A receptor β3 subunit have epilepsy, cleft palate, and hypersensitive behavior. *Proceedings of the National Academy of Sciences of the United States of America, 94,* 4143–4148.

Hoshino, Y., Yamamoto, T., Kaneko, M., Tachibana, R., Watanabe, M., Ono, Y., et al. (1984). Blood serotonin and free tryptophan concentration in autistic children. *Neuropsychobiology, 11*(1), 22–27.

Hsiung, S. C., Tamir, H., Thomas, F. F., & Liu, K-P. (2005). Roles of extracellular signal-regulated kinase and Akt signal in coordinating nuclear transcription factor-κB-dependent cell survival after serotonin 1A receptor activation. *Journal of Neurochemistry, 95,* 1653–1666.

Huang, Z. J., Kirkwood, A., Pizzorusso, T., Porciatti, V., Morales, B., Bear, M. F., et al. (1999). BDNF regulates the maturation of inhibition and the critical period of plasticity in mouse visual cortex. *Cell, 98,* 739–755.

Huntsman, M. M., Isackson, P. J., & Jones, E. G. (1994). Lamina-specific expression and activity-dependent regulation of seven GABAA receptor mRNAs in monkey visual cortex. *Journal of Neuroscience, 14,* 2236–2259.

Huntsman, M. M., Woods, T. M., & Jones, E.G.(1995). Laminar patterns of expression of GABAA receptor subunit mRNAs in monkey sensory motor cortex. *Journal of Comparative Neurology, 362,* 565–582.

Ide, S., Itoh, M., & Goto, Y. (2005). Defect in normal developmental increase of the brain biogenic amine concentration in the mecp2-null mouse. *Neuroscience Letters, 386,* 14–17.

Ikeda, K., Tojo, K., Otsubo, C., Udagawa, T., Kumazawa, K., Ishikawa, M., et al. (2005). 5-hydroxytryptamine synthesis in HL-1 cells and neonatal rat cardiocytes. *Biochemical and Biophysical Research Communications, 328*(2), 522–525.

Ji, S-P., Zhang, Y., Cleemput, J. V., Jiang, W., Liao, M., Li, L., et al. (2006). Disruption of PTEN coupling with 5-HT2C receptors suppresses behavioral responses induced by drugs of abuse. *Nature Medicine, 12*(3), 324–329.

Jones, M. B., Palmour, R. M., Zwaigenbaum, L.,& Szatmari, P. (2004). Modifier effects in autism at the MAO-A and DBH loci. *American Journal of Medical Genetics. Part B, Neuropsychiatric Genetics, 126,* 58–65.

Kaufman, D. L., Houser, C. R., & Tobin, A. J. (1991). Two forms of the gammaminobutyric acid synthetic enzyme glutamate decarboxylase have distinct intraneuronal distributions and cofactor intereactions. *Journal of Neurochemistry, 56,* 720–723.

Khawaja, X., Xu, J., Liang, J.-J., & Barrett, J. E. (2004). Proteomic analysis of protein changes developing in rat hippocampus after chronic antidepressant treatment: implications for depressive disorders and future therapies. *Journal of Neuroscience Research, 75,* 451–460.

Kishino, T., Lalande, M., & Wagstaff, J.(1997). UBE3A/E6-AP mutations cause Angelman syndrome. *Nature Genetics, 15*(1), 70–73.

Lam, K. S. L., Aman, M. G., & Arnold, L. E. (2006). Neurochemical correlates of autistic disorder: A review of the literature. *Research in Developmental Disabilities, 27,* 254–289.

Lambert, H. W., & Lauder, J. M. (1999). Serotonin receptor agonists that increases cyclic AMP positively regulate IGF-I in mouse mandibular mesenchymal cells. *Developmental Neuroscience, 21,* 105–112.

Lauder, J. M. (1993). Neurotransmitters as growth regulatory signals: role of receptors and second messengers. *Trends in Neurosciences, 16,* 233–240.

Leboyer, M., Philippe, A., Bouvard, M., Guilloud-Bataille, M., Bondoux, D., Tabuteau, F., et al. (1999). Whole blood serotonin and plasma beta-endorphin in autistic probands and their first-degree relatives. *Biological Psychiatry, 45(2),* 158–163.

Lebrand, C., Cases, O., Adelbrecht, C., Doye, A., Alvarez, C., Mestikawy, S. E., et al. (1996). Transient uptake and storage of serotonin in developing thalamic neurons. *Neuron, 17,* 823–835.

Lesch, K. P., Bengel, D., Heils, A., Sabol, S. Z., Greenberg, B. D., Petri, S., et al. (1996). Association of anxiety-related with a polymorphism in the serotonin transporter gene regulatory region. *Science, 274*(5292), 1527–1531.

Leventhal, B. L., Cook Jr., E. H., Morford, M., Ravitz, A., Freedman, D. X., (1990). Relationships of whole blood serotonin and plasma norepinephrine within families. *Journal of Autism and Developmental Disorders, 20*(4), 499–511.

Li, X., Zhu, W., Roh, M-S., Friedman, A. B., Rosborough, K., & Jope, R.S. (2004). In vivo regulation of glycogen synthase kinase-3β (GSK3β) by serotonergic activity in mouse brain. *Neuropsychopharmacology, 29*(8),1426–1431.

Lucignani, G., Panzacchi, A., Bosio, L., Moresco, R. M., Ravasi, L., Coppa, I., et al. (2004). GABA A receptor abnormalities in Prader-Willi syndrome assessed with positron emission tomography and [11C]flumazenil. *NeuroImage, 22*(1), 22–28.

Macdonald, R. L., & Olsen, R.W.(1994). GABAA receptor channels. *Annual Review of Neuroscience, 17*, 569–602.

Mahmoudi, M., Kang M-H., Tillakaratne, N., Tobin, A. J., & Olsen, R. W. (1997). Chronic intermittent ethanol treatment in rats increased GABAA receptor a4-subunit expression: Possible relevance to alcohol dependence. *Journal of Neurochemistry, 68*, 2485–2492.

Maragnoli, M. E., Fumagalli, F., Gennarelli, M., Racagni, G., & Riva, M. A. (2004). Fluoxetine and olanzapine have synergistic effects in the modulation of fibroblast growth factor 2 expression within the rat brain. *Biological Psychiatry, 55*, 1095–1102.

Marshall, S. E., Bird, T. G., Hart, K., & Welsh, K. I. (1999). Unified approach to the analysis of genetic variation in serotonergic pathways. *American Journal of Medical Genetics, 88*, 621–627.

Martin, E. R. Menold, M. M., Wolpert, C. M. Bass, M. P. Donelly, S. L., Ravan, S. A., et al. (2000). Analysis of linkage disequilibrium in γ-aminobutyric acid receptor subunit genes in autistic disorder. *American Journal of Medical Genetics, 96*, 43–48.

Matsuda, M., Imaoka, T., Vomachka, A. J., Gudelsky, G. A., Hou, Z., Mistry, M., et al. (2004). Serotonin regulates mammary gland development via an autocrine-paracrine loop. *Developmental Cell, 6*, 193–203.

McCauley, J. L., Olson, L. M., Delahanty, R., Amin, T., Nurmi, E. L., Organ, E. L., et al. (2004). A linkage disequilibrium map of the 1-Mb 15q12 GABA(A) receptor subunit cluster and association to autism. *American Journal of Medical Genetics. Part B, Neuropsychiatric Genetics, 131*, 51–59.

Menold, M. M., Shao, Y., Wolpert, C. M., Donnelly, S. L., Raiford, K. L., Martin, E. R., et al. (2001). Association analysis of chromosome 15 GABAA receptor subunit genes in autistic disorder. *Journal of Neurogenetics, 15*(3–4), 245–259.

Müller, C. P., & Carey, R. J. (2006, September). Intracellular 5-HT 2C-receptor dephosphorylation: A new target for treating drug addiction. *Trends in Pharmacological Sciences, 27*(9), 455–458.

Muller, R. A., Rothermel, R. D., Behen, M. E., Muzik, O., Chakraborty, P. K., & Chugani, H. T. (1999). Language organization in patients with early and late left-hemisphere lesion: A PET study. *Neuropsychologia, 37*, 545–557.

Munn, D. H., Zhou, M., Attwood, J. T., Bondarev, I., Conway, S. J., Marshall, B., et al. (1998). Inhibition of T cell proliferation by macrophage tryptophan catabolism. *Science, 281*, 1191–1193.

Nabi, R, Serajee, F. J., Chugani, D. C., Zhong, H, & Huq, A. H. (2004). Association of tryptophan 2,3 dioxygenase gene polymorphism with autism. *American Journal of Medical Genetics. Part B, Neuropsychiatric Genetics, 125*, 63–68.

Nayeem, N., Green, T. P., Martin I. L., & Barnard E. A. (1994). Quaternary structure of the native GABAA receptor determined by electron microscope image analysis. *Journal of Neurochemistry, 62*, 815–818.

Ni, W., Geddes, T. J., Priestley, J. R., Szasz, T., Kuhn, D. M., & Watts, S. W. (2008). The existence of a local5-hydroxytryptaminergic system in peripheral arteries. *British Journal of Pharmacology, 154*(3), 663–674.

Ni, W., & Watts, S. W. (2006). 5-hydroxytryptamine in the cardiovascular systems: focus on the serotonin transporter (SERT). *Clinical and Experimental Pharmacology and Physiology, 33*, 575–583.

Nibuya, M., Nestler E., J., & Duamn R. S. (1996). Chronic antidepressant administration increases the expression of a cAMP response element binding protein (CREB) in rat hippocampus. *Journal of Neuroscience, 16*, 2365–2372.

Nicholls R. D., & Knepper J. L. (2001). Genome organization: function and imprinting in Prader-Willi and Angelman syndromes. *Annual Review of Genomics and Human Genetics, 2*, 153–175.

Nishi, M., Whitaker-Azmitia, P. M., & Azmitia, E. C. (1996). Enhanced synaptophysin immunoreactivity in rat hippocampal culture by 5-HT 1A agonist, S100b, and corticosteroid receptor agonists *Synapse, 23*(1), 1–9.

Nocito, A., Dahm, F., Jochum, W., Jang, J. H., Georgiev, P., Bader, M., et al. (2007). Serotonin mediates oxidative stress and mitochondrial toxicity in a murine model of nonalcoholic steatohepatitis. *Gastroenterology, 133*(2), 608–618.

Nurmi, E. L., Bradford, Y., Chen, Y., Hall, J., Arnone, B., Gardiner, M. B., et al. (2001). Linkage disequilibrium at the Angelman syndrome gene UBE3A in autism families. *Genomics, 77*(1–2), 105–113.

Oblak, A., Gibbs, T. T., Blatt, G. J. (2009). Decreased GABAA receptors and benzodiazepine binding sites in the anterior cingulated cortex in autism. *Autism Research, 2*, 205–219.

Olsen, R. W., Sapp, D. W. (1995). Neuroactive steroid modulation of GABAA receptors. *Advances in Biochemical Psychopharmacology, 48*, 57–74.

Olsen, R. W., Sapp, D. W., Bureau, M. H., Turner, D. M., & Kokka, N. (1991). Allosteric actions of central nervous system depressants including anesthetics on subtypes of the inhibitory g -aminobutyric acid A receptor-chloride channel complex. *Annals of the New York Academy of Sciences, 625*, 145–154.

Oritz-Alvarado, R., Guzmán-Quevedo, O., Meracado-Camargo, R., Haertle, T., Vignes, C., & Bolaños-Jiménez, F. (2006). Expression of tryptophan hydroxylase in developing mouse taste papillae. *FEBS Letters, 580*, 5371–5376.

Osterheld-Haas, M. C., & Hornung, J. P. (1996). Laminar development of the mouse barrel cortex, effects of neurotoxins against monoamines. *Experimental Brain Research. Experimentelle Hirnforschung. Experimentation Cerebrale, 110*, 183–195.

Owens, D. F., Boyce, L. H., Davis, M. B. E., & Kriegstein, A. R. (1996). Excitatory GABA responses in embryonic and neonatal cortical slices demonstrated by gramicidin perforated patch recordings and calcium imaging. *Journal of Neuroscience, 16*, 6414–6423.

Pardridge, W. M. (1977). Kinetics of competitive inhibition of neutral amino acid transport across the blood-brain barrier. *Journal of Neurochemistry, 28*, 103–108.

Piven, J., & Palmer, P., (1999). Psychiatric disorder and the broad autism phenotype: evidence from a family study of multiple-incidence autism families. *American Journal of Psychiatry, 56*(4), 557–563.

Ramoa, A. S., Paradiso, M. A., & Freeman, R. D. (1988). Blockade of intracortical inhibition in kitten striate cortex: Effects on receptive field properties and associated loss of ocular dominance plasticity. *Experimental Brain Research. Experimentelle Hirnforschung. Experimentation Cerebrale, 73*, 285–298.

Rasmussen, T., Milner, B. (1977). The role of early left-brain injury in determining lateralization of cerebral speech functions. *Annals of the New York Academy of Sciences, 299*, 355–369.

Reiter, H. O., & Stryker, M. P. (1988). Neural plasticity without postsynaptic action potentials: Less active inputs become dominant when kitten visual cortical cells are pharmacologically inhibited. *Proceedings of the National Academy of Sciences of the United States of America, 85*, 3623–3627.

Rivera, C., Voipio, J, Payne, J. A., Ruusuvuori, E., Lahtenin, H., Lamsa, K., et al. (1999). The K+/Cl- co-transporter KCC2 renders GABA hyperpolarizing during neuronal maturation. *Nature, 397*, 251–255.

Rolf, L. H., Haarmann, F. Y., Grotemeyer, K. H., & Kehrer, H. (1993). Serotonin and amino acid content in platelets of autistic children. *Acta Psychiatrica Scandinavica, 87*, 312–316.

Sakowski, S. A., Geddes, T. J., Thomas, D. M., Levi, E., Hatfield, J. S., & Kuhn, D. M. (2006). Differential tissue distribution of tryptophan hydroxylase isoforms 1 and 2 as revealed with monospecific antibodies. *Brain Research, 1085*, 11–18.

Schain, R. J., & Freedman, D. X. (1961). Studies on 5-hydoxyindole metabolism in autism and other mentally retarded children. *Journal of Pediatrics, 59*, 315–320.

Silva, A. E., Vayego-Lourenco, S. A., Fett-Conte, A. C., Goloni-Bertollo, E. M., & Varella-Garcia, M. (2002). Tetrasomy 15q11-q13 identified by fluorescence in situ hybridization in a patient with autistic disorder. *Arquivos de neuro-psiquiatria, 60*(2-A), 290–294.

Sinkkonen, S. T., Homanics, G. E., & Korpi, E. R. (2003). Mouse models of Angelman syndrome, a neurodevelopmental disorder, display different brain regional GABA(A) receptor alterations *Neuroscience Letters, 340*(3), 205–208.

Slominski, A., Pisarchik, A., Semak, I., Sweatman, T., Worstman, J., Szczesniewski, A., et al. (2002). Serotoninergic and melatoninergic systems are fully expressed in human skin. *FASEB Journal, 16*, 896–898.

Smith, Q. R., Monna, S., Aoyagi, M., & Rapoport, S. I. (1987). Kinetics of neutral amino acid transport across the blood-brain barrier. *Journal of Neurochemistry, 49*, 1651–1658.

Stull, M. A., Pai, V, Vomachka, A. J., Marshall, A. M., Jacob, G. A., & Horseman, N. D. (2007). Mammary gland homeostasis employs serotonergic regulation of epithelial tight junctions. *Proceedings of the National Academy of Sciences of the United States of America, 104*(42), 16708–16713.

Suzuki, S., Tone, S., Takikawa, O., Kubo, T., Kohno, I., & Minatogawa, Y. (2001). Expression of indoleamine 2,3-dioxygenase and tryptophan 2,3-dioxygenase in early concepti. *Biochemical Journal, 355*, 425–429.

Varga, E. A., Pastore, M., Prior, T., Herman, G. E., & McBride, K.L. (2009). The prevalence of PTEN mutations in a clinical pediatric cohort with autism spectrum disorders, developmental delay, and macrocephaly. *Genetics in Medicine, 11*(2), 111–117.

Wassink, T. H., Hazlett, H. C., Epping, E. A., Arndt, S., Dager, S. R., Schellenberg, G. D., et al. (2007). Cerebral cortical gray matter overgrowth and functional variation of the serotonin transporter gene in autism. *Archives of General Psychiatry, 64*(6), 709–717.

Weiss, L. A., Kosova, G., Delahanty, R. J., Jiang, L., Cook, E. H., Ober, C., et al. (2006). Variation in ITGB3 is associated with whole-blood serotonin level and autism susceptibility. *European Journal of Human Genetics: EJHG, 14*(8), 923–931.

Weiss, L. A., Ober, C., Cook, E. H., Jr. (2006). ITGB3 shows genetic and expression interaction with SLC6A4. *Human Genetics, 120*(1), 93–100.

Whitaker-Azmitia, P. M., Druse, M., Walker, P., & Lauder, J. M. (1996). Serotonin as a developmental signal. *Behavioural Brain Research, 73*(1–2), 19–29.

Whiting, P. J. (1999). The GABA-A receptor gene family: new targets for therapeutic intervention. *Neurochemistry International, 34*, 387–390.

Wolf, W., Hicks, T. P., & Albus, K. (1986). The contribution of GABA-mediated inhibitory mechanisms to visual response properties of neurons in the kitten's striate cortex. *Journal of Neuroscience, 6*, 2779–2796.

Yan, W., Wilson, C. C., & Haring, J. H. (1997). Effects of neonatal serotonin depletion on the development of rat dentate granule cells. *Brain Research. Developmental Brain Research, 98*, 177–184.

Yip, J., Soghomonian, J. J., & Blatt, G. J. (2007). Decreased GAD67 mRNA levels in cerebellar Purkinje cells in autism: pathophysiological implications. *Acta Neuropathologica, 113*(5), 559–568.

Yip, J., Soghomonian, J. J., & Blatt, G. J. (2008). Increased GAD67 mRNA levels in cerebellar interneurons in autism: implications for Purkinje cell dysfunction. *Journal of Neuroscience Research, 86*, 525–530.

Yip, J., Soghomonian, J. J., & Blatt, G. J. (2009). Decreased GAD65 mRNA levels in select subpopulations in the cerebellar dentate nuclei in autism: an in situ hybridization study. *Autism Research, 2*(1), 50–59.

Yuste, R., & Katz, L.C.(1991). Control of postsynaptic Ca2+ influx in developing neocortex by excitatory and inhibitory neurotransmitters. *Neuron, 6*, 333–344.

Zhang, X., Beaulieu, J. M., Sotnikova, T. D., Gainetdinov, R. R., & Caron, M. G. (2004). Tryptophan hydroxylase-2 controls brain serotonin synthesis. *Science, 305*, 217.

Zhang, Y. Q., Friedman, D. B., Wang, Z., Woodruff, E., 3rd., Pan, L., O'Donnell, J., et al. (2005). Protein expression profiling of the drosophila fragile X mutant brain reveals up-regulation of monoamine synthesis. *Molecular and Cellular Proteomics: MCP, 4*, 278–290.

Zhao, X., Leotta, A., Kustanovich, V., Lajonchere, C., Geschwind, D. H., Law, K., et al. (2007). A unified genetic theory for sporadic and inherited autism. *Proceedings of the National Academy of Sciences of the United States of America, 104*, 12831–12836.

Zoghbi, H. Y., Milstien, S., Butler I. J., Smith, E. O., Kaufman, S., Glaze, D. G., et al. (1989). Cerebrospinal fluid biogenic amines and biopterin in Rett syndrome. *Annals of Neurology, 25*, 56–60.

33 Stephen R. Dager, Neva M. Corrigan, Todd L. Richards, Dennis W. Shaw

Brain Chemistry: Magnetic Resonance Spectroscopy

Points of Interest

- ^{1}H MRS is FDA-approved and uses the same equipment as MRI to noninvasively measure hydrogen-containing brain chemicals.
- The areas under the curve of individual peaks in a ^{1}H MRS spectrum used to calculate chemical concentrations also are influenced by pulse sequence and acquisition parameters (e.g., echo time) used to acquire the spectrum.
- The concurrent measurement of multiple chemicals by ^{1}H MRS provides relational information that can reveal patterns of chemical alterations associated with a specific pathophysiology.
- ^{1}H MRS can assess interactions between glutamate and GABA levels, the most abundant excitatory and inhibitory neurotransmitters, respectively, as well as other chemicals, such as choline, creatine, myoinositol and N-acetyl-aspartate, that provide information on the functionality or "health" of neuronal and glial cells.
- Among the more consistently observed chemical alterations associated with ASD, particularly in younger children, are reduced levels of chemicals, such as N-acetyl-aspartate and choline, that are consistent with emerging theories of decreased brain packing density or inflammatory processes early in the developmental course of ASD.

Background

The diagnosis of ASD, typically made in early childhood, is based on rigorous behavioral assessment (APA, 1994). With improvements in diagnostic instruments, the earliest age for reliable clinical diagnosis of ASD has been progressively pushed back to the range of 18 to 36 months of age (Dawson et al., 2002; Dawson et al., 2004; Lord et al., 2006; Zwaigenbaum et al., 2005; Watson et al., 2006; Bryson, McDermott, Rombough, & Zwaigenbaum, 2008; Landa & Garrett-Mayer, 2006). During this time frame, the brain reaches 80–90% of its adult volume, with the overall adult pattern of myelination, and elaboration of new synapses, well underway (Pfefferbaum et al, 1994; Sampaio & Truwit, 2001; Huttenlocher & Dabholkar, 1997). Concurrent with this period of rapid brain development is the development of a wide range of cognitive, social, and language abilities (Kagan, Herschkowitz, & Herschkowitz, 2005).

The pathogenesis of ASD remains little understood but is generally thought to reflect an alteration in the underlying complex interaction of genetic and environmental influences on normal brain development during the postnatal period (DiCicco-Bloom et al., 2006). Earlier imaging studies seeking to identify specific anatomical correlates to ASD have reported a wide array of structural findings that have been often inconsistently replicated, as reviewed elsewhere (Lyon & Rumsey, 1996; Williams & Minshew, 2007). Often reflecting pragmatic considerations of clinical feasibility, imaging studies of ASD typically have concentrated on small samples of older, high-functioning individuals who can cooperate with the imaging procedure. One limitation with this approach of studying only cooperative individuals is that those with mental retardation and seizures, a clinically important and very prevalent subgroup of individuals with ASD, have often gone unstudied. Additionally, a particular difficulty with interpreting brain imaging findings from studies of ASD, beyond such considerations as imaging or analytic techniques used and the sample power, is that a broad range of subject ages are frequently grouped together in individual studies. Wide age ranges within a sample can inadvertently obscure brain developmental alterations that may be present only at distinct age points in ASD, making interpretation of the imaging literature difficult.

More recently, there have been several MRI studies of young children with ASD having samples that comprise a relatively narrow age range of between 2 and 4 years of age. These studies have consistently found on average 10–15% cerebral enlargement after exclusion of cerebrospinal fluid (Courchesne et al., 2001; Sparks et al., 2002; Hazlett et al., 2005). Retrospective and prospective studies of the trajectory of head circumference growth in infants subsequently diagnosed with ASD also suggest normal head size at birth but more rapid increases in size than for typically developing children between 6 and 12 to 18 months of age (Courchesne et al., 2001; Hazlett et al., 2005; Davidovitch, Patterson, & Gartside, 1996; Lainhart et al., 1997; Dawson et al., 2007). Clinically defining features of ASD, such as social deficits, are generally not observed at 6 months of age in children subsequently diagnosed with ASD. Rather, symptom onset occurs sometime after the second half of the first year. Although there are variable patterns of symptom onset, most children diagnosed with an ASD demonstrate symptoms between 12 and 24 months (Dawson et al., 2002; Dawson et al., 2004; Lord et al., 2006; Zwaigenbaum et al., 2005; Watson et al., 2006; Bryson et al., 2008; Landa et al., 2006). Thus, the onset of cerebral enlargement in ASD appears to be a postnatal phenomenon that has an initial time course that converges with the time course for symptom onset (Hazlett et al., 2005; Dawson et al., 2007).

Whether or not cerebral enlargement has a primary role in the pathogenesis of ASD, characterizing the nature of this phenomenon has the potential to provide important insights toward understanding the pathogenesis of ASD. In this regard, it has been proposed that mechanisms underlying cerebral enlargement may also alter brain cytoarchitecture in ASD, with secondary disturbances of white matter tract development and resultant abnormalities of connectivity (Casanova & Tillquist, 2008). Specific components of the white matter circuitry, which predominantly involves short- and medium-range intrahemispheric association fibers rather than longer-range white matter tracts, may be differentially impacted by early overgrowth of the cerebrum (Herbert et al., 2004). In keeping with this consideration, MRI investigations of the corpus callosum in ASD, which connects the right and left cerebral hemispheres, variably find decreases in absolute size but, more consistently, demonstrate a disproportionate reduction in corpus callosum size when total cerebral volume is taken into account (Piven, Bailey, Ranson, & Arndt, 1997; Boger-Megiddo et al., 2006). If optimalization of synaptic organization during the early postnatal period fails to occur, this could result in disruption of vulnerable neural structures and circuits implicated in ASD (Sampaio et al., 2001; Huttenlocher et al., 1997; Belmonte et al., 2004). It has been further suggested that other neurodevelopmental disorders that also manifest during this period, and may have phenotypic overlap with ASD (e.g., Rett syndrome, Fragile X syndrome [FXS]), could also involve alterations of synaptic maturation in common with ASD (Zoghbi, 2003; Bagni & Greenough, 2005). That white matter alterations might be secondary to alterations of gray matter development, which are in turn due to some other process such as inflammation at earlier stages of brain development, has been suggested though not yet established (Petropoulos et al., 2006).

Research applications of highly resolved 2-D and 3-D structural MRI have demonstrated intriguing clinical relationships between brain anatomical alterations and ASD. For example, an inverse relationship between amygdalar volume at 3 years of age and the trajectory for social skills development between 3 and 6 years of age in children with ASD has been reported (Munson et al., 2006). These structural observations can help to focus research efforts, but do not directly address pathological mechanisms underlying those relationships. The factors that influence image intensity in conventional MRI are complex, and image intensity changes alone do not allow underlying pathological processes to be identified. Furthermore, although MRI is sensitive to changes in tissue water characteristics used to define anatomy at a macroscopic level, it is less sensitive to what is occurring at a cellular level (Petropoulos et al., 2006). In this regard, magnetic resonance spectroscopy (MRS), a complementary imaging technique, can provide useful insights into mechanisms that may account for brain structural alternations in ASD (Dager, Friedman, Petropoulos, & Shaw, 2008; Dager, Corrigan, Richards, & Posse, 2008).

Magnetic Resonance Spectroscopy

MRS was first described in the 1940s and thereafter rapidly applied to characterize chemical samples, in vitro (Purcell, Torrey, & Pound, 1946; Bloch, Hansen, & Packard, 1946; Proctor & Yu, 1950). There are comprehensive reference works available that describe the basic principles of MRS (Gadian, 1982; De Graaf, 2007). As a brief overview, certain atomic nuclei, which include hydrogen (^{1}H), lithium (^{7}Li), carbon (^{13}C), fluorine (^{19}F), sodium (^{23}Na), and phosphorus (^{31}P), have magnetic properties due to the presence of unpaired nucleons (protons or neutrons) that result in a dipole or magnetic orientation to the nuclei. These nuclei are not radioactive and are naturally occurring, although often in small physiologic concentrations. Innovative adaptation of existing in vitro MRS technology, primarily in vivo detection of the spatial distribution of hydrogen atoms (protons) incorporated into the structure of water and lipid, is what made MRI clinically feasible long before MRS was first applied to living systems (Lauterbur, 1973; Mansfield & Grannell, 1973).

Magnetic Resonance Spectroscopy (MRS): At one time referred to as nuclear magnetic resonance (NMR) imaging, this imaging technique is now called MRI in recognition of its noninvasive and nonionizing (nonradioactive) properties. As with MRI, MRS data is produced by perturbing hydrogen nuclei that are aligned with the scanner magnetic field by transmission of a radiofrequency (RF) pulse, which causes them to absorb and reemit energy. The hydrogen nuclei change orientation ("flip") during the absorption process and subsequently realign with the magnetic field. The signal emitted during realignment is termed the free-induction decay (FID), and is detected up by a receiver coil, digitized, and Fourier transformed to produce a frequency domain MRS spectrum.

MRS can be used in vivo to noninvasively measure brain chemical composition, characterize certain cellular features, and characterize tissue metabolic processes (for a recent review of psychiatric clinical applications, see Dager, Corrigan et al., 2008). Detection of tissue-based abnormalities in brain regions that appear normal by MRI, as well as elucidation of pathology underlying MRI-visible abnormalities, is possible with MRS (Friedman et al., 1999). Although numerous studies have utilized MRI to detect brain structural abnormalities associated with ASD, there have been relatively few studies using MRS to investigate ASD. Several MRS studies of ASD have used nuclei other than ^{1}H, such as ^{31}P to investigate cell membrane turnover (Minshew, Goldstein, Dombrowski, Panchalingam, & Pettegrew, 1993) or ^{19}F MRS to study the brain uptake, steady-state concentration, and elimination half-life of fluorine-containing psychotropic drugs (e.g., fluoxetine and fluvoxamine) used clinically to treat children with ASD (Strauss, Unis, Cowan, Dawson, & Dager, 2002). However, as most MRS research investigating ASD has employed ^{1}H MRS, this is the focus of the chapter.

^{1}H MRS utilizes the same scanner equipment as MRI and can noninvasively detect and quantify low-molecular-weight brain chemicals other than water that also contain hydrogen as part of their molecular structure. To obtain a usable ^{1}H MRS signal, suppression of the water signal, which otherwise would overwhelm the signal from these other hydrogen-containing chemicals, is required first. The ^{1}H spins of chemicals at equilibrium in the scanner's static magnetic field (typically 1.5 Tesla or 3 Tesla) are perturbed by transmitting a radiofrequency (RF) pulse at a specific frequency. This causes the ^{1}H spins to absorb energy by putting more of the spins into a higher energy state and then reemit energy (resonate) as those spins drop back into the parallel state. This reemission of energy varies in strength depending on the properties of the particular electron cloud shielding each chemical bond. Since the electron cloud that shields each nuclei is different due to unique molecular bond configurations of the chemical, each proton experiences a slightly different local magnetic field and, as a result, resonates at a slightly different frequency, referred to as its "chemical shift."

Chemical Shift: The shift in resonance frequency of the hydrogen nucleus of a given chemical as compared to the resonance frequency of a hydrogen nucleus in a water molecule. The chemical shift of the hydrogen nucleus in a chemical dictates the location of the peaks for that chemical on an MRS spectrum and is what makes ^{1}H MRS a useful investigative tool, as specific chemicals can be identified and measured.

The chemical shift for a given chemical is directly proportional to the magnitude of the magnetic field strength used for data acquisition. Frequency measurements for a given chemical are expressed as a dimensionless quantity, by convention given in units of parts per million (PPM), to allow standardization between scanners having different field strengths. This chemical shift measure allows for identification and quantification of specific chemicals that are further described below, In addition, the rate at which spins realign with the static magnetic field following perturbation by the RF pulse, termed T_1 relaxation, and the rate by which the spins lose coherence, termed T_2 relaxation, can also be measured. These measurements, typically of water but also other brain chemicals, can help to characterize features of the microenvironment, or cytoarchitecture, which has been found to be altered in ASD (Dager, Friedman, et al., 2008; Petropoulos et al., 2006; Friedman et al., 2003).

T1 and T2 Relaxation: T1 relaxation (longitudinal or spin-lattice relaxation) is the rate at which hydrogen nuclei realign with the static magnetic field after perturbation by an RF pulse. For a given chemical, the T1 relaxation rate is governed by the magnetic field strength and the composition of the surrounding cellular matrix. T2 relaxation (transverse or spin-spin relaxation) reflects the loss of signal following the RF pulse that is caused by interactions with hydrogen nuclei from nearby tissues, The T1 and T2 relaxation rates of tissues can provide information on many tissue properties, including neuronal maturation and myelination in the brain.

MRS chemical levels are determined by measuring the area under each spectral peak using commercially available MRS software fitting packages (e.g., Provencher, 1993; Provencher, 2009). Often, these chemical peak areas are referenced, or normalized, by the computation of ratios between peak areas from two chemical peaks simultaneously acquired. Reporting chemical ratios for ^{1}H MRS findings (e.g., NAA/Cre) can reduce the effect of individual acquisition differences on chemical measurements across studies. This approach also has the advantage of compensating for partial volume differences in individual voxels. Partial volume primarily reflects the variable inclusion of CSF in the voxel, as well as differences in gray-white tissue composition, as this also can influence the relative chemical proportions. A substantial drawback to using chemical ratios is the requirement that the denominator (often Cre but other chemicals, such as NAA or Cho, may instead be used) not be affected by the pathological process under investigation. This requirement is often not met.

More recent quantification approaches have utilized measurements from a separate water scan, using the unsuppressed water peak as an internal reference standard to control for SNR differences across studies. "Absolute" quantification approaches reference the chemical of interest to an internal reference (e.g., brain water measured from a separately acquired ^{1}H MRS scan) or external phantom (e.g., test-tube placed next to the head) in order to follow or compare chemical levels within and between individuals. However, if this quantification approach requires the acquisition of an additional scan, there can be problems when scanning under time constraints, as occurs in the study of sleeping children. Quantification techniques also are more difficult to implement and entail many assumptions, such as the stability or full visibility of brain water, but are generally the preferred approach for reporting MRS data. Using the water peak as an internal standard does necessitate a correction for partial volume effects, frequently not performed in published studies.

Reliability for brain chemical measurements using ^{1}H MRS has been clearly established, but due diligence is critical when applying this methodology, as numerous potential pitfalls exist, both in data acquisition and analysis (Dager & Steen, 1992; Brooks, Friedman, & Stidley, 1999). In practical terms, there are limitations in detecting chemicals at low concentrations, generally in the millimolar range, for in vivo ^{1}H MRS (Dager, Corrigan, et al., 2008; De Graaf, 2007; Ross & Michaelis, 1994; Gadian, 1982). Chemicals in the brain that can be detected and quantified by ^{1}H MRS include N-acetyl aspartate (NAA), most often measured as the total of NAA + N-acetyl aspartyl glutamate (NAAG); creatine (Cre), composed of creatine and phosphocreatine; choline (Cho), which has multiple resonances reflecting signal from four membrane/myelin related chemicals: phosphorylethanolamine (PE), phosphorylcholine (PC), glycerophosphorylethanolamine (GPE), and glycerophosphorylcholine (GPC); myoinositol (mI); and lactate, which is difficult to detect at rest in the normal brain. Glutamate (Glu), gamma-aminobutyric acid (GABA), and glutamine (Gln) have complicated peak shapes and resonate at overlapping spectral locations, resulting in the use of the term GLX as a common description of the combined peaks, although at higher field strength individual peaks can be resolved and quantified, as described further below (Dager, Corrigan et al., 2008; Posse et al., 2007; Lin et al., 2007; Schubert, Gallinat, Seifert, & Rinneberg, 2004; Hurd, Gurr, & Sailasuta, 1998; Behar & Ogino, 1991; Ryner, Sorenson, & Thomas, 1995).

Turning to some of the specific chemicals that have been studied in ASD, NAA is an amino acid that is found only in the nervous system, and primarily in neurons and axons (Tallan, Moore, & Stein, 1956). A complex NAA shuttle between neurons and oligodendrocytes suggests important roles for NAA in regulating synaptogenesis and synaptic maintenance, as well as myelination, cellular osmolarity, and neuronal metabolism (Coyle et al., 2000; Neale et al., 2000; Tsacopoulos & Magistretti, 1996; Baslow, 2000). During normal development, NAA levels increase dramatically over the first year of life, then variably increases across different brain regions, gradually plateauing in early adulthood (Kreis & Ross, 1993; van der Knaap et al., 1990; Huppi et al., 1991). Increases in NAA parallel myelination, and are thought to reflect neuronal maturation as a result of increasing synaptic complexity, as well as increased axonal projections. Available data further support a role for NAA as a sensitive marker of both neuronal integrity and neuronal-glial homeostasis (Birken & Oldendorf, 1989; Coyle & Schwarcz, 2000; Neale, Bzdega, & Wroblewska, 2000). For example, a ^{1}H MRS study of traumatic brain injury found that NAA brain levels were reduced in relation to severity of head trauma and higher NAA levels were predictive of improved clinical outcome (Friedman et al., 1999). NAA alterations characterized by ^{1}H MRS also have been reported to be useful for predicting clinical outcome in pediatric studies of developmental disorders. As shown in a study of neurologically at-risk children, those who subsequently manifested developmental disorders (DD) clinically had reduced NAA measures, reported as NAA/Cho or NAA/Cre ratios (Kimura, Fujii, & Itoh, 1995). These chemical alterations also were found to be a better outcome predictor than structural MRI features.

Chemical Ratios: Meaningful comparison of chemical differences using a ratio (e.g. NAA/Cho in the example of at-risk DD children) requires that the concentration of the chemical in the denominator be equivalent across diagnostic groups. As Cho might be expected to be altered in a direction opposite that of NAA in DD children, its use as the denominator in assessing NAA could amplify any NAA differences between groups. Because neurodevelopmental disorders, such as ASD, are likely to affect the concentrations of multiple brain chemicals, the use of ratios may obscure specific chemical abnormalities.

The Cho spectral peak reflects only the mobile fraction of choline-containing compounds present in tissue, with the larger fraction of Cho being incorporated into molecules in cell membranes and myelin, rendering them MR-invisible (Gadian, 1982; Ross et al., 1994). In contrast to NAA, Cho levels decrease rapidly over the first year of life, also paralleling myelination, and reflect decreases in the PE and PC components of the Cho peak; in contrast, smaller magnitude increases of GPE and GPC also occur (Kreis et al., 1993; van der Knaap et al., 1990). In many individuals with traumatic brain injury, Cho is increased in relation to severity of neuronal injury as a result of the addition of membrane and myelin breakdown products to the ^{1}H MRS signal (Friedman et al., 1999). Furthermore, in contrast to NAA reductions, ^{1}H MRS visible Cho is elevated, at least acutely, in most pathological CNS disease states with cellular disruption.

Bulk Cre in the ^{1}H spectrum provides some indication of energy metabolism and high energy phosphate storage, although ^{31}P MRS provides an unambiguous measure of phosphocreatine, a more straightforward measure of high-energy phosphate levels (Gadian, 1982; Ross et al., 1994). Cre levels also change during normal brain development, with ^{1}H MRS measures of Cre increasing from birth until around 2 years of age, in a direction opposite that of Cho (Kreis et al., 1993; van der Knaap et al., 1990; Huppi et al., 1991). Similarly to NAA, Cre is decreased in response to traumatic brain injury or in the setting of neuronal injury associated with many CNS disease states (Friedman, 1999).

An important regulator of brain osmotic balance, mI is also a putative marker for glial cells, in particular astrocytes, and a precursor for the phosphoinositides that are involved in the cell membrane second messenger system (Moore et al., 1999). In the setting of inflammatory processes, or acute stroke with associated cytotoxic edema, mI levels may be acutely altered as a measure of glial swelling (Rumpel, Lim, Chang, et al., 2003).

Lactate, at one time thought to be solely a by-product of cellular metabolism, has been found to have an important role in brain bioenergetics, including as an energy substrate for neuronal metabolism (Schurr, West, & Rigor, 1988). Elevated resting brain Lactate levels, often in conjunction with other chemical alterations such as elevated GLX or reduced NAA, may also reflect alterations of brain energy metabolism, such as a shift in redox state from oxidative metabolism toward glycolysis, and provide a potential marker for mitochondrial compromise, as has been observed in medication-free subjects with bipolar disorder (Dager et al., 2004) or individuals with mitochondrial genetic diseases (Dinopoulos et al., 2005; Kaufmann et al., 2004). However, it is important to recognize that moderate reductions in cerebral blood flow and/or increased brain metabolism, as occurs with hyperventilation (Dager et al., 1995) or caffeine ingestion (Dager et al., 1999), also can acutely increase brain lactate levels.

Brain levels of Glu and GABA, the major excitatory and inhibitory neurotransmitter, respectively, are of substantial interest in many neuropsychiatric conditions, including ASD. It is now quite feasible to separate and accurately measure these chemicals at scanner field strengths of 3 Tesla and higher. Whereas Glu can be accurately identified and measured at 3 Tesla using standard pulse sequences with specific acquisition parameters (Schubert, Gallinat, Seifert, et al., 2004), measurement of GABA requires the use of newer, specialized ^{1}H MRS acquisition and analytic techniques, as briefly described below.

Advances in Magnetic Resonance Spectroscopy

Recent technical advances in ^{1}H MRS have led to substantial improvements in spectral, spatial, and temporal resolution. Spectral resolution, the degree of separation or isolation of individual chemical peaks, improves as scanner field strength increases (Vaughan, et al., 2006; Otazo, Mueller, Ugurbil, Wald, Posse, et al., 2006). Better acquisition methods (pulse sequences) and analytic approaches, to be further discussed below, also can further enhance spectral resolution. There is generally a tradeoff between spatial and temporal resolution, with increased spatial resolution achieved at the expense of temporal resolution, or vice versa. Spatial resolution and temporal resolution are both functions of the signal-to-noise ratio (SNR), which is also a function of scanner field strength and coil sensitivity, chemical concentration, acquisition parameters (e.g., echo time), and magnetic resonance characteristics of the chemicals of interest. Pragmatically, the most practical approach for enhancing SNR is through increasing signal averaging or number of acquisitions, but the improvement is proportional only to the square root of the number of acquisitions (i.e., in order to double the SNR ratio, there must be 4-times the signal averaging). Although in practical terms, there are technical problems that mount as magnetic field strength increases, the SNR of singlet resonances increases linearly with increases with field strength (Vaughan et al., 2006; Otazo et al., 2006). Improvements in SNR also can be achieved with the use of a shorter echo time (TE) (Posse, Schuknecht, Smith, van Zijl, & Herschkowitz, 1993) and with improved head coil designs (Wald, Moyher, Day, Nelson, & Vigneron, 1995).

Initial MRS studies were limited to measuring chemicals within a single large volume of tissue, referred to as single-voxel techniques. With earlier ^{1}H MRS single-voxel techniques performed at 1.5 Tesla, in order to acquire a scan in a relatively short duration of time (e.g., 5 minutes) while at the same time allowing for measurement of chemicals at low natural abundance, such as lactate, voxel sizes as large as 27cc were required to achieve adequate SNR (Dager et al., 1995). Most ^{1}H MRS studies of ASD populations have employed single-voxel techniques that provide chemical information for only a single brain area and, due to large voxel sizes, there can be quite variable anatomical placement of the voxel. With technical advances, particularly in scanner and head coil hardware, voxel sizes can be substantially reduced. Thus, ^{1}H MRS with a voxel size of 0.18 cc (3.4 x 3.4 x 15 mm^{3}), or smaller, can be acquired at 3 Tesla field strength, albeit with a lower SNR that requires more signal averaging (Dager, Corrigan, et al., 2008; Lin et al., 2007).

A substantial advance in ^{1}H MRS research applications has been the implementation of rapid 2-D and 3-D ^{1}H MRS imaging techniques (^{1}H MRSI). ^{1}H MRSI allows for the mapping of anatomical distributions of chemical concentrations, similar to the mapping of anatomical distributions of ^{1}H water signal obtainable with MRI (Posse et al., 1997). In contrast to the substantial time required for performing repeated single-voxel ^{1}H MRS acquisitions to sample multiple individual regions, ^{1}H MRSI techniques, such as proton echo-planar spectroscopic imaging (PEPSI), use very rapid spectral-spatial encoding techniques for simultaneous spectral acquisitions across many anatomical voxels. For example, instead of a single 27cc voxel, a 32 x 32 spatial matrix [1024 voxels, individual voxel resolution = 1cc] can be acquired in the same 4–5 minute time frame across a single tissue slice at 1.5 Tesla (Posse et al., 1997). In Figure 33-1, a representative MRI axial slice (20 mm thick) is shown overlaid with a 32 x 32 2-D PEPSI voxel matrix (voxel resolution =1.0 cc). A subset of acquired spectra and the fitting of an individual spectrum are illustrated in Figure 33-2. More recently developed 3-D ^{1}H MRSI techniques can allow the simultaneous acquisition of multiple contiguous anatomical slices (e.g., 8192 voxels over 8 slices with 0.3 cc voxel resolution) within the same 4- to 5-minute time frame using a 3 Tesla scanner (Lin et al., 2007; Dager, Corrigan, et al., 2008). In Figure 33-3, example 3-D PEPSI acquisitions from a standard 3 Tesla clinical scanner are shown for a sleeping 6-month-old without a family history of ASD and for a 12-month-old at high risk for an ASD due to an older affected sibling.

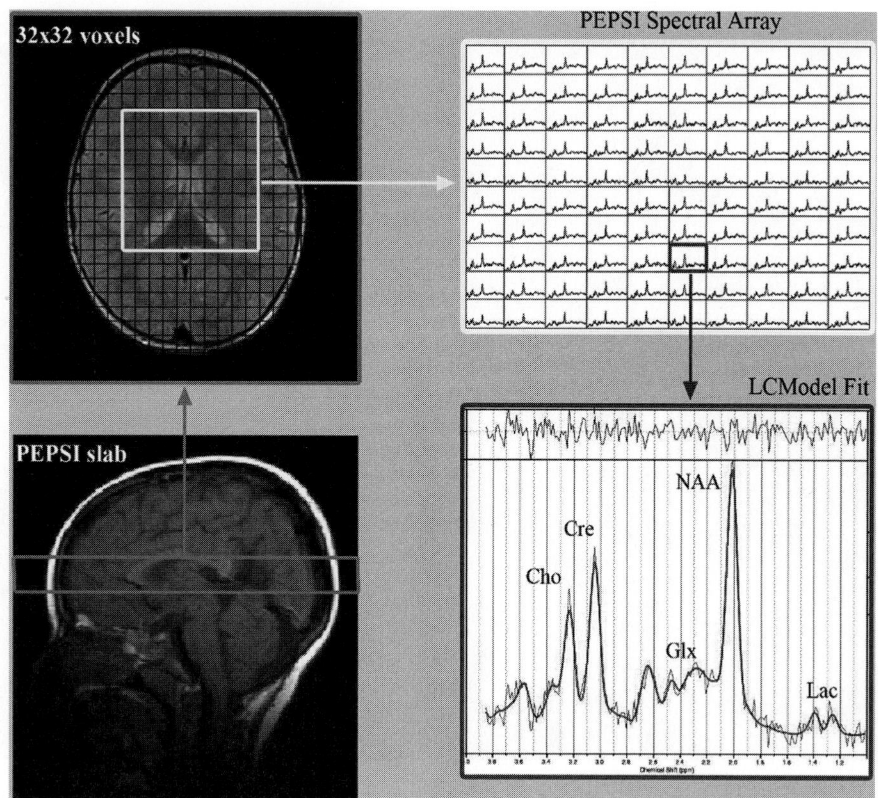

Figure 33–1. A ^{1}H magnetic resonance spectroscopy imaging (^{1}H MRSI) axial slab location (20 mm thick) overlaid with a 32 x 32 2-D MRSI voxel matrix. A subset of the acquired MRSI voxels is shown on the upper right-hand corner. An individual voxel with identified chemical peaks is shown in the lower right-hand corner.

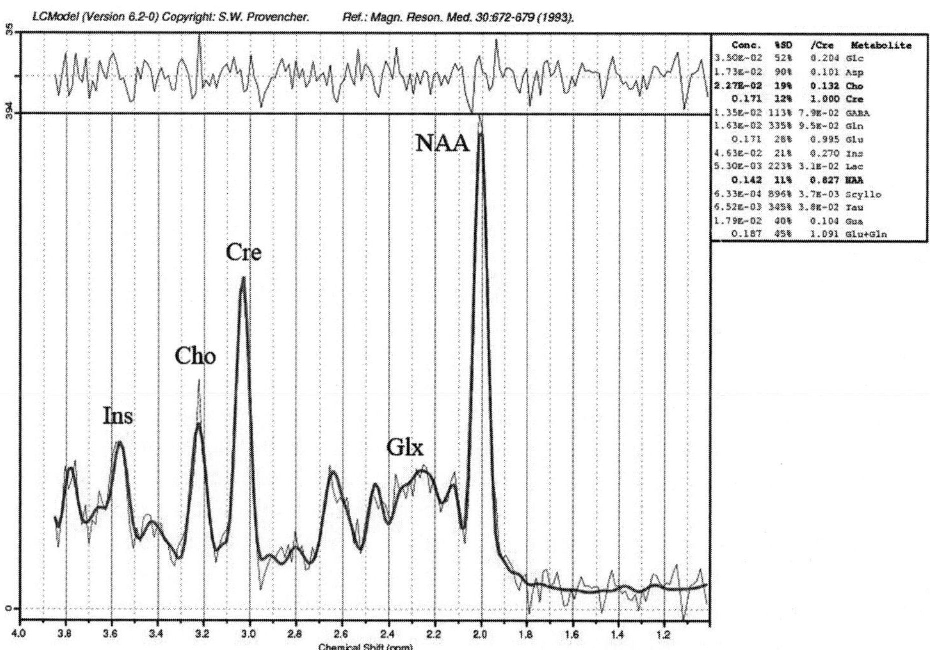

Conc.	%SD	/Cre	Metabolite
3.50E-02	52%	0.204	Glc
1.73E-02	90%	0.101	Asp
2.27E-02	**19%**	**0.132**	**Cho**
0.171	**12%**	**1.000**	**Cre**
1.35E-02	113%	7.9E-02	GABA
1.63E-02	335%	9.5E-02	Gln
0.171	28%	0.995	Glu
4.63E-02	21%	0.270	Ins
5.30E-03	223%	3.1E-02	Lac
0.142	**11%**	**0.827**	**NAA**
6.33E-04	896%	3.7E-03	Scyllo
6.52E-03	345%	3.8E-02	Tau
1.79E-02	40%	0.104	Gua
0.187	45%	1.091	Glu+Gln

Figure 33–2. LC Model fitting results for an individual spectrum acquired from the left frontal lobe. Shown are the raw absorption mode spectrum (lighter line) and corresponding LC Model fit based on a priori knowledge (darker line). The residuals, calculated as a subtraction of the fit from the spectrum, are plotted at the top. The table of chemical concentrations calculated from the fit is to the right. Cramer-Rao lower bound (%SD) also is shown on the right-hand side for each chemical concentration map. Cramer-Rao lower bounds provide information on the "goodness of fit" and can be used as an objective method for filtering out poor quality spectra.

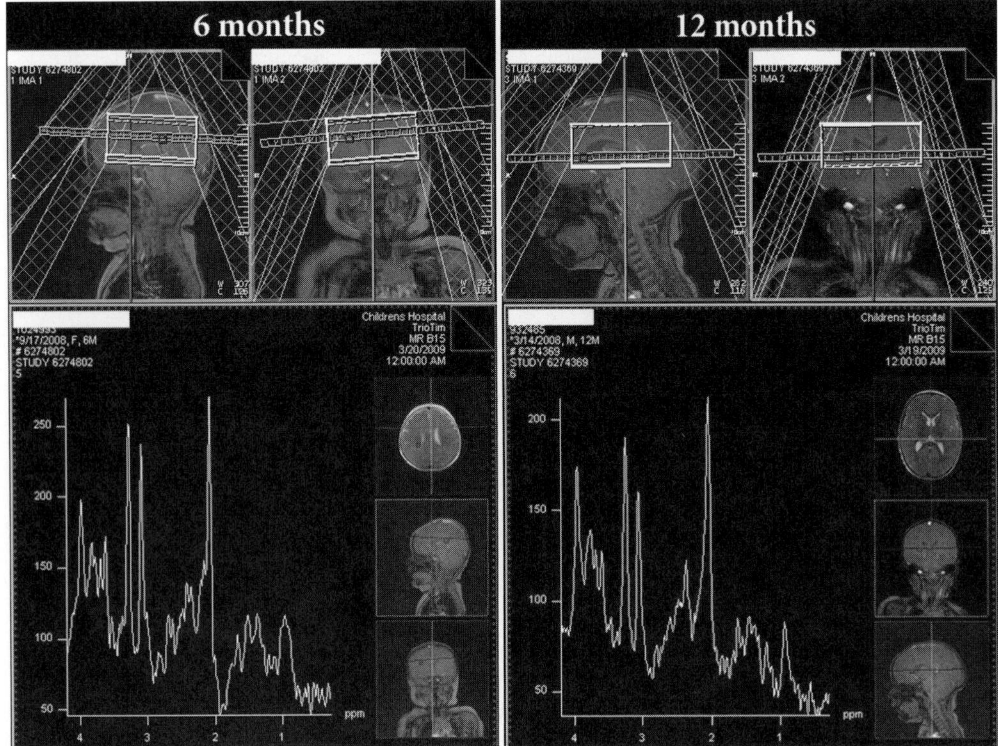

Figure 33–3. Example 3-D PEPSI spectra, acquired over 4.5 minutes on a clinical 3 Tesla scanner, showing the 3-D anatomical volume, individual voxel placement (blue box) and outer volume sat band positioning for a 6m infant without a family history of ASD and for a 12m infant at high risk for an ASD due to an older affected sibling. Each example shows one 0.3 cc voxel out of the 8,192 collected concurrently. (See Color Plate Section for a color version of this figure.)

Magnetic Resonance Spectroscopic Imaging (MRSI): MRSI represents an important advancement in MRS technology by acquiring spectra from multiple voxels simultaneously. This dramatically increases the number of brain regions that can be sampled in a single scan and allows for the creation of spatial maps of chemical distributions across brain regions or for gray/white matter.

^{1}H MRSI approaches have obvious clinical advantages for the study of populations that are difficult to image, such as agitated or sleeping subjects (such as young children), or for measuring anatomical relationship to changing metabolic states, such as in response to brain metabolic challenges (Dager et al., 1999). Coupled with volumetric MRI using regression analysis, one also can take advantage of the large number of voxel samples obtained with ^{1}H MRSI to calculate estimates of "pure" gray or white matter neurochemistry in studies of ASD (Friedman et al., 2006; DeVito et al., 2007). One substantial challenge associated with using ^{1}H MRSI techniques, however, is the necessity of an adequately uniform magnetic field over the anatomical volume scanned. This requirement of field uniformity, which can be partially compensated for with higher-order shimming, is much more stringent than that required for acquisition of structural MRI.

Shimming: Magnetic resonance data acquisition requires a uniform static magnetic field, which is provided by the main scanner magnet. Imperfections in scanner electronics and the introduction of a person's head inside the scanner can cause alterations in the static magnetic field. Shimming is a method by which scanner hardware is used to detect and compensate for magnetic field variations to make the static magnetic field as uniform as possible during data acquisition.

The use of the pulse sequences utilizing the most up-to-date technology, or optimization of existing product pulse sequences by using improved acquisition parameters (e.g., short echo times that maximize signal by reducing the effects of T2 decay), can substantially improve data quality. For example, very short echo times (e.g., 11 ms) can be used for some ^{1}H MRSI acquisitions to increase SNR and improve detection of chemicals with short T2s, such as mI or GLX, as well as alleviate some of the confounds associated with chemical quantification (Dager, Corrigan, et al., 2008; Friedman et al., 2003; Posse et al., 1993). Furthermore, acquisition of both short and long echo time chemical measurements can allow for estimation of chemical T2 relaxation, shown to be abnormal in ASD (Friedman et al., 2003).

Echo Time: The echo time, or TE, is the time following the RF pulse when acquisition of the FID signal is initiated.

Although ^{1}H MRS can detect a number of chemical signals, the spectra also contain a "forest" of multiple overlapping resonances that can substantially hinder the quantification of many of these chemicals (Dager, Corrigan, et al., 2008). Spectral editing techniques are increasingly being used to provide more specific information about chemical bond structure and to individually measure some chemicals that are not otherwise separable, such as Gln and GABA (Lin et al., 2007; Jensen, Frederick, & Renshaw, 2005; Jensen, Frederick, Wang, Brown, & Renshaw, 2005; Behar & Ogino, 1991; Ryner et al., 1995; Hurd et al., 1998; Hurd et al., 2004; Mescher, Merkle, Kirsch, Garwood, & Gruetter, 1998). An example two-dimensional spectral plot from a typical adult male acquired using J-resolved spectral editing is shown in Figure 33-4. Identification of chemical spectra that were acquired simultaneously demonstrates the separation of the coupled resonances of brain glutamine and glutamate, in addition to other typically measured chemicals. In Figure 33-5, results are shown using a MEGA-PRESS acquisition to isolate and identify the GABA resonance that would otherwise be obscured by the overlapping spectral peaks of other chemicals.

Spectral Editing Techniques: Spectral editing techniques are acquisition methods that vary the timing of specific data acquisition parameters to allow for measurement of chemicals that are difficult to distinguish due to overlapping peaks. MEGA-PRESS is a ^{1}H MRS spectral editing technique designed to measure chemicals such as GABA, glutamate, and glutamine. This technique requires separate acquisitions for measurement of each chemical of interest. Two-dimensional J-resolved ^{1}H MRS spectral editing techniques are designed to measure multiple chemicals during a single acquisition, allowing for simultaneous measurement of multiple chemicals, although separating some chemicals, such as GABA, can be analytically challenging.

Imaging research centers are increasingly utilizing higher field scanners (up to 9.4 Tesla), although scanner strengths beyond 3 Tesla are not yet approved for clinical use by the Food and Drug Administration. The use of high field scanners (3 Tesla and higher), in conjunction with advancing RF coil array technology, allows substantially improved measurement sensitivity and enhanced ability to resolve specific brain chemicals of particular importance in ASD investigations. By combining MRSI approaches with recent advances in parallel imaging, ^{1}H MRSI data acquisition times can be drastically reduced to under a minute for some applications, depending on the scanner field strength, to obtain single-average images of chemicals such as Cho, Cre, and NAA, as well as Glu, with acceptable spectral quality and localization (Lin et al., 2007; Posse, Otazo, Tsai, Yoshimoto, & Lin, 2008; Otazo, Tsai, Lin, & Posse, 2007; Tsai et al., 2008; Dager, Corrigan, et al., 2009). A further area of technical advancement, the development of ^{1}H MRS approaches for acquiring spectra from brain areas typically difficult to study due to susceptibility artifacts, will be useful for investigating brain regions important for understanding ASD, such as the amygdala (Josey, Al Sayyari, Buckley, & Coulthard, 2009).

MRS Findings in ASD

A substantial proportion of the available literature using ^{1}H MRS to investigate ASD must be considered descriptive since findings are based on only a limited number of cases. Also, as described above, the manner by which methodological factors have been handled, such as patient and control group selection criteria, including differences in diagnostic criteria, age ranges, autistic subtypes, and IQ inclusion parameters, has varied widely across studies. Comparison between studies can also be difficult due to differences in ^{1}H MRS data acquisition protocols, particularly since the field is continuously developing newer acquisition techniques and more powerful scanners are becoming increasingly available. ^{1}H MRS studies of ASD

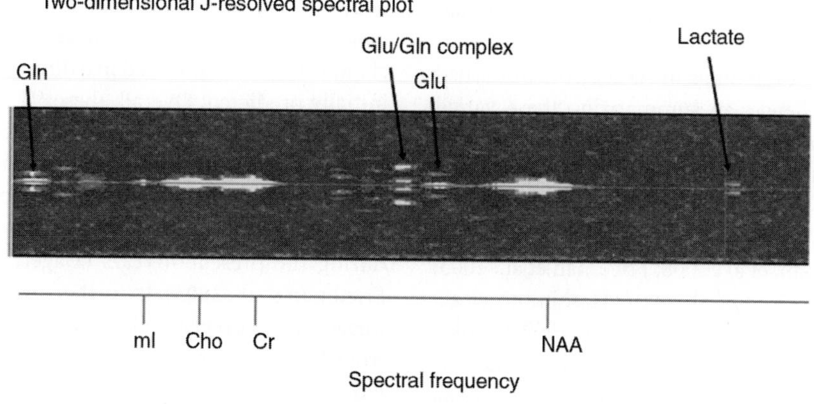

Figure 33–4. A 2-D J-resolved spectral image acquired over 20 minutes from a 64 cc volume at 3 Tesla. Spectral resonances for glutamine, glutamate, Glu/Gln complex, lactate, as well as myoinositol, choline, creatine, and NAA are shown. Data were acquired as a function of echo time, using progressively increasing echo times to record signal change that can differentiate between chemicals. (See Color Plate Section for a color version of this figure.)

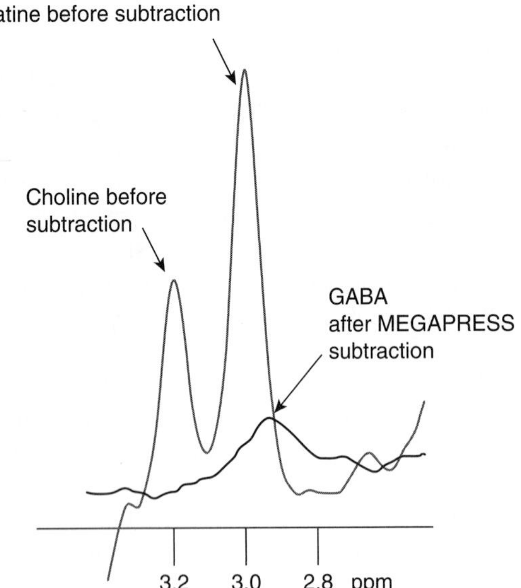

Figure 33–5. Separation and identification of the GABA resonance from the overlapping resonances of other chemicals using MEGAPRESS. These data were acquired over 13 minutes from a 18 cc voxel at 3 Tesla, using the interaction of neighboring ^{1}H within the GABA molecule to subtract out signal from other overlapping chemicals. A specific RF pulse is required for GABA signal acquisition with MEGAPRESS.

generally have been conducted using single-voxel techniques that typically involve the acquisition of data from only a few anatomical regions of relatively large volume (on the order of 2 x 2 x 2 = 8 cm^{3}). Importantly, the regions of interest chosen for study, and anatomical specificity, often vary substantially between studies. The analytic approaches used for quantification of chemical measures also are not well standardized and can substantially influence results. Moreover, MRS and MRSI are intrinsically low-resolution techniques that rely heavily on MRI-based partial volume correction of the different tissue types and relaxation time constants of water and chemicals with any propagation of small errors producing significant downstream effects on chemical quantification (Friedman et al., 2003).

Comparison of ^{1}H MRS findings in ASD across published studies, despite the challenges in summarizing these varied data, does reveal interesting patterns of chemical alterations. Abnormal ^{1}H MRS chemical patterns, most consistently reductions in NAA, found in many, though not all, studies of ASD suggest differences in tissue chemical composition or neuronal integrity (Dager, Friedman, et al., 2008; Friedman et al., 2003; Friedman et al., 2006; DeVito et al., 2007; Hashimoto et al., 1997; Chugani, Sundram, Behen, Lee, & Moore, 1999; Otsuka, Harada, Mori, Hisaoka, & Nishitani, 1999; Hisaoka, Harada, & Nishitani, 2001; Murphy et al., 2002; Page et al., 2006; Kleinhans, Schweinsburg, Cohen, Muller, & Courchesne, 2007; Endo et al., 2007; Zeegers, van der Grond, van Daalen, Buitelaar, & van Engeland, 2006; Vasconcelos et al., 2008; Gabis et al., 2008; Levitt et al., 2003; Oner et al., 2007; Hardan et al., 2008). Although findings have been more variable, perhaps reflecting greater regional specificity, reduced Cho found in some studies may reflect decreased membrane turnover, in a direction opposite to what would be expected due to neuronal injury from membrane or myelin breakdown. There is also some suggestion of age-related effects on ^{1}H MRS differences. For example, evidence for reduced NAA levels tend to be more consistently found in younger populations with ASD, although one study of adults with ASD also reports regional reductions of NAA (Kleinhans et al., 2007). A summary of published single-voxel ^{1}H MRS findings (Hashimoto et al., 1997; Chugani et al., 1999; Otsuka et al., 1999; Hisaoka et al., 2001; Murphy et al., 2002; Page et al., 2006; Kleinhans et al., 2007; Endo et al., 2007; Zeegers et al., 2006; Vasconcelos et al., 2008; Gabis et al., 2008) is shown in Table 33-1.

As illustrated in Table 33-2, there have been only a few published ^{1}H MRSI investigations of ASD (Friedman et al., 2003; Friedman et al., 2006; DeVito et al., 2007; Levitt et al., 2003; Oner et al., 2007; Hardan et al., 2008). Findings from these studies are generally consistent with ^{1}H MRS single-voxel evidence for widespread alterations of tissue chemical composition. Importantly, the integration of ^{1}H MRSI measurements and MRI anatomical findings can lead to a better understanding of mechanisms underlying specific brain structural alterations associated with ASD. For example, to explain the approximately 10% cerebral enlargement observed from structural MRI studies of ASD children at 3 to 4 years of age, we tested an exploratory hypothesis of regionally increased NAA concentrations posited to reflect increased numbers of neurons or more dense connections arising from a disturbance of normal neuronal apoptosis or synaptic pruning processes during early development in children with autism (Friedman et al., 2003). In this model, regional chemical concentrations were predicted to be increased, and chemical T2 relaxation times, estimated from acquisition of ^{1}H MRSI using two TE (20 ms and 272 ms), were predicted to be shortened as a result of densely packed molecules having increased interaction over time following excitation by the RF pulse. Results from this study instead revealed a pattern of widely distributed regional reductions in NAA, Cre, and mI concentrations (and Cho in gray matter), and prolonged chemical T2 relaxation, all in a direction opposite to what was initially predicted. Overall, these ^{1}H MRSI findings were not consistent with increased cellular packing density among the 3- to 4-year-old children with ASD and, thus, do not support models of abnormally reduced apoptosis and/or delayed synaptic pruning, nor provide evidence for neuronal "overgrowth" during the preschool years (Dager, Friedman, et al., 2008; Friedman et al., 2003). In further analyses of these data, MRSI images were coregistered to segmented tissue maps produced from MRI acquired at the same session, and regression analytic techniques were used to characterize the compartmental distribution of chemical alterations between white and gray matter (Friedman et al., 2006). Chemical abnormalities were predominantly observed in gray matter, supporting an altered gray matter cytoarchitecture for the 3- to 4-year-old ASD

Table 33–1.
Single voxel ¹H spectroscopy studies of autism spectrum disorders

Investigator	N	Age in years (mean±SD)	Population	Echo Time (ms)	Brain Region	Finding
Hashimoto, 1997	28 (20M,8F)	2–12 (5.6±2.2)	AD	270	Right parietal lobe	No differences in NAA/Cho, NAA/Cre, Cho/Cre
Chugani, 1999	9 (8M,1F)	3–12 (5.7±2.5)	AD	30	Frontal and temporal lobes, cerebellum	Reduced cerebellar NAA Increased frontal lobe lactate in 1 child
Otsuka, 1999	27 (21M,6F)	2–18	AD	18	Right hippocampus/amygdala, left cerebellum	Reduced hippocampus/amygdala and left cerebellar NAA
Hisaoka, 2001	55 (47M,8F)	2–21 (5.8)	AD	135	Bilateral frontal, parietal, and temporal lobes, cingulate, brain stem	Reduced bilateral temporal lobe NAA
Murphy, 2002	14 (all M)	(30±9)	ASP	136	Right medial prefrontal and parietal lobes	Increased right medial prefrontal NAA, Cho and Cre
Page, 2006	25 (20 M,5F)	(35.6±11.5)	ASD	35	Right hippocampus/amygdala, right parietal lobe	Increased right hippocampus/ amygdala Glu+Gln and Cre
Kleinhans, 2007	13 (all M)	15–44 (24.5±9.5)	ASD	35	Left middle frontal and superior parietal cortex, occipital cortex at calcarine fissure, cerebellum	Reduced left middle frontal cortex NAA Reduced NAA in combined brain regions
Endo, 2007	38 (32M,6F)	6–20 (12.9±3.8)	ASD	35	Right medial temporal and prefrontal lobes, cerebellar vermis	Reduced right medial temporal NAA/Cre
Zeegers, 2006	25 (all M)	AD: (3.6±0.6) PDD-NOS: (3.8±1.3)	ASD	144	Left frontal subcortical white matter, left hippocampus/ amygdala	No differences in NAA, Cho, Cre, NAA/Cre, NAA/Cho between children with ASD and developmentally delayed children without ASD
Vasconcelos, 2008	10 (all M)	median age 9.53±1.8	AD	30	Bilateral anterior cingulate, left striatum, cerebellum and frontal lobe	Increased anterior cingulate mI and Cho Increased anterior cingulate and left striatum mI/Cre
Gabis, 2008	13 (10M,3F)	7–16 (10±2.5)	ASD	40	Bilateral hippocampus/ amygdala and cerebellum	Reduced bilateral hippocampus/ amygdala NAA/Cre Increased bilateral hippocampus/ amygdala and cerebellar mI/Cre Increased left hippocampus/ amygdala and cerebellar Cho/Cre

children compared to age-matched typically developing and developmentally delayed children. A subsequent ¹H MRSI study of preadolescent children with ASD, which used different acquisition techniques but similar regression analytic approaches, also observed reduced NAA in gray matter, but not white matter, compared to typically developing controls (DeVito et al., 2007).

Overall, the direction and widespread anatomical distribution of chemical alterations observed from these ¹H MRSI studies, which primarily demonstrate reduced brain chemical concentrations per unit brain tissue volume, were not consistent with our a priori theoretical model of diffusely increased neuronal packing density in the children with ASD (Friedman et al., 2003). Furthermore, evidence from quantitative T2 relaxation measures of brain water, used as a temporal marker for brain maturational stage, does not support accelerated "normal" brain growth early in the developmental course of ASD (Petropoulos et al., 2006). Instead, evidence to date suggests a revised model characterized most simply as altered gray matter cytoarchitecture having a reduced unit density, at least at the 3- to 4-year-old age range in ASD (Dager, Friedman, et al., 2008).

In the postnatal developing brain, increased levels of whole blood and platelet serotonin, reported in an estimated 30% of affected individuals with ASD, may lead to abnormal development of serotonergic fibers with decreased numbers of

Table 33–2.
2-D ¹H spectroscopic imaging studies of ASD

Investigator	N	Age in years (mean±SD)	Population	Echo Time (ms)	Brain Region	Finding
Friedman, 2003	45 (38M,7F)	3–4 (4.0±0.4)	ASD	20/272	21 brain regions	Widespread regional reductions of NAA, Cre and mI Prolonged NAA T2 relaxation
Levitt, 2003	22 (18M,4F)	5–16 (10.4±3.4)	ASD	272	22 brain regions	Reduced left anterior cingulate Cho Reduced left caudate and right occipital cortex Cre Increased right caudate Cho and Cre
Friedman, 2006	45 (38M,7F) [same sample as Friedman, 2003]	3–4 (4.0±0.4)	ASD	20/272	21 brain regions	Gray matter reductions predominate over white matter reductions of NAA, Cho, Cre, and mI Prolonged gray matter Cho T2 relaxation
DeVito, 2007	26 (all M)	6–17 (9.8±3.2)	AD	135	Frontal, temporal, and occipital gray matter, cerebral white matter, cerebellum	Widespread reductions of NAA and Glx in cerebral gray matter and cerebellum
Oner, 2007	14 (all M)	17–38 (24.3±7.1)	ASP	270	Right dorsolateral prefrontal cortex, right anterior cingulate cortex [data from additional regions not reported]	Increased right anterior cingulate NAA/Cho
Hardan, 2008	18 (all M)	(11.9±2.2)	AD	20	Bilateral thalamus [data from additional regions not reported]	Reduced left thalamus NAA, Cre, and Cho

serotonin terminals, decreased synaptogenesis, and reduced synaptic density (Whitaker-Azmitia, 2005). This mechanism also has been implicated in aberrations in cortical columnar development and connectivity (Casanova et al., 2008; Chugani, 2004). As a possible mediator or alternative consideration, there is emerging evidence to suggest the possibility of early inflammatory processes in autism that, if present, might also contribute to findings of reduced tissue density. For example, microglial activity and elevated cytokines in various brain regions have been reported across a broad age range of individuals with autism (Vargas, Nascimbene, Krishnan, Zimmerman, & Pardo, 2005). Additionally, increased glial fibrillary acidic protein found in postmortem samples of frontal and parietal cerebral cortex and cerebellum from older (> 18 years old) individuals with autism also suggests abnormal CNS immune activity persisting from an earlier age-point (Laurence & Fatemi, 2005). These findings are intriguing, but any related model that might account for abnormal cortical development in ASD, perhaps reflecting altered serotonergic function and/or early inflammatory processes, awaits systematic investigation. Thus, ¹H MRSI findings for altered brain tissue cytoarchitecture point toward a substantially different explanatory model than cerebral overgrowth or abnormal apoptotic or synaptic pruning regulatory mechanisms for structural MRI findings of cerebral enlargement in very young children with ASD. However, newer explanatory models that potentially could address MRI and ¹H MRS findings at this time remain speculative (Dager, Friedman, et al., 2008).

¹H MRS studies of ASD at lower magnetic field strength scanners (1.5 Tesla) have not been able to satisfactorily resolve the Glx complex to separately quantify Glu, Gln, and GABA. The capability to individually measure these chemicals, now feasible with the availability of advanced spectral editing techniques at higher field strength, provides new opportunities to address specific hypothesis-driven theories such as competing theories of hypoglutamatergic (Carlsson, 1998) or reduced inhibitory balance (Belmonte et al., 2004) mechanisms in ASD. These theories could support alterations of either decreased or elevated Glu, Gln, and GABA, conceivably for different brain regions concurrently (Polleux & Lauder, 2004). Although ¹H MRS studies of children with ASD have found either no differences or lower levels of Glx, the possibility remains that diagnostic differences in individual constituent chemicals are lost in the overall GLX measurement, regional differences exist, or there are age-related differences. Keeping in mind the inherent difficulties in accurately measuring the large and broad Glx peak that comprises the overlapping resonances of Glu, Gln, and GABA at 1.5 Tesla, a single-voxel ¹H MRS study of a small sample of medication-naïve adults with ASD found regional elevations of GLX in the right amygdala-hippocampal region compared to a control brain region in the parietal lobe (Page et al., 2006). In consideration of this

finding, a ^{13}C MRS study that evaluated glutamate-glutamine cycling in patients with intractable temporal lobe epilepsy found significant slowing of the cycle and elevated hippocampal Glu levels (Petroff, Errante, Rothman, Kim, & Spencer, 2002). As proposed by those authors and others (During & Spencer, 1993; Maragakis & Rothstein, 2001), regionally increased Glu release, or impaired clearance, could contribute to an ongoing state of increased cerebral excitability/excitotoxicity that could potentially create conditions suitable for seizure generation. This model is of potential clinical relevance to ASD, as there is a substantial risk of seizures that has a bimodal pattern of onset either in the first 2 years of life or, more typically, as the child enters adolescence, with estimates of prevalence rates ranging between 15 and 38% (Volkmar & Nelson, 1990; Giovanardi, Posar, & Parmeggiani, 2000; Tuchman & Rapin, 2002). Although the finding of elevated GLX in older individuals with ASD remains to be replicated, in conjunction with a recent report that GLX levels in preadolescents with ASD were lower (DeVito et al., 2007), the possibility of GLX levels increasing as these children grow older has potential implications for seizure onset in adolescents with ASD and for new targeted treatment approaches as well (Niederhofer, 2007).

More recently, speculation has focused on the possible role of mitochondrial compromise in ASD (NIH, 2008). This interest, in part, has been stimulated by recent clinical reports of adverse reactions temporally related to vaccination that implicated mitochondrial deficits as the mediating factor. There also are important treatment considerations if evidence for a mitochondrial contribution to vulnerability or symptom expression in ASD were to be established. For example, therapeutic properties of lithium carbonate are hypothesized to be mediated via elevations of bcl-2, a neuroprotective protein that also has mitochondrial membrane-stabilizing effects (Manji et al., 2003).

To date, a standardized approach for medical assessment of mitochondrial abnormalities and objective criteria for diagnosis of mild mitochondrial dysfunction have yet to be established (NIH, 2008). As mitochondrial DNA is distinct from nuclear DNA, much less stable and with substantially different patterns of heritability, different genetic models are required to test for relationships to ASD (Pons et al., 2004). The wide variability of clinical and metabolic manifestations of mitochondrial dysfunction could reflect variable loading of mitochondrial DNA polymorphisms, and across tissue types, that exhibit differing threshold response to oxidative stress (Calabrese et al., 2001). Elevated brain lactate determined by ^{1}H MRS is considered to be a sensitive biomarker, and substantially more specific than blood lactate elevations, for establishing the presence of mitochondrial dysfunction (Dinopoulos et al., 2005; Kaufmann et al., 2004; NIH, 2008). However, the substantial brain lactate elevations that occur in healthy subjects in response to mild, event-dependent physiological alterations, such as hyperventilation or caffeine ingestion, illustrate the difficulties attributing specificity to increased brain lactate as a biomarker for mitochondrial compromise (Dager et al., 1995; Dager et al., 1999).

^{1}H MRS investigations of subtle evidence for brain mitochondrial abnormalities in other psychiatric disease processes, such as bipolar disorder, have sought to evaluate brain lactate elevations in conjunction with other brain chemical alterations, such as NAA reductions or GLX elevations (Dager et al., 2004). To date, there has been only a single ^{1}H MRS report of regional brain lactate elevations associated with ASD, for one individual within a case series of older children with ASD, who also had elevated blood lactate levels (Chugani et al., 1999). Furthermore, although a number of ^{1}H MRS studies of ASD have found reduced NAA, only one study has reported regionally elevated GLX in adults with ASD (Page et al., 2006). In contrast, a ^{1}H MRSI study of 3- to 4-year-old children with ASD ($N = 45$), that used acquisition parameters and a 1.5T scanner platform identical to that employed for a study that detected a generalized pattern of gray matter lactate and GLX elevations in medication-free bipolar subjects (Dager et al., 2004), found no such evidence for either lactate or GLX regional or gray matter elevations (Friedman et al., 2003; Friedman et al., 2006). For this later work, confounding effects of anxiety or hyperventilation that could have artificially elevated brain lactate were eliminated through the use of propofol anesthesia to conduct the study. It is conceivable that use of propofol in the ASD group could have obscured possible lactate differences between diagnostic groups, as the typically developing control group were not sedated but instead scanned late at night during natural sleep. The alternative consideration, that use of propofol might produce regional lactate elevations in conjunction with any compromise of cerebral blood flow, was evaluated for but not found (Amundsen et al., 2005).

Brain lactate can be difficult to detect or accurately measure under basal conditions. Increasing scanner magnetic field strength and improved spectral analytic methods offer the possibility of enhanced sensitivity for detecting subtle metabolic alterations (Dager, Corrigan, et al., 2010). It is also possible that physiological challenge approaches designed to "unmask" subtle metabolic alterations, as has been demonstrated for panic disorder subjects in response to regulated hyperventilation (Dager et al., 1995), could more fully address the potential occurrence of subtle mitochondrial dysfunction in ASD.

It is important to recognize that ^{1}H MRS or ^{1}H MRSI findings most frequently reported in association with ASD (e.g., reduced NAA) are not diagnostic of ASD or specific to symptom expression. Other disorders that have overlapping phenotypic expression as ASD, such as Rett syndrome, may also exhibit a similar ^{1}H MRS pattern of altered brain chemistry. For example, the majority of published ^{1}H MRS studies of Rett syndrome, albeit usually with very small sample sizes, also find reduced NAA or NAA/Cre (Nielsen et al., 1993; Hanefeld et al., 1995; Hashimoto et al., 1998; Pan, Lane, Hetherington, & Percy, 1999; Gokcay, Kitis, Ekmekci, Karasoy, & Sener, 2002; Khong, Lam, Ooi, Ko, & Wong, 2002; Horska et al., 2000). Also, reduced NAA is one of the more consistent ^{1}H MRS alterations associated with idiopathic developmental delay (Kimura et al., 1995). Other psychiatric disorders also may exhibit overlapping patterns of brain tissue chemical alterations as ASD. For example, the most robust ^{1}H MRS findings in adults with schizophrenia are substantial NAA reductions in frontal lobe, parietal lobe, and medial temporal lobe gray and white matter, along with a similar magnitude of reduced NAA in the cerebellum (Steen, Hamer, & Lieberman, 2005). As NAA increases are observed following both short-term and longer duration antipsychotic treatment of schizophrenia (Bertolino, Callicott, Mattay, Weidenhammer, Rakow, et al., 2001), it is unlikely that reduced baseline NAA levels in schizophrenia primarily reflects reduced neuronal density. These observations may instead reflect the effects of medication on NAA's role in synaptic maintenance, myelination, regulation of cellular osmolarity, and neuronal metabolism (Birken et al., 1989; Coyle et al., 2000; Neale et al., 2000).

Conclusions

^{1}H MRS is advancing our understanding of basic mechanisms underlying brain developmental abnormalities associated with ASD, such as the early cerebral enlargement observed by MRI. ^{1}H MRS findings, to date, from studies of ASD do not appear to be of diagnostic specificity but can be used to interrogate brain structural alterations in ASD and relationships to specific developmental time points. Studies of young children with ASD provide evidence for widespread reductions in NAA and other brain chemical levels, and alterations in the mobility of these chemicals (T2 relaxation), suggest early alterations in brain tissue development. This altered brain tissue cytoarchitecture is posited to reflect generalized reductions in neuronal density and/or alterations in neuronal and synaptic maintenance, and is found to primarily affect gray matter at earlier ages. Applications of ^{1}H MRS and quantitative T2 relaxation to test specific models hypothesized to account for early cerebral enlargement do not support accelerated cerebral overgrowth or abnormal apoptotic or synaptic pruning mechanisms. Instead, insights gained from ^{1}H MRS findings are contributing to the formulation of new explanatory models to account for multimodal imaging and related histopathological findings in ASD.

Challenges and Future Directions

- Current, widely available ^{1}H MRS/I methods can be used to characterize:
  - the timing of chemical changes in relationship to developmental course
  - anatomical localization of chemical alterations
  - relationships between chemical alterations and structural abnormalities
  - relationships between chemical alterations, clinical prognosis, and treatment response
- Advances in the field are improving:
  - isolation and quantification of chemicals of particular interest to ASD.
  - temporal resolution for better evaluation of active metabolic processes
  - spatial resolution and magnetic field homogeneity to allow for more precise interrogation of particular brain regions of interest in ASD, such as the amygdala, and even amygdalar subregions.
- Current methodological limitations include:
  - difficulties with between-site standardization of MRS measurements
  - lack of a standardized analytic methodology that avoids common pitfalls and yields accurate and reproducible MRS measurements.

SUGGESTED READINGS

Dager, S. R., Corrigan, N. M., Richards, T. L., & Posse, S. (2008). Research applications of magnetic resonance spectroscopy (MRS) to investigate psychiatric disorders. *Topics in Magnetic Resonance Imaging*, *19*, 81–96.

De Graaf, R. A. (2007). *In vivo NMR spectroscopy-2nd edition: Principles and techniques*. Chichester, UK: Wiley.

Gadian, D. F. (1982). *Nuclear magnetic resonance and its applications to living systems*. New York: Oxford University Press.

REFERENCES

American Psychiatric Association. (1994). *Diagnostic and statistical manual of mental disorders* (4th ed.; DSM-IV). Washington, DC: Author.

Amundsen, L. B., Artru, A. A., Dager, S. R., Shaw, D. W., Friedman, S., Sparks, B., et al. (2005). Propofol sedation for longitudinal pediatric neuroimaging research. *Journal of Neurosurgical Anesthesiology*, *17*, 180–192.

Bagni, C., & Greenough, W. T. (2005). From mRNP trafficking to spine dysmorphogenesis: The roots of Fragile X syndrome. *Nature Reviews Neuroscience*, *6*, 376–387.

Baslow, M. H. (2000). Functions of N-acetyl-L-aspartate and N-acetyl-L-aspartylglutamate in the vertebrate brain: Role in glial cell-specific signaling. *Journal of Neurochemistry*, *75*, 453–459.

Behar, K. L., & Ogino, T. (1991). Assignment of resonance in the ^{1}H spectrum of rat brain by two-dimensional shift correlated and j-resolved NMR spectroscopy. *Magnetic Resonance in Medicine*, *17*, 285–303.

Belmonte, M. K., Cook, E. H., Jr., Anderson, G. M., Rubenstein, J. L., Greenough, W. T., Beckel-Mitchener, A., et al. (2004). Autism as a disorder of neural information processing: Directions for research and targets for therapy. *Molecular Psychiatry*, *9*, 646–663.

Bertolino, A., Callicott, J. H., Mattay, V. S., Weidenhammer, K. M., Rakow R., Egan, M. F., et al. (2001). The effect of treatment with antipsychotic drugs on brain N-acetylaspartate measures in patients with schizophrenia. *Biological Psychiatry*, *49*, 39–46.

Birken, D. L., & Oldendorf, W. H. (1989). N-acetyl-L-aspartic acid: A literature review of a compound prominent in 1H NMR spectroscopic studies of brain. *Neuroscience and Biobehavioral Reviews, 13*, 23–31.

Bloch, F., Hansen, W. W., & Packard, M. E. (1946). Nuclear induction. *Physics Review, 69*, 127.

Boger-Megiddo, I., Shaw, D. W., Friedman, S. D., Sparks, B. F., Artru, A. A., Giedd, J. N., et al. (2006). Corpus callosum morphometrics in young children with autism spectrum disorder. *Journal of Autism and Developmental Disorders, 36*(6), 733–739.

Braus, D. F., Ende, G., Weber-Fahr, W., Demirakca, T., & Henn, F. A. (2001). Favorable effect on neuronal viability in the anterior cingulate gyrus due to long-term treatment with atypical antipsychotics: An MRSI study. *Pharmacopsychiatry, 34*, 251–253.

Brooks, W. M., Friedman, S. D., & Stidley, C. (1999). Reproducibility of ^{1}H MRS in vivo. *Magnetic Resonance in Medicine, 41*, 193–197.

Bryson, S. E., McDermott, C., Rombough, V., & Zwaigenbaum, L. (2008). The Autism Observational Scale for Infants: Scale development and assessment of reliability. *Journal of Autism and Developmental Disabilities, 38*(4), 731–738.

Calabrese, V., Seapagnini, G., Giuffrida, Stella, A. M., Bates, T. E., & Clark, J. B. (2001). Mitochondrial involvement in brain function and dysfunction: Relevance to aging, neurodegenerative disorders, and longevity. *Neurochemical Research, 26*, 739–764.

Carlsson, M. L. (1998). Hypothesis: Is infantile autism a hypoglutamatergic disorder? Relevance of glutamate serotonin interactions for pharmacotherapy. *Journal of Neural Transmission, 105*, 525–535.

Casanova, M. F., & Tillquist, C. R. (2008). Encephalization, emergent properties, and psychiatry: A minicolumnar perspective. *Neuroscientist, 14*(1), 101–118.

Chugani, D. (2004). Serotonin in autism and pediatric epilepsies. *Mental Retardation and Developmental Disabilities Research Reviews, 10*, 112–116.

Chugani, D. C., Sundram, B. S., Behen, M., Lee, M. L., & Moore, G. J. (1999). Evidence of altered energy metabolism in autistic children. *Progress in Neuropsychopharmacology and Biological Psychiatry, 23*, 635–641.

Corrigan, N. M., Richards, T. L., Friedman, S. D., Petropoulos, H., & Dager, S. R. (2010). Improving ^{1}H MRSI measurement of cerebral lactate for clinical applications. *Psychiatry Research, 182*, 40–47.

Courchesne, E., Karns, C. M., Davis, H. R., Ziccardi, R., Carper, R. A., Tigue, Z. D., et al. (2001). Unusual brain growth patterns in early life in patients with autistic disorder: An MRI study. *Neurology, 57*, 245–254.

Coyle, J. T., & Schwarcz, R. (2000). Mind glue: Implications of glial cell biology for psychiatry. *Archives of General Psychiatry, 57*, 90–93.

Dager, S. R., Corrigan, N. M., Richards, T. L., & Posse, S. (2008). Research applications of magnetic resonance spectroscopy (MRS) to investigate psychiatric disorders. *Topics in Magnetic Resonance Imaging, 19*, 81–96.

Dager, S. R., Friedman, S. D., Parow, A., Demopulos, C., Stoll, A. L., Lyoo, I. K., et al. (2004). Brain metabolic alterations in medication-free patients with bipolar disorder. *Archives of General Psychiatry, 61*, 450–458.

Dager, S. R., Friedman, S. D., Petropoulos, H., & Shaw, D. W. (2008). Imaging evidence for pathological brain development in autism spectrum disorders. In A. Zimmerman (Ed.), *Autism: Current theories and evidence* (pp. 361–379). Totowa, NJ: Humana.

Dager, S. R., Layton, M. E., Strauss, W., Richards, T. L., Heide, A., Friedman, S. D., et al. (1999). Human brain metabolic response to caffeine and the effects of tolerance. *American Journal of Psychiatry, 156*, 229–237.

Dager, S. R., Strauss, W. L., Marro, K. I., Richards, T. L., Metzger, G. D., & Artru, A. A. (1995). Proton magnetic resonance spectroscopy investigation of hyperventilation in subjects with panic disorder and comparison subjects. *American Journal of Psychiatry, 152*, 666–672.

Dager, S. R., & Steen, R. G. (1992). Applications of magnetic resonance spectroscopy to the investigation of neuropsychiatric disorders. *Neuropsychopharmacology, 6*(4), 249–266.

Davidovitch, M., Patterson, B., & Gartside, P. (1996). Head circumference measurements in children with autism. *Journal of Child Neurology, 11*, 389–393.

Dawson, G., Munson, J., Estes, A., Osterling, J., McPartland, J., Toth, K., et al. (2002). Neurocognitive function and joint attention ability in young children with autism spectrum disorder versus developmental delay. *Child Development, 73*, 345–358.

Dawson, G., Munson, J., Webb, S. J., Nalty, T., Abbott, R., & Toth, K. (2007). Rate of head growth decelerates and symptoms worsen in the second year of life in autism. *Biological Psychiatry, 61*(4), 458–464.

Dawson, G., Toth, K., Abbott, R., Osterling, J., Munson, J., Estes, A., et al. (2004). Early social attention impairments in autism: Social orienting, joint attention, and attention to distress. *Developmental Psychology, 40*, 271–283.

De Graaf, R. A. (2007). *In vivo NMR spectroscopy-2nd edition: Principles and techniques*. Chichester, UK: Wiley.

DeVito, T. J., Drost, D. J., Neufeld, R. W., Rajakumar, N., Pavlosky, W., Williamson, P., et al. (2007). Evidence for cortical dysfunction in autism: A proton magnetic resonance spectroscopic imaging study. *Biological Psychiatry, 61*(4), 465–473.

DiCicco-Bloom, E., Lord, C., Zwaigenbaum, L., Courchesne, E., Dager, S. R., Schmitz, C., et al. (2006). The developmental neurobiology of autism spectrum disorder. *Journal of Neuroscience, 26*, 6897–6906.

Dinopoulos, A., Cecil, K. M., Schapiro, M. B., Papadimitriou, A., Hadjigeorgiou, G. M., Wong, B., et al. (2005). Brain MRI and proton MRS findings in infants and children with respiratory chain defects. *Neuropediatrics, 36*, 290–301.

During, M. J., & Spencer, D. D. (1993). Extracellular hippocampal glutamate and spontaneous seizure in the conscious human brain. *Lancet, 341*, 1607–1610.

Endo, T., Shioiri, T., Kitamura, H., Kimura, T., Endo, S., Masuzawa, N., et al. (2007). Altered chemical metabolites in the amygdala-hippocampus region contribute to autistic symptoms of autism spectrum disorders. *Biological Psychiatry, 62*(9), 1030–1037.

Friedman, S. D., Brooks, W. M., Jung, R. E., Chiulli, S. J., Sloan, J. H., Montoya, B. T., et al. (1999). Quantitative proton MRS predicts outcome after traumatic brain injury. *Neurology, 52*, 1384–1391.

Friedman, S. D., Jensen, J., Frederick, B., Artru, A., Renshaw, P., Dager, S. R. (2007). Brain changes to hypocapnia using rapidly interleaved phosphorus-proton magnetic resonance spectroscopy at 4 Tesla. *Journal of Cerebral Blood Flow and Metabolism, 27*(3), 646–653.

Friedman, S. D., Shaw, D. W., Artru, A. A., Dawson, G., Petropoulos, H., & Dager, S. R. (2006). Gray and white matter brain chemistry in young children with autism. *Archives of General Psychiatry, 63*, 786–794.

Friedman, S. D., Shaw, D. W., Artru, A. A., Gardner, J. Dawson, G., & Dager, S. R. (2003). Regional brain chemical alterations in young children with autism spectrum disorder. *Neurology, 60*, 100–107.

Gabis, L., Huang, W., Azizian, A., DeVincent, C., Tudorica, A., Kesner-Baruch, Y., et al. (2008). ^{1}H-magnetic resonance spectroscopy markers of cognitive and language ability in clinical subtypes of autism spectrum disorders. *Journal of Child Neurology, 23*(7), 766–774.

Gadian, D. F. (1982). *Nuclear magnetic resonance and its applications to living systems*. New York: Oxford University Press.

Giovanardi, R., Posar, A., & Parmeggiani, A. (2000). Epilepsy in adolescents and young adults with autistic disorder. *Brain Development, 22*, 102–168.

Gökcay, A., Kitis, O., Ekmekci, O., Karasoy, H., & Sener, R. N. (2002). Proton MR spectroscopy in Rett syndrome. *Computerized Medical Imaging Graphics, 26*, 271–275.

Hanefeld, F., Christen, H. J., Holzbach, U., Kruse, B., Frahm, J., & Hänicke, W. (1995). Cerebral proton magnetic resonance spectroscopy in Rett syndrome. *Neuropediatrics, 26*, 126–127.

Hardan, A. Y., Minshew, N. J., Melhem, N. M., Srihari, S., Jo, B., Bansal, R., et al. (2008). An MRI and proton spectroscopy study of the thalamus in children with autism. *Psychiatry Research, 163*(2), 97–105.

Hashimoto, T., Kawano, N., Fukuda, K., Endo, S., Mori, K., Yoneda, Y., et al. (1998). Proton magnetic resonance spectroscopy of the brain in three cases of Rett syndrome: Comparison with autism and normal controls. *Acta Neurologica Scandinavica, 98*, 8–14.

Hashimoto, T., Tayama, M., Miyazaki, M., Yoneda, Y., Yoshimoto, T., Haradaet, M., et al. (1997). Differences in brain metabolites between patients with autism and mental retardation as detected by in vivo localized proton magnetic resonance spectroscopy. *Journal of Child Neurology, 12*, 91–96.

Hazlett, H. C., Poe, M., Gerig, G., Smith, R. G., Provenzale, J., Ross, A., et al. (2005). Magnetic resonance imaging and head circumference study of brain size in autism: Birth through age 2 years. *Archives of General Psychiatry, 62*, 1366–1376.

Herbert, M. R., Ziegler, D. A., Makris, N., Filipek, P. A., Kemper, T. L., Normandin, J. J., et al. (2004). Localization of white matter volume increase in autism and developmental language disorder. *Annals of Neurology, 55*, 530–540.

Hisaoka, S., Harada, M., Nishitani, H., & Mori, K. (2001). Regional magnetic resonance spectroscopy of the brain in autistic individuals. *Neuroradiology, 43*, 496–498.

Horská, A., Naidu, S., Herskovits, E. H., Wang, P. Y., Kaufmann, W. E., & Barker, P. B. (2000). Quantitative ^{1}H MR spectroscopic imaging in early Rett syndrome. *Neurology, 54*, 715–722.

Huppi, P. S., Posse, S., Lazeyras, F., Burri, R., Bossi, E., & Herschkowitz, N. (1991). Magnetic resonance in preterm and term newborns: ^{1}H-spectroscopy in developing human brain. *Pediatric Research, 30*, 574–578.

Hurd, R. E., Gurr, D., & Sailasuta, N. (1998). Proton spectroscopy without water suppression: The oversampled j-resolved experiment. *Magnetic Resonance in Medicine, 40*, 343–347.

Hurd, R., Sailasuta, N., Srinivasan, R., Vigneron, D. B., Pelletier, D., & Nelson, S. J. (2004). Measurement of brain glutamate using te-averaged press at 3t. *Magnetic Resonance in Medicine, 51*, 435–440.

Huttenlocher, P. R., & Dabholkar, A. S. (1997). Regional differences in synaptogenesis in human cerebral cortex. *Journal of Comprehensive Neurology, 387*, 167–178.

Jensen, J. E., Frederick, B. de B., & Renshaw, P. F. (2005). Grey and white matter gaba level differences in the human brain using two-dimensional, j-resolved spectroscopic imaging. *NMR in Biomedicine, 18*, 570–576.

Jensen, J. E., Frederick, B. D., Wang, L., Brown, J., & Renshaw, P. F. (2005). Two-dimensional, j-resolved spectroscopic imaging of gaba at 4 tesla in the human brain. *Magnetic Resonance in Medicine, 54*, 783–788.

Josey, L., Al Sayyari, A., Buckley, R., & Coulthard, A. (2009). Usefulness of susceptibility-weighted imaging for voxel placement in MR spectroscopy. *American Journal of Neuroradiology Research, 30*, 752–754.

Kagan, J., Herschkowitz, N., & Herschkowitz, E. (2005). *A young mind in a growing brain*. Mahwah, NJ: Erlbaum.

Kaufmann, P., Shungu, D. C., Sano, M. C., Jhung, S., Engelstad, K., Mitsis, E., et al. (2004). Cerebral lactic acidosis correlates with neurological impairment in MELAS. *Neurology, 62*, 1297–1302.

Khong, P. L., Lam, C. W., Ooi, C. G., Ko, C. H., & Wong, V. C. (2002). Magnetic resonance spectroscopy and analysis of MECP2 in Rett syndrome. *Pediatric Neurology, 26*, 205–209.

Kimura, H., Fujii, Y., Itoh, S., & Matsuda, T. (1995). Metabolic alterations in the neonate and infant brain during development: Evaluation with proton MR spectroscopy. *Radiology, 194*, 483–489.

Kleinhans, N. M., Schweinsburg, B. C., Cohen, D. N., Muller, R. A., & Courchesne, E. (2007). N-acetyl aspartate in autism spectrum disorders: Regional effects and relationship to fMRI activation. *Brain Research, 1162*, 85–97.

Kreis, R., Ernst, T., & Ross, B. D. (1993). Development of the human brain: In vivo quantification of metabolite and water content with proton magnetic resonance spectroscopy. *Magnetic Resonance in Medicine, 30*, 424–437.

Lainhart, J. E., Piven, J., Wzorek, M., Landa, R., Santangelo, S. L., Coon, H., et al. (1997). Macrocephaly in children and adults with autism. *Journal of American Academy of Child and Adolescent Psychiatry, 36*, 282–290.

Landa, R., & Garrett-Mayer, E. (2006). Development in infants with autism spectrum disorders: A prospective study. *Journal of Child Psychology and Psychiatry, 47*, 629–638.

Laurence, J. S., & Fatemi, S. (2005). Glial fibrillary acidic protein is elevated in superior frontal, parietal, and cerebellar cortices of autistic subjects. *Cerebellum, 4*, 206–210.

Lauterbur, P. C. (1973). Image formation by induced local interactions: Examples employing nuclear magnetic resonance. *Nature, 242*, 190–191.

Levitt, P. (2005). Disruption of interneuron development. *Epilepsia, 46*(7), 22–28.

Levitt, J. G., O'Neill, J., Blanton, R. E., Smalley, S., Fadale, D., McCracken, J. T., et al. (2003). Proton magnetic resonance spectroscopic imaging of the brain in childhood autism. *Biological Psychiatry, 54*, 1355–1366.

Lin, F. H., Tsai, S. Y., Otazo, R., Caprihan, A., Wald, L. L., Belliveau, J. W., et al. (2007). Sensitivity-encoded (SENSE) proton echo-planar spectroscopic imaging (PEPSI) in the human brain. *Magnetic Resonance in Medicine, 57*(2), 249–257.

Lord, C., Risi, S., DiLavore, P. S., Shulman, C., Thurm, A., & Pickles, A. (2006). Autism from 2 to 9 years of age. *Archives of General Psychiatry, 63*, 694–701.

Lymer, K., Haga, K., Marshall, I., Sailasuta, N., & Wardlaw, J. (2007). Reproducibility of gaba measurements using 2d j-resolved magnetic resonance spectroscopy. *Magnetic Resonance Imaging, 25*, 634–640.

Lyon, G. R., & Rumsey, J. M. (1996). *Neuroimaging studies of autism: Neuroimaging: a window to the neurological foundations of learning and behavior in children*. Baltimore: Brookes.

Manji, H. K., Quiroz, J. A., Sporn, J., Payne, J. L., Denicoff, K., Gray, A., et al. (2003). Enhancing neuronal plasticity and cellular resilience to develop novel, improved therapeutics for difficult-to-treat depression. *Biological Psychiatry, 53*, 707–742.

Mansfield, P., & Grannell, P. K. (1973). NMR diffraction in solids? *Journal of Physics. C. Solid State Physics, 6*, 422–426.

Maragakis, N. J., & Rothstein, J. D. (2001). Glutamate transporters in neurologic disease. *Archives of Neurology, 58*, 365–370.

Mescher, M., Merkle, H., Kirsch, J., Garwood, M., & Gruetter, R. (1998). Simultaneous in vivo spectral editing and water suppression. *NMR in Biomedicine, 11*, 266–272.

Minshew, N. J., Goldstein, G., Dombrowski, S. M., Panchalingam, K., & Pettegrew, J. W. (1993). A preliminary 31P MRS study of autism: Evidence for undersynthesis and increased degradation of brain membranes. *Biological Psychiatry, 33*(11–12), 762–773.

Moore, C. M., Breeze, J. L., Kukes, T. J., Rose, S. L., Dager, S. R., Cohen, B. M., et al. (1999). Effects of myo-inositol ingestion on human brain myo-inositol levels: A proton magnetic resonance spectroscopic imaging study. *Biological Psychiatry, 45*, 1197–1202.

Munson, J., Dawson, G., Abbott, R., Faja, S., Webb, S. J., Friedman, S. D., et al. (2006). Amygdalar volume and behavioral development in autism. *Archives of General Psychiatry, 63*(6), 686–693.

Murphy, D. G., Critchley, H. D., Schmitz, N., McAlonan, G., Van Amelsvoort, T., Robertson, D., et al. (2002). Asperger syndrome: A proton magnetic resonance spectroscopy study of brain. *Archives of General Psychiatry, 59*, 885–891.

Neale, J. H., Bzdega, T., & Wroblewska, B. (2000). N-Acetylaspartylglutamate: The most abundant peptide neurotransmitter in the mammalian central nervous system. *Journal of Neurochemistry, 75*, 443–452.

Niederhofer, H. (2007). Glutamate antagonists seem to be slightly effective in psychopharmacologic treatment of autism. *Journal of Clinical Psychopharmacol, 27*(3), 317–318.

Nielsen, J. B., Toft, P. B., Reske-Nielsen, E., Jensen, K. E., Christiansen, P., Thomsen, C., et al. (1993). Cerebral magnetic resonance spectroscopy in Rett syndrome. *Brain Development, 15*, 107–112.

NIH. (2008). Mitochondrial encephalopathies: Potential relationships to autism? *National Institutes of Neurological Disorders and Stroke*. Available at: http://www.ninds.nih.gov/news_and_events/proceedings/20090629_mitochondrial.htm

Oner, O., Devrimci-Ozguven, H., Oktem, F., Yagmurlu, B., Baskak, B., & Munir, K. M. (2007). Proton MR spectroscopy: Higher right anterior cingulate N-acetylaspartate/choline ratio in Asperger syndrome compared with healthy controls. *American Journal of Neuroradiology, 28*(8), 1494–1498.

Otazo, R., Mueller, B., Ugurbil, K., Wald, L., & Posse, S. (2006). Signal-to-noise ratio and spectral linewidth improvements between 1.5 and 7 Tesla in proton echo-planar spectroscopic imaging. *Magnetic Resonance in Medicine, 56*(6), 1200–1210.

Otazo, R., Tsai, S. Y., Lin, F. H., & Posse, S. (2007). Accelerated short-te 3d proton echo-planar spectroscopic imaging using 2d-sense with a 32-channel array coil. *Magnetic Resonance in Medicine, 58*, 1107–1116.

Otsuka, H., Harada, M., Mori, K., Hisaoka, S., & Nishitani, H. (1999). Brain metabolites in the hippocampus-amygdala region and cerebellum in autism: An 1 H-MR spectroscopy study. *Neuroradiology, 41*(7), 517–519.

Page, L. A., Daly, E., Schmitz, N., Simmons, A., Toal, F., Deeley, Q., et al. (2006). In vivo ^{1}H-magnetic resonance spectroscopy study of amygdala-hippocampal and parietal regions in autism. *American Journal of Psychiatry, 163*(12), 2189–2192.

Pan, J. W., Lane, J. B., Hetherington, H., & Percy, A. K. (1999). Rett syndrome: ^{1}H spectroscopic imaging at 4.1 Tesla. *Journal of Child Neurology, 14*, 524–528.

Petroff, O. A., Errante, L. D., Rothman, D. L., Kim, J. H., & Spencer, D. D. (2002). Glutamate-glutamine cycling in the epileptic human hippocampus. *Epilepsia, 43*, 703–710.

Petropoulos, H., Friedman, S. D., Shaw, D., Artru, A., Dawson, G., & Dager, S. R. (2006). T2 relaxometry reveals evidence for gray matter abnormalities in autism spectrum disorder. *Neurology, 67*, 632–636.

Pfefferbaum, A., Mathalon, D. H., Sullivan, E. V., Rawles, J. M., Zipursky, R. B., & Lim, K. O. (1994). A quantitative magnetic resonance imaging study of changes in brain morphology from infancy to late adulthood. *Archives of Neurology, 51*, 874–887.

Piven, J., Bailey, J., Ranson, B. J., & Arndt, S. (1997). An MRI study of the corpus callosum in autism. *American Journal of Psychiatry, 154*, 1051–1056.

Polleux, F., & Lauder, J. M. (2004). Toward a developmental neurobiology of autism. *Mental Retardation and Developmental Disabilities Research Reviews, 10*, 303–317.

Pons, R., Andreu, A. L., Checcarelli, N., Vilà, M. R., Engelstad, K., Sue, C. M., et al. (2004). Mitochondrial DNA abnormalities and autistic spectrum disorders. *Journal of Pediatrics, 144*, 81–85.

Posse, S., Dager, S. R., Richards, T. L., Yuan, C., Ogg, R., Artru, A. A., et al. (1997). In vivo measurement of regional brain metabolic response to hyperventilation using functional proton echo-planar spectroscopic imaging (PEPSI). *Magnetic Resonance Medicine, 37*, 858–865.

Posse, S., Otazo, R., Caprihan, A., Bustillo, J., Chen, H., Henry, P. G., et al. (2007). Proton echo-planar spectroscopic imaging of j-coupled resonances in human brain at 3 and 4 Tesla. *Magnetic Resonance in Medicine, 58*, 236–244.

Posse, S., Otazo, R., Tsai, S. Y., Yoshimoto, A. E., & Lin, F. H. (2008, December 18). Single-shot magnetic resonance spectroscopic imaging with partial parallel imaging. *Magnetic Resonance in Medicine* [Epub ahead of print].

Posse, S., Schuknecht, B., Smith, M. E., van Zijl, P. C., Herschkowitz, N., Moone, C. T., et al. (1993). Short echo time proton MR spectroscopic imaging. *Journal of Computer Assisted Tomography, 17*, 1–14.

Proctor, W. G., & Yu, F. C. (1950). The dependency of a nuclear magnetic resonance frequency upon chemical compound. *Physics Review, 77*, 717.

Provencher, S. (2009). *LCModel*. Available at: http://s-provencher.com/pages/ (accessed September 9, 2009).

Provencher, S. W. (1993). Estimation of metabolite concentrations from localized in vivo proton NMR spectra. *Magnetic Resonance in Medicine, 30*, 672–679.

Purcell, E. M., Torrey, H. C., & Pound, R. V. (1946). Resonance absorption by nuclear magnetic moments in a solid. *Physics Review, 69*, 37–38.

Ross, B., & Michaelis, T. (1994). Clinical applications of magnetic resonance spectroscopy. *Magnetic Resonance in Medicine, 10*, 191–247.

Ryner, L. N., Sorenson, J. A., & Thomas, M. A. (1995). Localized 2d j-resolved 1h mr spectroscopy: Strong coupling effects in vitro and in vivo. *Magnetic Resonance in Medicine, 13*, 853–869.

Rumpel, H., Lim, W. E. H., Chang, H. M., Chan, L. L., Ho, G. L., Wong, M. W., et al. (2003). Is Myo-inositol a measure of glial swelling after stroke? A magnetic resonance study. *Journal of Magnetic Resonance Imaging, 17*, 11–19.

Sampaio, R., & Truwit, C. (2001). Myelination in the developing human brain. In C. A. Nelson & M. Luciana (Eds.), *Handbook of developmental cognitive neuroscience* (pp. 35–44). Cambridge, MA: MIT Press.

Schubert, F., Gallinat, J., Seifert, F., & Rinneberg, H. (2004). Glutamate concentrations in human brain using single voxel proton magnetic resonance spectroscopy at 3 Tesla. *Neuroimage, 21*, 1762–1771.

Schurr, A., West C. A., & Rigor B. M. (1988). Lactate-supported synaptic function in the rat hippocampal slice preparation. *Science, 240*(4857), 1326–1328.

Sparks, B. F., Friedman, S. D., Shaw, D. W., Aylward, E. H., Echelard, D., Artru, A. A., et al. (2002). Brain structural abnormalities in young children with autism spectrum disorder. *Neurology, 59*, 184–192.

Steen, R. G., Hamer, R. M., & Lieberman, J. A. (2005). Measurement of brain metabolites by ^{1}H magnetic resonance spectroscopy in patients with schizophrenia: A systematic review and meta-analysis. *Neuropsychopharmacology, 30*(11), 1949–1962.

Strauss, W. L., Unis, A. S., Cowan, C., Dawson, G., & Dager, S. R. (2002). 19F measurement of brain fluvoxamine and fluoxetine in pediatric patients treated for pervasive developmental disorders. *American Journal of Psychiatry, 159*, 755–760.

Tallan, H. H., Moore, S., & Stein, W. H. (1956). N-acetyl-l-aspartic acid in brain. *Journal of Biological Chemistry, 219*, 257–264.

Tsacopoulos, M., & Magistretti, P. J. (1996). Metabolic coupling between glia and neurons. *Journal of Neuroscience, 16*, 877–885.

Tsai, S. Y., Otazo, R., Posse, S., Lin, Y. R., Chung, H. W., Wald, L. L., et al. (2008). Accelerated proton echo planar spectroscopic imaging (PEPSI) using grappa with a 32-channel phased-array coil. *Magnetic Resonance in Medicine, 59*, 989–998.

Tuchman, R., & Rapin, I. (2002). Epilepsy in autism. *Lancet Neurology, 1*, 352–358.

van der Knaap, M. S., van der Grond, J., van Rijen, P. C., Faber, J. A., Valk, J., & Willemse, K. (1990). Age-dependent changes in localized proton and phosphorus MR spectroscopy of the brain. *Radiology, 176*, 509–515.

Vargas, D. L., Nascimbene, C., Krishnan, C., Zimmerman, A. W., & Pardo, C. A. (2005). Neuroglial activation and neuroinflammation in the brain of patients with autism. *Annals of Neurology, 57*, 67–81.

Vasconcelos, M. M., Brito, A. R., Domingues, R. C., da Cruz, L. C., Jr., Gasparetto, E. L., Werner, J., Jr., et al. (2008). Proton magnetic resonance spectroscopy in school-aged autistic children. *Journal of Neuroimaging, 18*(3), 288–295.

Vaughan, T., DelaBarre, L., Snyder, C., Akgun, C. S. D., Liu, W. O. C., Strupp, G., et al. (2006). 9.4T human MRI: Preliminary results. *Magnetic Resonance in Medicine, 56*, 1274–1282.

Volkmar, F. R., & Nelson, D. S. (1990). Seizure disorders in autism. *Journal of American Academy of Child and Adolescent Psychiatry, 29*, 127–129.

Wald, L. L., Moyher, S. E., Day, M. R., Nelson, S. J., & Vigneron, D. B. (1995). Proton spectroscopic imaging of the human brain using phased array detectors. *Magnetic Resonance in Medicine, 34*, 440–445.

Watson, L. R., Baranek, G. T., Crais, E. R., Reznick, J. S., Dykstra, J., & Perryman, T. (2006). The First Year Inventory: Retrospective parent responses to a questionnaire designed to identify one-year-olds at risk for autism. *Journal of Autism Developmental Disorders, 37*, 49–61.

Whitaker-Azmitia, P. (2005). Behavioral and cellular consequences of increasing serotonergic activity during brain development: A role in autism? *International Journal of Developmental Neuroscience, 23*, 75–83.

Williams, D. L., & Minshew, N. J. (2007). Understanding autism and related disorders: What has imaging taught us? *Neuroimaging Clinics of North America, 17*(4), 495–509.

Zeegers, M., van der Grond, J., van Daalen, E., Buitelaar, J., & van Engeland, H. (2006). Proton magnetic resonance spectroscopy in developmentally delayed young boys with or without autism. *Journal of Neural Transmission, 114*(2), 289–295.

Zoghbi, H. Y. (2003). Postnatal neurodevelopmental disorders: Meeting at the synapse? *Science, 302*, 826–830.

Zwaigenbaum, L., Bryson, S., Rogers, T., Roberts, W., Brian, J., & Szatmari, P. (2005). Behavioral manifestations of autism in the first year of life. *International Journal of Developmental Neuroscience, 23*, 143–152.

34 Meera E. Modi, Larry J. Young

Oxytocin, Vasopressin, and Social Behavior: Implications for Autism Spectrum Disorders

Points of Interest

- Oxytocin and vasopressin are highly evolutionarily conserved modulators of reproductive and social behavior.
- Oxytocin and vasopressin modulate social motivation, social information processing, and social bonding in a variety of rodent species.
- Individual variation in the neuropeptide receptor systems has been associated with variation in social behavior in rodents.
- Oxytocin has been shown to modulate a variety of complex social behaviors in humans, such as trust, emotional perception, and face processing.
- Disregulation of peripheral peptide levels and polymorphisms in oxytocin, vasopressin, and their receptor genes have been associated with ASD.

Elucidation of the basic neurobiological mechanisms underlying social cognition and social behavior is pivotal for understanding the biology mediating normal human social behavior and may also provide valuable insights into the pathophysiology and potential treatment of disorders of social behavior. An extensive literature has implicated the neuropeptides oxytocin and vasopressin as being key modulators of species-typical social behavior. This chapter will review the evidence from animal and human research demonstrating that these neuropeptides modulate several aspects of social cognition and behavior, including social motivation, social information processing, and social attachment.

Oxytocin (OT) and arginine vasopressin (AVP) are evolutionarily conserved molecular modulators of complex social behavior (Donaldson & Young, 2008). These nine–amino acid peptides have been implicated in the regulation of many different aspects of affiliative behavior including social recognition and social memory in rodents, communication, parental care, and social bonding (Insel & Young, 2001). Variations in the OT and AVP systems have been linked with both interspecies and individual variation of sociality in animal models, which has inspired researchers to look for parallel relationships in human populations. Despite the complexity of human social behavior, OT and AVP have also been linked to trust, altruism, emotional expression and perception, and social bonding.

Due to their involvement in social behavior, it has been suggested that disregulation of these systems may contribute to the disruptions in the social domain in autism spectrum disorder (ASD) and other psychiatric disorders characterized by social impairment (Hammock & Young, 2006). Even if alterations in the OT and AVP systems are not involved in the etiology of ASD, pharmacological manipulation of these systems may be a viable strategy for enhancing social cognition and interpersonal relationships in this disorder (Bartz & Hollander, 2006). Social impairments are the most defining characteristic of ASD. In clinical populations, social impairments are seen as gaze aversion, limited affective expression, improper coordination of gestures with speech and impairment in interpreting these nonverbal cues in others (Bartz & Hollander, 2006). Animal models have shown that inhibition of the OT and AVP systems, either through genetic or pharmacological manipulation, results in impairments of social investigation, recognition, and motivation that are analogous to the deficits seen in individuals with autism. To understand the nature of the complex relationship between these neuropeptides and social behaviors, numerous studies have looked at their effect on three facets of affiliative behavior: social motivation, social information processing, and social attachment.

This chapter will examine the role that OT, AVP, and their related systems play in mediating the core components of social behavior. Their involvement in both normal social behavior and how their disregulation leads to disturbances in behavior will be discussed. Parallels will be drawn between the neurobiological findings in animal models and the genetic and imaging studies done in both typical and clinical human populations. Finally, the direct evidence implicating a role for these neuropeptide systems in autism spectrum disorders will be presented with a discussion of how these findings may shape the development of novel pharmacological therapies for treating social impairment.

Oxytocin and Vasopressin: The Social Peptides

Oxytocin

OT is a nine–amino acid peptide (nonapeptide) that is synthesized in the magnocellular neurons of the paraventricular nucleus (PVN) and the supraoptic nucleus (SON) of the hypothalamus and transported to the posterior pituitary, where it is stored and secreted into systemic circulation (Gimpl & Fahrenholz, 2001). Peripherally, OT acts as a reproductive hormone to facilitate uterine contractions during parturition and milk letdown during lactation. OT is released during orgasm and ejaculation in humans (Carmichael et al., 1987). OT functions centrally as a neuromodulator, acting at discrete receptor sites throughout the brain on a relatively slow time scale, mediating sociosexual behaviors (Landgraf & Neumann, 2004). In the brain, oxytocin is released both axonally and dendritically from the hypothalamic oxytocinergic neurons targeting a number of distant regions, including the septal region, nucleus accumbens, hippocampus, amygdala, medio-basal hypothalamus, and even the brain stem and spinal cord in rodents (see Figure 34-1) (Ross & Young, 2009) While the innervation of oxytocin fibers is conserved among species, OT receptor (OTR) distribution is highly species-specific, with significant inter- and intraspecies variation that may contribute to the variation in social behavior (Ross et al., 2009).

Vasopressin

Arginine vasopressin (AVP) is an evolutionarily homologous molecule that differs from the structure of OT at only two amino acid positions (See Figure 34-2). Like OT, AVP is also a neurohypophyseal peptide that is synthesized in the magnocellular neurons of the PVN and SON and is released from the posterior pituitary into peripheral circulation. Vasopressin is also released within the brain from neuronal projections arising from the parvocellular neurons of the PVN, the superchiasmatic nucleus, the bed nucleus of the stria terminalis (BNST), and the medial amygdala (MeA; see Figure 34-1; De Vries & Miller, 1998). The vasopressinergic neurons in the BNST and MeA are regulated by androgens, making the AVP system one of the most sexually dimorphic neurotransmitter systems (De Vries & Miller, 1998). Within specific brain regions, like the BNST and MeA, males have significantly more AVP than do females (Van Leeuwn, Caffe, & De Vries, 1985). Peripherally,

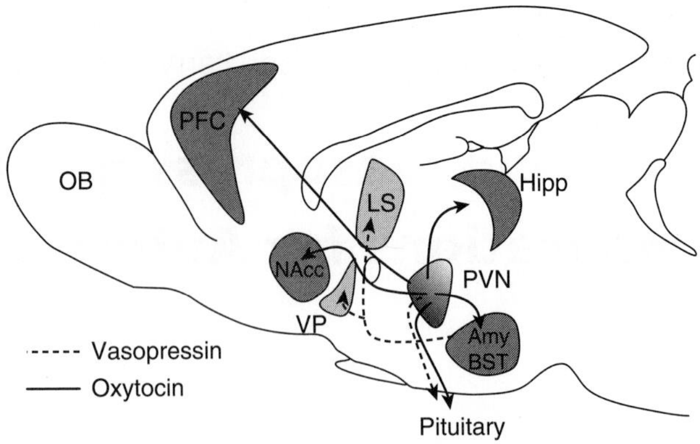

Figure 34–1. Localization of the oxytocin and vasopressin systems. In the prairie vole (*Microtus orchogaster*), oxytocin and vasopressin are synthesized in the paraventricular (PVN) and supraoptic nuclei (SON) of the hypothalamus. These neurons project directly to the pituitary gland for storage and release into the blood stream. In addition, the hypothalamic neurons also project both axonally and dendritically to discrete regions throughout the brain for local release. Oxytocin projections from the PVN and SON target OT receptors in a number of brain regions including the nucleus accumbens (NAcc), hippocampus (Hipp), and amygdala (Amy). Vasopressin from the PVN, the superchiasmatic nucleus of the hypothalamus, Amy, and the bed nucleus of the stria terminalis (BST) is released throughout the brain, primarily targeting V1a and V1b receptors.

AVP plays an important role in maintaining fluid homeostasis and blood pressure. AVP acts at three different receptor subtypes: vasopressin receptor 1a (V1aR), vasopressin receptor 1b (V1bR), and vasopressin receptor 2 (V2R). While all three receptors types are expressed in varying densities in both the brain and the periphery, V1aR is the most widely distributed AVP receptor in the brain and is thought to be the most behaviorally relevant. The V1b receptor is expressed primarily in the pituitary and some restricted brain regions, and the V2 receptor is expressed primarily in the kidney, where it regulates water balance (Caldwell, Wersinger, & Young, 2008). The similarity in structure of the AVP and OT molecules enables each to bind and activate the other's receptor, creating a degree of redundancy in these systems, which complicates the interpretation of experiments using these peptides (Figure 34-2).

Evolutionary Conservation of Neuropeptide Structure and Social Function

The OT and AVP family of neuropeptides have been inextricably linked with social behaviors throughout evolutionary history. Homologues of these peptides have been identified in animals as diverse as hydra, worms, insects, fish, amphibians, birds, and mammals and have been shown to

OT: Cys-Tyr-**Ile**-Gln-Asn-Cys-Pro-**Leu**-Gly-NH_2
AVP: Cys-Tyr-**Phe**-Gln-Asn-Cys-Pro-**Arg**-Gly-NH_2

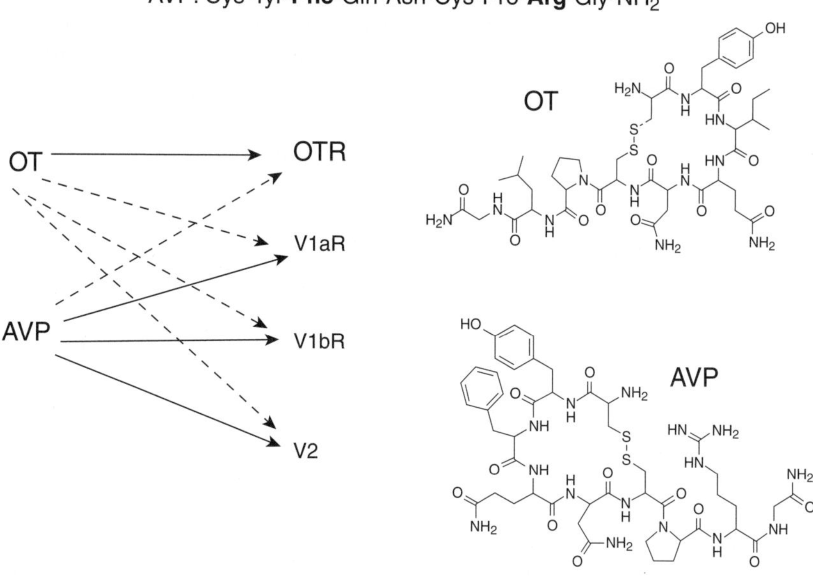

Figure 34–2. Oxytocin and Vasopressin. OT (oxytocin) and AVP (vasopressin) are closely related nine–amino acid peptides. OT has only one known receptor, while AVP binds to three known receptors: AVP-R1a, AVP-R1b, and AVP-R2. However, as the peptides differ at only two amino acids, there is some binding of each peptide at the other's receptor(s). Thus there is some degree of cross-reactivity of both endogenous peptides and in pharmacological studies.

regulate social and reproductive behaviors (Donaldson & Young, 2008). The genes encoding these two molecules are thought to be originally derived from a single common ancestral gene through a gene duplication event early in vertebrate evolution. Arginine vasotocin (AVT), an evolutionary antecedent of AVP, is present in all nonmammalian vertebrates examined to date, and may have been modulating social and reproductive behaviors as early as the Precambrian era, almost 600 million years ago (Acher, 1995). It is thought that the gene encoding AVT underwent duplication in the evolution of early fish approximately 450 million years ago, resulting in a second oxytocin-like peptide, isotocin, that is still present in bony fish. In male goldfish (*Carassius auratus*), both isotocin and vasotocin modulate social approach, and levels of these peptides have been associated with levels of sociality (Thompson & Walton, 2004). Isotocin was replaced by mesotocin during the water-to-land transition and is currently present in amphibians, reptiles, and birds. Mesotocin has been shown to regulate aggression differentially in songbirds, based on the social organization of the species (Goodson, 1998). OT is present in all utherian and protherian mammals and, despite the evolutionary divergence, still only differs from AVT by one amino acid. AVP also arose from a single peptide substitution in AVT in placental mammals. The conservation of the structure and function of these neuropeptides throughout evolution is quite remarkable, and the conservation of regulation of sociosexual behaviors in animals from goldfish to rodents suggests that OT and AVP may also play a role in regulating human social behavior.

Neuropeptides and Their Role in Mammalian Social Behavior

"Social behavior" is a complex term encompassing several different aspects of interaction between conspecifics. To better understand the complexities of social behavior, the social domain can be parsed into discrete, identifiable, and most importantly, analytical components. To be useful for scientific research, each of these components must consist of a specific behavioral phenotype that can be measured in a controlled laboratory setting, and must provide a reflection of the organism's total social repertoire. In both animals and humans, social motivation, social information processing, and social attachment have been indentified as subdomains contributing to the complexity of social behavior (Figure 34-3). The study of each of these components independently simplifies the examination of the biological underpinning of complex social behavior. Here we will examine each of these subdomains separately.

Social Motivation

The motivation to interact with conspecifics is the first step needed to engage in a successful social relationship. Inherent in every social encounter is the possibility of a negative outcome, such as indifference or aggression. Thus, there are strong pressures limiting engagement in social interactions. Social motivation is a measure of desire to overcome these

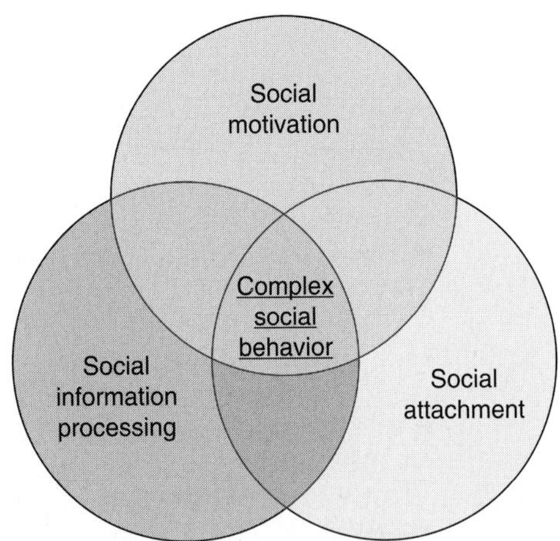

Figure 34–3. A conceptual model of complex social behavior. "Social behavior" is a broad term that encompasses any interaction between two conspecifics. To be able to study the biological mechanisms governing this behavior, it must be broken down into discrete subgroups of behavior that can be measured in a laboratory. Affiliative social behavior is comprised of three subdomains: social motivation, social information processing, and social attachment. Each of these domains contributes to the complexity of social behavior through separate but converging systems. The study of each of these components independently allows for the design and implementation of experiments that can more directly address the mechanisms. Social motivation can be studied through experiments of maternal motivation, social information processing through social recognition paradigms, and social attachment through pair bonding or maternal bonding.

negative factors to actively engage in a social interaction. OT is thought to play a role in enhancing social motivation. One potential mechanism for this is related to its anxiolytic actions. OT has been shown to reduce the behavioral and neuroendocrine responses to social stress enabling an animal to approach and interact with conspecifics. Alternatively, OT may alter the valence of social interactions, making them more rewarding and ultimately promoting social interaction.

In Rodents

In animal models, social motivation can be assessed by measuring behaviors that promote social contact, the latency of the subject to approach another individual and the amount of time spent in social contact with the individual. Social motivation can be measured in adult conspecific, offspring-parent, and parent-offspring interactions. For example, rodent pups emit ultrasonic vocalizations when separated from their nest or mother to protest social isolation. The role of OT in social motivation was examined using this offspring-parent paradigm through the comparison of vocalizations produced by wild type mice and OT knockout (OTKO) mice after separation. OTKO mice emit significantly fewer distress vocalizations than their wild type litter mates (Winslow et al., 2000). In a similar reunion task, where pups are separated from their mothers by a divider with small holes that allow the pups cross though but not the mothers, wild type mice quickly learn to cross through holes to reunite with their mothers while the OTKO mice do not. As both the mutant strain and the wild type strain are able to emit normal vocalizations and show similar locomotor activity, the data suggest that the knockout pups may not find social isolation as distressing or may lack the social motivation to engage in these behaviors.

Initiation of parental behavior, though, represents one of the most dramatic shifts in social motivation, as in many rodent species the female shifts from an aversion to an attraction to infants. Thus, maternal nurturing behavior may be a useful assay for understanding the neurobiology of social motivation. Maternal behavior, which for rodents includes nest building, licking and grooming of pups, and crouching over pups, is induced at the time of labor and parturition (see Figure 34-4). Virgin female rats find pups highly aversive and will avoid or attack them if encountered. Only after the birth of a female's first litter will she be motivated to interact with pups. Though after that moment, for the rest of her life, regardless of reproductive status, she will find all pups highly rewarding and can even be trained to lever press for access to the pups in the same way rats can be trained to work for drugs of abuse (Fleming & Anderson, 1987; Lee, Clancy, & Fleming, 1999). The switch from indifferent to nurturing behavior toward pups is thought to be mediated in part by OT. Lesions of the hypothalamic PVN prior to parturition, which effectively eliminates the brain oxytocin system, prevents the initiation of maternal behavior (Insel & Harbaugh, 1989). Correspondingly, infusion of OTR antagonists into the ventricles of psuedopregnant female rats, attenuates the expression of maternal behavior (Fahrbach, Morrell, & Pfaff, 1985). Specific infusions of the antagonist directly into the medial preoptic area (MPOA) and ventral tegmental area (VTA) also inhibit maternal behavior, indicating that OT in these regions is necessary for the normal expression of maternal behavior (Pedersen, Caldwell, Walkder, Ayers, & Mason, 1994). It was also shown that not only is OT necessary to promote maternal behavior in virgin rodents, but it is sufficient for inducing it. Ventricular injections of OT stimulates maternal behavior in females rats and mice independent of their sexual experience or hormonal state (McCarthy, 1990; Pedersen, Ascher, Monroe, & Prange, 1982).

The hormones of pregnancy are thought to prime the brain's ability to respond to the OT surge experienced at parturition, thus enabling OT to initiate the onset of maternal behavior. OTR expression is increased by changes in estrogen, such that during pregnancy when estrogen levels increase, OTR expression increases in the hypothalamus and preoptic area (Meddle, Bishop, Gkoumassi, Van Leeuwen, & Douglas, 2007). Individual variation in levels of OTR expression in brain regions such as the bed nucleus of the stria terminalis, the amygdala, and the MPOA have been correlated with variation in maternal care (Champagne, Diorio, Sharma, & Meaney, 2001; Francis, Champagne, & Meaney, 2000; Francis, Young, Meaney, & Insel, 2002).

While the switch to maternal care is based on the hormonal changes associated with pregnancy in mice and rats,

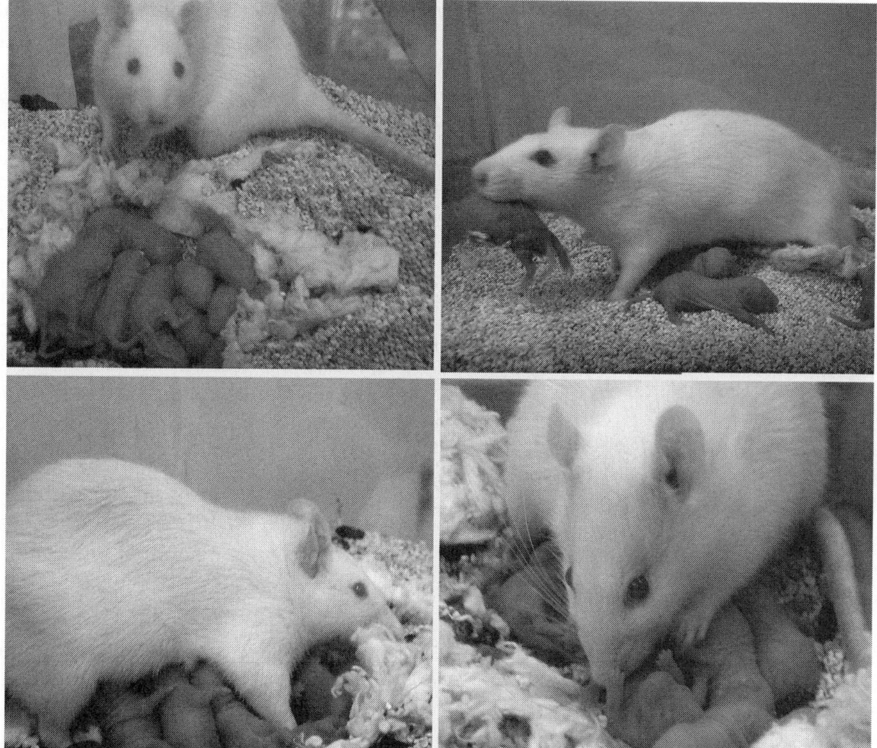

Figure 34–4. Maternal Behavior as a Model for Social Motivation. Maternal behavior for rodents, including rats, consists of nest-building (upper left panel), pup retrieval (upper right panel), crouched nursing (lower left panel), and licking and grooming (lower right panel). Female rats only express maternal behavior after giving birth to their first litter of pups; prior to this experience female rats are indifferent toward pups. This switch in behavior demonstrates the extremes of social motivation.

spontaneous parental behavior exists in other species like the prairie vole (*Microtus ochrogaster*). Prairie voles are highly social, monogamous rodents that display both biparental and alloparental behavior. Female prairie voles display spontaneous juvenile parental behavior in which nonreproductively active adolescent voles provide care for successive sibling litters (Solomon, 1991). This parental behavior recedes in approximately 50% of females once they reach sexual maturity. Spontaneous alloparental behavior is also thought to be OT dependent, as injections of OTR antagonist directly into the nucleus accumbens, an area of the brain that mediates reward and reinforcement, blocks the expression in adult nulliparious females (Olazabal & Young, 2006a). The expression of spontaneous alloparental behavior in both juvenile and adult prairie voles is positively correlated with the density of OTR binding in the nucleus accumbens (See Figure 34-5) (Olazabal & Young, 2006a, 2006b). Juvenile females with high levels of OTR binding show more time spent crouching over pups than those with low levels (Olazabal & Young, 2006b). Viral vector upregulation of OTR in the nucleus accumbens of adult female prairie voles, though, is not sufficient to increase the expression of spontaneous care, however it is sufficient to accelerate social bond formation (Ross et al., 2009). This suggests that the developmental influence of OTR in the nucleus accumbens, as opposed to simply receptor number in adulthood, may regulate this behavior.

As a biparental species, male prairie voles are also highly motivated to care for pups, unlike mice, rats, and nonmonogamous meadow voles. In males, it is thought that parental behavior is mediated by the AVP system. Injection of a V1aR antagonist prevents the expression of paternal care. Infusions of AVP into the lateral septum of male prairie voles increases time spent crouching over and licking and grooming pups (Wang, Ferris, & De Vries, 1994). Similar to the relationship between OTR levels in females and maternal behavior patterns, expression patterns of the V1aR corresponds to paternal behavior, in the form of licking and grooming of pups (Hammock & Young, 2006).

In Humans

Reduced social motivation is one of the defining and most debilitating features of ASD. The expression of social withdrawal is a dimension of diagnostic instruments, like the Aberrant Behavior Checklist. This makes characterization of the neurobiological mechanisms underlying this behavior central to developing novel treatment strategies for autism. Normal social motivation in humans, like in rodents, has been

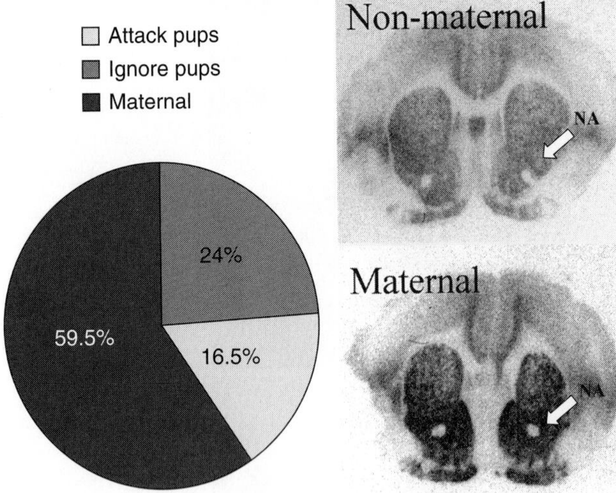

Figure 34–5. Variation in Maternal Behavior in Prairie Voles. Unlike mice or rats, about half of all virgin female prairie voles show spontaneous alloparental behavior. The expression of this behavior is positively correlated with the density of OTR in the nucleus accumbens (NA). Autoradiographic binding of brain sections shows high levels of receptors in maternal animals (lower panel). Adapted with permission from Olazabal, D. E., & Young, L. J. (2006a). Oxytocin receptors in the nucleus accumbens facilitate "spontaneous" maternal behavior in adult female prairie voles. *Neuroscience*, *141*(2), 559–568.

studied in mother-infant interactions. It has been suggested, though not directly shown, that OT influences some aspects of human maternal behavior. OT is released peripherally during the initiation of labor, the early postpartum period, and breastfeeding in human mothers (Carmichael et al., 1987; McNeilly, Robinson, Houston, & Howie, 1983; Nissen, Lilja, Widstrom, & Unvas-Moberg, 1995; Vasicka, Kumaresan, Han, & Kumaresan, 1978). About one third of women also see a spike in peripheral OT levels late in their third trimester of pregnancy, which interestingly has been correlated with higher ratings of maternal-infant bonding (Levine, Zagoory-Sharon, Feldman, & Weller, 2007). Maternal behavior in humans, though, is not entirely mediated by hormonal changes, as spontaneous parental behavior can be seen in families with adopted children. Despite this correlational evidence, precise role of OT in modulating maternal responsiveness in humans remains unknown.

Social Information Processing

After the initiation of interaction, social recognition and social memory are critical for stable functioning in social groups. Social memory, which enables an individual to distinguish between family, friends, and foes, and behave accordingly, is dependent on the processing of social information. The social impairments of autism are associated with deficits in face identity recognition and facial expression perception (Schultz, 2005). The ability to recognize individuals in animal models, referred to as social recognition, has been used to examine the neural mechanisms underlying social memory and social information processing.

In Rodents

Humans and other nonhuman primates primarily depend on visual and auditory cues to recognize conspecifics. Rodents, however, while employing similar mechanisms for discrimination, use an alternative modality; relying on olfactory and pheromonal cues to detect and recognize familiar individuals. Research into this field has shown that both OT and AVP are involved in the encoding and recall of olfactory-cued social memories. Social recognition can be modeled experimentally in rodents by utilizing their natural interest in novelty. Rats and mice will generally spend more time investigating a novel object or animal than a familiar one. To experimentally assay social recognition, an animal is allowed to investigate a conspecific for a period of time, thus becoming familiar with the animal. The animal is then reexposed to either the same familiar animal or a novel animal, and the amount of time the test animal spends sniffing the stimulus animal is measured (Ferguson, Young, Hearn, Insel, & Winslow, 2000). Typically, over multiple exposures to the same animal the amount of investigatory time will decrease and this is interpreted as recognition of the stimulus animal. If a novel animal is then introduced, the test animal should return to their original levels of investigation. Manipulations that disrupt social recognition will be reflected in a constant investigation time over multiple trials. OT enhances social recognition. OT infused into the olfactory bulbs (OB), lateral septum (LS) and medial preoptic area (MPOA) of male rats prolongs the duration of the social recognition response (Dluzen, Muraoka, Engelmann, & Landgraf, 1998). The generation of oxytocin knockout (OTKO) mice has provided an eloquent model for assessing the role of OT in social memory. Male OTKO mice are unable to recognize familiar conspecifics following a prolonged encounter (Ferguson et al., 2000). In OTKO mice, a novel female stimulus mouse elicits the same amount of olfactory investigatory behavior, as does a familiar mouse after multiple exposures, whereas control mice show a decrease in olfactory investigation of familiar individuals (See Figure 34-6). This deficit does not represent an impairment in either nonsocial sensory or memory processes, as the OTKO mice are able to discriminate between nonsocial scents. This suggests that the impairments of OTKO mice are specific to the recognition of socially important cues (Ferguson et al., 2000). Anatomical studies of c-Fos expression, a marker of neuronal activity, show that OTKO mice have decreased activation in the medial amygdala following a social encounter (see Figure 34-7). Furthermore, OT injection into the medial amygdala (MeA), but not into the olfactory bulb of OTKO mice restores social recognition. Complementarily, application of an OTR antagonist only to the MeA inhibits social recognition in wild type mice (Ferguson, Aldagm, Insel, & Young, 2001). The rescue effect of OT in OTKO mice is only effective if it is injected prior to initial encounter. This suggests OT may function in the processing of social information or memory acquisition rather than in social memory recall.

The AVP system has also been shown to play a significant role in mediating social recognition. Intracerebroventricular injection of AVP prolongs social recognition by activating the V1aR in the LS and in the OB. Site-specific injection of AVP into the LS enhances social recognition, while V1aR antagonist administration inhibits social recognition (Dantzer, Koob, Bluthe, & Moal, 1988). Downregulation of the V1aR through the use of antisense oligonucleotides reduces social recognition in normal rats (Landgraf et al., 1995). Conversely, upregulation of the V1aR using viral vector gene transfer enhances the duration of the animals' social recognition memory. Recently, the V1b receptors have also been implicated in mediating social recognition. Both V1aR and V1bR knockout mice show impairments in social memory. Characterization of the deficits in social recognition of V1bRKO mice, though, suggests they are more mild than in the V1aRKO and may be primarily due to deficits of social motivation. The mice can differentiate between male and female urine, but do not spend more time investigating the scent of the opposite sexed animal, thus behaving in a highly

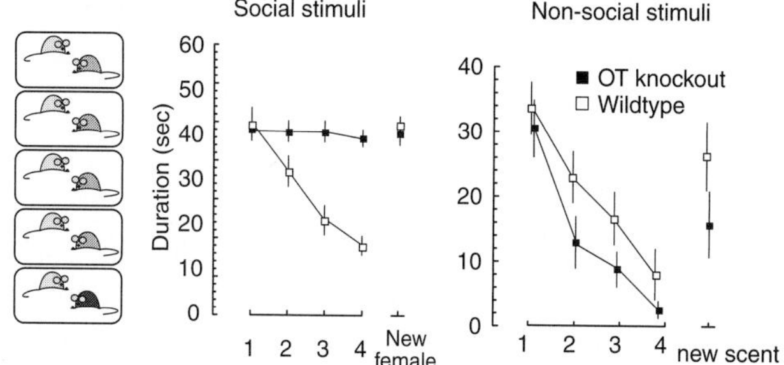

Figure 34–6. Social Amnesia in OTKO Mice. In Wild-Type Mice, Repeated Exposure to the Same Stimulus Animal Results in Decreased Duration of Olfactory Investigation. When Presented with a Novel Stimulus Animal, the Amount of Olfactory Investigation Returns to the Same Levels as Seen During the First Trial of Investigation of the Original Animal. In the OTKO Mice there is No Decrease in Investigation of the Stimulus Animal Over Multiple Trials. In Olfactory Investigation of a Nonsocial, Citrus Scent, though, both the Wild-Type and the OTKO Mice Both Show Decreased Investigation of the Odor, Indicating that the Deficits of the OTKO Mice are Specific to the Processing of Social Stimuli. Reprinted with Permission from Ferguson, J. N., Young, L. J., Hearn, E. F., Insel, T. R., & Winslow, J. T. (2000). Social Amnesia in Mice Lacking the Oxytocin Gene. *Nature Genetics, 25*, 284–288.

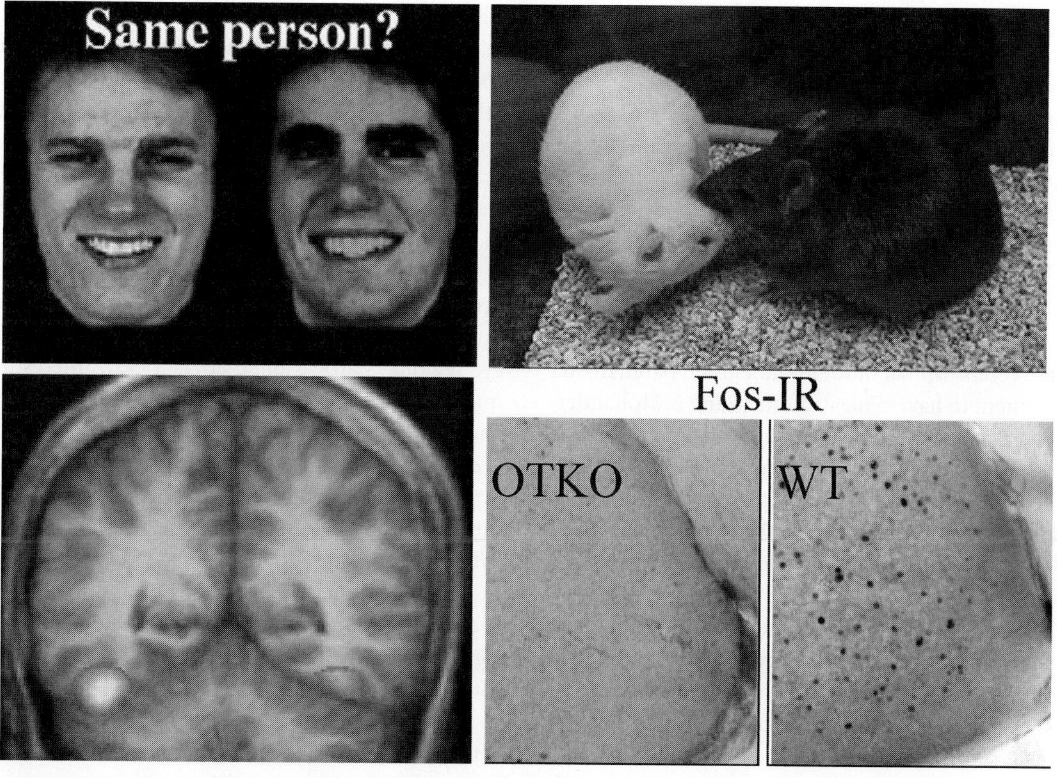

Figure 34–7. Social Information Processing in Humans and Rodents. Individuals with autism show reductions in the activation of the fusiform face area, a structure regulated by amygdala activation, as measured by fMRI, when viewing human faces compared to controls (Left Panel). Analogously, OTKO mice show reduced activity of the medial amygdala in response to olfactory investigation, as evidenced by the expression of c-Fos (a neuronal marker of activity), compared with wild-type mice (Right Panel). Adapted with permission from Schultz, R. T. (2005). Developmental deficits in social perception in autism: The role of the amygdala and the fusiform face area. *International Journal of Developmental Neuroscience, 23*(2–3), 125–141, and Ferguson, J. N., Aldagm, J. M., Insel, T. R., & Young, L. J. (2001). Oxytocin in the medial amygdala is essential for social recognition in the mouse. *Journal of Neuroscience*, *21*, 8278–8285. (See Color Plate Section for a color version of this figure.)

species atypical fashion. Thus, they can discriminate the odors but are not motivated to further investigate scents of sociosexual importance (Caldwell et al., 2008).

In Humans

The significant body of evidence linking OT with social recognition in rodents has spurred a number of studies looking at the effects of OT on face-processing in humans. A number of caveats exist in translating research on social behavior in rodents to humans, primarily related to how social information is differentially processed between the species. Social cognition in humans involves far more cortical processes than in rodents. Human social behavior is based on an integration of the visual and auditory systems with executive cortical regions, while in rodents the sensory systems are primarily connected to the limbic system. It is possible that the neuropeptides play a strong modulatory role in mediating olfactory or limbic responses and consequently may have less of an effect on human social behavior (Hammock & Young, 2006). However, it is likely that OT and AVP modulate the circuitry involved in processing of visual and auditory social information in humans analogously to its role in rodents (Domes, Heinrichs, Michel, Berger, & Herpertz, 2007; Guastella, Mitchell, & Dadds, 2008; Meyer-Lindenberg, 2008).

Research into the function of OT and AVP in the brains of humans is in its infancy and is limited in the types of experiments that can be undertaken. As a result, scientists are just coming to understand the role of neuropeptides in human social cognition. Currently, the most effective technique for studying the direct functional effects of the neuropeptides in the brain is through intranasal administration of the peptides. OT and AVP have low penetrance across the blood-brain barrier and consequently have limited efficacy when administered peripherally. However, it is thought that intranasally administered peptides are transported directly across the nasal mucosa to the cerebrospinal fluid, into the brain parenchyma thus allowing them to have central effects (Bartz & Hollander, 2008). To date, only one study has physiologically demonstrated the efficacy of this route of administration. In humans, AVP was shown to increase in CSF within 10 minutes after intranasal administration and remain elevated for at least 80 minutes (Born et al., 2002). Thus far, the equivalent study has not been done for OT.

Several recent studies have linked the functional effects of the neuropeptides with cognitive processes associated with social recognition and social information processing. Intranasal OT has been shown to enhance face recognition and interpretation of facial expression (Domes et al., 2007; Rimmele, Hediger, Heinrichs, & Klaver, 2009). OT administration preferentially enhanced memory of faces over memory of nonsocial stimuli (Rimmele et al., 2009). OT may also play a role in social memory consolidation as it has been shown to enhance memory for previously seen faces when administered after viewing the faces (Savaskan, Ernhardt, Schulz, Walter, & Schachinger, 2008). OT has even been shown to enhance emotional perception as seen in a test of "mind reading," a paradigm that requires individuals to infer the emotion of stimulus faces, by viewing images of only the eye regions (Domes et al., 2007). These findings are likely due to OT's ability to enhance facial and emotional recognition by increasing the amount of time an individual spends looking at the eye region of a conspecific (Guastella, Mitchell, & Mathews, 2008). OT also regulates social stimuli perception by modulating amygdala function in humans. Functional imaging studies have shown that strong amygdala activation is induced by fear-inducing visual stimuli. Administration of intranasal OT potently reduces the activation of the amygdala in response to these stimuli (Kirsch et al., 2005). Interestingly, fMRI studies have shown that application of intranasal OT specifically decreases the activation of the right amygdala typically associated with emotional facial recognition (Domes et al., 2007).

Individuals with ASD appear to have deficits in social recognition that are reminiscent of those seen in OTKO mice. Individuals with autism can identify faces in relation to basic objects; however, they do show impairments when asked to match unfamiliar faces on tests like the Benton Face Recognition Test (Barton, 2003; Davies, Bishop, Manstead, & Tantam, 1994). They also show deficits in perceiving facial expression, age, and sex (Hobson, 1987; Tantam, Monaghan, Nicholson, & Stirling, 1989). Patients with Turner's syndrome, which has a high comorbidity with autism, also show deficits in recognizing faces and facial expressions (Lawrence et al., 2003). This deficit may, in part, be attributed to decreased activation in the amygdala and the fusiform face area, the areas typically involved in face recognition, and increased activation of cortical regions when viewing images of human faces compared to normal subjects (Critchley et al., 2000; Pierce, Müller, Ambrose, Allen, & Courchesne, 2001; Schultz et al., 2000). Individuals with autism also fail to show amygdala activation typically seen in control subjects, when asked to interpret the expressions of face stimuli while viewing human eye regions (Baron-Cohen et al., 1999). Interestingly, OTKO mice show a similar pattern of decreased amygdala activation and increased cortical recruitment in social recognition tasks (Ferguson et al., 2001).

Currently only a limited number of studies have looked at the effects of AVP on human social information processing. Intranasal AVP modulates the perception of facial expression in a sexually dimorphic fashion. In animals, AVP modulates social communication, particularly the production of social signals involved in courtship and aggression. In human males, intranasal AVP modulates facial expressions in response to social stimuli. AVP administration in men decreases the perception of friendliness in unfamiliar male faces and stimulates the production of antagonistic facial expressions. However in females, the opposite effect is observed; AVP increases the perception of friendliness in female faces and stimulates affiliative facial motor patterns in response to those faces (Thompson, George, Walton, Orr, & Benson, 2006). It is possible that this dimorphic effect is due to the opposing strategies adopted by men and women to handle stressful social situations.

Social Attachment

Social bonding is a complex social behavior that requires social motivation and social information processing to develop an enduring attachment. A social bond is apparent when individuals demonstrate a preference for interaction with a specific conspecific. Impairments in social motivation and social information processing in individuals with autism likely contribute to difficulty in forming normal social relationships. The study of social attachment in animal models allows for the investigation of the neurobiological mechanisms underlying the attachment process and may be relevant to many types of social relationships. Two animal models have contributed significantly to our understanding of the neurobiological mechanisms underlying attachment, pair bonding in the prairie vole and maternal-infant bonding in sheep. Each of these models is discussed in detail below.

In Voles

The genus *Microtus* (voles) is an ideal model for the comparative study of social attachment as it contains both monogamous (prairie and pine voles) and polygamous (meadow and montane voles) species. Prairie and pine voles are highly social, monogamous animals that form long-lasting social bonds with a specific partner. In contrast, meadow and montane voles are asocial and polygamous, with males and females coming together only to mate. One difference between these species that contributes to their highly divergent social systems is the organization of their OT and AVP systems.

Because of the important role that OT plays in mother-infant relationships, the peptide was hypothesized to mediate pair bonding in prairie voles. OT infusions into the brains of female prairie voles induce pair bonds as measured by the development of a partner preference (See Figure 34-8) under conditions nonconducive to bond formation (Williams, Harbough, & Carter, 1994). Complementarily, application of an OTR antagonist intracerebroventricularly prevents the formation of social bonds even after long cohabitation periods with mating (Williams et al., 1994). Central OT receptor manipulation was able to directionally modulate social bond formation without having any impact on sexual behavior. These data suggest that the species differences in the ability to form a social bond between mates may be attributed to differences in the OT system. The distribution of OT fibers throughout the brain is well conserved throughout mammalian

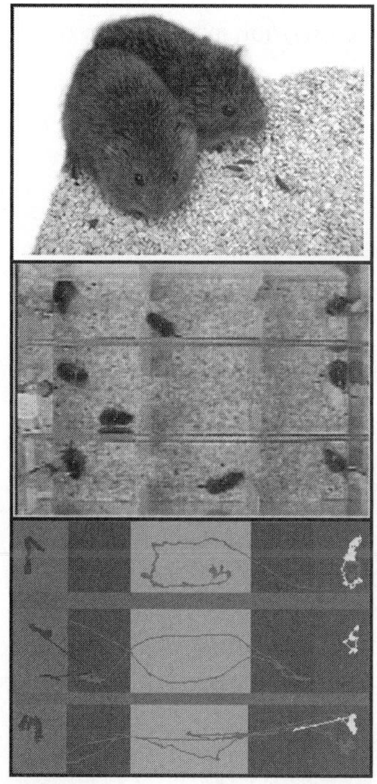

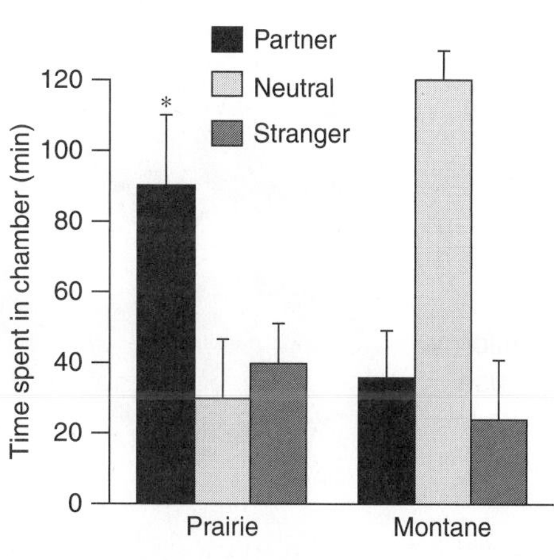

Figure 34–8. Partner Preference Test. Social attachment in prairie voles is measured using the partner preference test. In this behavioral test a male is paired with an unfamiliar female vole and allowed to cohabitate for a period of time (Upper Panel). The pair is then separated, and the partner female is tethered in the partner preference apparatus along with a stranger female. The male is then placed in the apparatus and allowed to wander freely for 3 hours (Middle Panel). The amount of time the male spends with either the partner female or the stranger female is recorded and analyzed using behavior analysis software (Lower Panel). If the male is shown to have spent twice as much time with the partner female than with the stranger female, he is said to have formed a partner preference. Partner preference is a marker of social attachment. Prairie voles easily form a partner preference after about 24 hours of cohabitation. Montane voles, however, fail to show a preference for their partner after as much as 2 weeks of cohabitation. (See Color Plate Section for a color version of this figure.)

species and both prairie and meadow voles have similar patterns of OT in the brain. There is, however, striking variation in the distribution of the OTR between the prairie and the meadow vole. Prairie voles have a significantly higher density of OTR in the caudate putamen and the nucleus accumbens than do the polygamous species. Application of OTR antagonists directly to the nucleus accumbens inhibits mating induced partner preference, implicating the accumbens particularly as a site necessary for pair bonding (Young, Lim, Gingrich, & Insel, 2001).

In males, OT plays a lesser role in pair bond formation (Liu, Curtis, & Wang, 2001). Instead AVP has primarily been implicated in mediating pair bonding. AVP's effect on male pair bonding parallels the role of OT in females, in that centrally infused AVP facilitates partner preference (without mating) while a V1aR antagonist inhibits mating-induced partner preference (Winslow, Hastings, Carter, Harbaugh, & Insel, 1993). Like OT, vasopressin innervation is consistent across mammalian species with dramatic differences in receptor densities apparently mediating inter and intraspecies variation (Wang, Zhou, Hulihan, & Insel, 1996). Considerable variation in the distribution of V1aR in the brain is seen between prairie and meadow voles, with higher densities of the receptor in the ventral pallidum in the monogamous voles. The ventral pallidum is a major efferent of the nucleus accumbens, and like the accumbens, mediates reward and reinforcement. Interestingly, the difference in receptor distribution between monogamous and polygamous species of voles is mirrored in other closely related species that have similar social organizations of other species of rodents and even in some nonhuman primates. For example, the monogamous marmoset has higher densities of V1aR in the ventral forebrain reward areas than do nonmonogamous rhesus macaques (see Figure 34-9) (Young, 1999). Despite the variation in receptor densities between the two microtine species, there are no species differences in the functional mechanics of the V1aR between the montane and prairie voles, and the protein coding region of the V1aR gene (*avpr1a*) is 99% genetically identical (Insel, Wang, & Ferris, 1994; Young, Nilsen, Waymire, MacGregor, & Insel, 1999). This implicated the promoter region of the gene encoding the V1aR (*avpr1a*) in the differential expression of the receptor and the subsequent differences in both paternal care and social bonding. Transgenic mice containing the regulatory region of prairie vole *avpr1* gene show a receptor expression profile very similar to that of prairie voles (Young et al., 1999). Furthermore, if these mice are given an injection of AVP they showed an increase in affiliative behavior. This led to comparison of the regulatory regions between prairie voles and montane voles. The prairie vole promoter region at the *avpr1a* locus contains a microsatellite element that consists of a repetitive sequence upstream of the transcriptional start site that is largely absent from the meadow vole. The differences in the microsatellite region, therefore, may in part regulate the species differences in receptor expression. Within prairie voles there is also great degree of variation in the density of V1aR expression in specific

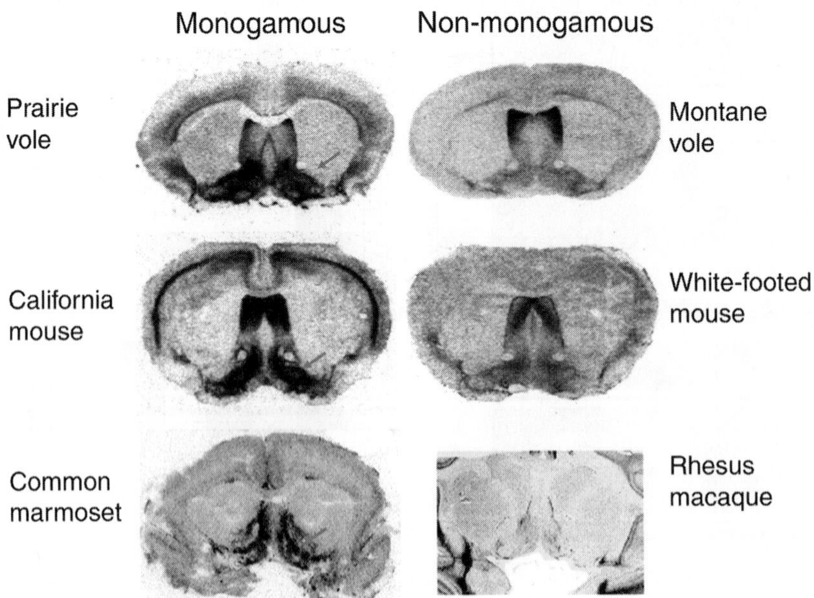

Figure 34–9. Distribution of V1aR in Monogamous and Nonmonogamous Species. The pattern of higher V1aR expression in the ventral pallidum of the prairie vole than in the montane vole is mirrored in several other species, including the monogamous California mouse and the closely related promiscuous white-footed mouse. This pattern is even seen in some primate species, with the monogamous marmoset showing higher levels of V1aR in the ventral forebrain than the nonmonogamous rhesus macaque. Reprinted with permission from Young, L. J. (1999). Frank A. Beach Award. Oxytocin and vasopressin receptors and species typical social behaviors. *Hormones and Behavior, 36*(3), 212–221.

brains regions, including the olfactory bulb, extended amygdala, thalamus, cingulate cortex, and the ventral pallidum. Furthermore, there is significant variation in the length of the repetitive microsatellite among individual prairie voles. To determine whether variation in the length of the microsatellite contributed to variation in V1aR expression and social behavior, two lines of prairie voles were generated, one with a long microsatellite repeat and one with the short repeat (Hammock & Young, 2005). The resulting animals had robust differences in V1aR expression in the brain, with the long-alleled animals showing greater expression in olfactory bulb and the lateral septum but with lower levels in the amygdala and the hippocampus than the short-alleled animals. Long-alleled male prairie voles also displayed a shorter latency to approach and investigate a novel juvenile male and developed partner preferences more quickly than short-alleled animals (Hammock & Young, 2005). These data suggest that the microsatellite polymorphism in the 5' regulatory region of the *avpr1a* gene alters the expression of the receptor throughout the brain and that the distribution of the receptor influences social behavior. The relationship between receptor density in specific brain regions and prosocial behavior was further tested by overexpressing the V1aR in the ventral pallidum of nonmonogamous meadow voles. Upregulation of the V1aR in the ventral pallidum enhances partner preference in prairie voles and can even induce partner preferences in nonmonogamous meadow voles (see Figure 34-10; Lim et al., 2004). Thus demonstrating that simply by increasing the density of receptors in a single brain region, social behavior can be radically changed.

In Sheep

Maternal-infant bonding in sheep has been used as a model to identify the mechanisms involved in social attachment as well. Unlike rodents, which are typically promiscuously maternal, ewes form a strong selective bond for their own lamb. Sheep live in large social groups and are constantly moving while they graze. They are synchronous breeders, which means many young are born in the herd at the same time, and they birth precocial young who are able to stand and run shortly after birth. These features require that ewes form a strong

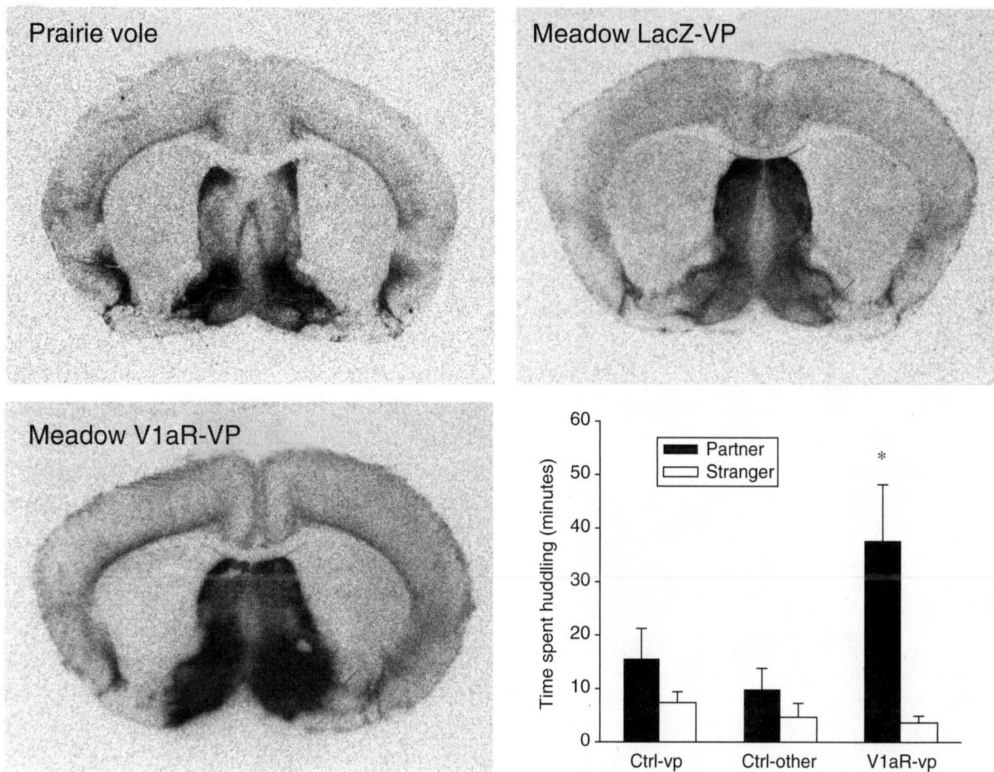

Figure 34–10. V1aR Gene Transfer in Meadow Voles. The monogamous male prairie vole shows high expression of the V1aR in the ventral pallidum (Upper Left Panel), which corresponds to high levels of partner preference. To induce the ability to form social attachments in the polygamous male meadow vole the V1aR was upregulated by the injection of a viral vector containing the *avpr1a* gene. When injected into a specific brain region the viral vector induces the production of its gene product, in this case causing the increased expression of the V1aR (Lower Left Panel). Upregulation of the V1aR but not a control molecule, LacZ (Upper Right Panel), induced partner preference in the male meadow vole (Lower Right Panel). Reprinted with permission from Lim, M. M., Wang, Z., Olazabal, D. E., Ren, X., Terwilliger, E. F., & Young, L. J. (2004). Enhanced partner preference in a promiscuous species by manipulating the expression of a single gene. *Nature, 429*(6993), 754–757.

selective bond shortly after birth to prevent the lamb from being lost (see Figure 34-11; Kendrick et al., 1997). Bond formation, like maternal behavior, in ewes is induced by the hormonal changes associated with pregnancy and the physiological feedback associated with labor and delivery. Ewes become maternal immediately after birth, and within a couple of hours postpartum they become selectively maternal toward one lamb and will allow only their own lamb to nurse. Vagino-cervical stimulation (VCS) can induce a ewe to accept an unfamiliar lamb even after she has bonded with her own lamb. Epidural anesthesia prevents VCS from inducing maternal bonding (Levy, Kendrick, Keverne, Piketty, & Poindron, 1992). OT infusion alone induces acceptance of an unfamiliar lamb even in a nonpregnant ewe (Kendrick, Keverne, & Baldwin, 1987). It is thought that in sheep VCS, which occurs naturally during parturition, sends sensory signals through the spinal cord to the PVN, which then releases large amounts of OT into the circulation and throughout the brain. OT release in limbic structures facilitates the onset of maternal nurturing behavior, while OT infusion in the olfactory bulb induces a reorganization resulting in selective responsiveness to their own lamb's odor. The specific odor of the lamb is encoded through plastic changes in the olfactory bulb that are permitted by OT and mediated by the neurotransmitters GABA and glutamate (Kendrick et al., 1997). In humans, selective kin recognition is primarily mediated by visual input, but remarkably it has also been reported that women are able to recognize the smell of their infant within hours of giving birth, suggesting a potentially conserved mechanism (Porter, Cernock, & McLaughlin, 1983).

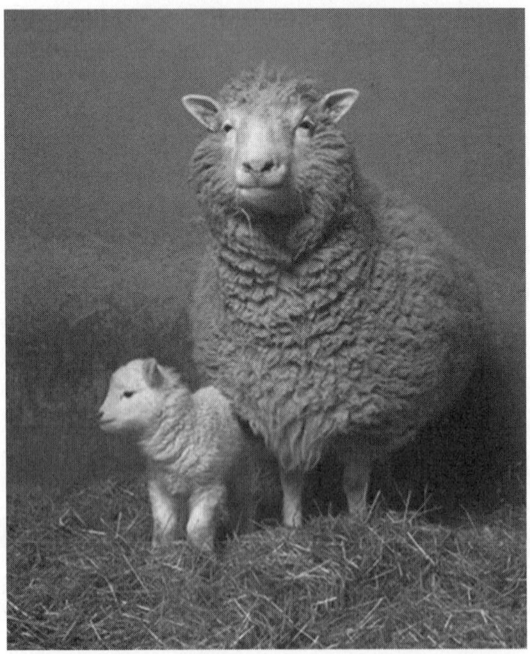

Figure 34–11. Maternal Infant Bonding in Sheep. Maternal bonding in sheep is a model of social attachment. Ewes form a strong selective bond specific for their own lamb soon after parturition. It is particularly important that the ewe learn to recognize their lamb, as sheep are synchronous breeders that give birth to precocial young, which prevents kin identification by proximity. The formation of this selective bond is dependent on OT. Photo courtesy of Keith Kendricks.

In Humans

Preliminary research in humans is consistent with the animal studies mentioned above and suggests that the OT and AVP systems may also be involved in human social attachments. Functional magnetic resonance imaging has shown there is a high degree of overlap between the distribution of OT receptors in the human brain and the regions of brain activation when viewing images of romantic partners or mothers viewing images of their infants (Bartels & Zeki, 2004). Plasma levels of OT have also been shown to increase in both males and females during sexual activity and intercourse (Blaicher et al., 1999; Carmichael et al., 1987; Uvnas-Moberg, 1998). As the most intense form of social contact, sexual intercourse is also likely to be the stimulus for OT release in the brain (Neumann, 2008). Women with high levels of OT report the occurrence of nonsexual tactile interaction between partners, like massage or hugging, at greater frequency than those with lower levels (Light, Grewen, & Amico, 2005). Perceived partner support has also been associated with higher levels of OT in both men and women (Grewen, Girdler, Amico, & Light, 2005). Conversely, negative social experiences, like early life abuse or neglect, result in decreased levels of OT in the CSF. OT levels are negatively correlated with the number and duration of abuses (Heim et al., 2008).

The opposite relationship was seen though, in associations between reports on relationship quality and levels of OT. Basal plasma levels of OT were negatively correlated with living situations, marriage quality, physical affection, and communication (Taylor et al., 2006; Turner, Altemus, Enos, Cooper, & McGuinness, 1999). However, it should be noted that plasma levels of neuropeptide should be interpreted with caution since peptides are released into the periphery and into the brain independently, and circulating peptides do not cross the blood-brain barrier.

A recent study demonstrated an association between a microsatellite element in the 5' flanking region of the human *avpr1a* gene, similar to the microsatellite seen in prairie voles, and several traits indicative of pair bonding behavior in men. One particular allele was associated with marital status, perceived marital problems, and even marital quality as perceived by their spouses. As would be predicted by the animal research, no association was found between women and this locus (Walum et al., 2008). This study provides remarkable evidence of a conserved mechanism regulating social cognition in rodents and man.

In humans, both neuropeptides may also promote interpersonal relationships by increasing perceptions of trust and altruism. The aforementioned microsatellite polymorphism of the human *avpr1a* gene has also been linked to prosocial behavior. Individuals with the short allele (308–325bp) are less generous in the Dictator game, an economic game of altruistic decision making, than those with the long allele (Knafo et al., 2008). In a similar game, intranasal OT was found to promote trust behavior, in that subjects that had received the peptide shared more money with their social partner than those that had not, even after being cheated by their social partner (Kosfeld, Heinrichs, Zak, Fischbacher, & Fehr, 2005).

Evidence for Disregulation of Neuropeptides Systems in Autism Spectrum Disorders

Genetic Evidence

It is clear that OT and AVP play a central role in the regulation of complex social behaviors. This, coupled with the high heritability of autism, has led many researchers to look at the possible link between mutations of the neuropeptides systems and ASD. To date several genetic association studies have implicated the OTR and V1aR in the etiology of autism. The human OTR is encoded by a 19 kbp gene located on chromosome 3p25 containing three introns and four exons (Inoue et al., 1994). Two genomewide scans have highlighted the 3p25 region as a linkage site for ASD (Lauritsen et al., 2006; McCauley et al., 2005). Four studies to date have found a positive association of the OTR gene with autism in three distinct populations. A study of the Chinese Han trios demonstrated an association between ASD and two single nucleotide polymorphisms (rs2254298 and rs53576) and several haplotypes involving one of the sites (Wu et al., 2005). A second study by Jacob et al. (2007) looked at whether these associations replicated in a Caucasian population and verified the association at the rs2254298 site. The two studies found overtransmission of opposing alleles in the affected population, the G allele in the Caucasian population and the A allele in the Chinese population. A third comprehensive association study was undertaken by Israel et al. (2008) of an Israeli population looking at all of the known labeled SNPs across the OTR gene region and found a strong association between a five locus haplotype block including the site found in both previous studies and ASD. This group also showed an association with IQ and daily living skills with SNPs in the OTR gene, suggesting this gene may play a role in other disorders and nonclinical populations (Israel et al., 2008). These findings reinforced the work done by Lerer et al. (2008), which showed similar association of ASD with specific loci in the OXTR gene in the Israeli population, as well as associations with IQ and the Vineland Adaptive Behavior Scales, a clinical measure of personal and social skills. The association of the OXTR gene with ASD found in the aforementioned targeted studies was also seen by Yrigollen et al. in a study of genes associated with affiliative behavior as candidate genes for autism (Yrigollen et al., 2008).

Single-subject cases have also implicated the OTR gene in the etiology of autism. A unique case study of a 9-year-old boy with pervasive developmental disorder was found to have a duplication of the chromosome region containing the OTR gene resulting in a 2- to 3-fold increase of OTR expression compared to control subjects (Bittel, Kibiryeva, Dasouki, Knoll, & Butler, 2006). The oxytocin gene has also been implicated in autism in a case study in which a child with Asperger's syndrome was found to have a 1.1Mb deletion of 20p13 a region with involves ~27 genes including the OT peptide gene (Bittel et al., 2006; Sebat et al., 2007).

Associations have also been made between the *avpr1a* gene and autism. In humans, the *avpr1a* gene located on chromosome 12q14-15, contains three microsatellite regions in the 5' flanking and one in the single intron, analogous to but different from the vole polymorphisms. Two microsatellites, RS1 and RS3, have been the focus of much investigation due to their highly polymorphic number of repeats. Three independent groups have found a possible link between polymorphisms in the *avpr1a* gene and autism. Studies have shown linkage disequilibrium between autism and the RS3 microsatellite in the *avpr1a* gene (Kim, 2001; Wassink et al., 2004; Yirmiya et al., 2006). The microsatellites in humans, as in voles, have been shown to have functional consequences. The number of microsatellite repeats in both the RS1 and RS3 sites is shown to have an effect on amygdala activity in response to fear stimuli. The long allele of the RS3 site is associated with extremely high levels of amygdala activation in response to the stimuli (Meyer-Lindenberg et al., 2008), which is particularly interesting as autistic individuals have been shown to have abnormal amygdala activation in fMRI studies (Dalton et al., 2005). The long RS3 allele has also been associated with higher levels of the *avpr1a* mRNA in human postmortem hippocampal tissue than the short RS3 allele, similar to what is seen in the vole literature (Knafo et al., 2008). Despite these numerous studies, there is no evidence that genetic variation in the OTR or V1aR genes are a major contributor to ASD. Rather, they suggest that variation in these genes may be one of many contributing factors in some small fraction of ASD cases.

Peripheral Evidence

Children with autism have been observed to have lower levels of peripheral OT in plasma than age-matched controls. Within the control group, levels of OT were found to be positively correlated with measures of social behavior including socialization, social coping, and interpersonal relationships. Unexpectedly, in the autistic group the lower baseline levels of OT were negatively correlated with these same measures of social behavior (Modahl et al., 1998). This difference could be the result of differential processing of OT in the brains of children with autism, as plasma samples of autistic children were also found to have higher levels of OT precursors as well as a higher ratio of OT precursor to OT (Green et al., 2001). These findings were replicated in a second independent study that also found autistic children to have lower peripheral levels of vasopressin (Al-Ayadhi, 2005). In adults the findings appear to be reversed, as individuals with ASD have higher plasma levels of OT compared to controls (Jansen et al., 2006). There is no apparent reason to account for the discrepancy in findings between the groups, suggesting there may be a developmental compensatory mechanism. However, it is important to note that peripheral levels of oxytocin and vasopressin do not necessarily reflect central levels (Bartz & Hollander, 2006).

Implications for Developing Pharmacological Therapies

Given the role of OT and AVP in modulating social motivation, social information processing, and social attachment, these systems may be viable targets for treating the social deficits associated with ASD. Indeed, some very preliminary studies have suggested that OT infusion may have positive effects in ASD patients, but more work is needed to draw any conclusions. Hollander et al. (2003) investigated the role of intravenous OT administration on the inhibition of repetitive behavior, one of the other core symptoms of ASD. A continuous 4-hour treatment with the Pitocin, a synthetic oxytocin, was found to significantly decrease repetitive behaviors over time as compared to placebo. A similar procedure was then used to look at the effect of OT on social cognition as assayed by a test of affective speech comprehension. Subjects who received the peptide prior to the first trial were shown to have enhanced retention of speech comprehension 2 weeks later compared to those who received it prior to the second trial. The study did, however, fail to observe a direct effect of OT on performance. Collectively these studies suggest that OT may have a therapeutic value for treating two of the three primary deficits of autism. One point of concern, though, is the issue of peripheral administration and brain penetration. Endogenous plasma OT is unable to efficiently cross the blood brain barrier (Landgraf & Neumann, 2004), which calls into question how intravenously administered OT can have a direct effect on behavior. It is hypothesized that high levels of exogenous administration allows for low levels of OT to be transported across the blood-brain barrier. As an alternative, intranasal OT has been proposed as a route of administration, as it has been used in many of the human behavioral studies. However, due to the relative inefficiency in the transmission of peripherally administered OT and the unknown efficacy of intranasally delivered OT, the development of small molecule OTR agonists that more easily cross the blood brain barrier is needed to explore the viability of peripherally administered OT drugs for the treatment of social deficits in autism.

Conclusion

OT and AVP are important regulators of complex social behaviors. These neuropeptides modulate three major components of social interaction: social motivation, social information processing, and social attachment. Individuals with ASD show impairments in each of these three subdomains, with reduced social interest, reduced perception of nonverbal social cues and reduced ability to form reciprocal social relationships. Social motivation to care for infants in many species is dependent on central release of OT. The proper processing of social information necessary for social recognition requires OT and AVP neurotransmission. Social attachment in monogamous species and the mother-infant bond are modulated by these neuropeptides. Even in humans it appears that OT systems may play some role in complex social behaviors such as attachment and interpersonal trust. Regardless of whether disregulation of these neuropeptide systems contributes to the etiology of social deficits in ASD, the OT and AVP systems may prove to be viable targets for novel pharmacotherapies to enhance social cognition in psychiatric disorders characterized by social deficits.

Challenges and Future Directions

- Animal models have already provided a great deal of insights into the role of OT and AVP in the regulation of social behavior and social cognition. A major challenge is to develop behavioral paradigms in animal models with face, construct, and predictive validity relevant to ASD to facilitate further studies on the potential of drugs that modulate the OT and AVP systems as therapies to treat the social cognitive deficits in ASD.
- Several studies have reported genetic associations between ASD phenotypes and polymorphisms in the OT and AVP systems. However, it will be important to explore in more detail the impact of early social experience on OT and AVP systems. For example, can social enrichment enhance these peptide systems?
- Animal studies have revealed relationships between OTR and V1aR densities in particular brain regions and social behavior. However, the examination of these receptor systems has been difficult in human tissue. It will be important to develop technologies, such as positron emission tomography (PET), that will allow visualization of these peptide receptors in living individuals to determine whether alterations in receptor systems in the brain are associated with social deficits in ASD.
- ASD is a multigenic disorder, and disruptions in OT and AVP related genes are clearly not a major risk factor for the disorder. However, it will be important to consider whether diverse etiologies may have a common impact on social cognition through disregulation of some aspect of the OT and AVP system. Regardless as to whether disregulation of OT and AVP are involved in the social deficits in ASD, these systems should be considered when developing pharmacotherapies to enhance social function in ASD.

SUGGESTED READINGS

Donaldson, Z. R., & Young, L. J. (2008). Oxytocin, vasopressin, and the neurogenetics of sociality *Science, 322*(5903), 900–904.

Hammock, E. A. D., & Young, L. J. (2006). Oxytocin, vasopressin, and pair bonding: implications for autism. *Philosophical Transactions of the Royal Society of London. Series B, Biological Sciences, 361*, 2187–2198.

Heinrichs, M., von Dawans, B., & Domes, G. (2009). Oxytocin, vasopressin, and human social behavior. *Frontiers in Neuroendocrinology, 30*(4), 548–557.

REFERENCES

Acher, R. (1995). The neurohypophysial endocrine regulatory cascade: precursors, mediators, receptors, and effectors. *Frontiers in Neuroendocrinology, 16*(3), 237–289.

Al-Ayadhi, L. Y. (2005). Altered oxytocin and vasopressin levels in autistic children in Central Saudi Arabia. *Neuroscience, 10*, 47–50.

Baron-Cohen, S., Ring, H. A., Wheelwright, S., Bullmore, E. T., Brammer, M. J., Simmons, A., et al. (1999). Social intelligence in the normal and autistic brain: an fMRI study. *European Journal of Neuroscience, 11*(6), 1891–1898.

Bartels, A., & Zeki, S. (2004). The neural correlates of maternal and romantic love. *NeuroImage, 21*, 1155–1166.

Barton, J. J. (2003). Disorders of face perception and recognition. *Neurologic Clinics, 21*(2), 521–548.

Bartz, J., & Hollander, E. (2006). The neuroscience of affiliation: forging links between basic and clinical research on neuropeptides and social behavior. *Hormones and Behavior, 50*(4), 518–528.

Bartz, J. A., & Hollander, E. (2008). Oxytocin and experimental therapeutics in autism spectrum disorders. *Progress in Brain Research, 170*, 451–462.

Bittel, D. C., Kibiryeva, N., Dasouki, M., Knoll, J. H., & Butler, M. G. (2006). A 9-year old male with a duplication of chromosome 3p25.3p26.2: clinical report and gene expression analysis. *American Journal of Medical Genetics. Part A, 140*(6), 573–579.

Blaicher, W., Gruber, D., Bieglmayer, C., Blaicher, A. M., Knogler, W., & Huber, J. C. (1999). The role of oxytocin in relation to female sexual arousal. *Gynecologic and Obstetric Investigation, 47*(2), 125–126.

Born, J., Lange, T., Kern, W., McGregor, G. P., Bickel, U., & Fehm, H. L. (2002). Sniffing neuropeptides: a transnasal approach to the human brain. *Nature Neuroscience, 5*, 514–516.

Caldwell, H. K., Wersinger, S. R., & Young, W. S. (2008). The role of vasopressin 1b receptor in aggression and other social behaviors. *Progress in Brain Research, 170*, 65–72.

Carmichael, M. S., Humbert, R., Dixen, J., Palmisano, G., Greenlead, W., & Davidson, J. M. (1987). Plasma oxytocin increases in the human sexual response. *Journal of Clinical Endocrinology and Metabolism, 64*, 27–31.

Champagne, F., Diorio, J., Sharma, S., & Meaney, M. J. (2001). Naturally occurring variations in maternal behavior in the rat are associated with differences in estrogen-inducible central oxytocin receptors. *Proceedings of the National Academy of Sciences of the United States of America, 98*(22), 1236–1241.

Critchley, H. D., Daly, E. M., Bullmore, E. T., Williams, S. C., Van Amelsvoort, T., Robertson, D. M., et al. (2000). The functional neuroanatomy of social behavior: changes in cerebral blood flow when people with autistic disorder process facial expressions. *Brain, 123*(11), 2203–2212.

Dalton, K. M., Nacewicz, B. M., Johnstone, T., Schaefer, H. S., Gernbacher, M. A., & Goldsmith, H. H. (2005). Gaze fixation and the neural circuitry of face processing in autism. *Nature Neuroscience, 8*, 519–526.

Dantzer, R., Koob, G., Bluthe, R., & Moal, M. L. (1988). Septal vasopressin modulates social memory in male rats. *Brain Research, 457*, 143–147.

Davies, S., Bishop, D., Manstead, A. S., & Tantam, D. (1994). Face perception in children with autism and Asperger's syndrome. *Journal of Child Psychology and Psychiatry, 35*(6), 1033–1057.

De Vries, G. J., & Miller, M. A. (1998). Anatomy and function of extrahypothalamic vasopressin systems in the brain. *Progress in Brain Research, 119*, 3–20.

Dluzen, D. E., Muraoka, S., Engelmann, M., & Landgraf, R. (1998). The effects of infusion of arginine vasopressin, oxytocin, or their antagonists into the olfactory bulb upon social recognition responses in male rats. *Peptides, 19*, 999–1005.

Domes, G., Heinrichs, M., Michel, A., Berger, C., & Herpertz, S. C. (2007). Oxytocin improves "mind reading" in humans. *Biological Psychiatry, 15*(61), 731–733.

Donaldson, Z. R., & Young, L. J. (2008). Oxytocin, vasopressin, and the neurogenetics of sociality. *Science, 322*(5903), 900–904.

Fahrbach, S. E., Morrell, J. I., & Pfaff, D. W. (1985). Possible role for endogenous oxytocin in estrogen-facilitated maternal behavior in rats. *Neuroendocrinology, 40*(6), 526–532.

Ferguson, J. N., Aldagm, J. M., Insel, T. R., & Young, L. J. (2001). Oxytocin in the medial amygdala is essential for social recognition in the mouse. *Journal of Neuroscience, 21*, 8278–8285.

Ferguson, J. N., Young, L. J., Hearn, E. F., Insel, T. R., & Winslow, J. T. (2000). Social amnesia in mice lacking the oxytocin gene. *Nature Genetics, 25*, 284–288.

Fleming, A. S., & Anderson, V. (1987). Affect and nurturance: mechanisms mediating maternal behavior in two female mammals. *Progress in Neuropsychopharmacology and Biological Psychiatry, 11*(2–3), 121–127.

Francis, D. D., Champagne, F. C., & Meaney, M. J. (2000). Variations in maternal behavior are associated with differences in oxytocin receptor levels in the rat. *Journal of Neuroendocrinology, 12*(12), 1145–1148.

Francis, D. D., Young, L. J., Meaney, M. J., & Insel, T. R. (2002). Natu-rally occurring differences in maternal care are associated with expression of oxytocin and vasopressin (V1a) receptors: gender differences. *Journal of Neuroendocrinology, 14*(5), 349–353.

Gimpl, G., & Fahrenholz, F. (2001). The oxytocin receptor system: structure, function, and regulation. *Physiology Review, 81*(2), 629–683.

Goodson, J. L. (1998). Vasotocin and vasoactive intestinal polypeptide modulate aggression in a territorial songbird, the violet-eared waxbill (Estrildidae: Uraeginthus granatina). *General Comparative Endocrinology, 111*(2), 233–244.

Green, L. A., Fein, D., Modahl, C., Feinstein, C. M., Waterhouse, L., & Morris, M. (2001). Oxytocin and autistic disorder: alterations in peptide forms. *Biological Psychiatry, 50*, 609–613.

Grewen, K. M., Girdler, S. S., Amico, J., & Light, K. C. (2005). Effects of partner support on resting oxytocin, cortisol, norepinephrin, and blood pressure before and after warm partner contact. *Psychosomatic Medicine, 67*(4), 531–583.

Guastella, A. J., Mitchell, P. B., & Dadds, M. R. (2008). Oxytocin increases gaze to the eye region of human faces. *Biological Psychiatry, 63*(1), 3–5.

Guastella, A. J., Mitchell, P. B., & Mathews, F. (2008). Oxytocin enhances the encoding of positive social memories in humans. *Biological Psychiatry, 64*(3), 256–258.

Hammock, E. A. D., & Young, L. J. (2005). Microsatellite instability generates diversity in brain and sociobehavioral traits. *Science, 308*, 1630–1634.

Hammock, E. A. D., & Young, L. J. (2006). Oxytocin, vasopressin, and pair bonding: implications for autism. *Philosophical Transactions of the Royal Society of London. Series B, Biological Sciences, 361*, 2187–2198.

Heim, C., Young, L. J., Newport, D. J., Mletzko, T., Miller, A. H., & Nemeroff, C. B. (2008). Lower CSF oxytocin concentrations in women with a history of childhood abuse. *Molecular Psychiatry, 14(10)*, 954–958.

Hobson, R. P. (1987). The autistic child's recognition of age- and sex-related characteristics of people. *Journal of Autism and Developmental Disorders, 17*(1), 63–79.

Hollander, E., Novotny, S., Hanratty, M., Yaffe, R., DeCaria, C. M., Aronowitz, B. R., et al. (2003). Oxytocin infusion reduces repetitive behaviors in adults with autism and Asperger's disorders. *Neuropsychopharmacology, 28*(1), 193–198.

Inoue, T., Kimura, T., Azuma, C., Takemura, M., Kubota, Y., Ogia, K., et al. (1994). Structural organization of the human oxytocin receptor gene. *Journal of Biological Chemistry, 269*(51), 32451–32456.

Insel, T. R., & Harbaugh, C. R. (1989). Lesions of the hypothalamic paraventricular nucleus disrupts the initiation of maternal behavior. *Physiology and Behavior, 45*(5), 1033–1041.

Insel, T. R., Wang, Z. X., & Ferris, C. F. (1994). Patterns of brain vasopressin receptor distribution associated with social organization in microtine rodents. *Journal of Neuroscience, 14*(9), 5381–5392.

Insel, T. R., & Young, L. J. (2001). The neurobiology of attachment. *Nature Reviews Neuroscience, 2*(2), 129–136.

Israel, S., Lerer, E., Shalev, I., Uzefovsky, F., Reibold, M., Bachner-Melman, R., et al. (2008). Molecular genetics studies of the arginine vasopressin 1a receptor (AVPR1a) and the oxytocin receptor (OXTR) in human behavior: from autism to altruism with some notes in between. *Progress in Brain Research, 170*, 435–449.

Jacob, S., Brune, C. W., Carter, C. S., Leventhal, B. L., Lord, C., & Cook, E. H. J. (2007). Association of the oxytocin receptor gene (OXTR) in Caucasian children and adolescents with autism. *Neuroscience Letters, 417*(1), 6–9.

Jansen, J. M., Gispen-de Wied, C. C., Weigant, V. M., Westernberg, H. G., Lahuis, B. E., & van Engeland, H. (2006). Autonomic and neuroendocrine responses to a psychosocial stressor in adults with autistic spectrum disorder. *Journal of Autism and Developmental Disorders, 36*(7), 891–899.

Kendrick, K. M., Costa, A. P. C. D., Broad, K. D., Ohkura, S., Guevara, R., Levy, F., et al. (1997). Neural control of maternal behavior and olfactory recognition of offspring. *Brain Research Bulletin, 44*, 383–395.

Kendrick, K. M., Guevara-Guzman, R., Zorilla, J., Hinton, M. R., Borad, K. D., Mimmack, M., et al. (1997). Formation of olfactory memories mediated by nitric oxide. *Nature, 388*(6643), 670–674.

Kendrick, K. M., Keverne, E. B., & Baldwin, B. A. (1987). Intracerebroventricular oxytocin stimulates maternal behavior in the sheep. *Neuroendocrinology, 46*(1), 56–61.

Kim, S. (2001). Transmission disequilibrium testing of arginine vasopressin receptor 1a (AVPR1A) polymorphisms in autism. *Molecular Psychiatry, 7*, 503–507.

Kirsch, P., Esslinger, C., Chen, Q., Mier, D., Lis, S., Siddhanti, S., et al. (2005). Oxytocin modulates neural circuitry for social cognition and fear in humans. *Journal of Neuroscience, 25*(49), 11489–11493.

Knafo, A., Israel, S., Darvasi, A., Bachner-Melman, R., Uzefovsky, F., Cohen, L., et al. (2008). Individual differences in allocation of funds in the dictator game associated with length of the arginine vasopressin 1a receptor RS3 promoter region and correlation between RS3 length and hippocampal mRNA. *Genes, Brain, and Behavior, 7*(3), 266–275.

Kosfeld, M., Heinrichs, M., Zak, P. J., Fischbacher, U., & Fehr, E. (2005). Oxytocin increases trust in humans. *Nature, 435*, 673–676.

Landgraf, R., Gerstberger, R., Montkowski, A., Probst, J. C., Wotjak, C. T., Holsboer, F., et al. (1995). V1 vasopressin receptor antisense oligodeoxynucleotide into septum reduces vasopressin binding, social discrimination abilities, and anxiety-related behavior in rats. *Journal of Neuroscience, 15*, 4250–4258.

Landgraf, R., & Neumann, I. D. (2004). Vasopressin and oxytocin release within the brain: a dynamic concept of multiple and variable modes of neuropeptide communication. *Frontiers in Neuroendocrinology, 25*(3–4), 150–176.

Lauritsen, M. B., Als, T. D., Dahl, H. A., Flint, T. J., Wang, A. G., Vang, M., et al. (2006). A genome-wide search for alleles and haplotypes associated with autism and related pervasive developmental disorders on the Faroe Islands. *Molecular Psychiatry, 11*(1), 37–46.

Lawrence, K., Campbell, R., Swettenham, J., Terstegge, J., Akers, R., Coleman, M., et al. (2003). Interpreting gaze in Turner syndrome: impaired sensitivity to intention and emotion, but preservation of social cueing. *Neuropsychologia, 41*(8), 894–905.

Lee, A., Clancy, S., & Fleming, A. S. (1999). Mother rats bar-press for pups: effects of lesions of the mpoa and limbic sites on maternal behavior and operant responding for pup-reinforcement. *Behavioural Brain Research, 100*(1–2), 15–31.

Lerer, E., Levi, S., Salomon, S., Darvasi, A., Yirmiya, N., & Ebstein, R. P. (2008). Association between the oxytocin receptor (OXTR) gene and autism: relationship to Vineland Adaptive Behavior Scales and cognition. *Molecular Psychiatry, 13*, 980–988.

Levine, A., Zagoory-Sharon, O., Feldman, R., & Weller, A. (2007). Oxytocin during pregnancy and early post-partum: individual patterns and maternal-fetal bonding. *Peptides, 28*(6), 1162–1169.

Levy, F., Kendrick, K. M., Keverne, E. B., Piketty, V., & Poindron, P. (1992). Intracerebral oxytocin is important for the onset of maternal behavior in inexperienced ewes delivered under peridural anesthesia. *Behavioral Neuroscience, 106*(2), 427–432.

Light, K. C., Grewen, K. M., & Amico, J. A. (2005). More frequent partner hugs and higher oxytocin levels are linked to lower blood pressure and heart rate in premenopausal women. *Biological Psychiatry, 69*(1), 5–21.

Lim, M. M., Wang, Z., Olazabal, D. E., Ren, X., Terwilliger, E. F., & Young, L. J. (2004). Enhanced partner preference in a promiscuous species by manipulating the expression of a single gene. *Nature, 429*(6993), 754–757.

Liu, Y., Curtis, J. T., & Wang, Z. X. (2001). Vasopressin in the lateral septum regulates pair bond formation in male prairie voles (Microtus ochrogaster). *Behavioral Neuroscience, 115*(4), 910–919.

McCarthy, M. M. (1990). Oxytocin inhibits infanticide in female house mice (Mus domesticus). *Hormones and Behavior, 24*(3), 365–375.

McCauley, J. L., Li, C., Jiang, L., Olson, L. M., Crockett, G., Gainer, K., et al. (2005). Genome-wide and ordered subset linkage analyses provide support for autism loci on 17q and 19p with evidence of phenotypic and interlocus genetic correlates. *BMC Medical Genetics, 6*(1), 1–11.

McNeilly, A. S., Robinson, I. C., Houston, M. J., & Howie, P. W. (1983). Release of oxytocin and prolactin in response to suckling. *British Medical Journal, 286*(6361), 257–259.

Meddle, S. L., Bishop, V. R., Gkoumassi, E., Van Leeuwen, F. W., & Douglas, A. J. (2007). Dynamic changes in oxytocin receptor expression and activation at parturition in the rat brain. *Endocrinology, 148*(10), 5095–5104.

Meyer-Lindenberg, A. (2008). Impact of prosocial neuropeptides on human brain function. *Progress in Brain Research, 170*, 463–470.

Meyer-Lindenberg, A., Kolachana, B., Gold, B., Olsh, A., Nicodemus, K. K., Mattay, V., et al. (2009). Genetic variants in AVPR1a linked to autism predicts amygdala activation and personality traits in healthy humans. *Molecular Psychiatry*, 1–8, *14*(10): 968–975.

Modahl, C., Green, L. A., Fein, D., Morris, M., Waterhouse, L., Feinstein, C., et al. (1998). Plasma oxytocin levels in autistic children. *Biological Psychiatry, 43*, 270–277.

Neumann, I. (2008). Brain oxytocin: a key regulator of emotional and social behaviors in both females and males. *Journal of Neuroendocrinology, 20*(6), 858–865.

Nissen, E., Lilja, G., Widstrom, A. M., & Unvas-Moberg, K. (1995). Elevation of oxytocin levels early post partum in women. *Acta Obstetricia et Gynecologica Scandinavica, 74*(7), 530–533.

Olazabal, D. E., & Young, L. J. (2006a). Oxytocin receptors in the nucleus accumbens facilitate "spontaneous" maternal behavior in adult female prairie voles. *Neuroscience, 141*(2), 559–568.

Olazabal, D. E., & Young, L. J. (2006b). Species and individual differences in juvenile female alloparental care are associated with oxytocin receptor density in the striatum and the lateral septum. *Hormones and Behavior, 49*(5), 681–687.

Pedersen, C. A., Ascher, J. A., Monroe, Y. L., & Prange, A. J. J. (1982). Oxytocin induces maternal behavior in virgin female rats. *Science, 216*(4546), 648–650.

Pedersen, C. A., Caldwell, J. D., Walkder, C., Ayers, G., & Mason, G. A. (1994). Oxytocin activates the postpartum onset of rat maternal behavior in the ventral tegmental and medial preoptic areas. *Behavioral Neuroscience, 108*(6), 1163–1171.

Pierce, K., Müller, R. A., Ambrose, J., Allen, G., & Courchesne, E. (2001). Face processing occurs outside the fusiform "face area" in autism: evidence from functional MRI. *Brain, 124*(10), 2059–2073.

Porter, R. H., Cernock, J. M., & McLaughlin, F. (1983). Maternal recognition of neonates through olfactory cues. *Physiology and Behavior, 30*, 151–154.

Rimmele, U., Hediger, K., Heinrichs, M., & Klaver, P. (2009). Oxytocin makes a face in memory familiar. *Journal of Neuroscience, 29*(1), 38–42.

Ross, H., Cole, C., Smith, Y., Neumann, I., Landgraf, R., & Young, L. (2009). Characterization of the oxytocin system regulating affiliative behavior in female prairie voles. *Neuroscience, 162*(4), 892–903.

Ross, H. E., Freeman, S. M., Speigel, L. L., Ren, X., Terwilliger, E. F., & Young, L. J. (2009). Variation in oxytocin receptor density in the nucleus accumbens has differential effects on affiliative behavior in monogamous and polygamous voles. *Journal of Neuroscience, 29*(5), 1312–1318.

Ross, H. E., & Young, L. J. (2009). Oxytocin and the neural mechanisms regulating social cognition and affiliative behavior. *Frontiers in Neuroendocrinology, 30*(4), 534–547.

Savaskan, E., Ernhardt, R., Schulz, A., Walter, M., & Schachinger, H. (2008). Post-learning intranasal oxytocin modulates human memory for facial identity. *Psychoneuroendocrinology, 33*(3), 368–374.

Schultz, R. T. (2005). Developmental deficits in social perception in autism: the role of the amygdala and the fusiform face area. *International Journal of Developmental Neuroscience, 23*(2–3), 125–141.

Schultz, R. T., Gauthier, I., Klin, A., Fulbright, R. K., Anderson, A. W., Volkmar, F., et al. (2000). Abnormal ventral temporal cortical activity during face discrimination among individuals with autism and Asperger syndrome. *Archives of General Psychiatry, 57*(4), 331–340.

Sebat, J., Lakshmi, B., Malhotra, D., Troge, J., Lese-Martin, C., Walsh, T., et al. (2007). Strong association of de novo copy number mutations with autism. *Science, 316*(5823), 445–449.

Solomon, N. G. (1991). Age of pairing affects reproduction in prairie voles. *Laboratory Animals, 25*(3), 232–235.

Tantam, D., Monaghan, L., Nicholson, H., & Stirling, J. (1989). Autistic children's ability to interpret faces: a research note. *Journal of Child Psychology and Psychiatry, 30*(4), 623–630.

Taylor, S. E., Gonzaga, G. C., Klein, L. C., Hu, P., Greendale, G. A., & Seema, T. E. (2006). Relation of oxytocin to psychological stress responses and hypothalamic-pituitary adrenocortical axis activity in older women. *Psychosomatic Medicine, 68*(2), 238–245.

Thompson, R. R., George, K., Walton, J. C., Orr, S. P., & Benson, J. (2006). Sex-specific influences of vasopressin on human social communication. *Proceedings of the National Academy of Sciences of the United States of America, 103*(20), 7889–7894.

Thompson, R. R., & Walton, J. C. (2004). Peptide effects on social behavior: effects of vasotocin and isotocin on social approach behavior in male goldfish (Carassius auratus). *Behavioral Neuroscience, 118*(3), 620–626.

Turner, R. A., Altemus, M., Enos, T., Cooper, B., & McGuinness, T. (1999). Preliminary research on plasma oxytocin in normal cycling women: investigating emotion and interpersonal distress. *Psychiatry, 62*(2), 97–113.

Uvnas-Moberg, K. (1998). Oxytocin may mediate the benefits of positive social interaction and emotions. *Psychoneuroendocrinology, 23*(8), 877–890.

Van Leeuwen, F. A., Caffe, A. R., & De Vries, G. J. (1985). Vasopressin cells in the bed nucleus of the stria terminalis of the rat: sex differences and the influence of androgens. *Brain Research, 325*, 391–394.

Vasicka, A., Kumaresan, P., Han, G. S., & Kumaresan, M. (1978). Plasma oxytocin in initiation of labor. *American Journal of Obstetrics and Gynecology, 130*(3), 263–273.

Walum, H., Westberg, L., Henningsson, S., Neiderhiser, J. M.,Reiss, D., Lgl, W., et al. (2008). Genetic variation in the vasopressin receptor 1a (AVPR1a) associates with pair-bonding behavior in humans. *Proceedings of the National Academy of Sciences of the United States of America, 105*(37), 14153–14156.

Wang, Z. X., Ferris, C. F., & De Vries, G. J. (1994). Role of septal vasopressin innervation in parental behavior in prairie voles. *Proceedings of the National Academy of Sciences of the United States of America, 91*(1), 400–404.

Wang, Z. X., Zhou, L., Hulihan, T. J., & Insel, T. R. (1996). Immunoreactivity of central vasopressin and oxytocin pathways in microtine rodents: a quantitative comparative study. *Journal of Comparative Neurology, 366*(4), 726–737.

Wassink, T. H., Piven, J., Vieland, V. J., Pietilia, J., Goedken, R. J., Folstein, S. E., et al. (2004). Examination of AVPR1a as an autism susceptibility gene. *Molecular Psychiatry, 9*, 968–972.

Williams, J. R., Harbough, C. R., & Carter, C. S. (1994). Oxytocin administered centrally facilitates formation of a partner preference in prairie voles. *Journal of Neuroendocrinology, 6*, 247–250.

Winslow, J. T., Hastings, N., Carter, C. S., Harbaugh, C. R., & Insel, T. R. (1993). A role for central vasopressin pair bonding in monogamous prairie voles. *Nature, 365*(6446), 545–548.

Winslow, J. T., Hearn, E. F., Ferguson, J. N., Young, L. J., Matzuk, M. M., & Insel, T. R. (2000). Infant vocalization, adult aggression, and fear behavior of an oxytocin null mutant mouse. *Hormones and Behavior, 37*, 145–155.

Wu, S., Jia, M., Ruan, Y., Liu, J., Gou, Y., Shaung, M., et al. (2005). Positive association of the oxytocin receptor gene (OXTR) with autism in the Chinese Han population. *Biological Psychiatry, 58*(1), 74–77.

Yirmiya, N., Rosenberg, C., Levi, S., Salomon, S., Shulman, C., Nemanov, L., et al. (2006). Association between the arginine vasopressin 1a receptor (AVPR1a) gene and autism in a family based study: medication by socialization skills. *Molecular Psychiatry, 11*(5), 488–494.

Young, L. J. (1999). Frank A. Beach Award. Oxytocin and vasopressin receptors and species typical social behaviors. *Hormones and Behavior, 36*(3), 212–221.

Young, L. J., Lim, M. M., Gingrich, B., & Insel, T. R. (2001). Cellular mechanisms of social attachment. *Hormones and Behavior, 40*(2), 133–138.

Young, L. J., Nilsen, R., Waymire, K. G., MacGregor, G. R., & Insel, T. R. (1999). Increased affiliative response to vasopressin mice expressing the V1a receptor from a monogamous vole. *Nature, 400*(6746), 766–768.

Yrigollen, C. M., Han, S. S., Kochetkova, A., Babitz, T., Chang, J. T., Volkmar, F. R., et al. (2008). Genes controlling affiliative behavior as candidate genes for autism. *Biological Psychiatry, 63*(10), 91–916.

35 Eric Courchesne, Sara Jane Webb, Cynthia M. Schumann

From Toddlers to Adults: The Changing Landscape of the Brain in Autism

Points of Interest

- Autism is due to abnormal brain development beginning early in life. The signature(s) of this early neural maldevelopment is far more likely to be detectable at the developmental time when behavioral symptoms first appear.
- Autism involves early brain overgrowth prior to 3 years of age followed by arrested growth and degeneration. This atypical neural development is pronounced in key structures such as the frontal lobe, temporal lobe, and amygdala; hypoplasia of subregions of cerebellar vermis also occurs during this early period of life in individuals with autism.
- Abnormal neural connectivity is hypothesized to be a downstream consequence of an earlier neural defect.

The behavioral signs and symptoms of autistic disorder and pervasive developmental disorder begin during later infancy and the toddler period in the majority of cases. Before 6–12 months of age, such signs are typically absent or, at most, very subtle, according to recent prospective studies (Wetherby, et al., 2004; Zwaigenbaum, et al., 2005; Ozonoff, Heung, et al., 2008; Pierce, Glatt, et al., 2009). The first red flags in older infants and toddlers include deficits in the development of higher-order social, language, communication, and emotion functions. Ritualistic and/or repetitive behaviors and cognitive deficits are not as consistently present but do occur in some individuals even at an early age. These behavioral deficits must necessarily be due to abnormal development of the brain at or before this early age period.

In humans, this very period from roughly 6–12 months to 3 years is a time of major cell growth, synaptogenesis, and circuit formation for the neural systems that mediate these higher-order functions. No other period in human development is its equal: Circuit formation and functional organization in these systems at this time create the single most astonishing expansion of human higher-order processing capacity of any age period in human life. Therefore, abnormal development of processes in these systems during this age period almost certainly underlies the emergence of autistic behavioral signs and symptoms in infants and toddlers. However, a major unknown is whether such maldevelopment began *before* this period or, instead, occurs for the very first time *during* this period. This gap in knowledge exists because these higher-order neural systems are not developed sufficiently before this period, even in the completely neurotypical infant, and so, behavioral indices of deviation from normal capacity in these systems can only be readily behaviorally detected after the age when these functions typically develop. Behavioral methodologies alone, therefore, cannot address this key gap in knowledge in the biological time of onset of autism. From the perspective of elucidating the causes of autism, identifying early markers will allow effective interventions to begin earlier or even the identification of plausible paths to preventing autism. There are few questions in the field of autism that are more important to answer.

Since autism is undeniably due to abnormal brain development beginning in early life, knowledge of this early brain abnormality is paramount. Clearly, the signature of this early maldevelopment is far more likely to be detectable, perhaps even vivid, at the developmental time when behavioral symptoms first appear. However, there is a lack of a clear developmental perspective in the literature. As highlighted in a recent review, more than 90% of all studies of neuroanatomy in autism have been on 10-, 20-, or 40-year-olds with autism, not on 1- to 3-year-olds (Courchesne, Pierce, et al., 2007). In the past, most but not all (Courchesne, Pierce, et al., 2007; Amaral et al., 2008) reviews of the neuroanatomy of autism have not considered age-related effects when seeking a coherent picture of the neuroanatomic defects that underlie the emergence of autism.

In the recent research of a few laboratories, however, early brain development in autism has been a focus of investigations (Courchesne, Karns, et al., 2001; Courchesne, Carper, et al., 2003;

Hazlett, Poe, et al., 2005; Dawson, Munson, et al., 2007; Mosconi, Cody-Hazlett, et al., 2009; Schumann, Barnes, et al., 2009; Schumann, Bloss, et al., 2010). Findings led to the theory that autism involves early brain overgrowth followed by arrested growth and potential degeneration (Courchesne & Pierce, 2005; Courchesne, Pierce, et al., 2007; see Figure 35-1), Support for this theory of an unusual brain growth trajectory across the lifespan in autism comes from a new longitudinal and cross-sectional MRI study of 586 autistic and typically subjects 1 to 50 years of age (Courchesne Campbell, 2010). This theory (Courchesne, Pierce, et al., 2007) argues that early brain growth pathology begins *before* the first detected signs of autism. If the early brain overgrowth theory of autism is valid, then it would provide a central organizing principle for a host of research into genetic and nongenetic causes, avenues for treatment, animal models, and early identification. In this chapter, we review the head circumference and MRI evidence relevant to this theory and highlight areas of evidence that remain to be gathered to refine or refute it. In addition, new information from functional neuroimaging and postmortem studies that speak to this theory are also discussed. Future directions in research into the early developmental neuroanatomical bases of autism are suggested, including research that aims to define relationships between brain growth abnormality in autism spectrum disorders (ASD) and clinical, treatment, and etiological factors.

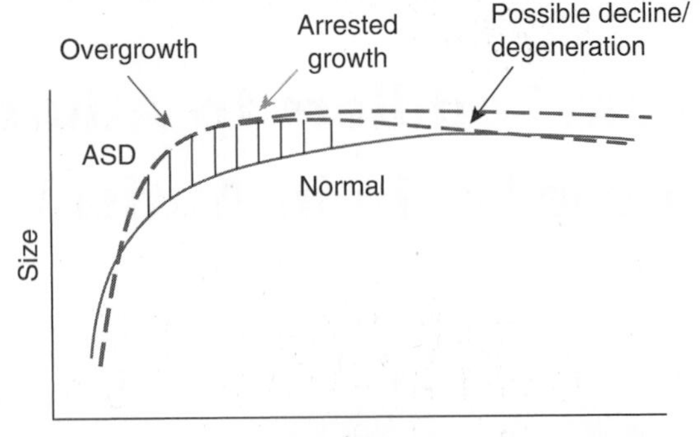

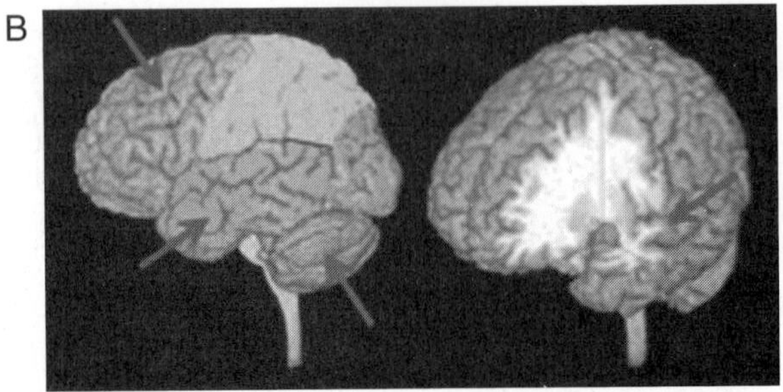

Figure 35–1. Three phases of growth pathology in ASD. (A) Model of early brain overgrowth that is followed by arrest of growth. Red line represents ASD, while blue line represents age-matched typically developing individuals. In some regions and individuals, the arrest of growth may be followed by degeneration, indicated by the red dashes that slope slightly downward. (B) Sites of regional overgrowth in ASD include frontal and temporal cortices, and amygdala. From Courchesne, E., Pierce, K., et al. (2007). Mapping early brain development in autism. *Neuron, 56*(2), 399–413. (See Color Plate Section for a color version of this figure.)

Discovery of Early Brain Overgrowth in Autism and Replication Studies

Head Circumference Evidence of Early Overgrowth in Autism

Abnormal brain enlargement in 2- to 3-year-old toddlers diagnosed with autism was first discovered using quantitative MRI a number of years ago (Courchesne, Karns, et al., 2001). Since autism begins before that age, the question remained as to whether this enlargement preceded or followed the onset of the first signs of autism. However, this same study also reported that autistic children with brain enlargement had normal to slightly smaller than normal head circumference (HC) at birth. That suggested the hypothesis that early brain overgrowth in autism begins sometime during the first 2 years of life.

To test that possibility, Courchesne et al. (2003) analyzed cross-sectional and longitudinal HC data using retrospective records from birth to 2 years of age in patients with autism from the Courchesne et al. (2001) study. To determine whether HC is a good retrospective index of brain size, Courchesne and colleagues additionally conducted a separate MRI-HC correlation study in autistic and typically developing toddlers and children (Bartholomeusz, Courchesne, et al., 2002). They found that HC at that early age (but not in adolescents or adults) is an excellent predictor of overall brain volume.

Courchesne et al. (2003) found that at birth, HC in infants who later went on to develop autism was typically near normal (by World Health Organization norms) or slightly below normal average (by Centers for Disease Control norms) with a mean of 34.6 cm; only about 6% of these newborns had excessively enlarged HC at birth (Figure 35-2A including Webb, Nalty, et al., 2007; Figure 35-2B Dementieva et al., 2005). However, by 6–14 months of age, HC had become enlarged, with 76% of infants across different studies (Courchesne et al., 2003; Dementieva et al., 2005; Webb et al., 2007) exceeding +1 standard deviation above normal average (Figure 35-2C). This finding of early overgrowth during the first years of life in autism based on HC has now been replicated by several independent research groups (Dementieva, Vance, et al., 2005; Hazlett, Poe, et al., 2005; Dissanayake, Bui, et al., 2005; Dawson et al., 2007; Webb et al., 2007). Further, Elder et al. (Elder, Dawson, et al., 2008) found that toddler siblings of children with ASD who had more rapid growth from birth to 12 months and showed a deceleration in head circumference growth from 12 to 24 months had more parent reported difficulties in social and communication behaviors.

In addition to these longitudinal and cross-sectional studies of HC across the first 2 years of life in autism, several older studies reported only on birth HC. Figure 35-3 showed that in every

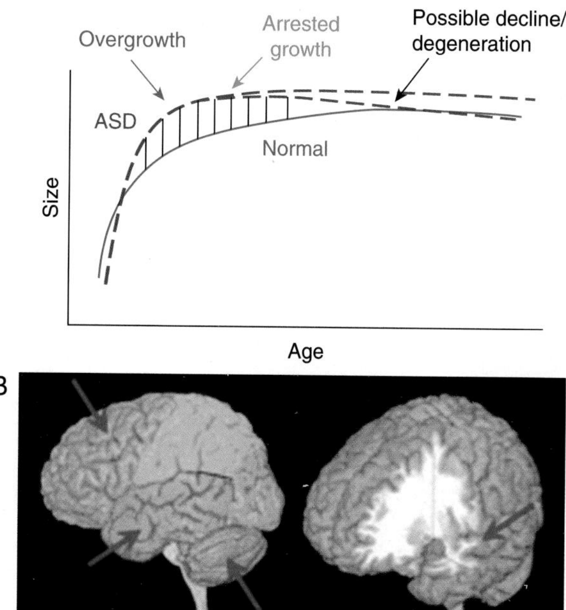

Figure 35–1. Three phases of growth pathology in ASD. (A) Model of early brain overgrowth that is followed by arrest of growth. Red line represents ASD, while blue line represents age-matched typically developing individuals. In some regions and individuals, the arrest of growth may be followed by degeneration, indicated by the red dashes that slope slightly downward. (B) Sites of regional overgrowth in ASD include frontal and temporal cortices, and amygdala. From Courchesne, E., Pierce, K., et al. (2007). Mapping early brain development in autism. *Neuron, 56*(2), 399–413.

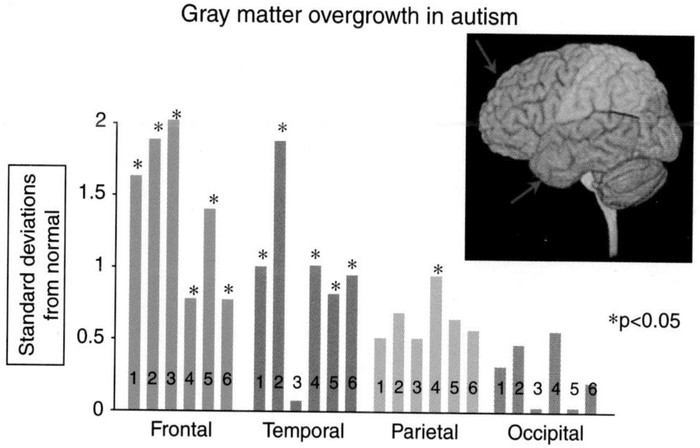

Figure 35–7. Summary of observed gray matter abnormalities (standard deviations from normal) from studies of children and adolescents with autism. Included data from: (1) Carper et al., 2002; (2) Bloss & Courchesne, 2007; (3) Kates et al., 2004; (4) Palmen et al., 2005; (5) Hazlett et al., 2005; (6) Schumann, Bloss et al., 2010. Note the general gradient of abnormality, with frontal and temporal regions most profoundly enlarged. Adapted from Courchesne, E., Pierce, K., et al. (2007). Mapping early brain development in autism. *Neuron, 56*(2), 399–413.

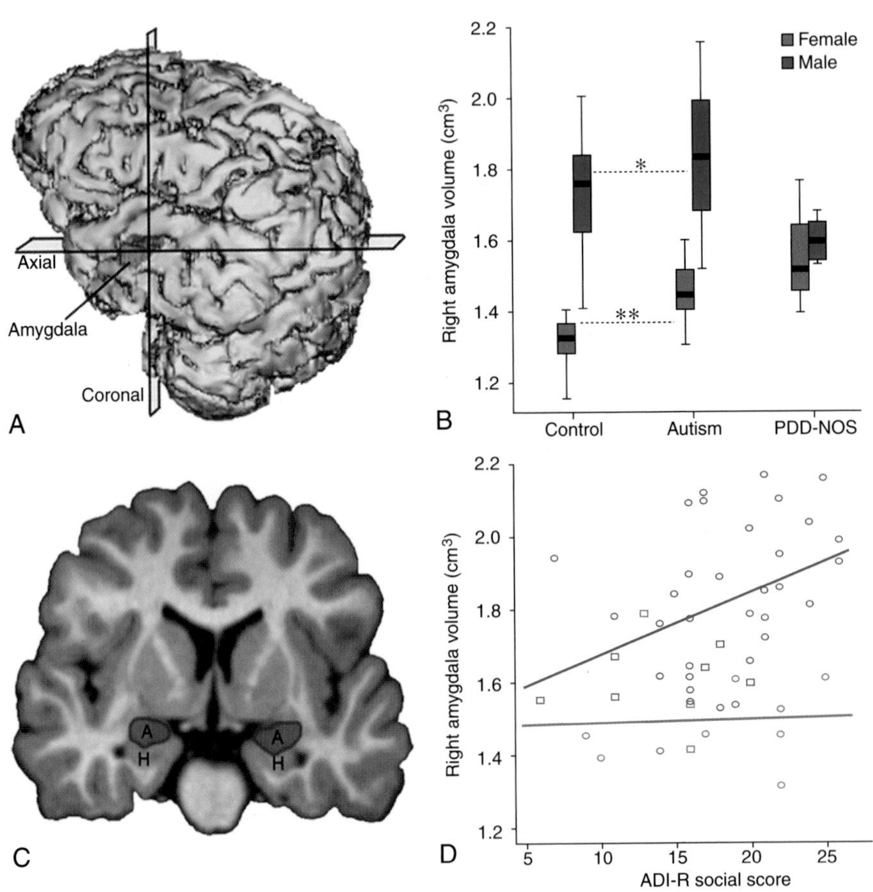

Figure 35–9. Amygdala enlargement in toddlers and young children with autism. (A) Three-dimensional reconstruction of MRI scan; (B) Right amygdala volume (in cm³) for children at about 3 years of age by diagnostic group (*$p < .05$; **$P < .01$ significantly different from sex-matched control); (C) Amygdala (A) and Hippocampus (H) in the coronal plane; (D) Linear regression scatter plot showing a positive correlation for right ($r = 0.52$, $p = .001$) amygdala volume (in cm³) and Autism Diagnostic Interview-Revised (ADI-R) social score in males with autism spectrum disorder. Adapted from Schumann, C. M., Barnes, C. C., et al. (2009). Amygdala enlargement in toddlers with autism related to severity of social and communication impairments. *Biological Psychiatry, 66*, 942–949.

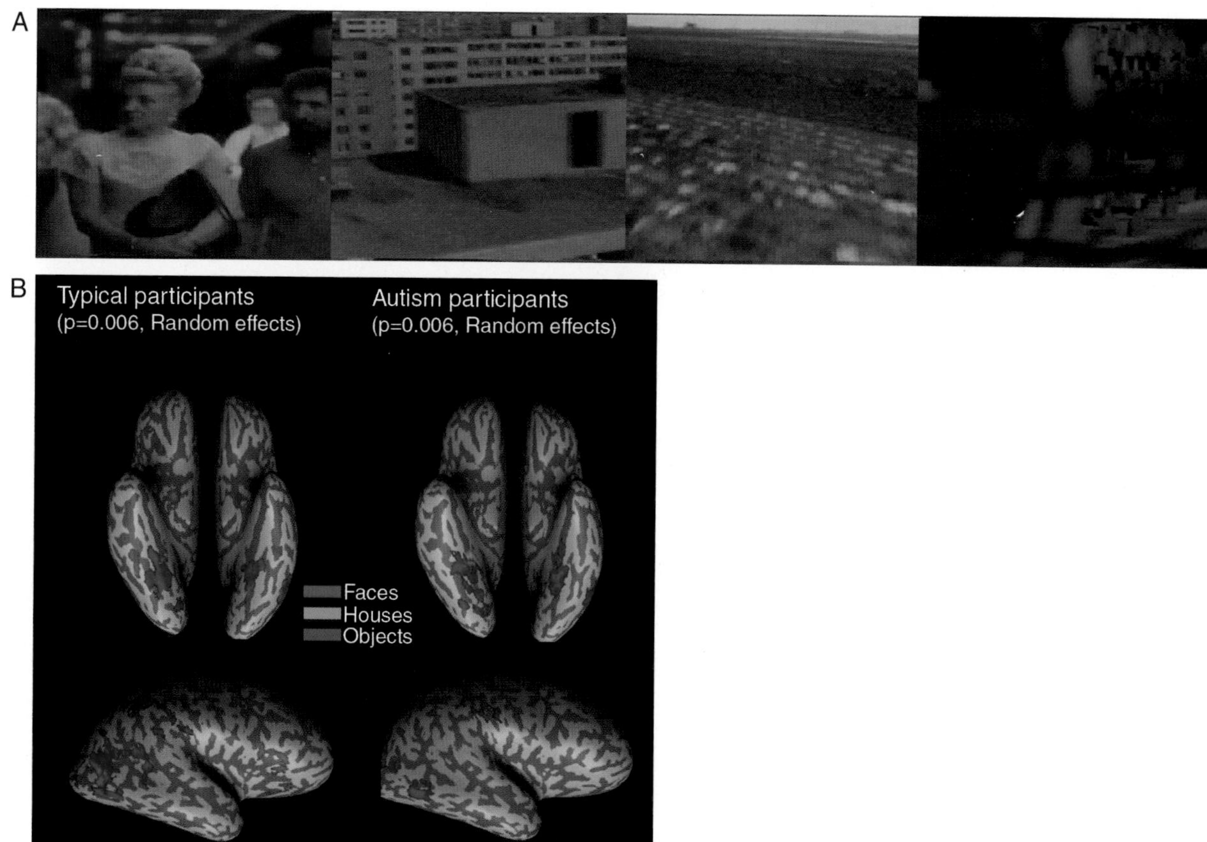

Figure 36–3. Functional MRI study using moving pictures of faces, buildings, scenes, and objects: (a) examples of the stimuli; (b) group averaged cortical maps from the typical and autism groups showing activation in response to faces, buildings, landscapes, and objects. The first map shows the average activation map for typical individuals and the second for individuals with autism.

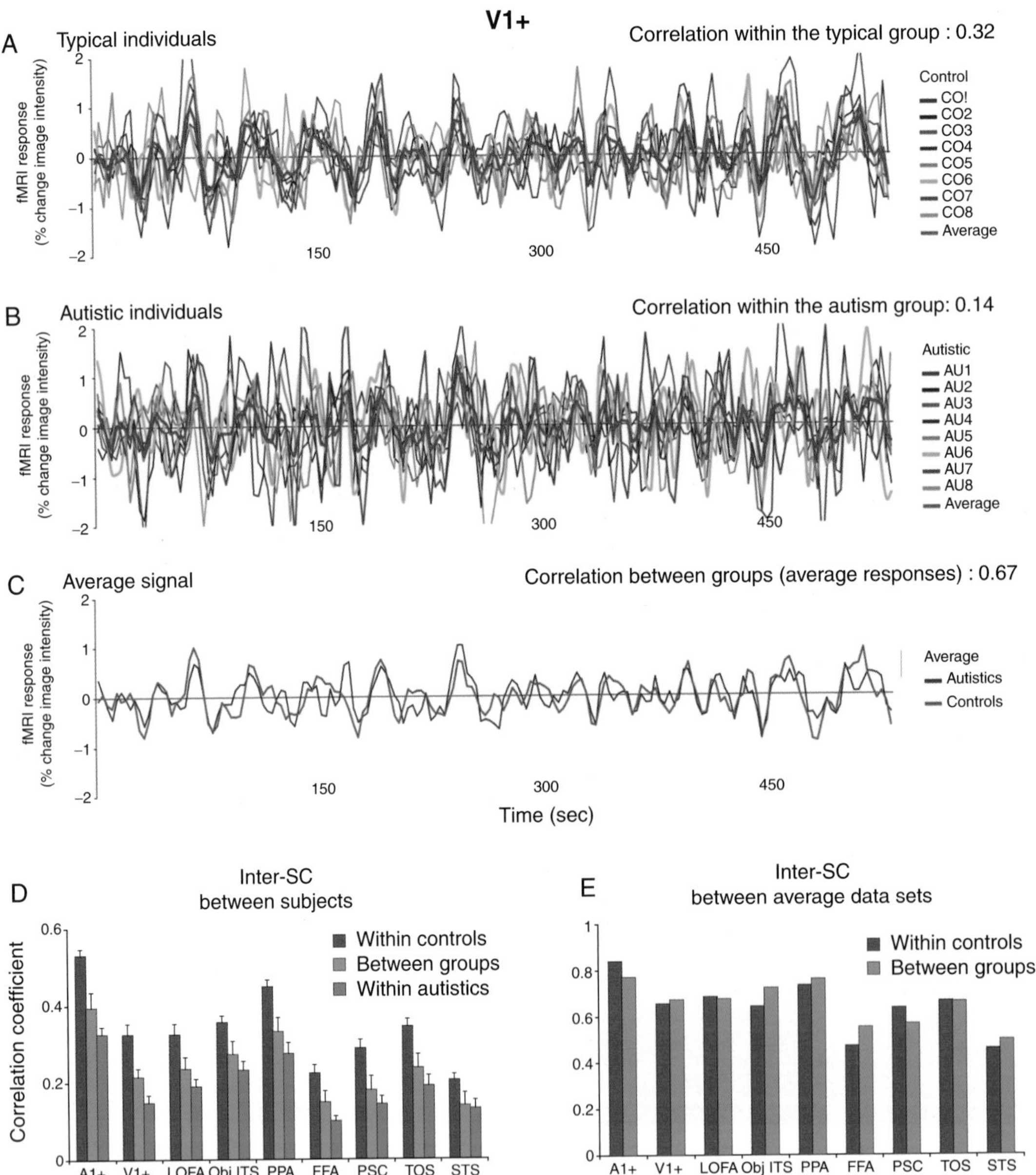

Figure 36–4. Signal fluctuations within ROIs. Visual cortex (V11) response time courses for (A) each typical subject and (B) each participant with autism. (C) The average signal for the typical group (red line) and autism (blue line) group. (D) The mean inter-SC values for the within-typical group (typical–typical, red bars), within-autism group (autism–autism, light green bars), and between the two groups (autism–typical, green bars) for selected ROIs. ROI abbreviations: A11, primary and secondary auditory cortices; V11, primary and secondary visual cortices; LOFA, lateral occipital cortex responsive to pictures of faces; Obj-ITS, object-related area in the inferior temporal sulcus; PPA, parahippocampal place area; FFA, fusiform face area; PCS, posterior central sulcus responsive to pictures of objects; TOS, transverse occipital sulcus responsive to pictures of places; STS-Face, area in superior temporal sulcus responsive to pictures of faces. (E) The inter-SC between the average autism–typical time courses (green bars) and the typical–typical time courses (red bars) in each ROI (same abbreviations as in D). Note the extent of variability in signal fluctuation in the autism individuals relative to the typical subjects. Moreover, note that by averaging the time courses within a group the responses become highly correlated across groups.

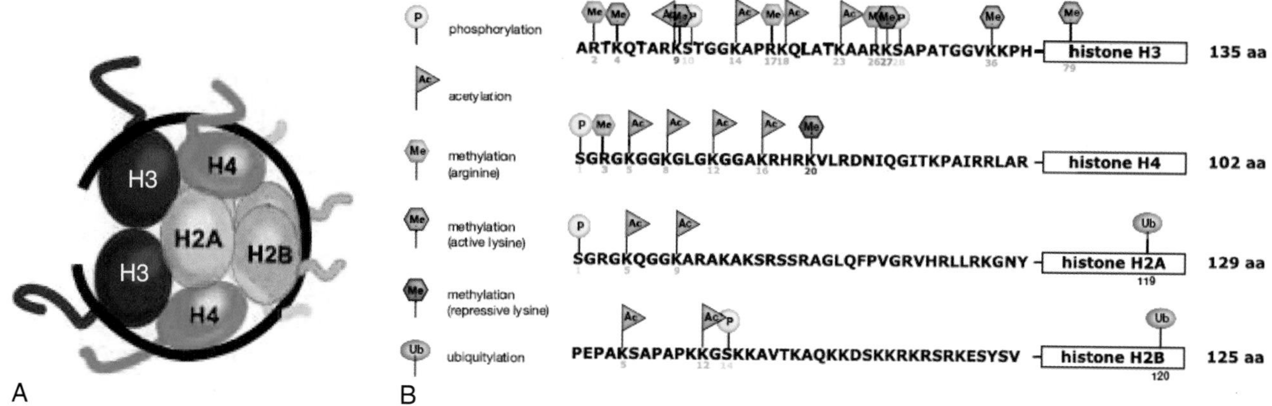

Figure 42–2. A (left). Nucleosome Structure. A schematic representation of histone organization within the octamer core around which the DNA (black line) is wrapped. Nucleosome formation occurs first through the deposition of an H3/H4 tetramer on the DNA, followed by two sets of H2A/H2B dimers. Unstructured animo-terminal histone tails extrude from the DNA-nucleosome core, and the core consists of structured globular domains of the eight histone proteins. Modified with permission from Chapter 3 in Allis, C. D., Jenuwein, T., & Reinberg, D. (2007). *Epigenetics.* Cold Spring Harbor, NY: Cold Spring Harbor Laboratory Press. B (Right). Sites of Histone Tail Modifications. The amino-terminal tails of histones host the vast majority of known covalent modification sites as illustrated. Modifications do occur in the globular domain (boxed), some of which are indicated. In general, active marks include acetylation (turquoise Ac flag), arginine methylation (yellow Me flag), and some lysine methylation such as H3K4 and H3K36 (green Me flag). H3K79 in globular domain has anti-silencing function. Repressive marks include H3K9, H3K27, and H4K20 (red Me flags) Green = active mark, red = repressive mark. Reproduced with permission from Chapter 3 in Allis, C. D., Jenuwein, T., & Reinberg, D. (2007). *Epigenetics.* Cold Spring Harbor, NY: Cold Spring Harbor Laboratory Press.

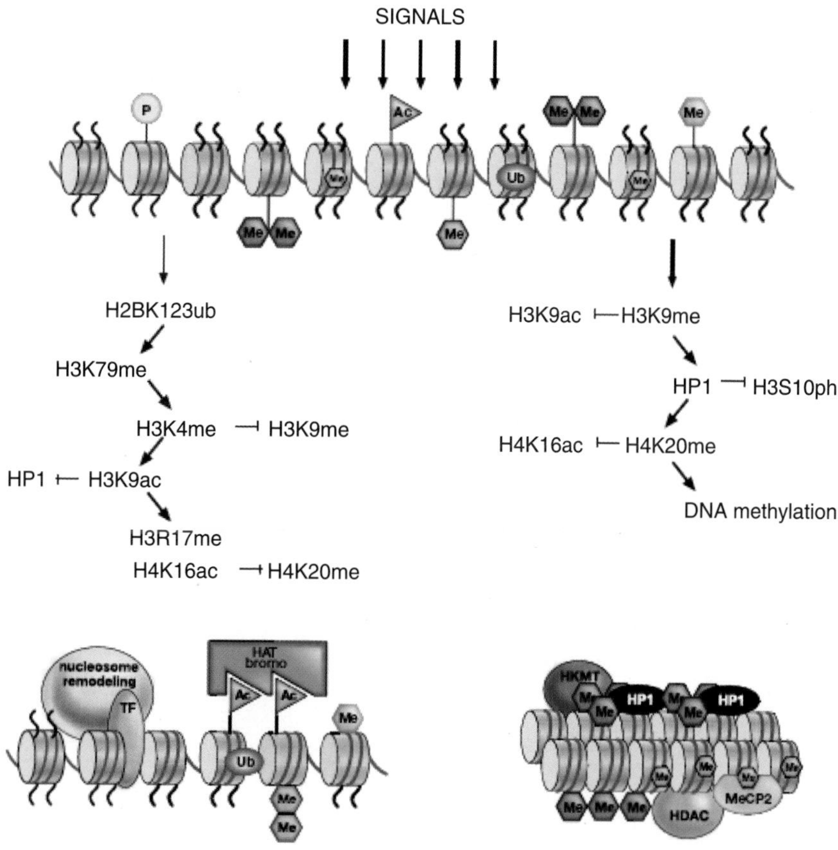

Figure 42–3. Coordinated Modification of Chromatin. The transition of a naive chromatin template to active euchromatin (left) or the establishment of repressive heterochromatin (right), involving a series of coordinated chromatin modifications. In the case of transcriptional activation, this is accompanied by the action of nucleosome remodeling complexes and the replacement of core histones with histone variants (yellow—namely, H3.3). Reproduced with permission from Chapter 3 in Allis, C. D., Jenuwein, T., & Reinberg, D. (2007). *Epigenetics.* Cold Spring Harbor, NY: Cold Spring Harbor Laboratory Press.

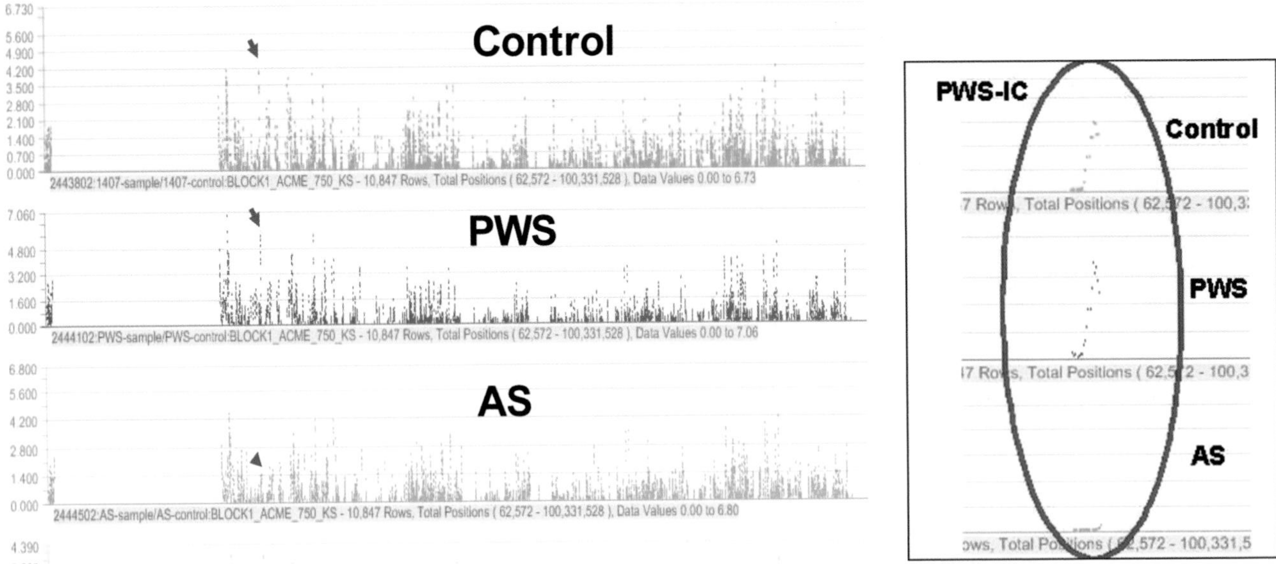

Figure 42–6. Analysis of DNA methylation using methylated DNA immunoprecipitation (MeDIP). Genomic DNA from control, PWS deletion, and Angelman deletion were first digested with *Mse*I restriction enzyme and then immunoprecipitated using an antibody against 5-methyl-cytosine (Weber et al., 2005). Precipitated DNA was co-hybridized with its respective input on the Nimblegen CpG island arrays. At the PWS-IC on chromosome 15, a peak of methylated DNA on the maternal chromosome is detected in control and PWS DNA but not Angelman DNA. Right panel is an expanded view of the region with the red arrows. X. Z., unpublished.

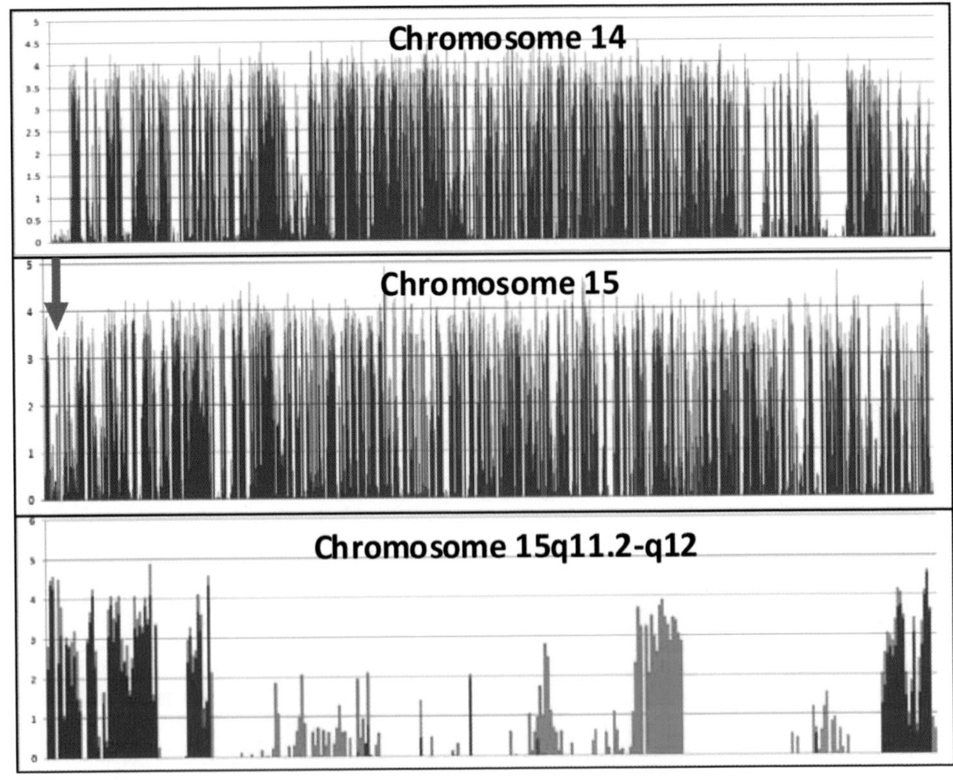

Figure 42–7. Native chromatin immunoprecipitation with microarray analysis (N-ChIP-chip). N-ChIP-chip was performed using an antibody against H3K4me3, in both a PWS-UPD and control cerebellum samples. H3K4me3, a mark indicative of transcription, is known to be absent at the SNRPN-DMR in PWS deletion and UPD samples. Immunoprecipitates were individually hybridized to an Agilent whole genome promoter array and plots of enrichment for two chromosomes superimposed (top two panels, green = control and pink = PWS). The largest difference of H3K4me3 enrichment genome-wide was detected at the *SNRPN* promoter evident by the presence of a single green peak on chromosome 15 (red arrow in middle panel). This finding was additionally confirmed by individually hybridizing samples to custom Agilent tiling arrays of 15q11-q13 (bottom panel). R.P., unpublished.

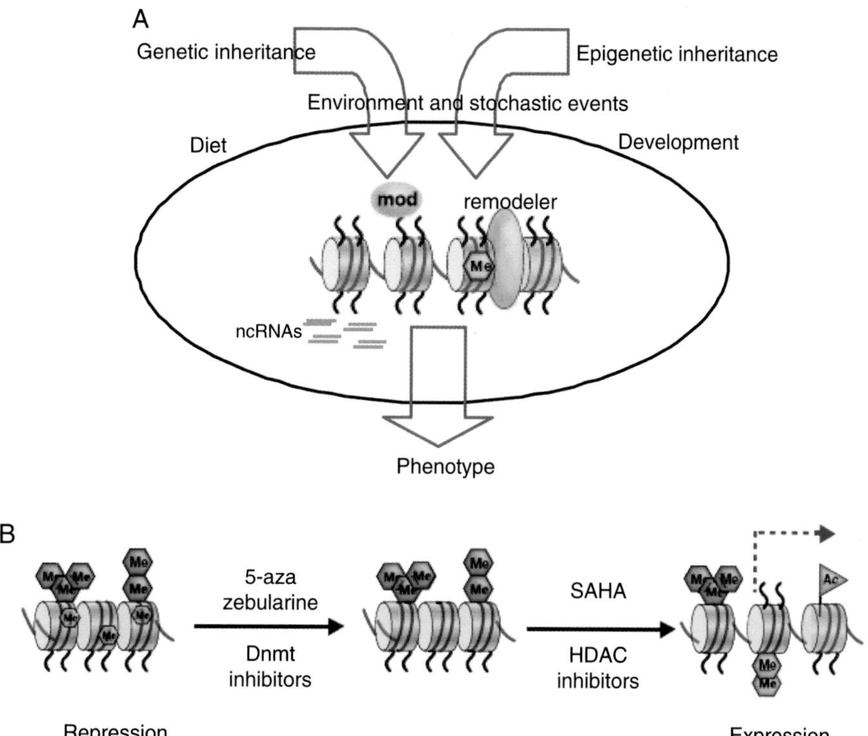

Figure 42–8. A (Upper panel). Interaction between genetics, epigenetics, and environment to give rise to phenotype. B (Lower Panel) Potential for pharmacologic modification of the epigenome. Exposure to Dnmt inhibitors such as 5-aza-cytidine (5-aza) or zebularine can result in a loss of DNA methylation, and exposure to HDAC inhibitors such as suberoylanilide hydroxamic acid (SAHA) can result in the acquisition of histone acetyl marks and subsequent downstream modifications, including active histone methyl marks and the incorporation of histone variants. The cumulative chromatin changes can lead to gene expression. Modified with permission from Chapter 3 in Allis, C. D., Jenuwein, T., & Reinberg, D. (2007). *Epigenetics*. Cold Spring Harbor, NY: Cold Spring Harbor Laboratory Press.

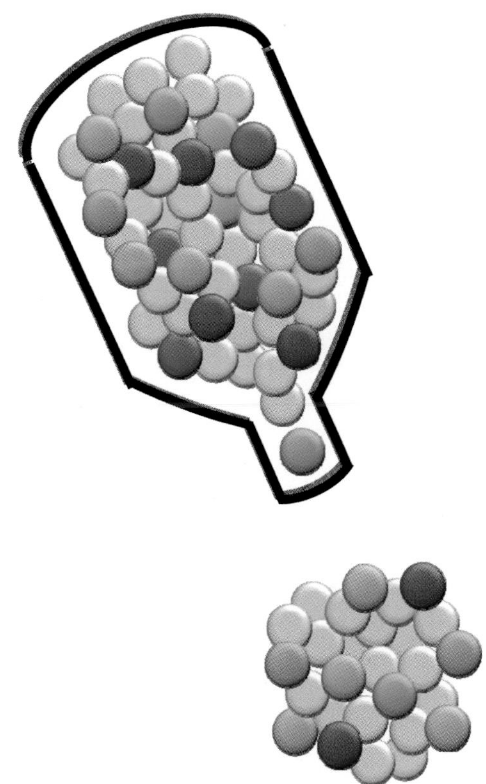

Figure 43–1. The genetic risk factors for complex traits are heterogenous in outbred populations (top). When an isolate is founded, the population goes through a genetic bottleneck, and a random selection of the original genetic risk factors are present in the new subpopulation. If the founder population is small, then random effects caused by genetic drift are accentuated. Some of the original genetic risk factors are eliminated and others are significantly enriched compared to the founder population.

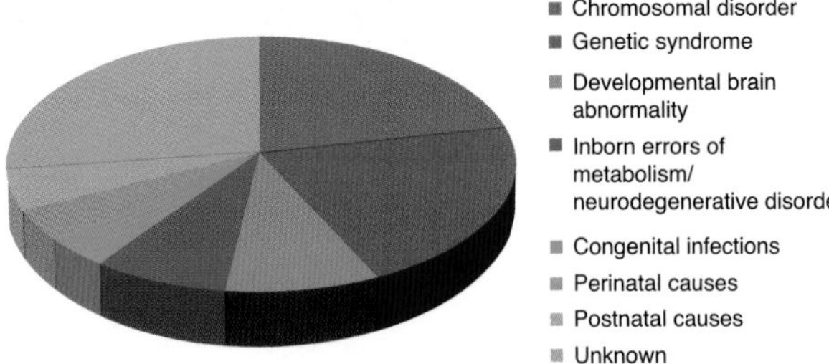

Figure 44–1. Causes of severe intellectual disability. The genetic architecture for ID may be helpful in conceptualizing at least a subset of autism. For ID, only 27% of cases cannot be accounted for by a discrete cause. 22% of diagnoses can be traced to a chromosomal disorder, and 21% of diagnoses are the result of a genetic syndrome. Other causes of intellectual disability include developmental brain abnormalities, metabolic/neurodegenerative disorders, congenital infections, and peri- and postnatal causes. Data from Stromme P and Hayberg G. (2000) Aetiology in severe and mild mental retardation: A population based study of Norwegian children. *Dev Med Child Neurol* 42: 76–86.

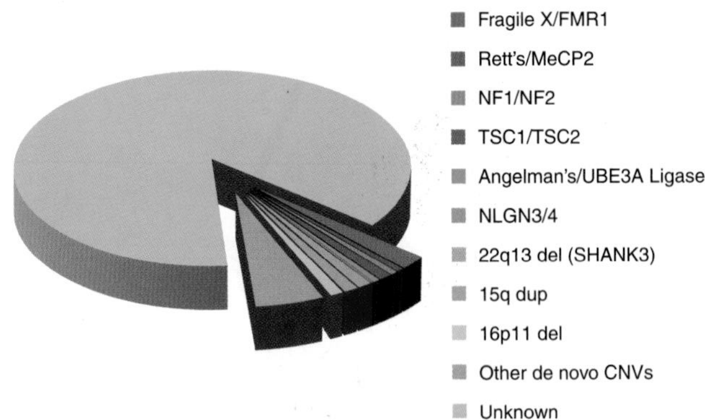

Figure 44–2. A subset of ASD has genetic architecture composed of diverse, individually-rare loci. The causes underlying ASDs are largely unknown: up to 87.4% of cases cannot be traced to a distinct genetic mechanism. Of the remaining 12.6% of cases, 5% may be attributed to de novo copy number variants (CNVs), and 2% may be attributed to silencing of the *FMR1* gene (associated with Fragile X mental retardation). The remaining cases suggest that aberrations in genes associated with Rett's Syndrome, tuberous sclerosis, and various synaptic proteins may contribute to the etiology of ASDs. Data from Abrahams, BD and Geschwind, DH. (2008) Advances in Autism Genetics: on the threshold of a new neurobiology. *Nat Rev* 9: 341–355.

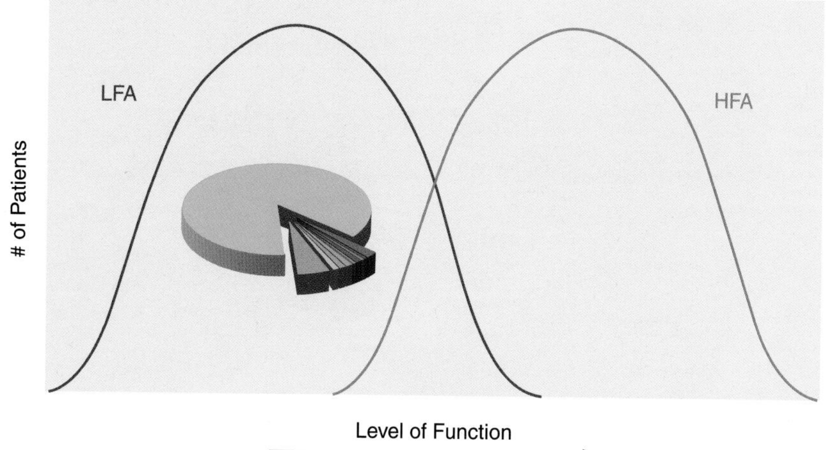

Figure 44–3. Hypothesis of the genetic architecture of ASD. ASDs may be conceptualized in a bimodal nature within the diagnosed population, with two populations of patients diagnosed: one at the low-functioning level (low-functioning autism [LFA]), which might have a genetic architecture similar to ID, and one at the high-functioning level (high-functioning autism [HFA]). which might have more complex genetic architecture. Naturally this is a straw-man hypothesis but this underlying conceptualization may have use in bringing together different schools of thought in the ASD genetics field.

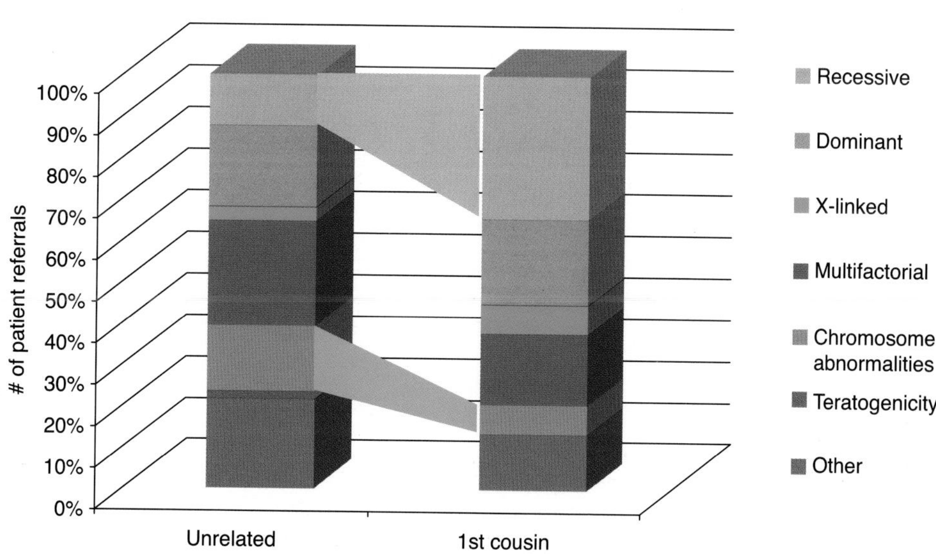

Figure 44–4. Consanguinity increases rate of recessive disorders. Causes of medical referrals between offspring with parental consanguinity versus offspring without. Autosomal recessive conditions are more than twice as common among offspring with parental consanguinity (1st cousin), than among those without (unrelated) (33.3% versus 12.4%), while chromosomal abnormalities are more than twice as common among offspring of unrelated unions in comparison with those of 1st cousin unions (15.7% versus 6.7%). Data from Hoodfar, E. and A. S. Teebi (1996). Genetic referrals of Middle Eastern origin in a western city: inbreeding and disease profile. *J Med Genet* **33**(3): 212–215.

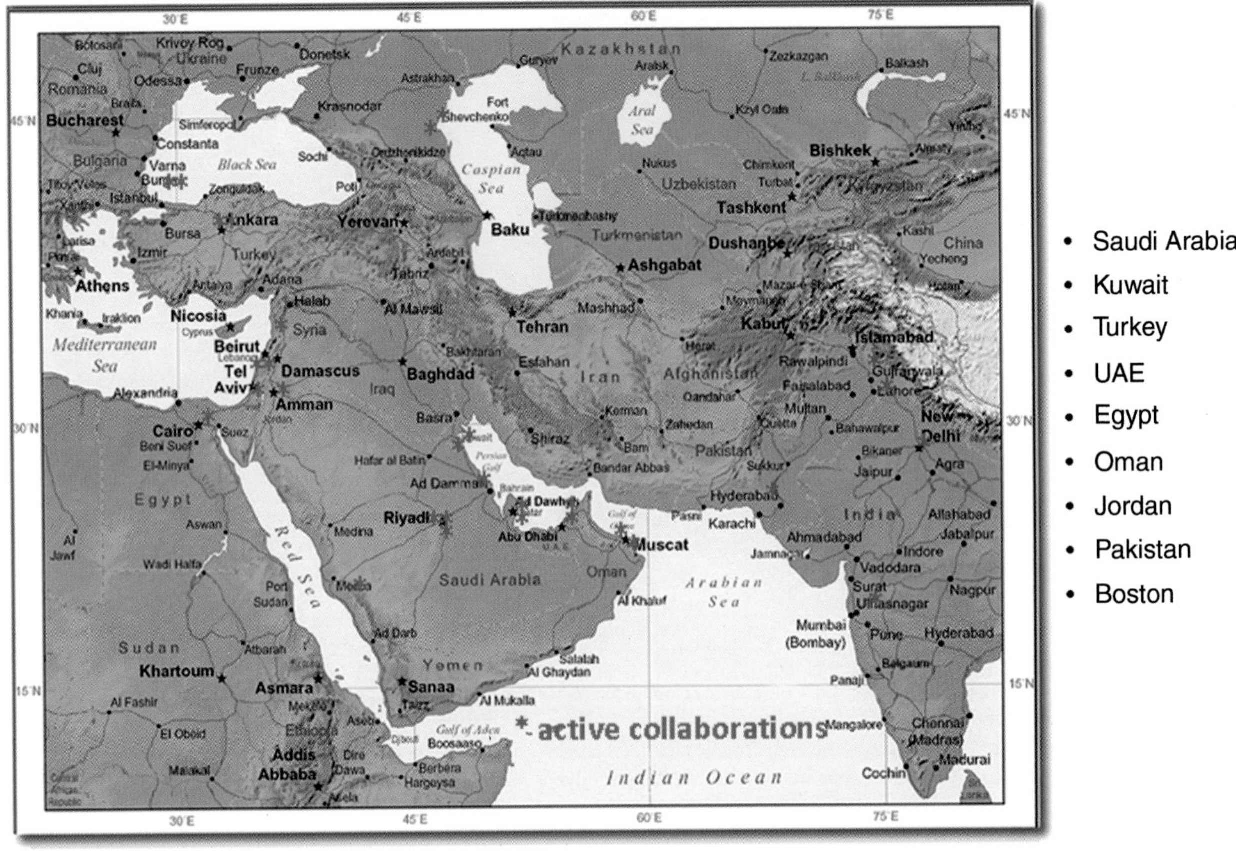

Figure 44–6. Homozygosity Mapping Collaborative for Autism (HMCA). The approach of the HMCA involves collaborators from around the world with a focus in the Middle East. Asterisks indicate locations of active collaborations. In these countries, traditions of marriage between cousins increase the prevalence of recessive disorders, which can be traced using homozygosity mapping.

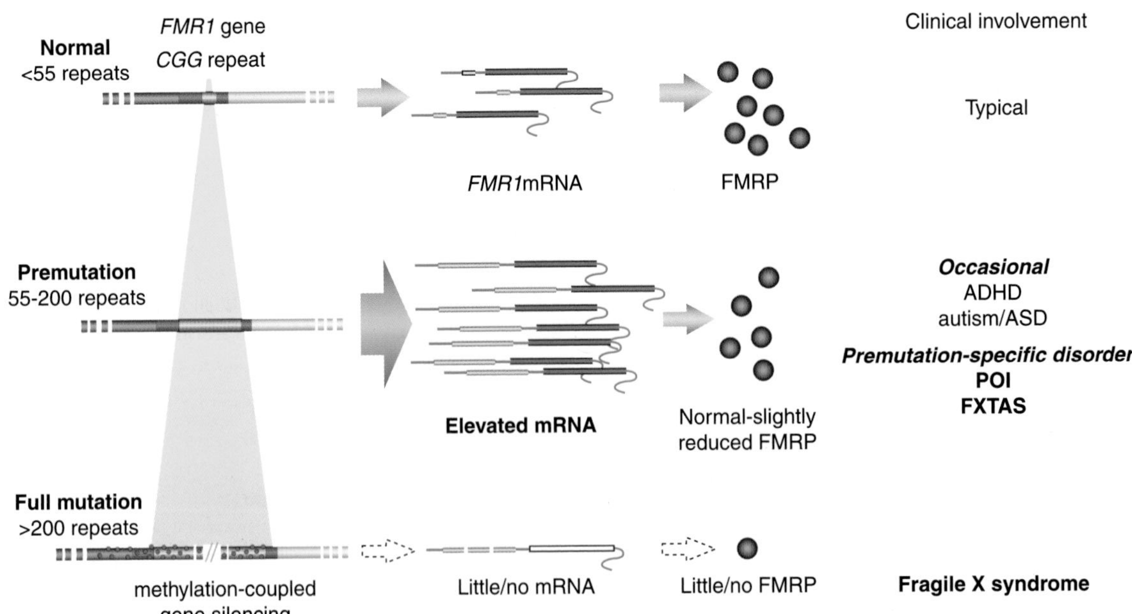

Figure 46–1. Dependence of *FMR1* expression on the length of the CGG repeat. Premutation alleles result in elevated mRNA levels (increased RNA synthesis); the increased CGG repeat in the mRNA partially blocks translation, resulting in slightly lowered protein levels in the premutation range. Full-mutation alleles are generally hypermethylated and silenced, thus producing little or no mRNA or protein. Elevated mRNA is now believed to give rise to the premutation-specific disorders, FXTAS and POI, and may also contribute to occasional children with developmental delays, ADHD, or autism. Fragile X Syndrome is caused by the absence of the protein FMRP.

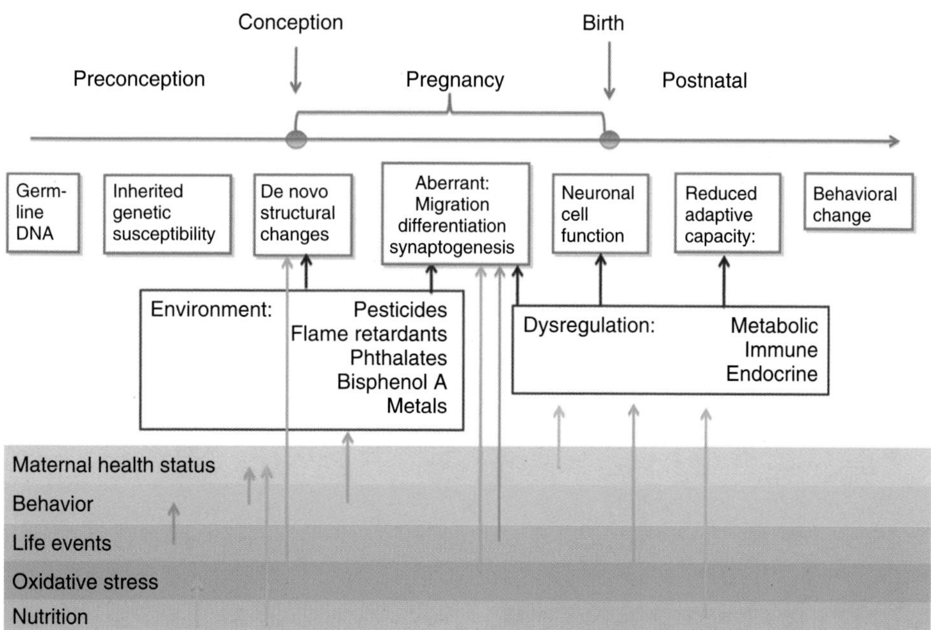

Figure 47–1. Environmental influences on development.

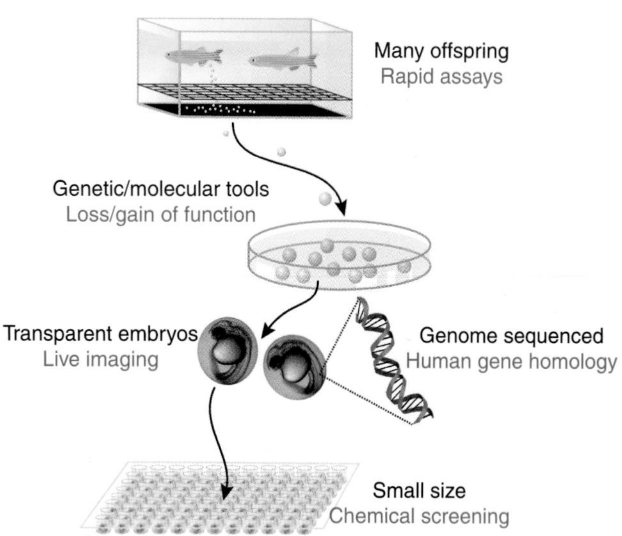

Figure 50–1. Attributes of the zebrafish. See text for details.

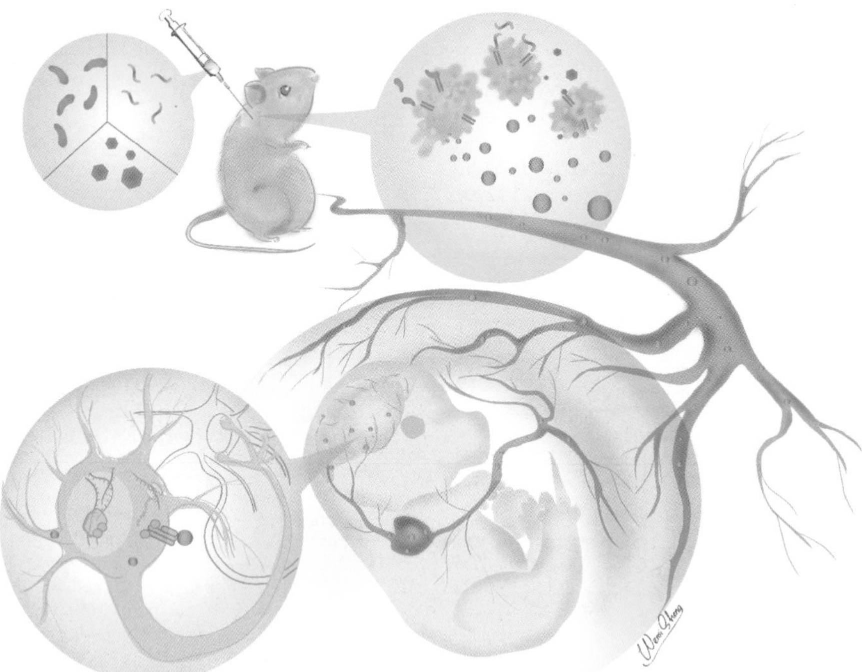

Figure 52–2. Cytokines produced by activation of the maternal immune system can alter fetal brain development. Various types of infection (bacteria, viruses, and parasites are illustrated) in pregnant rats or mice can be mimicked by injection of LPS or poly(I:C). These activate cells (pink in blue sphere) to produce cytokines (blue balls), which travel in the blood to the placenta, where they can activate cells. The cytokines can also cross the placenta into the fetal circulatory system and activate cells in the fetal brain. Illustration by Wensi Sheng.

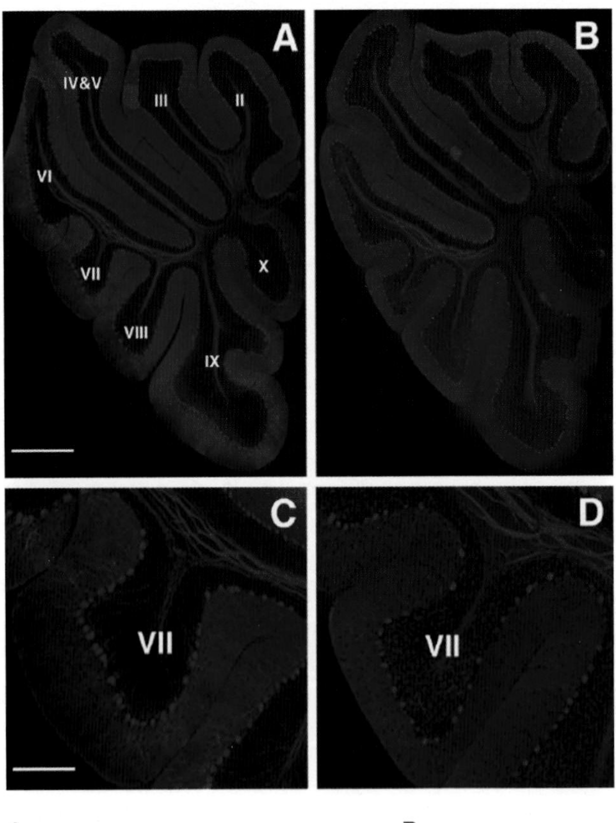

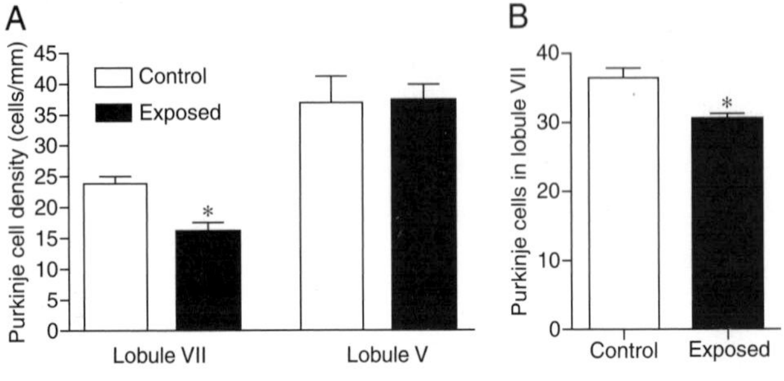

Figure 52–3. Maternal infection causes a spatially restricted Purkinje cell deficit. Adult offspring of mice given a respiratory infection with influenza virus at midgestation display a deficit in Purkinje cells in lobules VII but not in other lobules. Top: Calbindin staining of adult cerebella from offspring of control (A,C) and infected mothers (B,D) reveals a deficit in lobule VII of the latter. Panels C and D (bar = 200 μm) are higher magnification views of panels A and B (bar–800 μm). Bottom: (A) Quantification of the linear density of Purkinje cells reveals a 33% deficit in lobule VII of the adult offspring of infected mothers, while no difference from controls is found in lobule V. (B) A similar, localized deficit is observed in postnatal day 11 offspring of infected mothers. Reprinted from Shi, L., Smith, S. E., Malkova, N., Tse, D., Su, Y., & Patterson, P. H. (2009). Activation of the maternal immune system alters cerebellar development in the offspring. *Brain, Behavior, and Immunity, 23*, 116–123, with permission.

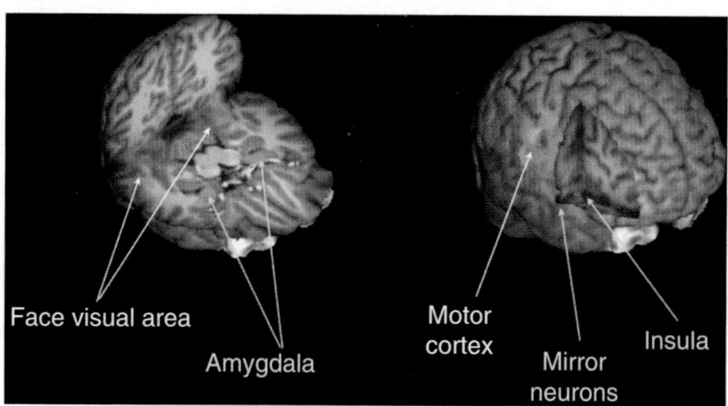

Figure 56–2. Neural Circuitry for Empathy. When subjects imitate or observe facial emotional expressions, they activate a complex network of areas. The activity in areas highlighted in yellow correlates with behavioral scales of empathy and social competence, suggesting that this neural circuit may represent a biomarker of sociality in humans.

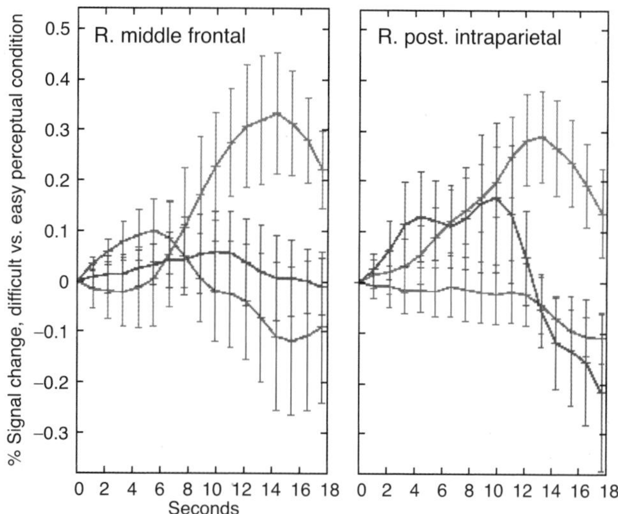

Figure 57–1. Top-down cognition in non-autistic individuals, bottom-up cognition in those with autism spectrum conditions. fMRI time-courses from prefrontal cortex (right middle frontal gyrus) and posterior, sensory-driven cortex (right posterior intraparietal sulcus at its junction with transverse occipital sulcus) illustrate that non-autistic children (red) respond rapidly to a difficult perceptual problem with additional frontal activation. In those with autism spectrum conditions (blue), this differential frontal activation is muted, delayed, and prolonged so far past the end of the experimental trial that it is of no use in rendering a response decision. Those with autism spectrum conditions seem rather to depend on bottom-up signaling from early activation of posterior cortices. Clinically unaffected sibs (magenta) of those with autism spectrum conditions manifest a similarly delayed and prolonged time-course of differential frontal activation, and a frontally driven, top-down activation of posterior cortex but not the autistic, bottom-up, early peak in posterior cortical activation. Reprinted with permission from Belmonte et al. (2010). Visual attention in autism families: "unaffected" sibs share atypical frontal activation. *Journal of Child Psychology and Psychiatry, 51*, 259–276, published by Blackwell Publishing on behalf of the Association for Child and Adolescent Mental Health.

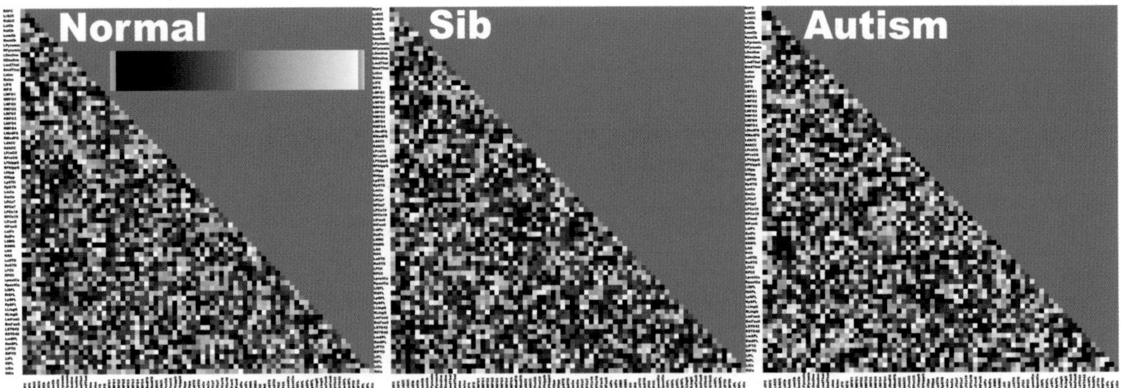

Figure 57–2. Functional connectivity among 76 brain regions (38 bilateral pairs) in children with autism spectrum conditions, clinically unaffected sibs of children with autism spectrum conditions, and unrelated non-autistic children. The axes are lists of brain regions; a colored dot indicates a statistically significant correlations between fMRI time-courses in the indicated region pair. Although no difference survives correction for the large number of multiple comparisons, when measures are collapsed across all regions pairs, the non-autistic and sib groups are statistically indistinguishable in their degrees of overall functional connectivity, whereas both groups are highly significantly distinct from the autism spectrum group. Reprinted with permission from Belmonte et al. (2010) Visual attention in autism families: "unaffected" sibs share atypical frontal activation. *Journal of Child Psychology and Psychiatry, 51*, 259–276, published by Blackwell Publishing on behalf of the Association for Child and Adolescent Mental Health.

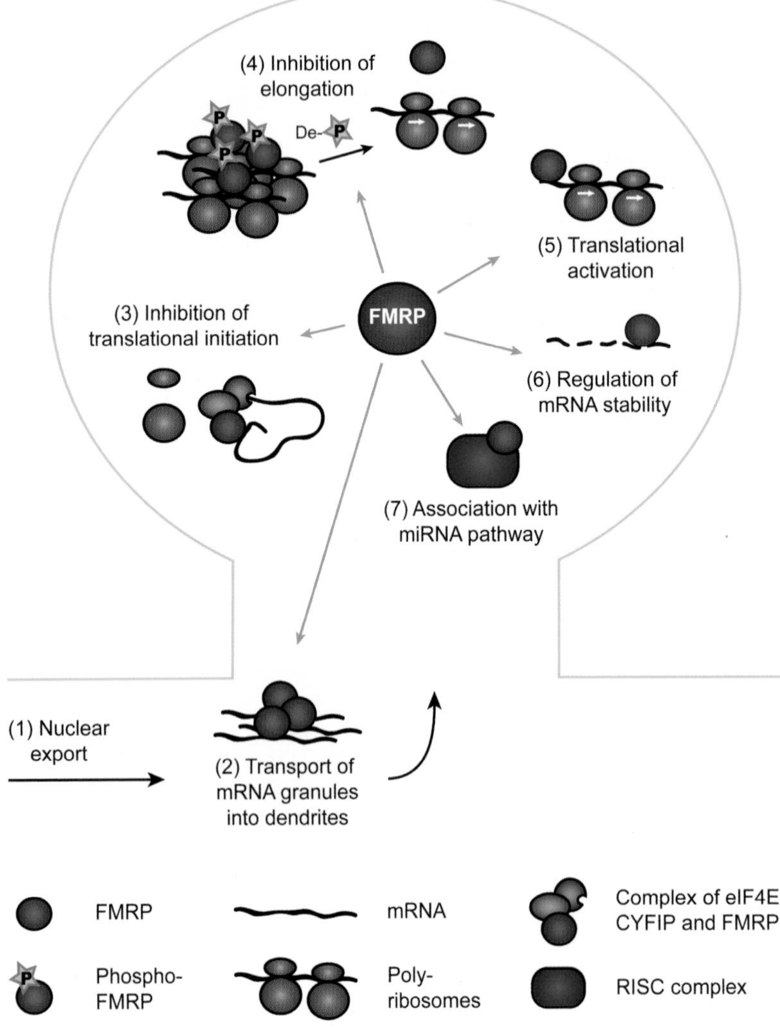

Figure 72–1. Putative roles of FMRP at the synapse. A number of different mechanisms have been proposed by which FMRP may regulate synaptic function and plasticity. These mechanisms include *(1)* Export of target mRNAs from the nucleus, *(2)* Trafficking of mRNA granules into dendrites and synapses, *(3)* Inhibition of translation initiation, *(4)* Inhibition of elongation in response to FMRP phosphorylation, possibly by sequestration of stalled ribosomes into translationally inactive mRNA granules, *(5)* Activation of translation of certain target mRNAs, *(6)* Regulation of stability of target mRNAs, and *(7)* Association with the microRNA pathway. To date, the relative contribution of each of these mechanisms to the regulation of synaptic structure and function remains unknown. It is conceivable that several of these functions occur in parallel at the same synapses or that different mechanisms may play differential roles depending on brain region, developmental stage, species, or other unknown factors.

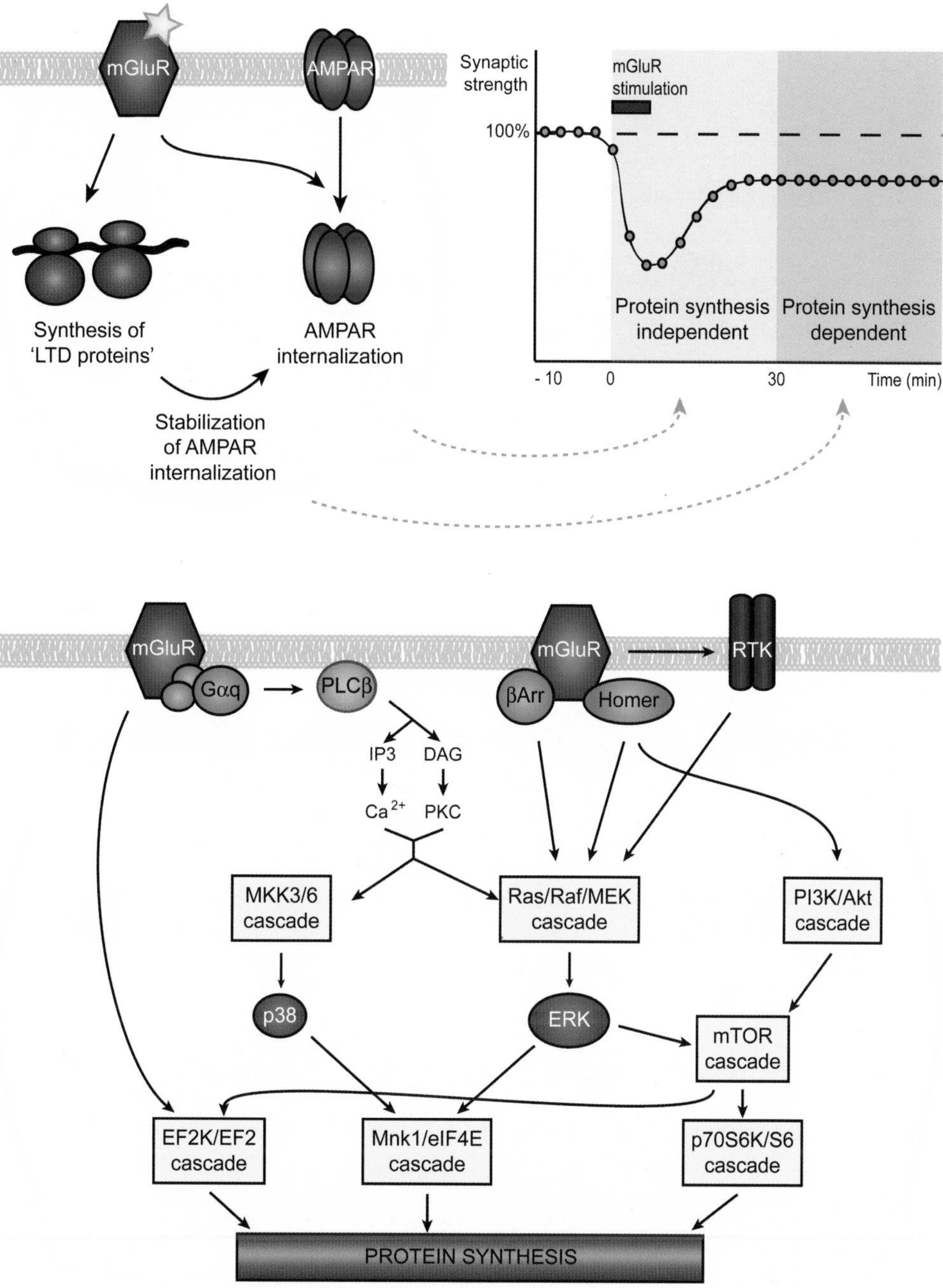

Figure 72–2. Function and signaling of group I mGluRs. *Upper panel*: Stimulation of group I mGluRs can result in the induction of long-term depression (LTD), a persistent reduction in synaptic strength. Activation of mGluRs causes a rapid internalization of postsynaptic AMPA receptor subunits, which is thought to underlie the initial, protein synthesis-independent, decrease in synaptic strength. Activation of mGluRs also stimulates synaptic protein synthesis, which results in the synthesis of "LTD proteins" that are believed to be required for stabilizing the internalized AMPA receptors. This stabilization of AMPAR internalization is believed to be the basis for the persistent, protein synthesis-dependent, decrease in synaptic strength following induction of LTD. *Lower panel:* Signaling pathways proposed to be activated upon group I mGluR stimulation. To date, the relative contribution of each of these signaling pathways to synaptic protein synthesis remains unknown and is likely to vary depending on factors such as brain region and developmental stage. It should also be noted that research into these signaling pathways is still actively ongoing, and that this schematic may therefore be incomplete.

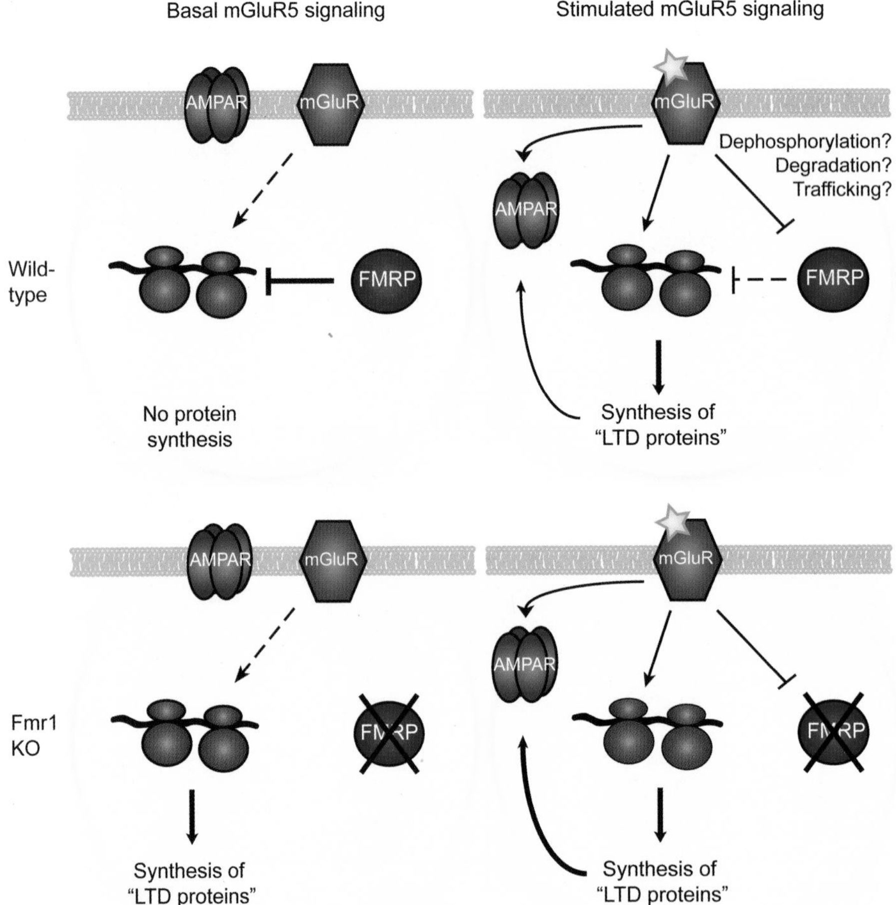

Figure 72–3. Model for the interaction between FMRP and group I mGluRs in translational regulation and LTD. *Upper left panel*: Under basal conditions in wild-type mice, FMRP acts as a repressor of protein synthesis. As a result, no protein synthesis occurs, despite low levels of basal mGluR signaling. *Upper right panel*: mGluR stimulation in wild-type mice is thought to trigger three events: *(1)* internalization of AMPA receptors, (2) upregulation of protein synthesis signaling pathways, and *(3)* relief of FMRP-mediated translational repression by dephosphorylation of FMRP, degradation of FMRP, or translocation of FMRP out of the synapse. This leads to the synthesis of "LTD proteins," which stabilize the internalized AMPA receptors, resulting in protein synthesis-dependent LTD. *Lower left panel*: In *Fmr1* KO mice, FMRP is not present to repress translation, and basal mGluR signaling is therefore sufficient to induce synthesis of LTD proteins. In the absence of AMPA receptor internalization, however, these proteins alone do not result in LTD. *Lower right panel*: Upon mGluR stimulation in *Fmr1* KO mice, AMPA receptors are internalized just as in wild-type mice. However, the LTD proteins are already present in excess, resulting in stabilization of internalized AMPA receptors and hence LTD that is both exaggerated compared to wild-type mice and independent of new protein synthesis.

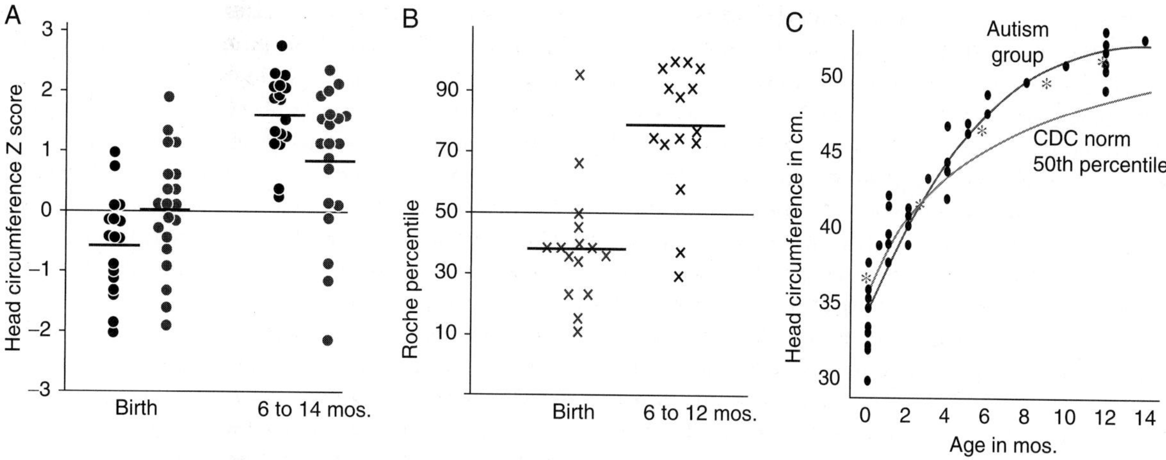

Figure 35–2. Abnormal growth of head circumference during infancy and the toddler years in autism. (A) Z scores from Courchesne et al. (2003) (in black circles) and Webb et al. (2007) (in gray circles) showing individual data points at birth and a second point between 6 and 14 months. Means represented by black lines. (B) Percentiles from Dementieva et al. (2005) showing mean and individual data points at birth and a second point between 6 and 12 months. Means represented by black lines. (C) Longitudinal data from N=14 babies who developed autism (black circles) and growth curve based on their data (darker top line) from Courchesne et al. (2003) and mean data from Webb et al. (2007) (in gray asterisks).

report of HC at birth in newborns who later go on to develop autism, it is typically near normal or slightly below normal average. What is remarkable about this evidence is the consistency of the absolute HC at birth in autism across studies and decades. Some previous reviews of the HC literature have failed to note this consistency; "differences" between studies have been due to the norms used and not to the actual size of the HC and therefore the brain at birth. Importantly, among the studies that provided individual subject HC data (Courchesne, Carper, et al., 2003; Dementieva, Vance, et al., 2005), only about 5–10% had excessively large HC at birth (Figure 35-2A and 35-2B).

Other major questions are whether HC growth patterns differ between domains of the autism spectrum (e.g., autistic disorder, PDD-NOS, and Asperger's syndrome) or vary in some other way in relation to symptom severity. Courchesne et al. (2003) reported that more abnormally accelerated HC growth at young ages was associated with more severe stereotyped and repetitive behaviors, later onset of first words, and greater likelihood of an autistic disorder rather than PDD-NOS diagnosis. In contrast, accelerated HC growth in early life in autism has been associated with higher levels of adaptive functioning (Dementieva, Vance, et al., 2005). Webb et al. (2007) did not find any association between a diagnosis of PDD-NOS versus autistic disorder or with history of regression. In one study, small and nonsignificant differences between autistic disorder and Asperger's groups in HC growth rates in the first years of life were detected, but sample sizes may have been too small to detect differences (Dissanayake, Bui, et al., 2006).

Perhaps less valuable are HC studies of older children, adolescents, and adults with ASD because with increasing age, HC becomes a progressively poorer index of the size of the brain (Aylward, Minshew, et al., 2002; Bartholomeusz, Courchesne, et al., 2002). MRI would clearly be the measure of choice at those ages, and results from such studies are reviewed below. Similarly, MRI will eventually become the measure of choice for even infants and toddlers at-risk for autism because of its greater accuracy and unparalleled resolution of living human brain anatomy.

Nonetheless, important gaps and ambiguity in information remain. While CDC or WHO norms remain the largest normative database against which to compare autism HC in early life, it is important to be able to additionally show effects in large samples of comparably recruited autistic and healthy, typically developing (nonpediatric patient) infants and toddlers. By doing so, it will be possible to test more complex and

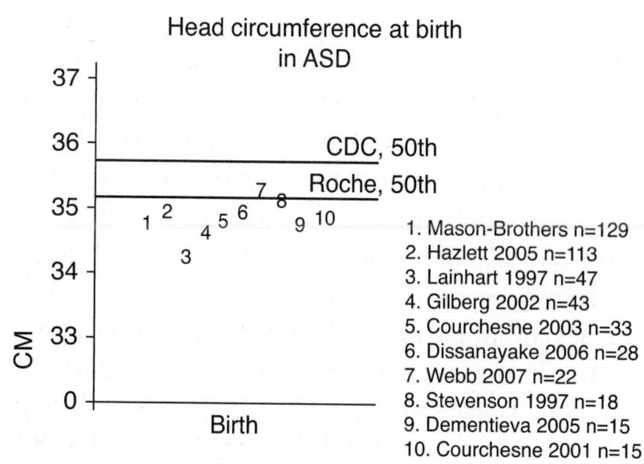

Figure 35–3. Summary of 10 reports of birth head circumference in neonates who were later diagnosed as having autism. Graph adapted from Courchesne, E., Pierce, K., et al. (2007). Mapping early brain development in autism. *Neuron, 56*(2), 399–413, and includes data means from Mason-Brothers et al., 1990; Lainhart et al., 1997; Stevenson et al., 1997; Courchesne et al., 2001; Gillberg & De Souza, 2002; Courchesne et al., 2003; Dementieva et al., 2005; Hazlett et al., 2005; Dissanayake et al., 2006; Webb et al., 2007.

clinically useful relations between growth rates of HC in early life and a variety of important biological and behavioral measures including genotype, diagnostic, prognostic, in vivo MRI and fMRI, blood biomarkers, treatment responsiveness, and so forth. To this end, a new study has developed a procedure that identifies in the general population (not just in younger siblings of autistic children) infants and toddlers who are at risk for ASD and then obtains at that early stage diagnostic, psychometric, biomarker, DNA, blood-based RNA, MRI, and fMRI measures along with HC (Pierce, Glatt et al., 2009).

The results raise the possibility that early brain overgrowth could be common across the autism spectrum, and as such may point to a common set of biological pathways that cause an ASD. Courchesne et al. (Courchesne, Pierce, et al., 2007) concluded that there was evidence that brain overgrowth occurs in the first 2-3 years of life in autism and that in many cases this growth pathology precedes the first clinical signs of the disorder (also see Courchesne, Carper, et al., 2003; Dementieva, Vance, et al., 2005; Dawson et al., 2007; Webb et al., 2007). This suggests that the neural defects that cause autism are present *before* the critical peak period of circuit formation and functional organization in higher-order social, communication, emotion, and language systems and as such cause circuit formation and function to proceed abnormally. Thus, abnormal connectivity and function was theorized to be the downstream consequence of an earlier neural defect. Finally, the authors pointed out that while a number of different cellular and molecular factors could underlie early brain overgrowth, the most obvious and likely candidates include excess neuron numbers due to dysregulation of neurogenesis and/or naturally occurring cell death and excess glial numbers (see Courchesne, Carper, et al., 2003; Courchesne & Pierce, 2005; Courchesne, Pierce, et al., 2007). The discovery of the common underlying neuropathology could be key to identification of the upstream causes of ASD. Equally important then, would be the question of whether clinical outcome differences along the spectrum (from low functioning to high) might reflect individual genetic or experiential differences that modify the impact of a common triggering neuropathology. While interesting, these possibilities remain largely conjectural, and much additional information is needed from future studies. For instance, are there clinical and/or biological differences related to age of onset, rate, duration, and magnitude of early brain overgrowth?

There is additional interest in how the accelerated postnatal HC growth in autism compares to other disorders that involve head and brain enlargement. Table 1 in Courchesne and Pierce (2005) summarizes a variety of neuroanatomical, physical, metabolic, behavioral, and/or other clinical characteristics that distinguish other disorders from autism. For example, autism does not typically involve pronounced ventricular enlargement, craniofacial abnormalities, or excessive head enlargement in utero and/or at birth, but one or another of these are common features of several other disorders presenting with excessive head size at birth as well as during infancy, such as Sotos syndrome, hydrocephaly, and macrocephaly-Cutis marmorata telangiectatica congenita (M-CMTC). Also presenting with HC enlargement at birth is familial macrocephaly (defined as absence of a clinical syndrome, normal radiographic brain development, parent or sibling with macrocephaly and/or macrocephaly traced through several generations; DeMyer, 1986). There are 164 conditions that are associated with macrocephaly (Williams, Dagli, & Battaglia, 2008). Most are extremely rare, with some having as few as 30 total cases worldwide. Thus, ASD, which occurs in 1 in 150 individuals, is the single most common condition associated with excessive head and brain size at young ages. On the other hand, unlike these other conditions—including familial macrocephaly, brain enlargement in the great majority of ASD individuals is developmentally restricted to the first several years of life, and, as discussed below, eventually most ASD individuals do *not* have excessive brain size by adolescent and adult years. Studies that have compared rates of macrocephaly in ASD to other types of mild developmental disorder (e.g., ADHD; see e.g., Rodier, Bryson, et al., 1997; Ghaziuddin, Zaccagnini, et al., 1999; Fidler, Bailey, et al., 2000) or to relatives of ASD individuals (Fidler, Bailey, et al., 2000; Miles, Hadden, et al., 2000) and have not found large differences, have not taken into account the latter fact that brain enlargement in autism is unusual in being relatively restricted to younger developmental age periods. This is reviewed further below.

MRI Evidence of Early Brain Overgrowth, Arrest, and Decline in Autism

As noted above, abnormal early brain overgrowth in autism was initially discovered in 2- to 3-year-olds with quantitative MRI nearly a decade ago (Courchesne, Karns, et al., 2001); overall brain size in the autistic toddlers was 10% larger than in typically developing toddlers (see Figure 35-4). In that study, abnormal enlargement in these very young autistic toddlers was also present for whole cerebral volume, cerebral gray matter volume, and cerebral white matter volume. This new phenomenon of pathological early brain and cerebrum overgrowth in autism has since been replicated in a number of other studies. First, in 3- to 4-year-olds, Sparks et al. (Sparks, Friedman, et al., 2002) reported a 9% larger cerebrum volume in autistic as compared to typically developing and developmentally delayed children. Then, in 2-year-olds, Hazlett et al. (Hazlett, Poe, et al., 2005) reported a significantly larger cerebrum, including cerebral gray and white matter in autism as compared to typically developing and developmentally delayed children. In the first MRI study of very young autistic girls, Bloss and Courchesne (2007) found abnormal enlargement of the brain and cerebrum volume in 2- to 5-year-old autistic girls compared to typical girls. Interestingly, this abnormal increase in brain and cerebrum size in the autistic girls was somewhat greater than that seen in age-, IQ-, and autism severity–matched autistic 2- to 5-year-old boys. Most recently, we have also found enlargement of cerebral, cerebral gray, and cerebral white volumes in 2- to 5-year-old autistic boys and girls (Schumann, Bloss, et al., 2010). As discussed below, Bloss

Brain or cerebral overgrowth in autism by 2 to 4 years of age

Courchesne et al., 2001
Sparks et al., 2002
Carper et al., 2002
Carper & Courchesne, 2005
Hazlett et al., 2005
Bloss & Courchesne, 2007
Schumann, Bloss, et al., 2010

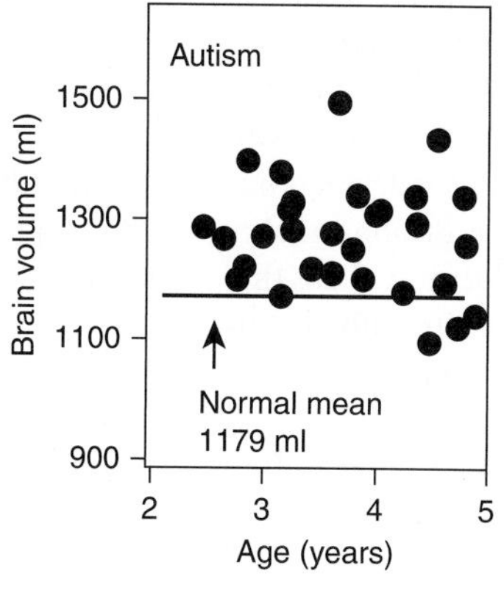

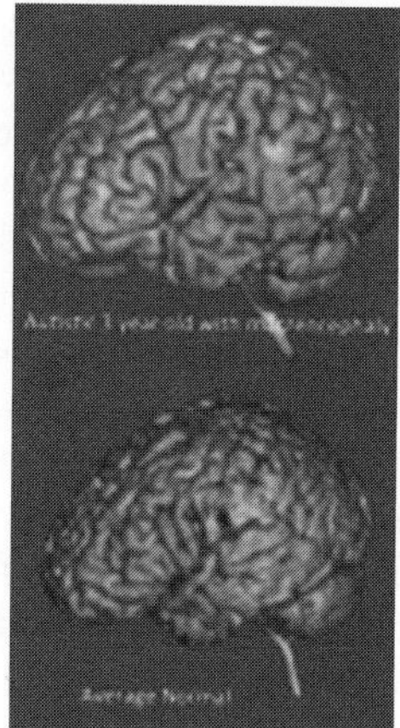

Figure 35–4. Studies showing abnormal brain or cerebral overgrowth in autism by age 2 to 4 years. Data plot shows individual MRI-based brain volumes in autistic 2- to 4-year-old males (black dots) as compared to the average volume of 1179 ml in typical 2- to 4-year-old males (from Courchesne et al., 2001). On the right, 3D reconstructions shown of a 3-year-old autistic boy with a brain volume of 1810 cc as compared to the brain of a typically developing 3-year-old boy with an average brain size. Adapted from Courchesne, E., Karns, C., et al. (2001). Unusual brain growth patterns in early life in patients with autistic disorder: An MRI study. *Neurology, 57,* 245–254.

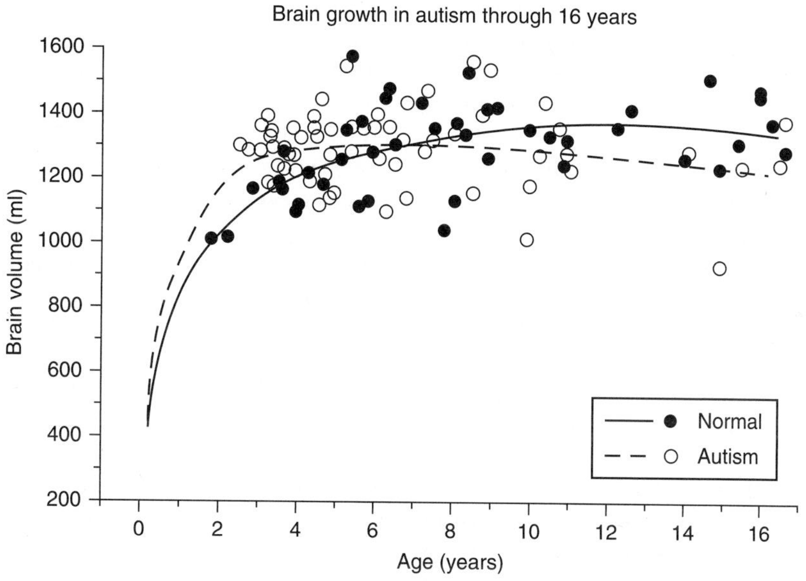

Figure 35–5. Unusual brain growth trajectory from early life to 16 years of age in autism. Data plotted from the only MRI study of age-related changes in brain size in autism from toddler years through to adolescent years. Each data point is the MRI-based brain volume from different autistic (open circles) or typically developing (closed circles) boys. Adapted from Courchesne, E., Karns, C., et al. (2001). Unusual brain growth patterns in early life in patients with autistic disorder: An MRI study. *Neurology, 57,* 245–254.

and Courchesne (2007) concluded that while abnormal early brain enlargement appears to be common to both girls and boys with autism, autistic girls may have more severe and possibly slightly different patterns of anatomic abnormality.

By quantifying MRI at all ages from 2 to 16 years, Courchesne et al. (2001) identified three different phases of pathological brain growth (see Figure 35-5). The first phase of pathology was accelerated brain overgrowth: Between the first year of life and 2–3 years of age, the autistic brain becomes abnormally enlarged. After that early period, a second phase of pathology was abnormally slow development or arrested growth: Between roughly 3–5 years and 8–9 years of age accelerated brain growth stops in most autistic children, and further growth is either abnormally slow or arrested. Finally, a third phase of pathology, less clear-cut and distinct than the first two, appeared to be premature decline, possibly due to degeneration. As discussed by Courchesne and Pierce (2005), this unusual and pathological pattern of age-related changes, which has also been found in a new lifespan study of 586 autistic and typical subjects (Courchesne, Campbell, et al., 2010), distinguishes autism from a large number of other developmental disorders that display enlarged brain size. While overgrowth of the brain as well as frontal and temporal cortices, cerebral white matter, and the amygdala in large samples of young children with autism has now been reported by several independent laboratories (see below), studies show the degree of abnormality varies across autistic children from a subset of individuals that differ little from normal average to the majority with significant enlargement including some with as much as a 50% increase in size (see Figure 35-5).

This first developmental MRI study of 2- to 16-year-olds as well as a recent study of 1 to 50 year olds (Courchesne, Campbell, et al., 2010) make clear one major and fundamental point about autism: The underlying neural pathological processes and structural abnormalities in autism change with age: That is, they are not the same at all ages, and so neural, functional, behavioral, and genetic study of the older autistic brain reflects *outcome,* not the original upstream events and defects that started the disorder. Consider that a host of evidence on the adolescent and adult autistic brain (review: Courchesne, Campbell, et al., 2010) shows reduced size and/or volume loss in cerebral, amygdala, callosum and cerebellar structures (see below), neuron loss in the amygdala, cerebellum and fusiform cortex (Bailey, Luthert, et al., 1998; Schumann & Amaral, 2006; van Kooten, Palmen, et al., 2008), decreased dendritic arbors and minicolumn size (Casanova, Buxhoeveden, et al., 2002; Mukaetova-Ladinska, Arnold, et al., 2004; Buxhoeveden, Semendeferi, et al., 2006; Casanova, van Kooten, et al., 2006; Morgan et al., submitted), the presence of proapoptotic molecules (Araghi-Niknam & Fatemi, 2003), and possible Purkinje cell degeneration with neuroinflammation (Vargas et al., 2005), none of which can account for early brain enlargement. Furthermore, these three separate phases of pathology indicate that autism almost certainly must involve multiple different underlying neural defects and processes and therefore genetic and nongenetic factors associated with each one (Courchesne & Pierce, 2005; Courchesne, Pierce, et al., 2007).

Three new longitudinal studies provide evidence consistent with this theory of three different phases of pathological brain growth in autism. One found significant cerebral enlargement and abnormal cerebral growth trajectories across the ages of 2–5 years in autism (Schumann, Bloss, et al., 2010), while another found evidence of a slightly accelerated rate of loss of cerebral gray matter in several regions including the frontal cortex in older autistic children and preadolescents (Hardan, Libove, et al., 2009). The third found evidence of brain overgrowth in the first years of life but an accelerated rate of loss of brain volume from preadolescence to 50 years of age (Courchesne, Campbell, et al., 2010). Interestingly, in the first quantitative study of age-related changes in the postmortem brain in autism, Morgan et al. (Morgan, Buxhoeveden, et al., submitted) found evidence of enlargement of neuropil space in cerebral gray matter in very young autistic cases but reduction in adolescent and adult cases, which parallels the developmental pattern of early cerebral enlargement and later decline seen via MRI. While there have been only two longitudinal MRI studies of cerebral growth, there have been a large number of MRI studies of adolescent and adult autism subjects. At these older ages, effects have been variable, with some studies reporting slightly larger cerebral gray matter volumes (Lotspeich, Kwon, et al., 2004; Palmen, Hulshoff Pol, et al., 2005; Hazlett, Poe, et al., 2006), but most reporting either slightly reduced volumes (Courchesne, Karns, et al., 2001) or no difference from normal (Herbert, Ziegler, et al., 2003; Rojas, Peterson, et al., 2006). Nonetheless, the pattern across these several studies is consistent with an overall decline in the difference between autism and normal with age. Further, one study of the distribution of cortical thickness shows widespread but patchy thinning or atrophy in autistic adults in regions involved in social cognition and emotion processing, including frontal, temporal, and parietal areas (Hadjikhani, Joseph, et al., 2006); cortical thinning was also correlated with autism symptom severity.

Because the Courchesne, Karns, et al. (2001) and Courchesne, Campbell, et al. (2010) MRI studies are the only ones to quantitatively and statistically analyze age-related anatomical changes in brain size from early toddler years to adolescence and adulthood, the best objective method for testing their results and conclusions at the present time is via a formal, statistical meta-analysis of all brain size data that has been reported in other more age-limited studies of autism (Redcay & Courchesne, 2005; Stanfield, McIntosh, et al., 2008).

Statistical Meta-Analyses of the Autism MRI and Postmortem Literature: Evidence of Overgrowth, Arrest, and Decline

To test this theory and the generality of age-related changes in MRI-based brain size observed from ages 2 to 16 years in autism, Redcay and Courchesne (2005) analyzed all brain size data available from the autism literature and showed the entire developmental course of brain size in autism. Data from 12 MRI studies on autism were included covering ages 2–46 years, head circumference data from three studies on autism in the first years of life, brain weight data from 55 postmortem autistic cases covering ages 3–65 years, and brain weight data from more than 8,000 postmortem cases from 10 studies covering ages from birth to 70 years. The strength of their meta-analysis was in its large autism subject sample size ($n = 531$) allowing for the power to detect age-related changes in brain size in autism and to concurrently examine the consistency of findings across measurement type (head circumference, MRI brain volume, postmortem brain weight) and research study.

Their analyses showed that early postnatal brain overgrowth is a phenomenon in autism that is detectable across multiple study samples and measurement methods (Figure 35-6). These findings suggest that "conflicting" reports of brain size may be largely an effect of age. Despite the method of acquisition, when brain size findings were organized according to age, a clear pattern of early brain overgrowth followed by normal brain size in adulthood emerged. Thus, this study confirmed that abnormal brain enlargement in autism is

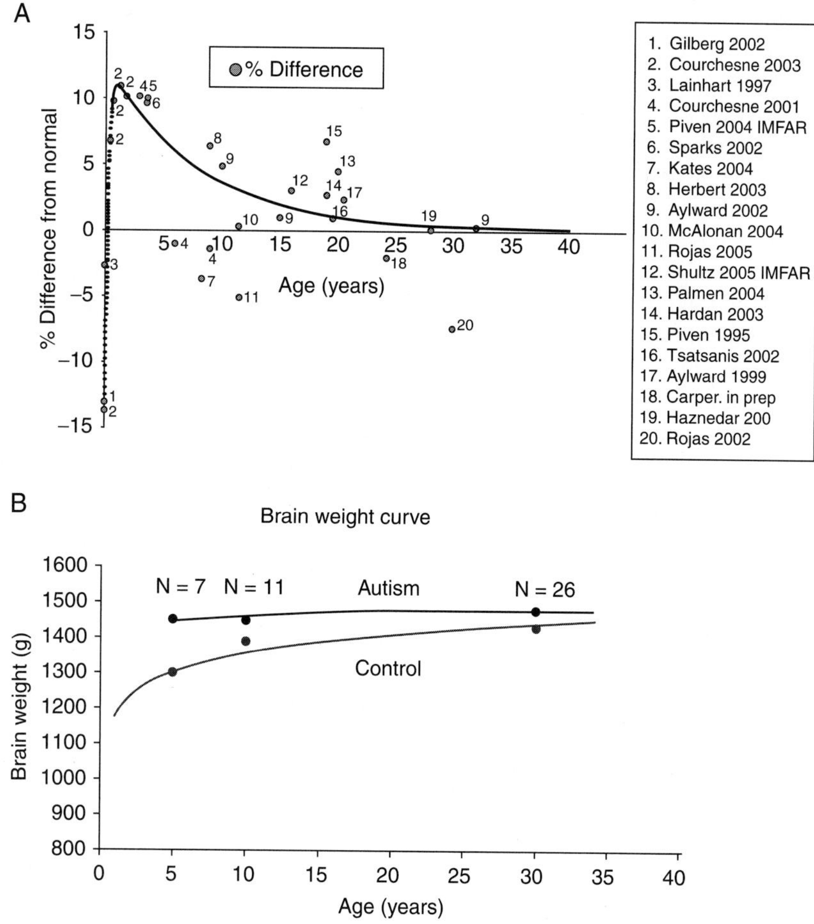

Figure 35–6. In autism the difference in brain size from normal diminishes with age. (A) Plot of a meta-analysis of 20 studies depicting brain size changes with age in ASD. Adapted with permission from Redcay, E. & Courchesne, E. (2005). When is the brain enlarged in autism? A meta-analysis of all brain size reports. *Biol Psychiatry, 58*(1), 1–9. (B) Autism and control mean brain weight by age. Means of postmortem brain weight values from individual autistic males and mean normative data were calculated for three age groups (3–5, 7–12, 13–70). Comparison of the two lines illustrates that while the normal brain continues to grow into adolescence, the autistic brain has already reached its near maximal weight by 3–5 years of age.

time-delimited to the first 2 to 3 years of life and is followed by arrested or abnormally slow growth, as shown in Figure 35-5. It is especially important to see that the two main but very different methods of measuring brain size—volume from MRI and weight from postmortem analyses—portray the very same picture of early overgrowth in the first years of life followed by arrested growth (compare panels A and B in Figure 35-6). Moreover, by the end of this first phase of growth pathology, the 3- to 5-year-old autistic brain has already reached a size not very different from a normal adult or adolescent (see panel B of Figure 35-6). So, in autism, full brain size is achieved 8 to 10 years prematurely, but unlike many other disorders involving macroencephaly, this excess size does not persist in most cases into the preadolescent, adolescent, and adult years. This demonstrates an important aspect of the unusual brain growth profile in autism. In addition, these analyses indicate that at the age of typical clinical diagnosis of the disorder (i.e., 3–4 years), the critical early period of pathological growth and arrest has likely already passed, leaving clinicians and researchers with an outcome, rather than process, of pathology for study and treatment intervention.

Stanfield and colleagues (Stanfield, McIntosh, et al., 2008) conducted another major meta-analyses of the entire autism MRI literature. Their results are consistent with those of Redcay and Courchesne (Redcay & Courchesne, 2005) and extend them in many important ways including the addition of 4 new MRI brain volume studies (for a total of N = 16 MRI studies) and the inclusion of calculations of effect sizes and age-effects for many other major regions of interest. Many key findings result from their work: First, they showed age-related changes in brain overgrowth with maximum abnormality at the youngest ages and then steadily decreasing differences thereafter with negligible differences by adulthood, a pattern that confirms the original cross-sectional findings of Courchesne, et al. (2001) and the Redcay and Courchesne (2005) brain development meta-analyses. In short, the abnormal brain size findings change with age in autism. Second, in the first formal meta-analyses of other brain regions in autism, Stanfield et al. also demonstrated that for many other structures, effects also change with age in autism. Like overall brain volume, amygdala volume is enlarged in 3- to 4-year-old autistic children, as first discovered by Dawson and colleagues (Sparks et al., 2002), but this difference declines with age so that by adulthood, the amygdala is *reduced* in size (see further discussion below). Third, in some regions that are significantly *smaller than normal at the youngest ages in autism*, such as the cerebellar vermis lobules VI–VII, there is an age-related change whereby they become *near normal in size by adulthood* (Stanfield, McIntosh, et al., 2008) (see further discussion below).

In sum, a major discovery in autism comes out of these cross-sectional, longitudinal, and meta-analysis studies of age-related changes in brain structure in autism: The landscape of neuroanatomic abnormality in autism changes significantly with age from birth through early childhood to adulthood. Effects should be *expected* to vary somewhat from study to study so that negative findings need to be considered in the larger frame of reference of the literature rather than as "contradictory" evidence, small sample sizes may not be as desirable as very large ones, and age is a major factor that must always be taken into account.

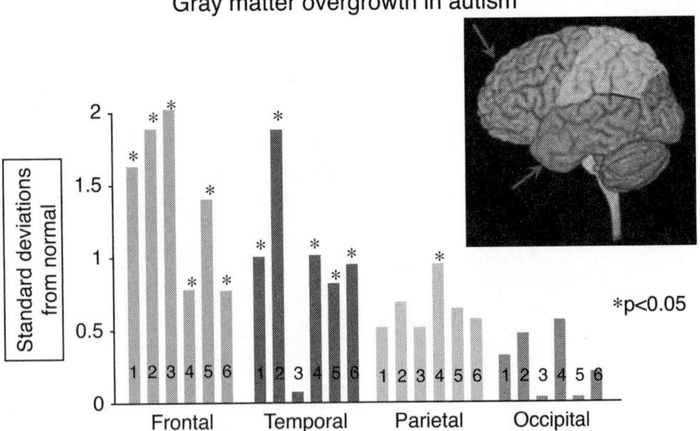

Figure 35–7. Summary of observed gray matter abnormalities (standard deviations from normal) from studies of children and adolescents with autism. Included data from: (1) Carper et al., 2002; (2) Bloss & Courchesne, 2007; (3) Kates et al., 2004; (4) Palmen et al., 2005; (5) Hazlett et al., 2005; (6) Schumann, Bloss et al., 2010. Note the general gradient of abnormality, with frontal and temporal regions most profoundly enlarged. Adapted from Courchesne, E., Pierce, K., et al. (2007). Mapping early brain development in autism. *Neuron, 56*(2), 399–413. (See Color Plate Section for a color version of this figure.)

Specific Regions Showing Early Overgrowth

The Frontal and Temporal Lobes

Signature abnormalities of autism in the first years of life are deficits in higher-order social, language, communication, and emotion functions, each one heavily dependent on frontal and temporal lobes. Conversely, relatively spared in autism are visual-spatial abilities mediated by posterior cortical areas, especially occipital cortex. To test the hypothesis that frontal and temporal lobes are indeed developmentally abnormal at the time of clinical onset, Carper et al. (Carper, Moses, et al., 2002) conducted the first autism MRI study to separately measure frontal, temporal, parietal, and occipital lobes. They found overgrowth of frontal and temporal, but not parietal and occipital, gray matter in autistic 2- to 4-year-olds as compared to typically developing children (Figure 35-7). Since then a number of MRI studies have also separately measured each of these lobes in autistic subjects. In the youngest age group studied to date, 2-year-olds with autism had enlargement of frontal, temporal, and cingulate cortices (Schumann, Bloss, et al., 2010). As seen in Figure 35-7, across multiple studies (Carper, Moses, et al., 2002; Kates, Burnette, et al., 2004; Hazlett, Poe, et al., 2005; Palmen, Hulshoff Pol, et al., 2005; Bloss & Courchesne, 2007; Schumann, Bloss, et al., 2010) frontal and temporal gray matter volumes are most abnormally enlarged while occipital is the least. Within frontal cortex, dorsolateral and mesial prefrontal gray matter volumes (Carper & Courchesne, 2005) and cingulate gray matter volume (Schumann, Bloss, et al., 2010) are most enlarged in very young autistic children, while orbital gray matter is little affected. Thus, frontal areas that mediate social, language, communication, and higher-order cognitive functions are most developmentally abnormal in autism.

These effects vary somewhat with gender. First, as compared to 2- to 5-year-old boys with autism, 2- to 5-year-old girls with autism show somewhat more severe enlargement in frontal and temporal cortices (Bloss & Courchesne, 2007; Schumann, Bloss, et al., 2010). Second, in 2- to 5-year-old girls with autism, the temporal cortex is much more abnormal than frontal cortex, while in young boys, abnormality may be slightly greater in frontal (Bloss & Courchesne, 2007; Schumann, Bloss, et al., 2010). In the first longitudinal MRI study of cerebral cortex during early development, 2- to 5-year-old boys and girls with autism had abnormal growth rates in multiple cortical regions (overall cerebral gray, frontal gray, temporal gray, cingulate gray, and parietal gray) except occipital gray, but the girls with autism had a more pronounced abnormal growth profile in more cerebral regions than did boys with autism.

White matter also shows striking regional differences, with both volumetric (Carper, Moses, et al., 2002) and DTI (Ben Bashat, Kronfeld-Duenias, et al., 2007) measures being most deviant in frontal regions and least in occipital lobe in 2- to 5-year-old children with autism. Roughly parallel to these regional differences, Herbert et al. (2003) report that the greatest deviation in their 7- to 11-year-old subjects with autism was in short-distance white matter immediately underlying frontal cortices and the least deviation in long-distance pathways and in occipital white matter.

Missing are studies of cortical folding patterns, surface area, and thickness in specific frontal and temporal regions at very young ages in autism. Such studies would provide invaluable clues to the neural and connectivity defects that underlie the early abnormal overgrowth. One study of sulcal patterns in 10-year-olds with autism (Levitt, Blanton, et al., 2003) found a tendency for some frontal and temporal sulci to be more posterior-superiorly positioned than normal—which could be consistent with frontal and temporal overgrowth. Another study (Nordahl, Dierker, et al., 2007) found significant cortical shape differences between autistic and control 7- to 12-year-olds, primarily in the inferior lateral frontal cortex. Because segmentation and surface reconstruction in the infant and toddler pose special challenges to most commonly used MRI analysis programs, studies of cortical thickness and surface area are susceptible to mismeasurement. Unfortunately, many such programs were originally developed to process adult gray, white, and CSF voxel signals that differ in important ways from the young developing brain, and they can make substantial errors when applied to young populations. Further, surface rendering algorithms that operate best in the mature brain whose sulci have much more CSF than the young developing brain, can make even more substantial errors in correctly finding the entire surface of deep sulci in young brains. Nonetheless, advances in this area will be crucial to discovery of the underlying neural and connectivity defects present in the abnormally enlarged frontal and temporal cortex in autistic babies and toddlers.

Arrested or abnormally slowed growth in frontal and temporal lobes occurs sometime during early to middle childhood, but there is too little information to be certain of the timing of this and how it might vary across autistic individuals and with clinical variables. To date, only two cross-sectional MRI studies provide information (Carper, Moses, et al., 2002; Carper & Courchesne, 2005). Carper, Moses, et al. (2002) show that between 2 and 4 years of age and later childhood, frontal and temporal lobes undergo robust increases in gray and white matter in typical children but little or no growth in children with autism. By late childhood, the autistic frontal and temporal lobe is marginally different in size compared to typical children.

If verified, this would mean that studies of the clinical and biological correlates of frontal and temporal anatomical abnormality should target infants and toddlers when the abnormality is most quantitatively evident. Since overgrowth effect sizes are small to medium for many of the measures reported for frontal and temporal lobes, it will be necessary to image large samples of both typically developing and autistic infants and toddlers in order to detect replicable anatomico-clinical and anatomico-biological correlations. The recent work by Piven and colleagues is currently the best example of a successful design aimed at testing specific brain overgrowth–genetic relationships. In a large sample of very young autistic children, they (Wassink, Losh, et al., 2007) found cerebral and frontal gray matter overgrowth related to a functional promoter polymorphism of a gene that modulates serotonin reuptake, SLC6A4. During early stages of development, serotonin plays an important role in neurite outgrowth and possibly synaptic stabilization, and so change in its availability for release at synapses could impact neurite growth and connectivity.

A major gap in knowledge in autism is the absence of data that explain the frontal and temporal overgrowth in the first years of life. While every paper reviewing the literature has made interesting speculations, virtually no evidence has been found to support any current conjecture. In brief, no cellular or molecular study of the young autistic postmortem brain has been published, with the exception of rare individual cases (e.g., Buxhoeveden, Semendeferi, et al., 2006; Kennedy, Semendeferi, et al., 2007). When one or two young autism cases have been included, statistical analyses have not examined age-effects. For instance, some have speculated that overgrowth is due to an excess number of minicolumns. However, the number of minicolumns in frontal or temporal regions has never been quantified. Further, while adult autism cases have been repeatedly shown to have abnormally narrow minicolumn widths, two recent studies do not find this abnormality in very young autism cases (Buxhoeveden, Semendeferi, et al., 2006; Morgan, Buxhoevede, et al., submitted), but instead find evidence of neuropil increases at young ages. A popular explanation for autism and overgrowth is abnormal, perhaps excess, synaptogenesis or failure of synaptic pruning and connections. However, synapse numbers and morphology have never been examined in the young autistic brain. Excess local connectivity and disproportionately reduced long-distance functional connectivity have been speculated in numerous papers (Belmonte, Cook, et al., 2004; Courchesne & Pierce, 2005; Just, Cherkassky, et al., 2007; Geschwind & Levitt, 2007), but this has never been verified by postmortem analyses, and no one has addressed how disconnection could produce excess growth in early life in autism.

There is a simple reason for this lack of key knowledge: Almost all of the more than 40 postmortem publications have examined the autistic brain at older ages, and so their observations may well reflect the *long-term outcome pathological process* rather than the original pathology that causes overgrowth and autism in the first place. Studying early defects is possible. For instance, Morgan et al. (submitted, personal communication), in frontal cortex minicolumns, has examined neural and glial spatial organization and microglial activation in autistic cases ages 3 to 50 and analyzed for age-related effects. In one of these studies, for instance, at the youngest ages, there was an increase in neuropil space, but with age there is a failure of further growth and eventually minicolumns become reduced. In another, at the youngest ages microglial density and size was already abnormally greater in autism than controls.

With the exception of Piven and colleagues (Wassink, Losh, et al., 2007; Davis, Hazlett, et al., 2008), there have been no studies aimed at identifying genes associated with early brain, including frontal and temporal lobe, white and gray matter overgrowth. Across genomewide association studies, CNV studies, specific gene association, and gene expression studies of autism, more than 400 genes have been implicated at one time or another in the disorder. A large number of these have to do with synaptic structure and function, neurite growth, apoptosis, and many other developmental and brain organization functions and would thus serve as a good beginning point for targeted brain-gene analyses, provided the brain data came from very young autism subjects and not only from adolescents or adults with autism whose brain measurements would not be a good index of early growth pathology.

The importance of establishing the genetic, molecular, and cellular bases of early frontal and temporal lobe maldevelopment in autism is very high because functional imaging studies (e.g., fMRI, EEG, and ERP) and core clinical symptoms all point to deficits in these regions, the amygdala (see below), and cerebellum (see below) as fundamental to autism.

The Amygdala

The amygdala has long been a site of intense interest in the search for neuropathology in the brains of people, given its well-established role in the production and recognition of emotions and modulatory role in social behavior (Adolphs, 2001). However, the heterogeneity and unknown etiologies of autism, variability of methods employed between laboratories, and different age groups studied have limited the consistency of results across structural MRI studies of amygdala volume (Schumann & Amaral, 2009). It was only when the age of the subject was considered to be a critical factor did an interesting pattern of amygdala development in children with autism emerge (Schumann, Hamstra, et al., 2004). Four studies of toddlers and young children with autism have found the amygdala to be enlarged by ~15% relative to age-matched controls (Sparks, Friedman, et al., 2002; Schumann, Hamstra, et al., 2004; Mosconi, Cody-Hazlett, et al., 2009; Schumann, Barnes, et al., 2009). However, studies of older adolescents, adults, or a wide age range of subjects, have found either no difference in (Schumann, Hamstra, et al., 2004; Palmen, Durston, et al., 2006) or even smaller (Aylward, Minshew, et al., 1999; Pierce, 2001; Nacewicz, Dalton, et al., 2006) amygdala volumes in individuals with autism. In addition, the amygdala continues to grow in size throughout adolescence in typically developing male children (Giedd, 1997), but this growth pattern does not seem to take place in male children with autism (Schumann, Hamstra, et al., 2004). Therefore, the amygdala appears to be initially larger than normal in children with autism, but does not undergo the same age-related increase in volume that takes place in typical children (Figure 35-8). This hypothesis parallels the general theory of early brain overgrowth, as discussed above (Courchesne, Karns, et al., 2001; Courchesne, Pierce, et al., 2007), although the aberrant growth trajectory of the amygdala may extend to a later age of development relative to cortical regions (Schumann, Hamstra, et al., 2004).

Sparks and colleagues were the first to suggest that the amygdala may be enlarged in young children with autism at 36–56 months of age (Sparks, Friedman, et al., 2002). In this same cohort of children, Munson et al. (Munson, Dawson, et al., 2006) found that the amygdala enlargement in the children with autism was associated with more severe social and communication impairments on the ADI and Vineland Adaptive Scales and poorer outcome at 6 years of age. In a recent longitudinal study of children at 2 and 4 years of age, bilateral amygdala enlargement was also observed in children with autism compared to a control group that consisted of typical and developmentally delayed children (Mosconi, Cody-Hazlett, et al., 2009).

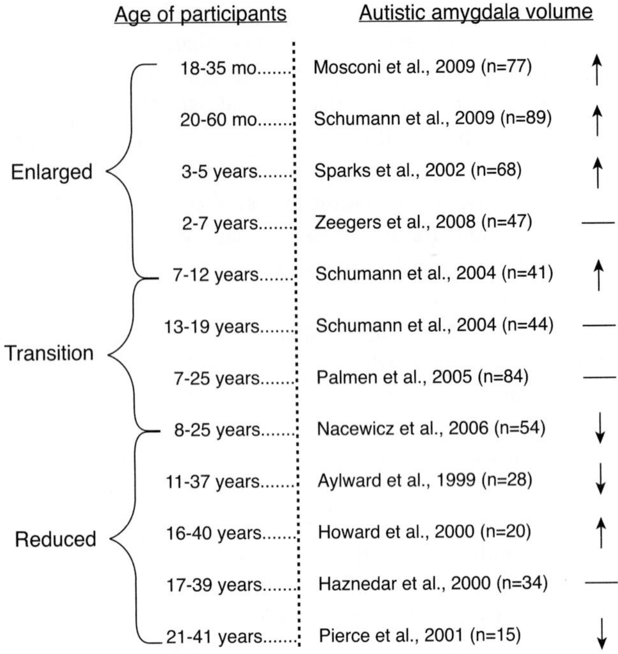

Figure 35–8. Summary of findings on amygdala volume in autism from 11 MRI studies showing age-related changes in differences from normal size. Upward arrows indicate studies that found greater amygdala volumes in autism compared to normal average; short horizontal lines indicates studies finding no amygdala volume differences between autism and normal; and downward arrows indicate studies findings smaller amygdala volumes in autism compared to normal average.

Schumann and colleagues (Schumann, Barnes, et al., 2009) recently carried out a prospective study to measure amygdala volume in toddlers at risk for autism at the age of first clinical detection compared to age-matched typically developing children; the children underwent an MRI around 3 years of age and returned later at 5 years of age for clinical diagnosis and testing. They found further evidence that the amygdala is enlarged in young children with autism and that the overgrowth must begin before 3 years of age, at about the time symptoms become clinically evident (Figure 35-9). As found in the Sparks (Sparks, Friedman, et al., 2002) and Mosconi (Mosconi, Cody-Hazlett, et al., 2009) studies, the amygdala was disproportionately enlarged relative to total cerebral volume at 3 years of age. This study differed from previous studies on amygdala volume in that one of the primary goals was to characterize the neuropathological and behavioral profiles of males and females with autism independently. Strikingly, amygdala enlargement in females with autism was found to be more severe, compared to age- and gender-matched typically developing counterparts, than in males with autism (Figure 35-9). This significant difference was present despite a group size of only 9 females with autism in their cohort. In male, but not female, toddlers who later received a diagnosis of autism, the degree of amygdala enlargement at 3 years of age was associated with the severity of the child's social

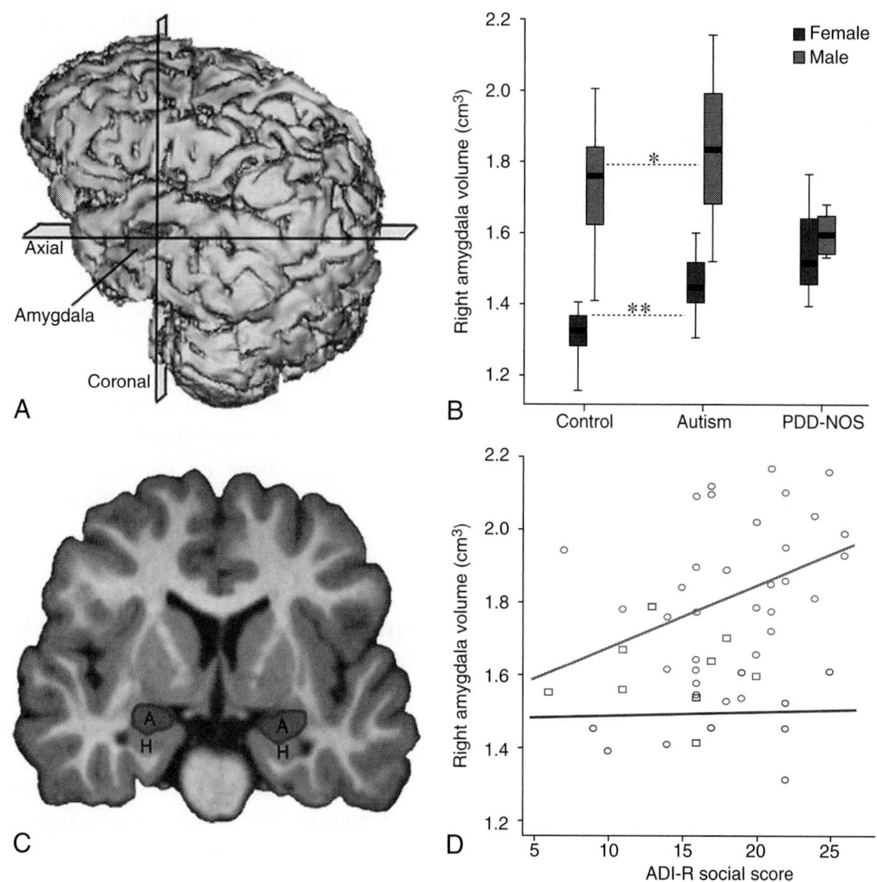

Figure 35–9. Amygdala enlargement in toddlers and young children with autism. (A) Three-dimensional reconstruction of MRI scan; (B) Right amygdala volume (in cm^3) for children at about 3 years of age by diagnostic group (*$p < .05$; **$P < .01$ significantly different from sex-matched control); (C) Amygdala (A) and Hippocampus (H) in the coronal plane; (D) Linear regression scatter plot showing a positive correlation for right ($r = 0.52$, $p = .001$) amygdala volume (in cm^3) and Autism Diagnostic Interview-Revised (ADI-R) social score in males with autism spectrum disorder. Adapted from Schumann, C. M., Barnes, C. C., et al. (2009). Amygdala enlargement in toddlers with autism related to severity of social and communication impairments. *Biol Psychiatry, 66*, 942–949. (See Color Plate Section for a color version of this figure.)

and communication impairments at final clinical evaluation at ~5 years of age (Figure 35-9). This finding is similar to reports of other brain regions, in which enlargement at 3–5 years of age is associated with the severity of symptoms at 5–8 years of age (Munson, Dawson, et al., 2006). Previous studies (Bloss & Courchesne, 2007), including our own longitudinal studies of this cohort (Schumann, Bloss, et al., 2010), have also found more robust differences in cortical volumes in females than males. Although speculative at present, the Schumann et al. (Schumann, Barnes, et al., 2009) study suggests that autistic males may be a more heterogeneous group in amygdala volume, which varies with the degree of clinical impairment, compared to autistic females, who may have a more homogeneous neuropathological profile of an enlarged amygdala regardless of the degree of their behavioral impairment.

Collectively, studies suggest that the amygdala is enlarged in young children with autism (Sparks, Friedman, et al., 2002; Schumann, Hamstra, et al., 2004; Mosconi, Cody-Hazlett, et al., 2009; Schumann, Barnes, et al., 2009). However, Schumann, Amaral, and colleagues (Schumann, Hamstra, et al., 2004) found that the period of amygdala enlargement in children with autism appears to be limited to early development, due to the continued growth of the amygdala in typically developing males which increases in size by 40% from 5 to 18 years of age (Giedd, Snell, et al., 1996; Giedd, 1997). Therefore, by adolescence, amygdala size in the typically developing child has caught up with, and likely surpassed, amygdala size in the child with autism (Schumann, Hamstra, et al., 2004). Studies of older populations have found that amygdala volume is actually smaller in adolescents and adults with autism relative to age-matched typical controls (Aylward, Minshew, et al., 1999; Pierce, 2001; Nacewicz, Dalton, et al., 2006). In one study by Nacewicz and colleagues (Nacewicz, Dalton, et al., 2006), a smaller amygdala volume was associated with gaze avoidance and more severe behavioral impairments as measured with the ADI-R. This relation is the opposite pattern of that observed in younger children in both the Munson et al. (Munson, Dawson, et al., 2006) and Schumann et al. (Schumann, Barnes, et al., 2009) studies. It remains unknown if autism subjects that demonstrate early overgrowth and more severe behavioral impairments also demonstrate reduced amygdala size later in adulthood, as preliminarily suggested by these findings; this awaits confirmation from a longitudinal study on brain growth throughout development in people with autism.

How might pathology in the amygdala relate to specific behavioral abnormalities? Pierce and colleagues (Pierce, Haist, et al., 2004; Pierce & Redcay, 2008) found that the amygdala in young autistic children as well as autistic adults can be responsive in the presence of stimuli that represent high reward value, such as mother's face or the face of children. Conversely, reduced activation to adult stranger faces may reflect reduced attention and interest. Diminished attention to faces early in development may be part of a developmentally early cascade of impairments that lead to later emotional and social deficits (Osterling & Dawson, 1994; Pierce & Redcay, 2008). An emerging hypothesis is that the amygdala may play a role in mediating or directing attention to the eye region of the face to detect emotion or danger (Adolphs, 2001). Indeed, autistic subjects show abnormal visual scan paths during eye-tracking studies when viewing faces, typically displaying less time attending to core social features such as the eyes (Klin, Jones, et al., 2002; Pelphrey, Sasson, et al., 2002). Dalton and colleagues (Dalton, Nacewicz, et al., 2005) utilized functional imaging and eye-tracking technology simultaneously while showing subjects familiar and unfamiliar faces; the amount of time persons with autism spent looking at the eye region of the face was strongly positively correlated with amygdala activation. Thus, more attention-getting, interesting, and perhaps socially rewarding stimuli may engender greater amygdala activation in autism, with uninteresting adult stranger faces triggering less activation than normal. Recently, Kleinhans and colleagues (Kleinhans, Johnson, et al., 2009) found evidence of reduced activation in the amygdala to neutral faces in autistic as compared to control subjects, but also less habituation to the faces; interestingly, more socially impaired autistic subjects showed less habituation.

No study to date has evaluated younger postmortem cases with autism to determine what cellular properties account for the early overgrowth in volume, but there is some evidence that a decreased number of neurons may be contributing to the reduction in volume later in adulthood. Schumann and Amaral (2006) carried out a stereological study to count the number of neurons in postmortem amygdala tissue from 9 male autism and 10 male control cases. In their cases ranging from 10 to 44 years of age, they found a reduction in the number of neurons in the autism cases relative to controls in the amygdala as a whole and in its lateral nucleus. Younger autism cases need to be evaluated with postmortem stereological techniques to determine at what stage of development the decrease of neurons occurs in relation to the overall abnormal growth trajectory.

How might pathology in the amygdala generate specific behavioral abnormalities? We and others have found that the volume of the amygdala in individuals with autism is associated with the severity of their social and nonverbal impairments as measured on the ADI and Vineland Adaptive Scales. Given that each score is comprised of several domains, the correlation analyses carried out are exploratory, and it would be inappropriate to make inferences on the effect of amygdala pathology on any specific behavior. There is also considerable overlap of the behaviors observed for the social and nonverbal communication scores on both algorithms. For example, both scores include observing social smiling, gaze direction, facial expressions, imaginative and imitative social play, and seeking to share enjoyment with others. Many of these behaviors are associated with amygdala function, and therefore it is not surprising that amygdala pathology might be associated with the severity of these impairments in people with autism. From human and nonhuman primate studies, a pathological amygdala can be associated with increased anxiety, unusual fear, gaze avoidance, social avoidance, and inappropriate modulation of social behavior (see Osterling & Dawson, 1994; for review Adolphs, 2010; Amaral, Bauman, & Schumann, 2003).

Age-Related Changes in Other Brain Regions in Autism

The Cerebellar Hemispheres and Vermis

The first hypothesis that cerebellar abnormality might play a part in autism was based on the recognition of its complex and important involvement in numerous functions known to be deficit in autism (Courchesne, Yeung-Courchesne, et al., 1988). As with anatomical studies of the cerebrum in autism, studies of the cerebellum and its subregions and output pathways highlight a major topic in MRI studies of autism: the potential for different patterns of growth across development in different regions within a larger structure. As mentioned above and highlighted by Courchesne et al. (Courchesne, Karns, et al., 2001), overall brain and cerebral volumes in individuals with autism peak early in development, potentially suggestive of aberrant excessive early growth with later slowing of growth during middle childhood and adolescence. Yet, within the cerebrum, some regions display this early overgrowth, while others do not (see Figure 35-7). Similarly, studies of the cerebellum also may be extremely sensitive to age-related factors, with potentially differing patterns of growth within the cerebellar hemispheres and the cerebellar vermis.

Overall cerebellar enlargement has been reported in autistic toddlers and young children (Courchesne, Karns, et al., 2001; Webb, Sparks, et al., 2009), but this enlargement may be related to cerebellar white matter, as 2- to 3-year-olds with ASD show volumes much larger than controls. Suggestive of atypical later growth, in one study (Courchesne, Karns, et al., 2001), increases in cerebellar white matter from 2–3 years to 12–16 years was only 7% in the ASD group as compared to 50% in typically developing children. Cross-sectional samples in older children are also supportive of this pattern of slowed later development resulting in volumes becoming more in-line with those seen in controls. Herbert et al. (Herbert, Ziegler, et al., 2004) found increased absolute volume but in proportion to overall increased head size in 7- to 11-year-olds (also see Kates, Burnette, et al., 2004 for 5- to 13-year-olds); in contrast, in slightly older samples, McAlonan et al. (McAlonan, Cheung, et al., 2005) found reduced white matter bilaterally in the cerebellum in children aged 8–14 years (also see Boddaert, Chabane, et al., 2004 for children 7–15 years) (see Figure 35-10).

In contrast to the development of the cerebellar hemispheres, analyses of the vermis suggest that some of its subregions are disproportionately smaller in young children with autism and remain so throughout the lifespan (e.g., Figure 35-10). One of the first quantitative MRI studies of autism targeted the superior posterior vermis (i.e., neocerebellar vermis lobules VI–VII) for quantitative analyses and found hypoplasia of this cerebellar subregion in a subset of autistic patients (Courchesne, Yeung-Courchesne, et al., 1988). Because MRI methodology and analytic approaches at the time were underdeveloped, several studies that attempted to replicate the discovery failed due to methodological and statistical errors. In more recent years, however, newer studies with higher quality methodologies, stronger analytic approaches, and larger sample sizes have reported that the vermis is indeed reduced in

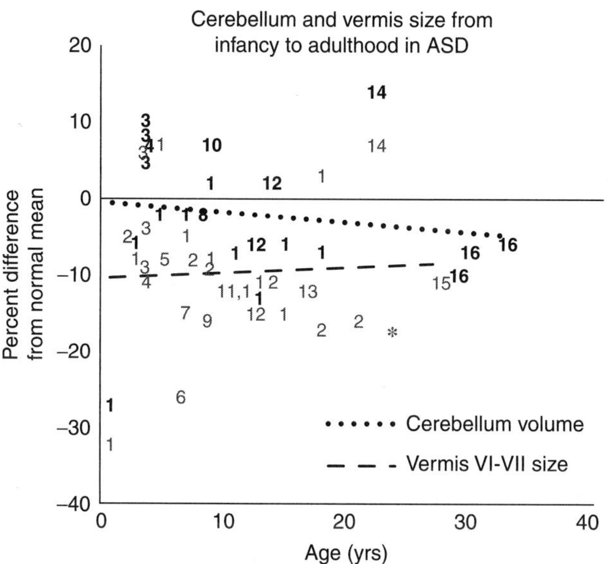

Figure 35–10. Changes in cerebellar volume and vermis lobules VI-VII size from infancy to adulthood in ASD. Percent differences from normal average in each study for autistic subjects are plotted for cerebellar volume (bold numbers) and vermis lobules VI–VII cross-sectional area (grey numbers) against age. Regression lines are shown for cerebellar volume (dotted line) and vermis lobules VI–VII area (dash line). The solid line represents normal average. Data originated from: (1) Hashimoto et al., 1995; (2) Courchesne et al., 2001; (3) Akshoomoff et al., 2004; (4) Webb et al., 2009; (5) Carper et al., 2000; (6) Kleiman et al., 1992; (7) Kaufmann et al., 2003; (8) Kates et al., 2004; (9) Mitchell et al., 2009; (10) Herbert et al., 2003; (11) Elia et al., 2000; (12) Cleavinger et al., 2008; (13) Ciesielski et al., 1997; (14) Hardan et al., 2001; (15) Piven et al., 1992; (16) Hallahan et al., 2009. Asterisk is from the first report of hypoplasia of vermis lobules VI–VII In autism (Courchesne, Yeung-Courchesne, et al., 1988).

size in autism (Kates, Mostofsky, et al., 1998; Carper & Courchesne, 2000; Courchesne, Karns, et al., 2001; Sparks, Friedman, et al., 2002; Kaufmann, Cooper, et al., 2003; Webb, Sparks, et al., 2009; Scott, Schumann, et al., 2009) for meta-analysis and review see (Stanfield, McIntosh, et al., 2008). Specifically addressing early autism, Webb et al. (Webb, Sparks, et al., 2009) found that total vermal areas were disproportionately smaller in children aged 3–4 years with ASD; when children with ASD were compared to children with developmental delays (age- and mental age–matched), the groups demonstrated similar smaller total vermal areas compared to chronological age–matched controls. Examining the development of the vermal areas, (Hashimoto, Tayama, et al., 1995), with a sample of 102 individuals with ASD from 6 months to 20 years, found that total vermal area was smaller in autism than controls but increased with age in a manner similar to controls.

One region within the vermis, however, has not shown the same consistency. Specifically, the anterior vermis (i.e., paleocerebellar vermis lobules I–V) in children with ASD has been found to be normal in 3- to 16-year-olds (Courchesne, Karns, et al., 2001), increased in 1.9- to 5.2-year-olds (Akshoomoff et al., 2004), and decreased in 3- to 4-year-olds (Webb, Sparks, et al., 2009). Hashimoto et al. (Hashimoto, Tayama, et al., 1995) also found that the anterior vermis was generally smaller during infancy and early childhood in ASD, but the regression slope was significantly steeper in early life in the ASD group than in the control group, suggesting that the size of this region "catches up" to typically developing individuals.

More consistently, the superior posterior midsagittal vermis (lobules VI–VII) has been found to be about 12% smaller in autistic as compared to typical subjects (Figure 35-10; Courchesne, Yeung-Courchesne, et al., 1988; Courchesne, Saitoh, et al., 1994; Hashimoto, Tayama, et al., 1995; Kates, Mostofsky, et al., 1998; Carper & Courchesne, 2000; Courchesne, Karns, et al., 2001; Kaufmann, Cooper, et al., 2003; Akshoomoff, Lord, et al., 2004; Webb, Sparks, et al., 2009). This pattern of decreased superior posterior vermis area may be a general anatomical finding associated with ASD, consistent with the results of older meta-analyses, which noted that between 84% and 92% of individuals with ASD exhibited vermal hypoplasia (Courchesne,1997), and with a more recent meta-analysis of all MRI studies of this vermis subregion in autism (Stanfield, McIntosh, et al., 2008). Hashimoto (Hashimoto, Tayama, et al., 1995) found that the regression slope was significantly steeper especially during infancy and toddler years in the ASD group than the control group, again suggesting that the size of this subregion "caught up" to typically developing individuals (also see Stanfield, McIntosh, et al., 2008). In contrast, Courchesne et al. (Courchesne, Karns, et al., 2001) did not find age-related changes in autism in this vermis subregion across ages 2–16 years. Hashimoto, Tayama, et al. (1995) was the first quantitative MRI study to examine a substantial number of ASD infant and toddler patients as well as young children, preadolescents, and adolescents, potentially suggesting that the inclusion of data from the early period of autism onset may change our understanding of the slope of neuroanatomic growth in this disorder. It will be important in future work to include sample sizes that will allow more sophisticated modeling of the growth associated with this vermis subregion.

Lastly, the inferior posterior vermis (vermis lobules VIII–X, which includes both paleocerebellum and vestibulocerebellum) has been found to be both decreased (Hashimoto, Tayama, et al., 1995; Levitt, Blanton, et al., 1999) and normal (Webb, Sparks, et al., 2009). Hashimoto et al. (Hashimoto, Tayama, et al., 1995) found this region to remain smaller across development, thus suggestive of little catch-up growth.

Why might there be differences in age-related growth in different vermis subregions? The enormity and diversity of afferent and efferent tracts, which connect neocerebellar, paleocerebellar, and vestibulocerebellar regions of both cerebellar hemispheres and vermis to brainstem, limbic, and neocortex regions likely results in multiple critical periods of circuitry formation (also see Hashimoto, Tayama, et al., 1995). This is supported by results from diffusion tensor imaging of the cerebellum in autism that indicates impairment in white matter microstructure in the cerebellar peduncles and intracerebellar fibers (Catani, Jones, et al., 2008; Brito, Vasconcelos, et al., 2009) resulting in alterations in intracerebellar circuitry. Abnormal functional connectivity between the cerebellum and frontal cortex in autism was also suggested by Carper and Courchesne (2000) based on evidence of an inverse relationship between frontal lobe size and cerebellar vermis measures.

Cerebellar abnormalities in autism have important implications for understanding many behavioral deficits in this disorder because the cerebellum plays a role in a wide range of functions including timing and coordination of movement, learning of complex motor skills, evaluation of the match between intention and action, providing feedback information to adjust the operations of the cortex and brain stem, motor learning, predictive learning, exploration of the environment and objects, behavioral inhibition, attention, and visual orienting. More specifically, the cerebellar vermis has been associated with modulation of limbic functions including emotion and sensory reactivity and salience detection, while the cerebellar hemispheres have been linked to numerous higher-order cerebral functions including language, working memory, planning, and behavioral sequencing (e.g., Courchesne & Allen, 1997; Steinlin, 2008; Stoodley & Schmahmann, 2009a, 2009b). It has been argued that the cerebellum is one of the single busiest neural intersections in the brain, receiving signals from and sending signals back to nearly every major neural system (Courchesne & Allen, 1997). In neurologically typical individuals, larger cerebellum size is correlated with better neurophysiological functioning, including memory, fine motor dexterity, and IQ (Andreasen, Cizadlo, et al., 1993; Paradiso, Andreasen, et al., 1997). In a recent functional connectivity study using fMRI methodology ("rs-fcMRI") in normal adults, Greicius et al. (Greicius, Supekar, et al., 2009) demonstrated that the neocerebellum participates in several higher-order functional networks via corticocerebellar loops involved in executive control, salience detection, and episodic memory/self-reflection. They argue that the largest portions of the neocerebellum take part in the executive control network implicated in higher cognitive functions such as working memory. Especially germane to autism is a new fMRI study that shows cerebellar involvement in the early stages of development of language perception in typically developing 1- to 3-year-olds (Redcay, Haist, et al., 2008).

While the theoretical implications of abnormalities of the cerebellar hemispheres and vermis are clear, the functional relation of abnormal anatomy to behavior in ASD has been less precise, although likely due to both age-related effects and the functional specialization of different regions of the cerebellum. Specifically focusing on motor behaviors that are known to involve the cerebellum, during sequential finger tapping, 8- to 12-year-old children with ASD showed decreased cerebellar activation (ipsilateral anterior cerebellum and contralateral cerebellum lobes IV–V), increased supplemental motor activation, and decreased functional connectivity within the motor network (Mostofsky, Powell, et al., 2009). In contrast, adults with ASD during a repetitive single finger-tapping task showed decreased premotor (Muller, Pierce, et al., 2001) and increased ipsilateral cerebellar activation (Allen, Muller, et al., 2004). In relation to eye movements, regions VI–VII (occulomotor vermis) were found to be related to saccade and smooth pursuit function in adults with autism (Takarae, Minshew, et al., 2004). Deficits in rapidly orienting visual spatial attention are associated with smaller vermal lobes VI–VII in ASD adults (Townsend, Courchesne, et al., 1999) and are predictive of later orienting deficits in ASD children (Harris, Courchesne, et al., 1999). Cerebellar volume has been related to performance IQ in 8- to 26-year-olds with ASD (Cleavinger, Bigler, et al., 2008). Pierce and Courchesne (2001) found that reduced vermal lobe VI–VII area in 3- to 7-year-old children was associated with less active exploration and more repetitive movements. Webb et al. (2009) did not find any relation between more general indices of symptom severity, IQ, or adaptive functioning and vermal area or cerebellum volume in 3- to 4-year-olds with autism (also see Harris, Courchesne, et al., 1999). In children aged 6–14 years, white matter abnormalities (as measured by fractional anisotropy using DTI) were found to be associated with repetitive behaviors assessed via the ADI (Cheung, Chua, et al., 2009); in adults, fractional anisotropy in the superior cerebellar peduncles was associated with social behaviors via the ADI (Catani, Jones, et al., 2008). Kates et al. (Kates, Burnette, et al., 2004) also found that cerebellar white matter, specifically the discrepancy in volume between twins, was associated with discrepancies in the twins' ADOS scores. Adults with ASD and psychosis compared to adults with ASD (without psychosis) also showed a reduction in grey and white matter volume in the cerebellum (Toal, Bloemen, et al., 2009).

What is the underlying neuropathology of cerebellar structural and functional abnormalities in autism? Postmortem studies have consistently reported reduction in the number of a vital type of cerebellar neuron, the Purkinje neuron, in the hemispheres and vermis in the majority of autism cases

(Bailey, Luthert, et al., 1998; Kemper & Bauman, 1998; for review Allen et al., 2005). Reduction in Purkinje numbers in autism is strikingly evident because these cells normally form a very distinctive monolayer (layer 2) within the 3-layer cerebellar cortex. In addition to being reduced in number, Purkinje neurons that do remain have, in some cases, abnormal morphological features. Degenerating Purkinje neurons have also been reported (Vargas et al., 2005), and new evidence shows that the reduction in number is not due to reduction in Purkinje genesis or abnormal migration during development, but instead is due to later loss of previously present Purkinje cells (Whitney et al., 2009). The amount of Purkinje cell loss varies widely across postmortem autism cases from extreme to little or none (Whitney, Kemper, et al., 2008). With the exception of very small focal sites of cerebellar cortical malformation in one postmortem autistic case (Lee, Martin-Ruiz, et al., 2002), gross cerebellar malformation does not appear to occur in autistic postmortem cases, unlike many other neurodevelopmental disorders of the cerebellum (Bolduc and Limperopolus, 2009).

Because Purkinje neurons are the *only* output from the cerebellar cortex (which when unfolded is about three quarters the size of the cerebral cortex), massive loss of Purkinje neurons effectively disconnects this huge and important multifunction processing structure from the rest of the brain. Purkinje neurons exert inhibitory control over deep cerebellar nuclei, and so their loss could cause unregulated and excessive excitatory signaling from the deep nuclei to brain stem, limbic, and cerebral structures. Interestingly, there has been one report observing what appear to be hypertrophied neurons in the deep nuclei in younger autism cases but then abnormally small deep neurons in older autism cases (Kemper & Bauman, 1998). This has raised the hypothesis that initially loss of Purkinje neuron inhibitory signals allows deep nuclei to be abnormally excitable stimulating abnormal growth but continued unregulated and aberrant activity eventually triggers synapse and process elimination in these same cells (Courchesne, Townsend, et al., 1994; Carper & Courchesne, 2000; Allen, McColl, et al., 2005). The combination of loss of this important processing system plus the injection of disruptive excitatory signals likely contributes to the abnormal functioning of limbic and cerebral systems (Allen, Buxton, et al., 1997; Courchesne & Allen, 1997).

The difficulty in establishing precise cerebellar-behavior and cerebellar-autism symptom correlations is due to the absence of studies mapping the distribution of Purkinje neuron loss in autistic cerebellar cortex. Like the cerebrum, the cerebellum has a complex functional representational map. Therefore, in the absence of quantitative and statistical information about precisely which functional locales have Purkinje loss, cerebellar-behavior and cerebellar-symptom correlations in autism will remain a challenge to establish.

The etiology of cerebellar abnormality in autism, including the age when Purkinje neuron loss begins, is largely unknown, although important clues have emerged recently. Of note, work has implicated engrailed 1 and 2 (EN1 and EN2) as potential candidates for cerebellar pathology in humans as well as in mice (e.g., Millonig, Graziadei, et al., 2004); human EN2 maps to a region of chromosome 7 that has been linked to ASD (e.g., Gharani, Benayed, et al., 2004); and the EN2 mouse mutants display cerebellar anatomical abnormalities that are similar to those seen in autism, such as reduced number of Purkinje cells (Millen, Wurst, et al., 1994; Kuemerle, Gulden, et al., 2007) and mild behavioral problems such as reduced exploratory behaviors (Cheh, Millonig, et al., 2006) similar to the findings of Pierce and Courchesne (2001). In addition, like the autistic cerebellar cortex, the cortex in the EN2 mouse model retains its basic 3-layer form despite the Purkinje neuron loss. The loss in the EN2 mouse occurs after Purkinje neurogenesis and early stages of cerebellar corticogenesis. In fact, in the EN2 mouse, Purkinje loss occurs after the first week of postnatal life. Such observations in various developmental cerebellar mouse models raise the question of whether Purkinje neuron loss in autism also occurs during the first years of life. While the Whitney et al. (2009) study indicates that reduction in Purkinje numbers in autism is due to secondary loss (and not to reduced developmental neurogenesis), the youngest case in that study was 19 years. However, except for a single case report of a 4-year-old autistic boy with no loss of Purkinje cells (Bailey, Luthert, et al., 1998), there is a lack of information about whether Purkinje loss is occurs in the very young autistic brain. Thus, the age when Purkinje loss begins in autism is unknown and, so, there is a need for quantitative stereological studies of Purkinje neuron numbers in the youngest autistic cases. Since MRI abnormalities in autism vary with cerebellar subregion and age, stereological studies would need to quantify Purkinje numbers separately in each of the vermis and hemisphere subregions and statistically test for age effects.

A second genetic link may be MET (transmembrane receptor tyrosine kinase of the hepotocyte growth factor/scatter factor), which is suppressed in the developing nervous system and implicated in neuronal development in the cerebellum (Ieraci, Forni, et al., 2002) and has been implicated in genetic analyses of 7q in autism families (IMGSAC, 1998; Sousa, Clark, et al., 2009). Another possibility is that Purkinje neuron loss in the cerebellum may result from neuroinflammatory reactions (i.e., neuroglial activation) associated with activation of the CNS immune system in the cerebellum (Vargas, Nascimbene, et al., 2005). In mouse models, prenatal viral infections result in dysregulation of myelin associated genes in the cerebellum (Mytl1, MAG, MAL, MBP, MobP, MOG), which leads to alterations in fractional anisotropy in the white matter of the cerebellum (Fatemi, Reutiman, et al., 2008; Fatemi, Folsom, et al., 2009).

Regions Less Studied During the Early Years of Development: Hippocampus, Thalamus, Brain Stem, Basal Ganglia

The investigation of other subcortical regions beyond the amygdala that may be affected in autism is limited. There is evidence of abnormalities in the hippocampus (though somewhat inconsistent), including increased volume in young autistic children 3–5 years of age (Sparks et al., 2002) and older children and adolescents (Schumann, et al., 2004), decreased cross-sectional area of the dentate gyrus (Saitoh et al., 2001) in autism subjects from 2 to 42 years of age, and more recently in atypical shape (Nicolson, DeVito, et al., 2006; Dager, Wang, et al., 2007). There is little evidence for abnormalities in the thalamus (Tsatsanis, Rourke, et al., 2003; Hardan, Girgis, et al., 2006; Hardan, Girgis, et al., 2008; Hardan, Minshew, et al., 2008) and inconsistent findings of either no difference or decreased brain stem gray matter volume in adults with autism (Hsu, Yeung-Courchesne, et al., 1991; Jou, Minshew, et al., 2009). There are currently no studies of thalamic or brain stem volume in very young children with autism.

The most interesting findings of these regions come from studies of the basal ganglia (Sears, Vest, et al., 1999; Hardan, Kilpatrick, et al., 2003; Hollander, Anagnostou, et al., 2005; Rojas, Peterson, et al., 2006; Langen, Durston, et al., 2007; Hazlett, Poe, et al., 2009) which have consistently found an increased caudate nucleus volume in adolescents and young adults with autism. These studies also suggest that an enlargement of the caudate nucleus may be correlated with the presence of repetitive and ritualistic behaviors (Sears, Vest, et al., 1999; Hollander, Anagnostou, et al., 2005; Rojas, Peterson, et al., 2006), although this has yet to be explored in young children with autism.

The Corpus Callosum

In the only MRI study of the corpus callosum in very young autistic children, *no* difference from normal was seen (Boger-Megiddo, Shaw, et al., 2006). The 3- to 4-year-old autistic children in this callosal study were from the same sample for whom abnormal enlargement of the cerebrum had been previously reported (Sparks, Friedman, et al., 2002). Not surprisingly, then, the ratio of the callosum to cerebrum in those autistic children was less than typical children, raising the question of whether cerebral enlargement was at the expense of a normal callosal connectivity or due to defects not directly related to callosal development. Clearly, additional studies of corpus callosum development during the first years of life in autism are needed. Because abnormal left-right asymmetry in fMRI and EEG activation patterns in very young as well as older autism subjects is commonly reported especially in studies of language processing (e.g., Redcay & Courchesne, 2008), it is possible that this abnormality of hemispheric specialization emerges from abnormal organization, size, or functioning of callosal axons.

In contrast, since the first MRI report of callosal reduction in autism (Egaas, Courchesne, et al., 1995), the great majority of subsequent studies of the callosum in older autistic children, adolescents, and adults have also found reductions in overall callosum size or in the size of specific callosal subregions (Piven, Bailey, et al., 1997; Manes, Piven, et al., 1999; Hardan, Minshew, et al., 2000; Chung, Dalton, et al., 2004; Vidal, Nicolson, et al., 2006; Alexander, Lee, et al., 2007). A few have found no abnormality (e.g., Rice, Bigler, et al., 2005). Nonetheless, the callosum may be one of the more consistent sites of anatomic abnormality in the autism literature. Hardan et al. (Hardan, Pabalan, et al., 2009) provide a comprehensive overview and meta-analysis of the corpus callosum in autism. Their analyses examined ten studies representing 253 autistic and 250 control subjects with mean ages across studies ranging from 10 to 27 years (except for the Boger-Megiddo, Shaw, et al., 2006). Results showed overall reduction in callosal size in autism across those ages. Callosal subregions that convey frontal and temporal axons, according to lesion-based (Moses, Egaas, et al., 2000) and DTI-based (Hofer & Frahm, 2006) studies, had the most reduction; callosal subregions that primarily convey occipital and parietal axons had the least. This pattern of greater anterior and lesser posterior callosal pathology parallels the distribution of early cortical gray matter overgrowth pathology in autism, with frontal and temporal cortices being most abnormal in this disorder.

Ideally, future autism studies would analyze data on the size of callosal subregions, DTI values in those same subregions and gray matter in specific cortical subregions all in the same autistic subjects during the first years of life when callosal growth, axon pruning and change is at a peak in normal children.

Functional Implications of Early Brain Overgrowth

Because of the extensive connectivity of the brain, disruption of the rate of growth in frontal, temporal, and amygdala structures has wide implications for connectivity in other regions. Abnormalities in brain growth in autism may be best characterized by an aberrant gradient of growth, with early atypical (broad based) acceleration of growth represented generally by increased brain, frontal lobe, temporal lobe, and amygdala volumes, and then a plateau or slowing of continual growth represented generally by volumes in abnormal regions normalizing in later childhood or adolescence. Thus, the slope of growth may be of critical importance in this disorder.

If development is represented by a pattern of change from variability to consolidation, this might be reflected in a more diverse neural response (anatomically and temporally) that becomes localized and efficient (or even automated). Development and learning result from a more consistent neural response with a greater signal relative to noise. Infants and toddlers at risk for autism may fail to show this pattern both anatomically and behaviorally. For example, the early phase of brain overgrowth occurs at a time when language should be both consolidating and expanding, represented by increased expertise for the child's own language, loss of the ability to distinguish nonnative language sounds, and concurrent with expression moving from babbling to functional single word production. Language may be critically disrupted by the early phase of overgrowth such that stable, functional circuits do not arise from the noise. That is, regions that should be engaged in ongoing pruning and stabilization of functional circuits may be overwhelmed with the growth of novel circuitry resulting in greater noise relative to signal.

This period of overgrowth seems to "end" in early childhood for children with autism, although specific timing is unknown and may differ by region, and is followed by relatively slowed growth over childhood and adolescents. This may also result in less opportunity for plasticity and responsive cortical tuning. That is, later in development, stable circuits are available, but these may be less functional circuits, represent earlier learning patterns, provide less flexibility in learning, and result in greater rigidity in the system. Potentially, differences in symptom trajectory, such as during childhood when many children make positive intellectual growth or adolescence where symptoms seem to worsen, may reflect the influence of this slowed growth period on short-term and long-term outcome.

A Sea Change In Biological Research On Autism

The above evidence shows three major discoveries in the past decade from autism MRI research: (1) early brain overgrowth occurs in autism in the first postnatal years and is most pronounced in frontal and temporal lobes and the amygdala, (2) the age of maximum MRI anatomic abnormality in autism is at this early age, and (3) MRI anatomic effects change with age requiring findings on autism to be organized and interpreted according to age. Given that overgrowth clearly begins before 2 years of age, future longitudinal studies would benefit from inclusion of infants and toddlers at-risk for autism.

This suggests that studies of autism at the youngest ages have the best chance of revealing the original biological bases of autism. Clearly, early biomarkers of risk for autism, diagnosis, prognosis, and treatment outcome will most likely come from studies of the youngest ages and not from studies of older subjects. Discovery of effective interventions addressing original neural and functional defects are also most likely to emerge from studies of autism during these early years of initial brain growth pathology.

The discovery of arrest of growth and possible premature decline is vital for all types of biological studies, especially those involving older autistic children and adults, to consider. This new phenomenon signals significant changes in underlying genetic and nongenetic factors and molecular mechanisms as well as changes in the pattern of neural circuits and their functioning. It could be an indication of changes in survival of neurons, connections, and synapses. This second stage of pathology in autism may reflect reactive changes in response to the original upstream defects that produce autism. As such, studies of older children and adults with autism are forewarned that abnormalities detected at that age could reflect this second stage of pathology. Therefore, theories of the possible causes and brain and behavioral bases of autism derived from older subjects should be considered with considerable caution.

The striking early brain growth changes in autism signal the need for a sea change in autism biological research. Autism is a disorder of early brain maldevelopment, and the best opportunity to identify the biology that causes it is at the youngest ages when the abnormality is first occurring and at its maximum expression. Even studies of the genetics of autism may benefit from this change in approach. That is, even though autism is understood to be a highly heritable disorder, the genes and genetic pathways involved have been elusive and a deeper guiding principle of the genetics underlying autism has yet to emerge. Instead, it sometimes appears that each new and larger genetic study of autism has challenged previous reports and introduced new candidate genes, genetic functions, and/or loci. Perhaps a different and more powerful approach to the genetic study of autism would employ early biological as well as behavioral phenotypic profiles.

Challenges And Future Directions

Future challenges include the following:

- establishing the underlying cellular, molecular, and genetic bases of early brain overgrowth and functional abnormalities in autism;
- defining the timing of aberrant growth and its specificity to autism outcomes; and
- characterizing the relationship between regional maldevelopment and formation of abnormal functional connectivity.

SUGGESTED READINGS

Amaral, Schumann & Nordahl, 2008Amaral, D. G., Schumann, C. M., & Nordahl, C. W. (2008). Neuroanatomy of autism. *Trends in Neurosciences, 31*, 137–145.

Courchesne, E., Pierce, K., et al. (2007). Mapping early brain development in autism. *Neuron, 56*, 399–413.

Schumann, C. M., Barnes, C. C., et al. (2009). Amygdala enlargement in toddlers with autism related to severity of social and communication impairments. *Biological Psychiatry. 66*, 942–949.

Webb, S. J., Sparks, B. F., et al. (2009). Cerebellar vermal volumes and behavioral correlates in children with autism spectrum disorder. *Psychiatry Research, 172*(1), 61–67.

ACKNOWLEDGMENTS

The writing of this chapter was supported by the UCSD-NIH Autism Center of Excellence (E. Courchesne, 1-P50-MH081755, 2-R01-MH036840), the UC Davis M.I.N.D. Institute (C. Schumann), the NIH University of Washington Autism Center of Excellence (S.J. Webb; P50-HD055782), and the NIH Shared Neurobiology of Autism and Fragile X (S.J. Webb; R03-HD057321). We send many thanks to all of the children and parents who participate in autism research.

REFERENCES

Adolphs, R. (2001). The neurobiology of social cognition. *Current Opinion in Neurobiology, 11*(2), 231–239.

Adolphs, R. (2010). What does the amygdala contribute to social cognition? *Annals of the New York Academy of Sciences. 1191*, 42–61.

Akshoomoff, N., Lord, C., et al. (2004). Outcome classification of preschool children with autism spectrum disorders using MRI brain measures. *Journal of the American Academy of Child and Adolescent Psychiatry, 43*(3), 349–357.

Alexander, A. L., Lee, J. E., et al. (2007). Diffusion tensor imaging of the corpus callosum in Autism. *NeuroImage, 34*(1), 61–73.

Allen, G., Buxton, R. B., et al. (1997). Attentional activation of the cerebellum independent of motor involvement. *Science, 275*(5308), 1940–1943.

Allen, G., McColl, R., et al. (2005). Magnetic resonance imaging of cerebellar-prefrontal and cerebellar-parietal functional connectivity. *NeuroImage, 28*(1), 39–48.

Allen, G., Muller, R. A., et al. (2004). Cerebellar function in autism: Functional magnetic resonance image activation during a simple motor task. *Biological Psychiatry, 56*(4), 269–278.

Amaral, D. G., Bauman, M. D., Schumann, C. M. (2003). The amygdala and autism: implications from non-human primate studies. *Genes, Brain, and Behavior, 2*(5), 295–302.

Amaral, D. G., Schumann, C. M., et al. (2008). Neuroanatomy of autism. *Trends in Neurosciences, 31*, 137–145.

Andreasen, N. C., Cizadlo, T., et al. (1993). Voxel processing techniques for the antemortem study of neuroanatomy and neuropathology using magnetic resonance imaging. *Journal of Neuropsychiatry and Clinical Neurosciences, 5*(2), 121–130.

Araghi-Niknam M. & Fatemi. SH. (2003). Levels of Bcl-2 and P53 are altered in superior frontal and cerebellar cortices of autistic subjects. *Cellular and Molecular Neurobiology, 23*, 945–952.

Aylward, E., Minshew, N., et al. (1999). MRI volumes of amygdala and hippocampus in non-mentally retarded autistic adolescents and adults. *Neurology, 53*(9), 2145–2150.

Aylward, E. H., Minshew, N. J., et al. (2002). Effects of age on brain volume and head circumference in autism. *Neurology, 59*(2), 175–183.

Bailey, A., Luthert, P., et al. (1998). A clinicopathological study of autism. *Brain, 121*, 889–905.

Baldacara, L., Borgio, J. G., et al. (2008). Cerebellum and psychiatric disorders. *Revista Brasileira de Psiquiatria, 30*(3), 281–289.

Bartholomeusz, H. H., Courchesne, E., et al. (2002). Relationship between head circumference and brain volume in healthy normal toddlers, children, and adults. *Neuropediatrics, 33*(5), 239–241.

Belmonte, M. J., Cook, E. H., et al. (2004). Autism as a disorder of neural information processing: Directions for research and targets for therapy. *Molecular Psychiatry*, online publication: 1–18.

Ben Bashat, D., Kronfeld-Duenias, V., et al. (2007). Accelerated maturation of white matter in young children with autism: a high b value DWI study. *NeuroImage, 37*(1), 40–47.

Bloss, C. S., & Courchesne, E. (2007). MRI neuroanatomy in young girls with autism: a preliminary study. *Journal of the American Academy of Child and Adolescent Psychiatry, 46*(4), 515–523.

Boddaert, N., Chabane, N., et al. (2004). Superior temporal sulcus anatomical abnormalities in childhood autism: a voxel-based morphometry MRI study. *NeuroImage, 23*(1), 364–369.

Boger-Megiddo, I., Shaw, D. W., et al. (2006). Corpus callosum morphometrics in young children with autism spectrum disorder. *Journal of Autism and Developmental Disorders, 36*, 733–739.

Brito, A. R., Vasconcelos, M. M., et al. (2009). Diffusion tensor imaging findings in school-aged autistic children. *Journal of Neuroimaging, 19*(4), 337–343.

Buxhoeveden, D. P., Semendeferi, K., et al. (2006). Reduced minicolumns in the frontal cortex of patients with autism. *Neuropathology and Applied Neurobiology, 32*(5), 483–491.

Carper, R. A., & Courchesne,E. (2000). Inverse correlation between frontal lobe and cerebellum sizes in children with autism. *Brain, 123*, 836–844.

Carper, R. A., & Courchesne, E. (2005). Localized enlargement of the frontal cortex in early autism. *Biological Psychiatry, 57*(2), 126–133.

Carper, R. A., Moses, P., et al. (2002). Cerebral lobes in autism: early hyperplasia and abnormal age effects. *NeuroImage, 16*(4), 1038–1051.

Casanova, M. F., Buxhoeveden, D. P., et al. (2002). Minicolumnar pathology in autism. *Neurology, 58*(3), 428–432.

Casanova, M. F., van Kooten, I. A., et al. (2006). Minicolumnar abnormalities in autism. *Acta Neuropathologica, 112*(3), 287–303.

Catani, M., Jones, D. K., et al. (2008). Altered cerebellar feedback projections in Asperger syndrome. *NeuroImage, 41*(4), 1184–1191.

Cheh, M. A., Millonig, J. H., et al. (2006). En2 knockout mice display neurobehavioral and neurochemical alterations relevant to autism spectrum disorder. *Brain Research, 1116*(1), 166–176.

Cheung, C., Chua, S. E., et al. (2009). White matter fractional anisotrophy differences and correlates of diagnostic symptoms in autism. *Journal of Child Psychology and Psychiatry, 50*(9), 1102–1112.

Chung, M. K., Dalton, K. M., et al. (2004). Less white matter concentration in autism: 2D voxel-based morphometry. *NeuroImage, 23*(1), 242–251.

Cleavinger, H. B., Bigler, E. D., et al. (2008). Quantitative magnetic resonance image analysis of the cerebellum in macrocephalic and normocephalic children and adults with autism. *Journal of the International Neuropsychological Society, 14*(3), 401–413.

Courchesne, E. (1997). Brainstem, cerebellar and limbic neuroanatomical abnormalities in autism. *Current Opinion in Neurobiology, 7*, 269–278.

Courchesne, E., Yeung-Courchesne, R., et al. (1988). Hypoplasia of cerebellar vermal lobules VI and VII in infantile autism. *New England Journal of Medicine, 318*, 1349–1354.

Courchesne, E., & Allen, G. (1997). Prediction and preparation, fundamental functions of the cerebellum. *Learning and Memory, 4*, 1–35.

Courchesne, E., Carper, R., et al. (2003). Evidence of brain overgrowth in the first year of life in autism. *Journal of the American Medical Association, 290*(3), 337–344.

Courchesne, E., Campbell, K., & Solso, S. (2010). Brain growth across the life span in autism: Age-specific changes in anatomical pathology. *Brain Research*, Oct 1. [Epub ahead of print].

Courchesne, E., Karns, C., et al. (2001). Unusual brain growth patterns in early life in patients with autistic disorder: An MRI study. *Neurology, 57*, 245–254.

Courchesne, E., & Pierce, K. (2005). Brain overgrowth in autism during a critical time in development: implications for frontal pyramidal neuron and interneuron development and connectivity. *International Journal of Developmental Neurosciences, 23*(2–3), 153–170.

Courchesne, E., & Pierce, K. (2005). Why the frontal cortex in autism might be talking only to itself: local over-connectivity but long-distance disconnection. *Current Opinion in Neurobiology, 15*(2), 225–230.

Courchesne, E., Pierce, K., et al. (2007). Mapping early brain development in autism. *Neuron, 56*(2), 399–413.

Courchesne, E., Saitoh, O., et al. (1994). Abnormality of cerebellar vermian lobules VI and VII in patients with infantile autism: identification of hypoplastic and hyperplastic subgroups with MR imaging. *American Journal of Roentgenology, 162*(1), 123–130.

Courchesne, E., Townsend, J., et al. (1994). A new finding: impairment in shifting attention in autistic and cerebellar patients. In M. L. Bauman & T. L. Kemper (Eds.), *The neurobiology of autism* (pp. 101–137). Baltimore: Johns Hopkins University Press.

Dager, S. R., Wang, L., et al. (2007). Shape mapping of the hippocampus in young children with autism spectrum disorder. *American Journal of Neuroradiology, 28*(4), 672–677.

Dalton, K. M., Nacewicz, B. M., et al. (2005). Gaze fixation and the neural circuitry of face processing in autism. *Nature Neuroscience, 8*(4), 519–526.

Davis, L. K., Hazlett, H. C., et al. (2008). Cortical enlargement in autism is associated with a functional VNTR in the monoamine oxidase A gene. *American Journal of Medical Genetics. Part B, Neuropsychiatric Genetics, 147B*(7), 1145–1151.

Dawson, G., Munson, J., et al. (2007). Rate of head growth decelerates and symptoms worsen in the second year of life in autism. *Biological Psychiatry, 61*(4), 458–464.

Dementieva, Y. A., Vance, D. D., et al. (2005). Accelerated head growth in early development of individuals with autism. *Pediatric Neurology, 32*(2), 102–108.

DeMyer, W. (1986). Megalencephaly: types, clinical syndromes, and management. *Pediatric Neurology, 2*, 321–328.

Dissanayake, C., Bui, Q. M., et al. (2006). Growth in stature and head circumference in high-functioning autism and Asperger disorder during the first 3 years of life. *Developmental Psychopathology, 18*(2), 381–393.

Egaas, B., Courchesne, E., et al. (1995). Reduced size of corpus callosum in autism. *Archives of Neurology, 52*(8), 794–801.

Elder, L. M., Dawson, G., et al. (2008). Head circumference as an early predictor of autism symptoms in younger siblings of children with autism spectrum disorder. *Journal of Autism and Developmental Disorders, 38*(6), 1104–1111.

Fatemi, S. H., Folsom, T. D., et al. (2009). Abnormal expression of myelination genes and alterations in white matter fractional anisotropy following prenatal viral influenza infection at E16 in mice. *Schizophrenia Research, 112*(1–3), 46–53.

Fatemi, S. H., Reutiman, T. J., et al. (2008). The role of cerebellar genes in pathology of autism and schizophrenia. *Cerebellum, 7*(3), 279–294.

Fidler, D. J., Bailey, J. N., et al. (2000). Macrocephaly in autism and other pervasive developmental disorders. *Developmental Medicine and Child Neurology, 42*(11), 737–740.

Geschwind, D. H., & Levitt, P. (2007). Autism spectrum disorders: developmental disconnection syndromes. *Current Opinion in Neurobiology, 17*(1), 103–111.

Gharani, N., Benayed, R., et al. (2004). Association of the homeobox transcription factor, ENGRAILED 2, *3*, with autism spectrum disorder. *Molecular Psychiatry, 9*(5), 474–484.

Ghaziuddin, M., Zaccagnini, J., et al. (1999). Is megalencephaly specific to autism? *Journal of Intellectual Disability Research, 43*(Pt 4), 279–282.

Giedd, J. N. (1997). Normal development. *Child and Adolescent Psychiatric Clinics of North America, 6*(2), 265–282.

Giedd, J. N., Snell, J. W., et al. (1996). Quantitative magnetic resonance imaging of human brain development: Ages 4–18. *Cerebral Cortex, 6*, 551–560.

Greicius, M. D., Supekar, K., et al. (2009). Resting-state functional connectivity reflects structural connectivity in the default mode network. *Cerebral Cortex, 19*(1), 72–78.

Hadjikhani, N., Joseph, R. M., et al. (2006). Anatomical differences in the mirror neuron system and social cognition network in autism. *Cerebral Cortex, 16*(9), 1276–1282.

Hardan, A. Y., Girgis, R. R., et al. (2006). Abnormal brain size effect on the thalamus in autism. *Psychiatry Research, 147*(2–3), 145–151.

Hardan, A. Y., Girgis, R. R., et al. (2008). Brief report: abnormal association between the thalamus and brain size in Asperger's disorder. *Journal of Autism and Developmental Disorders, 38*(2), 390–394.

Hardan, A. Y., Kilpatrick, M., et al. (2003). Motor performance and anatomic magnetic resonance imaging (MRI) of the basal ganglia in autism. *Journal of Child Neurology, 18*(5), 317–324.

Hardan, A. Y., Libove, R. A., et al. (2009). A preliminary longitudinal magnetic resonance imaging study of brain volume and cortical thickness in autism. *Biological Psychiatry, 66*(4), 320–326.

Hardan, A. Y., Minshew, N. J., et al. (2000). Corpus callosum size in autism. *Neurology, 55*(7), 1033–1036.

Hardan, A. Y., Minshew, N. J., et al. (2008). An MRI and proton spectroscopy study of the thalamus in children with autism. *Psychiatry Research, 163*(2), 97–105.

Hardan, A. Y., Pabalan, M., et al. (2009). Corpus callosum volume in children with autism. *Psychiatry Research.*

Harris, N. S., Courchesne, E., et al. (1999). Neuroanatomic contributions to slowed orienting of attention in children with autism. *Cognitive Brain Research, 8*, 61–71.

Hashimoto, T., Tayama, M., et al. (1995). Development of the brainstem and cerebellum in autistic patients. *Journal of Autism and Developmental Disorders, 25*(1), 1–18.

Hazlett, H. C., Poe, M., et al. (2005). Magnetic resonance imaging and head circumference study of brain size in autism: birth through age 2 years. *Archives of General Psychiatry, 62*(12), 1366–1376.

Hazlett, H. C., Poe, M. D., et al. (2006). Cortical gray and white brain tissue volume in adolescents and adults with autism. *Biological Psychiatry, 59*(1), 1–6.

Hazlett, H. C., Poe, M. D., et al. (2009). Teasing apart the heterogeneity of autism: Same behavior, different brains in toddlers with fragile X syndrome and autism. *Journal of Neurodevelopmental Disorders, 1*(1), 81–90.

Herbert, M. R., Ziegler, D. A., et al. (2003). Dissociations of cerebral cortex, subcortical, and cerebral white matter volumes in autistic boys. *Brain, 126*(Pt 5), 1182–1192.

Herbert, M. R., Ziegler, D. A., et al. (2004). Localization of white matter volume increase in autism and developmental language disorder. *Annals of Neurology, 55*(4), 530–540.

Hofer, S., & Frahm, J. (2006). Topography of the human corpus callosum revisited: Comprehensive fiber tractography using diffusion tensor magnetic resonance imaging. *NeuroImage, 32*(3), 989–994.

Hollander, E., Anagnostou, E., et al. (2005). Striatal volume on magnetic resonance imaging and repetitive behaviors in autism. *Biological Psychiatry, 58*(3), 226–232.

Hsu, M., Yeung-Courchesne, R., et al. (1991). Absence of magnetic resonance imaging evidence of pontine abnormality in infantile autism. *Archives of Neurology, 48*(11), 1160–1163.

Ieraci, A., Forni, P. E., et al. (2002). Viable hypomorphic signaling mutant of the Met receptor reveals a role for hepatocyte growth factor in postnatal cerebellar development.

Proceedings of the National Academy of Sciences of the United States of America, 99(23), 15200–15205.

Jou, R. J., Minshew, N. J., et al. (2009). Brainstem volumetric alterations in children with autism. *Psychological Medicine, 39*(8), 1347–1354.

Just, M. A., Cherkassky, V. L., et al. (2007). Functional and anatomical cortical underconnectivity in autism: Evidence from an fMRI study of an executive function task and corpus callosum morphometry. *Cerebral Cortex, 17*, 951–961.

Kates, W. R., Burnette, C. P., et al. (2004). Neuroanatomic variation in monozygotic twin pairs discordant for the narrow phenotype for autism. *American Journal of Psychiatry, 161*(3), 539–546.

Kates, W. R., Mostofsky, S. H., et al. (1998). Neuroanatomical and neurocognitive differences in a pair of monozygous twins discordant for strictly defined autism. *Annals of Neurology, 43*(6), 782–791.

Kaufmann, W. E., Cooper, K. L., et al. (2003). Specificity of cerebellar vermian abnormalities in autism: a quantitative magnetic resonance imaging study. *Journal of Child Neurology, 18*(7), 463–470.

Kemper, T., & Bauman, M. (1998). Neuropathology of infantile autism. *Journal of Neuropathology and Experimental Neurology, 57*(7), 645–652.

Kennedy, D. P., Semendeferi, K., et al. (2007). No reduction of spindle neuron number in frontoinsular cortex in autism. *Brain and Cognition, 64*(2), 124–129.

Kleinhans, N. M., Johnson, L. C., et al. (2009). Reduced neural habituation in the amygdala and social impairments in autism spectrum disorders. *American Journal of Psychiatry, 166*(4), 467–475.

Klin, A., Jones, W., et al. (2002). Visual fixation patterns during viewing of naturalistic social situations as predictors of social competence in individuals with autism. *Archives of General Psychiatry, 59*(9), 809–816.

Kuemerle B., Gulden F., Cherosky N., Williams E., & Herrup K. (2007). The mouse Engrailed genes: a window into autism. *Behavioral Brain Research, 176*, 121–132.

Lainhart, J. E., Piven, J., et al. (1997). Macrocephaly in children and adults with autism. *Journal of the American Academy of Child and Adolescent Psychiatry, 36*(2), 282–290.

Langen, M., Durston, S., et al. (2007). Caudate nucleus is enlarged in high-functioning medication-naive subjects with autism. *Biological Psychiatry, 62*(3), 262–266.

Lee, M., Martin-Ruiz, C., et al. (2002). Nicotinic receptor abnormalities in the cerebellar cortex in autism. *Brain, 125*(Pt 7), 1483–1495.

Levitt, J. G., Blanton, R., et al. (1999). Cerebellar vermis lobules VIII–X in autism. *Progress in Neuropsychopharmacology and Biological Psychiatry, 23*(4), 625–633.

Levitt, J. G., Blanton, R. E., et al. (2003). Cortical sulcal maps in autism. *Cerebral Cortex, 13*(7), 728–735.

Lotspeich, L. J., Kwon, H., et al. (2004). Investigation of neuroanatomical differences between autism and Asperger syndrome. *Archives of General Psychiatry, 61*(3), 291–298.

Manes, F., Piven, J., et al. (1999). An MRI study of the corpus callosum and cerebellum in mentally retarded autistic individuals. *Journal of Neuropsychiatry and Clinical Neurosciences, 11*(4), 470–474.

Mason-Brothers, A., Ritvo, E. R., et al. (1990). The UCLA-University of Utah epidemiologic survey of autism: prenatal, perinatal, and postnatal factors. *Pediatrics, 86*(4), 514–519.

McAlonan, G. M., Cheung, V., et al. (2005). Mapping the brain in autism: A voxel-based MRI study of volumetric differences and intercorrelations in autism. *Brain, 128*(Pt 2), 268–276.

Miles, J. H., Hadden, L. L., et al. (2000). Head circumference is an independent clinical finding associated with autism. *American Journal of Medical Genetics, 95*(4), 339–350.

Millen, K. J., Wurst, W., et al. (1994). Abnormal embryonic cerebellar development and patterning of postnatal foliation in two mouse Engrailed-2 mutants. *Development, 120*(3), 695–706.

Millonig, G., Graziadei, I. W., et al. (2004). Percutaneous management of a hepatic artery aneurysm: bleeding after liver transplantation. *Cardiovascular and Interventional Radiology, 27*(5), 525–528.

Morgan, J., Buxhoevede, D., et al. (submitted). Alterations in developmental minicolumn organization in the autistic dorsolateral prefrontal cortex.

Mosconi, M. W., Cody-Hazlett, H., et al. (2009). Longitudinal study of amygdala volume and joint attention in 2- to 4-year-old children with autism. *Archives of General Psychiatry, 66*(5), 509–516.

Moses, P., Egaas, B., et al. (2000). Regional size reduction in the human corpus callosum following pre and perinatal injury. *Cerebral Cortex, 10*, 1200–1210.

Mostofsky, S. H., Powell, S. K., et al. (2009). Decreased connectivity and cerebellar activity in autism during motor task performance. *Brain, 132*(Pt 9), 2413–2425.

Mukaetova-Ladinska, E. B., Arnold, H., et al. (2004). Depletion of MAP2 expression and laminar cytoarchitectonic changes in dorsolateral prefrontal cortex in adult autistic individuals. *Neuropathology and Applied Neurobiology, 30*(6), 615–623.

Muller, R.-A., Pierce, K., et al. (2001). Atypical patterns of cerebral motor activation in autism: a functional magnetic resonance study. *Biological Psychiatry, 49*, 665–676.

Munson, J., Dawson, G., et al. (2006). Amygdalar volume and behavioral development in autism. *Archives of General Psychiatry, 63*(6), 686–693.

Nacewicz, B. M., Dalton, K. M., et al. (2006). Amygdala volume and nonverbal social impairment in adolescent and adult males with autism. *Archives of General Psychiatry, 63*(12), 1417–1428.

Nicolson, R., DeVito, T. J., et al. (2006). Detection and mapping of hippocampal abnormalities in autism. *Psychiatry Research, 148*(1), 11–21.

Nordahl, C. W., Dierker, D., et al. (2007). Cortical folding abnormalities in autism revealed by surface-based morphometry. *Journal of Neuroscience, 27*(43), 11725–11735.

Osterling, J., & Dawson, G. (1994). Early recognition of children with autism: a study of first birthday home videotapes. *Journal of Autism and Developmental Disorders, 24*(3), 247–257.

Ozonoff, S., Heung, K., et al. (2008). The onset of autism: patterns of symptom emergence in the first years of life. *Autism Research, 1*(6), 320–328.

Palmen, S. J., Durston, S., et al. (2006). No evidence for preferential involvement of medial temporal lobe structures in high-functioning autism. *Psychological Medicine, 36*(6), 827–834.

Palmen, S. J., Hulshoff Pol, H. E., et al. (2005). Increased gray-matter volume in medication-naive high-functioning children with autism spectrum disorder. *Psychological Medicine, 35*(4), 561–570.

Paradiso, S., Andreasen, N. C., et al. (1997). Cerebellar size and cognition: correlations with IQ, verbal memory and motor dexterity. *Neuropsychiatry, Neuropsychology, and Behavioral Neurology, 10*(1), 1–8.

Pelphrey, K. A., Sasson, N. J., et al. (2002). Visual scanning of faces in autism. *Journal of Autism and Developmental Disorders, 32*(4), 249–261.

Pierce, K., & Courchesne, E. (2001). Evidence for a cerebellar role in reduced exploration and stereotyped behavior in autism. *Biological Psychiatry, 49*(8), 655–664.

Pierce, K., Glatt, S. J., et al. (2009). The power and promise of identifying autism early: insights from the search for clinical and biological markers. *Annals of Clinical Psychiatry, 21*(3), 132–147.

Pierce, K., Haist, F., et al. (2004). The brain response to personally familiar faces in autism: findings of fusiform activity and beyond. *Brain, 127*(Pt 12), 2703–2716.

Pierce, K., Müller, R-A., Ambrose, J., Allen, G. & Courchesne, E. (2001). People with autism process faces outside the fusiform face area: Evidence from fMRI. *Brain, 124*(10), 2059–2073.

Pierce K., & Redcay, E. (2008). Fusiform function in children with an autism spectrum disorder is a matter of who. *Biological Psychiatry, 64*(7), 552–560.

Piven, J., Bailey, J., et al. (1997). An MRI study of the corpus callosum in autism. *American Journal of Psychiatry, 154*(8), 1051–1055.

Redcay, E., & Courchesne, E. (2005). When is the brain enlarged in autism? A meta-analysis of all brain size reports. *Biological Psychiatry, 58*(1), 1–9.

Redcay, E. & Courchesne, E. (2008). Deviant functional magnetic resonance imaging patterns of brain activity to speech in 2-3-year-old children with autism spectrum disorder. *Biological Psychiatry, 64*(7), 589–598.

Redcay, E., Haist, F., et al. (2008). Functional neuroimaging of speech perception during a pivotal period in language acquisition. *Developmental Science, 11*(2), 237–252.

Rice, S. A., Bigler, E. D., et al. (2005). Macrocephaly, corpus callosum morphology, and autism. *Journal of Child Neurology, 20*(1), 34–41.

Rodier, P. M., Bryson, S. E., et al. (1997). Minor malformations and physical measurements in autism: data from Nova Scotia. *Teratology, 55*(5), 1.

Rojas, D. C., Peterson, E., et al. (2006). Regional gray matter volumetric changes in autism associated with social and repetitive behavior symptoms. *BMC Psychiatry, 6*, 56.

Schumann, C. M., & Amaral, D. G. (2006). Stereological analysis of amygdala neuron number in autism. *Journal of Neuroscience, 26*(29), 7674–7679.

Schumann, C. M., & Amaral, D. G. (2009). The human amygdala and autism. In P. J. Whalen & E. A. Phelps (Eds.), *The human amygdala*. New York: Guilford.

Schumann, C. M., Barnes, C. C., et al. (2009). Amygdala enlargement in toddlers with autism related to severity of social and communication impairments. *Biological Psychiatry, 66*, 942–949.

Schumann, C. M., Bloss, C., et al. (2010). Longitudinal MRI study of cortical development through early childhood in autism. *Journal of Neuroscience, 30*, 4419–4427.

Schumann, C. M., Hamstra, J., et al. (2004). The amygdala is enlarged in children but not adolescents with autism; the hippocampus is enlarged at all ages. *Journal of Neuroscience, 24*, 6392–6401.

Scott, J., Schumann, C. M., et al. (2009). A comprehensive volumetric analysis of the cerebellum in children and adolescents with autism spectrum disorder. *Autism Research*, 2(5), 246–257.

Sears, L. L., Vest, C., et al. (1999). An MRI study of the basal ganglia in autism. *Progress in Neuropsychopharmacology and Biological Psychiatry, 23*(4), 613–624.

Sousa, I., Clark, T. G., et al. (2009). MET and autism susceptibility: family and case-control studies. *European Journal of Human Genetics, 17*(6), 749–758.

Sparks, B. F., Friedman, S. D., et al. (2002). Brain structural abnormalities in young children with autism spectrum disorder. *Neurology, 59*(2), 184–192.

Stanfield, A. C., McIntosh, A. M., et al. (2008). Towards a neuroanatomy of autism: a systematic review and meta-analysis of structural magnetic resonance imaging studies. *European Psychiatry, 23*(4), 289–299.

Steinlin, M. (2008). Cerebellar disorders in childhood: cognitive problems. *Cerebellum, 7*(4), 607–610.

Stevenson, R. E., Schroer, R. J., et al. (1997). Autism and macrocephaly [letter]. *Lancet, 349*(9067), 1744–1745.

Stoodley, C. J., & Schmahmann, J. D. (2009a). The cerebellum and language: evidence from patients with cerebellar degeneration. *Brain and Language, 110*(3), 149–153.

Stoodley, C. J., & Schmahmann, J. D. (2009b). Functional topography in the human cerebellum: a meta-analysis of neuroimaging studies. *NeuroImage, 44*(2), 489–501.

Takarae, Y., Minshew, N. J., et al. (2004). Oculomotor abnormalities parallel cerebellar histopathology in autism. *Journal of Neurology, Neurosurgery, and Psychiatry, 75*(9), 1359–1361.

Toal, F., Bloemen, O. J., et al. (2009). Psychosis and autism: magnetic resonance imaging study of brain anatomy. *British Journal of Psychiatry, 194*(5), 418–425.

Townsend, J., Courchesne, E., et al. (1999). Spatial attention deficits in patients with acquired or developmental cerebellar abnormality. *Journal of Neuroscience, 19*, 5632–5642.

Tsatsanis, K. D., Rourke, B. P., et al. (2003). Reduced thalamic volume in high-functioning individuals with autism. *Biological Psychiatry, 53*(2), 121–129.

van Kooten, I. A., Palmen, S. J., et al. (2008). Neurons in the fusiform gyrus are fewer and smaller in autism. *Brain, 131*(Pt 4), 987–999.

Vargas, D. L., Nascimbene, C., et al. (2005). Neuroglial activation and neuroinflammation in the brain of patients with autism. *Annals of Neurology, 57*(1), 67–81.

Vidal, C. N., Nicolson, R., et al. (2006). Mapping corpus callosum deficits in autism: an index of aberrant cortical connectivity. *Biological Psychiatry, 60*(3), 218–225.

Wassink, T. H., Losh, M., et al. (2007). Systematic screening for subtelomeric anomalies in a clinical sample of autism. *Journal of Autism and Developmental Disorders, 37*(4), 703–708.

Webb, S. J., Nalty, T., et al. (2007). Rate of head circumference growth as a function of autism diagnosis and history of autistic regression. *Journal of Child Neurology, 22*(10), 1182–1190.

Webb, S. J., Sparks, B. F., et al. (2009). Cerebellar vermal volumes and behavioral correlates in children with autism spectrum disorder. *Psychiatry Research, 172*(1), 61–67.

Wetherby, A. M., Woods, J., et al. (2004). Early indicators of autism spectrum disorders in the second year of life. *Journal of Autism and Developmental Disorders, 34*, 473–493.

Whitney, E. R., Kemper, T. L., et al. (2008). Cerebellar Purkinje cells are reduced in a subpopulation of autistic brains: a stereological experiment using calbindin-D28k. *Cerebellum, 7*(3), 406–416.

Whitney, E. R., Kemper, T. L., et al. (2009). Density of cerebellar basket and stellate cells in autism: evidence for a late developmental loss of Purkinje cells. *Journal of Neuroscience Research, 87*(10), 2245–2254.

Williams, C. A., Dagli, A., & Battaglia, A. (2008). Genetic disorders associated with macrocephaly. *American Journal of Medical Genetics. Part A, 146A*, 2023–2037.

Zwaigenbaum, L., Bryson, S., et al. (2005). Behavioral manifestations of autism in the first year of life. *International Journal of Developmental Neuroscience, 23*, 143–152.

36 Nancy J. Minshew, K. Suzanne Scherf, Marlene Behrmann, Katherine Humphreys

Autism as a Developmental Neurobiological Disorder: New Insights from Functional Neuroimaging

Points of Interest

- A paradigm shift in autism research, involving conceptualizing the syndrome as a developmental *neurobiological disorder* rather than a behavioral disorder, is critical to reconcile a gulf between behaviorally oriented researchers, clinicians, geneticists, and developmental neurobiologists and to address the most pressing questions about the etiology, brain bases, and effective treatments for autism spectrum disorders (ASD).
- A developmental neurobiological approach emphasizes a search for the underlying brain mechanisms when examining the manifestations of a disorder, which includes *both* the pattern of deficits as well as intact, or even enhanced, abilities and "associated signs and symptoms."
- An emerging body of genetic, functional and structural neuroimaging, and behavioral work suggests that defects in early neuronal organizational events during brain development disrupt the *connectivity of neural systems.*
- There appears to be a trade-off such that there is enhanced local neural connectivity, leading to preserved and potentially enhanced elementary information processing abilities, and disrupted connectivity among more distributed and integrative regions of the brain at the systems level, which leads to a deficit in complex information processing across multiple domains of functioning.
- Our investigations into the psychological mechanisms of visual processing in autism reveal relative preservation (and perhaps even enhancement, on some accounts) in more elemental, simple, or featural processing, whereas information processing that requires the integration of the simple elements is disproportionately affected. The imaging data yield a similar profile: relative preservation of earlier parts of the visual system and more pronounced atypical activation in higher-order regions. These alterations have a profound impact on how the brain in autism processes information and, in turn, how individuals with autism "see" the world differently.

With the first evidence of neurologic dysfunction in autism spectrum disorders (ASDs) in the 1950s and 1960s, there have been "neurobehavioral" theories were proposed to explain autism. These early theories typically focused on a behavioral feature of the syndrome and then inferred its relation to a localized region of the brain. These behavioral symptoms, or neurobehavioral deficits, were posited to be causally related to all other manifestations for the entire syndrome. These kind of localized region and single primary deficit theories for the cause of autism dominated the field for nearly 70 years, despite the recent structural and functional imaging evidence implicating widespread involvement of the cerebral cortex and associated white matter, and disruptions to functional neural systems. Importantly, this historical approach was not informed by an understanding of developmental neurobiologic events, particularly neuronal organizational events, in the developing brain, nor of knowledge about how disease processes affect the developing brain. As a result, there exists a conceptual and pragmatic gulf in autism research between 1) behaviorally oriented researchers and clinicians, who attempt to identify a causative feature of the syndrome that is anchored to impaired behavior, and 2) geneticists and developmental neurobiologists, who study genetic risk factors linked to disruption in neuronal organizational events.

In this chapter, we argue that a paradigm shift is critical to the study of autism in order to reconcile this gulf and address the most pressing questions about how genetic and developmental neurobiological findings can be integrated with findings about the characterization of the behavioral syndrome, which has become increasingly well defined in the last few decades. We propose that this paradigm shift involves conceptualizing autism as a *developmental neurobiological disorder* rather than a behavioral disorder when considering its cause(s). The benefit of this approach is that it is informed by an understanding of basic principles of neurological disorders, including the notions that such disorders do not result in single primary deficits, that they typically have a genetic basis, and that, when they are nontraumatic or arise de novo, as in the case of ASDs, they are multiorgan system disorders. This approach also emphasizes a search for the underlying brain mechanisms when examining the manifestations, which includes *both* the pattern of deficits as well as intact, or even enhanced, abilities and "associated signs and symptoms." An emerging body of genetic, functional and structural neuroimaging, and behavioral work suggests that a potential underlying brain mechanism in autism is a disruption in the *connectivity of neural systems*. More specifically, due to defects in early neuronal organizational events, there may be a systematic trade-off between enhanced local neural connectivity within posterior and perhaps frontal regions of the brain, leading to preserved and potentially enhanced elementary information processing abilities, and disrupted neural connectivity among more distributed regions of the brain at the systems level, which may lead to a deficit in complex information processing across multiple domains of functioning. We review the evidence suggesting that a disruption in neural connectivity is fundamental in autism. Also, we highlight our own findings, particularly in the domain of visual processing, to illustrate the strength of our interdisciplinary approach that seeks to integrate and correlate genetic, neurobiological, and behavioral findings to understand the etiology, brain bases, and effective treatments for the complex disorder of ASD.

The chapter is organized as follows. First, we provide a brief review of the current "neurobehavioral" theories of autism. Second, we challenge these theories by reviewing current evidence, particularly from longitudinal studies of infants at high risk for developing autism, which challenges the notion of a single causative behavioral or cognitive feature of the syndrome or even a cluster of core causative behavioral or cognitive features. Third, we propose that research on ASDs would benefit enormously from taking the perspective that autism is a developmental neurobiological disorder, rather than a behavioral or single systems disorder. In this section, we describe the principles of neurologic disorders, the neuropsychological profile of autism, potential neural mechanisms of ASDs, including disruptions to neuronal events that fundamentally organize cortical systems during brain development, and the genetic factors that predispose individuals who go on to develop autism and are linked to disruptions in these early neuronal events. The key concept of this section is to demonstrate how this neurological approach to the study of autism leads directly to the search for underlying *brain mechanisms*, as opposed to behavioral phenotypes, that result in both the pattern of deficits and the intact abilities that are observed in ASD as well as the associated signs and symptoms of "comorbid disorders." Third, we review the evidence that a disruption in the connectivity of neural systems resulting from a disturbance early in neuronal organization is a likely candidate for such an underlying brain mechanism. Finally, we describe our program of research in the domain of visual processing that illustrates the strength of this interdisciplinary approach to uncover novel relations between the behavioral and brain bases of autism and that supports our claim that disruptions to neural connectivity are a fundamental contributing factor to the etiology of autism.

"Neurobehavioral" Theories of Autism and Challenges to Such Theories

The predominant single deficit models at present are the social primacy theories (e.g., Schultz, 2005; Klin et al., 2002; Dawson, 2008), and their alternative, the dimensional approaches (Happe & Ronald, 2008). The social primacy theories postulate that a social impairment comes first in time and is of sufficient severity to be viewed as causative of subsequent deficits, which are thus viewed as secondary to the social impairment. According to this model, autism is primarily, if not solely, a social-communication disorder both in terms of early etiological events and in terms of later presentation.

The dimensional hypotheses were proposed after investigators failed to find satisfactory evidence of a single or even a triad of primary deficits to account for the clinical syndrome, and hypothesized a cluster of independent core symptoms/signs that co-occur in autism but that are independently inherited (e.g., central coherence, theory of mind, executive function, repetitive behavior; Happe et al., 2006). These investigators tested their hypotheses by assessing typical populations for evidence of autism traits to ascertain their occurrence independently or in association with each other (Happe & Ronald, 2008; but see also Constantino et al., 2004).

Notice that both of these classes of "neurobehavioral" theories primarily focus on a functional analysis of *problematic behavior*. In other words, the central goal of these theories is to examine behavior to understand the cause of the disorder. A significant drawback of this approach is that focusing on describing an underlying mechanism is based on the behavioral impairments that present most severely, which may actually overestimate their significance in the etiology of the disorder. Furthermore, this approach does not emphasize an understanding of the abilities that are selectively preserved and even enhanced in the disorder. Our early work hinted that there are significant challenges to this approach and that the search for underlying brain mechanism(s) in autism must include an investigation of the profile of impaired *and* intact abilities.

Neuropsychological Studies Challenging Single Deficit and Dimensional Theories of Autism

Our initial approach to the investigation of autism was to pursue a comprehensive definition of the profile of functioning across all major neuropsychological domains, not just those that present with impairments in ASDs (Minshew et al., 1992; Minshew et al., 1997). We studied 33 individually matched pairs of adolescents and adults with and without high-functioning autism (HFA), and assessed a broad range of abilities within each domain from the most basic to higher-order skills. Our original hypothesis was that the brain dysfunction causing autism diffusely and symmetrically involved altered development of connections with association cortex. We therefore proposed that higher-order abilities across multiple domains would be selectively affected. For this reason, elementary and higher-order abilities in all domains were assessed. At the time, there were some proposals of primary deficits in basic skills like elementary sensory perception, various aspects of attention, and basic associative memory abilities (see Minshew et al., 1997, for review of early theories). Assessments of nonverbal language and social abilities were not included in this study, since tests of these abilities in verbal individuals were not widely available at that time.

We found deficits across a number of domains, which enabled us to describe a broader pattern of deficits than had been previously reported in autism. The results revealed deficits in: skilled motor movements, higher cortical sensory perception, memory for material that required use of an organizing strategy or identification of an organizing strategy, higher-order language meaning, and concept formation. Notice that we identified deficits in several affected domains that were not previously considered to be integral parts of the autism syndrome, including aspects of the sensory-perceptual, motor, and memory domains. Hence, the evidence suggested that autism affected the brain far more generally than the single deficit and dimensional theories indicated. We also reported evidence of intact and sometimes enhanced abilities across multiple domains, including attention, elementary motor abilities, elementary sensory abilities, basic associative memory abilities, formal language skills (vocabulary, spelling, fluency, decoding), and the rule-learning aspects of abstraction. Again, unlike any previously reported findings, we observed enhanced skills and impaired abilities within the same domains (e.g., language). We have since completed an additional study with a younger sample of 56 children with autism and 56 controls that replicated this pattern of results with appropriate developmental modifications in the abstract reasoning domain (Williams, Goldstein, & Minshew, 2006).

Finally, we also evaluated single deficit theories about the role of cerebellar dysfunction in autism. We performed a study of postural control in 79 individuals with autism and 61 typical controls between 5 and 52 years. We observed delayed maturation of postural control and failure to achieve adult levels (Minshew, Sung, Jones, & Furman, 2004). The impairments were related to inadequate multimodal sensory integration across vestibular, visual, and position senses by the brain. There was no evidence of a cerebellar or motor contribution to postural instability in autism. These findings reinforced the notion that autism impacts neural connectivity and information integration very broadly and provided further evidence for the need to reconceptualize autism to accommodate these findings.

We were able to draw several conclusions from this constellation of findings. First, in all domains that we tested, the deficits were not in the acquisition of information as reflected in intact performance on multiple measures of attention, elementary sensory perception, and associative memory. In fact, we found that more elementary skills in each of these domains were intact or enhanced. Instead, the deficits selectively involved the most demanding aspects of information processing within each domain. Because the subjects were matched on gender, age, and IQ scores, this pattern of results indicated that the individuals with autism were unable to perform the more challenging tasks that might have been predicted based on their age and IQ scores and on their enhanced performance on the simpler tasks. We argued that this pattern of impairments and preserved abilities could be summed up as follows. First, the abilities that placed the highest demands on information processing or integration within the affected domains were most likely to be impaired, and the domains with the most prominent symptoms (concept formation, thematic and idiomatic language) were those that had the highest information processing demands. Hence, we proposed that the common denominator of the impaired abilities was the higher-order or "complex" information processing demands. Second, the abilities that were most likely to be preserved required elementary information processing demands (see Minshew, Webb, Williams, & Dawson, 2006, for detailed explanation). In sum, our early work challenged the "neurobehavioral" theories of autism primarily on the basis that they could not account for the comprehensive pattern of both deficits and intact aspects of the disorder both within and across multiple domains.

Beyond the Neuropsychological Profile of Autism

Our characterization of autism, based on all the neuropsychological testing, was that its manifestations reflected a disorder of information processing that disproportionately impacted complex information processing while preserving, or even enhancing, elementary information processing skills. This led to a novel hypothesis that we should observe an inverse relation between the impairments and the intact abilities at a neurobiological level as well (Kuschner, Bodner, & Minshew, 2009; Damarla et al., 2011).

We then began to investigate difficulties in information processing as a general construct. We pursued two lines of research. Because concept formation appeared common to impairments in conceptual understanding, cognitive memory, story theme creation and detection, and face recognition (in the sense of the requirement to integrate information for configural processing), we explored concept formation extensively. This line of research led to forays into the development and maturation of object categorization, the development of face identity and emotion recognition, and later the study of the emergence of these abilities in infants at high risk for autism (e.g., Best et al., 2010; Gastgeb et al., 2009; Gastgeb et al., 2006; Gastgeb et al., 2011; Humphreys et al., 2007; Iverson & Goldin-Meadow, 2005; Iverson & Wozniak, 2007; Newell et al., in press; Rump et al., 2009; Scherf, Behrmann, Minshew, & Luna,

2008). The second line of research focused on the area of visual information processing and used microgenetic techniques and fMRI studies to carefully investigate information processing in children, adolescents, and adults with autism (e.g., Behrmann et al., 2006; Hasson et al., 2009; Humphreys et al., 2008; Scherf, Luna, Kimchi, Minshew, & Behrmann, 2008; Scherf, Luna, Minshew, & Behrmann, 2010). Throughout this research program, we have considered how the profile of results implicates neurobiological mechanisms of brain development that could lead to atypical cortical specialization and a proclivity to use local rather than distributed representations for information processing. This approach was novel in the way we extended the definition of the syndrome to the neurologic realm and framed the issue in terms of information processing and integration, which was readily translatable to mechanisms within the brain and neural systems.

However, our findings were somewhat limited in the sense that they were conducted in children, adolescents, and adults, in whom a significant amount of brain and behavioral development had occurred. Given that ASDs are a developmental disorder first manifest in the first two years of life, it was critical to obtain earlier developmental data to truly and fully evaluate the explanatory power of the early "neurobehavioral" theories of autism.

High Risk Infant Studies Challenge Single Deficit and Dimensional Theories of Autism

Very recently, longitudinal studies of infants at high risk for developing autism (because they have an older sibling who has already been diagnosed with autism) have provided this critical early developmental data. These studies have been able to document the earliest identifiable signs of autism as emerging between 9 and 12 months of age (Rogers, 2009). Interestingly, the earliest identifiable manifestations of autism are not in the form of a primary social impairment, as the social motivation theories had long predicted, but instead in the form of unusual responses to sensory stimuli, unusual but subtle odd motor movements, and unusual visual regard for objects (Rogers, 2009). These findings were also inconsistent with the predictions of the dimensional theories. For example, Rogers (2009) explained:

> not only the core symptoms like joint attention deficits, repetitive behaviors, and language delays appear at 12 months and grow more severe over time, but even what were previously considered secondary symptoms—irritability, sensory responsivity, activity level, and poor gross motor development, are on board, and in some cases appear well before the social problems! These findings do not support the view that autism is [etiopathophysiologically] primarily a social-communicative disorder and instead suggest that autism disrupts multiple aspects of development rather simultaneously. (p. 133)

These longitudinal studies indicate that social and language impairments, long considered the *causative* features of autism, emerge later between 12 and 24 months. Furthermore, in some children, the diagnosis of autism could not be made until 2 to 3 years of age, when the classic symptoms and signs were obviously observable, and "it was particularly notable that disturbances in temperament, self-regulation, and hyperactivity emerged along side of these core symptoms," (Rogers, 2009).

These findings provide direct and clear evidence that there is no single primary deficit, brain region, or neural system causing autism, but also that a causative set of "core" symptoms is equally unlikely. Rather, Roger finds that autism broadly affects many abilities at the same time and systematically from its earliest presentation and continuing throughout life. This is exactly the view that we proposed previously based on our work with children, adolescents, and adults with autism (Minshew et al., 1992; Minshew et al., 1997; Williams, Goldstein, & Minshew, 2007). Additionally, the concept of associated and comorbid symptoms as representing the co-occurrence of other conditions is also clearly not supported by these data. This integrated perspective was particularly evident in the early observation of presentation of mental retardation and various regulatory disturbances in these infants and toddlers later diagnosed with autism. Rather, the evidence suggests that these conditions are part and parcel of the same disorder, resulting from atypical developmental brain processes (i.e., neuronal organizational events) that cause all the signs and symptoms of ASDs. Rogers concluded, "autism is not a disorder that profoundly affects social development from the earliest months of life. Rather, it is a disorder involving symptoms across multiple domains with a gradual onset" (p. 135).

Rogers made two more comments directly relevant to the present discussion. She noted that the high rate of autism and related manifestations in the infant siblings was striking, which supporting the importance of genetic contributions to its etiopathophysiology. To this she added that the absence of discernable behavioral manifestations at or before 6 months was likely a reflection of the limitation of behavioral measures in infants and the need for biologic measures in these early months.

Autism as a Neurological Disorder Rather Than a Behavioral Disorder

Given that there is significant evidence to discredit the notion that a single behavioral deficit, or even a core set of deficits, cause autism, we argue that a paradigm shift is critical to the study of autism. We propose that this paradigm shift involves conceptualizing autism as a *neurological and developmental neurobiological disorder* rather than as a behavioral disorder. There are several benefits of this approach, including that it is guided by an understanding of basic principles of neurological disorders, brain development, and how disease processes affect brain development. In this section, we briefly review principles of neurological disorders, the neuropsychological profile of autism, potential neural mechanisms leading to

ASDs, and the genetic contributions that may affect these neural mechanisms.

Principles of Neurological Disorders

Neurological disorders tend to conform to a common set of well known principles. First, such disorders produce a pattern or constellation of deficits and intact abilities that reflects the underlying disease mechanism. In other words, neurological disorders do not result in single primary deficits. The search for a single primary causal deficit of a neurologic disorder at the behavioral or cognitive level is not compatible with mechanisms of neurologic disease or dysfunction. Second, neurologic disorders that develop de novo (i.e., absent trauma or other injury) typically have a genetic basis. Hence, idiopathic autism is likely to have its origins in complex genetics (superimposed on the background of individual familial inheritance), as do innumerable other childhood neurological disorders that appear to have a sudden onset (e.g. see neuronal ceroid lipofucsinosis, which has three forms expressed at very different developmental time points from the first month to adolescence). Thus the work investigating genetic vulnerabilities for autism is critical for understanding the etiology of the disorder. Third, most nontraumatic neurologic disorders are *multiorgan system disorders* because they result from genetic errors that are present in all tissues in the body though not necessarily functionally expressed (Campbell et al., 2009).

To this set of core principles, we also add the concept that symptoms of a pediatric neurological disorder are expressed at a developmentally appropriate time window (i.e., when the affected skills are developing). Our characterization of the syndrome of autism is consistent with an emerging body of work that suggests that autism is largely a disorder of what neurologists call "higher cortical functions." Based on this characterization, it is to be expected that disruption in these higher-order functions becomes much more apparent in the second year of life when complex information processing abilities and their underlying neural systems are emerging.

We argue that research investigating the etiology of autism must focus on identifying aspects of the disorder that are consistent with tenets of neurological disorders. Furthermore, based on the existing work, we suggest that the focus of such an approach should be on discerning known neurological and neurobiological mechanisms for disruption to the development of higher cortical brain functions.

Developmental Neurobiologic Mechanisms and the Clinical Syndrome of Autism

ASDs are becoming increasingly recognized as developmental neurobiological disorders (Geschwind & Levitt, 2007; Minshew, Williams, & McFadden, 2008; Volpe, 2008). The notion that a disturbance in a developmental neurobiological mechanism could cause autism is consistent with early reports of truncated dendritic tree development in hippocampal neurons (Bauman & Kemper, 1994), increased brain weight in children and decreased brain weight in adults (Bauman & Kemper, 1998), and premature acceleration in head growth at 9 months followed by a plateau in growth (Dawson et al., 2007). In particular, it is likely that a developmental neurobiological mechanism that guides or regulating *neuronal organizational* event is strongly implicated in the etiology of autism.

Neuronal organizational events are described in clinical neurology texts as "the sequence of organizational events that result in the intricate circuitry characteristic of the human brain" (Volpe 2008, p. 51). In fact, autism is now described as a clinical example of a neuronal organizational disorder (Volpe, 2008). Neuronal organizational events occur between 5 months gestation and many years if not decades after birth. The neuronal laminar pattern is established by 3 years of age, and the bulk of the cortical axonal density is present by 12 years of age. "The major developmental features of neuronal organization events include the following: 1) the establishment and differentiation of subplate neurons; 2) attainment of proper alignment, orientation and layering of cortical neurons, 3) the elaboration of dendritic and axonal ramifications, 4) establishment of synaptic contacts, 5) cell death and selective elimination of processes and 6) proliferation and differentiation of glia" (Volpe, 2008, p. 82). When reviewing histologic displays of cortical neurons and images of the whole brain and cortex undergoing maturational events from 22 weeks gestation through several years postnatal age, it becomes apparent that organizational events have a widespread impact throughout the cerebral cortex, and are more symmetric than not. The cerebral cortex goes from a nearly smooth surface to a highly folded surface in the last trimester; organizational changes in the cortex and brain continue long after birth. These events are responsible for the amazing capacity of cortical neurons to send and receive innumerable connections within and between hemispheres and to ultimately form the systems level organization responsible for the many specialized functions of the human forebrain.

The aspects of brain development that have been most clearly implicated in autism are neuronal organizational events, though some cases have also implicated neuronal migration events (Strauss et al., 2006; Volpe, 2008). In addition, ASD has been identified in 20–30% of young children with cerebral palsy who were extremely premature (born at or before 28 weeks gestational age) at birth (Moster et al., 2008), a time in brain development when neurons destined for the cerebral cortex are in the periventricular region. The periventricular region is also the premature infant's the watershed zone, or vulnerable region during compromised vascular perfusion of the brain in extreme premature infants. This pathophysiology raises the possibility that a stroke induced disturbance in neuronal number and/or in early neuronal migrational events during which neurons travel from the periventricular region to cortex might be the basis of the autism syndrome in association with cerebral palsy (Kuban et al., 2009; Minshew, 2010 in press, 2011; Volpe, 2008).

Though research studies have demonstrated widespread disturbances in cortical functioning in ASD, the disturbances are also somewhat selective. The cellular basis for this selectivity is not yet known other than that the disturbance involves cerebral cortical neurons that are involved in forming *distributed systems*. The developmental neurobiological events that produce the development of this circuitry are highly genetically regulated. It is reasonable to expect that the process of identifying genetic causes of ASD (and carrier status) will unfold the same way as did the causes in other child neurological disorders. That is, ASDs will be found to result from numerous related errors in the genetic code for a selected aspect of neuronal organization, just as many other childhood neurological disorders that develop de novo have been found to be the result of groups of abnormal genes. An error in the genetic code for a fundamental aspect of neuronal organization could potentially produce a broad profile of similar deficits (e.g. autism versus William's syndrome; Minshew, 2010; see also Volpe, 2008, pp. 82–102).

Genetic Foundations of ASDs

Developmental neurobiological events are extraordinarily complex, require precise guidance, and are known to be under strict genetic control (see Chapter 30 by J. Rubenstein, in this volume). Currently, approximately 20 or so mostly rare genes (and an occasional common gene or gene sequence) have been discovered that contribute to the cause up to 15–20% of cases of autism and ASD (Abrahams & Geschwind, 2008; Bolton, 2009; see also Commentary by Geschwind in this volume). Though "heterogeneous," these genes have in common a role in the development of connectivity among neurons and share common molecular signaling pathways (Geschwind & Levitt, 2007; Minshew, 2010a; Minshew, Williams, & McFadden, 2008).

The identification of these genes followed two decades of neuroimaging research establishing premature acceleration in brain growth as measured by total brain volume, including cerebral gray and white matter, followed by growth deceleration (reviewed in Levy et al., 2009; Mosconi, Zwaigenbaum, & Piven, 2006; and Chapter 35 in this volume). These are classic signs of disturbances in developmental neurobiological events. Furthermore, this research has also indicated disruptions in connectivity of cortical systems as a major etiopathophysiologic mechanism in autism and ASD (summarized in Minshew & Williams, 2007; and Chapter 54 in this volume). The convergence of genetic and neuroanatomical evidence for neuronal connectivity disturbances provides strong support for the notion of a developmental neurobiologically based model of autism and the ASDs. Imaging genetics, a comparison of genotype variability with imaging and behavioral phenotype variability, holds promise for additional insight into genetic contributions to the heterogeneity of the behavioral expression of the syndrome (see, for example, Raznahan et al., 2009; Wassink et al., 2007). In the discussion above, autism and ASD were referred to separately to indicate that the gene mutations were often found to be associated with both autism and ASD, often in the same families, supporting common underlying neurobiological and genetic mechanisms rather than separate etiologies for autism, Asperger's disorder, and Pervasive Developmental Disorders Not-Otherwise-Specified.

The identification of genes in autism has led to a number of major advances. The first is the development of a molecular pathophysiology for syndromic autism (e.g., tuberous sclerosis and TSC1 TSC2 genes, 22q deletion and SHANK3 gene, Rett syndrome and MECP2 gene, Fragile X syndrome and FMR1 gene, Timothy syndrome and CACNA1C gene), and some instances of nonsyndromic autism, (e.g., NRXN1, MET, and NLGN3; Abrahams & Geschwind, 2008). The development of animal models of these genes (primarily gene-neuroanatomical relationships with limited cognitive-behavioral correlates of autism) is enabling the development and study of neurobiological interventions (for example: Dolen et al., 2007; Ehninger & Silva, 2011; Silva & Ehninger, 2009), which confirm a connection between gene-to-brain development and autism-ASD phenotypes. This line of research has led directly to clinical trials with Rapamycin, an mTor inhibitor, for prevention of seizures, mental retardation, and ASD in infants and toddlers with genetically diagnosed tuberous sclerosis (Ess, 2009; Nie et al., 2010), providing clear proof of concept of the merits of uncovering molecular mechanisms for brain dysfunction in ASD. Animal models also provide opportunities for investigating potential molecular and cellular mechanisms of cortical dysfunction, such as the hypothesized role of an excitatory-inhibitory imbalance as a mechanism of cortical dysfunction and seizures in autism (Gogolla et al., 2009).

Another line of research supporting a developmental neurobiological model and connection between gene abnormality, cortical development, and manifestations of ASD has been the *MET* receptor research. This work was initiated as a result of reports of an increased association of the *MET* receptor CC allele with autism (Campbell, Sutcliffe, Ebert, et al., 2006; Campbell, Sutcliffe, Persico, & Levitt, 2008). Subsequently, researchers discovered increased *MET* mRNA expression levels in ASD brains (Campbell, D'Oronzio, Garbett et al., 2007), correspondence between *MET* mRNA levels in temporal lobe in ASD and language status (Campbell, Warren, Sutcliffe, et al., 2009), and correspondence between the presence of the *MET* gene and presence of gastrointestinal difficulties in ASD individuals (Campbell, Buie, Winter, et al., 2009) all provided additional support for a critical role of the MET receptor gene in autism. The *MET* receptor gene codes for cortical and cerebellar development, gastrointestinal repair, and immune competence (Campbell et al., 2006; Campbell et al., 2007), thus providing an example of a single genetic explanation for multiple organ involvement in ASD. Together, this body of imaging and genetic findings in ASD over the past decade has established a firm foundation for autism as a developmental neurobiological disorder and has identified a number of genetic abnormalities and mutations likely to be causative, which, though "heterogeneous," share signaling pathways at a molecular level involved in the development of neuronal connectivity (Levitt & Campbell, 2009).

The rapid growth in gene technology makes it highly likely that the list of ASD causative and associated genes will expand quickly and, with it, the delineation of a highly complex and heterogeneous molecular pathophysiology for autism. It is also likely that the growing number of gene variants and mutations discovered in ASD will nonetheless be found to contri-bute to a select number of common neuronal signaling pathways involved in developmental neurobiological events that result in the connectivity disturbances and growth dysregulation that is now well documented in autism (Minshew, 2010a). It is also likely that increasing knowledge about the variation in implicated genes will account for the variability in brain growth trajectories that has been observed in autism and ASD (Lainhart et al., 2006), as well as the variability in symptom severity. Greater genetic and developmental neurobiological diversity can be expected in very low functioning individuals with ASD, since there is less specification or restriction of events that can result in the absence of functional cortical connectivity compared to genes that are very selective in their impact on cortical connectivity.

With all of this in mind, the next question is how to connect the genetic and developmental neurobiological findings with the behavioral syndrome, which has been defined in growing detail over the past seven decades. Thus far, the answer has been found in altered development of cortical systems connectivity in autism.

Disruptions in Cortical Connectivity as the Brain Basis for Autism

Given 1) our previous findings of a simple-complex dissociation in the neuropsychological profile of autism with deficits in higher-order abilities across multiple domains and 2) the work implicating a disruption in neural organization events related to particular genes; we launched a program of research to investigate the role of disruptions in *cortical connectivity* as the brain basis of autism.

Language Domain

One of the simple-complex dissociations that we and many others have observed in autism in the language domain is that many individuals are superb spellers but have trouble understanding sentence meaning. Understanding this dissociation became the basis for our first functional neuroimaging study that resulted in a theory proposing cortical functional underconnectivity in autism (Just, Cherkassky, Keller, & Minshew, 2004). We used fMRI to measure brain activation in adults with high-functioning autism and typically developing, verbal, IQ-matched controls as they read sentences. The autism group exhibited increased activation in Wernicke's area, but reduced activation in Broca's area compared to controls. These findings map onto the behavioral profile of increased word knowledge and reduced sentence knowledge in the participants with autism. Furthermore, the functional connectivity (i.e., the degree of synchronization or correlation of the time series of the activation) between these cortical areas was consistently lower for the autism than the control participants. These findings suggested that the neural basis of disordered language in autism entails a lower degree of information integration and synchronization across the large-scale cortical network for language processing. This was the first of many subsequent studies showing a reduced collaboration among a network of cortical regions that support higher order function. It was a critical first step in support of our theory that connectivity within and between cortical systems is fundamentally underdeveloped and may be a central pathophysiologic mechanism for autism (see Chapter 54 in this volume).

Alterations in Connectivity More Broadly in the Brain

Subsequent studies also demonstrated reduced connectivity between posterior cortical regions and frontal cortex, and more bilateral activation within posterior visual and visuospatial cortex than occurs in typically developing individuals (Kana, Keller, Cherkassky, et al., 2009; Koshino, Kana, Keller, et al., 2008; Sahyoun, Belliveau, Soulieres, et al., 2010). We have proposed that these findings reflect underdevelopment of systems-level connectivity between cortical regions and frontal cortex, as well as enhanced local connectivity within visual cortex (see next sections on visual processing in autism). Other investigators have documented underdevelopment of cortical connectivity with amygdala and related circuits to account for the fundamental disturbances in affective contact in autism, and alterations in frontal-amygdala and striatal connections to account for difficulty in comprehending and regulating emotions (Gaigg & Bowler, 2007, 2008; Kleinhans et al., 2008). Analogous disturbances have been demonstrated in motor systems connectivity (Mostofsky et al., 2009).

Underconnectivity of cortical systems is now a widely accepted characterization of the structural and functional brain abnormality in autism. The initial index of functional underconnectivity was reduced synchronization between fMRI-measured activation in coactivating cortical areas during a sentence comprehension task (Just et al., 2004), which was subsequently demonstrated across a wide range of tasks to broadly involve cerebral association cortex (Just et al., 2007; Schipul et al., 2011). Over the course of many studies, *frontal-posterior* underconnectivity emerged as a common finding (Kana et al., 2009). The second characteristic of the altered task-related cortical connectivity in autism was enhanced activation of occipitoparietal areas. This activation pattern was hypothesized to result from *increased local connectivity* in posterior regions and to account for the unusual strengths also typical of autism. The dissociation between impaired higher order skills and intact basic skills was commonly characterized in the past in terms of a distinction between verbal and visuospatial abilities, rather than in terms of reduced frontal and enhanced posterior neural connectivity.

A recent fMRI study of the neural networks underlying visuospatial and linguistic reasoning has provided direct evidence that verbal individuals with average IQ scores and HFA have increased activation and connectivity of occipitoparietal and ventral temporal circuits, greater reliance on visuospatial skills for solving both visual and verbal problems, and reduced activation and connectivity of frontotemporal language areas (Sahyoun, Beliveasu, Soulieres, et al., 2010). The study concluded that the HFA group's engagement of posterior regions along with its weak connections to frontal language areas resulted in reliance on visual mediation even for higher order cognitive tasks. This study recapitulates the findings of the connectivity studies and adds some of the clearest evidence yet to support the neural basis of the visuospatial processing strengths in autism.

One outstanding and perhaps puzzling issue concerns the underconnectivity (defined here as reduced correlation in activation profile between two areas of cortex) between cortical regions and the concurrent evidence for increased white matter connectivity between disparate cortical regions in ASD. For example, in one of our recent studies with high functioning autistic adults, we observed an increase in white matter connectivity in long intrahemispheric fibers such as the inferior longitudinal fasciculus and the inferior fronto-occipital fasciculus, but not in the homotopic callosal fibers (Thomas et al., 2010). One might have predicted that an overproliferation or overabundance of white matters fibers would be associated with an increase in cross-areal correlation and yet the studies, such as Kana et al. (2009), suggest otherwise. A possible resolution to this apparent discrepancy between the reduced correlations and the increased white matter tracts is that the signal propagated across the increased tracts may not have sufficient fidelity with the consequence that the correlation across regions will be substantially impeded.

Understanding the Neurobiological Substrates of Autism Through Studies of Visual Information Processing

Many of our studies conducted over the last few years have focused on the cortical visual system of individuals with ASD and have provided converging evidence for the claim that sensory-perceptual function evinces the same simple-complex dissociation, as described in other more abstract domains such as language. Because the same dissociation between simpler versus more complex information processing is evident in the visual system in ASD, we think the same underlying neurobiological process is likely implicated. Thus, whereas more elementary visuoperceptual skills are preserved, or possibly even enhanced (Ashwin et al., 2009; Mottron et al., 2006; Mottron et al., 2009; Soulières et al., 2009) relative to typical controls, more complex information processing requiring the synthesis of disparate bits of information is disproportionately impacted. We begin this section by reporting data from visuoperceptual processing in adults and in children with autism and then turn to describe a series of recent imaging investigations conducted with the same populations. The associated imaging investigations, which we describe, also offer supportive evidence for a biological system in which local or short-range connectivity is better preserved but longer-range connectivity especially with multi-modal association cortex and in particular with frontal cortex, necessary for integration at the neural and information processing level, is compromised.

Visual Processing: Behavioral Studies

One of the most essential visuoperceptual skills for humans is face processing. Interestingly, impairments in face processing are a widely accepted aspect of the behavioral profile of autism. The impairment involves difficulty remembering faces (Boucher & Lewis, 1992), processing facial expressions (Ashwin, Baron-Cohen, Wheelwright, O'Riordan, & Bullmore, 2007), and knowing which components of faces convey especially important communicative information (Joseph & Tanaka, 2003). One of the key behavioral processes considered critical for intact face perception is the ability to perceptually organize, or integrate, disparate components of the input rapidly and efficiently. Moreover, the failure to do so impacts both facial identity and emotional expression recognition. Both face perception and perceptual organization have been shown to be compromised in autism, and the studies we describe below document the atypicalities in both domains and suggest an association between the difficulties in these processes in individuals with autism. We start off by examining the *local processing bias*, or enhancement, in individuals with autism and then discuss the difficulties in face perception.

In contrast with the documented difficulties in higher-order perceptual abilities, such as those engaged for face processing (Gastgeb et al., 2011; Klin et al., 2002; Joseph & Tanaka, 2003; Humphreys et al., 2008; Lahaie et al., 2006; Pellicano et al., 2007; Scherf, Behrmann, et al., 2008), individuals with autism have been shown to exhibit hyper- or enhanced sensitivity to the more simple local elements of the input (Mottron et al., 2009; Soulières et al., 2009). For example, compared to age-matched, typically developing individuals, those with autism exhibit superior abilities to detect local targets in visual search tasks (Plaisted et al., 1999), ignore the influence of increasing numbers of distracters during visual search (O'Riordan et al., 2001), and identify fine stimulus features in spatial tasks like the Wechsler block design and Embedded Figures Task (Shah & Frith, 1993; Jolliffe & Baron-Cohen, 1997), to name but a few such observations. At the same time, individuals with autism appear to be limited in their ability to derive organized wholes from perceptual parts, which has been linked to their limited use of gestalt grouping heuristics (Brosnan et al., 2004), the failure to process inter-element relationships (Behrmann et al., 2006), and/or the failure to consider the entire visual context (Happé, 1996). Several studies have argued that this focus on local features is specifically detrimental to face recognition processes (Hobson et al., 1988; Boucher & Lewis, 1992; Davies et al., 1994; Klin et al., 2002; Joseph & Tanaka, 2003; Lahaie et al., 2006), and we consider this further below.

Although there is general consensus that the perceptual abilities of individuals with ASD are atypical (for review see Behrmann et al., 2006; Dakin & Frith, 2005), there still remains some controversy both about the nature of the atypicality as well as the source of this atypicality. Some researchers have suggested that children with autism exhibit limited abilities to integrate local elements into a coherent global shape (Plaisted et al., 1999; Rinehart et al., 2000; Wang et al., 2007), whereas others have reported typical processing of both the global and local information in hierarchical visual stimuli (Ozonoff et al., 1994; Mottron et al., 2003; Iarocci et al., 2006; Plaisted et al., 2006).

To explore both the difficulty in global organization and perhaps the undue focus on local elements, in a recent study (Scherf, Luna et al., 2008b), we conducted two related investigations in children, adolescents, and adults with high-functioning autism (HFA) and age- and IQ-matched typically developing (TD) controls, using a well-known task of global/local processing with compound letter stimuli as well as a more novel, fine-grained microgenetic priming paradigm with hierarchical shapes including both few and many local elements.

In the first investigation, we employed the well-known hierarchical compound stimuli (Navon, 1977), which included global letters composed of smaller local letters that were either consistent or inconsistent with the global letter in identity (see Figure 36-1A). This design allows for performance measures, such as the speed of identification and asymmetric interference during inconsistent trials (for example, a global 'H' made of small 's's), to be used to infer the advantage of one level over the other (Navon, 1977, 1983). Participants were required to respond

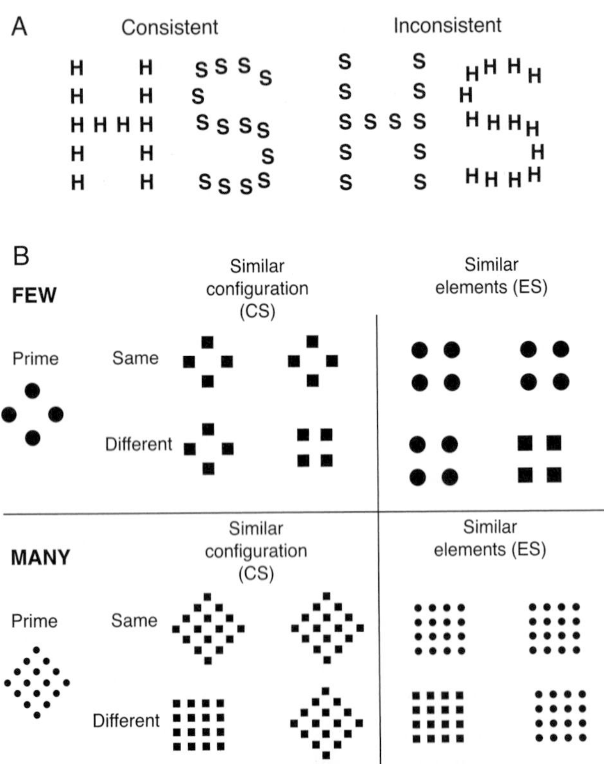

Figure 36–1. A) The compound letter stimuli used in the global/local task to evaluate developmental differences in sensitivity to global (big letter) and local (small letters) information. B) The hierarchical shape stimuli used in the microgenetic priming task (few- and many-element).

by key press (is an H or S present) to indicate letter identity. Identification of the global or local letter was required in different blocks of trials. As expected and as predicted from well-established findings, the typically developing (TD) adults were faster to identify letters at the global level (for example, a global 'H' made of small 's's) than at the local letter (for example, the small 's's in the global 'H'), reflecting the so-called forest before the trees finding and indicating a bias to perceptually organize the disparate local elements to perceive the global letter. Importantly, this bias to perceptually organize the local elements increased linearly with age in the TD group. This pattern of results was not true for the HFA group, who was faster to identify letters at the local level, clearly revealing the bias to perceive the local (trees) rather than global (forest) arrangement of the letters. These findings are consistent with the idea that the emergence of the local processing bias in autism becomes prominent in adolescence and never transitions into a global bias in adulthood as in the TD individuals.

To confirm these findings, we conducted a second study in the same participants and, in this investigation, we assessed the temporal evolution of the organized visual percept, instead of simply measuring reaction time to identify a global or local letter as we had done in the first investigation reported above. To do so, we adopted a paradigm developed by Kimchi (1998, Expt 1) to test perceptual organization processes in typical adults. In this paradigm, participants view (but ignore) an ambiguous prime (for example, a diamond made of four circles in the "few" element condition or a diamond made of many circles in the "many" element condition) followed immediately by a pair of test figures (probes). Participants are required to judge whether the two probe images are the same or different and to indicate their response by key press. As evident from Figure 36-1B, both the prime and probe stimuli include patterns (i.e., global diamonds composed of smaller circles) with few large elements or with many small elements. Each test stimulus includes two probes from one of two conditions, defined by their similarity to the prime stimulus (see Figure 36-1B). In the *element-similarity* (ES) condition, probes are similar to the prime in their local elements (circles), but differ in their global configuration (global square instead of global diamond). In the *configuration-similarity* (CS) condition, probes are similar to the prime in their global configuration (diamond), but differ in their local elements (local squares instead of local circles).

The (ignored) prime is presented at several durations, providing multiple temporal windows over which the representation evolves prior to the onset of the probe, and behavioral responses are compared across the prime durations. The expectation is that, at short prime durations, only the most dominant characteristic of the percept of the priming stimulus is represented (e.g., for the few element stimuli, only the local information may be represented this early). When the test figures share these entry-level or early characteristics with the prime stimulus, responses will be facilitated. At longer prime durations, it is possible that both local and global characteristics are represented, in which case the prime would enhance both of these dimensions in responses to the test figures. Because we know that grouping into a whole is easier when there are many local elements, we expect there to be an advantage for the configuration-similarity probes for the many versus few elements and this advantage may even manifest at early prime durations, reflecting the rapid organization into a gestalt in the typical visual process.

Unsurprisingly, we replicated the original Kimchi (1998) data, and showed that it takes longer (at longer prime durations) for the TD adults to evince an advantage for the "few" *configuration-similarity* (CS) condition both because the local elements are few and prominent in their own right, but also because they are somewhat spatially distant and have to be integrated to form a global whole and this is perceptually demanding. Of particular importance to us here, and again like the Kimchi data, these TD adults encode global shape information in the entry-level units (at very brief prime durations) of the representation for the "many" element displays, indicating the rapid and efficient integration of local information and access to global shape information. The question then is how individuals with ASD fare under these experimental conditions.

We found that HFA adults are faster to make similarity judgments about test figures that share local elements (ES trials) rather than global shape information (CS trials) with the prime, regardless of the prime duration or the number and size of the elements (Behrmann et al., 2006; also reported in Scherf, Luna et al., 2008). These results indicate that, in the HFA adults, both the entry-level units and the final percept of hierarchical visual stimuli are dominated by information about the local elements, regardless of whether the elements are few and large or small and many. This result is consistent with the data from the first investigation using compound stimuli in which the local bias dominated performance in the HFA individuals, even in the adults with HFA. The same investigation with CS and ES test trials conducted with HFA adolescents and children revealed a similar finding to that of the HFA adults: they are faster to say "same" to the *element-similarity* (ES) probes across nearly all exposure durations. Thus, not only do they **not** glean the advantage for the configuration at early prime durations, but, interestingly, they show a much greater advantage for the element similarity probes than do their matched controls, perhaps reflecting the hypersensitivity to the local elements (even though they are many and small).

In the few-element displays, children, adolescents, and adults in both groups were biased to encode the local elements, regardless of the prime duration, indicating that the ability to individuate elements presented in hierarchical displays with few, large items matures quite early in both TD and HFA populations. These results suggest that, beginning in childhood, local information dominates the formation of a percept in autism from the entry-level units to the longer-term visual representation, regardless of the stimulus characteristics of the local elements. Furthermore, the ability to group local elements perceptually in order to perceive a global shape does not appear to mature during the developmental transition from adolescence to adulthood in HFA as it does in TD individuals, as was apparent in the results from the many-element condition.

In sum, the findings from both the few- and many-element displays indicate that local information dominates the formation of a percept in children, adolescents, and adults with autism regardless of whether the local items are few and large or small and many. The local information is encoded in the entry-level units of the percept (results from short prime durations) and organizes the final percept (results from long prime durations). We only found evidence for superior processing of local information in the many-elements task, which is present by childhood. TD children, adolescents, and adults encode more global shape information from the many-element displays (as evidenced by their weaker ES advantage), while those with autism exhibit enhanced perception of the local elements. The atypical development of these perceptual organizational processes in ASD may contribute directly to disruptions in the processing of visually presented objects, which may, in turn, fundamentally influence the development of major aspects of the social and emotional deficits characteristic of autism (see New et al., 2010, for recent discussion of social deficit and complexity of this deficit). We go on now to explore the relationship between the obvious local bias and higher order pattern recognition in ASD.

These atypical perceptual organizational processes, we have argued, may contribute to the difficulties in more complex visual processing, such as face perception, in ASD. In particular, ASD individuals may be more focused on local elements of faces and less able to integrate the elements into a whole. This process of integration is thought to become even more critical when faces are similar and the featural differences themselves do not suffice for differentiation. The focus on local aspects of faces is well captured in this comment by Temple Grandin:

> I often get into embarrassing situations because I do not remember faces unless I have seen the people many times or they have a very distinct facial feature such as a big beard, thick glasses or a strange hairstyle. (*Thinking in Pictures and Other Reports from My Life with Autism* by Temple Grandin)

To evaluate whether the same HFA individuals who showed an undue local bias in the compound letter task and micro-genetic task described above also show a difficulty in face recognition, especially as faces become more similar to one another, the same adults with HFA who participated in the studies above, made same/different judgments to two faces presented alongside each other, for unlimited duration, in the center of a computer screen. On "different" trials, the faces could be either two faces from different genders or, in the more perceptually taxing case, two different faces of the same gender (see Figure 36-2a). It is in this latter condition that the reliance not only on featural information but also on the second-order relational information among the features becomes even more necessary. As shown in Figure 36-2b, not only were the ASD adults slow at making the similarity judgments, but they were disproportionately slower for judging the more

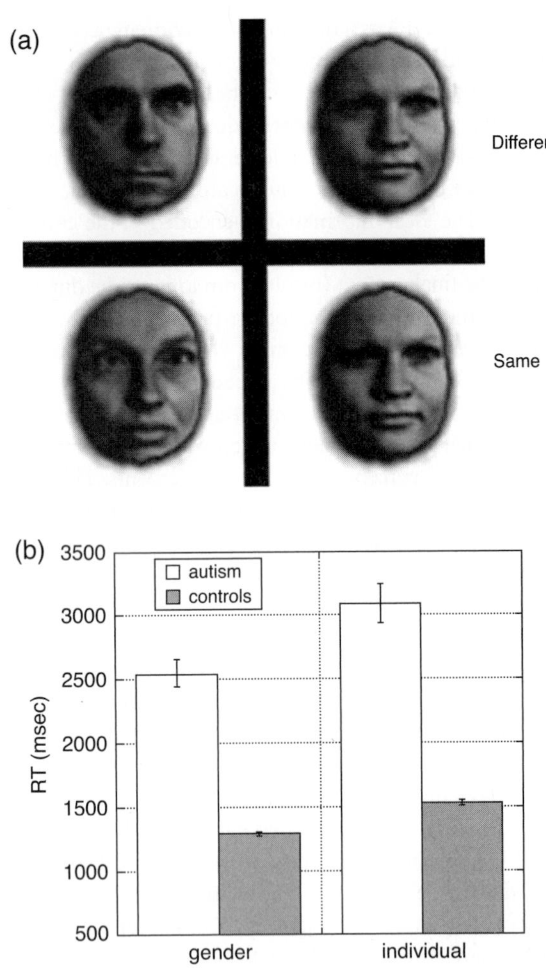

Figure 36–2. a. Examples of stimuli for face discrimination experiment, including one trial where faces differ on the basis of gender and one trial where faces differ on the basis of individual identity. b. Mean of median RT (and 1 SE) for correct different trials as a function of conditions of discrimination for autistic and control groups.

similar faces (albeit a "different" judgment). Taken together, these behavioral findings not only reveal the slow responses in face perception in the HFA adults, but also the disproportionate difficulty in the more demanding face task that requires perceptual binding of the elemental features.

We have shown atypical perceptual processing in tasks requiring holistic grouping or binding of elements and we have shown disproportionate slowing in face discrimination in the same individuals. To establish whether there is any association between performances on these two tasks, we took the median RT for each HFA individual on the "individually different/same gender" and correlated them with the local advantage from the compound hierarchical letter task. This analysis yielded a significant r^2 value of .61 ($p = 0.03$). Although correlation is not causation, the relationship between RT in face processing and the local bias is clear in the autistic adult individuals and is highly suggestive of some common atypicality.

In sum, the behavioral data we have reported here document not only the advantage for processing local elements in individuals with HFA across the age span but also the association between the local bias and the difficulty making fine-grained discrimination between faces. The view we have taken here is that the slowing in face processing in autism, a higher-order visual task that requires the integration of many local elements, might arise from a more fundamental visual (and possibly even sensory-independent) bias toward the local elements and perhaps simultaneous or resultant difficulty in integrating local components of a stimulus into a whole. We have also argued that this fundamental perceptual form of processing is likely not restricted to faces but may impact visual processing of other, nonface objects, too, when the demands for discrimination and recognition are high, as is true in the case of faces (Behrmann et al., 2006; Scherf, Behrmann, et al., 2008).

These findings are not easily accounted for by views that argue for a primary social, rather than perceptual, deficit in autism. The perceptual deficit that we and others have documented may exist independently of a social deficit. Alternatively, perceptual and social deficits may work in tandem: the lack of experience and the inadequate attention to faces may limit the acquisition of the normal configural perceptual skill and/or the perceptual deficit may constrain the ability to acquire typical face representations (see also Grelotti et al., 2005). Either way, there appears to be some fundamental dissociation between the ability to process local elements and the ability to integrate these elements efficiently for higher order pattern perception.

Visual Processing: Imaging Investigations

In our pursuit to understand the relation between the neurobiological and behavioral manifestations of autism, we have also undertaken several functional neuroimaging studies of visuoperceptual processing in adults and adolescents with autism.

Activation of Earlier Versus Later Visual Cortex.

One prediction that arises from the behavioral studies is that individuals with ASD should show reduced or minimal activation of those regions of visual cortex that support higher-order visual perception, while earlier parts of the visual system should remain intact. Our own experiments have focused on the former point, although there are good data to suggest that there is preservation (even if not totally normal activation) of the earlier parts of the visual system (Hadjikhani et al., 2004). We also note that some recent investigations have suggested enhancement of activation in earlier parts of the cortical system (Mottron et al., 2006), and a recent study reports an increase in grey matter in auditory and visual primary and associative perceptual areas. These last results demonstrating potential structural brain correlates of atypical auditory and visual perception in autism provides possible support for the enhanced perceptual functioning model (Mottron, Dawson, Soulières, Hubert, & Burack, 2006; Mottron, Dawson, & Soulières, 2009).

Consistent with the claim that higher-order regions of visual cortex (such as the fusiform gyrus or "fusiform face area"; FFA) are engaged in face processing, and that individuals with autism do not respond preferentially to faces, many studies (Corbett et al., 2009; Critchley et al., 2000; Schultz et al., 2000; Pierce et al., 2001; Hall et al., 2003; Hubl et al., 2003; Humphreys et al., 2008; Ogai et al., 2003; Piggot et al., 2004; Wang et al., 2004; Dalton et al., 2005; Grelotti et al., 2005; Deeley et al., 2007) have found reduced BOLD activation in the fusiform face area (FFA, Kanwisher et al., 1997). However, other studies have failed to replicate this finding (Hadjikhani et al., 2004; Hadjikhani et al., 2007; Pierce et al., 2004; Bird et al., 2006), and so there remains some controversy surrounding the brain-behavior correspondences in FFA and ASD.

To explore the integrity of higher-order visual cortex and to map out cortical activation for faces in a broader network that extends beyond the FFA to include the occipital face area (OFA) and superior temporal sulcus (STS), but also for other images such as places and objects, ASD and TD adult participants viewed naturalistic, real-time movies of unfamiliar faces, buildings, navigation through open fields, and objects in a blocked fMRI paradigm (Figure 36-3a; Humphreys et al., 2008). Rich, moving stimuli from multiple categories, such as these (see Figure 36-3a), have been shown to induce stronger activation in ventral cortex than do static, black and white images, and so we used them to increase our chances of uncovering robust cortical response profiles in the HFA group. We also note that this task has been used successfully to map category-selective activation in the ventral visual cortex in other populations (Hasson et al., 2004; Avidan et al., 2005; Scherf et al., 2007). There are no specific task demands in this investigation, and so performance differences between the autism and comparison groups cannot account for any different levels of functional activation.

Figure 36-3b shows the average activation maps for the autism and typical adults in this experiment projected into a single inflated brain with both lateral and ventral projections. Note that we group together the building and scene related activation, as both typically activate the parahippocampal place area (PPA) in the collateral sulcus (Scherf et al., 2007). The findings from the typical group largely replicate the standard findings with extensive activation for faces (red) and objects (blue). The building/scene-related activation (green) in PPA appears somewhat reduced, especially in the left hemisphere but this has been noticed in other studies as well (Avidan et al., 2005). The most marked feature is the clear

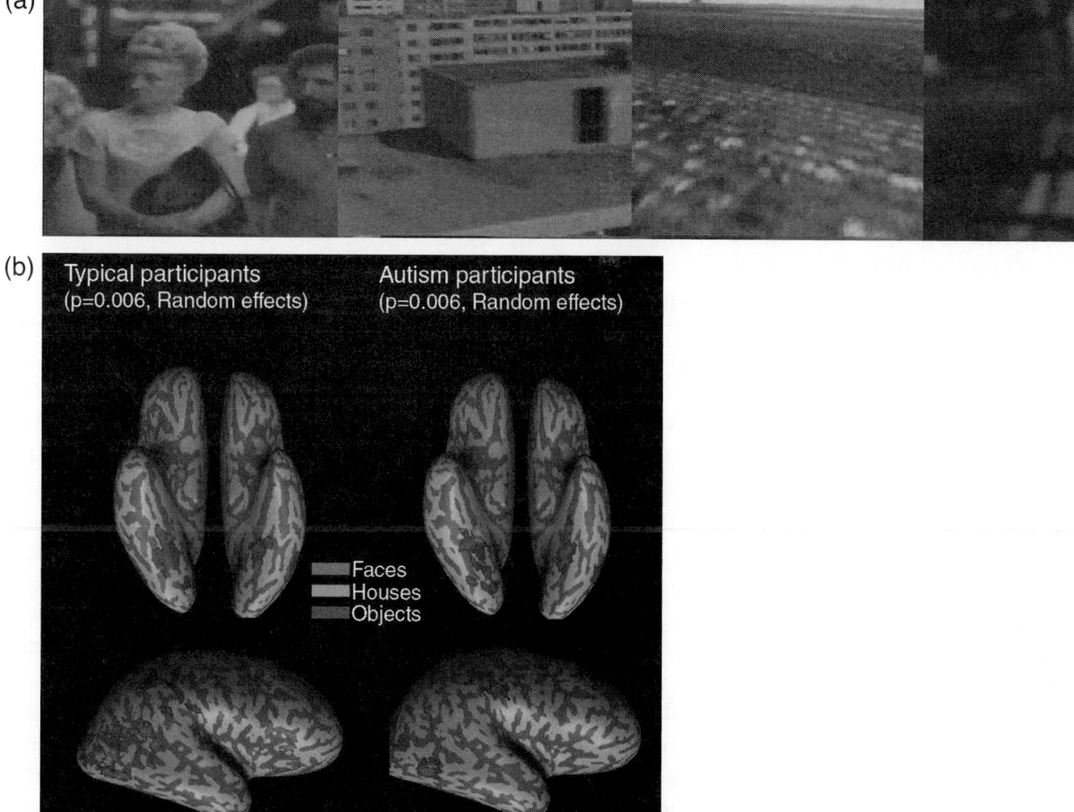

Figure 36–3. Functional MRI study using moving pictures of faces, buildings, scenes, and objects: (a) examples of the stimuli; (b) group averaged cortical maps from the typical and autism groups showing activation in response to faces, buildings, landscapes, and objects. The first map shows the average activation map for typical individuals and the second for individuals with autism. (See Color Plate Section for a color version of this figure.)

reduction in face-related activity in the ASD group and the only face-related activity at this threshold for the autism group is in the right OFA. In contrast, object-related activity in object-related lateral occipital cortex (LO) appears more extensive for the ASD than comparison group, this time in both hemispheres. Ventral visual cortex appears to be organized differently in high-functioning adults with autism, at least for face-selective regions, although subtle differences may also exist for other categories such as objects. These findings are compatible with the other studies that have demonstrated atypical activation in FFA and other face-related regions in ASD and are also compatible with those studies showing enhancement in object related activation (Baily et al., 2005).

Recently, we also evaluated whether functional organization in the ventral visual pathway is fundamentally disrupted in individuals with HFA during adolescence, the important period of visuoperceptual development when HFA individuals fail to develop mature perceptual organizational abilities (Scherf, Luna, Minshew, & Behrmann, 2010). We used the same fMRI paradigm described above to map face-, object-, and place-related activation in 10 high-functioning (FSIQ > 80) adolescents with autism (ages 11–14) and 10 age- and IQ-matched controls. Although the HFA adolescents exhibited typical organization in object- and place-related cortex, as a group they failed to show consistent face-selective activation in classical face regions (FFA, OFA, STS). These results suggest that the functional topography of face-related cortex is selectively disrupted in autism and that this alteration is present in early adolescence, an important stage of cortical specialization for TD adolescents. Furthermore, for those adolescents with autism who do exhibit face-selective activation, face-selective cortex tends to be located in traditionally object-related regions, which supports the hypothesis that perceptual processing of faces in autism may be more akin to the perceptual processing of common objects in typically developing individuals. Such alterations could result from direct pathology to regions within the face-processing network, like the fusiform gyrus (van Kooten et al., 2008), and/or to the structural and functional connections between such regions. Also, alterations in the visual experiences that individuals with autism have with faces as a result of social aversion and/or excessive focus on features may configure these regions in the face-processing network atypically (Grelotti et al., 2005).

Cortical Response Profile Under Naturalistic Conditions

The fMRI studies conducted with ASD individuals, to date, focus predominantly on documenting the cortical response profile of an area or subset of areas of cortex. To examine the claim that multiple higher-order areas, engaged more in integration of information, are more atypical than lower order areas, we have also explored whole brain activation in a group of ASD adults. In perhaps the most naturalistic imaging study we have run to date, we compared the functional connectivity between disparate regions of cortex from data obtained while adults with autism and typical controls lay in a MRI scanner watching a common, popular movie. We mapped the whole-brain activation profile by comparing the evoked fMRI response time courses across different subjects (inter-subject correlation, inter-SC; Hasson et al., 2004). Computing the inter-SC within the typical individuals (typical-typical), on a voxel-by-voxel basis, quantifies the reliability of the response time-courses in each brain area across members of the typical group. Recently, using this technique, Hasson et al. (2009) demonstrated that, across typical observers, approximately 30–65% of the cerebrum evinces similar shared reliable response time-courses under free-viewing of complex naturalistic stimuli, and this provides a benchmark against which to assess the inter-SC in ASD. Computing the inter-SC between the typical and the autism groups (typical-autism) provides a measure of similarity in the functional response in each brain areas across the two groups. Low inter-SC between the typical-autism group in conjunction with high inter-SC within the typical group would indicate that the response time course in a given brain area is markedly different in individuals with autism from that of the typical individuals. Moreover, computing the inter-SC within the autism group (autism-autism) alone can identify reliable response time courses, which are unique to the ASD group and are not observed in the typical subjects.

All participants watched a 10-minute excerpt from the popular movie, *The Good, the Bad, and the Ugly,* directed by Sergio Leone, and answered questions posed afterward to probe their comprehension of the plot and sequence of events. After normalizing all brains to the Talairach coordinate system, we calculated the inter-SC across the entire movie sequence within the typical group on a voxel-by-voxel basis (see Hasson et al., 2004; Hasson et al., 2009, for more details). This was done separately for every voxel. Figure 36-4A shows the activation profile sampled from the vicinity of the calcarine sulcus, which includes the primary visual cortex and nearby early visual areas (termed in the paper as area V1+) for each individual in each group, plotted across the entire movie sequence (600s). We also show the correlation among the typical individuals (0.32), reflecting strong similarity in the individual time courses, and among the ASD individuals (0.14), reflecting rather different time courses in each individual. This area was chosen as a clear illustrative example of the findings, but similar results were obtained in the other regions of cortex (see Figure 36-4D). In sum, the response time-courses in area V1+ were highly reliable across all typical subjects whereas the time-courses from the same area in the individuals with autism, although highly fluctuating, were poorly correlated across individuals.

The reduction in the correlation of the response time courses in individuals with autism held across large regions of posterior cortex. Figure 36-4D presents the average inter-SC values for the within- and between-group comparisons across the preselected ROIs. The high correlation values within the group of control subjects (typical-typical: red) replicate previous findings (Hasson et al., 2004). In all ROIs (including early and higher-order regions), the autism-autism analysis (dark green) and the autism-control analysis (light green) showed a substantially reduced correlation of about 40–50%,

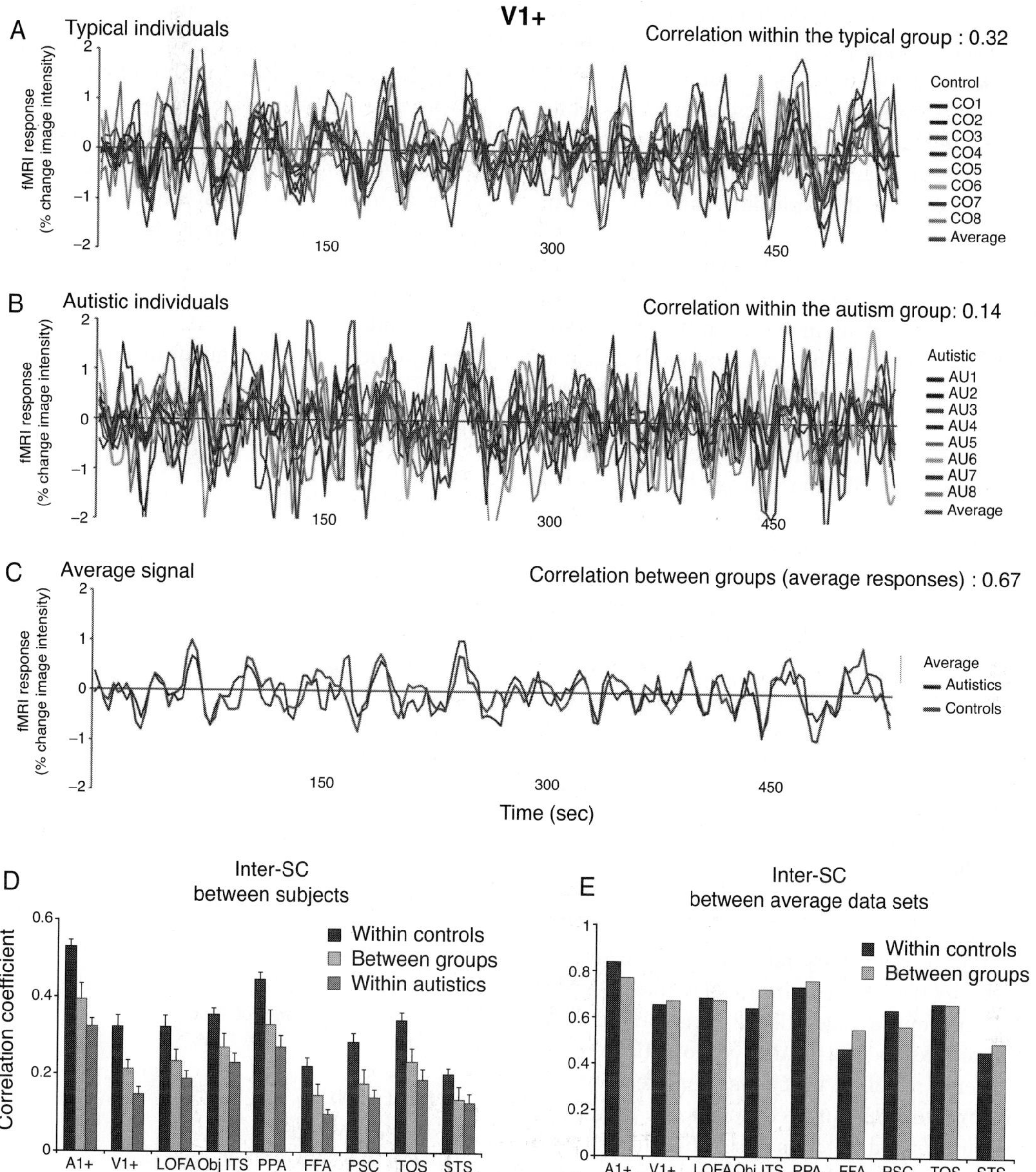

Figure 36–4. Signal fluctuations within ROIs. Visual cortex (V11) response time courses for (A) each typical subject and (B) each participant with autism. (C) The average signal for the typical group (red line) and autism (blue line) group. (D) The mean inter-SC values for the within-typical group (typical–typical, red bars), within-autism group (autism–autism, light green bars), and between the two groups (autism–typical, green bars) for selected ROIs. ROI abbreviations: A11, primary and secondary auditory cortices; V11, primary and secondary visual cortices; LOFA, lateral occipital cortex responsive to pictures of faces; Obj-ITS, object-related area in the inferior temporal sulcus; PPA, parahippocampal place area; FFA, fusiform face area; PCS, posterior central sulcus responsive to pictures of objects; TOS, transverse occipital sulcus responsive to pictures of places; STS-Face, area in superior temporal sulcus responsive to pictures of faces. (E) The inter-SC between the average autism–typical time courses (green bars) and the typical–typical time courses (red bars) in each ROI (same abbreviations as in D). Note the extent of variability in signal fluctuation in the autism individuals relative to the typical subjects. Moreover, note that by averaging the time courses within a group the responses become highly correlated across groups. (See Color Plate Section for a color version of this figure.)

relative to the typical subjects' inter-SC values. An important observation, however, is that the overall inter-SC values are higher in primary sensory cortices than in higher-order association cortex, consistent with the hypothesis that more primary regions of cortex, whose responsibility it is to mediate more simple forms of processing, might be better preserved in ASD than those regions whose role it is to integrate the higher-order statistics of the more complex input.

Visual Processing: Conclusions

Taken together, our investigations into the psychological and neural mechanisms of visual processing in high-functioning individuals with ASD reveal a similar pattern: there is relative preservation (and perhaps even enhancement, on some accounts) in more elemental, simple, or featural processing, whereas information processing that requires the integration of the simple elements is disproportionately affected. The imaging data yield a similar profile: relative preservation of earlier parts of the visual system and more pronounced atypical activation in higher-order regions. These alterations, while appearing subtle, nonetheless have a profound impact on how the brain in autism processes information, and, in turn, how individuals with autism "see" the world differently (Behrmann, Thomas, & Humphreys, 2006).

These findings exemplify some of the major advances that have occurred in delineating the neurobiological basis of neuropsychological functioning in autism in the past decade in large part due to the impact of numerous, carefully executed functional MRI studies in conjunction with equally meticulous cognitive studies. These findings have created a convergent and consistent picture of distinctive alterations in cortical functional connectivity in ASD characterized by intact and or increased local connectivity in posterior or occipital parietal regions (and probably other primary cortical regions too) and decreased systems connectivity that particularly impacts connectivity with frontal cortex. This distinctive alteration in circuitry has been shown to alter how the brain processes a broad range of social and nonsocial information, how the person with ASD perceives the world, and how the person with ASD thinks and feels.

General Conclusions

Across all domains impacted by autism, the common thread is the preservation of elementary skills and greatest impairments in those abilities that require on-line integration of information. In previous decades, this dissociation was characterized as a contrast between intact visuospatial abilities and impaired verbal abilities, which was considered nearly pathognomonic of autism. With technologic advances, this pattern is now understood in terms of selective disturbances in cortical connectivity. Recent genetic advances have identified a multitude of abnormal and mutated genes for ASD that all share a role in the development of neuronal connections and share common molecular signaling pathways. A little is known about the molecular pathophysiology of ASD but far from enough to explain the specific connection of these genes to the impact ASD has on cortical circuitry. These findings have produced a convergent developmental neurobiological model of autism as a disorder of neuronal organization and in some cases neuronal migration as well as the first neurobiologically based treatment for prevention of syndromic autism.

Challenges and Future Directions

- In the next 5 years, our hope is that investigators will work to advance the knowledge in their respective areas to diminish the gaps and increase the specificity of detail essential to designing treatments for autism.
- The focus on future work should strive to explain autism as a developmental neurobiological disorder with disturbances in cortical circuitry to create an integrated, multidimensional definition of the cause of autism from gene to behavioral variability.
- Interdisciplinary research that seeks to integrate and correlate genetic, neurobiological, neurological, and behavioral findings will be crucial for making progress in understanding the etiology, brain basis, and effective treatments for the complex disorder of ASD.

SUGGESTED READINGS

Minshew, N. J., Goldstein, G., & Siegel, D. J. (1997). Neuropsychologic functioning in autism: Profile of a complex information processing disorder. *Journal of the International Neuropsychological Society*, *3*, 303–316.

Behrmann, M., Thomas, C., & Humphreys, K. (2006). Seeing it differently: visual processing in autism. *Trends in Cognitive Sciences*, *10*(6), 258–264.

Geschwind, D. H., & Levitt, P. (2007). Autism spectrum disorders: developmental disconnection syndromes. *Current Opinion in Neurobiology*, *17*(1), 103–111.

ACKNOWLEDGMENTS

The work reported in this chapter was conducted under the auspices of research awards granted to NJM from NICHD #HD055748, an NIH Autism Center of Excellence, and to MB, KSS, and KH from Cure Autism Now and from the Pennsylvania Department of Health, State of Pennsylvania #4100047862.

REFERENCES

Abrahams, B. S., & Geschwind, D. H. (2008). Advances in autism genetics: on the threshold of a new neurobiology. *Nature Reviews Genetics*, *9*(5), 341–355.

Ashwin, C., Baron-Cohen, S., Wheelwright, S., O'Riordan, M., & Bullmore, E. T. (2007). Differential activation of the amygdala and the "social brain" during fearful face-processing in Asperger Syndrome. *Neuropsychologia*, *45*(1), 2–14.

Ashwin, C., Ricciardelli, P., & Baron-Cohen, S. (2009). Positive and negative gaze perception in autism spectrum conditions. *Social Neuroscience*, *4*(2), 153–164.

Avidan, G., Hasson, U., Malach, R., & Behrmann, M. (2005). Detailed exploration of face-related processing in congenital prosopagnosia: 2. Functional neuroimaging findings. *Journal of Cognitive Neuroscience*, *17*(7), 1150–1167.

Bailey, A. J., Braeutigam, S., Jousmäki, V., & Swithenby, S. J. (2005). Abnormal activation of face processing systems at early and intermediate latency in individuals with autism spectrum disorder: a magnetoencephalographic study. *European Journal of Neuroscience*, *21*(9), 2575–2585.

Bauman, M., & Kemper, T. L. (1998). Neuropathology of infantile autism. *Journal of Neuropathology and Experimental Neurology*, *57*(7), 645–652.

Bauman, M., & Kemper, T. (1994). Neuroanatomic observations of the brain in autism. In M. Bauman & T. Kemper, The neurobiology of autism. Baltimore: The Johns Hopkins University Press.

Behrmann, M., Avidan, G., Leonard, G. L., Kimchi, R., Luna, B., Humphreys, K., et al. (2006). Configural processing in autism and its relationship to face processing. *Neuropsychologia, 44*(1), 110–129.

Behrmann, M., Thomas, C., & Humphreys, K. (2006). Seeing it differently: visual processing in autism. *Trends in Cognitive Sciences, 10*(6), 258–264.

Best, C. A., Minshew, N. J., & Strauss, M. S. (2010). Gender discrimination of eyes and mouths by individuals with autism. *Autism Research, 3*, 88–93.

Bird, G., Catmur, C., Silani, G., Frith, C., & Frith, U. (2006). Attention does not modulate neural responses to social stimuli in autism spectrum disorders. *NeuroImage, 31*, 1614–1624.

Bolton, P. E. (2009). Medical conditions in autism spectrum disorders. *Journal of Neurodevelopmental Disorders, 1*, 102–113.

Boucher, J., & Lewis, V. (1992). Unfamiliar face recognition in relatively able autistic children. *Journal of Child Psychology and Psychiatry, 33*, 843–859.

Brosnan, M. J., Scott, F. J., Fox, S., & Pye, J. (2004). Gestalt processing in autism: Failure to process perceptual relationships and the implications for contextual understanding. *Journal of Child Psychology and Psychiatry, 45*, 459–469.

Campbell, D. B., Buie, T. M., Winter, H., Bauman, M., Sutcliffe, J. S., Perrin, J. M., et al. (2009). Distinct genetic risk based on association of MET in families with co-occurring autism and gastrointestinal conditions. *Pediatrics, 123*(3), 1018–1024.

Campbell, D. B., D'Oronzio, R., Garbett, K., Ebert. P. J., et al. (2007). Disruption of cerebral cortex MET signaling in autism spectrum disorder. *Annals of Neurology, 62*(3), 243–250.

Campbell, D. B., Li, C., Sutcliffe, J. S., Persico, A. M., & Levitt, P. (2008). Genetic evidence implicating multiple genes in the MET receptor tyrosine kinase pathway in autism spectrum disorder. *Autism Research, 1*(3), 159–168.

Campbell, D. B., Sutcliffe, J. S., Ebert, P. J., Militerni, R., et al. (2006). A genetic variant that disrupts MET transcription is associated with autism. *Proceedings of the National Academy of Sciences of the United States of America, 103*(45), 16834–16839.

Campbell, D. B., Warren, D., Sutcliffe, J. S., Lee, E. B., & Levitt, P. (2009). Association of MET with social and communication phenotypes in individuals with autism spectrum disorder. *American Journal of Medical Genetics. Part B, Neuropsychiatric Genetics*, (Epub ahead of print).

Constantino, J. N., Gruber, C. P., Davis, S., Hayes, S., Passanante, N., & Przybeck, T. (2004). The factor structure of autistic traits. *Journal of Child Psychology and Psychiatry, 4*(7), 19–26.

Corbett, B. A., Carmean, V., Ravizza, S., Wendelken, C., Henry, M. L., Carter, C., et al. (2009). A functional and structural study of emotion and face processing in children with autism. *Psychiatry Research, 173*(3), 196–205.

Critchley, H. D., Daly, E. M., Bullmore, E. T., Williams, S. C., Van Amelsvoort, T., Robertson, D. M., et al. (2000). The functional neuroanatomy of social behaviour: changes in cerebral blood flow when people with autistic disorder process facial expressions. *Brain, 123*, 2203–2212.

Dakin, S., & Frith, U. (2005). Vagaries of visual perception in autism. *Neuron, 48*(3), 497–507.

Dalton, K. M., Nacewicz, B. M., Johnstone, T., Shaefer, H. S., Gernsbacher, M. A., Goldsmith, H. H., et al. (2005). Gaze fixation and the neural circuitry of face processing in autism. *Nature Neuroscience, 8*, 519–526.

Damarla, S. R., Keller, T. A., Kana, R. K., Cherkassky, V. L., Williams, D. L., Minshew, N. J., & Just, M. A. (2010). Cortical underconnectivity coupled with preserved visuospatial cognition in autism: Evidence from an fMRI study of an embedded figures task. *Autism Research*, 3(5), 273–279.

Davies, S., Bishop, D., Manstead, A. S., & Tantam, D. (1994). Face perception in children with autism and Asperger's syndrome. *Journal of Child Psychology and Psychiatry, 35*(6), 1033–1057.

Dawson, G. (2008). Early behavioral intervention, brain plasticity, and the prevention of autism spectrum disorder. *Development and Psychopathology, 20*(3), 775–803. Review.

Dawson, G., Munson, J., Webb, S. J., Nalty, T., Abbott, R., & Toth, K. (2007). Rate of head growth decelerates and symptoms worsen in the second year of life in autism. *Biological Psychiatry, 61*(4), 458–464.

Deeley, Q., Daly, E. M., Surguladze, S., Page, L., Toal, F., Robertson, D., et al. (2007). An event-related functional magnetic resonance imaging study of facial emotion processing in Asperger Syndrome. *Biological Psychiatry, 62*, 207–217.

Dolen, G., Osterweil, E., Rao, B. S., Smith, G. B., Auerbach, B. D., Chattarji, S., et al. (2007). Correction of fragile X syndrome in mice. *Neuron, 56*(6), 955–962.

Ehninger, D., & Silva, A. J. (2011). Rapamycin for treating Tuberous sclerosis and Autism spectrum disorders. *Trends in Molecular Medicine, 17*(2), 78–87.

Ess, K. C. (2009). Tuberous sclerosis complex: everything old is new again. *Journal of Neurodevelopmental Disorders, 1*, 141–149.

Gaigg, S. B., & Bowler, D. M. (2007). Differential fear conditioning in Asperger's syndrome: implications for an amygdala theory of autism. *Neuropsychologia, 45*(9), 2125–2134.

Gaigg, S. B., & Bowler, D. M. (2008). Free recall and forgetting of emotionally arousing words in autism spectrum disorder. *Neuropsychologia, 46*(9), 2336–2343.

Gastgeb, H., Rump, K. M., Best, C. A., Minshew, N. J., & Strauss, M. S. (2009). Prototype formation in autism: Can individuals with autism abstract facial prototypes? *Autism Research, 2*, 232–236.

Gastgeb, H., Strauss, M. S., & Minshew, N. J. (2006). Do individuals with autism process categories differently: The effect of typicality and development. *Child Development, 77*, 1717–1729.

Gastgeb, H. Z., Wilkinson, D. A., Minshew, N. J., & Strauss, M. S. (2011 Epub ahead of print). Can individuals with autism abstract prototypes of natural faces? *Journal of Autism and Developmental Disorders.*

Geschwind, D. H., & Levitt, P. (2007). Autism spectrum disorders: developmental disconnection syndromes. *Current Opinion in Neurobiology, 17*(1), 103–111.

Gogolla, N., LeBlanc, J. J., Quast, K. B., Sudho, T. C., Fagiolini, M., & Hensch, T. K. (2009). Common circuit defect of excitatory-inhibitory balance in mouse models of autism. *Journal of Neurodevelopmental Disorders, 1*, 172–181.

Grandin, T. (1995). Thinking in pictures and other reports from my life with autism. New York: Doubleday.

Grelotti, D. J., Klin, A. J., Gauthier, I., Skudlarski, P., Cohen, D. J., Gore, J. C., et al. (2005). fMRI activation of the fusiform gyrus and amygdala to cartoon characters but not to faces in a boy with autism. *Neuropsychologia, 43*, 373–385.

Hadjikhani, N., Joseph, R. M., Snyder, J., Chabris, C. F., Clark, J., Steele, S., et al. (2004). Activation of the fusiform gyrus when individuals with autism spectrum disorder view faces. *NeuroImage, 22*, 1141–1150.

Hadjikhani, N., Joseph, R. M., Snyder, J., & Tager-Flusberg, H. (2007). Abnormal activation of the social brain during face perception in autism. *Human Brain Mapping, 28*, 441–449.

Hall, G. B., Szechtman, H., & Nahmias, C. (2003). Enhanced salience and emotion recognition in Autism: a PET study. *American Journal of Psychiatry, 160*, 1439–1441.

Happé, F. G. E. (1996). Studying weak central coherence at low levels: Children with autism do not succumb to visual illusions, a research note. *Journal of Child Psychology and Psychiatry, 37*, 873–877.

Happé, F., & Ronald, A. (2008). The "fractionable autism triad": A review of evidence from behavioural, genetic, cognitive and neural research. *Neuropsychology Review, 18*, 287–304.

Happé, F., Ronald, A., & Plomin, R. (2006). Time to give up on a single explanation for autism. *Nature Neuroscience, 9*(10), 1218–1220.

Hasson, U., Avidan, G., Gelbard, H., Vallines, I., Harel, M., Minshew, N., et al. (2009). Shared and idiosyncratic cortical activation patterns in autism revealed under continuous real-life viewing conditions. *Autism Research, 2*(4), 220–231.

Hasson, U., Nir, Y., Levy, I., Fuhrmann, G., & Malach, R. (2004). Intersubject synchronization of cortical activity during natural vision. *Science, 303*(5664), 1634–1640.

Hobson, R. P., Ouston, J., & Lee, A. (1988). What's in a face? The case of autism. *British Journal of Psychology, 79*, 441–453.

Hubl, D., Bolte, S., Feineis-Matthews, S., Lanfermann, H., Federspeil, A., Strik, W., et al. (2003). Functional imbalance of visual pathways indicates alternative face processing strategies in autism. *Neurology, 61*, 1232–1237.

Humphreys, K., Hasson, U., Avidan, G., Minshew, N., & Behrmann, M. (2008). Cortical patterns of category-selective activation for faces, places, and objects in adults with autism. *Autism Research, 1*, 52–63.

Humphreys, K., Minshew, N., Lee Leonard, G., & Behrmann, M. (2007). A fine-grained analysis of facial expression processing in autism. *Neuropsychologia, 45*, 685–695.

Iarocci, G., Burack, J. A., Shore, D. I., Mottron, L., & Enns, J. T. (2006). Global-local visual processing in high functioning children with autism: structural vs. implicit task biases. *Journal of Autism and Developmental Disorders, 36*(1), 117–129.

Iverson, J. M., & Goldin-Meadow, S. (2005). Gesture paves the way for language development. *Psychological Science, 16*(5), 367–371.

Iverson, J. M., & Wozniak, R. H. (2007). Variation in vocal-motor development in infant siblings of children with autism. *Journal of Autism and Developmental Disorders, 37*(1), 158–170.

Jolliffe, T., & Baron-Cohen, S. (1997). Are people with autism and Asperger syndrome faster than normal on the Embedded Figures Test? *Journal of Child Psychology and Psychiatry, 38*(5), 527–534.

Joseph, R. M., & Tanaka, J. (2003). Holistic and part-based face recognition in children with autism. *Journal of Child Psychology and Psychiatry, 44*(4), 529–542.

Just, M. A., Cherkassky, V. L., Keller, T. A., Kana, R. K., & Minshew, N. J. (2007). Functional and anatomical cortical underconnectivity in autism: Evidence from an fMRI study of an executive function task and corpus callosum morphometry. *Cerebral Cortex, 17*, 951–961.

Just, M. A., Cherkassky, V. L., Keller, T. A., & Minshew, N. J. (2004). Cortical activation and synchronization during sentence comprehension in high-functioning autism: evidence of underconnectivity. *Brain, 127*, 1811–1821.

Kana, R. K., Keller, T. A., Cherkassky, V. L., Minshew, N. J., & Just, M. A. (2009). Atypical frontal-posterior synchronization of theory of mind regions in autism during mental state attribution. *Social Neuroscience, 4*, 135–152.

Kanwisher, N., McDermott, J., & Chun, M. M. (1997). The fusiform face area: a module in human extrastriate cortex specialized for face perception. *Journal of Neuroscience, 17*, 4302–4311.

Kimchi, R. (1998). Uniform connectedness and grouping in the perceptual organization of hierarchical patterns. *Journal of Experimental Psychology. Human Perception and Performance, 24*(4), 1105–1118.

Kleinhans, N. M., Richards, T., Sterling, L., Stegbauer, K. C., Mahurin, R., et al. (2008). Abnormal functional connectivity in autism spectrum disorders during face processing. *Brain, 131*(Pt 4), 1000–1012.

Klin, A., Jones, W., Schultz, R., Volkmar, F., & Cohen, D. (2002). Visual fixation patterns during viewing of naturalistic social situations as predictors of social competence in individuals with autism. *Archives of General Psychiatry, 59*, 809–816.

Kuban, K. C., O'Shea, T. M., Allred, E. N., Tager-Flusberg, H., Goldstein, D. J., & Leviton, A. (2009). Positive screening on the Modified Checklist for Autism in Toddlers (M-CHAT) in extremely low gestational age newborns. *Journal of Pediatrics, 154*(4), 535–540.

Kuschner, E., Bodner, K., & Minshew, N. J. (2009). Local versus global approaches to reproducing the Rey Osterrieth complex figure by children, adolescents and adults with high functioning autism. *Autism Research, 2*(6), 348–358.

Lahaie, A., Mottron, L., Arguin, M., Berthiaume, C., Jemel, B., & Saumier, D. (2006). Face perception in high-functioning autistic adults: evidence for superior processing of face parts, not for a configural face-processing deficit. *Neuropsychology, 20*(1), 30–41.

Lainhart, J. E., Bigler, E. D., Bocian, M., Coon, H., Dinh, E., Dawson, G., et al. (2006). Head circumference and height in autism: a study by the Collaborative Program of Excellence in Autism. *American Journal of Medical Genetics. Part A, 140*(21), 2257–2274.

Levitt, P., & Campbell, D. B. (2009). The genetic and neurobiologic compass points toward common signaling dysfunctions in autism spectrum disorders. *Journal of Clinical Investigation, 119*(4), 747–754.

Levy, S. E., Mandell, D. S., & Schultz, R. T. (2009). Autism. *Lancet, 374*(9701), 1627–1638.

Minshew, N. J. (2010, in press). Chapter 36: Is the structure of the brain different in autism spectrum conditions? In S. Bölte & J. Hallmayer 1. Autism Spectrum Conditions: International Experts answer your Questions on Autism, Asperger syndrome and PDD-NOS. (pgs 118–124), Hogrefe Publishers, United Kingdom.

Minshew, N. J. (2011). Chapter 38: Neuroimaging of developmental disorders commentary: What Has The Study of Neurodevelopmental Disorders Taught Us? In M Shenton & B Turestsky. Understanding Neuropsychiatric Disorders: Insights from Neuroimaging (pgs 555–558).

Minshew, N. J., Goldstein, G., Muenz, L. R., & Payton, J. B. (1992). Neuropsychological functioning in nonmentally retarded autistic individuals. *Journal of Clinical and Experimental Neuropsychology, 14*(5), 749–761.

Minshew, N. J., Goldstein, G., & Siegel, D. J. (1997). Neuropsychologic functioning in autism: Profile of a complex information processing disorder. *Journal of the International Neuropsychological Society, 3*, 303–316.

Minshew, N. J., Sung, K., Jones, B., & Furman, J. M. (2004). Underdevelopment of the postural control system in autism. *Neurology, 63*(11), 2056–2061.

Minshew, N. J., Webb, J. S., Williams, D. L., & Dawson, G. (2006). Neuropsychology and neurophysiology of autism spectrum disorders. In F. S. Moldin & J. Rubenstein (Eds.), Understanding autism: From basic neuroscience to treatment (Vol. 1, pp. 380–398). New York: CRC.

Minshew, N. J., & Williams, D. L. (2007). The new neurobiology of autism. *Archives of Neurology, 64*(7), 945–950.

Minshew, N. J., Williams, D. L., & McFadden, K. (2008). Information processing, neural connectivity, and neuronal organization. In A. W. Zimmerman (Ed.), *Autism*. Totowa, NJ: Humana.

Mosconi, M., Zwaigenbaum, L., & Piven J. (2006). Structural MRI in autism: Findings and future directions. *Clinical Neuroscience Research, 6*, 135–144.

Mostofsky, S. H., Powell, S. K., Simmonds, D. J., Goldberg, M. C., Caffo, B., & Pekar, J. J. (2009). Decreased connectivity and cerebellar activity in autism during motor task performance. *Brain, 132*(Pt 9), 2413–2425.

Mottron, L., Burack, J. A., Iarocci, G., Belleville, S., & Enns, J. T. (2003). Locally oriented perception with intact global processing among adolescents with high-functioning autism: evidence from multiple paradigms. *Journal of Child Psychology and Psychiatry, 44*(6), 904–913.

Mottron, L., Dawson, M., & Soulières, I. (2009). Enhanced perception in savant syndrome: patterns, structure, and creativity. *Philosophical Transactions of the Royal Society of London. Series B, Biological Sciences, 364*(1522), 1385–1391. Review.

Mottron, L., Dawson, M., Soulières, I., Hubert, B., & Burack, J. (2006). Enhanced perceptual functioning in autism: an update, and eight principles of autistic perception. *Journal of Autism and Developmental Disorders, 36*(1), 27–43. Review.

Navon, D. (1977). Forest before trees: The precedence of global features in visual perception. *Cognitive Psychology, 9*, 353–383.

Navon, D. (1983). How many trees does it take to make a forest? *Perception, 12*(3), 239–254.

New, J. J., Schultz, R. T., Wolf, J., Niehaus, J. L., Klin, A., German, T. C., et al. (2010). The scope of social attention deficits in autism: prioritized orienting to people and animals in static natural scenes. *Neuropsychologia, 48*(1), 51–59.

Newell, L. C., Best, C. A., Gastgeb, H., Rump, K. M., & Strauss, M. S. (in press). The development of categorization and facial knowledge: Implications for the study of autism. In L. M. Oakes, C. H. Cashon, M. Casasola, & R. H. Rakison (Eds.), *Early Perceptual and Cognitive Development*. New York: Oxford University Press.

Nie, D., Di Nardo, A., Han, J. M., Baharanyi, H., Kramvis, I., et al. (2010). Tsc2-Rheb signaling regulates EphA-mediated axon guidance. *Nature Neuroscience*, (Epub ahead of print).

Ogai, M., Matsumoto, H., Suzuki, K., Ozawa, F., Fukada, R., Ichiyama, I., et al. (2003). fMRI study of recognition of facial expressions in high-functioning autistic patients. *Neuroreport, 14*, 559–563.

O'Riordan, M. A., Plaisted, K. C., Driver, J., & Baron-Cohen, S. (2001). Superior visual search in autism. *Journal of Experimental Psychology. Human Perception and Performance, 27*(3), 719–730.

Ozonoff, S., Strayer, D. L., McMahon, W. M., & Filloux, F. (1994). Executive function abilities in autism and Tourette syndrome: an information processing approach. *Journal of Child Psychology and Psychiatry, 35*(6), 1015–1032.

Pellicano, E., Jeffery, L., Burr, D., & Rhodes, G. (2007). Abnormal adaptive face-coding mechanisms in children with autism spectrum disorder. *Current Biology, 17*(17), 1508–1512.

Pierce, K., Haist, F., Sedaghat, F., & Courchesne, E. (2004). The brain response to personally familiar faces in autism: findings of fusiform activity and beyond. *Brain, 127*, 2703–2716.

Pierce, K., Muller, R. A., Ambrose, J., Allen, G., & Courchesne, E. (2001). Face processing occurs outside the fusiform "face area" in autism: evidence from functional MRI. *Brain, 124*, 2059–2073.

Piggot, J., Kwon, H., Mobbs, D., Blasey, C., Lotspeich, L., Menon, V., et al. (2004). Emotional attribution in high-functioning individuals with autistic spectrum disorder: a functional imaging study. *Journal of the American Academy of Child and Adolescent Psychiatry, 43*, 473–480.

Pinto, D., Klei, L., Anney, R., Pagnamenta, A., Regan, R., et al. (submitted). Genome-wide analysis identifies global rare variation in autism.

Plaisted, K., Dobler, V., Bell, S., & Davis, G. (2006). The microgenesis of global perception in autism. *Journal of Autism and Developmental Disorders, 36*(1), 107–116.

Plaisted, K., Swettenham, J., & Rees, L. (1999). Children with autism show local precedence in a divided attention task and global precedence in a selective attention task. *Journal of Child Psychology and Psychiatry, 40*, 733–742.

Raznahan, A., Pugliese, L., Barker, G. J., Daly, E., Powell, J., Bolton, P. F., et al. (2009). Serotonin transporter genotype and neuroanatomy in autism spectrum disorders. *Psychiatric Genetics, 19*(3), 147–150.

Rinehart, N. J., Bradshaw, J. L., Moss, S. A., Brereton, A. V., & Tonge, B. J. (2000). Atypical interference of local detail on global processing in high-functioning autism and Asperger's disorder. *Journal of Child Psychology and Psychiatry, 41*(6), 769–778.

Rogers, S. J. (2009). What are infant siblings teaching us about autism in infancy? *Autism Research, 2*(3), 125–137.

Rump, K. M, Giovannelli, J. L., Minshew, N. J., & Strauss, M. S. (2009). The development of emotion recognition in individuals with autism. *Child Development, 80*(5), 1434–1447.

Sahyoun, C. P., Belliveau, J. W., Soulières, I., Schwartz, S, & Mody, M. (2010). Neuroimaging of the functional and structural networks underlying visuospatial vs. linguistic reasoning in high-functioning autism. *Neuropsychologia, 48*(1), 86–95.

Scherf, K. S., Behrmann, M., Humphreys, K., & Luna, B. (2007). Visual category-selectivity for faces, places, and objects emerges along different developmental trajectories. *Developmental Science, 10*(4), F15–30.

Scherf, K. S., Behrmann, M., Minshew, N., & Luna, B. (2008). Atypical development of face and greeble recognition in autism. *Journal of Child Psychology and Psychiatry, 49*(8), 838–847.

Scherf, K. S., Luna, B., Kimchi, R., Minshew, N., & Behrmann, M. (2008). Missing the big picture: impaired development of global shape processing in autism. *Autism Research, 1*(2), 114–129.

Scherf, K. S., Luna, B., Minshew, N. J., & Behrmann, M. (2010). Location, location, location: Alterations in the functional topography of face- but not object- or place-related cortex in adolescents with autism. *Frontiers in Human Neuroscience, 22*(4), 26.

Schipul, S. E., Keller, T. A., & Just, M. A. (accepted 2011). Interregional brain communication and its disturbance in autism. *Frontiers in Systems Neuroscience.*

Schultz, R. T. (2005). Developmental deficits in social perception in autism: the role of the amygdala and fusiform face area. *International Journal of Developmental Neuroscience, 23*(2–3), 125–141.

Schultz, R. T., Gauthier, I., Klin, A., Fulbright, R. K., Anderson, A. W., Volkmar, F., et al. (2000). Abnormal ventral temporal cortical activity during face discrimination among individuals with autism and Asperger syndrome. *Archives of General Psychiatry, 57*(4), 331–340.

Shah, A., & Frith, U. (1993). Why do autistic individuals show superior performance on the block design task? *Journal of Child Psychology and Psychiatry, 34*, 1351–1364.

Silva, A. J., & Ehninger, D. (2009). Adult reversal of cognitive phenotypes in neurodevelopmental disorders. *Journal of Neurodevelopmental Disorders, 1*(2), 150–157.

Soulières, I., Dawson, M., Samson, F., Barbeau, E. B., Sahyoun, C. P., et al. (2009). Enhanced visual processing contributes to matrix reasoning in autism. *Human Brain Mapping, 30*(12), 4082–4107.

Strauss, K. A., Puffenberger, E. G., Huentelman, M. J., Gottlieb, S., Dobrin, S. E., Parod, J. M., et al. (2006). Recessive symptomatic focal epilepsy and mutant contactin-associated protein-like. *New England Journal of Medicine, 354*, 1370–1377.

van Kooten, I. A., Palmen, S. J., von Cappeln, P., Steinbusch, H. W., Korr, H., Heinsen, H., et al. (2008). Neurons in the fusiform gyrus are fewer and smaller in autism. *Brain, 131*(Pt 4), 987–999.

Volpe J. J. (2008). *Neurology of the newborn* (5th ed). Philadelphia: Elsevier.

Wang, A. T., Dapretto, M., Hariri, A. R., Sigman, M., & Bookheimer, S. Y. (2004). Neural correlates of facial affect processing in children and adolescents with autism spectrum disorder. *Journal of the American Academy of Child and Adolescent Psychiatry, 43*, 481–490.

Wang, L., Mottron, L., Peng, D., Berthiaume, C., & Dawson, M. (2007). Local bias and local-to-global interference without global deficit: A robust finding in autism under various conditions of attention, exposure time, and visual angle. *Cognitive Neuropsychology, 24*, 550–574.

Wassink, T. H., Hazlett, H. C., Epping, E. A., Arndt, S., Dager, S. R., Schellenberg, G. D., et al. (2007). Cerebral cortical gray matter overgrowth and functional variation of the serotonin transporter gene in autism. *Archives of General Psychiatry, 64*(6), 709–717.

Williams, D. L, Goldstein, G., & Minshew, N. J. (2006). The profile of memory function in children with autism. *Neuropsychology, 20*(1), 21–29.

Williams, D. L., Goldstein, G., & Minshew, N. J. (2007). Neuropsychologic functioning in children with autism: Further evidence for disordered complex information-processing. *Child Neuropsychology, 12*, 279–298.

37 Sara Jane Webb, Raphael Bernier, Karen Burner, Michael Murias

Electrophysiological Research on Autism

Points of Interest

- EEG activity is exquisitely sensitive to neural timing, on a resolution that is not matched by other methodologies, providing the ability to scrutinize physiological changes at a unique level of analysis.
- EEG/ERP paradigms can be designed for use both across the age continuum and across variable cognitive functioning.
- ERP components enable one to disentangle and differentiate sensory processing from integration and higher order cognitive abilities, which may be important in understanding autism.
- A failure or delay in activating neural structures that are normally specialized for a given process could result in a failure to integrate social information.

Electroencephalography (EEG) is the measurement of electrical activity produced by the brain. More specifically, scalp recorded EEG is a noninvasive method of measuring postsynaptic activity that is rhythmic and continuous, transient and episodic. While scalp EEG is not a direct measurement of brain activation, the recordings reflect the propagation of electrical activity to the scalp arising from the synchronous activation of a population of neurons that have a similar spatial organization. These generators or sources of scalp recorded activity are located parallel to each other and oriented radially to the scalp.

EEG can be examined in many different ways, providing valuable information about the functioning of the brain including: (1) EEG oscillatory activity, which is the frequency and amplitude of synchronized neural activity and characterizes the "state" of the brain; (2) evoked potentials (EPs) or event-related potentials (ERPs), which reflect measurements that are time-locked to the presentation of an external stimulus; and (3) coherence, in which functional connectivity in brain networks can be inferred from statistical relations between neurophysiological signals measured over spatially separated neuronal regions.

The benefits of this methodology are easy to identify. EEG is noninvasive, only requiring the participant to wear an electrode hat for the length of the experiment. In contrast to other neuroimaging methodologies, EEG generally does not necessitate adherence to strict behavioral requirements. Participant movement and compliance can be evaluated in real time and can be tolerated to a greater extent than in other imaging methods. EEG also has exquisite temporal resolution, with recordings reflecting electrical activity changes on the scale of milliseconds. Limitations have also been recognized including: poorer spatial resolution than other imaging modalities, increased sensitivity to generators that are closer to the surface, and insensitivity to sources that are located tangential to the skull, located in sulci, or located in deep structures (e.g., hippocampus).

Why Utilize Electrophysiology Measures for the Study of Autism?

EEG has been used to study both typical and atypical brain processes since its first recording in humans by Hans Berger in the 1920s; the first (published) reports focusing on autism emerged in the 1960s. The usefulness of EEG measurements in autism arises from both theoretical and methodological considerations. Theoretically, EEG allows the evaluation of hypotheses with respect to the timing of brain functioning, alterations in resting and active brain states, and the potential under- and overfunctional connectivity of the brain in individuals with autism. Methodologically, EEG paradigms can be created that reduce demands for behavioral compliance or manual/vocal responses. The implementation of passive paradigms, such as passive viewing of faces or listening to phonemes, allows the same paradigm to be used both across the age continuum and across variable cognitive functioning. This approach provides useful information about the whole of the autism spectrum. As well, some EEG technologies allow for the application of the scalp electrodes quickly and for recordings to be conducted over short time periods, accommodating limited attention or behavioral compliance.

Electrophysiology is a broad topic; we have chosen to focus on EEG and ERPs in response to visual stimuli during perceptual and attention processes, social processes, and background neural processes.

Event Related Potentials to Perceptual and Attention Processes

Theory and Methods

ERPs in response to visual stimulation can be recorded within a short time of stimulus onset. Basic level processing to black and white checkerboards can be characterized within milliseconds of stimulus onset over occipital electrodes and likely reflects the activity of the extrastriate visual cortex. More complex stimuli, which evoke more complicated "higher-level" perceptual and cognitive processes, likely reflect the activity and contributions of many different neural systems that overlap in time and spatial distribution. The resulting waveform is composed of multiple potentials, each with a characteristic latency range and spatial distribution.

A careful analysis of ERPs enables one to disentangle and differentiate sensory processing from integration and higher-order cognitive abilities, which may be important in understanding autism. If a sensory system is limited in its ability to perceive the environment, this would be represented in abnormal sensory ERPs such as brain stem evoked potentials or early visual evoked potentials. If autism, however, is better represented by a failure of integration or a limitation in overall capacity for information processing, this would be represented in abnormal endogenous, later cognitive components of the signal, or decreased coherence.

Visual Processing

While not specifically captured in the diagnostic criteria for autism, the existence of altered perceptual processing has been proposed as an important phenotype of the disorder. The early visual component C1 peaks approximately 60–100 ms after stimulus onset and is thought to be generated by the primary visual cortex (V1, area 17) (e.g., Clark et al., 1995; di Russo et al., 2001). During perception of Gabor patches, sinusoidal luminance patterns, children with pervasive developmental disorder (PDD) demonstrated shorter latency to the peak of C1 compared to matched typical controls. Higher Childhood Autism Rating Scale scores were correlated with faster latency (Milne, Scope, Pascalis, Buckley, & Makeig, 2009). Given the simplicity of the stimuli, the authors concluded that the faster neural response was consistent with the behavioral findings of faster visual detection in individuals with PDD and suggested that this behavior may be due to varying mechanisms of perception rather than attention.

In another simple visual paradigm using gratings, Boeschoten, Kenemnas, van Engeland, and Kemner (2007) found increased N80 responses to high spatial frequencies in children with PDD compared to controls but a failure to show differential sources of activity for high and low spatial frequencies (also see Milne et al., 2006). The P1, thought to be generated by the extrastriate cortex V2 (e.g., Mangun, Buonocore, Girelli, & Jha, 1998; Di Russo, Martinez, Sereno, Pitzalis, & Hillyard, 2002), was smaller in children with PDD than in controls, and the inferior medial sources were weaker with increased supplementary source activity in the superior lateral area. The authors concluded that this represented a failure of anatomical separation for the N80, decreased specialized processing of frequencies, and decreased extrastriate activity.

Visual boundary detection mechanisms, but not surface segregation, have been found to be abnormal in adults with ASD compared to typical controls. ERP results in adults with ASD suggested reduced perception of boundary detection starting 121 ms after stimulus presentation consistent with impaired (behavioral) identification of boundaries (Vandenbroucke, Scholte, van Engeland, Lamme, & Kemner, 2008). This was hypothesized to reflect a deficit in horizontal connections within visual areas; intact surface segregation was interpreted as associated with normal recurrent or feedback processes from higher-level areas.

While the number of early visual processing reports is relatively small, there are some general conclusions that can be made. First, activity within the primary visual cortex seems to be intact or potentially enhanced. Second, ERPs located originating from the extrastriate cortex demonstrate a pattern suggestive of perceptual impairment. Area V2 receives direct projections from V1 and shares many similar properties but is also modulated by more complex properties including figure/ground separation. Bertone et al. (2005) have suggested that individuals with autism have reduced efficiency of neurointegrative mechanisms within the perceptual systems, which would invariably impact the relatively more integrative processes of the extrastriate cortex. Both Milne et al. (2009) and Vandenbroucke et al. (2008) are consistent with this interpretation.

Attention

Central Attention: Target Processing

ERPs can be collected during selective attention paradigms in which a rare, novel, infrequent, or unattended stimulus is compared to a standard, frequent, or attended stimulus. This type of experiment results in a N1, P2, N2, and P3 complex (or LPC). The P3 is thought to reflect neural generators in the temporal, parietal, and frontal areas, and amplitude of the P3 is thought to be related to the amount of attention and processing capacity. Smaller P3 amplitudes are thought to reflect decreased processing capacity or allocation of resources, abnormal executive functions (e.g., Halgren, Marinkovic, & Chauvel, 1998), working memory (e.g., Donchin & Coles, 1988), or completion of perceptional processes and associated release of neural inhibition that follows task resolution (e.g., Kutas, McCarthy, & Donchin, 1977; Verleger, 1988). Of note, individuals with a wide range of conditions demonstrate abnormal P3 responses, including but not limited to schizophrenia, depression, ADD, dyslexia, alcoholism, multiple sclerosis, and normal aging (Picton, 1992; Polich & Criado, 2006).

During auditory/visual divided attention tasks, for example, when the participant is required to attend to a stimulus in a primary modality (e.g., tone) and ignore the presence of irrelevant (unattended) probe a in a second modality (e.g., square), reduced P3 amplitude to the attended stimuli is thought to reflect attention trade-offs. Several studies suggest that individuals with autism fail to reduce activation to the attended stimulus (Ciesielski et al., 1990; Hoeksma, Kemner, Verbaten, & van Engeland, 2004). For example, Hoeksma et al. (2004) found that when the task load was increased, children and adolescents with PDD showed increased early responses to unattended (visual) probes and failed to show normal reduction of processing to attended (auditory) probes. The authors suggested this represented abnormal allocation of attention but not necessarily a decreased processing capacity. This pattern of results was clearly found in the children but was less characteristic of the adolescents. It is unclear if this represents delayed development of the attention system or potentially subtle differences in subgroups of individuals with ASD.

Central Attention: Novelty Detection

Some findings suggest that late visual evoked parietal P3b to novel stimuli is abnormal in individuals with ASD (Novick et al., 1979; Verbaten, Roelofs, van Engeland, Kenemans, & Slangen, 1991), but that these responses to visual stimuli may be less impaired than responses to auditory stimuli (Courchesne et al., 1989; Courchesne, Lincoln, et al., 1985). Lincoln, Courchesne, Harms, and Allen (1993) propose that the decreased P3b amplitudes noted in ASD may reflect difficulty in changing expectancies in response to contextually relevant information. Furthermore, the authors suggest that a basic disturbance in the habituation process results in difficulties in discriminating novel information. An alternative hypothesis is that a failure to extract relevant information in order to create a "standard" category results in impairments in differentiating novel stimuli *to the same degree* as controls (Gastgeb, Strauss, & Minshew, 2006).

Shifting Attention from Central to Peripheral Stimuli

Behaviorally, individuals with autism demonstrate a number of impairments in orienting. Children with ASD, when attending to targets in the periphery, demonstrate reduced LPC amplitude and smaller P3b amplitudes accompanied by high variability in performance (Verbaten, Roelofs, van Engeland, Kenemans, & Slangen, 1991). Similarly, Townsend et al. (2001) found reduced accuracy to targets in the visual periphery, delayed or missing early LPC during attention to peripheral visual fields, and smaller amplitudes over the parietal cortex during conditions when context updating was of paramount importance. The authors interpreted this as a disruption of spatial attention networks and consistent with abnormalities in the cerebellar-frontal/parietal spatial attention systems. When the central stimulus overlapped with the peripheral target, Kawakubo et al. (2007) found increased amplitude activity during the presaccade period in adults with ASD as compared to neurotypical adults, which was interpreted as a difficulty in disengagement during visuospatial attention.

Summary

The studies reviewed here suggest that individuals with ASD may have subtle impairments in the integrative stages of visual processing and attention allocation. Abnormalities in these early stages of information processing have the potential to disrupt integrative cognitive processes that require complex information. For example, if visual stimuli are being encoded without correct figure-ground information or the correct balance of high/low spatial frequency information, then systems that must utilize this to identify and respond accordingly would organize around incorrect or degraded information. This might result in reduced attention to and differentiation of social stimuli.

Electrophysiology and Social Processes

Theory and Methods

Much of what we think of as social represents a dynamic interaction between two or more people. One of the constraints of ERP methodology is that social processes must be decomposed into time locked segments. These simple component parts can be presented as static images and contrasted to nonsocial categories or perceptual matches. However, EEG recordings in general do not have this temporal constraint, and more recent work has focused on changes in the state of brain activity during dynamic protocols.

Face Processing

A sizable amount of literature exists regarding the exploration of the neural circuitry of face processing via ERPs and other neuroimaging methods of individuals with typical development. One ERP component, called the N170, has been identified as a face sensitive component because it is greater in amplitude and shorter in latency to face stimuli relative to other types of stimuli (e.g., Bentin et al., 1996). Recorded over the posterior temporal region and peaking between 130 and 170 ms in response to faces, the N170 is larger in amplitude to eyes than inverted faces and upright faces. Likewise, these stimuli result in a larger N170 amplitude than the presentation of noses or mouths (e.g., Bentin et al., 1996).

In individuals with ASD, reports suggest abnormalities in the precursor N170 in 3- to 4-year-old children with ASD, and the N170 in adolescents and adults with ASD, as well as in parents of children with ASD (Dawson et al., 2005; McPartland, Dawson, Webb, Panagiotides, & Carver, 2004; Webb, Dawson, Bernier, & Panagiotides, 2006). Three- to 4-year-old children with autism showed a faster response to objects than faces (Webb et al., 2006). In contrast, children with typical development demonstrated a faster precursor N170 to faces than objects in the right hemisphere, while children with developmental delay (chronologic and mental age controls) failed to demonstrate any differential responses.

Adults with autism spectrum disorder (ASD) also show disruptions in face processing measured via ERPs. McPartland et al. (2004) found that 9 adolescents and adults with ASD had slower N170 responses to faces than objects (also O'Connor et al., 2007). O'Connor et al. (2005) found that the group with Asperger's (ASP) had slower P1 and N170 responses to facial expressions of emotions compared to controls Additionally, the ASP group had reduced amplitude at the N170 compared to the typical group. O'Connor et al. (2005, 2007) interpreted these results as reflecting impaired holistic and configural processing of faces, potentially due to decreased attention to internal features or a failure of expertise processing. In contrast, in a recent report that explicitly directed the subject's attention toward the eye region of the face, Webb et al. (2009) found that 32 high-functioning adults with ASD demonstrated P1 and N170 responses to faces that were greater in amplitude and faster in latency than to houses. This pattern is similar to that found in neurotypical adults. Adults with ASD, however, failed to show any inversion differences. Namely, they failed to differentiate upright and inverted faces at the ERP component level. This failure to differentiate upright and inverted faces in the temporal domain was related to self-reported social skills. Specifically, a faster response to upright vs. inverted faces, was correlated to less social anxiety and distress, greater social competence, and fewer autism social symptoms. Similar to Jemel et al. (2006), we concluded that if face processing was a pervasive and encompassing deficit in ASD, we would expect the results to be similar across reports.

It has been hypothesized that altered face processing ability might be an endophenotypic trait associated with autism. Parents of children with ASD failed to show a differential latency of the N170 to faces versus nonface stimuli and failed to show a right-lateralized N170 distribution (Dawson et al., 2005). During a task involving the processing of a facial emotion, again, parents of children with ASD failed to demonstrate differential latency of the N170 to neutral and happy faces versus fear faces and N170 (amplitude) hemispheric differences. Within the parent group, atypical hemispheric activation was associated with poorer performance on the Reading the Mind in the Eyes task (Dawson et al., 2008). These ERP findings parallel ERP responses to emotional faces in young children with autism (Dawson et al., 2004).

Face Memory

Several studies with infants and children have evaluated face and object memory processes using ERPs (e.g., Carver et al., 2003; de Haan & Nelson, 1997, 1999; Webb, Long & Nelson, 2005). In these studies a highly familiar stimulus, such as a picture of the child's mother or favorite object, is compared to a picture of an unfamiliar face or an unfamiliar object, respectively. In this paradigm, both image categories, familiar and unfamiliar, are presented in the same manner within the experimental setting, but differ in the child's a priori experience with them. By 45 to 54 months, typical children show a faster latency and increased amplitude response to unfamiliar faces than to familiar faces. In contrast, responses to familiar and unfamiliar objects are similar (Carver et al., 2003).

In 3- to 4-year-old children with ASD, the Nc does not differ in response to the mother's face versus an unfamiliar face, but does differ between a favorite toy as compared to an unfamiliar toy (Dawson et al., 2002). Chronologically age-matched typical children, demonstrated a greater Nc amplitude response to both the unfamiliar face compared to the familiar face and the unfamiliar object compared to the familiar object. By 6 years of age, both children with ASD and chronologically and mentally age matched children show differential temporal processing of familiar and unfamiliar faces at the Nc as well as the pr-N170. As seen in Figure 37-1, children with ASD continue to show delays in latency when processing face stimuli compared to control children—both children with developmental delay and neurotypical development (Webb, Dawson, Bernier, & Panagiotides, 2008).

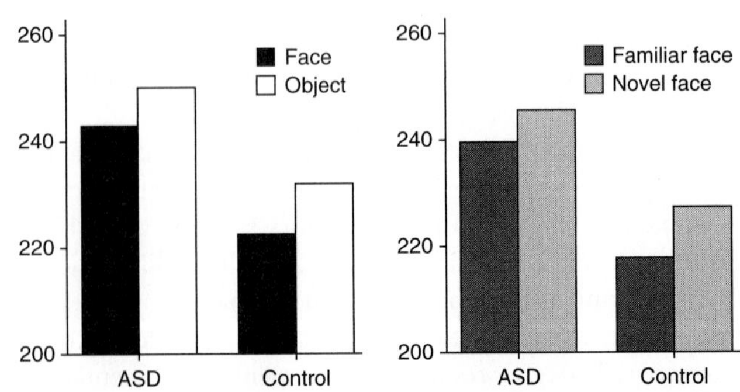

Figure 37–1. Latency (in milliseconds) of pr-N170 response to faces and objects (left) and familiar and novel face (right) in 6-year-old children with ASD or controls. Both groups demonstrate a faster response to faces than objects, and a faster response to familiar than novel face. However, the ASD group's responses remain significantly slower to all categories compared to those by the control group.

Emotion

Many researchers have suggested that the ability to use or understand information from faces is a core deficit in autism (e.g., Baron-Cohen, 1994; Dawson et al., 2002; Frith, 1989). Given that emotion is often displayed in the face, differentiating a deficit in face processing from impairments in understanding and recognizing facial expressions is difficult. However, studies have shown intact recognition of facial expressions despite significant deficits in facial recognition in patients with prosopagnosia (Shuttleworth et al., 1982). On the other hand, patients who underwent an amygdalectomy demonstrate the reverse pattern, i.e., exhibiting a deficit in expression recognition but retaining facial recognition processes (Adolphs et al., 1994). These findings suggest that the two abilities can be separated at the neural and theoretical level (Bruce & Young, 1986).

Differential ERPs to distinct facial expressions of emotion have also been shown in infants (Nelson & de Haan, 1996) and young children (Batty & Taylor, 2003), suggesting that some discrimination of facial expressions may occur at early processing stages. In preschoolers aged 3 to 4 years, with ASD or typical development, only the typical group displayed a faster and larger early (300 ms) ERP response and a larger slow wave amplitude ERP response to the fear face than the neutral face. In contrast, children with ASD did not differentiate the fear face at either stage of processing. These findings suggest that ASD is associated with abnormal processing of facial expressions of emotion and that these abnormalities originate during early stages of processing. Given that the processing of facial expression requires facial processing, it is likely that any abnormalities in the initial stages of face processing would disrupt further processing of the emotion displayed on the face.

Conflicting evidence exists for impairment in processing emotional expressions in children with ASD. In older children, differential processing of emotions via ERPs has not shown pervasive impairments in ASD. Wong et al. (2008) found normal patterns of ERP and behavioral responses to emotional expressions. However, using source localization, the children with autism displayed slower and weaker responses to emotional expressions in regions responsible for face perception and emotion processing (Wong, Fung, Chua, & McAlonan, 2008). Supporting this finding, another ERP study failed to find a difference in emotional face processing between high-functioning, 9-year-old children with ASD compared with mental-aged-matched typically developing children (Burner, Webb, & Dawson, 2008). In summary, these results suggest that further examination of factors such as age and verbal abilities in individuals with ASD is warranted in the area of facial emotion processing.

Eye Gaze

Eye contact and eye gaze serve as important functions in social interaction and communication. Individuals with autism often display atypical eye contact (Baranek, 1999; Charman et al., 1997; Osterling, Dawson, & Munson, 2002), atypical gaze fixation patterns (Klin, Jones, Schultz, Volkmar, & Cohen, 2002), and eye gaze processing impairments (Mundy et al., 1986; Dawson et al., 1998) that may contribute to their social cognitive deficits. These behavioral observations of eye gaze behavior have led to the examination of the neural basis of eye gaze processing in individuals with autism, which has produced inconsistent results. A few studies have found a larger response (measured by the N2, a face specific occipitotemporal component) to direct gaze than to averted gaze in children with ASD (Grice et al., 2005; Kylliainen, Braeutigam, Hietanen, Swithenby, & Bailey, 2006) while others have failed to find a difference in the N2 between direct and averted gaze in individuals with ASD (Senju, Hasegawa, & Tojo, 2005). In addition, response to eye gaze in the N2 was bilaterally distributed in children with ASD, whereas the response was lateralized on the right side in typically developing children (Senju et al., 2005).

Developmental and contextual factors may account for these different results since the Senju et al. (2005) study included older children and required attention to be paid to the direction of the gaze. Another possible interpretation of these contrasting findings comes from a recent behavioral examination of eye gaze detection. The study found that similarly to typically developing children, children with autism detect direct gaze faster and more efficiently than averted gaze. However, children with ASD tended to use featural information to detect direct gaze whereas typically developing children relied on configural information (Senju, Kikuchi, Hasegawa, Tojo, & Osanai, 2008). The authors interpreted these findings in the context of previous neuropsychological research showing that direct gaze elicits a larger ERP response than averted gaze in children with autism, but not typically developing children (Grice et al., 2005; Kyllianinen et al., 2006). This is possibly because the children with autism are using a featural strategy that may rely on low-level psychophysiological features in eye gaze detection.

Imitation

In the 30-year history of imitation research in autism, imitative deficits in individuals with ASD have consistently been observed, and several researchers have suggested that imitation deficits are one of the core impairments of autism (e.g., Rogers & Pennington, 1991; Williams, Whiten, Suddendorf & Perrett, 2001). Despite the variability in imitation testing methodologies, sample characteristics, and control groups employed, 19 of 21 well-designed studies have found imitative deficits in autism. This imitation impairment is most marked by deficits in imitation of nonmeaningful gestures and reversal errors (Williams et al., 2004).

The EEG mu rhythm, first observed by Gastaut and Bert in 1954, is believed to reflect activity of an execution/observation matching system—the mirror neuron system (Pineda, 2005; Muthukumaraswamy & Johnson, 2004). The EEG mu rhythm band falls between 8 and 13 Hz (generally the alpha frequency band) but is recorded from central electrodes. Underlying neurons fire synchronously when an individual is at rest, but during the execution and observation of an action, the underlying neurons activate, and this results in the attenuation of the mu rhythm amplitude. This attenuation pattern of the mu wave has been consistently observed in adults and children (e.g., recent papers include Babiloni et al., 2003; Cochin et al., 2001; Lepage & Theoret, 2006; Martineau & Cochin, 2003; Muthukumaraswamy, Johnson, & McNair, 2004).

Recent work analyzing the EEG mu rhythm in individuals with ASD suggests differential activation of mu related to action execution and observation (Bernier et al., 2007; Oberman et al., 2005; Oberman, Ramachandran, & Pineda, 2008). Oberman and colleagues reported on 10 males with ASD ranging from 6 to 47 years of age and 10 age- and gender-matched controls. Participants executed a simple hand movement or watched videos of a moving hand, two bouncing balls, or television static (Oberman et al., 2005). In the typical group, as expected, the authors found characteristic mu attenuation during the execution and observation of the hand movements but not during the two control conditions. However, the ASD group failed to show attenuation of the mu rhythm during the observation condition. In a second study of adults with ASD utilizing the EEG mu rhythm, Bernier and colleagues replicated Oberman's findings, using a paradigm in which participants executed a grasp of a wooden block and observed the experimenter grasping the block (Bernier et al., 2007). In this study of adults with ASD compared to age and cognitive ability matched adults with typical development, the typical adults showed attenuation of the mu rhythm during both the conditions of execution and observation. The adults with ASD showed mu attenuation only during the execution of the simple hand action. Additionally, the adults with ASD showed significant impairments in imitative ability behaviorally. However, imitation ability was also significantly correlated with degree of mu wave attenuation. As imitative ability increased so did the degree of mu rhythm attenuation when observing movement. This correlation was strongest for mu attenuation and the ability to imitate facial expressions (Figure 37-2).

Summary

Impairments in multiple aspects of face processing and imitation have been documented in individuals with ASD using both behavioral and EEG methods. Recent results examining the N170 suggest that early stages of face processing may be relatively more impaired in young children with autism, with variable impairments in adults. This pattern would suggest that performance of the face processing system may be influenced by associated processing related to the type of task (e.g., attention) and ultimately more amenable to developmental mechanisms or intervention. Similarly, our recent finding that mu attenuation during observation of action is correlated with behavioral performance suggests that there may be important neural variability within the autism phenotype. Given the heterogeneity within the social symptom domain in individuals with ASD, addressing this source of variability will be important.

Background Neural Processes

Theory and Methods

Most EEG research in ASD focuses on scalp recordings in awake human subjects. Cortical neural populations that exhibit a high degree of oscillatory synchrony over relatively large areas (on the order of at least 100–1000 mm^2) can generate electrical potentials that are measurable with electrodes placed on the scalp (Lopes da Silva & Pfurtsceller, 1999; Nunez & Srinivasan, 2006). This neuronal activity is spatially low-pass filtered by the poorly conducting skull, limiting the spatial resolution of scalp recorded EEG. Estimates of spatial resolution are dependant on the density of the electrode array employed, ranging from 20 cc^3 or more in low density (19 electrode arrays) to 6–8 cm cc^3 in higher density (128 channel) arrays (Ferree et al., 2001).

Epilepsy

A striking feature of ASD is the increased but variable risk of epilepsies among affected individuals. Seizure occurrence is common, with prevalence estimates ranging from 5% to 39% (Tuchman et al., 2002). These EEG instabilities are proposed to result from atypical cellular, molecular, and local excitatory-inhibitory neuronal circuits (Rubenstein & Merzenich, 2003) that result in imbalanced cortical function due either to increased excitatory glutamatergic signaling, or reduced inhibitory GABAergic activity. Proposed disruptions in

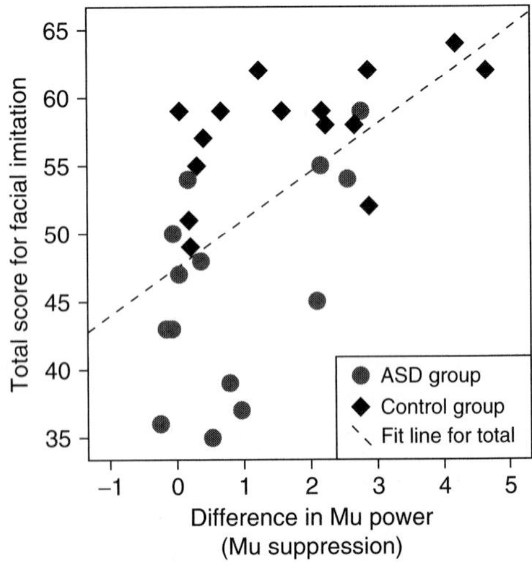

Figure 37–2. Mu suppression (difference in mu power between observe and baseline) and face summary score for the behavioral imitation measure. Greater mu suppression is correlated with higher (better) face imitation scores.

interneuron development (Levitt, 2005) that contribute to seizure activity may reduce neural synchrony, as coupling among interneurons underlies the generation of oscillatory and synchronous activity in the cerebral cortex (Buzsáki & Chrobak, 1995). At a larger scale, cortical minicolumns appear narrower and more numerous in ASD, with constituent neurons more dispersed, and a suspected coincident deficit of GABAergic inhibition (Casanova et al., 2002), which may serve to diminish local connectivity. Brain stem abnormalities may also play a role in atypical electrical activity. Welsh et al. (2005) suggested ASD may be associated with disruptions in synchronization among neural networks in the inferior olive, in which rhythmical oscillation in membrane potentials, mediated by altered connexin36 receptors, could contribute to reduced neural synchrony in ASD.

Spontaneous EEG Rhythms in ASD

Spontaneous EEG generally refers to recordings made without time locking to an external stimulus, often in an awake but resting subject (similar to "default mode") (e.g., Raichle, 2001). Spontaneous activity is typically interpreted across predefined frequency bands that represent the speed of neural oscillations: delta (< 4 Hz), theta (4–8 Hz), alpha (8–12 Hz), beta 1 (12–20 Hz), beta 2 (20–30 Hz), and gamma (30–80 Hz). These wide frequency bands are functionally defined in adults. Understanding the development of these rhythms poses a significant challenge for pediatric research, as functional reactivity in any particular frequency range can differ according to age. Spontaneous EEG is generally reported in terms of absolute or relative power. Relative power measures, which express amplitudes in a particular frequency band as a percentage of the wider power spectrum, serve to normalize the EEG and facilitate comparisons between subjects without bias from individual amplitude differences. However, relative power creates interdependencies across frequency bands. Optimally, both relative and absolute measurements should be analyzed.

Delta, Theta, and Alpha Range EEG in ASD

Accumulating evidence suggests elevated power in the theta range is frequently associated with ASD. Murias et al. (2007) found significantly increased relativez power in ASD adults compared to controls at theta range (3–6 Hz) frequencies. This appears consistent with Daoust et al.'s (2004) observations of elevated absolute frontal theta power among ASD subjects during sleep and waking states. Similarly, Coben et al. (2008) found relative, but not absolute, theta was greater and reduced relative delta amplitudes in the ASD group. Murias et al. (2007) found decreased relative power in the alpha (9–10 Hz) range, consistent with pediatric findings of Cantor et al. (1986) and Dawson et al. (1995), both of which noted decreased absolute alpha power in frontal regions among children with ASD.

Higher Frequency Rhythms

The higher frequency EEG bands beta 1, beta 2 and gamma span 12–80 Hz and are thought to be generated in neuronal networks that include excitatory pyramidal cells and inhibitory gamma-aminobutyric acid (GABA)-ergic interneurons (Whittington et al., 2000). Murias et al. (2007) discerned that a lower beta range (13–17 Hz) relative power increase existed at posterior scalp locations in adults with ASD. Orekhova et al. (2007) demonstrated a pathological increase of gamma (24.4–44.0 Hz) in two separate populations of boys with ASD. Consistent with the theory of imbalanced excitatory/inhibitory mechanisms in ASD (Rubenstein & Merzenich, 2003), the abnormally high levels of spontaneous gamma activity in autism suggests high levels of excitability, reflecting noisy cortical networks.

Lateralization

In participants with ASD, Dawson et al. (1982) found atypical patterns of cerebral lateralization, involving right-hemisphere dominance for both verbal and spatial functions, suggesting selective impairment of the left cerebral hemisphere. Stroganova et al. (2007) found abnormal lateralization in children with ASD, especially in the right temporal cortex. Resting anterior EEG asymmetry in high-functioning children with ASD who displayed right frontal asymmetry displayed more symptoms of social impairments and better visual analytic skills than did children who displayed left frontal asymmetry (Sutton et al., 2005).

Connectivity

Theoretical conceptions of ASD have postulated abnormalities in connections among distributed neural systems (Belmonte et al., 2004; Rippon et al., 2007; Courchesne & Pierce, 2005; Just et al., 2004). Anatomical support for disordered cortical connectivity includes the observation of increased white matter in ASD, with frontal lobe white matter showing the greatest increase (Herbert et al., 2004). Decreased volumes of the corpus callosum have been observed in adults (Hardan et al., 2000) and children (Boger-Megiddo et al., 2006; Manes et al., 1999; Vidal et al., 2006) with ASD. This suggests that the symptoms of ASD may be related to impaired interactions within brain networks, rather than impaired function of specialized cortical regions. Other factors beside white matter contribute to connectivity, for example, reduced cortical inhibition in ASD would tend to decrease the degree of synchrony of widely distributed regions (Courchesne & Pierce, 2005).

The levels of synchronization between neural populations can be estimated from EEG recordings via coherence measurements. The coherence statistic is a squared correlation coefficient that provides a measure of the linearity of the relation between two EEG electrodes at one particular frequency. High coherence between two EEG signals indicates the contribution of synchronized neuronal oscillations to each electrode, suggesting functional integration between neural populations, while low coherence suggests functional segregation. EEG coherence is primarily a measure of phase correlation and with a sufficient density of recording electrodes is believed to reflect functional cortical connectivity on a centimeter scale (Nunez & Srinivasan, 2006; Srinivasan et al., 1998) either directly via corticocortical fiber systems or indirectly through networks that include other cortical or subcortical structures. The dynamics of EEG coherence may be more sensitive to changes in the developing brains than power measures. Srinivasan et al. (1999) differentiated genuine spatial correlations from volume conduction and reference electrode effects, and found cortical areas contributing to the alpha rhythm to be far more weakly correlated with each other in preadolescent children than in adults.

In adults with ASD with the eyes closed in a resting state, Murias et al. (2007) reported globally reduced EEG coherence in the 8–10 Hz frequency range (Figure 37-3). Coherence was markedly diminished within frontal electrode sites, and between frontal and temporal, parietal, and occipital sites. In contrast to the globally reduced alpha rhythm, this study found local ASD increases in theta range (3–6 Hz) coherence in temporal regions that were independent of frontal lobe power findings. The nature of these findings suggests that the frontal lobe has weak functional connections with the rest of the cortex in the alpha frequency range and appears consistent with metabolic studies showing reduced correlated blood flow between frontal and other regions (Horwitz et al., 1988; Villalobos et al., 2005). Coben et al. (2008) reported decreased coherences in children with ASD in delta, theta, and alpha ranges.

Challenges

Methodology

Similar to other scientific domains, differences in analytical methods employed by different investigators make comparisons across EEG and ERP studies difficult. For EEG, of particular importance is the definition of frequency bands. Reports of EEG spectra averaged over broad frequency bands provide only coarse frequency resolution and allow for the possibility that frequency-specific effects within bands cancel out or go otherwise undetected.

Any choice of reference electrode placement distributes the signal at the reference site throughout the array of electrodes. For example, the use of either one ear potential or the average of two ear potentials as a reference confounds coherence estimates by redistributing the potentials at the reference site (Srinivasan et al., 1998; Nunez & Srinivasan, 2006). Historically, many ERP studies have shifted from low-density arrays using ear, nose, or vertex references to high-density average reference arrays. Specifically, recordings made from sparse electrode arrays with a linked-ears reference strategy limit interpretation of prior literature in developmental psychopathology. Depending on the nature of the (unknown) signals at "recording" and "reference" sites, changes in power or phase at the reference location can easily be reflected as changes in coherence or amplitude between two other recording electrodes. With a sufficiently large number of recording electrodes the average reference approximates reference independence.

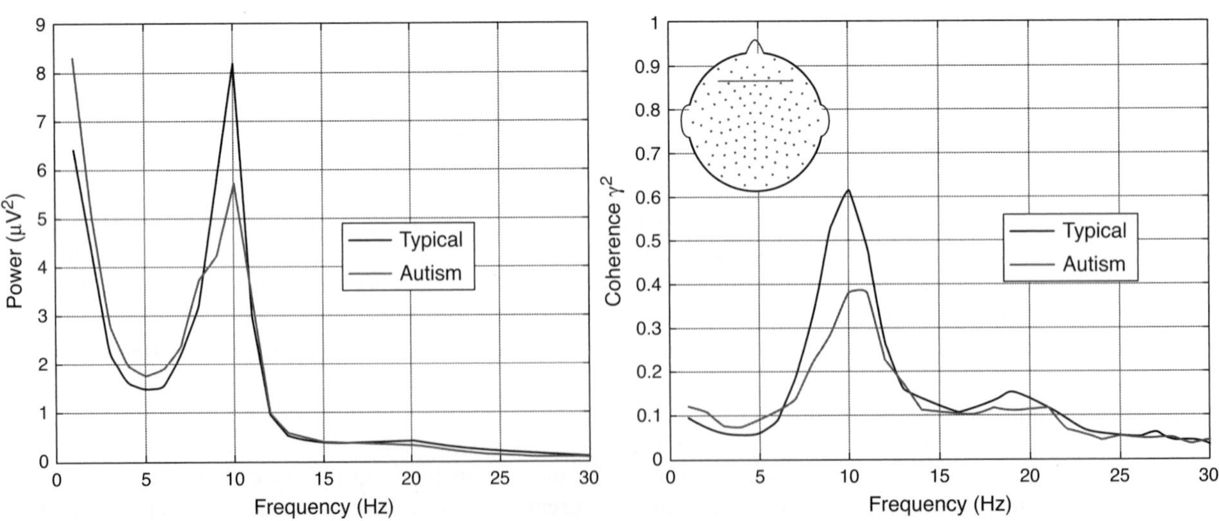

Figure 37-3. Eyes closed, resting EEG averages from 18 high functioning adults with autism, and 18 age- and IQ-matched controls. The power spectrum of frontal electrode Fz, shown at left, shows that groups do not differ in peak frequency of the alpha rhythm (10 Hz), but peak alpha amplitude is significant reduced in the ASD group. The coherence spectra between two frontal electrodes is shown at right, showing reduced coherence in the ASD group.

Volume conduction (the passive flow of current across the scalp, skull, and cerebrospinal fluid) also strongly influences scalp potential EEG coherence (Srinivasan et al., 1998; Nunez & Srinivasan, 2006), and has been shown in electrical models of the head to introduce artificial coherence between electrodes separated by less than 10–12 centimeters. Thus, EEG potential coherence measurements are only meaningful with regard to widely spaced electrode pairs. Coherence between closely spaced EEG electrodes is elevated even when the underlying brain sources are entirely uncorrelated, such that increases in the strength of one cortical source region will increase coherence between two electrodes located within 10 cm of the source region, confounding source strength with coherence. Spatial enhancement methodologies such as the Laplacian derivation (Nunez & Srinivasan, 2006) and finite element deblurring (Gevins & Illes, 1991) avoid spatial filtering by volume conduction, but may be insensitive to low spatial frequency source dynamics, especially those generated in broadly distributed cortical or subcortical regions.

Functioning of Subjects

Individuals with ASD have substantial adaptive functioning difficulties, including variable cognitive performance and sensory abnormalities. Behaviors related to verbal understanding, tactile hypersensitivity, hyperactivity, and inattention will impact compliance, which in turn can impede recording of quality data and lead to subject selection bias that can reduce the representativeness of the findings. Appropriate methodological and behavioral strategies in the EEG lab can mitigate these issues (Foote, 2004). Training in methods for desensitizing individuals with ASD to the EEG lab and methods for monitoring attention and compliance is essential. However, practical problems such as motion artifact and short recording times contribute substantially to difficulties in interpreting across studies.

Benefits and Risks of EEG/ERP

To a large degree, the risks and benefits of utilizing EEG/ERP methodologies to elucidate autism profiles are similar to other methodological domains. As stated previously, EEG (and MEG) activity is exquisitely sensitive to neural timing, on a resolution that is not matched by other methodologies, providing the ability to scrutinize physiological changes at a unique level of analysis. Benefits also include the ability to develop and utilize passive paradigms that are not reliant on the insight of participants, not under explicit control (i.e., most participants can not purposely alter brain activity), and may be less subjective to experimenter bias during data collection. Given the variability in the autism phenotype and the necessary focus on *development*, data can be collected under (relatively) similar paradigms across functioning levels and across the lifespan. Similarly, EEG can be utilized in other species, increasing our ability to model and evaluate similar neural processes under more tightly constrained circumstances.

With any methodology, risks are also present in the development, analysis, and interpretation of research findings. Primarily, behavioral compliance and resulting noise/error within EEG recordings is a significant issue. Second, known (and unknown) differences in anatomical architecture will impact and contribute to signal propagation and the scalp recording of EEG activity. These differences may reflect within and between group variability, as well as natural variability in the developmental trajectory of neural architecture. The spatial resolution of EEG may be improved with source localization methods, specifically when used in combination with MRI images. Third, similar to behavioral paradigms, researchers often assume that two individuals or two groups are "participating" in the same manner; that is, similar external behaviors reflect a similar internal strategy. Even under directed states, such as counting or resting with eyes closed, participants may have different strategies for completing the same task. Lastly, facility with EEG analysis can be varied and often the detection of noise, eye blinks or eye movements, and other noise signals is subjective or poorly defined across reports.

Conclusion

In the study of autism, EEG/ERP findings have demonstrated slowed neural speed, lack of stimulus or condition differentiation, both reduced and increased activation, and altered topographical distribution. Each of these results has independently contributed to our understanding of autism and has been used to redefine our understanding of the processes that contribute to autism behaviors. For example, a failure or delay in activating neural structures that are normally specialized for a given process such as the fusiform gyrus for faces, could result in a failure to interconnect information such as linking a facial movement to vocalization. Temporal asynchrony in processing has consequences for both the formation of neural circuits and the behaviors that directly result from the utilization of that circuitry (Dawson, Webb, & McPartland, 2005; Brock, Brown, Boucher, & Rippon, 2002). As well, alterations in coherence across the frequency spectrum may signal distinct patterns of over- and underconnectivity supporting neuroanatomical models of autism (Horwitz et al., 1988; Just et al., 2004) that may be directly assessed as risk factors, predictors, and measures of response to treatment.

Our current understanding of autism has benefited greatly from the integration of information across multiple levels of analysis. The EEG methodology provides information that allows us to get closer to neural functioning, to divide the behaviors of autism into meaningful endophenotypes that can be investigated across the spectrum of the disorder, and to characterize stages of cognitive and affective processing. This methodology is also well suited for developmental studies as it can be utilized with individuals from infancy through late adulthood. EEG has promise as an endophenotype or biological marker of variability, which will allow for more refined measurements and may yield greater precision in investigating the systems that contribute to risk and outcome in individuals affected by autism.

Challenges and Future Directions

- The risks of utilizing EEG/ERP methodologies to elucidate autism profiles are similar to other methodological domains and include within- and between-group variability, verbal understanding, tactile hypersensitivity, hyperactivity, and inattention.

SUGGESTED READING

Picton, T., Benton, S., Berg, P., Donchin, E., Hillyard, S., Johnson, R., et al. (2000). Guidelines for using human event-related potentials to study cognition: Recording standards and publication criteria. *Psychophysiology, 37,* 127–152.

Pineda, J. (2005). The functional significance of mu rhythms: Translating "seeing" and "hearing" into "doing." *Brain Research: Brain Research Reviews, 50*(1), 57–68.

Uhlhaas, P. J. & Singer, W. (2006). Neural synchrony in brain disorders: Relevance for cognitive dysfunctions and pathophysiology, *Neuron, 52*(1), 155–168.

ACKNOWLEDGMENT

Writing of this chapter was supported by the NIH University of Washington Autism Center of Excellence (Webb; P50 HD 055782), NIH Shared Neurobiology of Autism and Fragile X (Webb; R03 HD 057321), Autism Speaks and Cure Autism Now (Murias), the Simons Foundation (Bernier) and the support of the University of Washington Psychophysiology and Behavioral Systems lab. Most importantly, we thank all of the individuals with autism and their families who participated in the research reported in this chapter.

REFERENCES

Adolph, R., Tranel, D., Damasio, H., & Damasio, D. (1994). Impaired recognition of emotion in facial expressions following bilateral damage to the human amygdala. *Nature, 372,* 669–667.

Babiloni, C., Del Percio, C., Babiloni, F., Carducci, F., Cincotti, F., et al. (2003). Transient human cortical responses during the observation of simple finger movements: A high-resolution EEG study. *Human Brain Mapping, 20,* 148–157.

Baranek, G. T. (1999). Autism during infancy: A retrospective video analysis of sensory-motor and social behaviors at 9–12 months of age. *Journal of Autism and Developmental Disorders, 29,* 213–224.

Baron-Cohen, S. (1994). How to build a baby that can read minds: Cognitive mechanisms in mindreading. *Cahiers de Psychologie Cognitive/Current Psychology of Cognition, 13,* 513–552.

Batty, M., & Taylor, M. J. (2003). Early processing of the six basic facial emotional expressions. *Cognitive Brain Research, 17,* 613–620.

Belmonte, M. K., Allen, G., Beckel-Mitchener, A., Boulanger, L. M., Carper, R. A., & Webb, S. J. (2004). Autism and abnormal development of brain connectivity. *Journal of Neuroscience, 24,* 9228–9231.

Bentin, S, Allison, T, Puce, A., Perez, E., & McCarthy, G. (1996). Electrophysiological studies of face perception in humans. *Journal of Cognitive Neuroscience, 8*(6), 551–565.

Bernier, R., Dawson, G., Webb, S., & Murias, M. (2007). EEG mu rhythm and imitation impairments in individuals with autism spectrum disorder. *Brain and Cognition, 64,* 288–237.

Bertone, A., Mottron, L., Jelenic, P., & Faubert, J. (2005). Enhanced and diminished visuo-spatial information processing in autism depends on stimulus complexity. *Brain: American Journal of Neurology, 128,* 2430–2441.

Boeschoten, M. A., Kenemnas, J. L., van Engeland, H., & Kemner, C. (2007). Abnormal spatial frequency processing in high-functioning children with pervasive developmental disorder (PDD). *Clinical Neurophysiology, 118,* 2076–2088.

Boger-Megiddo, I., Shaw, D., Friedman, S., Sparks, B., Artru, A., Giedd, J., et al. (2006). Corpus callosum morphometrics in young children with autism spectrum disorder. *Journal of Autism and Developmental Disorders, 36*(6), 733–739.

Brock, J., Brown, C. C., Boucher, J., & Rippon, G. (2002). The temporal binding deficit hypothesis of autism. *Developmental Pathology, 14,* 209–224.

Bruce, V., & Young, A. (1986). Understanding face recognition. *British Journal of Psychology, 77,* 305–327.

Buzsáki, G., & Chrobak, J. J. (1995). Temporal structure in spatially organized neuronal ensembles: A role for interneuronal networks. *Current Opinion in Neurobiology, 4,* 504–510.

Cantor, D., Thatcher, R., Hrybyk, M., & Kaye, H. (1986). Computerized EEG analyses of autistic children. *Journal of Autism and Developmental Disorders, 16,* 169–187.

Carver, L. J., Dawson, G., Panagiotides, H., McPartland, J., Gray, J., & Munson, J. (2003). Age-related differences in neural correlates of face recognition during the toddler and preschool years. *Developmental Psychobiology, 42,* 148–159.

Casanova, M. F., Buxhoeveden, D. P., & Brown, C. (2002). Clinical and macroscopic correlates of minicolumnar pathology in autism. *Journal of Child Neurology, 17,* 692–695.

Charman, T., Swettenham, J., Baron-Cohen, S., Cox, A., Baird, G., & Drew, A. (1997). Infants with autism: An investigation of empathy, pretend play, joint attention, and imitation. *Developmental Psychology, 33,* 781–789.

Ciesielski, K.T., Courchesne, E., & Elmasian, R. (1990). Effects of focused selective attention tasks on event-related potentials in autistic and normal individuals. *Electroencephalography and Clinical Neurophysiology, 75,* 207–220.

Clark, V., Keil, K., Maisong, J., Courtney, S., Ungerleider, L., & Haxby, J. (1995). Functional magnetic resonance imaging of human visual cortex during face matching: A comparison with positron emission tomography. *Neuroimage, 4,* 1–15.

Cochin, S., Barthelemy, S., Rous, S., & Martineau, J. (2001). Electroencephalographic activity during perception of motion in childhood. *European Journal of Neuroscience, 13,* 1791–1796.

Courchesne, E., Lincoln, A. J., Kilman, B. A., & Galambos, R. (1985). Event-related brain potential correlates of the processing of novel visual and auditory information in autism. *Journal of Autism and Developmental Disorders, 15,* 55–76.

Courchesne, E., Lincoln, A. J., Yeung-Courchesne, R., Elmasian, R., & Grillon, C. (1989). Pathophysiologic findings in nonretarded autism and receptive developmental language disorder. *Journal of Autism and Developmental Disorders, 19*, 1–17.

Courchesne, E., & Pierce, K. (2005). Why the frontal cortex in autism might be talking only to itself: Local over-connectivity but long-distance disconnection. *Current Opinion in Neurobiology, 15*, 225–230.

Daoust, A. M., Limoges, E., Bolduc, C., Mottron, L., & Godbout, R. (2004). EEG spectral analysis of wakefulness and REM sleep in high functioning autistic spectrum disorders. *Clinical Neurophysiology, 115*(6), 1368–1373.

Dawson, G., Carver, L., Meltzoff, A., Panagiotides, H., McPartland, J., & Webb, S. (2002). Neural correlates of face and object recognition in young children with autism spectrum disorder, developmental delay, and typical development. *Child Development, 73*, 700–717.

Dawson, G., Meltzoff, A., Osterling, J., & Brown, E. (1998). Children with autism fail to orient to social stimuli. *Journal of Autism and Developmental Disorders, 28*, 479–485.

Dawson, G., Warrenburg, S., & Fuller, P. (1982). Cerebral lateralization in individuals diagnosed as autistic in early childhood. *Brain and Language, 15*, 353–368.

Dawson, G., Webb, S., Carver, L., Panagiotides, H., & McPartland, J. (2004). Young children with autism show atypical brain responses to fearful versus neutral facial expressions of emotion. *Developmental Science, 7*(3), 340–349.

Dawson, G., Webb, S. J., Estes, A., Munson, J., & Faja, S. (2008). Electrophysiological indices of altered emotional face processing in parents of children with autism. Unpublished manuscript.

Dawson, G., Webb, S. J., & McPartland, J. (2005). Understanding the nature of face processing impairment in autism: Insights from behavioral and electrophysiological studies. *Developmental Neuropsychology, 27*, 403–424.

de Haan, M., & Nelson, N. (1999). Electrocortical correlates of face and object recognition by 6-month-old infants. *Developmental Psychology, 35*, 1113–1121.

de Haan, M., & Nelson, C. (1997). Recognition of the mother's face by 6-month-old infants: A neurobehavioral study. *Child Development, 68*, 187–210.

di Russo, F., Martinez, A., Sereno, M. I., Pitzalis, S., & Hillyard, S. A. (2002). Cortical sources of the early components of the visual evoked potential. *Human Brain Mapping, 15*, 95–111.

di Russo, F., Spinelli, D., & Morrone, M. C. (2001). Automatic gain control contrast mechanisms are modulated by attention in humans: Evidence from visual evoked potentials. *Vision Research, 41*, 2435–2447.

Donchin, E., & Coles, M. G. (1988). Is the P300 component a manifestation of context updating? *Behavioral and Brain Sciences, 11*, 357–427.

Ferree, T. C., Clay, M. T., & Tucker, D. M. (2001). The spatial resolution of scalp EEG. *Neurocomputing, 38–40*, 1209–1216.

Foote, N. L. (2004). Challenges of testing autistic patients. *American Journal of Electroneurodiagnostic Technology, 44*, 103–107.

Friston, K. J. (1994). Functional and effective connectivity in neuroimaging: A synthesis. *Human Brain Mapping, 2*, 56–78.

Frith, U. (1989). A new look at language and communication in autism. *British Journal of Disorders of Communication, 24*, 123–150.

Gastaut, H., & Bert, J. (1954). EEG changes during cinematographic presentation: Moving picture activation of the EEG. *Electroencephalography Clinical Neurophysiology Supplement, 6*, 433–444.

Gastgeb, H., Strauss, M., & Minshew, N. (2006). Do individuals with autism process categories differently? The effect of typicality and development. *Child Development, 77*(6), 1717–1729.

Gevins, A. S., & Illes, J. (1991). Neurocognitive networks of the human brain. *Annals of the New York Academy of Sciences, 620*, 22–44.

Grice, S.J., Halit, H., Farroni, T., Baron-Cohen, S., Bolton, P., & Johnson, M. H. (2005). Neural correlates of eye-gaze detection in young children with autism. *Cortex, 41*, 1871–1875.

Halgren, E., Marinkovic, K., & Chauvel, P. (1998). Generators of the late cognitive potentials in auditory and visual oddball tasks. *Electroencephalography and Clinical Neurophysiology, 106*, 156–164.

Hardan, A., Minshew, N., & Keshavan, M. (2000). Corpus callosum size in autism. *Neurology, 55*, 1033–1036.

Herbert, M., Ziegler, D., Makris, N., Filipek, P., Kemper, T., Normandin, J., et al. (2004). Localization of white matter volume increases in autism and developmental language disorder. *Annals of Neurology, 55*, 530–540.

Hoeksma, M. R., Kemner, C., Verbaten, M., & van Engeland, H. (2004). Processing capacity in children and adolescents with pervasive developmental disorders. *Journal of Autism and Developmental Disorders, 34*, 341–354.

Horwitz, B., Rumsey, J., Grady, C., & Rapoport, S. (1988). The cerebral metabolic landscape in autism: Intercorrelations of regional glucose utilization. *Arch Neurol, 45*(7), 79–55.

Jemel, B., Mottron, L., & Dawson, M. (2006). Impaired face processing in autism: Fact or artifact? *Journal of Autism and Developmental Disorders, 36*, 91–106.

Just, M. A., Cherkassky, V. L., Keller, T. A., & Minshew, N. J. (2004). Cortical activation and synchronization during sentence comprehension in high-functioning autism: Evidence of underconnectivity. *Brain: American Journal of Neurology, 127*, 1811–1821.

Kawakubo, Y., Kasai, K., Okazaki, S., Hosokawa-Kakurai, M., Watanabe, K., Kuwabara, H., et al. (2007). Electrophysiological abnormalities of spatial attention in adults with autism during the gap overlap task. *Clinical Neurophysiology, 118*, 1464–1471.

Klin, A., Jones, W., Schulz, R., Volkmar, F., & Cohen, D. (2002). Visual fixation patterns during viewing of naturalistic social situations as predictors of social competence in individuals with autism and related disorders. *Archives of General Psychiatry, 59*, 809–816.

Kutas, M., McCarthy, G., & Donchin, E. (1977). Augmenting mental chronometry: The P300 as a measure of stimulus evaluation time. *Science, 197*, 792–795.

Kylliainen, A., Braeutigam, S., Hietanen, J. Swithenby, S., & Bailey, A. (2006). Face- and gaze-sensitive neural responses in children with autism: A magnetoencephalographic study. *European Journal of Neuroscience, 24*, 2679–2690.

Lepage, J., & Theoret, H. (2006). EEG evidence for the presence of an action observation-execution system in children. *European Journal of Neuroscience, 23*, 2505–2510.

Levitt, P. (2005). Disruption of interneuron development. *Epilepsia, 46*, 22–28.

Lincoln, A. J., Courchesne, E., Harms, L., & Allen, M. H. (1993). Contextual probability evaluation in autistic, receptive developmental language disorder, and control children: Event-related brain potential evidence. *Journal of Autism and Developmental Disorders, 23*, 37–58.

Lopes da Silva, F. H., & Pfurtscheller, G. (1999). Event-related EEG/MEG synchronization and desynchronization: Basic principles. *Clinical Neurophysiology, 110*, 1842–1857.

Manes, F., Piven, J., Vrancic, D., Nanclares, V., Plebst, C., & Starkstein, S. (1999). An MRI study of the corpus callosum and cerebellum in mentally retarded autistic individuals. *Journal of Neuropsychiatry Clinical Neuroscience, 11*, 470–474.

Mangun, G. R., Buonocore, M. H., Girelli, M., & Jha, A. P. (1998). ERP and fMRI measures of visual spatial selective attention. *Human Brain Mapping, 6*, 383–389.

Martineau, J., & Cochin, S. (2003). Visual perception in children: Human, animal, and virtual movement activates different cortical areas. *International Journal of Psychophysiology, 51*, 37–44.

McPartland, J., Dawson, G., Webb, S. J., Panagiotides, H., & Carver, L. J. (2004). Event-related brain potentials reveal anomalies in temporal processing of faces in autism spectrum disorder. *Journal of Child Psychology and Psychiatry, 45*, 1235–1245.

Milne, E., Scope, A., Pascalis, O., Buckley, D., & Makeig, S. (2009). Independent component analysis reveals electroencephalograph activity during visual perception in individuals with autism. *Biological Psychiatry, 65*, 22–30.

Milne, E., Scope, A., Vigon, L., Buckley, D., & Pascalis, O. (2006). Abnormal N1/P1responses in children with ASD elicited by both low and high spatial frequency gratings. Poster presented at the International Meeting For Autism Research; Program book, p. 183.

Mundy, P., Sigman, M., Ungerer, J., & Sherman, T. (1986). Defining the social deficits in autism: The contribution of nonverbal communication measures. *Journal of Child Psychology and Psychiatry, 27*, 657–669.

Murias, M., Webb, S. J., Greenson, J., & Dawson, G. (2007). Resting state cortical connectivity reflected in EEG coherence in individuals with autism. *Biol Psychiatry, 62*, 270–273.

Muthukumaraswamy, S., Johnson, B., & McNair, N. (2004). Mu rhythm modulation during observation of an object-directed grasp. *Cognitive Brain Research, 19*, 195–201.

Novick, B., Kurtzberg, D., & Vaughn, H. (1979). An electrophysiologic indication of defective information storage in childhood autism. *Psychiatry Research, 1*, 101–108.

Nunez, P. (1995). *Neocortical dynamics and human EEG rhythms.* New York: Oxford University Press.

Nunez, P., & Srinivasan, R. (2006). A theoretical basis for standing and traveling brain waves measured with human EEG with implications for an integrated consciousness. *Clinical Neurophysiology, 117*, 2424–2435.

Nunez, P., Wingeler, B., & Siberstein, R. (2001). Spatial-temporal structures of human alpha rhythms: Theory, microcurrent sources, multiscale measurements, and global binding of local networks. *Human Brain Mapping, 13*(3), 125–164.

Oberman, L., Hubbard, E., McCleery, J., Altschuler, E., Ramachandran, V., & Pineda, J. (2005). EEG evidence for mirror neuron dysfunction in autism spectrum disorders. *Cognitive Brain Research, 24*, 190–198.

Oberman, L., Ramachandran, V., & Pineda, J. (2008). Modulation of mu suppression in children with autism spectrum disorders in response to familiar or unfamiliar stimuli: The mirror neuron hypothesis. *Neuropsychologia, 46*, 1558–1565.

O'Connor, K., Hamm, J., & Kirk, I. (2005). The neurophysiological correlates of face processing in adults and children with Asperger's syndrome. *Brain and Cognition, 59*, 82–95.

O'Connor, K., Hamm, J. P., & Kirk, I. J. (2007). Neurophysiological responses to face, facial regions, and objects in adults with Asperger's syndrome: An ERP investigation. *International Journal of Psychophysiology, 63*, 283–293.

Orekhova, E. V., Stroganova, T. A., Nygren, G., Tsetlin, M. M., Posikera, I. N., Gillberg, C., et al. (2007). Excess of high frequency electroencephalogram oscillations in boys with autism. *Biological Psychiatry, 62*, 1022–1029.

Osterling, J., Dawson, G., & Munson, J. (2002). Early recognition of one-year-old infants with autism spectrum disorder versus mental retardation: A study of first birthday party home videotapes. *Development and Psychopathology, 14*, 239–251.

Picton, W. (1992). The P300 wave of the human event-related potential. *Journal of Clinical Neurophysiology, 4*, 456–479.

Pineda, J. (2005). The functional significance of mu rhythms: Translating "seeing" and "hearing" into "doing." *Brain Research Reviews, 50*, 57–68.

Polich, J., & Criado, J. (2006). Neuropsychology and neuropharmacology of P3a and P3b. *International Journal of Psychophysiology, 60*, 172–185.

Raichle, M. (2001). Cognitive neuroscience: Bold insights. *Nature, 12*(412), 128–130.

Rippon, G., Brock, J., Brown, C., & Boucher, J. (2007). Disordered connectivity in the autistic brain: Challenges for the "new psychophysiology." *International Journal of Psychophysiology, 63*, 164–172.

Rogers, S., & Pennington, B. (1991). A theoretical approach to the deficits in infantile autism. *Development and Psychopathology, 3*, 137–162.

Rubenstein, J. L. R., & Merzenich, M. M. (2003). Model of autism: Increased ratio of excitation/inhibition in key neural systems. *Genes, Brain, and Behavior, 2*, 255–267.

Senju, A., Kikuchi, Y., Hasegawa, T., Tojo, Y., & Osanai, H. (2008). Is anyone looking at me? Direct gaze detection in children with and without autism. *Brain and Cognition, 67*, 127–139.

Senju, A., Hasegawa, T., & Tojo, Y. (2005). Does perceived direct gaze boost detection in adults and children with and without autism? The stare-in-the-crowd effect revisited. *Visual Cognition, 12*, 1474–1496.

Shuttleworth, E., Syring, V., & Allen, N. (1982). Further observations on the nature of prosopagnosia. *Brain and Cognition, 1*, 307–322.

Srinivasan, R., Tucker, D. M., & Murias, M. (1998). Estimating the spatial Nyquist of the human EEG. *Behavior Research Methods, Instruments and Computers, 30*, 8–19.

Srinivasan, R. (1999). Spatial structure of the human alpha rhythm: Global correlation in adults and local correlation in children. *Clinical Neurophysiology, 110*, 1351–1362.

Stroganova, T., Nygren, G., Tsetlin, M. M., Posikera, I. N., Gillberg, C., Elam, M., et al. (2007). Abnormal EEG lateralization in boys with autism. *Clinical Neurophysiology, 118*, 1842–1854.

Sutton, S. K., Burnette, C. P., Mundy, P., Meyer, J., Vaughan, A. E., Sanders, C. E., et al. (2005). Resting cortical brain activity and social behavior in higher functioning children with autism. *Journal of Child Psychology and Psychiatry, 46*, 211–222.

Townsend, J., Westerfield, M., Leaver, E., Makeig, S., Jung, T., Pierce, K., et al. (2001). Event-related brain response abnormalities in autism: Evidence for impaired cerebello-frontal spatial attention networks. *Cognitive Brain Research, 11*, 127–145.

Tuchman R., & Rapin, I. (2002). Epilepsy in autism. *Lancet Neurology, 1*, 352–358.

Uhlhaas, P. J., & Singer, W. (2006). Neural synchrony in brain disorders: Relevance for cognitive dysfunctions and pathophysiology. *Neuron, 52*(1), 155–68.

Vandenbroucke, M. W. G., Scholte, H. S., van Engeland, H., Lamme, V. A. F., & Kemner, C. (2008). A neural substrate for atypical low-level visual processing in autism spectrum disorder. *Brain: American Journal of Neurology, 131*, 1013–1024.

Verbaten, M. N., Roelofs, J. W., van Engeland, H., Kenemans, J. K., & Slangen, J. L. (1991). Abnormal visual event-related potentials of autistic children. *Journal of Autism and Developmental Disorders, 21*, 449–470.

Verleger, R. (1988). Event-related potentials and cognition: A critique of the context updating hypothesis and an alternative interpretation of P3. *Behavioral and Brain Sciences, 11*, 343–356.

Vidal, C. N., Nicolson, R., DeVito, T. J., Hayashi, K. M., Geaga, J. A., Drost, D. J., et al. (2006). Mapping corpus callosum deficits in autism: An index of aberrant cortical connectivity. *Biological Psychiatry, 60*, 218–225.

Villalobos, M., Mizuno, A., Dahl, B., Kemmotsu, N., & Muller, R. (2005). Reduced functional connectivity between V1 and inferior frontal cortex associated with visuomotor performance in autism. *Neuroimage, 25*(3), 916–925.

Webb, S. J., Merkle, K., Murias, M., Todd, R., Aylward, E., & Dawson, G. (2009). ERP responses differentiate inverted but not upright face processing in adults with ASD. *Social Cognitive and Affective Neuroscience.*

Webb, S. J., Dawson, G., Bernier, R., & Panagiotides, H. (2006). ERP evidence of atypical face processing in young children with autism. *Journal of Autism and Developmental Disorders, 36*, 881–890.

Webb, S. J., Dawson, G., Bernier, R., & Panagiotides, H. (2008). Face and object memory in children with autism spectrum disorder: Developmental change and continuity in ERP responses. Unpublished manuscript.

Webb, S. J., Long, J. D., & Nelson, C. A. (2005). A longitudinal investigation of visual event-related potentials in the first year of life. *Developmental Science, 8*, 605–616.

Welsh, J. P., Ahn, E. S., & Placantonakis, D. G. (2005). Is autism due to brain desynchronization? *International Journal of Developmental Neuroscience, 23*, 253–263.

Whittington, M. A, Traub, R. D., Kopell, N., Ermentrout, B., & Buhl, E. H. (2000). Inhibition-based rhythms: Experimental and mathematical observations on network dynamics. *International Journal of Psychophysiology, 38*, 315–336.

Williams, J., Whiten, A., & Singh, T. (2004). A systematic review of action imitation in autistic spectrum disorder. *Journal of Autism and Developmental Disorders, 34*(3), 285–299.

Williams, J., Whiten, A., Suddendorf, T., & Perrett, D. (2001). Imitation, mirror neurons, and autism. *Neuroscience and Biobehavioral Reviews, 25*, 287–295.

Wong, T. K., Fung, P. C., Chua, S. E., & McAlonan, G. M. (2008). Abnormal spatiotemporal processing of emotional facial expressions in childhood autism: Dipole source analysis of event-related potential. *European Journal of Neuroscience, 28*, 407–416.

Commentary

Pat Levitt

Toward a Neurobiology of Autism

Careful examination of the major sections of *Autism Spectrum Disorders* epitomizes well the current understanding of the autisms (plural noun used here to emphasize the heterogeneous nature of the spectrum; see Geschwind & Levitt, 2007)—long on clinical description and characterization of the breadth of associated phenotypic features in fine detail and in cataloging the plethora of strategies used in diagnosis and treatment; short on neurobiological characterization and mechanisms that actually generate the spectrum disorders. The latter is challenged by the very nature of the disorder—targeting perhaps the most complex of human cognitive skill sets that are built developmentally through a hierarchical process in which elementary circuitry that mediates basic skills (homeostatic control, attention, motivation, and reward) are integrated with more complex networks that ultimately mediate the abilities and desire of an individual to interact with the outside world through social engagement and communication (Hammock & Levitt, 2006). For the neurobiologists among us, I highly recommend further examination of the other major sections of the book, because the chapters are illustrative of the high degree of clinical complexity beyond the three core domains used to diagnose a child on the spectrum. Co-occurring medical, psychiatric, sensory, and motor conditions are the norm, not the exception for children, adolescents, and adults on the spectrum (Geschwind, 2009). Thus, attempts to model the clinically defined autism spectrum disorders in biological systems more tractable than humans may not be the best use of time. Rather, a dimensional approach to examine specific neurobiological processes that one believes are disrupted developmentally (see Modi & Young, Chapter 34), with each being examined in great detail and with precision in experimental systems may be a more fruitful strategy as the field continues to move forward.

Challenges First

Of all the dimensions of the autisms covered in this book, understanding neurobiological mechanisms that cause the disorder remains the most deficient in a working knowledge base for the scientific field. However, the growth curve for accumulating data is rapidly accelerating, and that bodes well. It is important to emphasize that *development* in its simplest form can be defined by "change over time." Inherent to this equation, therefore, is a moving target of a genetic blueprint that lays out fundamental brain architecture prenatally, which is then acted on by experience to sculpt a homeostatically balanced set of circuits that perform sensory, motor, cognitive, and regulatory functions (Thompson & Levitt, 2010). Rubenstein, in Chapter 30, provides a brief summary of our state of knowledge in this area, and in fact, we know quite a lot about the progression of neurodevelopment, particularly in nonprimate species. He raises an interesting point that there are dramatic changes in scale in the developing primate brain, and perhaps this feature has created a stress on assembling a far more complex set of circuits. If this is the case, then we need to understand a great deal more about the intimate details of normal primate brain development, which to date has focused mostly on prenatal histogenic events (Rakic, 2006). Moreover, we recognize that risk for the autisms are highly heritable, as noted in great detail in the section on genetics and genomics in this book. Thus, there is a clear role for genetic mechanisms (though not to the exclusion of currently ill-defined environmental factors), and there are replicated findings of common polymorphisms, de novo copy number variations, and rare mutations that implicate genes involved in developmental processes (Abrahams & Geschwind, 2008; Geschwind, 2008; Levitt & Campbell, 2009). But most of the genome is expressed in the developing brain at some point in time, which means that most genes can be implicated when a variation is defined. Moreover, we have a very limited knowledge base from which to draw basic information regarding when and where risk genes even are expressed in the brain (and other organ systems) during development. It is likely to be insufficient to extrapolate from rodent datasets with regard to this issue, because of the fundamental differences in the time period over which neurogenesis, cell migration, synaptogenesis, and myelination occur in the primate

(Levitt, 2003), and the evolutionary advances in establishing primate-specific circuitry.

Current Thinking

So where are we with understanding the neurobiological basis of autism spectrum disorders? Our starting point is that the autisms collectively can be viewed as an alteration in the trajectory of neurodevelopment, and thus the current gene X environment puzzle is somehow impacting the *change over time* computation There is clear evidence for this, as recent accumulation of multiple structural imaging studies (highlighted by Courchesne et al., Chapter 35) is consistent with early changes in the events that contribute to brain growth. It is important to emphasize as with many other childhood or adult onset neurodevelopmental disorders, the impact on structural integrity is subtle (5–10% difference range), but it may be that the *absolute* values of increases in frontal, parietal and temporal gray and white matter, and reduced corpus callosum are less important than the *kinetics* of how the growth occurred. Thus, the *slope* of *change over time* becomes essential to monitor, as Giedd and colleagues have done for neurotypical populations in relation to IQ (Shaw et al., 2006). A very recent longitudinal structural imaging study emphasizes the issue regarding developmental trajectory (Schumann et al., 2010), an approach that is far more tractable in model systems, but rarely performed. It also is evident from neuropathological studies reviewed by Schumann et al. (Chapter 31, this volume), as challenging as these are to do because of small sample sizes and the spread of subject age (child to adult), that there are likely a multitude of very modest changes that occur (e.g., reduced cell number in the amygdala, altered cell packing density in neocortex) through primary and secondary adaptive processes. The latter is a hallmark of typical brain development, so the challenge will be to understand whether the plasticity and adaptation exhibited by children with autism spectrum disorders is qualitatively different from typically developing individuals. Compared to adult-onset neurodevelopmental disorders (e.g., schizophrenia) or neurodegenerative disorders, the fine details of neuropathological changes in the autisms are missing—even taking into account our knowledge of syndromic disorders such as Fragile X syndrome or tuberous sclerosis with a high prevalence of autism codiagnosis. Reported changes overall are sufficiently variable and very modest in scope across autistic disorders. For example, cortical excitation: inhibition imbalance has been suggested as a common neurobiological feature (P. Levitt, Eagleson, & Powell, 2004; Rubenstein & Merzenich, 2003), but this is based almost entirely on clinical data reporting high prevalence of seizure disorder in the autisms (estimates range from 10–60%) and syndromic disorders with known genetic etiology. We remain in the dark regarding the site(s) of action—altered interneuron number, GABA receptor subunit changes, glutamate receptor trafficking or expression changes, local circuit connectivity—all could be at risk in the autisms. The specific details are important to learn, of course, because strategies for intervention will vary depending on the therapeutic targets.

Is atypical brain wiring at the heart of the clinical phenomena? Neuropathological and structure imaging is consistent with this, with the very best neurobiological evidence to date coming from the use of modern imaging and psychophysiological tools in humans. Chugani, Webb et al., Minshew et al., and Dager et al., (in this volume, Chapters 32, 33, 36, and 37, respectively) suggest that indeed this is a core neurodevelopmental deficiency. Each chapter emphasizes different components of neural and neurochemical pathways that clearly are not functioning in individuals with autism spectrum disorders as they do in neurotypical individuals. The concept of the autisms likened to neurological disconnection syndromes (Geschwind & Levitt, 2007; Minshew, Goldstein, & Siegel, 1997) has face validity in the variety of combined neuropsychological, neuroimaging, and ERP studies that suggest long-range connections that are relevant for integrating information across sensory and cognitive domains are dysfunctional, whereas local connectivity in some neocortical regions, including frontal, temporal, and polysensory association regions may be enhanced (discussed by Minshew et al., Chapter 36). The imaging and ERP studies (Webb et al., Chapter 33) are consistent—there are local regions of greater responsiveness, coherence across domains that may be decreased or increased, and a disturbed topography. The latter is particularly important, because the current evidence suggests that the fundamental neurobiological substrate for dysfunction may be both quantitative (under- or overconnectivity of otherwise normally organized circuits) and qualitative (miswiring in cortico-cortical and cortico-subcortical circuits). Consistent as these findings may be, the situation grows more complex as an ever-increasing array of information is gathered. The Magnetic Resonance Spectroscopy findings to date (Dager et al., Chapter 33) suggest that there may be fundamental metabolic changes that are widespread in individuals on the spectrum. This could establish differential challenges for the maturation of specific circuits that are more sensitive than others to metabolic challenges. Thus, not all neural processes will be at great risk. Because dysfunction of information processing is a fundamental feature of the autisms, and the brain uses neurotransmitters to distribute and process information, it comes as no surprise that even cursory measures of specific neurochemicals are demonstrating changes (Chugani, Chapter 32). As with analyses of metabolic disruption, assigning specificity and functional relevance is problematic thus far, because neurotransmitter systems are so highly adaptive under normal and pathophysiological conditions. As attractive as the hypotheses may be, a specific neurobiological understanding of neurotransmitter dysfunction in the clinical syndrome remains distant. Finally, we are gaining steam in certain areas with regard to a developmentally relevant, molecular understanding of signaling pathways that may, more often than not, be direct targets in the autisms. This is discussed in other sections of *Autism Spectrum Disorders*, and is mentioned by Rubenstein in Chapter 30. It has relevance here because certain cell signaling pathways ultimately control the building of early brain architecture and guiding later growth through gene X environment mechanisms. Thus, syndromic disorders such as tuberous sclerosis, neurofibromatosis, Angelman syndrome, rare mutations in the genes encoding pTEN and Akt, and a convergence of genetic findings indicate that the PI3 Kinase/ERK pathways are common neurobiological targets in the autisms (Levitt & Campbell, 2009). More complex network analyses are beginning to bear fruit in identifying key elements of these pathways and others that we know are intimately involved in the control of cellular growth (Bill & Geschwind, 2009). From any view, the disruption of growth control, broadly defined neurobiologically (e.g., early regionalization of the neocortex, synapse formation, dendritic and spine growth, axon branching, myelination, and cell migration are all biological growth phenomena) is a primary defect in the autisms.

The Future of Neurobiological Discoveries

A recent Policy/Forum commentary by Akil et al. (2010) served as a call to arms for genomics and the neural sciences to integrate in a far more refined way, because the solutions to understanding brain disorders lie in defining the circuits that are at greatest risk for disruption, which we understand can likely occur through a variety of mechanisms. For developmental neurobiologists, this bodes well with regard to an increasing appreciation for careful studies in developing clinical populations and a more discerning and restricted set of strategies for developing a better biological understanding in animal models of dimensions that are targeting in the autisms. Here are a few suggestions for looking forward:

- define disrupted circuitry longitudinally (e.g., Schumann et al., 2010).
- clinical probes of function through ever-improving methods can provide greater insight when done in combination with approaches that define genetic risk (that make sense biologically) in the same study populations.
- moratorium on developing animal models of the autisms—replaced by an expanding effort to define far better the core mechanisms that underlie the *development* of specific behaviors and skills that are targeted in the autisms. For example, social behavior, of which we know little regarding ontogeny, can be examined across models in ethologically relevant contexts that will provide a new appreciation of developmental trajectory and how it can be disrupted (see Modi & Young, Chapter 34)–and ultimately improved through best intervention practices.
- The initial neuropathological studies in the field, with limited resolution and power, can be replaced by larger analyses with sufficient statistical power and appropriate specificity and sensitivity of the assays. To date, the replicable changes that have been discovered are small in size—thus assay quality control is essential to discern these subtle, yet functionally relevant alterations.
- this section of the book *Autism Spectrum Disorders* has a "cortical-centric" focus. The clinical picture is far more complex. As ill-defined as the neuropathology and structure/function disruptions are in the cerebral cortex, there is far less known regarding nonneocortical circuits. Renewed efforts here will pay dividends for neurobiologists who may have sensitive assays to probe functions that are at the beginning of the functional hierarchy of social behavior and communication.

REFERENCES

Abrahams, B. S., & Geschwind, D. H. (2008). Advances in autism genetics: On the threshold of a new neurobiology. *Nature Reviews Genetics*, *9*(5), 341–355.

Akil, H., Brenner, S., Kandel, E., Kendler, K. S., King, M.-C., Scolnick, E., et al. (2010). Medicine: The future of psychiatric research; Genomes and neural circuits. *Science*, *327*(5973), 1580–1581.

Bill, B. R., & Geschwind, D. H. (2009). Genetic advances in autism: Heterogeneity and convergence on shared pathways. *Current Opinion in Genetics and Development*, *19*(3), 271–278.

Geschwind, D. H. (2008). Autism: many genes, common pathways? *Cell*, *135*(3), 391–395.

Geschwind, D. H. (2009). Advances in autism. *Annual Review of Medicine*, *60*, 367–380.

Geschwind, D. H., & Levitt, P. (2007). Autism spectrum disorders: Developmental disconnection syndromes. *Current Opinion in Neurobiology*, *17*(1), 103–111.

Hammock, E. A. D., & Levitt, P. (2006). The discipline of neurobehavioral development: The emerging interface that builds processes and skills. *Human Development*, *49*, 294–309.

Levitt, P. (2003). Structural and functional maturation of the developing primate brain. *Journal of Pediatrics*, *143*(4 Suppl), S35–45.

Levitt, P., & Campbell, D. B. (2009). The genetic and neurobiologic compass points toward common signaling dysfunctions in autism spectrum disorders. *Journal of Clinical Investigation*, *119*(4), 747–754.

Levitt, P., Eagleson, K. L., & Powell, E. M. (2004). Regulation of neocortical interneuron development and the implications for neurodevelopmental disorders. *Trends in Neurosciences*, *27*(7), 400–406.

Minshew, N. J., Goldstein, G., & Siegel, D. J. (1997). Neuropsychologic functioning in autism: Profile of a complex information processing disorder. *Journal of the International Neuropsychological Society*, *3*(4), 303–316.

Rakic, P. (2006). A century of progress in corticoneurogenesis: From silver impregnation to genetic engineering. *Cerebral Cortex*, *16*(Suppl 1), i3–i17.

Rubenstein, J. L. R., & Merzenich, M. M. (2003). Model of autism: Increased ratio of excitation/inhibition in key neural systems. *Genes, Brain, and Behavior*, *2*(5), 255–267.

Schumann, C. M., Bloss, C. S., Barnes, C. C., Wideman, G. M., Carper, R. A., Akshoomoff, N., et al. (2010). Longitudinal Magnetic Resonance Imaging study of cortical development through early childhood in autism. *Journal of Neuroscience*, *30*(12), 4419–4427.

Shaw, P., Greenstein, D., Lerch, J., Clasen, L., Lenroot, R., Gogtay, N., et al. (2006). Intellectual ability and cortical development in children and adolescents. *Nature*, *440*(7084), 676–679.

Thompson, B. L., & Levitt, P. (2010). Now you see it, now you don't—Closing in on allostasis and developmental basis of psychiatric disorders. *Neuron*, *65*(4), 437–439.

Section VI

Etiology: Genetics

38 Janine A. Lamb

Whole Genome Linkage and Association Analyses

Points of Interest

- Autism is a behaviorally defined lifelong neurodevelopmental disorder, with strong evidence for a complex genetic predisposition.
- Many linkage and candidate gene association studies have been carried out over the last decade to identify genetic variants increasing risk of autism spectrum disorders, and have yielded ambiguous results.
- Recent advances in genomic technology now provide greater ability to assay genetic variation, enabling genomewide association and copy number variation studies.
- The results from these genomewide studies, together with other recent genetic findings, implicate both common and rare variants in genes involved in the postsynaptic density, synaptogenesis, and neuronal cell-adhesion in susceptibility to autism.
- These genetic variants often show incomplete penetrance and imperfect segregation and may also influence risk of mental retardation and other neurodevelopmental and psychiatric disorders, suggesting that considerable genetic and clinical heterogeneity is likely to underlie autism spectrum disorders.
- These results underscore the complex genetic architecture of autism, suggesting that interdisciplinary, convergent approaches, large sample sizes, and in-depth phenotyping may be required to further elucidate the risk variants and biological pathways involved.

Autism spectrum disorders (ASDs) are a group of behaviorally defined lifelong neurodevelopmental disorders. Several twin and family studies have indicated a high heritability for autism, with evidence for a strong genetic basis first reported from twin studies published 20–30 years ago (Folstein & Rutter, 1977; Steffenburg et al., 1989). The risk of autism in siblings of autistic individuals is reported as approximately 15–20%, which is considerably higher than the general population prevalence (Baird et al., 2006; Fombonne, 2005). Similarly, there is an increased risk for the Broader Autism Phenotype in relatives of individuals with autism (Bailey et al., 1998). However, despite this evidence for a genetic susceptibility to autism, only in approximately 10% of cases are the ASDs associated with a recognized cause ("syndromic" autism); in the remaining 90% of cases the cause is unknown ("idiopathic" autism). Increasingly intensive research has been carried out since the initial reports of a genetic basis with the aim of identifying the genetic variants predisposing to idiopathic autism. It is hoped that discovery of the etiological mechanisms will lead to an increased understanding of the disorder, offer improved diagnosis and the possibility of better intervention and treatment. It is now over a decade since the first whole genome screen for linkage in ASD was reported (International Molecular Genetic Study of Autism Consortium [IMGSAC], 1998). This chapter gives an overview of the linkage, association, and copy number variation studies that have been published during this period, and reflects on what has been learned about the probable genetic architecture of autism and how this theory impacts on the likely success of different strategies for variant discovery. It also considers the ways in which experimental technology and practice have evolved to meet these challenges.

Linkage and Association Analyses are Strategies for Identification of Genetic Risk Variants

In recent years typically the first strategy to identify susceptibility genes for common complex disease has been to conduct a whole-genome linkage scan using several hundred polymorphic genetic markers in families with more than one affected individual. Linkage aims to identify regions of the genome containing genetic marker alleles that are shared between affected relative pairs more often than expected by chance, or less often in the case of relative pairs discordant for the disease. This is based on the expectation that these regions have a higher probability of harboring genetic variants increasing susceptibility to the disorder, as the genetic markers map close to (are linked to) the disease locus. The likelihood of the observed sharing data is compared to the likelihood of the observed data due to chance alone, and the result expressed most commonly as the logarithm of the odds (LOD) score. This results in a genomewide LOD score profile, with a LOD score ≥ 2.2 accepted as suggestive evidence of linkage and a LOD score ≥ 3.6 giving genomewide significant evidence for linkage (Lander & Kruglyak, 1995). This method may enable mapping of the disease risk variant to a relatively small chromosomal interval, although considerable additional work is required after the genome screen to refine the linked region and to identify and confirm the risk alleles in affected individuals. Linkage is a powerful approach to detect rare, highly penetrant disease alleles, and has been used with great success in mapping monogenic disorders segregating in large families. Although this approach can be used successfully in the presence of allelic heterogeneity where there are many different disease causing alleles at the same locus, linkage rapidly loses power in the presence of locus heterogeneity when the same phenotype is caused by risk alleles at multiple different loci.

Monogenic: caused by a single gene.

Recently, due to rapid technological advances in high-throughput genotyping, association studies have become the method of choice to identify risk alleles for common complex diseases. In a case-control association study, the frequency of alleles or genotypes of polymorphic genetic markers—usually single nucleotide polymorphisms (SNPs)—are compared between affected individuals and unaffected controls to detect those that differ significantly between the two groups. This method assumes that a significant proportion of "unrelated" affected individuals carry one of a few, or the same, common ancestral mutations. Hence, marker alleles that differ in frequency between the affected and unaffected groups are presumed to be directly causative, or located close to the disease risk variant. Family-based association studies test for linkage in the presence of association by evaluating the number of alleles that are transmitted versus nontransmitted from parents to affected offspring. Association studies have more power than linkage to detect common variants of small effect that confer only a very modest disease risk. However, association is less powerful in the presence of extensive allelic heterogeneity where multiple variants at the same locus contribute to disease risk.

Single Nucleotide Polymorphism (SNP): a DNA sequence variation involving a single base pair.

Hence, linkage and association approaches have both potential advantages and disadvantages for identifying genetic variants underlying disease risk, with the relative strength and likely success of each approach depending on the unknown underlying genetic architecture.

Whole Genome Linkage Analyses

The first whole genome screen for linkage in autism was reported over a decade ago (IMGSAC, 1998). Since this initial publication, many genomewide linkage and follow-up studies have been carried out, and regions of nearly every chromosome have been linked with susceptibility to ASD (Auranen et al., 2002; Barrett et al., 1999; Buxbaum et al., 2001; Lamb et al., 2005; McCauley et al., 2005; Philippe et al., 1999; Risch et al., 1999; Schellenberg et al., 2006; Shao et al., 2002b; Yonan et al., 2003; and reviewed by Abrahams & Geschwind, 2008; and Gupta & State, 2007). These studies have generally used 350–400 microsatellite markers and tens to hundreds of largely Caucasian families. In studies of autism, the most widely used approach has been the affected sib pair approach, which looks at the sharing of markers between two or more affected siblings, although some studies have included more distantly related relative pairs such as cousins or avuncular pairs. Although several studies have been published reaching criteria for genomewide suggestive or significant evidence for linkage (for example, see Auranen et al., 2002; Liu et al., 2001; IMGSAC, 2001; Yonan et al., 2003; Barrett et al., 1999; and Auranen et al., 2002; Liu et al., 2001; IMGSAC, 2001; respectively), a unifying theme from these data is the lack of consistency in the linked regions between studies, and even within extended studies from the same group (IMGSAC, 2001; Lamb et al., 2005; Yonan et al., 2003; Liu et al., 2001). Several reasons have been posited for this lack of reproducibility, including the limited size of sample cohorts, sample heterogeneity resulting from differing diagnostic and inclusion criteria for subjects and cohort ascertainment between research groups, use of different genetic markers and statistical analyses, and the presence of false positives.

In an effort to identify rare founder mutations segregating in families, a small number of reports have focused on large, extended multiple-generation pedigrees from genetically isolated populations, for instance, from an isolated region of central Finland, in an approach resembling that of traditional linkage studies for monogenic disorders (Auranen et al., 2002; Auranen et al., 2003; Allen-Brady et al., 2008; see also Chapters by Rehnstöm & Peltonen, and Morrow & Walsh in this volume). A recent linkage analysis of a 6-generation pedigree from Utah with seven affected males using the Affymetrix 10k SNP array identified two regions on chromosome 3q and a region on chromosome 20q meeting criteria for genomewide significance, while regions on 7p and 9p met suggestive criteria for significance (Allen-Brady et al., 2008). Analysis of haplotype sharing within these five chromosomal regions showed that five of the seven affected cases shared multiple chromosome regions with other affected subjects. However, no single haplotype was shared between all seven affected individuals, suggesting genetic heterogeneity even within this single large pedigree.

Haplotype: a set of DNA sequence variations that are close together on the same chromosome and tend to be inherited as a unit.

Larger Sample Sizes May Increase Power to Detect Linkage Signals

In an effort to garner statistical power, two partial meta-analyses of the published linkage data have been carried out. The first study analyzed data from four studies and identified genomewide suggestive evidence for linkage to chromosomes 7q and 13q (Badner & Gershon, 2002). The second study applied a heterogeneity-based genome search meta-analysis approach to six of the published genome scans (including some of those in the previous meta-analysis) and identified significant evidence for linkage to chromosome 7q22-32, and suggestive evidence for linkage to the neighboring region 7q32-qter (Trikalinos et al., 2006).

Meta-analysis: a combined statistical analysis of several separate but related studies to test the pooled data for statistical significance.

However, the most definitive combined linkage analysis carried out to date is the study recently published by the Autism Genome Project (AGP) Consortium (Szatmari et al., 2007). This collaboration involved greater than 20 research institutions across the United States, Canada, and Europe, with a joint sample size of approximately 1500 families containing at least two individuals with ASD, thus creating a sample three times larger than any autism linkage study carried out previously. For the first phase of this project, 1181 families were genotyped using two sets of genomewide markers on two different genotyping platforms; the Affymetrix GeneChip® Human Mapping 10K SNP Array (Szatmari et al., 2007) and a panel of approximately 450 microsatellite markers. Using the Affymetrix 10k SNP Array, this study identified suggestive linkage to chromosome 11p12-p13 (Szatmari et al., 2007), a region not identified previously as significant by other genomewide scans. However, as none of the linkage results could be interpreted as statistically significant, this study demonstrates that despite the large increase in size of the sample cohort the significance of the linkage findings did not increase in parallel. In the AGP study, use of the same genetic markers and methods for statistical analysis argues against these reasons for the lack of consistency in the previously published linkage findings from the constituent groups making up the AGP. However, there are theoretical reasons why increasing the sample size in the presence of locus heterogeneity may actually decrease the LOD score at a true susceptibility locus (Vieland et al., 2001; Bartlett & Vieland, 2007). Nonetheless, the absence of more significant results from this large study and the fact that the genomewide linkage profile did not appear significantly different from those previously published by the smaller constituent groups suggests that extensive genetic heterogeneity underlies ASD, and only a small effect size may be attributable to any given variant contributing to ASD at the population level.

Autism Subphenotypes Offer Hope of Increased Sample Homogeneity

The lack of reproducibility of the linkage results and the suggestion of underlying genetic heterogeneity have led to sample cohort subdivision in an effort to identify more genetically informative phenotypes and illuminate biological pathways. Autism-related subphenotypes, or endophenotypes, have been used on the premise that they are more directly related to the underlying susceptibility variants than the psychiatric diagnosis and are therefore more tractable to genetic dissection than the disease state itself (Flint & Munafo, 2007). Anatomical, physiological, or developmental endophenotypes, such as head circumference, whole-blood serotonin levels, or language impairment, have been investigated in autism. Linkage analysis in a subset of families with more severe obsessive-compulsive behaviors resulted in stronger evidence for linkage to chromosome 1 than in the whole sample (Buxbaum et al., 2004). Studies incorporating diagnostic measures of language, for example, subsets of families containing probands meeting criteria for "delayed onset of phrase speech" have also demonstrated increased evidence for linkage to chromosomes 2q (Buxbaum et al., 2001; Shao, Raiford, et al., 2002) and 11p (Liu et al., 2008), and a study incorporating information on proband and parental language phenotypes showed increased linkage to chromosomes 7q and 13q (Bradford et al., 2001). Other classifications, for example using measures of IQ (Liu et al., 2008) and "strictness" of diagnostic criteria (Szatmari et al., 2007; IMGSAC, 2001; Yonan et al., 2003) have also been investigated. It has been suggested that the subclassification of affected sibling pairs according to their sex may index genetic heterogeneity, as one of the characteristics of autism is a gender bias of 4 times as many affected males as females and a higher reported recurrence risk for siblings of female versus male probands (Ritvo et al., 1989). Consistent with this, several studies have indicated increased evidence for linkage to specific genomic regions in male-only or female-containing affected sibling pairs (Lamb et al., 2005; Stone et al., 2004; Szatmari et al., 2007; Cantor et al., 2005; Ma et al., 2007), including a male-specific locus identified on chromosome 17q11q21 in families from the Autism Genetics Resource Exchange (Stone et al., 2004), which was subsequently replicated in an independent family sample (Cantor et al., 2005).

Endophenotype: a heritable simpler intermediate trait of a complex psychiatric disorder than the disease syndrome itself.

So, has categorizing samples using subphenotypes really increased cohort homogeneity, or is increased statistical significance in the linkage signals solely due to stochastic variation? Several studies that have examined subgroups have resulted in very small numbers of cases in each group, raising doubts about the robustness of the findings. Therefore, it is probable that, as with other linkage findings, the results reflect both true and false positives. The success of the use of subgroups or endophenotypes will depend on whether the distinct aspects of ASD are under independent genetic control or due to shared risk factors. A principal components factor analysis of data from the Social Responsiveness Scale in children with and without pervasive developmental disorders suggested the existence of a single, continuously distributed underlying factor contributing to multiple distinct aspects of the phenotype (Constantino et al., 2004). Conversely, a recent population-based study of 3000 twin pairs aged 7–9 from the Twins Early Development Study (TEDS) found high heritability for each of the three areas of the "triad of impairments" of autism; the social, communication, and repetitive and/or restrictive domains, both for children across the distribution and at the extremes of the distribution. However, there was only modest to low correlation between the three core areas of the triad, and individuals with extreme scores in one domain did not necessarily have extreme scores in the other domains (Ronald et al., 2006). This suggests that the majority of genes contributing to ASD have symptom specific action, and indicates that the use of cohorts of individuals showing extreme scores in one area of the triad of impairments may be more effective than looking for genes for autism as a whole (Happe et al., 2006). This view is supported by the observation that "unaffected" relatives of individuals with autism show only isolated traits of the Broader Autism Phenotype. Moreover, the relative ease of phenotyping subphenotypes may make them more amenable for collecting the large samples required for statistically reliable analysis of complex genetic traits using large population-based or epidemiological approaches. It seems likely that use of anatomical or physiological subphenotypes such as head circumference or presence/absence of seizures might provide a less subjective biomarker than measures, for example, of repetitive behavior or language ability. Indeed, examination of subgroups of individuals with autism and macrocephaly has led to identification of mutations in the *PTEN* gene (Butler et al., 2005; Buxbaum et al., 2007; Herman et al., 2007; Varga et al., 2009) (see Box 38-1).

Box 38–1

Mutations in *PTEN* are identified in individuals with autism and macrocephaly

Mutations in the *PTEN* (phosphatase and tensin homologue) tumour suppressor gene have been identified in individuals with autism and macrocephaly (Buxbaum et al., 2007; Butler et al., 2005; Herman et al., 2007; Varga et al., 2009). Previous research has shown that individuals with hamartoma disorders such as Cowden Syndrome, Bannayan-Riley-Ruvalcaba syndrome and Proteus syndrome, which are characterised by germline *PTEN* mutations, may have autistic behaviours as well as overgrowth and macrocephaly. Progressive macrocephaly is one of the most consistent findings in autism (reviewed in (Lainhart, 2006)). This overgrowth is usually not present at birth but develops during the first year of life, and is found in approximately 20% of individuals. Four studies of subsets of individuals with autism and macrocephaly (defined as head circumference ≥2 standard deviations above the mean) were carried out by mutation analysis and sequencing of the coding and putative regulatory regions of the *PTEN* gene. These studies identified germline mutations of the *PTEN* gene in 1.1-16.7% of individuals with autism, which were not found in control individuals (Buxbaum et al., 2007; Butler et al., 2005; Herman et al., 2007). These data suggest that there is an important role for *PTEN* in brain development. This is supported by the observation that conditional knockout mice which lack *Pten* in the cerebral cortex and hippocampus exhibit macrocephaly, neuronal hypertrophy and abnormal dendritic spine morphology (Kwon et al., 2006), and further research showing that *PTEN* is involved in mechanisms controlling synaptic function and myelination abnormalities (Fraser et al., 2008). Taken together, these data suggest that individuals with autism and pronounced macrocephaly should be screened for *PTEN* gene mutations.

Quantitative Linkage Analyses May Increase Power to Identify Autism Loci

Linkage studies to date have generally used a discrete binary trait approach for phenotype classification and subsequent analysis in cohorts of individuals with autism. However, the analysis of quantitative traits should offer improved power for linkage through added dimensionality of the phenotype leading to measurement of more subtle differences over a continuum, and the ability to include relatives previously classified as "unaffected." In contrast to the development of diagnostic instruments, the refinement of measures and application of quantitative traits to ASD are still in their infancy, despite the use of both univariate and multivariate (simultaneous analysis of several traits) quantitative trait approaches in other neurodevelopmental disorders, for example dyslexia (Fisher et al., 2002; Marlow et al., 2003) and specific language impairment (Specific Language Impairment Consortium (SLIC), 2004; Monaco, 2007).

In autism, quantitative approaches have most often been limited to "affected" individuals, for example, the Autism Genetic Resource Exchange (AGRE) Consortium found that use of "age at first word" as a quantitative trait in their genome scan analysis generated the strongest evidence for linkage on chromosomes 3q and 17q, with a subset of families linked to chromosome 7q (Alarcon et al., 2005). Analysis of five quantitative traits related to autism from the Broader Phenotype Autism Symptom Scale (BPASS) using multivariate models showed that social motivation and range of interest/flexibility had the highest heritabilities, as well as the highest genetic correlation (Sung et al., 2005). A further study using a measure of autistic-like behavior from the Social Responsiveness Scale evaluated in both affected and "unaffected" individuals identified a locus on chromosome 11 that reached the level of suggestive linkage (Duvall et al., 2007). The IMGSAC has recently developed and refined Family History Interview (FHI; Bolton et al., 1994; Folstein et al., 1999) based instruments using informant (FHI-I) and subject (FHI-S) interviews and an observational measure of autism related broader behavioral phenotypes (Bailey et al., 1998). However, a quantitative genome screen for the broader phenotype carried out using these measures yielded no significant evidence for linkage at a genomewide level (Falcaro, Lamb, & Pickles, unpublished data). The largest quantitative genomewide linkage analysis using total scores of the reciprocal social interaction and restricted, repetitive, and stereotyped patterns of behavior domains from the Autism Diagnostic Interview-Revised also failed to identify significant evidence for linkage in 976 multiplex families from the Autism Genome Project Consortium (Liu et al., 2008) (see also Chapter by Cantor in this volume).

How Much Faith Should We Place in Published Linkage Results?

Does the inability of numerous research groups to identify consistent and statistically robust linkage signals over the last decade suggest a lack of utility of this approach to identify risk variants for ASD? Are most of the published linkage findings really just noise? The relative value of this approach will be determined by the successful identification of disease risk alleles underlying the linked loci, and the subsequent elucidation of biological pathways. While the absence of more convincing linkage results from the large AGP study (Szatmari et al., 2007) suggests that only a small effect size may be attributable to any given variant contributing to ASD at the population level, there have been some successes using a linkage approach; methyl-CpG-binding protein 2 (*MECP2*) was identified as the gene mutated in Rett syndrome, an autism spectrum disorder (Amir et al., 1999), and more recently, variants in Contactin-Associated Protein-Like 2 (*CNTNAP2*) have been implicated in autism by linkage and subsequent association analysis (Alarcon et al., 2008; see below). Similarly, linkage and association mapping led to the identification of a risk haplotype in the *KIAA0319* gene associated with dyslexia (Fisher et al., 1999; Francks et al., 2004), which has subsequently been replicated in several independent studies (Cope et al., 2005; Harold et al., 2006; Paracchini et al., 2008). This risk haplotype was shown to reduce expression of the gene leading to impaired neuronal migration in the developing cerebral neocortex (Paracchini et al., 2006), and the putative causal regulatory variant has subsequently been identified (Dennis et al., 2009).

The likely success of a linkage approach will depend on the unknown genetic architecture underlying susceptibility to autism (covered in further detail below). In the meantime, it is the responsibility of authors and scientific journals to try to ensure publication of robust scientific data, both positive and negative, using well-designed studies.

Genetic Association Studies

The general inability of several research groups to refine linked intervals using extended sample sizes or subphenotypes over the last decade has led to follow-up genetic association studies targeting these linked regions using a positional candidate gene approach. The hypothesis that common complex diseases are likely to be caused by a combination of both common and rare variants has also led to an increase in the number of candidate gene association studies, as association offers more power than linkage to detect common variants of small effect that confer only a very modest disease risk.

Furthermore, as technologies for higher throughput SNP genotyping have evolved from the ability to genotype a single variant, to tens, hundreds, thousands, and currently over a million variants in a single experiment, so too have the regions targeted expanded from isolated genetic variants, to whole genes, genomic loci, and now even the whole genome can be investigated in a single experiment.

Candidate Gene Association Studies

To date, the majority of published association studies have been limited to the investigation of a relatively small number of candidate genes using a similarly small number of genetic variants. These genetic variants have typically been single nucleotide polymorphisms (SNPs), the most common form of variation in the human genome, but also microsatellites or insertion/deletions. Collectively, many candidate genes have been investigated using this approach. These studies have generally examined a combination of known genetic variants and novel variants identified through screening the coding and putative regulatory regions of candidate genes in a small subset of the sample cohort. These genes have been selected as they map to a region of linkage, or because they are plausible biological candidates for involvement in autism etiology based on putative gene function, or patterns of expression (see Abrahams & Geschwind, 2008, for review). A tacit assumption of the former approach is that both linkage and association are powered to detect the same genetic risk variants. Moreover, the candidate gene approach is reliant on an ability to select good functional candidates, based on imperfect knowledge of biological function.

A common limitation arising from these association studies, as with the linkage analyses, is a lack of replication between studies. Again, many reasons have been posited for this lack of reproducibility, including genetic and phenotypic heterogeneity between samples due to ascertainment differences and suboptimal sampling, heterogeneity in subject exposure to environmental influences, data overinterpretation, and disparity in sample sizes between research groups leading to false-positive or false-negative results because of differing power to detect real effects (Zondervan & Cardon, 2004). A further challenge in genetic association studies is the need to appropriately match cases and controls in order to avoid spurious results arising from population stratification. In retrospect, it is increasingly clear that the sample sizes used in early candidate gene studies were an order of magnitude too small to detect the moderate risks associated with common variants underlying complex disease. Furthermore, the first published study likely represents an overestimate of the true effect size due to a phenomena known as the "winner's curse," suggesting that replication of both association and linkage studies will require larger sample sizes than the initial detection study (Trikalinos et al., 2004; Zollner & Pritchard, 2007).

Population stratification: systematic differences in allele frequencies between subgroups of a population (in this context, cases and controls) that arise due to different ancestral and demographic histories between the two groups.

Nevertheless, as understanding of the pitfalls and limitations of association studies has improved, there has been a trend toward more methodologically robust experiments, using larger and better powered samples, more rigorous statistical thresholds and analytical methods, and with an increasing requirement for independent replication before publication and functional evidence to support the results. One such example of this is an investigation of the *MET* (proto-oncogene hepatocyte growth factor receptor) gene.

A Common Promoter Variant in the *MET* Gene is Associated with Autism

The *MET* gene is a proto-oncogene, but *MET* signaling also participates in cerebral cortex and cerebellar growth and maturation, immune system regulation, and peripheral organ development and repair (such as gastrointestinal), consistent with medical complications reported in some children with autism. *MET* maps to a region linked to autism on chromosome 7q31.2 (Lamb et al., 2005; Trikalinos et al., 2006; Badner & Gershon, 2002), and thus represents a good positional and functional candidate for involvement in autism susceptibility. In an initial study, association of the common allele of an SNP in the promoter region of the *MET* gene was identified in 204 families with autism ($P = 0.0005$; Campbell et al., 2006). This association was confirmed in a replication sample of 539 families with autism ($P = 0.001$) and in the combined sample ($P = 5 \times 10^{-6}$), with multiplex families exhibiting the strongest association. The authors subsequently carried out functional assays which showed that the associated allele resulted in a 2-fold decrease in *MET* promoter activity and altered binding of specific transcription factor complexes. In a follow-up study, the authors showed altered expression of *MET*, and three other genes that regulate *MET* signaling activity, in *post-mortem* cerebral cortex from ASD cases compared to matched controls (Campbell et al., 2007). However, despite the robust initial finding and replication in an independent cohort, a second group failed to replicate association of the common promoter variant in their independent sample of 325 multiplex families and 10 trio families, instead demonstrating association to a different SNP in intron 1 ($P < 0.004$; Sousa et al., 2008). These conflicting results between the two studies epitomize the challenges facing autism genetics researchers, and may indicate false negative or false positive results, the presence of allelic heterogeneity and the influence of different regulatory variants on *MET* expression, or differing ancestral histories between the two study samples.

Association Studies of Implicated Genomic Regions

Several groups have adopted a high-density SNP genotyping association approach to follow up regions identified by genomewide linkage studies. Three such examples are investigation of the linked regions on chromosomes 2q and 7q in the IMGSAC sample (Maestrini et al., 2009), and investigation of the chromosome 17 male-specific linked locus (Stone et al., 2004; Yonan et al., 2003; Cantor et al., 2005) and 7q35 language delay QTL (Alarcon et al., 2002; Alarcon et al., 2005) in the AGRE sample. In the first study, 3000 SNPs were genotyped in each ~40Mb genomic region targeting ~170 and 270 known genes and additional highly conserved noncoding sequences on chromosomes 2 and 7 respectively. Association analysis revealed association to several genes, including inner-mitochondrial membrane protease-like (*IMMP2L)* and dedicator of cytokinesis 4 (*DOCK4*), a guanine nucleotide exchange factor gene involved in dendritic morphogenesis, on chromosome 7. Evidence for a role of *DOCK4* in autism susceptibility was supported by replication of the results in an independent European sample and the finding of a submicroscopic deletion (copy number variant; see section on structural variation below) segregating to both affected siblings in one family. In the second study, a dense panel of 2053 SNPs with an average intermarker distance of 6.1kb was genotyped across the 13.7Mb chromosome 17 linkage interval, which contains ~180 known genes. These SNPs were analyzed in 219 independent families containing only affected male siblings using a parent-child trio based study design, but no single SNP or haplotype association survived correction for multiple comparisons or was sufficient to account for the initial linkage signal (Stone et al., 2007).

A Regional Association Approach Identifies Contactin-Associated Protein-Like 2 as a Susceptibility Gene for Autism Spectrum Disorders

A two-stage approach was used to test 2758 SNPs across the 15Mb 7q34-q36 region encompassing the language-related autism QTL (average intermarker distance of 5.6Kb) and containing approximately 200 known genes (Alarcon et al., 2008). In the first stage, 172 parent-child trios were tested for association to the quantitative trait "age at first word." These analyses identified association to four genes including Contactin-Associated Protein-Like 2 (*CNTNAP2*), primarily driven by the male-only affected sibling pair containing families, and this association to *CNTNAP2* was subsequently confirmed in 304 independent parent-child trios. A relatively large microdeletion within *CNTNAP2* was also identified in this study in a proband and his father, but not in his affected sibling or in 1000 control chromosomes. Regional gene expression analyses in eight human fetal brains demonstrated that *CNTNAP2* is enriched in regions of the brain that may be important for language development. These findings led the authors to suggest that common variation within *CNTNAP2* contributes to ASD and related conditions, and increases risk of language delay (Alarcon et al., 2008). *CNTNAP2* is one of the largest known genes in the genome and encodes a member of the neurexin family of neuronal cell adhesion molecules that are known to mediate cell-cell interactions in the nervous system, and may play a role in axon differentiation. As such, it is a good functional candidate for autism susceptibility. Two concurrent studies published in the same journal also reported a possible role for *CNTNAP2* in susceptibility to ASD (Arking et al., 2008; Bakkaloglu et al., 2008). The first study reported association of a common noncoding variant at the 5' end of the *CNTNAP2* gene in 72 families with a strict qualitative definition of autism (overlapping with the AGRE families reported above), which was supported in an independent sample of 1295 parent-child trios, albeit with a broader definition of autism than in the initial sample. This study also identified a parent-of-origin and gender effect for association of this common variant (Arking et al., 2008). The second study investigated the possible involvement of rare *CNTNAP2* variants in individuals with ASD, again from the AGRE Consortium (Bakkaloglu et al., 2008). In this study, a de novo chromosomal inversion that disrupted *CNTNAP2* in a child with cognitive and social delay led the authors to sequence the 24 coding exons of the gene in a large cohort of 635 ASD cases and 942 unselected controls, and those changes that were identified only in the case or the control group were genotyped in an additional control sample of 1073 unrelated Caucasian subjects. This identified 13 rare (defined as allele frequency less than 1 in 4000 in the combined control sample) and unique variants in the case group, eight of which were predicted to be deleterious to protein function by bioinformatic approaches and/or altered conserved residues across all species examined, and 11 rare or unique variants in the control group, of which six were predicted to be deleterious or conserved. However, despite this increase in mutation burden in the cases, this did not reach statistical significance. The possible involvement of rare *CNTNAP2* mutations in susceptibility to ASD is supported by the prior identification of a rare homozygous mutation in *CNTNAP2* in an extended Old Order Amish family with cortical dysplasia-focal epilepsy, in which affected individuals had seizures, relative macrocephaly, language regression, and 67% of affected individuals had pervasive developmental delay or autism (Strauss et al., 2006). Furthermore, a complex cytogenetic abnormality disrupting *CNTNAP2* was also identified in an affected father and his two affected children with Gilles de la Tourette syndrome and obsessive compulsive disorder (Verkerk et al., 2003), and deletions of varying size have been observed in individuals with epilepsy and schizophrenia (Friedman et al., 2008). However, a balanced translocation disrupting *CNTNAP2* has also been described in phenotypically normal individuals (Belloso et al., 2007), again highlighting the complexity of inferring causality of genetic variants in ASD.

Genomewide Association Studies

The pursuit of genomewide association studies (GWAS) has been facilitated largely by two major advances in molecular genetics: the rapid improvement in genotyping platforms, and

Box 38–2
Gene expression profiling in individuals with autism implicates biological pathways

Several recent studies have profiled gene expression in peripheral blood or lymphoblastoid cell lines derived from individuals with autism (Gregg et al., 2008; Hu et al., 2006; Nishimura et al., 2007), and it has been shown that differentially expressed genes are able to distinguish individuals with autism from controls, and to distinguish individuals with autism based on their genetic etiology due to a fragile X mutation or a 15q11-q13 duplication (Nishimura et al., 2007). Although these data require independent confirmation and there appears to be little overlap between the results emerging from separate studies, developing bioinformatic resources of gene and protein interactions and pathways enable researchers to make inferences about the underlying molecular and physiological mechanisms. These results suggest that several genes within the 15q11-q13 interval and genes from Gene Ontology pathways including ubiquitin conjugation, SH3 domain containing proteins, GTPase regulator activity, and alpha–protocadherin genes are over-represented within the differentially expressed genes in autism (Abrahams & Geschwind, 2008). These findings are supported by the results of a recent genomewide CNV study and the identification of neuronal cell-adhesion molecules as genes involved in ASD susceptibility. Nonetheless, these bioinformatic resources are currently far from complete, and time will determine whether the complex genetics of autism converges on a single genetic pathway, or multiple distinct pathways. The different developmental trajectories of ASD also emphasise the need for temporally and spatially restricted gene expression studies. The integration of gene expression data with high density SNP genotype data enables an expression QTL (eQTL) approach, whereby SNPs are investigated for association using gene transcript levels as the quantitative trait (Stranger et al., 2007; Dixon et al., 2007). This may provide a more direct correlate of risk than the neurobehavioural phenotype.

the advent of the International HapMap Consortium (2003). The innovation in genotyping platforms has been driven by the emergence of commercially available high density microarrays (chips) that can simultaneously characterize DNA sequence variation at hundreds of thousands of genetic variants at ever declining costs. Phases I and II of The HapMap Project have identified and genotyped over 3.1 million SNPs spread throughout the genome in 269 samples from four different ethnic populations (International HapMap Consortium, 2005; Frazer et al., 2007). This information has been made publically available through the HapMap website (www.hapmap.org). These advances have made it possible to attempt to survey all the variation in the human genome, including noncoding sequence, in a single experiment. However, even with current array density, it is still not feasible to directly genotype all known variants in the human genome, as this would be prohibitively expensive. This has led to the use of an "indirect" approach, which takes advantage of linkage disequilibrium (LD), whereby the genotypes of variants in strong LD are correlated, therefore creating redundancy between SNPs. Two general strategies for indirect GWAS have been taken: the first using a random set of SNPs spread across the genome; the second taking advantage of the LD data from the HapMap Project to select subsets of highly informative "tagging" SNPs based on the LD between them, which can then be used as a proxy to effectively capture the entire set of ungenotyped common SNPs throughout the genome. This latter tagging approach has been shown to provide greater coverage of ungenotyped common (minor allele frequency > 5%) variants throughout the genome (Barrett & Cardon, 2006; Pe'er et al., 2006). However, the development of imputation approaches to infer genotypes at ungenotyped loci (Burdick et al., 2006; Marchini et al., 2007) has reduced the drive to develop arrays of ever-increasing density.

International HapMap Project: aims to determine the common patterns of DNA sequence variation and common haplotypes in the human genome, as a resource for genetic association studies. This project initially investigated samples of African, Asian, and European ancestry, and is now being expanded to seven additional populations.

Linkage Disequilibrium (LD): the nonrandom association of alleles at two or more genetic loci.

These genomewide approaches are unbiased with regard to the likely biological candidacy of the genomic region tested, and rely less on the ability of the researcher to identify "good" biological candidates a priori. The parallel development of gene-based discovery projects such as the Seattle SNPs Variation Discovery Resource (http://pga.gs.washington.edu/) and Innate Immunity Programs (http://innateimmunity.net), which aim to identify all variation in candidate genes and pathways that underlie inflammatory responses and innate immunity respectively, enables a combination of gene-based and indirect genomewide association approaches.

Over the last 2 to 3 years, there has been a dramatic increase in the number of GWAS of common complex diseases published, facilitated by the development of large collaborative networks with access to thousands of samples (Wellcome Trust Case Control Consortium, 2007; Manolio et al., 2007). These studies have resulted in the identification of common genetic variants associated with disorders such as asthma (Moffatt et al., 2007; Himes et al., 2009), Type 2 diabetes (Sladek et al., 2007; Takeuchi et al., 2009; Wellcome Trust Case Control Consortium, 2007; Zeggini et al., 2007), coronary artery disease (Erdmann et al., 2009; Helgadottir et al., 2007; Samani et al., 2007; Wellcome Trust Case Control Consortium, 2007), breast cancer (Easton et al., 2007; Stacey et al., 2007; Stacey et al., 2008), and traits such as height (Weedon et al., 2008; Sanna et al., 2008; Lettre et al., 2008) and obesity (Frayling et al., 2007; Loos et al., 2008). Many of these associations have been convincingly replicated in independent sample cohorts. These studies are providing valuable insights into the genetic architecture of complex disease, and are uncovering potential new mechanistic connections between diseases, for example, the association of *PTPN22* and *IL2RA* with both type 1 diabetes and rheumatoid arthritis, and *JAZF1* with aggressive prostate cancer and type II diabetes. These studies have been reviewed by Iles (2008) and McCarthy et al. (2008) and cataloged online at the National Human Genome Research Institute (http://www.genome.gov/26525384).

Genomewide SNP Association Studies of Autism Spectrum Disorders

Two SNP GWAS of autism spectrum disorders have been very recently published, and further GWAS are currently underway by large collaborative groups such as the AGP. Wang et al., (2009) investigated a cohort of 780 families with 1299 affected children from AGRE, and a second cohort of 1204 affected individuals and 6491 control subjects, all of European ancestry. A meta-analysis of the two combined discovery cohorts identified six SNPs in a 100kb intergenic region between the cadherin 10 (*CDH10*) and cadherin 9 (*CDH9*) genes on chromosome 5p14.1 with strong association signals, the most significant result being a P value of 3.4×10^{-8}. These signals were replicated in two independent cohorts, and generated combined discovery and replication P values of 7.4×10^{-8} to 2.1×10^{-10}. These intergenic SNPs may have a regulatory effect on the expression of *CDH10* and *CDH9*. These genes encode neuronal cell-adhesion molecules, which are involved in cell adhesion and generation of synaptic complexity in the developing brain. Two pathway-based association approaches applied to the genotype data again suggested that cadherin genes are significantly associated with ASD, thus implicating these genes in the pathogenesis of ASD. Weiss et al. (2009) carried out a genomewide linkage and association study of 1553 affected offspring from 1031 multiplex families using more than 500,000 SNPs on Affymetrix arrays, with subsequent examination of the most significantly associated regions in additional families. Initial analysis of the discovery sample did not reveal any SNPs showing association with genomewide significance. However, a SNP on chromosome 5p15 between the semaphorin 5A (*SEMA5A*) and taste receptor type 2 (*TAS2R1*) genes was significantly associated with autism in the combined discovery and replication cohorts ($P = 2 \times 10^{-7}$). *SEMA5A* has been implicated in axon guidance during neuronal development, and expression of *SEMA5A* was subsequently shown to be reduced in brain tissue from individuals with autism compared to controls, hence implicating this gene in susceptibility to autism.

What Can We Learn from the Candidate Gene and Genomewide Association Studies of Complex Disease Published So Far?

A recent evaluation of GWAS and published linkage studies for Type II diabetes suggests that there is little concordance in the genomic location of the significantly associated variants and linked loci, again indicating that these approaches are powered to detect different variants (E. Zeggini, personal communication). Hence, with some exceptions such as *CNTNAP2* (Alarcon et al., 2008) and *KIAA0319* (Paracchini et al., 2006), linkage followed by association may have limited success to detect susceptibility variants for common complex disease. The extent to which variants identified by GWAS support those implicated by candidate gene association studies has yet to be formally investigated, but many GWAS suggest previously unsuspected biological pathways. Furthermore, in many cases the most strongly associated SNPs map to genes of unknown function or to intergenic regions far from the nearest coding sequence, again suggesting a limited ability to select good functional candidates for complex disease a priori. Given that known coding regions make up less than half of the evolutionarily conserved sequence in the human genome (Birney et al., 2007), this finding should not be surprising. Moreover, finding an association with an intragenic SNP does not mean that this SNP or gene is necessarily involved in disease pathogenesis, as it may be indirectly associated with the true functional variant outside the transcription unit.

As genotyping technologies have evolved, study designs and statistical methodologies have also become more robust—both by necessity and by design—with studies including larger samples with better power, more rigorous quality control and statistical thresholds, and analytical methods built on a combination of population and statistical genetics and epidemiology (Altshuler & Daly, 2007). The GWAS carried out to date have generally used a case-control design, as these samples are cheaper and easier to collect than those using a family-based approach due to the thousands of samples required. In addition, family-based association methods generally have reduced power, and several statistical methods to detect and adjust for population stratification between cases and controls have been developed, with minimal loss of power (Price et al., 2006; Devlin & Roeder, 1999).

A major challenge in GWAS is interpretation of the results and identification of variants that survive a stringent correction for multiple tests, due to the large number of genotype-phenotype associations investigated. Given that there are estimated to be in excess of ten million SNPs genomewide and few true associations for which GWAS are adequately powered, the prior probability of detecting a true association is low, and spurious associations will substantially outnumber true ones. Stringent *P*-value cut-offs, for example, $P < 5 \times 10^{-7}$, have therefore been applied (Wellcome Trust Case Control Consortium, 2007) in order to avoid an abundance of false positive associations. However, the confidence that can be attributed to any given significance level is a function of sample size, and Bayesian approaches, which incorporate prior information on the likely number of true associations, are increasingly being used. Typically, the most compelling signals identified have shown very modest effects in the disease samples investigated, with heterozygote odds ratios generally less than 1.5. However, due to imperfect LD, a modest GWAS finding might ultimately lead to identification of variants with larger effect sizes. Furthermore, the biological insight into disease pathogenesis provided by identification of associated loci is not necessarily correlated with the effect size of the variants identified.

Bayesian: statistical approaches, based on Bayes' theorem, that assess the probability of a hypothesis being correct by incorporating prior probabilities, which are then revised after obtaining experimental data.

The extent of reproducibility of GWAS for some disorders, especially psychiatric disorders, is still unknown, and limited statistical power is demonstrated by the tendency of different GWAS of the same phenotype to find partially overlapping association results. It has been suggested that the effect size of common variants underlying psychiatric disorders may be smaller than those detected for other complex diseases due to an adverse influence on reproductive fitness and subsequent elimination of variants conferring a high degree of risk from the population (Craddock et al., 2008). This suggestion is supported by the existing genomewide association data from studies of autism and other psychiatric disorders, and it is possible that ongoing and future GWAS of psychiatric disorders may yield a raft of nonreproducible associations, akin to those resulting from candidate gene association studies. However, some loci may be missed even by well-powered GWAS due to insufficient coverage of the causal variants by SNPs on the genotyping array. Therefore, the absence of an association signal does not necessarily mean that a gene or region can be excluded.

Recently, guidelines for the design, conduct, analysis, and publication of GWAS and replication studies have been suggested (Chanock et al., 2007), including those of a working group convened on replication in association studies (Chanock et al., 2007). This group suggested that claims of replication should be reserved for effects of a similar magnitude, with the same allele or haplotype (or those in perfect LD), analyzed for the same phenotype and population and using the same genetic model, and that equal preference for publication should be given to well-conducted negative studies.

Genetic model: model of how a genetic locus affects susceptibility to a disease or trait.

To date, most GWAS have reported single SNP analyses, and association of haplotypes or 2-locus or higher-order interaction between SNPs has not been explored. However, for N biallelic markers there are 2^N possible haplotypes, so the greater information offered by haplotypes or tests for epistasis is offset by the cost of multiple testing. Incorporation of longitudinal data on environmental exposures would enable assessment of modifying environmental variables. The large majority of GWAS also have been carried out in Caucasian samples, and there is a need to extend these studies to other populations. HapMap Phase 3 is carrying out genomewide SNP genotyping and targeted sequencing in 1,301 DNA samples from 11 human populations (including the 270 samples from the four populations originally genotyped in Phases I and II of the project), which should aid this endeavor. The large collaborative networks and expanding sample sizes provide investigators with the ability to study a range of phenotypes simultaneously using the rich sets of data available, and including information on peripheral traits such as height. New public data archives, such as the Database of Genotypes and Phenotypes (dbGaP; Mailman et al., 2007), have been introduced to facilitate analysis of existing datasets employing new hypotheses and methods by investigators carrying out approved research according to study principles. This presents the additional challenge, in common with candidate gene and regional association studies, of a retrospective and prospective need to correct for an unknown number of statistical tests when a successive series of analyses are published independently. Again, it is the responsibility of authors and journals to present a balanced and thoughtful interpretation of research data, both positive and negative.

Epistasis: a circumstance where the expression of one gene is affected by the expression of one or more other genes at a different locus.

Association Studies are Underpowered to Detect Rare Variation

A recent review of 54 genomewide association studies for 22 different diseases published to February 2008 suggests that the frequency distribution and effect size of alleles associated with common disease are more reflective of study power than of the true underlying disease allele frequency distribution; even when the causative genetic variants are mostly rare, the significantly associated alleles are expected to be common, as they are the easiest to detect (Iles, 2008). This may imply that the many, likely more common, intergenic associated variants identified is a reflection of statistical power, rather than true underlying disease biology. Although population theory models indicate that the allelic spectrum of variants contributing to common complex disease is likely to be small (the "common disease-common variant" hypothesis; Reich & Lander, 2001), several studies have suggested that multiple rare variants with an intermediate penetrance at a number of loci may have a considerable influence on disease susceptibility (Pritchard & Cox, 2002). These low-frequency variants may explain a significant proportion of the missing genetic risk identified by genomewide association studies. The involvement of rare variants in susceptibility to ASD has long been known from the presence of cytogenetic anomalies, and rare copy number variants and coding mutations have been recently identified (see structural variation below). The importance of rare variants is supported by empirical data identifying many rare variants in two candidate genes for neuropsychiatric phenotypes in an ethnically diverse reference sample (Glatt et al., 2001), in genes contributing to variation of triglyceride levels in a population-based cohort (Romeo et al., 2007) and in three renal salt handling genes contributing to blood pressure variation (Ji et al., 2008). Thus, common complex diseases are more likely to be caused by a combination of both common and rare variants.

These rare variants are not sufficiently high risk to be detected by linkage, and association approaches are unable to detect them due to poor coverage of rare variation by commercially available genotyping arrays, and the fact that even very large sample sizes do not provide the statistical power necessary to establish an association due to rare variant frequency (Zeggini et al., 2005). Hence, the definition and detection of common versus rare variation is largely determined by the study power, and a more extensive set of loci influencing common complex disease may be found by GWAS of greater power, or by meta-analysis of existing GWAS data, as has been demonstrated for several disorders including type 2 diabetes (Zeggini et al., 2007; Zeggini et al., 2008; Scott et al., 2007; Saxena et al., 2007).

Recent years have seen a proliferation of novel large-scale sequencing approaches, with dramatically increased throughput and reduced costs (Margulies et al., 2005; Service, 2006), enabling the detection of rare sequence variants. However, genome sequencing strategies are still considerably more expensive than those to detect common variation. The difficulty of establishing statistical significance for overrepresentation of a rare variant in cases versus controls has led to the use of mutation burden analysis, in which the collective rare variant frequency is compared in cases versus controls, as discussed for *CNTNAP2* above (Bakkaloglu et al., 2008). However, proving the relevance of rare variants may still take some time, and other methods are required to demonstrate causality, for example, evidence of a functional effect, demonstrating biological relevance in a model system, or finding additional rare variants in other genes in the same biological pathway or in the same gene in related phenotypes.

Structural Variation May Underlie Susceptibility to Common Complex Disease

Although estimates of the number of genes in the human genome have decreased as our knowledge of genome structure has evolved (International Human Genome Sequencing Consortium, 2004), our knowledge of the extraordinary variability and apparent structural complexity among human genomes is rapidly increasing. The recent technological advances in array-based genotyping and comparative genomic hybridization (array-CGH) now allow investigation of the genome for chromosomal imbalances at a resolution that is considerably higher than that offered by conventional karyotyping. Recent research has highlighted that structural variation is ubiquitous and common throughout the human genome (Eichler et al., 2007; Wong et al., 2007; Korbel et al., 2007; Conrad et al., 2009; Redon et al., 2006). These variants include deletions, insertions, inversions, and duplications, and encompass copy number variants (CNVs) as well as more complex variation, ranging from kilobases to megabases in size (see Feuk et al., 2006, for review). This structural variation comprises millions of nucleotides of sequence heterogeneity and is an important contributor to phenotypic diversity, evolution, and disease susceptibility. To date, over 8000 distinct regions of the reference human genome assembly have been annotated to harbor nearly 30,000 CNVs in healthy control individuals (see the Database of Genomic Variants (dGV) at http://projects.tcag.ca/variation/, version hg18, August 05, 2009). These CNVs may affect gene expression directly by disrupting genes and altering dosage or indirectly through a position effect or unmasking of recessive mutations or functional variants on the remaining allele in the case of a deletion.

Copy number variant: a submicroscopic structural variation that results in gain or loss of genomic material.

Copy Number Variants are Associated with Autism Spectrum Disorders

Much research published over the last 2 decades has shown that there is a high rate of microscopic chromosomal anomalies in individuals with autism spectrum disorders, which may contribute to autism in approximately 7% of cases (for an online catalog see http://projects.tcag.ca/autism/). The majority of these abnormalities arise de novo in simplex rather than multiplex families, with the majority found in syndromic forms of ASD. However, several recent studies have suggested that the proportion of cases of ASD attributable to rare submicroscopic structural variation may be even higher than the 7% identified by standard cytogenetic approaches. Thus, rapid advances in array technology coupled with an increase in knowledge of genetic structural variation have led to the search for copy number variants increasing risk of autism.

Syndromic autism: autism secondary to another known disorder.

The first genomewide array–CGH investigation of chromosomal rearrangements in autism was carried out in 29 karyotypically normal individuals presenting with syndromic forms of ASD using arrays at 1Mb resolution. In this study, unique rearrangements of 1.4–16Mb in size were observed in 27.5% of cases (Jacquemont et al., 2006). Since this publication, several genomewide studies of CNVs in autism using increasingly high resolution arrays have been carried out. An investigation of individuals with idiopathic autism from 118 singleton, 47 multiplex, and 99 control families, including families from the Autism Genetic Resource Exchange (AGRE), found that the cumulative frequency of de novo CNVs was higher in individuals with ASD than in unaffected individuals ($P = 0.0005$), and more common among female and sporadic cases than in multiplex families, with most of the CNVs detected being deletions (Sebat et al., 2007). This led the authors to suggest a causal role of de novo mutation in autism. This paper demonstrated for the first time that chromosomal anomalies are present in idiopathic individuals with ASD, rather than solely in those with mental retardation or syndromic forms of autism, a finding subsequently replicated by several other groups. The Autism Genome Project analyzed their Affymetrix 10k SNP data for linkage (see above) and CNVs in 1181 multiplex families (Szatmari et al., 2007). This revealed several recurrent or overlapping CNVs in multiple unrelated affected individuals and CNVs coincident with published autism rearrangements, suggesting that these CNVs may be involved in susceptibility to ASDs. A hemizygous deletion of coding exons of neurexin 1 (*NRXN1*), a neuronal cell-adhesion gene on chromosome 2p16.3, was also identified in two affected siblings. An array-CGH study using a 19K whole genome tiling path bacterial artificial chromosome (BAC) array with ~200kb resolution was carried out on 397 unrelated individuals with ASD from AGRE and 372 controls (Christian et al., 2008). This study identified 51 autism-specific CNVs in 46 ASD subjects (11.6%), of which 9 were de novo and 42 were inherited. Recurrent CNVs were identified at 3 loci: maternal duplications of 15q11-q13, duplications of 22q11, and de novo microdeletions of 16p11.2 (see below). The CNVs were present at a relatively higher frequency in the female subjects (M:F ratio of 0.84 in individuals with CNVs compared to 1.4 in the study population). A study using the Affymetrix 500k SNP array identified CNVs in 44% of 427 ASD families that were not present in 500 controls, or in a further 1152 controls subsequently examined (Marshall et al., 2008). Although most of these CNVs were inherited, de novo CNVs were again observed at a higher frequency in families having one child compared to those with two or more affected children (7.1% vs. 2% respectively), and recurrent or overlapping autism-specific CNVs were observed at 13 loci in unrelated cases. The most recent study of genomewide copy number variation examined a cohort of 859 ASD cases and 1409 healthy children of European ancestry using the

Illumina HumanHap550 SNP array (Glessner et al., 2009). A replication cohort of 1336 ASD cases from AGRE were subsequently investigated. In addition to the identification of CNVs in previously reported autism susceptibility genes such as *NRXN1* and contactin 4 (*CNTN4*), several new CNVs in neuronal cell-adhesion molecules including Neuroligin 1 (*NLGN1*) and astrotactin 2 (*ASTN2*) were enriched in ASD cases compared to controls ($P = 9.5 \times 10^{-3}$), again implicating these genes in susceptibility to ASD. CNVs in genes involved in ubiquitin pathways were also identified in cases, but not in controls.

In an innovative homozygosity linkage mapping and CNV approach, the Homozygosity Mapping Collaborative for Autism recently investigated 88 consanguineous families in which the parents were first cousins, to detect autosomal recessive alleles underlying susceptibility to ASD (Morrow et al., 2008). This approach has previously proved to be highly successful in mapping disease genes for autosomal recessive disorders, including autosomal recessive mental retardation (Noor et al., 2008; Alders et al., 2009). Using the Affymetrix 500k SNP array, Morrow et al. mapped several loci containing large, rare, inherited homozygous deletions within linked regions. These deletions were present in 5/88 (6.4%) of consanguineous pedigrees, ranging in size from 18kb to >800kb, and mapped to chromosomes 2q24, 3p12, 3q24, 4q28, and 6p12. Notably, this limited overlap of the linked regions between pedigrees suggests considerable genetic heterogeneity. Furthermore, the majority of these deletions did not contain known genes, suggesting that effects may be mediated through defective regulation of expression of nearby genes; these included solute carrier family 9 (*SLC9A9/NHE9*) protocadherin 10 (*PCDH10*), contactin 3 (*CNTN3*), and sodium channel, voltage-gated, type VII, alpha (*SCN7A*). Potential mutations of *SLC9A9* were also identified in cases with unrelated parents, with the finding of a nonsense mutation in two male siblings with autism that was not identified in greater than 3800 control chromosomes. Rare, nonconservative coding changes identified by resequencing were also more common in individuals with autism and epilepsy than in controls (5.95% versus 0.63%, Fisher's exact test $P = 0.005$), further implicating this gene in autism susceptibility.

Recurrent Copy Number Variants of *SHANK3* and Chromosome 16p11.2 are Identified in Autism

Two of the most notable recent genetic findings in ASD are the identification of a recurrent 16p11.2 copy number variable region spanning ~500kb and a copy number variant of chromosome 22q13 including the SH3 and multiple ankyrin repeat domains 3 (*SHANK3*) gene; a synaptic scaffolding protein involved in structural organization of the postsynaptic density (Sebat et al., 2007; Kumar et al., 2008; Weiss et al., 2008; Christian et al., 2008).

The recurrent microdeletion at 16p11.2 was first observed in 2/180 probands from the Autism Genetic Resource Exchange (AGRE), and was not present in 372 control subjects using a 19k whole genome tiling array (Kumar et al., 2008). Screening an additional 532 probands and 465 controls for this CNV identified two more cases but no controls with the microdeletion, indicating a combined frequency of 0.6% in autism (4/712 autism versus 0/837 controls). The reciprocal duplication of this region was observed in one individual with autism and in two controls. Bioinformatic analysis of the CNV region localized 12 of the 25 known genes to a single interaction network that included genes involved in cell-to-cell signaling and interaction, whereas pathways for 3 of the 25 genes included postsynaptic density genes (Kumar et al., 2008). A second higher-resolution study used the Affymetrix SNP array 5.0, which contains probes for ~500,000 SNPs and a similar number of nonpolymorphic probes for detection of copy number variation (Weiss et al., 2008). This study identified five individuals from 4/751 multiplex families, again from AGRE, with the same de novo deletion. This finding was followed up and observed in 5/512 children referred for developmental delay, mental retardation, or suspected ASD, as well as in 3/299 individuals with autism from the Icelandic population. Using three different control groups, the deletion was also observed in 3/2814 control samples, which included individuals with bipolar disorder but unscreened for ASD, and in 2/18,834 unscreened Icelandic control subjects, but not in 434 clinical samples from children where ASD, developmental delay, or mental retardation was not indicated. The 16p11.2 duplication occurred in 7 affected individuals from the AGRE families, in 4 of the 512 follow-up children and in 7 of the control individuals. Apart from the known maternal duplication of chromosome 15q11-q13, no other recurrent de novo events > 20kb were identified that were not present in control subjects. In total, deletion and duplication events at 16p11.2 were observed in nearly 1% of multiplex families with autism, in 1% of individuals with autism from a general population sample, and in more than 1.5% of clinical samples from individuals with a developmental or language delay, but at less than 0.1% in the general population. The Affymetrix 500k SNP array study by Marshall et al., (2008) also identified this 16p11.2 CNV at a frequency of ~1% in individuals with autism. Thus, the 16p11.2 deletion and reciprocal duplication appears to contribute to up to 1% of cases with autism, and suggests that one or more genes in the region may be dosage sensitive.

The CNVs and sequence variants observed in *SHANK3* also showed a combined frequency of ~1% in ASD cases and were observed in individuals with autism and Asperger's syndrome (Durand et al., 2007; Marshall et al., 2008; Moessner et al., 2007). Similarly, the deletion of 16p11.2 was also observed at a markedly increased rate in subjects with a psychiatric or language disorder, including schizophrenia, bipolar disorder, attention-deficit hyperactivity disorder (ADHD), dyslexia, and panic disorder, anxiety, depression, or addiction (Weiss et al., 2008). This 16p11.2 CNV is flanked by segmental duplications with >99% sequence identity, a characteristic common of genomic disorders. Although the 16p11.2 deletion appears to have more severe phenotypic consequences than the duplication, the finding of asymptomatic carriers and variable penetrance for both the 16p11.2 and *SHANK3* CNVs suggests that interpretation of their significance is complex.

Notably, some large, well-powered studies have failed to identify the 16p11.2 CNV at elevated frequency in cases compared to controls (Glessner et al., 2009). Nonetheless, the frequency of CNVs of *SHANK3* and 16p11.2 suggests that these variants should be given careful consideration in a clinical diagnostic setting.

Considerations for CNV findings in Autism Spectrum Disorders

The frequency of CNVs reported in the studies above probably represents an underestimate, as balanced rearrangements cannot be identified, and syndromic cases of autism were excluded from the majority of these studies. Although rare copy number variants can be detected by genomewide SNP arrays in contrast to rare SNPs, which are not well represented (see above), the resolution of detection is limited by current technology, and the semiquantitative methods for CNV detection may be more error prone than those for SNP genotyping. Furthermore, while common CNV associations can be identified as described above for SNPs, the same principles for demonstration of statistically significant association with disease apply for rare CNVs as for rare SNPs, leading several groups to adopt a cumulative CNV frequency or mutation burden approach. Moreover, it is not yet known whether CNVs are effectively a monogenic cause of ASD, or contribute only as risk factors in the presence of other susceptibility variants. Notably, several of these studies again report findings from overlapping patient cohorts, therefore further studies in independent samples are required. Hence, differentiating pathogenic from nonpathogenic CNVs will be challenging, and empirical evidence to demonstrate how a CNV affects gene function or expression will be required in order to identify CNVs that are causally related to disease.

Genetic Risk Variants Do Not Obey Diagnostic Boundaries

Autism spectrum disorders are a group of behaviorally defined heterogeneous disorders with diverse symptoms. A growing body of genetic research supports the concept of an ASD continuum, or "the autisms," with an increasingly blurred distinction of the relationship between ASDs, mental retardation (MR), and other psychiatric and neurodevelopmental disorders. This is supported by the observation of many individuals with isolated difficulties in one aspect of the triad of autistic impairments of a severity comparable to autism (Ronald et al., 2006). The current edition of the *Diagnostic and Statistical Manual of Mental Disorders* (DSM-IV) identifies nearly 300 subcategories of psychiatric disorder (Abbott, 2008), and the boundaries between these subcategories evolve with time. Indeed, a recent study of adults with a history of developmental language disorder supports evidence for diagnostic substitution in autism, as 8 of 38 individuals met criteria for autism using contemporary diagnostic instruments, and 4 met criteria for milder forms of ASD (Bishop et al., 2008).

The suggestion that the same genetic variants arising on a different genetic background may give rise to a different phenotype is illustrated by the *SHANK3* and 16p11.2 microdeletions described above. A rare 15q13.3 microdeletion between the distal breakpoints of the Prader-Willi/Angelman locus identified in approximately 0.3% of individuals with mental retardation (Sharp et al., 2008) was also observed in two studies of copy number variation in schizophrenia in 0.17% cases versus 0.02% population controls, and in nine cases and no controls (Stefansson et al., 2008; Stone et al., 2008). This microdeletion also segregates with autism in a family with three affected male siblings (Pagnamenta et al., 2009). Very rare nonsense and missense mutations have also been identified in individuals with nonsyndromic autism in the neuroligin genes *NLGN4* and *NLGN3* (Jamain et al., 2003), and in a pedigree with MR and ASD (Laumonnier et al., 2004), and a familial deletion of *NLGN4* was also observed in a family with autism, Tourette syndrome, ADHD, depression, and anxiety (Lawson-Yuen et al., 2008). Hence, the same copy number variants and rare variants may lead to an array of abnormal neurobehavioral phenotypes, and clinical presentation may be modulated by additional interacting factors such as common genetic variation. This suggests that combining data from multiple studies may enable researchers to leverage this genetic heterogeneity to identify phenotypic signatures related to the underlying genetics. The possible utility of this approach is hinted at by the identification of mutations and CNVs of chromosome 22q13 including *SHANK3*, where an individual with the deletion presented with autism and severe language delay, whereas her brother with the duplication had Asperger's syndrome and precocious language development (Durand et al., 2007). This necessitates a "bottom-up" approach to genetic homogeneity, rather than the "top-down" phenotypic approach suggested using autism subphenotypes above, and indicates that individuals within the grey areas of phenotypic overlap between disorders and mixed clinical samples may be required to identify genetic boundaries and commonalities. This latter approach is being explored by the Psychiatric Genomewide Association Study Consortium, which aims to carry out cross-disorder meta-analysis of genomewide association data of 59,000 individuals from studies of autism, bipolar disorder, ADHD, major depressive disorder, and schizophrenia to identify convincing genotype-phenotype associations common to two or more disorders, and associated comorbidities (The Psychiatric GWAS Consortium Steering Committee, 2009).

Should We Have Paid More Attention to Penetrant Monogenic Causes of Autism Spectrum Disorders?

There is a significant body of published research showing that autism is observed at a higher than expected frequency in disorders due to single genetic abnormalities, for example, in Fragile X syndrome or tuberous sclerosis (reviewed in Zafeiriou et al., 2007). Moreover, methyl-CpG-binding protein 2 (*MECP2*) was identified as the gene mutated in Rett syndrome, an autism spectrum disorder (Amir et al., 1999). The growing list of genetic abnormalities that appear to be sufficient to result in an ASD phenotype further supports the concept of a continuum of autisms, and fractionation of the ASD phenotype. This is similar to mental retardation, where the collective phenotype is attributable to many relatively rare penetrant mutations, each accounting for a small percentage of cases (Chelly et al., 2006). In the case of MR, array-CGH has a successful history of identification of de novo submicroscopic chromosome aberrations, and particularly in those individuals with dysmorphic features. This suggests that Mendelian disorders could contribute significantly to our understanding of genetic susceptibility to phenotypically related common complex disorders. Does this mean that most published genetic studies of ASD have minimized our chances of identifying risk variants by excluding those individuals, for example, with dysmorphology? The answer to this question depends on the unknown underlying genetic architecture, in which increased power from sample homogeneity is balanced against biological insight into disease pathogenesis offered by identification of more rare variants.

What Can Linkage, Association, and Copy Number Variation Studies Tell Us About the Genetic Architecture of Autism Spectrum Disorders?

As discussed previously, the unknown genetic architecture of ASDs impacts on the likely success of different approaches to identify risk variants. The question of how many variants contribute to ASD susceptibility within an individual, within a population, and between populations, and the relative frequency of these variants, is still largely unknown. The high heritability of the distinct core domains of ASD and the occurrence of related autistic traits and rapidly decreasing recurrence rates of autism in relatives with decreasing genetic relatedness supports the influence of several common genetic variants. However, the influence of a small number of genes should have been identified by linkage or association studies, even allowing for the presence of multiple disease alleles at each locus (allelic heterogeneity) in the case of linkage. In contrast, the difference in monozygotic to dizygotic twin concordance rates in autism (Bailey et al., 1995; Folstein & Rutter, 1977; Steffenburg et al., 1989) is consistent with the contribution of multiple rare variants (Risch, 1990). It has been suggested that the reduced fecundity associated with severe psychiatric disorders negatively selects against risk alleles, and this may explain why common variants that increase risk in disorders such as autism, schizophrenia, and mental retardation have not been consistently identified (Stefansson et al., 2008). This suggests that rare variants may account for a larger fraction of disease risk than previously assumed, and is supported by the identification of possible etiological CNVs at relatively low frequency.

The finding of increased de novo CNV rates in simplex compared to multiplex families (Sebat et al., 2007; Marshall et al., 2008) suggests that different genetic mechanisms may contribute to ASD risk in these families, namely spontaneous mutation and inherited variation, although the presence of identical de novo CNVs in multiple affected siblings suggests that paternal or maternal germline mosaicism may contribute to autism pathogenesis. This also raises the intriguing possibility of somatic mosaicism and the suggestion that CNVs may be differentially expressed in different tissue types. The relatively high incidence of de novo CNVs in autism (Sebat et al., 2007; Marshall et al., 2008) and schizophrenia (Stefansson et al., 2008; Stone et al., 2008; Xu et al., 2008), but relatively low population frequency again suggests the action of negative selection. A recent formal analysis of recurrence risk in multiplex families with autism suggested that the data is consistent with a significant contribution from two major risk categories: a majority of low-risk families in which autism is caused by de novo mutations with high penetrance in males and relatively poor penetrance in females, where there is little genetic risk for autism in other family members; and a minority of high-risk families in which there is dominant inheritance in males transmitted from these unaffected carrier females (Zhao et al., 2007).

It seems likely that the majority of nonsyndromic autism is caused by a combination of common and rare variants, with common variants exerting a subtle effect on the ASD phenotype and rare mutations exerting a more major effect. It is not yet known whether rare de novo events represent effectively monogenic forms of ASD, cause specific ASD endophenotypes, or interact as modifiers of common variant effects, as suggested by the variable phenotypic presentation. Similarly, it is not known whether the complex genetics of autism converges on a single genetic pathway, or multiple distinct pathways. Increased knowledge of two-locus or higher order interactions between variants will lead to better understanding of the mechanisms underlying autism pathogenesis. Studies of large multigenerational families are needed in order to assess the segregation and penetrance of putative risk variants and how distinct variants interact. The effects of gender and modifying variables such as environmental exposures or the influence of epigenetics, together with stochastic effects, also need to be incorporated into genetic models.

Epigenetic: heritable genetic variation that is not due to changes in DNA sequence.

Increasing Sample Sizes and the Challenge of Data Interpretation

In recent years, genetic research in autism has moved from the challenge of overinterpretation of too little data to the challenge of mining the wealth of data generated by increasingly high-throughput genomic technologies and expanding sample cohorts. This data must be collated, stored, and analyzed, posing a computational and statistical hurdle.

While the absence of more significant linkage results from the Autism Genome Project study (Szatmari et al., 2007) suggests that future increases in sample size may not lead to more significant linkage findings, genomewide association and CNV studies of common complex disease generally have illustrated that the more samples the better for detection of common variants of moderate effect and rare risk alleles. These studies are facilitated by large consortia and publically available resources such as the Autism Genetic Resource Exchange (AGRE). The drive by funding bodies and scientists toward a more holistic, interdisciplinary approach, the implementation of infrastructures to support data sharing between investigators, and the impetus to make biomaterials and genotype data available to the scientific community has both a positive and negative impact on scientific research. While publically available resources lead to a wealth of informative analyses using different approaches, this also leads to multiple reporting and nonindependence of results, so that repeated publication of the same or partially overlapping data becomes accepted "fact" in the autism literature. This is exacerbated by individuals with autism and their families who are motivated to participate in multiple studies, leading to resampling of the same individuals. The pressing need for sample sizes considerably larger than those currently available is supported by online resources such as the Interactive Autism Network (IAN: http://www.ianproject.org/). Population-based samples such as these and epidemiological cohorts allow exploration of the boundaries and overlap between genetic and clinical presentation, but lead to a conflict between broad-brush phenotyping and large samples via Web-based resources, versus the need for detailed diagnoses and phenotyping.

Conclusions

The last decade of research into the genetics of autism spectrum disorders has been notable for the general lack of reproducibility of results from whole genome linkage and candidate gene association studies. However, recent advances in genomic technology now provide greater ability to assay genetic variation, enabling genomewide association and copy number variation studies. It remains to be seen whether the findings of published and ongoing genomewide association studies will prove to be more consistent than those from previous candidate gene association studies. Nonetheless, several copy number variants and rare mutations that appear to increase risk of autism have been recently discovered by multiple groups. The identification of associated variants, structural variation, and rare sequence mutations in genes such as *CNTNAP2, CDH10, SHANK3, NRXN1,* and the neuroligin genes is beginning to offer insight into the underlying biology, suggesting that genes involved in the postsynaptic density, neuronal cell-adhesion, and glutamatergic synaptogenesis may be involved in susceptibility to ASD. Some of these genes are also implicated in mental retardation and other neurodevelopmental and psychiatric disorders. These findings have led to a clear shift in thinking about the genetic basis of autism, indicating extensive genetic heterogeneity with the likely contribution of both common and rare variation in multiple genes with diverse functions. As technologies emerge for genetic research into complex neurodevelopmental disorders, theories of causality also evolve, and the technologies and theories regarded as state of the art and complex today will probably be regarded as routine and simplistic tomorrow. In spite of this, significant progress in understanding the genetic variation underlying ASD has been made in the last 2 to 3 years. This suggests that despite major challenges, there is cause for optimism for continued discovery of autism risk variants and illumination of the etiological biological mechanisms.

Challenges and Future Directions

- The identification of multiple rare mutations and CNVs that are involved in ASD susceptibility suggests that large consortia and convergent interdisciplinary approaches will be required to further elucidate the risk variants and biological pathways involved. This need for large sample sizes conflicts with the need for improved phenotypic resolution.
- The real translational benefit from this genetic research is likely to come from an improved understanding of disease mechanisms and risk in the population.
- Considerable in vitro and in vivo functional evidence will be required to demonstrate causality of putative risk variants, and to understand how they influence clinical presentation.
- The likely etiological overlap with other neurodevelopmental and psychiatric disorders suggests that epidemiological and longitudinal studies will be required to identify additional genetic, epigenetic, environmental, and stochastic risk factors and to understand how these different risk factors interact functionally. This complicates potential therapeutic translation and hinders progress to effective generic or personalized clinical intervention.
- The rapid development of next generation sequencing technologies means that in the near future the genomes of individuals with autism will likely be investigated at nucleotide resolution, bringing with it the challenge of managing and interpreting this wealth of biological data.

SUGGESTED READING

O'Roak, B. J., & State, M. W. (2008). Autism genetics: Strategies, challenges, and opportunities. *Autism Research, 1*(1), 4–17.

McCarthy, M. I., Abecasis, G. R., Cardon, L. R., Goldstein, D. B., Little, J, Ioannidis, J. P., et al. (2008). Genome-wide association studies for complex traits: Consensus, uncertainty, and challenges. *Nature Reviews Genetics, 9*(5), 356–369.

Feuk, L., Marshall, C. R., Wintle, R. F., & Scherer, S. W. (2006). Structural variants: Changing the landscape of chromosomes, design of disease studies. *Human Molecular Genetics, 15* (Spec No 1), R57–66.

REFERENCES

Abbott, A. (2008). Psychiatric genetics: The brains of the family. *Nature, 454*, 154–157.

Abrahams, B. S., & Geschwind, D. H. (2008). Advances in autism genetics: on the threshold of a new neurobiology. *Nature Reviews Genetics, 9*, 341–355.

Alarcon, M., Abrahams, B. S., Stone, J. L., Duvall, J. A., Perederiy, J. V., Bomar, J. M., et al. (2008). Linkage, association, and gene-expression analyses identify CNTNAP2 as an autism-susceptibility gene. *American Journal of Human Genetics, 82*, 150–159.

Alarcon, M., Cantor, R. M., Liu, J., Gilliam, T. C., & Geschwind, D. H. (2002). Evidence for a language quantitative trait locus on chromosome 7q in multiplex autism families. *American Journal of Human Genetics, 70*, 60–71.

Alarcon, M., Yonan, A. L., Gilliam, T. C., Cantor, R. M., & Geschwind, D. H. (2005). Quantitative genome scan and ordered-subsets analysis of autism endophenotypes support language QTLs. *Molecular Psychiatry, 10*, 747–757.

Alders, M., Hogan, B. M., Gjini, E., Salehi, F., Al-Gazali, L., Hennekam, E. A., et al. (2009). Mutations in CCBE1 cause generalized lymph vessel dysplasia in humans. *Nature Genetics, 41*, 1272–1274.

Allen-Brady, K., Miller, J., Matsunami, N., Stevens, J., Block, H., Farley, M., et al. (2008). A high-density SNP genome-wide linkage scan in a large autism extended pedigree. *Molecular Psychiatry, 14*(6), 590–600.

Altshuler, D., & Daly, M. (2007). Guilt beyond a reasonable doubt. *Nature Genetics, 39*, 813–815.

Amir, R. E., Van den Veyver, I. B., Wan, M., Tran, C. Q., Francke, U., & Zoghbi, H. Y. (1999). Rett syndrome is caused by mutations in X-linked MECP2, encoding methyl-CpG-binding protein 2. *Nature Genetics, 23*, 185–188.

Arking, D. E., Cutler, D. J., Brune, C. W., Teslovich, T. M., West, K., Ikeda, M., et al. (2008). A common genetic variant in the neurexin superfamily member CNTNAP2 increases familial risk of autism. *American Journal of Human Genetics, 82*, 160–164.

Auranen, M., Vanhala, R., Varilo, T., Ayers, K., Kempas, E., Ylisaukko-Oja, T., et al. (2002). A genomewide screen for autism-spectrum disorders: evidence for a major susceptibility locus on chromosome 3q25-27. *American Journal of Human Genetics, 71*, 777–790.

Auranen, M., Varilo, T., Alen, R., Vanhala, R., Ayers, K., Kempas, E., et al. (2003). Evidence for allelic association on chromosome 3q25-27 in families with autism spectrum disorders originating from a subisolate of Finland. *Molecular Psychiatry, 8*, 879–884.

Badner, J. A., & Gershon, E. S. (2002). Regional meta-analysis of published data supports linkage of autism with markers on chromosome 7. *Molecular Psychiatry, 7*, 56–66.

Bailey, A., Le Couteur, A., Gottesman, I., Bolton, P., Simonoff, E., Yuzda, E., et al. (1995). Autism as a strongly genetic disorder: evidence from a British twin study. *Psychological Medicine, 25*, 63–77.

Bailey, A., Palferman, S., Heavey, L., & Le Couteur, A. (1998). Autism: the phenotype in relatives. *Journal of Autism and Developmental Disorders, 28*, 369–392.

Baird, G., Simonoff, E., Pickles, A., Chandler, S., Loucas, T., Meldrum, D., et al. (2006). Prevalence of disorders of the autism spectrum in a population cohort of children in South Thames: the Special Needs and Autism Project (SNAP). *Lancet, 368*, 210–215.

Bakkaloglu, B., O'Roak, B. J., Louvi, A., Gupta, A. R., Abelson, J. F., Morgan, T. M., et al. (2008). Molecular cytogenetic analysis and resequencing of contactin associated protein-like 2 in autism spectrum disorders. *American Journal of Human Genetics, 82*, 165–173.

Barrett, J. C., & Cardon, L. R. (2006). Evaluating coverage of genome-wide association studies. *Nature Genetics, 38*, 659–662.

Barrett, S., Beck, J. C., Bernier, R., Bisson, E., Braun, T. A., Casavant, T. L., et al. (1999). An autosomal genomic screen for autism. Collaborative linkage study of autism. *American Journal of Medical Genetics, 88*, 609–615.

Bartlett, C. W., & Vieland, V. J. (2007). Accumulating quantitative trait linkage evidence across multiple datasets using the posterior probability of linkage. *Genetic Epidemiology, 31*, 91–102.

Belloso, J. M., Bache, I., Guitart, M., Caballin, M. R., Halgren, C., Kirchhoff, M., et al. (2007). Disruption of the CNTNAP2 gene in a t(7;15) translocation family without symptoms of Gilles de la Tourette syndrome. *European Journal of Human Genetics, 15*, 711–713.

Birney, E., Stamatoyannopoulos, J. A., Dutta, A., Guigo, R., Gingeras, T. R., Margulies, E. H., et al. (2007). Identification and analysis of functional elements in 1% of the human genome by the ENCODE pilot project. *Nature, 447*, 799–816.

Bishop, D. V., Whitehouse, A. J., Watt, H. J., & Line, E. A. (2008). Autism and diagnostic substitution: evidence from a study of adults with a history of developmental language disorder. *Developmental Medicine and Child Neurology, 50*, 341–345.

Bolton, P., Macdonald, H., Pickles, A., Rios, P., Goode, S., Crowson, M., et al. (1994). A case-control family history study of autism. *Journal of Child Psychology and Psychiatry, 35*, 877–900.

Bradford, Y., Haines, J., Hutcheson, H., Gardiner, M., Braun, T., Sheffield, V., et al. (2001). Incorporating language phenotypes strengthens evidence of linkage to autism. *American Journal of Medical Genetics, 105*, 539–547.

Burdick, J. T., Chen, W. M., Abecasis, G. R., & Cheung, V. G. (2006). In silico method for inferring genotypes in pedigrees. *Nature Genetics, 38*, 1002–1004.

Butler, M. G., Dasouki, M. J., Zhou, X. P., Talebizadeh, Z., Brown, M., Takahashi, T. N., et al. (2005). Subset of individuals with autism spectrum disorders and extreme macrocephaly associated with germline PTEN tumour suppressor gene mutations. *Journal of Medical Genetics, 42*, 318–321.

Buxbaum, J. D., Cai, G., Chaste, P., Nygren, G., Goldsmith, J., Reichert, J., et al. (2007). Mutation screening of the PTEN gene in patients with autism spectrum disorders and macrocephaly. *American Journal of Medical Genetics. Part B, Neuropsychiatric Genetics, 144B*, 484–491.

Buxbaum, J. D., Silverman, J., Keddache, M., Smith, C. J., Hollander, E., Ramoz, N., et al. (2004). Linkage analysis for autism in a subset families with obsessive-compulsive behaviors: evidence for an autism susceptibility gene on chromosome 1 and further support for susceptibility genes on chromosome 6 and 19. *Molecular Psychiatry, 9*, 144–150.

Buxbaum, J. D., Silverman, J. M., Smith, C. J., Kilifarski, M., Reichert, J., Hollander, E., et al. (2001). Evidence for a susceptibility gene for autism on chromosome 2 and for genetic heterogeneity. *American Journal of Human Genetics, 68*, 1514–1520.

Campbell, D. B., D'Oronzio, R., Garbett, K., Ebert, P. J., Mirnics, K., Levitt, P., et al. (2007). Disruption of cerebral cortex MET signaling in autism spectrum disorder. *Annals of Neurology, 62*, 243–250.

Campbell, D. B., Sutcliffe, J. S., Ebert, P. J., Militerni, R., Bravaccio, C., Trillo, S., et al. (2006). A genetic variant that disrupts MET transcription is associated with autism. *Proceedings of the National Academy of Sciences of the United States of America, 103*, 16834–16839.

Cantor, R. M., Kono, N., Duvall, J. A., Alvarez-Retuerto, A., Stone, J. L., Alarcon, M., et al. (2005). Replication of autism linkage: fine-mapping peak at 17q21. *American Journal of Human Genetics, 76*, 1050–1056.

Chanock, S. J., Manolio, T., Boehnke, M., Boerwinkle, E., Hunter, D. J., Thomas, G., et al. (2007). Replicating genotype-phenotype associations. *Nature, 447*, 655–660.

Chelly, J., Khelfaoui, M., Francis, F., Cherif, B., & Bienvenu, T. (2006). Genetics and pathophysiology of mental retardation. *European Journal of Human Genetics, 14*, 701–713.

Christian, S. L., Brune, C. W., Sudi, J., Kumar, R. A., Liu, S., Karamohamed, S., et al. (2008). Novel submicroscopic chromosomal abnormalities detected in autism spectrum disorder. *Biological Psychiatry, 63*, 1111–1117.

Conrad, D. F., Pinto, D., Redon, R., Feuk, L., Gokcumen, O., Zhang, Y., et al. (2009). Origins and functional impact of copy number variation in the human genome. *Nature, 464*, 704–712.

Constantino, J. N., Gruber, C. P., Davis, S., Hayes, S., Passanante, N., & Przybeck, T. (2004). The factor structure of autistic traits. *Journal of Child Psychology and Psychiatry, 45*, 719–726.

Cope, N., Harold, D., Hill, G., Moskvina, V., Stevenson, J., Holmans, P., et al. (2005). Strong evidence that KIAA0319 on chromosome 6p is a susceptibility gene for developmental dyslexia. *American Journal of Human Genetics, 76*, 581–591.

Craddock, N., O'Donovan, M. C., & Owen, M. J. (2008). Genome-wide association studies in psychiatry: lessons from early studies of non-psychiatric and psychiatric phenotypes. *Molecular Psychiatry, 13*, 649–653.

Dennis, M. Y., Paracchini, S., Scerri, T. S., Prokunina-Olsson, L., Knight, J. C., Wade-Martins, R., et al. (2009). A common variant associated with dyslexia reduces expression of the KIAA0319 gene. *PLoS Genetics, 5*, e1000436.

Devlin, B., & Roeder, K. (1999). Genomic control for association studies. *Biometrics, 55*, 997–1004.

Dixon, A. L., Liang, L., Moffatt, M. F., Chen, W., Heath, S., Wong, K. C., et al. (2007). A genome-wide association study of global gene expression. *Nature Genetics, 39*, 1202–1207.

Durand, C. M., Betancur, C., Boeckers, T. M., Bockmann, J., Chaste, P., Fauchereau, F., et al. (2007). Mutations in the gene encoding the synaptic scaffolding protein SHANK3 are associated with autism spectrum disorders. *Nature Genetics, 39*, 25–27.

Duvall, J. A., Lu, A., Cantor, R. M., Todd, R. D., Constantino, J. N., & Geschwind, D. H. (2007). A quantitative trait locus analysis of social responsiveness in multiplex autism families. *American Journal of Psychiatry, 164*, 656–662.

Easton, D. F., Pooley, K. A., Dunning, A. M., Pharoah, P. D., Thompson, D., Ballinger, D. G., et al. (2007). Genome-wide association study identifies novel breast cancer susceptibility loci. *Nature, 447*, 1087–1093.

Eichler, E. E., Nickerson, D. A., Altshuler, D., Bowcock, A. M., Brooks, L. D., Carter, N. P., et al. (2007). Completing the map of human genetic variation. *Nature, 447*, 161–165.

Erdmann, J., Grosshennig, A., Braund, P. S., Konig, I. R., Hengstenberg, C., Hall, A. S., et al. (2009). New susceptibility locus for coronary artery disease on chromosome 3q22.3. *Nature Genetics, 41*, 280–282.

Feuk, L., Carson, A. R., & Scherer, S. W. (2006). Structural variation in the human genome. *Nature Reviews Genetics, 7*, 85–97.

Fisher, S. E., Francks, C., Marlow, A. J., MacPhie, I. L., Newbury, D. F., Cardon, L. R., et al. (2002). Independent genome-wide scans identify a chromosome 18 quantitative-trait locus influencing dyslexia. *Nature Genetics, 30*, 86–91.

Fisher, S. E., Marlow, A. J., Lamb, J., Maestrini, E., Williams, D. F., Richardson, A. J., et al. (1999). A quantitative-trait locus on chromosome 6p influences different aspects of developmental dyslexia. *American Journal of Human Genetics, 64*, 146–156.

Flint, J., & Munafo, M. R. (2007). The endophenotype concept in psychiatric genetics. *Psychological Medicine, 37*, 163–180.

Folstein, S., & Rutter, M. (1977). Infantile autism: a genetic study of 21 twin pairs. *Journal of Child Psychology and Psychiatry, 18*, 297–321.

Folstein, S. E., Santangelo, S. L., Gilman, S. E., Piven, J., Landa, R., Lainhart, J., et al. (1999). Predictors of cognitive test patterns in autism families. *Journal of Child Psychology and Psychiatry, 40*, 1117–1128.

Fombonne, E. (2005). Epidemiology of autistic disorder and other pervasive developmental disorders. *Journal of Clinical Psychiatry, 66*(Suppl 10), 3–8.

Francks, C., Paracchini, S., Smith, S. D., Richardson, A. J., Scerri, T. S., Cardon, L. R., et al. (2004). A 77-kilobase region of chromosome 6p22.2 is associated with dyslexia in families from the United Kingdom and from the United States. *American Journal of Human Genetics, 75*, 1046–1058.

Fraser, M. M., Bayazitov, I. T., Zakharenko, S. S., & Baker, S. J. (2008). Phosphatase and tensin homolog, deleted on chromosome 10 deficiency in brain causes defects in synaptic structure, transmission and plasticity, and myelination abnormalities. *Neuroscience, 151*, 476–488.

Frayling, T. M., Timpson, N. J., Weedon, M. N., Zeggini, E., Freathy, R. M., Lindgren, C. M., et al. (2007). A common variant in the FTO gene is associated with body mass index and predisposes to childhood and adult obesity. *Science, 316*, 889–894.

Frazer, K. A., Ballinger, D. G., Cox, D. R., Hinds, D. A., Stuve, L. L., Gibbs, R. A., et al. (2007). A second generation human haplotype map of over 3.1 million SNPs. *Nature, 449*, 851–861.

Freimer, N. B., & Sabatti, C. (2005). Guidelines for association studies in Human Molecular Genetics. *Human Molecular Genetics, 14*, 2481–2483.

Friedman, J. I., Vrijenhoek, T., Markx, S., Janssen, I. M., van der Vliet, W. A., Faas, B. H., et al. (2008). CNTNAP2 gene dosage variation is associated with schizophrenia and epilepsy. *Molecular Psychiatry, 13*, 261–266.

Glatt, C. E., DeYoung, J. A., Delgado, S., Service, S. K., Giacomini, K. M., Edwards, R. H., et al. (2001). Screening a large reference sample to identify very low frequency sequence variants: comparisons between two genes. *Nature Genetics, 27*, 435–438.

Glessner, J. T., Wang, K., Cai, G., Korvatska, O., Kim, C. E., Wood, S., et al. (2009). Autism genome-wide copy number variation reveals ubiquitin and neuronal genes. *Nature, 459*, 569–573.

Gregg, J. P., Lit, L., Baron, C. A., Hertz-Picciotto, I., Walker, W., Davis, R. A., et al. (2008). Gene expression changes in children with autism. *Genomics, 91*, 22–29.

Gupta, A. R., & State, M. W. (2007). Recent advances in the genetics of autism. *Biological Psychiatry, 61*, 429–437.

Happe, F., Ronald, A., & Plomin, R. (2006). Time to give up on a single explanation for autism. *Nature Neuroscience, 9*, 1218–1220.

Harold, D., Paracchini, S., Scerri, T., Dennis, M., Cope, N., Hill, G., et al. (2006). Further evidence that the KIAA0319 gene confers susceptibility to developmental dyslexia. *Molecular Psychiatry, 11*, 1085–91, 1061.

Helgadottir, A., Thorleifsson, G., Manolescu, A., Gretarsdottir, S., Blondal, T., Jonasdottir, A., et al. (2007). A common variant on chromosome 9p21 affects the risk of myocardial infarction. *Science, 316*, 1491–1493.

Herman, G. E., Butter, E., Enrile, B., Pastore, M., Prior, T. W., & Sommer, A. (2007). Increasing knowledge of PTEN germline mutations: Two additional patients with autism and macrocephaly. *American Journal of Medical Genetics. Part A, 143*, 589–593.

Himes, B. E., Hunninghake, G. M., Baurley, J. W., Rafaels, N. M., Sleiman, P., Strachan, D. P., et al. (2009). Genome-wide association analysis identifies PDE4D as an asthma-susceptibility gene. *American Journal of Human Genetics, 84*, 581–593.

Hu, V. W., Frank, B. C., Heine, S., Lee, N. H., & Quackenbush, J. (2006). Gene expression profiling of lymphoblastoid cell lines from monozygotic twins discordant in severity of autism reveals differential regulation of neurologically relevant genes. *BMC Genomics, 7*, 118.

Iles, M. M. (2008). What can genome-wide association studies tell us about the genetics of common disease? *PLoS Genetics, 4*, e33.

International HapMap Consortium. (2003). The International HapMap Project. *Nature, 426*, 789–796.

International HapMap Consortium. (2005). A haplotype map of the human genome. *Nature, 437*, 1299–1320.

International Human Genome Sequencing Consortium. (2004). Finishing the euchromatic sequence of the human genome. *Nature, 431*, 931–945.

International Molecular Genetic Study of Autism Consortium (IMGSAC). (1998). A full genome screen for autism with evidence for linkage to a region on chromosome 7q. *Human Molecular Genetics, 7*, 571–578.

International Molecular Genetic Study of Autism Consortium (IMGSAC). (2001). A genomewide screen for autism: strong evidence for linkage to chromosomes 2q, 7q, and 16p. *American Journal of Human Genetics, 69*, 570–581.

Jacquemont, M. L., Sanlaville, D., Redon, R., Raoul, O., Cormier-Daire, V., Lyonnet, S., et al. (2006). Array-based comparative genomic hybridisation identifies high frequency of cryptic chromosomal rearrangements in patients with syndromic autism spectrum disorders. *Journal of Medical Genetics, 43*, 843–849.

Jamain, S., Quach, H., Betancur, C., Rastam, M., Colineaux, C., Gillberg, I. C., et al. (2003). Mutations of the X-linked genes encoding neuroligins NLGN3 and NLGN4 are associated with autism. *Nature Genetics, 34*, 27–29.

Ji, W., Foo, J. N., O'Roak, B. J., Zhao, H., Larson, M. G., Simon, D. B., et al. (2008). Rare independent mutations in renal salt handling genes contribute to blood pressure variation. *Nature Genetics, 40*, 592–599.

Korbel, J. O., Urban, A. E., Affourtit, J. P., Godwin, B., Grubert, F., Simons, J. F., et al. (2007). Paired-end mapping reveals extensive structural variation in the human genome. *Science, 318*, 420–426.

Kumar, R. A., Karamohamed, S., Sudi, J., Conrad, D. F., Brune, C., Badner, J. A., et al. (2008). Recurrent 16p11.2 microdeletions in autism. *Human Molecular Genetics, 17*, 628–638.

Kwon, C. H., Luikart, B. W., Powell, C. M., Zhou, J., Matheny, S. A., Zhang, W., et al. (2006). Pten regulates neuronal arborization and social interaction in mice. *Neuron, 50*, 377–388.

Lainhart, J. E. (2006). Advances in autism neuroimaging research for the clinician and geneticist. *American Journal of Medical Genetics. Part C, Seminars in Medical Genetics, 142C*, 33–39.

Lamb, J. A., Barnby, G., Bonora, E., Sykes, N., Bacchelli, E., Blasi, F., et al. (2005). Analysis of IMGSAC autism susceptibility loci: evidence for sex limited and parent of origin specific effects. *Journal of Medical Genetics, 42*, 132–137.

Lander, E., & Kruglyak, L. (1995). Genetic dissection of complex traits: guidelines for interpreting and reporting linkage results. *Nature Genetics, 11*, 241–247.

Laumonnier, F., Bonnet-Brilhault, F., Gomot, M., Blanc, R., David, A., Moizard, M. P., et al. (2004). X-linked mental retardation and autism are associated with a mutation in the NLGN4 gene, a member of the neuroligin family. *American Journal of Human Genetics, 74*, 552–557.

Lawson-Yuen, A., Saldivar, J. S., Sommer, S., & Picker, J. (2008). Familial deletion within NLGN4 associated with autism and Tourette syndrome. *European Journal of Human Genetics, 16*, 614–618.

Lettre, G., Jackson, A. U., Gieger, C., Schumacher, F. R., Berndt, S. I., Sanna, S., et al. (2008). Identification of ten loci associated with height highlights new biological pathways in human growth. *Nature Genetics, 40*, 584–591.

Liu, J., Nyholt, D. R., Magnussen, P., Parano, E., Pavone, P., Geschwind, D., et al. (2001). A genomewide screen for autism susceptibility loci. *American Journal of Human Genetics, 69*, 327–340.

Liu, X.-Q., Paterson, A. D., Szatmari, P., & The Autism Genome Project Consortium (2008). Genome-wide linkage analyses of quantitative and categorical autism sub-phenotypes. *Biological Psychiatry, 64*, 561–570.

Loos, R. J., Lindgren, C. M., Li, S., Wheeler, E., Zhao, J. H., Prokopenko, I., et al. (2008). Common variants near MC4R are associated with fat mass, weight and risk of obesity. *Nature Genetics, 40*, 768–775.

Ma, D. Q., Cuccaro, M. L., Jaworski, J. M., Haynes, C. S., Stephan, D. A., Parod, J., et al. (2007). Dissecting the locus heterogeneity of autism: significant linkage to chromosome 12q14. *Molecular Psychiatry, 12*, 376–384.

Maestrini, E., Pagnamenta, A. T., Lamb, J. A., Bacchelli, E., Sykes, N. H., Sousa, I., et al. (2009). High-density SNP association study and copy number variation analysis of the AUTS1 and AUTS5 loci implicate the IMMP2L-DOCK4 gene region in autism susceptibility. *Molecular Psychiatry, 15*, 954–968.

Mailman, M. D., Feolo, M., Jin, Y., Kimura, M., Tryka, K., Bagoutdinov, R., et al. (2007). The NCBI dbGaP database of genotypes and phenotypes. *Nature Genetics, 39*, 1181–1186.

Manolio, T. A., Rodriguez, L. L., Brooks, L., Abecasis, G., Ballinger, D., Daly, M., et al. (2007). New models of collaboration in genome-wide association studies: the Genetic Association Information Network. *Nature Genetics, 39*, 1045–1051.

Marchini, J., Howie, B., Myers, S., McVean, G., & Donnelly, P. (2007). A new multipoint method for genome-wide association studies by imputation of genotypes. *Nature Genetics, 39*, 906–913.

Margulies, M., Egholm, M., Altman, W. E., Attiya, S., Bader, J. S., Bemben, L. A., et al. (2005). Genome sequencing in microfabricated high-density picolitre reactors. *Nature, 437*, 376–380.

Marlow, A. J., Fisher, S. E., Francks, C., MacPhie, I. L., Cherny, S. S., Richardson, A. J., et al. (2003). Use of multivariate linkage analysis for dissection of a complex cognitive trait. *American Journal of Human Genetics, 72*, 561–570.

Marshall, C. R., Noor, A., Vincent, J. B., Lionel, A. C., Feuk, L., Skaug, J., et al. (2008). Structural variation of chromosomes in autism spectrum disorder. *American Journal of Human Genetics, 82*, 477–488.

McCarthy, M. I., Abecasis, G. R., Cardon, L. R., Goldstein, D. B., Little, J., Ioannidis, J. P., et al. (2008). Genome-wide association studies for complex traits: consensus, uncertainty, and challenges. *Nature Reviews Genetics, 9*, 356–369.

McCauley, J. L., Li, C., Jiang, L., Olson, L. M., Crockett, G., Gainer, K., et al. (2005). Genome-wide and ordered-subset linkage analyses provide support for autism loci on 17q and 19p with evidence of phenotypic and interlocus genetic correlates. *BMC Medical Genetics, 6*, 1.

Moessner, R., Marshall, C. R., Sutcliffe, J. S., Skaug, J., Pinto, D., Vincent, J., et al. (2007). Contribution of SHANK3 mutations to autism spectrum disorder. *American Journal of Human Genetics, 81*, 1289–1297.

Moffatt, M. F., Kabesch, M., Liang, L., Dixon, A. L., Strachan, D., Heath, S., et al. (2007). Genetic variants regulating ORMDL3 expression contribute to the risk of childhood asthma. *Nature, 448*, 470–473.

Monaco, A. P. (2007). Multivariate linkage analysis of specific language impairment (SLI). *Annals of Human Genetics, 71*, 660–673.

Morrow, E. M., Yoo, S. Y., Flavell, S. W., Kim, T. K., Lin, Y., Hill, R. S., et al. (2008). Identifying autism loci and genes by tracing recent shared ancestry. *Science, 321*, 218–223.

Nishimura, Y., Martin, C. L., Vazquez-Lopez, A., Spence, S. J., Alvarez-Retuerto, A. I., Sigman, M., et al. (2007). Genome-wide expression profiling of lymphoblastoid cell lines distinguishes different forms of autism and reveals shared pathways. *Human Molecular Genetics, 16*, 1682–1698.

Noor, A., Windpassinger, C., Patel, M., Stachowiak, B., Mikhailov, A., Azam, M., et al. (2008). CC2D2A, encoding a coiled-coil and C2 domain protein, causes autosomal-recessive mental retardation with retinitis pigmentosa. *American Journal of Human Genetics, 82*, 1011–1018.

Pagnamenta, A. T., Wing, K., Akha, E. S., Knight, S. J., Bolte, S., Schmotzer, G., et al. (2009). A 15q13.3 microdeletion segregating with autism. *European Journal of Human Genetics, 17*, 687–692.

Paracchini, S., Steer, C. D., Buckingham, L. L., Morris, A. P., Ring, S., Scerri, T., et al. (2008). Association of the KIAA0319 dyslexia susceptibility gene with reading skills in the general population. *American Journal of Psychiatry, 165*, 1576–1584.

Paracchini, S., Thomas, A., Castro, S., Lai, C., Paramasivam, M., Wang, Y., et al. (2006). The chromosome 6p22 haplotype associated with dyslexia reduces the expression of KIAA0319, a novel gene involved in neuronal migration. *Human Molecular Genetics, 15*, 1659–1666.

Pe'er, I., de Bakker, P. I., Maller, J., Yelensky, R., Altshuler, D., & Daly, M. J. (2006). Evaluating and improving power in whole-genome association studies using fixed marker sets. *Nature Genetics, 38*, 663–667.

Philippe, A., Martinez, M., Guilloud-Bataille, M., Gillberg, C., Rastam, M., Sponheim, E., et al. (1999). Genome-wide scan for autism susceptibility genes. Paris Autism Research International Sibpair Study. *Human Molecular Genetics, 8*, 805–812.

Price, A. L., Patterson, N. J., Plenge, R. M., Weinblatt, M. E., Shadick, N. A., & Reich, D. (2006). Principal components analysis corrects for stratification in genome-wide association studies. *Nature Genetics, 38*, 904–909.

Pritchard, J. K., & Cox, N. J. (2002). The allelic architecture of human disease genes: common disease-common variant . . . or not? *Human Molecular Genetics, 11*, 2417–2423.

Redon, R., Ishikawa, S., Fitch, K. R., Feuk, L., Perry, G. H., Andrews, T. D., et al. (2006). Global variation in copy number in the human genome. *Nature, 444*, 444–454.

Reich, D. E., & Lander, E. S. (2001). On the allelic spectrum of human disease. *Trends in Genetics, 17*, 502–510.

Risch, N. (1990). Linkage strategies for genetically complex traits. I: Multilocus models. *American Journal of Human Genetics, 46*, 222–228.

Risch, N., Spiker, D., Lotspeich, L., Nouri, N., Hinds, D., Hallmayer, J., et al. (1999). A genomic screen of autism: evidence for a multilocus etiology. *American Journal of Human Genetics, 65*, 493–507.

Ritvo, E. R., Jorde, L. B., Mason-Brothers, A., Freeman, B. J., Pingree, C., Jones, M. B., et al. (1989). The UCLA-University of Utah epidemiologic survey of autism: recurrence risk estimates and genetic counseling. *American Journal of Psychiatry, 146*, 1032–1036.

Romeo, S., Pennacchio, L. A., Fu, Y., Boerwinkle, E., Tybjaerg-Hansen, A., Hobbs, H. H., et al. (2007). Population-based resequencing of ANGPTL4 uncovers variations that reduce triglycerides and increase HDL. *Nature Genetics, 39*, 513–516.

Ronald, A., Happe, F., Bolton, P., Butcher, L. M., Price, T. S., Wheelwright, S., et al. (2006). Genetic heterogeneity between the three components of the autism spectrum: a twin study. *Journal of the American Academy of Child and Adolescent Psychiatry, 45*, 691–699.

Samani, N. J., Erdmann, J., Hall, A. S., Hengstenberg, C., Mangino, M., Mayer, B., et al. (2007). Genomewide association analysis of coronary artery disease. *New England Journal of Medicine, 357*, 443–453.

Sanna, S., Jackson, A. U., Nagaraja, R., Willer, C. J., Chen, W. M., Bonnycastle, L. L., et al. (2008). Common variants in the GDF5-UQCC region are associated with variation in human height. *Nature Genetics, 40*, 198–203.

Saxena, R., Voight, B. F., Lyssenko, V., Burtt, N. P., de Bakker, P. I., Chen, H., et al. (2007). Genome-wide association analysis identifies loci for type 2 diabetes and triglyceride levels. *Science, 316*, 1331–1336.

Schellenberg, G. D., Dawson, G., Sung, Y. J., Estes, A., Munson, J., Rosenthal, E., et al. (2006). Evidence for multiple loci from a genome scan of autism kindreds. *Molecular Psychiatry, 11*, 1049–60, 979.

Scott, L. J., Mohlke, K. L., Bonnycastle, L. L., Willer, C. J., Li, Y., Duren, W. L., et al. (2007). A genome-wide association study of type 2 diabetes in Finns detects multiple susceptibility variants. *Science, 316*, 1341–1345.

Sebat, J., Lakshmi, B., Malhotra, D., Troge, J., Lese-Martin, C., Walsh, T., et al. (2007). Strong association of de novo copy number mutations with autism. *Science, 316*, 445–449.

Service, R. F. (2006). Gene sequencing. The race for the $1000 genome. *Science, 311*, 1544–1546.

Shao, Y., Raiford, K. L., Wolpert, C. M., Cope, H. A., Ravan, S. A., Ashley-Koch, A. A., et al. (2002a). Phenotypic homogeneity provides increased support for linkage on chromosome 2 in autistic disorder. *American Journal of Human Genetics, 70*, 1058–1061.

Shao, Y., Wolpert, C. M., Raiford, K. L., Menold, M. M., Donnelly, S. L., Ravan, S. A., et al. (2002b). Genomic screen and follow-up analysis for autistic disorder. *American Journal of Medical Genetics, 114*, 99–105.

Sharp, A. J., Mefford, H. C., Li, K., Baker, C., Skinner, C., Stevenson, R. E., et al. (2008). A recurrent 15q13.3 microdeletion syndrome associated with mental retardation and seizures. *Nature Genetics, 40*, 322–328.

Sladek, R., Rocheleau, G., Rung, J., Dina, C., Shen, L., Serre, D., et al. (2007). A genome-wide association study identifies novel risk loci for type 2 diabetes. *Nature, 445*, 881–885.

Sousa, I., Clark, T. G., Toma, C., Kobayashi, K., Choma, M., Holt, R., et al. (2009). *MET* and autism susceptibility: an analysis of family and case-control studies. *European Journal of Human Genetics, 17*, 749–758.

Specific Language Impairment Consortium. (SLIC) (2004). Highly significant linkage to the SLI1 locus in an expanded sample of individuals affected by specific language impairment. *American Journal of Human Genetics, 74*, 1225–1238.

Stacey, S. N., Manolescu, A., Sulem, P., Rafnar, T., Gudmundsson, J., Gudjonsson, S. A., et al. (2007). Common variants on chromosomes 2q35 and 16q12 confer susceptibility to estrogen receptor-positive breast cancer. *Nature Genetics, 39*, 865–869.

Stacey, S. N., Manolescu, A., Sulem, P., Thorlacius, S., Gudjonsson, S. A., Jonsson, G. F., et al. (2008). Common variants on chromosome 5p12 confer susceptibility to estrogen receptor-positive breast cancer. *Nature Genetics, 40*, 703–706.

Stefansson, H., Rujescu, D., Cichon, S., Pietilainen, O. P., Ingason, A., Steinberg, S., et al. (2008). Large recurrent microdeletions associated with schizophrenia. *Nature, 455*, 232–236.

Steffenburg, S., Gillberg, C., Hellgren, L., Andersson, L., Gillberg, I. C., Jakobsson, G., et al. (1989). A twin study of autism in Denmark, Finland, Iceland, Norway, and Sweden. *Journal of Child Psychology and Psychiatry, 30*, 405–416.

Stone, J. L., Merriman, B., Cantor, R. M., Geschwind, D. H., & Nelson, S. F. (2007). High density SNP association study of a major autism linkage region on chromosome 17. *Human Molecular Genetics, 16*, 704–715.

Stone, J. L., Merriman, B., Cantor, R. M., Yonan, A. L., Gilliam, T. C., Geschwind, D. H., et al. (2004). Evidence for sex-specific risk alleles in autism spectrum disorder. *American Journal of Human Genetics, 75*, 1117–1123.

Stone, J. L., O'Donovan, M. C., Gurling, H., Kirov, G. K., Blackwood, D. H., Corvin, A., et al. (2008). Rare chromosomal deletions and duplications increase risk of schizophrenia. *Nature, 455*, 237–241.

Stranger, B. E., Nica, A. C., Forrest, M. S., Dimas, A., Bird, C. P., Beazley, C., et al. (2007). Population genomics of human gene expression. *Nature Genetics, 39*, 1217–1224.

Strauss, K. A., Puffenberger, E. G., Huentelman, M. J., Gottlieb, S., Dobrin, S. E., Parod, J. M., et al. (2006). Recessive symptomatic focal epilepsy and mutant contactin-associated protein-like 2. *New England Journal of Medicine, 354*, 1370–1377.

Sung, Y. J., Dawson, G., Munson, J., Estes, A., Schellenberg, G. D., & Wijsman, E. M. (2005). Genetic investigation of quantitative traits related to autism: use of multivariate polygenic models with ascertainment adjustment. *American Journal of Human Genetics, 76*, 68–81.

Szatmari, P., Paterson, A. D., Zwaigenbaum, L., Roberts, W., Brian, J., Liu, X. Q., et al. (2007). Mapping autism risk loci using genetic linkage and chromosomal rearrangements. *Nature Genetics, 39*, 319–328.

Takeuchi, F., Serizawa, M., Yamamoto, K., Fujisawa, T., Nakashima, E., Ohnaka, K., et al. (2009). Confirmation of multiple risk loci and genetic impacts by a genome-wide association study of type 2 diabetes in the Japanese population. *Diabetes, 58*, 1690–1699.

The Psychiatric GWAS Consortium Steering Committee. (2009). A framework for interpreting genome-wide association studies of psychiatric disorders. *Molecular Psychiatry, 14*, 10–17.

Trikalinos, T. A., Karvouni, A., Zintzaras, E., Ylisaukko-oja, T., Peltonen, L., Jarvela, I., et al. (2006). A heterogeneity-based genome search meta-analysis for autism-spectrum disorders. *Molecular Psychiatry, 11*, 29–36.

Trikalinos, T. A., Ntzani, E. E., Contopoulos-Ioannidis, D. G., & Ioannidis, J. P. (2004). Establishment of genetic associations for complex diseases is independent of early study findings. *European Journal of Human Genetics, 12*, 762–769.

Varga, E. A., Pastore, M., Prior, T., Herman, G. E., & McBride, K. L. (2009). The prevalence of PTEN mutations in a clinical pediatric cohort with autism spectrum disorders, developmental delay, and macrocephaly. *Genetic Medicine, 11*, 111–117.

Verkerk, A. J., Mathews, C. A., Joosse, M., Eussen, B. H., Heutink, P., & Oostra, B. A. (2003). CNTNAP2 is disrupted in a family with Gilles de la Tourette syndrome and obsessive compulsive disorder. *Genomics, 82*, 1–9.

Vieland, V. J., Wang, K., & Huang, J. (2001). Power to detect linkage based on multiple sets of data in the presence of locus heterogeneity: comparative evaluation of model-based linkage methods for affected sib pair data. *Human Heredity, 51*, 199–208.

Wang, K., Zhang, H., Ma, D., Bucan, M., Glessner, J. T., Abrahams, B. S., et al. (2009). Common genetic variants on 5p14.1 associate with autism spectrum disorders. *Nature, 459*, 528–533.

Weedon, M. N., Lango, H., Lindgren, C. M., Wallace, C., Evans, D. M., Mangino, M., et al. (2008). Genome-wide association analysis identifies 20 loci that influence adult height. *Nature Genetics, 40*, 575–583.

Weiss, L. A., Shen, Y., Korn, J. M., Arking, D. E., Miller, D. T., Fossdal, R., et al. (2008). Association between microdeletion and microduplication at 16p11.2 and autism. *New England Journal of Medicine, 358*, 667–675.

Weiss, L. A., Arking, D. E., Gene Discovery Project of Johns Hopkins & the Autism Consortium, Daly, M. J., & Chakravarti, A. (2009). A genome-wide linkage and association scan reveals novel loci for autism. *Nature, 461*, 802–808.

Wellcome Trust Case Control Consortium. (2007). Genome-wide association study of 14,000 cases of seven common diseases and 3,000 shared controls. *Nature, 447*, 661–678.

Wong, K. K., deLeeuw, R. J., Dosanjh, N. S., Kimm, L. R., Cheng, Z., Horsman, D. E., et al. (2007). A comprehensive analysis of common copy-number variations in the human genome. *American Journal of Human Genetics, 80*, 91–104.

Xu, B., Roos, J. L., Levy, S., van Rensburg, E. J., Gogos, J. A., & Karayiorgou, M. (2008). Strong association of de novo copy number mutations with sporadic schizophrenia. *Nature Genetics, 40*, 880–885.

Yonan, A. L., Alarcon, M., Cheng, R., Magnusson, P. K., Spence, S. J., Palmer, A. A., et al. (2003). A genomewide screen of 345 families for autism-susceptibility loci. *American Journal of Human Genetics, 73*, 886–897.D

Zafeiriou, D. I., Ververi, A., & Vargiami, E. (2007). Childhood autism and associated comorbidities. *Brain and Development, 29*, 257–272.

Zeggini, E., Rayner, W., Morris, A. P., Hattersley, A. T., Walker, M., Hitman, G. A., et al. (2005). An evaluation of HapMap sample size and tagging SNP performance in large-scale empirical and simulated data sets. *Nature Genetics, 37*, 1320–1322.

Zeggini, E., Scott, L. J., Saxena, R., Voight, B. F., Marchini, J. L., Hu, T., et al. (2008). Meta-analysis of genome-wide association data and large-scale replication identifies additional susceptibility loci for type 2 diabetes. *Nature Genetics, 40*, 638–645.

Zeggini, E., Weedon, M. N., Lindgren, C. M., Frayling, T. M., Elliott, K. S., Lango, H., et al. (2007). Replication of genome-wide association signals in UK samples reveals risk loci for type 2 diabetes. *Science, 316*, 1336–1341.

Zhao, X., Leotta, A., Kustanovich, V., Lajonchere, C., Geschwind, D. H., Law, K., et al. (2007). A unified genetic theory for sporadic and inherited autism. *Proceedings of the National Academy of Sciences of the United States of America, 104*, 12831–12836.

Zollner, S., & Pritchard, J. K. (2007). Overcoming the winner's curse: estimating penetrance parameters from case-control data. *American Journal of Human Genetics, 80*, 605–615.

Zondervan, K. T., & Cardon, L. R. (2004). The complex interplay among factors that influence allelic association. *Nature Reviews Genetics, 5*, 89–100.

39 Autism Endophenotypes and Quantitative Trait Loci

Rita M. Cantor

Points of Interest

- Twin, linkage, and association studies indicate that ASD is genetically complex, and may be the result of different subsets of multiple risk genes interacting to produce this phenotype.
- Analytic strategies to reduce the complexity of ASD are needed to reveal its genetic etiology.
- Identification of ASD-related quantitative endophenotypes that are heritable and have sufficient variation is an important first step.
- Ascertaining study samples with ASD, measuring related endophenotypes in family members, genotyping, and conducting linkage analyses to detect quantitative trait loci (QTL) is an effective approach to reduce complexity.
- For ASD, QTL studies have been conducted and loci have been replicated. In one case quantitative association studies reveal the predisposing gene.

1.0 ASD: Genetic But Not Mendelian

During the 6 decades since ASD was defined there has been a growing recognition of the importance of genes in its etiology. This was first revealed by twin studies; the ASD concordance rate in monozygotic (MZ) twins who share all of their genes has been estimated at 90%, while that rate in dizygotic (DZ) twins, who share on average 50 percent of their genes, is much lower, at 10% (Bailey et al., 1995). Despite this substantive support for genetics, efforts to identify ASD genes exhibit inconsistent linkage results and weak association effects (Lamb, Parr, Bailey, & Monaco, 2002). These are likely to reflect its genetic complexity (Veenstra-Vanderweele, Christian, & Cook, 2004). In contrast, single-gene Mendelian disorders that exhibit clear family segregation ratios of 50 percent for dominant traits and 25 percent for recessive traits, yield linkage signals that are usually unambiguously significant at one locus, allowing the responsible genes and their predisposing alleles to be localized and then identified by positional cloning techniques. As an example, the single gene for cystic fibrosis, an autosomal recessive Mendelian disorder, was one of the first to be discovered using linkage studies followed by positional cloning. Even though follow-up studies in patients from around the world indicate that there are over 1000 causal mutations in this gene (Farrell et al., 2008), linkage analysis was successful in localizing it as well as those for other Mendelian disorders.

1.1 Linkage Analysis for Mendelian Disorders

Linkage studies are designed to find the chromosome regions harboring the genes that contribute to phenotypic differences among individuals. The statistical algorithms to test for linkage have evolved over time to accommodate changes in the nature and complexity of the phenotypes and the numbers of markers available for mapping. However, all linkage studies require the ascertainment of pedigrees with members that show variation in the phenotype and have genotypes at informative markers. The statistical algorithms and computer programs for linkage analysis identify where the cosegregation of trait values and marker alleles within pedigrees is greater than what one would expect by chance alone. Linkage results at each locus reflect the statistical information that has been combined across all pedigrees in the analysis (Cantor, 2006; Ott, 1999).

Initially the traits in linkage studies were binary, such as the presence or absence of disease, and the models of inheritance used in the analyses were Mendelian dominant or recessive. Using model based or classical linkage analysis, the statistical evidence for linkage is evaluated by LOD scores. The LOD score is the log of the odds of linkage compared to the null hypothesis of no linkage at a marker. The LOD is calculated by comparing the statistical likelihood of the observed cosegregation of trait values and marker alleles in the study pedigrees to the statistical likelihood of the cosegregation in the same pedigrees at the same marker that is expected by chance alone when there is no linkage. Traditionally, a LOD greater than 3 (odds of 1000 to 1) has been taken as evidence supporting linkage to the region containing the genetic marker. Significant linkage implies that the disease gene is in the chromosome region containing the marker. Following a successful linkage analysis, positional cloning, association analyses, or sequencing studies designed to detect predisposing genes and causal alleles are conducted in the linked regions.

1.2 ASD is Genetically Complex

In addition to inconsistent linkage and association results, the genetic complexity of ASD is revealed by the large discrepancy between the MZ and DZ twin concordance rates. That is, when there is a multigene model with no allelic or gene interactions, the DZ twin concordance rate is expected to be about one half that seen in MZ twins. The large difference estimated for ASD (90% vs. 10%) is explained by a model of inheritance that includes numerous interacting genes and alleles (Ijichi et al., 2008; Risch et al., 1999), with each making a small contribution to the ASD phenotype. The complex genetics of ASD is also likely to include significant genetic heterogeneity (Happe, Ronald, & Plomin, 2006; Ronald et al., 2006). Thus, a realistic model of inheritance might include 20 or more predisposing ASD genes, with each having numerous risk alleles. One individual with ASD might have a particular subset of those genes and alleles, while another with ASD could have a different but overlapping or completely different subset. In addition, the environment is likely to play an important role, and its effects may be unequal among the affected individuals.

In summary, there are a very large number of genetic models that could each be invoked to explain the genetic risk for ASD, with none being correct. Linkage analyses of ASD cannot employ simple models of inheritance such as the dominant and recessive ones used for Mendelian disorders, as the true model is very complex and remains unknown. Given this genetic complexity, designing an appropriate gene identification study remains a challenge. However investigators continue to feel a pressing need to use the current molecular and analytic tools to tackle gene identification for ASD and other common complex disorders that are clearly genetic, but not Mendelian. The trajectory of this endeavor has been accelerated by the molecular and bioinformatics tools developed and refined in conjunction with the Human Genome (Roberts, Davenport, Pennisi, & Marshall, 2001) and HapMap (Manolio, Brooks, & Collins, 2008) projects.

1.2.1 Model Free Linkage for Complex Traits

Linkage methods that do not require a genetic model have been developed to address the genetic complexity. They are referred to as model free methods, and some approaches used in QTL mapping are based on them. While no model of inheritance is put forth, the principle on which the methods are based is that if a chromosome region contains a disease gene, siblings or other relative pairs who both have the disease will share marker genotypes in the region containing a disease gene more often than one would expect by chance alone. Thus, chromosomal loci exhibiting excess marker allele sharing identical by descent (IBD) (or the same allele inherited from common ancestors) by affected sibling pairs are linked to the disorder. Marker allele sharing IBD is illustrated in Figure 39-1.

In this pedigree with a mother, a father, and their two children, the parents have genotypes A1A2 and A3A4 respectively. The mother passes A1 and the father passes A3 to their daughter. If the son gets A2 from the mother and A4 from the father, these two siblings share 0 alleles IBD, which is expected to occur 25% of the time. If the son gets A1 and A4, the siblings share one allele IBD. Sharing one allele could also occur if the son gets A2 and A3, so sharing one allele IBD is expected to occur 50% of the time. If, like the daughter, the son also gets A1 and A3 from their parents, the siblings share 2 alleles IBD, which is expected to happen 25% of the time. The null hypothesis of no linkage or no excess allele sharing has a probability distribution of 25%, 50%, and 25% for sharing 0, 1, or 2 alleles IBD. If, for example, in a panel of sibling pairs ascertained for ASD, an observed distribution of 15%, 40%, and 45% for a marker provides evidence of ASD linkage to the chromosome region containing the marker indicating the presence of an ASD gene at that locus.

Model free linkage analysis tests for deviations of the observed IBD distributions from the expected IBD sharing distribution under the null hypothesis of 25%, 50%, and 25%. Various statistics have been used to assess the significance of the deviations, and some methods provide a LOD score (Cantor, 2006; Ott, 1999). A threshold for significance should be set to declare linkage. Setting this threshold is not straightforward, but researchers often use a LOD score of 3 (or a p-value equivalent to it), which is the same as the one used for parametric linkage analysis. Replication in an independent sample is a hallmark of success in mapping complex traits.

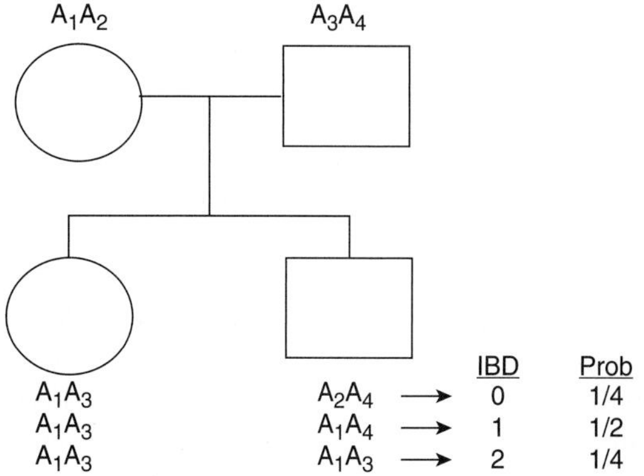

Figure 39-1. Illustration of allele-sharing identical by descent.

ASD, like many other genetically complex disorders, shows evidence of linkage to numerous chromosome loci, but only a few replications have been observed (Cantor et al., 2005). Thus, even model free linkage methods may not be adequate for a phenotype with this degree of genetic complexity. This suggests that ASD is appropriate for well-designed QTL studies.

1.3 Genomewide Association Studies

Currently, studies are employing an alternative to linkage analysis as the first step in gene detection. That is, preliminary linkage analyses are not conducted to localize genes, but the whole genome is tested for association with ASD or other complex disorders using 500,000 to one million single nucleotide polymorphisms (SNPs) to identify the predisposing genes and alleles (Simon-Sanchez & Singleton, 2008). The rationale is that linkage studies have some drawbacks, and the tools to identify risk genes through association analysis are now available (Frazer et al., 2007). One drawback is that linkage studies require the collection of families, which can be difficult to find and expensive to ascertain. Also, linkage analysis is not sensitive enough to detect the alleles that confer small risks.

Genomewide association studies (GWAS) conducted on large samples of cases and well-matched controls can identify alleles with small effects. They capitalize on the likely linkage disequilibrium between genetic risk variants and the nearby SNPs that have traveled with them on the same chromosome throughout the history of the population. It is thought that there are 10 million SNPs in humans, and that a large fraction of the genetic variants that contribute to the risk of disease will be captured by the commercial panels of 500,000 to 1,000,000 SNPs available for these studies. The mechanism by which fewer genotyped SNPs capture the variation of others is referred to as "tagging." GWAS has met with success in a number of complex disorders, but in many of those cases the associated variants explain very little of the genetic risk for the trait (Willer et al., 2009). ASD GWAS studies are currently being conducted. In preliminary findings, significant associations with common variants have not been observed, and the focus has been mainly on rare copy number variants. Although genetic models are not needed for GWAS studies, strategies to reduce genetic complexity will be important. As with linkage, methods are available to test quantitative endophenotypes for association with SNP panels.

2.0 ASD: Reducing Genetic Complexity

Identifying the genetic contributions to complex disorders such as ASD has not been straightforward. Study designs and analytic methods that have been suggested (Almasy & Blangero, 2001), indicate that a more successful path to gene identification would include the identification and analysis of traits with simpler genetic models. There are two straightforward strategies to reducing complexity. The first is to stratify the members of the study sample by a factor thought to contribute to genetic heterogeneity. For example, one could know or assume that those with ASD who are nonverbal have a different set of predisposing genes than those who are affected and verbal. Depending on the analysis conducted, the members of the ASD study sample are stratified by a feature of ASD and separate gene finding analyses are conducted in the two samples.

A second strategy is to analyze a quantitative trait or endophenotype that is associated with ASD and known or assumed to capture a single or reduced number of genetic dimensions of the disorder. It is anticipated that the endophenotype is likely to result from fewer genes and alleles acting with less complexity. This approach can be successful if there are common genetic variants serving as the basis of the endophenotype (Wijsman, 2007). Using this strategy, genes predisposing to features of ASD are mapped through QTL analyses, an approach that is addressed here. To clarify, the goal is to identify heritable traits that have substantial variance and are known to be associated with or can contribute to a diagnosis of ASD. A common example illustrates this point. The genes that contribute to triglyceride levels, a continuous and heritable trait, are also likely to contribute to the risk for coronary artery disease (CAD), as high triglycerides are seen in those with CAD. Therefore triglyceride levels provide a good CAD endophenotype for QTL mapping. Identifying appropriate quantitative traits associated with ASD poses a greater challenge, because our understanding of its biology is not as well developed as that for CAD.

2.1 Quantitative Endophenotypes

The goal is to distill the genetically complex phenotype into more specific heritable features. That is, for many complex disorders including ASD, the diagnosis of being affected results from positive responses on a checklist of observed features or behaviors. For example, a genetically complex autoimmune disease like systemic lupus erythematosus is diagnosed if any of four out of eleven criteria are met (Hochberg, 1997); metabolic syndrome, which is also complex, is associated with diabetes and coronary artery disease and diagnosed when several criteria involving disturbances in metabolism and lipids are met (Qiao et al., 2009). Most relevant to ASD, neurobiological disorders are diagnosed when an individual exhibits a pattern of behaviors consistent with criteria listed in the *Diagnostic and Statistical Manual* (American Psychiatric Association, 1994). Focusing on single traits from these checklists may reveal entities that derive from the major effects of fewer genes with a simpler genetic model. Also, since the analysis of quantitative traits is more statistically powerful than the analysis of discrete traits, identifying quantitative features of the ASD phenotype can provide a robust approach to gene identification.

2.1.1 A Quantitative Trait Model

The genetic contribution to a quantitative trait or endophenotype can be illustrated by a simple arbitrary model with 3 genes. While the genetics of any "real" quantitative trait will be more complex, the principles illustrated by this model can be applied. In this hypothetical model, there are 3 genes each with 2 alleles contributing to Trait1 in an additive fashion. The alleles are "A" and "a" for gene1, "B" and "b" for gene2, and "C" and "c" for gene 3, and each capital letter allele contributes 3 to the trait value, while each lower case letter allele contributes 1. Thus, a person with genotype AA, Bb, and cc would have a trait value of 12. The maximum and minimum trait values are 18 and 6, respectively. Complexities might include gene-gene or gene-environment interactions that would alter the trait values. If the alleles with capital letters exhibit dominance at each locus, someone with genotype AA, Bb, and cc would have a trait value of 14. Interactions among loci would produce a wider number of possible trait values. Ascertainment of an informative study sample is critical, and gene finding efforts are enhanced if the sample is drawn from families exhibiting the entire range of the trait. These related individuals are expected to be correlated in their trait values because they share common genes. Identifying the genes by QTL analyses capitalizes on the expected relationships of trait values and marker allele sharing by the relative pairs in the pedigrees.

2.1.2 Three Criteria for Good QTL Endophenotypes

QTL mapping, like linkage analysis, is directed toward finding the chromosomal loci that harbor genes contributing to a trait, however here the trait is a quantitative endophenotype. Specific criteria must be met for an endophenotype to be appropriate for QTL mapping. The first is that the endophenotype exhibit substantial variation in the study sample under analysis. Achieving this can sometimes be difficult. A powerful study design consists of genotyped individuals in pedigrees ascertained for those with the complex disorder, where both the affected and unaffected are measured. The contrast of these individuals provides good power to detect the correlation of trait value differences and allele sharing that is used to map the genes. Thus, pedigrees with a large number of affected individuals are more powerful.

Sometimes the trait can only be measured in those who are affected. An example is the age of onset of the disorder. A common design consists of multiplex nuclear families with at lease two affected members measured for the endophenotype. This design will provide less power than one including unaffected individuals from the families, but it may be necessary for the proposed endophenotype. For other disorders, the endophenotype can only be assessed effectively in unaffected individuals. This will reduce the statistical power to identify the predisposing genes, as it leads to an enrichment of alleles that have very small effects on the trait value, since the bigger effects are likely to occur in the affected who have the disturbed trait values. Trait variation can be continuous, such as IQ, or ordinal, such as the degree of dysfunction (mild, moderate, or severe). A statistical power calculation taking the nature of the study sample, level of significance, and distribution of the trait can be conducted. It will allow the investigator to estimate the detectable effect size of the predisposing alleles. Since there is no simple approach that can be used in every situation, it is important to evaluate the distribution of the quantitative trait in the choice of analytic method and interpretation of results.

The second criterion for effective QTL mapping is that the endophenotype should be associated with the binary definition of the disorder. That is, one should be able to subdivide the values of the trait so that it correlates with binary definition of the disorder. Figure 39-2 illustrates this point. Here, in Figure 39-2a, the horizontal axis reflects the observed values of the trait, and the vertical axis reflects the percent or probability of each of those values. Hypothetically, the vertical line that is drawn divides those who are affected from those who are not. This indicates there is a perfect relationship between the endophenotype and the binary disorder. In reality, the relationship will not be that strong. This is illustrated in Figure 39-2b, where, as in 39-2a, the white color reflects the trait values of those who are affected and the grey color reflects the trait values of those who are not affected, but a clean vertical line cannot be drawn. Since the quantitative trait is not used to diagnose the disorder directly, there are no strict rules regarding this expected relationship between quantitative values and diagnosis, and the judgment of the investigator as to the acceptability of this correlation is important.

The third critical criterion is that the endophenotype have a significant heritability. The heritability of a quantitative trait is the fraction of the trait variance that can be attributed to genes. Narrow heritability is operating if the genes act in an additive fashion, as illustrated by the example in section *2.1.1*. Broad heritability is the estimate that includes the interactive effects of genes, also discussed in that section. Because these interactions are difficult to identify or predict, investigators usually make the simplifying assumption that all gene effects are additive, and they estimate the narrow heritability. The closer the genetic model is to one that is additive, the easier it is to map the QTL.

2.1.2.1 Estimating Heritability

The heritability of a trait in a given population can be estimated by calculating the observed trait correlations in classes of relative pairs, such as siblings, and adjusting them for their degrees of relationship. The most informative pairs are MZ twins, as they share all of their genes and their correlation without an adjustment is a direct estimate of trait heritability. DZ twins share on average half of their genes and doubling their correlation provides an estimate of heritability. Their contrast, twice the difference in these correlations, provides a better estimate of heritability because it accounts for the sampling error and environmental correlations in these estimates. There are more complex methods to estimate heritability that involve analyses of trait variance (Rice, 2008).

Sometimes only sibling pairs are available for a heritability estimate. While the trait correlation for these pairs can be doubled for a rough estimate of trait heritability, it includes the effects of common family environment. Thus, it provides an upper bound for the heritability of the trait, which can be

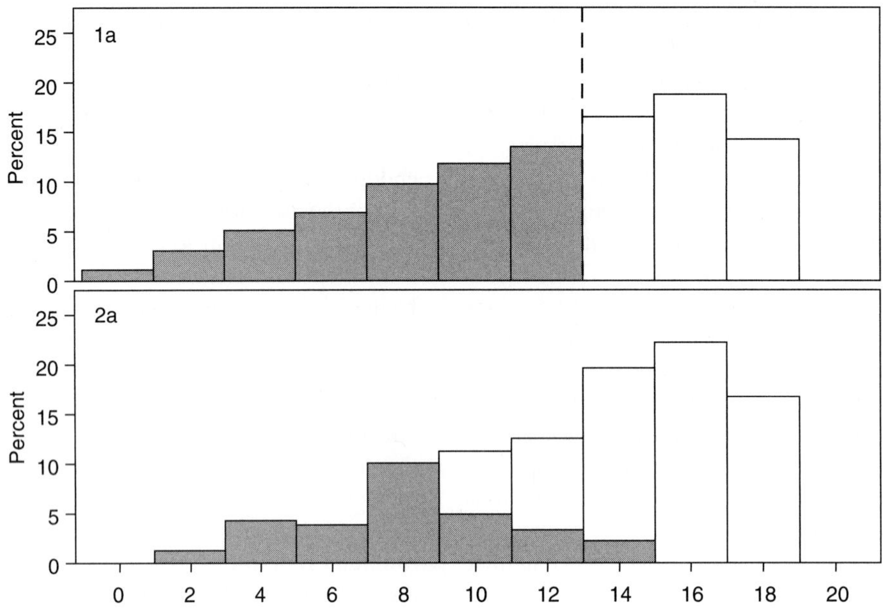

Figure 39–2. Relationships of a quantitative endophenotype and a binary diagnosis.

much smaller. Using multiple types of relative pairs provides a more refined estimate, but the "gold standard" is derived from data on MZ and DZ twin pairs. For most study designs, the heritability estimate has a standard error that can be used to test the null hypothesis that it is zero.

The heritability of a quantitative trait provides an upper bound for the heritability contributed by any one locus, referred to as the locus specific heritability. For example, if three genes contribute to the trait, the heritability will be divided among the three loci, although not necessarily evenly, giving some of the loci with bigger effects a better chance of detection by QTL analysis. If many genes contribute to the trait value, the heritability can be high and the locus specific heritabilities can all be low. Thus, a high heritability for a trait that is polygenic does not guarantee that a QTL will be identified. A well-defined study for a highly heritable trait, a sufficient sample size, and luck will all be important.

3.0 ASD: Quantitative Endophenotypes

The identification of quantitative endophenotypes for ASD is at an early stage of development, and QTL studies may be premature for many quantitative traits. However, several authors have addressed the value of identifying endophenotypes for general psychiatric disorders (Gottesman & Gould, 2003; Szatmari et al., 2007; Walters & Owen, 2007), and others provided general guidance for their definition in ASD (Allison et al., 2008; Chiu et al., 2008; Pickles et al., 2000; Viding & Blakemore, 2007; Wijsman, 2007). Their general guidelines for ASD suggest quantifying the features of a particular symptom and including normally functioning adults who also exhibit aspects of the trait, when this is feasible. The guidelines acknowledge that often the traits can only be assessed in those who are affected, limiting the range of variability. Suggested classes of traits include dimensions of mental skills that can explain features of ASD (Baron-Cohen, Wheelwright, Skinner, Martin, & Clubley, 2001). For example, employing an instrument to assess and measure the degree of central coherence could allow investigators to capture and quantify the skill that permits savant behavior, because it is thought to be explained by weak central coherence (Viding & Blakemore, 2007).

3.1 Behavioral Questionnaire Endophenotypes

Appropriate endophenotypes can come from instruments devised to assess the features of (Hoekstra, Bartels, Verweij, & Boomsma, 2007; Skuse, Mandy, & Scourfield, 2005) and diagnose ASD (Piven, Palmer, Landa et al., 1997). The Quantitative Checklist for Autism in Toddlers (QCHAT), a 25-item checklist with a score of 0–4 on each item provides a number of possible traits for analysis. These items are correlated with ASD, as the mean scores for those with ASD are significantly higher than for those who are unaffected (Allison et al., 2008). Additional analyses of the heritability or familiality of the scores would be important for further work. The broad autism phenotype (BAP) is described by features of language and personality, ranging from mild to severe. It is correlated with, but does not lead to autism, and can be quantified as a potential endophenotype (Losh & Piven, 2007; Piven, Palmer, Jacobi, Childress, & Arndt, 1997). The Broader Phenotype Autism Symptom Scale (BPASS) is a good source of endophenotypes. A trained clinician measures social motivation, social expressiveness, conversational skills, and flexibility in ASD-affected individuals and their family members along a quantitative continuum (Dawson et al., 2007; Dawson et al., 2002). Developers of this instrument anticipated the possibilities of QTL studies, as they identified BPASS traits that are familial (Sung et al., 2005) and correlated with ASD.

The Social Responsiveness Scale (SRS) (Constantino et al., 2006; Constantino & Todd, 2003) provides a quantitative score measuring the deficit in this defining feature of ASD. The SRS score is highly correlated with ASD and provides a measure of a single dimension of social skills. It has been validated, and found to be heritable in normal individuals, as assessed by twin studies. It can be administered to pedigree members and provides an excellent trait for QTL mapping. A small QTL study was conducted in nuclear families with ASD, which is discussed more extensively in section 5.0.

3.2 Behavioral Traits: Autism Diagnostic Instrument Revised (ADIR)

The ADIR, which has been used extensively to diagnose ASD (Lord, Rutter, & Le Couteur, 1994), provides a wealth of potential endophenotypes for QTL analyses. It assesses deficits in the domains of language and social skills and identifies the presence of stereotyped and repetitive behaviors. Quantification of these deficits and their specific features provides candidate endophenotypes for QTL analyses. These capture the global degree of deficit in language or social skills or focus on the quantitative assessment of a single dimension of language or social skills, such as the degree of delay in speech.

The ADIR is an assessment of approximately 100 ASD features by trained clinicians interrogating caregivers. Many questions address the levels at which the child exhibits particular deficits. The value for each item varies from 0 to 3, with a higher score reflecting a greater deficit. Thus, scores are elevated in those with ASD. A single item provides an ordinal score and combinations of items provide a more continuous range of values. Scores for item combinations can be achieved by direct addition or derived from multivariate statistical methods like factor analysis (Afifi, Clark, & May, 2004), which is applied to find a linear combination of the scores on individual items reflecting language deficits that are most correlated with each other in those with ASD. More sophisticated analytic methods are also available to find multivariate quantitative traits appropriate for QTL analysis (Kutner, Nachtsheim, & Neter, 2004).

3.3 Autism Diagnostic Observation Schedule (ADOS)

The ADOS is a semistructured assessment with diagnostic modules that are customized for both nonverbal and verbal patients and tailored for individuals that range in age from toddlerhood to adulthood. The assessment is open-ended, and an examiner uses a series of situations and interview questions to elicit behavior and verbal responses from the individual tested. An overall assessment is used to discriminate among forms of ASD, such as autism itself, pervasive developmental delay, or Asperger's syndrome. Since it involves direct observation of a person's behavior by an examiner who is taking careful note of traits and behaviors central to the diagnosis of autism, it is difficult to convert this instrument into a tool with quantitative traits. Thus, the ADOS is much less adaptable to QTL analyses than the ADI-R and the other instruments discussed in this chapter. These differences indicate that one must recognize that it is not only the quality of the traits that must be considered for QTL studies, but the nature of their measurement as well. An interactive tool for diagnosis may not adapt well to providing a consistent and well-defined phenotype.

3.4 Biological Endophenotypes

Although knowledge of the biology of ASD is currently limited, investigations suggest a number of ASD-correlated, heritable, and variable biological endophenotypes appropriate for QTL analyses. For example, an increased number of those with ASD exhibit a large head circumference for their age and sex (Fombonne, Roge, Claverie, Courty, & Fremolle, 1999; Lainhart et al., 2006; Sacco et al., 2007). Significant familial correlations in head circumference have been observed in family members of those with ASD, indicating this is a good ASD endophenotype for QTL analysis (Spence, Black, Miyamoto, & Geschwind, 2005). The sizes of certain structures of the brain have been implicated as causing the large head (Courchesne et al., 2007), and if the sizes are familial they may also be appropriate endophenotypes for QTL analysis. This endophenotype has already been associated with a genetic polymorphism (Conciatori et al., 2004). Increased blood serotonin levels have been reported in those with ASD (Cross et al., 2008; Weiss et al., 2006). The trait is familial, making it a good candidate for QTL analysis in pedigrees ascertained for individuals with ASD.

4.0 QTL Analyses

QTL analyses are conducted to localize genes that contribute to quantitative traits or endophenotypes. They were originally designed to localize genes in model organisms (Mackay, 2004) and in particular inbred strains of mice (Flint, Valdar, Shifman, & Mott, 2005). Inbred mouse strains are derived by breeding siblings for 20 generations until they are homozygous at almost every locus. Mating mice from two different inbred strains that differ significantly in their trait mean provides a straightforward approach to localizing genes contributing to that trait. Using this design, a significant test statistic identifies marker loci where mice differing in their genotypes also differ in their mean trait values. The differences are assessed by t-tests or Analyses of Variance (ANOVA) (Ott & Longnecker, 2000), and the loci with markers exhibiting significantly different trait means reveal the QTL. In inbred mice, gene identification at a QTL is a significant challenge, because they exhibit reduced genetic variability, making their QTL very broad, and thus encompassing many genes. Very large numbers of mice are needed to narrow the QTL by breeding, and complex study designs have been proposed to address this problem (Rockman & Kruglyak, 2008). After a QTL or gene is identified in mice, the human orthologs can be found using mouse/human comparative maps available at the Jackson Laboratories Web site (http://www.jax.org).

4.1 Methods of QTL Analyses in Humans

This method of QTL analysis for inbred mice has been extended to address gene localization in outbred humans. Multiple analytic approaches are available, and factors that influence the choice are the degree of distributional normality of the trait and the configuration of the study sample. QTL analyses differ when the trait is continuous with a normal distribution and studied in several large pedigrees compared to when it is ordinal with a few categories and studied in a large number of nuclear families. Table 39-1 outlines some of the options in QTL analysis.

4.1.1 Variance Components Analyses

If large pedigrees with most members measured for a normally distributed endophenotype are available, a variance component analysis is the most appropriate and statistically powerful approach. Computer programs that implement this method include SOLAR (Blangero & Almasy, 1996) (Almasy et al., 1999), MENDEL (Lange et al., 2001), and MERLIN (Abecasis, Cherny, Cookson, & Cardon, 2002; Heath, 1997). In each case, the trait variance is partitioned into components attributable to genes, the environment, and when appropriate, their interactions. The partition is achieved by comparing the degrees of the genetic relationships among the pedigree members and the covariances in their trait values, resulting in an estimate of trait heritability. Genetic markers are incorporated into the analysis to estimate marker allele sharing IBD among the relative pairs in the pedigrees and these IBD estimates are analyzed in relation to the covariances among the trait values. The QTL analysis tests whether including the effects of a gene contributing to the trait at that marker locus better explains the data. This is accomplished by a likelihood ratio test, which is similar to what is used by the LOD score linkage analysis. The test statistic compares the likelihood of the data with a trait influencing gene in the chromosome region included compared to the likelihood of the data without this gene. The loci with LOD scores exceeding a predetermined threshold are considered to be QTL, and the analysis allows for an estimate of the locus specific heritability at each QTL.

If the pedigrees under analysis have a large number of affected individuals, and the distribution of their trait values is bimodal, thus violating the normality assumption of this statistical method, transformation of the trait values to fit a normal distribution would satisfy the assumptions of the method. Alternatively, a nonparametric mapping method, such as those in given Table 39-1 may be more appropriate. Algorithms to conduct variance component QTL analyses can use a great deal of computer time, particularly if the analysis is multipoint, which incorporates the information from many markers to estimate the allele sharing IBD, rather than single point, where each marker is analyzed individually. Multipoint analyses consider more information simultaneously, and are thus more powerful statistically.

4.1.2 QTL Mapping for ASD Traits

Since individuals with ASD rarely have offspring, and their parents may respond to the burden of caring for a child with this disorder with stoppage (Slager, Foroud, Haghighi, Spence, & Hodge, 2001), ceasing to have children, it is difficult to identify large pedigrees with substantial numbers of

Table 39–1.
QTL mapping approaches

Study Sample	Genetic Markers	Analytic Method	Software	Comments
Large Pedigrees	Multiallelic Markers or SNPs	Analysis of Variance Components	SOLAR MENDEL MERLIN	The trait variance is partitioned into genetic and environmental components
Nuclear Families	Multiallelic Markers or SNPs	Haseman-Elston Kruskal Wallis test	Sibpal in SAGE Nonparametric in GENEHUNTER	Identity-by-descent allele sharing in siblings is correlated with their trait differences
Parent/Child Trios	SNPs	Family Based Association Test	FBAT	Preferential Transmission of alleles to those with higher trait values
Cases and/or Controls	SNPs	Quantitative Association Measured Genotype	Any General Statistical Package	Analysis of Variance or t-test

ASD-affected individuals for variance components QTL studies. In this case, sibpair analyses are appropriate and families with affected sibling pairs are most often available for QTL studies. Here, the analysis finds QTL contributing to trait variation in those with ASD (Spiker, Lotspeich, Dimiceli, Myers, & Risch, 2002). A more powerful QTL analysis can be derived from panels of ASD parent/affected child trio samples that are being collected for genomewide association studies. Including an unaffected sibling measured for the endophenotype in the study sample provides a powerful contrast to the affected sibling. QTL mapping in these nuclear families can also employ a variance components approach when the trait is normally distributed.

For traits that are not normally distributed, several algorithms are available for sibpair QTL analyses. All are based on IBD sharing in sibpairs. The algorithms compare trait differences and IBD allele sharing, combining the results over the sibling pairs. It is expected that IBD sharing and trait differences will be negatively correlated at a QTL, because for each pair, the greater their allele sharing, the closer their trait values should be. This approach was originally proposed by Haseman and Elston (1972), and it is still in use today. The Statistical Analysis of Genetic Epidemiodogy (SAGE) software conducts these analyses (http://darwin.cwru.edu/sage). Variations on this method include a nonparametric analysis in the GENEHUNTER software (Kruglyak, Daly, Reeve-Daly, & Lander, 1996). Using that algorithm, the trait differences are ranked over the complete sample of sibpairs and the differences are categorized by the observed IBD values in the pairs. The Kruskal Wallis test, a nonparametric ANOVA, is conducted (Ott & Longnecker, 2000). Consistent with other nonparametric statistical methods, using ranks as is done here prevents the undue influence of trait value outliers on the analysis.

4.2 Interpreting QTL Results

QTL are identified by setting a threshold for the test statistic that reflects the strength of the evidence at that locus. The test statistic follows a normal or t-distribution statistic or is reported as a LOD score, depending on the algorithm. Figure 39-3 illustrates the genomewide results of a QTL analysis in graphic form. The genome is represented across the horizontal axis, with the chromosomes listed from one to 22. The vertical axis is a value from the normal distribution. The test is one-sided, so that all the probability is in a single tail. The best result occurs on chromosome 1, with a z-score being a little greater than 3.5. The probability of observing this score or one that is larger when there is no endophenotype gene is approximately .000001, making this a likely QTL. If a z-score threshold is set at 3.0, QTL are also found on chromosomes 4 and 16.

Figure 39-4 illustrates the results of this QTL analysis on chromosome 1 in greater detail. The horizontal axis reflects the distance from the telomere of the chromosome in centimorgans (cM) and the vertical axis reflects the z-score at each point along the chromosome. As with all statistical tests, setting a less stringent p-value will provide more power to detect true signals, but will also permit more false signals to be included. Here we illustrate that QTL are usually wide and encompass many genes. Additional markers interspersed among those that are already in the analysis can often narrow the QTL. While it is more likely that the predisposing alleles are in genes under the peak of the QTL, stochastic variation in genotypes and trait values in the study sample may cause some variation in location of this peak. As with most linkage findings, replication is important. This principle is illustrated by the inclusion of a curve representing the QTL results on this chromosome in an independent sample.

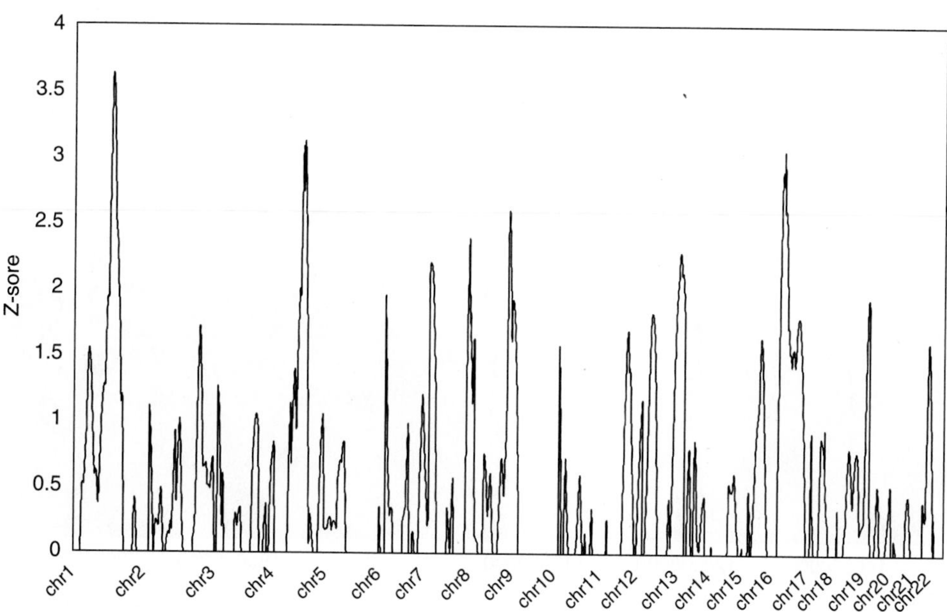

Figure 39–3. QTL along the genome.

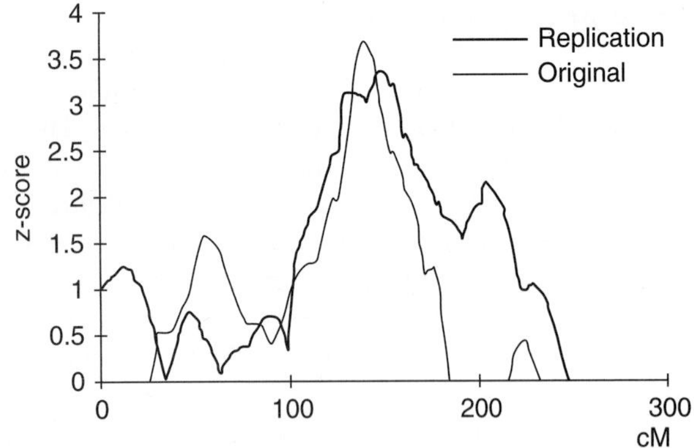

Figure 39–4. QTL in original and replication samples.

4.3 Association Studies at QTL

Once QTL have been identified, SNPs in the QTL can be genotyped for association analyses that can lead to gene identification. Table 39-1 gives information on two types of study designs for association analysis of quantitative traits. The first is to ascertain parent/child trios where the child is assessed for the endophenotype. The genotypes of both parents and the child are included to provide information on the alleles that are transmitted to the child and those that are not transmitted. The untransmitted alleles act as "controls" that are matched within each trio for ethnicity and other important factors. The Family Based Association Test (FBAT) (Horvath, Xu, & Laird, 2001) tests if the transmitted SNP alleles associate with high or low values of the endophenotype more than one would expect by chance alone, while taking into account the alleles that could have been transmitted. If additional members of a sibship are included with the trio, their associations will not be independent, and the level of significance of the association can be a false positive result. Corrections for non-independence of the siblings in a sibship can be achieved by using an empiric p-value or by adjusting the variance of the test, as is programmed in the FBAT software (Horvath et al., 2001). The last line of Table 39-1 refers to the simple design where parents and siblings of affected individuals are not studied. The association test for the quantitative trait is referred to as a measured genotype analysis, which is conducted using an one way ANOVA (Ott & Longnecker, 2000).

Figure 39-5 illustrates the results of association analyses at a QTL. The horizontal axis is the number of base pairs along the chromosome, from 80,000,000 to 220,000,000 and the vertical axis represents the p-values of the test statistics for each SNP. The plot uses the negative of the log of this p-value, where the log of a small p-value becomes a positive number that increases as the result get more significant. In this figure, four SNPs are associated with the endophenotype when the criterion is set at the Bonferroni corrected value of $p < .0001$, for 500 SNPs. These SNPs do not necessarily contribute to variation in the endophenotype directly, but are more likely to be in linkage disequilibrium with SNPs that do. Follow-up

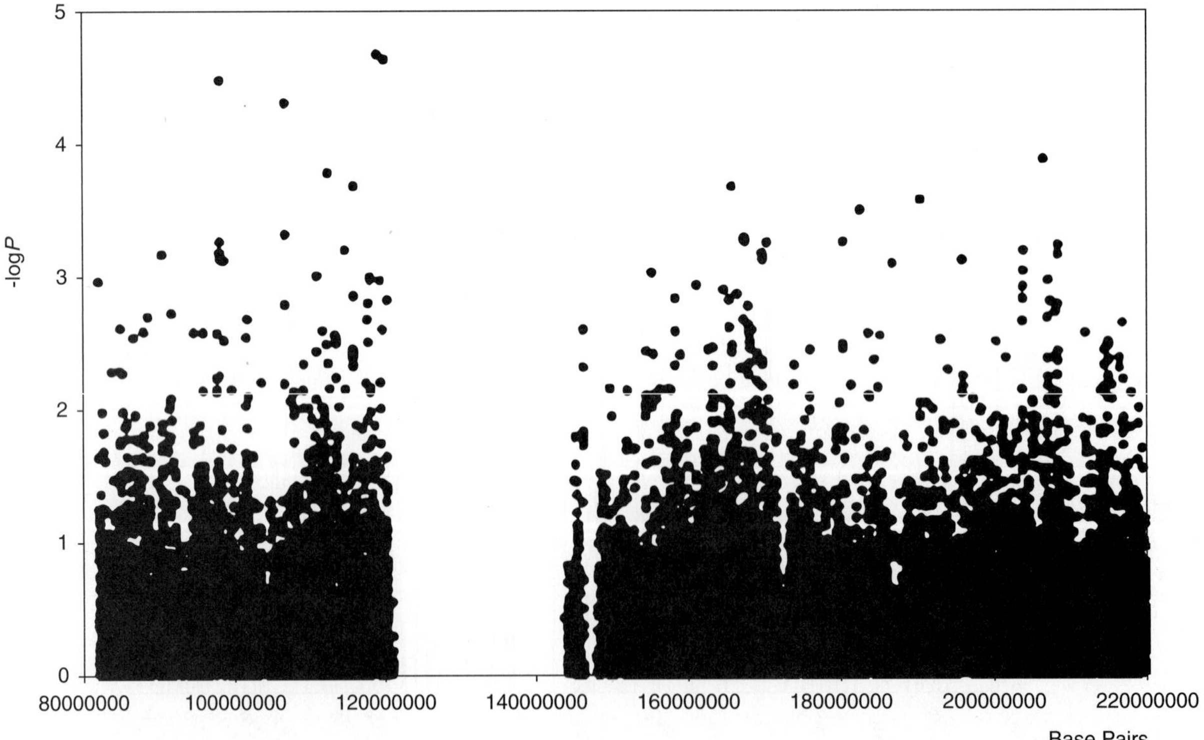

Figure 39–5. Association analysis of SNPs in the QTL.

studies might include replication in an independent sample and sequencing of a sample of those who have the associated variant to potentially identify the causal variants.

5.0 ASD QTL Analyses

Investigators are just beginning to develop sufficient study samples and identify appropriate endophenotypes for effective QTL analyses in ASD. As these evolve, substantial findings may begin to emerge. Currently, there are a number of published manuscripts and abstracts reporting QTL results, and they are summarized in Table 39-2.

Most of the QTL analyses reported in Table 39-2 have been conducted on samples of nuclear families drawn from the Autism Genetics Research Exchange (AGRE, www.agre.org) resource, from which trait and genotype data are freely available to interested investigators (Geschwind et al., 2001). The AGRE study sample currently has about 1400 multiplex families ascertained for two children affected with ASD. The children in this sample have been diagnosed with ASD by trained staff using the ADIR. The data have been developed over the last 10 years, and thus the QTL findings given in Table 39-2 report AGRE samples of differing sizes, depending on when they were conducted and when the quantitative measure were included in the protocol. More complete samples are in the process of being collected.

In addition to providing data on the individual items from the ADIR (Lord et al., 1994), the AGRE data set includes individual responses on the ADOS (Lord et al., 2000), parent and teacher scores on the SRS (Constantino & Todd, 2003), and measurements of head circumference, all discussed as potential endophenotypes in section 3. Multiallelic genotypes and SNP data are available for QTL analyses. Densely spaced SNPs genotyped on the Affymetrix and Illumina platforms are available for quantitative association analyses (http://www.agre.org).

5.1 QTL Analyses: "Age at First Word"

QTL analyses on data from the AGRE sample began in 2002 with the analysis of the ADIR caregiver report of "age at first word," which is provided for each child who has been verbal at some time in their childhood. Delayed speech is associated with ASD, and this endophenotype is measured in months, providing a correlated trait with sufficient variability. The sibling correlation is .33, which is significantly different from 0, making this endophenotype a good candidate for QTL analyses. The QTL analysis was conducted using the nonparametric option of the GENEHUNTER software, and the strongest evidence for a QTL was found on chromosome band 7q34-36 (Alarcon, Cantor, Liu, Gilliam, & Geschwind, 2002). This sample was expanded, and the same analysis was conducted in the larger sample in 2005. While there was no formal replication, evidence supporting this QTL was attenuated but remained significant (Alarcon, Yonan, Gilliam, Cantor, & Geschwind, 2005).

A QTL analysis of "age at first word" was subsequently conducted in a different collection of multiplex families, also reported in Table 39-2. Schellenberg and colleagues conducted their study on a sample of 222 ASD multiplex United States families from the NIH Collaborative Programs of Excellence in Autism (CPEA) collection (Schellenberg et al., 2006). Using

Table 39–2.
QTL and quantitative association results in ASD family panels

Trait	Reference	Design	Result (Location and p-Value)
ADIR Age at First Word	Alarcon et al., 2002 Alarcon et al., 2005	152 ASD AGRE Families	QTL 7q34-36 ($p<.001$)
ADIR Age at First Word	Schellenberg et al., 2006	222 CPEA Families	QTL 9q33-34 ($p<.0008$)
ADIR Age at First Word	Alarcon et al., 2008	172 and 304 AGRE Parent/ Child Trios	CNTNAP2 gene 7q35 Association ($p<.002$) Replication ($p<.005$)
Social Responsiveness Scale (SRS)	Duvall et al., 2007	99 AGRE Families	QTL 11p12-13 ($p<.0007$)
ADIR Nonverbal Communication (NVC)	Chen et al., 2005	228 AGRE Families	QTL 1p13-q12 ($p<.0001$)
ADIR Nonverbal Communication (NVC)	Yoon et al., 2008	219 AGRE Families	QTL 1p13-q12 Replication ($p<.0001$)
ADIR Social Interaction Domain (SOC) Behavioral Domain (BEH)	Liu et al., 2008	976 AGP Families	QTL 12q13 ($p<.002$) QTL 14q22 ($p<.001$)

the ADIR and the ADOS for diagnosis, the families each had two children meeting the criteria for autism, pervasive developmental disorder, or ASD, which makes the CPEA selection criteria somewhat different from the AGRE selection criteria. The QTL analyses were also conducted using a different analytic algorithm, as the CPEA sample was analyzed using a variance components approach, while the AGRE sample was analyzed using the nonparametric approach. This CPEA study did not replicate the QTL on 7q34-36, but found one at 9q33-34. The lack of replication for this particular trait while disappointing, can be attributed to a reduced sample size, differing clinical ascertainment criteria, and a different analytic method. Using the same diagnostic criteria and analytic methods would be important for a replication study.

5.2 QTL Analyses: The Social Responsiveness Scale

The SRS is an ASD endophenotype that covers a wide range of values and discriminates well among those who are socially adept and those who are not. Twin studies indicate that scores on the SRS are heritable in normal individuals (Constantino & Todd, 2003). A small study was conducted on 99 AGRE families, and a QTL was identified on 11p12-13. The locus was also found to also be linked to the binary trait of ASD in that sample, and the SRS provided greater power (Duvall et al., 2007). The AGRE sample is continuing to expand and include the SRS assessment in the protocol. Future studies in much larger samples may reveal important ASD loci through the analysis of this quantitative endophenotype. Quantitative association studies will be an important component.

5.3 QTL Analyses: "Nonverbal Communication"

The ADIR subscore assessing deficits in nonverbal communication (NVC) provides an appropriate endophenotype for ASD QTL analyses. The NVC score is composed of the individual scores on seven items from the ADIR, where the deficits are categorized in an ordinal fashion from 0 to 3. NVC skills would allow the child to engage with others by doing such things as pointing to share information. Deficits would reflect a lack in the ability to communicate with others that may be considered independent of language skills. This endophenotype is best measured in those who have ASD, and it exhibits the full range of values in that sample. The NVC correlation in ASD affected siblings is .21, indicating it is familial as well as correlated with ASD and variable in the sample under analysis. A nonparametric QTL analysis of 228 AGRE families identified a QTL on 1p13-q12 (Chen, Kono, Geschwind, & Cantor, 2006), which has been replicated in an independent sample of 213 AGRE families, using the same multiallelic genotyping, ascertainment scheme, and analytic approach (Yoon, Alarcon, Geschwind, & Cantor, 2008). The result of $p < .0001$ in the first sample and $p < .0001$ in the second provide consistent evidence of and NVC QTL in this region. This QTL is very broad, and targeted SNP association studies and follow-up sequencing studies are revealing the genes in the region that contribute to this endophenotype.

5.4 QTL Analyses: Autism Genome Project

Large-scale studies of multiple ASD samples are an important focus for the Autism Genome Project (AGP). The AGP conducted a QTL study on its combined sample of ASD multiplex families ascertained at 10 coordinating sites in the United States and Europe over a 30-year period. This sample includes the CPEA and AGRE samples. While genotyping was conducted on all AGP families, the QTL analyses were done on a subset of 976 for whom the quantitative data could be made compatible among the sites (Liu, Paterson, & Szatmari, 2008). In preliminary analyses, the data from the different sites with varying ascertainment and diagnostic criteria were combined to reflect the same phenotypes. Fortunately, the genotype platform and analytic method was the same for all of the families. Two ADIR derived endophenotypes were analyzed in this sample. They are the ADIR total scores on the reciprocal social interaction domain total (SOC), with a heritability estimate of .35 and the restricted, repetitive, and stereotyped patterns of behavior domain (BEH), with a heritability estimate of .52. Since the data were only collected in sibling pairs, these estimates reflect the effects of common family environment, which are likely to be nontrivial. The QTL analyses were conducted using the variance components approach as programmed in the Merlin software (Abecasis et al., 2002). The best QTL signals for these endophenotypes were on chromosomes 12q13.11 ($p = .002$) for SOC and 14q22.1 ($p = .001$) for BEH. These results, which exhibit marginal significance in the largest sample analyzed for an ASD QTL, can be explained in a few ways. First the heritability estimates derived from the sibling pairs in this sample include common family environment indicating the true trait heritabilities may be considerably lower than .33 and .52. In addition, there may be many genes contributing to these endophenotypes, each with small locus specific heritabilities that cannot be detected, even with a study sample of this size. It is anticipated that other endophenotype studies in this large sample will result in stronger QTL.

5.4.1 Association of "Age at First Word"

An association study in a sample of the AGRE families was conducted within the 7q34-36 QTL to find the gene influencing "age at first word" in children with ASD. The density of the SNPs was substantial, providing more information than what would be seen in microarray SNP panel. The SNPs were tested for association individually, and haplotypes in a moving window were also tested. While several associations were observed, replication studies in an independent sample of AGRE families implicated only one haplotype that was located in the CNTNAP2 gene (Alarcon et al., 2008). Remarkably, the same gene showed association with the binary ASD phenotype in the AGRE families (Arking et al., 2008).

These QTL studies followed by association analysis and replication for "age at first word" provides strong support for the QTL approach proposed herein. QTL studies with larger samples and more refined endophenotype are likely to reveal other ASD genes.

5.4.2 A Roadmap for QTL Discovery

From a statistical genetics perspective, the analytic tools for QTL studies are in place. These tools await the application of suitable ASD phenotypes that are variable within the population under analysis, correlated with ASD, and exhibit evidence of a reasonable nonzero heritability. The nature of the study sample and distribution of the trait will limit the feasible analytic approaches.

These same design principles have been successfully applied to the study of coronary artery disease (CAD) through QTL analyses of heritable quantitative traits such as serum cholesterol and triglycerides levels. An important advantage for CAD studies, however, is that long-term epidemiology studies revealed important quantitative risk factors before genomewide studies became feasible.

Thus, it becomes critical to identify the important ASD quantitative traits, although the epidemiology studies are only in their very early stages. Perhaps the best approach currently is to create an environment where experts in the clinical and research features of ASD can participate in collaborative studies with investigators having QTL expertise and epidemiologists focused on revealing important ASD risk factors. It is expected such endeavors are likely to create a synergy among investigators that will lead to success.

Conclusions

The genetic complexity of ASD can be addressed by studying correlated quantitative endophenotypes that have simpler modes of inheritance. Successful ASD endophenotypes will exhibit wide variation and substantial heritability. QTL studies of these endophenotypes involve selecting an appropriate study sample that captures sufficient variation in those who are affected and possibly those who are unaffected. The choice of statistical algorithm for QTL mapping will depend on the individuals who can be studied and the distribution of the endophenotype. Although QTL studies for ASD are at an early stage, its application to ASD led to initial successes. The QTL for deficits in nonverbal communication has been replicated in an independent sample and awaits effective association studies. The CNTNAP2 gene in a language related QTL shows association with the language-related quantitative trait and ASD. Application of this approach to more refined endophenotypes in larger samples can lead to a substantial increase in our understanding of the genetic etiology of ASD.

Challenges and Future Directions

The identification of the best quantitative endophenotypes for QTL mapping remains a challenge. New study samples of ASD affected children and their unaffected offspring provide opportunities to pursue this approach. Synergy among experts on the ASD phenotypes, ASD epidemiology, and QTL mapping could energize the field. Once QTL are identified, it will be an interesting challenge to integrate GWAS, copy number variation, and sequence data into studies of these endophenotypes.

SUGGESTED READINGS

Alarcon, M., Abrahams, B. S., Stone, J. L., Duvall, J. A., Perederiy, J. V., Bomar, J. M., et al. (2008). Linkage, association, and gene-expression analyses identify CNTNAP2 as an autism-susceptibility gene. *American Journal of Human Genetics, 82*(1), 150–159.

Abrahams, B. S., & Geschwind, D. H. (2008). Advances in autism genetics: On the threshold of a new neurobiology. *Nature Reviews Genetics, 9*, 341–355.

Lynch, M., & Walsh, B. (1998). *Genetics and the analysis of quantitative traits.* Sunderland, MA: Sinauer Associates.

REFERENCES

Abecasis, G. R., Cherny, S. S., Cookson, W. O., & Cardon, L. R. (2002). Merlin: rapid analysis of dense genetic maps using sparse gene flow trees. *Nature Genetics, 30*(1), 97–101.

Afifi, A., Clark, V. A., & May, S. (2004). *Computer-aided multivariate analysis* (4th ed.). Boca Raton, FL: CRC.

Alarcon, M., Abrahams, B. S., Stone, J. L., Duvall, J. A., Perederiy, J. V., Bomar, J. M., et al. (2008). Linkage, association, and gene-expression analyses identify CNTNAP2 as an autism-susceptibility gene. *American Journal of Human Genetics, 82*(1), 150–159.

Alarcon, M., Cantor, R. M., Liu, J., Gilliam, T. C., & Geschwind, D. H. (2002). Evidence for a language quantitative trait locus on chromosome 7q in multiplex autism families. *American Journal of Human Genetics, 70*(1), 60–71.

Alarcon, M., Yonan, A. L., Gilliam, T. C., Cantor, R. M., & Geschwind, D. H. (2005). Quantitative genome scan and ordered-subsets analysis of autism endophenotypes support language QTLs. *Molecular Psychiatry, 10*(8), 747–757.

Allison, C., Baron-Cohen, S., Wheelwright, S., Charman, T., Richler, J., Pasco, G., et al. (2008). The Q-CHAT (Quantitative CHecklist for Autism in Toddlers): a normally distributed quantitative measure of autistic traits at 18–24 months of age: preliminary report. *Journal of Autism and Developmental Disorders, 38*(8), 1414–1425.

Almasy, L., & Blangero, J. (2001). Endophenotypes as quantitative risk factors for psychiatric disease: rationale and study design. *American Journal of Medical Genetics, 105*(1), 42–44.

Almasy, L., Hixson, J. E., Rainwater, D. L., Cole, S., Williams, J. T., Mahaney, M. C., et al. (1999). Human pedigree-based quantitative-trait-locus mapping: localization of two genes influencing HDL-cholesterol metabolism. *American Journal of Human Genetics, 64*(6), 1686–1693.

American Psychiatric Association. (1994). *Diagnostic and statistical manual of mental disorders* (4th ed.; DSM-IV). Washington, DC: Author.

Arking, D. E., Cutler, D. J., Brune, C. W., Teslovich, T. M., West, K., Ikeda, M., et al. (2008). A common genetic variant in the neurexin superfamily member CNTNAP2 increases familial risk of autism. *American Journal of Human Genetics, 82*(1), 160–164.

Bailey, A., Le Couteur, A., Gottesman, I., Bolton, P., Simonoff, E., Yuzda, E., et al. (1995). Autism as a strongly genetic disorder: evidence from a British twin study. *Psychological Medicine, 25*(1), 63–77.

Baron-Cohen, S., Wheelwright, S., Skinner, R., Martin, J., & Clubley, E. (2001). The autism-spectrum quotient (AQ): evidence from Asperger syndrome/high-functioning autism, males and females, scientists and mathematicians. *Journal of Autism and Developmental Disorders, 31*(1), 5–17.

Blangero, J., & Almasy, L. (1996). *SOLAR: Sequential oligogenic linkage analysis routines.* Population Genetics Laboratory Technical Report No. 6. San Antonio, TX: Southwest Foundation for Biomedical Research.

Breiman L. (2001). Random forests. *Machine Learning, 45*, 5–32.

Cantor, R. M. (2006). Linkage analysis. In A. E. H. Emery & D. L. Rimoin (Eds.), *Principles and practice of medical genetics* (5th ed.). London: Churchill Livingstone.

Cantor, R. M., Kono, N., Duvall, J. A., Alvarez-Retuerto, A., Stone, J. L., Alarcon, M., et al. (2005). Replication of autism linkage: fine-mapping peak at 17q21. *American Journal of Human Genetics, 76*(6), 1050–1056.

Chen, G. K., Kono, N., Geschwind, D. H., & Cantor, R. M. (2006). Quantitative trait locus analysis of nonverbal communication in autism spectrum disorder. *Molecular Psychiatry, 11*(2), 214–220.

Chiu, P. H., Kayali, M. A., Kishida, K. T., Tomlin, D., Klinger, L. G., Klinger, M. R., et al. (2008). Self responses along cingulate cortex reveal quantitative neural phenotype for high-functioning autism. *Neuron, 57*(3), 463–473.

Conciatori, M., Stodgell, C. J., Hyman, S. L., O'Bara, M., Militerni, R., Bravaccio, C., et al. (2004). Association between the HOXA1 A218G polymorphism and increased head circumference in patients with autism. *Biological Psychiatry, 55*(4), 413–419.

Constantino, J. N., Lajonchere, C., Lutz, M., Gray, T., Abbacchi, A., McKenna, K., et al. (2006). Autistic social impairment in the siblings of children with pervasive developmental disorders. *American Journal of Psychiatry, 163*(2), 294–296.

Constantino, J. N., & Todd, R. D. (2003). Autistic traits in the general population: a twin study. *Archives of General Psychiatry, 60*(5), 524–530.

Courchesne, E., Pierce, K., Schumann, C. M., Redcay, E., Buckwalter, J. A., Kennedy, D. P., et al. (2007). Mapping early brain development in autism. *Neuron, 56*(2), 399–413.

Cross, S., Kim, S. J., Weiss, L. A., Delahanty, R. J., Sutcliffe, J. S., Leventhal, B. L., et al. (2008). Molecular genetics of the platelet serotonin system in first-degree relatives of patients with autism. *Neuropsychopharmacology, 33*(2), 353–360.

Dawson, G., Estes, A., Munson, J., Schellenberg, G., Bernier, R., & Abbott, R. (2007). Quantitative assessment of autism symptom-related traits in probands and parents: Broader Phenotype Autism Symptom Scale. *Journal of Autism and Developmental Disorders, 37*(3), 523–536.

Dawson, G., Webb, S., Schellenberg, G. D., Dager, S., Friedman, S., Aylward, E., et al. (2002). Defining the broader phenotype of autism: genetic, brain, and behavioral perspectives. *Developmental Psychopathology, 14*(3), 581–611.

Duvall, J. A., Lu, A., Cantor, R. M., Todd, R. D., Constantino, J. N., & Geschwind, D. H. (2007). A quantitative trait locus analysis of social responsiveness in multiplex autism families. *American Journal of Psychiatry, 164*(4), 656–662.

Farrell, P. M., Rosenstein, B. J., White, T. B., Accurso, F. J., Castellani, C., Cutting, G. R., et al. (2008). Guidelines for diagnosis of cystic fibrosis in newborns through older adults: Cystic Fibrosis Foundation consensus report. *Journal of Pediatrics, 153*(2), S4–S14.

Flint, J., Valdar, W., Shifman, S., & Mott, R. (2005). Strategies for mapping and cloning quantitative trait genes in rodents. *Nature Reviews Genetics, 6*(4), 271–286.

Fombonne, E., Roge, B., Claverie, J., Courty, S., & Fremolle, J. (1999). Microcephaly and macrocephaly in autism. *Journal of Autism and Developmental Disorders, 29*(2), 113–119.

Frazer, K. A., Ballinger, D. G., Cox, D. R., Hinds, D. A., Stuve, L. L., Gibbs, R. A., et al. (2007). A second generation human haplotype map of over 3.1 million SNPs. *Nature, 449*(7164), 851–861.

Geschwind, D. H., Sowinski, J., Lord, C., Iversen, P., Shestack, J., Jones, P., et al. (2001). The autism genetic resource exchange: a resource for the study of autism and related neuropsychiatric conditions. *American Journal of Human Genetics, 69*(2), 463–466.

Gottesman, I. I., & Gould, T. D. (2003). The endophenotype concept in psychiatry: etymology and strategic intentions. *American Journal of Psychiatry, 160*(4), 636–645.

Happe, F., Ronald, A., & Plomin, R. (2006). Time to give up on a single explanation for autism. *Nature Neuroscience, 9*(10), 1218–1220.

Haseman, J. K., & Elston, R. C. (1972). The investigation of linkage between a quantitative trait and a marker locus. *Behavior Genetics, 2*(1), 3–19.

Heath, S. C. (1997). LOKI, ver 2.3.5: Markov chain Monte Carlo segregation and linkage analysis for oligogenic models. *American Journal of Human Genetics, 61*(3), 748–760.

Hochberg, M. C. (1997). Updating the American College of Rheumatology revised criteria for the classification of systemic lupus erythematosus. *Arthritis and Rheumatism, 40*(9), 1725.

Hoekstra, R. A., Bartels, M., Verweij, C. J., & Boomsma, D. I. (2007). Heritability of autistic traits in the general population. *Archives of Pediatrics and Adolescent Medicine, 161*(4), 372–377.

Horvath, S., Xu, X., & Laird, N. M. (2001). The family based association test method: strategies for studying general genotype-phenotype associations. *European Journal of Human Genetics, 9*(4), 301–306.

Ijichi, S., Ijichi, N., Ijichi, Y., Kawamura, Y., Hashiguchi, T., & Morioka, H. (2008). For others: epistasis and the evolutionary survival of an extreme tail of the quantitative distribution of autistic assets. *Medical Hypotheses, 70*(3), 515–521.

Kruglyak, L., Daly, M. J., Reeve-Daly, M. P., & Lander, E. S. (1996). Genehunter, ver 2.1: Parametric and nonparametric linkage analysis: a unified multipoint approach. *American Journal of Human Genetics, 58*(6), 1347–1363.

Kutner, M. H., Nachtsheim, C. J., & Neter, J. (2004). *Applied linear regression models* (4th ed.). Boston: McGraw-Hill.

Lainhart, J. E., Bigler, E. D., Bocian, M., Coon, H., Dinh, E., Dawson, G., et al. (2006). Head circumference and height in autism: a study by the Collaborative Program of Excellence in Autism. *American Journal of Medical Genetics. Part A, 140*(21), 2257–2274.

Lamb, J. A., Parr, J. R., Bailey, A. J., & Monaco, A. P. (2002). Autism: in search of susceptibility genes. *Neuromolecular Medicine, 2*(1), 11–28.

Lange, K., Cantor, R. M., Horvath, S., Perola, M., Sabatti, C., Sinsheimer, J. S., et al. (2001). Mendel version 4.0: A complete package for the exact genetic analysis of discrete traits in pedigree and population data sets. *American Journal of Human Genetics 69*(supplement), 504.

Liu, X. Q., Paterson, A. D., & Szatmari, P. (2008). Genome-wide linkage analyses of quantitative and categorical autism subphenotypes. *Biological Psychiatry, 64*(7), 561–570.

Lord, C., Risi, S., Lambrecht, L., Cook, E. H., Jr., Leventhal, B. L., DiLavore, P. C., et al. (2000). The Autism Diagnostic Observation Schedule-Generic: a standard measure of social and communication deficits associated with the spectrum of autism. *Journal of Autism and Developmental Disorders, 30*(3), 205–223.

Lord, C., Rutter, M., & Le Couteur, A. (1994). Autism Diagnostic Interview-Revised: a revised version of a diagnostic interview for caregivers of individuals with possible pervasive developmental disorders. *Journal of Autism and Developmental Disorders, 24*(5), 659–685.

Losh, M., & Piven, J. (2007). Social-cognition and the broad autism phenotype: identifying genetically meaningful phenotypes. *Journal of Child Psychology and Psychiatry and Allied Disciplines, 48*(1), 105–112.

Mackay, T. F. (2004). The genetic architecture of quantitative traits: lessons from Drosophila. *Current Opinion in Genetics and Development, 14*(3), 253–257.

Manolio, T. A., Brooks, L. D., & Collins, F. S. (2008). A HapMap harvest of insights into the genetics of common disease. *Journal of Clinical Investigation, 118*(5), 1590–1605.

Ott, J. (1999). *Analysis of human genetic linkage* (3rd ed.). Baltimore: The Johns Hopkins University Press.

Ott, L., & Longnecker, M. (2000). *An introduction to statistical methods and data analysis* (6th ed.). Belmont, CA: Duxbury.

Pickles, A., Starr, E., Kazak, S., Bolton, P., Papanikolaou, K., Bailey, A., et al. (2000). Variable expression of the autism broader phenotype: findings from extended pedigrees. *Journal of Child Psychology and Psychiatry and Allied Disciplines, 41*(4), 491–502.

Piven, J., Palmer, P., Jacobi, D., Childress, D., & Arndt, S. (1997). Broader autism phenotype: evidence from a family history study of multiple-incidence autism families. *American Journal of Psychiatry, 154*(2), 185–190.

Piven, J., Palmer, P., Landa, R., Santangelo, S., Jacobi, D., & Childress, D. (1997). Personality and language characteristics in parents from multiple-incidence autism families. *American Journal of Medical Genetics, 74*(4), 398–411.

Qiao, Q., Laatikainen, T., Zethelius, B., Stegmayr, B., Eliasson, M., Jousilahti, P., et al. (2009). Comparison of definitions of metabolic syndrome in relation to the risk of developing stroke and coronary heart disease in Finnish and Swedish cohorts. *Stroke, 40*(2), 337–343.

Rice, T. K. (2008). Familial resemblance and heritability. *Advances in Genetics, 60*, 35–49.

Risch, N., Spiker, D., Lotspeich, L., Nouri, N., Hinds, D., Hallmayer, J., et al. (1999). A genomic screen of autism: evidence for a multilocus etiology. *American Journal of Human Genetics, 65*(2), 493–507.

Roberts, L., Davenport, R. J., Pennisi, E., & Marshall, E. (2001). A history of the Human Genome Project. *Science, 291*(5507), 1195.

Rockman, M. V., & Kruglyak, L. (2008). Breeding designs for recombinant inbred advanced intercross lines. *Genetics, 179*(2), 1069–1078.

Ronald, A., Happe, F., Bolton, P., Butcher, L. M., Price, T. S., Wheelwright, S., et al. (2006). Genetic heterogeneity between the three components of the autism spectrum: a twin study. *Journal of the American Academy of Child and Adolescent Psychiatry, 45*(6), 691–699.

Sacco, R., Militerni, R., Frolli, A., Bravaccio, C., Gritti, A., Elia, M., et al. (2007). Clinical, morphological, and biochemical correlates of head circumference in autism. *Biological Psychiatry, 62*(9), 1038–1047.

Schellenberg, G. D., Dawson, G., Sung, Y. J., Estes, A., Munson, J., Rosenthal, E., et al. (2006). Evidence for multiple loci from a genome scan of autism kindreds. *Molecular Psychiatry, 11*(11), 1049–1060, 1979.

Simon-Sanchez, J., & Singleton, A. (2008). Genome-wide association studies in neurological disorders. *Lancet Neurology, 7*(11), 1067–1072.

Skuse, D. H., Mandy, W. P., & Scourfield, J. (2005). Measuring autistic traits: heritability, reliability, and validity of the Social and Communication Disorders Checklist. *British Journal of Psychiatry, 187*, 568–572.

Slager, S. L., Foroud, T., Haghighi, F., Spence, M. A., & Hodge, S. E. (2001). Stoppage: an issue for segregation analysis. *Genetic Epidemiology, 20*(3), 328–339.

Spence, S., Black, D., Miyamoto, J., & Geschwind, D. H. (2005). *The occurrence of macrocephaly in autistic and non-autistic individuals from a large familial idiopathic autism sample (AGRE)*. 5th Annual International Meeting For Autism Research (IMFAR), Boston, MA (pp. S7.7).

Spiker, D., Lotspeich, L. J., Dimiceli, S., Myers, R. M., & Risch, N. (2002). Behavioral phenotypic variation in autism multiplex families: evidence for a continuous severity gradient. *American Journal of Medical Genetics, 114*(2), 129–136.

Sung, Y. J., Dawson, G., Munson, J., Estes, A., Schellenberg, G. D., & Wijsman, E. M. (2005). Genetic investigation of quantitative traits related to autism: use of multivariate polygenic models with ascertainment adjustment. *American Journal of Human Genetics, 76*(1), 68–81.

Szatmari, P., Maziade, M., Zwaigenbaum, L., Merette, C., Roy, M. A., Joober, R., et al. (2007). Informative phenotypes for genetic studies of psychiatric disorders. *American Journal of Medical Genetics. Part B, Neuropsychiatric Genetics*, 144B(5), 581–588.

Veenstra-Vanderweele, J., Christian, S. L., & Cook, E. H., Jr. (2004). Autism as a paradigmatic complex genetic disorder. *Annual Review of Genomics and Human Genetics, 5*, 379–405.

Viding, E., & Blakemore, S. J. (2007). Endophenotype approach to developmental psychopathology: implications for autism research. *Behavior Genetics, 37*(1), 51–60.

Walters, J. T., & Owen, M. J. (2007). Endophenotypes in psychiatric genetics. *Molecular Psychiatry*, *12*(10), 886–890.

Weiss, L. A., Kosova, G., Delahanty, R. J., Jiang, L., Cook, E. H., Ober, C., et al. (2006). Variation in ITGB3 is associated with whole-blood serotonin level and autism susceptibility. *European Journal of Human Genetics*, *14*(8), 923–931.

Wijsman, E. M. (2007). *Statistical genetic approaches for analysis of autism and autism endophenotypes.* 6th Annual International Meeting For Autism Research (IMFAR), Seattle, WA (pp. 84).

Willer, C. J., Speliotes, E. K., Loos, R. J., Li, S., Lindgren, C. M., Heid, I. M., et al. (2009). Six new loci associated with body mass index highlight a neuronal influence on body weight regulation. *Nature Genetics*, *41*(1), 25–34.

Yoon, J. L., Alarcon, M., Geschwind, D. H., & Cantor, R. M. (2008). *Replication and association analysis of a 1p13-q12 locus for non-verbal communication deficits in autism spectrum disorder.* 7th Annual International Meeting For Autism Research (IMFAR) London, United Kingdom (pp. 105–109).

40 Judith H. Miles

Autism Subgroups from a Medical Genetics Perspective

Points of Interest

- A first step in the quest for etiologically discrete autism subgroups is the identification of "phenotypic features" that are present in some but not all individuals with autism, are relatively discrete, quantifiable, and pathophysiologically relevant.
- Phenotypes may be physical (e.g., dysmorphology), medical (e.g., seizures), laboratory based (e.g., EEG abnormalities, pupillary light reflex parameters), clinical course elements (e.g., age of onset, regression, trajectory), and genetic indicators (e.g., gender, recurrence risk, family history of autism and related disorders).
- The terms "phenotype," "endophenotype," and "biomarker" are comparable.
- The core autism behavioral symptoms are less likely to separate out etiologically discrete subgroups because by definition they occur in all diagnosed individuals.
- A phenotype is presumed valuable when subgroups defined on that basis differ in clinical course, outcome, response to therapy, and/or genetic indicators.
- Subgroups of families with strong family histories of autism plus another neurologic disorder may allow us to identify shared biochemical pathways and genes.

To unravel the clinical and etiologic heterogeneity within autism or what is best termed the autism spectrum disorders (ASD) is an ambitious but compulsory goal. Because autism is a behavioral disorder with few physical and laboratory features, this has proven much more difficult than for the prototypic single gene disorders (reviewed in Fein et al., 1999; Spence, 2001). Reports of sibs discordant for their autism spectrum disorders led to the disheartening expectation that we would not be able to understand the heterogeneity until we found specific autism genes and we could not find the autism genes until we understand the heterogeneity (DeLong & Dwyer, 1988; Silverman, 2002).

Strategies for Defining Autism Subgroups

Historically, interest in subclassifying autism was focused on assessing validity of the classical autism diagnoses by seeing which clinical symptoms, adaptive behaviors, and cognitive skills occurred together (reviewed in Gillberg, 1992; Fein et al., 1999; Prior et al., 1998). To determine whether there were true diagnostic differences between putative subgroups, analyses considered all symptoms and their variations and used cluster analyses and other taxonomic techniques to see if and what groups of symptoms co-occurred. Many of these studies demonstrated real associations—such as Asperger's subjects were more likely to be male and autism-like subjects compared with autism subjects were more likely to be female—but did not actually identify discrete autism subgroups. And most of the differences identified related more to the level of cognitive and adaptive functioning, rather than distinctive diagnostic behavior patterns. More importantly, the behavioral profiles that were generated were not correlated with biological mechanisms or etiologies.

Recently, there has been a renewed interest in more refined taxometric methods to look at the heritability of autism's core symptoms (Beglinger & Smith, 2001; Constantino, Chapter 29 in this book; Happé & Ronald, 2008; Ingram, Takahashi, & Miles, 2007). The premise underlying all subtyping paradigms is that there is a phenotypic marker that has a taxonomic, i.e., categorical structure, which can identify discrete subgroups with different etiologies, outcomes, or therapeutic responses. In their 2008 review, Happé and Ronald presented evidence that alterations in the separate defining domains of social relatedness, language/communication, and restricted interest/repetitive behavior are separable and that approaches that consider autism as an entity may be ineffective. Ingram et al. (2007) used taxometric methods to look at both behavioral and physical phenotypes to see which varied categorically rather than only by degree. Their analyses support subgrouping subjects based on variation in social interaction/communication, intelligence, and the essential/complex phenotype; in contrast, subjects varied continuously in repetitive sensory and motor actions, language acquisition, and insistence on sameness. These studies not only highlight the importance of phenotypic clarity but indicate that continuous markers are less useful or at least more complicated to study.

The goal of a medical geneticist is to define subgroups that are etiologically discrete and do not overlap, such that a defined subgroup will not only be homogeneous, but its removal from the pool will leave a more homogeneous remainder. The standard approach to identifying homogeneous subsets of patients with any medical condition is to identify phenotypic features that occur in some but not all of the population. To be useful, the phenotypic features should be consistently present in most if not all autism populations, relatively discrete, quantifiable, and most importantly pathophysiologically relevant. Features that remain constant over time are particularly useful, while those that describe continuous variables are less helpful. Table 40-1 lists

Table 40–1.
Phenotypic variables that may define discrete autism (ASD) subgroups

Phenotypic Variables	Consistently Present in a Proportion of ASD Populations (% of ASD)	Discrete	Continuous or Categorical	Measurable	Constant Over Time	Pathophysiologically Relevant	May Suggest a Genetic Marker
Core Autism Symptoms							
Social functioning	No, 100%	Yes		Yes	No	Yes	Maybe
Communication	No, 100%	Yes	Categorical	Yes	No	Probably	Maybe
Repetitive, stereotypic behaviors and/or preoccupations, obsessions	Yes, but must be scored separately	Yes	Continuous	Yes	No	Probably	Maybe
Functionally Defined Variables							
IQ	Yes	No	Categorical	Yes	Yes/No	Yes	Maybe
Adaptive behaviors (Vineland)	Maybe	No	uk	Yes	No	Probably	No
Outcome measures	Poorly defined	No	uk	Yes, but takes years	No	Probably	No
Response to therapy	Yes	Yes	uk	Yes	Yes	Probably	Maybe
Clinical Course							
Age of onset	Yes	Yes	? Categorical	Yes	Yes	Yes	Yes
Regressive onset	Yes, ~ 30%	Yes	? Categorical	Yes	Yes	Yes	Yes
Adolescent/adult catatonic regression	Yes, ~17%	Yes	? Categorical	Yes	Yes	Yes	Yes
Medical/Neurological							
Seizures	Yes, ~ 25%	No	Categorical	Yes	No	Yes	Yes
EEG abn	Yes, ~ 50%	No	? Categorical	Yes	No	Yes	Yes
Sleep disorder	Yes, ~ 65%	No	Categorical	Yes	No	Yes	Yes
Savant skills	Yes, ~ 5%	?	Categorical	Yes	Yes	Probably	Maybe
Morphology & Growth							
Generalized Dysmorphology	Yes, 15%–20%	Yes	Categorical	Yes	Yes	Yes	Yes
Macrocephaly	Yes, ~ 30%	Yes	Continuous	Yes	Yes	Yes	Yes
Head growth trajectory	Probably	uk	uk	Yes	No	Yes	Yes
Microcephaly	Yes, ~ 5%	Yes	Categorical	Yes	Yes	Yes	Yes
Brain malformations	Yes, ~ 20%	Yes	Categorical	Yes	Yes	Yes	Yes

(Continued)

Table 40–1. (*Contd.*)

Phenotypic Variables	Consistently Present in a Proportion of ASD Populations (% of ASD)	Discrete	Continuous or Categorical	Measurable	Constant Over Time	Pathophysiologically Relevant	May Suggest a Genetic Marker
Significant Family History of Related Disorders							
ASD	Yes, 25%	Yes	uk	Yes	Yes	Yes	Yes
Affective Disorders	Probably	Yes	Categorical	Yes	Yes	Yes	Yes
Alcoholism	Yes, 30%	Yes	Categorical	Yes	Yes	Yes	Yes
ADHD	Probably	Yes	Categorical	Yes	Yes	Yes	Yes
Bipolar/Major Affective Disorder	Yes	Yes	Categorical	Yes	No	Yes	Yes

phenotypic variables that have been suggested or used to dissect out autism subgroups. The list is not inclusive, and the assessment of the usefulness of each phenotype is my generalization, since most have not been tested and rarely does a yes or no answer explain the complexity of the answer.

From this table we see that the core autism symptoms are less likely to easily separate out subtypes because by definition they occur in all of the diagnosed individuals, though recent taxometric analyses (Ingram et al., 2007) support the opinion that combined impairments in social interaction and communication into one domain may be a valuable phenotypic variable. A characteristic of the clinical course of autism, regression provides an a priori excellent candidate, though it is often difficult to categorize mild symptoms of regression. Regression is a relatively common phenomenon in many pediatric neurologic disorders and has been linked to genetic diagnoses, including Rett syndrome, mitochondrial disease, and metabolic enzyme deficiency and storage disorders (Clarke, 2005; Weissman et al., 2008). Family histories of autism and alcoholism are attractive candidates because of their clear association with known genetic markers, though phenotypic reliability can be imprecise when obtained through family history alone. Based on this analysis, it is the abnormalities of morphology and growth that emerge as highly likely candidates for subgrouping.

This identification of potentially informative phenotypic variables is only a first step; ultimately each potential variable must be carefully studied to determine its usefulness. This includes investigating the mechanistic basis of the variable to substantiate its biologic relevance. Once that is done, the population can be divided into two or more subgroups based on the study phenotype. Finally, the subgroups are analyzed to look for differences in outcome measures (language, cognitive, adaptive), physical phenotypes (growth, head size, general dysmorphology), clinical course measures (age of onset, type of onset with or without regression, developmental trajectory), medical/neurologic features (seizures, EEG abnormalities), and genetic features (male to female ratio, sib recurrence risk, family history of autism, alcoholism, affective disorders, cognitive and language impairments). Obviously, this list is incomplete and is constantly expanded as new phenotypic variables are recognized as useful vehicles with which to separate ASD into discrete etiologic subgroups.

Relationship Between Clinical Phenotypes and Endophenotypes

This is probably a good place to discuss the relationship between phenotypes as used by medical geneticists to subgroup populations and endophenotypes. Gottesman and Gould (2003) proposed that phenotypic features that would be most helpful be termed "endophenotypes"—i.e., phenotypes that were more biological and thus more proximally related to the underlying etiologic processes—and that endophenotypes in autism may provide an avenue for homing in on specific neuropsychological mechanisms of biological and genetic significance to autism. Piven, Palmer, Jacobi, Childress, and Arndt (1997) suggested that these endophenotypes might also be traceable in unaffected relatives of individuals with autism. Conceptually, there is no real difference between phenotypes and endophenotypes. From a medical perspective phenotypes may be thought of as clinical, observable symptoms of a disorder and endophenotypes as the results of laboratory tests that measure specific biological actions. Both are used to further describe the disorder in question, in our case autism. A review of the literature illustrates that many autism researchers use these terms interchangeably and consider any circumscribed symptom, such as insistence on sameness or savant skills, as an endophenotype (Spence et al., 2006). The introduction of the term "biomarkers" affords an excellent compromise that envelops the essence of both phenotype and endophenotype.

A few examples of phenotypes and endophenotypes are provided in Table 40-2. As we learn more, there will undoubtedly be many examples of phenotypes being described on a biological level, which can then be used in genetic studies (James et al., 2006). In all cases, the geneticist will try to link clinical phenotypes and endophenotypes with etiologies, outcomes, and responses to therapies.

Table 40–2.
Phenotypes, endophenotypes, and etiologies

Autism Related Phenotypes	Laboratory Tests & Measures as Endophenotypes	Genes/ Teratogens/Toxins
Aloof personality (Social-cognition). (This subset of ASD children are aloof, have poorer pragmatic language and poorer friendships)	Eyes Test[1] The Eyes Test is an endophenotype associated with aloof personality.	?
Seizures, sleep, hearing loss, vision loss, facial asymmetry	EEG, sMRI, SPEC Scan, PET scan, Evoked response, ERG, Pupillary light responses etc.	?
Regressive onset	Oxidative stress measures	?
Craniofacial dysmorphology	Facial anthropomorphic measures, Shape analysis of midline brain areas	Developmental genes

[1] Losh & Piven, 2007; Baron-Cohen & Hammer, 1997.

Autism Subgroups: Proposed and/or Analyzed

Most of these categories are based on a phenotypic variable that may or may not turn out to identify a distinct and biologically relevant ASD subgroup. Given current uncertainty over which phenotypes will be the most informative, it is appropriate that each phenotypic variable in Table 40-1 be assessed as part of any autism study.

Morphologically Defined Subgroups

In the 1970s and early 1980s a number of studies documented that, taken as a group, autistic children had physical features outside the norm (Mnukhin & Isaev, 1975; Campbell, Geller, Small, Petti, & Ferris, 1978; Walker, 1977; Links, 1980; Links, Stockwell, Abichandani, & Simeon, 1980; Steg & Rapoport, 1975; Gualtieri, Adams, Shen, & Loiselle, 1982). Walker, using the Waldrop weighted scoring scale (Waldrop & Halverson, 1971) for sixteen anomalies, studied 74 autistic and nonautistic children matched for age, sex, socioeconomic group, and geographic domicile, and found that the mean minor anomaly score of 5.76 for the autistic children was significantly higher than the control group score of 3.53. He concluded that this shift to a greater number of anomalies in the autistic subjects proved organicity in autism. Links et al. (1980) recognized that autistic children had more anomalies than their sibs, and that the autistic children with the higher anomaly scores had lower IQs, spent more time in the hospital, had less frequent family histories of psychotic illness, or drug or alcohol abuse. They concluded that the anomalies were the result of some unknown organic factor that played a role in the etiology of autism. Smalley, Asarnow, and Spence (1988) declared that minor physical anomalies (MPAs) result from insults, either genetic or environmental, that occur in the first trimester, and represent an indirect measure of an abnormality in fetal development. Full understanding of these studies was, however, hindered by the prevailing dogma that autism was homogeneous, and the authors did not speculate that there could be etiologically distinct groups within the autism behavioral diagnosis.

We hypothesized that physical dysmorphology would be a useful phenotypic feature which would allow us to divide autism into subgroups (Miles & Hillman, 2000). The premise was that individuals for whom there is evidence for some insult to early morphogenesis will be etiologically different. They would have developed their autistic behavioral disorder on a different basis than the individuals whose early morphogenesis proceeded normally. The group with evidence of abnormal morphogenesis was described as having complex autism, the remainder essential autism.

Generalized dysmorphology fits our criteria for a potentially useful phenotype. It occurs in a consistent proportion of ASD individuals, is constant over time and most importantly is biologically relevant. Though dysmorphic features used to characterize generalized dysmorphology are usually obvious to the geneticist, they can be subtle and are usually missed by therapists and clinicians not trained to look for them. However, we have been able to demonstrate that generalized dysmorphology is measurable, with good reliability (Miles, Takahashi, Hillman, & Martin, 2004, Miles et al., 2008). Most important, physical dysmorphology is a biologically based phenotype that suggests a developmental etiology.

The third step was to determine whether autistic individuals with generalized dysmorphology differ from those in whom there is no evidence of abnormal physical development. For all functional and outcome measures, the individuals with complex autism did less well. They are twice as likely to have IQ scores less than 55 (52% vs. 25%) and less than half as likely to have IQ scores in the normal range (22% vs. 46%). They are twice as likely to develop seizures (39% vs. 17%), and twice as likely to have abnormal brain structure (28% vs. 13%). Our outcome analyses, based on both the acquisition of functional language and IQ scores, show that though many features correlate with poor outcomes, the diagnosis of complex designation is the most sensitive test, yielding an 86% positive predictive value of poor outcome (Miles et al., 2005). This cross-sectional outcome data is consistent with our study of 19 children with autism who completed 1 year of one-on-one early intensive (22 hrs/wk) behavioral intervention (Stoelb et al., 2004). The most significant predictor of change in performance scores over the year of therapy was dysmorphic physical features ($p = .0009$). And the presence or absence of dysmorphic features predicted language acquisition for 90% of the nonverbal participants.

Step four is to determine whether the complex and essential subgroups are genetically different. This can be addressed in two ways. First, genetic consequences, including the sex ratio, recurrence risks, and family histories, are compared. Our data (Miles et al., 2005) found that individuals in the essential autism subgroup were twice as likely to be male (6.5:1 vs. 3.2:1), were more than twice as likely to have a family history of autism (20% vs. 9%), and had a sib recurrence risk of 4–6% compared with no recurrences in the 46 families of children with complex autism. The occurrence of lesser autistic traits in sibs of children with essential autism was twice that for complex autism families (12% vs. 6%). The small number of sibs limits the power of the calculations; however, the very similar magnitude of differences for all sibs, latter born sibs, and for classical autism and milder autistic traits illustrates a consistent pattern. The fact we did not observe any recurrence in sibs in these 46 children with complex autism is certainly a statistical aberration. We know that the risk of recurrence is not zero, since children with complex autism may have disorders such as Fragile X syndrome and familial chromosome disorders that confer explicit recurrence risks. Notwithstanding, we feel that parents of children with complex autism, once chromosome disorders, Fragile X syndrome, tuberous sclerosis, and other discrete genetic syndromes have been ruled out, may be counseled that their recurrence risk is lower than the 4–6% observed with essential autism. A number of observations by other laboratories are consistent with this model. Szatmari et al. (1996) noted that relatives of probands with higher IQs were at greater risk than those of probands with lower IQ.

An additional genetic and clinically practical consequence of the separation is that all of the individuals with recognizable syndromes fall in the complex autism diagnosis, or in the case of tuberous sclerosis can almost always be recognized by the dysmorphology examination (Miles et al., 2005). We have not identified any children with chromosome disorders, including the 15q duplications, who have not declared themselves on the dysmorphology examination. It is, however, expected that genome wide chromosomal array technology will discover copy number variants (CNVs) in children with both complex and essential autism, with specific CNVs associated with dysmorphology.

Major ramifications of this distinction come from studying the essential and complex autism subgroups independently. One example is studies attempting to understand the autism 4:1 male to female ratio. Analyzing essential autism has allowed us to make a number of significant observations. First, within the essential autism group, a regressive onset and macrocephaly have both emerged as stronger predictors of poorer outcomes. A history of regression in language at the onset of the autistic symptoms predicts a poor outcome with 46% sensitivity, 73% specificity, and a positive predictive value of 84%. An association between cognitive level and macrocephaly is consistent with a recent report that children with macrocephaly have greater discrepancies between verbal and nonverbal IQ scores (Tager-Flusberg & Joseph, 2003). Tager-Flusberg and Joseph hypothesize that macrocephaly indicates a more severe disturbance of neurocognitive development and organization. Though essential autism remains heterogeneous, with more children having poor than good outcomes, we find that limiting studies to the group of individuals with essential autism has allowed us to begin to identify outcome predictors that we couldn't see before we removed the complex group. Recognizing these outcome predictors is a first step toward designing treatments to improve outcomes. Furthermore, since essential autism is the more heritable subgroup, removing complex autism probands from analyses should improve the power of linkage and sib pair analyses.

The distinction between complex and essential autism represents the first pass at dissecting the etiologic heterogeneity within the autism diagnosis. The distinction fits our criteria for a phenotype we would predict as useful in the delineation of autism subgroups. Though each group remains heterogeneous, the functional and genetic differences indicate that essential and complex autism are inherently different subgroups with different etiologies. The distinction between essential and complex autism also illustrates the overlap between the terms "clinical phenotypes" and "endophenotypes." Complex autism captures the subgroup of children whose physical phenotype indicates a different embryological process. Analysis of specific morphologic abnormalities is expected to point our studies toward specific developmental pathways.

Brain-Size Defined Subgroups

In addition to generalized dysmorphology, specific malformations, especially those related to the brain, are important for delineating ASD subgroups. Macrocephaly, which occurs in 20–30% of ASD children and 37–45% of their nonautistic parents, is the best example (Miles, Hadden, Takahashi, & Hillman, 2000; Fombonne, Bolton, Prior, Jordan, & Rutter, 1999; Lainhart et al., 1997; Lainhart et al., 2006, Sacco et al., 2007, Vaccarino, Grigorenko, Smith, & Stevens, 2009). Its importance was underscored by Bolton's (1999) report, that infantile macrocephaly was a significant predictor (OR = 5.44) for the development of autism. However, the timing and mechanism responsible for increased head size is not well understood. Macrocephaly is generally a reflection of increased brain size in ASD (Stanfield et al., 2007; reviewed in Casanova, 2007), though Aylward, Minshew, Field, Sparks, and Singh (2002) found head circumference was only an accurate index of brain volume in young ASD children, and not in adolescents or adults. Tate, Bigler, McMahon, and Lainhart (2007) found that the relationship between head circumference and brain volume was not as highly correlated in ASD individuals as in typically developing individuals. Recent analyses of patterns of brain growth are refining our understanding of macrocephaly in autism. At birth, head circumference in infants later diagnosed with ASD has been found to be either similar to typically developing individuals or even reduced (McCaffery & Deutsch, 2005; Courchesne & Pierce, 2005; Pardo & Eberhart, 2007). Our studies indicate that the presence and number of surges in head size occurring throughout childhood in autism is more informative than ultimate head size, which may explain why macrocephaly itself is not an independent predictor of phenotypic or genetic traits or outcome measures (Miles, Hadden, Takahashi, & Hillman, 2000; Keegan, Takahashi, & Miles, 2007). This literature is still complicated by conflicting reports, which are likely due to the inherent heterogeneity within ASD, the scarcity of longitudinal data, and perhaps lack of correlation between head circumference and brain volume in some children.

Macrocephaly, in addition to being a common physical phenotype of idiopathic autism, is a key feature in a number of genetically well characterized syndromes that can cause autism, including Fragile X syndrome, PTEN syndromes, Sotos syndrome, and HOXA1 G alleles. Fragile X syndrome, which is due to expansion of the CGG trinucleotide repeat in the *FMR1* gene, causes many autistic behaviors, including avoidance of eye contact, language delays, repetitive behaviors, sleep disturbances, tantrums, self-injurious behaviors, hyperactivity, impulsiveness, inattention, and sound sensitivities. In one study of 63 males with Fragile X syndrome 30% met criteria for autistic disorder and 30% criteria for PDD-NOS (Harris et al., 2008). Molecular studies indicate the *FMR1* gene may cause the autism phenotype via two mechanisms, RNA toxicity to the neurons and gene silencing, which impacts neuronal connectivity (Schenck et al., 2003; Handa et al., 2005; Hagerman, Rivera, & Hagerman, 2008). Though these mechanisms are not the primary cause of autism, they can offer insight into its pathogenesis. For example, evidence suggests that some molecular defects in autism may interfere with synaptic protein synthesis, as in Fragile X, suggesting that this is one possible pathway leading to autistic phenotypes (Kelleher & Bear, 2008) The PTEN (phosphatase and tensin homolog) gene is a tumor suppressor gene associated with a broad group of disorders referred to as PTEN hamartoma tumor syndromes, which include Cowden syndrome, Bannayan-Riley-Ruvlacaba syndrome, Proteus syndrome, and Lhermitte-Duclos disease. Recently, *PTEN* gene mutations have been associated with autism and macrocephaly (Zori, Marsh, Graham, Marliss, & Eng, 1998; Parisi et al., 2001; Delatycki, Danks, Churchyard, Zhou, & Eng, 2003; Butler et al., 2005; Buxbaum et al., 2007). Correspondingly, *PTEN* is recognized to play an important role in brain development, including neuronal survival and synaptic plasticity. The frequency of *PTEN* mutations as a cause of ASD is unclear; results from studies of children with autism and macrocephaly range from 1% (Buxbaum et al., 2007) to 8.3% (Varga, Pastore, Prior, Herman, & McBride, 2009) to 17% (Butler et al., 2005). Both de novo and familial *PTEN* mutations have been identified in this population. It may be significant that more of the children studied by Buxbaum et al. (2007) were from multiplex families, whereas in the Butler et al. (2005) study all children were from simplex families. Children with ASD found to have a *PTEN* mutation generally have extreme macrocephaly ranging from +3.7 SD to +9.6 SD (average: +5.4 SD) (Buxbaum et al., 2007). In addition, mutation of *PTEN* is not specific for autism: Varga et al. (2009) found children with macrocephaly and mental retardation but not autism had a similar chance of having a *PTEN* mutation. Sotos syndrome, which is characterized by overgrowth (head circumference and height ≥ 2 SD), typical facial features, cognitive and behavioral problems including difficulty with peer group relationships and a lack of awareness of social cues, though not a significant cause of classic autism—it is caused by a mutation or deletion of NSD1 gene in 80–90% of cases—provides an additional avenue of investigation of the genesis of autistic behaviors. Conciatori et al. (2004) presented evidence that the *HOXA1* G allele correlates with larger head circumferences, explaining approximately 5% of the variance in head circumference in their population. Each of these disorders that overlap clinically and physically with autism has a known etiology. And, as the Fragile X studies of neurotransmission indicate, study of these related disorders is apt to provide insight into mechanisms underlying idiopathic autism. Other genes involved in brain overgrowth have recently been reviewed by McCaffery & Deutsch (2005).

Microcephaly, defined as head circumference at or below 2 standard deviations is also an informative phenotype. It occurs in 5–15% of children with autism and is highly predictive of poor outcome (Fombonne et al., 1999; Miles, Hadden, et al., 2000; Miles et al., 2005). Similar to generalized dysmorphology, microcephaly almost always indicates a neurodevelopmental etiology, especially chromosomal disorders. Though it is likely that some microcephaly/ASD syndromes will be identified, at this time the main use of microcephaly in subgrouping is to identify the complex autism subtype.

Brain-Malformation Defined Subgroups

Numerous lines of evidence suggest abnormalities in brain structure are closely related to the etiology of autism. In addition to brain volume studies (Courchesne et al., 2001; Courchesne, Carper, & Akshoomoff, 2003; Hazlett et al., 2005), there are numerous reports of structural malformations. Levitt et al. (2003) showed that cortical sulcal patterns were significantly different in control children and children with autism, and that these differences were mainly in the frontal and temporal sulci. Using a direct measurement of cortical thickness to examine the gray matter integrity, Hadjikhani et al. (2004) found local decreases of gray matter thickness in the ASD group in the inferior frontal gyrus, inferior parietal lobule, and the superior temporal sulcus (STS). In addition, cortical thinning in these regions correlated with

ASD symptom severity. Barnea-Goraly et al. (2004) found a significant disruption of white matter structures between brain regions implicated in social functioning that might contribute to impaired social cognition in autism, and provide an example of the abnormal brain connectivity theory in autism (Just, Cherkassky, Keller, & Minshew, 2004; Geschwind & Levitt, 2007). Other brain structures such as the brain stem (Hashimoto et al., 1993), thalamus (Tsatsanis, 2003), corpus callosum (Boger-Megiddo et al., 2006; Egaas, Courchesne, & Saitoh, 1995; Piven, Bailey, Ranson, & Arndt, 1997, Vidal et al., 2006), amygdala (Nacewicz et al., 2006), and hippocampus (Dager et al., 2007; Nicolson et al., 2006) have also been reported as abnormal in autism. Results have often ranged from inconclusive to contradictory. For example, Boddaert and colleagues (2004) investigated 21 autistic children and 12 children of normal intelligence and found a bilateral decrease in gray matter concentration in the superior temporal sulcus (STS) and a white matter concentration decrease in the right temporal pole and left cerebellar hemisphere in autistic children compared to control children. But Waiter et al. (2004) investigated 16 autistic children and 16 controls, finding total gray matter to be increased in the autism group, with local volume increases in the right fusiform gyrus, the right temporo-occipital region, and the left frontal pole. Limbic structures, specifically the amygdala and hippocampus have also been implicated with contradicting findings. Increased (Abell et al., 1999; Howard et al., 2000; Sparks et al., 2002; Juranek et al., 2006; Munson et al., 2006; Schumann et al., 2004), decreased (Aylward et al., 1999; Herbert et al., 2003; Pierce & Courchesne, 2001; Nacewicz et al., 2006), and "normal" amygdala volumes (Haznedar et al., 2000) have been reported. As in the amygdala studies, no consistent abnormalities have been reported in hippocampus. Increased (Sparks et al., 2002; Rojas et al., 2004; Schumann et al., 2004; Geuze, Vermetten, & Bremmer, 2005), decreased (Aylward et al., 1999; Herbert et al., 2003; Saitoh, Karns, & Courchesne, 2001; Nicolson et al., 2006), or "normal" (Haznedar et al., 2000; Howard et al., 2000; Piven, Bailey, Ranson, & Arndt,1998; Saitoh, Courchesne, Egaas, Lincoln, & Schreibman, 1995) hippocampal volumes have been reported in autism. These results call to mind the apparent disparities of the dysmorphology studies of the 1970s and early 1980s. It was not until individuals with and without dysmorphology and microcephaly were analyzed separately, that the inherent structural heterogeneity with ASD was appreciated. Based on these lessons from the past, it is suggested that efforts be launched to identify discrete brain morphology subgroups.

Family-History Defined Subgroups

The family pedigree, which consists of documenting the history for at least three generations, is an indispensible part of the clinical genetics evaluation. Data on multiple generations is essential for analysis of modes of transmission including autosomal versus X-linked, recessive versus dominant, and epigenetic patterns. Family ASD studies have revealed significant clustering of neuropsychiatric disorders including depression, manic depression, obsessive-compulsive disorder, social phobia, anxiety disorders, alcoholism and substance abuse, and motor tics, in addition to ASD phenotypes in relatives of autism probands. This genetic overlap between autism and other neuropsychiatric disorders suggests that at least for certain types of autism there are common biochemical and genetic aberrations. Lobascher, Kingerlee, and Gubbay (1970) compared the family histories of 23 autistic children with normal controls and found a greater incidence of alcoholism (35%), psychiatric illness (35%), and mental retardation (26%) in the parents of autistic children. DeLong and Dwyer (1988) reported that 55% of their 51 autism families had a first- or second-degree relative with alcoholism, though the overall incidence rate of alcoholism among all 929 first- and second-degree relatives was only 6.5%. Piven et al. (1991) reported that 12.3% of 81 parents of autistic children were alcoholic compared with 0% of 34 Down syndrome parents; the difference was not statistically significant. In a study of 36 autism families, Smalley, McCracken, and Tanguay (1995) compared the lifetime rates of psychopathology based on direct SADS-LA interviews of parents and adult siblings of autism probands versus controls who had either tuberous sclerosis or an unspecified seizure disorder. They found that 47% (17/36) of the autism families had a first-degree relative with substance abuse, including alcoholism, versus none in the 21 control families. And 22% of first-degree relatives reported substance abuse compared to none in the controls ($p = 0.002$). They also found increased rates of depression (32.3% vs. 11.1%; $p = 0.013$) and social phobia (20.2% vs. 2.4%; $p = 0.016$). Not all family studies have reported increased rates of alcoholism. Bolton, Pickles, Murphy, and Rutter (1998), using direct SADS-L interviews to assess the lifetime prevalence rates of psychopathology found a significant increase in major depression, but not alcoholism in first-degree relatives of an individual with autism.

In 2003 we reported family history analyses of 167 autism families (Miles, Takahashi, Haber, & Hadden, 2003). Families were ascertained through a child with autism and queried using the family history method (Andreasen, Rice, Endicott, Reich, & Coryell, 1986; Orvaschel, Thompson, Belanger, Prusoff, & Kidd, 1982; Yuan, Marazita, & Hill, 1996; Thompson, Orvaschel, Prusoff, & Kidd, 1982; Rice et al., 1995; Davies, Sham, Gilvarry, Jones, & Murray, 1997) to determine the prevalence and pedigree configuration of alcoholism and related neuropsychiatric disorders. Looking at the population as a whole, 13.5% of first-degree relatives and 13.6% of second-degree adults were reported to have alcoholism, including 6.6% of mothers, 20.4% of fathers, 8.4% of grandmothers, and 27.5% of grandfathers. Alcoholism rates in the autism ascertained families were compared to a control population ascertained through a child with Down syndrome and to lifetime alcohol prevalence data reported by three large United States alcoholism epidemiological studies, including a Missouri rural and suburban cohort (Eaton, Kramer, & Drywall, 1989;

Robins et al., 1984; Kessler et al., 1994; Grant, 1997). The Down syndrome families reported significantly less alcoholism in all family members ($p < 0.0001$). Compared to the 15.2% lifetime prevalence of alcoholism reported for suburban, small town, and rural Missouri (Robins et al., 1984), the overall 13.7% rate of alcoholism reported by the autism families was similar ($p = 0.19$). Women in our population, however, were significantly more likely to report alcoholism than all women in Missouri (6.6% vs. 4.3%) ($p = 0.008$).

Since alcoholism, like autism, is a heterogeneous disorder (Johnson et al., 2000; Cloninger, 1987; Brown, Seraganian, & Tremblay, 1994; Litt, Babor, DelBoca, Kadden, & Cooney, 1992; Hesselbrock & Hesselbrock, 2006; Edenberg & Faroud, 2006; Zucker, Ellis, Bingham, & Fitzgerald, 1996), we wanted to distinguish families with strongly genetic alcoholism from those with only sporadic or occasional cases that might be more environmentally induced. Using strict criteria to pick out the families with clusters of alcoholism, we classified 39% (65/167) of the families as having probable genetic alcoholism. A family history was rated as significant or "probably genetic" if the proband had (1) a first-degree relative with alcoholism (manifesting prior to concerns about the health of the proband), (2) a second-degree relative plus at least two additional individuals in the same family branch in a pattern suggesting Mendelian inheritance, or (3) alcoholism in at least four individuals all in the same branch of the family. The high alcoholism families had an elevated percentage of affected relatives in all categories, with 17% of mothers, 52% of fathers, 14% of maternal grandmothers, 41% of maternal grandfathers, 21% of paternal grandmothers, and 45% of paternal grandfathers reported as alcoholic. The remaining 102 families reported scattered individuals with alcoholism in unrelated branches of the family (less than 1% of females and less than 10% males).

Families and children whose pedigrees revealed an apparent genetic distribution of alcoholism (designated high alcoholism families) were compared with those that didn't (low alcoholism families). The family histories differed in two ways. First, the high alcoholism families had a significantly higher proportion of affected (alcoholic) females. In the high alcoholism families, the number of female alcoholics was 18 times the number in the low alcoholism families, whereas males were only 4 times more likely to be alcoholic (15.9% vs. 0.9% females; 38.2% vs. 8.7% males). The ratio of female to male alcoholics was significantly higher in the high alcoholism families compared to the low (0.46 vs. 0.052, $p = 0.0001$). And compared with unselected Missouri families (126), the females in our high alcohol families were 3.7 times more apt to be alcoholic. Second, high alcoholism families had more relatives with affective disorders, also distributed in a familial pattern (50.8% vs. 24%) ($p = 0.0006$). This is consistent with previous studies of alcoholism, which report an association between alcoholism and affective disorders in families (Kendler, Heath, Neale, Kessler, & Eaves, 1993; Bierut et al., 1998; Tsuang et al., 1998; Nurnberger et al., 2004). A significant family history of alcoholism did not associate preferentially with any other family history categories (cognitive, language, dyslexia, ADHD, or seizures).

Evaluation of the autism probands from the high and low alcoholism groups differed in two important autism phenotypes: macrocephaly and type of autism onset. Children from the high alcoholism families were 2.8 times less likely to be macrocephalic (14.7% vs. 40.6%) ($p = 0.0006$). The very significant inverse relationship between high alcoholism family histories and macrocephaly suggests that whatever the genes are that predispose to both autism and macrocephaly are different and operate independently from gene(s) that predispose to alcoholism and autism. The second difference between the autism probands from high versus low alcohol families was the clinical course of their autistic disorder. Children from high alcoholism families were 1.5 times more apt to present with a regressive onset (52.5% vs. 35.8%) ($p = 0.04$). This was found predominately in families where the mother was alcoholic (80% vs. 40%) ($p = 0.05$). There was no correlation with paternal alcoholism. This raised the question of a direct teratogenic effect of alcohol on the developing fetus. However, only one mother with a history of alcoholism reported drinking during the pregnancy. And in all of the children, fetal alcohol syndrome was ruled out by careful physical examinations. We believe that the connection between autism and familial alcoholism is consistent with the idea that there is an alcoholism subtype that is genetically mediated, highly penetrant, and predisposes to the development of autism.

The next step is to look for evidence of some shared biochemical pathways or genes. Theoretically, a maternal factor is of interest since recent studies have reported that autism is associated with the maternal dopamine β-hydroxylase alleles and that there is sib concordance for maternal, but not paternal, alleles linked to dopamine, serotonin, and norepinephrine transmitters (Robinson, Schutz, Macciardi, White, & Holden, 2001). Clarification of our association between regressive autism and maternal alcoholism will depend on replication of the studies in a larger sample of families. Nevertheless, it does recommend that for autism, like other complex disorders parental genotypes should be considered as possible risk factors (Labuda, Krajinovic, Sabbagh, Infante-Rivard, & Sinnett, 2002; DeLong, 2007).

Though the majority of autism candidate genes and regions do not overlap with biochemical pathways or genes implicated in alcoholism, there are common areas. Dysregulation of the major neurotransmitter systems for GABA and serotonin occur in autism and in alcoholism. And recently genes that encode structural cell adhesion molecule subfamilies which specify brain connectivity during development and in adulthood have been linked to both disorders (Geschwind & Levitt, 2007; Garber, 2007; Persico & Bourgeron, 2006; Uhl et al., 2008). Uhl et al. (2008) analyzed convergence data from genomewide association studies identifying 27 candidate genes that link addiction and co-occurring brain disorders ranging from smoking to Alzheimer's disease; three cell adhesion genes (Neurexin 1, Contactin-associated protein-like 2, and Contactin 4) previously linked to autism were identified in addictive disorder populations. Moreover, addiction and autism share associations with a number of cell adhesion gene subfamilies including nicotine dependence and autism with Neurexin 1 (Nussbaum et al., 2008), and alcoholism with Neurexin 3 (Hishimoto et al., 2007). These data support the concept that the same genetic variants can have overlapping or pleiotropic influences on more than one brain-based disorder.

Clinical Course Phenotypes

As with other medical and developmental disorders, the age of onset and clinical course are generally helpful in separating diseases that have similar symptomatology but different causes. For ASD the most intriguing separation is between children whose autism symptoms are noted from early infancy and those who regress from normal or near normal social and communicative development into autistic disorder, usually accompanied by the development of motor and other stereotypies (Lord, Schulman, & DiLavore, 2004; Stefanatos, 2008; Ozonoff, Williams, & Landa, 2005; Wilson, Djukic, Shinnar, Dharmani, & Rapin, 2003). Simultaneous cognitive declines have been documented (Bryson et al., 2007). Longitudinal studies, typically of the infant siblings of children with ASD, are poised to answer questions about the timing and patterns of early symptom developments (Baird et al., 2008; Rogers et al., 2008). Of equal interest will be results from extended longitudinal studies that permit us to identify which children drop into a prolonged developmental nadir, which undergo multiple periods of cognitive and communicative regression and which groups gradually improve in all areas, often irrespective of the intensity of developmental intervention. Once these developmental groups are better defined, they can be defined in terms of biologically and etiologically linked phenotypes which in turn should lead to the discovery of biological markers.

Core Autism Behavior Based Subgroups

Autism, like most if not all medical disorders, can be described on a variety of levels. Initially described as a psychiatric disorder of childhood, autism was defined by its behavioral variances in social interaction, language, and stereotypic interests and behaviors (Kanner, 1943). A number of behaviorally based autism subgroups were subsequently identified and cataloged by the American Psychiatric Association in the *Diagnostic and Statistical Manual of Mental Disorders* (DSM-IV-TR) manual as Autistic Disorder, Asperger's syndrome, Childhood Disintegrative Disorder, Rett syndrome, and Pervasive Developmental Disorders Not-Otherwise-Specified (PDD-NOS) (American Psychiatric Association, 2000). This remains the standard for definition of the behavioral autism diagnoses. Important research continues to refine diagnostic criteria for each clinical subtype, their boundaries, and treatment responses.

The most widely referenced clinical subgroups, proposed by Wing and Gould (1979), classify children based on the quality of their social interaction; "Socially aloof," "Passive interaction," or "Active-but-odd interaction." Aloof children reject most social contact and have atypical attachment to caregivers, lack pretend play and joint attention, have little eye contact, engage in inappropriate behaviors such as tantrums and are usually nonverbal. Passive children also do not initiate social interaction spontaneously, but accept other's approaches. Their play typically consists of imitative rather than imaginative activities, and their communication tends to be repetitive. Active-but-odd children seek interactions with others but these interactions are one-sided and peculiar. They use language communicatively but may have poor eye contact, speak in a monotone, lack conventional gestures, and have difficulty comprehending idiomatic statements. Based on the Wing Subgroups Questionnaire (Castelloe & Dawson, 1993), the literature supports the validity of the subtypes with most children falling into the aloof group, which correlates with lower IQs, and less change in IQ with early intensive behavioral intervention (Beglinger & Smith, 2001). Though Wing subgroups do correlate with some biological variables (Dawson, Klinger, Panagiotides, Lewy, & Castelloe, 1995), the classification is not always stable over time, with some children in the aloof group maturing into a passive social type. Some authors have questioned whether the Wing subtypes simply reflect IQ; however Volkmar, Cohen, Bregman, Hooks, and Stevenson (1989) found that only 53% of the variance in their study was accounted for by IQ, indicating the validity of this subgrouping paradigm. I am not aware of any association with etiology.

Other groups have focused on language variability to create more homogeneous subgroups. Language competence, like cognitive ability, is under significant genetic control, demonstrated by the robust language correlations reported within sibships, twins, and/or extended family members (Fombonne, Bolton, Prior, Jordan, & Ruter, 1997; Bailey et al., 1998; Piven & Palmer, 1997; Hughes, Plumet, & Leboyer, 1999; MacLean et al., 1999; Pickles et al., 2000; Spiker, Lotspeich, Dimiceli, Myers, & Risch, 2002; Silverman et al., 2002). Silverman et al. (2002) found reduced variance within sibships for speech delays and age at phrase speech. Likewise, in a study of 171 autism sibships Spiker et al. (2002) found a highly significant association within autism sib pairs for language delay and absence of phrase speech. Buxbaum et al. (2001) showed that concordance for delayed speech substantially increased the modestly positive evidence for linkage at loci on chromosomes 2 and 7. Hutcheson et al. (2003) found when presence or absence of language acquisition was used to segregate populations for linkage analysis, higher LOD scores for linkage to the AUT1 region on chromosome 7q region occurred in the more language impaired group. These were the first functional phenotypes to be successfully correlated with genetic linkage. Nevertheless, language development does not appear to be the primary autism genetic determinant, since many nonverbal autistic children have parents and/or siblings with high functioning autism or Asperger's (Eisenmajer et al., 1996; Gillberg, 1999; Gillberg & Wing,

1999; Volkmar, Klin, & Pauls, 1998). Miller and Ozonoff (2000) compared individuals with high-functioning autism with impaired language to individuals with Asperger's, with IQ differences controlled, and found no significant group differences in motor, visual spatial, or executive functions, suggesting language development is primarily IQ dependent.

Repetitive Behaviors

The presence of motor stereotypies together with preoccupations, rigidity, and restricted interests count as one criteria for a diagnosis of an ASD and thus are almost always reported in diagnosed children. However, the type, frequency, and intensity of repetitive behaviors, including stereotypic movements, inflexible routines, repetitive play, and perseverative speech in ASD vary widely. Stereotypies positively correlate with ASD severity and with cognitive deficiency (Bodfish, Symons, Parker, & Lewis, 2000; Bishop, Maybery, Wong, Maley, & Hallmayer, 2006; Goldman et al., 2009). And taken together they are the strongest predictor that an early ASD diagnosis will endure (Richler, Bishop, Kleinker, & Lord, 2007). Recent evidence, however, suggests that repetitive behaviors and interests are complex and probably stem from a number of sources (Beglinger & Smith, 2001; Happé & Ronald, 2008; Ingram et al., 2007). Whereas social and communication symptoms are closely associated and may even stem from the same biologic mechanism, repetitive behaviors, preoccupations, and restricted interests are not inextricably bound to those core symptoms (Happé & Ronald, 2008; Mandy & Skuse, 2008). Moreover, there is evidence that repetitive behaviors are etiologically distinct from restricted interests or obsessions (Goldman et al., 2009; Miles, Takahashi, & Mudrick, 2000b). In our study of 153 children with autistic disorder, those with no prominent motor repetitive behaviors had a lower sex ratio and less family history of ASD, but a greater family history of obsessive-compulsive behavior diagnoses. Recently Wiggins, Robins, Bakeman, and Adamson (2009) reported that tactile, auditory filtering and taste/smell hypersensitivity impairments in children with ASD correlate strongly with measures of stereotypic interests and behaviors. Lam, Bodfish, and Piven (2008), using exploratory factor analysis identified three distinct repetitive factors—repetitive motor behaviors, insistence on sameness, and circumscribed interests—each with distinct associations with subject characteristics such as IQ, age, social/communication impairments, presence of regression, and sib pair correlations. Based on these findings, it appears that repetitive behaviors could become a rich phenotypic trait for defining ASD subgroups. However, much more study is needed to separate this complex collection of symptoms into biologically homogeneous traits.

Cognitively and Functionally Defined Subgroups

A number of approaches for separating autism into subgroups based on function have been proposed. Variance in IQ has garnered the most attention, since between half and three quarters of autistic children have IQ scores below 70 (Lotter, 1966; Rutter & Garmezy, 1983; Steffenburg & Gillberg, 1986; Cohen, Paul, & Volkmar, 1987; Chakrabarti & Fombonne, 2001; Lincoln, Allen, & Kilman, 1995) and because cognitive levels measured in early childhood have been a strong predictor of outcome (Cohen et al., 1987; Lord & Schopler, 1989a, 1989b; Kobayashi, Murata, & Yoshinaga, 1992; Venter, Lord, & Schopler, 1992; Volkmar, 1992; Fein et al., 1999). However, it is clear that IQ is not a primary genetic variable in autism. Le Couteur et al. (1996) found that IQ scores can vary widely in identical twins. Jorde et al. (1990) found that dividing the Utah cohort by IQ revealed no significant differences in recurrence risks and gave no indications of inheritance patterns. Moreover, in the young child with autism, IQ assessment is difficult (reviewed in Bailey, Phillips, & Rutter, 1996), and IQ and DQ scores measured in early childhood may change over time and with therapy. Lord and Schopler (1989a) reported mean differences greater than 23 points comparing test scores prior to age 4 with those at age 8 and older, findings which have been replicated in other populations (Sigman et al., 1999). Even without special treatment, children first assessed in early preschool years are likely to show marked increases in IQ score by school age (Lord & Schopler, 1989b). There is however a correlation between IQ and genetics. In multiplex sibships, nonverbal IQ scores correlate positively (Spiker et al., 2002; Szatmari et al., 1996), indicating that cognitive abilities in autism, as in typically developing populations, were largely genetically determined. In addition, IQ levels have appeared to correlate with a fundamental genetic variable, the male to female ratio; the more severely retarded the population, the lower the male to female ratio (Wing, 1981; Gillberg, 1989; Szatmari, Bartolucci, Bremner, Bond, & Rich, 1989). The greatest male predominance occurs in Asperger's syndrome, as do the highest IQ scores. These examples illustrate the difficulty in determining which variables are primary when defining subgroups. Our studies indicate that it is the essential/complex autism distinction that provides the primary subgroup separation. Individuals with complex autism as a group have lower IQ scores than those with essential autism. When controlled for this distinction IQ scores do not correlate with sex ratios, recurrence risks, family histories of autism, or type of onset (Miles, unpublished data). This, of course, is not surprising since the complex/essential autism is based on the premise that dysmorphology and microcephaly are indicators of disruptions of early embryogenesis and thus more closely related to etiology.

Neurologically and Medically Defined Subgroups

Neurologic and medical symptoms are important variables affecting outcome and quality of life for children with autism. Seizures develop in approximately 25% of children with autism and the rate of electroencephalographic abnormalities is increased even when there is no history of seizures

(Kim, Donnelly, Tournay, Book, & Filipek, 2006; Spence & Schneider, 2009). And though individuals with autism plus seizures are more apt to have moderate to severe mental retardation, motor deficits, and poorer adaptive, behavioral, and social outcomes (Tuchman & Rapin, 2002; Hara, 2007), seizures by themselves are not a sensitive outcome predictor. Seizures and EEG abnormalities, though they fit many of the criteria for a promising subgroup defining phenotypic variable (Table 40-1), have not been successful phenotypic subgroup indicators. This is not surprising since, like autism, seizures are etiologically heterogeneous and are symptomatic of many underlying neurologic mechanisms.

Similar to seizures, sleep disorders and gastrointestinal symptoms are not pathophysiologically discrete entities and thus are too vague to define discrete autism subgroups. That is not to say, however, that future definition of discrete types of seizures, sleep disorders, or GI disorders, with clear linkages to biological mechanisms may not become useful in defining etiologic autism subgroups.

Conclusions: The Nosology of Autism as a Biologically Based Disorder

The transition of autism from a diagnostically inclusive behaviorally defined disorder to an etiological based nosology mirrors the history of mental retardation in the 1960s and cerebral palsy in the 1970s, as well as many less common disorders like X-linked muscular dystrophy (Darras, Korf, & Urion, 2009) and lissencephaly (Barkovich, Koch, & Carrol, 1991; Norman, McGillivray, Kalousek, Hill, & Poskitt, 1995; Dobyns & Das, 2009). In each case, a disorder that had originally been clinically defined was divided into subgroups based on recognition of phenotypic differences plus the introduction of new technologies. Mental retardation's demise as a diagnosis began in the 1950s with the introduction of two "new" techniques; clinical cytogenetics and physical dysmorphology (Jones, 2006). Redefinition of the cerebral palsies began when CT scans became available in the mid-1970s. Subsequently, molecular genetic analysis of subgroups of each of these descriptive diagnoses have resulted in the identification of hundreds of etiology specific diagnoses.

Relative to autism, the history of mental retardation is perhaps most informative, since the successes were based on breaking up hundreds of similar phenotypes into broad categories based on associated symptoms, such as MR plus craniofacial anomalies (Cohen, 2006), MR plus regression versus the static encephalopathies, MR with early overgrowth, or MR plus skin pigment changes, etc. For the geneticist, separating a broad heterogeneous disorder into its separate homogeneous diagnoses, usually depends on finding a "hook." This is a biologically discrete feature or phenotype found in a small proportion of individuals with the general diagnosis. A feature not commonly associated with the general descriptive diagnosis provides specificity to the subgroup. Thus, every sign, symptom, or oddball phenotype that occurs in children with ASDs must be noted and reported, so researchers can assemble putative, etiologically discrete subgroups for fresh and innovative investigations.

Challenges and Future Directions

- Discover the neurologic, biologic, and molecular bases behind the phenotypes that define discrete autism subgroups.
- Develop large autism research populations that are studied jointly by behavioralists, clinical geneticists, neuroanatomists, molecular biologists, and other neuroscientists.
- Pursue longitudinal studies of these same populations to answer the practical translational question "Which phenotypic features or biomarkers are most closely linked to recovery?"

SUGGESTED READINGS

Gottesman, I. I., & Gould, T. D. (2003). The endophenotype concept in psychiatry: Etymology and strategic intentions. *American Journal of Psychiatry, 160*, 636–645.

Miles, J. H., Takahashi, T. N., Bagby, S., Sahota, P. K., Vaslow, D. F., Wang, C. H., et al. (2005). Essential versus complex autism: Definition of fundamental prognostic subtypes. *American Journal of Medical Genetics A, 135*, 171–180.

Szatmari, H., Maziade, M., Zwaigenbaum, L., Merette, C., Roy, M., Ridham, J., et al. (2007). Informative phenotypes for genetic studies of psychiatric disorders. *American Journal of Medical Genetics B, 144B*, 581–588.

REFERENCES

Abell, F., Krams, M., Ashburner, J., Passingham, R., Friston, K., Frackowiak, R., et al. (1999). The neuroanatomy of autism: a voxel-based whole based analysis of structural scans. *Neuroreport, 10*, 1647–1651.

American Psychiatric Association. (2000). *Diagnostic and statistical manual of mental disorders* (4th ed., text rev.; DSM-IV-TR). Washington DC: Author.

Andreasen, N. C., Rice, J., Endicott, J., Reich, T., & Coryell, W. (1986). The family history approach to diagnosis: How useful is it? *Archives of General Psychiatry, 43*, 421–429.

Aylward, E. H., Minshew, N. J., Field, K., Sparks, B. F., & Singh, N. (2002). Effects of age on brain volume and head circumference in autism. *Neurology, 59*, 175–183.

Aylward, E. H., Minshew, N. J., Goldstein, G., Honeycutt, N. A., Augustine, A. M., Yates, K. O., et al. (1999). MRI volumes of amygdala and hippocampus in non-mentally retarded autistic adolescents and adults. *Neurology, 53*, 2145–2150.

Babor, T. F., Hofmann, M., DelBoca, F. K., Hesselbrock, V., Meyer, R. E., Dolinsky, Z. S., et al. (1992). Types of alcoholics: I. Evidence for an empirically derived typology based on indicators of vulnerability and severity. *Archives of General Psychiatry, 49*, 599–608.

Bailey, A., Luthert, P., Dean, A., Harding, B., Janota, I., Montgomery, M., et al. (1998). A clinicopathological study of autism. *Brain, 121*, 889–905.

Bailey, A., Phillips, W., & Rutter, M. (1996). Autism: towards an integration of clinical, genetic, neuropsychological, and neurobiological perspectives. *Journal of Child Psychology and Psychiatry and Allied Disciplines, 37*, 89–126.

Baird, G., Charman, T., Pickles, A., Chandler, S., Loucas, T., Meldrum, D., et al. (2008). Regression, developmental trajectory, and associated problems in disorders in the autism spectrum: the SNAP study. *Journal of Autism and Developmental Disorders, 38*, 1827–1836.

Barkovich, A. J., Koch, T. K., & Carrol, C. L. (1991). The spectrum of lissencephaly: report of ten patients analyzed by magnetic resonance imaging. *Annals of Neurology, 30*, 139–146.

Barnea-Goraly, N., Kwon, H., Menon, V., Eliez, S., Lotspeich, L., & Reiss, A. L. (2004). White matter structure in autism: preliminary evidence from diffusion tensor imaging. *Biological Psychiatry, 55*, 323–326.

Baron-Cohen, S., & Hammer, J. (1997). Parents of children with Asperger syndrome: What is the cognitive phenotype? *Journal of Cognitive Neuroscience, 9*, 548–554.

Beglinger, L. J., & Smith, T. H. (2001). A review of subtyping in autism and proposed dimensional classification model. *Journal of Autism and Developmental Disorders, 31*, 411–422.

Bierut, L. J., Dinwiddie, S. H., Begleiter, H., Crowe, R. R., Hesselbrock, V., Nurnberger, J. I., Jr., et al. (1998). Familial transmission of substance dependence: alcohol, marijuana, cocaine, and habitual smoking: a report from the Collaborative Study on the Genetics of Alcoholism. *Archives of General Psychiatry, 55*, 982–988.

Bishop, D. V., Maybery, M., Wong, D., Maley, A., & Hallmayer, J. (2006). Characteristics of the broader phenotype in autism: a study of siblings using the children's communication checklist-2. *American Journal of Medical Genetics. Part B, Neuropsychiatric Genetics, 141*, 117–122.

Boddaert, N., Chabane, N., Gervais, H., Good, C. D., Bourgeois, M., Plumet, M. H., et al. (2004). Superior temporal sulcus anatomical abnormalities in childhood autism: a voxel-based morphometry MRI study. *NeuroImage, 23*, 364–369.

Bodfish, J. W., Symons, F. J., Parker, D. E., & Lewis, M. H. (2000). Varieties of repetitive behavior in autism: comparisons to mental retardation. *Journal of Autism and Developmental Disorders, 30*, 237–243.

Boger-Megiddo, I., Shaw, D. W., Friedman, S. D., Sparks, B. F., Artru, A. A., Giedd, J. N., et al. (2006). Corpus callosum morphometrics in young children with autism spectrum disorder. *Journal of Autism and Developmental Disorders, 36*, 733–739.

Bolton, P. F., Pickles, A., Murphy, M., & Rutter, M. (1998). Autism, affective, and other psychiatric disorders: patterns of familial aggregation. *Psychological Medicine, 28*, 385–395.

Bolton, P. F., Roobol, M., Allsopp, L., & Pickles, A. (2001). Association between idiopathic infantile macrocephaly and autism spectrum disorders. *Lancet, 358*, 726–727.

Brown, T. G., Seraganian, P., & Tremblay, J. (1994). Alcoholics also dependent on cocaine in treatment: do they differ from "pure" alcoholics? *Addictive Behaviors, 19*, 105–112.

Bryson, S. E., Zwaigenbaum, L., Brian, J., Roberts, W., Szatmari, P., Rombough, V., et al. (2007). A prospective case series of high-risk infants who developed autism. *Journal of Autism and Developmental Disorders, 37*, 12–24.

Butler, M. G., Dasouki, M. J., Zhou, X. P., Talebizadeh, Z., Brown, M., Takahashi, T. N., et al. (2005). Subset of individuals with autism spectrum disorders and extreme macrocephaly associated with germline PTEN tumour suppressor gene mutations. *Journal of Medical Genetics, 42*, 318–321.

Buxbaum, J. D., Cai, G., Chaste, P., Nygren, G., Goldsmith, J., Reichert, J., et al. (2007). Mutation screening of the PTEN gene in patients with autism spectrum disorders and macrocephaly. *American Journal of Medical Genetics. Part B, Neuropsychiatric Genetics, 144B*, 484–491.

Buxbaum, J. D., Silverman, J. M., Smith, C. J., Kilifarski, M., Reichert, J., Hollander, E., et al. (2001). Evidence for a susceptibility gene for autism on chromosome 2 and for genetic heterogeneity. *American Journal of Human Genetics, 68*, 1514–1520.

Campbell, M., Geller, B., Small, A. M., Petti, T. A., & Ferris, S. H. (1978). Minor physical anomalies in young psychotic children. *American Journal of Psychiatry, 135*, 573–575.

Casanova, M. F. (2007). The neuropathology of autism. *Brain Pathology, 17*, 422–433.

Castelloe, P., & Dawson, G. (1993). Subclassification of children with autism and pervasive developmental disorder: a questionnaire based on Wing's subgrouping scheme. *Journal of Autism and Developmental Disorders, 23*, 229–241.

Chakrabarti, S., & Fombonne, E. (2001). Pervasive developmental disorders in preschool children. *Journal of the American Medical Association, 285*, 3093–3099.

Clarke, J. T. R. (2005). *A clinical guide to inherited metabolic diseases.* New York: Cambridge University Press.

Cloninger, C. R. (1987). Neurogenetic adaptive mechanisms in alcoholism. *Science, 236*, 410–416.

Cohen, D. J., Paul, R., & Volkmar, F. R. (1987). Issues in the classification of pervasive developmental disorders and associated conditions. In D. J. Cohen & A. M. Donnellan (Eds.), *Handbook of autism and pervasive developmental disorders* (pp. 20–40). New York: Wiley.

Cohen, M. M. (2006). *Perspectives on the face.* New York: Oxford University Press.

Conciatori, M., Stodgell, C. J., Hyman, S. L., O'Bara, M., Militerni, R., Bravaccio, C., et al. (2004). Association between the HOXA1 A218G polymorphism and increased head circumference in patients with autism. *Biological Psychiatry, 55*, 413–419.

Courchesne, E., Carper, R., & Akshoomoff, N. (2003). Evidence of brain overgrowth in the first year of life in autism. *Journal of the American Medical Association, 290*, 337–344.

Courchesne, E., Karns, C. M., Davis, H. R., Ziccardi, R., Carper, R. A., Tigue, Z. D., et al. (2001). Unusual brain growth patterns in early life in patients with autistic disorder: An MRI study. *Neurology, 57*, 245–254.

Courchesne, E., & Pierce, K. (2005). Brain overgrowth in autism during a critical time in development: implications for frontal pyramidal neuron and interneuron development and connectivity. *International Journal of Developmental Neuroscience, 23*, 153–170.

Dager, S. R., Wang, L., Friedman, S. D., Shaw, D. W., Constantino, J. N., Artru, A. A., et al. (2007). Shape mapping of the hippocampus in young children with autism spectrum disorder. *AJNR. American Journal of Neuroradiology, 28*, 672–677.

Darras, B. T., Korf, B. R., & Urion, D. K. (2009). *Dystrophinopathies.* Gene Reviews at GenetTests: Medical Genetics

Information Resource [On-line]. Retrieved from http://www.genetests.org

Davies, N. J., Sham, P. C., Gilvarry, C., Jones, P. B., & Murray, R. M. (1997). Comparison of the family history with the family study method: report from the Camberwell Collaborative Psychosis Study. *American Journal of Human Genetics, 74*, 12–17.

Dawson, D. A., & Grant, B. F. (1998). Family history of alcoholism and gender: their combined effects on DSM-IV alcohol dependence and major depression. *Journal of Studies on Alcohol, 59*, 97–106.

Dawson, G., Klinger, L. G., Panagiotides, H., Lewy, A., & Castelloe, P. (1995). Subgroups of autistic children based on social behavior display distinct patterns of brain activity. *Journal of Abnormal Child Psychology, 23*, 569–583.

Delatycki, M. B., Danks, A., Churchyard, A., Zhou, X. P., & Eng, C. (2003). De novo germline PTEN mutation in a man with Lhermitte-Duclos disease which arose on the paternal chromosome and was transmitted to his child with polydactyly and Wormian bones. *Journal of Medical Genetics, 40*, e92.

DeLong, G. R., & Dwyer, J. T. (1988). Correlation of family history with specific autistic subgroups: Asperger's syndrome and bipolar affective disease. *Journal of Autism and Developmental Disorders, 18*, 593–600.

DeLong, R. (2007). GABA(A) receptor alpha5 subunit as a candidate gene for autism and bipolar disorder. *Autism, 11*, 135–147.

Dobyns, W. B., & Das, S. (2009). *LIS1-associated lissencephaly/subcortical band heterotopia*. Gene Reviews at GenetTests: Medical Genetics Information Resource [On-line]. Retrieved from http://www.genetests.org.

Eaton, W. W., Kramer, M., Anthony, J. C., & Dryman, A. (1989). The incidence of specific DIS/DSM-III mental disorders: Data from the NIMH Epidemiologic Catchment Area program. *Acta Psychiatrica Scandinavica, 79*, 163–178.

Edenberg, H. J., & Foroud, T. (2006). The genetics of alcoholism: identifying specific genes through family studies. *Addiction Biology, 11*, 386–396.

Egaas, B., Courchesne, E., & Saitoh, O. (1995). Reduced size of corpus callosum in autism. *Archives of Neurology, 52*, 794–801.

Eisenmajer, R., Prior, M., Leekam, S., Wing, L., Gould, J., Welham, M., et al. (1996). Comparison of clinical symptoms in autism and Asperger's disorder. *Journal of the American Academy of Child and Adolescent Psychiatry, 35*, 1523–1531.

Fein, D., Stevens, M. C., Dunn, M., Waterhouse, L., Allen, D., Rapin, I., et al. (1999). Subtypes of pervasive developmental disorder: clinical characteristics. *Child Neuropsychology, 5*, 1–23.

Fombonne, E., Bolton, P., Prior, J., Jordan, H., & Rutter, M. (1997). A family study of autism: cognitive patterns and levels in parents and siblings. *Journal of Child Psychology and Psychiatry and Allied Disciplines, 38*, 667–683.

Fombonne, E., Roge, B., Claverie, J., Courty, S., & Fremolle, J. (1999). Microcephaly and macrocephaly in autism [In Process Citation]. *Journal of Autism and Developmental Disorders, 29*, 113–119.

Garber, K. (2007). Neuroscience: Autism's cause may reside in abnormalities at the synapse. *Science, 317*, 190–191.

Geschwind, D. H., & Levitt, P. (2007). Autism spectrum disorders: developmental disconnection syndromes. *Current Opinion in Neurobiology, 17*, 103–111.

Geuze, E., Vermetten, E., & Bremner, J. D. (2005). MR-based in vivo hippocampal volumetrics: 2. Findings in neuropsychiatric disorders. *Molecular Psychiatry, 10*, 160–184.

Gillberg, C. (1989). Asperger syndrome in 23 Swedish children. [Review] [24 refs]. *Developmental Medicine and Child Neurology, 31*, 520–531.

Gillberg, C. (1992). Subgroups in autism: are there behavioural phenotypes typical of underlying medical conditions? *Journal of Intellectual Disability Research, 36*(Pt 3), 201–214.

Gillberg, C. (1999). Autism and its spectrum disorders. In N. Bouras (Ed.), *Psychiatric and behavioral disorders in developmental disabilities and mental retardation* (pp. 73–95). Cambridge, MA: Cambridge University Press.

Gillberg, C., & Wing, L. (1999). Autism: Not an extremely rare disorder. *Acta Psychiatrica Scandinavica, 99*, 399–406.

Goldman, S., Wang, C., Salgado, M. W., Greene, P. E., Kim, M., & Rapin, I. (2009). Motor stereotypies in children with autism and other developmental disorders. *Developmental Medicine and Child Neurology, 51*, 30–38.

Gottesman, I. I., & Gould, T. D. (2003). The endophenotype concept in psychiatry: etymology and strategic intentions. *American Journal of Psychiatry, 160*, 636–645.

Grant, B. F. (1997). Prevalence and correlates of alcohol use and DSM-IV alcohol dependence in the United States: results of the National Longitudinal Alcohol Epidemiologic Survey. *Journal of Studies on Alcohol, 58*, 464–473.

Grice, D. E., & Buxbaum, J. D. (2006). The genetics of autism spectrum disorders. *Neuromolecular Medicine, 8*, 451–460.

Gualtieri, C. T., Adams, A., Shen, C. D., & Loiselle, D. (1982). Minor physical anomalies in alcoholic and schizophrenic adults and hyperactive and autistic children. *American Journal of Psychiatry, 139*, 640–643.

Hadjikhani, N., Joseph, R. M., Snyder, J., Chabris, C. F., Clark, J., Steele, S., et al. (2004). Activation of the fusiform gyrus when individuals with autism spectrum disorder view faces. *NeuroImage, 22*, 1141–1150.

Hagerman, R. J., Rivera, S. M., & Hagerman, P. J. (2008). The fragile X family of disorders: A model for autism and targeted treatments. *Current Pediatric Reviews, 4*, 40–52.

Handa, V., Goldwater, D., Stiles, D., Cam, M., Poy, G., Kumari, D., et al. (2005). Long CGG-repeat tracts are toxic to human cells: implications for carriers of Fragile X premutation alleles. *FEBS Letters, 579*, 2702–2708.

Happe, F., & Ronald, A. (2008). The "fractionable autism triad": a review of evidence from behavioural, genetic, cognitive, and neural research. *Neuropsychology Review, 18*, 287–304.

Hara, H. (2007). Autism and epilepsy: a retrospective follow-up study. *Brain and Development, 29*, 486–490.

Harris, S. W., Hessl, D., Goodlin-Jones, B., Ferranti, J., Bacalman, S., Barbato, I., et al. (2008). Autism profiles of males with fragile X syndrome. *American Journal of Mental Retardation, 113*, 427–438.

Hashimoto, T., Tayama, M., Miyazaki, M., Murakawa, K., Shimakawa, S., Yoneda, Y., et al. (1993). Brainstem involvement in high functioning autistic children. *Acta Neurologica Scandinavica, 88*, 123–128.

Hazlett, H. C., Poe, M., Gerig, G., Smith, R. G., Provenzale, J., Ross, A., et al. (2005). Magnetic resonance imaging and head circumference study of brain size in autism: birth through age 2 years. *Archives of General Psychiatry, 62*, 1366–1376.

Haznedar, M. M., Buchsbaum, M. S., Wei, T. C., Hof, P. R., Cartwright, C., Bienstock, C. A., et al. (2000). Limbic circuitry in patients with autism spectrum disorders studied with positron emission tomography and magnetic resonance imaging. *American Journal of Psychiatry, 157*, 1994–2001.

Herbert, M. R., Ziegler, D. A., Deutsch, C. K., O'Brien, L. M., Lange, N., Bakardjiev, A., et al. (2003). Dissociations of cerebral cortex, subcortical, and cerebral white matter volumes in autistic boys. *Brain, 126*, 1182–1192.

Hesselbrock, V. M., & Hesselbrock, M. N. (2006). Are there empirically supported and clinically useful subtypes of alcohol dependence? *Addiction, 101*(Suppl 1), 97–103.

Hishimoto, A., Liu, Q. R., Drgon, T., Pletnikova, O., Walther, D., Zhu, X. G., et al. (2007). Neurexin 3 polymorphisms are associated with alcohol dependence and altered expression of specific isoforms. *Human Molecular Genetics, 16*, 2880–2891.

Howard, M. A., Cowell, P. E., Boucher, J., Broks, P., Mayes, A., Farrant, A., et al. (2000). Convergent neuroanatomical and behavioural evidence of an amygdala hypothesis of autism. *Neuroreport, 11*, 2931–2935.

Hughes, C., Plumet, M. H., & Leboyer, M. (1999). Towards a cognitive phenotype for autism: increased prevalence of executive dysfunction and superior spatial span amongst siblings of children with autism. *Journal of Child Psychology and Psychiatry, 40*, 705–718.

Hutcheson, H. B., Bradford, Y., Folstein, S. E., Gardiner, M. B., Santangelo, S. L., Sutcliffe, J. S., et al. (2003). Defining the autism minimum candidate gene region on chromosome 7. *American Journal of Medical Genetics, 117B*, 90–96.

Ingram, D. G., Takahashi, T. N., & Miles, J. H. (2007). Defining autism subgroups: A taxometric solution. *Journal of Autism and Developmental Disorders, 38*, 950–960.

James, S. J., Melnyk, S., Jernigan, S., Cleves, M. A., Halsted, C. H., Wong, D. H., et al. (2006). Metabolic endophenotype and related genotypes are associated with oxidative stress in children with autism. *American Journal of Medical Genetics. Part B, Neuropsychiatric Genetics, 141B*, 947–956.

Johnson, B. A., Roache, J. D., Javors, M. A., DiClemente, C. C., Cloninger, C. R., Prihoda, T. J., et al. (2000). Ondansetron for reduction of drinking among biologically predisposed alcoholic patients: A randomized controlled trial. *Journal of the American Medical Association, 284*, 963–971.

Jones, K. L. (2006). *Smith's recognizable patterns of human malformation* (6th ed.). Philadelphia: Elsevier Saunders.

Jorde, L. B., Mason-Brothers, A., Waldmann, R., Ritvo, E. R., Freeman, B. J., Pingree, C., et al. (1990). The UCLA-University of Utah epidemiologic survey of autism: genealogical analysis of familial aggregation. *American Journal of Human Genetics, 36*, 85–88.

Juranek, J., Filipek, P. A., Berenji, G. R., Modahl, C., Osann, K., & Spence, M. A. (2006). Association between amygdala volume and anxiety level: magnetic resonance imaging (MRI) study in autistic children. *Journal of Child Neurology, 21*, 1051–1058.

Just, M. A., Cherkassky, V. L., Keller, T. A., & Minshew, N. J. (2004). Cortical activation and synchronization during sentence comprehension in high-functioning autism: evidence of underconnectivity. *Brain, 127*, 1811–1821.

Kanner, L. (1943). Autistic disturbances of affective contact. *Nervous Child, 2*, 217–250.

Keegan, M. M., Takahashi, T. N., & Miles, J. H. (2007). Macrocephaly in autism is not a homogeneous marker phenotype. *American Journal of Human Genetics*, 171. Abstract retrieved November 30, 2009, from http://www.ashg.org/genetics/ashg/annmeet/2007/call/abstractbook.pdf.

Kelleher, R. J., III, & Bear, M. F. (2008). The autistic neuron: troubled translation? *Cell, 135*, 401–406.

Kendler, K. S., Heath, A. C., Neale, M. C., Kessler, R. C., & Eaves, L. J. (1993). Alcoholism and major depression in women: A twin study of the causes of comorbidity. *Archives of General Psychiatry, 50*, 690–698.

Kessler, R. C., McGonagle, K. A., Zhao, S., Nelson, C. B., Hughes, M., Eshleman, S., et al. (1994). Lifetime and 12-month prevalence of DSM-III-R psychiatric disorders in the United States: Results from the National Comorbidity Survey. *Archives of General Psychiatry, 51*, 8–19.

Kim, H. L., Donnelly, J. H., Tournay, A. E., Book, T. M., & Filipek, P. (2006). Absence of seizures despite high prevalence of epileptiform EEG abnormalities in children with autism monitored in a tertiary care center. *Epilepsia, 47*, 394–398.

Kobayashi, R., Murata, T., & Yoshinaga, K. (1992). A follow-up study of 201 children with autism in Kyushu and Yamaguchi areas, Japan. *Journal of Autism and Developmental Disorders, 22*, 395–411.

Labuda, D., Krajinovic, M., Sabbagh, A., Infante-Rivard, C., & Sinnett, D. (2002). Parental genotypes in the risk of a complex disease. *American Journal of Human Genetics, 71*, 193–197.

Lainhart, J. E., Bigler, E. D., Bocian, M., Coon, H., Dinh, E., Dawson, G., et al. (2006). Head circumference and height in autism: a study by the Collaborative Program of Excellence in Autism. *American Journal of Medical Genetics. Part A, 140*, 2257–2274.

Lainhart, J. E., Piven, J., Wzorek, M., Landa, R., Santangelo, S. L., Coon, H., et al. (1997). Macrocephaly in children and adults with autism. *Journal of the American Academy of Child and Adolescent Psychiatry, 36*, 282–290.

Lam, K. S., Bodfish, J. W., & Piven, J. (2008). Evidence for three subtypes of repetitive behavior in autism that differ in familiality and association with other symptoms. *Journal of Child Psychology and Psychiatry, 49*, 1193–1200.

Lasser, K., Boyd, J. W., Woolhandler, S., Himmelstein, D. U., McCormick, D., & Bor, D. H. (2000). Smoking and mental illness: A population-based prevalence study. *Journal of the American Medical Association, 284*, 2606–2610.

Le Couteur, A., Bailey, A., Goode, S., Pickles, A., Robertson, S., Gottesman, I., et al. (1996). A broader phenotype of autism: the clinical spectrum in twins. *Journal of Child Psychology and Psychiatry and Allied Disciplines, 37*, 785–801.

Levitt, J. G., O'Neill, J., Blanton, R. E., Smalley, S., Fadale, D., McCracken, J. T., et al. (2003). Proton magnetic resonance spectroscopic imaging of the brain in childhood autism. *Biological Psychiatry, 54*, 1355–1366.

Lincoln, A. J., Allen, M. H., & Kilman, A. (1995). The assessment and interpretation of intellectual abilities in people with autism. In E. Schopler & G. B. Mesibov (Eds.), *Learning and cognition in autism*. New York and London: Plenum.

Links, P. S. (1980). Minor physical anomalies in childhood autism, Part II: Their relationship to maternal age. *Journal of Autism and Developmental Disorders, 10*, 287–292.

Links, P. S., Stockwell, M., Abichandani, F., & Simeon, J. (1980). Minor physical anomalies in childhood autism, Part I: Their relationship to pre- and perinatal complications. *Journal of Autism and Developmental Disorders, 10*, 273–285.

Lintas, C., & Persico, A. M. (2009). Autistic phenotypes and genetic testing: state-of-the-art for the clinical geneticist. *Journal of Medical Genetics, 46*, 1–8.

Litt, M. D., Babor, T. F., DelBoca, F. K., Kadden, R. M., & Cooney, N. L. (1992). Types of alcoholics, II: Application of an empirically derived typology to treatment matching. *Archives of General Psychiatry, 49*, 609–614.

Lobascher, M. E., Kingerlee, P. E., & Gubbay, S. S. (1970). Childhood autism: an investigation of aetiological factors in twenty- five cases. *British Journal of Psychiatry, 117*, 525–529.

Lord, C., & Schopler, E. (1989a). Stability of assessment results of autistic and non-autistic language-impaired children from preschool years to early school age. *Journal of Child Psychology and Psychiatry and Allied Disciplines, 30*, 575–590.

Lord, C., & Schopler, E. (1989b). The role of age at assessment, developmental level, and test in the stability of intelligence scores in young autistic children. *Journal of Autism and Developmental Disorders, 19*, 483–499.

Lord, C., Shulman, C., & DiLavore, P. (2004). Regression and word loss in autistic spectrum disorders. *Journal of Child Psychology and Psychiatry, 45*, 936–955.

Losh, M., & Piven, J. (2007). Social-cognition and the broad autism phenotype: identifying genetically meaningful phenotypes. *Journal of Child Psychology and Psychiatry, 48*, 105–112.

Lotter, V. (1966). Epidemiology of autistic conditions in young children. *Social Psychiatry, 1*, 124–137.

MacLean, J. E., Szatmari, P., Jones, M. B., Bryson, S. E., Mahoney, W. J., Bartolucci, G., et al. (1999). Familial factors influence level of functional in pervasive developmental disorder. *Journal of the American Academy of Child and Adolescent Psychiatry, 38*, 746–753.

Mandy, W. P., & Skuse, D. H. (2008). Research review: What is the association between the social-communication element of autism and repetitive interests, behaviours, and activities? *Journal of Child Psychology and Psychiatry, 49*, 795–808.

McCaffery, P., & Deutsch, C. K. (2005). Macrocephaly and the control of brain growth in autistic disorders. *Progress in Neurobiology, 77*, 38–56.

Miles, J. H., Hadden, L., Takahashi, T. N., & Hillman, R. E. (2000). Head circumference is an independent clinical finding associated with autism. *American Journal of Medical Genetics, 95*, 339–350.

Miles, J. H., & Hillman, R. E. (2000). Value of a clinical morphology examination in autism. *American Journal of Medical Genetics, 91*, 245–253.

Miles, J. H., Takahashi, T. N., Bagby, S., Sahota, P. K., Vaslow, D. F., Wang, C. H., et al. (2005). Essential versus complex autism: definition of fundamental prognostic subtypes. *American Journal of Medical Genetics. Part A, 135*, 171–180.

Miles, J. H., Takahashi, T. N., Haber, A., & Hadden, L. (2003). Autism families with a high incidence of alcoholism. *Journal of Autism and Developmental Disorders, 33*, 403–415.

Miles, J. H., Takahashi, T. N., Hillman, R. E., & Martin, K. L. (2004, October). Autism symptoms are less severe in girls with essential autism. Poster session presented at the annual meeting of the American Society of Human Genetics, Toronto, Canada.

Miles, J. H., Takahashi, T. N., Hong, J., Munden, N., Flournoy, N., Braddock, S. R., et al. (2008). Development and validation of a measure of dysmorphology: useful for autism subgroup classification. *American Journal of Medical Genetics. Part A, 146A*, 1101–1116.

Miles, J. H., Takahashi, T. N., & Mudrick, J. (2000). Repetitive behaviors differentiate autism subgroups [Abstract]. *American Journal of Human Genetics, 67*, 117.

Miller, J. N., & Ozonoff, S. (2000). The external validity of Asperger disorder: lack of evidence from the domain of neuropsychology. *Journal of Abnormal Psychology, 109*, 227–238.

Mnukhin, S. S., & Isaev, D. N. (1975). On the organic nature of some forms of schizoid or autistic psychopathy. *Journal of Autism and Childhood Schizophrenia, 5*, 99–108.

Munson, J., Dawson, G., Abbott, R., Faja, S., Webb, S. J., Friedman, S. D., et al. (2006). Amygdalar volume and behavioral development in autism. *Archives of General Psychiatry, 63*, 686–693.

Nacewicz, B. M., Dalton, K. M., Johnstone, T., Long, M. T., McAuliff, E. M., Oakes, T. R., et al. (2006). Amygdala volume and nonverbal social impairment in adolescent and adult males with autism. *Archives of General Psychiatry, 63*, 1417–1428.

Nicolson, R., DeVito, T. J., Vidal, C. N., Sui, Y., Hayashi, K. M., Drost, D. J., et al. (2006). Detection and mapping of hippocampal abnormalities in autism. *Psychiatry Research, 148*, 11–21.

Norman, M. G., McGillivray, B. C., Kalousek, D. K., Hill, A., & Poskitt, K. J. (1995). *Congenital malformations of the brain: pathological, embryological, clinical, radiological, and genetic aspects.* New York: Oxford University Press.

Nurnberger, J. I., Jr., Wiegand, R., Bucholz, K., O'Connor, S., Meyer, E. T., Reich, T., et al. (2004). A family study of alcohol dependence: coaggregation of multiple disorders in relatives of alcohol-dependent probands. *Archives of General Psychiatry, 61*, 1246–1256.

Nussbaum, J., Xu, Q., Payne, T. J., Ma, J. Z., Huang, W., Gelernter, J., et al. (2008). Significant association of the neurexin-1 gene (NRXN1) with nicotine dependence in European- and African-American smokers. *Human Molecular Genetics, 17*, 1569–1577.

Orvaschel, H., Thompson, W. D., Belanger, A., Prusoff, B. A., & Kidd, K. K. (1982). Comparison of the family history method to direct interview: Factors affecting the diagnosis of depression. *Journal of Affective Disorders, 4*, 49–59.

Ozonoff, S., Williams, B. J., & Landa, R. (2005). Parental report of the early development of children with regressive autism: the delays-plus-regression phenotype. *Autism, 9*, 461–486.

Pardo, C. A., & Eberhart, C. G. (2007). The neurobiology of autism. *Brain Pathology, 17*, 434–447.

Parisi, M. A., Dinulos, M. B., Leppig, K. A., Sybert, V. P., Eng, C., & Hudgins, L. (2001). The spectrum and evolution of phenotypic findings in PTEN mutation positive cases of Bannayan-Riley-Ruvalcaba syndrome. *Journal of Medical Genetics, 38*, 52–58.

Persico, A. M., & Bourgeron, T. (2006). Searching for ways out of the autism maze: genetic, epigenetic, and environmental clues. *Trends in Neurosciences, 29*, 349–358.

Pickles, A., Starr, E., Kazak, S., Bolton, P., Papanikolaou, K., Bailey, A., et al. (2000). Variable expression of the autism broader phenotype: findings from extended pedigrees. *Journal of Child Psychology and Psychiatry and Allied Disciplines, 41*, 491–502.

Pierce, K., & Courchesne, E. (2001). Evidence for a cerebellar role in reduced exploration and stereotyped behavior in autism. *Biological Psychiatry, 49*, 655–664.

Piven, J., Bailey, J., Ranson, B. J., & Arndt, S. (1997). An MRI study of the corpus callosum in autism. *American Journal of Psychiatry, 154*, 1051–1056.

Piven, J., Bailey, J., Ranson, B. J., & Arndt, S. (1998). No difference in hippocampus volume detected on magnetic resonance imaging in autistic individuals. *Journal of Autism and Developmental Disorders, 28*, 105–110.

Piven, J., Chase, G. A., Landa, R., Wzorek, M., Gayle, J., Cloud, D., et al. (1991). Psychiatric disorders in the parents of autistic individuals. *Journal of the American Academy of Child and Adolescent Psychiatry, 30*, 471–478.

Piven, J., & Palmer, P. (1997). Cognitive deficits in parents from multiple-incidence autism families. *Journal of Child Psychology and Psychiatry and Allied Disciplines, 38*, 1011–1021.

Piven, J., Palmer, P., Jacobi, D., Childress, D., & Arndt, S. (1997). Broader autism phenotype: evidence from a family history study of multiple-incidence autism families. *American Journal of Psychiatry, 154*, 185–190.

Prior, M., Eisenmajer, R., Leekam, S., Wing, L., Gould, J., Ong, B., et al. (1998). Are there subgroups within the autistic spectrum? A cluster analysis of a group of children with autistic spectrum disorders. *Journal of Child Psychology and Psychiatry, 39*, 893–902.

Rice, J. P., Reich, T., Bucholz, K. K., Neuman, R. J., Fishman, R., Rochberg, N., et al. (1995). Comparison of direct interview and family history diagnoses of alcohol dependence. *Alcoholism: Clinical and Experimental Research, 19*, 1018–1023.

Richler, J., Bishop, S. L., Kleinke, J. R., & Lord, C. (2007). Restricted and repetitive behaviors in young children with autism spectrum disorders. *Journal of Autism and Developmental Disorders, 37*, 73–85.

Robins, L. N., Helzer, J. E., Weissman, M. M., Orvaschel, H., Gruenberg, E., Burke, J. D. J., et al. (1984). Lifetime prevalence of specific psychiatric disorders in three sites. *Archives of General Psychiatry, 41*, 949–958.

Robinson, P. D., Schutz, C. K., Macciardi, F., White, B. N., & Holden, J. J. (2001). Genetically determined low maternal serum dopamine beta-hydroxylase levels and the etiology of autism spectrum disorders. *American Journal of Medical Genetics, 100*, 30–36.

Rogers, S. J., Young, G. S., Cook, I., Giolzetti, A., Ozonoff, S., Rogers, S. J., et al. (2008). Deferred and immediate imitation in regressive and early onset autism. *Journal of Child Psychology and Psychiatry and Allied Disciplines, 49*, 449–457.

Rojas, D. C., Smith, J. A., Benkers, T. L., Camou, S. L., Reite, M. L., & Rogers, S. J. (2004). Hippocampus and amygdala volumes in parents of children with autistic disorder. *American Journal of Psychiatry, 161*, 2038–2044.

Rutter, M., & Garmezy, N. (1983). Developmental psychopathology. In I Handbook of Child Psychology, I ed. E. M. Hetherington, Vol. 4. New York: Wiley.

Sacco, R., Militerni, R., Frolli, A., Bravaccio, C., Gritti, A., Elia, M., et al. (2007). Clinical, morphological, and biochemical correlates of head circumference in autism. *Biological Psychiatry, 62*, 1038–1047.

Saitoh, O., Courchesne, E., Egaas, B., Lincoln, A. J., & Schreibman, L. (1995). Cross-sectional area of the posterior hippocampus in autistic patients with cerebellar and corpus callosum abnormalities. *Neurology, 45*, 317–324.

Saitoh, O., Karns, C. M., & Courchesne, E. (2001). Development of the hippocampal formation from 2 to 42 years: MRI evidence of smaller area dentata in autism. *Brain, 124*, 1317–1324.

Sauer, C. D., Takahashi, T. N., & Miles, J. H. (2005). Autism and alcoholism: Quest for genetic linkage. Abstract obtained from http://www.ashg.org/cgi-bin/ashg05s/ashg05?author=Miles&sort=pgmnums&sbutton=Detail&absno=593&sid=787312, Abstract No. 593.

Schenck, A., Bardoni, B., Langmann, C., Harden, N., Mandel, J. L., & Giangrande, A. (2003). CYFIP/Sra-1 controls neuronal connectivity in Drosophila and links the Rac1 GTPase pathway to the fragile X protein. *Neuron, 38*, 887–898.

Schumann, C. M., Hamstra, J., Goodlin-Jones, B. L., Lotspeich, L. J., Kwon, H., Buonocore, M. H., et al. (2004). The amygdala is enlarged in children but not adolescents with autism; the hippocampus is enlarged at all ages. *Journal of Neuroscience, 24*, 6392–6401.

Sigman, M., Ruskin, E., Arbeile, S., Corona, R., Dissanayake, C., Espinosa, M., et al. (1999). Continuity and change in the social competence of children with autism, Down syndrome, and developmental delays. *Monographs of the Society for Research in Child Development, 64*, 1–114.

Silverman, J. M., Smith, C. J., Schmeidler, J., Hollander, E., Lawlor, B. A., Fitzgerald, M., et al. (2002). Symptom domains in autism and related conditions: evidence for familiality. *American Journal of Medical Genetics, 114*, 64–73.

Smalley, S. L., Asarnow, R. F., & Spence, M. A. (1988). Autism and genetics. A decade of research. *Archives of General Psychiatry, 45*, 953–961.

Smalley, S. L., McCracken, J., & Tanguay, P. (1995). Autism, affective disorders, and social phobia. *American Journal of Human Genetics, 60*, 19–26.

Sparks, B. F., Friedman, S. D., Shaw, D. W., Aylward, E. H., Echelard, D., Artru, A. A., et al. (2002). Brain structural abnormalities in young children with autism spectrum disorder. *Neurology, 59*, 184–192.

Spence, M. A. (2001). The genetics of autism. *Current Opinion in Pediatrics, 13*, 561–565.

Spence, S. J., Cantor, R. M., Chung, L., Kim, S., Geschwind, D. H., & Alarcon, M. (2006). Stratification based on language-related endophenotypes in autism: attempt to replicate reported linkage. *American Journal of Medical Genetics. Part B, Neuropsychiatric Genetics, 141B*, 591–598.

Spence, S. J., & Schneider, M. T. (2009). The role of epilepsy and epileptiform EEGs in autism spectrum disorders. *Pediatric Research, 65*, 599–606.

Spiker, D., Lotspeich, L. J., Dimiceli, S., Myers, R. M., & Risch, N. (2002). Behavioral phenotypic variation in autism multiplex families: evidence for a continuous severity gradient. *American Journal of Medical Genetics, 114*, 129–136.

Stanfield, A. C., McIntosh, A. M., Spencer, M. D., Philip, R., Gaur, S., & Lawrie, S. M. (2007). Towards a neuroanatomy of autism: A systematic review and meta-analysis of structural magnetic resonance imaging studies. *European Psychiatry, 23*, 289–299.

Stefanatos, G. A. (2008). Regression in autistic spectrum disorders. *Neuropsychology Review, 18*, 305–319.

Steffenburg, S., & Gillberg, C. (1986). Autism and autistic-like conditions in Swedish rural and urban areas: a population study. *British Journal of Psychiatry, 149*, 81–87.

Steg, J. P., & Rapoport, J. L. (1975). Minor physical anomalies in normal, neurotic, learning disabled, and severely disturbed children. *Journal of Autism and Childhood Schizophrenia, 5*, 299–307.

Stoelb, M., Yarnal, R., Miles, J. H., Takahashi, T. N., Farmer, J., & McCathren, R. (2004). Predicting responsiveness to treatment of children with autism: the importance of physical dysmorphology. *Focus on Autism and Other Developmental Disabilities, 19*, 66–77.

Szatmari, P., Bartolucci, G., Bremner, R., Bond, S., & Rich, S. (1989). A follow-up study of high-functioning autistic children. *Journal of Autism and Developmental Disorders, 19*, 213–225.

Szatmari, P., Jones, M. B., Holden, J., Bryson, S., Mahoney, W., Tuff, L., et al. (1996). High phenotypic correlations among siblings with autism and pervasive developmental disorders. *American Journal of Medical Genetics, 67*, 354–360.

Szatmari, P., Maziade, M., Zwaigenbaum, L., Merette, C., Roy, M. A., Joober, R., et al. (2007). Informative phenotypes for genetic studies of psychiatric disorders. [Review] [66 refs]. *American Journal of Medical Genetics. Part B, Neuropsychiatric Genetics*, 581–588.

Tager-Flusberg, H., & Joseph, R. M. (2003). Identifying neurocognitive phenotypes in autism. *Philosophical Transactions of the Royal Society of London. Series B, Biological Sciences, 358*, 303–314.

Tate, D. F., Bigler, E. D., McMahon, W., & Lainhart, J. (2007). The relative contributions of brain, cerebrospinal fluid-filled structures, and non-neural tissue volumes to occipital-frontal head circumference in subjects with autism. *Neuropediatrics, 38*, 18–24.

Thompson, W. D., Orvaschel, H., Prusoff, B. A., & Kidd, K. K. (1982). An evaluation of the family history method for ascertaining psychiatric disorders. *Archives of General Psychiatry, 39*, 53–58.

Tsatsanis, K. D. (2003). Outcome research in Asperger syndrome and autism. *Child and Adolescent Psychiatric Clinics of North America, 12*, 47–63, vi.

Tsuang, M. T., Lyons, M. J., Meyer, J. M., Doyle, T., Eisen, S. A., Goldberg, J., et al. (1998). Co-occurrence of abuse of different drugs in men: the role of drug-specific and shared vulnerabilities. *Archives of General Psychiatry, 55*, 967–972.

Tuchman, R., & Rapin, I. (2002). Epilepsy in autism. *Lancet Neurology, 1*, 352–358.

Uhl, G. R., Drgon, T., Johnson, C., Li, C. Y., Contoreggi, C., Hess, J., et al. (2008). Molecular genetics of addiction and related heritable phenotypes: genome-wide association approaches identify "connectivity constellation" and drug target genes with pleiotropic effects. *Annals of the New York Academy of Sciences, 1141*, 318–381.

Vaccarino, F. M., Grigorenko, E. L., Smith, K. M., & Stevens, H. E. (2009). Regulation of cerebral cortical size and neuron number by fibroblast growth factors: implications for autism. *Journal of Autism and Developmental Disorders, 39*, 511–520.

Vandeleur, C. L., Rothen, S., Jeanpretre, N., Lustenberger, Y., Gamma, F., Ayer, E., et al. (2008). Inter-informant agreement and prevalence estimates for substance use disorders: direct interview versus family history method. *Drug and Alcohol Dependence, 92*, 9–19.

Varga, E. A., Pastore, M., Prior, T., Herman, G. E., & McBride, K. L. (2009). The prevalence of PTEN mutations in a clinical pediatric cohort with autism spectrum disorders, developmental delay, and macrocephaly. *Genetics in Medicine, 11*, 111–117.

Venter, A., Lord, C., & Schopler, E. (1992). A follow-up study of high-functioning autistic children. *Journal of Child Psychology and Psychiatry and Allied Disciplines, 33*, 489–507.

Vidal, C. N., Nicolson, R., DeVito, T. J., Hayashi, K. M., Geaga, J. A., Drost, D. J., et al. (2006). Mapping corpus callosum deficits in autism: an index of aberrant cortical connectivity. *Biological Psychiatry, 60*, 218–225.

Volkmar, F. R. (1992). Childhood disintegrative disorder: issues for DSM-IV. *Journal of Autism and Developmental Disorders, 22*, 625–642.

Volkmar, F. R., Cohen, D. J., Bregman, J. D., Hooks, M. Y., & Stevenson, J. M. (1989). An examination of social typologies in autism. *Journal of the American Academy of Child and Adolescent Psychiatry, 28*, 82–86.

Volkmar, F. R., Klin, A., & Pauls, D. (1998). Nosological and genetic aspects of Asperger syndrome. *Journal of Autism and Developmental Disorders, 28*, 457–463.

Waiter, G. D., Williams, J. H., Murray, A. D., Gilchrist, A., Perrett, D. I., & Whiten, A. (2004). A voxel-based investigation of brain structure in male adolescents with autistic spectrum disorder. *NeuroImage, 22*, 619–625.

Waldrop, M. F., & Halverson, C. F. (1971). Minor physical anomalies and hyperactive behavior in young children. In J. Hellmuth (Ed.), *Exceptional infant: Studies in abnormalities* (pp. 343–381). New York: Brunner/Mazel.

Walker, H. A. (1977). Incidence of minor physical anomaly in autism. *Journal of Autism and Childhood Schizophrenia, 7*, 165–176.

Weissman, J. R., Kelley, R. I., Bauman, M. L., Cohen, B. H., Murray, K. F., Mitchell, R. L., et al. (2008). Mitochondrial disease in autism spectrum disorder patients: a cohort analysis. *PLoS ONE, 3*, e3815.

Wiggins, L. D., Robins, D. L., Bakeman, R., & Adamson, L. B. (2009). Brief report: sensory abnormalities as distinguishing symptoms of autism spectrum disorders in young children. *Journal of Autism and Developmental Disorders, 39*, 1087–1091.

Wilson, S., Djukic, A., Shinnar, S., Dharmani, C., & Rapin, I. (2003). Clinical characteristics of language regression in children. *Developmental Medicine and Child Neurology, 45*, 508–514.

Wing, L. (1981). Sex ratios in early childhood autism and related conditions. *Psychiatry Research, 5*, 129–137.

Wing, L., & Gould, J. (1979). Severe impairments of social interaction and associated abnormalities in children: epidemiology and classification. *Journal of Autism and Developmental Disorders, 9*, 11–29.

Yuan, H., Marazita, M. L., & Hill, S. Y. (1996). Segregation analysis of alcoholism in high density families: a replication. *American Journal of Medical Genetics, 67*, 71–76.

Zori, R. T., Marsh, D. J., Graham, G. E., Marliss, E. B., & Eng, C. (1998). Germline PTEN mutation in a family with Cowden syndrome and Bannayan-Riley-Ruvalcaba syndrome. *American Journal of Medical Genetics, 80*, 399–402.

Zucker, R. A., Ellis, D. A., Bingham, C. R., & Fitzgerald, H. E. (1996). The development of alcoholic subtypes: Risk variation among alcoholic families during the early childhood years. *Alcohol Health and Research World, 20*, 46–55.

41 Hande Kaymakçalan, Matthew W. State

Rare Genetic Variants and Autism Spectrum Disorders

Points of Interest

- The study of rare variation offers important avenues to expand the understanding of autism and related conditions. The investigation of rare genetic syndromes may generalize and shed light on the pathophysiology of autism spectrum disorders (ASDs); the study of unusual families or individuals with ASD may reveal basic biological mechanisms and molecular pathways, resulting in novel conceptual approaches to treating ASD; and new genomic technologies will soon reveal whether individually rare variations may account for a significant proportion of the population risk for social disability.
- Highly productive studies of rare variation have been ongoing for decades with regard to developmental syndromes and ASDs, with key early findings emerging from the study of chromosomal abnormalities.
- Recent advances in technology in the area of copy number variation has offered high-resolution detection of rare variation at a genome-wide scale and has been the basis of a series of key advances in the past several years;
- Next generation sequencing is currently being applied to studies of ASDs and the increasing resolution of genome-wide detection of rare variation will dramatically expand the possibilities for gene discovery in ASDs.
- A key distinction must be drawn between rare variation and "simple" inheritance. Recent CNV analyses and resequencing studies have challenged previous assumptions regarding the manner in which individually rare mutations might contribute to complex common syndromes such as ASDs.
- Recent findings point to a strong likelihood that specific genes associated with ASDs may also be involved with risks not only for mental retardation, specific language impairment, and seizure but potentially a wide array of neuropsychiatric disorders, including schizophrenia. The latter findings, if replicated, will fundamentally challenge the current psychiatric diagnostic nosology.

The evidence for a genetic contribution to ASDs is incontrovertible. However, the underlying composition or architecture of the genetic variation contributing to social disability as well as the identity of specific changes in DNA sequence or structure accounting for the lion's share of risk remains largely a mystery (O'Roak & State, 2008; State, 2010). This is not to suggest that there has not been dramatic and important progress in elucidating the biological underpinnings of these devastating syndromes (Abrahams & Geschwind, 2008; O'Roak & State, 2008; Toro et al., 2010). Indeed, engendered in part by rapidly advancing genomic technologies, there have been equally remarkable strides in developmental neurobiology and a highly effective collaboration among advocacy groups, researchers, and the federal government. In fact there are few areas in psychiatric genetics where the pace of progress has been as rapid as it has been with regard to ASD over the past several years.

Over this period of time, interest in the potential contribution of rare variation (or alleles), defined as having a frequency of 1% to 5%, and very rare alleles (minor allele frequency <1%) has taken center stage. This transition has been motivated by converging factors: *(1)* the increasing appreciation of the relevance of the phenotypic overlap observed between ASD and rare single-gene developmental disorders such as Fragile X and tuberous sclerosis complex (Abrahams & Geschwind, 2008; Johnson & Myers, 2007; O'Roak & State, 2008); *(2)* the development of technologies that enable the detection of a new class of variation involving submicroscopic changes in chromosomal structure, known as CNVs (Iafrate et al., 2004; Redon et al., 2006; Sebat et al., 2004), an advance that has made affordable high-resolution genome-wide discovery of rare variation; *(3)* the recognition that common variation is likely to account for a smaller fraction of inter-individual variability in common complex disorders than previously anticipated (Altshuler & Daly, 2007); and *(4)* the rapid pace of advance in the development of next-generation sequencing technology, which will soon allow for genome-wide detection of rare sequence variation to a degree that would have been difficult to conceive of as recently as the end of the past century.

This chapter will elaborate on these developments and focus on the issue of the contribution of rare and very rare genetic variation to ASD. In addition to dividing the discussion broadly based on a dichotomy between common and low-frequency alleles, it is also useful to distinguish three overlapping but distinct areas of investigation in this latter area: *(1)* the study of known rare genetic syndromes that show overlap with ASD; *(2)* the investigation of unusual, or outlier, individuals and families in search of rare variation that may shed light on the pathophysiology of ASD; and *(3)* research into the hypothesis that ASD *writ large* is the result of the accumulation, within the population, of multiple individually rare genetic variations. As other chapters in this volume address issues related to ASD and established genetic syndromes, the ensuing discussion will restrict its focus to the latter two topics.

This discussion will be divided into five sections: the first will provide a basic background into the nature of genetic variation and distinctions between common and rare alleles; the second will describe two competing, but not necessarily mutually exclusive, hypotheses about the genomic underpinnings of ASD, the common-variant: common-disease hypothesis and the rare-variant: common-disease hypothesis; the third will address the so-called "outlier strategy" of gene discovery, in which the focus is on rare and very rare alleles irrespective of their overall contribution to population risk (see Table 41-1); and the fourth will address the emerging evidence regarding the cumulative contribution of rare variation to ASD, including a consideration of opportunities and challenges facing current efforts to tackle this question. Finally, the chapter will close with a consideration of recent rare variant discoveries that have raised the prospect that a given specific genetic mutation may contribute to a broad spectrum of neuropsychiatric and neurodevelopmental outcomes (Eichler & Zimmerman, 2008; McCarthy et al., 2009; Mefford et al., 2008; Stefansson et al., 2008; Weiss et al., 2008) ranging from ASD to mental retardation, seizure, and schizophrenia.

Genetic Variation and Allelic Architecture of Autism Spectrum Disorder

Sequence Variation

The vast majority of the sequence of DNA is identical between any two people. Nonetheless, it is the variation among and between individuals that is most interesting to those studying the relationship of genes to disease risk. Although the biological processes that protect the genetic code from variation are robust, both environmental factors and intrinsic imperfections in the process of DNA replication and maintenance also lead to a slow but steady accumulation of variations over time.

Sequence variation is a change at a specific position within the genetic code of the constituent parts of the DNA molecule, known as bases or nucleotides. These are: A (adenosine), T (thymidine), G (guanine), and C (cytosine). Thus a sequence variation commonly involves either a substitution of one base for another, the loss or gain of a single or small number of bases (referred to as "in-dels" for "insertion-deletion"), or a variation in the number of repeats of a particular sequence motif. In addition, there can be rearrangements of genetic material in the human genome, such as inversions and translocations, which disrupt the expected order of the DNA sequence without leading to a net gain or loss of genetic material. If any of these changes occur in sperm or egg cells, they have the potential to be passed from generation to generation. In addition, if there is a germline mosaicism (i.e., the genetic mutation is present in only the germline of the parent but not in the parental somatic cells), an apparently new, or de novo, mutations may be found in more than one of the offspring. This possibility is one reason that de novo disease-causing mutations may be found in multiple affected individuals in one generation within a family as well as in pedigrees with only a single affected child.

The "life cycle" of germline variation—that is, what happens to an allele once it is introduced into the human genome in a manner that can be passed from generation to generation—is dictated by the interplay of natural selection, time, the mechanics of DNA transmission from generation to generation, and the history of human migration and population growth. Although all of these factors are important, this brief introduction will focus largely on the first—namely, natural selection—as recent evidence has underscored the relevance of this process for understanding the dynamics of human disease genetics.

Recall that the Darwinian notion is that in general, sequence variation that either has no biological consequence or is advantageous to the species will, over time and given reasonable opportunity, rise in frequency within a population and become common. At present, geneticists define this threshold as a minor (meaning the lesser of the two sequence options) frequency of greater than 5%. Alternatively, any variation that finds its way into an individual's germline and is deleterious will be subject, over time, to purifying selection, which will either eliminate the change from the population or drive it to low frequencies. For the sake of this discussion, the notion of good (neutral or advantageous) versus bad (deleterious) variation is very narrowly defined, referring only to the impact on reproductive fitness—that is, the ability of the organism to procreate and thus to pass the DNA from one generation to the next.

Although this dichotomy is a significant oversimplification, the relationship between the impact of a genetic variation on reproductive fitness and its likely frequency within the

Table 41–1.
Genes disrupted by rare variation via several different mechanisms (rare deletions, inversions, point mutations, duplications, translocations, de novo and transmitted CNVs) that are implicated in autism spectrum disorders and discussed in detail in the chapter

Gene Symbol	Chromosome Location	Gene Function	Study Type	Reference
GRPR	Xp22.2	Regulates gastrointestinal and central nervous system function	Molecular cytogenetics	Brush et al. (Seidita et al.)
AUTS2	7q11.22	Unknown	Molecular cytogenetics, CNV analysis	Sultana et al., Kalscheuer et al., Bakkaloglu et al., Redon et al.
NLGN4X, NLGN3	Xp22.3, Xq13	Members of neuroligin family of proteins. Involved in formation of functional synapses	Molecular cytogenetics, linkage analysis	Jamain et al., Thomas et al., Laumonnier et al.
SHANK3	22q13.3	Synaptic scaffolding protein	Molecular cytogenetics	Meyer et al., Moessner et al.
NRXN1	2p16	Neurotransmitter release	Molecular cytogenetics, linkage analysis, CNV analysis	Szatmari et al., Feng et al., Kim et al., Glessner et al.
CNTN4	3p14	Neuronal cell adhesion molecule	Molecular cytogenetics, CNV analysis	Fernandez et al., Roohi et al., Glessner et al.
CNTNAP2	7q36.1	Neuronal cell adhesion molecule	Molecular cytogenetics, linkage analysis	Bakkaloglu et al., Strauss et al., Alarcon et al., Arking et al.
DIA1,NHE9 PCDH10,CNTN3	22q13.2, 3q24, 4q28.3, 3p12.3	Involved in cell migration, sodium/proton exchanger, neuronal cell adhesion molecules	Linkage analysis	Morrow et al.
A2BP1	16p13.2	Neuronal splicing enhancer	CNV analysis, molecular cytogenetics	Martin et al., Bhalla et al.
DPP6, DPP10, PCDH9, ANKRD11, DPYD, PTCHD1	7q36.2, 2q14.1, 13q21.32, 16q24.3, 1p21.3, Xp22.11	Modulation of calcium and potassium channels, cell adhesion molecule, transcriptional initiator, pyrimidine metabolism, participates in cell interaction	CNV analysis	Marshall et al.
NLGN1, ASTN2, UBE3A, PARK2, RFWD2, FBXO40	3q26.31, 9q33.1, 15q11.2, 6q26, 1q25.1-q25.2, 3q13.33	Neuronal cell adhesion molecule, makes enzyme ubiquitin protein ligase 3A, ubiquitin protein ligase Parkin, degradation of proteins, protein interaction	CNV analysis	Glessner et al., Vrijenhoek et al., Kahler et al.

population is an important touchstone for understanding contemporary arguments regarding the allelic architecture of childhood developmental disorders. For example, if a phenotype is subject to strong purifying selection, alleles of large effect are likely to be rare. Conversely, common alleles are likely to carry smaller effects compared to very low frequency variations influencing the same phenotype.

Before launching into a discussion of the major competing hypotheses with regard to the allelic contributions to ASD, several related points deserve mention. First, "rare" variation and "deleterious" variation are not synonymous. As suggested above, time, the mechanics of DNA transmission, and the dynamics of human migration and population history influence allele frequencies. For example, any mutation that has occurred recently is likely to be rare, having not had the time to flourish within a population. Consequently, a highly deleterious mutation is likely to be rare, but a rare variation is not necessarily highly deleterious. Moreover, even if a mutation is deleterious, it may be able to become common by "hitchhiking" through the generations due to its residing very near to an allele that provides survival advantages. Another important caveat is that it can be quite difficult to anticipate what types of phenotypic characteristics will or will not be subject to negative or purifying selection, particularly with regard to common disease. For example, although it is not difficult to predict that a mutation that inalterably leads to fetal demise will be found at low frequency, the manner in which natural selection will act on alleles contributing to adult-onset disorders or childhood syndromes that are not life-threatening may be impossible to anticipate. It is important to recall that such arguments must presuppose the interplay between a phenotypic trait and environmental factors that may have changed over evolutionary time. Third, rare variation is not rare. Although geneticists classify variation based on allele frequency, these categories are not a comment on the overall prevalence of a *class* of variation within an individual or a population. For example, in any given person, a very large percentage of sequence changes will be found to consist of alleles with frequency of less than 5% (Kidd, Pakstis, Speed, & Kidd, 2004; Meigs et al., 2007; Wang et al., 2008).

Common-Variant: Common-Disease

For most of the past decade, gene discovery in ASD has largely focused on common genetic variation. The presumption that common alleles will carry most of the genetic load for a common disorder is known as the "common-variant: common-disease" hypothesis. It is based on the notion that a conspiracy of genetic variations of relatively subtle effect, in combination with environmental factors, is likely to carry the majority of risk for prevalent clinical conditions (including ASD).

This hypothesis emerged in part as a result of the failure of early single-gene models to account for the genetics of common disorders. The earliest successes in gene discovery were the result of mapping rare alleles carrying very large effects for clearly defined (often relatively homogenous) clinical entities, mutations for which there is essentially a one-to-one relationship between possessing the variation and demonstrating a disease phenotype. As genetic tools became increasingly powerful, it was quickly apparent that this model did not hold for neuropsychiatric disorders *writ large* or for most common medical conditions.

Alternative hypotheses shifted the focus from Mendelian mutations carrying very large effects to common variations carrying more subtle risks. It was posited that individual alleles might carry such small risks as to be able to escape purifying selection because only a conspiracy of alleles would result in a phenotype that would impair fitness. Moreover, variation that might have enhanced fitness at one time in history, and thus gained a foothold in terms of allele frequency, could, in a different environmental context, lead to disease. Several additional related ideas support a role for common variation even for a disorder that *prima face* would appear to reduce reproductive fitness: the first involves so-called "balancing selection" in which genetic changes might enhance fitness in one manner while reducing it in another. Another is that a deleterious variation might be present in sufficiently close proximity to a fitness-enhancing genetic variation that the two alleles would often be passed together from generation to generation, yielding a so-called "hitchhiking allele." Finally, it is worth noting that the overall hypothesis of common variants underlying common disease fits nicely with the Out-of-Africa theory of human history: one can construct a strong theoretical case that in a situation in which there was a very small initial population followed by very rapid growth, it would be likely that at the current stage in human evolution, most common diseases would be accounted for by the same variations that were present in the initial population.

A detailed history of methods to test for the contribution of common variation to common disease is beyond the scope of this chapter. However, it is useful to keep in mind that in general, such studies have involved some variation on a case–control design, performing comparisons of allele frequencies in these groups. Until the last few years, it was only technically feasible to test the relative abundance of alleles by focusing on a small amount of variation at time—for example, investigating one or several common variants located in or near a single or small numbers of candidate genes.

However, with the advent of high-density micro-arrays, it has recently become possible to test many alleles simultaneously. The technology has rapidly advanced from assaying tens to hundreds of thousands and now typically more than a million known alleles in a single rapid and inexpensive experiment. This technology has led to a remarkable proliferation of genome-wide association studies (GWAS), in which variations in and near every gene in the genome are tested simultaneously for association with a phenotype.

This shift, which eliminated the need to specify a gene of interest *a priori*, has had a striking effect, leading to the definitive discovery of many common alleles contributing to common medical conditions, including diabetes (Meigs et al., 2007), inflammatory bowel disease (Weersma et al., 2009), asthma (Moffatt et al., 2007), and intracranial aneurysm (Bilguvar et al., 2008). The rapid maturation of methods for common variant studies has allowed an empirical reappraisal of the common variant common disease hypothesis, leading to the following observations: first, the majority of disorders that have so far yielded to GWAS have shown genotype-relative risks that fall within the range of a 10% to 40% increase in cases versus controls for a given allele, far short of the two- to threefold change that was generally thought to represent a reasonable lower bound for powering common variant studies (Manolio, Brooks, & Collins, 2008). Moreover, this appears to hold true for adult-onset conditions, even when the manner in which the disorder might impair fitness is not clear (e.g., intracranial aneurysm). This observation does not prove, but is consistent with, the notion that natural selection is a powerful factor in human disease genetics. The fact that only alleles carrying very small risks are found at high frequency in affected populations suggests that alleles carrying larger risks must have been driven down in frequency in the population and have been either eliminated or become rare. A second key observation emerging from the recent rash of GWAS successes is that the total amount of genetic risk that is explained by common alleles has so far also been quite small. Now that studies of some disorders (such as diabetes) have been completed on very large samples (large enough to detect effects in the range of 10%–15%) and multiple risk alleles have been confirmed, it is notable that less than 10% of interindividual variability has been accounted for, compared to the 40%–60% thought to be relevant in most common conditions (Altshuler, Daly, & Lander, 2008; Zeggini et al., 2008). These results suggests several alternatives: *(1)* genetic risks have been vastly overestimated across all of medicine; *(2)* studies of hundreds of thousands of patients will be needed to identify the hundreds of additional alleles that will ultimately be found to carry fleetingly small individual risks; *(3)* new methodologies and approaches will need to be developed to better detect the interactive contributions of multiple genes and environmental factors; and/or *(4)* rare variation accounts for a more substantial population burden of common disease than expected based on the common variant common disease hypothesis.

Rare-Variant: Common-Disease

The early failure of Mendelian genetics to account for a significant proportion of the risk for common conditions did not lead the entire genetics field to abandon the study of rare variation. Indeed, many of the most important advances in human genetics in the contemporary era have come from the search for rare examples of common disorders, including in breast cancer (Miki et al., 1994), Alzheimer's disease (Bertram et al., 2000), and hypertension (Simon et al., 1996).

One of the driving rationales for these studies was that some proportion of the genetic architecture of a common condition would be accounted for by rare, highly penetrant mutations. And, moreover, these variations would be more amenable to mapping using traditional methods *and* more tractable to study in vitro and in vivo given the relative large effect sizes. Most importantly, the studies shared the hypothesis that the insights into molecular mechanisms and disease pathophysiology could be transformative regardless of whether the specific genes discovered accounted for significant population genetic risk. In fact, for many complex disorders, this has turned out to be the case.

A second rational motivating such studies has been the recognition that rare variation could, in addition to accounting for disease in outliers, accumulate in the population to account for an appreciable proportion of common disease (Cohen et al., 2006; Ji et al., 2008). One could imagine that if variations in multiple different genes or multiple variations in the same gene could lead to similar clinical outcomes, over time, an accumulation of rare variation could accrue, accounting for a significant proportion of a commonly occurring disorder. Moreover, for conditions in which de novo mutation played a significant role, this would obtain—and one would expect to see—a considerable number of apparently sporadic cases (in which only the proband in the family was affected) and a very high rate of monozygotic concordance versus dizygotic (DZ) concordance.

Until very recently, for practical reasons, it has been difficult to test this hypothesis. Evaluating individuals for sequence variation that has previously been discovered, as is typically the case with common variation, is relatively inexpensive and is now both economically and technically feasible to carry out on a genome-wide scale. In brief, once a variation is known, binary assays can be developed that are quite inexpensive, investigating the presence or absence of a given base without having to sequence the corresponding DNA. Conversely, the identification of rare variation often requires some degree of direct DNA sequencing to identify which of the four possible bases is present at each position in the genetic code. This is an order of magnitude more expensive than most binary common variant detection schemes. Consequently, studies at a genome-wide scale have not been yet conducted, and it is only recently, with the advent of "massively parallel" "next generation" sequencing technologies, that such studies are emerging as within reach of the typical genetics laboratories.

Nonetheless, for some time, both the outlier approach as well as the question of the overall contribution of rare variation to common disease risk has been of great interest among a group of investigators (Abelson et al., 2005; Jamain et al., 2003; Marshall et al., 2008; McClellan, Susser, & King, 2007) and has recently become a major area of preoccupation in psychiatry, particularly with regard to autism and schizophrenia, as discussed below.

Rare Variation in Autism Spectrum Disorder

Presently, there is evidence supporting *both* common and rare variation contributing to ASDs. The former is discussed in considerable detail elsewhere in this volume. In fact there are multiple lines of evidence to support the contribution of rare variants to ASDs, both with regard to the relevance of outliers as well as supporting the rare-variant: common-disease hypothesis. For example: *(1)* over the past two decades, microscopic chromosomal abnormalities have been identified at a far greater rate in ASDs than in the typically developing population (Vorstman et al., 2006); *(2)* several recurrent contiguous-gene microscopic chromosomal rearrangements are either known or suspected to increase the risk for ASDs, including maternally-inherited duplications of 15q11-13 and deletions of 22q11; *(3)* rare monogenic syndromes show phenotypic overlap with ASDs, and, not infrequently, the ASD diagnosis precedes recognition and molecular confirmation of the syndrome (Schaefer & Mendelsohn, 2008); *(4)* recent studies have demonstrated that, as is the case with microscopic cytogenetic abnormalities, large submicroscopic copy number variations are also more commonly identified in individuals with autism than in controls (Sebat et al., 2007) and that such CNVs may either be individually rare or recurrent (Kumar et al., 2008; Weiss et al., 2008); and finally, *(5)* individually rare variations in both chromosome structure and DNA sequence have been either associated with or found to be linked to so-called "idiopathic ASD."

Recent evidence supporting both the utility of outlier approaches as well as evidence supporting the overall contribution of rare variation to the prevalence of ASDs is discussed below.

Rare Variants and Outlier Approaches

Historically, outlier approaches have relied on the characterization of chromosomal abnormalities or the use of traditional multigenerational (parametric) linkage analyses to identify highly penetrant mutations in rare individuals or families. These two approaches are discussed in turn. In addition, over the past several years, the analysis of CNV has become an important means both to expand the search for outliers (discussed here) as well as to assess the overall contribution of rare variation to ASDs (discussed in the subsequent section).

In recent years, it has become commonplace to follow on the characterization of a candidate transcript identified through any of these approaches by re-sequencing the gene or genes of interest in a larger group of individuals. Such an approach is intuitively attractive, but presents some methodological and conceptual challenges that are highlighted below. In addition as suggested above, new sequencing technologies have rapidly emerged as a means to identify most or all rare variation in an individual, a topic which will be addressed in the penultimate section of the chapter.

Molecular Cytogenetics

The earliest studies addressing the question of rare structural variation used the light microscope and converged on an estimated consensus of approximately 3% to 7% burden of balanced translocations, inversions, and aneuploidies in cases of autism that had passed screening for "known" etiologies, a rate that is estimated to be 50- to 100-fold higher than for developmentally typical children (Nielsen & Sillesen, 1975; Nielsen et al., 1982).

More than a decade ago, the first reports describing fine mapping of chromosomal abnormalities in individuals with autism emerged, coincident with the development of molecular cytogenetic techniques (Speicher, Gwyn Ballard, & Ward, 1996). In 1997, Ishikawa-Brush and colleagues (Ishikawa-Brush et al., 1997) reported a chromosome X;8 translocation in a 27-year-old female with multiple exostoses, autism, MR, and epilepsy that disrupted the gene *gastrin-releasing peptide receptor* (*GRPR*) on the X-chromosome and mapped approximately 30 kilobases from the gene *Syndecan-2* gene (*SDC2* on chromosome 8). The authors were particularly interested in *GRPR* given its position on the X chromosome and disruption by the rearrangement. Moreover, subsequent studies have demonstrated that the receptor is present on GABAergic interneurons of the lateral nucleus of the amygdala (Shumyatsky et al., 2002). So far, additional functional mutations have not been found in either gene clearly associated with developmental delay or autism (Seidita et al., 2008).

Using a similar strategy, Sultana et al. (2002) reported on a chromosomal breakpoint in a pair of twins with ASDs, mapping this to a previously uncharacterized transcript they dubbed *AUTS2*. Interestingly, several subsequent investigations have found CNVs at this locus in individuals with MR and ASDs (Kalscheuer et al., 2007; Sultana et al., 2002) (Bakkaloglu et al., 2007) as well as in normal controls (Redon et al., 2006).

However, the most notable early discovery based on cytogenetic findings was the result of work by Jamain and colleagues in the laboratory of Thomas Buergeron. They were motivated to study transcripts mapping to chromosome Xp22.3 because of the prior finding of deletions of this interval in three females with autism (Thomas et al., 1999). Within this region, they identified the transcript *KIAA1260*, corresponding to *NLGN4X*, a member of the neuroligin family of proteins, later found to be essential for the formation of functional synapses (Lisé & El-Husseini, 2006). They sequenced the gene, as well as the related transcripts *NLGN3* and *NLGN4Y*, in 36 pairs of affected siblings and 122 trios with autism or AS. Within *NLGN4X*, they identified a nonsense mutation that segregated with both autism and AS in a single family, marking the first observation of a clearly deleterious point mutation identified in individuals with apparently idiopathic or nonsyndromic ASDs. In addition, in the transcript *NLGN3*, they identified a missense substitution at a highly conserved residue in a second family. Although subsequent mutation screening studies of relatively small numbers of patients have not identified additional clearly functional mutations in either of these transcripts (confirming their status as outlier findings), the *NLGN4X* finding was confirmed shortly after initial publication by an independent lab investigating a multigenerational family affected with both MR and ASDs using parametric linkage analysis (discussed below) (Laumonnier et al., 2004).

As the technology for mapping chromosomal abnormalities has improved and the identification of genes at chromosomal breakpoint become routine, multiple examples of de novo abnormalities or chromosomal rearrangements have been found disrupting or mapping near brain expressed transcripts in individuals and families with social disability (Borg et al., 2002; Collins et al., 2006; Roohi et al., 2009; Savelyeva et al., 2006; Vincent et al., 2000). The challenges that accompany determining which of these are incidental findings and which are truly involved in disease risk are considered in subsequent sections of this chapter.

Interestingly, in the wake of the *NGLN4X* findings, several recent studies have provided support for the involvement of synaptic and/or neuronal adhesion molecules in ASDs. For example, in families with ASDs, the Buergeron lab identified rare de novo and transmitted structural and sequence variations in the gene *SHANK3*, a protein present in the postsynaptic density that interacts with a binding partner of *NLGN4* (Meyer et al., 2004). Moreover, in a second study of *SHANK3*, four de novo abnormities and nine inherited missense variants were identified among 400 families (Moessner et al., 2007). Three of the de novo events were large-scale deletions, encompassing 277 kb, 3.2 Mb, 4.36 Mb, whereas the fourth was a missense variant. The high rate of de novo mutations involving coding segments of *SHANK3* in individuals with ideopathic ASDs identified in independent studies, the finding of developmental delay and autistic features in patients with the 22q13 deletion syndrome (the region in which *SHANK3* resides), and the shared molecular pathway with *NLGN4X* provide strong convergent evidence for the importance of rare mutations in this transcript for ASDs. In addition, two very recent publications found evidence for the association of the gene SHANK2, a closely related scaffolding molecule, with ASD (Pinto et al. Nature. 2010 Jul 15;466(7304):368-72.; Berkel et al Nat Genet. 2010 Jun;42(6):489-91).

Several recent papers have also suggested that variations in *Neurexin 1* (*NRXN1*) a trans-synaptic binding partner for neuroligins (Lisé & El-Husseini, 2006) carries risks for ASDs. The Autism Genome Project Consortium (2007; Szatmari & Consortium, 2007) reported a combined linkage and copy number analysis involving 1168 subjects. This early investigation was one of the first to address the issue of CNVs in autism but was confined to an analysis of only large-scale variations because of the use of a first generation array with 10,000 probes. Nonetheless, one family was identified in which two affected siblings had the same 300-kb deletion, encompassing the coding region of *NRXN1*. This was not present in the parents, again highlighting the phenomena of germline mosaicism. Subsequently, rare missense variants, balanced chromosomal abnormities disrupting *NRXN1* and an over-representation of micro-deletions in cases versus control have all been reported (Feng et al., 2006; Kim et al., 2008; Glessner et al., 2009; Bucan et al., 2009).

Cytogenetic approaches have also highlighted a role for contactin and contactin-associated neuronal adhesion molecules in ASDs (as have common variant studies discussed in detail elsewhere in this volume). Fernandez and colleagues (T. Fernandez et al., 2004; T. V. Fernandez et al., 2008) identified a child with features of a rare deletion syndrome on the short arm of chromosome 3 who also presented with social disability. They identified and mapped a balanced translocation that disrupted the coding segment of the gene *Contactin 4*. Several subsequent studies of CNVs have supported a role for this molecule in ideopathic ASDs (Glessner et al., 2009; Roohi et al., 2009).

In a similar vein, Bakkaloglu et al. (2007) mapped a de novo chromosomal abnormality in the only affected member of a pedigree and found the rearrangement disrupted both the neuronal adhesion molecule *contactin-associated protein 2* (*CNTNAP2;* a.k.a. *Caspr2* in the mouse) and the previously identified transcript *AUTS2* (Sultana et al., 2002). Based on prior evidence implicating contactin molecules in ASDs and a previous study demonstrating that rare recessive mutations in this gene lead to seizures, developmental delay and autism (Strauss et al., 2006), the authors chose to prioritize the evaluation of *CNTNAP2* and comprehensively resequenced this molecule in 635 patients and 942 controls. Among patients, they identified 13 very rare variants, 8 of which mapped to highly conserved sites and/or were predicted to be deleterious by bioinformatics approaches. However, they also identified 11 rare variants, 6 of which were presumed deleterious among the larger group of controls. Among the affected individuals, the majority of very rare variants showed partial penetrance (i.e., as expected for complex disease, some individuals who had the mutation did not appear to be affected), but most of the identified variants did segregate among the affected individuals within a family (i.e., all presumed affected individuals in a nuclear family carried the same putative mutation). One variant at a highly conserved position, 1869T, was inherited by 4 affected children in 3 unrelated families and was not present in 4010 control chromosomes ($p = 0.014$), although the authors were not able to rule out the confound of occult ancestral differences between cases and controls given the data available at that time.

Overall, this large-scale resequencing effort demonstrated a twofold increase in the burden of rare variants in cases versus controls, which did not reach statistical significance. Subsequent deep sequencing studies have highlighted the importance of differentiating rare variation that is deleterious to protein function versus that which is neutral (Ji et al. Nat Genet. 2008 May;40(5):592-9), an effort that is currently underway with regard to CNTNAP2. Nonetheless, as noted below and in other chapters of this volume, work from other groups of investigators has implicated both common and rare variation in *CNTNAP2* with ASDs and language development. In this light, the cytogenetic and resequencing screening data presented in Bakkaloglu et al. (2007) suggest that individually, very rare variants in this transcript may also contribute to the pathophysiology of idiopathic ASDs.

Parametric Linkage Analyses

If the mode of inheritance of a gene is known or suspected, as is often the case for Mendelian conditions, genome-wide parametric linkage analysis is a highly effective approach to gene discovery. Genetic data are analyzed in multiple generations within a family or group of families searching for chromosomal segments that contain (or are linked to) a disease locus and that fit a proposed model (the parameters) of inheritance. The likelihood of observing the data based on the proposed model is compared to likelihood of the same set of observations being made by chance. This method has been used infrequently in studies of autism, as the mode of inheritance is typically not straightforward. However, when such a strategy has been employed in unusual outlier families or special populations, the results have been striking.

For example, shortly after the publication by Jamain et al. (2003), which reported a truncating *NLGN4X* mutation in ASDs, Laumonnier et al. (2004) described a parametric linkage analysis performed on a single large family with probands affected either with mental retardation, ASDs, or both. They observed segregation in this family consistent with an X-linked mode of inheritance and identified a statistically significant region on the X-chromosome yielding evidence for genome-wide linkage. Within this interval, fine mapping revealed a nonsense substitution in *NLGN4X* that was quite similar, but not identical, to the previous reported mutation (Jamain et al., 2003). This result provided a critical confirmation of the earlier observation.

More recently, a particular type of parametric linkage known as homozygosity mapping has been undertaken in Old Order Amish families displaying a syndrome of intractable epilepsy, MR, and autism. This approach relies on intermarried families to increase the statistical power available to identify rare recessive mutations. In this case, the analysis led to the discovery of a truncating mutation in the transcript *CNTNAP2* (Strauss et al., 2006). As mentioned above, a role for this gene in idiopathic autism and language development was subsequently identified by four independent groups of investigators (Alarcon et al., 2008; Arking et al., 2008; Bakkaloglu et al., 2007; Vernes et al., 2008).

Finally, a recent intensive search for rare recessive mutations based on homozygosity mapping was reported by Morrow and colleagues (2008; *see also* Chapter 44). The authors recruited and carefully phenotyped 88 consanguineous families. They identified multiple, mostly nonoverlapping regions of homozygosity (i.e., regions of the genome in which, as a result of the fact that parents share a common ancestor, a single identical chromosomal segment is inherited from both mother and father). Although the resulting statistical scores did not quite achieve genome-wide significance, several rare, large (18 kbp to >880 kbp), inherited homozygous deletions were found disrupting either the coding or potential regulatory regions of brain-expressed transcripts, including *deleted in autism-1* (*DIA1*) (*c3orf58*), *sodium/proton exhanger 9* (*NHE9*), *protocadherin 10* (*PCDH10*), and *contactin 3* (*CNTN3*). The authors then found additional strong evidence supporting a role for the gene *NHE9*, the (Na^+, K^+)/H^+ exchanger, in ASDs through the identification of a rare nonsense mutation in two male siblings with autism, one of whom had epilepsy and the other with probable seizures, in a non-consanguineous family. Overall, they identified rare amino acid changes in *NHE9* in almost 6% of patients with both autism and epilepsy versus only 0.63% of controls. Interestingly, based on an independent series of studies reported in the same publication, three of the genes located within or closest to the two largest deletions (*DIA1*, *NHE9*, *PCDH10*) were found to either be regulated by neural activity and/or were the targets of activity-induced transcription factors, suggesting that activity-regulated gene expression during early brain development may be a common mechanism contributing to ASDs.

Rare-Variants: Common-Disease?

Copy Number Variants

Copy number variants refer to variations in chromosome structure that generally fall below the resolution of the light microscope. This type of cytogenetic variability was identified as a potential cause of developmental disorders in the mid-1990s (Folstein, 1996; Lipska & Weinberger, 1995), but it was not until 2004 that several groups (Lucito et al., 2003; Sebat et al., 2004; Iafrate et al., 2004) first identified CNVs as being widespread in apparently unaffected individuals. These discoveries both marked the development of technology that could identify previously cryptic rare chromosomal rearrangements as the cause of disease, but also suggested that assumptions regarding the biological requirement for an "intact" genome for normal development would need to be re-evaluated.

In the wake of these influential papers, the technology to detect CNVs with increasing resolution quickly followed. Moreover, given the longstanding appreciation of the potential role of gross chromosomal abnormalities to ASDs, there seemed to be a real possibility that this increasing resolution would dramatically expand the understanding of the genetic underpinnings of autism.

In 2007, Both the Autism Genome Project (AGP; as discussed previously) (Szatmari & Consortium, 2007) and Sebat et al. (2007) reported the first genome-wide detection of CNVs in patients with autism (Sebat et al., 2007). Findings from both papers were notable: first, as suggested above, several of the single observations reported in these papers have turned out to map to genomic intervals that have later been found to harbor recurrent rare abnormalities showing evidence for association with disease (Eichler & Zimmerman, 2008; Kumar et al., 2008; Miller et al., 2009; Morrow et al., 2008; Rujescu et al., 2009; Weiss et al., 2008; Glessner et al., 2009; Bucan et al., 2009; Pinto et al., 2010); second, the Sebat paper highlighted a distinction between so-called "simplex families" (those with only a single affected child), in which approximately 11% were found to carry large de novo CNVs, versus "multiplex families" (with more than one affected child), in which only 2% were found to carry similar events and controls, which had a rate of 1%. Subsequent studies have consistently replicated this finding and placed this burden in simplex families at between 3.4 and 11 percent (Itsara et al., 2010; Marshall et al., 2008; Pinto et al., 2010).

Notably, the precise results of different CNV studies may be difficult to compare. The number of CNVs identified in any investigation will depend in part on the number and distribution of probes on the array, which contribute to the resolution of the detection platform, on whether the authors rely on predictions versus confirmations using a "gold standard" method, and on the manner in which authors categorize CNVs (e.g., studies may use different methods for defining "rare," "large," or even "de novo" CNVs). Any or all of these variables may lead to somewhat different results from groups studying identical samples.

The contribution of recurrent rare CNVs as risk factors for autism were further highlighted in reports by Marshall et al. (2008); Kumar et al. (2008) and Weiss and colleagues (2008). in which these groups nearly simultaneously identified deletions and/or duplications in the region 16p11.2 in families with autism.These and subsequent findings underscored the contribution of this region to disease and, at the same time, highlighted the issue of complex inheritance in ASDs, even in the context of searching for rare variation. As expected, many of the CNVs that were transmitted showed incomplete penetrance, which is a well-accepted phenomenon even for monogenetic traits. However, in addition, neither the de novo mutations nor the inherited duplications initially identified were found consistently in all affected members of a individual nuclear families (Bucan et al., 2009). For a rare Mendelian trait, this observation would be taken as evidence against a causal relationship for the variant. However, in complex disorders, the finding is consistent with the hypothesis that multiple risk alleles are present within these families.

A final note with regard to this very interesting region of the genome: a subsequent large-scale study of CNVs in autism (Glessner et al., 2009) did not replicate the 16p11.2 most likely due to a comparatively high rate of CNVs in this region among their control groups. The result highlights several potentially important methodological issues, including the inherent difficulties in assessing the precise frequencies of CNV from multiple array platforms using predictions alone; the impact of false-negative prediction rates; and the possible confound of population stratification (cryptic differences in the ethnic make-up of cases and controls leading to varying allele frequencies). Of note, very recent data from a large simplex autism cohort, which controlled for these confounds, strongly replicate the association of both duplications and deletions at 16p11.2 for autism spectrum disorders.

CNV analyses are currently the most practical high-resolution approach to identifying rare variation across the genome and, consequently, are both the most practical approach to testing the rare-variant: common-disease hypothesis as well as to generating leads for outlier studies. Several large scale studies have identified a variety of interesting candidate genes and molecular pathways of interest. For example, Glessner et al. (2009) reported a whole-genome CNV study of 859 ASD cases and 1409 healthy children of European ancestry and a replication sample consisting of 1336 ASD cases and 1110 controls from the AGRE sample, which consisted largely of multiplex families. They reported positive associations in previously identified candidate genes, including *NRXN1* and *CNTN4*, as well as several new putative susceptibility genes encoding neuronal cell-adhesion molecules, including *neuroglin 1* (*NLGN1*) *and astrotactin 2* (*ASTN2*). These genes harbored recurrent CNVs that were not observed in controls. Other recurrent CNVs were found within or nearby genes involved in the ubiquitin pathway, including *UBE3A, PARK2, RFWD2*, and *FBXO40* that also were not observed in controls.

The authors noted the biological plausibility of involvement of this latter pathway in ASDs and other developmental neurogenetic disorders based on several lines of evidence including that known mutations in *ubiquitin protein ligase 3A* (*UBE3A*) are seen in 5% to 10% of Angelman Syndrome cases, *astrotactin 2* (*ASTN2*) deletions have recently been associated with schizophrenia (Vrijenhoek et al., 2008; Kahler et al., 2008), and *PARK2* (Mefford et al., 2008) mutations lead to autosomal recessive juvenile Parkinson's disease. Ring finger and W repeat domain 2 (*RFWD2*) and F box protein 40 (*FBXO40*) have not previously associated with disease-causing mutations.

Similarly, Bucan et al. (2009) performed CNV analyses using arrays with approximately 550,000 probes in 912 multiplex families from the AGRE collection and 1488 healthy controls. They identified hundreds of loci harboring rare deletions and/or duplications in unrelated probands that were not seen in the unaffected group. Moreover, they tested their findings in an additional independent cohort of 859 cases and 1051 controls. This rigorous two-step study identified previously implicated loci including the genes *NRXN1* and *UBE3A*, and pathway analysis provided further support for the involvement of neuronal adhesion molecules in ASDs. In addition, the study identified evidence for the involvement of several interesting novel transcripts, including the *benzodiazapine receptor (peripheral) associated protein 1* (*BZRAP1*) and *MAM domain-containing glycosylphosphatidylinositol anchor 2M* (*MDGA2*), which, as the authors note, shows a strikingly high similarity to *Contactin 4*.

More recently, Pinto et al. (2010) reported on a sample of 996 ASD individuals of European ancestry to 1,287 matched controls and found evidence for the involvement of *SYNGAP1, DLGAP2, SHANK2*, and the X-linked *DDX53-PTCHD1* locus. The findings with regard to SHANK2 emerged nearly simultaneously with a description of rare de novo mutations in this gene among individuals with ASD (Berkel et al., 2010) and a second subsequent report identified multiple rare protein altering sequence variants in *PTCHD1* that were transmitted from mothers to affected sons and were not found in controls (Noor et al., 2010).

Cause and Effect: Association Strategies and Rare Variants

The extremely interesting data emerging from both resequencing and CNV studies have also underscored important challenges in confirming cause-and-effect relationships between rare variants and developmental syndromes. These issues are likely to become even more pressing in the next epoch of rare variant analyses, which will undoubtedly include a comprehensive assessment of rare variation through the simultaneous sequencing of all, or a large portion, of the human genome.

As many of the aforementioned studies have demonstrated both rare structural and sequence variation is plentiful in unaffected as well as affected individuals. This observation reinforces a point made at the outset: although highly deleterious variations are likely to be rare, rare variations are not necessarily deleterious. Clearly, in the early stages of gene discovery in Mendelian disorders, a tendency to assign pathogenecity to rare deleterious variation in a single or small number of cases was well-justified. However, as gene discovery efforts involving rare variation have been applied to complex common disorders, this conventional wisdom is being supplanted by the recognition that no class of variation is uniformly disease-related and that rare variation may contribute to ASDs in a non-Mendelian fashion.

Indeed, to date, the vast majority of findings with regard to rare recurrent CNVs and autism have been based on population association, an approach that is suited to characterizing complex patterns of inheritance. As noted above, even with regard to chromosome 16p11.2 CNVs, which are presently among the most replicated finding in this area, these variations do not exhibit the type of one-to-one relationship with affected status within pedigrees that is expected for single-gene disorders.

Given the longstanding tendency to equate rare mutation with Mendelian inheritance and common variation with complex inheritance, it is worthwhile to reflect on the increasing likelihood that rare and very rare alleles for ASDs will be found carrying risks exceeding those of common variants but falling short of those previously attributed to simple genetic diseases. To the extent that this is the case, it will be essential for researchers to confirm association of rare variation by contending with the same types of issues now recognized as critical for successful studies of common variants. These include acknowledging the superiority of genome-wide compared to candidate gene studies for initial efforts at gene discovery; establishing appropriate statistical thresholds for these types of investigations; avoiding a deluge of underpowered analyses resulting from overestimation of effect sizes; controlling for the confound of occult ethnic stratification; and ensuring that the technical quality and consistency of CNV typing, as non-random technical errors have clearly been a significant issue in common variant studies.

Some of these issues will be easier to address than others. For example, in some cases very large samples sizes, similar to those currently estimated to be required for common variant studies will be sufficient to ensure adequate power for CNV analyses, particularly for those recurrent CNVs that fall close to the threshold of 5% minor allele frequency. However, for some extremely rare variants, it simply may not be practical to ascertain a sample size that is sufficiently large to support allelic association analyses, unless one is focussed on recurrent de novo events.

Moreover, it is important to recall that for very rare sequence variants, once a single observation is made either in a case or control, the allele is not be likely to ever be seen again in samples of the size typically employed in such studies. Therefore, the identification of individually very rare mutations in a case group followed by the search for those same variants in a control group does not provide strong evidence for association. Instead, studies focusing on variants with allele frequencies far below 5% will likely need to be pursued by investigating the totality of rare functional sequence variants in cases versus controls, examining each group in an identical fashion—an approach commonly referred to as a mutation burden study.

The foregoing arguments point to the high value of identifying recurrent risk alleles in the 1%- to 5%-frequency range: they are of sufficiently low frequency to suggest that they may carry large effects, but they are also sufficiently common that standard allelic association strategies may be employed in attainable sample sizes. When mutation burden approaches are employed, a central challenge is presented by the sheer volume of normal rare variation throughout the genome, which may then obscure true associations. As noted above, recent studies have underscored the limitations of current bioinformatics approaches to determining the consequences of amino acid substitutions and have highlighted the value, in these analyses, of being able to truly distinguish between those rare alleles that alter protein function and those that do not (Ji et al., 2008).

The issue of statistical thresholds is also an important one for rare variant studies that has not yet been resolved. For GWAS common variant studies, it has been possible over time to arrive at commonly accepted levels for genome-wide significance. This has played an important part in transforming allelic association from a strikingly unreliable approach to one that is now leading to highly reproducible findings across all fields in medicine. With regard to rare variants, a similar consensus has not been reached. Not surprisingly, some early studies relied on nominal p-values. However, as the number of published studies grows, the resolution of array platforms increases and the numbers of CNVs found in individuals proliferate, it is increasingly important to address the issue to avoid a flood of nonverifiable findings of the type that plagued early efforts at candidate gene single nucleotide polymorphism association. Given the focus on rare and very rare variation and the expected small number of observations likely at any given locus, it may turn out be quite challenging for any study (even those with very large samples) to correct for the total number of genome-wide comparisons and still reach statistical significance. A combination of statistical analyses of the likelihood of recurrence of *de novo* events, simulation studies, and two-stage designs are likely play a role in addressing this issue.

Finally, whether one is studying rare or very rare variants, it is clear that one must consider the issue of ethnic mismatch or population stratification. There is ample evidence that recurrent CNVs show differences in frequency based on the ethnic composition of the population under study in a manner similar to that seen for common variants (Redon et al., 2006). The early history of common variant analysis was plagued by case–control mismatch leading to false-positive results.

There is every reason to expect that CNV studies involving transmitted recurrent variants are liable to the same difficulties. Fortunately, the tools are now available to derive genomic profiles of ethnic origin that can be used to match individuals and minimize the liability for this confound. This will likely be recognized in the future as an essential component of methodologically sound studies of rare sequence and structural variation, as it is now for common variant studies.

Copy Number Variants: Rethinking Genotype/Phenotype Relationships

One of the most interesting results of investigations of CNVs has been the degree to which recent findings have challenged the traditional diagnostic boundaries in psychiatry. For example, as noted, 16p11.2 CNVs have been associated with autism but have also been observed in individuals with schizophrenia, mental retardation, and seizure disorder (Marshall et al., 2008). Recent studies have found CNVs at 1q21.1, 15q11.2, and 15q13.3 that are strongly associated with schizophrenia, and these too have been encountered in individuals with autism and mental retardation (Burbach & van der Zwaag, 2009; Mefford et al., 2008). In addition, both the region 22q11.2 and 16p11.2 have been associated with both psychosis and ASDs (Weiss et al., 2008; McCarthy et al., 2009).

The chromosome 1q21.1 region has been associated with a particularly wide range of phenotypic manifestations. An initial study by the International Schizophrenia Consortium reported deletions in this region among 0.26% of patients with schizophrenia versus 0.002% in controls. Subsequent studies have identified both deletions and duplication in this region in a range of phenotypes including congenital heart defects (Christiansen et al., 2004), developmental delay (Shaffer, 2006), mild-to-moderate mental retardation, learning difficulties, and ASDs. For example, Brunetti-Pierri et al. (2008) performed array based comparative genomic hybridization on 16,577 patients with mental retardation, autism, and congenital anomalies. They identified 27 subjects with 1q21.1 deletions (0.16%) and 17 with duplications (0.1%). The deletions were compared to the rate observed in the aforementioned International Schizophrenia Consortium Study and were found to be increased. It is important to note, however, that CNV detection platforms differed between the two studies, and there was no control for population stratification.

However, a second study of this region by Mefford et al. (2008) came to similar conclusions: their sample consisted of 5218 patients referred for genetic testing, predominantly for evaluation of mental retardation (95%). Both de novo and inherited deletions and duplications were identified at similar rates to those described above. Moreover, deletions were not present among 4737 controls ($p = 1.1 \times 10^{-7}$). The reciprocal duplication was found among nine children with mental retardation or an ASD, which again was noted to be higher than the rate observed in unaffected individuals ($p = 0.02$).

Chromosome 15q11-13 duplications of the maternal chromosome are the most common microscopic abnormalities reported among individuals with ASDs. Recently, Stefansson et al. (2008) showed statistical evidence for 15q11.2 and 15q13.3 deletions associated with schizophrenia in their large sample of 1433 schizophrenia patients and 33,250 controls.

The chromosome 22q11.2 region is the best-known region for CNVs that predispose to psychosis. Deletions in this region show variable phenotypes, including velo-cardiofacial syndrome and DiGeorge syndrome, and there are hundreds of reports documenting new findings from polymicrogyria to juvenile rheumatoid arthritis related to variations in this region. The list of associated findings has grown to more than 180 (Robin & Shprintzen, 2005). Individuals with chromosome 22q11.2 deletion syndrome have consistently been noted to be at elevated risk to develop psychiatric difficulties, especially psychosis (Murphy, Jones, & Owen, 1999). In the study by Stefansson et al., 22q11.2 deletions were present in 8 of 3838 cases of schizophrenia, but absent in 39,299 controls ($p = 4.2 \times 10^{-5}$). Similarly, a number of case series have pointed to elevated rates of ASD among individuals carrying the 22q11 deletion (Fine et al., 2005; Vorstman et al., 2006).

Finally, a recent large-scale study of the 16p11.2 region demonstrated an association of duplications but not deletions in the region with schizophrenia (McCarthy et al., 2009), whereas a meta-analysis of several recently published studies, reported in the same manuscript, continued to support an association between both duplications and deletions in this interval and ASDs. As noted, the frequency of both duplications and deletions in controls has varied in recent investigations. However, as additional large-scale studies confirm these results, it will have a significant impact on our conceptualization of the current diagnostic nosology.

Although these studies are not an exhaustive listing of findings in which mutations in a region or gene has led to widely varying neuropsychiatric and developmental disorders, they clearly point to the possibility that a single genetic variation may result in multiple development outcomes. This, of course, has been observed for decades with regard to the overlap of mental retardation and autism. However, the range of phenotypic variability suggested in the current literature is far more extensive, including diagnostic categories, such as schizophrenia, that were previously thought to be entirely distinct from developmental delay. These findings may be accounted for by a variety of factors, ranging from epigenetic or environmental mechanisms, to ascertainment bias, to pleiotropic effects of CNVs. Collectively, these recent findings underscore the limitations in our understanding of the link between biology and diagnostic nosology and suggest that our notions of "clear" categorical boundaries will continue to be challenged. In addition to raising very interesting questions regarding the possible convergence of biological mechanisms involved in multiple disorders, these overlaps begin to raise important practical questions regarding how one assigns affected (or unaffected status) to individuals in genetic studies.

Summary and Conclusions

Overall, it is evident that findings from rare variant studies have played a leading role in elaborating the genetics of ASDs. From the early observations of increased rates of chromosomal abnormalities in children with these disorders to the identification of CNVs and the application of deep sequencing approaches, the study of outliers has provided the first extremely important and illuminating insights into the biology of these complex devastating syndromes.

Although the elegant and paradigm-challenging studies of rare genetic *syndromes* are discussed in other chapters, it is nonetheless interesting to note that "nonsyndromic" rare variant findings have begun to converge in some senses. As previously noted, early data suggests that some ASDs are likely the result of synaptic pathology (Zoghbi, 2003) and/or the consequence of variations in neuronal adhesion molecules including Cadherins, Contactins, Neuroligins, and Neurexins. However, it is also a near certainty that these findings are just the tip of iceberg, and a variety of processes important for establishing the basic architecture and maintaining the function of the human CNS will also be implicated in the etiology of ASDs (Page et al., 2009).

It is not at all surprising that the first biological insights into ASDs have emerged from studies of Mendelian syndromes. Given the relatively early discovery of genes underlying syndromes that overlap with ASDs, these have provided the best opportunity so far to move from gene identification to an understanding of protein function, to establishing protein–protein interactions and their roles in brain development and function, to the identification of novel therapeutic targets. Clearly, the current challenge for the field, which is already being undertaken in earnest, is to move this process of translational neuroscience from Mendelian syndromes showing features of ASDs squarely into the realm of the complex common and heterogeneous set of syndromes collectively referred to as ideopathic ASDs.

So far, the early evidence suggests that this will require a re-orientation, moving away from conceiving of rare mutations as synonymous with "Mendelian" inheritance and expecting unequivocal one-to-one relationships to embracing the notion of probabilitistic outcomes, multiple rare variant "hits" in a single individual or family and gene environment interactions—phenomena that are already well-accepted with regard to common variants.

Challenges and Future Directions

On an optimistic note, despite the methodological challenges that arise with regard to studying rare variants in complex disorders, all roads appear to lead in the same direction. The practical implications of the foregoing discussion are clear:

- Rare variant gene discovery will require large sample sizes, rigorous statistical threshold, the elaboration of appropriate genome-wide analytic methodologies, an appreciation of the central importance of ethnicity in genomic variation, and a continuing and realistic appraisal of effect sizes. Fortunately, all or nearly all of these issues have been solved with regard to genome-wide common variant studies, boding well for the future of investigations aimed at clarifying and elaborating the contribution of rare variants to autism and related conditions.
- The rapid pace of technological development in genomics provides a glimpse of where the field is headed in the future. Next-generation sequencing has already made practical the interrogation of a large percentage of the coding regions of the genome in groups of individuals.
- Sequencing of complete genomes applied to large samples of cases, family members, and controls is clearly just over the horizon. This transition will not only fuel gene discovery in ASDs but will undoubtedly presage a far better understanding of the formerly "dark," noncoding regions of the genome.
- It is likely that there will be substantial contribution of rare variation to ASDs via its influence on gene regulation and expression, topics that have so far been difficult to broach using previous generation technologies.
- The convergence of large patient collections, the increasing ability to detect rare variation both in the form of CNVs and at single base resolution, and the concomitant advances in the study of developmental neurobiology described elsewhere in this text suggest that the next few years will be a remarkable era of discovery.

REFERENCES

Abelson, J. F., Kwan, K. Y., O'Roak, B. J., Baek, D. Y., Stillman, A. A., Morgan, T. M., et al. (2005). Sequence variants in SLITRK1 are associated with Tourette's syndrome. *Science, 310*(5746), 317–320.

Abrahams, B. S., & Geschwind, D. H. (2008). Advances in autism genetics: On the threshold of a new neurobiology. *Nature Reviews Genetics, 9*(5), 341–355.

Alarcon, M., Abrahams, B. S., Stone, J. L., Duvall, J. A., Perederiy, J. V., Bomar, J. M., et al. (2008). Linkage, association, and gene-expression analyses identify CNTNAP2 as an autism-susceptibility gene. *American Journal of Human Genetics, 82*(1), 150–159.

Altshuler, D., & Daly, M. (2007). Guilt beyond a reasonable doubt. *Nature Genetics, 39*(7), 813–815.

Altshuler, D., Daly, M. J., & Lander, E. S. (2008). Genetic mapping in human disease. *Science, 322*(5903), 881–888.

Arking, D. E., Cutler, D. J., Brune, C. W., Teslovich, T. M., West, K., Ikeda, M., et al. (2008). A common genetic variant in the neurexin superfamily member CNTNAP2 increases familial risk of autism. *American Journal of Human Genetics, 82*(1), 160–164.

Bakkaloglu, B., Klin, A., Lifton, R. P., Morgan, T. M., Geshwind, D. H., Abrahams, B. S., et al. (2007). Molecular Cytogenetic Analysis and Resequencing of Contactin Associated Protein-Like 2 in Autism Spectrum Disorders. *American Journal of Human Genetics, 82*, 165–173.

Bertram, L., Blacker, D., Mullin, K., Keeney, D., Jones, J., Basu, S., et al. (2000). Evidence for genetic linkage of Alzheimer's disease to chromosome 10q. *Science, 290*(5500), 2302–2303.

Bhalla, K., Phillips, H. A., Crawford, J., McKenzie, O. L., Mulley, J. C., Eyre, H., et al. (2004). The de novo chromosome 16 translocations of two patients with abnormal phenotypes (mental retardation and epilepsy) disrupt the A2BP1 gene. *Journal of Human Genetics, 49*(6), 308–311.

Bijlsma, E. K., Gijsbers, A. C., Schuurs-Hoeijmakers, J. H., van Haeringen, A., Fransen van de Putte, D. E., Anderlid, B. M., et al. (2009). Extending the phenotype of recurrent rearrangements of 16p11.2: Deletions in mentally retarded patients without autism and in normal individuals. *European Journal of Medical Genetics, 52*(2–3), 77–87.

Bilguvar, K., Yasuno, K., Niemela, M., Ruigrok, Y. M., von Und Zu Fraunberg, M., van Duijn, C. M., et al. (2008). Susceptibility loci for intracranial aneurysm in European and Japanese populations. *Nature Genetics, 40*(12), 1472–1477.

Bodmer, W., & Bonilla, C. (2008). Common and rare variants in multifactorial susceptibility to common diseases. *Nature Genetics, 40*, 695–701.

Borg, I., Squire, M., Menzel, C., Stout, K., Morgan, D., Willatt, L., et al. (2002). A cryptic deletion of 2q35 including part of the PAX3 gene detected by breakpoint mapping in a child with autism and a de novo 2;8 translocation. *Journal of Medical Genetics, 39*(6), 391–399.

Brunetti-Pierri, N., Berg, J. S., Scaglia, F., Belmont, J., Bacino, C. A., Sahoo, T., et al. (2008). Recurrent reciprocal 1q21.1 deletions and duplications associated with microcephaly or macrocephaly and developmental and behavioral abnormalities. *Nature Genetics, 40*(12), 1466–1471.

Bucan, M., Abrahams M., Wang K., Glessner J., Herman E., Sonnenblick L. et al. (2009). Genome-Wide Analyses of Exonic Copy Number Variants in a Family-Based Study Point to Novel Autism Susceptibility Genes. *PLoS Genetics, 5*(6), e1000536.

Burbach, J. P., & van der Zwaag, B. (2009). Contact in the genetics of autism and schizophrenia. *Trends in Neurosciences, 32*(2), 69–72.

Christiansen, J., Dyck, J. D., Elyas, B. G., Lilley, M., Bamforth, J. S., Hicks, M., et al. (2004). Chromosome 1q21.1 contiguous gene deletion is associated with congenital heart disease. *Circulation Research, 94*(11), 1429–1435.

Cohen, J. C., Pertsemlidis, A., Fahmi, S., Esmail, S., Vega, G. L., Grundy, S. M., et al. (2006). Multiple rare variants in NPC1L1 associated with reduced sterol absorption and plasma low-density lipoprotein levels. *Proceedings of the National Academy of Sciences of the United States of America, 103*(6), 1810–1815.

Collins, A. L., Ma, D., Whitehead, P. L., Martin, E. R., Wright, H. H., Abramson, R. K., et al. (2006). Investigation of autism and GABA receptor subunit genes in multiple ethnic groups. *Neurogenetics, 7*(3), 167–174.

Eichler, E. E., & Zimmerman, A. W. (2008). A hot spot of genetic instability in autism. *New England Journal of Medicine, 358*(7), 737–739.

Feng, J., Schroer, R., Yan, J., Song, W., Yang, C., Bockholt, A., et al. (2006). High frequency of neurexin 1beta signal peptide structural variants in patients with autism. *Neuroscience Letters, 409*(1), 10–13.

Fernandez, T., Morgan, T., Davis, N., Klin, A., Morris, A., Farhi, A., et al. (2004). Disruption of contactin 4 (CNTN4) results in developmental delay and other features of 3p deletion syndrome. *American Journal of Human Genetics, 74*(6), 1286–1293.

Fernandez, T. V., Garcia-Gonzalez, I. J., Mason, C. E., Hernandez-Zaragoza, G., Ledezma-Rodriguez, V. C., Anguiano-Alvarez, V. M., et al. (2008). Molecular characterization of a patient with 3p deletion syndrome and a review of the literature. *American Journal of Medical Genetics. Part A, 146A*(21), 2746–2752.

Folstein, S. (1996). Twin and adoption studies in child and adolescent psychiatric disorders. *Current Opinion in Pediatrics, 8*(4), 339–347.

Ghebranious, N., Giampietro, P. F., Wesbrook, F. P., & Rezkalla, S. H. (2007). A novel microdeletion at 16p11.2 harbors candidate genes for aortic valve development, seizure disorder, and mild mental retardation. *American Journal of Medical Genetics. Part A, 143A*(13), 1462–1471.

Glessner, J. T., Wang, K., Cai, G., Korvatska, O., Kim, C. E., Wood, S., et al. (2009). Autism genome-wide copy number variation reveals ubiquitin and neuronal genes. *Nature, 459*(7246), 569–573.

Iafrate, A. J., Feuk, L., Rivera, M. N., Listewnik, M. L., Donahoe, P. K., Qi, Y., et al. (2004). Detection of large-scale variation in the human genome. *Nature Genetics, 36*(9), 949–951.

Ishikawa-Brush, Y., Powell, J. F., Bolton, P., Miller, A. P., Francis, F., Willard, H. F., et al. (1997). Autism and multiple exostoses associated with an X;8 translocation occurring within the GRPR gene and 3' to the SDC2 gene. *Human Molecular Genetics, 6*(8), 1241–1250.

Itsara, A., et al. (2010). De novo rates and selection of large copy number variation. *Genome Research, 20*(11), 1469–1481.

Jamain, S., Quach, H., Betancur, C., Rastam, M., Colineaux, C., Gillberg, I. C., et al. (2003). Mutations of the X-linked genes encoding neuroligins NLGN3 and NLGN4 are associated with autism. *Nature Genetics, 34*(1), 27–29.

Ji, W., Foo, J. N., O'Roak, B. J., Zhao, H., Larson, M. G., Simon, D. B., et al. (2008). Rare independent mutations in renal salt handling genes contribute to blood pressure variation. *Nature Genetics, 40*(5), 592–599.

Johnson, C. P., & Myers, S. M. (2007). Identification and evaluation of children with autism spectrum disorders. *Pediatrics, 120*(5), 1183–1215.

Kahler, A. K., Djurovic, S., Kulle, B., Jonsson, E. G., Agartz, I., Hall, H., et al. (2008). Association analysis of schizophrenia on 18 genes involved in neuronal migration: MDGA1 as a new susceptibility gene. *American Journal of Medical Genetics. Part B, Neuropsychiatric Genetics, 147B*(7), 1089–1100.

Kalscheuer, V. M., FitzPatrick, D., Tommerup, N., Bugge, M., Niebuhr, E., Neumann, L. M., et al. (2007). Mutations in autism susceptibility candidate 2 (AUTS2) in patients with mental retardation. *Human Genetics, 121*(3-4), 501–509.

Kidd, K. K., Pakstis, A. J., Speed, W. C., & Kidd, J. R. (2004). Understanding human DNA sequence variation. *Journal of Heredity, 95*(5), 406–420.

Kim, H., Kishikawa, S., Higgins, A., Seong, I., Donovan, D., Shen, Y., et al. (2008). Disruption of Neurexin 1 Associated with Autism Spectrum Disorder. *American Journal of Human Genetics, 82*, 199–207.

Kumar, R. A., KaraMohamed, S., Sudi, J., Conrad, D. F., Brune, C., Badner, J. A., et al. (2008). Recurrent 16p11.2 microdeletions in autism. *Human Molecular Genetics, 17*(4), 628–638.

Laumonnier, F., Bonnet-Brilhault, F., Gomot, M., Blanc, R., David, A., Moizard, M. P., et al. (2004). X-linked mental retardation and autism are associated with a mutation in the NLGN4 gene, a member of the neuroligin family. *American Journal of Human Genetics, 74*(3), 552–557.

Lipska, B. K., & Weinberger, D. R. (1995). Genetic variation in vulnerability to the behavioral effects of neonatal hippocampal damage in rats. *Proceedings of the National Academy of Sciences of the United States of America, 92*(19), 8906–8910.

Lisé, M., & El-Husseini, A. (2006). The neuroligin and neurexin families: From structure to function at the synapse. *Cellular and Molecular Life Sciences, 63*, 1833–1849.

Lucito, R., Healy, J., Alexander, J., Reiner, A., Esposito, D., Chi, M., et al. (2003). Representational oligonucleotide microarray analysis: A high-resolution method to detect genome copy number variation. *Genome Research, 13*(10), 2291–2305.

Manolio, T. A., Brooks, L. D., & Collins, F. S. (2008). A HapMap harvest of insights into the genetics of common disease. *Journal of Clinical Investigation, 118*(5), 1590–1605.

Marshall, C. R., Noor, A., Vincent, J. B., Lionel, A. C., Feuk, L., Skaug, J., et al. (2008). Structural variation of chromosomes in autism spectrum disorder. *American Journal of Human Genetics, 82*(2), 477–488.

Martin, C. L., Duvall, J. A., Ilkin, Y., Simon, J. S., Arreaza, M. G., Wilkes, K., et al. (2007). Cytogenetic and molecular characterization of A2BP1/FOX1 as a candidate gene for autism. *American Journal of Medical Genetics. Part B, Neuropsychiatric Genetics, 144B*(7), 869–876.

McClellan, J. M., Susser, E., & King, M. C. (2007). Schizophrenia: A common disease caused by multiple rare alleles. *British Journal of Psychiatry, 190*, 194–199.

McCarthy et al. (2009). *Nature Genetics, 41*(11), 1223–1227.

Mefford, H. C., Sharp, A. J., Baker, C., Itsara, A., Jiang, Z., Buysse, K., et al. (2008). Recurrent rearrangements of chromosome 1q21.1 and variable pediatric phenotypes. *New England Journal of Medicine, 359*(16), 1685–1699.

Meigs, J. B., Manning, A. K., Fox, C. S., Florez, J. C., Liu, C., Cupples, L. A., et al. (2007). Genome-wide association with diabetes-related traits in the Framingham Heart Study. *BMC Medical Genetics, 8*(Suppl 1), S16.

Meyer, G., Varoqueaux, F., Neeb, A., Oschlies, M., & Brose, N. (2004). The complexity of PDZ domain-mediated interactions at glutamatergic synapses: A case study on neuroligin. *Neuropharmacology, 47*(5), 724–733.

Miki, Y., Swensen, J., Shattuck-Eidens, D., Futreal, P. A., Harshman, K., Tavtigian, S., et al. (1994). A strong candidate for the breast and ovarian cancer susceptibility gene BRCA1. *Science, 266*(5182), 66–71.

Miller, D. T., Shen, Y., Weiss, L. A., Korn, J., Anselm, I., Bridgemohan, C., et al. (2009). Microdeletion/duplication at 15q13.2q13.3 among individuals with features of autism and other neuropsychiatric disorders. *Journal of Medical Genetics, 46*(4), 242–248.

Moessner, R., Marshall, C. R., Sutcliffe, J. S., Skaug, J., Pinto, D., Vincent, J., et al. (2007). Contribution of SHANK3 mutations to autism spectrum disorder. *American Journal of Human Genetics, 81*(6), 1289–1297.

Moffatt, M. F., Kabesch, M., Liang, L., Dixon, A. L., Strachan, D., Heath, S., et al. (2007). Genetic variants regulating ORMDL3 expression contribute to the risk of childhood asthma. *Nature, 448*(7152), 470–473.

Morrow, E. M., Yoo, S. Y., Flavell, S. W., Kim, T. K., Lin, Y., Hill, R. S., et al. (2008). Identifying autism loci and genes by tracing recent shared ancestry. *Science, 321*(5886), 218–223.

Murphy, K. C., Jones, L. A., & Owen, M. J. (1999). High rates of schizophrenia in adults with velo-cardio-facial syndrome. *Archives of General Psychiatry, 56*(10), 940–945.

Nielsen, J., & Sillesen, I. (1975). Incidence of chromosome aberrations among 11,148 newborn children. *Humangenetik, 30*(1), 1–12.

Nielsen, J., Wohlert, M., Faaborg-Andersen, J., Hansen, K. B., Hvidman, L., Krag-Olsen, B., et al. (1982). Incidence of chromosome abnormalities in newborn children: Comparison between incidences in 1969–1974 and 1980–1982 in the same area. *Human Genetics, 61*(2), 98–101.

Noor, A., et al. (2010). Disruption at the PTCHD1 Locus on Xp22.11 in autism spectrum disorder and intellectual disability. *Science Translational Medicine, 2*, 49–68.

O'Roak, B. J., & State, M. W. (2008). Autism genetics: Strategies, challenges, and opportunities. *Autism Research, 1*(1), 4–17.

Page, D. T., Kuti, O. J., Prestia, C., & Sur, M. (2009). Haploinsufficiency for Pten and Serotonin transporter cooperatively influences brain size and social behavior. *Proceedings of the National Academy of Sciences of the United States of America, 106*(6), 1989–1994.

Pinto, D., et al. (2010). Functional impact of global rare copy number variation in autism spectrum disorders. *Nature, 466*(7304), 368–372.

Redon, R., Ishikawa, S., Fitch, K. R., Feuk, L., Perry, G. H., Andrews, T. D., et al. (2006). Global variation in copy number in the human genome. *Nature, 444*(7118), 444–454.

Robin, N. H., & Shprintzen, R. J. (2005). Defining the clinical spectrum of deletion 22q11.2. *Journal of Pediatrics, 147*(1), 90–96.

Roohi, J., Montagna, C., Tegay, D. H., Palmer, L. E., DeVincent, C., Pomeroy, J. C., et al. (2009). Disruption of contactin 4 in three subjects with autism spectrum disorder. *Journal of Medical Genetics, 46*(3), 176–182.

Rujescu, D., Ingason, A., Cichon, S., Pietilainen, O. P., Barnes, M. R., Toulopoulou, T., et al. (2009). Disruption of the neurexin 1 gene is associated with schizophrenia. *Human Molecular Genetics, 18*(5), 988–996.

Savelyeva, L., Sagulenko, E., Schmitt, J. G., & Schwab, M. (2006). The neurobeachin gene spans the common fragile site FRA13A. *Human Genetics, 118*(5), 551–558.

Schaefer, G. B., & Mendelsohn, N. J. (2008). Clinical genetics evaluation in identifying the etiology of autism spectrum disorders. *Genetics in Medicine, 10*(4), 301–305.

Sebat, J., Lakshmi, B., Malhotra, D., Troge, J., Lese-Martin, C., Walsh, T., et al. (2007). Strong association of de novo copy number mutations with autism. *Science, 316*(5823), 445–449.

Sebat, J., Lakshmi, B., Troge, J., Alexander, J., Young, J., Lundin, P., et al. (2004). Large-scale copy number polymorphism in the human genome. *Science, 305*(5683), 525–528.

Seidita, G., Mirisola, M., D'Anna, R. P., Gallo, A., Jensen, R. T., Mantey, S. A., et al. (2008). Analysis of the gastrin-releasing peptide receptor gene in Italian patients with autism spectrum disorders. *American Journal of Medical Genetics. Part B, Neuropsychiatric Genetics, 147B*(6), 807–813.

Shaffer, L. G. (2006). Targeted genomic microarray analysis for identification of chromosomal abnormalities in 1500 consecutive clinical cases. *Journal of Pediatrics, 149*, 98–102.

Sharp, A. J., Selzer, R. R., Veltman, J. A., Gimelli, S., Gimelli, G., Striano, P., et al. (2007). Characterization of a recurrent 15q24 microdeletion syndrome. *Human Molecular Genetics, 16*(5), 567–572.

Shumyatsky, G. P., Tsvetkov, E., Malleret, G., Vronskaya, S., Hatton, M., Hampton, L., et al. (2002). Identification of a signaling network in lateral nucleus of amygdala important for inhibiting memory specifically related to learned fear. *Cell, 111*(6), 905–918.

Simon, D. B., Karet, F. E., Hamdan, J. M., DiPietro, A., Sanjad, S. A., & Lifton, R. P. (1996). Bartter's syndrome, hypokalaemic alkalosis with hypercalciuria, is caused by mutations in the Na-K-2Cl cotransporter NKCC2. *Nature Genetics, 13*(2), 183–188.

Speicher, M. R., Gwyn Ballard, S., & Ward, D. C. (1996). Karyotyping human chromosomes by combinatorial multi-fluor FISH. *Nature Genetics, 12*(4), 368–375.

State, M. W. (2010). The genetics of child psychiatric disorders: Focus on autism and tourette syndrome, *Neuron, 68*, 254–269.

Stefansson, H., Rujescu, D., Cichon, S., Pietilainen, O. P., Ingason, A., Steinberg, S., et al. (2008). Large recurrent microdeletions associated with schizophrenia. *Nature, 455*(7210), 232–236.

Strauss, K. A., Puffenberger, E. G., Huentelman, M. J., Gottlieb, S., Dobrin, S. E., Parod, J. M., et al. (2006). Recessive symptomatic focal epilepsy and mutant contactin-associated protein-like 2. *New England Journal of Medicine, 354*(13), 1370–1377.

Sultana, R., Yu, C. E., Yu, J., Munson, J., Chen, D., Hua, W., et al. (2002). Identification of a novel gene on chromosome 7q11.2 interrupted by a translocation breakpoint in a pair of autistic twins. *Genomics, 80*(2), 129–134.

Szatmari, P., & Consortium, T. A. G. P. (2007). Mapping autism risk loci using genetic linkage and chromosomal rearrangements. *Nature Genetics, 39*, 319–328.

Thomas, N. S., Sharp, A. J., Browne, C. E., Skuse, D., Hardie, C., & Dennis, N. R. (1999). Xp deletions associated with autism in three females. *Human Genetics, 104*(1), 43–48.

Toro et al., (2010). *Trends Genetics, 26*(8), 363–372.

Vernes, S. C., Newbury, D. F., Abrahams, B. S., Winchester, L., Nicod, J., Groszer, M., et al. (2008). A functional genetic link between distinct developmental language disorders. *New England Journal of Medicine, 359*(22), 2337–2345.

Vincent, J. B., Herbrick, J. A., Gurling, H. M., Bolton, P. F., Roberts, W., & Scherer, S. W. (2000). Identification of a novel gene on chromosome 7q31 that is interrupted by a translocation breakpoint in an autistic individual. *American Journal of Human Genetics, 67*(2), 510–514.

Vorstman, J. A., Staal, W. G., van Daalen, E., van Engeland, H., Hochstenbach, P. F., & Franke, L. (2006). Identification of novel autism candidate regions through analysis of reported cytogenetic abnormalities associated with autism. *Molecular Psychiatry, 11*(1), 1, 18–28.

Vrijenhoek, T., Buizer-Voskamp, J. E., van der Stelt, I., Strengman, E., Sabatti, C., Geurts van Kessel, A., et al. (2008). Recurrent CNVs disrupt three candidate genes in schizophrenia patients. *American Journal of Human Genetics, 83*(4), 504–510.

Wang, J., Wang, W., Li, R., Li, Y., Tian, G., Goodman, L., et al. (2008). The diploid genome sequence of an Asian individual. *Nature, 456*(7218), 60–65.

Weersma, R. K., Stokkers, P. C., Cleynen, I., Wolfkamp, S. C., Henckaerts, L., Schreiber, S., et al. (2009). Confirmation of multiple Crohn's disease susceptibility loci in a large Dutch-Belgian cohort. *American Journal of Gastroenterology, 104*(3), 630–638.

Weiss, L. A., Shen, Y., Korn, J. M., Arking, D. E., Miller, D. T., Fossdal, R., et al. (2008). Association between microdeletion and microduplication at 16p11.2 and autism. *New England Journal of Medicine, 358*(7), 667–675.

Zeggini, E., Scott, L. J., Saxena, R., Voight, B. F., Marchini, J. L., Hu, T., et al. (2008). Meta-analysis of genome-wide association data and large-scale replication identifies additional susceptibility loci for type 2 diabetes. *Nature Genetics, 40*(5), 638–645.

Zoghbi, H. Y. (2003). Postnatal neurodevelopmental disorders: Meeting at the synapse? *Science, 302*(5646), 826–830.

42

Richard Person, Xinna Zhang, Soeun Kim, Marwan Shinawi, Arthur L. Beaudet

Known and Possible Roles of Epigenetics in Autism

Points of Interest

- Research into the role of epigenetics in the etiology of autism has been neglected compared to the extensive genetic studies.
- For the most part, neither *de novo* mutations nor epigenetic abnormalities are detectable by linkage and association studies.
- Epigenetic mechanisms could contribute modestly to any missing causality or missing heritability of autism.
- Epigenetic analysis using chromatin-immunoprecipitation (ChIP) and analysis of DNA methylation can be used to assess the importance of epigenetics in the etiology of forms of autism that remain idiopathic—especially in milder forms of autism.
- Analysis of postmortem brain may be required to detect some epigenetic abnormalities, whereas others may be detectable in leukocytes.

The objective of this chapter is to review the known and hypothetical roles of epigenetics in the etiology of autism. Epigenetics in this medical context is commonly defined as the regulatory changes in gene function that are stable and heritable (or potentially heritable as in terminally differentiated neurons) and do not entail a change in DNA sequence. Bird (2007) provides an up-to-date discussion of how the term *epigenetics* has been used very differently within biology, and he proposes what he believes "could be a unifying definition of epigenetic events: the structural adaptation of chromosomal regions so as to register, signal or perpetuate altered activity states." This definition is intended to apply whether the effect is of long or short duration and whether inherited or not. The first definition emphasizes stability and heritability, and the heritability might be either somatic or germ-line. Although epigenetics usually involves transcriptional regulation, the first definition would include protein-based heritability (Feinberg, 2007; Wickner et al., 2008), RNA-mediated inheritance (Rassoulzadegan et al., 2006), and stochastic, potentially heritable effects on gene expression. Stochastic contributions to etiology refers to the role of noise, or variation, in the process of gene expression in contributing to phenotypic variability, with transcriptional infidelity being one source of such noise (Raser & O'Shea, 2005; Gordon et al., 2009). The second definition is narrower in terms of mechanism but more open regarding the possibility of epigenetic changes occurring in nondividing, long-lived cells such as neurons. Both definitions involve a stable change in gene expression in the absence of a change in nucleotide sequence.

Epigenetic change: alterations in chromosome structure that cause a stable change in gene expression in the absence of a change in nucleotide sequence.

Epimutation: a stable change in the epigenotype or in gene expression that does not involve a change in DNA sequence.

As an example of epigenetic changes of short duration, the role of epigenetics in regulation across the various stages of the cell cycle has been reviewed (Probst, Dunleavy, & Almouzni, 2009). The terms *epigenotype* and *epigenome* are now often used to describe the epigenetic state (chromatin in all its complexities) of part or all of the genome. Although each of us has essentially one genome identical in all of our cells apart from somatic mutations, there are hundreds of eipgenomes/epigenotypes in the various cell types in our tissues (Fig. 42-1A). Numerous reviews regarding epigenetics generally (Jaenisch & Bird, 2003; Bird, 2007; Suzuki & Bird, 2008) and as it relates to disease states are available (Jiang, Bressler, & Beaudet, 2004; Jirtle & Skinner, 2007; Kaminsky, Wang, & Petronis, 2006; van, Oates, & Whitelaw, 2007; Feinberg, 2007; Hatchwell & Greally, 2007). An excellent book entitled *Epigenetics* (Allis, Jenuwein, & Reinberg, 2007)—authored by experts in the field—is available, with many chapters on different aspects of

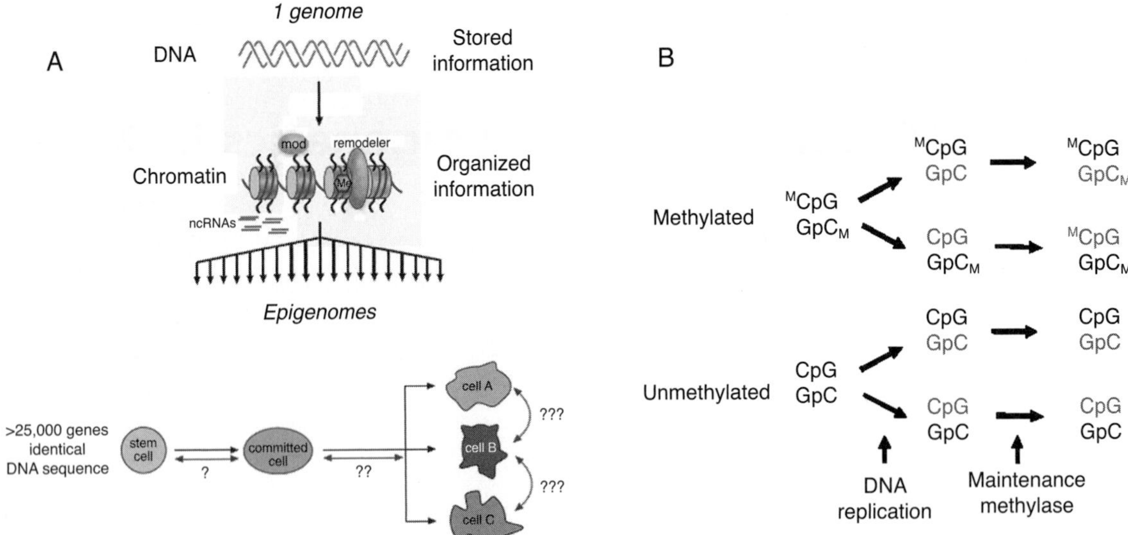

Figure 42–1. (A) (left). DNA versus Chromatin. The genome: Invariant DNA sequence (double helix) of an individual. The epigenome: The overall chromatin composition, which indexes the entire genome in any given cell. It varies according to cell type, and response to internal and external signals it receives. (Lower panel) Epigenome diversification occurs during development in multicellular organisms as differentiation proceeds from a single stem cell (the fertilized embryo) to more committed cells. Reversal of differentiation or transdifferentiation (bottom lines) requires the reprogramming of the cell's epigenome. Modified with permission from Chapter 3 in Allis, C. D., Jenuwein, T., & Reinberg, D. (2007). *Epigenetics.* Cold Spring Harbor, NY: Cold Spring Harbor Laboratory Press. (B) (Right). DNA methylation. The maintenance methylase system preserves methylation status of CpG dinucleotides through mitosis. The parental strand of DNA is in black with the daughter strand highlighted in gray. M = methyl group on C nucleotide. Reproduced with permission from Jiang, Y., Bressler, J., & Beaudet, A. L. (2004). Epigenetics and Human Disease. *Annual Review of Genomics and Human Genetics, 5,* 479–510.

epigenetics, including a thorough review of the biochemistry and molecular biology of epigenetics (Chapter 3) and a discussion of the role of epigenetics in human disease (Chapter 23).

Genomic imprinting: a form of epigenetic regulation by which the activity of a gene is reversibly modified, depending on the sex of the parent that transmits it.

Genomic imprinting leads to unequal expression from the maternal and paternal alleles for a diploid locus. Genomic imprinting is well-described in plants and mammals, but it appears to be less frequent, if not absent, in egg-laying vertebrates. Perhaps the most striking evidence for a role of epigenetics in autism involves genomic imprinting as described below for interstitial duplications of chromosome 15q11-q13. In its simplest form, genomic imprinting involves one parental allele with high gene expression, whereas the other parental allele has low or absent expression. Imprinted genes typically occur in clusters with oppositely imprinted genes within the imprinted domain. Imprinted domains characteristically include an imprinting center with differential DNA methylation and differential histone modifications; regulation of imprinting usually spreads over hundreds of kilobases (kb) from the imprinting center. The terminology stating that a gene is maternally imprinted or paternally imprinted is sometimes used to imply maternal or paternal repression, respectively, but it seems preferable to refer to a gene as imprinted with maternal repression or paternal repression for greater clarity. Thus, one would state that a gene is imprinted with maternal repression rather than that a gene is maternally imprinted. Numerous reviews of genomic imprinting in its role in human disease are available (Reik & Walter, 2001; Morgan et al., 2005; Hore, Rapkins, & Graves, 2007; Ubeda & Wilkins, 2008; Bartolomei, 2009; Butler, 2009).

Biochemistry and Molecular Biology of Epigenetic Regulation

The best characterized and most straightforward aspect of molecular epigenetics is the role of DNA methylation. DNA methylation is often associated with transcriptional silencing as on the inactive X chromosome and in regions of repetitive sequence. DNA within CpG islands located at promoters of genes is typically unmethylated whether or not the gene is expressed in a given cell type. Increasing attention is being given to differential DNA methylation within and near genes but outside of CpG islands (Meissner et al., 2008; De et al., 2009). There is also a suggestion that differential DNA methylation at "shores" of CpG islands may be important (Doi et al., 2009). A novel conversion of 5-methylcytosine to 5-hydroxymethylcytosine was described recently (Tahiliani et al., 2009), but its biological significance is unknown at present.

Box 42–1

The great majority of DNA methylation in mammalian genomes involves methylation of cytosine residues in CpG dinucleotides, although there is some methylation of non-CpG sequences, especially in embryonic stem (ES) cells (Lister, et al., 2009). A large proportion of CpG dinucleotides occur in repetitive DNA sequences where they are usually methylated, and the regions are transcriptionally silent. Another substantial proportion of CpGs occur in so-called "CpG islands," which are DNA segments with increased CpG sequence content. The CpG islands are often associated with promoters of genes and are usually in the unmethylated state, although exceptions occur as seen below for regions of genomic imprinting. A clear mechanism is available to preserve the methylated or unmethylated status of a CpG dinucleotide across DNA replication and mitosis (Fig. 42-1B). DNA replication leads to the production of two, hemi-methylated copies of the daughter DNA strands, and there exists a maintenance methylation mechanism, which will methylate the diagonally opposite C in a hemi-methylated substrate. Thus a methylated CpG can give rise to two methylated daughter strands of DNA. When an unmethylated CpG dinucleotide is replicated, the two daughter strands are both unmethylated and not recognized by the maintenance methylase system, thus leading to two daughter strands both unmethylated.

A second well-defined aspect of epigenetic biochemistry involves the covalent modification of histone proteins. The DNA is, to a large extent, wrapped around nucleosomes comprised of a histone core (Fig. 42-2A). Various histones—particularly H3 and H4—are subject to many such covalent modifications, including lysine acetylation, lysine methylation, arginine methylation, and serine phosphorylation (Figure 42-2B), which are collectively referred to as the *histone code* (Jenuwein & Allis, 2001).

Histone code: covalent modifications of histones, including acetylation, methylation or phosphorylation that modify histone binding to DNA and alter chromatin structure and function.

Covalent modification of lysine is particularly complex with mono-methyl, di-methyl, and tri-methyl forms. This complex modification of lysine-4 in histone H3 is often denoted as H3K4me1, H3K4me2, H3K4me3. These histone modifications, also referred to as histone marks, are typically associated with chromatin regions having a particular function. For example, H3K4me3 and lysine acetylation are commonly associated with active promoters, whereas H3K9me3 and H3K27me3 are commonly associated with repressed promoters. Histone modifications are particularly relevant to studies of disease, because techniques are available to interrogate histone marks across the entire genome to compare disease samples to normal controls. This typically depends on the availability of antibodies that uniquely recognize a particular chromatin mark, such as H3K4me3. The histones are very tightly associated with DNA in the form of nucleosomes, and it is feasible to carry out ChIP and analyze the DNA that is precipitated by the antibody. The relationships between histone marks and chromatin functionality are quite complex and are reviewed in Chapter 10 of *Epigenetics* (Allis et al., 2007) and elsewhere (Ruthenburg et al., 2007).

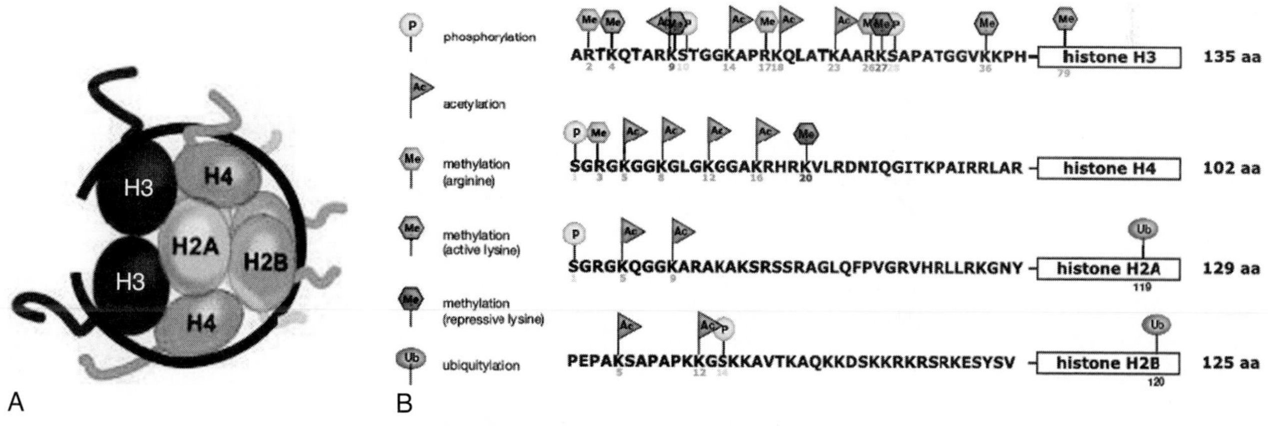

Figure 42–2. A (left). Nucleosome structure. A schematic representation of histone organization within the octamer core around which the DNA (black line) is wrapped. Nucleosome formation occurs first through the deposition of an H3/H4 tetramer on the DNA, followed by two sets of H2A/H2B dimers. Unstructured animo-terminal histone tails extrude from the DNA-nucleosome core, and the core consists of structured globular domains of the eight histone proteins. Modified with permission from Chapter 3 in Allis, C. D., Jenuwein, T., & Reinberg, D. (2007). *Epigenetics*. Cold Spring Harbor, NY: Cold Spring Harbor Laboratory Press. B (Right). Sites of Histone Tail Modifications. The amino-terminal tails of histones host the vast majority of known covalent modification sites as illustrated. Modifications do occur in the globular domain (boxed), some of which are indicated. In general, active marks include acetylation (turquoise Ac flag), arginine methylation (yellow Me flag), and some lysine methylation such as H3K4 and H3K36 (green Me flag). H3K79 in globular domain has anti-silencing function. Repressive marks include H3K9, H3K27, and H4K20 (red Me flags). Green = active mark, red = repressive mark. Reproduced with permission from Chapter 3 in Allis, C. D., Jenuwein, T., & Reinberg, D. (2007). *Epigenetics*. Cold Spring Harbor, NY: Cold Spring Harbor Laboratory Press. (See Color Plate Section for a color version of this figure.)

There are also many non-histone proteins that become stably or transiently associated with chromatin. These include various transcription factors, repressors, and large complexes of proteins that mediate replication and transcription. There are also large complexes of proteins referred to as histone remodeling complexes that play a major role in placing and removing various histone marks, as discussed in Chapters 11 and 12 of *Epigenetics* (Allis et al., 2007) (Fig. 42-3). As an example, these include various histone methylases, histone demethylases, and histone deacetylases (HDACs) (Aalfs & Kingston, 2000). The biochemistry of these histone remodeling complexes is the subject of rapidly progressing research.

Biology and Heritability of Epigenetics

The heterogeneity of the epigenotype in different cell types within a single individual is enormous compared to the lack of heterogeneity of the genomic sequence in a single individual. Except for somatic mutation, every cell in the body has the same genomic sequence. In contrast, the epigenotypes of cells across tissues and across development differ dramatically. There is evidence that the epigenotype changes with age (Gravina & Vijg, 2009). Indeed, it is the epigenetic information that causes a hepatocyte to be stably different than a neuron. Reviews of the role of epigenetics in development are available (Reik, 2007). Epigenetic errors in brain development could theoretically contribute to the etiology of autism. Given the tens of millions of sites for potential differences in DNA methylation and histone modification and the diploid nature of the genome, one could reasonably argue that no two cells in the body have precisely the same detailed epigenotype at any given moment in time, although functionally equivalent genotypes are probably relatively common within a single cell type. There certainly are millions of epigenetic differences between a hepatocyte and a neuron. Although the term *epigenome* has been used loosely to describe epigenetic variation, it seems likely that there are as many functional epigenotypes or epigenomes as there are cell types in the body.

The heritability of genetic and epigenetic information also differs dramatically. The vast majority of mutations are

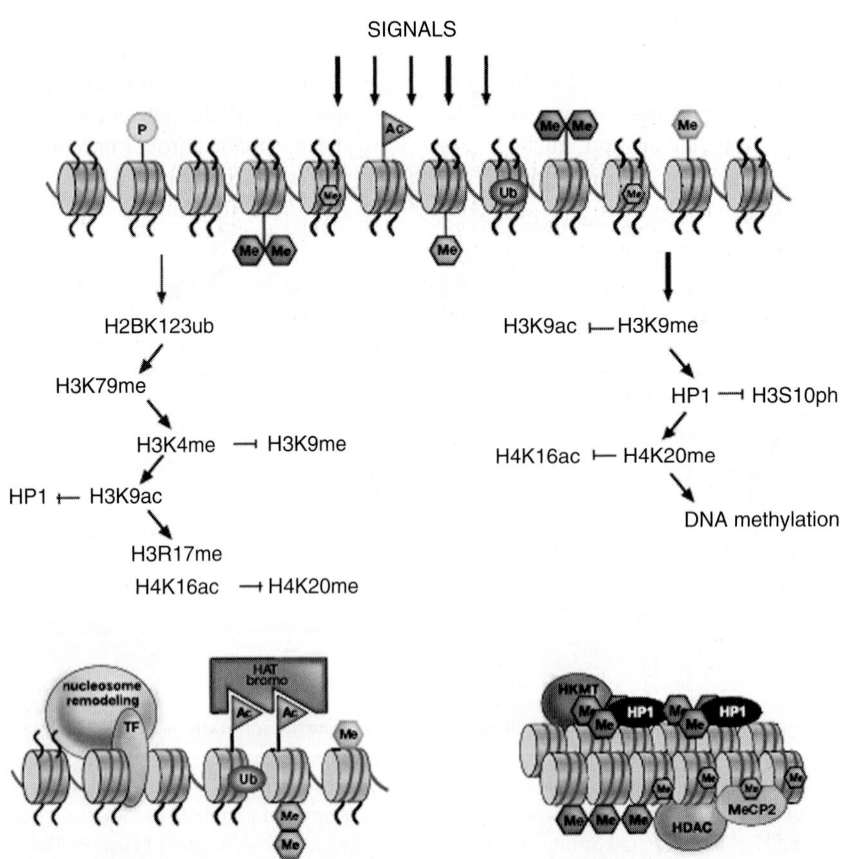

Figure 42–3. Coordinated Modification of Chromatin. The transition of a naive chromatin template to active euchromatin (left) or the establishment of repressive heterochromatin (right), involving a series of coordinated chromatin modifications. In the case of transcriptional activation, this is accompanied by the action of nucleosome remodeling complexes and the replacement of core histones with histone variants (yellow—namely, H3.3). Reproduced with permission from Chapter 3 in Allis, C. D., Jenuwein, T., & Reinberg, D. (2007). *Epigenetics*. Cold Spring Harbor, NY: Cold Spring Harbor Laboratory Press. (See Color Plate Section for a color version of this figure.)

inherited, but germline de novo point mutations have been appreciated for decades, although de novo copy number variations (CNVs) have only been appreciated more recently. Despite these de novo germline mutations, the genomic sequence is highly heritable in transmission from parent to offspring. In contrast, epigenetic information has the potential to be entirely heritable or entirely nonheritable. There is compelling evidence that certain epigenetic marks can be transmitted from a parent to offspring both in plants (Chandler & Stam, 2004) and in mammals (Morgan et al., 1999; Rassoulzadegan et al., 2006). In contrast, other epigenetic marks can be completely erased and reset in the course of transmission from parent to offspring, as occurs at every generation for sites of genomic imprinting. In fact, within genomic imprinting, both extremes are simultaneously present. In the mother, the state of all maternally derived alleles will be entirely heritable and all paternally derived alleles will be erased and reset. The reciprocal is true for paternal inheritance. Thus, one might say that epigenetic information or the epigenotype is semi-heritable or variably heritable. Although genomic imprinting displays the ability for the epigenotype at a locus to be relatively completely heritable on one parental allele while at the same time being nonheritable on the other allele, presumably intermediate states of heritability can occur as well, such as partial erasure and resetting of the epigenotype in the course of germline transmission. This relatively unpredictable behavior of the epigenotype as regards heritability creates significant challenges for the interpretation of complex data from human control and disease populations.

Does epigenetics contribute to any missing heritability in autism? The puzzle of missing heritability (McCarthy & Hirschhorn, 2008; Maher, 2008; Manolio et al., 2009) is exemplified by the evidence that the heritability of height is very high, yet the putative loci identified by genome-wide association studies (GWAS) account for only a tiny fraction of this heritability. In the case of autism, one puzzle is that concordance is very high in monozygous twins (MZ) but low in dizygous (DZ) twins. This seeming contradiction is likely explained primarily by the role of de novo mutations, which will cause concordance in MZ but not DZ twins, although de novo epimutations could contribute as well. Recent mutations occurring in the last few generations in a family with reduced penetrance can also contribute to heritability in siblings that will not be detected efficiently by GWAS (Shinawi et al., 2009). There are multiple possible sources for "missing heritability" (Maher, 2008), but epigenetics is certainly among them. Purely epigenetic effects will generally not be detected by GWAS, although they might be detected if they were heritable over many generations, but this is unlikely given the semi-heritable nature of epigenotypes. Epigenetic contributions might be abrupt and precise, as in a de novo epimutation that silences a single gene. Alternatively, they might be incremental and affect the genome more broadly if, for example, cumulative nutritional changes over decades and centuries altered DNA or histone methylation.

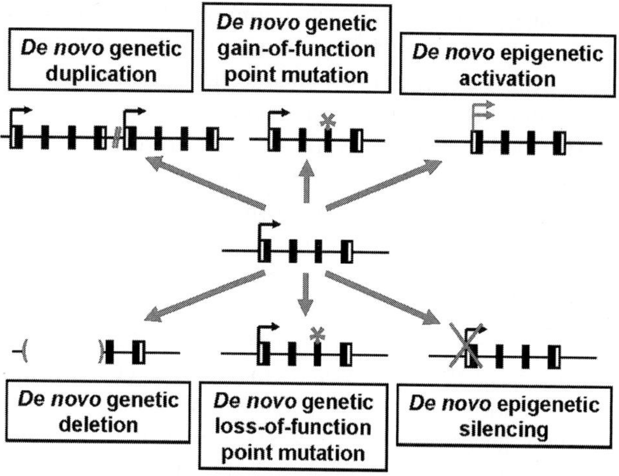

Figure 42-4. Large mutations, small mutations, and epimutations. Large mutations (copy number variants; CNVs) typically delete or duplicate a complete copy of a gene resulting in under- or overexpression, although position effects on regulatory elements can have unpredictable outcomes. Point mutations can inactivate a gene (nonsense or frameshift), increase or decrease or otherwise alter (e.g., dominant negative) the function of a transcribed RNA or the resulting protein. Epimutations can up- or down-regulate expression, most often at a transcriptional level.

Epimutations and Transgenerational Inheritance

Any known genetic mutation has the potential to provide a precedent for a similarly acting epimutation (Fig. 42-4). We know large deletions and duplications can cause decreases or increases, respectively, in the abundance of a protein, and we know of point mutations that can cause loss of function or gain of function. Analogous epimutations are possible. Figure 42-4 depicts a circumstance for dominant mutations and epimutations. One can imagine recessive epimutations analogous to recessive mutations and perhaps speculatively even an individual with a recessive mutation on one chromosome and a recessive epimutation on the other chromosome. This might be considered as a compound heterozygous mixed genetic and epigenetic genotype/epigenotype.

The potential for inheritance of epigenetic states has been referred to as *transgenerational inheritance* (Pembrey, 1996). Sex-specific, male-line transgenerational effects in humans and transgenerational effects related to nutrition, early life circumstances, and longevity have been discussed (Pembrey et al., 2006; Kaati et al., 2007). Nadeau (2009) has reviewed how "many studies showed that a remarkable variety of factors including environmental agents, parental behaviors, maternal physiology, xenobiotics, nutritional supplements and others lead to epigenetic changes that can be transmitted to subsequent generations without continued exposure." A proposed distinction between heritable germ-line epimutation and transgenerational epigenetic inheritance has been suggested (Chong, Youngson, & Whitelaw, 2007), whereby the first is envisioned as an "atypical" (perhaps disease-causing) epigenetic state and the second represents more of a continuum of common epigenetic states.

The Barker hypothesis focuses on how the *in utero* environment—specifically reduced fetal growth—is associated with a number of chronic conditions later in life. The Barker hypothesis does not necessarily invoke transgenerational heritability of epigenetic effects, but it is commonly believed to imply an epigenetic mechanism (Waterland & Michels, 2007). Numerous reports have emphasized the potential for harmful, epigenetically mediated effects such as adverse environmental effects (Franklin & Mansuy, 2009), a metabolic ghetto effect (Wells, 2009), and the potential epigenetic impact of abuse and neglect (Neigh, Gillespie, & Nemeroff, 2009). Meaney and colleagues have published multiple studies suggesting that maternal licking behaviors in rats alters hippocampal glucocorticoid receptor gene expression in the pups by altering the acetylation of H3K9 and the DNA methylation at the promoter (Fish et al., 2004). These data argue that maternal postnatal behavior can alter the epigenotype of offspring. More recently, these investigators have presented data suggesting epigenetic differences in postmortem brain from suicide victims with a history of childhood abuse compared to brain from either suicide victims with no childhood abuse or controls (McGowan et al., 2009).

Box 42–2

Here, chromatin is isolated from cells or tissue usually with formaldehyde cross-linking and is fragmented to yield material with a DNA length of 150–500 bp; ~150 bp of DNA wraps around one nucleosome. ChIP can be performed with formaldehyde cross-linking (X-ChIP) or without cross-linking (native ChIP, N-ChIP) for tightly associated proteins such as histones. For more loosely associated non-histone chromatin proteins, X-ChIP is ordinarily required. An antibody is used to precipitate the chromatin fragments with a particular epitope. Initially, ChIP was performed using PCR amplification of target regions to identify DNA segments which were immunoprecipitated by a particular antibody. Subsequently, analysis of precipitates was performed on microarrays for quantification of large numbers of sites in the genome (ChIP-chip). More recently, DNA precipitates are commonly analyzed by high throughput parallel DNA sequencing (ChIP-seq). In 2008, the U.S. National Institutes of Health funded a series of Reference Epigenome Mapping Centers; *see* NIH Roadmap for Medical Research, Roadmap Initiatives, Epigenomics (http://nihroadmap.nih.gov/epigenomics/). The pros and cons of the Roadmap initiative are debated (Madhani et al., 2008; Henikoff, Strahl, & Warburton, 2008).The mapping centers have all adopted ChIP-seq as the standard methodology for analysis of histone modifications. Although new covalent modifications are still being defined, and better antibodies are sorely needed, it can be anticipated that ChIP-seq will be applied widely in the studies of control compared to disease samples. In September 2009, the NIH Roadmap Initiative funded as series of grants focused on the epigenomics of human health and disease.

Methods for Epigenetic Analysis

One approach to the study of epigenetic differences in disease compared to control tissues is to analyze gene expression at the transcript or protein level, which reflects the combined genetic and epigenetic effects, and then try to deduce whether any differences are of genetic or epigenetic origin. Alternatively, one can attempt to study the epigenotype directly. The methods for analysis of covalent histone modifications are well-developed and quite satisfactory, although they are by no means mature (*see* Box 42-2).

The methodology for genome-wide analysis of DNA methylation is much more problematic than that for analysis of histone modifications. There are numerous restriction enzymes that will digest DNA differentially depending on its state of methylation. Many procedures have been developed using these methylation-dependent restriction enzymes to deduce the DNA methylation status at specific CpG dinucleotides. A variety of methods utilize these restriction enzymes to enrich for methylated or unmethylated DNA, and these selected DNAs are then quantified often using array technology. Methods based on the use of restriction enzymes detect polymorphisms in recognition sites, which may appear as false-positive evidence of methylation differences. Another powerful technique is the use of bisulfite sequencing to distinguish methyl C residues from C residues in DNA. Although the molecular details are relatively complex as explained elsewhere (Xi & Li, 2009), this method uses a chemical modification of DNA such that in subsequent sequencing methyl-C will be retained as C and unmethylated-C residues will be converted to T in the sequence. One foreseeable optimal bisulfite strategy will be to perform genome-wide bisulfite shotgun sequencing (BS-seq) (Lister et al., 2009), but this is currently cost-prohibitive for large-scale, high-throughput studies. Meanwhile, alternative strategies, such as reduced representation BS-seq (RRBS) (Smith et al., 2009), comprehensive high-throughput arrays for relative methylation (Irizarry et al., 2008), and other restriction enzymes methodologies are being used to compare control and disease samples. The methodology to be employed to analyze DNA methylation in disease research projects is likely to continue to evolve rapidly. If the cost of genome-wide BS-Seq were to drop by two orders of magnitude, as some experts predict, it might become feasible to use this strategy for disease studies. Another very useful method is array-based analysis of the percent methylation at individual CpG positions (Bibikova et al., 2006), and a recent improvement with the ability to analyze 450,000 CpG sites in a single array analysis (HumanMethylation450 DNA Analysis BeadChip; Illumina Inc. San Diego, CA) makes this a very attractive option for disease projects at present.

The computational methods necessary for genome-wide epigenetic analysis are extremely challenging and in a relatively early stage of development. The ability to compare the genome-wide epigenotype between cell types and between individuals is being refined. In addition, various analyses of DNA methylation and ChIP are being performed on mixed cell populations, such as mixed leukocytes isolated from blood or mixtures of neuronal and non-neuronal cells in brain tissue, and there is no method, at present, to assign the data to individual cell types within the populations other than prior fractionation of cell populations.

Although ChIP for the analysis of histone modifications is widely performed, ChIP analysis for proteins more loosely associated with chromatin is less well-standardized, but there are numerous demonstrations of the feasibility for such analysis—for example, using antibodies to methyl-CpG binding proteins. ChIP can be used to distinguish transcription initiation from transcription elongation using antibodies against RNA polymerase II (Gilchrist, Fargo, & Adelman, 2009). ChIP-seq using antibodies against CCCTC-binding factor has been used to characterize chromatin barriers and their tissue specificity (Cuddapah et al., 2009). ChIP-seq using an antibody against enhancer-associated protein p300 is useful in localizing enhancers and defining their tissue specificity (Visel et al., 2009; Heintzman et al., 2009). This analysis has the potential to discover both genetic and epigenetic abnormalities affecting enhancers. ChIP was used to study the polycomb group (PcG) and trithorax group (trxG) proteins in Drosophila (Schuettengruber et al., 2009), and similar studies will be important in mice and humans.

Difficulties Encountered in Epigenetic Studies of Human Disease

The major obstacle in epigenetic studies of human disease lies in the fact that all cell types can differ from each other and that only a limited number of cell types are easily accessible from living patients and controls. In the context of autism, one could hypothesize that there might be epigenetic changes in specific neural cell types, such as Purkinje cells, various classes of hippocampal neurons, and so forth. The epigenetic differences of disease importance may be present in all cells of the body or they may be unique to individual cell types. Examples of epigenetic differences detectable in all cell types and epigenetic differences restricted to selected populations are both available from disorders of genomic imprinting, such as Prader-Willi syndrome (PWS), Angelman syndrome, Beckwith-Wiedemann syndrome (BWS), and others. For example, the differential DNA methylation at the imprinting center for the PWS/Angelman syndrome domain is detectable in all cell types that have been studied, and it is stable in cultured cells. In contrast, the imprinted expression of the Angelman syndrome gene (*UBE3A*) is prominent in many neurons, but expression is not imprinted or at least not as dramatically differential in glia and somatic cell types (Yamasaki et al., 2003). In genetic studies, one can safely assume that the genomic sequence is similar in leukocytes to that in other parts of the body, and even DNA from cultured lymphoblasts is quite useful for large studies because of the unlimited amounts of DNA available, although cell culture artifacts—particularly involving aneuploidy—are found in lymphoblast cultures (Redon et al., 2006). Thus, utilization of blood leukocytes, cultured skin fibroblasts, and cultured lymphoblasts all have a very substantial risk that epigenetic abnormalities present in brain may not be reflected in these cell types.

One additional option has emerged with the emphasis on stem cell research. It is now possible to develop induced pluripotent stem cells (iPSCs) from cultured skin fibroblasts (Byrne, Nguyen, & Reijo Pera, 2009), and this offers the possibility that such cells can be induced to differentiate toward a neural pathway. These differentiated iPSCs might provide an opportunity to study neural-specific properties of cells from living patients. For example, there is a report of attempts to model the pathogenesis and treatment of familial dysautonomia using patient-specific iPSCs (Lee et al., 2009). This strategy has some potential to greatly facilitate studies of epigenetics in autism.

If one resorts to epigenetic analysis of postmortem brain tissue, there are still numerous obstacles, including the limited number of samples available and the potential for agonal and postmortem artifacts. Although disease-specific brain banks exist, there are important limitations and cautions in their utilization particularly as regards heterogeneous preservation of specific RNAs and proteins (Ferrer et al., 2008). Agonal effects on gene expression profiles occur (Tomita et al., 2004), although the levels of miRNAs may be less susceptible to artifact (Zhang et al., 2008). The pH of the postmortem tissue is a helpful index of agonal effects (Vawter et al., 2006). Studies of histone modifications using ChIP (Huang et al., 2006) and studies of DNA methylation (Ernst et al., 2008; Byun et al., 2009) in postmortem tissues are believed to be relatively resistant to artifact. Premortem effects of medications, diet, age, smoking, and other factors, such as epilepsy, also could lead to secondary changes not related to the causative factors for autism. In the case of point mutations and CNVs causing autism, it is feasible to collect blood samples from hundreds and even thousands of affected patients for comparison to appropriate controls. This is important because of the presence of extreme heterogeneity in autism such that mutations in any one locus will likely account for less than 1% of all cases. In comparison, brain tissue is available for perhaps a few hundred cases or less, and the ability to obtain strong statistical evidence that a particular epigenetic abnormality found in brain is associated with autism will be extremely difficult. In addition, it usually is not feasible to study the heritability of any brain-specific epimutations. If one finds an epigenetic abnormality in neurons from postmortem brain in a case of autism, then there is usually no ability to obtain similar data from living or deceased parents. The presence of cellular heterogeneity within most brain regions provides another important challenge. For example, epigenetic abnormalities restricted to Purkinje cells and not affecting cells in the granular or molecular layer cells are likely to be difficult to detect in a fragment of cerebellum containing all cell types.

Epigenetics and Disease States

Epigenetic abnormalities may occur through a variety of mechanisms that include both primary and secondary effects, as enumerated in Table 42-1. There are many examples of primary genetic mutations causing secondary epigenetic abnormalities associated with intellectual disability and/or autism. Most of these involve trans-acting effects on all the chromosomes in the genome as is the case for Rett syndrome and other disorders as listed in Table 42-1 (*see* reviews for disease-specific information; Ausio et al., 2003; Bickmore & van der Maarel, 2003; Urdinguio, Sanchez-Mut, & Esteller, 2009). Another example that could provide a precedent for autism is a report of homozygous mutation in *NLRP2* in a mother resulting in multiple offspring with BWS (Meyer et al., 2009). Given the numerous genes involved in chromatin modification, many more such disorders will certainly be described.

In contrast to genome-wide effects, primary genetic mutations may be cis-acting—that is, they may have secondary epigenetic effects only on the chromosome on which the abnormality occurs, as is the case for Fragile X syndrome and deletions of imprinting centers. There are also numerous examples of combined co-primary genetic and epigenetic effects giving rise to phenotypes. This is particularly well-demonstrated by disorders involving genomic imprinting. Deletions of the paternal copy of chromosome 15q11-q13 cause PWS, whereas the same deletion on the maternal chromosome causes Angelman syndrome (Fig. 42-5). The available data regarding PWS and Angelman syndrome are particularly instructive regarding the potential for epigenetic abnormalities causing human disease, because duplication of this same region is one of the more common genetic/epigenetic abnormalities causing autism. The data from PWS and Angelman syndrome provide numerous lessons. The most common cause of these disorders is a 5- to 6-Mb deletion whose phenotype depends on the chromosomal parent of origin. Thus, the primary abnormality is entirely genetic, although the expression of the phenotype entirely depends on the epigenetic state of the chromosome. In contrast, the PWS can be caused by maternal uniparental disomy (UPD), and Angelman syndrome can be caused by paternal UPD. In these cases, there is usually an initial genetic abnormality, such as

Table 42–1.
Secondary and primary epigenetic abnormalities associated with human disease

A. Primary Genetic with Secondary Trans-Acting Epigenetic Effects
1. Rett syndrome, MECP2 duplication, immunodeficiency–centromeric instability–facial anomalies (ICF) syndrome, alpha-thalassemia/intellectual disability syndrome X-linked (ATRX), Rubinstein–Taybi syndrome, Coffin–Lowry syndrome, and mutations in *JARID1C, EHMT1, NRLP2, NRLP7, ZFP57*
B. Primary Genetic with Cis-Acting Secondary Genetic Effects
1. Fragile X syndrome, deletions of imprinting centers, PWS, Angelman Syndrome
C. Combined Co-Primary Genetic and Epigenetic Interaction
1. Parent-of-origin dependent PWS or Angelman Syndrome for the same deletion 15q11-q13
2. Parent-of-origin-dependent autism with duplication of chromosome 15q11-q13
3. Uniparental disomy where genetic trisomy or monosomy is rescued to result in UPD.
D. Pure Epigenetic Mechanism Spontaneous or Environment-Induced
1. Imprinting defect causing PWS, Angelman Syndrome, or BWS with no imprinting center deletion or mutation with or without assisted reproductive technology.
2. Epimutation of HNPCC
3. Possible epimutation of UBE3A, hypothetical epimutation silencing of known autism genes such as *NRXN1, SHANK3, NLGN4X/Y*
4. Hypothetical similar to licking behavior induced epigenetic changes in rat
5. Hypothetical similar to folic acid effects on Agouti locus in mouse and *SYBL1* in human

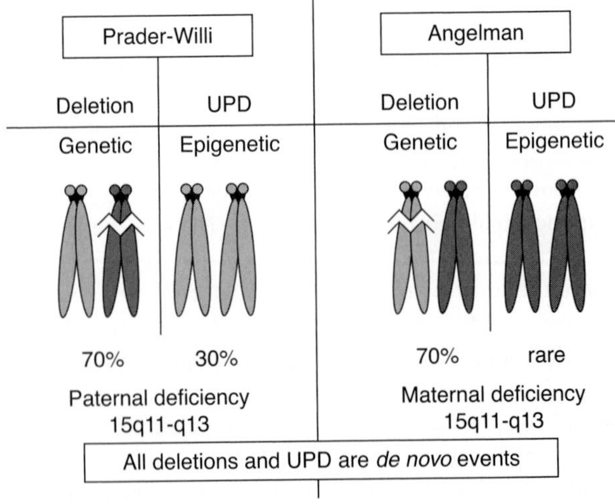

Figure 42–5. Genetic deletion or epigenetic uniparental disomy (UPD) give rise to indistinguishable phenotypes. UPD = uniparental disomy. Modified with permission from Jiang, Y., Bressler, J., & Beaudet, A. L. (2004). Epigenetics and Human Disease. *Annual Review of Genomics and Human Genetics, 5*, 479–510.

monosomy or trisomy conception, followed by genetic rescue to disomy status but with both chromosomes coming from a single parent. In this case, the genetic abnormalities result in a final product that is entirely epigenetic in that there is no abnormality of nucleotide sequence. Another important lesson is that both of these forms of genetic and epigenetic PWS/Angelman syndrome are of de novo origin. For the most part, neither genetic nor epigenetic de novo events will be detected by linkage or association studies, unless the genotyping detects the mutation itself, as can occur when arrays used to analyze single nucleotide polymorphisms (SNPs) detect large deletions or duplications. There are also two forms of imprinting defects causing PWS and Angelman syndrome. There are genetic forms involving small deletions of the imprinting center with secondary epigenetic effects. There are also imprinting defects with no evidence of any genetic mutation, and these are believed to be strictly epigenetic imprinting defects. There is some evidence that assisted reproductive technologies may increase the risk of epigenetic imprinting defects, causing Angelman syndrome and BWS (Owen & Segars, Jr., 2009). Thus, the experience from PWS and Angelman syndrome demonstrates that there can be extremely complex mixtures of genetic and epigenetic abnormalities causing a single phenotype and that many of the events may be of de novo, rather than inherited, origin. We have suggested that this fits a mixed epigenetic and genetic and mixed de novo and inherited (MEGDI) model for the etiology of a phenotype, and we have suggested that de novo and epigenetic abnormalities might explain the relative lack of success in using linkage and association studies to identify autism genes (Jiang et al., 2004).

Finally, there is the possibility of a pure epigenetic abnormality, such as the silencing of a single gene. Figure 42-4 depicts the potential for de novo point mutations to cause loss-of-function or gain-of-function for a gene. Similarly, a CNV may delete or duplicate a gene with corresponding reduced or increased expression, respectively. Finally, a strictly epigenetic abnormality might cause silencing of a gene, which ordinarily should be active, or activation of expression of a gene, which ordinarily should be silenced. All of these mechanisms can lead to increased or decreased function for a particular gene product. It now appears relatively clear that a very large fraction of autism associated with intellectual disability and dysmorphic features is caused by recent or de novo CNVs or point mutations (Jacquemont et al., 2006; Sebat et al., 2007; Marshall et al., 2008). These mutations are typically deleterious in terms of reproductive fitness, and the mutations ordinarily persist for only one or a few generations in the family. If a genotype is incompatible with reproduction, all cases will be of de novo origin (e.g., *SHANK3* deletion). If a mutation is highly penetrant but compatible with reproduction, one may see a parent-to-child transmission of a phenotype such as intellectual disability and/or autism affecting both parent and child. This is common for deletion of chromosome 15q13.3 (Shinawi et al., 2009). If a mutation is incompletely penetrant, then one may see a parent with the mutation and a normal phenotype, whereas the child has the mutation with an autism phenotype. For those genes where a loss-of-function mutation with the resulting haploinsufficiency causes an autism phenotype, it is always theoretically possible that an epimutation silencing one allele of the gene would also cause autism. There is one report of what may be an epimutation causing autism involving methylation of the CpG island at the promoter for *UBE3A* (Jiang et al., 2004), but no similar cases have been found. There is evidence of epimutations causing mismatch repair defects, leading to hereditary nonpolyposis colon cancer (*see* below). For the severe portion of the autism spectrum associated with intellectual disability and dysmorphic features, it now seems that de novo and recent deleterious mutations account for the majority of cases. Presumably, many loss-of-function point mutations will be discovered in similar patients without CNV mutations. It is possible that a smaller fraction of cases could be caused by epigenetic abnormalities of individual genes, but this has yet to be clearly documented.

For the milder end of the autism spectrum, typically associated with more normal cognitive function and absence of dysmorphic features, the etiology remains much less clear. For this population, the dividing line between affected versus unaffected status is more difficult to define. To the extent that genetic abnormalities are involved, we might speculate that these abnormalities could be more subtle, involving lesser degrees of dysregulation; if a single mutation or epimutation confers a major risk, then this may be associated with relatively low penetrance and variable expression. Factors with low penetrance may be difficult to detect in linkage and association studies. The large body of data from studies of linkage and association suggests that no one individual gene with highly penetrant mutations has a particularly large role in this population. One widely tested hypothesis to explain this milder portion of the autism spectrum is a multilocus epistatic model (Bonora et al., 2006). In this model, multiple loci would contribute to the autism risk in a single individual. This hypothesis generally would assume that the genotypes involved are ancient and might be detected by linkage disequilibrium, as in genome-wide association studies. The multilocus epistatic model remains a viable possibility for the milder portion of the autism spectrum, but many other etiological mechanisms also are possible. One can hypothesize that epigenetic abnormalities might be important, and these might be heritable, partially heritable, or not at all heritable. One can hypothesize environmental effects, and it is attractive to consider the possibility of environmental effects being mediated through epigenetic mechanisms.

Epimutations That Cause Disease

Errors in erasing and resetting the genomic imprint during gameteogenesis could cause epimutations.

Gametogenesis: process by which diploid precursor cells undergo cell division and differentiation to form mature haploid gametes (egg and sperm).

Maternal mutations in *NLRP7* that cause recurrent biparental complete hydatidiform molar pregnancies (Murdoch et al., 2006) and maternal mutations in *NLRP2* that cause recurrent BWS (Meyer et al., 2009) represent genetic mutations that cause secondary epimutations. Imprinting defects associated with BWS can be either germline or de novo, and UPD is often mosaic (Riccio et al., 2009; Weksberg, Shuman, & Beckwith, 2010) Epimutations of chromosome 11p15 that affect the *H19* and/or *IGF2* genes are the most common cause of Silver-Russell syndrome (Bartholdi et al., 2009). Mutations in *ZFP57* are associated with transient neonatal diabetes and a global imprinting disorder compatible with life (Mackay et al., 2008).

Primary epimutations with no apparent genetic precursor that affect the mismatch repair genes *MLH1* or *MSH2*, resulting in hereditary nonpolyposis colon cancer and other cancers (Suter, Martin, & Ward, 2004; Chan et al., 2006), represent convincing and compelling examples of how epimutations could theoretically be occurring in autism. Initial and subsequent reports (Cropley, Martin, & Suter, 2008) demonstrate how these epimutations may be inherited or de novo and affect a single locus. De novo epimutations may be mosaic or may be present in all cells tested, with the latter implying a germline origin. One can easily hypothesize that epimutations silencing genes such as *NRXN1, NLGN4X/Y, SHANK3, CNTNAP2*, or others (Sutcliffe, 2008) could cause autism and that these epimutations might be brain- or neuron-specific and quite difficult to detect.

Epigenetics and Autism, Schizophrenia, and Related Phenotypes

The etiology of autism and schizophrenia are increasingly viewed as intertwined. Deletions of single regions can cause a wide spectrum of phenotypic abnormalities, as exemplified by the ability of deletions of 15q13.3 and *CHRNA7* to cause intellectual disability, autism, schizophrenia, epilepsy, and bipolar disorder with incomplete penetrance (Shinawi et al., 2009). Data of this type has led to the suggestion that schizophrenia, and by inference autism, might be described as: "one disorder, multiple mutations; one mutation, multiple disorders" (Sebat, Levy, & McCarthy, 2009). For other CNVs involving chromosome 16p11.2, there is the suggestion that deletions cause autism and intellectual disability (Weiss et al., 2008), whereas duplications cause schizophrenia (McCarthy et al., 2009b).

Crespi and colleagues have suggested that imprinted genes may play an important role in both autism and schizophrenia (Crespi, 2008; Badcock & Crespi, 2008). The possibility that schizophrenia and autism might have some diametrically opposite and/or overlapping biochemical or physiological components to their etiology has been discussed (Crespi, Stead, & Elliot, 2009), and these could involve a complex mixture of genetic and epigenetic mechanisms.

It has been suggested that epigenetic abnormalities may be important in the etiology of schizophrenia (Oh & Petronis, 2008). This might be compatible with suggestions that epigenetic mechanisms may play a role in memory formation and that DNA methylation and histone acetylation may work in concert to regulate memory formation and synaptic plasticity (Levenson & Sweatt, 2005; Miller, Campbell, & Sweatt, 2008).

There are some intriguing data suggesting that *in utero* exposure to famine during the Dutch Hunger Winter at the end of World War II increased the risk of schizophrenia and schizophrenia spectrum personality disorders (Hoek, Brown, & Susser, 1998). Similar data from a Chinese famine support the notion that *in utero* exposure to famine increases the risk of schizophrenia (St. Clair et al., 2005). Epigenetic studies of the Dutch cohort performed six decades after the famine found less DNA methylation of the imprinted *IGF2* gene compared with their unexposed, same-sex siblings (Heijmans et al., 2008) and found that the differences depended on the sex of the exposed individual and the gestational timing of the exposure (Tobi et al., 2009). Given the increasing examples where the same CNV is associated with both autism and schizophrenia (Sebat et al., 2009), and the sex ratio in autism relative to the differential effect of famine dependent on fetal sex, the possibility of a link between *in utero* nutrition and autism is intriguing.

The famine connection is easily linked to the possible role of folic acid deficiency, because the famine increased the risk of neural tube defects as well as schizophrenia (Hoek et al., 1998). It is known that folic acid and intake of related metabolites can influence one-carbon metabolism and DNA methylation in vivo. Methylation of DNA and methylation of histones both play important roles in epigenetic regulation. There is evidence that folic acid and metabolite intake can influence gene expression in mice and humans. In mice, the widely cited example of the effect of diet on expression of the agouti viable yellow allele has been studied extensively (Wolff et al., 1998; Waterland & Jirtle, 2003). There is limited analogous evidence in humans that folic acid and metabolite intake can affect gene expression (Ingrosso et al., 2003). From the possibility of opposite biochemical mechanisms for autism and schizophrenia, one can speculate that folate deficiency might increase the risk of schizophrenia and that folate excess might increase the risk of autism. The apparent increase in the diagnosis of autism has occurred over an interval when folic acid intake in many countries started increasing in the mid-1970s and increased progressively to include fortification in the late 1990s. This has led to discussion of the relevance of folic acid intake to autism (Jiang, Bressler, & Beaudet, 2004) and to speculation that increased folic acid intake may increase the risk of autism (Leeming & Lucock, 2009). In contrast, data from Schmidt et al. (Abstract 2009 IMFAR Meeting http://imfar.confex.com/imfar/2009/webprogram/Paper4182.html) suggest the increased folic acid intake may reduce the risk of autism. There is some evidence that autism is associated with impaired methylation capacity and increased oxidative stress (James et al., 2004) and that treatment with methylcobalamin and folic acid might improve glutathione redox status (James et al., 2009).

Examples of Studies of PostMortem Brain in Autism

The LaSalle laboratory has published numerous studies of autism brain including evidence that MeCP2 expression is reduced in autism brain in association with aberrant *MECP2* promoter methylation (Nagarajan et al., 2008; Hogart et al., 2009). There is a report that reduced expression of the oxytocin receptor is associated with significant increases in the DNA methylation in the peripheral blood cells and temporal cortex in autism (Gregory et al., 2009). Detailed genome-wide analyses of the epigenotype in postmortem brain are just beginning to appear. In a first-of-its-kind study, DNA methylation changes were described in the frontal cortex and in the germline associated with schizophrenia and bipolar disorder (Mill et al., 2008). The results suggested that systemic epigenetic dysfunction may be associated with major psychosis. The authors also found that DNA methylation of the *BDNF* gene in frontal cortex was correlated with genotype at a nearby nonsynonymous SNP previously associated with major psychosis. Two earlier reports of gene-specific analyses found increased methylation of the reelin promoter in schizophrenia brain (Abdolmaleky et al., 2005) and decreased methylation of the *COMT* promoter in schizophrenia and bipolar disorder brain (Abdolmaleky et al., 2006).

We have performed genome-wide analyses of postmortem brains from PWS, Angelman syndrome, and controls to demonstrate the feasibility of detecting known epigenetic abnormalities using genome-wide methods. Using methyated DNA immunoprecipitation, we found the expected absence of methylated DNA at the PWS imprinting center (PWS-IC) in Angelman syndrome brains, but PWS brains were not detectably different from controls (Fig. 42-6). Using restriction enzyme methods that detect enrichment of unmethylated DNA, we found the expected absence of the unmethylated DNA at the PWS-IC in PWS brains, but Angelman syndrome brains appeared normal (unpublished and not shown). These results demonstrate that two methods—one each to detect methylated and unmethylated DNA—may be required to detect all abnormalities. Bisulfite sequencing has the potential to quantify methylated and unmethylated sites in a single analysis.

We have performed similar studies using ChIP-chip and ChIP-seq to compare PWS and Angelman syndrome brains to controls. ChIP analysis using an antibody to H3K4me3 detects the difference in the active promoter for *SNRPN*, which is present in controls but absent in PWS brains (Fig. 42-7), but Angelman syndrome brains are not distinguished from controls. ChIP-chip using an antibody to H3K9me3 detects the absence of this mark in Angelman syndrome brains compared to controls but does not detect any difference between PWS brains and controls (unpublished and not shown). Thus, ChIP must use multiple antibodies to different histone marks to detect all abnormalities.

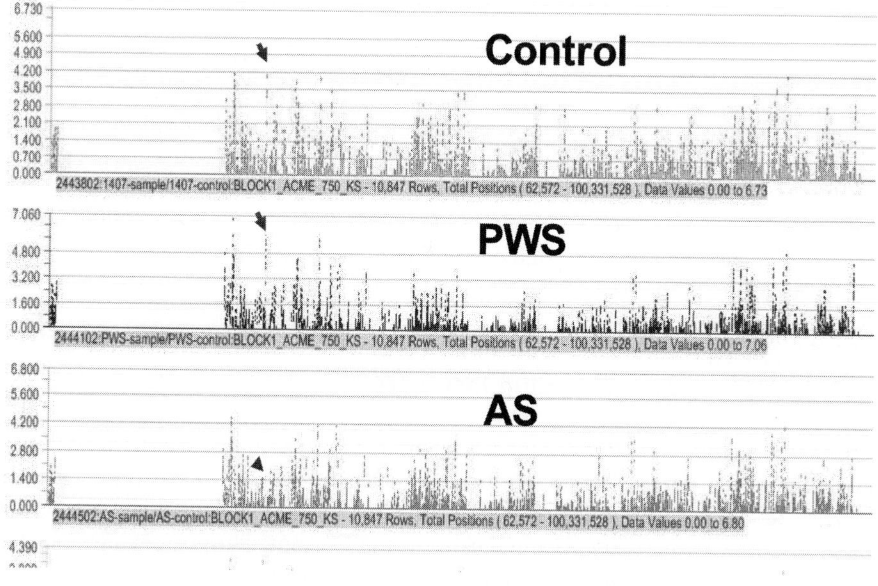

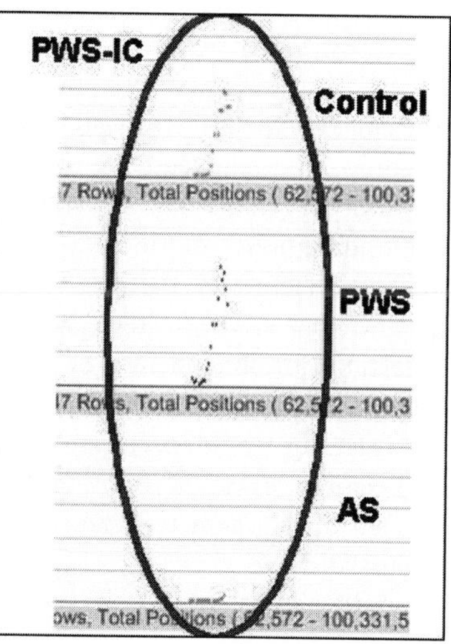

Figure 42–6. Analysis of DNA methylation using methylated DNA immunoprecipitation (MeDIP). Genomic DNA from control, PWS deletion, and Angelman deletion were first digested with *MseI* restriction enzyme and then immunoprecipitated using an antibody against 5-methyl-cytosine (Weber et al., 2005). Precipitated DNA was co-hybridized with its respective input on the Nimblegen CpG island arrays. At the PWS-IC on chromosome 15, a peak of methylated DNA on the maternal chromosome is detected in control and PWS DNA but not Angelman DNA. Right panel is an expanded view of the region with the red arrows. X. Z., unpublished. (See Color Plate Section for a color version of this figure.)

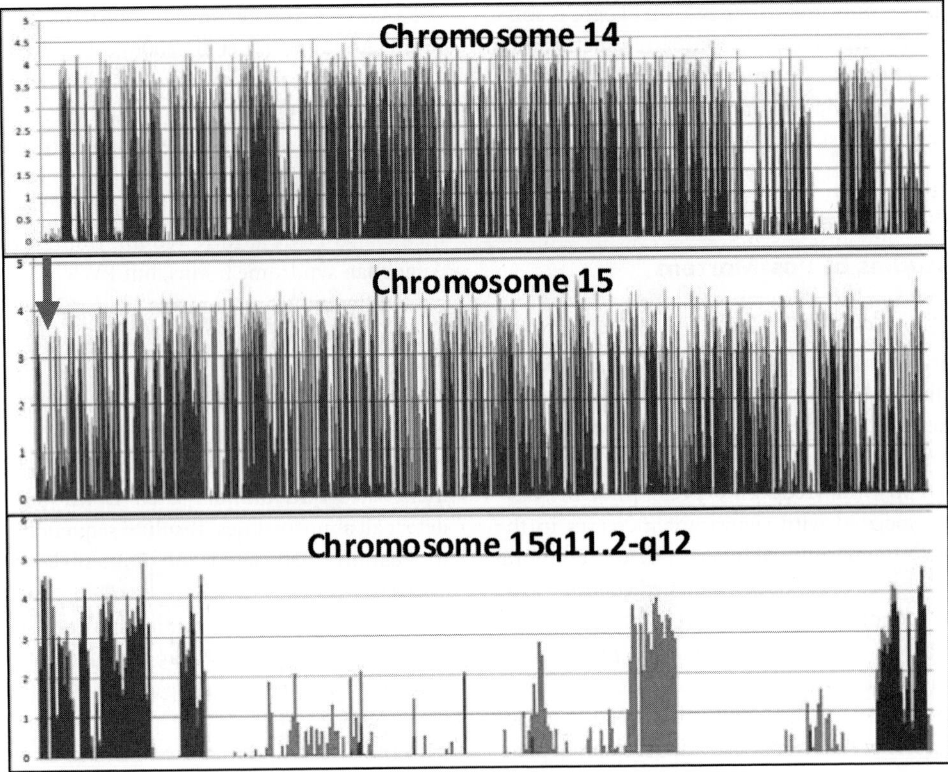

Figure 42–7. Native chromatin immunoprecipitation with microarray analysis (N-ChIP-chip). N-ChIP-chip was performed using an antibody against H3K4me3, in both a PWS-UPD and control cerebellum samples. H3K4me3, a mark indicative of transcription, is known to be absent at the SNRPN-DMR in PWS deletion and UPD samples. Immunoprecipitates were individually hybridized to an Agilent whole genome promoter array and plots of enrichment for two chromosomes superimposed (top two panels, green = control and pink = PWS). The largest difference of H3K4me3 enrichment genome-wide was detected at the *SNRPN* promoter evident by the presence of a single green peak on chromosome 15 (red arrow in middle panel). This finding was additionally confirmed by individually hybridizing samples to custom Agilent tiling arrays of 15q11-q13 (bottom panel). R.P., unpublished. (See Color Plate Section for a color version of this figure.)

Epimutations: Genetic, Epigenetic, Environment, and Stochastic Interactions

The epigenotype is intrinsically more variable and more plastic compared to the sequence of the genome (Fig. 42-8A). The epigenotype can dramatically alter gene expression. Thus there is abundant potential for the genotype, the environment, and stochastic factors to alter the epigenotype. There must be a specific epigenotype for the egg and the sperm at the moment of fertilization, but there is evidence that the epigenotype is changing even in the fertilized oocyte (Reik, 2007), and epimutations could occur prior to and immediately after fertilization. Errors in erasing and resetting the genomic imprint during gameteogenesis could cause epimutations as discussed above.

Potential for Epigenetic Therapy

The fact that the epigenotype is potentially alterable during life opens the possibility at least for epigenetic pharmacotherapy (Szyf, 2009). There are numerous histone deacetylase inhibitors, and there are animal studies exploring effects on gene expression in brain. The most widely studied HDAC inhibitors are trichostatin A and suberoylanilide hydroxamic acid (Fig. 42-8B). Data are also available for histone methyltransferase inhibitors and DNA demethylating agents such as 5-aza-cytidine and zebularine. There is a report of long-term oral administration of zebularine to mice with minimal side effects and prevention of intestinal tumors (Yoo et al., 2008).

Changing Incidence?

There has been extensive debate as to whether the incidence of autism has increased over the last 20 years as is discussed in other chapters in this book. Although there is definitely an increase in the diagnosis of autism, the apparent increase may be partially or completely explained by diagnostic substitution, diagnosis of milder phenotypes, and/or increased awareness (King & Bearman, 2009; Fombonne, 2009). If there is a true increase, this is of enormous importance, as this would suggest that some change in the environment is affecting the incidence of autism and that reversal of this environmental effect should lower the incidence of autism. Understanding

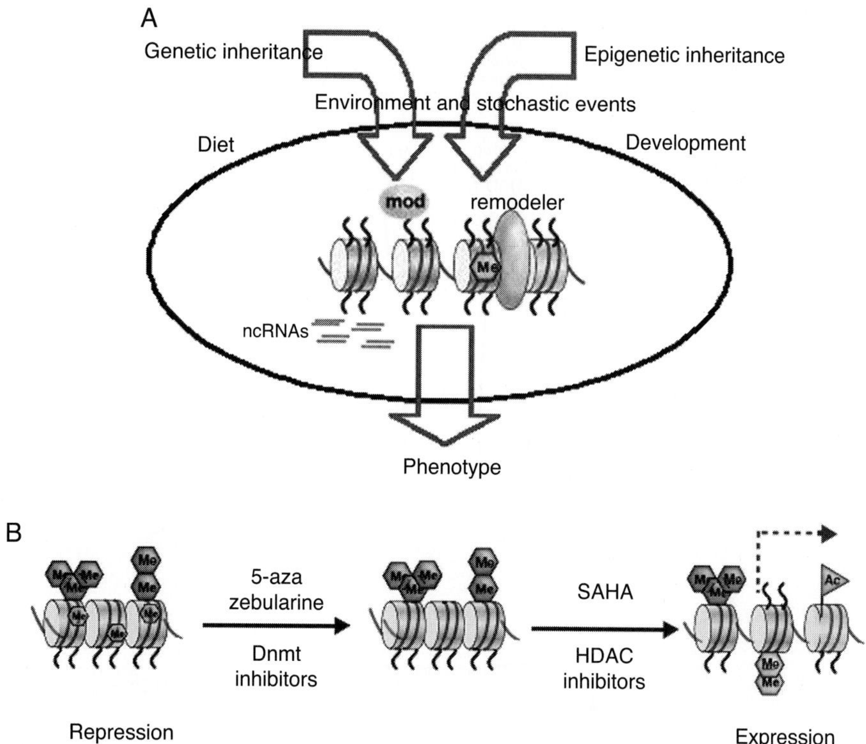

Figure 42–8. A (Upper panel). Interaction between genetics, epigenetics, and environment to give rise to phenotype. B (Lower panel) Potential for pharmacologic modification of the epigenome. Exposure to Dnmt inhibitors such as 5-aza-cytidine (5-aza) or zebularine can result in a loss of DNA methylation, and exposure to HDAC inhibitors such as suberoylanilide hydroxamic acid (SAHA) can result in the acquisition of histone acetyl marks and subsequent downstream modifications, including active histone methyl marks and the incorporation of histone variants. The cumulative chromatin changes can lead to gene expression. Modified with permission from Chapter 3 in Allis, C. D., Jenuwein, T., & Reinberg, D. (2007). *Epigenetics*. Cold Spring Harbor, NY: Cold Spring Harbor Laboratory Press. (See Color Plate Section for a color version of this figure.)

the basis for a true increase in incidence, if it exists, would also likely have benefits in terms of both treatment and prevention of autism generally. The possibility of a true increase in incidence is interesting from a general perspective, as some environmental effect would be implied, and environmental factors such as maternal diet at the time of pregnancy, prenatal ultrasound, prenatal or postnatal exposure to chemical toxins, and many other factors changing over the decades can be hypothesized to affect the risk of autism. Vaccines and mercury exposure have been widely debated (Baker, 2008) and like most other environmental factors can be hypothesized to act through epigenetic mechanisms. From an epigenetic perspective, the fact that folic acid intake increased substantially in many countries from the late 1970s through the 1990s is interesting, because it can affect DNA methylation and gene expression as discussed above.

An Overall Synthesis

In 2004, we proposed a mixed epigenetic and genetic and MEGDI model (Fig. 42-9) that might apply to autism (Jiang et al., 2004). In this context, de novo includes mutations or epimutations arising in the affected individual or in the preceding few generations but excludes ancient mutations. This model is in sharp contrast to a multilocus epistatic model in which the causative factors are hypothesized to be ancient mutations that would be discoverable through linkage and association studies including GWAS. The MEGDI model would predict that GWAS would not, for the most part, detect de novo or epigenetic abnormalities, although some might be detected if the mutation or epimutation were inherited for a few generations. The MEGDI model was proposed at a time when chromosome abnormalities were known to cause a small fraction of cases of autism (Vorstman et al., 2006), but the role of CNVs was yet to be recognized (Sebat et al., 2007). Deletions with modest reductions in fitness may yield virtually any ratio of de novo to inherited cases among probands. Numerous reciprocal duplications of well-known deletion syndromes are commonly associated with autism with reduced penetrance (e.g., duplications of the regions deleted in DiGeorge, Willams, and Smith-Magenis syndromes). The recognition of the role of CNVs in the etiology of autism and the implications for point mutations in genes within the CNVs is the most dramatic advance in understanding the cause of autism over the last few years, and the data fit well within the MEGDI model but not with the multilocus epistatic model. For severe autism phenotypes associated with intellectual disability, birth defects, and dysmorphic features, CNVs may be found in as much as a

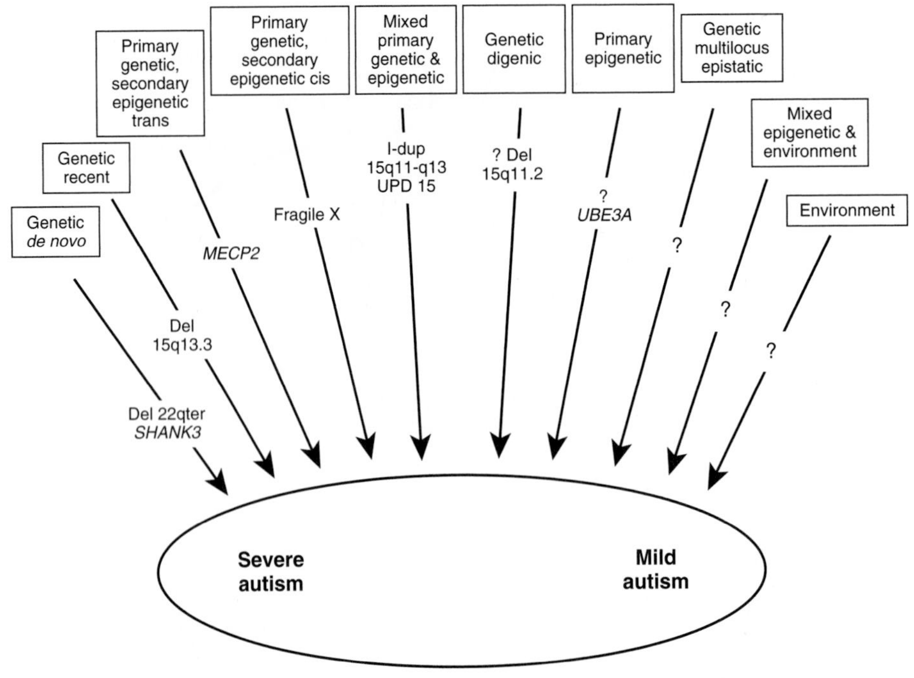

Figure 42–9. A *m*ixed *e*pigenetic and *g*enetic and mixed *d*e novo and *inherited* (MEGDI) plus environment model for autism. *SHANK3* and *MECP2* refer to mutations in these genes and *UBE3A* refers to possible epimutation. I-dup 15q11-q13 is interstitial duplications which cause autism when maternal but usually not when paternal.

one-fourth of patients (Jacquemont et al., 2006). The general experience in diagnostic laboratories is that disease-causing CNVs are found in very few higher functioning, nondysmorphic patients or in those diagnosed with Asperger's syndrome.

Do the studies of the role of CNVs in severe autism leave any role for epigenetics in this population? Presumably, epimutations will not account for a large fraction of cases in this cohort of patients, although a few may yet be discovered, and a significant contribution is still possible. The CNVs and small mutations in the causative genes therein are generally expected to account for the majority of cases of severe autism, and whole-genome or whole-exome sequencing is widely expected to identify many additional mutations in this population. The association of advanced paternal age with autism (Reichenberg et al., 2006) could be compatible with a role of de novo point mutations, although the effects are small, and maternal age may be important as well (Durkin et al., 2008; King et al., 2009), perhaps through nondisjunction contributing to confined placental mosaicism (Leschot et al., 1996) or uniparental disomy. There are no data regarding the possibility of a parental age effect on the risk of epimutations.

How might the MEGDI model fit for the etiology of the higher functioning, nondysmorphic autism population? This population has a much higher male:female ratio compared to the lower functioning dysmorphic population. Certainly mutations contributing to this group are likely to be less penetrant and be associated with significant reproductive fitness, although such mutations need not be ancient. In general, the etiology of high-functioning autism is much less understood, with ancient mutations, recent mutations, epimutations, and environmental factors all remaining very feasible. The sex ratio could be explained by changes in genes mapping to the X or Y chromosome (sex-linked effects) or to sex-limited effects on autosomal genes. Sex-limited effects are mediated by the genes that directly cause sex determination, primarily *SRY* that cause maleness in humans. For severe autism, mutations in X-linked genes may be sufficient to explain the modest increase in male:female ratio. A good example of a sex-limited effect is provided by mutations in *BRCA1* and *BRCA2* that cause breast cancer with a much higher penetrance in females than in males. A proposal for a unified genetic theory for sporadic and inherited autism (Zhao et al., 2007) is equivalent to a sex-limited effect on autosomal genes. A recent review of sex-limited gene expression (Williams & Carroll, 2009) is thought-provoking regarding the sex bias in milder forms of autism. The authors concluded, "A common theme emerging from these studies is that the integration of sex determination and other transcriptional inputs by cis-regulatory elements is central to the development and evolution of sexually dimorphic traits." This is consistent with the precedent for a sex-dependent mutation in an enhancer associated with Hirschsprung disease (Emison et al., 2005) and is of interest regarding the sex bias in mild autism. The epigenetics of sex differences in the brain was reviewed recently (McCarthy et al., 2009a). There is no obvious basis to hypothesize that the prominent sex effect in mild autism is primarily genetic or epigenetic or primarily of de novo or inherited origin. A moderately or highly penetrant inherited genetic effect involving a single X-linked, Y-linked, or autosomal locus in a large fraction of cases is essentially ruled out by the failure to detect such an effect using linkage and association studies. A multilocus epistatic hypothesis remains very viable and would likely involve primarily autosomal genes. An epigenetic hypothesis involving sex-linked or sex-limited effects also remains very viable. Epimutations might be inherited in some cases or entirely erased and corrected with germline transmission. The full role of epigenetics in the etiology of autism remains to be delineated.

Conclusions

There are many disorders that cause autism in which primary genetic abnormalities are associated with secondary epigenetic abnormalities in trans affecting the entire genome (e.g., *MECP2* mutations) or in cis on the mutated chromosome (e.g., Fragile X syndrome). There is at least one case where genetic and epigenetic factors work in concert such that maternal interstitial duplication of chromosome 15q11-q13 cause autism but paternal duplications are usually benign. Although single-gene epimutations have been described for a few genes, no examples of single-gene epimutations have been described convincingly to date. Because the etiology of severe autism with intellectual disability and dysmorphic features is increasingly documented to be caused by recent and de novo mutations, there is the potential for some analogous epimutations in some of these patients. The etiology of mild autism and Asperger's syndrome is much less clear, and epigenetic and other mechanisms all deserve further study.

Challenges and Future Directions

- Either global or single-gene epigenetic abnormalities could contribute to the etiology of autism as primary, secondary, or modifier factors.
- Environmental effects including nutritional factors could play a role in the etiology of autism mediated by epigenetic mechanisms.
- Epigenetic analysis is challenging because key abnormalities may be brain-specific or even cell-specific, as would be the case if epigenetic changes were limited to hippocampal or Purkinje neurons.
- Epigenetic analysis of DNA methylation and chromatin structure in postmortem autism compared to control brain is now feasible and should be carried out for both mild autism and severe autism.

SUGGESTED READINGS

Allis, C. D., Jenuwein, T., & Reinberg, D. (2007). *Epigenetics*. Cold Spring Harbor, NY: Cold Spring Harbor Laboratory Press. 1. (In particular, Chapters 3 and 23).

Feinberg, A. P. (2007). Phenotypic plasticity and the epigenetics of human disease. *Nature, 447*, 433–440.

Mill, J., Tang, T., Kaminsky, Z., Khare, T., Yazdanpanah, S., Bouchard, L. et al. (2008). Epigenomic profiling reveals DNA-methylation changes associated with major psychosis. *American Journal of Human Genetics, 82*, 696–711.

Suzuki, M. M. & Bird, A. (2008). DNA methylation landscapes: provocative insights from epigenomics. *Nature Reviews Genetics, 9*, 465–476.

REFERENCES

Aalfs, J. D. & Kingston, R. E. (2000). What does "chromatin remodeling" mean? *Trends in Biochemical Sciences, 25*, 548–555.

Abdolmaleky, H. M., Cheng, K. H., Faraone, S. V., Wilcox, M., Glatt, S. J., Gao, F., et al. (2006). Hypomethylation of MB-COMT promoter is a major risk factor for schizophrenia and bipolar disorder. *Human Molecular Genetics, 15*, 3132–3145.

Abdolmaleky, H. M., Cheng, K. H., Russo, A., Smith, C. L., Faraone, S. V., Wilcox, M., et al. (2005). Hypermethylation of the reelin (RELN) promoter in the brain of schizophrenic patients: a preliminary report. *American Journal of Medical Genetics. Part B, Neuropsychiatric Genetics, 134B*, 60–66.

Allis, C. D., Jenuwein, T., & Reinberg, D. (2007). *Epigenetics*. Cold Spring Harbor, NY: Cold Spring Harbor Laboratory Press.

Ausio, J., Levin, D. B., De Amorim, G. V., Bakker, S., & MacLeod, P. M. (2003). Syndromes of disordered chromatin remodeling. *Clinical Genetics, 64*, 83–95.

Badcock, C. & Crespi, B. (2008). Battle of the sexes may set the brain. *Nature, 454*, 1054–1055.

Baker, J. P. (2008). Mercury, vaccines, and autism: one controversy, three histories. *American Journal of Public Health, 98*, 244–253.

Bartholdi, D., Krajewska-Walasek, M., Ounap, K., Gaspar, H., Chrzanowska, K. H., Ilyana, H., et al. (2009). Epigenetic mutations of the imprinted IGF2-H19 domain in Silver-Russell syndrome (SRS): results from a large cohort of patients with SRS and SRS-like phenotypes. *Journal of Medical Genetics, 46*, 192–197.

Bartolomei, M. S. (2009). Genomic imprinting: employing and avoiding epigenetic processes. *Genes and Devevelopment, 23*, 2124–2133.

Bibikova, M., Lin, Z., Zhou, L., Chudin, E., Garcia, E. W., Wu, B., et al. (2006) High-throughput DNA methylation profiling using universal bead arrays. *Genome Research, 16*, 383–93.

Bickmore, W. A. & van der Maarel, S. M. (2003). Perturbations of chromatin structure in human genetic disease: recent advances. *Human Molecular Genetics, 12 Spec No 2*, R207–R213.

Bird, A. (2007). Perceptions of epigenetics. *Nature, 447*, 396–398.

Bonora, Lamb, Barnby, G., Bailey, A. J., & Monaco (2006). Genetic Basis of Autism. In Moldin, S. O., & Rubenstein, J. L. (Eds.), *Understanding autism: From basic neuroscience to treatment* (pp. 49–67). Boca Raton: CRC Press.

Butler, M. G. (2009). Genomic imprinting disorders in humans: a mini-review. *Journal of Assisted Reproduction and Genetics, 26*, 477–86.

Byrne, J. A., Nguyen, H. N., & Reijo Pera, R. A. (2009). Enhanced generation of induced pluripotent stem cells from a subpopulation of human fibroblasts. *PLoS ONE, 4*, e7118.

Byun, H. M., Siegmund, K. D., Pan, F., Weisenberger, D. J., Kanel, G., Laird, P. W., et al. (2009). Epigenetic profiling of somatic tissues from human autopsy specimens identifies tissue-and individual-specific DNA methylation patterns. *Human Molecular Genetics, 18*, 4808–4817.

Chan, T. L., Yuen, S. T., Kong, C. K., Chan, Y. W., Chan, A. S., Ng, W. F., et al. (2006). Heritable germline epimutation of MSH2 in a family with hereditary nonpolyposis colorectal cancer. *Nature Genetics, 38*, 1178–1183.

Chandler, V. L. & Stam, M. (2004). Chromatin conversations: mechanisms and implications of paramutation. *Nature Reviews Genetics, 5*, 532–544.

Chong, S., Youngson, N. A., & Whitelaw, E. (2007). Heritable germline epimutation is not the same as transgenerational epigenetic inheritance. *Nature Genetics, 39*, 574–575.

Crespi, B. (2008). Genomic imprinting in the development and evolution of psychotic spectrum conditions. *Biological Reviews of the Cambridge Philosophical Society, 83*, 441–493.

Crespi, B., Stead, P., & Elliot, M. (2009). Evolution in Health and Medicine Sackler Colloquium: Comparative genomics of autism and schizophrenia. *Proceedings of the National Academy of Sciences of the United States of America. 107*(Suppl 1), 1736–1741.

Cropley, J. E., Martin, D. I., & Suter, C. M. (2008). Germline epimutation in humans. *Pharmacogenomics, 9*, 1861–1868.

Cuddapah, S., Jothi, R., Schones, D. E., Roh, T. Y., Cui, K., & Zhao, K. (2009). Global analysis of the insulator binding protein CTCF in chromatin barrier regions reveals demarcation of active and repressive domains. *Genome Research, 19*, 24–32.

De, B. C., Ramos, E., Young, J. M., Tran, R. K., Menzel, U., Langford, C. F., et al. (2009). Tissue-specific variation in DNA methylation levels along human chromosome 1. *Epigenetics and Chromati, 2*, 7.

Doi, A., Park, I. H., Wen, B., Murakami, P., Aryee, M. J., Irizarry, R., et al. (2009). Differential methylation of tissue- and cancer-specific CpG island shores distinguishes human induced pluripotent stem cells, embryonic stem cells and fibroblasts. *Nature Genetics, 41*, 1350–1353.

Durkin, M. S., Maenner, M. J., Newschaffer, C. J., Lee, L. C., Cunniff, C. M., Daniels, J. L., et al. (2008). Advanced parental age and the risk of autism spectrum disorder. *American Journal of Epidemiology, 168*, 1268–1276.

Emison, E. S., McCallion, A. S., Kashuk, C. S., Bush, R. T., Grice, E., Lin, S., et al. (2005). A common sex-dependent mutation in a RET enhancer underlies Hirschsprung disease risk. *Nature, 434*, 857–863.

Ernst, C., McGowan, P. O., Deleva, V., Meaney, M. J., Szyf, M., & Turecki, G. (2008). The effects of pH on DNA methylation state: In vitro and post-mortem brain studies. *Journal of Neuroscience Methods, 174*, 123–125.

Feinberg, A. P. (2007). Phenotypic plasticity and the epigenetics of human disease. *Nature, 447*, 433–440.

Ferrer, I., Martinez, A., Boluda, S., Parchi, P., & Barrachina, M. (2008). Brain banks: benefits, limitations and cautions concerning the use of post-mortem brain tissue for molecular studies. *Cell and Tissue Banking, 9*, 181–194.

Fish, E. W., Shahrokh, D., Bagot, R., Caldji, C., Bredy, T., Szyf, M., et al. (2004). Epigenetic programming of stress responses through variations in maternal care. *Annals of the New York Academy of Sciences, 1036*, 167–180.

Fombonne, E. (2009). Commentary: on King and Bearman. *International Journal of Epidemiology, 38*, 1241–1242.

Franklin, T. B. & Mansuy, I. M. (2010). Epigenetic inheritance in mammals: Evidence for the impact of adverse environmental effects. *Neurobiological Disease, 39*, 61–65.

Gilchrist, D. A., Fargo, D. C., & Adelman, K. (2009). Using ChIP-chip and ChIP-seq to study the regulation of gene expression: genome-wide localization studies reveal widespread regulation of transcription elongation. *Methods, 48*, 398–408.

Gordon, A. J., Halliday, J. A., Blankschien, M. D., Burns, P. A., Yatagai, F., & Herman, C. (2009). Transcriptional infidelity promotes heritable phenotypic change in a bistable gene network. *PLoS Biology, 7*, e44.

Gravina, S. & Vijg, J. (2009). Epigenetic factors in aging and longevity. *Pflugers Archives, 459*, 247–258

Gregory, S. G., Connelly, J. J., Towers, A. J., Johnson, J., Biscocho, D., Markunas, C. A., et al. (2009). Genomic and epigenetic evidence for oxytocin receptor deficiency in autism. *BMC Medicine, 7*, 62.

Hatchwell, E. & Greally, J. M. (2007). The potential role of epigenomic dysregulation in complex human disease. *Trends in Genetics, 23*, 588–595.

Heijmans, B. T., Tobi, E. W., Stein, A. D., Putter, H., Blauw, G. J., Susser, E. S., et al. (2008). Persistent epigenetic differences associated with prenatal exposure to famine in humans. *Proceedings of the National Academy of Sciences of the United States of America, 105*, 17,046–17,049.

Heintzman, N. D., Hon, G. C., Hawkins, R. D., Kheradpour, P., Stark, A., Harp, L. F., et al. (2009). Histone modifications at human enhancers reflect global cell-type-specific gene expression. *Nature, 459*, 108–112.

Henikoff, S., Strahl, B. D., & Warburton, P. E. (2008). Epigenomics: a roadmap to chromatin. *Science, 322*, 853.

Hoek, H. W., Brown, A. S., & Susser, E. (1998). The Dutch famine and schizophrenia spectrum disorders. *Social Psychiatry and Psychiatric Epidemiology, 33*, 373–379.

Hogart, A., Leung, K. N., Wang, N. J., Wu, D. J., Driscoll, J., Vallero, R. O., et al. (2009). Chromosome 15q11-13 duplication syndrome brain reveals epigenetic alterations in gene expression not predicted from copy number. *Journal of Medical Genetics, 46*, 86–93.

Hore, T. A., Rapkins, R. W., & Graves, J. A. (2007). Construction and evolution of imprinted loci in mammals. *Trends in Genetics, 23*, 440–448.

Huang, H. S., Matevossian, A., Jiang, Y., & Akbarian, S. (2006). Chromatin immunoprecipitation in postmortem brain. *Journal of Neuroscience Methods, 156*, 284–292.

Ingrosso, D., Cimmino, A., Perna, A. F., Masella, L., De Santo, N. G., De Bonis, M. L., et al. (2003). Folate treatment and unbalanced methylation and changes of allelic expression induced by hyperhomocysteinaemia in patients with uraemia. *Lancet, 361*, 1693–1699.

Irizarry, R. A., Ladd-Acosta, C., Carvalho, B., Wu, H., Brandenburg, S. A., Jeddeloh, J. A., et al. (2008). Comprehensive high-throughput arrays for relative methylation (CHARM). *Genome Research, 18*, 780–790.

Jacquemont, M.-L., Sanlaville, D., Redon, R., Raoul, O., Cormier-Daire, V., Lyonnet, S., et al. (2006). Array- based comparative genomic hybridization identifies high frequency of cryptic chromosomal rearrangements in patients with syndromic autism spectrum disorders. *Journal of Medical Genetics., 43*, 843–849.

Jaenisch, R. & Bird, A. (2003). Epigenetic regulation of gene expression: how the genome integrates intrinsic and environmental signals. *Nature Genetics., 33 Suppl*, 245–254.

James, S. J., Cutler, P., Melnyk, S., Jernigan, S., Janak, L., Gaylor, D. W., et al. (2004). Metabolic biomarkers of increased oxidative stress and impaired methylation capacity in children with autism. *American Journal of Clinical Nutrition, 80*, 1611–1617.

James, S. J., Melnyk, S., Fuchs, G., Reid, T., Jernigan, S., Pavliv, O., et al. (2009). Efficacy of methylcobalamin and folinic acid treatment on glutathione redox status in children with autism. *American Journal of Clinical Nutrition, 89*, 425–430.

Jenuwein, T. & Allis, C. D. (2001). Translating the histone code. *Science, 293*, 1074–1080.

Jiang, Y. H., Sahoo, T., Michaelis, R. C., Bercovich, D., Bressler, J., Kashork, C. D., et al. (2004). A mixed epigenetic/genetic model for oligogenic inheritance of autism with a limited role for UBE3A. *American Journal of Medical Genetics, 131A*, 1–10.

Jiang, Y., Bressler, J., & Beaudet, A. L. (2004). Epigenetics and Human Disease. *Annual Review of Genomics and Human Genetics, 5*, 479–510.

Jirtle, R. L. & Skinner, M. K. (2007). Environmental epigenomics and disease susceptibility. *Nature Reviews Genetics, 8*, 253–262.

Kaati, G., Bygren, L. O., Pembrey, M., & Sjostrom, M. (2007). Transgenerational response to nutrition, early life circumstances and longevity. *European Journal of Human Genetics, 15*, 784–790.

Kaminsky, Z., Wang, S. C., & Petronis, A. (2006). Complex disease, gender and epigenetics. *Annals of Medicine, 38*, 530–544.

King, M. & Bearman, P. (2009). Diagnostic change and the increased prevalence of autism. *International Journal of Epidemiology, 38*, 1224–1234.

King, M. D., Fountain, C., Dakhlallah, D., & Bearman, P. S. (2009). Estimated autism risk and older reproductive age. *American Journal of Public Health, 99*, 1673–1679.

Lee, G., Papapetrou, E. P., Kim, H., Chambers, S. M., Tomishima, M. J., Fasano, C. A., et al. (2009). Modelling pathogenesis and treatment of familial dysautonomia using patient-specific iPSCs. *Nature, 461*, 402–406.

Leeming, R. J. & Lucock, M. (2009). Autism: Is there a folate connection? *Journal of Inherited Metabolic Disease, 32*, 400–402.

Leschot, N. J., Schuring-Blom, G. H., Van Prooijen-Knegt, A. C., Verjaal, M., Hansson, K., Wolf, H., et al. (1996). The outcome of pregnancies with confined placental chromosome mosaicism in cytotrophoblast cells. *Prenatal Diagnosis, 16*, 705–712.

Levenson, J. M. & Sweatt, J. D. (2005). Epigenetic mechanisms in memory formation. *Nature Reviews Neuroscience, 6*, 108–118.

Lister, R., Pelizzola, M., Dowen, R. H., Hawkins, R. D., Hon, G., Tonti-Filippini, J., et al. (2009). Human DNA methylomes at base resolution show widespread epigenomic differences. *Nature, 462*, 315–322.

Mackay, D. J., Callaway, J. L., Marks, S. M., White, H. E., Acerini, C. L., Boonen, S. E., et al. (2008). Hypomethylation of multiple imprinted loci in individuals with transient neonatal diabetes is associated with mutations in ZFP57. *Nature Genetics, 40*, 949–951.

Madhani, H. D., Francis, N. J., Kingston, R. E., Kornberg, R. D., Moazed, D., Narlikar, G. J., et al. (2008). Epigenomics: a roadmap, but to where? *Science, 322*, 43–44.

Maher, B. (2008). Personal genomes: The case of the missing heritability. *Nature, 456*, 18–21.

Manolio, T. A., Collins, F. S., Cox, N. J., Goldstein, D. B., Hindorff, L. A., Hunter, D. J., et al. (2009). Finding the missing heritability of complex diseases. *Nature, 461*, 747–753.

Marshall, C. R., Noor, A., Vincent, J. B., Lionel, A. C., Feuk, L., Skaug, J., et al. (2008). Structural variation of chromosomes in autism spectrum disorder. *American Journal of Human Genetics, 82*, 477–488.

McCarthy, M. I. & Hirschhorn, J. N. (2008). Genome-wide association studies: potential next steps on a genetic journey. *Human Molecular Genetics, 17*, R156–R165.

McCarthy, M. M., Auger, A. P., Bale, T. L., De Vries, G. J., Dunn, G. A., Forger, N. G., et al. (2009a). The epigenetics of sex differences in the brain. *Journal of Neuroscence, 29*, 12815–12823.

McCarthy, S. E., Makarov, V., Kirov, G., Addington, A. M., McClellan, J., Yoon, S., et al. (2009b). Microduplications of 16p11.2 are associated with schizophrenia. *Nature Genetics, 41*, 1223–1227.

McGowan, P. O., Sasaki, A., D'Alessio, A. C., Dymov, S., Labonte, B., Szyf, M., et al. (2009). Epigenetic regulation of the glucocorticoid receptor in human brain associates with childhood abuse. *Nature Neuroscience, 12*, 342–348.

Meissner, A., Mikkelsen, T. S., Gu, H., Wernig, M., Hanna, J., Sivachenko, A., et al. (2008). Genome-scale DNA methylation maps of pluripotent and differentiated cells. *Nature, 454*, 766–770.

Meyer, E., Lim, D., Pasha, S., Tee, L. J., Rahman, F., Yates, J. R., et al. (2009). Germline mutation in NLRP2 (NALP2) in a familial imprinting disorder (Beckwith-Wiedemann Syndrome). *PLoS Genetics, 5*, e1000423.

Mill, J., Tang, T., Kaminsky, Z., Khare, T., Yazdanpanah, S., Bouchard, L., et al. (2008). Epigenomic profiling reveals DNA-methylation changes associated with major psychosis. *American Journal of Human Genetics, 82*, 696–711.

Miller, C. A., Campbell, S. L., & Sweatt, J. D. (2008). DNA methylation and histone acetylation work in concert to regulate memory formation and synaptic plasticity. *Neurobiology of Learning and Memory, 89*, 599–603.

Morgan, H. D., Santos, F., Green, K., Dean, W., & Reik, W. (2005). Epigenetic reprogramming in mammals. *Human Molecular Genetics, 14 Spec No 1*, R47–R58.

Morgan, H. D., Sutherland, H. G., Martin, D. I., & Whitelaw, E. (1999). Epigenetic inheritance at the agouti locus in the mouse. *Nature Genetics, 23*, 314–318.

Murdoch, S., Djuric, U., Mazhar, B., Seoud, M., Khan, R., Kuick, R., et al. (2006). Mutations in NALP7 cause recurrent hydatidiform moles and reproductive wastage in humans. *Nature Genetics, 38*, 300–302.

Nadeau, J. H. (2009). Transgenerational genetic effects on phenotypic variation and disease risk. *Human Molecular Genetics, 18*, R202–R210.

Nagarajan, R. P., Patzel, K. A., Martin, M., Yasui, D. H., Swanberg, S. E., Hertz-Picciotto, I., et al. (2008). MECP2 promoter methylation and X chromosome inactivation in autism. *Autism Research, 1*, 169–178.

Neigh, G. N., Gillespie, C. F., & Nemeroff, C. B. (2009). The neurobiological toll of child abuse and neglect. *Trauma, Violence, and Abuse, 10*, 389–410.

Oh, G. & Petronis, A. (2008). Environmental studies of schizophrenia through the prism of epigenetics. *Schizophrenia Bulletin, 34*, 1122–1129.

Owen, C. M. & Segars, J. H., Jr. (2009). Imprinting disorders and assisted reproductive technology. *Seminars in Reproductive Medicine, 27*, 417–428.

Pembrey, M. (1996). Imprinting and transgenerational modulation of gene expression; human growth as a model. *Acta Geneticae Medicae et Gemellologiae (Roma), 45*, 111–125.

Pembrey, M. E., Bygren, L. O., Kaati, G., Edvinsson, S., Northstone, K., Sjostrom, M., et al. (2006). Sex-specific, male-line transgenerational responses in humans. *European Journal of Human Genetics, 14*, 159–166.

Probst, A. V., Dunleavy, E., & Almouzni, G. (2009). Epigenetic inheritance during the cell cycle. *Nature Reviews Molecular Cell Biology, 10*, 192–206.

Raser, J. M. & O'Shea, E. K. (2005). Noise in gene expression: origins, consequences, and control. *Science, 309*, 2010–2013.

Rassoulzadegan, M., Grandjean, V., Gounon, P., Vincent, S., Gillot, I., & Cuzin, F. (2006). RNA-mediated non-mendelian inheritance of an epigenetic change in the mouse. *Nature, 441*, 469–474.

Redon, R., Ishikawa, S., Fitch, K. R., Feuk, L., Perry, G. H., Andrews, T. D., et al. (2006). Global variation in copy number in the human genome. *Nature, 444*, 444–454.

Reichenberg, A., Gross, R., Weiser, M., Bresnahan, M., Silverman, J., Harlap, S., et al. (2006). Advancing paternal age and autism. *Archives of General Psychiatry, 63*, 1026–1032.

Reik, W. (2007). Stability and flexibility of epigenetic gene regulation in mammalian development. *Nature, 447*, 425–432.

Reik, W. & Walter, J. (2001). Genomic imprinting: Parental influence on the genome. *Nature Reviews Genetics, 2*, 21–32.

Riccio, A., Sparago, A., Verde, G., De, C. A., Citro, V., Cubellis, M. V., et al. (2009). Inherited and Sporadic Epimutations at the IGF2-H19 locus in Beckwith-Wiedemann syndrome and Wilms' tumor. *Endocrine Development, 14*, 1–9.

Ruthenburg, A. J., Li, H., Patel, D. J., & Allis, C. D. (2007). Multivalent engagement of chromatin modifications by linked binding modules. *Nature Reviews Molecular Cell Biology, 8*, 983–994.

Schuettengruber, B., Ganapathi, M., Leblanc, B., Portoso, M., Jaschek, R., Tolhuis, B., et al. (2009). Functional anatomy of polycomb and trithorax chromatin landscapes in Drosophila embryos. *PLoS Biology, 7*, e13.

Sebat, J., Lakshmi, B., Malhotra, D., Troge, J., Lese-Martin, C., Walsh, T., et al. (2007). Strong association of de novo copy number mutations with autism. *Science, 316*, 445–449.

Sebat, J., Levy, D. L., & McCarthy, S. E. (2009). Rare structural variants in schizophrenia: one disorder, multiple mutations; one mutation, multiple disorders. *Trends in Genetics, 25*, 528–535.

Shinawi, M., Schaaf, C. P., Bhatt, S. S., Xia, Z., Patel, A., Cheung, S. W., et al. (2009). A small recurrent deletion within 15q13.3 is associated with a range of neurodevelopmental phenotypes. *Nature Genetics, 41*, 1269–1271.

Smith, Z. D., Gu, H., Bock, C., Gnirke, A., & Meissner, A. (2009). High-throughput bisulfite sequencing in mammalian genomes. *Methods, 48*, 226–232.

St. Clair, Xu, M., Wang, P., Yu, Y., Fang, Y., Zhang, F., et al. (2005). Rates of adult schizophrenia following prenatal exposure to the Chinese famine of 1959-1961. *Journal of the American Medical Association, 294*, 557–562.

Sutcliffe, J. S. (2008). Genetics. Insights into the pathogenesis of autism. *Science, 321*, 208–209.

Suter, C. M., Martin, D. I., & Ward, R. L. (2004). Germline epimutation of MLH1 in individuals with multiple cancers. *Nature Genetics, 36*, 497–501.

Suzuki, M. M. & Bird, A. (2008). DNA methylation landscapes: provocative insights from epigenomics. *Nature Reviews Genetics, 9*, 465–476.

Szyf, M. (2009). Epigenetics, DNA methylation, and chromatin modifying drugs. *Annual Review of Pharmacology and Toxicology, 49*, 243–263.

Tahiliani, M., Koh, K. P., Shen, Y., Pastor, W. A., Bandukwala, H., Brudno, Y., et al. (2009). Conversion of 5-methylcytosine to 5-hydroxymethylcytosine in mammalian DNA by MLL partner TET1. *Science, 324*, 930–935.

Tobi, E. W., Lumey, L. H., Talens, R. P., Kremer, D., Putter, H., Stein, A. D., et al. (2009). DNA methylation differences after exposure to prenatal famine are common and timing- and sex-specific. *Human Molecular Genetics, 18*, 4046–4053.

Tomita, H., Vawter, M. P., Walsh, D. M., Evans, S. J., Choudary, P. V., Li, J., et al. (2004). Effect of agonal and postmortem factors on gene expression profile: quality control in microarray analyses of postmortem human brain. *Biological Psychiatry, 55*, 346–352.

Ubeda, F. & Wilkins, J. F. (2008). Imprinted genes and human disease: an evolutionary perspective. *Advances in Experimental Medicine and Biology, 626*, 101–115.

Urdinguio, R. G., Sanchez-Mut, J. V., & Esteller, M. (2009). Epigenetic mechanisms in neurological diseases: genes, syndromes, and therapies. *Lancet Neurology, 8*, 1056–1072.

van, V. J., Oates, N. A., & Whitelaw, E. (2007). Epigenetic mechanisms in the context of complex diseases. *Cellular and Molecular Life Sciences, 64*, 1531–1538.

Vawter, M. P., Tomita, H., Meng, F., Bolstad, B., Li, J., Evans, S., et al. (2006). Mitochondrial-related gene expression changes are sensitive to agonal-pH state: implications for brain disorders. *Molecular Psychiatry, 11, 615*, 663–679.

Visel, A., Blow, M. J., Li, Z., Zhang, T., Akiyama, J. A., Holt, A., et al. (2009). ChIP-seq accurately predicts tissue-specific activity of enhancers. *Nature, 457*, 854–858.

Vorstman, J. A. S., Staal, W. G., van, D. E., van, E. H., Hochstenbach, P. F. R., & Franke, L. (2006). Identification of novel autism candidate regions through analysis of reported cytogenetic abnormalities associated with autism. *Molecular Psychiatry, 11*, 18–28.

Waterland, R. A. & Jirtle, R. L. (2003). Transposable elements: targets for early nutritional effects on epigenetic gene regulation. *Molecular and Cellular Biology, 23*, 5293–5300.

Waterland, R. A. & Michels, K. B. (2007). Epigenetic epidemiology of the developmental origins hypothesis. *Annual Review of Nutrition, 27*, 363–388.

Weber, M. Davies, J. J., Wittig, D., Oakeley, E. J., Haase, M., Lam, W. L. (2005). Chromosome-wide and promoter-specific analyses identify sites of differential DNA methylation in normal and transformed human cells. *Nature Genetics, 37*, 853–862.

Weiss, L. A., Shen, Y., Korn, J. M., Arking, D. E., Miller, D. T., Fossdal, R., et al. (2008). Association between microdeletion and microduplication at 16p11.2 and autism. *New England Journal of Medicine, 358*, 667–675.

Weksberg, R., Shuman, C., & Beckwith, J. B. (2010). Beckwith-Wiedemann syndrome. *European Journal of Human Genetics, 18*, 8–14.

Wells, J. C. (2009). Maternal capital and the metabolic ghetto: An evolutionary perspective on the transgenerational basis of health inequalities. *American Journal of Human Biology, 22*, 1–17.

Wickner, R. B., Shewmaker, F., Kryndushkin, D., & Edskes, H. K. (2008). Protein inheritance (prions) based on parallel in-register beta-sheet amyloid structures. *Bioessays, 30*, 955–964.

Williams, T. M. & Carroll, S. B. (2009). Genetic and molecular insights into the development and evolution of sexual dimorphism. *Nature Reviews Genetics, 10*, 797–804.

Wolff, G. L., Kodell, R. L., Moore, S. R., & Cooney, C. A. (1998). Maternal epigenetics and methyl supplements affect agouti gene expression in Avy/a mice. *FASEB Journal, 12*, 949–957.

Xi, Y. & Li, W. (2009). BSMAP: whole genome bisulfite sequence MAPping program. *BMC Bioinformatics, 10*, 232.

Yamasaki, K., Joh, K., Ohta, T., Masuzaki, H., Ishimaru, T., Mukai, T., et al. (2003). Neurons but not glial cells show reciprocal imprinting of sense and antisense transcripts of Ube3a. *Human Molecular Genetics, 12*, 837–847.

Yoo, C. B., Chuang, J. C., Byun, H. M., Egger, G., Yang, A. S., Dubeau, L., et al. (2008). Long-term epigenetic therapy with oral zebularine has minimal side effects and prevents intestinal tumors in mice. *Cancer Prevention Research (Philadelphia, PA), 1*, 233–240.

Zhang, X., Chen, J., Radcliffe, T., Lebrun, D. P., Tron, V. A., & Feilotter, H. (2008). An array-based analysis of microRNA expression comparing matched frozen and formalin-fixed paraffin-embedded human tissue samples. *Journal of Molecular Diagnostics, 10*, 513–519.

Zhao, X., Leotta, A., Kustanovich, V., Lajonchere, C., Geschwind, D. H., Law, K., et al. (2007). A unified genetic theory for sporadic and inherited autism. *Proceedings of the National Academy of Sciences of the United States of America, 104*, 12,831–12,836.

43 Isolated Populations and Common Variants

Karola Rehnström, Leena Peltonen†

Points of Interest

- Isolated populations are characterized by a decrease in genetic heterogeneity, and this has been successfully used to identify genes underlying Mendelian disorders.
- The genetic risk for common disorders is conferred by a multitude of variants of which each only increases the risk of the disease marginally. These genetic variants are often common in the population and can be detected using genome-wide association studies (GWAS).
- Genome-wide association analyses have shown that for some complex disorders and traits, the genetic risk factors are more uniform in population isolates compared to outbred populations, thereby increasing the statistical power to detect them.
- Many of the genetic susceptibility factors identified in isolated populations have also been shown to confer risk in outbred populations, suggesting that the genetic risk factors for at least some phenotypes are similar in isolates and other populations.

Isolated Populations

Isolated populations are defined as populations originating from a small number of founders, experiencing only limited immigration, and where expansion has primarily taken place through population growth. The lack of immigration often results from either geographical or cultural isolation. These populations are also sometimes termed *founder populations.* The value of isolated populations in the identification of genes for Mendelian disorders can be considered to be undisputed, as numerous Mendelian genes have been identified in these special populations (*see also* Chapters 44 and 41, this volume). Examples include identification mutations in the connexin 26 gene in nonsyndromic deafness in the Bedouin population and genes for 35 Mendelian disorders in the Finns (Guilford et al., 1994; Carrasquillo et al., 1997; Norio, 2003a; Norio, 2003c). However, the possible advantage of using isolated populations in identification of genetic risk factors for complex traits has been highly debated, and only recent successes have validated the place of isolated populations in complex trait-mapping approaches.

Genetic Characteristics of Isolated Populations

The identifying characteristic of isolated populations is the reduced genetic diversity, which can be observed using uniparentally inherited mitochondrial DNA and Y chromosomal genetic markers, as well as autosomal data. The decrease of genetic diversity, which can still be observed in isolates today, is a direct consequence of the genetic bottleneck caused by the limited number of founders. Many population isolates have undergone multiple bottlenecks caused by famines, war, or internal migrations subsequent to founding. Recent, rapid population growth is a prerequisite for the population to be useful for genetic mapping, as an adequate number of affected individuals are available for genetic mapping of disorders or traits that have a low frequency in the population. The same demographic phenomena that give rise to decreased genetic diversity also result in extended linkage disequilibrium (LD) and increased homozygosity. The drastic reduction in population size in the form of one or several genetic bottlenecks during the population history has resulted in changes in the allele frequencies caused by genetic drift. In addition to differences in allele frequencies, the bottlenecks together with random drift have, in some populations, resulted in a distinctive pattern of disorders (Morton et al., 2003; Norio, 2003a; Charrow, 2004).

Linkage disequilibrium (LD) is the non-random association of alleles at two or more loci. Linkage disequilibrium can be observed as pairwise correlation between the allele frequencies of genetic markers.

Genetic bottleneck is an event in which the population size is drastically reduced. A type of genetic bottleneck termed a *founder effect* is an event in which a new population is established by a small random sample of the original population.

Genetic drift is the random change in relative frequency of alleles. Genetic drift is especially emphasized in small populations, where it can lead to drastic changes in allele frequency or even to fixation or total elimination of alleles.

Environmental Factors

In addition to genetic homogeneity, environmental and cultural factors often are also less heterogeneous in isolates compared to large, admixed populations. Factors such as shared language and religion increase social cohesion, which, in addition to a common education system, health care, and similar diet, minimizes the environmental heterogeneity. In many isolated populations, lifestyle choices can be affected by cultural customs or restrictions, which can in some cases be used beneficially in genetic mapping. In a study of genetic risk factors for asthma in the Hutterite population, the fact that smoking is prohibited and very rare reduced the variability in this environmental risk factor for the phenotype of interest (Ober et al., 2008). In many isolated populations, population registries or church parish records are available for genealogical studies, and allow construction of extended pedigrees with multiple affected individuals and identification of common founders for distantly related individuals.

Finland as an Example of the Archetypal Isolate

Finland is an example of a typical founder population that has undergone many of the population history events typical for isolates. The population history of Finns is well-known and corresponds well with the genetic substructure observed today (Sajantila et al., 1996; Kittles et al., 1999; Jakkula et al., 2008). The population was originally founded by a small number of individuals and has undergone multiple consecutive bottlenecks, resulting in reduction of genetic diversity. For thousands of years, only the coastal regions of the country were inhabited, settled originally thousands of years ago by two small settling groups with European and eastern Uralic origin. An internal migration, which took place only 500 to 600 years ago, resulted in the inhabitation of the sparsely populated eastern and northern regions of the country termed the *late settlement region* (Peltonen et al., 1999; Norio, 2003b). The youngest subisolates in northeastern Finland were first inhabited 300 to 400 years ago by a few dozen families and have remained almost entirely isolated until World War II. The Finnish population experienced a famine that, together with subsequent epidemics, killed approximately one-third of the 400,000 strong population in 1696 through 1698. After this, population growth has been rapid, starting from 250,000 in the late seventeenth century to the present population of more than 5 million. Population growth has occurred in relative isolation without major immigration because of the remote location of Finland, as well as cultural reasons resulting from the Finnish language, a part of the Uralic language family, which is not spoken elsewhere in Europe, with the exception of Hungary and Estonia (Varilo et al., 2000; Varilo et al., 2003). As groups inhabiting the late settlement region have been small, and new settlements were geographically isolated, the internal migration has formed classical bottleneck effects, which together with isolation have resulted in significant population structure observed today (Jakkula et al., 2008).

The unique population history of Finland has led to enrichment of certain alleles and extinction of others by genetic drift. This has resulted in a unique pattern of disorders, consisting of 36 Mendelian, mostly recessive disorders that are overrepresented compared to any other population. These disorders are often referred to as the Finnish disease heritage. The genes for all but one of these disorders have been identified, and for most disorders one major mutation accounting for all—or a significant subset of—cases have been identified. Further, some Mendelian disorders common in European populations, such as phenylketonuria and cystic fibrosis, are absent from Finland (Norio, 2003a). The publicly available health-care system provides equal health care across the country and detailed, standardized medical records for careful delineation of the phenotype of interest. The training in medical schools across the country is highly uniform, resulting in highly standardized diagnostic criteria in all hospitals across the country. Population registries cover several centuries and make it possible to trace genealogical connections across dozens of generations as well as information about geographical origins of the genetic variants.

Complex Disorders

Complex, or common, disorders are caused by multiple genetic risk factors, of which each only increases risk marginally, but a large number of genetic susceptibility variants together with environmental risk factors result in the disorder. The first steps in the elucidation of the genetic mechanisms responsible for complex disorders were taken when the Human Genome Project deciphered the sequence of the human genome (Lander et al., 2001; Venter et al., 2001). Following the completion of the human sequence, another colossal project, the International HapMap project, aimed to characterize the variation in the human genome in European, African, and Asian populations (The International HapMap Consortium, 2005; Frazer et al., 2007). As a result of these efforts, millions of variants in the human genome, termed *single nucleotide polymorphisms* (SNPs), have been identified. The HapMap project mainly aimed to characterize SNPs that are commonly observed in populations, but genome-wide sequencing efforts feasible today have drastically increased the rate at SNP detection and also have enabled the identification of SNPs that are rare in the population or even private to single individuals (Levy et al., 2007; Wang et al., 2008; Wheeler et al., 2008).

Single nucleotide polymorphism (SNP) is a form of DNA sequence variation where two nucleotides differing between individuals in a population occur at the same position in the genome.

The International HapMap project is a large collaborative project aiming to identify and characterize genetic similarities and differences in human beings (www.hapmap.org). In the first stage, four populations (a population with Northern European descent, a Japanese population, a Chinese population, and the African Yoruba population) were included, but in subsequent stages, several populations have been added to the project.

The term common SNP refers to a SNP with a high minor allele frequency (>5%) in the population, whereas SNPs with a low (<1%) minor allele frequency are termed *rare*. Current genetic mapping methods enable identification of rare variants with a high impact on the phenotype of interest, as well as SNPs with a small impact on the phenotype if they are common enough in the population. A multitude of rare SNPs probably also confer small effects on susceptibility to disorders, but statistical power of current methods does not allow for identification of this type of variation.

Genetic Architecture of Complex Disorders

Primarily, two opposing but complementary hypotheses exist concerning the genetic model of complex disorders (Reich & Lander, 2001; Bodmer & Bonilla, 2008). The role of rare variants in common disorders proposes that the disorders are caused by a small number of variants, each with a large effect on the phenotype with a low frequency (<1%) in the population (*see* Chapter 41, this volume). Rare variants are often population-specific, as founder effects have established different rare variants in each population. Approaches to identify rare variants include linkage analysis and resequencing of interesting candidate genes in large families with multiple affected individuals and possibly other distinct clinical features such as early age of onset. A review of 61 rare variants identified in complex disorders has shown that rare variants are associated with odds ratios ranging from 1.1 to more than 5, with the percentage of variants increasing toward the high end of the odds ratio spectrum, and the mean odds ratio is 3.74 (Bodmer & Bonilla, 2008).

Odds ratio is a measure of effect size. In genetic studies, the odds ratio often refers to the odds of having a disorder for an individual carrying a specific genetic variant relative to individuals not carrying the genetic variant.

The common variant hypothesis proposes that common disorders are caused by the interaction of numerous small effect variants, which are all common in the population. The assumption that common variants comprise risk factors for common disorders has been termed the *common disease-common variant hypothesis* (Lander, 1996; Chakravarti, 1999). The smaller the effect size of the SNP, the larger the study set needed to obtain statistically significant results. Of 217 common variants affecting complex phenotypes summarized by Bodmer and Bonilla (2008), most odds ratios are smaller than 2, and the mean odds ratio is 1.36.

Usually the genetic architecture for complex disorders displays components of both rare and common risk variants (*see also* Chapter 38, this volume). Here, isolates can offer a significant advantage as pedigrees with multiple affected individuals can be ascertained, suggesting inheritance closer to a monogenic model, with rare high-impact variants, implicating candidate genes that can subsequently be tested in the general population. This approach was used to identify genes underlying familial combined hyperlipidemia, a disorder where multiple types of dyslipidemia co-occur and result in significant risk of premature coronary heart disease. Initially, linkage to 1q21 through q23 was identified in Finnish families with familial combined hyperlipidemia (Pajukanta et al., 1998). Finmapping using SNPs in three genes in the linked region identified *USF1* as the susceptibility gene for familial combined hyperlipidemia (Pajukanta et al., 2004). Subsequently, variants in *USF1* have been shown to confer susceptibility for common disorders such as coronary heart disease and metabolic phenotypes in both Finns and other populations (Komulainen et al., 2006; Holzapfel et al., 2008; Kristiansson et al., 2008; Meex et al., 2008).

Dyslipidemia is an abnormal level of lipids in the blood.

Genome-Wide Association Studies

During the last few years, the combination of novel, high-throughput genotyping methods and careful characterization of the variation in the genome have made it possible to conduct hypothesis-free GWAS in large populations to identify genetic determinants for common disorders, as proposed by Risch and Merikangas (1996) more than a decade ago in a seminal paper. The results obtained from the HapMap project in the form of catalogs of frequencies of variants in the genome and their pairwise correlation (LD) have been imperative for the progress of this gene-mapping method. By screening a sufficiently large number of SNPs (usually hundreds of thousands or millions), the common variants in the whole genome can be tagged by these SNPs through LD. SNPs where allele frequencies show statistically significant deviations between cases and controls indicate genes or chromosomal regions affecting the trait of interest. This is referred to as a GWAS, and it enables identification of genetic risk factors for disorders and traits without *a priori* hypothesis of the genes or biological processes involved in the phenotype. Although the early GWAS did not always produce reproducible results, when sample sizes were increased to provide adequate power to detect the common, low-impact variants, replicated genetic risk factors were identified for a multitude of phenotypes, and meta-analysis of existing data sets provided further novel susceptibility variants (Wellcome Trust Case Control Consortium (WTCCC), 2007; Cooper et al., 2008; Zeggini et al., 2008; Aulchenko et al., 2009).

Successes in Identification of Common Variants in Isolated Populations

Before GWAS became standard practice, the biggest advantage conferred by isolated populations was envisaged to be the increased LD, as a smaller number of markers would be needed to tag the entire genome (Shifman & Darvasi, 2001; Service et al., 2006). However, today this gain is mostly theoretical, as genotyping is performed using predesigned SNP sets, which have been chosen to tag the majority of allelic variation in the genomes of outbred European populations. It is therefore not surprising that tagSNPs chosen using the HapMap European population perform well in several isolates (Service et al., 2007). However, it has been suggested that the tagging power of these SNPs, even for rare haplotypes, is better in isolated populations because of the excess of information provided by the off-the-shelf genotyping chips in populations with high LD.

The more significant value of isolated populations in genetic mapping of complex disorders is the reduced genetic variability, which has resulted in enrichment of a subset of susceptibility alleles in the population compared to outbred populations. As isolates have undergone bottlenecks during the population history, the susceptibility variants often reside on a more homogenous haplotypic background compared to mixed populations (Figure 43-1). The enrichment of certain susceptibility variants will require fewer individuals to find theses shared genetic factors. In the following, as well as in Table 43-1, a few examples illustrating the power of isolated populations in complex gene identification are presented.

Haplotype is the combination of alleles at multiple loci, which are transmitted together on the same chromosome.

One of the success-stories of common variant mapping in isolates have been provided by data from the Icelandic company deCODE genetics. The combination of extensive genotype and phenotype data from a significant proportion of the inhabitants of the entire country with extensive genealogical records has led to the identification of numerous susceptibility variants for complex disorders and traits. Iceland was populated approximately 1000 years ago, and the genetic roots of the current population can be traced back to Scandinavia and the British Isles, resulting in admixture at the time of founding (Helgason et al., 2001). The population has undergone several bottlenecks caused by diseases and famine and has grown rapidly in the last 100 years to the present size of 320,000. Data from studies of mitochondrial DNA suggests that the population has undergone considerable and rapid genetic drift, resulting in decrease of genetic diversity characteristic of isolated populations (Helgason et al., 2003, 2009). Genome-wide linkage analysis and GWAS have identified common genetic risk variants for multiple phenotypes, including atrial fibrillation and ischemic stroke (Gudbjartsson et al., 2007; Gretarsdottir et al., 2008), bone mineral density and fractures (Styrkarsdottir et al., 2008, 2009), essential tremor (Stefansson et al., 2009), glaucoma (Thorleifsson et al., 2007), multiple types of cancer (Gudmundsson et al., 2007a, 2007b; Stacey et al., 2007; Goldstein et al., 2008; Gudmundsson et al., 2008; Stacey et al., 2008; Rafnar et al., 2009), pigmentation (Sulem et al., 2008), myocardial infarction and aneurysms (Helgadottir et al., 2007, 2008), and type 2 diabetes (Grant et al., 2006). In these studies, the genomic control method was used to control for population structure and relatedness (Helgason et al., 2005). In some studies, previously identified linkage peaks in the same population were used to prioritize regions for follow-up in cases where no genome-wide significant results were identified in the primary stage of the GWAS.

In a study utilizing the combined power of linkage and association, individuals from the Croatian island of Vis were

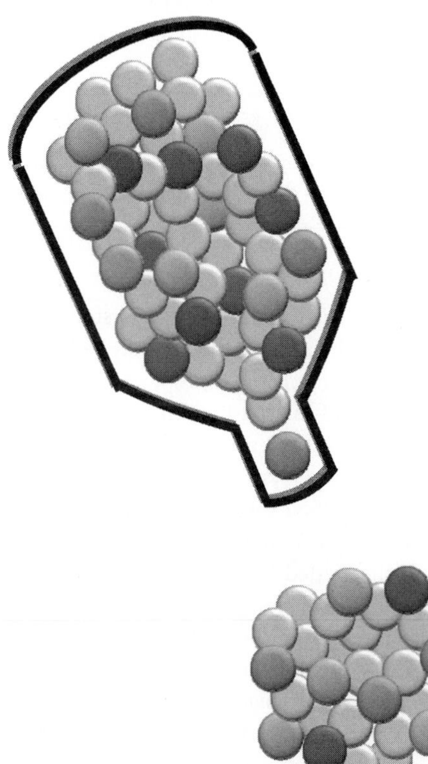

Figure 43–1. The genetic risk factors for complex traits are heterogenous in outbred populations (top). When an isolate is founded, the population goes through a genetic bottleneck, and a random selection of the original genetic risk factors are present in the new subpopulation. If the founder population is small, then random effects caused by genetic drift are accentuated. Some of the original genetic risk factors are eliminated and others are significantly enriched compared to the founder population. (See Color Plate Section for a color version of this figure.)

Table 43–1.
Examples of isolates used in genome-wide linkage or association studies of complex phenotypes

Population	Age	Phenotypes	References
Amish	250	Bipolar disorder, blood pressure, type 2 diabetes	Ginns et al., 1996; Hsueh et al., 2000; Rampersaud et al., 2007; McArdle et al., 2008
Antioquia (Colombia), Central Valley of Costa Rica	300–400	Bipolar disorder	Herzberg et al., 2006; Jasinska et al., 2009
Ashkenazi	2000	Breast cancer	Gold et al., 2008
Azores (Portugal)	650	Schizophrenia	Sklar et al., 2004
Finland	300–2000	Schizophrenia, multiple sclerosis, familial combined hyperlipidemia, asthma, fasting glucose levels, height	Hovatta et al., 1999; Laitinen et al., 2004; Pajukanta et al., 2004; Chen et al., 2008; Sanna et al., 2008; Kallio et al., 2009
French Canadians	300–400	Coronary heart disease, Crohn's disease	Raelson, et al., 2007; Engert et al., 2008
Hutterites	100	Asthma	Ober et al., 1998; Ober et al., 2008
Iceland	1000	Bone mineral density, breast cancer, myocardial infarction, exfoliation glaucoma, height, prostate cancer, type 2 diabetes	Gudmundsson et al., 2007; Helgadottir et al., 2007; Steinthorsdottir et al., 2007; Thorleifsson et al., 2007; Gudbjartsson et al., 2008; Stacey et al., 2008; Styrkarsdottir et al., 2008
Northern Sweden	350	Familial prostate cancer, affective disorders	Berthon et al., 1998; Venken et al., 2005
Pima Indians	>10,000	Diabetes, BMI, early onset type 2 diabetes	Hanson et al., 1998; Hanson et al., 2007
Sardinia	3000	Asthma, height, obesity, fasting gluciose levels	Balaci et al., 2007; Scuteri et al., 2007; Chen et al., 2008; Sanna et al., 2008
The Netherlands, subisolate	<400	Parkinsons	Bertoli-Avella et al., 2006
Vis (Croatia)	>1000	Systolic blood pressure, serum urate concentration, serum creatinine, anthropometric traits	Vitart et al., 2009; Barbali et al., 2009; Polašek et al., 2009

used to identify genetic variants affecting systolic and diastolic blood pressure, as this isolated population had a high prevalence of hypertension (Kolcic et al., 2006). Vis is a remote island in the Adriatic Sea off the coast of Croatia, which has experienced several bottlenecks during its history. In this study, first a genome-wide QTL analysis for systolic blood pressure was performed, and then SNPs were tested for association in the linkage peaks in the Vis population. The 15 most significant SNPs were further tested for association in the British 1958 Birth Cohort, and association was replicated for two SNPs. The SNP showing most significant association to systolic blood pressure, located close to potassium voltage gate channel gene (*KCNB1*), showed a much bigger effect size in the Vis data than in the British 1958 Birth Cohort (Barbalic et al., 2009).

The identification of genetic risk factors for complex disorders in isolated populations has raised the question of the validity of these risk variants in outbred populations. GWAS have shown that many of the genetic susceptibility factors identified in GWASs conducted in isolated populations can be replicated in outbred populations. The North American Hutterite population was founded by only 62 individuals, and current individuals can be linked to these founders through multiple lines of descent in a 13-generation pedigree. This population has remained genetically isolated through cultural isolation from the rest of the North American population. The communal lifestyle of the Hutterites ensures a highly similar environment, decreasing the variance in any environmental risk factors. A GWAS was performed in 753 Hutterites to identify genetic factors affecting the serum level of chitinase-like protein (YKL-40), which is linked with asthma. The most significantly associated SNP was found in the promoter of the *CHI3L1* gene encoding the YKL-40 protein. This SNP was subsequently shown to be associated with asthma, bronchial hyperresponsiveness, and measures of pulmonary function in very small data sets consisting of 63 to 121 individuals from the Hutterite population. Further, the same SNP was found to be associated with asthma in two bigger data sets from populations of European descent (Ober et al., 2008).

Similar results, suggesting that genetic risk factors identified in isolates can be extended to other populations, were obtained in a GWAS for lipid levels comprising close to 5000 individuals from the late-settlement region of Finland. Several of the identified risk loci had been reported previously in other populations. In addition, six novel loci were identified. Larger data sets will be needed to determine whether these variants represent isolate specific risk variants or if they can be replicated in larger data sets (Sabatti et al., 2009).

Careful characterization of the population structure is imperative for the most efficient study design for GWAS. The available genetic data, combined with careful genealogical data, have shown distinct substructure in isolates such as Finns and Icelanders (Helgason et al., 2005; Jakkula et al., 2008). In Finland, the aggregation of grandparents of individuals affected with rare Mendelian disorders is well-documented, but some subisolates also have shown higher frequencies of complex disorders (Hovatta et al., 1997; Sumelahti et al., 2001). With proper selection of cases and controls, this approach has proved successful in mapping genetic risk factors for complex disorders. The prevalence of multiple sclerosis (MS) is twice as high in an internal subisolate of Finland compared to the rest of the country (Sumelahti et al., 2001). Using available genealogical data and carefully matched controls originating from the same, geographically limited region, two risk genes were identified using only 68 individuals connected to two large pedigrees having common ancestors 14 to 16 generations ago. The first risk haplotype, located under a previously identified linkage peak at chromosome 5p, identified complement component 7 (C7) as a genetic risk factor for MS. The haplotype association was replicated in an independent sample from the same Finnish subisolate, and the risk haplotype correlates with increased expression of C7. A trend toward association was also observed in other European populations, suggesting that the risk variant has been enriched in the internal isolate but conferring susceptibility to MS in other populations as well (Kallio et al., 2009). Subsequently, the same Finnish subisolate was used to identify a SNP in signal transducer and activator of transcription 3 (*STAT3*) gene conferring susceptibility to MS. This finding was replicated in several data sets, including MS cases both from Finland and other populations (Jakkula et al., 2009). In these studies, the careful selection of geographically matched cases and controls was imperative for the identification of the risk loci, as preliminary analysis using less strictly matched controls did not result in findings that could be replicated in other data sets.

The successes of these studies are all based on careful study design utilizing the enrichment of certain susceptibility alleles that have been originally carried to the isolates by random founder effect and enriched by genetic drift. The power of combining linkage with association, in the form of extended haplotypes or IBD sharing, has enabled identification of risk variants in relatively small sample sizes. Although many of the identified risk variants have also been identified to confer susceptibility in outbred populations, the enrichment of the risk allele in the isolates enabled their identification using relatively small sample sizes.

Challenges in Genetic Mapping in Isolates

Although isolated populations provide excellent opportunities for identification of genetic risk factors for genetic disorders, there are some drawbacks that need to be considered in the study design stage. As isolated populations are usually smaller than outbred populations, it should be established that a large enough cohort of affected individuals can be ascertained from the population, considering the frequency of the trait of interest and the size of the population. One of the drawbacks often encountered when the initial region of interest has been identified is the LD structure. Although extended LD can be helpful in initial localization of the risk loci, it can make it harder to identify causative variants within the block of strong LD. Therefore, it might be beneficial to include a more admixed population in the fine mapping stage of the study where LD blocks are shorter. Replication of initial findings can prove to be challenging, especially if the isolate is small and the disorder is rare, as all available samples have already been used in the initial mapping effort. It should also be noted that replication will not be observed using highly strict criteria for statistical significance if the risk variant is significantly enriched in the isolate, and only confers a small risk in the replication population. However, even if the effect of the variant is limited to the isolate, characterization of these risk variants can prove to be beneficial in other populations, as it could help understanding of the underlying biology of the trait.

The assumption that high-impact variants are enriched in founder populations is not always true. A recent study of genetic risk factors with metabolic phenotypes in the Kosrae population revealed a similar spectrum of genetic risk variants compared to other, more outbred, populations. The Kosrae, a native population of the Federated States of Micronesia, display both decreased genetic diversity and extended LD resulting from founder effects and multiple bottlenecks (Bonnen et al., 2006). In common with many other populations worldwide, the prevalence of obesity and metabolic disorders is increasing in this population (Shmulewitz et al., 2001). An effort was initiated to identify genes for these disorders in the Kosrae hypothesizing that founder effects, bottlenecks, and genetic drift have concentrated a small number of high-impact genetic risk variants in this population. In the study, simulation studies showed that the study design provided ample power to identify common alleles explaining 5% or more of the variation in the phenotype. However, no common genetic risk factors for metabolic traits were identified in this population. The results suggest that even in a highly inbred population such as the Kosrae, for many quantiative phenotypes, common alleles only have a modest effect and no enriched risk variants exist (Lowe et al., 2009).

Conclusions

Isolated populations have been used successfully in genetic mapping of Mendelian disorders because of the reduced genetic heterogeneity. Emerging results from GWAS suggest that for some phenotypes, isolated populations also offer advantages in mapping of common genetic risk factors. As each isolate is uniquely different because of different demographic histories, careful characterization of the population substructure is crucial for optimal study design. Encouragingly, several studies have shown that the genetic risk factors originally identified in the isolates were replicated in outbred populations, validating the role of isolated populations as a useful tool in genetic mapping studies.

Challenges and Future Directions

- It is already clear from the GWAS performed to date that the genetic architecture for complex traits ranges from being controlled by highly penetrant rare variants to common, low-risk variants. The characterization of the genetic architecture of specific traits and disorders is incomplete, and future studies will show if it will differ between populations.
- Although many studies have shown that genetic risk factors for complex disorders identified in isolates can be generalized to more outbred populations, the role of isolate specific risk variants remains poorly understood. It will also be challenging to replicate isolate-specific findings, as sample sizes are usually limited.
- The characterization of genetic risk factors for complex disorders using GWAS is only the first step of understanding the role these variants play in the etiology of the disease. The next step will be to pinpoint the actual causative variants and to functionally characterize their role in the biological processes involved in the phenotype of interest. Whether isolated populations can aid in this step as well (e.g., as a result of the homogenous environmental factors) remains to be discovered.

SUGGESTED READING

Arcos-Burgos M, Muenke M. (2002). Genetics of population isolates. *Clinical Genetics, 61*, 233–247.

Kristiansson K, Naukkarinen J, Peltonen L. (2008). Isolated populations and complex disease gene identification. *Genome Biology, 9*, 109.

Peltonen L, Palotie A, Lange K. (2000). Use of Population Isolates for Mapping Complex Traits. *Nature Reviews Genetics, 1*, 182–190.

REFERENCES

Aulchenko YS, Ripatti S, Lindqvist I, Boomsma D, Heid IM, Pramstaller PP, et al. (2009). Loci influencing lipid levels and coronary heart disease risk in 16 European population cohorts. *Nature Genetics, 41*, 47–55.

Balaci L, Spada MC, Olla N, Sole G, Loddo L, Anedda F, et al. (2007). IRAK-M is involved in the pathogenesis of early-onset persistent asthma. *American Journal of Human Genetics, 80*, 1103–1114.

Barbali M, Smolej Narani N, Kari-Juri T, Perii Salihovi M, Martinovi Klari E, Bara Lauc L, et al. (2009). A Quantitative Trait Locus for SBP Maps Near KCNB1 and PTGIS in a Population Isolate. *American Journal of Hypertension, 22*, 663–668.

Barbalić M, Narancić NS, Skarić-Jurić T, Salihović MP, Klarić IM, Lauc LB, et al. (2009). A quantitative trait locus for SBP maps near KCNB1 and PTGIS in a population isolate. *American Journal of Hypertension, 22*, 663–668.

Berthon P, Valeri A, Cohen-Akenine A, Drelon E, Paiss T, Wöhr G, et al. (1998). Predisposing gene for early-onset prostate cancer, localized on chromosome 1q42.2-43. *American Journal of Human Genetics, 62*, 1416–1424.

Bertoli-Avella AM, Dekker MC, Aulchenko YS, Houwing-Duistermaat JJ, Simons E, Testers L, et al. (2006). Evidence for novel loci for late-onset Parkinson's disease in a genetic isolate from the Netherlands. *Human Genetics, 119*, 51–60.

Bodmer W, Bonilla C. (2008). Common and rare variants in multifactorial susceptibility to common diseases. *Nature Genetics, 40*, 695–701.

Bonnen PE, Pe'er I, Plenge RM, Salit J, Lowe JK, Shapero MH, et al. (2006). Evaluating potential for whole-genome studies in Kosrae, an isolated population in Micronesia. *Nature Genetics, 38*, 214–217.

Carrasquillo MM, Zlotogora J, Barges S, Chakravarti A. (1997). Two different connexin 26 mutations in an inbred kindred segregating non-syndromic recessive deafness: implications for genetic studies in isolated populations. *Human Molecular Genetics, 6*, 2163–2172.

Chakravarti A. (1999). Population genetics—making sense out of sequence. *Nature Genetics, 21*, 56–60.

Charrow, J. (2004). Ashkenazi Jewish genetic disorders. *Familial Cancer, 3*, 201–206.

Chen WM, Erdos MR, Jackson AU, Saxena R, Sanna S, Silver KD, et al. (2008). Variations in the G6PC2/ABCB11 genomic region are associated with fasting glucose levels. *European Journal of Clinical Investigation, 118*, 2620–2628.

Cooper JD, Smyth DJ, Smiles AM, Plagnol V, Walker NM, Allen JE, et al. (2008). Meta-analysis of genome-wide association study data identifies additional type 1 diabetes risk loci. *Nature Genetics, 40*, 1399–1401.

Engert JC, Lemire M, Faith J, Brisson D, Fujiwara TM, Roslin NM, et al. (2008). Identification of a chromosome 8p locus for early-onset coronary heart disease in a French Canadian population. *European Journal of Human Genetics, 16*, 105–114.

Frazer KA, Ballinger DG, Cox DR, Hinds DA, Stuve LL, Gibbs RA, et al. (2007). A second generation human haplotype map of over 3.1 million SNPs. *Nature, 449*, 851–861.

Ginns EI, Ott J, Egeland JA, Allen CR, Fann CS, Pauls DL, et al. (1996). A genome-wide search for chromosomal loci linked to bipolar affective disorder in the Old Order Amish. *Nature Genetics, 12*, 431–435.

Gold B, Kirchhoff T, Stefanov S, Lautenberger J, Viale A, Garber J, et al. (2008). Genome-wide association study provides evidence for a breast cancer risk locus at 6q22.33. *Proceedings of National Academy of Sciences of the United States of America, 105*, 4340–4435.

Goldstein AM, Stacey SN, Olafsson JH, Jonsson GF, Helgason A, Sulem P, et al. (2008). CDKN2A mutations and melanoma risk in the Icelandic population. *Journal of Medical Genetics, 45*, 284–289.

Grant SF, Thorleifsson G, Reynisdottir I, Benediktsson R, Manolescu A, Sainz J, et al. (2006). Variant of transcription factor 7-like 2 (TCF7L2) gene confers risk of type 2 diabetes. *Nature Genetics, 38*, 320–323.

Gretarsdottir S, Thorleifsson G, Manolescu A, Styrkarsdottir U, Helgadottir A, Gschwendtner A, et al. (2008). Risk variants for atrial fibrillation on chromosome 4q25 associate with ischemic stroke. *Annuals of Neurology*, *64*, 402–409.

Gudbjartsson DF, Arnar DO, Helgadottir A, Gretarsdottir S, Holm H, Sigurdsson A, et al. (2007). Variants conferring risk of atrial fibrillation on chromosome 4q25. *Nature*, *448*, 353–357.

Gudbjartsson DF, Walters GB, Thorleifsson G, Stefansson H, Halldorsson BV, Zusmanovich P, et al. (2008). Many sequence variants affecting diversity of adult human height. *Nature Genetics*, *40*, 609–615.

Gudmundsson J, Sulem P, Manolescu A, Amundadottir LT, Gudbjartsson D, Helgason A, et al. (2007a). Genome-wide association study identifies a second prostate cancer susceptibility variant at 8q24. *Nature Genetics*, *39*, 631–637.

Gudmundsson J, Sulem P, Steinthorsdottir V, Bergthorsson JT, Thorleifsson G, Manolescu A, et al. (2007b). Two variants on chromosome 17 confer prostate cancer risk, and the one in TCF2 protects against type 2 diabetes. *Nature Genetics*, *39*, 977–983.

Gudmundsson J, Sulem P, Rafnar T, Bergthorsson JT, Manolescu A, Gudbjartsson D, et al. (2008). Common sequence variants on 2p15 and Xp11.22 confer susceptibility to prostate cancer. *Nature Genetics*, *40*, 281–283.

Guilford P, Ben Arab S, Blanchard S, Levilliers J, Weissenbach J, Belkahia A, et al. (1994). A non-syndrome form of neurosensory, recessive deafness maps to the pericentromeric region of chromosome 13q. *Nature Genetics*, *6*, 24–28.

Hanson RL, Bogardus C, Duggan D, Kobes S, Knowlton M, Infante AM, et al. (2007). A search for variants associated with young-onset type 2 diabetes in American Indians in a 100K genotyping array. *Diabetes*, *56*, 3045–3052.

Hanson RL, Ehm MG, Pettitt DJ, Prochazka M, Thompson DB, Timberlake D, et al. (1998). An autosomal genomic scan for loci linked to type II diabetes mellitus and body-mass index in Pima Indians. *American Journal of Human Genetics*, *63*, 1130–1138.

Helgadottir A, Thorleifsson G, Magnusson KP, Grétarsdottir S, Steinthorsdottir V, Manolescu A, et al. (2008). The same sequence variant on 9p21 associates with myocardial infarction, abdominal aortic aneurysm and intracranial aneurysm. *Nature Genetics*, *40*, 217–224.

Helgadottir A, Thorleifsson G, Manolescu A, Gretarsdottir S, Blondal T, Jonasdottir A, et al. (2007). A common variant on chromosome 9p21 affects the risk of myocardial infarction. *Science*, *316*, 1491–1493.

Helgason A, Hickey E, Goodacre S, Bosnes V, Stefánsson K, Ward R, et al. (2001). mtDna and the islands of the North Atlantic: estimating the proportions of Norse and Gaelic ancestry. *American Journal of Human Genetics*, *68*, 723–737.

Helgason A, Lalueza-Fox C, Ghosh S, Sigurethardóttir S, Sampietro ML, Gigli E, et al. (2009). Sequences from first settlers reveal rapid evolution in Icelandic mtDNA pool. *PLoS Genetics*, *5*, e1000343.

Helgason A, Nicholson G, Stefánsson K, Donnelly P. (2003). A reassessment of genetic diversity in Icelanders: strong evidence from multiple loci for relative homogeneity caused by genetic drift. *Annual Human Genetics*, *67*, 281–297.

Helgason A, Yngvadóttir B, Hrafnkelsson B, Gulcher J, Stefánsson K. (2005). An Icelandic example of the impact of population structure on association studies. *Nature Genetics*, *37*, 90–95.

Herzberg I, Jasinska A, García J, Jawaheer D, Service S, Kremeyer B, et al. (2006). Convergent linkage evidence from two Latin-American population isolates supports the presence of a susceptibility locus for bipolar disorder in 5q31-34. *Human Molecular Genetics*, *15*, 3146–3153.

Holzapfel C, Baumert J, Grallert H, Müller AM, Thorand B, Khuseyinova N, et al. (2008). Genetic variants in the USF1 gene are associated with low-density lipoprotein cholesterol levels and incident type 2 diabetes mellitus in women: results from the MONICA/KORA Augsburg case-cohort study, 1984-2002. *European Journal of Endocrinology*, *159*, 407–416.

Hovatta I, Terwilliger JD, Lichtermann D, Mäkikyrö T, Suvisaari J, Peltonen L, et al. (1997). Schizophrenia in the genetic isolate of Finland. *American Journal of Medical Genetics*, *74*, 353–360.

Hovatta I, Varilo T, Suvisaari J, Terwilliger JD, Ollikainen V, Arajärvi R, et al. (1999). A genomewide screen for schizophrenia genes in an isolated Finnish subpopulation, suggesting multiple susceptibility loci. *American Journal of Human Genetics*, *65*, 1114–1124.

Hsueh WC, Mitchell BD, Schneider JL, Wagner MJ, Bell CJ, Nanthakumar E, et al. (2000). QTL influencing blood pressure maps to the region of PPH1 on chromosome 2q31-34 in Old Order Amish. *Circulation*, *101*, 2810–2816.

Jakkula E, Rehnström K, Varilo T, Pietiläinen OP, Paunio T, Pedersen NL, et al. (2008). The Genome-wide Patterns of Variation Expose Significant Substructure in a Founder Population. *American Journal of Human Genetics*, *83*, 787–794.

Jakkula E, Leppä V, Sulonen A, Varilo T, Kallio S, Kemppinen A, et al. (2010). Genome-wide association study in a high-risk isolate for multiple sclerosis reveals associated variants in STAT3 gene. *American Journal of Human Genetics*, 86, 285–291.

Jasinska AJ, Service S, Jawaheer D, DeYoung J, Levinson M, Zhang Z, et al. (2009). A narrow and highly significant linkage signal for severe bipolar disorder in the chromosome 5q33 region in Latin American pedigrees. *American Journal of Medical Genetics. Part B, Neuropsychiatric Genetics*, *150B*, 998–1006.

Kallio SP, Jakkula E, Purcell S, Suvela M, Koivisto K, Tienari PJ, et al. (2009). Use of a Genetic Isolate to Identify Rare Disease Variants: C7 on 5p associated with MS. *Human Molecular Genetics*, *18*, 1670–1683.

Kittles RA, Bergen AW, Urbanek M, Virkkunen M, Linnoila M, Goldman D, et al. (1999). Autosomal, mitochondrial, and Y chromosome DNA variation in Finland: evidence for a male-specific bottleneck. *American Journal of Physical Anthropology*, *108*, 381–399.

Kolcić I, Vorko-Jović A, Salzer B, Smoljanović M, Kern J, Vuletić S. (2006). Metabolic syndrome in a metapopulation of Croatian island isolates. *Croatian Medical Journal*, *47*, 585–592.

Komulainen K, Alanne M, Auro K, Kilpikari R, Pajukanta P, Saarela J, et al. (2006). Risk alleles of USF1 gene predict cardiovascular disease of women in two prospective studies. *PLoS Genetics*, *2*, e69.

Kristiansson K, Ilveskoski E, Lehtimäki T, Peltonen L, Perola M, Karhunen PJ. (2008). Association analysis of allelic variants of USF1 in coronary atherosclerosis. *Arteriosclerosis, Thrombosis, and Vascular Biology*, *28*, 983–989.

Laitinen T, Polvi A, Rydman P, Vendelin J, Pulkkinen V, Salmikangas P, et al. (2004). Characterization of a common susceptibility locus for asthma-related traits. *Science*, *304*, 300–304.

Lander ES. (1996). The new genomics: global views of biology. *Science*, *274*, 536–359.

Lander ES, Linton LM, Birren B, Nusbaum C, Zody MC, Baldwin J, et al. (2001). Initial sequencing and analysis of the human genome. *Nature, 409*, 860–921.

Levy S, Sutton G, Ng PC, Feuk L, Halpern AL, Walenz BP, et al. (2007). The diploid genome sequence of an individual human. *PLoS Biology*, 5, e254.

Lowe JK, Maller JB, Pe'er I, Neale BM, Salit J, Kenny EE, et al. (2009). "Genome-wide association studies in an isolated founder population from the Pacific Island of Kosrae." *PLoS Genetics* 5(2), e1000365.

McArdle PF, Rutherford S, Mitchell BD, Damcott CM, Wang Y, Ramachandran V, et al. (2008). Nicotinic acetylcholine receptor subunit variants are associated with blood pressure; findings in the Old Order Amish and replication in the Framingham Heart Study. *BMC Medical Genetics, 9*, 67.

Meex SJ, van Vliet-Ostaptchouk JV, van der Kallen CJ, van Greevenbroek MM, Schalkwijk CG, Feskens EJ, et al. (2008). Upstream transcription factor 1 (USF1) in risk of type 2 diabetes: association study in 2000 Dutch Caucasians. *Molecular Genetics and Metabolism, 94*, 352–355.

Morton DH, Morton CS, Strauss KA, Robinson DL, Puffenberger EG, Hendrickson C, et al. (2003). Pediatric medicine and the genetic disorders of the Amish and Mennonite people of Pennsylvania. *American Journal of Medical Genetics. Part C, Seminars in Medical Genetics, 121C*, 5–17.

Norio, R. (2003a). Finnish Disease Heritage I: characteristics, causes, background. *Human Genetics, 112*, 441–456.

Norio, R. (2003b). Finnish Disease Heritage II: population prehistory and genetic roots of Finns. *Human Genetics, 112*, 457–469.

Norio, R. (2003c). The Finnish Disease Heritage III: the individual diseases. *Human Genetics, 112*, 470–526.

Ober C, Cox NJ, Abney M, Di Rienzo A, Lander ES, Changyaleket B, et al. (1998). Genome-wide search for asthma susceptibility loci in a founder population. The Collaborative Study on the Genetics of Asthma. *Human Molecular Genetics, 7*, 1393–1398.

Ober C, Tan Z, Sun Y, Possick JD, Pan L, Nicolae R, et al. (2008). Effect of variation in CHI3L1 on serum YKL-40 level, risk of asthma, and lung function. *New England Journal of Medicine, 358*, 1682–1691.

Pajukanta P, Lilja HE, Sinsheimer JS, Cantor RM, Lusis AJ, Gentile M, et al. (2004). Familial combined hyperlipidemia is associated with upstream transcription factor 1 (USF1). *Nature Genetics, 36*, 371–376.

Pajukanta P, Nuotio I, Terwilliger JD, Porkka KV, Ylitalo K, Pihlajamäki J, et al. (1998). Linkage of familial combined hyperlipidaemia to chromosome 1q21-q23. *Nature Genetics, 18*, 369–373.

Peltonen L, Jalanko A, Varilo T. (1999). Molecular genetics of the Finnish disease heritage. *Human Molecular Genetics, 8*, 1913–1923.

Polasek O, Marusić A, Rotim K, Hayward C, Vitart V, Huffman J, et al. (2009). Genome-wide association study of anthropometric traits in Korcula Island, Croatia. *Croatian Medical Journal, 50*, 7–16.

Raelson JV, Little RD, Ruether A, Fournier H, Paquin B, Van Eerdewegh P, et al. (2007). Genome-wide association study for Crohn's disease in the Quebec Founder Population identifies multiple validated disease loci. *Proceedings of National Academy of Sciences of the United States of America, 104*, 14,747–14,752.

Rafnar T, Sulem P, Stacey SN, Geller F, Gudmundsson J, Sigurdsson A, et al. (2009). Sequence variants at the TERT-CLPTM1L locus associate with many cancer types. *Nature Genetics, 41*, 221–227.

Rampersaud E, Damcott CM, Fu M, Shen H, McArdle P, Shi X, et al. (2007). Identification of novel candidate genes for type 2 diabetes from a genome-wide association scan in the Old Order Amish: evidence for replication from diabetes-related quantitative traits and from independent populations. *Diabetes, 56*, 3053–3062.

Reich DE, Lander ES, (2001). On the allelic spectrum of human disease. *Trends in Genetics, 17*, 502–510.

Risch N, Merikangas K. (1996). The future of genetic studies of complex human diseases. *Science, 273*, 1516–1517.

Sabatti C, Service SK, Hartikainen AL, Pouta A, Ripatti S, Brodsky J, et al. (2009). Genome-wide association analysis of metabolic traits in a birth cohort from a founder population. *Nature Genetics, 41*, 35–46.

Sajantila A, Salem AH, Savolainen P, Bauer K, Gierig C, Pääbo S. (1996). Paternal and maternal DNA lineages reveal a bottleneck in the founding of the Finnish population. *Proceedings of National Academy of Sciences of the United States of America, 93*, 12,035–12,039.

Sanna S, Jackson AU, Nagaraja R, Willer CJ, Chen WM, Bonnycastle LL, et al. (2008). Common variants in the GDF5-UQCC region are associated with variation in human height. *Nature Genetics, 40*, 198–203.

Scuteri A, Sanna S, Chen WM, Uda M, Albai G, Strait J, et al. (2007). Genome-wide association scan shows genetic variants in the FTO gene are associated with obesity-related traits. *PLoS Genetics, 3*, e115.

Service S, DeYoung J, Karayiorgou M, Roos JL, Pretorious H, Bedoya G, et al. (2006). Magnitude and distribution of linkage disequilibrium in population isolates and implications for genome-wide association studies. *Nature Genetics, 38*, 556–560.

Service S; International Collaborative Group on Isolated Populations, Sabatti C, Freimer N. (2007). Tag SNPs chosen from HapMap perform well in several population isolates. *Genetic Epidemiology, 31*, 189–194.

Shifman S, Darvasi A. (2001). The value of isolated populations. *Nature Genetics, 28*, 309–310.

Shmulewitz D, Auerbach SB, Lehner T, Blundell ML, Winick JD, Youngman LD, et al. (2001). Epidemiology and factor analysis of obesity, type II diabetes, hypertension, and dyslipidemia (syndrome X) on the Island of Kosrae, Federated States of Micronesia. *Human Heredity, 51*, 8–19.

Sklar P, Pato MT, Kirby A, Petryshen TL, Medeiros H, Carvalho C, et al. (2004). Genome-wide scan in Portuguese Island families identifies 5q31-5q35 as a susceptibility locus for schizophrenia and psychosis. *Molecular Psychiatry, 9*, 213–218.

Stacey SN, Gudbjartsson DF, Sulem P, Bergthorsson JT, Kumar R, Thorleifsson G, et al. (2008). Common variants on 1p36 and 1q42 are associated with cutaneous basal cell carcinoma but not with melanoma or pigmentation traits. *Nature Genetics, 40*, 1313–1318.

Stacey SN, Manolescu A, Sulem P, Rafnar T, Gudmundsson J, Gudjonsson SA, et al. (2007). Common variants on chromosomes 2q35 and 16q12 confer susceptibility to estrogen receptor-positive breast cancer. *Nature Genetics, 39*, 865–869.

Stefansson H, Steinberg S, Petursson H, Gustafsson O, Gudjonsdottir IH, Jonsdottir GA, et al. (2009). Variant in the sequence of the LINGO1 gene confers risk of essential tremor. *Nature Genetics, 41*, 277–279.

Steinthorsdottir V, Thorleifsson G, Reynisdottir I, Benediktsson R, Jonsdottir T, Walters GB, et al. (2007). A variant in CDKAL1 influences insulin response and risk of type 2 diabetes. *Nature Genetics, 39*, 770–775.

Styrkarsdottir U, Halldorsson BV, Gretarsdottir S, Gudbjartsson DF, Walters GB, Ingvarsson T, et al. (2008). Multiple genetic loci for bone mineral density and fractures. *New England Journal of Medicine, 358*, 2355–2365.

Styrkarsdottir U, Halldorsson BV, Gretarsdottir S, Gudbjartsson DF, Walters GB, Ingvarsson T, et al. (2009). New sequence variants associated with bone mineral density. *Nature Genetics, 41*, 15–17.

Sulem P, Gudbjartsson DF, Stacey SN, Helgason A, Rafnar T, Jakobsdottir M, et al. (2008). Two newly identified genetic determinants of pigmentation in Europeans. *Nature Genetics, 40*, 835–837.

Sumelahti ML, Tienari PJ, Wikström J, Palo J, Hakama M. (2001). Increasing prevalence of multiple sclerosis in Finland. *Acta Neurologica Scandinavica, 103*, 153–158.

The International HapMap Consortium (2005). A haplotype map of the human genome. *Nature, 437*, 1299–1320.

Thorleifsson G, Magnusson KP, Sulem P, Walters GB, Gudbjartsson DF, Stefansson H, et al. (2007). Common sequence variants in the LOXL1 gene confer susceptibility to exfoliation glaucoma. *Science, 317*, 1397–1400.

Varilo T, Laan M, Hovatta I, Wiebe V, Terwilliger JD, Peltonen L. (2000). Linkage disequilibrium in isolated populations: Finland and a young sub-population of Kuusamo. *European Journal of Human Genetics, 8*, 604–612.

Varilo T, Paunio T, Parker A, Perola M, Meyer J, Terwilliger JD, et al. (2003). The interval of linkage disequilibrium (LD) detected with microsatellite and SNP markers in chromosomes of Finnish populations with different histories. *Human Molecular Genetics, 12*, 51–59.

Venken T, Claes S, Sluijs S, Paterson AD, van Duijn C, Adolfsson R, et al. (2005). Genomewide scan for affective disorder susceptibility Loci in families of a northern Swedish isolated population. *American Journal of Human Genetics, 76*, 237–248.

Venter JC, Adams MD, Myers EW, Li PW, Mural RJ, Sutton GG, et al. (2001). The sequence of the human genome. *Science, 291*, 1304–1351.

Vitart V, Rudan I, Hayward C, Gray NK, Floyd J, Palmer CN, et al. (2009). SLC2A9 is a newly identified urate transporter influencing serum urate concentration, urate excretion and gout. *Nature Genetics, 40*, 437–442.

Wang J, Wang W, Li R, Li Y, Tian G, Goodman L, et al. (2008). The diploid genome sequence of an Asian individual. *Nature, 456*, 60–65.

Wheeler DA, Srinivasan M, Egholm M, Shen Y, Chen L, McGuire A, et al. (2008). The complete genome of an individual by massively parallel DNA sequencing. *Nature, 452*, 872–876.

WTCCC (2007). Genome-wide association study of 14,000 cases of seven common diseases and 3,000 shared controls. *Nature, 447*, 661–678.

Zeggini E, Scott LJ, Saxena R, Voight BF, Marchini JL, Hu T, et al. (2008). Meta-analysis of genome-wide association data and large-scale replication identifies additional susceptibility loci for type 2 diabetes. *Nature Genetics, 40*, 638–645.

44 Eric M. Morrow, Christopher A. Walsh

Isolate Populations and Rare Variation in Autism Spectrum Disorders

Points of Interest

- Autism is highly heterogeneous at the genetic level.
- Forward genetics offers important opportunity for progress as it relates to the neurobiology of the condition.
- Rare variation may play an important role, and loci of major effect have been previously reported.
- Recessive mutations may play an important role by analogy to intellectual disability, and pedigrees with recent shared ancestry offer increased power for mapping such loci.
- Loci discovered by these approaches may be generalizable to populations without recent shared ancestry.
- Studies in isolate populations and of rare variation offer an important approach to gene discovery, which is complementary to other ongoing efforts to studies of common variation.

Autism is one of the most severe neuropsychiatric conditions emerging in childhood. Autistic symptoms include complex behavioral and cognitive deficits that appear prior to age 3 years (American Psychiatric Association and American Psychiatric Association Task Force on DSM-IV, 2000). These symptoms include abnormal communication and social interaction, rigid and repetitive stereotyped behaviors, and atypical information processing. There are core deficits in social reciprocity—that is, expressing emotions and understanding the emotions of others known as "theory of mind" (Baron-Cohen et al., 1985). Children with autism have uneven cognitive profiles, with strengths in some areas—that is, "splinter domains"—yet general weaknesses in executive function and seeing the big picture known as "central coherence" (Happe & Frith, 2006). Approximately 50% of autistic individuals have some degree of intellectual disability (ID, formerly mental retardation) (Fombonne, 1999), and approximately 25% have epilepsy (Danielsson et al., 2005); therefore autism, ID, and epilepsy are likely to share some biological links with autism. Intellectual disability ranks first among all chronic conditions causing disability in the United States (U.S. National Center for Health Statistics, 1996). Autistic disorder is one of several neurodevelopmental conditions categorized in the DSM-IV as the pervasive developmental disorders (PDDs), which also include Asperger's Syndrome, Rett's Syndrome, Childhood Disintegrative Disorder, and PDD-not otherwise specified (PDD-NOS) (American Psychiatric Association and American Psychiatric Association Task Force on DSM-IV, 2000). The prevalence of autism is high and at least four times more common in boys than girls. Prevalence estimates vary across studies but are approximately 1:300–800 for autistic disorder and 1:200 for all PDD, which appears to be a 10-fold increase in the last 10 to 20 years (Fombonne, 1999; Fombonne, 2003). Some degree of this increase is likely attributable to increased awareness and broadening the diagnostic spectrum; however, the prevalence is high and may be increasing. As most autistic individuals require lifelong assistance, the financial costs to society are very high, whereas the emotional costs to family members cannot even be estimated (Ganz, 2007).

The Options for Diagnosis and Treatment of Autism are Limited

Currently, there are a small number of genetic tests (i.e., array comparative genomic hybridization [aCGH], or Fragile X Syndrome) and metabolic tests that may provide a biological diagnosis (Martin & Ledbetter, 2007; Beaudet & Belmont, 2008). Otherwise, diagnosis is limited to neuropsychological assessments alone. Treatments for autism are similarly limited. Behavioral and educational training has partial efficacy in a subset of children, particularly when started early. Indeed, this has led to the proposal of using "developmental medicines" in a time-restricted fashion to augment response to behavior treatments during development, as is being pursued for Fragile X (Dolen & Bear, 2005). However, psychopharmacological studies thus far have been largely limited to antipsychotics (mostly risperidone) and antidepressants for behavior symptoms. Indeed, children with PDD have been traditionally excluded from pharmacotherapeutic trials. Overall, advances in diagnostic subtyping and a deeper, translational understanding of pathophysiology is an important foundation for future treatment trials (Geschwind, 2009).

Autism is Highly Genetic and "Forward Genetics" Offers Opportunity for Progress

Our understanding of the neurobiology of autism is rudimentary (Abrahams & Geschwind, 2008). Perhaps the most established fact is that autism is highly genetic. Autistic disorder is the most strongly genetically influenced, childhood neuropsychiatric disorder (Bailey et al., 1995). There is a 60% to 90% concordance rate of autism in monozygotic twins as opposed to a 0% to 10% rate in dizygotic twins. Autism has an approximately 45-fold higher recurrence risk in families versus the general population. Given this fact, "forward genetics" (taking whole-genome approaches with patients and families, and moving from the phenotype to identifying specific genes and mutations) is an extremely important approach for discovering the core patholobiology of autism.

The disease causing mutations in *Presinilin* and *APP* were found in a relatively rare early-onset form of Alzheimer's disease in large, highly informative pedigrees (Tanzi et al., 1996; Tanzi & Bertram, 2005). As with the forward genetics approach of Alzheimer's disease, this approach has been taken with autism with some success (explained below for the *Neuroligin* gene), yet the opportunities from this approach have not been systematically exhausted for autism. The subject of this chapter is to outline the hypotheses central to the forward genetic approaches of isolate populations and rare variants. This chapter will outline these hypotheses and provide a rationale for this approach—particularly from the point of view of populations with recent shared ancestry that may be enriched for autosomal recessive loci. Finally, this chapter will outline some of the early data in this area of autism spectrum disorder (ASD) genetics.

The central hypotheses of the rare variant and isolate population approach in ASDs are outlined below. To stress, we contend that this approach to mutation discovery in autism represents an important complementary approach. Given the complex and heterogeneous genetic architecture of ASDs, this approach, together with a variety of additional approaches (including rare and common copy number studies as well as rare and common sequence association studies) are required to develop a full understanding of the genetic underpinning of this profound and complex condition (Geschwind, 2008; Walsh et al., 2008).

The central hypotheses of the rare variant and isolate population approach in ASDs as discussed in this chapter are outlined below:

1. ASDs are genetically heterogeneous.
2. A subset of ASDs worldwide will result from individually rare, highly penetrant loci.
3. As a syndrome of neurodevelopmental conditions, ASD genetics will be informed by two other syndromes of neurodevelopment—namely, intellectual disability (ID) and epilepsy.
4. As ASDs (at least for lower-functioning autism) appear to decrease reproductive fitness, a subset of loci are likely to be de novo and/or recessive (X-linked or autosomal recessive).
5. Autosomal recessive loci underlying autism susceptibility will be enriched in populations with recent shared ancestry.
6. Although genome-wide association studies are undoubtably important, linkage studies may remain as an important complementary approach, particularly in special founder populations.
7. Pedigrees with rare, highly penetrant loci may involve syndromic forms of autism that may involve ID or epilepsy.
8. Pedigrees from isolate populations or with syndromic forms of autism may be highly informative to other forms of ASDs with more complex genetic architecture.

Autism Spectrum Disorders Display Genetic Heterogeneity With Some Cases Caused by Loci of Major Effect

We hypothesize that at least for lower-functioning autism, a subset of the genetic architecture may resemble that for ID. Intellectual disability naturally is caused by a large number of chromosomal anomalies, submicroscopic copy number variants (CNVs), and a large number of Mendelian forms—particularly de novo, X-linked, and autosomal recessive (Figure 44-1) (Stromme, 2000). To date, 90 of the 818 (11%) annotated genes on the X chromosome have been found to harbor mutations in X-linked recessive ID, some of which have autistic symptoms (Gecz et al., 2009). Based on these findings, one may hypothesize that autosomal recessive causes of ID and autism will also be common, particularly in pedigrees with recent shared ancestry; however, systematic searches for autosomal recessive genes are in the very early stages.

The genetic architecture of autism is highly heterogeneous. Up to 3% of cases of autism are caused by microscopically detectable chromosomal anomalies. Chromosomal anomalies are common in autism, of major effect, and found throughout the genome (Abrahams & Geschwind, 2008). Some of the chromosomal regions, such as chromosome 7 and 15q11-13, have shown overlap with loci from linkage and association studies.

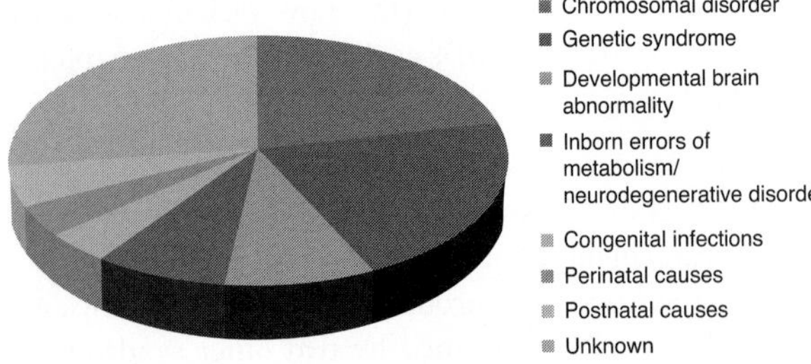

Figure 44–1. Causes of severe intellectual disability. The genetic architecture for ID may be helpful in conceptualizing at least a subset of autism. For ID, only 27% of cases cannot be accounted for by a discrete cause. 22% of diagnoses can be traced to a chromosomal disorder, and 21% of diagnoses are the result of a genetic syndrome. Other causes of intellectual disability include developmental brain abnormalities, metabolic/neurodegenerative disorders, congenital infections, and peri- and postnatal causes. Data from Stromme P and Hayberg G. (2000) Aetiology in severe and mild mental retardation: A population based study of Norwegian children. *Developmental Medicine and Child Neurology 42*, 76–86. (See Color Plate Section for a color version of this figure.)

Other regions include 2q37, 5p15, 11q25, 16q22.3, 17p11.2, 18q21.1, 18q23, 22q11.2, 22q13.3, and Xp22.2-22.3. One prominent example of genomic rearrangements in autism is the inverted duplication of proximal chromosome 15q11-13 (Cook et al., 1997). Given the frequency of chromosomal anomalies, novel high-resolution methodologies for analyzing genomic copy number variants (duplications/insertions and deletions), such as array CGH (aCGH) or high-density SNP chips, are currently being employed to study autism. Indeed, estimates of up to 10% of autism may be explainable by known genetic causes, including chromosomal anomalies, submicroscopic copy number variants or known genetic syndromes with autistic symptoms—that is, "syndromic autism," such as Fragile X syndrome (Martin & Ledbetter, 2007). Notably, a significant fraction of children who present with ASDs without clear syndromic features of Fragile X (in some studies up to 2%, although it is likely lower in the majority of clinics) will test positive for Fragile X syndrome (Reddy, 2005). In addition, a small number of Mendelian forms of autism, mostly X-linked, have been identified, such as mutations in the *Neuroligin* genes (Jamain et al., 2003; Laumonnier et al., 2004).

Many genetic syndromes are associated with ASDs, including Fragile X Syndrome, Tuberous Sclerosis, Angelman Syndrome, Rett Syndrome, Timothy's Syndrome, Joubert Syndrome, or MR syndromes resulting from mutations in *HoxA1* or *ARX* (Muhle et al., 2004; Moss & Howlin, 2009). All of these conditions are caused by loci of major effect, are generally X-linked and frequently de novo, or are autosomal recessive. These conditions may give clues as to the biological etiology of autistic symptoms. Fragile X syndrome is particularly significant. Approximately 2% of boys with idiopathic autism (i.e., without any syndromic features of Fragile X Syndrome) test positive for mutations at the Fragile X locus (Reddy, 2005), and the condition may be particularly frequent in populations with ASD (Brown et al., 1986); therefore, this genetic test already serves as a tool for diagnostic subtyping in autism.

Finally, there are a large number of cases of ASD wherein CNVs (most prominently de novo CNVs) represent highly penetrant susceptibility loci (Cook & Scherer, 2008). Finally, the remaining majority of autism is idiopathic. The majority of idiopathic autism is likely polygenic—that is, caused by the combination of multiple genes of small effect—or even epigenetic. A core debate in autism genetics is whether autism is caused by the complex interaction of common disadvantageous alleles, or rare, highly penetrant deleterious lesions. Given heterogeneity, these models likely co-exist and thereby may be complementary, and studies to explore each mechanism (rare families with highly penetrant lesions as well as association studies) must be undertaken. However, for at least a subset of ASDs (including both syndromic and lower-functioning ASDs) a large number of individually rare, highly penetrant loci may be implicated with a genetic architecture that resembles intellectual disability (Figure 44-2). Indeed, several of these known loci may be shared or found in a range of conditions, including ID and ASDs but also others such as epilepsy (15q13 CNVs [Helbig et al., 2009; Miller et al., 2009]) and schizophrenia (multiple CNVs, with the longest standing example including 22q11 deletions [2008]).

Figure 44-3 demonstrates our hypotheses for the genetic architecture of ASDs, whereby at least a subset of the lower-functioning cohort has a genetic architecture resembling that of ID, and the remainder—particularly that of the higher functioning cohort—may have more complex genetic architecture. To stress, this is only a model at this stage, and the presentation

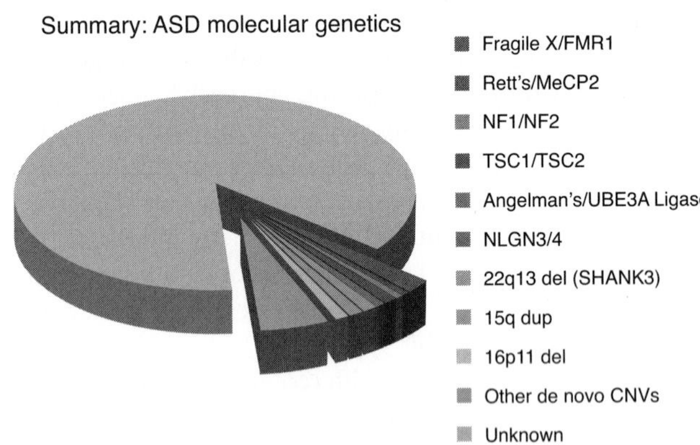

Figure 44–2. A subset of ASD has genetic architecture composed of diverse, individually-rare loci. The causes underlying ASDs are largely unknown: up to 87.4% of cases cannot be traced to a distinct genetic mechanism. Of the remaining 12.6% of cases, 5% may be attributed to de novo copy number variants (CNVs), and 2% may be attributed to silencing of the *FMR1* gene (associated with Fragile X mental retardation). The remaining cases suggest that aberrations in genes associated with Rett's Syndrome, tuberous sclerosis, and various synaptic proteins may contribute to the etiology of ASDs. Data from Abrahams, BD and Geschwind, DH. (2008) Advances in Autism Genetics: On the threshold of a new neurobiology. *Nature Reviews Genetics, 9*, 341–355. (See Color Plate Section for a color version of this figure.)

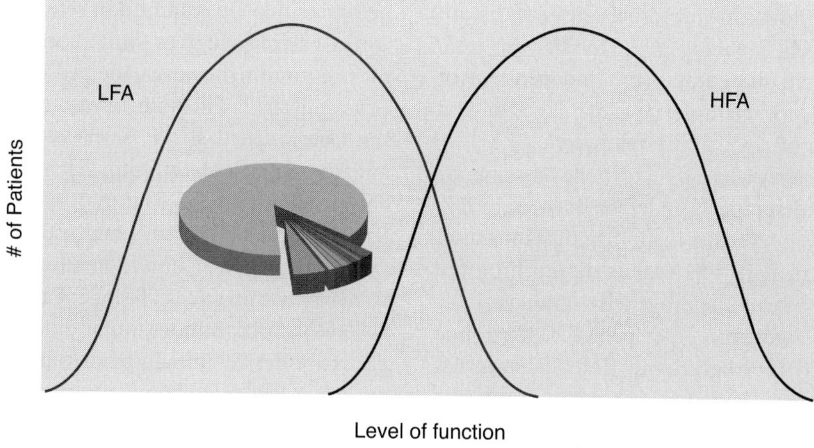
Hypothesis
• Syndromic autism
• Individually rare, monogenic or oligogenic
• Highly penetrant loci
• Non-syndromic autism
• Complex
• Multigenic
• Common, low-penetrant alleles
LFA
HFA
# of Patients
Level of function

Figure 44–3. Hypothesis of the genetic architecture of ASD. ASDs may be conceptualized in a bimodal nature within the diagnosed population, with two populations of patients diagnosed: one at the low-functioning level (low-functioning autism [LFA]), which might have a genetic architecture similar to ID, and one at the high-functioning level (high-functioning autism [HFA]), which might have more complex genetic architecture. Naturally this is a straw-man hypothesis but this underlying conceptualization may have use in bringing together different schools of thought in the ASD genetics field. (See Color Plate Section for a color version of this figure.)

of the ASD population as falling into two dichotomous groups is likely an oversimplification. Further, although the examples of common variants in ASDs that have been substantiated or replicated with whole-genome significance or through meta-analysis are few, there are a few examples of even higher-functioning autism being caused by rare, highly penetrant loci such as NLGN3 and NLGN4 mutations, although these examples are exceedingly rare (Jamain et al., 2003).

Genes and Loci Implicated by Linkage

Relatively few genes have been definitively identified for idiopathic, nonsyndromic autism. Indeed, for the majority of situations wherein loci have been found in ASDs, similar mutations have also been found in ID. Carefully designed genome-wide linkage screens in autistic disorder have identified heterogeneous linkage peaks, on 1q21-22, 2q21-33, 3q25-27, 7q11-12, 7q31-36, 13q14.1-14.2, 15q11-13, 16p13, 17q21, and others. Candidate genes have also been tested by association, however because of heterogeneity and limited power of available samples, examples of strong associations are few (Campbell et al., 2006; Alarcon et al., 2008; Arking et al., 2008). Among the most convincing evidence implicating a gene in autism has been obtained from single pedigrees— namely, the recent studies implicating *Neuroligin3* and *Neuroligin4* in ASDs (Jamain et al., 2003; Laumonnier et al., 2004). Laumonnier et al. (2004) described an extended French pedigree segregating three distinct phenotypes: autism alone, MR alone, or autism with MR. This example of *NLGN* mutations in autism represents another example of a locus of major effect in autistic symptomology, although the occurance of these mutations are exceedingly rare.

Recent Shared Ancestry Facilitates Mapping Autosomal Recessive Conditions

Although many studies have assumed a modified form of dominant inheritance, some segregation analyses of autism suggest that affected individuals represent about 0.16 to 0.2 of all offspring, more suggestive of recessively inherited loci (Ritvo et al., 1985); however, existing evidence does not allow a clear choice. Recessive inheritance characterizes vast numbers of metabolic, developmental, and degenerative diseases of the nervous system, many of which can cause autistic symptoms. If we accept the likelihood that autosomal recessive genes cause some ASDs, then conducting homozygosity mapping offers a powerful, systematic way for finding such loci by enrolling families with consanguinity. Populations in which there is a high prevalence of recent shared ancestry within pedigrees (such as the Middle Eastern Arabic countries, Turkey, and Pakistan) have a different spectrum of genetic disease from populations where recent shared ancestry is less common (2006; Teebi & El-Shanti, 2006). In Saudi Arabia, Jordan, and many other Gulf countries, 40% to 60% of marriages involve first cousins (Teebi & Farag, 1997). Populations with a high degree of recent shared ancestry show rates of congenital neurological disease that are two- to threefold higher than Western populations, and this increased incidence has been attributed repeatedly to the action of recessive genes (Teebi & Farag, 1997) (Figure 44-4). There is also a reduced rate of de novo chromosomal causes of disease in these populations (Teebi & Farag, 1997; Hoodfar & Teebi, 1996). Parents with recent shared ancestry (independent of socioeconomic factors)—for example, cousins may also be a risk factor for disorders of cognitive development (Morton, 1978). Recent shared ancestry also facilitates gene mapping by allowing homozygosity mapping (Lander & Botstein, 1987; Kruglyak et al., 1995). Homozygosity mapping offers increased power from individual pedigrees as well as diminishing the problems imposed by locus heterogeneity and variable expressivity. With increased power per pedigree, there is a reduced need to pool across pedigrees and, potentially, across heterogeneous conditions. In addition, some countries wherein recent shared ancestry is prevalent in pedigrees also have very high fertility rates, with large families (on average ≥6 children per mother) also simplifying genetic linkage analysis and allowing gene mapping to be often accomplished using just one or two extended families.

The power of consanguineous pedigrees for mapping recessive genes is illustrated (Figure 44-5A) by showing the maximal theoretical LOD score for genetic linkage in a pedigree with unrelated parents (left), first-cousin parents (middle), and second-cousin parents (right). The LOD score triples when we go from unrelated to first-cousin parents and increases further when parents are more distantly related. This effect reflects the fact that the consanguinity includes more individuals from the pedigree in the linkage calculation (Lander & Botstein, 1987; Kruglyak et al., 1995). Also shown in Figure 44-5B are two pedigrees with equal power (i.e., number of of meioses) for mapping autosomal recessive traits. The one at the left represents a pedigree in which parents are second cousins. Such pedigrees may be common in referral clinics in regions of the world where pedigrees with recent shared ancestry may be more common; however, the pedigree on the right, which has equal power, is fairly uncommon worldwide. In addition to the factors listed above, some countries with recent shared ancestry—particularly Saudi Arabia—tend to have a remarkably tribal structure. The majority of the 16 million ethnic Saudi people belong to 8 major tribes (consisting of up to 1 million people each) and 12 smaller tribes, with high tendencies to marry within tribes (Teebi & Farag, 1997). Each tribe tends to have its own founder mutations resulting from the fact that each tribe derives initially from founder populations equivalent to just a few tents of people. Even where definable shared ancestry is absent, the likelihood of homozygosity for founder mutations is high. These patterns make mapping of recessive autism loci feasible, whereas the possibility of founder mutations makes fine mapping and gene identification a realistic possibility. As described with the example of the Amish described below, studying founder populations in genetics is not new, and many of the features of the populations described above for those with recent shared ancestry are true to a degree for other populations around the world that have also been studied by geneticists, such as the Ashkenazi Jewish population, the French Canadian population, the Icelandic population, or the Old Order Amish population.

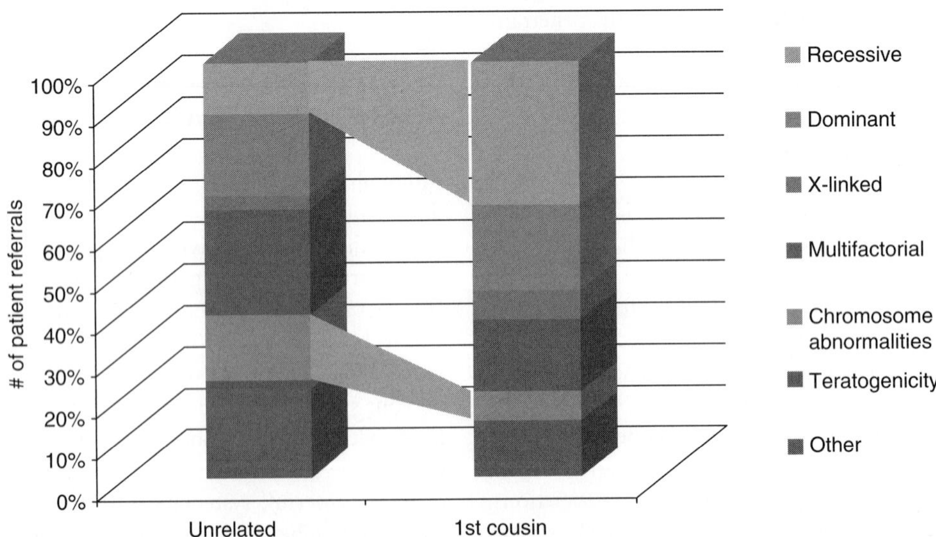

Figure 44–4. Consanguinity increases rate of recessive disorders. Causes of medical referrals between offspring with parental consanguinity versus offspring without. Autosomal recessive conditions are more than twice as common among offspring with parental consanguinity (1st cousin), than among those without (unrelated) (33.3% versus 12.4%), while chromosomal abnormalities are more than twice as common among offspring of unrelated unions in comparison with those of 1st cousin unions (15.7% versus 6.7%). Data from Hoodfar, E. and A. S. Teebi (1996). Genetic referrals of Middle Eastern origin in a western city: inbreeding and disease profile. *Journal of Medical Genetics*, **33**(3), 212–215. (See Color Plate Section for a color version of this figure.)

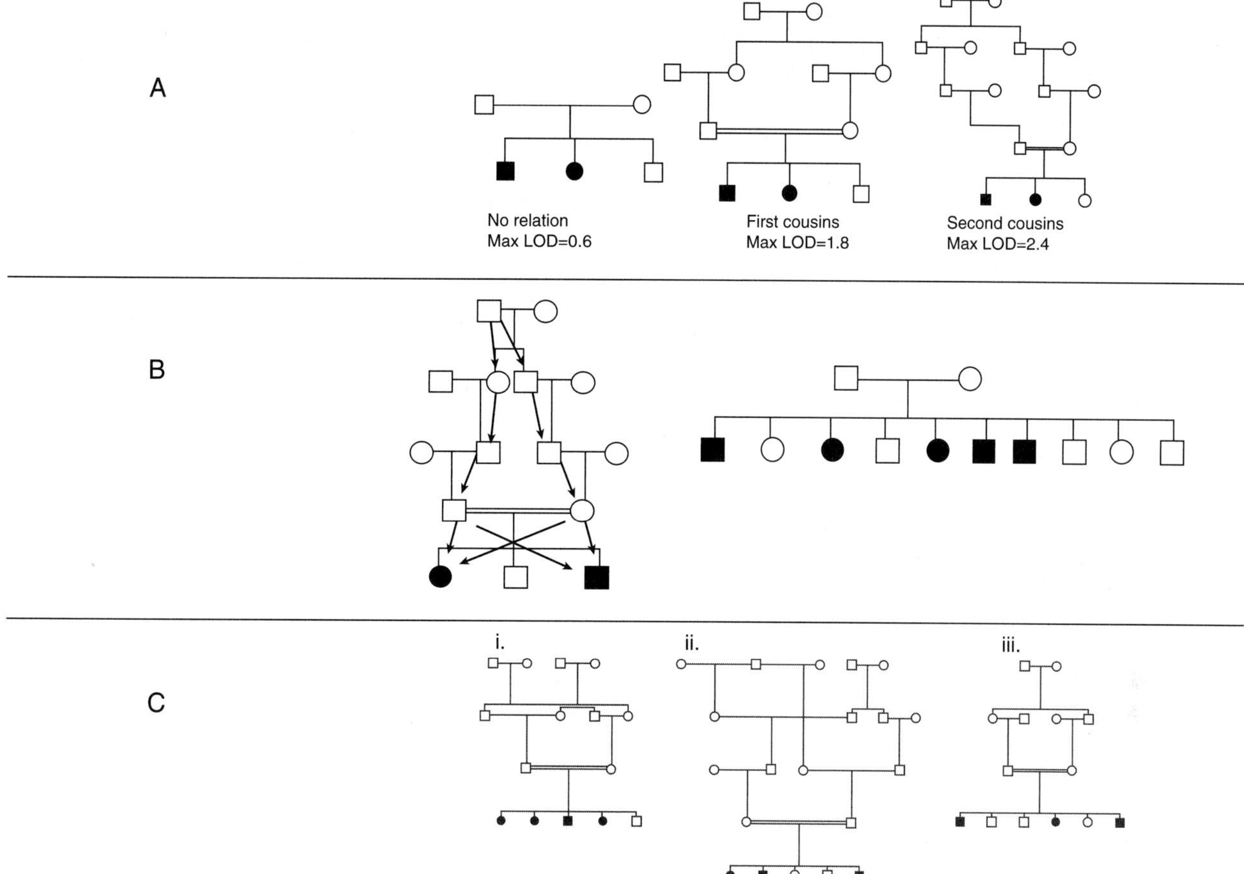

Figure 44–5. Consanguineous pedigrees have increased power for mapping autosomal recessive loci. A. Simulated LOD scores from families with two affected offspring segregating a recessive trait when the parents are unrelated (left), first cousins (center), or second cousins (right). B. Model pedigrees each with equal power for mapping autosomal recessive loci. The consanguineous pedigree as drawn is common in regions of the world wherein consanguinity is common. The pedigree without parental consanguinity is exceedingly challenging to find anywhere in the world. **C.** Pedigrees with ASD with parental consanguinity from the Homozygosity Mapping Collaborative for Autism. In many cases, not all unaffected siblings have been included in the pedigree.

Lessons From Autosomal Recessive Loci for Brain Malformations Such as Joubert Syndrome

One hypothesis outlined above for the approach taken in rare isolate populations (hypothesis 7 above) is that genes and loci found in pedigrees from isolate populations may be relevant to non-syndromic autism or "complex" autism. Indeed this hypothesis has been tested, and a recent report has confirmed that a common haplotype of *AHI1* (a gene mutated in some forms of Joubert syndrome as discovered by homozygosity mapping) in populations without recent shared ancestry appears to be associated with ASDs (Alvarez Retuerto et al., 2008). This same haplotype had been previously implicated in schizophrenia. Overall, these data suggest that *AHI1* may have rare highly penetrant mutations in Joubert syndrome (which is associated with autistic symptoms) and common variation in the same gene may be associated with neuropsychiatric disorders with cognitive and developmental components such as ASD and/or schizophrenia. This is early evidence to support the hypothesis (#7) that loci from rare syndromic forms of autism may yield important clues in non-syndromic or "complex" autism.

Lessons From a Rare Autosomal Recessive Mutation in the Old Order Amish in Focal Epilepsy

Given recent shared ancestry in the U.S. Older Amish population, there are several examples of autosomal recessive conditions that have been reported in this population and an important example of a mutation in a cohort with focal epilepsy, relative macrocephaly, and focal dysplasia was reported (Strauss et al., 2006). Affected individuals in the pedigree were also identified to have a high rate of PDD-NOS. Using homozygosity mapping, Strauss et al. identified a homozygous mutation in the contactin-associated protein-like 2 (CASPR2), which is encoded by CNTNAP2.

Based in part of the identification of a translocation that disrupted this gene, and also on the PDD symptoms in the

Amish epilepsy pedigree, CNTNAP2 became the subject of intense study through gene resequencing and gene association studies (Alarcon et al., 2008; Arking et al., 2008; Bakkaloglu et al., 2008). Again, these findings provide support for the notion that syndromic forms of autism may provide critical clues for loci in non-syndromic ASDs.

Lessons From Genetic Studies of Non-Syndromic MR in Populations With Recent Shared Ancestry

To date, although homozygosity mapping has been very successful for rare neuromedical conditions with distinctive brain malformations and other syndromic features (Barkovich et al., 2005), genes have also been identified for non-syndromic MR (NSMR) using homozygosity mapping (Basel-Vanagaite et al., 2007). Also, promising loci for other non-syndromic neurologic conditions, such as deafness (Tariq et al., 2006), or complex neurologic traits, such as stuttering, are under active study (Riaz et al., 2005). For NSMR, Basel et al. (2006) successfully identified mutations in CC2D1A in autosomal recessive NSMR by homozygosity mapping (Basel-Vanagaite et al., 2006). Some cases of autism are highly related to NSMR (Laumonnier et al., 2004), and thereby the successful use of homozygosity mapping for NSMR is strong preliminary support for its application to familial ASDs.

A Systematic Search for Autosomal Recessive Loci in Populations with Recent Shared Ancestry: The Homozygosity Mapping Collaborative for Autism

Given the hypotheses, rationale, and data described above, in 2005, a systematic approach for studying autosomal recessive loci in populations with recent shared ancestry was started through international collaboration. Clinician research collaborators in several centers began to enroll pedrigees with children affected by autism and with recent shared ancestry. These efforts are ongoing and the initial studies have been published by Morrow et al. (2008). Figure 44-6 demonstrates the locations of the most active centers of the collaboration.

The study plan for the HMCA is described in Figure 44-7. Pedigrees were enrolled through clinician collaborators and examples are shown in Figure 44-5C. To establish thorough research diagnoses, international participating clinicians received training in accepted autism research scales. When research scales were not available in the language of their country, these clinicians enrolled patients and family members

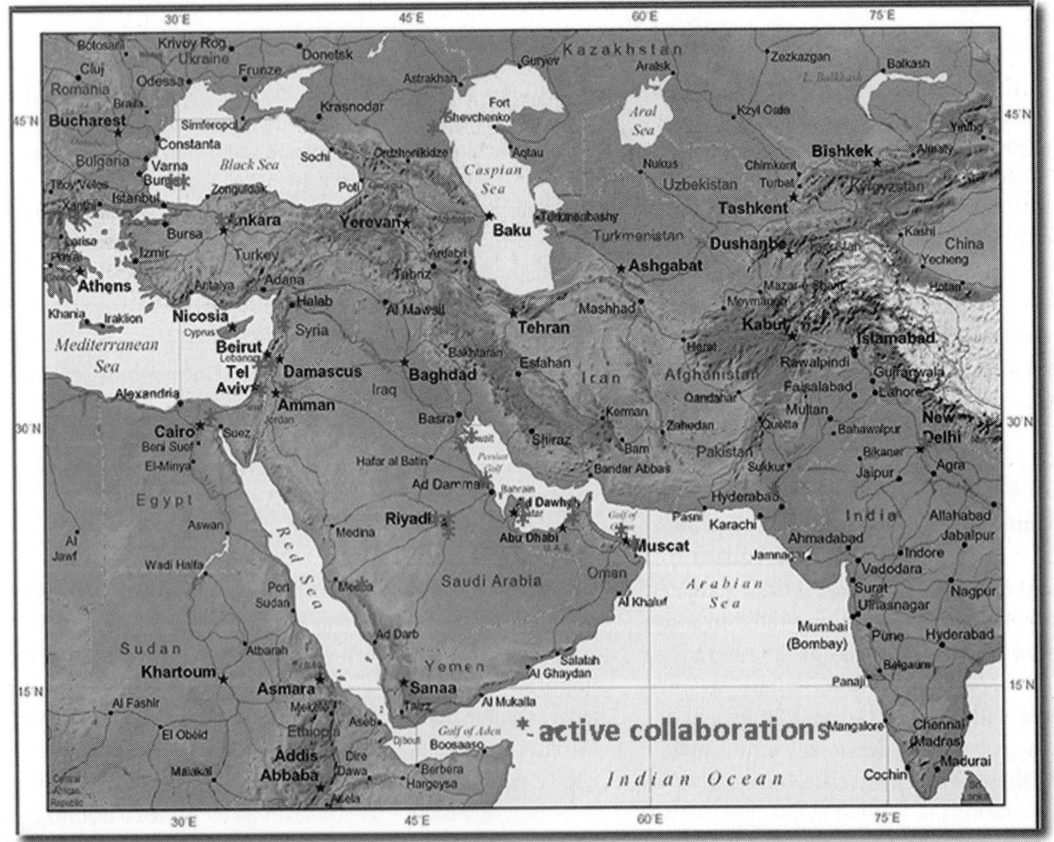

Figure 44–6. Homozygosity Mapping Collaborative for Autism (HMCA). The approach of the HMCA involves collaborators from around the world with a focus in the Middle East. Asterisks indicate locations of active collaborations. In these countries, traditions of marriage between cousins increase the prevalence of recessive disorders, which can be traced using homozygosity mapping. (See Color Plate Section for a color version of this figure.)

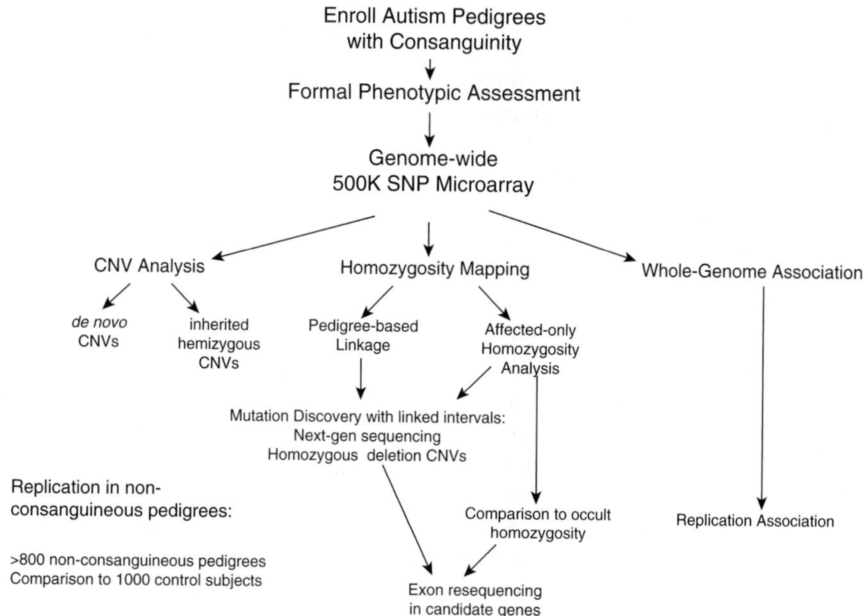

Figure 44–7. HMCA Study Plan. The approach taken by the Homozygosity Mapping Collaborative for Autism (HMCA) involves enrollment of subjects from consanguineous families affected by autism, phenotypic assessment, and genome-wide SNP micro-array analysis.

based on DSM-IV-TR diagnoses that were informed by these clinicians' experiences with validated research scales. Additional direct assessments of patients were conducted by clinical members of the Boston team, which included a multidisciplinary group, such as developmental psychologists, pediatric neurologists, a clinical geneticist, and a neuropsychiatrist. Reliability between clinician assessments was high; a description of clinical assessment is available.

An increased role for inherited factors in autism with shared ancestry was suggested by a low rate of de novo CNVs (Morrow et al., 2008). Additionally, in the multiplex families (which provided support for linkage through homozygosity mapping), implicated loci were heterogeneous, with each pedigree providing support for distinct loci. This latter data-point again underscores the heterogeneity of the condition even in this special founder population. Notably, several loci were mapped that contained large, inherited homozygous deletions that are likely mutations. The largest deletions implicated genes, including *PCDH10* (protocadherin 10); *DIA1* (deleted in autism1, or c3orf58), and *NHE9*. A subset of genes—particularly *NHE9* (Na^+/H^+ exchanger 9)—was studied in pedigrees without recent shared ancestry through resequencing, and additional potential mutations in patients with unrelated parents were found. Interestingly, the proportion of patients with *NHE9* gene alterations that were likely deleterious was only slightly higher in autistic children than in normals overall but was significantly higher in patients with autism and comorbid epilepsy. The initial patient in the pedigree with recent shared ancestry also had autism with epilepsy. This finding, as for AHI1 and CNTNAP2, provided further support that loci implicated in special populations may be generalized, albeit in this case an intermediate phenotype of autism (autism with epilepsy). As shown in Figure 44-7, in addition to homozygosity studies, these samples were included in the recent whole-genome association study and linkage studies. This collaborative, which is ongoing, is now also involved in a major deep resequencing study utilizing next-generation sequencing methods. Overall, the initial results of the HMCA have provided important clues and insights. Nonetheless, it is evident that the genetic dissection of ASDs, even in these special founder populations, is only at the beginning stages, and there is a great deal more work to be done. In particular, larger epidemiologic sampling of these special populations combined with novel, more high-throughput methods will capitalize further on this approach, which stands in complement to other ongoing, critical efforts in ASD genetics.

Conclusion

In conclusion, "forward" genetics efforts in ASDs offer a critical opportunity to tackle this profound and costly problem. Given the heterogeneity of ASD genetics, it is without a doubt that multiple concurrent approaches to dissecting the genetic susceptibility of the condition is necessary. Examination of isolate populations and rare variants is one such complementary and important approach. Stemming from the notion that rare, highly penetrant genetic factors may explain a subset of the genetic architecture, this approach draws heavily from the field of ID and epilepsy genetics, syndromic forms of autism, and rare pedigrees. It is based on the following hypotheses: *(1)* ASD is genetically heterogeneous; *(2)* a subset of

ASDs worldwide will be caused by individually rare, highly penetrant loci; *(3)* As a syndrome of neurodevelopmental conditions, ASD genetics will be informed by two other syndromes of neurodevelopment—namely, ID and epilepsy; *(4)* as ASD (at least for lower-functioning autism) appears to decrease reproductive fitness, a subset of loci are likely to be de novo and/or recessive (X-linked or autosomal recessive); *(5)* autosomal recessive loci underlying autism susceptibility will be enriched in populations with recent shared ancestry; *(6)* although genome-wide association studies are undoubtedly important, linkage studies may remain as an important complementary approach, particularly in special founder populations; *(7)* pedigrees with rare, highly penetrant loci may involve syndromic forms of autism that may involve ID or epilepsy; and *(8)* pedigrees from isolate populations or with syndromic forms of autism may be highly informative to other forms of ASDs with more complex genetic architecture. Although this endeavor for ASDs is in the very early stages, and there is much work ahead, there are some initial clues and loci that are being followed up extensively, as the field moves forward with expanded study-sized and novel genomic methods.

Challenges and Future Directions

- Large epidemiologic studies of autism in special populations with recent shared ancestry.
- High-throughput sequencing of linkage peaks and genome-wide in samples with recent shared ancestry to characterize full extent of recessive genetic changes, which may be associated with disease.
- Large-scale sequencing of candidate targets emerging from above studies in populations without recent shared ancestry to test possibility of general significance of loci to non-founder populations.

SUGGESTED READING

Basel-Vanagaite, L., Taub, E., Halpern, G. J., Drasinover, V., Magal, N., Davidov, B., et al. (2007). Genetic screening for autosomal recessive nonsyndromic mental retardation in an isolated population in Israel. *European Journal of Human Genetics: EJHG, 15*, 250–253.

Morrow, E. M., Yoo, S. Y., Flavell, S. W., Kim, T. K., Lin, Y., Hill, R. S., et al. (2008). Identifying autism loci and genes by tracing recent shared ancestry. *Science, 321*, 218–223.

Strauss, K. A., Puffenberger, E. G., Huentelman, M. J., Gottlieb, S., Dobrin, S. E., Parod, J. M., et al. (2006). Recessive symptomatic focal epilepsy and mutant contactin-associated protein-like 2. *New England Journal of Medicine, 354*, 1370–1377.

ACKNOWLEDGMENTS

Supported by the NIMH (R01 MH083565), the NLM Family Foundation, the Simons Foundation, and the Manton Center for Orphan Disease Research. EMM is supported by the NIMH (K23 MH080954) and the Career Award for Medical Scientists from the Burroughs Wellcome Fund. C.A.W. is an Investigator of the Howard Hughes Medical Institute.

REFERENCES

Abrahams, B. S., & Geschwind D. H. (2008). Advances in autism genetics: On the threshold of a new neurobiology. *Nature Reviews Genetics, 9*(5), 341–355.

Alarcon, M., Abrahams, B. S., Stone, J. L., Duvall, J. A., Perederiy, J. V., Bomar, J. M. et al. (2008). Linkage, association, and gene-expression analyses identify CNTNAP2 as an autism-susceptibility gene. *American Journal of Human Genetics, 82*(1), 150–159.

Alvarez Retuerto, A. I., Cantor, R. M., Gleeson, J. G., Ustaszewska, A., Schackwitz, W. S., Pennacchio, L. A. et al. (2008). Association of common variants in the Joubert syndrome gene (AHI1) with autism. *Human Molecular Genetics, 17*(24), 3887–3896.

American Psychiatric Association. (2000). *Diagnostic and statistical manual of mental disorders* (4th ed., text rev.; DSM-IV-TR). Washington, DC: Author.

Arking, D. E., Cutler, D. J., Brune, C. W., Teslovicha, T. M., West, K., Ikeda, M. (2008). A common genetic variant in the neurexin superfamily member CNTNAP2 increases familial risk of autism. *American Journal of Human Genetics, 82*(1), 160–164.

Bailey, A., Le Couteur, A., Gottesman, I., Bolton, P., Simonoff, E., Yuzda, E., et al. (1995). Autism as a strongly genetic disorder: Evidence from a British twin study. *Psychological Medicine, 25*(1), 63–77.

Bakkaloglu, B., O'Roak, B. J., Louvi, A., Gupta, A. R., Abelson, J. F., Morgan, T. M. (2008). Molecular cytogenetic analysis and resequencing of contactin associated protein-like 2 in autism spectrum disorders. *American Journal of Human Genetics, 82*(1), 165–173.

Barkovich, A. J., Kuzniecky, R. I., Jackson, G. D., Guerrini, R., & Dobyns, W. B. (2005). A developmental and genetic classification for malformations of cortical development. *Neurology, 65*(12), 1873–1887.

Baron-Cohen, S., Leslie, A. M. & Frith, U. (1985). Does the autistic child have a theory of mind? *Cognition, 21*(1), 37–46.

Basel-Vanagaite, L., Attia, R., Yahav, M., Ferland, R. J., Anteki, L., Walsh, C. A. (2006). The CC2D1A, a member of a new gene family with C2 domains, is involved in autosomal recessive non-syndromic mental retardation. *Journal of Medical Genetics, 43*(3), 203–210.

Basel-Vanagaite, L., Taub, E., Halpern, G. J., Drasinover, V., Magal, N., Davidov, B. et al. (2007). Genetic screening for autosomal recessive nonsyndromic mental retardation in an isolated population in Israel. *European Journal of Human Genetics: EJHG, 15*(2), 250–253.

Beaudet, A. L., & Belmont J. W. (2008). Array-based DNA diagnostics: Let the revolution begin. *Annual Review of Medicine, 59*, 113–129.

Brown, W. T., Jenkins, E. C., Cohen, I. L., Fisch, G. S., Wolf-Schein, E. G., Gross, A., et al. (1986). Fragile X and autism: A multicenter survey. *American Journal of Medical Genetics, 23*(1–2), 341–352.

Campbell, D. B., Sutcliffe, J. S., Ebert, P. J., Militerni, R., Bravaccio, C., Trillo, S., et al. (2006). A genetic variant that disrupts MET transcription is associated with autism.

Proceedings of National Academy of Sciences of the United States of America, 103(45), 16,834–16,839.

Cook, E. H., Jr., Lindgren, V., Leventhal, B. L., Courchesne, R., Lincoln, A., Shulman, C., et al. (1997). Autism or atypical autism in maternally but not paternally derived proximal 15q duplication. *American Journal of Human Genetics, 60*(4), 928–934.

Cook, E. H., Jr., & Scherer, S. W. (2008). Copy-number variations associated with neuropsychiatric conditions. *Nature, 455*(7215), 919–923.

Danielsson, S., Gillberg, I. C., Billstedt, E., Gillberg, C., & Olsson, I. (2005). Epilepsy in young adults with autism: A prospective population-based follow-up study of 120 individuals diagnosed in childhood. *Epilepsia, 46*(6), 918–923.

Dolen, G., & Bear, M. F. (2005). Courting a cure for fragile X. *Neuron, 45*(5), 642–644.

Fombonne, E. (1999). The epidemiology of autism: A review. *Psychological Medicine, 29*(4), 769–786.

Fombonne, E. (2003). Epidemiological surveys of autism and other pervasive developmental disorders: An update. *Journal of Autism and Developmental Disorders, 33*(4), 365–382.

Ganz, M. L. (2007). The lifetime distribution of the incremental societal costs of autism. *Archives of Pediatrics and Adolescent Medicine, 161*(4), 343–349.

Gecz, J., Shoubridge, C., & Corbett, M. (2009). The genetic landscape of intellectual disability arising from chromosome X. *Trends in Genetics, 25*(7), 308–316.

The germinating seed of Arab genomics. (2006). *Nature Genetics, 38*(8), 851.

Geschwind, D. H. (2008). Autism: Many genes, common pathways? *Cell, 135*(3), 391–395.

Geschwind, D. H. (2009). Advances in autism. *Annual Review of Medicine, 60*, 367–380.

Happe, F., & Frith, U. (2006). The weak coherence account: Detail-focused cognitive style in autism spectrum disorders. *Journal of Autism and Developmental Disorders, 36*(1), 5–25.

Helbig, I., Mefford, H. C., Sharp, A. J., Guipponi, M., Fichera, M., Franke, A., et al. (2009). 15q13.3 microdeletions increase risk of idiopathic generalized epilepsy. *Nature Genetics, 41*(2), 160–162.

Hoodfar, E., & Teebi, A. S. (1996). Genetic referrals of Middle Eastern origin in a western city: Inbreeding and disease profile. *American Journal of Medical Genetics, 33*(3), 212–215.

Jamain, S., Quach, H., Betancur, C., Rastam, M., Colineaux, C., Gillberg, I. C., et al. (2003). Mutations of the X-linked genes encoding neuroligins NLGN3 and NLGN4 are associated with autism. *Nature Genetics, 34*(1), 27–29.

Kruglyak, L., Daly, M. J., & Lander, E. S. (1995). Rapid multipoint linkage analysis of recessive traits in nuclear families, including homozygosity mapping. *American Journal of Human Genetics, 56*(2), 519–527.

Lander, E. S., & Botstein, D. (1987). Homozygosity mapping: A way to map human recessive traits with the DNA of inbred children. *Science, 236*(4808), 1567–1570.

Laumonnier, F., Bonnet-Brilhault, F., Gomot, M., Blanc, R., David, A., & Moizard, M. P. (2004). X-linked mental retardation and autism are associated with a mutation in the NLGN4 gene, a member of the neuroligin family. *American Journal of Human Genetics, 74*(3), 552–557.

Martin, C. L., & Ledbetter, D. H. (2007). Autism and cytogenetic abnormalities: Solving autism one chromosome at a time. *Current Psychiatry Reports, 9*(2), 141–147.

Miller, D. T., Shen, Y., Weiss, L. A., Korn, J., Anselm, I., Bridgemohan, C., et al. (2009). Microdeletion/duplication at 15q13.2q13.3 among individuals with features of autism and other neuropsychiatric disorders. *American Journal of Medical Genetics, 46*(4), 242–248.

Morrow, E. M., Yoo, S. Y., Flavell, S. W., Kim, T. K., Lin, Y., Hill, R. S., et al. (2008). Identifying autism loci and genes by tracing recent shared ancestry. *Science, 321*(5886), 218–223.

Morton, N. E. (1978). Effect of inbreeding on IQ and mental retardation. *Proceedings of National Academy of Sciences of the United States of America, 75*(8), 3906–3908.

Moss, J., & Howlin, P. (2009). Autism spectrum disorders in genetic syndromes: Implications for diagnosis, intervention and understanding the wider autism spectrum disorder population. *Journal of Intellectual Disability Research, 53*(10), 852–873.

Muhle, R., Trentacoste, S. V., & Rapin, I. (2004). The genetics of autism. *Pediatrics, 113*(5), e472–486.

National Center for Health Statistics (U.S.). (1996). National Health Interview Survey on Disability, phase 1.

Rare chromosomal deletions and duplications increase risk of schizophrenia. (2008). *Nature, 455*(7210), 237–241.

Reddy, K. S. (2005). Cytogenetic abnormalities and fragile-X syndrome in Autism Spectrum Disorder. *BMC Medical Genetics, 6*, 3.

Riaz, N., Steinberg, S., Ahmad, J., Pluzhnikov, A., Riazuddin, S., Cox, N. J., et al. (2005). Genomewide significant linkage to stuttering on chromosome 12. *American Journal of Human Genetics, 76*(4), 647–651.

Ritvo, E. R., Spence, M. A., Freeman, B. J., Mason-Brothers, A., Mo, A., & Marazita, M. L. (1985). Evidence for autosomal recessive inheritance in 46 families with multiple incidences of autism. *American Journal of Psychiatry, 142*(2), 187–192.

Strauss, K. A., Puffenberger, E. G., Huentelman, M. J., Gottlieb, S., Dobrin, S. E., Parod, J. M., et al. (2006). Recessive symptomatic focal epilepsy and mutant contactin-associated protein-like 2. *New England Journal of Medicine, 354*(13), 1370–1377.

Stromme, P. (2000). Aetiology in severe and mild mental retardation: A population-based study of Norwegian children. *Developmental Medicine and Child Neurology, 42*(2), 76–86.

Tanzi, R. E., & Bertram, L. (2005). Twenty years of the Alzheimer's disease amyloid hypothesis: A genetic perspective. *Cell, 120*(4), 545–555.

Tanzi, R. E., Kovacs, D. M., Kim, T. W., Moir, R. D., Guenette, S. Y., & Wasco, W. (1996). The gene defects responsible for familial Alzheimer's disease. *Neurobiology of Disease, 3*(3), 159–168.

Tariq, A., Santos, R. L., Khan, M. N., Lee, K., Hassan, M. J., Ahmad, W., et al. (2006). Localization of a novel autosomal recessive nonsyndromic hearing impairment locus DFNB65 to chromosome 20q13.2-q13.32. *Journal of Molecular Medicine, 84*(6), 484–490.

Teebi, A. S., & El-Shanti, H. I. (2006). Consanguinity: Implications for practice, research, and policy. *Lancet, 367*(9515), 970–971.

Teebi, A. S., & Farag, T. I. (1997). *Genetic disorders among Arab populations.* New York, Oxford University Press.

Walsh, C. A., Morrow, E. M., & Rubenstein, J. L. (2008). Autism and brain development. *Cell, 135*(3), 396–400.

45 Jeffrey L. Neul

Rett Syndrome and *MECP2*-Related Disorders

Points of Interest

- RTT is a clinical diagnosis that predicts genetic alterations, but a fraction of individuals do not have any identified genetic alterations.
- Mutations in *MECP2* are found in the majority of people with typical RTT. Some defined atypical variant forms of RTT have mutations in other loci (e.g., *CDKL5, FOXG1*).
- Mutations in *MECP2* have been identified in neurodevelopmental disorders that do not have the distinctive clinical features of RTT.
- Both loss of MeCP2 function and increasing the amount of MeCP2 protein leads to neurodevelopmental disorders in people as well as distinct phenotypic abnormalities in mice. Thus, the precise level of MeCP2 with a cell is critical for the normal functioning of the nervous system.
- Because the spectrum of phenotypic and neuroanatomic abnormalities that occur as a result of alterations in MeCP2 protein level display similarities to a number of neurodevelopmental disorders, understanding these *MECP2*-related disorders and the functional changes that occur at a molecular and cellular level will likely provide insight into a number of neurodevelopmental disorders such as autism.

In the 1960s, Andreas Rett, an Austrian pediatrician, noticed two markedly impaired girls in his waiting room with similar relentless hand-wringing. He recognized that these girls also shared a number of additional clinical features. By reviewing his charts, he identified a cohort of girls with this unique condition, which he reported in a German language journal (Rett, 1966). The condition was not routinely recognized until 1983, when Bengt Hagberg and colleagues published a series of 35 similar cases (B. Hagberg et al., 1983) in English and gave it the eponym by which it is commonly referred, Rett Syndrome (RTT; OMIM 312750). Since that time, not only have a large number of additional cases been identified, but mutations in *Methyl-CpG-binding protein 2* (*MECP2*) have been determined to cause RTT (Amir et al., 1999). Although this is a relatively rare condition, affecting 1.09 per 10,000 females by age 12 years (Laurvick et al., 2006), broad interest in this disorder exists because clinical features found in RTT are also seen in a number of other neurodevelopmental disorders, as well as adult neurological and psychiatric conditions. Additionally, the spectrum of clinical disorders caused by either decreasing or increasing MeCP2 function (*MECP2*-related disorders) has grown to include autism, Angelman Syndrome-like features, intellectual disability in boys with associated neuropsychiatric features, and neuropsychiatric features such as anxiety and depression in women. The fact that alterations in MeCP2 function can cause such a wide range of clinical features with similarities to many other neurological and psychiatric disorders both in children and adults argues for a common pathogenic mechanism. This chapter provides a brief outline of the clinical features of typical RTT and describes the genetic locus mutated in the majority of typical RTT. The clinical aspects and genetics of atypical forms of RTT and other *MECP2*-related disorders are presented, followed by an introduction to the molecular function of MeCP2 and animal models of RTT and *MECP2*-related disorders.

Typical Rett Syndrome

Diagnosis of Rett Syndrome

Typical, or classic, RTT is a clinical diagnosis based on the presence of clinical features that meet defined consensus criteria (Table 45-1) (Neul et al., 2010). The diagnosis of typical RTT requires a period of regression, specifically of hand and spoken language skills, the development of gait abnormalities (or the failure to walk), and the onset of characteristic hand stereotypies. In a previous consensus criteria published in

2002 (B. Hagberg, Hanefeld, Percy, & Skjeldal et al., 2002), acquired microcephaly was a necessary criteria, however it has been recognized that a significant fraction of people with RTT do not have acquired microcephaly, therefore this requirement has been removed in the recent criteria. However, because it is a clinical feature that can alert a clinician to the potential diagnosis and it is a distinctive feature in the disorder, acquired microcephaly is included as a preamble to the criteria as a feature that should raise suspicion for the diagnosis. In addition to the above listed required features, the diagnosis of typical RTT also requires grossly normal development in the first six months of life and the exclusion of any other possible known causes of neurological dysfunction.

It has long been recognized that some individuals present with many of the features of RTT but do not exhibit all the necessary criteria for the diagnosis of typical RTT. Consequently, a separate set of criteria, derived from the criteria for typical RTT, were devised for these "atypical" cases (Table 45-1). (Neul et al., 2010). Such persons may have a more severe presentation than typical RTT, with no period of normal development (known as the congenital variant), or may have a greater degree of preserved function (known as the preserved speech variant [PSV]). As these atypical variants demonstrate important features concerning both the clinical and genetic heterogeneity found in RTT, the specific clinical and genetic features will be discussed at length later.

Despite the fact that the majority of cases of typical RTT have mutations in *MECP2* (discussed below), RTT remains a clinical diagnosis. This may strike some as anachronistic. If most cases of RTT have mutations in a *MECP2*, why not define the disease by the presence of a mutation in *MECP2*? There are two important reasons that a *MECP2* mutation does not equal the clinical condition and vice versa. First, although the majority of individuals with typical RTT have a *MECP2* mutation, at least 5% do not, despite clearly having the clinical condition (Neul et al., 2008). Therefore, having a *MECP2* mutation is not *necessary* for the clinical diagnosis. In fact, some people with features of RTT have mutations in other genetic loci (discussed later). Second, *MECP2* mutations can also be found in people who do not manifest the clinical features of RTT. Therefore, mutations in this locus are not *sufficient* to make the diagnosis. Throughout the course of this chapter, the clinical and genetic knowledge to demonstrate this argument will be presented. In light of the importance of both the clinical condition and the details of the genetic alterations, when characterizing individuals, it is worthwhile to state *both* the clinical condition and the genetic mutations—for example, typical RTT with a disease-causing mutation in *MECP2*, atypical RTT with a disease-causing mutation in *CDKL5*, and so forth.

Table 45–1.
Consensus criteria for diagnosis of RTT

RTT Diagnostic Criteria
Consider diagnosis when postnatal deceleration of head growth observed.
Required for Typical or Classic RTT
1. A period of regression followed by recovery or stabilization
2. All main criteria and all exclusion criteria
3. Supportive criteria are not required, although often present in typical RTT
Required for Atypical or Variant RTT
1. A period of regression followed by recovery or stabilization
2. 2 out of the 4 main criteria
3. 5 out of 11 supportive criteria
Main Criteria
1. Partial or complete loss of acquired purposeful hand skills
2. Partial or complete loss of acquired spoken language
3. Gait abnormalities: Impaired (dyspraxic) or absence of ability
4. Stereotypic hand movements such as hand wringing/squeezing, clapping/tapping, mouthing and washing/rubbing automatisms
Exclusion Criteria for Typical RTT
1. Brain injury secondary to trauma (peri- or postnatally), neurometabolic disease, or severe infection that causes neurological problems
2. Grossly abnormal psychomotor development in first 6 months of life
Supportive Criteria for Atypical RTT
1. Breathing disturbances when awake
2. Bruxism when awake
3. Impaired sleep pattern
4. Abnormal muscle tone
5. Peripheral vasomotor disturbances
6. Scoliosis/kyphosis
7. Growth retardation
8. Small cold hands and feet
9. Inappropriate laughing/screaming spells
10. Diminished response to pain
11. Intense eye communication - "eye pointing"

Adapted with permission from Neul et al., 2010.

Clinical Features of Rett Syndrome

Early Development

RTT is a neurodevelopmental disorder that primarily affects girls, causing intellectual disability, loss of purposeful hand use and spoken language, stereotypic hand movements, and a particular gait abnormality. The clinical course follows a specific disease progression. Individuals with RTT initially undergo apparently normal development after a normal pregnancy and delivery (B. Hagberg et al., 1983) with normal height, weight, and head size. In retrospect, they are considered "good" babies, typically relatively placid (A. M. Kerr, Montague, & Stephenson, 1987; Leonard & Bower, 1998; Naidu, 1997; Nomura & Segawa, 1990b; Witt-Engerstrom, 1987). Individuals who ultimately develop RTT reach typical developmental screening milestones appropriately, and no concerns with development at this time are noted (A. M. Kerr & Stephenson, 1985; Witt-Engerstrom & Gillberg, 1987), although retrospective review of early family videos revealed subtle movement abnormalities (Einspieler, Kerr, & Prechtl, 2005a, 2005b; A. M. Kerr et al., 1987; Witt-Engerstrom, 1987). Development begins to stagnate between 6 to 18 months without clear developmental regression.

Regression

After this period of developmental stagnation, dramatic and relatively rapid regression prominently affecting hand and spoken language skills occurs between approximately 1 to 4 years of life over a variable interval of several days to a year. The loss of skills is relative to the degree that specific skills had previously been acquired. For example, a child who previously had at best achieved nuanced babbling may become essentially mute, whereas a child who had distinct spoken words may revert to babbling. Social interaction and communication become impaired with the development of autistic features such as a dislike for being held, avoidance of eye contact, or unresponsiveness to human contact. Some children display screaming episodes in which they appear to be in pain, sometimes raising concern for an infectious encephalitic process. Before the onset of additional typical clinical features of the disorder, individuals may be diagnosed with an autistic spectrum disorder or a neurodegenerative condition. Some of the distinctive clinical features, such as hand stereotypies, may manifest at this stage, but they often are not apparent until regression has ended. A history of regression is considered to be an essential criteria for the diagnosis of classic, or typical, RTT (B. Hagberg, 2002).

Stabilization

After the period of distinct regression of developmental skills, a period of relative stability ensues. Notably, the children show improvement in mood, eye contact, and general sociability in affected individuals, which clearly distinguishes RTT from other relentless neurodegenerative conditions or typical autism. Communication using intense eye gaze and eye pointing begins, which is a very prominent and distinctive feature of RTT (B. Hagberg, 2002) and distinguishes this condition from classic autism. Hand stereotypies and other characteristic features of the disorder become prominent and clearly mark affected individuals as having the specific disorder. In the era before the discovery of the genetic basis of RTT, the diagnosis of RTT was rarely made until this stage.

Distinct Clinical Features

Hand Stereotypies

Probably the most readily recognized feature of RTT is the repetitive hand-wringing, washing-like motion, or hand-clapping behavior. These movements are typically midline but may also be lateral, on the head, or behind the back (Temudo et al., 2007). They occur only during wakefulness and vary in frequency both between and within individuals, often worsened with anxiety or stress. These stereotypies appear to inhibit volitional hand use, as mild improvement in volitional hand use occurs after splinting of the arms at the elbows (Aron, 1990; Bumin et al., 2002; Kubas, 1992; Sharpe, 1992; Sharpe & Ottenbacher, 1990). With age, the movements become slower and simpler in concert with increased rigidity (FitzGerald et al., 1990; Nomura & Segawa, 1990a; Temudo et al., 2007). Notably, although hand-washing stereotypies are often considered to be pathognomonic of RTT, recent work has indicated that such behaviors may not be specific to RTT (Temudo et al., 2007).

Gait and Movement Abnormalities

Although some individuals never learn to walk or completely lose the ability during regression, many are able to walk. However, all have some degree of gait abnormality with a characteristic dyspraxic, wandering quality. Elements of ataxia are also present and the stance is typically wide-based. Affected individuals also have a variety of movement abnormalities including dystonia, tremor, myoclonus, and bruxism. Muscle tone is initially hypotonic with the development of increased limb tone and rigidity as the child ages.

Growth Failure

Although birth head size, weight, and height are typically normal, individuals with RTT suffer from pervasive growth failure. The rate of head growth declines as early as 2 months and may result in frank acquired microcephaly (G. Hagberg, Stenbom, & Engerstrom, 2001). Most individuals with RTT are markedly underweight and short, despite apparently normal appetite, although a subset have increased body mass indices (Renieri et al., 2008). Hand and foot growth are also impaired. Although objectively their hands are small, they often appear long and slender because of decreased muscle mass of the intrinsic muscles of the hands and fingers, likely secondary to decreased volitional hand use (personal observation). Additionally, bone mineral density is low (Budden & Gunness, 2003; Motil et al., 2008), and some individuals have increased bone fractures (Motil et al., 2008), which may be identified on routine X-ray without any clear proximate cause.

Seizures and Nonepileptic Spells

All affected individuals have abnormal electroencephalograms (EEGs) after age 2 years with slowing of background activity, spike, and slow spike and wave activity (Glaze, 2002). Seizures are present in some individuals, but the reported prevalence of seizures varies widely, from 30% to 80% (Glaze et al., 1987; Glaze, Schultz, & Frost, 1998; Hagne, Witt-Engerstrom, & Hagberg, 1989; Steffenburg, Hagberg, & Hagberg, 2001). The source of this variation is likely the spectrum of nonepileptic events that can be confused with true epileptic seizures. These nonepileptic events can manifest as vacant spells associated with breath-holding (Cooper, Kerr, & Amos, 1998), dystonic posturing, or paroxysmal dyskinesias (personal observation). Video EEG recordings during these spells show no electrographic seizure activity (Cooper et al., 1998). It has been proposed that these nonepileptic events may result from brain stem dysfunction. In general, typical anti-seizure medications do not show significant efficacy toward these nonepileptic spells; however, use of topirimate reduced breathing irregularity in individuals being treated for epilepsy (Goyal, O'Riordan, & Wiznitzer, 2004). The frequency of these nonepileptic spells, the potential for confusion with cortical seizures, and the inherent increased risk of seizures in this population demonstrate the importance of careful evaluation with video EEG monitoring to determine the exact nature of such spells.

Autonomic Dysfunction

A serious clinical issue in RTT is the high incidence of sudden unexpected death, which accounts for up to 25% of the deaths of affected individuals (A. M. Kerr et al., 1997). Although the exact nature of such deaths is unknown, the variety of autonomic abnormalities found in girls and women with RTT suggests that this autonomic dysfunction may be a factor (Guideri et al., 1999; Julu et al., 1997; Sekul et al., 1994). Evidence of cardiac rhythm abnormalities exist including decreased beat-to-beat variability of their heart rate (Guideri et al., 1999; Julu et al., 2001), tachycardia (Rohdin et al., 2007; Weese-Mayer et al., 2006), and bradycardia (Madan et al., 2004; Rohdin et al., 2007). Furthermore, the electrocardiograms of a significant fraction of affected individuals have a prolonged corrected QT interval (Ellaway et al., 1999; Sekul et al., 1994).

Respiration is altered in the majority of girls and women with RTT, and many have markedly irregular breathing with periods of hyperventilation and/or apnea (Julu et al., 2001; Rohdin et al., 2007; Weese-Mayer et al., 2006). The breathing irregularities are exaggerated in novel, stress-inducing environments. Detailed analysis of respiratory patterns during wakefulness (Weese-Mayer et al., 2006) has revealed that breathing in RTT is more irregular, faster, and deeper than in control individuals even in "normal" non-apneic periods. In contrast to previous reports of complete normalization of respiration during sleep, prolonged in-home studies have shown both an equal number of apneas during daytime and nighttime (Rohdin et al., 2007) and faster, more irregular breathing during nighttime (Weese-Mayer et al., 2008). Although these studies lack coincident EEG measurements to unequivocally determine the sleep–wake state, the overall findings suggest some degree of breathing dysfunction during sleep and wakefulness.

Analysis of the relationship between breathing and heart rate has revealed a lack of coordination between the two, suggesting alteration in the medullary network that controls and integrates these systems (Julu et al., 2001; Rohdin et al., 2007; Weese-Mayer et al., 2008). This notion is supported by evidence from mouse models and human pathological studies of alterations in both the serotoninergic and noradrenergic systems within the medulla, both critical in the modulation of cardiorespiratory rhythms (Paterson et al., 2005; Viemari et al., 2005).

Nearly all affected individuals have cool extremities—especially their feet, which at times can be cold and mottled (A. M. Kerr & Julu, 1999). Interestingly, an anecdotal report indicates that the cool extremities likely have a sympathetic nervous system origin. An accidental unilateral sympathectomy was performed in an affected individual undergoing spinal fusion for scoliosis,. After recovery, the foot on the sympathectomy side was warmer, despite the opposite foot remaining as cool as presurgically (Naidu et al., 1987).

The gastrointestinal system shows significant alterations. Most girls and women with RTT have disrupted oromotor function and difficulty swallowing, with frequent choking and gagging on food (Motil et al., 1999). Furthermore, many are afflicted with severe gastroesophageal reflux and constipation (B. Hagberg et al., 1983), two issues that cause significant morbidity in affected individuals. Additionally, the motility of the esophagus, stomach, and duodenum is uncoordinated (Motil et al., 1999).

Late Motor Decline

As they enter their teens and twenties, many affected individuals show a protracted decline in motor skills and develop a hypoactive pattern of behavior ("couch potatoes"). Parkinsonian features such as rigidity, hypomimia, and retropulsion also become more prominent (FitzGerald, Jankovic, Glaze et al., 1990; FitzGerald, Jankovic, & Percy, 1990; B. Hagberg, 2005). Associated musculoskeletal alterations such as scoliosis and contractures can become serious enough to warrant surgical intervention (Smeets, Schrander-Stumpel, & Curfs, 2008). Although this motor decline sometimes impairs independent ambulation, a number of affected individuals continue to walk throughout their lives (Smeets et al., 2008). Although previously considered to be fatal by the teenage years, survival into at least middle age is typical and should be anticipated (Kirby et al., 2009). This improvement in survival likely reflects the greater attention currently paid to monitoring nutritional status and providing additional nutritional support when needed (Motil et al., 2009).

Neuropathology

The brains of individuals with RTT are small, as expected from the small head size, but neuropathology has revealed no gross abnormalities, gliosis, or migrational defects (D. D. Armstrong, 2005b). However, there is decreased synaptic density (Belichenko et al., 1994), decreased dendritic arborization (D. Armstrong et al., 1995), and increased neuronal cell packing in the hippocampus (Kaufmann & Moser, 2000). Importantly, no signs of cell loss or neurodegeneration have been observed (Jellinger et al., 1988), indicating that RTT is not a neurodegenerative process.

Genetics of Rett Syndrome

Because RTT typically manifests in females, the hypothesis arose that it was the result of an X-linked dominant genetic alteration with male lethality (B. Hagberg et al., 1983). The majority of cases are sporadic; however, rare familial cases have allowed exclusion mapping of the X-chromosome and localization to Xq27-qter. Analyzing candidate transcripts within the region has revealed mutations in *MECP2*, located at Xq28, in both familial as well as sporadic cases (Amir et al., 1999). The vast majority (95%) of people with typical RTT have mutations in *MECP2* (Neul et al., 2008). Most of the mutations found in sporadic cases arise from the parental germline (Trappe et al., 2001) and often occur at CpG mutational hotspots by deamination of methylated cytosines, which creates a C-T transition.

The coding sequence of *MECP2* spans four exons that encode two splice isoforms of the protein that differ in their amino-terminus (Kriaucionis & Bird, 2004; Mnatzakanian et al., 2004). Additional mRNA species complexity exists because *MECP2* has a large 3′untranslated region (3′UTR) that contains multiple polyadenylation sites. Alternative use of these polyadenylation sites generates four 3′UTR isoforms, with the longest transcript being the dominant species in the brain (Coy et al., 1999). There are highly conserved sequence regions within the 3′UTR (B. Kerr et al., 2008), suggesting a role in regulation of MeCP2 expression, and recently a micro-RNA (miR132) was found to bind to the 3′UTR and regulate MeCP2 translation (Klein et al., 2007).

An interesting genetic feature of the rare familial cases of RTT is the presence of the pathogenic mutation in *MECP2* in asymptomatic carrier mothers and other female relatives. Because *MECP2* resides on the X-chromosome, one source of this variation in expressivity is the pattern of X-chromosome inactivation (XCI). In females, only one X-chromosome is active in any cell whereas the other is inactivated. The process of inactivation occurs during development and usually results in a random pattern, with half the cells in her body expressing the maternal X-chromosome and half expressing the paternal X-chromosome. In most girls with typical RTT, the XCI pattern is random, with half of the cells expressing a wild-type copy of *MECP2* and half expressing the mutated version. However, the asymptomatic carriers have markedly skewed XCI, with most of the cells in their body expressing the wild-type copy of *MECP2* (Wan et al., 1999). It should be noted that there are rare boys who have the clinical features of RTT. The majority of these have mutations in *MECP2* and additional genetic abnormalities such as X-chromosomal aneupleudy or somatic mosaicism, which allows mosaic expression of wild-type and mutant alleles of *MECP2* similar to that which results in girls with RTT secondary to XCI. Although these cases are presented in the section titled "*MECP2*-related disorders," it should be noted that they do have typical RTT, despite being boys.

X Chromosome Inactivation (XCI): In females, only one X-chromosome is active in any cell, whereas the other is inactivated. The process of inactivation occurs during development and usually results in a random pattern, with half the cells of the body expressing the maternal X-chromosome and half expressing the paternal X-chromosome.

Skewed XCI: In most girls and women, XCI is a random process that results in roughly the same percentage of cells expressing genes from the maternal chromosome as from the paternal chromosome. However, in some people, non-random skewing of XCI is observed with a larger fraction of cells expressing genes from one of the parental chromosomes than the other. This may be the result of selective pressure during development favoring cells expressing one parental X-chromosome over the other. In people with mutations in *MECP2*, all informative examples of skewed XCI have been shown to favor the "good" X-chromosome containing the non-mutated copy of *MECP2*. This suggests that cells that express a mutated version of MeCP2 may be at a developmental disadvantage compared with cells expressing a normal version of MeCP2.

Phenotypic Variation in Rett Syndrome

Although RTT is defined by a distinct set of clinical features, clinical severity varies considerably among individuals. One explanation for the difference in expressivity of the atypical cases, as well as variation in typical cases, is variation in the degree of XCI skewing. As mentioned above, this is most apparent in the extreme case of an asymptomatic mother with complete XCI skewing. In the same way, incomplete XCI skewing can explain some of the variation seen in individuals with RTT (Amir et al., 2000); however, it accounts for only 20% of the clinical variability seen in typical RTT (Archer, Evans, Leonard et al., 2006).

Another possible source of variation is the molecular nature of the specific mutation in *MECP2*. Hundreds of pathogenic mutations in *MECP2* have been associated with RTT (Christodoulou et al., 2003), including missense, nonsense, frameshift, and large DNA rearrangements that typically remove large regions of the coding sequence (Archer, Whatley et al., 2006; Pan et al., 2006; Ravn et al., 2005). The fact that large DNA rearrangements that completely disrupt gene expression and point mutations result in the same clinical condition implies that these point mutations are loss-of-function mutations. Despite the large number of pathogenic mutations, eight common missense and nonsense mutations (Figure 45-1)—all the result of C-T transitions—account for approximately 70% of all typical RTT cases (Bebbington et al., 2008; Neul et al., 2008). Additionally, a number of small insertions and deletions in the carboxy-terminal domain (CTD) result in frameshift mutations that lead to similar truncations late in the protein. As a group, these CTD truncations account for approximately 7% to 12% of all typical RTT cases (Bebbington et al., 2008; Neul et al., 2008). Finally, large DNA rearrangements account for approximately 7% of typical RTT cases (Neul et al., 2008). Thus, in total, more than 80% of individuals with typical RTT have 1 of these 10 mutations.

This fact has allowed genotype/phenotype correlation studies to be performed. In general, mutations that truncate the protein before the nuclear localization sequence (NLS) are more severe than missense mutations or truncations after the NLS (Huppke et al., 2002; Smeets et al., 2005). Recent studies have had the power to detect phenotypic differences between the common mutations and have found that p.Arg168X, p.Arg255X, p.Arg270X, and large rearrangements are more severely affected, whereas p.Arg133Cys, p.Arg294X, p.Arg306Cys, and CTD truncations are milder (Bebbington et al., 2008; Neul et al., 2008).

Atypical Forms of Rett Syndrome

Individuals who have regression and cardinal features of RTT but do not meet the consensus criteria for the disorder are termed *atypical variants*. These variants may have clinical features more severe than typical RTT, present with milder manifestations, or have features not commonly associated with typical RTT (B. A. Hagberg & Skjeldal, 1994). Although the majority of individuals with typical RTT have mutations in *MECP2* (Neul et al., 2008), only 58% of atypical cases have

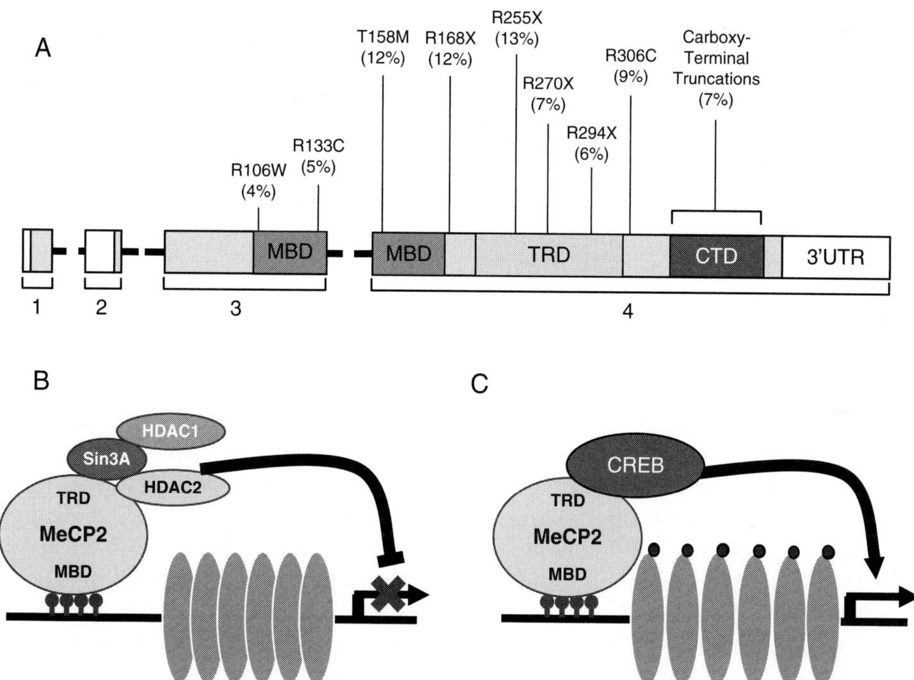

Figure 45–1. *MECP2* genetic locus, common mutations, and proposed function of MeCP2 protein (A) *MECP2* coding sequence spans four exons and encodes a protein that contains at least three molecular domains, the Methyl-Binding Domain (MBD), the Transcriptional Repression Domain (TRD), and the Carboxy-Terminal Domain (CTD). The gene also contains a large 3′ untranslated region (3′UTR, not drawn to scale), which has highly conserved areas that likely represent a major region of regulation of gene transcription and translation. Several hundred disease-causing mutations have been identified in *MECP2* but there are hot-spots for mutations. The eight most common point mutations and the frequency these mutations are present in typical RTT (Neul et al., 2008) are shown above the gene illustration. In addition to the common point mutations, a number of small insertions and deletions are found that cause frame-shift mutations and thus truncations in the CTD. As a group, these Carboxy-Terminal Truncations are found in approximately 7% of typical RTT cases. Not shown are large DNA deletions that disrupt most or all of the coding sequence of *MECP2* and account for an additional 7% of typical RTT cases. The protein product of this locus, MeCP2, is believed to function primarily as a regulator of gene transcription. The MBD binds methylated cytosines incorporated in DNA (B). The Transcriptional Repression Domain (TRD) interacts and recruits histone deacetylase complexes (B) containing Sin3A and Histone Deacetylase 1 and 2 (HDAC1,2). These HDAC complexes remove acetyl groups (small balls) from histones (large ovals) which causes the chromatin to adopt a tight closed structure that represses local gene transcription (B). Recent work has found that MeCP2 also forms a complex with the transcriptional activator CREB (Chahrour et al., 2008). This interaction is believed to increase local gene expression (C). An additional role (not shown) for MeCP2 as a regulator of RNA splicing has been proposed (Young et al., 2005), possibly by interactions between the CTD and splicing factors (Buschdorf & Stratling, 2004).

mutations in *MECP2* (A. K. Percy et al., 2007). Recent genetic studies have demonstrated that certain atypical forms are commonly associated with *MECP2* mutations, whereas mutations in other loci are associated with other distinct clinical forms of RTT (Table 45-2).

Forme Fruste Variant

Clinical Features and Genetics of Forme Fruste Variant of Rett Syndrome

One bridge between the typical RTT presentation and asymptomatic female carriers is the "forme fruste" variant (B. Hagberg & Rasmussen, 1986; B. A. Hagberg & Skjeldal, 1994). In this variant, the presence of a clear history of regression of hand skills and language is present, but the regression may occur later or be milder than that typically seen in RTT. Furthermore, the degree of retained or regained skills may be increased compared with typical RTT, and the distinct hand stereotypies found in typical RTT may be absent or less severe. In the evaluation of 12 forme fruste individuals, 9 were identified with mutations in *MECP2* (Huppke et al., 2003; Huppke et al., 2006; Smeets et al., 2003). Eight of these are pathogenic mutations commonly associated with typical RTT (p.Arg133Cys, p.Thr158Met, p.Pro225Arg, p.Arg306Cys, c.1164del44). One had a missense mutation of uncertain significance (p.Glu10Gln) not found in typical RTT. Skewing was observed in 5 of these 9 cases.

Preserved Speech Variant

Clinical Features of Preserved Speech Variant

One of the most interesting and possibly the most common variant of RTT is the PSV, also known as the Zapella variant. These individuals experience a post-regression restoration of some spoken language. This variant has been reported in more than 90 cases (Fukuda et al., 2005; Huppke et al., 2000; A. M. Kerr et al., 2006; Nielsen, Ravn, & Schwartz, 2001; Oexle et al., 2005; Renieri et al., 2008; Yamashita et al., 2001; Zappella, Gillberg, & Ehlers, 1998; Zappella et al., 2003; Zappella et al., 2001). Affected individuals develop hand stereotypies and undergo the typical progression of the disease; however, regression may be very gradual such that it is only noticed in retrospect (Zappella et al., 1998). The amount of spoken language regained varies from multiple single words to multiple word sentences. The speech pattern is abnormal with pronoun reversal (using third person), echolalia, and perseverative repetition of particular phrases.

In contrast to typical RTT, a large percentage of people with PSV have no evidence of head growth deceleration (Renieri et al., 2008), and, in fact, a subset have macrocephaly (Oexle et al., 2005; Renieri et al., 2008). Further, many people with PSV do not show growth failure—rather, some PSV individuals are overweight and a fraction are obese (Renieri et al., 2008). Although uncommon in typical RTT, some individuals with PSV show increased aggression both toward themselves and others.

Many PSV individuals will show autistic traits and some will fulfill criteria for autism (Zappella et al., 2003). In contrast to typical RTT in which these autistic features are mostly restricted to the regression period, some PSV individuals may continue to show some autistic features after the regression. The autistic features that have been noted are decreased facial expression, poor reciprocal interaction, decreased ability to share emotions, absence of symbolic or imaginative play, and repetitive, echolalic speech. Without attention to the history of regression and the recognition of hand stereotypies (which may have disappeared later in life), the diagnosis of a variant of RTT may be overlooked.

Genetics of Preserved Speech Variant

PSV is allelic with typical RTT, with the majority of the reported cases having mutations in *MECP2*. Many of the specific mutations identified in PSV are also found in typical RTT, although there is a bias toward particular mutations in PSV. In the 64 reported cases of PSV with MECP2 mutations (Fukuda et al., 2005; Huppke et al., 2000; A. M. Kerr et al., 2006; Nielsen, Henriksen et al., 2001; Petel-Galil et al., 2006; Renieri et al.,

Table 45–2.
Atypical forms of RTT

Variant Name	Clinical Features	Genetic Associations	
		MECP2 Mutations	Other Loci
Forme Fruste	Delayed regression, retained skills	9 of 12 cases (75%)*	None identified
Preserved Speech	Post-regression restoration of some language	64 of 92 cases (~70%)**	None identified
Early Seizure	Seizures within the first six months, or seizures before regression	Very Rare (<0.1%)#	*CDKL5* *NTNG1*
Congenital	No period of normal development. Hypotonia and delayed from birth	Very Rare (only 4 reported cases)##	*FOXG1*

*(Huppke et al., 2003; Huppke et al., 2006; Smeets et al., 2003).
**(Renieri et al., 2008).
#(Archer, Evans, Edwards et al., 2006).
##(Huppke et al., 2000; Monros et al., 2001; Smeets et al., 2003).

2008; Scala et al., 2007; Smeets et al., 2003; Yamashita et al., 2001; Zappella et al., 2001), 25 have p.Arg133Cys (39%) and 21 have CTD truncations (33%). In comparison, although these two mutation groups are commonly found in typical RTT, they only represent 5% and 7%, respectively (Neul et al., 2008). It is useful to note that in typical RTT, these mutations display the least severe clinical symptoms. This supports the notion that the PSV is on the mild end of a phenotypic continuum with typical RTT. However, a small number of cases with PSV have p.Arg168X, which results in more severe cases of typical RTT (Neul et al., 2008). Thus, the specific *MECP2* mutation cannot entirely account for the presentation of the mild PSV condition. Although XCI skewing is one possible mechanism by which the phenotypic manifestations of a specific mutation could be altered, the majority (22 of 26) of the reported cases of PSV for which XCI has been analyzed and informative show random XCI (<80% skewing). Therefore, other mechanisms such as genetic modifiers need to be considered to explain the mild PSV phenotype in the face of random XCI.

Early Seizure Variant

Clinical Features of Early Seizure Variant

Although a number of individuals with typical RTT have seizures during their lifetime, it is uncommon to have seizures during the first 6 months of life (Steffenburg et al., 2001). However, a subset of individuals who have features of RTT and are plagued by early onset of severe seizures (Goutieres & Aicardi, 1986; Hanefeld, 1985). These cases have been described as an early seizure variant, also known as the Hanefeld variant. Some of these individuals have myoclonic spasms that appear similar to infantile spasms, although not necessarily with the characteristic hypsarrythmic pattern on EEG (Goutieres & Aicardi, 1987). A major issue in terms of the classification of these individuals with a variant form of RTT is regression. Many people with this early seizure variant do have a period of regression; however, this is often in the midst of severe, intractable epilepsy. Because loss of previously acquired skills can be seen in other conditions with severe intractable epilepsy, it is not clear if the regression found in these individuals shares the same etiology as that seen in typical RTT (Goutieres & Aicardi, 1987).

Genetics of Early Seizure Variant

CDKL5

Few early seizure variant cases have been associated with mutations in *MECP2*—less than 1 out of 345 in a large British cohort (Archer, Evans, Edwards et al., 2006). Recently, mutations in a different X-linked locus, *CDKL5*, have been associated with some of these cases (Bahi-Buisson et al., 2008; Evans et al., 2005; Mari et al., 2005; Nectoux et al., 2006; Rosas-Vargas et al., 2008; Scala et al., 2005; Tao et al., 2004; Weaving et al., 2004). From these reported cases, a general clinical pattern is emerging. These individuals do not have a period of normal cognitive development, and all have seizures in the first 3 months of life. Many have some of the features found in RTT, such as acquired deceleration of head growth, impaired hand skills, impaired language, and some form of hand stereotypies. However, most of these cases lack some of the most critical features of RTT: a clear history of regression and the typical disease progression. Furthermore, autistic features are present in 85% with reduced social interaction and poor eye fixation (Bahi-Buisson et al., 2008). This is in contrast to the intense eye gaze found in girls with typical RTT. As the number of individuals identified with CDKL5 mutations grows, it is becoming clear that the clinical features found in these individuals are distinct from those people with typical RTT, and the ongoing diagnosis of these individuals with RTT is questionable. As in typical RTT with *MECP2* mutations, the majority of reported individuals are girls, with the few reported boys with *CDKL5* mutations showing a much more severe clinical course with Lennox-Gastaut type epilepsy, spastic quadriplegia, cortical blindness, and profound intellectual disability (Weaving et al., 2004).

An initial report suggested that CDKL5 protein directly interacts with and phosphorylates MeCP2 (Mari et al., 2005). Because MeCP2 is phosphorylated in an activity-dependent fashion (W. G. Chen et al., 2003; Martinowich et al., 2003), this was proposed to be the molecular link that explained the phenotypic similarities of individuals with mutations in *MECP2* and those with mutations in *CDKL5*. However, a subsequent study failed to show the physical association or the phosporylation of MeCP2 by CDKL5 (Lin, Franco, & Rosner, 2005), and in fact recent work indicates that CDKL5 protein is localized to the cytoplasm and interacts with a Rho GTPase signalling pathway to modulate neuronal morphogenesis (Chen et al., 2010).

Congenital Variant

Clinical Features of the Congenital Variant

A subset of individuals with features of RTT has been identified, with evidence of developmental delay and hypotonia from birth (Goutieres & Aicardi, 1987; Rolando, 1985); this subset has been classified as a congenital variant of RTT. The reported cases have hand stereotypies, hyperventilation, gait abnormalities, hand dysfunction, and autistic features. A major challenge in individuals with such a presentation is determining whether they have evidence of regression, a cardinal feature of RTT (Goutieres & Aicardi, 1987). Dr. Hagberg described congenital RTT as "very rare and should be regarded with skeptism" (B. Hagberg, 2002) because of the difficulty in determining whether there is a true developmental regression in these individuals.

Genetics of the Congenital Variant

Similarly to the early seizure variant, most cases with the congenital variant have no mutations in *MECP2* or in *CDKL5*

(Erlandson et al., 2003; Scala et al., 2007). In total, *MECP2* mutations have only been identified in four individuals with the congenital variant of RTT (Huppke et al., 2000; Monros et al., 2001; Smeets et al., 2003). However, recent reports have identified mutations in another locus, *FOXG1*, in people with the congenital variant (Ariani et al., 2008; Papa et al., 2008; Jacob et al., 2009; Mencarelli et al., 2010). These cases are marked by severe early psychomotor delay, microcephaly by 3 months, stereotypic hand movements, no acquisition of spoken language, and corpus callosum hypoplasia (Ariani et al., 2008).

MECP2-Related Disorders

The recognition that mutations in *MECP2* cause RTT led to the discovery of *MECP2* sequence changes in a variety of neurodevelopmental conditions in both females and males. These individuals clearly do not have clinical features of RTT, so it would be inappropriate describe them as "Rett Syndrome." Rather they represent the broad group of *MECP2*-related disorders. The clinical features as well as the molecular details of these various disorders vary and will be presented in detail.

Girls With *MECP2* Mutations and Non-Rett Syndrome Clinical Features

Three non-RTT clinical presentations have been observed in girls and women with mutations in *MECP2*: girls with Angelman Syndrome-like features, girls with autism, and individual cases of girls with other neurological or psychiatric features (Table 45-3).

Girls With Angelman-Like Features

Similarities between Angelman Syndrome and RTT were recognized before the identification of the specific genetic cause of RTT (Scheffer et al., 1990); however, a major distinguishing feature is the absence in Angelman Syndrome of a period of normal development followed by developmental regression (Jedele, 2007). The similarity between these two neurodevelopmental conditions led to the molecular investigation of *MECP2* in individuals with clinical features of Angelman Syndrome but no molecular changes at 15q11-13 (Hitchins et al., 2004; Milani et al., 2005; Turner et al., 2003; Watson et al., 2001). Mutations in *MECP2* were identified in a fraction of these individuals; however, careful review of clinical history after the discovery of *MECP2* mutations revealed that these people had clinical features more consistent with a diagnosis of RTT. However, four cases with RTT disease-causing mutations in *MECP2* did not have evidence of regression and were felt to meet the criteria for Angelman Syndrome (Milani et al., 2005; Turner et al., 2003; Watson et al., 2001). In total, *MECP2* mutations are not a common cause of Angelman Syndrome (Hitchins et al., 2004; Milani et al., 2005; Turner et al., 2003; Watson et al., 2001), but some individuals with *MECP2* mutations can present with features more compatible with a diagnosis of Angelman Syndrome than RTT.

Autism in Girls With Mutations in *MECP2*

From early on, it has been recognized that there are features (such as apparently normal development followed by loss of skills, decreased eye contact and avoidance of social contact) present during regression in RTT that are similar to those observed in idiopathic autism. In the 1980s, Gillberg and colleagues noted that a large percentage (80%) of people ultimately diagnosed with RTT were initially characterized as having autism (Gillberg, 1987, 1989; Witt-Engerstrom & Gillberg, 1987), leading to the prediction that a common neurobiological substrate exists for the two disorders (Gillberg, 1989). A recent report found a smaller but significant percentage (17.6%) of individuals with RTT receiving an initial diagnosis of autism (D. J. Young et al., 2008). This overlap in clinical features led investigators to look for mutations in *MECP2* in cases with autism and no clear features of RTT. Screening a cohort of 69 girls with autism identified two individuals with mutations in *MECP2* (Carney et al., 2003). Both alterations are changes previously found in girls with typical RTT (c.1157del41 and p.Arg294X) and are clearly pathogenic. In contrast, a number of studies have attempted to identify pathogenic sequence changes within the coding sequence for *MECP2* in individuals with autism without success (Beyer et al., 2002; Coutinho et al., 2007; Harvey et al., 2007; Li et al., 2005;

Table 45–3.
***MECP2* mutations in girls with other neurodevelopmental disorders**

Clinical Presentation	*MECP2* Mutations	Frequency of *MECP2* Mutations
Angelman Syndrome-like	Loss of function mutations seen in RTT	Isolated cases
Autism	Loss of function mutations seen in RTT	Rare (0.5%)
Various clinical features		
Electrical Status Epilepticus of Sleep	c.880del8	Isolated case
Learning disability	c.1164del44	Isolated case
Learning disability, obese, aggressive	p.P152A[#]	Isolated case

[#]Mutation shared with father.

Lobo-Menendez et al., 2003; Shibayama et al., 2004; Vourc'h et al., 2001; Xi et al., 2007). In total, 1119 individuals (378 females, 741 males) were screened, and only three potential mutations in *MECP2* coding sequence or introns were identified—all within girls. Only two are clearly pathogenic, giving a frequency of 2 of 378 (0.5%) in girls and 0 of 741 in boys.

Recently, analysis of the UTRs of *MECP2*—specifically the large, well-conserved 3′UTR—identified sequence changes within the 3′UTR of *MECP2* in boys and girls with autism (Coutinho et al., 2007; Shibayama et al., 2004) and a boy with attention deficit and hyperactivity disorder (Shibayama et al., 2004). These sequence changes were not found in normal controls (Coutinho et al., 2007; Shibayama et al., 2004), and *MECP2* mRNA expression was reduced in peripheral monocytes from four individuals with these 3'UTR sequence changes (Coutinho et al., 2007). Interestingly, these 3′UTR sequence changes are in concert with recent experiments (described below) in a mouse model (Samaco et al., 2008) and in cell culture (Klein et al., 2007) that demonstrate that the 3′UTR is critical for controlling MeCP2 levels and that subtle changes in MeCP2 level may result in neurodevelopmental disorders. The 3′UTR alterations observed in autism (Coutinho et al., 2007; Shibayama et al., 2004) may disrupt these critical regions. A detailed dissection of the critical regions within the 3'UTR is needed to conclusively determine this hypothesis. With such knowledge, methods for systematic screening of human cases of neurodevelopmental problems could be undertaken.

Other Clinical Conditions in Girls Associated With MECP2 Mutations

The recognition that pathogenic mutations in *MECP* can present asymptomatically in familial cases as a result of dramatically skewing of the XCI to favor the chromosome of the wild-type allele led to the notion that variation in XCI skewing could alter the clinical presentation of individuals with pathogenic mutations. These individuals might show cognitive and/or neurological impairments but lack distinctive features of RTT. A number of individuals with various neurological features and sequence changes have been identified, and they can be clustered into two groups—those with clearly pathogenic mutations in *MECP2* and those with sequence changes in *MECP2* of uncertain significance.

A subset of individuals with sequence changes in *MECP2* and intellectual disability (ID) but lacking a clear history of regression have been identified. In two cases, clearly pathogenic mutations in *MECP2* were identified (Huppke et al., 2003; Huppke et al., 2006). In the first, a frameshift mutation (c.880del8) was found in a girl with electrical status epilepticus of sleep who previously had no history of regression, slow development of single spoken words, microcephaly, stereotyped hand movements, but normal gait and good hand function (Huppke et al., 2003). A later frameshift mutation (c.1164del44) was found in an older child with learning disabilities and episodes of uncontrolled aggression, the ability to read, write, and perform simple mathematics (Huppke et al., 2006). She was able to ride a bike and inline skate. She did have bouts of hand stereotypies and hyperventilation when in stressful situations but not otherwise and had no history of regression. She had evidence of skewing of her XCI (84:16). Three other cases have been presented that have mutations in *MECP2* in affected girls with no history of regression; however, they were between ages 2 and 4 years at evaluation, and it is possible that they had not yet undergone regression (Kammoun et al., 2004), which can occur as late as age 6 years (Huppke et al., 2006). A report identified a sequence change in *MECP2* (p.Pro152Ala) in an obese girl with a learning disability, normal hand use, aggressive outbursts, and a diagnosis of PDD-NOS (Adegbola et al., 2008); however, the pathogenic nature of this mutation was unclear because although it alters in vitro biochemical features of MECP2, it was also present in the girl's father who had a milder clinical condition.

Finally, although most familial cases have been reported to have "asymptomatic" female carriers, no systematic formal evaluation has ever been undertaken. In one of the families used to identify the genetic cause of RTT, the mother of an affected individual was found to have motor-coordination issues, mild learning disability, and skewed XCI (Wan et al., 1999). One mother who shared a large deletion of the *MECP2* locus with her daughter with RTT and a son with congenital encephalopathy was reported to have a history of attention problems at school, longstanding severe depression and anxiety, and infrequent hand tremors (Hardwick et al., 2007). Although these could have been present as coincident conditions, the recent finding of consistent neuropsychiatric features in the female carriers of a duplication of *MECP2* (Ramocki et al., 2009) raises the issue that similar subtle changes may exist within the "asymptomatic" female carriers of loss-of-function mutations in *MECP2*. Detailed neuropsychiatric evaluations of these individuals are needed to identify such psychiatric features.

Boys With *MECP2* Mutations

Because RTT was originally recognized only in girls, a genetic explanation was proposed that RTT was the result of an X-linked dominant mutation that resulted in male lethality. An alternative hypothesis is that the sporadic nature of RTT could be explained by a mechanism in which mutations occur on an X-linked gene during spermatogenesis. The identification of mutations in MECP2 has demonstrated that this hypothesis is partially correct, with the majority of MECP2 mutations occurring spontaneously during spermatogenesis (Girard et al., 2001; Trappe et al., 2001). However, a number of boys with mutations in *MECP2* have been identified. They fall into three general categories: boys with clinical features of RTT, boys with congenital encephalopathy, and boys with other neurodevelopmental features (Table 45-4). These three classes of clinical features in boys are the result of specific genetic abnormalities in *MECP2*.

Table 45–4.
***MECP2* mutations in boys**

Clinical Category	*MECP2* Mutation Type	Frequency	Unique Aspects
Typical or atypical RTT	Loss-of-function mutations seen in RTT	14 cases reported*	Mosaicism of X-chromosome due to X-chromosomal aneuploidy or somatic mosaicism (similar to females), rare cases without mosaicism
Congenital Encephalopathy	Loss-of-function mutations seen in RTT	17 cases reported**	Severe, death resulting from cardiorespiratory failure
ID with neurological features	Mutations not found in typical RTT	4 of 1559 from population screening*** 20 cases with p.Ala140Val#	XLMR families, psychotic features, spasticity, tremor
ID with recurrent infections	Duplications of *MECP2*	1%–2% males with XLMR or severe encephapathy##	Female carriers display subtle neuropsychiatric features

*(Budden et al., 2005; Dayer et al., 2007; Kleefstra et al., 2004; Masuyama et al., 2005; Moog et al., 2003; Ravn et al., 2003) and references therein.
**(Kankirawatana et al., 2006; Lundvall et al., 2006; Schule et al., 2008) and references therein.
***(Bourdon et al., 2003; Donzel-Javouhey et al., 2006; Lesca et al., 2007; Ylisaukko-Oja et al., 2005).
#(Cohen et al., 2002; Couvert et al., 2001; Klauck et al., 2002; Orrico et al., 2000; Winnepenninckx et al., 2002).
##(Lugtenberg et al., 2009).

Boys With Rett Syndrome

A handful of cases have been reported of boys who meet the clinical criteria for typical or variant RTT. In many of these cases, mutations in *MECP2* that are associated with typical RTT in girls have been identified. The majority of the boys with typical RTT and mutations in *MECP2* have either complete X-chromosome aneuploidy (Kleinfelter Syndrome 47, XXY) (Hoffbuhr et al., 2001; Schwartzman et al., 2001), mosaic X-chromosome aneuploidy (47XXY/46XY) (Leonard et al., 2001; Vorsanova et al., 2001), or somatic mosaicism for the *MECP2* mutation (J. Armstrong et al., 2001; Clayton-Smith et al., 2000; Topcu et al., 2002). In all of these cases, the presence of these unusual genetic features allows for mosaic expression of the mutant *MECP2* allele in these boys, similar to the mosaicism that is found as a result of normal XCI in girls with typical RTT.

Interesting reports exist involving boys who appeared to have normal chromosomes (46 XY), no evidence of somatic mutation, and features of RTT (Budden, Dorsey, & Steiner, 2005; Dayer et al., 2007; Masuyama et al., 2005). These three cases share clinical features. The *MECP2* mutation found in the boys were all inherited from their mothers. In two of the cases (Budden et al., 2005; Dayer et al., 2007), the mothers were completely asymptomatic and had skewed XCI. In the third case (Masuyama et al., 2005), the mother had mild MR and microcephaly. The causative *MECP2* mutation was also found in affected sisters with RTT in two of the families (Budden et al., 2005; Masuyama et al., 2005). An interesting similarity in these cases is the presence of mutations of *MECP2* (p.Arg133Cys, p. Ser134Cys, and c.1158del44) that confer a milder phenotype in typical RTT girls (Neul et al., 2008) and are common in PSV (*see* above). This suggests that *MECP2* mutations that confer a milder phenotype in girls can, when present in boys, create a phenotype that is very similar to typical RTT in girls. In contrast, boys who have *MECP2* mutations that confer increased clinical severity in typical RTT girls (i.e., p.R168X) display severe infantile encephalopathy (described below). One exception to this general trend has been reported: a boy who meets the criteria for typical RTT, has a normal male karyotype with no evidence of mosaicism, and has a c.816dup7 mutation in *MECP2* (Ravn et al., 2003). Such unusual cases could provide material for future studies to identify genetic modifiers.

Boys With Congenital Encephalopathy

Boys with *MECP2* mutations and a distinct clinical picture of congenital encephalopathy have been found in families with a sister who has typical RTT (Geerdink et al., 2002; Hardwick et al., 2007; Milunsky et al., 2001; Venancio et al., 2007; Villard et al., 2000; Wan et al., 2001; Zeev et al., 2002), families with multiple affected boys (Hoffbuhr et al., 2001; Lundvall, Samuelsson, & Kyllerman, 2006), and sporadically (Kankirawatana et al., 2006; Leuzzi et al., 2004; Lundvall et al., 2006; Lynch et al., 2003; Schule et al., 2008). In total, 17 cases of male congenital encephalopathy have been identified with *MECP2* mutations, and a clinical and molecular picture of this disorder is evolving.

First, the type of *MECP2* mutations associated in nearly all the cases of male congenital encephalopathy are either found in girls with typical RTT or are predicted to disrupt the protein in a manner similar to those mutations found in typical RTT. Second, the clinical features and course is consistent among these affected individuals and is distinct from the clinical features found in RTT. In general, affected individuals present with evidence of severe neonatal hypotonia and poor feeding. Many show respiratory abnormalities shortly after birth that continue throughout life, manifesting as periodic breathing, central hypoventilation, apnea, and respiratory insufficiency. Most affected individuals die within the first 3 years of life, often because of respiratory arrest, although the oldest reported case was alive and ventilatory-dependent at 6 years of life (Milunsky et al., 2001). Interestingly, in one case it was noted that at the end of life, the affected individual had marked bradycardia (Schule et al., 2008). Acquired deceleration of head growth is common, with many affected individuals ultimately developing microcephaly. Cognitive development is severely impaired, with most gaining few skills. Affected individuals have severe axial hypotonia with limb rigidity. Additionally, many affected individuals are reported to show various movement abnormalities such as myoclonus, tremor, chorea, and dyskinesias.

Although only a relatively small number of cases of boys with congenital encephalopathy and *MECP2* mutations have been identified, consideration for *MECP2* testing should be made when presented with a boy with neonatal or early encephalopathy, respiratory abnormalities, hypotonia with developing limb rigidity, and abnormal movements. An estimation of the de novo maternal mutation frequency in *MECP2* suggests that the incidence of boys with these mutations should be approximately 1:50,000 to 1:100,000, indicating that this may be an under-recognized condition.

Intellectual Disability in Boys With Additional Neurological Features

Mutations in *MECP2* have been discovered in families that display an X-linked mental retardation (XLMR) pattern with multiple affected boys (Couvert et al., 2001; Klauck et al., 2002; Meloni et al., 2000; Orrico et al., 2000; Winnepenninckx et al., 2002; Yntema, Oudakker et al., 2002) and in boys with ID without a clear family pattern (Bourdon et al., 2003; Campos et al., 2008; Couvert et al., 2001; Kleefstra et al., 2002; Laccone et al., 2002; Moog et al., 2003; Moog et al., 2006; Xi et al., 2007). The clinical features present in these individuals are variable, with cognitive skills ranging from moderate to severe ID. Additional features include obesity, tremor, spasticity, and neuropsychiatric problems, including mood instability, psychosis, and mania.

A pattern emerged that the sequence alterations observed in these boys were never seen in girls with typical RTT. Although some of the sequence alterations result in clear changes to the coding sequence of *MECP2*, such as nonsense mutations (p.Gln406X), frameshift mutations (c.1411del2), or large in-frame deletions (c.1161del240), a number caused missense mutations of uncertain significance are also found (Bourdon et al., 2003; Campos et al., 2008; Couvert et al., 2001; Klauck et al., 2002; Laccone et al., 2002; Moog et al., 2003; Moog et al., 2006; Orrico et al., 2000; Winnepenninckx et al., 2002), many of which appear to be benign polymorphisms (Laccone et al., 2002; Yntema, Kleefstra et al., 2002). Multiple population studies have been conducted in boys with ID assessing for pathogenic alterations in *MECP2* with little success (Bourdon et al., 2003; Donzel-Javouhey et al., 2006; Lesca et al., 2007; Ylisaukko-Oja et al., 2005; Yntema, Kleefstra et al., 2002). In total, of the 1559 individuals tested in these studies, four sequence changes have been identified, with only one clearly altering the coding sequence (c.1161del240 [Yntema, Oudakker et al., 2002]), one missense mutation that has been recurrently identified in boys with ID (p.Ala140Val, *see* below), and two mutations of uncertain significance (p.Arg435Gln and p.Lys284Glu). These findings indicate that care must be taken to determine the functional significance of sequence alterations in *MECP2* associated with intellectual disability in boys, preferably by pedigree analysis to determine that the change is only found in affected individuals.

Although not necessarily definitive genetic proof of causality, *de novo* sequence changes suggest a higher likelihood of pathogenesis. Three *de novo* mutations in *MECP2* have been found in boys with ID: p.Pro225Leu, p.ProP405Leu, and c.1141del2 (Campos et al., 2008; Kleefstra et al., 2002). Both the p.Pro225Leu and the p.Pro405Leu alterations are found in severely affected boys, and p.Pro405Leu has also been identified in a boy who inherited it from his mother who has borderline IQ (Moog et al., 2006), which supports the notion that this is a pathogenic change. The frameshift mutation (c.1141del2) causes a late truncation (p.379fs) similar to the frameshift mutations found in girls with typical RTT, which is consistent with the notion that late truncating mutations represent a hypomorphic allele with the production of a partially functional protein (Neul et al., 2008).

Besides p.Pro405Leu, the only other recurrent *MECP2* mutation identified in boys with ID is p.Ala140Val, identified in a total of 17 affected individuals from three families (Klauck et al., 2002; Orrico et al., 2000; Winnepenninckx et al., 2002) and three sporadic cases (Cohen et al., 2002; Couvert et al., 2001). Aside from ID, many of these individuals also have tremor, spasticity, and neuropychiatric features such as hypomania or frank psychosis (Cohen et al., 2002). In all cases identified to date, the mutation was maternally inherited; however, the clinical phenotype of the carrier females is variable, with reports of mild ID (Orrico et al., 2000), below average intelligence (Klauck et al., 2002), or normal intelligence (Couvert et al., 2001; Winnepenninckx et al., 2002) despite random XCI in all informative cases. This variability has led some to question the pathogenic nature of this mutation (Laccone et al., 2002). In vitro analysis of molecular function indicates that this molecular change alters the ability of the protein to repress transcription, allowing promiscuous transcriptional repression from nonmethylated promoter sequences (Kudo et al., 2002; Kudo et al., 2003). Mice expressing this p.Ala140Val mutation have neuronal abnormalities such as increased cell-packing and decreased dentric branching, supporting the notion that this is a pathogenic change to *MECP2* (Jentarra et al., 2010)

Duplications of *MECP2*

The identification of behavioral and epileptic phenotypes in mice that overexpress MeCP2 (Collins et al., 2004) led to the prediction that genomic duplications of *MECP2* would result in neurodevelopmental abnormalities in humans. Subsequently, duplication of *MECP2* was identified in a boy with ID and features of RTT, including hand stereotypies and loss of hand skills (Meins et al., 2005). This led to the identification of a duplication in a large XLMR family in which all affected boys had progressive spasticity in addition to ID (Van Esch et al., 2005). The prominent XLMR and spasticity led to the identification of a number of additional XLMR families (Clayton-Smith et al., 2008; Friez et al., 2006; Lugtenberg et al., 2009), which when combined suggested that *MECP2* duplications may have accounted for 1% of XLMR cases (Lugtenberg et al., 2009). Additional cases of boys with *MECP2* duplications were identified through chromosomal micro-array analysis of individuals with ID (del Gaudio et al., 2006; Smyk et al., 2008) or by screening boys with a history of encephalopathy (Lugtenberg et al., 2009). The size of the duplicated region varies and contains a number of coding regions; however, in aggregate, the critical region can be refined to a region containing *MECP2* and the closely linked gene *interleukin receptor-associated kinase I* (*IRAK1*) (Van Esch et al., 2005).

Aside from the common feature of ID, generally in the moderate-to-severe range, other consistent clinical features have emerged. Individuals present with distinct infantile hypotonia, and then many develop progressive spasticity (Lugtenberg et al., 2009). Acquisition of the ability to walk is delayed and most have markedly impaired speech.

One of the most striking features of people with duplications is the history of recurrent infections, primarily respiratory (del Gaudio et al., 2006; Friez et al., 2006; Van Esch et al., 2005; Lugtenberg et al., 2009; Smyk et al., 2008; Ramocki et al., 2009). A significant percentage of affected individuals (40%) die before 25 years of life (Lugtenberg et al., 2009). In one study, four of five individuals who survived more than 15 years required tracheostomies secondary to recurrent pneumonias. Although swallowing problems might contribute to the recurrent respiratory infections, evidence exists for specific immunological deficits that might contribute to the propensity toward recurrent infections. Although detailed analysis of the immune system in many cases has not been performed, low serum IgA levels were detected in 4 of 10 cases evaluated in one study (Friez et al., 2006). Additional research is needed to determine whether low serum IgA is a consistent finding with duplications of this region and whether it is the result of duplication of *MECP2* or duplication of a linked locus.

Autistic Features in MECP2 Duplications

Autistic features were noted in a fraction of the individuals reported in one study (del Gaudio et al., 2006), but formal clinical evaluation for autism was not performed in that or previous studies. When eight boys with genomic duplications containing *MECP2* were formally evaluated using the Autism Diagnostic Observational Schedule, seven met or exceeded the criteria for autism and the remaining individual met the criteria for autistic spectrum disorder (ASD) and all exceeded the cutoff criteria for autism using the Autism Diagnostic Inventory (Ramocki et al., 2009). With consistent clinical characterization, it is likely that autism or autistic features will be present in the majority of boys with genomic duplications including *MECP2*, but currently no studies have been performed to determine the percentage of individuals with ASD who have increased copy number variations of *MECP2*.

All carrier females of duplications including *MECP2* whose XCI status was evaluated displayed markedly skewed XCI, with many showing complete (100%) skewing. Most of these individuals have been characterized as "asymptomatic" or "normal"; however, limited or no clinical evaluation was presented on these individuals. When formal neuropsychological analysis was performed on a cohort of female carriers, an interesting constellation of neuropsychiatric features emerged (Ramocki et al., 2009). There was variation in the IQ, as assessed using the Wechsler Abbreviated Scale of Intelligence with two women in the low average range, two women in the average range, one woman with high average intelligence, and two women with superior range intelligence. On the other hand, all of the women reported symptoms consistent with anxiety, compulsive behaviors, and inflexible personality when assessed with the Symptom Checklist-90-R. Notably, many had been diagnosed with anxiety and depressive symptoms before the birth of the affected son. None of the carrier mothers had autism, but four of seven evaluated with the Broad Autism Phenotype Questionnaire (BAPQ) exceeded the cutoff for the broad autism phenotype. These results suggest that an extra copy of *MECP2* in females may cause various psychiatric features including features identified using the BAPQ. Although this finding was identified in families with more severely affected boys, it is possible that *de novo* duplications in this genomic region might be present in females with sporadic presentation of anxiety, depression, or features identified by the BAPQ. This finding warrants further investigation to determine whether duplications or other alterations in *MECP2* expression or function contribute to these clinical features.

Biological Insights from Basic Studies of Rett Syndrome and *MECP2*-Related Disorders

Molecular Function of MECP2

MeCP2 belongs to the methyl-CpG-binding domain family of proteins (Hendrich & Bird, 1998). These proteins have a conserved methyl-CpG-binding domain (Figure 45-1) that binds methylated CpG dinucleotides (Lewis et al., 1992; Nan, Meehan, & Bird, 1993). In addition, MeCP2 contains two other molecular domains: a transcriptional repression domain (Nan, Campoy, & Bird, 1997), which recruits corepressors such as histone deacetylases (Jones et al., 1998; Nan, Cross, & Bird, 1998), and a carboxy-terminal domain (Chandler et al.,

1999), which may interact with splicing factors (Buschdorf & Stratling, 2004) to regulate RNA splicing (J. I. Young et al., 2005).

Because MeCP2 binds methylated CpG dinucleotides and can recruit corepressors, the function has been considered to be a repressor of gene transcription (Figure 45-1). However, recent experiments have indicated that MeCP2 can also act as a transcriptional activator (Chahrour et al., 2008; Yasui et al., 2007) and is associated with a well-known transcriptional activator, CREB1. Within the hypothalamus, MeCP2 activates a number of neuropeptides such as *Corticotropin-releasing hormone* and *oxytocin* (Chahrour et al., 2008). Given the role of various neuropeptides in the regulation of stress responses and social behavior (Meyer-Lindenberg, 2008; Winslow, 2005; Winslow & Insel, 2002), the alteration in expression of these molecules may help explain particular phenotypes as well as offer possible therapeutic targets.

An interesting target of MECP2, *brain-derived neurotrophic factor* (*Bdnf*), was identified using a candidate gene approach (W. G. Chen et al., 2003; Martinowich et al., 2003), which indicated that *Bdnf* expression was repressed by MECP2. However, in vivo analysis revealed the BDNF protein levels are decreased in animals lacking Mecp2 (Chahrour et al., 2008; Chang et al., 2006; Wang et al., 2006) and increased in an animal model that overexpressed MeCP2 (Chahrour et al., 2008). Chang and colleagues demonstrated that increasing *Bdnf* expression in *Mecp2*$^{null/Y}$ partially rescued the phenotype (Chang et al., 2006). Thus, modulation of *Bdnf* activity may be a useful therapeutic modality in the treatment of RTT.

Transcriptional regulator: Gene expression (transcription) is controlled by a variety of protein and non-protein factors and mechanisms. Factors that increase gene expression are called transcriptional activators and those that decrease gene expression are transcriptional repressors. Evidence exists that MeCP2 functions as a regulator of gene transcription, both as an activator by recruiting repressors and as an activator by recruiting activators.

Animal Models of MeCP2 Dysfunction

Mouse Models of Rett Syndrome

Mouse models of RTT have been generated that reproduce features of the human disorder (R. Z. Chen et al., 2001; Guy et al., 2001; Lawson-Yuen et al., 2007; Pelka et al., 2006; M. Shahbazian et al., 2002). Male animals that lack MeCP2 develop severe neurological abnormalities and die between 8 and 12 weeks of life (R. Z. Chen et al., 2001; Guy et al., 2001; Pelka et al., 2006). Heterozygous female mice lacking one copy of *Mecp2* develop similar phenotypes as the hemizygous male mice, albeit at a much later time period and with increased variability (R. Z. Chen et al., 2001; Guy et al., 2001). This variability in phenotypic expression in heterozygous female animals likely results from nonrandom XCI in individual animals (J. I. Young & Zoghbi, 2004). There is evidence of decreased synapse formation in neurons from animals that lack MeCP2 function (Chao, Zoghbi, & Rosenmund, 2007).

Two additional mouse models of RTT have been created with the intention of mimicking human disease-causing mutations. Recently, a mouse was generated that contains the most common human allele, p.Arg168X. This allele behaves like the null allele and the animals display very similar phenotypes, including early death (Lawson-Yuen et al., 2007). On the other hand, a mouse that expresses more of the protein, truncated at amino acid 308 (M. Shahbazian et al., 2002), shows a slower progression of phenotypes including increased anxiety, memory problems, social behavior abnormalities, and hypoactivity (McGill et al., 2006; Moretti et al., 2005; Moretti et al., 2006; M. Shahbazian et al., 2002). Strikingly, these mice develop forepaw stereotypies that appear very similar to affected girls (M. Shahbazian et al., 2002).

A conditional allele of *MECP2* was generated by placing DNA sequences (loxP) around the majority of the *Mecp2* coding sequence. When this flanked-loxP ("floxed") allele is crossed to a transgenic animal that expresses the site-specific recombinase Cre, recombination occurs between the loxP sites removing the *Mecp2* coding sequence generating a null allele of *Mecp2* (R. Z. Chen et al., 2001; Guy et al., 2001). Using this conditional knockout (CKO) strategy has revealed that animals lacking MeCP2 function in the postmitotic neurons reproduce some of the features seen in the complete null animals, such as weight abnormalities and impaired social behavior, demonstrating the critical role of MeCP2 function in postmitotic neurons (R. Z. Chen et al., 2001; Gemelli et al., 2006).

Because *Crh* is misregulated within the PVN in a mouse model of RTT (McGill et al., 2006), the role of MeCP2 within the PVN was assessed using the CKO strategy outlined above (Fyffe et al., 2008). Animals lacking MeCP2 function in the PVN, supraoptic hypothalamic nuclei, posterior hypothalamic nuclei, and the nucleus of the lateral olfactory tract of the amygdala are markedly obese because of hyperphagia and have novelty-induced aggression. Interestingly, although most people with RTT are not aggressive and are underweight, the combination of increased aggressiveness and weight is observed in a number of people with the PSV (Renieri et al., 2008).

Concentrations of spinal fluid biogenic amine metabolites are reduced in RTT, therefore Samaco and colleages (Samaco et al., 2009) selectively removed MeCP2 function from either the serotoninergic neurons or neurons expressing tyrosine hydroxylase, which produce dopamine and norepinephrine. Animals lacking MeCP2 within the serotoninergic neurons showed a reduction in serotonin and were aggressive, whereas animals lacking MeCP2 in the tyrosine hydroxylase neurons had a reduction in dopamine and norepinephrine and had movement abnormalities.

MECP2 Misexpression Mouse Models

Twofold overexpression of MeCP2 in wild-type mice resulted in a progressive neurological phenotype (Collins et al., 2004;

Luikenhuis et al., 2004). Overexpression of MeCP2 results in decreased survival, aggressiveness, motor dysfunction, and seizures (Collins et al., 2004). These results indicated that tight control of MeCP2 levels is critical within neurons and only a twofold increase in expression is detrimental. The discovery that twofold excess of *MECP2* causes a progressive neurological abnormality in mice preceded the identification of humans with a duplication of this locus, demonstrating the value of mouse models not only in the understanding of pathogenesis of human disease but also in the prediction of genetic causes of disease. Interestingly, neurons from these transgenic mice overexpressing Mecp2 seem to form excessive synapses when grown in culture, the opposite phenotype to that observed in animals lacking Mecp2 function (Chao et al., 2007).

Further reinforcing the notion that tight regulation of MeCP2 levels are critical for normal neuronal function, reduction of MeCP2 by approximately 50% of mice caused a variety of neurological phenotypes including learning problems, motor dysfunction, altered pain recognition, and breathing irregularities (B. Kerr et al., 2008; Samaco et al., 2008). The reduction in *Mecp2* mRNA expression in these mice is likely secondary to genetic engineering that introduced a *neomycin* cassette into the 3′UTR of the endogenous *Mecp2* locus (Guy et al., 2001), disrupting the primary 3′UTR *Mecp2* isoform that predominates within the brain (Coy et al., 1999; B. Kerr et al., 2008). Within the region disrupted in the binding site for miR132, a microRNA has been shown to repress *Mecp2* translation (Klein et al., 2007). Although this is the opposite of what was observed when this region was disrupted, it emphasizes the importance of the 3′UTR in the regulation of MeCP2 levels. Just as the phenotypes observed from overexpression of MeCP2 in mice predicted a human disorder, it is likely that a human neurodevelopmental disorder will result from reduction of MeCP2 levels by half, similarly to that observed in mice. Suggestively, Coutinho and colleagues identified sequence changes in the 3′UTR of *MECP2* from people with autism and found decreased expression of *MECP2* mRNA in leukocytes from some of those samples (Coutinho et al., 2007).

Genetic Rescue in Animal Models

The fact that gross brain formation is normal in RTT and there is no evidence of neurodegeneration led to the hypothesis that restoring MeCP2 function after the development of disease would ameliorate symptoms. The possibility of disease reversal would be extremely important in the treatment of this disorder. Two research endeavors have demonstrated that in mouse models, postnatal restoration of MeCP2 function partially or completely rescues the disease process (Giacometti et al., 2007; Guy et al., 2007). Strikingly, restoring MeCP2 function, even after clear onset of disease phenotypes, is sufficient to reverse the disease process (Guy et al., 2007). Although these experiments do not provide a direct method of therapy for humans with RTT, they do provide hope that reversibility in this disorder is possible.

Cellular Requirement for MeCP2 Function

MeCP2 protein is highly expressed in the brain, specifically in neurons. In fact, previous work has suggested that it is only expressed within neurons and not expressed in glial (Shahbazian et al., 2002), which has led to the hypothesis that the primary function of MeCP2 resides within neurons. This hypothesis is supported by experiments showing that removing *Mecp2* from postmitotic neurons in mice reproduces neuronal phenotypes, albeit later in life and to a lesser degree (R. Z. Chen et al., 2001). Furthermore, inducing expression of *Mecp2* in postmitotic neurons in mice that otherwise lack *Mecp2* partially rescues the phenotype present in these animals (Luikenhuis et al., 2004). In fact, there is no survival difference when *Mecp2* expression is restored in both neurons and glia compared with expression in neurons alone (Giacometti et al., 2007). However, recent work has shown that MeCP2 has important function in astrocytes as well as neurons and that MeCP2 may have a cell non-autonomous role in these non-neuronal cells. *Mecp2* expression is observed within glial lineages at a much lower level than in neurons (Ballas et al., 2009; Maezawa et al., 2009). Astrocytes that lack MeCP2 grow more slowly in vitro, express higher levels of *Bdnf*, and do not support the growth of wild-type neurons in vitro as well as wild-type astrocytes (Maezawa et al., 2009). Surprisingly, in vitro growth of wild-type neurons in conditioned media from astrocytes lacking MeCP2 is inhibited; similarly, neurons lacking MeCP2 appear to have improved growth and development when grown in conditioned media from wild-type astrocytes (Ballas et al., 2009). Thus, these results indicate that MeCP2 may have an important function within astrocytes as well as in neurons. Further work will be required to determine the in vivo significance of these results and to determine the relative contribution of these two lineages in the nervous system.

Treatment

No cure for RTT or *MECP2*-related disorders exist and treatment is directed toward symptomatic amelioration using a combination of pharmacotherapy, nutritional supplementation, physical and speech therapy, and surgical intervention. Successful interventions include anti-epileptic drugs or vagal nerve stimulator (Wilfong & Schultz, 2006) for seizures and aggressive nutritional support for growth failure (Motil et al., 2009). Future symptom-directed therapies are targeting breathing dysfunction (Roux et al., 2007), anxiety, and dystonias.

Genetic and molecular knowledge are allowing the conceptual development of therapies targeted to specific molecular defects identified in these disorders. For example, determination of altered BDNF protein levels has led to interest in chemical compounds that can increase the level of BDNF, which in animal models can improve respiration (Ogier et al., 2007). Recent work has suggested that treatment with a tripeptide from insulin-like growth factor 1 can improve

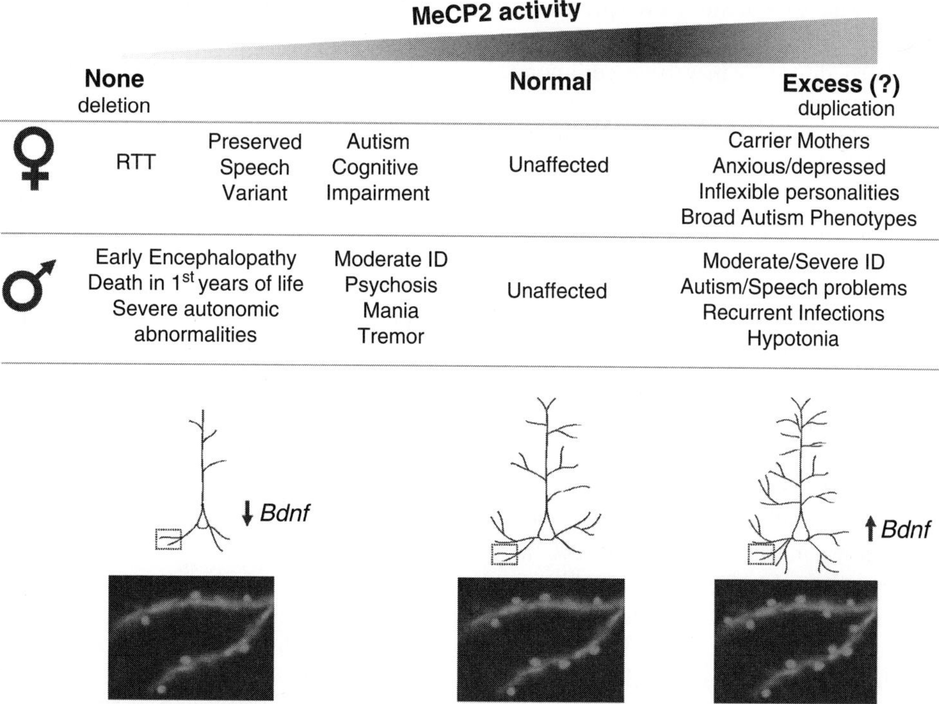

Figure 45–2. Clinical, cellular, and molecular abnormalities caused by changes in MeCP2 activity. Along the top of the figure is a representation of increasing MeCP2 activity ranging from no activity (None) on the left of the figure, through "Normal" activity in the middle of the figure, to "Excess" activity (putatively, although it is possible that increasing the amount of MeCP2 protein might generate new functional activity not typically seen by MeCP2 or even interfere with normal MeCP2 function) on the right side. Below are the clinical features that are found in both girls and boys. In girls, decreased or loss of MeCP2 activity leads to Rett Syndrome (RTT). Some people with milder loss of function mutations or other factors such as skewing of XCI display milder clinical features such as autism and intellectual disability (ID). On the other side of the activity gradient are women with duplication of the *MECP2* locus, putatively leading to excessive MeCP2 activity. These individuals are mothers of boys with similar duplications. On careful neuropsychological testing, these carrier mothers show evidence of depression, anxiety, and meet criteria for the Broad Autism Phenotype. Alterations in MeCP2 activity also cause a variety of clinical features in boys ranging from severe early encephalopathy with decreased MeCP2 function to autistic features, recurrent infections, and ID in boys with an excess of MeCP2 activity due to a duplication in the *MECP2* locus. Below the clinical phenotypes is a cartoon representation of neurons showing the alterations in the dendritic arbors that occur as a result of changes in MeCP2 activity. The drawings below are diagrams showing the changes in synaptic density (represented by dots) along dendrites within the small dotted boxes on the neuron drawing. Decreased MeCP2 activity leads to decreased dendritic arborization, decreased synaptic density, and decreased expression of activity dependent genes such as *Bdnf*. On the other extreme, overexpression of MeCP2 leads to increased *Bdnf* expression and increased synaptic density, and likely will lead to increased dendritic arborization, although this has not yet been characterized. The neuron arborization drawings for decreased and normal MeCP2 activity were modeled after (Schule et al., 2008) and the drawings illustrating the increased synaptic density were modeled after (Chao et al., 2007).

lifespan in male null animals (Tropea et al., 2009). As additional molecular changes are identified, further preclinical and possibly clinical trials will be developed.

Recently, clinical trials on two genetic disorders, cystic fibrosis (CF) and Duchenne Muscular Dystrophy (DMD), have started using a novel chemical compound, PTC124, that allows "read-through" of premature stop codons resulting from point mutations (Welch et al., 2007). Preclinical trials on animal models of both DMD and CF demonstrated efficacy in improving function (Du et al., 2008; Welch et al., 2007). Because a significant percentage of individuals with RTT have mutations that cause such premature stop codons, many families and clinicians have become interested in the prospect of using this or a related compound in RTT. Given the additional complication of crossing the blood–brain barrier and the importance of tight regulation of MeCP2 protein levels within neurons, detailed preclinical testing on animal models will be needed prior to any clinical study.

Conclusion

Despite the identification of the genetic cause of RTT, the diagnosis of RTT remains a clinical diagnosis because a mutation in *MECP2* is neither necessary nor sufficient to make the diagnosis. Although loss-of-function mutations in *MECP2* can cause the well-defined clinical condition RTT, growing evidence exists that a wide spectrum of clinical disorders can occur in both boys and girls from a loss or decrease of MeCP2 function as well as a putative increase of MeCP2 function as a result of duplication of *MECP2* locus (Figure 45-2). As a group, these *MECP2*-related disorders may be a common cause of neurodevelopmental, neurological, and psychiatric disorders; furthermore, *MECP2* may be involved in common molecular systems disrupted by a variety of neurodevelopmental disorders.

One possible explanation for the manifestation of various neurodevelopmental problems as a result of alterations in MeCP2 function may be the fact that these alterations appear to affect synaptic development. Decreased MeCP2 activity leads to decreased dendritic arborization (Figure 45-2) in girls with RTT (D. D. Armstrong, 2005a) and boys with congenital encephalopathy (Schule et al., 2008) and decreased synapse formation in neurons from mice lacking *Mecp2* grown in culture (Chao et al., 2007). In a complementary fashion, increasing *Mecp2* dosage in transgenic mice leads to increased synapse formation when neurons are grown in culture (Chao et al., 2007). Although detailed neuropathological studies have not yet been done in people with duplication of *MECP2* or in transgenic animals that overexpress MeCP2, it is likely that an increase in dendritic arborization will be present in these situations.

Gene expression changes that result from alterations in MeCP2 function also show a monotonic relationship to such alterations, with decreased MeCP2 activity leading to decreased expression of genes such as *Bdnf* and *Crh* and increased MeCP2 activity leading to increased expression of the same genes. Similarly, a different set of genes show increased expression when MeCP2 function is lost and decreased expression when MeCP2 protein levels are increased (not shown). Although not all gene expression changes identified are in genes that show distinct activity dependent expression, the identification of such gene expression changes leads to the hypothesis that MeCP2 function may be critical for the interpretation and integration of stimuli that causes activity-dependent gene expression. The generation of an appropriate immediate and long-term response may be one of the key roles of MeCP2, and when this system is altered either by decreased or increased function, aberrant adaptation may occur. In the nervous system, aberrant adaptation is potentially manifested by alterations in synaptic and dendritic formation. Because one of the common pathological features identified in many neurodevelopmental disorders is alterations in dendritic arborization and synapse formation (Belichenko et al., 1994; Huttenlocher, 1974, 1991, 2000; Irwin, Galvez, & Greenough, 2000; Jay et al., 1991; Raymond, Bauman, & Kemper, 1996), understanding these *MECP2*-related disorders may provide insight into many disorders of cognition and neuronal function.

Challenges and Future Directions

- What are the additional factors that modify the clinical features resulting from *MECP2* mutations other than mutation type and XCI?
- What is the incidence of *MECP2* mutations in non-RTT neurodevelopmental disorders?
- What methods can be used or developed to test the functional consequence of sequence changes in *MECP2* of uncertain significance?
- What is the common underlying relationship between RTT and other neurodevelopmental disorders?
- How can biological knowledge of MeCP2 function and animal models be used to design and test treatments for RTT and other *MECP2*-related disorders?
- What is the relative contribution to the disease phenotype from MeCP2 dysfunction within specific cells (neurons versus glia) and within different regions of the nervous system?

SUGGESTED READING

Hagberg, B., Aicardi, J., Dias, K., & Ramos, O. (1983). A progressive syndrome of autism, dementia, ataxia, and loss of purposeful hand use in girls: Rett's syndrome: report of 35 cases. *Annals of Neurology, 14*(4), 471–479.

Amir, R. E., Van den Veyver, I. B., Wan, M., Tran, C. Q., Francke, U., & Zoghbi, H. Y. (1999). Rett syndrome is caused by mutations in X-linked MECP2, encoding methyl-CpG-binding protein 2. *Nature Genetics, 23*(2), 185–188.

Bebbington, A., Anderson, A., Ravine, D., Fyfe, S., Pineda, M., de Klerk, N., et al. (2008). Investigating genotype-phenotype relationships in Rett syndrome using an international data set. *Neurology, 70*(11), 868–875.

Neul, J. L., Fang, P., Barrish, J., Lane, J., Caeg, E. B., Smith, E. O., et al. (2008). Specific mutations in methyl-CpG-binding protein 2 confer different severity in Rett syndrome. *Neurology, 70*(16), 1313–1321.

Ramocki, M., Peters, S. U., Tavyev, Y. J., Zhang, F., Carvhalho, C. M. B., Fang, P., et al. (2009). High Penetrance of Autism and other Neuropsychiatric Symptoms in Individuals with *MECP2* Duplications. *Annals of Neurology, 66*(6), 771–782.

ACKNOWLEDGEMENTS

I thank Drs. Alan Percy, Kathleen Motil, and Daniel Glaze for sharing unpublished data and observations and providing useful discussions and advice on the clinical features of RTT, Drs. Melissa Ramocki and Rodney Samaco for assistance and advice on the preparation of this chapter, and the International Rett Syndrome Foundation for ongoing support. Furthermore, I am grateful to all the families and children with RTT that I have had the privilege to meet and I dedicate this work to you.

REFERENCES

Adegbola, A. A., Gonzales, M. L., Chess, A., Lasalle, J. M., & Cox, G. F. (2008). A novel hypomorphic MECP2 point mutation is associated with a neuropsychiatric phenotype. *Human Genetics, 124*(6), 615–623.

Amir, R. E., Van den Veyver, I. B., Schultz, R., Malicki, D. M., Tran, C. Q., Dahle, E. J., et al. (2000). Influence of mutation type and X chromosome inactivation on Rett syndrome phenotypes. *Annals of Neurology, 47*(5), 670–679.

Amir, R. E., Van den Veyver, I. B., Wan, M., Tran, C. Q., Francke, U., & Zoghbi, H. Y. (1999). Rett syndrome is caused by mutations in X-linked MECP2, encoding methyl-CpG-binding protein 2. *Nature Genetics, 23*(2), 185–188.

Archer, H. L., Evans, J., Edwards, S., Colley, J., Newbury-Ecob, R., O'Callaghan, F., et al. (2006). CDKL5 mutations cause infantile spasms, early onset seizures, and severe mental retardation in female patients. *Journal of Medical Genetics, 43*(9), 729–734.

Archer, H. L., Evans, J., Leonard, H., Colvin, L., Ravine, D., Christodoulou, J., et al. (2006). Correlation between clinical severity in Rett syndrome patients with a p.R168X or p.T158M MECP2 mutation and the direction and degree of skewing of X chromosome inactivation. *Journal of Medical Genetics, 11*, 11.

Archer, H. L., Whatley, S. D., Evans, J. C., Ravine, D., Huppke, P., Kerr, A., et al. (2006). Gross rearrangements of the MECP2 gene are found in both classical and atypical Rett syndrome patients. *Journal of Medical Genetics, 43*(5), 451–456.

Ariani, F., Hayek, G., Rondinella, D., Artuso, R., Mencarelli, M. A., Spanhol-Rosseto, A., et al. (2008). FOXG1 is responsible for the congenital variant of Rett syndrome. *American Journal of Human Genetics, 83*(1), 89–93.

Armstrong, D., Dunn, J. K., Antalffy, B., & Trivedi, R. (1995). Selective dendritic alterations in the cortex of Rett syndrome. *Journal of Neuropathology and Experimental Neurology, 54*(2), 195–201.

Armstrong, D. D. (2005a). Can we relate MeCP2 deficiency to the structural and chemical abnormalities in the Rett brain?. *Brain and Development, 27* Suppl *1*, S72–S76.

Armstrong, D. D. (2005b). Neuropathology of Rett syndrome. *Journal of Child Neurology, 20*(9), 747–753.

Armstrong, J., Pineda, M., Aibar, E., Gean, E., & Monros, E. (2001). Classic Rett syndrome in a boy as a result of somatic mosaicism for a MECP2 mutation. *Annals of Neurology, 50*(5), 692.

Aron, M. (1990). The use and effectiveness of elbow splints in the Rett syndrome. *Brain and Development, 12*(1), 162–163.

Bahi-Buisson, N., Nectoux, J., Rosas-Vargas, H., Milh, M., Boddaert, N., Girard, B., et al. (2008). Key clinical features to identify girls with CDKL5 mutations. *Brain, 131(10)*, 2647–2661

Ballas, N., Lioy, D. T., Grunseich, C., & Mandel, G. (2009). Non-cell autonomous influence of MeCP2-deficient glia on neuronal dendritic morphology. *Nature Neuroscience, 12*(3), 311–317.

Bebbington, A., Anderson, A., Ravine, D., Fyfe, S., Pineda, M., de Klerk, N., et al. (2008). Investigating genotype-phenotype relationships in Rett syndrome using an international data set. *Neurology, 70*(11), 868–875.

Belichenko, P. V., Oldfors, A., Hagberg, B., & Dahlstrom, A. (1994). Rett syndrome: 3-D confocal microscopy of cortical pyramidal dendrites and afferents. *Neuroreport, 5*(12), 1509–1513.

Beyer, K. S., Blasi, F., Bacchelli, E., Klauck, S. M., Maestrini, E., & Poustka, A. (2002). Mutation analysis of the coding sequence of the MECP2 gene in infantile autism. *Human Genetics, 111*(4-5), 305–309.

Bourdon, V., Philippe, C., Martin, D., Verloes, A., Grandemenge, A., & Jonveaux, P. (2003). MECP2 mutations or polymorphisms in mentally retarded boys: diagnostic implications. *Molecular Diagnosis, 7*(1), 3–7.

Budden, S. S., Dorsey, H. C., & Steiner, R. D. (2005). Clinical profile of a male with Rett syndrome. *Brain and Development, 27 Suppl 1*, S69–S71.

Budden, S. S., & Gunness, M. E. (2003). Possible mechanisms of osteopenia in Rett syndrome: bone histomorphometric studies. *Journal of Child Neurology, 18*(10), 698–702.

Bumin, G., Uyanik, M., Kayihan, H., Duger, T., & Topcu, M. (2002). The effect of hand splints on stereotypic hand behavior in Rett's syndrome. *Turkish Journal of Pediatrics, 44*(1), 25–29.

Buschdorf, J. P., & Stratling, W. H. (2004). A WW domain binding region in methyl-CpG-binding protein MeCP2: impact on Rett syndrome. *Journal of Molecular Medicine, 82*(2), 135–143.

Campos, M. Jr., Abdalla, C. B., Santos, A. V., Pestana, C. P., Santos, J. M., Santos-Reboucas, C. B., et al. (2008). A MECP2 mutation in a highly conserved aminoacid causing mental retardation in a male. *Brain and Development, 31(2)*, 176–178.

Carney, R. M., Wolpert, C. M., Ravan, S. A., Shahbazian, M., Ashley-Koch, A., Cuccaro, M. L., et al. (2003). Identification of MeCP2 mutations in a series of females with autistic disorder. *Pediatric Neurology, 28*(3), 205–211.

Chahrour, M., Jung, S. Y., Shaw, C., Zhou, X., Wong, S. T., Qin, J., et al. (2008). MeCP2, a key contributor to neurological disease, activates and represses transcription. *Science, 320*(5880), 1224–1229.

Chandler, S. P., Guschin, D., Landsberger, N., & Wolffe, A. P. (1999). The methyl-CpG binding transcriptional repressor MeCP2 stably associates with nucleosomal DNA. *Biochemistry, 38*(22), 7008–7018.

Chang, Q., Khare, G., Dani, V., Nelson, S., & Jaenisch, R. (2006). The disease progression of Mecp2 mutant mice is affected by the level of BDNF expression. *Neuron, 49*(3), 341–348.

Chao, H. T., Zoghbi, H. Y., & Rosenmund, C. (2007). MeCP2 controls excitatory synaptic strength by regulating glutamatergic synapse number. *Neuron, 56*(1), 58–65.

Chen, Q., Xhu, Y. C., Yu, J., Miao, S., Zheng, J., Xu, L., et al. (2010). CDKL5, a protein associated with Rett syndrome, regulates neuronal morphogenesis via Racl signaling. *Journal of Neuroscience, 30(38)*,12777–12786.

Chen, R. Z., Akbarian, S., Tudor, M., & Jaenisch, R. (2001). Deficiency of methyl-CpG binding protein-2 in CNS neurons results in a Rett-like phenotype in mice. *Nature Genetics, 27*(3), 327–331.

Chen, W. G., Chang, Q., Lin, Y., Meissner, A., West, A. E., Griffith, E. C., et al. (2003). Derepression of BDNF transcription involves calcium-dependent phosphorylation of MeCP2. *Science, 302*(5646), 885–889.

Christodoulou, J., Grimm, A., Maher, T., & Bennetts, B. (2003). RettBASE: The IRSA MECP2 variation database-a new mutation database in evolution. *Human Mutation, 21*(5), 466–472.

Clayton-Smith, J., Walters, S., Hobson, E., Burkitt-Wright, E., Smith, R., Toutain, A., et al. (2008). Xq28 duplication presenting with intestinal and bladder dysfunction and a distinctive facial appearance. *European Journal of Human Genetics.*

Clayton-Smith, J., Watson, P., Ramsden, S., & Black, G. C. (2000). Somatic mutation in MECP2 as a non-fatal neurodevelopmental disorder in males. *Lancet, 356*(9232), 830–832.

Cohen, D., Lazar, G., Couvert, P., Desportes, V., Lippe, D., Mazet, P., et al. (2002). MECP2 mutation in a boy with language disorder and schizophrenia. *American Journal of Psychiatry, 159*(1), 148–149.

Collins, A. L., Levenson, J. M., Vilaythong, A. P., Richman, R., Armstrong, D. L., Noebels, J. L., et al. (2004). Mild overexpression of MeCP2 causes a progressive neurological disorder in mice. *Human Molecular Genetics*, *13*(21), 2679–2689.

Cooper, R. A., Kerr, A. M., & Amos, P. M. (1998). Rett syndrome: critical examination of clinical features, serial EEG and video-monitoring in understanding and management. *European Journal of Paediatric Neurology*, *2*(3), 127–135.

Coutinho, A. M., Oliveira, G., Katz, C., Feng, J., Yan, J., Yang, C., et al. (2007). MECP2 coding sequence and 3'UTR variation in 172 unrelated autistic patients. *American Journal of Medical Genetics. Part B, Neuropsychiatric Genetics*, *144B*(4), 475–483.

Couvert, P., Bienvenu, T., Aquaviva, C., Poirier, K., Moraine, C., Gendrot, C., et al. (2001). MECP2 is highly mutated in X-linked mental retardation. *Human Molecular Genetics*, *10*(9), 941–946.

Coy, J. F., Sedlacek, Z., Bachner, D., Delius, H., & Poustka, A. (1999). A complex pattern of evolutionary conservation and alternative polyadenylation within the long 3"-untranslated region of the methyl-CpG-binding protein 2 gene (MeCP2) suggests a regulatory role in gene expression. *Human Molecular Genetics*, *8*(7), 1253–1262.

Dayer, A. G., Bottani, A., Bouchardy, I., Fluss, J., Antonarakis, S. E., Haenggeli, C. A., et al. (2007). MECP2 mutant allele in a boy with Rett syndrome and his unaffected heterozygous mother. *Brain and Development*, *29*(1), 47–50.

del Gaudio, D., Fang, P., Scaglia, F., Ward, P. A., Craigen, W. J., Glaze, D. G., et al. (2006). Increased MECP2 gene copy number as the result of genomic duplication in neurodevelopmentally delayed males. *Genetics in Medicine*, *8*(12), 784–792.

Donzel-Javouhey, A., Thauvin-Robinet, C., Cusin, V., Madinier, N., Manceau, E., Dipanda, D., et al. (2006). A new cohort of MECP2 mutation screening in unexplained mental retardation: careful re-evaluation is the best indicator for molecular diagnosis. *American Journal of Medical Genetics. Part A*, *140*(14), 1603–1607.

Du, M., Liu, X., Welch, E. M., Hirawat, S., Peltz, S. W., & Bedwell, D. M. (2008). PTC124 is an orally bioavailable compound that promotes suppression of the human CFTR-G542X nonsense allele in a CF mouse model. *Proceedings of the National Academy of Sciences of the United States of America*, *105*(6), 2064–2069.

Einspieler, C., Kerr, A. M., & Prechtl, H. F. (2005a). Abnormal general movements in girls with Rett disorder: the first four months of life. *Brain and Development*, *27* (Suppl *1*), S8–S13.

Einspieler, C., Kerr, A. M., & Prechtl, H. F. (2005b). Is the early development of girls with Rett disorder really normal? *Pediatric Research*, *57*(5 Pt 1), 696–700.

Ellaway, C. J., Sholler, G., Leonard, H., & Christodoulou, J. (1999). Prolonged QT interval in Rett syndrome. *Archives of Disease in Childhood*, *80*(5), 470–472.

Erlandson, A., Samuelsson, L., Hagberg, B., Kyllerman, M., Vujic, M., & Wahlstrom, J. (2003). Multiplex ligation-dependent probe amplification (MLPA) detects large deletions in the MECP2 gene of Swedish Rett syndrome patients. *Genetic Testing*, *7*(4), 329–332.

Evans, J. C., Archer, H. L., Colley, J. P., Ravn, K., Nielsen, J. B., Kerr, A., et al. (2005). Early onset seizures and Rett-like features associated with mutations in CDKL5. *European Journal of Human Genetics*, *13*(10), 1113–1120.

FitzGerald, P. M., Jankovic, J., Glaze, D. G., Schultz, R., & Percy, A. K. (1990). Extrapyramidal involvement in Rett's syndrome. *Neurology*, *40*(2), 293–295.

FitzGerald, P. M., Jankovic, J., & Percy, A. K. (1990). Rett syndrome and associated movement disorders. *Movement Disorders*, *5*(3), 195–202.

Friez, M. J., Jones, J. R., Clarkson, K., Lubs, H., Abuelo, D., Bier, J. A., et al. (2006). Recurrent infections, hypotonia, and mental retardation caused by duplication of MECP2 and adjacent region in Xq28. *Pediatrics*, *118*(6), e1687–1695.

Fukuda, T., Yamashita, Y., Nagamitsu, S., Miyamoto, K., Jin, J. J., Ohmori, I., et al. (2005). Methyl-CpG binding protein 2 gene (MECP2) variations in Japanese patients with Rett syndrome: pathological mutations and polymorphisms. *Brain and Development*, *27*(3), 211–217.

Fyffe, S. L., Neul, J. L., Samaco, R. C., Chao, H. T., Ben-Shachar, S., Moretti, P., et al. (2008). Deletion of Mecp2 in Sim1-expressing neurons reveals a critical role for MeCP2 in feeding behavior, aggression, and the response to stress. *Neuron*, *59*(6), 947–958.

Geerdink, N., Rotteveel, J. J., Lammens, M., Sistermans, E. A., Heikens, G. T., Gabreels, F. J., et al. (2002). MECP2 mutation in a boy with severe neonatal encephalopathy: clinical, neuropathological and molecular findings. *Neuropediatrics*, *33*(1), 33–36.

Gemelli, T., Berton, O., Nelson, E. D., Perrotti, L. I., Jaenisch, R., & Monteggia, L. M. (2006). Postnatal loss of methyl-CpG binding protein 2 in the forebrain is sufficient to mediate behavioral aspects of Rett syndrome in mice. *Biological Psychiatry*, *59*(5), 468–476.

Giacometti, E., Luikenhuis, S., Beard, C., & Jaenisch, R. (2007). Partial rescue of MeCP2 deficiency by postnatal activation of MeCP2. *Proceedings of the National Academy of Sciences of the United States of America*, *104*(6), 1931–1936.

Gillberg, C. (1987). Autistic symptoms in Rett syndrome: the first two years according to mother reports. *Brain and Development*, *9*(5), 499–501.

Gillberg, C. (1989). The borderland of autism and Rett syndrome: five case histories to highlight diagnostic difficulties. *Journal of Autism and Developmental Disorders*, *19*(4), 545–559.

Girard, M., Couvert, P., Carrie, A., Tardieu, M., Chelly, J., Beldjord, C., et al. (2001). Parental origin of de novo MECP2 mutations in Rett syndrome. *European Journal of Human Genetics*, *9*(3), 231–236.

Glaze, D. G. (2002). Neurophysiology of Rett syndrome. *Mental Retardation and Developmental Disabilities Research Reviews*, *8*(2), 66–71.

Glaze, D. G., Frost, J. D., Jr., Zoghbi, H. Y., & Percy, A. K. (1987). Rett's syndrome. Correlation of electroencephalographic characteristics with clinical staging. *Archives of Neurology*, *44*(10), 1053–1056.

Glaze, D. G., Schultz, R. J., & Frost, J. D. (1998). Rett syndrome: characterization of seizures versus non-seizures. *Electroencephalography and Clinical Neurophysiology*, *106*(1), 79–83.

Goutieres, F., & Aicardi, J. (1986). Atypical forms of Rett syndrome. *American Journal of Medical Genetics. Supplement*, *1*, 183–194.

Goutieres, F., & Aicardi, J. (1987). New experience with Rett syndrome in France: the problem of atypical cases. *Brain and Development*, *9*(5), 502–505.

Goyal, M., O'Riordan, M. A., & Wiznitzer, M. (2004). Effect of topiramate on seizures and respiratory dysrhythmia in Rett syndrome. *Journal of Child Neurology*, *19*(8), 588–591.

Guideri, F., Acampa, M., Hayek, G., Zappella, M., & Di Perri, T. (1999). Reduced heart rate variability in patients affected with Rett syndrome. A possible explanation for sudden death. *Neuropediatrics, 30*(3), 146–148.

Guy, J., Gan, J., Selfridge, J., Cobb, S., & Bird, A. (2007). Reversal of Neurological Defects in a Mouse Model of Rett Syndrome. *Science, 8*, 8.

Guy, J., Hendrich, B., Holmes, M., Martin, J. E., & Bird, A. (2001). A mouse Mecp2-null mutation causes neurological symptoms that mimic Rett syndrome. *Nature Genetics, 27*(3), 322–326.

Hagberg, B. (2002). Clinical manifestations and stages of Rett syndrome. *Mental Retardation and Developmental Disabilities Research Reviews, 8*(2), 61–65.

Hagberg, B. (2005). Rett syndrome: long-term clinical follow-up experiences over four decades. *Journal of Child Neurology, 20*(9), 722–727.

Hagberg, B., Aicardi, J., Dias, K., & Ramos, O. (1983). A progressive syndrome of autism, dementia, ataxia, and loss of purposeful hand use in girls: Rett's syndrome: report of 35 cases. *Annals of Neurology, 14*(4), 471–479.

Hagberg, B., Hanefeld, F., Percy, A., & Skjeldal, O. (2002). An update on clinically applicable diagnostic criteria in Rett syndrome. Comments to Rett Syndrome Clinical Criteria Consensus Panel Satellite to European Paediatric Neurology Society Meeting, Baden Baden, Germany, September 11, 2001. *European Journal of Paediatric Neurology, 6*(5), 293–297.

Hagberg, B., & Rasmussen, P. (1986). "Forme fruste" of Rett syndrome—a case report. *American Journal of Medical Genetics Supplement, 1*, 175–181.

Hagberg, B. A., & Skjeldal, O. H. (1994). Rett variants: a suggested model for inclusion criteria. *Pediatric Neurology, 11*(1), 5–11.

Hagberg, G., Stenbom, Y., & Engerstrom, I. W. (2001). Head growth in Rett syndrome. *Brain and Development, 23*(Suppl 1), S227–229.

Hagne, I., Witt-Engerstrom, I., & Hagberg, B. (1989). EEG development in Rett syndrome. A study of 30 cases. *Electroencephalography and Clinical Neurophysiology, 72*(1), 1–6.

Hanefeld, F. (1985). The clinical pattern of the Rett syndrome. *Brain and Development, 7*(3), 320–325.

Hardwick, S. A., Reuter, K., Williamson, S. L., Vasudevan, V., Donald, J., Slater, K., et al. (2007). Delineation of large deletions of the MECP2 gene in Rett syndrome patients, including a familial case with a male proband. *European Journal of Human Genetics, 15*(12), 1218–1229.

Harvey, C. G., Menon, S. D., Stachowiak, B., Noor, A., Proctor, A., Mensah, A. K., et al. (2007). Sequence variants within exon 1 of MECP2 occur in females with mental retardation. *American Journal of Medical Genetics. Part B, Neuropsychiatric Genetics, 144B*(3), 355–360.

Hendrich, B., & Bird, A. (1998). Identification and characterization of a family of mammalian methyl-CpG binding proteins. *Molecular and Cellular Biology, 18*(11), 6538–6547.

Hitchins, M. P., Rickard, S., Dhalla, F., Fairbrother, U. L., de Vries, B. B., Winter, R., et al. (2004). Investigation of UBE3A and MECP2 in Angelman syndrome (AS) and patients with features of AS. *American Journal of Medical Genetics. Part A, 125*(2), 167–172.

Hoffbuhr, K., Devaney, J. M., LaFleur, B., Sirianni, N., Scacheri, C., Giron, J., et al. (2001). MeCP2 mutations in children with and without the phenotype of Rett syndrome. *Neurology, 56*(11), 1486–1495.

Huppke, P., Held, M., Hanefeld, F., Engel, W., & Laccone, F. (2002). Influence of mutation type and location on phenotype in 123 patients with Rett syndrome. *Neuropediatrics, 33*(2), 63–68.

Huppke, P., Held, M., Laccone, F., & Hanefeld, F. (2003). The spectrum of phenotypes in females with Rett Syndrome. *Brain and Development, 25*(5), 346–351.

Huppke, P., Laccone, F., Kramer, N., Engel, W., & Hanefeld, F. (2000). Rett syndrome: analysis of MECP2 and clinical characterization of 31 patients. *Human Molecular Genetics, 9*(9), 1369–1375.

Huppke, P., Maier, E. M., Warnke, A., Brendel, C., Laccone, F., & Gartner, J. (2006). Very mild cases of Rett syndrome with skewed X inactivation. *Journal of Medical Genetics, 43*(10), 814–816.

Huttenlocher, P. R. (1974). Dendritic development in neocortex of children with mental defect and infantile spasms. *Neurology, 24*(3), 203–210.

Huttenlocher, P. R. (1991). Dendritic and synaptic pathology in mental retardation. *Pediatric Neurology, 7*(2), 79–85.

Huttenlocher, P. R. (2000). The neuropathology of phenylketonuria: human and animal studies. *European Journal of Pediatrics, 159 Suppl 2*, S102–106.

Irwin, S. A., Galvez, R., & Greenough, W. T. (2000). Dendritic spine structural anomalies in fragile-X mental retardation syndrome. *Cerebral Cortex, 10*(10), 1038–1044.

Jacob, F. D., Ramaswamy, V., Andersen, J., & Bolduc, F. V., (2009). Atypical Rett syndrome with selective FOXG1 deletion detected by comparative genomic hybridization: case report and review of literature. *European Journal of Human Genetics, 17*(12), 1577–1581.

Jay, V., Becker, L. E., Chan, F. W., & Perry, T. L., Sr. (1991). Puppet-like syndrome of Angelman: a pathologic and neurochemical study. *Neurology, 41*(3), 416–422.

Jedele, K. B. (2007). The overlapping spectrum of rett and angelman syndromes: a clinical review. *Seminars in Pediatric Neurology, 14*(3), 108–117.

Jellinger, K., Armstrong, D., Zoghbi, H. Y., & Percy, A. K. (1988). Neuropathology of Rett syndrome. *Acta Neuropathologica (Berlin), 76*(2), 142–158.

Jentarra, G. M., Olfers, S. L., Rice, S. G., Srivastava, N., Homanics, G. E., Blue, M., et al. (2010). Abnormalities of cell packing density and dendritic complexity in the MeCP2 A140V mouse model of Rett syndrome/X-linked. *BMC Neuroscience, 11*(19).

Jones, P. L., Veenstra, G. J., Wade, P. A., Vermaak, D., Kass, S. U., Landsberger, N., et al. (1998). Methylated DNA and MeCP2 recruit histone deacetylase to repress transcription. *Nature Genetics, 19*(2), 187–191.

Julu, P. O., Kerr, A. M., Apartopoulos, F., Al-Rawas, S., Engerstrom, I. W., Engerstrom, L., et al. (2001). Characterisation of breathing and associated central autonomic dysfunction in the Rett disorder. *Archives of Disease in Childhood, 85*(1), 29–37.

Julu, P. O., Kerr, A. M., Hansen, S., Apartopoulos, F., & Jamal, G. A. (1997). Immaturity of medullary cardiorespiratory neurones leading to inappropriate autonomic reactions as a likely cause of sudden death in Rett's syndrome. *Archives of Disease in Childhood, 77*(5), 464–465.

Kammoun, F., de Roux, N., Boespflug-Tanguy, O., Vallee, L., Seng, R., Tardieu, M., et al. (2004). Screening of MECP2 coding sequence in patients with phenotypes of decreasing likelihood for Rett syndrome: a cohort of 171 cases. *Journal of Medical Genetics, 41*(6), e85.

Kankirawatana, P., Leonard, H., Ellaway, C., Scurlock, J., Mansour, A., Makris, C. M., et al. (2006). Early progressive encephalopathy in boys and MECP2 mutations. *Neurology, 67*(1), 164–166.

Kaufmann, W. E., & Moser, H. W. (2000). Dendritic anomalies in disorders associated with mental retardation. *Cerebral Cortex, 10*(10), 981–991.

Kerr, A. M., Archer, H. L., Evans, J. C., Prescott, R. J., & Gibbon, F. (2006). People with MECP2 mutation-positive Rett disorder who converse. *Journal of Intellectual Disability Research, 50*(Pt 5), 386–394.

Kerr, A. M., Armstrong, D. D., Prescott, R. J., Doyle, D., & Kearney, D. L. (1997). Rett syndrome: analysis of deaths in the British survey. *European Child and Adolescent Psychiatry, 6*(Suppl 1), 71–74.

Kerr, A. M., & Julu, P. O. (1999). Recent insights into hyperventilation from the study of Rett syndrome. *Archives of Disease in Childhood, 80*(4), 384–387.

Kerr, A. M., Montague, J., & Stephenson, J. B. (1987). The hands, and the mind, pre- and post-regression, in Rett syndrome. *Brain and Development, 9*(5), 487–490.

Kerr, A. M., & Stephenson, J. B. (1985). Rett's syndrome in the west of Scotland. *British Medical Journal (Clinical Research Ed.), 291*(6495), 579–582.

Kerr, B., Alvarez-Saavedra, M., Saez, M. A., Saona, A., & Young, J. I. (2008). Defective body-weight regulation, motor control and abnormal social interactions in Mecp2 hypomorphic mice. *Human Molecular Genetics, 17*(12), 1707–1717.

Kirby, R., Percy, A., Lane, J., Glaze, D., Skinner, S., MacLeod, P., et al. (2009). Longevity in Rett Syndrome: Probing the North American Database. *Journal of Pedatrics,* in press.

Klauck, S. M., Lindsay, S., Beyer, K. S., Splitt, M., Burn, J., & Poustka, A. (2002). A mutation hot spot for nonspecific X-linked mental retardation in the MECP2 gene causes the PPM-X syndrome. *American Journal of Human Genetics, 70*(4), 1034–1037.

Kleefstra, T., Yntema, H. G., Nillesen, W. M., Oudakker, A. R., Mullaart, R. A., Geerdink, N., et al. (2004). MECP2 analysis in mentally retarded patients: implications for routine DNA diagnostics. *European Journal of Human Genetics, 12*(1), 24–28.

Kleefstra, T., Yntema, H. G., Oudakker, A. R., Romein, T., Sistermans, E., Nillessen, W., et al. (2002). De novo MECP2 frameshift mutation in a boy with moderate mental retardation, obesity and gynaecomastia. *Clinical Genetics, 61*(5), 359–362.

Klein, M. E., Lioy, D. T., Ma, L., Impey, S., Mandel, G., & Goodman, R. H. (2007). Homeostatic regulation of MeCP2 expression by a CREB-induced microRNA. *Nature Neuroscience, 10*(12), 1513–1514.

Kriaucionis, S., & Bird, A. (2004). The major form of MeCP2 has a novel N-terminus generated by alternative splicing. *Nucleic Acids Research, 32*(5), 1818–1823.

Kubas, E. S. (1992). Use of splints to develop hand skills in a woman with Rett syndrome. *American Journal of Occupational Therapy, 46*(4), 364–368.

Kudo, S., Nomura, Y., Segawa, M., Fujita, N., Nakao, M., Hammer, S., et al. (2002). Functional characterisation of MeCP2 mutations found in male patients with X linked mental retardation. *Journal of Medical Genetics, 39*(2), 132–136.

Kudo, S., Nomura, Y., Segawa, M., Fujita, N., Nakao, M., Schanen, C., et al. (2003). Heterogeneity in residual function of MeCP2 carrying missense mutations in the methyl CpG binding domain. *Journal of Medical Genetics, 40*(7), 487–493.

Laccone, F., Zoll, B., Huppke, P., Hanefeld, F., Pepinski, W., & Trappe, R. (2002). MECP2 gene nucleotide changes and their pathogenicity in males: proceed with caution. *Journal of Medical Genetics, 39*(8), 586–588.

Laurvick, C. L., de Klerk, N., Bower, C., Christodoulou, J., Ravine, D., Ellaway, C., et al. (2006). Rett syndrome in Australia: a review of the epidemiology. *Journal of Pediatrics, 148*(3), 347–352.

Lawson-Yuen, A., Liu, D., Han, L., Jiang, Z. I., Tsai, G. E., Basu, A. C., et al. (2007). Ube3a mRNA and protein expression are not decreased in Mecp2R168X mutant mice. *Brain Research, 1180*, 1–6.

Leonard, H., & Bower, C. (1998). Is the girl with Rett syndrome normal at birth? *Developmental Medicine and Child Neurology, 40*(2), 115–121.

Leonard, H., Silberstein, J., Falk, R., Houwink-Manville, I., Ellaway, C., Raffaele, L. S., et al. (2001). Occurrence of Rett syndrome in boys. *Journal of Child Neurology, 16*(5), 333–338.

Lesca, G., Bernard, V., Bozon, M., Touraine, R., Gerard, D., Edery, P., et al. (2007). Mutation screening of the MECP2 gene in a large cohort of 613 fragile-X negative patients with mental retardation. *European Journal of Medical Genetics, 50*(3), 200–208.

Leuzzi, V., Di Sabato, M. L., Zollino, M., Montanaro, M. L., & Seri, S. (2004). Early-onset encephalopathy and cortical myoclonus in a boy with MECP2 gene mutation. *Neurology, 63*(10), 1968–1970.

Lewis, J. D., Meehan, R. R., Henzel, W. J., Maurer-Fogy, I., Jeppesen, P., Klein, F., et al. (1992). Purification, sequence, and cellular localization of a novel chromosomal protein that binds to methylated DNA. *Cell, 69*(6), 905–914.

Li, H., Yamagata, T., Mori, M., Yasuhara, A., & Momoi, M. Y. (2005). Mutation analysis of methyl-CpG binding protein family genes in autistic patients. *Brain and Development, 27*(5), 321–325.

Lin, C., Franco, B., & Rosner, M. R. (2005). CDKL5/Stk9 kinase inactivation is associated with neuronal developmental disorders. *Human Molecular Genetics, 14*(24), 3775–3786.

Lobo-Menendez, F., Sossey-Alaoui, K., Bell, J. M., Copeland-Yates, S. A., Plank, S. M., Sanford, S. O., et al. (2003). Absence of MeCP2 mutations in patients from the South Carolina autism project. *American Journal of Medical Genetics. Part B, Neuropsychiatric Genetics, 117*(1), 97–101.

Lugtenberg, D., Kleefstra, T., Oudakker, A. R., Nillesen, W. M., Yntema, H. G., Tzschach, A., et al. (2009). Structural variation in Xq28: MECP2 duplications in 1% of patients with unexplained XLMR and in 2% of male patients with severe encephalopathy. *European Journal of Human Genetics, 17*(4), 444–453.

Luikenhuis, S., Giacometti, E., Beard, C. F., & Jaenisch, R. (2004). Expression of MeCP2 in postmitotic neurons rescues Rett syndrome in mice. *Proceedings of the National Academy of Sciences of the United States of America, 101*(16), 6033–6038.

Lundvall, M., Samuelsson, L., & Kyllerman, M. (2006). Male Rett Phenotypes in T158M and R294X MeCP2-mutations. *Neuropediatrics, 37*(5), 296–301.

Lynch, S. A., Whatley, S. D., Ramesh, V., Sinha, S., & Ravine, D. (2003). Sporadic case of fatal encephalopathy with neonatal onset associated with a T158M missense mutation in MECP2. *Archives of Disease in Childhood. Fetal and Neonatal Edition, 88*(3), F250–252.

Madan, N., Levine, M., Pourmoghadam, K., & Sokoloski, M. (2004). Severe sinus bradycardia in a patient with Rett syndrome: a new cause for a pause? *Pediatric Cardiology, 25*(1), 53–55.

Maezawa, I., Swanberg, S., Harvey, D., LaSalle, J. M., & Jin, L. W. (2009). Rett syndrome astrocytes are abnormal and spread MeCP2 deficiency through gap junctions. *Journal of Neuroscience, 29*(16), 5051–5061.

Mari, F., Azimonti, S., Bertani, I., Bolognese, F., Colombo, E., Caselli, R., et al. (2005). CDKL5 belongs to the same molecular pathway of MeCP2 and it is responsible for the early-onset seizure variant of Rett syndrome. *Human Molecular Genetics, 14*(14), 1935–1946.

Mencarelli, M. A., Spanhol-Rosseto, A., Artuso, R., Rondinella, D., De Filippis, R., Bahi-Buisson, N., et al. (2010). Novel FOXG1 mutations associated with the congenital variant of Rett syndrome. *Journal of Medical Genetics, 47*(1), 49–53.

Martinowich, K., Hattori, D., Wu, H., Fouse, S., He, F., Hu, Y., et al. (2003). DNA methylation-related chromatin remodeling in activity-dependent BDNF gene regulation. *Science, 302*(5646), 890–893.

Masuyama, T., Matsuo, M., Jing, J. J., Tabara, Y., Kitsuki, K., Yamagata, H., et al. (2005). Classic Rett syndrome in a boy with R133C mutation of MECP2. *Brain and Development, 27*(6), 439–442.

McGill, B. E., Bundle, S. F., Yaylaoglu, M. B., Carson, J. P., Thaller, C., & Zoghbi, H. Y. (2006). Enhanced anxiety and stress-induced corticosterone release are associated with increased Crh expression in a mouse model of Rett syndrome. *Proceedings of the National Academy of Sciences of the United States of America, 103*(48), 18267–18272.

Meins, M., Lehmann, J., Gerresheim, F., Herchenbach, J., Hagedorn, M., Hameister, K., et al. (2005). Submicroscopic duplication in Xq28 causes increased expression of the MECP2 gene in a boy with severe mental retardation and features of Rett syndrome. *Journal of Medical Genetics, 42*(2), e12.

Meloni, I., Bruttini, M., Longo, I., Mari, F., Rizzolio, F., D'Adamo, P., et al. (2000). A mutation in the rett syndrome gene, MECP2, causes X-linked mental retardation and progressive spasticity in males. *American Journal of Human Genetics, 67*(4), 982–985.

Meyer-Lindenberg, A. (2008). Impact of prosocial neuropeptides on human brain function. *Progress in Brain Research, 170*, 463–470.

Milani, D., Pantaleoni, C., D'Arrigo, S., Selicorni, A., & Riva, D. (2005). Another patient with MECP2 mutation without classic Rett syndrome phenotype. *Pediatric Neurology, 32*(5), 355–357.

Milunsky, J. M., Lebo, R. V., Ikuta, T., Maher, T. A., Haverty, C. E., & Milunsky, A. (2001). Mutation analysis in Rett syndrome. *Genetic Testing, 5*(4), 321–325.

Mnatzakanian, G. N., Lohi, H., Munteanu, I., Alfred, S. E., Yamada, T., MacLeod, P. J., et al. (2004). A previously unidentified MECP2 open reading frame defines a new protein isoform relevant to Rett syndrome. *Nature Genetics, 36*(4), 339–341.

Monros, E., Armstrong, J., Aibar, E., Poo, P., Canos, I., & Pineda, M. (2001). Rett syndrome in Spain: mutation analysis and clinical correlations. *Brain and Development, 23*(Suppl 1), S251–253.

Moog, U., Smeets, E. E., van Roozendaal, K. E., Schoenmakers, S., Herbergs, J., Schoonbrood-Lenssen, A. M., et al. (2003). Neurodevelopmental disorders in males related to the gene causing Rett syndrome in females (MECP2). *European Journal of Paediatric Neurology, 7*(1), 5–12.

Moog, U., Van Roozendaal, K., Smeets, E., Tserpelis, D., Devriendt, K., Buggenhout, G. V., et al. (2006). MECP2 mutations are an infrequent cause of mental retardation associated with neurological problems in male patients. *Brain and Development, 28*(5), 305–310.

Moretti, P., Bouwknecht, J. A., Teague, R., Paylor, R., & Zoghbi, H. Y. (2005). Abnormalities of social interactions and home-cage behavior in a mouse model of Rett syndrome. *Human Molecular Genetics, 14*(2), 205–220.

Moretti, P., Levenson, J. M., Battaglia, F., Atkinson, R., Teague, R., Antalffy, B., et al. (2006). Learning and memory and synaptic plasticity are impaired in a mouse model of Rett syndrome. *Journal of Neuroscience, 26*(1), 319–327.

Motil, K. J., Ellis, K. J., Barrish, J. O., Caeg, E., & Glaze, D. G. (2008). Bone Mineral Content and Bone Mineral Density Are Lower in Older than in Younger Females with Rett Syndrome. *Pediatric Research, 64*(4),435–439.

Motil, K. J., Morrissey, M., Caeg, E., Barrish, J. O., & Glaze, D. G. (2009). Gastrostomy placement improves height and weight gain in girls with Rett syndrome. *Journal of Pediatric Gastroenterology and Nutrition, 49*(2), 237–242.

Motil, K. J., Schultz, R. J., Browning, K., Trautwein, L., & Glaze, D. G. (1999). Oropharyngeal dysfunction and gastroesophageal dysmotility are present in girls and women with Rett syndrome. *Journal of Pediatric Gastroenterology and Nutrition, 29*(1), 31–37.

Naidu, S. (1997). Rett syndrome: a disorder affecting early brain growth. *Annals of Neurology, 42*(1), 3–10.

Naidu, S., Chatterjee, S., Murphy, M., Uematsu, S., Phillapart, M., & Moser, H. (1987). Rett syndrome: new observations. *Brain and Development, 9*(5), 525–528.

Nan, X., Campoy, F. J., & Bird, A. (1997). MeCP2 is a transcriptional repressor with abundant binding sites in genomic chromatin. *Cell, 88*(4), 471–481.

Nan, X., Cross, S., & Bird, A. (1998). Gene silencing by methyl-CpG-binding proteins. *Novartis Foundation Symposium, 214*, 6–16; discussion 16–21, 46–50.

Nan, X., Meehan, R. R., & Bird, A. (1993). Dissection of the methyl-CpG binding domain from the chromosomal protein MeCP2. *Nucleic Acids Research, 21*(21), 4886–4892.

Nectoux, J., Heron, D., Tallot, M., Chelly, J., & Bienvenu, T. (2006). Maternal origin of a novel C-terminal truncation mutation in CDKL5 causing a severe atypical form of Rett syndrome. *Clinical Genetics, 70*(1), 29–33.

Neul, J. L., Fang, P., Barrish, J., Lane, J., Caeg, E. B., Smith, E. O., et al. (2008). Specific mutations in methyl-CpG-binding protein 2 confer different severity in Rett syndrome. *Neurology, 70*(16), 1313–1321.

Neul, J. L., Kaufmann, W. E., Glaze, D. G., Christodoulou, J., Clarke, A. J., Bahi-Buisson, N., et al. for the RettSearch Consortium (2010). Rett Syndrome: Revised Diagnostic Criteria and Nomenclature. *Annals of Neurology, 68*(6), 944–950.

Nielsen, J. B., Henriksen, K. F., Hansen, C., Silahtaroglu, A., Schwartz, M., & Tommerup, N. (2001). MECP2 mutations in Danish patients with Rett syndrome: high frequency of mutations but no consistent correlations with clinical severity or with the X chromosome inactivation pattern. *European Journal of Human Genetics, 9*(3), 178–184.

Nielsen, J. B., Ravn, K., & Schwartz, M. (2001). A 77-year-old woman and a preserved speech variant among the Danish Rett patients with mutations in MECP2. *Brain and Development, 23*(Suppl 1), S230–232.

Nomura, Y., & Segawa, M. (1990a). Characteristics of motor disturbances of the Rett syndrome. *Brain and Development, 12*(1), 27–30.

Nomura, Y., & Segawa, M. (1990b). Clinical features of the early stage of the Rett syndrome. *Brain and Development, 12*(1), 16–19.

Oexle, K., Thamm-Mucke, B., Mayer, T., & Tinschert, S. (2005). Macrocephalic mental retardation associated with a novel C-terminal MECP2 frameshift deletion. *European Journal of Pediatrics, 164*(3), 154–157.

Ogier, M., Wang, H., Hong, E., Wang, Q., Greenberg, M. E., & Katz, D. M. (2007). Brain-derived neurotrophic factor expression and respiratory function improve after ampakine treatment in a mouse model of Rett syndrome. *Journal of Neuroscience, 27*(40), 10,912–10,917.

Orrico, A., Lam, C., Galli, L., Dotti, M. T., Hayek, G., Tong, S. F., et al. (2000). MECP2 mutation in male patients with non-specific X-linked mental retardation. *FEBS Letters, 481*(3), 285–288.

Pan, H., Li, M. R., Nelson, P., Bao, X. H., Wu, X. R., & Yu, S. (2006). Large deletions of the MECP2 gene in Chinese patients with classical Rett syndrome. *Clinical Genetics, 70*(5), 418–419.

Papa, F. T., Mencarelli, M. A., Caselli, R., Katzaki, E., Sampieri, K., Meloni, I., et al. (2008). A 3 Mb deletion in 14q12 causes severe mental retardation, mild facial dysmorphisms and Rett-like features. *American Journal of Medical Genetics. Part A, 146A*(15), 1994–1998.

Paterson, D. S., Thompson, E. G., Belliveau, R. A., Antalffy, B. A., Trachtenberg, F. L., Armstrong, D. D., et al. (2005). Serotonin transporter abnormality in the dorsal motor nucleus of the vagus in Rett syndrome: potential implications for clinical autonomic dysfunction. *Journal of Neuropathology and Experimental Neurology, 64*(11), 1018–1027.

Pelka, G. J., Watson, C. M., Radziewic, T., Hayward, M., Lahooti, H., Christodoulou, J., et al. (2006). Mecp2 deficiency is associated with learning and cognitive deficits and altered gene activity in the hippocampal region of mice. *Brain, 129*(Pt 4), 887–898.

Percy, A., Lee, H., Neul, J. L., Lane, J., Skinner, S., Geerts, S., et al. (2009). Profiling Scoliosis in Rett Syndrome. *Pediatric Research. 67(4)*, 435–439.

Percy, A. K., Lane, J. B., Childers, J., Skinner, S., Annese, F., Barrish, J., et al. (2007). Rett syndrome: North American database. *Journal of Child Neurology, 22*(12), 1338–1341.

Petel-Galil, Y., Benteer, B., Galil, Y. P., Zeev, B. B., Greenbaum, I., Vecsler, M., et al. (2006). Comprehensive diagnosis of Rett's syndrome relying on genetic, epigenetic and expression evidence of deficiency of the methyl-CpG-binding protein 2 gene: study of a cohort of Israeli patients. *Journal of Medical Genetics, 43*(12), e56.

Ramocki, M., Peters, S. U., Tavyev, Y. J., Zhang, F., Carvhalho, C. M. B., Fang, P., et al. (2009). High Penetrance of Autism and other Neuropsychiatric Symptoms in Individuals with *MECP2* Duplications. *Annals of Neurology,66*(6), 771–782.

Ravn, K., Nielsen, J. B., Skjeldal, O. H., Kerr, A., Hulten, M., & Schwartz, M. (2005). Large genomic rearrangements in MECP2. *Human Mutation, 25*(3), 324.

Ravn, K., Nielsen, J. B., Uldall, P., Hansen, F. J., & Schwartz, M. (2003). No correlation between phenotype and genotype in boys with a truncating MECP2 mutation. *Journal of Medical Genetics, 40*(1), e5.

Raymond, G. V., Bauman, M. L., & Kemper, T. L. (1996). Hippocampus in autism: a Golgi analysis. *Acta Neuropathologica, 91*(1), 117–119.

Renieri, A., Mari, F., Mencarelli, M. A., Scala, E., Ariani, F., Longo, I., et al. (2008). Diagnostic criteria for the Zappella variant of Rett syndrome (the preserved speech variant). *Brain and Development. 31*(3), 208–216.

Rett, A. (1966). [On a unusual brain atrophy syndrome in hyperammonemia in childhood]. *Wiener Medizinische Wochenschrift, 116*(37), 723–726.

Rohdin, M., Fernell, E., Eriksson, M., Albage, M., Lagercrantz, H., & Katz-Salamon, M. (2007). Disturbances in cardiorespiratory function during day and night in Rett syndrome. *Pediatric Neurology, 37*(5), 338–344.

Rolando, S. (1985). Rett syndrome: report of eight cases. *Brain and Development, 7*(3), 290–296.

Rosas-Vargas, H., Bahi-Buisson, N., Philippe, C., Nectoux, J., Girard, B., N'Guyen Morel, M. A., et al. (2008). Impairment of CDKL5 nuclear localisation as a cause for severe infantile encephalopathy. *Journal of Medical Genetics, 45*(3), 172–178.

Roux, J. C., Dura, E., Moncla, A., Mancini, J., & Villard, L. (2007). Treatment with desipramine improves breathing and survival in a mouse model for Rett syndrome. *European Journal of Neuroscience, 25*(7), 1915–1922.

Samaco, R. C., Fryer, J. D., Ren, J., Fyffe, S., Chao, H. T., Sun, Y., et al. (2008). A partial loss of function allele of methyl-CpG-binding protein 2 predicts a human neurodevelopmental syndrome. *Human Molecular Genetics, 17*(12), 1718–1727.

Samaco, R. C., Mandel-Brehm, C., Chao, H. T., Ward, C. S., Fyffe-Maricich, S. L., Ren, J., et al. (2009). Loss of MeCP2 in aminergic neurons causes cell-autonomous defects in neurotransmitter synthesis and specific behavioral abnormalities. *Proceedings of the National Academy of Sciences of the United States of America, 106*(51), 21966–21971.

Scala, E., Ariani, F., Mari, F., Caselli, R., Pescucci, C., Longo, I., et al. (2005). CDKL5/STK9 is mutated in Rett syndrome variant with infantile spasms. *Journal of Medical Genetics, 42*(2), 103–107.

Scala, E., Longo, I., Ottimo, F., Speciale, C., Sampieri, K., Katzaki, E., et al. (2007). MECP2 deletions and genotype-phenotype correlation in Rett syndrome. *American Journal of Medical Genetics. Part A, 143A*(23), 2775–2784.

Scheffer, I., Brett, E. M., Wilson, J., & Baraitser, M. (1990). Angelman's syndrome. *Journal of Medical Genetics, 27*(4), 275–276.

Schule, B., Armstrong, D. D., Vogel, H., Oviedo, A., & Francke, U. (2008). Severe congenital encephalopathy caused by MECP2 null mutations in males: central hypoxia and reduced neuronal dendritic structure. *Clinical Genetics, 74*(2), 116–126.

Schwartzman, J. S., Bernardino, A., Nishimura, A., Gomes, R. R., & Zatz, M. (2001). Rett syndrome in a boy with a 47,XXY karyotype confirmed by a rare mutation in the MECP2 gene. *Neuropediatrics, 32*(3), 162–164.

Sekul, E. A., Moak, J. P., Schultz, R. J., Glaze, D. G., Dunn, J. K., & Percy, A. K. (1994). Electrocardiographic findings in Rett syndrome: an explanation for sudden death? *Journal of Pediatrics, 125*(1), 80–82.

Shahbazian, M., Young, J., Yuva-Paylor, L., Spencer, C., Antalffy, B., Noebels, J., et al. (2002). Mice with truncated MeCP2 recapitulate many Rett syndrome features and display hyperacetylation of histone H3. *Neuron, 35*(2), 243–254.

Shahbazian, M. D., Antalffy, B., Armstrong, D. L., & Zoghbi, H. Y. (2002). Insight into Rett syndrome: MeCP2 levels display tissue- and cell-specific differences and correlate with neuronal maturation. *Human Molecular Genetics, 11*(2), 115–124.

Sharpe, P. A. (1992). Comparative effects of bilateral hand splints and an elbow orthosis on stereotypic hand movements and toy play in two children with Rett syndrome. *American Journal of Occupational Therapy, 46*(2), 134–140.

Sharpe, P. A., & Ottenbacher, K. J. (1990). Use of an elbow restraint to improve finger-feeding skills in a child with Rett syndrome. *American Journal of Occupational Therapy, 44*(4), 328–332.

Shibayama, A., Cook, E. H., Jr., Feng, J., Glanzmann, C., Yan, J., Craddock, N., et al. (2004). MECP2 structural and 3'-UTR variants in schizophrenia, autism and other psychiatric diseases: a possible association with autism. *American Journal of Medical Genetics. Part B, Neuropsychiatric Genetics, 128*(1), 50–53.

Smeets, E., Schollen, E., Moog, U., Matthijs, G., Herbergs, J., Smeets, H., et al. (2003). Rett syndrome in adolescent and adult females: clinical and molecular genetic findings. *American Journal of Medical Genetics. Part A, 122*(3), 227–233.

Smeets, E., Schrander-Stumpel, C., & Curfs, L. (2008). Rett Syndrome and long-term disorder profile. *Journal of Intellectual Disability Research, 52*(10), 818.

Smeets, E., Terhal, P., Casaer, P., Peters, A., Midro, A., Schollen, E., et al. (2005). Rett syndrome in females with CTS hot spot deletions: a disorder profile. *American Journal of Medical Genetics. Part A, 132*(2), 117–120.

Smyk, M., Obersztyn, E., Nowakowska, B., Nawara, M., Cheung, S. W., Mazurczak, T., et al. (2008). Different-sized duplications of Xq28, including MECP2, in three males with mental retardation, absent or delayed speech, and recurrent infections. *American Journal of Medical Genetics. Part B, Neuropsychiatric Genetics, 147B*(6), 799–806.

Steffenburg, U., Hagberg, G., & Hagberg, B. (2001). Epilepsy in a representative series of Rett syndrome. *Acta Paediatrica, 90*(1), 34–39.

Tao, J., Van Esch, H., Hagedorn-Greiwe, M., Hoffmann, K., Moser, B., Raynaud, M., et al. (2004). Mutations in the X-linked cyclin-dependent kinase-like 5 (CDKL5/STK9) gene are associated with severe neurodevelopmental retardation. *American Journal Human Genetics, 75*(6), 1149–1154.

Temudo, T., Oliveira, P., Santos, M., Dias, K., Vieira, J., Moreira, A., et al., (2007). Stereotypies in Rett syndrome: analysis of 83 patients with and without detected MECP2 mutations. *Neurology, 68*(15), 1183–1187.

Topcu, M., Akyerli, C., Sayi, A., Toruner, G. A., Kocoglu, S. R., Cimbis, M., et al. (2002). Somatic mosaicism for a MECP2 mutation associated with classic Rett syndrome in a boy. *European Journal Human Genetics, 10*(1), 77–81.

Trappe, R., Laccone, F., Cobilanschi, J., Meins, M., Huppke, P., Hanefeld, F., et al. (2001). MECP2 mutations in sporadic cases of Rett syndrome are almost exclusively of paternal origin. *American Journal Human Genetics, 68*(5), 1093–1101.

Tropea, D., Giacometti, E., Wilson, N. R., Beard, C., McCurry, C., Fu, D. D., et al. (2009). Partial reversal of Rett Syndrome-like symptoms in MeCP2 mutant mice. *Proceedings of the National Academy of Sciences of the United States of America, 106*(6), 2029–2034.

Turner, H., MacDonald, F., Warburton, S., Latif, F., & Webb, T. (2003). Developmental delay and the methyl binding genes. *Journal of Medical Genetics, 40*(2), E13.

Van Esch, H., Bauters, M., Ignatius, J., Jansen, M., Raynaud, M., Hollanders, K., et al. (2005). Duplication of the MECP2 region is a frequent cause of severe mental retardation and progressive neurological symptoms in males. *American Journal of Human Genetics, 77*(3), 442–453.

Venancio, M., Santos, M., Pereira, S. A., Maciel, P., & Saraiva, J. M. (2007). An explanation for another familial case of Rett syndrome: maternal germline mosaicism. *European Journal of Human Genetics, 15*(8), 902–904.

Viemari, J. C., Roux, J. C., Tryba, A. K., Saywell, V., Burnet, H., Pena, F., et al. (2005). Mecp2 deficiency disrupts norepinephrine and respiratory systems in mice. *Journal of Neuroscience, 25*(50), 11,521–11,530.

Villard, L., Kpebe, A., Cardoso, C., Chelly, P. J., Tardieu, P. M., & Fontes, M. (2000). Two affected boys in a Rett syndrome family: clinical and molecular findings. *Neurology, 55*(8), 1188–1193.

Vorsanova, S. G., Yurov, Y. B., Ulas, V. Y., Demidova, I. A., Sharonin, V. O., Kolotii, A. D., et al. (2001). Cytogenetic and molecular-cytogenetic studies of Rett syndrome (RTT): a retrospective analysis of a Russian cohort of RTT patients (the investigation of 57 girls and three boys). *Brain and Development, 23*(Suppl 1), S196–201.

Vourc'h, P., Bienvenu, T., Beldjord, C., Chelly, J., Barthelemy, C., Muh, J. P., et al. (2001). No mutations in the coding region of the Rett syndrome gene MECP2 in 59 autistic patients. *European Journal of Human Genetics, 9*(7), 556–558.

Wan, M., Lee, S. S., Zhang, X., Houwink-Manville, I., Song, H. R., Amir, R. E., et al. (1999). Rett syndrome and beyond: recurrent spontaneous and familial MECP2 mutations at CpG hotspots. *American Journal of Human Genetics, 65*(6), 1520–1529.

Wan, M., Zhao, K., Lee, S. S., & Francke, U. (2001). MECP2 truncating mutations cause histone H4 hyperacetylation in Rett syndrome. *Human Molecular Genetics, 10*(10), 1085–1092.

Wang, H., Chan, S. A., Ogier, M., Hellard, D., Wang, Q., Smith, C., et al. (2006). Dysregulation of brain-derived neurotrophic factor expression and neurosecretory function in Mecp2 null mice. *Journal of Neuroscience, 26*(42), 10,911–10,915.

Watson, P., Black, G., Ramsden, S., Barrow, M., Super, M., Kerr, B., et al. (2001). Angelman syndrome phenotype associated with mutations in MECP2, a gene encoding a methyl CpG binding protein. *Journal of Medical Genetics, 38*(4), 224–228.

Weaving, L. S., Christodoulou, J., Williamson, S. L., Friend, K. L., McKenzie, O. L., Archer, H., et al. (2004). Mutations of CDKL5 cause a severe neurodevelopmental disorder with infantile spasms and mental retardation. *American Journal of Human Genetics, 75*(6), 1079–1093.

Weese-Mayer, D. E., Lieske, S. P., Boothby, C. M., Kenny, A. S., Bennett, H. L., & Ramirez, J. M. (2008). Autonomic dysregulation in young girls with Rett Syndrome during nighttime in-Home recordings. *Pediatric Pulmonology. 43(11)*, 1045–1060.

Weese-Mayer, D. E., Lieske, S. P., Boothby, C. M., Kenny, A. S., Bennett, H. L., Silvestri, J. M., et al. (2006). Autonomic nervous system dysregulation: breathing and heart rate perturbation during wakefulness in young girls with Rett syndrome. *Pediatric Research, 60*(4), 443–449.

Welch, E. M., Barton, E. R., Zhuo, J., Tomizawa, Y., Friesen, W. J., Trifillis, P., et al. (2007). PTC124 targets genetic disorders caused by nonsense mutations. *Nature, 447*(7140), 87–91.

Wilfong, A. A., & Schultz, R. J. (2006). Vagus nerve stimulation for treatment of epilepsy in Rett syndrome. *Developmental Medicine and Child Neurology, 48*(8), 683–686.

Winnepenninckx, B., Errijgers, V., Hayez-Delatte, F., Reyniers, E., & Frank Kooy, R. (2002). Identification of a family with nonspecific mental retardation (MRX79) with the A140V mutation in the MECP2 gene: Is there a need for routine screening? *Human Mutation, 20*(4), 249–252.

Winslow, J. T. (2005). Neuropeptides and non-human primate social deficits associated with pathogenic rearing experience. *International Journal of Developmental Neuroscience, 23*(2-3), 245–251.

Winslow, J. T., & Insel, T. R. (2002). The social deficits of the oxytocin knockout mouse. *Neuropeptides, 36*(2-3), 221–229.

Witt-Engerstrom, I. (1987). Rett syndrome: a retrospective pilot study on potential early predictive symptomatology. *Brain and Development, 9*(5), 481–486.

Witt-Engerstrom, I., & Gillberg, C. (1987). Rett syndrome in Sweden. *Journal of Autism and Developmental Disorders, 17*(1), 149–150.

Xi, C. Y., Ma, H. W., Lu, Y., Zhao, Y. J., Hua, T. Y., Zhao, Y., et al. (2007). MeCP2 gene mutation analysis in autistic boys with developmental regression. *Psychiatric Genetics, 17*(2), 113–116.

Yamashita, Y., Kondo, I., Fukuda, T., Morishima, R., Kusaga, A., Iwanaga, R., et al. (2001). Mutation analysis of the methyl-CpG-binding protein 2 gene (MECP2) in Rett patients with preserved speech. *Brain and Development, 23*(Suppl 1), S157–160.

Yasui, D. H., Peddada, S., Bieda, M. C., Vallero, R. O., Hogart, A., Nagarajan, R. P., et al. (2007). Integrated epigenomic analyses of neuronal MeCP2 reveal a role for long-range interaction with active genes. *Proceedings of the National Academy of Sciences of the United States of America, 104*(49), 19,416–19,421.

Ylisaukko-Oja, T., Rehnstrom, K., Vanhala, R., Kempas, E., von Koskull, H., Tengstrom, C., et al. (2005). MECP2 mutation analysis in patients with mental retardation. *American Journal of Medical Genetics. Part A, 132*(2), 121–124.

Yntema, H. G., Kleefstra, T., Oudakker, A. R., Romein, T., De Vries, B. B., Nillesen, W., et al. (2002). Low frequency of MECP2 mutations in mentally retarded males. *European Journal of Human Genetics, 10*(8), 487–490.

Yntema, H. G., Oudakker, A. R., Kleefstra, T., Hamel, B. C., van Bokhoven, H., Chelly, J., et al. (2002). In-frame deletion in MECP2 causes mild nonspecific mental retardation. *American Journal of Medical Genetics, 107*(1), 81–83.

Young, D. J., Bebbington, A., Anderson, A., Ravine, D., Ellaway, C., Kulkarni, A., et al. (2008). The diagnosis of autism in a female: could it be Rett syndrome? *European Journal of Pediatrics, 167*(6), 661–669.

Young, J. I., Hong, E. P., Castle, J. C., Crespo-Barreto, J., Bowman, A. B., Rose, M. F., et al. (2005). Regulation of RNA splicing by the methylation-dependent transcriptional repressor methyl-CpG binding protein 2. *Proceedings of the National Academy of Sciences of the United States of America, 102*(49), 17,551–17,558.

Young, J. I., & Zoghbi, H. Y. (2004). X-chromosome inactivation patterns are unbalanced and affect the phenotypic outcome in a mouse model of rett syndrome. *American Journal of Human Genetics, 74*(3), 511–520.

Zappella, M., Gillberg, C., & Ehlers, S. (1998). The preserved speech variant: a subgroup of the Rett complex: a clinical report of 30 cases. *Journal of Autism and Developmental Disorders, 28*(6), 519–526.

Zappella, M., Meloni, I., Longo, I., Canitano, R., Hayek, G., Rosaia, L., et al. (2003). Study of MECP2 gene in Rett syndrome variants and autistic girls. *American Journal of Medical Genetics. Part B Neuropsychiatric Genetics, 119*(1), 102–107.

Zappella, M., Meloni, I., Longo, I., Hayek, G., & Renieri, A. (2001). Preserved speech variants of the Rett syndrome: molecular and clinical analysis. *American Journal of Medical Genetics, 104*(1), 14–22.

Zeev, B. B., Yaron, Y., Schanen, N. C., Wolf, H., Brandt, N., Ginot, N., et al. (2002). Rett syndrome: clinical manifestations in males with MECP2 mutations. *Journal of Child Neurology, 17*(1), 20–24.

46 Fragile X: A Molecular and Treatment Model for Autism Spectrum Disorders

Randi J. Hagerman, Vivien Narcisa, Paul J. Hagerman

Points of Interest

- FMRP is a regulator of translation for many messages important for synaptic plasticity, including the messages of genes implicated in autism.
- Lack of FMRP in individuals with FXS is associated with enhanced downstream activity of the metabotropic glutamate receptor 5 (mGluR5) system, which causes enhanced long-term depression (LTD) and weak synaptic connections.
- Use of mGluR5 antagonists rescues the synaptic deficits, the behavior problems, and the cognitive deficits of the fragile X knock-out mouse.
- Preliminary studies in humans suggest that an mGluR5 antagonist, fenobam, is helpful for behavior and prepulse inhibition with no significant side effects.
- Minocycline lowers the elevated MMP9 levels in the fragile X mouse, rescues synaptic abnormalities, and improves behavior and cognition with 1 month of treatment after birth. Studies of minocycline treatment have begun in children with FXS.

Overview

Both the premutation (55-200 CGG repeats) and the full mutation (>200 repeats) of the fragile X (*fragile X mental retardation 1*; *FMR1*) gene are associated with autism or autism spectrum disorders (ASDs), although these associations occur through different molecular mechanisms (Farzin et al., 2006; R. J. Hagerman, 2006; Hatton et al., 2006; Kaufmann et al., 2004; Rogers, Wehner, & Hagerman, 2001). The full mutation typically causes methylation of the promoter region of the *FMR1* gene, disrupting transcription, translation, and *FMR1* protein (FMRP) production. It is the lack or deficiency of FMRP that leads to fragile X syndrome (FXS). The premutation causes an elevation of the *FMR1* mRNA, leading to a gain-of-function effect and toxicity to the cells and causing both neurodevelopmental and neurodegenerative effects (Figure 46-1).

Full-mutation females and males with mosaicism (either CGG-size mosaicism or methylation mosaicism) produce a varied range of FMRP levels (Tassone et al., 1999). The range of overall intellectual abilities correlates with FMRP levels (Loesch, Huggins, & Hagerman, 2004). Individuals with a mild FMRP deficiency present with a normal or borderline IQ and also experience learning disabilities, social deficits, and emotional problems, such as anxiety; this latter group represents about 15% of males and 70% of females with FXS (de Vries et al., 1996; R. J. Hagerman, 1992). Those individuals who produce little or no FMRP fall on the other end of the FXS spectrum and experience moderate-to-severe intellectual disability. Those patients with FXS and a lower IQ are more likely to have autism (Bailey et al., 2001; Kaufmann et al., 2004; Rogers et al., 2001). A new FMRP ELISA measure has been developed that quantitates the level of FMRP and demonstrates significant variability, even in the normal populations (Iwahashi et al., 2009). The FMRP ELISA will be studied in normals, in those with autism without the *FMR1* mutation, and in those with *FMR1* mutations to see if levels correlate with social deficits.

Approximately 30% of those with FXS have autism, and another 20% to 30% have pervasive developmental disorder-not otherwise specified (PDD-NOS; Harris et al., 2008); the remaining individuals do not meet criteria for ASDs but exhibit autistic-like features, including hand-flapping, hand-biting, and poor eye contact (Hatton et al., 2006; Kaufmann et al., 2004; Rogers et al., 2001). Although the level of FMRP may initially correlate with the presence of autism (Hatton et al., 2006), this relationship disappears when controlled for IQ (Loesch et al., 2007).

Although the level of FMRP is usually normal among individuals with the premutation (also called "carriers"

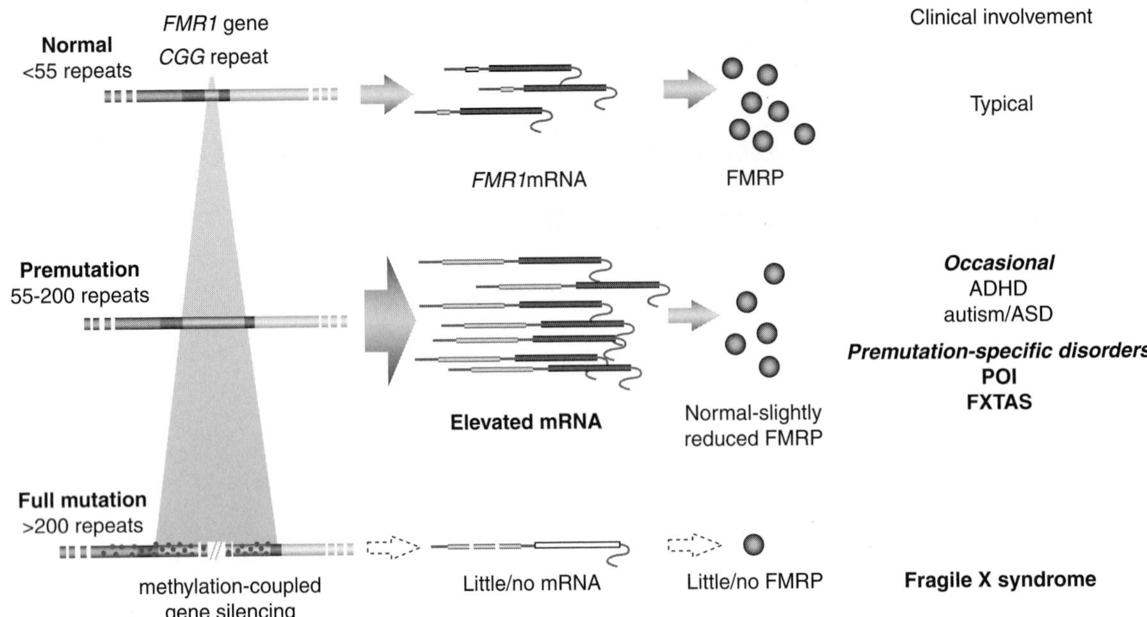

Figure 46–1. Dependence of *FMR1* expression on the length of the CGG repeat. Premutation alleles result in elevated mRNA levels (increased RNA synthesis); the increased CGG repeat in the mRNA partially blocks translation, resulting in slightly lowered protein levels in the premutation range. Full-mutation alleles are generally hypermethylated and silenced, thus producing little or no mRNA or protein. Elevated mRNA is now believed to give rise to the premutation-specific disorders, FXTAS and POI, and may also occasionally contribute to children with developmental delays, ADHD, or autism. Fragile X Syndrome is caused by the absence of the protein FMRP. (See Color Plate Section for a color version of this figure.)

because these individuals were once thought to be clinically unaffected), the level of *FMR1* mRNA is elevated from two to eight times normal levels (Tassone et al., 2000). The elevated, expanded-CGG-repeat mRNA leads to a "toxic" gain of function that results in neuronal and astrocytic dysfunction, leading in turn to early cell death and dysregulation of specific proteins (P. J. Hagerman & Hagerman, 2004b). Clinical involvement in carriers can take several forms, which are all distinct from FXS. In approximately 40% of older male carriers and 8% of older female carriers, ascertained through known fragile X families, a neurodegenerative disorder known as fragile X-associated tremor/ataxia syndrome (FXTAS) develops (Coffey et al., 2008; Jacquemont et al., 2004). FXTAS is characterized by tremor, ataxia, cognitive decline, autonomic dysfunction, neuropathy, brain atrophy, and white matter disease (Berry-Kravis et al., 2007; Leehey et al., 2007; Sullivan et al., 2005). Also, in 20% of adult females with the premutation, primary ovarian insufficiency (POI) develops.

In some children with the premutation, developmental problems occur, including autism or ASDs, and attention deficit hyperactivity disorder (ADHD; Aziz et al., 2003; Clifford et al., 2007; Farzin et al., 2006; S. W. Harris et al., 2005). These neurodevelopmental problems also appear to be related to RNA toxicity during early development, although there may be additional contributing factors of environmental and genetic origin. Nevertheless, these problems are common in carriers who present clinically; they are, however, less common in those with the premutation who are identified by cascade testing in a family tree (Farzin et al., 2006).

For those with FXS, recent advances in understanding the neurobiology of the disorder have led to the development of new targeted treatments. These treatments can reverse the brain abnormalities in the animal models of FXS, leading to rescue of the dendritic spine defects, behavioral problems, and cognitive deficits (Dolen & Bear, 2008; Nakamoto et al., 2007).

The key to understanding the relationship between FXS and autism is the fact that FMRP is an RNA transport protein that also regulates the translation of many mRNAs. Most of the proteins that FMRP regulates are involved with synaptic plasticity. FMRP normally inhibits the translation of these proteins until a glutamate signal is received at the postsynaptic terminus, resulting in stimulation of metabotropic glutamate receptors. FMRP is then briefly dephosphorylated (several minutes)—releasing the translational inhibition—followed by subsequent rephosphorylation of FMRP and reinhibition of protein synthesis (Antion et al., 2008; Narayanan et al., 2007). In the absence of FMRP, there is significant dysregulation of a number of pathways that have been associated with autism, including upregulation of the mGluR5 pathway (Bear et al., 2004; Huber et al., 2002), upregulation of the mTOR pathway, downregulation of the PTEN pathway (Klann, personal communication, 2008), downregulation of the $GABA_A$ receptors (D'Hulst et al., 2006; D'Hulst et al., 2007), and downregulation of the dopamine pathway (Wang et al., 2008). The following chapter details the clinical, molecular, and treatment aspects of the association between fragile X mutations and ASDs.

Phenotypic Features of Fragile X Syndrome

FXS occurs as a result of a deficiency or absence of FMRP. In the full mutation, this occurs when the *FMR1* gene is fully methylated, inhibiting transcription of the gene. In approximately 20% of cases of the full mutation, the gene is incompletely methylated and a small percentage of cells are able to transcribe mRNA (Tassone et al., 2000). This incomplete methylation, also known as methylation mosaicism, enables individuals to typically produce greater than 10% but less than 50% of normal FMRP levels, as measured in blood (Tassone et al., 1999a).

Another molecular variation is size mosaicism, where some cells have the premutation and other cells have full-mutation alleles. In these cases, cells with the premutation will produce FMRP. The higher the percentage of premutation cells to full-mutation cells, the higher the level of FMRP produced. Therefore, individuals with size mosaicism typically have a higher IQ and fewer physical characteristics typical of FXS (Loesch et al., 2004).

Most individuals with FXS have prominent ears, a high-arched palate, a long face, hyperextensible finger joints and flat feet (R. J. Hagerman, 2002b), but typically the physical appearance is normal (*see* Figure 46-2). These features relate to a connective tissue problem in FXS that is most obvious in young children. Although the lack of FMRP appears to disrupt the elastin fibers of connective tissue (R. J. Hagerman, 2002a), most individuals do not look dysmorphic. Other common physical features include soft, velvet-like skin and a long face, which is common in adulthood. Greater than 90% of adult males with FXS also present with macroorchidism (large testicles). In early puberty, testicle size increases dramatically. By age 15 years, testicular volume stabilizes at two to four times normal size (Butler et al., 1991). There is a greater amount of connective tissue in the large testicles, but fertility is normal.

As FXS is an X-linked disorder and sperm only house the premutation and not the full mutation, daughters of men with FXS will receive only the premutation allele from their fathers. Sons of men with FXS will be unaffected because they receive the unaffected Y-chromosome. Each child of a woman with the full mutation will have a 50% chance of inheriting the full mutation because the mother has two X-chromosomes—one with the full mutation and one normal. More commonly, mothers of children with FXS have the premutation; the premutation will expand to a full mutation when passed on by the mother at a rate that depends on the size of the premutation. For example, 70 repeats will expand to a full mutation about 40% of the time, but 90 repeats or higher will almost always expand to a full mutation when this allele is passed on through a female to the next generation (Gane & Cronister, 2002; McConkie-Rosell et al., 2007).

Often children with FXS will not be diagnosed until they are 3 years or older, when delays (especially in language) are brought to medical attention and the child is referred for a developmental evaluation (Bailey, Skinner, & Sparkman, 2003). Children with FXS also have an enhanced response to sensory stimuli, as documented by electrophysiological studies (Miller et al., 1999; Roberts et al., 2001). Their sympathetic response is upregulated, leading to enhanced anxiety, and their vagal response is deficient particularly with transitions. These altered responses occur more in those with autism and FXS compared to those without autism and FXS

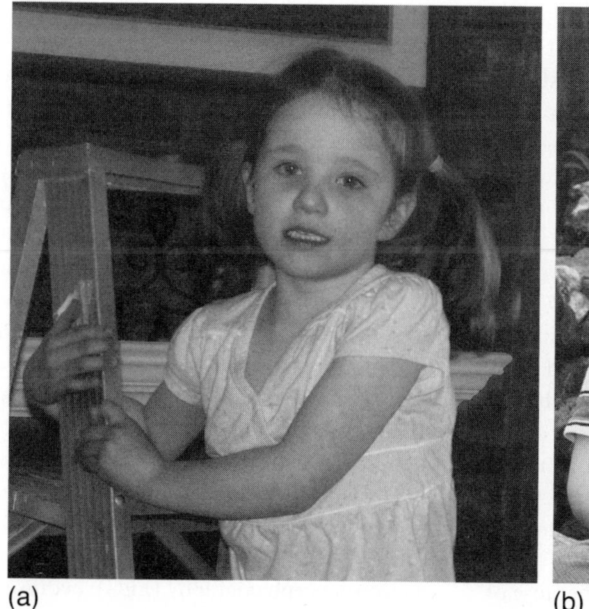
(a)

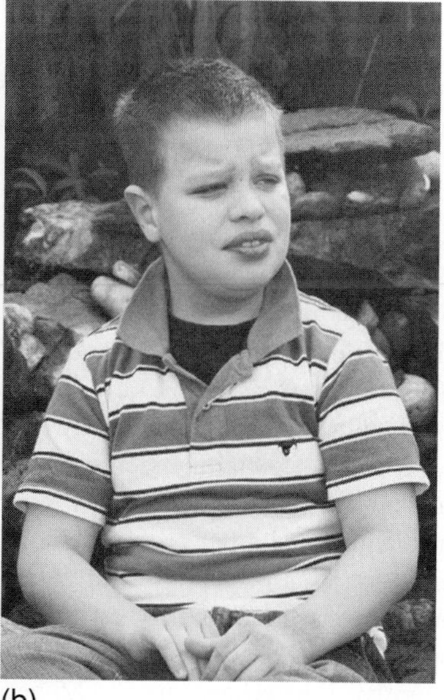
(b)

Figure 46–2. A girl (a) and a boy (b) with the full mutation and Fragile X Syndrome. Notice that the girl has no obvious physical features suggesting Fragile X Syndrome.

(Roberts et al., 2001; Roberts et al., 2006). Boys with FXS have been found to have an enhanced cortisol release after stress (Hessl et al., 2002), which may also be related to the enhanced sympathetic activity and anxiety. Hall et al. (2006) found that the enhanced cortisol release was correlated with increased eye aversion in FXS. However, in a more recent report, the increase in autistic behaviors in FXS was associated with lowered cortisol levels (Hall et al., 2008).

Although the majority of patients with FXS hand-flap, hand-bite, and have poor eye contact, the diagnosis of autism is not related to these behavioral features. The studies in the Kaufmann lab have eloquently demonstrated that autism in FXS is related to an impairment in complex social interactions and language deficits rather than an impairment in nonverbal behaviors (Budimirovic, 2006; Kau et al., 2004; Kaufmann et al., 2004). Social withdrawal is a key element in the development of autism in FXS, which is somewhat different from idiopathic autism that demonstrates more social aloofness and social indifference rather than social avoidance (Budimirovic, 2006). The social avoidance may be related to the sensory and autonomic issues described above, and it is (relating to social avoidance, rather than autonomic issues) typically manifested as anxiety. These features constitute an important subtype of autism related to FXS, and the anxiety features are likely to improve with targeted treatments described below. In addition to language deficits involving verbal reasoning, recognition of emotions and labeling of emotions are associated with ASDs in FXS (Budimirovic et al., 2006). Other studies have also documented language deficits in those with FXS and ASDs (Lewis et al., 2006; Philofsky et al., 2004). Overall, both IQ and adaptive behavior are lower in those with FXS and autism compared to those with FXS alone (Hatton et al., 2006; Kau et al., 2004; Kaufmann et al., 2004; Rogers et al., 2001).

It is difficult to assess autism in FXS because the phenotype may change at different times of the day or with different evaluators, even when standardized instruments are used. In our studies that utilize the ADOS-G, the ADI-R, and DSMIV-R criteria, we convene a conference of all of the evaluators/clinicians to review the data and reach consensus on the diagnosis (S. W. Harris et al., 2008). To address these problems, Roberts and colleagues (Roberts et al., 2007) developed a novel social approach scale (SAS) to measure the modulation of social interactions over time in patients with FXS. They coded aspects of social interaction, including eye contact, physical movement, and facial expressions over a few hours in two encounters. Although almost all patients with FXS had difficulty with all three aspects of social interaction initially, the individuals with autism and FXS did not become more sociable over time. They maintained a flat profile, demonstrating continued problems in all aspects of social interactions. Improved eye contact over time was the best predictor for lowered autistic behavior in FXS (Roberts et al., 2007).

The autism phenotype is heterogeneous in FXS because of a number of medical and genetic factors. The presence of additional medical problems affecting the CNS can increase the risk of autism in the FXS population. For example, seizures occur in about 12% of children with FXS without ASDs but increase to 28% in those with FXS and ASDs (Garcia-Nonell et al., 2008). Presence of a second genetic condition in addition to FXS, such as Down syndrome, also increases the likelihood of autism (Roberts, Chapman, & Warren, 2008).

The most remarkable secondary genetic condition involved in predisposing a child with FXS to autism is the Prader-Willi Phenotype (PWP) of FXS. Approximately 70% of those with the PWP of FXS have ASDs (Nowicki et al., 2007). In the PWP of FXS, individuals exhibit symptoms of hyperphagia, lack of satiation after meals, obesity, and hypogenitalia. Recently, expression levels of cytoplasmic *FMR1* interacting protein (CYFIP), coded within the 15q deletion region of the PWP, were lower in PWP of FXS compared to FXS without PWP and typically developing individuals (Nowicki et al., 2007). Because CYFIP interacts with the Rac GTPase, it has an additional impact on synaptic plasticity that may explain why lowered CYFIP expression predisposes an individual with FXS to autism. However, CYFIP expression has also been found to be upregulated in individuals with autism and the 15q11-13 duplications but not FXS (Nishimura et al., 2007). Studies exploring changes in the serotonin transporter (*5HTT*) and *BDNF* genes are also underway to assess whether other allelic changes in individuals with FXS that may increase the prevalence of autism.

There are a number of similarities between idiopathic autism and FXS. Individuals with either disorder have large heads with rapid brain growth in early childhood (Chiu et al., 2007; Courchesne, Carper, & Akshoomoff, 2003). Chiu et al. (2007) have demonstrated that the head size in those with FXS plus autism grows faster in early childhood than for those with FXS without autism. Approximately 18% of those patients with idiopathic autism and extreme macrocephaly have a *PTEN* mutation (Butler et al., 2005). The *PTEN* gene regulates cell growth, and studies are now underway to assess how the absence of FMRP may dysregulate *PTEN* activity. In FXS, there is also enhanced phosphorylation of the PTEN protein, leading to its lowered function and (possibly) the large brains in children with FXS, particularly those with autism and FXS (Chiu et al., 2007). Other systems that are dysregulated in FXS include the GABA pathway, which is downregulated, and the mTOR pathway, which is upregulated (Bassell & Warren, 2008; Zupan & Klann, personal communication 2009). The mTOR pathway is also upregulated in individuals with tuberous sclerosis, which is a frequent cause of autism. The overlap of neurobiological pathways between those individuals with FXS and those with other forms of autism is important to elucidate because targeted treatments may be helpful for more than one cause of autism, as described below.

As mentioned, a subgroup of individuals with FXS and idiopathic autism have seizures (Berry-Kravis, 2002; Musumeci et al., 1999). Seizure activity is important to identify early with an electroencephalography (EEG), because treatment with an anticonvulsant can dramatically improve a child's language and social responsiveness (R. J. Hagerman, 2002a). For many individuals, anticonvulsant treatment prevents the disruption of connectivity caused by abnormal spike wave discharges and subsequently enables an individual to engage in their environment and avoid emerging social deficits (Garcia-Nonell et al., 2008).

Prepulse inhibition (PPI) deficits occur in individuals with FXS and in individuals with autism (Frankland et al., 2004; Hessl et al., 2008; Perry et al., 2007). PPI is a measure of frontal gating or inhibition, and it is likely related to abnormalities in the GABA and the mGluR5 systems. In both autism and FXS, there are GABA and glutamate abnormalities that are described below (El Idrissi et al., 2005; Gruss & Braun, 2004). The PPI deficit is a consistent abnormality with test–retest reliability in FXS, and it is therefore a good quantitative measure to be used in medication studies in FXS (Berry-Kravis et al., 2009).

Interesting similarities and differences have been seen in neuroimaging studies of both FXS and autism. Both disorders have a large cerebrum, and in FXS the caudate and thalamus are large, whereas the cerebellar vermis is small (Mostofsky et al., 1998; Reiss & Dant, 2003). In a direct comparison of young children with FXS and young children with idiopathic autism compared to controls, Hazlett et al. (2009) found that the amygdala was significantly larger in those with autism compared to FXS and controls, whereas the caudate was larger in those with FXS compared to autism and controls. In girls with FXS, the smaller the size of the cerebellar vermis, the more severe the autistic behaviors (Mazzocco et al., 1997). Girls with FXS also have reduced basal forebrain and hippocampal activation, which are two areas of the brain important to memory encoding and attention (Greicius et al., 2004). Hoeft et al. (2007) used tasks to test executive functioning and found that the FXS group had reduced activation in the right ventrolateral prefrontal cortex (VLPFC) compared to both autistic and typically developing individuals. They also found increased left VLPFC activation in those with FXS, suggesting possible compensation for this right fronto-striatal deficit (Hoeft et al., 2007). Dalton et al. (2008) compared face processing and gaze fixation in FXS and autism groups and found that both groups had similar deficits in gaze fixation to human faces, with decreased activation patterns in the fusiform gyrus. The FXS group, however, had greater activation than the autism and control groups in brain regions associated with fear and emotional face processing including the left hippocampus, the right insula, the left postcentral gyrus, and the left superior temporal gyrus, suggesting a divergent neural cause for face-processing deficits between FXS and idiopathic autism groups (Dalton et al., 2008).

Involvement in Premutation Carriers

Individuals with the premutation have 55 to 200 CGG repeats. Methylation does not occur in the premutation range, so FMRP levels are usually normal or close to normal. However, the higher the repeat size, the higher the level of mRNA. In individuals with more than 150 CGG repeats, the level of FMRP can be mildly decreased, and subtle physical features of full FXS may be observed, such as prominent ears, loose connective tissue with hyperextensible finger joints, and macroorchidism (R. J. Hagerman, 2006; Tassone et al., 2000). Some behavioral features are also similar to FXS, including ADHD symptoms, poor eye contact, shyness, and social anxiety (Farzin et al., 2006).

Occasionally a patient in the premutation range will present with cognitive deficits, autism, or ASDs—characteristics more commonly found in those with a full mutation and FXS (Aziz et al., 2003; Farzin et al., 2006; Goodlin-Jones et al., 2004). Often in these cases, a significant FMRP deficit can be documented, but not always (Tassone et al., 2000). However, for the most part, premutation carriers have a normal IQ.

The most significant problem in the premutation range is the elevation of mRNA, which can lead to an RNA toxicity that does not occur in the full mutation. The excess mRNA binds to other proteins and causes dysregulation of proteins essential to normal neuronal functioning (P. J. Hagerman & Hagerman, 2004a). As premutation carriers age, inclusions form in neurons and astrocytes and are eosinophilic and intranuclear. Inclusions are a hallmark of the fragile X-associated tremor/ataxia syndrome (FXTAS) (Greco et al., 2006). As previously mentioned, this disorder occurs in approximately 40% of older adult male carriers and 8% of aging female carriers, ascertained through families with known FXS probands, and is characterized by intention tremor, gait ataxia, neuropathy, brain atrophy, and white matter disease on MRI (Coffey et al., 2008; Jacquemont et al., 2003; Jacquemont et al., 2004). The RNA toxicity also has an impact on the ovary in female carriers and approximately 16% to 20% experience POI, with menstruation ceasing before age 40 years (Sullivan et al., 2005; Wittenberger et al., 2007).

Recently, a study of 146 adult female carriers was conducted, and the cohort was divided into those with FXTAS and those without FXTAS. Approximately 50% of those with FXTAS had thyroid disease—particularly hypothyroidism—and 42% had fibromyalgia, both significantly different from age-matched controls (Coffey et al., 2008). Muscle pain was also common in those who did not have a medical diagnosis of fibromyalgia and even in those without FXTAS. Zhang et al. (2005) have reported three cases of multiple sclerosis (MS) in 106 cases of premutation females, which is a higher rate than the general population. A woman who had a severe case of MS over a 15-year period was diagnosed with the premutation 1 week before she died. At autopsy, she had the inclusions of FXTAS in addition to MS lesions with neuroinflammation (Greco et al., 2008). These studies suggest an association between the premutation and autoimmune disease that requires further investigation. This association may be related to the proteins that become dysregulated in the premutation neuron, including upregulation of the heat-shock proteins hnRNP A2, myelin basic protein, lamin A/C and alpha-B-crystallin (which may be an important antigen for MS) (Greco et al., 2008). It is also possible that the elevation of mRNA may stimulate toll receptors that may, in turn, stimulate autoimmunity (Greco et al., 2008).

The increased prevalence of autism and ASDs in boys with the premutation who present clinically (73%), compared to their premutation brothers identified through cascade testing (8%) and normal brothers without the premutation (0%), suggests that the premutation can predispose an individual to autism (Farzin et al., 2006). Emerging evidence suggests that the RNA toxicity mechanism may also affect early development. Cultures of neurons with the premutation have reductions in branching and larger synaptic size compared to normal neurons (Chen et al., 2009). This mechanism is distinct from the decreased FMRP mechanism found in FXS. Placement of the premutation in cultured neural cells alters cellular morphology, including formation of intranuclear inclusions, and leads to reduced cell viability (Arocena et al., 2005). Because neuronal death occurs more readily in FXTAS cases, neural cells are likely to be more vulnerable to environmental toxicity, which can further exacerbate cell loss. An example of this vulnerability to environmental toxins was seen in a carrier woman who developed tremor and ataxia while undergoing chemotherapy for cancer (O'Dwyer et al., 2005). This effect, however, disappeared once the patient ended her chemotherapy. Further study of environmental toxicity in the young premutation carrier may shed light on why there is such a high frequency of ASDs in male carriers.

Neurobiological Mechanism Leading to Targeted Treatments in FXS

Because FMRP inhibits the translation of many messages, the absence or deficiency of FMRP leads to a dramatic upregulation of proteins throughout the brain but especially in the hippocampus and amygdala (Qin et al., 2005). A number of these proteins have been identified, including MAP1B and PSD95, which are involved in the postsynaptic complex (R. J. Hagerman, Rivera, & Hagerman, 2008). FMRP also regulates additional proteins known to be involved with autism when their genes are mutated, such as SHANK, neuroligen 3 and 4, CYFIP, Arc, Sema3F, and neurorexins (J. C. Darnell, 2005; Darnell personal communication 2010; Nowicki et al., 2007). Therefore, the cascade of dysregulated proteins triggered by the lack of FMRP provides a molecular link between autism and FXS. The resulting changes in synaptic plasticity, glutamate, GABA and dopamine pathways represent the overlap between FXS and idiopathic autism or autism caused by other mutations (Belmonte & Bourgeron, 2006) (*see* Figure 46-3).

Autism is a behavioral diagnosis defined by DSMIV-TR and is known to be attributable to a number of different gene mutations, with possible environmental overlays to vulnerable genetic conditions. The goal of the clinician is to determine the genetic diagnosis responsible for the behavioral diagnosis in a child with autism. Although FXS is a specific genetic diagnosis, it is the most common known single gene cause of autism (Persico & Bourgeron, 2006; Reddy, 2005; Wassink, Piven, & Patil, 2001). Because of this connection, the fragile X DNA test should be carried out in all children who are diagnosed with autism or ASDs (R. J. Hagerman et al., 2008). This testing is particularly important now that targeted treatments are becoming available to ameliorate the neurobiological abnormalities present in FXS.

The most important pathway upregulated by the absence of FMRP is the mGluR5 pathway (Huber et al., 2002). This pathway mediates the weakening of synaptic function (long-term depression; LTD) in the brain, particularly in the hippocampus. Changes affecting the mGluR5 system are considered to be the primary cause of intellectual deficiency in FXS; this relationship between FMRP, LTD, and FXS is known as the mGluR5 model of FXS (Bear, Huber, & Warren, 2004; Dolen & Bear, 2008). FMRP normally inhibits protein translation in this pathway, which controls LTD. FMRP deficits cause internalization of the AMPA receptors and has been directly demonstrated in hippocampal slices (Nakamoto et al., 2007), leading to enhanced LTD in FXS. The normalization of FMRP levels or the use of mGluR5 antagonists can reverse these changes both in vitro and in vivo (de Vrij et al., 2008; Dolen et al., 2007; Nakamoto et al., 2007). In the mouse, fly, and even zebrafish models of FXS, the use of mGluR5 antagonists or cross-breeding with an mGluR5 deficit animal can improve the behavioral and cognitive phenotype of FXS (Dolen et al., 2007; McBride et al., 2005; Nakamoto et al., 2007; Tucker, Richards, & Lardelli, 2006; Yan et al., 2005).

Initial studies of mGluR5 antagonists utilized 2-methyl-6-phenylethynyl-pyridine (MPEP) in the animal models of FXS. MPEP rescued the seizure phenotype in the fragile X knockout mouse (KO) (Yan et al., 2005), and it also normalized the mating behavior and the overall life-span of the *Drosophila* model of FXS (McBride et al., 2005). However, MPEP is genotoxic to humans so it cannot be used with individuals with FXS. Lithium has some mGluR5 antagonist effects and has also been utilized in the *Drosophila* model and in the KO mouse with effects similar to MPEP (McBride et al., 2005; Yan et al., 2005). An open trial of lithium was tried in several patients with FXS, and benefits were seen in behavior over several months. In addition, some cognitive improvements were also noted (Berry-Kravis et al., 2008). Therefore, further controlled studies should be carried out to understand if lithium benefits cognition and behavior problems, including autism in FXS. Lithium is neuroprotective in aging, so it may have beneficial effects on the neurological problems associated with aging in carriers experiencing FXTAS.

Recently, researchers (Porter et al., 2005) found that fenobam, an anti-anxiety agent that demonstrated efficacy in phase II trials in the 1980s, acts as an mGluR5 antagonist. It has therefore become a candidate for a targeted treatment for FXS. A recent study of pharmacokinetics and toxicity has been completed in 12 adults with FXS who were given a dose of 50 to 150 mg orally (Berry-Kravis et al., 2009). We found the peak blood level at 3 hours after oral dosing, and no significant side effects were seen at any dose. We also found that the deficit in PPI (a measure of frontal gating) typically seen in FXS (Frankland et al., 2004; Hessl et al., 2008) was significantly

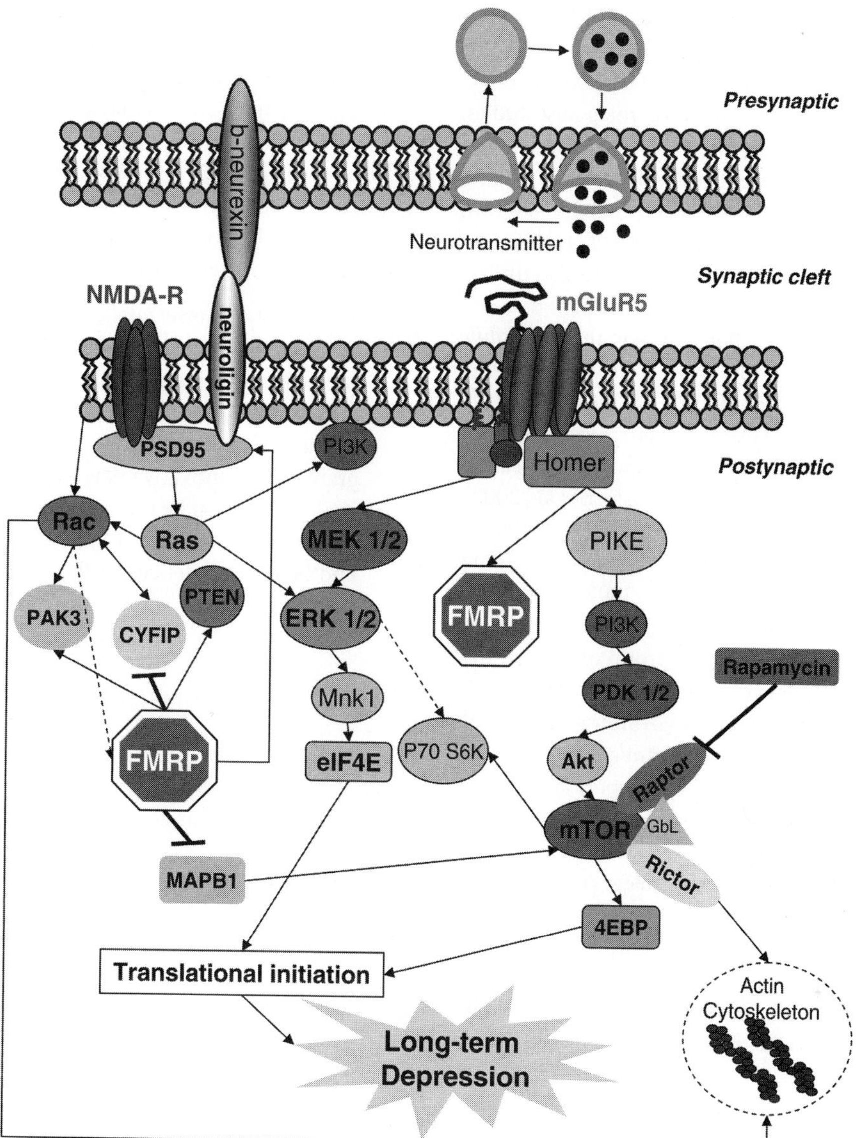

Figure 46–3. The interactions of FMRP and other proteins in neurons. Akt – protein kinase B (PKB); CYFIP – cytoplasmic interacting *FMR1* protein; elF4E – E74-like factor 4; ERK – extracellular signal-regulated kinases, synonym for mitogen-activated protein kinase (MAPK); FMRP – fragile X mental retardation protein; Homer – scaffolding protein; MAPB1 – microtubule-associated protein 1B; MEK – mitogen-activated protein kinase (MAPK); mGluR – metabotropic glutamate receptor; Mnk – MAP kinase integrating kinase; mTOR – mammalian target of rapamycin/FK506 binding protein 12-rapamycin associated protein 1 (FRAP1); NMDA-R – ionotropic *N*-methyl-D-aspartic acid receptor; P70 S6K – p70 ribsomal S6 protein kinase; PAK3 – P21 (CDKN1A)-activated kinase 3; PDK – 3-phosphoinositide-dependent protein kinase; PI3K – class I phosphoinositide 3-kinses; PIKE – PI 3-kinase enhancer; PSD95 – postsynaptic density protein; PTEN – phosphatase and tensin homolog; Rac/Ras – small guanosine triphosphatases. Figure drawn by Dr Andrea Schneider, MIND Institute, UC Davis Medical Center.

improved on fenobam (Berry-Kravis et al., 2009). After a single dose of fenobam, many individuals, demonstrated a decrease in hyperactivity and anxiety with a calming effect that lasted about 4 hours. Additional mGluR5 antagonists are currently being developed by several pharmaceutical companies, and these, too, will be studied in patients with FXS. Recently a controlled trial has been initiated with Arbaclofen, an R isomer of Baclofen. Arbaclofen acts as a GABA agonist and has been used in patients with cerebral palsy and significant spasticity. The R isomer has significant mGluR5 antagonist effects, so it is being studied in phase III trials in FXS at multiple centers. Anecdotal evidence has shown that Baclofen and Arbaclofen are also helpful in some patients with idiopathic autism (Berry-Kravis, 2008). Arbaclofen controlled trials are taking place in both children and adults with FXS and idiopathic autism.

The development of biomarkers distinct from the behavioral phenotype is in progress to tease out those individuals in the autism group who would benefit from mGluR5 antagonists. Patients with autism who have PPI deficits similar to those with FXS may be one possible subgroup (Hessl et al., 2008).

One promising biomarker may involve the rate of ERK phosphorylation, which is slowed in FXS. This rate has been shown to improve in the lithium open trial in FXS (Berry-Kravis et al., 2008), and it will be studied in other mGluR5 antagonist studies.

Fragile X KO mouse studies have also demonstrated abnormalities in the GABAergic pathways. Decreased expression of the $GABA_A$ receptor, particularly the delta subunit, has been noted by D'Hulst and colleagues (D'Hulst et al., 2006; D'Hulst & Kooy, 2007). Other subunits are also underexpressed in the KO mouse, including the alpha, beta, and gamma subunits (D'Hulst et al., 2006). Even in the *Drosophila* model of FXS, the GABA receptors show approximately 50% reduction (D'Hulst et al., 2006). FMRP has been shown to bind the delta subunit of the GABA receptor, so it is postulated that FMRP is responsible for its transport and localization, which would be disrupted in FXS (Miyashiro et al., 2003). Decreased GABAergic function has been shown to interfere with cholinergic function in electrophysiological studies in the KO mouse (D'Antuono, Merlo, & Avoli, 2003). Therefore, treatments that can target the GABAergic abnormalities in FXS may also be beneficial to a broader group of neurotransmitter abnormalities, including cholinergic function.

Another treatment possibility for the GABAergic abnormalities in FXS is the neurosteroid anticonvulsant ganaxolone. This medication is a modulator of the $GABA_A$ receptor and an agonist—particularly for the delta receptor. Ganaxolone is a synthetic analog of allopregnanolone; however, it does not have any active hormonal effects (Monaghan, McAuley, & Data, 1999). It is an anticonvulsant that has demonstrated efficacy in infantile spasms through phase II studies without significant side effects, with the exception of mild sedation, even in young children. A controlled trial in patients with FXS will hopefully take place in the future to assess efficacy in behavior and cognition.

Conclusion

FXS is the most common inherited cause of intellectual disability and autism known. There is an absence or deficiency of FMRP in FXS leading to the upregulation of many proteins and pathways important for other forms of autism. All children with ASDs should be tested for mutations in the *FMR1* gene and both premutations and full mutations can lead to ASDs. Presently, a variety of targeted treatments are being tested for efficacy in children and adults with FXS. It is likely that targeted treatments for FXS will lead the way for new treatments in idiopathic autism, including the use of mGluR5 antagonists.

Challenges and Future Directions

The field of targeted treatments is just beginning for many neurodevelopmental disorders, and it holds the promise of reversing both intellectual disability and autism. At this time, fragile X is leading the way because of the advances in the neurobiology for this disorder. At the National Fragile X Foundation International Conference in 2008, Nelson reported that an mGluR5 antagonist demonstrated reversal of the brain structural abnormalities in the adult KO mouse (Nelson et al., 2008). This leads to the hope that even in adulthood, these medications will make a significant difference for patients with FXS and perhaps for those with autism and other neurodevelopmental disorders.

- To actually reverse intellectual disability and autism in those with FXS, the targeted treatments need to be coupled with learning programs that will give the appropriate stimulation to the synapse, particularly in adults.
- The use of computer programs, brain rehabilitation programs, and innovative new learning approaches are necessary, and must be utilized simultaneously with targeted treatments to reach the goal of reversing the cognitive and behavioral deficits of those with FXS both with and without autism.

ACKNOWLEDGMENTS

This work was supported by NICHD grants HD036071, HD02274, NIDCR grant DE019583, NIA grant AG032115, NINDS grant NS062412, and 90DD0596 from the Health and Human Services Administration on Developmental Disabilities.

REFERENCES

Antion, M. D., Hou, L., Wong, H., Hoeffer, C. A., & Klann, E. (2008). mGluR-dependent long-term depression is associated with increased phosphorylation of S6 and synthesis of elongation factor 1A but remains expressed in S6K-deficient mice. *Molecular and Cell Biology, 28*, 2996–3007.

Arocena, D. G., Iwahashi, C. K., Won, N., Beilina, A., Ludwig, A. L., Tassone, F., et al. (2005). Induction of inclusion formation and disruption of lamin A/C structure by premutation CGG-repeat RNA in human cultured neural cells. *Human Molecular Genetics, 14*(23), 3661–3671.

Aziz, M., Stathopulu, E., Callias, M., Taylor, C., Turk, J., Oostra, B., et al. (2003). Clinical features of boys with fragile X premutations and intermediate alleles. *American Journal of Medical Genetics, 121B*(1), 119–127.

Bailey, D. B., Jr., Hatton, D. D., Skinner, M., & Mesibov, G. B. (2001). Autistic behavior, *FMR1* protein, and developmental trajectories in young males with fragile X syndrome. *Journal of Autism and Developmental Disorders, 31*(2), 165–174.

Bailey, D. B., Jr., Skinner, D., & Sparkman, K. L. (2003). Discovering fragile X syndrome: family experiences and perceptions. *Pediatrics, 111*(2), 407–416.

Bear, M. F., Huber, K. M., & Warren, S. T. (2004). The mGluR theory of fragile X mental retardation. *Trends in Neurosciences, 27*(7), 370–377.

Belmonte, M. K., & Bourgeron, T. (2006). Fragile X syndrome and autism at the intersection of genetic and neural networks. *Nature Neuroscience, 9*(10), 1221–1225.

Berry-Kravis, E. (2002). Epilepsy in fragile X syndrome. *Developmental Medicine and Child Neurology, 44*(11), 724–728.

Berry-Kravis, E. (2008). Chicago, IL.

Berry-Kravis, E., Hessl, D., Coffey, S., Hervey, C., Schneider, A., Yuhas, J., et al. (2009). A pilot open label, single dose trial of fenobam in adults with fragile X syndrome. *Journal of Medical Genetics, 46*(4), 266–271.

Berry-Kravis, E., Sumis, A., Hervey, C., Nelson, M., Porges, S. W., Weng, N., et al. (2008). Open-label treatment trial of lithium to target the underlying defect in fragile X syndrome. *Journal of Developmental and Behavioral Pediatrics, 29*(4), 293–302.

Budimirovic, D. B., Bukelis, I., Cox, C., Gray, R.M., Tierney, E., & Kaufmann, W.E. (2006). Autism spectrum disorder in Fragile X syndrome: Differential contribution of adaptive socialization and social withdrawal. *American Journal of Medical Genetics. Part A, 140A*(17), 1814–1826.

Butler, M. G., Allen, G. A., Haynes, J. L., Singh, D. N., Watson, M. S., & Breg, W. R. (1991). Anthropometric comparison of mentally retarded males with and without the fragile X syndrome. *American Journal of Medical Genetics, 38*(2-3), 260–268.

Butler, M. G., Dasouki, M. J., Zhou, X. P., Talebizadeh, Z., Brown, M., Takahashi, T. N., et al. (2005). Subset of individuals with autism spectrum disorders and extreme macrocephaly associated with germline PTEN tumour suppressor gene mutations. *Journal of Medical Genetics, 42*(4), 318–321.

Chen, Y., Tassone, F., Berman, R. F., Hagerman, P. J., Hagerman, R. J., Willemsen, R., et al. (2009). Murine hippocampal neurons expressing *Fmr1* gene premutations show early developmental deficits and late degeneration. *Human Molecular Genetics*, doi:10.1093/hmg/ddp479

Chiu, S., Wegelin, J. A., Blank, J., Jenkins, M., Day, J., Hessl, D., et al. (2007). Early acceleration of head circumference in children with fragile x syndrome and autism. *Journal of Developmental and Behavioral Pediatrics, 28*(1), 31–35.

Clifford, S., Dissanayake, C., Bui, Q. M., Huggins, R., Taylor, A. K., & Loesch, D. Z. (2007). Autism spectrum phenotype in males and females with fragile X full mutation and premutation. *Journal of Autism and Developmental Disorders, 37*(4), 738–747.

Coffey, S. M., Cook, K., Tartaglia, N., Tassone, F., Nguyen, D. V., Pan, R., et al. (2008). Expanded clinical phenotype of women with the *FMR1* premutation. *American Journal of Medical Genetics. Part A, 146*(8), 1009–1016.

Courchesne, E., Carper, R., & Akshoomoff, N. (2003). Evidence of brain overgrowth in the first year of life in autism. *Journal of the American Medical Association, 290*(3), 337–344.

D'Antuono, M., Merlo, D., & Avoli, M. (2003). Involvement of cholinergic and gabaergic systems in the fragile X knockout mice. *Neuroscience, 119*(1), 9–13.

D'Hulst, C., De Geest, N., Reeve, S. P., Van Dam, D., De Deyn, P. P., Hassan, B. A., et al. (2006). Decreased expression of the GABAA receptor in fragile X syndrome. *Brain Research, 1121*(1), 238–245.

D'Hulst, C., & Kooy, R. F. (2007). The GABAA receptor: a novel target for treatment of fragile X? *Trends in Neurosciences, 30*(8), 425–431.

de Vries, B. B., Wiegers, A. M., Smits, A. P., et al. (1996). Mental status of females with an *FMR1* gene full mutation. *American Journal of Human Genetics, 58*(5), 1025–1032.

de Vrij, F. M., Levenga, J., van der Linde, H. C., Koekkoek, S. K., De Zeeuw, C. I., Nelson, D. L., et al. (2008). Rescue of behavioral phenotype and neuronal protrusion morphology in *Fmr1* KO mice. *Neurobiology of Disease, 31*(1), 127–132.

Dolen, G., & Bear, M. F. (2008). Role for metabotropic glutamate receptor 5 (mGluR5) in the pathogenesis of fragile X syndrome. *Journal of Physiology, 586*(6), 1503–1508.

Dolen, G., Osterweil, E., Rao, B. S., Smith, G. B., Auerbach, B. D., Chattarji, S., et al. (2007). Correction of fragile X syndrome in mice. *Neuron, 56*(6), 955–962.

El Idrissi, A., Ding, X. H., Scalia, J., Trenkner, E., Brown, W. T., & Dobkin, C. (2005). Decreased GABA(A) receptor expression in the seizure-prone fragile X mouse. *Neuroscience Letters, 377*(3), 141–146.

Farzin, F., Perry, H., Hessl, D., Loesch, D., Cohen, J., Bacalman, S., et al. (2006). Autism spectrum disorders and attention-deficit/hyperactivity disorder in boys with the fragile X premutation. *Journal of Developmental and Behavioral Pediatrics, 27*(2 Suppl), S137–144.

Frankland, P. W., Wang, Y., Rosner, B., Shimizu, T., Balleine, B. W., Dykens, E. M., et al. (2004). Sensorimotor gating abnormalities in young males with fragile X syndrome and *FMR1*-knockout mice. *Molecular Psychiatry, 9*(4), 417–425.

Gane, L., & Cronister, A. (2002). Genetic Counseling. In R. J. Hagerman & P. J. Hagerman (Eds.), *The fragile X syndrome: Diagnosis, treatment, and research* (3rd ed.). Baltimore: Johns Hopkins University Press: 251–286.

Garcia-Nonell, C., Ratera, E. R., Harris, S., Hessl, D., Ono, M. Y., Tartaglia, N., et al. (2008). Secondary medical diagnosis in fragile X syndrome with and without autism spectrum disorder. *American Journal of Medical Genetics. Part A, 146A*(15), 1911–1916.

Goodlin-Jones, B., Tassone, F., Gane, L. W., & Hagerman, R. J. (2004). Autistic spectrum disorder and the fragile X premutation. *Journal of Developmental and Behavioral Pediatrics, 25*(6), 392–398.

Greco, C. M., Berman, R. F., Martin, R. M., Tassone, F., Schwartz, P. H., Chang, A., et al. (2006). Neuropathology of fragile X-associated tremor/ataxia syndrome (FXTAS). *Brain, 129*(Pt 1), 243–255.

Greco, C. M., Tassone, F., Garcia-Arocena, D., Tartaglia, N., Coffey, S. M., Vartanian, T. K., et al. (2008). Clinical and neuropathologic findings in a woman with the *FMR1* premutation and multiple sclerosis. *Archives of Neurology, 65*(8), 1114–1116.

Gruss, M., & Braun, K. (2004). Age- and region-specific imbalances of basal amino acids and monoamine metabolism in limbic regions of female *Fmr1* knock-out mice. *Neurochemistry International, 45*(1), 81–88.

Hagerman, P. J., & Hagerman, R. J. (2004a). The fragile-X premutation: a maturing perspective. *American Journal of Human Genetics, 74*(5), 805–816.

Hagerman, P. J., & Hagerman, R. J. (2004b). Fragile X-associated Tremor/Ataxia Syndrome (FXTAS). *Mental Retardation and Developmental Disabilities Research Reviews, 10*(1), 25–30.

Hagerman, R. J. (1992). Clinical conundrums in fragile X syndrome [news]. *Nature Genetics, 1*(3), 157–158.

Hagerman, R. J. (2002a). Medical follow-up and pharmacotherapy. In R. J. Hagerman & P. J. Hagerman (Eds.), *Fragile X syndrome: Diagnosis, treatment and research* (3rd ed., pp. 287–338). Baltimore: The Johns Hopkins University Press.

Hagerman, R. J. (2002b). Physical and behavioral phenotype. In R. J. Hagerman & P. J. Hagerman (Eds.), *Fragile X syndrome: Diagnosis, treatment and research* (3rd ed., pp. 3–109). Baltimore: The Johns Hopkins University Press.

Hagerman, R. J. (2006). Lessons from fragile X regarding neurobiology, autism, and neurodegeneration. *Journal of Developmental and Behavioral Pediatrics, 27*(1), 63–74.

Hagerman, R. J., Rivera, S. M., & Hagerman, P. J. (2008). The fragile X family of disorders: A model for autism and targeted treatments. *Current Pediatrics in Review, 4*, 40–52.

Harris, S. W., Goodlin-Jones, B., Nowicki, S. T., Bacalman, S., Hessl, D., Tassone, F., et al. (2005). *Autism profiles in males with fragile X syndrome.* Paper presented at the Presented at SRCD biennial meeting, Atlanta, GA, April 7-10.

Harris, S. W., Goodlin-Jones, B., et al. (2008). Autism profiles of young males with fragile X syndrome. *American Journal of Mental Retardation, 113*, 427–438.

Hatton, D. D., Sideris, J., Skinner, M., Mankowski, J., Bailey, D. B., Jr., Roberts, J. E., et al. (2006). Autistic behavior in children with fragile X syndrome: Prevalence, stability, and the impact of FMRP. *American Journal of Medical Genetics. Part A, 140*(17), 1804–1813.

Hazlett, H. C., Poe, M. D., Lightbody, A. A., Gerig, G., MacFall, J. R., Ross, A. K., et al. (2009). Teasing apart the heterogeneity of autism: Same behavior, different brains in toddlers with fragile X syndrome and autism. *Journal of Neurodevelopmental Disorders, 1*, 81–90.

Hessl, D., Berry-Kravis, E., Cordeiro, L., Yuhas, J., Ornitz, E. M., Campbell, A., et al. (2008). Prepulse inhibition in fragile X syndrome: Feasibility, reliability, and implications for treatment. *American Journal of Medical Genetics. Part B, Neuropsychiatric Genetics, 150B*, 545–553.

Hessl, D., Glaser, B., Dyer-Friedman, J., Blasey, C., Hastie, T., Gunnar, M., et al. (2002). Cortisol and behavior in fragile X syndrome. *Psychoneuroendocrinology, 27*(7), 855–872.

Huber, K. M., Gallagher, S. M., Warren, S. T., & Bear, M. F. (2002). Altered synaptic plasticity in a mouse model of fragile X mental retardation. *Proceedings of the National Academy of Sciences of the United States of America, 99*(11), 7746–7750.

Iwahashi, C., Tassone, F., Hagerman, R. J., Yasui, D., Parrott, G., Nguyen, D., et al. (2009). A quantitative ELISA assay for the fragile x mental retardation 1 protein. *Journal of Molecular Diagnostics, 11*(4), 281–289.

J. C. Darnell, Mostovetsky, O., Darnell, R. B. (2005). FMRP RNA targets: identification and validation. *Genes, Brain, and Behavior, 4*, 341–349.

Jacquemont, S., Hagerman, R. J., Leehey, M., Grigsby, J., Zhang, L., Brunberg, J. A., et al. (2003). Fragile X premutation tremor/ataxia syndrome: molecular, clinical, and neuroimaging correlates. *American Journal of Human Genetics, 72*(4), 869–878.

Jacquemont, S., Hagerman, R. J., Leehey, M. A., Hall, D. A., Levine, R. A., Brunberg, J. A., et al. (2004). Penetrance of the fragile X-associated tremor/ataxia syndrome in a premutation carrier population. *Journal of the American Medical Association, 291*(4), 460–469.

Kau, A. S. M., Tierney, E., Bukelis, I., Stump, M. H., Kates, W. R., Trescher, W. H., et al. (2004). Social behavior profile in young males with fragile X syndrome: Characteristics and specificity. *American Journal of Medical Genetics, 126A*, 9–17.

Kaufmann, W. E., Cortell, R., Kau, A. S., Bukelis, I., Tierney, E., Gray, R. M., et al. (2004). Autism spectrum disorder in fragile X syndrome: communication, social interaction, and specific behaviors. *American Journal of Medical Genetics, 129A*(3), 225–234.

Lewis, P., Abbeduto, L., Murphy, M., Richmond, E., Giles, N., Bruno, L., et al. (2006). Cognitive, language and social-cognitive skills of individuals with fragile X syndrome with and without autism. *Journal of Intellectual Disability Research, 50*(Pt 7), 532–545.

Loesch, D. Z., Bui, Q. M., Dissanayake, C., Clifford, S., Gould, E., Bulhak-Paterson, D., et al. (2007). Molecular and cognitive predictors of the continuum of autistic behaviours in fragile X. *Neuroscience and Biobehavioral Reviews, 31*, 315–326.

Loesch, D. Z., Huggins, R. M., & Hagerman, R. J. (2004). Phenotypic variation and FMRP levels in fragile X. *Mental Retardation and Developmental Disabilities Research Reviews, 10*(1), 31–41.

Mazzocco, M. M., Kates, W. R., Baumgardner, T. L., Freund, L. S., & Reiss, A. L. (1997). Autistic behaviors among girls with fragile X syndrome. *Journal of Autism and Developmental Disorders, 27*(4), 415–435.

McBride, S. M., Choi, C. H., Wang, Y., Liebelt, D., Braunstein, E., Ferreiro, D., et al. (2005). Pharmacological rescue of synaptic plasticity, courtship behavior, and mushroom body defects in a Drosophila model of fragile X syndrome. *Neuron, 45*(5), 753–764.

McConkie-Rosell, A., Abrams, L., Finucane, B., Cronister, A., Gane, L. W., Coffey, S. M., et al. (2007). Recommendations from multi-disciplinary focus groups on cascade testing and genetic counseling for fragile X-associated disorders. *Journal of Genetic Counseling, 16*(5), 593–606.

Miller, L. J., McIntosh, D. N., McGrath, J., Shyu, V., Lampe, M., Taylor, A. K., et al. (1999). Electrodermal responses to sensory stimuli in individuals with fragile X syndrome: a preliminary report. *American Journal of Medical Genetics, 83*(4), 268–279.

Miyashiro, K. Y., Beckel-Mitchener, A., Purk, T. P., Becker, K. G., Barret, T., Liu, L., et al. (2003). RNA cargoes associating with FMRP reveal deficits in cellular functioning in *Fmr1* null mice. *Neuron, 37*(3), 417–431.

Monaghan, E. P., McAuley, J. W., & Data, J. L. (1999). Ganaxolone: a novel positive allosteric modulator of the GABA(A) receptor complex for the treatment of epilepsy. *Expert Opinion on Investigational Drugs, 8*(10), 1663–1671.

Mostofsky, S. H., Mazzocco, M. M., Aakalu, G., Warsofsky, I. S., Denckla, M. B., & Reiss, A. L. (1998). Decreased cerebellar posterior vermis size in fragile X syndrome: correlation with neurocognitive performance. *Neurology, 50*(1), 121–130.

Musumeci, S. A., Hagerman, R. J., Ferri, R., Bosco, P., Dalla Bernardina, B., Tassinari, C. A., et al. (1999). Epilepsy and EEG findings in males with fragile X syndrome. *Epilepsia, 40*(8), 1092–1099.

Nakamoto, M., Nalavadi, V., Epstein, M. P., Narayanan, U., Bassell, G. J., & Warren, S. T. (2007). Fragile X mental retardation protein deficiency leads to excessive mGluR5-dependent internalization of AMPA receptors. *Proceedings of the National Academy of Sciences of the United States of America, 104*(39), 15,537–15,542.

Narayanan, U., Nalavadi, V., Nakamoto, M., Pallas, D. C., Ceman, S., Bassell, G. J., et al. (2007). FMRP phosphorylation reveals an immediate-early signaling pathway triggered by group I mGluR and mediated by PP2A. *Journal of Neuroscience, 27*, 14,349–14,357.

Nishimura, Y., Martin, C. L., Vazquez-Lopez, A., Spence, S. J., Alvarez-Retuerto, A. I., Sigman, M., et al. (2007). Genome-wide expression profiling of lymphoblastoid cell lines distinguishes different forms of autism and reveals shared pathways. *Human Molecular Genetics, 16*(14), 1682–1698.

Nowicki, S. T., Tassone, F., Ono, M. Y., Ferranti, J., Croquette, M. F., Goodlin-Jones, B., et al. (2007). The Prader-Willi phenotype of fragile X syndrome. *Journal of Developmental and Behavioral Pediatrics, 28*(2), 133–138.

Perry, W., Minassian, A., Lopez, B., Maron, L., & Lincoln, A. (2007). Sensorimotor gating deficits in adults with autism. *Biological Psychiatry, 61*(4), 482–486.

Persico, A. M., & Bourgeron, T. (2006). Searching for ways out of the autism maze: genetic, epigenetic and environmental clues. *Trends in Neurosciences, 29*(7), 349–358.

Philofsky, A., Hepburn, S. L., Hayes, A., Hagerman, R. J., & Rogers, S. J. (2004). Linguistic and cognitive functioning and autism symptoms in young children with fragile X syndrome. *American Journal of Mental Retardation, 109*(3), 208–218.

Porter, R. H., Jaeschke, G., Spooren, W., Ballard, T. M., Buttelmann, B., Kolczewski, S., et al. (2005). Fenobam: A clinically validated nonbenzodiazepine anxiolytic is a potent, selective, and non-competitive mGlu5 receptor antagonist with inverse agonist activity. *Journal of Pharmacology and Experimental Therapeutics, 315*(2), 711–721.

Qin, M., Kang, J., Burlin, T. V., Jiang, C., & Smith, C. B. (2005). Postadolescent changes in regional cerebral protein synthesis: an in vivo study in the *FMR1* null mouse. *Journal of Neuroscience, 25*(20), 5087–5095.

Reddy, K. S. (2005). Cytogenetic abnormalities and fragile-X syndrome in Autism Spectrum Disorder. *BMC Medical Genetics, 6*(1), 3.

Reiss, A. L., & Dant, C. C. (2003). The behavioral neurogenetics of fragile X syndrome: analyzing gene-brain-behavior relationships in child developmental psychopathologies. *Development and Psychopathology, 15*(4), 927–968.

Roberts, J. E., Boccia, M. L., Bailey, D. B., Hatton, D., & Skinner, M. (2001). Cardiovascular indices of physiological arousal in boys with fragile X syndrome. *Developmental Psychobiology, 39*(2), 107–123.

Roberts, J. E., Boccia, M. L., Hatton, D. D., Skinner, M. L., & Sideris, J. (2006). Temperament and vagal tone in boys with fragile X syndrome. *Journal of Developmental and Behavioral Pediatrics, 27*(3), 193–201.

Roberts, J. E., Chapman, R. S., & Warren, S. F. (2008). *Speech and language development and intervention in Down syndrome and fragile X syndrome.* Baltimore, MD: Paul H. Brookes Publishing Co.

Roberts, J. E., Price, J., Barnes, E., Nelson, L., Burchinal, M., Hennon, E. A., et al. (2007). Receptive vocabulary, expressive vocabulary, and speech production of boys with fragile X syndrome in comparison to boys with down syndrome. *American Journal of Mental Retardation, 112*(3), 177–193.

Rogers, S. J., Wehner, E. A., & Hagerman, R. J. (2001). The behavioral phenotype in fragile X: Symptoms of autism in very young children with fragile X syndrome, idiopathic autism, and other developmental disorders. *Journal of Developmental and Behavioral Pediatrics, 22*(6), 409–417.

Sullivan, A. K., Marcus, M., Epstein, M. P., Allen, E. G., Anido, A. E., Paquin, J. J., et al. (2005). Association of *FMR1* repeat size with ovarian dysfunction. *Human Reproduction, 20*(2), 402–412.

Tassone, F., Hagerman, R. J., Iklé, D. N., Dyer, P. N., Lampe, M., Willemsen, R., et al. (1999). FMRP expression as a potential prognostic indicator in fragile X syndrome. *American Journal of Medical Genetics, 84*(3), 250–261.

Tassone, F., Hagerman, R. J., Taylor, A. K., Gane, L. W., Godfrey, T. E., & Hagerman, P. J. (2000). Elevated levels of *FMR1* mRNA in carrier males: a new mechanism of involvement in the fragile-X syndrome. *American Journal of Human Genetics, 66*(1), 6–15.

Tassone, F., Hagerman, R. J., Taylor, A. K., Mills, J. B., Harris, S. W., Gane, L. W., et al. (2000). Clinical involvement and protein expression in individuals with the *FMR1* premutation. *American Journal of Medical Genetics, 91*(2), 144–152.

Tucker, B., Richards, R. I., & Lardelli, M. (2006). Contribution of mGluR and *Fmr1* functional pathways to neurite morphogenesis, craniofacial development and fragile X syndrome. *Human Molecular Genetics, 15*(23), 3446–3458.

Wassink, T. H., Piven, J., & Patil, S. R. (2001). Chromosomal abnormalities in a clinic sample of individuals with autistic disorder. *Psychiatric Genetics, 11*(2), 57–63.

Wittenberger, M. D., Hagerman, R. J., Sherman, S. L., McConkie-Rosell, A., Welt, C. K., Rebar, R. W., et al. (2007). The *FMR1* premutation and reproduction. *Fertility and Sterility, 87*(3), 456–465.

Yan, Q. J., Rammal, M., Tranfaglia, M., & Bauchwitz, R. P. (2005). Suppression of two major fragile X syndrome mouse model phenotypes by the mGluR5 antagonist MPEP. *Neuropharmacology, 49*(7), 1053–1066.

Zhang, L., Coffey, S., Apperson, M., Agius, M., Nowicki, S. T., Tartaglia, N., et al. (2005). *Symptoms or diagnosis of MS in premutation females: A variant of Fragile X-Associated Tremor Ataxia Syndrome (FXTAS)?* Paper presented at the American Academy of Neurology 2005 Annual Meeting, Miami, FL.

Commentary

Daniel H. Geschwind

Autism Genetics and Genomics: A Brief Overview and Synthesis

Autism genetics has been one of the most exciting and dynamic fields in psychiatric genetics over the last decade. The field has moved from having virtually no significant leads about the genetic etiology of autism to knowing the molecular genetic basis of ASD in between 10 and 20% of cases (Abrahams & Geschwind, 2008; Kaymakçalan & State, Chapter 41; Lamb, Chapter 38; Morrow & Walsh, Chapter 44, this volume). Despite these advances and all of the surrounding hype and excitement, however, there are many unanswered questions and looming controversies. Therefore, it is very reasonable to take a philosophical perspective, asking circa 2010, "Where has autism genetics led us?" After all, the major reason for finding genes is to understand the biology and pathophysiology of the disorder, so as to lead to better diagnosis and treatment. For more in-depth coverage of specific topics in autism genetics, I refer the reader to the far more comprehensive chapters on whole genome linkage and association (Lamb, chapter 38), medical genetics and intellectual disability (Dykens & Lense, chapter 15; Miles, chapter 40), quantitative endophenotypes (Cantor, chapter 39), the role of rare variation (Kaymakçalan & State, chapter 41), the study of common variation in genetic isolates (Rehnström & Peltonen, chapter 43), homozygosity mapping in genetic isolates (Morrow & Walsh, chapter 44), epigenetics (Person et al., chapter 42), and the overlap of autism with model syndromes such as Fragile X and Rett syndrome (Hagerman et al., chapter 46; Neul, chapter 45).

One of the major themes of autism genetic research has been the acceleration of progress in finding genes over the last decade, and certainly the last five years, primarily due to technology. In fact, one could take the position that technological advances have had as much or more influence than careful consideration of phenotype or overriding genetic theories, and therefore technology and marketing has guided much work in autism genetics.

In the 1980s, the development and refinement of the autism diagnosis using modern tools such as the Autism Diagnostic Interview Revised (ADI-R) and the Autism Diagnostic Observation Schedule (ADOS) permitted international and cross-institutional collaborations to employ a common diagnostic rubric. This was essential for growing the samples to sizes necessary for international genetic studies. However, since that time, with a few exceptions, relatively little has been done to delineate phenotype-genotype relationships, especially when seen in the context of many of the large-scale genetic studies that have been done. This is not meant as a criticism, but an observation based on the fact that molecular technology has expanded and has done much to permit the prevalent culture of "genotyping large numbers and seeing what we find" that now predominates. In fact, in support of the "genotype first" approach, one can reasonably argue that it is cheaper to genotype now and phenotype later, after one identifies a set of contributory or causal mutations that can be used to define cases with genetically homogeneous etiologies (so-called inverse-mapping).

So, if we relate the major progress in autism genetics to the prevailing technologies (Figure C6-1, adapted from Abrahams & Geschwind, 2010), we can see that, early in the field, karyotyping and light-microscope resolution cytogenetic analysis predominated, identifying mostly rare cytogenetic rearrangements that were visible by eye, and an occasional molecularly defined cytogenetic lesion (Cook et al., 1997). At the same time, whole-genome linkage studies (Table C6-1; see Lamb, Chapter 38) were being developed and planned. The advent of linkage was permitted by the development of what, at the time, were relatively high-resolution linkage maps of the human genome and commercial platforms on which such markers could be typed. Subsequent to this, in the late 1990s, it became feasible to perform candidate gene association studies, testing single nucleotide polymorphisms (SNPs; Table C6-1), one gene at a time. Candidate gene studies, even those under linkage peaks, quickly fell out of favor, as it became possible to do whole-genome studies. Once dense SNP maps of the human genome were established, based on the HapMap (Table C6-1) project and microarray based assays became widely available

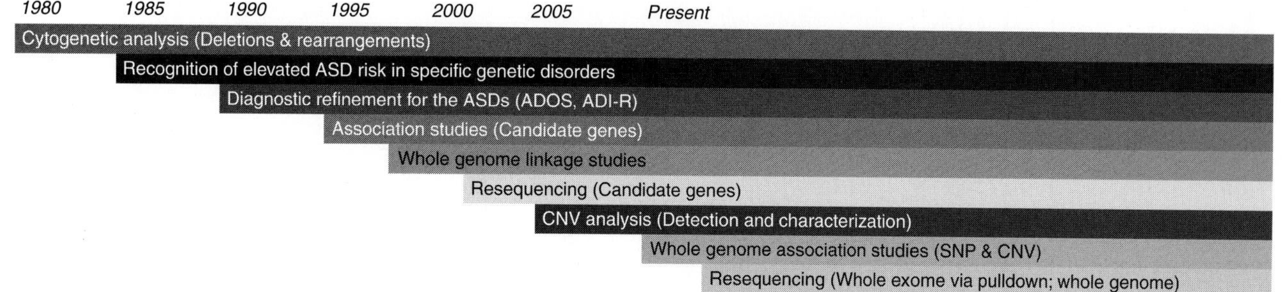

Figure C6–1. Methodological changes have accelerated progress in ASD genetics. Collection of large cohorts via international collaboration together with array-based technologies enabling genomewide interrogation of variation has resulted in major advances. Similar progress will come from massively parallel sequencing of partial and whole genomes. Although such experiments are soon likely to become routine, interpretation of results, particularly in the context of diverse phenotype data, will require massive computational infrastructure. Adaptation of Figure 23.4.1 from Abrahams, B. S., & Geschwind, D. H. (2010). Autism genetics. In M. Speicher, S. E. Antonarakis, and A. G. Motulsky (Eds.), *Vogel and Motulsky's human genetics* (chapter 23, pp. 699–714). Berlin, Springer, with authors' permissions.

from commercial entities, efficient whole genome association and analysis of copy number variation (CNV) became possible. Now, NextGen (Table C6-1) sequencing is becoming available in major academic centers, so that whole-exome (Table C6-1) or whole genome sequencing of individual patients and controls is being planned. All of these advances and changes in approach, although potentially related to underlying differences in hypotheses or the theoretical underpinnings of the genetics of complex traits, have nevertheless been mostly driven by widespread platform availability and hence feasibility of such genomewide studies. There is no arguing that each new method is more powerful than what has come before. But, as the field has been carried in this tide of technology, we may have failed to adequately address many critical issues of disease phenotypes and disease boundaries that now currently face us.

Prominent Genetic Models

Common Variation (Polymorphisms) Versus Rare Variation (Mutations)

Common genetic polymorphisms, are defined as those with a population frequency of at least, a relatively arbitrary threshold that depends on who is drawing the bar. Such variants are presumed to act incrementally to increase risk for disease, as they have been propagated over generations and have not been selected against by evolution (hence their relatively high population frequency). Therefore, common genetic polymorphisms are thought to be factors that act in combination with other genetic, environmental, or epigenetic influences to increase one's risk for a disease (Lamb, chapter 38; Rehnström & Peltonen, chapter 43, Cantor, chapter 39). Rare variants, or mutations, in contrast, undergo purifying selection (Table C6-1) and are typically considered causal, or having a major effect (Kaymakçalan & State, chapter 41; Lamb, chapter 38; Morrow & Walsh, chapter 44). Most whole genomewide association approaches have relied on the concept that common variation modulates risk in common diseases such as autism (Lamb, chapter 38; Rehnström & Peltonen, chapter 43). Even in population isolates, where inbreeding could be conceived as enriching for recessive mutations (Morrow & Walsh, chapter 44), the use of northern European population isolates has been championed as an efficient way to reduce genetic heterogeneity and increase power to find common ASD-related variation (Rehnström & Peltonen, 2010). Thus, "common disease is caused by common variation" has been the prevailing model until recently.

However, over the last two years, identification of rare variants has become the new mantra in neuropsychiatric genetics (Kaymakçalan & State, chapter 41; Morrow & Walsh, chapter 44). This change is driven by several factors. These include: (1) the small effect size observed in whole genome association studies, which are only well powered to detect common variation (Lamb, chapter 38; Wang et al., 2009; Weiss et al., 2009); (2) that association signals from common variation do not appear to account for major linkage signals, or overlap with major linkage peaks (Stone et al., 2007; Strom et al., 2009; Wang et al., 2009; Weiss et al., 2009; As linkage can detect signals from both rare and common variation, the lack of association signals large enough to explain the overlying linkage peaks implies that rare variants therefore underlie linkage peaks); and (3) the emerging recognition of the role of rare, de novo, and recurrent structural chromosomal variation (Kaymakçalan & State, chapter 41; Sebat et al., 2007). Although rare single base pair mutations (Jamain et al., 2003; Laumonnier et al., 2004) and large chromosomal structural variation were identified, the latter in conjunction with intellectual disability (Jacquemont et al., 2006; Vorstman et al., 2006), the broader role of rare variants in autism was really fueled by the initial finding that de novo copy number variants (CNV) contributed up to 10% of autism cases without severe intellectual disability (Marshall et al., 2008; Sebat et al., 2007). Based on these data and modeling of family data, it was suggested that rare, Mendelian mutations with lower penetrance

Table C6–1.
Biological functions implicated in ASD.

	Genes	References
Cell adhesion molecules	*CNTN4, CNTNAP2, MDGA2 (CNTN4 related), MADCAM1, CDH9, CDH10, ITGB3*	(Fernandez, Morgan, et al., 2004; Wang, Zhang, et al., 2009) (Strauss, Puffenberger, et al., 2006; Alarcon, Abrahams, et al., 2008; Arking, Cutler, et al., 2008; Poot, Beyer, et al., 2009) (Bucan, Abrahams, et al., 2009) (Wang, Zhang, et al., 2009) (Weiss, Kosova, et al., 2006; Coutinho, Sousa, et al., 2007)
Vesicle release/ neurotransmission	*CACNA1C* (Timothy Syndrome), CACNA1H, CACNA1G, BZRAP1, GABRB3, CADPS2, *SCN2A, SLC6A4*	(Splawski, Timothy, et al., 2004) (Splawski, Yoo, et al., 2006) (Strom, Stone, et al., 2009) (Cook, Courchesne, et al., 1998; Buxbaum, Silverman, et al., 2002; Samaco, Hogart, et al., 2005; Kim, Kim, et al., 2006) (Bucan, Abrahams, et al., 2009) (Sadakata, Washida, et al., 2007) (Weiss, Escayg, et al., 2003)
Synaptic development and function	*NLGN3, NLGN4X, NRXN1, SHANK3, GRIK2* *Many of those above could probably fit here.*	(Jamain, Quach, et al., 2003; Gauthier, Bonnel, et al., 2004; Laumonnier, Bonnet-Brilhault, et al., 2004; Lawson-Yuen, Saldivar, et al., 2008) (Bucan, Abrahams, et al., 2009; Wang, Zhang, et al., 2009) (Wilson, Wong, et al., 2003; Durand, Betancur, et al., 2007; Moessner, Marshall, et al., 2007) (Kim, Kim, et al., 2007; Motazacker, Rost, et al., 2007)
Hormonal control of social behavior	*AVPR1A, DHCR7, OXT*	(Wu, Jia, et al., 2005; Jacob, Brune, et al., 2007; Lerer, Levi, et al., 2007) (Kim, Young, et al., 2002; Wassink, Piven, et al., 2004; Yirmiya, Rosenberg, et al., 2006; Meyer-Lindenberg, Kolachana, et al., 2008) (Tierney, Nwokoro, et al., 2001)
Activity dependent translation:	*FMR1, CYFIP1, JAKMIP1, NHE9*	(Morrow, Yoo, et al., 2008) (Nishimura et al., 2007) (Hatton, Sideris, et al., 2006)
Ubiquitin and related	*UBE3A, FBOX, PARK2*	(Cook, Lindgren, et al., 1997) (Wang, Zhang, et al., 2009)
RNA splicing and processing	*FOX1/A2BP1, MECP2*	(Martin, Duvall, et al., 2007) (Amir, Van den Veyver, et al., 1999; Watson, Black, et al., 2001; Samaco, Nagarajan, et al., 2004; Milani, Pantaleoni, et al., 2005; Samaco, Hogart, et al., 2005; Van Esch, Bauters, et al., 2005; del Gaudio, Fang, et al., 2006; Nagarajan, Hogart, et al., 2006)

Neurodevelopmental patterning, migration	*EN2*	(Gharani, Benayed, et al., 2004; Benayed, Gharani, et al., 2005; Brune, Korvatska, et al., 2007; Wang, Jia, et al., 2007; Benayed, Choi, et al., 2009)
	DISC1	(Kilpinen, Ylisaukko-Oja, et al., 2007)
	RELN	(Skaar, Shao, et al., 2005; Li, Li, et al., 2007)
	CNTN4	(Fernandez, Morgan, et al., 2004; Christian, Brune, et al., 2008; Glessner, Wang, et al., 2009; Roohi, Montagna, et al., 2009)
	(Entries from many/most categories probably fit here; is there some way to make less broad)	
Multiple functions including dendritic arborizations, signaling, or cytokinesis/cell cycle.	*MET*	(Campbell, D'Oronzio, et al., 2007; Campbell, Buie, et al., 2009; Sousa, Clark, et al., 2009)
	PTEN	(Butler, Dasouki, et al., 2005; Orrico, Galli, et al., 2009; Page, Kuti, et al., 2009; Varga, Pastore, et al., 2009)
	TSC1	(Baker, Piven, et al., 1998)
	TSC2	(Dixon-Salazar, Silhavy, et al., 2004; Ferland, Eyaid, et al., 2004; Valente, Brancati, et al., 2006; Alvarez Retuerto, Cantor, et al., 2008)
	AHI	
Other/Undefined	*DOCK4*	(Maestrini, Pagnamenta, et al., 2009)
	PRKCB	(Philippi, Roschmann, et al., 2005; Lintas, Sacco, et al., 2008)

Here we summarize the putative functions of some of the current ASD candidate genes. Assignment of genes to functional categories is relatively arbitrary and is just meant to emphasize the heterogeneity of molecular and biological functions implicated. It must be acknowledged that many of the genes have multiple functions and their categorization, based on current knowledge, is incomplete. Abreviations are as follows: *AHI1* Jouberin; ASD autism spectrum disorder; *ASMT* acetylserotonin *O*-methyltransferase; *AVPR1A* vasopressin V1a receptor; *BZRAP1* benzodiazapine receptor (peripheral), associated protein 1; *CACNA1C* calcium channel, voltage-dependent, L type, alpha 1Csubunit; *CACNA1G* calcium channel, voltage-dependent, T type, alpha 1G subunit; *CACNA1H* calcium channel, voltage-dependent, Ttype, alpha 1H subunit; *CDH9* cadherin 9; *CDH10* cadherin 10; *CADPS2* calcium-dependent secretion activator, 2; *CNTN4* contactin4; *CNTNAP2* contactin-associated protein-like 2 precursor; *DHCR7* 7-dehydrocholesterol reductase; *DISC1* disrupted in schizophrenia1; *DOCK4* dedicator of cytokinesis 4; *EN2* homeobox protein engrailed-2; *FMR1* fragile X mental retardation 1 protein; *GABRB3*gamma aminobutyric acid receptor subunit beta-3 precursor; *GRIK2* glutamate receptor, ionotropic kainate 2 precursor; *ITGB3* integrinbeta-3 precursor; *MDGA2* MAM domain containing glycosylphosphatidylinositol anchor 2; *MECP2* methyl-CpG-binding protein 2; *MET* met proto-oncogene; *MR* mental retardation; *NLGN3* Neuroligin 3; *NLGN4X* Neuroligin-4, X-linked precursor; *NRXN1*Neurexin-1; *OXTR* oxytocin receptor, PDDs pervasive developmental disorders; *PRKCB* protein kinase C, beta, *PTEN* phosphataseand tensin homolog, *RELN* Reelin precursor, *SCN2A* sodium channel, voltage-gated, type II, alpha subunit; *SEMA5A* sema domain, seven thrombospondin repeats (type 1 and type 1-like), transmembrane domain (TM) and short cytoplasmic domain, (semaphorin) 5A; *SHANK3* SH3 and multiple ankyrin repeat domains protein 3; *SLC6A4* sodium-dependent serotonin transporter; *SLC25A12* calciumbindingmitochondrial carrier protein Aralar1; *TSC1* hamartin; *TSC2* tuberin; *UBE3A* ubiquitin-protein ligase E3A.a. Table and data adapted with permission from Abrahams, B. S., & Geschwind, D. H. (2008). Advances in autism genetics: On the threshold of a new neurobiology. *Nature Reviews. Genetics, 9,* 341–355.

in females would potentially be the cause in a majority of ASD cases (Zhao et al., 2007).

Certainly, a rare, major gene model is consistent with other developmental disorders, such as X-linked intellectual disability (ID), where rare or even private Mendelian-acting mutations in nearly 100 genes have been identified (Chiurazzi et al., 2008; Gecz et al., 2009) and there is little support for the role of common variation in this condition. One prediction from this model would be that as the resolution of CNV detection methods increases, a larger proportion of ASD would be found attributable to these specific mutations, especially in simplex autism cases. Here, the data are still being analyzed but the data so far has not shown an increase in the number of causal variants in parallel with increases in resolution. Additionally, CNV are just one form of rare mutation. Single base pair mutations, although thought to be less frequent than CNV, could formally account for the majority of ASD. Further, it is plausible that rare variants even underlie some or many of the association signals to common variants (Dickson et al., 2010). So, until whole exome resequencing is completed on a large number of cases, the Mendelian or de novo rare variant model will not be fully tested and the extent of the contribution of rare variants to ASD will remain hotly debated.

Another set of observations to be considered when weighing the relevance of Mendelian models of ASD is the presence of less severe aspects of the core features of autism observed in many families with ASD probands, the so-called broader phenotype of autism. Aspects of social cognition, developmental language impairment, and rigid personality characteristics are all observed at higher frequency in first-degree relatives of ASD probands than in the general population (Bailey et al., 1998; Bolton et al., 1994; Bolton et al., 1998; Constantino et al., 2004; Constantino & Todd, 2000; Fombonne et al., 1997; Le Couteur et al., 1996; Pickles et al., 2000; Piven & Palmer, 1999; Piven et al., 1997; Tager-Flusberg, 2004; Tager-Flusberg & Joseph, 2003). This would suggest that common alleles of smaller effects are segregating in families and modulate individual aspects of ASD observed in unaffected first-degree relatives (see discussion on endophenotypes below). Furthermore, twin studies of the core domains underlying ASD demonstrate that they are separable, distinct domains that quantitatively relate to the normal distribution of these traits in the population (Happe & Ronald, 2008; Ronald et al., 2006a). This apparent tension between de novo or major Mendelian mutation models can be simply resolved if one accepts that there are different classes of families, those in which the ASD presents in a de novo or Mendelian fashion, those predominantly segregating common variation and those with a mixture of the above, sprinkled with intermediate effect-size alleles. The existence of different classes of families is supported both by family studies (Losh et al., 2008; Virkud et al., 2009), and genetic modeling (Zhao et al., 2007), which is consistent with the growing appreciation for the extraordinary heterogeneity in ASDs' etiologies and the likely presence of a range of genetic and gene-environment models (Abrahams & Geschwind, 2010).

Are de novo or Rare Inherited CNV "Causal?": A Merging of Models

Even in our current state of relative ignorance, a potentially informative picture is emerging with regard to CNVs and their inheritance patterns. First, it must be acknowledged that many of the known causes of ASD, such as cases of rare genetic syndromes or certain forms of large recurrent CNV have variable expressivity (Table C6-1) and markedly reduced penetrance (Table C6-1) with regard to the phenotype of autism. The majority of these mutations cause a variety of syndromes, ranging from global developmental delay, syndromic epilepsy, intellectual disability, and autism to schizophrenia (Abrahams & Geschwind, 2008, 2010). The usual Mendelian model that underlies typical rare variant models must be modified to include the notion of intermediate alleles with intermediate effect sizes. So, the genetic models now have to be modified to include a wide range of risk alleles from rare mutations with large to intermediate effect sizes, as well as common variants, albeit common variants with very small effect sizes, typically under 1.3 (see Lamb, chapter, for overview). Thus, one can envision a continuous distribution of familial risk, ranging from alleles of small and intermediate effect size to major mutations.

A very salient example of data supporting this notion is the recent work by Bucan et al. (2009), who performed a genomewide analysis of copy number variation to identify those involving exons. The rationale behind this is that, analogous to the case for single base pair changes, CNV involving changes in protein sequence are most likely to be functional. Strong support for this contention comes from the observations that CNVs involving exons have been shown to be deleterious based on evidence of strong negative selection, which is most evident for deletions, but also holds for duplications, as both are under significantly more negative selection than intronic CNVs. Therefore, on aggregate, CNVs involving exons (eDels) are the most likely CNV to be pathogenic. Using a very stringent approach requiring any eDels to be identified in three independent cases from different families and none in more than 2500 controls, approximately a dozen new potential autism loci were identified (Bucan et al., 2009). In contrast to several earlier studies, these investigators were able to obtain statistical support for individual CNVs. Several of these, including BZRAP1, a benzodiazepine receptor associated protein, as well as MADCAM1, which shows high homology to CNTN4, are thought to regulate synaptic transmission, and were replicated in independent samples. Similarly, CNV involving UBE3A and NRXN1, both relatively established autism risk loci, were also identified.

However, even these known loci showed complex transmission patterns consistent with reduced penetrance and multifactorial inheritance. In NRXN1, for example, there was incomplete segregation with disease and a control carrier frequency of nearly 50%. This again suggests that even at these presumed major functional loci, these mutations cannot be considered causal and they are not acting in a purely Mendelian fashion. For CNVs in NRXN1, it is not just the case of variable expressivity, but very reduced penetrance, as a significant fraction of neurotypical individuals carry the deletions. This is similar to the case of 15q13 deletions, which were originally associated with autism (Pagnamenta et al., 2009). Subsequent investigations found these CNV in unaffected subjects, as well as those with a wide range of neurodevelopmental phenotypes from epilepsy to developmental delay, ID, and autism (Ben-Shachar et al., 2009; Shinawi et al., 2009; van Bon et al., 2009).

Mendelian mutations leading to neurodevelopmental disorders that encompass autism, most of which are rare, now include over a dozen disorders (Abrahams & Geschwind, 2008). In some of these, such as Beckwith-Wiedemann syndrome or Fragile X, the percentage of children having the syndrome and autism is under 25%. In others, such as the cortical dysplasia-focal epilepsy syndrome due to recessive mutations in CNTNAP2, or 3p deletion duplications involving CNTN4, maternally inherited duplication at 15q, and 16p deletions, the proportion of children having autism may be greater than 50%. Some argue that this is no different than other known Mendelian causes of ID, or neurological disorders, such as the inherited frontotemporal dementias (FTD). In FTD, dominantly inherited mutations in one gene lead to a very wide range of neurodegenerative diseases, including motor neuron disease and Parkinson's disease, not infrequently, within the same family (Chow et al., 1999; Rademakers et al., 2007). However, this still begs the question as to whether the large variability in phenotype, which includes being essentially unaffected with respect to autism, is modulated by stochastic factors in the environment, or modifier genes of smaller effect size (e.g., see Figure C6-2).

Does this complexity limit the power of studying these rare disorders to gain a foothold in understanding autism pathophysiology? On the contrary, since these rare alleles have a major effect, they provide a great opportunity for connecting genotype to phenotype. Here one has the advantage of starting with a relatively genetically homogeneous population, which opens up the possibility of performing inverse mapping—that is, rather than the usual genetics paradigm of defining a phenotype and then searching for genotype, one starts with the genotype and carefully studies the phenotype. This may be especially powerful in circumstances where a significant proportion with a given recurrent mutation do not have autism. These individuals can be used as a comparison group with those that are autistic, to identify any neurobiologically

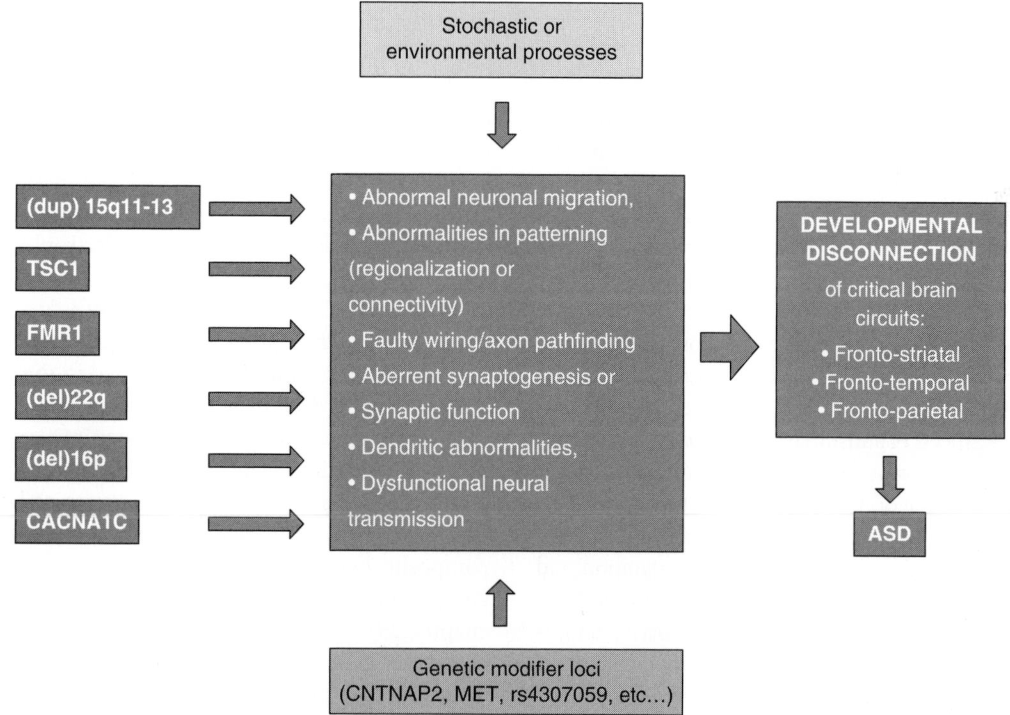

Figure C6–2. Convergence of genes on neural systems. Here we illustrate a working model for how major affect autism risk alleles, such as those shown at the left, might act to lead to autism. Since these Mendelian conditions are not specific for ASD (perhaps with the exception of (dup)15q11-13 syndrome), and typically lead to ID, either environmental or genetic factors must modify their affects on brain development. The biological pathways through which such genes are known to act (shown in the middle box) are myriad. We hypothesize that, while certainly these or other molecular and biological pathways provide potential source of convergence, the ultimate convergence must lie in neural systems. At a neural systems level, the convergent process will likely be disconnection of the circuits outlined in the far right box, since these systems are thought to underlie the core deficits of ASD.

relevant phenotypes that distinguish those with autism from those without the diagnosis. So, studying the cognitive, neuroimaging, or gene expression profile phenotypes in rare "single gene" disorders provides one potentially powerful means for trying to understand the range of phenotypes associated with a particular mutation and how a particular genetic abnormality leads to specific nervous system dysfunction at the cell, synapse, and circuit level.

The key issue for the clinician, neurobiologist, practitioner, and therapist is, how do these rare variants contribute to phenotype? How are they modified? Is there any specificity, and do particular variants or affected pathways lead to specific forms of autism for which a specific treatment or trajectory can be predicted? This is hard work, and will require identification of variants in very large sample sizes and concerted comprehensive efforts to phenotype clinical samples. Such an effort has already begun (Christa Leese-Martin and David Ledbetter, personal communication) and will be critical in such mobilization of clinical populations, either in the United States or in countries with more centralized or public health care, as it provides an efficient means for understanding the roles of these variants in autism pathophysiology.

How Might Common Variation Influence the Development of ASDs?: The Endophenotype Model

The absence of strong association signals for common variants in studies of ASD genetics has been taken as evidence for rare, causal mutations, as discussed above. However, an alternative (and potentially complementary) model considers that the broad phenotype of autism, while highly heritable, is not itself related as strongly to specific genetic risk factors as its component cognitive or behavioral domains. Given the presence of the broader phenotype of ASD in first-degree relatives of those with an ASD, and the evidence from twins, it seems very reasonable to test whether common genetic risk factors are related to more elemental, heritable aspects of autism, such as language, social cognition, or any other relevant biomedical measurements, rather than the broad syndrome of ASD itself. Such a model considers autism as the outcome of a set of risk alleles that modulate the normal continuum of quantitative variation of cognition and behavior in humans (Cantor, chapter 39; Constantino, 2010; Happe et al., 2006; Ronald et al., 2006b). This approach attempts to increase power by focusing on more elemental, presumably less heterogeneous, quantitative phenotypes.

From this perspective, autism-related traits should be measured, and are presumed to be present even in those who are unaffected within families, but to a lesser extent. This notion is supported by numerous family studies that have observed subthreshold social and language related traits in both siblings and parents (i.e., first-degree relatives) of autistic probands as referenced above. Furthermore, the neural circuitry underlying these distinct neuropsychological domains, while sharing some common elements, are also distinct, especially at a cortical level. Since genes act during development to orchestrate the development of these brain structures and circuits, genetic variation would therefore be expected to have domain-specific effects, in addition to effects shared across domains. For example, development of specific frontal lobe structures might be under the influence of specific sets of genes, in which variation would affect the specific cognitive and behavioral domains served by the particular frontal lobe circuits. In contrast, ubiquitously expressed synaptic genes would be expected to have more widespread effects on intellectual functioning; mutations in such genes would be more likely to cause general intellectual disability (ID).

In support of this model, we found that common variation in the gene CNTNAP2, whose expression is enriched in human frontal-striatal circuits during development, was found to modulate variation in language delay in families with two or more probands with ASD (Alarcon et al., 2008). Subsequently, the same region of CNTNAP2 was related to quantitative endophenotypes, such as nonword repetition, in subjects with specific language impairment (Alarcon et al., 2008; Vernes et al., 2008; see also Cantor, Chapter 39, and Lamb, Chapter 38, this volume).

The identification of common variation that contributes to phenotypic variation across two distinct neurodevelopmental disorders involving language provides one clear example that supports the quantitative endophenotype model of ASD (Cantor, chapter 39). However, the major stumbling block in applying such a quantitative trait locus (QTL) approach is defining the appropriate intermediate traits or endophenotypes to be used in such analyses. Very few family studies have been done using modern phenotyping methods, as well as assessment of phenotypes appropriate for modern cognitive neuroscience such as neuroimaging, electrophysiology, as well as more advanced, more localizing cognitive tasks (Bilder, 2008; Bilder et al., 2009). There are many issues and challenges facing studies attempting to apply quantitative measures to identify autism risk loci, as highlighted in the chapter in this volume by Rita Cantor (Cantor, chapter 39). However, the inherent power in QTL methodology mitigates against the potential difficulties identifying and measuring relevant heritable phenotypes. For example, measures of language delay, quantitative measures of social cognition, as well as a simple composite heritable measure of nonverbal communication (NVC) derived from the ADI-R, appear promising (Cantor, chapter 39). These endophenotypes, such as NVC or ADI-measured language delay, are not the most sophisticated measures that modern cognitive neuroscience has to offer; however, they are heritable traits and clearly related to the diagnosis of ASD, and so represent a reasonable starting point for such studies. It will be critical to develop sophisticated approaches grounded in a contemporary conception of brain-behavior relationships to the identification of appropriate autism-related traits or endophenotypes and to apply these in large-scale studies. This is one of the very important frontiers in neurobehavioral genetics (Bilder, 2008; Freimer & Sabatti,

2003; Sabb et al., 2009), as it will take us closer to defining more specific neurobiological entities that underlie ASD pathophysiology.

A Synthesis/Where Are We Now?

Does the Genetics Point to Specific Molecular Pathways and What Might That Mean for Treatment?

Now that whole genome association, whole genome linkage studies, and whole genome copy number analyses have been performed in several thousand cases and controls, we can certainly say that individual common alleles clearly have small effect sizes and can not account for the linkage signals in most cases. At the same time, rare variants have been identified, but very few, if any, are entirely specific for autism, again consistent not only with heterogeneity, but with extreme complexity. These data implicate gene-gene and gene-environment interactions in molding the phenotype in most cases of autism, leading to a very complex picture, even in the individual. This means significant heterogeneity not only in the genes involved, but also in the mode of inheritance of ASD. In some individuals, a single major gene may interact with environmental or other common genetic factors, and in others, multiple common or rare genetic factors may interact, with or without environmental or epigenetic factors to cause an ASD (Geschwind, 2008).

What does this genetic heterogeneity mean for treatment? One promise of genetics is to identify potentially treatable etiologies. So, despite the heterogeneity, is there evidence for convergence on one or a group of final common molecular pathways that could be targets for therapeutic development? Here, if we begin to agglomerate the findings from multiple sources, it seems that many potential categories of molecular or biological function emerge, ranging from cell adhesion, vesicle release and neurotransmission, synaptic development and function, to RNA splicing and brain patterning (Table C6-1; see also Abrahams & Geschwind, 2008; Bill & Geschwind, 2009). Perhaps specific pharmacologic therapies could be tailored to ameliorate the problems caused by etiologically similar pathways, such as those highlighted above. Similarly, knowing this degree of etiological heterogeneity may allow one to design treatment studies that use knowledge of genetic etiology to understand how different forms of ASD respond to treatment.

Autism vs. ID: At What Level Is the Specificity of Autism Derived?

Since many of the genes now known or suspected to contribute to ASD were initially discovered as causes of intellectual disability, another obvious, but important question is raised: why do mutations that frequently cause ID also lead to a proportion with autism? Although almost half of patients with ASD have ID, the two are distinct disorders. Many patients with ASD not only have intact functions such as memory, but indeed may have superiority in certain cognitive arenas, including visuo-spatial skills. Furthermore, most patients with mild ID do not suffer from the same social disabilities as those with an ASD.

From a neurologic and a cognitive neuroscience perspective, the behavioral and cognitive specificity of the syndrome of autism must be due to the maldevelopment or injury to specific brain circuits that underlie the core cognitive and behavioral features of ASD (Figure C6-2; Abrahams & Geschwind, 2008; Geschwind & Levitt, 2007). This model predicts that the largest point of convergence in the ASDs will be on neural systems, rather than on a few specific molecular pathways or one anatomical feature, such as the synapse (Figure C6-2). These neural systems are certainly those involved in social cognition and language, which implicates areas of frontal, anterior temporal, and cingulate cortex, and their major connections in the posterior superior temporal and parietal lobes, as well as subcortical regions, such as the striatum (Abrahams et al., 2007; Geschwind & Levitt, 2007; Mundy, 2003). The developmental expression pattern of genes such as CNTNAP2 (Abrahams et al., 2007) and Met (Mukamel and Geschwind, unpublished) supports this model, but this hypothesis sorely needs to be explored in a more systematic manner. So, as more and more autism genes are identified, putting them within a rubric of both molecular pathways (e.g., Konopka et al., 2009; Vernes et al., 2008) and brain circuitry (e.g., Abrahams et al., 2007) will be critical to understand how they lead to autism and other related neurodevelopmental disabilities.

This effort to understand how genes influence brain development and function to cause ASD will require going beyond conventional pathway analysis to network biology, so as to understand the systems level organization of gene and protein networks (Geschwind & Konopka, 2009; Figure C6-3). A necessary foundation for understanding how such a complex phenotype emerges will require integrating genomewide protein and gene interaction data with temporal and spatial expression data that relates individual molecules and functional pathways to specific brain regions or circuits.

So too, is it necessary to carefully integrate animal model work, along with a consideration of evolutionary issues. A mouse brain is not merely a small human brain, and yet there is much we can learn from mouse genetics and behavior, as well as basic in vitro cell biology to inform our understanding of human brain development and autism. The optimal multipronged approach needs to involve genomic approaches along with high throughput assays to screen rare and common variants for functionality (Geschwind & Konopka, 2009). In turn, these data will need to be integrated within an emerging understanding of the neurobiology of human brain evolution and development, finally connecting these molecules to the development of language and social cognition, key core elements that are disrupted in autism.

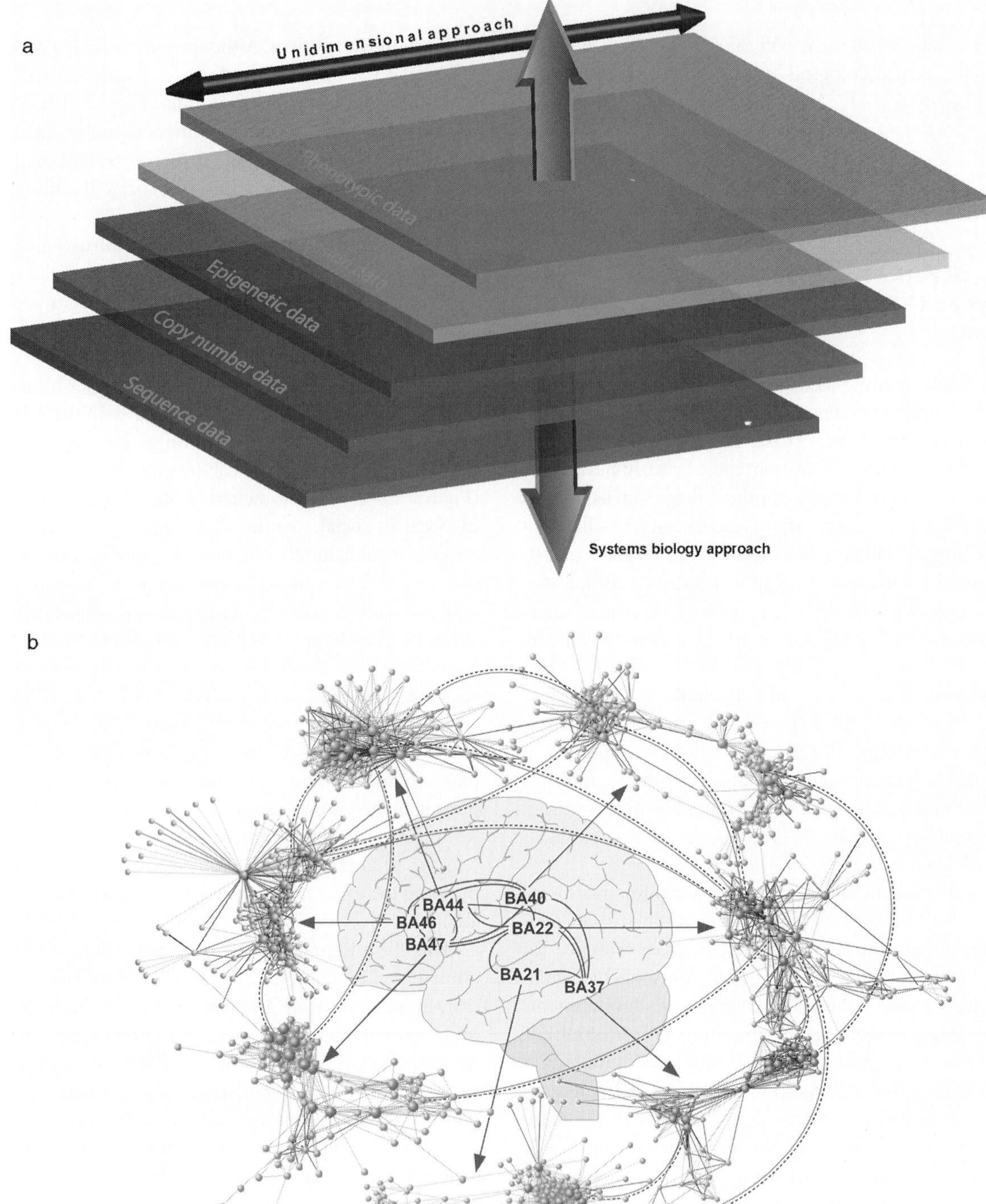

Figure C6–3. A systems biology approach for integration of genetic, genomic, and phenotype data. (a) The traditional experimental approach to the complexity of neuronal systems and diseases usually encompasses one or two layers of information. Typically, efforts are directed toward genetic (sequence variants, epigenetic modifications), genomic (gene expression), or phenotypic (electrophysiological, clinical) data. The systems biology approach strives, within reason, to consider all of these aspects concurrently, via the creation of comprehensive relational databases. The identification of a higher structure in high-dimensional datasets (for example via network methods) facilitates the connection between different types of information (e.g., genetic vs. genomic data). (b) Here, we illustrate a potential systems level integration of regional brain gene expression, coupled with network-based analysis methods and imaging data, to provide insights into brain connectivity. This is a stylized imagining of combining diffusion tensor imaging data for language areas with gene expression and WGCNA analysis to uncover integration of gene coexpression across brain areas, as well as novel brain region wiring. The lines suggest information flow in both directions, and can also be extrapolated to suggest excitatory and inhibitory interconnections. The integration of network analysis, gene expression data, and imaging analysis will elucidate the relationships among key genetic drivers in distinct regions and their relationship to brain regional connectivity in normal conditions and in disease. Adapted from Konopka, G. & Geschwind, D. H. (2009). Neuroscience in the era of functional genomics and systems biology. *Nature, 461*(7266), 908–915, with permission.

ACKNOWLEDGMENTS

The author is grateful to his colleagues in the UCLA Center for Autism Research and Treatment and AGRE for their collaborations and insights. The UCLA CART is supported by the National Institute of Mental Health P50 HD055784 and the original research described in this chapter by the author was also supported by NIMH R21 MH075028, R01 MH081754, R01 MH71425, R37 MH60233, as well as the generosity of the Guerin Foundation.

REFERENCES

Abrahams, B. S., & Geschwind, D. H. (2008). Advances in autism genetics: On the threshold of a new neurobiology. *Nature Reviews Genetics, 9*, 341–355.

Abrahams, B. S., & Geschwind, D. H. (2010). Autism genetics. In M. Speicher, S. E. Antonarakis, and A. G. Motulsky (Eds.), *Vogel and Motulsky's human genetics* (pp. 699–714). Berlin, Springer.

Abrahams, B. S., Tentler, D., Perederiy, J. V., Oldham, M. C., Coppola, G., & Geschwind, D. H. (2007). Genome-wide analyses of human perisylvian cerebral cortical patterning. *Proceedings of the National Academy of Sciences of the United States of America, 104*, 17849–17854.

Alarcon, M., Abrahams, B. S., Stone, J. L., Duvall, J. A., Perederiy, J. V., Bomar, J. M., et al. (2008). Linkage, association, and gene-expression analyses identify CNTNAP2 as an autism-susceptibility gene. *American Journal of Human Genetics, 82*, 150–159.

Alvarez Retuerto, A. I., Cantor, R. M., et al. (2008). Association of common variants in the Joubert syndrome gene (AHI1) with autism. *Human Molecular Genetics, 17*(24), 3887–3896.

Amir, R. E., Van den Veyver, I. B., et al. (1999). Rett syndrome is caused by mutations in X-linked MECP2, encoding methyl-CpG-binding protein 2. *Nature Genetics, 23*(2), 185–188.

Arking, D. E., Cutler, D. J., et al. (2008). A common genetic variant in the neurexin superfamily member CNTNAP2 increases familial risk of autism. *American Journal of Human Genetics, 82*(1), 160–164.

Bailey, A., Palferman, S., Heavey, L., & Le Couteur, A. (1998). Autism: the phenotype in relatives. *Journal of Autism and Developmental Disorders, 28*, 369–392.

Baker, P., Piven, J., et al. (1998). Autism and tuberous sclerosis complex: prevalence and clinical features. *Journal of Autism and Developmental Disorders, 28*(4), 279–285.

Benayed, R., Choi, J., et al. (2009). Autism-associated haplotype affects the regulation of the homeobox gene, ENGRAILED 2. *Biological Psychiatry, 66*, 911–917.

Benayed, R., Gharani, N., et al. (2005). Support for the homeobox transcription factor gene ENGRAILED 2 as an autism spectrum disorder susceptibility locus. *American Journal of Human Genetics, 77*(5), 851–868.

Ben-Shachar, S., Lanpher, B., German, J. R., Qasaymeh, M., Potocki, L., Nagamani, S. C., et al. (2009). Microdeletion 15q13.3: a locus with incomplete penetrance for autism, mental retardation, and psychiatric disorders. *Journal of Medical Genetics, 46*, 382–388.

Bilder, R. M. (2008). Phenomics: building scaffolds for biological hypotheses in the post-genomic era. *Biological Psychiatry, 63*, 439–440.

Bilder, R. M., Sabb, F. W., Cannon, T. D., London, E. D., Jentsch, J. D., Parker, D. S., et al. (2009). Phenomics: the systematic study of phenotypes on a genome-wide scale. *Neuroscience, 164*, 30–42.

Bill, B. R., & Geschwind, D. H. (2009). Genetic advances in autism: heterogeneity and convergence on shared pathways. *Current Opinion in Genetics and Development, 19*, 271–278.

Bolton, P., Macdonald, H., Pickles, A., Rios, P., Goode, S., Crowson, M., et al. (1994). A case-control family history study of autism. *Journal of Child Psychology and Psychiatry and Allied Disciplines, 35*, 877–900.

Bolton, P. F., Pickles, A., Murphy, M., & Rutter, M. (1998). Autism, affective and other psychiatric disorders: patterns of familial aggregation. *Psychological Medicine, 28*, 385–395.

Brune, C. W., Korvatska, E., et al. (2007). Heterogeneous association between engrailed-2 and autism in the CPEA network. *American Journal of Medical Genetics. Part B, Neuropsychiatric Genetics, 147B*, 187–193.

Bucan, M., Abrahams, B. S., Wang, K., Glessner, J. T., Herman, E. I., Sonnenblick, L. I., et al. (2009). Genome-wide analyses of exonic copy number variants in a family-based study point to novel autism susceptibility genes. *PLoS Genetics, 5*, e1000536.

Butler, M. G., Dasouki, M. J., et al. (2005). Subset of individuals with autism spectrum disorders and extreme macrocephaly associated with germline PTEN tumour suppressor gene mutations. *Journal of Medical Genetics, 42*(4), 318–321.

Buxbaum, J. D., Silverman, J. M., et al. (2002). Association between a GABRB3 polymorphism and autism. *Molecular Psychiatry, 7*(3), 311–316.

Cai, G., Edelmann, L., et al. (2008). Multiplex ligation-dependent probe amplification for genetic screening in autism spectrum disorders: Efficient identification of known microduplications and identification of a novel microduplication in ASMT. *BMC Medical Genomics, 1*, 50.

Campbell, D. B., Buie, T. M., et al. (2009). Distinct genetic risk based on association of MET in families with co-occurring autism and gastrointestinal conditions. *Pediatrics, 123*(3), 1018–1024.

Campbell, D. B., D'Oronzio, R., et al. (2007). Disruption of cerebral cortex MET signaling in autism spectrum disorder. *Annals of Neurology, 62*(3), 243–250.

Cantor, R. M. (2011). Autism endophenotypes and quantitative trait loci. In D. G. Amaral, G. Dawson, & D. H. Geschwind (Eds.), *Autism spectrum disorders.* New York, Oxford University Press.

Chiurazzi, P., Schwartz, C. E., Gecz, J., & Neri, G. (2008). XLMR genes: update 2007. *European Journal of Human Genetics: EJHG, 16*, 422–434.

Chow, T. W., Miller, B. L., Hayashi, V. N., & Geschwind, D. H. (1999). Inheritance of frontotemporal dementia. *Archives of Neurology, 56*, 817–822.

Christian, S. L., Brune, C. W., et al. (2008). Novel submicroscopic chromosomal abnormalities detected in autism spectrum disorder. *Biological Psychiatry, 63*(12), 1111–1117.

Constantino, J. N. (2011). Autism as a quantitative trait. In D. G. Amaral, G. Dawson, & D. H. Geschwind (Eds.), *Autism spectrum disorders.* New York, Oxford University Press.

Constantino, J. N., Gruber, C. P., Davis, S., Hayes, S., Passanante, N., & Przybeck, T. (2004). The factor structure of autistic traits. *Journal of Child Psychology and Psychiatry and Allied Disciplines, 45*, 719–726.

Constantino, J. N., & Todd, R. D. (2000). Genetic structure of reciprocal social behavior. *American Journal of Psychiatry, 157*, 2043–2045.

Cook, E. H., Jr., Courchesne, R. Y., et al. (1998). Linkage-disequilibrium mapping of autistic disorder, with 15q11-13 markers. *American Journal of Human Genetics, 62*(5), 1077–1083.

Cook, E. H., Jr., Lindgren, V., Leventhal, B. L., Courchesne, R., Lincoln, A., Shulman, C., et al. (1997). Autism or atypical autism in maternally but not paternally derived proximal 15q duplication. *American Journal of Human Genetics, 60*, 928–934.

Cook, E. H., Jr., & Scherer, S. W. (2008). Copy-number variations associated with neuropsychiatric conditions. *Nature, 455*, 919–923.

Coutinho, A. M., Sousa, I., et al. (2007). Evidence for epistasis between SLC6A4 and ITGB3 in autism etiology and in the determination of platelet serotonin levels. *Human Genetics, 121*(2), 243–256.

del Gaudio, D., Fang, P., et al. (2006). Increased MECP2 gene copy number as the result of genomic duplication in neurodevelopmentally delayed males. *Genetics in Medicine, 8*(12), 784–792.

Dickson, S. P., Wang, K., Krantz, I., Hakonarson, H., & Goldstein, D. B. (2010). Rare variants create synthetic genome-wide associations. *PLoS Biology, 8*, e1000294, 1000291–1000212.

Dixon-Salazar, T., Silhavy, J. L., et al. (2004). Mutations in the AHI1 gene, encoding jouberin, cause Joubert syndrome with cortical polymicrogyria. *American Journal of Human Genetics, 75*(6), 979–987.

Durand, C. M., Betancur, C., et al. (2007). Mutations in the gene encoding the synaptic scaffolding protein SHANK3 are associated with autism spectrum disorders. *Nature Genetics, 39*(1), 25–27.

Dykens, E. M., & Lense, M. (2011). Intellectual disabilities and autism spectrum disorder: A cautionary note. In D. G. Amaral, G. Dawson, & D. H. Geschwind (Eds.), *Autism spectrum disorders*. New York: Oxford University Press.

Ferland, R. J., Eyaid, W., et al. (2004). Abnormal cerebellar development and axonal decussation due to mutations in AHI1 in Joubert syndrome. *Nature Genetics, 36*(9), 1008–1013.

Fernandez, T., Morgan, T., et al. (2004). Disruption of contactin 4 (CNTN4) results in developmental delay and other features of 3p deletion syndrome. *American Journal of Human Genetics, 74*(6), 1286–1293.

Fombonne, E., Bolton, P., Prior, J., Jordan, H., & Rutter, M. (1997). A family study of autism: cognitive patterns and levels in parents and siblings. *Journal of Child Psychology and Psychiatry and Allied Disciplines, 38*, 667–683.

Freimer, N., & Sabatti, C. (2003). The human phenome project. *Nature Genetics, 34*, 15–21.

Gauthier, J., Bonnel, A., et al. (2004). NLGN3/NLGN4 gene mutations are not responsible for autism in the Quebec population. *American Journal of Medical Genetics. Part B, Neuropsychiatric Genetics, 132B*(1), 74–75.

Gecz, J., Shoubridge, C., & Corbett, M. (2009). The genetic landscape of intellectual disability arising from chromosome X. *Trends in Genetics: TIG, 25*, 308–316.

Geschwind, D. H. (2008). Autism: many genes, common pathways? *Cell, 135*, 391–395.

Geschwind, D. H., & Konopka, G. (2009). Neuroscience in the era of functional genomics and systems biology. *Nature, 461*, 908–915.

Geschwind, D. H., & Levitt, P. (2007). Autism spectrum disorders: developmental disconnection syndromes. *Current Opinion in Neurobiology, 17*, 103–111.

Gharani, N., Benayed, R., et al. (2004). Association of the homeobox transcription factor, ENGRAILED 2, 3, with autism spectrum disorder. *Molecular Psychiatry, 9*(5), 474–484.

Glessner, J. T., Wang, K., et al. (2009). Autism genome-wide copy number variation reveals ubiquitin and neuronal genes. *Nature, 459*(7246), 569–573.

Hagerman, R., Narcisa, V., & Hagerman, P. J. (2011). Fragile X: A molecular and treatment model for autism spectrum disorders. In D. G. Amaral, G. Dawson, & D. H. Geschwind (Eds.), *Autism spectrum disorders*. New York, Oxford University Press.

Happe, F., & Ronald, A. (2008). The fractionable autism triad: a review of evidence from behavioural, genetic, cognitive and neural research. *Neuropsychology Review, 18*, 287–304.

Happe, F., Ronald, A., & Plomin, R. (2006). Time to give up on a single explanation for autism. *Nature Neuroscience, 9*, 1218–1220.

Hatton, D. D., Sideris, J., et al. (2006). Autistic behavior in children with fragile X syndrome: prevalence, stability, and the impact of FMRP. *American Journal of Medical Genetics. Part A, 140*(17), 1804–1813.

Jacob, S., Brune, C. W., et al. (2007). Association of the oxytocin receptor gene (OXTR) in Caucasian children and adolescents with autism. *Neuroscience Letters, 417*(1), 6–9.

Jacquemont, M. L., Sanlaville, D., Redon, R., Raoul, O., Cormier-Daire, V., Lyonnet, S., et al. (2006). Array-based comparative genomic hybridisation identifies high frequency of cryptic chromosomal rearrangements in patients with syndromic autism spectrum disorders. *Journal of Medical Genetics, 43*, 843–849.

Jamain, S., Quach, H., Betancur, C., Rastam, M., Colineaux, C., Gillberg, I. C., et al. (2003). Mutations of the X-linked genes encoding neuroligins NLGN3 and NLGN4 are associated with autism. *Nature Genetics, 34*, 27–29.

Kaymakçalan, H., & State, M. (2011). Rare genetic variants and autism spectrum disorders. In D. G. Amaral, G. Dawson, & D. H. Geschwind (Eds.), *Autism spectrum disorders*. New York, Oxford University Press.

Kilpinen, H., Ylisaukko-Oja, T., et al. (2007). Association of DISC1 with autism and Asperger syndrome. *Molecular Psychiatry, 13*, 187–196.

Kim, S. A., Kim, J. H., et al. (2006). Association of GABRB3 polymorphisms with autism spectrum disorders in Korean trios. *Neuropsychobiology, 54*(3), 160–165.

Kim, S. A., Kim, J. H., et al. (2007). Family-based association study between GRIK2 polymorphisms and autism spectrum disorders in the Korean trios. *Neuroscience Research, 58*(3), 332–335.

Kim, S. J., Young, L. J., et al. (2002). Transmission disequilibrium testing of arginine vasopressin receptor 1A (AVPR1A) polymorphisms in autism. *Molecular Psychiatry, 7*(5), 503–507.

Konopka, G., Bomar, J. M., Winden, K., Coppola, G., Jonsson, Z. O., Gao, F., et al. (2009). Human-specific transcriptional regulation of CNS development genes by FOXP2. *Nature, 462*, 213–217.

Lamb, J. A. (2011). Whole genome linkage and association analyses. In D. G. Amaral, G. Dawson, & D. H. Geschwind (Eds.), *Autism spectrum disorders*. New York, Oxford University Press.

Laumonnier, F., Bonnet-Brilhault, F., Gomot, M., Blanc, R., David, A., Moizard, M. P., et al. (2004). X-linked mental retardation and autism are associated with a mutation in the NLGN4 gene, a member of the neuroligin family. *American Journal of Human Genetics, 74*, 552–557.

Lawson-Yuen, A., Saldivar, J. S., et al. (2008). Familial deletion within NLGN4 associated with autism and Tourette syndrome. *European Journal of Human Genetics: EJHG, 16*(5), 614–618.

Le Couteur, A., Bailey, A., Goode, S., Pickles, A., Robertson, S., Gottesman, I., et al. (1996). A broader phenotype of autism: the clinical spectrum in twins. *Journal of Child Psychology and Psychiatry, and Allied Disciplines, 37*, 785–801.

Lerer, E., Levi, S., et al. (2007). Association between the oxytocin receptor (OXTR) gene and autism: relationship to Vineland

Adaptive Behavior Scales and cognition. *Molecular Psychiatry, 13*, 980–988.

Li, H., Li, Y., et al. (2007). The association analysis of RELN and GRM8 genes with autistic spectrum disorder in Chinese Han population. *American Journal of Medical Genetics. Part B, Neuropsychiatric Genetics, 147B*, 194–200.

Lintas, C., Sacco, R., et al. (2008). Involvement of the PRKCB1 gene in autistic disorder: significant genetic association and reduced neocortical gene expression. *Molecular Psychiatry, 14*, 705–718.

Losh, M., Childress, D., Lam, K., & Piven, J. (2008). Defining key features of the broad autism phenotype: a comparison across parents of multiple- and single-incidence autism families. *American Journal of Medical Genetics. Part B, Neuropsychiatric Genetics, 147B*, 424–433.

Maestrini, E., Pagnamenta, A. T., et al. (2009). High-density SNP association study and copy number variation analysis of the AUTS1 and AUTS5 loci implicate the IMMP2L-DOCK4 gene region in autism susceptibility. *Molecular Psychiatry, 15*, 954–968.

Marshall, C. R., Noor, A., Vincent, J. B., Lionel, A. C., Feuk, L., Skaug, J., et al. (2008). Structural variation of chromosomes in autism spectrum disorder. *American Journal of Human Genetics, 82*, 477–488.

Martin, C. L., Duvall, J. A., et al. (2007). Cytogenetic and molecular characterization of A2BP1/FOX1 as a candidate gene for autism. *American Journal of Medical Genetics. Part B, Neuropsychiatric Genetics, 144*(7), 869–876.

Meyer-Lindenberg, A., Kolachana, B., et al. (2008). Genetic variants in AVPR1A linked to autism predict amygdala activation and personality traits in healthy humans. *Molecular Psychiatry, 14*, 968–975.

Milani, D., Pantaleoni, C., et al. (2005). Another patient with MECP2 mutation without classic Rett syndrome phenotype. *Pediatric Neurology, 32*(5), 355–357.

Miles, J. H. (2011). Autism subtypes from a medical genetics perspective. In D. G. Amaral, G. Dawson, & D. H. Geschwind (Eds.), *Autism spectrum disorders*. New York, Oxford University Press.

Moessner, R., Marshall, C. R., et al. (2007). Contribution of SHANK3 mutations to autism spectrum disorder. *American Journal of Human Genetics, 81*(6), 1289–1297.

Morrow, E. M., & Walsh, C. A. (2011). Isolate populations and rare variation in autism spectrum disorders. In D. G. Amaral, G. Dawson, & D. H. Geschwind (Eds.), *Autism spectrum disorders*. New York, Oxford University Press.

Morrow, E. M., Yoo, S. Y., et al. (2008). Identifying autism loci and genes by tracing recent shared ancestry. *Science (New York, N.Y.), 321*(5886), 218–223.

Motazacker, M. M., Rost, B. R., et al. (2007). A defect in the ionotropic glutamate receptor 6 gene (GRIK2) is associated with autosomal recessive mental retardation. *American Journal of Human Genetics, 81*(4), 792–798.

Mundy, P. (2003). Annotation: the neural basis of social impairments in autism: the role of the dorsal medial-frontal cortex and anterior cingulate system. *Journal of Child Psychology and Psychiatry and Allied Disciplines, 44*, 793–809.

Nagarajan, R. P., Hogart, A. R., et al. (2006). Reduced MeCP2 expression is frequent in autism frontal cortex and correlates with aberrant MECP2 promoter methylation. *Epigenetics: Official Journal of the DNA Methylation Society, 1*(4), e1–11.

Neul, J. L. (2011). Rett syndrome and MECP2-related disorders. In D. G. Amaral, G. Dawson, & D. H. Geschwind (Eds.), *Autism spectrum disorders*. New York, Oxford University Press.

Orrico, A., Galli, L., et al. (2009). Novel PTEN mutations in neurodevelopmental disorders and macrocephaly. *Clinical Genetics, 75*(2), 195–198.

Page, D. T., Kuti, O. J., et al. (2009). Haploinsufficiency for Pten and serotonin transporter cooperatively influences brain size and social behavior. *Proceedings of the National Academy of Sciences of the United States of America, 106*(6), 1989–1994.

Pagnamenta, A. T., Wing, K., Akha, E. S., Knight, S. J., Bolte, S., Schmotzer, G., et al. (2009). A 15q13.3 microdeletion segregating with autism. *European Journal of Human Genetics: EJHG, 17*, 687–692.

Person, R., Zhang, X., Kim, S., Shinawi, M., & Beaudet, A. L. (2011). Known and hypothetical roles of epigenetics in autism. In D. G. Amaral, G. Dawson, & D. H. Geschwind (Eds.), *Autism spectrum disorders*. New York, Oxford University Press.

Philippi, A., Roschmann, E., et al. (2005). Haplotypes in the gene encoding protein kinase c-beta (PRKCB1) on chromosome 16 are associated with autism. *Molecular Psychiatry, 10*(10), 950–960.

Pickles, A., Starr, E., Kazak, S., Bolton, P., Papanikolaou, K., Bailey, A., et al. (2000). Variable expression of the autism broader phenotype: findings from extended pedigrees. *Journal of Child Psychology and Psychiatry and Allied Disciplines, 41*, 491–502.

Piven, J., & Palmer, P. (1999). Psychiatric disorder and the broad autism phenotype: evidence from a family study of multiple-incidence autism families. *American Journal of Psychiatry, 156*, 557–563.

Piven, J., Palmer, P., Jacobi, D., Childress, D., & Arndt, S. (1997). Broader autism phenotype: evidence from a family history study of multiple-incidence autism families. *American Journal of Psychiatry, 154*, 185–190.

Poot, M., Beyer, V., et al. (2009). Disruption of CNTNAP2 and additional structural genome changes in a boy with speech delay and autism spectrum disorder. *Neurogenetics, 11*, 81–89.

Rademakers, R., Baker, M., Gass, J., Adamson, J., Huey, E. D., Momeni, P., et al. (2007). Phenotypic variability associated with progranulin haploinsufficiency in patients with the common 1477C—>T (Arg493X) mutation: an international initiative. *Lancet Neurology, 6*, 857–868.

Ronald, A., Happe, F., Bolton, P., Butcher, L. M., Price, T. S., Wheelwright, S., et al. (2006a). Genetic heterogeneity between the three components of the autism spectrum: a twin study. *Journal of the American Academy of Child and Adolescent Psychiatry, 45*, 691–699.

Ronald, A., Happe, F., Price, T. S., Baron-Cohen, S., & Plomin, R. (2006b). Phenotypic and genetic overlap between autistic traits at the extremes of the general population. *Journal of the American Academy of Child and Adolescent Psychiatry, 45*, 1206–1214.

Roohi, J., Montagna, C., et al. (2009). Disruption of contactin 4 in three subjects with autism spectrum disorder. *Journal of Medical Genetics, 46*(3), 176–182.

Sabb, F. W., Burggren, A. C., Higier, R. G., Fox, J., He, J., Parker, D. S., et al. (2009). Challenges in phenotype definition in the whole-genome era: multivariate models of memory and intelligence. *Neuroscience, 164*, 88–107.

Sadakata, T., Washida, M., et al. (2007). Autistic-like phenotypes in Cadps2-knockout mice and aberrant CADPS2 splicing in autistic patients. *Journal of Clinical Investigation, 117*(4), 931–943.

Samaco, R. C., Hogart, A., et al. (2005). Epigenetic overlap in autism-spectrum neurodevelopmental disorders: MECP2 deficiency causes reduced expression of UBE3A and GABRB3. *Human Molecular Genetics, 14*(4), 483–492.

Samaco, R. C., Nagarajan, R. P., et al. (2004). Multiple pathways regulate MeCP2 expression in normal brain development and exhibit defects in autism-spectrum disorders. *Human Molecular Genetics, 13*(6), 629–639.

Sebat, J., Lakshmi, B., Malhotra, D., Troge, J., Lese-Martin, C., Walsh, T., et al. (2007). Strong association of de novo copy number mutations with autism. *Science (New York, N.Y.), 316*, 445–449.

Shinawi, M., Schaaf, C. P., Bhatt, S. S., Xia, Z., Patel, A., Cheung, S. W., et al. (2009). A small recurrent deletion within 15q13.3 is associated with a range of neurodevelopmental phenotypes. *Nature Genetics, 41*, 1269–1271.

Skaar, D. A., Shao, Y., et al. (2005). Analysis of the RELN gene as a genetic risk factor for autism. *Molecular Psychiatry, 10*(6), 563–571.

Sousa, I., Clark, T. G., et al. (2009). MET and autism susceptibility: family and case-control studies. *European Journal of Human Genetics: EJHG, 17*(6), 749–58.

Splawski, I., Timothy, K. W., et al. (2004). Ca(V)1.2 calcium channel dysfunction causes a multisystem disorder including arrhythmia and autism. *Cell, 119*(1), 19–31.

Splawski, I., Yoo, D. S., et al. (2006). CACNA1H mutations in autism spectrum disorders. *Journal of Biological Chemistry, 281*(31), 22085–22091.

Stone, J. L., Merriman, B., Cantor, R. M., Geschwind, D. H., & Nelson, S. F. (2007). High density SNP association study of a major autism linkage region on chromosome 17. *Human Molecular Genetics, 16*, 704–715.

Strauss, K. A., Puffenberger, E. G., et al. (2006). Recessive symptomatic focal epilepsy and mutant contactin-associated protein-like 2. *New England Journal of Medicine, 354*(13), 1370–1377.

Strom, S. P., Stone, J. L., Ten Bosch, J. R., Merriman, B., Cantor, R. M., Geschwind, D. H., et al. (2009). High-density SNP association study of the 17q21 chromosomal region linked to autism identifies CACNA1G as a novel candidate gene. *Molecular Psychiatry, 16*, 704–715.

Tager-Flusberg, H. (2004). Strategies for conducting research on language in autism. *Journal of Autism and Developmental Disorders, 34*, 75–80.

Tager-Flusberg, H., & Joseph, R. M. (2003). Identifying neurocognitive phenotypes in autism. *Philosophical Transactions of the Royal Society of London. Series B, Biological Sciences, 358*, 303–314.

Tierney, E., Nwokoro, N. A., et al. (2001). Behavior phenotype in the RSH/Smith-Lemli-Opitz syndrome. *American Journal of Medical Genetics, 98*(2), 191–200.

Valente, E. M., Brancati, F., et al. (2006). AHI1 gene mutations cause specific forms of Joubert syndrome-related disorders. *Annals of Neurology, 59*(3), 527–534.

van Bon, B. W., Mefford, H. C., Menten, B., Koolen, D. A., Sharp, A. J., Nillesen, W. M., et al. (2009). Further delineation of the 15q13 microdeletion and duplication syndromes: a clinical spectrum varying from non-pathogenic to a severe outcome. *Journal of Medical Genetics, 46*, 511–523.

Van Esch, H., Bauters, M., et al. (2005). Duplication of the MECP2 region is a frequent cause of severe mental retardation and progressive neurological symptoms in males. *American Journal of Human Genetics, 77*(3), 442–453.

Varga, E. A., Pastore, M., et al. (2009). The prevalence of PTEN mutations in a clinical pediatric cohort with autism spectrum disorders, developmental delay, and macrocephaly. *Genetics in Medicine, 11*(2), 111–117.

Vernes, S. C., Newbury, D. F., Abrahams, B. S., Winchester, L., Nicod, J., Groszer, M., *et al.*, (2008). A functional genetic link between distinct developmental language disorders. *New England Journal of Medicine, 359*, 2337–2345.

Virkud, Y. V., Todd, R. D., Abbacchi, A. M., Zhang, Y., & Constantino, J. N. (2009). Familial aggregation of quantitative autistic traits in multiplex versus simplex autism. *American Journal of Medical Genetics. Part B, Neuropsychiatric Genetics, 150B*, 328–334.

Vorstman, J. A., Staal, W. G., van Daalen, E., van Engeland, H., Hochstenbach, P. F., & Franke, L. (2006). Identification of novel autism candidate regions through analysis of reported cytogenetic abnormalities associated with autism. *Molecular Psychiatry, 11, 1*, 18–28.

Wang, K., Zhang, H., Ma, D., Bucan, M., Glessner, J. T., Abrahams, B. S., et al. (2009). Common genetic variants on 5p14.1 associate with autism spectrum disorders. *Nature, 459*, 528–533.

Wang, L., Jia, M., et al. (2007). Association of the ENGRAILED 2 (EN2) gene with autism in Chinese Han population. *American Journal of Medical Genetics. Part B, Neuropsychiatric Genetics, 147B*, 434–438.

Wassink, T. H., Piven, J., et al. (2004). Examination of AVPR1a as an autism susceptibility gene. *Molecular Psychiatry, 9*(10), 968–972.

Watson, P., Black, G., et al. (2001). Angelman syndrome phenotype associated with mutations in MECP2, a gene encoding a methyl CpG binding protein. *Journal of Medical Genetics, 38*(4), 224–228.

Weiss, L. A., Arking, D. E., Daly, M. J., & Chakravarti, A. (2009). A genome-wide linkage and association scan reveals novel loci for autism. *Nature, 461*, 802–808.

Weiss, L. A., Escayg, A., et al. (2003). Sodium channels SCN1A, SCN2A and SCN3A in familial autism. *Molecular Psychiatry, 8*(2), 186–194.

Weiss, L. A., Kosova, G., et al. (2006). Variation in ITGB3 is associated with whole-blood serotonin level and autism susceptibility. *European Journal of Human Genetics: EJHG, 14*(8), 923–931.

Wilson, H. L., Wong, A. C., et al. (2003). Molecular characterisation of the 22q13 deletion syndrome supports the role of haploinsufficiency of SHANK3/PROSAP2 in the major neurological symptoms. *Journal of Medical Genetics, 40*(8), 575–584.

Wu, S., Jia, M., et al. (2005). Positive association of the oxytocin receptor gene (OXTR) with autism in the Chinese Han population. *Biological Psychiatry, 58*(1), 74–77.

Yirmiya, N., Rosenberg, C., et al. (2006). Association between the arginine vasopressin 1a receptor (AVPR1a) gene and autism in a family-based study: mediation by socialization skills. *Molecular Psychiatry, 11*(5), 488–494.

Zhao, X., Leotta, A., Kustanovich, V., Lajonchere, C., Geschwind, D. H., Law, K., et al. (2007). A unified genetic theory for sporadic and inherited autism. *Proceedings of the National Academy of Sciences of the United States of America, 104*, 12831–12836.

Section VII

Etiology: Environmental Factors

47 Irva Hertz-Picciotto

Environmental Risk Factors in Autism: Results from Large-Scale Epidemiologic Studies

Points of Interest

- Advanced parental age is a consistent indicator of higher risk for autism, with contributions from both the mother and father. However, it should not be construed as a cause but rather a marker of biologic processes yet to be discovered.
- A few studies have observed greater risk for children of recent immigrants into developed countries from less developed ones.
- Some infections during pregnancy appear to confer increased risk, with no particular specificity to these findings, suggesting that a maternal inflammatory response rather than the microbiologic agent may influences brain development.
- Research on obstetric and perinatal factors has been sparse and has often produced mixed results, perhaps arising from weaknesses in the analytic approaches used.
- Much attention has addressed mercury, but no rigorous studies have indicated an elevated risk either from prenatal or postnatal exposures to this metal.
- Residence close to freeways near the time of delivery is associated with higher risks, suggesting a possible role for toxic chemicals in vehicle exhaust.
- Pesticide exposures during the prenatal period have been associated with increased risk for autistic behaviors, with studies identifying several different classes of compounds.
- Other exogenous factors that plausibly could increase risk include several nutrients, endocrine-disrupting chemicals, certain air pollutants, and medically related exposures, along with geneXenvironment interactions.

The multifactorial etiology of autism is now well-accepted. This concept applies both across the population and within the individual, such that multiple events or exposures contribute to surpassing the threshold beyond which the organism can simply no longer adapt. Although inherited gene profiles confer susceptibility and may, for a small percentage of cases, be sufficient by themselves to cause autism, numerous lines of evidence support a critical role for environmental factors. The lack of complete concordance in monozygotic twins (Steffenburg et al., 1989; Bailey et al., 1995), as well as variation in severity in concordant pairs, leaves little room for doubt that nongenetic exposures contribute to the neuropathology of autism. Even where chromosomal rearrangements, mutations, and copy number variants are identified, these alterations are often de novo events and hence may be attributable to upstream environmental insults. The strong link between congenital rubella and autism, with a relative risk (RR) of 100 or higher (Chess, 1977) calculated using estimates of background prevalence of 4 per 10,000 for that time period (Fombonne, 2003), provides concrete evidence that the risk for this complex neurodevelopmental disorder can be profoundly influenced by the prenatal environment, though clearly this specific factor plays little if any role in the present period.

Mechanisms by which environmental insults may alter the course of CNS development, resulting in the final behaviorally defined syndrome of autism, are manifold. Figure 47-1 presents a schemata, in which the developing organism is subject to a variety of exposures over time, with susceptibility factors such as behavior, life events, nutrition, and so forth, moderating or exacerbating the effects. Exposures, whether chemical, physical, or microbiological, may act directly upon neural cells, interfering with critical processes of proliferation, migration, differentiation, synaptogenesis, programmed apoptosis, and myelination, or may affect the expression of genes that regulate such embryonic/fetal/infant processes (e.g., by interacting with the genome to alter methylation), resulting in activation or suppression of such genes. They operate during sensitive periods of gestation by disrupting endocrine systems and altering the hormonal milieu necessary for fetal brain development.

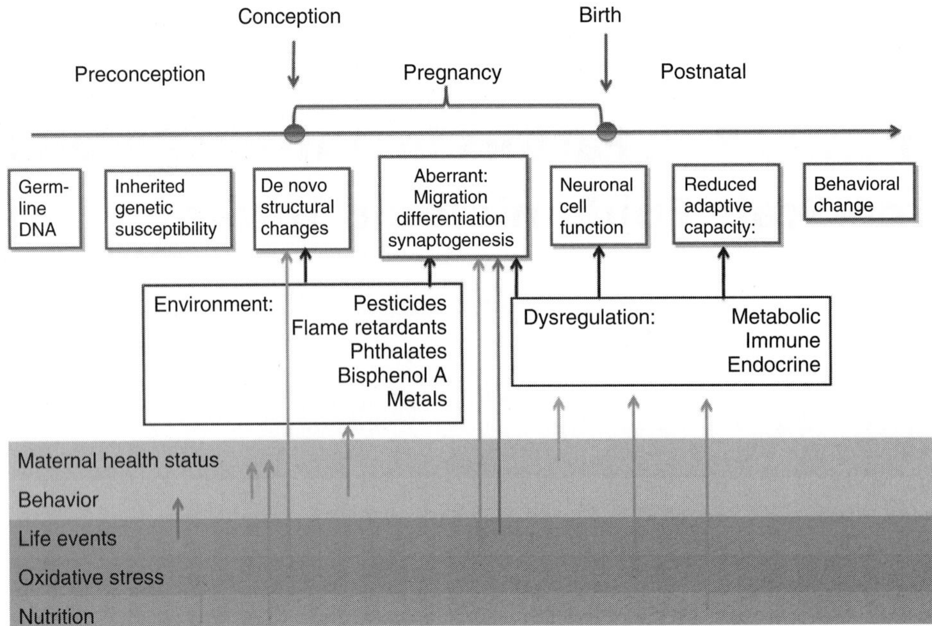

Figure 47–1. Environmental influences on development. (See Color Plate Section for a color version of this figure.)

Environmental exposures could contribute to a dysregulated immune system that interacts at the molecular level with glial cells and astrocytes, creating a neuroinflammatory condition. This list is not an exhaustive one. Moreover, none of these mechanisms need be exclusive, nor does one sensitive time period preclude another. The complexity and plasticity in brain development dictate that if multiple insults are necessary to the pathogenesis of autism, then critical events could occur before or at the time of conception, during embryogenesis, throughout gestation, at the time of parturition, and during the first year or so of life. In other words, the search for etiologic clues should not be limited to a single time window.

In comparison with the predictors of other adverse outcomes in early life such as deficits in cognitive development, perinatal mortality, or suboptimal birth characteristics (low birth weight, preterm delivery), the literature on environment and its etiologic role in autism is, on the whole, rather sparse. This chapter presents findings from large-scale epidemiologic studies that address risk and protective factors for autism. Rather than a simple summary of findings, this exposition synthesizes the literature through critical evaluation of both methods and evidence, highlighting areas in need of further investigation. Here environment is broadly defined to include exogenous factors ranging from chemicals in household products or ambient air to dietary nutrients, and from infections to injections and other medical treatments and procedures, with the exposure periods covering the periconceptional period through infancy and up until the symptoms have fully manifested. We will not concern ourselves with risk markers such as birth weight or APGAR scores. We define large-scale as a study with a minimum of 100 subjects and a minimum of 50 cases of autism.

Conducting large-scale epidemiologic studies that are entirely free of bias is virtually impossible. Nevertheless, rigorous methods applied during all three of the design, data collection, and statistical analysis phases can minimize those biases. For a summary of epidemiologic study designs and their advantages/disadvantages, see Box 47-1. A variety of textbooks can be consulted regarding data collection methodology, and similarly for statistical analysis of observational data. Ultimately, the standard by which one judges the quality of a study and hence the credibility of the findings is the degree to which the investigators have reduced the chances of confounding, selection bias, and information bias, and have conducted an analysis that is valid. In turn, validity of the statistical methods requires that they are appropriate to the design, selection process of the study participants, and data collection, and especially, to the hypothesis and aim of the investigation. A *null association*, which is the lack of a link between an exposure and an outcome, is difficult to establish and requires multiple studies (each of which is large enough and sufficiently free of bias) that together result in the weight of evidence being adequate to be deemed definitive.

Much has been written about epidemiologic study designs (Rothman, 2002; Rothman et al., 2008), but a few issues are of special concern for studies of autism: *(1)* the abundance of ecologic studies on autism, reflecting the immature state of autism epidemiology. An ecologic design and the corresponding analysis correlate rates of exposure with rates of an outcome, and are inherently the weakest approach for etiologic research (they are better suited to generating hypotheses); *(2)* the principles of control selection for etiologic epidemiology (e.g., Wacholder, McLaughlin et al., 1992; Wacholder, Silverman et al., 1992a, 1992b). The use of an

Box 47–1.
Study designs in epidemiology

Study Designs in Epidemiology	Description	Advantages	Disadvantages	Strength of Evidence
Case series	Assembly of a group of patients with similar disease or health condition profiles. Description of attributes, usually obtained cross-sectionally.	Can be conducted within a clinic, using patient population. Simple, inexpensive.	Does not provide a control group for comparison (although in some instances comparative population data may be accessible).	Very weak.
Ecologic	Division of a population, often by geographic or temporal distribution into groups. Comparison of rates of an exposure with rates of a health condition to look for correlation.	Can be conducted using pre-existing data collected for other, e.g., administrative, purposes. Inexpensive to conduct.	Lacks individual data and hence is subject to serious biases: Assumes factors not examined remain constant over time and/or across geographic regions. Control for confounders at ecologic level is usually inadequate. Ecologic fallacy can occur, whereby the subjects with exposure within a group are not those with the disease or health condition, even though exposure and disease are correlated across groups.	Weak.
Cross-sectional	Study population is selected irrespective of exposure or disease. Prevalence of exposure conditional on disease or vice versa can be calculated. Comparison of disease is made between exposed and unexposed or by level of exposure.	Data can be collected at one point or during one period of time, on both exposure and health outcome. At most, one contact with a participant is required. Individual-level data are collected on health outcomes and confounders.	Temporality of the relationship between exposure and outcome may not be discernible. Because temporality is required for causal inference, no causal inference can be made from cross-sectional studies, unless outside data on timing of exposure is available.	Moderate.
Case-control	Study population is sampled separately for cases and controls (i.e., different sampling probabilities are applied). Inclusion criteria (other than health status) must be equivalent. Associations are measured as odds ratios, representing the comparison of the odds of exposure in cases to the odds of exposure in controls. For rare health conditions, this is equivalent to the relative risk: risk of disease in the exposed vs. risk of disease in the unexposed.	Individual data are collected. Often characterized by high quality data on health outcomes. Useful for health conditions with multifactorial etiology, as many risk factors can be examined simultaneously. Similar to the cross-sectional study, data can be collected at virtually one time point or period of time, usually requiring only one contact with participant. Strengthened by collection of data on multiple potential confounding variables, especially if obtained from objective sources.	Because this is a retrospective study, obtaining high quality exposure data can be difficult. This design is subject to "reporting bias" whereby persons with a health condition may recollect their past differently than others who are not affected. Use of objective measures of exposure, such as medical records, exposure databases, or biological or environmental samples representing past exposures is recommended whenever possible.	Moderate. Can be strong if data on exposures are obtained from objective sources, or other evidence of lack of "reporting bias" can be obtained, and if outcome data are of high quality.

(*Continued*)

Box 47–1. *(Contd.)*

Study Designs in Epidemiology	Description	Advantages	Disadvantages	Strength of Evidence
Cohort	Cohort at start of the study must be free of the health condition under investigation. Cohort may be defined through a cross-sectional study (ignoring exposure distribution), or by sampling strata with and without exposure (or at different levels). Rates of incidence of the health condition are compared (using rate ratios or related derivations thereof) for those with and without exposure.	Individual data are collected. Cohort studies ensure that the exposure information is generally obtained prior to the occurrence of the outcome, permitting inference related to causality. Also, they ensure that exposure data is collected in a manner that is not influenced by the health outcome of the individual. Can be used to examine multiple health outcomes in the same study, as well as multiple exposures. Permit prospective collection of data on multiple potential confounding variables.	Depending on the length of follow-up required before sufficient numbers of cases occur, losses to follow-up can induce bias under certain conditions. Because cohort studies can assess multiple outcomes, attention to each specific outcome may be lower than in some case-control studies.	Strong. Can be moderate if quality of exposure or outcome data is weak.
Randomized clinical trial	Participants are randomly allocated to a treatment/exposure (yes/no), which is then administered, preferably in a blinded manner for the participant and the investigator. To achieve blinding, some type of placebo is necessary. Comparison of incidence of health outcome in the treated vs. placebo groups, measured by the rate ratio (or related derivation).	Provides basis for causal inference, since treatment/exposure is assigned independently of risk factors for the health outcome. If the trial is sufficiently large, random allocation can protect against major confounding.	Not an ethical design to study an exposure with potential for harm that outweighs benefits. Some participants will refuse to be in a study if they can't choose the treatment or know which group they are assigned. If treatment is complex, invasive, or causes serious side effects, compliance may be low and may give rise to confounding.	Very high, particularly if sample size is adequate to ensure that random allocation achieves even distribution of confounders across treatment groups.

inappropriate control group in a case-control study can lead to invalid results when the likelihood of an exposure in the controls differs from that of the general population that produced the cases. A single control group of children with other developmental disorders, therefore, may not be appropriate, regardless of whether the subjects are aware of their exposures. For example, pesticide exposures from proximally located agricultural fields may also be associated with other developmental deficits or conditions. Use of friend controls would similarly be inappropriate when examining any exposure that is associated with, for instance, socioeconomic status or geography because friendships tend to be formed with persons who are of similar socioeconomic level. In the extreme this would result in identical or very similar exposure distributions in controls and cases, biasing toward the null any true association with autism.

Other considerations arise during the fieldwork and analytic phases. During data collection, epidemiologists are concerned about blinding the team obtaining exposure data or conducting laboratory analyses of samples, and the degree to which recall may be influenced by an interviewer or by parents' knowledge of their child's diagnosis. Notably, biases can arise through omission and/or commission in data collection, but also in the analysis, e.g, when subjects with missing data items are excluded. Whereas the broader need for explicit conceptual models to guide analysis is recognized in many disciplines, less well-appreciated is the bias introduced by inappropriate adjustment for intermediate or marker variables. (Only under certain defined conditions will this strategy provide a valid measure of association (Petersen et al., 2006).) Understanding the conditions for generalizability is fundamental to interpreting the results and their applicability more broadly than the study source population. In assessing the adherence to sound epidemiologic principles, the abilities to transcend significance testing, to give proper relative weight to random vs. systematic error, and to distinguish the small from large biases, are paramount.

The remainder of the chapter provides a synthetic overview of the extant literature relevant to the noninherited etiologic factors in autism, highlighting promising leads that may point to causal and modifiable exposures. It is not intended, in the space available, to be comprehensive, and many relevant topics have been omitted, such as research conducted on environmental factors in relation to other neurodevelopmental impairments or psychiatric conditions. We begin with the literature on sociodemographic characteristics, focusing on how variables such as parental age, ethnicity, social class, and seasonality are a source of clues about etiology, including environmental exposures. The second section concerns medical exposures, and comprises infections and immunology, fertility treatments, obstetric factors, and vaccines. The third section in this chapter addresses traditional environmental exposures, most of which are, to some extent, involuntary: metals, pesticides, air pollutants, endocrine-disrupting chemicals, and other compounds we breathe, ingest, or absorb dermally. Finally, the limited research on lifestyle, including smoking, alcohol, nutrients, and diet, is described, along with topics holding for future work. Throughout this chapter, the methodologic hurdles, unresolved discrepancies, and types of mechanisms implied by the results are woven into the text.

Sociodemographic Factors: Clues about Environmental Exposures

The association between sociodemographic characteristics and autism appeared early in the history of autism research, with the first descriptions of Leo Kanner (1943), who wrote that the parents of the children with autism were highly educated and very successful professionals. Since then, epidemiological studies have investigated further the associations between autism and socioeconomic status, as well as race/ethnicity, place and season of birth, parental age, and child's sex. In most of these areas, the research has produced conflicting results. Salient studies on several of these sociodemographic factors are summarized in Table 47-1.

Socioeconomic Level

The association of higher socioeconomic status (SES) with autism has been widely reported but the results are not uniform. Markers of SES included maternal education in a cohort study involving over 4,000 autism cases from California (Croen et al., 2002) and family income of a large group of cases and controls in metropolitan Atlanta (Bhasin & Schendel, 2007). Children of mothers with a postgraduate education were twice as likely to have a diagnosis of autism compared to children of mothers who did not graduate from high school, after adjustment for multiple factors, and risk rose incrementally with each increase in level of education (Croen et al., 2002). In multivariate-adjusted models for the Atlanta study, however, whenever race was significant, education was not, and the association with family income was attenuated; conversely, in models where education was significant, race was not. This co-confounding suggests the study sample had limited power to disentangle the influences of race, education, and income. Durkin and colleagues reported no association of maternal education with risk of autism after adjustment for a large number of factors (Durkin et al., 2008).

Several European studies failed to show evidence of an association with socioeconomic indicators. Fombonne and du Mazaubrun reported no difference comparing social class distribution of 134 cases in four French regions with data from the census (Fombonne & du Mazaubrun, 1992), or in a larger birth cohort study with case identification through review of medical records (Fombonne et al., 1997). In an active screening project of a birth cohort in Sweden, Gillberg et al. (1991) found no variation in rates of autism by social class, based on father's occupation. In a larger study, encompassing all births in Denmark after 1972 and diagnoses until 1999, no association was seen for either maternal education or parental wealth

Table 47–1.
Selected demographic factors and autism

Demographic Factor	Major Studies*	Design	Findings (95% Confidence Intervals)**	Strengths & Limitations: Bias, Confounding	Notes on Interpretation of Findings
Socioeconomic status	Fombonne et al. (1997)	Birth cohort, 174 cases in 1985 birth cohort, from population of 325,000.	No differences in three regions: chi-square statistics (df) were 7.3 (5), 10.9 (5), and 2.9 (4). No excess of higher SES occupations.	Occupation of the head of household was categorized based on national classification system.	Cases identified through special education records and confirmed by psychiatrist.
	Croen et al. (2002)	Birth cohort, 4,381 cases of autism from population of 3.5 million live births.	Compared with < high school education: OR = 1.4 (1.3, 1.6) for high school education OR = 1.9 (1.7, 2.1) for college education OR = 2.0 (1.7, 2.3) for postgraduate education.	SES variable was maternal education from birth certificate. Cases from California DDS*** database, derived from a passive surveillance system. Adjusted for downstream variable and multiple highly correlated variables, which may have introduced bias.	Probable underascertainment of cases among those with low education resulting from lack of active case-finding in DDS*** system. Control for birth weight, an intermediate variable, could have distorted true association in an unpredictable direction.
	Bhasin & Schendel (2007)	Case-control, 617 cases from MADDSP****, 617 population-based controls.	Median family income, (referent = middle): OR = 0.5 (0.3, 0.6) for low income, OR = 1.6 (1.2, 2.3) for high income. Maternal education (referent = 12 years) OR = 0.9 (0.6, 1.5) for <12 years, OR = 0.9 (0.6, 1.2) for 13 to 15 years, OR = 0.9 (0.6, 1.3) for 16 years, OR = 1.3 (0.8, 1.6) for 16+ years.	SES variables were: maternal education (individual-level) and family income (median in Census tract of mother's residence). Strong association with income but not education in adjusted models (but not unadjusted) may have been a result of high correlation between these variables and also with maternal age and race.	Although difficult to tease apart which SES factor is most related, SES does show a strong association with autism diagnoses, even in this population-based study that used active case finding from review of existing medical and school records.
	Durkin et al. (2008)	Birth cohort from CDC's ADDM***** network; 1,251 cases from a population of 250,000 births.	Compared with high school graduates, OR = 1.0 (0.8 or 0.9, 1.2) for each of the other levels of education.	Large multisite study with standardized criteria for case definition. SES variable = maternal education. Adjusted for numerous covariates. Adjusted for downstream (potentially intermediate) variables (gestational age and birth weight for gestational age), which may have introduced bias.	Large study with standardized case definition and active case-finding methods. Lack of association between maternal education and autism may be a result of high correlation with maternal age and adjustment for potential intermediate variables.
	Larsson et al. (2005)	Case-control, 698 cases, 17,450 controls from all births in Denmark in the year 1972.	Compared with elementary education, OR = 0.92 (0.75, 1.13) for high school or some college, OR = 0.89 (0.67, 1.19) for baccalaureate, master's or doctoral degree. Compared with highest quartile of wealth, OR = 0.83 (0.67, 1.02) for high-middle wealth, OR = 1.09 (0.85, 1.38) for low-middle wealth, OR = 1.30 (0.97, 1.75) for lowest quartile.	SES variables were parental income and maternal education. Adjusted for birth characteristics (APGAR score, birth weight for gestational age, gestational age), as well as prenatal care; these variables could have been intermediates on a causal pathway, potentially resulting in biased ORs.	Large study. Provides marginal evidence for higher risk among children of lower-income families. This and the lack of association between maternal education and autism may have stemmed from adjustment for intermediate variables and/or close association of income, education and both parental ages. Alternatively, there may be no association in a country with a high level of access for all.

	Baird et al. (2006)	Population cohort in South Thames, UK, 81 cases of autism.	Compared with children whose parents had not completed secondary education, OR = 5.0 (1.99, 12.7) for those whose parents had at least a secondary education.	Two-stage case ascertainment beginning with screening from special needs register for child health services. Study assessed proportion of identified cases that had been previously identified by locally based assessment.	Study design was able to identify significantly lower ascertainment of ASD in children born to parents of low education using records based on existing diagnoses made locally. In contrast, the complete ascertainment indicated no SES association with ASD.
Immigrant status	Lauritsen et al. (2005)	Population cohort, with 818 incident autism cases from Danish Psychiatric Central Register of population of 944,000 births.	Compared with children whose mothers were born in Denmark, OR = 1.42 (1.10, 1.83) for maternal birthplace outside Europe.	Adjusted for child's age, gender, calendar year of diagnosis, age of each parent, history of psychiatric disorders in the mother, father, or sibling, and urbanicity of residence.	Large sample size, and relatively thorough adjustment for covariates. Provides some evidence for parental place of birth effect, but some of the adjustment variables could have been downstream, potentially biasing the results.
	Hultman et al. (2002)	Case-control: 408 cases 2,040 controls, population-based in Sweden and matched on sex, year, and hospital of birth.	RR = 3.0 (1.7, 5.2) for maternal birth outside Europe or North America.	Linked Swedish national registries for births and inpatients. Adjusted for numerous confounders such as maternal age, parity, country of birth, smoking, hypertensive diseases, etc. Unclear whether results shown were also adjusted for some downstream factors such as delivery type, birth weight, and child's APGAR score.	Population-based study with comprehensive data on maternal medical conditions and labor and delivery factors. Based on inpatient records for autism spectrum disorders, and hence may include only most severe cases. Controlled for confounders; may have inappropriately adjusted for downstream variables, which could have biased the RR.
	Gillberg et al. (1991)	Population cohort of children born 1975 through 1984 in city of Goteborg or county of Bohuslan, and residing in the same locale in 1988, n = 77,000.	RRs not given, explicitly: 11.6/10,000 prevalence in Goteborg, vs. 7.2/10,000 in rural area where no immigration was said to occur.	No clear denominator data on immigration in the population. Immigrants were from a variety of regions: other Nordic countries, Central and Southern Europe, England, Asia, Africa, and South America.	Authors assert that the increase in prevalence from a previous survey was accounted for by autism diagnoses in immigrant children.
Parental age (maternal, paternal, or both)	Lauritsen et al. (2005)	Population cohort, with 818 incident autism cases from Danish Psychiatric Central Register of population of 944,000 births.	Compared with mothers 25 to 29 years of age, OR = 1.68 (1.07, 2.63) for ages <20 years, OR = 1.19 (0.96, 1.47) for ages 20 to 24, OR = 1.08 (0.89, 1.29) for ages 30 to 34, OR = 1.18 (0.92, 1.53) for ages 35 to 39, OR = 1.17 (0.90, 1.97) for ages 40+. Compared with fathers 25 to 29 years of age, OR = 0.81 (0.60, 1.09) for ages <25 years, OR = 1.08 (0.89, 1.29) for ages 30 to 34, OR = 1.35 (1.07, 1.70) for ages 35 to 39, OR = 1.61 (1.19, 2.18) for ages 40 to 44, OR = 1.21 (0.78, 1.86).	Adjusted for child's age, gender, calendar year of diagnosis, parental education, history of psychiatric disorders in the mother, father, or sibling, and urbanicity of residence.	Relatively large sample size and thorough adjustment for confounders. If ages of the two parents were highly correlated, ability to distinguish independent effects of either one would have been limited. Demonstrates increasing risk with advancing age for both mothers and fathers.

(*Continued*)

Table 47–1. (Contd.)

Demographic Factor	Major Studies*	Design	Findings (95% Confidence Intervals)**	Strengths & Limitations: Bias, Confounding	Notes on Interpretation of Findings
Parental age (con't)	Larsson et al. (2005)	Case-control, 698 cases, 17,450 controls from all births in Denmark in the year 1972.	Compared with mothers 25 to 29 years of age, OR = 1.54 (0.87, 2.74) for ages <20 years, OR = 1.03 (0.80, 1.34) for ages 20 to 24, OR = 1.18 (0.95, 1.48) for ages 30 to 34, OR = 1.07 (0.76, 1.52) for ages 35 to 39, OR = 1.55 (0.87, 2.74) for ages 40+. Compared with fathers 25 to 29 years of age, OR = 0.61 (0.42, 0.89) for ages <25, OR = 1.10 (0.88, 1.38) for ages 30 to 34, OR = 1.28 (0.96, 1.69) for ages 35 to 39, OR = 1.36 (0.96, 1.93) for ages 40+.	SES variables were parental income and maternal education. Analysis of age of each parent adjusted for age of the other. Adjusted for birth characteristics (APGAR score, birth weight for gestational age, gestational age), as well as prenatal care; these variables could have been intermediates on a causal pathway, potentially resulting in biased ORs.	Large study. Appears to suggest a U-shaped relationship of maternal age with autism risk. However, adjustment for intermediate variables or for multiple variables correlated with parental age may have constituted overadjustment, potentially leading to attenuated ORs. High correlation between the two parents' ages may have hampered ability to accurately measure independent effects.
	Reichenberg et al. (2006)	Cohort of military conscriptees, n=319,000 for paternal age analysis, n=132,000 for maternal age analysis, born over 6 consecutive years (dates not specified) in Israel.	Compared with mothers 15 to 29 years of age, OR = 0.87 (0.54, 1.41) for ages 30 to 39, OR = 2.68 (0.81, 8.96) for ages 40+. Compared with fathers 15 to 29 years of age, OR = 1.62 (0.99, 2.65) for ages 30 to 39, OR = 5.75 (2.65, 12.46) for ages 40 to 49.	Diagnoses generally made by clinical team. Analysis of age of each parent adjusted for age of the other. Maternal age available for less than half the cohort; paternal age for 84%. Adjusted for socioeconomic status, but this variable was not defined. Wide age range for the referent group. Small cell sizes for parents over age 40 years, especially mothers.	High proportion missing maternal information, which may have been related to parents' ages. Small cell sizes resulted in large random error. High correlation between the two parents' ages and the wide age range of the referent group limited ability to accurately measure independent effects. Adequacy of adjustment for SES is indeterminate.
	Croen et al. (2007)	Cohort of 133,000 births 1995 through 1999 in a northern California HMO. Autism/ASD cases diagnosed by April 2005.	Compared with mothers 25 to 29 years of age, OR = 0.62 (0.30, 1.27) for ages <20 years, OR = 0.86 (0.62, 1.18) for ages 20 to 24, OR = 1.04 (0.83, 1.31) for ages 30 to 34, OR = 1.18 (0.92, 1.53) for ages 35-39, OR = 1.27 (0.83, 1.95) for ages 40+. Compared with fathers 25 to 29 years of age, OR = 0.45 (0.15, 1.41) for ages <20, OR = 0.86 (0.57, 1.30) for ages 20 to 24, OR = 1.14 (0.89, 1.48) for ages 30 to 34, OR = 1.38 (1.04, 1.84) for ages 35 to 39, OR = 1.52 (1.10, 2.10) for ages 40+.	Diagnoses based on ICD criteria applied to medical records. Used proportional hazards model to adjust for differences in length of follow-up by date of birth. Adjustment for four socioeconomic factors (both parents' educational levels, both parents' race ethnicity), and adjustment for the other parent's age may have constituted overadjustment, given that these six variables may have had strong correlations among them. This could have biased estimates of some of these variables, including parental ages.	For ASD, results of each parent's age, modeled as a continuous variable and adjusted for the other, were similar. For autistic disorder, paternal age appeared to have a stronger effect. High quality, carefully constructed and consistent diagnostic criteria applied for ASD definition. Authors correctly refrained from adjusting for birth characteristics. The use of proportional hazards models assumes that censoring is independent of outcome, which may not be the case, given the strong temporal trend of autism in California.

Durkin et al. (2008)	Birth cohort from CDC's ADDM***** network; 1,251 cases from a population of 250,000 births.	Compared with mothers 25 to 29 years of age, OR = 0.7 (0.5, 1.0) for ages <20 years, OR = 0.9 (0.8, 1.1) for ages 20 to 24, OR = 1.1 (0.9, 1.3) for ages 30 to 34, OR = 1.3 (1.1, 1.6) for ages 35+. Compared with fathers 25 to 29 years of age, OR = 0.6 (0.4, 1.0) for ages <20, OR = 0.9 (0.7, 1.1) for ages 20 to 24, OR = 1.0 (0.9, 1.2) for ages 35 to 39, OR = 1.4 (1.1, 1.8) for ages 40+.	Large multisite study with standardized criteria for case definition. Analysis of age of each parent adjusted for age of the other and for numerous SES factors, as well as for site. Adjusted for downstream (potentially intermediate) variables (gestational age and birth weight for gestational age), which may have introduced bias.	Large study with standardized case definition and active case-finding methods lends confidence in the data quality. Some attenuation of the associations for both maternal and paternal age could have occurred because of adjustment for intermediate variables. Nevertheless, provides strong evidence that both maternal and paternal age contribute to increased risk for autism in offspring.
Shelton et al. (2010)	Population cohort of 5 million births 1990 through 1999, in California. ASD cases, n = 12,000 from statewide DDS* system.	Compared with mothers 25 to 29 years of age, OR = 0.86 (0.80, 0.92) for ages <25, OR = 1.12 (1.06, 1.19) for ages 30 to 34, OR = 1.31 (1.22, 1.41) for ages 35 to 39, OR = 1.51 (1.35, 1.70) for ages 40+. Compared with fathers 25 to 29 years of age, OR = 0.76 (0.71, 0.82) for ages <25, OR = 1.10 (1.04, 1.18) for ages 30 to 34, OR = 1.24 (1.15, 1.33) for ages 35 to 39, OR = 1.36 (1.26, 1.47) for ages 40+. However, these values were heterogeneous for fathers, depending on the mothers' age. For mothers 30+ years of age, paternal age was not a significant risk factor for ASD.	Very large cohort of 5 million births, data on covariates quite complete. DDS ascertainment is estimated to be 75 to 80% complete. Father's age missing for 9.6% of controls, 7.0% of cases.	Extremely large cohort with small percentage of missing data. Finely stratified analysis with adjustment for covariates indicated consistent increases in ASD risk as maternal age increased, regardless of paternal age. Similar analysis showed increases in ASD risk for paternal age only when mother was <30 years of age. This study was unique in assessing heterogeneity of age effects of each parent's age stratified on other parent's age.

*Major studies included those with at least 50 cases and 100 total subjects. However, no attempt was made to be comprehensive or complete.
**All findings shown in this table are multivariate adjusted associations.
***DDS = Department of Developmental Services of the State of California, an agency that coordinates services for persons with developmental disorders who have functional disabilities, but does not conduct active case finding.
****MADDSP = Metropolitan Atlanta Developmental Disabilities Surveillance Program, which conducts active case finding using school and medical records.
*****ADDM = Autism and Developmental Disabilities Monitoring Network, a CDC program that conducts active surveillance in various selected states within the United States.

(Larsson et al., 2005). Baird and colleagues, reporting results from the UK using an active case finding through screening and assessment, noted that existing local records showed a strong underascertainment of autism cases among children from parents with low education: children of parents who completed secondary education had fivefold higher odds of having a previous diagnosis of autism, among those identified from the active screening program (Baird et al., 2006).

Taken as a whole, evidence supporting an association with higher SES largely comes from the United States or from databases with passive surveillance and the resultant underascertainment. Where cases are identified through active screening, population-wide surveillance is conducted, or access to health care is universal (Denmark, France, and Sweden), socioeconomic differentials tend not to be found (Larsson et al., 2005; Fombonne et al., 1997; Gillberg et al., 1991). Associations with social class therefore may represent a greater rate of success when parents with higher education advocate for their children as compared with those having less education. Based on the evidence to date, socioeconomic differences seem unlikely to reveal clues about environmental factors in the development, as opposed to the clinical diagnosis, of autism.

Race/Ethnicity

Reported differences in prevalence by race and ethnicity have not been consistent. In California, one report found African-American children were at higher risk for autism compared with Caucasian children (Croen et al., 2002). As a high percentage of African-Americans in California reside in Los Angeles, where overall reporting of autism in the Department of Developmental Services (DDS) system is greater than elsewhere in the state, this finding may be spurious as a result of confounding by geography. In addition, Hispanic children in California were less likely than Caucasians to have an autism diagnosis, possibly due to language barriers and reluctance of families with an undocumented parent or other relative to report to centers affiliated with DDS, a state agency. In contrast, Yeargin-Allsopp et al. (2003) did not find any association between race and autism in a study from metropolitan Atlanta using all sources, with results varying by source of diagnostic information (health records, schools). In a study of Medicaid-eligible children who later were diagnosed with autistic disorder (AD), African-Americans were far less likely to receive an ASD diagnosis on their first visit (Mandell et al., 2007) and were more than 1.5 years older at diagnosis with AD than Caucasian children (Mandell et al., 2002). Most recently, based on ASD prevalent cases at 8 years of age, confirmed by the CDC's Autism and Developmental Disabilities Monitoring multisite network that reviewed records from multiple sources, Mandell and colleagues (Mandell et al., 2009) determined that after adjustment for confounders, African-Americans, Hispanics and other races/ethnicities were less likely to have documentation of an ASD diagnosis in their records; for Hispanics and other racial/ethnic groups, this was especially true for children with intellectual disabilities.

It appears that race differences in autism rates may stem from differences in care-seeking and clinician practices. Combined with evidence of an ASD diagnostic artifact associated with socioeconomic level and the correlation of race/ethnicity with SES, this line of inquiry seems to have a low probability of yielding true etiologic leads but can 'underscore' concerns related to access.

Place of Birth and of Residence (Immigration and Geography)

Place of birth or residence has been reported to be associated with autism. Living in an urban, as compared with rural, area is associated with a higher prevalence of autism (Gillberg et al., 1991; Lauritsen et al., 2005; Hultman et al., 2002). Because health providers tend to be concentrated in urban centers, this phenomenon is likely an artifact of greater access to qualified diagnosticians.

An effect of immigration has been reported from several parts of the world. In Denmark, children of mothers born outside of Europe (Lauritsen et al., 2005) or with non-Danish citizenship (Maimburg & Vaeth, 2006) were at increased risk; a British study found a greater risk for autism among second generation Afro-Caribbean immigrants than among other British-born children (Goodman & Richards, 1995); in Australia, children whose mother was born outside the country were at increased risk (Williams et al., 2008), with the highest risk in those from southeast or northeast Asia. In Sweden, an early study suggested that increases in autism risk in an urban area resulted from immigration (Gillberg et al., 1991). More recently children in Sweden whose mothers' birthplace was outside Europe and the United States had an elevated risk of autism (Hultman et al., 2002).

The principal environmental hypotheses that have emerged from these studies are: mothers born elsewhere may be more susceptible to unfamiliar microbial exposures in their newer place of residence; or social stresses associated with emigration and subsequent social integration may put the fetus/infant at higher risk, possibly mediated by placental enzymes involved in cortisol metabolism (O'Donnell et al., 2009).

Parental Age

Inconsistent results have been reported regarding the association between parental age and autism. A number of large studies reported an association with advanced maternal age (Bhasin & Schendel, 2007; Croen et al., 2002; Durkin et al., 2008; Glasson, 2002) and/or advanced paternal age after adjustment for maternal age (Reichenberg et al., 2006; Lauritsen et al., 2005; Croen et al., 2007; Glasson, 2002; Durkin et al., 2008). However, one found a significant inverse relationship (Burd et al., 1999) and another found neither parent's age to be predictive (Larsson et al., 2005). Investigations used variable approaches to adjusting for the other parent's age, or other factors. Interpretation of studies is hampered, in part by adjustment for variables that are on the causal pathway or serve as intermediate markers for high risk (e.g., obstetric or fetal conditions); this approach is common and may, rather than control bias in estimated age effects, actually create bias in either direction (towards or away from the null value).

Moreover, the high correlation between advanced maternal and paternal age at procreation is difficult to disentangle and some studies lacked the statistical power to do so, despite having conducted multivariate analyses. Shelton et al., however, in a study that was far larger than any other on this topic, implemented tight control by examining each parent's age after restricting to relatively narrow age strata of the other parent. This analysis showed a consistent maternal age effect. In contrast, paternal age was influential only in younger mothers, those below 30 years of age (Shelton et al., 2010). This study thus demonstrated an independent effect of maternal age, regardless of the paternal age, and an effect of paternal age that was dependent on maternal age.

Notably, paternal age is more frequently missing than maternal age, and the analyses that mutually adjust are therefore limited to the subset of births with a nonmissing value for paternal age. If data absence is more common in younger fathers (e.g., Mouridsen et al., 1993) and less common for cases (for instance, if men on the broader spectrum who have children, do so later), then the paternal age association may be overestimated.

Most importantly, the effects of maternal and paternal age raise the issue: what is it about older mothers and fathers that is disadvantageous for the offspring? That advancing maternal and paternal age are each associated with chromosomal aberrations, low birth weight, and congenital malformations is certainly relevant (Berkowitz et al., 1990; Djahanbakhch et al., 2007; Meacham & Murray, 1994; Reichman & Teitler, 2006). Older mothers, who often have older fathers as partners, are more likely to use fertility treatments or other assisted reproductive technologies and even if conceived naturally, the ova are older and more biologically vulnerable to chromosomal aberrations. Paternal de novo mutations or epigenetic dysregulation of spermatogonia cells have been hypothesized to underlie the association of schizophrenia with increasing paternal age (Perrin et al., 2007). The ever-increasing number of spermatogonial divisions offers multiple opportunities for age-related de novo chromosomal aberrations and possible changes in methylation patterns (Sartorius & Nieschlag, 2010). Older age of fathers is associated with increased telomere length in spermatozoa. Whether these vulnerabilities for both maternal and paternal age are programmed or result from an accumulation of insults remains unclear.

Other mechanisms suggested by maternal aging include: placental insufficiency or an increased prevalence of cardiovascular conditions such as chronic or gestational hypertension, both of which could lead to hypoxia; a less favorable hormonal milieu than occurs with younger mothers; a higher body burden of toxic chemicals; and/or a less efficient development of tolerance for "nonself" stemming from age-related increased tendency toward autoimmune responses. Specific classes of environmental exposures worthy of further investigation based on the evidence regarding parental age include reproductive technologies (see section of this chapter "Medical Factors," subsection "Medical Intervention"), endocrine disruptors and compounds that bioaccumulate or are persistent in human tissues (see section of this chapter: "Chemicals in the Environment," subsection "Endocrine Disruptor"), as well as factors influencing vascular function, or immune toxins.

Sex

One of the consistent demographic findings in autism is a higher prevalence among males as compared with females. Typically, the ratio is around 4:1, with sizeable variation from study to study (Fombonne, 2003). Mechanisms hypothesized to be responsible for this skewed sex ratio include endogenous hormones (Knickmeyer & Baron-Cohen, 2006) or epigenetic alterations such as X-chromosome inactivation (Nagarajan et al., 2008). By extension, exogenous endocrine disruptors might also play a role. An altered sex ratio at birth, favoring females, has been associated with several persistent endocrine-disrupting chemicals such as 2-, 3-, 7-, 8-tetrachlorodibenzodioxin (dioxin)(Mocarelli et al., 2000), and polychlorinated biphenyl ethers (PCBs) (Hertz-Picciotto et al., 2008); the PCBs are also associated with intrauterine growth restriction in males but not in females (Vartiainen et al., 1998; Hertz-Picciotto et al., 2005; Sonneborn et al., 2008). Thus, male sperm, embryos, or fetuses appear to be more susceptible to certain types of preconceptional, periconceptional, or prenatal insults, respectively. Other childhood conditions in which males are disproportionately affected are ADHD, childhood leukemia, and childhood asthma, all of which have seen increases in the last decades.

Seasonality

Seasonality of births has been well-studied for other developmental and psychiatric conditions, particularly schizophrenia (Boyd et al., 1986; Torrey et al., 1977; Parker & Neilson, 1976). An excess of winter births suggested an etiologic role for infectious agents, and indeed, a higher rate of schizophrenia was confirmed for children exposed during their second trimester *in utero* to an influenza epidemic in Helsinki (Mednick et al., 1988). Brown and coworkers reported serological evidence that maternal influenza infections in the first half of pregnancy were more prevalent for cases of schizophrenia than for controls (Brown et al., 2004).

Several research groups have examined seasonal birth patterns in autism. Two separate teams reported March and August to be months of excess births of children who developed autism. One was a case-control study in North Carolina of 810 children with autism and 768 unaffected controls (Bartlik, 1981), and another used the birth registry in Israel (Barak et al., 1995). Two other studies found excess births in March but not in August (Gillberg, 1990;

Mouridsen et al., 1994). Larger studies using more sophisticated methods found discrepant results and no evidence for a March or August excess (Bolton et al., 1992; Landau et al., 1999). A new analysis based on a very large dataset from the California DDS showed November to be a high risk birth month. Reports that focused on season rather than month gave inconsistent results (Atladottir et al., 2007; Tanoue et al., 1988), though two found winter to be a low-risk period (Konstantareas et al., 1986; Lee et al., 2008).

Methodologically, the lack of consistency in findings across studies could be a result of geographic variation in seasonality, but may also be a result of misclassification resulting from differing definitions of season, small sample sizes, and variation in lengths of gestation. With respect to the latter, if there is a critical window during the prenatal developmental period when the insult predisposes to aberrant development, then dates of conception rather than births would provide a more accurate measure of the relevant period. The finding by Lee et al. (2008) that the peak excess for multiple births was 2 to 3 weeks earlier than for singletons supports the notion that dating from conception would be less error-prone, as multiple births tend to deliver earlier than singletons. Using the California DDS data, Zerbo and colleagues found higher risks for children who were conceived in the winter months, December through March (Zerbo et al., in press).

What etiologic clues do these studies provide? Although the March birth excess is a recurrent finding, the inconsistent results underscore the need for more rigorous research, either using season of conception or through investigation of seasonally variable factors in tandem with mechanistic biologic studies. Just as parental age is a surrogate for numerous possible causal factors, seasonality represents variation in the meteorologic (temperature, rainfall), infectious, allergenic (pollen), dietary, and chemical (e.g., pesticides in agriculture and for home pest control) environments. Several of these exposures are discussed in later sections of this chapter.

Medical Factors: Infections and Immunology, Fertility Treatment, Obstetric Factors, Medications, and Vaccines

The higher risk for autism after complicated pregnancy, labor, or delivery or in association with neonatal suboptimality is a recurring theme. The literature is not, however, entirely consistent about which of these conditions or events is informative. A recent meta-analysis based on 40 investigations that evaluated a wide range of maternal factors (sociodemographic, as well as medical) concluded that evidence was insufficient for any single prenatal factor (Gardener et al., 2009). In practical terms, the origins of maternal and perinatal conditions may be ill-defined: microbiological insults, pregnancy complications, medical interventions, characteristics of labor and delivery, and infant attributes may influence each other, as well as early child neurobehavioral trajectory but could also be influenced by aberrant CNS development. Thus, the findings presented regarding medical factors are fundamentally descriptive, yet all pertain to fetal stress, in the broad sense of the term. For this chapter, the specific medically related stressors covered are: infection; immunologic development; medical interventions for subfertility, diagnostic ultrasonography, or to facilitated delivery, medical conditions of the mother; and vaccines in childhood. The focus is on upstream factors rather than measures of infant health status such as APGAR scores or low birth weight. Table 47-2 summarizes prominent studies on maternal health conditions, both acute and chronic, as well as on medical procedures.

Infections and Immunology

Early evidence about infections as a cause of autism arose from an epidemic of rubella several decades ago. Data from two separate studies of 243 and 64 congenital rubella cases, respectively, found risks of autism between 4% and 12% (Chess, 1971, 1977; Desmond et al., 1967), in a time period when prevalences were reported at less than five per 10,000 (Fombonne, 2003). Thus, the relative risk could well have been over 100. Deykin and MacMahon conducted a case-control study comparing children with autism to their siblings, adjusting for sibship size, using interviews and medical record reviews to assess encephalitic infections. They examined the hypotheses of associations between autism and clinical infections of the mother during the gestational period, of the child in the first 18 months of life, or of another household member during these periods (Deykin & MacMahon, 1979). The mothers were more likely, during gestations of cases as compared with siblings, to have had or been exposed to rubella ($RR = 3.3$, $p = 0.004$), measles ($RR = 5.5$, $p = 0.04$), mumps ($RR = 5.5$, $p = 0.04$), or influenza ($RR = 4.1$, $p = 0.0006$). The cases themselves were more likely than their siblings, during the first 18 months of life, to have had or been exposed to mumps ($RR = 2.8$, $p = 0.007$), chicken pox ($RR = 2.1$, $p = 0.02$), ear infections ($RR = 1.2$, $p = 0.0003$), or fever of unknown origin ($RR = 2.1$, $p = 0.0003$). A comparison of medical records vs. parental reports showed differences in reporting of exposures of cases vs. siblings, but they were small, with cases sometimes more often and sometimes less often exposed; hence any bias from differential recall is unlikely to have been large. Notably, reliance on medical records alone missed a large proportion of illnesses reported by the parents; this has implications for interpretation of medical databases. Information on timing of illnesses was not available but published data suggest congenital rubella is less probable when the maternal infection occurs late in pregnancy (Peckham, 1985). Because of effective vaccination programs, most of the aforementioned illnesses are extremely rare today; however, ear infections, influenza, and unexplained fevers are still relevant. A meta-analysis of studies through March 1994 found maternal infections to be significantly associated with autism in four studies that controlled for covariates, but not in seven studies that did not (Gardener et al., 2009).

Table 47–2.
Medical factors and autism

	Major Studies*	Design	Findings**	Strengths & Limitations: Bias, Confounding	Notes
Medical Interventions in Preconception or Pregnancy					
Assisted conception	Maimburg & Vaeth (2007)	Case-control; 461 cases, 461 controls.	OR = 0.37 (0.14, 0.98).	Sample size was borderline adequate as only 10 assisted conceptions among cases. Analysis inappropriately adjusted for factors potentially influenced by the exposure: multiplicity, birth weight, gestational age, and birth defect.	Multiplicity is a common consequence of assisted conception and therefore adjustment may have strongly biased the OR.
Antenatal ultrasound	Grether et al. (2009)	Case-control; 362 cases, 393 controls.	OR = 1.06 (0.95, 1.20) for each additional scan at any time during pregnancy.	Analysis adjusted for potential confounders. Elevated risk was observed for females in relation to second trimester ultrasounds.	Number of ultrasounds may not measure the dose to the fetus based on intensity and duration of scan, and location of transducer relative to fetal tissue of concern.
Rhogam	Miles & Takahashi (2007)	Case series; diverse comparison populations, 214 cases.	OR = 1.00 (0.47, 2.16) using de novo chromosomal disorder as controls. OR = 1.02 (0.7, 1.48), OR = 0.85 (0.61, 1.27) using larger populations as controls.	Cases confirmed. Small or poorly defined comparison groups. No confounder adjustment.	Only one analysis was for anti-D immunoglobulin, with four exposed controls (i.e., statistical power was low). Race/ethnicity potentially confounded the comparison with a large control group.
Infections in Pregnancy					
Rubella	Chess (1971, 1977)	Case series; 243 cases implicit comparison with general population.	RR = 100 assuming population background prevalence of 4/10,000.	Formal diagnostic criteria not applied. Children with congenital rubella have a wide range of developmental conditions (e.g., hearing impairments, cognitive deficits, etc.), making autism diagnosis difficult.	Some of the children appeared to recover. The RR is based on only those showing no recovery.
Rubella, measles, mumps, influenza	Deykin & MacMahon (1979)	Case-control; 163 cases, 355 sibling controls.	RR = 3.3 for rubella, RR = 5.5 for measles, RR = 5.5 for mumps, RR = 4.1 for influenza.	Study used sibling controls. High proportion of obstetric records obtained for both the cases and sibling controls, and confirmation of parental report in medical records was similar for cases and sibling controls. Careful screening of confounders. Possible exaggerated p-values due to multiple siblings per family.	Well conducted. Rubella finding confirms results from case series. Consistency across viral conditions with known encephalitic sequelae could support an inflammatory mechanism. Excellent response rate and validity of data appears high, with little evidence of reporting differences for case vs. sibling pregnancies.
Miscellaneous infections	Gardener et al. (2009)	Meta-analysis of various demographic, reproductive and obstetric factors.	OR = 1.82 (1.01, 3.30 in four studies that controlled for covariates or used sibling controls. OR = 0.89 (0.56, 1.42) in seven studies that did not.	Unclear which studies or which infections were included in the calculations, whether they combined several infections from the same study, nor whether the same infections were examined in multiple studies or not.	This meta-analysis suggests maternal infections during pregnancy may play a role, but the findings are nonspecific and may include both viral and bacterial.

(*Continued*)

Table 47–2. (Contd.)

	Major Studies*	Design	Findings**	Strengths & Limitations: Bias, Confounding	Notes
Medical Conditions					
Diabetes	Hultman et al. (2002)	Case-control; 408 cases, 2,040 controls, population-based and matched on sex, year, and hospital of birth.	RR = 1.2 (0.3, 5.7).	Linked Swedish national registries for births and inpatients. Adjusted for numerous confounders such as maternal age, parity, country of birth, smoking, hypertensive diseases, etc. Unclear whether results shown were also adjusted for some downstream factors such as delivery type, birth weight, and child's APGAR score.	Population-based study. Comprehensive data on maternal medical conditions, and labor and delivery factors. Low prevalence of diabetes was main weakness. Possible bias from controlling for intermediate factors. Based on inpatient records for autism spectrum disorders, and hence may include only most severe cases.
Preeclampsia	Glasson et al. (2004)	Case-control; 465 cases, 481 sibling controls, 1,313 population-based controls.	Unadjusted analysis,*** using population controls: RR = 0.99 (0.66, 1.50).	Large study using Western Australian state medical database for 14 years, covering 90% of diagnoses. Diagnostic reports were reviewed by pediatrician, and in last few years, by pediatrician, speech pathologist, and clinical psychologist.	Similar results were found using sibling controls. Lack of control for confounders, especially parity, hampers interpretation due to likely confounding.
	Hultman et al. (2002)	Case-control; 408 cases, 2,040 controls, population-based and matched on sex, year, and hospital of birth.	RR = 1.6 (0.9, 2.9) for "hypertensive diseases," ICD8 codes 401 and 637 (essential benign hypertension, and eclampsia, preeclampsia and toxemia) and ICD9 code 642 hypertensive disorders affecting pregnancy, childbirth and the postpartum period).	Linked Swedish national registries for births and inpatients. Adjusted for numerous confounders such as maternal age, parity, country of birth, smoking, etc., but also for some downstream factors such as delivery type and gestational age.	Population-based study. Comprehensive data on maternal medical conditions, and labor and delivery factors. Possible bias from controlling for intermediate factors. Based on inpatient records for autism spectrum disorders, and hence may include only most severe cases.
	Wallace et al. (2008)	AGRE database; (n = 228). Study of predictors of severity of autism signs.	Higher scores on communication domain of ADI-R for those with: preeclampsia (2.71 pts, SE = 1.16), hypertension (2.42 pts, SE = 0.75), generalized edema (2.25 pts, SE = 0.87).	Medical histories were self-reported. Used mixed effects model to account for correlations of twins and siblings within families.	Multiplex families only. Specificity of findings for the communication but not social domain.

Labor & Delivery					
Delivery: C-sections	Glasson et al. (2004)	Case-control; 465 cases, 481 sibling controls, 1,313 population-based controls.	RR = 1.83 (1.32, 2.54) for elective C-sections. No adjusted analyses were presented for emergency C-sections.	Large study using Western Australian state medical database for 14 years, covering 90% of diagnoses. Diagnostic reports were reviewed by pediatrician, and in last few years, by pediatrician, speech pathologist, and clinical psychologist. Adjusted for maternal age, birth order, birth year, threatened abortion, and fetal distress.	Sample size adequate. Appropriate control group. Systematic review of diagnoses. Potential residual confounding if birth years were not well-matched between cases and controls, especially since use of C-sections may have been rising sharply during this time period. An adjusted analysis of emergency C-sections was not presented.
	Hultman et al. (2002)	Case-control; 408 cases, 2,040 controls, population-based and matched on sex, year, and hospital of birth.	RR = 1.6 (1.1, 2.3).	Linked Swedish national registries for births and inpatients. Adjusted for numerous confounders such as maternal age, parity, country of birth, smoking, hypertensive diseases, etc., but also for some downstream factors such as child's APGAR score.	Population-based study. Controlled for confounders. Comprehensive data on maternal medical conditions and labor and delivery. Possible bias from controlling for intermediate factors. Based on inpatient records for autism spectrum disorders, and hence may include only most severe cases.
Induction of labor	Glasson et al. (2004)	Same as above.	Unadjusted analysis*** using population controls: RR = 1.40 (1.03, 1.90) using sibling controls, RR = 1.43 (1.12, 1.83) using population controls.	Same as above.	
Postnatal Medical Factors					
MMR vaccines	DeStefano et al. (2004)	Case-control; 624 cases, 1,824 controls, matched on age, gender and school.	OR = 0.93 (0.66, 1.30) for first MMR vaccine before 18 months of age, OR = 0.99 (0.63, 1.55) for first MMR vaccine before 24 months of age.	Adjusted for maternal age, education, multiplicity and birth weight. Assessed timing of MMR.	Earlier vs. later MMR vaccine was not associated with development of autism.

(*Continued*)

Table 47–2. (Contd.)

	Major Studies*	Design	Findings**	Strengths & Limitations: Bias, Confounding	Notes
Postnatal Medical Factors					
MMR vaccines (con't)	Taylor et al. (1999)	Case series; 498 cases	Fold differences in mean age at diagnosis: 0.93 (0.81, 1.08) for children vaccinated after 18 months of age, 0.91 (0.79, 1.05) for children vaccinated before 18 months of age, where referents were unvaccinated.	No control group. Prevalence rates were reported but methods for calculation and definition of denominator were absent.	No comparison of those with vs. without autism. Focus, instead, was on age at diagnosis. Because it was a case series, calculation of an RR comparing incidence in children receiving vaccinations late, early or never, was not possible.
	Smeeth et al. (2004)	Case-control; 1,294 cases, 4,469 controls matched on year of birth, sex, and practice.	All children: OR = 0.86 (0.68, 1.09). Children who joined GPRD*** by 1 year of age: OR = 1.47 (0.84, 2.57). Children who joined later: OR = 0.75 (0.57, 0.97).	Blind review of medical records for vaccine status. No adjustment for demographic confounders such as parental age or social class; no adjustment for calendar time.	Large study with sensitivity analyses of timing of MMR. Blinded record abstraction. Large difference in OR for children who joined GPRD after 1 year of age (majority of children in study) suggests misclassification bias from unknown vaccinations obtained prior to joining GPRD. Confounding uncontrolled.
	Madsen et al. (2002)	Full population cohort; (n = 537,303; vaccinated n = 440,655; unvaccinated n = 96,658).	OR = 0.92 (0.68, 1.24) for autistic disorder, OR = 0.83 (0.65, 1.07) for other ASDs.	Controlled for many confounders but not for maternal age, and control for calendar time was crude. Extremely high percentage missing gestational age at delivery (51% of unvaccinated, 27% of vaccinated); method of adjustment for missingness known to bias other associations.	Large study comparing those who did vs. did not receive MMR. Unclear whether the unvaccinated varied by birth year. Possible confounding and bias resulting from analytic strategies.

*Major studies included those with at least 50 cases and 100 total subjects. However, no attempt was made to be comprehensive or complete.

**All findings shown in this table are multivariate adjusted associations, unless otherwise noted.

***For these outcomes, Glasson et al. did not report any adjusted analyses.

****GPRD = General Practice Research Database, a consortium of pediatric practices across the UK.

A study that recruited cases through the Autism Society of America found self-reports of viral infections were far more common for mothers of children with autism, as compared with mothers of controls who were participants in a previous study of perinatal complications (Wilkerson et al., 2002). Additionally, urinary tract infections distinguished case from control mothers. Key information about the control group, however, was not reported, and at the time of data collection, some of the children were well into adulthood, raising concerns about quality of long-term recall. A recent study on early childhood infections recorded in medical records showed scant evidence of differences between cases and controls, although cases were less likely, overall, to have been diagnosed with any infection in the first 2 years of life (Rosen et al., 2007). Since parents frequently do not visit a physician for mild illnesses, it is plausible that the lower incidence was a function of care-seeking behaviors. As birth order strongly influences parental health-care seeking, this variable would have been useful to explore, especially in relation to the milder infections. Genitourinary infections were more common in the case children, possibly a result of case-control differences in risk factors for urinary tract infections, most of which were not controlled.

Because of the heterogeneity of kinds of viruses associated with neurodevelopmental and psychiatric illnesses, currently it is thought that the specific micro-organism is less important than the inflammatory response it produces. This concept is supported by a number of animal studies. Experiments in rodents show that introduction of influenza infection in pregnant dams results in behavioral deficits in offspring (Shi et al., 2003), and injection of poly(I:C) or lipopolysaccharide to induce inflammatory responses produces similar behavioral aberrations with no infection (Smith et al., 2007). Some evidence indicates that earlier exposures have greater impact (Meyer et al., 2007) while other research supports mid- and late-gestational effects of immune challenges (Meyer et al., 2006).

Corresponding research in humans indicates immune dysregulation is commonly observed in autism. Neuroinflammation has been suggested to modulate cortical and cerebellar function through activation of microglia and astroglia and production of proinflammatory cytokines in some proportion of autism cases (Vargas et al., 2005). A wide range of markers of immune abnormalities has been reported in autism: alterations in plasma immunoglobulins and cytokines (Ashwood et al., 2008; Enstrom et al., 2009; Heuer et al., 2008), aberrant NK cell activity (Enstrom et al., 2009; Vojdani et al., 2008), increased mast cells (Castellani et al., 2009), maternal IgG antibodies directed against fetal brain (Braunschweig et al., 2008), proinflammatory cytokines in brain tissue (Li et al., 2009) and altered inflammatory markers in cerebrospinal fluid (Zimmerman et al., 2005). Whether early immune changes lead to neuropathology, or alternatively, deviant brain development results in immune aberrations, or possibly neither (e.g., both are downstream sequelae of a shared but unknown initiating event), remains to be delineated. Nevertheless, these observations provide the key insight, namely, that mechanisms by which environmental exposures adversely affect CNS development might include disruption of immune developmental and maturation processes at critical junctures (Hertz-Picciotto, Park, et al., 2008). In other words, direct insult to neuronal tissue is not necessarily required, and both infectious and other agents should be evaluated in this broader perspective.

Medical Interventions

Use of assisted reproductive technology to achieve conception has been rising. In vitro fertilization (IVF) and intracellular sperm injection (ICSI) have been hypothesized to increase the risk of autism. In a large series of ICSI pregnancies resulting in 5,891 neonates, of whom 811 were followed to 3 years of age, over 10% were developmentally delayed (Palermo et al., 2008), but power was inadequate to examine autism as an outcome. Several other studies conducted to date were also underpowered to address this link (Pinborg et al., 2003; Stromberg et al., 2002). Middelburg et al. conducted a systematic review of studies of developmental outcomes of ICSI and IVF conceptions (Middelburg et al., 2008). They identified 23 reports that were judged to be of "good quality," which included rigorous criteria for a naturally conceived control group, and adequacy of follow-up and sample size. Cerebral palsy and epilepsy were frequently observed to be higher in assisted vs. natural conceptions, but only one study assessed autism (Maimburg & Vaeth, 2007). In this well-designed large study comparing 461 autism cases with matched controls, Maimburg and Vaeth reported a deficit of ICSI or IVF conceptions. However, their crude analysis (OR = 0.41) did not control for maternal or paternal age, country of origin, or plurality—four likely confounders. Their adjusted analysis (OR = 0.37) inappropriately controlled for numerous intermediate variables such as multiplicity (a direct consequence of fertility treatments), and other potentially downstream factors: birth weight, gestational age, and birth defects. As a result, both odds ratios would be expected to be biased (Cole & Hernan, 2002).

Ultrasonography is widely used to estimate gestational age, determine the number of fetuses, and screen for congenital anomalies, and the technology and equipment have undergone changes over the last few decades. Ultrasonography delivers a high frequency sound wave that can heat soft tissue, including at diagnostic levels. An HMO-based case-control study reviewed medical records to determine the number of ultrasounds taken during pregnancy and found that about 87% of women in the study had at least one ultrasound and over 20% received three or more (Grether et al., 2010). Results from fitting a logistic regression model (adjusted for potential confounders) indicated that the odds of autism did not rise exponentially as a function of number of ultrasounds taken during gestation, but second trimester scans of female fetuses were associated with an elevated risk. The possibility of a threshold response was not investigated. A challenge in studying ultrasounds during pregnancy is the greater number of ultrasound scans performed in response to an observed abnormality.

Obstetric Conditions

Large-scale studies of obstetric factors in relation to autism have used existing medical databases from national registries, health maintenance organizations, or conglomerates of medical practices. Two major studies were from Sweden (Hultman et al., 2002) and Australia (Glasson, 2002), and a smaller one was from Denmark (Eaton et al., 2001). Hultman and coworkers drew data from the linked Swedish Medical Birth Register and Inpatient Registry to conduct a case-control study of diagnoses of "infantile autism (ICD-9 code of 299A)" (n = 408) in the years 1987 through 1994. Controls with no autism diagnosis (n = 2,040) were matched 5:1 on sex and on year and hospital of birth. Multivariate analysis was performed with several obstetric conditions, with control for certain birth and infant characteristics. A team from Australia (Glasson, 2002) similarly used the Maternal and Child Health Research Database of Western Australia which covers all births in that state's population of 1.9 million residents, and diagnoses that are made at five state centers providing services in the same region. Births in 1980 through 1995 and autism diagnoses from 1986 until 1999 were included, with earlier diagnoses reviewed by a qualified pediatric expert on autism, and later diagnoses made by a team of three (clinical psychologist, speech pathologist, and pediatrician). A total of 465 ASD cases, 481 unaffected siblings, and 1,313 population-based controls were included; maternal age and other factors were controlled in some analyses. In Denmark, two studies were conducted using national registry linkage, one with 116 cases of autism, 279 of Asperger's Syndrome, and a 10% sample of births (Eaton et al., 2001), the other with 473 cases of autism and 10 controls for each case (Maimburg & Vaeth, 2006). Diagnoses for both studies were based on ICD codes in the Danish Psychiatric Case Register.

With regard to labor and delivery, the Swedish study found Cesarean section delivery significantly more frequently in case births, OR = 1.6 (95% CI = 1.1, 2.3) (Hultman et al., 2002), and the Australian study observed this to be true for both emergency OR = 1.6 (1.1, 2.2), and elective OR = 2.0 (1.5, 2.8) procedures (Glasson et al., 2004). Nonsignificantly elevated risks for autism but not for Asperger's Disorder were associated with C-sections when adjusted for only gender and year of birth in one of the Danish studies (Eaton et al., 2004); the other study adjusted for APGAR, which could be influenced by the C-section, potentially biasing the results (Maimburg & Vaeth, 2006). In the Australian cohort, elective C-section was associated with elevated risk for autism in a multivariate model that adjusted for fetal distress, maternal age, year of birth and other factors, but emergency C-section was not. Although multivariate analyses were not conducted using sibling controls, in the univariate analysis, fewer risk factors were identified with these than with population controls, reinforcing the view that sibling may be too similar to cases to provide valid referents. Thus, pregnancy-specific exposures may operate by intensifying susceptibility to other insults, be they inherited or environmentally induced.

Neither the Swedish nor the Australian study saw an elevated risk from preeclampsia, although hypertensive disorders were associated with a somewhat imprecise but elevated risk, OR = 1.6 (0.9, 2.9) in the former (Hultman et al., 2002). Within a sample of 228 multiplex families of children with autism in the Autism Genetic Resource Exchange (AGRE) study, hypertension, preeclampsia and edema were all associated with higher Autism Diagnostic Inventory Revised (ADI-R) communication scores (Wallace et al., 2008). Preeclampsia was not reported by Eaton and colleagues in the sample from Denmark, but placental insufficiency was strongly associated with autism in models adjusted only for gender and year of birth (Eaton et al., 2001), with similar results for "any complication."

For medications taken during pregnancy, few were examined in more than one study, effectively precluding definitive conclusions, according to a meta-analysis (Gardener et al., 2009). However, strong evidence of links to autism have been observed in small studies for thalidomide and valproic acid (Rodier et al., 1997). Fetal/infant characteristics such as low APGAR scores (Glasson et al., 2004; Hultman & Sparen, 2004; Larsson et al., 2005), breech presentation (Bilder et al., 2009), and fetal distress (Glasson et al., 2004), have been observed in autism. Current thinking regarding mechanistic implications of stress markers is that prenatal or birth hypoxia, the former being inducible by infection and the latter by C-section, may alter structural or functional features of CNS development, with permanent consequences through mechanisms such as: delayed neuronal migration (Zechel et al., 2005), degeneration and chromatolysis in the striatum (Zhuravin et al., 2006), reduced myelination (Wang et al., 2007), increased dopamine D1 receptor binding (Boksa et al., 2002), astrocytic fibroblast growth factor (Flores et al., 2002), and binding of insulin-like growth factors I and II (Boksa et al., 2006).

Vaccines and Autism

A hypothesized link between childhood vaccines and autism has stirred considerable controversy. Several distinct hypotheses have emerged. One specific conjecture is that the measles, mumps, rubella (MMR) vaccine has been a cause of autism; another is that vaccines containing the preservative thimerosal, which contains ethyl mercury, increase the risk of autism. This latter hypothesis is addressed below in the section "Chemicals in the Environment." A third theory is that the number of different vaccine antigens administered to infants is too large for some subset of children whose immune systems may not be sufficiently matured, leading ultimately to autism. Virtually no research has addressed this question. Here we synthesize the scientific literature on the MMR vaccine.

First articulated by Andrew Wakefield, who treated children for gastrointestinal symptoms, the MMR hypothesis focused on intestinal disturbances, including possible inflammation or increases in permeability that could lead to excess absorption of opioids, in the form of food-derived peptides (Wakefield & Montgomery, 1999; Wakefield et al., 1998). Various follow-up investigations have since been published, of which we present the stronger and larger ones; these did not primarily address the GI comorbidity. One ecologic analysis evaluated the relationship between rates of autism and years in which the MMR was and was not administered. Between 1980, when MMR almost completely replaced the separate measles, mumps, and rubella vaccines, and 1994, the increase in California in uptake of the combined MMR vaccine by 24 months of age rose from 72% to 82% (Dales et al., 2001). In contrast, during this same period, the rise in cumulative incidence of autism in California's DDS database, based on children born in those years and diagnosed with autism, went from just under 200 to nearly 1,200. As factors other than MMR vaccine uptake changed during this period, including the proportion of the population of affected children who were enrolled in the DDS system, conclusions from this ecologic analysis would necessarily be limited.

In Japan, the history of MMR vaccinations provided an opportunity to examine the impact of cessation of use of the MMR combined vaccine, which occurred in April 1993. After that time, the Immunization Law specified it be replaced with three separate vaccines, and that there be a 4-week period between administrations. Honda and colleagues therefore examined cumulative incidence of ASD up to 7 years of age in one Yokohama ward from 1988 through 1996 (Honda et al., 2005). Outcomes were derived from population-based screening for developmental disorders using a standardized tool at 18 and 36 months of age and summarized as annual cumulative incidence proportions. These incidence proportions rose from 1988 to 1990 while uptake of MMR declined from 70% to 34%, dropped in 1991 and 1992, and then rose higher, peaking in 1994. With a continued rise in incidence after MMR was withdrawn, the data are inconsistent with MMR having played a predominant role in the upward trajectory prior to that time. This time trend analysis, similar to other ecologic studies, presumes that other causal factors are held constant, and did not adjust for individual-level confounders.

Of studies utilizing individual-level data, a few evaluated whether cases with autism were more likely to have received the MMR; others conducted an analysis of age at vaccination to determine whether cases received their vaccinations earlier than controls or if they developed autism symptoms or regressed within a short time of the vaccinations.

CDC investigators (DeStefano et al., 2004) addressed the hypothesis that children receiving their first MMR vaccination at an earlier age (<18, <24, or <36 months old) would be more likely to develop autism, using prevalent cases aged 3 to 10 years from the population-based Metropolitan Atlanta Developmental Disabilities Surveillance Program. Controls were matched 3:1 to cases, and selected from the same school or a regular school that served the same residential area as that of a case child attending a special needs school. Age at first MMR vaccination was similar in cases and controls. Of those vaccinated *after* 36 months of age, 78% had documented developmental delays prior to 36 months of age, suggesting that age at vaccination may, for some children, be a consequence of, rather than a cause, of developmental conditions. This issue also arises in relation to thimerosal exposures, discussed in the section "Chemicals in the Environment".

The other study focusing on timing was based on a large case series of autism diagnoses in eight health districts of England among births in 1979 through 1992 (Taylor et al., 1999). Against an ongoing trend of increasing diagnoses of autism, Taylor and colleagues found no observable step-function in childhood autism incidence after introduction of the MMR vaccine. As compared with unvaccinated children, those vaccinated by 18 months of age, and those vaccinated at 18 months of age or later had similar mean ages at diagnosis, but the data did not permit examination of rates of autism. Different lag-times between the age at vaccination and age of parental concern (<1, <2, <3,...<12 month intervals) indicated a significantly higher proportion for one interval (<6 months), but not for any other in this case-only analysis. Additionally, no excess of regression occurred within 2, 4, or 6 months of receiving the MMR vaccine. In short, the results give little indication that autism diagnoses or regression clusters in specified time intervals after vaccination. Deficiencies in this study include: lack of control for factors related to age at diagnosis, such as social class (Baird et al., 2006); lack of a control group with comparable data on timing of vaccines—this was a *case-only* analysis; and, as discussed above, age at vaccination may itself be influenced by developmental status. Methodologically, this study also highlights the problem of time-to-onset analysis when onset itself is difficult to pinpoint and a common acute exposure routinely occurs shortly before typical recognition of a rare but severe disease.

The remaining studies examined those receiving vs. not receiving an MMR vaccine. Clinic records for the UK General Practice Research Database (GRPD), which contain diagnoses for pervasive developmental delay (PDD) as well as vaccination information and dates, were used to address the MMR hypothesis in a large case-control study (Smeeth et al., 2004). Abstractors were blind to the developmental outcome and up to 5 controls were matched to each case. The adjusted odds ratio for MMR was 1.47 (95% CI = 0.84, 2.57) if they joined the GPRD before their first birthday, and otherwise, 0.75 (95% CI = 0.57, 0.97). The study provides no evidence for increased risk with MMR vaccination, although potential confounders (including social class, maternal and paternal age, and birth weight) were uncontrolled, and heterogeneity by age at entry into the GPRD indicated potential bias.

In Denmark, a cohort study of all children born in 1991 through 1998 was conducted to examine associations with the MMR vaccine (Madsen et al., 2002). The authors compared vaccinated vs. unvaccinated children. Diagnoses were obtained from the Danish Psychiatric Registry and a validation substudy indicated that 92% of those with an autism diagnosis met the operational criteria used by the CDC in the Brick Township, New Jersey prevalence study, with the remaining 8% having other ASDs. The MMR vaccine used in Denmark was "identical to that used in the United States." The adjusted relative risk was 0.92 (95% CI = 0.68, 1.24). This study was impressive in that close to 100,000 children were in the unvaccinated group, though they were far outnumbered by those who did receive the vaccine. Individual-level data on vaccine administration was collected prospectively and independently of diagnostic information and the multivariate analysis adjusted tightly for an array of potential confounders, and did not adjust for intermediate variables, lending some confidence to the validity of results. Nevertheless, because of variable follow-up depending on year of birth, a survival analysis should have been conducted. At least 1/4 of the children were too young at the end of the study period to have a diagnosis of autism spectrum disorder, and vaccination status by year of birth was not shown. Some bias may also have been introduced by the use of an ad hoc method to adjust for the unusually large percentage of subjects with missing gestational age, which were unevenly distributed between vaccinated (28%) and unvaccinated (51%); it is known that adjustment for a "missing" category of a covariate inevitably biases results for other factors in a multivariate model (Vach & Blettner, 1991). Although this Danish study is, in many respects, the strongest investigation of MMR vaccines and autism, the potential for and direction of bias in those results is difficult to assess.

By and large, the evidence does not support the contention that MMR vaccines played a major role in the rise in autism during the 1990s. Studies comparing earlier vs. later receipt of the MMR found no differences in risk for autism. Only two studies with adequate control groups directly addressed vaccinated vs. unvaccinated children. The study from Denmark compared a very large sample of children who did not receive the MMR vaccine with an even larger group of children who did, controlled for risk factors that were antecedents of both the receipt of vaccines and the diagnosis of autism, and refrained from adjusting for intermediate variables. Methodologic concerns pertain to residual confounding resulting from crude control for calendar time (during a period of increasing diagnoses); nonuniform follow-up periods; and inappropriate comparisons involving inpatients in some years and both in- and outpatients in other years. Similar, as well as other issues regarding lack of adequate vaccination data in the children who joined the GPRD after their first birthday also limit the interpretation of the UK study of MMR. Although establishing a "null" finding (i.e., a lack of association) presents challenges from the statistical point of view, the evidence to date, which includes large studies, provides no indication that MMR vaccines, regardless of the age at administration, increase risk for autism. Nevertheless, stronger studies would be desirable to enhance conclusiveness. No studies attempted to identify susceptible subgroups of children in whom vaccines might contribute to risk of an ASD.

Chemicals in the Environment: Metals, Air Pollutants, Pesticides, and Endocrine Disruptors

Quite a number of environmental toxins affect critical CNS developmental processes. Proliferation and migration are sensitive to methyl mercury and ethanol; an organophosphate pesticide (chlorpyrifos) has been shown to influence proliferation as well as apoptosis (Rice et al., 2007). Methyl mercury and nicotine affect differentiation; several pesticides can alter synaptogenesis; and thyroid hormones or malnutrition adversely impact myelination. As the neuropathologic pathways in autism are yet to be delineated, any of these or similar observations may be relevant to autism.

As discussed earlier, besides direct insult to the CNS, another potential etiologic pathway leading to autism is via dysregulation of immune development or function. Interestingly, several classes of compounds are not only neurotoxins but also have demonstrated adverse effects on prenatal or postnatal markers of immune status, including metals, pesticides, air pollutants, and some endocrine disruptors (Dietert & Piepenbrink, 2006; Luebke et al., 2006; Hertz-Picciotto, Park, et al., 2008; Desi et al., 1986; Institoris et al., 1999; Park et al., 2008). Other mechanisms to be considered include disruption of thyroid hormones, sex steroids, or energy metabolism.

Many of the persistent organic pollutants (POPs) are endocrine disruptors. POPs are defined as meeting four criteria: *(1)* highly toxic; *(2)* stable or persistent, lasting years or decades before degrading; *(3)* transported long distances through air and water; *(4)* bioaccumulative in fatty tissue of humans and wildlife. Worldwide concern about POPs culminated in a global (intergovernmental) treaty known as the Stockholm Convention (United Nations Environment Programme, 2001); a dozen compounds were listed in the initial treaty, including nine pesticides and a few industrial chemicals or their by-products, and more have been added since that time. Although many are slated for elimination, this process is slow, and the United States, a major producer and polluter of POPs, was a signatory but did not ratify the Stockholm Convention.

In epidemiologic studies of environmental chemicals, the assessment of exposure can be quite complex. Some chemicals have extremely short half-lives of minutes or hours, while others may remain in the human body for years. Strategies to assess exposure include measurements in the environment, linkage of information from databases with emissions inventories, incorporation of data from monitoring systems for pollutant levels in given geographic areas, questions about behaviors and use of products known to contain specific chemicals, and biologic markers such as blood levels or metabolites in urine. Of critical importance for this research is the susceptible time period during which exposures can influence the development of autism. On the one hand, in the context of multifactorial etiology whereby each of multiple "hits" contributes to reducing the resilience of the fetus or child, there is no reason to preclude adverse effects at any point prior to the full manifestation of diagnosable autism or ASD. On the other hand, if a specific target tissue is sensitive during a narrow critical window, the use of broader time intervals (because of incomplete understanding of mechanism) may hamper the ability to detect effects of relevant exposures (Hertz-Picciotto et al., 1996), as shown in a study of fetal deaths with chromosomal anomalies (Bell et al., 2001a, 2001b). Inaccurate assignment of exposure timing could be somewhat less of a problem for the POPs, especially if new sources of exposure have been eliminated, rendering temporal variability more predictable.

This section synthesizes the research base on mercury, air pollutants, endocrine-disrupting chemicals, and pesticides. Table 47-3 describes the salient studies.

Mercury

Most of the literature on metals has focused on mercury, though some reports have measured cadmium, lead, or others. A few investigations have assessed mercury emissions from industrial sources in relation to risk of autism. However, the vast majority of studies on mercury have examined thimerosal from childhood vaccines. Thimerosal is 49% mercury by weight, in the form of ethylmercury attached to thiosalicylate. Further sources of thimerosal are injections for rhesus negative (Rh-) pregnant women and personal care products (e.g., nasal sprays, contact lens solutions). Sources of *other* forms of mercury, which are major contributors to human body burdens, are fish consumption (methyl Hg), dental amalgams, and industrial emissions (inorganic Hg). No research has yet been conducted that comprehensively evaluated all sources of mercury in relation to autism. Despite in vivo metabolism to inorganic Hg, the different forms appear to have different toxicologic effects (Clarkson et al., 2003). The next subsections discuss studies of autism and thimerosal exposures in the prenatal and postnatal periods, followed by other forms of mercury.

Thimerosal in Immunoglobulin Injections to Rh- Women during Pregnancy

Several investigations in the U.S. examined whether maternal Rh- status or receipt of thimerosal-containing anti-D immunoglobulin, administered to Rh- mothers to prevent serious neurodevelopmental damage to future children, might be associated with increased risk of autism. Miles and Takahashi (2007) enrolled 305 families identified from the Autism Clinic at the University of Missouri and obtained obstetric medical records from 214 to ascertain Rh- status and receipt of Rh anti-D immunoglobulin. Childhood Autism Rating Scale (CARS) and ADI-R scores were used to confirm case status. Prevalence of Rh- status was 15.4%, very close to that expected (15.4%, 15.2%, 17.7%) based on various comparison populations, although these comparison populations were small, potentially unsuitable, and/or not well-defined. Moreover, no information was provided on race/ethnicity or other relevant demographic or medical factors. A larger and better-defined comparison series for the thimerosal analysis would have provided more convincing evidence. This study also did not adjust for any confounders.

The investigation by Croen et al., involved 400 cases and 410 age- and gender-matched controls who were members of the Kaiser Permanente medical system for at least 2 years after birth. (Croen et al., 2008). Medical records were reviewed for Rh status, anti-D immunoglobulin, and thimerosal-containing vaccines for influenza. Unlike Miles and Takahashi, these authors adjusted for maternal age, race/ethnicity, and education, and child's sex, birth order, and plurality. The OR for Rh- status was 1.1 (95% CI = 0.7, 1.7) and for receiving anti-D immunoglobulin, 1.0 (0.6, 1.7). Rh- prevalence varied markedly by race/ethnicity, being much higher in Caucasian non-Hispanics and lower in other groups, particularly Hispanics. Since the latter were underrepresented in cases relative to controls, any bias would have been toward overestimation of the association with Rh status. Bias might also have arisen if undiagnosed cases among controls who left the Kaiser Permanente system shortly after the second birthday (before being diagnosed) were more or less likely to be Rh- than the ascertained cases, but moving a few subjects from the control to case group would have had little impact, given the size of this study.

This study would appear to be solid, if it were not for one fact, apparently not widely appreciated (Bernard et al., 2008): not all formulations of anti-D immunoglobulin contained thimerosal during the study periods. Pharmaceutical sales data (IMS, 2001) indicate that although somewhere between 31% and 51% of the market share from 1996 to 2000 was for Rhogam™, which did contain thimerosal, a similarly sized share of the market (from 44% to over 60%) was captured by BayRho™ and WinRho™ combined, both of which contained no thimerosal. Thus, a comparison across brands would have been the optimal comparison to answer the question of whether gestational thimerosal is associated with later autism in the child. Whether the medical records would be accurate with regard to the manufacturer or whether Kaiser's purchases were available is unclear, as the word "Rhogam" has come to be used generically, like the word "Kleenex," irrespective of the actual brand.

Thimerosal from Vaccines in the Postnatal Period

Thimerosal was introduced into U.S. vaccines as a preservative beginning in the 1930s. Both ecological and more rigorous epidemiologic studies using individual-level data on thimerosal-containing vaccine exposures have addressed a possible role for this mercuric compound in autism.

Three ecologic studies were conducted in Denmark, Canada, and California. Each examined time trends covering periods when thimerosal was in or had been removed from vaccines. In Denmark, the period studied was 1971 through 2000; thimerosal was used in vaccines from the 1950s until 1992 (Madsen et al., 2003). Autism rates did not begin to rise

Table 47–3.
Environmental chemicals and autism

	Major Studies*	Design	Findings (95% Con-fidence Intervals)**	Strengths & Limitations: Bias, Confounding	Notes on Interpretation of Findings
Mercury					
Thimerosal in anti-D immunoglobulin	Miles & Takahashi (2007)	Case series; diverse comparison populations; 214 cases.	OR = 0.93 (0.30, 2.89) for receipt of anti-D immunoglobulin.	Cases confirmed. Comparison groups poorly defined or of questionable validity. No confounder adjustment.	Only one analysis was for anti-D immunoglobulin, with four exposed controls (i.e., statistical power was low). Confounding likely a problem.
	Croen et al. (2008)	Case-control; 400 cases, 400 controls.	OR = 1.0; (0.6, 1.7) for receipt of anti-D immunoglobulin.	Confounders well controlled. Possible misclassification of 60% or more in the exposed category (estimated 40% PPV*** of exposure assignment).	Possible strong downward bias resulting from high misclassification, as many Rhogam manufacturers did not use thimerosal.
Thimerosal in vaccines	Hviid et al. (2003)	Full population cohort (n = 467,450) 1,227 cases.	RR = 0.85 (0.6, 1.2) for autism, RR = 1.12 (0.88, 1.43) for ASD.	Case ascertainment may have differed for exposed vs. unexposed due to changes in use of outpatients over the study period. Possible residual confounding because time was categorized in one year blocks with steep rise of autism (24% per year). Sensitivity analysis of 1991 through 1993 did not adjust for calendar time.	Brief report omitted many details. Analysis of vaccinated with and without thimerosal controls confounding by health-seeking behavior. Substantial downward bias from low ascertainment during thimerosal-exposed period. Likely residual confounding from time trend.
	Verstraeten et al. (2003)	Cohort; (n = 110,833 term infants in HMO B; other HMOs too small for meaningful analysis).	Three-month cumulative thimerosal dose: RR = 1.06 (0.88, 1.28); seven-month cumulative thimerosal dose: RR = 1.00 (0.90, 1.09).	Exclusions of infants with perinatal conditions of any type, or whose mothers had any complication of pregnancy or labor; this removed a disproportionate number with susceptibility to autism. In HMO B (the largest one), 24% of births were thereby excluded. Medical records not validated, hence case underascertainment possible.	Low birth weight, anomalies, birth hypoxia and other perinatal conditions are risk factors for autism, suggesting that the children most at risk for autism were excluded. Hence population-based estimates of thimerosal effects not possible from this analysis.
	Andrews et al. (2004)	Cohort; (n = 100,572 term infants). Hypothesis examined was early vs. late timing of vaccinations.	For each dose by 3 months of age: HR = 0.89 (0.65, 1.21); by 4 months of age: HR = 0.94 (0.73, 1.24); for time-adjusted dose by 6 months of age: HR = 0.99 (0.88, 1.12).	Compared early vs. late vaccinations, when both had thimerosal. Analysis controlled for follow-up time but not for confounders. Unvaccinated were excluded but were a small percentage of children, selection bias would be low. Significantly reduced risk was observed for general developmental delay, unspecified developmental delay, and ADD, suggesting systematic differences between those receiving vaccinations on time vs. later.	Addressed early vs. late vaccinations among those receiving three DPTs by 12 months of age. Restricted to those who received three DPT doses by 12 months of age. Unclear why other developmental delays and related conditions (Attention Deficit Disorder) show significantly lower risk in those receiving early vaccines.

Mercury					
	Heron et al. (2004)	Cohort; (n = 12,956, but 6610 for prosocial behavioral problems)	Outcome at 47 months of age: HR = 1.12 (1.01, 1.23) per dose by 3 months of age; HR = 1.05 (0.97, 1.15) per dose by 4 months of age; HR = 1.03 (0.98, 1.08) for time-adjusted dose by 6 months of age. Outcome at 81 months of age: HRs ranged from 0.97 to 0.99, with all confidence intervals including 1.0.	Conducted analysis in identical manner as Andrews et al. Controlled for a wide range of potential confounders. Small study for cohort analysis of autism, hence insufficient statistical power to address autism.	Because of small sample size, did not address autism or ASD diagnoses. Instead used continuous variables on behavioral scales. Control for confounders had little impact on results.
Inorganic mercury in air pollution	Windham et al. (2006)	Case-control; 284 cases, 657 controls.	RR = 1.31 (0.91,1.88) for third quartile of Hg emissions; RR = 1.92 (1.36,2.71) for fourth quratile.	Choice of exposures was based on biologic relevance. Estimated exposures were for second year of life. Cases from the California DDS**** were confirmed by thorough record review.	Used individual-level data. Adjusted for sociodemographic factors. Relevance of exposures in second year of life is unknown. Origins of autism are likely earlier, but triggers as late as second year cannot be excluded.
Other Air Pollutants					
Endocrine disruptors					
Chlorinated solvents	Windham et al. (2006)	Case-control; 284 cases, 657 controls.	RR = 1.33 (0.93, 1.88) for third quartile of exposures; RR = 1.55 (1.08, 2.23) for fourth quartile.	Same as above.	Same as above.
Aromatic solvents	Windham et al. (2006)	Case-control; 284 cases, 657 controls.	RR = 0.84 (0.59, 1.20) for third quartile of exposures; RR = 1.15 (0.80, 1.65) for fourth quartile.	Same as above.	Same as above.
	Windham et al. (2006)	Case-control; 284 cases, 657 controls.	RR = 1.33 (0.94, 1.88) for third quartile of exposures; RR = 1.28 (0.88, 1.85) for fourth quartile.	Same as above.	Same as above. Notably, primary exposures to endocrine disruptors occur through food and household products, not from ambient air pollution. Many endocrine-disrupting compounds not examined by Windham et al. are ubiquitous in the home environment and disrupt thyroid and sex hormones critical to neurodevelopment. Examples include: PCBs, PBDEs, phthalates, bisphenol A.

(Continued)

Table 47–3. (Contd.)

	Major Studies*	Design	Findings (95% Confidence Intervals)**	Strengths & Limitations: Bias, Confounding	Notes on Interpretation of Findings
Pesticides					
Organochlorines	Roberts et al. (2007)	Case-control; 465 cases, 6,975 controls.	A priori hypotheses, exposure 7 days preconception to 49 days post-LMP: RR = 4.2 (1.7, 10.9) for fourth quartile of nonzero exposure, 500m buffer RR = 2.4 (0.7, 8.2) for third quartiles of nonzero exposure, 500m buffer A posteriori hypotheses, exposure days 40–95 post-LMP: maximum RR = 7.6 Above RRs for 500m buffer.	DDS**** cases not confirmed; DDS estimated at 75% complete. Adjusted for sociodemographic confounders. Adjusted for multiple comparisons. A priori hypotheses based on biologically based time windows.	Careful assessment of exposure, analysis of specific time windows and dose–response relationships. Dicofol and endosulfan were the principal organochlorines.
Pyrethroids (bifenthrin)	Roberts et al. (2007)	See above.	RR = 4.8 (no CI given) for fourth nonzero quartile, 250m buffer, exposure from LMP to delivery.	See above.	Careful assessment of exposure, analysis of specific time windows, and dose–response relationships.
Organophosphates	Roberts et al. (2007)	See above.	RR = 1.6 (no CI given) for fourth nonzero quartile, 250m buffer, exposure from LMP to delivery.	See above.	Careful assessment of exposure, analysis of specific time windows, and dose–response relationships.
	Eskenazi et al. (2007)	Cohort; (n = 372), population of mainly Latino farmworkers.	RR = 2.25 (0.99, 5.16) for 10-fold increase in maternal urinary metabolites; RR = 1.71 (1.02, 2.87) for 10-fold increase in child's urinary metabolites.	Adjusted for age, sex, breastfeeding, HOME score, income, parity, maternal intelligence, and maternal depression. High prevalence of PDD***** may suggest overreporting of signs.	Prospective study with individual urinary measurements of DAPs (di-alkylphosphate) metabolites of organophosphates. Outcome was PDD subscale on the Child Behavior Checklist.

*Major studies included those with at least 50 cases and 100 total subjects. However, no attempt was made to be comprehensive or complete.
**All findings shown in this table are multivariate adjusted associations, unless otherwise noted.
***PPV = Positive predictive value.
****DDS = Department of Developmental Services of the State of California.
*****PDD = Pervasive Developmental Delay.

until 1991, and continued rising following removal of thimerosal from vaccines. A similar analysis was conducted using the California Department of Developmental Services data (Schechter & Grether, 2008) covering the period 1995 to 2007, which also found no fall-off in incidence after the removal of thimerosal from most U.S. vaccines. A Canadian study (Fombonne et al., 2006) using school-district-identified PDDs and assigning thimerosal doses based on grade level and immunization schedules for Quebec found that neither a continuous nor categorical ecologic measure of thimerosal exposure predicted autism incidence. The authors of the California study concluded, quite reasonably, that the "DDS data do not support the hypothesis that exposure to thimerosal during childhood is a *primary cause of autism* [italics added]." These studies provide evidence that a strong, predominant effect on risks for autism from thimerosal in vaccines is unlikely to have occurred.

In all three studies, the ecologic fallacy may have affected the findings because linkage between exposure and disease is not present, and hence, theoretically, cases could have been largely among the unexposed, yet the associations observed would be identical. More importantly, for time-trend studies, results can only be interpretable *when all other predictors of autism are held constant.* Since changes in ascertainment, relevant environmental exposures, and other risk factors contributing to incidence of autism are entirely plausible, ecologic studies are uninformative for assessing smaller contributions to risk from single factors.

Researchers from several countries, including Denmark, the United Kingdom, and the United States have retrospectively examined the link between thimerosal-containing vaccines in childhood and autism, using individual-level vaccine histories from medical records. Hviid et al. (2003) examined diagnoses for autism in a cohort of births spanning the period from 1990 to 1996, with follow-up through December 31, 2000. This analysis took advantage of the national Danish medical record system, whereby all vaccinations and all diagnoses can be linked. Follow-up for over 450,000 eligible children covered, collectively, nearly three million person-years and gave rise to 440 cases of autism and 787 cases of other autism spectrum disorders. During the time period of interest, only the pertussis vaccine contained thimerosal, and doses were calculated based on the number of pertussis vaccines received (1, 2, or 3) and the known composition of the formulation (50 μg of thimerosal, equal to ~25 μg of ethylmercury). Analyses adjusted for child's age and calendar period, or additionally for child's sex, place of birth, birth weight, 5-minute APGAR score, gestational age, mother's age at delivery, and mother's country of birth showed no elevated risk for autism, or for other autism spectrum disorders, regardless of the dose received. Despite control for numerous individual-level confounders, use of broad categories of calendar time against the backdrop of a steep, steady rise in incidence leaves open the possibility of residual confounding. Moreover, as described in the ecologic study by Madsen and colleagues, case ascertainment methods were inconsistent, involving inpatients only during the period prior to 1995 but both inpatients and outpatients afterward. As a result, the differential source of cases may have introduced misclassification bias.

Two major papers from the UK pertain to thimerosal from vaccines. Andrews et al. (Andrews et al., 2004) utilized a cohort of over 100,000 children born in 1988 through 1997 in a consortium of general practices in the UK. The second study, though smaller, involved an in-depth characterization of a birth cohort (Avon Longitudinal Study of Parents and Children or ALSPAC), with a broad spectrum of outcomes and covariates collected prospectively and systematically (Heron & Golding, 2004). Of the vaccines routinely administered to infants in the UK during the 1970s and 1980s, thimerosal was only used in diphtheria-tetanus-whole-cell pertussis (DTP), diphtheria-tetanus (DT), and combination vaccines containing these two, with doses similar to those used in the pertussis vaccine in Denmark. In 1990, the UK changed from a 3-, 5-, 10-month schedule to a 2-, 3-, 4-month schedule, leading to a dose of 75 μg mercury by 4 months of age in infants receiving the recommended dose on schedule.

The focus of the analysis in both investigations was to compare those with earlier vs. later receipt of thimerosal-containing vaccines. Exposure was defined as number of doses by 3 months of age, by 4 months of age, and a constructed scale for combined doses to 6 months of age. To account for wide variability in durations of follow-up, both studies appropriately performed survival analysis using Cox proportional hazards models. Andrews and coworkers (Andrews et al., 2004) found no increased incidence of autism, comparing those who received their DPT or DT vaccines earlier vs. later; the hazard ratios for autism ranged from 0.89 to 0.99. Of the nine developmental conditions examined in the consortium of general practices, only tics were significantly elevated in those with greater doses at an early age, but incidences of general developmental disorder, ADD, unspecified developmental delay, and autism were all significantly *reduced* in those who received earlier doses of thimerosal. A similar analysis in the ALSPAC study showed, among the 23 adverse developmental outcomes (with fewer than 10,000 in the cohort, autism diagnoses were too rare for analysis), the only significantly elevated risk for an adverse outcome was for poor scores on prosocial behaviors; five other significant results showed positive outcomes associated with early life thimerosal exposure (Heron & Golding, 2004). Data on potential confounding variables such as maternal and paternal age were not available in the Andrews study, and autism diagnoses were not validated, whereas in the ALSPAC study, numerous potential confounders were controlled (birth weight, gestational age, maternal education, parity, midpregnancy smoking status, breastfeeding, child's gender and ethnicity, and housing).

The authors of two studies (Andrews et al., 2004; Heron & Golding, 2004) do not comment on the unexpectedly high proportion of outcomes showing reduced incidence or improved scores. One interpretation is that early vaccines benefit several domains of neurodevelopment. An alternative possibility is that of reverse causation. In other words, the healthiest babies would be those who were given the earliest vaccines, while vaccines may have been withheld for later administration to those not thriving or with indications of problems predictive of developmental delays. Similar to the "healthy worker effect," this may represent a "healthy vaccinee effect."

Thimerosal was used in a wider range of vaccines in the U.S., resulting in infant doses of up to 187.5μg by 7 months of age as compared with a maximum of 75μg in Denmark and the UK. The Centers for Disease Control and Prevention in the United States sponsored a retrospective study (Verstraeten et al., 2003) that took advantage of computerized databases from three health maintenance organizations (HMOs), which are combined into the Vaccine Safety Datalink. This combined database includes medical event information, specific vaccine history, including manufacturer and lot number, and selected demographic variables. Exposures were estimated from DTP, hepatitis B, and Haemophilus influenza type B (Hib) vaccines.

Only one of the three HMOs had adequate statistical power to examine the association with autism, and no significant elevation in risk was found for cumulative dose at 1 month of age, nor for doses at 3 or 7 months of age (Verstraeten et al., 2003). A considerable limitation in this study was the exclusion of a relatively large proportion of children. In the largest HMO, 24% of births were excluded on the basis of low birth weight or congenital, perinatal, or maternal complications or medical problems. Since several of these factors, and neonatal suboptimality in general, are indicators of increased risk for autism, it is possible that the authors excluded the most vulnerable children. Further concerns about the Vaccine Safety Database were discussed by an expert panel convened by the U.S. National Institutes of Health (NIH) (Hertz-Picciotto et al., 2006).

A small study of thimerosal exposure and neurodevelopmental outcomes was carried out using a subset of participants from a previously conducted randomized trial of two acellular diphtheria-tetanus vaccines in Italy (Tozzi et al., 2009), one with and one without thimerosal. With only one case of autism identified in about 1,700 children, this research was extremely underpowered and did not meet our criteria for "large-scale" epidemiologic studies.

From the public health viewpoint, it is clear that these vaccines are essential to the core mission of protecting our population from life-threatening diseases. A National Academy of Sciences panel concluded that "the evidence is inadequate to accept or reject a causal relationship between exposure to thimerosal from vaccines and the neurodevelopmental disorders of autism...." They also recommended that action to remove thimerosal from vaccines and other pharmaceutical products "might be warranted to ensure that exposures to thimerosal do not contribute to combined mercury exposures that could exceed guidelines for safe exposure." (Stratton et al., 2001). At the time of the report, there were no published epidemiologic studies examining the hypothesis that exposure to thimerosal-containing vaccines was associated with autism. By now, four studies of adequate sample size have now appeared, each of which provides evidence for a "null" conclusion. Nevertheless, none is free from serious inherent limitations.

To summarize, multiple investigations have assessed the association between thimerosal-containing vaccines given to infants and the risk for autism. The continuing trend toward increased incidence of autism, even after the removal of thimerosal from vaccines, demonstrates that the steep rise in diagnoses of the last 15 to 20 years cannot be explained by this preservative. If thimerosal has played any role, it likely has been a small one. Yet misclassification and other uncertainties in data quality, inadequate control for confounding in the analysis, and/or systematic biases in the study populations have reduced the ability of these studies to validly test the theory, underscoring the need for stronger science on this question. Although the extant literature does not rule out a contribution of thimerosal as one of many risk factors for autism, possibly acting on a susceptible subset of the population, at present there are no published studies supporting this hypothesis.

Mercury from Other Sources

Other major sources of mercury exposures include dental amalgams (inorganic Hg), industrial emissions leading to air or water pollution (elemental Hg), and fish or seafood (methylmercury). Hair Hg is known to be an excellent biomarker, consisting of about 80% organic Hg (primarily methyl) with about 20% inorganic Hg (Clarkson & Magos, 2006). An autopsy study of brain Hg levels in neonates who died of natural causes showed that either biomarker, maternal blood or maternal hair, correlates with the infant brain levels (Cernichiari et al., 1995).

Several studies have compared hair measurements of Hg in cases and controls. One group reported lower concentrations in the first haircut from children with autism (Holmes et al., 2003). However, the mean hair concentration in their control series was unusually high: 16-fold greater than the mean from the National Health and Nutrition Examination Survey (NHANES) representative sample of children 1 to 5 years of age. In fact, the vast majority of measurements on the controls were above the 95th percentile in the NHANES sample, whereas the concentrations in the children with the greatest severity of autism were very close to the national average (McDowell et al., 2004). These issues combined with absent information regarding whether cases and controls were analyzed simultaneously on the same instruments, whether the laboratory personnel were blinded, and how contamination was addressed, raise concerns about validity of the findings.

Other studies conducted measurements in specimens collected *postdiagnosis* and therefore do not directly address the role of Hg as a causal factor in autism, although differences in concentrations have been argued to indicate altered metabolism, distribution and/or excretion. However, without quantification of and control for intake (e.g., via diet and other routes), such conclusions are not warranted. A study of post diagnosis blood concentration in children from the CHARGE (Childhood Autism Risks from Genetics and Environment Study), after adjustment for dietary and other Hg sources, observed no differences comparing children with autism to typically developing controls (Hertz- Picciotto et al., 2010).

Exposures to mercury in ambient air are discussed in the next section.

Ambient Air Pollutants

Investigators in two states have examined air pollutants in relation to autism. In an ecologic design, rates of autism were related to industrial emissions of mercury and mercury compounds in school districts in Texas (Palmer et al., 2006), but besides the problem of ecologic fallacy, incomplete confounder control likely occurred. The coefficient for mercury emissions was substantially lowered by adjustment for numbers of special education students (influenced by availability of special education classes), and addition of other socioeconomic or educational variables might have further reduced it. Also, the handling of zero or small event cells could have induced bias (Bartell & Lewandowski, in press). The large reduction in the coefficient for mercury emissions after adjustment for numbers of special education students (often influenced by availability of special education classes) suggests that inclusion of a few other socioeconomic or educational variables might have reduced the association even further. Moreover, exposure data was concurrent with autism cases (i.e., occurring when children have already reached school age and hence unlikely to be etiologically relevant since autism, by definition, develops before 36 months of age).

A second study examining emissions into ambient air was conducted in the San Francisco Bay Area (Windham et al., 2006). Analyses focused on 19 compounds having sufficient exposure variability within this region and with known or suspected developmental, neurologic or endocrine-disrupting toxicity. Using a case-control design, the authors confirmed diagnoses through an expert review of DDS case records, and selected controls from birth records, matching 2:1 to cases by county and month of birth. Residential address at the time of delivery was geocoded and linked to Census tract. Census-tract-specific average annual exposures for each compound were derived from models of Hazardous Air Pollutants (HAPs) emissions based on locations of large polluting industries, smaller area emitters, and mobile sources. Exposures for each child were ranked, and analysis compared the upper two quartiles with those below the median. Other analyses grouped compounds by structure (aromatic solvents, chlorinated solvents, metals) or mechanism (endocrine disruptors, developmental toxicants).

After adjusting for maternal age, education and race, Windham and colleagues found significantly elevated odds ratios for 3rd or 4th quartile exposures for several individual HAPs, (namely methylene chloride, trichloroethylene, vinyl chloride, cadmium, mercury and nickel) and also for chlorinated solvents and metals. Many of these exposures were strongly intercorrelated and hence the individual results require further follow-up to determine which, if any, of these compounds might play a role in autism etiology. This problem, combined with the use of long-term (annual) modeled estimates of ambient air concentrations that corresponded to postnatal year 2 or 3 of the child's life, complicate the interpretation of findings. Nevertheless, despite these caveats, the report by Windham et al. took a commendably evenhanded approach to generating useful leads about environmental causes of autism, and is a refreshing contrast to the many ecologic studies on autism that lack individual-level information on confounding factors and/or use databases with major biases (e.g., related to funding of educational services).

Volk and colleagues (2010) also conducted a study with individual level data, investigate exposure to traffic, a surrogate for air pollution rom vehicle emission. In this case-control study from California (the CHARGE study), addresses of mothers at the time of delivery or during pregnancy were geocoded and distance to the closest freeway was calculated. Those children born to mothers residing within 309 m of the nearest freeway had a 1.9-fold greater risk for autism. All cases in this study were clinically confirmed using the ADI-R and the Autism Diagnostic Obsevation Schedule. Exposures to pollutants decline to background at about 300 m from a freeway, supporting plausibility of a true association.

Pesticides

Major classes of pesticides include organochlorines (OCs), organophosphates (OPs), carbamates, and pyrethroids. Their mechanisms of action differ in the details, but many insecticides are designed to kill insects by acting directly on the CNS. The primary acute effect of OPs, used largely for cockroaches, is acetylcholinesterase inhibition, but at subacute levels, especially in the prenatal period, noncholinergic mechanisms may be most relevant (Rauh et al., 2006). Most OCs are endocrine disruptors, and many dysregulate thyroid homeostasis or have estrogenic, antiestrogenic, androgenic, or antiandrogenic activity. Several large investigations into pesticide exposures as a risk factor for autism have produced intriguing results.

Roberts and colleagues (Roberts et al., 2007) used record linkage among California's DDS system, Vital Statistics birth records and Pesticide Use Reporting System. The study population was based on births in 19 highly agricultural counties. Pesticide exposures were compared for DDS autism or ASD cases, with 15 controls matched to each case based on last menstrual period in birth records. Three time periods of exposure were examined, corresponding to neural tube closure, CNS development during embryogenesis, and the entire pregnancy period. For a total of 249 combinations of chemicals/chemical compounds, time periods of application, and distances of pesticide application to the residential address at the time of birth, the authors compared those at the highest quartile of nonzero exposure to the unexposed. After adjustment for multiple testing, the most significant findings were for organochlorine pesticides, with an adjusted odds ratio of 4.2 (95% CI = 1.7, 10.9) for applications during embryonic CNS development. The third-quartile exposures were elevated but not as strikingly. Dicofol and endosulfan were the primary compounds in this class. Several other associations were also significant: bifenthrin, a pyrethroid pesticide, with an adjusted OR of 4.8 (p = 0.005) for exposure at any time during gestation; and the class of organophosphates, with an adjusted OR of 1.6 (p = 0.006) for exposure at any time during gestation.

OPs are used not only in agriculture but also for home applications. Eskenazi and colleagues (Eskenazi et al., 2007) followed a birth cohort of primarily Hispanic families living in the Salinas Valley and evaluated metabolites of OP pesticides in urine collected during pregnancy and postnatally in relation to neurodevelopmental tests, including a subscale for Pervasive Developmental Disorders on the Child Behavior Check List for ages 1.5 to 5 years of age (Achenbach & Rescorla, 2000). Items resemble behaviors from the ADI-R, including: "avoids eye contact," "rocks head, body," and "unresponsive to affection." Urine specimens were analyzed for six nonspecific dialkyl phosphate (DAP) metabolites, representing the bulk of agricultural OP pesticides used in the California Salinas Valley, and previously reported to be associated with shorter gestation and abnormal neonatal reflexes (Eskenazi et al., 2004; Young et al., 2005). In this study, a 10-fold increase in total DAPs was associated with an approximate 2.2-fold higher odds of scoring in the clinical or borderline clinical range for PDD. Of 355 children, 14.4% scored above the 97th percentile on the PDD subscale, and another 29.6% were above the 93rd percentile. With a total of 44% affected, the ORs would be overestimates of the corresponding relative risks. Additionally, the high scores on the PDD subscale suggest that the administration of this subscale possibly was not reliable, and/or the translation into Spanish might not have appropriately captured the intent with regard to scoring of behaviors. Nevertheless, these findings, combined with the results mentioned above (Roberts et al., 2007) related to commercially applied organophosphates in the central valley suggest further investigation of these compounds in relation to autism or ASD is warranted.

Other supporting evidence regarding OPs comes from a comparative study of gene variants in autism family trios in Italy and North America (D'Amelio et al., 2005). OPs are detoxified by paraoxonase, an enzyme encoded by the gene PON1. Using four different statistical approaches, a significant association between autism and PON1 variants that were less active in in vitro tests was found in the North American sample but not the Italian one. This finding is consistent with a causal role for OP pesticides since they are far more widely used in North American than Italian households.

Since the banning of most organophosphates for home uses, pyrethroid and pyrethrin pesticides are increasingly used for control of household insects, recently reported to account for 17% of world insecticide sales (Davies et al., 2007). Pyrethrins are present in pet shampoos for fleas and ticks; pyrethroids, which are a synthetic version engineered for greater toxicity to insects, are widely used in household sprays and foggers for ants, flies, and cockroaches. In insects, they interfere with voltage-sensitive sodium channels (Davies et al., 2007; Shafer et al., 2005), although rodent studies also suggest glutamergic, and mechanisms GABA-mediated (Hossain et al., 2008), BDNF-gene expression changes (Imamura et al., 2006) and compromise of the blood brain barrier (Sinha et al., 2004). Pyrethroids are immunotoxic in experimental animals, causing decreased thymic weight (Garg et al., 2004; Prater et al., 2003), suppressed cellular immunity (Blaylock et al., 1995), altered macrophage, T cell and neutrophil function and lower IgG (Liu et al., 2006; Righi & Palermo-Neto, 2005) and reduced antibody production (Punareewattana et al., 2001). Two years after acute pyrethroid intoxication, patients had autoimmune disorders, deficient cellular and humoral immunity, and opportunistic infections (Muller-Mohnssen, 1999). These compounds have received little attention in human studies, but concern is raised by the presence of metabolites of pyrethroids in urine of most U.S. adults. Metabolites of pyrethroids are found in most U.S. adults (NHANES, 1999; Riederer et al., 2008).

Endocrine Disruptors

To date, little research has directly addressed any role of these compounds in autism etiology, but the critical contributions of various hormones to prenatal CNS development has led to numerous hypotheses. Many organochlorines are known to disrupt thyroid hormone homeostasis, as well as sex steroids, and the pesticides identified by Roberts & colleagues to be associated with autism (Roberts et al., 2007), endosulfan and dicofol are no exceptions. Thyroid hormones and sex steroids are of particular interest, and disruption of these endocrine systems by environmental pollutants has been studied extensively, including polychlorinated and polybrominated compounds, dioxins, pesticides, phthalates, bisphenol A, lead, and mercury. Thyroid hormones, specifically tri-iodothyronine, are required for differentiation and neuronal migration in early to mid-prenatal life, with common outcomes of hypothyroidism being mental retardation, deafness and speech problems (Porterfield, 1994). PCBs and other thyroid-disrupting chemicals have been shown to reduce levels of free and total thyroxine, inhibit sulfation, bind to thyroxine transport proteins, alter thyroid enzyme activity in the brain and/or increase levels of TSH in experimental animals (Brouwer, 1989; Brouwer et al., 1998; Crofton, 2008; Morse et al., 1993; Zoeller & Crofton, 2000; Abdelouahab et al., 2009). Roman has proposed that even a transient disruption in thyroid hormone homeostasis of a few days during prenatal development could underlie some cases of autism (Roman, 2007).

Numerous pollutants, including PCBs, dioxins, dichlorodiphenyltrichloroethane (DDT), phthalates, bisphenol A, and polybrominated diphenl ethers (PBDEs), and/or their metabolites (OH-PCBs, OH-dioxins, OH-BPA, etc.) have estrogenic, antiestrogenic, androgenic, or antiandrogenic properties

(Kester et al., 2002; Darnerud, 2008; Moore et al., 1997; Hamers et al., 2008; Meeker et al., 2009; Wilson et al., 2008). Human PBDE concentrations were found to be associated with free androgen index, as well as luteinizing hormone and follicle-stimulating hormone (Meeker et al., 2009). Baron-Cohen and colleagues have hypothesized that sex steroids, especially fetal testosterone concentrations in prenatal life, may alter autism-related behaviors and play a role in the sex ratio of autism diagnoses (Baron-Cohen et al., 2005; Knickmeyer et al., 2006). If this hypothesis is confirmed, some of the aforementioned compounds could operate through such a mechanism. PBDE concentrations in human tissues have been increasing over the last few decades (Sjodin et al., 2004). Phthalates operate as antiandrogens, and bisphenol A is estrogenic (Talsness et al., 2009). In a nationally representative sample of adults from the U.S., 92% had detectable levels of bisphenol A (Lang et al., 2008).

Lifestyle

Few studies have addressed potential risk factors such as smoking, alcohol, diet, or other aspects of lifestyle. The large-scale Swedish case-control study by Hultman et al., described above, observed daily smoking to be associated with a modest increase in risk for autism, OR = 1.4 (95% CI = 1.1, 1.8), whereas a population-based Danish study (Maimburg & Vaeth, 2006) did not find an association comparing smokers to nonsmokers based on maternal report at her first prenatal visit. The few case reports on alcohol do not represent real evidence of a link to autism, as discussed by Fombonne (2002).

Over the last few years, a number of nutritional hypotheses have been proposed for factors that might contribute to autism or explain its rise. At a fundamental level, nutritional factors have been shown to affect epigenetics, which in turn influences gene expression. Muskiet and Kemperman (2006) hypothesize that both autism and schizophrenia are influenced by early folate. Evidence cited in support of this theory comes from those exposed prenatally to the Dutch hunger, in which both schizophrenia and neural tube defects were increased, and elevated prevalence of MTHFR 677C→T homozygotes among schizophrenics. Data from the California-based CHARGE Study also indicate the use of prenatal supplements during the 3 months prior to conception or first month after conception may reduce the risk of autism (Schmidt et al., in press). Evidence also supports interactions between maternal intake of prenatal supplements and variants in folate metabolism genes. Rodier argues for an initial event occurring near the time of neural tube closure (Rodier et al., 1997). Folate may function epigenetically by ensuring sufficient methyl groups on DNA, or may promote methylation of proteins, phospholipids, and neurotransmitters in the prenatal period and beyond (Moretti et al., 2004).

Muskiet and Kemperman further postulate that these neuropsychiatric disorders are characterized by deficiency in long chain polyunsaturated fatty acids such as arachidonic acid and docosahexanoic acid (DHA), essential in the phospholipids layer of cell membranes and critical to cell signaling. One report from the large CHARGE study (Wiest et al., 2009) and several smaller studies (Bell et al., 2000; Vancassel et al., 2001) provide supportive data regarding a deficiency of DHA in children with autism or ASD.

Another micronutrient proposed to be influential in autism etiology is zinc, which plays an essential role in preventing oxidative damage and ensuring expression of genes that direct embryonic development of the cerebral cortex and adrenal glands (Johnson, 2001).

Concern has been raised regarding reduced levels of vitamin D (Cannell, 2008). Also known as calcitriol, vitamin D is both a nutrient and a hormone. It is suggested that over the last few decades, vitamin D deficiency has increased as a result of increased use of sunscreens and reduced time spent outdoors. A remarkably high percentage of pregnant women are deficient in calcitriol (Bodnar et al., 2007). Prenatally, the vitamin D receptor appears in the brain very early in gestation, and vitamin D deficiency is associated with altered expression of proteins involved in neurotransmission, synapse formation, and calcium homeostasis (Almeras et al., 2007).

Based on the hypothesis that transient hypothyroxinemia early in gestation contributes to autism, Roman (2007) catalogs the many dietary, pharmacologic, and environmental chemical exposures that could operate through this pathway. These include soy-based flavonoids, pearl millet, and plants rich in thiocyanate, such as cabbage, cauliflower, and lima beans. Besides natural food sources, chemicals with antithyroid activity are found in tobacco smoke, many herbicides, PCBs, perchlorate, mercury, and phthalates.

Conclusion

From all the evidence gathered at this point in time, the etiology of autism appears to be highly multifactorial, complex in regard to timing of insults, influenced by susceptibility genes, and dependent on synergistic effects of combined exposures. From large epidemiologic studies, the data currently provide clues but few definitive results. The consistent increases in risk with advanced parental age might indicate a wide array of types of mechanisms. Strong associations with infectious agents, specifically viral infections during pregnancy, are intriguing; however, most of these are today quite rare because of vaccinations. The one exception is influenza. A number of investigations implicate one or another obstetric condition or medical intervention, but methodologic flaws impart the need for caution in interpretation. Studies on the MMR vaccine have not supported any major role, though more rigorous studies could enhance definitiveness of results. Investigations into thimersal have similarly shown no evidence of association with autism, but significant weaknesses in their design, and/or deficiencies in the analysis leave open the possibility of effects in susceptible subgroups. Suggestive data on pesticides and sources of fetal stress should be pursued, including ambient air pollutants, such as from vehicle emissions. Additionally, mechanistic and toxicity studies provide the bases for future studies on a wide range of environmental chemicals, especially persistent organic compounds with endocrine-disrupting capacity. Nutritional factors also deserve serious attention.

To date, no gene has been identified that accounts for more than a few percent of autism cases, whereas linkage has been found to regions on virtually every chromosome. It is likely that the situation for environmental factors will similarly uncover dozens of factors each contributing to a relatively small proportion of cases. To the extent that the field assumes a "smoking gun," progress will appear disappointingly slow. Nevertheless, casting a wide net, linking large-scale epidemiologic investigations with state-of-the-art molecular science, "omics" or high-throughput technologies and mechanistic studies, and pursuing exploration of interactions—geneX-environment, geneXgene, and environmentXenvironment—are strategies that can be expected, with high probability, to bear fruit.

Challenges & Future Directions

- Autism etiology is multifactorial and the specific factors involved are likely quite heterogeneous, with each playing a relatively small role.
- Interactions of environmental, modifiable factors with common gene polymorphisms, or possibly sequence variants, may be involved in the vast majority of autism cases, dictating that large sample sizes are need to unravel these causes.
- Future studies should seek integration across disciplines and across mechanisms of investigation, from the molecular genetic, epigenetic, or signaling pathway to disruption of cellular or physiologic function, to the organismic, behavioral, and social levels of human responses.
- Molecular epidemiology is a particularly fruitful strategy, linking state-of-the-art bench science with large-scale human studies collecting biospecimens and a wide array of phenotypic, medical, environmental, social, and behavioral measurements.
- Attention to timing of exposures is critical, as there may be windows of vulnerability corresponding to specific mechanisms, developmental stages, or types of insult.

SUGGESTED READING

Daniels, J. (2006). Autism and the environment. *Environmental Health Perspectives, 114*, A396. PMID: 16835036.

Hertz-Picciotto, I., Croen, L., Hansen, R., Jones, C., & Pessah, I. N. (2006). The CHARGE Study: An epidemiologic investigation of genetic and environmental factors contributing to autism. *Environmental Health Perspectives, 114*(7), 1119–1125. Retrieved from http://www.ehponline.org/members/2006/8483/8483.pdf.

Newschaffer, C. J., Croen, L. A., Daniels, J., Giarelli, E., Grether, J. K., Levy, S. E., et al. (2007). *Annual Review of Public Health, 28*, 235–258. Review. PMID: 17367287.

REFERENCES

Abdelouahab, N., Suvorov, A., Pasquier, J. C., Langlois, M. F., Praud, J. P., & Takser, L. (2009). Thyroid disruption by low-dose BDE-47 in prenatally exposed lambs. *Neonatology, 96*(2), 120–124.

Achenbach, T., & Rescorla, L. (2000). *Manual for the ASEBA preschool forms and profiles.*

Almeras, L., Eyles, D., Benech, P., Laffite, D., Villard, C., Patatian, A., et al. (2007). Developmental vitamin D deficiency alters brain protein expression in the adult rat: Implications for neuropsychiatric disorders. *Proteomics, 7*(5), 769–780.

Andrews, N., Miller, E., Grant, A., Stowe, J., Osborne, V., & Taylor, B. (2004). Thimerosal exposure in infants and developmental disorders: a retrospective cohort study in the United Kingdom does not support a causal association. *Pediatrics, 114*(3), 584–591.

Ashwood, P., Enstrom, A., Krakowiak, P., Hertz-Picciotto, I., Hansen, R. L., Croen, L. A., et al. (2008). Decreased transforming growth factor beta1 in autism: A potential link between immune dysregulation and impairment in clinical behavioral outcomes. *Journal of Neuroimmunology, 204*(1–2), 149–153.

Atladottir, H. O., Parner, E. T., Schendel, D., Dalsgaard, S., Thomsen, P. H., & Thorsen, P. (2007). Variation in incidence of neurodevelopmental disorders with season of birth. *Epidemiology, 18*(2), 240–245.

Bailey, A., Le Couteur, A., Gottesman, I., Bolton, P., Simonoff, E., Yuzda, E., et al. (1995). Autism as a strongly genetic disorder: evidence from a British twin study. *Psychological Medicine, 25*(1), 63–77.

Baird, G., Simonoff, E., Pickles, A., Chandler, S., Loucas, T., Meldrum, D., et al. (2006). Prevalence of disorders of the autism spectrum in a population cohort of children in South Thames: The Special Needs and Autism Project (SNAP). *Lancet, 368*(9531), 210–215.

Barak, Y., Ring, A., Sulkes, J., Gabbay, U., & Elizur, A. (1995). Season of birth and autistic disorder in Israel. *American Journal of Psychiatry, 152*(5), 798–800.

Baron-Cohen, S., Knickmeyer, R. C., & Belmonte, M. K. (2005). Sex differences in the brain: Implications for explaining autism. *Science, 310*(5749), 819–823.

Bartell, S. M., Lewandowski, T. A. (in press). Administrative censoring in ecological analyses of autism, and a Bayesian solution. *Journal of Environmental and Public Health.*

Bartlik, B. D. (1981). Monthly variation in births of autistic children in North Carolina. *Journal of the American Medical Women's Association, 36*(12), 363–368.

Bell, E. M., Hertz-Picciotto, I., & Beaumont, J. J. (2001a). A case-control study of pesticides and fetal death due to congenital anomalies. *Epidemiology, 12*(2), 148–156.

Bell, E. M., Hertz-Picciotto, I., & Beaumont, J. J. (2001b). Pesticides and fetal death due to congenital anomalies: Implications of an erratum. *Epidemiology, 12*(5), 595–596.

Bell, J. G., Sargent, J. R., Tocher, D. R., & Dick, J. R (2000). Red blood cell fatty acid compositions in a patient with autistic spectrum disorder: A characteristic abnormality in neurodevelopmental disorders? *Prostaglandins, Leukotrienes, and Essential Fatty Acids, 63*(1–2), 21–25.

Berkowitz, G. S., Skovron, M. L., Lapinski, R. H., & Berkowitz, R. L. (1990). Delayed childbearing and the outcome of pregnancy. *New England Journal of Medicine, 322*(10), 659–664.

Bernard, S., Blaxill, M., & Redwood, L. (2008). Re: Miles & Takahashi paper on RhIg and autism. *American Journal of Medical Genetics. Part A, 146*(3), 405–406; author reply 407.

Bhasin, T. K., & Schendel, D. (2007). Sociodemographic risk factors for autism in a U.S. metropolitan area. *Journal of Autism and Developmental Disorders, 37*(4), 667–677.

Bilder, D., Pinborough-Zimmerman, J., Miller, J., & McMahon, W. (2009). Prenatal, perinatal, and neonatal factors associated with autism spectrum disorders. *Pediatrics, 123*(5), 1293–1300.

Blaylock, B. L., Abdel-Nasser, M., McCarty, S. M., Knesel, J. A., Tolson, K. M., Ferguson, P. W., et al. (1995). Suppression of cellular immune responses in BALB/c mice following oral exposure to permethrin. *Bulletin of Environmental Contamination and Toxicology, 54*(5), 768–774.

Bodnar, L. M., Simhan, H. N., Powers, R. W., Frank, M. P., Cooperstein, E., & Roberts, J. M. (2007). High prevalence of vitamin D insufficiency in black and white pregnant women residing in the northern United States and their neonates. *Journal of Nutrition, 137*(2), 447–452.

Boksa, P., Zhang, Y., Amritraj, A., & Kar, S. (2006). Birth insults involving hypoxia produce long-term increases in hippocampal [125I] insulin-like growth factor-I and -II receptor binding in the rat. *Neuroscience, 139*(2), 451–462.

Boksa, P., Zhang, Y., & Bestawros, A. (2002). Dopamine D1 receptor changes due to caesarean section birth: Effects of anesthesia, developmental time course, and functional consequences. *Experimental Neurology, 175*(2), 388–397.

Bolton, P., Pickles, A., Harrington, R., Macdonald, H., & Rutter, M. (1992). Season of birth: Issues, approaches and findings for autism. *Journal of Child Psychology and Psychiatry and Allied Disciplines, 33*(3), 509–530.

Boyd, J. H., Pulver, A. E., & Stewart, W. (1986). Season of birth: Schizophrenia and bipolar disorder. *Schizophrenia Bulletin, 12*(2), 173–186.

Braunschweig, D., Ashwood, P., Krakowiak, P., Hertz-Picciotto, I., Hansen, R., Croen, L. A., et al. (2008). Autism: Maternally derived antibodies specific for fetal brain proteins. *Neurotoxicology, 29*(2), 226–231.

Brouwer, A. (1989). Inhibition of thyroid hormone transport in plasma of rats by polychlorinated biphenyls. *Archives of toxicology. Supplement. = Archiv fur Toxikologie. Supplement, 13*, 440–445.

Brouwer, A., Morse, D. C., Lans, M. C., Schuur, A. G., Murk, A. J., Klasson-Wehler, E., et al. (1998). Interactions of persistent environmental organohalogens with the thyroid hormone system: Mechanisms and possible consequences for animal and human health. *Toxicology and Industrial Health, 14*(1–2), 59–84.

Brown, A. S., Begg, M. D., Gravenstein, S., Schaefer, C. A., Wyatt, R. J., Bresnahan, M., et al. (2004). Serologic evidence of prenatal influenza in the etiology of schizophrenia. *Archives of General Psychiatry, 61*(8), 774–780.

Burd, L., Severud, R., Kerbeshian, J., & Klug, M. G. (1999). Prenatal and perinatal risk factors for autism. *Journal of Perinatal Medicine, 27*(6), 441–450.

Cannell, J. J. (2008). Autism and vitamin D. *Medical Hypotheses, 70*(4), 750–759.

Castellani, M. L., Conti, C. M., Kempuraj, D. J., Salini, V., Vecchiet, J., Tete, S., et al. (2009). Autism and immunity: Revisited study. *International Journal of Immunopathology and Pharmacology, 22*(1), 15–19.

Cernichiari, E., Brewer, R., Myers, G. J., Marsh, D. O., Lapham, L. W., Cox, C., et al. (1995). Monitoring methylmercury during pregnancy: Maternal hair predicts fetal brain exposure. *Neurotoxicology, 16*(4), 705–710.

Chess, S. (1971). Autism in children with congenital rubella. *Journal of Autism and Childhood Schizophrenia, 1*(1), 33–47.

Chess, S. (1977). Follow-up report on autism in congenital rubella. *Journal of Autism and Childhood Schizophrenia, 7*(1), 69–81.

Clarkson, T. W., & Magos, L. (2006). The toxicology of mercury and its chemical compounds. *Critical Reviews in Toxicology, 36*(8), 609–662.

Clarkson, T. W., Magos, L., & Myers, G. J. (2003). The toxicology of mercury: Current exposures and clinical manifestations. *New England Journal of Medicine, 349*(18), 1731–1737.

Cole, S. R., & Hernan, M. A. (2002). Fallibility in estimating direct effects. *International Journal of Epidemiology, 31*(1), 163–165.

Croen, L. A., Grether, J. K., & Selvin, S. (2002). Descriptive epidemiology of autism in a California population: Who is at risk? *Journal of Autism and Developmental Disorders, 32*(3), 217–224.

Croen, L. A., Matevia, M., Yoshida, C. K., & Grether, J. K. (2008). Maternal Rh D status, anti-D immune globulin exposure during pregnancy, and risk of autism spectrum disorders. *American Journal of Obstetrics and Gynecology, 199*(3), e231–236.

Croen, L. A., Najjar, D. V., Fireman, B., & Grether, J. K. (2007). Maternal and paternal age and risk of autism spectrum disorders. *Archives of Pediatrics and Adolescent Medicine, 161*(4), 334–340.

Crofton, K. M. (2008). Thyroid disrupting chemicals: Mechanisms and mixtures. *International Journal of Andrology, 31*(2), 209–223.

D'Amelio, M., Ricci, I., Sacco, R., Liu, X., D'Agruma, L., Muscarella, L. A., et al. (2005). Paraoxonase gene variants are associated with autism in North America, but not in Italy: Possible regional specificity in gene-environment interactions. *Molecular Psychiatry, 10*(11), 1006–1016.

Dales, L., Hammer, S. J., & Smith, N. J. (2001). Time trends in autism and in MMR immunization coverage in California. *Journal of the American Medical Association, 285*(9), 1183–1185.

Darnerud, P. O. (2008). Brominated flame retardants as possible endocrine disrupters. *International Journal of Andrology, 31*(2), 152–160.

Davies, T. G., Field, L. M., Usherwood, P. N., & Williamson, M. S. (2007). DDT, pyrethrins, pyrethroids and insect sodium channels. *IUBMB Life, 59*(3), 151–162.

Desi, I., Dobronyi, I., & Varga, L. (1986). Immuno-, neuro-, and general toxicologic animal studies on a synthetic pyrethroid: cypermethrin. *Ecotoxicology and Environmental Safety, 12*(3), 220–232.

Desmond, M. M., Wilson, G. S., Melnick, J. L., Singer, D. B., Zion, T. E., Rudolph, A. J., et al. (1967). Congenital rubella encephalitis. Course and early sequelae. *Journal of Pediatrics, 71*(3), 311–331.

DeStefano, F., Bhasin, T. K., Thompson, W. W., Yeargin-Allsopp, M., & Boyle, C. (2004). Age at first measles-mumps-rubella vaccination in children with autism and school-matched control subjects: A population-based study in metropolitan Atlanta. *Pediatrics, 113*(2), 259–266.

Deykin, E. Y., & MacMahon, B. (1979). Viral exposure and autism. *American Journal of Epidemiology, 109*(6), 628–638.

Dietert, R. R., & Piepenbrink, M. S. (2006). Perinatal immunotoxicity: Why adult exposure assessment fails to predict risk. *Environmental Health Perspectives, 114*(4), 477–483.

Djahanbakhch, O., Ezzati, M., & Zosmer, A. (2007). Reproductive aging in women. The Journal of Pathology, *211*(2), 219–231.

Durkin, M. S., Maenner, M. J., Newschaffer, C. J., Lee, L. C., Cunniff, C. M., Daniels, J. L., et al. (2008). Advanced parental age and the risk of autism spectrum disorder. *American Journal of Epidemiology, 168*(11), 1268–1276.

Eaton, W. W., Mortensen, P. B., Thomsen, P. H., & Frydenberg, M. (2001). Obstetric complications and risk for severe psychopathology in childhood. *Journal of Autism and Developmental Disorders, 31*(3), 279–285.

Enstrom, A. M., Lit, L., Onore, C. E., Gregg, J. P., Hansen, R. L., Pessah, I. N., et al. (2009). Altered gene expression and function of peripheral blood natural killer cells in children with autism. *Brain, Behavior, and Immunity, 23*(1), 124–133.

Eskenazi, B., Harley, K., Bradman, A., Weltzien, E., Jewell, N. P., Barr, D. B., et al. (2004). Association of in utero organophosphate pesticide exposure and fetal growth and length of gestation in an agricultural population. *Environmental Health Perspectives, 112*(10), 1116–1124.

Eskenazi, B., Marks, A. R., Bradman, A., Harley, K., Barr, D. B., Johnson, C., et al. (2007). Organophosphate pesticide exposure and neurodevelopment in young Mexican-American children. *Environmental Health Perspectives, 115*(5), 792–798.

Flores, C., Stewart, J., Salmaso, N., Zhang, Y., & Boksa, P. (2002). Astrocytic basic fibroblast growth factor expression in dopaminergic regions after perinatal anoxia. *Biological Psychiatry, 52*(4), 362–370.

Fombonne, E. (2002). Is exposure to alcohol during pregnancy a risk factor for autism? *Journal of Autism and Developmental Disorders, 32*(3), 243.

Fombonne, E. (2003). Epidemiological surveys of autism and other pervasive developmental disorders: An update. *Journal of Autism and Developmental Disorders, 33*(4), 365–382.

Fombonne, E., & Du Mazaubrun, C. (1992). Prevalence of infantile autism in four French regions. *Social Psychiatry and Psychiatric Epidemiology, 27*(4), 203–210.

Fombonne, E., Du Mazaubrun, C., Cans, C., & Grandjean, H. (1997). Autism and associated medical disorders in a French epidemiological survey. *Journal of the American Academy of Child and Adolescent Psychiatry, 36*(11), 1561–1569.

Fombonne, E., Zakarian, R., Bennett, A., Meng, L., & McLean-Heywood, D. (2006). Pervasive developmental disorders in Montreal, Quebec, Canada: Prevalence and links with immunizations. *Pediatrics, 118*(1), e139–150.

Gardener, H., Spiegelman, D., & Buka, S. L. (2009). Prenatal risk factors for autism: comprehensive meta-analysis. *British Journal of Psychiatry: The Journal of Mental Science, 195*(1), 7–14.

Garg, U. K., Pal, A. K., Jha, G. J., & Jadhao, S. B. (2004). Haemato-biochemical and immuno-pathophysiological effects of chronic toxicity with synthetic pyrethroid, organophosphate and chlorinated pesticides in broiler chicks. *International Immunopharmacology, 4*(13), 1709–1722.

Gillberg, C. (1990). Do children with autism have March birthdays? *Acta Psychiatrica Scandinavica, 82*(2), 152–156.

Gillberg, C., Steffenburg, S., & Schaumann, H. (1991). Is autism more common now than ten years ago? *The British Journal of Psychiatry: The Journal of Mental Science, 158*, 403–409.

Glasson, E. J. (2002). The Western Australian register for autism spectrum disorders. *Journal of Paediatrics and Child Health, 38*(3), 321.

Glasson, E. J., Bower, C., Petterson, B., de Klerk, N., Chaney, G., & Hallmayer, J. F. (2004). Perinatal factors and the development of autism: a population study. *Archives of General Psychiatry, 61*(6), 618–627.

Goodman, R., & Richards, H. (1995). Child and adolescent psychiatric presentations of second-generation Afro-Caribbeans in Britain. *The British Journal of Psychiatry: The Journal of Mental Science, 167*(3), 362–369.

Grether, J. K., Li, S. X., Yoshida, C. K., & Croen, L. A. (2010). Antenatal ultrasound and risk of autism spectrum disorders. *Journal of Autism and Developmental Disorders, 40*(2), 238–245.

Hamers, T., Kamstra, J. H., Sonneveld, E., Murk, A. J., Visser, T. J., Van Velzen, M. J., et al. (2008). Biotransformation of brominated flame retardants into potentially endocrine-disrupting metabolites, with special attention to 2,2', 4,4'-tetrabromodiphenyl ether (BDE-47). *Molecular Nutrition and Food Research, 52*(2), 284–298.

Heron, J., & Golding, J. (2004). Thimerosal exposure in infants and developmental disorders: A prospective cohort study in the United Kingdom does not support a causal association. *Pediatrics, 114*(3), 577–583.

Hertz-Picciotto, I., Charles, M. J., James, R. A., Keller, J. A., Willman, E., & Teplin, S. (2005). In utero polychlorinated biphenyl exposures in relation to fetal and early childhood growth. *Epidemiology, 16*(5), 648–656.

Hertz-Picciotto, I., Green, P. G., Delwiche, L., Hansen, R., Walker, C., Pessah, N. (2010). Blood mercury concentrations in CHARGE Study children with and without autism. *Environmental Health Perspectives, 118*(1), 161–166. doi: 10.1289/ehp.0900736. http://www.ehponline.org/members/2009/0900736/0900736.pdf.

Hertz-Picciotto, I., Jusko, T. A., Willman, E. J., Baker, R. J., Keller, J. A., Teplin, S. W., et al. (2008). A cohort study of in utero polychlorinated biphenyl (PCB) exposures in relation to secondary sex ratio. *Environmental Health: A Global Access Science Source, 7*, 37.

Hertz-Picciotto, I., Park, H. Y., Dostal, M., Kocan, A., Trnovec, T., & Sram, R. (2008). Prenatal exposures to persistent and non-persistent organic compounds and effects on immune system development. *Basic and Clinical Pharmacology and Toxicology, 102*(2), 146–154.

Hertz-Picciotto, I., Pastore, L. M., & Beaumont, J. J. (1996). Timing and patterns of exposures during pregnancy and their implications for study methods. *American Journal of Epidemiology, 143*(6), 597–607.

Hertz-Picciotto, I., Bartell, S., Burbacher, T., Daniels, J., Davidson, P. W., Factor-Litvak, P., et al. (2006). *Report of the expert panel to the National Institute of Environmental Health Sciences. Thimerosal exposure in pediatric vaccines: Feasibility of studies using the vaccine safety datalink*. Department of Health and Human Services, National Institutes of Health.

Heuer, L., Ashwood, P., Schauer, J., Goines, P., Krakowiak, P., Hertz-Picciotto, I., et al. (2008). Reduced levels of immunoglobulin in children with autism correlates with behavioral symptoms. *Autism Research, 1*(5), 275–283.

Holmes, A. S., Blaxill, M. F., & Haley, B. E. (2003). Reduced levels of mercury in first baby haircuts of autistic children. *International Journal of Toxicology, 22*(4), 277–285.

Honda, H., Shimizu, Y., & Rutter, M. (2005). No effect of MMR withdrawal on the incidence of autism: a total population study. *Journal of Child Psychology and Psychiatry and Allied Disciplines, 46*(6), 572–579.

Hossain, M. M., Suzuki, T., Unno, T., Komori, S., & Kobayashi, H. (2008). Differential presynaptic actions of pyrethroid insecticides on glutamatergic and GABAergic neurons in the hippocampus. *Toxicology, 243*(1–2), 155–163.

Hultman, C. M., & Sparen, P. (2004). Autism: Prenatal insults or an epiphenomenon of a strongly genetic disorder? *Lancet, 364*(9433), 485–487.

Hultman, C. M., Sparen, P., & Cnattingius, S. (2002). Perinatal risk factors for infantile autism. *Epidemiology, 13*(4), 417–423.

Hviid, A., Stellfeld, M., Wohlfahrt, J., & Melbye, M. (2003). Association between thimerosal-containing vaccine and autism. *Journal of the American Medical Association, 290*(13), 1763–1766.

Imamura, L., Yasuda, M., Kuramitsu, K., Hara, D., Tabuchi, A., & Tsuda, M. (2006). Deltamethrin, a pyrethroid insecticide, is a potent inducer for the activity-dependent gene expression of brain-derived neurotrophic factor in neurons. *Journal of Pharmacology and Experimental Therapeutics, 316*(1), 136–143.

IMS. (2001). *IMS health report* (www.imshealth.com).

Institoris, L., Undeger, U., Siroki, O., Nehez, M., & Desi, I. (1999). Comparison of detection sensitivity of immuno- and genotoxicological effects of subacute cypermethrin and permethrin exposure in rats. *Toxicology, 137*(1), 47–55.

Johnson, S. (2001). Micronutrient accumulation and depletion in schizophrenia, epilepsy, autism and Parkinson's disease? *Medical Hypotheses, 56*(5), 641–645.

Kanner, L. (1943). Autistic disturbances of affective contact. *Nervous Child, 2*, 217–250.

Kester, M. H., Bulduk, S., van Toor, H., Tibboel, D., Meinl, W., Glatt, H., et al. (2002). Potent inhibition of estrogen sulfotransferase by hydroxylated metabolites of polyhalogenated aromatic hydrocarbons reveals alternative mechanism for estrogenic activity of endocrine disrupters. *Journal of Clinical Endocrinology and Metabolism, 87*(3), 1142–1150.

Knickmeyer, R. C., & Baron-Cohen, S. (2006). Fetal testosterone and sex differences in typical social development and in autism. *Journal of Child Neurology, 21*(10), 825–845.

Konstantareas, M. M., Hauser, P., Lennox, C., & Homatidis, S. (1986). Season of birth in infantile autism. *Child Psychiatry and Human Development, 17*(1), 53–65.

Landau, E. C., Cicchetti, D. V., Klin, A., & Volkmar, F. R. (1999). Season of birth in autism: A fiction revisited. *Journal of Autism and Developmental Disorders, 29*(5), 385–393.

Lang, I. A., Galloway, T. S., Scarlett, A., Henley, W. E., Depledge, M., Wallace, R. B., et al. (2008). Association of urinary bisphenol A concentration with medical disorders and laboratory abnormalities in adults. *Journal of the American Medical Association, 300*(11), 1303–1310.

Larsson, H. J., Eaton, W. W., Madsen, K. M., Vestergaard, M., Olesen, A. V., Agerbo, E., et al. (2005). Risk factors for autism: Perinatal factors, parental psychiatric history, and socioeconomic status. *American Journal of Epidemiology, 161*(10), 916–925; discussion 926–918.

Lauritsen, M. B., Pedersen, C. B., & Mortensen, P. B. (2005). Effects of familial risk factors and place of birth on the risk of autism: A nationwide register-based study. *Journal of Child Psychology and Psychiatry and Allied Disciplines, 46*(9), 963–971.

Lee, L. C., Newschaffer, C. J., Lessler, J. T., Lee, B. K., Shah, R., & Zimmerman, A. W. (2008). Variation in season of birth in singleton and multiple births concordant for autism spectrum disorders. *Paediatric and Perinatal Epidemiology, 22*(2), 172–179.

Li, X., Chauhan, A., Sheikh, A. M., Patil, S., Chauhan, V., Li, X. M., et al. (2009). Elevated immune response in the brain of autistic patients. *Journal of Neuroimmunology, 207*(1–2), 111–116.

Liu, P., Song, X., Yuan, W., Wen, W., Wu, X., Li, J., et al. (2006). Effects of cypermethrin and methyl parathion mixtures on hormone levels and immune functions in Wistar rats. *Archives of Toxicology, 80*(7), 449–457.

Luebke, R. W., Chen, D. H., Dietert, R., Yang, Y., King, M., & Luster, M. I. (2006). The comparative immunotoxicity of five selected compounds following developmental or adult exposure. *Journal of Toxicology and Environmental Health. Part B, Critical Reviews, 9*(1), 1–26.

Madsen, K. M., Hviid, A., Vestergaard, M., Schendel, D., Wohlfahrt, J., Thorsen, P., et al. (2002). A population-based study of measles, mumps, and rubella vaccination and autism. *New England Journal of Medicine, 347*(19), 1477–1482.

Madsen, K. M., Lauritsen, M. B., Pedersen, C. B., Thorsen, P., Plesner, A. M., Andersen, P. H., et al. (2003). Thimerosal and the occurrence of autism: Negative ecological evidence from Danish population-based data. *Pediatrics, 112*(3 Pt 1), 604–606.

Maimburg, R. D., & Vaeth, M. (2006). Perinatal risk factors and infantile autism. *Acta psychiatrica Scandinavica, 114*(4), 257–264.

Maimburg, R. D., & Vaeth, M. (2007). Do children born after assisted conception have less risk of developing infantile autism? *Human Reproduction, 22*(7), 1841–1843.

Mandell, D. S., Ittenbach, R. F., Levy, S. E., & Pinto-Martin, J. A. (2007). Disparities in diagnoses received prior to a diagnosis of autism spectrum disorder. *Journal of Autism and Developmental Disorders, 37*(9), 1795–1802.

Mandell, D. S., Listerud, J., Levy, S. E., & Pinto-Martin, J. A. (2002). Race differences in the age at diagnosis among Medicaid-eligible children with autism. *Journal of the American Academy of Child and Adolescent Psychiatry, 41*(12), 1447–1453.

Mandell, D. S., Wiggins, L. D., Carpenter, L. A., Daniels, J., DiGuiseppi, C., Durkin, M. S., et al. (2009). Racial/ethnic disparities in the identification of children with autism spectrum disorders. *American Journal of Public Health, 99*(3), 493–498.

McDowell, M. A., Dillon, C. F., Osterloh, J., Bolger, P. M., Pellizzari, E., Fernando, R., et al. (2004). Hair mercury levels in U.S. children and women of childbearing age: Reference range data from NHANES 1999–2000. *Environmental Health Perspectives, 112*(11), 1165–1171.

Meacham, R. B., & Murray, M. J. (1994). Reproductive function in the aging male. *Urologic Clinics of North America, 21*(3), 549–556.

Mednick, S. A., Machon, R. A., Huttunen, M. O., & Bonett, D. (1988). Adult schizophrenia following prenatal exposure to an influenza epidemic. *Archives of General Psychiatry, 45*(2), 189–192.

Meeker, J. D., Johnson, P. I., Camann, D., & Hauser, R. (2009). Polybrominated diphenyl ether (PBDE) concentrations in house dust are related to hormone levels in men. *Science of the Total Environment, 407*(10), 3425–3429.

Meyer, U., Nyffeler, M., Engler, A., Urwyler, A., Schedlowski, M., Knuesel, I., et al. (2006). The time of prenatal immune challenge determines the specificity of inflammation-mediated brain and behavioral pathology. *Journal of Neuroscience, 26*(18), 4752–4762.

Meyer, U., Yee, B. K., & Feldon, J. (2007). The neurodevelopmental impact of prenatal infections at different times of pregnancy: The earlier the worse? *Neuroscientist, 13*(3), 241–256.

Middelburg, K. J., Heineman, M. J., Bos, A. F., & Hadders-Algra, M. (2008). Neuromotor, cognitive, language and behavioural outcome in children born following IVF or ICSI: A systematic review. *Human Reproduction Update, 14*(3), 219–231.

Mocarelli, P., Gerthoux, P. M., Ferrari, E., Patterson, D. G., Jr., Kieszak, S. M., Brambilla, P., et al. (2000). Paternal concentrations of dioxin and sex ratio of offspring. *Lancet, 355*(9218), 1858–1863.

Moore, M., Mustain, M., Daniel, K., Chen, I., Safe, S., Zacharewski, T., et al. (1997). Antiestrogenic activity of hydroxylated polychlorinated biphenyl congeners identified in human serum. *Toxicology and Applied Pharmacology, 142*(1), 160–168.

Moretti, R., Torre, P., Antonello, R. M., Cattaruzza, T., Cazzato, G., & Bava, A. (2004). Vitamin B12 and folate depletion in cognition: A review. *Neurology India, 52*(3), 310–318.

Morse, D. C., Groen, D., Veerman, M., van Amerongen, C. J., Koeter, H. B., Smits van Prooije, A. E., et al. (1993). Interference of polychlorinated biphenyls in hepatic and brain thyroid hormone metabolism in fetal and neonatal rats. *Toxicology and Applied Pharmacology, 122*(1), 27–33.

Mouridsen, S. E., Nielsen, S., Rich, B., & Isager, T. (1994). Season of birth in infantile autism and other types of childhood psychoses. *Child Psychiatry and Human Development, 25*(1), 31–43.

Mouridsen, S. E., Rich, B., & Isager, T. (1993). Brief report: parental age in infantile autism, autistic-like conditions, and borderline childhood psychosis. *Journal of Autism and Developmental Disorders, 23*(2), 387–396.

Muller-Mohnssen, H. (1999). Chronic sequelae and irreversible injuries following acute pyrethroid intoxication. *Toxicology Letters, 107*(1–3), 161–176.

Muskiet, F. A., & Kemperman, R. F. (2006). Folate and long-chain polyunsaturated fatty acids in psychiatric disease. *Journal of Nutritional Biochemistry, 17*(11), 717–727.

Nagarajan, R. P., Patzel, K. A., Martin, M., Yasui, D. H., Swanberg, S. E., Hertz-Picciotto, I., et al. (2008). MECP2 promoter methylation and X chromosome inactivation in autism. *Autism Research, 1*(3), 169–178.

O'Donnell, K., O'Connor, T. G., & Glover, V. (2009). Prenatal stress and neurodevelopment of the child: Focus on the HPA axis and role of the placenta. *Developmental Neuroscience, 31*(4), 285–292.

Palermo, G. D., Neri, Q. V., Takeuchi, T., Squires, J., Moy, F., & Rosenwaks, Z. (2008). Genetic and epigenetic characteristics of ICSI children. *Reproductive Biomedicine Online, 17*(6), 820–833.

Palmer, R. F., Blanchard, S., Stein, Z., Mandell, D., & Miller, C. (2006). Environmental mercury release, special education rates, and autism disorder: An ecological study of Texas. *Health and Place, 12*(2), 203–209.

Park, H. Y., Hertz-Picciotto, I., Petrik, J., Palkovicova, L., Kocan, A., & Trnovec, T. (2008). Prenatal PCB exposure and thymus size at birth in neonates in Eastern Slovakia. *Environmental Health Perspectives, 116*(1), 104–109.

Parker, G., & Neilson, M. (1976). Mental disorder and season of birth: A southern hemisphere study. *British Journal of Psychiatry: The Journal of Mental Science, 129*, 355–361.

Peckham, C. (1985). Congenital rubella in the United Kingdom before 1970: The prevaccine era. *Reviews of Infectious Diseases, 7 Suppl 1*, S11–16.

Perrin, M. C., Brown, A. S., & Malaspina, D. (2007). Aberrant epigenetic regulation could explain the relationship of paternal age to schizophrenia. *Schizophrenia Bulletin, 33*(6), 1270–1273.

Petersen, M. L., Sinisi, S. E., & van der Laan, M. J. (2006). Estimation of direct causal effects. *Epidemiology, 17*(3), 276–284.

Pinborg, A., Loft, A., Schmidt, L., & Andersen, A. N. (2003). Morbidity in a Danish national cohort of 472 IVF/ICSI twins, 1132 non-IVF/ICSI twins and 634 IVF/ICSI singletons: Health-related and social implications for the children and their families. *Human Reproduction, 18*(6), 1234–1243.

Porterfield, S. P. (1994). Vulnerability of the developing brain to thyroid abnormalities: Environmental insults to the thyroid system. *Environmental Health Perspectives, 102 Suppl 2*, 125–130.

Prater, M. R., Gogal, R. M., Jr., Blaylock, B. L., & Holladay, S. D. (2003). Cis-urocanic acid increases immunotoxicity and lethality of dermally administered permethrin in C57BL/6N mice. *International Journal of Toxicology, 22*(1), 35–42.

Punareewattana, K., Smith, B. J., Blaylock, B. L., Longstreth, J., Snodgrass, H. L., Gogal, R. M., Jr., et al. (2001). Topical permethrin exposure inhibits antibody production and macrophage function in C57Bl/6N mice. *Food and Chemical Toxicology, 39*(2), 133–139.

Rauh, V. A., Garfinkel, R., Perera, F. P., Andrews, H. F., Hoepner, L., Barr, D. B., et al. (2006). Impact of prenatal chlorpyrifos exposure on neurodevelopment in the first 3 years of life among inner-city children. *Pediatrics, 118*(6), e1845–1859.

Reichenberg, A., Gross, R., Weiser, M., Bresnahan, M., Silverman, J., Harlap, S., et al. (2006). Advancing paternal age and autism. *Archives of General Psychiatry, 63*(9), 1026–1032.

Reichman, N. E., & Teitler, J. O. (2006). Paternal age as a risk factor for low birthweight. *American Journal of Public Health, 96*(5), 862–866.

Rice, C. E., Baio, J., Van Naarden Braun, K., Doernberg, N., Meaney, F. J., & Kirby, R. S. (2007). A public health collaboration for the surveillance of autism spectrum disorders. *Paediatric and Perinatal Epidemiology, 21*(2), 179–190.

Riederer, A. M., Bartell, S. M., Barr, D. B., & Ryan, P. B. (2008). Diet and nondiet predictors of urinary 3-phenoxybenzoic acid in NHANES 1999–2002. *Environmental Health Perspectives, 116*(8), 1015–1022.

Righi, D. A., & Palermo-Neto, J. (2005). Effects of type II pyrethroid cyhalothrin on peritoneal macrophage activity in rats. *Toxicology, 212*(2–3), 98–106.

Roberts, E. M., English, P. B., Grether, J. K., Windham, G. C., Somberg, L., & Wolff, C. (2007). Maternal residence near agricultural pesticide applications and autism spectrum disorders among children in the California Central Valley. *Environmental Health Perspectives, 115*(10), 1482–1489.

Rodier, P. M., Ingram, J. L., Tisdale, B., & Croog, V. J. (1997). Linking etiologies in humans and animal models: Studies of autism. *Reproductive Toxicology, 11*(2–3), 417–422.

Roman, G. C. (2007). Autism: Transient in utero hypothyroxinemia related to maternal flavonoid ingestion during pregnancy and to other environmental antithyroid agents. *Journal of the Neurological Sciences, 262*(1–2), 15–26.

Rosen, N. J., Yoshida, C. K., & Croen, L. A. (2007). Infection in the first 2 years of life and autism spectrum disorders. *Pediatrics, 119*(1), e61–69.

Rothman, K. J. (2002). *Epidemiology: An introduction.* New York, NY: Oxford University Press.

Rothman, K. J., Greenland, S., & Lash, T. (2008). *Modern epidemiology* (3rd ed.). Philadelphia, PA: Lippincott, Williams & Wilkins.

Sartorius, G. A., & Nieschlag, E. (2010). Paternal age and reproduction. *Human Reproduction Update, 16*(1), 65–79.

Schechter, R., & Grether, J. K. (2008). Continuing increases in autism reported to California's developmental services system: Mercury in retrograde. *Archives of General Psychiatry, 65*(1), 19–24.

Schmidt, R. J., Hansen, R. L., Hartiala, J., ALlayee, H., Schmidt, L. C., Tassone, F., et al. (in press). The combined effects of maternal prenatal vitamin intake and common functional gene variants in folate and transmethylation pathways on risk for autism spectrum disorders in the CHARGE Study. *Epidemiology.*

Shafer, T. J., Meyer, D. A., & Crofton, K. M. (2005). Developmental neurotoxicity of pyrethroid insecticides: Critical review and future research needs. *Environmental Health Perspectives, 113*(2), 123–136.

Shelton, J., Tancredi, D., Hertz-Picciotto, I. (2010). Independent and dependent contributions of advanced maternal and paternal ages for autism risk. *Autism Research, 3*(1), 30–39.

Shi, L., Fatemi, S. H., Sidwell, R. W., & Patterson, P. H. (2003). Maternal influenza infection causes marked behavioral and pharmacological changes in the offspring. *Journal of Neuroscience, 23*(1), 297–302.

Sinha, C., Agrawal, A. K., Islam, F., Seth, K., Chaturvedi, R. K., Shukla, S., et al. (2004). Mosquito repellent (pyrethroid-based) induced dysfunction of blood-brain barrier permeability in developing brain. *International Journal of Developmental Neuroscience, 22*(1), 31–37.

Sjodin, A., Jones, R. S., Focant, J. F., Lapeza, C., Wang, R. Y., McGahee, E. E., III, et al. (2004). Retrospective time-trend study of polybrominated diphenyl ether and polybrominated and polychlorinated biphenyl levels in human serum from the United States. *Environmental Health Perspectives, 112*(6), 654–658.

Smeeth, L., Cook, C., Fombonne, E., Heavey, L., Rodrigues, L. C., Smith, P. G., et al. (2004). MMR vaccination and pervasive developmental disorders: A case-control study. *Lancet, 364*(9438), 963–969.

Smith, S. E., Li, J., Garbett, K., Mirnics, K., & Patterson, P. H. (2007). Maternal immune activation alters fetal brain development through interleukin-6. *Journal of Neuroscience, 27*(40), 10695–10702.

Sonneborn, D., Park, H. Y., Petrik, J., Kocan, A., Palkovicova, L., Trnovec, T., et al. (2008). Prenatal polychlorinated biphenyl exposures in eastern Slovakia modify effects of social factors on birthweight. *Paediatric and Perinatal Epidemiology, 22*(3), 202–213.

Steffenburg, S., Gillberg, C., Hellgren, L., Andersson, L., Gillberg, I. C., Jakobsson, G., et al. (1989). A twin study of autism in Denmark, Finland, Iceland, Norway and Sweden. *Journal of Child Psychology and Psychiatry and Allied Disciplines, 30*(3), 405–416.

Stratton K., Gable A., & McCormick M.C. (Eds.). (2001). *Immunization safety review: Thimerosal-containing vaccines and neurodevelopmental disorders.* Washington, DC: National Academy Press.

Stromberg, B., Dahlquist, G., Ericson, A., Finnstrom, O., Koster, M., & Stjernqvist, K. (2002). Neurological sequelae in children born after in-vitro fertilisation: A population-based study. *Lancet, 359*(9305), 461–465.

Talsness, C. E., Andrade, A. J., Kuriyama, S. N., Taylor, J. A., & vom Saal, F. S. (2009). Components of plastic: Experimental studies in animals and relevance for human health. *Philosophical Transactions of the Royal Society of London. Series B, Biological Sciences, 364*(1526), 2079–2096.

Tanoue, Y., Oda, S., Asano, F., & Kawashima, K. (1988). Epidemiology of infantile autism in southern Ibaraki, Japan: Differences in prevalence in birth cohorts. *Journal of Autism and Developmental Disorders, 18*(2), 155–166.

Taylor, B., Miller, E., Farrington, C. P., Petropoulos, M. C., Favot-Mayaud, I., Li, J., et al. (1999). Autism and measles, mumps, and rubella vaccine: No epidemiological evidence for a causal association. *Lancet, 353*(9169), 2026–2029.

Torrey, E. F., Torrey, B. B., & Peterson, M. R. (1977). Seasonality of schizophrenic births in the United States. *Archives of General Psychiatry, 34*(9), 1065–1070.

Tozzi, A. E., Bisiacchi, P., Tarantino, V., De Mei, B., D'Elia, L., Chiarotti, F., et al. (2009). Neuropsychological performance 10 years after immunization in infancy with thimerosal-containing vaccines. *Pediatrics, 123*(2), 475–482.

United Nations Environment Programme (2001). *Resolution of the Stockholm Convention on Persistent Organic Pollutants.* Stockholm, Sweden: United Nations.

Vach, W., & Blettner, M. (1991). Biased estimation of the odds ratio in case-control studies due to the use of ad hoc methods of correcting for missing values for confounding variables. *American Journal of Epidemiology, 134*(8), 895–907.

Vancassel, S., Durand, G., Barthelemy, C., Lejeune, B., Martineau, J., Guilloteau, D., et al. (2001). Plasma fatty acid levels in autistic children. *Prostaglandins, Leukotrienes, and Essential Fatty Acids, 65*(1), 1–7.

Vargas, D. L., Nascimbene, C., Krishnan, C., Zimmerman, A. W., & Pardo, C. A. (2005). Neuroglial activation and neuroinflammation in the brain of patients with autism. *Annals of Neurology, 57*(1), 67–81.

Vartiainen, T., Jaakkola, J. J., Saarikoski, S., & Tuomisto, J. (1998). Birth weight and sex of children and the correlation to the body burden of PCDDs/PCDFs and PCBs of the mother. *Environmental Health Perspectives, 106*(2), 61–66.

Verstraeten, T., Davis, R. L., DeStefano, F., Lieu, T. A., Rhodes, P. H., Black, S. B., et al. (2003). Safety of thimerosal-containing vaccines: A two-phased study of computerized health maintenance organization databases. *Pediatrics, 112*(5), 1039–1048.

Vojdani, A., Mumper, E., Granpeesheh, D., Mielke, L., Traver, D., Bock, K., et al. (2008). Low natural killer cell cytotoxic activity in autism: The role of glutathione, IL-2 and IL-15. *Journal of Neuroimmunology, 205*(1–2), 148–154.

Volk, H.E., Hertz-Picciotto, I., Delwiche, L., Lurmann, F., McConnell, R., (2010). [Epub ahead of print]. Residential proximity to freeways and autism in the CHARGE Study. *Environmental Health Perspectives,* Online 16 Dec 2010 | doi:10.1289/ehp.1002835.

Wacholder, S., McLaughlin, J. K., Silverman, D. T., & Mandel, J. S. (1992). Selection of controls in case-control studies. I. Principles. *American Journal of Epidemiology, 135*(9), 1019–1028.

Wacholder, S., Silverman, D. T., McLaughlin, J. K., & Mandel, J. S. (1992a). Selection of controls in case-control studies. II. Types of controls. *American Journal of Epidemiology, 135*(9), 1029–1041.

Wacholder, S., Silverman, D. T., McLaughlin, J. K., & Mandel, J. S. (1992b). Selection of controls in case-control studies. III. Design options. *American Journal of Epidemiology, 135*(9), 1042–1050.

Wakefield, A. J., & Montgomery, S. M. (1999). Autism, viral infection and measles-mumps-rubella vaccination. *Israel Medical Association Journal: IMAJ, 1*(3), 183–187.

Wakefield, A. J., Murch, S. H., Anthony, A., Linnell, J., Casson, D. M., Malik, M., et al. (1998). Ileal-lymphoid-nodular hyperplasia, non-specific colitis, and pervasive developmental disorder in children. *Lancet, 351*(9103), 637–641.

Wallace, A. E., Anderson, G. M., & Dubrow, R. (2008). Obstetric and parental psychiatric variables as potential predictors of autism severity. *Journal of Autism and Developmental Disorders, 38*(8), 1542–1554.

Wang, X., Hagberg, H., Nie, C., Zhu, C., Ikeda, T., & Mallard, C. (2007). Dual role of intrauterine immune challenge on neonatal and adult brain vulnerability to hypoxia-ischemia. *Journal of Neuropathology and Experimental Neurology, 66*(6), 552–561.

Wiest, M. M., German, J. B., Harvey, D. J., Watkins, S. M., & Hertz-Picciotto, I. (2009). Plasma fatty acid profiles in autism: A case-control study. *Prostaglandins, Leukotrienes, and Essential Fatty Acids, 80*(4), 221–227.

Wilkerson, D. S., Volpe, A. G., Dean, R. S., & Titus, J. B. (2002). Perinatal complications as predictors of infantile autism. *International Journal of Neuroscience, 112*(9), 1085–1098.

Williams, K., Helmer, M., Duncan, G. W., Peat, J. K., & Mellis, C. M. (2008). Perinatal and maternal risk factors for autism spectrum disorders in New South Wales, Australia. *Child: Care, Health, and Development, 34*(2), 249–256.

Wilson, V. S., Blystone, C. R., Hotchkiss, A. K., Rider, C. V., & Gray, L. E., Jr. (2008). Diverse mechanisms of anti-androgen action: Impact on male rat reproductive tract development. *International Journal of Andrology, 31*(2), 178–187.

Windham, G. C., Zhang, L., Gunier, R., Croen, L. A., & Grether, J. K. (2006). Autism spectrum disorders in relation to distribution of hazardous air pollutants in the San Francisco bay area. *Environmental Health Perspectives, 114*(9), 1438–1444.

Yeargin-Allsopp, M., Rice, C., Karapurkar, T., Doernberg, N., Boyle, C., & Murphy, C. (2003). Prevalence of autism in a U.S. metropolitan area. *Journal of the American Medical Association, 289*(1), 49–55.

Young, J. G., Eskenazi, B., Gladstone, E. A., Bradman, A., Pedersen, L., Johnson, C., et al. (2005). Association between in utero organophosphate pesticide exposure and abnormal reflexes in neonates. *Neurotoxicology, 26*(2), 199–209.

Zechel, J. L., Gamboa, J. L., Peterson, A. G., Puchowicz, M. A., Selman, W. R., & Lust, W. D. (2005). Neuronal migration is transiently delayed by prenatal exposure to intermittent hypoxia. *Birth Defects Research. Part B, Developmental and Reproductive Toxicology, 74*(4), 287–299.

Zhuravin, I. A., Tumanova, N. L., Ozirskaya, E. V., Vasil'ev, D. S., & Dubrovskaya, N. M. (2006). Formation of the structural and ultrastructural organization of the striatum in early postnatal ontogenesis of rats in altered conditions of embryonic development. *Neuroscience and Behavioral Physiology, 36*(5), 473–478.

Zimmerman, A. W., Jyonouchi, H., Comi, A. M., Connors, S. L., Milstien, S., Varsou, A., et al. (2005). Cerebrospinal fluid and serum markers of inflammation in autism. *Pediatric Neurology, 33*(3), 195–201.

Zoeller, R. T., & Crofton, K. M. (2000). Thyroid hormone action in fetal brain development and potential for disruption by environmental chemicals. *Neurotoxicology, 21*(6), 935–945.

48 Patricia M. Rodier

Environmental Exposures That Increase the Risk of Autism Spectrum Disorders

Points of Interest

- More is known about environmental risk factors for autism than for other developmental disabilities.
- The risk factors that have been established are all potent teratogens, which cause many different birth defects.
- The relative risk for each of the exposures is extremely high.
- The critical period for exposure for each environmental risk factor is during the first trimester.
- Phenotypic features that accompany the autism outcome after exposure are shared by several exposed groups and are seen in idiopathic cases and genetic syndromes, as well.

Autism spectrum disorders are unique among the conditions described in the *Diagnostic and Statistical Manual of the American Psychiatric Association* (DSM), in that several environmental exposures have been determined to increase the risk of ASDs. Although the etiology of autism is known to have a strong genetic component (e.g., Bailey et al., 1995), these environmental factors offer other avenues by which the nature of ASDs can be investigated. For example, they offer scientists the opportunity to create animal models based on exposures to risk factors, just as genetic discoveries offer the opportunity to create models by manipulating animal genotypes.

The environmental factors identified thus far account for a very small proportion of autism cases, but that does not diminish the importance of their contribution to our understanding of ASDs. The purpose of this chapter is to summarize our present knowledge of the environmental factors that are known to increase autism risk.

Rubella

Evidence and Relative Risk

The first environmental factor associated with autism was rubella infection (Chess et al., 1978; Chess & Fernandez, 1980). Because rubella exposure of the embryo has long been known to be a cause of birth defects including brain damage (Gregg, 1941; Ariens Kappers, 1957), it is hardly surprising that it might produce injuries that lead to autism. What is more remarkable is that a significantly elevated rate of autism was found using the very narrow criteria of Kanner (1943). It seems likely that the same population of rubella-exposed children, if examined with today's much broader definition of ASDs, would have shown an effect that was even more striking. However, comparing the 18 autism cases out of 243 rubella-exposed cases (Chess et al., 1978) to modern rates for autistic disorder (16.8/10,000, from Chakrabarti & Fombonne, 2001) gives a relative risk greater than 40. This is an enormous effect.

As we consider each of the known risk factors for autism, it will become apparent that each has a relative risk that is much higher than those familiar from toxicology studies. For example, the National Institutes of Health (NIH) recognizes a relative risk of 2 to 4 for the effect of smoking in increasing the risk of heart disease, and this is considered a large effect. It is worthwhile to pause here and consider what makes the risk factors for ASDs' relative risks dramatically higher. The effects of teratogens on development are different from the effects of toxic agents to which we are exposed over long periods. For example, in the case of rubella, postnatal exposure or exposure late in pregnancy cannot cause any of the permanent defects we associate with this virus. Instead, there is a brief window during development when exposure leads to injury. This is called the critical period, and it differs for different teratogens and different defects. Notice that Chess ascertained cases exposed to rubella in an institutionalized population. That is, all the cases were severely injured. Therefore, only cases exposed during the critical period were represented in the 243 cases examined. The relative risk of 40 does not represent the risk associated with exposure to rubella at any time, or even with exposure at any time during pregnancy; it is the risk of autism among cases exposed during the critical period for severe injury. Throughout this chapter, the reader will find more examples of cases ascertained from selected groups of exposed populations. Often, there is no other way to identify exposed cases.

The reports from Chess' group did not consider the timing of exposure to rubella that resulted in autism, but critical periods for various rubella sequelae have been studied by others. Ueda, Nishida, Oshima, and Shepard (1979) investigated a sample of cases in which the time of appearance of the rash associated with the disease was known, and they described the outcome for eye defects, deafness, mental retardation, and heart malformations. They concluded that the period from the second to the fifth week postconception was associated with severe cognitive limitation, and cases with multiple defects had been exposed within the first 8 weeks. Because the autism cases reported by Chess and others all had multiple defects, it is likely that they had been exposed during the first 8 weeks postconception.

Fortunately, because of the development of a vaccine against rubella, we should no longer face the prospect of epidemics of this disease followed by epidemics of offspring with severe birth defects. As long as vaccination rates remain near 100%, this cause of autism has been eliminated.

Ethanol

Evidence and Relative Risk

In a clinic for children with Fetal Alcohol Syndrome (FAS) or Fetal Alcohol Effects (FAE), Nanson (1992) identified six who scored as severely autistic on the Childhood Autism Rating Scale (Schopler et al., 1988) in a sample of 326 cases. Each was also diagnosed with FAS, which requires facial dysmorphology, growth retardation, and dysfunction of the central nervous system. Subsequent papers (Harris et al., 1995; Aronson et al., 1997) have supported the conclusion that ASDs can coexist with FAS and perhaps with FAE. The additional cases described in these papers all shared the facial anomalies characteristic of FAS. The relative risk, based on the first study and again using Chakrabarti and Fombonne's data for autistic disorder, is over 10. Fombonne (2002) has pointed out several difficulties that make the ethanol studies hard to interpret. None is based on the kinds of diagnostic measures for autism that are commonly used today. Furthermore, FAS and FAE are very common, so it is likely that they would occur in concert with autism occasionally by chance. However, the relative risk of 10 is still high, even with those caveats.

Rather than depending completely on the epidemiological findings, a teratologist might ask other questions to determine whether an association of ethanol exposure with autism makes biological sense. For example, "Is the critical period for FAS similar to any critical period associated with autism?" The critical period for FAS is thought to be in the third to fifth week postconception (Sulik et al., 1986). This period overlaps with the one we have just discussed for rubella, making it seem reasonable that ethanol exposures leading to FAS are occurring at a developmental stage that is sensitive to autism outcomes, as well. Another question might be, "Do children with FAS and autism share any dysmorphic features with autism after other exposures?" Yes, the facial dysmorphologies that characterize FAS (epicanthal folds, short palpebral fissures, underdeveloped maxillary region [Jones & Smith, 1973]) include features observed in autism subsequent to valproate exposure (to be discussed below). This suggests that the critical periods for autism after ethanol exposure and valproate exposure are similar. Thus, from an embryological standpoint, an FAS–autism association makes sense.

FAS and ASD Compared

Could it be that the behavioral phenotypes of ASDs and FAS are so similar that the autism diagnoses within FAS represent diagnostic substitution? First, let us consider the behavioral characteristics attributed to cases exposed to ethanol in utero. In the earliest description of FAS, based on eight severe cases in very young children (Jones et al., 1973), cognitive limitation was evident in all. Subsequent studies (e.g., Streissguth, et al., 1991) have examined a broader range of degrees of injury and included adolescents and adults, allowing a more detailed examination of cognitive abilities. The average IQ in this sample was 68, but almost half of the subjects fell in or near the normal range. Academic testing revealed that the subjects had particular difficulty with arithmetic, as compared to reading and spelling. Vineland (Sparrow et al., 1984) scores on daily living skills averaged age 9 years although the chronological age was 17 years. Socialization scores were the most affected, averaging 6 years of age. The patients in this study were not just deficient in adaptive behaviors, but exhibited a remarkable level of maladaptive behaviors. Of 31 subjects, none had a maladaptive behavior score in the insignificant range. The most common maladaptive behaviors cited were "poor concentration and attention, dependency, stubbornness or sullenness, social withdrawal, teasing or bullying, crying or laughing too easily, impulsivity, and periods of high anxiety."

After many years of recording caregivers' descriptions of the behavior of patients with prenatal alcohol injury, Streissguth, Bookstein, Barr, Press, and Sampson (1998) attempted to determine the descriptors most characteristic of offspring exposed to ethanol and evaluate descriptors for the strength of their association with other items on the list. The result is a 36-item checklist, the Fetal Alcohol Behavior Scale, with some predictive value for identifying people exposed to maternal drinking.

This set of behaviors is a list of features of FAS/FAE, just as the diagnostic behaviors of autism are a list of features of ASDs. Starting with the behavior most highly correlated with the scale as a whole, the list includes: *(1)* overreacting to situations, *(2)* chatting with little content, *(3)* bringing up unusual topics, *(4)* demanding attention, and *(5)* not aware of consequences of actions. Of 36 items, only a few sound similar to the behaviors seen in autism. Many of the behaviors are more like the opposite of autism (e.g., likes to talk, interrupts, wants to be the center of attention, physically loving, overly friendly).

Bishop, Gahagan, and Lord (2007) have compared children with ASD diagnoses to children with FAS/FAE diagnoses, in an attempt to determine the core features of autism that separate this diagnosis from other disabilities. They used the AutismDiagnostic Inventory Revised (ADI-R) (Lord et al., 1994) and the Autism Diagnostic Observation Schedule (ADOS) (Lord et al., 2000) to evaluate sample groups of children with autism, pervasive developmental disorder, and FAS/FAE who were matched for age and full-scale IQ. The results are presented as sets of items on which the groups show great differences and ones on which they are more similar. ADI items from all domains were among those that discriminated between the groups. For example, subjects with autism were much more likely to have problems with pointing to express interest, using gestures, and imitative social play. These are from the communications domain. From the social domain, difficulties on items such as range of facial expressions, sharing enjoyment, and offering comfort were more than twice as common in children with autism as in those with FAS/FAE. The one behavior from the restricted and repetitive behavior domain with reported difficulties strongly favoring the autistic group was hand and finger mannerisms.

Direct observation with the ADOS also showed striking differences across domains for children with autism compared to the Fetal Alcohol spectrum. These included problems with eye contact, directed facial expressions, amount of reciprocal social communication, and unusual sensory interests. The authors have pointed out that even categories of behavior for which the groups seem to have similar degrees of difficulty may reflect different kinds of behavior. For example, abnormalities of group play with peers could be scored for a child who ignores the approaches of peers, or for one who is loud, bossy, and demanding (the second list is borrowed from the Fetal Alcohol Behavior Scale, described above). Bishop et al. (2007) suggest that reduced propensity for and frequency of social interactions seem to be core features of autism, but the quality of such interactions may be disturbed in too many ways to be as useful for diagnosis.

In summary, it seems unlikely that investigators could mistake the behavioral characteristics of FAS for those of autism. It seems more likely that a subset of FAS/FAE cases exhibits a different behavioral phenotype consistent with an autism diagnosis. It remains to be seen whether that behavioral pattern arises from ethanol exposure alone, perhaps with slightly different timing, or on a different genetic background, from the more typical pattern, or whether the subset results from dual etiologies, with ethanol leading to the physical features by which FAS is diagnosed and some other factor leading to the behaviors diagnostic of autism. This author favors the view that high doses of ethanol early in pregnancy increase the risk of autism spectrum disorders.

Thalidomide

Evidence and Relative Risk

The description of autism among people exposed to thalidomide in utero (Strömland et al., 1994) is part of a remarkable study that offers a very specific time of origin for the injuries that resulted in autism. More extensive reporting of the ophthalmological results of the study can be found in work by Miller (1991) and by Miller & Strömland (1991). Work by Strömland & Miller (1993) provides a detailed description of the physical anomalies that characterized the patients. Of about 100 cases in the Swedish registry of thalidomide victims, Miller and Strömland were able to enroll 86 and personally examine them for a host of ophthalmological measures, for physical malformations, and for cranial neurological dysfunctions. In the course of their investigation, they noted four cases with obvious mental retardation and psychiatric disturbances. With the assistance of a psychiatrist, the cases with mental retardation were diagnosed as having autistic disorder, using the criteria of DSM III-R. Four cases in a sample of 86 suggest a relative risk of almost 30. However, the authors collected other data that show that the risk is even greater than this.

Each of the 86 subjects was examined for physical malformations. Strömland and Miller (1993) summarized earlier work on the specific stages of development when thalidomide results in particular physical effects. The earliest defects are those of the ears (starting at day 20 postconception) and cranial nerves, followed by those of the upper limb (starting at day 24) and then the lower limb (starting at day 27). Among the 86 cases studied in Sweden, only 17 had been injured in the earliest part of the critical period for thalidomide embryopathy, as evidenced by ear anomalies and cranial nerve dysfunctions without limb anomalies (Strömland & Miller, 1993). Each of the cases with autism had ear anomalies and cranial nerve dysfunction, indicating early exposure. One also had an upper limb effect, and none had malformations of the lower limb. Therefore, the period of injury that results in an autism outcome must be between days 20 and 24. If we use the 17 cases injured early as our denominator for our relative risk calculation, rather than including the whole thalidomide-exposed sample, then the relative risk for autism after exposure during the critical period is 140 times the risk in the general population.

For readers not familiar with the field of teratology, the finding of a very narrow window when a particular defect can arise is not unusual, but typical, of birth defects in general. In most cases we don't have supporting data to define a critical period as specific as the one in this study, but it is clear that such periods exist and that they depend on the coincidence of a particular exposure with particular events in development.

The critical period identified in this study is the time when the neural tube is closing and the first neurons are forming (Bayer et al., 1993). Those neurons are the motor neurons that make up the cranial nerve motor nuclei. The cranial nerve dysfunctions observed in the thalidomide study are evidence that some of these earliest-forming neurons were affected by the teratogen, offering another line of support to the critical period determined from physical malformations. Duane syndrome (a type of strabismus with lack of innervation from the abducens nerve to the lateral rectus muscle of the eye and reinnervation of the muscle by the oculomotor nerve) was seen in two of the cases with autism and in 24 cases altogether. Four others had some limitation of abduction. One case with autism had gaze paresis, as did six others in the total sample. Six patients had esotropia. Three of the patients with autism had palsy of the VIIth cranial nerve (the facial nerve) and 14 from the rest of the sample were affected. Abnormal lacrimation (lack of emotional tearing and/or crying to gustatory stimuli) was present in a total of 17 cases, including two of the cases with autism (Strömland et al., 1994; Strömland & Miller, 1993).

Mechanism of Action

The mechanism of action of thalidomide is not well-known. Recent hypotheses about mechanisms have focused on explaining the limb anomalies and may not explain the effects on the nervous system. It has long been known that the thalidomide-induced limb anomalies seen in primates and rabbits do not occur in rodents (Shumacher et al., 1968), but recent studies suggest that central nervous system (CNS) effects do occur in rodents (e.g., Myazaki et al., 2005; Hallene et al., 2006). Thus, it is possible that the mechanistic pathways involved in thalidomide teratogenicity may differ for different terata.

A recent series of studies in chick embryos indicates that thalidomide's disruption of limb development may have its origin in disturbances of the expression of bone morphogenetic proteins, leading to overexpression of the gene Dickkopf1, which inhibits *Wnt* signaling (Knobloch et al., 2007). Because thalidomide is a potent antiangiogenic agent (Folkman, 1995), another hypothesis has focused on the effects of the drug on angiogenic factors, such as insulin growth factor1 and fibroblast growth factor 2 (Stephens et al., 2000). Another idea is that the drug's induction of oxidative stress alters limb outgrowth by way of its effect on nuclear factor kappa B, a redox-sensitive transcription factor (Hansen et al., 2002). The authors have shown that thalidomide effects on this pathway differ between sensitive species (e.g., rabbit) and insensitive species (e.g., rat).

In summary, the Swedish thalidomide study, although carried out in humans, offers the kind of specificity and powerful conclusions usually seen only in animal studies. This is the result of many features of the study; for example, the fact that thalidomide's effects include very rare anomalies made it relatively easy to identify cases. Additionally, medical record keeping in Sweden is so thorough that exposures could be documented retrospectively. The discovery of autism among the subjects was serendipitous, but it occurred because the investigators devoted so much time to interacting with each subject and family, completing exhaustive examinations of each case. It is also a tribute to the scientific acumen of these expert clinicians that they did not confine their curiosity to their specialty (pediatric ophthalmology). It was the additional data on somatic defects and cranial nerve dysfunction that allowed them to understand the meaning of the autism cases.

Valproic Acid

Evidence and Relative Risk

All the antiseizure medications are teratogenic to some degree (reviewed in Holmes, 2002). They are frequently given in combination. The reader should be aware that these drugs tend to interfere with one another. The result is that patients taking more than one medication tend to be on higher doses of each drug than patients who are taking only one.

The first report of autism in a child exposed in utero to valproic acid (Christianson et al., 1994) appeared in the same issue of Developmental Medicine and Child Neurology as Strömland et al. (1994). The paper discusses two sibling pairs with classic features of Fetal Valproate Syndrome (Di Liberti et al., 1984; Jager-Roman et al., 1986; Ardinger et al., 1988; Kozma, 2001), such as epicanthal folds, hypertelorism, broad nasal bridge; long upper lip with flat filtrum, ear malformations, and "pinched" finger tips. One of the four children tested positive for autism. Developmental delay, and especially delay in expressive language, had been reported earlier (Ardinger et al., 1988) but those cases were not tested for pervasive developmental disorder. Soon, another case of autism in Fetal Valproate Syndrome was described (Williams & Hersh, 1997), then five more (Williams et al., 2001). One of the five had a performance IQ of 100 and a verbal IQ of 81, suggesting that the autism risk in Fetal Valproate Syndrome is not dependent on the mental retardation sometimes seen in the syndrome.

More recent studies have examined larger populations of children exposed to valproic acid in utero and offer information on the risk of autism after exposure to this teratogen. In the first (Moore et al., 2000), 52 cases were ascertained through a parent support group for children diagnosed with a fetal anticonvulsant syndrome and five came from referrals to the local genetics service. The main purpose of the study was to document and compare the dysmorphologies of the various anticonvulsant exposures. In essence, the dysmorphologies of the valproate cases were similar to those described in the earlier case reports. Many other data were collected directly, as well, but behavioral diagnoses were ascertained from parental reports. As one might guess from the method of ascertainment, there was a very high degree of developmental delay or behavioral problems among children in the sample, with only four of the families reporting no problems.

Among the whole group, 34 had been exposed to valproate alone and 12 to valproate plus one or more other drugs. Among these 46 cases, there were three previously diagnosed with autism and two previously diagnosed with Asperger's Syndrome. There was one case with an autism diagnosis in which the individual had been exposed to carbamazepine and diazepam. Assuming that the reported clinical diagnoses were accurate, the five in 46 rate of ASDs appears to be very high. Because of the Asperger's cases, we must calculate the relative risk using Chakrabarti and Fombonne's value of 62.6/10,000 for pervasive developmental disorder (PDD) as the denominator, so the relative risk is about 17. However, in this study, with its subjects selected from a group already known to have behavioral problems, we have no way to estimate the true risk of ASDs among all children exposed to valproate in utero.

Rasalam et al. (2005) carried out a population-based study using records over a 20-year period to identify all local children known to have been exposed to antiepileptic drugs in utero. Their mothers had been referred to Aberdeen Maternity Hospital because of their high-risk pregnancies. There were 398 mothers who had 626 exposed children at the facility. From this pool, 159 mothers with 260 children agreed to participate in the study. Families were interviewed by a trained research nurse. The structured interview included questions about behavioral and social issues.

From the responses, 26 children were identified for an extensive review of their medical records, and 14 of these had indications of ASDs. The investigators accessed this group's complete records, including reports from specialists who had examined their behavior. A child psychiatrist then studied these notes for items specified in the DSM IV criteria for autism, and found that 12 met the criteria for ASD. Among those who had been exposed to valproate alone, five of 56 were positive and among those exposed to valproate alone or in combination with other drugs, nine of 77 were positive. Eight qualified for a diagnosis of autism and one for a diagnosis of Asperger's Syndrome. Comparing this rate to Chakrabarti and Fombonne's rate for PDD, the relative risk is about 19.

There may be a remaining selection bias in this study, even though it was a serious attempt to assess the whole exposed population. It seems possible that families of children with behavioral difficulties might be more likely to agree to recruitment than families of children developing normally. Unfortunately, we don't know whether this was the case, nor do we know how many children of the initial 626 children exposed to antiseizure medication were exposed to valproate. We don't know how many were lost to follow-up (their appearance in the unenrolled group does not represent a refusal of recruitment). However, assuming that the proportion exposed to valproate was the same in the unenrolled cases as in those who were enrolled, then even if we include those lost to follow-up and assume that there were no cases of ASDs in the unenrolled group, the risk associated with valproate would still be substantial. In fact, it is 7.72 with a confidence interval of 3.90 to 15.29. This is significantly different from 1.00 (no effect) at $p = < .0001$.

Now let us consider some other characteristics of the children evaluated in this study. For some variables, the authors describe the children with ASD diagnoses subsequent to exposure to antiseizure medications as a group, without separating out those exposed to valproic acid, but since most of the cases (9/12) had been exposed to valproate, these generalizations are of interest. The mean IQ of those with ASDs was below average, but most cases were in the normal range. No child had any evidence of regression or loss of skills. Results specific to the children exposed to valproate included: head circumference above average, a male to female ratio of 3:6, and an assortment of birth defects (e.g., strabismus, pyloric stenosis, hypospadias).

Children with autism after in utero exposure to valproate share the many dysmorphologies of Fetal Valproate Syndrome with exposed children who do not meet the diagnostic criteria for autism. Some of these features appear in other environmental etiologies as well. For example, epicanthal folds and maxillary hypoplasia are typical of Fetal Alcohol Syndrome as well as Fetal Valproate Syndrome. Strabismus and ear anomalies characterize children exposed to thalidomide as well as those exposed to valproate. These common features suggest that the critical periods for valproate teratogenicity must be similar to those for ethanol and thalidomide.

Mechanism of Action

The mechanism of action of valproic acid in teratogenesis cannot be described completely at this time, but at least two mechanisms have been identified. First, valproate is a direct inhibitor of histone deacetylase (HDAC) (Phiel et al., 2002). The HDACs have a role in the folding of chromatin, and their inhibition can unfold chromosomes, making some genes more available for transcription. Other HDAC inhibitors are also teratogenic, so there is good reason to think that this mechanism is one of the ways valproic acid alters development. It has been proposed that increases in *Wnt* gene signaling after HDAC inhibition are one of the mechanisms by which valproic acid leads to birth defects (reviewed in Wiltse, 2005).

A second mechanism, which may be related to the first (see Gurvich et al., 2005), is the ability of valproate to drive the expression of the gene, *Hoxa1* (Stodgell et al., 2006). This gene is critical to the development of the early embryo when the neural plate is developing into the neural tube, and it plays a special role in hindbrain development (Chisaka et al., 1992). Its expression is dependent on levels of retinoic acid and both high and low levels of retinoic acid are extremely teratogenic, presumably because of their effect on the levels of *Hoxa1* expression (e.g., Means & Gudas, 1995; White et al., 2000).

A number of analogs of valproic acid have been synthesized and tested for antiseizure activity and teratogenicity (e.g., Hauck & Nau, 1989; Bojic et al., 1996). These studies have demonstrated that the antiseizure property of the drug and the teratogenic property do not share the same mechanism. Stodgell and others (2006) made use of these analogs in their studies of gene expression in rat embryos after exposure to valproate. They found that compounds with high teratogenicity had strong effects on *Hoxa1* expression, although those with no teratogenic action had no effect on the expression of the gene. Thus, the effect on *Hoxa1* may be one mechanism of action of the drug. These effects on the gene's expression can be seen only during its normal period of expression (the time of neural tube closure) and very brief periods before and after normal expression.

Animal Model

More than the other environmental factors discussed above, valproate has proven useful in the creation of animal models relevant to autism (reviewed in Arndt et al., 2006). Rats exposed to the drug around the time of neural tube closure exhibit several neuroanatomical features similar to ones reported in histological studies of brains from people with autism. For example, the rat model has low Purkinje cell counts and small cerebellar volume (Ingram et al., 2000). The same features have been reported in human autism cases (e.g., Bauman & Kemper, 1985; Ritvo et al., 1986; Bailey et al., 1998; Whitney et al., 2008; Courchesne et al., 1988).

The rat model has also been found to express a variety of behavioral abnormalities (e.g., Schneider et al., 2001; Schneider & Przewlocki, 2005; Stanton et al., 2007; Schneider et al., 2007; Markram et al., 2008). Many of the behavioral effects are in general categories of behavior that are related to autism (e.g., nociception, social behavior) but a few are in very specific behaviors known to be affected in the same way as in autism. One is a decrement in prepulse inhibition of the acoustic startle response. This was first reported in subjects with ASDs by McAlonan and colleagues (2002) and more recently by Perry and colleagues (2007). The same depression of prepulse inhibition has been demonstrated in rats exposed to valproate around the time of neural tube closure (Schneider & Przewlocki, 2005). This measure of sensory gating in the CNS could be related to failures of inhibition as seen in repetitive thoughts and actions in autism.

Eyeblink conditioning is a second very specific behavior affected similarly in both human autism and the valproic acid rat model. This basic paradigm of association learning, in which a tone is paired repeatedly with a stimulus to the eye that causes a blink until the blink occurs to the tone alone, has been studied in many neurological and psychiatric conditions. For example, children with FAE or dyslexia are severely impaired in acquisition of the conditioned eyeblink response (Coffin et al., 2005), as are people with Alzheimer's disease (Woodruff-Pak & Papka, 1996a). People with Huntington's disease have normal acquisition of the learned response, although the timing of their blinks is abnormal (Woodruff-Pak & Papka, 1996b). In contrast to all the other conditions that have been studied, autism results in an enhancement of conditioning (Sears et al., 1994; Arndt et al., 2006). The same enhancement has been demonstrated in the rat model exposed to valproate (Stanton et al., 2001). Thus, the rat exposed to valproate around the time of neural tube closure has both anatomic and behavioral parallels to autism.

Misoprostol

Evidence and Relative Risk

Misoprostol is a prostaglandin with various legitimate uses in medicine. In South America, it is used illegally by the poor as an abortifacient. Exposure causes uterine contractions, which may or may not expel the conceptus. When the drug fails and the conceptus comes to term there is a risk of birth defects consistent with ischemia in utero (Gonzalez et al., 1998). One of these is Moebius sequence, a bilateral or unilateral diplegia of the facial nerve and the abducens nerve. Investigations of familial cases of Moebius sequence indicate that anomalies of multiple genes can produce the deficit (Verzijl et al., 1999). There is also evidence that environmental factors play a role (Lipson et al., 1989). Ischemia was suggested as a possible cause of Moebius sequence long before the teratology of misoprostol was recognized (Bavinck & Weaver, 1986). The rate of autism is high among idiopathic cases of Moebius sequence (e.g., Johansson et al., 2001).

Bandim and colleagues (2003) recruited children diagnosed with Moebius sequence in Brazil, queried their mothers regarding misoprostol use, and tested the Moebius cases for autism. In the 23 cases under study, 14 had been exposed to misoprostol, according to the mothers' statements. Among these, three met the criteria for an autism diagnosis under DSM IV. Of the nine children whose mothers denied misoprostol use, two met the criteria for an autism diagnosis. Thus, the relative risk for autism in misoprostol-induced Moebius sequence is 128. Notice that this incredible risk does not apply to misoprostol exposure in general, but only to exposures with dose and timing adequate to cause Moebius sequence. Unfortunately, at this time, we have no way to tell whether misoprotol exposure has occurred unless it has caused an obvious but rare birth defect such as Moebius sequence. The results in cases not exposed to misoprostol support earlier findings that idiopathic cases of Moebius sequence have a high rate of autism. Indeed, the 2/9 rate is just what other studies would predict. For example, the rate in the study by Johansson and colleagues (2001) was about 25%.

Why is Moebius sequence related to autism? The fact that ischemia of the brain stem appears to be the etiology of the misoprostol cases suggests that it may be the location of injury that links the two conditions. All the mothers who reported using misoprostol in studies by Bandim et al. (2003) exposed the embryo in the sixth week postconception, so the timing is slightly later than that discussed for other teratogens that increase autism risk. Further, the proposed mechanism, ischemia, seems unrelated to the mechanisms proposed for other factors. But we know from the neurological symptoms of valproate-exposed cases and thalidomide-exposed cases that brain stem nuclei were affected and animal studies show that valproate exposure can injure the developing cranial nerve motor nuclei (e.g., Rodier et al., 1996). Thus, location of injury appears to be the one obvious common feature shared by Moebius sequence and autism associated with environmental etiologies.

What Can We Learn from Environmental Etiologies?

Early Origins and Neurobiology

The fact that all the environmental factors recognized thus far share critical periods in embryonic life (the first 9 weeks postconception) is an important contribution to our understanding of autism etiologies. Table 48-1 summarizes the critical periods for all the known environmental risk factors. At the time these studies began to appear, few scientists were thinking that autism's origins might occur so early in development. But in retrospect it seems obvious that very early injuries are the ones with the potential to explain the histology and connectivity observed in the brains of people with autism. For example, low numbers of Purkinje cells have been reported by many investigators, as discussed above, and Ingram et al. (2000), demonstrated that this condition could be reproduced in rats exposed to valproic acid during neural tube closure. Interestingly, the exposure used in this study occurred before the Purkinje cells form, so they were not injured directly. This reminds us that insults to a developing brain can have consequences for later-forming structures.

Table 48–1.
Exposure period associated with an autism outcome for five known environmental risk factors

Environmental Risk Factor	Critical Period (Postconception)
Rubella	< 8 weeks
Ethanol	2 to 5 weeks
Thalidomide	20 to 24 days
Valproic acid	3 to 4 weeks
Misoprostal	6th week

The deep nuclei of the cerebellum have been studied in a number of brains from people with autism (Bauman & Kemper, 1994; Bailey et al., 1998). The globose and emboliform nuclei were especially altered, although the dentate nucleus was less affected. These nuclei form just before the Purkinje cells (Bayer et al., 1993), again suggesting an early injury.

Rodier et al. (1996) reported a case of autism in which the superior olive was virtually absent. This very early-forming complex of nuclei (Bayer et al., 1993) is the first point in the auditory pathway where information from both ears converges on the same neurons, and plays a role in sound localization. Recently, experts on the structure examined five brains from people with ASDs and found that the medial superior olive was abnormal in every case (Kulesza & Mangunay, 2008). The normal strict orientation of the neurons was deranged, even in cases where the number of neurons appeared to be unaffected.

Early loss of neurons can alter the connections formed subsequently by other neurons. Duane syndrome, as seen in thalidomide-exposed subjects (Strömland & Miller, 1993) is a good example. Many theories of the neurobiology of autism focus on abnormalities of connections (e.g., Just et al., 2004; Kana et al., 2007), and it is easy to see how projections might go to the wrong places when tissue that provides axonal guidance to them is missing or altered. In the case reported by Rodier et al. (1996), fibers that normally go up or down the neuroaxis were seen going in all directions in the region where they would typically form a capsule around the facial nucleus. In its absence, they appear to have lost their orientation. In Bailey et al. (1998), one case of autism exhibited an extra brain stem tract never seen in controls. All these findings fit well with the idea of a disruption of development in the early embryo.

Early Origins and Early Developmental Genes

In retrospect, we now know that a number of the genes thought to play a role in autism are ones whose main or only period of expression occurs in embryonic life. These include *Engrailed 2*, which organizes aspects of early cerebellar development (Joyner et al., 1991; Kuemerle et al., 1997). Several alleles of the human gene have been shown to be associated with autism, although the causal variants have not been identified (Gharani et al., 2004; Benayed et al., 2005).

Individuals who inherit two copies of a truncating mutation of *HOXA1* have a high rate of autism, as well as deafness, vascular malformations, large head size, Duane syndrome, and facial hypotonia (Tischfield et al., 2005; Bosley et al., 2007; Bosley et al., 2008). This is called the Bosley-Salih-Alorainy syndrome (BSAS). Homozygous inheritance of another truncating mutation of the same gene (Holve et al., 2003; Bosley et al., 2008) leads to many of the same symptoms, but not autism.

Several theories of the mechanisms of action of valproate involve the *Wnt* gene pathway, and there is some evidence that

WNT2 might be a susceptibility gene for autism (Wassink et al., 2001). The involvement of early developmental genes in the etiology of autism makes the early critical periods found for teratologic risk factors seem logical, rather than surprising.

Communalities Across Etiologies

It would be exciting if all the environmental risk factors shared similar mechanisms of action, but they do not. Although their critical periods are similar, they are not exactly the same. Yet this review demonstrates that patients with these different etiologies do share many characteristics. Table 48-2 summarizes some characteristics shared across different conditions leading to autism. For example, there are some common facial features shared across several risk factors, such as malformed ears, epicanthal folds, and maxillary hypoplasia. There are dysfunctions of cranial nerves, such as strabismus and Moebius sequence.

In addition, some individuals exposed to environmental risk factors have symptoms also observed in cases with disruptions of early developmental genes. Hearing impairments are typical of rubella-induced autism, thalidomide-induced autism, and of both syndromes traced to homozygous inheritance of truncating mutations of *HOXA1*. The large head size reported in valproate-associated autism is also present in BSAS (Tischfield et al., 2005). Duane syndrome is typical of thalidomide-induced autism and of both syndromes arising from deficient expression of the HOXA1 protein.

Do idiopathic cases of autism share any of the symptoms reviewed for environmental exposure etiologies and early developmental gene etiologies? Obviously, they do. The high rate of minor craniofacial malformations in idiopathic ASDs has been recognized for many years (e.g., Steg & Rapoport, 1975; Walker, 1977). Because these can only arise during early stages of development, their presence suggests that many idiopathic cases have been subject to some early disturbance of development.

Table 48–2.
Craniofacial anomalies reported in individuals with autism subsequent to four environmental exposures and one genetic syndrome

	Thalidomide	VPA	FAS	Misoprostol	BSAS
Large head size		yes	no		yes
Moebius sequence or facial hypotonia	yes			yes	yes
Duane syndrome or other strabismus	yes	yes		yes	yes
Abnormal tearing	yes			yes	
Epicanthal folds		yes	yes		
Ear abnormalities	yes	yes			yes
Hearing deficits	yes				yes
Hypoplasia of the midface or maxilla		yes	yes		

Strabismus, which we have seen to occur after exposure to thalidomide and valproate, and after homozygous inheritance of truncating mutations of *HOXA1*, has been noted to occur at elevated rates in idiopathic cases of autism as well (e.g., Sharre & Creedon, 1992). Similarly, the comorbidity of Moebius sequence or facial hypotonia with autism is seen in idiopathic cases (e.g., Johansson et al., 2001), as well as in cases associated with environmental risk factors and genetic syndromes reviewed here.

Large head size is a particularly interesting characteristic of a substantial number of people with ASDs that has received much attention. It appears that overgrowth of the brain and head begins soon after birth and tapers off in the second year of life (e.g., Courchesne et al., 2003; Dawson et al., 2007). One might speculate that postnatal overgrowth reflects some untoward influence on postnatal development occurring during the period of excessive growth. However, the fact that prenatal exposure to valproic acid also results in large head size (Rasalam et al., 2005), suggests that it may not be necessary to propose any postnatal events to account for this phenomenon. Indeed, the presence of large head size in Bosley-Salih-Alorainy syndrome proves that genetic activity altered only in the embryonic period can lead to large head size later in life. Even a single nucleotide polymorphism of *HOXA1* has been shown to be associated with the quantitative trait of head size in autism (Conciatori et al., 2004). The same polymorphism influences head growth rates in typically developing children as well (Muscarella et al., 2007). Even though large heads occur after birth, the conditions that create them may be set in motion much earlier in development.

Does Cognitive Limitation Play a Part in Environmental Etiologies of Autism?

The question has often been raised as to whether the cognitive impairment associated with many teratogenic exposures creates the apparent association of ASDs with environmental factors. In some situations, as when sample cases are collected from institutional settings, the patients are almost certain to have cognitive deficits, but this may not be true of all autism cases with the same etiology. A good example comes from two studies of autism in Moebius sequence. In the first, subjects were recruited from institutional care, and all the autism cases had cognitive limitation (Johansson et al., 2001). In the second study, subjects were recruited from families attending an international meeting of support groups for people with a Moebius sequence diagnosis (McConnell et al., 2002). In this sample, the rate of autism was slightly higher than in the first study, but more than half of the autism cases had IQs in the normal range. Among the studies of environmental exposures discussed in this chapter, several have provided data on IQ. Rasalam et al. (2005) reported IQ data for all their subjects exposed to valproate. Although the mean IQ was significantly lower in subjects with ASDs than in those without, most subjects with ASDs had IQs within the normal range. The four thalidomide cases studied in Strömland et al. (1994) had cognitive limitation, but a fifth case, whom the investigators were unable to recruit, was known from her records to have autism and a normal IQ. Additional data from the Brazilian misoprostol study has been shared with the author, and suggests that three of seven autism cases tested for IQ fell in the normal range (personal communication from Liana Ventura, 2009). Taken together, the available data do not rule out a role for cognitive limitation as a contributing factor in the autism rates observed after environmental exposures, but they do indicate that cognitive limitation is not a requirement for the development of autism after environmental exposures.

In summary, the discovery of environmental factors that increase the risk of autism has given us information that helps to explain many histological findings in this spectrum of disorders. An early origin for autism fits well with the issues of connectivity that seem to be part of the neurobiology of ASDs. Cases with different environmental etiologies are related to one another in symptoms and the same symptoms can be seen in some cases with known genetic etiologies. Similarly, those same symptoms often occur in idiopathic cases. Rather than being a set of rare etiologies unrelated to the much greater number of cases of unknown origin, cases associated with environmental risks appear to represent different developmental pathways to similar phenotypes.

Conclusions

The discovery of environmental exposures that increase the risk of autism spectrum disorders has provided the field with new ideas regarding the etiology of autism and new approaches to understanding its neurobiology. The idea that autism arises in early stages of development is a strong message from studies of environmental risk factors. Animal models, such as the one based on early exposure to valproic acid, promise to add to our understanding of both anatomy and behavior in autism. Comparing cases whose autism arose after environmental exposures to idiopathic cases and to some genetic syndromes suggests that different etiologies often result in similar outcomes. Not only are the diagnostic behaviors similar across etiologies, but so are some neurological and somatic anomalies that occur with increased frequency in people with autism. Although we need ways to stratify cases to advance our understanding of the genetics of autism, we also need to recognize phenotypic features that are shared by different etiologies.

Challenges and Future Directions

- It is no accident that the first five environmental risk factors identified are a virus and four drugs. It is much easier to identify these kinds of exposures and determine dose levels for them than for many potential teratogens. Can we recognize the association between terata and exposures to agents that are widespread in the environment? This is a much greater challenge, especially when individual doses are unknown.
- Susceptibility genes that interact with environmental exposures should vary from one risk factor to another. Can we identify these genes?

SUGGESTED READINGS

Arndt, T. L., Stodgell, C. J., & Rodier, P. M. (2005). The teratology of autism. *International Journal of Developmental Neuroscience, 23*, 189–199.

Rasalam, A. D., Hailey, H., Williams, J. H., Moore, S. J., Turnpenny, P. D., & Lloyd, D. J., et al. (2005). Characteristics of fetal anticonvulsant syndrome associated autistic disorder. *Developmental Medicine and Child Neurology, 47*, 551–555.

Strömland, K., Nordin, V., Miller, M., Akerstrom, B., & Gillberg, C. (1994). Autism in thalidomide embryopathy: A population study. *Developmental Medicine and Child Neurology, 36*, 351–356.

REFERENCES

Ardinger, H. H., Atkin, J. F., Blackston, R. D., Elsas, L. J., Clarren, S. K., Livingstone, S., et al. (1988). Verification of the fetal valproate syndrome phenotype. *American Journal of Medical Genetics, 29*, 171–185.

Ariens Kappers, J. (1957). Developmental disturbance of the brain induced by German measles in an embryo of the 7th week. *Acta Anatomica, 31*, 1–20.

Arndt, T. L., Chadman, K. K., Watson, D. J., Tsang, V., Rodier, P. M., & Stanton, M. E. (2006). Long delay eyeblink conditioning inautism [Abstract]. *Birth Defects Research, Part A, 76*, 323.

Arndt, T. L., Stodgell, C. J., & Rodier, P. M. (2005). The teratology of autism. *International Journal of Developmental Neuroscience, 23*, 189–199.

Aronson, M., Hagberg, B., & Gillberg, C. (1997). Attention deficits and autism spectrum problems in children exposed to alcohol during gestation: A follow-up study. *Developmental Medicine and Child Neurology, 39*, 583–587.

Bailey, A., Le Couteur, A., Gottesman, I., Bolton, P., Simonoff, E, Yuzda, E., et al. (1995). Autism as a strongly genetic disorder: Evidence from a British twin study. *Psychological Medicine, 25*, 63–77.

Bailey, A., Luthert, P., Dean, A., Harding, B., Janota, I., Mongomery, M., et al. (1998). A clinicopathological study of autism. *Brain, 121*, 889–905.

Bandim, J. M., Ventura, L. O., Miller, M. T., Almeida, H. C., & Costa, A. E. (2003). Autism and Mobius sequence: An exploratory study of children in northeastern Brazil. *Arquivos de Neuro-Psiquiatria, 61*, 181–185.

Bauman, M. L. & Kemper, T. L. (1985). Histoanatomic observations of the brain in early infantile autism. *Neurology, 35*, 866–874.

Bauman, M. L. & Kemper, T. L. 1994. Neuroanatomic observations in autism. In M. L. Bauman & T. L. Kemper (Eds.), *The neurobiology of autism* (pp. 119–145). Baltimore, MD: Johns Hopkins University Press.

Bavinck, J. N. B. & Weaver, D. D. (1986). Subclavian artery supply disruption sequence: Hypothesis of a vascular etiology for Poland, Kippel-Feil, and Moebius anomalies. *American Journal of Medical Genetics, 23*, 903–919.

Bayer, S. A., Altman, J., Russo, R. J., Zhang, X. (1993). Timetables of neurogenesis in the human brain based on experimentally determined patterns in the rat. *Neurotoxicology, 14*, 83–144.

Benayed, R., Gharani, N., Rossman, I., Mancuso, V., Lazar, G., Kamdar S, et al. (2005). Support for the homeobox transcription factor gene ENGRAILED 2 as an autism spectrum disorder susceptibility locus. *American Journal of Human Genetics, 77*, 851–868.

Bishop, S., Gahagan, S., & Lord, C. (2007). Re-examining the core features of autism spectrum disorder and fetal alcohol spectrum disorder. *Journal of Child Psychology and Psychiatry, 48*, 1111–1121.

Bojic, U., Elmazar, M. M., Hauck, R. S. & Nau, H. (1996). Further branching of valproate-related carboxylic acids reduces the teratogenic activity, but not the anticonvulsant effect, *Chemical Research in Toxicology, 9*, 866–870.

Bosley, T. M., Alorainy, I. A., Salih, M. A., Aldhalaan, H. M., Abu-Amero, K. K., Oystreck, D.T., et al. (2008). The clinical spectrum of homozygous HOXA1 mutations. *American Journal of Medical Genetics, 146*, 1235–1240.

Bosley, T.M., Salih, M. A., Alorainy, I. A., Oystreck, D.T., Nester, M., Abu-Amero, K. K., et al., (2007). Clinical characterization of the HOXA1 syndrome BSAS variant. *Neurology, 69*, 1245–1253.

Chakrabarti, S. & Fombonne, E. (2001). Pervasive developmental disorders in preschool children. *Journal of the American Medical Association, 285*, 3093–3099.

Chess, S., Fernandez, P., & Korn, S. (1978). Behavioral consequences of congenital rubella. *Journal of Pediatrics, 93*, 699–703.

Chess, S. & Fernandez, P. (1980). Neurologic damage and behavior disorder in rubella children. *American Annals of Deafness, 125*, 998–1001.

Chisaka, O., Musci, T. S., & Cappechi, M. R. (1992). Developmental defects of the ear, cranial nerves, and hindbrain resulting from targeted disruption of the mouse homeobox gene Hox1.6. *Nature, 355*, 516–520.

Christianson, A. L., Chesler, N., & Kromberg. J. G. R. (1994). Fetal valproate syndrome: Clinical and neurodevelopmental features in two sibling pairs. *Developmental Medicine and Child Neurology, 36*, 357–369.

Coffin, J. M,. Baroody, S., Schneider, K., & O'Neill, J. (2005). Impaired cerebellar learning in children with prenatal alcohol exposure: a comparative study of eyeblink conditioning in children with ADHD and dyslexia. *Cortex, 41*, 389–398.

Conciatori, M., Stodgell, C. J., Hyman, S. L., O'Bara, M., Militerni, R., Bravaccio, C., et al. (2004). Association between the HOXA1 A218G polymorphism and increased head circumference in patients with autism. *Biological Psychiatry, 55*, 413–419.

Courchesne, E., Carper, R., & Akshoomoff, N. (2003). Evidence of brain overgrowth in the first year of life in autism. *Journal of the American Medical Association, 290*, 337–344.

Courchesne, E., Yeung-Courschesne, R., Press, G. A., Hesselink, J. R., & Jernigan, T. L. (1988). Hypoplasia of cerebellar vermal lobules VI and VII in autism. *New England Journal of Medicine, 318*, 1349–1354.

Dawson, G., Munson, J., Webb, S. J., Nalty, T., Abbott, R., & Toth, K. (2007). Rate of head growth decelerates and symptoms worsen in the second year of life in autism. *Biological Psychiatry, 61*, 458–464.

DiLiberti, J. H., Farndon, P. A., Dennis, N. R., & Curry, C. J. R. (1984). The fetal valproate syndrome. *American Journal of Medical Genetics, 19*, 473–481.

Folkman, J. (1995). Clinical applications of research on angiogenesis. *New England Journal of Medicine, 333*, 1757–1763.

Fombonne, E. (2002). Is exposure to alcohol during pregnancy a risk factor for autism? *Journal of Autism and Developmental Disorders, 32*, 243.

Gharani, R., Benayed, V., Mancuso, L. M., Brzustowicz, L., & Millonig, J. H. (2004). Association of the homeobox transcription factor, ENGRAILED 2, with autism spectrum disorder. *Molecular Psychiatry, 9*, 474–484.

Gonzalez, C. H., Marques-Dias, M. J., Kim, C. A., Sugayama, S. M. M., Da Paz, J. A., Huson, S. M., et al. (1998). Congenital anomalies in Brazilian children associated with misoprostol misuse in first trimester of pregnancy. *Lancet, 351*, 1624–1627.

Gregg, N. M. (1941). Congenital cataract following German measles in the mother. *Transactions of the Ophthalmologic Society of Australia, 3*, 35–46.

Gurvich, N., Berman, M. G., Wittner, B. S., Gentleman, R. C., Klein, P. S., & Green, J. B. A. (2005). Association of valproate-induced teratogenesis with histone deacetylase inhibition in vivo. *FASEB Journal, 19*, 1166–1187.

Hallene, K. L., Oby, E., Lee, B. J., Santaguida, S., Bassanini, S., & Cipolla, M. (2006). Prenatal exposure to thalidomide, altered vasculogenesis, and CNS malformations. *Neuroscience, 142*, 267–283.

Hansen, J. M., Harris, K. K., Philbert, M. A., & Harris, C. (2002). Thalidomide modulates nuclear redox status and preferentially depletes glutathione in rabbit limb versus rat limb. *Journal of Pharmacology and Experimental Therapeutics, 300*, 768–776.

Harris, S. R., MacKay, L. L., & Osborn, J. A. (1995). Autistic behaviors in offspring of mothers abusing alcohol and other drugs: A series of case reports. *Alcoholism: Clinical and Experimental Research, 19*, 660–665.

Hauck, R. S. & Nau, H. (1989). Asymmetric synthesis and enantioselective teratogenicity of 2-*n*-propyl-4-pentenoic acid (4-en-VPA), an active metabolite of the anticonvulsant drug, valproic acid. *Toxicology Letters, 49*, 41–48.

Holmes, L. B. (2002). The teratogenicity of anticonvulsant drugs: A progress report. *Journal of Medical Genetics, 39*, 245–247.

Ingram, J. L., Peckham, S. M., Tisdale, B., & Rodier, P. M. (2000). Prenatal exposure of rats to valproic acid reproduces the cerebellar anomalies associated with autism. *Neurotoxicology and Teratology, 22*, 319–324.

Jager-Roman, E., Deichl, A., Jakob, S., Hartmann, A. M., Koch, S., Rating, D., et al. (1986). Fetal growth, major malformations, and minor anomalies in infants born to women receiving valproic acid. *Journal of Pediatrics, 108*, 997–1004.

Johansson, M., Wentz, E., Fernell, E., Strömland, K., Miller, M. T, & Gillberg, C. (2001). Autistic spectrum disorder in Mobius sequence: A comprehensive study of 25 individuals. *Developmental Medicine and Child Neurology, 43*, 338–345.

Jones, K. L. & Smith, D. W. (1973). Recognition of the Fetal Alcohol Syndrome in early infancy. *Lancet, 836*, 999–1001.

Jones, K. L., Smith, D. W., Ulleland, C. N., & Streissguth, A. P. (1973). Pattern of malformation in the offspring of chronic alcoholic mothers. *Lancet, 815*, 1267–1271.

Joyner, A. L., Herrup, K., Auerbach, B.A., Davis, C.A., & Rossant, J. (1991). Subtle cerebellar phenotype in mice homozygous for a targeted deletion of the En-2 homeobox, *Science, 251*, 1239–1243.

Just, M. A., Cherkassy, V. L., Keller, T. A., & Minshew, N. J. (2004). Cortical activation and synchronization during sentence comprehension in high-functioning autism: Evidence of underconnectivity. *Brain, 127*, 1811–1821.

Kana, R. K., Keller, T. A., Minshew, N. J., & Just, M. A. (2007). Inhibitory control in high-functioning autism. *Biological Psychiatry, 62*, 198–206.

Kanner, L. (1943). Autistic disturbances in affective contact. *Nervous Child, 2*, 217–250.

Knobloch, J., Shaughnessy, J. D., & Ruther, U. (2007). Thalidomide induces limb deformities by perturbing the Bmp/Dkk1/Wnt signaling pathway. *FASEB Journal, 21*, 1410–1421.

Kozma, C. (2001). Valproic acid embryopathy: Report of two siblings with further expansion of the phenotypic abnormalities and a review of the literature. *American Journal of Medical Genetics, 98*, 168–175.

Kuemerle, B., Zanjani, H., Joyner, A., & Herrup, K. (1997). Pattern deformities and cell loss in *Engrailed-2* mutant mice suggest two separate patterning events during cerebellar development. *Journal of Neuroscience, 17*, 7881–7889.

Kulesza, R. J., & Mangunay, K. (2008). Morphological features of the medial superior olive in autism. *Brain Research, 1200*, 132–137,

Lipson, A. H., Webster, W. S., Brown-Woodman, P. D. C., & Osborn, R. A. (1989). Moebius syndrome: Animal model–human correlations and evidence for a brainstem vascular etiology. *Teratology, 40*, 339–350.

Lord, C., Risi, S., Lambrecht, L., Cook, E. H., Leventhal, B. L., DiLavore, P. S., et al. (2000). The Autism Diagnostic Schedule-Generic: A standard measure of social and communication deficits associated with the spectrum of autism. *Journal of Autism and Developmental Disorders, 30*, 205–223.

Lord, C., Rutter, M., & Le Couteur, A. (1994). Autism Diagnostic Interview-Revised: A revised version of a diagnostic interview for caregivers of individuals with possible pervasive developmental disorders. *Journal of Autism and Developmental Disorders, 24*, 659–685.

Markram, K., Rinaldi, T., La Mendola, D., Sandi, C., & Markram, H. (2008). Abnormal fear conditioning and amygdala processing in an animal model of autism. *Neuropsychopharmacology, 33*, 901–912.

McAlonan, G. M., Daly, E., Kumari, V., Critchley, H. D., van Amelsvoort, T., Suckling, et al. (2002). Brain anatomy and sensorimotor gating in Asperger's syndrome. *Brain,127*, 1594–1606.

McConnell, B., Drmic, I., Roberts, W., Miller, M. T., & Bryson, S. E. (2002, November 2). *The co-occurrence of autistic spectrum disorders and Moebius syndrome*: Data *from the ADI-R and ADOS.* Poster session at the International Meeting for Autism Research, Orlando FL.

Means, A. L. & Gudas, L. J. (1995). The role of retinoids in vertebrate development. *Annual Review of Biochemistry, 64*, 201–233.

Miller, M. T. (1991). Thalidomide embryopathy: A model for the study of congenital incomitant horizontal strabismus. *Transactions of the American Ophthalmological Society, 89*, 623–674.

Miller, M. T. & Strömland, K. (1991). Ocular motility in thalidomide embryopathy. *Journal of Pediatric Ophthalmology and Strabismus, 28*, 47–54.

Miyazaki, K., Narita, N., & Narita, M. (2005). Maternal administration of thalidomide or valproic acid causes abnormal serotonergic neurons in the offspring: Implication for pathogenesis of autism. *International Journal of Developmental Neuroscience, 23*, 287–297.

Moore, S. J., Turnpenny, P., Quinn, A., Glover, S., Lloyd, D. J., Montgomery, T., et al. (2000). A clinical study of 57 children with fetal anticonvulsant syndrome. *Journal of Medical Genetics, 37*, 489–497.

Muscarella, L. A., Guarnieri, V., Sacco, R., Militerni, R., Bravaccio, C., Trillo, S., et al. (2007). HOXA1 gene variants influence head growth rates in humans. *American Journal of Medical Genetics, Part B, 144*, 388–390.

Nanson, J. L. (1992). Autism in fetal alcohol syndrome: A report of six cases. *Alcoholism: Clinical and Experimental Research, 16*, 558–565.

Perry, W., Minassian, A., Lopez, B., Maron, L., & Lincoln, A. (2007). Sensorimotor gating deficits in adults with autism. *Biological Psychiatry, 61*, 482–486.

Phiel, C. J., Zhang, F., Huang, E. Y., Guenther, M. G., Lazar, M. A., & Klein, P. S. (2001). Histone deacetylase is a direct target of valproic acid, a potent anticonvulsant, mood stabilizer, and teratogen. *Journal of Biological Chemistry, 276*, 36734–36741.

Rasalam, A. D., Hailey, H., Williams, J. H., Moore, S. J., Turnpenny, P. D., Lloyd, D. J., et al. (2005). Characteristics of fetal anticonvulsant syndrome associated autistic disorder. *Developmental Medicine and Child Neurology, 47*, 551–555.

Ritvo, E. R., Freeman, B. J., Scheibel, A. B., Duong, T., Robinson, H., Guthrie, D., et al. (1986). Lower Purkinje cell counts in the cerebella of four autistic subjects: Initial findings of the UCLA-NSAC autopsy research report. *American Journal of Psychiatry, 146*, 862–866.

Rodier, P. M., Ingram, J. L., Tisdale, B., Nelson, S., & Romano, J. (1996). An embryological origin for autism: Developmental anomalies of the cranial nerve motor nuclei. *Journal of Comparative Neurology, 370*, 247–261.

Scharre, J. E., & Creedon, M. P. (1992). Assessment of visual function in autistic children. *Optometry and Visual Science, 69*, 433–439.

Sears, L. L., Finn, P. R., & Steinmetz, J. E. (1994). Abnormal classical eye-blink conditioning in autism. *Journal of Autism and Developmental Disorders, 24*, 737–751.

Schneider, T., Labuz, D., & Przewlocki, R. (2001). Nociceptive changes in rats after prenatal exposure to valproic acid. *Polish Journal of Pharmacology, 53*, 531–534.

Schneider, T. & Przewlocki, R. (2005). Behavioral alterations in rats prenatally exposed to valproic acid. *Neuropsychopharmacology, 30*, 80–89.

Schneider, T., Ziolkowska, B., Gierik, A., Tyminska, A., & Przewlocki, R. (2007). Prenatal exposure to valproic acid disturbs the enkephalinergic system functioning, basal hedonic tone, and emotional responses in an animal model of autism. *Psychopharmacology, 193*, 547–555.

Schopler, E. Reichler, R. J., DeVellis, R. F., & Daly, K. (1988). Towards objective classification of childhood autism: Childhood Autism Rating Scale (CARS). *Journal of Autism and Developmental Disorders, 10*, 91–103.

Schumacher, H. J., Terpane, J., Jordan, R. L., & Wilson, J. G. (1968). The teratogenic activity of a thalidomide analogue, EM12, in rabbits, rats, and monkeys. *Teratology, 5*, 233–240.

Sparrow, S. S., Bella, D. A., & Cicchetti, D. V. (1984). *A manual for the Vineland.* Circle Pines, MN: American Guidance Services.

Stanton, M. E., Erwin, R. J., Rush, A. N., Robinette, B. L., & Rodier, P. M. (2001). Eyeblink conditioning in autism and a developmental rodent model [Abstract]. *Neurotoxicology and Teratology, 23*, 297.

Stanton, M. E., Peloso, E., Brown, K. L., & Rodier, P. M. (2007). Discrimination learning and reversal of the conditioned eyeblink reflex in a rodent model of autism. *Behavioral Brain Research, 176*, 133–140.

Steg, J. P., & Rapoport, J. L. (1975). Minor physical anomalies in normal, neurotic, learning disabled, and severely disturbed children. *Journal of Autism and Childhood Schizophrenia, 5*, 299–307.

Stephens, T. D., Bundy, C. J., & Fillmore, B. J. (2000). Mechanism of action in thalidomide teratogenesis. *Biochemical Pharmacology, 59*, 1489–1499.

Streissguth, A. P., Aase, J. M., Clarren, S. K., Randels, R. N., LaDue, R., & Smith, D. W. (1991). Fetal Alcohol Syndrome in adolescents and adults. *Journal of the American Medical Association, 265*, 1961–1967.

Streissguth, A. P., Bookstein, F. L., Barr, H. M, Press, S., & Sampson, P. D. (1998). A fetal alcohol behavior scale. *Alcoholism: Clinical and Experimental Research, 22*, 325–333.

Strömland, K. & Miller, M.T. 1993. Thalidomide embryopathy: Revisited 27 years later. *Acta Ophthalmologica, 71*, 238–245.

Strömland, K., Nordin, V., Miller, M., Akerstrom, B., & Gillberg, C. (1994). Autism in thalidomide embryopathy: A population study. *Developmental Medicine and Child Neurology, 36*, 351–356.

Sulik, K. K., Johnston, M. C., Daft, P. A., Russell, W. F., & Dehart, D. B. (1986). Fetal alcohol syndrome and DiGeorge anomaly: Critical ethanol exposure periods for craniofacial malformations as illustrated in an animal model. *American Journal of Medical Genetics, Suppl. 2*, 97–112.

Tischfield, M. A., Bosley, T. H., Salih, M. A., Alorainy, I. A., Sener, E. C., Nester, M. J., et al. (2005). Homozygous HOXA1 mutations disrupt human brainstem, inner ear, cardiovascular and cognitive development. *Nature Genetics, 37*, 1035–1037.

Ueda, K., Nishida,Y., Oshima, K., & Shepard, T. H. (1979). Congenital rubella syndrome: Correlations of gestational age at time of maternal rubella with type of defect. *Journal of Pediatrics, 94*, 763–765.

Verzijl, H. T., van den Helm, B., Veldman, B., Hamel, B. C., Kuyt, L. P., Padberg, G. W., et al. (1999). A second gene for autosomal dominant Mobius syndrome is localized to chromosome 10q, in a Dutch family. *American Journal of Human Genetic, 65*, 752–756.

Walker, H. A. (1977). Incidence of minor physical anomaly in autism. *Journal of Autism and Childhood Schizophrenia, 7*, 165–176.

Wassink, T. H., Piven, J., Vieland, V. J., Huang, J., Swiderski, R. E., Pietila, J., et al. (2001). Evidence supporting WNT2 as an autism susceptibility gene. *American Journal of Medical Genetics, 105*, 406–413.

White, J. C., Highland, M., Kaiser, M., & Claggett-Dame, M. (2000). Vitamin A deficiency results in the dose-dependent acquisition of anterior character and shortening of the caudal hindbrain of the rat embryo. *Developmental Biology, 220*, 263–264.

Whitney, E. R., Kemper, T. L., Bauman, M. L., Rosene, D. L., & Blatt, G. J. (2008). Cerebellar Purkinje cellsare reduced on a subpopulation of autistic brains: Astereological experiment using calbindin-D28k. *Cerebellum, 7*, 406–416.

Williams, P. G., & Hersh, J. H. (1997). A male with fetal valproate syndrome and autism. *Developmental Medicine and Child Neurology, 39*, 632–634.

Williams, P. G., King, J., Cunningham, M., Stephan, M., Kerr, B., & Hersh, J. H. (2001). Fetal valproate syndrome and autism: Additional evidence of an association. *Developmental Medicine and Child Neurology, 43*, 202–206.

Wiltse, J. (2005). Mode of action: Inhibition of histone deacetylase, altering WNT-dependent gene expression, and regulation of beta-catenin—developmental effects of valproic acid. *Critical Reviews in Toxicology, 35*, 727–738.

Woodruff-Pak, D. S., & Papka, M. (1996a). Alzheimer's Disease and eyeblink conditioning: 750 ms trace vs. 400 ms delay paradigm. *Neurobiology of Aging, 17*, 397–404.

Woodruff-Pak, D. S., & Papka, M. (1996b). Huntington's disease and eyeblink classical conditioning: Normal learning but abnormal timing. *Journal of the International Neuropsychology Society, 2*, 323–334.

49 Mark A. Corrales, Martha R. Herbert

Autism and Environmental Genomics: Synergistic Systems Approaches to Autism Complexity

Points of Interest

- Genomic and environmental factors work together in determining risk and severity of ASDs. Four mechanisms are highlighted:
  - Gene–environment interactions (GxE) (genetic susceptibility to environmental exposures).
  - Environmental factors causing genetic damage in germ cells (including point mutations or structural changes).
  - Environmental factors acting via heritable epigenetic modifications.
  - Genetic traits influencing environmental exposure via behavior (sometimes called *gene–environment correlation*).
- The apparently high heritability of ASDs is often misinterpreted as ruling out a large role for environmental risk factors. In fact, common, preventable environmental factors might be just as necessary as genetic factors for the occurrence of ASDs, despite high heritability, because of gene–environment interplay:
  - Heritability estimates mistakenly count gene–environment interaction as purely genetic for environmental exposures shared by twins.
  - Many genetic contributors may actually depend upon environmental exposures to have an impact, making the exposures the root cause.
  - Heritable epigenetic causes also may result from environmental exposures as the root cause.
  - Shared placentas are an environmental factor that may boost monozygotic (MZ) twin concordance and apparent heritability (through a different sort of gene–environment correlation). Genetic effects on a child's individual (nonshared) social environment (traditional gene–environment correlations) also inflate apparent heritability.
- Genetic findings in ASDs should inform research on environmental pollutants (or other risk factors) and vice versa, since genes and pollutants may have common targets. Greater collaboration, synthesis, and prioritization of risk factors based on toxicology and population attributable fraction (PAF) would be valuable. A systems and pathway-based approach, using bioinformatics and toxicogenomics tools would also benefit ASD research.

Introduction

What is "environmental genomics" and why is it important in research on autism spectrum disorders? The title of this chapter is meant to suggest that both environment and genetics are important in ASDs, and that studying the genome and environment together, in an integrated, systems approach, can drive a fruitful research and intervention agenda.

Genetics is obviously important in ASDs. But the investigation of genetic influences has run into frustrating limitations, including a realization that genome-wide association studies suffer from a high rate of false positive findings (Ioannidis, 2005; Moonesinghe et al., 2007), as well as generally modest-to-small odds ratios (typically less than 1.5) (Wellcome Trust Case Control Consortium, 2007; Allen et al., 2008; Harrison & Weinberger, 2005). In cases where larger odds ratios are suggested in autism gene candidates, the risk-associated variants are rare, so the PAF is still small, meaning that no single genetic factor has been able to account for even 50% of all cases of ASDs. Even all de novo copy number variants (CNVs) combined may be a critical factor in roughly 6% (Sebat et al., 2007) or speculatively perhaps up to 30% or more of ASDs (Zhao et al., 2007; Guilmatre et al., 2009). Genetics research is in need of new approaches that can explain and ultimately treat or prevent a larger share of all cases of ASD.

A simple focus on environmental factors alone is likewise unable to provide an adequate explanation for autism. Although various lines of evidence implicate environmental risk factors in ASDs (Institute of Medicine, 2008; Newschaffer et al., 2007; Lathe, 2006; Pessah & Lein, 2008) no specific environmental factor as yet has been verified with a large PAF. This may be because each important environmental factor mainly affects some genetic subgroup, or because many environmental factors converge upon common biological targets; either would make detection of specific culprits unlikely, because (partly resulting from sample size requirements) almost no studies of environmental factors in autism have examined risk stratified by genetic subgroup or biological mechanism of impact.

Although many research groups are still focused on either genes or environmental risk factors alone, striking progress has been made by those who study how genome and environment work together to cause disease. As explained in this chapter, they work together in several important ways, and four mechanisms are highlighted here:

Environmental factors causing genetic damage in germ cells (including point mutations or structural changes).
Environmental factors acting through epigenetic modifications.
Genetic traits influencing environmental exposure via behavior (sometimes called *gene–environment correlation*).
Gene–environment interactions (GxE).

These four general mechanisms cover a broad range of potential routes by which environmental and genetic or epigenetic factors may work together to either cause or affect the severity and phenotypic diversity of complex conditions such as ASDs. These four types of causal routes may provide a useful overarching framework for considering the many specific mechanisms that may contribute to the risk and severity of various aspects of ASDs. The advantage of this simple framework is that it calls attention to a very broad range of ways in which environmental and inherited risk factors may jointly contribute to ASDs. In particular, this perspective extends beyond narrowly defined gene–environment interaction (as discussed below), to highlight the potential importance of environment in causing de novo genetic and also epigenetic alterations, both of which have received little attention in ASD research until very recently.

There has been substantial confusion in the general public about the relative importance of environment and genetics in autism. A critical factor underlying the debate has been the widespread citation of extremely high heritability estimates. In the face of these estimates many have considered the residual role for environmental factors to be so small as not to merit serious attention. However, upon examination it becomes apparent that these heritability estimates, as well as related estimates of PAF, can be misleading and lead to erroneous conclusions about the contributions of genetics and environment (Visscher et al., 2008). In general, there is a long history of misinterpretation of estimates of the share of cases attributable to environmental (or other) causes, as emphasized at the start of the authoritative textbook, *Modern Epidemiology*, by Rothman and Greenland (1998). As these authors point out,

> "There is a tendency to think that the sum of the fractions of disease attributable to each of the causes of the disease should be 100%... it is clear on a priori grounds that 100% of any disease is environmentally caused.... Similarly, one can show that 100% of any disease is inherited.... Many researchers have spent considerable effort in developing heritability indices that are supposed to measure the fraction of disease that is inherited. Unfortunately, these indices only assess the relative roles of environmental and genetic causes of disease in a particular setting."

The significance of this point is further developed later in this chapter, but the essential point is that a disease can be simultaneously 100% genetic and 100% environmental. Another way of putting it is that genetics may be essential, but not sufficient, to cause autism. An implication for public health is that if environmental factors are also essential, then environmental changes may be able to prevent disease or reduce its severity.

The mechanisms by which genome and environment work together in ASDs are still unclear for the most part. What is clear, however, is that the simplistic dichotomy of nature versus nurture is largely obsolete, and that both are essential.

Just as viewing genome and environment separately limits progress, a piecemeal approach to risk factors and biological avenues of inquiry may be insufficient. Given the limited findings from attempts to find single strong causes, shifting to a systems biology perspective (Kitano, 2002) (i.e., genomics and epigenomics rather than genetics, and multiple environmental factors rather than one chemical at a time) may allow us most effectively to synthesize and reconcile findings related to multiple genes and multiple environmental risk factors that seem disparate and inconsistent when considered separately. It is important to note that this does not mean ASDs should be treated as a monolithic disorder whose many and varied features can be explained by a unified set of causes. On the contrary, it is essential to recognize the heterogeneity of ASDs' features and causes (Happé et al., 2006), and a key goal should be synthesis at the population level, where various features are influenced by various causes across various individuals, forming a complete picture that accounts for the wide range of conditions.

Finally, autism research also would benefit from greater integration of findings across biological levels and areas of expertise, linking new data from genetics, toxicology, physiology, epidemiology, and other fields. The next phase of progress will require greater application of high-throughput data along with tools from systems biology and bioinformatics, to study more comprehensive sets of molecules, genomic features, microbiota, physiological functions, cell types, brain regions, systems, and symptoms.

Part One: Mechanisms by which Genome and Environment Work Together

To help transcend the historical polarization, it will be useful to consider four ways environment and genome/epigenome can work together. These four causal routes are sketched in Figure 49-1.

Genetic Damage (E→ G→ D)

Some recent evidence has suggested that a substantial percentage of cases of autism—perhaps on the order of 6%, though some have suggested the majority of cases—may be attributable to de novo genetic changes (Sebat et al., 2007; Zhao et al., 2007). To the extent this is true, it becomes critical to determine the cause of these genetic alterations. Many authors have referred to de novo genetic changes as "sporadic" or as resulting from "stochastic processes." This may imply they occur for no particular reason or with no identifiable cause. But in fact environmental factors can cause genetic damage, and susceptibility to such damage is also influenced by nutrition (Bagnyukova et al., 2008) and by genetic factors, including genes involved in xenobiotic metabolism (Dorne, 2007) and DNA repair (Spry et al., 2007). Particularly if a substantial share of autism is attributable to de novo changes, this has important implications for etiology and possibly prevention.

DNA damage can be passed on to the next generation if it occurs in germ cells (sperm or oocytes), rather than just in somatic cells (as in cancer). The effects of germ line damage are initially seen as de novo mutations; but in subsequent generations, assuming the carrier reproduces, they are inherited and seem to be simply genetic causes of disease even if they originally resulted from environmental exposures.

Recent work suggests oxidative damage is a major cause of increased recombination and mutation in germ cells (Ohno et al., 2006). This hypothesis has profound implications for the study of genetic and environmental causes of disease, and suggests the need for research focused on environmental agents causing oxidative stress and subsequent DNA damage.

Numerous environmental factors result in DNA damage, including environmental toxicants, infectious agents, radiation, and some medications (Elespuru & Sankaranarayana, 2007). Given reported associations of ASDs with urban birth (Lauritsen et al., 2005; Williams et al., 2006), the link between urban air pollution and DNA damage may be relevant. Although hundreds of genotoxic chemicals are found in urban air samples, the components most often studied and implicated as causing DNA damage are components of particulate matter (a complex mixture of substances), particularly polycyclic aromatic hydrocarbons (PAHs) (DeMarini & Claxton, 2006; Tovalin et al., 2006). The urban environment, however, contains thousands of chemicals in addition to air pollutants, and a review of these candidates is beyond the scope of this discussion. The urban environment also differs from rural settings in terms of exposures to infectious agents and allergens in

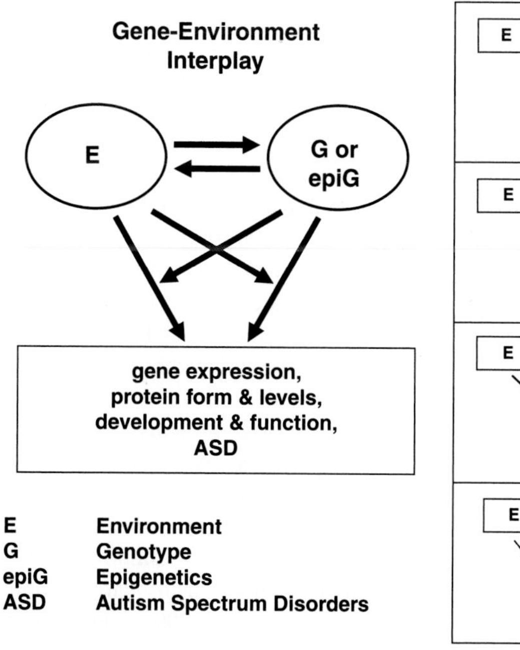

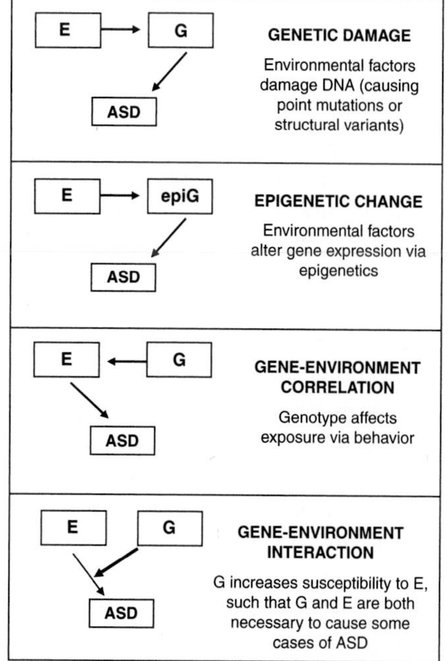

Figure 49–1. Potential direct and interactive effects of environment, genes, and the epigenome on disease.

ways that increase risk, for example of allergies among certain genotypes (Becker, 2007; Martinez, 2007).

There are substantial gender differences in germ cell mutagenesis, in type and risk of mutation, which in cases of de novo mutations may provide clues about which parent was exposed and at what age (Crow, 2000; Eichenlaub-Ritter et al., 2007). Paternal age is a risk factor for ASDs (Croen et al., 2007; Kolevzon et al., 2007; Grether et al., 2009), and genetic damage in sperm cells does increase with the father's age (Wyrobek et al., 2006). Some recent research, though not specific to ASDs, suggests that >80% of de novo structural chromosomal abnormalities in live births are paternally derived, and most spontaneous point mutations also are of paternal origin, according to work cited by Eichenlaub-Ritter, Adler, Carere, and Pacchierotti (2007). Maternal age is a risk factor for aneuploidy (Hassold et al., 2007). Although full-blown aneuploidy does not appear to play a major role in ASDs, in one recent study 16% of 116 boys with idiopathic autism reportedly had greatly elevated rates of mosaic aneuploidy (mostly gains of the X chromosome) (Yurov et al., 2007).

Although dozens of germ line genotoxins have been identified in animal models, definitive identification of germ line mutagens in humans has been elusive for a variety of reasons (Wyrobek et al., 2007). The strongest evidence suggesting environmentally caused germ line genotoxicity in humans includes recent studies showing increased chromosomal aberrations and other forms of DNA damage in sperm following exposure to chemotherapeutic agents or radiation, and germ line mutations found in children born in heavily polluted areas following the Chernobyl accident (Wyrobek et al., 2007). Germ cell mutagens are defined and classified by the United Nations globally harmonized system (GHS) and other national approaches (Morita et al., 2006). There are well over 100 substances classified by the GHS as *Class 1B germ cell mutagens*, which are chemicals that "should be regarded as if they produce heritable mutations in the germ cells of humans." (United Nations, 2003)

A substantial body of evidence beginning in 1975 has shown that urban outdoor air pollution causes DNA damage, and more recent work has extended findings to heritable (germ line) mutations in male mice (Somers et al., 2004; Samet et al., 2004), with lower rates of DNA damage in rural areas or when urban air is first filtered to remove fine particulate matter, and these findings have been reviewed recently (Claxton & Woodall, 2007). Interestingly, DNA damage in human sperm now has been linked to elevated levels of air pollution, particularly in a high-risk GSTM1 genotype (Rubes et al., 2007), such that the preceding 90-day-average particulate matter concentration predicted elevated sperm DNA damage. Additional environmental factors including folate intake may affect susceptibility to germ line DNA damage (Boxmeer et al., 2008).

Environmental genotoxins can cause various types of point mutations, structural changes (deletions, insertions), or aneuploidy, through a variety of mechanisms (Salnikow & Zhitkovich, 2008; Schins & Knaapen, 2007; Husgafvel-Pursiainen, 2004). Different types of environmental mutagens cause differing types of DNA changes, and to some extent leave signatures. For example, as discussed in the very useful review by Claxton and Woodall (2007), G $\rightarrow$ T base substitutions are the main type of mutation produced by PAHs and nitroarenes. Research may be able to identify certain types of DNA alterations that occur more often in autism, and this might provide clues regarding the causes of those alterations. A recent study demonstrated the great potential of genome-wide analysis of various types of genetic damage and their connection with disease, in a comprehensive analysis of multiple tumors in human breast and colorectal cancer (Wood et al., 2007), where the two cancer types had different types of mutations, interpreted as suggesting exposure to different mutagens or differences in the DNA repair process.

Epigenetic Change/Damage (E→ epiG→ D)

Inherited epigenetic (epiG) alterations may be one explanation for why genetic factors identified to date have been unable to explain most cases of ASD, despite high heritability (although rare or multiple interacting factors are also possible explanations). In fact, it is very possible that the careful regulation of gene expression and more importantly protein levels, not the DNA sequence itself, is what really matters most often in ASDs. In any event, it is increasingly recognized that gene or protein dosage, not just function, can be critical in neurodevelopment.

Epigenetic change and damage in ASDs have thus far been little studied, so their potentially important roles have not yet been elucidated. A significant role for epigenetic factors in autism has been proposed in recent years (Jiang et al., 2004), and is supported by several findings related to MECP2 and MBD1 (Hogart, 2007; Cukier et al., 2008; Allan et al., 2008; Nagarajan et al., 2006), as well as evidence that methylation is impaired in some fraction of ASD cases (James et al., 2006; Deth et al., 2008) and possibly the fact that valproic acid (a risk factor for autism and used to create an animal model of autism) causes epigenetic changes, via its action as a histone deacetylase (HDAC) inhibitor (Schneider et al., 2008; Moore et al., 2000; Khan et al., 2008). Genetic disruptions of normal epigenetic mechanisms also appear to be important in causing mental retardation (Kramer, & van Bokhoven, 2008), and their importance in the nervous system has been reviewed (Colvis et al., 2005). Knowledge is rapidly evolving in this area, and it must be noted that the practical significance of these environmental influences on the epigenome in human health and disease overall remains to be established.

A number of environmental factors are known to alter DNA methylation patterns, including certain dietary factors, such as the intake of methyl donors (folates, choline, methionine), and DNA methyltransferase inhibitors (e.g., polyphenols and perhaps isothiocyanates from plants) (Johnson & Belshaw, 2008; Edwards & Myers, 2007). Furthermore, environmentally caused genetic damage can disrupt mechanisms of epigenetic control in some cases: oxidative damage to methyl-CpG sites on DNA has been shown to impair the ability of MECP2 to bind to these target sites (Valinluck et al., 2004).

We also note that microRNAs and other forms of ribonucleic acid (RNA) are another aspect of the genome that is relatively understudied but may be important in mediating the effects of environment (Service, 2008; Riddihough et al., 2008; Bao et al., 2007) and in ASDs specifically (Abu-Elneel et al., 2008). For example, the 15q11 to 15q13 autism locus includes a locus coding for a small nucleolar RNA (snoRNA) that regulates serotonin 2c receptor splicing (Kishore & Stamm, 2006).

A group of major studies of cancer genomics has revealed that epigenetic changes, point mutations, and copy number variants all contribute to disruption of key pathways in various types of tumors (Jones et al., 2008; Parsons et al., 2008; Chan et al., 2008; The Cancer Genome Atlas Research Network et al., 2008; Wood et al., 2007). Of particular note, the mechanism of disruption varied across tumors and genes, sometimes involving point mutations, and in other cases CNVs or altered methylation. A pathway-based, comprehensive analysis including epigenetics was essential to illuminating all relevant genes and pathways.

Strikingly, some similar findings have been reported in ASD research. Different types of defects may alter MECP2 protein levels or function in different cases, including genetic (exon or promoter mutations) and epigenetic (promoter hypermethylation) (Nagarajan et al., 2006). One study of protein and mRNA expression in frontal cortex tissue from autistic and other patients revealed that multiple pathways, including apparently both transcriptional and posttranslational mechanisms, account for variation in expression of different MECP2 transcripts within different neuronal subsets (Samaco et al., 2004). Epigenetics rather than genetics explained the majority of cases of reduced MECP2 expression in autism cases in this study, although only 14 autism cases were analyzed. More recently, a similar pattern has been observed for the oxytocin receptor gene, where promoter methylation was increased in ASD cases relative to controls, in addition to some cases of deletions involving this gene (Gregory, 2009).

A further complexity is that some individuals or families are genetically predisposed to greater epigenetic stability versus lability over time in response to environment: the amount of change in global methylation over an 11- or 16-year interval clustered within families (Bjornsson et al., 2008). This might result in a gene–environment interaction in which certain gene variants make an individual's epigenome more susceptible to environmental exposures, resulting in substantially increased risk of disease when such gene variants and exposures co-occur.

Epigenetics is a relatively new field, and the mechanisms and implications are still being explored. Epigenetic changes can act like a strange hybrid of genetic and environmental risk factors, in that they can reflect the effects of the environment but also be inherited as relatively stable multigenerational factors. This complicates the way genes and environment work together to cause disease, and is not accounted for in most models of heritability or environmental risk. If epigenetic changes are actually a frequent cause of ASDs, this will have major implications for the types of genetic/epigenetic and environmental studies that should be undertaken. Resources are becoming available to investigate these issues more comprehensively, including the Human Epigenome Project, which has been attempting to catalog genome-wide DNA methylation patterns in all major tissues (Brena et al., 2006). Genome-wide epigenetic scans are becoming feasible (Berman et al., 2009), and it is clear they will add significantly to our understanding of the full range of causes of certain diseases.

Gene–Environment Correlation (G→ E→ D)

Gene–environment correlation is the situation where genotype affects one's social environment or one's exposure to environmental risk factors. To the extent that genes influence social environment or environmental exposures, it is possible that some genes increase the risk of autism by acting via environment. In other words, environment may be mediating some of the effects of genetics on autism risk. This is an underrecognized but important route of environmental influence, and one that needs to be understood in order to appropriately interpret heritability.

Genes can influence a child's exposure to environmental factors through various mechanisms, as discussed by Scarr and McCartney (1983) and Purcell (2002). There are at least three general routes by which genes could affect a child's social environment and exposure to physical/chemical environmental factors: *(1)* parental genes affecting parental behaviors that determine social and physical environmental exposure, *(2)* the child's genes affecting the child's behaviors, altering exposure to the social and physical environment, and *(3)* the child's genes affecting the child's behaviors, in turn affecting parental behavioral responses and the social environment.

Gene–environment correlation may be important to consider in autism research. Failure to take it into account can result in incorrect estimates of heritability and an incomplete picture of the prospects for intervention. If a genotype increases risk of autism, it is generally assumed that complete prevention is impossible, at least without gene therapy. However, if the genotype is actually causing autism partly by influencing the child's environment, interventions may be able to alter that environment and prevent some or all of the harm. For example, interventions focused on parenting practices (i.e., the social environment) can improve ADHD outcomes (Nigg, 2006), despite estimated heritability of 60% to 70% or even 90% (Nigg, 2006) and twin studies that identify almost no effects of shared environment. Gene–environment interactions and/or correlations could explain such seemingly conflicting findings.

Gene–Environment Interaction (GxE → D)

The term *GxE* is used here as shorthand for gene–environment interaction. The mechanisms underlying GxE, and even the basic definition of what is meant by GxE, are still unclear in many cases. The term *gene–environment interaction* has been used in a variety of ways, sometimes referring to biological interactions and in other cases describing statistical interactions, for example (Khoury et al., 1993). As used here, GxE refers to genetic susceptibility, where the effects of environmental exposures differ depending on genotype. Of particular interest is the case where an added environmental exposure increases the risk of disease more in a high-susceptibility genotype subgroup than in the low-susceptibility genotype.

It has become very clear from research in a variety of fields that genetics and environment clearly can and do interact (Rieder et al., 2008; Kelada et al., 2003), including in some neurodevelopmental diseases (Genc & Schantz-Dunn, 2007; Caspi & Moffitt, 2006; Thapar et al., 2007; Tsuang et al., 2004).

The possibility of gene–environment interaction in ASDs has been raised (Lawler et al., 2004; Newschaffer et al., 2002). Hints of such interaction may be starting to emerge in autism research, such as in findings related to PON1 (Pasca et al., 2008; D'Amelio et al., 2005), glutathione-related factors (James et al., 2006), immune system alterations (Enstrom et al., 2008; Ashwood et al., 2008), and pathways involving the MET gene (Sheng et al., 2010; Campbell et al., 2008).

GxE may be an important concept in ASD research for a variety of reasons:

- Studying GxE may help the field progress more rapidly in finding larger relative risk (RR) values and perhaps larger PAF values (Rutter, 2008).
- Studying GxE may identify important genes and medical intervention targets that would have been overlooked otherwise.
- Identifying environmental factors would be useful because some are avoidable or preventable in the near term, in contrast with genetic risk factors.
- Identifying genetic factors that create susceptibility to environment may enable targeted prevention efforts focused on a genetic subpopulation.

Two simple scenarios may demonstrate how genes and environment can interact to increase risk of disease. Table 49-1 shows the nomenclature used to refer to four combinations of genotype and environmental exposure, and Figure 49-2 illustrates two simple scenarios. It is critical to note that if E is ubiquitous, both scenarios appear to be simple cases of genetic causation.

Scenario 1: Gene and environment are both necessary (Figure 49-2A).

The simplest type of GxE is the case where both G and E are necessary for any impact on risk (Scenario 1).

Scenario 2: Gene simply increases susceptibility to environment (Figure 49-2B).

In this case, the risk allele (G) alone (without E) has no effect, but E alone (in the low risk genotype, g) has some effect. The combination of G and E has a much larger effect on risk than E with the low-risk genotype (g). If, for example, G controls metabolism of a toxicant, in that capacity it has no effect on ASD risk on its own, and thus it only matters when E (the toxicant) is present. E has some modest impact on ASDs in the low-risk genotype (g), but much more effect in the high-risk genotype (G).

There are, in fact, several general types of GxE, with typologies proposed by Ottman (1990, 1996) and Khoury et al. (1988). An extensive discussion of gene–environment research, including study designs and other key issues, was provided in the report, *Genes, Behavior, and the Social Environment: Moving Beyond the Nature/Nurture Debate* (National Research Council, 2006). Standard nomenclature denoting various combinations of genotype and exposure has been applied in the context of risk analysis (Cullen et al., 2008). In some cases, G and E each have direct effects on risk, apart from their interaction; in other cases only G has direct effects. Impacts on risk might be nonlinear or even nonmonotonic. It is also important to distinguish between interaction on additive and multiplicative scales. The nature of the interaction in GxE also can be expressed in the "component causes" framework (Greenland & Robins, 1986; Rothman & Greenland, 2005). These complexities have been well-covered elsewhere, albeit not in the context of autism research (National Research Council, 2006).

Table 49–1.
Nomenclature used to refer to four combinations of genotype and environmental exposure

Relative Risk (vs. Baseline, Which is Low-Risk Genotype and no Exposure)	g: (Genotype A: Low Sensitivity to E)	G: (Genotype B: High Sensitivity to E)
E (exposed to environmental risk factor)	gE (E has some direct effect, even in low-risk genotype)	GE (GxE means that RR is much larger among those with the high-risk combination of G and E)
e: (not exposed)	ge (baseline: no increased risk)	Ge (gene has some direct effect, even without E)

Toxicokinetics and Toxicodynamics

A critical research goal is to elucidate the types of mechanisms underlying GxE. It may be useful to consider two broad areas where GxE can arise: toxicokinetics (TK) and toxicodynamics (TD). Toxicokinetic variability refers to differences between individuals in the extent to which an external dose (ambient environmental concentration outside the body) results in a biologically available dose at the target organ(s). Toxicokinetics involves absorption, distribution, metabolism, and elimination

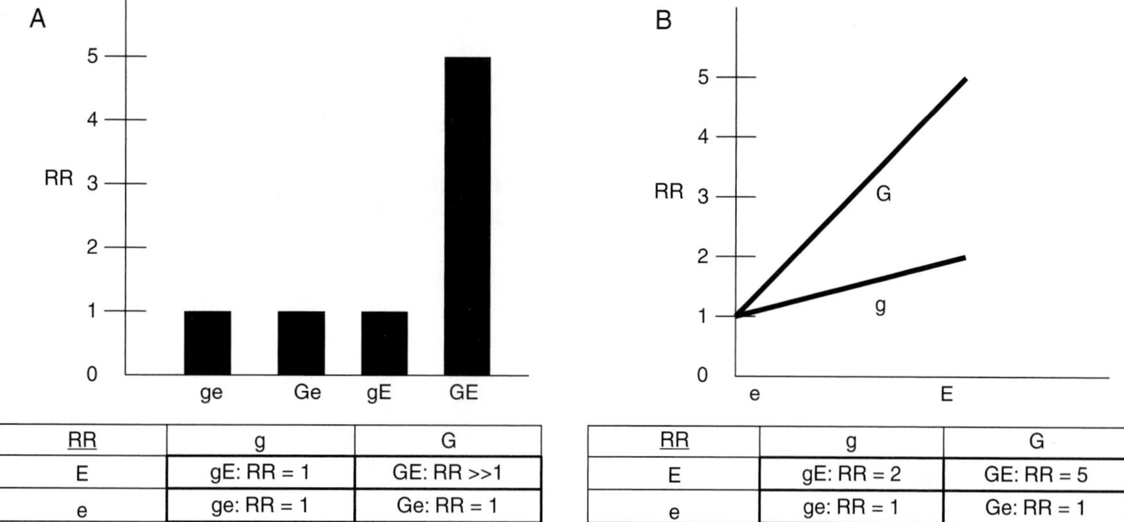

RR	g	G
E	gE: RR = 1	GE: RR >>1
e	ge: RR = 1	Ge: RR = 1

RR	g	G
E	gE: RR = 2	GE: RR = 5
e	ge: RR = 1	Ge: RR = 1

Figure 49–2. Scenarios for the interaction of gene and environment on disease risk. Explanation in text.

(ADME) of toxicants and their metabolites. Toxicokinetics has been studied intensively in the field of toxicology, and numerous models have been developed to quantify interindividual TK variability, describing how some individuals receive a larger effective internal dose for the same external exposure. Toxicodynamics, in contrast, refers to the extent to which the available dose at the target organ(s) results in adverse effects on health.

The vast majority of genes studied in autism so far are not related to TK vulnerability, partly because candidate gene studies have prioritized "brain genes" rather than genes that might result in the brain being exposed to higher levels of environmental agents or being vulnerable at lower levels of exposure (Herbert et al., 2006). Research and data in TK variability could inform the search for and analysis of potential environmental risk factors in ASDs. Research on autism's relationship with the PON1 gene that is important for organophosphate metabolism is one example (D'Amelio et al., 2005), and ASDs have been associated with two genes involved in metal metabolism (MTF1 and SLC11A3) (Serajee et al., 2004), but many other opportunities remain untapped. It is known that TK differences across the population can be caused by age, health status, infection and immune status, and genetic differences in a range of TK genes.

Genes that regulate metabolism of environmental chemicals: Numerous genes are thought to affect sensitivity to xenobiotics by altering metabolism of various compounds. These are reviewed relatively comprehensively and quantitatively by Dorne (2007).

Genetically sensitive individuals may have a given biological response or risk associated with a much lower ambient concentration of a chemical, compared with the average individual. Viewed in another way, genetically sensitive individuals may be at substantially higher risk than the average individual, when exposed to a given ambient concentration. TK variability in some major metabolic pathways may result in a twofold to even a tenfold or sometimes much greater increase in the effective dose experienced by individuals at the high end of the population distribution of TK variability (Dorne, 2007). TD factors would provide additional variability, resulting in even greater sensitivity for some individuals.

Genes relevant to infection: There are numerous genes known to control susceptibility to infection (Kaslow et al., 2008). If infection (or the maternal immune response to infection) is a risk factor for autism, then immune defense genes may be an important determinant of autism risk. This is an avenue of investigation that appears to be untapped in autism research.

Genes involved in DNA repair: Approximately 150 human genes involved in DNA repair have been identified, and mutations in many of these are known to increase the likelihood of DNA damage and cancer (Spry et al., 2007).

Genes upregulated or downregulated in response to environmental exposures: A recent review summarized gene expression changes seen in response to multiple air pollutants, including particulate matter, diesel exhaust, secondhand smoke from tobacco, and others. Key categories of genes upregulated by exposure to multiple air pollutant mixtures included genes related to xenobiotic metabolism (e.g., CYP1B1), oxidative stress response (e.g., glutathione-related genes, heme oxygenase 1, metallothioneins), and immune response (e.g. IL-6 and IL-1b) (Sen et al., 2007).

Part Two: Methodological Pitfalls in Assessing Relative Contributions of Genes, Environment, and Gene–Environment Interactions in a Disorder with High Heritability

One of the obstacles to a serious consideration of environmental contributors to ASDs has been the high heritability calculated for this condition, and how heritability has been misinterpreted in some cases. How can environment play a major role in autism if heritability is so high? This is a critical question that arises in discussions of research on environmental risk factors. As explained here, high heritability does not preclude a major role for environmental factors, contrary to common misinterpretations of heritability. Furthermore, there are other ways heritability may be overestimated. For these reasons, population attributable fraction is recommended as a more useful metric for describing the importance of environmental factors in ASDs.

Heritability Is Overestimated Since It Counts GxE as G, and Is Misinterpreted as Ruling out Environment

A heritability estimate describes the percentage of observed phenotypic variance that can be explained by genetic variation in the study. This generally involves taking 100% of the variance in symptoms and splitting it up between genes and environment. Such heritability estimates may be taken to imply that the "impacts" of genes and environment are separable and must sum to 100%.

In particular, twin studies overestimate heritability (and underestimate the role of environment) when genes interact with environmental risk factors that are shared within twin pairs (Nigg, 2006). To the extent a disease is caused by the interaction of genes and shared environment, the importance of shared environment is invisible in such a study design, and all the combined impact of genes and shared environment is misleadingly assigned to genes alone. The direction of bias does depend on whether shared or nonshared environmental effects are involved (Nigg, 2006). Environmental exposures shared by twins may be more common than nonshared exposures during prenatal or perinatal periods, suggesting overestimated heritability is more likely if such exposures are important sources of GxE in ASDs.

Michael Rutter has emphasized the importance of GxE eloquently (2008). GxE may be part of the explanation for the difficulty in finding obvious major causes in either genetics or environment research, despite high heritability estimates.

PAF Is a More Useful Metric for Comparing Interacting Risk Factors

Unfortunately, a heritability estimate of 90% has sometimes been misinterpreted as meaning that only 10% of cases are caused or even influenced by environmental factors. PAF is a more useful metric than heritability if the goal is to describe the proportion of disease burden that could be alleviated through research and interventions focused on a particular risk factor. PAF values estimated for various individual risk factors are not expected to sum to 100%, because the PAF values will overlap where two or more risk factors share responsibility for causation (Ezzati, 2006). Each PAF value accounts for all the cases that might be avoided if the risk factor were removed, even if some of those cases could also be prevented by removal of a different risk factor instead. Autism research would benefit from greater use of PAF estimates.

Heritability May be Overestimated in Other Ways

In addition to GxE, another cause of overestimated heritability may be the impact of shared placentas. Monozygotic (MZ) twins usually share one placenta (*monochorionic, MC*), but sometimes have different placentas (*dichorionic, DC*). Monochorionic twins are more likely to share exposure to certain environmental factors, including pathogens, than dichorionic twins. In this regard it is notable that concordance rates for schizophrenia are higher for monochorionic than for dichorionic twins: "...concordances for MZ twins without MC markers averaged 10.7 percent. In contrast, concordances for MZ twins with one or more MC markers averaged 60 percent." (Davis et al., 1995). This suggests many MZ twins may be concordant because they share a placental environment, not just because they share genes, and heritability may be overestimated.

A heritable change caused by the environment also appears to be a genetic cause, in subsequent generations (once no longer de novo), whether via DNA sequence damage or heritable epigenetic changes. Furthermore, traits influenced by inherited epigenetic modifications appear to be genetic and add to estimates of heritability, when in reality they might result from environmental factors, and could be altered through interventions.

Gene–environment correlation may also affect heritability. It tends to bias heritability estimates upward in the case of nonshared environment, the opposite of how GxE operates. If genes influence a child's behavior and social environment in ways that in turn increase risk of developing an ASD, such environmental factors are again counted as purely genetic and inflate heritability.

Finally, heritability estimates fail to quantify any impacts that lower levels of environmental exposure would have on disease, unless such lower levels are already represented in the study sample. Estimates of the importance of environment in twin studies are limited by the amount of variance in the environment experienced by the study population. Heritability estimates take existing environmental levels and their impacts as a given, and are not designed to measure the baseline impacts of ubiquitous environmental factors.

The Need for Rethinking Heritability

Given the likelihood of GxE, environmentally caused genetic and epigenetic alterations, and other issues raised, it is incumbent upon us to rethink how we have estimated and interpreted heritability, and the roles of genes and environment, in ASDs. PAF could be a valuable metric to use more often in comparisons among risk factors in ASD research.

Part Three: Research Directions and Resources

This chapter has suggested that investigating the combined effects of multiple genes and multiple environmental influences has more potential than studying individual factors in isolation, particularly if the goal is to identify targets for intervention accounting for a larger share of all cases.

Given what is known so far, what next steps might be most productive? Several related approaches are outlined here that may speed advances in autism research, categorized using the framework of four basic causal paths developed in Part One for the ways in which genes and environmental factors may work together in autism. Although a focus on genes within environmentally responsive pathways was introduced and illustrated in Herbert et al. (2006), an expansion is suggested here, to include identifying and studying the combined impacts of both: *(A)* environmental risk factors implicated by autism genetics, and *(B)* genes suggested by environmental risk factors. In other words, genetic findings should inform the focus of environmental research, and vice versa, especially through collaborative studies of combined effects.

(A) Given a candidate autism gene or pathway, identify and study environmental factors that may relate to the key candidate gene or pathway:

1. E→ D: seek environmental factors (e.g., mutagens) that could be a cause of the observed genetic alteration.
2. E→ epiG: seek environmental factors (e.g., nutrition) causing epigenetic changes affecting gene expression (and environment-caused changes in gene expression through other mechanisms).
3. G→ E: seek environmental conditions influenced by the gene (e.g. gaze avoidance, or dietary habits).
4. GxE: seek environmental factors that could interact with the given gene or pathway (GxE), including environmental factors affecting the same pathway already disrupted and made vulnerable by the genetic variant (e.g., pollutants affecting redox status and related metabolic pathways). This approach actually can apply to more than genes or pathways—one might select any alteration found in autism (e.g., alterations in a key brain region, cell type, or biomarker), and then investigate environmental factors reported to affect this parameter. This chapter, however, focuses only on genetic changes, with reported alterations at other levels of biological organization as the starting point for investigating potential environmental factors being beyond the present scope.

(B) Given a candidate environmental factor implicated in autism, identify and study genes and ideally pathways that may relate to the key environmental factor:

1. E→ G: seek genes/pathways most vulnerable to damage by such environmental factors.
2. E→ epiG: seek genes/pathways most vulnerable to epigenetic change resulting from the environmental factor (and genes with altered expression in response to the environmental factor, through any mechanism, not just epigenetic).
3. G→ E: seek genes/pathways that might influence exposure to the environmental factor (e.g., identify any genotypes associated with urban birth or advanced parental age at conception).
4. GxE: seek genes/pathways likely to interact with the environmental factor (GxE), including:
   a. genes in the pathways acutely or permanently disrupted by the environmental factor (e.g., studying acute and permanent gene expression changes that result from the implicated environmental risk factor) or more generally any genes with known roles in some function disrupted by the environmental factor;
   b. genes controlling toxicokinetic parameters (controlling the effective dose of a toxicant resulting from exposure to a given ambient level, through absorption, distribution, metabolism, or elimination of the toxicant and metabolites, such as PON1 or glutathione-related pathways);
   c. genes influencing likelihood of maternal infection or nature of response to infection (e.g., TGFB1);
   d. genes directly affecting sensitivity of genome integrity to environment, including DNA repair genes;
   e. genes affecting genome's sensitivity to epigenetic change caused by environment (e.g., DNA methyltransferases);
   f. genes in stress response pathways in general.

Research opportunities based on the above framework are suggested below. These are followed by some brief references to new informatics resources and research methods that will be helpful in pursuing these opportunities. A conclusion reiterates the importance of shifting from a search for individual genes or single environmental contributors to genomics, combinations of environmental contributors, and systems approaches.

Genetic Implications of Environmental Findings

The environmental factors implicated in autism by studies published to date are likely to be an incomplete and biased list of candidate factors, because a discovery-based approach has not been used to identify potential environmental factors in autism.

A comprehensive, authoritative, standard database summarizing the environmental risk factors implicated in autism does not exist, although this would be a valuable resource. In the absence of such a database, the most comprehensive listing of implicated risk factors may be found in review articles and textbooks Newschaffer et al., 2007; Pessah & Lein, 2008; Lathe, 2006). Environmental risk factors implicated by at least some evidence include maternal infection, urban birth, exposure to certain heavy metals, pesticides, solvents, PCBs, and other pollutants. Medications and treatments have also been studied as candidate risk factors, including valproic acid and the use of various anticonvulsants for other indications, thalidomide, and assisted reproductive technology. Also implicated are maternal and/or paternal age, which may in turn suggest germ line genetic damage that could partly result from environmental factors such as genotoxins. The few environmental factors implicated to date already provide some leads and suggest the types of genes that may interact with these environmental factors.

The framework discussed above should be applied to environmental findings, as a way to prioritize candidate genes, pathways, and environmental factors for further study. General principles may be useful here as well—a subset of genes can be referred to as *environmentally responsive* genes. These tend to fall in a few key functional categories: cell cycle, DNA repair, cell division, cell signaling, cell structure, gene expression, apoptosis, and metabolism (Herbert et al., 2006; Wilson and Olden, 2004).

Environmental Implications of Genetic and Pathway Findings

In contrast with environmental risk factors, there arguably do exist reasonably comprehensive databases listing the genetic risk factors implicated so far in autism (although no list can claim to include all genomic alterations actually contributing to autism). These genes are one source of information that may suggest candidate environmental risk factors (Corrales, 2009a). Some of the relevant database resources are reviewed in Table 49-2.

Belmonte and Bourgeron (2006) highlight four brain-related features that may contribute to subgroups of ASDs: excess neuronal growth and macrocephaly, abnormal neuromodulatory function, underconnectivity, and overexcitability relative to inhibition (Belmonte & Bourgeron, 2006). From an environmental vantage point, the list would be updated to include oxidative stress, immune system dysregulation, and gender-specific factors, which are environmentally modulated phenomena that may be important in a large percentage of ASD cases, since they are reported in a substantial share of ASD cases but relatively few controls (James et al., 2008; Enstrom et al., 2008). The ASD literature provides many additional clues about potential gene–environment interaction, including findings related to zinc metabolism (Faber et al., 2009; Li et al., 2003), oxytocin (Bartz & Hollander, 2008), steroids (Auyeung et al., 2008; Nakayama et al., 2007), cholesterol synthesis (Tierney et al., 2006; Zecavati & Spence, 2009), circadian rhythms (Melke et al., 2008), and key receptors and pathways including calcium channels and homeostasis (Palmieri et al., 2008; Krey & Dolmetsch, 2007; Pessah, Seegal, et al., 2008). Additionally much can be learned from studying the more extensive research on environmental factors that may influence comorbid disorders (Corrales et al., 2008).

These broad pathways or specific findings in ASDs have implications for the study of environmental risk factors. In general, next steps in pursuing these leads could involve prioritization based on potential for a large population attributable fraction (based on exposure and risk ratio when available), replication in larger samples, and testing for gene–environment interaction in cell-based, animal toxicology, and human epidemiological studies.

Methodologies and Data

In general, biological and environmental databases are multiplying and growing very rapidly. Today, it is far easier to find data on multiple biological molecules or multiple environmental chemicals, and synthesize across databases, than it was just 5 years ago. Table 49-2 reviews some of the resources. Given the paucity of our knowledge, there is a need for discovery-based approaches, which should be applied to screen very broadly, ideally comprehensively, across the full range of genomic/epigenomic factors and environmental factors that might be involved. High-throughput methods and predictive models will be helpful in this regard, and some relevant resources such as the Comparative Toxicogenomics Database (CTD) (Mattingly et al., 2006a, 2006b; Davis et al., 2008) and the Aggregated Computational Toxicology Resource (ACToR) database (Judson et al., 2008) are already useful in compiling available information generated by these methods on gene–toxin interactions. Databases of genes, pathways, and xenobiotics can provide useful tools for network analysis of multiple factors and their potential interactions (see Table 49-2).

Methodological advances are also providing many new opportunities for ASD research. Approaches to identifying gene–environment interactions have been reviewed (Moffitt et al., 2005), and a variety of models are available. Only a very limited number of environmental factors and susceptibilities have been tested so far in such models (Corrales, 2009b), so there is great potential for advances here.

In screening the full range of potential environmental risk factors to determine which ones are worthy of further study, it will be important to consider not only potential toxicity but also the magnitude and timing of exposure. Unfortunately, exposure estimation remains a significant obstacle (Wild, 2005; Cohen-Hubal, 2009), and clearly will require ongoing attention.

Furthermore, the importance of applying a complex systems approach to studying and classifying human diseases is becoming increasingly apparent (Loscalzo et al., 2007; Wu et al., 2008; Sieberts, & Schadt, 2007). Systems biology approaches have been applied to toxicology, and models have been constructed to predict metabolism and toxicity of new chemicals, accounting for genetic variability (Ekins et al., 2006). One important methodological question is what level of detail will be most useful for modeling interactions and causal paths within networks of genes or gene–environment networks. Small to moderately sized networks of genes can be simplified and represented using binary interactions where genes turn other genes on or off, but larger predictive networks, still out of reach with current computational methods,

Table 49–2.
Selected informatics resources related to environment and/or genetics

Database	Location
Exposure and Body Burden Data	
National Health and Nutrition Examination Survey (NHANES) at CDC	http://www.cdc.gov/nchs/nhanes.htm
ExpoCast at EPA (Hubal, 2009)	http://www.epa.gov/ncct/expocast/
Databases at EPA	http://www.epa.gov/epahome/data.html
Gene–Environment Initiative (GEI) at NIH	http://www.gei.nih.gov/exposurebiology/index.asp
ChemIDPlus at NIH ChemIDPlus includes links to databases on household products, food ingredients, medications, illegal drugs, and environmental pollutants.	http://chem.sis.nlm.nih.gov/chemidplus/
Human Microbiome Project at NIH (Turnbaugh et al., 2007)	http://nihroadmap.nih.gov/hmp/
Epidemiology and Toxicology Data	
ACToR and ToxCast databases at EPA's National Center for Computational Toxicology (NCCT) (Judson et al., 2008; Judson et al., 2009; Kavlock et al., 2008)	http://www.epa.gov/comptox/
Office of Environmental Information (OEI), Office of Prevention, Pesticides, and Toxic Substances (OPPTS), and other databases at EPA	http://www.epa.gov/oei/ http://www.epa.gov/oppt/existingchemicals/ http://www.epa.gov/epahome/data.html
Human Genetic Epidemiology (HuGE) Navigator at CDC (including gene–environment interaction literature) (Lin et al., 2006)	http://hugenavigator.net/
Review of NCBI databases at NIH (Sayers et al., 2009)	http://nar.oxfordjournals.org/content/38/suppl_1/D5.abstract
PubChem at NIH (Wang et al., 2009)	http://pubchem.ncbi.nlm.nih.gov/
Comparative Toxicogenomics Database (CTD) The CTD compiles data on and infers relationships between genes, environmental factors, and disorders. (Mattingly, Rosenstein, Colby et al., 2006; Mattingly, Rosenstein, Davis, et al., 2006; Davis et al., 2009)	http://ctd.mdibl.org
National Institute of Environmental Health Sciences databases (including links to the Environmental Polymorphism Registry and the Environmental Genome Project, and Chemical Effects in Biological Systems [CEBS] database)	http://www.niehs.nih.gov/research/resources/databases/index.cfm
European eChemPortal	http://www.echemportal.org/
Toxipedia	http://toxipedia.org
Genetic Variant Databases	
Review of top 26 autism gene candidates (Abrahams & Geschwind, 2008)	http://www.ncbi.nlm.nih.gov/pubmed/18414403
Database of genomic variants in autism (Xu et al., 2004; Zhang et al., 2006)	http://projects.tcag.ca/variation/
Autism genetics database (AGD) (includes approximately 226 autism candidate genes as of December 2010) (Matuszek & Talebizadeh, 2009)	http://wren.bcf.ku.edu/
Comparative Toxicogenomics Database (CTD) (includes approximately 220 genes directly related to autism as of December 2010) (Mattingly, Rosenstein, Colby, et al., 2006; Mattingly, Rosenstein, Davis, et al., 2006; Davis, et al., 2009)	http://ctd.mdibl.org/
Autism genetics database (AutDB) (includes approximately 219 autism candidate genes as of December 2010) (Basu et al., 2009)	http://www.mindspec.org/autdb.html
Harvard University project on autism genetics (includes approximately 700 genes with potential relevance to autism as of December 2010) (Wall et al., 2009)	http://autworks.hms.harvard.edu/

(Continued)

Table 49–2. (Contd.)

Database	Location
Sullivan Lab Evidence Project (SLEP), Psychiatric Genetics database. Compiles data from unbiased genome-wide studies (expression, linkage, association, etc.), so candidate gene studies are not included, nor are studies focused on particular regions of DNA. (Konneker et al., 2008)	http://slep.unc.edu
Genetic Association Database (GAD) at NIH (lists approximately 160 genes studied in autism as of December 2010) (Becker et al., 2004)	http://geneticassociationdb.nih.gov
Human Genetic Epidemiology (HuGE) Gene Prospector at U.S. Centers for Disease Control and Prevention (CDC) (Lists approximately 437 genes that may have been studied in connection with autism as of December 2010). (Yu et al., 2008)	http://hugenavigator.net
Online Mendelian Inheritance in Man (OMIM) at NIH	http://www.ncbi.nlm.nih.gov/omim

will require modeling that clusters genes into functional modules (Bornholdt, 2005).

Systems biology approaches are starting to be applied in the context of ASD research. For example, key signaling pathways are being identified through gene expression analysis of blood-derived lymphoblastoid cells, and are demonstrating that certain key genes or proteins (e.g., excess CYFIP1 and altered levels of JAKMIP1 and GPR155) are consistently dysregulated in autism cases caused by two entirely different causal genetic mutations (FMR1 and 15qdup) (Nishimura et al., 2007). Notably, immune response and mRNA processing were functions impacted by many of the dysregulated genes, and genes implicated in gastrointestinal disease and lipid metabolism were notably overrepresented. Other studies have also analyzed gene expression in ASDs and have implicated immune-related pathways among others (Hu et al., 2006; Gregg et al., 2008; Garbett et al., 2008). Given the influence of environment on so many of these pathways, a GxE approach to further research is strongly indicated.

Conclusion

Future discussions of genetic or environmental risk factors should be motivated by the public and clinical health importance of identifying and prioritizing among all possible contributors, and especially malleable contributors, to ASDs. From this point of view, it is important to make certain that we are turning every stone worth turning, and setting priorities rationally. This chapter has outlined how genetic and environmental factors may converge on common mechanisms pertinent to neurodevelopmental disorders, and the ways that high heritability can involve not only high genetic but also high environmental contributions. This material points toward the strong need for collaboration between genetic and environmental investigators, since this is in the best interests of both. This review has attempted to provide a glimpse of the breadth of substantive arguments for this synergistic approach, and also the many resources that already exist to facilitate it.

Both from an environmental and a medical point of view, ASDs are not only developmental disorders but also chronic conditions. For virtually all major common chronic conditions, finding clear causes, either genetic or environmental, has been difficult, raising fundamental questions about what we are trying to do (Buchanan et al., 2006). Recent systems analyses are finding that not only are there a plethora of interacting causes, but surprisingly there appear to be many core similarities among apparently different diseases (Torkamani et al., 2008). In the face of the prevalence of autism, we should remember as we seek causes that our primary purpose should be to help people with autism; our overriding goal must be to translate our findings into preventing or treating the problems associated with ASDs, and to move eventually to individualized treatments when systems assessments can be integrated into medical practice. At the population level, research should facilitate learning how to provide the greatest improvement in the largest number of cases in the shortest timeframe. This means we need to consider, of the many risk factors, which are most preventable or treatable in the near term and which have the largest impacts (high prevalence of exposure combined with high relative risk results in a high population attributable fraction). There may be important clues gained from rare factors like MECP2, certainly, but their importance at the population level is only in proportion to the extent that they may suggest actionable targets important for most cases of autism.

Michael Rutter argues that our efforts may indeed move faster if we pursue GxE effects:

> "... it is very striking that the G×E effects that have been found are of moderate size and by no means are as small as the main effects of single genes considered independently of the environment. Moreover, the G×E has been found with a sample size of about 1,000. There are a variety of reasons why that is probably rather smaller than is optimal, but it does not necessarily follow that it

is necessary to move to samples of 500,000 as some geneticists have sought to argue." (Rutter, 2008)

Just as there are causes and mechanisms at multiple levels, there will be multiple levels of benefits from going forth and integrating genetic and environmental efforts. The more thorough and rapid generation of results should hasten our ability to provide treatment and prevention.

Challenges and Future Directions

- Misinterpretation of heritability estimates has created the impression that environmental factors play only a minor role in ASDs. Ongoing discussion of gene–environment interaction, mutagens, epigenetics, and gene–environment correlation could help correct any misconceptions.
- Greater collaboration across disciplines would be helpful, particularly between geneticists, toxicologists, and epidemiologists.
- Systematic review and integration across research findings from different disciplines, including PAF calculations, would be helpful in assessing priorities across possible risk factors, biomarkers, and avenues of inquiry.
- Exposure assessment and sample size are substantial obstacles to the study of gene–environment interaction, and deserve ongoing attention. Emerging exposure measurement tools will be extremely helpful, as will large cohort studies such as the National Children's Study.

SUGGESTED READINGS

Judson, R., Richard, A., Dix, D. J., Houck, K., Martin, M., Kavlock, R., et al. (2009). The toxicity data landscape for environmental chemicals. *Environmental Health Perspectives, 117*(5), 685–695. Epub December 20, 2008.

Rutter, M. (2006). *Genes and behavior: Nature-nurture interplay explained.* Malden, MA: Blackwell Publishing.

Nigg, J. T. (2006). *What causes ADHD?* New York: The Guilford Press.

Disclaimer: The opinions expressed in this chapter are the authors' and do not necessarily represent those of the United States Environmental Protection Agency.

REFERENCES

Abrahams, B. S., & Geschwind, D. H. (2008). Advances in autism genetics: On the threshold of a new neurobiology. *Nature Review Genetics, 9*(5), 341–355.

Abu-Elneel, K., Liu, T., Gazzaniga, F. S., Nishimura, Y., Wall, D. P., Geschwind, D. H., et al. (2008). Heterogeneous dysregulation of microRNAs across the autism spectrum. *Neurogenetics, 9,* 153–161.

Allan, A. M., Liang, X., Luo, Y., Pak, C., Li, X., Szulwach, K. E., et al. (2008). The loss of methyl-CpG binding protein 1 leads to autism-like behavioral deficits. *Human Molecular Genetics, 17,* 2047–2057.

Allen, N. C., Bagade, S., McQueen, M. B., Ioannidis, J. P., Kavvoura, F. K., Khoury, M. J., et al. (2008). Systematic meta-analyses and field synopsis of genetic association studies in schizophrenia: The SzGene database. *Nature Genetics, 40,* 827–834.

Ashwood, P., Enstrom, A., Krakowiak, P., Hertz-Picciotto, I., Hansen, R. L., Croen, L. A., et al. (2008). Decreased transforming growth factor beta1 in autism: A potential link between immune dysregulation and impairment in clinical behavioral outcomes. *Journal of Neuroimmunology,* August 30, 2008. [Epub ahead of print]

Auyeung, B., Baron-Cohen, S., Ashwin, E., Knickmeyer, R., Taylor, K., & Hackett, G. (2008). Fetal testosterone and autistic traits. *British Journal of Psychology,* June 20, 2008, 10. [Epub ahead of print]

Bagnyukova, T. V., Powell, C. L., Pavliv, O., Tryndyak, V. P., & Pogribny, I. P. (2008). Induction of oxidative stress and DNA damage in rat brain by a folate/methyl-deficient diet. *Brain Research,* July 29, 2008. [Epub ahead of print]

Bao, L., Zhou, M., Wu, L., Lu, L., Goldowitz, D., Williams, R. W., et al. (2007). The polymorphism in microRNA target site (PolymiRTS) database is a collection of DNA variations in putative microRNA target sites. *Nucleic Acids Research, 35,* D51–54.

Bartz, J. A., & Hollander, E. (2008). Oxytocin and experimental therapeutics in autism spectrum disorders. *Progress in Brain Research, 170,* 451–462.

Basu, S. N., Kollu, R., & Banerjee-Basu, S. (2009). AutDB: A gene reference resource for autism research. *Nucleic Acids Research, 37*(Database issue), D832–836.

Becker, K. G., Barnes, K. C., Bright, T. J., & Wang, S. A. (2004). The genetic association database. *Nature Genetics, 36*(5), 431–432.

Becker, K. G. (2007). Autism, asthma, inflammation, and the hygiene hypothesis. *Medical Hypotheses, 69,* 731–740.

Belmonte, M. K., & Bourgeron, T. (2006). Fragile X syndrome and autism at the intersection of genetic and neural networks. *Nature Neuroscience, 9,* 1221–1225.

Berman, B. P., Weisenberger, D. J., & Laird, P. W. (2009). Locking in on the human methylome. *Nature Biotechnology, 27*(4), 341–342.

Bjornsson, H. T., Sigurdsson, M. I., Fallin, M. D., Irizarry, R. A., Aspelund, T., Cui, H., et al. (2008). Intra-individual change over time in DNA methylation with familial clustering. *Journal of the American Medical Association, 299,* 2877–2883.

Bornholdt, S. (2005). Systems biology. Less is more in modeling large genetic networks. *Science, 310,* 449–451.

Boxmeer, J. C., Smit, M., Utomo, E., Romijn, J. C., Eijkemans, M. J., Lindemans, J., et al. (2008). Low folate in seminal plasma is associated with increased sperm DNA damage. *Fertility and Sterility,* August 21, 2008. [Epub ahead of print]

Brena, R. M., Huang, T. H., & Plass, C. (2006). Toward a human epigenome. *Nature Genetics, 38,* 1359–1360.

Buchanan, A. V., Weiss, K. M., & Fullerton, S. M. (2006). Dissecting complex disease: The quest for the Philosopher's Stone? *International Journal of Epidemiology, 35,* 562–571.

Campbell, D. B., Li, C., Sutcliffe, J. S., Persico, A. M., & Levitt, P. (2008). Genetic evidence implicating multiple genes in the MET receptor tyrosine kinase pathway in autism spectrum disorder. *Autism Research, 1*(3), 159–168.

Cancer Genome Atlas Research Network, et al. (2008). Comprehensive genomic characterization defines human glioblastoma genes and core pathways. *Nature, 455,* 7209.

Caspi, A., & Moffitt, T. E. (2006). Gene-environment interactions in psychiatry: Joining forces with neuroscience. *Nature Reviews Neuroscience, 7*, 583–590.

Centers for Disease Control and Prevention (CDC) (2007). Prevalence of Autism Spectrum Disorders–Autism and Developmental Disabilities Monitoring Network, 14 Sites, United States, 2002. *Surveillance Summaries Morbidity and Mortality Weekly Report 56, SS-1*, 12–28.

Chan, T. A., Glockner, S., Yi, J. M., Chen, W., Van Neste, L., Cope, L., et al. (2008). Convergence of mutation and epigenetic alterations identifies common genes in cancer that predict for poor prognosis. *PLoS Medicine, 5*, e114.

Claxton, L. D., & Woodall, G. M. Jr. (2007). A review of the mutagenicity and rodent carcinogenicity of ambient air. *Mutation Research, 636*(1–3), 36–94.

Cohen-Hubal, E. A. (2009). Biologically-relevant exposure science for 21st century toxicity testing. *Toxicological Sciences, 111*(2), 226–232.

Colvis, C. M., Pollock, J. D., Goodman, R. H., Impey, S., Dunn, J., Mandel, G., et al. (2005). Epigenetic mechanisms and gene networks in the nervous system. *Journal of Neuroscience, 25*, 10379–10389.

Corrales, M. A., Ringer, A. P., & Herbert, M. (2008). Potential autism research gaps suggested by analysis of literature and comorbidities. Abstract presented at International Meeting for Autism Research (London, May 15–17, 2008). http://imfar.confex.com/imfar/2008/webprogram/Paper2999.html

Corrales, M. A. (2009a). Chemicals that interact with autism gene candidates - Identifying candidate environmental risk factors for autism via bioinformatics databases of reported gene-chemical interactions. Abstract presented at International Meeting for Autism Research (Chicago, IL, May 7–9, 2009).

Corrales, M. A. (2009b). Data availability for analyzing sensitive groups defined by genetic variability in environmental health risk assessment. Symposium presentation at Society for Risk Analysis Annual Meeting (Baltimore, MD, December 8, 2009).

Croen, L. A., Najjar, D. V., Fireman, B., & Grether, J. K. (2007). Maternal and paternal age and risk of autism spectrum disorders. *Archives of Pediatrics and Adolescent Medicine, 161*(4), 334–340.

Crow, J. F. (2000). The origins, patterns and implications of human spontaneous mutation. *Nature Reviews Genetics, 1*(1), 40–47.

Cukier, H. N., Perez, A. M., Collins, A. L., Zhou, Z., Zoghbi, H. Y., & Botas, J. (2008). Genetic modifiers of MeCP2 function in Drosophila. *PLoS Genetics, 4*, e1000179.

Cullen, A. C., Corrales, M. A., Kramer, C. B., & Faustman, E. M. (2008). The application of genetic information for regulatory standard setting under the clean air act: A decision-analytic approach. *Risk Analysis, 28*, 877–890.

D'Amelio, M., Ricci, I., Sacco, R., Liu, X., D'Agruma, L., Muscarella, L. A., et al. (2005). Paraoxonase gene variants are associated with autism in North America, but not in Italy: Possible regional specificity in gene-environment interactions. *Molecular Psychiatry, 10*, 1006–1016.

Davis, A. P., Murphy, C. G., Saraceni-Richards, C. A., Rosenstein, M. C., Wiegers, T. C., & Mattingly, C. J. (2008). Comparative Toxicogenomics Database: A knowledgebase and discovery tool for chemical-gene-disease networks. *Nucleic Acids Research*, September 9, 2008. [Epub ahead of print]

Davis, A. P., Murphy, C. G., Saraceni-Richards, C. A., Rosenstein, M. C., Wiegers, T. C., & Mattingly, C. J. (2009). Comparative Toxicogenomics Database: a knowledgebase and discovery tool for chemical-gene-disease networks. *Nucleic Acids Research, 37*(Database issue), D786–792.

Davis, J. O., Phelps, J. A., & Bracha, H. S. (1995). Prenatal development of monozygotic twins and concordance for schizophrenia. *Schizophrenia Bulletin, 21*(3), 357–366.

DeMarini, D. M., & Claxton, L. D. (2006). Outdoor air pollution and DNA damage. *Occupational and Environmental Medicine, 63*, 227–229.

Deth, R., Muratore, C., Benzecry, J., Power-Charnitsky, V. A., & Waly, M. (2008). How environmental and genetic factors combine to cause autism: A redox/methylation hypothesis. *Neurotoxicology, 29*, 190–201.

Dorne, J. L. (2007). Human variability in hepatic and renal elimination: implications for risk assessment. *Journal of Applied Toxicology, 27*, 411–420.

Edwards, T. M., & Myers, J. P. (2007). Environmental exposures and gene regulation in disease etiology. *Environmental Health Perspectives, 115*, 1264–1270.

Eichenlaub-Ritter, U., Adler, I. D., Carere, A., & Pacchierotti, F. (2007). Gender differences in germ-cell mutagenesis and genetic risk. *Environmental Research, 104*, 22–36.

Ekins, S., Bugrim, A., Brovold, L., Kirillov, E., Nikolsky, Y., Rakhmatulin, E., et al. (2006). Algorithms for network analysis in systems: ADME/Tox using the MetaCore and MetaDrug platforms. *Xenobiotica, 36*(10), 877–901.

Elespuru, R. K., & Sankaranarayanan, K. (2007). New approaches to assessing the effects of mutagenic agents on the integrity of the human genome. *Mutation Research, 616*, 83–89.

Enstrom, A. M., Lit, L., Onore, C. E., Gregg, J. P., Hansen, R. L., Pessah, I. N., et al. (2008). Altered gene expression and function of peripheral blood natural killer cells in children with autism. *Brain, Behavior, and Immunity*, August 20, 2008, 14. [Epub ahead of print]

Faber, S., Zinn, G. M., Kern, J. C. II, Kingston, H. M. (2009). The plasma zinc/serum copper ratio as a biomarker in children with autism spectrum disorders. *Biomarkers, 14*(3), 171–180.

Gardener, H., Spiegelman, D., & Buka, S. L. (2009). Prenatal risk factors for autism: Comprehensive meta-analysis. *British Journal of Psychology, 195*, 7–14.

Garbett, K., Ebert, P. J., Mitchell, A., Lintas, C., Manzi, B., Mirnics, K., et al. (2008) Immune transcriptome alterations in the temporal cortex of subjects with autism. *Neurobiology of Disease, 30*, 303–311.

Genc, M. R., & Schantz-Dunn, J. (2007). The role of gene-environment interaction in predicting adverse pregnancy outcome. *Best Practice and Research: Clinical Obstetrics and Gynaecology, 21*, 491–504.

Greenland, S., & Robins, J. M. (1986). Identifiability, exchangeability, and epidemiological confounding. *International Journal of Epidemiology, 15*, 413–419.

Gregg, J. P., Lit, L., Baron, C. A., Hertz-Picciotto, I., Walker, W., Davis, R. A., et al. (2008). Gene expression changes in children with autism. *Genomics, 91*, 22–29.

Gregory, S. G., Connelly, J. J., Towers, A. J., Johnson, J., Biscocho, D., Markunas, C. A., et al. (2009). Genomic and epigenetic evidence for oxytocin receptor deficiency in autism. *BMC Medicine, 7*, 62.

Grether, J. K., Anderson, M. C., Croen, L. A., Smith, D., & Windham, G. C. (2009). Risk of autism and increasing maternal and paternal age in a large north American population. *American Journal of Epidemiology, 170*(9), 1118–1126.

Guilmatre, A., Dubourg, C., Mosca, A. L., Legallic, S., Goldenberg, A., Drouin-Garraud, V., et al. (2009). Recurrent rearrangements in synaptic and neurodevelopmental genes and shared biologic pathways in schizophrenia, autism, and mental retardation. *Archives of General Psychiatry*. *66*(9), 947–956.

Happé, F., Ronald, A., & Plomin, R. (2006). Time to give up on a single explanation for autism. *Nature Neuroscience*, *9*, 1218–1220.

Harrison, P. J., & Weinberger, D. R. (2005). Schizophrenia genes, gene expression, and neuropathology: On the matter of their convergence. *Molecular Psychiatry*, *10*, 40–68.

Hassold, T., Hall, H., & Hunt, P. (2007). The origin of human aneuploidy: Where we have been, where we are going. *Human Molecular Genetics*, *16*(Spec No. 2), R203–8.

Herbert, M. R., Russo, J. P., Yang, S., Roohi, J., Blaxill, M., Kahler, S. G., et al. (2006). Autism and environmental genomics. *Neurotoxicology*, *27*, 671–684.

Hogart, A., Nagarajan, R. P., Patzel, K. A., Yasui, D. H., & Lasalle, J. M. (2007). 15q11-13 GABAA receptor genes are normally biallelically expressed in brain yet are subject to epigenetic dysregulation in autism spectrum disorders. *Human Molecular Genetics*, *16*(6), 691–703. Epub March 5, 2007.

Houck, K. A., & Kavlock, R. J. (2008). Understanding mechanisms of toxicity: Insights from drug discovery research. *Toxicology and Applied Pharmacology*, 227, 163–178.

Hu, V. W., Frank, B. C., Heine, S., Lee, N. H., & Quackenbush, J. (2006) Gene expression profiling of lymphoblastoid cell lines from monozygotic twins discordant in severity of autism reveals differential regulation of neurologically relevant genes. *BMC Genomics*, *7*, 118.

Hubal, E. A. (2009). Biologically relevant exposure science for 21st century toxicity testing. *Toxicological Sciences*, *111*(2), 226–232.

Husgafvel-Pursiainen, K. (2004). Genotoxicity of environmental tobacco smoke: A review. *Mutation Research*, *567*(2–3), 427–445.

Institute of Medicine (IOM) (2008). *Autism and the environment: Challenges and opportunities for research.* Workshop proceedings. Washington, DC: National Academies Press.

Ioannidis, J. P. (2005). Why most published research findings are false. *PLoS Medicine*, *2*, e124.

James, S. J., Melnyk, S., Jernigan, S., Hubanks, A., Rose, S., & Gaylor, D. W. (2008). Abnormal transmethylation/transsulfuration metabolism and DNA hypomethylation among parents of children with autism. *Journal of Autism and Developmental Disorders*, *38*(10), 1976.

James, S. J., Melnyk, S., Jernigan, S., Cleves, M. A., Halsted, C. H., Wong, D. H., et al. (2006). Metabolic endophenotype and related genotypes are associated with oxidative stress in children with autism. *American Journal of Medical Genetics. Part B, Neuropsychiatric Genetics*, *141B*, 947–956.

Jiang, Y. H., Sahoo, T., Michaelis, R. C., Bercovich, D., Bressler, J., Kashork, C. D., et al. (2004). A mixed epigenetic/genetic model for oligogenic inheritance of autism with a limited role for UBE3A. *American Journal of Medical Genetics. Part A*, *131*, 1–10.

Johnson, I. T., & Belshaw, N. J. (2008). Environment, diet and CpG island methylation: Epigenetic signals in gastrointestinal neoplasia. *Food and Chemical Toxicology*, *46*, 1346–1359.

Jones, S., Zhang, X., Parsons, D. W., Lin, J. C., Leary, R. J., Angenendt, P., et al. (2008). Core signaling pathways in human pancreatic cancers revealed by global genomic analyses. *Science*, *321*, 1801–1806.

Judson, R., Richard, A., Dix, D., Houck, K., Elloumi, F., Martin, M., et al. (2008). ACToR–Aggregated Computational Toxicology Resource. *Toxicology and Applied Pharmacology*, *233*(1), 7–13. Epub July 11, 2008.

Judson, R., Richard, A., Dix, D. J., Houck, K., Martin, M., Kavlock, R., et al. (2009). The toxicity data landscape for environmental chemicals. *Environmental Health Perspectives*, *117*(5), 685–695. Epub December 20, 2008.

Kaslow, R. A., McNicholl, J., & Hill, A. V. S. (Eds.) (2008). *Genetic susceptibility to infectious diseases.* New York, Oxford University Press.

Kavlock, R. J., Ankley, G., Blancato, J., Breen, M., Conolly, R., Dix, D., et al. (2008). Computational toxicology: A state of the science mini review. *Toxicological Sciences*, *103*(1), 14–27.

Kelada, S. N., Eaton, D. L., Wang, S. S., Rothman, N. R., & Khoury, M. J. (2003). The role of genetic polymorphisms in environmental health. *Environmental Health Perspectives*, *111*(8), 1055–1064.

Khan, N., Jeffers, M., Kumar, S., Hackett, C., Boldog, F., Khramtsov, N., et al. (2008). Determination of the class and isoform selectivity of small-molecule histone deacetylase inhibitors. *Biochemistry Journal*, *409*, (2), 581–589.

Khoury, M. J., Beaty, T. H., & Cohen, B. H. (1993). *Fundamentals of genetic epidemiology*. Oxford University Press, New York.

Khoury, M. J., Adams, M. J. Jr., & Flanders, W. D. (1988). An epidemiologic approach to ecogenetics. *American Journal of Human Genetics*, *42*, 89–95.

Kishore, S., & Stamm, S. (2006). The snoRNA HBII-52 regulates alternative splicing of the serotonin receptor 2C. *Science*, *311*, 230–232.

Kitano, H. (2002). Systems biology: A brief overview. *Science*, *295*(5560), 1662–1664.

Kolevzon, A., Gross, R., & Reichenberg, A. (2007). Prenatal and perinatal risk factors for autism: A review and integration of findings. *Archives of Pediatrics and Adolescent Medicine. 161*(4), 326–333.

Konneker, T., Barnes, T., Furberg, H., Losh, M., Bulik, C. M., & Sullivan, P. F. (2008). A searchable database of genetic evidence for psychiatric disorders. *American Journal of Medical Genetics. Part B, Neuropsychiatric Genetics*, *147B*(6), 671–675.

Kramer, J. M., & van Bokhoven, H. (2008). Genetic and epigenetic defects in mental retardation. *International Journal of Biochemistry and Cell Biology*, August 20 2008, 13. [Epub ahead of print]

Krey, J. F., & Dolmetsch, R. E. (2007). Molecular mechanisms of autism: A possible role for Ca2+ signaling. *Current Opinion in Neurobiology*, *17*, 112–119.

Lathe, R. (2006). *Autism, brain, and environment.* London: Jessica Kingsley Publishers.

Lauritsen, M. B., Pedersen, C. B., & Mortensen, P. B. (2005). Effects of familial risk factors and place of birth on the risk of autism: A nationwide register-based study. *Psychological Psychiatry*, *46*(9), 963–971.

Lawler, C. P., Croen, L. A., Grether, J. K., & Van de Water, J. (2004). Identifying environmental contributions to autism: Provocative clues and false leads. *Mental Retardation and Developmental Disabilities Research Reviews*, *10*, 292–302.

Li, Y. V, Hough, C. J., & Sarvey, J. M. (2003). Do we need zinc to think? *Science Signaling*, *182*, pe 19.

Lin, B. K., Clyne, M., Walsh, M., Gomez, O., Yu, W., Gwinn, M., et al. (2006). Tracking the epidemiology of human genes in the literature: The HuGE Published Literature database. *American Journal of Epidemiology*, *164*(1), 1–4.

Loscalzo, J., Kohane, I., & Barabasi, A. L. (2007). Human disease classification in the postgenomic era: A complex systems approach to human pathobiology. *Molecular Systems Biology*, *3*, 124.

Martinez, F.D. (2007). CD14, endotoxin, and asthma risk: actions and interactions. *Proceedings of the American Thoracic Society 4*(3), 221–225.

Mattingly, C. J., Rosenstein, M. C., Davis, A. P., Colby, G. T., Forrest, J. N. Jr., & Boyer, J. L. (2006a). The comparative toxicogenomics database: A cross-species resource for building chemical-gene interaction networks. *Toxicological Sciences, 92*, 587–595.

Mattingly, C. J., Rosenstein, M. C., Colby, G. T., Forrest, J. N. Jr., & Boyer, J. L. (2006b). The Comparative Toxicogenomics Database (CTD): A resource for comparative toxicological studies. *Journal of Experimental Zoology. Part A, Comparative Experimental Biology, 305*(9), 689–692.

Matuszek, G., & Talebizadeh, Z. (2009). Autism Genetic Database (AGD): A comprehensive database including autism susceptibility gene-CNVs integrated with known noncoding RNAs and fragile sites. *BMC Medical Genetics, 10*, 102.

Melke, J., Goubran Botros, H., Chaste, P., Betancur, C., Nygren, G., Anckarsater, H., et al. (2008). Abnormal melatonin synthesis in autism spectrum disorders. *Molecular Psychiatry, 13*, 90–98.

Moffitt, T. E., Caspi, A., & Rutter, M. (2005). Strategy for investigating interactions between measured genes and measured environments. *Archives of General Psychiatry, 62*, 473–481.

Moonesinghe, R., Khoury, M. J., & Janssens, A. C. (2007) Most published research findings are false-but a little replication goes a long way. *PLoS Medicine, 4*, e28.

Moore, S. J., Turnpenny, P., Quinn, A., Glover, S., Lloyd, D. J., Montgomery, T., et al. (2000). A clinical study of 57 children with fetal anticonvulsant syndromes. *Journal of Medical Genetics, 37*(7), 489–497.

Morita, T., Hayashi, M., & Morikawa, K. (2006). Globally harmonized system on hazard classification and labeling of chemicals and other existing classification systems for germ cell mutagens. *Genes and Environment, 28*, 141–152.

Nagarajan, R. P., Hogart, A. R., Gwye, Y., Martin, M. R., & LaSalle, J. M. (2006). Reduced MeCP2 expression is frequent in autism frontal cortex and correlates with aberrant MECP2 promoter methylation. *Epigenetics, 1*, e1–11.

Nakayama, Y., Takahashi, T., Wakabayashi, A., Oono, H., & Radford, M. H. (2007). Sex differences in the relationship between cortisol levels and the empathy and systemizing quotients in humans. *Neuroendocrinology Letters, 28*(4), 445–448.

National Research Council, Committee on Assessing Interactions among Social, Behavioral, Genetic Factors in Health, Board on Health Sciences Policy. Hernandez, L.M. & Blazer, D.G. (Eds.) (2006). *Genes, behavior, and the social environment: Moving beyond the nature/nurture debate.* Washington, DC: National Academies Press.

Newschaffer, C. J., Croen, L. A., Daniels, J., Giarelli, E., Grether, J. K., Levy, S. E., et al. (2007). The epidemiology of autism spectrum disorders. *Annual Review of Public Health, 28*, 235–258.

Newschaffer, C. J., Fallin, D., & Lee, N. L. (2002). Heritable and nonheritable risk factors for autism spectrum disorders. *Epidemiologic Reviews, 24*, 137–153.

Nigg, J. T. (2006). *What causes ADHD?* New York: The Guilford Press.

Nishimura, Y., Martin, C. L., Vazquez-Lopez, A., Spence, S. J., Alvarez-Retuerto, A. I., Sigman, M., et al. (2007). Genome-wide expression profiling of lymphoblastoid cell lines distinguishes different forms of autism and reveals shared pathways. *Human Molecular Genetics 16*, 1682–1698.

Ottman, R. (1990). An epidemiologic approach to gene-environment interaction. *Genetic Epidemiology, 7*, 177–185.

Ottman, R. (1996). Gene-environment interaction: Definitions and study designs. *Preventive Medicine, 25*, 764–770.

Ovsyannikova, I. G., Jacobson, R. M., Dhiman, N., Vierkant, R. A., Pankratz, V. S., & Poland, G. A. (2008). Human leukocyte antigen and cytokine receptor gene polymorphisms associated with heterogeneous immune responses to mumps viral vaccine. *Pediatrics, 121*, e1091–1099.

Palmieri, L., Papaleo, V., Porcelli, V., Scarcia, P., Gaita, L., Sacco, R., et al. (2008). Altered calcium homeostasis in autism-spectrum disorders: Evidence from biochemical and genetic studies of the mitochondrial aspartate/glutamate carrier AGC1. *Molecular Psychiatry*, July 8, 2008. [Epub ahead of print]

Parsons, D. W., Jones, S., Zhang, X., Lin, J. C., Leary, R. J., Angenendt, P., et al. (2008). An integrated genomic analysis of human glioblastoma multiforme. *Science, 321*, 1807–1812.

Pasca, S. P., Dronca, E., Nemes, B., Kaucsar, T., Endreffy, E., Iftene, F., et al. (2008). Paraoxonase 1 activities and polymorphisms in autism spectrum disorders. *Journal of Cellular and Molecular Medicine*, June 20, 2008, 28. [Epub ahead of print]

Pessah, I., & Lein, P. (2008). Evidence for environmental susceptibility in autism: What we need to know about gene x environment interactions. In A. W. Zimmerman (Ed.), *Autism: Current theories and evidence* (pp. 409–428). Totowa, NJ: Humana Press.

Pessah, I. N., Seegal, R. F., Lein, P. J., LaSalle, J., Yee, B. K., Van De Water, J., et al. (2008). Immunologic and neurodevelopmental susceptibilities of autism. *Neurotoxicology, 29*, 532–545.

Purcell, S. (2002). Variance components models for gene-environment interaction in twin analysis. *Twin Research, 5*, 554–571.

Riddihough, G., Purnell, B. A., & Travis, J. (2008). Freedom of expression. Introduction to special issue. *Science, 319*, 1781.

Rieder, M. J., Livingston, R. J., Stanaway, I. B., & Nickerson, D. A. (2008). The environmental genome project: Reference polymorphisms for drug metabolism genes and genome-wide association studies. *Drug Metabolism Reviews, 40*(2), 241–261.

Rothman, K. J., & Greenland, S. (1998). *Modern epidemiology.* Philadelphia, PA: Lippincott Williams & Wilkins.

Rothman, K. J., & Greenland, S. (2005). Causation and causal inference in epidemiology. *American Journal of Public Health, 95*(Suppl 1), S144–150.

Rubes, J., Selevan, S. G., Sram, R. J., Evenson, D. P., & Perreault, S. D. (2007). GSTM1 genotype influences the susceptibility of men to sperm DNA damage associated with exposure to air pollution. *Mutation Research, 625*(1–2), 20–28. Epub July 13, 2007.

Rutter, M. (2006). *Genes and behavior: Nature-nurture interplay explained.* Malden, MA: Blackwell Publishing.

Rutter, M. (2008). Biological implications of gene-environment interaction. *Journal of Abnormal Child Psychology, 36*, 969–975.

Salnikow, K., & Zhitkovich, A. (2008). Genetic and epigenetic mechanisms in metal carcinogenesis and cocarcinogenesis: Nickel, arsenic, and chromium. *Chemical Research in Toxicology, 21*(1), 28–44. Epub October 20, 2007.

Samaco, R. C., Nagarajan, R. P., Braunschweig, D., & LaSalle, J. M. (2004). Multiple pathways regulate MeCP2 expression in normal brain development and exhibit defects in autism-spectrum disorders. *Human Molecular Genetics, 13*, 629–639.

Samet, J. M., DeMarini, D. M., & Malling, H. V. (2004). Biomedicine: Do airborne particles induce heritable mutations? *Science, 304*, 971–972.

Sayers, E. W., Barrett, T., Benson, D. A., Bolton, E., Bryant, S. H., Canese, K., et al. (2009). Database resources of the National

Center for Biotechnology Information. *Nucleic Acids Research, 38*(Database issue) D5-D16.

Scarr, S., & McCartney, K. (1983). How people make their own environments: a theory of genotype greater than environment effects. *Child Development, 54*, 424–435.

Schins, R. P., & Knaapen, A. M. (2007). Genotoxicity of poorly soluble particles. *Inhalation Toxicology, 19*(Suppl 1), 189–198.

Schneider, T., Roman, A., Basta-Kaim, A., Kubera, M., Budziszewska, B., Schneider, K., et al. (2008). Gender-specific behavioral and immunological alterations in an animal model of autism induced by prenatal exposure to valproic acid. *Psychoneuroendocrinology, 33*(6), 728–740. Epub April 8, 2008.

Sebat, J., Lakshmi, B., Malhotra, D., Troge, J., Lese-Martin, C., Walsh, T., et al. (2007). Strong association of de novo copy number mutations with autism. *Science, 316*, 445–449.

Sen, B., Mahadevan, B., & DeMarini, D. M. (2007) Transcriptional responses to complex mixtures: A review. *Mutation Research, 636*, 144–177.

Serajee, F. J., Nabi, R., Zhong, H., & Huq, M. (2004). Polymorphisms in xenobiotic metabolism genes and autism. *Journal of Child Neurology, 19*, 413–417.

Service, R. F. (2008). Proteomics. Proteomics ponders prime time. *Science, 321*, 1758–1761.

Sheng, L., Ding, X., Ferguson, M., McCallister, M., Rhoades, R., Maguire, M., et al. (2010). Prenatal polycyclic aromatic hydrocarbon exposure leads to behavioral deficits and downregulation of receptor tyrosine kinase, MET. *Toxicological Sciences, 118*(2), 625–634.

Sieberts, S. K., & Schadt, E. E. (2007). Moving toward a system genetics view of disease. *Mammalian Genome, 18*, 389–401.

Somers, C. M., McCarry, B. E., Malek, F., & Quinn, J. S. (2004). Reduction of particulate air pollution lowers the risk of heritable mutations in mice. *Science, 304*, 1008–1010.

Spry, M., Scott, T., Pierce, H., & D'Orazio, J. A. (2007). DNA repair pathways and hereditary cancer susceptibility syndromes. *Frontiers in Bioscience, 12*, 4191–4207.

Thapar, A., Harold, G., Rice, F., Langley, K., & O'Donovan, M. (2007). The contribution of gene-environment interaction to psychopathology. *Development and Psychopathology, 19*, 989–1004.

Tierney, E., Bukelis, I., Thompson, R. E., Ahmed, K., Aneja, A., Kratz, L., et al. (2006). Abnormalities of cholesterol metabolism in autism spectrum disorders. *American Journal of Medical Genetics. Part B, Neuropsychiatric Genetics, 141B*(6), 666–668.

Torkamani, A., Topol, E. J., & Schork, N. J. (2008). Pathway analysis of seven common diseases assessed by genome-wide association. *Genomics*, September 20, 08, 15. [Epub ahead of print]

Tovalin, H., Valverde, M., Morandi, M. T., Blanco, S., Whitehead, L., & Rojas, E. (2006). DNA damage in outdoor workers occupationally exposed to environmental air pollutants. *Occupational and Environmental Medicine, 63*, 230–236.

Trovato, M., D'Armiento, M., Lavra, L., Ulivieri, A., Dominici, R., Vitarelli, E., et al. (2007). Expression of p53/HGF/c-met/STAT3 signal in fetuses with neural tube defects. *Virchows Archiv, 450*(2), 203–210.

Tsuang, M. T., Bar, J. L., Stone, W. S., & Faraone, S. V. (2004). Gene-environment interactions in mental disorders. *World Psychiatry, 3*, 73–83.

Turnbaugh, P. J., Ley, R. E., Hamady, M., Fraser-Liggett, C. M., Knight, R., & Gordon, J. I. (2007). The human microbiome project. *Nature, 449*(7164), 804–810.

United Nations (2003). *Globally harmonized system of classification and labelling of chemicals (GHS)*. http://www.osha.gov/dsg/hazcom/ghs.html

Valinluck, V., Tsai, H. H., Rogstad, D. K., Burdzy, A., Bird, A., & Sowers, L.C. (2004). Oxidative damage to methyl-CpG sequences inhibits the binding of the methyl-CpG binding domain (MBD) of methyl-CpG binding protein 2 (MeCP2). *Nucleic Acids Research, 32*(14), 4100–4108.

Visscher, P. M., Hill, W. G., & Wray, N. R. (2008). Heritability in the genomics era: Concepts and misconceptions. *Nature Reviews Genetics, 9*, 255–266.

Wall, D. P., Esteban, F. J., Deluca, T. F., Huyck, M., Monaghan, T., Velez de Mendizabal, N., et al. (2009). Comparative analysis of neurological disorders focuses genome-wide search for autism genes. *Genomics, 93*(2), 120–129.

Wang, Y., Bolton, E., Dracheva, S., Karapetyan, K., Shoemaker, B. A., Suzek, T. O., et al. (2009). An overview of the PubChem BioAssay resource. *Nucleic Acids Research*, November 20, 2009, 19. [Epub ahead of print]

Wellcome Trust Case Control Consortium (2007). Genome-wide association study of 14,000 cases of seven common diseases and 3,000 shared controls. *Nature, 447*, 661–678.

Wild, C. P. (2005). Complementing the genome with an "exposome": The outstanding challenge of environmental exposure measurement in molecular epidemiology. *Cancer Epidemiology, Biomarkers and Prevention, 14*(8), 1847–1850.

Williams, J. G., Higgins, J. P., & Brayne, C. E. (2006). Systematic review of prevalence studies of autism spectrum disorders. *Archives of Disease in Childhood, 91*(1), 8–15.

Wilson, S. H., & Olden, K. (2004). The environmental genome project: Phase I and beyond. *Molecular Interventions, 4*(3), 147–156.

Wood, L. D., Parsons, D. W., Jones, S., Lin, J., Sjoblom, T., Leary, R. J., et al. (2007). The genomic landscapes of human breast and colorectal cancers. *Science, 318*, 1108–1113.

Wu, X., Jiang, R., Zhang, M. Q., & Li, S. (2008). Network-based global inference of human disease genes. *Molecular Systems Biology, 4*, 189.

Wyrobek, A. J., Eskenazi, B., Young, S., Arnheim, N., Tiemann-Boege, I., Jabs, E. W., et al. (2006). Advancing age has differential effects on DNA damage, chromatin integrity, gene mutations, and aneuploidies in sperm. *Proceedings of the National Academy of Sciences of the United States of America, 103*(25), 9601–9606. Epub June 9, 2006.

Wyrobek A. J., Mulvihill, J. J., Wassom, J. S., Malling, H. V., Shelby, M. D., Lewis, S. E., et al. (2007). Assessing human germ-cell mutagenesis in the postgenome era: A celebration of the legacy of William Lawson (Bill) Russell. *Environmental and Molecular Mutagenesis, 48*(2), 71–95.

Xu, J., Zwaigenbaum, L., Szatmari, P., & Scherer, S. W. (2004). Molecular cytogenetics of autism. *Current Genomics, 5*(4), 347–364.

Yu, W., Wulf, A., Liu, T., Khoury, M. J., & Gwinn, M. (2008). Gene prospector: An evidence gateway for evaluating potential susceptibility genes and interacting risk factors for human diseases. *BMC Bioinformatics, 9*, 528.

Yurov, Y. B., Vorsanova, S. G., Iourov, I. Y., Demidova, I. A., Beresheva, A. K., Kravetz, V. S., et al. (2007). Unexplained autism is frequently associated with low-level mosaic aneuploidy. *Journal of Medical Genetics, 44*(8), 521–525. Epub May 4, 2007.

Zecavati, N., & Spence, S. J. (2009). Neurometabolic disorders and dysfunction in autism spectrum disorders. *Current Neurology and Neuroscience Report, 9*, 129–136.

Zhang, J., Feuk, L., Duggan, G. E., Khaja, R., & Scherer, S. W. (2006). Development of bioinformatics resources for display and analysis of copy number and other structural variants in the human genome. *Cytogenetic and Genome Research, 115*(3–4), 205–214.

Zhao, X., Leotta, A., Kustanovich, V., Lajonchere, C., Geschwind, D.H., Law, K., et al. (2007). A unified genetic theory for sporadic and inherited autism. *Proceedings of the National Academy of Sciences of the United States of America, 104*, 12831–12836.

Section VIII

Animal Models and Theoretical Perspectives

50

Alicia Blaker-Lee, Gianluca DeRienzo, Hazel Sive

Zebrafish As a Tool to Study Autism

Points of Interest

- Given the multitude of genes associated with autism and other mental health disorders, a whole animal system that can be used to screen candidate genes and potential therapeutics is in demand.
- An animal tool provides useful insight into a disorder without attempting to recapitulate all aspects of the disorder.
- The zebrafish-tool provides rapid, clear, relatively high-throughput analyses of candidate genes in an organism with high conservation in genetics and in brain development.
- Rapid and efficient manipulation of zebrafish gene expression can be easily attained by loss-of-function and gain-of-function strategies.
- Many characterized mutants and morphants can be useful in understanding nervous system development, including nervous system patterning, neural tube shaping, neuroepithelial junction formation, and neuronal differentiation.
- The zebrafish-tool can be applied to the study of autism, in circumstances where human genes associated with the disorder have been identified, where the genes are important early in brain development and where the genes have clear zebrafish homologs.

Introduction

Autism spectrum disorders (ASDs) include an array of behavioral and neurodevelopmental symptoms with considerable variation in severity and time of onset. Despite the phenotypic complexity, clear evidence indicates a strong genetic component. Recently, genes associated with autism have begun to be identified. These include common and rare gene variants (Kim et al., 2008; Miller et al., 2009; Persico et al., 2001; Steffenburg et al., 1996), as well as copy number variants (CNVs). One clear CNV associated with autism lies on chromosome 16, in the 16p11.2 interval (Christian et al., 2008; Kumar et al., 2008; Weiss et al., 2008). Consideration of the 16p11.2 interval highlights some of the challenges of analyzing ASD candidate susceptibility genes. This interval is approximately 500kb in length and includes 30 genes or putative open reading frames. Which of these genes is connected with ASDs? Is just one gene pivotal, or are several? And how can this knowledge be used to develop potential therapeutics that will ameliorate the disorder?

Two key questions must be addressed in analyzing CNVs that include many genes or in analyzing the many common or rare variants associated with ASDs. First, how can one screen through many genes to define candidates that are most closely associated with ASDs? One way is association studies using large numbers of human patient and control samples. Another way is to study homologs of human genes in an animal system. Mice display behaviors such as anxiety, hyperactivity, and enhanced spatial learning, which may describe a subset of behaviors included in ASD diagnosis and can be assayed directly for neuronal abnormalities. However, constructing and analyzing dozens or hundreds of mutations in transgenic mice is extremely cumbersome, time-consuming, and expensive. As we will discuss, the zebrafish embryo can be used as a relatively high-throughput system to assay gene function more rapidly and inexpensively than the mouse.

Second, how will knowledge of gene function lead to development of therapeutics, a major goal of autism research? Known or new psychoactive medications can be assayed for efficacy. Alternately, small-molecule screens focusing on mutations of interest as the targets may be successful. The zebrafish embryo is one of the few vertebrate systems that can be used for whole-animal, small-molecule screening, as will be discussed below.

The Zebrafish As a Tool

The zebrafish is a powerful system for the study of disease-associated gene function. In some cases, zebrafish may be a direct disease model. For example, zebrafish cancer models are proving useful for recapitulation of human cancer (Amatruda & Patton, 2008; Ceol et al., 2008). However, in the study of autism, zebrafish do not display the complex behaviors present in humans and cannot be used to recapitulate the disorder. Nonetheless, the fish can be useful for analyzing function of genes associated with autism or other mental health disorders.

We have therefore developed the idea of an *animal "tool"* as distinct from an animal *"model."* Whereas a model recapitulates the human disorder and can be used in a one-to-one fashion to study the disorder, a tool does not recapitulate the disorder. Nonetheless, a tool can be used to provide insight into the disorder. Specifically, we suggest that an animal tool can be used for its attributes, which may not be available in a more conventional model. In the case of the zebrafish, the attributes useful for analysis of genes implicated in autism and other mental health disorders include ability to perform rapid loss- and gain-of-function assays, ability to assay function of human gene variants rapidly, and ability to use embryos and larvae in chemical screens (Figure 50-1).

Zebrafish Attributes

Conservation of Brain Structure

Vertebrate brain development is highly conserved, and the zebrafish brain possesses significant structural and functional homology to the human brain (Hakryul Jo, 2005; Lowery & Sive, 2009; Tropepe & Sive, 2003). The overall organization of the zebrafish brain is conserved in humans. This includes, for example, the presence of ventricle spaces, many common projections in the olfactory and visual pathways, and common descending and premotor pathways (Tropepe & Sive, 2003; Wulliman, 1998). Neurulation results from neural plate movements to form the neural tube that will become the brain and spinal cord, and as indicated by fate mapping, the neural plate movements are conserved in mammals (Lowery et al., 2009; Papan & Campos-Ortega, 1999). Opening of the lumen follows, forming the ventricles, which are often abnormal in autistic patients (Hardan et al., 2001). These anatomical features make the fish an appropriate organism for studying brain development.

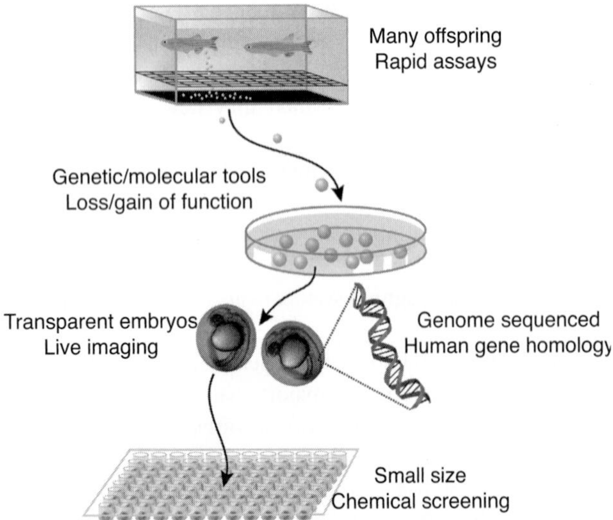

Figure 50-1. Attributes of the zebrafish. See text for details. (See Color Plate Section for a color version of this figure.)

Neurulation: the development of the neural plate and the processes involved with its subsequent closure to form the neural tube during the early stages of embryonic development.

Husbandry and Accessibility

Zebrafish are relatively small (3–4 cm), making their husbandry relatively inexpensive. Embryos develop external to the mother, allowing accessibility to all stages of development. A single mating can yield 200 embryos, and experiments can therefore be designed to test multiple conditions with a large sample size. Development is rapid, with distinct brain regions and functional neurons developing by 24 hours post-fertilization and therefore facilitating rapid analyses. Embryos are small, approximately 0.2 mm, making relatively high-throughput assays feasible. In addition to convenience and cost benefits, large sample sizes, and ease of manipulation and analysis, a complete generation time is 3 months, which makes genetic mutant screens practical and expedient.

Imaging

Zebrafish embryos are transparent and develop externally, facilitating visualization of the brain *in vivo*, especially in conjunction with expression of fluorescent marker proteins. This feature is particularly useful to monitor the effects of loss of gene function on nervous system development. Brain structure and axon outgrowth can be captured as digital images that can be used for further analysis, including high-resolution whole-embryo images, sophisticated confocal images, and 3D reconstructions. Thus, the early consequences of changes in gene function can be studied (e.g., Gutzman et al., 2008).

Genome Project

The *Danio rerio* genome sequencing project is a collaboration between the Wellcome Trust Sanger Institute and the zebrafish community; including contributions from ZFIN, Ensembl, and Vega (http://www.sanger.ac.uk/Projects/D_rerio/). The Sanger Institute began sequencing the zebrafish genome in

2001, and the ninth annotated version is currently available on Ensembl or Vega. The Human Genome Project was assembled using a similar strategy and completed in 2003, thus it is available for comparison with the zebrafish genome (www.sanger.ac.uk/HGP/overview.shtml). In a 2000 analysis of zebrafish and human genomes, 523 zebrafish genes and expressed sequence tags (ESTs) contained mapped human orthologs (Barbazuk et al., 2000). Eighty percent of the human and zebrafish genes had conserved synteny, which was defined as two or more linked genes. Conserved syntenic regions between the human genome and the zebrafish genome suggest there may be some orthology between the species (Barbazuk et al., 2000). However, as variability in the gene sequences, gene duplications, and homologs may exist in humans or zebrafish, gene function in either organism should be analyzed more specifically. For this task, the full-length and EST sequences of interest are available for order online, and their order pages are often links from the NCBI webpage. If a human homolog can restore gene function of a zebrafish loss-of-function mutant, then there must be conservation in the function of these two genes.

Ortholog: A gene in two or more species that has evolved from a common ancestor

Homolog: A gene similar in structure and evolutionary origin to a gene in another species

Loss-of-Function Analyses

Multiple strategies can be used to create loss-of-function phenotypes including mutagen-induced screening, insertional mutagenesis, targeting induced local lesion in genomes (TILLING), zinc finger nuclease targeting, and morpholino knockdown. The choice of loss-of-function strategy depends on the specific gene. For a gene with a characterized genetic mutant, analysis of the mutant line is the most definitive way to proceed. However, most genes will not have a cognate genetic mutant, and some other strategy to ablate function must be taken. Use of antisense morpholino-modified oligonucleotides (MOs) are the most rapid and effective approach but can be used only to analyze embryonic phenotypes. Targeted mutagenesis, either by searching through random mutations (TILLING) or by use of zinc finger nucleases allow analysis of older animals, as is the case for all stable genetic mutants.

Mutagenesis Screens

Large-scale mutant screening in zebrafish, using N-ethyl-nitrosourea (ENU), has produced thousands of mutations that disrupt a wide range of genes involved in the early steps of development (Driever et al., 1996; Haffter et al., 1996; Solnica-Krezel et al., 1994). Following mutagenesis, many affected genes have been identified by a positional cloning strategy, and many mutants resembling human disease states have been useful tools to study human pathologies (Hinkes et al., 2006; Shin & Fishman, 2002; Xu et al., 2002). Insertional mutagenesis, using retrovirus to disrupt gene sequences, has also been used to identify genes involved in early development (Amsterdam & Hopkins, 1999; Golling et al., 2002). This strategy offers the advantage of identifying the affected gene by inverse polymerase chain reaction through an associated tag at the insertion site, thus reducing cloning time. Use of stable mutants is the best way to analyze phenotypes in the adult and of enormous use in the embryo. Some mutants may be hypomorphs and retain some function, and the extent of this can be difficult to determine.

Antisense Morpholino-Modified Oligonucleotides

In zebrafish, gene expression can be knocked down using the MO strategy (Summerton & Weller, 1997), where MOs target specific mRNA at either a start or a splice site to prevent translation or to produce aberrant proteins. Morpholine rings replace the sugar-phosphate backbone of the antisense oligonucleotides, a modification that stabilizes the oligos, allowing inhibition of gene function until at least 48 hours post-fertilization. Designing the MO to the start site is beneficial if the maternal contribution of already splice-processed mRNA is a complicating factor in the experiment. However, designing the MO to target a splice site in the RNA will result in an mRNA product that can be monitored by PCR (Draper et al., 2001). Specificity of the phenotype is determined by comparison with a control MO and, most importantly, by rescue of the phenotype with injected mRNA engineered to lack the MO binding site. In our hands, rescue is achieved with at least 80% of MOs tested. The development of photo-activatable MOs provide the possibility of using MOs to achieve conditional gene silencing (Ando et al., 2001; Shestopalov et al., 2007). "Caged" MOs are synthesized with a complementary oligomer tethered to the MO by a photo-cleavable linker. Because the embryos are transparent, upon exposure to 360-nm light, the linker is cleaved and the MO is active. MOs are an outstanding tool for ablation of gene function where there is no corresponding genetic mutant. This is especially true for splice site MOs, where amount of normal RNA remaining can be monitored. Caged MOs hold enormous promise but are still under development and not commercially available at this time. MO technology is very useful for embryonic phenotypes, but beyond 48 hours of development, the MO will be diluted as cells divide and MOs cannot, therefore, be used to study adult phenotypes.

Morpholino: a molecule used to modify gene expression. MOs are an antisense technology used to block access of other molecules to specific sequences within nucleic acid.

TILLING

TILLING is a reverse genetic strategy, which involves random chemical mutagenesis (by N-ethyl-N-nitrosourea) followed by DNA screening for point mutation of a specific target gene of interest (Skromne & Prince, 2008; Wienholds et al., 2003). After exposure to ENU, PCR using fluorescently labeled primers results in heteroduplex formation. Then, mismatch cleavage by Cell is used to identify rare ENU-induced mutations. TILLING can then proceed by a variety of approaches, including sequencing, agarose gels, denaturing high-performance liquid chromatography, and capillary electrophoresis (Sood et al., 2006). Using this technique, it is possible to create mutations in a gene of interest, facilitating the identification of functional or critical regions in the protein. TILLING is of proven use, especially where a null mutation is identified. A new TILLING consortium coordinates efforts in the United States, making this approach more accessible. However, it may prove difficult to isolate a mutation in a specific gene, and the lag from request to definition of the mutant may be many months.

Zinc Finger Nucleases

Zinc finger nucleases are used for targeted modification of the genome (Cathomen & Joung, 2008; Foley et al., 2009; Porteus & Carroll, 2005). These enzymes bind double-stranded DNA and cause a double-stranded break. The nuclease domain is nonspecific, but the zinc finger domain can be designed to target and bind a specific DNA sequence. Resulting double-stranded breaks are repaired by non-homologous end-joining of the DNA and can therefore be used for targeted insertions or deletions. The gene modification is transmitted through the germline, so after appropriate screening for founders of the desired modification, the transgenic fish line can be maintained and studied (Foley et al., 2009). This technique holds promise but has not been extensively proven in the zebrafish system.

Gain-of-Function Analyses

Gain-of-function analyses assess the effects of protein over-expression, or expression of a variant form of the protein.

mRNA Injection

This is the simplest gain-of-function approach, where mRNA encoding a protein of interest is injected into an early embryo and thereby expressed. Temporal control can be achieved by using a hormone inducible fusion protein (Kolm & Sive, 1995) or a tissue-specific promoter (Ju et al., 1999).

Stable Transgenics

Stable transgenic insertion can be achieved using the I-SceI restriction endonuclease, for example, which also "escorts" DNA into the chromosome (Soroldoni et al., 2009). Transgenic expression can be studied in the F0 as mosaic expression or in the F1 in case of genomic integration of the DNA into the germ cells. The Tol2 system is a useful method for gene and enhancer trapping in zebrafish, and it can result in identification of genes that are developmentally regulated (Asakawa et al., 2008; Parinov et al., 2004). The enhancer trap system requires a transposable element such as Tol2 for random insertion into the genome, a promoter that is sensitive and can be activated by the enhancer of interest, and a reporter gene such as Gal4 or GFP (Bellen, 1999). Genes affected by the insertion can be identified by PCR amplification of genomic sequences flanking the Tol2 insertion site followed by sequencing reactions. Expression of the reporter genes in enhancer trap fish lines can be used to identify tissue-specific expression of the associated genes (Parinov et al., 2004).

Chemical Screening

The classical drug discovery approach is a screen for small molecules that bind *in vitro* to a target of interest. Such screens require a specific target, and a detailed molecular understanding of a process. Forward chemical genetics involves screening for small molecules that alter the function of a biological pathway, resulting in the induction or rescue of a specific phenotype. This approach uses a library of compounds that may be very large (~10^5 compounds) and functionally uncharacterized, or smaller (~10^3 compounds), but with annotation as to likely targets, based on preliminary assays *in vitro* or in cell lines.

Whole animals offer several advantages over cell lines for chemical screens, indicating effects on the whole animal, toxicity, and tissue specificity. Use of the whole animal can also allow the screening of processes that are not easily replicated in vitro, such as organ development. Whole-animal chemical screens are only feasible in invertebrates and in very small vertebrates. The latter include embryos and larvae of the zebrafish or the frog Xenopus, where large numbers of embryos can easily be obtained, and exclude any mammal. The zebrafish, particularly, has been used extensively in chemical screens (Macrae & Peterson, 2003; Murphey & Zon, 2006). The ease of waterborne compound application and their closer evolutionary relationship to humans make zebrafish the system of choice relative to invertebrates.

Several approaches have been developed to screen small molecules in zebrafish, taking advantage of its attributes described above (Peterson, 2008; Peterson et al., 2000; Pichler et al., 2003). Chemical screens for developmental modifiers involve arraying embryos into the wells of microtiter plates (ranging from 24– to 96-well), adding small molecules from a chemical library, and allowing development to proceed. At various stages of development, the embryos are screened visually for perturbations in the system(s) of interest. Zebrafish mutants can be screened for rescue or modulation of the mutant phenotype (Murphey & Zon, 2006), a powerful method that may be extremely useful in analysis of gene function associated with autism.

Lessons from Mutants and Morphants

Mutant Phenotypes

The embryonic zebrafish has an accessible and relatively simple nervous system, with many of its components formed and functioning as early as 24 hours post-fertilization. To help facilitate studies on the nervous system, mutagenesis screens have produced mutations that affect nervous system development. The first examples of large-scale mutagenesis screens were conducted in two independent experiments using ENU as a mutagen and produced many mutants grouped in different classes according to the affected embryonic organs (Driever et al., 1996; Haffter et al., 1996). Successively different strategies were used to produce mutagenesis by viral insertion (Amsterdam & Hopkins, 1999; Wiellette et al., 2004) or by gene trapping using the Tol2 transposable element (Kawakami, 2004). The characterization of these mutants has revealed that many aspects of vertebrate nervous system development are well-conserved in zebrafish. In this section, we describe some mutants isolated in these screens and corresponding genes that have been useful in understanding the complexity of nervous system development (Table 50-1).

Genes Affecting Nervous System Patterning

Spiel-ohne-grenzen (spg)

The mutant phenotype caused by disruption of the gene *pou2,* which is the ortholog of the human *oct4. spg/pou2* expression is essential for proper development of the midbrain, hindbrain, ear, and body axis (Burgess et al., 2002). *spg/pou2* functions during the establishment and maintenance of these brain regions. In addition, *spg/pou2* functions also during development of the forebrain—particularly the diencephalon—and in differentiation of the paraxial mesoderm and endoderm. In zebrafish, *spg/pou2* is the first example of a tissue specific competence factor for Fgf8 signaling (Reim & Brand, 2002).

Bozozok

The *bozozok* locus encodes the homeodomain protein Dharma, which is a regulator of cell fate determination. *boz* inhibits the Wnt pathway, aiding formation of the gastrula organizer. In the early gastrula, *boz* positively regulates the expression of Chordin and other BMP antagonists dorsally, which in turn inhibit BMP signaling and induce anterior neuroectoderm. In the late gastrula, *boz* dorsally inhibits the posteriorizing activity of Wnt

Table 50–1.
Zebrafish mutant phenotypes in the nervous system

Class	Locus	Gene	Nervous System Defects	References
Early patterning				
	SPG	pou2	midbrain and hindbrain organization	1, 2, 3
	bozozok	dharma	Abnormal neuroectoderm size	1, 4
	Parachute	N-cadherin	Loss of neuroepithelium cell adhesion	5, 6
Neural tube shaping				
Laminin mutants				
	Bashful	Laminin α1	Reduced ventricles, MHB folding	7, 8
	Sleepy	Laminin γ1	Reduced ventricles, MHB folding	7, 9, 10, 11
	Grumpy	Laminin β1	Reduced ventricles, MHB folding	7, 9, 11
Epithelial apicobasal polarity				
	Nagie oko	Mpp5a	Midline opening	1, 12, 11
	Oko meduzy	crb2	Midline opening	1, 13, 11
	Heart and soul	prkci	Midline opening	1, 14, 11
	Mosaic eyes	Epb4.1/5	Midline opening	15
Neuronal Differentiation				
	Motionless	Med12	NA neurons, cranial sensory ganglia	1, 16, 11
	Unplugged	MuSK	Motor neurons pathfinding	17, 18, 19
	No soul	Foxi1	Visceral sensory neurons	17, 20
	Zieharmonika	AChE	Rohon-Beard sensory neuron	17, 21

1. Schier et al., 1996; 2. Burgess et al., 2002; 3. Reim & Brand, 2002; 4. Fekany-Lee et al., 2000; 5. Jiang et al., 1996; 6. Lele et al., 2002; 7. Karlstrom et al., 1996; 8. Paulus & Halloran, 2006; 9. Parsons et al., 2002; 10. Gutzman et al., 2008; 11. Lowery et al., 2009; 12. Wei & Malicki, 2002; 13. Omori & Malicki, 2006; 14. Horne-Badovinac et al., 2001; 15. Hsu et al., 2006; 16. Wang et al., 2006; 17. Granato et al., 1996; 18. Zhang et al., 2004; 19. Lefebvre et al., 2007; 20. Lee et al., 2003; 21. Downes & Granato, 2004.

and/or other factors, whereas in the lateral blastoderm margin these posteriorizing factors transform some of the anterior neuroectoderm into more posterior neural fates. This results in specification of appropriately sized forebrain, MHB, and hindbrain anlagen in the neural plate (Fekany-Lee et al., 2000).

Parachute

The mutant phenotype is characterized by loss of the corresponding protein, N-cadherin. In zebrafish, it has a crucial role in the control of neural tube morphogenesis, maintenance of neural tube integrity by loss of neuroepithelium cell adhesion, axonal pathfinding, and neural cell proliferation (Lele et al., 2002).

Genes Affecting Neural Tube Shaping

Laminin mutants—*bashful, sleepy,* and *grumpy*—show reduced brain ventricle size relative to wild-type. Additionally, the MHB does not form normally. The *bashful, sleepy* and *grumpy* loci encode components of the extracellular matrix (ECM) proteins, Laminin α1, Laminin γ1 and Laminin β1, respectively. These genes have previously been shown to play roles during zebrafish development that include retinotectal axon pathfinding (Karlstrom et al., 1996), notochord differentiation (Parsons et al., 2002), blood vessel formation (Pollard et al., 2006), and retinal morphogenesis (Biehlmaier et al., 2007). Loss of Laminin in the basement membrane prevents normal neuroepithelial morphogenesis, particularly at the midbrain–hindbrain boundary constriction, where we have described the novel process of basal constriction (Gutzman et al., 2008; Lowery et al., 2009).

Junction Mutants

Epithelial apicobasal polarity mutants—*nagie oko, oko meduzy, heart and soul,* and *mosaic eyes*—correspond to genes previously implicated in epithelial polarity and junction formation. The *nagie oko* locus encodes the MAGUK protein Mpp5a (Wei & Malicki, 2002). *Oko meduzy* animals have a mutation in the *crb2* gene (encoding a Crumbs homolog), *heart and soul* mutants correspond to *prkci* (encoding atypical protein kinase C), and *mosaic eyes* to Epb4.1/5 (a FERM protein). The Mpp5, Crb2a, Prkci, and the FERM proteins colocalize at the apical surface of the neuroepithelium and control apical junction formation and epithelial apicobasal polarity (Horne-Badovinac et al., 2001; Hsu et al., 2006; Omori & Malicki, 2006). All these mutants have defects in neural tube midline separation, perhaps because of apicobasal polarity defects (Lowery et al., 2009).

Genes Affecting Specific Differentiated Neurons

Motionless

The mutant phenotype is caused by the disruption of a gene encoding the Mediator subunit Med12. Mutants exhibit deficits of certain neuronal subtypes, including monoaminergic neurons and cranial sensory ganglia but not GABAergic neurons. Overexpression of *mot/med12* is capable of inducing premature neuronal differentiation and an increased production of brain dopaminergic, noradrenergic, and serotonergic neurons (Wang et al., 2006). Moreover, polymorphisms of the *med12* gene in humans are associated with an increased risk for schizophrenia (Philibert et al., 2007).

Unplugged

The *unplugged* gene encodes a muscle-specific kinase (MuSK). In zebrafish, MuSK is important for motor neuron pathfinding, and it is critical for the assembly of focal synapses by cooperating with dystroglycan and also in the formation of nonfocal myoseptal and distributed synapses (Lefebvre et al., 2007; Zhang et al., 2004).

No soul

No soul encodes Foxi1, a winged helix domain-containing transcriptional regulator that is expressed in the placodal progenitor cells. Foxi1 activity is required for the coordinated expression of both neuronal fate and subtype identity genes in the visceral sensory lineage (Lee et al., 2003).

Zieharmonika

This locus encodes for enzyme acetylcholinesterase (AChE). AChE is indispensable for muscle fiber development and Rohon-Beard sensory neuron growth and survival. In absence of AChE, the acetylcholine receptor clusters at neuromuscular junctions initially assemble, but these clusters are not maintained. AChE is required for muscle fiber formation and sensory neuronal development and regulates stability of neuromuscular synapses (Downes & Granato, 2004).

Morphant Phenotypes

Morphants are animals in which gene function has been decreased by injection of a MO (Summerton & Weller, 1997). To date, most of the mutations that have been mapped are successfully phenocopied by the respective MO, making this a powerful alternate to genetic mutants, during embryonic development. MO knockdowns are rapid and effective, making zebrafish a powerful tool to study autism by selectively and easily knocking down the candidate genes emerging from genetic studies.

Recently, several risk genes for mental health disorders (including autism, schizophrenia, and mental retardation) have been intensively studied in zebrafish.

Disrupted in schizophrenia-1 (DISC-1)

The *DISC-1* gene was identified as a locus that was translocated in an extended Scottish family with psychotic illness and major depression (Millar et al., 2000). *DISC-1* loss of function in dentate gyrus neurons causes an abnormal neurite formation (Mao et al., 2009). In zebrafish, two independent studies demonstrate different functions during fish development. In early stages of embryonic development, *DISC-1* is required for development of the forebrain by modulating the canonical Wnt pathway (DeRienzo & Sive, submitted; Brandon et al., 2009). In later stages of zebrafish development, *DISC-1* is required for normal oligodentrocytes and cerebellar neurons (Wood et al., 2009).

Reelin

There is considerable evidence for involvement of Reelin protein in autism, by association of a polymorphism in the untranslated region of its mRNA with susceptibly to autism (Fatemi, 2001). Costagli et al. have shown in the developing zebrafish embryo that reelin dynamically localizes in the central nervous system, particularly in the dorsal telencephalon and in the thalamic and hypothalamic regions, demonstrating many similarities with Reelin localization in mammals (Costagli et al., 2002).

Abelson-Helper Integration Site One (Ahi1)

Mutations in the *Ahi1* gene are correlated with Joubert Syndrome (JBTS), a developmental brain disorder characterized by autism, seizures, and mental retardation. The cerebellum and brainstem are malformed, suggesting a role for this gene in midbrain–hindbrain development (Dixon-Salazar et al., 2004; Ferland et al., 2004). Comparisons of the expression pattern between human, mouse, and zebrafish demonstrated high similarity between fish and human, showing *Ahi1* expression in the developing cerebellum that is not present in mouse (Doering et al., 2008).

Using the Fish-Tool to Study Autism

How does one put together the attributes of the zebrafish tool in a useful way to address gene function leading to autism? Figure 50-2 indicates a flowchart outlining what we consider to be a productive approach. The approach rests on the hypotheses that *(1)* zebrafish homologs of human autism risk genes can be identified; *(2)* these genes function early during brain development; and *(3)* human and zebrafish genes will show orthologous functions. We use the 16p11.2 region of chromosome 16 as an example of a set of autism risk genes to be analyzed (Weiss et al., 2008).

The first step is to identify zebrafish homologs of human risk genes, using information from the zebrafish and human genome projects. In some cases, there is a single zebrafish homolog, whose projected protein sequence matches closely with that of human protein. In the simplest case, this single gene is also syntenic (on a preserved chromosomal segment) in human and fish, suggesting not simply homology (sequence equivalence) but also orthology (functional equivalence).

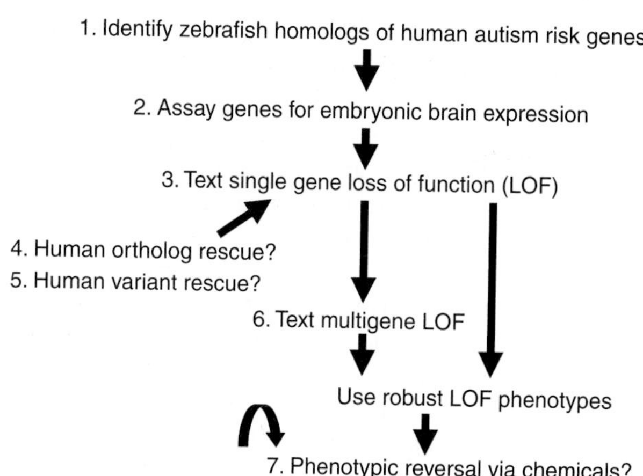

Figure 50–2. Scheme for analysis of autism risk genes in the zebrafish tool. See text for details.

However, because the teleost genome is partially duplicated, in some cases, two zebrafish homologs correspond to one mammalian gene. These may have redundant function or may have diverged sufficiently to assume non-overlapping function (Mcclintock et al., 2002). In other cases, there may be several genes with equal levels of similarity to the human gene. In rare cases, there may be no corresponding zebrafish gene, suggesting that the human gene encodes a mammalian-specific function. How does one best decide which of two or more zebrafish genes are likely to be orthologs? One way is to ask for synteny of the location of a fish gene with human chromosome 16; however, this may not indicate similar function (Catchen et al., 2008). Another way is to address expression pattern, as genes with both similar sequence and expression pattern in fish and human are likely to be orthologous. A third level of analysis is to directly test whether the human gene can substitute for the function of the fish gene. Together with sequence identity, this last is the strongest criterion for orthology. Thus, in the 16p11.2 region, we have identified 17 genes in the 16p11.2 region with a single zebrafish homolog, three with two or more homologs and five with no fish homologs (Blaker-Lee, Gupta, & Sive, unpublished).

A second step is to assess expression patterns, where expression in the developing brain suggests genes that may function during early neurogenesis or brain morphogenesis. The third step, then, is to assess the function of each gene. The quickest way to do this is to inject MOs into the one- to two-cell embryo and assay the "morphant" phenotype at 24 to 48 hours post-fertilization, after the nervous system has formed. Antisense oligos that target either the translational start site or a splice donor or acceptor site can be used. However, the latter are most useful, as successful targeting of a target almost always results in aberrant splicing, which can be monitored and quantified by reverse-transcription polymerase chain reaction (RT-PCR). Because the 16p11.2 region is generally hemizygous in autistic patients, dosage of one or more genes in this region is likely to be very important. This dosage correlation can be addressed using different amounts of injected MO to give differing amounts of normally and abnormally spliced target RNA. The splice site MO choice also ensures that maternally stored RNAs can get the embryo through very early stages, so that only zygotic gene function is assayed, often being required at the onset of neurogenesis and brain morphogenesis.

Injection of a "control" oligo indicates MO specificity, however the key control, and the fourth step in this assay scheme, is a "rescue" experiment, which corrects the morphant phenotype to a more normal one. Thus, injection of mRNA encoding the target gene, but lacking the oligo binding site, should rescue the phenotype of the morphant. At this point, we suggest using the human homolog to perform the rescue. Not only does this confirm antisense specificity—it indicates orthology between fish and human genes. We estimate that 80% to 90% of MO oligos tested are specific—that is, resulting phenotypes will be rescued by either fish or human cognate mRNA. This sets the stage for the fifth step, which is assay of human gene variants. The functional significance of gene variants identified in autism and other mental health disorder risk genes is unclear. However, the morphant rescue assay is very sensitive and rapid, allowing analysis of scores of gene variants. Confirming the usefulness of this approach, we have shown that mutants in the *DISC-1* schizophrenia risk gene rescue the loss of function phenotype with distinct efficacy (DeRienzo & Sive, submitted). Once single-gene, loss-of-function analysis has been performed, a sixth step is analysis of synergy between 16p11.2 genes via inhibiting function of two or more. In particular, this has the potential to define whether interactions between genes in this interval may contribute to autism etiology.

Finally, a risky, but high-payoff, seventh step is to screen morphants with robust (reliable and clear) phenotypes for small molecules that can reverse morphant phenotypes. Chemical screening is well-established in the zebrafish; however, few screens have not addressed phenotypic reversal (Kokel & Peterson, 2008). Phenotypic reversal may result from changing remaining gene activity or may result from commandeering a different, compensatory pathway. Such screens can be performed using small and plentiful zebrafish embryos, where screens of similar magnitude with mammalian embryos are impossible. Such screens would be moderate throughput, of the order of several thousand compounds, prescreened on cell lines, or purified proteins. Identification of compounds that modulate activity of a gene or pathway implicated in autism could provide important directions toward therapeutics.

We emphasize that this scheme does not try to address all manifestations of autism phenotypes but, rather, uses the fish as a tool to gain insight into aspects of gene function, which will be useful in more direct models.

Challenges and Future Directions

In conclusion, we have outlined the notion of the zebrafish as a "tool" to study the activity of genes implicated in autism and other mental health disorders. This tool will be extremely useful in meeting the challenge of assaying activity of human gene variants connected to autism. In addition, the fish provides an outstanding whole animal vertebrate system, which can be used in small molecule screens for modulation of gene function associated with autism. This attribute will be of major importance in the first steps of defining potential therapeutics that may ameliorate or reverse symptoms of autism and other mental health disorders.

SUGGESTED READINGS

Hakryul Jo, L. A. L., Tropepe, V., & Sive, H. (2005). The zebrafish as a model for analyzing neural tube defects. In Wyszynski, D. F. (Ed.), *Neural tube defects: From origin to treatment.* New York: Oxford University Press.

Peterson, R. T. (2008). Chemical biology and the limits of reductionism. *Nature Chemical Biology*, *4*, 635–638.

Weiss, L. A., Shen, Y., Korn, J. M., Arking, D. E., Miller, D. T., Fossdal, R., et al. (2008). Association between microdeletion and microduplication at 16p11.2 and autism. *New England Journal of Medicine*, *358*, 667–675.

ACKNOWLEDGMENTS

We thank our colleagues for helpful discussion. This work was supported by a grant from the Simons Foundation (SFARI 95091 to H.S.), and also from the Stanley Medical Research Institute, via their grant to the Stanley Center for Psychiatric Research at the Broad Institute.

REFERENCES

Amatruda, J. F. & Patton, E. E. (2008). Genetic models of cancer in zebrafish. *International Review of Cell and Molecular Biology*, *271*, 1–34.

Amsterdam, A. & Hopkins, N. (1999). Retrovirus-mediated insertional mutagenesis in zebrafish. *Methods of Cellular Biology*, *60*, 87–98.

Ando, H., Furuta, T., Tsien, R. Y. & Okamoto, H. (2001). Photo-mediated gene activation using caged RNA/DNA in zebrafish embryos. *Nature Genetics*, *28*, 317–325.

Asakawa, K., Suster, M. L., Mizusawa, K., Nagayoshi, S., Kotani, T., Urasaki, A., et al. (2008). Genetic dissection of neural circuits by Tol2 transposon-mediated Gal4 gene and enhancer trapping in zebrafish. *Proceedings of the National Academy Sciences of the United States of America*, *105*, 1255–1260.

Barbazuk, W. B., Korf, I., Kadavi, C., Heyen, J., Tate, S., Wun, E., Bedell, J. A., McPherson, J. D. & Johnson, S. L., et al. (2000). The syntenic relationship of the zebrafish and human genomes. *Genome Research*, *10*, 1351–1358.

Bellen, H. J. (1999). Ten years of enhancer detection: lessons from the fly. *Plant and Cell Physiology*, *11*, 2271–2281.

Biehlmaier, O., Makhankov, Y. & Neuhauss, S. C. (2007). Impaired retinal differentiation and maintenance in zebrafish laminin mutants. *Investigative Ophthalmology and Visual Science*, *48*, 2887–2894.

Brandon, N. J., Millar, J. K., Korth, C., Sive, H., Singh, K. K. & Sawa, A. (2009). Understanding the Role of DISC1 in Psychiatric Disease and during Normal Development. *Journal of Neuroscience*, *29*(41), 12768–12775.

Burgess, S., Reim, G., Chen, W., Hopkins, N. & Brand, M. (2002). The zebrafish spiel-ohne-grenzen (spg) gene encodes the POU domain protein Pou2 related to mammalian Oct4 and is essential for formation of the midbrain and hindbrain, and for pre-gastrula morphogenesis. *Development*, *129*, 905–916.

Catchen, J. M., Conery, J. S. & Postlethwait, J. H. (2008). Inferring ancestral gene order. *Methods of Molecular Biology*, *452*, 365–383.

Cathomen, T. & Joung, J. K. (2008). Zinc-finger nucleases: the next generation emerges. *Molecular Therapy*, *16*, 1200–1207.

Ceol, C. J., Houvras, Y., White, R. M. & Zon, L. I. (2008). Melanoma biology and the promise of zebrafish. *Zebrafish*, *5*, 247–255.

Christian, S. L., Brune, C. W., Sudi, J., Kumar, R. A., Liu, S., Karamohamed, S., et al. (2008). Novel submicroscopic chromosomal abnormalities detected in autism spectrum disorder. *Biological Psychiatry*, *63*, 1111–1117.

Costagli, A., Kapsimali, M., Wilson, S. W. & Mione, M. (2002). Conserved and divergent patterns of Reelin expression in the zebrafish central nervous system. *Journal of Comparative Neurology*, *450*, 73–93.

Dixon-Salazar, T., Silhavy, J. L., Marsh, S. E., Louie, C. M., Scott, L. C., Gururaj, A., et al. (2004). Mutations in the AHI1 gene, encoding jouberin, cause Joubert syndrome with cortical polymicrogyria. *American Journal of Human Genetics*, *75*, 979–987.

Doering, J. E., Kane, K., Hsiao, Y. C., Yao, C., Shi, B., Slowik, A. D., et al. (2008). Species differences in the expression of Ahi1, a protein implicated in the neurodevelopmental disorder Joubert syndrome, with preferential accumulation to stigmoid bodies. *Journal of Comparative Neurology*, *511*, 238–256.

Downes, G. B. & Granato, M. (2004). Acetylcholinesterase function is dispensable for sensory neurite growth but is critical for neuromuscular synapse stability. *Developmental Biology*, *270*, 232–245.

Draper, B. W., Morcos, P. A. & Kimmel, C. B. (2001). Inhibition of zebrafish fgf8 pre-mRNA splicing with morpholino oligos: a quantifiable method for gene knockdown. *Genesis*, *30*, 154–156.

Driever, W., Solnica-Krezel, L., Schier, A. F., Neuhauss, S. C., Malicki, J., Stemple, D. L., et al. (1996). A genetic screen for mutations affecting embryogenesis in zebrafish. *Development*, *123*, 37–46.

Fatemi, S. H. (2001). Reelin mutations in mouse and man: from reeler mouse to schizophrenia, mood disorders, autism and lissencephaly. *Molecular Psychiatry*, *6*, 129–133.

Fekany-Lee, K., Gonzalez, E., Miller-Bertoglio, V. & Solnica-Krezel, L. (2000). The homeobox gene bozozok promotes anterior neuroectoderm formation in zebrafish through negative regulation of BMP2/4 and Wnt pathways. *Development*, *127*, 2333–2345.

Ferland, R. J., Eyaid, W., Collura, R. V., Tully, L. D., Hill, R. S., Al-Nouri, D., et al. (2004). Abnormal cerebellar development and axonal decussation due to mutations in AHI1 in Joubert syndrome. *Nature Genetics*, *36*, 1008–1013.

Foley, J. E., Yeh, J. R., Maeder, M. L., Reyon, D., Sander, J. D., Peterson, R. T. et al. (2009). Rapid mutation of endogenous zebrafish genes using zinc finger nucleases made by Oligomerized Pool ENgineering (OPEN). *PLoS ONE*, *4*, e4348.

Golling, G., Amsterdam, A., Sun, Z., Antonelli, M., Maldonado, E., Chen, W., Burgess, S., et al. (2002). Insertional mutagenesis in zebrafish rapidly identifies genes essential for early vertebrate development. *Nature Genetics*, *31*, 135–140.

Granato, M., van Eeden, F. J., Schach, U., Trowe, T., Brand, M., Furutani-Seiki, M., et al. (1996). Genes controlling and mediating locomotion behavior of the zebrafish embryo and larva. *Development*, *123*, 399–413.

Gutzman, J. H., Graeden, E. G., Lowery, L. A., Holley, H. S. & Sive, H. (2008). Formation of the zebrafish midbrain-hindbrain boundary constriction requires laminin-dependent basal constriction. *Mechanisms of Development*, *125*, 974–983.

Haffter, P., Granato, M., Brand, M., Mullins, M. C., Hammerschmidt, M., Kane, D. A., et al. (1996). The identification of genes with unique and essential functions in the development of the zebrafish, Danio rerio. *Development*, *123*, 1–36.

Hakryul Jo, L. A. L., Tropepe, V., & Sive, H. (2005). The zebrafish as a model for analyzing neural tube defects. In Wyszynski, D. F. (Ed.), *Neural tube defects: From origin to treatment*. New York: Oxford University Press.

Hardan, A. Y., Minshew, N. J., Mallikarjuhn, M., & Keshavan, M. S. (2001). Brain volume in autism. *Journal of Child Neurology*, *16*, 421–424.

Hinkes, B., Wiggins, R. C., Gbadegesin, R., Vlangos, C. N., Seelow, D., Nurnberg, G., et al. (2006). Positional cloning uncovers mutations in PLCE1 responsible for a nephrotic syndrome variant that may be reversible. *Nature Genetics*, *38*, 1397–1405.

Horne-Badovinac, S., Lin, D., Waldron, S., Schwarz, M., Mbamalu, G., Pawson, T., et al. (2001). Positional cloning of heart and soul reveals multiple roles for PKC lambda in zebrafish organogenesis. *Current Biology*, *11*, 1492–1502.

Hsu, Y. C., Willoughby, J. J., Christensen, A. K., & Jensen, A. M. (2006). Mosaic Eyes is a novel component of the Crumbs complex and negatively regulates photoreceptor apical size. *Development*, *133*, 4849–4859.

Jiang, Y. J., Brand, M., Heisenberg, C. P., Beuchle, D., Furutani-Seiki, M., Kelsh, R. N., et al. (1996). Mutations affecting neurogenesis and brain morphology in the zebrafish, Danio rerio. *Development*, *123*, 205–216.

Ju, B., Xu, Y., He, J., Liao, J., Yan, T., Hew, C. L., et al. (1999). Faithful expression of green fluorescent protein (GFP) in transgenic zebrafish embryos under control of zebrafish gene promoters. *Developmental Genetics*, *25*, 158–167.

Karlstrom, R. O., Trowe, T., Klostermann, S., Baier, H., Brand, M., Crawford, A. D., et al. (1996). Zebrafish mutations affecting retinotectal axon pathfinding. *Development*, *123*, 427–438.

Kawakami, K. (2004). Transgenesis and gene trap methods in zebrafish by using the Tol2 transposable element. *Methods of Cellular Biology*, *77*, 201–222.

Kim, H. G., Kishikawa, S., Higgins, A. W., Seong, I. S., Donovan, D. J., Shen, Y., et al. (2008). Disruption of neurexin 1 associated with autism spectrum disorder. *American Journal of Human Genetics*, *82*, 199–207.

Kokel, D. & Peterson, R. T. (2008). Chemobehavioural phenomics and behaviour-based psychiatric drug discovery in the zebrafish. *Briefings in Functional Genomics and Proteomics*, *7*, 483–490.

Kolm, P. J. & Sive, H. L. (1995). Efficient hormone-inducible protein function in Xenopus laevis. *Developmental Biology*, *171*, 267–272.

Kumar, R. A., KaraMohamed, S., Sudi, J., Conrad, D. F., Brune, C., Badner, J. A., et al. (2008). Recurrent 16p11.2 microdeletions in autism. *Human Molecular Genetics*, *17*, 628–638.

Lee, S. A., Shen, E. L., Fiser, A., Sali, A., & Guo, S. (2003). The zebrafish forkhead transcription factor Foxi1 specifies epibranchial placode-derived sensory neurons. *Development*, *130*, 2669–2679.

Lefebvre, J. L., Jing, L., Becaficco, S., Franzini-Armstrong, C., & Granato, M. (2007). Differential requirement for MuSK and dystroglycan in generating patterns of neuromuscular innervation. *Proceedings of the National Academy Sciences of the United States of America, 104*, 2483–2488.

Lele, Z., Folchert, A., Concha, M., Rauch, G. J., Geisler, R., Rosa, F., et al. (2002). parachute/n-cadherin is required for morphogenesis and maintained integrity of the zebrafish neural tube. *Development, 129*, 3281–3294.

Lowery, L. A., De Rienzo, G., Gutzman, J. H., & Sive, H. (2009). Characterization and classification of zebrafish brain morphology mutants. *Anatomical Record (Hoboken), 292*, 94–106.

Lowery, L. A. & Sive, H. (2009). Totally tubular: the mystery behind function and origin of the brain ventricular system. *Bioessays, 31*, 446–458.

MacRae, C. A. & Peterson, R. T. (2003). Zebrafish-based small molecule discovery. *Chemical Biology, 10*, 901–908.

Mao, Y., Ge, X., Frank, C. L., Madison, J. M., Koehler, A. N., Doud, M. K., et al. (2009). Disrupted in schizophrenia 1 regulates neuronal progenitor proliferation via modulation of GSK3beta/beta-catenin signaling. *Cell, 136*, 1017–1031.

McClintock, J. M., Kheirbek, M. A., & Prince, V. E. (2002). Knockdown of duplicated zebrafish hoxb1 genes reveals distinct roles in hindbrain patterning and a novel mechanism of duplicate gene retention. *Development, 129*, 2339–2354.

Millar, J. K., Wilson-Annan, J. C., Anderson, S., Christie, S., Taylor, M. S., Semple, C. A., et al. (2000). Disruption of two novel genes by a translocation co-segregating with schizophrenia. *Human Molecular Genetics, 9*, 1415–1423.

Miller, D. T., Shen, Y., Weiss, L. A., Korn, J., Anselm, I., Bridgemohan, C., et al. (2009). Microdeletion/duplication at 15q13.2q13.3 among individuals with features of autism and other neuropsychiatric disorders. *Journal of Medical Genetics, 46*, 242–248.

Murphey, R. D. & Zon, L. I. (2006). Small molecule screening in the zebrafish. *Methods, 39*, 255–261.

Omori, Y. & Malicki, J. (2006). oko meduzy and related crumbs genes are determinants of apical cell features in the vertebrate embryo. *Current Biology, 16*, 945–957.

Papan, C. & Campos-Ortega, J. A. (1999). Region-specific cell clones in the developing spinal cord of the zebrafish. *Development Genes and Evolution, 209*, 135–144.

Parinov, S., Kondrichin, I., Korzh, V., & Emelyanov, A. (2004). Tol2 transposon-mediated enhancer trap to identify developmentally regulated zebrafish genes in vivo. *Developmental Dynamics, 231*, 449–459.

Parsons, M. J., Pollard, S. M., Saude, L., Feldman, B., Coutinho, P., Hirst, E. M. et al. (2002). Zebrafish mutants identify an essential role for laminins in notochord formation. *Development, 129*, 3137–3146.

Paulus, J. D. & Halloran, M. C. (2006). Zebrafish bashful/laminin-alpha 1 mutants exhibit multiple axon guidance defects. *Developmental Dynamics, 235*, 213–224.

Persico, A. M., D'Agruma, L., Maiorano, N., Totaro, A., Militerni, R., Bravaccio, C., et al. (2001). Reelin gene alleles and haplotypes as a factor predisposing to autistic disorder. *Molecular Psychiatry, 6*, 150–159.

Peterson, R. T. (2008). Chemical biology and the limits of reductionism. *Nature Chemical Biology, 4*, 635–638.

Peterson, R. T., Link, B. A., Dowling, J. E. & Schreiber, S. L. (2000). Small molecule developmental screens reveal the logic and timing of vertebrate development. *Proceedings of the National Academy Sciences of the United States of America, 97*, 12965–12969.

Philibert, R. A., Bohle, P., Secrest, D., Deaderick, J., Sandhu, H., Crowe, R. et al. (2007). The association of the HOPA(12bp) polymorphism with schizophrenia in the NIMH Genetics Initiative for Schizophrenia sample. *American Journal of Medical Genetics. Part B, Neuropsychiatric Genetics, 144B*, 743–747.

Pichler, F. B., Laurenson, S., Williams, L. C., Dodd, A., Copp, B. R. & Love, D. R. (2003). Chemical discovery and global gene expression analysis in zebrafish. *Nature Biotechnology, 21*, 879–883.

Pollard, S. M., Parsons, M. J., Kamei, M., Kettleborough, R. N., Thomas, K. A., Pham, V. N., et al. (2006). Essential and overlapping roles for laminin alpha chains in notochord and blood vessel formation. *Developmental Biology, 289*, 64–76.

Porteus, M. H. & Carroll, D. (2005). Gene targeting using zinc finger nucleases. *Nature Biotechnology, 23*, 967–973.

Reim, G. & Brand, M. (2002). Spiel-ohne-grenzen/pou2 mediates regional competence to respond to Fgf8 during zebrafish early neural development. *Development, 129*, 917–933.

Schier, A. F., Neuhauss, S. C., Harvey, M., Malicki, J., Solnica-Krezel, L., Stainier, D. Y., et al. (1996). Mutations affecting the development of the embryonic zebrafish brain. *Development, 123*, 165–178.

Shestopalov, I. A., Sinha, S. & Chen, J. K. (2007). Light-controlled gene silencing in zebrafish embryos. *Nature Chemical Biology, 3*, 650–651.

Shin, J. T. & Fishman, M. C. (2002). From Zebrafish to human: modular medical models. *Annual Reviews of Genomics and Human Genetics, 3*, 311–340.

Skromne, I. & Prince, V. E. (2008). Current perspectives in zebrafish reverse genetics: moving forward. *Developmental Dynamics, 237*, 861–882.

Solnica-Krezel, L., Schier, A. F. & Driever, W. (1994). Efficient recovery of ENU-induced mutations from the zebrafish germline. *Genetics, 136*, 1401–1420.

Sood, R., English, M. A., Jones, M., Mullikin, J., Wang, D. M., Anderson, M., et al. (2006). Methods for reverse genetic screening in zebrafish by resequencing and TILLING. *Methods, 39*, 220–227.

Soroldoni, D., Hogan, B. M., & Oates, A. C. (2009). Simple and efficient transgenesis with meganuclease constructs in zebrafish. *Methods of Molecular Biology, 546*, 117–130.

Steffenburg, S., Gillberg, C. L., Steffenburg, U. & Kyllerman, M. (1996). Autism in Angelman syndrome: a population-based study. *Pediatric Neurology, 14*, 131–136.

Summerton, J. & Weller, D. (1997). Morpholino antisense oligomers: design, preparation, and properties. *Antisense and Nucleic Acid Drug Development, 7*, 187–195.

Tropepe, V. & Sive, H. L. (2003). Can zebrafish be used as a model to study the neurodevelopmental causes of autism? *Genes, Brain and Behavior, 2*, 268–281.

Wang, X., Yang, N., Uno, E., Roeder, R. G. & Guo, S. (2006). A subunit of the mediator complex regulates vertebrate neuronal development. *Proceedings of the National Academy of Sciences of the United States of America, 103*, 17284–17289.

Wei, X. & Malicki, J. (2002). nagie oko, encoding a MAGUK-family protein, is essential for cellular patterning of the retina. *Nature Genetics, 31*, 150–157.

Weiss, L. A., Shen, Y., Korn, J. M., Arking, D. E., Miller, D. T., Fossdal, R.,et al. (2008). Association between microdeletion and microduplication at 16p11.2 and autism. *New England Journal of Medicine, 358*, 667–675.

Wiellette, E., Grinblat, Y., Austen, M., Hirsinger, E., Amsterdam, A., Walker, C., et al. (2004). Combined haploid and insertional mutation screen in the zebrafish. *Genesis, 40*, 231–240.

Wienholds, E., van Eeden, F., Kosters, M., Mudde, J., Plasterk, R. H. & Cuppen, E. (2003). Efficient target-selected mutagenesis in zebrafish. *Genome Research, 13*, 2700–2707.

Wood, J. D., Bonath, F., Kumar, S., Ross, C. A., & Cunliffe, V. T. (2009). Disrupted-in-schizophrenia 1 and neuregulin 1 are required for the specification of oligodendrocytes and neurones in the zebrafish brain. *Human Molecular Genetics, 18*, 391–404.

Wulliman, M. F. (1998). The central nervous system. In Evans, D. H. (Ed.), *The physiology of fishes*. New York: CRC Press LLC, pp. 245–281.

Xu, X., Meiler, S. E., Zhong, T. P., Mohideen, M., Crossley, D. A., Burggren, W. W., et al. (2002). Cardiomyopathy in zebrafish due to mutation in an alternatively spliced exon of titin. *Nature Genetics, 30*, 205–209.

Zhang, J., Lefebvre, J. L., Zhao, S., & Granato, M. (2004). Zebrafish unplugged reveals a role for muscle-specific kinase homologs in axonal pathway choice. *Nature Neuroscience, 7*, 1303–1309.

51

Mu Yang, Maria Luisa Scattoni, Kathryn K. Chadman, Jill L. Silverman, Jacqueline N. Crawley

Behavioral Evaluation of Genetic Mouse Models of Autism

Points of Interest

- Animal models provide essential translational tools for studying mechanisms underlying human genetic disorders and for developing treatment strategies. An effective mouse model should incorporate face validity (i.e., strong analogies to the endophenotypes of the human syndrome); construct validity (i.e., the same biological dysfunction that causes the human disease, such as a gene mutation or anatomical abnormality); and predictive validity (i.e., the analogous response to treatments that prevent or reverse symptoms in the human disease). It is essential to keep in mind that no animal model will ever fully recapitulate a uniquely human disorder such as the autism spectrum disorders (ASDs).
- Mouse models have been extordinarily useful in identifying genetic factors underlying human disorders. Reverse genetic approaches test mice with mutations in candidate genes for autism, such as the genes for engrailed 2, reelin, neurexins, neuroligins, shanks, and contactins; chromosomal deletions and duplications such as 15q11-13; and comorbid monogenic disorders such as Fragile X and tuberous sclerosis. Forward genetic approaches identify inbred strains of mice with phenotypes relevant to autism and explore mechanisms responsible for the phenotypes. Quantitative trait loci (QTL) analysis in recombinant inbred strains could lead to the discovery of novel genetic factors relevant to autism-like phenotypes.
- Because autism is diagnosed by behavioral symptoms, analogous behavioral assays are needed to phenotype mouse models of autism. The primary diagnostic symptom of autism is impaired reciprocal social interactions. Mouse social behaviors have been studied by ethologists and behavioral neuroscientists for many years. Recently, specific behavioral tasks have been developed to quantitiate simple social approach behaviors toward a novel mouse, reciprocal social interaction behaviors between two unfamiliar mice, preference for social novelty, social dominance, and tests of home cage social behaviors to model the types of social deficits seen in autistic individuals. These tasks represent the beginning of a new frontier, which has yet to be fully explored. New tasks need to be developed to study social behaviors in complex situations, subtle deficits in the social domain, Theory of Mind, and other aspects of social abnormalities that are common to ASDs. Social communication, repetitive behaviors, and restricted interests are components of the mouse repertoire for which assays are being developed to maximize relevance to the second and third diagnostic symptoms of autism.
- Although humans and nonhuman primates rely primarily on visual and auditory information to discriminate individuals, mice mainly utilize olfactory cues for the same purposes. Care must be taken to distinguish physical defects in a sensory modality from abnormalities in higher-order processing of sensory information. Although the sensory organs used to receive and transmit social cues differ between mice and humans, the critical integration and interpretation of social stimuli that appears to be problematic in autism may be processed in similar cortical regions across species.
- Mice emit vocalizations within the ultrasonic range in various social contexts and across developmental ages. Neonatal mice emit distress calls when separated from the mother. Adult mice of both sexes produce complex USV patterns in different social situations. The communicative property of USVs is under intense investigations, and the potential to use USVs to assay communication deficits in mice is being explored.

Introduction

Autism is a complex neurodevelopmental disorder with extraordinarily high heritability. Intense efforts are now focusing on identifying genetic causes of autism. Animal models provide essential translational tools to investigate hypotheses about the biological causes of ASDs, including candidate genes, synaptic and neuroanatomical abnormalities, environmental toxins, prenatal insults, and immune dysfunctions (Smith et al., 2007; Abrahams & Geschwind, 2008; Berman et al., 2008; Buxbaum, 2009; James et al., 2009; Singer et al., 2009). Robust phenotypes in model organisms offer translational tools to identify causes and to seek putative treatments for autism. This chapter discusses the most promising mouse models of autism and strategies to phenotype new genetic lines of mice.

It is important to recognize that no model system will ever fully recapitulate the uniquely human qualities of ASDs. Rather, the optimal animal model will incorporate *(1)* face validity (i.e., strong analogies to the endophenotypes of the human syndrome); *(2)* construct validity (i.e., the same causes as in the human syndrome); and *(3)* predictive validity (i.e., prevention and/or reversal of phenotypes by treatments that prevent or reverse components of the human syndrome). Because the causes of autism remain unknown, and as yet no treatments consistently improve the core symptoms, it is presently not possible to incorporate definitive construct and predictive validity into an animal model of autism. In the absence of consistent biological markers, the diagnosis of ASDs is currently based on well-defined behavioral symptoms, and animal models therefore focus on behavioral phenotypes with face validity to the diagnostic symptoms of autism. Behavioral neuroscientists are in the early stages of elaborating a set of behavioral assays with face validity to the defining symptoms of autism.

The first DSM-IV diagnostic criterion for autism, qualitative impairments in reciprocal social interactions (American Psychiatric Association, 1994; Piven et al., 1997; Lord et al., 2000; Dawson et al., 2002; Volkmar & Pauls, 2003; Lord et al., 2006; London, 2007; Landa, 2008; Rapin & Tuchman, 2008; Lord & Bishop, 2009; Volkmar et al., 2009), is perhaps the most easily modeled in rodents. Mice and rats are social species (Grant & MacIntosh, 1963; Carter et al., 1992; Young et al., 2002; Terranova & Laviola, 2005). Standard methods for scoring adult social approaches, reciprocal social interactions, nesting, sexual interactions, parental behaviors, and aggressive encounters are available in the behavioral neuroscience literature (Hofer et al., 1996; Miczek et al., 2001; Winslow, 2003; Wrenn et al., 2003; Keller et al., 2006; Champagne et al., 2007; Panksepp & Lahvis, 2007; Wersinger et al., 2007; Burgdorf et al., 2008; McFarlane et al., 2008; Scattoni et al., 2008b; Yang et al., 2009; Yang & Crawley, 2009). Our laboratory and others have developed more specialized behavioral assays using dedicated equipment to rate the types of social interactions that are most analogous to the lack of spontaneous seeking of interactions with others, lack of social reciprocity, and failure to develop peer relationships appropriate to developmental ages (Crawley, 2007a, 2007b; Crawley, 2007c), as listed in Tables 51-1 and 51-2 and described below.

Social approach is assayed in an automated apparatus that compares time that the subject mouse spends with a novel mouse versus time spent with a nonsocial novel object (Figure 51-1) (Moy et al., 2004; Nadler et al., 2004; Kwon et al., 2006; Mineur et al., 2006; Crawley et al., 2007; Moy et al., 2007; Yang et al., 2007a; Yang et al., 2007b; Jamain et al., 2008; McFarlane et al., 2008; Moy et al., 2008a; Chadman et al., 2008a; Moy et al., 2009; Yang et al., 2009, 2010; Silverman et al., 2010a).

> Sociability in our automated three-chambered social approach task is defined as the subject mouse spending more time in the side chamber with a novel mouse than in the side chamber with a novel object.

Most strains of mice spend more time with the novel mouse, representing normal sociability. Equal or less time spent with the novel mouse and the novel object would represent the absence of sociability in this task. Investigating the novel object instead of the novel mouse may be analogous to the tendency of individuals with autism to engage in nonsocial activities such as playing with one toy train, repeatedly assembling a jigsaw puzzle, excellence at a video game, rock collecting, or comprehensive knowledge of baseball statistics (Frith, 2003; Frith & Happe, 2005). Because mice investigate novel conspecifics by sniffing, an important corroborative parameter in the social approach task is significantly more time spent sniffing the novel mouse than the novel object. Sniffing is directed to the face, nose, anogenital, or other body region, depending on the relative positions of the two animals. Sniffing tends to decline after several minutes, as the subject grows familiar with the novel mouse. Mouse models displaying lack of sociability are described below and in Tables 51-1 and 51-2.

Reciprocal Social Interaction is Assayed in a Neutral Arena

> Reciprocal social interactions are scored between a pair of two age-matched mice unfamiliar to each other. Parameters scored include nose-to-nose sniffing, nose-to-anogenital sniffing, approaching from the front, following, pushing past and crawling over, as well as nonsocial behaviors such as self-grooming and arena exploration.

Behaviors exhibited by two unfamiliar age-matched mice are detected with automated videotracking equipment or rated by an observer from videotapes. The same scoring method is applicable to animals of both sexes tested at all post-weaning ages. A standard test session is 10 to 20 minutes long, a period when intense social interactions occur

Table 51–1.
Examples of candidate gene mutation mouse models with phenotypes relevant to autism

Section 1, Genes Implicated in Single-Gene Disorders with High Rate of Autism

Gene	Chromosomal Locus	Protein	Behavioral Tasks Relevant to Autism	Findings	References
Fmr1	Xq27.3	Fragile X mental retardation protein	Social approach Partition test Social dominance test Social recognition test	*Fmr1* –/– generated on B6 or B6 x FVB/NJ background exhibited normal sociability. *Fmr1* –/– generated on a FVB/129 background show deficits in sociability. *Fmr1* –/– showed altered social behaviors as compared to +/+ in these tasks	Spencer et al., 2005; McNaughton et al., 2008; Moy et al., 2009 Spencer et al., 2005; Mineur et al., 2006; Spencer et al., 2008
Mecp2	Xq28	Methyl-CpG-binding protein-2	Partition test Social approach and social recognition Nest building Separation-induced USV	$MeCP^{Floxy/y}$ mice (with partial loss of MeCP2 protein) showed altered behaviors in the partition test. Mice with conditional forebrain Mecp 2 knockout showed deficits in social approach and social recognition $Mecp2^{308/y}$ mice showed poor nesting behavior $Mecp2^{1lox}$ +/– and –/– pups showed increased separation-induced vocalizations	Samaco et al., 2008 Gemelli et al., 2006; Moretti et al., 2005 Picker et al., 2006
Gabrb3	15q11-q13	GABA A receptor beta3 subunit	Social approach and repetitive behaviors	*Gabrb3* –/– mice showed a lack of sociability, poor nesting behavior, and stereotyped circling.	DeLorey et al., 2008
15q11-13 duplication	15q11-13 (Human) 7 (mouse)	Contains a cluster of imprinted genes	Social approach and perseverative behaviors	Chromosome segment duplication mice showed sociability deficit sin the three-chambered task and persevarative behaviors in the Morris Water Maze	Nakatani et al., 2009
Tsc1	9q34	Hamartin	Learning and memory Social behavior Nest building	*Tsc1*+/– mice were impaired in spatial learning and contextual fear conditioning, but not cued fear conditioning *Female Tsc1*+/– mice showed reduced social interaction and poor nest-building	Goorden et al., 2007
Tsc 2	16p13		Learning and memory Social approach	*Tsc2* +/– mice showed learning and memory deficits *Tsc2* +/– mice showed normal social approach behavior	Ehninger et al., 2008

Section 2, Synaptic Cell-Adhesion Molecules

Gene	Chromosomal Locus	Protein	Behaviors Relevant to Autism	Findings	References
Nlgn2	17p13	Neuroligin 2	Social approach and repetitive behaviors	*Nlgn2* –/– mice exhibited normal sociability Mice with *Nlgn2* overexpression showed a lack of sociability and stereotyped behaviors	Blundell et al. 2008; Hines et al., 2008
Nlgn3	X	Neuroligin 3	Social approach	*Nlgn3* knockin mice showed normal sociability	Chadman et al., 2008 a
			Social approach	*Nlgn3* knockin mice showed minor deficits	Tabuchi et al., 2007

(*Continued*)

Table 51-1. (Contd.)

Gene	Chromosomal Locus	Protein	Behaviors Relevant to Autism	Findings	References
			Preference for social novelty	*Nlgn3* –/– showed normal sociability but a lack of preference for social novelty, which might due to olfactory deficits	Radyushkin et al., 2009
Nlgn4	X	Neuroligin 4	Adult male vocalizations Social approach and reciprocal social interaction	The original cohort of *Nlgn4* –/– mice showed deficits in ultrasonic vocalizations The original cohort of *Nlgn4* –/– mice showed a lack of sociability and reduced social interaction	Jamain et al., 2008
Shank1	19q13.3	Shank1	Social approach	*Shank1* –/– show normal sociability *Shank1* –/– show increased anxiety-like behaviors and impaired fear conditioning responses	Barkan et al., 2009; Hung et al., 2008

Section 3, Signaling, Transcription, Methylation, and Neurotrophic Factors

Gene	Chromosomal locus	Protein	Behaviors relevant to autism	Findings	References
En2	7q32	Engrailed-2	Social behaviors	*En2* –/– mice showed reduced reciprocal social interactions at juvenile age and adult age	Cheh et al., 2006
Foxp2	7q31	Forkhead box P2	Ultrasonic vocalizations	*Foxp2* +/– showed reduced separation-induced pup vocalizations Mice with R552H knockin mutations displayed impaired USV on postnatal day 10	Shu et al., 2005 Fujita et al., 2008
Pten	10	Phosphatase and tensin homolog on chromosome 10	Social behaviors	Mice with conditional forebrain inactivation of *Pten* showed reduced reciprocal social interactions and a lack of sociability	Kwon et al., 2006

Section 4, Neurotransmitters

Gene	Chromosomal locus	Protein	Behaviors relevant to autism	Findings	References
Oxt	20	Oxytocin	Social approach	*Oxt* –/– mice generated in two independent groups exhibited normal sociability	Crawley et al., 2007
Avpr1a	12q14-q15	Arginine vasopressin receptor 1a	Social behavior	*Avpr1a* –/– showed impaired social recognition	Bielsky et al., 2004
Avpr1b	12q14–15	Arginine vasopressin receptor 1b	Social recognition Resident - intruder vocalizations	*Avpr1b* –/– mice displayed impaired social memory *Avpr1b* –/– mice emitted fewer USVs	Wersinger et al., 2002 Scattoni et al., 2008 b
Vip	6p21	Vasoactive intestinal peptide	Social approach	Male offspring of *Vip* +/– showed sociability deficits regardless of their own genotypes	Stack et al., 2008
Cadps2	7q31.32	Ca2+ dependent activator protein for secretion 2	Social interaction	*Cadps2* –/– show reduced social interactions	Sadakata et al., 2007

(Nadler et al., 2004; Cheh et al., 2006; Bolivar et al., 2007; Yang et al., 2007b; McFarlane et al., 2008; Scearce-Levie et al., 2008; Yang et al., 2009a). Tables 51-1 and 51-2 below describe rodent models displaying decreased reciprocal social interactions.

When two unfamiliar mice are placed in a neutral arena simultaneously, they quickly begin to sniff each other, mainly around the nose/face region (nose-to-nose sniff) and the anogenital region (anogenital sniff) (Figure 51-2). Nose-to-nose sniff could conceivably be analogous to social greeting in

Table 51–2.
Examples of behaviors relevant to autism in inbred strains of mice

Strain	Sociability Detected in the Three Chambered Social Approach Task		Reciprocal Social Interactions	References
129S1/SvImJ	Low	Moy et al., 2007	Normal social interaction	Bolivar et al., 2007
129X1/SvJ	High	Delorey et al., 2008	Normal social investigation; Normal nesting	Harms et al., 2008
129/SvEv	N/A		Normal social transmission of food preference Normal nesting and social behaviors; low stereotypies	Mayeux-Portas et al., 2000 Moretti et al., 2005
129/SvEvTac	N/A		Normal social huddling in the home cage	Long et al., 2004
A/J	Low	Brodkin et al., 2004; Moy et al., 2007	Low social interaction time Normal social reward in juveniles	Bolivar et al., 2007 Panksepp & Lahvis, 2007
AKR	High	Brodkin et al., 2004 ; Moy et al., 2007		
B6	High	Brodkin et al., 2004 ; McFarlane et al., 2008 ; Moy et al., 2007, 2008 a, b; Yang et al., 2009 a, b	High sociability Normal juvenile social reward; High juvenile play	Bolivar et al., 2007 ; McFarlane et al., 2008 ; Panksepp & Lahvis, 2007; Ryan et al., 2008 ; Yang et al., 2007b
BALB/c	No	Brodkin et al., 2004 ; Moy et al., 2007; Sankoorikal et al., 2005	Low social reward in juveniles; Low social investigation	Panksepp et al., 2007;Panksepp & Lahvis, 2007
BTBR	Low	Moy et al., 2007; McFarlane et al., 2008; Yang et al., 2007 a, b; Yang et al., 2009 a, b	Low social interaction time; Poor social transmission of food preference; Low juvenile play	Bolivar et al., 2007; Yang et al., 2007 a, b; Moy et al., 2007; McFarlane et al., 2008; Yang et al., 2009 a, b
C3H	High	Moy et al., 2007		
C57L	High	Moy et al., 2007		
C58	Low	Moy et al., 2008		
DBA	Low	Moy et al., 2007, 2008 b		
DBA2	Low High	Moy et al., 2008 b Moy et al., 2007	Normal social interaction Normal social reward in juveniles	Bolivar et al., 2007 Panksepp & Lahvis, 2007
FVB/NJ	High	Moy et al., 2008 b	High social interaction	Brodkin et al., 2004; Bolivar et al., 2007
NOD	Low	Moy et al., 2008 b		
NZB	Low	Moy et al., 2008 b		
PL/J	High	Moy et al., 2008 b		
SJL	Low	Moy et al., 2008 b		
SWR	High	Moy et al., 2008 b		

Notes: An optimal model strain incorporates social deficits replicated in multiple cohorts and across different laboratories. Additional autism-like phenotypes such as unusual social olfactory or vocalization responses, repetitive behaviors, and restricted interests, along with normal physical and procedural abilities, increase the value of the strain as a model for autism. High = sociability present; Low = sociability absent; N/A = the strain has not been tested in the three-chambered social approach test.

humans. Other measures of social interaction are front approach, follow, push and crawl, and allogrooming (McFarlane et al., 2008; Yang et al., 2009). These basic, non-aggressive social behaviors are present in animals of both sexes and at all post-weaning ages, making them suitable parameters for studying developmental trajectory of social behaviors relevant to autism. Aggressive behaviors are unique to sexually mature male mice, including chasing, offensive attacking, and defensive postures. Aggressive behaviors are not as relevant to modeling the diagnostic symptoms of autism but might reflect altered social behaviors caused by genetic mutations and/or pharmacological treatments (Jamain et al., 2008; Navarro et al., 2008). An important control measure of this task is bouts of general arena exploration, locomotor activity, and

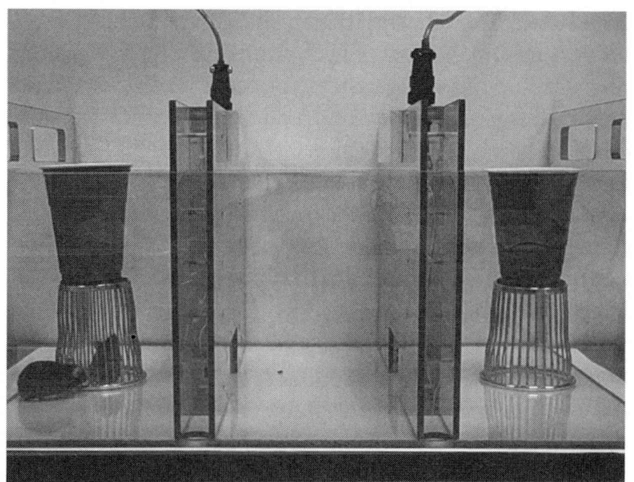

Figure 51–1. Illustration of the automated three-chambered social approach apparatus to assay sociability in mice.

general investigation toward nonsocial stimuli (Yang et al., 2009).

The second DSM-IV diagnostic criterion, qualitative impairments in communication (Lord et al., 2000; Frith, 2003; Tager-Flusberg & Caronna, 2007), may be the most difficult domain to model in rodents. The extent to which mice communicate concrete information to each other is a question that requires a great deal more investigation. As described below, olfaction is the primary sense used by mice and rats for individual recognition. However, the exact pheromonal messages being emitted by one mouse, and the correct responses to the olfactory information by the other mouse, are not yet sufficiently well-explicated in the literature to be employed as quantitative assays for communication. Besides pheromonal communication, mice also emit vocalizations in the ultrasonic range in some social situations (Maggio & Whitney, 1985; White et al., 1998; Branchi et al., 2001; D'Amato & Moles, 2001; Hofer et al., 2001; Gourbal et al., 2004; Holy & Guo, 2005; Panksepp et al., 2007; Wang et al., 2008; Scattoni et al., 2008b; Hammerschmidt et al., 2009; Scattoni et al., 2009, 2010).

Mice emit vocalizations in the ultrasonic range in some social situations, indicating potential communicative values of USVs. Ultrasonic vocalizations emitted by pups separated from the mother and nest, and juveniles or adults during social interactions, are recorded by an ultrasonic microphone and scored for total number of calls and properties of the calls.

Pups separated from the nest emit calls that the parents use to locate the straying pup and retrieve it to the nest (Zippelius & Schleidt, 1956; Winslow et al., 2000; D'Amato & Moles, 2001; Hofer et al., 2001; Shu et al., 2005). Adult rats emit 22 kHz distress calls and 50 kHz calls during aggressive and sexual behaviors (Blanchard et al., 1991; Brudzynski et al., 1993; Panksepp & Burgdorf, 2000; Brudzynski & Pniak, 2002; Brudzynski, 2005; Burgdorf et al., 2008). Mice communicate by emitting USVs during juvenile social interactions and during the appetitive phases of sexual behavior (Holy & Guo, 2005; Cai et al., 2006; Panksepp et al., 2007; Wang et al., 2008). Playback of recorded vocalizations during social encounters and scoring of socially appropriate responses to the calls will be needed to understand the role of USVs in rodent communication (Hammerschmidt et al., 2009).

The third DSM-IV diagnostic criterion, stereotyped, repetitive, and restricted patterns of behavior, interests, and activities (Bodfish et al., 2000; Lord et al., 2000; Cuccaro et al., 2003; Frith, 2003; South et al., 2005; Morgan et al., 2008), can be broken down into components that have analogies in the rodent behavioral repertoire. Motor stereotypies in mice and rats include high levels of vertical jumping, backflipping, circling, digging, marble burying, rearing, repeated sniffing of one location or object, barbering, excessive self-grooming, and excessive running (Creese & Iversen, 1975; Powell et al., 1999; Turner et al., 2001; Lee et al., 2002; Pogorelov et al., 2005; Korff & Harvey, 2006; Lewis et al.,

A

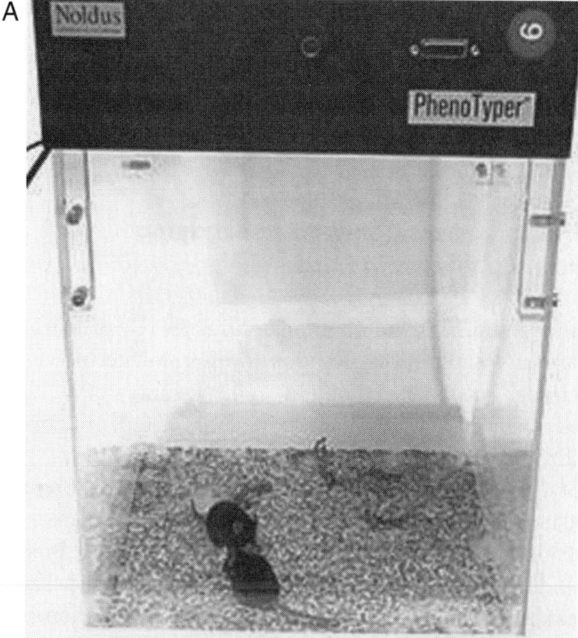

B

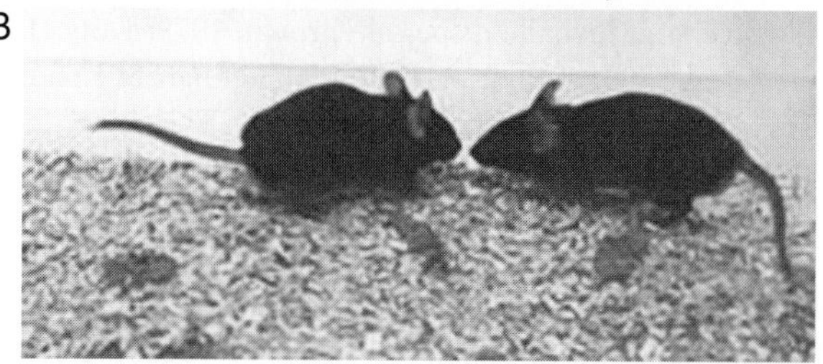

Figure 51–2. (**A**) Reciprocal social interaction test, illustrating the Noldus PhenoTyper 3000 apparatus used for videotaping pairs of mice engaged in social interactions. (**B**) A nose-to-nose sniff between two juvenile mice.

2007; Crawley, 2007c; McFarlane et al., 2008; Moy et al., 2008b; Yang et al., 2009, 2010). Perseverative patterns include the inability to change to a new search strategy, or an excessive focus on one component of a complex environment (Ralph et al., 2001; Brigman et al., 2006; Chen et al., 2007; Moy et al., 2008a). Tasks analogous to restricted interests or activities are under development, including restricted interest in a subset of holes in an open-field holeboard array (Moy et al., 2008a) and deficits in reversal learning in a T-maze task (Tanimura et al., 2008).

Analysis of multiple control parameters is essential in animal models to rule out physical and procedural abnormalities that would interfere with performance on the behaviors of interest (Crawley, 2007c). Simple physical disabilities could impair the ability of animals to conduct the procedures of the tasks that define autism-like phenotypes. For example, if a gene mutation directly affects olfactory functions, subject mice may engage in less social interaction because they are unable to detect the pheromonal cues emanating from a novel mouse. If a drug treatment induces sedation, then it is likely that impaired scores on social, communication, and exploratory tests will reflect low overall activity rather than a meaningful deficit in social approach or repetitive traits relevant to autism. Therefore, careful analyses of general health, neurological reflexes, sensory abilities, and motor functions are incorporated into the experimental design to avoid the overinterpretation of artifacts (Crawley, 2007c).

Olfactory Tasks Relevant to Studying Social Behaviors in Mice

Although humans and nonhuman primates rely primarily on visual and auditory information to discriminate individuals (Schaefer et al., 2001; Adolphs, 2002; Pelphrey et al., 2002; Hadjikhani et al., 2007; Chawarska & Shic, 2009), mice mainly utilize olfactory cues for the same purposes (Brown, 1979; Doty, 1986; Schellinck et al., 1993; Isles et al., 2001; Brennan, 2004; Keverne, 2004; Restrepo et al., 2004; Kavaliers et al., 2005; Brennan & Zufall, 2006; Arakawa et al., 2008b; Bredy & Barad, 2009). Odor cues influence a wide range of social activities in mice, including kin recognition, bond formation, mate recognition and selection, sexual maturation, inbreeding avoidance, and juvenile dispersal (Brown, 1979; Doty, 1986; Hurst et al., 2001; Hurst et al., 2005; Brennan & Kendrick, 2006; Sanchez-Andrade & Kendrick, 2009). The ability to differentiate familiar and unfamiliar individuals has advantages in many social contexts, enabling animals to form and maintain affiliative relationships while avoiding potential conspecific threats (Luo et al., 2003; Brennan & Keverne, 2004; Mombaerts, 2004; Brennan & Kendrick, 2006; Dulac & Wagner, 2006; Spehr et al., 2006).

The mouse olfactory system includes two anatomically distinct pathways (Buck, 2000; Luo et al., 2003; Brennan, 2004; Brennan & Kendrick, 2006; Kang et al., 2009; Martel & Baum, 2009). The main olfactory system consists of the main olfactory epithelium, which connects to the main olfactory bulb. The accessory olfactory system consists of the vomeronasal organ whose sensory neurons send signals to the accessory olfactory bulb. Recent advances have shown complementary roles of the main and the accessory systems. The two systems respond to overlapping social chemosignals, and both are connected to neural systems (such as the medial amygdala) that are important for social behaviors (Trinh & Storm, 2003; Baum, 2009; Kang et al., 2009).

Basic Olfactory Tests Used to Check for Anosmia (Loss of Sense of Smell)

Table 51-3 summarizes some of the widely used mouse olfactory tasks. The buried food test measures the latency to uncover a piece of odorous food, such as cookies, cereals, chocolate chips, or food pellets, which are hidden underneath a layer of bedding. The olfactory habituation/dishabituation test (Figure 51-3) measures the ability to detect and differentiate different odors. Almond and vanilla extracts (1:100 dilution) can be used as nonsocial odors, and soiled cage bedding or fresh urine can be used as social odors (Alberts & Galef, 1971; Klein et al., 1996; Yamada et al., 2001; Del Punta et al., 2002; Trinh & Storm, 2003; Woodley & Baum, 2003; Wersinger et al., 2007; Yang & Crawley, 2009). Habituation, a progressive decrease in olfactory investigation (sniffing) following repeated exposure to the same odor stimulus, indicates that the subject can recognize that identical odors are the same. Dishabituation, a reinstatement of sniffing when a novel odor is presented, reflects that the subject can differentiate a new odor from a now-familiar odor. The peaks of the habituation/dishabituation curves reflect the animal's interests in the each odor (Wersinger & Rissman, 2000; Bielsky et al., 2004; Yang & Crawley, 2009).

Social recognition, social memory, and preference for social novelty tests rely on the intrinsic tendency to investigate other individuals, especially *novel ones* (Winslow, 2003; Sanchez-Andrade & Kendrick, 2009). *Social recognition* is usually studied using a habituation/dishabituation task or the discrimination paradigm. For the habituation/dishabituation task, the subject is presented with a same-stimulus animal for multiple times. Then a novel stimulus animal is presented. Social recognition is demonstrated by a decline in investigation following repeated exposure to a same-stimulus animal (habituation) (Bielsky et al., 2004; Bielsky & Young, 2004; Bielsky et al., 2005; Sanchez-Andrade et al., 2005; Wersinger et al., 2007) and by a reinstatement of high levels of sniffing when a novel stimulus animal is introduced (dishabituation) (Bielsky & Young, 2004; Richter et al., 2005; Sanchez-Andrade et al., 2005; Wanisch et al., 2008). The same habituation/dishabituation presentations are employed in *social memory* tests, except that a time interval delay is introduced between presentations. For the discrimination test, the subject is given a simultaneous choice of two stimulus animals, one that the subject has previously encountered and one completely

Table 51–3.
Some basic olfactory tests relevant to investigating social behaviors in rodents

Test Category	Tests	References
General olfactory abilities	Buried food test	Crawley et al., 2007; Wersinger et al., 2007; Lu et al., 2008; Moy et al., 2009
	Olfactory habituation/ dishabituation	Isles et al., 2001; Crawley et al., 2007; Wersinger et al., 2007; Fleming et al., 2008; Wesson et al., 2008
Social recognition and social memory	Social memory	Richter et al., 2005; Sanchez-Andrade et al., 2005; Wanisch et al., 2008
	Social recognition (habituation-dishabituation paradigm)	Bielsky et al., 2004; Sanchez-Andrade et al., 2005; Juch et al., 2009
	Social recognition (preference for social novelty)	Crawley et al., 2007; Chadman et al., 2008a; McFarlane et al., 2008; Moy et al., 2008; Moy et al., 2009
	Scent marking (counter marking)	Arakawa et al., 2008 a; Roullet et al., 2009
Discrimination and preference for social odors	Olfactometry	Slotnick & Restrepo, 2005; Slotnick, 2007; Wesson et al., 2008
	Social odor discrimination test	Wersinger & Rissman, 2000; Woodley et al., 2004; Keller et al., 2006; Wesson et al., 2008

unfamiliar to the subject. Significantly more investigation of the new-stimulus animal compared to the original-stimulus animal indicates normal recognition memory (Engelmann et al., 1995; Wanisch et al., 2008). The interval before the novel animal is introduced can be varied to study neural mechanisms of social memory. The social recognition and social memory paradigms described above can be combined into a comprehensive social olfaction test (Sanchez-Andrade et al., 2005; Sanchez-Andrade & Kendrick, 2009). In addition, the automated three-chambered social approach test, which was designed as an assay for sociability, can also be used to test social recognition, as indicated by a significant preference for social novelty. After the 10-minute sociability test in which the subject investigates a novel mouse in one side chamber and a novel object in the other side chamber, a second novel mouse is brought into the side chamber formerly containing the novel object and simultaneously presented with the first novel mouse. More time spent investigating the new novel mouse than the original novel mouse is interpreted as the ability to differentiate the two sequentially introduced social stimuli (McFarlane et al., 2008; Moy et al., 2008b; Chadman et al., 2008).

Besides tests in which olfactory investigation is the main behavioral parameter, several paradigms evaluate scent-marking behavior (Humphries et al., 1999; Hurst et al., 2001; Hurst & Beynon, 2004; Hurst et al., 2005; Arakawa et al., 2008b; Roullet et al., 2009) or behavioral responses toward scent marks (Cheetham et al., 2007) to study social recognition. Scent-marking tasks are based on the fact that urinary odors are distinct among genetically diverse individuals and that a male mouse tends to countermark new scent marks deposited in its territory by other males (Hurst et al., 2001; Hurst & Beynon, 2004). Arakawa and colleagues (Arakawa et al., 2008a) showed that male mice gradually reduce countermarking behavior toward a repeatedly introduced stimulus mouse, and increase countermarking when a novel stimulus mouse that is genetically different from the first stimulus mouse is introduced. These findings indicate that countermarking behavior might be useful for studying the ability to discriminate different individuals based on unique molecular components contained in urinary deposits.

Odor Discrimination Tests

Social odors used in this test derive urine samples from awake or anesthetized mice, soiled bedding from a cage of group-housed mice, or nesting material from a cage of mice (Wersinger & Rissman, 2000; Woodley et al., 2004). In the non-conditioned form of the discrimination test, the subject is simultaneously presented with different social odors. More time spent sniffing one odor over the other indicates preference (Wersinger & Rissman, 2000; Isles et al., 2001; Bakker et al., 2002). Quantitation is by an observer scoring time spent

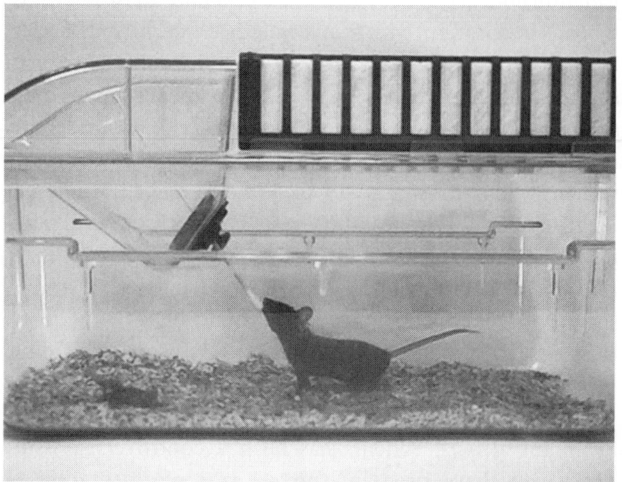

Figure 51–3. Olfactory habituation/dishabituation test, showing a mouse sniffing a cotton-tipped applicator saturated with a social odor.

sniffing each stimulus, with a stopwatch, event recorder, or videotracking software, in real time or from videotapes (Schellinck et al., 2001). In the conditioning versions of the discrimination test, subjects are first trained to associate two odors, one paired with a reinforcer (CS+) and the other one not (CS−). During the subsequent discrimination test, in which the two odors are copresented in the absence of the reinforcer, more time spent investigating the previously reinforced odor indicates the ability to differentiate the two odors (Bodyak & Slotnick, 1999; Petrulis et al., 2005; Wesson et al., 2006; Wersinger et al., 2007). Olfactometer tasks are more elaborate and sensitive discrimination tests that employ an operant chamber that delivers up to eight individual odors. The subject is trained to respond to odors paired with reinforcement versus non-reinforced odors. High levels of performance accuracy indicate the ability to differentiate odors. Delays between presentations are introduced to evaluate olfactory memory. Odorant concentrations and training schedules can be adjusted to study subtle differences in olfactory sensitivity (Slotnick & Restrepo, 2005).

Ultrasonic Vocalizations

A wide range of rodents, including mice, rats, hamsters, and gerbils belonging to the family Muridae, emit ultrasonic calls in a variety of situations. Calls have been detected from neonates at the time of birth, from pups removed from the nest, from adults during courtship and mating, and from adults during aggression and/or exploration (Bell et al., 1972; Robinson & D'Udine, 1982; Hofer & Shair, 1993; Moles & D'Amato F, 2000; Nyby, 2001; Panksepp, 2003; Venerosi et al., 2006; Moles et al., 2007; Scattoni et al., 2008b).

Separated Pup Vocalizations

Isolation-induced USVs in mice are generally 10 to 140 milliseconds in duration, with frequencies between 40 and 90 kHz. USV production follows a clear ontogenetic profile from birth through the second week of life, thus allowing longitudinal analysis during very early postnatal ontogeny. Considerable differences in this ontogenetic profile have been found among strains (Roubertoux et al., 1996). For example, C57BL/6 and BALB/c strains show peak USV rates very early, around postnatal days (PNDs) 3 to 4 (Bell et al., 1972; Robinson & D'Udine, 1982), as compared to SEC, C3H, or outbred strains, such as CD-1, which show a peak around PNDs 6 to 7 (Bell et al., 1972; Elwood & Keeling, 1982; Robinson & D'Udine, 1982; Branchi et al., 1998).

Since the early 1970s, the functional role of USVs emitted by infant altricial rodents has been a controversial issue. These calls have been interpreted as a representation of emotional state and as a communicatory act designed to elicit maternal behavior. Alternatively, USV was believed to be a byproduct of the physiological response to a thermal challenge, through laryngeal braking or an abdominal compression reaction to cold temperature (Blumberg & Alberts, 1990; Blumberg & Sokoloff, 2001). However, a considerable amount of data indicates that USV is modulated by maternal cues and reflects higher integrative processes (Hofer & Shair, 1993; Panksepp, 2003), offering evidence against the interpretation by Blumberg and Sokoloff (2001). For example, Hofer and Shair (1993) reported an immediate reduction in USVs produced by isolated rat pups when they were placed back in contact with the mother (Hofer & Shair, 1993). When rat pups were re-isolated after a brief reunion with an active or anesthetized mother, calling rate increased approximately twofold above the baseline rate measured during the first isolation.This phenomenon, called *maternal potentiation* of the separation vocalization response, indicates that the separation call does not depend exclusively on thermal factors (Hofer et al., 1994; Hofer et al., 1998). Further, qualitative changes in ultrasonic emission are detected with maternal potentiation (Myers et al., 2004).

To investigate the functional role of USVs, the emission profile has been studied by monitoring several physiological parameters, by manipulating the environmental/social context, and by characterizing maternal behavior in response to USVs. The results showed that USVs elicit approach and retrieval (Noirot, 1972; Smotherman et al., 1974; Cohen-Salmon et al., 1985; Ehret & Bernecker, 1992) and reduce attacks or rough manipulation by the dam (Noirot, 1966; Ihnat, 1995). One report demonstrated that the number of calls emitted by normal hearing pups strongly decreased when these pups were cross-fostered to deaf dams, suggesting that the number of ultrasonic calls uttered by the pups in social isolation conditions is modulated by the behavior of the mother (D'Amato & Populin, 1987). A relationship between maternal responsiveness and pup calling rate has been confirmed more recently in a study comparing C57BL/6 and BALB/c maternal responsiveness to USV (D'Amato et al., 2005).

USV analysis has been employed in several studies using mouse models of neurodevelopmental disorders (Branchi & Ricceri, 2002; Ricceri et al., 2007). In the *Ts65Dn* mouse model of Down syndrome, which carries a partial trisomy of chromosome 16 that includes the region homologous to the human chromosome 21, the ontogenetic profile of USV emissions appeared delayed by 4 days, with *Ts65Dn* mice showing a peak of emission on PND 9, as compared to PND 5 in the wild-type controls (Holtzman et al., 1996). Jimpy, a shortened life-span (PND 30) mutant line showing recessive sex-linked inheritance with a point mutation in the proteolipid protein *(PLP)* gene, displays a severe CNS myelin deficiency that is associated with a variety of complex abnormalities affecting all glial populations (Vela et al., 1998). Jimpy males produced fewer USVs than their normal male littermates, beginning at PND 2 and persisting throughout the first postnatal week (Bolivar & Brown, 1994). As observed in *Ts65Dn* mice, the USV deficit is accompanied by a delay in reaching developmental milestones, delayed body weight gain, and reduced locomotor activity. The reduced vocalization rate had no consequences on maternal retrieval behavior (Bolivar & Brown, 1995). Oxytocin-null mice displayed a decrease in calling (Winslow et al., 2000), although exogenously administered oxytocin also decreased calling in rat pups and prairie voles (Insel & Winslow, 1991; Kramer et al., 2003). Oxytocin receptor gene KO mice showed a decrease in USV at PND 7 (Takayanagi et al., 2005), consistent with the hypothesis that oxytocin neurotransmission is necessary for the perception of social separation and the subsequent USV response. Vasopressin receptor 1b (*Avpr1b*) gene KO mouse pups showed a deficit in USVs but only in the maternal potentiation of USV paradigm (Scattoni et al., 2008b). Adult female *Avp1b*-null mutants also emitted fewer USVs during social interaction with an unfamiliar female partner (Scattoni et al., 2008b). Reeler mice, which carry a mutation in the gene for reelin, an extracellular-matrix protein involved in plasticity of dendritic spines and synaptic transmission, showed alterations in USV patterns with a clear gene-dose dependency (Laviola et al., 2006). Null reeler mice emitted fewer calls than wild-type controls, and heterozygotes emitted USVs at an intermediate level (Laviola et al., 2006) associated with body weight decreases. Vocalizations in reeler mice were reversed by prenatal exposure to an organophosphate (Laviola et al., 2006) and repeated maternal separations (Ognibene et al., 2007). *Dvl1* mutant mice deficient for *dishevelled-1*, a developmental gene in mammalian brain that regulates segment polarity in Drosophila, showed no differences in separated pup calling rate (Long et al., 2004). Mice deficient for fibroblast growth Factor 17 (*Fgf17*), a trophic factor involved in neural embryonic development and regional organization of cortical layers in cerebellum, inferior colliculus, and frontal cortex in rodents (Cholfin & Rubenstein, 2007), displayed selective alterations in the social domain, including a general deficit in USVs and decreased reactivity to social novelty in a social recognition task associated with reduced frontal cortex activation (Scearce-Levie et al., 2008).

Some of the most intriguing USV patterns are seen in mutant mouse models of human genetic disorders (Shu et al., 2005; Fujita et al., 2008; Groszer et al., 2008). Mutations in *FOXP2*, a gene that encodes the forkhead box transcription factor, was thought to be responsible for the rare disorders seen in the KE family, including verbal dyspraxia, dysphasia, and other severe language and speech disorders (Vargha-Khadem et al., 2005). Mouse pups heterozygous for *Foxp2* showed a selective decrease in USVs emitted after neonatal isolation on PNDs 6 and 10 (Shu et al., 2005). Mice with a knock-in R552H mutation in *Foxp2*, which corresponds to the human *FOXP2* R553H mutation, showed severe impairments in USVs at PND 10 (Fujita et al., 2008). These results were interpreted as supporting the role for *Foxp2* in regulating neural development and social communication. Somatic growth, somatosensory reflexes, and USVs have been examined in *Mecp2*^{1lox} mutant mice, a mouse model of Rett Syndrome (RTT) (Picker et al., 2006). Somatic development is similar to wild-type controls in both *Mecp2*-null male and *Mecp2* heterozygous female mice. However, beginning at PND 5, both *Mecp2*-null males and heterozygous females exhibited dramatic increases in USVs in response to social isolation. This is the earliest and most prominent sign detected in *Mecp2* mutant mice. Elevated USV levels might indicate either an altered response to social isolation or altered respiratory function, a question that has been receiving increasing attention in mouse models of RTT in recent years (Viemari et al., 2005; Ogier et al., 2007). Pharmacological studies showed that the muscarinic cholinergic agonist oxotremerine increased USVs in rat pups, and the antagonist atropine decreased USVs (Kehoe et al., 2001), offering evidence that might be relevant to the cholinergic deficits that have been reported for RTT individuals (Wenk & Hauss-Wegrzyniak, 1999). These data have translational significance, because they suggest that the early deficits noted in RTT individuals may be mimicked in the mouse models and that USVs can be used as a neonatal behavioral response to evaluate therapeutic interventions at an early age. The ontogenetic profile of USVs has been characterized in knock-in mice with a humanized mutation in the cell adhesion protein gene *Nlgn3*. Male mice with the human R451C mutation in the mouse *Nlgn 3* gene showed less USV on PND 8 than wild-type controls, whereas the emission profile in female knock-in mice was normal (Chadman et al., 2008). Developmental differences were detected between R451C knock-in mice and control groups, including slightly different rates of growth, slower righting reflexes at infancy, and faster homing responses in females (Chadman et al., 2008).

Adult Mouse Vocalizations

USVs in adult rats have been extensively described, including a 22 kHz call during stressors and aggressive interactions, and a 50 kHz call during social interactions such as sexual behaviors, juvenile interaction, and tickling (Blanchard et al., 1991; Brudzynski et al., 1993; Panksepp & Burgdorf, 2000; Brudzynski & Pniak, 2002; Brudzynski, 2005). Adult mice emit USVs with frequencies ranging from 20 to 70 kHz. The USV emission of adult mice has been primarily reported during sexual interactions (Nyby, 2001), with males responsible for most of the calls (Whitney & Nyby, 1979; Maggio et al., 1983). Unlike in rats, USVs during adult male–male encounters has not yet been extensively studied in laboratory settings (Nyby, 2001). Exposure to a female partner or to female mouse urine induces a clear USV response in adult male mice with previous reproductive experience (Whitney and Nyby, 1979; Maggio et al., 1983; Nyby, 2001; Holy and Guo, 2005; Wang et al., 2008). The quantitative analysis by Holy and Guo illustrated for the first time that the male vocalizations are characterized by temporal sequences that are specific for each individual (Holy & Guo, 2005). Female-induced male vocalization responses were reported in a study of muscarinic and dopamine receptor KO mice focused on the reward mechanisms underlying male/female recognition and sexual reward (Wang et al., 2008). USVs during adult female–female encounters have been reported by several laboratories (Maggio & Whitney, 1985; Moles & D'Amato F, 2000; Venerosi et al.,

2006; Scattoni et al., 2008b, 2010). For example, null mutation of the vasopressin *Avpr1b* gene resulted in reduced USV emission by adult females during the resident–intruder test, whereas social sniffing levels were unaltered (Scattoni et al., 2008b). Female–female calls appear to serve as communication signals, enhancing physical proximity and enabling social information gathering (Pomerantz et al., 1983; Maggio & Whitney, 1985; D'Amato & Moles, 2001; Moles et al., 2007).

A recent study reported that mouse USV was detected in adolescent C57BL/6J and BALB/cJ mice of both sexes during social interaction after 4 days of social housing followed by 1 day of social isolation (Panksepp et al., 2007). Detailed qualitative analysis revealed significant strain differences in frequency distribution of waveforms with prevalence of downward and complex sonograms in C57BL/6J mice and prevalence of upward and inverted U-shaped sonograms in BALB/cJ mice (Panksepp et al., 2007). The first generation of mice with a loss-of-function mutation in the murine *NLGN4* ortholog *Nlgn4*, which encodes the synaptic cell adhesion protein neuroligin 4, were found to exhibit deficits in reciprocal social interactions and communication (Jamain et al., 2008). Latency to start calling, upon contact with a female mouse in estrous, was 3.2 times longer in *Nlgn4*-null mutants as compared to wild-type littermate controls, and the total number of calls per session was reduced by 48% in *Nlgn4* mutants as compared to wild-type controls. These results showed that *Nlgn4* mutants were either less responsive to the social stimuli eliciting the calling or were otherwise inhibited in their propensity to vocalize.

The growing literature on USVs in mice suggests that this assay could be useful to characterize communication between the pup and the mother, and between adults of the same and opposite sex, in some inbred strains and in some lines of mutant mice. Playback experiments, in which previously recorded calls are played to a subject mouse, could be used to evaluate responses by the subject and will be necessary to determine the communicative function of various vocalizations in mice.

Mutant Mouse Models of Autism

One robust experimental approach to systematically evaluate the roles of each of the many candidate genes for autism susceptibility (Abrahams & Geschwind, 2008) is to generate mouse models with targeted mutations in genes homologous or orthologous to the human candidate gene. Table 51-1 presents a summary of autism-relevant behavioral phenotypes in some prominent genetic mouse models of autism(Silverman et al., 2010b).

Comorbidities With Single-Gene Neurodevelopmental Disorders

Growing evidence associates single-gene mutations, copy number variations, and epigenetic factors with increased risk for autism, indicating that multiple genetic pathways are involved in the disease onset. Single-gene neurodevelopmental disorders in which a high proportion of individuals meet the diagnostic criteria for autism might offer insights into the genetic mechanisms underlying autism. Fragile X Syndrome (FXS) is caused by silencing of *FMR1*, an X-linked gene that codes for the Fragile X mental retardation protein (FMRP). FXS is the most common genetic cause of mental retardation and is frequently comorbid with autism symptoms (Turner et al., 1996). As compared to wild-type controls, mice deficient for the *Fmr1* gene display impairments in reversal learning in the Morris water maze (The Dutch-Belgian Fragile X Consortium, 1994; D'Hooge et al., 1997; Bakker et al., 2002), increased startle response (Nielsen et al., 2002), increased exploratory activity, lowered anxiety (Peier et al., 2000; Yan et al., 2005), and sensorimotor gating abnormalities (Paylor et al., 2008). Social approach behavior in *Fmr1* null mice appears to be influenced by background strains on which the mutation was generated. Although KO mice generated on a B6 background (Spencer et al., 2005; Moy et al., 2009) and a B6 x FVB/NJ background (McNaughton et al., 2008) exhibited normal sociability, null mutants on a FVB/129 background were found to have deficits in the three-chambered social approach task (Moy et al., 2009). Altered social behaviors in *Fmr1* null mice have been found in other social tasks, including the mirrored chamber test, the tube test for social dominance, and direct social interaction test (Spencer et al., 2005; Mineur et al., 2006).

Rett Syndrome, a neurodevelopmental disorder caused by a mutation in the X-linked *MECP2* gene that encodes the methyl-CpG-binding protein 2 (MeCP2), is found mostly in females (Wan et al., 1999; Moretti & Zoghbi, 2006; Chahrour & Zoghbi, 2007). Individuals with this disorder are characterized by severe problems in language and communication development, muscle strength, motor functions, decreased somatic growth, mental retardation, and pronounced autism-like symptoms, including stereotyped hand movements, lack of facial expression, avoidance of eye contact, and unresponsiveness to social cues (Nomura, 2002; Chahrour & Zoghbi, 2007). Several mouse models have been generated to study the effects of *Mecp2* mutation. *Mecp2*$^{\mathrm{Flox/y}}$ mice, which have a partial loss of MeCP, exhibited motor coordination deficits, impaired learning and memory, poor nesting behaviors, and altered social behaviors in a partition test (Samaco et al., 2008). *Mecp2*$^{308/\mathrm{y}}$ mice, which carry a mutation similar to common RTT-causing alleles, showed abnormal homecage circadian activity, poor nesting behaviors, and impaired social interactions (Moretti et al., 2005). Mice with deletion of the exon 3 of the *Mecp2* gene (*Mecp2*$^{\mathrm{1lox}}$) show increased separation-induced pup vocalizations. Genotype differences in USVs were significant on PND 5 for males and on PND 7 for females (Picker et al., 2006). Mice with a forebrain conditional KO of *Mecp2* exhibited hindlimb clasping, impaired motor coordination, increased anxiety-like behaviors, and deficits in sociability and social memory, indicating that selective loss of *Mecp2* in the forebrain is sufficient to induce behavioral abnormalities seen in RTT (Gemelli et al., 2006).

Human chromosome 15q11-13 contains a cluster of imprinted genes essential for neurodevelopment. Lack of a functional paternal copy of 15q11-13 causes Prader-Willi Syndrome; lack of a functional maternal copy of 15q11-13 causes Angelman Syndrome (Donlon, 1988; Baker et al., 1994; Browne et al., 1997; Dykens et al., 2004; Veltman et al., 2005; Hogart et al., 2009). Strong evidence suggests duplication of the 15q11-13 region as a cytogenetic aberration in autism (Bolton et al., 2004; Dykens et al., 2004; Koochek et al., 2006; Cook & Scherer, 2008). A mouse genetic model for the human 15q11-13 duplication condition was created by generating a duplication of a conserved linkage group on mouse chromosome 7. These transgenic mice exhibited an absence of sociability and lack of preference for social novelty in the three-chambered social approach task, and perseverative behaviors in the Morris water maze and Barnes Maze tests. Pups displayed reduced maternal-separation induced USV on PNDs 7 and 14 (Nakatani et al., 2009). Two genes in the 15q11-13 region, *GABRB3* and *UBE3A*, are suggested as candidate genes for autism (Buxbaum et al., 2002; Bonati et al., 2007; Nakatani et al., 2009). Mice heterozygous for the *Gabrb3* subunit exhibit several autism-like phenotypes, including absence of sociability in the three-chambered task, poor nest-building behaviors, and stereotyped circling behaviors (DeLorey et al., 2008). These mice also display features with face validity to Angelman Syndrome, including learning and memory deficits, poor motor coordination, hyperactivity, altered rest–active cycle, (Liljelund et al., 2005; Dolen et al., 2007). Mice with a maternally inherited *Ube3a* deficiency showed impaired motor functions in a number of tests and deficits in spatial learning in the Morris water maze test (Miura et al., 2002; Heck et al., 2008).

Tuberous sclerosis is a single-gene disorder caused by heterozygous mutations in the *TSC1* (9q34) or *TSC2* (16p13.3) gene (Consortium, 1993; van Slegtenhorst et al., 1997). Besides physical dysfunctions in brain, skin, heart, kidneys, and lung; epilepsy; and cognitive impairments, tuberous sclerosis is characterized by a high prevalence of autism (25%–60%) (Wiznitzer, 2004; Napolioni & Curatolo, 2008). Mice heterozygotes for *Tsc1* and *Tsc2* displayed learning and memory impairments (Goorden et al., 2007; Ehninger et al., 2008). Male *Tsc2* +/- mice exhibited normal social approach toward an ovariectomized female novel mouse in the three-chambered task (Ehninger et al., 2008). Female *Tsc1* +/- mice exhibited reduced social interaction behaviors with a novel stimulus mouse in a neutral arena and poor nest-building behaviors (Goorden et al., 2007).

Cell Adhesion Proteins Mediating Synapse Development

Several rare mutations in genes encoding synaptic cell-adhesion molecules, including neurexins, neuroligins, contactins, cadherins, and shanks, have each been identified in a small number of individuals with autism, Asperger's Syndrome, and related neurodevelopmental disorders (Jamain et al., 2003; Laumonnier et al., 2004; Jeffries et al., 2005; Lise & El-Husseini, 2006; Autism Genome Project Consortium, 2007; Durand et al., 2007; Garber, 2007; Moessner et al., 2007; Alarcon et al., 2008; Arking et al., 2008; Jamain et al., 2008; Kim et al., 2008; Lawson-Yuen et al., 2008; Bucan et al., 2009; Gauthier et al., 2009; Sykes et al., 2009), prompting the hypothesis that the mechanisms in the early stages of synapse development contribute to the pathogenesis of autism (Bourgeron, 2007; Betancur et al., 2009; Bourgeron, 2009). Transgenic mice overexpressing neuroligin 2 displayed social deficits and high levels of repetitive jumping (Hines et al., 2008). *Nlgn2* null mutant mice displayed normal social behaviors, decreased pain sensitivity, and increased anxiety-like behaviors (Blundell et al., 2009). One line of transgenic mice with a knock-in human R451C point mutation in the *Nlgn3* gene exhibited normal social interactions and social approach behaviors, as well as normal spatial learning and memory performance (Chadman et al., 2008), whereas minor social reductions and improved performance in the spatial learning and memory task were found in another line (Tabuchi et al., 2007). *Nlgn3* null mutant mice exhibited reduced USVs by adult males contacting estrus females, normal sociability in the three-chambered task, and a lack of preference for social novelty, which might have resulted from their olfactory deficits (Radyushkin et al., 2009). The original cohort of *Nlgn4*-null mutant mice exhibited deficits in social interaction and social approach tests, as well as reduced USVs (Jamain et al., 2008). *Shank1* null mutant mice displayed hypoactivity, increased anxiety-like behaviors, and impaired fear conditioned memory but enhanced radial arm maze spatial learning and memory (Hung et al., 2008).

Signalling, Transcription, Methylation, and Neurotrophic Factors

Engrailed 2 (*EN2*) is a homeobox transcription factor that is critical for the development of the cerebellum and many serotonergic, noradrenergic, and dopaminergic nuclei (Benayed et al., 2005). *En2* null mice showed deficits in social interaction, hyperactivity, impaired motor coordination, and impaired spatial learning (Cheh et al., 2006). *FOXP2* encodes for a forkhead box DNA-binding domain. Disruption of this gene has been associated with speech and language deficits of varying severity in humans (Lai et al., 2001). Deletion and point mutations of the *Foxp2* gene has resulted in an absence (deletion) or reduction (point mutation) of separation-induced USVs in mouse pups, as well as gross developmental delays (Shu et al., 2005; Fujita et al., 2008; Groszer et al., 2008). Calcium-dependent activator protein for secretion 2 (CADPS2) is involved in the release of several trophic factors implicated in autism, such as neurotrophin 3 and brain-derived neurotrophic factor (BDNF) (Katoh-Semba et al., 2007; Sadakata et al., 2007b).

Cadps2 null mutant mice have displayed impairments in spatial learning and social behaviors (Sadakata et al., 2007a; Sadakata et al., 2007b). Phosphatase and tensin homolog on chromosome 19 (*PTEN*) is a lipid phosphatase implicated in many cancers and brain disorders (Zhou et al., 2009). Mutations in *PTEN* have been found in a small number of autistic individuals (Goffin et al., 2001; Buxbaum et al., 2007; Herman et al., 2007). Mice with a conditional Pten mutation in forebrain neurons have displayed impaired social behaviors, along with changes in locomotor activities, anxiety-like behaviors, increased startle responses, and impaired spatial learning (Kwon et al., 2006). Mice haploinsufficient for *Pten* have displayed deficits in sociability, which is exacerbated in mice haploinsufficient for both *Pten* and *Sclc6a4* (Page et al., 2009). *Pten* KO mice treated with rapamycin, which inhibits the signaling protein mammalian target of rapamycin complex 1 (mTOR), have displayed fewer seizures and increased social interactions (Zhou et al., 2009).

Neurotransmitters

Genes encoding the serotonin transporter, oxytocin and vasopressin receptors, and GABA receptor subunit β3 have been implicated in autism (Buxbaum et al., 2002; Lam et al., 2006; Anderson et al., 2009; Hranilovic et al., 2009). Mice null for the oxytocin gene (*Oxt*) display deficits in social memory and separation-induced pup vocalizations (Winslow & Insel, 2002; Takayanagi et al., 2005). Social approach was normal in two independent lines (Crawley et al., 2007). Mice deficient for the vasopressin receptor 1a gene (*Avr1a*) have demonstrated lower levels of anxiety-like behaviors, impaired social behavior, and intact learning and memory (Bielsky et al., 2004; Egashira et al., 2007). *Avr1b* null mutants exhibit some changes in social behaviors, including fewer USVs during social interaction with an unfamiliar partner (Scattoni et al., 2008), lower levels of aggression, and social recognition deficits (Wersinger et al., 2002). Social approach behaviors were normal in *Avr1b* null mutants (Yang et al., 2007a). *Slc6a4* null mutants displayed normal social approach behavior but a lack of preference for social novelty in the automated three-chambered task (Moy et al., 2009). Vasoactive intestinal peptide (VIP) regulates embryonic growth and development (Hill et al., 1996). Mouse dams heterozygous for *Vip* produce offspring with impairments in social behaviors that are independent of the pups' genotype (Lim et al., 2008; Stack et al., 2008).

Inbred Mouse Strain Models of Autism

Inbred strains of mice are generated by at least 20 generations of brother × sister matings to create a genetically stable line of individuals that are homozygous at greater than 99% of their genetic loci (Beck et al., 2000; Goios et al., 2007). The Jackson Laboratory, a major supplier of laboratory mice in North America, currently carries more than 400 inbred mouse strains (http://www.informatics.jax.org/external/festing/mouse/STRAINS.shtml), among which 40 genetically diverse strains have been intensively phenotyped (Mouse Phenome Database, http://phenome.jax.org/pub-cgi/phenome/mpdcgi?rtn=docs/home). The genomes of 16 strains of JAX mice have been partially or completely sequenced (C57BL/6J,129S1/SvImJ, A/J, AKR/J, BALB/cByJ, BTBR *T*+ *tf*/J, C3H/HeJ, CAST/EiJ, DBA/2J, FVB/NJ, MOLF/EiJ, KK/HlJ, NOD/ShiLtJ, NZW/LacJ, PWD/PhJ, and WSB/EiJ) and the single nucleotide polymorphism (SNP) data of these strains are publicly available (Mouse SNP Database (http://phenome.jax.org/pub-cgi/phenome/mpdcgi?rtn=snps/door). With relevance to autism, large strain differences in social behaviors exist among commonly used inbred mouse strains (McFarlane et al., 2007; Moy et al., 2007; Yang et al., 2007b; Moy et al., 2008b; Yang et al., 2009). The intra-strain homogeneity, cross-strain diversity, and heritable nature of mouse social phenotypes make inbred mice ideal for discovering genes mediating social, communication, and repetitive behavioral traits relevant to autism. The inbred strain "forward genetics" strategy is analogous to human linkage studies for discovery of genes linked to autism (Volkmar et al., 2005; Geschwind & Levitt, 2007; Abrahams & Geschwind, 2008).

Table 51-2 summarizes and references reports of autism-like behavioral traits across a growing number of inbred strains of mice. Lack of sociability was reported in 11 strains (129/SvImJ, A/J, BALB/c, BTBR *T*+ *tf*/J, C58/J, DBA, DBA/2J, NOD/LtJ, NZB/B1NJ, SJL/J).

BTBR T+tf/J is a genetically homogenous inbred strain that displays behavioral phenotypes with face validty to major symptoms of autism, including deficits in social approach and social interaction, unusual vocalization patterns, and high levels of repetitive self-grooming.

Among these, 4 strains have been tested in multiple studies. A/J, BALB/c, and BTBR consistently failed to display sociability in multiple laboratories (Bolivar et al., 2007; Brodkin, 2007; Moy et al., 2007; Yang et al., 2007 a; Yang et al., 2007b; McFarlane et al., 2008; Yang et al., 2009). A/J and BTBR displayed low scores on reciprocal social interactions (Bolivar et al., 2007), indicating good cross-paradigm consistencies in adult social behaviors for A/J and BTBR. At juvenile ages, social interaction was low in BTBR and BALB/c as compared to B6 (Panksepp & Lahvis, 2007; Yang et al., 2007a; Yang et al., 2007b; McFarlane et al., 2008; Yang et al., 2009). DBA2 exhibited sociability in two of the three studies. 129Sv/ImJ showed normal sociability in a reciprocal social interaction test (Bolivar et al., 2007) but low sociability in the three-chambered task, probably related to their low levels of general exploratory locomotion (Moy et al., 2007).

Repetitive behaviors in inbred strains of mice are conceptually relevant to the third diagnostic domain of autism. Excessive self-grooming is a prominent phenotype in BTBR and is among the most replicable findings of this strain (Yang et al., 2007a; Yang et al., 2007b; McFarlane et al., 2008; Yang et al., 2009). High levels of self-grooming begin at early juvenile ages and remain high in adults, leading to hair loss but not skin lesions (McFarlane et al., 2008). In addition, repetitive self-grooming is observed within a social test apparatus when another mouse is present (Yang et al., 2009) and also when the subject is alone in a bare cage. Repetitive self-grooming is equally high in BTBR adults raised as pups with their own dams, cross-fostered with B6 dams, or cross-fostered with B6 dams (Yang et al., 2007b), indicating that their high self-grooming is a stable trait rather than a consequence of behavioral response to early maternal environment. Excessive spontaneous self-grooming has also been observed in several mutant mouse lines. *Sapap3* (Welch et al., 2007) and *Hoxb8* mutant mice (Greer & Capecchi, 2002) exhibit extreme self-grooming that leads to hair loss and skin injuries. *Hoxb8* KO mice also groom their cagemates, suggesting that the high levels of self-grooming in these mutant mice is not likely the result of a skin disorder that caused itching. Other repetitive and stereotyed behaviors reported in mice include water mist-induced grooming (Moretti et al., 2005), repetitive rearing (Pogorelov et al., 2005), somersaulting, jumping, leaping, tail-chasing, cage top twirling, and object chewing (Lewis et al., 2007).

Investigators often ask which inbred strain provides the benchmark scores for "normal" social behaviors, against which potential mouse models of autism can be compared. As illustrated in Table 51-2, B6 and FVB strains have consistently been found to display high social behaviors and low repetitive behaviors in all paradigms in which they have been tested.

Treatment Strategies

As described above, several robust behavioral phenotypes in mice—including low social interaction, high repetitive behaviors, and unusual patterns of communication—present reasonable face validity to the symptoms of autism (Crawley, 2007a; Crawley, 2007c). Mouse models of autism offer translational tools to evaluate potential treatment strategies. Because there are no confirmed biological markers for autism at present, but many candidate genes, models with construct validity based on candidate gene mutations may prove useful in the development of biological intervention strategies. The single-gene mutations and chromosomal copy number variants described above could become targets for pharmacological interventions and/or gene therapies (Abrahams & Geschwind, 2008; Beaulieu et al., 2008; Campbell et al., 2008; Kelleher & Bear, 2008; Bourgeron, 2009). At the time of this writing, behavioral interventions are the only effective methods to treat social deficits in autism. Intervention studies using mouse genetic models with robust autism-like phenotypes could facilitate the development of pharmacological, genetic, and behavioral treatments for autism. Table 51-4 summarizes the most promising pharmacological, genetic, and behavioral interventions in the currently available mouse models.

Drug Treatments

Pharmacological treatments, including selective serotonin reuptake inhibitors (SSRIs) and oxytocin, have been reported to modestly reduce some symptoms in individuals with autism (Hollander et al., 2000; Kolevzon et al., 2006). A recent multicenter clinical trial reported that citalopram, a prominent SSRI, produced no significant behavioral improvements and had some adverse side effects in children (King et al., 2009; Volkmar, 2009). At present, the antipsychotic risperidone, which is a dopamine receptor (D2) and serotonin ($5HT_{2A}$) receptor antagonist, is the only drug approved by the U.S. Food and Drug Administration for autism, specifically for treating the irritability associated with autism, which includes

Table 51–4.
Examples of intervention strategies in mouse models of autism

Pharmacologic Intervention	Mechanism of Action	Animal Model	Resulting Behavioral Improvements	References
2-methyl-6-phenylethynyl-pyridine hydrochloride (MPEP)	Noncompetitive antagonists to the mGluR5 receptor	*Fmr1 –/–*	Reduced susceptibility to audiogenic seizures Reduced open field hyperactivity Rescued abnormal spine morphology Reversed prepulse inhibition deficits	Yan et al., 2005 Chuang et al., 2005 De Vrij et al., 2008
Fenobam		BTBR	Reduced repetitive self-grooming behavio	Silverman et al., 2009
BDNF	Neurotrophin	*Fmr1 –/–*	Restored synaptic plasticity	Lauterborn et al., 2007
Rapamycin or RAD001	Inhibitors of mTOR Translational regulation	*Pten*	Reduced morphological abnormalities Improved social interaction Increased open field center time Reduced duration and frequency of seizures	Kwon et al., 2006 Zhou et al., 2007 Zhou et al., 2009

(*Continued*)

Table 51–4. (Contd.)

Pharmacologic Intervention	Mechanism of Action	Animal Model	Resulting Behavioral Improvements	References
		Tsc1 –/– (neuronal)	Increased survival rates Reduced tremors Improved gait function Improved neuronal morphology Restored myelination	Meikle et al., 2008 Ehninger et al., 2008
		Tsc1 –/– (glial)	Normalized weight gain Reduced seizure frequency	Zeng et al., 2008
		Tsc2 –/–	Reversed contextual discrimination impairment in fear conditioning Rescued spatial learning deficits	Ehninger et al., 2008
Oxytocin	Neuropeptide	*OT–/–*	Facilitated social recognition	Ferguson et al., 2001
CX546	Increases AMPA receptor activation	*Mecp2 –/–*	Improved respiratory function	Ogier et al., 2007
Genetic Intervention	**Mechanism of Action**	**Animal Model**	**Resulting Behavioral Improvements**	**References**
YAC transgene replacement *FMR1*	Cell specific expression of human Fragile X mental retardation protein (FMRP) 10- to 15-fold greater than endogenous levels	*Fmr1 –/–*	Rescued hyperactivity in open field Reversed excessive approaches in social partition task Normalized duration of social behavior	Spencer et al., 2008
			Rescued hyperactivity in open field Reduced high open field center time Reversed hypoanxiety-like phenotype in the light ↔ dark task	Peier et al., 2000
Dominant negative expression of p21-activated kinase (PAK)	Interaction with the (FMRP) Actin polymerization and spine morphogenesis	*Fmr1 –/–*	Rescued hyperactivity in open field Reduced high open field center time Reduced repetitive behavior and stereotypy Enhanced performance on trace fear conditioning task	Hayashi et al., 2007
Genetic Mutation of mGluR5	Double knockouts of Fmr1 and mGluR5 (Knockdown to 50% mGluR5 expression)	*Fmr1 –/–*	Rescue of ocular dominance plasticity Rescued inhibitory avoidance learning Rescued memory retention and acquisition	Dolen et al., 2007
Activation of *Mecp2* expression	Re-express MeCP2 using a fusion transgene activated by tamoxifen injections	*Mecp2* $^{lox\text{-}Stop}$	Improved gait Reduced tremors General poor health condition improved Reduced hindlimb clasping	Guy et al., 2007
Targeted delivery of *Mecp2* transgene	Double mutant of mice overexpressing MeCP2 in cortex crossed with Mecp2 +/– mice	*Mecp2 +/–*	Rescued open field mobility	Jugloff et al., 2008
Behavioral intervention	**Mechanism of action**	**Animal model**	**Resulting behavioral improvements**	**References**
Enriched environment	Increased spine density Increased BDNF Increased cytochrome oxidase activity	Deer mice	Reduction of stereotypy including back flipping and jumping	Turner & Lewis 2003 Lewis 2004
Peer enrichment	Unknown	BTBR mice	Improved sociability in the social approach task Juvenile play?	Yang et al., 2009

self-injury, aggression, and tantrums (West et al., 2009b). Although some studies demonstrated mild improvements in eye contact and other measures relevant to social behaviors after risperidone (McDougle et al., 1997; McDougle et al., 2000; Barnard et al., 2002; Chavez et al., 2006; Posey et al., 2008), other studies found minimal or no improvements in social relatedness after risperidone treatment (McDougle et al., 2005; Chavez et al., 2006). Pharmacological treatments to reverse social deficits remain to be discovered (Kratochvil et al., 2005; West et al., 2009b). In a preclinical study, it was found that mice expressing a mutant form of *Tph2*, a rate-limiting enzyme for serotonin synthesis, showed increased depressive- and anxiety-like behaviors, as well as high levels of aggressive behaviors. The depressive-like phenotypes were alleviated by treatment with TDZD-8, a pharmacological agent that inactivates Gsk3β, an intracellular signaling molecule, and by genetic inactivation of GSK3β in *Tph2* mutants. Genetic inactivation of GSK3β also reduced aggressive behaviors and increased non-aggressive social investigation in *Tph2* mutant mice (Beaulieu et al., 2008). Social recognition deficits in oxytocin KO mice were rescued by low-dose oxytocin microinjections into the medial amygdala (Ferguson et al., 2001).

Recent studies in several mouse mutant models of neurodevelopmental disorders indicate abnormal functional and structural synaptic connectivity in autism and FXS (Silva & Ehninger, 2009). This evidence prompts the hypothesis that regulators of synaptic plasticity, including metabatropic glutamate receptor antagonists (mGluRs), AMPA receptor activators, and antagonists of the mTOR, might be promising molecular targets for pharmacological interventions (Parsons et al., 2006; Hayashi et al., 2007; Ogier et al., 2007; Blundell et al., 2008; Dolen & Bear, 2008; Ehninger et al., 2008; Garber et al., 2008; Meikle et al., 2008; Silva & Ehninger, 2009; Zhou et al., 2009). In the mouse model of FXS, pharmacological treatment with 2-methyl-6-phenylethynyl-pyridine (MPEP), a potent mGluR5 antagonist, rescued behavioral phenotypes, including seizures, hyperactivity, anxiety-like behavior, PPI deficits (Yan et al., 2005; de Vrij et al., 2008), and restored deficits in synaptic plasticity and spine morphology in *Fmr1* mutant mice (de Vrij et al., 2008). An in vitro study showed that the impaired hippocampal LTP in fragile X mice was fully restored by BDNF infusion, indicating a possible mechanism for treating synaptic deficits associated with FXS (Lauterborn et al., 2007). A single intraperitoneal injection of MPEP significantly reduced repetitive self-grooming behaviors in the BTBR T+tf/J mice, the robust mouse model that displays endophenotypes relevant to all three core symptoms of autism (Silverman et al., 2010a). mGluR5 antagonists may have therapeutic potential for a variety of neurodevelopmental disorders and are in clinical trials for FXS, (Rorick-Kehn et al., 2007; Berry-Kravis et al., 2009), which has a high comorbidity with autism. Chronic rapamycin treatment normalized several neuronal morphology deficits, seizures, and alleviated social deficits in *Pten* mutant mice (Zhou et al., 2007). Treatment with rapamycin or the mTOR inhibitor RAD001 significantly increased survival, decreased tremors, and prevented seizures in the *Tsc1* mutant mouse model of tuberous sclerosis, a single-gene disorder with a high autism comorbidity (Meikle et al., 2008). Cognitive deficits were reversed by rapamycin treatment in the *Tsc2* heterozygote mouse model of tuberous sclerosis (Ehninger et al., 2008). Treatment with the AMPA activator CX546 improved respiratory abnormalities and increased BDNF levels in the *Mecp2* mutant mouse model of RTT (Ogier et al., 2007).

Genetic Rescues

The mGluR5 receptor, one of the pharmacological targets described above, was found to be an effective target for genetic intervention. Breeding mGluR5-deficient mice with fragile X mice reduced the mGluR5 overexpression in *Fmr1* mice, and rescued several *Fmr1* phenotypes, including amelioration of audiogenic seizures and cognitive impairments (Dolen et al., 2007). p21-activated kinase (PAK) is a kinase known to play a critical role in actin polymerization and dendritic spine morphogenesis. Postnatal expression of a dominant negative transgene for PAK in *Fmr1* mice partially rescued reduced cortical LTP deficits and overgrowth of dendritic spines and partially normalized several behavioral phenotypes associated with *Fmr1* mutation, including low anxiety-like behaviors, hyperactivity, and high levels of stereotypy in an open field, as well as deficits in fear conditioning (Hayashi et al., 2007). Overexpression of human *FMRP* in *Fmr1* mice, using yeast artificial chromosomes, normalized the overactive social responses in *Fmr1* mice in the partition test (Spencer et al., 2008) and reversed and overcorrected several *Fmr1* phenotypes, resulting in hypolocomotion and high anxiety-like phenotypes (Peier et al., 2000).

Behavioral Intervention

Early behavioral interventions remain the most effective treatment for the symptoms of autism (Landa, 2007; Williams White et al., 2007; Dawson, 2008; Rao et al., 2008). Effective behavioral interventions have been demonstrated in two robust mouse models. Deer mice reared in standard laboratory housing have exhibited abnormalities in social behaviors and repetitive jumping (Turner & Lewis, 2003; Turner et al., 2003). Environmental enrichment ameliorated these stereotypies, improved behavioral performance on learning and memory and anxiety-related tasks, reduced seizure vulnerability, and increased BDNF levels and neurogenesis in deer mice (Powell et al., 2000; Lewis, 2004). BTBR mice reared with social B6 cagemates after weaning exhibited significant improvements in sociability as adults (Yang et al., 2010).

Challenges and Future Directions

The multiple assays described above are likely to be useful in analyzing behaviors in emerging mouse models of autism.

Methods are in place for many social tasks, measures relevant to communication, and parameters of repetitive and perseverative behaviors. The literature cited in the tables represents a growing body of literature on the generation of tasks relevant to the symptoms of autism spectrum disorders, and their applications to lines of mice with mutations in candidate genes for autism spectrum disorders.

- The second diagnostic domain, impaired communication, requires considerably more task development. Behavioral neuroscientists will need to confirm the communicative nature of olfactory and vocal cues during various types of social interactions in mice. Further methods development is needed to quantitate reciprocal scent marking, and to evaluate playback experiments for auditory communication in mice. A fundamental question is whether the very different sensory modalities used for communication in humans and mice share common cortical mechanisms for higher levels of information processing. In addition, mice may use other sensory modalities for communication, including visual cues and tactile body contact, for which assays remain to be invented. Diagnostic domains such as joint attention and Theory of Mind may be difficult to model in mice. Task development to determine whether mice display observational learning may be helpful, perhaps using methods previously developed for rats and other species (White & Barfield, 1989; Brudzynski & Chiu, 1995; Sadananda et al., 2008; Wohr & Schwarting, 2009).
- Associated symptoms of autism include mental retardation, seizures, anxiety, hyperreactivity to sensory stimuli, gastrointestinal distress, and sleep disturbances. These associated symptoms occur only in some autistic individuals and are therefore not considered diagnostic. To what extent should behavioral neuroscientists attempt to include associated endophenotypes in mouse models of ASDs? This is an open question for which animal modelers need considerable input from clinical experts. There is a technical complication in some cases, wherein mouse phenotypes relevant to an associated symptom domain would directly confound the detection of phenotypes in a core symptom domain. For example, although seizures are an associated symptom of autism, a line of mice with severe seizures may not survive to ages at which behavioral testing occurs, as seen in the GABA-A receptor unit β3 KOs, which have an approximately 10% survival rate (DeLorey et al., 2008). A line of mice with high anxiety-like traits would likely display low locomotor activity in a social environment, confounding the interpretation of low social approach scores, as seen in adult BALB/c (Brodkin, 2007). If clinical investigators strongly recommend including associated symptoms in mouse models of autism, one solution is to focus on heterozygotes in which the protein reduction is partial and the phenotype may be milder, or conditional mutants in which the mutation is neuroanatomically restricted and appears later in development, or inducible mutants in which the mutation is activated only at the time of behavioral testing. Knockdowns, using anatomically discrete gene delivery with viral vectors, and RNA silencing, represent technologies that allow highly specific expression of a mutation in a brain region of interest.
- A point that cannot be made too often is the need for replicating mouse behavioral findings. A single finding in one experiment may be spurious, as in any field of science. Experimental designs in mouse behavioral genetics must plan for at least two cohorts of mice, each of sufficient numbers of littermates for each genotype and sex (Crawley, 2007b; Crawley, 2007c). Statistical analyses must adhere to the standards in the behavioral neuroscience literature. A Two-Way or Three-Way Repeated Measures ANOVA, with subsequent *post hoc* tests such Tukey's, Dunnett's, Newman-Keuls, and Bonferroni-Dunn, determine which genotypes differ from their wild-type littermate controls. Significant findings replicated in two cohorts, and then replicated across two laboratories, will contribute the best evidence to the literature on mouse models of autism.
- As described above, a strong behavioral phenotype in a mutant line of mice offers a model system for investigating biological causes and testing treatments. Definitive biological markers for autism have not yet been identified (Carrona et al., 2008). However, several neuroanatomical abnormalities have been reported, including larger head circumference and larger volumes of some brain regions at early ages (Courchesne et al., 2001; Hazlett et al., 2005), reduced white matter and pathway connectivity (Geschwind & Levitt, 2007; Minshew & Williams, 2007; Sundaram et al., 2008), reductions in specific brain structures such as cortical minicolumns, gray matter containing mirror neurons, amygdala, and Purkinje neurons in the cerebellum (Casanova, 2006; Hadjikhani et al., 2007; Amaral et al., 2008), reduced activation of the amygdala and fusiform gyrus during social tasks (Pierce et al., 2001; Pelphrey et al., 2002), and less activation of the anterior cingulate and posterior parietal cortex during set-shift tasks (Shafritz et al., 2008). Multiple rare variants continue to emerge from whole-genome scans, association studies, and sequencing of chromosomal loci identified in linkage studies of family pedigrees (Abrahams & Geschwind, 2008; Campbell et al., 2008; Rapin & Tuchman, 2008; Buxbaum, 2009; Glessner et al., 2009; Lintas & Persico, 2009). Future investigations will determine whether similar biological markers appear in various model organisms. Experiments with animal models can be designed to reveal which of these neuroanatomical and genetic abnormalities are causal in nature—that is, which represent the mechanisms responsible for the relevant behavioral traits. When the true causes of autism are identified, then the identical mutation, neuroanatomical abnormality, neuropharmacological disruption, environmental toxin, immunological dysfunction, and other mechanisms can be

generated in model organisms. Models with face validity for the diagnostic symptoms and construct validity for the underlying causes then become valuable translational research tools to test potential treatments for autism. At present, several robust and well-replicated behavioral phenotypes in mouse models of autism spectrum disorders are available as preclinical translational tools, toward developing drugs and behavioral interventions to reverse autism-relevant traits.

SUGGESTED READING

Abrahams, B. S., & Geschwind, D. H. (2008). Advances in autism genetics: On the threshold of a new neurobiology. *Nature Reviews Genetics, 9*, 341–355. Comprehensive overview of the genes implicated in autism, and the available mouse models incorporating candidate gene mutations.

Crawley, J. N. (2007). *What's Wrong With My Mouse? Behavioral Phenotyping of Transgenic and Knockout Mice.* Second ed. Hoboken, NJ: John Wiley & Sons, Inc., A comprehensive overview of theory and methodology for the most commonly used mouse behavioral assays, including illustrations of necessary control experiments for reliable mouse behavioral phenotyping.

Scattoni, M. L., Crawley, J., & Ricceri, L. (2009). Ultrasonic vocalizations: A tool for behavioural phenotyping of mouse models of neurodevelopmental disorders. A detailed review that emphasizes the importance of qualitative evaluation. *Neuroscience and Biobehavioral Reviews, 33*, 508–515.

Silverman, J., Yang, M., Lord, C., & Crawley, J. N. (2010). Behavioural phenotyping assays for mouse models of autism. *Nature Reviews Neuroscience, 11*(7), 490–502. A concise review that covers topics similar to those in this chapter.

ACKNOWLEDGMENTS

Supported by the National Institute of Mental Health Intramural Research Program.

REFERENCES

Aarnoudse, J. G., Crawley, J. C., Flecknell, P. A., & Hytten, F. E. (1983). Scalp blood flow measured by the xenon clearance technique and transcutaneous PO2 in the fetal lamb. *Pediatric Research, 17*, 982–985.

Abbott, L. C., Conforti, M. L., Isaacs, K. R., Crawley, J. N., & Sterchi, D. (1994). A simplified technique for histologic analysis of central nervous system tissues using glycol-methacrylate plastic coupled with pre-embedding immunocytochemistry. *Journal of Neuroscience Methods, 54*, 23–29.

Abrahams, B. S., & Geschwind, D. H. (2008). Advances in autism genetics: On the threshold of a new neurobiology. *Nature Reviews Genetics, 9*, 341–355.

Abramson, R. K., Wright, H. H., Carpenter, R., Brennan W., Lumpuy O., Cole E., et al. (1989). Elevated blood serotonin in autistic probands and their first-degree relatives. *Journal of Autism and Developmental Disorders, 19*, 397–407.

Adolphs, R. (2002). Recognizing emotion from facial expressions: Psychological and neurological mechanisms. *Behavioral and Cognitive Neuroscience Reviews, 1*, 21–62.

Ajdukiewicz, A. B., Bassett, N., & Crawley, J. C. (1985). The diagnostic value of liver scanning in The Gambia. *Transactions of the Royal Society of Tropical Medicine and Hygiene, 79*, 462–463.

Al-Aloul, M., Crawley, J., Winstanley, C., Hart, C. A., Ledson, M. J., & Walshaw, M. J. (2004). Increased morbidity associated with chronic infection by an epidemic Pseudomonas aeruginosa strain in CF patients. *Thorax, 59*, 334–336.

Alarcon, M., Abrahams, B. S., Stone, J. L., Duvall, J. A., Perederiy, J. V., Bomar, J. M., et al. (2008). Linkage, association, and gene-expression analyses identify CNTNAP2 as an autism-susceptibility gene. *American Journal of Human Genetics, 82*, 150–159.

Albeck, D. S., McKittrick, C. R., Blanchard, D. C., Blanchard, R. J., Nikulina, J., McEwen, B. S., et al. (1997). Chronic social stress alters levels of corticotropin-releasing factor and arginine vasopressin mRNA in rat brain. *Journal of Neuroscience, 17*, 4895–4903.

Alberts, J. R., & Galef, B. G., Jr. (1971). Acute anosmia in the rat: A behavioral test of a peripherally-induced olfactory deficit. *Physiology Behavior, 6*, 619–621.

Albrecht, U., Sun, Z. S., Eichele, G., & Lee, C. C. (1997). A differential response of two putative mammalian circadian regulators, mper1 and mper2, to light. *Cell, 91*, 1055–1064.

Altschuler, R. A., Dolan, D. F., Ptok, M., Gholizadeh, G., Bonadio J., & Hawkins, J. E. (1991). An evaluation of otopathology in the MOV-13 transgenic mutant mouse. *Annals of the New York Academy of Sciences, 630*, 249–252.

Amaral, D. G., Schumann, C. M., & Nordahl, C. W. (2008). Neuroanatomy of autism. *Trends in Neurosciences, 31*, 137–145.

American Psychiatric Association. (1994). *Diagnostic and statistical manual of mental disorders* (4th ed.; DSM-IV). Washington, DC: Author.

Amir, R. E., Van den Veyver, I. B., Wan, M., Tran, C. Q., Francke, U., & Zoghbi, H. Y. (1999). Rett syndrome is caused by mutations in X-linked MECP2, encoding methyl-CpG-binding protein 2. *Nature Genetics, 23*, 185–188.

Amir, R., Dahle, E. J., Toriolo, D., & Zoghbi, H. Y. (2000). Candidate gene analysis in Rett syndrome and the identification of 21 SNPs in Xq. *American Journal of Medical Genetics, 90*, 69–71.

Amir, R. E., Van den, Veyver, I. B., Schultz, R., Malicki, D. M., Tran, C. Q., Dahle, E. J., et al. (2000). Influence of mutation type and X chromosome inactivation on Rett syndrome phenotypes. *Annals of Neurology, 47*, 670–679.

Amir, R. E., & Zoghbi, H. Y. (2000). Rett syndrome: Methyl-CpG-binding protein 2 mutations and phenotype-genotype correlations. *American Journal of Medical Genetics, 97*, 147–152.

Amir, R. E., Fang, P., Yu, Z., Glaze, D. G., Percy, A. K., Zoghbi, H. Y., et al.(2005). Mutations in exon 1 of MECP2 are a rare cause of Rett syndrome. *Journal of Medical Genetics, 42*, e15.

Amir, R. E., Sutton, V. R., & Van den Veyver, I. B. (2005). Newborn screening and prenatal diagnosis for Rett syndrome: Implications for therapy. *Journal of Child Neurology, 20*, 779–783.

Amuasi, J. H., Crawley, J. C., Veall, N., Wilkins, H. A., & Cronquist, A. G. (1983). Estimation of mean transit times from semiquantitative indices derived from standard renograms. *Clinical Physics and Physiological Measurement, 4*, 211–216.

Analytis, J. G., Ardavan, A., Blundell, S. J., Owen, R. L., Garman, E. F., Jeynes, C., et al. (2006). Effect of irradiation-induced disorder on the conductivity and critical temperature of the organic superconductor kappa-(BEDT-TTF)2Cu(SCN)2. *Physical Review Letters, 96*, 177002.

Anderson, G. M., Horne, W. C., Chatterjee, D., & Cohen, D. J. (1990). The hyperserotonemia of autism. *Annals of New York Academy of Sciences, 600*, 331–340; discussion 341–332.

Anderson, B. M., Schnetz-Boutaud, N. C., Bartlett, J., Wotawa, A. M., Wright, H. H., Abramson, R. K., et al. (2009). Examination of association of genes in the serotonin system to autism. *Neurogenetics, 10*, 209–216.

Angel, I., Kiss, A., Stivers, J. A., Skirboll, L., Crawley, J. N., & Paul, S. M. (1986). Regulation of [3H]mazindol binding to subhypothalamic areas: Involvement in glucoprivic feeding. *Brain Research Bulletin, 17*, 873–877.

Angel, I., Stivers, J. A., Paul, S. M., & Crawley, J. N. (1987). Site of action of anorectic drugs: Glucoprivic- versus food deprivation-induced feeding. *Pharmacology, Biochemistry, and Behavior, 27*, 291–297.

Ansorge, M., Tanneberger, C., Davies, B., Theuring, F., & Kusserow, H. (2004). Analysis of the murine 5-HT receptor gene promoter in vitro and in vivo. *European Journal of Neuroscience, 20*, 363–374.

Arac, D., Boucard, A. A., Ozkan, E., Strop, P., Newell, E., Sudhof, T. C., et al. (2007). Structures of neuroligin-1 and the neuroligin-1/neurexin-1 beta complex reveal specific protein-protein and protein-Ca2+ interactions. *Neuron, 56*, 992–1003.

Arakawa, H., Arakawa, K., Blanchard, D. C., & Blanchard, R. J. (2007). Scent marking behavior in male C57BL/6J mice: Sexual and developmental determination. *Behavioural Brain Research, 182*, 73–79.

Arakawa, H., Blanchard, D. C., & Blanchard, R. J. (2007). Colony formation of C57BL/6J mice in visible burrow system: Identification of eusocial behaviors in a background strain for genetic animal models of autism. *Behavioural Brain Research, 176*, 27–39.

Arakawa, H., Arakawa, K., Blanchard, D. C., & Blanchard, R. J. (2008). A new test paradigm for social recognition evidenced by urinary scent marking behavior in C57BL/6J mice. *Behavioural Brain Research, 190*, 97–104.

Arakawa, H., Blanchard, D. C., Arakawa, K., Dunlap, C., & Blanchard, R. J. (2008). Scent marking behavior as an odorant communication in mice. *Neuroscience and Biobehavioral Reviews, 32*, 1236–1248.

Arking, D. E., Cutler, D. J., Brune, C. W., Teslovich, T. M., West, K., Ikeda, M., et al. (2008). A common genetic variant in the neurexin superfamily member CNTNAP2 increases familial risk of autism. *American Journal of Human Genetics, 82*, 160–164.

Arndt, T. L., Stodgell, C. J., & Rodier, P. M. (2005). The teratology of autism. *International Journal of Developmental Neuroscience, 23*, 189–199.

Asaka, Y., Jugloff, D. G., Zhang, L., Eubanks, J. H., & Fitzsimonds, R. M. (2006). Hippocampal synaptic plaşticity is impaired in the Mecp2-null mouse model of Rett syndrome. *Neurobiology of Diseases, 21*, 217–227.

Austin, M. C., Cottingham, S. L., Paul, S. M., & Crawley, J. N. (1990). Tyrosine hydroxylase and galanin mRNA levels in locus coeruleus neurons are increased following reserpine administration. *Synapse, 6*, 351–357.

Austin, M. C., Schultzberg, M., Abbott, L. C., Montpied, P., Evers, J. R., Paul, S. M., et al. (1992). Expression of tyrosine hydroxylase in cerebellar Purkinje neurons of the mutant tottering and leaner mouse. *Brain Research. Molecular Brain Research, 15*, 227–240.

Autism Genome Project Consortium. (2007). Mapping autism risk loci using genetic linkage and chromosomal rearrangements. *Nature Genetics, 39*, 319–328.

Babovic, D., O'Tuathaigh, C. M., O'Sullivan, G. J., Clifford, J. J., Tighe, O., Croke, D. T., et al. (2007). Exploratory and habituation phenotype of heterozygous and homozygous COMT knockout mice. *Behavioural Brain Research, 183*, 236–239.

Bailey, K. R., Rustay, N. R., & Crawley, J. N. (2006). Behavioral phenotyping of transgenic and knockout mice: Practical concerns and potential pitfalls. *ILAR Journal, 47*, 124–131.

Bailey, K. R., Pavlova, M. N., Rohde, A. D., Hohmann, J. G., & Crawley, J. N. (2007). Galanin receptor subtype 2 (GalR2) null mutant mice display an anxiogenic-like phenotype specific to the elevated plus-maze. *Pharmacology, Biochemistry, and Behavior, 86*, 8–20.

Bainbridge, N. K., Koselke, L. R., Jeon, J., Bailey, K. R., Wess, J., Crawley, J. N., et al. (2008). Learning and memory impairments in a congenic C57BL/6 strain of mice that lacks the M(2) muscarinic acetylcholine receptor subtype. *Behavioural Brain Research, 190*(1), 50–58.

Baker, P., Piven, J., Schwartz, S., & Patil, S. (1994). Brief report: Duplication of chromosome 15q11-13 in two individuals with autistic disorder. *Journal of Autism and Developmental Disorders, 24*, 529–535.

Bakker, C. E., Verheij, C., Williamsen, R., Vanderhelm, R., Oerlemans, F., Vermey, M., et al. (1994). Fmr1 knockout mice: A model to study fragile X mental retardation. The Dutch-Belgian Fragile X Consortium. *Cell, 78*, 23–33.

Bakker, J., Honda, S., Harada, N., & Balthazart, J. (2002). The aromatase knock-out mouse provides new evidence that estradiol is required during development in the female for the expression of sociosexual behaviors in adulthood. *Journal of Neuroscience, 22*, 9104–9112.

Barkan, C. L., Tolu, S. S., Hung, A. Y., Sheng, M., Silverman, J. L., & Crawley, J. N. (2009). Comprehensive behavioral phenotyping of Shank1 mutant mice Society for Neuroscience Annual Conference, Chicago, IL.

Barnard, L., Young, A. H., Pearson, J., Geddes, J., & O'Brien, G. (2002). A systematic review of the use of atypical antipsychotics in autism. *Journal of Psychopharmacology, 16*, 93–101.

Baum, M. J. (2009). Sexual differentiation of pheromone processing, links to male-typical mating behavior and partner preference. *Hormones and Behavior, 55*, 579–588.

Bear, M. F. (2005). Therapeutic implications of the mGluR theory of fragile X mental retardation. *Genes, Brain, and Behavior, 4*, 393–398.

Beaulieu, J. M., Zhang, X., Rodriguiz, R. M., Sotnikova, T. D., Cools, M. J., Wetsel, W. C., et al. (2008). Role of GSK3 beta in behavioral abnormalities induced by serotonin deficiency. *Proceedings of the National Academy of Sciences of the United States of America, 105*, 1333–1338.

Beck, J. A., Lloyd, S., Hafezparast, M., Lennon-Pierce, M., Eppig, J. T., Festing, M. F., et al. (2000). Genealogies of mouse inbred strains. *Nature Genetics, 24*, 23–25.

Bell, R. W, Nitschke, W., & Zachman, T. A. (1972). Ultra-sounds in three inbred strains of young mice. *Behavioral Biology, 7*, 805–814.

Benayed, R., Gharani, N., Rossman, I., Mancuso, V., Lazar, G., Kamdar, S., et al. (2005). Support for the homeobox transcription factor gene ENGRAILED 2 as an autism spectrum disorder susceptibility locus. *American Journal of Human Genetics, 77*, 851–868.

Berman, R. F., Pessah, I. N., Mouton, P. R., Mav, D, & Harry, J. (2008). Low-level neonatal thimerosal exposure, further evaluation of altered neurotoxic potential in SJL mice. *Toxicological Sciences, 101*, 294–309.

Berry-Kravis, E., Hessl, D., Coffey, S., Hervey, C., Schneider, A., Yuhas, J., et al. (2009). A pilot open label, single dose trial of fenobam in adults with fragile X syndrome. *Journal of Medical Genetics, 46*, 266–271.

Betancur, C., Sakurai, T., & Buxbaum, J. D. (2009). The emerging role of synaptic cell-adhesion pathways in the pathogenesis of autism spectrum disorders. *Trends in Neurosciences, 32*, 402–412.

Bielsky, I. F., Hu, S. B., Szegda, K. L., Westphal, H., & Young, L. J. (2004). Profound impairment in social recognition and reduction in anxiety-like behavior in vasopressin V1a receptor knockout mice. *Neuropsychopharmacology, 29*, 483–493.

Bielsky, I. F., & Young, L. J. (2004). Oxytocin, vasopressin, and social recognition in mammals. *Peptides, 25*, 1565–1574.

Bielsky, I. F., Hu, S. B., Ren, X., Terwilliger, E. F., & Young, L. J. (2005). The V1a vasopressin receptor is necessary and sufficient for normal social recognition: A gene replacement study. *Neuron, 47*, 503–513.

Blanchard, R. J., Blanchard, D. C., Agullana, R., & Weiss, S. M. (1991). Twenty-two kHz alarm cries to presentation of a predator, by laboratory rats living in visible burrow systems. *Physiology and Behavior, 50*, 967–972.

Blumberg, M. S., & Alberts, J. R. (1990). Ultrasonic vocalizations by rat pups in the cold: An acoustic by-product of laryngeal braking? *Behavioral Neuroscience, 104*, 808–817.

Blumberg, M. S., & Sokoloff, G. (2001). Do infant rats cry? *Psychological Review, 108*, 83–95.

Blundell, J., Hoang, C. V., Potts, B., Gold, S. J., & Powell, C. M. (2008). Motor coordination deficits in mice lacking RGS9. *Brain Research, 1190*, 78–85.

Blundell, J., Kouser, M., & Powell, C. M. (2008). Systemic inhibition of mammalian target of rapamycin inhibits fear memory reconsolidation. *Neurobiology of Learning and Memory, 90*(1), 28–35.

Blundell, J., Tabuchi, K., Bolliger, M. F., Blaiss, C. A., Brose, N., Liu, X., et al. (2009). Increased anxiety-like behavior in mice lacking the inhibitory synapse cell adhesion molecule neuroligin 2. *Genes, Brain, and Behavior, 8*, 114–126.

Bodfish, J. W., Symons, F. J., Parker, D. E., & Lewis, M. H. (2000). Varieties of repetitive behavior in autism, comparisons to mental retardation. *Journal of Autism and Developmental Disorders, 30*, 237–243.

Bodyak, N., & Slotnick, B. (1999). Performance of mice in an automated olfactometer: Odor detection, discrimination and odor memory. *Chemical Senses, 24*, 637–645.

Bolivar, V. J., & Brown, R. E. (1994). The ontogeny of ultrasonic vocalizations and other behaviors in male jimpy (jp/Y) mice and their normal male littermates. *Developmental Psychobiology, 27*, 101–110.

Bolivar, V. J., & Brown, R. E. (1995). Selective retrieval of jimpy mutant pups over normal male littermates by lactating female B6CBACa-Aw-J/A-Ta jp mice. *Behavior Genetics, 25*, 75–80.

Bolivar, V. J., Walters, S. R., & Phoenix, J. L. (2007). Assessing autism-like behavior in mice: Variations in social interactions among inbred strains. *Behavioural Brain Research, 176*, 21–26.

Bolton, P. F., Veltman, M. W., Weisblatt, E., Holmes, J. R., Thomas, N. S., Youings, S. A., et al. (2004). Chromosome 15q11-13 abnormalities and other medical conditions in individuals with autism spectrum disorders. *Psychiatric Genetics, 14*, 131–137.

Bonati, M. T., Russo, S., Finelli, P., Valsecchi, M. R., Cogliati, F., Cavalleri, F., et al. (2007). Evaluation of autism traits in Angelman syndrome: A resource to unfold autism genes. *Neurogenetics, 8*, 169–178.

Bourgeron, T. (2007). The possible interplay of synaptic and clock genes in autism spectrum disorders. *Cold Spring Harbor Symposia on Quantitative Biology, 72*, 645–654.

Bourgeron, T. (2009). A synaptic trek to autism. *Current Opinion in Neurobiology, 19*, 231–234.

Bowers, J. M. & Alexander, B. K. (1967). Mice: Individual recognition by olfactory cues. *Science, 158*, 1208–1210.

Branchi, I., Santucci, D., Vitale, A., & Alleva, E. (1998). Ultrasonic vocalizations by infant laboratory mice: A preliminary spectrographic characterization under different conditions. *Developmental Psychobiology, 33*, 249–256.

Branchi, I., Santucci, D., & Alleva, E. (2001). Ultrasonic vocalisation emitted by infant rodents: A tool for assessment of neurobehavioural development. *Behavioural Brain Research, 125*, 49–56.

Branchi, I. & Ricceri, L. (2002). Transgenic and knock-out mouse pups: The growing need for behavioral analysis. *Genes, Brain, and Behavior, 1*, 135–141.

Bredy, T. W. & Barad, M. (2009). Social modulation of associative fear learning by pheromone communication. *Learning and Memory, 16*, 12–18.

Brennan, P. A. (2004). The nose knows who's who: Chemosensory individuality and mate recognition in mice. *Hormones and Behavior, 46*, 231–240.

Brennan, P. A. & Zufall, F. (2006). Pheromonal communication in vertebrates. *Nature, 444*, 308–315.

Brennan, P. A. & Kendrick, K. M. (2006). Mammalian social odours: Attraction and individual recognition. *Philosophical Transactions of the Royal Society of London. Series B, Biological Sciences, 361*, 2061–2078.

Brigman, J. L., Padukiewicz, K. E., Sutherland, M. L., & Rothblat, L. A. (2006). Executive functions in the heterozygous reeler mouse model of schizophrenia. *Behavioral Neuroscience, 120*, 984–988.

Brodkin, E. S., Hagemann, A., Nemetski, S. M., & Silver, L. M. (2004). Social approach-avoidance behavior of inbred mouse strains towards DBA/2 mice. *Brain Research, 1002*, 151–157.

Brodkin, E. S. (2007). BALB/c mice: Low sociability and other phenotypes that may be relevant to autism. *Behavioural Brain Research, 176*, 53–65.

Brown, R. E. (1979). Mammalian social odors. *Advances in the Study of Behavior, 10*, 107–161.

Brudzynski, S. M., Bihari, F., Ociepa, D., & Fu, X. W. (1993). Analysis of 22 kHz ultrasonic vocalization in laboratory rats: Long and short calls. *Physiology and Behavior, 54*, 215–221.

Brudzynski, S. M. & Chiu, E. M. (1995). Behavioural responses of laboratory rats to playback of 22 kHz ultrasonic calls. *Physiology and Behavior, 57*, 1039–1044.

Brudzynski, S. M. & Pniak, A. (2002). Social contacts and production of 50-kHz short ultrasonic calls in adult rats. *Journal of Comparative Psychology, 116*, 73–82.

Brudzynski, S. M. (2005). Principles of rat communication: Quantitative parameters of ultrasonic calls in rats. *Behavior Genetics, 35*, 85–92.

Bucan, M., Abrahams, B. S., Wang, K., Glessner, J. T., Herman E. I., Sonnenblick, L. I., et al. (2009). Genome-wide analyses of exonic copy number variants in a family-based study point to novel autism susceptibility genes. *PLoS Genetics, 5*, e1000536.

Buck, L. B. (2000). The molecular architecture of odor and pheromone sensing in mammals. *Cell, 100*, 611–618.

Burgdorf, J., Kroes, R. A., Moskal, J. R., Pfaus, J. G., Brudzynski, S. M., & Panksepp, J. (2008). Ultrasonic vocalizations of rats (Rattus norvegicus) during mating, play, and aggression: Behavioral concomitants, relationship to reward, and self-administration of playback. *Journal of Comparative Psychology, 122*, 357–367.

Buxbaum, J. D., Silverman, J. M., Smith, C. J., Greenberg, D. A., Kilifarski, M., Reichert, J., et al. (2002). Association between a GABRB3 polymorphism and autism. *Molecular Psychiatry, 7*, 311–316.

Buxbaum, J. D., Cai, G., Chaste, P., Nygren, G., Goldsmith, J., Reichert, J., et al. (2007). Mutation screening of the PTEN gene in patients with autism spectrum disorders and macrocephaly. *American Journal of Medical Genetics. Part B, Neuropsychiatric Genetics, 144*, 484–491.

Buxbaum, J. D. (2009). Multiple rare variants in the etiology of autism spectrum disorders. *Dialogues in Clinical Neuroscience, 11*, 35–43.

Cai, W. H., Blundell, J., Han, J., Greene, R. W., & Powell, C. M. (2006). Postreactivation glucocorticoids impair recall of established fear memory. *Journal of Neuroscience, 26*, 9560–9566.

Campbell, D. B., Li, C., Sutcliffe, J. S., Persico, A. M., & Levitt, P. (2008). Genetic evidence implicating multiple genes in the MET receptor tyrosine kinase pathway in autism spectrum disorder. *Autism Research, 1*, 159–168.

Carrona, E. B., Milunsky, J. M., & Tager-Flusberg, H. (2008). Autism: Clinical and research frontiers. *Archives of Disease in Childhood, 93*(6), 518–523.

Carter, C. S., Williams, J. R., Witt, D. M., & Insel, T. R. (1992). Oxytocin and social bonding. *Annals of the New York Academy of Sciences, 652*, 204–211.

Casanova, M. F. (2006). Neuropathological and genetic findings in autism: The significance of a putative minicolumnopathy. *Neuroscientist, 12*, 435–441.

Chadman, K. K., Gong, S., Scattoni, M. L., Boltuck, S. E., Gandhy, S. U., Heintz, N., et al. (2008). Minimal aberrant behavioral phenotypes of neuroligin-3 R451C knockin mice. *Autism Research, 1*, 147–158.

Chadman, K. K., Yang, M., & Crawley, J. N. (2009). Criteria for validating mouse models of psychiatric diseases. *American Journal of Medical Genetics. Part B, Neuropsychiatric Genetics, 150*B(1), 1–11.

Chahrour, M. & Zoghbi, H. Y. (2007). The story of Rett syndrome: From clinic to neurobiology. *Neuron, 56*, 422–437.

Chavez, B., Chavez-Brown, M., & Rey, J. A. (2006). Role of risperidone in children with autism spectrum disorder. *Annals of Pharmacotherapy, 40*, 909–916.

Chawarska, K. & Shic, F. (2009). Looking But Not Seeing, Atypical Visual Scanning and Recognition of Faces in 2 and 4-Year-Old Children with Autism Spectrum Disorder. *Journal of Autism and Developmental Disorders, 39*, 1663–1672.

Cheetham, S. A., Thom, M. D., Jury, F., Ollier, W. E., Beynon, R. J., & Hurst, J. L. (2007). The genetic basis of individual-recognition signals in the mouse. *Current Biology, 17*, 1771–1777.

Cheh, M. A., Millonig, J. H., Roselli, L. M., Ming, X., Jacobsen, E., Kamdar, S., et al. (2006). En2 knockout mice display neurobehavioral and neurochemical alterations relevant to autism spectrum disorder. *Brain Research, 1116*, 166–176.

Cholfin, J. A. & Rubenstein, J. L. (2007). Genetic regulation of prefrontal cortex development and function. *Novartis Foundation Symposium, 288*, 165–173; discussion 173-167, 276-181.

Chuang, S. C., Zhao, W., Bauchwitz, R., Yan, Q., Bianchi, R., & Wong, R. K. (2005). Prolonged epileptiform discharges induced by altered group I metabotropic glutamate receptor-mediated synaptic responses in hippocampal slices of a fragile X mouse model. *Journal of Neuroscience, 25*, 8048–8055.

Cohen-Salmon, C., Carlier, M., Roubertoux, P., Jouhaneau, J., Semal, C., & Paillette, M. (1985). Differences in patterns of pup care in mice. V—Pup ultrasonic emissions and pup care behavior. *Physiology and Behavior, 35*, 167–174.

Consortium TECTS. (1993). Identification and characterization of the tuberous sclerosis gene on chromosome 16. *Cell, 75*, 1305–1315.

Cook, E. H., Jr. & Scherer, S. W. (2008). Copy-number variations associated with neuropsychiatric conditions. *Nature, 455*, 919–923.

Courchesne, E., Karns, C. M., Davis, H. R., Ziccardi, R., Carper, R. A., Tigue, Z. D., et al. (2001). Unusual brain growth patterns in early life in patients with autistic disorder: An MRI study. *Neurology, 57*, 245–254.

Crawley, J. N. (2003). Behavioral phenotyping of rodents. *Comparative Medicine, 53*, 140–146.

Crawley, J. N. (2004). Designing mouse behavioral tasks relevant to autistic-like behaviors. *Mental Retardation and Developmental Disabilities Research Reviews, 10*, 248–258.

Crawley, J. N., Chen, T., Puri, A., Washburn, R., Sullivan, T. L., Hill, J. M., et al. (2007). Social approach behaviors in oxytocin knockout mice: Comparison of two independent lines tested in different laboratory environments. *Neuropeptides, 41*, 145–163.

Crawley, J. N. (2007a). Mouse behavioral assays relevant to the symptoms of autism. *Brain Pathology, 17*, 448–459.

Crawley, J. N. (2007b). Medicine. Testing hypotheses about autism. *Science, 318*, 56–57.

Crawley, J. N. (2007c). *What's wrong with my mouse? Behavioral phenotyping of transgenic and knockout mice* (2nd ed.). Hoboken, NJ., John Wiley & Sons, Inc.

Creese, I. & Iversen, S. D. (1975). The pharmacological and anatomical substrates of the amphetamine response in the rat. *Brain Research, 83*, 419–436.

Cuccaro, M. L., Shao, Y., Grubber, J., Slifer, M., Wolpert, C. M., Donnelly, S. L., et al. (2003). Factor analysis of restricted and repetitive behaviors in autism using the Autism Diagnostic Interview-R. *Child Psychiatry and Human Development, 34*, 3–17.

D'Amato, F. R. & Populin, R. (1987). Mother-offspring interaction and pup development in genetically deaf mice. *Behavior Genetics, 17*, 465–475.

D'Amato, F. R. & Moles, A. (2001). Ultrasonic vocalizations as an index of social memory in female mice. *Behavioral Neuroscience, 115*, 834–840.

D'Amato, F. R., Scalera, E., Sarli, C., & Moles, A. (2005). Pups call, mothers rush: Does maternal responsiveness affect the amount of ultrasonic vocalizátions in mouse pups? *Behavior Genetics, 35*, 103–112.

Dawson, G., Webb, S., Schellenberg, G. D., Dager, S., Friedman, S., Aylward, E., et al. (2002). Defining the broader phenotype of autism: Genetic, brain, and behavioral perspectives. *Development and Psychopathology, 14*, 581–611.

Dawson, G. (2008). Early behavioral intervention, brain plasticity, and the prevention of autism spectrum disorder. *Development and Psychopathology, 20*, 775–803.

de Vrij, F. M., Levenga, J., van der Linde, H. C., Koekkoek, S. K., De Zeeuw, C. I., Nelson, D. L., et al. (2008). Rescue of behavioral phenotype and neuronal protrusion morphology in Fmr1 KO mice. *Neurobiology of Disease, 31*, 127–132.

Del Punta, K., Leinders-Zufall, T., Rodriguez, I., Jukam, D., Wysocki, C. J., Ogawa, S., et al. (2002). Deficient pheromone responses in mice lacking a cluster of vomeronasal receptor genes. *Nature, 419*, 70–74.

DeLorey, T. M., Sahbaie, P., Hashemi, E., Homanics, G. E., & Clark, J. D. (2008). Gabrb3 gene deficient mice exhibit impaired social and exploratory behaviors, deficits in non-selective attention and hypoplasia of cerebellar vermal lobules: A potential model of autism spectrum disorder. *Behavioural Brain Research, 187*, 207–220.

D'Hooge, R., Nagels, G., Franck, F., Bakker, C. E., Reyniers, E., Storm, K., et al. (1997). Mildly impaired water maze performance in male Fmr1 knockout mice. *Neuroscience, 76*, 367–376.

Dolen, G., Osterweil, E., Rao, B. S., Smith, G. B., Auerbach, B. D., Chattarji, S., et al. (2007). Correction of fragile X syndrome in mice. *Neuron, 56*, 955–962.

Dolen, G. & Bear, M. F. (2008). Role for metabotropic glutamate receptor 5 (mGluR5) in the pathogenesis of fragile X syndrome. *Journal of Physiology, 586*, 1503–1508.

Doty, R. L. (1986). Odor-guided behavior in mammals. *Experientia, 42*, 257–271.

Dulac, C. & Wagner, S. (2006). Genetic analysis of brain circuits underlying pheromone signaling. *Annual Review of Genetics, 40*, 449–467.

Durand, C. M., Betancur, C., Boeckers, T. M., Bockmann, J., Chaste, P., Fauchereau, F., et al. (2007). Mutations in the gene encoding the synaptic scaffolding protein SHANK3 are associated with autism spectrum disorders. *Nature Genetics, 39*, 25–27.

Dykens, E. M., Sutcliffe, J. S., & Levitt, P. (2004). Autism and 15q11-q13 disorders: Behavioral, genetic, and pathophysiological issues. *Mental Retardation and Developmental Disabilities Research Reviews, 10*, 284–291.

Egashira, N., Tanoue, A., Matsuda, T., Koushi, E., Harada, S., Takano, Y., et al. (2007). Impaired social interaction and reduced anxiety-related behavior in vasopressin V1a receptor knockout mice. *Behavioural Brain Research, 178*, 123–127.

Ehninger, D., Han, S., Shilyansky, C., Zhou, Y., Li, W., Kwiatkowski, D. J., et al. (2008). Reversal of learning deficits in a Tsc2+/- mouse model of tuberous sclerosis. *Nature Medicine, 14*, 843–848.

Ehret, G. & Bernecker, C. (1992). Categorical perception of mouse-pup ultrasounds in the temporal domain. *Animal Behaviour, 43*, 409–416.

Elwood, R. W. & Keeling, F. (1982). Temporal organization of ultrasonic vocalizations in infant mice. *Developmental Psychobiology, 15*, 221–227.

Engelmann, M., Wotjak, C. T., & Landgraf, R. (1995). Social discrimination procedure: An alternative method to investigate juvenile recognition abilities in rats. *Physiology and Behavior, 58*, 315–321.

Ferguson, J. N., Aldag, J. M., Insel, T. R., & Young, L. J. (2001). Oxytocin in the medial amygdala is essential for social recognition in the mouse. *Journal of Neuroscience, 21*, 8278–8285.

Fleming, S. M., Tetreault, N. A., Mulligan, C. K., Hutson, C. B., Masliah, E., & Chesselet, M. F. (2008). Olfactory deficits in mice overexpressing human wildtype alpha-synuclein. *European Journal of Neuroscience, 28*, 247–256.

Frith, U. (2003). *Autism: Explaining the Enigma*. Blackwell Publishing. Oxford, UK: Wiley–Blackwell.

Frith, U. & Happe, F. (2005). Autism spectrum disorder. *Current Biology: CB, 15*, R786–790.

Fujita, E., Tanabe, Y., Shiota, A., Ueda, M., Suwa, K., Momoi, M. Y., et al. (2008). Ultrasonic vocalization impairment of Foxp2 (R552H) knockin mice related to speech-language disorder and abnormality of Purkinje cells. *Proceedings of the National Academy of Sciences of the United States of America, 105*, 3117–3122.

Garber, K. (2007). Neuroscience. Autism's cause may reside in abnormalities at the synapse. *Science, 317*, 190–191.

Garber, K. B., Visootsak, J., & Warren, S. T. (2008). Fragile X syndrome. *European Journal of Human Genetics: EJHG, 16*, 666–672.

Gauthier, J., Spiegelman, D., Piton, A., Lafreniere, R. G., Laurent, S., St-Onge, J., et al. (2009). Novel de novo SHANK3 mutation in autistic patients. *American Journal of Medical Genetics. Part B, Neuropsychiatric Genetics, 150B*, 421–424.

Gemelli, T., Berton, O., Nelson, E. D., Perrotti, L. I., Jaenisch, R., & Monteggia, L. M. (2006). Postnatal loss of methyl-CpG binding protein 2 in the forebrain is sufficient to mediate behavioral aspects of Rett syndrome in mice. *Biological Psychiatry, 59*, 468–476.

Geschwind, D. H. & Levitt, P. (2007). Autism spectrum disorders: Developmental disconnection syndromes. *Current Opinion in Neurobiology, 17*, 103–111.

Glessner, J. T., Wang, K., Cai, G., Korvatska, O., Kim, C. E., Wood, S., et al. (2009). Autism genome-wide copy number variation reveals ubiquitin and neuronal genes. *Nature, 459*, 569–573.

Goffin, A., Hoefsloot, L. H., Bosgoed, E., Swillen, A., & Fryns, J. P. (2001). PTEN mutation in a family with Cowden syndrome and autism. *American Journal of Medical Genetics, 105*, 521–524.

Goios, A., Pereira, L., Bogue, M., Macaulay, V., & Amorim, A. (2007). mtDNA phylogeny and evolution of laboratory mouse strains. *Genome Research, 17*, 293–298.

Goorden, S. M., van Woerden, G. M., van der Weerd, L., Cheadle, J. P., & Elgersma, Y. (2007). Cognitive deficits in Tsc1+/- mice in the absence of cerebral lesions and seizures. *Annals of Neurology, 62*, 648–655.

Gourbal, B. E., Barthelemy, M., Petit, G., & Gabrion, C. (2004). Spectrographic analysis of the ultrasonic vocalisations of adult male and female BALB/c mice. *Die Naturwissenschaften, 91*, 381–385.

Grant, E. C. & MacIntosh, J. H. (1963). A comparison of the social postures of some common laboratory rodents. *Behaviour, 21*, 246–259.

Greer, J. M. & Capecchi, M. R. (2002). Hoxb8 is required for normal grooming behavior in mice. *Neuron, 33*, 23–34.

Groszer, M., Keays, D. A., Deacon, R. M., de Bono, J. P., Prasad-Mulcare, S., Gaub, S., et al. (2008). Impaired synaptic plasticity and motor learning in mice with a point mutation implicated in human speech deficits. *Current Biology: CB, 18*, 354–362.

Guy, J., Hendrich, B., Holmes, M., Martin, J. E., & Bird, A. (2001). A mouse Mecp2-null mutation causes neurological symptoms that mimic Rett syndrome. *Nature Genetics, 27*, 322–326.

Hadjikhani, N., Joseph, R. M., Snyder, J., & Tager-Flusberg, H. (2007). Abnormal activation of the social brain during face perception in autism. *Human Brain Mapping, 28*, 441–449.

Hammerschmidt, K., Radyushkin, K., Ehrenreich, H., & Fischer, J. (2009). Female mice respond to male ultrasonic "songs" with approach behaviour. *Biology Letters, 5*, 589–592.

Hayashi, M. L., Rao, B. S., Seo, J. S., Choi, H. S., Dolan, B. M., Choi, S. Y., et al. (2007). Inhibition of p21-activated kinase rescues symptoms of fragile X syndrome in mice. *Proceedings of the National Academy of Sciences of the United States of America, 104*, 11489–11494.

Hazlett, H. C., Poe, M., Gerig, G., Smith, R. G., Provenzale, J., Ross, A., et al. (2005). Magnetic resonance imaging and head circumference study of brain size in autism: Birth through age 2 years. *Archives of General Psychiatry, 62*, 1366–1376.

Herman, G. E., Butter, E., Enrile, B., Pastore, M., Prior, T. W., & Sommer, A. (2007). Increasing knowledge of PTEN germline mutations: Two additional patients with autism and macrocephaly. *American Journal of Medical Genetics. Part A, 143*, 589–593.

Hill, J. M., McCune, S. K., Alvero, R. J., Glazner, G. W., & Brenneman, D. E. (1996). VIP regulation of embryonic growth. *Annals of the New York Academy of Sciences, 805*, 259–268; discussion 268–259.

Hines, R. M., Wu, L., Hines, D. J., Steenland, H., Mansour, S., Dahlhaus, R., et al. (2008). Synaptic imbalance, stereotypies, and impaired social interactions in mice with altered neuroligin 2 expression. *Journal of Neuroscience, 28*, 6055–6067.

Hofer, M. A. & Shair, H. N. (1993). Ultrasonic vocalization, laryngeal braking, and thermogenesis in rat pups: A reappraisal. *Behavioral Neuroscience, 107*, 354–362.

Hofer, M. A., Brunelli, S. A., & Shair, H. N. (1994). Potentiation of isolation-induced vocalization by brief exposure of rat pups to maternal cues. *Developmental Psychobiology, 27*, 503–517.

Hofer, M. A., Brunelli, S. A., Masmela, J., & Shair, H. N. (1996). Maternal interactions prior to separation potentiate isolation-induced calling in rat pups. *Behavioral Neuroscience, 110*, 1158–1167.

Hofer, M. A., Masmela, J. R., Brunelli, S. A., & Shair, H. N. (1998). The ontogeny of maternal potentiation of the infant rats' isolation call. *Developmental Psychobiology, 33*, 189–201.

Hofer, M. A., Shair, H. N., Masmela, J. R., & Brunelli, S. A. (2001). Developmental effects of selective breeding for an infantile trait: The rat pup ultrasonic isolation call. *Developmental Psychobiology, 39*, 231–246.

Hollander, E., Kaplan, A., Cartwright, C., & Reichman, D. (2000). Venlafaxine in children, adolescents, and young adults with autism spectrum disorders: An open retrospective clinical report. *Journal of Child Neurology, 15*, 132–135.

Hollander, E., Bartz, J., Chaplin, W., Phillips, A., Sumner, J., Soorya, L., et al. (2007). Oxytocin increases retention of social cognition in autism. *Biological Psychiatry, 61*, 498–503.

Holtzman, D. M., Santucci, D., Kilbridge, J., Chua-Couzens, J., Fontana, D. J., Daniels, S. E., et al. (1996). Developmental abnormalities and age-related neurodegeneration in a mouse model of Down syndrome. *Proceedings of the National Academy of Sciences of the United States of America, 93*, 13,333–13,338.

Holy, T. E. & Guo, Z. (2005). Ultrasonic songs of male mice. *PLoS Biology, 3*, e386.

Hranilovic, D., Bujas-Petkovic, Z., Tomicic, M., Bordukalo-Niksic, T., Blazevic, S., & Cicin-Sain, L. (2009). Hyperserotonemia in autism: Activity of 5HT-associated platelet proteins. *Journal of Neural Transmission, 116*, 493–501.

Humphries, R. E., Robertson, D. H., Beynon, R. J., & Hurst, J. L. (1999). Unravelling the chemical basis of competitive scent marking in house mice. *Animal Behaviour, 58*, 1177–1190.

Hung, A. Y., Futai, K., Sala, C., Valtschanoff, J. G., Ryu, J., Woodworth M. A., et al. (2008). Smaller dendritic spines, weaker synaptic transmission, but enhanced spatial learning in mice lacking Shank1. *Journal of Neuroscience, 28*, 1697–1708.

Hurst, J. L., Payne, C. E., Nevison, C. M., Marie, A. D., Humphries, R. E., Robertson, D. H., et al. (2001). Individual recognition in mice mediated by major urinary proteins. *Nature, 414*, 631–634.

Hurst, J. L. & Beynon, R. J. (2004). Scent wars: The chemobiology of competitive signalling in mice. *BioEssays, 26*, 1288–1298.

Hurst, J. L., Thom, M. D., Nevison, C. M., Humphries, R. E., & Beynon, R. J. (2005). MHC odours are not required or sufficient for recognition of individual scent owners. *Proceedings. Biological sciences/The Royal Society, 272*, 715–724.

Insel, T. R., & Winslow, J. T. (1991). Central administration of oxytocin modulates the infant rat's response to social isolation. *European Journal of Pharmacology, 203*, 149–152.

Isles, A. R., Baum, M. J., Ma, D., Keverne, E. B., & Allen, N. D. (2001). Urinary odour preferences in mice. *Nature, 409*, 783–784.

Jamain, S., Quach, H., Betancur, C., Rastam, M., Colineaux, C., Gillberg, I. C., et al. (2003). Mutations of the X-linked genes encoding neuroligins NLGN3 and NLGN4 are associated with autism. *Nature Genetics, 34*, 27–29.

Jamain, S., Radyushkin, K., Hammerschmidt, K., Granon, S., Boretius, S., Varoqueaux, F., et al. (2008). Reduced social interaction and ultrasonic communication in a mouse model of monogenic heritable autism. *Proceedings of the National Academy of Sciences of the United States of America, 105*, 1710–1715.

James, S. J., Rose, S., Melnyk, S., Jernigan, S., Blossom, S., Pavliv, O., & Gaylor, D. W. (2009). Cellular and mitochondrial glutathione redox imbalance in lymphoblastoid cells derived from children with autism. *FASEB Journal, 23*, 2374–2383.

Jeffries, A. R., Curran, S., Elmslie, F., Sharma, A., Wenger, S., Hummel, M., et al. (2005). Molecular and phenotypic characterization of ring chromosome 22. *American Journal of Medical Genetics. Part A, 137*, 139–147.

Juch, M., Smalla, K. H., Kahne, T., Lubec, G., Tischmeyer, W., Gundelfinger, E. D., et al. (2009). Congenital lack of nNOS impairs long-term social recognition memory and alters the olfactory bulb proteome. *Neurobiology of Learning and Memory, 92*, 469–484.

Jugloff, D. G., Vandamme, K., Logan, R., Visanji, N. P., Brotchie, J. M., Eubanks, J. H. (2008). Targeted delivery of an Mecp2 transgene to forebrain neurons improves the behavior of female Mecp2-deficient mice. *Human Molecular Genetics, 17*, 1386–1396.

Kang, N., Baum, M. J., & Cherry, J. A., (2009). A direct main olfactory bulb projection to the "vomeronasal" amygdala in female mice selectively responds to volatile pheromones from males. *European Journal of Neuroscience, 29*, 624–634.

Kavaliers, M., Choleris, E., & Pfaff, D. W. (2005). Recognition and avoidance of the odors of parasitized conspecifics and predators: Differential genomic correlates. *Neuroscience and Biobehavioral Reviews, 29*, 1347–1359.

Kehoe, P., Callahan, M., Daigle, A., Mallinson, K., & Brudzynski, S. (2001). The effect of cholinergic stimulation on rat pup ultrasonic vocalizations. *Developmental Psychobiology, 38*, 92–100.

Kelleher, R. J., 3rd, & Bear, M. F. (2008). The autistic neuron: Troubled translation? *Cell, 135*, 401–406.

Keller, M., Douhard, Q., Baum, M. J., & Bakker, J. (2006). Sexual experience does not compensate for the disruptive effects of zinc sulfate—lesioning of the main olfactory epithelium on sexual behavior in male mice. *Chemical Senses, 31*, 753–762.

Kendrick, K. M. (2004). The neurobiology of social bonds. *Journal of Neuroendocrinology, 16*, 1007–1008.

Kim, H. G., Kishikawa, S., Higgins, A. W., Seong, I. S., Donovan, D. J., Shen, Y., et al. (2008). Disruption of neurexin 1 associated with autism spectrum disorder. *American Journal of Human Genetics, 82*, 199–207.

King, B. H., Hollander, E., Sikich, L., McCracken, J. T., Scahill, L., Bregman, J. D., et al. (2009). Lack of efficacy of citalopram in children with autism spectrum disorders and high levels of repetitive behavior: Citalopram ineffective in children with autism. *Archives of General Psychiatry, 66*, 583–590.

Klein, S. L., Kriegsfeld, L. J., Hairston, J. E., Rau, V., Nelson, R. J., & Yarowsky, P. J. (1996). Characterization of sensorimotor performance, reproductive and aggressive behaviors in segmental trisomic 16 (Ts65Dn) mice. *Physiology and Behavior, 60*, 1159–1164.

Kolevzon, A., Mathewson, K. A., & Hollander, E. (2006). Selective serotonin reuptake inhibitors in autism: A review of efficacy and tolerability. *Journal of Clinical Psychiatry, 67*, 407–414.

Koochek, M., Harvard, C., Hildebrand, M. J., Van Allen, M., Wingert, H., Mickelson, E., et al. (2006). 15q duplication associated with autism in a multiplex family with a familial cryptic translocation t(14;15)(q11.2;q13.3) detected using array-CGH. *Clinical Genetics, 69*, 124–134.

Korff, S. & Harvey, B. H. (2006). Animal models of obsessive-compulsive disorder: Rationale to understanding psychobiology and pharmacology. *Psychiatric Clinics of North America, 29*, 371–390.

Kramer, K. M., Cushing, B. S., & Carter, C. S. (2003). Developmental effects of oxytocin on stress response: Single versus repeated exposure. *Physiology and Behavior, 79*, 775–782.

Kratochvil, C. J., Findling, R. L., McDougle, C. J., Scahill, L., & Hamarman, S. (2005). Pharmacological management of agitation and aggression in an adolescent with autism. *Journal of the American Academy of Child and Adolescent Psychiatry, 44*, 829–832.

Kriaucionis, S., Paterson, A., Curtis, J., Guy, J., Macleod, N., & Bird, A. (2006). Gene expression analysis exposes mitochondrial abnormalities in a mouse model of Rett syndrome. *Molecular and Cellular Biology, 26*, 5033–5042.

Kusserow, H., Davies, B., Hortnagl, H., Voigt, I., Stroh, T., Bert, B., et al. (2004). Reduced anxiety-related behaviour in transgenic mice overexpressing serotonin 1A receptors. *Brain Research. Molecular Brain Research, 129*, 104–116.

Kwon, C. H., Luikart, B. W., Powell, C. M., Zhou, J., Matheny, S. A., Zhang, W., et al. (2006). Pten regulates neuronal arborization and social interaction in mice. *Neuron, 50*, 377–388.

Lai, C. S., Fisher, S. E., Hurst, J. A., Vargha-Khadem, F., & Monaco, A. P. (2001). A forkhead-domain gene is mutated in a severe speech and language disorder. *Nature, 413*, 519–523.

Lam, K. S., Aman, M. G., & Arnold, L. E. (2006). Neurochemical correlates of autistic disorder: A review of the literature. *Research in Developmental Disabilities, 27*, 254–289.

Landa, R. (2007). Early communication development and intervention for children with autism. *Mental Retardation and Developmental Disabilities Research Reviews, 13*, 16–25.

Landa, R. J. (2008). Diagnosis of autism spectrum disorders in the first 3 years of life. *Nature Clinical Practice Neurology, 4*, 138–147.

Laumonnier, F., Bonnet-Brilhault, F., Gomot, M., Blanc, R., David, A., Moizard, M. P., et al. (2004). X-linked mental retardation and autism are associated with a mutation in the NLGN4 gene, a member of the neuroligin family. *American Journal of Human Genetics, 74*, 552–557.

Lauterborn, J. C., Rex, C. S., Kramar, E., Chen, L. Y., Pandyarajan, V., Lynch, G., et al. (2007). Brain-derived neurotrophic factor rescues synaptic plasticity in a mouse model of fragile X syndrome. *Journal of Neuroscience, 27*, 10685–10694.

Laviola, G., Adriani, W., Gaudino, C., Marino, R., & Keller, F. (2006). Paradoxical effects of prenatal acetylcholinesterase blockade on neuro-behavioral development and drug-induced stereotypies in reeler mutant mice. *Psychopharmacology, 187*, 331–344.

Lawson-Yuen, A., Saldivar, J. S., Sommer, S., & Picker, J. (2008). Familial deletion within NLGN4 associated with autism and Tourette syndrome. *European Journal of Human Genetics, 16*, 614–618.

Lewis, M. I., Sieck, G. C., Fournier, M., & Belman, M. J. (1986). Effect of nutritional deprivation on diaphragm contractility and muscle fiber size. *Journal of Applied Physiology, 60*, 596–603.

Lewis, M. H. (2004). Environmental complexity and central nervous system development and function. *Mental Retardation and Developmental Disabilities Research Reviews, 10*, 91–95.

Lewis, M. H., Tanimura, Y., Lee, L. W., & Bodfish, J. W. (2007). Animal models of restricted repetitive behavior in autism. *Behavioural Brain Research, 176*, 66–74.

Liljelund, P., Handforth, A., Homanics, G. E., & Olsen, R. W. (2005). GABAA receptor beta3 subunit gene-deficient heterozygous mice show parent-of-origin and gender-related differences in beta3 subunit levels, EEG, and behavior. *Brain Research. Developmental Brain Research, 157*, 150–161.

Lim, M. A., Stack, C. M., Cuasay, K., Stone, M. M., McFarlane, H. G., Waschek, J. A., et al. (2008). Regardless of genotype, offspring of VIP-deficient female mice exhibit developmental delays and deficits in social behavior. *International Journal of Developmental Neuroscience, 26*, 423–434.

Lintas, C. & Persico, A. M. (2009). Autistic phenotypes and genetic testing: State-of-the-art for the clinical geneticist. *Journal of Medical Genetics, 46*, 1–8.

Lise, M. F. & El-Husseini, A. (2006). The neuroligin and neurexin families: From structure to function at the synapse. *Cellular and Molecular Life Sciences: CMLS, 63*, 1833–1849.

London, E. (2007). The role of the neurobiologist in redefining the diagnosis of autism. *Brain Pathology, 17*, 408–411.

Long, J. M., LaPorte, P., Paylor, R., & Wynshaw-Boris, A. (2004). Expanded characterization of the social interaction abnormalities in mice lacking Dvl1. *Genes, Brain, and Behavior, 3*, 51–62.

Lord, C., Risi, S., Lambrecht, L., Cook, E. H., Jr., Leventhal, B. L., DiLavore, P. C., et al. (2000). The autism diagnostic observation schedule-generic: A standard measure of social and communication deficits associated with the spectrum of autism. *Journal of Autism and Developmental Disorders, 30*, 205–223.

Lord, C., Risi, S., DiLavore, P. S., Shulman, C., Thurm, A., & Pickles, A. (2006). Autism from 2 to 9 years of age. *Archives of General Psychiatry, 63*, 694–701.

Lord, C. & Bishop, S. L. (2009). The autism spectrum: Definitions, assessment and diagnoses. *British Journal of Hospital Medicine (London, England: 2005), 70*, 132–135.

Lu, D. C., Zhang, H., Zador, Z., & Verkman, A. S. (2008). Impaired olfaction in mice lacking aquaporin-4 water channels. *FASEB Journal, 22*, 3216–3223.

Luo, M., Fee, M. S., & Katz, L. C. (2003). Encoding pheromonal signals in the accessory olfactory bulb of behaving mice. *Science, 299*, 1196–1201.

Maggio, J. C., Maggio, J. H., & Whitney, G. (1983). Experience-based vocalization of male mice to female chemosignals. *Physiology and Behavior, 31*, 269–272.

Maggio, J. C. & Whitney, G. (1985). Ultrasonic vocalizing by adult female mice (Mus musculus). *Journal of Comparative Psychology, 99*, 420–436.

Martel, K. L. & Baum, M. J. (2009). A centrifugal pathway to the mouse accessory olfactory bulb from the medial amygdala conveys gender-specific volatile pheromonal signals. *European Journal of Neuroscience, 29*, 368–376.

Mayeux-Portas, V., File, S. E., Stewart, C. L., & Morris, R. J. (2000). Mice lacking the cell adhesion molecule Thy-1 fail to use socially transmitted cues to direct their choice of food. *Current Biology: CB, 10*, 68–75.

McDonald, M. P., Wong, R., Goldstein, G., Weintraub, B., Cheng, S. Y., & Crawley, J. N. (1998). Hyperactivity and learning deficits in transgenic mice bearing a human mutant thyroid hormone beta1 receptor gene. *Learning and Memory, 5*, 289–301.

McDougle, C. J., Holmes, J. P., Bronson, M. R., Anderson, G. M., Volkmar, F. R., Price, L. H., et al. (1997). Risperidone treatment of children and adolescents with pervasive developmental disorders: A prospective open-label study. *Journal of the American Academy of Child and Adolescent Psychiatry, 36*, 685–693.

McDougle, C. J., Scahill, L., McCracken, J. T., Aman, M. G., Tierney, E., Arnold, L. E., et al. (2000). Research Units on Pediatric Psychopharmacology (RUPP) Autism Network. Background and rationale for an initial controlled study of risperidone. *Child and Adolescent Psychiatric Clinics of North America, 9*, 201–224.

McDougle, C. J., Scahill, L., Aman, M. G., McCracken, J. T., Tierney, E, Davies, M., et al. (2005). Risperidone for the core symptom domains of autism: Results from the study by the autism network of the research units on pediatric psychopharmacology. *American Journal of Psychiatry, 162*, 1142–1148.

McFarlane, H. G., Kusek, G. K., Yang, M., Phoenix, J. L., Bolivar, V. J., & Crawley, J. N. (2008). Autism-like behavioral phenotypes in BTBR T+tf/J mice. *Genes, Brain, and Behavior, 7*, 152–163.

McManus, J., Perry, P., Sumner, A. T., Wright, D. M., Thomson, E. J., Allshire, R. C., et al. (1994). Unusual chromosome structure of fission yeast DNA in mouse cells. *Journal of Cell Science, 107*(Pt 3), 469–486.

McNaughton, C. H., Moon, J., Strawderman, M. S., Maclean, K. N., Evans, J., & Strupp, B. J. (2008). Evidence for social anxiety and impaired social cognition in a mouse model of fragile X syndrome. *Behavioral Neuroscience, 122*, 293–300.

Meikle, L., Pollizzi, K., Egnor, A., Kramvis, I., Lane, H., Sahin, M., et al. (2008). Response of a neuronal model of tuberous sclerosis to mammalian target of rapamycin (mTOR) inhibitors: Effects on mTORC1 and Akt signaling lead to improved survival and function. *Journal of Neuroscience, 28*, 5422–5432.

Miczek, K. A., Maxson, S. C., Fish, E. W., & Faccidomo, S. (2001). Aggressive behavioral phenotypes in mice. *Behavioural Brain Research, 125*, 167–181.

Mineur, Y. S., Huynh, L. X., & Crusio, W. E. (2006). Social behavior deficits in the Fmr1 mutant mouse. *Behavioural Brain Research, 168*, 172–175.

Minshew, N. J. & Williams, D. L. (2007). The new neurobiology of autism: Cortex, connectivity, and neuronal organization. *Archives of Neurology, 64*, 945–950.

Miura, K., Kishino. T., Li, E., Webber, H., Dikkes, P., Holmes, G. L., et al. (2002). Neurobehavioral and electroencephalographic abnormalities in Ube3a maternal-deficient mice. *Neurobiology of Disease, 9*, 149–159.

Moles, A. & D'Amato, F. R. (2000). Ultrasonic vocalization by female mice in the presence of a conspecific carrying food cues. *Animal Behaviour, 60*, 689–694.

Moles, A., Costantini, F., Garbugino, L., Zanettini, C., & D'Amato, F. R. (2007). Ultrasonic vocalizations emitted during dyadic interactions in female mice: A possible index of sociability? *Behavioural Brain Research, 182*, 223–230.

Mombaerts, P. (2004). Genes and ligands for odorant, vomeronasal and taste receptors. *Nature Reviews Neuroscience, 5*, 263–278.

Moretti, P., Bouwknecht, J. A., Teague, R., Paylor, R., & Zoghbi, H. Y. (2005). Abnormalities of social interactions and home-cage behavior in a mouse model of Rett syndrome. *Human Molecular Genetics, 14*, 205–220.

Moretti, P., Levenson, J. M., Battaglia, F., Atkinson, R., Teague, R., Antalffy, B., et al. (2006). Learning and memory and synaptic plasticity are impaired in a mouse model of Rett syndrome. *Journal of Neuroscience, 26*, 319–327.

Moretti, P. & Zoghbi, H. Y. (2006). MeCP2 dysfunction in Rett syndrome and related disorders. *Current Opinion in Genetics and Development, 16*, 276–281.

Morgan, L., Wetherby, A. M., & Barber, A. (2008). Repetitive and stereotyped movements in children with autism spectrum disorders late in the second year of life. *Journal of Child Psychology and Psychiatry, and Allied Disciplines, 49*, 826–837.

Moy, S. S., Nadler, J. J., Perez, A., Barbaro, R. P., Johns, J. M., Magnuson, T. R., et al. (2004). Sociability and preference for social novelty in five inbred strains: An approach to assess autistic-like behavior in mice. *Genes, Brain, and Behavior, 3*, 287–302.

Moy, S. S., Nadler, J. J., Young, N. B., Perez, A., Holloway, L. P., Barbaro, R. P., et al. (2007). Mouse behavioral tasks relevant to autism: Phenotypes of 10 inbred strains. *Behavioural Brain Research, 176*, 4–20.

Moy, S. S., & Nadler, J. J. (2008). Advances in behavioral genetics: Mouse models of autism. *Molecular Psychiatry, 13*, 4–26.

Moy, S. S., Nadler, J. J., Poe, M. D., Nonneman, R. J., Young, N. B., Koller, B. H., et al. (2008a). Development of a mouse test for repetitive, restricted behaviors: Relevance to autism. *Behavioural Brain Research, 188*, 178–194.

Moy, S. S., Nadler, J. J., Young, N. B., Nonneman, R. J., Segall, S. K., Andrade, G. M., et al. (2008b). Social approach and repetitive behavior in eleven inbred mouse strains. *Behavioural Brain Research, 191*, 118–129.

Moy, S. S., Nadler, J. J., Young, N. B., Nonneman, R. J., Grossman, A. W., Murphy, D. L., et al. (2009). Social approach in genetically engineered mouse lines relevant to autism. *Genes, Brain, and Behavior 8*, 129–142.

Moy, S. S., Nonneman, R. J., Young, N. B., Demyanenko, G. P., & Maness, P. F. (2009). Impaired sociability and cognitive function in Nrcam-null mice. *Behavioural Brain Research, 205*, 123–131.

Myers, M. M., Ali, N., Weller, A., Brunelli, S. A., Tu, A. Y., Hofer, M. A., et al. (2004). Brief maternal interaction increases number, amplitude, and bout size of isolation-induced ultrasonic vocalizations in infant rats (Rattus norvegicus). *Journal of Comparative Psychology, 118*, 95–102.

Nadler, J. J., Moy, S. S., Dold, G., Trang, D., Simmons, N., Perez, A., et al. (2004). Automated apparatus for quantitation of social approach behaviors in mice. *Genes, Brain, and Behavior, 3*, 303–314.

Nakatani, J., Tamada, K., Hatanaka, F., Ise, S., Ohta, H., Inoue, K., et al. (2009). Abnormal behavior in a chromosome-engineered mouse model for human 15q11-13 duplication seen in autism. *Cell, 137*, 1235–1246.

Napolioni, V. & Curatolo, P. (2008). Genetics and molecular biology of tuberous sclerosis complex. *Current Genomics, 9*, 475–487.

Navarro, J. F., De Castro, V., & Martin-Lopez, M. (2008). JNJ16259685, a selective mGlu1 antagonist, suppresses isolation-induced aggression in male mice. *European Journal of Pharmacology, 586*, 217–220.

Nielsen, D. M., Derber, W. J., McClellan, D.A., & Crnic, L. S. (2002). Alterations in the auditory startle response in Fmr1 targeted mutant mouse models of fragile X syndrome. *Brain Research, 927*, 8–17.

Noirot, E. (1966). Ultra-sounds in young rodents. I. Changes with age in albino mice. *Animal Behaviour, 14*, 459–462.

Noirot, E. (1972). Ultrasounds and maternal behavior in small rodents. *Developmental Psychobiology, 5*, 371–387.

Nomura, Y. (2002). Pathophysiology of Rett syndrome from the standpoints of clinical characteristics and clinical neurophysiological findings. *No To Hattatsu, 34*, 200–206.

Nyby, J. (2001). Auditory communication among adults. In Willott J. F., ed. *Handbook of mouse auditory research: From behavior to molecular biology*. Boca Raton, FL: CRC Press.

Ogier, M., Wang, H., Hong, E., Wang, Q., Greenberg, M. E., & Katz, D. M. (2007). Brain-derived neurotrophic factor expression and respiratory function improve after ampakine treatment in a mouse model of Rett syndrome. *Journal of Neuroscience, 27*, 10912–10917.

Ognibene, E., Adriani, W., Macri, S., & Laviola, G. (2007). Neurobehavioural disorders in the infant reeler mouse model: Interaction of genetic vulnerability and consequences of maternal separation. *Behavioural Brain Research, 177*, 142–149.

Page, D. T., Kuti, O. J., Prestia, C., & Sur, M. (2009). Haploinsufficiency for Pten and Serotonin transporter cooperatively influences brain size and social behavior. *Proceedings of the National Academy of Sciences of the United States of America, 106*, 1989–1994.

Panksepp, J. & Burgdorf, J. (2000). 50-kHz chirping (laughter?) in response to conditioned and unconditioned tickle-induced reward in rats: Effects of social housing and genetic variables. *Behavioural Brain Research, 115*, 25–38.

Panksepp, J. (2003). Can anthropomorphic analyses of separation cries in other animals inform us about the emotional nature of social loss in humans? Comment on Blumberg and Sokoloff (2001). *Psychological Review, 110*, 376–388; discussion 389–396.

Panksepp, J. B. & Lahvis, G. P. (2007). Social reward among juvenile mice. *Genes, Brain, and Behavior, 6*, 661–671.

Panksepp, J. B., Jochman, K. A., Kim, J. U., Koy, J. J., Wilson, E. D., Chen, Q., et al. (2007). Affiliative behavior, ultrasonic communication and social reward are influenced by genetic variation in adolescent mice. *PLoS ONE, 2*, e351.

Parsons, R. G., Gafford, G. M., & Helmstetter, F. J. (2006). Translational control via the mammalian target of rapamycin pathway is critical for the formation and stability of long-term fear memory in amygdala neurons. *Journal of Neuroscience, 26*, 12977–12983.

Paylor, R., Yuva-Paylor, L. A., Nelson, D. L., & Spencer, C. M. (2008). Reversal of sensorimotor gating abnormalities in Fmr1 knockout mice carrying a human Fmr1 transgene. *Behavioral Neuroscience, 122*, 1371–1377.

Peier, A. M., McIlwain, K. L., Kenneson, A., Warren, S. T., Paylor, R., & Nelson, D. L. (2000). (Over)correction of FMR1 deficiency with YAC transgenics: Behavioral and physical features. *Human Molecular Genetics, 9*, 1145–1159.

Pelphrey, K. A., Sasson, N. J., Reznick, J. S., Paul, G., Goldman, B. D., & Piven, J. (2002). Visual scanning of faces in autism. *Journal of Autism and Developmental Disorders, 32*, 249–261.

Petrulis, A., Alvarez, P., & Eichenbaum, H. (2005). Neural correlates of social odor recognition and the representation of individual distinctive social odors within entorhinal cortex and ventral subiculum. *Neuroscience, 130*, 259–274.

Picker, J. D., Yang, R., Ricceri, L., & Berger-Sweeney, J. (2006). An altered neonatal behavioral phenotype in Mecp2 mutant mice. *Neuroreport, 17*, 541–544.

Pierce, K., Muller, R. A., Ambrose, J., Allen, G., & Courchesne, E. (2001). Face processing occurs outside the fusiform "face area" in autism: Evidence from functional MRI. *Brain: A Journal of Neurology, 124*, 2059–2073.

Piven, J., Palmer, P., Jacobi, D., Childress, D., & Arndt, S. (1997). Broader autism phenotype: Evidence from a family history study of multiple-incidence autism families. *American Journal of Psychiatry, 154*, 185–190.

Pogorelov, V. M., Rodriguiz, R. M., Insco, M. L., Caron, M. G., & Wetsel, W. C. (2005). Novelty seeking and stereotypic activation of behavior in mice with disruption of the Dat1 gene. *Neuropsychopharmacology, 30*, 1818–1831.

Posey, D. J., Erickson, C. A., & McDougle, C. J. (2008). Developing drugs for core social and communication impairment in autism. *Child and Adolescent Psychiatric Clinics of North America, 17*, 787–801, viii–ix.

Powell, S. B., Newman, H. A., Pendergast, J. F., & Lewis, M. H. (1999). A rodent model of spontaneous stereotypy: Initial characterization of developmental, environmental, and neurobiological factors. *Physiology and Behavior, 66*, 355–363.

Powell, S. B., Newman, H. A., McDonald, T. A., Bugenhagen, P., & Lewis, M. H. (2000). Development of spontaneous stereotyped behavior in deer mice: Effects of early and late exposure to a more complex environment. *Developmental Psychobiology, 37*, 100–108.

Radyushkin, K., Hammerschmidt, K., Boretius, S., Varoqueaux, F., El-Kordi, A., Ronnenberg, A., et al. (2009). Neuroligin-3-deficient mice: Model of a monogenic heritable form of autism with an olfactory deficit. *Genes, Brain, and Behavior, 8*, 416–425.

Ralph, R. J., Paulus, M. P., Fumagalli, F., Caron, M. G., & Geyer, M. A. (2001). Prepulse inhibition deficits and perseverative motor patterns in dopamine transporter knock-out mice: Differential effects of D1 and D2 receptor antagonists. *Journal of Neuroscience, 21*, 305–313.

Rao, P. A., Beidel, D. C., & Murray, M. J. (2008). Social skills interventions for children with Asperger's syndrome or high-functioning autism: A review and recommendations. *Journal of Autism and Developmental Disorders, 38*, 353–361.

Rapin, I. & Tuchman, R. F. (2008). Autism: Definition, neurobiology, screening, diagnosis. *Pediatric Clinics of North America, 55*, 1129–1146, viii.

Restrepo, D., Arellano, J., Oliva, A. M., Schaefer, M. L., & Lin, W. (2004). Emerging views on the distinct but related roles of the main and accessory olfactory systems in responsiveness to chemosensory signals in mice. *Hormones and Behavior, 46*, 247–256.

Ricceri, L., Moles, A., & Crawley, J. (2007). Behavioral phenotyping of mouse models of neurodevelopmental disorders: Relevant social behavior patterns across the life span. *Behavioural Brain Research, 176*, 40–52.

Richter, K., Wolf, G., & Engelmann, M. (2005). Social recognition memory requires two stages of protein synthesis in mice. *Learning and Memory, 12*, 407–413.

Robinson, D. & D'Udine, B. (1982). Ultrasonic calls produced by three laboratory strains of Mus musculus. *Journal of Zoology London, 197*, 383–389.

Rorick-Kehn, L. M., Johnson, B. G., Knitowski, K. M., Salhoff, C. R., Witkin, J. M., Perry, K. W., et al. (2007). In vivo pharmacological characterization of the structurally novel, potent, selective mGlu2/3 receptor agonist LY404039 in animal models of psychiatric disorders. *Psychopharmacology, 193*, 121–136.

Roubertoux, P. L., Martin, B., Le Roy, I., Beau, J., Marchaland, C., Perez-Diaz, F., et al. (1996). Vocalizations in newborn mice: Genetic analysis. *Behavior Genetics, 26*, 427–437.

Roullet, F. I., Wohr, M., & Crawley, J. N. (2009). Scent marking and countermarking behaviors as a measure of olfactory communication in the BTBR T+tf/J inbred strain, a mouse model of autism Society for Neuroscience Annual Conference, Chicago, IL.

Ryan, B. C., Young, N. B., Moy, S. S., & Crawley, J. N. (2008). Olfactory cues are sufficient to elicit social approach behaviors but not social transmission of food preference in C57BL/6J mice. *Behavioural Brain Research, 193*, 235–242.

Sadakata, T., Washida, M., Iwayama, Y., Shoji, S., Sato, Y., Ohkura, T., et al. (2007). Autistic-like phenotypes in Cadps2-knockout mice and aberrant CADPS2 splicing in autistic patients. *Journal of Clinical Investigation, 117*, 931–943.

Sadakata, T., Kakegawa, W., Mizoguchi, A., Washida, M., Katoh-Semba, R., Shutoh, F., et al. (2007). Impaired cerebellar development and function in mice lacking CAPS2, a protein involved in neurotrophin release. *Journal of Neuroscience, 27*, 2472–2482.

Samaco, R. C., Fryer, J. D., Ren, J., Fyffe, S., Chao, H. T., Sun, Y., et al. (2008). A partial loss of function allele of methyl-CpG-binding protein 2 predicts a human neurodevelopmental syndrome. *Human Molecular Genetics, 17*, 1718–1727.

Sanchez-Andrade, G., James, B. M., & Kendrick, K. M. (2005). Neural encoding of olfactory recognition memory. *Journal of Reproduction and Development, 51*, 547–558.

Sanchez-Andrade, G. & Kendrick, K. M. (2009). The main olfactory system and social learning in mammals. *Behavioural Brain Research, 200*, 323–335.

Scattoni, M. L., Gandhy, S. U., Ricceri, L., & Crawley, J. N. (2008a). Unusual repertoire of vocalizations in the BTBR T+tf/J mouse model of autism. *PLoS ONE, 3*, e3067.

Scattoni, M. L., McFarlane, H. G., Zhodzishsky, V., Caldwell, H. K., Young, W. S., Ricceri, L., et al. (2008b). Reduced ultrasonic vocalizations in vasopressin 1b knockout mice. *Behavioural Brain Research, 187b*, 371–378.

Scattoni, M. L., Crawley, J., & Ricceri, L. (2009). Ultrasonic vocalizations: A tool for behavioural phenotyping of mouse models of neurodevelopmental disorders. *Neuroscience and Biobehavioral Reviews, 33*, 508–515.

Scattoni, M. L., Ricceri, L., Crawley, J. N. (2010). Unusual repertoire of vocalizations in adult BTBR T+tf/J mice during three types of social encounters. *Genes, Brain, and Behavior*. doi: 10.1111/j.1601-183X.2010.00623.x. [Epub ahead of print].

Scearce-Levie, K., Roberson, E. D., Gerstein, H., Cholfin, J. A., Mandiyan, V. S., Shah, N. M., et al. (2008). Abnormal social behaviors in mice lacking Fgf17. *Genes, Brain, and Behavior, 7*, 344–354.

Schellinck, H. M., Forestell, C. A., & LoLordo V. M. (2001). A simple and reliable test of olfactory learning and memory in mice. *Chemical Senses, 26*, 663–672.

Shafritz, K. M., Dichter, G. S., Baranek, G. T., & Belger, A. (2008). The neural circuitry mediating shifts in behavioral response and cognitive set in autism. *Biological Psychiatry, 63*, 974–980.

Shu, W., Cho, J. Y., Jiang, Y., Zhang, M., Weisz, D., Elder, G. A., et al. (2005). Altered ultrasonic vocalization in mice with a disruption in the Foxp2 gene. *Proceedings of the National Academy of Sciences of the United States of America, 102*, 9643–9648.

Silva, A. J. & Ehninger, D. (2009). Adult reversal of cognitive phenotypes in neurodevelopmental disorders. *Journal of Neurodevelopmental Disorders, 1*, 150–157.

Silverman, J. L., Tolu, S. S., Barkan, C. L., & Crawley, J. N. (2010a). Repetitive self-grooming behavior in the BTBR mouse model of autism is blocked by the mGluR5 antagonist MPEP. *Neuropsychopharmacology, 35*(4), 976–989.

Silverman, J., Yang, M., Lord, C., & Crawley, J. N. (2010b). Behavioural phenotyping assays for mouse models of autism. *Nature Reviews Neuroscience, 11*(7), 490–502. Review.

Singer, H. S., Morris, C., Gause, C., Pollard, M., Zimmerman, A. W., & Pletnikov, M. (2009). Prenatal exposure to antibodies from mothers of children with autism produces neurobehavioral alterations: A pregnant dam mouse model. *Journal of Neuroimmunology, 211*, 39–48.

Slotnick, B. (2007). Odor-sampling time of mice under different conditions. *Chemical Senses, 32*, 445–454.

Smith, S. E., Li, J., Garbett, K., Mirnics, K., & Patterson, P. H. (2007). Maternal immune activation alters fetal brain development through interleukin-6. *Journal of Neuroscience, 27*, 10695–10702.

Smotherman, W. P., Bell, R. W., Starzec, J., Elias, J., & Zachman, T. A. (1974). Maternal responses to infant vocalizations and olfactory cues in rats and mice. *Behavioral Biology, 12*, 55–66.

Soorya, L., Kiarashi, J., & Hollander, E. (2008). Psychopharmacologic interventions for repetitive behaviors in autism spectrum disorders. *Child and Adolescent Psychiatric Clinics of North America, 17*, 753–771, viii.

South, M., Ozonoff, S., & McMahon, W. M. (2005). Repetitive behavior profiles in Asperger syndrome and high-functioning autism. *Journal of Autism and Developmental Disorders, 35*, 145–158.

Spehr, M., Spehr, J., Ukhanov, K., Kelliher, K. R., Leinders-Zufall, T., & Zufall, F. (2006). Parallel processing of social signals by the mammalian main and accessory olfactory systems. *Cellular and Molecular Life Sciences: CMLS, 63*, 1476–1484.

Spencer, C. M., Alekseyenko, O., Serysheva, E., Yuva-Paylor, L. A., & Paylor, R. (2005). Altered anxiety-related and social behaviors in the Fmr1 knockout mouse model of fragile X syndrome. *Genes, Brain, and Behavior, 4*, 420–430.

Spencer, C. M., Serysheva, E., Yuva-Paylor, L. A., Oostra, B. A., Nelson, D. L., & Paylor, R. (2006). Exaggerated behavioral phenotypes in Fmr1/Fxr2 double knockout mice reveal a functional genetic interaction between Fragile X-related proteins. *Human Molecular Genetics, 15*, 1984–1994.

Spencer, C. M., Graham, D. F., Yuva-Paylor L. A., Nelson, D. L., & Paylor, R. (2008). Social behavior in Fmr1 knockout mice carrying a human FMR1 transgene. *Behavioral Neuroscience, 122*, 710–715.

Stack, C. M., Lim, M. A., Cuasay, K., Stone, M. M., Seibert, K. M., Spivak-Pohis, I., et al. (2008). Deficits in social behavior and reversal learning are more prevalent in male offspring of VIP deficient female mice. *Experimental Neurology, 211*(1), 67–84.

Steiner, R. A., Hohmann, J. G., Holmes, A., Wrenn, C. C., Cadd, G., Jureus, A., et al. (2001). Galanin transgenic mice display cognitive and neurochemical deficits characteristic of Alzheimer's disease. *Proceedings of the National Academy of Sciences of the United States of America, 98*, 4184–4189.

Sundaram, S. K., Kumar, A., Makki, M. I., Behen, M. E., Chugani, H. T., & Chugani, D. C. (2008). Diffusion tensor imaging of frontal lobe in autism spectrum disorder. *Cerebral Cortex, 18*(11), 2659–2665.

Sy, M. (1991). Reasons for Senegalese migration determined by ethnic background and social status. *Pop Sahel, 16*, 29–35.

Sykes, N. H., Toma, C., Wilson, N., Volpi, E. V., Sousa, I., Pagnamenta, A. T., et al. (2009). Copy number variation and association analysis of SHANK3 as a candidate gene for autism in the IMGSAC collection. *European Journal of Human Genetics: EJHG, 17*, 1347–1353.

Tabuchi, K., Blundell, J., Etherton, M. R., Hammer, R. E., Liu, X., Powell, C. M., et al. (2007). A neuroligin-3 mutation implicated in autism increases inhibitory synaptic transmission in mice. *Science, 318*, 71–76.

Tager-Flusberg, H. & Caronna, E. (2007). Language disorders, autism and other pervasive developmental disorders. *Pediatric Clinics of North America, 54*, 469–481, vi.

Takayanagi, Y., Yoshida, M., Bielsky, I. F., Ross, H. E., Kawamata, M., Onaka, T., et al. (2005). Pervasive social deficits, but normal parturition, in oxytocin receptor-deficient mice. *Proceedings of the National Academy of Sciences of the United States of America, 102*, 16096–16101.

Tanimura, Y., Yang, M. C., & Lewis, M. H. (2008). Procedural learning and cognitive flexibility in a mouse model of restricted, repetitive behaviour. *Behavioural Brain Research, 189*, 250–256.

Terranova, M. L. & Laviola, G. (2005). Scoring of social interactions and play in mice during adolescence. *Current Protocols in Toxicology, 13*, 10.1–10.10.

Trinh, K. & Storm, D. R. (2003). Vomeronasal organ detects odorants in absence of signaling through main olfactory epithelium. *Nature Neuroscience, 6*, 519–525.

Turner, G., Webb, T., Wake, S., & Robinson, H. (1996). Prevalence of fragile X syndrome. *American Journal of Medical Genetics, 64*, 196–197.

Turner, C. A., Presti, M. F., Newman, H. A., Bugenhagen, P., Crnic, L., & Lewis, M. H. (2001). Spontaneous stereotypy in an animal model of Down syndrome: Ts65Dn mice. *Behavior Genetics, 31*, 393–400.

Turner, C. A., Yang, M. C., & Lewis, M. H. (2002). Environmental enrichment: Effects on stereotyped behavior and regional neuronal metabolic activity. *Brain Research, 938*, 15–21.

Turner, C. A. & Lewis, M. H. (2003). Environmental enrichment: Effects on stereotyped behavior and neurotrophin levels. *Physiology and Behavior, 80*, 259–266.

van Slegtenhorst, M., de Hoogt, R., Hermans, C., Nellist, M., Janssen, B., Verhoef, S., et al. (1997). Identification of the tuberous sclerosis gene TSC1 on chromosome 9q34. *Science, 277*, 805–808.

Vargha-Khadem, F., Gadian, D. G., Copp, A., & Mishkin, M. (2005). FOXP2 and the neuroanatomy of speech and language. *Nature Reviews Neuroscience, 6*, 131–138.

Vela, J. M., Gonzalez, B., & Castellano, B. (1998). Understanding glial abnormalities associated with myelin deficiency in the jimpy mutant mouse. *Brain Research. Brain Research Reviews, 26*, 29–42.

Veltman, M. W., Thompson, R. J., Craig, E. E., Dennis, N. R., Roberts, S. E., Moore, V., et al. (2005). A paternally inherited duplication in the Prader-Willi/Angelman syndrome critical region: A case and family study. *Journal of Autism and Developmental Disorders, 35*, 117–127.

Venerosi, A., Calamandrei, G., & Ricceri, L. (2006). A social recognition test for female mice reveals behavioral effects of developmental chlorpyrifos exposure. *Neurotoxicology and Teratology, 28*, 466–471.

Viemari, J. C., Roux, J. C., Tryba, A. K., Saywell, V., Burnet, H., Pena, F., et al. (2005). Mecp2 deficiency disrupts norepinephrine and respiratory systems in mice. *Journal of Neuroscience, 25*, 11,521–11,530.

Volkmar, F. R. & Pauls, D. (2003). Autism. *Lancet, 362*, 1133–1141.

Volkmar, F., Chawarska, K., & Klin, A. (2005). Autism in infancy and early childhood. *Annual Review of Psychology, 56*, 315–336.

Volkmar, F. R. (2009). Citalopram treatment in children with autism spectrum disorders and high levels of repetitive behavior. *Archives of General Psychiatry, 66*, 581–582.

Volkmar, F. R., State, M., & Klin, A. (2009). Autism and autism spectrum disorders: Diagnostic issues for the coming decade. *Journal of Child Psychology and Psychiatry, and Allied Disciplines, 50*, 108–115.

Wan, M., Lee, S. S., Zhang, X., Houwink-Manville, I., Song, H. R., Amir, R. E., et al. (1999). Rett syndrome and beyond: Recurrent spontaneous and familial MECP2 mutations at CpG hotspots. *American Journal of Human Genetics, 65*, 1520–1529.

Wang, H., Liang, S., Burgdorf, J., Wess, J., & Yeomans, J. (2008). Ultrasonic vocalizations induced by sex and amphetamine in M2, M4, M5 muscarinic and D2 dopamine receptor knockout mice. *PLoS ONE, 3*, e1893.

Wanisch, K., Wotjak, C. T., & Engelmann, M. (2008). Long-lasting second stage of recognition memory consolidation in mice. *Behavioural Brain Research, 186*, 191–196.

Welch, J. M., Lu, J., Rodriguiz, R. M., Trotta, N. C., Peca, J., Ding, J. D., et al. (2007). Cortico-striatal synaptic defects and OCD-like behaviours in Sapap3-mutant mice. *Nature, 448*, 894–900.

Wenk, G. L. & Hauss-Wegrzyniak, B. (1999). Altered cholinergic function in the basal forebrain of girls with Rett syndrome. *Neuropediatrics, 30*, 125–129.

Wersinger, S. R. & Rissman, E. F. (2000). Oestrogen receptor alpha is essential for female-directed chemo-investigatory behaviour but is not required for the pheromone-induced luteinizing hormone surge in male mice. *Journal of Neuroendocrinology, 12*, 103–110.

Wersinger, S. R., Ginns, E. I., O'Carroll, A. M., Lolait, S. J., & Young, W. S., 3rd (2002). Vasopressin V1b receptor knockout reduces aggressive behavior in male mice. *Molecular Psychiatry, 7*, 975–984.

Wersinger, S. R., Caldwell, H. K., Martinez, L., Gold, P., Hu, S. B., & Young, W. S., 3rd (2007). Vasopressin 1a receptor knockout mice have a subtle olfactory deficit but normal aggression. *Genes, Brain, and Behavior, 6*, 540–551.

Wesson, D. W., Keller, M., Douhard, Q., Baum, M. J., & Bakker, J. (2006). Enhanced urinary odor discrimination in female aromatase knockout (ArKO) mice. *Hormones and Behavior, 49*, 580–586.

Wesson, D. W., Donahou, T. N., Johnson, M. O., & Wachowiak, M. (2008). Sniffing behavior of mice during performance in odor-guided tasks. *Chemical Senses, 33*, 581–596.

West, L., Brunssen, S. H., & Waldrop, J. (2009a). Review of the evidence for treatment of children with autism with selective serotonin reuptake inhibitors. *Journal for Specialists in Pediatric Nursing: JSPN, 14*, 183–191.

West, L., Waldrop, J., & Brunssen, S. (2009b). Pharmacologic treatment for the core deficits and associated symptoms of autism in children. *Journal of Pediatric Health Care, 23*, 75–89.

White, N. R. & Barfield, R. J. (1989). Playback of female rat ultrasonic vocalizations during sexual behavior. *Physiology and Behavior, 45*, 229–233.

White, N. R., Prasad, M., Barfield, R. J., & Nyby, J. G. (1998). 40- and 70-kHz vocalizations of mice (Mus musculus) during copulation. *Physiology and Behavior, 63*, 467–473.

Whitney, G. & Nyby, J. (1979). Cues that elicit ultrasounds from adult male mice. *American Zoologist, 19*, 457–463.

Williams White, S., Keonig, K., & Scahill, L. (2007). Social skills development in children with autism spectrum disorders: A review of the intervention research. *Journal of Autism and Developmental Disorders, 37*, 1858–1868.

Winslow, J. T., Hearn, E. F., Ferguson, J., Young, L. J., Matzuk, M. M., & Insel, T. R. (2000). Infant vocalization, adult aggression, and fear behavior of an oxytocin null mutant mouse. *Hormones and Behavior, 37*, 145–155.

Winslow, J. T. & Insel, T. R. (2002). The social deficits of the oxytocin knockout mouse. *Neuropeptides, 36*, 221–229.

Winslow, J. T. (2003). Mouse social recognition and preference. *Current Protocols in Neuroscience, 8*, Unit 8 16.

Wiznitzer, M. (2004). Autism and tuberous sclerosis. *Journal of Child Neurology, 19*, 675–679.

Wohr, M., & Schwarting, R. K. (2007). Ultrasonic communication in rats: Can playback of 50-kHz calls induce approach behavior? *PLoS ONE, 2*, e1365.

Woodley, S. K. & Baum, M. J. (2003). Effects of sex hormones and gender on attraction thresholds for volatile anal scent gland odors in ferrets. *Hormones and Behavior, 44*, 110–118.

Woodley, S. K., Cloe, A. L., Waters, P., & Baum, M. J. (2004). Effects of vomeronasal organ removal on olfactory sex discrimination and odor preferences of female ferrets. *Chemical Senses, 29*, 659–669.

Wrenn, C. C., Harris, A. P., Saavedra, M. C., & Crawley, J. N. (2003). Social transmission of food preference in mice: Methodology and application to galanin-overexpressing transgenic mice. *Behavioral Neuroscience, 117*, 21–31.

Wrenn, C. C., Kinney, J. W., Marriott, L. K., Holmes, A., Harris, A. P., Saavedra, M. C., et al. (2004). Learning and memory performance in mice lacking the GAL-R1 subtype of galanin receptor. *European Journal of Neuroscience, 19*, 1384–1396.

Wu, W. L., Wang, C. H., Huang, E. Y., & Chen, C. C. (2009). Asic3(-/-) female mice with hearing deficit affects social development of pups. *PLoS ONE, 4*, e6508.

Xiang, F., Buervenich, S., Nicolao, P., Bailey, M. E., Zhang, Z., & Anvret, M. (2000). Mutation screening in Rett syndrome patients. *Journal of Medical Genetics, 37*, 250–255.

Yamada, K., Wada, E., & Wada, K. (2000). Male mice lacking the gastrin-releasing peptide receptor (GRP-R) display elevated preference for conspecific odors and increased social investigatory behaviors. *Brain Research, 870*, 20–26.

Yamada, K., Wada, E., & Wada, K. (2001). Female gastrin-releasing peptide receptor (GRP-R)-deficient mice exhibit altered social preference for male conspecifics: Implications for GRP/GRP-R modulation of GABAergic function. *Brain Research, 894*, 281–287.

Yan, Q. J., Rammal, M., Tranfaglia, M., & Bauchwitz, R. P. (2005). Suppression of two major Fragile X Syndrome mouse model phenotypes by the mGluR5 antagonist MPEP. *Neuropharmacology, 49*, 1053–1066.

Yang, M., Scattoni, M. L., Zhodzishsky, V., Chen, T., Caldwell, H. K., Young, W. S., et al. (2007a). Similar social approach behaviors in BTBR T+ tf/J, C57BL/6J, and vasopressin receptor 1B knockout mice tested on conventional versus reverse light cycles, and in replications across cohorts. *Frontiers in Behavioral Neuroscience, 1*, 9.

Yang, M., Zhodzishsky, V., & Crawley, J. N. (2007b). Social deficits in BTBR T+tf/J mice are unchanged by cross-fostering with C57BL/6J mothers. *International Journal of Developmental Neuroscience, 25*, 515–521.

Yang, M. & Crawley, J. N. (2009). Simple behavioral assessment of mouse olfaction. *Current Protocols in Neuroscience, 48*, 8.24.1–8.24.12.

Yang, M., Clarke, A. M., & Crawley, J. N. (2009a). Postnatal lesion evidence against a primary role for the corpus callosum in mouse sociability. *European Journal of Neuroscience, 29*, 1663–1677.

Yang, M., Weber, M. D., Perry, K., Katz, A. M., & Crawley, J. N. (2009b). Social Peers Rescue Autism-like Phenotypes in Adolescent Mice. Society for Neuroscience Annual Conference, Chicago, IL.

Yang, M., Perry, K., Weber, M., Katz, A., & Crawley, J. N. (2010). Social peers rescue autism-like phenotypes in adolescent mice. *Autism Research*, Epub ahead of print.

Young, L. J., Pitkow, L. J., & Ferguson, J. N. (2002). Neuropeptides and social behavior: Animal models relevant to autism. *Molecular Psychiatry 7 Suppl, 2*, S38–39.

Zeng, L. H., Xu, L., Gutmann, D. H., & Wong, M. (2008). Rapamycin prevents epilepsy in a mouse model of tuberous sclerosis complex. *Annals of Neurology, 63*, 444–453.

Zhou, J., Blundell, J., Ogawa, S., Zhang, W., Kwon, C. H., Sinton, C. M., et al. (2007). Dysregulation of the PI3K/AKT pathway, Mouse models for social interaction deficits and for ASD with macrocephaly. In, Society for Neuroscience Annual Meeting San Diego, CA.

Zhou, J., Blundell, J., Ogawa, S., Kwon, C. H., Zhang, W., Sinton, C., et al. (2009). Pharmacological inhibition of mTORC1 suppresses anatomical, cellular, and behavioral abnormalities in neural-specific Pten knock-out mice. *Journal of Neuroscience, 29*, 1773–1783.

Zippelius, H. M. & Schleidt, W. M. (1956). Ultraschall-aute bei jungen Mausen. *Die Naturwissenschaften, 43*, 502–503.

52 Elaine Y. Hsiao, Catherine Bregere, Natalia Malkova, Paul H. Patterson

Modeling Features of Autism in Rodents

Points of Interest

- A number of abnormal behaviors found in autism can be produced in rodent models. None of these behaviors are specific for autism, however.
- Human disorders caused by single-gene mutations that exhibit features of autism provide proof-of-principle for the role of genetics in autism. Similarly, studies showing that maternal thalidomide, valproate, or infection can increase the risk for features of autism in the offspring provide proof-of-principle for the role of environmental factors. Both the environmental and genetic factors can be very effectively modelled in mice.
- Certain neuropathologies that are relatively common in autism can be reproduced in rodent models.

Introduction

Animal models of many neurological diseases (Alzheimer's, Parkinson's, Huntington's, multiple sclerosis) have proven enormously useful for determining the roles of genes and environment, for understanding pathogenesis, and for testing potential therapeutic approaches. There is some skepticism, however, concerning models of psychiatric or mental illnesses (e.g., autism, schizophrenia, depression). After all, can cognitive abnormalities or language deficits be detected in animals? However, to give up on this approach would deny the application of powerful genetic and molecular tools to these critical illnesses. Moreover, animal models need not be perfect mimics of human diseases to be valuable. This is clear from the extensive and productive use of genetic mouse models for Huntington's and other neurodegenerative diseases, which do not exhibit the severe loss of particular types of neurons that characterize these disorders. The power of animal models is in the examination of key features of a disease, and the relevance of an animal model should be judged by how well it reflects one or more features of that disease, which may include genetics, neuropathology, behavior, etiology, electrophysiology, or molecular changes.

Autism is a particularly difficult case for animal studies because it has a heterogeneous behavioral phenotype, the susceptibility genes have not been firmly identified, and it does not have a pathognomonic histology that allows definitive diagnosis. Nonetheless, autism does have generally agreed upon features that are distinctive, such as a deficit of Purkinje cells (PCs), decreased hippocampal γ-aminobutyric acid ($GABA_A$) receptors, and elevated levels of brain-derived neurotrophic factor (BDNF) and platelet serotonin (5-HT) (Palmen et al., 2004; Pardo & Eberhart, 2007; Amaral et al., 2008). There is also striking evidence for immune dysregulation in the autistic brain and cerebrospinal fluid (Pardo et al., 2006; Arion et al., 2007; Chez et al., 2007; Pardo & Eberhart, 2007; Morgan et al., 2010). Moreover, some of the characteristic behavioral features of autism can be assayed in animals, such as neophobia, abnormal social interactions, stereotyped and repetitive motor behaviors, communication deficits (ultrasonic vocalizations; USVs), enhanced anxiety, abnormal pain sensitivity, disturbed sleep patterns, abnormal eye blink conditioning, and deficits in sensorimotor gating (prepulse inhibition; PPI) (Silverman et al., 2010).

Although autism has a strong genetic basis, it is not a monogenic disorder, and thus it is not possible to establish an immediately relevant genetic mouse model, as was done with Huntington's disease. Nonetheless, there are several genetic changes that do entail an elevated risk for autism, and mouse models of these changes share some features with the human disorder. There are also several human disorders caused by single gene mutations that display autistic features and mouse mutants of these mutations display behavior or neuropathology relevant to autism. In addition, models based on autism etiology are valuable, and there are several known environmental risk factors that are being successfully modeled in rodents. Finally, there are brain lesion models of interest. Therefore, even at this early stage of analysis, it is clear that various models can be used to study how particular genes influence certain autism endophenotypes, and how known environmental risk factors influence such endophenotypes. It will also be interesting to determine how a particular genotype influences the response to an environmental risk factor, and vice versa. There are currently very few examples of such gene-environment interactions in mouse models. This chapter discusses current genetic, environmental risk factor and lesion models. Several other authors have reviewed various aspects of animal models related to autism (Murcia et al., 2005; Tordjman et al., 2007; Moy & Nadler, 2008).

Environmental Manipulations

Thalidomide and Valproic Acid

Prenatal or early postnatal drug exposure can increase autism risk. Comorbidity of Moebius syndrome and autism support a correlation between autism and the use of the prostaglandin misoprostol, a drug historically administered for labor induction or abortion (Miller et al., 2004). Case studies of fetal alcohol syndrome also suggest that prenatal exposure to ethanol increases risk for autism (Nanson, 1992). Perhaps most clearly associated with autism, however, are the teratogens thalidomide (Stromland et al., 1994) and valproic acid (VPA; valproate) (Christianson et al., 1994). Not only can these drugs cause an array of birth defects, they also increase the incidence of autism when administered early in human pregnancy (Miyazaki et al., 2005).

The use of thalidomide led to the discovery of a window of vulnerability for the development of autism (Figure 52-1). During the 1950s and 60s, thalidomide treatment of morning sickness resulted in thousands of offspring with severe malformations. Since the timing of drug exposure leads to specific types of craniofacial defects, the defects seen in the autistic offspring could be used to determine when these offspring were exposed. In this way, vulnerability to autism was pinpointed to days 20 to 24 of gestation, the time of neural tube closure and formation of motor nuclei and cranial nerves. Importantly, there is some evidence that idiopathic autism cases may also exhibit abnormalities in the cranial nerve nuclei and other neuropathologies that originate during fetal brain development (Schneider & Przewlocki, 2005; Palmen et al., 2004).

A few laboratories have translated maternal thalidomide exposure into rodent models. Exposure of rats to thalidomide on embryonic day 9 (E9) yields adult offspring with hyperserotonemia in the plasma (as in autism), hippocampus, and frontal cortex (Narita et al., 2002), with altered distribution of serotonergic neurons in the raphe nuclei (Miyazaki et al., 2005). These offspring also display hyperactivity in the open field and decreased learning in the radial maze (Narita et al., 2010). Exposure on E15 inhibits vasculogenesis and alters cortical and hippocampal morphology (Fan et al., 2008). Furthermore, daily maternal injection of rats from E7 to E18 yields adult offspring with altered learning and memory as measured by increased errors and latency in the Cincinnati water maze (Vorhees et al., 2001). Clearly, much more could be done with this model to establish its relevance for autism.

Because VPA retains its teratogenicity in rodents, its administration during the time of neural tube closure has proven useful as a rodent model. VPA was first introduced in the 1960s as an anticonvulsant and later as a mood-stabilizing drug for treatment of epilepsy and bipolar disorder (Markram et al., 2007). Like thalidomide, use of VPA during early human pregnancy significantly elevates the incidence of autism and the development of craniofacial defects in exposed offspring. Both case and epidemiological studies have confirmed the association between fetal valproate syndrome and autism (Hyman et al., 2006; Fan et al., 2008). Although women who are prescribed VPA for treatment of epilepsy often take the drug throughout pregnancy, it is unclear whether brain regions other than the brain stem are vulnerable to VPA insult at later stages of development (Rinaldi et al., 2007a).

Fetal valproate syndrome—rare congenital disorder caused by exposure of the fetus to valproic acid during the first trimester of pregnancy; characterized by symptoms of spina bifida, dysmorphic features, musculoskeletal malformations and developmental delay

In animal studies, a single injection of VPA in a pregnant rat results in striking neuropathology and behavioral abnormalities. Offspring of rats injected with VPA show brain defects resembling those sometimes found in autism, including

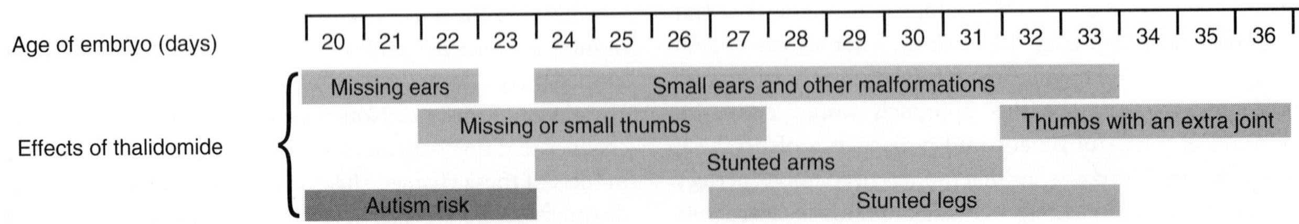

Figure 52–1. Timeline of birth defects caused by thalidomide, and the critical period of vulnerability to autism. The specific dysmorphologies in the offspring depend on the precise timing of drug ingestion. The fact that autistic features were only seen in offspring of a particular set of dysmorphologies indicates that the period of thalidomide-induced autistic features corresponds to days 20–23 of human gestation. Graphic after Rodier, PM. (2000) The early origins of autism. Scientific American, *282*(2), 56–63.

reduced number of motor nuclei and PCs (Schneider & Przewlocki, 2005), hyperserotonemia, and disorganized migration of 5-HT neurons in the dorsal raphe nuclei (Miyazaki et al., 2005). Fetuses from VPA-injected mothers display hypoplasia of the cortical plate, abnormal migration of dopaminergic and serotonergic neurons, and abnormal pons pathology (Kuwagata et al., 2009). VPA is a histone deacetylase inhibitor that is thought to impede neuronal differentiation and migration by interfering with the sonic hedgehog signaling pathway.

Interestingly, offspring of rats injected with VPA on E12.5 develop behavioral abnormalities that appear before puberty, a feature that distinguishes this model from behavioral changes seen in schizophrenia (Schneider & Przewlocki, 2005). VPA offspring display lower sensitivity to pain and higher sensitivity to nonpainful sensory stimuli, which parallels reported changes in endogenous opioid systems in some autistic patients. These offspring also exhibit impaired sensorimotor gating as measured by acoustic PPI, elevated anxiety as evidenced by decreased open field exploration, increased stereotypic/repetitive activity, decreased social interaction, impaired reversal learning, altered eyeblink conditioning patterns, and enhanced fear memory processing, all of which are consistent with results in autistic children (Stanton et al., 2007; Murawski et al., 2008; Markram et al., 2008; Dufour-Rainfray et al., 2010; Roullet et al., 2010) (Table 52-1). A sexual dimorphism has been reported for some of these parameters, with abnormalities seen only in male offspring, which is also consistent with the very significant male bias in autism

Sonic hedgehog signaling pathway—signal transduction pathway initiated by the binding of Hedgehog ligand to Patched; plays an important role in embryonic patterning and cell fate decisions

Table 52–1.
Behavioral assays used in rodent models of autistic features

Behavioral Paradigm	Testing Environment	Dependent Variables
SOCIAL BEHAVIOR		
sociability	three-chambered cage with inanimate object versus social object (mouse)	time spent in each chamber; number of approaches
preference for social novelty	three-chambered cage with familiar mouse versus unfamiliar mouse	time spent in each chamber; number of approaches
ultrasonic vocalizations	empty cage; pups are briefly isolated from mothers	number of calls, frequency of calls, type of call
LEARNING AND MEMORY		
Cincinnati water maze (multiple T maze)	maze design consisting of nine interlinked T-units submerged in water; mice are trained to swim to the escape platform	latency to find platform; time spent swimming in the trained quadrant of the pool as compared to time spent in the other quadrants
Morris water maze	circular pool of opaque water; mice are initially trained to swim to visible platform and then to submerged hidden platform	latency to find platform; time spent swimming in the trained quadrant as compared to time spent in the other three quadrants
eyeblink conditioning	chamber with tone generator for administration of a series of tones (conditioned stimulus, CS) followed by a periorbital shock (unconditioned stimulus)	occurrence of eyeblink as measured by EMG eyeblink signal (conditioned response, CR); amplitude of CR; latency between CS and onset of CR; latency between CS and peak of CR
novel object exploration	brightly lit open arena; in first trial, mice are exposed to two objects; in the second trial, one of the two objects is exchanged for a novel object	investigation of novel object; time spent with the novel object
novel location exploration	brightly lit open arena; in the first trial, mice are exposed to two objects; in the second trial, one of the two objects is moved to a new location	investigation of moved object; time spent with moved object
latent inhibition	chamber with tone generator for administration of a series of tones followed by an adversive stimulus (mild foot shock)	whole body flinch amplitude; freezing in context environment and after tonal cues
SENSORIMOTOR GATING		
acoustic prepulse inhibition	cage with tone generator for administration of a series of prepulse tones followed by startle stimulus	whole body flinch amplitude; freezing
ANXIETY/LOCOMOTION		
open field exploration	brightly lit open arena	center duration, number of center entries, total distance traveled, horizontal activity, vertical activity (rearing)
amphetamine-induced locomotion	brightly lit open arena	total distance traveled, horizontal activity, vertical activity (rearing)

(Schneider et al., 2008). It will also be interesting to look for communication deficits (USVs) in this model.

Electrophysiological studies indicate that offspring of VPA-treated mothers exhibit abnormal microcircuit connectivity in the neocortex and amygdala. Exposure to VPA results in over-expression of CaMKII and the NR2A and NR2B NMDA receptor subunits in the neocortex (Rinaldi et al., 2007b). These observations are consistent with observed increases in NMDA receptor-mediated synaptic transmission and enhanced postsynaptic long-term potentiation in neocortical pyramidal neurons. Adult VPA offspring also show increased connection probability of layer 5 pyramidal cells but decreased excitability and decreased putative pyramidal cell synaptic contacts (Rinaldi et al., 2008). These results relate to MRI studies showing impaired long-range functional connectivity in autistic individuals (Just et al., 2004).

CaMKII—calcium/calmodulin-dependent protein kinase II; a member of a family of serine/threonine-specific protein kinases that is known for its role in regulating long-term potentiation

NR2A and NR2B NMDA receptor subunits—two out of several isoforms of NMDA receptor subunits that combine with other subunits to form a NMDA receptor. NR2A contains a binding site for glutamate and continues to increase in expression throughout development. NR2B contains a binding site for the inhibitor ifenprodil and is expressed mainly in immature neurons of the early postnatal brain

Recordings from neurons in the lateral amygdaloid nucleus demonstrate hyper-reactivity to electrical stimulation, elevated long-term potentiation and impaired stimulus inhibition that may contribute to the deficient fear extinction and high anxiety seen in VPA offspring (Markram et al., 2008). These results suggest molecular and synaptic alterations in VPA mice that are relevant for the alterations in amygdala morphology observed in autism (Amaral et al., 2008). Dysfunction in the amygdala may contribute to the decreased social interaction and/or abnormal fear processing characteristic of autistic pathology (Markram et al., 2008). While deficits in social play and exploration have been reported in VPA rodent offspring (Schneider et al., 2008), an important gap in the behavioral analysis of social interaction is in the analysis of social preference and USVs.

Although the mechanisms underlying the effects of prenatal VPA on fetal brain development are largely unknown, neural inflammation and gene regulation could be involved. Immunological alterations have been reported in offspring of VPA-treated mice (Schneider et al., 2008; Bennett et al., 2000), and *in vitro* studies indicate that VPA promotes astrocyte proliferation, inhibits microglial and macrophage activation, and induces microglial apoptosis (Peng et al., 2005; Dragunow et al., 2006). This is consistent with the finding that VPA can regulate epigenetic modifications through three mechanisms: inhibiting histone deacetylases, enhancing histone acetylation, and promoting demethylase activity (Chen et al., 2007). The ability of VPA to alter HOX gene expression is of particular interest, as HOXa1 is expressed during the time of neural tube closure and regulates development of the facial nucleus and superior olive (c.f., Finnell et al., 2002). Moreover, VPA treatment may actually promote neurogenesis of GABAergic neurons and facilitate neurite outgrowth (Dragunow et al., 2006). These neuroprotective effects occur after chronic VPA treatment rather than the acute exposure administered in the maternal VPA model, however (Hao et al., 2004; Ren et al., 2004).

Although maternal VPA and thalidomide exposure are responsible for only a small fraction of autism cases, the extremely high risk for autism in the offspring provides proof-of-principle for environmental influences on autism incidence. Moreover, the similarities in neuropathology and behavior between the rodent models and human autism support the utility of environment-based models for defining relevant pathways of developmental dysregulation. It will be important to extend the VPA model to mice carrying genetic variants associated with increased risk for autism, which would provide a test of the gene x environment paradigm. Interestingly, prenatal VPA exposure has been linked to altered expression of neuroligin3, a genetic susceptibility factor for autism (Kolozsi et al., 2009).

HOX—group of related genes defined by the presence of a DNA sequence known as the homeobox; they code for a class of homeodomain-carrying transcription factors that serve as regulators of embryonic development

Maternal Infection

Maternal infection is an environmental risk factor for the development of several neuropsychiatric disorders in the offspring. As is the case for schizophrenia (Patterson, 2007; Brown & Derkits, 2010), maternal viral infection is linked to higher incidence of autism by clinical, epidemiological, and case studies. Early evidence for this came from the 1964 rubella pandemic, in which the incidence of autistic features was increased more than 200-fold in the offspring of infected mothers (Chess, 1977). Case studies have linked autism to several other prenatal viral infections, including varicella, rubeola, and cytomegalovirus (Ciaranello & Ciaranello, 1995). Bacterial and protozoan infections have also been associated with autism (Nicolson et al., 2007; Bransfield et al., 2008). The most compelling evidence linking maternal infection with autism comes from a very large study utilizing the Danish Medical Birth Register. An examination of over 10,000 autism cases found a very significant association with maternal viral infection in the first trimester (Atladottir et al., 2010). In sum, the diversity of micro-organisms implicated in autism, along with the fact that several of these infections do not involve direct transmission into the fetus, suggests that the maternal immune response, rather than microbial pathogenesis, is responsible for increasing the risk for autism in the offspring (Figure 52-2). Animal models of maternal infection further

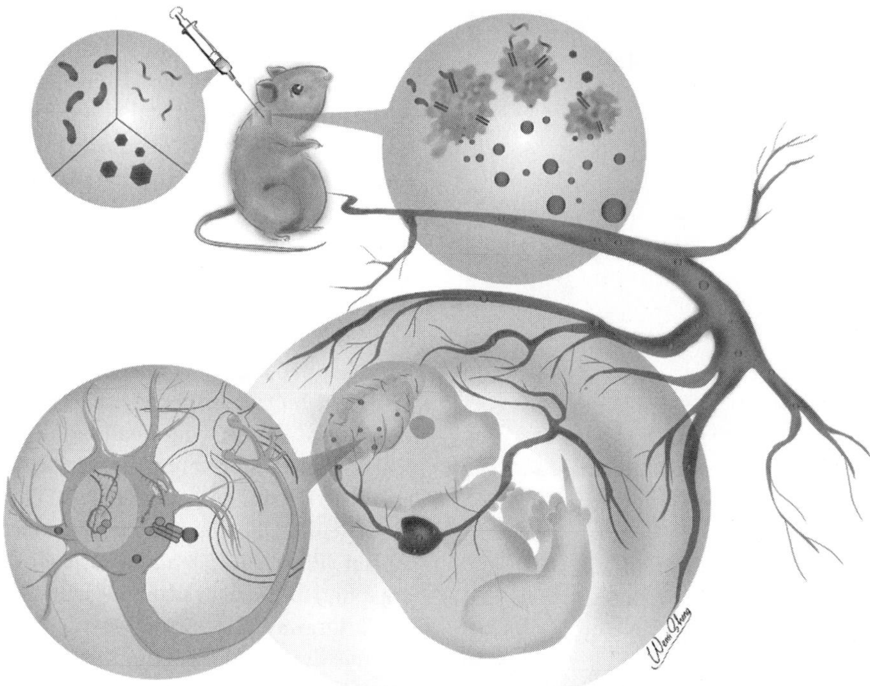

Figure 52–2. Cytokines produced by activation of the maternal immune system can alter fetal brain development. Various types of infection (bacteria, viruses, and parasites are illustrated) in pregnant rats or mice can be mimicked by injection of LPS or poly(I:C). These activate cells (pink in blue sphere) to produce cytokines (blue balls), which travel in the blood to the placenta, where they can activate cells. The cytokines can also cross the placenta into the fetal circulatory system and activate cells in the fetal brain. Illustration by Wensi Sheng. (See Color Plate Section for a color version of this figure.)

support the idea that maternal immune activation (MIA) and the production of pro-inflammatory cytokines are what unite the various types of maternal infection as risk factors for autism. There are three primary rodent models for MIA: maternal influenza infection, poly(I:C) injection, and lipopolysaccharide (LPS) injection.

Pregnant mice intranasally infected with influenza yield offspring with behavioral and neuropathological abnormalities that parallel those seen in autism. Abnormal behaviors include heightened anxiety during open-field exploration, deficient PPI, decreased novel object exploration, and reduced social interaction (Shi et al., 2003). These offspring display spatially selective PC loss in lobules VI and VII (Figure 52-3) (Shi et al., 2009), which is a common neuropathology in autism (Palmen et al., 2004; Amaral et al., 2008). There is also macrocephaly, delayed cerebellar granule cell migration, reduced Reelin immunoreactivity in the cortex, thinning of the neocortex and hippocampus, and altered expression of neuronal nitric oxide synthase and synaptosome-associated protein-25 (Fatemi et al., 2002; Shi et al., 2009). Infection on E16 or E18 causes altered expression of several genes associated with autism, white matter thinning in the corpus callosum, widespread brain atrophy, and altered levels of cerebellar 5-HT but not dopamine (Fatemi et al., 2008, 2009; Winter et al., 2008).

Because maternal influenza infection is largely confined to the respiratory tract, it is unlikely that these neurological defects are caused by direct viral infection of the fetus.

Reelin—a secreted extracellular matrix glycoprotein that regulates neuronal migration in the developing brain and synaptic plasticity in the adult brain

Nitric oxide synthase (NOS)—a class of dimeric, calmodulin-associated enzymes that catalyze the formation of nitric oxide

Synaptosome-associated protein-25 (SNAP-25)—a membrane-bound component of the neurotramsmitter vesicle release mechanism

There are, however, conflicting reports as to whether viral mRNA or protein is present in fetal tissues (Aronsson et al., 2002; Shi et al., 2005). Nonetheless, the fact that stimulating the maternal immune system with poly(I:C) (mimicking viral infection) and LPS (mimicking bacterial infection) causes neuropathogical and behavioral defects in the offspring similar to those seen with maternal influenza infection supports the idea that MIA is the causative event, as no pathogen is required. Poly(I:C) is a synthetic, double-stranded RNA that generates an antiviral immune response in the absence of virus. Depending on the dosage, mode of injection (intraperitoneal or intravenous) and timing of maternal poly(I:C) administration, offspring display deficits in PPI, latent inhibition, open field exploration, working memory, social interaction and USVs, while reversal learning and amphetamine-induced

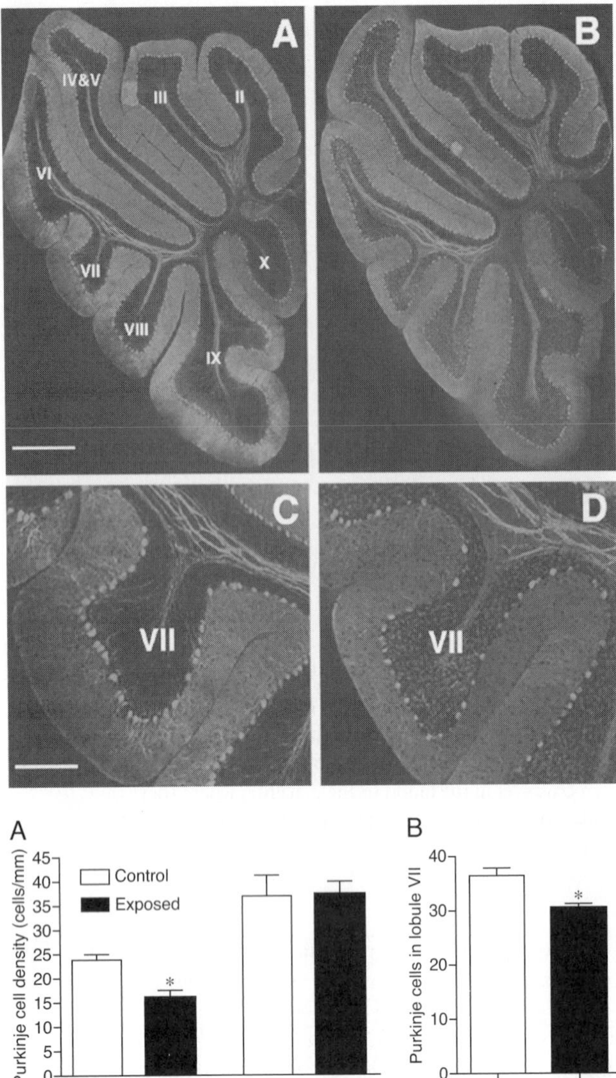

Figure 52–3. Maternal infection causes a spatially restricted Purkinje cell deficit. Adult offspring of mice given a respiratory infection with influenza virus at midgestation display a deficit in Purkinje cells in lobules VII but not in other lobules. Top: Calbindin staining of adult cerebella from offspring of control (A,C) and infected mothers (B,D) reveals a deficit in lobule VII of the latter. Panels C and D (bar = 200 μm) are higher magnification views of panels A and B (bar–800 μm). (See Color Plate Section for a color version of this figure.) Bottom: (A) Quantification of the linear density of Purkinje cells reveals a 33% deficit in lobule VII of the adult offspring of infected mothers, while no difference from controls is found in lobule V. (B) A similar, localized deficit is observed in postnatal day 11 offspring of infected mothers. Reprinted from Shi, L., Smith, S. E., Malkova, N., Tse, D., Su, Y., & Patterson, P. H. (2009). Activation of the maternal immune system alters cerebellar development in the offspring. *Brain, Behavior, and Immunity, 23*, 116–123, with Permission.

locomotion are enhanced (Shi et al., 2003; Zuckerman et al., 2003, 2005; Lee et al., 2007; Meyer et al., 2007; Smith et al., 2007; Winter et al., 2009; Malkova & Patterson, 2010). A single poly(I:C) injection also causes histopathological changes similar to those seen in autism, including increased $GABA_A$ receptor, spatially-restricted reduction in PCs, and delayed myelination, and decreased cortical neurogenesis (Nyffeler et al., 2006; Shi et al., 2009; Makinodan et al, 2008; De Miranda et al., 2010). A cardinal pathology in schizophrenia, enlarged lateral ventricles, is also observed (Li et al., 2009; Piontkewitz, Assaf, & Weiner, 2009). In addition, there is evidence of physiological abnormalities in the hippocampus. In slices from adult offspring of poly(I:C)-treated mothers, oscillations in CA1 are less rhythmic than in controls, and CA1 pyramidal neurons display reduced frequency and increased amplitude of miniature excitatory postsynaptic currents. Differing results have been reported regarding a deficit in long term potentiation (Ito et al., 2010; Oh-Nishi et al., 2010). Interestingly, the specific component of the temporoammonic pathway that mediates object-related information displays significantly increased sensitivity to dopamine (Lowe et al., 2009; Ito et al., 2010). There are a few studies describing abnormal dopamine levels in autism (Previc, 2007), and a variety of changes in dopamine are found in the maternal poly(I:C) model (Zuckerman et al., 2003; Ozawa et al., 2006; Meyer et al., 2008a). However, whether dysregulation of the dopaminergic system is an important feature of autism is unknown. Dopamine pathology is very important in schizophrenia, where maternal infection is also a risk factor. Another finding consistent with both schizophrenia and autism is a disruption in long-range synchrony of neuronal firing. Adult MIA offspring display significant reduction in medial prefrontal cortex-hippocampal EEG coherence (Dickerson, Wolff & Bilkey, 2010).

Intraperitoneal injection—administration of material into the peritoneum (body cavity)

Intravenous injection—in mice, this is typically done through the lateral tail veins

Further supporting the role of MIA in altering fetal brain development is the use of maternal LPS injection to simulate bacterial infection. Although poly(I:C) and LPS act through different toll-like receptors, their effects on the behavior and brain pathology in offspring often overlap. For example, a single injection of LPS in a pregnant rat yields offspring with elevated anxiety, aberrant social behavior, reduced play behavior and USVs, reduced PPI, enhanced amphetamine-induced locomotion, and abnormal learning and memory (Borrell et al., 2002; Fortier et al., 2004; Golan et al., 2005; Hava et al., 2006; Basta-Kaim et al., 2010; Baharnoori et al., 2010; Hao et al., 2010; Kirsten et al., 2010), many of which parallel behaviors seen in autism. There is also evidence of hyperactivity in the hypothalamus-pituitary-adrenal axis in the LPS offspring, and some of the abnormal behaviors can be reversed by anti-psychotic drug treatment (Basta-Kaim et al., 2010), as is the case for the poly(I:C) offspring. Recall that maternal infection is a risk factor for schizophrenia as well as autism.

Histological findings include smaller, more densely packed neurons in the hippocampus, increased numbers of pyknotic cells in the cortex, fewer tyrosine hydroxylase-positive (TH+)

Toll-like receptors (TLRs)—a class of transmembrane pattern recognition receptors that bind to structurally conserved molecules on microbes (pathogen-associated molecular patterns [PAMPs]); when activated by PAMP ligands, TLR signal transduction leads to the stimulation of innate immune responses

neurons in the substantia nigra, and increased TH+ cells in the nucleus accumbens (Golan et al., 2005; Ling et al., 2004; Borrell et al., 2002). Further studies indicate that changes in dendritic length, dendritic branching, spine structure, and spine density in the medial prefrontal cortex and hippocampus, suggesting dysregulated neuronal connections formed during embryogenesis (Baharnoori et al., 2008). Some of these effects, including increased cell density and limited dendritic arbors in the hippocampus, have been found in MRI and post mortem brain studies in autism (Amaral et al., 2008). Electrophysiological recordings reveal reduced synaptic input to CA1 of the hippocampus, heightened excitability of pyramidal neurons, enhanced postsynaptic glutamatergic response, and impaired NMDA-induced synaptic plasticity (Lowe et al., 2008; Lante et al., 2008). Interestingly, many of these effects are prevented by pretreatment of pregnant rats with N-acetyl-cysteine (Lante et al., 2008), which increases calcium influx when binding to glutamate receptors in combination with the transmitter. Brain imaging studies of the hippocampus and of particular neurotransmitter systems in autism have yielded inconsistent results, so no definite statement can be made about their exact roles in autism (Palmen et al., 2004).

Tyrosine hydroxylase—an enzyme that catalyzes the conversion of L-tyrosine into dihydroxyphenylalanine (DOPA), a precursor for dopamine

N-acetyl-cysteine—a glutathione precursor with antioxidant and anti-inflammatory properties; FDA-approved drug for treatment of respiratory conditions, renal impairment, interstitial lung disease and acetaminophen overdose

In addition to the behavioral deficits and neuropathology, the MIA models also share with autism dysregulation of immune status in the brain. Post mortem brain and cerebrospinal fluid samples from autistic individuals exhibit marked astrogliosis, microglial activation, dysregulation of immune-related genes, and high levels of pro-inflammatory cytokines and chemokines (Vargas et al., 2005; Garbett et al., 2008; Chez et al., 2007; Tetreault et al., 2009; Patterson, 2009). Although LPS itself does not cross the placental barrier, maternal LPS injections yield offspring with MHC II induction along with increased GFAP and microglial staining in various adult (Borrell 2002; Ling et al., 2004) and fetal (Paintlia et al., 2004) brain regions. While several cytokines are elevated in the placenta and amniotic fluid after MIA, mRNA transcripts for a number of cytokines are also elevated in the fetal brain following maternal LPS or poly(I:C) (Urakubo et al., 2001; Cai et al., 2000; Paintlia et al., 2004; Liverman et al., 2006; Golan et al., 2005; Meyer et al., 2008b; Elovitz et al., 2006; Hsiao & Patterson, 2010). The importance of cytokines as soluble mediators of the effects of MIA on fetal brain development was demonstrated using cytokine knockout (KO) mice and mice injected with recombinant cytokines or cytokine-neutralizing antibodies. Interleukin (IL)-6 is necessary and sufficient for mediating the effects of MIA on the development of neurological, behavioral, and transcriptional changes in poly(I:C)-exposed offspring (Figure 52-2; Samuelsson et al., 2006; Smith et al., 2007). In a converse approach, overexpression of the anti-inflammatory cytokine IL-10 suppresses the effects of maternal poly(I:C) on the fetus (Meyer et al., 2008c). Perturbation of IL-10, IL-1, or TNFα can also significantly influence the outcome of MIA in the LPS MIA model (Girard et al., 2010; reviewed in Patterson, 2011).

MHC II—major histocompatibility complex class II; cell surface protein heterodimers found on professional antigen-presenting cells; responsible for presenting extracellular peptides to helper CD4+ T cells to stimulate an immune response

GFAP—glial fibrillary acidic protein; an intermediate filament protein that is used as a marker for astrocytes in the central nervous system

How cytokines induced by MIA alter the course of fetal brain development is largely unknown. The most obvious possibility is by direct action on the developing brain, as both cytokines and chemokines are key modulators of astrogliosis, neurogenesis, microglial activation, and synaptic pruning (Bauer et al., 2007; Deverman & Patterson, 2009), and some maternal cytokines have been reported to cross the placenta (Dahlgren et al., 2006; Zaretsky et al., 2004). A second possibility is that MIA alters the endocrine function and/or the immunological state of the placenta. In fact, poly(I:C) MIA increases maternally-derived IL-6 protein as well as IL-6 mRNA in the placenta. Such placentas exhibit increases in CD69+ decidual macrophages, granulocytes and uterine NK cells, indicating elevated early immune activation. Moreover, maternally-derived IL-6 mediates activation of the JAK/STAT3 pathway in the placenta, which parallels an IL-6-dependent disruption of the growth hormone-insulin-like growth factor axis (Hsiao & Patterson, 2010). Such endocrine changes could affect the development of the fetal brain and immune system, with permanent consequences. It is notable that a greater occurrence of placental trophoblast inclusions is observed in placental tissue from births of children who develop autism spectrum disorder compared to non-ASD controls (Anderson et al., 2007). Moreover, chorioamnionitis and other obstetric complications are significantly associated with socialization and communication deficits in autistic infants (Limperopoulos, 2008).

In this context, it is of interest that several studies have reported that the sera of some mothers of autistic children contain antibodies that bind fetal human, monkey, or rat brain antigens (Zimmerman et al., 2007; Braunschweig et al., 2008; Martin et al., 2008). Most relevant to this review is the further finding that injection of such maternal sera into pregnant mice (Dalton et al., 2003) or purified maternal IgG into pregnant Rhesus monkeys (Martin et al., 2008) yields offspring with several behavioral abnormalities, including hyperactivity and stereotopies in the case of the monkeys. That something is different about the immune system of in the mothers of autistic offspring is further supported by the observation that these mothers are more likely to have a history of autoimmune disease or asthma (e.g., Altadottir et al., 2009). There is also evidence that the peripheral immune system of autistic subjects is abnormal (Pardo & Eberhart, 2007; Enstrom, Van de Water, & Ashwood, 2009). In that light it is interesting that, compared to controls, CD4+ T cells from the spleen and mesenteric lymph nodes of adult mouse MIA offspring display significantly elevated IL-6 and IL-17 responses to in vitro stimulation (Hsiao et al., 2010; Mandal et al., 2010). Furthermore, adult MIA offspring display reduced T cell responses to CNS-specific antigens, despite elevated proliferation of nonspecific T cells (Cardon et al., 2009).

Although it is commonly stated that autism can result from an environmental stimulus acting on a susceptible genetic background, there is little support for this hypothesis thus far. Thus, it is of interest that mice heterozygous for the tuberous sclerosis 2 (*TSC2*) gene display a social interaction deficit only when they are born to mothers treated with poly (I:C) (Ehninger et al., 2010). That is, this deficit is most severe when the MIA environmental risk factor is combined with a genetic defect that, in humans, also carries a very high risk for ASD. In addition, there is an excess of TSC-ASD individuals born during the peak influenza season, an association that is not seen for TSC individuals not displaying ASD symptoms (Ehninger et al., 2010).

Postnatal Vaccination

Although there is currently no convincing evidence that postnatal vaccination is a cause of autism, the occasional coincidence in the timing of routine childhood immunizations with the appearance of autistic symptoms continues to fuel public concern. The measles-mumps-rubella (MMR) vaccine is of particular interest because of the use of live, attenuated virus, but there are currently no rodent models for the effects of MMR on neural development. Moreover, many epidemiological studies have failed to substantiate a connection between MMR vaccination and autism (DeStefano, 2007).

There has been investigation of the effects of thimerosal-containing vaccines (TCVs) on neurodevelopment in rodents. Increased mercury burden from this sodium ethylmercurithiosalicylate preservative is of concern because of known neurotoxic properties of methylmercurials. One study reported that immunogenetic factors can render mice susceptible to thimerosal-induced neurotoxicity (Hornig et al., 2004). The autoimmune-prone SJL/J (H-2^s) strain developed neuropathology and abnormal behavior. However, a recent study failed to replicate the histological and behavioral results (Berman et al., 2008). This latter paper is consistent with several epidemiological studies failing to support a link between thimerosal and autism (Andrews et al., 2004; Schechter & Grether, 2008; Gerber & Offit, 2008 Price et al., 2010).

Terbutaline

The β2 adrenergic receptor is expressed early in fetal brain development, and its activation affects cell proliferation and differentiation. Terbutaline is a selective β2 adrenergic receptor agonist that is used to relax uterine smooth muscle to prevent premature labor and birth. A study of dizygotic twins found an increased rate of concordance for autism if the mother was given terbutaline for 2 weeks (Conners et al., 2005). Further implicating the β2 adrenergic receptor is the finding that certain functional variants of this gene are associated with increased risk for autism (Cheslack-Postava et al., 2007). In modeling this risk factor in rats, neonates are given subcutaneous injections of terbutaline daily, from postnatal days 2 through 5, a time meant to mimic the stage of human brain development at which the drug is given. A significant deficit in PCs was found, but no mention of any spatial restriction of this change was made. Histological changes were reported in the hippocampus and somatosensory cortex as well, including microglial activation in cortex and cerebellum (Rhodes et al., 2004; Zerrate et al., 2007). Also of interest in terms of autism is a finding of increased 5-HT turnover (Slotkin & Seidler, 2007). Behavioral analysis of this model is somewhat disappointing thus far, with female-specific hyperactivity and no change in PPI (Zerrate et al., 2007).

Genetic Manipulations

X-Linked and Autosomal Lesions

Fmr1 Knockout Mice

Fragile X Syndrome (FXS) is an X-linked condition that is the leading genetic cause of mental retardation (Hatton et al., 2006). It is caused by the loss of expression of FMRP, an mRNA-binding protein that is highly expressed in hippocampal and cortical synapses, where it regulates translation of its target mRNAs and thus plays a key role in protein synthesis-dependent functions (Bassell & Warren, 2008). It is estimated that 90% of FXS patients present some autistic-like behaviors, and that 15% to 33% meet the full diagnostic criteria of autism (Cohen et al., 1988; Bailey et al., 1998). Overall, FXS accounts for about 5% of the autistic population (Li et al., 1993). *Fmr1* KO mice display some anatomical features of FXS, such as macro-orchidism and abnormal dendritic development and morphology (The Dutch-Belgian Fragile X Consortium, 1994) and spines are altered in idiopathic autism (Zoghbi, 2003). These mice also display some core behavioral features relevant to autism, including impaired social interaction (McNaughton et al., 2008) and repetitive behaviors. Whether they display learning and memory deficits is unclear (Dobkin et al., 2000; Frankland et al., 2004) and whether they show other autism-related symptoms such as anxiety and hyperactivity depends on the genetic background (Bernardet & Crusio, 2006). The observations that both cognitive performance and behaviors relevant to autistic traits are affected by genetic background is of interest given the genetic variability in humans and the phenotypic heterogeneity in FXS. Although overall resemblance to autism is partial, the presence of two core features of autism indicates that molecular investigation of *Fmr1* KO mice may further our understanding of the genetic etiology of FXS and autistic traits.

The signaling pathways for metabotropic glutamate receptor 5 (mGluR-5) and PAK, a kinase involved in actin remodeling and regulation of synapse structure, represent two plausible therapeutic targets for FXS and autism. A 50% reduction of mGluR-5 expression in *Fmr1* KO mice normalizes dendrite morphology, seizure susceptibility, and inhibitory avoidance extinction (Dolen et al., 2007) (Table 52-2). This supports the mGluR theory, which posits that upregulation of group I mGluR leads to exaggerated protein synthesis-dependent functions, such as long-term depression, and therefore underlies the neuropathology and behavioral traits associated with FXS (Bear, Huber, & Warren, 2004). Interestingly, postnatal inhibition of PAK in the forebrain of *Fmr1* KO mice normalizes dendrite morphology and restores locomotion, repetitive behavior, and anxiety (Hayashi et al., 2007). In addition, in a *Drosophila* model, treatment with

Table 52–2.
Amelioration (orange) or rescue (yellow) of some features of the autism-like phenotype in double mouse mutants phenotypic improvements or reversals indicate functional (direct or indirect) interactions between the targeted genes, whereas persistence of one phenotype (blue) suggests that additional genes contribute to the full phenotype. Investigation of genetic interactions provides insight into the molecular pathways underlying particular facets of autism, and may suggest novel therapeutic targets

Mouse Mutant Relevant to Autism	Rescuer Mouse Mutant	Phenotype of the Double Mutant		
		Behavior	Neuropathology	Additional Parameters
FMR1 knockout (*FMR1* KO) mice	**Dominant negative PAK transgenic mice** 40% inhibition of the catalytic activity of PAK (Hayashi et al., 2007)	Hyperactivity, stereotypy, and hypoanxiety in open field are rescued	Spine density partially restored	
		Memory deficits restored	Spine length comparable to WT	
			Reduced cortical LTP is rescued	
	***Grm5* mutant mice** 50% reduction in mGluR5 expression (Dolen et al., 2007)	Exaggerated inhibitory avoidance extinction rescued	Spine density comparable to WT	Ocular dominance plasticity rescued
			Increased protein synthesis in the hippocampus is prevented	Growth increase at P30 rescued
			Audiogenic seizures attenuated	Macroorchidism not rescued
Germline *Mecp2* mutant	**Conditional BDNF-over-expressing transgenic mice** Increase in BDNF expression (Chang et al., 2006)	Improvement in the running wheel assay (locomotor function)	Neuronal activity indistinguishable from WT	Extension of the lifespan
			Modest increase in brain weight	
Angelman syndrome mutant	**CaMKII-T305V/T306A mutant mice** Mutations in CaMKII that prevent its autophosphorylation (Van Woerden et al., 2007)	Rotarod performance indistinguishable from WT	Absence of audiogenic seizures	Increase in body weight rescued
			75% reduction of propensity for seizures	
		Context-dependant memory restored (hippocampal learning deficit rescued)	Long-term potentiation rescued	
		Improved water maze performance		

mGluR antagonists or protein synthesis inhibitors in adulthood can partially restore deficits in courtship behavior and improve memory (McBride et al., 2005; Bolduc et al., 2008). Two small, open label human trials based on these findings yielded promising results (Berry-Kravis et al., 2008, 2009; Paribello et al., 2010), supporting the use of FXS animal models for preclinical purposes.

Methyl-CpG-Binding Protein-Null, Mutant, and Overexpressing Mice

Rett syndrome is another X-linked disorder that causes mental retardation, primarily affecting females. It is estimated that 95% of Rett syndrome cases are caused by mutations in the methyl-CpG-binding protein (*MECP2*) gene (Chahrour & Zoghbi, 2007), leading to deficiency in this global transcriptional regulator, whose targets include BDNF. During the regression phase of the disease, affected girls display autistic-like behaviors, such as stereotypies as well as reduced social contact and communication. Association between *MECP2* variants and autism have also been reported (Loat et al., 2008). Both *Mecp2*-null mice, and mice in which *Mecp2* is deleted in mature neurons only, exhibit a neurological phenotype consistent with Rett, including hypoactivity, ataxic gait, tremor, limb-clasping, and reduced brain size with smaller neuronal cell bodies in cortex and hippocampus (Chen et al., 2001; Guy et al., 2001). BDNF levels are also reduced in comparison to wild-type (WT) animals, and deletion or over-expression of *Bdnf* in the *Mecp2* mutant brain either accelerates or delays the onset of the symptoms, suggesting a functional interaction between MECP2 and BDNF *in vivo* (Chang et al., 2006). Male mice that carry the truncating mutation, *Mecp2*$^{308/y}$, a common variant observed in Rett patients, display a milder Rett-like phenotype (Shahbazian et al., 2002). Increased synaptic transmission and impaired LTP induction is observed in the mutant mice, whereas spine morphology, BDNF levels, and synaptic biochemical composition are not altered. Behavioral deficits in these mice include enhanced anxiety in the open field, reduced nest-building, and aberrant social interactions. Genetic background modifies performance in the Morris water maze, latent inhibition, and long-term memory tasks (Moretti et al., 2005; Moretti et al., 2006). Mice over-expressing *Mecp2* also develop a progressive neurological disorder with, surprisingly, an enhancement in synaptic plasticity, motor and contextual learning skills between age 10 and 20 weeks, and, at an older age, hypoactivity, seizures, and abnormal forelimb-clasping, all of which are reminiscent of human Rett syndrome (Collins et al., 2004). These results with the various *Mecp2* mouse models indicate that this gene must be tightly regulated under normal conditions. These mice should aid in the search for genes that are regulated by MECP2 (Chahrour et al., 2008) and possibly the various behavioral abnormalities. These mice are also providing reason for optimism regarding the testing of potential treatments for Rett syndrome. In a conditional KO model, it was shown that restoring *Mecp2* expression in immature or even in mature mice results in reversal of the disease phenotype, as measured by behavioral and electrophysiological tests (Guy et al., 2007). Thus, despite the fact that MECP2 function was disrupted during fetal and postnatal development, the disease symptoms can be reversed. In one test of a potential treatment, administration of an active peptide fragment of insulin-like growth factor 1 to *Mecp2* mutant mice extends life span, improves locomotor, heart and breathing functions, and stabilizes a measure of cortical plasticity (Tropea et al., 2009). Such results provide proof-of-principle that these mice can be used to screen candidate treatments of autism-related disorders.

Angelman and Prader-Willi Syndromes

Loss of function of maternal or paternal genes in the imprinted chromosomal region 15q11-q13 causes Angelman Syndrome and Prader-Willi Syndrome (PWS), respectively. Although clinically distinct, both syndromes are behavioral disorders presenting with some autistic traits as well as other diverse symptoms (Veltman et al., 2005). Linkage studies have also associated the 15q11-q13 locus with autism, and maternal duplications of this region account for rare cases of autism (Wassink & Piven, 2000). 70% of Angelman Syndrome patients carry large maternal deletions of 15q11-q13, and display a severe phenotype; yet, mutations in a single gene, *UBE3A*, are sufficient to cause major clinical manifestations of the syndrome. By contrast, PWS is clearly a multigenic syndrome involving 10 imprinted genes, whose individual significance in the etiology of the disorder is not yet fully clarified (Nicholls & Knepper, 2001). *UBE3A* encodes E6-AP, an enzyme that has ubiquitin protein ligase and transcriptional coactivator activities (Nawaz et al., 1999). Two different KO mouse strains with maternally inherited mutations in *Ube3a* display a phenotype consistent with human Angelman Syndrome: motor dysfunction, propensity for seizures, defective learning and memory, and abnormal electroencephalograms (Jiang et al., 1998; Miura et al., 2002). These mice also display deficits in hippocampal LTP and decreased hippocampal CaMKII activity, which may contribute to learning problems in Angelman Syndrome (Weeber et al., 2003). When crossed to mice carrying a mutation in CaMKII that prevents its autophosphorylation, the double mutants no longer exhibit the Angelman Syndrome phenotype (van Woerden et al., 2007). This suggests that increased inhibitory autophosphorylation may provide a molecular basis for deficits in LTP, motor coordination, and seizure propensity. Studies of another Angelman Syndrome mouse model, the *Ube3a*^{YFP} knock-in (KI) reporter mouse, reveal that E6-AP is found in synapses and the nucleus (Dindot et al., 2008). These mice display decreased spine density, an interesting finding because altered spine morphology is observed in Rett and FXS patients, as well as in *Fmr1* KO mice (Kaufmann & Moser, 2000). Thus, the neuropathology in this KI suggests that E6-AP could play a role in spine development and synaptic plasticity. It is relevant that loss of UBE3A activity or its overexpression in *Drosophila* reduces dendritic branching and affects dendrite morphogenesis

(Lu et al., 2009). It remains to be determined whether similar neuropathology is present in the KO mouse lines and Angelman Syndrome patients and whether it contributes to cognitive dysfunction and behavioral abnormalities.

More recently, mutant mice carrying a large maternal deletion from *Ube3a* to *Gabrb3* were generated (Jiang et al., 2010). Similar to the *Ube3a* KO mice, these mutants display increased spontaneous seizure activity, abnormal electroencephalograms, as well as impairments in learning and memory. Additional behavioral tests reveal that they display anxiety traits in the light-dark box, but no difference in pain sensitivity or in PPI. Mutant newborn pups emit more USVs than control mice. This latter observation is of interest, since Angelman syndrome patients show a happy disposition that is currently interpreted as increased signaling behavior. Relevance to autism is also possible, as increased USVs have been reported in *Mecp2* mutant and BTBR pups. However, one would expect to see fewer USVs in an autism model, given the deficits in communication in ASD. Comparative studies of the various mouse models of Angelman syndrome should yield new insights into the contribution of additional, maternally imprinted genes of this region, or biallelically expressed genes such as *Gabrb3* or *Atp10a*. Mouse models for PWS with deletion of the corresponding murine imprinted locus have been generated, but early postnatal lethality has precluded behavioral characterization (Yang et al., 1998). Among the mice engineered to carry a mutation in one candidate gene of the imprinted region, *Necdin* (*Ndn*), paternally-deficient mice display some behavioral traits reminiscent of PWS, such as skin-scraping, improved performance in Morris water maze, and reduced numbers of hypothalamic oxytocin- and LHRH-producing neurons (Muscatelli et al., 2000). Serotonergic alterations are also observed in these mice and are linked to respiratory deficiency (Zanella et al., 2008). All these findings might be relevant to autism, because repetitive self-injury, enhanced visual-spatial skills, oxytocin abnormalities, and alterations in serotonin levels have been described in autism. As with Angelman syndrome mice, *Necdin* mutant mice require further behavioral characterization.

Pten Mutant Mice

Phosphatase and tensin homolog on chromosome 10, PTEN, is a tumor suppressor that negatively regulates phosphatidylinositol 3-kinase PI3K/Akt signaling, a pathway that promotes cell growth, proliferation, and survival. Germline mutations in *PTEN* cause Cowden and Bannayan–Riley–Ruvalcaba syndromes (CS and BRRS, respectively). CS and BRRS are characterized by benign and malignant tumors in multiple organs as well as brain disorders such as macrocephaly, mental retardation, and seizure. Association between these syndromes—particularly CS—and autism has occasionally been reported (Zori et al., 1998; Goffin et al., 2001; Pilarski & Eng, 2004). Moreover, genetic screening identified *PTEN* mutations in a subset of autistic individuals who display macrocephaly (Butler et al., 2005; Buxbaum et al., 2007), an anatomical anomaly also present in 15% to 20% of autistic patients (Lainhart et al., 2006). Of particular interest is the mouse strain Nse-cre-*Pten*$^{loxP/loxP}$, in which a *Pten* deletion is restricted to differentiated neurons in the cerebral cortex and hippocampus (Kwon et al., 2006). These mutants develop forebrain macrocephaly resulting from neuronal hypertrophy in the cortex and hippocampus. In addition, analysis of the hippocampus shows increased dendritic and axonal growth, ectopic positioning of axons and dendrites of granule neurons and elevated synapse number.

Abnormalities in *Pten*-deleted neurons correlate with enhanced levels of phosphorylated Akt and its downstream effectors, mTOR and S6. Components of the mTOR/S6K/S6 pathway are present in dendrites, where they are involved in the regulation of protein synthesis. Protein synthesis in dendrites is believed to modulate synapse morphology and function and thus is involved in synapse plasticity. These mice display behaviors reminiscent of autism, such as deficits in social interaction, exaggerated responses to sensory stimuli, decreased PPI (but only at one prepulse stimulus intensity), anxiety-like behavior in the open field, and learning deficits in the Morris water maze. However, no impairments in fear conditioning, elevated plus maze, or motor activity are observed. Increased spine density and social deficits are also observed in the *Fmr1* KO. In this context, it is relevant that ribosomal S6 kinase (S6K1), a component of the mTOR/PI3K signaling cascade, was recently identified as a major *Fmrp* kinase (Narayanan et al., 2008). Because the phosphorylation status of FMRP may govern translational regulation of its target mRNAs, upstream modulators of the mTOR/PI3K pathway such as PTEN may modulate synaptic function by affecting FMRP phosphorylation status (Bassell & Warren, 2008). Thus, FMRP phosphorylation may be affected in CS, BRRS, and also tuberous sclerosis (TSC), another human disorder associated with autism, caused by mutations in the *TSC1/2* complex. Indeed, hamartin and tuberin, the gene products of *TSC1* and *TSC2*, can inhibit mTOR (Yates, 2006). Moreover, mTOR signaling is dysregulated in the *Fmrp*-deficient mouse (Sharma et al., 2010). Taken together, these data support the hypothesis that synaptic alteration may underlie autistic-like behaviors (Zoghbi, 2003) and highlight the mTOR pathway as a key regulator of synaptic function. In addition, as in the case of the *Mecp2* mice, the *Tsc2+/-* mouse model responds to treatment in adulthood. Brief administration of the mTOR inhibitor rapamycin rescues synaptic plasticity and the behavioral deficits in the TSC model (Ehninger et al., 2009). Moreover, early phase clinical trials suggest that cognitive features of TSC may be reversible in adult humans (De Vries, 2010).

Autism Candidate Genes

Neuroligins 3 and 4

Recent findings in autism genetics have revealed several, rare causal variants that are associated with ASD (Betancur,

Sakurai, & Buxbaum, 2009). Neuroligins (NLGNs) constitute a family of transmembrane postsynaptic proteins, which, together with their presynaptic and intracellular binding partners, the β-neurexins and SHANK3, respectively, play a key role in synaptic maturation and transmission. *NLGN3* and *-4* were identified in two X-chromosome loci previously associated with ASDs (Jamain et al., 2003). Thus far, one missense mutation in *NLGN3* and four missense and two nonsense mutations in *NLGN4* have been identified in a very small number of individuals with ASDs (Jamain et al., 2003; Laumonnier et al., 2004; Yan et al., 2005), supporting the hypothesis that synaptic dysfunction is important in ASDs. Mutations in neurexin and *SHANK3* are also found in ASD probands, but whether they are involved in ASD etiology is controversial (Sudhof, 2008). There is currently no KO for *Shank3*, but a KO for *Shank1*, the closest relative to *Shank3*, was recently created. These mutants display morphological alterations in hippocampal neurons that are associated with a reduction in basal synaptic transmission, but no change in several other electrophysiological parameters (LTP, LTD, and L-LTP). Behaviorally, *Shank1* KO mice exhibit increased anxiety, impaired contextual fear memory, and, surprisingly, enhanced performance in a spatial learning task but impaired memory retention of that task (Hung et al., 2008). Additional behavioral tasks relevant to the three core symptoms have yet to be reported.

Results with *Nlgn3* and *-4* mutant mice confirm the functional significance of NLGNs in synaptic function. A *Nlgn3* KI mouse was engineered with a point mutation in the endogenous mouse gene that is identical to the relevant human NLGN-3 gene (Tabuchi et al., 2007). These mice display increased inhibitory synaptic transmission without a change in excitatory transmission, a phenotype not observed in *Nlgn3* KO mice, emphasizing the disparity between missense and nonsense mutations. It will be of interest to characterize the behavior of the KO mice to check for differential phenotypes. The augmentation in inhibitory synaptic transmission in the *Nlgn3* KI mice is accompanied by a deficit in social interaction and, as observed in the *Shank1* KO, enhanced spatial learning ability. These results are surprising because *(1)* a loss, rather than a gain of inhibition in different neural systems was hypothesized to contribute to ASDs (Hussman, 2001; Rubenstein & Merzenich, 2003), and *(2)* the individuals identified with mutations in *NLGN3* and *-4* do not exhibit potentiated learning skills. The latter observations are consistent with a report of minimal aberrant behaviors in the *Nlgn-3* KI mice (Chadman et al., 2008). Nevertheless, the results suggesting that a disequilibrium between excitatory and inhibitory synapses can affect social behavior (Sudhof, 2008) and that decreasing inhibitory transmission may be an effective therapy in some autism patients are worth pursuing. In fact, administration of the NMDA receptor partial co-agonist D-cycloserine can rescue the excessive grooming behavior in adult *Nlgn1* KO mice (Blundell et al., 2010).

Unlike humans, the rodent *Nlgn4* gene localizes to a still unknown autosome. Although there is only a 57% homology between the two species, the protein is found in synapses in both. Although *Nlgn4* KO mice display abnormalities in two of the three core autistic symptoms, reciprocal social interaction, and impaired communication, as approximated by measuring USVs, they do not display repetitive behavior or impairments in some of the other autism symptoms such as sensory ability, sensorimotor gating, locomotion, exploratory activity, anxiety, or learning and memory (Jamain et al., 2008). These observations are consistent with those seen in patients with the *NLGN4* mutation, who do not show these comorbid features. MRI analysis of the brains of *Nlgn4* KO mice show a slight reduction in size of the total brain, cerebellum, and brain stem, and some of these neuroanatomical changes are reminiscent of autism.

To summarize, several *Nlgn* models exhibit strong construct validity with the rare human mutations associated with human ASDs. Moreover, the face validity of the *Nlgn4* KO mice is fairly good at the behavioral level, but much remains to be done on its neuropathology.

CNTNAP2

One of the most validated susceptibility genes is contactin associated protein-like2 (*CNTNAP2*). This gene encodes a member of the neuronal neurexin superfamily that is involved in neuron-glial interactions and is very likely to be important in brain development (Abrahams et al., 2008b). An intriguing feature of CNTNAP2 is its enriched expression in circuits in the human cortex that are important for language development. Moreover, its expression is enriched in song nuclei important for vocal learning in the zebra finch, and feature is male-specific, as is the song behavior (Panaitof et al., 2010). In addition, (*CNTNAP2*) polymorphisms are associated with language disorders, and the expression of this gene can be regulated by FOXP2, a transcription factor that, when mutated, can cause language and speech disorders (Vernes et al., 2008). In light of these associations, it is important that recent study of the *Cntnap2* KO mouse reveals a deficit in USVs. Moreover, these mice display the other core features of autism, repetitive behavior and a social interaction deficit. They also exhibit several other features of ASD: seizures, mild cortical laminar disorganization and hyperactivity (D. H. Geschwind, personal communication).

EN2

Engrailed homeobox 1 (*EN1*) and 2 encode transcription factors expressed during embryonic and postnatal stages that regulate the development of the cerebellum. *EN2* localizes in proximity to an autism susceptibility locus on chromosome 7 (Liu et al., 2001; Alarcon et al., 2002), and genetic variations in *EN2* have also been reported to associate with ASDs (Petit et al., 1995; Gharani et al., 2004; Benayed et al., 2005; Wang et al., 2008; Yang et al., 2008), although one report could not replicate such association (Zhong et al., 2003). Although mice homozygous for a mutation in *En-1* lack a cerebellum and die shortly after birth (Wurst, Auerbach, & Joyner, 1994), *En2* KO mice are viable and display some cerebellar pathologies resembling those reported in the brains of some autistic individuals, such as a decreased PC number, hypoplasia, and abnormal foliation (Kuemerle et al., 1997; Amaral, Schumann, & Nordahl, 2008). The juvenile KO mice display reduced social and play behaviors, and abnormal social behavior and repetitive self-grooming as adults (Cheh et al., 2006). In addition, although *En2* KO mice display normal locomotor activity in the open field, motor deficits are observed in specific tasks such as mid-air righting, hanging-wire grip strength, and rotorod. Learning and memory impairments are also evident in the water maze and modified open field with objects. At the neurochemical level, mutant mice exhibit increased cerebellar serotonin compared to controls but no alteration in dopamine levels in hippocampus, striatum, and frontal cortex or cerebellum. Thus, *En2* KO mice display face validity for autism, except for the motor deficits, which can interfere with some behavioral tests. It will be of interest to examine USVs in this model.

Serotonin

Several lines of evidence indicate that changes in serotonin signaling may contribute to autism pathogenesis. Serotonin levels in platelets are elevated in autistic patients (Cook & Leventhal, 1996), and numerous polymorphisms in genes implicated in 5-HT signaling or metabolism have been reported in autism, including the serotonin-transporter gene *SLC6A4* (*SERT*), monoamine oxidase A (*MAOA*), tryptophan 2,3 dioxygenase gene, and two serotonin receptors, 5-HT2A (*HTR2A*) and 5-HT7 (*HTR7*). Pharmacological modulation of the serotonin system using the 5-HT receptor antagonist risperidone improves ritualistic behavior and irritability of autistic children and, similarly, selective 5-HT reuptake inhibitors ameliorate repetitive thoughts and behaviors as well as mood disturbances. Conversely, depletion of tryptophan, a serotonin precursor, aggravates autistic symptoms (Hollander et al., 2005). Abnormalities in brain serotonin synthesis at different ages, as well as cortical asymmetries in serotonin synthesis, have been reported in children with autism (Chugani et al., 1997; Chugani et al., 1999). These alterations could be linked to abnormalities in cortical minicolumn organization in autism (Casanova & Tillquist, 2008). Serotonin signaling modulates various aspects of pre- and postnatal brain development (Gaspar, Cases, & Maroteaux, 2003), and some mouse lines with disruption in the 5-HT system show neuropathology consistent with those observed in autism. Behavioral changes observed in these mutants relate to mood, aggression, anxiety, depression, seizure, and learning and memory, all of which are relevant to autism.

A mouse line in which serotonin signaling is impaired is the *Dhcr7* mutant. DHCR7 (7-dehydrocholesterol reductase) is an enzyme required for the biosynthesis of cholesterol, and mice lacking functional *Dhcr7* display an increase in the area and intensity of serotonin immunoreactivity in the embryonic hindbrain (Waage-Baudet et al., 2003). Unfortunately, *Dhcr7* KO mice die shortly after birth, precluding behavioral studies. In humans, *DHCR7* deficiency causes the Smith–Lemli–Opitz syndrome (SLOS), a disease characterized by dysmorphic facial features, mental retardation, and limb defects (Yu & Patel, 2005). Approximately 50% of patients with SLOS are also diagnosed with autism (Tierney et al., 2001). Levels of cholesterol are decreased in some idiopathic autistic children (Tierney et al., 2006), and cholesterol dietary supplementation improves autistic-like behavior of patients with SLOS (Aneja & Tierney, 2008). Presently, the mechanisms by which cholesterol deficiency affects serotonin pathways are not fully elucidated, but it is known that cholesterol can modulate the functional activity of MAO (Caramona et al., 1996) and SERT (Scanlon, Williams, & Schloss, 2001). Investigation of *Dhcr7* heterozygous mice or development of conditional mutants could further the understanding of the role of cholesterol in autism.

Bdnf-deficient mice also display alterations in the serotonin system. Signaling mediated by BDNF and its receptor tyrosine kinase (TrkB) is crucial for serotonergic neuronal development, as well as a wide variety of other neuronal functions. Variants in the *BDNF* gene have been associated with autism (Nishimura et al., 2007), and post mortem analysis of brains from autistic adults show enhanced levels of BDNF (Perry et al., 2001), whereas blood and serum levels in autism are controversial (cf. Croen et al., 2008). Various *Bdnf* or *TrkB* mutant mouse lines are available, including heterozygous null mice (homozygous KOs are not viable), conditional, and inducible *Bdnf* KO mice. Presence and severity of behavioral alterations in these mice depends on the stage at which BDNF is depleted, the brain regions targeted for BDNF deficiency, and the gender of the mutants (cf. Monteggia et al., 2004). Autistic-like behavioral impairments commonly reported are heightened aggression, hyperactivity, depression-like traits, and, in some instances, altered locomotor activity. Hyperphagia is reported in some *Bdnf* mutant lines, a finding inconsistent with autism *per se* but also observed in PWS. Despite behavioral deficits, surprisingly, dendritic morphology and GAD67 are not altered in brains from fetal and postnatal KOs (Hashimoto et al., 2005; Hill et al., 2005). In contrast, double *Bdnf +/-* x *Sert -/-* mutants display exacerbated anxiety in the elevated plus maze, greater elevation in plasma ACTH after stressful stimulus, and reduction in the size of dendrites of hippocampal and hypothalamic neurons in comparison to WT, *Sert+/+* x *Bdnf+/-* and *Sert-/-*x *Bdnf +/+* mice (Ren-Patterson et al., 2005). Because autism is often considered to be a multigenic disorder, investigation of gene/gene interaction is a logical approach.

Urokinase Plasminogen Activator Receptor Knockout Mice

Variations in the *MET* gene encoding a receptor tyrosine kinase are associated with autism (Campbell et al., 2006). Moreover, post mortem analysis of cortical tissue from autistic individuals reveals decreased levels of MET protein in comparison to matched controls (Campbell et al., 2007). Disruption in signaling mediated by MET and its ligand, hepatocyte growth factor/scatter factor (HGF/SF), may be particularly relevant to the etiology of the disorder because, in addition to playing a key role in the CNS during development and adulthood, it is also involved in gastrointestinal repair and regulation of the immune system, two other systems that are altered in autism (Vargas et al., 2005). The PI3K/Akt pathway is one of the prominent signaling cascades activated by MET, which thereby antagonizes PTEN function. In the CNS, HGF/SF-MET signaling promotes the migration of cortical interneurons during development (Powell, Mars, & Levitt, 2001), contributes to cerebellar development and function (Leraci, Forni, & Ponzetto, 2002), stimulates dendritic growth in cortical neurons (Gutierrez et al., 2004), and induces protein clustering at excitatory synapses (Tyndall & Walikonis, 2006). Although genetic deletion of *Met* causes embryonic lethality, the KO of urokinase plasminogen activator receptor (*uPAR*), which exhibits reduced uPA activity (the protease required for the activation of HGF), is viable and displays a diminution in HGF levels and, as observed in autism, in MET levels. The *uPAR* KO mice display increased anxiety and are prone to seizures (Powell et al., 2003), features that are relevant to autism (Tuchman & Rapin, 2002). Whether these mice display deficits in any core symptoms of the disorder has not been reported. Gastrointestinal and immune pathology also needs to be assessed in these mutants.

Disrupted in Schizophrenia-1

A balanced translocation between chromosome 1 and 11 t(1;11) (q42.2;q14.1) cosegregates with schizophrenia and related disorders in a large Scottish family (St Clair et al., 1990; Blackwood et al., 2001). Disrupted in Schizophrenia-1 (*DISC1*) is altered by this translocation (Muir et al., 1995; Millar et al., 2000; Millar et al., 2001), and there is an association between variations within the *DISC* locus and autism and Asperger syndrome (Kilpinen et al., 2008). DISC1 is a scaffold protein, which, through interactions with various proteins (e.g., PDE4B, LIS1, NDEL1, NDE1, CIT, MAP1A), regulates cAMP signaling, cortical neuron migration, neurite outgrowth, glutamatergic neurotransmission, and synaptogenesis (Muir, Pickard, & Blackwood, 2008). There are a number of *Disc1* mouse variants currently available: mice carrying a truncated version of the endogenous *Disc1* ortholog, transgenic lines with inducible expression of mutant human DISC1 (hDISC1), and lines carrying N-ethyl-N-nitrosourea-induced mutations in *Disc1* (Chubb et al., 2008). Hippocampal neurons in mice with mutations of endogenous *Disc1* display dendritic misorientation and reduced number of spines, as observed in the *Fmr1* KO mice. These mice display a working memory deficit but do not show deficits in PPI or latent inhibition (Koike et al., 2006; Kvajo et al., 2008). Transgenic mice expressing hDISC1 in forebrain regions show a mild enlargement of the lateral ventricles in comparison to WT animals, and neurite outgrowth is decreased in primary cortical neurons from these mutants. These neuropathologies are associated with altered social interaction and enhanced spontaneous locomotor activity in male hDISC1 mice and with mild impairment in spatial memory in females (Pletnikov et al., 2008). Tests assessing repetitive behavior and ultrasonic vocalizations remain to be reported. Further study of neuropathology in the various strains will also be important.

Oxytocin and Vasopressin

Neuropeptides and their associated receptors play a central role in the regulation of complex social behaviors. Several lines of evidence suggest that functional alterations in these systems may contribute not only to social deficits in autism but also to repetitive behaviors. *(1)* A reduction in oxytocin (OXT) plasma levels, associated with an elevation in the prohormone form, is observed in autistic children (Modahl et al., 1998; Green et al., 2001). Mixed results have been reported for OXT plasma levels in high-functioning adult autistic patients(Jansen et al., 2006; Andari et al., 2010). *(2)* Intranasal infusion of OXT reduces stereotyped behavior and improves eye contact, social memory and use of social information in high functioning autistic patients (Hollander et al., 2003, 2007; Guastella et al., 2009; Andari et al., 2010). *(3)* Genetic variations in OXT receptor and vasopressin receptor V1aR can be associated with autism (Donaldson & Young, 2008; Israel et al., 2008; Gregory et al., 2009). *(4)* Oxytocin receptor mRNA is decreased in post-mortem autism temporal cortex (Gregeory et al., 2009).

Current knowledge derived from studies in *Oxt* and *Oxt* receptor (*Oxtr*) KO mice underscore the subtle role of this system in aggression and anxiety. Thus, *Oxt* KO adult male progeny from homozygous crosses display high levels of aggression, whereas levels of aggression in *Oxt* KO adult male progeny from heterozygous crosses are either less pronounced or similar to WT mice, suggesting that absence of *OXT* during prenatal stages modulates the development of aggression in adulthood (Ferguson et al., 2000; Winslow et al., 2000; Takayanagi et al., 2005). *Oxt* KO female mice also display exaggerated aggression under controlled stress conditions designed to mimic the natural environment, indicating a possible interaction between the postnatal environment and the *OXT* system (Ragnauth et al., 2005). Similarly, *Oxtr* KO adult males display elevated aggressive behavior, as well as deficits in social discrimination (Takayanagi et al., 2005). *Oxt* KO adult mice nevertheless display reduced anxiety in the plus maze and acoustic startle reflex, a finding inconsistent with autism. In addition, as infants, both *Oxt* and *Oxtr* KO males emit fewer USVs in the isolation test than WT animals, which is also suggestive of decreased anxiety during maternal separation, but is also consistent with the lack of communication in ASD. The *Oxt* KO mice fail to recognize familiar conspecifics upon repeated social encounters, although olfactory and nonsocial memory are intact (Winslow & Insel, 2002). This has been interpreted as an autism-like social deficit, although social amnesia has not been described in autism. Comprehensive neuropathology remains to be reported in these strains. Given the implications for ASD in the human findings, further study of *Oxt* mutant mice is warranted, although striking species differences are apparent for *OXT* and vasopressin, and their receptors (Insel, 2010).

Male *V1aR* KO mice exhibit deficits in olfactory social recognition and social interaction (Bielsky et al., 2004; Egashira et al., 2007). Similarly to *Oxt* and *Oxtr* KO mice, *V1aR* KO mice show reduced anxiety-like behavior in the elevated plus maze and the open field and the light/dark box, although high levels of anxiety are observed in the WT animals in comparison to other reports. No deficits in learning and memory in the Morris water maze or in PPI are detected, indicating that the face validity of this model is partial. *V1bR* KO adult females emit fewer USVs in a resident-intruder test. Although the number of USVs emitted by infant mutants is not affected during the conventional pup separation test, mutant pups fail to display maternal potentiation of USVs, which could suggest either a defect in a cognitive component or reduced anxiety (Scattoni et al., 2008). Although reduced anxiety is inconsistent with autism, V1bR antagonists could be tested to lower anxiety.

BTBR Mice

The BTBR mouse strain exhibits low levels of sociability at juvenile and adult ages, as well as abnormal social learning in the transmission of food preference test. Moreover, BTBR mice show a high level of spontaneous repetitive grooming, poor shift performance in a hole-board task, and a deficit in the water maze reversal task, which can be interpreted as the resistance to change in routine that is observed in autism (Bolivar, Walters, & Phoenix, 2007; Moy et al., 2007; Yang, Zhodzishsky, & Crawley, 2007; McFarlane et al., 2008; Moy et al., 2008). Finally, BTBR pups separated from their mother emit more and longer USVs in comparison to C57 pups (Scattoni et al., 2008). Their repertoire of vocalizations is also narrower in comparison to pups from standard mouse strains. The latter observation is significant, as human infants later diagnosed with autism make unusual vocalizations (Johnson, 2008). However, one might expect to see lower rates of USVs in pups if modeling the ASD communication deficit. Such a deficit is reported in adult BTBR mice (Wohr et al., 2010). Detailed study of the fine structure of USVs, as well as their behavioral functions in adult mice, is an important area for future studies of animal models of psychiatric disease.

A recent study indicates that BTBR mice display an exaggerated response to stress that is associated with high blood levels of corticosterone in comparison to C57 mice (Benno et al., 2009). Thus, it is not clear whether enhanced stress causes or aggravates the behavioral phenotype of these mice. Key anatomical features of BTBR mice are the absence of the corpus callosum and a reduced hippocampal commissure. These deficits correlate with impaired contextual fear memory, which could arise from an increased susceptibility to de-potentiation. Otherwise, electrophysiological properties of hippocampal slices from BTBR (LTP, paired pulse facilitation, and basal synaptic transmission) are similar to those of C57 (MacPherson et al., 2008). Thus, several BTBR behaviors are consistent with autism, and the most striking anatomical feature in this strain is consistent with many, but not all, studies of the corpus callosum in autism (Amaral, Schumann, & Nordahl, 2008).

A difficulty with this line is that comparisons are necessarily made to other, unrelated mouse lines, and it is not clear to which line(s) BTBR should be compared. For instance, similar to BTBR mice, but unlike C57 mice, BALB/c mice display low social behavior, reduced USVs and reduced empathy-like behavior (Silverman et al., 2010). Because it is likely that there is a wide variety of genetic differences between such strains, comparing their behaviors is not equivalent to comparing behaviors and neuropathology between mutant and WT mice of the same genetic background. Nonetheless, the search for the genes causing behavioral phenotypes is ongoing, and a single nucleotide polymorphism in *Kmo*, which encodes kynurenine 3-hydroxylase, has been found in BTBR mice when compared to unrelated strains (McFarlane et al., 2008). This enzyme regulates the synthesis of kynurenic acid, a neuroprotective compound for which levels are abnormal in other neuropsychiatric diseases, including schizophrenia.

Myocyte Enhancer Factor 2 KO mice

A recent homozygosity mapping study of autism loci identified several candidate genes that are regulated by myocyte enhancer factor 2 (MEF2) transcription factors (Morrow et al., 2008). MEF2 factors mediate synapse elimination. Conditional KO of *Mef2c* at the neural stem cell stage yields mice with fewer, smaller, and more compacted neurons that exhibit what is interpreted as immature electrophysiological network properties. It is of interest that these mice display marked paw-clasping stereotypy, possibly altered spatial memory, and complex changes in anxiety tests when tested as adults (Li et al., 2008). Indeed, such behaviors resemble those observed in *Mecp2* mutants. In addition, a recent study revealed that active FMRP is required for MEF2-dependant synapse elimination, thus further pinpointing the molecular factors at play in regulating synapse number (Pfeiffer et al., 2010).

Copy Number Variations

Copy number variations (CNVs) are DNA fragments whose number is altered by deletion or duplication between various individuals. They are thought to account for a significant proportion of normal phenotypic variation within the human population (Freeman et al., 2006). Several recent studies have indicated that de novo CNVs associate with autism. Interestingly, some of the genes identified within the loci subject to CNVs in autism are related to synaptic or neuronal activity (e.g., *SHANK3*, *NLGN4*, and *NRXN1*) (for reviews, *see* Abrahams & Geschwind, 2008a; Cook & Scherer, 2008). Thus, genome-wide investigation of CNVs might further implicate or reveal novel candidate genes in autism, for which rodent mutant lines can be developed.

Lesions

Autism is a common occurrence in children with brain lesions caused by hemorrhage or tumor (Asano et al., 2001; Limperopoulos et al., 2007). One example of this is TSC, a genetic disorder that causes benign lesions or tumors to form in many different organs, including the brain. MRI and positron emission tomography (PET) demonstrate correlations between abnormalities in the cortex and communication deficits, whereas changes in subcortical circuits correlate with stereotypies and lack of social interaction (Asano et al., 2001). Therefore, the study of autism in children with TSC and the development of animal lesion models may provide clues about autistic behavior.

Tuberous sclerosis complex (TSC)—a genetic disorder that causes tumors to form in many different organs, including the brain; associated with developmental delay, mental retardation and autism and attributed to two genes: *TSC1* gene (harmartin) located on chromosome 9 and *TSC2* gene (tuberin) located on chromosome 16

Although brain lesions have commonly been used in animal models to study the circuitry underlying behaviors (Lavond & Steinmetz, 2003), interpretation of such results can be complex. First, the loss of a behavior does not prove that the lesioned brain area is the originating source for brain activity associated with that behavior. Second, lesions often damage axons passing through the brain area of interest, giving rise to erroneous conclusions about that brain region's importance in the behavior. Third, behavioral testing is necessarily performed on subjects responding to injury with various inflammatory and regenerative mechanisms whose influence on behavior is poorly understood. More recent advances in the ability to silence particular neuronal populations using genetic techniques promise much greater sophistication in unraveling the circuitry underlying behavior.

Amygdala

The amygdala has reciprocal connections with many areas, including the orbital and medial prefrontal cortex and the hippocampus, which are implicated in autism. Several post mortem studies have demonstrated amygdala abnormalities in autistic subjects, such as altered developmental trajectory and fewer neurons (Amaral et al., 2008). In case reports, children with severe temporal lobe damage resulting from viral encephalitis, tumors, or other factors developed autistic symptoms (Sweeten et al., 2002). In children with TSC, symptoms of autism are strongly related to the presence of tubers in the temporal lobe (Gillberg et al., 1994). These findings, along with recent functional neuroimaging data, led Baron-Cohen to develop an "amygdala theory of autism" (2000), which suggests a crucial role for the amygdala in the impairment of social behavior. In addition, patients with amygdala lesions (Adolphs, 2003) and individuals with autism (Adolphs et al., 2001) appear to have similar deficits in recognizing complex emotions in facial expressions. Neonatal ibotenic acid lesion of the amygdala in the rat has been proposed as an animal model of neurodevelopmental disorders such as autism (Daenen et al., 2001; 2002a; 2002b; Diergaarde et al., 2004). In this model, animals display increased latency to play with social partners, decreased duration of contact, and hyperactivity as well as decreased adaptation and habituation to the open field, which is interpreted as locomotor stereotypy and low anxiety (Daenen et al., 2001; 2002a). Thus, excitotoxic lesions of the amygdala in the neonatal rat produce multiple behavioral abnormalities relevant to autism. This conclusion differs from that found in similar nonhuman primate studies (Amaral et al., 2003). Moreover, humans with amygdala lesions do not display deficits in social interaction like those seen in autism (Amaral et al., 2003).

Ibotenic acid—a powerful neurotoxin that occurs in the mushrooms Amanita muscaria and Amanita pantherina, among others

Hippocampus

Limbic system dysfunction is fundamental to autism (Amaral et al., 2008). Neonatal ibotenic acid lesion of the hippocampus in the rat causes locomotor stereotypy in the open field test, but there are mixed results concerning deficits in social behavior early in life or in adulthood (Daenen et al., 2002b; Silva-Gomez et al., 2003) In rodent models, hippocampal lesions grossly impair memory, and autistic subjects display a selective deficit in hippocampal-dependent memory (Lathe, 2006). Because there are only a few studies analyzing social behavior in hippocampus-lesioned rats, and the damage in this area has no, or only a temporary, effect in monkeys (Amaral et al., 2003), more research is required in this area.

Prefrontal Cortex

Patients who suffer damage to the prefrontal cortex have problems in making decisions and in behaving appropriately in social situations where empathy and social and moral reasoning are appropriate (Anderson et al., 1999; Koenigs et al., 2007). There is also evidence that both the medial temporal lobe and dorsolateral prefrontal cortex are implicated in autism (Amaral et al., 2008). Moreover, lesions to the orbital and medial prefrontal cortex in nonhuman primates cause abnormal social personality expression, decision making, and loss of position within the social group (Butter & Snyder, 1972). Lesioning prefrontal cortex also provokes a decrease in positive social behaviors (grooming, huddling, and near-body contact) and socially communicative facial, vocal, and postural behaviors, as well as an increase in inappropriate social interactions (Myers et al., 1973). Consistent with these results are ibotenic acid lesion studies of the medial prefrontal cortex in rats (Schneider & Koch, 2005). In addition, the lesion-induced disturbances of juvenile play behavior in rodents may also contribute to the social deficits observed in adult animals, because play-fighting is important for the development of communicative skills and appropriate behavioral patterns. Further work on the rodent model showed that neonatal lesion of the medial prefrontal cortex leads to reduced anxiety in the elevated plus maze, increased motor activity in open field, and, more interestingly, perseverative behavior in a reward-related test of operant behavior (Schwabe et al., 2006). This is in line with the behavioral changes reported for cerebellum lesion models.

Perseverative behavior—common feature of autism, expressed as "insistence on sameness"; believed to result from the inability to understand and cope with novel situations.

Cerebellum

The cerebellum is involved not only in the regulation of motor skills but also in higher functions, including cognition, language, and emotional expression (Turner et al., 2007). Adults and children with cerebellar lesions have high social isolation, communicative disturbance, and deficits in cognitive processing (Eluvathingal et al., 2006; Limperopoulos et al., 2007). A common finding in autism is a loss of PCs (72% of cases; Palmen et al., 2004; 79% of cases; Amaral et al., 2008). Therefore, surgical or toxin lesions of the cerebellum are of particular interest in studying animal models of autism. In addition to cognitive dysfunction reported in a rat model of cerebellum lesion (Gaytan-Tocaven & Olvera-Cortes, 2004), there are two rat models displaying perseverative behavior, which is common in autism and is expressed as insistence on sameness as well as inability to understand and cope with novel situations. This kind of behavior is found in a rat model of early (P10) midline cerebellar lesion (Bobee et al., 2000). In addition, these animals display elevated spontaneous motor activity and exhibit lack of attention to environmental distractors. Unlike the autism phenotype, however, the lesioned animals are neophilic and less anxious than controls. Vermis-lesioned rats show a decreased coefficient of learning during extended training of an instrumental task, which is interpreted as perseverative behavior (Callu et al., 2007).

In sum, the lesion models support dysfunction in autism in several areas: the prefrontal cortex, the temporal lobe and the cerebellum. This may be because an early defect in the functioning of these areas of the brain alters the development of multiple other areas, however. Behavioral analysis has focused primarily on motor tasks and anxiety. These lesion models display hyperactivity and low anxiety in the open field, which is unlike the autism phenotype (Lathe, 2006). No changes, or decreased general social activity, are reported for rodent models with lesions in the amygdala, prefrontal cortex, or hippocampus. Early damage to the amygdala or the prefrontal cortex results in altered juvenile play behavior, the earliest form of non-mother-directed social behavior in rodents. Thus far, these lesion models display two types of behaviors impaired in autism—namely, a deficit in social behavior and stereotypy. It will be important to assay other types of social and communicative behavior (for example, ultrasonic vocalizations in different social contexts), as well as to compare the changes in brain pathology, biochemistry, and gene expression to those seen in autism.

Conclusions

Given that the background genotypes of the rat and mouse strains that are used for experiments are somewhat arbitrary, and that genotype is very important in autism, it is remarkable that both behaviors and neuropathology consistent with autism can be reproduced in rodents. This issue of background genotype could potentially become increasingly important as more sophisticated models incorporating human genetic variants are introduced. Although no single rodent model has yet been thoroughly studied at all levels of investigation, several models have already been explored in some depth. Among those that display face and construct validity are the maternal valproate and maternal infection models of environmental risk factors, as well as the NLGN-4, Frmr1, CNTNAP2, and MeCP2 models of genetic risk factors. Nonetheless, no model has been thoroughly investigated with all available experimental tools, including behavior, histology, biochemistry, electrophysiology, and imaging.

Challenges and Future Directions

- The fine structure of ultrasonic vocalizations, as well as their behavioral functions in adult mice, are intriguing areas for future study of potential communication abnormalities.
- Theory of mind, the ability to intuit another's thinking, is an important deficit in autism. An analogous test of empathy can be done in mice, where observing cage mates experience stressful experiences can alter the witness' responses to later tests (Langford et al., 2006; Chen, Panksepp & Lahvis, 2009). This assay should be widely tested in the available environmental and genetic models.
- To reach their full potential in mimicking the human situation, models of candidate genes should carry the variant identified in the human studies, not just a KO of the gene.
- It is now possible to test the hypothesis that the full autism phenotype may emerge from environmental risk factors acting on susceptibility genotypes.

- Multi-electrode recording, functional imaging, and immediate early gene activation studies will be important for mapping patterns of functional activity in rodent models and comparing it to fMRI data from human subjects.
- Translational, preclinical studies in several mouse models have already stimulated small clinical trials in ASD-related disorders. Although this will likely accelerate in the near future, significant species differences will undoubtedly lead to failures along the way.

SUGGESTED READINGS

Patterson, P. H. (2009). Immune involvement in schizophrenia and autism: Etiology, pathology and animal models. *Behavioural Brain Research, 204*, 313–321.

Patterson, P. H. (2011). *Infectious behavior: Brain-immune connections in autism, schizophrenia and depression*, Cambridge, MA: MIT Press.

Silverman, J. L., Yang, M., Lord, C., & Crawley, J. N. (2010). Behavioral phenotyping assays for mouse models of autism. *Nature Reviews Neuroscience, 11*, 490–502.

ACKNOWLEDGMENTS

Research related to autism from the authors' laboratory was supported by a McKnight Foundation Neuroscience of Brain Disorder Award, the Stanley Medical Research Institute, the National Institute of Mental Health, and the Binational Science, International Rett Syndrome, Cure Autism Now, Simons and Autism Speaks Foundations.

REFERENCES

Abrahams, B. S., & Geschwind, D. H. (2008a). Advances in autism genetics: On the threshold of a new neurobiology. *Nature Reviews Genetics, 9*, 341–355.

Abrahams, A. M., Stone, J. L., Duvall, J. A., Perederly, J. V., Bomar, J. M., Sebat, J. et al. (2008) Linkagae, association, and gene-expression analyses identify CNTNAP2 as an autism-susceptibility gene. *American Journal of Human Genetics, 82*, 150–159.

Adolphs, R., Sears, L., & Piven, J. (2001). Abnormal processing of social information from faces in autism. *Journal of Cognitive Neuroscience*, 13, 232–240.

Adolphs, R. (2003). Is the human amygdala specialized for processing social information? *Annals of the New York Academy of Sciences, 985*, 326–340.

Alarcon, M., Cantor, R. M., Liu, J., Gilliam, T. C., & Geschwind, D. H. (2002). Evidence for a language quantitative trait locus on chromosome 7q in multiplex autism families. *American Journal of Human Genetics, 70*, 60–71.

Amaral, D. G., Bauman, M. D., & Schumann, C. M. (2003). The amygdala and autism: Implications fro non-human primate studies. *Genes, Brain, and Behavior, 2*, 295–302.

Amaral, D. G., Schumann, C. M., & Nordahl, C. W. (2008). Neuroanatomy of autism. *Trends in Neurosciences, 31*, 137–145.

Andari, E., Duhamel, J. R., Zalla, T., Herbrecht, E., Leboyer, M., & Sirigu, A. (2010). Promoting social behavior with oxytocin in high-functioning autism spectrum disorders. *Proceedings of the National Academy of Sciences of the United States of America, 107*, 4389–4394.

Anderson, G. M., Jacobs-Stannard, A., Chawarska, K., Volkmar, F. R. & Kliman, H. J. (2007). Placental trophoblast inclusions in autism spectrum disorder. *Biological Psychiatry, 61*, 487–491.

Anderson, S. W., Bechara, A., Damasio, H., Tranel, D., & Damasio, A. R. (1999). Impairment of social and moral behavior related to early damage in human prefrontal cortex. *Nature Neuroscience, 2*, 1032–1037.

Andrews, N., Miller, E., Grant, A., Stowe, J., Osborne, V., & Taylor, B. (2004). Thimerosal exposure in infants and developmental disorders: A retrospective cohort study in the United Kingdom does not support a causal association. *Pediatrics, 114*, 584–591.

Aneja, A., & Tierney, E. (2008). Autism: The role of cholesterol in treatment. *International Review of Psychiatry, 20*, 165–170.

Aronsson, F., Lannebo, C., Paucar, M., Brask, J., Kristensson, K., & Karlsson, H. (2002). Persistence of viral RNA in the brain of offspring to mice infected with influenza A/WSN/33 virus during pregnancy. *Journal of Neurovirology, 4*, 353–357.

Asano, E., Chugani, D. C., Muzik, O., Behen, M., Janisse, J., Rothermel, R. et al. (2001). Autism in tuberous sclerosis complex is related to both cortical and subcortical dysfunction. *Neurology, 57*, 1269–1277.

Atladottir, H.O., Pedersen, M.G., Thorsen, P., Mortensen, P.B., Deleuran, B., Eaton, W.W., Parner, E.T. (2009). Association of family history of autoimmune diseases and autism spectrum disorders. *Pediatrics, 124*, 687–694.

Atladottir, H. O., thorson, P., Ostergaard, L., Schendel, D. E., Lemcke, S., Abdallah, M. & Parner, E. T. (2010). Maternal infection requiring hospitalization during pregnancy and autism spectrum disorders. *Journal of Autism and Developmental Disorders, 40*, 1423–1430.

Baharnoori, M., Brake, W. G., & Srivastava, L. K. (2009). Prenatal immune challenge induces developmental changes in the morphology of pyramidal neurons of the prefrontal cortex and hippocampus of rats. *Schizophrenia Research, 107*, 99–109.

Baharnoori, M., Bhardwaj, S. K. & Srivastava, L. K. (2010). Neonatal behavioral changes in rats with gestational exposure to lipopolysaccharide: A prenatal infection model for developmental neuropsychiatric disorders. *Schizophrenia Bulletin*, doi: 10.1093/schbul/sbq098.

Bailey, D. B., Jr., Mesibov, G. B., Hatton, D. D., Clark, R. D., Roberts, J. E., & Mayhew, L. (1998). Autistic behavior in young boys with fragile X syndrome. *Journal of Autism and Developmental Disorders, 28*, 499–508.

Baron-Cohen, S., Ring, H. A., Bullmore, E. T., Wheelwright, S., Ashwin, C., & Williams S. C. R. (2000). The amygdala theory of autism. *Neuroscience and Biobehavioral Reviews, 24*, 355–364.

Bassell, G. J., & Warren, S. T. (2008). Fragile X syndrome: Loss of local mRNA regulation alters synaptic development and function. *Neuron, 60*, 201–214.

Basta-Kaim, A., Budziszewska, B., Leskiewicz, M., Fijal, K., Regulska, M., Kubera, M. et al. (2010). Hyperactivity of the hypothalamus-pituitary-adrenal axis in lipopolysaccharide-induced neurodevelopmental model of schizophrenia in rats: Effects of antipsychotic drugs. *European Journal of Pharmacology, 650*, 586–595.

Bauer, S., Kerr, B. J., & Patterson, P. H. (2007). The neuropoietic cytokine family in development, plasticity, disease and injury. *Nature Reviews Neuroscience, 8*, 221–232.

Bear, M. F., Huber, K. M., & Warren, S. T. (2004). The mGluR theory of fragile X mental retardation. *Trends in Neurosciences, 27*, 370–377.

Benayed, R., Gharani, N., Rossman, I., Mancuso, V., Lazar, G., Kamdar, S., et al. (2005). Support for the homeobox transcription factor gene ENGRAILED 2 as an autism spectrum disorder susceptibility locus. *American Journal of Human Genetics, 77*, 851–868.

Bennett, G. D., Wlodarczyk, B., Calvin, J. A., Craig, J. C., & Finnell, R. H. (2000). Valproic acid-induced alterations in growth and neurotrophic factor gene expression in murine embryos. *Reproductive Toxicology, 14*, 1–11.

Benno, R., Smirnova, Y., Vera, S., Liggett, A., & Schanz, N. (2009). Exaggerated responses to stress in the BTBR T+tf/J mouse: An unusual behavioral phenotype. *Behavioural Brain Research, 197*, 462–465.

Berman, R. F., Pessah, I. N., Mouton, P. R., Mav, D., & Harry, J. (2008). Low-level neonatal thimerosal exposure: Further evaluation of altered neurotoxic potential in SJL mice. *Toxicological Sciences, 101*, 294–309.

Bernardet, M., & Crusio, W. E. (2006). Fmr1 KO mice as a possible model of autistic features. *ScientificWorldJournal, 6*, 1164–1176.

Berry-Kravis, E., Hessl, D., Coffey, S., Hervey, C., Schneider, A., Yuhas, J., Hutchison, J., Snape, M., Tranfaglia, M., Nguyen, D.V., & Hagerman, R. (2009). A pilot open label, single dose trial of fenobam in adults with fragile X syndrome. *Journal of Medical Genetics, 46*, 266–271.

Berry-Kravis, E., Sumis, A., Hervey, C., Nelson, M., Porges, S.W., Weng, N., et al. (2008). Open label trial to target the underlying defect in fragile X syndrome. *Journal of Developmental and Behavioral Pediatrics, 29*, 293–302.

Betancur, C., Sakurai, T., & Buxbaum, J.D. (2009). The emerging role of synaptic cell-adhesion pathways in the pathogenesis of autism spectrum disorders. *Trends in Neurosciences, 32*, 402–412.

Bielsky, I. F., Hu, S. B., Szegda, K. L., Westphal, H., & Young, L. J. (2004). Profound impairment in social recognition and reduction in anxiety-like behavior in vasopressin V1a receptor knockout mice. *Neuropsychopharmacology, 29*, 483–493.

Blackwood, D. H., Fordyce, A., Walker, M. T., St Clair, D. M., Porteous, D. J., & Muir, W. J. (2001). Schizophrenia and affective disorders—cosegregation with a translocation at chromosome 1q42 that directly disrupts brain-expressed genes: Clinical and P300 findings in a family. *American Journal of Human Genetics, 69*, 428–433.

Blundell, J., Blaiss, C.A., Etherton, M.R., Espinosa, F., Tabuchi, K., Walz, C., et al. (2010). Neuroligin-1 deletion results in impaired spatial memory and increased repetitive behavior. *Journal of Neuroscience, 30*, 2115–2129.

Bobee, S., Mariette, E., Tremblay-Leveau, H., & Caston, J. (2000). Effects of early midline cerebellar lesion on cognitive and emotional functions in the rat. *Behavioural Brain Research, 112*, 107–117.

Bolduc, F.V., Bell, K., cox, H., Broadie, K.S., & Tully, T. (2008). Excess protein synthesis in Drosophila Fragile X mutants impairs long-term memory. *Nature Neuroscience, 11*, 1143–1145.

Bolivar, V. J., Walters, S. R., & Phoenix, J. L. (2007). Assessing autism-like behavior in mice: Variations in social interactions among inbred strains. *Behavioural Brain Research, 176*, 21–26.

Borrell, J., Vela, J. M., Arevalo-Martin, A., Molina-Holgado, E., & Guaza, C. (2002). Prenatal immune challenge disrupts sensorimotor gating in adult rats- implications for the etiopathogenesis of schizophrenia. *Neuropsychopharmacology, 26*, 204–215.

Bransfield, R. C., Wulfman, J. S., Harvey, W. T., & Usman, A. I. (2008). The association between tick-borne infections, Lyme borreliosis and autism spectrum disorders. *Medical Hypotheses, 70*, 967–974.

Braunschweig, D., Ashwood, P., Krakowiak, P., Hertz-Picciotto, I., Hansen, R., Croen, L.A., et al. (2008). Autism: Maternally derived antibodies specific for fetal brain proteins. *Neurotoxicology, 29*, 226–231.

Brown, A. S. & Derkits, E. J. (2010). Prenatal infection and schizophrenia: A review of epidemiologic and translational studies. *American Journal of Psychiatry, 167*, 261–280.

Butler, M. G., Dasouki, M. J., Zhou, X. P., Talebizadeh, Z., Brown, M., Takahashi, T. N., et al. (2005). Subset of individuals with autism spectrum disorders and extreme macrocephaly associated with germline PTEN tumour suppressor gene mutations. *Journal of Medical Genetics, 42*, 318–321.

Butter, C. M. & Snyder, D. R. (1972). Alterations in aversive and aggressive behaviors following orbital frontal lesions in rhesus monkeys. *Acta Neurobiologiae Experimentalis, 32*, 525–565.

Buxbaum, J. D., Cai, G., Chaste, P., Nygren, G., Goldsmith, J., Reichert, J., et al. (2007). Mutation screening of the PTEN gene in patients with autism spectrum disorders and macrocephaly. *American Journal of Medical Genetics. Part B, Neuropsychiatric Genetics, 144B*, 484–491.

Cai, Z., Pan, Z. L., Pang, Y., Evans, O. B., & Rhodes, P. G. (2000). Cytokine induction in fetal rat brains and brain injury in neonatal rats after maternal lipopolysaccharide administration. *Pediatric Research, 47*, 64–72.

Callu, D., Puget, S., Faure, A., Guegan, M., & El Massioui, N. (2007). Habit learning dissociation in rats with lesions to the vermis and the interpositus of the cerebellum. *Neurobiology of Disease, 27*, 228–237.

Campbell, D. B., D'Oronzio, R., Garbett, K., Ebert, P. J., Mirnics, K., Levitt, P., et al. (2007). Disruption of cerebral cortex MET signaling in autism spectrum disorder. *Annals of Neurology, 62*, 243–250.

Campbell, D. B., Sutcliffe, J. S., Ebert, P. J., Militerni, R., Bravaccio, C., Trillo, S., et al. (2006). A genetic variant that disrupts MET transcription is associated with autism. *Proceedings of the National Academy of Sciences of the United States of America, 103*, 16,834–16,839.

Caramona, M. M., Cotrim, M. D., Figueiredo, I. V., Tavares, P., Ribeiro, C. A., Beja, M. L., et al. (1996). Influence of experimental hypercholesterolemia on the monoamine oxidase activity in rabbit arteries. *Pharmacological Research, 33*, 245–249.

Cardon, M., Ron-Harel, N., Cohen, H., Lewitus, G. M., & Schwartz, M. (2009). Dysregulation of kisspeptin and neurogenesis at adolescence link inborn immune deficits to the late onset of abnormal sensorimotor gating in congenital psychological disorders. *Molecular Psychiatry, 15*, 415–425.

Casanova, M. F. & Tillquist, C. R. (2008). Encephalization, emergent properties, and psychiatry: A minicolumnar perspective. *Neuroscientist, 14*, 101–118.

Chahrour, M., Jung, S. Y., Shaw, C., Zhou, X., Wong, S. T., Qin, J., et al. (2008). MeCP2, a key contributor to neurological disease, activates and represses transcription. *Science, 320*, 1224–1229.

Chahrour, M., & Zoghbi, H. Y. (2007). The story of Rett syndrome: From clinic to neurobiology. *Neuron, 56*, 422–437.

Chang, Q., Khare, G., Dani, V., Nelson, S., & Jaenisch, R. (2006). The disease progression of Mecp2 mutant mice is affected by the level of BDNF expression. *Neuron, 49*, 341–348.

Cheh, M. A., Millonig, J. H., Roselli, L. M., Ming, X., Jacobsen, E., Kamdar, S., et al. (2006). En2 knockout mice display neurobehavioral and neurochemical alterations relevant to autism spectrum disorder. *Brain Research, 1116*, 166–176.

Chen, P. S., Wang, C. C., Bortner, C. D., Peng, G. S., Wu, X., Pang, H., et al. (2007). Valproic acid and other histone deacetylase inhibitors induce microglial apoptosis and attenuate lipopolysaccharide induced dopaminergic neurotoxicity. *Neuroscience, 149*, 203–212.

Chen, Q., Panksepp, J.B., & Lahvis, G.P. (2009). Empathy is moderated by genetic background in mice. *PLoS One, 4*, e4387.

Chen, R. Z., Akbarian, S., Tudor, M., & Jaenisch, R. (2001). Deficiency of methyl-CpG binding protein-2 in CNS neurons results in a Rett-like phenotype in mice. *Nature Genetics, 27*, 327–331.

Cheslack-Postava, K., Fallin, M. D., Avramopoulos, D., Connors, S. L., Zimmerman, A. W., Eeberhart, C. G., et al. (2007). Beta(2)-adrenergic receptor gene variants and risk for autism in the AGRE cohort. *Molecular Psychiatry, 12*, 283–291.

Chess, S. (1977). Follow-up report on autism in congenital-rubella. *Journal Autism and Childhood Schizophrenia*, 7, 69–81.

Chez, M. G., Dowling, T., Patel, P. B., Khanna, P., & Kominsky, M. (2007). Elevation of tumor necrosis factor-alpha in cerebrospinal fluid of autistic children. *Pediatric Neurology, 36*, 361–365.

Christianson, A. L., Chesler, N., & Kromberg, J. G. (1994). Fetal valproate syndrome: Clinical and neuro-developmental features in two sibling pairs. *Developmental Medicine and Child Neurology, 36*, 361–369.

Chubb, J. E., Bradshaw, N. J., Soares, D. C., Porteous, D. J., & Millar, J. K. (2008). The DISC locus in psychiatric illness. *Molecular Psychiatry, 13*, 36–64.

Chugani, D. C., Muzik, O., Behen, M., Rothermel, R., Janisse, J. J., Lee, J., et al. (1999). Developmental changes in brain serotonin synthesis capacity in autistic and nonautistic children. *Annals of Neurology, 45*, 287–295.

Chugani, D. C., Muzik, O., Rothermel, R., Behen, M., Chakraborty, P., Mangner, T., et al. (1997). Altered serotonin synthesis in the dentatothalamocortical pathway in autistic boys. *Annals of Neurology, 42*, 666–669.

Ciaranello, A. L., & Ciarenello, R. D. (1995). The neurobiology of infantile autism. *Annual Reviews Neuroscience*, 18, 101–128.

Chadman, K.K., Gong, S., Scattoni, M.L., Boltuck, S.E., Gandhy, S.U., Heintz, N. & Crawley, J.N. (2008). Minimal aberrant behavioral phenotypes of neuroligin-3 R451C knockin mice. *Autism Research, 1*, 147–158.

Cohen, I. L., Fisch, G. S., Sudhalter, V., Wolf-Schein, E. G., Hanson, D., Hagerman, R., et al. (1988). Social gaze, social avoidance, and repetitive behavior in fragile X males: A controlled study. *American Journal of Mental Retardation, 92*, 436–446.

Collins, A. L., Levenson, J. M., Vilaythong, A. P., Richman, R., Armstrong, D. L., Noebels, J. L., et al. (2004). Mild overexpression of MeCP2 causes a progressive neurological disorder in mice. *Human Molecular Genetics, 13*, 2679–2689.

Connors, S. L., Crowell, D. E., Eberhart, C. G., Copeland, J., Newschaffer, C. J., & Zimmerman, A. W. (2005). Beta(2)-adrenergic receptor activation and genetic polymorphisms in autism: Data from dizygotic twins. *Journal of Child Psychiatry, 20*, 876–884.

Cook, E. H., Jr., & Scherer, S. W. (2008). Copy-number variations associated with neuropsychiatric conditions. *Nature, 455*, 919–923.

Cook, E. H., & Leventhal, B. L. (1996). The serotonin system in autism. *Current Opinion in Pediatrics, 8*, 348–354.

Silverman, J. L., Yang, M., Lord, C. & Crawley, J. N. (2010) Behavioral phenotyping assays for mouse models of autism. *Nature Reviews Neuroscience, 11*, 490–502.

Croen, L. A., Goines, P., Braunschweig, D., Yolken, R., Yoshida, C. K., Grether, J. K., et al. (2008). Brain-derived neurotrophic factor and autism: Maternal and infant peripheral blood levels in the Early Markers for Autism (EMA) Study. *Autism Research, 1*, 130–137.

Daenen, E. W. P. M., Van der Heyden, J. A., Kruse, C. G., Wolterink, G., & Van Ree, J. M. (2001). Adaptation and habituation to an open field and responses to various stressful events in animals with neonatal lesions in the amygdala or ventral hippocampus. *Brain Research, 918*, 153–165.

Daenen, E. W. P. M., Wolterink, G., Gerrits, M. A. F. M., & Van Ree, J. M. (2002a). Amygdala or ventral hippocampal lesions at two early stages of life differentially affect open field behavior later in life; an animal model of neurodevelopmental psychopathological disorders. *Behavioural Brain Research, 131*, 67–78.

Daenen, E. W. P. M., Wolterink, G., Gerrits, M. A. F. M., & Van Ree, J. M. (2002b). The effect of neonatal lesions in the amygdala or ventral hippocampus on social behaviour later in life. *Behavioural Brain Research, 136*, 571–582.

Dahlgren, J., Samuelsson, A. M., Jansson, T., Halmang, A. (2006). Interleukin-6 in the maternal circulation reaches the rat fetus in mid-gestation. *Pediatric Research, 60*, 147–151.

Dalton, P., Deacon, R., Blamire, A., Pike, M., McKinlay, I., Stein, J., et al. (2003). Maternal neuronal antibodies associated with autism and a language disorder. *Annals of Neurology, 53*, 533–537.

De Miranda, J., Yaddanapudi, K., Hornig, M., Villar, G., Serge, R. & Lipkin, W. I. (2010). Induction of toll-like receptor 3-mediated immunity during gestation inhibits cortical neurogenesis and causes behavioral disturbances. *MBio, 1*, e00176–10.

DeStefano, F. (2007). Vaccines and autism: Evidence does not support a causal association. *Clinical Pharmacology and Therapeutics, 82*, 756–759.

Deverman, B. E. & Patterson, P. H. (2009) Cytokines and CNS development. *Neuron 64*, 61–78.

de Vries, P.J. (2010). Targeted treatments for cognitive and neurodevelopmental disorders in turberous sclerosis complex. *Neurotherapeutics, 7*, 275–282.

Dickerson, D. D., Wolff, A. R. & Bilkey, D. K. (2010). Abnormal long-range neural synchrony in a maternal immune activation animal model of schizophrenia. *Journal of Neuroscience, 30*, 12424–12431.

Diergaarde, L., Gerrits, M., Stuy, A., Spruijt, B. M., & van Ree, J. M. (2004). Neonatal amygdala lesions and juvenile isolation in the rat: Differential effects on locomotor and social behavior later in life. *Behavioral Neuroscience, 118*, 298–305.

Dindot, S. V., Antalffy, B. A., Bhattacharjee, M. B., & Beaudet, A. L. (2008). The Angelman syndrome ubiquitin ligase localizes to the synapse and nucleus, and maternal deficiency results in abnormal dendritic spine morphology. *Human Molecular Genetics, 17*, 111–118.

Dobkin, C., Rabe, A., Dumas, R., El Idrissi, A., Haubenstock, H., & Brown, W. T. (2000). Fmr1 knockout mouse has a distinctive strain-specific learning impairment. *Neuroscience, 100*, 423–429.

Donaldson, Z. R., & Young, L. J. (2008). Oxytocin, vasopressin, and the neurogenetics of sociality. *Science, 322*, 900–904.

Dragunow, M., Greenwood, J. M., Cameron, R. E., Narayan, P. J., O'Carroll, S. J., Pearson, A. G., et al. (2006). Valproic acid induces caspase 3- mediated apoptosis in microglial cells. *Neuroscience, 140*, 1149–1156.

Dufour-Rainfray, D., Vourc'h, T., Le Guisquet, A. M., Garreau, L., Ternant, D., Bodard, S., et al. (2010). Behavior and serotonergic disorders in rats exposed prenatally to valproate: A model for autism. *Neuroscience Letters, 470*, 55–59.

The Dutch-Belgian Fragile X Consortium (1994). Fmr1 knockout mice: A model to study fragile X mental retardation. *Cell, 78*, 23–33.

Egashira, N., Tanoue, A., Matsuda, T., Koushi, E., Harada, S., Takano, Y., et al. (2007). Impaired social interaction and reduced anxiety-related behavior in vasopressin V1a receptor knockout mice. *Behavioural Brain Research, 178*, 123–127.

Ehninger, D., de Vries, P.J., & Silva, A.J. (2009). From mTOR to cognition: Molecular and cellular mechanisms of cognitive impairments in tuberous sclerosis. *Journal of Intellectual Disability Research, 53*, 838–851.

Ehninger, D., Sano, Y., De Vries, P. J., Dies, K., Franz, D., Geschwind, D. H., et al. (2010). Gestational immune activation and *TSC2* haploinsufficiency cooperate to disrupt social behavior in mice. *Molecular Psychiatry*, on line.

Elovitz, M. A., Mrinalini, C., & Sammel, M. D. (2006). Elucidating the early signal transduction pathways leading to fetal brain injury in preterm birth. *Pediatric Research, 59*, 50–55.

Eluvathingal, T. J., Behen, M. E., Chugani, H. T., Janisse, J., Bernardi, B., Chakraborty, P. et al. (2006). Cerebellar lesions in tuberous sclerosis complex. *Journal of Child Neurology, 21*, 846–851.

Enstrom, A. M., Van de Water, J. A., & Ashwood, P. (2009). Autoimmunity in autism. *Current Opinion in Investigative Drugs, 10*, 463–473.

Fan, Q., Ramakrishna, S., Marchi, N., Fazio, V., Hallene, K., & Janigro, D. (2008). Combined effects of prenatal inhibition of vasculogenesis and neurogenesis on rat brain development. *Neurobiology of Disease*, doi:10.1016/j.nbd.2008.09.007.

Fatemi, S.H., Earle, J., Kanodia, R., Kist, D., Emamian, E. S., Patterson, P. H., et al. (2002). Prenatal viral infection leads to pyramidal cell atrophy and macrocephaly in adulthood: Implications for genesis of autism and schizophrenia. *Cellular and Molecular Neurobiology, 22*, 25–33.

Fatemi, S. H., Folsom, T. D., Reutiman, T. J., Abu-Odeh, D., Mori, S., Huang. H., et al. (2009). Abnormal expression of myelination genes and alterations in white matter fractional anisotropy following prenatal viral influenza infection at E16 in mice. *Schizophrenia Research, 112*, 46–53.

Fatemi, S. H., Reutiman, T. J, Folsom, T. D., Huang, H., Oishi, K., Mori, S., et al. (2008). Maternal infection leads to abnormal gene regulation and brain atrophy in mouse offspring: Implications for genesis of neurodevelopmental disorders. *Schizophrenia Research, 99*, 56–70.

Ferguson, J. N., Young, L. J., Hearn, E. F., Matzuk, M. M., Insel, T. R., & Winslow, J. T. (2000). Social amnesia in mice lacking the oxytocin gene. *Nature Genetics, 25*, 284–288.

Finnell, R. H., Waes, J. G., Eudy, J. D., & Rosenquist, T. H. (2002). Molecular basis of environmentally induced birth defects. *Annual Review of Pharmacology and Toxicology, 42*, 181–208.

Fortier, M. E., Joober, R., Luheshi, G. N., & Boksa, P. (2004). Maternal exposure to bacterial endotoxin during pregnancy enhances amphetamine-induced locomotion and startle responses in adult rat offspring. *Journal of Psychiatric Research, 38*, 335–345.

Frankland, P. W., Wang, Y., Rosner, B., Shimizu, T., Balleine, B. W., Dykens, E. M., et al. (2004). Sensorimotor gating abnormalities in young males with fragile X syndrome and Fmr1-knockout mice. *Molecular Psychiatry, 9*, 417–425.

Freeman, J. L., Perry, G. H., Feuk, L., Redon, R., McCarroll, S. A., Altshuler, D. M., et al. (2006). Copy number variation: New insights in genome diversity. *Genome Research, 16*, 949–961.

Garbett, K., Ebert, P. J., Mitchell, A., Lintas, C., Manzi, B., Mirnics, K., et al. (2008). Immune transcriptome alterations in the temporal cortex of subjects with autism. *Neurobiology of Disease, 30*, 303–311.

Gaspar, P., Cases, O., & Maroteaux, L. (2003). The developmental role of serotonin: News from mouse molecular genetics. *Nature Reviews Neuroscience, 4*, 1002–1012.

Gaytan-Tocaven, L., & Olvera-Cortes, M. E. (2004). Bilateral lesion of the cerebellar-dentate nucleus impairs egocentric sequential learning but not egocentric navigation in the rat. *Neurobiology of Learning and Memory, 82*, 120–127.

Gerber, J. S. & Offit, P. A. (2008) Vaccines and autism: A tale of shifting hypotheses. *Vaccines, 48*, 456–461.

Gillberg, C., Gillberg, I. C., & Ahlsen, G. (1994). Autistic behavior and attention deficits in tuberous sclerosis: A population-based study. *Developmental Medicine and Child Neurology, 36*, 50–56.

Girard, S., Tremblay, L., Lepage, M. & Sébire, G. (2010). IL-1 receptor antagonist protects against placental and neurodevelopmental defects induced by maternal inflammation. *Journal of Immunology, 84*, 3997–4005.

Goffin, A., Hoefsloot, L. H., Bosgoed, E., Swillen, A., & Fryns, J. P. (2001). PTEN mutation in a family with Cowden syndrome and autism. *American Journal of Medical Genetics, 105*, 521–524.

Golan, H. M., Lev, V., Hallak, M., Sorokin, Y., & Huleihel, M. (2005). Specific neurodevelopmental damage in mice offspring following maternal inflammation during pregnancy. *Neuropharmacology, 48*, 903–917.

Green, L., Fein, D., Modahl, C., Feinstein, C., Waterhouse, L., & Morris, M. (2001). Oxytocin and autistic disorder: Alterations in peptide forms. *Biological Psychiatry, 50*, 609–613.

Gregory, S. G., Connelly, J. J., Towers, A. J., Johnson, J., Bisocho, D., Markunas, C. A., et al. (2009). Genomic and epigenetic evidence for oxytocin receptor deficiency in autism. *BMC Medicine, 7*, 62.

Guastella, A. J., Einfeld, S. L., Gray, K. M., Rinehart, N. J., tonge, B. J., Lambert, T. J., et al. (2009). Intransal oxytocin improves emotion recognition for youth with autism spectrum disorders. *Biological Psychiatry, 67*, 692–694.

Gutierrez, H., Dolcet, X., Tolcos, M., & Davies, A. (2004). HGF regulates the development of cortical pyramidal dendrites. *Development, 131*, 3717–3726.

Guy, J., Hendrich, B., Holmes, M., Martin, J. E., & Bird, A. (2001). A mouse Mecp2-null mutation causes neurological symptoms that mimic Rett syndrome. *Nature Genetics, 27*, 322–326.

Guy, J., Gan, J., Selfridge, J., Cobb, S., & Bird, A. (2007). Reversal of neurological defects in a mouse model of Rett syndrome. *Science, 315*, 1143–1147.

Hao, Y., Creson, T., Zhang, L., Li, P., Du, F., Yuan, P., et al. (2004). Mood stabilizer valproate promotes ERK pathway dependent cortical neuronal growth and neurogenesis. *Journal of Neuroscience, 24*, 6590–6599.

Hao, L. Y., Hao, X. Q., Li, S. H. & Li, X. H. (2010) Prenatal exposure to lipopolysaccharide results in cognitive deficits in age-increasing offspring rats. *Neuroscience, 166*, 763–770.

Hashimoto, T., Bergen, S. E., Nguyen, Q. L., Xu, B., Monteggia, L. M., Pierri, J. N., et al. (2005). Relationship of brain-derived neurotrophic factor and its receptor TrkB to altered inhibitory prefrontal circuitry in schizophrenia. *Journal of Neuroscience, 25*, 372–383.

Hatton, D. D., Sideris, J., Skinner, M., Mankowski, J., Bailey, D. B., Jr., Roberts, J., et al. (2006). Autistic behavior in children with fragile X syndrome: Prevalence, stability, and the impact of FMRP. *American Journal of Medical Genetics. Part A, 140A*, 1804–1813.

Hava, G., Vered, L., Yael, M., Mordechai, H., & Mahoud, H. (2006). Alterations in behavior in adult offspring mice following maternal inflammation during pregnancy. *Developmental Psychobiology, 48*, 162–168.

Hayashi, M. L., Rao, B. S., Seo, J. S., Choi, H. S., Dolan, B. M., Choi, S. Y., et al. (2007). Inhibition of p21-activated kinase rescues symptoms of fragile X syndrome in mice. *Proceedings of the National Academy of Sciences of the United States of America, 104*, 11489–11494.

Hill, J. J., Kolluri, N., Hashimoto, T., Wu, Q., Sampson, A. R., Monteggia, L. M., et al. (2005). Analysis of pyramidal neuron morphology in an inducible knockout of brain-derived neurotrophic factor. *Biological Psychiatry, 57*, 932–934.

Hollander, E., Novotny, S., Hanratty, M., Yaffe, R., DeCaria, C. M., Aronowitz, B. R., et al. (2003). Oxytocin infusion reduces repetitive behaviors in adults with autistic and Asperger's disorders. *Neuropsychopharmacology, 28*, 193–198.

Hollander, E., Phillips, A., Chaplin, W., Zagursky, K., Novotny, S., Wasserman, S., et al. (2005). A placebo controlled crossover trial of liquid fluoxetine on repetitive behaviors in childhood and adolescent autism. *Neuropsychopharmacology, 30*, 582–589.

Hollander, E., Bartz, J., Chaplin, W., Phillips, A., Sumner, J., Soorya, L., et al. (2007). Oxytocin increases retention of social cognition in autism. *Biological Psychiatry, 61*, 498–503.

Hornig, M., Chian, D., & Lipkin, W. I. (2004). Neurotoxic effects of postnatal thimerosal are mouse strain dependent. *Molecular Psychiatry, 9*, 833–845.

Hsiao, E. Y., Chow, J., Mazmanian, S. K., & Patterson, P. H. (2010). Modeling an autism risk factor in mice leads to permanent changes in the immune system. Program No. 130.124. Philadelphia, PA: International Society for Autism Research.

Hsiao, E. Y. & Patterson, P. H. (2010). Activation of the maternal immune system induces endocrine changes in the placenta via IL-6. *Brain, Behavior, and Immunity*, doi: 10.1016/j.bbi.2010.12.017.

Hung, A. Y., Futai, K., Sala, C., Valtschanoff, J. G., Ryu, J., Woodworth, M. A., et al. (2008). Smaller dendritic spines, weaker synaptic transmission, but enhanced spatial learning in mice lacking Shank1. *Journal of Neuroscience, 28*, 1697–1708.

Hussman, J. P. (2001). Suppressed GABAergic inhibition as a common factor in suspected etiologies of autism. *Journal of Autism and Developmental Disorders, 31*, 247–248.

Hyman, S. L., Arndt, T. L., & Rodier, P. M. (2006). Environmental agents and autism: Once and future associations. *International Review of Research in Mental Retardation, 30*, 171–194.

Ieraci, A., Forni, P. E., & Ponzetto, C. (2002). Viable hypomorphic signaling mutant of the Met receptor reveals a role for hepatocyte growth factor in postnatal cerebellar development. *Proceedings of the National Academy of Sciences of the United States of America, 99*, 15200–15205.

Insel, T.R. (2010). The challenge of translation in social neuroscience: A review of oxytocin, vasopressin, and affiliative behavior. *Neuron, 65*, 768–779.

Israel, S., Lerer, E., Shalev, I., Uzefovsky, F., Reibold, M., Bachner-Melman, R., et al. (2008). Molecular genetic studies of the arginine vasopressin 1a receptor (AVPR1a) and the oxytocin receptor (OXTR) in human behaviour: From autism to altruism with some notes in between. *Progress in Brain Research, 170*, 435–449.

Ito, H. T., Smith, S. E. P., Hsiao, E. & Patterson, P. H. (2010). Maternal immune activation alters nonspatial information processing in the hippocampus of the adult offspring. *Brain, Behavior, and Immunity, 24*, 930–941.

Jamain, S., Quach, H., Betancur, C., Rastam, M., Colineaux, C., Gillberg, I. C., et al. (2003). Mutations of the X-linked genes encoding neuroligins NLGN3 and NLGN4 are associated with autism. *Nature Genetics, 34*, 27–29.

Jamain, S., Radyushkin, K., Hammerschmidt, K., Granon, S., Boretius, S., Varoqueaux, F., et al. (2008). Reduced social interaction and ultrasonic communication in a mouse model of monogenic heritable autism. *Proceedings of the National Academy of Sciences of the United States of America, 105*, 1710–1715.

Jansen, L. M., Gispen-de Wied, C. C., Wiegant, V. M., Westenberg, H. G., Lahuis, B. E., & van Engeland, H. (2006). Autonomic and neuroendocrine responses to a psychosocial stressor in adults with autistic spectrum disorder. *Journal of Autism and Developmental Disorders, 36*, 891–899.

Jiang, Y. H., Armstrong, D., Albrecht, U., Atkins, C. M., Noebels, J. L., Eichele, G., et al. (1998). Mutation of the Angelman ubiquitin ligase in mice causes increased cytoplasmic p53 and deficits of contextual learning and long-term potentiation. *Neuron, 21*, 799–811.

Jiang, Y.H., Pan, Y., Zhu, L., Landa, L., Yoo, J., Spencer, C., et al. (2010). Altered ultrasonic vocalization and impaired learning and memory in Angelman syndrome mouse model with a large maternal deletion from Ube3a to Gabrb3. *PLoS ONE, 5*, e12278.

Johnson, C. P. (2008). Recognition of autism before age 2 years. *Pediatrics in Review, 29*, 86–96.

Just, M. A., Cherkassky, V. L., Keller, T. A., & Minshew, N. J. (2004). Cortical activation and synchronization during sentence comprehension in high-functioning autism: Evidence of underconnectivity. *Brain, 127*, 1811–1821.

Kaufmann, W. E., & Moser, H. W. (2000). Dendritic anomalies in disorders associated with mental retardation. *Cerebral Cortex, 10*, 981–991.

Kilpinen, H., Ylisaukko-Oja, T., Hennah, W., Palo, O. M., Varilo, T., Vanhala, R., et al. (2008). Association of DISC1 with autism and Asperger syndrome. *Molecular Psychiatry, 13*, 187–196.

Kirsten, T. B., Taricano, M., Maiorka, P. C., Palermo-Neto, J. & Bernardi, M. M. (2010). Prenatal lipopolysaccharide reduces social behavior in male offspring. *Neuroimmunomodulation 17*, 240–251.

Koenigs, M., Young, L., Adolphs, R., Tranel, D., Cushman, F., Hauser, M. et al. (2007). Damage to the prefrontal cortex increases utilitarian moral judgements. *Nature, 446*, 908–911.

Koike, H., Arguello, P. A., Kvajo, M., Karayiorgou, M., & Gogos, J. A. (2006). Disc1 is mutated in the 129S6/SvEv strain and modulates working memory in mice. *Proceedings of the National Academy of Sciences of the United States of America, 103*, 3693–3697.

Kolozsi, E., Mackenzie, R. N., Roullet, F. I., deCatanzaro, D. & Foster, J. A. (2009). Prenatal exposure to valproic acid leads to reduced expression of synaptic adhesion molecule neuroligin 3 in mice. *Neuroscience, 163*, 1201–1210.

Kuemerle, B., Zanjani, H., Joyner, A., & Herrup, K. (1997). Pattern deformities and cell loss in Engrailed-2 mutant mice suggest two separate patterning events during cerebellar development. *Journal of Neuroscience, 17*, 7881–7889.

Kuwagata, M., Ogawa, T., Shioda, S. & Nagata, T. (2009). Observation of fetal brain in rat valproate-induced autism model: A developmental neurotoxicity study. *International Journal of Developmental Neuroscience, 27*, 399–405.

Kvajo, M., McKellar, H., Arguello, P. A., Drew, L. J., Moore, H., MacDermott, A. B., et al. (2008). A mutation in mouse Disc1 that models a schizophrenia risk allele leads to specific alterations in neuronal architecture and cognition. *Proceedings of the National Academy of Sciences of the United States of America, 105*, 7076–7081.

Kwon, C. H., Luikart, B. W., Powell, C. M., Zhou, J., Matheny, S. A., Zhang, W., et al. (2006). Pten regulates neuronal arborization and social interaction in mice. *Neuron, 50*, 377–388.

Lainhart, J. E., Bigler, E. D., Bocian, M., Coon, H., Dinh, E., Dawson, G., et al. (2006). Head circumference and height in autism: A study by the Collaborative Program of Excellence in Autism. *American Journal of Medical Genetics. Part A, 140*, 2257–2274.

Langford, D. J., Crager, S. E., Shehzad, Z., Smith, S. B., Sotocinal, S. G., Levenstadt, J. S., et al. (2006). Social modulation of pain is evidence for empathy in mice. *Science, 312*, 1967–1970.

Lante, F., Meunier, J., Guiramand, J., De Jesus Rerreira, M. C., Cambonie, G., Aimar, R., et al. (2008). Late N-acetylcysteine treatment prevents the deficits induced in the offspring of dams exposed to an immune stress during gestation. *Hippocampus, 18*, 602–609.

Lathe, R. (2006). *Autism, Brain, and Environment*. London, UK: Jessica Kingsley Publishers.

Laumonnier, F., Bonnet-Brilhault, F., Gomot, M., Blanc, R., David, A., Moizard, M. P., et al. (2004). X-linked mental retardation and autism are associated with a mutation in the NLGN4 gene, a member of the neuroligin family. *American Journal of Human Genetics, 74*, 552–557.

Lavond, D. G., & Steinmetz, J. E. (2003). *Handbook of classical conditioning*. New York, USA: Kluwer Academic Publishers.

Lee, K. H., Smith, S. E. P., Kim, S., Patterson, P. H. & Thompson, R. F. (2007). Maternal immune activation impairs extinction of the conditioned eyeblink response in the adult offspring. Program No. 209.4, *Neuroscience Meeting Planner, San Diego: Society for Neuroscience*, on line.

Li, H., Radford, J. C., Ragusa, M. J., Shea, K. L., McKercher, S. R., Zaremba, J. D., et al. (2008). Transcription factor MEF2C influences neural stem/progenitor cell differentiation and maturation in vivo. *Proceedings of the National Academy of Sciences of the United States of America, 105*, 9397–9402.

Li, S. Y., Chen, Y. C., Lai, T. J., Hsu, C. Y., & Wang, Y. C. (1993). Molecular and cytogenetic analyses of autism in Taiwan. *Human Genetics, 92*, 441–445.

Li, Q., Cheung, C., Wei, R., Hui, E. S., Feldon, J., Meyer, U., et al. (2009). Prenatal immune challenge is an environmental risk factor for brain and behavior change relevant to schizophrenia: Evidence from MRI in a mouse model. *PLoS ONE, 4*, e6354.

Limpeopoulos, C., Bassan, H., Gauvreau, K., Robertson, R. L. Jr., Sullivan, N. R., Benson, C. B. et al. (2007). Does cerebellar injury in premature infants contribute to the high prevalence of long-term cognitive, learning, and behavioral disability in survivors? *Pediatrics, 120*, 584–593.

Limperopoulos, C., Bassan, H., Sullivan, N. R., Soul, J. S., Robertson, R. L. Jr., Moore, M., et al. (2008). Positive screening for autism in ex-preterm infants: Prevalence and risk factors. *Pediatrics, 121*, 758–765.

Ling, Z., Chang, Q. A., Tong, C. W., Leurgans, S. E., Lipton, J. W., & Carvey, P. M. (2004). Rotenone potentiates dopamine neuron loss in animals exposed to lipopolysaccharide prenatally. *Experimental Neurology, 190*, 373–383.

Liu, J., Nyholt, D. R., Magnussen, P., Parano, E., Pavone, P., Geschwind, D., et al. (2001). A genomewide screen for autism susceptibility loci. *American Journal of Human Genetics, 69*, 327–340.

Liverman, C. S., Kaftan, H. A., Cui, L., Hersperger, S. G., Taboada, E., Klein, R. M., et al. (2006). Altered expression of pro-inflammatory and developmental genes in the fetal brain in a mouse model of maternal infection. *Neuroscience Letters, 399*, 220–225.

Loat, C., Curran, S., Lewis, C., Abrahams, B., Duvall, J., Geschwind, D., et al. (2008). Methyl - CpG - binding protein (MECP2) polymorphisms and vulnerability to autism. *Genes, Brain, and Behavior, 7*, 754–760.

Lowe, G., Jackson, J., Goutagny, R., & Williams, S. (2009). Altered oscillatory activity in the hippocampus after prenatal infection: Possible relevance to schizophrenia. Program No. 425.21, *Neuroscience Meeting Planner. Chicago, IL: Society for Neuroscience*, 2009. Online.

Lowe, G. C., Luheshi, G. N., & Williams, S. (2008). Maternal infection and fever during late gestation are associated with altered synaptic transmission in the hippocampus of juvenile offspring rats. *American Journal of Physiology. Regulatory, Integrative, and Comparative Physiology, 295*, R1563–1571.

Lu, Y., Wang, F., Li, Y., Ferris, J., Lee, J. A., & Gao, F. B. (2009). The Drosophila homologue of the Angelman syndrome ubiquitin ligase regulates the formation of terminal dendritic branches. *Human Molecular Genetics, 18*, 454–462.

MacPherson, P., McGaffigan, R., Wahlsten, D., & Nguyen, P. V. (2008). Impaired fear memory, altered object memory and modified hippocampal synaptic plasticity in split-brain mice. *Brain Research, 1210*, 179–188.

Makinodan, M., Tatsumi, K., Manabe, T., Yamauchi, T., Makinodan, E., Matsuyoshi, H., et al. (2008). Maternal immune activation in mice delays myelination and axonal development in the hippocampus of the offspring. *Journal of Neuroscience Research, 86*, 2190–2200.

Malkova, N. V. & Patterson, P. H. (2010). Maternal immune activation causes a deficit in social and communicative behavior in male mouse offspring. Program No. 561.29, *Neuroscience Meeting Planner, San Diego: Society for Neuroscience*, online.

Mandal, M., Marzouk, A. C., Donnelly, R. & Ponzio, N. M. (2010). Maternal immune stimulation during pregnancy affects adaptive immunity in offspring to promote development of TH17 cells. *Brain, Behavior, and Immunity*, in press.

Markram, K., Rinaldi, T., La Mendola, D., Sandi, C., & Markram, H. (2008). Abnormal fear conditioning and amygdala processing in an animal model of autism. *Neuropsychopharmacology, 33*, 901–912.

Markram, H., Rinaldi, T., & Markram K. (2007). The intense world syndrome: An alternative hypothesis for autism. *Frontiers in Neuroscience, 1*, 77–96.

Martin, L. A., Ashwood, P., Braunschweig, D., Cabanlit, M., Van de Water, J., & Amaral, D. G. (2008). Stereotypies and hyperactivity in rhesus monkeys exposed to IgG from mothers of children with autism. *Brain, Behavior, and Immunity, 22*, 806–816.

McBride, S.M.J., Choi, C.H., Wang, Y., Liebelt, D., Braunstein, E., Ferreiro, D., et al. (2005). Pharmacological rescue of synaptic plasticity, courtship behavior, and mushroom body defects in a Drosophila model of fragile X syndrome. *Neuron, 45*, 753–764.

McFarlane, H. G., Kusek, G. K., Yang, M., Phoenix, J. L., Bolivar, V. J., & Crawley, J. N. (2008). Autism-like behavioral phenotypes in BTBR T+tf/J mice. *Genes, Brain, and Behavior, 7*, 152–163.

McNaughton, C. H., Moon, J., Strawderman, M. S., Maclean, K. N., Evans, J., & Strupp, B. J. (2008). Evidence for social anxiety and impaired social cognition in a mouse model of fragile X syndrome. *Behavioral Neuroscience, 122*, 293–300.

Meyer, U., Yee, B. K., & Feldon, J. (2007). The neurodevelopmental impact of prenatal infections at different times of pregnancy: The earlier the worse? *Neuroscientist, 13*, 241–256.

Meyer, U., Engler, A., Weber, L., Schedlowski, M., & Feldon, J. (2008a). Preliminary evidence for a modulation of fetal dopaminergic development by maternal immune activation during pregnancy. *Neuroscience, 154*, 701–709.

Meyer, U., Nyffeler, M., Yee, B. K., Kneusel, I., & Feldon, J. (2008b). Adult brain and behavioral pathological markers of prenatal immune challenge during early/middle and late fetal development in mice. *Brain, Behavior, and Immunity, 22*, 469–486.

Meyer, U., Murray, P. J., Urwyler, A., Yee, B. K., Schedlowski, M., & Feldon, J. (2008c). Adult behavioral and pharmacological dysfunctions following disruption of the fetal brain balance between pro-inflammatory and IL-10-mediated anti-inflammmatory signaling. *Molecular Psychiatry, 13*, 208–221.

Millar, J. K., Christie, S., Anderson, S., Lawson, D., Hsiao-Wei Loh, D., Devon, R. S., et al. (2001). Genomic structure and localisation within a linkage hotspot of Disrupted In Schizophrenia 1, a gene disrupted by a translocation segregating with schizophrenia. *Molecular Psychiatry, 6*, 173–178.

Millar, J. K., Wilson-Annan, J. C., Anderson, S., Christie, S., Taylor, M. S., Semple, C. A., et al. (2000). Disruption of two novel genes by a translocation co-segregating with schizophrenia. *Human Molecular Genetics, 9*, 1415–1423.

Miller, M. T., Stromland, K., Ventura, L., Johansson, M., Bandim, J. M., & Gillberg, C. (2004). Autism associated with conditions characterized by developmental errors in early embryogenesis: A mini review. *International Journal of Developmental Neuroscience, 23*, 201–219.

Miura, K., Kishino, T., Li, E., Webber, H., Dikkes, P., Holmes, G. L., et al. (2002). Neurobehavioral and electroencephalographic abnormalities in Ube3a maternal-deficient mice. *Neurobiology of Disease, 9*, 149–159.

Miyazaki, K., Narita, N., & Narita, M. (2005). Maternal administration of thalidomide of valproic acid causes abnormal serotonergic neurons in the offspring: Implication for pathogenesis of autism. *International Journal of Developmental Neuroscience, 23*, 287–297.

Modahl, C., Green, L., Fein, D., Morris, M., Waterhouse, L., Feinstein, C., et al. (1998). Plasma oxytocin levels in autistic children. *Biological Psychiatry, 43*, 270–277.

Monteggia, L. M., Barrot, M., Powell, C. M., Berton, O., Galanis, V., Gemelli, T., et al. (2004). Essential role of brain-derived neurotrophic factor in adult hippocampal function. *Proceedings of the National Academy of Sciences of the United States of America, 101*, 10827–10832.

Morgan, J. T., Chana, G., Pardo, C. A., Achim, C., Semendeferi, K., Buckwalter, J., et al. (2010). Microglial activation and increased density observed in the dorsolateral prefrontal cortex in autism. *Biological Psychiatry, 68*, 368–376.

Moretti, P., Bouwknecht, J. A., Teague, R., Paylor, R., & Zoghbi, H. Y. (2005). Abnormalities of social interactions and home-cage behavior in a mouse model of Rett syndrome. *Human Molecular Genetics, 14*, 205–220.

Moretti, P., Levenson, J. M., Battaglia, F., Atkinson, R., Teague, R., Antalffy, B., et al. (2006). Learning and memory and synaptic plasticity are impaired in a mouse model of Rett syndrome. *Journal of Neuroscience, 26*, 319–327.

Morrow, E. M., Yoo, S. Y., Flavell, S. W., Kim, T. K., Lin, Y., Hill, R. S., et al. (2008). Identifying autism loci and genes by tracing recent shared ancestry. *Science, 321*, 218–223.

Moy, S. S., & Nadler, J. J. (2008). Advances in behavioral genetics: Mouse models of autism. *Molecular Psychiatry, 13*, 4–26.

Moy, S. S., Nadler, J. J., Poe, M. D., Nonneman, R. J., Young, N. B., Koller, B. H., et al. (2008). Development of a mouse test for repetitive, restricted behaviors: Relevance to autism. *Behavioural Brain Research, 188*, 178–194.

Moy, S. S., Nadler, J. J., Young, N. B., Perez, A., Holloway, L. P., Barbaro, R. P., et al. (2007). Mouse behavioral tasks relevant to autism: Phenotypes of 10 inbred strains. *Behavioural Brain Research, 176*, 4–20.

Muir, W. J., Gosden, C. M., Brookes, A. J., Fantes, J., Evans, K. L., Maguire, S. M., et al. (1995). Direct microdissection and microcloning of a translocation breakpoint region, t(1;11)(q42.2;q21), associated with schizophrenia. *Cytogenetics and Cell Genetics, 70*, 35–40.

Muir, W. J., Pickard, B. S., & Blackwood, D. H. (2008). Disrupted-in-Schizophrenia-1. *Current Psychiatry Reports, 10*, 140–147.

Murawski, N. J., Brown, K. L., & Stanton, M. E. (2008). Interstimulus interval (ISI) discrimination of the conditioned eyeblink response in a rodent model of autism. *Behavioural Brain Research*, doi:10.1016/j.bbr.2008.09.020.

Murcia, C. L., Gulden, F., & Herrup, K. (2005). A question of balance: A proposal for new mouse models of autism. *International Journal of Developmental Neuroscience, 23*, 265–275.

Muscatelli, F., Abrous, D. N., Massacrier, A., Boccaccio, I., Le Moal, M., Cau, P., et al. (2000). Disruption of the mouse Necdin gene results in hypothalamic and behavioral alterations reminiscent of the human Prader-Willi syndrome. *Human Molecular Genetics, 9*, 3101–3110.

Myers, R. E., Swett, C., & Miller, M. (1973). Loss of social group affinity following prefrontal lesions in free-ranging macaques. *Brain Research, 64*, 257–269.

Nanson, J. L. (1992). Autism in fetal alcohol syndrome: A report of six cases. *Alcoholism: Clinical and Experimental Research, 16*, 558–565.

Narayanan, U., Nalavadi, V., Nakamoto, M., Thomas, G., Ceman, S., Bassell, G. J., et al. (2008). S6K1 phosphorylates and regulates fragile X mental retardation protein (FMRP) with the neuronal protein synthesis-dependent mammalian target of rapamycin (mTOR) signaling cascade. *Journal of Biological Chemistry, 283*, 18,478–18,482.

Narita, N., Kato, M., Tazoe M., Miyazaki, K., Narita, M., & Okado, N. (2002). Increased monoamine concentration in the brain and blood of fetal thalidomide- and valproic acid-exposed rat: Putative animal models for autism. *Pediatric Research, 52*, 576–579.

Narita, M., Oyabu, A., Imura, Y., Kamada, N. Yokoyama, T., Tano, K. et al. (2010). Nonexploratory movement and behavioral alterations in a thalidomide or valproic acid-induced autism model rat. *Neuroscience Research, 66*, 2–6.

Nawaz, Z., Lonard, D. M., Smith, C. L., Lev-Lehman, E., Tsai, S. Y., Tsai, M. J., et al. (1999). The Angelman syndrome-associated protein, E6-AP, is a coactivator for the nuclear hormone receptor superfamily. *Molecular and Cellular Biology, 19*, 1182–1189.

Nicholls, R. D., & Knepper, J. L. (2001). Genome organization, function, and imprinting in Prader-Willi and Angelman syndromes. *Annual Review of Genomics and Human Genetics, 2*, 153–175.

Nicolson, G. L., Gan, R., Nicolson, N. L., & Haier, J. (2007). Evidence for Mycoplasma ssp., Chlamydia pneumoniae, and human herpes virus-6 coinfections in the blood of patients with autistic spectrum disorders. *Journal of Neuroscience Research, 85*, 1143–1148.

Nishimura, K., Nakamura, K., Anitha, A., Yamada, K., Tsujii, M., Iwayama, Y., et al. (2007). Genetic analyses of the brain-derived neurotrophic factor (BDNF) gene in autism. *Biochemical and Biophysical Research Communications, 356*, 200–206.

Nyffeler, M., Meyer, U., Yee, B. K., Feldon, K., & Kneusel, I. (2006). Maternal immune activation during pregnancy increases limbic GABAA receptor immunoreactivity in the adult offspring: Implications for schizophrenia. *Neuroscience, 143*, 51–62.

Oh-Nishi, A., Obayashi, S., Sugihara, I., Minamimoto, T., & Suhara, T. (2010). Maternal immune activation by polyriboinosinic-polyribocytidilic acid injection produces synaptic dysfunction but not neuronal loss in the hippocampus of juvenile offspring. *Brain Research*, in press.

Ozawa, K., Hashimoto, K., Kishimoto, T., Shimizu, E., Ishikura, H., & Iyo, M. (2006). Immune activation during pregnancy in mice leads to dopaminergic hyperfunction and cognitive impairment in the offspring: A neurodevelopmental animal model of schizophrenia. *Biological Psychiatry, 59*, 546–554.

Paribello, C., Tao, L., Folino, A., Berry-Kravis, E., Tranfaglia, M., Ethell, E.M., et al. (2010). Open-label add-on treatment trial of minocycline in fragile X syndrome. *BMC Neurology, 10*, 91.

Paintlia, M. K., Paintlia, A. S., Barbosa, E., Singh, I, & Singh, A. K. (2004). N-acetylcysteine prevents endotoxin-induced degeneration of oligodendrocyte progenitors and hypomyelination in developing rat brain. *Journal of Neuroscience Research, 78*, 347–361.

Palmen, S., van Engeland, H., Hof, P. R., & Schmitz, C. (2004). Neuropathological findings in autism. *Brain, 127*, 2572–2583.

Panaitof, S. C., Abrahams, B. S., Dong, H., Geschwind, D. H. & White, S. A. (2010) Language-related Cntnap2 gene is differentially expressed in sexually dimorphic nuclei essential for vocal learning in songbirds. *Journal of Comparative Neurology, 518*, 1995–2018.

Pardo, C. A., & Eberhart, C. G. (2007). The neurobiology of autism. *Brain Pathology, 17*, 434–447.

Pardo, C. A., Vargas, D. L., & Zimmerman, A. W. (2006). Immunity, neuroglia and neuroinflammation in autism. *International Review of Psychiatry, 17*, 485–495.

Patterson, P. H. (2007). Maternal effects on schizophrenia risk. *Science, 318*, 576–577.

Patterson, P. H. (2009). Immune involvement in schizophrenia and autism: Etiology, pathology and animal models. *Behavioural Brain Research, 204*, 313–321.

Patterson, P. H. (2011). Modeling autistic features in animals. *Pediatric Research*, in press.

Peng, G. S., Li, G., Tzengc N. S., Chen, P. S., Chuange, D. M., Hsua Y. D., et al. (2005). Valproate pretreatment protects dopaminergic neurons from LPS-induced neurotoxicity in rat primary midbrain cultures: Role of microglia. *Brain Research. Molecular Brain Research, 24*, 162–169.

Perry, E. K., Lee, M. L., Martin-Ruiz, C. M., Court, J. A., Volsen, S. G., Merrit, J., et al. (2001). Cholinergic activity in autism: Abnormalities in the cerebral cortex and basal forebrain. *American Journal of Psychiatry, 158*, 1058–1066.

Petit, E., Herault, J., Martineau, J., Perrot, A., Barthelemy, C., Hameury, L., et al. (1995). Association study with two markers of a human homeogene in infantile autism. *Journal of Medical Genetics, 32*, 269–274.

Pfeiffer, B. E., Zang, T., Wilkerson, J. R., Taniguchi, M., Maksimova, M. A., Smith, L. N., et al. (2010). Fragile X mental retardation protein is required for synapse elimination by the activity-dependent transcription factor MEF2. *Neuron, 66*, 191–197.

Pilarski, R., & Eng, C. (2004). Will the real Cowden syndrome please stand up (again)? Expanding mutational and clinical spectra of the PTEN hamartoma tumour syndrome. *Journal of Medical Genetics, 41*, 323–326.

Piontkewitz, Y., Assaf, Y. & Weiner, I. (2009). Clozapine administration in adolescence prevents postpurbertal emergence of brain structural pathology in an animal model of schizophrenia. *Biological Psychiatry, 66*, 1038–1046.

Pletnikov, M. V., Ayhan, Y., Nikolskaia, O., Xu, Y., Ovanesov, M. V., Huang, H., et al. (2008). Inducible expression of mutant human DISC1 in mice is associated with brain and behavioral abnormalities reminiscent of schizophrenia. *Molecular Psychiatry, 13*, 173–186, 115.

Powell, E. M., Campbell, D. B., Stanwood, G. D., Davis, C., Noebels, J. L., & Levitt, P. (2003). Genetic disruption of cortical interneuron development causes region- and GABA cell type-specific deficits, epilepsy, and behavioral dysfunction. *Journal of Neuroscience, 23*, 622–631.

Powell, E. M., Mars, W. M., & Levitt, P. (2001). Hepatocyte growth factor/scatter factor is a mitogen for interneurons migrating from the ventral to dorsal telencephalon. *Neuron, 30*, 79–89.

Previc, F. H. (2007). Prenatal influences on brain dopamine and their relevance to the rising incidence of autism. *Medical Hypotheses, 68*, 46–60.

Price, C. S., Thompson, W. W., Goodson, B., Weintraub, E. S., Croen, L. A., Hinrichsen, V. L., et al. (2010). Prenatal and infant exposure to thimerosal from vaccines and immunoglobulins and risk of autism. *Pediatrics, 126*, 656–664.

Ragnauth, A. K., Devidze, N., Moy, V., Finley, K., Goodwillie, A., Kow, L. M., et al. (2005). Female oxytocin gene-knockout mice, in a semi-natural environment, display exaggerated aggressive behavior. *Genes, Brain, and Behavior, 4*, 229–239.

Raymond, G. V., Bauman, M. L., & Kemper, T. L. (1996). Hippocampus in autism: A Golgi analysis. *Acta Neuropathologica, 91*, 117–119.

Ren, M., Leng, Y., Jeong, M., Leeds, P. R., & Chuang, D. M. (2004). Valproic acid reduces brain damage induced by transient focal cerebral ischemia in rats: Potential roles of histone deacetylase inhibition and heat shock protein induction. *Journal of Neurochemistry, 89*, 1358–1367.

Ren-Patterson, R. F., Cochran, L. W., Holmes, A., Sherrill, S., Huang, S. J., Tolliver, T., et al. (2005). Loss of brain-derived neurotrophic factor gene allele exacerbates brain monoamine deficiencies and increases stress abnormalities of serotonin transporter knockout mice. *Journal of Neuroscience Research, 79*, 756–771.

Rhodes, M. C., Seidler,. J., Abdel-Rahman, A., Tate, C. A., Nyska, A., Rincavage, H. L., et al. (2004). Terbutaline is a neurotoxicant: Effects on neuroproteins and morphology in cerebellum, hippocampus, and somatosensory cortex. *Journal of Pharmacology and Experimental Therapeutics, 308*, 529–537.

Rinaldi, T., Kulangara, K., Antoniello, K., & Markram, H. (2007a). Elevated NMDA receptor levels and enhanced postsynaptic long-term potentiation induced by prenatal exposure to valproic acid. *Proceedings of the National Academy of Sciences of the United States of America, 104*, 13501–13506.

Rinaldi, T., Silberberg, G., & Markram, H. (2007b). Hyperconnectivity of local neocortical microcircuitry induced by prenatal exposure to valproic acid. *Cerebral Cortex, 18*, 763–770.

Roullet, F. I., Wollaston, L., Decantanzaro, D. & Foster, J. A. (2010). Behavioral and molecular changes in the mouse in response to prenatal exposure to the anti-epileptic drug valproic acid. *Neuroscience, 170*, 514–522.

Rubenstein, J. L., & Merzenich, M. M. (2003). Model of autism: Increased ratio of excitation/inhibition in key neural systems. *Genes, Brain, and Behavior, 2*, 255–267.

Samuelsson, A. M., Jennische, E., Hansson, H. A., & Holmang, A. (2006). Prenatal exposure to interleukin-6 results in inflammatory neurodegeneration in hippocampus with NMDA/GABA(A) dysregulation and impaired spatial learning. *American Journal of Physiology- Regulatory, Integrative, and Comparative Physiology, 290*, 1345–1356.

Scanlon, S. M., Williams, D. C., & Schloss, P. (2001). Membrane cholesterol modulates serotonin transporter activity. *Biochemistry, 40*, 10507–10513.

Scattoni, M. L., Gandhy, S. U., Ricceri, L., & Crawley, J. N. (2008). Unusual repertoire of vocalizations in the BTBR T+tf/J mouse model of autism. *PLoS ONE, 3*, e3067.

Scattoni, M. L., McFarlane, H. G., Zhodzishsky, V., Caldwell, H. K., Young, W. S., Ricceri, L., et al. (2008). Reduced ultrasonic vocalizations in vasopressin 1b knockout mice. *Behavioural Brain Research, 187*, 371–378.

Schechter, R., & Grether, J. K. (2008). Continuing increases in autism reported to California's developmental services system. *Archives of General Psychiatry, 65*, 19–24.

Schneider, M., & Koch, M. (2005). Deficient social and play behavior in juvenile and adult rats after neonatal cortical lesion: Effects of chronic pubertal cannabinoid treatment. *Neuropsychopharmacology, 30*, 944–957.

Schneider, T., & Przewlocki, R. (2005). Behavioral alterations in rats prenatally exposed to valproic acid: Animal model of autism. *Neuropsychopharmacology, 30*, 80–89.

Schneider, T., Roman, A., Basta-Kaim, A., Kubera, M., Budziszewska, B., & Schneider, K. (2008). Gender specific behavioral and immunological alterations in an animal model of autism induced by prenatal exposure to valproic acid. *Psychoneuroendocrinology, 33*, 728–740.

Schwabe, K., Klein, S., & Koch, M. (2006). Behavioural effects of neonatal lesions of the medial prefrontal cortex and subchronic pubertal treatment with phencyclidine of adult rats. *Behavioural Brain Research, 168*, 150–160.

Shahbazian, M., Young, J., Yuva-Paylor, L., Spencer, C., Antalffy, B., Noebels, J., et al. (2002). Mice with truncated MeCP2 recapitulate many Rett syndrome features and display hyperacetylation of histone H3. *Neuron, 35*, 243–254.

Sharma, A., Hoeffer, C. A., Takayasu, Y., Miyawaki, T., McBride, S. M., Klann, E., et al. (2010). Dysregulation of mTOR signaling in fragile X syndrome. *Journal of Neuroscience, 30*, 694–702.

Shi, L., Fatemi, S. H., Sidwell, R. W., & Patterson, P. H. (2003). Maternal influenza infection causes marked behavioral and pharmacological changes in the offspring. *Journal of Neuroscience, 23*, 297–302.

Shi, L., Smith, S. E., Malkova, N., Tse, D., Su, Y., & Patterson, P. H. (2009). Activation of the maternal immune system alters cerebellar development in the offspring. *Brain, Behavior, and Immunity, 23*, 116–123.

Shi, L., Tu, N., & Patterson, P.H. (2005). Maternal influenza infection is likely to alter fetal brain development indirectly: The virus is not detected in the fetus. *International Journal of Developmental Neuroscience, 23*, 299–305.

Silva-Gomez, A. B., Bermudez, M., Quirion, R., Srivastava, L. K., Picazo, O., & Florez, G. (2003). Comparative behavioral changes between male and female postpubertal rats following neonatal excitoxic lesions of the ventral hippocampus. *Brain Research, 973*, 285–292.

Slotkin, T. A., & Seidler, F. J. (2007). Developmental exposure to terbutaline and chlorpyrifos, separately or sequentially, elicits presynaptic serotonergic hyperactivity in juvenile and adolescent rats. *Brain Research Bulletin, 73*, 301–309.

Smith, S. E., Li J., Garbett, K., Mirnics, K., & Patterson, P. H. (2007). Maternal immune activation alters fetal brain development through interleukin-6. *Journal of Neuroscience, 27*, 10695–10702.

St Clair, D., Blackwood, D., Muir, W., Carothers, A., Walker, M., Spowart, G., et al. (1990). Association within a family of a balanced autosomal translocation with major mental illness. *Lancet, 336*, 13–16.

Stanton, M. E., Peloso, E., Brown, K. L., & Rodier, P. (2007). Discrimination learning and reversal of the conditioned eyeblink reflex in a rodent model of autism. *Behavioural Brain Research, 176*, 133–140.

Stromland, K., Nordin, V., Miller, M., Akerstrom, B., & Gillberg, C. (1994). Autism in thalidomide embryopathy: A population study. *Developmental Medicine and Child Neurology, 36*, 351–356.

Sudhof, T. C. (2008). Neuroligins and neurexins link synaptic function to cognitive disease. *Nature, 455*, 903–911.

Sweeten, T. L., Posey, D. J., Shekhar, A., & McDougle, C. J. (2002). The amygdala and related structures in the pathophysiology of autism. *Pharmacology, Biochemistry, and Behavior, 71*, 449–455.

Tabuchi, K., Blundell, J., Etherton, M. R., Hammer, R. E., Liu, X., Powell, C. M., et al. (2007). A neuroligin-3 mutation implicated in autism increases inhibitory synaptic transmission in mice. *Science, 318*, 71–76.

Takayanagi, Y., Yoshida, M., Bielsky, I. F., Ross, H. E., Kawamata, M., Onaka, T., et al. (2005). Pervasive social deficits, but normal parturition, in oxytocin receptor-deficient mice. *Proceedings of the*

National Academy of Sciences of the United States of America, 102, 16,096–16,101.

Tetreault, N. A., Williams, B. A., Hasenstaub, A., Hakeem, A. Y., Liu, M., Abelin, A. C. T., et al. (2009). RNA-Seq studies of gene expression in fronto-insular cortex in autistic and control subjects reveal gene networks related to inflammation and synaptic function. Program No. 473.3. 2009 *Neuroscience Meeting Planner. Chicago, IL: Society for Neuroscience*. Online.

Tierney, E., Bukelis, I., Thompson, R. E., Ahmed, K., Aneja, A., Kratz, L., et al. (2006). Abnormalities of cholesterol metabolism in autism spectrum disorders. *American Journal of Medical Genetics. Part B, Neuropsychiatric Genetics, 141B*, 666–668.

Tierney, E., Nwokoro, N. A., Porter, F. D., Freund, L. S., Ghuman, J. K., & Kelley, R. I. (2001). Behavior phenotype in the RSH/Smith-Lemli-Opitz syndrome. *American Journal of Medical Genetics, 98*, 191–200.

Tordjman, S., Drapier, D., Bonnot, O., Graignic, R., Fortes, S., Cohen, D., et al. (2007). Animal models relevant to schizophrenia and autism: Validity and limitations. *Behavior Genetics, 37*, 61–78.

Tropea, D., Giacometti, E., Wilson, N. R., Beard, C., McCurry, C., Fu, D. D., et al. (2009). Partial reversal of Rett Syndrome-like symptoms in MeCP2 mutant mice. *Proceedings of the National Academy of Sciences of the United States of America, 106*, 2029–2034.

Tuchman, R., & Rapin, I. (2002). Epilepsy in autism. *Lancet Neurology, 1*, 352–358.

Turner, B. M., Paradiso, S., Marvel, C. L., Pierson, R., Boles Ponto, L. L., Hichwa, R. D. et al. (2007). The cerebellum and emotional experience. *Neuropsychologia, 45*, 1331–1341.

Tyndall, S. J., & Walikonis, R. S. (2006). The receptor tyrosine kinase Met and its ligand hepatocyte growth factor are clustered at excitatory synapses and can enhance clustering of synaptic proteins. *Cell Cycle, 5*, 1560–1568.

Urakubo, A., Jarskog, L. F., Lieberman, J. A., & Gilmore, J. H. (2001). Prenatal exposure to maternal infection alters cytokine expression in the placenta, amniotic fluid, and fetal brain. *Schizophrenia Research, 47*, 27–36.

van Woerden, G. M., Harris, K. D., Hojjati, M. R., Gustin, R. M., Qiu, S., de Avila Freire, R., et al. (2007). Rescue of neurological deficits in a mouse model for Angelman syndrome by reduction of alphaCaMKII inhibitory phosphorylation. *Nature Neuroscience, 10*, 280–282.

Vargas, D. L., Nascimbene, C., Krishnan, C., Zimmerman, A. W., & Pardo, C. A. (2005). Neuroglial activation and neuroinflammation in the brain of patients with autism. *Annals of Neurology, 57*, 67–81.

Veltman, M. W., Craig, E. E., & Bolton, P. F. (2005). Autism spectrum disorders in Prader-Willi and Angelman syndromes: A systematic review. *Psychiatric Genetics, 15*, 243–254.

Vernes, S. C., Newbury, D. F., Abrahams, B. S., Winchester, L., Nicod, J., Groszer, M., Alarcon, M. et al. (2008). A functional genetic link between distinct developmental language disorders. *New England Journal of Medicine, 359*, 2337–2345.

Vorhees, C. V., Weisenburger, W. P., & Minck, D. R. (2001). Neurobehavioral teratogenic effects of thalidomide in rats. *Neurotoxicology and Teratology, 23*, 255–264.

Waage-Baudet, H., Lauder, J. M., Dehart, D. B., Kluckman, K., Hiller, S., Tint, G. S., et al. (2003). Abnormal serotonergic development in a mouse model for the Smith-Lemli-Opitz syndrome: Implications for autism. *International Journal of Developmental Neuroscience, 21*, 451–459.

Wang, L., Jia, M., Yue, W., Tang, F., Qu, M., Ruan, Y., et al. (2008). Association of the ENGRAILED 2 (EN2) gene with autism in Chinese Han population. *American Journal of Medical Genetics. Part B, Neuropsychiatric Genetics, 147B*, 434–438.

Wassink, T. H., & Piven, J. (2000). The molecular genetics of autism. *Current Psychiatry Reports, 2*, 170–175.

Weeber, E. J., Jiang, Y. H., Elgersma, Y., Varga, A. W., Carrasquillo, Y., Brown, S. E., et al. (2003). Derangements of hippocampal calcium/calmodulin-dependent protein kinase II in a mouse model for Angelman mental retardation syndrome. *Journal of Neuroscience, 23*, 2634–2644.

Winslow, J. T., Hearn, E. F., Ferguson, J., Young, L. J., Matzuk, M. M., & Insel, T. R. (2000). Infant vocalization, adult aggression, and fear behavior of an oxytocin null mutant mouse. *Hormones and Behavior, 37*, 145–155.

Winslow, J. T., & Insel, T. R. (2002). The social deficits of the oxytocin knockout mouse. *Neuropeptides, 36*, 221–229.

Winter, C., Reutiman, T. J., Folsom, T. D., Sohr, R., Wolf, R. J., Juckel, G., et al. (2008). Dopamine and serotonin levels following prenatal viral infection in mouse - implications for psychiatric disorders such as schizophrenia and autism. *European Neuropsychopharmacology, 18*, 712–716.

Wohr, M., Roullet, F., & Crawley, J. (2010). Reduced scent marking and ultrasonic vocalizations in the BRBR T+tf/J inbred strain mouse model of autism. *Genes, Brain, and Behavior, PMID: 20345893.*

Wurst, W., Auerbach, A. B., & Joyner, A. L. (1994). Multiple developmental defects in Engrailed-1 mutant mice: An early mid-hindbrain deletion and patterning defects in forelimbs and sternum. *Development, 120*, 2065–2075.

Yan, J., Oliveira, G., Coutinho, A., Yang, C., Feng, J., Katz, C., et al. (2005). Analysis of the neuroligin 3 and 4 genes in autism and other neuropsychiatric patients. *Molecular Psychiatry, 10*, 329–332.

Yang, M., Zhodzishsky, V., & Crawley, J. N. (2007). Social deficits in BTBR T+tf/J mice are unchanged by cross-fostering with C57BL/6J mothers. *International Journal of Developmental Neuroscience, 25*, 515–521.

Yang, P., Lung, F. W., Jong, Y. J., Hsieh, H. Y., Liang, C. L., & Juo, S. H. (2008). Association of the homeobox transcription factor gene ENGRAILED 2 with autistic disorder in Chinese children. *Neuropsychobiology, 57*, 3–8.

Yang, T., Adamson, T. E., Resnick, J. L., Leff, S., Wevrick, R., Francke, U., et al. (1998). A mouse model for Prader-Willi syndrome imprinting-centre mutations. *Nature Genetics, 19*, 25–31.

Yates, J. R. (2006). Tuberous sclerosis. *European Journal of Human Genetics, 14*, 1065–1073.

Yu, H., & Patel, S. B. (2005). Recent insights into the Smith-Lemli-Opitz syndrome. *Clinical Genetics, 68*, 383–391.

Zanella, S., Watrin, F., Mebarek, S., Marly, F., Roussel, M., Gire, C., et al. (2008). Necdin plays a role in the serotonergic modulation of the mouse respiratory network: Implication for Prader-Willi syndrome. *Journal of Neuroscience, 28*, 1745–1755.

Zaretsky, M. V., Alexander, J. M., Byrd, W., & Bawden, R. E. (2004). Transfer of inflammatory cytokines across the placenta. *Obstetrics and Gynecology, 103*, 546–550.

Zerrate, M. C., Pletnikov, M., Connors, S. L., Vargas, D. L., Seidler, F. J., Zimmerman, A. W., et al. (2007). Neuroinflammation and behavioral abnormalities after neonatal terbutaline treatment in rats. *Journal of Pharmacology and Experimental Therapeutics, 322*, 16–22.

Zhong, H., Serajee, F. J., Nabi, R., & Huq, A. H. (2003). No association between the EN2 gene and autistic disorder. *Journal of Medical Genetics, 40*, e4.

Zimmerman, A. W., Connors, S. L., Matteson, K. J., Lee, L. C., Singer, H. S., Castaneda, J. A., et al. (2007). Maternal antibrain antibodies in autism. *Brain, Behavior, and Immunity, 21*, 351–357.

Zoghbi, H. Y. (2003). Postnatal neurodevelopmental disorders: Meeting at the synapse? *Science, 302*, 826–830.

Zori, R. T., Marsh, D. J., Graham, G. E., Marliss, E. B., & Eng, C. (1998). Germline PTEN mutation in a family with Cowden syndrome and Bannayan-Riley-Ruvalcaba syndrome. *American Journal of Medical Genetics, 80*, 399–402.

Zuckerman, L., Rehavi, M., Nachman, R. & Weiner, I. (2003) Immune activation during pregnancy in rats leads to a postpubertal emergence of disrupted latent inhibition, dopaminergic hyperfunction, and altered limbic morphology in the offspring: A novel neurodevelopmental model of schizophrenia. *Neuropsychopharmacology, 28*, 17781–1789.

Zuckerman, L. & Weiner, I. (2005). Maternal immune activation leads to behavioral and pharmacological changes in the adult offspring. *Journal of Psychiatric Research, 39*, 311–323.

53 Melissa. D. Bauman, David. G. Amaral

Nonhuman Primate Models of Autism

Points of Interest

- Rhesus macaque monkeys live in a sophisticated social environment and use gestures of social communication, such as facial expressions, that are very similar to those used by humans. Many of these behaviors that macaque monkeys share with humans are impaired in autism.
- The neuroanatomy of the rhesus monkey brain more closely approximates that of the human brain than does the rodent brain. The frontal cortex, for example, a region that likely mediates many facets of social cognition, includes regions that are prominent in the human brain but are lacking in the rodent brain.
- Primate models based on lesions of brain regions such as the amygdala do not demonstrate construct, face, or predictive validity.
- Although few models based on known etiologies of human autism exist in the nonhuman primate, recent efforts at modeling potential immune etiologies have demonstrated provocative results.
- There is currently a great need for behavioral probes for nonhuman primate models of autism that are more sensitive to the core features of the deficit.

What Can We Learn from Nonhuman Primate Models of Human Disorders?

An animal model is defined as "an animal sufficiently like humans in its anatomy, physiology, or response to a pathogen to be used in medical research in order to obtain results that can be extrapolated to human medicine" (Merriam-Webster Online Dictionary, n.d.). Although animal models usually do not replicate all aspects of a human disorder, they do provide an experimental system to evaluate hypotheses that, for ethical and practical reasons, are impossible to test using human subjects. Nonhuman primates share many features of human physiology, anatomy, and behavior, thus making the nonhuman primate an ideal species to study a variety of human disorders (J. P. Capitanio & Emborg, 2008). For example, nonhuman primate models have revolutionized the understanding of Parkinson's disease by providing insight into the neural circuitry underlying this disorder (Burns et al., 1983; DeLong, 1990). This, in turn, led to the development of new therapies for humans such as targeted surgical ablation and deep brain stimulation (Bergman, Wichmann, & DeLong, 1990). Nonhuman primates have also played a key role in understanding the neural underpinnings of Alzheimer's disease (Wenk, 1993) and provided a model system for evaluating novel therapeutic interventions for this disorder (Lemere et al., 2004; Lemere, Maier, Jiang, Peng, & Seabrook, 2006; Nagahara et al., 2009; Tuszynski & Blesch, 2004; Tuszynski, Roberts, Senut, U, & Gage, 1996). More recently, a primate transgenic model of Huntington's disease has provided important links between the underlying cellular pathology and the behavioral symptoms of this disorder (Yang et al., 2008). Although we are in the very early stages of developing valid animal models of autism, it is likely that nonhuman primate models will play an important role in identifying biological underpinnings of autism and facilitating the development of future treatment and prevention strategies.

What Constitutes a Good Animal Model of Autism?

The strength of an animal model depends on its resemblance to the human disorder in question. Three criteria are commonly used to evaluate animal models: *(1)* Construct validity—the extent to which the model reproduces the etiology and/or pathophysiology of the disorder; *(2)* Face validity—the degree to which the model resembles symptoms of the disorder; and *(3)* Predictive validity—the extent to which treatment of the animal model provides insight into therapeutic options for the human condition (Crawley, 2004; McKinney, 1984). The role of these three criteria in establishing animal models of autism is described in detail below.

Construct Validity

Construct validity refers to the degree of similarity between the experimental manipulation used to create the animal model and the underlying cause(s) of the human disease being studied. Construct validity of animal models of autism can be evaluated by asking the following questions: *Does the experimental manipulation stem from findings in human autism research? Does the model stem from a putative etiology of human autism?*

We suggest that for an animal model to provide a valuable contribution to autism research, it must stem from hypotheses that are directly related to the human disorder. This has proven particularly challenging for the field of autism where the underlying cause(s) of the disease for most cases remain unknown. However, as potential causes of autism are identified, animal models will play a critical role in translating results from human autism research into testable hypotheses. For example, recent research with human subjects has identified putative genetic, immunological, environmental and neurobiological markers for autism (Abrahams & Geschwind, 2008; Amaral, Schumann, & Nordahl, 2008; Ashwood, Wills, & Van de Water, 2006; Hertz-Picciotto et al., 2008; Pessah et al., 2008). Although such studies from human subjects shed light on potential biological mechanisms and plausible causes of autism, it is not possible to determine if these findings are causally involved with autism or simply an epiphenomenon of the disease. Animal models provide a means of experimentally evaluating these findings from human studies. This translational approach produces animal models with high construct validity.

Face Validity

Animal models may produce changes in gene expression, brain anatomy and chemistry, and ultimately behavior. Face validity is the extent to which these changes resemble the phenotype of the human disorder. Because autism is a behaviorally defined disorder, the assessment of face validity of animal models is currently focused on changes in behavior that resemble symptoms of autism. The following questions provide a framework to evaluate the face validity of an animal model of autism: *Is it reasonable to hypothesize that the experimental manipulation may result in behavioral changes that resemble autistic symptomatology? Are the changes in behaviors relevant to human autism? Have appropriate behavioral tests been used to evaluate behavior in this particular species? Have other factors that may influence the behavioral data been controlled for?*

For behaviorally defined disorders such as autism, it is important to relate the behavioral outcome of the animal model to the hallmark features of the human disorder. Diagnosis of autism is based on qualitative impairments in social interaction and communication, with the presence of restricted repetitive and stereotyped patterns of behavior, interests, and activities. Table 53-1 outlines the DSM-IV criteria for autism diagnosis as well as the ADOS Module 1 items that are used to diagnose autism for individuals who are pre-verbal or only produce single-word utterances. Table 53-1 also includes a list of nonhuman primate behavioral assays that can be used to assess comparable behaviors in nonhuman primate models of autism. Although some features of autism cannot be successfully modeled in animal species (i.e., language, deficits in theory of mind etc.), it is possible to examine fundamental changes in species-typical behaviors relevant to autistic symptomatology. An ideal animal model with high face validity would produce behavioral changes in the three diagnostic domains of autism: *(1)* social development, *(2)* communication, and *(3)* repetitive behaviors. However, it is important to emphasize that the goal is not necessarily to create "autistic animals." Rather, the goal is to model one or more *features* of human autism in another species so as to enable experimental approaches to understanding its biological underpinnings. Thus, it may not be realistic to expect an animal model of autism to involve behavioral changes in all three symptom domains.

This leads to the second question regarding the appropriateness of the behavioral tests that are used to evaluate the model. Face validity is enhanced by utilizing tests that tap into species-specific behaviors that are related to the symptoms of autism. This requires knowledge of autistic symptomatology, as well as an understanding of the natural behavior of the species being studied. Typical social behavior for a human child will certainly differ from typical social behavior of any model species. It is critical to keep these differences in mind when designing tests to evaluate animal models of autism. For example, diminished eye contact may be characteristic of many individuals with autism (Klin, Jones, Schultz, Volkmar, & Cohen, 2002; J. Osterling & Dawson, 1994; J. A. Osterling, Dawson, & Munson, 2002; Pelphrey et al., 2002; Swettenham et al., 1998). However, species such as rhesus macaques naturally avoid making direct eye contact because it is considered to be a threatening gesture. Thus, it would be inappropriate to use direct eye contact as a measure of social attention/interest in rhesus monkeys. Instead, we must look to other measures of social attention that reflect species-typical social interest in rhesus monkeys (i.e., trying to engage another animal in grooming, etc.). Testing behaviors that are relevant to autism and designing tests that are appropriate for the model species are critical components of creating a valid animal model of autism.

Finally, we must also control for other factors known to trigger autistic-like behaviors in laboratory animals. For example, it is well-known that restricted environments (i.e., small cages, lack of social interaction, etc.) are associated with motor stereotypies and atypical social development in a variety of species (J. Capitanio, 1986; C. Lutz, Well, & Novak, 2003). Given that atypical social development and stereotypies are

Table 53–1.
Diagnostic criteria of autism and relevant behavioral assays for nonhuman primates

DSM-IV diagnosis: six (or more) items from (1), (2), and (3), with at least two from (1), and one each from (2) and (3)	ADOS Module 1 *items included in ADOS algorithm for autism diagnosis	Comparable behavioral assays for nonhuman primate models of autism
(1) Qualitative impairments in social interaction Marked impairment in the use of multiple nonverbal behaviors such as eye-to-eye gaze, facial expression, body postures, and gestures to regulate social interaction Failure to develop peer relationships appropriate to developmental level Lack of spontaneous seeking to share enjoyment, interests, or achievements with other people (e.g., by a lack of showing, bringing, or pointing out objects of interest) Lack of social or emotional reciprocity	**Reciprocal social interaction** Unusual eye contact* Responsive social smile Facial expressions directed to others* Integration of gaze and other behaviors Shared enjoyment in interactions* Response to name Requesting Giving Showing* Spontaneous initiation of joint attention* Response to joint attention* Quality of social overtures*	Quantification of species-typical social behaviors (Bauman, M. D. et al., 2004a, 2004b) Social attention/motivation modeled after (Rudebeck et al., 2006) Neonatal facial imitation (Ferrari et al., 2006) Assessment of dominance hierarchy (Bauman M. D. et al., 2006)
(2) Qualitative impairments in communication Delay in, or total lack of, the development of spoken language In individuals with adequate speech, marked impairment in the ability to initiate or sustain a conversation with others Stereotypes or repetitive use of language or idiosyncratic language Lack of varied, spontaneous make-believe play or social imitative play	**Language and communication** Level of non-echoed language Frequency of vocalization directed to others* Intonation of vocalizations Immediate echolalia Stereotyped/idiosyncratic use of words* Use of other's body to communicate* Pointing* Gestures*	Quantification of species-typical vocalizations (Bauman M. D. et al., 2004a, 2004b) Quantification of vocalizations during separation from mother (Bauman M. D. et al., 2004a) Response to mother's vocalization (Masataka, 1985)
(3) Restricted repetitive and stereotyped patterns of behavior, interests, and activities Encompassing preoccupation with one or more stereotyped and restricted patterns of interest that is abnormal either in intensity or focus Apparently inflexible adherence to specific, nonfunctional routines or rituals Stereotyped and repetitive motor manners (e.g., hand or finger flapping or twisting, or complex whole-body movements) Persistent preoccupation with parts of objects	**Stereotyped behaviors and restricted interests** Unusual sensory interest in play material/ person* Hand and finger and other complex mannerisms* Self-injurious behaviors Unusually repetitive interests or stereotyped behaviors	Quantitative assessment of repetitive and stereotyped behaviors (Bauman M. D. et al., 2008) Restricted patterns of interests (modeled after (Moy et al., 2008)
	Play Functional play with objects* Imagination/creativity*	Atypical toy play (modeled after Ozonoff et al., 2008).
	Other abnormal behaviors Overactivity Tantrums, aggression, negative or disruptive behaviors Anxiety	Activity monitoring (Martin et al., 2008) Responsiveness to fear-inducing objects (Prather et al., 2001)

hallmark features of autism, it is essential to control for these behaviors in any animal model of the disorder. Every effort must be made to raise and house animal subjects in a way that assures the development of species-typical social behavior. This includes providing adequate cage sizes, maternal rearing, and opportunities to engage in social interactions with conspecifics. Appropriate control groups are necessary to ensure that changes in behavior can be attributed to the experimental manipulation, rather than to any aspect of the experimental environment (or to a combination of the experimental manipulation and environment). Changes in behavior related to autism that are observed after selecting species-appropriate behavioral assays and utilizing proper controls result in a model with strong face validity.

Predictive Validity

The ultimate goal of any animal model is to develop a means of preventing or treating the human disorder. Predictive validity refers to treatment discoveries in an animal model that provides insight into therapeutic options for the human condition. Although we are just beginning to develop valid animal models of autism, the information gained through these models will ultimately help us move toward the goal of developing preventative strategies and/or novel therapies to reduce the incidence of autism.

Advantages and Limitations of Nonhuman Primate Models

Mouse models have certain advantages over nonhuman primate models. Mouse models can be used for a variety of approaches, including genetic manipulation, environmental manipulation, and alterations in central nervous system function (*see* Chapters 51 and 52). Mouse models are also less expensive, and because of the shorter gestation and larger litters produced by rodents, a greater number of experiments can be completed in a shorter time (mouse gestation = approximately 20 days; rhesus monkey gestation = 165-days). This allows for more extensive pilot and experimental work to be conducted with mouse models than would be practical with nonhuman primate models. Mouse models, however, are also faced with the challenges of relating the rodent brain to the human brain and rodent behavior to human behavior. Portions of the human brain, such as the prefrontal cortex, that are believed to be heavily impacted by autism, are not well-developed in the rodent brain. Given that autism is a disorder defined by changes in complex human behaviors, many of which are mediated by the frontal lobe, developing a mouse model with strong face validity has posed a considerable challenge. It is possible that a uniquely human disorder such as autism may ultimately require the use of animal species that are more closely related to humans, such as nonhuman primates. This may be particularly germane to attempts at developing new therapies. Both the advantages and the limitations of the nonhuman primate model are discussed in detail below.

Advantages

In this chapter, we focus our descriptions on research utilizing the rhesus macaque (*Macacca mulatta*), often considered to be the model species of choice for biomedical research. However, it is notable that other nonhuman primate species may also be used to study human neurodevelopmental disorders. Vervet monkeys, for example, have been used to study the complex interactions among genes, brain, and behavior (Fairbanks et al., 2004; Fears et al., 2009) and may provide an alternative approach to modeling complex human disorders in nonhuman primates.

Compared with rodents, which are separated from humans by more than 70 million years (Gibbs et al., 2004; Kumar & Hedges, 1998), macaques exhibit greater similarity to human physiology, neurobiology, behavior, and susceptibility to diseases. This is not surprising, given that macaques shared a common ancestor with humans some 25 million years ago (Kay, Ross, & Williams, 1997) and that the macaque genome demonstrates a 90% to 93% alignment of nucleotide sequences with the human genome (Gibbs et al., 2007). The genetic similarities between humans and macaques are further demonstrated by more subtle comparisons of macaque and human genome. For example, polymorphisms in the serotonin transporter gene that have been associated with temperamental differences and susceptibility to psychiatric disorders are similar in humans and rhesus monkeys but not other nonhuman primates (Champoux et al., 2002; Lesch et al., 1997; Trefilov, Krawczak, Berard, & Schmidtke, 1999). In addition to the genetic similarities between macaques and humans, there are compelling similarities between brain and behavior that make rhesus macaques the model of choice for studying complex human disorders such as autism. The neuroanatomical and behavioral complexity of rhesus monkeys is described below in detail.

Neuroanatomical Complexity of Rhesus Monkeys

Despite the fact that the macaque monkey brain is only one-tenth the size of the human brain, the neural organization of the macaque monkey brain is remarkably similar to the human brain (Fig. 53-1). Although it is beyond the scope of this chapter to provide a detailed review of the comparative neuronanatomy of the rodent, macaque monkey and human brains, one or two examples will suffice to make the point that the macaque monkey brain is more similar to that of the human than the rodent.

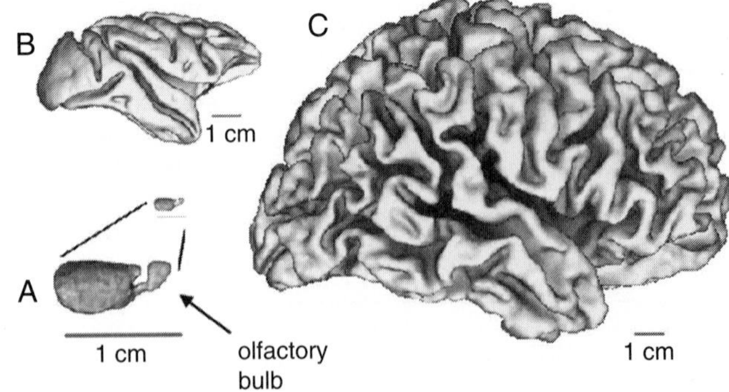

Figure 53–1. Lateral surface of the (A) mouse, (B) macaque monkey, and (C) human brain. The sulci of the monkey and human have been expanded to show gyral and sulcal patterns. Although the mouse has a relatively large olfactory bulb (hidden from view on the orbital surface of the monkey and human brain), the frontal lobe by comparison is much larger in the monkey and human brain. Images courtesy of Dr. David Van Essen.

Perhaps the frontal lobe is the best regions to explore these differences. The frontal lobe has demonstrated the greatest phylogenetic advancement of any cortical area. There is substantial evidence, in fact, that the demands of living in a social environment (Byrne & Whiten, 1988; Jolly, 1966) have spurred on the evolutionary development of the nonhuman and human frontal lobes—particularly of the increased complexity of connections of these regions (Semendeferi, Lu, Schenker, & Damasio, 2002). Put simply, there are cytoarchitectonic divisions of the frontal lobe that are identifiable in the human brain and in the macaque monkey brain but are not identifiable in the mouse or rat brain (T. Preuss, 1995). As Preuss has argued (Box 53-1), based on cytoarchitectonic, connectional, and neurotransmitter distribution grounds, it is unlikely that rats have cortical homologs of the human dorsolateral prefrontal cortex that is also a prominent component of the monkey brain (T. M. Preuss, 2000). Because the frontal lobe appears to be one of the brain regions most commonly implicated in the neuropathology of autism (Carper & Courchesne, 2005), it raises the concern of whether any rodent model of autism could truly have face validity.

Others have argued that even the rhesus monkey may not be an appropriate model for the human brain. Allman and colleagues have demonstrated a unique type of cortical neuron (the Von Economo Cell [VENs]) located in medial frontal cortex of humans, all of the great ape species, four cetacean species, and African and Indian elephants (Hakeem et al., 2009). These neurons do not appear to be in the rhesus monkey brain. Allman has noted that the VENs emerge mainly after birth in humans and increase in number for the first 4 years of life. He has proposed (Allman, Watson, Tetreault, & Hakeem, 2005) that in autism spectrum disorders, the VENs fail to develop normally and that this failure might be partially responsible for the associated social disabilities that result.

Box 53–1

Comparison of the frontal cortex of the macaque monkey (A) with that of the rat (B and C). Panels B and C present two different interpretations of the organization of the rat frontal cortex. As reviewed by Preuss (2007), traditional views of the rat organization (B) identify the cortex occupying the medial wall of the frontal cortex with the dorsolateral prefrontal cortex (DLPFC) of primates. Traditional descriptions of the rat frontal cortex either make no attempt to identify homologues of the cingulate cortex (grey patterned region—medial view, panel A) or treat medial cortex as containing a mixture of DLPFC and cingulate characteristics. Preuss's interpretation (2007) shown in C, identifies the medial prefrontal cortex of rats with the medial frontal areas of primates. In particular, the areas in rats situated immediately anterior and dorsal to the corpus callosum are identified with subdivisions of the primate cingulate cortex, specifically the anterior cingulate (AC), prelimbic (PL), and infralimbic (IL) areas (grey patterned region—medial view, panel C). Under this interpretation, rats lack cortex homologous to primate DLPFC.

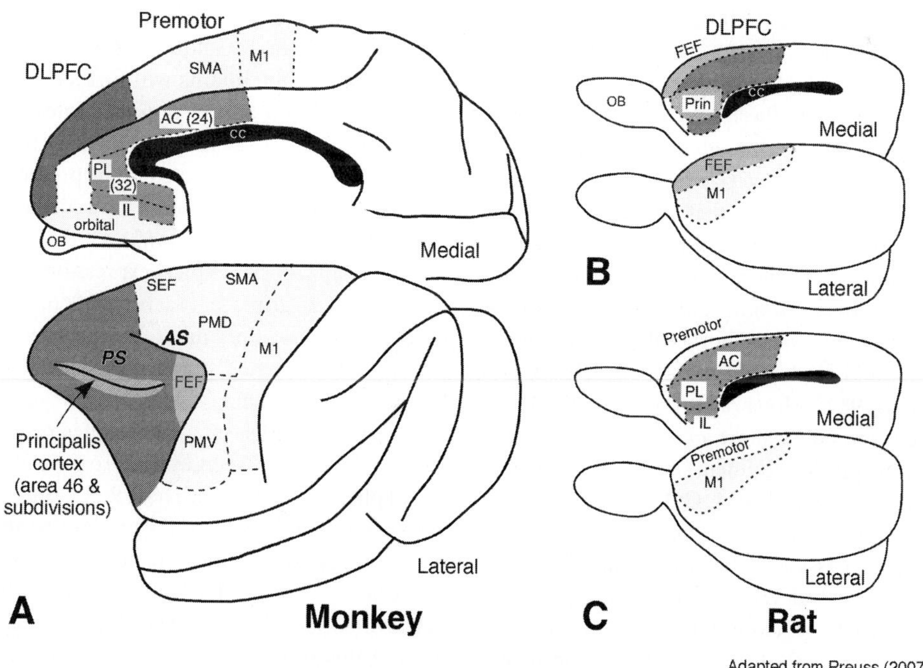

Additional abbreviations: frontal eye field (FEF), olfactory bulb (OB), primary motor area (M1), dorsal and ventral premotor cortex (PMD, PMV), supplementary motor area (SMA), supplementary eye field (SEF)

If this were true, neither the mouse not the rhesus monkey would be an entirely appropriate model for the syndrome. However, in a recent study of the number and size of VENs in the anterior cingulate cortex of brains from individuals with autism and typically developing controls, there were no overall differences in the number or size of VENs in the autistic brains compared to controls (Simms et al., 2009).

Social Behavior Complexity of Rhesus Monkeys

In addition to the neuroanatomical similarities with humans, rhesus monkeys also display sophisticated social behavior that resembles many features of human social behavior. Much like humans, macaques spend their lives in complex societies where survival depends on their ability to quickly and accurately interpret and respond to a variety of social signals. Macaque females from several generations live together and form long-lasting social networks or matrilines (S. Altmann, 1967; Wrangham, 1980). These matrilines are organized into dominance hierarchies where prediction of social rank is closely linked to the dominance status of kin (i.e., high-ranking mothers produce high-ranking offspring) (Bernstein & Mason, 1963; Drickamer, 1975; Missakian, 1972; Sade, 1967). This complex system of social organization requires an equally sophisticated social communication system. Much like humans, macaques use a variety of vocalizations, facial expressions, and body postures to communicate with conspecifics. The sophisticated use of social signals makes rhesus monkeys an ideal species to model complex disorders of social behavior such as autism. Moreover, the well-defined sequence of macaque monkey social development provides a rich context in which to model features of human autism.

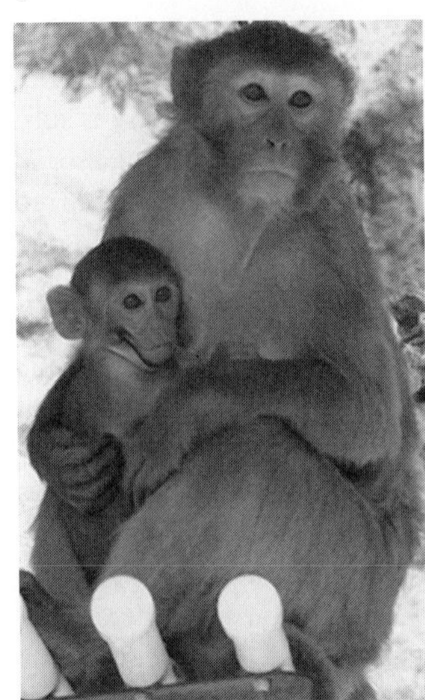
Rhesus monkey social development
0–3 Months
• Display a variety of reflexive behaviors
• Transient ability to imitate faces
• Show preference for face-like stimuli
• Averts gaze in response to stare
• Increased exploration away from mother
3–6 Months
• Produces fear grimaces
• Displays fear of strangers
• Develops ability to regulate fear responses
6–9 Months
• Peer play is most common activity
• Social grooming increases
• Transition to weaning begins
• Expression of social rank
9–12 Months
• Reduced maternal care
• Social integration into mother's network
• Birth of new sibling

Figure 53–2. Mother and infant rhesus macaques (Image courtesy of the California National Primate Research Center).

Infant macaques must rapidly learn to interpret and produce social signals to successfully interact with members of their social group. A well-characterized sequence of social development in many ways parallels that of human infants (Figure 53-2), although at a maturational rate approximately four times faster (i.e., a 1-month-old monkey is roughly developmentally comparable to a 4-month-old human) (Suomi, 1999). Infant macaque monkeys are born with largely functional sensory systems and display an array of reflexive motor responses (Mendelson, 1982a; Mowbray & Cadell, 1962). Like human infants, infant macaques show a clear preference for face-like stimuli very early in development (Kuwahata, Adachi, Fujita, Tomonaga, & Matsuzawa, 2004; C. K. Lutz, Lockard, Gunderson, & Grant, 1998) and demonstrate a transient ability to imitate facial expression in the early postnatal period (Ferrari et al., 2006). The early developmental period of rhesus monkeys is characterized by close physical contact and frequent social interactions with their mother (C. I. Berman, 1980; Ferrari et al., 2006; Hansen, 1966; R. A. Hinde & Spencer-Booth, 1967). Around two weeks of age, infant macaques begin to explore the surrounding environment and interact with their mother's close female kin and other related offspring (C. M. Berman, 1982). Like human infants, the macaque infant uses the mother as a secure base and will return to her immediately if alarmed or distressed (C. I. Berman, 1980; R.A. Hinde, Rowell, & Spencer-Booth, 1964). At this critical stage of development, the infant macaque must acquire the ability to correctly evaluate social signals, particularly signals that may convey potential aggression and predict potential harm. Indeed, by age 3 weeks, infants make fewer fixations on faces of conspecifics staring at them (a potential threat) compared to faces looking away (Mendelson, 1982b; Mendelson, Haith, & Goldman-Rakic, 1982). Between 2 and 4 months of age, the infants will further develop the ability to correctly interpret and respond to potential danger by regulating their responses to direct versus indirect danger (e.g., freezing to remain undetected in the presence of danger versus producing threats when threatening stimuli are being directed at them) (Kalin & Shelton, 1989). During this time, the infants also develop a species-typical expression of fear or subordination, the fear grimace (Sackett, 1966; Suomi, 1999), and develop a fear of unfamiliar conspecifics, a behavior that is possibly akin to the "stranger anxiety" observed in human infants (Suomi, 1999).

At age 3 months, infant macaques regularly explore away from their mothers, spending approximately 50% of their time out of physical contact with her (R. A. Hinde & Spencer-Booth, 1967). Social play becomes the predominant activity between 4 and 8 months of age and is believed to facilitate development of species-typical social behaviors (Ruppenthal, Harlow, Eisele, Harlow, & Suomi, 1974). Social grooming skills also emerge around this time and play an important role in establishing and maintaining social relationships (R. A. Hinde & Spencer-Booth, 1967; Matheson & Bernstein, 2000). During the second half of the first year, infants begin to express their social rank by directing aggression to group members who are lower in rank than their mothers, while deferring to group members who are higher ranking than their mother (Datta, 1984). The mother–infant relationship begins to transition into weaning at 5 to 7 months (Hansen, 1966). Following the birth of a sibling, macaques continue to develop more independence from their mothers and progress from infant to juvenile social behavior (Devinney, Berman, & Rasmussen, 2001).

Limitations

Despite the neuroanatomical and behavioral advantages of using nonhuman primates to model features of autism, there are important limitations to consider as well. There are certainly ethical issues that must be considered, and research involving nonhuman primates is not undertaken lightly. As described above, nonhuman primates share remarkable similarities with humans in both neuroanatomical organization and social behavior complexity. Although these qualities make them an ideal model species for human disorders, it also raises concerns with humane treatment and minimizing both the number of animals used and the kinds of procedures that are performed. As a result, nonhuman primate models of human disorder rely on very low sample sizes (usually 4–8 subjects per experimental condition). Even with these low sample sizes, research involving nonhuman primates is inherently costly. Obtaining an adequate number of subjects, providing husbandry and veterinary care, and acquiring large enclosures for housing and testing is cost-prohibitive for many investigators. Finally, it is important to recognize that progress is also much slower for nonhuman primate models. This is especially true for developmental models that require 165 days for gestation followed by years of behavioral assessments of the offspring.

In addition, not all human behaviors can be modeled in nonhuman primates. Complex behaviors associated with autism, such as theory of mind, empathy, and even imitation abilities may not be present in all species of nonhuman primates. For example, although macaques can use information about where an experimenter is looking in order to successfully "steal" an item of food (Flombaum & Santos, 2005), chimpanzees demonstrate much more sophisticated use of this social information. Through a series of experiments in which a dominant and subordinate chimpanzee compete for food, Tomasello and colleagues have demonstrated that chimpanzees not only have knowledge of what others see, they also know something about intention in action (Tomasello, Call et al., 2003). Moreover, chimpanzees also are able to draw inferences from other's behaviors, as evidenced by different reactions to behaviors that occur accidentally versus behaviors that are performed with a purpose (Call, Hare, Carpenter, & Tomasello, 2004; Call & Tomasello, 1998). Current practice, however, precludes the use of chimpanzees from invasive biomedical research.

There are also nonprimate species that may prove to be useful models of social processing. Tomasello and colleagues, for example, have found that domestic dogs can use human social and communicative behavior (i.e., pointing) to find hidden food, whereas all nonhuman primates tested (including chimpanzees) demonstrated little ability to solve the same task (Brauer, Kaminski, Riedel, Call, & Tomasello, 2006; Hare, Brown, Williamson, & Tomasello, 2002; Hare & Tomasello, 2005; Riedel, Buttelmann, Call, & Tomasello, 2006). These examples illustrate that although macaques may be the biomedical species of choice, there are important limitations to their behavioral repertoire that must be considered when designing species-appropriate tasks.

Finally, our inability to effectively utilize transgenic technologies in nonhuman primates poses another major obstacle in establishing nonhuman primate models of human disorders. Although transgenic mice models for human diseases have become common, the low efficiency of conventional gene transfer protocols has hindered the progress of developing transgenic nonhuman primates. As a result, attempts to model human diseases in nonhuman primates has been restricted to behavioral, pharmacological, cognitive, or biochemical experimental manipulations. However, as technology advances, so too does our ability to utilize genetic modification in nonhuman primates. The feasibility of applying transgenic approaches to nonhuman primates was recently established by transgene introduction of green fluorescent protein into the macaque monkey (Chan, Chong, Martinovich, Simerly, & Schatten, 2001). This breakthrough has led to the first transgenic nonhuman primate model of Huntington's disease (Yang et al., 2008). The transgenic monkeys display key features of Huntington's disease, thereby demonstrating the power of this technique in studying human disorders with a known genetic cause. Although these studies have established that genetic manipulations in nonhuman primates are possible, future work is needed to refine the techniques (Chan & Yang, 2009).

Modeling Features of Autism in Nonhuman Primates

Given that autism is a behaviorally defined disorder, current efforts to model features of autism focus primarily on inducing changes in behavior in the animal model that resemble behavioral symptoms of human autism. In the following section, we discuss current behavioral assessments used in nonhuman primate models and suggest directions to expand these behavioral assays into more autism specific probes.

Current Behavioral Assessments

One way of assessing the behavior of an animal model of autism is to observe and quantify the emergence of species-typical social and communication behaviors, while screening for the presence of atypical behaviors, such as abnormal motor patterns or stereotypies. Sophisticated analysis of behavior should include: *(1)* a comprehensive catalogue of species-typical behaviors (an ethogram), *(2)* quantitative assessments of both frequency and duration of these behaviors recorded by reliable observers, and *(3)* assessments of subjects at different time-points in development.

This approach requires extensive knowledge of primate behavior and highly trained observers to identify and record a catalog of species-typical facial expressions, vocalizations, and body postures. In our laboratory, we have consulted with primatologists to create a catalog of 56 species-typical behaviors (M. D. Bauman, Lavenex, Mason, Capitanio, & Amaral, 2004a, 2004b; M. D. Bauman, Toscano, Babineau, Mason, & Amaral, 2008; M. D. Bauman, Toscano, Mason, Lavenex, & Amaral, 2006). The frequency and duration of these behaviors is quantified for one focal subject at a time (J. Altmann, 1974), resulting in a detailed record of the use of species-typical behaviors. In addition to frequencies and durations of discrete behaviors, observers also record the identity of the second subject and direction of the interaction (initiate or receive), thus providing insight into the appropriateness of each individual's use of social communication. In our laboratory, all observations are collected with The Observer (Noldus, 1991) behavioral data collection software by trained observers who demonstrate a predetermined interobserver concordance of better than 90%. It is important to emphasize that observers remain blind to the experimental condition of each infant for the duration of the study.

Because autism is a developmental disorder, the majority of animal models focus on prenatal or early postnatal manipulations. To screen for changes in behaviors associated with a developmental model, it is essential to monitor behavior at different time-points in development. In our laboratory, each subject is observed daily in their individual cages to screen for abnormal behaviors, weekly in their rearing groups to document the emergence of species-typical social behavior within a familiar group, and at specific time-points in development to provide more comprehensive assessments of social behavior under more challenging conditions (i.e., response to novel conspecifics, etc.).

Our current behavioral assays focus heavily on quantifying the development of species-specific behaviors and then relating these changes to human autism. By measuring the frequency and duration of macaque social signals we are able to determine whether the infant monkeys exhibit appropriate social signals at the correct developmental time-points, whether they have developed a complete repertoire of social signals, and whether they are using these behaviors in a species-typical way. We are also able to screen for the presence of atypical behaviors, such as motor stereotypies. Although this approach provides a wealth of data regarding species-typical development, it does not specifically probe for behavioral changes that are observed in humans with autism. The addition of specific probes for behaviors directly related to human autism would result in a powerful assessment of nonhuman primate models of autism.

Future Directions for Nonhuman Primate Behavioral Assessments

In recent years, rodent models of autism have undergone substantial changes spearheaded by Crawley and colleagues (Crawley, 2004, 2007a, 2007b) reviewed in Chapter 51. The result is a standardized battery of behavioral tests for rodents that focus on behaviors most directly related to autistic symptomatology. This has undoubtedly improved the quality of rodent models of autism. Future nonhuman primate models of autism will also benefit from designing behavioral probes that focus on behaviors most directly related to human autism. Indeed, the complex social behaviors exhibited by rhesus monkeys may allow them to model features of autism that are simply not present in rodent models. We are in the process of developing a series of nonhuman primate behavioral tests that can be adapted to probe for behaviors more directly related to human autism. Our strategy is to take findings from human autism research and translate these into species-appropriate behavioral tasks for our nonhuman primate models. It is fair to say that these types of tests do not currently exist because the interest in developing primate models of autism and other neurodevelopmental disorders is a relatively recent phenomenon. These behavioral assays include tests for each of the three diagnostic domains of autism:

Probes of Social Behavior Deficits Related to Autism

Recent studies have focused on two early components of social development that may be impaired in young children who go on to develop autism: *(1)* social attention and *(2)* social imitation. Many individuals with autism do not attend to salient social information (i.e., faces, eyes, etc.) in a typical fashion. For example, infants who are later diagnosed with autism look less at the face early in development compared to typically developing or developmentally delayed infants (J. Osterling & Dawson, 1994; J. A. Osterling et al., 2002; Swettenham et al., 1998). This pattern of abnormal face processing persists into adolescence and adulthood (Pelphrey et al., 2002) and may affect the ability to perceive social information (Klin et al., 2002). In addition to social orienting, individuals with autism may also have difficulty imitating the actions of others (Williams, Whiten, & Singh, 2004).

Tests of social attention and imitation that are currently used for young children could readily be modified for use in nonhuman primate models. Indeed, a test of social attention and motivation has recently been developed for rhesus monkeys (Rudebeck, Buckley, Walton, & Rushworth, 2006). Briefly, adult rhesus monkeys are placed in a cognitive testing cage where they are shown still images of salient social information (i.e., pictures of an alpha male monkey) as well as nonsocial images (i.e., objects, etc.). Social attention is measured by the amount of time spent looking at the screen, and a rough estimate of social motivation is measured by recording the amount of time it takes for the monkeys to retrieve a small food reward in front of the screen. When monkeys are presented with nonsocial images, they immediately retrieve the food reward. In contrast, monkeys delay retrieving the food reward when presented with social images. Presumably, the monkeys find the social images more interesting and choose to attend to the social images rather than glancing down and retrieving the food reward. This task could easily be modified to assess social motivation and attention in young rhesus monkeys by creating an age-appropriate social stimulus set. This test would provide important information on how infant rhesus monkeys respond to specific probes of salient social information and provide rough assessments of social attention and motivation.

In addition to social attention, individuals with autism may also demonstrate impairments in imitation of others (Colombi et al., 2009). This combined with the discovery of "mirror neurons" in the macaque brain that fire both when an animal is in action as well as when it observes the same action by another individual has led to a hypothesis that dysfunction of the mirror neuron system might be a core deficit in autism (Iacoboni, 2005; Iacoboni & Dapretto, 2006). Recording of mirror neurons requires invasive electrophysiological experiments that are not compatible with naturalistic housing strategies. However, there are other means of evaluating imitation processing in rhesus monkeys. In the past, such experiments have been hindered by the traditional view from primate behavioral studies that apes imitate, and monkeys do not. However, it has recently been demonstrated that infant macaques possess a transient ability to imitate human facial expressions during the first week of life (Ferrari et al., 2006). This ability bears many similarities to the same abilities demonstrated in newborn humans and apes and may prove to be a sensitive assay of early imitative abilities for animal models of autism.

Probes for Communication Deficits Related to Autism

Recent developments in autism research have highlighted an infant's lack of response to their own name at 12 months as a possible developmental abnormality (Nadig et al., 2007). This study found that decreased response to name at 12 months discriminates children at risk for autism from a control group, suggesting that poor response to name may be an early feature of autism. Although it is not possible to test "response to name" in macaque monkeys, it is feasible to evaluate the infant's ability to differentiate important vocal communications. Rhesus mothers respond to separation from their infant with a species-typical "coo call," and the infants are able to discriminate maternal versus non-maternal vocalizations (Masataka, 1985). Determining whether infant monkeys respond to their own mothers coo call in a species-typical fashion may provide insight into the infants' ability to respond to salient social communication, paralleling the human infants' response to their own name.

Probes for Repetitive Behavior and Restricted Interests

Young children with autism display unusual repetitive behavior and/or restricted interests that may be modeled in nonhuman primates. Given the overlap between motor stereotypies in human disorders and animal models, we have focused much of our attention on screening animals for the presence of any atypical motor behaviors. However, we have not screened for other aspects of repetitive behaviors that are extremely common in children with autism, such as persistent preoccupation with parts of objects or toys. Moreover, we have not developed tests to assess "higher order" repetitive behaviors that are often characteristic of individuals with autism, including insistence on sameness as well as patterns of restricted interests. It is entirely feasible to adapt tests from human autism research to probe for these behaviors in the nonhuman primate model.

For example, Ozonoff and colleagues have recently demonstrated that 12-month-old infants who are later diagnosed with autism display atypical patterns of object exploration compared to control groups (Ozonoff et al., 2008). Specifically, the infants who were later diagnosed with autism displayed more spinning, rotating, and unusual visual exploration of objects compared to individuals who were typically developing. This toy play paradigm could readily be modeled to assess lower level repetitive behaviors in infant rhesus monkeys. Higher order restricted interests could be assessed by modifying a task of novel object exploration used in young children with autism. When allowed free access to a room filled with novel toys, children with autism spend less time exploring novel objects compared to typically developing subjects (Pierce & Courchesne, 2001). These data suggest that the restricted patterns of interest characteristic of many children with autism may interfere with their ability to explore novel environments. Bodfish and colleagues have recently modified this paradigm for use in rodent models of autism (Moy et al., 2008). This paradigm could easily be modified for use in nonhuman primates.

What is the Status of Nonhuman Primate Models of Autism?

There are many possible approaches to creating an animal model of autism. Distinctions should be drawn among models that are designed to elicit behavioral symptoms, those designed to study underlying neurobiological mechanisms, and those designed to test a specific etiological theory. We have selected nonhuman primate studies from each of these approaches to discuss in detail below. Each model is evaluated based on construct, face and predictive validity to determine their value as a potential animal model of autism.

Isolate Rearing Models

We have chosen to include historical studies using isolate reared monkeys in our discussion of nonhuman primate models of autism. Although these studies were not intended as animal models of autism, the isolate rearing paradigm elicits behavioral changes in nonhuman primates that are strikingly similar to human autism. Nonhuman primates reared in isolation from

Table 53–2.
Evaluation of nonhuman primate models of autism

Nonhuman Primate Models of Autism	Construct Validity	Face Validity	Predictive Validity	Interpretation
Isolate-rearing	Moderate: requires further investigation	High	Moderate	The model exhibits high face validity because the behavioral outcome resembles many features of human autism. The construct validity is unclear—extreme social isolation may produce autistic like behaviors in children, although it is unclear how this relates to idiopathic autism. The nonhuman primate isolate-rearing model does, however, provide evidence that restricting access to social information early in development results in an animal model that in many ways resembles human autism. This lends support to current hypotheses suggesting that children who go on to develop autism are not able to obtain and process social information at critical developmental time-points. Moreover, exposing the isolate-reared monkeys to peer at specific time-points in development can "rescue" the effects of isolate-rearing. Thus, this model may provide general insight in means of rescuing atypical social development.
Neonatal amygdala lesion models	Low	Low	Not tested	Current evidence suggests that the amygdala may undergo atypical development in children with autism. However, individuals with autism do not have bilateral amygdala damage, and patients with bilateral amygdala damage are not autistic (the model has low construct validity). The behavioral outcome of neonatal amygdala lesions depends on the lesion technique, rearing conditions, and quality of behavioral observations. However, the most current evidence indicates that nonhuman primates with neonatal amygdala damage do not demonstrate autistic symptomotology early in development.
Maternal antibody model	High	Moderate	Not tested	The immunological challenge utilized in this model was derived from mothers who have produced multiple children with autism, thus identifying a putative human cause of autism (the model has high construct validity). This model has created an animal with a clear neurodevelopmental disorder (characterized by motor stereotypies) following prenatal exposure to antibodies from mothers of children with autism. Although alterations in social development were not observed in this pilot study (moderate face validity), efforts are underway to replicate and expand upon this promising model.

conspecifics will direct filial responses such as ventral clasping and nursing to their own bodies, resulting in abnormal behaviors such as self-clasping, huddling, self-orality, and rocking with stereotypic movements (Griffin & Harlow, 1966; Harlow, 1965; Harlow & Zimmermann, 1959). Even more striking, nonhuman primates reared in complete isolation for the first 6 months of life fail to develop species-typical social behaviors (Harlow, 1965; Harlow, Dodsworth, & Harlow, 1965) as evidenced by their failure to initiate or reciprocate play and grooming behaviors (Harlow & Harlow, 1962; Harlow & Harlow, 1965; Harlow, Rowland, & Griffin, 1964) and by their inability to respond to a variety of species-specific social signals (Mason, 1960). In addition to the deficits in social behavior, restricted rearing or housing practices are also associated with abnormal behaviors, such as self-directed (Champoux, Metz, & Suomi, 1991) and self-injurious behavior (C. Lutz et al., 2003).

Deficits in social and communication development, combined with the presence of self-directed repetitive behaviors, in many ways parallels symptoms of human autism. This is not at all to suggest that restricted rearing practices are a common cause of autism. We know that children with autism are not raised in substandard conditions. If anything, parents and therapists put forth heroic efforts to create an environment that will help a young child with autism acquire social and communication skills. It is, however, possible that extreme social deprivation conditions such as those found in substandard orphanages, may predispose children to develop autistic like behaviors. A 1999 study by Rutter and colleagues reported that 6% of 111 children adopted from Romanian orphanages showed autistic-like patterns of behavior between 4 and 6 years of age (Rutter et al., 1999). The findings by Rutter suggest that early deprivation of social stimuli may alter brain development and result in behavioral symptoms that resemble autism.

The parallels between primate deprivation studies and autistic-like behaviors associated with substandard human orphanages warrants further discussion as a possible animal model of autism. Both the isolate reared nonhuman primate studies and the reports of children raised in substandard orphanages indicate that there are critical periods of development when social interaction is required to develop species-typical social behavior.

If social interaction is withheld during these critical periods, the resulting behavior resembles autistic symptomatology. Clearly, social interaction is not intentionally withheld from children who go on to develop autism. However, it is possible that autism is caused by a failure to develop the neural circuitry required for infants to attend to and engage in social interaction during these critical periods. Thus, a disruption in the neural circuitry required to engage in early social interactions may mimic the effects of early social deprivation. Indeed, Schultz and colleagues have proposed that early abnormalities in visual attention mediated by the amygdala result in an inability to identify salient signals, which in turn alters overall development of social perception and knowledge of others (Schultz, 2005). Another hypothesis argues that a primary deficit in social motivation mediated by dopamenergic reward systems underlies early inattention to social signals that is characteristic of autism (Dawson, Webb, & McPartland, 2005; Dawson et al., 2005). Either a disruption in processing capabilities or a deficit in social reward systems could conceivably lead to an inability to attend to social information early in development. The same brain systems that mediate these behaviors in human children may be altered in the nonhuman primate rearing models. Thus, there is a potential similarity between isolate rearing and the underlying cause(s) of human autism; however, more research is needed to determine the construct validity of this model.

In addition to high face validity, the nonhuman primate isolate rearing studies may also demonstrate high predictive validity by providing valuable insight into therapeutic interventions. Subsequent studies of the isolate reared monkeys revealed that recovery of social behavior was possible under specific circumstances. Although young isolate reared monkeys exposed to age-matched peers showed only limited recovery of social responses, it was later shown that 6-month-old isolates exposed to much younger monkeys achieved almost complete recovery of social behaviors (Harlow & Suomi, 1971). The authors suggested that the younger monkeys posed no threat to the isolate reared subjects, thus allowing the isolate reared monkeys to "learn" species-typical social behaviors as the younger monkeys passed through their own stages of socialization. Interestingly, peer-mediated play has also been used as an effective social intervention for young children with autism (Rogers, 2000). In peer-mediated therapies, typically developing peers are taught to initiate play behaviors using common play materials and activities (Odom & Strain, 1986; Oke & Schreibman, 1990). This approach has proved effective in increasing the social interactions in young children with autism, thus demonstrating another parallel between human autism and the primate isolation research.

Amygdala Lesion Models

In the early 1990s, much attention was focused on the potential role of amygdala pathology in autism. This "amygdala theory of autism" was based on several findings: *(1)* reports of abnormal cell density in the amygdala of autistic brains (M. L. Bauman, 1991; M. L. Bauman, Filipek, & Kemper, 1997); *(2)* atypical patterns of amygdala activation in human subjects with autism (Baron-Cohen et al., 2000; Baron-Cohen et al., 1999); and *(3)* a putative animal model of autism resulting from neonatal amygdala damage in rhesus monkeys (Bachevalier, 1994, 1996).

The nonhuman primate model of autism developed by Bachevalier and colleagues was based primarily on a study of six peer-reared monkeys that received aspiration lesions of the amygdala within the first postnatal month (Bachevalier, 1994). When placed in social dyads at age 2 months, the neonatal amygdala-lesioned infants showed less overall activity, exploration, and social behavior initiation than age-matched controls. At age 6 months, activity levels were relatively normal, but social interactions were reduced in amygdalectomized infants compared to the controls. The authors also reported that more extensive lesions of the medial temporal lobe, including the amygdala, hippocampus, and ventromedial temporal cortex produced a more profound effect on social interactions, including lack of social skills, flat affect, and increased stereotypic behaviors. Given that impaired social communication and a lack of social interest hallmark features of autism, the authors proposed that lesions of the medial temporal lobe, specifically the amygdala, might provide an animal model of autism (Bachevalier, 1994, 2000).

The studies by Bachevalier et al. were some of the first attempts to use the nonhuman primate to model features of autism. It is possible, however, that the behavioral changes in these monkeys may have been influenced by unintended collateral damage of neural tissue surrounding the amygdala and/or by the restricted rearing practices that were employed. To address the potential limitations of the Bachevalier study, our laboratory designed a series of experiments to evaluate the effects of more selective neonatal amygdala lesions on the development of socially reared rhesus monkeys. We utilized the injectable neurotoxin ibotenic acid which selectively removes neurons, while sparing surrounding cortex and fibers of passage (Meunier, Bachevalier, Murray, Malkova, & Mishkin, 1999). Unlike the Bachevalier subjects that were reared with access to peers only, we raised our subjects with their mothers and provided them daily access to larger social groups consisting of several mother–infant pairs and an adult male. This semi-naturalistic rearing strategy facilitates the development of species-typical social behavior and decreases the presence of abnormal repetitive behaviors. We predicted that if the amygdala is a core component of the social brain, then removal of the amygdala early in development would profoundly alter fundamental features of social behavior, including social attention and the ability to produce and interpret social signals. However, if these core features of social behavior remain intact following amygdala damage, then it is reasonable to conclude that the amygdala is not essential for the development of fundamental aspects of social behavior.

In our studies, 24 rhesus monkeys were given selective ibotenic acid-induced lesions of the amygdala or hippocampus or a sham lesion procedure at age 2 weeks. We then observed the social development of these animals during the first year of life by systematically quantifying social interactions with their mothers, familiar peers, and novel peers. When observed at age 3 months, the amygdala-lesioned monkeys spent the same amount of time nursing and in contact or proximity with their mothers as did control or hippocampus-lesioned subjects (M. D. Bauman et al., 2004a). There were no differences among the experimental groups in the frequency of mother–infant behaviors, and none of the infants engaged in maladaptive behaviors in the first year of life, such as self-clasping, crouching, rocking, or motor stereotypies, which are indicative of abnormal social behavior development (J. Capitanio, 1986). After the amygdala-lesioned subjects were weaned from their mothers at age 6 months, they continued to develop a species-typical repertoire of social behavior (M. D. Bauman et al., 2004b). They were observed successfully interacting with members of their social rearing group, with familiar conspecifics at ages 6 and 9 months, and with novel conspecifics at age 1 year. These studies demonstrated that infant macaques with neonatal amygdala lesions are able to *(1)* form filial bonds; *(2)* develop a species-typical repertoire of social behavior; *(3)* display interest in conspecifics; and*(4)* interact with conspecifics in various social contexts.

Although the amygdala-lesioned subjects developed fundamental aspects of social behavior, they differed from control and hippocampus-lesioned subjects in some significant ways. The most striking abnormality of the amygdala-lesioned subjects was their inappropriate fear behaviors in various contexts. We observed that amygdala-lesioned subjects produced fear behaviors more frequently than control or hippocampus-lesioned subjects during social interactions with both novel and familiar social partners (M. D. Bauman et al., 2004b). We have proposed that through its mediation of fear, the amygdala plays a modulatory—rather than essential—role in social processing. It is plausible that the absence of social interaction observed by Bachevalier was not the result of "autistic-like" symptomatology but rather the result of abnormal social fear response that is characteristic of amygdala-lesioned monkeys. This explanation is consistent with the view that the amygdala is not essential for fundamental aspects of social behavior, such as producing social signals and interacting with conspecifics. However, the amygdala may indirectly modulate social behavior by detecting danger within a social context and orchestrating an appropriate behavioral response.

Observations of these animals are ongoing, and we have observed additional changes in their behavior over time. For example, the amygdala-lesioned subjects are lower ranking in their social groups compared to hippocampus-lesioned or control subjects (M. D. Bauman et al., 2006). Interestingly, both the amygdala- and hippocampus-lesioned subjects developed repetitive behaviors in the second year of life (M. D. Bauman et al., 2008). The emergence of stereotypies after a period of relatively normal development bears some resemblance to developmental disorders, such as autism, where abnormal behaviors may become apparent or worsen following seemingly typical developmental trajectory.

In spite of these later changes in behavior, the absence of pronounced social deficits or repetitive behaviors early in development indicates that neonatal amygdala lesions do not result in an animal model of autism with high face validity. To produce a model with high face validity, we would have expected to see pronounced changes in social behavior and communication by the time the monkeys reached age 12 months (roughly equivalent to a 4-year-old human). Moreover, the construct validity of an amygdala lesion model is questionable. Although there is compelling evidence for structural and functional amygdala abnormalities in individuals with autism (K. M. Dalton, Nacewicz, Alexander, & Davidson, 2007; K. M. Dalton et al., 2005; Schumann & Amaral, 2005; Schumann et al., 2004), complete amygdala lesions do not replicate this pathophysiology. Likewise, human subjects who do suffer from bilateral amygdala damage display subtle deficits in social processing but clearly are not autistic (Adolphs et al., 2005; Adolphs & Tranel, 2003; Adolphs, Tranel, & Damasio, 1998; Adolphs, Tranel, Damasio, & Damasio, 1994; Adolphs, Tranel, Damasio, & Damasio, 1995). The low construct and face validity of the neonatal amygdala lesion model would argue against this approach as a valid animal model of autism.

Maternal Auto-Antibody Model

Converging evidence indicates that immune dysfunction may play an important role in a subset of autism cases (van Gent, Heijnen, & Treffers, 1997). Some patients with autism demonstrate abnormalities and/or deficits of immune system function, including inappropriate immune response to pathogen challenge (Ashwood, Anthony, Torrente, & Wakefield, 2004), recurrent infections (Stern et al., 2005), peripheral immune abnormalities (Ashwood et al., 2003; Croonenberghs, Bosmans, Deboutte, Kenis, & Maes, 2002; Singh, 1996) and neuroinflammatory responses in the central nervous system (CNS; Vargas, Nascimbene, Krishnan, Zimmerman, & Pardo, 2005). In addition to general immune system dysfunction, recent evidence suggests that certain forms of autism are associated with autoimmune conditions (Ashwood & Van de Water, 2004). Autoimmunity occurs when the immune system inappropriately identifies and reacts to "self" components. Several studies have also reported that autoimmune disorders are more common in family members of individuals with autism compared to typically developing controls (Comi, Zimmerman, Frye, Law, & Peeden, 1999; Richler et al., 2006; Sweeten, Bowyer, Posey, Halberstadt, & McDougle, 2003). Moreover, antibodies directed against CNS proteins have been found in the sera of children with autism (Cook, Perry, Dawson, Wainwright, & Leventhal, 1993; Plioplys, Greaves, Kazemi, & Silverman, 1994; Singh & Rivas, 2004; Singh, Warren, Averett, & Ghaziuddin, 1997; Singh, Warren, Odell, Warren, & Cole, 1993; Todd & Ciaranello, 1985).

In addition to the presence of auto-antibodies in individuals with autism, recent evidence raises the possibility that maternal auto-antibodies to fetal brain tissue may play a role in a subset of autism cases (Vincent, Dalton, Clover, Palace, & Lang, 2003). Antibodies from serum of mothers who have children with autism have been shown to react to antigens on lymphocytes from their affected children (Warren et al., 1990). Given that antigens expressed on lymphocytes are also found on cells of the CNS, these authors proposed that aberrant maternal immunity may be associated with the development of some cases of autism. In support of this, the presence of antibodies against brain tissue was recently identified in the serum of a mother whose child has autism (P. Dalton et al., 2003), and Van de Water and colleagues have identified a common pattern of auto-antibody production to fetal brain tissue in the serum of mothers who have two or more children with autism (Braunschweig et al., 2008). Collectively, these studies suggest that an atypical maternal antibody response directed against the fetal brain during pregnancy may be present in a subset of autism cases.

Although evidence for pathogenic maternal antibodies is very suggestive, it is not feasible to establish a causal relationship in human subjects. Animal models are needed to evaluate the effects of prenatal exposure to potentially pathogenic antibodies. A preliminary rodent model of developmental disorders reported behavioral abnormalities in mice prenatally exposed to serum from a woman whose children have autism and other developmental disorders (P. Dalton et al., 2003). Similarly, Martin et al. (Martin et al., 2008) recently published a study on the effects of exposing gestating rhesus monkeys to IgG class antibodies obtained from human mothers of multiple children with autism. Behavioral observations of monkeys prenatally exposed to purified IgG from mothers of children with autism revealed more whole body stereotypies than both untreated control monkeys and monkeys prenatally exposed to purified IgG from mothers of typically developing children. Importantly, the increased stereotypies were observed consistently across several different testing paradigms over a 7-month period. These testing situations are described in detail below.

One month following weaning, each subject was observed for behavioral differences either while alone or while paired with a familiar conspecific from their social rearing group. Behaviors were scored in real time using a catalog of normal and abnormal behaviors commonly displayed by rhesus monkeys. Results demonstrated significantly higher frequencies of whole-body stereotypies in the maternal autism IgG treated monkeys compared to the control IgG treated and control untreated monkeys in both solo and paired conditions. When the subject was engaged in a particular stereotypy for more than 6 seconds, an extended stereotypy was scored. Significant differences were observed in the frequency and duration of extended stereotypies when animals were in the paired condition. A similar pattern of whole body stereotypies was also observed during dyadic interactions with unfamiliar conspecifics. One month following the pairings with familiar peers, monkeys were removed from their social groups and placed with one of four unfamiliar monkeys in the same large testing enclosures. Once again, results demonstrated a higher frequency of whole-body stereotypies in the maternal autism IgG treated monkeys compared to control IgG treated and control untreated monkeys.

In addition to these three behavioral settings, the autism IgG-exposed monkeys produced an increased number of midline crossings (an indication of hyperactivity) in the mother preference task that is administered over the first 4 days following weaning. In this task, infants are provided access to their mothers or to another familiar adult female. The species-typical response is to identify the location of the mother and then to remain in proximity for the remainder of the trial. In contrast, the autism IgG-treated animals demonstrated significantly more cross-cage pacing and did not settle in proximity with their mothers. Finally, all animals in this pilot study were fitted with actimeters that measured activity throughout 3 weeks of testing. No differences in activity were detected when the animals remained in their social groups. However, during the individual housing condition, the autism IgG-treated group demonstrated significantly higher levels of activity than the control group.

These preliminary data indicate that prenatal exposure to IgG class antibodies from mothers of children with autism alters the behavioral development of rhesus monkeys. Profound stereotypies were observed in several behavioral settings across 7 months of testing. In addition to these striking results, this study provides evidence for the feasibility of examining the effects of potentially pathological maternal antibodies in nonhuman primate models. Although these results are provocative, it is clearly premature to consider these findings indicative of an animal model of autism. We are currently conducting a larger-scale study attempting to replicate the results of this pilot study. We are also aware that repetitive stereotypies only represent one facet of autistic symptomatology. We have thus far not observed robust deficits in social behavior and communication in the pilot animals. Thus, we may have succeeded in modeling one feature of autistic symptomotology rather than the entire disorder. It is also noteworthy that repetitive behaviors are not specific to autism. Indeed, motor stereotypies are a common feature of many developmental disorders, including Rett syndrome and mental retardation (Berkson, 1983; Berkson, Gutermuth, & Baranek, 1995; Bodfish, Symons, Parker, & Lewis, 2000; Wales, Charman, & Mount, 2004). Despite these limitations, we find the results obtained from the pilot study promising for several reasons:

1. The model demonstrates high construct validity. The proposed model comes directly from families of children with autism. The immunological challenge utilized in our pilot study was derived from mothers who have produced multiple children with autism, thus identifying a putative human cause of autism.
2. The model demonstrates moderate face validity. At the very least, this immunological model has created an animal that demonstrates one of the core features of autism (motor stereotypies). Given the prevalence of repetitive behaviors across a wide range of neurodevelopmental disorders, this research may provide

important information regarding the neurobiology of abnormal repetitive behaviors.

3. There is a potential for high predictive validity. If we are successful in replicating and extending the findings from our pilot study, we foresee important clinical implications. The focus of concurrent studies is to identify the relevant fetal brain auto-antigens. This would allow us to use the identified auto-antigen to break tolerance, establish the behavioral model, and extend this immunological model using immunomodulation to alter the developmental outcome of the infants. These future studies may provide directions for treatment of human mothers. For example, screening for brain-directed antibodies may provide an indication of risk factors for women who intend to become pregnant. This information may be particularly important to women who have had previous children with autism since the probability of having a second child with autism is substantially higher than risk for a first child with autism. More importantly, the detection of brain-directed auto-antibodies may lead to therapeutic interventions that may decrease the risk of producing children with serious neurodevelopmental disorders.

Conclusions

It is likely that future animal models will play an important role in evaluating the biological underpinnings of autism and facilitating the development of future treatment and prevention strategies. The validity of animal models is based on: *(1)* construct validity (degree of similarity between the experimental manipulation and the underlying cause of the human disease), *(2)* face validity (the extent to which the resulting model resembles the phenotype of the human disorder), and *(3)* predictive validity (treatment discoveries in an animal model which may provide insight into therapeutic options for the human condition). Nonhuman primates closely resemble humans in both sophistication of social behavior, (e.g., they use facial expressions for social communication) and neural organization, (e.g., they have all of the regions of the frontal lobe identified in the human brain), thus making the nonhuman primate an ideal species to model features of autism. Coe and colleagues (Short et al., 2010; Willette et al., 2010) have recently capitalized on these similarities by including assessments of both behavior and brain development in nonhuman primate models of prenatal exposure to infection. While these studies were not specifically proposed as animal models of autism, their findings demonstrate the power of pairing sophisticated behavioral assessments with structural MRI to systematically evaluate the effects of a prenatal insult on both brain and behavior development. Future efforts to evaluate the validity of nonhuman primate models will require increasingly sophisticated behavioral probes that are sensitive to the core features of autism, as well as research tools, such as eye tracking and functional neuroimaging, that bridge the gap between human and animal studies. A current limitation to the development of additional primate models of autism is the dearth of convincing evidence on specific etiologies of autism. Assuming this information will be forthcoming in the near future, it will also be essential to develop behavioral probes for nonhuman primates that are sensitive to the core features autism. With these developments, the nonhuman primate can provide a valuable test bed for evaluating preventative measures and innovative treatments.

Challenges and Future Directions

- Developing nonhuman primate models of autism with high construct validity (e.g., models that stem from hypotheses that are directly related to causes of the human disorder).
- Improving face validity of nonhuman primate models by developing assays of nonhuman primate behavior that are relevant to symptoms of human autism.
- Establishing collaborative efforts between rodent and nonhuman primate models of autism to make use of the unique advantages each approach offers.
- Translating results from nonhuman primate models into preventative strategies and/or novel therapies to reduce the incidence of autism.

SUGGESTED READINGS

Capitanio, J. P., & Emborg M. E. (2008). Contributions of nonhuman primates to neuroscience research. *Lancet, 371*(9618), 1126–1135.

Crawley, J. N. (2007). Mouse behavioral assays relevant to the symptoms of autism. *Brain Patholology, 17*(4), 448–459.

Suomi, S. J. (1999). Attachment in rhesus monkeys. In J. Cassidy & P. R. Shaver (Eds.), *Handbook of attachment: Theory, research, and clinical application* (pp. 181–197). New York: The Guilford Press.

ACKNOWLEDGMENTS

Original research described in this chapter was supported by a grant from the National Institute of Mental Health (R37MH57502) and by the base grant (RR00169) of the California National Primate Research Center (CNPRC). This work was also supported through the Early Experience and Brain Development Network of the MacArthur Foundation.

REFERENCES

Abrahams, B. S., & Geschwind, D. H. (2008). Advances in autism genetics: On the threshold of a new neurobiology. *Nature Reviews Genetics, 9*(5), 341–355.

Adolphs, R., Gosselin, F., Buchanan, T. W., Tranel, D., Schyns, P., & Damasio, A. R. (2005). A mechanism for impaired fear recognition after amygdala damage. *Nature, 433*(7021), 68–72.

Adolphs, R., & Tranel, D. (2003). Amygdala damage impairs emotion recognition from scenes only when they contain facial expressions. *Neuropsychologia, 41*(10), 1281–1289.

Adolphs, R., Tranel, D., & Damasio, A. R. (1998). The human amygdala in social judgment. *Nature, 393*(6684), 470–474.

Adolphs, R., Tranel, D., Damasio, H., & Damasio, A. (1994). Impaired recognition of emotion in facial expressions following bilateral damage to the human amygdala. *Nature, 372*(6507), 669–672.

Adolphs, R., Tranel, D., Damasio, H., & Damasio, A. R. (1995). Fear and the Human Amygdala. *Journal of Neuroscience, 15*(9), 5879–5891.

Allman, J. M., Watson, K. K., Tetreault, N. A., & Hakeem, A. Y. (2005). Intuition and autism: A possible role for Von Economo neurons. *Trends in Cognitive Sciences, 9*(8), 367–373.

Altmann, J. (1974). Observational study of behavior: Sampling methods. *Behaviour, 49*(3–4), 227–267.

Altmann, S. (1967). The structure of primate social communication. In S. Altmann (Ed.), *Social communication among primates.* Chicago: University of Chicago Press.

Amaral, D. G., Schumann, C. M., & Nordahl, C. W. (2008). Neuroanatomy of autism. *Trends in Neurosciences, 31*(3), 137–145.

Ashwood, P., Anthony, A., Pellicer, A. A., Torrente, F., Walker-Smith, J. A., & Wakefield, A. J. (2003). Intestinal lymphocyte populations in children with regressive autism: Evidence for extensive mucosal immunopathology. *Journal of Clinical Immunology, 23*(6), 504–517.

Ashwood, P., Anthony, A., Torrente, F., & Wakefield, A. J. (2004). Spontaneous mucosal lymphocyte cytokine profiles in children with autism and gastrointestinal symptoms: Mucosal immune activation and reduced counter regulatory interleukin-10. *Journal of Clinical Immunology, 24*(6), 664–673.

Ashwood, P., & Van de Water, J. (2004). Is autism an autoimmune disease? *Autoimmunity Reviews, 3*(7–8), 557–562.

Ashwood, P., Wills, S., & Van de Water, J. (2006). The immune response in autism: A new frontier for autism research. *Journal of Leukocyte Biology, 80*(1), 1–15.

Bachevalier, J. (1994). Medial Temporal Lope Structures and Autism – a Review of Clinical and Experimental Findings. *Neuropsychologia, 32*(6), 627–648.

Bachevalier, J. (1996). Brief Report - Medial Temporal Lobe and Autism – a Putative Animal Model in Primates. *Journal of Autism and Developmental Disorders, 26*(2), 217–220.

Bachevalier, J. (2000). The amygdala, social cognition, and autism. In J. P. Aggleton (Ed.), *The Amygdala: A functional analysis* (pp. 509–543). New York: Oxford University Press.

Baron-Cohen, S., Ring, H. A., Bullmore, E. T., Wheelwright, S., Ashwin, C., & Williams, S. C. (2000). The amygdala theory of autism. *Neuroscience and Biobehavioral Reviews, 24*(3), 355–364.

Baron-Cohen, S., Ring, H. A., Wheelwright, S., Bullmore, E. T., Brammer, M. J., Simmons, A., et al. (1999). Social intelligence in the normal and autistic brain: An fMRI study. *European Journal of Neuroscience, 11*(6), 1891–1898.

Bauman, M. D., Lavenex, P., Mason, W. A., Capitanio, J. P., & Amaral, D. G. (2004a). The development of mother-infant interactions after neonatal amygdala lesions in rhesus monkeys. *Journal of Neuroscience, 24*(3), 711–721.

Bauman, M. D., Lavenex, P., Mason, W. A., Capitanio, J. P., & Amaral, D. G. (2004b). The development of social behavior following neonatal amygdala lesions in rhesus monkeys. *Journal of Cognitive Neuroscience, 16*(8), 1388–1411.

Bauman, M. D., Toscano, J. E., Babineau, B. A., Mason, W. A., & Amaral, D. G. (2008). Emergence of stereotypies in juvenile monkeys (Macaca mulatta) with neonatal amygdala or hippocampus lesions. *Behavioral Neuroscience, 122*(5), 1005–1015.

Bauman, M. D., Toscano, J. E., Mason, W. A., Lavenex, P., & Amaral, D. G. (2006). The expression of social dominance following neonatal lesions of the amygdala or hippocampus in rhesus monkeys (Macaca mulatta). *Behavioral Neuroscience, 120*(4), 749–760.

Bauman, M. L. (1991). Microscopic neuroanatomic abnormalities in autism. *Pediatrics, 87*(5 Pt 2), 791–796.

Bauman, M. L., Filipek, P. A., & Kemper, T. L. (1997). Early infantile autism. *International Review of Neurobiology, 41*, 367–386.

Bergman, H., Wichmann, T., & DeLong, M. R. (1990). Reversal of experimental parkinsonism by lesions of the subthalamic nucleus. *Science, 249*(4975), 1436–1438.

Berkson, G. (1983). Repetitive stereotyped behaviors. *American Journal of Mental Deficiency, 88*(3), 239–246.

Berkson, G., Gutermuth, L., & Baranek, G. (1995). Relative prevalence and relations among stereotyped and similar behaviors. *American Journal of Mental Retardation, 100*(2), 137–145.

Berman, C. I. (1980). Mother-infant relationships among free-ranging rhesus monkeys on Cayo Santiago: A comparison with captive pairs. *Animal Behaviour, 28*, 860–873.

Berman, C. M. (1982). The ontogeny of social relationships with group companions among free-ranging rhesus monkeys: I. Social networks and differentiation. *Animal Behaviour, 30*, 149–162.

Bernstein, I. S., & Mason, W. A. (1963). Group Formation by Rhesus Monkeys. *Animal Behaviour, 11*(1), 28–31.

Bodfish, J. W., Symons, F. J., Parker, D. E., & Lewis, M. H. (2000). Varieties of repetitive behavior in autism: Comparisons to mental retardation. *Journal of Autism and Developmental Disorders, 30*(3), 237–243.

Brauer, J., Kaminski, J., Riedel, J., Call, J., & Tomasello, M. (2006). Making inferences about the location of hidden food: Social dog, causal ape. *Journal of Comparative Psychology, 120*(1), 38–47.

Braunschweig, D., Ashwood, P., Krakowiak, P., Hertz-Picciotto, I., Hansen, R., Croen, L. A., et al. (2008). Autism: Maternally derived antibodies specific for fetal brain proteins. *Neurotoxicology, 29*(2), 226–231.

Burns, R. S., Chiueh, C. C., Markey, S. P., Ebert, M. H., Jacobowitz, D. M., & Kopin, I. J. (1983). A primate model of parkinsonism: Selective destruction of dopaminergic neurons in the pars compacta of the substantia nigra by N-methyl-4-phenyl-1,2,3,6-tetrahydropyridine. *Proceedings of the National Academy of Sciences of the United States of America, 80*(14), 4546–4550.

Byrne, R., & Whiten, A. (1988). *Machiavellian intelligence: Social expertise and the evolution of intellect in monkeys, apes, and humans.* Oxford: Clarendon Press.

Call, J., Hare, B., Carpenter, M., & Tomasello, M. (2004). "Unwilling" versus "unable": Chimpanzees' understanding of human intentional action. *Developmental Science, 7*(4), 488–498.

Call, J., & Tomasello, M. (1998). Distinguishing intentional from accidental actions in orangutans (Pongo pygmaeus), chimpanzees (Pan troglodytes), and human children (Homo sapiens). *Journal of Comparative Psychology, 112*(2), 192–206.

Capitanio, J. (1986). Behavioral pathology. In G. Mitchell & J. Erwin (Eds.), *Comparative primate biology: Behavior, conservation, and ecology* (Vol. 2A, pp. 411–454). New York: Alan R. Liss.

Capitanio, J. P., & Emborg, M. E. (2008). Contributions of nonhuman primates to neuroscience research. *Lancet, 371*(9618), 1126–1135.

Carper, R. A., & Courchesne, E. (2005). Localized enlargement of the frontal cortex in early autism. *Biological Psychiatry, 57*(2), 126–133.

Champoux, M., Metz, B., & Suomi, S. J. (1991). Behavior of nursery/peer-reared and mother-reared rhesus monkeys from birth through 2 years of age. *Primates, 32*(4), 509–514.

Chan, A. W., Chong, K. Y., Martinovich, C., Simerly, C., & Schatten, G. (2001). Transgenic monkeys produced by retroviral gene transfer into mature oocytes. *Science, 291*(5502), 309–312.

Chan, A. W., & Yang, S. H. (2009). Generation of transgenic monkeys with human inherited genetic disease. *Methods, 49*(1), 78–84.

Colombi, C., Liebal, K., Tomasello, M., Young, G., Warneken, F., & Rogers, S. J. (2009). Examining correlates of cooperation in autism: Imitation, joint attention, and understanding intentions. *Autism, 13*(2), 143–163.

Comi, A. M., Zimmerman, A. W., Frye, V. H., Law, P. A., & Peeden, J. N. (1999). Familial clustering of autoimmune disorders and evaluation of medical risk factors in autism. *Journal of Child Neurology, 14*(6), 388–394.

Cook, E. H., Jr., Perry, B. D., Dawson, G., Wainwright, M. S., & Leventhal, B. L. (1993). Receptor inhibition by immunoglobulins: Specific inhibition by autistic children, their relatives, and control subjects. *Journal of Autism and Developmental Disorders, 23*(1), 67–78.

Crawley, J. N. (2004). Designing mouse behavioral tasks relevant to autistic-like behaviors. *Mental Retardation and Developmental Disabilities Research Reviews, 10*(4), 248–258.

Crawley, J. N. (2007a). Medicine. Testing hypotheses about autism. *Science, 318*(5847), 56–57.

Crawley, J. N. (2007b). Mouse behavioral assays relevant to the symptoms of autism. *Brain Pathology, 17*(4), 448–459.

Croonenberghs, J., Bosmans, E., Deboutte, D., Kenis, G., & Maes, M. (2002). Activation of the inflammatory response system in autism. *Neuropsychobiology, 45*(1), 1–6.

Dalton, K. M., Nacewicz, B. M., Alexander, A. L., & Davidson, R. J. (2007). Gaze-fixation, brain activation, and amygdala volume in unaffected siblings of individuals with autism. *Biological Psychiatry, 61*(4), 512–520.

Dalton, K. M., Nacewicz, B. M., Johnstone, T., Schaefer, H. S., Gernsbacher, M. A., Goldsmith, H. H., et al. (2005). Gaze fixation and the neural circuitry of face processing in autism. *Nature Neuroscience, 8*(4), 519–526.

Dalton, P., Deacon, R., Blamire, A., Pike, M., McKinlay, I., Stein, J., et al. (2003). Maternal neuronal antibodies associated with autism and a language disorder. *Annals of Neurology, 53*(4), 533–537.

Datta, S. B. (1984). Relative power and the acquisition of rank. In R. A. Hinde (Ed.), *Primate social relationships: An integrated approach* (pp. 93–103). Oxford: Blackwells Scientific Publishers.

Dawson, G., Webb, S. J., & McPartland, J. (2005). Understanding the nature of face processing impairment in autism: Insights from behavioral and electrophysiological studies. *Developmental Neuropsychology, 27*(3), 403–424.

Dawson, G., Webb, S. J., Wijsman, E., Schellenberg, G., Estes, A., Munson, J., et al. (2005). Neurocognitive and electrophysiological evidence of altered face processing in parents of children with autism: Implications for a model of abnormal development of social brain circuitry in autism. *Development and Psychopathology, 17*(3), 679–697.

DeLong, M. R. (1990). Primate models of movement disorders of basal ganglia origin. *Trends in Neurosciences, 13*(7), 281–285.

Devinney, B. J., Berman, C. M., & Rasmussen, K. L. (2001). Changes in yearling rhesus monkeys' relationships with their mothers after sibling birth. *American Journal of Primatology, 54*(4), 193–210.

Drickamer, L. C. (1975). Quantitative observation of behavior in free-ranging Macaca mulatta: Methodology and aggression. *Behaviour, 55*(3–4), 209–236.

Ferrari, P. F., Visalberghi, E., Paukner, A., Fogassi, L., Ruggiero, A., & Suomi, S. J. (2006). Neonatal imitation in rhesus macaques. *PLoS Biology, 4*(9), e302.

Flombaum, J. I., & Santos, L. R. (2005). Rhesus monkeys attribute perceptions to others. *Current Biology, 15*(5), 447–452.

Gibbs, R. A., Weinstock, G. M., Metzker, M. L., Muzny, D. M., Sodergren, E. J., Scherer, S., et al. (2004). Genome sequence of the Brown Norway rat yields insights into mammalian evolution. *Nature, 428*(6982), 493–521.

Griffin, G. A., & Harlow, H. F. (1966). Effects of three months of total social deprivation on social adjustment and learning in the rhesus monkey. *Child Development, 37*(3), 533–547.

Hakeem, A. Y., Sherwood, C. C., Bonar, C. J., Butti, C., Hof, P. R., & Allman, J. M. (2009). Von Economo neurons in the elephant brain. *Anatomical Record (Hoboken), 292*(2), 242–248.

Hansen, E. W. (1966). The Development of Maternal and Infant Behavior in the Rhesus Monkey. *Behaviour, 27*(1–2), 107–149.

Hare, B., Brown, M., Williamson, C., & Tomasello, M. (2002). The domestication of social cognition in dogs. *Science, 298*(5598), 1634–1636.

Hare, B., & Tomasello, M. (2005). Human-like social skills in dogs? *Trends in Cognitive Sciences, 9*(9), 439–444.

Harlow, H. F. (1965). Total Social Isolation: Effects on Macaque Monkey Behavior. *Science, 148*(3670), 666.

Harlow, H. F., Dodsworth, R. O., & Harlow, M. K. (1965). Total social isolation in monkeys. *Proceedings of the National Academy of Sciences of the United States of America, 54*(1), 90–97.

Harlow, H. F., & Harlow, M. (1962). Social deprivation in monkeys. *Scientific American, 207*, 136–146.

Harlow, H. F., & Harlow, M. K. (1965). The effect of rearing conditions on behavior. *International Journal of Psychiatry in Medicine, 1*, 43–51.

Harlow, H. F., Rowland, G. L., & Griffin, G. A. (1964). The effect of total social deprivation on the development of monkey behavior. *Psychiatric Research Reports American Psychiatric Association, 19*, 116–135.

Harlow, H. F., & Suomi, S. J. (1971). Social recovery by isolation-reared monkeys. *Proceedings of the National Academy of Sciences of the United States of America, 68*(7), 1534–1538.

Harlow, H. F., & Zimmermann, R. R. (1959). Affectional responses in the infant monkey; orphaned baby monkeys develop a strong and persistent attachment to inanimate surrogate mothers. *Science, 130*(3373), 421–432.

Hertz-Picciotto, I., Park, H. Y., Dostal, M., Kocan, A., Trnovec, T., & Sram, R. (2008). Prenatal exposures to persistent and non-persistent organic compounds and effects on immune system development. *Basic and Clinical Pharmacology and Toxicology, 102*(2), 146–154.

Hinde, R. A., Rowell, T. E., & Spencer-Booth, Y. (1964). Behavior of socially living rhesus monkeys in their first six months. *Proceedings of the Zoological Society London, 143*, 609–649.

Hinde, R. A., & Spencer-Booth, Y. (1967). The behaviour of socially living Rhesus monkeys in their first two and a half years. *Animal Behaviour, 15*(1), 169–196.

Iacoboni, M. (2005). Neural mechanisms of imitation. *Current Opinion in Neurobiology, 15*(6), 632–637.

Iacoboni, M., & Dapretto, M. (2006). The mirror neuron system and the consequences of its dysfunction. *Nature Reviews Neuroscience, 7*(12), 942–951.

Jolly, A. (1966). Lemur social behavior and primate intelligence. *Science, 153*(735), 501–506.

Kalin, N., & Shelton, S. (1989). Defensive behaviors in infant Rhesus monkeys: Environmental cues and neurochemical regulation. *Science, 243*, 1718–1721.

Klin, A., Jones, W., Schultz, R., Volkmar, F., & Cohen, D. (2002). Visual fixation patterns during viewing of naturalistic social situations as predictors of social competence in individuals with autism. *Archives of General Psychiatry, 59*(9), 809–816.

Kumar, S., & Hedges, S. B. (1998). A molecular timescale for vertebrate evolution. *Nature, 392*(6679), 917–920.

Kuwahata, H., Adachi, I., Fujita, K., Tomonaga, M., & Matsuzawa, T. (2004). Development of schematic face preference in macaque monkeys. *Behavioural Processes, 66*(1), 17–21.

Lemere, C. A., Beierschmitt, A., Iglesias, M., Spooner, E. T., Bloom, J. K., Leverone, J. F., et al. (2004). Alzheimer's disease abeta vaccine reduces central nervous system abeta levels in a non-human primate, the Caribbean vervet. *American Journal of Pathology, 165*(1), 283–297.

Lemere, C. A., Maier, M., Jiang, L., Peng, Y., & Seabrook, T. J. (2006). Amyloid-beta immunotherapy for the prevention and treatment of Alzheimer disease: Lessons from mice, monkeys, and humans. *Rejuvenation Research, 9*(1), 77–84.

Lutz, C., Well, A., & Novak, M. (2003). Stereotypic and self-injurious behavior in rhesus macaques: A survey and retrospective analysis of environment and early experience. *American Journal of Primatology, 60*(1), 1–15.

Lutz, C. K., Lockard, J. S., Gunderson, V. M., & Grant, K. S. (1998). Infant monkeys' visual responses to drawings of normal and distorted faces. *American Journal of Primatology, 44*(2), 169–174.

Martin, L. A., Ashwood, P., Braunschweig, D., Cabanlit, M., Van de Water, J., & Amaral, D. G. (2008). Stereotypies and hyperactivity in rhesus monkeys exposed to IgG from mothers of children with autism. *Brain, Behavior, and Immunity, 22*(6), 806–816.

Masataka, N. (1985). Development of vocal recognition of mothers in infant Japanese macaques. *Developmental Psychobiology, 18*(2), 107–114.

Mason, W. A. (1960). The effects of social restriction on the behavior of rhesus monkeys: I. Free social behavior. *Journal of Comparative and Physiological Psychology, 53*, 582–589.

Matheson, M. D., & Bernstein, I. S. (2000). Grooming, social bonding, and agonistic aiding in rhesus monkeys. *American Journal of Primatology, 51*(3), 177–186.

McKinney, W. T. (1984). Animal models of depression: An overview. *Psychiatric Developments, 2*(2), 77–96.

Mendelson, M. J. (1982a). Clinical examination of visual and social responses in infant rhesus monkeys. *Developmental Psychology, 18*(5), 658–664.

Mendelson, M. J. (1982b). Visual and social responses in infant rhesus monkeys. *American Journal of Primatology, 3*, 333–340.

Mendelson, M. J., Haith, M. M., & Goldman-Rakic, P. S. (1982). Face scanning and responsiveness to social cues in infant rhesus monkeys. *Developmental Psychology, 18*(2), 222–228.

Meunier, M., Bachevalier, J., Murray, E. A., Malkova, L., & Mishkin, M. (1999). Effects of aspiration versus neurotoxic lesions of the amygdala on emotional responses in monkeys. *European Journal of Neuroscience, 11*(12), 4403–4418.

Missakian, E. A. (1972). Genealogical and cross-genealogical dominance relations in a group of free ranging rhesus monkeys (Macaca mulatta) on Cayo Santiago. *Primates, 13*(2), 169–180.

Mowbray, J. B., & Cadell, T. E. (1962). Early behavior patterns in rhesus monkeys. *Journal of Comparative and Physiological Psychology, 55*, 350–357.

Moy, S. S., Nadler, J. J., Poe, M. D., Nonneman, R. J., Young, N. B., Koller, B. H., et al. (2008). Development of a mouse test for repetitive, restricted behaviors: Relevance to autism. *Behavioural Brain Research, 188*(1), 178–194.

Nadig, A. S., Ozonoff, S., Young, G. S., Rozga, A., Sigman, M., & Rogers, S. J. (2007). A prospective study of response to name in infants at risk for autism. *Archives of Pediatric and Adolescent Medicine, 161*(4), 378–383.

Nagahara, A. H., Merrill, D. A., Coppola, G., Tsukada, S., Schroeder, B. E., Shaked, G. M., et al. (2009). Neuroprotective effects of brain-derived neurotrophic factor in rodent and primate models of Alzheimer's disease. *Nature Medicine, 15*(3), 331–337.

Noldus, L. P. (1991). The Observer: A software system for collection and analysis of observational data. *Behavior Research Methods, Instruments & Computers, 23*, 415–429.

Odom, S. L., & Strain, P. S. (1986). A comparison of peer-initiation and teacher-antecedent interventions for promoting reciprocal social interaction of autistic preschoolers. *Journal of Applied Behavior Analysis, 19*(1), 59–71.

Oke, N. J., & Schreibman, L. (1990). Training social initiations to a high-functioning autistic child: Assessment of collateral behavior change and generalization in a case study. *Journal of Autism and Developmental Disorders, 20*(4), 479–497.

Osterling, J., & Dawson, G. (1994). Early recognition of children with autism: A study of first birthday home videotapes. *Journal of Autism and Developmental Disorders, 24*(3), 247–257.

Osterling, J. A., Dawson, G., & Munson, J. A. (2002). Early recognition of 1-year-old infants with autism spectrum disorder versus mental retardation. *Development and Pscyhopathology, 14*(2), 239–251.

Ozonoff, S., Macari, S., Young, G. S., Goldring, S., Thompson, M., & Rogers, S. J. (2008). Atypical object exploration at 12 months of age is associated with autism in a prospective sample. *Autism, 12*(5), 457–472.

Pelphrey, K. A., Sasson, N. J., Reznick, J. S., Paul, G., Goldman, B. D., & Piven, J. (2002). Visual scanning of faces in autism. *Journal of Autism and Developmental Disorders, 32*(4), 249–261.

Pessah, I. N., Seegal, R. F., Lein, P. J., LaSalle, J., Yee, B. K., Van De Water, J., et al. (2008). Immunologic and neurodevelopmental susceptibilities of autism. *Neurotoxicology, 29*(3), 532–545.

Pierce, K., & Courchesne, E. (2001). Evidence for a cerebellar role in reduced exploration and stereotyped behavior in autism. *Biological Psychiatry, 49*(8), 655–664.

Plioplys, A. V., Greaves, A., Kazemi, K., & Silverman, E. (1994). Lymphocyte function in autism and Rett syndrome. *Neuropsychobiology, 29*(1), 12–16.

Prather, M. D., Lavenex, P., Mauldin-Jourdain, M. L., Mason, W. A., Capitanio, J. P., Mendoza, S. P., et al. (2001). Increased social fear and decreased fear of objects in monkeys with neonatal amygdala lesions. *Neuroscience, 106*(4), 653–658.

Preuss, T. (1995). Do rats have a prefrontal cortex? The Rose-Woolsey-Akert reconsidered. *Journal of Cognitive Neuroscience* (7), 1–24.

Preuss, T. M. (2000). Taking the measure of diversity: Comparative alternatives to the model-animal paradigm in cortical neuroscience. *Brain, Behavior, and Evolution, 55*(6), 287–299.

Richler, J., Luyster, R., Risi, S., Hsu, W. L., Dawson, G., Bernier, R., et al. (2006). Is There a "Regressive Phenotype" of Autism Spectrum Disorder Associated with the Measles-Mumps-Rubella Vaccine? A CPEA Study. *Journal of Autism and Developmental Disorders*.

Riedel, J., Buttelmann, D., Call, J., & Tomasello, M. (2006). Domestic dogs (Canis familiaris) use a physical marker to locate hidden food. *Animal Cognition*, *9*(1), 27–35.

Rogers, S. J. (2000). Interventions that facilitate socialization in children with autism. *Journal of Autism and Developmental Disorders*, *30*(5), 399–409.

Rudebeck, P. H., Buckley, M. J., Walton, M. E., & Rushworth, M. F. (2006). A role for the macaque anterior cingulate gyrus in social valuation. *Science*, *313*(5791), 1310–1312.

Ruppenthal, G. C., Harlow, M. K., Eisele, C. D., Harlow, H. F., & Suomi, S. J. (1974). Development of peer interactions of monkeys reared in a nuclear-family environment. *Child Development*, *45*(3), 670–682.

Rutter, M., Andersen-Wood, L., Beckett, C., Bredenkamp, D., Castle, J., Groothues, C., et al. (1999). Quasi-autistic patterns following severe early global privation. English and Romanian Adoptees (ERA) Study Team. *Journal of Child Psychology and Psychiatry*, *40*(4), 537–549.

Sackett, G. P. (1966). Monkeys reared in isolation with pictures as visual input: Evidence for an innate releasing mechanism. *Science*, *154*(3755), 1468–1473.

Sade, D. S. (1967). Determinants of dominance in a group of free-ranging rhesus monkeys. In S. A. Altmann (Ed.), *Social communication among primates* (pp. 99–114). Chicago: University of Chicago Press.

Schultz, R. T. (2005). Developmental deficits in social perception in autism: The role of the amygdala and fusiform face area. *International Journal of Developmental Neuroscience*, *23*(2–3), 125–141.

Schumann, C. M., & Amaral, D. G. (2005). Stereological estimation of the number of neurons in the human amygdaloid complex. *Journal of Comparative Neurology*, *491*(4), 320–329.

Schumann, C. M., Hamstra, J., Goodlin-Jones, B. L., Lotspeich, L. J., Kwon, H., Buonocore, M. H., et al. (2004). The amygdala is enlarged in children but not adolescents with autism; the hippocampus is enlarged at all ages. *Journal of Neuroscience*, *24*(28), 6392–6401.

Semendeferi, K., Lu, A., Schenker, N., & Damasio, H. (2002). Humans and great apes share a large frontal cortex. *Nature Neuroscience*, *5*(3), 272–276.

Short, S. J., Lubach, G. R., Karasin, A. L., Olsen, C. W., Styner, M., Knickmeyer, R. C., Gilmore, J. H., Coe, C. L. (2010). Maternal influenza infection during pregnancy impacts postnatal brain development in the rhesus monkey. *Biological Psychiatry*, *67*(10), 965–973.

Singh, V. K. (1996). Plasma increase of interleukin-12 and interferon-gamma. Pathological significance in autism. *Journal of Neuroimmunology*, *66*(1–2), 143–145.

Singh, V. K., & Rivas, W. H. (2004). Prevalence of serum antibodies to caudate nucleus in autistic children. *Neuroscience Letters*, *355*(1–2), 53–56.

Singh, V. K., Warren, R., Averett, R., & Ghaziuddin, M. (1997). Circulating autoantibodies to neuronal and glial filament proteins in autism. *Pediatric Neurology*, *17*(1), 88–90.

Singh, V. K., Warren, R. P., Odell, J. D., Warren, W. L., & Cole, P. (1993). Antibodies to myelin basic protein in children with autistic behavior. *Brain, Behavior, and Immunity*, *7*(1), 97–103.

Stern, L., Francoeur, M. J., Primeau, M. N., Sommerville, W., Fombonne, E., & Mazer, B. D. (2005). Immune function in autistic children. *Annals of Allergy, Asthma, and Immunology*, *95*(6), 558–565.

Suomi, S. J. (1999). Attachment in rhesus monkeys. In J. Cassidy & P. R. Shaver (Eds.), *Handbook of attachment: Theory, research, and clinical applications* (pp. 181–197). New York: The Guilford Press.

Sweeten, T. L., Bowyer, S. L., Posey, D. J., Halberstadt, G. M., & McDougle, C. J. (2003). Increased prevalence of familial autoimmunity in probands with pervasive developmental disorders. *Pediatrics*, *112*(5), e420.

Swettenham, J., Baron-Cohen, S., Charman, T., Cox, A., Baird, G., Drew, A., et al. (1998). The frequency and distribution of spontaneous attention shifts between social and nonsocial stimuli in autistic, typically developing, and nonautistic developmentally delayed infants. *Journal of Child Psychology and Psychiatry*, *39*(5), 747–753.

Todd, R. D., & Ciaranello, R. D. (1985). Demonstration of inter- and intraspecies differences in serotonin binding sites by antibodies from an autistic child. *Proceedings of the National Academy of Sciences of the United States of America*, *82*(2), 612–616.

Tuszynski, M. H., & Blesch, A. (2004). Nerve growth factor: From animal models of cholinergic neuronal degeneration to gene therapy in Alzheimer's disease. *Progress in Brain Research*, *146*, 441–449.

Tuszynski, M. H., Roberts, J., Senut, M. C., U, H. S., & Gage, F. H. (1996). Gene therapy in the adult primate brain: Intraparenchymal grafts of cells genetically modified to produce nerve growth factor prevent cholinergic neuronal degeneration. *Gene Therapy*, *3*(4), 305–314.

van Gent, T., Heijnen, C. J., & Treffers, P. D. (1997). Autism and the immune system. *Journal of Child Psychology and Psychiatry*, *38*(3), 337–349.

Vargas, D. L., Nascimbene, C., Krishnan, C., Zimmerman, A. W., & Pardo, C. A. (2005). Neuroglial activation and neuroinflammation in the brain of patients with autism. *Annals of Neurology*, *57*(1), 67–81.

Vincent, A., Dalton, P., Clover, L., Palace, J., & Lang, B. (2003). Antibodies to neuronal targets in neurological and psychiatric diseases. *Annals of the New York Academy of Sciences*, *992*, 48–55.

Wales, L., Charman, T., & Mount, R. H. (2004). An analogue assessment of repetitive hand behaviours in girls and young women with Rett syndrome. *Journal of Intellectual Disability Research*, *48*(Pt 7), 672–678.

Warren, R. P., Cole, P., Odell, J. D., Pingree, C. B., Warren, W. L., White, E., et al. (1990). Detection of maternal antibodies in infantile autism. *Journal of the American Academy of Child and Adolescent Psychiatry*, *29*(6), 873–877.

Wenk, G. L. (1993). A primate model of Alzheimer's disease. *Behavioural Brain Research*, *57*(2), 117–122.

Willette, A. A., Lubach, G. R., Knickmeyer, R., C., Short, S. J., Styner, M., Gilmore, J. H., Coe, C. L. (2010). Brain enlargement and increased behavioral and cytokine reactivity in infant monkeys following acute prenatal endotoxemia. *Behavioural Brain Research*, *(2010)*, doi:10.1016/j.bbr.2010.12.023.

Williams, J. H., Whiten, A., & Singh, T. (2004). A systematic review of action imitation in autistic spectrum disorder. *Journal of Autism and Developmental Disorders*, *34*(3), 285–299.

Wrangham, R. W. (1980). An ecological model of female-bonded primate groups. *Behaviour*, *75*, 262–300.

Yang, S. H., Cheng, P. H., Banta, H., Piotrowska-Nitsche, K., Yang, J. J., Cheng, E. C., et al. (2008). Towards a transgenic model of Huntington's disease in a non-human primate. *Nature*, *453*(7197), 921–924.

54 Autism as a Disorder of Functional Brain Connectivity

Rajesh K. Kana, Marcel Adam Just

Points of Interest

- Autism is not localized to a single place in the brain, but rather is a neural systems level disorder.
- Cortical Underconnectivity Theory proposes that the connectivity between frontal and posterior brain areas is compromised in autism, lowering the communication bandwidth between these regions. The underconnectivity is manifested as aberrant white matter (measured with MRI morphometry and diffusion tensor imaging) and reduced synchronization of brain activity between frontal and posterior areas.
- The reduced availability of frontal areas in autism may lead to increased reliance on posterior areas, particularly visual areas.
- Cognitive and other behavioral intervention programs may be able to strengthen the connections among relevant brain areas by training in thought processes that require frontal-posterior collaboration. The use of explicit instructions and selective reinforcements would be a starting point in such programs designed for children with autism.

"During the last couple of years, I have become more aware of a kind of electricity that goes on between people. I have observed that when several people are together and having a good time, their speech and laughter follow a rhythm. They will all laugh together and they talk quietly until the next laughing cycle. I have always had a hard time fitting in with this rhythm, and I usually interrupt conversations without realizing my mistake. The problem is that I can't follow the rhythm." Grandin (1995, pp. 89–92)

The above words from Temple Grandin provide lucid testimony of how casual social interaction in daily life is alien territory for people with autism. The complex nature of the functioning of the world, especially the social world, is enigmatic to people with autism just as the disorder itself is intriguing to families and researchers. Whereas human interactions are the products of a carefully orchestrated symphony of understanding and accessing minds, the conductor of it, the human brain, carries out this coordinated venture with utmost precision and with regular rhythm. Temple Grandin points out that she can't follow the rhythm of human interactions, but what lies beneath the struggle is a brain trying to keep up with the symphony. This chapter is about how the brain coordinates the orchestra of cognitive and social functions, the symphony of the organization and the functioning of the brain, and how an aberrant brain communication system in autism produces thought processes and behaviors that are atypical.

The symptoms of autism are extremely widespread such that it manifests itself as a multidimensional (social, cognitive, linguistic, and information processing) disorder. Researchers, especially neuroscientists who study autism, have long been in the hunt for finding the dysfunction of a single region in the brain that could explain the complexities of autism. The commonly asked, although implicit, question is, "Where in the brain is autism located?" Obviously, there has been no single convincing answer to this question. Considering the complexity, breadth of symptoms, and the intriguing nature of autism, any attempt to localize the disorder to a single cortical structure seems unlikely to succeed. Studies seeking such localized abnormalities have not demonstrated a consistent pattern of brain dysfunction in autism (Jacobson et al., 1988; Sears et al., 1999; Piven & Arndt, 1995). On the other hand, this difficulty in finding a single structural culprit in autism attests to the complex nature of the disorder and calls for an explanation at a more comprehensive and global level. A relatively novel approach to answer the questions related to the neural basis of autism would be to consider the brain as a system of coordinated components, a network in which different parts function together collaboratively to accomplish a goal. This approach to studying the brain in autism has resulted in a theory called the Cortical Underconnectivity Theory of autism (Just et al., 2004), according to which, the communication between frontal and posterior brain regions is impaired in autism, negatively affecting the coordinated network functioning during task performance. In other words, the brain is functionally and structurally underconnected in autism, particularly when complex cognitive and social functions are processed. In this chapter, we will discuss cortical underconnectivity as an emerging theory of autism and its potential implications at the neural and behavioral domains. In addition, we will also relate the underconnectivity theory to various other neuropathological findings in autism research.

Cortical Underconnectivity Theory of Autism

The performance of any task is associated with the co-activation of multiple cortical and subcortical regions, and successful task performance depends on the effective integration of neural output from the distinct brain regions involved (Tononi, Edelman, & Sporns, 1998). This integrative functioning of cortical regions may be compromised in individuals with autism. According to the Cortical Underconnectivity Theory (Just et al., 2004), autism is a cognitive and neurobiological disorder marked by underconnectivity among cortical regions that results in a deficit of integration of information at the neural and, therefore, cognitive levels. The first-discovered indication of the underconnectivity was the reduced synchronization between the functional MRI (fMRI)-measured activation in co-activating cortical areas, referred to as *functional underconnectivity* (See Box 54-1). More recent elaborations of the underconnectivity theory localize the functional underconnectivity to frontal-posterior synchronization (Just et al., 2007), relate the underconnectivity to properties of cortical white matter, and construe the underconnectivity as a limitation on frontal-posterior bandwidth. Bandwidth is a critical factor in the performance of a computational network, referring to the amount of information that can be transmitted between the nodes of the network per unit time. Neuroimaging research has been very clear that human thought involves a network of cortical areas whose activity is coordinated (Just & Varma, 2007), and that coordination has to be based on inter-regional communication, using the white matter tracts that provide the anatomical connectivity.

The fMRI findings emerging in the last few years indicate that the synchronization between frontal and posterior areas is lower in autism in many diverse tasks, such as sentence comprehension (Just et al., 2004), verbal working memory (Koshino et al., 2005), executive functioning (Just et al., 2007), attribution of mental states to animated shapes (Kana et al., 2009), visuomotor coordination (Villalobos et al., 2005), visual imagery in sentence comprehension (Kana et al., 2006), response inhibition (Kana et al., 2007), processing of fearful faces (Welchew et al., 2005), discourse processing (Mason et al., 2008), and working memory for faces (Koshino et al., 2008). In brief, functional imaging studies are providing evidence of underconnectivity in the distributed networks of cortical centers that subserve the core symptoms in autism, including social cognition, language comprehension, and reasoning. The synchronization across time-points is independent of the absolute levels of activation in the two areas, and vice versa, so the fMRI findings of functional underconnectivity are providing an entirely different and richer account of the coordination of activation across brain areas.

A particularly interesting case of underconnectivity occurs in people who are just relaxing when their brain goes into what is called *a resting state* or a *default mode*. Even in that state, the degree of synchronization between the frontal and posterior parts of the default mode network is lower in people with autism (Cherkassky et al., 2006). This result shows that the brain characteristics of autism are manifest not just when a person is performing a particular cognitive or social task, but even when they are just relaxing. The brain marker of underconnectivity in autism is present in the resting state.

The common finding of cortical underconnectivity across all of the studies mentioned earlier highlights the pervasiveness

Box 54–1
Measurement of functional connectivity

Functional connectivity (the temporal correlation of brain activity in spatially separated areas) can be measured by several different approaches. In our approach, it is usually computed separately for each participant, as a correlation between the activation time-course averaged over all of the activated voxels in each member of a pair of activated regions of interest. In our approach, the following steps are used: *(1)* Functional regions of interest (ROIs) are manually defined on the group activation map to encircle the main clusters of activation. A sphere is defined for each cluster (with a radius of approx. 8–14mm) that best captures each cluster of activation in the activation map. *(2)* The time-course of the fMRI signal from each ROI is extracted from individual subjects' data based on the normalized and smoothed images. The activation time-course is based on the mean activation level of only the activated voxels within the ROI (minus their baseline level established during "rest" periods). *(3)* The functional connectivity between two ROIs is computed as the correlation between their activation time-courses, which is then converted to Fisher's "z"-score to test for statistical differences. Further analyses can be carried out by grouping the ROIs into different sets of ROI pairs (such as frontal-parietal pairs, or temporal-occipital pairs, etc.) to compare the functional connectivity between autism and control groups for a given set of ROI pairs. It is in the frontal-posterior pairs where the functional connectivity has usually been found to be lower in autism during the performance of high-level tasks.

of the frontal-posterior undersynchronization of brain regions in autism. In addition to the findings from brain imaging studies, results of several behavioral studies of autism provide evidence for an information processing style relying on reduced frontal-posterior integration and coordination. For example, people with autism are not impaired when processing the meaning of individual words (Eskes, Bryson, & McCormick, 1990; Frith & Snowling, 1983) but have difficulty in integrating the meaning of different words in a sentence (Goldstein, Minshew, & Siegel, 1994). In these cases, the trouble seems to be not at the level of comprehending individual word meanings but at the level of integrating these word meanings to form a more complex representation. This type of focusing on unintegrated components may stand in the way of comprehending complex linguistic discourse (such as irony, metaphor, ambiguity, and puns) and understanding complex social situations (such as face processing, gaze processing, and joint attention), all of which require a coordination among the psychological processes that operate on the components of a larger array of information. At the same time, the focus on the processing of components of an array may be advantageous when the properties of the larger array may interfere with processing of a component (as might occur in finding an embedded figure whose presence is occluded by the larger array). The Cortical Underconnectivity Theory attempts to explain not only the deficits in autism but also the relative sparing of some functions.

Underconnectivity theory also provides an alternative framing for previous theories of autism, providing a link between the behavioral characteristics of autism to the underlying biological substrate. For example, both the weak central coherence theory (Frith, 1989; Happe & Frith, 2006) and the enhanced perceptual functioning proposal (Mottron et al., 2001; 2006) emphasize that people with autism have difficulty integrating parts of information into a meaningful whole. Underconnectivity theory also predicts this weak coherence among ongoing processes, by virtue of poorer communication and collaboration among brain areas associated with such processes. The complex information processing deficit approach (Minshew et al., 1997) attributed autism to a fundamental inability in handling information in complex tasks requiring abstraction. Tasks that are considered more complex typically require more participation of frontal areas, and the postulated underconnectivity to frontal areas would account for the impaired performance in such tasks.

Cortical Underconnectivity Theory is also in agreement with other neural models such as the temporal binding deficit hypothesis of autism (Brock et al., 2002). According to this hypothesis, it is the impairment of temporal binding *between* local networks that results in the deficits found in autism, whereas temporal binding mechanisms *within* local networks may be intact or possibly enhanced. Binding entails communication, and an impairment in communication will impair binding. Overall, the theme of several cognitive and neurological theories points to an underlying deficit in cortical connectivity in autism.

The Generality and Specificity of Underconnectivity

Investigations into the generality and specificity of the manifestation of underconnectivity in autism have found that underconnectivity is more pronounced in the communication to and from the frontal lobe. Again, one area of difference in functional connectivity found between autism and control participants is between frontal and parietal networks. Frontal-parietal underconnectivity has been reported in executive functioning (Just et al., 2007), in visual imagery in sentence comprehension (Kana et al., 2006), in a response-inhibition task (Kana et al., 2007), and in working memory for faces (Koshino et al., 2008). Hence, the theory posits that the communication bandwidth between frontal and posterior cortical regions is lower in participants with autism than in typical participants.

Reduced functional connectivity is not confined to a particular domain or task but is likely to be a general phenomenon at least across the neural systems involved in high-level cognition. At the cognitive level, the demand for communication between frontal and posterior regions is greater in relatively complex tasks, such as problem-solving, working memory, attribution of mental states, and language comprehension.

By contrast, functional connectivity within and between the relatively posterior brain areas has been found to be intact or sometimes superior in people with autism. This intact functional connectivity is centered mainly in the occipital-parietal areas (e.g., Villalobos et al., 2005). The higher connectivity in autism, seen mainly in the visual or visuospatial brain areas, is not surprising considering the behavioral findings of relative preservation of visuospatial ability in autism (Shah & Frith, 1983; Caron et al., 2004, Ring et al., 1999; Mottron & Burack, 2001). People with high-functioning autism might resort to an information processing style that is less reliant on frontal participation and more reliant on posterior visuospatial processing. In this perspective, this is not an information processing style chosen as a preference by people with autism but a brain systems adaptation to reduced frontal input. It is possible that people with autism have difficulty in solving tasks that have high cognitive and social processing demands that are normally accomplished with the involvement of frontal regions, and to compensate for this limitation, they rely on visuospatial processing that draws more on posterior cortical regions.

Informational connectivity with the frontal lobe may be impaired in autism because of several structural and functional abnormalities found in this region (discussed later in this chapter). These structural and functional abnormalities might be the underlying problem that results in underconnectivity between the frontal lobe and other regions in autism (although other causal interpretations cannot be dismissed). In the following sections, we will discuss how the autistic brain responds to cortical underconnectivity and also how structural abnormalities in autism might affect functional connectivity.

How Does the Autistic Brain Adapt to Underconnectivity?

If autism is characterized by decreased frontal-posterior communication bandwidth, then one might expect to see concomitant adaptations in cortical functioning. Just et al. (submitted) propose a computational model of an executive functioning task that accounts for the some of the autism brain activation findings in fMRI studies. One of the main contributions of the model is the insight it provides into how a bandwidth constraint could bring about a consequent adaptation. The model is instantiated within a computational theory of the cortical neuroarchitecture, 4CAPS, which characterizes cognitive functioning as the emergent product of the collaborative activity of a set of co-activating brain centers that are in communication with each other (Just & Varma, 2007). In the autism model, the bandwidth limitation is implemented as a limitation on the amount of information that can be communicated per unit time between any frontal center and any posterior center. (This limitation could result from compromised structural integrity of some of the white matter tracts that carry the communication [Keller et al., 2007].) In addition to modeling the decreased frontal-posterior bandwidth, the model also implements an increase in parietal autonomy in autism. This adaptation may arise in response to the decreased frontal-parietal bandwidth. In particular, the task that the participants were performing was a visuospatial problem-solving task (Tower of London), which evokes substantial frontal and parietal activation. Because the input from the frontal center is slow in coming (because of the bandwidth limitation), the system, in some straightforward cases, proceeds to make a move in the task without the benefit of the frontal input. In effect, this adaptation accords greater autonomy to the parietal centers.

More generally, the cortical infrastructure of thought could adapt to a lower frontal-posterior bandwidth by relying less on collaboration with frontal nodes and instead functioning more autonomously of the frontal nodes. This would be an instance of a resource limitation exerting a shaping influence on the functional architecture of the network.

The proposal of greater reliance on posterior cortical regions in autism is reflected in the brain activity observed in autism. Several fMRI studies have shown a decrease in frontal activation in autism with an increase or no difference in activation in posterior regions, such as parietal and occipital areas (e.g., Ring et al., 1999; Kana et al., 2006; Kana et al., 2007; Koshino et al., 2005). Another possible form of adaptation in autism to frontal-posterior underconnectivity is higher connectivity between other pairs of other regions, such as cortical and subcortical regions (Mizuno et al., 2006). It is extremely likely that whatever the initial biological impact that autism imposes on the brain, the subsequent development and learning in the dynamic brain system establishes widespread adaptations to the system.

Structural and White Matter Correlates of Functional Underconnectivity in Autism

Could the functional underconnectivity in autism (the limited frontal-posterior bandwidth) result from an underlying structural abnormality? Structural limits on communication between regions in the brain may cause computational changes to evolve to deal with a pattern of reduced connectivity. Two different MRI-based methods have been used for the investigation of structural abnormalities in autism: *(1)* MRI morphometry examining the volumes of various gray and white matter structures and *(2)* diffusion tensor imaging (DTI) to examine the structural integrity of white matter. As mentioned earlier in this chapter, some of the autism volumetric results have been inconsistent. However, one of the more consistent volumetric findings is the abnormality in brain volume in autism. For example, an increase in brain size (Aylward et al., 2002; Piven et al., 1995) with substantial size difference in early development (Courchesne, Carper, & Akshoomoff, 2003; Sparks et al., 2002; Courchesne et al., 2001) has been reported in autism. The greater brain size in early childhood in autism might well be related to compromised interconnectivity between specialized neural systems, giving rise to a more fragmented processing structure (Herbert, 2005; Schultz, 2001).

Another relatively consistent morphometric finding in autism is the smaller size of the corpus callosum (Vidal et al., 2003; Hardan et al., 2000; Manes et al., 1999; Piven et al., 1997; Egaas et al., 1995). Because the corpus callosum is a major white matter tract, an abnormality of its volume may be an index of a more general compromise of white matter. Such white matter abnormalities may contribute to diminished functional connectivity patterns in autism. In a comparison of structural and functional measures of cortical connectivity, we reported that across individuals with autism, the lower frontal-posterior functional connectivity (i.e., lower synchronization) was correlated with the (relatively reduced) size of the corpus callosum (Just et al., 2007; Kana et al., 2006). The findings suggest the possibility that in autism, the compromised properties of the white matter (measured indirectly in terms of corpus callosum size) constrain the communication between frontal and posterior regions (measured by the functional connectivity). By contrast, in control participants, the white matter is assumed not to constrain the normal range of functional connectivity, and accordingly, there is no correlation between corpus callosum size and functional connectivity in control participants. Later in this section, we will further discuss the role white matter structures may play in functional connectivity.

Underconnectivity theory brings to light the role of the frontal cortex by postulating its impaired communication with the rest of the cortex. (Impaired executive function theory [Hughes et al., 1994; Pennington et al., 1998] and impaired complex information processing theories of autism [Minshew et al., 1997] are also suggestive of a compromised role of frontal cortex.) Evidence concerning brain structure is consistent with this emphasis. Abnormalities such as delayed maturation of the frontal lobe (Zilbovicius et al., 1995), increased frontal cortical folding (Hardan et al., 2004), anatomical shifting of major sulci in the frontal lobe (Levitt et al., 2003), localized enlargement of the frontal lobe (Carper & Courchesne, 2005), and maldevelopment in minicolumns in the frontal cortex (Buxhoeveden et al., 2004; Casanova et al., 2002) have been reported in autism. White matter abnormalities have also been reported in the radiate compartment of the frontal lobe (Herbert et al., 2004).

The structural abnormalities of the frontal lobe raise interesting questions about the causal pathway through which underconnectivity enters into autism. It may be that abnormalities in the white matter connecting frontal to posterior areas are the primary cause and that the changes in frontal gray matter are a consequence of its inability to communicate normally with posterior parts of the brain. This causal account stands in contrast to (and is difficult to empirically distinguish from) the possibility that the primary abnormality is in the frontal gray matter, an abnormality that leads to decreased attempts to communicate with posterior areas, which in turn may lead to less use of frontal-posterior white matter tracts and hence to their deterioration. Because the system develops dynamically, with interplay between gray and white matter, it is difficult to determine which facet is primary and which is a consequence.

Taking into consideration several structural abnormalities observed in the frontal lobe in autism, Courchesne and Pierce (2005) have suggested that the connectivity *within* the frontal lobe may be excessive, disorganized, and inadequately selective, whereas connectivity between frontal cortex and other systems may be poorly synchronized, weakly responsive, and informationally impoverished. The frontal cortex may be functioning abnormally in itself, or it may be abnormal in its interaction with posterior collaborating centers. Abnormal interaction could result from a failure to develop, modify, or prune various connections during the development of the neuropil (Zilbovicius et al., 1995). In brief, the structural and developmental abnormalities in the frontal lobe may contribute to underconnectivity in autism. The prefrontal cortex, an area that has been consistently implicated in the etiology of behavioral disorders, has profuse afferent and efferent axonal connections with multiple neocortical, subcortical, and limbic regions (Fuster, 2001; Mesulam, 1985). Several of these connections are reciprocal and provide the anatomic substrate for the prefrontal lobe to temporally coordinate its functioning with other cortical areas in performing functions like language, problem-solving, and memory. Results of functional MRI studies have consistently reported atypical activation and synchronization of brain areas (especially frontal-posterior) in autism during the performance of higher cognitive functions.

The findings of abnormalities in brain structures in autism suggest that the connectivity between cortical regions could be altered in autism in several ways (Boddaert & Zilbovicius, 2002). Findings of delayed maturation of frontal lobe circuitry in autism (Zilbovicius et al., 1995), decreased functional connections within the cerebral cortex and between the cortex and subcortical regions (Horwitz et al., 1988), and abnormalities of the dentato-thalamo-cortical pathways (Chugani et al., 1997) suggest that connection abnormalities could be the basis of autism.

Another facet of structural abnormality in autism is related to the integrity of the white matter fibers. Widespread white matter volumetric abnormalities (increased volumes in some areas and decreased volumes in other areas) have been found in individuals with autism (Herbert et al., 2003), indicating connectivity disruption. A recent DTI study of autism involving a large sample size and a wide age range (Keller, Kana, & Just, 2007) demonstrated reductions in the structural integrity of white matter, measured by fractional anisotropy (FA), in the corpus callosum area and in frontal lobe areas near the corpus callosum in child and adult participants with autism. FA of water diffusion refers to the directional selectivity of the random motion of water molecules within a tissue (Basser, 1994; Pierpaoli & Basser, 1996). Lower FA values may reflect decreased fiber density, reduced myelination of fiber tracts, or less directionally coherent organization of fibers within a voxel (Basser, 1995; Pierpaoli & Basser, 1996; Beaulieu, 2002), all of which could reflect decreased anatomical connectivity in autism. At least one study (Ben Bashat et al., 2007) found increased FA in two young children with autism spectrum disorder (ASD). However, the age range in that study was 1.8 to 3.3 years, which is around the same time increased brain volume is first seen in ASDs. Our study as well as others (e.g., Barnea-Goraly et al., 2004) used children older than age 8 years, and the results show reduction in FA in ASD.

Note that the white matter abnormalities in autism include not only smaller white matter volumes in some regions but also larger white matter volumes in other regions (Herbert et al., 2002; Courchesne et al., 2001). For example, Carper et al. (2002) found both frontal and parietal increased white matter volumes in children with autism compared to typically developing children.

Based on studies of white matter differences in autism, several researchers have recently proposed disconnection as a key characteristic of autism, such as Belmonte et al. (2004), Courchesne & Pierce (2005), Herbert et al. (2004), and Rippon et al. (2006). This proposal converges with the findings of functional connectivity abnormalities in autism (Just et al., 2004). The findings of morphometric abnormalities, white matter abnormalities, and aberrant activation in complex tasks in autism all suggest that autism is a neural systems disorder that involves the development of abnormal systems connectivity.

Microstructural Abnormalities in Autism and Their Relation to Cortical Underconnectivity

The lower frontal-posterior functional connectivity observed in autism in multiple social and cognitive tasks could possibly result from several underlying microstructural abnormalities.

Earlier we discussed one such possibility: abnormalities related to the structural integrity of white matter. In addition, several early neurodevelopmental processes (such as neuronal migration and axonal pathfinding) could be abnormal. The period of initial cortical plate formation in the human telencephalon is 7 to 10 gestational weeks; neuronal proliferation, 8 to 16 gestational weeks; neuronal migration, 12 to 20 weeks; and development of six-layered cortex, following migration (Volpe, 2001). Neuronal migration abnormalities have been reported in postmortem cases of autism (Bailey et al., 1998). Developmental alterations in axon number, axon pathfinding, synaptogenesis, and subsequent pruning of axons could result in abnormalities in white matter tracts involving selective disruption of both long-range as well as local connections (Geschwind & Levitt, 2007). Thus, the alterations found in functional and structural connectivity in the autistic brain could be the consequence of at least one neurodevelopmental process.

Abnormalities associated with glial cells may also play a role in maldevelopment of brain structure and connections. Specialized glial cells called *oligodendrocytes* support neurons by creating an insulating myelin sheath around some axons, increasing its bandwidth by a factor of 10. If these cells were in some way underfunctioning, they could fail to adequately build up the myelin sheath that enables higher-bandwidth transmission of information through bundles of axons and provides connectivity between cortical centers. Evidence of astroglial and microglial activation and neuroinflammation in gray and white matter (in samples taken from the middle frontal gyrus, anterior cingulate gyrus, and posterior cerebellar hemispheres) have been found in studies of autistic postmortem cases (Vargas et al., 2005). Glial cells are also involved in neural migration, structural formation of the minicolumn, minicolumn function, and apoptosis (Marin-Teva et al., 2004). Defects associated with the organization of minicolumns in autism could be the result of abnormalities in neuronal migration. Migration abnormalities could alter the fundamental vertical organization of the minicolumns, which would lead to fractionated and incompletely or aberrantly formed minicolumn vertical circuitry, as well as an imbalance between excitation and inhibition within and between minicolumns (Courchesne et al., 2005). Minicolumn abnormalities (more numerous and abnormally narrow minicolumns in frontal and temporal cortex) have been reported in autism (Casanova et al., 2002). This would create an abundance of short connective fibers relative to long ones, which may indicate a deficiency in long distance (inter-regional) connectivity.

Yet another possibility is that abnormalities in neurochemistry could lead to abnormal brain development. Studies using magnetic resonance spectroscopy have been helpful in examining the brain neurochemistry in autism. Regionally specific reductions in N-acetylaspartate (NAA; an amino acid present predominantly in neurons and axons [Baslow, 2003] that impacts the neuronal integrity) have been reported in autism. Some of the regions with NAA reduction include cingulate gyrus, temporal gray matter, frontal and parietal white matter, hippocampal-amygdaloid complex, and cerebellum (Friedman et al., 2003; Hisaoka et al., 2001; Levitt et al., 2003; Otsuka et al., 1999). Several researchers have proposed that dysfunction of another amino acid, glutamate, could be of etiological relevance to autism (Carlsson, 1998; Polleux & Lauder, 2004; Rubenstein & Merzenich, 2003). Glutamate plays an important role in neurodevelopmental processes, including neuronal migration, differentiation, axon genesis, and plasticity (Coyle, Leski, & Morrison, 2002). Thus, irregularities in brain neurochemistry could be a potential factor in the abnormal development of connections and, hence, atypical brain functioning in people with autism.

Relevance to Intervention and Training

With converging findings of brain connectivity abnormalities emerging in the field of autism research, an obvious question, especially from parents, families, and educators, is how this new understanding of brain function in autism might lead to a potential remedy or treatment program. The effectiveness of behavioral training programs in modifying brain function has been documented previously in studies of stroke patients using constraint-induced therapy (Taub, Uswatte, & Morris, 2003; Liepert et al., 2000) and in children with reading disability using instructional training (Temple et al., 2003; Meyler et al., 2008). The main target of such an approach in autism would be the improvement of communication among brain areas or improving the strength and integrity of white matter fibers connecting various brain regions. One possible treatment research direction is to develop a training regimen in a task that requires extensive repeated frontal-posterior communication, as many executive tasks do. Functional and structural brain imaging techniques could assess the brain activation, functional connectivity, and white matter connectivity before, during, and after training. One study that provided 100 hours of intensive remedial reading instruction over 6 months to 8- to 10-year-old children who were poor readers produced a reliable increase in the structural integrity of their white matter in a region that had shown lower-than-normal integrity prior to the intervention (Keller & Just, 2009). Specifically, DTI measures showed improvement of the white matter after behavioral remediation treatment. Moreover, the amount of white matter improvement in an individual child was correlated with the amount of improvement in their reading performance, indicating the relevance of the white matter change to the cognitive functioning. These remediation findings in children who were poor readers are a promising harbinger for ameliorating connectivity deficits in autism with analogous therapy programs.

Cognitive and behavior-based intervention programs can attempt to strengthen the connections among relevant brain areas. The use of explicit instructions and selective reinforcements would be a starting point in such programs. For example, one of the key findings in the domain of face processing is that people with autism tend not to look at the eye region or the whole face but focus on isolated features, such as the mouth or ear. Such an isolated or detailed processing style would mean a failure to view the face in an integrated and holistic manner, which typically would be facilitated by the coordinated functioning of the face processing area in the brain and the frontal regions and emotion-related regions. For example, the connections among the fusiform face area (face perception), amygdala (emotion), and inferior frontal gyrus (semantic coding) may play a role in processing face information within a social context. However, in autism, the fragmented processing style is accompanied by weaker functional connectivity among these regions (Koshino et al., 2007), suggesting that in autism, there may be a lack in coordinating different types of information about a face. Intervention programs that encourage integrated, coordinated processing could possibly improve the connectivity. And to the extent that a particular neurobiological substrate of underconnectivity is eventually identified (say, possibly, oligodendrocyte activity), pharmacological agents could be developed to regulate that activity. More generally, deeper scientific understanding of the nature of autism inherently provides new clues for possible therapeutic approaches.

Conclusion

Cortical Underconnectivity Theory provides a compelling framework for explaining the cognitive and behavioral impairments in people with ASDs. The theory explains not only the deficits of people with autism (cognitive, social, and complex language) but also their strengths (visuospatial processing). The theory also provides accounts for many of the phenomena prior theoretical accounts of autism have focused on, such as the complex information processing deficit, executive dysfunction hypothesis, and the theory-of-mind account. The underconnectivity theory encourages the design of training programs for children with autism that focus on targeting and improving the cross-communication between different areas of the brain.

Challenges and Future Directions

- **Developmental studies:** Because autism is a developmental disorder, the connection abnormalities found in autism might either be a disruption of previously connected regions or a failure in the normal development of connections among the regions (Geschwind & Levitt, 2007). Future studies might focus on longitudinal as well as cross-sectional studies examining connectivity across different age groups. Functional MRI and DTI studies at very early ages in autism (DTI studies are quite possible in infancy), as well as at later stages, can trace the developmental trajectory of cortical connectivity in autism in comparison to control groups.
- **Novel measurement techniques:** Functional connectivity in autism has been examined mainly by the use of functional MRI. Because functional connectivity measures the synchronization of brain activation, future studies and some in progress will use techniques such as magnetoencephalography (MEG) and electroencephalography, which both have much higher temporal resolution than fMRI. As of now, there are very few MEG studies in the field of autism. In addition, the measures of functional connectivity can be supplemented by measures of white matter integrity (using DTI) and brain neurochemistry (using magnetic resonance spectroscopy). Furthermore, using these varied approaches in conjunction with each other may provide an enriched characterization of cortical connectivity in autism.

SUGGESTED READINGS

Courchesne, E. & Pierce, K. (2005). Why the frontal cortex in autism might be talking only to itself: local over-connectivity but long-distance disconnection. *Current Opinion in Neurobiology, 15*(2), 225–230.

Herbert, M. R. (2005). Large brains in autism: the challenge of pervasive abnormality. *Neuroscientist, 11*(5), 417–440.

Just, M. A., Cherkassky, V. L., Keller, T. A., Kana, R. K., & Minshew, N. J. (2007). Functional and anatomical cortical underconnectivity in autism: Evidence from an fMRI study of an executive function task and corpus callosum morphometry. *Cerebral Cortex, 17*(4), 951–961.

Just, M. A., Cherkassky, V. L., Keller, T. A., & Minshew, N. J. (2004). Cortical activation and synchronization during sentence comprehension in high-functioning autism: Evidence of underconnectivity. *Brain, 127,* 1811–1821.

Kana, R. K., Keller, T. A., Cherkassky, V. L., Minshew, N. J., & Just, M. A. (2006). Sentence comprehension in autism: Thinking in pictures with decreased functional connectivity. *Brain, 129,* 2484–2493.

REFERENCES

Akshoomoff, N., Pierce, K., & Courchesne, E. (2002). The neurobiological basis of autism from a developmental perspective. *Development and Psychopathology, 14,* 613–634.

Aylward, E. H., Minshew, N. J., Field, K., Sparks, B. F., & Singh, N. (2002). Effects of age on brain volume and head circumference in autism. *Neurology, 59,* 175–183.

Barnea-Goraly, N., Kwon., H., Menon, V., Eliez, S., Lotspeich, L., & Reiss, A. L. (2004). White matter structure in autism: Preliminary evidence from diffusion tensor imaging. *Biological Psychiatry, 55,* 323–326.

Baslow, M. H (2003). N-acetylaspartate in the vertebrate brain: Metabolism and function. *Neurochemical Research, 28,* 941–953.

Basser, P. J. (1995). Inferring microstructural features and the physiological state of tissues from diffusion-weighted images. *NMR in Biomedicine, 8*(7–8), 333–344.

Basser, P. J. (1994). Focal magnetic stimulation of an axon. *IEEE Transactions on Biomedical Engineering, 41*(6), 601–606.

Beaulieu, C. (2002). The basis of anisotropic water diffusion in the nervous system - a technical review. *NMR in Biomedicine, 1,5* (7–8), 435–455.

Belmonte, M. K., Allen, G., Beckel-Mitchener, A., Boulanger, L. M., Carper, R. A., & Webb, S. J. (2004). Autism and Abnormal development of brain connectivity. *Journal of Neuroscience, 24*(42), 9228–9231.

Ben Bashat, D., Kronfeld-Duenias, V., Zachor, D. A., Ekstein, P. M., Hendler, T., Tarrasch, R., et al. (2007). Accelerated maturation of white matter in young children with autism: A high b value DWI study. *NeuroImage, 37(*1), 40–47.

Boddaert, N., & Zilbovicius, M. (2002). Functional brain imaging in childhood autism. *Pediatric Radiology, 32*(1), 1–7.

Brock, J., Brown, C. C., Boucher, J., & Rippon, G. (2002). The temporal binding deficit hypothesis of autism. *Development and Psychopathology, 14*, 209–224.

Carlsson, M. L. (1998). Hypothesis: Is infantile autism a hypoglutamatergic disorder? Relevance of glutamate - serotonin interactions for pharmacotherapy. *Journal of Neural Transmission, 105*, 525–535.

Caron, M. J., Mottron, L., Rainville, C., & Chouinard, S. (2004). Do high functioning persons with autism present superior spatial abilities? *Neuropsychologia, 42*, 467–481.

Casanova, M. F., Buxhoeveden, D. P., Switala, A. E., & Roy, E. (2002). Minicolumnar pathology in autism. *Neurology, 58*, 428–432.

Castelli, F., Frith, C., Happe, F., & Frith, U. (2002). Autism, Asperger syndrome and brain mechanisms for the attribution of mental states to animated shapes. *Brain, 125* (Pt 8), 1839–1849.

Chugani, D. C., Muzik, O., Rothermel, R., Behen, M., Chakraborty, P., Mangner, T et al. (1997). Altered serotonin synthesis in the dentatothalamocortical pathway in autistic boys. *Annals of Neurology, 42*(4), 666–669.

Cohen, I. L. (1994). An artificial neural network analogue of learning in autism. *Biological Psychiatry, 36*, 5–20.

Courchesne, E., Carper, R. A., & Akshoomoff, N. A. (2003). Evidence of brain overgrowth in the first year of life in autism. *Journal of the American Medical Association, 290*, 337–344.

Courchesne, E., Karns, C. M., Davis, H. R., Ziccardi, R., Carper, R. A., Tigue, Z. D, et al. (2001). Unusual brain growth patterns in early life in patients with autistic disorder: an MRI study. *Neurology, 57*, 245–254.

Courchesne, E. & Pierce, K. (2005). Why the frontal cortex in autism might be talking only to itself: local over-connectivity but long-distance disconnection. *Current Opinion in Neurobiology, 15*(2), 225–230.

Coyle, J. T., Leski, M. L., & Morrison, J. H. (2002). The diverse roles of L-glutamic acid in brain signal transduction. In: Davis KL, Charney D, Coyle JT, Nemeroff C, editors. *Neuropsychopharmacology, The fifth generation of progress.* Philadelphia: Lippincott, Williams, and Wilkins, 71–90.

Egaas, B., Courchesne, E., & Saitoh, O. (1995). Reduced size of the corpus callosum in autism. *Archives of Neurology, 52*, 794–801.

Eskes, G., Bryson, S., & McCormick, T. (1990). Comprehension of concrete and abstract words in autistic children. *Journal of Autism and Developmental Disorders, 20*, 61–73.

Friedman, S. D., Shaw, D. W., Artru, A. A., Richards, T. L., Gardner, J., Dawson, G., et al. (2003). Regional brain chemical alterations in young children with autism spectrum disorder. *Neurology, 60*, 100–107.

Frith, U. (1989). *Autism: Explaining the enigma*. Oxford: Blackwell.

Frith U., & Snowling M. (1983). Reading for meaning and reading for sound in autistic and dyslexic children. *British Journal of Developmental Psychology, 1*, 329–342.

Fuster, J. M. (2001). The prefrontal cortex–an update: Time is of the essence. *Neuron, 30*, 319–333.

Geschwind, D. H. & Levitt, P. (2007). Autism spectrum disorders: developmental disconnection syndromes. *Current Opinion in Neurobiology, 17*, 103–111.

Goldstein, G., Minshew, N., & Siegel, D. (1994). Age differences in academic achievement in high-functional autistic individuals. *Journal of Clinical Experimental Neuropsychology, 16*, 671–680.

Grandin, T. (1995). *Thinking in pictures* (pp. 89–92). New York: Vintage Press (Division of Random House).

Gustafsson, L. (1997). Inadequate cortical feature maps: A neural circuit theory of autism. *Biological Psychiatry, 42*, 1138–1147.

Happé F. & Frith U. (2006). The weak coherence account: Detail-focused cognitive style in autism spectrum disorders. *Journal of Autism and Developmental Disorders, 36*, 5–25.

Hardan, A. Y., Jou, R. J., Keshavan, M. S., Varma, R., & Minshew, N. J. (2004). Increased frontal cortical folding in autism: A preliminary MRI study. *Psychiatry Research, 131*, 263–268.

Hardan, A. Y., Minshew, N. J., & Keshavan, M. S. (2000). Corpus callosum size in autism. *Neurology, 55*, 1033–1036.

Herbert, M. R. (2005). Large brains in autism: the challenge of pervasive abnormality. *Neuroscientist, 11*(5), 417–440.

Herbert, M. R., Ziegler, D. A., Deutsch, C. K., O'Brien, L. M., Lange, N., Bakardjiev, A. et al. (2003). Dissociations of cerebral cortex, subcortical and cerebral white matter volumes in autistic boys. *Brain, 126*, 1182–1192.

Herbert, M. R., Ziegler, D. A., Makris, N., Filipek, P. A., Kemper, T. L., Normandin, J. J., et al. (2004). Localization of white matter volume increase in autism and developmental language disorder. *Annals of Neurology, 55*, 530–540.

Hisaoka, S., Harada, M., Nishitani, H., & Mori, K. (2001). Regional magnetic resonance spectroscopy of the brain in autistic individuals. *Neuroradiology, 43*, 496–498.

Horwitz, B., Rumsey, J. M., Grady, C. L., & Rapoport, S.I. (1988). The cerebral metabolic landscape in autism. Intercorrelations of regional glucose utilization. *Archives of Neurology, 45*, 749–755.

Hughes, C., Russell, J., & Robbins, T. W. (1994). Evidence for executive dysfunction in autism. *Neuropsychologia, 32*, 477–492.

Jacobson, R., Le Couteur, A., Howlin, P., & Rutter, M. (1988). Selective subcortical abnormalities in autism. *Psychological Medicine, 18*, 39–48.

Just, M. A., Cherkassky, V. L., Keller, T. A., Kana, R. K., & Minshew, N. J. (2007). Functional and anatomical cortical underconnectivity in autism: Evidence from an fMRI study of an executive function task and corpus callosum morphometry. *Cerebral Cortex, 17*(4), 951–961.

Just, M. A., Cherkassky, V. L., Keller, T. A., & Minshew, N. J. (2004). Cortical activation and synchronization during sentence comprehension in high-functioning autism: Evidence of underconnectivity. *Brain, 127*, 1811–1821.

Kana, R. K., Keller, T. A., Cherkassky, V. L., Minshew, N. J., & Just, M. A. (2006). Sentence comprehension in autism: Thinking in pictures with decreased functional connectivity. *Brain, 129*, 2484–2493.

Kana, R. K., Keller, T. A., Minshew, N. J., & Just, M. A. (2007). Inhibitory control in high-functioning autism: decreased activation and underconnectivity in inhibition networks. *Biological Psychiatry, 62*(3), 198–206.

Kana, R. K., Keller, T. A., Cherkassky, V. L., Minshew, N. J., & Just, M. A. (2008). Atypical frontal-posterior synchronization of Theory of Mind regions in autism during mental state attribution. *Social Neuroscience, 4*(2), 135–152.

Keller, T. A., Kana, R. K., and Just, M. A. (2007). A developmental study of the structural integrity of white matter in autism. *NeuroReport, 18*(1), 23–27.

Koshino, H., Carpenter, P. A., Minshew, N. J., Cherkassky, V. L., Keller, T. A., & Just, M. A. (2005). Functional connectivity in an fMRI working memory task in high-functioning autism. *NeuroImage, 24*, 810–821.

Koshino, H., Kana, R. K., Keller, T. A., Cherkassky, V. L., Minshew, N. J., & Just, M. A. (2008). fMRI Investigation of Working Memory for Faces in Autism: Visual Coding and Underconnectivity with Frontal Areas. *Cerebral Cortex, 18*, 289–300.

Levitt, J. G., Blanton, R. E., Smalley, S., Thompson, P. M., Guthrie, G., & McCracken, J. T. (2003). Cortical sulcal maps in autism. *Cerebral Cortex, 13*, 728–735.

Lewis, J. D., & Elman, J. L. (2008). Growth-related neural reorganization and the autism phenotype: A test of the hypothesis that altered brain growth leads to altered connectivity. *Developmental Science, 11*, 135–155.

Liepert, J., Bauder, H., Miltner, W. H. R., Taub, E., & Weiller, C. (2000). Treatment-induced massive cortical reorganization after stroke in humans. *Stroke, 31*, 1210–1216.

Manes, F., Piven, J., Vrancic, D., Nanclares, V., Plebst, C., & Starkstein, S. E. (1999). An MRI study of the corpus callosum and cerebellum in mentally retarded autistic individuals. *Journal of Neuropsychiatry and Clinical Neuroscience, 11*, 470–474.

Marin–Teva, J. L., Dusart, I., Colin, C., Gervais, A., van Rooijen, N., & Mallat, M. (2004). Microglia promote the death of developing Purkinje cells. *Neuron, 41*, 535–547.

Mason, R. A., Williams, D. L., Kana, R. K., Minshew, N. J., & Just, M. A. (2008). Theory of Mind disruption and the recruitment of the right hemisphere during narrative comprehension in autism. *Neuropsychologia, 46*(1), 269–280.

Mesulam, M. (1985). *Principles of behavioral neurology*. Philadelphia: Davis.

Meyler, A., Keller, T. A., Cherkassky, V. L., Gabrieli, J. D. E., & Just, M. A. (2008). Modifying the brain activation of poor readers during sentence comprehension with extended remedial instruction: A longitudinal study of neuroplasticity. *Neuropsychologia, 46*, 2580–2592.

Minshew, N. J., Goldstein, G., & Siegel, D. J. (1997). Neuropsychologic functioning in autism: Profile of a complex information processing disorder. *Journal of the International Neuropsychological Society, 3*, 303–316.

Mizuno, A., Villalobos, M. E., Davies, M. M., Dahl, B. C., & Müller, R.-A. (2006). Partially enhanced thalamo-cortical functional connectivity in autism. *Brain Research, 1104* (1), 160–174.

Mottron, L. & Burack, J. A. (2001). Enhanced perceptual functioning in the development of autism. In J. A. Burack, T. Charman, N. Yirmiya, & P. R. Zelazo (Eds.), *The development of autism: Perspectives from theory and research* (pp. 131–148). Mahwah, NJ: Lawrence Erlbaum Associates.

Mottron, L., Burack, J., Iarocci Belleville, G. S., & Enns, J. (2003). Locally oriented perception with intact global processing among adolescents with high functioning autism: Evidence from Multiple Paradigms. *Journal of Child Psychology and Psychiatry, 44*, 904–913.

Mottron, L., Dawson, M., Soulieres, I., Huvert, B., & Burack, J. A. (2006). Enhanced perceptual functioning in autism: An update, and eight principles of autistic perception. *Journal of Autism and Developmental Disorders, 36*, 27–43.

Otsuka, H., Harada, M., Mori, K., Hisaoka, S., & Nishitani, H. (1999). Brain metabolites in the hippocampus-amygdala region and cerebellum in autism: An 1H-MR spectroscopy study. *Neuroradiology, 41*, 517–519.

Pennington, B., Rogers, S., Bennetto, L., Griffith, E., Reed, D., & Shyu, V. (1998). Validity test of the executive dysfunction hypothesis of autism. In *Autism as an executive disorder*, ed. J. Russel (pp. 143–178). Oxford: Oxford University Press.

Pierpaoli, C. & Basser, P. J. (1996). Toward a quantitative assessment of diffusion anisotropy. *Magnetic Resonance in Medicine, 36* (6), 893–906.

Piven J., & Arndt S. (1995). The cerebellum and autism. *Neurology, 45*, 398: 402.

Piven, J. Bailey, J., Ranson, B. J., & Arndt. S. (1997). An MRI study of the corpus callosum in autism. *American Journal of Psychiatry, 154*, 1051–1056.

Polleux, F. & Lauder, J. M. (2004). Toward a developmental neurobiology of autism. *Mental Retardation and Developmental Disabilities Research Reviews, 10*, 303–317.

Quigley, M., Cordes, D., Wendt, G., Turski, P., Moritz, C., Haughton, V., & Meyerand, M.E. (2001). Effect of focal and nonfocal cerebral lesions on functional connectivity studies with MR imaging. *American Journal of Neuroradiology, 22*, 294–300.

Ring, H. A., Baron-Cohen, S., Wheelwright, S., Williams, S. C., Brammer, M., Andrew, C., et al. (1999). Cerebral correlates of preserved cognitive skills in autism: a functional MRI study of embedded figures task performance. *Brain, 122*, 1305–1315.

Rippon, G., Brock, J., Brown, C., & Boucher, J. (2006). Disordered connectivity in the autistic brain: challenges for the "new psychophysiology." *International Journal of Psychophysiology, 63*, 164–172.

Rubenstein, J. L. R. & Merzenich, M. M. (2003). Model of autism: Increased ratio of excitation/inhibition in key neural systems. *Genes, Brain, and Behavior, 2*, 255–267.

Schultz, R. T. (2001). The neural basis of autism. In N. J. Smelser & P. B. Baltes (Eds.) *International encyclopedia of the social and behavioral sciences*. New York: Elsevier Science, 983–987.

Sears, L. L., Vest, C., Mohamed, S., Bailey, J., Ranson, B. J., & Piven, J. (1999). An MRI study of the basal ganglia in autism. *Progress in Neuropsychopharmacology and Biological Psychiatry, 23*, 613–624.

Shah A. & Frith U. (1983). An islet of ability in autistic children: A research note. *Journal of Child Psychology and Psychiatry, 24*, 613–620.

Sparks, B. F., Friedman, S. D., Shaw, D. W., Aylward, E. H., Echelard, D., Artru, A. A., et al. (2002). Brain structural abnormalities in young children with autism spectrum disorder. *Neurology, 59*, 184–192.

Taub, E., Uswatte, G., & Morris, D. M. (2003). Improved motor recovery after stroke and massive cortical reorganization following constraint-induced movement therapy. *Physical Medicine and Rehabilitation Clinics of North America, 14*, S77–S91.

Temple, E., Deutsch, G. K., Poldrack, R. A., Miller, S. L., Tallal, P., Merzenich, M. M., et al. (2003). Neural deficits in children with dyslexia ameliorated by behavioral remediation: evidence from functional MRI. *Proceedings of the National Academy of Sciences of the United States of America, 100*(5), 2860–2865.

Tononi, G., Edelman, G. M., & Sporns, O. (1998). Complexity and coherency: integrating information in the brain. *Trends in Cognitive Sciences, 2*, 474–484.

Vargas, D. L., Nascimbene, C., Krishnan, C., Zimmerman, A. W., & Pardo, C. A. (2005). Neuroglial activation and neuroinflammation in the brain of patients with autism. *Annals of Neurology, 57*, 67–81.

Villalobos, M. E., Mizuno, A., Dahl, B. C., Kemmotsu, N., & Muller, R. A. (2005). Reduced functional connectivity between V1 and inferior frontal cortex associated with visuomotor performance in autism. *NeuroImage, 25*, 916–925.

Volpe, J. J. (2001). *Neurology of the newborn.* Philadelphia: WB Saunders.

Welchew, D. E., Ashwin, C., Berkouk, K., Salvador, R., Suckling, J., Baron-Cohen, S., et al. (2005). Functional disconnectivity of the medial temporal lobe in Asperger's syndrome. *Biological Psychiatry, 57*, 991–998.

Zilbovicius, M., Garreau, B., Samson, Y., Remy, P., Barthelemy, C., & Syrota, A. (1995). Delayed maturation of the frontal cortex in childhood autism. *American Journal of Psychiatry, 152*, 248–252.

55

Simon Baron-Cohen, Bonnie Auyeung, Emma Ashwin, Rebecca Knickmeyer, Michael Lombardo, Bhismadev Chakrabarti

The Extreme Male Brain Theory of Autism: The Role of Fetal Androgens

Points of Interest

- There are sex differences in neuroanatomy, neural function, cognition, and behavior in the general population.
- People with ASD show an extreme of the typical male profile in terms of empathy and systemizing.
- Whether such hyper-masculinization is evident at the level of neuroanatomy and neural function in ASD remains to be tested.
- Fetal testosterone (fT) is known from animal research to play an organizing role in brain development.
- fT associated with individual differences in eye contact, vocabulary development, empathy, systemizing, attention to detail, and autistic traits in typically developing children.
- It remains to be tested whether fT is elevated in children who go on to develop an ASD.

Autism and Asperger Syndrome (AS) are autism spectrum disorders (ASDs). The diagnosis rests on the presence of difficulties in reciprocal social interaction and communication, along with strongly repetitive behavior and unusually narrow interests (A.P.A., 1994). The prevalence of ASD is currently estimated to be 1% (Scott et al., 2002). Autism spectrum disorder is biased toward males (Fombonne, 2005) with a 4:1 (male:female) ratio for classic autism (Chakrabarti & Fombonne, 2001) and 8:1 for AS (Scott et al., 2002). Classic autism and AS differ in terms of the presence of additional learning difficulties and language delay (in classic autism only). Autism spectrum disorders are neurobiological and genetic (Stodgell et al., 2001), but the specific factors responsible for the higher male incidence in ASDs remain unclear. One possible factor is that ASDs may be an extreme of the male brain (Baron-Cohen, 2002).

The Extreme Male Brain: Psychology

The extreme male brain (EMB) theory of autism is an extension of the empathizing-systemizing (E-S) theory of typical sex differences (Baron-Cohen, 2003). The latter theory proposes that females, on average, have a stronger drive to *empathize* (to identify another person's thoughts and feelings and to respond to these with an appropriate emotion), whereas males, on average, have a stronger drive to *systemize* (to analyze or construct rule-based systems) (Baron-Cohen, 2003). Evidence relevant to this is as follows: Individuals with ASD score higher on the systemizing quotient (SQ), an instrument on which typical males score higher than typical females (Baron-Cohen et al., 2003; Auyeung et al., 2006; Wheelwright et al., 2006). Individuals with ASDs have intact or superior functioning on tests of intuitive physics (Baron-Cohen et al., 2001; Lawson et al., 2004), a domain that shows a sex difference in favor of males (Lawson et al., 2004). Individuals with ASDs are faster and more accurate than controls on the Embedded Figures Task (EFT), a task on which typical males perform better than typical females (Shah & Frith, 1983; Jolliffe & Baron-Cohen, 1997). The EFT requires good attention to detail, a prerequisite for systemizing. All of these are relevant to systemizing.

On the empathizing quotient (EQ) (Baron-Cohen & Wheelwright, 2004), individuals with ASDs score lower than control groups, whereas typical females score higher than typical males (Baron-Cohen & Wheelwright, 2004). Individuals with ASDs score lower than typical males on the "Reading the Mind in the Eyes" task (Baron-Cohen et al., 1997), the Social Stories Questionnaire (Lawson et al., 2004), on tests of recognizing complex emotions from videos of facial expressions or audios of vocalizations (Golan et al., 2006), and on the Friendship and Relationship Questionnaire (which tests the importance of emotional intimacy and sharing in relationships)

(Baron-Cohen & Wheelwright, 2003). All of these are tests of empathy. On the Childhood Autism Spectrum Test (CAST) (Scott et al., 2002; Scott et al., 2002), boys score higher than girls (Williams et al., 2008), and children with ASDs score higher than controls (Williams et al., 2005). On the autism spectrum quotient (AQ) (Baron-Cohen et al., 2001a), individuals with ASDs score higher than those without a diagnosis (Baron-Cohen et al., 2001). Among controls, males score higher than females (Baron-Cohen et al., 2001; Baron-Cohen et al., 2006; Auyeung et al., 2008), a finding that has been reported cross-culturally (Wakabayashi et al., 2004; Wakabayashi et al., 2006; Wakabayashi et al., 2007; Hoekstra et al., 2008). Similar results have been found using the Social Responsiveness Scale (SRS), finding that individuals with an ASD diagnosis score higher than typical males, who in turn score higher than typical females (Constantino & Todd, 2005). All of these are measures of autistic traits.

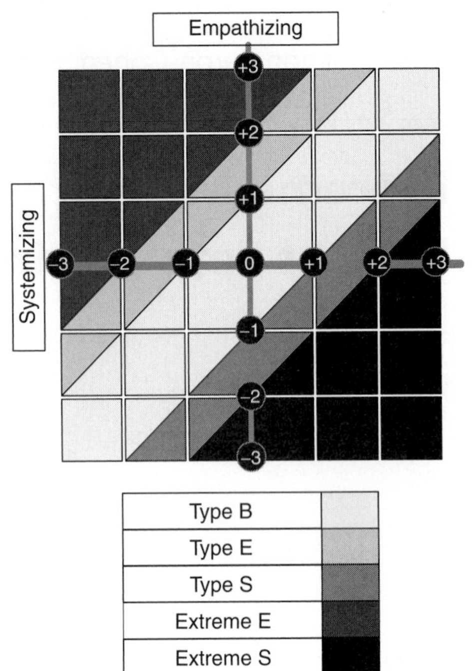

Figure 55–1. The Empathizing-Systemizing Model of Typical Sex Differences. The main brain types are illustrated on axes of Empathising (E) and Systemising (S) dimensions (numbers represent standard deviations from the mean). Balanced brain (Type B); female brain (Type E), male brain (Type S); the extreme Types E and S lie at the outer borders. According to the 'extreme male brain' theory of autism, people with ASD will generally fall in the darkest region. Modified with permission from Baron-Cohen, S. (2002). The extreme male brain theory of autism. *Trends in Cognitive Science, 6*, 248–254.

The Extreme Male Brain: Biology

Characteristics of neurodevelopment in autism may also represent an exaggeration of typical sex differences in brain development (Baron-Cohen et al., 2005). For example, there is larger overall brain volume in males during childhood (Giedd et al., 1996), and in ASDs, this may be even more extreme (Courchesne et al., 2004). There is greater growth of the amygdala in males during childhood (Merke et al., 2003), and in ASDs, this may be even more extreme (Sparks et al., 2002). The posterior section of the corpus callosum is thicker in females than males (Jancke et al., 1997) and in ASDs is even thinner than is typical (Herbert et al., 2004). These are all volumetric measures of the brain. Using fMRI, typical females show increased activity in the extrastriate cortex during the EFT and increased activity bilaterally in the inferior frontal cortex during the "Reading the Mind in the Eyes" Test compared to typical males (Baron-Cohen et al., 2006). People with ASDs show even less activity in each of these regions during these tasks (Baron-Cohen et al., 1999; Ring et al., 1999). Parents of children with ASDs also show hyper-masculinization of brain activity (Baron-Cohen et al., 2006), suggesting that this may be part of the broader autism phenotype. These are all functional neuroimaging measures of the brain. It remains important to identify the biological mechanisms that cause such sexual dimorphism. One possible biological mechanism is the effect of fetal testosterone (fT) (Geschwind & Galaburda, 1985), reviewed in the next section.

The Role of Fetal Testosterone in Brain Development

Fetal gonadal hormones (including the androgens [e.g., testosterone, dihydrotestosterone], estrogens [e.g., estradiol, estrone, estriol], and progestins [e.g., progesterone]) lead to the differentiation of the male and female phenotype (Fuchs & Klopper, 1983; Tulchinsky & Little, 1994; Kimura, 1999; Hines, 2004). If androgens and the androgen receptors are present, the male genital phenotype will develop. If not (as seen in Complete Androgen Insensitivity Syndrome), the female genital phenotype will develop (Jost, 1961; Jost, 1970, 1972; George et al., 1992). Fetal gonadal hormones are essential for sexual differentiation of both the body and the brain (Goy, 1980; Fitch & Denenberg, 1998). In what follows, we summarize some key points in this process. Three surges in testosterone levels are known to occur. The first surge is between weeks 8 and 24 of gestation (Collaer & Hines, 1995; Baron-Cohen et al., 2004; Hines, 2004). Most of the prenatal androgen effects occur between 7 and 12 weeks of gestation (Rommerts, 2001). Then, after birth, a second peak in circulating testosterone occurs in human male infants. Usually the levels remain in the pubertal range for a few months and then drop to the barely detectable levels observed in childhood by age 4 to 6 months (Smail et al., 1981). Finally, the third surge is associated with puberty. Individuals vary both in the levels of hormones to which they are exposed and in their sensitivity to those hormones. Variations in androgen responsivity (caused by mutations in the human androgen receptor gene) can result in complete insensitivity to androgens (and thus female differentiation) or to infertility and minor undervirilization (Casella et al., 2001). The timing of hormonal effects influences whether effects are organizational or activational (Goy, 1980). Organizational effects produce *permanent* changes in the brain (Phoenix et al., 1959) and are most likely to occur during early development when most neural structures are becoming established. The discovery of such organizational effects of fT came from animal research (mostly rodents), and to date, these have only looked at neuroanatomy or limited aspects of behavior (spatial ability and mating). Activational effects occur later and are associated with concurrent changes in circulating hormone levels (Kimura & Hampson, 1994; Cooke et al., 1999).

Fetal Androgens Affect Brain and Behavior: Evidence from Rare Medical Conditions

Although animal research provides strong evidence for the effect of hormones in development, the direct manipulation of hormones in human fetuses is unethical. Instead, researchers have studied people, in whom for medical reasons the sex hormones are higher or lower than expected for a person's sex (Money & Ehrhardt, 1972). Two examples are *Congenital Adrenal Hyperplasia (CAH)* and *Complete Androgen Insensitivity Syndrome (CAIS)*. Congenital Adrenal Hyperplasia is a condition in which an enzymatic defect (usually caused by mutations in the gene coding for 21-hydroxylase) results in high levels of adrenal androgens, beginning very early in gestation. It has an incidence of 1 in 10,000 to 1 in 15,000 live births (Grumbach et al., 2003). Females with CAH differ from unaffected females (their siblings or age- and sex-matched controls) in spatial orienting, visualization, and targeting (Resnick et al., 1986; Hampson et al., 1998; Hines et al., 2003b). Females with CAH are also more likely than controls to be left-handed (Nass et al., 1987), although the difference is small and inconsistent. Females with CAH are more interested in male-typical activities and less interested in female-typical activities (Ehrhardt & Baker, 1974; Berenbaum & Hines, 1992; Berenbaum & Snyder, 1995; Berenbaum, 1999; Hines et al., 2004). Girls with CAH score lower than sex-matched controls on measures assessing empathy, intimacy, and the need for close social relationships (Mathews et al., 2009; Helleday et al., 1993; Resnick, 1982; Kuhnle & Bullinger, 1997). Individuals with CAH showed higher levels of language and learning difficulties than unaffected family members (Resnick et al., 1986). All these changes can be interpreted as masculinization.

Complete Androgen Insensitivity Syndrome is a second example of a rare medical condition affecting prenatal endocrine responses. It occurs when there is a complete deficiency of working androgen receptors. It is an X-linked recessive disorder and hence occurs more often in genetic males. Prevalence is between 1 in 20,000 and 1 in 60,000 live male births. At birth, genetic male infants with CAIS are phenotypically female, despite an XY complement, and are usually raised as girls. At puberty, breasts develop under the influence of estrogen derived from testicular androgens. Diagnosis usually takes place when menarche fails to occur (Nordenstrom et al., 2002; Grumbach et al., 2003). In studies, gender identity has not differed between genetic males with CAIS and control women (Quadagno et al., 1977; Hines et al., 2003a). Individuals with CAIS perform in a female-typical fashion on tests of visuo-spatial ability (Money et al., 1984).

These findings suggest that two X chromosomes or functioning ovaries are not required for feminine-typical psychological development in humans and highlight the role of androgen receptors in influencing masculine-typical psychological development. However, existing studies have not examined all sexually dimorphic aspects of neurobiology and cognition in these populations. Therefore, one cannot rule out an effect of X-chromosome genes or ovarian hormones on some aspects of sex-typical neurodevelopment.

Fetal Androgens Affect Brain and Behavior: Evidence from Amniotic Fluid Testosterone

Another approach to testing if fetal androgens affect brain and behavior is to measure fT in amniotic fluid obtained during routine diagnostic amniocentesis. An advantage of this approach is its timing. It is typically performed during the second trimester of pregnancy (usually 14–20 weeks of gestation) that coincides with the serum testosterone peak period in male fetuses. Several studies have documented a large sex difference in amniotic androgen levels (Judd et al., 1976; Dawood, 1977; Robinson et al., 1977; Nagami et al., 1979; Finegan et al., 1989). The origin of androgens in amniotic fluid is the fetus itself. Hormones enter the amniotic fluid via diffusion through the fetal skin in early pregnancy and via fetal urine in later pregnancy (Judd et al., 1976; Schindler, 1982). Testosterone obtained in amniotic fluid is thought to be a good reflection of the levels in the fetus (van de Beek et al., 2004) and represents an alternative to direct assay of fetal serum that would be unnecessarily invasive. In the Cambridge Fetal Androgen Project, children whose mothers had amniocentesis during pregnancy (but who were otherwise typically developing children) were followed-up after birth at ages 12, 18, 24, 48, and 96 months (Baron-Cohen et al., 2004). Evidence that amniotic testosterone affects cognitive development includes the following. Fetal testosterone is inversely associated with eye contact in males at age 12 months (Lutchmaya et al., 2002). Fetal testosterone is inversely associated with size of vocabulary development at ages 18 and 24 months (Lutchmaya et al., 2002). Fetal testosterone is inversely associated with quality of social relationships, and positively associated with narrow interests, at age 48 months (Knickmeyer et al., 2005). Fetal testosterone is inversely associated with empathy at ages 48 and 96 months (Chapman et al., 2006; Knickmeyer et al., 2006). Fetal testosterone is positively associated with "systemizing" at age 96 months (Auyeung et al., 2006). Fetal testosterone is positively associated with performance on the EFT, as a measure of attention to detail, at age 96 months (Auyeung et al., submitted). The effect sizes in these studies range from 0.2 to 0.4. Because all of these domains of behavior (eye contact, language development, quality of social relationships, narrow interests, empathy, systemizing, and embedded figures/attention to detail) show sexual dimorphism and may be hyper-masculinized in ASDs, it raises the question as to whether fetal testosterone plays a role in the development of autism. In the final section, we review evidence that androgens—especially fetal testosterone—may play a role in autism or autistic traits.

The Role of Sex Steroid Hormones in Autism Spectrum Disorders or Autistic Traits

Evidence that supports a role for hormones in the development of ASDs is preliminary and includes the following: Androgen-related medical conditions such as polycystic ovary syndrome (PCOS), ovarian growths, and hirsutism occur with elevated rates in women with AS and in mothers of children with autism (Ingudomnukul et al., 2007). Girls with CAH have a higher AQ score than their unaffected sisters (Knickmeyer et al., 2006c). Children with AS and children with classic autism have lower 2D:4D ratios than typical developing children (Manning et al., 2001; Milne et al., 2006). The ratio of the second digit to the fourth digit (2D:4D ratio) is lower in men than in women. The 2D:4D ratio is fixed by week 14 of fetal life (Garn et al., 1975) and is influenced by testosterone (Manning et al., 2002). This suggests children with ASD have been exposed to higher amounts of androgens. A subset of male adolescents with autism show hyper-androgeny, or elevated levels of androgens, and precocious puberty (Tordjman et al., 1997). Delayed menarche has also been found in females with AS (Knickmeyer et al., 2006; Ingudomnukul et al., 2007). Puberty timing reflects hormonal programming of the hypothalamic-pituitary-gonadal axis during gestation (Grumbach & Shaw, 1998).

Left-handedness and ambidexterity are more common in typical males (Peters, 1991) and individuals with autism (Gillberg, 1983). Body asymmetries are related to prenatal sex hormones and breast or testis size on the left versus right sides of the body are related to cognition (Kimura, 1999). Fetal testosterone is implicated in left-handedness and asymmetric lateralization (Fein et al., 1985; Satz et al., 1985; Soper et al., 1986; McManus et al., 1992). The typical male brain is heavier than the female brain, a difference that partly results from fT exposure (Hines, 2004). Individuals with autism have even heavier brains than typical males (Hardan et al., 2001). Amniotic fT levels are positively associated with higher scores (indicating greater number of autistic traits) on the CAST and on the child autism spectrum quotient (AQ-C) (Auyeung et al., 2008). These findings are consistent with the fetal androgen theory of autism, although the ultimate test of this theory will require testing between fetal testosterone and clinically diagnosed ASDs. The latter will require much larger samples than have previously been tested.

It is important in a review chapter such as this to summarize criticisms of the fetal androgen theory of ASDs. First, if autism is an extreme of the typical male behavioral profile, why do people with ASD not show high levels of aggression or a strong interest in competitive sports? We suspect this criticism reflects a misunderstanding of the different roles that fetal as opposed to current (circulating) testosterone play. The latter may well affect aggression and competitiveness, but fetal androgens may selectively affect very different aspects of cognition such as attention to detail and empathy. This remains to be tested. Second, given that testosterone interacts with multiple systems in the body, why single it out for a special role? We acknowledge that if fT plays a role in ASDs, it is likely to do this in complex ways, as testosterone modulates neurotransmitters (such as GABA) as well as peptide hormones (such as oxytocin), to name just two examples. Understanding such relationships will require testing of multiple systems within the same experiment. Third, given that amniotic testosterone is currently only studied in humans via amniocentesis and only 6% of pregnant women undergo amniocentesis, does this not lead to potentially biased samples? We acknowledge this bias but would note that currently this is the only ethical way to study fT because amniocentesis itself carries a risk of inducing miscarriage (in 2% of cases) and so cannot be justified purely for research on a randomly selected, and therefore representative, sample of pregnant women. The main risk of bias comes from higher maternal age because this is one reason why women are referred for an amniocentesis (being older than 35 years old). For this reason, maternal age is entered as a variable in the regression analysis. All fT effects that have been found remain significant after removing any variance because of maternal age.

A further criticism is that if sex differences in the population are only found when one compares equal numbers of males and females, and if studies of ASDs tend to be biased toward males, is the extreme male brain theory really just a reflection that ASDs affect more males than females? This is a valid concern, but it is interesting that where it is possible to compare equal numbers of males and females with ASDs, typical sex differences are absent, which argues against any risk of circularity. Also, when fT effects are found on behavior, these are seen *within* sex, not just when the sexes are combined. This suggests these are hormone effects rather than a redescription of sex differences. Finally, Skuse and others have pointed out that sex-linked neural and behavioral phenotypes could emerge not just because of hormone effects but genetic effects. We agree that fT is only one of many mechanisms that are likely candidates for giving rise to such sex differences, and indeed our recent candidate gene study identified 10 genes involved in the sex steroid hormone pathway that were nominally associated with either autistic traits, empathy, or an ASD (Chakrabarti et al., 2009).

Conclusions

The higher incidence of autism in male individuals might provide important clues to the etiology of the condition, which has been described as an "extreme of the male brain" (Baron-Cohen, 2002). The studies reviewed here suggest that prenatal testosterone could be involved in the sex differences in key areas of behavior in the general population (social development, language development, empathy, systemizing, and attention to detail) and to the male vulnerability to autism. These studies suggest that variations in fetal testosterone are related to individual differences in cognition and behavior in typically developing children, but caution needs to be taken when extrapolating these results to individuals with autism. Our ongoing collaboration with the biobank in Denmark that has thousands of amniotic samples will enable a test of the fetal testosterone theory in clinically diagnosed cases of ASD.

Challenges and Future Directions

- Testing the fetal testosterone theory in relation to diagnosed ASD will require tens of thousands of amniotic samples because only 1 in 100 of these are expected to go on to develop an ASD.
- It is an assumption that amniotic testosterone reflects testosterone levels in the brain, but this remains untested.
- Ethically, if it were established that in ASD there are elevated fetal testosterone levels, this does not mean a treatment implication is to block fT, as fT is likely to be involved in many systems, not just the development of autistic traits.

SUGGESTED READINGS

Baron-Cohen, S. (2002). The extreme male brain theory of autism. *Trends in Cognitive Science, 6*, 248–254.

Baron-Cohen, S., Lutchmaya, S., & Knickmeyer, R. (2004). Prenatal testosterone in mind: Amniotic fluid studies. Cambridge, MA: MIT/Bradford Books.

Baron-Cohen, S., Knickmeyer, R., & Belmonte M. K. (2005). Sex differences in the brain: Implications for explaining autism. *Science, 310*, 819–823.

ACKNOWLEDGMENTS

SBC was supported by grants from the Nancy Lurie Marks Family Foundation and the MRC UK during the period of this work. We are grateful to Svetlana Lutchmaya, Bhismadev Chakrabarti, and Mike Lombardo for valuable discussions.

REFERENCES

A.P.A. (1994). DSM-IV Diagnostic and Statistical Manual of Mental Disorders, 4th Edition. Washington DC: American Psychiatric Association.

Auyeung, B., Baron-Cohen, S., Chapman, E., Knickmeyer, R., Taylor, K., & Hackett, G. (2006). Fetal testosterone and the Child Systemizing Quotient (SQ-C). *European Journal of Endrocrinology, 155*, 123–130.

Auyeung, B., Baron-Cohen, S., Chapman, E., Knickmeyer, R., Taylor, K., & Hackett, G. (2008). Fetal testosterone and autistic traits. *British Journal of Psychology*. online.

Auyeung, B., Baron-Cohen, S., Wheelwright, S., Samarawickrema, N., & Atkinson, M. (2009). The Children's Empathy Quotient (EQ-C) and Systemizing Quotient (SQ-C): Sex differences in typical development and of autism spectrum conditions. *Journal of Autism and Developmental Disorders, 39*, 1509–1521.

Auyeung, B., Baron-Cohen, S., Ashwin, E., Knickmeyer, R., Taylor, K., Hackett, G., et al. (2009). Fetal testosterone predicts sexually differentiated childhood behavior in girls and in boys. *Psychological Science, 20*, 144–148.

Baron-Cohen, S. (2002). The extreme male brain theory of autism. *Trends in Cognitive Science, 6*, 248–254.

Baron-Cohen, S. (2003). The Essential Difference: Men, Women and the Extreme Male Brain. London: Penguin.

Baron-Cohen, S. & Wheelwright, S. (2003). The Friendship Questionnaire (FQ): An investigation of adults with Asperger Syndrome or High Functioning Autism, and normal sex differences. *Journal of Autism and Developmental Disorders, 33*, 509–517.

Baron-Cohen, S. & Wheelwright, S. (2004). The Empathy Quotient (EQ). An investigation of adults with Asperger Syndrome or High Functioning Autism, and normal sex differences. *Journal of Autism and Developmental Disorders, 34*, 163–175.

Baron-Cohen, S., Lutchmaya, S., & Knickmeyer, R. (2004). Prenatal testosterone in mind: Amniotic fluid studies. Cambridge, MA: MIT/Bradford Books.

Baron-Cohen, S., Knickmeyer, R., & Belmonte, M. K. (2005). Sex differences in the brain: Implications for explaining autism. *Science, 310*, 819–823.

Baron-Cohen, S., Jolliffe, T., Mortimore, C., & Robertson, M. (1997). Another advanced test of theory of mind: Evidence from very high functioning adults with autism or Asperger Syndrome. *Journal of Child Psychology and Psychiatry, 38*, 813–822.

Baron-Cohen, S., Hoekstra, R. A., Knickmeyer, R., & Wheelwright, S. (2006). The Autism-Spectrum Quotient (AQ)-Adolescent version. *Journal of Autism and Developmental Disorders, 36*, 343–350.

Baron-Cohen, S., Ring, H., Wheelwright, S., Bullmore, E., Brammer, M., Simmons, A., & Williams, S. (1999). Social intelligence in the normal and autistic brain: An fMRI study. *European Journal of Neuroscience, 11*, 1891–1898.

Baron-Cohen, S., Wheelwright, S., Skinner, R., Martin, J., & Clubley, E. (2001). The Autism Spectrum Quotient (AQ): Evidence from Asperger Syndrome/High Functioning Autism, Males and Females, Scientists and Mathematicians. *Journal of Autism and Developmental Disorders, 31*, 5–17.

Baron-Cohen, S., Wheelwright, S., Scahill, V., Lawson, J., & Spong, A. (2001). Are intuitive physics and intuitive psychology independent? *Journal of Developmental and Learning Disorders, 5*, 47–78.

Baron-Cohen, S., Richler, J., Bisarya, D., Gurunathan, N., & Wheelwright, S. (2003). The Systemising Quotient (SQ): An investigation of adults with Asperger Syndrome or High Functioning Autism and normal sex differences. *Philosophical Transactions of the Royal Society, 358*, 361–374.

Baron-Cohen, S., Ring, H., Chitnis, X., Wheelwright, S., Gregory, L., et al. (2006). fMRI of parents of children with Asperger Syndrome: A pilot study. *Journal of Brain Cognition, 61*, 122–130.

Berenbaum, S. & Hines, M. (1992). Early androgens are related to childhood sex-typed toy preferences. *Psychological Medicine, 3*, 203–206.

Berenbaum, S. A. (1999). Effects of early androgens on sex-typed activities and interests in adolescents with congenital adrenal hyperplasia. *Hormones and Behavior, 35*(1), 102–110.

Berenbaum, S. A. & Snyder, E. (1995). Early hormonal influences on childhood sex-typed activity and playmate preferences: Implications for the development of sexual orientation. *Developmental Psychology, 31*, 31–42.

Casella, R., Maduro, M. R., Lipshultz, L. I., & Lamb, D. J. (2001). Significance of the polyglutamine tract polymorphism in the androgen receptor. *Urology, 58*, 651–656.

Chakrabarti, S. & Fombonne, E. (2001). Pervasive Developmental Disorders in pre-school children. *Journal of the American Medical Association, 285*, 3093–3099.

Chapman, E., Baron-Cohen, S., Auyeung, B., Knickmeyer, R., Taylor, K., & Hackett, G. (2006). Fetal testosterone and empathy: Evidence from the Empathy Quotient (EQ) and the "Reading the Mind in the Eyes" Test. *Social Neuroscience, 1*, 135–148.

Clark, M. M. & Galef, B. G. (1998). Effects of intraurine positioin on the behaviour and genital morphology of litter-bearing rodents. *Developmental Neurology, 14*, 197–211.

Collaer, M. & Hines, M. (1995). Human behavioural sex differences: A role for gonadal hormones during early development? *Psychological Bulletin, 118*, 55–107.

Constantino, J. N. & Todd, R. D. (2005). Intergenerational transmission of subthreshold autistic traits in the general population. *Biological Psychiatry, 57*(6), 655–660.

Cooke, B. M., Tabibnia, G., & Breedlove, S. M. (1999). A brain sexual dimorphism controlled by adult circulating androgens. *Proceedings of the National Academy of Sciences of the United States of America, 96*(13), 7538–7540.

Courchesne, E., Redcay, E., & Kennedy, D. P. (2004). The autistic brain: Birth through adulthood. *Current Opinion in Neurology, 17*(4), 489–496.

Dawood, M. Y. (1977). Hormones in amniotic fluid. *American Journal of Obstetrics and Gynecology, 128*, 576–583.

Ehrhardt, A. A. & Bakerm, S. W. (1974). Fetal androgens, human central nervous system differentiation, and behavior sex differences. In R. C. Freidman, R. R. Richart, R. L. Van de Wiele (Eds.), *Sex differences in behavior* (pp. 33–51). New York: Wiley.

Fein, D., Waterhouse, L., Lucci, D., Pennington, B., & Humes, M. (1985). Handedness and cognitve functions in pervasive developmental disorders. *Journal of Autism and Developmental Disorders, 15*, 323–333.

Finegan, J. A., Bartleman, B., & Wong, P. Y. (1989). A window for the study of prenatal sex hormone influences on postnatal development. *Journal of Genetic Psychology, 150*(1), 101–112.

Fitch, R. H. & Denenberg, V. (1998). A role for ovarian hormones in sexual differentiation of the brain. *Behavioral and Brain Sciences, 21*, 311–352.

Fombonne, E. (2005). The changing epidemiology of autism. *Journal of Applied Research in Intellectual Disabilities: JARID, 18*, 281–294.

Fuchs, F. & Klopper, A. (1983). *Endocrinology of Pregnancy*. Philadelphia: Harper & Row.

Garn, S. M., Burdi, A. R., Babler, W. J., & Stinson, S. (1975). Early prenatal attainment of adult metacarpal-phalangeal rankings and proportions. *American Journal of Physical Anthropology, 43*(3), 327–332.

George, M., Costa, D., Kouris, K., Ring, H., & Ell, P. (1992). Cerebral blood flow abnormalities in adults with infantile autism. *Journal of Nervous and Mental Diseases, 180*, 413–417.

Geschwind, N. & Galaburda, A. M. (1985). Cerebral lateralization: Biological mechanisms, associations and pathology. III. A hypothesis and a program for research. *Archives of Neurology, 42*, 634–654.

Giedd, J. N., Snell, J. W., Lange, N., Rajapakse, J. C., Casey, B. J., Kozuch, P. L., et al. (1996). Quantitative magnetic resonance imaging of human brain development: ages 4-18. *Cerebral Cortex, 6*, 551–560.

Gillberg, C. (1983). Autistic children's hand preferences: Results from an epidemiological study of infantile autism. *Psychiatry Research, 10*(1), 21–30.

Golan, O., Baron-Cohen, S., & Hill, J. (2006). The Cambridge Mindreading (CAM) Face-Voice Battery: Testing complex emotion recognition in adults with and without Asperger syndrome. *Journal of Autism and Developmental Disorders, 36*, 169–183.

Goy, R. W. (1980). *Sexual Differentiation of the Brain*. Cambridge, MA: The MIT Press.

Grimshaw, G., Sitarenios, G., & Finegan, J. (1995). Mental rotation at 7 years: Relations with prenatal testosterone levels and spatial play experiences. *Brain and Cognition, 29*, 85–100.

Grumbach, M. M. & Shaw, E. B. (1998). Further studies on the treatment of congenital adrenal hyperplasia with cortisone: IV. Effect of cortisone and compound B in infants with disturbed electrolyte metabolism, by John F. Crigler Jr, MD, Samuel H. Silverman, MD, and Lawson Wilkins, MD, Pediatrics, 1952;10:397–413. *Pediatrics, 102*, 215–221.

Grumbach, M. M., Hughes, I. A., & Conte, F. A. (2003). Disorders of sex differentiation. In P. R. Larsen, H. M. Kronenburg, S. Melmed, K. S. Polansky (Eds.), *Williams Textbook of Endocrinology*. Philadelphia: Saunders.

Hampson, E., Rovet, J. F., & Altmann, D. (1998). Spatial reasoning in children with congenital adrenal hyperplasia due to 21-hydroxylase deficiency. *Developmental Neuropsychology, 14*, 299–320.

Hardan, A. Y., Minshew, N. J., Harenski, K., & Keshavan, M. S. (2001). Posterior Fossa Magnetic Resonance Imaging in Autism. *Journal of the American Academy of Child and Adolescent Psychiatry, 40*(6), 666–672.

Helleday, J., Edman, G., Ritzen, E. M., & Siwers, B. (1993). Personality characteristics and platelet MAO activity in women with congenital adrenal hyperplasia (CAH). *Psychoneuroendocrinology, 18*, 343–354.

Herbert, M. R., Ziegler, D. A., Makris, N., Filipek, P. A., Kemper, T. L., Normandin, J. J. et al. (2004). Localization of white matter volume increase in autism and developmental language disorder. *Annals of Neurology, 55*(4), 530–540.

Hines, M. (2004). *Brain Gender*. Oxford & New York: Oxford University Press.

Hines, M., Ahmed, S. F., & Hughes, I. A. (2003a). Psychological outcomes and gender-related development in complete androgen insensitivity syndrome. *Archives of Sexual Behavior, 32*, 93–101.

Hines, M., Brook, C., & Conway, G. S. (2004). Androgen and psychosexual development: Core gender identity, sexual orientation and recalled childhood gender role behavior in women and men with congenital adrenal hyperplasia (CAH). *Journal of Sex Research, 41*(1), 75–81.

Hines, M., Fane, B. A., Pasterski, V. L., Mathews, G. A., Conway, G. S., Brook, C. (2003b). Spatial abilities following prenatal androgen abnormality: Targeting and mental rotations performance in individuals with congenital adrenal hyperplasia. *Psychoneuroendocrinology, 28*, 1010–1026.

Hoekstra, R. A., Bartels, M., Cath, D. C., & Boomsma, D. I. (2008). Factor Structure, Reliability and Criterion Validity of the Autism-Spectrum Quotient (AQ): A Study in Dutch Population and Patient Groups. *Journal of Autism and Developmental Disorders*.

Ingudomnukul, E., Baron-Cohen, S., Knickmeyer, R., & Wheelwright, S. (2007). Elevated rates of testosterone-related disorders in a sample of women with autism spectrum conditions. *Hormones and Behavior, 51*, 597–604.

Jancke, L., Staiger, J. F., Schlaug, G., Huang, Y., & Steinmetz, H. (1997). The relationship between corpus callosum size and forebrain volume. *Cerebral Cortex, 7*(1), 48–56.

Jolliffe, T. & Baron-Cohen, S. (1997). Are people with autism or Asperger's Syndrome faster than normal on the Embedded Figures Task? *Journal of Child Psychology and Psychiatry, and Allied Disciplines, 38*, 527–534.

Jost, A. (1961). The role of fetal hormones in prenatal development. *Harvey Lectures, 55*, 201–226.

Jost, A. (1970). Hormonal factors in the sex differentiation of the mammalian foetus. *Philosophical Transactions of the Royal Society of London, 259*(828), 119–130.

Jost, A. (1972). A new look at the mechanisms controlling sex differentiation in mammals. *The Johns Hopkins Medical Journal, 130*, 38–53.

Judd, H. L., Robinson, J. D., Young, P. E., & Jones, O. W. (1976). Amniotic fluid testosterone levels in midpregnancy. *Obstetrics and Gynecology, 48*(6), 690–692.

Kimura, D. (1999). *Sex and Cognition*. Cambridge, MA: MIT Press.

Kimura, D. & Hampson, E. (1994). Cognitive pattern in men and women is influenced by fluctuations in sex hormones. *Current Directions in Psychological Science, 3*, 57–61.

Knickmeyer, R., Baron-Cohen, S., Raggatt, P., & Taylor, K. (2005). Fetal testosterone, social cognition, and restricted interests in children. *Journal of Child Psychology and Psychiatry, and Allied Disciplines, 45*, 1–13.

Knickmeyer, R., Baron-Cohen, S., Hoekstra, R., & Wheelwright, S. (2006). Age of menarche in females with autism spectrum conditions. *Developmental Medicine and Child Neurology, 48*, 1007–1008.

Knickmeyer, R., Baron-Cohen, S., Raggatt, P., Taylor, K., & Hackett, G. (2006). Fetal testosterone and empathy. *Hormones and Behavior, 49*(3), 282–292.

Knickmeyer, R., Baron-Cohen, S., Fane, B. A., Wheelwright, S., Mathews, G. A., et al. (2006). Androgens and autistic traits: A study of individuals with congenital adrenal hyperplasia. *Hormones and Behavior, 50*, 148–153.

Kuhnle, U. & Bullinger, M. (1997). Outcome of congenital adrenal hyperplasia. *Pediatric Surgery International, 12*, 511–515.

Lawson, J., Baron-Cohen, S., & Wheelwright, S. (2004). Empathising and systemising in adults with and without Asperger Syndrome. *Journal of Autism and Developmental Disorders, 34*, 301–310.

Lutchmaya, S., Baron-Cohen, S., & Raggatt, P. (2002). Fetal testosterone and vocabulary size in 18- and 24-month-old infants. *Infant Behavior and Development, 24*(4), 418–424.

Lutchmaya, S., Baron-Cohen, S., & Raggatt, P. (2002). Fetal testosterone and eye contact in 12 month old infants. *Infant Behavior and Development, 25*, 327–335.

Mallin, S. R. & Walker, F. A. (1972). Effects of the XYY karyotype in one of two brothers with congenital adrenal hyperplasia. *Clinical Genetics, 3*, 490–494.

Manning, J., Baron-Cohen, S., Wheelwright, S., & Sanders, G. (2001). Autism and the ratio between 2nd and 4th digit length. *Developmental Medicine and Child Neurology, 43*, 160–164.

Manning, J. T., Martin, S., Trivers, R. L., & Soler, M. (2002). 2nd to 4th digit ratio and offspring sex ratio. *Journal of Theoretical Biology, 217*(1), 93–95.

Mathews, G. A., Fane, B. A., Conway, G. S., Brook, C. G., & Hines, M. (2009). Personality and congenital adrenal hyperplasia: Possible effects of prenatal androgen exposure. *Hormones and Behavior, 55*, 285–291.

McManus, I. C., Murray, B., Doyle, K., & Baron-Cohen, S. (1992). Handedness in childhood autism shows a dissociation of skill and preference. *Cortex, 28*, 373–381.

Merke, D. P., Fields, J. D., Keil, M. F., Vaituzis, A. C., Chrousos, G. P., & Giedd, J. N. (2003). Children with classic congenital adrenal hyperplasia have decreased amygdala volume: Potential prenatal and postnatal hormone effects. *Journal of Clinical Endocrinology and Metabolism, 88*, 1760–1765.

Milne, E., White, S., Campbell, R., Swettenham, J., Hansen, P., & Ramus, F. (2006). Motion and Form Coherence Detection in Autistic Spectrum Disorder: Relationship to Motor Control and 2:4 Digit Ratio. *Journal of Autism and Developmental Disorders, 36*, 1–13.

Money, J. & Ehrhardt, A. A. (1972). *Man and Woman, Boy and Girl*. Baltimore: Johns Hopkins University Press.

Money, J., Schwartz, M., & Lewis, V. G. (1984). Adult erotosexual status and fetal hormonal mASDulinization and demASDulinization: 46,XX congenital virilizing adrenal hyperplasia and 46,XY androgen-insensitivity syndrome compared. *Psychoneuroendocrinology, 9*, 405–414.

Nagami, M., McDonough, P., Ellegood, J., & Mahesh, V. (1979). Maternal and amniotic fluid steroids throughout human pregnancy. *American Journal of Obstetrics and Gynaecology, 134*, 674–680.

Nass, R., Baker, S., Speiser, P., Virdis, R., Balsamo, A., Cacciari, E., et al. (1987). Hormones and handedness: Left-hand bias in female adrenal hyperplasia patients. *Neurology, 37*, 711–715.

Nordenstrom, A., Servin, A., Bohlin, G., Larsson, A., & Wedell, A. (2002). Sex-typed toy play behavior correlates with the degree of prenatal androgen exposure assessed by CYP21 genotype in girls with congenital adrenal hyperplasia. *Journal of Clinical Endocrinology and Metabolism, 87*, 5119–5124.

Peters, M. (1991). Sex, handedness, mathematical ability, and biological causation. *Canadian Journal of Psychology, 45*(3), 415–419.

Phoenix, C. H., Goy, R. W., Gerall, A. A., & Young, W. C. (1959). Organizing action of prenatally administered testosterone propionate on the tissues mediating mating behavior in the female guinea pig. *Endocrinology, 65*, 369–382.

Quadagno, D. M., Briscoe, R., & Quadagno, J. S. (1977). Effect of perinatal gonadal hormones on selected nonsexual behavior patterns: A critical assessment of the nonhuman and human literature. *Psychological Bulletin, 84*, 62–80.

Resnick, S. M. (1982). Psychological functioning in individuals with congenital adrenal hyperplasia: Early hormonal influences on cognition and personality. Minneapolis: University of Minnesota.

Resnick, S., Berenbaum, S., Gottesman, I., & Bouchard, T. (1986). Early hormonal influences on cognitive functioning in congenital adrenal hyperplasia. *Developmental Psychology, 22*, 191–198.

Ring, H., Baron-Cohen, S., Williams, S., Wheelwright, S., Bullmore, E., Brammer, M., et al. (1999). Cerebral correlates of preserved cognitive skills in autism. A functional MRI study of Embedded Figures Task performance. *Brain, 122*, 1305–1315.

Robinson, J. D., Judd, H. L., Young, P. E., Jones, O. W., & Yen, S. S. (1977). Amniotic fluid androgens and estrogens in midgestation. *Journal of Clinical Endocrinology and Metabolism, 45*(4), 755–761.

Rohde Parfet, K. A., Ganjam, V. K., Lamberson, W. R., Rieke, A. R., Vom Saal, F. S., & Day, B. N. (1990). Intrauterine position effects in female swine: Subsequent reproductive performance and social and sexual behaviour. *Applied Animal Behaviour Science, 26*, 349–362.

Rommerts, F. F. G., Gromoll, J., Cato, A. C. B., Hiort, O., Zitzmann, M., Christiansen, K., et al. (2001). *Testosterone: Action, deficiency, substitution*. In E. Nieschlag, H. Behre (Eds.). Cambridge: Cambridge University Press.

Satz, P., Soper, H., Orsini, D., Henry, R., & Zvi, J. (1985). Handedness subtypes in autism. *Psychiatric Annals, 15*, 447–451.

Schindler, A. E. (1982). Hormones in human amniotic fluid. *Monographs on Endocrinology, 21*, 1–158.

Scott, F., Baron-Cohen, S., Bolton, P., & Brayne, C. (2002). Prevalence of autism spectrum conditions in children aged 5-11 years in Cambridgeshire, UK. *Autism, 6*(3), 231–237.

Scott, F., Baron-Cohen, S., Bolton, P., & Brayne, C. (2002). The CAST (Childhood Asperger Syndrome Test): Preliminary development of UK screen for mainstream primary-school children. *Autism, 6*(1), 9–31.

Shah, A. & Frith, U. (1983). An islet of ability in autism: A research note. *Journal of Child Psychology and Psychiatry, and Allied Disciplines, 24*, 613–620.

Smail, P. J., Reyes, F. I., Winter, J. S. D., & Fairman, C. (1981). The fetal hormonal environment and its effect on the morphogenesis of the genital system. In S. J. Kogan, E. S. E. Hafez (Eds.), *Pediatric Andrology* (pp. 9–19). The Hague: Martinus Nijhoff.

Soper, H., Satz, P., Orsini, D., Henry, R., Zvi, J., & Schulman, M. (1986). Handedness patterns in autism suggests subytpes. *Journal of Autism and Developmental Disorders, 16*, 155–167.

Sparks, B. F., Friedman, S. D., Shaw, D. W., Aylward, E. H., Echelard, D., Artru, A. A., et al. (2002). Brain structural abnormalities in young children with autism spectrum disorder. *Neurology, 59*, 184–192.

Stodgell, C. J., Ingram, J. I., & Hyman, S. L. (2001). The role of candidate genes in unravelling the genetics of autism. *International Review of Research in Mental Retardation, 23*, 57–81.

Tordjman, A., Ferrari, P., Sulmont, V., Duyme, M., & Roubertoux, P. (1997). Androgenic Activity in Autism. *American Journal of Psychriatry, 154*, 11.

Tulchinsky, D. & Little, A. B. (1994). *Maternal-fetal Endocrinology*. Philadelphia & London: W B Saunders.

Wakabayashi, A., Baron-Cohen, S., & Wheelwright, S. (2004). The Autism Spectrum Quotient (AQ) Japanese version: Evidence from high-functioning clinical group and normal adults. *Japanese Journal of Psychology, 75*, 78–84.

Wakabayashi, A., Baron-Cohen, S., Wheelwright, S., & Tojo, Y., (2006). The Autism-Spectrum Quotient (AQ) in Japan: A cross-cultural comparison. *Journal of Autism and Developmental Disorders, 36*, 263–270.

Wakabayashi, A., Baron-Cohen, S., Uchiyama, T., Yoshida, Y., Tojo, Y., Kuroda, M., et al. (2007). The autism-spectrum quotient (AQ) children's version in Japan: A cross-cultural comparison. *Journal of Autism and Developmental Disorders, 37*, 491–500.

Wheelwright, S., Baron-Cohen, S., Goldenfeld, N., Delaney, J., Fine, D., Smith, R., et al. (2006). Predicting Autism Spectrum Quotient (AQ) from the Systemizing Quotient-Revised (SQ-R) and Empathy Quotient (EQ). *Brain Research, 1079*, 47–56.

Williams, J., Scott, F., Allison, C., Bolton, P., Baron-Cohen, S., et al. (2005). The CAST (Childhood Asperger Syndrome Test): Test accuracy. *Autism*, 45–68.

Williams, J. G., Allison, C., Scott, F. J., Bolton, P. F., Baron-Cohen, S., et al. (2008). The Childhood Autism Spectrum Test (CAST): Sex Differences. *Journal of Autism and Developmental Disorders.*

56 Marco Iacoboni

The Mirror Neuron System and Imitation

Points of Interest

- Mirror neurons provide a functional matching between a motor response during the action of the self and a perceptual response to the actions of others.
- Mirror neurons have been recorded in many different areas of the primate brain as well as in songbirds.
- The functional properties of mirror neurons suggest that they are relevant to imitation, a pervasive form of learning and nonverbal communication and affiliation.
- Brain imaging studies have also revealed reduced mirroring responses in patients with autism.
- The reduced mirroring responses in autism have behavioral relevance, because they correlate with the severity of the condition.
- Mirroring responses may be used as biomarker of intervention efficacy.

Imitation is a pervasive form of learning and transmission of culture and has been strongly associated with higher cognitive functions in humans, such as language and the ability to understand other minds (Hurley & Chater, 2005). Reports on imitation deficits in children with autism date back to at least the early 1950s (Ritvo & Provence, 1953). For many years, however, these early findings had little impact on the research on autism. Recently, interest on imitation deficits in patients with autism has been revived by the work of Rogers and Pennington (Rogers & Pennington, 1991). At the same time, recent neuroscience discoveries have revealed neuronal mechanisms that seem ideally suited for imitation. Inevitably, these two lines of research recently merged and provided the first wave of data on the neural mechanisms of imitation in patients with autism.

Cellular Mechanisms of Mirroring

Macaques: Hand-and-Mouth Actions

Less than 20 years ago, depth electrode recordings in macaques demonstrated unexpected sensory properties in neurons located in motor areas and thus discharging—as expected—while the monkey performed a variety of actions. The unexpected sensory properties of some of these motor neurons were such that the neurons would also fire at the sight of someone else's action (di Pellegrino et al., 1992). Thus, the properties of these cells were as if the monkey was watching her own actions reflected by a mirror. Hence, because the discharges of these neurons seem to "reflect" the perceptual aspects of actions of others onto the motor repertoire of the observer, they were called *mirror neurons* (Gallese et al., 1996).

The initial recordings of mirror neurons were obtained in motor areas that coded for hand-and-mouth actions (di Pellegrino et al., 1992; Gallese et al., 1996; Rizzolatti & Craighero, 2004). Neurons in these cortical areas code for a variety of goal-oriented hand actions, such as grasping, holding, manipulating, tearing, bringing to the mouth, and so on. They also code for a variety of mouth actions, such as biting and sucking, and even communicative actions such as lip-smacking, a facial gesture of positive valence. For many years, recordings on mirror neurons have been restricted to two specific brain regions coding these kinds of actions. However, a recent wave of studies has revealed mirroring neural mechanisms in a variety of brain areas and for other kinds of actions, as discussed below. This recent wave of studies has suggested that neural mirroring is not restricted to specific brain regions and specific actions but, rather, may represent a widespread functional mechanism for learning and social interactions.

The mirror neurons for hand-and-mouth action that have been more heavily studied have been divided in two main categories: *strictly congruent* mirror neurons and *broadly congruent* mirror neurons (Rizzolatti & Craighero, 2004). Strictly congruent mirror neurons (approximately one-third of all recorded hand-and-mouth mirror neurons) discharge for the same action, either performed or observed (e.g., a precision grip—i.e., a hand-grasping action using only two fingers to grasp a tiny object). Broadly congruent mirror neurons (approximately two-thirds of all recorded mirror neurons) do not discharge for the same action during action execution and action observation but, rather, for similar actions achieving the same goal or for logically related actions—for example, the observation of placing an object (say, on a table) and the action execution of grasping it. The fact that broadly congruent mirror neurons outnumber strictly congruent ones is important, because it gives the mirror neuron system enough flexibility to be critically activated during a variety of social interactions. Although imitation is a fundamental human ability and it is critical for social interactions, it is often also useful not to imitate others but rather act in a complementary fashion (Newman-Norlund et al., 2007). Furthermore, a flexible imitative behavior does not necessarily result in copying faithfully all aspects of an action. Sometimes it is useful to copy only some elements of an action and creatively integrate those elements with one's own motor repertoire. Broadly congruent mirror neurons seem ideal cells to support these flexible forms of imitation.

Furthermore, mirror neurons seem to code action-related information in a fairly abstract way. Very often, in real-life situations, we are not able to observe the actions of other people in their entirety, because many objects may occlude our sight. Indeed, mirror neurons are able to code observed actions even though the action is not fully in sight. They are also able to discriminate between an action and its pantomime even when both action and its pantomime are visually identical. Indeed, if a screen occludes, in part, the sight of the animal, and the animal observes a human experimenter reaching behind the screen, then the cell will discharge when the animal knows that there is a graspable object behind the screen but will not discharge when the animal knows that there is no object to be grasped behind the screen (Umiltà et al., 2001).

Mirror neurons are able to code the actions of other people even in absence of visual stimulation. Actions are often associated with sounds (footsteps, clapping, breaking peanuts, etc.). We are typically able to recognize the actions of others by simply listening to those sounds. In monkeys, mirror neurons fire at the sound of an action (say, breaking a peanut) even when the action is not seen at all (Kohler et al., 2002).

Taken together, the properties of mirror neurons suggest that these cells provide a fairly abstract coding of the actions of others. The most compelling evidence in support of this interpretation is a study that, by adopting a clever experimental design, demonstrated that mirror neurons are able to discriminate between two identical grasping actions associated with different intentions (Fogassi et al., 2005). In this study, which included control conditions not described here, the presence or absence of a container indicated whether the experimenter was going to grasp food and place it in the container (grasping-for-placing) or was going to grasp food and eat it (grasping-for-eating). At the sight of the grasping action (i.e., well before observing what happened after grasping), the majority of mirror neurons discharged differentially for grasping-for-placing and grasping-for-eating, whereas only a minority discharged equally for both conditions. Most mirror neurons discharged for grasping-for-eating, although some preferred grasping-for-placing.

The experiment on coding intentions suggests that mirror neurons may actually code more the goal of the action than the action itself. A dramatic demonstration of this concept has been provided by a recent study (Umiltà et al., 2008). Monkeys were trained to grasp with normal pliers (i.e., requiring finger closing for grasping) and "reverse pliers" that required finger opening (a completely opposite finger movement!) for grasping. Mirror neurons discharged at the sight of the grasping actions with both normal and reverse pliers, confirming that these neurons code the goal of the grasping action rather than the finger movement itself. This finding also suggests that mirror neurons can rapidly change their functional properties, a concept that has potentially important implications for treatment, because it suggests that it may be possible to improve the functions of mirror neurons in patients with a deficit in the mirror neuron system (*see* below).

Two recent studies on grasping mirror neurons have demonstrated new properties in this neuronal population. Approximately half of the cells recorded in one of these studies (Caggiano et al., 2009) had preferential discharges for observed grasping actions in specific sectors of space. Some neurons discharged only for observed actions that occurred in the peri-personal space of the monkey (the space surrounding the body of the animal), whereas others discharged only for observed actions that were performed in the extra-personal space of the monkey (the sector of space outside the peri-personal space). The encoding of the space sectors in which the observed actions occur is also dynamical. If a transparent panel is interposed between the monkey and the observed action, an action in peri-personal space becomes unreachable by the monkey, although the action is still visible. Thus, from a pragmatic standpoint, this action is in extra-personal space, although it occurs near the body of the observing animal, because the animal cannot intervene on it. Mirror neurons coding for peri-personal space actions stop discharging when an action near the body is observed through a transparent panel. In contrast, mirror neurons coding for extra-personal space actions start discharging for peri-personal space actions when the actions are observed through a transparent panel that makes it impossible for the monkey to act on the observed action (Caggiano et al., 2009). Taken together, these findings suggest that the functional properties of mirror neurons allow an analysis of the actions of other people in terms of potential interactions with them.

However, one of the potential problems with premotor neurons that fire at the sight of somebody else's actions is that we might find ourselves imitating others all the time. This behavior is not desirable. A recent study in monkeys has revealed one of possibly many mechanisms of control of unwanted imitation (Kraskov et al., 2009). Some mirror neuron for grasping discharged when the monkey performed the grasping action but completely suppressed their activity during grasping observation. This suppression of activity in these mirror cells may represent a neuronal mechanism of control of unwanted imitation during action observation.

Macaques: Other Types of Mirror Neurons

Recently, a variety of mirroring responses in single neurons was recorded in cortical areas that code for reaching and ocular movements. In dorsal premotor cortex, neurons discharge when the monkey makes reaching movements toward a target by using a cursor and when the monkey observes the same cursor, operated by the experimenter, reaching the target (Cisek & Kalaska, 2005; Cisek & Kalaska, 2004). A similar finding was reported in a later study recording from both dorsal premotor cortex and primary motor cortex (Tkach et al., 2007). In addition, this later study demonstrated that watching the cursor movement in absence of the target did not elicit any discharge in the mirror cells, suggesting again a primary coding of the action goals in these cells. An even more recent study has confirmed that the primary motor cortex contains mirror neurons for reaching movements (Dushanova & Donoghue, 2010).

In the lateral intraparietal area (LIP), there are mirror neurons for ocular movements and attention. These neurons discharge both when the monkey gazes in the preferred direction of the neuron and when the monkey observes another monkey gazing in the preferred direction of the neuron (Shepherd et al., 2009). These mirroring mechanisms for ocular movements may be important neural mechanisms for shared attention.

These recent studies demonstrate that mirror neurons are not restricted to the areas coding for hand-and-mouth movements in which they were originally discovered by the group of Rizzolatti. Neural mirroring may be a pervasive mechanism in the primate brain, facilitating social learning and social interactions. An important evolutionary question involves whether neural mirroring is restricted to primates. Imitative vocal learning in songbirds is an obvious case to start investigating this question.

Audio-Vocal Mirror Neurons in Songbirds

The concept that communication requires a correspondence, or common code, between the sensory and motor codes representing the signal is not new (Liberman & Whalen, 2000; Liberman & Mattingly, 1985; Liberman et al., 1967; Liberman et al., 1957). In neural terms, the most compelling implementation of such a concept would be to establish this correspondence at the level of single cells. A recent study has demonstrated that neurons in the swamp sparrow forebrain provide a precise auditory-vocal correspondence, displaying nearly identical patterns of activity when the songbird is listening to the birdsong and when the songbird sings the birdsong. Importantly, the disruption of auditory feedback during singing does not alter this pattern of activity, demonstrating that this activity is of motor nature (Prather et al., 2008). Furthermore, the neurons displaying these functional properties input onto anatomical structures in the avian brain that are known to be important for learning.

Similar results have also been obtained in the juvenile zebra finch (Keller & Hahnloser, 2009). The demonstration of auditory-vocal mirror neurons in songbirds is important, because it suggests that neural mirroring may be a parsimonious, optimized neural mechanism for action-perception coupling that the evolutionary process exploits at many levels. If this is true, a question that naturally follows is whether mirroring is also anatomically and functionally pervasive. Recent depth electrode recordings in humans suggest that this is indeed the case.

Mirror Neurons in Humans

The typical practice of neuroscience is to study cellular mechanisms in animals and neural systems in humans. Neural systems in human are generally studied by investigating the behavior of patients with brain lesions and by using a variety of methods in healthy subjects and in patients, including brain imaging and brain stimulation techniques. Why do neuroscientists use animal models to study cellular mechanisms in the brain? There are two primary reasons. First of all, the study of cellular mechanisms is highly invasive and cannot be performed in humans unless rare clinical opportunities allow it. Second, it is assumed that the cellular mechanisms observed in animal models are mostly preserved in humans. Hence, the animal data have inferential validity with regard to cellular mechanisms in humans. For example, visual-cortical cells such as the simple and complex visual cells discovered by Hubel and Wiesel in the cat (Hubel & Wiesel, 1959; the authors received the Nobel Prize for Physiology and Medicine for this work; this was the first time that neurophysiologists received the award) have never been recorded in humans. However, there is no visual neuroscientist that challenges the notion that such cells are also present in the human brain. Indeed, when brain imaging data fail to show results compatible with the presence of such cells in the human visual cortex, the scientists interpret the findings not as a challenge to this notion but only as suggesting some limitations of brain imaging techniques (Boynton & Finney, 2003).

Curiously, mirror neurons have been treated quite differently, especially among non-neuroscientists. For mysterious reasons, the existence of mirror neurons in humans has been challenged on the grounds that mirror neurons had been recorded only in animals and not in humans and that brain imaging cannot unequivocally establish their existence in the human brain. The discussion of this issue is an oddity in neuroscience debates. This argument had never before been made, and hopefully it won't be made in the future. Indeed, it is quite irresponsible to challenge the inferential validity of neurophysiological data in animals, because such position undermines the ethical grounds of performing neurophysiology on animals. Although the recent report on individual mirror neurons in humans (Mukamel et al., 2010), recorded with depth electrode in patients with epilepsy, should end such a peculiar debate, it is important not to forget how irresponsible it has been to raise this issue, given the potential policy consequences of such an odd claim.

The proof of the existence of mirror neurons in humans is actually a relatively trivial achievement. The conceptual advancement of the data obtained with depth electrodes in humans is that these cells seem to be located in many neural systems. But let's first look at the results of this study (Mukamel et al., 2010). The action potentials of more than a thousand human neurons were recorded in a series of 21 patients implanted with depth electrodes. The patients were implanted to localize precisely the focus of epilepsy, such that only pathological brain tissue—and not healthy tissue—was subsequently removed during surgery. The location of the implanted electrodes was obviously determined only on the basis of clinical considerations. Thus, the modified clinical electrodes that were also able to record action potentials from individual neurons (for clinical purposes the electroencephalography [EEG] signal is obviously the key) were not located in human brain areas that were homologs of the macaque brain areas where mirror neurons had been recorded by monkey neurophysiologists. During the days preceding the localization of the epileptic focus (which generally happens when the patients seize), the patients were tested while performing and observing grasping actions and facial emotional expressions and also while performing some control tasks. Mirror neurons were found in the medial frontal cortex (in an area called the supplementary motor area [SMA], a brain area important for movement initiation and selection) and in the medial temporal cortex, a brain structure important for memory processes. These are brain areas where mirror neurons had not been previously recorded.

Taken together, the new human data and the recent monkey data suggest that the function of the mirroring neural mechanism depends on the functions of the neural system in which mirror neurons are embedded. The critical feature, and the common denominator, of mirror neurons is the functional matching between a motor response for actions of the self and a perceptual response to the actions of others. The mirror neurons initially recorded in areas coding for the goals of hand-and-mouth actions most likely mirror the goal of the action. The mirror neurons in SMA most likely mirror movement initiation. Mirror neurons in the medial temporal cortex most likely mirror the memory trace of executing the observed actions. Thus, when the patient performs the action, medial temporal cells encode the memory trace of making a grasping action. When the patient observes someone else performing the action, that memory trace is re-activated by the firing of the neuron. Thus, neural mirroring provides a pervasive and rich mapping of the actions of others onto our own actions and the experiences associated with performing them.

Because the mapping between the actions of self and others provided by mirror neurons is so rich, there must also be mechanisms of control and differentiation between actions of the self and actions of others. The depth electrode recordings in humans has revealed that a contingent of mirror neurons had opposite firing rate changes during action execution and action observation. The majority of this subset of mirror neurons increased their firing rate during action execution and suppressed entirely their activity during action observation. This pattern of activity, as for the mirror neurons recorded in monkeys with the same pattern of activity (Kraskov et al., 2009), may help inhibiting unwanted imitation. However, another function of these cells, especially the ones located in the medial temporal lobe, may be the important distinction between the actions of the self and the actions of others.

Mirroring Neural Systems and Their Role in Imitation

From Single-Unit Recordings to Brain Imaging

The neural systems for imitation in humans are typically studied with techniques that cannot record the activity of individual neurons but, rather, measure the integrated activity of large populations of cells, as in EEG, magnetoencephalography (MEG), and transcranial magnetic stimulation (TMS), or changes in blood flow and blood oxygenation that are thought to be related to changes in large populations of cells, as in positron emission tomography (PET) and functional magnetic resonance imaging (fMRI). An alternative way of studying the neural correlates of imitation is by investigating the effect of brain lesions, which also obviously involves a large number of neurons. The classical approach is the neuropsychological study of imitation deficits in patients with either naturally occurring lesions or surgical resections. A more recent approach has been the use of repetitive TMS to induce transient "lesions" in the stimulated brain areas and measure the resulting behavior.

A fundamental issue here is obviously how to translate the findings from single-cell recordings to the investigation of neuronal ensembles. The practice of interpreting human brain imaging data on the basis of single-cell neurophysiological data in nonhuman primates is well-established and has been adopted since the very early days of brain imaging. The exciting proliferation of fMRI experimental designs and analysis methods, however, has promised to circumvent this practice, which relies heavily on the scientists' interpretation of the imaging data on the basis of neuronal properties described in the animal literature. The hope was that these new brain imaging techniques would provide more "objective" measures of activity in specific neuronal populations.

This was indeed the promise of adaptation paradigms in fMRI. Adaptation fMRI paradigms exploit a neurophysiological property exhibited by many neurons—that is, the habituation to repeated presentation of the same stimulus or to repeated execution of the same action. The general idea of fMRI adaptation paradigms is that by using clever experimental designs, it is possible to image the action potentials of a specific neuronal population that discharge selectively for specific stimuli or during specific actions, even though fMRI obviously does not have the technical capability of imaging single neurons (Tootell et al., 1995). Although the idea was clever, it relied on insufficient knowledge of the neuronal mechanisms of adaptation (Bartels et al., 2008). Indeed, the changes that adaptation induces in the adapting neuron appear to happen at the level of its input, rather than its output, thus making it impossible to claim that fMRI adaptation can image the action potential activity of specific neuronal populations. For example, direction-selective adaptation in visual direction-selective neurons occurs in specific sectors of the receptive field of the adapting neuron and not throughout its receptive field (Kohn & Movshon, 2003). This seemingly odd finding can only be interpreted as showing that the changes in neuronal activity that determine adaptation occur in early visual neurons that input onto the adapting direction-selective neuron. Indeed, these earlier visual neurons are known to have smaller receptive fields than motion-direction selective neurons. Furthermore, neurons that are not selective and discharge equally for two stimuli (e.g., stimulus A and B) still show adaptation for repeated presentation of stimulus A or stimulus B but do not show adaptation for successive presentation of stimulus A followed by B or vice versa (Sawamura et al., 2006). The most likely explanation of this phenomenon is that the nonselective but adapting neuron receives separate inputs from neurons responding to stimulus A and B and that adaptation most likely happens at synaptic level (once again, at input level). This is extremely important for two reasons. First, it demonstrates that adaptation and neuronal selectivity do not go together, even though the basic assumption of fMRI adaptation is that they must go together to make the results interpretable. Second, it makes a specific type of adaptation, repeatedly adopted to test for the existence of mirror neurons in humans—the so-called "cross-modal adaptation—substantially untestable.

Although there is no evidence yet that mirror neurons adapt, many fMRI studies have used the adaptation paradigm to test for mirror neuron responses in humans. In light of the absence of evidence for adaptation in mirror neurons and in light of the neurophysiological evidence discussed above that suggest that the changes producing adaptation occur at the input level, rather than at the level of action potentials of the adapting neuron, the choice of fMRI adaptation designs applied to the study of mirror neurons is already odd. At any rate, one of these early papers made the argument that mirror neurons should adapt not only for performing or observing repeatedly the same action but also for cross-modal adaption—that is, performing and then observing the same action, or vice versa. Cross-modal adaptation in mirror neurons should occur because these cells respond selectively to the execution and observation of the same action (Dinstein et al., 2007). However, as we have seen above, selectivity and adaptation do not go together, making this assumption problematic. Furthermore, if adaptation happens at synaptic level, cross-modal adaptation in mirror neurons is difficult to obtain, because the neuron most likely receives input from frontal areas during action execution and from visual areas during action observation. Indeed, four studies using fMRI adaptation during execution and observation of actions (Dinstein et al., 2007; Chong et al., 2008; Lingnau et al., 2009; Kilner et al., 2009) have consistently demonstrated adaptation for repeatedly executed and for repeatedly observed actions, but the results of cross-modal adaptation have been inconsistent. One study failed to show cross-modal adaptation (Dinstein et al., 2007), two studies demonstrated cross-modal adaptation only in one condition (and they were inconsistent with each other!) (Chong et al., 2008; Lingnau et al., 2009), and only one study (admittedly, the most carefully designed of the whole series) demonstrated cross-modal adaptation for both the executed action following the observed one and vice versa (Kilner et al., 2009).

Another emerging trend in human functional brain imaging is the use of multivariate statistics (or classifiers) to look for reproducible patterns of brain activity over cortical areas. With this approach, patterns of activity in some trials presenting, for example, stimulus A are expected to correlate with patterns of activity in other trials also presenting stimulus A but not with patterns of activity in trials presenting stimulus B. This technique has produced beautiful studies of visual perception (Haxby et al., 2001). However, those studies applied this method to areas in which many neurons exhibit similar neurophysiological properties—that is, they are characterized by what is called "population coding." It makes sense that pattern recognition methods demonstrate robust results in these areas, given that in these areas a large number of neurons have similar responses. As we have seen in the section on single neuron recordings in monkeys, mirror neurons are only a subset of neurons in the brain areas in which they are recorded. It is almost inevitable that pattern recognition methods fail to reveal mirroring responses in paradigms of action execution and action observation, whereby action execution and action observation are assumed to yield similar patterns of activity. When these analysis techniques are coupled with an adaptation paradigm, a negative result must be expected, and indeed it has been reported (Dinstein et al., 2008). The significance of this negative result, however, is extremely limited. Furthermore, classifiers are inherently difficult to interpret even when positive results are obtained, as discussed in detail elsewhere (Bartels et al., 2008).

Given that spiking activity (the firing of neurons—i.e., their action potentials), local field potential (which is currently believed to represent the integrated synaptic input), and blood oxygenation level dependent (BOLD) fMRI signals tend to go together in many cases (Logothetis et al., 2001) (although dissociations have been observed, showing that BOLD and local field potential (LFP) tend to be coupled more than BOLD and spiking activity; Logothetis & Wandell, 2004), a much more effective strategy to investigate mirroring properties of human brain areas using fMRI is by manipulating specific parameters that are known to activate mirror neurons selectively while keeping constant some other parameters. This strategy has indeed produced a series of successful studies that have revealed the strong links between human mirror neuron areas and imitation.

Brain Imaging and Transcranial Magnetic Stimulation Data on Human Imitation

In an early fMRI study of human imitation, we based our prediction on the BOLD activity of human brain areas containing mirror neurons and on the single-cell recordings performed in the monkey with depth electrodes. Those data have indicated that mirror neurons discharge more vigorously during action execution compared to action observation. Indeed, the firing rate increase of mirror neurons during action observation is approximately half the firing rate increase during action execution. Thus, we predicted a higher BOLD increase compared to baseline during action execution than during action observation. Furthermore, given that during imitation subjects are both seeing and performing the action, we also predicted that the BOLD increase during imitation should approximately be the sum of the BOLD increases measured during action execution and during action observation. The fMRI results obtained in an experiment on imitation and observation of finger movements confirmed these predictions. Two areas of the human brain, the inferior frontal cortex and the anterior part of the posterior parietal cortex, displayed the predicted pattern of activity (Iacoboni et al., 1999). Furthermore, these areas corresponded fairly well (in anatomical terms) with the areas of the monkey brain in which mirror neurons were originally recorded. These results indicated not only homologies between the monkey and the human mirror neuron areas but also that these areas are important for imitation.

In a subsequent study, we tested whether the activity in the two human brain areas we had previously identified was modulated by action goals. Developmental psychology data have suggested that imitation in children is especially tuned to imitating the goals of other people's actions (Bekkering et al., 2000). In an fMRI experiment, we adopted a paradigm that was previously used in the developmental psychology experiments. The results demonstrated that among the two previously identified brain regions, the inferior frontal area was particularly sensitive to imitating the goal of the action (Koski et al., 2002). Indeed, a later study also demonstrated that this region codes the intention associated with the observed action, rather than the action itself (Iacoboni et al., 2005; Figure 56-1).

The inferior frontal area identified in these two imaging studies on imitation overlaps with the posterior part of Broca's area in the left hemisphere, a prominent brain area for language. This overlap is theoretically important. After the discovery of mirror neurons in macaques, it had been suggested that these cells may represent neural mechanisms that are the evolutionary precursors of neural systems for language (Rizzolatti & Arbib, 1998). Indeed, the macaque brain area in which mirror neurons were originally discovered is believed to be the homolog of Broca's area in the human brain (Rizzolatti & Arbib, 1998). Thus, our fMRI studies, which demonstrate mirror-like patterns of activation during imitation experiments in Broca's area, seem to corroborate the evolutionary hypothesis of mirror neurons as neuronal elements precursors of neural systems for language in humans. However, activation of a language area in a nonlanguage task in a brain imaging experiment may be ambiguous. Indeed, brain imaging gives us only correlational information between brain activity and behavior. In principle, an activation of a language area during

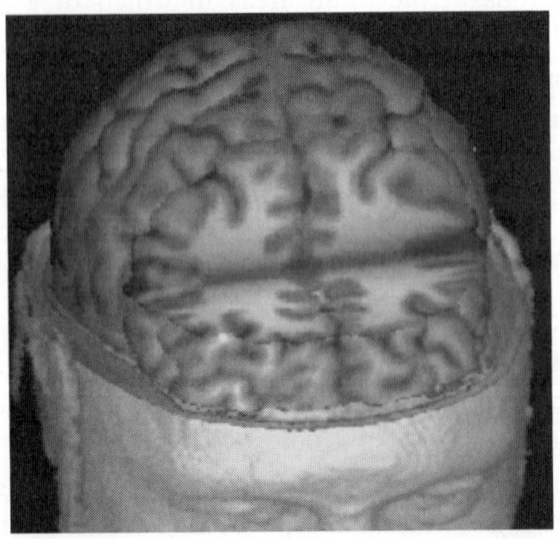

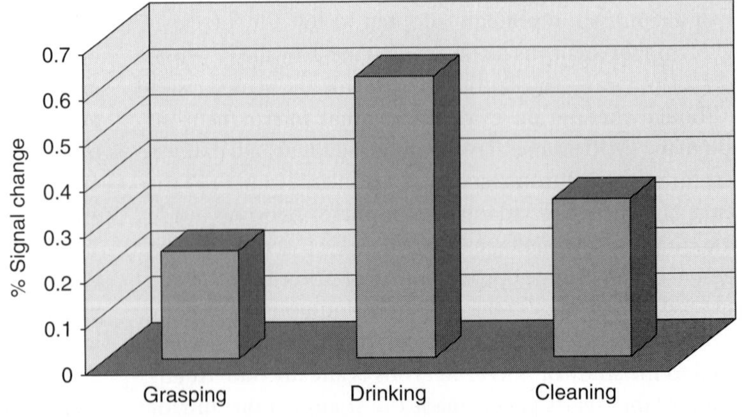

Figure 56–1. Mirror Neuron Areas and Intention Understanding. When subjects observe the same grasping action associated with different intentions (as suggested by the context in which the action is embedded), mirror neuron areas activate differently. Grasping the intentions of others with one's own mirror neuron system. *PLoS Biology, 3*(3), e79), the frontal mirror neuron area in humans is less active for a grasping action with no context and maximally active for a grasping action embedded in a context that suggests drinking. In this study (Iacoboni, M., Molnar-Szakacs, I., Gallese, V., Buccino, G., Mazziotta, J. C., & Rizzolatti, G. [2005].

a nonlanguage task may simply represent covert verbalization during the task. This alternative explanation is rather unlikely, because there is no apparent reason why subjects should covertly verbalize a little during action observation, a bit more during action execution, and even more during imitation (the pattern of activity we measured in the posterior part of Broca's area). At any rate, we decided to test the relationships between Broca's area and imitation directly by using repetitive TMS over the posterior part of Broca's area while subjects were imitating finger movements. The rationale behind this experiment was to produce a transient "lesion" in the posterior part of Broca's area to test whether its functioning is essential to imitation. To control for nonspecific effects, subjects also performed a visuo-motor control task and were stimulated in a control site. The results demonstrated a selective impairment for imitation but not for the control visuomotor task only when subjects were stimulated over the posterior part of Broca's area but not when they were stimulated over the control site (Heiser et al., 2003). These data demonstrate a causal link between activity in the posterior part of Broca's area and imitation, ruling out that the activation in imaging studies represented epiphenomenal activity.

In the monkey, neurons in the superior temporal sulcus (STS) demonstrate visual properties similar to the visual properties of mirror neurons. They respond to the sight of object-oriented actions and more generally to biological motion (Perrett et al., 1989; Jellema et al., 2000; Puce & Perrett, 2003). The STS neurons, however, are only higher-order visual neurons, do not activate during action execution, and thus do not have mirror properties. However, given their visual properties, they likely feed visual information into the fronto-parietal mirror neuron system. Indeed, there are well-established anatomical connections between STS and the posterior parietal mirror neuron area (Seltzer & Pandya, 1994). The brain imaging studies on imitation and action observation we have performed in the last 10 years have confirmed the role of human posterior STS in visual processing of observed and imitated actions (Iacoboni et al., 2001; Koski et al., 2002; Koski et al., 2003; Iacoboni et al., 2004; Iacoboni et al., 2005; Molnar-Szakacs et al., 2006; Kaplan and Iacoboni, 2006). Taken together, the imaging studies on human imitation suggest a core neural circuitry for imitation composed of three major cortical areas: the STS, the posterior parietal human mirror neuron area, and the inferior frontal human mirror neuron area. Within this circuitry, the processing of information necessary for imitation is likely implemented as follows: the STS provides a higher-order visual description of the action to be imitated and the parietal mirror neuron area is concerned with the copying of the detailed motor aspects of the action, whereas the inferior frontal mirror neuron area codes the goal of the action. When the imitative action is planned, an efferent copy of the imitative action is sent back to the STS, where there is a matching process between the visual description of the action and the prediction of the sensory consequences of the planned imitative action. If there is a good matching, then the imitative actions are executed. If not, then appropriate corrections are implemented until a good matching is achieved (Iacoboni, 2005). This core neural circuitry for imitation is presumed to interact with other neural systems to facilitate social cognitive skills. For example, there is evidence supporting the hypothesis that the interactions between the core neural circuitry for imitation and the limbic system are important for empathy, as we will see in the next section.

The Face of Empathy

Many notable authors have emphasized the links between imitation and empathy (de Montaigne, 1575; Smith, 1759; Poe, 1982; Nietzsche, 1881; Wittgenstein, 1980). More recently, quantitative studies have established strong correlations between the tendency to automatically imitate others during social interactions (a phenomenon known as "The Chameleon Effect") and the tendency to empathize, to be concerned about the mental and emotional states of others (Hatfield et al., 1994; Chartrand & Bargh, 1999). The relationships between imitation and empathy suggests strong functional interactions between the core neural circuitry for imitation and classical emotional brain areas belonging to the limbic system, such as the amygdala. Anatomically, these structures are connected in the primate brain through the dysgranular sector of the insular lobe (Augustine, 1996). A plausible hypothesis about the interactions between the neural circuitry for imitation and limbic areas during imitation that leads to empathy is as follows:

1. Neurons in STS code the higher-order visual description of facial expressions, actions, and body postures of other people.
2. This information is sent to the fronto-parietal mirror neuron areas that initiate the imitative process.
3. Signals from the mirror neuron areas are sent—via the insula—to limbic areas.
4. The activity in the limbic areas triggers the mental and/or emotional states often associated with those actions and/or facial expressions—for example, smiling.

This plausible series of neural events has also a neural counterpart during simple observation of the facial expressions, actions, and body postures of other people. Indeed, mirror neurons also fire during the mere observation of the actions of others. This firing can, in principle, initiate a similar cascade of neural activations that may lead to an inner imitation of the facial expressions, actions, and body postures of other people and eventually also to empathy for others by simulating the emotional states associated with the facial expressions, actions, and body postures of other people.

To test this model, we performed an fMRI experiment in which subjects were asked to observe and to imitate facial emotional expressions. The model makes two general predictions: First, during both observation and imitation, there should be activation of the core neural circuitry for imitation (STS and fronto-parietal mirror neuron areas), of the insula, and of limbic structures such as the amygdala. Second, during

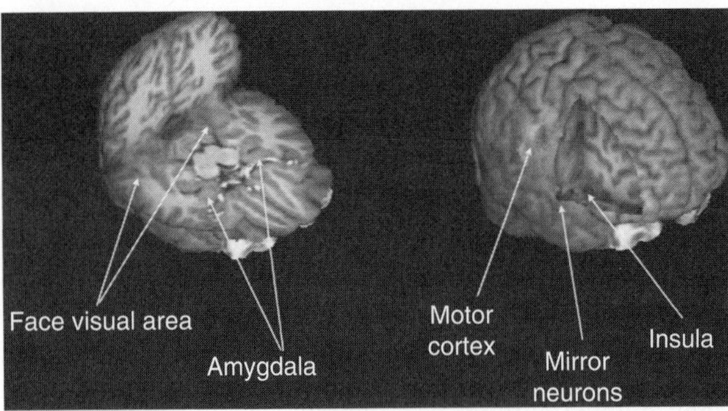

Figure 56–2. Neural Circuitry for Empathy. When subjects imitate or observe facial emotional expressions, they activate a complex network of areas. The activity in areas highlighted in yellow correlates with behavioral scales of empathy and social competence, suggesting that this neural circuit may represent a biomarker of sociality in humans. (See Color Plate Section for a color version of this figure.)

imitation, the activity throughout this large-scale neural network should be higher than during observation, if it is triggered by mirror neuron areas: indeed, mirror neuron areas had displayed this pattern of activity in our previous brain imaging experiments. The brain imaging results supported both predictions (Carr et al., 2003), suggesting that one way of empathizing with others is through bodily enactment of the actions of others or through the simulation of such enactment (during observation only; Figure 56-2).

This study described a large-scale network with functional properties that may plausibly explain the links between imitation and empathy. The lack of behavioral data correlating the tendency to empathize of the experimental subjects with the activity in this large-scale network, however, made it impossible to test more stringently the hypothesis that the functional properties of this network are important for empathy. A series of subsequent brain imaging studies, in both adults and children, and both from our lab and others labs, have tested and supported this hypothesis by providing strong correlations between the empathy scores of the experimental subjects and activity in mirror neuron areas (Kaplan & Iacoboni, 2006; Gazzola et al., 2006) and also in the insula and amygdala (Pfeifer et al., 2008).

The Mirror Neuron Hypothesis of Autism

Because mirror neurons have been implicated in a variety of functions that are cornerstones of social behavior, some authors have hypothesized that autism may be associated with a mirror neuron dysfunction (Williams et al., 2001). Evidence in support of this hypothesis has been obtained in different labs and using different methods. Some studies have shown anatomical differences between subjects with and without autism in mirror neuron areas (Hadjikhani et al., 2005). Other studies have shown EEG differences in the suppression of the mu rhythm (Oberman et al., 2005), a parameter taken to reflect mirror neuron activity (Hari et al., 1998). A MEG study has demonstrated that cortical activation during imitation is delayed in Asperger's Syndrome (Nishitani et al., 2004). Using fMRI and our paradigm on imitation of finger movements (Iacoboni et al., 1999), another group also found differences between subjects with and without autism in levels of activation in mirror neuron areas (Williams et al., 2006).

We used fMRI to test the hypothesis that the large-scale neural network composed of mirror neuron areas, insula, and limbic areas whose activity correlates with empathy (and other parameters of social competence) is impaired in patients with autism. Two groups of children were studied with fMRI while the children were both observing and imitating facial emotional expressions, as in the previously described study. One group was composed of typically developing children (TD) and the other was composed of children diagnosed with autism spectrum disorder (ASD). The brain imaging data revealed indeed that the group of children with ASD had reliably less activity in mirror neuron areas, insula, and amygdala during both imitation and observation of facial emotional expressions. Furthermore, and probably even more compellingly in support of the hypothesis that this circuitry is critically impaired in the ASD group, we found a correlation between the activity in these areas and the severity of the disease, as assessed by widely used scales. This correlation was such that the more reduced the activity in these areas (and especially so in mirror neuron areas), the more impaired was the social functioning of the subject (Dapretto et al., 2006).

Taken together, the correlations between brain imaging data and behavioral scales suggest that mirror neuron areas, the core neural circuitry for imitation, and even more broadly the large-scale network that includes also insula and limbic structures, may represent biomarkers of sociality. Future studies, especially if coupled with successful interventions, as briefly discussed in the conclusions, will further explore this exciting hypothesis.

Before concluding, however, it is important to address some criticisms to the mirror neuron hypothesis of autism. Despite the wealth of neurophysiological and brain imaging data supporting this hypothesis, some behavioral studies that demonstrated that children with ASD can understand action goals (Hamilton et al., 2007) dismissed the brain data and concluded that the "broken mirror" hypothesis of autism must be wrong (Southgate & de C Hamilton, 2008). This criticism rests on the assumption that there is a one-to-one correspondence between behavior and brain systems, so that one can infer the functioning of brain systems on the basis of human behavior. The behavioral data, however, can be easily explained with the idea that tasks can be successfully performed in many different ways, adopting different cognitive strategies and using different neural systems. Indeed, a recent study demonstrates that subjects with ASD understand the intentions of others' actions by relying on contextual and object semantic cues, whereas subjects without ASD rely on the observed motor behavior (Boria et al., 2009). These are two rather different strategies indeed, most likely relying on different neural systems.

Conclusions

To conclude, a potential application of the neuroscience studies discussed in this chapter is a wider use of imitation-based interventions in children with autism. Indeed, such interventions are already underway, and the preliminary results are rather promising (Ingersoll, 2010; Ingersoll et al., 2007; Ingersoll & Gergans, 2007; Ingersoll & Schreibman, 2006). The social behavior of subjects with autism undergoing relatively simple interventions based on reciprocal imitation between the patient and the therapist (indeed, these techniques can be taught to the parents of the children) ameliorates visibly (Ingersoll, 2010; Ingersoll et al., 2007; Ingersoll & Gergans, 2007; Ingersoll & Schreibman, 2006), thus promising to be an effective intervention.

Challenges and Future Directions

- Integrate single-unit data and brain imaging data on neural mirroring.
- Use activity in mirror neuron areas as a biomarker predicting the effectiveness of interventions.
- Make brain imaging laboratories more patient-friendly so that more data can be gathered in more naturalistic settings of imitation and action observation.

SUGGESTED READINGS

Iacoboni, M., & Mazziotta, J. C. (2007). Mirror neuron system: basic findings and clinical applications. *Annals of Neurology, 62*(3), 213–218.

Iacoboni, M. (2009). Imitation, empathy, and mirror neurons. *Annual Review of Psychology, 60*, 653–670.

Rizzolatti, G., & Sinigaglia, C. (2010). The functional role of the parieto-frontal mirror circuit: interpretations and misinterpretations. *Nature Reviews Neuroscience, 11*(4), 264–274.

ACKNOWLEDGMENTS

For generous support the author thanks the Brain Mapping Medical Research Organization, Brain Mapping Support Foundation, Pierson-Lovelace Foundation, The Ahmanson Foundation, William M. and Linda R. Dietel Philanthropic Fund at the Northern Piedmont Community Foundation, Tamkin Foundation, Jennifer Jones-Simon Foundation, Capital Group Companies Charitable Foundation, Robson Family and Northstar Fund.

REFERENCES

Augustine, J. R. (1996). Circuitry and functional aspects of the insular lobe in primates including humans. *Brain Research Brain Research Reviews, 22*(3), 229–244.

Bartels, A., Logothetis, N. K., & Moutoussis, K. (2008). fMRI and its interpretations: an illustration on directional selectivity in area V5/MT. *Trends in Neurosciences, 31*(9), 444–453.

Bekkering, H., Wohlschläger, A., & Gattis, M. (2000). Imitation of gestures in children is goal-directed. *Quarterly Journal of Experimental Psychology A, 53*(1), 153–164.

Boria, S., Fabbri-Destro, M., Cattaneo, L., Sparaci, L., Sinigaglia, C., Santelli, E., et al. (2009). Intention understanding in autism. *PLoS ONE, 4*(5), e5596.

Boynton, G. M., & Finney, E. M. (2003). Orientation-specific adaptation in human visual cortex. *Journal of Neuroscience, 23*(25), 8781–8787.

Caggiano, V., Fogassi, L., Rizzolatti, G., Thier, P., & Casile, A. (2009). Mirror neurons differentially encode the peripersonal and extrapersonal space of monkeys. *Science, 324*(5925), 403–406.

Carr, L., Iacoboni, M., Dubeau, M. C., Mazziotta, J. C., & Lenzi, G. L. (2003). Neural mechanisms of empathy in humans: a relay from neural systems for imitation to limbic areas. *Proceedings of the National Academy of Science U S A, 100*(9), 5497–5502.

Chartrand, T. L., & Bargh, J. A. (1999). The chameleon effect: The perception-behavior link and social interaction. *Journal of Personality & Social Psychology, 76*(6), 893–910.

Chong, T. T., Cunnington, R., Williams, M. A., Kanwisher, N., & Mattingley, J. B. (2008). fMRI Adaptation Reveals Mirror Neurons in Human Inferior Parietal Cortex. *Current Biology, 18*(20), 1576–1580.

Cisek, P., & Kalaska, J. F. (2004). Neural correlates of mental rehearsal in dorsal premotor cortex. *Nature, 431*(7011), 993–996.

Cisek, P., & Kalaska, J. F. (2005). Neural correlates of reaching decisions in dorsal premotor cortex: specification of multiple direction choices and final selection of action. *Neuron, 45*(5), 801–814.

Dapretto, M., Davies, M. S., Pfeifer, J. H., Scott, A. A., Sigman, M., Bookheimer, S. Y., et al. (2006). Understanding emotions in others: mirror neuron dysfunction in children with autism spectrum disorders. *Nature Neuroscience, 9*(1), 28–30.

di Pellegrino, G., Fadiga, L., Fogassi, L., Gallese, V., & Rizzolatti, G. (1992). Understanding motor events: a neurophysiological study. *Experimental Brain Research, 91*(1), 176–180.

Dinstein, I., Gardner, J. L., Jazayeri, M., & Heeger, D. J. (2008). Executed and observed movements have different distributed representations in human aIPS. *Journal of Neuroscience, 28*(44), 11,231–11,239.

Dinstein, I., Hasson, U., Rubin, N., & Heeger, D. J. (2007). Brain areas selective for both observed and executed movements. *Journal of Neurophysiology, 98*(3), 1415–1427.

Dushanova, J., & Donoghue, J. (2010). Neurons in primary motor cortex engaged during action observation. *European Journal of Neuroscience, 31*, 386–398.

Fogassi, L., Ferrari, P. F., Gesierich, B., Rozzi, S., Chersi, F., & Rizzolatti, G. (2005). Parietal lobe: from action organization to intention understanding. *Science, 308*(5722), 662–667.

Gallese, V., Fadiga, L., Fogassi, L., & Rizzolatti, G. (1996). Action recognition in the premotor cortex. *Brain, 119*(Pt 2), 593–609.

Gazzola, V., Aziz-Zadeh, L., & Keysers, C. (2006). Empathy and the somatotopic auditory mirror system in humans. *Current Biology*, *16*(18), 1824–1829.

Hadjikhani, N., Joseph, R. M., Snyder, J., & Tager-Flusberg, H. (2005). Anatomical Differences in the Mirror Neuron System and Social Cognition Network in Autism. *Cerebral Cortex*, *16*(9), 1276–1282.

Hamilton, A. F., Brindley, R. M., & Frith, U. (2007). Imitation and action understanding in autistic spectrum disorders: How valid is the hypothesis of a deficit in the mirror neuron system? *Neuropsychologia*, *45*(8), 1859–1868.

Hari, R., Forss, N., Avikainen, S., Kirveskari, E., Salenius, S., & Rizzolatti, G. (1998). Activation of human primary motor cortex during action observation: a neuromagnetic study. *Proceedings of the National Academy of Science U S A*, *95*(25), 15,061–15,065.

Hatfield, E., Cacioppo, J. T., & Rapson, R. L. (1994). *Emotional contagion*. Paris: Cambridge University Press.

Haxby, J. V., Gobbini, M. I., Furey, M. L., Ishai, A., Schouten, J. L., & Pietrini, P. (2001). Distributed and overlapping representations of faces and objects in ventral temporal cortex. *Science*, *293*(5539), 2425–2430.

Heiser, M., Iacoboni, M., Maeda, F., Marcus, J., & Mazziotta, J. C. (2003). The essential role of Broca's area in imitation. *European Journal of Neuroscience*, *17*(5), 1123–1128.

Hubel, D. H., & Wiesel, T. N. (1959). Receptive fields of single neurones in the cat's striate cortex. *Journal of Physiology*, *148*, 574–591.

Hurley, S., & Chater, N. (2005). *Perspective on imitation: From neuroscience to social science*. Cambridge, MA: MIT Press.

Iacoboni, M. (2005). Neural mechanisms of imitation. *Current Opinion in Neurobiology*, *15*(6), 632–637.

Iacoboni, M., Koski, L. M., Brass, M., Bekkering, H., Woods, R. P., Dubeau, M. C., et al. (2001). Reafferent copies of imitated actions in the right superior temporal cortex. *Proceedings of the National Academy of Science U S A*, *98*(24), 13,995–13,999.

Iacoboni, M., Lieberman, M. D., Knowlton, B. J., Molnar-Szakacs, I., Moritz, M., Throop, J., et al. (2004). Watching social interactions produces dorsomedial prefrontal and medial parietal BOLD fMRI signal increases compared to a resting baseline. *NeuroImage*, *21*(3), 1167–1173.

Iacoboni, M., Molnar-Szakacs, I., Gallese, V., Buccino, G., Mazziotta, J. C., & Rizzolatti, G. (2005). Grasping the intentions of others with one's own mirror neuron system. *PLoS Biology*, *3*(3), e79.

Iacoboni, M., Woods, R. P., Brass, M., Bekkering, H., Mazziotta, J. C., & Rizzolatti, G. (1999). Cortical mechanisms of human imitation. *Science*, *286*(5449), 2526–2528.

Ingersoll, B. (2010). Brief Report: Pilot Randomized Controlled Trial of Reciprocal Imitation Training for Teaching Elicited and Spontaneous Imitation to Children with Autism. *Journal of Autism and Developmental Disorders*, *40*, 1154–1160.

Ingersoll, B., & Gergans, S. (2007). The effect of a parent-implemented imitation intervention on spontaneous imitation skills in young children with autism. *Research on Developmental Disabilities*, *28*(2), 163–175.

Ingersoll, B., & Schreibman, L. (2006). Teaching reciprocal imitation skills to young children with autism using a naturalistic behavioral approach: effects on language, pretend play, and joint attention. *Journal of Autism and Developmental Disorders*, *36*(4), 487–505.

Ingersoll, B., Lewis, E., & Kroman, E. (2007). Teaching the imitation and spontaneous use of descriptive gestures in young children with autism using a naturalistic behavioral intervention. *Journal of Autism and Developmental Disorders*, *37*(8), 1446–1456.

Jellema, T., Baker, C. I., Wicker, B., & Perrett, D. I. (2000). Neural representation for the perception of the intentionality of actions. *Brain and Cognition*, *44*(2), 280–302.

Kaplan, J. T., & Iacoboni, M. (2006). Getting a grip on other minds: mirror neurons, intention understanding, and cognitive empathy. *Social Neuroscience*, *1*(3-4), 175–183.

Keller, G. B., & Hahnloser, R. H. (2009). Neural processing of auditory feedback during vocal practice in a songbird. *Nature*, *457*(7226), 187–190.

Kilner, J. M., Neal, A., Weiskopf, N., Friston, K. J., & Frith, C. D. (2009). Evidence of mirror neurons in human inferior frontal gyrus. *Journal of Neuroscience*, *29*(32), 10153–10159.

Kohler, E., Keysers, C., Umiltà, M. A., Fogassi, L., Gallese, V., & Rizzolatti, G. (2002). Hearing sounds, understanding actions: action representation in mirror neurons. *Science*, *297*(5582), 846–848.

Kohn, A., & Movshon, J. A. (2003). Neuronal adaptation to visual motion in area MT of the macaque. *Neuron*, *39*(4), 681–691.

Koski, L., Iacoboni, M., Dubeau, M. C., Woods, R. P., & Mazziotta, J. C. (2003). Modulation of cortical activity during different imitative behaviors. *Journal of Neurophysiology*, *89*(1), 460–471.

Koski, L., Wohlschläger, A., Bekkering, H., Woods, R. P., Dubeau, M. C., Mazziotta, J. C., et al. (2002). Modulation of motor and premotor activity during imitation of target-directed actions. *Cerebral Cortex*, *12*(8), 847–855.

Kraskov, A., Dancause, N., Quallo, M. M., Shepherd, S., & Lemon, R. N. (2009). Corticospinal neurons in macaque ventral premotor cortex with mirror properties: a potential mechanism for action suppression? *Neuron*, *64*(6), 922–930.

Liberman, A. M., & Mattingly, I. G. (1985). The motor theory of speech perception revised. *Cognition*, *21*, 1–36.

Liberman, A. M., & Whalen, D. H. (2000). On the relation of speech to language. *Trends in Cognitive Sciences*, *4*, 187–196.

Liberman, A. M., Cooper, F. S., Shankweiler, D. P., & Studdert-Kennedy, M. (1967). Perception of the speech code. *Psychological Review*, *74*, 431–461.

Liberman, A. M., Harris, K. S., Hoffman, H. S., & Griffith, B. C. (1957). The discrimination of speech sounds within and across phoneme boundaries. *Journal of Experimental Psychology*, *54*, 358–368.

Lingnau, A., Gesierich, B., & Caramazza, A. (2009). Asymmetric fMRI adaptation reveals no evidence for mirror neurons in humans. *Proceedings of the National Academy of Science U S A*, *106*(24), 9925–9930.

Logothetis, N. K., & Wandell, B. A. (2004). Interpreting the BOLD signal. *Annual Review of Physiology*, *66*, 735–769.

Logothetis, N. K., Pauls, J., Augath, M., Trinath, T., & Oeltermann, A. (2001). Neurophysiological investigation of the basis of the fMRI signal. *Nature*, *412*(6843), 150–157.

Molnar-Szakacs, I., Kaplan, J., Greenfield, P. M., & Iacoboni, M. (2006). Observing complex action sequences: The role of the fronto-parietal mirror neuron system. *NeuroImage*, *33*(3), 923–935.

de Montaigne, M. (1575). *Essays*. Harmondsworth, UK: Penguin.

Mukamel, R., Ekstrom, A. D., Kaplan, J., Iacoboni, M., & Fried, I. (2010). Single-Neuron Responses in Humans during Execution and Observation of Actions. *Current Biology*, *20*, 750–756.

Newman-Norlund, R. D., van Schie, H. T., van Zuijlen, A. M., & Bekkering, H. (2007). The mirror neuron system is more active during complementary compared with imitative action. *Nature Neuroscience, 10*(7), 817–818.

Nietzsche, F. (1881). *Daybreak.* Cambridge, UK: Cambridge University Press.

Nishitani, N., Avikainen, S., & Hari, R. (2004). Abnormal imitation-related cortical activation sequences in Asperger's syndrome. *Annals of Neurology, 55*(4), 558–562.

Oberman, L. M., Hubbard, E. M., McCleery, J. P., Altschuler, E. L., Ramachandran, V. S., & Pineda, J. A. (2005). EEG evidence for mirror neuron dysfunction in autism spectrum disorders. *Brain Research Cognitive Brain Research, 24*(2), 190–198.

Perrett, D. I., Harries, M. H., Bevan, R., Thomas, S., Benson, P. J., Mistlin, A. J., et al. (1989). Frameworks of analysis for the neural representation of animate objects and actions. *Journal of Experimental Biology, 146*, 87–113.

Pfeifer, J. H., Iacoboni, M., Mazziotta, J. C., & Dapretto, M. (2008). Mirroring others' emotions relates to empathy and interpersonal competence in children. *NeuroImage, 39*(4), 2076–2085.

Poe, E. A. (1982). *The Tell-Tale Heart and Other Writings.* New York: Bantam Books.

Prather, J. F., Peters, S., Nowicki, S., & Mooney, R. (2008). Precise auditory-vocal mirroring in neurons for learned vocal communication. *Nature, 451*(7176), 305–310.

Puce, A., & Perrett, D. (2003). Electrophysiology and brain imaging of biological motion. *Philosophical Transactions of the Royal Society of London, B Biological Sciences, 358*(1431), 435–445.

Ritvo, S., & Provence, S., (1953). From perception and imitation in some autistic children: Diagnostic findings and their contextual interpretation. *Psychoanalitic Study of the Child, VIII*, 155–161.

Rizzolatti, G., & Arbib, M. A. (1998). Language within our grasp. *Trends in Neurosciences, 21*(5), 188–194.

Rizzolatti, G., & Craighero, L. (2004). The mirror-neuron system. *Annual Review of Neuroscience, 27*, 169–192.

Rogers, S. J., & Pennington, B. F. (1991). A theoretical approach to the deficits in infantile autism. *Developmental Psychology, 3*, 137–162.

Sawamura, H., Orban, G. A., & Vogels, R. (2006). Selectivity of neuronal adaptation does not match response selectivity: a single-cell study of the FMRI adaptation paradigm. *Neuron, 49*(2), 307–318.

Seltzer, B., & Pandya, D. N. (1994). Parietal, temporal, and occipital projections to cortex of the superior temporal sulcus in the rhesus monkey: a retrograde tracer study. *Journal of Comparative Neurology, 343*(3), 445–463.

Shepherd, S. V., Klein, J. T., Deaner, R. O., & Platt, M. L. (2009). Mirroring of attention by neurons in macaque parietal cortex. *Proceedings of the National Academy of Science U S A, 106*(23), 9489–9494.

Smith, A. (1759). *The theory of moral sentiments.* Oxford, UK: Clarendon Press.

Southgate, V., & de C Hamilton, A. F. (2008). Unbroken mirrors: challenging a theory of Autism. *Trends in Cognitive Sciences, 12*(6), 225–229.

Tkach, D., Reimer, J., & Hatsopoulos, N. G. (2007). Congruent activity during action and action observation in motor cortex. *Journal of Neuroscience, 27*(48), 13241–13250.

Tootell, R. B., Reppas, J. B., Dale, A. M., Look, R. B., Sereno, M. I., Malach, R., et al. (1995). Visual motion aftereffect in human cortical area MT revealed by functional magnetic resonance imaging. *Nature, 375*(6527), 139–141.

Umiltà, M. A., Escola, L., Intskirveli, I., Grammont, F., Rochat, M., Caruana, F., et al. (2008). When pliers become fingers in the monkey motor system. *Proceedings of the National Academy of Science U S A, 105*(6), 2209–2213.

Umiltà, M. A., Kohler, E., Gallese, V., Fogassi, L., Fadiga, L., Keysers, C., et al. (2001). I know what you are doing. a neurophysiological study. *Neuron, 31*(1), 155–165.

Williams, J. H., Waiter, G. D., Gilchrist, A., Perrett, D. I., Murray, A. D., & Whiten, A. (2006). Neural mechanisms of imitation and "mirror neuron" functioning in autistic spectrum disorder. *Neuropsychologia, 44*(4), 610–621.

Williams, J. H., Whiten, A., Suddendorf, T., & Perrett, D. I. (2001). Imitation, mirror neurons and autism. *Neuroscience and Biobehavioral Reviews, 25*(4), 287–295.

Wittgenstein, L. (1980). *Remarks on the Philosophy of Psychology.* Oxford, UK: Blackwell.

57 Keith J. Yoder, Matthew K. Belmonte

Information Processing and Integration

Points of Interest

- The autistic brain is characterized by abnormal network architecture (increase in short-range connections and decrease or perturbation in long-range connections) and abnormal network recruitment.
- Network disruptions in autism manifest as intact or enhanced low-level information processing and dysfunctional or disengaged complex information processing.
- Deficits in complex information processing affect all domains of perception and cognition.
- Diagnostically salient social abnormalities may arise in combination with, or even partially as a consequence of, disordered perceptual processing.
- Some of these antecedent network abnormalities appear to be familial traits.

Developmental Disorders and Neural Information Processing

Much like the people whom it seeks to understand, autism research is prone to a sort of "weak central coherence," with a multiplicity of hypotheses targeted at particular systems or levels of analysis. The most vexing problem often is not identifying the observational details but assembling these details into a single, coherent theory. The challenge of autism research is that its work has been fractionated within many separate models of dysfunction, reflecting the many separate perspectives and approaches of cognitive and systems neuroscience that have been brought to bear on it. These models only now are beginning to be combined. Focusing on autism's social deficits, some have characterized autism as a dysfunction in a cognitive module for "theory of mind" (ToM), the ability to think in terms of social partners' beliefs and desires (Baron-Cohen et al., 1985, 2002). Others explain both social and nonsocial phenomena as consequences of a more general dysfunction of executive control (Hill, 2004), shifting and distribution of attention (Allen & Courchesne, 2001), "central coherence" of gestalt or global-level percepts (Frith & Happé, 1994; Happé & Frith, 2006), or an enhancement of local processing, often at the expense of engaging intact global-level processing (Mottron et al., 2006). Although each of these theories seems to contain at least a piece of the picture, the process of putting these pieces together has begun only recently (Belmonte et al., 2004b; Mottron et al., 2006).

In science, as in any human endeavor, what is discovered is constrained by what is looked for. All too often, experiments are framed so as to confirm or to refute hypotheses within one theoretical framework. ToM studies show deficits in tasks of attributing false belief (Baron-Cohen et al., 1985), executive function studies show deficits in tasks of planning (Hughes et al., 1994) and inhibition of prepotent responses (Ozonoff et al., 1994), attention studies show slowed shifting (Courchesne et al., 1994a) and abnormal distribution (Townsend & Courchesne, 1994; Burack, 1994) of attention, studies of central coherence show facilitation on tasks of perceptual disembedding (Shah & Frith, 1993; Plaisted et al., 1998), and perceptual studies show enhanced discrimination of first-order stimuli (Plaisted et al., 2003; Bertone et al., 2003, 2005). Each of these foundational results has been individually confirmed by further explorations, but each has remained largely unintegrated with other findings.

Significantly, within each of these domains of exploration, there is very appreciable variance in behavioral and physiological measures: many children with autism pass tasks of first-order or even second-order belief attribution (Frith & Happé, 1994); deficits in executive function vary across task paradigms, executive subdomains, and individuals (Hill, 2004); attention varies between abnormally narrow "spotlight" and abnormally broad distributions (Townsend & Courchesne, 1994); central coherence as measured by the Embedded

Figures Test varies substantially within the autism population and, in fact, correlates with similarly variable performance on ToM tests (Jarrold et al., 2000); and perceptual variation in motion coherence thresholds is very large, with a third of the autism population within the normal range (Milne et al., 2002; Belmonte, 2005). Despite this richness of variance within perceptual and cognitive domains, with a few notable exceptions (e.g., Jarrold et al., 2000), the covariance structure between domains remains unexplored. Linking these investigations is important because in illuminating pervasive abnormalities of neural information processing that span cognitive domains, one can explain how these domains normally relate to one another computationally and developmentally—in both abnormal and normal developmental contexts (Valla et al., 2010).

Recent theoretical constructions of autism have converged on the notion of a systems-level dysfunction in neural computation (Belmonte et al., 2004a, b), one whose interactions with normal programs of brain and cognitive development may result in perturbations at many levels of processing. Autistic deficits in complex social and communicative skills are comparatively well-studied, as these deficits are the most obvious, the most diagnostic, and the most debilitating. However, the relevance of abnormalities at lower levels of function (Rogers & Ozonoff, 2005) ought not to be ignored, as perturbations at these simpler, more tractable levels of processing may offer insights at the systems level. In particular, correlation between behavioral and physiological studies of sensory and attentional phenomena on the one hand, and complex social cognitive processes on the other, may illuminate abnormal modes of development in which a systems-level abnormality perturbs both low and high levels of processing, and/or abnormal developmental cascades in which dysfunction at low levels of processing perturbs activity-dependent development at higher levels. Support for the notion of such multilevel cascades of perturbed development comes from the success of interventions addressing rapid auditory sequence processing in language and communication disorders (Tallal et al., 1996, 2004; Fitch & Tallal, 2003), from studies of schizophrenia demonstrating deficits in early sensory processing (Butler & Javitt, 2005; Uhlhaas & Silverstein, 2005; Butler et al., 2007) and relating auditory frequency discrimination to deficits in affect recognition (Leitman et al., 2007) and visual size discrimination to deficits in ToM (Uhlhaas et al., 2006), from physiological studies of autism suggesting compensatory processing for dysfunctions in early sensory and attentional computations (Belmonte & Yurgelun-Todd, 2003) and behavioral studies linking joint attention to ToM and pretense (Charman, 1997), and even from studies of normal development and aging showing that deficits in automatic, early processing evoke downstream, compensatory abnormalities in later, more effortful stages of neuro-cognitive processing (Townsend et al., 2006). In each of these instances, what seems on face an alteration of higher-order cognition is seen to be related to, and in some cases a consequence of, perturbations at lower levels of processing.

Abnormal Complex Information Processing in Autism

The beginnings of a conception of autism as abnormal complex information processing arose from neurological evaluations of children with autism (e.g., Minshew & Payton, 1998). Many of the characteristic behavioral abnormalities in autism (e.g., seizures, mental retardation, and deficits in higher-order cognition and complex behaviors) are consistent with abnormal function of association cortex and cerebral gray matter. At the same time, autism is not characteristically associated with deficits in sensorimotor cortex (e.g., cerebral palsy, blindness, deafness). These findings led Minshew et al. initially to conclude that autism was characterized by an intact sensorimotor cortex but an abnormal association cortex.

Further, many children with autism have no difficulties learning new words (supporting the hypothesis that autism is not the result of focal brain dysfunction) and are quite capable of repeating words or phrases (e.g., in immediate echolalia) but seem to have problems with comprehension and the production of novel, spontaneous expressive language. These observations suggest that dysfunction in autism results primarily from an abnormal development of brain connectivity, affecting functional relationships between association cortex and sensorimotor cortex. This neuropsychologically driven view of autism as a disorder of neural connectivity has garnered support from physiological data and is consistent with therapeutic views of autism as a disconnection between cognitive and affective systems (Greenspan et al., 2001).

This integrative, neural-systems view of autism differs fundamentally from theories that have posited a single core deficit in some specific domain or sensory modality (Minshew et al., 1997), such as empathizing, executive function, ToM, or central coherence. In this view, the domain-specific deficits integral to the diagnostic triad of autism become manifestations of a general deficit in complex information processing. Autism then can be characterized by an abnormal balance between decreased or perturbed long-range connectivity and perhaps enhanced local connectivity. This perturbation of *neural* connectivity is reflected in *cognitive* connectivity, manifesting as intact or enhanced abilities in simple perceptual or cognitive tasks and deficits in complex cognitive tasks.

Deficits and Superiorities Beyond the Triad

Because autism is behaviorally defined, it is not surprising that many investigations of autism begin by examining those behaviors that are most diagnostically relevant. However, mature cognition is but the endpoint of a process of interactive specialization during which complex cognitive capacities emerge from simpler antecedents (Johnson et al., 2002). Thus, profound and pervasive deficits in social communication could be secondary to more primary neurological abnormalities. Systems-neuroscience models attempt to avoid this pitfall by seeking a broader, underlying abnormality in information processing in general.

Minshew et al. (1997) evaluated this hypothesis of complexity-dependent deficits by giving 33 adults with autism and age-matched controls a battery of neuropsychological tests to assess performance in nine domains: attention, sensory perception, motor skills, simple language, complex language, simple memory, complex memory, reasoning, and visual-spatial skills. Typically developing controls demonstrated better performance in the domains of motor skills, complex language, complex memory, and reasoning. The groups were indistinguishable in the domains of attention, sensory perception, simple memory and visual-spatial skills. The autism group demonstrated significantly better performance in the simple language domain.

The pattern of decreased performance in complex domains with intact or enhanced performance in relatively simple domains strongly supports the complexity-dependent information processing deficits hypothesis. However, a deficit in complex information processing could be expected also to produce abnormalities beyond the diagnostic triad. This prediction was confirmed by a later, large study, which found that individuals with autism develop postural control later than typically visual input with auditory or tactile information (Bonneh et al., 2008), or to combine ongoing cognitive developing children and do not attain the level of function observed in typically developing adults (Minshew et al., 2004). In further support of abnormal complex information processing, these authors found that the unusual postural development was related to a decreased ability to integrate visual, vestibular, and somatosensory information. This theme of a lack of ability to combine processing with visual input from direct gaze (Chen et al., 2010) has been cited in studies of "low-functioning" autism and has been elaborated by a recent finding of an autistic deficit in combining visual and proprioceptive feedback during a motor control task (Haswell et al., 2009). In general, autism seems marked by a lack of ability to integrate or to shift focus rapidly among distinct perceptual channels—for example, information from distinct sensory modalities (Akshoomoff & Courchesne, 1992), distinct spatial locations (Townsend et al., 1996), or even distinct perceptual channels within a sensory modality (e.g., speech content vs. speech prosody; Courchesne et al., 1994a)—and by a lack of ability to integrate such perceptual information with ongoing cognitive processing; thus individual perceptual and cognitive processes may be intact but not coordinated with each other, a realization that carries significant implications for psychological and educational therapies (Chen et al., 2010).

Minshew and colleagues repeated their initial neuropsychological profile of autism by giving 112 children (56 individuals who met diagnostic criteria for autism, 56 age- and IQ-matched controls) a similar battery of tests (Williams et al., 2006). The findings were similar in that the autism group showed decreased performance in the domains that put greater demands on information processing and integration. Unlike results from the earlier study, the children with autism did not show decreased performance in the reasoning domain or increased performance in the simple language domain. Additionally, the children with autism showed decreased performance in the sensory perception domain. Such age-related performance differences highlight the importance of understanding autism as a developmental disorder and the need to examine early stages of development to investigate its etiology.

Neurobiological Foundations of Autistic Information Processing

Just as many theories of autism have posited a single core deficit in a single domain, anatomical investigations of autism have tended to focus on localized neurobiological abnormalities. Previous research has identified specific, focal abnormalities in the brain stem (Hashimoto, 1995; Rodier et al., 1996), amygdala (Aylward et al., 1999), hippocampus (Aylward et al., 1999; Saitoh et al., 2001), cerebellum (Courchesne et al., 1988; Murakami et al., 1989; Courchesne, Townsend, & Saitoh, 1994b; Hashimoto, 1995), parietal lobes (Courchesnet et al., 1993), temporal lobes (Redcay, 2008), and frontal lobes (Carper & Courchesne, 2000; Courchesne et al., 2001; Sparks et al., 2002; Aylward et al., 2002). However, only recently have explanations begun to be offered as to how all of these anatomical abnormalities might be related, both to each other and to the complex symptomatology of autism.

This synthesis is complicated by autism's developmental nature. Many of the studies identifying specific abnormalities, whether in biology or behavior, have pragmatically investigated adult or adolescent populations. However, such an approach is ill-equipped to distinguish between a core deficit and a compensatory mechanism. As suggested earlier, many of the behaviors diagnostically essential to autism may, in fact, be secondary dysfunctions resulting from adaptive processing strategies that help normalize cognition (Belmonte et al., 2004b). Maintaining restricted interests, for example, can be an effective strategy for keeping a chaotic and unmodulated sensorium somewhat predictable and therefore cognitively tractable (Belmonte, 2008), and in fact childhood repetitive behaviors correlate with childhood fears and anxieties even in the context of normal early development (Evans et al., 1999). Any satisfying explanation of the etiology of autism must include developmentally early structure and function in the autistic brain.

Network Perturbations of Neural Information Processing

Twentieth-century neuroscience was marked by great successes at single-variable problems. Human and animal studies elucidated the effects of focal lesions affecting single brain regions and identified those regions with circumscribed cognitive capacities, resulting in clinical and basic understandings of focal brain disorders such as well-characterized frontal and temporal aphasias, parietal hemi-neglect, and medial temporal anterograde amnesia. Nearly coeval with these advances in the understanding of isolated brain regions came an understanding of the effects of isolated genes: errors in single genes give rise to well-characterized brain disorders as diverse as Huntington's disease and Rett Syndrome. As difficult as these problems were to solve, they were in some sense the low-hanging fruit. Twentieth-century, univariate neuroscience has been supplanted by the multivariate, integrative neuroscience of the twenty-first century, and the canonical multivariate neuroscientific problems are complex neuropsychiatric conditions that perturb networks of cooperating cognitive capacities, networks of communicating brain regions, and networks of interacting genes. Single-gene dysfunctions (e.g., Fragile X Syndrome [Pieretti et al., 1991], Timothy Syndrome [Amir et al., 1999], or the aforementioned Rett Syndrome [Splawski et al., 2004]) may mimic multivariate disorders, in that they involve dysfunctions in single genes whose protein products interact with many other genes and/or proteins, either by regulating transcription (Rett Syndrome and *MECP2*) or translation (Fragile X Syndrome and *FMR1*) or by perturbing the kinetics of ubiquitous cellular signaling mechanisms (Timothy Syndrome and *CACNA1C*). In these specific cases, however, what is in one sense a single-gene disorder is more proximally the result of network perturbations affecting the many genes and proteins whose regulation is directly or indirectly disrupted. In the general case, then, complex neuropsychiatric conditions arise from multiple interacting genetic factors—and, no doubt, environmental ones too.

Human cognition, including scientists' cognition, operates by constructing fetishes, in the anthropological sense of the term. That is, we think by attaching meanings to concrete artifacts that function as symbols. In the domain of neuroscience, these artifacts are brain regions, genes, proteins. Because our minds are structured for symbolic manipulations, it's easy for us to think of the anatomy of a piece of the brain or the structure of a gene or a protein. It becomes more difficult to wrap our heads around a problem, however, when the problem is defined not in terms of concrete objects but in terms of abstract networks. This preference for the concrete—ironically, given scientists' descriptions of autism's detail-oriented perception and trouble with abstraction—is why neuroscience and neuroscientists still enjoy pretending that complex disorders boil down to single brain regions in fMRI studies or to single susceptibility genes. The true picture certainly is more complicated: fMRI studies that show neatly delimited activations may be looking only at the major node or nodes within distributed networks of functional anatomy, and genetic studies that associate autism with a single allele may be looking only at an entry point to a complex graph structure of genetic interactions. Univariate projections of these complex networks are useful insofar as they provide such entry points from which the rest of the network connectivity graph can be explored.

The complexity-dependent pattern of deficits and intact or enhanced abilities, then, is the result of abnormal networks, both at the genetic and neuronal level. The topic of networks of interacting genes is covered elsewhere in this volume and will be reprised briefly at the end of this chapter. For now, the focus will turn to networks of interacting neurons. Work in the fields of graph theory and dynamical systems theory can be applied to neural networks to provide useful insights.

Dynamical Systems Theory. Mathematically defining the behaviors of networks is of interest to researchers in many fields, including physics, mathematics, and computer science (and increasingly, neuroscientists), and many of their insights are particularly relevant to neurobiology. Three concepts especially applicable to the brain are *(1)* synchronicity, *(2)* "small-world" networks, and *(3)* "scale-free" networks. (For a more thorough review, *see* Strogatz, 2001.)

Synchronicity is the extent to which oscillators in a network are related in terms of frequency and amplitude. Kuramoto (1984) discovered that a fairly simple mathematical equation can predict the number of edges that must be added to a collection of oscillators before some of the oscillators in that network synchronize. As the number of "edges" (connections) in the network increases past this connectivity threshold, more and more "nodes" (cells or columns or functional regions, depending on one's anatomical level of analysis) synchronize until the network is fully interconnected and all of the nodes are oscillating in unison. A biological example of a fully synchronized network is the sinoatrial node (Peskin, 1975). In this "natural pacemaker," even if the cells are not initially synchronized, the networked structure of the node causes the cells to synchronize over time.

"Small-world" networks are characterized by short average path lengths and high clustering. A classic example of a small-world network is the network of co-authors within a given discipline (e.g., Strogatz, 2001), where authors are the nodes and collaboration on a paper defines the edges—that is, if A and B have written a paper together, then (A, B) is an edge in the graph structure. Authors that are affiliated with the same institutions tend to be co-authors on each other's papers, creating many intramural edges (clustering). When researchers from different institutions collaborate, a shortcut is created between these institutional clusters (short path length). In a neurobiological context, small-world networks are interesting because it has been argued that such networks might have been selected for as an adaptation to a sensory-rich environment.

The "degree" of a node is the number of edges (connections) attached to that node. **"Scale-free" networks** have mostly low-degree (sparsely connected) nodes but a few high-degree (densely connected) nodes, or "hubs" (Barbási & Albert, 1999). These high-degree hubs can act as gateways for the shortcuts of a small-world network, and so many networks exhibit both small-world and scale-free properties. Scale-free networks are particularly interesting because they are resistant to random failure: intact function of neural and cognitive networks does not depend on the functional integrity of any particular subgroup of neurons. On the other hand, scale-free networks are very susceptible to targeted attacks—that is, if a hub is disrupted, then the entire network could be disrupted (Albert, Jeong, & Barbási, 2000; Barbási, Albert, & Jeong, 1999; Cohen, Erez, ben-Avraham, & Havlin, 2000). These properties may hold important implications for the developmental role of frontal-lobe hub abnormalities in autism.

The Brain As a Network

A great deal of research has shown that the nervous systems in biological organisms follow a scale-free and small-world organizational scheme. This characteristic holds even for relatively simple organisms such as the worm *Caenorhabditis elegans* (Strogatz, 2001). Before recent developments in neuroimaging, neurologists were positing small-world structural networks (using different terminology) based on lesion studies. Mesulam (1990) proposed that behavior and cognition arose from a collection of parallel distributed processing networks in the brain, each comprising several "widely separated and interconnected local networks." Using data gleaned from lesion studies, it was possible to identify the cortical and subcortical regions (local networks) necessary for a given behavior or cognitive task. Importantly, this work helped to highlight the fact that an observed deficit in some complex emergent capability could be arrived at from multiple, distinct mechanistic pathways (i.e., insult to any of the relevant hubs—highly connected cortical areas—could produce downstream disruption of the entire network).

With the advent of new technologies, it has become possible to begin to examine these systems in healthy individuals, allowing researchers to investigate normal variation in neural and cognitive networks. More recent research has directly shown that the human brain also follows a small-world organizational scheme at several levels of analysis (e.g., Supekar, Musen, & Menon, 2009). Many have argued that the human brain is also a scale-free network (e.g., Heuvel et al., 2008), although some are not convinced (Achard et al., 2006). Regardless, few would argue with the assertion that the vehicle by which diverse cortical and subcortical areas collaborate is synchronization. As discussed above, the synchronicity of a network depends in part on the connectivity of the network. *Connectivity*, however, is an overloaded term, susceptible to various theoretical definitions and to various experimental measures. Special care must be taken to specify the type of connectivity being discussed.

The Confusion of *Connectivity*

At a gross level, one can make a distinction between *structural connectivity* (i.e., nodes and edges of the network are physical structures) and *functional connectivity*, wherein the nodes are still physical structures, but the edges of a functional network are statistical relationships (usually measures of correlation or covariance). Functional connectivity, for its part, can be defined in raw terms of the degree to which one neuron or one neural assembly activates another or in terms of the degree to which information is transferred between neurons or neural assemblies. The first sense of this term—that of simple co-activation—is easily captured by statistical measures of correlation or covariation between two spike trains or two electroencephalography (EEG) or fMRI time series. The second sense is more complex and often of greater practical import. The capacity of a neural assembly—or of any computational system—to represent information depends on the number of distinct states in which it can exist. For example, a railway signal in operation can exist in three distinct states conveying three distinct pieces of information: red (stop), amber (caution), and green (go). The information-theoretic measure of entropy is a quantitative measure of this tendency of a computing system to exist in multiple states. This discussion will avoid mathematical definitions, focusing instead on the intuitive concept.

Consider, as a simplified example, the representation of information on a whiteboard. Each patch of the whiteboard can be either filled or unfilled by ink from a marker. In normal use, the whiteboard has a very high entropy because there are many possible distinct configurations (states) of filled or unfilled patches, and these many configurations each can represent characters or graphics. In the case where the marker dries out, however, the board is left with only one state—all white. Entropy is consequently zero, and no information can be represented. This case is analogous to that of pathologically weak neural connections in which neural assemblies remain in an all-off state regardless of the inputs with which they're presented. In the converse case where the marker bleeds all over the board the moment it touches the surface, again there is only one state, this time all black, and again the entropy is zero. This case is analogous to that of pathologically strong neural connections in which neural assemblies activate at the drop of a hat and remain activated. From this simple example, it can be seen that connectivity in terms of information transfer is not necessarily the same as connectivity measured in terms of mutual activations: the greatest degree of mutual activation evokes the least information capacity. In particular, overconnectivity at a neural level (or in general at the level of relatively local cell assemblies) may evoke underconnectivity at a cognitive level (Belmonte et al., 2004a)—a relationship that may be very significant for autism, as we shall see.

Entropy also exists in structural networks. Recall that for small-world networks, there exists a connectivity threshold for synchronicity. In a network whose connectivity is below this threshold, none of the neurons will synchronize. At the other extreme, a network whose connectivity greatly exceeds this threshold could become entirely synchronized. As in the case of the malfunctioning marker board, such a network loses its selectivity. Rather than pairing activation patterns with distinct stimuli, the overconnected network responds indiscriminately to any stimulus.

A growing body of research has found that individuals with autism exhibit abnormalities in functional (task-related and resting-state) networks as well as structural networks (Noonan et al., 2009), characterized by an increase in short-range, small-scale connections at the expense of long-range, large-scale connections (Courchesne et al., 2007; Hasson et al., 2009; Kennedy & Courchesne, 2008; Minshew & Williams, 2007). These findings lend support to the notion that disruptions in the finely tuned balance between underconnectivity and overconnectivity, perhaps associated in some cases with an imbalance at the neural level between inhibition and excitation (Rubenstein & Merzenich, 2003) may produce the wide-ranging symptomatology of autism spectrum conditions.

Further evidence for disordered neural networks comes from the investigations of abnormal neural structure and function associated with autism. The cortex of the autistic cerebellum contains abnormally few Purkinje cells and granule cells (Williams et al., 1980; Ritvo et al., 1986; Bauman & Kemper, 1985; Bauman & Kemper, 1994), which could allow disinhibition in the cerebellar deep nuclei causing downstream overexcitation of the thalamus and its cerebral cortical projections. At a cerebral cortical level, one report has noted that densities of dendritic spines in autism are generally increased (Hutsler & Zhang, 2010), although this increase occurred with an idiosyncratic anatomical distribution in different individuals: on average across individuals and across the several anatomical regions sampled, autistic spine densities exceed non-autistic densities; however, this relationship has been pinned down to a single region only in the case of output layer 5 in temporal cortex (Brodmann area 22). An increase in spine densities at the neural level is consistent with abnormalities of information transfer at the computational level of analysis, and the idiosyncratic distributions are consistent with similar individual variations in patterns of functional activation detected by fMRI in contexts of motor (Müller et al., 2001), visuomotor (Müller et al., 2003), free viewing (Hasson et al., 2009), and face perception tasks (Pierce et al., 2001) and suggest an interaction between individual experience and a systems-level perturbation of some general mechanism for synaptic plasticity or learning. Notable in this connection is the raft of recent results on autism-associated disorders, suggesting that alteration of activity-dependent synaptic plasticity may be one route into the neural computational differences that can produce autism (Kelleher & Bear, 2008; Sharma et al., 2010; Hoeffer & Klann, 2010); these results begin with Fragile X Syndrome but may generalize to other autism-associated pathophysiologies.

Finally, because brain networks exhibit at least some scale-free properties, and thus should be resilient to randomly located failures within the network but not to failures at network hubs, another crucial question is whether individuals with autism demonstrate structural or functional abnormalities of the hubs of networks that subserve behaviors associated with autism, both within and beyond the diagnostic triad. Based on the current literature, the answer appears to be "yes." When shown pictures of eyes and asked to infer mental states, individuals with autism show enhanced activation of the superior temporal gyrus, accompanied by reduced activations in prefrontal and medial temporal areas (Baron-Cohen et al., 1999). Further, the connectivity between extrastriate visual areas and prefrontal and temporal areas normally associated with inferring mental states is reduced. When given the Embedded Figures Test (a task that relies on visually separating local details from a gestalt whole), individuals with autism show enhanced activation of ventral visual areas in the occipital cortex, despite reduced activations in parietal and prefrontal areas (Ring et al., 1999). When viewing faces, activation in the fusiform gyrus is reduced, yet areas outside the "face area" of the fusiform gyrus (Pierce et al., 2001), including inferior temporal gyrus (Schultz et al., 2000) and peristriate cortex (Critchley et al., 2000), show enhanced activation.

Prefrontal cortex (PFC) plays an important role in many higher-order cognitive functions. Gilbert et al. (2008) found that individuals with autism showed task-specific atypical recruitment of medial PFC during an executive function task; of the many areas examined in the study, medial PFC was the only area that distinguished between the autism and control groups. The same result has been obtained in the case of a task of auditory change detection in which anterior cingulate activation nearly completely differentiated autism-spectrum and non-autism-spectrum boys (Gomot et al., 2005) and in the case of a complex task of visual attention, in which boys with autism spectrum conditions did not differentially activate anterior cingulate cortex as a function of task complexity and showed a delayed and prolonged activation of dorsolateral prefrontal cortex (Belmonte et al., 2010), echoing at a physiological level many behavioral findings of long latency to disengage and to shift attention (e.g. Courchesne et al., 1994a; Townsend et al., 1996, 1999; Belmonte, 2000; Landry & Bryson, 2004)—a phenomenon that constitutes one of autism's earliest behavioral signs (Zwaigenbaum et al., 2005). Significantly, many of the clinically unaffected siblings of children with autism spectrum conditions show attentional function intermediate between that of normal and autism spectrum groups and a typically autistic time-course of delayed and prolonged differential frontal activation when attention-demanding and less demanding task conditions are compared (Belmonte et al., 2010), suggesting that this delayed frontal discrimination may be a familial endophenotype permissive, but not determinative, of autistic development.

In autism, it seems, perception and cognition are driven in a bottom-up manner, with stimulus discrimination depending on early activation of posterior cortical regions subserving sensory and perceptual organization (e.g., Belmonte & Yurgelun-Todd, 2003) and frontal discrimination being brought to bear only much later (Figure 57-1), often too late for the demands of timed tasks that require quick-response decisions. This pattern stands in contrast to the physiology of nonautistic perception and cognition, in which discrimination is driven strongly and early by top-down signals from frontal cortex. Despite this strong difference between autistic and nonautistic populations, at an individual level it becomes somewhat more difficult to distinguish autistic and nonautistic people on the basis of brain physiology: in fact, the degree of delay in differential frontal activation correlates with psychometric measures of autistic traits, not only in those with autism spectrum disorders but also in their clinically unaffected siblings, even in unrelated children without any autism spectrum conditions in the family! It may be the case, then, that this dimensional variation in the degree of frontally based, top-down information processing represents a continuum of cognitive variation in all human beings, autistic or not.

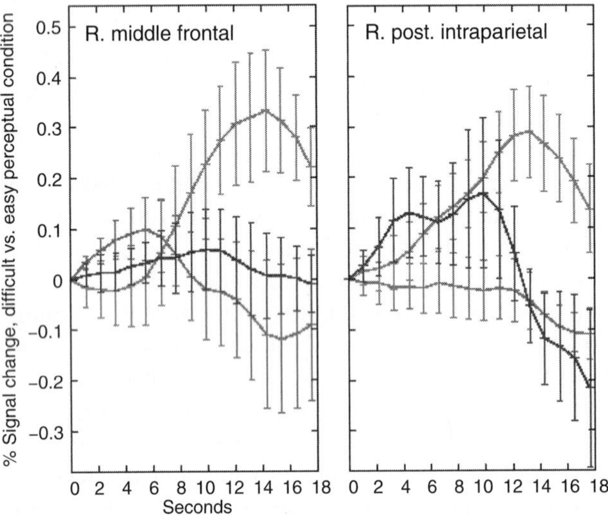

Figure 57–1. Top-down cognition in non-autistic individuals, bottom-up cognition in those with autism spectrum conditions. fMRI time-courses from prefrontal cortex (right middle frontal gyrus) and posterior, sensory-driven cortex (right posterior intraparietal sulcus at its junction with transverse occipital sulcus) illustrate that non-autistic children (red) respond rapidly to a difficult perceptual problem with additional frontal activation. In those with autism spectrum conditions (blue), this differential frontal activation is muted, delayed, and prolonged so far past the end of the experimental trial that it is of no use in rendering a response decision. Those with autism spectrum conditions seem rather to depend on bottom-up signaling from early activation of posterior cortices. Clinically unaffected sibs (magenta) of those with autism spectrum conditions manifest a similarly delayed and prolonged time-course of differential frontal activation, and a frontally driven, top-down activation of posterior cortex but not the autistic, bottom-up, early peak in posterior cortical activation. Reprinted with permission from Belmonte et al. (2010). Visual attention in autism families: "unaffected" sibs share atypical frontal activation *Journal of Child Psychology and Psychiatry*, *51*, 259–276, published by Blackwell Publishing on behalf of the Association for Child and Adolescent Mental Health. (See Color Plate Section for a color version of this figure.)

What may differentiate clinically affected and unaffected individuals, then, is the developmental translation of this dimensional, anatomically localized abnormality, within the frontal connectivity hub, to a more generalized, categorical degradation of functional connectivity throughout the brain: autism spectrum probands manifest this whole-brain connectivity degradation, whereas unaffected siblings do not (Belmonte et al., 2010)—or at least not to any similar degree (Figure 57-2). Future longitudinal studies of younger sibs at risk for autism spectrum conditions may usefully examine this question of the relationship between familial frontal-lobe abnormality and anatomically generalized disruption of functional connectivity.

Connectivity in Autism

To identify abnormalities in connectivity, it is essential to understand connectivity in typically developing individuals. For more than a decade, resting-state fMRI has been applied to investigate functional connectivity in humans. The first of this work applied low-frequency (<0.1 Hz) fluctuations in BOLD signal to identify functionally connected areas of motor cortex, which were later shown to be associated with motor function (Biswal et al., 1995). More recently, this method has been employed to assess the resting-state "default" network in healthy adults.

A recent study employing resting-state fMRI distinguished a "salience network" and "cognitive-control network" in healthy adults (Seeley et al., 2007). The "salience network" comprises superior temporal pole, anterior insula, and paracingulate and anterior cingulate cortices, with functional connections to temporal, parietal opercular, dorsolateral PFC, and subcortical areas, including parts of the thalamus, hypothalamus, extended amygdala, striatopallidum, substantia nigra, and periaqueductal gray. Activation of this network, specifically dorsolateral PFC and dorsal anterior cingulate cortex (ACC), correlates with reported levels of anxiety prior to scanning. The "executive-control network" comprises left frontoinsular areas and lateral PFC and dorsomedial PFC, with subcortical functional connections extending into anterior thalamus and dorsal caudate. Activations in this functional network are positively correlated with performance on a cognitively demanding task (the Trail Making Test).

Cherkassky et al. (2006) compared the resting-state functional networks in autism and control groups and found that both networks comprised similar areas, but the autistic resting-state network was less strongly connected. In another study (Just et al., 2004), subjects were asked to read and answer questions about sentences. Individuals with autism showed greater activations in left lateral superior temporal areas (classically defined Wernicke's area) and reduced activation in left inferior frontal gyrus (classically defined Broca's area). They also exhibited reduced functional connectivity between the two regions, indicating reduced synchronization between

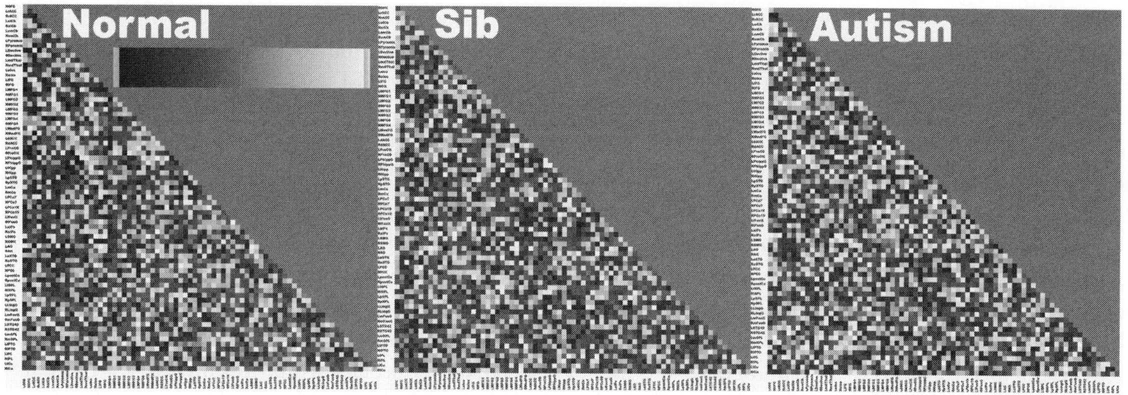

Figure 57–2. Functional connectivity among 76 brain regions (38 bilateral pairs) in children with autism spectrum conditions, clinically unaffected sibs of children with autism spectrum conditions, and unrelated non-autistic children. The axes are lists of brain regions; a colored dot indicates a statistically significant correlations between fMRI time-courses in the indicated region pair. Although no difference survives correction for the large number of multiple comparisons, when measures are collapsed across all regions pairs, the non-autistic and sib groups are statistically indistinguishable in their degrees of overall functional connectivity, whereas both groups are highly significantly distinct from the autism spectrum group. Reprinted with permission from Belmonte et al. (2010) Visual attention in autism families: "unaffected" sibs share atypical frontal activation. *Journal of Child Psychology and Psychiatry, 51*, 259–276, published by Blackwell Publishing on behalf of the Association for Child and Adolescent Mental Health. (See Color Plate Section for a color version of this figure.)

the broad cortical areas termed Broca's and Wernicke's. Cortical networks appear to demonstrate small-world and scale-free properties. Achard et al. (2006) defined a functional network with 90 cortical and subcortical regions. This network satisfied small-world criteria, with highly connected hubs located mainly in association areas of neocortex. They contrasted this "core" with the "periphery" of paralimbic areas that were less highly connected. By employing diffusion tensor imaging (DTI), they also identified white matter tracts underlying these functionally connected cortical regions. Moreover, these small-world anatomical networks closely mirror those already identified in cat and macaque cortex.

More recently, van den Heuvel et al. (2008) applied a similar methodology to investigate resting-state functionally connected networks in 28 healthy adults. They found small-world and scale-free characteristics in their voxel-based analysis and identified potential hub regions in bilateral anterior cingulate cortex, bilateral superior temporal lobe, bilateral thalamus, and bilateral posterior cingulate cortex. A follow-up study by DTI and fMRI confirmed that anatomically connected cortical areas on either end of well-known white matter tracts (e.g., genu and splenium of the corpus callusom, bilateral fronto-occipital, and parietal fasiculi) also exhibited functional connectivity (van den Heuvel et al., 2009).

Until quite recently, there have been almost no studies examining how functional networks in the brain change developmentally. Understanding the developmental trajectory of typically developing individuals is important because of the developmental nature of autism. Following the precedent set by Mesulam (2000), Supekar, Musen, and Menon (2009) parcellated the brain into five regions: primary sensory, subcortical, limbic, paralimbic, and association. Assaying differences between children and young adults with respect to small-world characteristics of these functional networks as defined by resting-state fMRI, they found that resting-state functional networks exhibit small-world properties (high clustering and low average path length) in both adults and children. However, the adults exhibited increased functional connectivity for cortico-cortical connections relative to children. These developmental changes in functional correlation were also related to changes in anatomy. DTI revealed that the child group was characterized by a greater number of short-range structural connections. In the adult group, these short-range connections were fewer and long-range connections became much more prevalent. Further, functional connectivity between anatomically close brain regions was greater in children than in adults, whereas functional connectivity between distant regions (whether measured by Euclidian distance or fiber-tract length) was greater in adults than in children. Supekar et al. concluded that normal development is a dynamic processes, wherein the brain is initially (at least by age 6 years) overconnected, both structurally and functionally. Subsequent pruning and rewiring reduce short-range structural and functional connections and increase long-range connections. Future anatomical and physiological studies of autism can usefully address, longitudinally or even simply cross-sectionally, this issue of the developmental relation between short-range and long-range connectivity.

These developmental abnormalities of connectivity may relate to more commonly measured developmental abnormalities of tissue volume. Because of the timing of diagnosis, little is known about autistic brain volume perinatally. By the second year of life, however, white matter and gray matter volumes have increased relative to typically developing controls (Courchesne et al., 1999; Ben Bashat et al., 2007). White matter increases, driven by premature myelination in frontal regions (Ben Bashat et al., 2007) are most pronounced in later developing, anterior regions of the brain, specifically in frontal and temporal lobes but not the posterior occipital lobe (Carper & Courchesne, 2005; Carper et al., 2002; Courchesne et al., 2001, Hazlett et al., 2005; Sparks et al., 2002). Gray matter development follows a similar pattern, with early overgrowth in frontal and temporal lobes but not in the occipital lobe (Bloss & Courchesne, 2007; Carper et al., 2002, Hazlett et al., 2006; Keats et al., 2004; Palmer et al., 2005). Later decreases in gray matter volumes are evidenced by cortical thinning and abnormal white matter development in frontal, temporal, and superior temporal areas in adults with autism (Hadjikhani et al., 2006; Lee et al., 2007). These changes are especially relevant to the connectivity paradigm; some have suggested that the developmental trajectory of brain volume is more strongly linked to performance on cognitive tasks than measures of static brain volume (Shaw et al., 2006).

This issue of brain size is important because it constrains the ratio of short-range to long-range anatomical connections. An increase in long-range connections is associated with a smaller brain, both in the context of brain imaging of normal adults (Lewis et al., 2009) and in a computational model based on anatomical observations of autism (Lewis & Elman, 2008). This relationship is thought to have been established evolutionarily because it helps to maximize cellular efficiency and to minimize conduction delays (Ringo, 1991; Ringo et al., 1994; Lewis et al., 2009). An increase in overall brain volume should be accompanied by an increase in short-range, intrahemispheric, and cortico-cortical connections and a reduction in long-range and inter-hemispheric connections. Thus, it should come as no surprise that autism is marked by a reduction in corpus callosum volume (e.g., Egaas et al., 1995; Alexander et al., 2007; Just et al., 2007) and abnormal white matter growth specific to short-range connections such as the corona radiata and intrahemispheric corticocortical connections (Herbert et al., 2004). Such an increase in local structural connectivity could degrade the signal-to-noise ratio of those networks by pushing the interconnectedness of the neurons too far past their synchronization threshold—a possibility consistent with the strong comorbidity of autism and epilepsy (Ballaban-Gil & Tuchman, 2000).

Manifestations of Abnormal Information Processing in Autism

These long-range connections, especially to and from frontal and parietal areas, are essential for large-scale networks subserving the unique computational complexities of social cognition, such as the resting or "default" network and the oft-cited "mirror neurone system" (Courchesne et al., 2007). Large-scale networks that additionally involve parietal areas have been postulated to mediate perspective-taking, both in a physical visuo-spatial sense and in a social ToM sense (Frith & Frith, 2006). Autism is often conceptualized from the perspective of cognitive modularism as though it were a selective deficit in a module for ToM, the ability to represent others' beliefs and desires as separate from one's own and to act on such separable representations. However, this exclusive conceptualization in terms of ToM cannot explain autism's characteristic pattern of superiorities and deficits in nonsocial domains, such as those described by the notion of "weak central coherence" (Frith & Happé, 1994). Key to unifying autism's social and nonsocial symptoms domains is understanding autism as a *developmental* condition—developmental not only in terms of its nosology but in terms of its etiology, in which complex social cognitive traits may unfold from more subtle abnormalities in simpler, nonsocial capacities, or in which both social and nonsocial symptoms may arise from common disruptions at the level of the underlying neural systems and substrates on which these capacities are built and refined as development proceeds. Thus, although autism's social and communicative deficits are its most obvious, most diagnostic, and most debilitating symptoms, they are not necessarily its most etiologically primary.

A possible computational connection between ToM or perspective-taking in general and the more sensory and perceptual qualities of weak central coherence is provided by a reframing of perspective-taking as the translation of egocentric into allocentric perspectives (Frith & de Vignemont, 2005). In this view, the core computational issue is described not in social terms but in the more perceptual terms of the transformation of egocentric coordinates (those centered on the observer) to allocentric ones (those centered on the surrounding space—-whether concrete physical or more abstract social space—and those who occupy it). This unifying view has links, too, with the notion of enhanced perceptual function in autism (Mottron et al., 2006) in that imagining an allocentric perspective demands suppressing one's own, veridical, perceptually immediate, and salient egocentric perspective on the world (Belmonte, 2008). Whereas this replacement of a detail-oriented, disconnected veridical percept with a more abstract, bound, and contextualized symbolic representation was described by Frith and Happé (1994) in the context of autism as "central coherence," Trope describes exactly the same concept as "level of construal" (Liberman & Trope, 2008) and relates it to the concept of psychological distance, which spans both simple spatial or geometric distance and social distance. In normal subjects, the spatial distance from which events are perceived is associated with more social and abstract forms of psychological distance such as perception of goal-directedness and use of abstract rather than concrete language (Fujita et al., 2006). Thus, autism's social, linguistic, and perceptual abnormalities may be all pieces, related to each other computationally in the same way in which less extreme variations in these abilities are inter-related in typically developing people.

Studies of complex cognitive traits tend to place experimental control at odds with ecological validity, and it usually is experimental control that wins. A simple Posner attention paradigm, for example, is a very specific assay for the disengagement, shifting, and engagement of attention, but its repetitive trials may so fail to engage the experimental subject's interest and excitement that the experiment fails to measure the levels to which these capacities are engaged in everyday behavior. Many investigators are attempting to find a way between the horns of this dilemma of experimental control versus ecological validity by embedding well-controlled stimuli in more naturalistic contexts (e.g., Valla et al., 2010).

A 2009 study (Cohen et al.) has helped to elucidate how social and spatial perspective-taking might be differentiated neurologically. Five adults with pharmacoresistant epilepsy (but not autism) were asked to provide responses that required either spatial or social perspective-taking. Four of the subjects had presurgical electrodes implanted on the surface of temporal cortex, and the fifth subject had a lesion in pSTS. The individual with a lesion to pSTS was significantly slower and less accurate at the social perspective-taking condition. Additionally, the four individuals with intracranial electrodes demonstrated significantly greater gamma power over pSTS during social perspective-taking as compared to spatial perspective-taking. These results suggest that pSTS is an important component of a cortical network utilized to assess the desires of others.

Gamma: frequencies greater than 30 Hz. Gamma power has been suggested as an electrophysiological indication of perceptual binding (Engel & Singer, 2001).

STS has also been implicated in the identification of biological motion in a point light display (PLD; Blake et al., 2002). Individuals with autism seem able to identify actions but have difficulties identifying and describing emotion in the biological motion depicted by PLDs (Moore, Hobson, & Lee, 1997; Hubert et al., 2007). A biological explanation for this surprising result may come from two recent fMRI studies that examined subjects' abilities to identify intact and scrambled PLDs (Herrington et al., 2007; Freitag et al., 2008). The intact versus baseline condition produced reduced activations in middle temporal gyrus and, in Freitag et al., was accompanied by increased activations in postcentral gyri, left hippocampus, and middle frontal gyrus. Moreover, it seems that individuals with autism may be recruiting a different neural network to identify intact human movements in PLDs. Freitag et al. compared intact and scrambled conditions and found that controls activated a network involving bilateral frontal, temporal (especially STS), and parietal areas, as well as insula and basal ganglia. The autism group did not demonstrate such widespread activations. Rather, they seemed to rely on the parietal-temporal junction and frontal areas in the left hemisphere and limbic areas and thalamus in the right hemisphere. Given that autism is associated with a reduction in the white matter tracts that lie next to parietal-temporal junction and STS (Barnea-Goraly et al., 2004), biological motion abnormalities in autism provide one further example of how atypical behavior associated with autism is related to atypical recruitment of an abnormally structured brain.

Point light display (PLD): a collection of moving points of light representing points on a single moving figure. These can be generated by attaching markers to important joints on actors.

Abnormal cortical recruitment was also found in a recent study examining functional networks during adult subjects' viewing of a film clip (Hasson et al., 2009). Whereas typically developing controls exhibited a consistent activation pattern relative to the film, subjects with autism manifested neither the same activation pattern as the controls nor the same activation pattern as each other. However, subsequent analysis revealed that the observed differences in the autism group (both between groups and within group) arose because of idiosyncratic fluctuations in cortical activity in the individuals with autism. In other words, typically developing adults recruit similar cortical areas that exhibit similar activations across time during the passive viewing of a film. Individuals with autism exhibit the same pattern, but it is obscured by superposition of idiosyncratic activations throughout this network, including high-order areas and primary sensory cortices. High test–retest reliability for these idiosyncratic activation patterns indicate that they are not transient abnormalities. Rather, these findings suggest that autism is marked by individually unique neural networks. Such idiosyncrasies help explain why one of the most consistent findings in autism research, regardless of the methodology or variables of interest, has been a much greater variance in the autism group than in controls.

Atypical cortical recruiment is not limited to the visual domain. For example, a recent fMRI study used a self-paced sequential finger-tapping paradigm to examine online cortical motor function in 13 right-handed children with high-functioning autism and 13 right-handed control children (Mostofsky et al., 2009). Although the behavioral results did not differ, the autism group demonstrated reduced activations in contralateral and ipsilateral anterior cerebellum relative to controls, with increased activations in posterior supplementary motor area (SMA). The functional connections between bilateral thalamus and SMA were also reduced in the autism group. The researchers noted that because the demands of the motor task were driving the correlations below "rest-level," it was likely advantageous for the individuals with high-functioning autism to treat SMA and right and left thalamus as independent processors.

This decreased connectivity may also help explain why individuals with autism seem to rely to a greater extent on proprioceptive feedback, rather than visual feedback, for updating and modulating motor programs. In a recent study (Haswell et al., 2009), individuals with autism were asked to move a lever hidden by a horizontal screen toward a target animal on a monitor in front of them. By applying force orthogonally to the intended direction of movement, it was possible to assess reliance on visual feedback and proprioceptive feedback. The individuals with autism relied much more strongly on intrinsic (proprioceptively defined) coordinates. Moreover, increased reliance on proprioceptive feedback was correlated with higher scores on the SRS and the Reciprocal Social Interaction Score on the ADOS-G, as well as greater impairment on the Physical and Neurological Examination of Subtle Signs (PANESS). PANESS scores are interesting because they not only distinguish children with autism (Jansiewicz et al., 2006) but correlate with increased white matter volume in left motor cortex (Mostofsky et al., 2007).

Perception in Autism

Across modalities, abnormal connectivity in autism manifests as intact or enhanced perception of simple stimuli with deficits in perception of complex stimuli. Further, individuals with autism seem to preferentially recruit computationally early stage information processing centers. It is important to note that for our purposes, a stimulus is more "complex" if it requires the recruitment of a greater number of interacting functional capacities. For example, Bertone and colleagues (e.g., Bertone et al., 2003) use luminance-defined (additive contrast) and texture-defined (multiplicative contrast) visual stimuli. The luminance-defined stimuli are "simple" because they can be processed in V1, whereas texture-defined stimuli require the integrative capacities of V5.

Individuals with autism show deficits in complex motion processing, as evidenced by abnormally high perceptual thresholds for coherent motion (e.g., Spencer et al., 2000). These findings have been taken by some to indicate that autism is characterized by a "dorsal stream vulnerability" because of impairments in abilities subserved by the magnocellular pathway (Spencer et al., 2000; Milne et al., 2002), possibly because of a decreased signal-to-noise ratio. However, as Bertone and Faubert (2006) have noted, these results could also be explained in terms of complexity-dependent deficits. When using computationally simple first-order and computationally complex second-order tasks, individuals with autism demonstrate decreased performance only on second-order motion perception tasks (Bertone et al., 2003). More recently, Pellicano et al. (2005) have found deficits in global motion coherence in autism with intact low-level (e.g. subcortical areas, thalamus) flicker sensitivity in the dorsal stream, suggesting that magnocellular function is relatively unaffected. Abnormally "noisy" networks may affect the ability of individuals with autism to perform integrative tasks, which might manifest only during complex, higher-order tasks (Minshew & Williams, 2007; Simmons et al., 2009).

Further evidence for complexity-dependent visual processing abnormalities in autism comes from research into contrast sensitivity. Some studies have found intact dynamic (Bertone et al., 2005; Pellicano et al., 2005) and static (Behrmann et al., 2006; de Jonge et al., 2007; Milne et al., 2009) contrast sensitivity in individuals with autism. Yet two studies have found that autism is associated with a higher contrast threshold for second-order stimuli (Bertone et al., 2003, 2005). Contrast sensitivity seems to be intact for dynamic first-order stimuli (Bertone et al., 2003) and enhanced when first-order stimuli are static (Bertone et al., 2005). These results were recently replicated in a small population of unaffected 6-month-olds whose older siblings had been diagnosed with autism (McCleery et al., 2007), suggesting that complexity-dependent perceptual processing may be an endophenotype of autism. This constellation of intact or enhanced perception of simple visual stimuli with decreased perception of complex visual stimuli could serve to differentiate between autism spectrum conditions (extending to clinically unaffected family members) and related neurodevelopmental disorders such as Fragile X Syndrome (Bertone et al., 2006).

Autism is associated with both hypersensitivies and hyposensitivities (e.g., Bogdashina, 2003) to a wide variety of stimuli. Moreover, these unusual sensitivities may interfere with an individual's ability to communicate, as in the case of the potential effect of cross-modal extinction (Bonneh et al., 2008) on perception of multimodal social and nonsocial stimuli. Given reports of unusual sensory sensitivities in autism, sensory gating might be expected to be disrupted. Yet people with autism spectrum conditions have intact auditory (Kemner et al., 2002) and audio-visual (Magnée et al., 2009) P50 suppression (a hallmark of sensory gating). A 2008 study (Orekhova et al.) did find impaired auditory P50 suppression but only in a low-IQ autism subgroup. Further, in the low-IQ subgroup only, P50 suppression was correlated with mean spontaneous gamma power, implicating abnormal perceptual binding. Because the studies that found intact P50 suppression did not include low-IQ subjects, these results suggest that relatively simple sensory gating may be disrupted only on the extreme end of the autism spectrum.

Consistent with the complexity-dependent hypothesis, some studies have found enhanced early stage perception in autism. For example, in an auditory mismatch study, N1 latency was reduced (Ferri et al., 2003). When viewing Gabor patches, autism has recently been associated with earlier, exogenous activation of right posterior intraparietal sulcus (Belmonte et al., 2010) and reduced P1 latencies and earlier alpha-band peaks (Milne et al., 2009). In Milne et al., P1 latency was significantly negatively correlated with CARS score, suggesting that the severity of autistic symptoms may be associated, more generally, with faster low-level information processing.

Milne and colleagues (2009) also found that the individuals with autism exhibited a less specialized visual processing network. They used Gabor patches with four different spatial frequencies. For the higher frequencies, the control group showed increased gamma power. This stimulus-dependent increase was depressed in the autism group, suggesting that at least for contrast sensitivity, individuals with autism possess a network with reduced entropy—that is, one that responds indiscriminately strongly to all types of inputs.

Not surprisingly, reduced selectivity (resulting from connectivity-driven reductions in network entropy) has been observed in several other EEG studies. If children with autism are asked to respond to an auditory stimulus, their P3 is abnormally distributed into occipital areas associated with visual processing (Kemner et al., 1994). In the same population, novel visual stimuli, even if they are task-irrelevant, reliably produce an enhanced N2 response (Kemner et al., 1994). In autistic adults, the evoked P1 response is either overgeneralized to stimuli far away from an attended location or unusually enhanced at the attended location (Townsend & Courchesne, 1994). Finally, during attentional shifts between hemifields, individuals with autism show indiscriminate activations, rather than spatially specific augmentation of the visual steady-state potentials observed in typically developing populations (Belmonte, 2000). These unusual evoked responses are consistent with primary sensory areas that suffer from degraded signal-to-noise ratio, perhaps resulting from overconnectedness of local structural and functional neural networks.

Networks of Neurons, Networks of Genes, and Proteins

A brief discussion of autism genetics is appropriate to the topic of autistic neural information processing insofar as the same network issues arise. Autism genetics, like autism physiology, has suffered from the distraction of twentieth-century, univariate approaches. Single-gene studies of complex neuropsychiatric disorders are valuable insofar as they highlight points of entry into networks of interacting genes, but it is these network-level disruptions that are the meat of the matter. The risk for autism arises not only in the protein product of an individual gene but, rather, in that protein product's many interactions with other genes and proteins that themselves carry individual differences. Many of these interacting susceptibility alleles vary greatly in their prevalance between distinct populations. For example, the G/T SNP rs3813034 in the 3' UTR of *SLC6A4* has been selected for the T-allele in African and European populations but for the G-allele in Asian (Chinese, Japanese, and eastern Indian) populations (Guhathakurta et al., 2008), and in the case of *RELN*, 16% of Indians but only 6% of Europeans carry an expanded sequence of 11 or more CGG repeats in the 5' UTR (Dutta et al., 2007). These are but two examples of a phenomenon that is likely widespread among populations and among individual autism risk factors. Because autism susceptibility or protection alleles individually produce only small increments or multiples of risk, we can expect that the risk level and perhaps even the very identity of an allele as an autism risk factor, within a specific population, may depend on the population-genetic context consisting of all the genes with which that putative risk factor interacts. Contrasts between genotypically and (endo)phenotypically well-characterized populations from different regions or other stratifications (e.g., castes; *see* Reich et al., 2009) therefore may have much to say about the nature of the genetic networks involved in autism susceptibility or protection. Candidate-gene studies in eastern Indian populations, for example (Dutta et al., 2007, 2008; Guhathakurta et al., 2008, 2009; Sen et al., 2010), have revealed tantalizing contrasts, both positive and negative, with findings from the more often studied populations of Europe and North America. Why is it germane, and important, to talk about genetics in the context of a chapter on information processing? As we hope that this brief discussion has shown, genetic networks and their associated environmental factors cannot be separated from their effects on neural networks. The answers to autism, and to other complex neurodevelopmental disorders, will come from an integrative style of neuroscience and an integrative sort of neuroscientist that deals in both these domains.

Conclusion

During the past decade, the neurobiological study of neuropsychiatric disorders has benefited from this new focus on connectivity between brain regions (Frith, 2003; Fusar-Poli & Broome, 2006). In particular, the systems-level dysfunction in autism has been characterized as a network perturbation possibly comprising abnormally strong and undifferentiated connectivity within local networks and a resultant failure to develop normal patterns of long-range connectivity among brain regions and among cognitive subsystems (Brock et al., 2002; Belmonte et al., 2004a; Courchesne & Pierce, 2005). This idea is consistent with an emerging collage of autism susceptibility genes that perturb neural connectivity by altering neuron numbers, synaptic structure, or neurotransmission (Belmonte & Bourgeron, 2006)—many of which may be responsible for dimensions of normal as well as abnormal cognitive variation (Ronald et al., 2006a, b; Valla et al., 2010)—and has been supported by functional imaging results in autism demonstrating abnormally strong activation within brain regions that subserve low levels of processing along with abnormally weak activation within higher-order, integrative regions (Belmonte & Yurgelun-Todd, 2003) and abnormally weak functional connectivity between brain regions (Just et al., 2004; Belmonte et al., 2010), as well as by anatomical studies of high local and low bridging white matter volume (Herbert et al., 2004) and low-diffusion anisotropy in white-matter regions subserving integrative processing (Barnea-Goraly et al., 2004).

The recency of interest in neural connectivity in autism arises in the context of the historical focus of neuroscience on single-variable problems. Science as a matter of course directs its enquiries toward well-framed and tractable hypotheses in which one independent variable is manipulated while all other factors are somehow held constant. Historically, this single-variable focus has produced great advances in the understanding of the effects of brain lesions (in which a single anatomical structure is silenced) and single-gene disorders (in which one gene is silenced or gains function). Complex neuropsychiatric conditions, however, are anything but single-variable problems. In autism in particular, the one truth that has become clear from decades of study is that this behaviorally defined condition converges from many possible etiological factors and combinations thereof and diverges into a welter of endophenotypic variability (Belmonte et al., 2004b). The lesion model is as poor a one as the single-gene model for understanding developmental disorders, as the experience-expectant maturation of any one brain structure depends on its receiving properly patterned inputs from the structures with which it communicates, and thus a perturbation of any one region becomes a perturbation of the entire network of interacting brain regions (Johnson et al., 2002), just as variants in a collection of genes combine to produce emergent variation in networks of interacting genes (Belmonte & Bourgeron, 2006). Instead, research into autism ought to proceed with the understanding that the ultimate etiological explanation of autism will involve complex genetic processes that produce unique brain anatomy and associated unique function, and that the very same genetic factors that underlie autism also produce a broad range of cognitive diversity in the nonautistic population and many cognitively beneficial traits in people with autism spectrum conditions. An eventual prevention and cure for autism will succeed insofar as it can ameliorate autistic deficits while preserving autism's unique, detail-oriented perceptual insights and confer the social and communicative abilities that will allow people with autism to share those insights with the broader social world (Belmonte, 2008). This volume, then, should more properly and generally to be titled not "Autism Spectrum Disorders" but "Autism Spectrum Conditions"—for the autism spectrum encompasses a wide range of phenotypes and may well turn out to be inseparable from the state of being human.

Challenges and Future Directions

- Distinguish between dimensional and categorical aspects of autism spectrum conditions.
- Investigate what factors affect bifurcation between diagnosis of autism and subclinical autistic traits (both additional risk factors in clinical populations and protective factors in nonclinical populations); develop targets for preventive treatments.
- Investigate how systems-level abnormalities of the neural computational substrate might give rise developmentally to diagnostic characteristics of autism; characterize covariation of low-level and high-level perceptual and cognitive abnormalities in autism spectrum conditions.
- Characterize the developmental relationship between short-range and long-range structural and functional connectivities in autism spectrum conditions.
- Integrate univariate conceptions of autism into multivariate, multilevel constructs.

SUGGESTED READINGS

Belmonte, M. K., Cook, E. H., Jr, Anderson, G. M., Rubenstein, J. L., Greenough, W. T., Beckel-Mitchener, A., et al. (2004). Autism as a disorder of neural information processing: Directions for research and targets for therapy. *Molecular Psychiatry, 9*, 646–663. Unabridged edition at http://www.cureautismnow.org/conferences/summitmeetings/.

Mottron, L., Dawson, M., Soulières, I., Hubert, B., & Burack, J. A. (2006). Enhanced perceptual functioning in autism: An update, and eight principles of autistic perception. *Journal of Autism and Developmental Disorders, 36*, 27–43.

Simmons, D. R., Robertson, A. E., McKay, L. S., Toal, E., McAleer, P., & Pollick, F. E. (2009). Vision in autism spectrum disorders. *Vision Research, 49*, 2705–2739.

REFERENCES

Achard, S., Salvador, R., Whitcher, B., Suckling, J., & Bullmore, E. (2006). A resilient, low-frequency, small-world human brain functional network with highly connected association cortical hubs. *Journal of Neuroscience, 26*, 63–72.

Akshoomoff, N. A., & Courchesne, E. (1992). A new role for the cerebellum in cognitive operations. *Behavioral Neuroscience, 106*, 731–738.

Albert, R., Jeong, H. & Barbasi, A. L. (2000). Error and attack tolerance of complex networks. *Nature, 406*, 378–382.

Alexander, A. L., Lee, J. E., Lazar, M., Boudos, R., DuBray, M. B., Oakes, T. R., et al. (2007). Diffusion tensor imaging of the corpus callosum in Autism. *NeuroImage, 34*, 61–73.

Allen, G. & Courchesne, E. (2001). Attention function and dysfunction in autism. *Frontiers in Bioscience, 6*, D105–119.

Amir, R. E., van den Veyver, I. B., Wan, M., Tran, C. Q., Francke, U., & Zoghbi, H. Y. (1999). Rett syndrome is caused by mutations in X-linked MECP2, encoding methyl-CpG-binding protein 2. *Nature Genetics, 23*, 185–188.

Aylward, E. H., Minshew, N. J., Field, K., Sparks, B. F., & Singh, N. (2002). Effects of age on brain volume and head circumference in autism. *Neurology, 59*, 175–183.

Aylward, E. H., Minshew, N. J., Goldstein, G., Honeycutt, N. A., Augustine, A. M., Yates, K. O., et al. (1999). MRI volumes of amygdala and hippocampus in non-mentally retarded autistic adolescents and adults. *Neurology, 53*, 2145–2150.

Ballaban-Gil, K. & Tuchman, R. (2000). Epilepsy and epileptiform EEG: Association with autism and language disorders. *Mental Retardation and Developmental Disabilities Research Reviews, 6*, 300–308.

Barabási, A. L., & Albert, R. (1999). Emergence of scaling in random networks. *Science, 286*, 509–512.

Barnea-Goraly, N., Kwon, H., Menon, V., Eliez, S., Lotspeich, L., & Reiss, A. L. (2004). White matter structure in autism: Preliminary evidence from diffusion tensor imaging. *Biological Psychiatry, 55*, 323–326.

Baron-Cohen, S. (2002). The extreme male brain theory of autism. *Trends in Cognitive Sciences, 6*, 248–254.

Baron-Cohen, S., Leslie, A. M., & Frith, U. (1985). Does the autistic child have a "theory of mind"? *Cognition, 21*, 37–46.

Baron-Cohen, S., Ring, H. A., Wheelwright, S., Bullmore, E. T., Brammer, M. J., Simmons, A., et al. (1999). Social intelligence in the normal and autistic brain: An fMRI study. *European Journal of Neuroscience, 11*, 1891–1898.

Bauman, M. L. & Kemper, T. L. (1985). Histoanatomic observations of the brain in earlyinfan tile autism. *Neurology, 35*, 866–874.

Bauman, M. L. & Kemper, T. L. (1994). Neuroanatomic observations of the brain in autism. In M. L. Bauman, & T. L. Kemper, eds.

The neurobiology of autism (pp. 119–145). Baltimore, MD: Johns Hopkins University Press.

Behrmann, M., Avidan, G., Leonard, G. L., Kimchi, R., Luna, B., Humphreys, K., et al. (2006). Configural processing in autism and its relationship to face processing. *Neuropsychologia, 44*, 110–129.

Belmonte, M. K. (2000). Abnormal attention in autism shown by steady-state visual evoked potentials. *Autism, 4*, 269–285.

Belmonte, M. K. (2005). Abnormal visual motion processing as a neural endophenotype of autism. *Cahiers de Psychologie Cognitive/Current Psychology of Cognition, 23*, 65–74.

Belmonte, M. K. (2008). Human, but more so: What the autistic brain tells us about the process of narrative. In M. Osteen, ed. *Autism and representation* (pp. 166–179). New York: Routledge.

Belmonte, M. K., Allen, G., Beckel-Mitchener, A., Boulanger, L. M., Carper, R. A., & Webb, S. J. (2004a). Autism and abnormal development of brain connectivity. *Journal of Neuroscience, 24*, 9228–9231.

Belmonte, M. K. & Bourgeron, T. (2006). Fragile X syndrome and autism at the intersection of genetic and neural networks. *Nature Neuroscience, 9*, 1221–1225.

Belmonte, M. K., Cook, E. H. Jr, Anderson, G. M., Rubenstein, J. L., Greenough, W. T., Beckel-Mitchener, A., et al. (2004b). Autism as a disorder of neural information processing: Directions for research and targets for therapy. *Molecular Psychiatry, 9*, 646–663. http://www.cureautismnow.org/conferences/summitmeetings/.

Belmonte, M. K., Gomot, M., & Baron-Cohen, S. (2010). Visual attention in autism families: "Unaffected" sibs share atypical frontal activation. *Journal of Child Psychology and Psychiatry, 51*, 259–276.

Belmonte, M. K. & Yurgelun-Todd, D. A. (2003). Functional anatomy of impaired selective attention and compensatory processing in autism. *Cognitive Brain Research, 17*, 651–664.

Ben Bashat, D., Kronfeld-Duenias, V., Zachor, D. A., Ekstein, P. M., Hendler, T., Tarrasch, R., et al. (2007). Accelerated maturation of white matter in young children with autism: A high b value DWI study. *NeuroImage, 37*, 40–47.

Bertone, A. & Faubert, J. (2006). Demonstrations of decreased sensitivity to complex motion information not enough to propose an autism-specific neural etiology. *Journal of Autism and Developmental Disorders, 36*, 55–64.

Bertone, A., Mottron, L., Jelenic, P., & Faubert, J. (2005). Enhanced and diminished visuo-spatial information processing in autism depends on stimulus complexity. *Brain, 128*, 2430–2441.

Bertone, E., Mottron, L., Jelenic, P., & Faubert, J. (2003). Motion perception in autism: A "complex" issue. *Journal of Cognitive Neuroscience, 15*, 226–235.

Biswal, B., Yetkin, F. Z., Haughton, V. M., & Hyde, J. S. (1995). Functional connectivity in the motor cortex of resting human brain using echo-planar MRI. *Magnetic Resonance in Medicine, 34*, 537–541.

Bloss, C. S. & Courchesne, E. (2007). MRI neuroanatomy in young girls with autism: A preliminary study. *Journal of the American Academy of Child and Adolescent Psychiatry, 46*, 515–523.

Bogdashina, O. (2003). In *Sensory perceptual issues in autism: Different sensory experiences–Different perceptual worlds*. London, UK: Jessica Kingsley.

Bonneh, Y. S., Belmonte, M. K., Pei, F., Iversen, P. E., Kenet, T., Akshoomoff, N., et al. (2008). Cross-modal extinction in a boy with severely autistic behaviour and high verbal intelligence. *Cognitive Neuropsychology, 25*, 635–652.

Brock, J., Brown, C. C., Boucher, J., & Rippon, G. (2002). The temporal binding deficit hypothesis of autism. *Development and Psychopathology, 14*, 209–224.

Burack, J. A. (1994). Selective attention deficits in persons with autism: Preliminary evidence of an inefficient attentional lens. *Journal of Abnormal Psychology, 103*, 535–543.

Butler, P. D. & Javitt, D. C. (2005). Early-stage visual processing deficits in schizophrenia. *Current Opinion in Psychiatry, 18*, 151–157.

Butler, P. D., Martinez, A., Foxe, J. J., Kim, D., Zemon, V., Silipo, G., et al. (2007). Subcortical visual dysfunction in schizophrenia drives secondary cortical impairments. *Brain, 130*, 417–430.

Carper, R. A. & Courchesne, E. (2000). Inverse correlation between frontal lobe and cerebellum sizes in children with autism. *Brain, 123*, 836–844.

Carper, R. A. & Courchesne, E. (2005). Localized enlargement of the frontal cortex in early autism. *Biological Psychiatry, 57*, 126–133.

Carper, R. A., Moses, P., Tigue, Z. D., & Courchesne, E. (2002). Cerebral lobes in autism: Early hyperplasia and abnormal age effects. *NeuroImage, 16*(4), 1038–1051.

Charman, T. (1997). The relationship between joint attention and pretend play in autism. *Development and Psychopathology, 9*, 1–16.

Chen, G. M., Yoder, K. Y., Ganzel, B. L., Goodwin, M. S., & Belmonte, M. K. (in revision). Harnessing repetitive behaviours to engage attention and learning in a novel therapy for autism.

Cohen, M. X., David, N., Vogeley, K., & Elger, C. E. (2009). Gamma-band activity in the human superior temporal sulcus during mentalizing from nonverbal social cues. *Psychophysiology, 46*, 43–51.

Cohen, R., Erez, K., ben-Avraham, D., & Havlin, S. (2000). Resilience of the Internet to random breakdowns. *Physical Review Letters, 85*, 4626–4628.

Courchesne, E., Karns, C., Davis, H. R., Ziccardi, R., Carper, R. A., Tigue, Z. D., et al. (2001). Unusual brain growth patterns in early life in patients with autistic disorder: An MRI study. *Neurology, 57*, 245–254.

Courchesne, E., Müller, R. A., & Saitoh, O. (1999). Brain weight in autism: Normal in the majority of cases, megalencephalic in rare cases. *Neurology, 52*, 1057–1059.

Courchesne, E. & Pierce, K. (2005). Why the frontal cortex in autism might be talking only to itself: Local over-connectivity but long-distance disconnection. *Current Opinion in Neurobiology, 15*, 225–230.

Courchesne, E., Pierce, K., Schumann, C. M., Redcay, E., Buckwalter, J. A., Kennedy, D. P., et al. (2007). Mapping early brain development in autism. *Neuron, 56*, 399–413.

Courchesne, E., Press, G., & Yeung-Courchesne, R. (1993). Parietal lobe abnormalities detected with MR in patients with infantile autism. *American Journal of Roentgenology, 160*, 387–393.

Courchesne, E., Townsend, J., Akshoomoff, N. A., Saitoh, O., Yeung-Courchesne, R., Lincoln, A. J., et al. (1994a). Impairment in shifting attention in autistic and cerebellar patients. *Behavioral Neuroscience, 108*, 848–865.

Courchesne, E., Townsend, J., & Saitoh, O. (1994b). The brain in infantile autism: Posterior fossa structures are abnormal. *Neurology, 44*, 214–223.

Courchesne, E., Yeung-Courchesne, R., Press, G., Hesselink, J. R., & Jernigan, T. L. (1988). Hypoplasia of cerebellar vermal lobules

VI and VII in autism. *New England Journal of Medicine, 318*, 1349–1354.

Critchley, H. D., Daly, E. M., Bullmore, E. T., Williams, S. C. R., van Amelsvoort, T., Robertson, D. M., et al. (2000). The functional neuroanatomy of social behaviour: Changes in cerebral blood flow when people with autistic disorder process facial expressions. *Brain, 123*, 2203–2212.

de Jonge, M. V., Kemner,., de Haan, E. H., Coppens, J. E., van den Berg, J. T. P., & van Engelund, H. (2007). Visual information processing in high-functioning individuals with autism spectrum disorders and their parents. *Neuropsychology, 21*(1), 65–73.

Dutta, S., Guhathakurta, S., Sinha, S., Chatterjee, A., Ahmed, S., Ghosh, S., et al. (2007). Reelin gene polymorphisms in the Indian population: A possible paternal 5'UTR-CGG-repeat-allele effect in autism. *American Journal of Medical Genetics. Part B, Neuropsychiatric Genetics, 144*, 106–112.

Dutta, S., Sinha, S., Ghosh, S., Chatterjee, A., Ahmed, S., & Rajamma, U. (2008). Genetic analysis of reelin gene (RELN) SNPs: No association with autism spectrum disorder in the Indian population. *Neuroscience Letters, 441*, 56–60.

Egaas, B., Courchesne, E. & Saitoh, O. (1995). Reduced size of corpus callosum in autism. *Archives of Neurology, 52*, 794–801.

Engel, A. K. & Singer, W. (2001). Temporal binding and the neural correlates of sensory awareness. *Trends in Cognitive Sciences, 5*(1), 16–25.

Evans, D. W., Gray, F. L. & Leckman, J. F. (1999). The rituals, fears, and phobias of young children: Insights from development, psychopathology, and neurobiology. *Child Psychiatry and Human Development, 29*, 261–276.

Ferri, R., Elia, M., Agarwal, H., Lanuzza, B., Musumeci, S. A., & Pennisi, G. (2003). The mismatch negativity and the P3a components of the auditory event-related potentials in autistic low-functioning subjects. *Clinical Neurophysiology, 114*(9), 1671–1680.

Fitch, R. H. & Tallal, P. (2003). Neural mechanisms of language-based learning impairments: Insights from human populations and animal models. *Behavioral and Cognitive Neuroscience Reviews, 2*, 155–178.

Freitag, C. M., Konrad, C., Häberlein, M., Kleser, C., von Gontard, A., Reith, W., et al. (2008). Perception of biological motion in autism spectrum disorders. *Neuropsychologia, 46*, 1480–1494.

Frith, C. D. (2003). What do imaging studies tell us about the neural basis of autism? *Novartis Foundation Symposia, 251*, 149–166.

Frith, C. D. & Frith, U. (2006). The neural basis of mentalizing. *Neuron, 50*, 531–534.

Frith, U. & Happé, F. (1994). Autism: Beyond "theory of mind." *Cognition, 50*, 115–132.

Frith, U. & de Vignemont, F. (2005). Egocentrism, allocentrism, and Asperger syndrome. *Consciousness and Cognition, 14*, 719–738.

Fujita, K., Henderson, M. D., Eng, J., Trope, Y., & Liberman, N. (2006). Spatial distance and mental construal of social events. *Psychological Science, 17*, 278–282.

Fusar-Poli, P. & Broome, M. R. (2006). Conceptual issues in psychiatric neuroimaging. *Current Opinion in Psychiatry, 19*, 608–612.

Gilbert, S. J., Bird, G., Brindley, R., Frith, C. D., & Burgess, P. W. (2008). Atypical recruitment of medial prefrontal cortex in autism spectrum disorders: An fMRI study of two executive function tasks. *Neuropsychologia, 46*, 2281–2291.

Gomot, M., Bernard, F. A., Davis, M. H., Belmonte, M. K., Ashwin, C., Bullmore, E. T., et al. (2005). Change detection in children with autism: An auditory event-related fMRI study. *NeuroImage, 29*, 475–484.

Greenspan, S. I. (2001). The affect diathesis hypothesis: The role of emotions in the core deficit in autism and the development of intelligence and social skills. *Journal of Development and Learning Disorders, 5*, 1–45.

Guhathakurta, S., Asem, S. S., Sinha, S., Chatterjee, A., Ahmed, S., Ghosh, S., et al. (2009). Analysis of serotonin receptor 2A gene (HTR2A): Association study with autism spectrum disorder in the Indian population and investigation of the gene expression in peripheral blood leukocytes. *Neurochemistry International, 55*, 754–759.

Guhathakurta, S., Sinha, S., Ghosh, S., Chatterjee, A., Ahmed, S., Gangopadhyay, P. K., et al. (2008). Population-based association study and contrasting linkage disequilibrium pattern reveal genetic association of SLC6A4 with autism in the Indian population from West Bengal. *Brain Research, 1240*, 12–21.

Hadjikhani, N., Joseph, R. M., Snyder, J., & Tager-Flusberg, H. (2006). Anatomical differences in the mirror neuron system and social cognition network in autism. *Cerebral Cortex, 16*, 1276–1282.

Happé, F. & Frith, U. (2006). The weak coherence account: Detail-focused cognitive style in autism spectrum disorders. *Journal of Autism and Developmental Disorders, 36*, 5–25.

Hashimoto, T., Tayama, M., Murakawa, K., Yoshimoto, T., Miyazaki, M., Harada, M., et al. (1995). Development of the brainstem and cerebellum in autistic patients. *Journal of Autism and Developmental Disorders, 25*, 1–18.

Hasson, U., Avidan, G., Gelbard, H., Vallines, I., Harel, M., Minshew, N. J., et al. (2009). Shared and idiosyncratic cortical activation patterns in autism revealed under continuous real-life viewing conditions. *Autism Research, 2*, 220–231.

Haswell, C. C., Izawa, J., Dowell, L. R., Mostofsky, S. H., & Shadmehr, R. (2009). Representation of internal models of action in the autistic brain. *Nature Neuroscience, 12*, 970–972.

Hazlett, H. C., Poe, M., Gerig, G., Smith, R. G., Provenzale, J., Ross, A., et al. (2005). Magnetic resonance imaging and head circumference study of brain size in autism: Birth through age 2 years. *Archives of General Psychiatry, 62*, 1366–1376.

Herbert, M. R., Ziegler, D. A., Makris, N., Filipek, P. A., Kemper, T. L., Normandin, J. J., et al (2004). Localization of white matter volume increase in autism and developmental language disorder. *Annals of Neurology, 55*, 530–540.

Herrington, J. D., Baron-Cohen, S., Wheelwright, S. J., Singh, K. D., Bullmore, E. T., Brammer, M., et al. (2007). The role of MT+/V5 during biological motion perception in Asperger syndrome: An fMRI study. *Research in Autism Spectrum Disorders, 1*, 14–27.

Hill, E. L. (2004). Executive dysfunction in autism. *Trends in Cognitive Sciences, 8*, 26–32.

Hoeffer, C. A., & Klann, E. (2010). mTOR signaling: At the crossroads of plasticity, memory and disease. *Trends in Neurosciences, 33*, 67–75.

Hubert, B., Wicker, B., Moore, D. G., Monfardini, E., Duverger, H., Da Fonséca, D., et al. (2007). Brief report: Recognition of emotional and non-emotional biological motion in individuals with autistic spectrum disorders. *Journal of Autism and Developmental Disorders, 37*, 1386–1392.

Hughes, C., Russell, J., & Robbins, T. W. (1994). Evidence for executive dysfunction in autism. *Neuropsychologia, 32*, 477–492.

Hutsler, J. J. & Zhang, H. (2010). Increased dendritic spine densities on cortical projection neurons in autism spectrum disorders. *Brain Research, 1309*, 83–94.

Jansiewicz, E., Goldberg, M. C., Newschaffer, C. J., Denckla, M. B., Landa, R. J., & Mostofsky, S. H. (2006). Motor signs distinguish children with high functioning autism and Asperger's syndrome from controls. *Journal of Autism and Developmental Disorders, 36*(5), 613–621.

Jarrold, C., Butler, D. W., Cottington, E. M., & Jimenez, F. (2000). Linking theory of mind and central coherence bias in autism and in the general population. *Developmental Psychology, 36*, 126–138.

Johnson, M. H., Halit, H., Grice, S. J., & Karmiloff-Smith, A. (2002). Neuroimaging of typical and atypical development: A perspective from multiple levels of analysis. *Development and Psychopathology, 14*, 521–536.

Just, M. A., Cherkassky, V. L., Keller, T. A., Kana, R. K., & Minshew, N. J. (2007). Functional and anatomical cortical underconnectivity in autism: Evidence from an FMRI study of an executive function task and corpus callosum morphometry. *Cerebral Cortex, 17*, 951–961.

Just, M. A., Cherkassky, V. L., Keller, T. A., & Minshew, N. J. (2004). Cortical activation and synchronization during sentence comprehension in high-functioning autism: Evidence of underconnectivity. *Brain, 127*, 1811–1821.

Kelleher, R. J. III, & Bear, M. F. (2008). The autistic neuron: Troubled translation? *Cell, 135*, 401–406.

Kemner, C., Oranje, B., Verbaten, M. N., & van Engeland, H. (2002). Normal P50 gating in children with autism. *Journal of Clinical Psychiatry, 63*, 214–217.

Kemner, C., Verbaten, M. N., Cuperus, J. M., Camfferman, G., & van Engeland, H. (1994). Visual and somatosensory event-related brain potentials in autistic children and three different control groups. *EEG and Clinical Neurophysiology, 92*, 225–237.

Kennedy, D. P. & Courchesne, E. (2008). Functional abnormalities of the default network during self- and other-reflection in autism. *Social Cognitive and Affective Neuroscience, 3*, 177–190.

Kuramoto, Y. (1984). *Chemical oscillations, waves, and turbulence.* Berlin: Springer.

Landry, R. & Bryson, S. E. (2004). Impaired disengagement of attention in young children with autism. *Journal of Child Psychology and Psychiatry, 45*, 1115–1122.

Lee, J. E., Bigler, E. D., Alexander, A. L., Lazar, M., DuBray, M. B., Chung, M. K., et al. (2007). Diffusion tensor imaging of white matter in the superior temporal gyrus and temporal stem in autism. *Neuroscience Letters, 424*, 127–132.

Leitman, D. I., Hoptman, M. J., Foxe, J. J., Saccente, E., Wylie, G. R., Nierenberg, J., et al. (2007). The neural substrates of impaired prosodic detection in schizophrenia and its sensorial antecedents. *American Journal of Psychiatry, 164*, 474–482.

Lewis, J. D. & Elman, J. L. (2008). Growth-related neural reorganization and the autism phenotype: A test of the hypothesis that altered brain growth leads to altered connectivity. *Developmental Science, 11*, 135–155.

Lewis, J. D., Theilmann, R. J., Sereno, M. I., & Townsend, J. (2009). The relation between connection length and degree of connectivity in young adults: A DTI analysis. *Cerebral Cortex, 19*, 554–562.

Liberman, N. & Trope, Y. (2008). The psychology of transcending the here and now. *Science, 322*, 1201–1205.

Magnée, M. J. C. M., Oranje, B., van Engeland, H., Kahn, R. S., & Kemner, C. (2009). Cross-sensory gating in schizophrenia and autism spectrum disorder: EEG evidence for impaired brain connectivity? *Neuropsychologia, 47*, 1728–1732.

McCleery, J. P., Allman, E., Carver, L. J., & Dobkins, K. R. (2007). Abnormal magnocellular pathway visual processing in infants at risk for autism. *Biological Psychiatry, 62*, 1007–1014.

Mesulam, M. M. (1990). Large-scale neurocognitive networks and distributed processing for attention, language, and memory. *Annals of Neurology, 28*, 597–613.

Mesulam, M. M. (2000). *Principles of behavioral and cognitive neurology* (2nd ed., pp. 439–522). Oxford: Oxford University Press.

Milne, E., Scope, A., Pascalis, O., Buckley, D., & Makeig, S. (2009). Independent component analysis reveals atypical electroencephalographic activity during visual perception in individuals with autism. *Biological Psychiatry, 65*, 22–30.

Milne, E., Swettenham, J., Hansen, P., Campbell, R., Jeffries, H., & Plaisted, K. (2002). High motion coherence thresholds in children with autism. *Journal of Child Psychology and Psychiatry, 43*, 255–263.

Minshew, N. J., Goldstein, G., & Siegel, D. J. (1997). Neuropsychologic functioning in autism: Profile of a complex information processing disorder. *Journal of the International Neuropsychological Society, 3*, 303–316.

Minshew, N. J. & Payton, J. B. (1988). New perspectives in autism, part II: The differential diagnosis and neurobiology of autism. *Current Problems in Pediatrics, 18*, 613–694.

Minshew, N. J., Sung, K., Jones, B., & Furman, J. (2004). Underdevelopment of the postural control system in autism. *Neurology, 63*, 2056–2061.

Minshew, N. J. & Williams, D. L. (2007). The new neurobiology of autism: Cortex, connectivity, and neuronal organization. *Archives of Neurology, 64*, 945–950.

Moore, D. G., Hobson, R. P., & Lee, A. (1997). Components of person perception: An investigation with autistic, non-autistic retarded and typically developing children and adolescents. *British Journal of Developmental Psychology, 15*, 401–423.

Mostofsky, S. H., Burgess, M. P., & Gidley Larson, J. C. (2007). Increased motor cortex white matter volume predicts motor impairment in autism. *Brain, 130*, 2117–2122.

Mostofsky, S. H., Powell, S. K., Simmonds, D. J., Goldberg, M. C., Caffo, B., & Pekar, J. J. (2009). Decreased connectivity and cerebellar activity in autism during motor task performance. *Brain, 132*, 2413–2425.

Mottron, L., Dawson, M., Soulières, I., Hubert, B., & Burack, J. A. (2006). Enhanced perceptual functioning in autism: An update, and eight principles of autistic perception. *Journal of Autism and Developmental Disorders, 36*, 27–43.

Müller, R-A., Kleinhans, N., Kemmotsu, N., Pierce, K., & Courchesne, E. (2003). Abnormal variability and distribution of fucntional maps in autism: An fMRI study of visuomotor learning. *American Journal of Psychiatry, 160*, 1847–1862.

Müller, R-A., Pierce, K., Ambrose, J. B., Allen, G., Courchesne, E. (2001). Atypical patterns of cerebral motor activation in autism: A functional magnetic resonance study. *Biological Psychiatry, 49*.

Murakami, J., Courchesne, E., Press, G., Yeung-Courchesne, R., & Hesselink, J. (1989). Reduced cerebellar hemisphere size and its relationship to vermal hypoplasia in autism. *Archives of Neurology, 46*, 689–694.

Noonan, S. K., Haist, F., & Müller, R.-A. (2009). Aberrant functional connectivity in autism: Evidence from low-frequency BOLD signal fluctuations. *Brain Research, 1262*, 48–63.

Orekhova, E. V., Stroganova, T. A., Prokofyev, A. O., Nygren, G., Gillberg, C., & Elam, M. (2008). Sensory gating in young children with autism: Relation to age, IQ, and EEG gamma oscillations. *Neuroscience Letters, 434*, 218–223.

Ozonoff, S., Strayer, D. L., McMahon, W. M., & Filloux, F. (1994). Executive function abilities in autism and Tourette syndrome: An information processing approach. *Journal of Child Psychology and Psychiatry, 35*, 1015–1032.

Pellicano, E., Gibson, L., Maybery, M., Durkin, K., & Badcock, D. R. (2005). Abnormal global processing along the dorsal pathway in autism: A possible mechanism for weak visuospatial coherence? *Neuropsychologia, 43*, 1044–1053.

Peskin, C. S. (1975). *Mathematical aspects of heart physiology* (pp. 268–278). New York: Courant Institute of Mathematical Sciences.

Pierce, K., Müller, R.-A., Ambrose, J., Allen, G., & Courchesne, E. (2001). Face processing occurs outside the fusiform "face area" in autism: Evidence from functional MRI. *Brain, 124*, 2059–2073.

Pieretti, M., Zhang, F. P., Fu, Y. H., Warren, S. T., Oostra, B. A., Caskey, C. T., et al. (1991). Absence of expression of the FMR-1 gene in fragile X syndrome. *Cell, 23*, 817–822.

Plaisted, K., O'Riordan, M., & Baron-Cohen, S. (1998). Enhanced visual search for a conjunctive target in autism: A research note. *Journal of Child Psychology and Psychiatry, 39*, 777–783.

Plaisted, K., Saksida, L., Alcantara, J., & Weisblatt, E. (2003). Towards an understanding of the mechanisms of weak central coherence effects: Experiments in visual configural learning and auditory perception. *Philosophical Transactions of the Royal Society of London. Series B, Biological Sciences, 358*, 375–386.

Redcay, E. (2008). The superior temporal sulcus performs a common function for social and speech perception: Implications for the emergence of autism. *Neuroscience and Biobehavioral Reviews, 32*, 123–142.

Reich, D., Thangaraj, K., Patterson, N., Price, A. L. & Singh, L. (2009). Reconstructing Indian population history. *Nature, 461*, 489–494.

Ring, H. A., Baron-Cohen, S., Wheelwright, S., Williams, S. C. R., Brammer, M. J., Andrew, C., et al. (1999). Cerebral correlates of preserved cognitive skills in autism. *Brain, 122*, 1305–1315.

Ringo, J. L. (1991). Neuronal interconnection as a function of brain size. *Brain, Behavior, and Evolution, 38*(1), 1–6.

Ringo, J. L., Doty, R. W., Demeter, S., & Simard, P. Y. (1994). Time is of the essence: A conjecture that hemispheric specialization arises from interhemispheric conduction delay. *Cerebral Cortex, 4*(4), 331–343.

Ritvo, E. R., Freeman, B. J., Scheibel, A. B., Duong, T., Robinson, H., Guthrie, D., & et al. (1986). Lower Purkinje cell counts in the cerebella of four autistic subjects: Initial findings of the UCLA-NSAC autopsy research report. *American Journal of Psychiatry, 143*, 862–866.

Rodier, P. M., Ingram, J. L., Tisdale, B., Nelson, S., & Romano, J. (1996). Embryological origin for autism: Developmental anomalies of the cranial nerve motor nuclei. *Journal of Comparative Neurology, 370*, 247–261.

Rogers, S. J. & Ozonoff, S. (2005). What do we know about sensory dysfunction in autism? A critical review of the empirical evidence. *Journal of Child Psychology and Psychiatry, 46*, 1255–1268.

Ronald, A., Happé, F., Bolton, P., Butcher, L. M., Price, T. S., Wheelwright, S., et al. (2006a). Genetic heterogeneity between the three components of the autism spectrum: A twin study. *Journal of the American Academy of Child and Adolescent Psychiatry, 45*, 691–699.

Ronald, A., Happé, F., Price, T. S., Baron-Cohen, S., & Plomin, R. (2006b). Phenotypic and genetic overlap between autistic traits at the extremes of the general population. *Journal of the American Academy of Child and Adolescent Psychiatry, 45*, 1206–1214.

Rubenstein, J. L. & Merzenich, M. M. (2003). Model of autism: Increased ratio of excitation/inhibition in key neural systems. *Genes, Brain, and Behavior, 2*, 255–267.

Saitoh, O., Karns, C. M., & Courchesne, E. (2001). Development of the hippocampal formation from 2 to 42 years: MRI evidence of smaller area dentata in autism. *Brain, 124*, 1317–1324.

Schultz, R. T., Gauthier, I., Klin, A., Fulbright, R. K., Anderson, A. W., Volkmar, F., et al. (2000). Abnormal ventral temporal cortical activityduring face discrimination among individuals with autism and Asperger syndrome. *Archives of General Psychiatry, 57*, 331–340.

Seeley, W. W., Menon, V., Schatzberg, A. F., Keller, J., Glover, G. H., Kenna, H., et al. (2007). Dissociable intrinsic connectivity networks for salience processing and executive control. *Journal of Neuroscience, 27*, 2349–2356.

Sen, B., Asem, S. S., Sinha, S., Chatterjee, A., Ahmed, S., Ghosh, S., et al. (2010). Family-based studies indicate association of Engrailed 2 gene with autism in an Indian population. *Genes, Brain, and Behavior*. doi:10.1111/j.1601-183X.2009.00556.x.

Shah, A. & Frith, U. (1993). Why do autistic individuals show superior performance on the block design task? *Journal of Child Psychology and Psychiatry, 34*, 1351–1364.

Sharma, A., Hoeffer, C. A., Takayasu, Y., Miyawaki, T., McBride, S. M., Klann, E., et al. (2010). Dysregulation of mTOR signaling in fragile X syndrome. *Journal of Neuroscience, 30*, 694–702.

Shaw, P., Greenstein, D., Lerch, J., Clasen, L., Lenroot, R., Gogtay, N. et al. (2006). Intellectual ability and cortical development in children and adolescents. *Nature, 440*, 676–679.

Simmons, D. R., Robertson, A. E., McKay, L. S., Toal, E., McAleer, P., & Pollick, F. E. (2009). Vision in autism spectrum disorders. *Vision Research, 49*, 2705–2739.

Sparks, B. F., Friedman, S. D., Shaw, D. W., Aylward, E. H., Echelard, D., Artru, A. A., et al. (2002). Brain structural abnormalities in young children with autism spectrum disorder. *Neurology, 59*, 184–192.

Spencer, J., O'Brien, J., Riggs, K., Braddick, O., Atkinson, J., & Wattam-Bell, J. (2000). Motion processing in autism: Evidence for a dorsal stream deficiency. *Neuroreport, 11*, 2765–2767.

Splawski, I., Timothy, K., Sharpe, L., Decher, N., Kumar, P., Bloise, R., et al. (2004). Ca(V)1.2 calcium channel dysfunction causes a multisystem disorder including arrhythmia and autism. *Cell, 119*, 19–31.

Strogatz, S. (2001). Exploring complex networks. *Nature, 410*, 268–276.

Supekar, K., Musen, M., & Menon, V. (2009). Development of large-scale functional brain networks in children. *PLoS Biology, 7*, 1–15.

Tallal, P., Miller, S. L., Bedi, G., Byma, G., Wang, X., Nagarajan, S. S., et al. (1996). Language comprehension in language-learning impaired children improved with acoustically modified speech. *Science, 271*, 81–84.

Tallal, P. (2004). Improving language and literacy is a matter of time. *Nature Reviews Neuroscience, 5*, 721–728.

Townsend, J., Adamo, M., & Haist, F. (2006). Changing channels: An fMRI study of aging and cross-modal attention shifts. *NeuroImage, 31*, 1682–1692.

Townsend, J. & Courchesne, E. (1994). Parietal damage and narrow "spotlight" spatial attention. *Journal of Cognitive Neuroscience, 6*, 220–232.

Townsend, J., Courchesne, E., Covington, J., Westerfield, M., Harris, N. S., Lyden, P., et al. (1999). Spatial attention deficits in patients with acquired or developmental cerebellar abnormality. *Journal of Neuroscience, 19*, 5632–5643.

Townsend, J., Harris, N. S., & Courchesne, E. (1996). Visual attention abnormalities in autism: Delayed orienting to location. *Journal of the International Neuropsychological Society, 2*, 541–550.

Uhlhaas, P. J. & Silverstein, S. M. (2005). Perceptual organization in schizophrenia spectrum disorders: A review of empirical research and associated theories. *Psychological Bulletin, 131*, 618–632.

Uhlhaas, P. J., Phillips, W. A., Schenkel, L. S., & Silverstein, S. M. (2006). Theory of mind and perceptual context-processing in schizophrenia. *Cognitive Neuropsychiatry, 11*, 416–436.

Valla, J. M., Ganzel, B. L., Yoder, K. J., Chen, G. M., Lyman, L. T., Sidari, A. P., et al. (in press). More than maths and mindreading: Sex differences in empathising/systemising covariance. *Autism Research*.

van den Heuvel, M. P., Stam, C. J., Boersma, M., & Hulshoff Pol, H. E. (2008). Small-world and scale-free organization of voxel-based resting-state functional connectivity in the human brain. *NeuroImage, 43*, 528–539.

van den Heuvel, M. P., Mandl, R. C. W., Kahn, R. S., & Hulshoff Pol, H. E. (2009). Functionally linked resting-state networks reflect the underlying structural connectivity architecture of the human brain. *Human Brain Mapping, 30*, 3127–3141.

Williams, R. S., Hauser, S. L., Purpura, D. P., DeLong, G. R., & Swisher, C. N. (1980). Autism and mental retardation: Neuropathologic studies performed in four retarded persons with autistic behavior. *Archives of Neurology, 37*, 749–753.

Williams, D. L., Goldstein, G., & Minshew, N. J. (2006). Neuropsychologic functioning in children with autism: Further evidence for disordered complex information-processing. *Child Neuropsychology, 12*, 279–298.

Zwaigenbaum, L., Bryson, S., Rogers, T., Roberts, W., Brian, J., & Szatmari, P. (2005). Behavioral manifestations of autism in the first year of life. *International Journal of Developmental Neuroscience, 23*, 143–152.

Commentary

Francesca Happé

Translation Between Different Types of Model

Inspired by the chapters in this section, the present commentary discusses possible relationships and interplay between animal models and neurocognitive accounts of autism spectrum disorders (ASD). It begins with a recap of types of validation possible for animal models in general. After brief comments on construct and predictive validity in models of ASD, face validity is discussed at a number of distinct levels. Face validity concerning behavior or symptom pattern has been the primary focus for this behaviorally diagnosed spectrum of conditions. What should be the aim of animal models of ASD focused on behavioral face validity? At least two possible approaches exist; to attempt to model the full syndrome (as advocated by Tordjman et al., 2007, for example), or to identify and target "fractionable" elements, ideally intermediate phenotypes, which need not be unique to ASD. These different approaches are discussed, and evidence is presented for fractionating the triad of ASD characteristics. Lastly, possible contributions from cognitive theories to animal models of ASD are considered.

Assessing Animal Models: Different Types of Validity

As several authors in this section (e.g., Yang, Scattoni, Chadman, Silverman, & Crawley, Chapter 51) remind us, animal models can be assessed in terms of three broad types of validity: "face validity" or analogy to human syndrome, "construct validity" or similarity of cause or pathogenesis, and "predictive validity" or similarity of prevention, reversal, or treatment effects. In our ongoing ethical consideration of the use of animal models, a clear rationale and justification of validity is imperative.

In human conditions where the genetic basis is known, such as Fragile X or Rett syndrome, **construct validity** can be achieved simply in, for example, knockout mice. In the case of ASD, as Hsiao, Bregere, Malkova, and Patterson point out (Chapter 52), the etiology is unknown, and so establishing construct validity is a huge challenge. That ASDs are highly heritable is not disputed: twin and family studies (reviewed elsewhere in this volume) suggest heritability as high or higher than for any other developmental disorder (although see Corrales & Herbert, Chapter 49, for cogent arguments about why heritability estimates might be inflated by, for example, unknown gene-environment interaction or placentation effects). The genes involved in vulnerability in most cases of ASD are as yet unknown (Abrahams & Geschwind, 2008). In a small minority of cases of ASD, a known chromosomal abnormality will be identified, or a rare single gene mutation. Such cases are the focus of much investigation, for example mouse models of FraX are studied to illuminate ASD, because of the raised rate of ASD in FraX children. Such research (e.g., Spencer, Graham, Yuva-Paylor, Nelson, & Paylor, 2008) has highlighted the important influence of the genetic background on which the knockout is made. This reminds us that in the human case, too, the identified single gene mutation may not be the sufficient cause of the individual's autism, even in this small minority. Similarly, the causal role of raised copy number variation (CNV) in autism (e.g., Sebat et al., 2007), and other psychiatric conditions, has been debated (e.g., Joober & Boksa, 2009).

Animal models are key to exploring putative *environmental* causal factors in ASD. These, which include in utero factors such as exposure to neurotoxins (e.g., valproic acid), maternal infection (e.g., rubella) or maternal autoantibodies, are well described in the Chapters in section VII, by Hertz-Picciotto, Rodier, and Corrales and Herbert (Chapters 47, 48, and 49, respectively). Rodier and Hertz-Picciotto highlight similarities between the study of environmental factors and the study of genetic contributions to ASD: extremely rare cases with known cause (e.g., thalidomide) may shed light on some final common pathway of effect relevant to ASD more widely, but apart from these only rather weak links can be made to many hundreds of possible environmental factors.

Animal models are vital for testing the causal role of environmental factors associated with autism in epidemiological studies (reviewed by Hertz-Picciotto, Chapter 47). As the authors in section VII note, however, even identifying reliably associated environmental risk factors is complicated by the likely gene-environment interaction—that is, only some individuals will be vulnerable to the key environmental factors (or, genetic vulnerability will only be seen in certain environments). This requires studies stratifying environment by genetic group or vice versa. Since, at present, we know neither the key environmental factors nor the key genetic factors, one might be forgiven for a certain pessimism about discovering the causes of autism "bottom up." Corrales and Herbert suggest, however, that the study of biomarkers that aggregate multiple environmental risk factors would be one way forward in the absence of knowledge of specific teratogens (Chapter 49). Animal models exploring gene-environment interaction will be essential; seeing how a particular genetic variant develops under different environmental circumstances may elucidate not only causal mechanisms of pathology but also possible paths of intervention.

The process of translational research is, ideally, one of iteration between clinical/human and nonhuman/lab work. **Predictive validity** is often tested, for example, by looking at the effect of clinically useful drug treatments on animal models of disorder. In the case of ASD, it is striking that there is no targeted drug therapy known to affect the core symptoms. Drugs may be given for aggression, anxiety, self-injury, and so forth, but no drug has been shown to alter social, communication, or repetitive/restricted behavioral aspects of the core phenotype. While this may change in the years ahead (note for example, recent work suggesting improved social processing during oxytocin administration, reviewed by Posey, Erickson, & McDougle, 2008), the most effective interventions for ASD to date are behavioral and educational (see Rogers & Wallace, Chapter 61; Kasari & Locke, Chapter 66; and others in this volume). These have not been "back-translated" into animal models relevant to ASD—although it is notable that social effects of maternal deprivation in monkeys can be reversed in some cases by peer contact (as discussed in Bauman & Amaral, Chapter 53). The effects of specific educational "environmental enrichment" deserve to be studied at the neuronal and epigenetic levels. It is interesting that individual differences, for example, in drug response within an inbred strain are typically regarded as "noise" in the data—whereas a clinical perspective might find drug nonresponders of particular interest. Even within inbred strains of lab animals (whose members are genetically identical), clear behavioral differences can be seen by handlers, in, for example, social hierarchy and cage stereotypy. These presumably reflect gene-environment interaction and epigenetic effects, important for understanding clinical heterogeneity.

The study of treatment effects highlights an important aspect of ASD that animal modelers need to note; developmental course. Studies of genetically at-risk infants, through the baby sib projects now underway in several centers (see Zwaigenbaum, Chapter 5, this volume), are providing more accurate information about how ASDs unfold. Animal models, and particularly possible future animal models of treatment effects, need to capture the profile of typically unexceptional very early development, followed by first signs of reduced social orienting (e.g., turn to name, preferential gaze to face, and eye contact) around 9–12 months. Recent research also suggests nonsocial symptoms emerging relatively early, such as peculiar visual exploration of objects (Ozonoff, Macari, Young, Goldring, Thompson, & Rogers, 2008) and repetitive behavior (Watt, Wetherby, Barber, & Morgan, 2008). Regression, ranging from relatively sudden "loss" of skills to increasing divergence from the typical developmental trajectory, appears to be common throughout the spectrum (see Ozonoff, Heung, & Thompson, Chapter 4, this volume).

Importantly, however, some individuals with ASD make good progress in later childhood or adulthood, and compensation can be dramatic, at least within structured and "scaffolding" settings. Thus the demands of the environment importantly modify the presentation of ASD—in line with gene-environment interaction effects discussed above (and in detail in Corrales & Herbert, Chapter 49, and Hertz-Picciotto, Chapter 47). Since laboratory conditions typically strive to limit "noise" due to variable environment, limited environmental variance may mask relevant genetic variance in animal models. Similarly, quantitative genetic research with humans has shown the snowballing effect of gene-environment (G-E) correlation; that many environmental factors are "heritable" in the sense that genetically influenced traits evoke and search out certain sorts of environments (see review by Jaffee & Price, 2007). If lab animals have little chance to seek out, choose, or influence elements of their environment, these G-E correlation effects (and hence heightening of heritability) will not be seen. Lastly, the final part of the developmental trajectory, that is, old age in ASD, has barely been charted and remains a key area for future research. Tracing brain changes during aging in putative animal models of ASD may give clues for future clinical studies of ASD in old age.

The remaining type of validity, **face validity**, has perhaps been the main focus for discussion of animal models: is autism a quintessentially human condition? Could a mouse, for example, ever be "autistic"? However, face validity can be examined at a number of levels, much as Morton and Frith's (1995) causal modeling framework suggests any condition can be described and explained at behavioral, cognitive, and biological (neural, genetic, etc.) levels. Thus, for example, face validity of an animal model of the *neuropathology* of autism would depend on the homology between the human and model neural organization. While no single or sufficient neuropathology has been identified as causal in ASD, better-replicated brain features include reduced Purkinje cells in the cerebellar vermis, accelerated brain growth in infancy, and increased platelet serotonin, as well as the more recent suggestion of abnormal long-range connectivity—all of which are discussed in contributions to the present volume. Each of these could be interestingly modeled in nonhuman animals (see Chapter 52, by Hsiao et al.). Blaker, DeRienzo, and Sive's chapter on the use of the zebrafish to investigate ASD (Chapter 50), also reminds us that an "animal tool" may shed light on human pathology *without* approximating a match to the human disorder.

Face validity has received most discussion, however, in relation to the behavioral level, perhaps because autism is a behaviorally defined diagnosis. Here it is pertinent to ask, what should be the focus for animal modelers seeking behavioral face validity? Should the aim be to mimic the full syndrome of ASD (as advocated by, for example, Tordjman et al., 2007), or to focus on one symptom of the disorder (e.g., Miczek & de Wit, 2008)? In the next section, I'd like to suggest that useful pointers may come from studies of ASD and ASD-like traits in human quantitative genetic studies.

The "Fractionable Triad"?

Autism is only diagnosed in the presence of qualitative impairments in social and communication skills, and rigid and repetitive behavior/interests (RRBI). However, when one looks outside core autism, it appears that the "autistic triad" is not monolithic but rather "fractionable" (Happé, Ronald, & Plomin, 2006). Four types of evidence are relevant to summarize here (for fuller discussion of the "fractionated triad" view, see Happé & Ronald, 2008; Mandy & Skuse, 2008; and for a contrary view, Constantino et al., 2004). First, studies of ASD-like traits in the general population suggest that traits reflecting the three parts of the triad are only moderately correlated; correlations in middle childhood in large samples of twins (N > 6,000) suggest correlation coefficients around .3 or .4 (e.g., Ronald et al., 2006). Even in a sample meeting diagnostic criteria for an ASD (autism, Asperger's syndrome, or atypical autism; N = 189), social and communication impairments correlated around .5, and each correlated with RRBIs around .2 (Dworzynski, Ronald, Happé, & Bolton, 2009). Second, twin modeling suggests genetic influence on each of the triad traits is largely distinct and nonoverlapping with genetic influences on the other traits (genetic correlations range from less than .2 to .5; Ronald et al., 2006).

Third, many children can be found in the general population who have parent-reported levels of impairment as high as do children with ASD diagnoses, but in just *one* area of the triad. Taking the most impaired 5% in the Twins Early Development Study (TEDS) sample at age 8, the expected and actual overlap of difficulties can be examined. Clustering of difficulties is seen (Wing & Gould, 1979), with many more children falling into the two- and three-impairments groups than would be expected by chance co-occurrence alone (1.9% rated as showing 2 impairments across the three areas versus expected 0.75%; 0.7% rated as showing impairment in all three areas, plus 0.5% with preexisting diagnosis of ASD, versus expected rate of co-occurrence by chance 0.0125%). However, the largest numbers of impaired children (10% in total) remain those who have difficulty in only *one* area (social, communication, or RRBI) from the ASD triad. Item analysis does not suggest any qualitative difference between the behaviors prompting high impairment scores in these "single impairment" groups compared with children (with or without existing diagnosis of ASD) showing the full triad of difficulties (Happé & Ronald, 2008). Further study using cognitive tests would be informative, and one might hypothesize that using cognitive rather than behavioral probes will lower still further the interrelation between the different aspects of ASD.

Lastly, these results from the general population and twin analyses (which should be viewed in the light of contrary findings from, e.g., Constantino et al., 2003, using a different measure of social skills), find support from quite independent research on the broader autism phenotype. Family studies have shown that relatives of ASD probands show elevated rates of subclinical ASD-like traits, and may show difficulties in just one area of the triad (e.g., rigid traits without social difficulties, or vice versa; Pickles et al., 2000; Szatmari et al., 2000). This suggests that distinct genetic contributions, underlying separate parts of the ASD triad, are contributed by different relatives, coming together in the proband to make the particular "catalytic" mixture that is ASD. It is interesting in this regard that recent genetic work has made a distinction between "familial" versus "de novo" cases of ASD (see, e.g., Abrahams & Geschwind, 2008). It may be that the fractionated triad view proposed above holds true primarily for familial ASD—and that phenotypic and genetic correlations between aspects of the triad will be higher in de novo cases and even lower in familial cases than those values reported above.

On the basis of these four types of data, the fractionated triad view would suggest that animal models of *specific* aspects of ASD (e.g., social abilities/difficulties), ideally of valid intermediate phenotypes, is likely to be the most helpful approach, and that modeling of the full syndrome or symptom profile is unnecessary and possibly unhelpful.

Using Cognitive Accounts to Help Refine the Behavioral Phenotype

One of the challenges to establishing behavioral-level face validity of an animal model is that the manifestation of the core symptoms in ASD is so heterogeneous, as reflected in the use of the term "spectrum." Thus, social impairment is not a simple lack of sociability, and social approach can range from aloof to "active-but-odd," with eye contact, for example, varying from avoidant to staring. Similarly, communication impairment is not "just" delay or lack of spoken language, but lack of compensation with communicative gesture, and abnormal pragmatics even in the face of excellent vocabulary and perfect syntax. Rigid/repetitive interests and activities also vary widely, ranging from rocking, to spinning objects, to abstruse fact collection. It is probably also important to note the "fractionation" within RRBIs apparent in, for example, factor analytic studies (e.g., Lam, Bodfish, & Piven, 2009). One facet of these varied manifestations is that some aspects of development are found to be at age-typical or even superior levels in ASD. Thus our models (animal or otherwise) need to allow for uneven profiles of skills. For example, models of social impairment in ASD need to allow for attachment to parent that appears to be no different from that of other children of the same developmental level (Rutgers, Bakermans-Kranenburg, van IJzendoorn, & Van Berckelaer-Onnes, 2004). Similarly, while intellectual disability is strongly associated with ASD, a good model of ASD would allow for typical or superior levels of intelligence alongside specific social difficulty. In this context, it is exciting to see possible mouse models with areas of *superior* ability: faster eye blink conditioning in the valproate model (reviewed by Rodier, Chapter 48); enhanced spatial learning/water maze in some knockout mouse models focused on autism candidate genes (reviewed in Hsiao et al., Chapter 52).

A second challenge in considering behavioral face validity of ASD models is the essential ambiguity of behavior. Consider, for example, a knockout mouse who fails to explore his environment. This single measure of behavior could reflect several alterative underlying factors: for example, high anxiety, difficulty switching attention from current focus, or sensory sensitivities. Another model animal who fails to approach a conspecific may do so due to reduced social interest, but might instead be demonstrating abnormally high interest in nonsocial aspects of his environment, or misrecognition of dominance or aggression cues. Behavior alone is ambiguous: is self-injury in a nonverbal child with ASD well modeled in an animal who shows excessive self-grooming? Do cage stereotypies in animals capture anything relevant to repetitive coin spinning in a young adult with ASD?

Cognitive theories help make sense of behavioral ambiguity and heterogeneity, by positing and testing core processing abnormalities. They draw together apparently disparate behavioral manifestations to triangulate on latent cognitive factors that may be invariant but displayed through a range of manifestations across ages and ability levels. Do these accounts offer any promise to those using animal models to understand the causes of ASD? Animal models are vital for testing the causal status of putative biological (including environmental and genetic) factors, which cannot be manipulated in studies with human participants. By contrast, cognitive level theories typically do not *need* animal models for testing their hypotheses, and cognitive factors can be manipulated through good task design (what Frith has called the method of "fine cuts"; Frith & Happé, 1998). However, cognitive theories may be useful in the process of so-called reverse translation, by, for example, suggesting novel behavioral assays. Bauman and Amaral highlight the need for behavioral probes sensitive to the core features of ASD in animals (Chapter 53). Cognitive accounts may help with this. For example, Klin, Lin, Gorrindo, Ramsay, and Jones (2009) found insensitivity to biological motion and increased sensitivity to audiovisual synchrony in toddlers with ASD. Since preferential attention to biological motion can be found in a variety of species (Johnson, 2006), this might prove a useful focus for behavioral assays of animal models—although perhaps only at certain stages of development.

Another strand of cognitive accounts takes as its focus the uneven profile of skills and difficulties, as well as the narrow focus of interests in ASD. Several current theories suggest superior featural processing in ASD (e.g., weak coherence, Happé & Frith, 2006; Happé & Booth, 2008; enhanced perceptual functioning, Mottron et al., 2006; enhanced discrimination/reduced generalization, Plaisted, 2001). While there is debate as to the precedence of global versus local processing in nonhuman animals (using classic paradigms such as Navon hierarchical figures, e.g., Goto et al., 2004), these accounts provide plenty of scope for developing novel behavioral assays for animal models. For example, the superior eye for detail that in ASD appears to contribute to distress at "tiny" changes, might in an animal model be probed by recognition or habituation paradigms incorporating minor featural changes. Baron-Cohen's recent work on hypersensitive perceptual discrimination (Baron-Cohen et al., 2009) would suggest that a mouse able, for example, to discriminate odors more sensitively than is typical, might be of interest in relation to ASD.

Considering superior featural processing in ASD also illustrates again the importance of cognitive theory and the potential ambiguity of behavior alone. For example, recognition memory for faces is poor in ASD (e.g., Blair, Frith, Smith, Abell, & Cipolotti, 2002). A candidate behavioral homologue in the mouse might be conspecific identity recognition by smell, since olfaction is the key sense in this species. Testing social sniffing behavior is a good probe, then, if your cognitive model of ASD is that identity recognition is disrupted secondary to a primary lack of social interest. However, if face processing is disrupted in ASD because of a featural processing bias (as suggested by reduced inversion decrement for faces), olfactory recognition may not be an appropriate assay.

The fractionated triad account, which suggests that different aspects of the phenotype have distinct and separable cognitive (as well as etiological) underpinnings, also promotes the study of aspects of ASD that are not necessarily unique to ASD. This is relevant to cognitive accounts of nonsocial features of ASD, such as the executive dysfunction account (see, e.g., Hill, 2004, for review). One criticism of this account has been that executive impairments are seen in a number of other clinical groups (e.g., ADHD), who do not show the striking social deficits seen in ASD. This was taken as detracting from the dysexecutive account of ASD because executive impairment could not explain the core social difficulties. However, on the fractionated triad account, executive dysfunction may be critical to ASD, even if it overlaps entirely with that seen in ADHD, because it is the *combination* of deficits that gives ASD its particular flavor and manifestation, not necessarily the uniqueness of any one of its components. This should be encouraging for researchers developing animal and other causal models of ASD: what has been discovered about response selection and action in response to novelty (e.g., Eagle, Bari, & Robbins, 2008), whatever the target clinical group or disorder, could prove relevant to understanding RRBI in ASD. The implication is that, for example, the lack of social impairment in the primate maternal autoantibody model of ASD, described by Bauman and Amaral in Chapter 53, in no way detracts from the importance of their successful modeling of stereotypies— and that the latter need not be specific to ASD to be highly informative.

Consideration of the executive dysfunction account also raises an important point about animal models. In human clinical groups, notably in those with acquired frontal lobe damage, there is often a significant discrepancy between performance on tests and adaptive functioning in real life (Mesulam, 1986; Shallice & Burgess, 1991). That is, tests may fail to capture real-life difficulties, because of the structured nature of tests, the reduction of timing demands, or the scaffolding of generative skills by the test situation. Similarly a verbal and intelligent child with ASD may be seen at his best in one-to-one discussion with a clinician, but appear very much less well adapted in the unstructured context of the school playground. Common tests of, for example, mouse social skills often do not extend beyond interacting with one or at most two peers, which may not tap complex naturalistic interaction. Yang et al.'s Chapter (51) discusses possibly more sensitive methods such as home cage observation of sleeping in a huddle.

It is notable that the theoretical models included in this section explicitly bridge and merge cognitive and neural data. Thus, Kana and Just (Chapter 54) link cognitive work showing good featural processing and poor integration of information, with neuroimaging data on functional and structural connectivity. Further links could be made to animal models; for example, Rinaldi, Perrodin, and Markram (2008) have reported abnormal frontal (hyper)connectivity in a valproate model of ASD. Baron-Cohen and colleagues (Chapter 55) propose high fetal testosterone as a factor influencing both superior featural processing and inferior social cognition in ASD. Iacoboni (Chapter 56) links the somewhat complex results on imitation deficits in ASD (for evidence and argument contra the mirror neuron account of ASD see Hamilton, Brindley, & Frith, 2007; Southgate & Hamilton, 2008) to single cell recording work in monkeys showing the existence of mirror neurons that link action recognition and production.

With their clear links to biological cause, these models would seem well placed to inspire animal models. It is interesting, however, that each appears to attempt to explain the whole of the autism symptom profile, in contrast to the suggestion from the fractionated triad hypothesis discussed above. Kana and Just suggest that "reduced functional connectivity is not confined to a particular domain or task, but is likely to be a general phenomenon at least across the neural systems involved in high-level cognition"—which would seem to predict a monolithic rather than fractionable triad of impairments in ASD (Chapter 54). In addition, a strong interpretation of their account would seem to render impossible the high intelligence seen in some ASD individuals. Abnormal functional connectivity is also not specific to ASD (e.g., dysconnection explanations of schizophrenia; Stephan, Friston, & Frith, 2009)—which is not a problem if it forms only one part of the neurocognitive underpinnings of the disorder (see above), but is problematic if proposed as a sole explanation for the full triad of symptoms.

Baron-Cohen et al. (Chapter 55) describe a sequence of findings linking fetal testosterone to both reduced social/communicative skills (e.g., less eye contact in boys at 1, lower vocabulary at 2, poorer social relationships and empathy at 4 years) and increased RRBI (more narrow interests at 4, higher "systemizing" ratings and EFT at 8 years). This contrasts with the prediction from the fractionated triad view, and the finding that ASD-like social difficulties can be found without accompanying RRBI traits, in the general population and in relatives of those with autism. Clearly animal models could be useful in testing the fetal testosterone account of ASD: if the "origin of fetal testosterone in amniotic fluid is the fetus itself" (Baron-Cohen et al., Chapter 55; but see Gitau, Adams, Fisk, & Glover, 2005 for positive correlation between maternal and fetal plasma testosterone levels), establishing the causal effects of high testosterone in utero will require experimental manipulation in randomized designs. Such research seems especially promising in light of Corrales and Herbert's (Chapter 49) reminder that some environmental factors (e.g., toxins, oxidative stress) differ in their effects by gender.

Do Animal Models Need to Consider *Associated* Features?

There are a number of behavioral and cognitive features strongly associated with ASD that are not part of the diagnostic criteria (discussed by Yang et al. in relation to practical difficulties with some animal models). These include epilepsy, intellectual disability, sensory abnormalities (sensory fascinations and sensory sensitivities), anxiety, and savant skills. All of these are found at greatly raised rates in ASD groups compared to other populations, but are neither universal nor specific to ASD. Should these associated features form part of the target for models of ASD, be they animal models, theoretical neurocognitive accounts or models of environmental factors?

At least some of these associated features show the interesting pattern that, despite high prevalence in ASD probands, they are not found at elevated rates in the first-degree relatives of those with ASD—i.e., they do not appear to be part of the broader autism phenotype. Thus epilepsy, seen in up to 30% of those with ASD, is not increased in rate in parents and siblings of ASD probands compared to the general population (e.g., Mourisden et al., 2008). How should we interpret this pattern? It would seem that epilepsy, and perhaps also intellectual impairment, arise only in the context of the full triad of impairments, but do not accompany individual parts of the triad. Anderson (2009) has suggested this pattern marks out "emergent" traits, arising from multiplicative effects between several genetic and/or environmental factors. Such "emergent phenomena" ("those phenomena that are sensitive to a particular configuration of risk alleles, factors, or traits", Anderson, 2009, 25) may be far harder to model than core features of ASD. Anderson also refers to the mirror image of emergence—submergence, where a typical developmental feature or skill fails to develop because one or more of the multiplicative collection of factors necessary for its development is disrupted. Such a process would be open to disruption from a large range of possible causes, since it involves many coacting healthy systems, contributing to one final common pathway. On a more optimistic note, Anderson points out that remediation of such an emergent process might be tractable: "The potential for small changes to produce large non-linear effects on emergent phenotypes is exciting and should provide impetus to this area of research" (2009, 25). In this regard it is interesting that Yang et al. (Chapter 51) report that environmental enrichment can not only reduce stereotypies in lab-reared deer-mice, but also improve learning and reduce seizure vulnerability.

Cognitively inspired twin modeling may be helpful in unpicking possible relationships between core and associated features of ASD, and in turn guide animal models of genetic and environmental effects. For example, Vital, Ronald, Wallace, and Happé (2009) have explored parent-reported special abilities (in music, math, art, or memory), because of the greatly raised rate of special skills in ASD (Happé & Frith, 2010). Their study in typically developing twins showed significant phenotypic and genetic correlation between reported special abilities and ASD-like RRBI traits (Happé & Vital, 2009). One implication of this might be that animal models of the RRBI part of the triad should search for signs of superior skills, memory and/or discrimination of stimuli.

Another possibility is that some of these associated features are secondary or downstream effects of core aspects of ASD. For example, work by Hallett and colleagues, again using twin modeling, has suggested that individual differences in ASD-like traits and in internalizing (anxiety and depression) in the general population are not linked by shared genetic effects, but over time show phenotypic links (Hallett, Ronald, Rijsdijk, & Happé, 2010). Thus, children's social and communication difficulties at age 7, for example, predict their traits of anxiety and depression at age 12, even controlling for their original level of internalizing at 7 years. In principle, downstream effects might not be key targets for animal models, unless the hypothesized "domino effect" is one that could be itself modeled closely enough to allow conclusions concerning relevant clinical intervention. For example, it has been suggested that low measured IQ in ASD may reflect downstream effects of lack of social insight (affecting social routes to skill and knowledge acquisition, despite good general processing efficiency as reflected in short inspection times; Schueffgen, Happé, Anderson, & Frith, 2000); since socially mediated learning is so much more important for human infants than probably any other species, this domino effect is better studied (and ameliorated) in clinical/cognitive studies than in animal models.

Conclusions

Cognitive accounts of autism have an important part to play in the search for the etiology and neural basis of this puzzling condition. Not only can intermediate phenotypes aid genetic research (and thereby the search for environmental factors), and inspire neuroimaging studies, they may also provide new behavioral assays for animal models. Twin modeling suggests that the different aspects of the ASD triad are "fractionable," and this might encourage the study of isolated aspects of the phenotype (e.g., social cognition), and of aspects that may not be unique to ASD. Translation from "bedside to bench" and back is needed, to create real cross-talk between those studying ASD through genetic, epidemiological, animal modeling, neuroimaging, cognitive, and clinical methods.

ACKNOWLEDGMENTS

The writing of this commentary was influenced and aided by the discussion at the EMBL workshop "Translating Behaviour" (December 2009) and I am grateful to the participants and organizers. Thanks also to Uta Frith, as ever, for her helpful comments on an earlier draft.

REFERENCES

Abrahams, B. S., & Geschwind, D. H. (2008). Advances in autism genetics: On the threshold of a new neurobiology. *Nature Reviews Genetics*, *9*, 341–355.

Anderson, G. M. (2009). Conceptualizing autism: The role for emergence. *Journal of the American Academy of Child and Adolescent Psychiatry*, *48*, 688–691.

Baron, Cohen, S., Ashwin, E., Ashwin, C., Tavassoli, T., & Chakrabarti, B. (2009). Talent in autism: Hyper-systemizing, hyper-attention to detail and sensory hypersensitivity. *Philosophical Transactions of the Royal Society of London. Series B, Biological Sciences*, *364*, 1377–1383.

Blair, R. J. R., Frith, U., Smith, N., Abell, F., & Cipolotti, L. (2002). Fractionation of visual memory: Agency detection and its impairment in autism. *Neuropsychologia*, *40*, 108–118.

Constantino, J. N., & Todd, R. D. (2003). Autistic traits in the general population: A twin study. *Archives of General Psychiatry*, *60*, 524–530.

Constantino, J. N., Gruber, C. P., Davis, S., Hayes, S., Passanante, N., & Przybeck, T. (2004). The factor structure of autistic traits. *Journal of Child Psychology and Psychiatry*, *45*, 719–726.

Dworzynski, K., Happe, F., Bolton, P., & Ronald, A. (2009). Relationship between symptom domains in autism spectrum disorders: A population based twin study. *Journal of Autism and Developmental Disorders*, *39*, 1197–1210.

Eagle, D. M., Bari, A., & Robbins, T. W. (2008). The neuropsychopharmacology of action inhibition: Cross-species translation of the stop-signal and go/no-go tasks. *Psychopharmacology*, *199*, 439–456.

Frith, U., & Happé, F. (1998). Why specific developmental disorders are not specific: On-line and developmental effects in autism and dyslexia. *Developmental Science*, *1*, 267–272.

Gitau, R., Adams, D., Fisk, N. M., & Glover, V. (2005). Fetal plasma testosterone correlates positively with cortisol. *Archives of Disease in Childhood: Fetal and Neonatal Edition*, *90*, F166–F169.

Goto, K., Wills, A. J., & Lea, S. E. G., (2004). Global-feature classification can be acquired more rapidly than local-feature classification in both humans and pigeons. *Animal Cognition*, *7*, 109–113.

Hallett, V., Ronald, A., Rijsdijk, F., & Happé, F. (2010). Association of autistic-like and internalizing traits during childhood: A longitudinal twin study. *American Journal of Psychiatry*, *167*, 809–817.

Hamilton, A. F., Brindley, R. M., & Frith, U. (2007). Imitation and action understanding in autistic spectrum disorders: How valid is the hypothesis of a deficit in the mirror neuron system? *Neuropsychologia, 45*, 1859–1868.

Happé, F., Ronald, A., & Plomin, R. (2006). Time to give up on a single explanation for autism. *Nature Neuroscience, 9*, 1218–1220.

Happe, F. G. E., & Booth, R. D. L. (2008). The power of the positive: Revisiting weak coherence in autism spectrum disorders. *Quarterly Journal of Experimental Psychology, 61*, 50–63.

Happé, F., & Ronald, A. (2008). 'Fractionable Autism Triad': A Review of Evidence from Behavioural, Genetic, Cognitive and Neural Research. *Neuropsychology Review, 18*, 287–304.

Happé, F., & Vital, P. (2009). What aspects of autism predispose to talent? *Philosophical Transactions of the Royal Society of London. Series B, Biological Sciences, 364*, 1369–1375.

Hill, E. L. (2004). Evaluating the theory of executive dysfunction in autism. *Developmental Review, 24*, 189–233.

Jaffee, S. R., & Price, T. S. (2007). Gene–environment correlations: A review of the evidence and implications for prevention of mental illness. *Molecular Psychiatry, 12*, 432–442.

Johnson, M. H. (2006). Biological motion: A perceptual life detector? *Current Biology, 16*, R376–R377.

Joober, R., & Boksa, P. (2009). A new wave in the genetics of psychiatric disorders: The copy number variant tsunami. *Journal of Psychiatry and Neuroscience, 34*, 55–59.

Klin, A., Lin, D. J., Gorrindo, P., Ramsay, G., & Jones, W. (2009). Two-year-olds with autism orient to non-social contingencies rather than biological motion. *Nature, 459*, 257–263.

Lam, K. S. L., Bodfish, J., & Piven, J. (2009). Evidence for three subtypes of repetitive behavior in autism that differ in familiality and association with other symptoms. *Journal of Child Psychology and Psychiatry, 49*, 1193–1200.

Mandy, W. P., & Skuse, D. H. (2008). Research review: What is the association between the social-communication element of autism and repetitive interests, behaviours and activities? *Journal of Child Psychology and Psychiatry, 49*, 795–808.

Mesulam, M. M. (1986). Frontal cortex and behavior. *Annals of Neurology, 19*, 320–325.

Mouridsen, S. E., Rich, B., & Isager, T. (2008). Epilepsy and other neurological diseases in the parents of children with infantile autism: A case control study. *Child Psychiatry and Human Development, 39*, 1–8.

Miczek, K. A., & de Wit, H. (2008). Challenges for translational psychopharmacology research some basic principles. *Psychopharmacology, 199*, 291–301.

Morton, J., & Frith, U. (1995). Causal modelling: A structural approach to developmental psychopathology. In D. Cicchetti & D. J. Cohen (Eds.), *A manual of developmental psychopathology* (Vol. 1, pp. 357–390). New York: John Wiley & Sons.

Mottron, L., Dawson, M., Soulières, I., Hubert, B., & Burack, J. A. (2006). Enhanced perceptual functioning in autism: An updated model, and eight principles of autistic perception. *Journal of Autism and Developmental Disorders, 36*, 27–43.

Posey, D. J., Erickson, C. A., & McDougle, C. J. (2008). Developing drugs for core social and communication impairment in autism. *Child and Adolescent Psychiatric Clinics of North America, 17*, 787–801.

Ozonoff, S., Macari, S., Young, G. S., Goldring, S., Thompson, M., & Rogers, S. J. (2008). Atypical object exploration at 12 months of age is associated with autism in a prospective sample. *Autism, 12*, 457–472.

Pickles, A., Starr, E., Kazak, S., Bolton, P., Papanikolaou, K., Bailey, A., et al. (2000). Variable expression of the autism broader phenotype: Findings from extended pedigrees. *Journal of Child Psychology and Psychiatry, 41*, 491–502.

Plaisted, K. C. (2001). Reduced generalization in autism: An alternative to weak central coherence. In J. A. Burack, T. Charman, N. Yirmiya & P. R. Zelazo (Eds.), *The development of autism: Perspectives from theory and research.* (pp. 149–169). Mahwah, NJ: Lawrence Erlbaum.

Rinaldi, T., Perrodin, C., & Markram, H. (2008). Hyper-connectivity and hyper-plasticity in the medial prefrontal cortex in the valproic acid animal model of autism. *Frontiers in Neural Circuits, 2*, 4.

Ronald, A., Happé, F., Bolton, P., Butcher, L. M., Price, T. S., Wheelwright, S., et al. (2006). Genetic heterogeneity between the three components of the autism spectrum: A twin study. *Journal of the American Academy of Child and Adolescent Psychiatry, 45*, 691–699.

Rutgers, A. H., Bakermans-Kranenburg, M. J., van IJzendoorn, M. H., & Van Berckelaer-Onnes, I. A. (2004). Autism and attachment: A meta-analytic review. *Journal of Child Psychology and Psychiatry, 45*, 1123–1134.

Schueffgen, K., Happé, F., Andersen, M., & Frith, U. (2000). High "intelligence," low "IQ"? Speed of processing and measured IQ in children with autism. *Development and Psychopathology, 12*, 83–90.

Sebat, J., Lakshmi, B., Malhotra, D., et al. (2007). Strong association of de novo copy number mutations with autism. *Science, 316*, 445–449.

Shallice, T., & Burgess, P. W. (1991). Deficits in strategy application following frontal lobe damage in man. *Brain, 114*, 727–741.

Southgate, V., & Hamilton, A. (2008). Unbroken mirrors: Challenging a theory of autism. *Trends in Cognitive Sciences, 12*, 225–229.

Spencer, C. M., Graham, D. F., Yuva-Paylor, L. A., Nelson, D. L., & Paylor, R. (2008). Social behavior in Fmr1 knockout mice carrying a human FMR1 transgene. *Behavioural Neuroscience, 122*, 710–715.

Stephan, K. E., Friston, K. J., & Frith, C. D. (2009). Dysconnection in schizophrenia: From abnormal synaptic plasticity to failures of self-monitoring. *Schizophrenia Bulletin, 35*, 509–527.

Szatmari, P., MacLean, J. E., Jones, M. B., Bryson, S. E., Zwaigenbaum, L., Bartolucci, G., et al. (2000). The familial aggregation of the lesser variant in biological and nonbiological relatives of PDD probands: A family history study. *Journal of Child Psychology and Psychiatry and Allied Disciplines, 41*(5), 579–586.

TordjmanS.,Drapier,D.,Bonnot,O.,Graignic,R.,Fortes,S.,Cohen,D., et al. (2007). Animal models relevant to schizophrenia and autism: Validity and limitations. *Behavior Genetics, 37*, 61–78.

Vital, P., Ronald, A., Wallace, G. L., & Happé, F. (2009). Relationship between special abilities and autistic-like traits in a large population-based sample of typically-developing 8-year-olds. *Journal of Child Psychology and Psychiatry, 50*, 1093–1101.

Watt, N., Wetherby, A. M., Barber, A., & Morgan, L. (2008). Repetitive and stereotyped behaviors in children with autism spectrum disorders in the second year of life. *Journal of Autism and Developmental Disorders, 38*, 1518–1533.

Wing, L., & Gould, J. (1979). Severe impairments of social interaction and associated abnormalities in children: Epidemiology and classification. *Journal of Autism and Developmental Disorders, 9*(1), 11–29.

Section IX

Treatment Approaches

58 Tristram Smith

Tristram Smith

Applied Behavior Analysis and Early Intensive Behavioral Intervention

Points of Interest

- Applied behavior analysis (ABA) is a discipline of research and practice within the helping professions. ABA interventions are implemented in many settings, with many different clinical and nonclinical populations.
- ABA interventions for individuals with autism spectrum disorders (ASD) primarily involve strategies based on operant conditioning, such as systematically reinforcing target behaviors and teaching individuals to distinguish between different cues in their environments.
- In both research and practice settings, ABA interventions are routinely evaluated with single-case experimental designs in which each individual serves as his or her own control.
- One ABA intervention format, discrete trial training (DTT), is designed to help individuals with ASD master new skills rapidly by breaking down instruction into a series of short, simple learning units, each of which lasts only a few seconds and has a clear beginning and end. Other ABA intervention formats are more loosely structured and are used to promote generalization from the teaching situation to everyday settings.
- Research suggests that when implemented intensively (20–40 hours per week) and early (beginning prior to age 4 years), ABA may enable some children to make significant gains in IQ and other standardized test scores.
- Many studies indicate that ABA interventions can help individuals with ASD learn new skills, but these studies have involved small numbers of subjects, most of whom are young, developmentally delayed, or both. Thus, larger studies that include a broader range of individuals with ASD are needed.

ABA draws on principles of learning theory to help people learn new skills and overcome behavior problems (Cooper, Heron, & Heward, 2007). ABA has become an important intervention strategy for persons with ASD, but, more generally, it is an applied science and profession that is practiced in diverse contexts. Examples include general and special education at all grade levels (Heward et al., 2005), psychotherapy for a variety of behavioral disorders (Woods & Kanter, 2007), safety programs at job sites and other locations (Geller, 2001), management of business organizations (MacWhinney, Redmon, & Johnson, 2001), and interventions to promote health and well-being (Cummings, O'Donahue, & Ferguson, 2003).

In ABA, the term *applied* refers to a focus on socially relevant outcomes (Baer, Wolf, & Risley, 1968). For individuals with autism, ABA practitioners and researchers (referred to as behavior analysts) have emphasized outcomes such as moving out of institutions into the community (Lovaas et al., 1973), entering general education classes (Lovaas, 1987), strengthening relationships with typically developing peers (Strain & Schwartz, 2001), and enabling caregivers to become effective teachers for their children (Johnson et al., 2007).

The term *behavioral* in ABA reflects an emphasis on measurable outcomes. Behavior analysts consider any action that can be measured to be a behavior (Baer et al., 1968). Thus, the defining features of ASD (problems with reciprocal social interaction, limited social communication, and intense repetitive behaviors or narrow interests) are all considered behaviors. Associated features of ASD, such as delays in cognitive and self-help skills, are also viewed as behaviors. Because internal states such as thoughts and feelings are associated with observable actions such as verbalizations, facial expressions, and body language, they too are deemed to be behaviors.

Analysis indicates that decisions about interventions derive from a systematic data-based evaluation. Data collection usually involves direct observations that are repeated on multiple occasions with the same individual over time. These observations are often supplemented by assessments of the acceptability of interventions and outcomes to consumers and caregivers (Wolf, 1978), as gauged from ratings or interviews.

Key Concepts

Behavior analysts recognize that ASD are biological syndromes and that research on genetic and neurological etiologies is necessary to advance understanding of the disorder (Smith, McAdam, & Napolitano, 2007). However, they also believe that it is possible to develop effective interventions without knowing the precise etiologies of ASD (Lovaas & Smith, 2003). They posit that whatever the etiologies turn out to be, the biological functioning in individuals with ASD leads them to be "ill-fitted" to typical environments (Bijou & Ghezzi, 1999; Lovaas & Smith, 1989) and that environmental modifications can promote behavior changes that improve their functioning and quality of life.

ABA emphasizes careful assessment of how environmental events influence the behavior of an individual. ABA studies show that many significant events involve operant learning, which occurs in all humans and many other organisms. This kind of learning takes place when an antecedent event sets the occasion for a behavior and a consequent event either increases or decreases the likelihood that the behavior will occur again. An antecedent event is a change within the individual or in the external environment that occurs just prior to the behavior and acts as a trigger. A *consequent event* is a change that immediately follows the behavior. Consequent events that increase behavior are called *reinforcers*; consequent events that decrease behavior are said to result in extinction. For example, when an individual with ASD sees a peer (*antecedent event*), she may make eye contact and say "Hi." If the consequence is a smile and praise from the peer (a reinforcer), the student is likely to greet the peer in the future. However, if the peer walks by without acknowledging the greeting, the student may not greet the peer on subsequent occasions because the behavior was not reinforced. Behavior analysts use the term *three-term contingency* to describe this relationship among the antecedent, behavior, and consequence.

Behavior analysts note that humans can acquire a three-term contingency without experiencing it directly. Through modeling, an individual learns a contingency by observing others. Thus, an individual with ASD might be taught how to make greetings by watching two people greet each other. In rule-governed behavior, the individual is merely told about the antecedent–behavior–consequence relationship. For example, a person with ASD might learn greetings by hearing an instructor explain, "When you greet others, it's important to make eye contact and say 'Hi' or 'Hello' to show you're interested." In equivalence class formation, an individual may learn that stimuli are associated with one another even if they have never been presented together. If an individual finds out that the spoken word "ball" corresponds to a picture of a ball, and that this spoken word also corresponds to the written word "ball," he is likely to associate the picture with written word, despite never being taught this association (Sidman, 1994).

As individuals learn new three-term contingencies, it becomes important for them to discriminate among antecedents. Discrimination learning involves giving different responses to different antecedents. For example, if a teacher holds up a ball and asks "What is it?," the correct response is to say "ball." However, if the teacher holds up a cup and asks "What is it?," the correct response is to say "cup" (and not "ball"). To help individuals make discriminations, behavior analysts systematically use prompting procedures such as providing physical, gestural, or verbal guidance to perform a behavior in response to an antecedent. Prompts are gradually reduced and eventually eliminated as the individual masters the discrimination. Throughout this instruction, correct responses may be reinforced immediately.

In ABA, an establishing operation (EO) is an event that alters the reinforcement value of a consequence. An EO also may alter the frequency of behaviors that the individual uses to obtain the consequence. For example, placing a favorite toy in sight but out of reach may increase both the reinforcement value of the toy and the rate at which an individual requests the toy. This situation creates opportunities to expand the individual's communication skills in ways such as requiring the individual to add more words to the request or to coordinate the request with eye contact. Systematic use of EOs is a central component of the incidental or "naturalistic" teaching approaches described in the next chapter.

Another common ABA procedure is task analysis, which consists of breaking down a complex skill into its component steps. For example, most self-help skills require completion of a series of steps. To wash hands, an individual must turn on the water, place her hands under the tap, apply soap, rub her hands together, and so on. Once behavior analysts have identified the steps, they can teach the skill with chaining procedures, in which steps are taught separately and subsequently linked together; and shaping, in which successive approximations of a behavior are taught (e.g., drying hands more and more completely).

Application of Applied Behavior Analysis Concepts to Autism Spectrum Disorders

In all, behavior analysts emphasize a rather small number of key concepts—mainly, the three-term contingency (antecedent–behavior–consequence), reinforcement, discrimination learning, and a handful of others. To behavior analysts, this short list has the virtue of parsimony (Lovaas & Smith, 1989). To many others, however, it seems too reductionistic to give an adequate account of ASD and support appropriate interventions (Greenspan, 2000). One reason for skepticism is that although most ABA concepts apply to humans and nonhumans alike, the defining features of ASD involve difficulties with skills that are unique to humans, such as reciprocal communication, creativity, and social interaction.

Behavior analysts have attempted to describe these difficulties in ABA terms. In ABA, communication is a particular kind of operant learning referred to as *verbal behavior* (Skinner, 1957). From this perspective, communication can be classified into different categories based on its function. In ABA terminology, mands include requests, questions, commands, and advice whose primary controlling variable is an EO, such as deprivation. For example, either stating a request or having a tantrum to obtain a favorite object could be a mand in which the reinforcer is receiving the object from another person and the establishing operation is lack of access to the object. Communication that occurs in the presence of a nonverbal discriminative stimulus is called a tact. Opinions, observations, replies to many questions, and verbal reports are all examples of tacts. Intraverbals are another class of communication that consist of verbal responses to a verbal discriminative stimulus, as occur in conversations between two people. An autoclitic is a unit of verbal behavior that clarifies or alters the meaning of other verbal behavior. Examples include plurals and verb tenses, which specify the number and timing, respectively, of other sentence structures and words such as *not*, which reverse the meaning of phrases.

From this perspective, many individuals with ASD make frequent mands, but the mands tend to be limited in variety or complexity (or both). Other classes of communication (tacts, intraverbals, etc.) may occur less often or may be inappropriate to the situation. (In ABA terms, the antecedents may differ from the antecedents for communication by typically developing individuals). The analysis of verbal behavior has had a strong influence on ABA interventions for enhancing communication skills (e.g., Bondy, Tincani, & Frost, 2004; Sundberg & Michael, 2001).

Creativity is defined in ABA in terms of fluency (number of responses), originality (novelty of responses), variability (differences between responses), flexibility (use of a stimulus for multiple purposes), and divergent thinking (problem solving) (Neuringer, 2004). By reinforcing responses with these characteristics, ABA practitioners seek to increase creativity (e.g., Lee, McComas, & Jawor, 2002).

Social interaction similarly can be characterized in terms of discriminative stimuli and reinforcers. For example, joint attention, which is an area of particular difficulty for young children with ASD, involves sharing an experience with another person (Mundy & Crawson, 1997). An example is looking at an adult, then looking at a toy, and then looking back at the adult. From an ABA standpoint, joint attention requires that the adult and toy each function both as discriminative stimuli and as reinforcers (Dube et al., 2004). ABA teaching methods for systematically establishing these functions may increase joint attention (Whalen & Schreibman, 2003). For older and more advanced individuals with ASD, problems with social interaction are often attributed to a lack of "theory of mind" (Baron-Cohen, 1995). That is, they struggle to explain, predict, and interpret the behavior of people in terms of mental states such as desires, beliefs, feelings, and thoughts. To behavior analysts, this problem may reflect an inability to detect social cues or a limited repertoire of responses to those cues.

Behavior analysts suggest that individuals with ASD tend to have learning styles that contribute to their difficulties in communication, social interaction, and overly repetitive or restrictive activities. For example, stimulus overselectivity, which is the tendency to focus on only one element of a complex antecedent, may interfere with generalizing communication skills to novel situations (Wilkerson & McIlvane, 1997), establishing joint attention, and detecting social cues (Koegel & Koegel, 2006). Inability to form equivalence classes may impede acquisition of abstract concepts (Wilkerson & McIlvane, 1997). A need for consistent, immediate reinforcement may deter individuals with ASD from engaging in social situations, which often have unpredictable outcomes (Bijou & Ghezzi, 1999).

In sum, relying on just a few concepts, behavior analysts have offered descriptions of the defining features of ASD. Of course, the adequacy of these descriptions is open to debate, but they have provided the basis for a large number of intervention studies, to which this chapter now turns.

Research Methods

Although other interventions such as psychotropic medications are also tested scientifically, a distinctive feature of ABA is that the same methodology is routinely used in both research and applied settings. This methodology is largely one of single-case research design in which individuals serve as their own controls, and interventions are evaluated for each person to whom they are applied (Bailey & Burch, 2002). Typically, the design involves comparing a baseline phase in which individuals receive no intervention to one or more intervention phases, with data collected continuously through all phases. If the behavior improves relative to the baseline phase each time that the intervention is introduced, one can conclude that the treatment may have produced this improvement. If the behavior does not improve, the intervention is refined or changed.

One single-case methodology is the alternating treatment design, also called a multi-element design (Barlow & Hersen, 1984). In this design, intervention is implemented on alternate days or sessions; on the other days or sessions, there is no intervention. This design is used when the effects of an intervention are expected to occur immediately. It also can be deployed as an assessment tool. For example, in a procedure called analog functional analysis, different experimental conditions are presented in an alternating treatment design to identify factors that may be maintaining a problem behavior. As an illustration, Ahearn et al. (2007) examined vocal stereotypy displayed by four children with autism. Following a standard functional analysis procedure developed by Iwata et al. (1994), participants' rates of vocal stereotypy were compared across four conditions, each of which was implemented in 5-minute sessions. In the alone condition, the participant was left by him- or herself. In the play condition, the participant was given the opportunity to play freely with toys. In the attention condition, the participant again played with toys, and the experimenter provided attention to the participant whenever the participant engaged in vocal stereotypy. In the demand condition, the experimenter made routine requests of the participants but withheld requests for 15 seconds in response to participants' stereotypy. Figure 58-1 presents data for one participant, Mitch. Each line in the figure corresponds to one of the four experimental conditions. The data reveal that Mitch's stereotypy occurred with the greatest frequency during the alone condition. This funding suggests that intervention strategies such as arranging the environment to minimize unstructured, alone time might be effective. The remaining participants showed different patterns in their data, indicating that appropriate interventions for them might not be the same as those for Mitch.

When an intervention might take longer to have an impact, the alternating treatment design may not be suitable, but another option is the reversal design, in which a baseline of several sessions, days, or weeks is followed by an intervention, followed by a return to the baseline phase, and so on. A reversal design can yield particularly strong evidence that an intervention causes behavior change for an individual participant (Barlow & Hersen, 1984). For example, Anglesea, Hoch, and Taylor (2008) used a reversal design to test an intervention for slowing down three teenagers with ASD who ate too rapidly. During the baseline condition, participants wore the pager, but it did not vibrate. During the intervention condition, the pager vibrated at 10- to 30-second intervals. Figure 58-2 shows data for one participant, Mark. As indicated in the figure, the baseline condition (pager prompt absent) was in effect for seven sessions, followed by six sessions of the intervention condition (pager prompt present), back to the baseline condition for another seven sessions, and finally back to the intervention condition for seven sessions. The black line shows the average number of seconds that Mark took to consume each bite during the session, whereas the gray line shows the total number of bites per session.

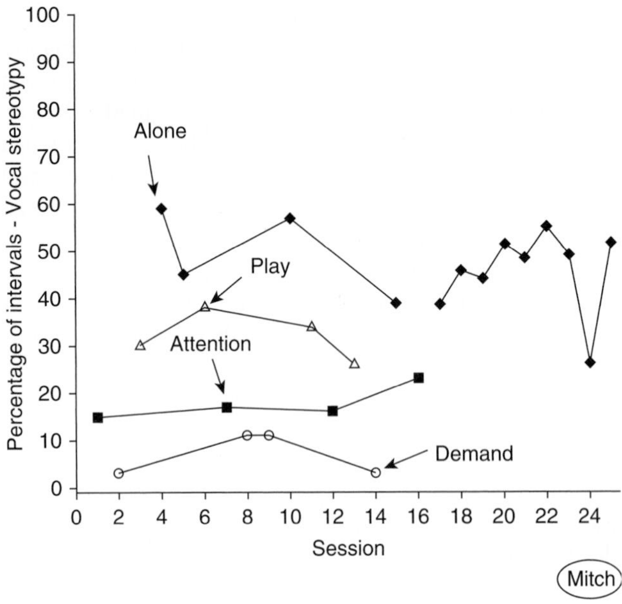

Figure 58–1. Example of an alternating treatment (multi-element) design. Percentage of observation intervals with stereotypic behavior for Mitch across four experimental conditions: Alone, Play, Attention, and Demand. Reprinted with permission from Ahearn, W. H., Clark, K. M., MacDonald, R. P. F., & Chung, B. I. (2007). Assessing and treating vocal stereotypy in children with autism. *Journal of Applied Behavior Analysis, 40*, 263–275. © Society for the Experimental Analysis of Behavior, 2007.

It can be seen that, going from the first baseline condition to the first intervention condition, Mark's time to consume each bite greatly increased, and the number of bites decreased. When he returned to the baseline condition, he reverted to the rates he had shown during the first baseline condition. However, re-introduction of the intervention replicated the gains made in the first intervention condition. This result

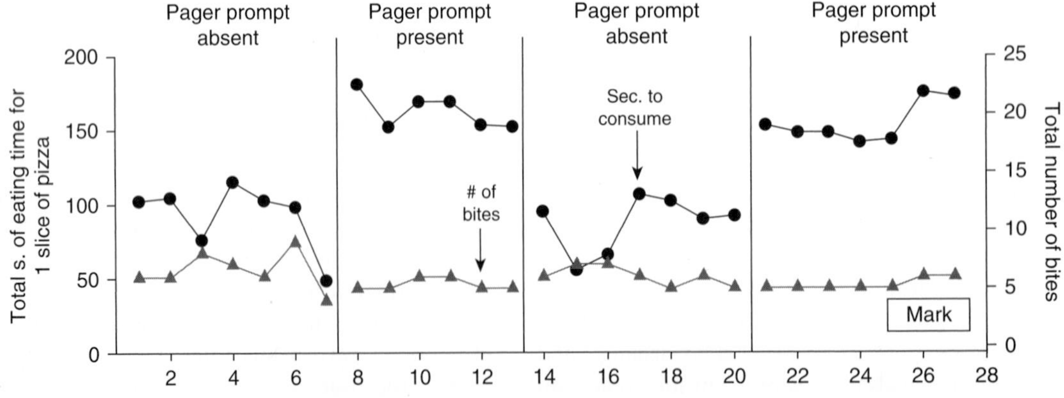

Figure 58–2. Example of a reversal design. Total eating time in seconds and number of bites to consume target foods for Mark across sessions. "Pager Prompt Absent" is the baseline condition. "Pager Prompt Present" is the intervention condition. Reprinted with permission from Anglesea, M. M., Hoch, H., & Taylor, B. A. (2008). Reducing rapid eating in teenagers with autism: Use of a pager prompt. *Journal of Applied Behavior Analysis, 41*, 107–111. © Society for the Experimental Analysis of Behavior, 2008.

demonstrates that the vibrating pager was effective in bringing down Mark's rate of eating.

Although useful for testing whether an intervention alters an already acquired behavior, alternating treatment and reversal designs are usually not appropriate for evaluating interventions intended to teach new skills. Such interventions should produce long-lasting increases in skill levels rather than gains that disappear as soon as intervention is withdrawn. A single-case methodology that allows for testing of more permanent effects is the multiple baseline design, which involves having two or more baseline phases that are of varying lengths and then applying treatment to one baseline at a time (Barlow & Hersen, 1984). For example, Betz, Higbee, and Reagon (2008) incorporated a multiple baseline design to evaluate an intervention for increasing peer interactions in three pairs of preschool children with autism. The intervention involved teaching each participant to follow a schedule that consisted of a series of photographs depicting games. The study included four phases: baseline, teaching, maintenance, re-scheduling (when the sequence of photographs was varied), and generalization (when new games were introduced). Figure 58-3 displays the results. The thinner line represents the percentage of intervals during which interaction occurred. The heavier line depicts the percentage of intervals during which instructors provided prompts for interaction. The first pair, Ali and Dillon (top of Figure 58-3), rapidly increased their rate of peer interaction and maintained this increase for the remainder of the study. At the same time, the rate of prompting decreased. A similar pattern emerged for the second pair, Brady and David (middle of Figure 58-3). This pair also participated in a reversal probe session during which the photographic activity schedule was removed (between the re-sequencing and generalization phases, as indicated in Figure 58-3). They seldom interacted during that session and thus appeared to depend on having the schedule available. However, they did interact during novel games in the generalization phase (with the schedule present). The third pair, Nathan and Jackson (bottom of Figure 58-3), also made gains when they were taught to follow the schedule. Overall, then, the schedule increased interactions across all three pairs of children with autism. Moreover, gains endured over time and extended to novel games, provided that teachers continued to provide a schedule.

Despite their extensive use in ABA, single-case designs remain somewhat controversial. Many psychologists and educators regard such designs as rigorous tests of the efficacy of an intervention. The clinical psychology division of the American Psychological Association suggests designating interventions as evidence-based if there are either two randomized clinical trials (RCTs) or a series of nine or more independent, well-designed single-case studies (Chambless & Hollon, 1998). The Council on Exceptional Children requires only six such studies, but with more stringent methodological benchmarks (Horner et al., 2005). Some investigators use single-case designs to evaluate interventions that originated outside of ABA (e.g., Rogers et al., 2006).

In contrast, criteria for identifying evidence-based medical interventions characterize single-case experiments as weak forms of evidence, on a par with uncontrolled case studies (Guyatt et al., 2008; Higgins & Green, 2006). According to this perspective, single-case experiments offer little more than anecdotal information, and other methodologies—particularly RCTs—are necessary to establish an intervention as evidence-based.

A working group that was convened by the National Institute of Mental Health proposed a middle ground (Smith et al., 2007; *see also* Reichow, Volkmar, & Cicchetti, 2008). The group noted that single-case experiments have greater methodological rigor than case studies because they provide continuous measures of the outcome variable and systematic replication of intervention effects. The group also suggested that there are some circumstances under which single-case experiments might stand alone as evidence for an intervention, but other circumstances under which it would be important to conduct further evaluations in RCTs. Single-case studies are best suited for evaluating the immediate effects of a specific intervention on a particular behavior for an individual participant. As such, they often suffice for testing interventions such as procedures to teach a new self-help skill. However, they may need to be followed by RCTs if it is important to look at more long-term and global outcomes, test combinations of interventions or compare alternate interventions, or evaluate outcomes across large groups of participants. For example, it might be useful to compare ABA interventions for problem behavior to psychotropic medication or to a combination of ABA and medication. Also, it might be informative to put together a package of ABA interventions to increase peer interactions and assess outcomes on general indices of social functioning such as reductions in core features of autism and increases in the quality of friendships and relationships with family members (Smith et al., 2007).

Applied Behavior Analysis Intervention Strategies

Many ABA interventions for individuals with ASD have support from multiple single-case studies. These interventions focus on either overcoming behavioral deficits (increasing the skillfulness or frequency of a behavior) or reducing behavioral excesses (decreasing the rate or severity of challenging behavior). Interventions for overcoming behavioral deficits range from highly structured teaching methods to more loosely structured methods and incidental teaching in which instruction is embedded in the context of everyday activities. (Incidental teaching methods are described in more detail in Chapter 59). Interventions for reducing behavioral excesses are based on an assessment of antecedents that may trigger a behavior and consequences that may reinforce it. The focus is mainly on preventing the occurrence of such behavior, but it

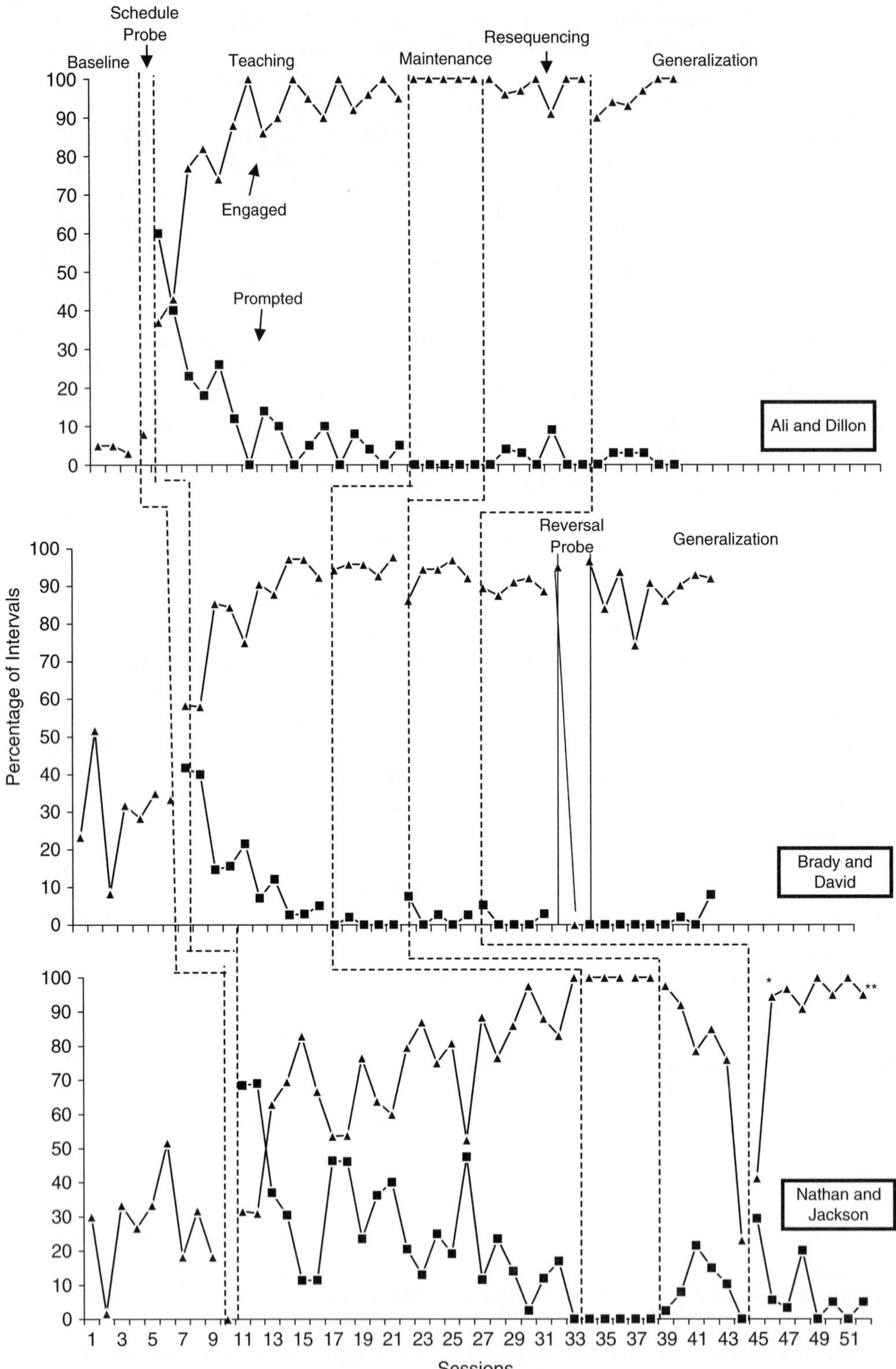

Figure 58–3. Example of a multiple baseline design. Results of the joint activity schedule intervention for Ali and Dillon (top), Brady and David (middle), and Nathan and Jackson (bottom). The intervention is introduced in the teaching phase and extended across subsequent phases of data collection. Reprinted with permission from Betz, A., Higbee, T. S., & Reagon, K. A. (2008). Using joint activity schedules to promote peer engagement in preschoolers with autism. *Journal of Applied Behavior Analysis, 41*, 237–241. © Society for the Experimental Analysis of Behavior, 2008.

is usually also necessary to consider how to respond when the behavior is displayed.

Discrete Trial Training

An especially distinctive ABA intervention is discrete trial training (DTT), which is a highly structured teaching format characterized by *(1)* one-to-one interaction between the practitioner and the child in a distraction free environment; *(2)* clear and concise instructions from the practitioner; *(3)* highly specific procedures for prompting and fading; and *(4)* immediate reinforcement such as praise or a preferred toy for correct responding (Smith, 2001). As a learner masters a new skill in DTT, interventionists aim to promote generalization of the skill to everyday environments by systematically loosening the format. For example, they may conduct sessions in many different settings, vary the instructions, reduce the frequency of reinforcement, and spread out the times when they ask the learner to practice the skill.

DTT is commonly implemented to shape new behaviors that were not previously in the repertoire of an individual with ASD, such as new speech sounds or motor skills. It is also emphasized in discrimination learning tasks such as imitating actions performed by another individual, matching identical objects or pictures to each other, labeling objects expressively or receptively, comprehending language concepts such as opposite pairs (e.g., big/little) and prepositions, and completing cognitive or preacademic tasks (e.g., counting objects or sequencing pictures).

DTT has been found to be effective in many single-case experiments (Goldstein, 2002) and outcome studies of early intervention programs in which DTT is a primary intervention procedure (reviewed later in this chapter). Behavior analysts offer several reasons why DTT may work (Smith, 2001). First, it breaks the continuous flow of social interaction into separate units that have a clear beginning and end (Newson, 1998). This simplification may help individuals with ASD—particularly those who are young or developmentally delayed—to learn the basic structure of an interaction between two people. Also, the trials have a predictable structure, and DTT sessions often involve repeating an instruction multiple times while systematically reducing prompts. This format may fit the preference that many individuals with ASD have for routine over novelty. In addition, DTT often involves breaking down a skill into small steps and teaching steps individually. Such an approach may be consistent with the detail-oriented learning style of individuals with ASD. Further, because each trial is relatively short (usually 5–20 seconds), DTT affords a large number of learning opportunities, thereby promoting rapid acquisition of new skills. Finally, the one-to-one instruction allows close monitoring of an individual's progress and careful tailoring of the instruction for the individual (Smith, 2001).

However, DTT also has important limitations (Smith, 2001). Because it requires setting up a tightly controlled environment with very specific cues, prompts, and instructional materials, skills may not generalize from DTT to everyday settings such as home or school even after interventionists systematically loosen the format. In addition, because it involves having children with ASD respond to cues from the interventionist, children may not initiate the use of skills that they acquire in DTT. Also, DTT is labor-intensive in that it consists of one-to-one instruction with the interventionist continually providing cues.

A more general concern is that DTT differs in many respects from the kinds of situations in which most children learn social and communication skills (Koegel & Koegel, 1995; Prizant & Wetherby, 2005). During the toddler and preschool years, most typically developing children learn these and other skills in the context of playful routines with caregivers, interactive games with peers and adults, make-believe activities, and independent exploration (Prizant & Wetherby, 2005). They seldom learn from being drilled. Moreover, typically developing children often learn by initiating activities to which others respond, rather than the other way around, as occurs in DTT. Although structured teaching becomes increasingly important as children grow older, unstructured times remain crucial for their development (Elkind, 2001).

For behavior analysts who rely on DTT, however, the differences between DTT and typical learning situations are precisely the point (Smith, 2001). Children with ASD present for treatment because, to varying degrees, they have been unsuccessful in learning social and communication skills in the same way that other children do. Although it sometimes may be possible to help individuals with ASD by finding or creating teachable moments during everyday activities, it may be necessary at other times to design an environment that better suits their learning styles (Lovaas & Smith, 1989).

DTT remains a central component of many long-established ABA programs, particularly for young children with ASD (Stahmer, Collings, & Palinakas, 2005). It is used in all comprehensive ABA programs that have been described in a manual and tested in published, controlled outcome studies of toddlers and preschoolers with ASD (cf. Rogers & Vismara, 2008). However, research indicates that it can be less effective than incidental or naturalistic teaching approaches (described in the next chapter) under some circumstances (Delprato, 2001), and outcome studies of comprehensive ABA models that place a greater emphasis on such approaches are currently underway. Also, as discussed, the highly structured format of DTT has both advantages and disadvantages. Therefore, DTT is not a standalone intervention for individuals with ASD. Rather, it needs to be implemented in conjunction with other intervention methods (Smith, 2001). In addition, there may be individual differences in how children with ASD respond to DTT as compared to incidental teaching. For example, Sherer and Schreibman (2005) found that although some children with ASD responded well to incidental teaching, others did not and might have fared better in an intervention program that emphasized structured teaching such as DTT.

Other Structured Intervention Methods

Other structured intervention methods in ABA have a more flexible format than DTT but still involve having the interventionist set the agenda, choose the skills to be taught, and provide direct instruction to the individual with ASD. One extensively studied set of approaches is called *peer-mediated social skills training* (Strain & Schwartz, 2001). These approaches involve coaching typically developing peers on how to engage individuals with ASD in social interactions and then having the peers and individuals with ASD play or work together in pairs or small groups. Research indicates that peer-mediated social skills training can significantly increase the rate of social interaction (McConnell, 2002) and also can be used to promote learning of academic skills (Kamps et al., 1999). Another set of approaches involves teaching individuals with ASD to follow a script, then fading out the script and systematically cuing individuals to use the script in appropriate contexts. A script might consist of a series of related conversational statements that the individual with ASD can make when talking with another person about a topic, a sequence of role-playing or make-believe activities, or a succession of actions involved in completing a self-help skill or activity of daily living. There are a variety of formats for presenting scripts. In video modeling, two or more models act out the script, and it is recorded for repeated viewing by the individual with ASD. A meta-analysis of single-case studies indicated that video modeling qualifies as an evidence-based intervention for enhancing skills in the areas of social communication, self-help, and on-task behavior during instructional activities (Bellini & Akullian, 2007). Alternatively, modeling can be provided in vivo, and some research indicates that this approach also can be effective in promoting skill acquisition (e.g., Coe et al., 1990). Additional formats for presenting scripts include pictorial schedules, in which each picture corresponds to a part of the script (McClannahan & Krantz, 1998), or simply written words or picture symbols (McClannahan & Krantz, 2005). A number of single-case studies support the use of pictorial schedules or written scripts to promote social communication and independent completion of activities of daily living (McClannahan & Krantz, 2005).

Interventions to Reduce Challenging Behaviors

Behavior analysts hypothesize that in most instances, challenging behavior is maintained (often inadvertently) by reinforcement from environmental or physiological events such as attention from others, opportunities to obtain preferred activities, or pain relief (Iwata et al., 2002). The environmental and physiological factors that are associated with challenging behavior are evaluated using a process called functional assessment, functional behavioral assessment, or functional analysis. This evaluation assists in designing interventions. For example, if an individual engages in challenging behavior to gain attention, a target for intervention might be to teach the individual to recruit attention through a simple request and ignore the problem behavior when it occurs. If, however, the challenging behavior serves to avoid an activity, the intervention might involve either skipping the activity or teaching the individual to request a break.

The quickest approach to conducting a functional assessment is simply to administer checklists such as the Motivation Assessment Scale (Durand & Crimmins, 1988) or the Questions About Behavioral Function (Matson & Vollmer, 1995) to ask caregivers why they believe that an individual engages in challenging behavior. Interviews such as the Functional Assessment Interview (O'Neill et al., 1997) can provide more extensive information. Another option is to observe the individual directly in his or her everyday environment. Finally, experimental or analog functional analysis can be conducted. This approach involves systematically introducing and withdrawing the antecedents and consequences for problem behavior in a clinical, home, or school setting (Iwata et al., 1994), as illustrated in the study by Ahearn et al. (2007) described in the section on Research Methods.

The choice of prevention or intervention procedure depends on the function or functions the behavior serves for the individual. Common prevention strategies include practicing activities beforehand (priming or preteaching) or presenting visual schedules to help individuals with ASD anticipate upcoming events (Koegel, Koegel, & Frea, 2003; McClannahan & Krantz, 1998). Another approach is to use differential reinforcement, which involves reinforcing adaptive replacement behaviors for the challenging behavior. For example, in differential reinforcement for alternative behavior (DRA), an individual with ASD might be reinforced for saying, "I need help," but ignored for flopping down to the floor. In differential reinforcement of incompatible behavior, behavior that is topographically incompatible with the target behavior is reinforced. For example, to reduce the frequency with which an individual with ASD gets up and leaves a teaching situation, in-seat behavior would be reinforced. Based on a systematic review of single-case studies, Odom et al. (2003) identified differential reinforcement as an evidence-based strategy for young children with ASD.

Strategies for responding to a challenging behavior and reducing the likelihood that it will recur include extinction (withholding reinforcement for previously reinforced behavior), time-out (placing an individual in a situation in which reinforcement is unavailable), and response cost (taking away preferred objects or activities). Another reductive procedure, overcorrection, consists of restitution (restoring the environment to a better state than it was in before the challenging behavior occurred) and positive practice. For example, if an individual with ASD throws a plate of food on the floor, she may be required not only to pick up the food but also to clean the surrounding areas and to practice throwing out food in the garbage. Until the mid-1980s, contingent aversives such as low doses of electric shock were sometimes used for severe challenging behavior such as self-injury that was causing significant tissue damage. Although research indicates that aversives often decrease challenging behavior rapidly (Matson & Taras, 1989), they are no longer implemented in the large majority of ABA programs because of ethical concerns, the potential for misuse, and the availability of non-aversive strategies (National Research Council, 2001). Behavior analysts currently recommend that if any reductive procedure is used, it should be based on a functional assessment and implemented as part of a multicomponent treatment plan that includes methods for preventing the occurrence of challenging behavior and increasing alternative, appropriate behaviors (Autism Special Interest Group, 2004). When implemented with these safeguards, single-case studies indicate that reductive procedures based on a functional assessment are often effective in decreasing challenging behavior, although additional studies are needed to examine the extent to which these improvements are maintained over time (Horner et al., 2002).

Applications of Applied Behavior Analysis to Teach Specific Skills to Individuals with Autism Spectrum Disorders

Social, Play, and Leisure Skills

Instruction on imitation is a standard feature of ABA and other intervention programs for toddlers and preschoolers with ASD (Dawson & Osterling, 1997; Rogers, 1998). The ability to imitate a verbal or physical action is an important prerequisite for learning more complex skills and is itself an important part of social interactions. ABA interventions to teach imitation usually involve one-to-one instruction in a DTT format. Instruction begins with a focus on imitation of simple gross motor actions (e.g., clapping hands) or actions with objects (e.g., putting a block in a bucket) and gradually progresses to more subtle actions (e.g., speech sounds) and chains of actions (e.g., sequences of motor movements). This approach can result in generalized imitation to new models (Young et al., 1994).

After an individual with ASD has acquired imitation skills, in vivo or video modeling can be used to teach a variety of social and play skills such as conversing with others, playing creatively, and taking turns during games (Bellini & Akullian, 2007). Peer-mediated social skills training also can boost such skills (Strain & Schwartz, 2001). Peers who are the same age as or slightly younger than the individual with ASD may be more effective than older peers (Lord & Hopkins, 1986).

Although these strategies produce immediate gains in social skills, generalizing these gains to new situations and maintaining them over time pose a challenge (Stahmer, Ingersoll, & Carter, 2003). Possible ways to improve generalization and maintenance include teaching individuals with ASD to self-monitor their interactions with others (Koegel et al., 1992), involving an entire class in implementing interventions (Kamps et al., 1994), providing scripts or cues of social interactions that the individual can use across a variety of peers or situations (Krantz & McClannahan, 1993) or systematically expanding on social initiations that some individuals with ASD spontaneously direct toward peers (Kennedy & Shukla, 1995).

Most of these interventions were developed for preschool and school-age children with ASD. Given that social demands change across the lifespan, it is unclear how effective the interventions are for adolescents and adults with ASD. Also, because the focus has been on specific target behaviors, the extent to which they produce more global improvements in core features of ASD and lead to improved quality of life (e.g., meaningful friendships with peers) requires further investigation.

Another important subpopulation that has received relatively little scientific study is children with high-functioning autism or Asperger's Syndrome. Peer tutoring may be beneficial (Kamps et al., 1992; Thiemann & Goldstein, 2004). Preliminary evidence suggests that self-monitoring and contingency contracting also may be successful (Mruzek, Cohen, & Smith, 2007). Behavioral social skills training in a clinic is another potentially beneficial intervention (Barry et al., 2003), but results thus far have generally been disappointing (Bellini et al., 2007). A possible way to increase efficacy is to provide intervention within the context of a classroom throughout the school day (Lopata et al., 2006).

Communication

DTT is often used to establish communication skills in nonverbal individuals with ASD (Lovaas, 2003). Instruction usually begins with a focus on receptive language, particularly following simple requests such as "sit down" or "come here" and identifying familiar objects or people. Once an individual has established imitation skills, he or she may be taught to imitate saying individual words and then to use basic expressive communication such as saying a word to label an object.

For individuals with ASD who have limited or no expressive vocal language, ABA interventions may focus on augmentative and alternative communication systems. In the 1980s, most research focused on sign language and indicated that many individuals with ASD were successful in learning to sign despite making slow progress in acquiring vocal communication (Carr & Dores, 1981). In the 1990s, the focus shifted to systems in which individuals selected pictures to indicate what they wanted—notably, the Picture Exchange Communication System (Bondy & Frost, 2001). Research indicates that this too can be an effective strategy for establishing communication (Howlin et al., 2007; Yoder & Stone, 2006).

Enhancing an individual's communication skills concurrently may decrease problem behavior. Functional Communication Training is an approach in which instructors teach or reinforce a functionally equivalent communicative response that can replace problem behavior (Carr & Durand, 1985). For example, an individual with ASD may learn to make a verbal request for a preferred object or activity instead of displaying aggression and may then begin to apply this new skill across settings (Durand & Carr, 1992).

Although ABA interventions have been developed to teach social communication skills such as conversing with others, repairing breakdowns in communication, and inferring implied meanings (e.g., Taylor & MacDonough, 2001), there is little research on the efficacy of such interventions. Also, as is true of interventions on social and play skills, the research that is available on interventions for social communication has focused mainly on preschool and school-age children with ASD and developmental delays. Consequently, research on adolescents and adults with ASD, as well as on individuals with high-functioning autism or Asperger's Syndrome, is a priority.

Repetitive Behaviors, Circumscribed Interests, and Other Problem Behavior

Functional assessments of stereotypic or repetitive behavior indicate that many individuals with ASD display such behavior at high rates regardless of environmental factors (Fisher et al., 1998). In some cases, however, the behavior may increase in response to specific events such as presentation of demands (Durand & Carr, 1987) or entry into an unfamiliar situation (Runco, Charlop, & Schreibman, 1986). Only a few studies have tested ABA interventions for reducing repetitive behavior. Simply increasing the availability of competing activities such as toys is one potentially effective strategy (Eason, White, & Newsom, 1982). Another approach is to interrupt the behavior and immediately redirect the individual to another activity (Ahearn et al., 2007). However, additional research is needed to confirm the utility of these interventions and test whether improvements are maintained over time. Unfortunately, even less information is available on ABA interventions for higher-order repetitive behavior such as an insistence on following routines or an intense preoccupation with a particular topic (Bodfish, 2004).

Daily Living, Community, and Vocational Skills

ABA interventions are often implemented to teach daily living skills such as toileting, dressing, brushing teeth, and food preparation (Matson et al., 1996). These interventions usually involve conducting a task analysis and then using chaining procedures to teach each step of an activity. The use of visual schedules, in which steps of an activity are displayed in separate pictures or photographs, appears especially useful (McClanahan & Krantz, 1998). ABA interventions also have been implemented to establish appropriate community behaviors such as crossing the street, but generalization of skills outside of the training context has been inconsistent (Haring et al., 1987). In addition, ABA curricula have been developed to teach academic and vocational skills. These curricula are based on a task analysis of the skills and involve developing the skills in a series of carefully planned, small steps (Engelmann et al., 1988). However, because evaluations of the efficacy of these curricula for individuals with ASD have been sparse, this is an area that merits further research.

Comprehensive Applied Behavior Analysis Programs: EIBI

In addition to conducting studies on focal interventions for specific target behaviors, behavior analysts also have developed comprehensive intervention packages. One comprehensive strategy is EIBI. EIBI is characterized by 20 to 40 hours per week of treatment for 2 years or longer, beginning prior to age 5 years. EIBI involves carefully structured, one-on-one, and small group intervention based on a broad curriculum that emphasizes communication, social skills, cognition, and pre-academics (e.g., colors, shapes, letters, and numbers; Leaf & McEachin, 1999).

There are also comprehensive ABA models for older children and adults with ASD throughout the lifespan (Handleman & Harris, 2006; Holmes, 1997). These programs take place in specialized classrooms, residential living programs, or occupational settings. They differ from EIBI in that they focus less on intensive, individualized, structured teaching and more on fostering participation in group activities and independent completion of tasks (without direct supervision).

Research shows that many individuals with ASD in comprehensive ABA programs successfully learn a variety of new skills (e.g., McClannahan, Macduff, & Krantz, 2002). At present, however, EIBI is the only type of comprehensive ABA program for individuals with ASD to have been tested in studies of long-term outcome. Research on EIBI suggests that ASD may be remarkably malleable in some cases during the first years of life (Rogers & Vismara, 2008).

The UCLA Young Autism Project

In the first study to draw widespread attention to EIBI, Lovaas (1987) and his colleagues at UCLA (McEachin, Smith, & Lovaas, 1993) evaluated an intervention that consisted of an average of 40 hours per week of individualized ABA instruction for 2 years or longer. Children with ASD began intervention when they were 2 or 3 years old. Intervention initially took place in children's homes and was conducted by teams of undergraduate students under close supervision by Lovaas, his graduate students, and other personnel who had 2 years of experience or more in Lovaas's intervention model.

During the first year of intervention, DTT was the primary intervention technique. An emphasis was placed on teaching skills considered necessary for subsequent progress, including compliance to elementary directions, imitation of others, and discrimination between instructional stimuli i.e., selecting a correct item from among a field of items, such as matching colors or pointing to objects or pictures called out by the examiner). At the same time, interventions were implemented to reduce behaviors that interfered with learning (e.g., tantrums or aggression) through procedures such as extinction or time-out. More controversially, as a last resort, contingent aversives such as a slap on the thigh were occasionally used.

The second year focused on expressive and receptive language skills, including abstract language concepts (e.g., adjectives and other qualifiers, prepositions, pronouns), as well as generalization of new skills to preschool and other community settings. The third year emphasized pre-academics such as early reading and writing skills, observational learning (learning by watching other children learn), and peer interaction. Also, children spent increasing amounts of time in preschool or kindergarten. DTT was gradually reduced and replaced with more naturalistic instructional approaches.

Lovaas (1987) compared a group of 19 children with ASD who received this EIBI intervention to two control groups: a group of 19 children with ASD who received less intensive ABA based on the same intervention manual (Lovaas, 1981) and a group of 21 children with ASD who received services in the community. Assignment to groups was based on therapist availability. If sufficient therapists were available at intake to provide EIBI, a subject entered the EIBI group; otherwise, the subject entered the less intensive ABA group. Although the groups had similar IQs at intake, the EIBI group had a mean IQ of 83 at age 7 years, much higher than the mean IQ of 52 in the low-intensity intervention group and 57 in the community-intervention group that received community intervention. Nine children from the EIBI group (47%) achieved average intellectual functioning (IQ >85) and unsupported placements in general education classrooms. Lovaas (1987) concluded that these 9 children could be described as "normal functioning" and possibly even "recovered." A follow-up evaluation took place when children averaged age 13 years (McEachin et al., 1993). This evaluation indicated that the EIBI group maintained its gains and also outperformed the low-intensity group on measures of adaptive behavior and psychopathology. (The community-intervention group was unavailable for follow-up.)

Some investigators hailed these findings as a breakthrough and identified a number of strengths in the study, including groups that appeared well-matched on most intake variables, use of an intervention manual, and outcome evaluations conducted by blind examiners (Baer, 1993). However, others pointed out many possible flaws, notably nonrandom assignment to groups, use of different IQ measures at intake and follow-up, failure to measure some potentially important outcomes such as changes in behaviors associated with ASD, and impracticality of implementing aspects of the intervention in community settings (e.g., 40 hours of intervention per week and occasional use of contingent aversives) (Gresham & MacMillan, 1997; Schopler, Short, & Mesibov, 1989). Lovaas and colleagues disputed these critiques but concurred that replications with improved methodological design were required (Lovaas, Smith, & McEachin, 1989; Smith & Lovaas, 1997; Smith, Lovaas, & McEachin, 1993).

Subsequent Early Intensive Behavioral Intervention Studies

Following the initial report by Lovaas and colleagues, a number of other studies on EIBI began to appear. At this writing, the literature totals 21 studies of ABA intervention in which toddlers or preschoolers received 15 hours or more of instruction per week, and outcomes were assessed on standardized tests. Table 58-1 lists these studies. Two studies were RCTs and are summarized in the first two rows of the table. Next, the table lists 10 quasi-experimental studies. In these studies, procedures other than random assignment were used (e.g., basing assignment on therapist availability or family preference). However, the EIBI group was matched to control groups on subject characteristics such as age and IQ. Finally, the table includes one study with a multiple baseline design and eight studies in which pre- and post-intervention scores were compared but that had no experimental controls.

In eight studies, including both RCTs and three quasi-experiments, intervention was described as adhering to the manual developed for Lovaas's UCLA Young Autism Project (Lovaas, 1981, 2003). These studies are identified by an asterisk in the table. All of the studies on the UCLA model differed from Lovaas's (1987) investigation in that contingent aversives were not used. With two exceptions (Cohen, Amerine-Dickens, & Smith, 2005; Sallows & Graupner, 2005), the studies also differed in that children received fewer intervention hours per week. The most common outcome measures, presented in the three rows at the right of the table, were IQ (assessed with a variety of measures), adaptive behavior (usually tested with the Vineland Adaptive Behavior Scales; Sparrow, Balla, & Cicchetti, 1984), and unassisted placement in general education classes (ascertained from school records).

One RCT (Sallows & Graupner, 2005) compared EIBI directed by clinic personnel to EIBI directed by parents. (State funding was available for parents to hire and supervise therapists.) There were few differences between the clinic-directed and parent-directed groups, but both made gains from pre- to post-intervention that were comparable to those in the study by Lovaas (1987). For example, 11 of 23 subjects (48%) obtained average IQs and unassisted placement in general education at follow-up, similar to the rate of 47% reported by Lovaas (1987).

The other RCT (Smith et al., 2000a) compared EIBI to in-home parent training on ABA techniques. At follow-up, the EIBI group obtained an average IQ score that was 16 points higher than the average in the control group. The EIBI group also had a higher rate of unassisted placement in general education (4 of 15 children, compared to 0 of 13 in the control group). These differences were statistically significant but were only about half the size of the effects reported by Lovaas (1987). The EIBI group also obtained higher scores than the control group on measures of nonverbal skills and academic achievement, although the groups did not differ significantly on measures of adaptive behavior, language, or level of behavior problems. Thus, the EIBI group made substantial gains

Table 58–1.
Peer-refereed studies on early intensive behavioral intervention for children with autism

Study	*N*	EIBI *N*	*M* Intake Age (months)	*M* intake IQ	Design	Control	Tx Site	*M* Tx Hrs/week	Follow-up	*M* IQ change	*M* Adaptive Behavior Change	General Ed Placement
Sallows & Graupner, 2005*	23	23	33	51	RCT	Parent-directed EIBI	Home	36	Age 7-8 years	+23	+9	11 of 23
Smith et al., 2000b*	28	15	36	51	RCT	Parent training	Home & School	25	4 years tx	+16	–2	4 of 15
Cohen et al., 2006*	42	21	31	62	Quasi Exp	Community Tx	School	35-40	3 years tx	+25	+20	6 of 21
Eikeseth et al., 2002; 2007*	25	13	63	63	Quasi Exp	Community Tx of equal intensity	School	18	Age 8 years	+25	+12	0 of 13
Howard et al., 2005	61	29	31	59	Quasi Exp	"	Center	35-40	14 months tx	+30	+11	–
Magiati et al., 2007	44	28	38	83	Quasi Exp	"	Home	33	2 years tx	-5	–2	23 of 28
Reed et al., 2007a*	27	14	43	57	Quasi Exp	Low intensity ABA	Home	30	10 months tx	+15	+2	–
Reed et al. 2007b	48	12	40	56	Quasi Exp	Community Tx	Home		9 months tx	+13	+3	–
Remington et al., 2007	44	23	36	61	Quasi Exp	Community Tx	Home	20-30	2 years tx	+12	**	–
Sheinkopf & Siegel, 1998	22	11	34	62	Quasi Exp	Community Tx	Home	20	20 months tx	+27	–	5 of 11
Smith et al., 1997*	21	11	37	28	Quasi Exp	Low-intensity ABA	Home	30	Age 5-20 years	+7	–	0 of 11
Zachor et al., 2007	39	20	29	76	Quasi Exp	Community Tx	Center	35	1 year tx	+2	–	–
Smith et al., 2000a*	6	6	36	50	Mult. Baseline	–	Home & Schonol	26	2-3 years tx	+4n	+5	5 of 6
Anderson et al., 1987*	14	14	43	58	Pre-Post	–	Center	15-25	2 years tx***	+14	10 months	0 of 14
Bibby et al., 2001	75	75	43	51	Pre-Post	–	Home	30		+1	+10	–
Birnbrauer & Leach, 1993	9	9	39	51	Pre-Post	–	Home & School	19	2 years tx	+14	+8	–
Harris et al., 1991	7	7	50	59	Pre-Post	–	Center	<30	1 year tx	+19	–	–
Handleman et al., 1991	6	6	40	47	Pre-Post	–	Center	<30	10 months tx	+11	–	–
Harris & Handleman, 2000	27	27	40	68	Pre-Post	–	Center	<30	4-6 years post-tx	+18	–	11 of 27
Perry et al., 2008	322	322	54	47	Pre-Post	–	Home & Center	20-40	18 months tx	+12	+1	–
Weiss, 1999	20	20	42	–	Pre-Post	–	Home	40	2 years tx	–	+34	15 of 20

* Study based on UCLA treatment manual, ** Raw scores reported, ***Year 1 results analyzed because of missing data at Year 2

Note. RCT = randomized clinical trial. Quasi Exp = Quasi-experimental design. Mult. Baseline - Multiple baseline design. Pre-Post = Comparison of pre- and post-intervention scores. Tx = treatment relative to the control group on some measures, but the gains were more modest and circumscribed than in the Lovaas study (1987).

The three quasi-experiments on the UCLA Model (Cohen, Amerine-Dickens, & Smith, 2006; Eikeseth et al., 2002, 2007; Smith et al., 1997) yielded positive results on measures of IQ. Cohen et al. (2006) and Eikeseth et al. (2007) also reported gains in adaptive behavior, but this variable was not assessed in the study by Smith et al. (2007). In addition, Cohen et al. (2006) also found that children in the EIBI group were more likely than control children to have unassisted placements in general education, although Eikeseth et al. (2007) and Smith et al. (1997) did not obtain this result. These studies are noteworthy because they extended the UCLA Model in various respects: Cohen et al. (2006) provided intervention in a community agency rather than a university setting. Smith et al. (1997) focused on lower functioning children with ASD and severe developmental delay. Although children remained quite delayed following intervention, they made gains on two variables (IQ and acquisition of communicative speech). Eikeseth et al. (2007) studied children who were older than those in Lovaas's (1987) study (age 4–7 years at intake), implemented intervention at school instead of in the home, and included a comparison group that received the same number of intervention hours as the EIBI group. Results were comparable to those obtained with younger children. The three remaining studies on the UCLA Model also yielded positive results (Anderson et al., 2007; Birnbrauer & Leach, 1993; Smith, Buch, & Gamby, 2000a), although Smith et al. (2000a) found more evidence of progress during the first few months of treatment than at a follow-up 2 to 3 years later.

Considering all eight studies on the UCLA Model, some investigators have classified the model as an efficacious treatment (Rogers & Vismara, 2008). Meta-analyses by Reichow and Wolery (2009) and Eldevik et al. (2009) also support this conclusion. However, another meta-analysis (Boyd & Spreckley, 2009) found that the evidence remains insufficient to support clear conclusions, and writers such as Howlin, Magiati, and Charman (2009) have identified many methodological limitations. For example, both RCTs had small numbers of participants. The control group in the Sallows and Graupner (2005) study received nearly the same intervention as the EIBI group. Concerns also have been raised about the procedures for monitoring fidelity to the intervention protocols, and the focus on developmental tests such as IQ (e.g., Kasari, 2002). Potentially important outcomes such as reductions in behaviors associated with ASD and the impact of intervention on the family have received relatively little attention. For such reasons, some investigators have classified the UCLA Model as only possibly efficacious (Faja & Dawson, 2006).

Some other models have support from studies without a control group (e.g., Harris & Handleman, 2000; Perry et al., 2008) or studies with quasi-random assignment (Howard et al., 2005; Reed, Osborne, & Corness, 2007a, b; Remington et al., 2007) but not studies with random assignment. As such, they have been regarded as promising but not yet established as efficacious or possibly efficacious (Rogers & Vismara, 2008). However, it should be noted that there are also studies that have failed to show benefits from EIBI (Bibby et al., 2002; Magiati, Charman, & Howlin, 2007). A possible reason is that these studies did not include procedures for assuring high-quality intervention (e.g., regular supervision of therapists), but in any event, they reveal that EIBI is not always effective.

Given that most EIBI studies have yielded positive outcomes, perhaps the next question is whether they have confirmed Lovaas's (1987) assertion that some children with autism achieve "normal functioning" after EIBI. None of the EIBI studies published before 2000 identified any such children. In contrast, more recent studies have indicated that a substantial minority of children (ranging from 27% to 48%) do perform in the average range in post-treatment assessments (Cohen et al., 2006; Howard et al., 2005; Sallows & Graupner, 2005; Smith et al., 2000b). However, Cohen et al. (2006) pointed out that they did not have enough data to describe the children in their study as normal-functioning. For example, they did not have information on whether children showed reductions in characteristics of autism.

Overall, despite some conflicting findings, EIBI—especially the UCLA Model—has substantial scientific support. Initial assertions that some children could be described as normal-functioning following intervention have not been replicated, but nearly all reports have described significant gains in IQ and other measures. These results provide reason for optimism. Nevertheless, it would be premature to conclude that its efficacy has been definitively proven. Additional research, especially large studies with random assignment to groups, remains a high priority (Lord et al., 2005).

Areas for Future Research on Early Intensive Behavioral Intervention

EIBI studies have incorporated a relatively narrow range of outcome measures, focusing mainly on IQ and other measures of children's level of functioning. Only three studies in Table 58-1 included tests of whether characteristics of autism were alleviated in EIBI. Remington et al. (2007) found an increase in joint attention following EIBI. Weiss (1999) and Zachor et al. (2007) reported a reduction in autism characteristics, but Sheinkopf and Siegel (1998) did not. Smith, McEachin, and Lovaas (1993) argued that tests such as the Vineland Adaptive Behavior Scales (Sparrow et al., 1984) could serve as proxy measures of autism characteristics. However, it is now known that many children with ASD perform well on such tests yet still display autism characteristics that interfere with their functioning (Klin, Volkmar, & Sparrow, 2000). Thus, more detailed assessments of autism characteristics will be necessary (Lord et al., 2005).

Little is known about "active ingredients" in EIBI, such as the choice of intervention procedures, dose or intensity of treatment, and content of the curriculum (Kasari, 2002). For example, regarding intervention procedures, two studies indicated that EIBI was more effective than community treatment of equal intensity (Eikeseth et al., 2002, 2007; Howard et al., 2005). These findings may indicate that the use of ABA procedures is an important component of intervention. However, in a third study, outcomes did not differ significantly between the EIBI group and the community treatment group (Magiati et al., 2007). Another issue pertaining to intervention method is that all EIBI studies in Table 58-1 emphasized DTT. No studies have been conducted comparing DTT-based EIBI to ABA approaches that rely more on incidental teaching (described in the next chapter) or to developmental models (Chapter 60).

Findings on intensity of intervention are similarly limited and inconsistent. The studies with the most number of intervention hours per week (Cohen et al., 2006; Sallows & Graupner, 2005) have yielded the most favorable outcomes, but a study in which children received nearly as many hours (Magiati et al., 2007) produced null findings. Apart from a small study by Reed et al. (2007a), direct comparisons of different levels of intervention intensity have not been conducted. Comparisons of interventions with different curriculum content also have not been performed.

Even in studies in which children with ASD showed large improvements following EIBI, there have been major individual differences in outcome. For example, the nine children who achieved the best outcomes in the Lovaas study (1987) made an average of 37 IQ points, but the remaining 10 children showed little change. However, it has been difficult to identify factors that predict differential response to interventions. For example, some studies suggest that intake IQ is positively correlated with outcome (e.g., Handleman & Harris, 2000; Sallows & Graupner, 2005), but other studies have not obtained evidence for such an association (Cohen et al., 2006; Smith et al., 2000b). Because EIBI requires considerable effort and resources, identifying factors that are associated with favorable outcomes has considerable practical importance.

Smith et al. (2007) recommended that following carefully designed RCTs to test efficacy and identify active ingredients, investigators should proceed to studies of effectiveness in community settings. This will be necessary for EIBI, which has already become widely available from community providers in many regions. For example, the Ontario Intensive Behavioral Intervention program was set up to provide services to children with ASD in the entire province of Ontario, Canada. A review of data on 322 children with ASD in this program indicated that children made gains on standardized tests and other measures from pretreatment to follow-up (Perry et al., 2008). Still, additional evaluations of such ambitious programs will be necessary to determine whether behavior analysts can "go to scale" and implement EIBI for much larger numbers of children than they have in the past.

Conclusion

ABA has become the most extensively studied psycho-educational intervention for individuals with ASD. On a practical level, ABA research has generated a number of potentially useful intervention techniques and comprehensive intervention packages—notably, EIBI—that may greatly enhance the functioning of individuals with ASD. On a theoretical level, ABA research has led to broad (although not universal) acceptance of single-case experiments as an appropriate strategy for evaluating interventions, increased understanding of the learning style of individuals with ASD, and suggested that ASD may be malleable if intervention begins early.

Challenges and Future Directions

- Extending ABA research to older and higher-functioning individuals with ASD: Almost all ABA intervention studies have focused on individuals with ASD who are young, developmentally delayed, or both. Obviously, these individuals are deserving of attention. However, older and higher-functioning individuals with ASD have been somewhat neglected, and increased efforts to develop and test ABA interventions for such individuals are warranted.
- Disseminating ABA teaching techniques: Some ABA intervention techniques have been refined over the course of many single-case studies but never presented in a format such as a published manual that would be accessible to non-specialists. Examples include peer-mediated social skills training and video modeling. These interventions also have not been tested in RCTs that would provide information on which individuals with ASD benefit most from them and what the long-term outcomes are. As a result, the interventions may be underutilized.
- Addressing core features of ASD: Along with the focus in individuals with ASD who have developmental delays, behavior analysts have emphasized accelerating overall rates of learning. In EIBI studies, the primary outcome measures have been cognitive tests such as IQ. Certainly, speeding up skill acquisition in individuals who have delays is a reasonable goal. However, alleviating difficulties that are core features of ASD (e.g., reciprocal interactions with others and social communication) is also crucial. A more systematic effort to create and test interventions for such difficulties is vital, and collaborations between behavior analysts and experts on the ASD phenotype could facilitate this effort.
- Conducting larger, more rigorous outcome studies: ABA research has involved either single-case experiments with small numbers of subjects or studies of EIBI at a single site. This state of affairs has allowed behavior analysts to work separately from one another and from other researchers. However, definitive tests of EIBI will require a concerted effort on the part of behavior analysts, probably in collaboration with investigators who have expertise in multisite RCTs and statisticians who can perform sophisticated analyses (e.g., to identify "active ingredients").

SUGGESTED READINGS

Cooper, J. O., Heron, T. E., & Heward, W. L. (2007). *Applied behavior analysis* (2nd ed.). Upper Saddle Hill, NJ: Prentice-Hall.

National Autism Center (2009). National Standards Report. Retrieved September 24, 2009, from http://www.nationalautismcenter.org/pdf/NAC%20Standards%20Report.pdf.

Sturmey, P., & Fitzer, A. (Eds.). *Autism spectrum disorders: Applied behavior analysis, evidence, and practice.* Austin, TX: Pro-Ed.

REFERENCES

Ahearn, W. H., Clark, K. M., MacDonald, R. P. F., & Chung, B. I. (2007). Assessing and treating vocal stereotypy in children with autism. *Journal of Applied Behavior Analysis, 40,* 263–275.

Anderson, S. R., Avery, D. L., DiPietro, E. K., Edwards, G. L., & Christian, W. P. (1987). Intensive home-based early intervention with autistic children. *Education and Treatment of Children, 10,* 352–366.

Anglesea, M. M., Hoch, H., & Taylor, B. A. (2008). Reducing rapid eating in teenagers with autism: Use of a pager prompt. *Journal of Applied Behavior Analysis, 41,* 107–111.

Autism Special Interest Group: Association for Behavior Analysis (2004). *Revised guidelines for consumers of applied behavior analysis services to individuals with autism and related disorders.* Retrieved August 14, 2008, from http://www.behavior.org/autism/index.cfm?page=http%3A//www.behavior.org/autism/autism_consumers_guide.cfm.

Baer, D. M. (1993). Quasi-random assignment can be as convincing as random assignment. *American Journal of Mental Retardation, 97,* 373–375.

Baer, D. M., Wolf, M. M., & Risley, T. R. (1968). Some current dimensions of applied behavior analysis. *Journal of Applied Behavior Analysis, 1,* 91–97.

Bailey, J. B., & Burch, M. R. (2002). *Research methods in applied behavior analysis.* Thousand Oaks, CA: Sage.

Baron-Cohen, S. (1995). *Mindblindness: An essay on autism and theory of mind.* Cambridge, MA: MIT Press.

Barlow, D. H., & Hersen, M. (1984). *Single case experimental designs: Strategies for discussing behavior change* (2nd ed.). New York: Pergamon.

Barry, T. D., Klinger, L. G., Lee, J. M., Palardy, N., Gilmore, T., & Bodin, S. D. (2003). Examining the effectiveness of an outpatient clinic-based social skills group for high-functioning children with autism. *Journal of Autism and Developmental Disorders, 33,* 685–701.

Bellini, S., & Akullian, J. (2007). A meta-analysis of video modeling and video self-modeling interventions for children and adolescents with autism spectrum disorders. *Exceptional Children, 73,* 264–287.

Bellini, S., Peters, J. K., Benner, L., & Hopf, A. (2007). A meta-analysis of school-based social skils interventions for children with autism spectrum disorders. *Remedial and Special Education, 28,* 153–162.

Betz, A., Higbee, T. S., & Reagon, K. A. (2008). Using joint activity schedules to promote peer engagement in preschoolers with autism. *Journal of Applied Behavior Analysis, 41,* 237–241.

Bibby, P., Eikeseth, S., Martin, N. T., Mudford, O. C., & Reeves, D. (2002). Progress and outcomes for children with autism receiving parent-managed intensive interventions. *Research in Developmental Disabilities, 23,* 81–104.

Bijou, S. W., & Ghezzi, P. M. (1999). The behavior interference theory of autistic behavior in young children. In P. M. Ghezzi, W. L. Williams, & J. E. Carr (Eds.), *Autism: Behavior-analytic perspectives* (pp. 33–43). Reno, NV: Context Press.

Birnbrauer, J. S., & Leach, D. J. (1993). The Murdoch early intervention program after 2 years. *Behavior Change, 10,* 63–74.

Bodfish, J. W. (2004). Treating the core features of autism: Are we there yet? *Mental Retardation and Developmental Disabilities Research Reviews, 10,* 318–326.

Bondy, A., & Frost, L. (2001). The Picture Exchange Communication System. *Behavior Modification, 25,* 725–744.

Bondy, A., Tincani, M., & Frost, L. (2004). Multiply controlled verbal operants: An analysis and extension to the Picture Exchange Communication System. *Behavior Analyst, 27,* 247–261.

Carr, E. G., & Dores, P. A. (1981). Patterns of language acquisition following simultaneous communication with autistic children. *Analysis and Intervention in Developmental Disabilities, 1,* 347–361.

Carr, E. G., & Durand, V. M. (1985). Reducing behavior problems through functional communication training. *Journal of Applied Behavior Analysis, 18,* 111–126.

Chambless, D. L., & Hollon, S. D. (1998). Defining empirically supported therapies. *Journal of Consulting and Clinical Psychology, 66,* 7–18.

Coe, D., Matson, J., Fee, V., Manikam, R., & Linarello, C. (1990). Training nonverbal and verbal play skills to mentally retarded and autistic children. *Journal of Autism and Developmental Disorders, 20,* 17–187.

Cohen, H. Amerine-Dickens, M., & Smith, T. (2006). Early intensive behavioral treatment: Replication of the UCLA Model in a community setting. *Journal of Developmental and Behavioral Pediatrics, 27,* S145–S155.

Cohen, H., Amerine-Dickens, M., & Smith, T. (2006). Early intensive behavioral treatment: Replication of the UCLA Model in a community setting. *Journal of Developmental and Behavioral Pediatrics, 27,* S145–S155.

Cooper, J. O., Heron, T. E., & Heward, W. L. (2007). *Applied behavior analysis* (2nd ed.). Upper Saddle Hill, NJ: Prentice-Hall.

Cummings, N., O'Donahue, W. T., & Ferguson, K. (Eds.). (2003). *Behavioral health as primary care: Beyond efficacy to effectiveness.* Reno, NV: Context Press.

Dawson, G., & Osterling, J. (1997). Early intervention in autism. In Guralnick M. (Ed.), *The effectiveness of early intervention* (pp. 307–326). Baltimore: Paul H. Brookes.

Delprato, D. J. (2001). Comparisons of discrete-trial and normalized behavioral intervention for young children with autism. *Journal of Autism and Developmental Disorders, 31,* 315–325.

DeMyer, M. K., Hingtgen, J. N., & Jackson, R. K. (1981). Infantile autism reviewed: A decade of research. *Schizophrenia Bulletin, 7*(3), 388–451.

Dube, W. V., MacDonald, R. P. F., Mansfield, R. C., Holcomb, W. L., & Ahearn, . H. (2004). Toward a behavioral analysis of joint attention. *Behavior Analyst, 27,* 197–208.

Durand, V. M., & Carr, E. G. (1987). Social influences on "self-stimulatory" behavior: Analysis and treatment application. *Journal of Applied Behavior Analysis, 20,* 119–132.

Durand, V. M., & Carr, E. G. (1992). An analysis of maintenance following functional communication training. *Journal of Applied Behavior Analysis, 25,* 777–794.

Durand, V. M., & Crimmins, D. B. (1988). Identifying the variables maintaining self-injurious behavior. *Journal of Autism and Developmental Disorders, 18*, 99–117.

Eason, L. J., White, M. J., & Newsom, C. (1982). Generalized reduction of self-stimulatory behavior: An effect of teaching appropriate play to autistic children. *Analysis and Intervention in Developmental Disabilities, 2*, 157–169.

Eikeseth, S., Smith, T., Eldevik, S., & Jahr, E. (2007). Outcome for children with autism who began intensive behavioral treatment between age four and seven: A comparison controlled study. *Behavior Modification, 31*, 264–278.

Eldevik, S., Hastings, R. P., Hughes, J. C., Jahr, E., Eikeseth, S., & Cross, S (2009). Meta-analysis of Early Intensive Behavioral Intervention for children With autism. *Journal of Clinical Child and Adolescent Psychology, 38*, 439–450.

Elkind, D. (2001). *The hurried child: Growing up too fast too soon* (25th Anniversary Ed.). Cambridge, ME: Da Capo Press.

Engelmann, S., Becker, W. C., Carnine, D. W., & Gersten, R. (1988). The direct instruction follow through model: Design and outcomes. *Education and Treatment of Children, 11*, 303–317.

Faja, S., & Dawson, G. (2006). Early intervention for autism. In Luby J. L. (Ed.), *Handbook of preschool mental health: Development, disorders, and treatment* (pp. 388–416). New York: Guilford Press.

Fisher, W. W., Lindauer, S. E., Alterson, C. J., & Thompson, R. H. (1998). Assessment and treatment of destructive behavior maintained by stereotypic object manipulation. *Journal of Applied Behavior Analysis, 31*, 513–527.

Geller, E. S. (2001). *Working safe: How to help people actively care for health and safety* (2nd ed.). Boca Raton, FL: CRC Press.

Goldstein, H. (2002). Communication interventions for children with autism: A review of treatment efficacy. *Journal of Autism and Developmental Disorders, 32*, 373–396.

Greenspan, S. I. (Ed.). (2000). *ICDL guidelines for assessment, diagnosis and treatment.* Bethesda, MD: Interdisciplinary Council for Developmental and Learning Disorders.

Gresham, F. M., & MacMillan, D. L. (1997). Autistic recovery? an analysis and critique of the empirical evidence on the early intervention project. *Behavioral Disorders, 22*, 185–201.

Guyatt, G. H., Oxman, A. D., Vist, G. E., Kunz, R., Falck-Ytter, Y., Alonso-Coello, P., et al. (2008). *British Medical Journal, 336*, 924–926.

Handleman, J. S., & Harris, S. L. (Eds.). (2006). *School-age education programs for children with autism.* Austin, TX: Pro-Ed.

Handleman, J. S., Harris, S. L., Celiberti, D., Lillehelt, E., & Tomchek, L. (1991). Developmental changes of preschool children with autism and normally developing peers. *Infant-Toddler Intervention, 1*, 137–143.

Haring, T. G., Kennedy, C. H., Adams, M. J., & PittsConway, V. (1987). Teaching generalization of purchasing skills across community settings to autistic youth using videotape modeling. *Journal of Applied Behavior Analysis, 20*, 89–96.

Harris, S. L., & Handleman, J. S. (2000). Age and IQ at intake as predictors of placement for young children with autism: A four- to six-year follow-up study. *Journal of Autism and Developmental Disorders, 30*, 137–142.

Harris, S. L., Handleman, J., Gordon, R., Kristoff, B., & Fuentes, F. (1991). Changes in cognitive and language functioning of preschool children with autism. *Journal of Autism and Developmental Disabilities, 21*, 281–290.

Harris, S., Handleman, J. S., Kristoff, B., Bass, L., & Gordon, R. (1990). Changes in language developmental among autistic and peer children in segregated and integrated preschool settings. *Journal of Autism and Developmental Disorders, 20*, 23–31.

Heward, W. L., Heron, T. E., Neef, N. A., Peterson, S. M., Sainato, D. M., Cartledge, G. Y., et al. (2005). *Focus on behavior analysis in education.* Upper Saddle Hill, NJ: Prentice-Hall.

Higgins, J. P. T., & Green, S. (Eds.). (2006). *Cochrane Handbook for Systematic Reviews of Interventions 4.2.6* [updated September 2006]. Accessed August 14, 2008, at http://www.cochrane.org/resources/handbook/hbook.htm.

Holmes, D. L. (1997). *Autism through the lifespan: The Eden Model.* Bethesda, MD: Woodbine House.

Horner, R. H., Carr, E. G., Halle, J., McGee, G., Odom, S., & Wolery, M. (2005). The use of single-subject research to identify evidence-based practice in special education. *Exceptional Children, 71*, 165–179.

Horner, R. H., Carr, E. G., Strain, P. S., Todd, A. W., & Reed, H. K. (2002). Problem behavior interventions for young children with autism: A research synthesis. *Journal of Autism and Developmental Disorders, 32*, 423–446.

Howard, J. S., Sparkman, C. R., Cohen, H. G., Green, G., & Stanislaw, H. (2005). A comparison of intensive behavior analytic and eclectic treatments for young children with autism. *Research in Developmental Disabilities, 26*, 359–383.

Howlin, P., Gordon, R. K., Pasco, G., Wade, G., & Charman, T. (2007). *Journal of Child Psychology and Psychiatry, 48*, 473–481.

Howlin, P., Magiati, I., & Charman, T. (2009). Systematic review of early intensive behavioral interventions for children with autism. *American Journal on Intellectual Disabilities, 114*, 23–41.

Iwata, B. A., Dorsey, M. F., Slifer, K. J., Bauman, K. E., Richman, G. S. (1994). Towards a functional analysis of self-injury. *Journal of Applied Behavior Analysis, 27*, 197–209. (Reprinted from *Analysis and Intervention in Developmental Disabilities, 2*, 3–20, 1982).

Iwata, B. A., Roscoe, E. M., Zarcone, J. R., & Richman, D. M. (2002). Environmental determinants of self-injurious behavior. In Schroeder S. R., Oster-Granite M. L. & Thompson T. (Eds.), *Self-injurious behavior: Gene-brain-behavior relationships* (pp. 93–103). Washington, DC: American Psychological Association.

Johnson, C. R., Handen, B. L., Butter, E., Wagner, A., Mulick, J., Sukhodolsky, D. G., et al. (2007). Development of a parent training program for children with pervasive developmental disorders. *Behavioral Interventions, 22*, 201–221.

Kamps, D. M., Barbetta, P. M., Leonard, B. R., & Delquadri, J. (1994). Classwide peer tutoring: An integration strategy to improve reading skills and promote peer interactions among students with autism and general education peers. *Journal of Applied Behavior Analysis, 27*, 49–61.

Kamps, D. M., Dugan, E., Potucek, J., & Collins, A. (1999). Effects of cross-age peer tutoring networks among students with autism and general education students. *Journal of Behavioral Education, 9*, 97–115.

Kamps, D. M., Leonard, B. R., Vernon, S., & Dugan, E. P. (1992). Teaching social skills to students with autism to increase peer interactions in an integrated first-grade classroom. *Journal of Applied Behavior Analysis, 25*, 281–288.

Kasari, C. (2002). Assessing change in early intervention programs for children with autism. *Journal of Autism and Developmental Disorders, 32*, 447–462.

Kennedy, C. H., & Shukla, S. (1995). Social interaction research for people with autism as a set of past, current, and emerging propositions. *Behavioral Disorders, 21*, 21–35.

Klin, A., Volkmar, F. R., & Sparrow, S. S. (Eds.). (2000). *Asperger syndrome*. New York: Guilford Press.

Koegel, L. K., Koegel, R. L., Frea, W., & GreenHopkins, I. (2003). Priming as a method of coordinating educational services for students with autism. *Language, Speech, and Hearing Services in Schools, 34*, 228–235.

Koegel, L. K., Koegel, R. L., Hurley, C., & Frea, W. D. (1992). Improving social skills and disruptive behavior in children with autism through self-management. *Journal of Applied Behavior Analysis, 25*, 341–353.

Koegel, R. L., & Koegel, L. K. (Eds.), *Teaching children with autism: Strategies for initiating positive interactions and improving learning opportunities* (pp. 17–32). Baltimore: Paul H. Brookes.

Koegel, R. L., & Koegel, L. K. (2006). *Pivotal response treatments for autism: Communication, social, and academic development*. Baltimore: Paul H. Brookes.

Krantz, P. J., & McClannahan, L. E. (1993). Teaching children with autism to initiate to peers: Effects of a script-fading procedure. *Journal of Applied Behavior Analysis, 26*, 121–132.

Leaf, R. B., & McEachin, J. J. (1999). *A work in progress: Behavior management strategies and a curriculum for intensive behavioral treatment of autism*. New York: DRL Books.

Lee, R., McComas, J. J., & Jawor, J. (2002). The effects of differential and lag reinforcement schedules on varied verbal responding by individuals with autism. *Journal of Applied Behavior Analysis, 35*, 391–402.

Lopata, C., Thomeer, M. L., Volker, M. A., & Nida, R. E. (2006). Effectiveness of a cognitive-behavioral treatment on the social behaviors of children with asperger disorder. *Focus on Autism and Other Developmental Disabilities, 21*, 237–244.

Lord, C., & Hopkins, J. M. (1986). The social behavior of autistic children with younger and same-age nonhandicapped peers. *Journal of Autism and Developmental Disorders, 16*, 249–262.

Lord, C., Wagner, A., Rogers, S., Szatmari, P., Aman, M., Charman, T., et al. (2005). Challenges in evaluating psychosocial interventions for autistic spectrum disorders. *Journal of Autism and Developmental Disorders, 35*, 696–708.

Lovaas, O. I. (1981). *Teaching developmentally disabled children: The Me book*. Baltimore, MD: University Park Press.

Lovaas, O. I. (1987). Behavioral treatment and normal educational and intellectual functioning in young autistic children. *Journal of Consulting and Clinical Psychology, 55*, 3–9.

Lovaas, O. I. (2003). *Teaching individuals with developmental delays: Basic intervention techniques*. Austin, TX: Pro–Ed.

Lovaas, O. I., & Smith, T. (1989). A comprehensive behavioral theory of autistic children: Paradigm for research and treatment. *Journal of Behavior Therapy and Experimental Psychiatry, 20*, 17–29.

Lovaas, O. I., & Smith, T. (2003). Early and intensive behavioral intervention in autism. In A. E. Kazdin & J. Weisz (Eds.), *Evidence-based psychotherapies for children and youth* (pp. 325–340). New York: Guilford.

Lovaas, O. I., Smith, T., & McEachin, J.J. (1989). Clarifying comments on the Young Autism Study. *Journal of Consulting and Clinical Psychology, 57*, 165–167.

Lovaas, O. I., Koegel, R., Simmons, J. Q., & Long, J. S. (1973). Some generalization and follow-up measures on autistic children in behavior therapy. *Journal of Applied Behavior Analysis, 6*, 131–166.

MacWhinney, T. C., Redmon, W. K., & Johnson, C. M. (2001). *Handbook of organizational performance*. New York: Routledge.

Magiati, I., Charman, T., & Howlin, P. (2007). A two-year prospective follow-up study of community-based early intensive behavioural intervention and specialist nursery provision for children with autism spectrum disorders. *Journal of Child Psychology and Psychiatry, 48*, 803–812.

Matson J. L., & Vollmer, T. R. (1995). *Questions about behavioral functions manual*. Baton Rouge, LA: Scientific Publishers.

Matson, J. L., & Taras, M. E. (1989). A 20 year review of punishment and alternative methods to treat problem behaviors in developmentally delayed persons. *Research in Developmental Disabilities, 10*, 85–104.

Matson, J. L., Benavidez, B. A., Compton, L. S., Packlawskyj, T, & Baglio, C., (1996). Behavioral treatment of autistic persons: A review of research from 1980 to the present. *Research in Developmental Disabilities, 17*, 433–465.

McClannahan, L. E., & Krantz, P. J. (1998). *Activity schedules for children with autism: Teaching independent behavior*. Bethesda, MD: Woodbine.

McClannahan, L. E., & Krantz, P. J. (2005). *Teaching conversation to children with autism: Scripts and script fading*. Bethesda, MD: Woodbine House.

McClannahan, L. E., MacDuff, G. S., & Krantz, P. J. (2002). Behavior analysis and intervention for adults with autism. *Behavior Modification, 26*, 9–26.

McConnell, S. (2002). Interventions to facilitate social interaction for young children with autism: Review of available research and recommendations for educational intervention and future research. *Journal of Autism and Developmental Disorders, 32*, 351–372.

McEachin, J. J., Smith, T., & Lovaas, O. I. (1993). Long-term outcome of children with autism who received early intensive behavioral treatment. *American Journal of Mental Retardation, 97*, 359–372.

Mruzek, D. W., Cohen, C., & Smith, T. (2007). Contingency contracting with students with autism spectrum disorders. *Journal of Developmental and Behavioral Disabilities, 19*, 103–114.

National Research Council (2001). *Educating children with autism*. Committee on Educational Interventions for Children with Autism. Division of Behavioral and Social Sciences and Education. Washington, DC: National Academy Press.

Neuringer, A. (2004). Reinforced variability in animals and people: Implications for adaptive action. *American Psychologist, 59*, 891–906.

Newsom, C. (1998). Autistic disorder. In Mash E. J. & Barkley R. A. (Eds.), *Treatment of childhood disorders* (2nd ed., pp. 416–467). New York: Guilford.

O'Neill, R. E., Story, K., Sprague, J. R. Horner, R. H., & Albin, R. W. (1997). *Functional assessment and program development for problem behavior: A practical handbook* (2nd ed.). Pacific Grove, CA: Brooks/Cole.

Odom, S. L., Brown, W. H., Frey, T., Karasu, N., Smith-Canter, L. L., & Strain, P. S. (2003). Evidence-based practices for young children with autism: Contributions from single-subject design research. *Focus on Autism and Other Developmental Disabilities, 18*, 166–175.

Perry, A., Cummings, A., Dunn Geier, J., Freeman, N. L., Hughes, S., LaRose, L., et al. (2008). Effectiveness of Intensive Behavioral Intervention in a large, community-based program. *Research on Autism Spectrum Disorders, 2*, 621–642.

Prizant, B. M., & Wetherby, A. M. (2005). Critical issues in enhancing communication abilities for persons with autism spectrum disorders. In Volkmar F. R., Paul R., Klin A. & Cohen D. (Eds.), *Handbook of autism and pervasive developmental disorders, vol. 2: Assessment, interventions, and policy* (3rd ed.) (pp. 925–945). Hoboken, NJ: John Wiley & Sons.

Reed, P., Osborne, L. A., & Corness (2007a). The real-world effectiveness of early teaching interventions for children with autism spectrum disorder. *Exceptional Children, 73,* 417–433.

Reed, P., Osborne, L. A., & Corness (2007b). Brief report: Relative effectiveness of different home-based behavioral approaches to early teaching intervention. *Journal of Autism and Developmental Disorders, 37,* 1815–1821.

Reichow, B., & Wolery, M. (2008). Comprehensive synthesis of early intervention behavioral interventions for young children with autism based on the UCLA Young Autism Project model. *Journal of Autism and Developmental Disorders, 39,* 23–41.

Reichow, B., Volkmar, F. R., & Cicchetti, D. V. (2008). Development of the evaluative method for evaluating and determining evidence-based practices in autism. *Journal of Autism and Developmental Disorders, 38,* 1311–1319.

Remington, B., Hastings, R. P., Kovshoff, H., degli Espinosa, F., Jahr, W., Brown, T., et al. (2007). A field effectiveness study of early intensive behavioral intervention: Outcomes for children with autism and their parents after two years. *American Journal of Mental Retardation, 112,* 418–438.

Rogers, S. J. (1998). Neuropsychology of autism in young children and its implications for early intervention. *Mental Retardation & Developmental Disabilities Research Reviews, 4,* 104–112.

Rogers, S. J., & Vismara, L. A. (2008). Evidence-based comprehensive treatments for early autism. *Journal of Clinical Child and Adolescent Psychology, 37,* 8–38.

Rogers, S. J., Hayden, D., Hepburn, S., Charlifue-Smith, R., Hall, T., & Hayes, A. (2006). Teaching young nonverbal children with autism useful speech: A pilot study of the Denver Model and the PROMPT interventions. *Journal of Autism and Developmental Disorders, 36,* 1007–1024.

Runco, M. A., Charlop, M. H., & Schreibman, L. (1986). The occurrence of autistic children's self-stimulation as a function of familiar versus unfamiliar stimulus conditions. *Journal of Autism and Developmental Disorders, 16,* 31–44.

Sallows, G., & Graupner, T. (2005). Intensive behavioral treatment for autism: Four-year outcome and predictors. *American Journal of Mental Retardation, 110,* 417–436.

Sherer, M. R., & Schreibman, L. (2005). Individual behavioral profiles and predictors of treatment effectiveness for children with autism. *Journal of Consulting and Clinical Psychology, 75,* 525–538.

Spreckley, M., & Boyd, R. (2009). Efficacy of applied behavioral intervention in preschool children with autism for improving cognitive, language, and adaptive behavior: A systematic review and meta-analysis. *Journal of Pediatrics, 154,* 338–344.

Schopler, E., Short, A., & Mesibov, G. (1989). Relation of behavioral treatment to "normal functioning": Comment on Lovaas. *Journal of Consulting and Clinical Psychology, 57,* 162–164.

Sheinkopf, S. J., & Siegel, B. (1998). Home-based behavioral treatment of young children with autism. *Journal of Autism and Developmental Disorders, 28,* 15–23.

Sidman, M. (1994). *Equivalence relations and behavior: A research story.* Sarasota, FL: Authors Cooperative.

Skinner, B. F. (1957). *Verbal behavior.* New York: Appleton-Century-Crofts.

Smith, T. (2001). Discrete trial training in the treatment of autism. *Focus on Autism and Related Disorders, 16,* 86–92.

Smith, T., & Lovaas, O. I. (1997). The UCLA Young Autism Project: Reply to Gresham and MacMillan. *Behavioral Disorders, 22,* 202–218.

Smith, T., Buch, G.A., & Evslin, T. (2000a). Parent-directed, intensive early intervention for children with pervasive developmental disorder. *Research in Developmental Disabilities, 21,* 297–309.

Smith, T., Eikeseth, S., Klevstrand, M., & Lovaas, O.I. (1997). Outcome of early intervention for children with pervasive developmental disorder and severe mental retardation. *American Journal of Mental Retardation, 102,* 228–237.

Smith, T., Groen, A., & Wynn, J. W. (2000b). Randomized trial of intensive early intervention for children with pervasive developmental disorder. *American Journal of Mental Retardation, 104,* 269–285.

Smith, T., McAdam, D., & Napolitano, D. (2007). Autism and applied behavior analysis. In Sturmey P. & Fitzer A. (Eds.), *Autism spectrum disorders: Applied behavior analysis evidence and practice* (pp. 1–29). Austin, TX: Pro-Ed.

Smith, T., McEachin, J. J., & Lovaas, O. I. (1993). Comments on replication and evaluation of outcome. *American Journal of Mental Retardation, 97,* 385–381.

Smith, T., Scahill, L., Dawson, G., Guthrie, D., Lord, C., Odom, S., Rogers, S., et al. (2007). Designing research studies on psychosocial interventions in autism. *Journal of Autism and Developmental Disorders, 37,* 354–366.

Sparrow, S. S., Balla, D. A., & Chicchetti, D. V. (1984). *Vineland Adaptive Behavior Scales.* Minnesota: American Guidance Service.

Stahmer, A. C., Collings, N. M., & Palinkas, L. A. (2005). Early intervention practices for children with autism: Descriptions from community providers. *Focus on Autism and Other Developmental Disabilities, 20,* 66–79.

Stahmer, A. C., Ingersoll, B., & Carter, C. (2003). Behavioral approaches to promoting play. *Autism, 7,* 401–413.

Strain, P. S., & Schwartz, I. (2001). ABA and the development of meaningful social relations for young children with autism. *Focus on Autism and Other Developmental Disabilities, 16,* 120–128.

Sundberg, M. L., & Michael, J. (2001). The benefits of Skinner's analysis of verbal behavior for children with autism. *Behavior Modification, 25,* 698–724.

Taylor, B. A., & Jasper, S. (2001). Teaching programs to increase peer interaction. In Maurice C., Green G. & Foxx R. M. (Eds.), *Making a difference: Behavioral intervention for autism* (pp. 97–162). Austin, TX: Pro-Ed.

Thiemann, K. S., & Goldstein, H. (2004). Effects of peer training and written text cueing on social communication of school-age children with pervasive developmental disorder. *Journal of Speech, Language, and Hearing Research, 47,* 126–144.

Weiss, M. J. (1999). Differential rates of skill acquisition and outcomes of early intensive behavioral intervention for autism. *Behavioral Interventions, 14,* 3–22.

Whalen, C., & Schreibman, L. (2003). Joint attention training for children with autism using behavior modification procedures. *Journal of Child Psychology and Psychiatry and Allied Disciplines, 44,* 456–468.

Wilkinson, K. M., & McIlvane, W. J. (1997). Contributions of stimulus control perspectives to psycholinguistic theories of vocabulary development and delay. In Adamson L. B. & Romski M. A. (Eds.), *Communication and language acquisition: Discoveries from atypical development* (pp. 25–48). Baltimore, MD: Paul H. Brookes.

Wolf, M. M. (1978). Social validity: The case for subjective measurement or how applied behavior analysis is finding its heart. *Journal of Applied Behavior Analysis, 11*, 203–214.

Woods, D., & Kanter, J. (Eds.). (2007). *Understanding behavior disorders: A contemporary behavioral perspective.* Reno, NV: Context Press.

Yoder, P., & Stone, W. L. (2006). Randomized comparison of two communication interventions for preschoolers with autism. *Journal of Consulting and Clinical Psychology, 74*, 426–425.

Young, J. M., Krantz, P. J., McClannahan, L. E., & Poulson, C. L. (1994). Generalized imitation and response-class formation in children with autism. *Journal of Applied Behavior Analysis, 27*, 685–698.

Zachor, D. A., Ben-Itzhak, E., Rabinovitz, A-L., & Lahat, E. (2007). Change in core symptoms with intervention. *Research in Autism Spectrum Disorders, 1*, 304–317.

59 Laura Schreibman, Brooke Ingersoll

Naturalistic Approaches to Early Behavioral Intervention

Points of Interest

- Naturalistic behavioral interventions use specific behavioral teaching strategies such as prompting, shaping, chaining, and reinforcement, to teach skills during child-directed activities.
- Naturalistic behavioral interventions were developed specifically to increase the generalization and maintenance of skills.
- These interventions have been found to be effective for increasing a range of social communication skills in young children with ASDs, including expressive language, play, imitation, and joint attention.
- This intervention approach has been used successfully by a range of intervention providers, including teachers, parents, siblings, and peers.
- Several child and parent characteristics have been identified to predict those children who are likely to respond best to this intervention approach.

There is now a large corpus of data supporting the effectiveness of behavioral interventions for the treatment of children with autism spectrum disorders (ASDs). In fact, treatments based upon a behavioral (learning theory) model are the only treatments with a strong empirical basis supporting substantial improvement in many of these children (e.g., National Research Council, 2001; Schreibman, 1997; Schreibman, 2005). Developed via the methodology of applied behavior analysis and based primarily on operant discrimination learning, these interventions involve the systematic application of the principles of learning to human behavior. The data-driven nature of behavioral technology and treatment development has ensured our constant evaluation of effectiveness, allowing for the identification of both treatment strengths and weaknesses. The early behavioral interventions applied to children with autism involved a highly structured format called *Discrete Trial Training* or DTT, which provided us with the first successful tools to teach individuals with ASDs (e.g., Baer, Peterson, & Sherman, 1967; Lovaas, 1987; Lovaas, Berberich et al., 1966; Lovaas, Koegel et al., 1973; Maurice, Green, & Luce, 1996; Metz, 1965; Schroeder & Baer, 1972).

DTT involves presentation of discrete trials that are small units of instruction composed of a discriminative stimulus provided by a therapist, the child's response, and an immediate consequence contingent upon the child's response. Each trial is followed by a short intertrial interval before presentation of the discriminative stimulus for the next trial. Trials are presented in blocks, with all trials focusing on the same target skill (e.g., discriminating red from blue). Complex behaviors are typically broken down into smaller component behaviors, and these components are taught one at a time until the complex behavior is learned. Over time and trials, more comprehensive behavioral repertoires are established. To summarize, programs using this procedure share these basic components: *(1)* the learning environment is highly structured; *(2)* target behaviors are broken down into a series of discrete subskills and taught successively; *(3)* teaching episodes, or trials, are initiated by the therapist and presented in a massed manner; *(4)* teaching materials are selected by the therapist and are often held constant within a task; *(5)* the child's production of the target response is explicitly prompted; *(6)* reinforcers, albeit functional, may be indirect in that they are not directly related to the target response; and *(7)* the child receives reinforcement only for correct responding or successive approximations (e.g., Lovaas, 2003; Maurice, Green, & Luce, 1996; Smith, 2001).

The contribution of this form of intervention cannot be overstated, as it represents the first form of treatment available that allowed children with autism to acquire a wide range of appropriate behaviors. A large body of literature attests to the substantial gains that these techniques may facilitate in children with autism (Cohen, Amerine-Dickens, & Smith, 2006; Goldstein, 2002; Green, 1996; Lovaas, 1987; McEachin,

Smith, & Lovaas, 1993; Miranda-Linne & Melin, 1992; Sallows & Graupner, 2005; Smith, Groen, & Wynn, 2000). Yet as effective as these early interventions proved to be, it was the case that continued study and evaluation of this original highly structured form of intervention exposed several significant limitations to their effectiveness (e.g., Schreibman, 2005).

The major identified limitations to these early DTT strategies related to the issue of generalization. Behaviors learned via this highly structured, repetitive-practice protocol often failed to generalize across people, situations, and settings (stimulus generalization); were not accompanied by changes in related behaviors (response generalization); and tended not to be durable (maintenance). Other problems noted included a lack of spontaneity, inflexible ("robotic") responding, and prompt dependency. In addition, the specific technique of DTT required treatment providers (clinicians, teachers, parents) to use a highly structured set of rules, which often made it difficult for parents to learn because these rules resulted in parent–child interactions that were quite different than the natural interactions one typically has with children. Further, these drill strategies were often not pleasant for the treatment provider and not usually fun for the child. Because the child might not be enjoying the teaching, often escape- and avoidance-motivated problem behaviors, such as tantrums, occurred (Koegel, O'Dell, & Dunlap, 1988). This could make the DTT approach less attractive for both adult and child (Koegel et al., 1988; Schreibman, Kaneko, & Koegel, 1991).

In response to the generalization and spontaneity issues that accompanied DTT training and also to address the fact that the implementation of this strategy was sometimes unpleasant for the child and treatment provider, more naturalistic forms of behavioral intervention were developed. Interestingly, a number of different laboratories across the country independently developed empirically based naturalistic behavioral strategies that are remarkably similar, as they involve some of the same features. These new naturalistic interventions were influenced by a seminal article by Stokes and Baer (1977), which described specific strategies for establishing generalization of learned behavior. The incorporation of these generalization strategies is evident in these interventions. They share the following components (note contrast with components of DTT described above): *(1)* the learning environment is loosely structured; *(2)* teaching occurs within ongoing interactions between the child and therapist; *(3)* the child initiates the teaching episode by indicating interest in an item or activity; *(4)* teaching materials are selected by the child and varied often; *(5)* the child's production of the target behavior is explicitly prompted; *(6)* a direct relationship exists between the child's response and the reinforcer; and *(7)* the child receives reinforcement for attempts to respond, not only correct responses or successive approximations (*see* Koegel et al., 1989). Thus, there is an emphasis on capitalizing on child motivation, fostering spontaneity, and bringing behavior under naturally occurring environmental contingencies. The goal is to promote generalization of treatment effects with strategies that therapists will find more pleasant and thus be more likely to use. (*See* Delprato, 2001, for a direct comparison of discrete trial versus naturalistic behavioral strategies.)

The most commonly used of these naturalistic behavioral interventions go by the names of *incidental teaching* (Hart & Risley, 1968; McGee et al., 1983), *milieu teaching* (Alpert & Kaiser, 1992; Kaiser, Yoder, & Keetz, 1992), *the natural language paradigm* (Koegel et al., 1988), and *pivotal response training* (Koegel et al., 1989).

A more detailed description of PRT will serve to illustrate naturalistic behavioral interventions.

Pivotal Response Training

Pivotal Response Training (PRT) focuses on the training of "pivotal" behaviors that are assumed to lead to widespread changes in other behaviors (hence, the term *pivotal*). Motivation and responsivity to multiple environmental cues are each pivotal behaviors, and both are known to be problematic in the ASD population (e.g., Schreibman & Koegel, 2005). Enhancing motivation leads to increased responding and thus learning opportunities. Increased responsivity helps to "normalize" the child's attention to the environment and thus increase the likelihood of successful learning. (Sometimes additional pivotal behaviors are included, such as self-initiations [Koegel, Carter, & Koegel, 2003] and self-management [Schreibman & Koegel, 1996; Schreibman & Koegel, 2005] because each of these will likely be associated with widespread enhancement of learning and generalization.)

To enhance the pivotal behavior of *motivation*, several specific treatment components are utilized. These include the following (*see* Koegel et al., 1989, for a more detailed description of specific procedures):

1. *Child choice and shared control.* To maximize the child's interest in the learning situation, he/she is given a great deal of input in determining the specific stimuli and the nature of the learning interaction. A variety of materials (e.g., toys, games, snacks) is presented and the child is allowed to select an activity or object around which the learning interaction will occur. Throughout the session, the therapist is alert to the child's changing interests and allows the child to change to another preferred activity. During the teaching interaction, the therapist and child take turns with the materials and activity, thus sharing control. This allows the child to become accustomed to the back-and-forth nature of verbal and social interaction while also allowing opportunities for the therapist to model appropriate and/or more sophisticated responses.
2. *Intersperse maintenance tasks.* To enhance motivation by keeping the overall success and reinforcement level high, previously mastered tasks are interspersed frequently among new (acquisition) tasks, which are more difficult for the child.

3. *Direct/natural reinforcers.* Direct, rather than indirect, reinforcers are used. Direct reinforcers are consequences that are directly related to the response they follow. A direct reinforcer for the verbal response "car" might be access to a toy car as opposed to a food or token reinforcer. Access to a toy car is a direct and natural consequence of saying "car," whereas food is not.
4. *Reinforcement of attempts.* To maximize reinforcement and therefore enhance the child's motivation to respond, therapists reinforce all reasonable attempts made by the child to respond. Thus, reinforcers are contingent upon attempts that may not be completely correct and may not be quite as good as previous attempts but are within a broader range of correct responses. Again, this serves to keep the overall level of reinforcement high.
5. *Responsivity to multiple cues.* Research has indicated that for many children with autism who are overselective in their responding, training on a series of successive *conditional discriminations* teaches them to respond to simultaneous multiple cues. A conditional discrimination is one that *requires* response to multiple cues (e.g., Koegel & Schreibman, 1977; Schreibman, Charlop, & Koegel, 1982). For example, asking a child to go get her red sweater is a conditional discrimination task. This is because the child undoubtedly has more than one red item of clothing and more than one sweater. Correct responding depends on attention to *both* color and object. To enhance the child's responsivity to multiple cues, the therapist presents the child with tasks involving conditional discriminations. It is assumed that as the child learns to respond on the basis of multiple cues, his or her attention is more normalized, allowing for more environmental cues to become functional. Because stimulus control of behavior is no longer as restricted, enhanced generalization should result.

An important caveat regarding teaching response to simultaneous stimulus input is that typically developing children are not skilled at such responding until approximately 3 or 4 years of age (Lovaas, Koegel, & Schreibman, 1979; Schreibman, 1997); thus, if the child with autism is functioning at a mental age below this, teaching responding to multiple cues is not recommended.

Naturalistic Behavioral Interventions and Specific Target Behaviors

Naturalistic behavioral interventions such as PRT initially targeted language behaviors, and it is in this area where much of the literature is focused. The emphasis on vocal communication skills is certainly understandable, as it is a hallmark deficit area in this population. Subsequent foci have included other hallmark deficits including social behaviors, nonverbal communication, imitation, and play.

Language

As noted above, expressive language has been the primary target behavior in the majority of research reports involving naturalistic behavioral strategies such as PRT, and it is now well-supported that this form of intervention is very effective in increasing spoken communication in children with ASDs (e.g., Delprato, 2001; Koegel & Koegel, 2006; Laski, Charlop, & Schreibman, 1988; National Research Council, 2001). Multiple single-subject and long-term outcome studies have confirmed that naturalistic behavioral language interventions facilitate the functional use of language for many children with autism, including verbal imitation (Laski, Charlop, & Schreibman, 1988), labeling (Koegel et al. 1998), question asking (Koegel et al., 1998), spontaneous speech (Laski et al., 1988), speech intelligibility (Koegel et al., 1998), conversational communication (Koegel et al., 1998), and rapid acquisition of functional speech in previously nonverbal children (Sze et al., 2003). Further, as will be noted in some of the above cited studies, this class of interventions has been shown to be effective for children who enter treatment essentially nonverbal. Moreover, when compared to more highly structured behavioral strategies, such as DTT, the specific components of naturalistic behavioral interventions facilitate relatively greater increases in verbalizations and spontaneous language use (Delprato, 2001; Koegel & Williams, 1980; Koegel, O'Dell, & Dunlap, 1988; Williams, Koegel, & Egel, 1981). Also, when these components are combined into a single naturalistic intervention (e.g., PRT, incidental teaching), they lead to more generalized speech and language skills (e.g., Charlop-Christy & Carpenter, 2000; Delprato, 2001; Koegel et al., 1998, McGee, Krantz, & McClannahan, 1985, Miranda-Linne & Melin, 1992). The fact that interventions involving naturalistic strategies lead to increased generalization is not surprising, given that these strategies were specifically developed to address the generalization limitations noted with the more highly structured forms of behavioral intervention.

Over the past 15 years, naturalistic behavioral interventions have been adapted to teach nonverbal social communication skills, such as joint attention, imitation, and pretend play (Schreibman & Ingersoll, 2005; Whalen & Schreibman, 2003). Interest in teaching these skills has gained popularity for two main reasons. First, these behaviors have been identified as autism-specific deficits (APA, 2001); thus, they have been targeted in their own right as an attempt to lessen the symptoms of autism. Second, these behaviors have *developmental potential.* A number of studies have shown that joint attention (e.g., Bates et al., 1979), imitation (Bates et al., 1988), and pretend play (Fein, 1981) are associated with the development of language and other social communication skills in typical development. Thus, research has focused on teaching these skills to children with autism in an attempt to promote social communication development more broadly (Ingersoll & Schreibman, 2006; Kasari, Freeman, & Paparella, 2006; Stahmer, 1995; Whalen, Schreibman, & Ingersoll, 2006).

Joint Attention

One of the earliest forms of social communication involves joint attention. There have been several studies using a naturalistic behavioral intervention to teach children to respond to the joint attention (RJA) bids of others as well as to initiate joint attention (IJA). For example, Whalen and Schreibman (2003) used a multiple-baseline design across five young children with autism to examine the efficacy of a naturalistic behavior modification technique for teaching response to increasingly complex bids for joint attention (i.e., placing child's hand on object, tapping an object, showing an object, following a point to an object, following a gaze shift to an object) and initiation of joint attention (i.e., showing and pointing). In their study, all five children increased their ability to respond to the therapist's bid for joint attention, and four of the children maintained this skill at a 3-month follow-up. After RJA training, the children showed an improvement in their RJA ability on Loveland and Landry's (1986) joint attention assessment but did not increase their use of IJA, necessitating IJA training. In the second phase of their study, four of the five children increased their ability to initiate joint attention with the therapist. In addition, improvements were found in the children's use of coordinated joint attention with their caregivers, indicating some generalization of skills. However, maintenance of IJA behaviors was somewhat limited at 3 months post-treatment. Jones, Carr, and Feeley (2006) used a multiple-baseline design across behaviors to examine the effect of a related procedure on improving RJA and IJA when implemented by the children's preschool teachers (5 children) and mothers (2 children). In both cases, in response to intervention the children exhibited an increase in their ability to respond to, and initiate, joint attention. Similarly to Whalen and Schreibman (2003), the children did not begin to use IJA during RJA training; rather, they required specific instruction in initiating joint attention.

Two additional single-subject design studies have focused on teaching RJA alone to examine whether improvements in RJA lead to gains in IJA. Rocha and Schreibman (2007) replicated and extended Whalen and Schreibman's (2006) results using a parent-implemented approach with three young children with autism. They found that parents were able to implement the intervention effectively and the children increased their response to their parents' bids for joint attention. Interestingly, although not directly targeted, the children also showed an increase in their use of coordinated joint attention, indicating some generalization to IJA. Using a related procedure, Martins and Harris (2006) taught three preschoolers with autism to follow the gaze of the therapist. Again, all three children exhibited an increase in their ability to respond the therapist's bids. In contrast to Rocha and Schreibman (2007), they did not find collateral changes in IJA, suggesting that for some children, joint attention initiations must be targeted directly. However, Martins and Harris (2006) defined IJA as showing and pointing, which are more complex behaviors than coordinated joint attention. This difference might suggest that coordinated joint attention is more responsive to intervention than showing and pointing.

In a larger, randomized controlled trial, Kasari and colleagues (2006) examined the effectiveness of a naturalistic behavioral intervention to teach joint attention skills. This study compared the effect of a short-term naturalistic behavioral intervention that targeted joint attention skills to a naturalistic behavioral symbolic play intervention (*see* below) and a control. They found that the children who had received training in joint attention made greater gains in RJA and IJA skills as measured on the Early Social Communication Scales (ESCS; Mundy et al., 2003) than the children in the symbolic play intervention and control group. Further, children who had received training in joint attention made greater gains in language 1 year post-treatment than the children in the control group (Kasari et al., 2008), suggesting that teaching joint attention skills using a naturalistic behavioral approach can have long-term effects on language learning.

It should be noted that in all of the above mentioned studies, joint attention training was taught with a combined structured and naturalistic behavioral approach, with initial training typically conducted at the table in a structured fashion, followed by practice during child-led activities. However, in keeping with the naturalistic focus, all stimuli and reinforcement were natural (highly preferred toys) to the interaction. This use of structure during the initial training episodes differs somewhat from the naturalistic behavioral interventions that have been used to teach imitation and pretend play and may be indicative of the difficulty in teaching joint attention episodes or the fact that joint attention training is less easily incorporated into unstructured play. However, it is unclear whether the initial structure is necessary or whether joint attention can be taught in more natural contexts from the beginning. Further, RJA has been typically targeted before IJA, as it emerges earlier in development and is an easier skill for children to master (Whalen & Schreibman, 2003). However, it is unclear whether RJA is necessary to teach before IJA, whether they can be taught concurrently, or whether teaching IJA would lead to gains in RJA without direct training.

Imitation

There have been several studies that have taught imitation skills to young children with autism using a naturalistic behavioral approach. In a series of single-subject design studies, Ingersoll and colleagues have examined teaching spontaneous, generalized imitation skills to preschool-aged children with autism during play. The first study used a multiple-baseline design across five young children with autism to examine the effectiveness of this approach for teaching object imitation (Ingersoll & Schreibman, 2006). In response to treatment, all children showed substantial gains in their use of object imitation. Follow-up data obtained after 1 month indicated that all children maintained their gains of object imitation, which generalized to novel settings, materials, and a therapist. Changes in object imitation were also evident on a structured imitation assessment and during a naturalistic, structured observation with the therapist and the caregiver. Perhaps more exciting was the finding that naïve observers blind to participants' treatment status rated the participants as exhibiting significantly more appropriate social communication skills and appearing more typically developing at post-treatment than pretreatment.

A second study targeted the imitation of meaningful gestures (Ingersoll, Lewis, & Kroman, 2007). This study used a multiple-baseline design across five young children with autism who had difficulty with the imitation and spontaneous use of descriptive gestures (e.g., spreading arms out for "big" or putting arms out at sides for "airplane"). All children showed an increase in their imitation of gestures, which generalized to novel environments and was maintained at a 1-month follow-up. In addition, three of the children exhibited substantial gains in their spontaneous use of gestures, whereas the other two exhibited small but consistent gains. Finally, naïve observers blind to treatment status rated the children as using more appropriate social communication during treatment than baseline.

In a third study, a multiple-baseline design was implemented, and three mothers were taught to implement the intervention techniques with their child (Ingersoll & Gergans, 2007). The mothers of the two nonverbal children were taught to use the intervention strategies to teach object imitation, and the mother of the verbal child was taught to target both object and gesture imitation. Results indicated that the parents learned to use the intervention strategies and their children improved their imitation skills. Importantly, the children's and parents' skills both generalized to the home and maintained over time.

Taken together, these studies indicate that imitation can be directly taught using a naturalistic behavioral intervention. Further, there is evidence that teaching imitation skills in this manner can lead to improvements in other social communication skills, including language, pretend play, and coordinated joint attention (Ingersoll & Schreibman, 2006), supporting the potential role that imitation plays in the developmental of more advanced social communication skills and its importance as a treatment target.

Pretend Play

Several studies have explicitly targeted pretend play skills in children with autism using a naturalistic behavioral approach. In the first of its kind, Stahmer (1995) used a multiple-baseline design across seven verbal children with autism to examine the effects of teaching symbolic play skills using a modified version of PRT. The results indicated that all children were able to engage in symbolic play skills with an adult at levels similar to those of language-age-matched typical peers. Generalization to new toys and new adults was also impressive, and these behavioral changes remained stable over time. Further, when rated by naive observers for creativity, spontaneity, and "typical" play, children with autism improved significantly after PRT play training; however, their play remained qualitatively distinguishable from the play of the typical children (Stahmer, Schreibman, & Palardy, 1994). One area of difficulty for the children that continued after play training was play with another peer, which did not improve. In a related study, Thorp, Stahmer, and Schreibman (1995) taught three children with autism to engage in socio-dramatic play with an adult. Again, children made gains in their ability to carry out socio-dramatic play schemes, and these gains generalized to novel materials and settings and maintained over a period of 3 months. In both of these studies, the children had some initial appropriate play skills and had expressive language ages of at least 2.5 years.

Kasari and colleagues (2006) used a randomized design to examine the effect of a naturalistic behavioral symbolic play intervention with preschool-aged children with autism. In their study, children were randomly assigned to a symbolic play intervention, joint attention intervention, or control group. Their results indicated that the children who received training in symbolic play made greater gains in their overall level of play on a structured play assessment than children in the control group and had a higher number of symbolic play schemes and overall play level during an unstructured parent–child interaction than children in the control group and children who received training in joint attention, both immediately (Kasari et al., 2006) and 1-year post-treatment (Kasari et al., 2008). This finding provides strong evidence that naturalistic behavioral interventions are effective for teaching symbolic play. Further, in their study, the average expressive language age of the participants at pretreatment was 21 months, indicating that symbolic play skills can be taught to children with lower language ages than in previous studies.

Taken together, these findings suggest that naturalistic behavioral interventions are effective for increasing a range of play skills found to be deficient in children with autism. In some cases, these skills were found to be similar in rate to the play of typically developing children of the same language age (Stahmer, 1995). In addition, the generalization and maintenance of the play skills may be indicative of the reinforcing nature of play itself. These findings have led others to conclude that the naturalistic behavioral approach may indeed produce meaningful changes in play skills that are spontaneous and flexible and thus meet the true definition of play (Luckett, Bundy, & Roberts, 2007). Despite these positive outcomes, the evidence suggests that the children's play remained qualitatively distinguishable from the play of the typical children (Stahmer et al., 1994) and that generalization to typical peers was not evident, suggesting that social play may need to be explicitly taught (*see* section on peer-mediated intervention below).

Further, in all three studies, children also made improvements in nontargeted skills, including joint engagement (Kasari et al., 2006; Stahmer, 1995; Thorp et al., 1995), coordinated joint attention (Kasari et al., 2006; 2008), and language skills, both concurrently (Thorp et al., 1995) and 1 year later

(Kasari et al., 2008). These findings support the developmental potential hypothesis that teaching pretend play skills using a naturalistic behavioral intervention can lead to improvements in other social communication skills.

In sum, there is a growing body of evidence indicating that children with autism can be taught nonverbal social communication skills via naturalistic behavioral interventions. There is also some indication that training in these nonverbal behaviors can also lead to collateral changes in other, nontargeted social communication skills. These finding are particularly true for language skills, which have been shown to increase as a result of teaching joint attention (Kasari et al., 2006; Whalen & Schreibman, 2003), imitation (Ingersoll & Schreibman, 2006), and pretend play (Kasari et al., 2006; Thorp et al., 1995). Interestingly, although there is some evidence that joint attention training (Kasari et al., 2006) and language training (Gillett & LeBlanc, 2007) using naturalistic behavioral methods may lead to improvements in functional play, symbolic play skills have been found to be unaffected by joint attention (Kasari et al., 2006; 2008) or language teaching (Stahmer, 1995). There is also evidence that gains in general social engagement and coordinated joint attention result from teaching a variety of social communication skills using a naturalistic behavioral approach, including RJA (Rocha et al., 2007), imitation (Ingersoll & Schreibman, 2006), symbolic play (Kasari et al., 2006; 2008; Stahmer, 1995; Thorp et al., 1995), and even language (Bruinsma, 2004). However, changes in more advanced IJA skills, such as showing and pointing, require specific training (Jones et al., 2006; Kasari et al., 2006; Whalen & Schreibman, 2003). These findings suggest that you "get what you teach" (Kasari et al., 2006); however, there appears to also be some general treatment effects—particularly in the area of social responsiveness, functional play, and language. Further, these general treatment effects may become more pronounced over time (Kasari et al., 2008).

The possibility of general treatment effects is exciting, as it suggests that wide-ranging positive effects on development can occur in response to teaching a pivotal skill. One possible explanation for the general treatment effects seen across nonverbal social communication interventions is the use of naturalistic behavioral interventions that, through the use of following the child's lead and natural reinforcement (usually toys), may increase social engagement, functional play, and language skills. It is also possible that some nonverbal social communication skills require the same underlying ability (such as the ability to attend to another person), such that teaching one skill (e.g., imitation) improves a related skill (e.g., coordinated joint attention), whereas others do not (e.g., IJA and symbolic play). This possibility may explain why there is less "spill-over" with these treatment targets. It is also possible that increasing one skill directly affects another skill, as it appears to do with language (Kasari et al., 2008).

In conclusion, the naturalistic behavioral approach has been used to target a range of social communication skills found to be deficient in children with autism. These skills, when targeted early in development appear to confer a wide range of benefits. However, it is still unclear which skills are most important to teach and at what point in development. Further research focused on the most efficient and effective way to teach social communication is needed.

Interventionists

Because naturalistic intervention strategies involve interactions that are more typical in terms of how individuals interact with children in the natural environment, it is not surprising that such techniques have been successfully implemented by a variety of treatment providers, including parents, teachers, and peers. Given that one of the main goals of naturalistic strategies is to enhance generalization of treatment effects, incorporating individuals with whom the child is likely to interact during his or her natural day makes perfect sense and has, in fact, proved to achieve these goals.

Parents

Naturalistic behavioral approaches, such as PRT, have been commonly utilized as a vocal language training program with an emphasis on parent training (Koegel et al., 1989). Indeed, parent involvement in the treatment of children with autism has been associated with increased maintenance and generalization of treatment (particularly language) gains both with highly structured (Crockett et al., 2007; Koegel et al., 1982) and naturalistic behavioral interventions (Hester et al., 1995; Schreibman & Koegel, 1996, 2005.). However, although both highly structured and naturalistic treatment strategies have been taught to parents who can subsequently use them effectively, it appears that naturalistic strategies are associated with other positive effects. For example, Schreibman, Kaneko, and Koegel (1991) had naïve observers view videotapes of parent–child dyads in which the parent was conducting a therapy session with the child. In one condition, parents were using a highly structured intervention (DTT), and in the other condition, parents were using a naturalistic intervention (PRT). The observers were asked to rate how happy, interested, and enthusiastic the therapist (parent) appeared when working with the child. Results indicated that parents were rated as having significantly more positive affect when using PRT. Further, Koegel, Bimbela, and Schreibman (1996) using a similar methodology asked naïve observers to rate the level of positive interactions during the family dinnertimes of families where the parents had been trained in DTT versus families where the parent had been trained in PRT. Pre- and post-parent training videotapes of the dinnertime family interactions were rated on four interactional scales (level of happiness, interest, stress, and general communication style). Both groups of families initially scored in the neutral range at pretreatment; this did not change significantly at post-treatment for the DTT group. However, at post-training, the PRT group showed a level of positive interaction on all four scales, suggesting high degrees of happiness and interest, low stress during the interactions, and more positive communication. It is noteworthy that these studies support one of the main rationales for the development of more naturalistic teaching strategies: Such forms of intervention would be more pleasant for the treatment provider (in this case the parent) and as such would be more likely to be implemented.

Another benefit of naturalistic strategies is that they can—and indeed should—be implemented in naturally occurring situations. These strategies have the advantage of lending themselves quite well to integration into a family's daily routines. For example, parents are taught how to use everyday activities such as sorting laundry, shopping, playing in a park, and so forth, as teaching opportunities. This encourages the parents to use the effective treatment in a variety of settings and with a variety of target behaviors, both of which promote generalization. Further, parents find these strategies less disruptive than more highly structured teaching as they do not necessarily have to set up specific teaching times and set up special teaching environments. All of these benefits likely make naturalistic strategies more positive for parents and thus more likely to be implemented on an ongoing basis.

Teachers and Classrooms

Incidental teaching, a naturalistic behavioral strategy, was originally designed for use in preschool classrooms for disadvantaged but typically developing children (Hart & Risley, 1968). This approach has subsequently been used as the primary intervention approach in a number of research-based inclusive classroom programs for 2- to 4-year-old children with autism. These programs have demonstrated gains in language, play, and social interaction skills (e.g., McGee, Morrier, & Daly, 1999; Stahmer & Ingersoll, 2004). However, as with other research-based practices, the use of naturalistic interventions in classroom settings is a fairly recent phenomenon. Arick and colleagues (2003) developed a public school program that included PRT along with other research-supported behavioral practices. Reporting on outcome data for more than 100 children participating in the program, these investigators reported that the majority of children made significant progress in the areas of social interaction, expressive speech, and use of language concepts. The children in the program gained, on average, more than 1 month of language age for every month of instruction. Also, they displayed significant decreases in inappropriate and disruptive behaviors. McNerney (2003) used videotapes to show parents interacting with their children with autism to regular education preschool teachers. The parents were implementing techniques to promote expressive verbalizations via PRT. She found that, indeed, the teachers showed increases in their use of PRT procedures and also the number of opportunities they provided for their students to verbalize. Importantly, the children showed increases in the number of functional verbalizations made at school.

Although the use of PRT and similar approaches obviously hold promise in educational settings and those provided by teachers, it is still the case that such approaches are not yet used extensively in classrooms, and teachers who often report using such procedures (and believe they are) are simply not doing it well (Stahmer, Collings, and Palinkas, 2005). It is hoped that upcoming research will help bridge the gap between research and practice in this area.

Peers

To promote generalization of treatment effects, it is important that treatment be conducted in as many environments as possible and by others with whom the child with autism interacts on a regular basis. Peers are an obvious choice of interventionist because they are a naturally occurring part of the child's environment and because multiple trained peers mean multiple treatment providers are available. Indeed, peers have been taught to successfully use naturalistic behavioral interventions to increase language, play, and social skills in their peers with autism. McGee et al. (1992) used a multiple-baseline design to demonstrate the effectiveness of peer incidental teaching to increase the reciprocal interactions of three preschoolers with autism (age 3–5 years) and three typically developing children (age 4 years). After training as peer-tutors, the typically developing children used incidental teaching in the classroom setting to facilitate the use of verbal labels of preferred toys by their peers with autism. Maintenance of increased reciprocal interactions was demonstrated after adult supervision was withdrawn. One of the children with ASD generalized the increased interactions in free-play periods. Pierce and Schreibman (1995) used modeling, role, playing, and didactic instruction to teach typical peers of two 10-year-old boys with autism to implement PRT in a classroom setting. After peer implementation of PRT, the two children with autism maintained prolonged interactions with the peers, initiated play and conversation, and increased engagement in language and joint attention behaviors. These results were replicated and extended by subsequent investigations (Pierce & Schreibman, 1997a,b) showing that PRT training of peers led to collateral improvements in social behaviors, language complexity, and play complexity and that training of multiple peers led to increased generalization of treatment effects.

In a more indirect application of behavioral teaching in a naturalistic manner, the literature supports the effectiveness of "integrated" preschool and classroom environments for children with autism. Typically these are classrooms in which children with ASDs are placed with typically developing children (usually a ratio of two typically developing peers per child with ASD) and where naturalistic behavioral strategies are embedded in activities with the peers (McGee, Daly, & Jacobs, 1994; McGee, Morrier, & Daly, 1999; Stahmer & Ingersoll, 2004; Strain & Cordisco, 1994; Strain, McGee, & Kohler, 2001). The rationale for such integrated classroom environments includes the obvious potential of typical peers as both intervention agents (either specifically trained or as part of normal interactions), behavior models, and as part of the type of environment within which we want these children to function (i.e., least restrictive environment). For example, Stahmer and Ingersoll (2004) report the outcomes for 20 toddlers with autism who participated in an inclusive program for children under age 3 years. (The program utilized both naturalistic and more highly structured interventions.) Outcomes on both standardized assessments and functional behaviors were compared for the children at program entry and at program exit (approximately 6 months later). The results of this program are impressive. Although only 11% of the toddlers with ASDs at intake scored in the typical range on standardized assessments, 37% of the children scored in this range at program exit. Further, although at intake, 50% of the ASD toddlers had a functional communication system, 90% of the children did at exit. The investigators also reported substantial increases in social and play behaviors.

Current Issues in Naturalistic Behavioral Strategy Implementation

Although the literature makes a convincing argument for the use of naturalistic behavioral strategies (such as PRT for children with autism), research continues with the goal of improving the overall effectiveness of such procedures and, importantly, determining which individuals will show the most positive treatment outcome. Naturalistic strategies have been found to be superior to more highly structured behavioral techniques (DTT) in terms of producing spontaneous and generalized social communication; however, it is unclear whether they are superior for teaching the wide range of skills children with autism need to learn, because comparative studies have examined only specific language skills (e.g., preposition use). It is possible that certain skills, such as spontaneous, social communication skills, are best taught using a naturalistic behavioral approach, whereas others are better taught using different teaching strategies. For example, it has been proposed that naturalistic behavioral approaches are more effective for teaching expressive language, whereas structured behavioral approaches are superior for teaching receptive language (Arick et al., 2003). Similarly, it has been suggested that naturalistic behavioral approaches are superior for teaching requesting skills, whereas developmental interventions may be more effective for improving commenting skills (Ingersoll, in press). Research that can examine which skills are best taught using a naturalistic behavioral approach is likely to be fruitful.

As is true of all interventions with this population, there is a wide heterogeneity of responding such that some children respond dramatically well, whereas others respond to a lesser degree, and a minority show no positive response. This renowned heterogeneity in response to treatment strongly suggests that other variables are interacting with treatment to affect response to intervention. Examples of such variables are child characteristics (including behaviors and neurobiological factors), parent/family variables (e.g., depression, stress), cultural variables (different cultures place emphasis on different behaviors and may find different forms of treatment differentially acceptable), and treatment/behavior interactions (i.e., some behaviors may be best targeted by different forms of behavioral intervention).

Sherer and Schreibman (2005) focused on child behaviors and identified a specific behavioral profile that predicted PRT treatment outcome of 4- to 6-year-old children with autism. These investigators first looked retrospectively at the treatment outcome of 28 children who had received PRT treatment. Identifying those children who showed the best response to treatment and those that showed the poorest response, the investigators identified a "responder profile" versus a "nonresponder profile" that characterized the different outcomes. During a structured observation with toys and an adult present, those children who were treatment "responders," when compared to "nonresponders," showed more interest in toys/activities, less social avoidance, more social approach behavior, more verbal stereotypy, and less nonverbal stereotypy. Next a prospective study was conducted wherein six children (age range 3–5.5 years) were identified where three matched the "responder" profile and three matched the "nonresponder" profile identified in the retrospective analysis. The children were matched on IQ, language age, and symptom severity to exclude these potential variables from accounting for outcome differences. Children were subsequently given intense PRT treatment for approximately 6 months. Within a multiple-baseline-across-subjects design, the investigators looked at communication, play, and social behaviors as dependent measures. As expected, the predicted "responders" evidenced substantial improvements in all behaviors, whereas the predicted "nonresponders" showed minimal or no gains.

Schreibman et al. (2008) conducted a subsequent study designed to determine whether all of the Sherer and Schreibman (2005) profile behaviors were required for treatment outcome prediction and if the predictive profile was specific to PRT as opposed to response to ANY treatment. In this study, investigators studied six children with autism (age 2–4 years) matching the original nonresponder profile on all but one of the profile behaviors (toy contact or avoidance) and then assessed their response to PRT. In addition, participants received a course of DTT to determine whether the profile predicted child response to this intervention. Results suggested that altering the original profile behavior of toy contact led to improved response to PRT, altering the profile behavior of high avoidance had little impact on treatment response, and the profile was not predictive of response to DTT.

Yoder and Stone (2006) compared a naturalistic behavioral language intervention, Responsive Education and Prelinguistic Milieu Teaching (RPMT), to a more structured augmentative communication intervention, the Picture Exchange Communication System (PECS; Bondy & Frost, 2001) in young, nonverbal children with autism. They found that that children who initiated joint attention at pretreatment made more gains in the RPMT, whereas the children with little joint attention made more gains in PECS.

There is also evidence to suggest that the effectiveness of naturalistic behavioral interventions vary based on the characteristics of the child's caregiver. For example, Yoder and Warren (2001) found that children whose mothers were initially more responsive and had more formal education made more progress in a naturalistic behavioral intervention (prelinguistic milieu teaching), whereas children whose mothers were less responsive and had less education made more gains in a developmental intervention (responsive interaction). Additional research that can identify for whom naturalistic behavioral interventions are likely to be most effective would likely improve child outcomes.

Although they are based on different underlying philosophies, naturalistic behavioral interventions share many similarities in their implementation with developmental and relationship-based interventions reviewed in this volume that make them highly compatible (*see* Ingersoll, 2010, for review). This compatibility has led some researchers to combine components from each approach in an effort to make more effective interventions. The resulting approaches, Enhanced Milieu Teaching (Kaiser & Hester, 1994), RPMT (Yoder & Warren, 2002), Project ImPACT (Ingersoll & Dvortcsak, 2006, 2010), and Roger and Dawson's Early Start Denver Model (Smith, Rogers, & Dawson, 2008) have been shown to be effective for teaching social communication skills to children with ASDs (Hancock & Kaiser, 2002; Kaiser, Hancock, & Nietfeld, 2000) and other developmental delays (Kaiser & Hester, 1994). However, it is unclear whether they are more effective than naturalistic behavioral interventions by themselves.

These research directions are necessary to determine for which skills, children, and families naturalistic behavioral interventions may be best-suited. Such work will also likely lead to information about how such treatment strategies may be refined and altered so as to lead to positive treatment outcome for more children overall.

Conclusions

Naturalistic behavioral interventions now enjoy a substantial empirical foundation for affecting a wide range of skills in children with autism. Although initially developed primarily in response to identified limitations to the highly structured discrete trial teaching format, naturalistic strategies such as PRT have been expanded to focus directly on behaviors such as communication, social involvement, imitation, and pretend play. Further, these strategies have been shown to be effectively implemented by a variety of treatment providers including parents, teachers, and peers. Although the potential for naturalistic behavioral strategies to target a comprehensive set of skills exists, the fact remains that children's response to treatment can be highly idiosyncratic and heterogenous. Thus current and future research must address for which children and for which behaviors such intervention strategies are most suited.

Challenges and Future Directions

- Compare effectiveness of this approach to other evidence-based interventions for children with ASDs for teaching a wide range of skills.
- Better characterize and identify treatment responders and nonresponders to this intervention approach.
- Further identify characteristics of effective intervention providers using this approach.
- Examine whether adding techniques from the developmental and relationship-based literatures can increase the effectiveness of this approach.

SUGGESTED READINGS

Delprato, D. J. (2001). Comparisons of discrete-trial and normalized behavioral intervention for young children with autism. *Journal of Autism and Developmental Disorders, 31*, 315–325.

Koegel, L. K., Koegel, R. L., Harrower, J. K., & Carter, C. M. (1999). Pivotal response intervention I: Overview of approach. *Journal of Association for Persons with Severe Handicaps, 24*, 174–185.

Schreibman, L. (2005). *The science and fiction of autism*. Cambridge, MA: Harvard University Press.

ACKNOWLEDGMENTS

The authors wish to acknowledge grants from the National Institute of Mental Health (#MH39434, Schreibman, P.I.), Autism Speaks (Schreibman, P.I., Ingersoll, P.I.), and Michigan State University's Families And Communities Together (FACT) Coalition Grant (Ingersoll, P.I.), which all served to facilitate the preparation of this chapter.

REFERENCES

Albert, C. L., & Kaiser, A. P. (1992). Training parents as milieu language teachers. *Journal of Early Intervention, 16*, 31–52.

Arick, J., Young, H. E., Falco, R. A., Loos, L. M., Krug, D. A., Gense, M. H., et al. (2003). Designing an outcome study to monitor the progress of students with autism spectrum disorder. *Focus on Autism and Other Developmental Disabilities, 18*, 75–87.

Baer, D. M., Peterson, R. F., & Sherman, J. A. (1967). The development of imitation by reinforcing behavior similarity to a model. *Journal of the Experimental Analysis of Behavior, 10*, 405–416.

Bates, E., Benigni, L., Bretherton, I., Camaioni, L., & Volterra, V. (1977). From gesture to the first word: On cognitive and social prerequisites. In Lewis, M. M. & Rosenblum, L. A. (Eds.), *Interaction, conversation, and the development of language*, (pp. 247–307.) New York: Wiley.

Bates, E., Benigni, L., Bretherton, I., Camaioni, L., & Volterra, V. (1979). *The emergence of symbols: cognition and communication in infancy*. New York: Academic Press.

Bates, E., Bretherton, I., Snyder, L., Beeghly, M., Shore, C., McNew, S., et al. (1988). *From first words to grammar: Individual differences and dissociable mechanisms*. New York: Cambridge University Press.

Bondy, A. S., & Frost, L. A. (1994). The picture exchange communication system. *Focus on Autistic Behavior, 9*, 1–19.

Bondy, A., & Frost, L. (2001). The picture exchange communication system. *Behavior Modification, 25*, 725–744.

Bruinsma, Y. E. M. (2004). Increases in joint attention: Behavior of eye gaze attention to share enjoyment as a collateral effect of pivotal response treatment for three children with autism. Doctoral dissertation, University of California, Santa Barbara). *Dissertation Abstracts International, 65*(9-B), 4811.

Cohen, H., Amerine-Dickens, M., & Smith, T. (2006). Early intensive behavioral treatment: Replication of the UCLA model in a community setting. *Journal of Developmental and Behavioral Pediatrics, 27*, S145–S155.

Crockett, J. L., Fleming, R. K., Doepke, K. J., & Stevens, J. S. (2007). Parent training: Acquisition and generalization of discrete trials teaching skills with parents of children with autism. *Research in developmental Disabilities, 28*, 23–36.

Delprato, D. J. (2001). Comparisons of discrete-trial and normalized behavioral intervention for young children with autism. *Journal of Autism and Developmental Disorders, 31*, 315–325.

Fein, G. G. (1981). Pretend play in childhood: an integrative review. *Child Development, 52*, 1095–1118.

Gillett, J. N., & LeBlanc, L. A. (2007). Parent-implemented natural language paradigm to increase language and play in children with autism. *Research in Autism Spectrum Disorders, 1*, 247–255.

Green, G. (1996). Early behavioral intervention for autism: What does research tell us? In Maurice, C ., Green, G., & Luce, S. C. (Eds.) (1996). *Behavioral intervention for young children with autism: A manual for parents and professionals* (pp. 29–44). Austin, TX: Pro-Ed.

Hancock, T. B., & Kaiser, A. P. (2002). The effects of trainer-implemented enhanced milieu teaching on the social communication of children with ASD. *Topics in Early Childhood Special Education, 22*, 39–55.

Hart, B., & Risley, T. R. (1968). Developing correspondence between the non-verbal and verbal behavior of preschool children. *Journal of Applied Behavior Analysis, 1*, 267–281.

Hart, B., & Risley, T. R. (1980). In vivo language intervention: Unanticipated general effects. *Journal of Applied Behavior Analysis, 13*, 407–423.

Ingersoll, B. (2010). Teaching social communication: A comparison of naturalistic behavioral and development, social pragmatic approaches for children with autism spectrum disorders. *Journal of Positive Behavior Interventions, 12*, 33–43.

Ingersoll, B. (in press). The differential effect of three of naturalistic language interventions on language use in children with autism. *Journal of Positive Behavioral Interventions.*

Ingersoll, B., & Dvortcsak, A. (2010). *Teaching social-communication: A practitioner's guide to parent training for children with autism.* New York, NY: Guilford Press.

Ingersoll, B., & Dvortcsak, A. (2006). Including parent training in the early childhood special education curriculum for children with autism spectrum disorders. *Journal of Positive Behavior Interventions, 8*, 79–87.

Ingersoll, B., & Gergans, S. (2007). The effect of a parent-implemented imitation intervention on spontaneous imitation skills in young children with autism. *Research in Developmental Disabilities, 28*, 163–175.

Ingersoll, B., Lewis, E., & Kroman, E. (2007). Teaching the imitation and spontaneous use of descriptive gestures in young children with autism using a naturalistic behavioral intervention. *Journal of Autism and Developmental Disorders, 37*, 1446–1456.

Ingersoll, B., & Schreibman, L. (2006). Teaching reciprocal imitation skills to young children with autism using a naturalistic behavioral approach: Effects on language pretend play, and joint attention. *Journal of Autism and Developmental Disorders, 36*, 487–505.

Jones, E. A., Carr, E. G., & Feeley, K. M. (2006). Multiple effects of joint attention intervention for children with autism. *Behavior Modification, 30*, 782–834.

Kaiser, A. P., Hancock, T. B., & Nietfeld, J. P. (2000). The effects of parent-implemented enhanced milieu teaching on the social communication of children who have ASD. *Early Education and Development, 11*, 423–446.

Kaiser, A. P., & Hester, P. P. (1994). Generalized effects of enhanced milieu teaching. *Journal of Speech and Hearing Research, 37*, 1320–1340.

Kaiser, A. P., Yoder, P. J., & Keetz, A. (1992). Evaluating milieu training. In S. F. Warren & J. Reichle (Eds.). *Causes and effects in communication and language intervention* (pp. 9–47). Baltimore, MD: P. H. Brookes Publishing Company.

Kasari, C., Freeman, S., & Paparella, T. (2006). Joint attention and symbolic play in young children with autism: a randomized controlled intervention study. *Journal of Child Psychology and Psychiatry, 47*, 611–620.

Kasari, C., Paparella, T., Freeman, S., & Jahromi, L. B. (2008). Language outcome in autism: randomized comparison of joint attention and play interventions. *Journal of Consulting and Clinical Psychology, 76*, 125–137.

Koegel, R. L., Bimbela, A., & Schreibman, L. (1996). Collateral effects of parent training on family interactions. *Journal of Autism and Developmental Disorders, 26*, 347–359.

Koegel, R., Camarata, S., Koegel, L., Ben-Tall, A., & Smith, A. (1988). Increasing speech intelligibility in children with autism. *Journal of Autism and Developmental Disorders, 28*, 241–251.

Koegel, L. K., Carter, C. M., & Koegel, R. L. (2003). Teaching children with autism self-initiations as a pivotal response. *Topics in Language Disorders, 23*, 134–145.

Koegel, R. L., & Koegel, L. K. (2006). *Pivotal response treatments for autism: Communication, social and academic development.* Baltimore, MD: Paul H Brookes Publishing.

Koegel, R. L., O'Dell, M., & Dunlap. G . (1988). Producing speech use in nonverbal autistic children by reinforcing attempts. *Journal of Autism and Developmental Disorders, 18*, 525–538.

Koegel, R. L., O'Dell, M. C., & Koegel, L. K. (1987). A natural language teaching paradigm for nonverbal autistic children. *Journal of Autism and Developmental Disorders, 17*, 187–200.

Koegel, R. L., & Schreibman, L. (1977). Teaching autistic children to respond to simultaneous multiple cues. *Journal of Experimental Child Psychology, 24*, 299–311.

Koegel, R. L., Schreibman L., Britten, K. R. Burke, J. C., & O'Neill, R. E. (1982). A comparison of parent training to direct clinic treatment. In R. L. Koegel, A. Rincover, & A. L. Egel (Eds.), *Educating and understanding autistic children* (pp. 260–279). San Diego: College Hill Press.

Koegel, R. L., Schreibman, L., Good, A., Cerniglia, L., Murphy, C., & Koegel, L. K. (1989). *How to teach pivotal behavior to children with autism: A training manual.* University of California, Santa Barbara.

Laski, K. E., Charlop, M. H., & Schreibman, L. (1988). Training parents to use the Natural Language Paradigm to increase their autistic children's speech. *Journal of Applied Behavior Analysis, 21*, 391–400.

Lovaas, O. I. (1987). Behavioral treatment and normal educational and intellectual functioning in young autistic children. *Journal of Consulting and Clinical Psychology, 55*, 3–9.

Lovaas, O. I. (2003). *Teaching individuals with developmental delays: Basic intervention techniques.* Austin, TX: Pro-Ed.

Lovaas, O. I., Berberich, J. P., Perloff, B. F., & Schaeffer, B. (1966). Acquisition of imitative speech in schizophrenic children. *Science, 151*, 705–707.

Lovaas, O. I., Koegel, R. L., & Schreibman, L. (1979). Stimulus overselectivity in autism: A review of research. *Psychological Bulletin, 86*, 1236–1254.

Lovaas, O. I., Koegel, R., Simmons, J. Q., & Long, J. S. (1972). Some generalization and follow-up measures on autistic children in behavior therapy. *Journal of Applied Behavior Analysis, 6*, 131–166.

Loveland, K. A., & Landry, S. H. (1986). Joint attention and language in autism and developmental language delay. *Journal of Autism and Developmental Disorders, 16*, 335–349.

Luckett, T., Bundy, A., & Roberts, J. (2007). Do behavioural approaches teach children with autism to play or are they pretending? *Autism, 11*, 365–388.

Martins, M. P., & Harris, S. L. (2006). Teaching children with autism to respond to joint attention initiations. *Child and Family Behavior Therapy, 28*, 51–67.

Maurice, C., Green, G., & Luce, S. C. (Eds) (1996). *Behavioral intervention for young children with autism: A manual for parents and professionals.* Austin, TX: Pro-Ed.

McEachin, J. J., Smith, T., & Lovaas, O. I. (1993). Long-term outcome for children with autism who received early intensive behavioral treatment. *American Journal of Mental Retardation, 97*, 359–372.

McGee, G. G., Almeida, M. C., Sulzer-Azaroff, B., & Feldman, R. S. (1992). Promoting reciprocal interactions via peer incidental teaching. *Journal of Applied Behavior Analysis, 25*, 117–126.

McGee, G. G., Daly, T., & Jacobs, H. (1994). The Walden preschool. In J. S. Handleman & S. L. Harris (Eds.). *Preschool education programs for children with autism* (2nd ed., pp. 157–190). Austin, TX: Pro-Ed.

McGee, G. G., Krantz, P. J., Mason, D., & McClannahan, L. E. (1983). A modified incidental-teaching procedure for autistic youth: Acquisition and generalization of receptive object labels. *Journal of Applied Behavior Analysis, 16*, 329–338.

McGee, G. G., Krantz, P. J., & McClannahan, L. E. (1985). The facilitative effects of incidental teaching on preposition use by autistic children. *Journal of Applied Behavior Analysis, 18*, 17–31.

McGee, G. G., Morrier, M. J., & Daly, T. (1999). An incidental teaching approach to early intervention for toddlers with autism. *Journal of the Association for Persons with Severe Handicaps, 24*, 133–146.

Metz, J. R. (1965). Conditioning generalized imitation in autistic children. *Journal of Experimental Child Psychology, 2*, 389–399.

Miranda-Linne & Melin, L. (1992). Acquisition, generalization, and spontaneous use of color adjectives: A comparison of incidental teaching and traditional discrete-trial procedures for children with autism. *Research in Developmental Disabilities, 13*, 191–210.

Mundy, P., Delgado, C. Block, J., Venezia, M., Hogan, A., & Seibert, J. (2003). *Early Social Communication Scales (ESCS).* Miami, FL: University of Miami.

National Research Council (2001). *Educating children with autism.* Committee on Educational Interventions for Children with Autism. Catherine Lord and James P. McGee, Eds. Division of Behavioral and Social Sciences and Education. Washington, DC: National Academy Press.

Pierce, K., & Schreibman, L. (1995). Increasing complex social behaviors in children with autism: Effects of peer-implemented pivotal response training. *Journal of Applied Behavior Analysis, 28*, 285–295.

Pierce, K., & Schreibman, L. (1997a). Multiple peer use of Pivotal Response Training to increase social behaviors of classmates with autism: Results from trained and untrained peers. *Journal of Applied Behavior Analysis, 30*, 157–160.

Pierce, K., & Schreibman, L. (1997b). Using peer trainers to promote social behavior in autism: Are they effective at enhancing multiple social domains? *Focus on Autism and Other Developmental Disabilities, 12*, 207–218.

Rocha, M. L., Schreibman, L., & Stahmer, A. C. (2007). Effectiveness of training parents to teach joint attention in children with autism. *Journal of Early Intervention, 29*, 154–172.

Sallows, G. O., & Graupner, T. D. (2005). Intensive behavioral treatment for children with autism: Four-year outcome and predictors. *American Journal of Mental Retardation, 110*, 417–438.

Schreibman, L. (1997). The study of stimulus control in autism. In D. M. Baer & E. M. Pinkston (Eds.) *Environment and behavior.* (pp. 203–209). Boulder, CO: Westview Press.

Schreibman, L. (2005). *The science and fiction of autism.* Cambridge, MA: Harvard University Press.

Schreibman, L. (1997). Theoretical perspectives on behavioral intervention for individuals with autism. In D. J. Cohen & F. R. Volkmar (Eds.). *Handbook of autism and pervasive developmental disorders, 2nd edition* (pp. 920–933) New York: John Wiley & Sons, Inc.

Schreibman, L., Charlop, M. H., & Koegel, R. L. (1982). Teaching autistic children to use extra-stimulus prompts. *Journal of Experimental Child Psychology, 33*, 475–491.

Schreibman, L., & Ingersoll, B. (2005). Behavioral interventions to promote learning in individuals with autism. In F. Volkmar, A., Klin, R. Paul, & D. Cohen (Eds.), *Handbook of autism and pervasive developmental disorders, Volume 2: Assessment, interventions, and policy* (pp. 882–896). New York: Wiley.

Schreibman, L., Kaneko, W. M., & Koegel, R. L. (1991). Positive affect of parents of autistic children: A comparison across two teaching techniques. *Behavior Therapy, 22*, 479–490.

Schreibman, L., & Koegel, R. L. (1996). Fostering self-management: Parent-delivered pivotal response training for children with autistic disorder. In E. D. Hibbs & P. S. Jensen (Eds.). *Psychosocial treatments for child and adolescent disorders: Empirically based strategies for clinical practice*, (pp. 525–552). Washington, DC: American Psychological Association.

Schreibman, L., & Koegel, R. L. (2005). Training for parents of children with autism: Pivotal responses, generalization, and individualization of interventions. In E. D. Hibbs & P. S. Jensen (Eds.). *Psychosocial treatments for child and adolescent disorders: Empirically based strategies for clinical practice* (2nd ed., pp. 605–631). Washington, DC: American Psychological Association.

Schreibman, L., Stahmer, A. C., Cestone-Barlett, V., & Dufek, L. (2009). Brief report: Toward refinement of a predictive behavioral profile for treatment outcome in children with autism. *Research in Autism Spectrum Disorders, 3*, 163–172.

Schroeder, G. L., & Baer, D. M. (1972). Effects of concurrent ad serial training on generalized vocal imitation in retarded children. *Developmental Psychology, 6*, 293–301.

Sherer, M. R., & Schreibman, L. (2005). Individual behavioral profiles and predictors of treatment effectiveness for children with autism. *Journal of Consulting and Clinical Psychology, 73*, 525–538.

Smith, T. (2001). Discrete trial training in the treatment of autism. *Focus on Autism and Other Developmental Disabilities, 16*, 86–92.

Smith, T., Groen, A. D ., & Wynn, J. W. (2000). Randomized trial of intensive early intervention for children with pervasive developmental disorder. *American Journal on Mental Retardation, 105*, 269–285.

Stahmer, A. C. (1995). Teaching symbolic play skills to children with autism using Pivotal Response Training. *Journal of Autism and Developmental Disorders, 25*, 123–141.

Stahmer, A . C., Collings, N. M., & Palinkas, L. (2005). Early intervention practices for children with autism: Descriptions from community providers. *Focus on Autism and Other Developmental Disabililties, 20*, 66–79.

Stahmer, A. C., & Ingersoll, B. (2004). Inclusive programming for toddlers with autistic spectrum disorders: Outcomes from the children's toddler school. *Journal of Positive Behavioral Interventions, 6*, 67–82.

Stahmer, A. C., Schreibman, L., & Palardy, N. (1994, May) Social validation of symbolic play training for children with autism. Paper presented at the meeting of the Association for Behavior Analysis, Atlanta, GA.

Strain, P., & Cordisco, K. (1994). The LEAP preschool. In S. L. Harris & J. S. Handleman (Eds.), *Preschool education programs for children with autism* (pp. 115–126). Austin, TX: Pro-Ed.

Strain, P. S., McGee, G. G., & Kohler, F. W. (2001). Inclusion of children with autism in early intervention settings: An examination of rationale, myths, and procedures. In M. J. Guralnick (Ed.), *Early childhood inclusion: Focus on change* (pp. 337–364). Baltimore: Brookes.

Stokes, T. F., & Baer, D. M. (1977). An implicit technology of generalization. *Journal of Applied Behavior Analysis, 10*, 349–367.

Thorp, D. M., Stahmer, A. C., & Schreibman, L. (1995). Effects of sociodramatic play training on children with autism. *Journal of Autism and Developmental Disorders, 25*, 265–282.

Whalen, C., & Schreibman, L. (2003). Joint attention training for children with autism using behavior modification procedures. *Journal of Child Psychology and Psychiatry, 44*, 456–468.

Whalen, C., Schreibman, L., & Ingersoll, B. (2006). The collateral effects of joint attention training on social initiations, positive affect, imitation, and spontaneous speech for young children with autism. *Journal of Autism and Developmental Disorders, 36*, 655–664.

Yoder, P., & Stone, W. L. (2006). Randomized comparison of two communication interventions for preschoolers with autism spectrum disorders. *Journal of Consulting and Clinical Psychology, 74*, 426–435.

Yoder, P. J., & Warren, S. F. (2001). Intentional communication elicits language-facilitating maternal responses in dyads with children who have developmental disabilities. *American Journal of Mental Retardation, 106*, 327–335.

Yoder, P. J., & Warren, S. F. (2002). Effects of prelinguistic milieu teaching and parent responsivity education on dyads involving children with intellectual disabilities. *Journal of Speech, Language, and Hearing Research, 45*, 1158–1174.

60 Stanley I. Greenspan†, Serena Wieder

Relationship-Based Early Intervention Approach to Autistic Spectrum Disorders: The Developmental, Individual Difference, Relationship-Based Model (The DIR Model)

Key Points

- The DIR Model *(1)* focuses on functional emotional capacities—joint attention, engagement, two-way communication, problem solving, and symbolic thought—which provide the foundation for development and *(2)* treats impeding sensory motor and regulatory challenges—auditory, visual-spatial, motor—through interactive learning relationships with parents, teachers, and therapists. These interactive experiences are believed to improve the connectivity of cortical neurons that process sensory motor information. This improvement, as a mechanism of improvement, is consistent with the current view of autism as a disorder of connectivity between different parts of the brain.
- Central to the DIR Model is the role of the child's natural emotions and interests. Studies have shown that they are essential for engagement and interaction between children and caregivers. These interactions improve the neural connectivity and thus enable successively higher levels of social, emotional, and intellectual capacities.
- Deficits associated with autism stem from compromises in an infant's ability to connect emotions (or intent) to motor planning and sequencing, to sensations, and later, to early forms of symbolic expression.
- With caregivers' creating states of heightened pleasurable and other affects tailored to the child's unique motor and sensory-processing profile, the child can develop and strengthen the connection between sensation, affect, and motor action, which leads to more purposeful affective behavior. This, in turn, leads to reciprocal signaling, a sense of self, symbolic functioning, and higher-level thinking skills.
- Clinical outcome reports have long described the benefits of DIR intervention, and new research is confirming the importance of developmental models of assessment and very early intervention, which can change the course of the disorder.

Relationship-based approaches are part of a broader category of developmental approaches that help children with autistic spectrum disorders (ASDs) and related special needs conditions. Based on a modern understanding of human development, these approaches recognize the importance of relationships; interactions with primary caregivers, therapists, and peers; and individual differences in infants' and children's ability to process sensations and plan actions. Developmental approaches call for early identification and early and intensive intervention.

A feature common to most developmental-relationship-based approaches is the focus on human interactions as a primary learning path. The Developmental, Individual-Difference, Relationship-Based Floortime Model (DIR Model) presented in this chapter systematizes an understanding of the child and his family and culture, including diagnostic profiles. This comprehensive framework enables clinicians, parents, and educators to construct a program tailored to the child's unique challenges and strengths.

Central to the DIR Model is the role of the child's natural emotions and interests. Studies have shown that they are essential for engagement and interaction between children and caregivers. These interactions improve the neural connectivity and thus enable successively higher levels of social, emotional, and intellectual capacities.

Floortime, derived from the DIR Model, is a specific intervention technique in which parents and other members of the intervention team follow the child's natural emotional interests while challenging the child to master richer social, emotional, and intellectual capacities. Floortime emphasizes the child's initiation, reciprocity, continuous flow of interactions, reasoning, and empathy. With young children, these playful interactions often occur on the "floor," but they expand to include conversations and interactions in other places.

The DIR Model guides a team that often includes speech therapists, occupational therapists, educators, mental health (developmental-psychological) professionals, and, where appropriate, biomedical personnel. Parents and other family members and caregivers are vital in developmental, relationship-based approaches because of the importance of their emotional relationships with the child. This chapter will describe the DIR Model in greater detail.

The Developmental, Individual-Difference, Relationship-Based Model

The "D" of DIR: Functional Emotional Developmental Capacities

Table 60-1 lists the six Functional Emotional Developmental levels, which explain how children integrate all their capacities (motor, cognitive, language, visual-spatial, sensory) to carry out emotionally meaningful goals. The support for these levels is reviewed elsewhere (Greenspan, 1979, 1989, 1992, 1997b).

The "I" of DIR: Individual Differences in Sensory Modulation, Sensory Processing, Sensory Affective Processing, and Motor Planning and Sequencing

These biologically based individual differences are the result of genetic, prenatal, perinatal, and maturational variations and/or deficits. They can be characterized in at least four ways:

1. Sensory modulation, including hypo- and hyper-reactivity in each sensory modality (touch, sound, smell, vision, and movement in space).
2. Sensory processing in each sensory modality, including auditory processing and language and visual-spatial processing. Processing includes the capacity to register, decode, and comprehend sequences and abstract patterns.
3. Sensory-affective processing in each modality (e.g., the ability to process and react to affect, including the capacity to connect "intent" or affect to motor planning and sequencing, language, and symbols). This processing capacity may be especially relevant for ASD (Greenspan & Wieder, 1997, 1998).
4. Motor planning and sequencing, including the capacity to sequence actions, behaviors, and symbols, such as symbols in the form of thoughts, words, visual images, and spatial concepts.

The "R" of DIR: Relationships and Interactions

Affective interaction patterns include developmentally appropriate, or inappropriate, relationships with the caregiver, parent, and family. These interaction patterns bring the child's biology into the larger developmental progression and can contribute to the child's functional developmental capacities. Developmentally appropriate interactions with a child mobilize his intentions and affects and enable him both to broaden his range of experience at each level of development and to move from one functional developmental level to the next. In contrast, interactions that do not deal with the child's functional developmental level or individual differences can undermine progress. For example, a reserved caregiver may not be able to easily engage an infant who is under-reactive and self-absorbed. A child who does not have the interactive support of a parent to explore negative emotions symbolically can have anxiety, rigidities, obsessions, and constricted affect.

The Importance of Affect

Explorations of the types of thinking that are part of skillful social interactions (i.e., emotional intelligence) and concepts of multiple intelligences have supported and increased interest in the role of emotions (Gardner, 1983; Goleman, 1995; Committee on Integrating the Science of Early Childhood Development, 2000; Kasari et al., 2006). A clinical outcome report study on DIR suggests that with an emphasis on emotional interactions, a subgroup of children diagnosed with ASDs can learn to engage with others; think creatively, logically, and reflectively; enjoy peers; and do well academically in regular classes (Greenspan & Wieder, 1998; Greenspan, 1999; Interdisciplinary Council on Developmental and Learning Disorders Clinical Practice Guidelines Workgroup, 2000).

Despite this support for and greater interest in the role of emotions in human development, there has not been sufficient understanding of how emotions and emotional interactions impact intelligence and related cognitive and language abilities as well as many complex social and self-regulation skills. There has also not been an understanding of the psychological or neurological mechanisms of action by which emotions shape these different aspects of the mind. Because of this lack of understanding, emotions have taken a back seat to cognition, language, and memory. Therefore, the question remains: What role does emotion play in the developmental steps and pathways through which such distinctly human capacities as symbol formation, language, and reflective thinking emerge in the life of each new infant and child?

The Core Psychological Deficit in Autism and the Developmental Pathways to Joint Attention, Pattern Recognition, Theory of Mind, Language, and Thinking

Suggested autism-specific developmental deficits include those in the following abilities: *(1)* empathy and seeing the world from another person's perspective (Baron-Cohen,

Table 60–1.
The six functional emotional developmental levels

Level	Description
1. Shared attention and regulation	Attends to multisensory affective experience and, at the same time, organizes a calm, regulated state (e.g., looks at, listens to, follows the movement and voice of a caregiver, and moves purposefully).
2. Engagement and relating	Engages with caregivers and expresses affective preference and pleasure (e.g., shows joyful smiles and warm affection with a familiar caregiver). Engagement evolves to include tolerating wider ranges of emotions, such as anger, frustration, disappointment, and fairness, within the relationship.
3. Purposeful emotional interactions	Initiates and responds to two-way presymbolic gestural communication (opens and closes circles of communication, e.g., back-and-forth smiles, sounds, and gestures that build around a common theme, such as reaching for and grasping a rattle in the caregiver's hand and then returning it when the caregiver reaches out).
4. Shared, social problem-solving (joint attention)	Organizes chains of two-way communication to solve social problems (opens and closes many circles of communication in a row); maintains communication across space; integrates affective polarities; and synthesizes an emerging prerepresentational organization of self and other (e.g., taking Dad by the hand to get a toy on the shelf). Here, aware of what he can and cannot do (self) to get the toy he wants, the child seeks the help of someone else (other). Prior to representing intent or ideas in words, the child does so through gestures and actions.
5. Creating ideas	Creates and functionally uses ideas as a basis for creative or imaginative thinking, giving meaning to symbols (e.g., engaging in pretend play, using words to meet needs, "Juice!").
6. Building bridges between ideas (logical thinking)	Build bridges between ideas as a basis for logic, reality testing, thinking, and judgment (e.g., answer "Wh" questions, including "Why"; engage in debates opinion-oriented conversations; elaborate pretend dramas).

1994); *(2)* higher-level abstract thinking, including making inferences (Minshew, Goldstein, & Siegel, 1997); *(3)* shared attention, including social referencing and problem-solving (Mundy, Sigman, & Kasari, 1990); *(4)* emotional reciprocity (Dawson & Galpert, 1990; Baranek, 1999); and *(5)* functional (pragmatic) language (Wetherby & Prizant, 1993). Neuropsychological models that have been proposed to account for the clinical features of autism further elaborate these autism-specific developmental deficits (Baron-Cohen, Leslie, & Frith, 1985; Sperry, 1985; Baron-Cohen, 1989; Frith, 1989; Bowler, 1992; Klin, Volkmar, & Sparrow, 1992; Dahlgren & Trillingsgaard, 1996; Pennington & Ozonoff, 1996; Ozonoff, 1997; Dawson et al., 1998; Greenspan, 2001). However, do deficits in these abilities actually occur downstream from other primary deficits?

Clinical work and current research (Greenspan, 2001; Greenspan & Shanker, 2004; Greenspan & Shanker, 2007; Wieder & Greenspan, 2003) suggest that the deficits described above stem from an earlier capacity that is compromised in children with ASDs. This earlier capacity is an infant's ability to interconnect emotions or intent, motor planning and sequencing, and sensations. It evolves into early forms of symbolic expression of their intent or emotions, such as pretending to have a tea party or act mad, which later lead to more elaborate use of symbols to create ideas (Greenspan, 1979, 1989; Greenspan, 1997b). It is hypothesized that the biological differences associated with ASDs may express themselves through the derailing of this connection, leading to both the primary and secondary features of ASDs.

The Sensory-Affect-Motor Connections

In healthy development, an infant connects the sensory system to the motor system through affect (e.g., turning to look at a caregiver's smiling face and wooing voice rather than scowling face and harsh voice). With caregivers' creating states of heightened pleasurable and other affects tailored to the child's unique motor and sensory-processing profile, the child can develop and strengthen the connection between sensation, affect, and motor action (e.g., simultaneously looking, listening, and moving while engaging in meaningful problem-solving interactions). This leads to more purposeful affective behavior, which, in turn, leads to reciprocal signaling, a sense of self, symbolic functioning, and higher-level thinking skills.

As the infant negotiates the first four Functional Emotional Developmental levels (*see* Table 60-1; shared attention and regulation, engagement, two-way communication, and shared social problem solving), she engages in progressively more complex patterns of affective signaling with caregivers (Greenspan & Shanker, 2004). These long chains of coregulated affective gesturing enable the child to recognize various patterns involved in satisfying her emotional needs. She learns, for example, how to solicit a caregiver's assistance to obtain some out-of-reach desired object. This solicitation becomes finely tuned, back-and-forth interactions requiring joint attention (through vocalizations and facial expressions) in a coregulated solution. She learns what different gestures or facial expressions signify—the connection between certain kinds of facial expressions, tones of voice, or behavior and an individual's mood or intentions. Recognizing when her dad is grumpy, she waits to ask for what she wants. This ability to read the patterns of others and, through recognition of one's own patterns, form a sense of self, is the basis for what is called *intention reading* or *theory of mind.*

This ability to read patterns is also essential if a child is to have and act on expectations—to know when to expect different kinds of responses from his caregiver or to know what love, anger, respect, and shame feel like. It is equally essential if the toddler is to know how to grasp the intentions of others. Pattern recognition, intention reading, and joint attention emerge from and require mastery of the first three Functional Emotional Developmental levels, as shown in Table 60-1 (Greenspan & Shanker, 2007).

Understanding the complexity of this process has led to the early identification of challenges and to the formulation of interventions that are tailored to the child's biological profile and vulnerabilities. This early intervention increases the likelihood that the child will achieve some relative mastery of these critical early affective transformations and of the subsequent abilities for joint attention, theory of mind, and higher levels of language and symbolic thinking. When affect is brought into the treatment of sensory motor processing challenges in language comprehension and visual-spatial knowledge, affective transformations convert labels into meanings. Thus begins the process of comprehending symbolic imagery as well as communicating thoughts and feelings, promoting more complex and abstract reasoning, shades of gray and multicausal thinking, as well as reflective capacities of self and others (Greenspan & Wieder, 1998).

Theory into Practice: DIR Assessment and Intervention Model

The theory outlined above was assessed on a representative population of more than 1,500 children whose parents were administered the Greenspan Social-Emotional Growth Chart (Greenspan, 2004). The results of this assessment suggests that mastery of the early stages of functional emotional development is necessary for children's social referencing and joint-attention capacities (such as reciprocal, shared social problem solving) and for progression to the subsequent stages of symbol formation, pragmatic language, and higher-level thinking (including theory-of-mind capacities such as empathy) (Bayley, 2005). This data set, supportive of the DIR Model, opens the door to further research on the central nervous system and compromises in these early emotional interactions.

Many of the core elements in the DIR Model have a long tradition in early interventions, having been used in speech and language therapy, occupational therapy, visual-spatial cognitive therapy, special and early childhood education, and playful interactions with parents (which is consistent with the developmentally appropriate practice guidelines of the National Association for the Education of Young Children [NAEYC]; Bredekamp & Copple, 1997). The DIR Model contributes to these traditional practices by further defining the child's developmental level, individual processing differences, and the need for certain types of affective interactions in terms of a comprehensive program where all the elements can work together toward common goals.

In this model, the therapeutic program should begin as early as possible so that the children can re-engage in emotional interactions that use their emerging, but not fully developing, capacities for communication (often initially with gestures rather than words). Recent improvement in early identification now makes it possible to screen and identify challenges for a child at risk for ASDs who is less than 1 year old. However, the DIR Model can be applied to any age, as it is a developmental framework useful across the lifespan.

The Functional Developmental Profile

Implementation of an appropriate assessment of all the relevant functional areas requires a number of sessions with the child and family. These sessions must begin with discussions with the caregivers and observations. The assessment process, which is described in detail elsewhere (Greenspan, 1992; Greenspan & Wieder, 1998), includes: *(1)* two or more 45-minute clinical observations of child–caregiver and/or clinician–child interactions; *(2)* developmental history and review of current functioning; *(3)* review of family and caregiver functioning; *(4)* review of standard diagnostic assessments, current programs, and patterns of interaction; *(5)* consultation with speech pathologists, occupational and physical therapists, educators, and mental health colleagues, including the use of structured tests on an as-needed, rather than routine, basis; and *(6)* biomedical evaluation (*see* Figure 60-1).

The assessment then leads to an individualized functional profile that captures each child's unique developmental features outlined above in the description of DIR and creates individually tailored intervention programs (i.e., tailoring the program to the child rather than fitting the child to a general program). The profile describes each of the child's functional developmental capacities and contributing biological processing differences and environmental interactive patterns, including the different interaction patterns available to the child at home, at school, with peers, and in other settings.

The DIR Intervention Program

The DIR Model enables the formation of a comprehensive intervention program for infants, toddlers, and preschoolers with ASDs and other developmental challenges. The program helps them to re-establish the developmental sequence that went awry (with a special focus on helping them become affectively connected and intentional). The program is built on *(1)* determining which of the functional emotional levels described earlier have been mastered fully, partially, or not at all; *(2)* understanding children's individual differences in sensory modulation, processing, and motor planning; and

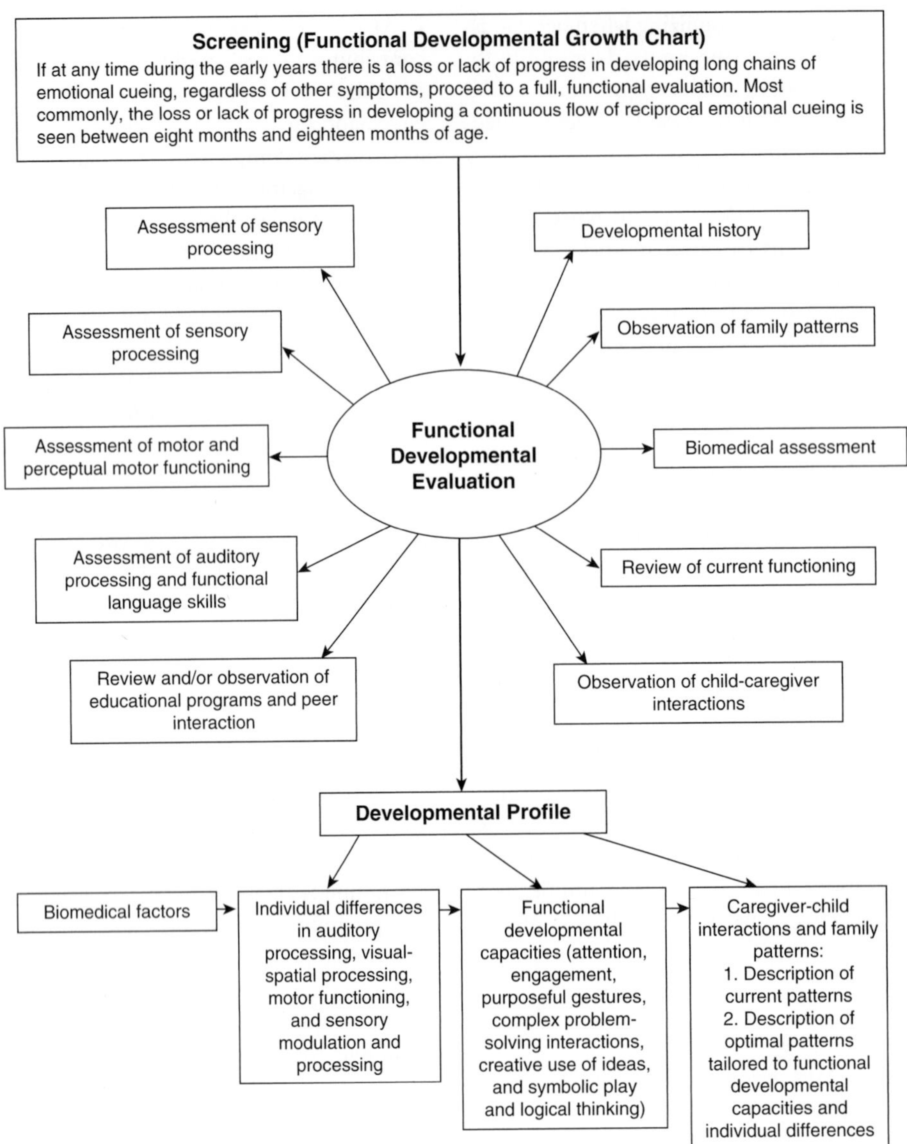

Figure 60–1. Outline of the DIR approach to assessment and evaluation.

(3) establishing a relationship that creates interactive, affective opportunities to negotiate the partially mastered or unmastered functional emotional developmental process. Rather than focus only on isolated behaviors or skills, the DIR-based approach focuses on the more essential functional emotional developmental processes and differences that underlie particular symptoms or behaviors. The goal is to pinpoint what is compromised and construct the developmental foundations for healthy emotional, social, intellectual functioning.

The DIR-based intervention is fundamentally different from behavioral, skill-building, play therapy, or psychotherapy. The primary goal of this intervention is to enable children to form a sense of themselves as intentional, interactive individuals; to develop cognitive, language, and social capacities from this basic sense of intentionality; and to progress through the six Functional Emotional Developmental capacities.

The DIR-based Intervention Model can be conceptualized as a pyramid, with each of the components of the pyramid building on one another (*see* Figure 60-2).

As shown in Figure 60-2, elements of a comprehensive program include home-based and educational elements, clinic-based therapies for both child and caregivers, as well as nutritional and biomedical components. Most children require most, if not all, of the following components for a comprehensive program as each addresses a major area requiring further development, and each component provides the countless opportunities for successful spontaneous and semi-structured interactions that have been derailed.

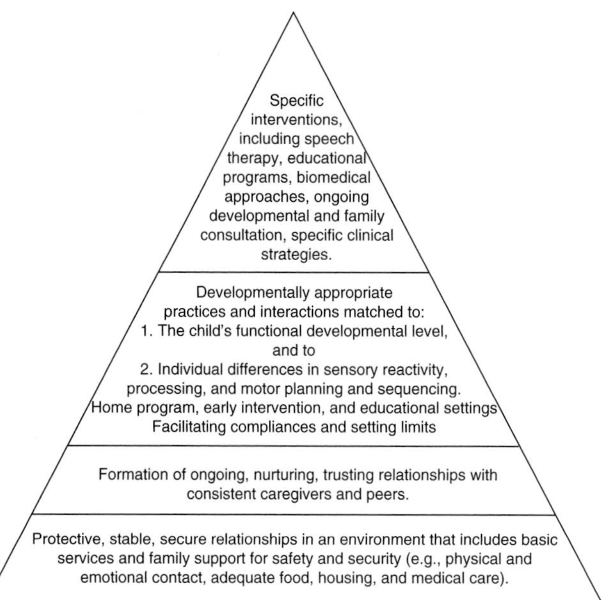

Figure 60–2. DIR-based intervention pyramid for children with ASD.

1. Home-based, developmentally appropriate interactions and practices:
   - Spontaneous interactions (Floortime) that follow the child's lead to focus on joint attention and engagement. The interactions eventually become a continuous flow and then advance to problem solving. The subsequent progression into creative pretend play supports mastering the full range of emotional and cognitive abilities and prepares the child for higher levels of abstract thinking. As the child gets older, Floortime becomes more reality-based conversations and reflective talk-time (20- to 30-minute sessions, eight or more times a day; as children improve, they can usually engage in longer sessions).
   - Semi-structured, affect-based problem solving, such as dealing with real-life situations where the child encounters problems throughout relevant daily experiences where he or she must interact with the parent to solve (e.g., finding his favorite crackers that are in a plastic bag, finding the tub empty when asked if ready for a bath, searching for daddy who is calling from somewhere in the house, negotiating with a sibling for a toy, or working on tasks together to support reasoning, planning and sequencing, etc.). These incidental learning opportunities require back-and-forth, problem-solving discussions or nonverbal interactions that promote logical reasoning when relevant to the child's experience or desire. If it is a problem for the child, it is affect-based. When relevant and meaningful to the child, these opportunities lead to interactions that support interconnectivity between different areas of the brain and the sequences necessary for execution.
   - Visual-spatial, motor, and sensory activities prescribed by OT, PT and visual-spatial cognitive therapists (VCTs) for 15 to 30 minutes or more, four times a day. These semi-structured activities or games may include running and changing direction, jumping, spinning, swinging, deep tactile pressure, perceptual motor challenges, including looking-and-doing games, visual-spatial movement, discrimination, visual thinking and logic games, including treasure hunts and obstacle courses. For some children, the above activities can become integrated with the pretend play of Floortime.
   - Play dates with older or younger peers who are natural play partners and will pursue and interact with the child or respond to the adult's coaching and mediation. The number of play dates a week should match the age of the child (i.e., a 3-year-old should have three play dates a week. Later, these can expand to small groups and semi-structured activities with other children in clubs and music, art, drama, and sports activities.
2. Clinic-Based Therapies
   - Speech therapy—developmentally based models or semi-structured models when indicated (e.g., the Developmental Social-Pragmatic Model [DSPM] [Gerber, 2003], the Affect-Based Language Curriculum [ABLC] [Greenspan & Lewis, 2002] and the Social Communication, Emotional Regulation and Transactional Support [SCERTS] [Prizant et al., 2003]).
   - Sensory integration and sensory motor-based occupational therapy and/or physical therapy.
   - Family consultation and counseling to help parents design and implement their comprehensive programs, support family functioning, and provide advocacy where needed.
3. Educational program, daily, with parent collaboration
   - For children who can interact and imitate gestures and/or words and engage in preverbal problem solving, the program can be either an integrated inclusion program or a regular preschool program with an aide.
   - For children not yet able to engage in preverbal problem solving or imitation, a special education program where the major focus is on engagement, preverbal purposeful gestural interaction, preverbal problem solving (a continuous flow of back-and-forth communication), and movement is needed.
   - As children prepare for academic learning, some may require individualized instruction or tutoring in reading, mathematics, visual thinking, as well specific learning techniques—for example, the Lindamood-Bell Learning Process (www.lindamoodbell.com) and visual-spatial exercises from *Thinking Goes to School: Piaget's Theory in Practice* (Furth & Wachs, 1975). The other considerations involve smaller class size and

facilitative environments that do not overwhelm the child.

4. Consideration of nutrition and diet, biomedical interventions, and, when indicated, medications that address regulation and anxiety, possible seizures, and enhance motor planning and sequencing, concentration, and learning.
5. Augmentative technologies geared to improve communication, auditory and visual-spatial processing, sensory modulation, and motor planning.

DIR-based intervention is a dynamic program, and the frequency or changes in the program depend on their progress, although Floortime, and later reflective Talktime, remain constant. In some cases, therapies and other program components can be modified if a strong home program guided by the therapists is implemented. In addition, specific techniques or tools may be indicated, such as augmentative communication, assistive technology, and activities to support imitative and ritualized learning such a social games, drama, sports, etc. As the child progresses, various activities will become part of a child's social activities, such as clubs, sports, music, and drama. During the early years, a comprehensive program of intensive intervention is very important but then can transition into more typical activities as the child progresses.

Floortime

Floortime is the most important element of this comprehensive program. Floortime refers to unstructured "play" sessions, where the child is in the lead and initiates the ideas and the adult both follows and gently challenges the child to support spontaneous, purposeful, and flowing reciprocal interactions at both pre-symbolic and symbolic levels. In addition to Floortime "play," the Floortime principles of follow the lead, engage, challenge, and expand inform all the child's therapies so that children are maximally interested and engaged in learning interactions.

In Floortime, the caregiver first enters into the child's world by showing interest in the child's activity and then engages with the child. Once the child and caregiver have established a rhythm—a back-and-forth communication (gesturally and verbally with deference to the child's sensory profile)—the caregiver next, gently and carefully, expands on the child's activity. The expansion occurs when the caregiver creates a challenge within the context of the child's interest.

Floortime Example

A nonverbal and unengaged child was fixated with four crayons—touching, rolling, and lining them up. To become a partner in this activity, Mom sat next to her daughter and, following her lead, touched and rolled the crayons too, carefully and non-intrusively. After being accepted as a partner in the activity, Mom moved to the next phase—challenge and expand. Staying with the crayons because this was the child's interest, she gently rolled the crayons into a small bag, which she then set on her head. Intrigued, the child reached up and grabbed the bag off Mom's head. A beginning—the child related Mom to the crayons—shared attention. Mom put the bag on her head again, and the child pulled it off a second time. Some back and forth. The third and fourth times, the child smirked a little as she got the bag off Mom's head. Now for a more complex challenge. Mom had to think about how to change the game slightly to expand the interaction without taking over and dampening the child's engagement. Mom hid the bag in her hand and showed the child the backs of both fists. Sure enough, the child opened Mom's hands to discover which one held the crayons. Upon finding them, she beamed with delight.

The principle is to increase the complexity of the child's motor behavior, such as searching in Mom's hand, while maintaining the shared attention. The same holds for increasing the complexity of the sensory input. Mom can add sound—wow's, eee's, woooo's, whatever—as her child searches for the crayons in slightly more difficult places. Then the child combines emotion, shared attention, motor planning and sequencing, visual-spatial thinking, and auditory processing, all which started with the child's fixation with four crayons and a Mom who followed the child's lead, engaged, challenged, and expanded.

Challenges and Principles in the DIR-Based Intervention Model

The critical principle in each aspect of a comprehensive intervention program is to engage the child at his or her level and to help the child master that level and subsequent levels. Often, teams are working at multiple levels at one time. A child, for example, who has partial mastery of using ideas but is not fully engaged or interactive, still needs work at the earlier levels.

As focus and engagement are fostered, attention must be paid to the children's profile of individual processing differences (regulatory profile), as described earlier. For example, if they are over-reactive to sound, talking to them in a loud voice may lead them to become more aimless and withdrawn. If they are over-reactive to sights, bright lights and even very animated facial expressions may be overwhelming for them. On the other hand, if they are under-reactive to sensations of sound and visual-spatial input, talking in a strong voice and using animated facial expressions in a well-lit room may help them attend. Similarly, in terms of their receptive language skills, if they are already at the point where they can decode a complex rhythm, making interesting sounds in complex patterns may be helpful. On the other hand, if they can only decode very simple, two-sequence rhythms, simpler rhythms will be better. One may find that children remain relatively better focused in motion, such as when they are being swung. Certain movement rhythms may be more effective than others.

It is especially difficult to foster a sense of intimacy. As children are encouraged to attend and engage, it is critically important to take advantage of their own natural interests. It is most helpful to follow their lead and look for opportunities for that visceral sense of pleasure and intimacy that leads them to want to relate to the human world. Intimacy is further supported as children are helped to form simple, and then more complex, gestural communications.

Illustration

A father was continually struggling to get his very withdrawn son to interact with him. When the father tried to draw him out by asking questions, the child ignored him. In a therapy session, the therapist suggested trying simple gestural interactions first.

While his son was exploring a toy car, the father put his finger on it very gently and pointed to a particular part, as though to say, "What's that?" In touching it, the father actually moved the car so the son felt the car moving in his hands and noticed, without upset, his father's involvement. The son pulled the car closer to him and looked at where the father had put his finger.

This more physical, gestural communication sparked at least a faint circle of communication: opening—the father's building on the son's interest in the car by touching a spot; closing—the son's looking at that particular spot and pulling the car towards him.

This circle created a foundation for more complex communication. After this minimal interaction, the son began to move his car back and forth. The father got another one and started first moving it back and forth next to his son's and then toward his son's car but not crashing into it. The son initially pulled his car away but then engaged by moving it faster toward his father's. A few circles were closed in a row, and real interaction was beginning.

As their gestural interaction became complex—the father hiding his son's car and his son pointing, vocalizing, and searching for it—it fostered expanding from gestures to symbols. During this gesturing, the father started to describe his own action by saying, "fast" and "slow." After he repeated these words several times, the boy zoomed his car past his father's and uttered a close approximation to "fast." The father beamed, amazed that his son could learn a new word and use it appropriately so quickly.

A major challenge is children's tendency to perseverate. One child would only repeatedly open and close a door. Another would only bang blocks together. The key is to transform the perseveration into an interaction. Caregivers can use children's intense motivation to their advantage to get gestural circles of communication opened and closed. For example, they can get stuck in a door or have their hands caught between some blocks. They can be gentle and playful as the child tries to get them out of the way (like a cat-and-mouse game). As gestural interactions occur, behavior becomes purposeful and affective. When doing "playful obstructions," "fencing in," or "playing dumb," they can modulate child's feelings of annoyance and can help soothe and comfort as well use affect cues and joint problem solving to "help," although often children find "playful obstruction" amusing.

As children become more purposeful and guided by their own initiation and intent, they can imitate gestures and sounds more readily and start simple but emotionally meaningful symbolic actions such as feeding a doll or kissing a bear. With continuing challenges to be intentional, they copy complex patterns and imitate sounds and words, often gradually beginning to use words and "pretend" on their own.

As one moves toward more representational or symbolic elaboration, it can be challenging to help children differentiate their experiences. They need to learn cause-and-effect communication at the level of ideas and to make connections between various representations or ideas. Caregivers become the representation for reality and the ability of clinicians or parents to enter the symbolic world of children and become "players" becomes the critical vehicle for fostering emotional differentiation and higher levels of abstract and logical thinking.

Relating to children when they are feeling strong affects is critical. They are connecting words to underlying affects that give them purpose and meaning. When children are motivated—for example, in trying to negotiate to get a certain kind of food or to go outside—there is often an opportunity to open and close many symbolic circles. The child who tries to open the door to go outside and is angry that he cannot may, in the midst of feeling annoyed, open and close 20 circles of communication if the adult soothingly tries to find out what he wants to do outside.

Children with ASDs find it especially difficult to shift from concrete to abstract modes of thinking because they do not easily generalize from a specific experience to other similar experiences. There is a temptation to teach them answers and repeat the same question by scripting the dialogue or providing scaffolding so they might guess and fill in the blank. However, they can only learn to abstract and generalize through active, emotionally meaningful experiences that help them connect affects or desires to reasoning and actions. Long conversations with debates are most helpful as it helps the child express his or her own opinions and the reasons for them (e.g., "I like juice because it tastes good") rather than memorized elaborations of rote facts (e.g., "The juice is orange") (Greenspan & Wieder, 1997).

As children develop, becoming symbolic and abstract is most often derailed by anxiety, which occurs secondary to poor language and visual-spatial processing. The child who may already have words to express what he wants and even why may not adequately understand what someone else is saying and may become anxious about feelings and ideas outside his comfort zone. Sometimes the child tries to respond, but his comments become tangential, associative, or off topic and the conversation becomes fragmented. Poor visual-spatial knowledge also derails the child's making sense of what he sees and knowing where he is in space. Without these abilities, he cannot respond purposefully to situations at hand. When both language and visual-spatial weaknesses interact, the child may appear distracted, inattentive, and/or illogical. Children who get stuck at concrete levels of language and thought derive security from what they see. Dependent on visual anchors and rituals, they have difficulty developing flexibility and logical abstracting abilities.

Summary

In summary, as the child progresses through the Functional Emotional Developmental levels of regulation and joint attention, engagement, two-way communication, shared social problem solving, creating ideas, and logical thinking (*see* Table 60-1), the therapeutic program works on mobilizing all levels at the same time in each and every interaction. The therapeutic program often evolves to a point where the child and family are involved in three types of activities: *(1)* spontaneous, creative interactions (Floortime); *(2)* semi-structured, problem-solving interactions to learn new skills, concepts, and master academic work (e.g., creating problems to solve, like negotiating for cookies or mastering spatial concepts, such as "behind" and "next to," by discovering where the favorite toy is located); and *(3)* motor, sensory, language, and visual-spatial play to strengthen fundamental processing skills. It is important to note that the DIR Model and intervention program apply as children get older when the different dimensions of development continue to be uneven and/or when the focus needs to shift to emotional development, learning challenges, and anxiety and mood regulation. The DIR Model can guide the intervention of each child and family and his or her unique profile as development unfolds across the lifespan.

Selected Research and Outcome Studies on the DIR-Floortime Model

In the following section, we briefly review selected studies relevant to the DIR approach. Built on years of research in developmental psychology (Greenspan & Wieder, 1998; Greenspan & Shanker, 2004) that underscores the importance of early relationships and family functioning (Greenspan, 1992), the DIR Model also integrates research contributions from various disciplines, such as speech and language pathology (Tannock, Girolametto, & Siegal, 1992; Wetherby & Prizant, 1995; Gerber & Prizant, 2000), occupational therapy (Ayres, 1979; Williamson & Anzalone, 1997; Case-Smith & Miller, 1999), and social work (Shahmoon-Shanok, 2000). Neuroscience research lends further support to developmental interventions (Mundy, Sigman, & Kasari, 1990; Minshew & Goldstein, 2000).

Centers for Disease Control and Prevention

A survey conducted by the National Center for Health Statistics of the Centers for Disease Control and Prevention of over 15,000 families nationwide included emotional variables from the DIR Functional Emotional Developmental Levels. This survey identified 30% more infants and children at risk (most of whom were not receiving services) than prior health surveys (Simpson, Colpe, & Greenspan, 2003).

National Research Council

Importantly, the National Research Council of the National Academy of Sciences, in their 2001 landmark report, *Educating Children with Autism* (Committee on Educational Interventions for Children with Autism, 2001), called for tailoring the treatment approach to unique features of the individual child and recommended to give priority to interventions that promote functional, spontaneous communication.

200 Case Chart Reviews

The first study to show initial evidence for the DIR Model was published in 1997 (Greenspan & Wieder, 1997). Greenspan and Wieder reviewed charts of 200 children who were diagnosed with ASDs and who were part of a cohort of children seen by the authors over a period of 8 years. All children met the criteria of autism or pervasive developmental disorder not otherwise specified (PDD-NOS) as described in DSM-III-R and DSM-IV, and scored in the autism range on the Childhood Autism Rating Scale (Western Psychology Services, 1988). All 200 cases received a comprehensive relationship and developmentally based intervention program for at least 2 years, under the supervision of Dr. Stanley Greenspan and/or Dr. Serena Wieder. The children ranged in age from 22 months to 4 years, with the majority between 2.5 and 3.5 at the initial evaluation. The goal of the review was to reveal patterns in presenting symptoms, underlying processing difficulties, early development, and response to intervention to generate hypotheses for future studies.

The study identified sensory processing and modulation difficulties in all the children, and the authors hypothesized that different underlying processing patterns seemed to include a difficulty in connecting affect and sequencing capacities and could be a possible common denominator, suggesting that difficulties with relating and intimacy are often secondary to underlying processing disturbances. (*See* Table 60-2.) They also suggested that the difficulty in engaging in complex purposeful gestural communication could be an early marker and that contrary to traditional beliefs, a significant number of children may have relatively better functioning in the first year with a regression in the second and third years when these more complex skills are required for social interaction.

According to the authors, the chart review suggested that a number of children with ASDs are, with an appropriate intervention program, capable of empathy, affective reciprocity, creative thinking, and healthy peer relationships. The authors also concluded that focusing on individual differences,

Table 60–2.
Presenting conditions of 200 cases of children with autistic spectrum disorders

Functional Developmental Component	Patients with Mild-to-Severe Impairment	Description of Functional Developmental Component
Presenting functional, emotional, developmental level	24%	Partially engaged and purposeful with limited use of symbols (ideas)
	40%	Partially engaged with limited complex problem-solving interactive sequences (half of this group evidenced only simple purposeful behavior)
	31%	Partially engaged with only fleeting purposeful behavior
	5%	No affective engagement
Sensory modulation	19%	Over-reactive to sensation
	39%	Under-reactive to sensation (with 11% craving sensation)
	36%	Mixed reactivity to sensation
	6%	Not classified
Motor planning dysfunction	52%	Mild-to-moderate motor planning dysfunction
	48%	Severe motor planning dysfunction
Low muscle tone	17%	Motor planning dysfunction with significant degree of low muscle tone
Visual-spatial processing dysfunction	22%	Relative strength (e.g., can find toys, good sense of direction)
	36%	Moderate impairment
	42%	Moderate-to-severe impairment
Auditory processing and language	45%	Mild-to-moderate impairment with intermittent abilities to imitate sounds and words or use selected words
	55%	Moderate-to-severe impairment with no ability to imitate or use words

developmental level, and affective interaction could be especially promising.

Greenspan and Wieder described that after 2 years of intervention, 58% of treated children no longer met the criteria for ASDs. They became warm and interactive, relating joyfully with appropriate, reciprocal preverbal gestures; could engage in lengthy, well-organized, and purposeful social problem-solving and share attention on various social, cognitive, or motor-based tasks; used symbols and words creatively and logically, based on their intent and desires, rather than using rote sequences; and progressed to higher levels of thinking, including making inferences and experiencing empathy. Some children in this group developed precocious academic abilities two or three grade levels above their ages. They all mastered basic capacities such as reality testing, impulse control, organization of thoughts and emotions, differentiated sense of self, and ability to experience a range of emotions, thoughts, and concerns. Finally, they no longer showed symptoms such as self-absorption, avoidance, self-stimulation, or perseveration. On the Childhood Autism Rating Scale (CARS), they shifted into the non-autistic range, although some still evidenced auditory or visual-spatial difficulties (which were improving), and most had some degree of fine or gross motor planning challenges.

Furthermore, children who made progress tended to improve in a certain sequence. First, within several months, they began showing more emotion and pleasure in relating to others. Contrary to the stereotypes of autism, they seemed eager for emotional contact. The problem was that they had trouble figuring out how to achieve it. They seemed grateful when their parents helped them express their desire for interaction. After parents learned to draw them out by various Floortime approaches, even children who had been very avoidant and self-absorbed began seeking out their parents for relatedness.

In 2005, Greenspan and Wieder published a 10- to 15-year follow-up study (since the start of treatment) of 16 children diagnosed with ASDs that were part of the first 200 case series and were part of the 58% of children who showed great improvements (Greenspan & Wieder, 2005). The children were all boys and ranged in age between 12 and 17 years, with a mean of 13.9 years. All these children had received a comprehensive relationship and developmentally based intervention program, including Floortime at home and DIR consultation, for at least 2 years (maximum 5), between ages 2 and 8.5 years. The authors described that after 10 to 15 years since receiving the intervention, these children became empathetic, creative, and reflective adolescents, with healthy peer relationships and solid academic skills. Based on these findings, the authors suggested that some children with ASDs can master the core deficits and reach levels of development formerly thought unattainable.

Social-Emotional Growth Chart

The DIR Model also served as the theoretical framework to develop the Greenspan Social-Emotional Growth Chart (SEGC) (Greenspan, 2004). This norm-referenced surveillance and screening of key social-emotional milestones in infants and children from birth to age 42 months is now part of the new Bayley Scales Kit of Infant and Early Childhood Development. Published by PsychCorp, the SEGC was field-tested on a representative sample of 1,500 infants and young children, and it is now offered as a surveillance and screening instrument for ASDs, with a sensitivity of 87% and specificity of 90%.

The P.L.A.Y. Project

In 2007, Dr. Richard Solomon and colleagues published an evaluation of The PLAY Project Home Consultation (PPHC), a widely disseminated program that trains parents of children with ASDs in the DIR Model (Solomon et al., 2007). Sixty-eight children from age 2 to 6 years (average 3.7 years) completed an 8- to 12-month program where parents were encouraged to deliver 15 hours per week of 1:1 interaction. Pre/post ratings of videotapes by blind raters using the Functional Emotional Assessment Scale (FEAS) showed significant increases ($p \leq 0.0001$) in child subscale scores. That is, 45.5% of children made good to very good functional developmental progress. Overall parents' satisfaction with PPHC was 90%. Average cost of intervention was $2,500/year. Despite some limitations, the pilot study of The PLAY Project Home suggests that the model has potential to both enhance developmental progress of young children with autism and to be a cost-effective intervention. The PLAY model has evolved from a small, university-based, clinical program into a low-cost train-the-trainer model that has the capacity to be disseminated nationally. [1]Dr. Solomon is now conducting an NIMH-funded randomized, controlled, community-based clinical trial of the PLAY Project (Phase II SBIR grant), including 3-to 5-year-old children with ASD.

Related Research

A recent article published by Zwaigenbaum and colleagues highlights the challenges related to early detection, diagnosis, and treatment of ASDs in very young children (Zwaigenbaum, et al., 2009). The authors outline the principles of effective intervention for infants and toddlers with suspected or confirmed diagnosis of ASDs, including responsive and sensitive caretaking, enriched language environments using responsive rather than directive interaction styles, environments that provide opportunities for toddlers to take initiative in their learning, and interventions that are individualized and targeted to specific skills. Furthermore, the authors underscore that existing programs for older children "cannot simply be extrapolated" to younger children.

In addition, other developmental relationship-based approaches have shown to have positive effects, including the work of Gerald Mahoney, Ph.D., and Frida Perales, M.Ed. (Mahoney & Perales, 2005), and Sally Rogers (The University of Colorado model) (Rogers & DiLalla, 1991; Rogers et al., 2000).

In 2010, Dawson, Rogers, and colleagues reported the results of a randomized controlled trial of a comprehensive developmental behavioral intervention for improving outcomes of toddlers (18–30 months) with ASDs using the Early Start Denver Model in a 2-year program (Dawson et al., 2010). They found significant improvement in IQ, adaptive behavior, and change in the autism diagnosis. Their cohort maintained growth in adaptive behavior compared with a normative sample reflecting the benefits of early intervention. Adaptive behaviors are most reflective of the benefits of the developmentally based interventions.

Conclusion

This chapter presents a brief overview of the DIR Model and discusses its implications for assessment, intervention, and understanding the developmental pathways leading to ASDs. It also presents studies that support the DIR Model and other related research findings. A developmental, relationship-based approach can change not only the way we think about developmental disabilities, including ASDs, but what is included in the research base to improve assessment and interventions. At this time the field is expanding, beginning to go beyond reporting outcomes according to IQ scores and educational placement. But it still needs research standards for studying developmental models that are defined by the relevant areas of developmental functioning as described here and the primary goals for each child and family.

Future Directions

- Research that captures the complexity of developmental disorders and differentiates the interventions and outcomes of children with different profiles.
- Integrated educational models that utilize affect-based developmental curricula to make learning experiences meaningful and build the foundations for higher level emotional and cognitive functioning, including ongoing training of those working in school settings.
- Long-term outcome studies that focus on the critical junctures of development for different subtypes along the autism spectrum and identify the opportunities and ongoing processing interventions that will support continued development.
- Long-term studies of parent and sibling experiences and their relationships with children on the autism spectrum.
- Expansion of social and community relationship models in various childhood settings, which extend into adulthood and identify the variables and interventions which provide continuity.

SUGGESTED READINGS

Greenspan, S. I., & Shanker, S. G. (2004). *The first idea: How symbols, language and intelligence evolved in early primates and humans.* Reading, MA: Perseus Books.

Cordero, J., Greenspan, S. I., Bauman, M., Brazelton, T. B., Dawson, G., Dunbar, B., et al. (2007). *CDC/ICDL Collaboration report on a framework for early identification and preventive intervention of emotional and developmental challenges.* Bethesda, MD: ICDL.

Solomon, R., Necheles, J., Ferch, C., & Bruckman, D. (2007). Pilot study of a parent training program for young children with autism: The P.L.A.Y. Project Home Consultation program. *Autism 11*(3), 205–224.

NOTES

1 The state of Michigan Autism Workgroup, convened by the Dept of Health, includes the PLAY Project among the accepted therapies. The PLAY Project, available in a dozen regions of the state, serves hundreds of children in Michigan and is supported by such well-respected agencies as Easter Seals and Mott Children's Health Center in Flint. Furthermore, Easter Seals Crossroads has contracted with P.L.A.Y. Project and is beginning to implement this intervention into all of its charter locations.

REFERENCES

Achenbach, T. M. (1991). *Integrative guide to the 1991 CBCL/4-18, YSR, and TRF profiles.* Burlington, VT: University of Vermont; Department of Psychiatry.

Ayres, J. (1979). *Sensory integration and the child.* Los Angeles, CA: Western Psychological Services.

Baranek, G. T. (1999). Autism during infancy: A retrospective video analysis of sensory-motor and social behaviors at 9-12 months of age. *Journal of Autism and Developmental Disorders, 29,* 213–224.

Baron-Cohen, S. (1989). The theory of mind hypothesis of autism: a reply to Boucher. *The British Journal of Disorders of Communication, 24,* 199–200.

Baron-Cohen, S. (1994). *Mindblindness: An essay on autism and theories of mind.* Cambridge, MA: MIT Press.

Baron-Cohen, S., Leslie, A. M., & Frith, U. (1985). Does the autistic child have a "theory of mind"? *Cognition, 21,* 37–46.

Bayley, N. (2005). *Bayley scales of infant and toddler development, third edition (Bayley-III).* Bulverde, TX: Psychological Corp.

Bowler, D. M. (1992). Theory of mind in Asperger's syndrome. *Journal of Child Psychology and Psychiatry, and Allied Disciplines, 33,* 877–893.

Bredekamp, S., & Copple, C. (1997). *Developmentally appropriate practices in early childhood programs.* Washington, DC: National Association for the Education of Young Children (NAEYC).

Case-Smith, J., & Miller, H. (1999). Occupational therapy with children with pervasive developmental disorders. *American Journal of Occupational Therapy, 53,* 506–513.

Committee on Educational Interventions for Children with Autism, National Research Council (2001). C. Lord & J. McGee (Eds.). *Educating children with autism.* Washington, DC: National Academy Press.

Committee on Integrating the Science of Early Childhood Development, National Research Council (2000). *From neurons to neighborhoods: The science of early childhood development.* J. Shonkoff & D. Phillips (Eds.). Washington, DC: National Academy Press.

Dahlgren, S., & Trillingsgaard, A. (1996). Theory of mind in non-retarded children with autism and Asperger's syndrome: a research note. *Journal of Child Psychology and Psychiatry, and Allied Disciplines, 37,* 759–763.

Dawson, G., & Galpert, I. (1990). Mother's use of imitative play for facilitating social responsiveness and toy play in young autistic children. *Developmental Psychopathology, 2,* 151–162.

Dawson, G., Meltzoff, A., Osterling, J., & Rinaldi, J. (1998). Neuropsychological correlates of early symptoms of autism. *Child Development, 69,* 1276–1285.

Dawson, G., Rogers, S., Munson, J., Smith, M., Winter, J., Greenson, J., et al. (2010). Randomized, controlled trial of an intervention for toddlers with autism: The Early Start Denver Model. *Pediatrics, 125,* e17–e23.

Frith, U. (1989). *Autism: Explaining the enigma.* London: Blackwell.

Furth, G., & Wachs, H. (1975). *Thinking goes to school: Piaget's theory in practice.* New York: Oxford University Press.

Gardner, H. (1983). *Frames of mind: The theory of multiple intelligences.* New York: Basic.

Gerber, S., & Prizant, B. (2000). Speech, Language and Communication Assessment and Intervention for Children. In *ICDL clinical practice guidelines: Redefining the standards of care for infants, children, and families with special needs.* Bethesda, MD: The Interdisciplinary Council on developmental and Learning Disorders.

Gerber, S. (2003). A developmental perspective on language assessment and intervention for children on the autistic spectrum. *Top Lang Disorders, 23,* 74–94.

Goleman, D. (1995). *Emotional intelligence: Why it can matter more than IQ.* New York: Bantam.

Greenspan, S. (2001). The affect diathesis hypothesis: The role of emotions in the core deficit in autism and the development of intelligence and social skills. *J Dev Learning Disord, 5,* 1–45.

Greenspan, S. (2004). *Greenspan Social-Emotional Growth Chart.* Bulverde, TX: The Psychological Corporation.

Greenspan, S. (1979). Intelligence and adaptation: An integration of psychoanalytic and Piagetian developmental psychology. *Psychological Issues. Monograph No. 47–48.* New York: International Universities Press.

Greenspan, S. (1989). *The development of the ego: Implications for personality theory, psychopathology, and the psychotherapeutic process.* New York: International Universities Press.

Greenspan, S. (1992). *Infancy and early childhood: The practice of clinical assessment and intervention with emotional and developmental challenges.* Madison, CT: International Universities Press.

Greenspan, S. (1997a). *Developmentally based psychotherapy.* Madison, CT: International Universities Press.

Greenspan, S. (1997b). *The growth of the mind and the endangered origins of intelligence.* Reading, MA: Addison Wesley Longman.

Greenspan, S. (1999). *Building healthy minds: The six experiences that create intelligence and emotional growth in babies and young children.* Cambridge, MA: Perseus Books.

Greenspan, S. (2004). *The Greenspan Social Emotional Growth Chart: A screening questionnaire for infants and young children.* PsychCorp (Hartcourt Assessment).

Greenspan S., DeGangi, G., & Wieder, S. (2001). *The functional emotional assessment scale (FEAS) for infancy and early childhood: Clinical and research applications.* Bethesda, MD: Interdisciplinary Council on Developmental and Learning Disorders.

Greenspan, S., & Lewis, D. (2002). *The affect-based language curriculum: An intensive program for families, therapists and teachers*. Bethesda, MD: The Interdisciplinary Council on Developmental and Learning Disorders.

Greenspan, S., & Shanker S. (2004). *The first idea: How symbols, language and intelligence evolved from our primate ancestors to modern humans*. Reading, MA: Perseus Books.

Greenspan, S., & Wieder, S. (1997). Developmental patterns and outcomes in infants and children with disorders in relating and communicating: A chart review of 200 cases of children with autistic spectrum diagnoses. *Journal of Developmental and Learning Disorders, 1*, 87–141.

Greenspan, S., & Wieder, S. (1998). *The child with special needs: Encouraging intellectual and emotional growth*. Reading, MA: Perseus Books.

Greenspan, S., & Wieder, S. (2005). Can children with autism master the core deficits and become empathetic, creative and reflective? A ten to fifteen year follow-up of a subgroup of children with autism spectrum disorders (ASD) who received a comprehensive Developmental, Individual-Difference, Relationship-Based (DIR) approach. *Journal of Developmental and Learning Disorders, 9*, 39–61.

Greenspan, S., & Wieder, S. (2006). *Engaging autism: The Floortime approach to helping children relate, communicate, and think*. Cambridge, MA: DaCapo Press/Perseus Books.

Interdisciplinary Council on Developmental and Learning Disorders Clinical Practice Guidelines Workgroup, SIGC (2000). *Clinical practice guidelines: Redefining the standards of care for infants, children, and families with special needs*. Bethesda, MD: Interdisciplinary Council on Developmental and Learning Disorders.

Kasari, C., Freeman, S., & Paparella, T. (2006). Joint attention and symbolic play in young children with autism: A randomized controlled intervention study. *Journal of Child Psychology and Psychiatry, and Allied Disciplines, 47*, 611–620.

Klin, A., Volkmar, F., & Sparrow, S. (1992). Autistic social dysfunction: Some limitations of the theory of mind hypothesis. *Journal of Child Psychology and Psychiatry, and Allied Disciplines, 33*, 861–876.

Mahoney, G., & Perales, F (2005). Relationship-focused early intervention with children with pervasive developmental disorders and other disabilities: A comparative study. *Journal of Developmental and Behavioral Pediatrics, 26*, 77–85.

McGee, G., Krantz, P., & McClannahan, L. (1985). The facilitative effects of incidental teaching on preposition use by autistic children. *Journal of Applied Behavior Analysis, 18*, 17–31.

Minshew, N., & Goldstein, G. (2000). Autism as a disorder of complex information processing. In *ICDL clinical practice guidelines: Redefining the standards of care for infants, children, and families with special needs*. Bethesda, MD: The Interdisciplinary Council on developmental and Learning Disorders.

Minshew, N., Goldstein, D., & Siegel, D. (1997). Neuropsychologic functioning in autism: Profile of a complex information processing disorder. *Journal of the International Neuropsychological Society, 3*, 303–316.

Mundy, P., Sigman, M., & Kasari, C. (1990). A longitudinal study of joint attention and language development in autistic children. *Journal of Autism and Developmental Disorders, 20*, 115–128.

Ozonoff, S. (1997). Causal mechanisms of autism: Unifying perspectives from an information-processing framework. In D. Cohen & F. Volkmar (Eds.), *Handbook of autism and pervasive developmental disorders* (pp. 868–879). New York: John Wiley.

Pennington, J., & Ozonoff, S. (1996). Executive functions and developmental psychopathology. *Journal of the International Neuropsychological Society, 37*, 51–87.

Prizant, B., Wetherby, A., Rubin, E., & Laurent, A. (2003). The SCERTS Model: A transactional, family-centered approach to enhancing communication and socio-emotional abilities of children with autism spectrum disorder. *Infants, Young Children, 16*, 296–316.

Rogers, S., & DiLalla, D. (1991). A comparative study of the effects of a developmentally based instructional model on young children with autism and young children with other disorders of behavior and development. *Topics in Early Childhood Special Education, 11*, 29–47.

Rogers, S., Hall, T., Osaki, D., Reaven, J., & Herbison, J. (2000). The Denver model: A comprehensive, integrated educational approach to young children with autism and their families. In J. Handleman & S. Harris (Eds.), *Preschool education programs for children with autism* (2nd Ed) (pp. 95–133). Austin, TX: Pro-Ed.

Shahmoon-Shanok, R. (2000). The action is in the interaction: Clinical practice guidelines for work with parents of children with developmental disorders. In *ICDL clinical practice guidelines: Redefining the standards of care for infants, children, and families with special needs*. Bethesda, MD: The Interdisciplinary Council on developmental and Learning Disorders.

Shanker, S., & Greenspan, S. (2007). The developmental pathways leading to pattern-recognition, joint attention, language and cognition. *New Ideas in Psychology, 25*, 128–142.

Simpson, G., Colpe, L., & Greenspan, S. (2003). Measuring functional developmental delay in infants and young children: Prevalence rates from the NHIS-D. *Paediatric and Perinatal Epidemiology, 17*, 68–80.

Solomon, R., Necheles, J., Ferch, D., & Bruckman, D. (2007). Pilot study of a parent training program for young children with autism: The P.L.A.Y. Project Home Consultation model. *Autism: The International Journal of Research and Practice, 11*, 205–224.

Sparrow, S., Balla, D., & Cicchetti, D. (1984). *Vineland Adaptive Behavior Scales*. American Guidance Service.

Sperry, R. (1985). Consciousness, personal identity, and the divided brain. In F. Benson & E. Zaidel (Eds.), *The Dual Brain* (pp. 11–27). New York: Guilford.

Tannock, R., Girolametto, L., & Siegal, L. (1992). Language intervention with children who have developmental delays: Effects of an interactive approach. *American Journal of Mental Retardation, 97*, 145–160.

Wieder, S., & Greenspan, S. (2003). Climbing the symbolic ladder in the DIR model through floortime/interactive play. *Autism, 7*, 425–436.

Western Psychology Services (1988). *Childhood Autism Rating Scale (CARS)*. Los Angeles, CA.

Wetherby, A., & Prizant, B.(1993). Profiling communication and symbolic abilities in young children. *Journal of Childhood Common Disorder, 15*, 23–32.

Wetherby, A., & Prizant, B. (1995). Facilitating language and communication in autism: Assessment and intervention guidelines. In D. Berkell (Ed.), *Autism: Identification, education, and treatment* (pp. 107–133). Hillsdale, NJ: Erlbaum.

Williamson, G., & Anzalone, M. (1997). Sensory integration: A key component of the evaluation and treatment of young children with severe difficulties in relating and communicating. *Zero to Three, 17*, 29–36.

Zwaigenbaum, L., Bryson, S., Lord, C., Rogers, S., Carter, A., Carver, L., et al. (2009). Clinical assessment and management of toddlers with suspected autism spectrum disorder: Insights from studies of high-risk infants. *Pediatrics, 123*, 1383–1391.

61

Sally J. Rogers, Katherine S. Wallace

Intervention for Infants and Toddlers with Autism Spectrum Disorders

Points of Interest

- Current knowledge about infant–toddler treatments and their efficacy, both in ASDs and in other clinical groups.
- Characteristics of children in this age group that might respond most favorably to such treatment.
- Characteristics of treatments for this age group that have the greatest empirical support.

One of the most exciting areas of current autism science involves the search for infant behavioral markers of incipient autism. Prospective studies of high-risk infants have now identified several behavioral risk markers for autism spectrum disorders (ASDs) risk as early as age 12 months (Nadig et al., 2007; Ozonoff et al., 2008a; Zwaigenbaum et al., 2005). The most recently funded studies are homing in on the 6- to 9-month period, with optimism that predictive markers of risk will be identified before developmental delays and aberrant behavior patterns of social and communicative development take hold.

However, the primary purpose of early detection of ASDs is to prevent or mitigate the full onset of autism and its associated severe disabilities in multiple domains. Early detection science requires that early treatment science develop in parallel, so that tested treatments are ready for infants identified by early detection. As our ability to identify infants and toddlers with suspected or confirmed ASDs improves, the need for research on the efficacy of very early intervention or prevention approaches for autism becomes critical (Rogers, 2009). Although a variety of evidence-based interventions exist for preschoolers with autism (*see* Rogers & Vismara, 2008 for a recent review), it is not at all clear that such interventions would be equally beneficial, or even appropriate, for children under age 2 years. There is currently very little empirical research on efficacious treatments for children with autism who are 24 months and younger, although a number of intervention approaches for children in the 12- to 24-month range are currently being investigated.

Current Interventions in Autism Spectrum Disorders

Efficacious interventions have been identified for children with autism in the 2- to 5-year age range. In fact, well-structured, long-term interventions delivered in early childhood appear to be the most effective interventions that currently exist for decreasing the level of disability associated with ASDs (Lovaas, 1987; McEachin et al., 1993; *see* review in Rogers & Vismara, 2008). Current delivery of early intervention for ASDs tends to follow one of three main approaches. One involves the application of principles of applied behavior analysis (ABA) delivered 1:1 to increase target skills and decrease problem behaviors. ABA-based interventions may be delivered in a mass trial, didactic style of teaching, most often based on Discrete Trial Teaching (Lovaas, 2002), or they may be delivered in a more interactive, child-centered style focused especially on communication and behavior interventions, as typified by the work on Pivotal Response Training (PRT) (Koegel et al., 1999) and incidental teaching (McGee et al., 1999; Sundberg & Michael, 2001).

The second main approach—the developmental approach—applies the principles of developmental science and follows the sequences of typical child development. Developmentally based approaches focus great attention on communicative, cognitive, and social development and deliver interventions in a child-centered, interactive style that emphasizes the quality of the adult–child relationship and adult sensitivity and responsivity to children's cues. Developmental approaches have been tested and found to be beneficial in short-term controlled designs (Aldred et al., 2004; Drew et al., 2002; Mahoney & Perales, 2003, 2005). The most widely known interventions associated with a developmental approach include Social Communication, Emotional Regulation and Transactional Support (SCERTS; Prizant et al., 2006); Floortime (Greenspan et al., 1997); Relationship Development Intervention (RDI) (Gutstein, 2005); Early Start Denver Model (Rogers & Dawson, 2009); and Hanen (McConachie et al., 2005), although the empirical support for these approaches is limited at this time. Some approaches combine a developmental approach with teaching strategies that are based on ABA. These include Milieu Therapy (Warren et al., 2006; Yoder & Stone, 2006) and the Early Start Denver Model (Smith et al., 2006); both combine a developmental curriculum with play-based interactive teaching approaches that integrate teaching methods from ABA.

The third widely used approach is Treatment and Education of Autistic and Related Communication-handicapped Children (TEACCH; Schopler et al., 1995), and its principles of structured teaching are widely used in specialized preschool classrooms for children with ASDs, in the United States and in many other countries as well. The TEACCH approach follows a developmental curriculum that particularly emphasizes cognitive and adaptive development. What sets TEACCH apart is its emphasis on delivery in a very structured group environment, with visual and other environmental accommodations based on a neuropsychological model of autism that emphasizes difficulties with auditory processing and communication development, working memory, top-down control of attention, and altered sensory perception. The TEAACH approach differs from the above approaches with its emphasis on adapting the environment by providing external support to promote focused attention to learning tasks, development of independent work habits, and use of a variety of visual systems to organize one's activities and one's time.

Although there is some empirical evidence supporting all three of these approaches, the most well studied approach (*see* Rogers & Vismara, 2008, for a review of the evidence and the standards) is the Discrete Trial Teaching method described by Lovaas (1987). Several controlled trials by different investigators have demonstrated that groups of preschool-aged children receiving at least 20 hours a week of Lovaas's intervention, delivered 1:1 by highly trained and carefully supervised staff for a year or longer, make significantly greater gains in IQ—and sometimes in other areas as well—than do comparison groups of children. The evidence from that approach, however, involves children who are mostly ages 2 years to 4 years. There is no published evidence of this approach when used with children below age 2 years, other than one case study (Green et al., 2002).

To summarize, current practices in early intervention for preschoolers with ASDs include *(1)* traditional intensive behavioral intervention based on Discrete Trial Teaching; *(2)* developmental approaches that can also incorporate ABA teaching strategies but emphasize developmental science and the adult–child relationship; and *(3)* the TEACCH model involving structured teaching to maximize independent learning within a group context. Research has not yet addressed whether optimal outcomes are tied to a specific intervention type or to a specific number of hours of intervention. However, there is evidence that pretreatment child characteristics are the best predictors of outcome—particularly the child's level of language, IQ, social engagement, and degree of stereotypies (Sallows & Graupner, 2005; Sherer & Schreibman, 2005). The common elements across the various approaches with the best evidence suggest that the critical elements of treatments related to better outcomes include: the earliest possible start of intervention; delivery of interventions for 25 hours or more per week using 1:1 ratios; use of teaching strategies based on ABA; emphasis on language development, social development, play, imitation, and joint attention; and family involvement (National Research Council, 2001). To date, there have been no comparative effectiveness studies of early intervention in autism—a great need in the autism early intervention field.

Differences Between Preschool and Infant Learning

To what extent can the existing approaches for preschoolers with autism be directly applied to infants and toddlers under age 2 years? Although there is a strong temptation to take existing treatments and simply apply them to younger and younger children, there are compelling reasons for resisting. Research on child development has taught us that infants are qualitatively different learners than preschoolers in a number of ways (Kagan, 2008). Socially, the preschool period is a time to learn to interact with peers, to develop parallel and interactive play skills, to use language as a tool for social interaction, and to learn to participate in small groups of children. Preschoolers relate to parents as both play partners and as authority figures, and they are learning to respond to directions and interactions from unfamiliar adults. Preschoolers can play together without adult interaction for significant periods of time.

In contrast, infancy and toddlerhood is a period in which infants are developing secure attachments to consistent caregivers through dyadic exchanges (Belsky & Fearon, 2002; Bowlby, 1969; Sroufe et al., 1999). Communication between the partners is carried out largely via affective cues and nonverbal gestures (Bruner, 1977), and much of the baby's early communication is nonintentional and depends on adults' sensitive interpretation and responses for success. Infants ages 9 to 12 months and older are typically wary and avoidant of unfamiliar adults and interact freely only with familiar, responsive caregivers. Infants are in dyadic interaction with a caregiving adult through most of their waking hours, and a great deal of this interaction involves caretaking experiences —holding, feeding, changing, bathing, carrying, playing. Furthermore, this type of interaction occurs during a period of rapid brain development, and this kind of social engagement plays a key role in facilitating cortical specialization and the development of perception and representational systems for social and language development (Dawson, 2008). Significant deprivation of this type of interaction during the infant period has severe long-term effects on child development, as seen in a long line of studies on the effects of institutional care on infants, the latest of which involves infants from Romanian orphanages (Rutter, 1999).

Preschoolers have developed the capacity to understand that objects and actions can be used to represent other objects. They readily grasp that photos represent known people and things, that actions in play can represent other events, and that words represent things, people, feelings, thoughts, actions, and events. They have a sophisticated ability to learn by watching others via observational learning skills, even without opportunities to practice. They are acquiring the conventional symbol systems of their culture, and they use these symbols to establish shared reference to topics of conversation, play, and learning. Thus, although object manipulation is important for preschoolers' learning, objects are tied to symbols, and preschoolers move fluidly between objects and representations, as seen in their pretend play, interactions with books, conversations, and efforts to draw representationally.

Infants' relations with objects are quite different than preschoolers'. Infants learn through visual and motor experiences involving direct, hands-on experiences with objects. They do not easily grasp the relationship between actual objects and their visual representations through photos, drawing, and so forth (Zack et al., 2009). Although there is evidence of some mental representation in infancy, as seen in deferred imitation and memory (Meltzoff, 1988), infants do not use representational systems in their play or communication until later in the second year of life. They are instead constructing prototypes of actual objects, people, and events from their day-to-day experiences. Although infants appear capable of a few imitative acts early on (Meltzoff & Moore, 1977), they do not appear to learn new behaviors readily through observation of others until the second year of life, and even then, imitative learning occurs most easily for meaningful actions on objects, gestures, and words that are embedded in ongoing social activities and intentionally modeled by a social partner.

Interestingly, even repetitive behaviors occur differently in these two age periods. Repetitive motor behaviors are commonly seen in infants, and they are considered to have important roles in motor development and cognitive development (Piaget, 1966; Thelen, 1979, 1996). Among other things, repetitive motor behaviors provide the infant with experiences involving the effects of their acts on the environment, and they appear to involve a practice period for movement aspects of emerging motor skills. "These movements appear to be manifestations of inherent motor patterning characteristics of neuromuscular pathways at certain stages of maturation" (Thelen, 1981, p. 9), not functionally related but motorically related. These motor stereotypies tend to drop off toward the end of the first year of life as the infants gain intentional control of their bodies and action patterns.

A different type of repetitive behavior emerges in the preschool period: rituals and habits, seen as "just right" behaviors when distressed (Evans et al., 1999). These ritualized behaviors appear to help children cope with anxiety, and this relationship strengthens over the childhood period (Pietrefesa & Evans, 2007).

Zwaigenbaum and colleagues summarize these points well:

> "The social and learning characteristics of infants and toddlers contrast sharply with those of preschool-aged children, whose experience involves higher levels of autonomy, increased influence of peers, less contextualized learning and memory, and greater facility with symbolic thought and communication. Interventions that address the learning characteristics of infants and toddlers need to focus on natural learning environments and contexts, child initiative and sensory-motor exploration, and the development of nonverbal intentional communicative acts and reciprocal play with social partners." (Zwaigenbaum et al., in press)

Existing Studies of Infant–Toddler Autism Spectrum Disorder Interventions

Until recently, published intervention research for children with autism ages 24 months and younger was limited to descriptive studies (Green et al., 2002; McGee et al., 1999). There are now several published treatment studies of ASD for 2-year-olds using group designs with some type of comparison group. In contrast to the Lovaas model, none of these interventions have used the discrete trial teaching method. Instead, they use a more responsive and child-centered approach, and they focus on work with parents to follow children's leads, embed interventions into daily routines, and stimulate joint attention, imitation, and play (Aldred et al., 2004; Carter et al., in press; Drew et al., 2002; Green et al., 2010; Kasari et al., 2010; Landa et al., 2010; Mahoney & Perales, 2003, 2005; Oosterling et al., 2010). This change in approach fits well with current research findings emerging from the autism literature that demonstrate the impact of caregiver sensitivity and following children's leads in language development. Both longitudinal studies (Siller & Sigman, 2002) and treatment studies (Mahoney & Perales, 2003, 2005) have documented the specific contribution of this type of interaction on child gains, both short and long term. Let us turn to the published studies for infants and toddlers with ASDs.

The first set of studies published, mostly between 2002 and 2009, documented positive outcomes related to treatments. One of the first studies from this period was provided by Drew et al. (2002), who tested the effects of a home-based, parent-delivered developmental intervention in a pilot randomized controlled study involving 24 toddlers with autism (mean age: 23 months) who met full criteria for autistic disorder.

Children were assigned to an experimental parent training group or to a community services control group. The parents were trained during 3-hour home visits by a speech pathologist every 6 weeks in two main areas: the pragmatics of social communication and behavior management. The behavior management intervention involved using operant reinforcement approaches, interruption of unwanted behavior, and reinforcing alternative behaviors for promoting compliance during joint action interactions. The pragmatics interventions involved development of joint action routines involving books, mirrors, and toys and other objects within which the parents carried out explicit teaching of joint attention, play, imitation, turn taking, use of visual supports for communication, and stimulation of nonverbal gestural communication in their interactions with their children. Parents were to use the techniques daily in their home routines and also in joint play sessions with their children for 30 to 60 minutes daily in set-aside activities. After 12 months of treatment, significantly more children in the treated group developed speech (8 of 12) than in the comparison group (3 of 12), and the only children who acquired phrase speech during the year were in the treated group. There was also a trend toward significance for the treated group to understand more words. Unfortunately, however, the treated group had a significantly higher nonverbal IQ than controls at the start of the study (88 vs. 66), which may have contributed to their greater language gain. The treated group lost 11 IQ points on the nonverbal measure over the course of the treatment, whereas the IQ scores of controls remained stable. Thus, the evidence presented in this study provides some support for the efficacy of this intervention in fostering language development over a 12-month period. Furthermore, the study was replicated in another RCT by Aldred et al. (2004).

Mahoney and Perales (2003, 2005) published two outcome studies involving a group of children with ASDs, most of whom were 2 years or younger at the time of enrollment, in a relationship-based intervention called "Responsive teaching." The focus of the intervention is to increase parental responsivity to children's "pivotal developmental behaviors," which in this model include attention, persistence, interest, initiation, cooperation, joint attention, and affect. Parent–child dyads were provided with an hour per week of intervention for a year, although on the average, 32 hours were provided over the treatment year. The intervention focused on play-based interactions and natural routines. Parents were found to significantly increase responsiveness and positive affect after the intervention, with parents of children with ASDs showing more changes than a comparison group of parents of children with developmental delays without ASDs. Children with ASDs made greater progress in communication and cognitive abilities in the temperamental-behavioral domain than did a comparison group of children. Furthermore, child change was, in part, related to parental changes in responsiveness, supporting the conceptual model.

Wetherby and Woods (2006) reported on an intervention for 17 toddlers with a mean age of 18 months at the start of a parent-delivered intervention consisting of two home visits per week from a professional staff member and one parent–toddler play group per week. Individualized social-communication goals were established for each child, and parents were taught to incorporate interventions using naturalistic techniques into daily play and caretaking activities. Outcomes involved two analyses: pre–post comparisons without control for expected developmental changes, which yielded significant changes in virtually all social-communicative domains, and a comparison to a community group matched for age and diagnosis at outcome. Significant differences were found in number of words, gestures, and consonants in the treated group compared to the comparison group, but the methodological problems in the research design prevented assessment of any intervention-specific effects on children's development.

Finally, Dawson, Rogers, and colleagues conducted a randomized controlled trial of the Early Start Denver Model (ESDM; Rogers & Dawson, 2009) on 48 infants ages 18 to 30 months (Dawson et al., 2010). Children were randomly assigned to one of two groups: *(1)* the intervention group who received, on average, 25 hours of the ESDM weekly for 2 years, with an average of 15 hours per week delivered in the home by trained therapists and another 10 to 15 hours delivered by parents; *(2)* the community treatment group who received ongoing assessment and monitoring and standard community-based treatments. The ESDM is a developmental, relationship-based intervention approach that uses teaching techniques consistent with applied behavior analysis (ABA) to foster social-communicative, cognitive, and language gains in young children with autism and to reduce atypical behaviors associated with ASDs. The content of intervention for each child comes from assessment using the ESDM Curriculum Checklist (Rogers & Dawson, 2009). Adults delivering ESDM focus on behaviors involved in capturing and holding children's attention; fostering their motivation for social interaction through highly enjoyable routines; use of joint play activities as the medium for treatment; developing nonverbal and verbal communication, imitation, and joint attention; and the use of reciprocal, turn-taking exchanges inside joint activity routines to foster social learning. At 2 years after the baseline assessment, the ESDM group showed significantly improved developmental and adaptive behavior scores compared to the community treatment group, with language measures showing particularly large group differences. A significantly higher proportion of children in the ESDM group also showed changes in diagnostic classification involving milder autism symptoms compared to the community treatment group. The size of the group differences was favorably comparable to those coming from studies using the Lovaas model. However, as this is the initial study of this approach, independent replication is needed before one can assess the efficacy of this model—a statement that applies to all the studies above other than Mahoney and Perales' work.

Two additional randomized controlled studies just published deserve mention here. Kasari et al. (2010) conducted an RCT involving 38 families, half of whom carried out a specific joint attention intervention during 24 weeks of weekly treatment, and were followed up one year later. Those receiving the intervention demonstrated moderate to large differences compared to the wait-list condition on both measures of joint engagement and joint attention, and also on diversity of play skills, both at the end of treatment and at a one year follow-up point. Landa and colleagues (2010) carried out a randomized controlled trial with 50 toddlers examining the effects of an enhanced imitation, joint attention, and affect sharing intervention carried out within a group program over a six month period of time. The intervention resulted in significantly improved imitation skills in the experimental group which were maintained over a six month period.

However, in contrast to these positive findings, some important negative findings have also recently been published. All three involve parent implemented interventions and used very high quality designs, including randomized assignments and blind assessors, to examine intervention effects. The British PACT study by Green et al. (2010) examined the treatment previously tested in small trials by Drew (2002) and Aldred (2004). This large, multi-site RCT found no effect of the intervention on expressive or receptive language, or on ADOS scores, tested in the lab, nor in teacher ratings involving social communicative skills in the classroom. The only significant effect occurred in improved ratings in the treatment group involving ratings of parent synchrony and of child shared attention to parent (similar to the findings in the Kasari et al. [2010] study). Two other groups also failed to find effects on standardized testing of parent-implemented interventions compared to community treatment groups. Carter and colleagues (in press) found no overall group effect of the Hanen More than Words treatment, and they found an interaction of language ability with treatment outcomes, in which those children with more language skills at the start of Hanen intervention did less well than community controls, while those with minimal language at the start did better than community controls. Oosterling et al. (2010) conducted a Dutch study of parent-implemented intervention with sessions carried out across a year's time. This group found no differences in child skill level or parent skill level compared to community controls at the end of the study.

How do we reconcile these differences? Future research will help us, and a number of additional, large, well-controlled studies of parent implemented interventions for toddlers will be published soon. At this point, perhaps the most important take-home message is that the effect of early intervention for ASD is not a slam-dunk. Not all interventions make as much of a difference as they seem. Most children progress over time, including those with ASD, and progress seen during an intervention cannot be confidently attributed to the intervention unless there is a comparison group to model the effects of time and other experiences on skills. Children with autism progress, and some interventions lead to much more progress than expected. We will have to wait for the next round of studies to start to interpret what crucial ingredients of toddler interventions stimulate large effects on language, social development, and cognition. Soon, the field should have enough efficacy data for the extraction of key variables for effective intervention for toddlers with autism.

Prospective studies of infants who will develop autism have been invaluable in defining the earliest symptoms that appear in infants (*see* Rogers, 2009, for a recent review) and are now consistently documenting differences in children by age 12 months who will later develop autism (Landa & Garrett-Mayer, 2006; Ozonoff et al., 2008a; Ozonoff et al., 2008b ; Zwaigenbaum et al., 2005). The newest autism screening tools are also targeting the 12- to 14-month period (Resnick et al., 2007; Swinkels et al., 2006; Wetherby et al., 2008). Although many infants who will later develop autism do not show symptoms at 6 months (Zwaigenbaum et al., 2005), case studies have shown that some do, as described in a series of case studies by Bryson et al. (2007). The characteristics that appear in the 6- to 11-month period, described by Bryson and colleagues (2007), include unusual visual examination and fixations, unusual repetitive patterns of object exploration, delays in motor development, temperamental fussiness and difficulty with transitions, and, for infants closer to 12 months, decreases in eye contact, social initiative, joint attention, and emotion sharing, as well as a failure to respond to name.

Studies with long-term data indicate that only a subset, perhaps half, of infants who will develop ASDs are symptomatic in the first year. However, for the group that has symptoms by 12 months, the course of onset appears more rapid, and the degree of delay and atypicality more severe, than those infants whose onset is more prolonged and occurs later than 12 months, excluding those with frank regression (*see* review by Rogers, 2009). However, there is only one paper describing an intervention approach for infants at risk for ASDs in the 6- to 11-month range, and this is a single case study (Vismara & Rogers, 2008).

A long line of studies of the early phenotype of ASDs has clearly identified the key characteristics that differentiate autism in toddlerhood: imitation, joint attention, emotion sharing, language development, nonverbal gestural communication, and repetitive behaviors with objects (Lord, 1995; Rogers, 1998; Stone et al., 1997a; Stone et al., 1997b; Wetherby et al., 1998). These characteristics at age 12 months also predict autism in infant sibling studies (Landa & Garrett-Mayer, 2006; Zwaigenbaum et al., 2005), and this well-documented profile provides for intervention targets in the toddler period. However, before age 12 to 15 months, these skills are not part of a typical developmental repertoire, and interventions for the 6- to 11-month-old period will need to draw from both the symptom presentation of these infants and existing infant intervention literature from other disorders.

We recently conducted a thorough review of the infant intervention literature in other developmental disorders to extract main intervention principles (Wallace & Rogers, 2010). Because some of the symptoms that define autism at these early ages are also seen in infants and toddlers with other developmental and medical disorders (e.g., language delays, regulatory problems, repetitive behaviors), design of efficacious interventions for such symptoms in ASDs may be helped by reports of efficacious interventions for these symptoms in other groups in the 6- to 11-month period. It is to this literature that we now turn.

Effective Aspects of Infant Interventions in Other Groups

A variety of studies have examined effects of various interventions and caretaking strategies for both infants with developmental risk and those with typical development. We will review the most powerful variables isolated in these literatures.

Interventions for Infants with Developmental Risk or Disability

Thirty-four Level 1 or Level 2 studies (those involving the use of comparison groups or randomized control trials) (Nathan & Gorman (1998)) were identified that focused on infants and toddlers in the 0- to 3-year chronological age range and found positive effects of their interventions. The interventions involved infants with prematurity, Down syndrome (DS), or those at risk for intellectual disability (ID) resulting from ID in the mother and low socioeconomic status. Seven characteristics of the interventions appeared linked to better outcomes either through manipulations in the research design or through commonalities across those approaches that yielded improved outcomes in the experimental groups.

First, the majority of effective interventions involved **parent coaching**, including parental use of the interventions daily at home, therapist modeling of the intervention to the parent, and/or the provision of activities through the parent that matched the individual child's developmental profile. Parental use of specific developmental activities was a major component of the majority of these studies. In many (Ross, 1984, with very premature infants; Sanz et al., 1996, 2002, 2003, with Down Syndrome; and Sloper et al., 1986, with Down Syndrome), parents and infants had regular sessions with a therapist and then carried out specific activities at home daily between sessions. Even the two center-based studies involving infants at high risk for ID (Ramey & Campbell, 1984; Ramey & Smith, 1977) strongly involved parents via the use of frequent home visits. Furthermore, Sanz and colleagues (1996, 2003) experimentally demonstrated the superiority of therapist modeling and coaching of parents versus use of written materials for parents in supporting progress of infants with Down Syndrome on measures of motor, verbal, social adaptation, and social relationships.

A second feature affecting outcomes involves the **frequency and length of the intervention.** The majority of the effective studies involved weekly sessions in the clinic or at home across a substantial portion of the 0- to 3-year age range (Aronson & Fallstrom, 1977; Infant Health and Development Program [IHDP], 1990; Resnick et al., 1987; Sanz, 1996; Sanz Aparicio & Balana, 2002, 2003). In contrast, many ineffective interventions or those which had only short-lasting positive effects in the literature were short-term interventions that consisted of few or widely spaced contacts (e.g., Palmer et al., 1988; Piper & Pless, 1980).

Third, most of the effective interventions involved **individualized activities designed to meet the developmental needs of each child.** Many were based on a manualized curriculum and approach (*see* IHDP, 1990) that allowed for individualization of the parent activities and adjustments based on child progress (i.e., Response to Treatment [RTI]; Resnick et al., 1988; Sanz et al., 2002).

The fourth characteristic of the effective studies involves **beginning the interventions as early as possible** after diagnosis. Outcomes from these early delivered interventions were strong and long-lasting. Brooks-Gunn et al. (1992), for example, found long-term differences in several areas of development, including both verbal and nonverbal skills, in a very large network intervention study for premature infants. Sanz and colleagues (2002) experimentally demonstrated the benefit of earlier intervention for infants with DS involving greater gains in motor, verbal, social adaptation, and social relationships.

Fifth, several studies demonstrated the positive effects of interventions focused on **increasing parental sensitivity and responsivity to infant cues**, including following children's leads for decreasing infant fussiness and negative temperamental qualities (Seifer et al., 1992) and improving infant social competence (Barrera et al., 1990). Promoting First Relationships (Kelly & Barnard, 1999) is a well-articulated example of a relationship-focused parent education approach that focuses on dyadic relations and parental responsivity and sensitivity.

Sixth, many of the effective early interventions were **broad-based**, in that they focused on improving many areas of the child's functioning, such as language, motor skills, and self-help skills (Aronson & Fallstrom, 1977; Field et al., 1980; IHDP, 1990; Kelly & Barnard, 1999; Ramey, Mulvihill, & Ramey, 1997; Ramey & Smith, 1977; Resnick et al., 1987; Ross, 1984). Rather than narrowing in on one or two areas, these interventions took a broader approach to helping the child.

Finally, many effective interventions **offered parents support** above and beyond that provided via the intervention itself. For example, in many studies of effective interventions, parents were offered support in the form of group therapy, psychosocial therapy, or material assistance and case management. A great majority of these provided a forum wherein parents could freely express grief and frustration, as well as assisting with more practical, tangible concerns (Bidder, Bryant, & Gray, 1975; Connolly et al., 1980; Gianni et al., 2006; Greenberg, Calderon, & Kusche, 1984; IHDP, 1990; Olafsen et al., 2006; Resnick, Armstrong, & Carter, 1988; Resnick et al., 1987).

Data from Typical Infant Development Research

Further guidance comes from studies involving effects of caregiver variables on typical infant development, including research on parental affect, following children's leads, parental sensitivity, elaboration, scaffolding, and motherese.

Situation-appropriate and contingent parental affect is considered vital to infants' development of emotion regulation. Infants are unable to regulate their emotions independently and depend on parental interventions to help with regulation and to learn self-regulation. Nichols, Gergely, and Fonagy (2001) have described the process wherein infants come to elicit appropriate affective responses from caregivers. Human infants show an initial species-specific sensitivity and propensity to engage in affective interactions with their caregivers. As parents provide contingent appropriate facial and vocal affective reactions to infants' positive and negative emotional displays, infants come to develop an increased awareness of their own emotions. An important component of this affective reflection, according to the authors, is that parents reflect back to infants their own behavior at a pace and activity level that is in tune with their behavior.

Adults' following of the child's lead in play and language has been shown to contribute positively to many aspects of development, including language development. McCathren, Yoder, and Warren (1995) concluded that providing follow-in directives to children (i.e., following their lead in play and language) contributes positively to language development, while providing directives against the child's lead (i.e., redirectives) contributes negatively to some aspects of children's language development. The authors propose that follow-in directives contribute positively to children's language development because they maintain established joint attention episodes. They also report studies demonstrating that following a child's lead contributes positively to the development of joint attention, vocabulary, and verbal responses. Similarly, Rocissano, Slade, and Lynch (1987) discovered that toddler compliance and maintenance of joint attention episodes were more optimal during moments when parents followed their child's lead, rather than broke the engagement by providing asynchronous directives, for example. Thus, among both typically developing youngsters and children with developmental delays, following a child's lead in play activities can prove vital for the learning opportunities presented within an episode.

Similarly, caregiver sensitivity has been shown to be important to infant mood and affect, as well as maternal–infant attachment quality (Lohaus et al., 2004). Aspects of sensitivity include perception of infant cues, correct interpretation of such cues, prompting, and appropriate reaction. Additional related components include warmth and behavioral contingency. These factors are closely related to following a child's lead as they involve mothers adjusting their responses and behaviors to the needs of their children. Appropriateness of maternal sensitivity is a frequent intervention target for special needs populations, especially for mothers and infants born prematurely (e.g., Barrera, Doucet, & Kitching, 1990; Barrera, Rosenbaum, & Cunningham 1986; Rauh et al., 1988).

Being sensitive to children's cues and following their leads does not preclude parents from elaborating on their children's play and vocalizations. Appropriate elaboration techniques, including modeling and praising of novel vocalizations during play, is an important component of parental teaching of infants. Hursh and Sherman (1973) have found that appropriate modeling in the form of vocal elaboration and positive reinforcement increases children's vocalizations already in their repertoire, as well as increases usage of novel vocalizations. These techniques provide children with opportunities to acquire novel skills within child-directed, elaborated activities.

Deeply imbedded in successful parent–infant learning opportunities are episodes of scaffolding. According to Stevens et al. (1998), scaffolding consists of the adult controlling elements of a task that are initially beyond an infant's capacity. To scaffold successfully for their children, parents simplify the task, maintain attention and motivation, demonstrate, and mark critical features. As the infant's skills mature, the parent diminishes support. Research suggests that parental scaffolding positively affects infant development in a multitude of realms, including game learning (Hodapp, Goldfield, & Boyatzis, 1984), attention, and problem-solving (Findji, 1994).

A final caregiver variable that appears to have a positive effect on the language development of typical infants is the use of motherese. A way of speaking to infants with increased prosody, increased pitch, slowed production, exaggerated pitch contours, simplified vocabulary, and repetition, motherese is typically utilized with exaggerated positive affect by parents (Sokol et al., 2005; Weppelman et al., 2003). Infants appear to prefer listening to motherese, rather than to typical, adult-directed speech (Weppelman et al., 2003). The use of motherese thus serves to increase infants' attention to communication by making speech more interesting. In addition, the use of motherese appears to facilitate many language-learning tasks. Because in motherese focused words tend to be placed on pitch peaks and in salient positions, such as at sentence end, this type of speech may assist infants in learning salient words (Weppelman et al., 2003). Kemler Nelsen et al. (1989) have found that infants are sensitive to segment-marking cues in motherese but not in adult-directed speech. Motherese may also facilitate associative learning for nonlinguistic information and aid listeners in separating speech from background noise (Weppelman et al., 2003).

Guidelines for Infant–Toddler Treatment

To summarize, the literature from the few studies of infant–toddler ASD intervention and from both the clinical and the typical infant–toddler literature suggest that autism-specific interventions for infants and toddlers should focus on the importance of particular characteristics of the child's ongoing social environment and experiences. Sensitive caretaking, enriched language environments using responsive rather than directive interaction styles, environments that provide opportunities for infants to have an active role in their own learning, and interventions that are individualized and targeted to specific skills in infants and parents (rather than a more general support or service coordination model) appear to characterize efficacious infant/toddler interventions. Because infants at risk of autism are, first and foremost, developing infants, variables that positively affect infant outcomes in other groups of infants should also characterize interventions for infants at risk of autism until future empirical evidence indicates otherwise. The literature suggests that although interventions designed for older children with autism can certainly inform research and practice focused on infants and toddlers, existing efficacious models for preschoolers with autism should not be applied to infants and toddlers without significant adaptation.

Interventions are culturally determined and typically reflect the value system, philosophy, and practices of the originators. The intervention models described above have at their core a particular cultural style of interacting with infants and young children. However, cultures vary markedly in the ways that adults talk to and interact with children (Goldin-Meadow & Saltzman, 2000; Rabain-Jamin & Sabeau-Jouannet, 1997). Cross-cultural psychology stresses the importance of goodness of fit between culturally based interaction styles and value systems of those providing help and those seeking help.

Delivery of a specific treatment approach without considering the cultural appropriateness of the parent–child interactive style, expectations, and values of the approach and those of the family seeking help may limit or prevent its acquisition and use by parents and other family members (Dyches et al., 2004). Cultural fittedness includes both the language being used and the values and priorities being discussed with the family. Is the intervention being delivered in the dominant language of the family (Harry et al., 1995)? If this is not occurring, then one is virtually assured that the intervention is not culturally fitted to the family. However, the concepts of race and of socioeconomic status are often confused with the concept of culture. To understand families' cultural value systems and culturally defined behavioral and interaction patterns, both researchers and clinicians must be careful to discuss families' views and preferences directly rather than relying on assumptions based on physical features or demographic information (Brown & Rogers, 2003). Suggestions for this type of dialogue can be found in Mandell and Novak (2005). Expectations such as being videotaped, learning interventions within a parent group, coming to a clinic, or sharing family information with persons outside of the family's cultural group violate cultural norms for some groups and may be barriers for participation (Birkin et al., 2008). Even the core promise of early intervention—of treating a disability and possibly facilitating a different outcome than would have occurred without the intervention—is at odds with some families' needs to accept the child as he or she is (King et al., 2006) and other families' needs to be private about the child's differences (Dyches et al., 2004). It may also be at odds with cultural ideas involving the degree of control individuals have over life outcomes (Mandell & Novak, 2005). Clinician values concerning child outcomes involving autonomy in decision making, personal independence, and self-assertion may not be values shared by the family, and in the case of children with more severe disabilities, cultural clashes between parents and professionals may be particularly evident (Brown & Rogers, 2003). Assuring that intervention goals reflect family priorities, rather than clinician priorities, allows for important points of dialogue between families and interventionists.

Because infant–toddler intervention (and indeed, intervention for children of every age) is mediated via family interactions, it is necessary that interventionists work with families to actively assess and evaluate the aspects of a specific intervention approach that "fit" the family and those that do not. Doing so requires that the interventionists are aware of the cultural biases—habits, values, practices—in the intervention approach and that they are aware of their own cultural values and behaviors. Once the fit is evaluated and potential difficulties identified, the interventionist has the responsibility of either tailoring the chosen intervention approach to improve the fit or considering other approaches that might be a better fit. The assumption is that intervention approaches for infants and toddlers must be congruent with family lifestyle, interaction styles, values, and priorities to provide maximum benefit.

Adjusting particular aspects of interventions to accommodate cultural differences, however, presents its own set of problems, because changing the intervention means that the tested and manualized intervention is not what is being delivered, and in making the needed changes, one may, in fact, alter the variables that have led to its efficacy in clinical trials. There is no simple solution to this dilemma. At the individual level, ongoing tracking of children's progress and learning rate and of parental fidelity of delivery of the intervention will indicate when changes to the intervention plan and/or procedures need to be made to enhance child learning. On a larger scale, as intervention groups seek to adopt established interventions and apply them in cultures other than the one in which they were developed and tested, there arises a need for efficacy research to determine whether outcomes in the new culture mirror outcomes in the culture of origin. Finally, interventionists who are culturally fitting interventions to specific cultural needs of families or groups should write up the adaptations and provide them to others, so that practices develop that can then be tested.

Discussions of interventions for 6- to 11-month-olds need to be carried out within the context of public support for such interventions. Public laws pertaining to infant and toddler interventions differ from those pertaining to children ages 3 years and older. The legislation involving infant–toddler interventions appears to have been influenced by the research literature in a number of ways. Let us briefly review the specifications of public law as it pertains to infant interventions.

The Individual with Disabilities Education Act, Part C: Early Intervention for Infants and Toddlers with Disabilities

Infants' and toddlers' access to publically funded interventions was legislated most recently in the IDEA: Individuals with Disabilities Education Act, Part C: Early Intervention Program for Infants and Toddlers with Disabilities, Federal Register,

May 8, 2007 (Dept of Education, Office of Special Education and Rehabilitative Services [OSERS] 34CFR Part 303). The purpose of this act was to provide financial assistance to states that offer early intervention services to children under age 3 years who are at risk of developmental delays because of biological and environmental factors. Such funds were to be used only for services that a child needs but that are not paid for by other public or private sources (payor of last resort).

Several Requirements Were Placed on Service Providers, Summarized Below

1. Such services were to be multidisciplinary (two or more) and comprehensive and were to meet the developmental needs of the infant in cognition, communication, motor, social or emotional, and adaptive domains. Services were also to meet the needs of the family as they request for them to assist their infant's development.
2. The service delivery process must begin with an evaluation of child and family needs from two or more disciplines, either from the service team or from previous assessment. The evaluation is followed by the development of a written Individualized Family Service Plan (IFSP) in a meeting with the family, to be reviewed at least every 6 months. The IFSP must contain clear and measurable goals and outcomes for the intervention. It also defines the services to be delivered, which may include assistive technology, audiology, family training including counseling and home visits, health and medical services, occupational therapy, physical therapy, psychological services involving assessment, interpretation, and planning, service coordination, social work services, special instruction, speech and language pathology, transportation, and vision services. Other needed services can also be included if identified in the IFSP.
3. Families must consent to the plan before services are delivered, and once consent is obtained, all services consented to must be delivered. Progress is to be reviewed and plans modified as needed to achieve the stated goals during these meetings.
4. Child interventions are to be carried out in environments that would be natural for infants without a disability and include the home to the maximum extent possible.

Missing from IDEA is any description or requirement regarding the intensity or frequency of services to be delivered, which instead is left to the discretion of the agencies and/or IFSP team. As such, the delivery of services to infants and toddlers with autism can vary tremendously from one state to the next. Currently, in Sacramento, CA, a 24-month-old with ASD may receive as many as 35 hours per week of 1:1 intervention in his or her home and may also receive a session or two of individual speech/language therapy and occupational therapy per week. In other regions within the same state, services may consist of a 1-hour visit weekly by a professional, and a 1.5-hour play group with several toddlers and parents biweekly. Thus, publicly provided services vary tremendously for families, both within and across states. Many families pay out of pocket to fund services of appropriate intensity and content for their children. Out-of-pocket expenses can involve as many as $40,000 to $50,000 or more per year. Families sell their homes, use college savings funds, and incur great debt to purchase services for their children. Furthermore, service delivery typically requires the parent's presence and often parental transportation. One parent may need to end employment, thereby reducing family income, to support intervention for the child.

Thus, the current public service delivery systems addressing Part C requirements have as strengths a family-based model, an orientation that focuses on child development, child health needs, and family supports and involvement, interventions occurring in natural environments, and multidisciplinary teams. However, decisions about the nature and intensity of services for infants and toddlers at risk for ASD are entirely at the discretion of the public service agency and IFSP team delivering care. Without definition of appropriate services for infants and toddlers with ASD either through the public service system or in the empirical literature currently available, families and practitioners are left to make decisions in the absence of information. Given the increase in infants and toddlers being identified with autism risk, and the strong statements by the American Academy of Pediatrics and the American Academy of Neurology about the need for autism screening during the first two years of life, empirical information about treatment efficacy is badly needed (American Association of Pediatrics, 2003; Filipek et al., 2000).

Conclusion

Whereas research programs in infant screening and diagnosis of autism are moving rapidly forward, research programs in infant treatment of autism have only just begun. Although beginning trials assessing the efficacy of infant–toddler intervention have been conducted, the science is still at an early stage and we currently have no identified infant–toddler interventions that meet the criteria necessary to consider them empirically supported interventions. The current published literature is limited to case studies, uncontrolled studies, and a few controlled but as yet unreplicated findings. However, this is presently an active area of research, with a number of controlled studies in progress. Data is beginning to appear from these studies for 12- to 24-month olds. Interventions for even younger infants have only just begun.

Although we lack data from autism infant–toddler intervention studies to define the key ingredients of efficacious interventions, the intervention research from other infant and toddler groups provides some well-replicated findings, the consistency of which suggests that they should be incorporated into the design of intervention approaches for infants and toddlers with ASDs. These include: *(1)* focus on parent–infant interactions as a main delivery system for the intervention; *(2)* use of the infant's direct, active experience rather than computerized, pictorial, or video content as the basis for intervention; and *(3)* a style of interaction characterized by adult following of child's focus of attention and interests rather than directing infant attention as the vehicle for communication interventions. However, individual differences in terms of both infant and family characteristics, as well as a cultural perspective, need to be taken into consideration when developing or delivering manualized interventions, both for parents and for children.

In addition to the need for models, there is the need for measures to assess both autism risk and progress during infancy. The research on screening and assessment instruments for infants as young as age 12 months is currently in progress, and the search for valid autism risk markers below age 12 months is underway. We need both teaching curricula and measures of core constructs like joint attention, repetitive behavior, imitation, functional play, emotion sharing, and gesture use—the behavioral variables that define the autism phenotype in this period—that are psychometrically sound and simple and fast to administer and score, for clinical use. We currently rely on autism diagnostic instruments as measures of treatment-related change as well as diagnostic status; more sensitive instruments are needed if we are to measure intervention associated changes in infant and toddlers over the short term—necessary for evaluating treatment efficacy and making needed adjustments for individual children.

Finally, we need studies of well-articulated, manualized intervention approaches for 6- to 15-month-olds at risk of ASDs that detail the content of the intervention as well as the teaching procedures used to impart the intervention to parents and to children. Content needs to be clearly defined, assessment tools described or provided, and decision-making approaches detailed. Teaching procedures need to be described in detail, and measures for examining adherence to the model—treatment fidelity instruments—need to be provided. Fidelity measures need to address each set of interactions that deliver the intervention. How is the interventionist to impart the intervention to the parent? To the child? How is the parent to impart the intervention to the child? Each of these interactions delivers the intervention, and the intervention model should define these and then report the degree of adherence that occurred. Finally, these methods need to be scalable and exportable if they are going to address the needs of the many children who are now diagnosed with ASDs.

The promise of early intervention for enhancing the skills and lives of children with ASDs first appeared in 1987, and now, 24 years later, we have the opportunity to intervene as symptoms first appear. Based on what is known about infant learning and infant brain development, delivering interventions in infancy has maximal likelihood of optimized outcomes, of perhaps stopping autism in its tracks. Our capacity to deliver on this promise depends on the speed and quality of early identification science to highlight autism risk and early intervention science to guide treatment.

Challenges and Future Directions

To support infant intervention for ASD, future research agenda must focus on the following:

- Development of programs of research on infant intervention for ASD risk
- Development of treatment models that allow for individual differences among families
- Development of models that allow for cultural fittedness
- Development of psychometrically sound measures that assess autism risk
- Development of psychometrically sound measures to assess changes in core symptoms
- Development of efficacious manualized interventions for 6- to 15-month-olds with ASD symptoms.

SUGGESTED READINGS

Bruner, J. S. (1977). Early social interaction and language acquisition. In H. R. Schaffer (Ed.), *Studies in mother-infant interaction* (pp. 271–289). New York: Academic Press.

Kagan, J. (2008). In defense of qualitative changes in development. *Child Development, 79*, 1606–1624.

Kelly, J. F., & Barnard, K. E. (1999) Parent education within a relationship-focused model. *Topics in Early Childhood Special Education, 19*, 151–157.

McCathren, R. B., Yoder, P. J., & Warren, S. F. (1995). The role of directives in early language intervention. *Journal of Early Intervention, 19*(2), 91–101.

Siller, M., & Sigman, M. (2002). The behaviors of parents of children with autism predict the subsequent development of their children's communication. *Journal of Autism and Developmental Disorders, 32*, 77–89.

REFERENCES

Aldred, C., Green, J., & Adams, C. (2004). A new social communication intervention for children with autism: Pilot randomised controlled treatment study suggesting effectiveness. *Journal of Child Psychology and Psychiatry, 45*, 1–11.

American Association of Pediatrics. (2003). Practice Parameter: Screening and diagnosis of autism. Internet Communication.

Aronson, M., & Fallstrom, K. (1977). Immediate and long-term effects of developmental training in children with Down's syndrome. *Developmental Medicine and Child Neurology, 19*(4), 489–494.

Barrera, M. E., Doucet, D. A., & Kitching, K. J. (1990). Early home intervention and socio-emotional development of preterm infants. *Infant Mental Health Journal, 11*(2), 142–157.

Barrera, M. E., Rosenbaum, P. L., Cunningham, C. E. (1986). Early home intervention with low-birth-weight infants and their parents. *Child Development, 57*(1), 20–33.

Belsky, J., & Fearon, R. M. (2002). Infant-mother attachment security, contextual risk, and early development: A moderational analysis. *Development and Psychopathology, 14*, 293–310.

Bidder, R. T., Bryant, G., & Gray, O. P. (1975). Benefits to Down syndrome children through training their mothers. *Archives of Disease in Childhood, 50*, 383–386.

Birkin, C., Anderson, A., Seymour, F., & Moore, D. W. (2008). A parent-focused early intervention program for autism: Who gets access? *Journal of Intellectual and Developmental Disabilities, 33*, 108–116.

Bowlby, J. (1969). *Attachment and loss: Volume I, attachment.* New York: Basic Books.

Brooks-Gunn, J., Gross, R. T., Kraemer, H. C., Spiker, D., & Shapiro, S. (1992). Enhancing the cognitive outcomes of low birth weight, premature infants: For whom is the intervention most effective?, *Pediatrics, 89*, 1209–1215.

Brown, J. R., & Rogers, S. J. (2003). Cultural issues in autism. In S. Ozonoff, S. J. Rogers, & R. L. Hendren (Eds.), *Autism spectrum disorders: A research review for practitioners* (pp. 209–226). Washington, DC: American Psychiatric Publishing.

Bruner, J. S. (1977). Early social interaction and language acquisition. In H. R. Schaffer (Ed.), *Studies in mother-infant interaction* (pp. 271–289). New York: Academic Press.

Bryson, S. E., Zwaigenbaum, L., Brian, J., Roberts, W., Szatmari, P., Rombough, V., et al. (2007). A prospective case series of high-risk infants who developed autism. *Journal of Autism and Developmental Disorders, 37*(1), 12–24.

Carter, A., Stone, W., Messinger, D., Celimli, S., Nahmias, A., & Yoder, P. (in press). A randomized control trial of Hanen's "More Than Words" in toddlers with early autism. *Association for Child and Adolescent Mental Health.*

Connolly, B., Morgan, S., Russell, F. F., & Richardson, B. (1980). Early intervention with Down syndrome children: Follow-up report. *Physical Therapy, 60*(11), 1405–1408.

Coulter, L., & Gallagher, C. (2001). Evaluation of the Hanen Early Childhood Educators Programme. *International Journal of Language and Communication Disorders, 36*, 264–269.

Dawson, G. (2008). Early behavioral intervention, brain plasticity, and the prevention of autism spectrum disorder. *Development and Psychopathology, 20*, 775–803.

Dawson, G., Rogers, S., Munson, J., Smith, M., Winter, J., Greenson, J., et al. (2010). Randomized, controlled trial of an intervention for toddlers with autism: The Early Start Denver Model. *Pediatrics, 125*(1), e17–e23.

Drew, A., Baird, G., Baron-Cohen, S., Cox, A., Slonims, V., Wheelwright, S., et al. (2002). A pilot randomized control trial of a parent training intervention for pre-school children with autism: Preliminary findings and methodological challenges. *European Child and Adolescent Psychiatry, 11*, 266–272.

Dyches, T. T., Wilder, L. K., Sudweeks, R. R., Obiakor, F. E., & Algozzine, B. (2004). Multicultural issues in autism. *Journal of Autism and Developmental Disorders, 34*, 211–222.

Evans, D. W., Gray, F. L., & Leckman, J. F. (1999). The rituals, fears and phobias of young children: Insights from Development, Psychopathology and Neurobiology. *Child Psychiatry and Human Development, 29*, 261–276.

Field, T. M., Widmayer, S. M., Stringer, S., & Ignatoff, E. (1980). Teenage, lower-class, black mothers and their preterm infants: An intervention and developmental follow-up. *Child Development, 51*(2), 426–436.

Filipek, P. A., Accardo, P. J., Ashwal, S., Baranek, G. T., Cook, E. H., Jr., Dawson, G., et al. (2000). Practice parameter: Screening and diagnosis of autism: Report of the Quality Standards Subcommittee of the American Academy of Neurology and the Child Neurology Society. *Neurology, 55*, 468–479.

Findji, F. (1994). Attentional abilities and maternal scaffolding in the first year of life. *International Journal of Psychology, 28*(5), 681–692.

Gianni, M. L., Picciolini, O., Ravasi, M., Gardon, L., Vegni, C., Fumagalli, M., et al. (2006). The effects of an early developmental mother-child intervention program on neurodevelopment outcome in very low birth-weight infants: A pilot study. *Early Human Development, 82*(10), 691–695.

Goldin-Meadow, S., & Saltzman, J. (2000). The cultural bounds of maternal accomodation: How Chinese and American mothers communicate with deaf and hearing children. *Psychological Science, 11*, 307–314.

Green, G., Brennan, L. C., & Fein, D. (2002). Intensive behavioral treatment for a toddler at high risk for autism. *Behavior Modification, 26*, 69–103.

Green, J., Charman, T., McConachie, H., Aldred, C., Slonims, V., Howlin, P., et al. (2010). Parent-mediated communication-focused treatment in children with autism (PACT): A randomized controlled trial. *Lancet, 375*(9732), 2152–2160.

Greenberg, M. T., Calderon, R., & Kusche, C. (1984). Early intervention using simultaneous communication with deaf infants: The effect on communication development. *Child Development, 55*(2), 607–616.

Greenspan, S. I., Kalmanson, B., Shahmoon-Shanok, R., Wieder, S., Gordon-Williamson, G., & Anzalone, M. (1997). *Assessing and treating infants and young children with severe difficulties in relating and communicating.* Washington, DC: Zero to Three.

Gutstein, S. E. (2005). Relationship development intervention: Developing a treatment program to address the unique social and emotional deficits in autism spectrum disorders. *Autism Spectrum Quarterly*, Winter, 8–12.

Harry, B., Grenot-Scheyer, M., Smith-Lewis, M., et al. (1995). Developing culturally inclusive services for individuals with severe disabilities. *Journal of the Association for Persons with Severe Handicaps, 20*, 99–195.

Hodapp, R. M., Goldfield, E. C., & Boyatzis, C. J. (1984). The use and effectiveness of maternal scaffolding in mother-infant games. *Child Development, 55*(3), 772–781.

Hursh, D. E., & Sherman, J. A. (1973). The effects of parent-presented models and praise on the vocal behavior of their children. *Journal of Experimental Child Psychology, 15*(2), 328–329.

IHDP. (1990). Enhancing the outcomes of low-birth-weight, premature infants. *Journal of the American Medical Association, 263*(22), 3035–3042.

Kagan, J. (2008). In defense of qualitative changes in development. *Child Development, 79*, 1606–1624.

Kasari, C., Gulsrud, A. C., Wong, C., Kwon, S., & Locke, J. (2010). Randomized controlled caregiver mediated joint engagement intervention for toddlers with autism. *Journal of Autism and Developmental Disorders, 40*(9), 1045–1056.

Kelly, J. F. & Barnard, K. E. (1999). Parent education within a relationship-focused model. *Topics in Early Childhood Special Education, 19*, 151–157.

Kemler Nelson, D. G., Hirsh-Paske, K., Jusczyk, P. W., & Cassidy, K. W. (1989). How the prosodic cues in motherese might assist language learning. *Journal of Child Language, 16*(1), 55–68.

King, G. A., Zwaigenbaum, L., King, S., Baxter, D., Rosenbaum, P., & Bates, A. (2006). A qualitative investigation of changes in the belief systems of families of children with autism or Down syndrome. *Child: Care, Health, and Development, 32*, 352–369.

Koegel, L. K., Koegel, R. L., Harrower, J. K., & Carter, C. M. (1999). Pivotal response intervention 1: Overview of approach. *Journal of the Association for Persons with Severe Handicaps, 24*, 174–185.

Landa, R., & Garrett-Mayer, E. (2006). Development in infants with autism spectrum disorders: A prospective study. *Journal of Child Psychology and Psychiatry, 47*(6), 629–638.

Landa, R. J., Holman, K. C., O'Neill, A. H., & Stuart, E. A. (2010). Intervention targeting development of socially synchronous engagement in toddlers with autism spectrum disorder: A randomized controlled trial. *Journal of Child Psychology and Psychiatry, 52*(1), 13–21.

Lohaus, A., Keller, H., Ball, J., Voelker, S., & Elben, C. (2004). Maternal sensitivity in interactions with three- and 12-month-old infants: Stability, structural composition, and developmental consequences. *Infant and Child Development, 13*(3), 235–252.

Lord, C. (1995). Follow-up of two-year-olds referred for possible autism. *Journal of Child Psychology and Psychiatry, 36*, 1365–1382.

Lovaas, O. I. (1987). Behavioral treatment and normal educational and intellectual functioning in young autistic children. *Journal of Consulting and Clinical Psychology, 55*, 3–9.

Lovaas, O. I. (2002). *Teaching individuals with developmental delays: Basic intervention techniques*. Austin, TX: PRO-ED.

Mahoney, G., & Perales, F. (2003). Using relationship-focused intervention to enhance the social-emotional functioning of young children with autism spectrum disorders. *Topics in Early Childhood Special Education, 23*, 77–89.

Mahoney, G., & Perales, F. (2005). The impact of relationship focused intervention on young children with autism spectrum disorders: A comparative study. *Journal of Developmental and Behavioral Pediatrics, 26*, 77–85.

Mandell, D. S., & Novak, M. (2005). The role of culture in families' treatment decisions for children with autism spectrum disorders. *Mental Retardation and Developmental Disabilities, 11*, 110–115.

McCathren, R. B., Yoder, P. J., & Warren, S. F. (1995). The role of directives in early language intervention. *Journal of Early Intervention, 19*(2), 91–101.

McConachie, H., Randle, V., Hammal, D., & Le Couteur, A. (2005). A controlled trial of a training course for parents of children with suspected autism spectrum disorder. *Journal of Pediatrics, 147*, 335–340.

McEachin, J. J., Smith, T., & Lovaas, I. O. (1993). Long-term outcome for children with autism who received early intensive behavioral treatment. *American Journal of Mental Retardation, 97*, 359–372.

McGee, G. G., Morrier, M. J., & Daly T. (1999). An incidental teaching approach to early intervention for toddlers with autism. *Journal of the Association for Persons with Severe Handicaps, 24*, 133–146.

Meltzoff, A. (1988). Infant imitation and memory: Nine month olds in immediate and deferred tests. *Child Development, 59*, 217–225.

Meltzoff, A., & Moore, M. K. (1977). Imitation of facial and manual gestures by human neonates. *Science, 198*, 75–78.

Oosterling, I., Visser, J., Swinkels, S., Rommelse, N., Donders, R., Woudenberg, T., et al. (2010). Randomized controlled trial of the focus parent training for toddlers with autism: 1-year outcome. *Journal of Autism and Developmental Disorders, 40*(12), 1447–1458.

Nadig, A. S., Ozonoff, S., Young, G. S., Rozga, A., Sigman, M., & Rogers, S. J. (2007). A prospective study of response-to-name in infants at risk of autism. *Archives of Pediatrics and Adolescent Medicine, 161*, 378–383.

Nathan, P. E., & Gorman, J. (1998). *A guide to treatments that work*. New York: Oxford University Press.

National Research Council. (2001). *Educating children with autism*. Washington, DC: National Academy Press.

Nichols, K., Gergely, G., & Fonagy, P. (2001). Experimental protocols for investigating relationships among mother-infant interaction, affect regulation, physiological markers of stress responsiveness, and attachment. *Bulletin of the Menninger Clinic, 65*, 371–379.

Office of Special Education and Rehabilitative Services, Department of Education. (2004). *Individuals with Disabilities Education Act, 34 CFR Part 303*. Washington, DC.

Olafsen, K. S., Ronning, J. A., Kaaresen, P. I., Ulvund, S. E., Handegard, B. H., & Dahl, L. B. (2006). Joint attention in term and preterm infants at 12 months corrected age: The significance of gender and intervention based on a randomized controlled trial. *Infant Behavior and Development, 29*(4), 554–563.

Ozonoff, S., Macari, S., Young, G. S., Goldring, S., Thompson, M., & Rogers, S. J. (2008a). Atypical object exploration at 12 months of age is associated with autism in a prospective sample. *Autism, 12*, 457–472.

Ozonoff, S., Young, G. S., Goldring, S., Greiss-Hess, L., Herrera, A. M., Steele, J., et al. (2008b). Gross motor development, movement abnormalities, and early identification of autism. *Journal of Autism and Development Disorders, 38*, 644–656.

Palmer, F. B., Shapiro, B. K., Wachtel, R. C., Allen, M. C., Hiller, J. E., Harryman, S. E., et al. (1988). The effects of physical therapy on cerebral palsy. A controlled trial in infants with spastic diplegia. *New England Journal of Medicine, 318*(13), 803–808.

Piaget, J. (1966). *Psychology of intelligence*. Totowa, NJ: Littlefield, Adams, & Co.

Pietrefesa, A. S., & Evans, D. W. (2007). Affective and neuropsychological correlates of children's rituals and compulsive-like behaviors: Continuities and discontinuities with obsessive–compulsive disorder. *Brain and Cognition, 65*, 36–46.

Piper, M. C., & Pless, I. B. (1980). Early intervention for infants with Down Syndrome: A controlled trial. *Pediatrics, 65*(3), 463–468.

Prizant, B. M., Wetherby, A. M., Rubin, E., Laurent, A. C., & Rydell, P. J. (2006). *The SCERTS Model: A comprehensive educational approach for children with autism spectrum disorders*. Baltimore: Paul H. Brookes.

Rabain-Jamin, J., & Sabeau-Jouannet, E. (1997). Maternal speech to 4-month-old infants in two cultures: Wolof and French. *International Journal of Behavioral Development, 20*, 425–451.

Ramey, C. T., & Campbell, F. A. (1984). Preventive education for high-risk children: Cognitive consequences of the Carolina Abecedarian Project. *American Journal of Mental Deficiency, 88*(5), 515–523.

Ramey, C. T., Mulvihill, B. A., & Ramey, S. L. (1997). Prevention: Social and educational factors and early intervention. In J. W. Jacobson and J. A. Mulick (Eds.), *Manual of diagnosis and professional practice in mental retardation* (pp. 215–227). Washington DC: American Psychological Association.

Ramey, C. T., & Smith, B. (1977). Assessing the intellectual consequences of early intervention with high-risk infants. *American Journal of Mental Deficiency, 81*, 319–324.

Rauh, V. A., Achenbach, T. M., Nurcombe, B., Howell, C. T., & Teti, D. M. (1988). Minimizing adverse effects of low birthweight: Four-year results of an early intervention program. *Child Development, 59*(3), 544–553.

Resnick, M. B., Armstrong, S., & Carter, R. L. (1988). Developmental intervention program for high-risk premature infants: Effects on development and parent- infant interactions. *Journal of Developmental and Behavioral Pediatrics, 9*(2), 73–78.

Resnick, J. S., Baranek, G. T., Reavis, S., Watson, L. R., & Crais, E. R. (2007). A parent-report instrument for identifying one-year-olds at risk for an eventual diagnosis of autism: The First Year Inventory. *Journal of Autism and Developmental Disorders, 37*(9), 1691–1710.

Resnick, M. B., Eyler, F. D., Nelson, R. M., Eitzman, D. V., & Bucciarelli, R. L. (1987). Developmental intervention for low birth weight infants: Improved early developmental outcome. *Pediatrics, 80*, 68–74.

Rocissano, L., Slade, A., & Lynch, V. (1987). Dyadic synchrony and toddler compliance. *Developmental Psychology, 23*(5), 698–704.

Rogers, S. J. (1998). Neuropsychology of autism in young children and its implications for early intervention. *Mental Retardation and Developmental Disabilities Research Reviews, 4*, 104–112.

Rogers, S. J., & Dawson, G. (2009). *Early Start Denver Model for young children with autism: Promoting language, learning, and engagement.* New York: Guilford.

Rogers, S. J., & Vismara, L. A. (2008). Evidence-based comprehensive treatments for early autism. *Journal of Clinical Child and Adolescent Psychology, 37*, 8–38.

Rogers, S. J., Estes, A., Lord, C., Young, G. S., Vismara, L., Winters, J. et al. (in preparation). Parent implementation of the Early Start Denver Model for one year olds with ASD : A randomized controlled study.

Rogers, S. J. (2009). What are infant siblings teaching us about autism in infancy? *Autism Research, 2*(3), 125–137.

Ross, G. S. (1984). Home intervention for premature infants of low-income families. *American Journal of Orthopsychiatry, 54*(2), 263–270.

Rutter, M. , Andersen-Wood, L., Beckett, C., Bredenkamp, D., Castle, J., Groothues, C. et al. (1999). Quasi-autistic patterns following severe early global privation. *Journal of Child Psychology and Psychiatry, 40*, 537–549.

Sallows, G. O., & Graupner, T. D. (2005). Intensive behavioral treatment for children with autism: Four-year outcome and predictors. *American Journal of Mental Retardation, 110*, 417–438.

Sanz Aparicio, M. T., & Balana, J. M. (2002). Early language stimulation of Down's syndrome babies: A study on the optimum age to begin. *Early Child Development and Care, 176*, 651–656.

Sanz Aparicio, M. T., & Balana, J. M. (2003). Social early stimulation of trisomy-21 babies. *Early Child Development and Care, 173*(5), 557–561.

Sanz, M. T., & Menendez, J. (1996). A study of the effect of age of onset of treatment on the observed development of Down Syndrome babies. *Early Child Development and Care, 118*, 93–101.

Schopler, E., Mesibov, G. B., & Hearsey, K. A. (1995). Structured teaching in the TEACCH system. In E.Schopler & G. B. Mesibov (Eds.), *Learning and cognition in autism* (pp. 243–268). New York: Plenum Press.

Seifer, R., Sameroff, A. J., Anagnostopolou, R., & Elias, P. K. (1992). Mother-infant interaction during the first year: Effects of situation, maternal mental illness, and demographic factors. *Infant Behavior and Development, 15*(4), 405–426.

Sherer, M. R., & Schreibman, L. (2005). Individual behavioral profiles and predictors of treatment effectiveness for children with autism. *Journal of Consulting and Clinical Psychology, 73*, 1–14.

Siller, M., & Sigman, M. (2002). The behaviors of parents of children with autism predict the subsequent development of their children's communication. *Journal of Autism and Developmental Disorders, 32*, 77–89.

Sloper, P., Glenn, S. M., & Cunningham, C.C. (1986). The effect of intensity of training on sensori-motor development in infants with Down's Syndrome. *Journal of Intellectual Disability Research, 30*(2), 149–162.

Smith, C. M., Rogers, S. J., & Dawson, G. (2006). The Early Start Denver Model: A comprehensive early intervention approach for toddlers with autism. In J.S. Handleman & S. L. Harris (Eds.), *Preschool education programs for children with autism: Third edition.* Austin, TX: Pro-Ed.

Sokol, R. I., Webster, K. L., Thompson, N. S., & Stevens, D. A. (2005). Whining as mother-directed speech. *Infant and Child Development, 14*(5), 478–490.

Sroufe, L. A., Carlson, E. A., Levy, A. K., & Egeland, B. (1999). Implications of attachment theory for developmental psychopathology. *Development and Psychopathology, 11*, 1–13.

Stevens, E., Blake, J., Vitale, G., & Macdonald, S. (1998). Mother-infant object involvement at 9 and 15 months: Relation to infant cognition and early vocabulary. *First Language, 18*(53), 203–222.

Stone, W. L., Ousley, O. Y., & Littleford, C. D. (1997a). Motor imitation in young children with autism: What's the object?. *Journal of Abnormal Child Psychology, 25*, 475–485.

Stone, W. L., Ousley, O. Y., Yoder, P. J., Hogan, K. L., & Hepburn, S. L. (1997b). Nonverbal communication in two and three-year-old children with autism. *Journal of Autism and Developmental Disorders, 27*, 677–696.

Sundberg, M. L., & Michael, J. (2001). The benefits of Skinner's analysis of verbal behavior for children with autism. *Behavior Modification, 25*, 698–724.

Swinkels, S. H. N., Dietz, C., van Daalen, E., Kerkhof, I., van Engeland, H., & Buitelaar, J. K. (2006). Screening for autistic spectrum in children aged 14 to 15 months. I: The development of the Early Screening of Autistic Traits Questionnaire (ESAT). *Journal of Autism and Developmental Disorders, 37*, 723–732.

Thelen, E. (1979). Rhythmical stereotypies in normal human infants. *Animal Behaviour, 27*, 699–715.

Thelen, E. (1981). Kicking, rocking, and waving: Contextual analysis of rhythymical stereotypies in normal human infants. *Animal Behavior, 29*, 3–11.

Thelen, E. (1996). Normal infant stereotypes: A dynamic systems approach. In R. L. Sprague & K. M. Newell (Eds.), *Stereotyped movements: Brain and behavior relationships* (pp. 139–166). Washington, DC: American Psychological Association.

Vismara, L. A., & Rogers, S. J. (2008). The Early Start Denver Model: A case study of an innovative practice. *Journal of Early Intervention, 31*(1), 91–108.

Wallace, K. S., & Rogers, S. J. (2010). Intervening in infancy: implications for autism spectrum disorders. *Journal of Child Psychology and Psychiatry, 51*(12), 1300–1320.

Warren S., Bredin-Oja, S., Fairchild, M., Finestack, L. H., Fey, M. E., & Brady, N. C. (2006). Responsivity education/prelinguistic milieu teaching. In R. McCauley & M. Fey (Eds.),

Treatment of language disorders in children (pp. 47–77). Baltimore: Brookes.

Weppelman, T. L., Bostow, A., Schiffer, R., Elbert-Perez, E., & Newman, R. S. (2003). Children's use of the prosodic characteristics of infant-directed speech. *Language and Communication, 23*(1), 63–80.

Wetherby, A. M., Brosnan-Maddox, S., Peace, V., & Newton, L. (2008). Validation of the Infant-Toddler Checklist as a broadband screener for autism spectrum disorders from 9 to 24 months of age. *Autism, 12*, 487–511.

Wetherby, A. M., Prizant, B. M., & Hutchinson, T. A. (1998). Communicative, social/affective, and symbolic profiles of young children with autism and pervasive developmental disorders. *American Journal of Speech-Language Pathology, 7*, 79–91.

Wetherby, A. M., & Woods, J. J. (2006). Early Social Interaction Project for children with autism spectrum disorders beginning in the second year of life: A preliminary study. *Topics in Early Childhood Special Education, 26*, 67–82.

Yoder, P., & Stone, W. L. (2006). Randomized comparison of two communication interventions for preschoolers with autism spectrum disorders. *Journal of Consulting and Clinical Psychology, 74*, 426–435.

Zack, E., Barr, R., Gerhardstein, P., Dickerson, K., & Melttzoff, A. N. (2009). Infant imitation from television using novel touch screen technology. *British Journal of Developmental Psychology, 27*, 13–26.

Zwaigenbaum, L., Bryson, S., Rogers, T., Roberts, W., Brian, J., & Szatmari, P. (2005). Behavioral manifestations of autism in the first year of life. *International Journal of Developmental Neuroscience, 23*, 143–152.

Zwaigenbaum, L., Bryson, S., Lord, C., Rogers, S., et al (in press). Insights from the study of high-risk infants. *Journal of Pediatrics.*

62 Lynn Kern Koegel, Rosy M. Fredeen, Robert L. Koegel, C. Enjey Lin

Relationships, Independence, and Communication in Autism and Asperger's Disorder

Points of Interest

- Motivation
- Social Interaction
- Psychological Health
- Initiations
- Communication
- Pivotal Response Treatment
- Behavioral Intervention
- Outcomes
- Generalization

Linguistic aptitude and communicative competence are critical to healthy relationships, gainful employment, and independence in adulthood. For individuals with autism spectrum disorders (ASDs), these are core deficits; therefore effective treatment in these areas is essential for positive long-term outcomes (Alpern & Zager, 2007; Howlin, Mawhood, & Rutter, 2000; Koegel et al., 1999; Koegel & LaZebnik, 2009). A lack of communicative competency can lead to significant problems, including a decreased number of social relationships (Howlin, 2000; Jobe & White, 2007; Orsmund, Krauss, & Seltzer, 2004), increased feelings of loneliness (Howlin, 2000; Jobe & White, 2007; Jennes-Coussens, Magill-Evans, & Koning, 2006; Jones & Meldal, 2001), social isolation and withdrawal, and poorer quality of friendships, (Strain & Schwartz, 2001; Bauminger & Kasari, 2000; Stewart et al., 2006). In fact, although individuals with ASDs may experience a range of comorbid conditions (Gadow DeVincent, Pomeroy, Azizian, 2004; Green et al., 2000; Klin et al., 2005; Meyer et al., 2006; Tantam, 2000), depression and anxiety disorders appear to be the most prevalent (Matson & Nebel-Schwalm, 2007; Ghaziuddin, Ghaziuddin, & Greden, 2002; Gillott & Standen, 2007; Shtayermman, 2007; Sterling et al., 2008; Tsakanikos et al., 2007). Therefore, it seems that social factors may play an important role, as individuals who lack adequate social communication have been found to be five times more likely to develop a comorbid diagnosis of depression in adulthood (Stewart et al., 2006). This interplay between ASD-related deficits and comorbid features has been linked to disruptions in underlying brain development (Amaral, Schumann, & Nordahl, 2008; Geschwind & Levitt, 2007), adding to the complexity of ensuring successful outcomes in this population. Therefore, given evidence that deficits in social and communicative competence can contribute to poorer psychological health, these factors appear to a play a pivotal role for later outcome and intervention.

Although a failure to develop age-appropriate peer relationships is a primary diagnostic criterion of autism and Asperger's Syndrome (American Psychological Association, 2000), research suggests that contrary to beliefs that people with ASDs prefer to be alone, most have a desire for meaningful friendships and romantic relationships (Jobe & White, 2007; Jones & Meldal, 2001; Jennes-Coussens et al., 2006; Howlin, 2000). When examining the broader autism phenotype, regardless of the desire for social relationships, the degree of ASD symptoms has been significantly correlated with a fewer number of and shorter duration of friendships (Jobe & White, 2007). This has significant implications given that depression is frequently related to loneliness and impacted by lack of successful social communication skills (cf., Howlin, 2000).

Despite evidence indicating that individuals with autism and Asperger's Syndrome desire both casual and intimate social relationships, and the association between dissatisfactory social relationships and comorbid conditions, there is an unfortunate paucity of research addressing this area. Outcome studies are particularly lacking. A review of the literature suggests that only a minority of individuals on the spectrum, even with a diagnosis of autism and few support needs or Asperger's Syndrome, achieve any remote semblance of integration into what most people would consider to be a desired lifestyle in adulthood (Alpern & Zager, 2007; Cederlund et al., 2008;

Howlin et al., 2004; Larson, Doljanac, & Lakin, 2005; Muller et al., 2003; Seltzer et al., 2004).

Specifically, in a summary of the literature, Howlin (2000) reported that only 16% to 50% of individuals with ASDs were living semi-independently, whereas 5% to 55% held paid work positions. Perhaps most tragically, despite their desire for meaningful romantic relationships, only up to 14.3% of adults on the spectrum were married. In contrast, almost 95% of typical adults are employed (U. S. Department of Labor, 2008), and 70% of adults are married (U. S. Census Bureau, 2006). More recently, Seltzer et al. (2003) corroborated these trends based on a study in which data were collected on ASD symptom patterns exhibited by 405 adolescents and adults. Similarly, Orsmund et al. (2004) assessed the peer relationships and social activities of 235 adolescents and adults with autism. They documented that only a small percentage of participants had relationships that met the ADI-R criteria for friendship, which was defined as a "same-aged friend with whom varied, mutually responsive and reciprocal activities were engaged in outside of organized settings" (p. 250).

It is important to emphasize that although individuals with ASDs continue to face long-term needs and challenges (Alpern & Zager, 2007; Howlin, 2000), the above findings should motivate, and serve as a base for, research in these areas. If anything has been learned from research conducted with this population over the past four decades, it is that very little is permanently unchangeable. The purpose of this chapter is to discuss research findings, best practices, and future directions that are necessary to move toward these goals. Because comprehensive socio-communication interventions need to begin early, this chapter will discuss interventions for early childhood that may be of particular importance to achieving long-term positive outcomes.

Defining and Measuring Communication

It is important to begin by discussing a few issues that complicate research in the area of communication. One area relates to the accurate nomenclature of communication and communicative acts. In particular, numerous definitions have been employed to describe a hallmark of social communication—namely, spontaneous (as compared to prompted) communication. Although researchers have emphasized the importance of spontaneous communication, particularly among children on the spectrum, definitions of "spontaneous" greatly differ, resulting in confusion and lack of consistency in terminology across the language literature (Chiang & Carter, 2008). Clear and uniform definitions are necessary for the identification and conceptual understanding of spontaneous language, given evidence that spontaneous communication is significantly related to independence and reduced need for support (Carter & Grunsell, 2001; Sigafoos & Reichle, 1993). Additionally, given that individuals on the spectrum may be highly prompt-dependent, defining exactly what constitutes spontaneity is challenging.

Furthermore, Carter and Hotchkis (2002) point out there exists in the literature two conceptually opposing views of spontaneous language—binary and continuum. A binary conceptualization of spontaneous communication refers to an "all-or-none" phenomenon (i.e., either the behavior is spontaneous or not; Chiang & Carter, 2008, p. 695), with numerous studies in the literature employing this model (Charlop & Trasowech, 1991; Koegel, O'Dell, & Koegel, 1987; Krantz & McClannahan, 1993).

However, while some studies view spontaneity as binary (Carter & Hotchkis, 2002; Chiang & Carter, 2007), most would agree that the degree of spontaneity an individual exhibits is multifaceted and may be associated with both the conversational partner and environmental cues. These findings have led to support for a tiered or continuum model of defining spontaneity. Halle (1987) argues that communication is always cued by environmental antecedents; therefore, a conceptualization that takes into account the potential influence of these controlling stimuli may be necessary to understand and describe spontaneous communication. Further complications for describing spontaneous language arise when taking into account the possible impact of state events (e.g., hunger, thirst, etc.) on spontaneous language. In addition, delayed echolalia can arguably be viewed as evidence for spontaneous language, even though it may be inappropriate and associated with previous antecedent cues. It seems, therefore, that a variety of important considerations are necessary when reporting results of spontaneous language across communication intervention programs. Factors such as the degree to which the natural cues in the environment trigger communication, the presence and level of influence of natural cues drawing the speaker's attention (Carter & Hotchkis, 2002), the type of speech acts the individual initiates (Koegel, Carter, & Koegel, 2003), and the association between spontaneous utterances within the existing social setting are extremely important variables. Moreover, these considerations should be clearly defined in research articles.

Vocal imitation within a communicative context is a common strategy for typical language learners but occurs at a significantly lower rate in children with autism (cf. Knott, Lewis, & Williams, 2007). In contrast, echolalic utterances, which may or may not have communicative intent, are common among individuals with ASDs. Given that some individuals exhibit high levels of echolalia, it may be important to assess whether it is being used in appropriate contexts and whether it is functional in any way. This is important given evidence that different types of echolalia exist (e.g., delayed and immediate) and may serve a variety of communicative functions (Wetherby & Prizant, 1987). Carefully defining echolalic or imitative utterances as a communication tool, assessing the appropriate or inappropriate spontaneous use of these utterances and considering the possibility of echolalia as a language learning strategy among individuals with ASD should be carefully analyzed for consistency across the literature.

Finally, although communication is relatively easy to measure in clinical and controlled settings, it is more challenging in natural settings—particularly in the context of intimate relationships, such as friendships and dating. Research exploring these issues and interventions to target socialization is warranted given that untreated, these deficits can lead to a large array of problems, including lack of intimate relationships and successful employment (Howlin, 2000). As children with ASDs mature and as more individuals are fully included in educational and community settings, social validation of interventions and feedback regarding intimate relationships require the continued development of effective monitoring and measurement systems in the context of natural settings.

In general, the above issues have led to a shift from interventions provided in isolated contexts to teaching functional communication and pragmatics in relevant social contexts (Stone & Caro-Martinez, 1990), but the bulk of the studies have focused on younger children. Future research on defining and measuring social communication in natural contexts, as well as intervention procedures to help individuals develop long-term social relationships, attain meaningful employment, and address mental health issues, is urgently needed across various developmental stages. The remainder of this chapter discusses empirically validated procedures for improving language and social communication. Although not exhaustively, we will discuss various interventions for individuals with high to low support needs and their applicability for different age ranges.

Communication and Typical Development

Researchers have long discussed the necessity of using typical development as benchmarks for ASD intervention. This principle makes especially good sense when it comes to communication. The typical development of communication is one of the most vastly researched areas in human development, providing the perfect context by which communicative needs of ASDs can be evaluated (Tager-Flusberg, Paul, & Lord, 2005).

Given the seemingly quick pace of communicative development in typically developing individuals, it is not a surprise that many parents find themselves in awe of their child's ability to acquire such important skills (Paul, 2008). From the very beginning, typically developing children are communicators. Stark (1979) identified five stages of infant vocalizations. The first 2 months of life are comprised of reflexive cries and vegetative sounds, whereas the second through fifth months consist of cooing and laughing vocalizations. Paul (2008) discusses the emergence of cooing and laughing as important for the development of communication because these behaviors primarily occur in response to social interactions, setting the stage for the inextricably social nature of communication.

Between 4 and 8 months of age, infants appear to engage in purposeful vocal play and this stage is marked by the beginning of babbling (Stark, 1979). Simple babbling then quickly develops into reduplicated babbling (e.g., bababa) between age 6 and 9 months (Stark, 1979). The ways in which babies use their babbling to both initiate and respond to back-and-forth interactions with adults has been described by some as "proto-conversations" (Bateson, 1975). In fact, researchers who have examined these proto-conversations have found that they are marked by turn-taking and reciprocity, components of advanced conversations seen in later development (Locke, 1995; McTear, 1985; Paul, 2008). The period between 9 and 18 months is marked by jargon babbling, and it is during this time that joint attention emerges (Bakeman & Adamson, 1984) and first words become consistent (Bates, 1979; Linder, 1993; Stark, 1979). Despite a relatively small vocabulary during this period, toddlers are by no means passive communicators. On the contrary, they are active social communicators (Paul, 2008), as evidenced by their use of pointing, holding out objects, and/or gesturing to initiate social communicative interactions (McLaughlin, 1998).

By around age 15 months, typical children have a receptive vocabulary of an average of 50 words. This period is followed by an ever-increasing expressive vocabulary, with the average 18-month-old toddler using approximately 50 to 100 words. Communication then seems to "explode" with children developing expressive and receptive use of hundreds of words by their second birthday (Fenson et al., 1993; Paul, 2008). As if this "explosion" in vocabulary were not impressive enough, this period is also marked by growth in the quality of communication. That is, young children's communicative acts, both initiations and responses, begin to serve a variety of functions including requesting, protesting, commenting, calling attention to oneself, greetings, and question-asking (Bates, 1979; Linder, 1993; Wetherby et al., 1988). The development of question-asking is especially noteworthy because it marks the first time that children use communication to direct their own learning (Fredeen & Koegel, 2006; Halliday, 1975; Meyer & Shane, 1973).

Children's communication skills continue to develop dramatically during the preschool years as they begin to expand the length and complexity of their utterances to develop conversational skills. For example, children ages 2 to 3 years can initiate a subject of conversation and take a few turns in exchanging information and details (McTear, 1985). Although lacking in sophistication, children between ages 5 and 6 years have developed discourse skills that resemble those of adults (Cook-Gumprez & Kyratzis, 2001; Fredeen & Koegel, 2006). In fact, by the time children reach adolescence, their conversations are fast-paced and remarkably complex (e.g., contain abstract topics, idioms, metaphors; Brinton, Robinson, & Fujiki, 2004). Although there are obvious differences between the communication skills of toddlers, preschoolers, adolescents, and adults, there is also an undeniable commonality of an inherent social function (Landa, 2008). Furthermore, social ability impacts communicative outcomes (Bono, Daley, & Sigman, 2004); thus, these early benchmarks provide guidance in working with the ASD population.

Communication, Socialization, and Diagnostic Criteria for Autism Spectrum Disorders

As Landa (2007) notes, "communication is a broad concept, encompassing linguistic, paralinguistic, and pragmatic aspects of functioning" (p. 16). Each of these domains consists of a variety of components. For example, the domain of linguistics comprises elements such as phonology, morphology, syntax, and semantics, whereas the paralinguistic domain includes components such as proxemics, intonation, and gestures. Finally, the pragmatic domain consists of a variety of elements related to discourse management. Interestingly, Landa further discusses how diagnostic criteria for autism related to socialization is inherently intertwined with symptoms manifested in the communication domain. That is, despite separate symptom categories, "some of the criteria specified for social impairment are intimately involved in the pragmatic aspects of communication" (p. 17), including the nonverbal lack of sharing interest and spontaneous enjoyment or the lack of social or emotional reciprocity (American Psychiatric Association, 2000; Landa, 2007). It is not surprising that without intervention in pragmatic areas, even adolescents and adults with fewer support needs continue to have difficulty with overall social communication (Alpern & Zager, 2007). For example, Brinton and colleagues (2004) discuss how conversations of typically developing adolescents include many social elements that require individuals to be able to take the perspectives of others. In the past, such skills seem to have been achieved by relatively few individuals with ASDs, often resulting in unintentional miscommunications and misunderstandings (Alpern & Zager, 2007; Hurbutt & Chalmers, 2004). These findings underscore that future interventions need to be designed to incorporate the natural social factor of communication.

In sum, Paul (2008) captures the essence of communicative development when she states that it is a dynamic process between the person and their social environment. This notion seems especially true for designing and assessing interventions for individuals with ASDs. As such, the remainder of this chapter will focus on discussing interventions designed to improve not just communicative functions but also the overall social communicative well-being of individuals with ASDs.

History of Intervention and Pivotal Response Teaching

The first scientifically documented effective interventions for instating first words and improving language use in children with autism were conducted in the 1960s (Ferster & DeMyer, 1961; Hewitt, 1965; Lovaas et al., 1966). These interventions were based on the principles of operant conditioning (Newsom & Rincover, 1998) and were implemented in highly structured settings that focused on teaching the child with autism to imitate first sounds or syllables, then several sounds or syllable reduplication, which subsequently focused on the semantic meaning of words (Landa, 2007; cf. Lovaas, 1987). These early studies resulted in a teaching method commonly known as Traditional Discrete Trial Training and/or Early Intensive Behavioral Intervention (Landa, 2007; Smith, 2001). In the original Applied Behavior Analysis (ABA) studies, as with the more current standard Discrete Trial models, communication was taught serially using drills in mass trials that were implemented in the context of stimulus-response-consequence chains, using arbitrary rewards (e.g., edibles and social praise), and often these rewards were not related to the child's specific behavioral response. Generally, intervention was implemented in a clinical room, free from distracting stimuli with the adult maintaining tight control over interactions, selecting stimuli/materials, and initiating instruction (Landa, 2007). Although effective for initial acquisition of speech for a large portion of children (Lovaas, 1987), generalization and spontaneity were considerable problems. Thus, a great deal of subsequent research focused on strategies promoting generalization, spontaneity, and maintenance of newly learned behaviors (Koegel & Koegel, 2006).

Using these original studies as a basis, researchers expanded upon these procedures to produce a more efficient intervention (Koegel & Koegel, 2006), resulting in what is now commonly referred to as "Contemporary ABA Approaches" or "Naturalistic Behavioral Interventions" (Landa, 2007; Koegel et al., 2008). Unlike more traditional models, contemporary or naturalistic behavioral approaches modify the principles of standard Discrete Trial Teaching so that instruction is centered on the child's interests and incorporated into meaningful daily routines. A variety of teaching methods fall under this category of contemporary/naturalistic ABA, including Incidental Teaching (McGee, Morrier, & Daly, 1999), Milieu Teaching (Warren & Bambara, 1989), and Pivotal Response Teaching (PRT; Koegel & Koegel, 2006). As a whole, the above-mentioned teaching methods are not only based on the scientific procedures of applied behavioral analysis but also incorporate elements of developmental and pragmatic approaches (Landa, 2007).

Researchers examining the limitations of the original Traditional Discrete Trial studies found that spontaneous and generalized improvements in first words and language were greater if intrinsic motivational components were incorporated into the intervention. That is, when motivational components were included in the intervention, children's rate of responsivity and correct responses improved, thereby creating a more efficient treatment approach. Furthermore, several individual components have been documented to be effective, such as providing child choice of stimulus materials or topics (Koegel, Dyer, & Bell, 1987), reinforcing communicative attempts (Koegel, O'Dell, & Dunlap, 1988), using task variation, incorporating maintenance tasks (Dunlap, 1984), and providing direct and natural rewards (Koegel, Egel, &

Williams, 1980; Koegel & Williams, 1980). When combined as a package, these variables were comparatively more effective in incurring change than the traditional Discrete Trial approach (Koegel, O'Dell, & Koegel, 1987). Initially the use of these intrinsic, motivational procedures were coined *The Natural Language Paradigm* (NLP) because they closely resembled the manner in which typical children were taught to use language in their natural environments. Incidental teaching approaches are similar to the NLP/PRT paradigm in that they rely on arranging the natural environment to attract children to desired activities and materials. The approach involves waiting for the child to initiate the teaching process, using this initiation to prompt communication, and then providing the item, activity, or topic contingent upon the child's response (McGee et al., 1983; McGee, Krantz, & McClannahan, 1985; McGee & Morrier, 2003). Such teaching strategies have changed the framework of traditional teaching models. Learning conditions using natural consequences have not only been documented to result in less avoidance and escape-motivated behavior (Koegel, Koegel, & Surratt, 1992) but have been shown to lead to increased improvements in the children's interest, happiness, and engagement (Dunlap, 1984) relative to approaches involving drilling children and then providing verbal praise or potentially unrelated small edibles.

The motivational strategies originally focused on language development, but since then they have been extended and shown to be effective across other areas, such as academics (Dunlap, Kern, & Worcester, 2001), speech intelligibility (Koegel et al., 1998), peer socialization (Harper, Simon, & Frea, 2008), joint attention (Bruinsma, Koegel, & Koegel, 2004; Vismara & Lyons, 2007), and socio-dramatic play (Thorp, Stahmer, & Schreibman, 2005). Additionally the procedures have been effective with improving communication in adults (LeBlanc et al., 2007). As a whole, rather than targeting individual behaviors one-by-one, procedures that focused on the core pivotal area of motivation resulted in widespread changes in a variety of other untargeted areas. Consequently, the core targeted areas were identified as "pivotal" in the learning process and thus the term *PRT* was coined (Koegel & Koegel, 2006).

In addition to improvements in the acquisition of first words and language, the benefits of PRT intervention included evidence that children demonstrated far lower levels of escape and avoidance-based disruptive behaviors when motivational procedures were incorporated (Koegel, Koegel, & Surratt, 1992). Simply put, when these motivational and naturalistic procedures were implemented, there were dramatic widespread positive improvements in the children's symptomology in a variety of areas including behavior, communication, and overall affect.

With an understanding of the historical trajectory of educating individuals with ASDs, the subsequent sections of this chapter will identify areas in communication requiring intervention and how those areas interact with an individual's ability to build relationships and independence.

Intervention

Initiations

The effectiveness of motivational procedures in teaching first words and language to children with autism has resulted in significantly more children learning to talk. In fact, although earlier procedures resulted in about only 50% of the children becoming verbal (Lord & Paul, 1997; Prizant, 1983), as many as 80% to 95% of the children become verbal when motivational procedures are incorporated at an early age (Koegel, 2000; Koegel & Koegel, 1995; McGee et al., 1999). However, in much of the literature, the use of highly desired items primarily has been used for teaching requests. Undeniably, requests are critical in communication, but many children with autism remain limited in the variation of their communicative functions (Wetherby et al., 1988). That is, language samples show that children with autism use their communication primarily, or exclusively, for requests and protests (Wetherby & Prutting, 1984). This lack of variety and restricted use of communication functions, coupled with the lack of spontaneity, and infrequent expressive communication in natural settings (Hauck et al., 1995), results in children getting very little practice with meaningful communication. Compounding these issues are findings that children with autism develop very few, if any, social initiations that have the function of information-seeking or curiosity. This varies considerably from typical language learners who demonstrate queries and initiations within their first lexicon (Owens, 2008). For example, prior to age 18 months, typical language learners generally use "that?" (first produced as an approximation, such as/da/?) as a prompt for parents to label items (Meyer & Shane, 1973). The intentions of these early verbalizations are both social and initiative, requesting a response from the communicative partner (Owens, 2008). Furthermore, these verbalizations are generally accompanied by nonverbal gestures such as eye contact, joint attention, and pointing (McLaughlin, 1998).

A number of researchers have undertaken the goal of teaching initiations to children on the spectrum to encourage the variety of language functions and to teach self-initiated strategies that the children can use to gain linguistic information and seek social interaction (Koegel et al., 2008). Early studies on initiations focused on teaching deictic questions to individuals with autism. In particular, teaching "wh-" questions has been of interest to researchers. Not only do many children on the spectrum fail to use questions at all, the small percentage of children who do often use them incorrectly and, specifically, not as requests for information (Hurtig, Ensrud, & Tomblin, 1982). In an early attempt to systematically teach question-asking, Hung (1977) taught children with autism to ask "What is ___ for?" and "What is/are _____ doing?" Assessments for generalization of the question outside of the clinic setting indicated that the questions could be programmed to occur if reinforcement was provided, but without reinforcement, the children did not demonstrate use of the questions for the purpose of "curiosity" or information seeking. In another study, Taylor and Harris (1995) taught question-asking to elementary school children with autism using picture cards. To assess generalization, new unknown items were placed around the school and the children were taken on walks and stopped at the new items. The children generalized question-asking without verbal prompting; however, the act of stopping may have functioned as a nonverbal prompt. Another study (Koegel et al., 1998) focused on producing spontaneous use of question-asking by incorporating motivational items into the intervention. Specifically, the researchers began with highly desired items, placed them in an opaque bag, and prompted the children to ask "What's that?" Following the query, the children were provided with a highly desired item from the bag. Gradually and systematically, the items were faded and replaced with unfamiliar items the child did not label at baseline. Following the intervention, the children demonstrated generalization of question-asking across settings, people, and to novel items. Additional questions, such as "Where is it?" and "Whose is it?", were taught with a similar methodology using desired items and generalization of these questions was also observed (Koegel & Koegel, 2006). Finally, the use of verbs and verb conjugations was improved by teaching children with autism to ask "What's happening?" and "What happened?" during storybook activities (Koegel, Carter, & Koegel, 2003). In a longitudinal study, children who used, or were taught to use, these types of communicative initiations had better long-term outcomes and were perceived to appear more developmentally appropriate on normalcy scale ratings than adolescents and young adults with autism who did not use these self-initiated queries (Koegel et al., 1999).

Along with responding to peer initiations, initiations have also been taught in the context of play, such as approaching a peer or commenting on a joint activity. In one study, Pierce and Schreibman (1995) explored the use of peer-mediated strategies to increase social behaviors in children with autism. In particular, these authors taught typically developing peers how to use the motivational procedures of PRT with classmates diagnosed with autism. They found that not only were the typically developing peers able to successfully use the PRT procedures, but the students with autism exhibited generalized gains in both maintaining and initiating social interactions. Shabani et al. (2002) also attempted to increase verbal initiations in children with autism toward their typically developing peers during free-play episodes. They found that prior to intervention, although the children with autism responded to questions and initiations from adults, they seldom initiated communication with their peers. By using a tactile prompting device (i.e., vibrating pager), all the participating children increased their frequency of communicative initiations with their peers. Unfortunately, once the prompting device was faded, only one participant demonstrated maintained improvements in initiations. In a more recent study, Licciardello, Harchik, and Luiselli (2008) used preteaching, prompting, and rewards to encourage children with autism to initiate with their peers. Specifically, prior to play periods, the children were provided with instructions, demonstrations, and behavioral rehearsal. Then, they were provided with child-choice to select both the activity and the play partner. The children briefly practiced the play initiation prior to each play session, and during the play periods, the children were verbally prompted if more than a minute elapsed without any play initiations. In addition, the children were praised and provided with rewards for appropriate play. The intervention resulted in the children demonstrating increases in both social initiations and within their natural free-play settings with their aides. However, no generalization or maintenance data were collected.

As a whole, these studies highlight the importance of child initiations. The positive long-term outcomes of children who initiate suggest that all children on the spectrum should have social verbal initiations as an integral part of their communication goals. Further, the improvements in socialization associated with interventions explicitly targeting initiations suggest that child initiations may function as another pivotal area for intervention based on evidence for widespread positive effects on other untreated areas.

Peer Interactions

School settings are ideal environments for social interventions because peers are abundant. However, research suggests that even with IEP social communication goals, children with autism rarely interact with their peers (Koegel et al., 2001). In fact, the most common communicative functions of children with autism in school settings appear to be requests, attention-seeking, and engaging in social routines; however, even these limited functions occur very infrequently, ranging from three to four times per hour (Stone & Caro-Martinez, 1990). Even more alarming are data collected in naturalistic settings, suggesting that teachers elicit expressive communication only an average of once per hour, despite recommendations that communication be elicited at a high rate (Chiang, 2008). Lack of communication opportunities has significant implications for children on the spectrum who will likely benefit from frequent and repeated practice (Hwang & Hughes, 2000).

Despite the fact that most children receive little intervention for socialization at school, a number of studies have described effective interventions with peers. For example, integrated play groups in which an adult monitors play initiations, provides scaffolding, structures the play, provides support when needed, and guides social communication can be helpful in promoting social interaction (Wolfberg & Schuler, 1999). Peer-buddy dyads in which children are taught to "stay with, play with, and talk to" a buddy have been shown to be effective in increasing appropriate social skills such as asking for objects, getting the attention of another child, turn-taking, and improving eye contact, even in the absence of an adult interventionist (Laushey & Heflin, 2000). Social skills training with peers can also be incorporated into academic learning tasks. For example, Kamps et al. (1999) conducted peer tutoring sessions in which academic tasks were provided in the context of group learning, wherein the children learned to share ideas, correct each other's work, give praise, react calmly, provide encouragement, and help others. The procedures resulted in improved academic engagement and attention, as well as significantly higher levels of social engagement for the students with autism as well as their peers.

PRT (described above) also has been taught to typically developing peers in the context of full-inclusion classrooms (Harper et al., 2008). Specifically, triads consisting of two typically developing children successfully learned to implement the intervention during recess with a child with autism. Another study using PRT technique that included getting the child with autism's attention, varying the activities, narrating play, reinforcing attempts, and turn-taking were taught in school settings. These procedures, along with providing the typical peers with cue cards to take on the playground, resulted in improving both the amount of social play between the peers and the number of social initiations exhibited by the classmate with autism (Pierce & Schreibman, 1997).

Fortunately, minimal effort for staff training in these strategies can produce large changes in peer behavior and, subsequently, the child on the spectrum. As little as a few hours of training regarding friendships and specific procedures for working with the child with autism and Asperger's Syndrome has been shown to greatly increase the number of peer initiations and the child with autism's interactions with peers (Owen-DeSchryver et al., 2008).

Priming

Priming involves previewing or practicing activities before they are presented. Research in the area of academics has shown that if activities are presented to the child the evening before they are introduced in class, children with autism engage in significantly lower levels of disruptive behavior and much higher levels of academic engagement and performance (Koegel et al., 2003; Wilde, Koegel, & Koegel, 1992). Although priming was originally developed for improving academics, the effectiveness of this strategy has also been demonstrated in social areas. For example, Zanolli, Daggett, and Adams (1996) taught preschool children with autism to request toys, show items, and use requests to see another child's item. Three 5-minute priming sessions were implemented per week for 6 to 12 weeks with 10 to 14 trials provided during each session. The procedure was conducted first with dyads, then later with the whole class, and eventually faded. Priming resulted in increased play initiations by the child with autism toward typical peers, with as many as six different initiation topographies, including novel behaviors (e.g., saying the peer's name, smiling, and saying "I want that"). However, the authors indicated that generalization to new activities did not occur. Thus, more research assessing whether multiple exemplars or implementation of priming in more contexts would result in durable, widespread gains is warranted. Yet this initial work underscored that priming is effective in increasing social initiations and can be conducted within the context of peer dyads as well as with an entire classroom.

Moreover, in another study, Sawyer et al. (2005) showed that priming, in the form of verbal instruction, was effective when used as a component of an intervention package. The package included prompting and rewards for targeted verbal comments and physical sharing in an integrated preschool classroom. The study demonstrated that with a package intervention that incorporated priming, preschoolers could learn to share and request to share toys with their peers.

In an adaptation of the original priming procedures, Schreibman, Whalen, and Stahmer (2000) used short, 1- to 4-minute video clips to prime children with autism who demonstrated disruptive behavior during transitions into community settings. The tapes did not show models engaging in the transition but simply successfully entering the community setting that was problematic for the child with autism. Results indicated that the procedure was effective with maintenance and some generalization observed across activities.

More recently, Gengoux (2007) used priming to increase the verbal initiations of children with autism during play episodes in natural settings with their typically developing peers. This study used short, low-demand practice sessions during which the child with autism practiced a preferred play activity before it was introduced at the child's full-inclusion setting. The study showed that although all of the participants exhibited low levels of initiations toward peers prior to the study, with priming, children on the spectrum significantly increased their rates to levels comparable to that of their typical peers.

Priming techniques are particularly promising as they do not require the interventions to be implemented in the setting where the problem behaviors are occurring. That is, if individuals engage in disruptive or asocial behavior, they may develop a negative history with peers or other community members that can reduce their likelihood of being welcomed into that environment. Furthermore, for older individuals and adults on the spectrum, this procedure has the advantage of decreasing stigmatization that may occur when an interventionist is present and intervening in natural settings. Overall, such antecedent interventions decrease the possibility of these potential adverse consequences by programming the positive behavior to occur *a priori.*

Incorporating Ritualistic Themes and Using Perseverative Interests

Many individuals with autism (particularly those with fewer support needs) and Asperger's Syndrome demonstrate circumscribed interests. In fact, it appears to be the norm rather than the exception, with 75% of younger children and 88% of older children on the spectrum engaging in circumscribed interests (Klin et al., 2007). The interests usually focus around memorization of facts and can greatly interfere with everyday activities and socialization (Klin et al., 2007). One successful area of intervention research has focused on incorporating these highly motivational individual topics or themes into socially appropriate games. For example, Baker, Koegel, and Koegel (1998) selected children who showed little to no social interaction with their peers at lunch recess and exhibited areas of extreme restricted and repetitive interests. The children were taught a socially appropriate game using these perseverative interests by developing them into themes of an activity that could only be played with a group of children (e.g., one child who was highly interested in maps and knew all his states was taught to play a variation of tag on a large outline of a U.S. map that was painted on his playground). These activities increased the social interactions of the children with autism, and generalization across other activities following the implementation of intervention. Also the intervention capitalized on the child with autism's interests and areas of knowledge such that the child was eventually perceived as a highly valued member of the peer group.

In a related study, Baker (2000) showed that the procedure was also effective for increasing socialization between children with autism and their typically developing siblings. The intervention resulted in the generalization and maintenance of socialization between the siblings, joint attention, and improved affect. Interestingly, although the ritualistic behaviors were used as the basis of the social game, no increases in the frequency of the ritualistic behaviors were noted during other times of the day. Thus, these findings underscore that incorporating circumscribed interests into intervention may be especially promising given that there appears to be a collateral gain in the improvement of other untargeted pro-social behaviors. These additional gains are important given that even among young nonverbal children or children with limited language, joint attention increased in these circumstances (Vismara & Lyons, 2007). Since joint attention is a precursor to the onset of verbal communication (Mundy & Crowson, 1997; Toth et al., 2006), is social in nature, and is often limited or absent in children with autism interventions that have the collateral effect of improving untreated behaviors, such as joint attention, are especially worthy of study (Bruinsma, 2005; Vismara, 2006).

Clubs

A number of studies have recruited a group of typically developing students to support students with autism in their natural environments. In the 1980s, the Circle of Friends (CoF) program was developed for individuals who were moving from institutions into community settings but eventually was adapted for use in mainstream school settings (Haring & Breen, 1992). The procedure involves enlisting a group of classmates during a classwide meeting and then setting up a "circle" of friends who help provide support for a child with special needs. The group also sets up, monitors, and reviews weekly targets in regular meetings that are facilitated by an adult (Frederickson, Warren, & Turner, 2005). One persistent issue that has arisen in these short-term programs and clubs is the lack of generalization and maintenance over time (Frederickson, Warren, & Turner, 2005). However, some have suggested that simultaneously targeting peers *and* the child on the spectrum may create more durable improvements in socialization (Kamps et al., 1992). In another study, Talebi (2008) formed lunch clubs at school based around the individualized interests of adolescents on the spectrum. These motivational activities resulted in improved social engagement, higher levels of social initiations, and generalization of these gains at later times and across other contexts. Thus, it appears that the most effective programs involving groups of children consist of targeting both typically developing peers and children on the spectrum, building on activities that will be mutually motivating to the child on the spectrum and the peers, and are conducted over a long period of time. The continued use of interventions involving groups of peers appears vital, given evidence that long-term generalization in the absence of clubs or "circles" has been elusive.

Video Modeling

Relatively recently, researchers have begun to incorporate video modeling technology in social interventions. Video modeling requires participants to watch videotaped demonstrations of a target behavior being performed (Charlop & Milstein, 1989) or videotaped segments of themselves (Falk, Dunlap, & Kern, 1996). The goal of these interventions is to teach individuals to either imitate the behaviors they observe or receive feedback on their own behavior. Video modeling may be especially effective among individuals with autism who have particular difficulty with picking up social cues in the complex, everyday environment. Specifically, video modeling may help the individual with autism identify who to imitate and what behaviors to model within specific contexts, as the clips can provide clear and appropriate frames of reference (McCoy & Hermansen, 2007). The success of video modeling interventions for children with ASDs may be attributed to their strengths in visual processing skills. Other benefits include the increased capability to gain a participant's attention while minimizing irrelevant features, thereby reducing the likelihood of problems associated with overselectivity (Bellini & Akullian, 2007).

In fact, video modeling interventions have been shown to be effective in teaching individuals on the spectrum a variety of social skills, including social initiations, play, perspective taking, compliment-giving, and conversational skills. For example, one study by Nikopoulos & Keenan (2004) examined the effects of video modeling on social initiations and play behaviors in three children with autism. Participants viewed a videotape of a typically developing peer and an experimenter engaged in social interactive play. After watching these clips, the participants were observed during a play session. Results showed that both social interactions and reciprocal play skills improved, and the effects were maintained even after a 3-month follow-up period. Another study by LeBlanc et al. (2003) used video modeling and reinforcement to teach perspective-taking skills to three children with ASDs. The children viewed a video of an adult successfully completing two target tasks that included an explanation of why the model's behavior was correct. After viewing the video, each participant was asked perspective-taking questions until the participant provided three consecutive correct responses. At baseline, all children failed the tasks; however, video modeling with reinforcement was associated with all three children mastering the tasks and two of the three children generalizing these behaviors to other similarly related tasks.

An additional benefit of video modeling is that it may also be time- and cost-efficient, especially in comparison to in vivo modeling. A study by Charlop-Christy, Le, and Freeman (2000) compared the effectiveness of video modeling versus in vivo modeling for teaching social, communication, and daily living skills to five children (ages 7–11 years) with autism ASDs. The study used adult models performing various tasks at an exaggeratedly slow pace, either live or on video. Results demonstrated that video modeling led to faster acquisition of skills and greater generalization effects relative to in vivo intervention. Moreover, video modeling has been associated with maintenance and generalization of behavioral gains. For example, Charlop and Milstein (1989) demonstrated that video modeling not only served as an effective intervention strategy for increasing conversational speech in three children with ASDs but the skills maintained and generalized for all three participants at a 15-month follow-up.

Like most interventions, studies have suggested that video modeling is most successful when other interventions such as practice, self-management, or peer training are also simultaneously incorporated (Scattone, 2007). For example, Apple, Billingsley, and Schwartz (2005) focused on teaching compliment-giving responses and initiations to two boys with autism (age 5 years) through video modeling. Their study showed that there was limited generalization with the single strategy, but the employment of tangible reinforcement and self-management strategies served to improve treatment and maintenance effects.

The results of several studies have shown that both the nature of the model/learner relationship and the length of the model/learner relationship are particularly important factors in the degree of success of video modeling interventions (Jones & Schwartz, 2004). The literature indicates that when a video model is familiar to a participant, the intervention is more likely to be effective. Given this finding, some researchers believe that video self-modeling (VSM), which involves the observation of videotapes of oneself performing desirable target behaviors, may be an effective form of intervention.

A meta-analysis by Bellini and Akullian (2007) reviewed 23 single-subject design studies assessing the effectiveness of VSM for children and adolescents with ASDs. Intervention effectiveness was determined by examining the direct effect of intervention, maintenance, and generalization of behavior gains of both video modeling and VSM interventions. The overall results suggest that video modeling and VSM are effective intervention strategies for addressing social communication skills and behavioral functioning in children and adolescents with ASDs. Three of four studies that used video modeling and VSM to address social/conversation skills demonstrated that video modeling and VSM interventions both effectively foster conversation skills and promote the maintenance of skills over time and across different situations. The review included a study by Buggey (2005), which examined the effects of VSM with older elementary school children with autism. The participants watched a 3-minute video showing themselves engaging in positive and typical social interactions prior to the start of class. Following VSM, significant gains in the frequency of social interactions within the school setting were observed and maintenance of skills was shown to be 100%.

Moreover, Thiemann, and Goldstein (2001) incorporated video feedback with other intervention techniques to teach young children (ages 7–12 years) peer-directed social communication skills. Target behaviors included securing attention, initiating comment, initiating request, and contingent responses. Participants received 10 minutes of visual instruction using social stories, text cues, and pictures of social skills. The children engaged in 10 minutes of social interaction and subsequently participated in 10 minutes of video feedback. In these video feedback sessions, participants evaluated unedited videotapes of themselves from the previous social interaction. The participants demonstrated improved and consistent rates of social interactions compared to baseline. Following intervention, all raters reported improvements in reciprocal social behaviors between the participants and their peers. In particular, the participant's active involvement in the interaction, use of comments or questions, and responses to peers' utterances increased.

Although effective, the issue of long-term generalization of video modeling effects is always a concern, particularly when scripted utterances are taught. For example, Taylor, Levin, and Jasper (1999) used video modeling to increase play-related statements of two children with autism to their siblings. Although scripted comments improved significantly for each participant, unscripted comments did not increase using only the video modeling. Yet, as mentioned above, a combination of programs may enhance generalization. The use of multiple exemplars may also improve generalization. Maione and Mirenda (2006) assessed the effectiveness of video modeling and video feedback in instructing a child with autism (age 5 years) to use peer-directed social language during play. Results suggested that video modeling was effective in significantly increasing social language in two of the three play activities. Additional intervention consisting of the participant evaluating appropriate and inappropriate verbalizations, providing examples of appropriate verbalizations, and prompting by the clinician resulted in a significant change in social language. Increases in the desired unscripted verbalizations and initiations were also noted. Thus, to increase and extend generalization effects, video modeling studies may benefit from the inclusion of individualized multiple exemplars.

Self-Management

Self-management is a procedure that teaches individuals to monitor their own behaviors (Quinn & Swaggart, 1994). Following appropriate engagement in targeted desired behaviors, individuals are taught to self-monitor the behavior. The individual is then rewarded by others or they are taught to deliver self-reinforcement. The value of self-management is that it is an instructional strategy, whereby the locus of control for the behavior is shifted from an external source, such as a teacher, therapist, or parent, to the individual (c.f., Jones, Nelson, & Kazdin, 1977).

Self-management and self-control, and the lack thereof in individuals, has long been discussed in the psychological literature, but systematic interventions using self-management only began to appear in the literature in the early 1970s. These early studies generally focused on typical adults addressing behaviors such as weight reduction (Horan & Gilmore, 1971), cigarette smoking (Chapman, Smith, & Layden, 1971), depression and other psychological difficulties (Mahoney, 1971), poor study habits, addictions, stress, and so on (*see* Yager, 1975). It wasn't until the late 1970s that research began to emerge suggesting that self-management may be a viable option for individuals with disabilities, such as mental retardation (Horner & Brigham, 1979; Wheeman, 1978) and learning disabilities (Edwards, 1976). In the mid-1980s, the procedures began to be implemented with individuals with more severe disabilities (Morrow & Presswood, 1984; Shapiro et al., 1984).

Finally in 1990, self-management procedures began being applied to individuals with autism. Koegel and Koegel (1990) showed that stereotypic behavior could be reduced by using self-management during academic tasks in a full-inclusion classroom and in community settings. This study was particularly important because in addition to demonstrating the effectiveness of the procedure among children with autism, it provided a framework for the programming of desired behavior in the absence of a treatment provider. Following this study, the procedures were replicated for improving play (Stahmer & Schreibman, 1992), and a 1-month maintenance of behavioral gains was observed even after removal of the interventionist and self-management device. In regard to communication, self-management procedures also have been adapted for use with social interactions in children with autism. Koegel et al. (1992) taught elementary-aged children, who initially were unresponsive to others, to monitor their social responsiveness to questions. All children improved their responsiveness and the behaviors generalized to home, school, and community settings in the absence of a treatment provider. Further, when the children were self-managing their behavior, concomitant decreases in untreated disruptive behaviors were evidenced.

Loftin, Odom, and Lance (2008) used a combination of self-management and peer training strategies to teach social initiations to three children with autism to target social conversation. Results demonstrated improvements in peer social interactions, collateral changes in the reduction of self-stimulatory behaviors, and generalization of these behaviors. In another study, Koegel and Frea (1993) showed that pragmatic behavior could be improved and that response classes appeared to be positively affected during intervention. Specifically, they targeted one or two pragmatic behaviors, such as eye gaze and nonverbal inappropriate mannerisms or topic perseveration, in children with autism who had mild support needs. The study showed that other, nontreated, pragmatic behaviors improved as a result of the self-management. This suggests that some pragmatic behaviors may function as a response class and that interventions targeting individual behaviors within a class may not be necessary.

Similarly, self-management has been successfully used in full-inclusion school settings, with demonstrated decreases in inappropriate and challenging behaviors and improvement in on-task behaviors (Harrower & Dunlap, 2001; Koegel, Harrower, & Koegel, 1999; Koegel et al., 1999). Appropriate question-asking using self-management also has been effective among teens and young adults with autism. Palmen, Didden, and Arts (2008) showed that question-asking improved after a relatively short intervention program of weekly 1-hour sessions for a duration of 6 weeks. These effects were maintained after a 1-month follow-up period.

Although self-management can indeed be a useful tool for individuals on the spectrum, fading of the self-management may be more challenging in individuals with greater support needs (Koegel et al., 1992). However, although there is a need for additional research, it appears that as individuals become more fluent with the targeted behavior, systematic fading may be possible (Boettcher, 2004).

Conclusion

The importance of communication and socialization for typically developing individuals is well-documented in the literature, and research over the past six decades has given us invaluable information about how these processes develop and interact (Landa, 2008; Paul, 2008). Evidence for the myriad of difficulties individuals with ASDs experience in social communication is also robust (Alpern & Zager, 2007; Paul et al., 2005). Addressing social communication issues to ensure that individuals on the spectrum have healthy and long-term friendships and relationships needs to be a priority in the area of ASDs. As previously discussed in this chapter, communication and socialization are inextricably intertwined, and recent research has confirmed that the linguistic outcomes of individuals with autism explicitly affect social ability (Bono et al., 2004). This is important given research indicating that individuals with ASDs may be prone to poorer long-term outcomes. Individuals with disabilities have been found to be involved in the criminal justice system at much higher rates than persons without disabilities (Mayes, 2003; National Research Council, 2001). Overall, these findings highlight that social and communicative interventions may contribute to better outcomes.

It is apparent that several important themes emerge in the literature on language and social communication. First, a combination of inter-related programs that are simultaneously implemented may be more effective than single, isolated interventions.

Second, frequent exposure to social communication opportunities and prompting (with subsequent fading) of targeted linguistic structures appears to be important. Children on the spectrum who are learning language and social communication skills may need frequent engagement in these behaviors. Unfortunately, opportunities for expressive social communication are infrequently elicited by teachers of children with autism (Chiang, 2008). Training teachers to evoke language and communication on an ongoing basis may potentially improve the socialization of children on the spectrum with ongoing carryover to the home through parent education (Koegel et al., 2005). Further, models that rely solely on pull-out approaches for language and social intervention are not likely to result in generalization and maintenance. However, developing comprehensive models in which school speech/language pathologists, teachers, aides, and other interventionists implement sessions in the natural environment, while also training relevant peers and adults in those environments, should result in more effective generalized intervention results.

Along with providing frequent, regular, and systematic opportunities for social communication, intervention should focus on the positive occurrences and strengths of the child with autism (Cosden et al., 2006). Expanding on the child's strengths results in improved affect and increased generalization (Baker et al., 1998).

There is no doubt that inclusion with typical peers in natural and community settings is essential. Not only do children with autism have more frequent social interactions when they are included with typical peers rather than segregated settings (Brookman et al., 2003; Kamps et al., 2002; Kennedy & Shukla, 1995; Koegel et al., 1999), but issues of generalization do not arise when intervention takes place in inclusion and community settings (Albin & Horner, 1988; Koegel & Koegel, 1988; Licciardello et al., 2008). Further, ecologically valid social goals can be developed, increasing the likelihood that they will be used by the individuals and peers in those specific environments (Frederickson et al., 2005).

Moreover, within these natural settings, targeting both the child with autism *and* the typical peers has tended to be more effective than targeting either separately. Typical children can be of great support and role models for children on the spectrum (Harper et al., 2008; Pierce & Schreibman, 1997). Teaching specific procedures to typical peers to enhance socio-communication goals has proven to be beneficial to both typically developing children and those on the spectrum.

Finally, spontaneity has emerged as an important pivotal area for children with Asperger's Syndrome and autism (Koegel & Koegel, 2006; Koegel & LaZebnik, 2009). Historically, intervention has been primarily adult-driven and adult-structured (Landa, 2007; Koegel et al., 1987). Teaching and creating opportunities for spontaneous self-generated communication (Koegel & LaZebnik, 2004) seems to result in more pragmatically appropriate interactions and improved long-term outcomes (Koegel et al., 1999).

In conclusion, most children with autism or Asperger's Syndrome receive little to no intervention for social communication throughout the day in school settings where peers are readily available. It has been clearly documented that multi-component interventions targeting both the child on the spectrum and the typically developing peers are effective in improving social communication and social interaction. Although longitudinal studies are still necessary, comprehensive interventions beginning in the preschool years and throughout the lifespan positively improve the social interactions of individuals on the spectrum. When individuals on the spectrum engage in improved social interactions, loneliness and isolation are likely to be reduced, sexual victimization and perpetration resulting from naïveté may become less frequent. That is, intervention may act as a potential barrier against the development of comorbid conditions, including depression and anxiety. There is evidence showing that interventions targeting the development of positive social interaction among children with ASDs and their peers can have an immediate effect on increasing positive affect (Baker et al., 1998; Koegel et al., 2005) and reports on self-esteem (Elder et al., 2006). Continued research on the long-term impact of social skills-based interventions—particularly using measurements of psychological well-being (i.e., symptoms of depression, anxiety, self-worth)—will undoubtedly be a growing area of clinical and theoretical exploration. In the meantime, the impact of social skills training in other populations may provide some insight into this matter. For example, in assessing the effects of a social problem-solving skills training program in adults with intellectual disabilities, Anderson and Kazantzis (2008) found that intervention was associated with an improvement in not only social-problem solving skills but also, for two of the three participants, symptoms of depression as well. The study is promising given that changes in symptoms of depression were observed after a relatively short duration of 15 sessions and suggests that a more long-term intervention in this domain may have widespread benefits on psychological well-being. In addition, there is some evidence supporting the notion that psychosocial interventions incorporating social skills training may prevent and improve symptoms of depression in typically developing children (Garber, 2006). Additionally, according to a review by Segrin (2000), most effective interventions for treating depression involve an emphasis on augmenting the social skills. Therefore, there appears to be a unique relationship between social skills difficulties and psychological distress that may help guide the future direction of research and, particularly, the measurement of outcomes of intervention in the ASD population.

Challenges and Future Directions

Longitudinal studies indicate that many adolescents and adults on the spectrum experience poor psychological health and continued dependence on their parents or other care providers. In an effort to alter this problematic trajectory, future theoretical and intervention research should focus on pivotal areas to ensure that individuals on the spectrum achieve a life of independence with meaningful social relationships. Continued research to assure that interventions are systematically implemented and to define areas that have the greatest long-term impact is needed. Comprehensive intervention packages, and their longitudinal effect, are undoubtedly an important area of future research. Inclusion in school and community settings has proven to be superior in regards to academic and social progress. In addition, multicomponent intervention programs, targeting both the individual on the spectrum and the typical peers, has also resulted in greater outcomes. However, more research on specific target behaviors that, when targeted, yield the greatest generalize effects, specific teaching strategies that are most effective, preparation and success in the work setting, and understanding the development and creation of durable friendships and intimate relationships will need to be studied and understood in future research. Below is a list of challenges and ideas for future research directions.

- There is still a great need for the development and investigation of outcome measures to accompany intervention research to more comprehensively reflect changes in social and communication symptoms as well as collateral gains in other meaningful psychosocial variables, such as emotional functioning.
- As discussed above, many individuals with ASDs do not develop relationships, despite their desire to do so. Research focused on identification of additional social communication skills that may contribute to enhancing immediate and long-term social success continues to be an area of need.
- Related, research is needed to both appropriately assess and target social communicative skills according to the developmental demands present in different age groups, which will have the greatest impact on long-term development, so that adolescents and adults with autism can more easily adjust as socialization becomes more complex.
- Similarly, intervention components and procedures that contribute to the long-term maintenance of treatment gains over time, once intervention has been completed, is critically important. For example, given that the data from many interventions for social areas suggest that these effects may not entirely generalize and maintain over time, in addition to the fact that developing "friendships" are often more difficult for individuals with ASDs, intervention components that may be more helpful with such long-term gains would be helpful.
- Understanding the motivational or behavioral characteristics of children who generalize social or communication skills compared to those who have more difficulty with generalizing treatment gains over time or across contexts would help inform the development of specialized interventions to address the different needs of children with ASDs. Doing so may also prove helpful in providing more robust findings of intervention effects across different children.
- Further examination of the interplay between the three core ASD symptoms, how such effects can contribute to social and communicative impairments, and the development interventions to address these contributing difficulties is important. For example, additional research on the impact of restricted interests on the overall functioning of ASDs and interventions to address these symptoms may an important factor in improving social difficulties.
- Expanding the application and conceptualization of existing interventions, such as those that are effective in improving for initiations and the use of priming for activities, to further develop and identify strategies to improve social and communicative functioning.
- Further development and understanding the role of motivational variables on early social and communicative functioning and how to use existing intervention strategies to tap into the development of successful social interactions may be helpful.
- Research that examines the longitudinal effect of targeted social communicative interventions on the development of romantic relationships in people with ASDs may help individuals with ASDs lead more fulfilling lives.

SUGGESTED READINGS

Koegel. R. L. & Koegel, L. K. (2006). *Pivotal Response Treatments.* Baltimore, MD: Paul H. Brookes Publishing Co.

Koegel, L. & LaZebnik, C. (2004) *Overcoming Autism.* New York: Viking/Penguin.

Koegel, L. & LaZebnik, C. (April, 2009). *Growing Up on the Spectrum: A Guide to Life, Love, and Learning for Teens and Young Adults with Autism and Asperger's.* New York: Viking/Penguin.

Koegel, R. L., Koegel, L. K., & McNerney, E. (2001). Pivotal behaviors in intervention for autism. *Journal of Child Clinical Psychology, 30*, 1, 19–32.

ACKNOWLEDGMENTS

We would like to thank the Eli and Edythe L. Broad Foundation, the Kelly Family Foundation, and the Kind World Foundation for their generous support of our research. In addition funding from the National Institutes of Health (grant #DC010924) helped support this work. These donations and grant funds have allowed us to work toward creating better lives for individuals with autism and Asperger's Disorder.

REFERENCES

Albin, R. W., & Horner, R. H. (1988). Generalization with precision. In R. H. Horner, G. Dunlap, & R. L. Koegel (Eds.), *Generalization and maintenance: Life-style changes in applied settings* (pp. 99–120). Baltimore, MD, England: Paul H. Brookes Publishing.

Alpern, C. S., & Zager, D. (2007). Addressing communication needs of young adults with autism in a college-based inclusion program. *Education and Training in Developmental Disabilities*, *42*, 428–436.

Amaral, D. G., Schumann, C. M., & Nordahl, C. W. (2008). Neuroanatomy of autism. *Trends in Neurosciences*, *31*(3), 137–145.

American Psychiatric Association (2000). *Diagnostic and statistical manual of mental disorders*, 4th ed. Text Revision. Washington, DC: American Psychiatric Association.

Anderson, G., & Kazantzis, N. (2008). Social problem-solving skills training for adults with mild intellectual disability: A multiple case study. *Behaviour Change*, *25*(2), 97–108.

Apple, A. L., Billingsley, F., & Schwartz, I. S. (2005). Effects of video modeling alone and with self-management on compliment-giving behaviors of children with high-functioning ASD. *Journal of Positive Behavior Interventions*, *7*(1), 33–46.

Baker, M. J. (2000). Incorporating the thematic ritualistic behaviors of children with autism into games: Increasing social play interactions with siblings. *Journal of Positive Behavior Interventions*, *2*(2), 66–84.

Baker, M. J., Koegel, R. L., & Koegel, L. K. (1998). Increasing the social behavior of young children with autism using their obsessive behavior. *The Journal of* the *Association for Persons* with *Severe Handicaps*, *23*, 4, 300–308

Bakeman, R., & Adamson, L.B. (1984). Coordinating attention to people and objects in mother infant and peer-infant interaction. *Child Development*, *55*, 1278–1289.

Bates, E. (1979). *The emergence of symbols: Cognition and communication in infancy*. San Diego: Academic Press.

Bateson, M. C. (1975). Mother-infant exchanges: The epigenesis of conversational interaction. *Annals of the New York Academy of Sciences*, *263*, 101–113.

Bauminger, N., & Kasari, C. (2000). Loneliness and friendship in high-functioning children with autism. *Child Development*, *71*(2), 447–456.

Bellini, S., & Akullian, J. (2007). A meta-analysis of video modeling and video self-modeling interventions for children and adolescents with autism spectrum disorders. *Exceptional Children*, *73*(3), 264–287.

Boettcher, M. A. (2004). Teaching social conversation skills to children with autism through self management: An analysis of treatment gains and meaningful outcomes. Unpublished Doctoral Dissertation. University of California, Santa Barbara.

Bono, M., Daley, T., & Sigman, M. (2004). Relations among joint attention, amount of intervention, and language gain in autism. *Journal of Autism and Developmental Disorders*, *34*, 495–505.

Brinton, B., Robinson, L. A., & Fujiki, M. (2004). Description of a program for social language intervention: "If you can have a conversation, you can have a relationship." *Language, Speech, and Hearing Services in Schools*, *35*, 283–290.

Brookman, L., Boettcher, M., Klein, E., Openden, D., Koegel, R. L., & Koegel, L. K. (2003). Facilitating social interactions in a community summer camp setting for children with autism. *Journal of Positive Behavior Interventions*, *5*(4), 249–252.

Bruinsma, Y. E. M. (2005). Increases in the joint attention behavior of eye gaze alternation to share enjoyment as a collateral effect of pivotal response treatment for three children with autism. *Dissertation Abstracts International: Section B: The Sciences and Engineering*, *65* (9–B).

Bruinsma, Y., Koegel, R. L., & Koegel, L. K. (2004). Joint attention and children with autism: A review of the literature. *Mental Retardation and Developmental Disabilities Research Reviews*, *10*(3), 169–175.

Buggey, T. (2005). Video self-modeling applications with students with autism spectrum disorder in a small private school setting. *Focus on Autism and Other Developmental Disabilities*, *20*(1), 52–63.

Carter, M., & Grunsell, J. (2001). The behavior chain interruption strategy: A review of research and discussion of future directions. *Journal of the Association for Persons with Severe Handicaps*, *26*(1), 37–49.

Carter, M. & Hotchkis, G. D. (2002). A Conceptual Analysis of Communicative Spontaneity. *Journal of Intellectual & Developmental Disability*, *27*(3), 168–190.

Cederlund, M., Hagberg, B., Billstedt, E., Gillberg, I. C., & Gillberg, C. (2008). Asperger syndrome and autism: A comparative longitudinal follow-up study more than 5 years after original diagnosis. *Journal of Autism and Developmental Disorders*, *38*(1), 72–85.

Chapman, R. F., Smith, J. W., & Layden, T. (1971). Elimination of cigarette smoking by punishment and self-management training. *Behaviour Research and Therapy*, *9*(3), 255- 264.

Charlop, M. H., & Trasowech, J.E. (1991). Increasing autistic children's spontaneous speech. *Journal of Applied Behavior Analysis*, *24*, 747–761.

Charlop-Christy, M. H., Le, L., & Freeman, K. A. (2000). A comparison of video modeling with in vivo modeling for teaching children with autism. *Journal of Autism and Developmental Disorders*, *30*(6), 537–552.

Charlop, M. H., & Milstein, J. P. (1989). Teaching autistic children conversational speech using video modeling. *Journal of Applied Behavior Analysis*, *22*(3), 275–285.

Chiang, H. (2008). Communicative spontaneity of children with autism: A preliminary analysis. *Autism*, *12*(1), 9–21.

Chiang, H-M., & Carter, M. (2008). Spontaneity of communication in individuals with autism. *Journal of Autism and Developmental Disorders*, *38*, 693–705.

Cook-Gumprez, J., & Kyratzis, A. (2001). Child discourse. In D. Schiffrin, D. Tannen, & H. Hamilton (Eds.) *A handbook of discourse analysis* (pp. 590–611). Malden, MA: Blackwell Publishers.

Cosden, M., Koegel, L. K., Koegel, R. L., Greenwell, A., & Klein, E. (2006). Strength-based assessment for children with autism spectrum disorders. *Research and Practice for Persons with Severe Disabilities*, *31*(2), 134–143.

Dunlap, G. (1984). The influence of task variation and maintenance tasks on the learning and affect of autistic children. *Journal of Experimental Child Psychology*, *37*(1), 41–64.

Dunlap, G., Kern, L., & Worcester, J. A. (2001). ABA and academic instruction. *Focus on Autism and Other Developmental Disabilities*, *16*(2), 129–136.

Edwards, J. S. (1976). Self-management in children labeled learning disabled. *Bulletin of the Psychonomic Society, 8*(1), 51–53.

Falk G., Dunlap, G., & Kern, L. (1996). An analysis of self-evaluation and videotape feedback for improving the peer interactions of students with externalizing and internalizing behavioral challenges. *Behavioral Disorders, 21*, 261–276.

Fensen, L., Dale, P., Reznick, J., Thal, D., Bates, E., Hartung, J.P., et al. (1993). *The MacArthur Communicative Development Inventories: User's guide and technical manual.* San Diego: Singular.

Ferster, C. B., & DeMyer, M. K. (1961). The development of performances in autistic children in an automatically controlled environment. *Journal of Chronic Diseases, 13*, 312–345.

Fredeen, R. M., & Koegel, R. L. (2006). The pivotal role of initiations in habilitation. In R. L. Koegel, & L. K., Koegel (Eds.), *Pivotal response treatments for autism* (pp.166–186). Baltimore: Brookes.

Frederickson, N., Warren, L., & Turner, J. (2005). "Circle of friends"—an exploration of impact over time. *Educational Psychology in Practice, 21*(3), 197–217.

Garber, J. (2006). Depression in children and adolescents: Linking risk research and prevention. *American Journal of Preventive Medicine, 31*(61), S104–S125.

Gadow, K. D., DeVincent, C. J., Pomeroy, J., & Azizian, A. (2004). Psychiatric symptoms in preschool children with PDD and clinic and comparison samples. *Journal of Autism and Developmental Disorders, 34*(4), 379–393.

Gengoux, G. W. (2007). Priming for cooperative opportunities for children with autism: Effects on social interactions with typically developing peers. Unpublished Doctoral Dissertation. University of California, Santa Barbara.

Geschwind, D. H., & Levitt, P. (2007). Autism spectrum disorders: Developmental disconnection syndromes. *Current Opinion in Neurobiology, 17*(1), 103–111.

Ghaziuddin, M., Ghaziuddin, N., & Greden, J. (2002). Depression in persons with autism: Implications for research and clinical care. *Journal of Autism and Developmental Disorders, 32*(4), 299–306.

Green, J., Gilchrist, A., Burton, D., & Cox, A. (2000). Social and psychiatric functioning in adolescents with Asperger syndrome compared with conduct disorder. *Journal of Autism and Developmental Disorders, 30*(4), 279–293.

Halle, J. W. (1987). Teaching language in the natural environment: An analysis of spontaneity. *Journal of the Association for Persons with Severe Handicaps, 12*(1), 28–37.

Halliday, M. A. K. (1975). *Learning how to mean: Explorations in the development of language.* New York: Arnold.

Haring, T. G., & Breen, C. G. (1992). A peer-mediated social network intervention to enhance the social integration of persons with moderate and severe disabilities. *Journal of Applied Behavior Analysis, 25*(2), 319–333.

Harper, C. B., Symon, J. B. G., & Frea, W. D. (2008). Recess is time-in: Using peers to improve social skills of children with autism. *Journal of Autism and Developmental Disorders, 38*, 815–826.

Harrower, J. K., & Dunlap, G. (2001). Including children with autism in general education classrooms: A review of effective strategies. *Behavior Modification. Special Issue: Autism*, Part 1, *25*(5), 762–784.

Hauck, M., Fein, D., Waterhouse, L., & Feinstein, C. (1995). Social initiations by autistic children to adults and other children. *Journal of Autism and Developmental Disorders, 25*(6), 579–595.

Hewitt, F. M. (1965). Teaching speech to autistic children through operant conditioning. *American Journal of Orthopsychiatry, 34*, 927–936.

Horan, J. J., & Johnson, R. G. (1971). Coverant conditioning through a self-management application of the premack principle: Its effect on weight reduction. *Journal of Behavior Therapy and Experimental Psychiatry, 2*(4), 243–249.

Horner, R. H., & Brigham, T. A. (1979). The effects of self-management procedures on the study behavior of two retarded children. *Education and Training of the Mentally Retarded, 14*, 1, 18–24.

Howlin, P. (2000). Outcome in adult life for more able individuals with autism or Asperger syndrome. *Autism. Special Issue: Asperger Syndrome, 4*(1), 63–83.

Howlin, P., Goode, S., Hutton, J., & Rutter, M. (2004). Adult outcome for children with autism. *Journal of Child Psychology and Psychiatry, 45*(2), 212–229.

Howlin, P., Mawhood, L., & Rutter, M. (2000). Autism and developmental receptive language disorder—A follow-up comparison in early adult life. II: Social, behavioural, and psychiatric outcomes. *Journal of Child Psychology and Psychiatry, 41*(5), 561–578.

Hung, D. W. (1977). Generalization of "curiosity" questioning behavior in autistic children. *Journal of Behavior Therapy and Experimental Psychiatry, 8*(3), 237–245.

Hurbutt, K., & Chalmers, L. (2004). Employment and adults with Aspergers syndrome. *Focus on Autism and Other Developmental Disabilities, 19*, 215–222.

Hurtig, R., Ensrud, S., & Tomblin, J. B. (1982). The communicative function of question production in autistic children. *Journal of Autism and Developmental Disorders, 12*(1), 57–69.

Hwang, B., & Hughes, C. (2000). The effects of social interaction training on early social communicative skills of children with autism. *Journal of Autism and Developmental Disorders, 30*, 331–343.

Jennes-Coussens, M., Magill-Evans, J., & Koning, C. (2006). The quality of life of young men with Asperger syndrome: A brief report. *Autism, 10*(4), 403–414.

Jobe, L. E., & White, S. W. (2007). Loneliness, social relationships, and a broader autism phenotype in college students. *Personality and Individual Differences, 42*(8), 1479–1489.

Jones, C. D., & Schwartz, I. S. (2004). Siblings, peers, and adults: Differential effects of models for children with autism. *Topics in Early Childhood Special Education, 24*(4), 187–198.

Jones, R. S. P., & Meldal, T. O. (2001). Social relationships and Asperger's syndrome. *Journal of Learning Disabilities, 5*(1), 35–41.

Jones, R. T., Nelson, R. E., & Kazdin, A. E. (1977). The role of external variables in self reinforcement: A review. *Behavior Modification, 1*(2), 147–178.

Kamps, D. M., Dugan, E., Potucek, J., & Collins, A. (1999). Effects of cross-age peer tutoring networks among students with autism and general education students. *Journal of Behavioral Education, 9*(2), 97–115.

Kamps, D. M., Leonard, B. R., Vernon, S., Dugan, E. P., Delquadri, J. C., Gershon, B., et al. (1992). Teaching social skills to students with autism to increase peer interactions in an integrated first-grade classroom. *Journal of Applied Behavior Analysis, 25*(2), 281–288.

Kamps, D., Royer, J., Dugan, E., Kravits, T., Gonzalez-Lopez, A., Garcia, J., et al. (2002). Peer training to facilitate social interaction for elementary students with autism and their peers. *Exceptional Children, 68*(2), 173–187.

Kennedy, C. H., & Shukla, S. (1995). Social interaction research for people with autism as a set of past, current, and emerging propositions. *Behavioral Disorders. Special Issue: Autism, 21*(1), 21–35.

Klin, A., Danovitch, J. H., Merz, A. B., & Volkmar, F. (2007). Circumscribed interests in higher functioning individuals with autism spectrum disorders: An exploratory study. *Research and Practice for Persons with Severe Disabilities, 32*(2), 89–100.

Klin, A., Pauls, D., Schultz, R., & Volkmar, F. (2005). Three diagnostic approaches to Asperger syndrome: Implications for research. *Journal of Autism and Developmental Disorders, 35*(2), 221–234.

Knott, F., Lewis, C., & Williams, T. (2007). Sibling interaction of children with autism: Development over 12 months. *Journal of Autism and Developmental Disorders, 37*(10), 1987–1995.

Koegel, L. K. (2000). Interventions to facilitate communication in autism. *Journal of Autism and Developmental Disorders, 30*(5), 383–391.

Koegel, L. K., & LaZebnik (2004). *Overcoming Autism.* New York: Penguin Books.

Koegel, L. K., & LaZebnik (2009). *Growing up on the Spectrum.* New York: Penguin Books.

Koegel, L. K., Camarata, S. M., Valdez-Menchaca, M., & Koegel, R. L. (1998). Setting generalization of question-asking by children with autism. *American Journal on Mental Retardation, 102*(4), 346–357.

Koegel, L. K., Carter, C. M., & Koegel, R. L. (2003). Teaching children with autism self initiations as a pivotal response. *Topics in Language Disorders, 23*(2), 134–145.

Koegel, L. K., Harrower, J. K., & Koegel, R. L. (1999). Support for children with developmental disabilities in full inclusion classrooms through self-management. *Journal of Positive Behavior Interventions, 1*, 26–34.

Koegel, L. K., Koegel, R. L., Frea, W. D., & Fredeen, R. M. (2001). Identifying early intervention targets for children with autism in inclusive school settings. *Behavior Modification. Special Issue: Autism, Part 1, 25*(5), 745–761.

Koegel, L. K., Koegel, R. L., Frea, W. & Green-Hopkins, I. (2003). Priming as a method of coordinating educational services for students with autism. *Language, Speech, and Hearing Services in Schools, 34*, 228–235.

Koegel, L. K., Koegel, R. L., Fredeen, R. M., & Gengoux, G. W. (2008). Naturalistic behavioral approaches to treatment. In Chawarska, K., Klin, A. & Volkmar, F. R. (Eds.), *Autism spectrum disorders in infants and toddlers: Diagnosis, assessment, and treatment* (pp. 207–242). New York: Guilford Press.

Koegel, L. K., Koegel, R. L., Harrower, J. K., & Carter, C. M. (1999). Pivotal response intervention I: Overview of approach. *Journal of the Association for Persons with Severe Handicaps, 24*(3), 174–185.

Koegel, L. K., Koegel, R. L., Hurley, C., & Frea, W. D. (1992). Improving social skills and disruptive behavior in children with autism through self-management. *Journal of Applied Behavior Analysis, 25*(2), 341–353.

Koegel, L. K., Koegel, R. L., Shoshan, Y., & McNerney, E. (1999). Pivotal response intervention II: Preliminary long-term outcome data. *The Journal of the Association for Persons with Severe Handicaps. 24*(3), 186–198.

Koegel, R. L., Camarata, S., Koegel, L. K., Ben-Tall, A., & Smith, A. E. (1998). Increasing speech intelligibility in children with autism. *Journal of Autism and Developmental Disorders, 28*(3), 241–251.

Koegel, R. L., Dyer, K., & Bell, L. K. (1987). The influence of child-preferred activities on autistic children's social behavior. *Journal of Applied Behavior Analysis, 20*(3), 243–252.

Koegel, R. L., Egel, A. L., & Williams, J. A. (1980). Behavioral contrast and generalization across settings in the treatment of autistic children. *Journal of Experimental Child Psychology, 30*(3), 422–437.

Koegel, R. L., & Frea, W. D. (1993). Treatment of social behavior in autism through the modification of pivotal social skills. *Journal of Applied Behavior Analysis, 26*(3), 369–377.

Koegel, R. L., & Koegel, L. K. (1988). Generalized responsivity and pivotal behaviors. In R. H. Horner, G. Dunlap & R. L. Koegel (Eds.), *Generalization and maintenance: Life-style changes in applied settings* (pp. 41–66). Baltimore, MD: Paul H. Brookes Publishing.

Koegel, R. L., & Koegel, L. K. (1990). Extended reductions in stereotypic behaviors through self-management in multiple community settings. *Journal of Applied Behavior Analysis, 1*, 119–127.

Koegel, R. L., & Koegel, L. K. (1995). *Teaching children with autism.* Baltimore: Brookes Publishing.

Koegel, R. L., & Koegel, L. K. (2003). Improving social skills and disruptive behavior in children with autism through self-management. Pivotal response intervention I: Overview of approach.

Koegel, R. L., & Koegel, L. K. (2006). *Pivotal response treatments for autism: Communication, social, and academic development.* Baltimore, MD: Paul H. Brookes Publishing.

Koegel, R. L., Koegel, L. K., & Surratt, A. (1992). Language intervention and disruptive behavior in preschool children with autism. *Journal of Autism and Developmental Disorders, 22*(2), 141–153.

Koegel, R. L., O'Dell, M., & Dunlap, G. (1988). Producing speech use in nonverbal autistic children by reinforcing attempts. *Journal of Autism and Developmental Disorders, 18*(4), 525–538.

Koegel, R. L., O'Dell, M. C., & Koegel, L. K. (1987). A natural language teaching paradigm for nonverbal autistic children. *Journal of Autism and Develpmental Disorders, 17*, 187–200.

Koegel, R. L., Werner, G. A., Vismara, L. A., & Koegel, L. K. (2005). The effectiveness of contextually supported play date interactions between children with autism and typically developing peers. *Research and Practice for Persons with Severe Disabilities. 30*, 93–102.

Koegel, R. L., & Williams, J. A. (1980). Direct versus indirect response-reinforcer relationships in teaching autistic children. *Journal of Abnormal Child Psychology, 8*(4), 537–547.

Krantz, P. J., & McClannahan, L. E. (1993). Teaching children with autism to initiate to peers: Effects of a script-fading procedure. *Journal of Applied Behavior Analysis, 26*, 121–132.

Landa, R. (2007). Early communication development for children with autism. *Mental Retardation and Developmental Disabilities Research Reviews, 13*, 16–25.

Larson, S. A., Doljanac, R., & Lakin, K. C. (2005). United States living arrangements of people with intellectual and/or developmental disabilities in 1995. *Journal of Intellectual and Developmental Disability, 30*(4), 236–239.

Laushey, K. M., & Heflin, L. J. (2000). Enhancing social skills of kindergarten children with autism through the training of multiple peers as tutors. *Journal of Autism and Developmental Disorders, 30*(3), 183–193.

LeBlanc, L. A., Coates, A. M., Daneshvar, S., Charlop-Christy, M. H., Morris, C., & Lancaster, B. M. (2003). Using video modeling and reinforcement to teaching perspective-taking skills to children with autism. *Journal of Applied Behavior Analysis, 36*(2), 253–257.

LeBlanc, L. A., Geiger, K. B., Sautter, R. A., & Sidener, T. M. (2007). Using the natural language paradigm (NLP) to increase vocalizations of older adults with cognitive impairments. *Research in Developmental Disabilities, 28*, 437–444.

Licciardello, C. C., Harchik, A. E., & Luiselli, J. K. (2008). Social skills intervention for children with autism during interactive play at a public elementary school. *Education and Treatment of Children, 31*(1), 27–37.

Linder, T. W. (1993). *Transdisciplinary play-bases assessment: A functional approach to working with young children* (Rev. ed.). Baltimore: Paul H. Brookes Publishing Co.

Locke, J. L. (1995). Development of the capacity for spoken language. In P. Fletcher & B. MacWhinney (Eds.), *The handbook of child language* (pp. 278–302). Malden, MA: Blackwell Publishers.

Loftin, R. L., Odom, S. L., & Lantz, J. F. (2008). Social interaction and repetitive motor behaviors. *Journal of Autism and Developmental Disorders, 38*(6), 1124–1135.

Lord, C., & Paul, R. (1997). Language and communication in autism. In D. Cohen & F. Volkmar (Eds.), Handbook of autism and pervasive developmental disorders (2nd ed., pp. 195–225). New York: Wiley.

Lovaas, O. I., Reitag, G., Kinder, M. I., Rubenstein, B. D., Schaeffer, B., & Simmons, J. Q. (1966). Establishment of social reinforcers in two schizophrenic children on the basis of food. *Journal of Experimental Child Psychology, 4*, 109–125.

Lovaas, O. I. (1987). Behavioral treatment and normal educational and intellectual functioning in young autistic children. *Journal of Consulting, Clinical Psychiatry, 55*, 3–9.

Mahoney, M. J. (1971). The self-management of covert behavior: A cast study. *Behavior Therapy, 2*(4), 575–578.

Maione, L., & Mirenda, P. (2006). Effects of video modeling and video feedback on peer- directed social language skills of a child with autism. *Journal of Positive Behavior Interventions, 8*(2), 106–118.

Mayes, T. A. (2003). Persons with autism and criminal justice: Core concepts and leading cases. *Journal of Positive Behavior Interventions, 5*(2), 92–100.

McCoy, K., & Hermansen, E. (2007). Video modeling for individuals with autism: A review of model types and effects. *Education & Treatment of Children. Special Issue: Papers Presented at the 30th Annual Teachers Educators for Children with Behavioral Disorders (TECBD) Conference in November 2006, 30*(4), 183–213.

McGee, G. G., Krantz, P. J., Mason, D., & McClannahan, L. E. (1983). A modified incidental- teaching procedure for autistic youth: Acquisition and generalization of receptive object labels. *Journal of Applied Behavior Analysis, 16*, 329–338.

McGee, G. G., Krantz, P. J., & McClannahan, L. E. (1985). The facilitative effects of incidental teaching on preposition use by autistic children. *Journal of Applied Behavior Analysis, 18*, 17–31.

McGee, G., & Morrier, M. (2003). Clinical implications of research in nonverbal behavior of children with autism. In P. Philippot, R. S. Feldman & E. J. Coats (Eds.). *Nonverbal behavior in clinical settings* (pp. 287–317). New York: Oxford University Press.

McGee, G. G., Morrier, M. J., & Daly, T. (1999). An incidental teaching approach to early intervention for toddlers with autism. *Journal of the Association for Persons with Severe Handicaps, 24*, 133–146.

McLaughlin, S. (1998). *Introduction to language development*. San Diego: Singular Publishing Group.

McTear, M. F. (1985). *Children's conversations*. Malden, MA: Blackwell Publishers.

Meyer, W. J., & Shane, J. (1973). The form and function of children's questions. *Journal of Genetic Psychology, 123*(2), 285–296.

Meyer, J. A., Mundy, P. C., van Hecke, A. V., & Durocher, J. S. (2006). Social attribution processes and comorbid psychiatric symptoms in children with Asperger syndrome. *Autism, 10*(4), 383–402.

Morrow, L. W., & Presswood, S. (1984). The effects of a self-control technique on eliminating three stereotypic behaviors in a multiply-handicapped institutionalized adolescent. *Behavioral Disorders, 9*(4), 247–253.

Muller, E., Schuler, A., Burton, B. A., & Yates, G. B. (2003). Meeting the vocational needs of individuals with Asperger's syndrome and other autism spectrum disabilities. *Journal of Vocational Rehabilitation, 18*, 163–175.

Mundy, P., & Crowson, M. (1997). Joint attention and early social communication: Implications for research on intervention with autism. *Journal of Autism and Developmental Disorders. Special Issue: Preschool Issues in Autism, 27*(6), 653–676.

National Research Council (2001). *Crime victims with developmental disabilities. Report of a workshop*. Washington, DC: National Academy Press.

Newsom, C., & Rincover, A. (1998). Autism. In: Mash, E. J., Barkley, R. A., (Eds.) *Treatment of childhood disorders* (pp. 286–346). New York: Guilford.

Nikopoulos, C. K., & Keenan, M. (2004). Effects of video modeling on social initiations by children with autism. *Journal of Applied Behavior Analysis, 37*(1), 93–96.

Orsmond, G. I., Krauss, M. W., Seltzer, M. M. (2004). Peer relationships and social and recreational activities among adolescents and adults with autism. *Journal of Autism and Developmental Disorders, 3*, 245–256.

Owen-DeSchryver, J. S., Carr, E. G., Cale, S. I., & Blakeley-Smith, A. (2008). Promoting social interactions between students with autism spectrum disorders and their peers in inclusive school settings. *Focus on Autism and Other Developmental Disabilities, 23*(1), 15–28.

Owens, R. E. (2008). *Language Development: An Introduction 7th Edition*. Boston: Allyn & Bacon.

Palmen, A., Didden, R., & Arts, M. (2008). Improving question asking in high functioning adolescents with autism spectrum disorders: Effectiveness of small group training. *Autism, 12*(1), 83–98.

Paul, R. (2008). Communication development and assessment. In K. Chawarska, A. Klin, & F.R. Volkmar (Eds.), *Autism spectrum disorders in infants and toddlers* (pp. 76–103). New York: Guilford.

Paul, R., Shriberg, L. D., McSweeny, J., Cicchetti, D., Klin, A., & Volkmar, F. (2005). Brief report: Relations between prosodic performance and communication and socialization ratings in high functioning speakers with autism spectrum disorders. *Journal of Autism and Developmental Disorders, 35*(6), 861–869.

Pierce, K., & Schreibman, L. (1995). Increasing complex social behaviors in children with autism: Effects of peer-implemented pivotal response training. *Journal of Applied Behavior Analysis, 28*(3), 285–295.

Pierce, K., & Schreibman, L. (1997). Using peer trainers to promote social behavior in autism: Are they effective at enhancing multiple social modalities? *Focus on Autism and Other Developmental Disabilities, 12*(4), 207–218.

Prizant, B. M. (1983). Language acquisition and communicative behavior in autism: Toward an understanding of the "whole" of it. *Journal of Speech and Hearing Disorders, 48*(3), 296–307.

Prizant, B. M., & Wetherby, A. M. (1987). Communicative intent: A framework for understanding social-communicative behavior in autism. *Journal of the American Academy of Child and Adolescent Psychiatry, 26*(4), 472–479.

Quinn, C., Swaggart, B. L., & Myles, B. S. (1994) Implementing cognitive behavior management programs for persons with *autism*: Guidelines for practitioners. *Focus on Autistic Behavior, 9*(4), 1–13.

Sawyer, L. M., Luiselli, J. K., Ricciardi, J. N., & Gower, J. L. (2005). Teaching a child with autism to share among peers in an integrated preschool classroom: Acquisition, maintenance, and social validation. *Education and Treatment of Children, 28*(1), 1–10.

Scattone, D. (2007). Social skills interventions for children with autism. *Psychology in the Schools. Special Issue: Autism Spectrum Disorders, 44*(7), 717–726.

Schreibman, L., Whalen, C., & Stahmer, A. C. (2000). The use of video priming to reduce disruptive transition behavior in children with autism. *Journal of Positive Behavior Interventions, 2*(1), 3–11.

Segrin, C. (2000). Social skills deficits associated with depression. *Clinical Psychology Review, 20*(3), 379–403.

Seltzer, M. M., Shattuck, P., Abbeduto, L., & Greenberg, J. S. (2004). Trajectory of development in adolescents and adults with autism. *Mental Retardation and Developmental Disabilities Research Reviews, 10*(4), 234–247.

Seltzer, M. M., Krauss, M. W., Shattuck, P. T., Orsmond, G., Swe, A., & Lord, C. (2003). The symptoms of autism spectrum disorder in adolescence and adulthood. *Journal of Autism and Developmental Disorders, 33*, 565–581.

Shapiro, E. S., Browder, D. M., & D'Huyvetters, K. K. (1984). Increasing academic productivity of severely multi-handicapped children with self-management: Idiosyncratic effects. *Analysis and Intervention in Developmental Disabilities, 4*(2), 171–188.

Shtayermman, O. (2007). Peer victimization in adolescents and young adults diagnosed with Asperger's syndrome: A link to depressive symptomatology, anxiety symptomatology and suicidal ideation. *Issues in Comprehensive Pediatric Nursing, 30*(3), 87–107.

Shabani, D. B., Katz, R. C., Wilder, D. A., Beauchamp, K., Taylor, C. R., & Fischer, K. J. (2002). Increasing social initiations in children with autism: Effects of a tactile prompt. *Journal of Applied Behavior Analysis, 35*, 79–83.

Sigafoos, J., & Reichle, J. (1993). Establishing spontaneous verbal behavior. In R. A. Gable & S. F. Warren (Eds.), *Strategies for teaching students with mild to severe mental retardation* (pp. 191–230). Baltimore, MD: Paul H Brookes Publishing.

Smith, T. (2001). Discrete trial training in the treatment of autism. *Focus on Autism and Other Developmental Disabilities, 16*, 86–92.

Stahmer, A. C., & Schreibman, L. (1992). Teaching children with autism appropriate play in unsupervised environments using a self-management treatment package. *Journal of Applied Behavior Analysis, 25*(2), 447–459.

Stark, R. (1979). Prespeech segmental feature development. In P. Fletcher & M. Garman (Eds.), *Language acquisition* (pp. 149–173). New York: Cambridge University Press.

Sterling, L., Dawson, G., Estes, A., & Greenson, J. (2008). Characteristics associated with presence of depressive symptoms in adults with autism spectrum disorder. *Journal of Autism and Developmental Disorders, 38*(6), 1011–1018.

Stewart, M. E., Barnard, L., Pearson, J., Hasan, R., & O'Brien, G. (2006). Presentation of depression in autism and Asperger syndrome: A review. *Autism, 10*(1), 103–116.

Strain, P. S., & Schwartz, I. (2001). ABA and the development of meaningful social relations for young children with autism. *Focus on Autism and Other Developmental Disabilities, 16*(2), 120–128.

Stone, W. L., & Caro-Martinez, L. M. (1990). Naturalistic observations of spontaneous communication in autistic children. *Journal of Autism and Developmental Disorders, 20*(4), 437–453.

Tager-Flusberg, H., Paul, R., & Lord, C. (2005). Language and Communication in Autism. *Handbook of Autism and Pervasive Developmental Disorders, 1*, pp. 335–364.

Talebi, J. L. (2008). Using a motivational extracurricular activity to improve the social interactions of adolescents with Asperger syndrome or high-functioning autism. *Dissertation Abstracts International Section A: Humanities and Social Sciences, 68*(10– A).

Tantam, D. (2000). Psychological disorder in adolescents and adults with Asperger syndrome. *Autism. Special Issue: Asperger Syndrome, 4*(1), 47–62.

Taylor, B. A., & Harris, S. L. (1995). Teaching children with autism to seek information: Acquisition of novel information and generalization of responding. *Journal of Applied Behavior Analysis, 28*(1), 3–14.

Taylor, B. A., Levin, L., & Jasper, S. (1999). Increasing play-related statements in children with autism toward their siblings: Effects of video modeling. *Journal of Developmental and Physical Disabilities, 11*(3), 253–264.

Thiemann, K. S., & Goldstein, H. (2001). Social stories, written text cues, and video feedback: Effects on social communication of children with autism. *Journal of Applied Behavior Analysis, 34*(4), 425–446.

Thorp, D. M., Stahmer, A. C., & Schreibman, L. (2005) Effects of sociodramatic play training on children with autism. *Journal of Autism and Developmental Disorders*, 25(3), 265–282.

Toth, K., Munson, J., Meltzoff, A. N., & Dawson, G. (2006). Early predictors of communication development in young children with autism spectrum disorder: Joint attention, imitation, and toy play. *Journal of Autism and Developmental Disorders, 36*(8), 993–1005.

Tsakanikos, E., Sturmey, P., Costello, H., Holt, G., & Bouras, N. (2007). Referral trends in mental health services for adults with intellectual disability and autism spectrum disorders. *Autism, 11*(1), 9–17.

United States Department of Labor (2008). Retrieved August 22, 2008, from http://www.dol.gov/dol/topic/statistics/employment.htm.

United States Census Bureau (2006). Retrieved August 22, 2008, from http://www.census.gov/popest/archives/2000s/vintage_2006/.

Vismara, L. A. (2006). Understanding the role of motivation in joint attention behaviors for children with autism. *Dissertation Abstracts International Section A: Humanities and Social Sciences 66*(10–A).

Vismara, L. A., & Lyons, G. L. (2007). Using perseverative interests to elicit joint attention behaviors in young children with autism: Theoretical and clinical implications to understanding motivation. *Journal of Positive Behavior Interventions, 9*, 214–228.

Warren, S. F., & Bambara, L. M. (1989) An experimental analysis of milieu language intervention: Teaching the action-object form. *Journal of Speech and Hearing Disorders, 54*, 448–461.

Wehman, P. (1978). Self-management programmes with mentally retarded workers: Implications for developing independent vocational behaviour. *British Journal of Social and Clinical Psychology, 17*(1), 57–64.

Wetherby, A. M., Cain, D. H., Yonclas, D. G., & Walker, V. G. (1988). Analysis of intentional communication of normal children from the prelinguistic to the multiword stage. *Journal of Speech and Hearing Research, 31*, 240–252.

Wetherby, A. M., & Prutting, C. A. (1984). Profiles of communicative and cognitive-social abilities in autistic children. *Journal of Speech and Hearing Research, 27*(3), 364–377.

Wilde, L. D., Koegel, L. K., & Koegel, R. L. (1992). *Increasing success in school through priming: A training manual.* Santa Barbara, California: University of California.

Wolfberg, P. J., & Schuler, A. L. (1999). Fostering peer interaction, imaginative play and spontaneous language in children with autism. *Child Language Teaching and Therapy, 15*(1), 41–52.

Yager, G. A. (1975). New behavioral emphasis: Turning the inside out. *Personnel and Guidance Journal, 53*(8), 585–591.

Zanolli, K., Daggett, J., & Adams, T. (1996). Teaching preschool age autistic children to make spontaneous initiations to peers using priming. *Journal of Autism and Developmental Disorders, 26*(4), 407–422.

63 Occupational Therapy

Linn Wakeford, Grace T. Baranek

Points of Interest

- Occupational therapy intervention for individuals with ASDs acknowledges the strengths and needs of the individual as embedded in and inseparable from the larger whole of meaningful daily life activities and social relationships.
- Individuals with ASDs and their larger social and cultural environments (e.g., families, school or work settings) are in constant interaction, each influencing and being influenced by the other. Therefore, those social and cultural contexts must be included in occupational therapy assessment and intervention processes.
- Similarly, the physical and temporal contexts of participation must be acknowledged and considered to ascertain how the individual with ASD "fits" into the particular situation and so that intervention strategies can be designed to address lack of fit.
- The meaning or value that an individual with ASD finds in various occupations and daily routines may differ significantly from that of persons without ASD, warranting careful attention to patterns in behavior that reveal motivation or purpose, and support intervention.
- Empirically supported strategies and approaches used by occupational therapists in addressing the needs of individuals with ASDs may be based on work from both occupational therapy and other fields, including education, psychology, and speech/language pathology. These strategies combine with a deep understanding of occupation and the wide array of factors that influence successful participation in daily life and result in individualized, comprehensive approaches to support participation for individuals with ASDs.
- Ongoing and future research endeavors for occupational therapists include work toward early identification, development of valid assessment tools, investigation of efficacious intervention approaches, as well as the further examination of the occupational experiences, values, and goals of people with ASDs and their families and significant others across the lifespan.

Introduction

Children, youth, and adults with autism spectrum disorders (ASDs) often find it difficult to participate successfully in one or more daily life activities or routines and to participate socially in family and community life. In addition, family members and other primary caregivers of individuals with ASDs often find their own participation in daily life difficult to orchestrate (Lee et al., 2008). Research indicates that both individuals with ASDs and their families often experience poorer quality of life, more social isolation, and/or a narrower range of life activities than do those who do not have ASDs (Donovan et al., 2005; Lee et al., 2008; Cederlund et al., 2008). Because occupational therapists are concerned with the ability of people, both individually and collectively, to participate meaningfully in these daily life activities and routines (occupations), as well as the social connections they imply, they are able to offer support and services to people with autism and their families in a variety of ways. Settings for occupational therapy service delivery may vary across the lifespan but often include early intervention settings, schools, family home, group homes, supported employment, outpatient clinics, mental health settings, and community-based programs.

The scope of occupational therapy practice includes a primary focus on enhancing participation in personal activities of daily living (e.g., basic self-care tasks), instrumental activities of daily living (e.g., meal preparation, financial management, care of pets), formal and informal education, work (including volunteering), play (e.g., constructive, social, symbolic, and outdoor play), and leisure (e.g., hobbies, restorative activities), and social participation at the levels of community, family, and friendships. Patterns, routines, and habits in these areas of occupation are addressed, as are the social, communication, sensory processing, cognitive, emotional, and motor aspects of occupational performance. In working specifically with people with ASDs, occupational therapists consider both core and associated features of the disorder in terms of their influence on patterns of and participation in occupation and identify strengths as well as areas of need in an effort to optimize engagement and participation in these occupations.

The DSM-IV-TR (APA, 2000) identifies core characteristics of autism as qualitative impairments in social interactions, qualitative impairments in communication, and restricted, repetitive, and stereotyped patterns of behavior, interests, and activities. Differences in sensory processing have also been documented as an associated feature in many individuals with ASDs (Kientz & Dunn, 1997; Baranek et al., 2006; Tomchek & Dunn, 2007) and appear correlated to core features (Ben-Sasson et al., 2009; Boyd et al., 2010; Gabriels et al., 2008; Hilton, Graver, & LaVesser, 2007). The influences of these core features and commonly associated characteristics on occupational participation can be significant. For example, tooth brushing may be a very difficult and unsatisfactory routine for both parent and child because of sensory processing difficulties and communication deficits that exacerbate the problem by limiting the ways the child has to let the parent know about the specific problem (i.e., is it the bristles of the brush, the texture, smell or taste of the toothpaste, or the echo of the parent's voice in the small tiled bathroom that are aversive?). Similarly, the inclusion of a 10-year-old with autism in outdoor play with his class may be quite limited by the child's insistence on repetitive play sequences, an overfocus on one particular aspect of the play, and/or difficulty managing the spontaneous nature of social interactions during the play.

The role of occupational therapists working with people with ASDs may include the following:

- Assessing the participation of those with ASDs in the occupations that are meaningful to them and/or to others involved with them, levels of satisfaction with that participation, and the contributions of that participation to quality of life. Both strengths and needs should be identified in the assessment process.
- Planning, implementation, and review (evaluation) of intervention (individual-, group-, or population oriented) that facilitates successful participation in daily life occupations
- Using educational and consultative models of service delivery to support families, teachers, other service providers, friends, and others in the community (coaches, religious leaders, scout leaders, etc.) who live, work, or play with individuals with ASDs
- Developing, contributing to, and/or disseminating results of programs of research that focus on early identification, development of relevant, functional assessment tools, trajectories of life participation and assessment of needs across the lifespan, and both early and lifespan interventions.

The remainder of this chapter will focus primarily on the occupational therapy processes of assessment and planning, implementing, and reviewing intervention for people with ASDs, as well as the use of education and consultation to support family members and others. The role of occupational therapists in research will be addressed briefly at the end of the chapter and under "Future Directions." We begin with the presentation of a conceptual framework that informs the delivery of occupational therapy services, and the ways in which this framework may be applied in practice to individuals with ASDs and their families and caregivers. A number of empirically supported strategies are included in the discussion of intervention and in case examples, but an extensive examination of the wide variety of specific intervention approaches and strategies that may be used by occupational therapy practitioners is beyond the scope of this chapter. (For more information on specific intervention approaches, please *see* Miller-Kuhanek, 2004; Baranek, Wakeford, & David, 2008; and Case-Smith & Arbesman, 2008.) Also, much of the discussion that follows addresses occupational therapy intervention for an individual with ASD, but because that individual is part of an important social context (e.g., family) the word "client system" in this chapter will be used to denote the individual and those key others as a single entity.

Participation in Occupational Situations

We use the term *occupational situation* to denote not only the daily life activity or routine (occupation) in which the individual needs or wants to participate but also the conditions surrounding that occupation, such as the physical, social, and cultural environments, as well as the temporal context (e.g., time of day, sequence of steps within the activity). Figure 63-1 shows the components of the occupational situation in relationship to one another, with participation in the occupation at the center, embedded in the contextual components. Because the occupational situation is a transactional (or dynamic) system, the two larger sets of arrows are used to represent the ongoing transactions that occur among contexts and participation (i.e., one's participation in an activity is influenced by context, and context is ultimately influenced by the fact that one is participating in something within it). There is a similar transaction that occurs that links all the individuals in the social context with one another and with all other contexts, as well as with the occupation itself, and these are represented by the smaller arrows to and from the person symbols. When considering the participation of a particular individual (the lighter person symbol in Figure 63-1), that individual is still embedded in the social context rather than

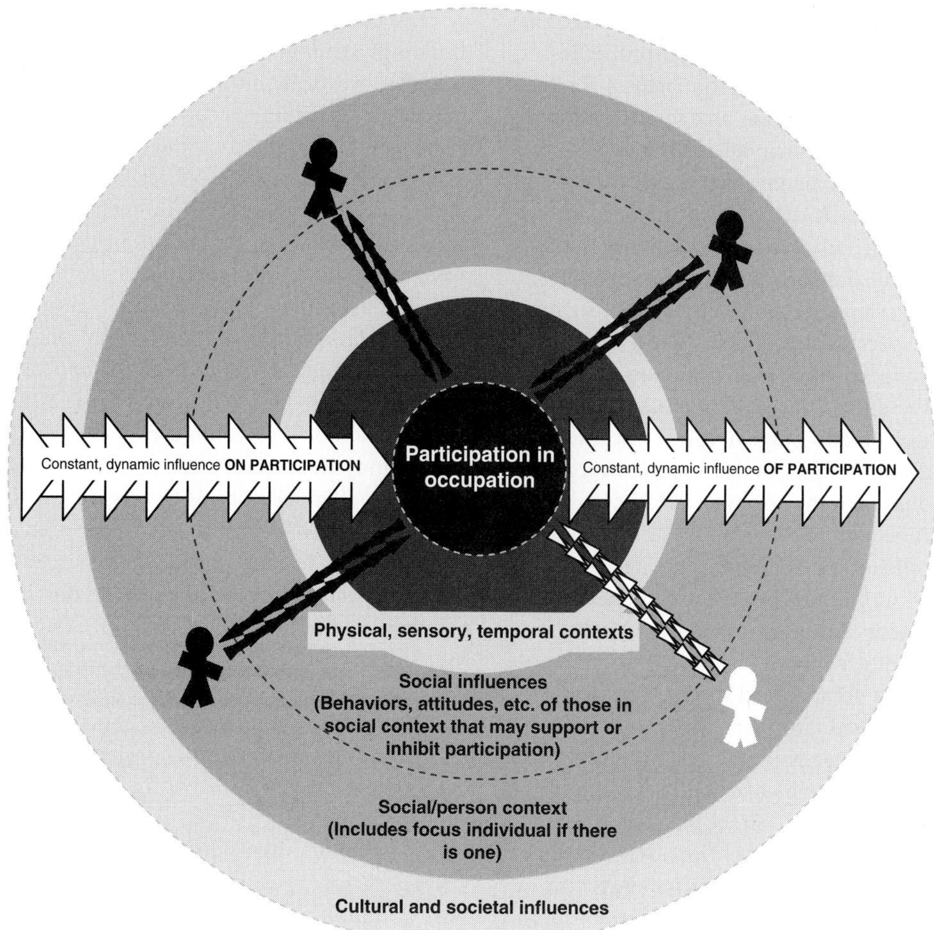

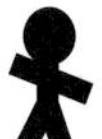
"PERSON" figure represents people in the situation, including likes/dislikes, preferences, perceptions, temperament, motivations, cognitive, communication, social, and sensory processing potential, as well as any individually expressed characteristics of ASD if present. The PERSON figure in white is the client (when the process is focused on an individual).

Figure 63–1. Participation in Occupational Situations (POS). "Person" figure represents people in the situation, including likes/dislikes, preferences, perceptions, temperament, motivations, cognitive, communication, social, and sensory processing potential, as well as any individually expressed characteristics of ASDs if present. The person figure in white is the client (when the process is focused on an individual).

separated from it. Although the Participation in Occupational Situations (POS) framework represents a conceptualization of occupational participation in general (i.e., it is not a "disability model"), its use to guide intervention for individuals with ASDs enables a perspective that views strengths or successes as easily as it does weaknesses or needs and allows for the use of a broader range of empirically supported interventions and translational research initiatives than does the use of approaches that target specific factors within the individual. More specific approaches (e.g., sensory processing, behavioral models, etc.) might be helpful as a part of overall intervention planning but are limited in their ability to provide a foundation for reasoning about *all* the contexts and factors that contribute to the ability of the person to participate in meaningful daily life activities.

From Conceptualization to Practice

The bridge between the conceptual foundations of occupational therapy and the practice itself is the practitioner's use of the most reliable, valid, and relevant evidence available, in concert with his/her own clinical reasoning and experience. Evidence-based practice in occupational therapy for people with ASDs includes the use of research, other relevant literature, information directly obtained from the client, and the expertise of the practitioner in areas that include the diagnosis itself and related or comorbid factors, tools, and methods for assessment; intervention strategies; methods of service delivery; family or caregiver concerns; specific occupations/activities; and/or the influence of contextual issues on occupational performance. The assessment process is informed by information about the development and psychometric properties of evaluation tools to determine their appropriateness for use with an individual with ASD. Many tools used for evaluation of people with other diagnoses or functional difficulties were not developed or standardized in a manner that makes them relevant or useful for those with ASDs, making the selection of evaluation tools a key first step in the occupational therapy process for this population. Similarly, intervention planning is incomplete without the examination of the evidence that supports action plans and specific intervention strategies, and this examination extends to information shared and recommendations made when the therapist is engaged in consultative modes of service delivery as well (Tickle-Degnen, 2002). The evidence may come from a variety of sources, and although research literature is typically considered the strongest evidence, all evidence should be examined for its integrity and its applicability to the specific client situation in question. In a recent study supported by the American Occupational Therapy Association's Evidence-Based Literature Review project, Case-Smith and Arbesman (2008) present a synthesis and review of interventions that may be used in occupational therapy practice with people with ASDs, categorized into six areas (sensory integration and sensory-based interventions; relationship-based, interactive interventions; developmental skill-based interventions; social-cognitive skills training, parent-directed or parent-mediated approaches; and intensive behavioral intervention). When tools, approaches, or strategies for which there is little or no solid evidence are included in an assessment of intervention plan, that plan should also include the systematic, well-documented collection of data to determine the efficacy of those strategies for the particular client. In addition, reliable, relevant evidence should be used not only in the planning of assessment and intervention but also as part of the ongoing process of re-evaluating and revising those plans (Tickle-Degnen, 2000).

Assessment

Although the occupational therapy assessment process may begin with a referral based on a specific need, the practitioner typically is interested in gathering as holistic a perspective on the client, typical environments, and desired or necessary occupations as possible. This is accomplished through a combination of interview methods (directly with the client and/or caregivers), structured and unstructured observations, and, at times, the administration of standardized assessment tools. Adherence to recommended practices that include client- and family-centered approaches dictates that the concerns, priorities, and desired outcomes of the individual and family/caregivers be considered central to the occupational therapy process (AOTA, 2008), so identifying those priorities and goals during the assessment is critical. Occupations that may be identified as challenging for young children with ASDs include many self-care activities, such as brushing teeth, washing hands, toileting and feeding, as well as constructive (building), symbolic, social and outdoor play, and, as children get older, pre-academic and academic tasks such as coloring, drawing, and writing may be added to the list of occupational challenges. Outings and errands in community settings such as a restaurant, the grocery store, or public library may be difficult, as may participation in religious events and family activities such as birthday parties or going to watch a sibling play basketball. Adolescents and adults with ASDs may have difficulty with many of these same types of occupations that comprise family, school, and community life (Cederlund et al., 2008) and may be in need of support to participate in leisure activities (Hilton, Crouch, & Israel, 2008) and to find and maintain paid or volunteer types of work. Social participation and the development of friendships are challenges faced by individuals with ASDs, regardless of age. Challenges for parents and other family members often include trying to integrate ways to meet their own needs for participation in various aspects of life with the need to provide structure, support (social, emotional, and financial), and treatment opportunities for their family member (DeGrace, 2004).

As the priority occupations are identified, the therapist can also begin to ascertain what current occupations are successful (as it is important to understand what is creating that success), determine the role of the environment in supporting or inhibiting the performance of occupations, and assess the extent to which individual likes, dislikes, temperament, abilities, and characteristics of autism (as expressed in that individual) support or inhibit occupational performance. Elements of occupational engagement and participation that are successful or satisfying and the interests, strengths, and resources of the client can be used both to provide motivation and to support intervention for areas of need.

Examination of the occupational situation (contexts or environments in which key occupations take place) should include consideration of the physical environment (e.g., arrangement and availability of objects, materials, built structures, elements of nature), the sensory characteristics (e.g., the frequency, duration, intensity, novelty, and complexity of different types of sensory input that may occur), the social environment (e.g., who is present, what they are doing and what role they have, how they relate to the client), the temporal context (e.g., time of day, sequences of activity, habitual or routine aspects of what happens in that environment), and cultural context, including broader cultural influences such as behaviors expected from workers in customer service jobs in the United States, as well as group or setting-specific manifestations of culture, such as a preschool teacher's use of the word "friend" for all children in the class, whether or not real friendships are evident among them all.

The individual also brings to the situation his or her own personality, temperament, preferences, perceptions, abilities (including cognitive, motor, sensory processing and communication), learning history, and needs, in addition to the specific characteristics of autism that are individually expressed. To the extent that they influence the performance of various activities or occupations, these characteristics of the individual should be included in the assessment process. Because the dynamics of participation in occupation are so embedded in the social context, the extent to which the individual is aware of, attends to, and interacts with others should be examined carefully during assessment. Observation and interview methods may yield sufficient information about the individual, but the therapist may administer standardized measures, such as those related to sensory processing and also may use the results of assessments conducted by other members of the team (e.g., speech-language pathologists and psychologists). In addition, the specific likes, dislikes, obsessions, habits, and routines of the individual should be determined, as they not only influence the performance of specific occupations but also provide insight into how occupations may hold meaning. This information is particularly salient for the design of intervention strategies that align with the motivation and strengths of the individual. Table 63-1 lists resources that may be helpful in conducting an occupational therapy assessment for individuals with autism, although not all of them have been specifically validated for this population.

Table 63–1.
Assessment tools

Assessment tools
Canadian Occupational Performance Measure
Law, Baptiste, McColl, Opzoomer, Polatajko, & Pollock, 1990 Law, Baptiste, Carswell, McColl, Polatajko, & Pollock, 1998
Children Helping Out: Responsibilities, Expectations, and Supports (CHORES)
Dunn, 2004
Child-Initiated Pretend Play Assessment
Stagnitti & Unsworth, 2004
Revised Knox Preschool Play Scale
Knox, 2008
Short Child Occupational Profile (SCOPE)
Bowyer, Kramer, Kielhofner, Maziero-Barbosa, & Girolami, 2007
School Function Assessment
Coster, Deeney, Haltiwanger, & Haley, 1998
Sensory Profile (Child, Infant-Toddler, Adolescent/Adult)
Dunn, 1999, 2002; Brown & Dunn, 2002
Sensory Processing Measure
Miller-Kuhaneck, Henry, & Glennon, 2007; Parham & Ecker, 2007; Miller-Kuhaneck, Henry, Glennon, & Mu, 2007
Sensory Experiences Questionnaire
Baranek, David, Poe, Stone, & Watson, 2006
Sensory Processing Assessment
Baranek, Boyd, Poe, David, & Watson, 2007
Test of Playfulness (Top) and Test of Environmental Supportiveness (TOES)
Skard & Bundy, 2008

Of particular importance to the assessment process is an analysis of occupational performance (AOTA, 2008), and this should be included in the assessment process whenever possible. As noted by Polatajko, Mandich, and Martini (2000), consideration of the individual's motivation for, understanding of, and actual ability to perform all or part of an activity must occur during direct observation of the individual performing the occupation in question in a natural context. In addition, the efficiency of performance, the amount and types of assistance needed, and the spoken and unspoken expectations regarding that performance must be understood by the therapist. This direct observation can offer valuable insights into difficulties and successes experienced by the individual and those participating with him/her that are not readily available with other methods of assessment. First, the occupation may hold different meaning for the individual with autism than it would for an individual without autism. Second, the way in which the individual understands or goes about the occupation to be performed may be affected by factors such as overfocus on particular parts of the activity and lack of attention to the activity as a whole, a need for sameness that makes it difficult to try something new, or difficulty expressing verbally what is or isn't understood about the task. Third, the interaction of the individual and the environment may be influenced by subtle or overt factors to which the individual has heightened, diminished, or unusual responses. This applies particularly to the sensory qualities of that environment and may include the frequency, intensity, duration, rhythm, novelty, and/or complexity of sounds, visual stimuli, movement and touch sensations, aromas, and tastes. Performance analysis allows the occupational therapist to observe facial expressions, eye gaze, gestures and other body movements as well as hear verbal communications from the client, all of which yield a much greater understanding of the client's actual experience of the occupation than is available when only interviews or standardized measures are used for assessment. This understanding by the therapist leads, in turn, to the harpist generating intervention strategies that are individualized and contextually relevant, using strengths, and targeting the observed, rather than "imagined," difficulties in performance.

Case Example:

Harold, a charming and relatively easy-going 3-year-old boy with autism, was usually cooperative in basic self-care occupations and particularly loved bath time. He had little expressive language, although receptively he was more competent, and he was able to follow simple routine one-step directions fairly consistently. He demonstrated aversion to high-pitched or sudden loud sounds and was a "picky eater" but otherwise tended to be hypo-responsive to sensory experiences, often needing significant movement, visual, and auditory (such as singing or "silly noises") input to get his attention. One of the difficulties noted by his mother, Maria, was getting his hair cut. She reported that although she took him to a salon that specifically catered to children, as soon as they pulled into the parking lot, Harold began to get upset and was often hard to get into the salon. Once inside, he could be distracted by the engaging toy play areas in which children and parents could wait or by looking at the selection of DVDs from which children could choose something to watch while getting their hair cut. However, when it was actually his turn and he was encouraged to climb into one of the four barber chairs (which were shaped like animals or vehicles), he began to cry and tantrum, and this often persisted throughout the haircut. Maria questioned whether or not this was a sensory processing issue, although she noted that he didn't mind having his hair combed or washed. Despite what seemed like a rather thorough conversation about this situation between the therapist and Maria, and the generation of several possible intervention strategies, the therapist still felt that until she had actually observed the situation, efficient intervention would be difficult to implement. Therefore, the therapist scheduled one of her next appointments with Harold and his mom for a morning on which Harold was scheduled to get a haircut.

Harold's behavior on arriving at and entering the salon was much as Maria had reported. Although there were other children there playing in the waiting area and getting their hair cut, Harold did not seem to attend to them, even when those in the play area were pointed out to him. As the therapist observed Harold at the DVD rack, she noted that he became over-focused on the Little Einstein™ videos (which he particularly liked), looking at and touching them one by one on the rack, repeatedly. When it came time for him to choose one, however, he had difficulty shifting his attention away from this activity and choosing only one. Maria eventually selected one for him, choosing the one that was his favorite and that he also had at home. Once he was seated in the "truck" seat and the DVD was playing on the small screen in front of him, Harold calmed down. The hair stylist then began cutting his hair with scissors, starting at the back. As she moved to the side, however, Harold began to get upset and swipe at the scissors with his hand. As she backed off, he again calmed down. Observing his facial expressions and eye movements as the hair stylist again tried to cut the hair near Harold's ears, the therapist noted that Harold seemed to catch the stylist in his peripheral vision, disrupting his attention to the video and creating a subtle startle reaction. It seemed that when all his visual attention was on the video, he essentially could "ignore" the stylist. When the therapist noted this out loud, the stylist picked up on the cue, and stayed behind Harold to finish cutting his hair. Harold had no further difficulty until it was time to leave, as he had to stop watching the DVD and give back the case, which he had been holding.

As a result of this performance analysis, the therapist recommended the following beginning intervention strategies:

1. Allow Harold to choose a DVD from among two of his favorites at home, take it with him to the salon, watch it there, and then bring it home again.

2. Have the stylist stay behind Harold to cut his hair (out of his peripheral view).

Four weeks later, at his next hair cut, these strategies were used, and Harold participated in the process without having a tantrum or getting upset. As time went on, the stylist was able to also use an electric razor on the hair on Harold's neck and over his ears, which hadn't been tried before because of concerns about his potential responses to this. Using only Maria's description of the haircut scenario, enhanced by the therapist's questioning, any number of intervention strategies may have been generated, many of which may not have led to a more successful trip to the hair salon. However, given the opportunity to observe and really see how Harold was participating in and reacting to this whole situation allowed the therapist to suggest strategies that targeted the specific problems noted, resulting in an efficient resolution of the problem.

In this example in which "getting a haircut" is the occupational routine, larger socio-cultural influences about grooming and appearance intersected with the values and preferences within Harold's family, creating a situation in which Harold was expected to get his hair cut fairly short every 4 weeks or so. This "haircut" situation also included the social, physical, and sensory characteristics of the environment in the hair salon, some aspects of which were actually supportive of Harold's participation. Harold was good at focusing on the movies he really liked, was careful with the DVD case, and, because of his typical low levels of arousal, was perfectly happy to sit still in the barber chair and watch TV. However, his past experience in this environment was not particularly positive, he didn't attend to the other children (and so wasn't able to use them as models), he had difficulty with the transitions that involved the DVD, and his heightened awareness of things in his peripheral visual field created difficulty for Harold. In addition, neither his mother nor the hair stylist, despite good intentions, had been able to change the situation, including their own behavior, to create a more successful performance. Harold's participation in getting a haircut was being created by all of these factors interacting with one another, and the therapist had to recognize and consider all aspects of this transaction in both assessment and intervention. The POS framework emphasizes that the potential for success in occupational participation is not housed in the characteristics of the individual alone but rather is the result of a working transaction within the situation as a whole. Therefore, all of these factors must be considered and examined in the assessment process, and that examination should include performance analysis whenever possible.

Intervention

Occupational therapy intervention occurs in three parts: planning, implementation, and review (AOTA, 2008). Although these may occur in a single discrete sequence at times, particularly in the initial process with a client system, they frequently "cycle" with some variability, depending on factors such as the methods and length of service delivery, desired outcomes of intervention, and documentation requirements. Intervention planning, implementation, and review should occur as a collaborative process that includes, at the least, the individual, family/caregivers, and the occupational therapist. Depending on the specific practice setting, a larger team may be involved (teachers, speech-language pathologist, psychologist, employer, coach, etc.), affording more collaboration for the benefit of the client.

Planning

Optimal intervention planning evolves naturally from the assessment process described above and takes into consideration not only the strengths and needs of the individual but also the concerns, expectations, strengths, resources and limitations of those living or working with that individual on a regular basis, as well as the situations in which the occupations typically occur. As the POS framework implies, the transactional nature of all participation in occupation means that a change or strategy inserted in one aspect of the action will have an effect on all other aspects, so intervention is planned with this understanding in mind. In addition, intervention plans must take into account the core and associated features of autism, particularly as they are expressed in the individual.

Plans for intervention begin with the establishment of goals that reflect the outcomes desired by the client, stated in measurable terms and targeting change in occupational performance, social participation, quality of life, and/or client satisfaction with one of more of these. Based on these stated goals, more specific plans for action can be designed and optimal methods of service delivery chosen. Action plans may include any or all of the following types of occupational therapy intervention: therapeutic use of self, use of occupation and purposeful activity, consultation, and education (AOTA, 2008), as they are appropriate to the client and situation. (Further discussion of these types of intervention and their specific application to people with ASDs follows below.) Although methods of service delivery in general occupational therapy practice may range from segregated (one-on-one or "pull-out") to integrated (within the natural contexts, activities and routines of the client), use of the POS framework and of performance analysis as a key assessment method, and the difficulties many people with ASDs demonstrate with generalization, should lead to the use of the most integrated models of service delivery possible in any given situation. Specifically planned, intentional uses of more segregated models may be appropriate at times, but plans should include transitions to more natural situations as quickly as possible.

Although it may seem premature to some, occupational therapy intervention planning should encompass discharge planning as well. Because occupational therapy is indicated for situations in which there is not a good "fit" among the individual/client, important occupations, and the contexts in which those occupations occur, the need for occupational therapy services may come and go for any particular client. As a part of intervention planning, the therapist discusses with the entire client system how often progress and goals will be reviewed, what will happen when goals are met, and what resources may be available in the community or elsewhere during times when occupational therapy services are not needed. This type of planning also takes into account the need for and process of transitions that may occur when occupational therapy services will be provided in a different manner or setting. The integration of intervention planning and discharge planning does not necessarily limit the course or scope of occupational therapy services provided in the present, nor does it preclude the re-institution of services when the need arises, but it allows all involved to be prepared for what follows the current course of intervention.

Implementation

Implementation of occupational therapy intervention is the enactment of the plan designed by the therapist, client, and others in collaboration with one another. As noted above, intervention strategies may fall into one or more of the following categories of intervention type: therapeutic use of self, use of occupation, and purposeful activity, consultation, and education.

Therapeutic use of self refers to the intentional use, by the therapist, of his or her interactive style, personality, perceptions, or insights as supports to the therapeutic process. The most common uses of this type of intervention are to develop rapport with the individual or entire client system and/or to enhance motivation. The therapist's role is to support the relationship between him- or herself and client (individual or entire system), help establish and maintain trust, and ideally create a relationship in which the client feels safe and willing to take on challenges. The importance of the therapist–child relationship in working with individuals with ASDs cannot be overstated. The willingness and ability of the therapist to attend to and be present with the individual allows significant opportunities to read subtle cues as intentional communication, to try to discern and understand motivations that are not obvious, and to respond with respect and reasonable expectation. Given the difficulties that most with children with ASDs have communicating with others and establishing social connectedness, the effort of the therapist to establish a relationship is an exceptionally important aspect of intervention.

Another role of the therapist is to elicit specific behaviors in the individual. The body of literature on relationship-based interventions for individuals with ASDs is particularly relevant to this type of occupational therapy intervention (Case-Smith & Arbesman, 2008). For example, research on the use of responsive interaction strategies with children with autism indicates that when parents, through their own behaviors, encourage and support their children in engaging in reciprocal social interactions, the children are able to develop pivotal behaviors such as joint attention, turn-taking, and imitation, all of which are key to learning and further participation in a variety of occupations (Greenspan & Weider, 1997; Baranek, Reinhartsen, & Wannamaker, 2001; Mahoney & Perales, 2003, 2005). In addition, Nadel et al. (2008) found that children with autism were more likely to approach adults who were imitative and playful than adults that were not. Although there is no significant research specifically targeting the use of these types of responsiveness by therapists, the use of interpersonal strategies that include sensitive attention to an individual's cues, and responses to those cues in ways that are contingent, reciprocal, and affectively appropriate, are well in line with the occupational therapist's role. Most responsive strategies can be embedded incidentally in a variety of occupational situations, as noted in the example below. These behaviors may include the positioning of the therapist relative to the individual, following the individual's lead in the activity, reinforcing all efforts at intentional communication, imitation of the individual's actions or vocalizations, and scaffolding behaviors (Mahoney & MacDonald, 2007). Returning to the POS framework, the therapist's goal is to create change in occupational participation through intentional change in the social context. Later in the chapter, further discussion of other types of intervention will examine how changes in the behaviors of others in the social context also can be used to support participation.

Case Example

Sarah is a 6-year-old girl with autism and minimal verbal skills who likes painting with a brush on large sheets of paper while vocalizing to herself in a low sing-song voice. She often uses repetitive actions to dip her brush and to make single slow strokes on the paper. If the teacher sits behind her in an effort to help her, Sarah actually waits for the teacher to give her a physical prompt to dip her brush in the paint again. Sarah doesn't attend to children or adults around her and doesn't look at the teacher even if the teacher is giving her physical prompts. The occupational therapist, Thomas, understands that Sarah may find it easier to interact with an adult initially, although his ultimate goal is to support Sarah's participation in the occupation of painting with classmates. Therefore, Thomas chooses several behaviors he can enact to elicit more social interaction and sense of shared engagement from Sarah and help her build more variety in her approach to painting. The first is to position himself in front of her, so that face to face interaction is possible, and he can read her facial expressions and follow her eye gaze. The second is to imitate her actions and vocalizations, using his own brush and paint, painting at the top of her paper. Attending carefully to small changes in her facial expression and posture, he sees that she's noticed what he's doing, although she hasn't looked up at him yet. He continues to imitate her, and she looks up at him briefly before returning to her own painting. He continues to imitate her actions and vocalizations but speeds them up a bit, becoming slightly more animated in his behavior. Sarah looks up at him with heightened interest, so he repeats his action. He sees that Sarah is very alert to his presence and actions, which is a nice change, but she isn't yet changing her own activity-related behaviors, so he alternates imitating her exact actions with animating his actions and vocalizations. Eventually Sarah takes turns with Thomas, imitating him interspersed with his imitation of her. Thomas is now able to introduce "new ways" of painting, such as using different colors and making different strokes with her brush. Her participation in this occupation has now changed to include "doing with," and her understanding and performance of painting has changed. Although her goal of painting with her classmates, as a shared experience, has not yet been met, she is closer to it than she was, and her occupational therapist can now work to connect her with the other children who are also painting.

Use of purposeful activity and occupation is a core foundation of occupational therapy intervention, and although certainly the choice of specific occupations and activities is a key element of this, the context, structure, and process of the occupation are of equal importance. It should be noted that the intervention strategies that are discussed in the following section may have been specifically validated for people with autism, but others may have been designed more generally to support the participation of people with many different abilities and disabilities. A combination of these two approaches may be considered. In a commentary published in the *Journal of Autism and Developmental Disorders*, Wolery (2000) made an astute statement that perhaps still holds true today: "To date, we have no strategies that are effective for all children with autism and are contraindicated for all other children with disabilities. Thus, the research on teaching other students with disabilities...may have relevance for students with autism." A similar stance seems appropriate for occupational therapists working with people with autism of all ages—using empirically supported strategies developed for other populations or by other professions broadens the possibilities for finding a combination of strategies that work well for any individual or client system in a particular occupational situation. The use of reasonable but relatively "uninvestigated" strategies may be undertaken with regular collection of data and re-assessment to assure efficacy of the intervention and satisfaction of the client system.

Because participation in occupation is intended, at most times, to be both the means *and* the end of occupational therapy intervention, the continuity between goals and intervention strategies should be evident. Thus the selection of the occupation or activity during which intervention will be embedded is based on specific goals and the routines and daily life activities of the entire client system. At times, opportunities for new occupations or for participating in familiar occupations in different settings will be included in intervention, again based on the needs of the individual and of the client system as a whole.

Another element to be considered in the selection of activities/occupations is meaning: the meaning of the activity/occupation for the individual and the meaning for the family or other significant social system. The meaning perceived by the individual may differ slightly or significantly from that perceived by family or others, and clarity about the purpose of participation and the expectations of all involved are important considerations. Spitzer (2004) expands on this idea and emphasizes the need to attend to the perception or subjective experience of the individuals in the occupational situation. In the example of Harold and the haircut situation, the meaning to Harold of getting a haircut is difficult to know with certainty but likely was significantly different from that of his mother, Maria, for whom the meaning involved the appearance of her child and her role as a mother who cared appropriately for her children.

The context, structure, and process of occupation used in a therapeutic setting offer significant opportunity for variation and for creating a situation that "fits" the client well.

Using the POS framework as a guide, the occupational therapist may consider intervention that targets or uses the various contexts (cultural, social, physical, sensory, and/or temporal) that create the occupational situation and may also make adaptations to the structure or process of the occupation itself. It should be noted that although these elements are addressed separately below, they are essentially inseparable, and strategies are typically used in combination to provide an individualized intervention designed to support participation in the specific occupational situation, as a whole.

In each occupational situation, cultural context may be a broad construct that reflects values and beliefs thought to be representative of a large group of people (e.g., U.S. citizens, Latino immigrants, Catholics) or may be more localized or specific, representing the values and beliefs of a much smaller group of people, such as a school, workplace, classroom, or family. Because "culture," regardless of its expanse, is often enacted through routines and rituals and often relies on interpersonal interaction for its perpetuation (Bonder, 2004; Iwama, 2005), it is an important context to consider when working with individuals with ASDs. The extent to which the individual's rituals and routines are consistent or in conflict with the rituals and routines of the identified culture will affect group membership of the individual and participation in occupation (Spitzer, 2004; Iwama, 2005). Similarly, the ability of the individual to engage in the types of social exchanges in which cultural norms are shared will effect participation. Occupational therapy intervention then must address the "fit" between the individual (including both strengths and challenges) and cultural context, either using the norms of the culture to support occupational participation or seeking change to create a better fit when necessary. This also includes work within family culture, as the previous rituals, routines, and meaningful daily life activities of the family may be restricted or abandoned to meet the needs of the individual with autism (DeGrace, 2004).

Adaptations to or constructions of the social context are particularly difficult to describe as separate from the occupation itself because they are inherently embedded in one another. The social context provides the "venue" for the learning, doing, changing, and terminating of occupation, and occupation, or activity, simultaneously does the same for social participation. This creates the opportunity for various roles in the social context, such as partner, learner, and teacher. For example, Humphry and Wakeford (2006) relate the interchange between Matthew, a preschooler with autism, and the social context of his classroom as he develops interest and participation in building with blocks. His interest evolves from encouragement from his mother and teacher to see what other children are doing with blocks, and then his own spontaneous peripheral participation (i.e., watching) as classmates build with blocks. As his interest builds his willingness to participate actively, he's drawn in to the "block building situation." As he is supported to participate on a more active level, his actions affect those of his peers and vice versa, and his participation expands to use of other types of materials for building, which then leads to another type of social opportunity—that is, shared construction of a structure. As evidenced in part by this example, occupational therapists may work to support the social participation of the individual to facilitate participation in a "group occupation," further develop or refine performance of a particular occupation, and/or support the development of friendships.

Peer-mediated interventions are well-researched and have significant empirical support as successful strategies for enhancing social interactions for individuals with ASDs. DiSalvo and Oswald (2002) present a review of a variety of tested methods to support peer interactions for children with autism, and these methods range from group (e.g., integrated peer groups) to one-on-one (e.g., peer tutors) contexts and represent a continuum from direct teaching of peers to direct teaching of the target child. Peer-mediated approaches have been documented not only to support the development of social skills but also to support participation in particular occupational situations, such as outdoor play (Kern, 2006; Harper, Symon, & Frea, 2007), other play settings (Bass & Mulick, 2007; Lee, Odom, & Loftin, 2007), and a variety of self-care and classroom routine behaviors (Kohler et al., 1997). Friendship clubs (Kampa et al., 2003), peers as on-camera subjects in video-modeling strategies, and the use of peer "buddies" are among the ways in which peers may be used to support occupational participation.

A number of strategies mentioned previously may be used in addition to or combination with peer-mediated strategies. Social Stories may be used to support engagement in occupation and peer interactions simultaneously. For example, Sandt (2008) outlines how social stories may help children with ASDs participate in both the activities and social interactions that occur in physical education classes, and Barry and Burlew (2004) describe a study in which social stories were successful in changing both object and peer play skills of two children with severe autism. In a description of a low-tech adaptation to support outdoor play for a preschooler with ASD, Wakeford (2008) discusses the use of visual supports in a book format with pictures of both activities and playmates from which the child could make choices. She also describes the use of the book strategy as a setting for collaboration between children in both the creation and the later reading of the book. The use of music in combination with peer-mediated approaches is examined by Kern (2006) and found helpful in establishing increased peer interaction and participation in an outdoor play activity. Danko and Buysse (2002) recommend the identification of special skills and potential common interests as a way to facilitate opportunities for social interaction between children with ASDs and their peers, as well as assuring that the environment contains materials for activities that encourage mutual engagement. Occupational therapists may guide or implement such intervention based on relevant information obtained during the occupational therapy assessment about both the individual and the environment. In addition, occupational engagement may be used to develop or enhance social connections, as in Reynold's (2006) case report regarding the participation of an older child with ASD on a lacrosse team and the ways in which her engagement in the game led to increased social interaction and group membership with her teammates.

Adaptations to or modifications of the physical and sensory environment may be designed to support desired behaviors, to inhibit undesired behaviors, or both. For example, Yuill et al. (2007) found that the expanse of space and arrangement of structures in a playground setting had significant effects on the play and social behaviors of eight boys with ASDs. Similarly, Duker and Rasing (1989) demonstrated that changes made in the arrangement of a classroom environment resulted in more on-task behaviors and fewer self-stimulatory behaviors for three young men with autism. The identification of a "home-base" is described as a modification to the physical environment that allows children with autism a place to "regroup" when the environment becomes too challenging (Dunn, Saiter, & Rinner, 2002). Considerations for the safety of the individual may also lead to adaptations to the physical environment, including placement of gates or barriers or installation of alarm systems to alert caregivers if the individual tries to leave a particular area independently. As noted in a chapter by Baranek, Wakeford, & David (2008), research on environmental modifications to address sensory processing issues is scarce, but those environments may be adapted to provide more opportunities for movement or other types of sensation or to decrease the amount or type of sensation present, depending on the needs of the individual. For example, the carpet, pillows, and bookshelves for a preschool reading corner were moved to a corner of the room near a large window. This allowed 4-year-old Katie to take advantage of the comfort and opportunities available in the reading corner without having to cope with her aversion to the visual and vibratory sensations created by the fluorescent light over the area in which the reading corner once resided.

In addition to these kinds of larger changes in the layout and use of physical space, the addition and location of objects and materials in the environment may also be used to support participation in various ways. Introducing new items or materials by placing them in view but not as focal objects may have a "priming" affect, allowing the individual to accommodate to the new item before interacting with it directly (Dunn et al., 2002). Locating all the scissors at the end of the table where the child with autism is sitting sets up a situation in which others interact with him or her to obtain a pair of scissors during art class. Adding visual supports to the environment (Ball, 1999; Odom et al., 2003), such as step-by-step pictures for toothbrushing at the sink (Pilebro & Bäckman, 2005), may increase on-task behaviors and independence in self-care routines.

Temporal context includes not only the time of day but also the duration and frequency of the occupation, what activities or routines have come before and what will come after the occupation in question, and transitions. The significantly temporal nature of habits and routines makes them important as well, and this is particularly true when parents, teachers, employers, friends, and others have routines and expectations about the use of time that are different from those of the individual. In addition, temporal considerations intersect with cycles of hunger, thirst, and fatigue, and all of these in turn affect the ability of the individual to process sensory information, communicate optimally, and pay attention to that which is salient to the current activity. Intervention strategies that target the temporal context may include addressing how long the activity lasts, how often it occurs (e.g., frequency of opportunities), the duration and frequency of transitions, the sequence of activities, the extent to which the creation of a routine or habit is encouraged, and/or ways to assure that the individual's needs for food, drink, and rest are met within the sequence of activity. Common strategies include the use of timers, teaching first-then concepts, musical or visual "warnings" about or signifiers of transition times, alternation of active and sedentary activities, giving the individual a "job" to have a socially acceptable reason for moving about, and establishing consistent, predictable routines for basic self-care tasks. Strategies with empirical support include the use of visual supports to communicate about time use (e.g., picture schedules, written list of the order of activities) (Ball, 1999; Dettmer et al., 2000) and the use of musical elements to support the timing and sequencing of self-care (Kern, Wakeford, & Aldridge, 2007) and classroom activities (Register & Humpal, 2007). Transitions are often particularly difficult for people with ASDs, and a combination of strategies (i.e., to increase salience of cues about and predictability of transitions) is often necessary for there to be a successful move from participation in one occupation or activity to participation in the next (Sterling-Turner & Jordan, 2007). These strategies, however, typically affect one or more other people, as illustrated in the case example below, and collaboration to assure satisfactory outcomes for the client system as a whole is important.

Case Example

Josh, a 17-year-old youth with ASD, has been working at a diner-style restaurant every weekday morning before school for 2 months. His parents alternate dropping him off at the restaurant based on their own work schedules, so that his mom drops him off 3 days, and his dad drops him off on 2 days. After he's completed all his work tasks, he catches the school bus in front of the diner. Josh has a list for each day on which he marks off each task as it gets done. For the first month of the job, an occupational therapist provided on-site support for Josh, starting on a daily basis and by the end of the month dropping to once a week or as needed. Since he's had the job, the first task on the list has been to help the manager bring all the large garbage cans from outside into the back part of the kitchen. Other tasks include taking all the chairs down off the tables and making sure that each table has full containers of salt, pepper, sugar packets, and ketchup. Josh is a good worker and the manager is very pleased to have him. However, over the last several weeks Josh has been arriving a little earlier at work the days his dad drops him off because of changes in his dad's work schedule. This has become a problem because the manager has things he needs to do before he's ready to help Josh get the trash cans into the kitchen. This means Josh has to wait for the manager, and this makes him anxious. Josh paces, touching things in the kitchen rhythmically as he walks, and he sings, getting louder and louder over time. The manager gets distracted, trying to reassure Josh, and then takes longer to complete his own tasks, prolonging even further Josh's waiting time, and escalating the situation. Although there are a number of possible interventions that would address the temporal dissonances here, the solution that caused the least disruption and was possible for all involved was to move the trash can task to last on Josh's list and have him begin taking chairs off tables first, as that was a task he could do on his own, whether the manager was available or not. Because he works five mornings a week, Josh had frequent opportunities to learn the new sequence of tasks, supported by the visual reminder of the list and minimal coaching by the therapist, and within a little over a week was initiating his "new" first task on his own.

As noted previously, the structure and process of occupation may also be adapted in a variety of ways to support participation. A number of empirically supported strategies for adapting the structure or process of occupation are discussed in some detail in publications by Baranek, Wakeford, and David (2008), Case-Smith and Arbesman (2008), and Dunn, Saiter, and Rinner (2002). The use of visual supports in the form of activity schedules, choice boards, step-by-step task sequences (Bryan & Gast, 2000), work systems (Hume & Odom, 2007), Social Stories™ (Gray & Garand, 1993; Kuoch & Mirenda, 2003), and variations on social stories (Brownell, 2002; Marr et al., 2007) are among the most successful means of adapting the structure or process of occupational participation. The addition of musical elements, mentioned previously, and the use of priming (Dunn, Saiter, & Rinner, 2002; Koegel et al., 2003), are supported in the research literature as effective augmentations that support participation of those with ASDs, and video modeling has been used by both occupational therapists (Kashman, Mora, & Glaser, 2000) and other professionals (McCoy & Hermansen, 2007) to teach both social and functional skills. Adaptations to the sensory qualities of a routine, activity, or occupation may support those who need more or less intensity, predictability, novelty or complexity of sensation to participate optimally (Dunn, Saiter, & Rinner, 2002; Baranek & Wakeford, 2000). For example, for some children who need enhanced sensory input to maintain an appropriate arousal level, sitting on an inflatable cushion or therapy ball during tabletop work may be helpful, as may standing up to work. Using textured surfaces for drawing activities, singing rather than saying task directions, adding sand to paints in art class, or using brightly colored tape to mark work areas may also be useful for other children. For some children who tend to be over-responsive to one or more types of sensory input, clearly delineated spaces in which to sit or stand may be helpful (thus diminishing the chances of unexpected touch by others), as may being first or last in a line. Allowing the individual to explore new materials or processes by watching others (a form of priming) and visual supports or songs that create predictability about the task may also be helpful. Some individuals who demonstrate sensory-seeking behaviors may benefit from some of the strategies listed above related to enhancing sensation, as well as to having objects or "fidget" toys, and opportunities to engage in "heavy work" activities, such as carrying a laundry basket, raking, vacuuming, or pushing a cart loaded with work supplies. The field of special education offers other naturalistic intervention measures that may support occupational participation for people with autism, including the use of positive reinforcement, prompting, time delay, and incidental teaching (Cowan & Allen, 2007; Vuran, 2007; Liber, Frea, & Symon, 2008; Kurt & Tekin-Iftar, 2008). The use of alternative and augmentative communication and other types of technology have been documented as a way to support functional communication and overall participation as well (More, 2008).

Consultation and education are methods of service delivery that can be used to support parents, siblings, other family members, and a wide variety of possible others who are involved with the individual with autism. These methods of service delivery may occur simultaneously with, in addition to, or even in the absence of the occupational therapist's work directly with an individual and may also be used to address the needs of a client that is not an individual but rather is a group, organization, or population. Consultation typically involves the occupational therapist in a collaborative relationship centered on making recommendations or generating solutions to identified problems but not as the party responsible for implementing the actual plan or for the results of the plan. For example, an occupational therapist may help the mother of child with autism generate ideas for a playroom environment that maximizes the child's opportunities for functional toy and social play; the mother then implements all or some of the ideas. Education typically involves the therapist in providing information or instruction to others, but without immediate or specific changes in the occupational participation or performance of a client. For example, an occupational therapist may provide a workshop on sensory processing in autism and its potential effect on worker behaviors for staff of a job training program.

Both consultation and education draw on the ability of the therapist to use themselves and their knowledge therapeutically, to develop rapport, to maintain good relationships, and to create an environment that facilitates willingness to learn, to accept challenges and potentially to make changes. This is particularly important given the increasing use of natural environments and integrated models of service delivery in early intervention and school settings and the rise in parent-mediated intervention approaches that are being investigated and used for children with autism. Team and collaborative approaches are recognized as optimal to develop the strengths and meet the needs of people with autism in a variety of settings, and the ways in which the occupational therapist provides consultation and education to others can affect the overall efficacy of intervention.

Parents and siblings of an individual with autism may require particular attention in terms of consultation and education services for a number of reasons. Despite both anecdotal and scientific reports that include positive parent perspectives on living with and loving a child with autism, the difficulties of this situation also are well-documented. Parents of newly diagnosed or young children may need help with a variety of issues, including finding community, educational, and therapy resources; beginning to understand their child's ASD; and learning the basic, ongoing types of intervention strategies that are likely to support their child's participation in a variety of environments and activities. Parents of young, adolescent, and adult children with autism report significant concerns about issues such as sleeping and eating patterns, pre-academic and academic success, social skills and development of friendships, sexuality, financial stability, independent living skills, and, ultimately, what will happen to their child when one or both parents die. Parenting stress in this population is variable, depending on a number of factors, but depression is not uncommon, especially among mothers. Also, given the research examining the genetic factors linked to autism, there is the possibility that siblings of the individual are also on the autism spectrum and/or that one or both parents have subthreshold characteristics of autism (broader autism phenotype). Although this may not be true in the majority of cases, it speaks to the need for occupational therapists to consider carefully the perspective, learning and interaction style, and coping mechanisms (internal and external resources) of the parents and family members to whom they may be providing consultation or education.

Review and Outcome Measurement

During and after the implementation of intervention, the occupational therapist reviews and evaluates, with the client, the effectiveness of chosen strategies and the outcomes of the intervention process. As noted previously, assessment and intervention should be planned and implemented based on a combination of client input, the most reliable evidence available, and the experience and reasoning of the occupational therapist. Intervention review is conducted as a part of evidence-based practice and in regard for ethical obligations to make the best and most appropriate use of the client's resources. Methods of review may include re-evaluation using assessment tools that were used on initial evaluation, the accomplishment of outcomes stated in short- or long-term goals, and/or the use of quantifiable measures of progress such as goal attainment scaling. Outcomes may include changes in the actual performance of targeted occupations, level of participation in occupational situations as a whole, satisfaction of the client, and/or quality of life. Intervention review and measurement of outcomes allows the client and the therapist to determine which interventions are working and how quickly progress is being made and to determine whether there is a need for changes in the intervention plan or initiation of a discharge plan.

Research

The contributions of occupational therapists to research evolve from unique perspectives on occupation and on the wide array of factors that influence the many behaviors that comprise daily life and participation in occupation. For example, an emphasis on the "lived experience" of the client as a central theme in occupation has led to research examining the meaning of occupation for children with autism (Spitzer, 2003) and the orchestration of daily life for families of children with autism (DeGrace, 2004). Occupational experiences were also the focus of a study conducted by Hilton, Crouch, and Israel (2008), who investigated the extent to which children with high-functioning autism participate in leisure or social events outside of school. In addition, an understanding of the mechanisms that underlie the ability of the individual to process and use sensory information, and the relationship among sensory processing, self-regulation, and participation occupational situations, has led to research focused on early identification of autism (Baranek, 1999; Reznick et al., 2007), a better understanding of the difference in sensory processing in people with autism relative to those with other disabilities or typically developing persons (Baranek et al., in revision, Watson et al., 2007; Watling, Dietz, & White, 2001), the development of assessment tools that help discriminate between those with ASDs and those with other disabilities or typical development (Kientz & Dunn, 1997; Baranek et al., 2006), and the influence of sensori-motor differences on the performance of self-care tasks in preschoolers with autism (Jasmin et al., 2009). To date, much of the intervention research related to occupational therapy approaches for children with autism focuses on sensory integration or sensory-based methods and has been criticized for lack of scientific rigor, small sample sizes, lack of focus on functional or occupational outcomes, and lack of transparency or replicability (Baranek, 2002; Mulligan, 2003; Schaff & Miller, 2005). Therefore, in addition to the continuation of programs of research already being conducted by occupational therapists working with and for people with autism, there is a particular need for scientifically rigorous research that addresses occupational experiences and outcomes for people with ASDs and their families across the lifespan, is developed in collaboration with stakeholders and an interdisciplinary team, is replicable, and includes dissemination to consumers, service-providers, and other researchers. This is consistent with calls for a different approach to research from within the profession of occupational therapy (Kielhofner et al., 2004) and for translational research initiatives coming from the National Institutes for Health (2008) and the nteragency Autism Coordinating Committee (2009).

Challenges and Future Directions

Occupational therapists are spearheading a wide range of studies that will lead to continuation and further development of translational ASD research programs related to early identification, tool development, and intervention approaches, as well as the further examination of the occupational experiences, values, and goals of those with ASDs and their families and significant others across the lifespan. However, challenges that must be faced and important future directions include the following:

- Addressing a need for more collaborative involvement from consumer populations (people with ASDs and their family members) in processes of assessment, intervention, and research, by
  - developing a variety of ways in which people with ASDs and their families can effectively and comfortably provide information, opinions, and ideas in research, educational, and intervention processes, and
  - continuing to work with client/consumer populations to develop a greater understanding of the spectrum of autism, and the life experiences of those on that spectrum and their families.
- Addressing a need for effective and appropriate identification and assessment tools, by
  - continuing contributions to research on early identifiers of ASDs, and
  - developing and validating occupational therapy assessment tools that are relevant for those with ASDs.
- Addressing a need for intervention methods that are evidence-based and easily replicable, by
  - continuing to develop methods for effective intervention with very young children and their families,
  - creating new approaches to consultation that support client systems as a whole,
  - becoming more innovative in the use of technology,
  - further examining and using strength-based models of intervention,
  - developing and testing of intervention "packages" (approaches that combine a variety of strategies and/or in which occupational therapy is one of several components in a comprehensive program), and
  - developing model approaches or programs that specifically support those with ASDs in the development of friendships.

SUGGESTED READINGS

Baranek, G. T., Wakeford, C. L., & David, F. J. (2008). Understanding, assessing, and treating sensory-motor issues in young children with autism. In Chawarska K., Klin A. & Volkmar F. (Eds.), *Autism spectrum disorders in infancy and early childhood.* New York: Guilford Press.

Case-Smith, J., & Arbesman, M. (2008). Evidence-based review of interventions for autism used in or of relevance to occupational therapy. *American Journal of Occupational Therapy, 62,* 416–429.

Miller-Kuhanek, H. (Ed.) (2004). *Autism: A comprehensive occupational therapy approach* (2nd ed.). Bethesda, MD: American Occupational Therapy Association.

REFERENCES

American Occupational Therapy Association. (2008). Occupational therapy practice framework: Domain and process (2nd ed.). *American Journal of Occupational Therapy, 62,* 625–683.

American Psychiatric Association. (2000). Pervasive developmental disorders. In *Diagnostic and statistical manual of mental disorders* 4th ed., text rev.; (DSM-IV-TR). (pp. 69–70) Washington, DC: Author.

Ball, D. (1999). Visual supports: Helping children with autism. *OT Practice, 4*(8), 37–40.

Baranek, G. T. (1999). Autism during infancy: A retrospective video analysis of sensory-motor and social behaviors at 9-12 months of age. *Journal of Autism and Developmental Disorders, 29,* 213–224.

Baranek, G. & Wakeford, L. (2000). Children with Autism: Legitimizing O. T. Practice. Presented at the North Carolina Conference on Exceptional Children Occupational Therapy Institute, July 17, 2000.

Baranek, G. T., Reinhartsen, D. B., & Wannamaker, S. W. (2001). Play: Engaging children with autism. In T. Huebner (Ed.). *Autism: A sensorimotor approach to management.* Philadelphia: F.A. Davis.

Baranek, G. T. (2002). Efficacy of sensory and motor interventions for children with autism. *Journal of Autism and Developmental Disorders, 5*(32), 397–422.

Baranek, G. T., David, F. J., Poe, M. D., Stone, W. L., & Watson, L. R. (2006). Sensory Experiences Questionnaire: discriminating sensory features in young children with autism, developmental delays, and typical development. *Journal of Child Psychology and Psychiatry, 47,* 591–601.

Baranek, G. T., Boyd, B. A., Poe, M. D., David, F. J., & Watson, L. R. (2007). Hyperresponsive sensory patterns in young children with autism, developmental delay, and typical development. *American Journal of Mental Retardation, 112*, 233–245.

Baranek, G. T., Wakeford, C. L., & David, F. J. (2008). Understanding, assessing, and treating sensory-motor issues in young children with autism. In K. Chawarska, A. Klin & F. Volkmar (Eds.), *Autism spectrum disorders in infancy and early childhood.* Guilford Press.

Baranek, G. T., Watson, L. R., Boyd, B. A., Poe, M. D., David, F. J., & McGuire, L. (in revision). Hyporesponsiveness to social and nonsocial sensory stimuli in young children with autism, developmental delays, and typical development. *Development and Psychopathology.*

Barry, L. M. & Burlew, S. B. (2004). Using social stories to teach choice and play skills to children with autism. *Focus on Autism and Other Developmental Disabilities, 19*, 45–51.

Bass, J. D. & Mulick, J. A. (2007). Social play skill enhancement of children with atusim using peers and siblings as therapists. *Psychology in the Schools, 44*, 727–735.

Ben-Sasson, A., Hen, L., Fluss, R., Cermak, S. A., Engel-Yeger, B., & Gal, E. (2009). A meta-analysis of sensory modulation symptoms in individuals with autism spectrum disorders. *Journal of Autism and Developmental Disorders, 39*(1), 1–11.

Bonder, B. R., Martin, L. & Miracle, A. W. (2004). Culture emergent in occupation. *American Journal of Occupational Therapy, 58*, 159–168.

Bowyer, P. L., Kramer, J., Kielhofner, G., Maziero-Barbosa, V., & Girolami, G. (2007). Measurement properties of the Short Child Occupational Profile (SCOPE). *Physical and Occupational Therapy in Pediatrics, 27*, 67–85.

Boyd, B. A., Baranek, G. T., Sideris, J., Poe, M., Watson, L. R., Patten, E., et al. (2010,). Relationship between sensory features and repetitive behaviors in children with autism and developmental delays. *Autism Research, 3*, 1-10.

Brown, C. & Dunn, W. (2002). *Adolescent/Adult Sensory Profile manual.* San Antonio, TX: The Psychological Corporation.

Brownell, M. K.(2002). Musically adapted social stories to modify behaviors in students with autism: Four case studies. *Journal of Music Therapy, 39* (2), 117–144.

Bryan, L. C. & Gast, D. L. (2000). Teaching on-task and on-schedule behaviors to high-functioning children with autism via picture activity schedules. *Journal of Developmental Disorders, 30*(6), 553–567.

Case-Smith, J. & Arbesman, M. (2008). Evidence-based review of interventions for autism used in or of relevance to occupational therapy. *American Journal of Occupational Therapy, 62*, 416–429.

Cederlund, M., Hagberg, B., Billstedt, E., Gillberg, I. C., & Gillberg, C. (2008). Asperger syndrome and autism: A comparative longitudinal follow-up study more than 5 years after original diagnosis. *Journal of Autism and Developmental Disorders, 38*, 72–85.

Coster, W. J., Deeney, T., Haltiwanger, J., & Haley, S. M. (1998). *The School Function Assessment: Standardized version.* Boston: Boston University.

Cowan, R. J. & Allen, K. D. (2007). Using naturalistic procedures to enhance learning in individuals with autism: A focus on generalized teaching within the school setting. *Psychology in the Schools, 44*, 701–715.

Danko, C. D. & Buysse, V. (2002). Thank you for being a friend. *Young Exceptional Children, 6*, 2–9.

DeGrace, B. W. (2004). Everyday occupations of families with children with autism. *American Journal of Occupational Therapy, 58*, 543–550.

Dettmer, S., Simpson, R. L., Myles, B. S., & Ganz, J. B. (2000). The use of visual supports to facilitate transitions of students with autism. *Focus on Autism and Other Developmental Disabilities, 15*, 163–169.

DiSalvo, C. A. & Oswald, D. P. (2002). Peer-mediated interventions to increase the social interaction of children with autism: Consideration of peer expectancies. *Focus on Autism and Other Developmental Disabilities, 17*(4), 198–207.

Donovan, J. M., Van Leit, B. J., Crowe, T. K., & Keefe, E. B. (2005). Occupational goals of mothers of children with disabilities: Influence of temporal, social, and emotional contexts. *American Journal of Occupational Therapy, 59*, 249–261.

Duker, P. C., & Rasing, E. (1989). Effects of redesigning the physical environment on self-stimulation and on-task behavior in three autistic-type developmentally disabled individuals. *Journal of Autism and Developmental Disorders, 19*(3), 449–460.

Dunn, L. (2004). Validation of the CHORES: A measure of school-aged children's participation in household tasks. *Scandinavian Journal of Occupational Therapy, 11*, 179–190.

Dunn, W. (1999). *Sensory Profile user's manual.* San Antonio, TX: The Psychological Corporation.

Dunn, W. (2002). *The Infant/Toddler Sensory Profile manual.* San Antonio, TX: The Psychological Corporation.

Dunn, W., Saiter, J., & Rinner, L. (2002). Asperger syndrome and sensory processing: A conceptual model and guidance for intervention planning. *Focus on Autism and Other Developmental Disabilities, 17*(3), 172–185.

Gabriels, R. L., Agnew, J. A., Miller, L. J., Gralla, J., Pan, Z., Goldson, E., et al. (2008). Is there a relationship between restricted, repetitive, stereotyped behaviors and interests and abnormal sensory response in children with autism spectrum disorders? *Research in Autism Spectrum Disorders, 2*(4), 660–670.

Gray, C. A. & Garand, J. D. (1993). Social stories: Improving responses of students with autism with accurate social information. *Focus on Autistic Behavior, 8*, 1–10.

Greenspan, S. & Wieder, S. (1997). Developmental patterns and outcomes in infants and children with disorders in relating and communicating: A chart review of 200 cases of children with autistic spectrum diagnoses. *Journal of Developmental and Learning Disorders, 1*, 87–141.

Harper, C. B., Symon, J. B. G., & Frea, W. D. (2007). Recess is time in: Using peers to imrove social skills of children with autism. *Journal of Autism and Developmental Disorders, 38*, 815–826.

Hilton, C. L., Crouch, M. C., & Israel, H. (2008). Out-of-school participation patterns in children with high-functioning autism spectrum disorders. *American Journal of Occupational Therapy, 62*, 54–563.

Hilton, C., Graver, K., & LaVesser, P. (2007). Relationship between social competence and sensory processing in children with high functioning autism spectrum disorders. *Research in Autism Spectrum Disorders, 1*, 164–173.

Hume, K. & Odom, S. (2007). Effects of an individual work system on the independent function of students with autism. *Journal of Autism and Developmental Disorders, 37*, 1166–1180.

Humphry, R. & Wakeford, L. (2006). An occupation-centered discussion of development and implications for practice. *American Journal of Occupational Therapy, 60*, 258–267.

Interagency Autism Coordinating Committee. (2009). Interagency Autism Coordinating Committee Strategic Plan for Autism Spectrum Disorder Research. Retrieved March 2, 2009 from http://iacc.hhs.gov/strategic-plan/

Iwama, M. K. (2005). Situated meaning: An issue of culture, inclusion, and occupational therapy. In F. Kronenberg, S. S. Algado, & N. Pollard (Eds.), *Occupational therapy without borders: Learning from the spirit of survivor* (pp. 127–139). Philadelphia: Elsevier.

Jasmin, E., Couture, M., McKinley, P., Reid, G., Fombonne, E., & Gisel, E. (2009). Sensori-motor and daily living skills of preschool children with autism spectrum disorder. *Journal of Autism and Developmental Disorders, 39*, 231–241.

Kampa, A., Kennedy, J., Velde, B., & Wittman, P. (October 20, 2003). The Friendship Club: Developing reciprocal relationships in children with Asperger's syndrome. *OT Practice, 8*, 25–27.

Kashman, N., Mora, J., & Glaser, T. (2000). Using videotapes to help children with autism. *OT Practice, 5*(July 3), 13–15.

Kern, P. (2006). Using embedded music therapy interventions to support outdoor play of young children with autism in an inclusive community-based child care program. *Journal of Music Therapy, 43*(4), 270–294.

Kern, P., Wakeford, L., & Aldridge, D. (2007). Improving the performance of a young child with autism during self-care tasks using embedded song interventions: A case study. *Music Therapy Perspectives, 25* (1), 43–51.

Kielhofner, G., Hammel, J., Finlayson, M., Helfrich, C., & Taylor, R. R. (2004). Documenting outcomes of occupational therapy: The Center for Outcomes Research and Education. *American Journal of Occupational Therapy, 58*, 15–23.

Kientz, M. A. & Dunn, W. (1997). A comparison of the performance of children with and without autism on the Sensory Profile. *American Journal of Occupational Therapy, 51*, 530–537.

Knox, S. (2008). Development and current use of the revised Knox Preschool Play Scale. In L. D. Parham & L. S. Fazio (Eds). *Play in occupational therapy for children* (2nd ed.) (pp. 55–70). St. Louis: Mosby.

Koegel, L. K., Koegel, R. L., Frea, W., & Green-Hopkins, I. (2003). Priming as a method of coordinating educational services for students with autism. *Language, Speech, and Hearing Services in Schools, 34*(3), 228–235.

Kohler, F. W., Strain, P. S., Hoyson, M., & Jamieson, B. (1997). Merging naturalistic teaching and peer-based strategies to address the IEP objectives of preschoolers with autism: An examination of structural and child behavior outcomes. *Focus on Autism and Other Developmental Disabilities, 12*, 196–206, 218.

Kuoch, H. & Mirenda, P. (2003). Social story interventions for young children with autism spectrum disorders. *Focus on Autism and Other Developmental Disabilities, 18*(4), 219–227.

Kurt, O. & Tekin-Iftar, E. (2008). A comparison of constant time delay and simultaneous prompting within embedded instruction on teaching leisure skills to children with autism. *Topics in Early Childhood Special Education, 28*, 53–64.

Law, M., Baptiste, S., Carswell, A., McColl, M. A., Polatajko, H., & Pollock, N. (1998). *Canadian Occupational Performance Measure* (2nd ed. Rev.) Ottawa, ON: CAOT Publications ACE.

Law, M., Baptiste, S., McColl, M., Opzoomer, A., Polatajko, H., & Pollock, N. (1990). The Canadian Occupational Performance Measure: An outcome measure for occupational therapy. *Canadian Journal of Occupational Therapy, 57*, 82–87.

Lee, L.-C., Harrington, R. A., Louis, B. B., & Newschaffer, C. J. (2008). Children with autism: Quality of life and parental concerns. *Journal of Autism and Developmental Disorders, 38*, 1147–1160.

Lee, S., Odom, S. L., & Loftin, R. (2007). Social engagement with peers and stereotypic behavior in children with autism. *Journal of Positive Behavior Interventions, 9*, 67–79.

Liber, D. B., Frea, W. D., & Symon, J. B. G. (2007). Using time-delay to improve social play skills with peers for children with autism. *Journal of Autism and Developmental Disorders, 38*, 312–323.

Mahoney, G. & Perales, F. (2003). Using relationship-focused intervention to enhance the social–emotional functioning of young children with autism spectrum disorders. *Topics in Early Childhood Special Education, 23*, 77–89.

Mahoney, G. & Perales, F. (2005). Relationship-focused early intervention with children with pervasive developmental disorders and other disabilities: A comparative study. *Journal of Developmental and Behavioral Pediatrics, 26*(2), 77–85.

Mahoney, G. J. & MacDonald, J. (2007). *Autism and developmental delays in young children: The responsive teaching curriculum for parents and professionals manual.* Austin, TX: PRO-ED.

Marr, D., Mika, H., Miraglia, J., Roerig, M., & Sinnott, R. (2007). The effect of sensory stories on targeted behaviors in preschool children with autism. *Physical and Occupational Therapy in Pediatrics, 27*(1), 63–79.

McCoy, K. & Hermansen, E. (2007). Video modeling for individuals with autism: A review of model types and effects. *Education and Treatment of Children, 30*, 183–213.

Miller-Kuhanek, H. (Ed.) (2004). *Autism: A comprehensive occupational therapy approach* (2nd ed.). Bethesda, MD: American Occupational Therapy Association.

Miller-Kuhaneck, H., Henry, D. A., Glennon, T. J., & Mu, K. (2007). Development of the Sensory Processing Measure–School: Initial studies of reliability and validity. *American Journal of Occupational Therapy, 61*, 170–175.

Miller-Kuhaneck, H., Henry, D. A., & Glennon, T. J. (2007). *Sensory Processing Measure: Main Classroom Form and School Environments Forms.* Los Angeles: Western Psychological Services.

More, C. (2008). Digital stories targeting social skills for children with disabilities: Multidimensional learning. *Intervention in School and Clinic, 43*, 168–177.

Mulligan, S. (2003, June). Examination of the evidence for occupational therapy using a sensory integration framework with children: Part two. *Sensory Integration Special Interest Section Quarterly, 26*, 1–5.

Nadel, J., Marini, M., Field, T., Escalona, A., & Lundy, B. (2008). Children with autism approach more imitative and playful adults. *Early Child Development and Care, 178*, 461–465.

National Institutes of Health. (2008). *NIH roadmap for medical research: Re-engineering the clinical research enterprise: Translational research.* Retrieved March 2, 2009 from http://nihroadmap.nih.gov/clinicalresearch/overview-translational.asp.

Odom, S. L., Brown, W. H., Frey, T., Karasu, N., Smith-Canter, L. L. & Strain, P. S. (2003). Evidence-based practices for young children with autism: Contributions for single-subject design research. *Focus on Autism and Other Developmental Disabilities, 18*, 166–175.

Pilebro, C. & Bäckman, B. (2005). Teaching oral hygiene to children with autism. *International Journal of Paediatric Dentistry, 15*, 1–9.

Polatajko, H. J., Mandich, A., & Martini, R. (2000). Dynamic performance analysis: A framework for understanding occupational performance. *American Journal of Occupational Therapy, 54*, 65–72.

Register, D. & Humpal, M. (2007). Using musical transitions in early childhood classrooms: Three case examples. *Music Therapy Perspectives, 25*, 25–31.

Reynolds, S. (2006). Get in the game! Participation in sports for children on the autism spectrum. *OT Practice, 11*(November 13), 13–17.

Reznick, J. S., Baranek, G. T., Reavis, S., Watson, L. R., Crais, E. R. (2007). A parent-report instrument for identifying one-year-olds at risk for an eventual diagnosis of autism: The first year inventory. *Journal of Autism and Developmental Disorders, 37*, 1691–1710.

Sandt, D. (2008). Social stories for students with autism in physical education. *Journal of Physical Education, Recreation, and Dance, 79*, 42–45.

Schaaf, R. C. & Miller, L. J. (2005). Occupational therapy using a sensory integrative approach for children with developmental disabilities. *Mental Retardation and Developmental Disabilities Research Review, 11*, 143–148.

Skard, G. & Bundy, A. C. (2008). Test of playfulness. In L. D. Parham & L. S. Fazio (Eds). *Play in occupational therapy for children* (2nd ed.) (pp. 71–93). St. Louis: Mosby.

Spitzer, S. (2003). Using participant observation to study the meaning of occupations of young children with autism and other developmental disabilities. *American Journal of Occupational Therapy, 57*, 66–76.

Spitzer, S. (2004). Common and uncommon daily activities in individuals with autism: Challenges and opportunities for supporting occupation. In H. Miller-Kuhanek (Ed.), *Autism: A comprehensive occupational therapy approach* (2nd ed.) (pp. 83–106). Bethesda, MD: American Occupational Therapy Association.

Stagnitti, K. & Unsworth, C. (2004). The test–retest reliability of the Child-Initiated Pretend Play Assessment. *American Journal of Occupational Therapy, 58*, 93–99.

Sterling-Turner, H. E. & Jordan, S. S. (2007). Interventions addressing transition difficulties for individuals with autism. *Psychology in the Schools, 44*, 681–690.

Tickle-Degnen, L. (2000). Evidence-based practice forum: Monitoring and documenting evidence during assessment and intervention. *American Journal of Occupational Therapy, 54*, 434–436.

Tickle-Degnen, L. (2002). Evidence-based practice forum: Client-centered practice, therapeutic relationship, and use of research evidence. *American Journal of Occupational Therapy, 56*, 470–474.

Tomchek, S. D. & Dunn, W. (2007). Sensory processing in children with and without autism: A comparative study using the Short Sensory Profile. *American Journal of Occupational Therapy, 61*, 190–200.

Vuran, S. (2007). Empowering leisure skills in adults with autism: An experimental investigation through the most to least prompting procedure. *International Journal of Special Education, 22*, 174–181.

Wakeford, L. (2008). Baggie books. *Journal of Occupational Therapy, Schools, and Early Intervention, 1*, 283–288.

Watling, R., Deitz, J., & White., O. (2001). Comparison of Sensory Profile scores of young children with and without autism spectrum disorders. *American Journal of Occupational Therapy, 55*, 416–423.

Watson, L. R., Baranek, G. T., Crais, E. R., Reznick, J. S., Dykstra, J., & Perryman, T. (2007). The First Year Inventory: Retrospective parent responses to a questionnaire designed to identify one-year-olds at risk for autism. *Journal of Autism and Developmental Disabilities, 37*, 49–61.

Wolery, M. (2000). Commentary: The environment as a source of variability: Implications for research with individuals who have autism. *Journal of Autism and Developmental Disorders, 30*, 379–381.

Yuill, N., Strieth, S., Roake, C., Aspden, R., & Todd, B. (2007). Brief report: Designing a playground for children with autistic spectrum disorders–effects on playful peer interactions. *Journal of Autism and Developmental Disorders, 37*, 1192–1196.

64 Augmentative and Alternative Communication Systems

Marjorie H. Charlop, Alissa L. Greenberg, Gina T. Chang

Points of Interest

- It is important to consider presentation format and stimulus duration when using AAC systems with persons with autism.
- A visual-constant system (i.e., one in which the stimuli are visual and always present) may best complement the strengths of this population.
- Research suggests that a variety of AAC systems can be effective in teaching communication to persons with autism.
- However, the most effective AAC system for a specific child needs to be individually chosen.
- When choosing an AAC system for an individual, practitioners should consult the literature as well as consider both individual and environmental characteristics.

Introduction

Much attention has been placed on the development of communication in persons with autism. By definition, autism is a social communicative disorder, including qualitative impairments in both verbal and nonverbal communication (APA, 2000; Schreibman, 2005). Approximately one-third of persons diagnosed with an autism spectrum disorder (ASD) will not develop functional natural speech by adulthood (National Research Council, 2001). If speech does occur, onset is usually delayed and it is often characterized by abnormalities such as echolalia, idiosyncratic words or phrases, monotonous intonation, and an inability to sustain reciprocal conversation (Howlin, 2006; Kanner, 1943). Although communication interventions for children with autism have a long history of targeting verbal speech (Baer et al., 1968; Risley & Wolf, 1967), progress is often extremely slow and limited (Lovaas, 1977; Howlin, 1989). Poor outcomes have led interventionists to turn to other means, including augmentative and alternative communication (AAC) (Howlin, 2006).

Augmentative and Alternative Communication Systems

The American Speech-Language-Hearing Association defines *augmentative and alternative communication (AAC) systems* as "an integrated group of components, including the symbols, aids, strategies and techniques used by individuals to enhance communication. The system serves to supplement any gestural, spoken, and/or written communication abilities." (ASHA, 1991, pp. 9–10.) *Augmentative* refers to the process of supplementing existing speech to increase communication, and *alternative* refers to the use of technology other than natural verbal speech to communicate (e.g., sign language, picture cards). Application of AAC has extended to people with sensory and motor deficits (e.g., individuals with visual and hearing impairments and cerebral palsy), intellectual and developmental disabilities (e.g., Down syndrome, Fragile X Syndrome, fetal alcohol syndrome, and autism), and physical disabilities (e.g., Amyotrophic Lateral Sclerosis) (Beukelman & Mirenda, 2005).

Autism and Augmentative and Alternative Communication Systems

AAC systems have been used to address the communicative deficits of persons with autism since the 1970s (Ogletree & Harn, 2001). Early applications focused on manual signs, tangible symbols, lexograms, and orthographic symbols. In the 1980s, the use of visual-spatial symbols gained popularity.

More recently, advances in technology have led to an increase in the use of computer software programs and voice-output communication aids for persons with autism (Mirenda & Erickson, 2000).

In this chapter we will review the different AAC systems that have been used with persons with autism, along with the relevant research for each system. Although several different categorizations can be used when presenting AAC systems (e.g., aided versus unaided, input versus output), we have chosen to categorize AAC systems along two dimensions that are relevant for this population: presentation format and stimulus duration. This format, adapted from Charlop-Christy and Jones (2006), will guide our discussion of the potential benefits and limitations for using each type of AAC system with persons with autism.

Presentation Format

Since Kanner (1943) first described children with autism, it has been well-documented that although these children's verbal skills are significantly impaired, their visual-spatial skills may be normal or even advanced (Hermellin, 1976). For example, many of these children perform quite well on embedded figures and block design tests (*see Mitchell & Ropar, 2004 for a review of visual-spatial abilities in persons with autism*).

This discrepancy between visual and verbal skills has been empirically validated by several studies. Lincoln, Courchesne, Kilman, Elmasian, and Allen (1988) assessed the intellectual functioning of 33 individuals with autism ranging in age from 8 to 29 years with the Wechsler Intelligence Scale for Children–Revised (WISC-R) (Wechsler, 1974) or the Wechsler Adult Intelligence Scale–Revised (WAIS-R) (Wechsler, 1981). Participants received the lowest scores on the Comprehension and Vocabulary subtests, which require the most verbal reasoning, and the highest scores on the Block Design and Object Assembly subtests, which require the most visual skills.

Other studies have found that when compared to typically developing controls, persons with autism show deficits in their verbal skills but not in their visual skills. Rumsey and Hamburger (1988) compared the performance of 10 men with infantile autism and average verbal and nonverbal intelligence, ages 18 to 39 years, with normal controls on a range of neuropsychological tests that measured language and visual-spatial abilities. Results indicated that although the men with autism did not perform differently from the controls on the visual-perceptual measures, they performed much worse than the controls on simple and complex verbal problem-solving tasks. A similar pattern of results was found in Ozonoff, Pennington, and Rogers' (1991) comparison of 23 people with ASD, ranging in age from 8 to 20 years, with 23 controls matched for IQ, age, sex, and socioeconomic status.

These results have also been replicated in studies that focus on children with autism. In Williams, Goldstein, and Minshew (2006), 56 high-functioning children with autism were compared to 56 control children matched for age and IQ. The children with autism performed worse than the controls on the complex language tasks but not on the visual-spatial tasks.

Although the previous studies were conducted with high-functioning persons with autism, this cognitive profile is also found in low-functioning children with autism (Quill, 1997). In addition to demonstrating higher abilities on nonverbal problem-solving tasks than on verbal reasoning problems, low-functioning persons with autism also have severe receptive and expressive language impairments (Bristol et al., 1996). In fact, as the overall degree of mental retardation increases, so does the gap between verbal and nonverbal abilities (Quill, 1997).

If persons with autism have advanced visual skills, then visually based interventions should have high rates of success with this population. Quill and Grant (1996) found that language comprehension increased for four nonverbal children with autism when both oral and graphic instructions were presented simultaneously. For example, although the children did not initially respond to purely oral questions, such as "Which one is [*attribute*]," they were able to correctly respond when the verbal question was paired with a picture that depicted the attribute. Other successful visual interventions include video modeling (e.g. Chalrop-Christy et al., 2000; Sherer et al., 2001), cue cards (e.g., Charlop-Christy & Kelso, 2003), and photographic activity schedules (e.g., MacDuff et al., 1993). This research implies that visual AAC systems might be effective systems for persons with autism.

Stimulus Duration

The issue, however, is more complex than presentation format. Research indicates that stimulus duration is also an important consideration. In the studies previously mentioned (Lincoln et al., 1988; Ozonoff et al., 1991; Rumsey & Hamburger, 1988; Williams et al., 2006) the participants with autism performed best on the tasks in which the stimuli were visible for the entire duration of the task (e.g., form discrimination, matching, block design, object assembly, and pattern analysis). These results suggest that constant visual stimuli may be preferable to transient visual stimuli.

Research on attention and memory processes further support this conclusion. Children with autism demonstrate impairments in rapidly shifting attention (Courchesne et al., 1994) This suggests that children would have difficulty attending to, and therefore encoding, a series of rapidly spoken words or rapidly presented visual stimuli, such as gestures or pictures. Visually constant stimuli, on the other hand, would be easier to attend to, and children could attend to the stimuli until they were successfully encoded (Quill, 1997). Research on memory in persons with autism also supports the use of visually constant stimuli. Persons with autism perform better on cued-recall memory tasks than on free-recall memory tasks (Quill, 1997). Therefore, constant visual stimuli may enhance memory because they can serve as visible retrieval cues.

Presentation Format and Stimulus Duration Applied to Communication

When applied to communication, the two dimensions of presentation format and stimulus duration yield three different modalities of communication training. Communication training may be *auditory-transient*, *visual-transient*, or *visual-constant* (Charlop-Christy & Jones, 2006). In auditory-transient AAC systems, the stimuli are presented auditorily and do not persist in time. Once a word is spoken, the stimulus is gone. Clearly, there would not be an auditory-constant system. Visual-transient AAC systems present information visually for brief periods of time. For example, in sign language, the stimuli consist of body movements, which, once they are performed, are no longer available. In contrast, in visual-constant AAC systems, the stimuli are also visual, but they are always available. For example, a picture is a visual stimulus that, unless removed, is always available to the AAC user.

Table 64-1 depicts these modalities, along with providing AAC examples for each category. In the following sections, we will review each modality and the relevant AAC systems, referring back to their potential advantages or disadvantages for persons with autism given our previous discussion on presentation format and stimulus duration.

Auditory-Transient

In the auditory-transient modality, stimuli are presented in the auditory modality and only last for brief periods of time. For example, in speech, the sounds of words do not persist over time. Therefore, a child with autism needs to "hear" speech, attend to it, remember it, and then figure out its meaning (Charlop-Christy & Jones, 2006). These steps may be difficult given the population's difficulties with encoding verbal information and may partially explain why communication interventions that focus on verbal imitation have limited success (Charlop-Christy et al., 2008; Lovaas, 1977). Computer-generated vocalizations, unless paired with a visual stimulus, have the same limitations as speech.

Table 64–1.
Augmentative and alternative communication systems categorized by stimulus duration and presentation format

	Presentation Format	
Stimulus Duration	*Auditory*	*Visual*
Transient	*Auditory-transient*: Speech; Computer-generated vocalization.	*Visual-transient*: Sign-language; Gestures.
Constant	*Auditory-constant*: N/A.	*Visual-constant*: Picture Exchange Communication System (PECS); Voice-output communication aids (VOCAs).

Visual-Transient

In visual-transient communication, information is presented visually but it also does not persist through time (Charlop-Christy & Jones, 2006). Sign language is an example of a visual-transient AAC system. The body movements that are used in sign language are presented visually, but they do not last. Studies that report on the use of signs with persons with autism first appeared in the 1970s (e.g., Bonvillian & Nelson, 1976; Fulwiler & Fouts, 1976; Konstantareas et al., 1978). After we review this area of research we will return to the potential problems with using a visual-transient system with persons with autism.

Sign Language

Although initial sign-language programs were based on formal systems, such as American Sign Language (ASL), today abridged versions are often used with persons with autism. These versions may incorporate simpler hand movements or a modified vocabulary (Howlin, 2006). Initial studies with persons with autism compared the effects of presenting speech and sign language together on receptive vocabulary (Brady & Smouse, 1978; Carr & Dores, 1981; Carr et al., 1984), expressive vocabulary (Barrera et al., 1980; Barrera & Sulzer-Araroff, 1983; Layton, 1988; Yoder & Layton, 1988), or both expressive and receptive vocabulary (Layton, 1988). The results of these studies demonstrate that, for many participants, total communication training generates faster and more complete learning of vocabulary in comparison with speech alone conditions. These findings were especially robust for participants who demonstrated low verbal-imitation skills (Carr & Dores, 1981; Carr et al., 1984; Yoder & Layton, 1988). Although these findings seem to support the use of sign language for children with autism, almost all of these studies taught receptive or expressive labels in response to questions such as, "What is this?" or, "Show me the sign for [object label]." That is, the participants were not using sign language to communicate functionally in the natural environment. It is unclear if the participants in these studies would use sign language to request preferred items. Unfortunately, little research has examined the use of total communication to teach communication that is functional (i.e., can be used to spontaneously request a variety of items; Mirenda, 2003).

One study, conducted by Richman, Wacker, and Winborn (2001), compared the use of signing with a picture communication system in a functional communication training (FCT) program. A highly aggressive 3-year-old boy with pervasive developmental disorder (PDD) learned both to sign "please" and to exchange a generic picture for "please" when requesting preferred items. The child acquired both systems, and aggression decreased when reinforcers were presented for either exchanging a card or signing "please." When reinforcement was provided concurrently for both systems, the child showed a preference for signing. From these results, researchers concluded that signing may have been more efficient (i.e., required less effort) for this particular child. Keep in mind, however, that this study had one participant and that heterogeneity and individual differences are common for this population. Also, the child in this study learned only one sign. Other studies, which target multiple signs, suggest that even after extensive training, students with autism are likely to acquire only a few functional signs (Layton & Watson, 1995). Clearly, more research based on the principles of best evidence is needed to empirically investigate the use of sign language as a means of teaching communication to persons with autism.

In the meantime, interventionists considering the use of sign language with persons with autism should evaluate certain characteristics of this AAC system. First, remember that sign language is a visual-transient modality (Charlop-Christy & Jones, 2006). Processing sign language requires both attention to the visual stimulus and an ability to hold the visual stimulus in one's memory after the sign is no longer being displayed. The transient form of sign-based communication requires faster processing speed of visual stimuli than of visual stimuli that are constant (e.g., a picture) (Charlop-Christy & Jones, 2006). Furthermore, when generating communication, sign formation requires a two-stage recall memory process: *(1)* a search of one's memory for potential signs, and *(2)* a discrimination process to decide which of the potential signs is correct (Light & Lindsay, 1991). In contrast, visually constant systems, which rely on recognition memory, do not require users to search their memory for the correct stimuli; the visuals are always present, thus lowering the processing demands placed on the system user (Mirenda, 2003).

In addition to the limitations of a visual-transient system, sign language has other features that may make it difficult for persons with autism. First, one of the prerequisites of symbolic communication, such as sign language, is the use of more basic communication forms, such as gestures (Miranda & Erickson, 2000). Persons with autism characteristically lack the use of complex gesturing to communicate (Schreibman, 2005). Many children with ASDs do not demonstrate gestures beyond taking a person by the arm to the item they want. Extensive training with basic gesturing (including proximal and distal pointing) would be required to develop an ability to understand the use of gestures prior to sign-language training (Miranda & Erickson, 2000).

Second, not everyone is familiar with sign language. Unless primary communicative partners, such as family members, are willing to learn sign language, the ability of nonverbal persons with ASDs to communicate is limited (Weitz et al., 1997; Wilkinson & Hennig, 2007). Furthermore, even if primary communicative partners do learn to sign, communication is still not completely functional because the user may be unable to communicate with unfamiliar persons (Mirenda & Erickson, 2000). The need for a translator for community outings thus makes independent living less likely.

Lastly, sign language requires that participants possess manual dexterity (Sundberg & Sundberg, 1990; Wraikat et al., 1991). Unfortunately, persons with ASDs often demonstrate difficulties with fine-motor actions, coordination, and gross-motor imitation, making the process of learning signs difficult (Seal & Bonvillian, 1997; National Research Council, 2001). As a result, persons with ASDs often develop idiosyncratic signs. Communication partners must not only know sign language, but they must also know how the specific person's signs differ from standard signs (Wilkinson & Hennig, 2007).

The benefits of sign language should not be discounted before future research further explores the applications of this AAC system to persons with autism. Better methodology, larger sample sizes, and replications of present research are needed. Thus, much more exploration into the use of sign language is suggested before a conclusion about this AAC with children with ASDs can be reached.

Visual-Constant

Information in the visual-constant modality is presented visually and persists over time (Charlop-Christy & Jones, 2006). The majority of AAC systems fall under this category, including orthography, picture schedules, Aided Language Simulation (ALS), System for Augmenting Language (SAL), voice-output communication aids (VOCAs), and the Picture Exchange Communication System (PECS). As we review each AAC system, remember the benefits that the visual-constant modality may have for persons with autism. Because these visual stimuli persist over time, they accommodate the potential need for longer periods of processing time (Ogletree & Oren, 2006). Furthermore, visual-constant stimuli are easier to attend to, enhance encoding, and may serve as a memory aid during retrieval processes (Charlop-Christy & Jones, 2006).

Orthography

Orthography refers to written stimuli. Research on orthography has focused on using the written word as an AAC *input*. That is, children are shown a word, and then taught to respond appropriately. In an early study, three nonverbal adolescents with autism were taught three words both expressively and receptively (La Vigna, 1977). In the expressive task, the participants were shown an object and taught to choose the corresponding word card. In the receptive task, the participants were shown the word card and taught to choose the corresponding object. It took the participants an average of 1,471 trials to master three words both expressively and receptively.

Given the slow rate of acquisition, orthography may be more appropriate for higher-functioning persons (Howlin, 2006). In fact, research findings indicate that written scripts can be used to teach complex social behaviors to children with autism in elementary and middle school. For example, Charlop-Christy and Kelso (2003) taught conversational skills to three children with autism, ages 8 to 10 years, who were verbal and literate. In this study, children successfully responded to a conversational question and asked a contextually appropriate question after just two to four presentations with the cue cards. After training, this skill was generalized across setting and conversation topic, in the absence of cue cards. Similarly, Krantz and McLannahan (1993) used written scripts to facilitate social initiations. During an art project, four children with autism were given a card with 10 single-line social initiations (e.g., "John, did you like to swing outside today?"). Initially, the children were physically prompted to read each script and then cross it off when finished. The scripts were then faded one word at a time. After training, the children's initiations had increased to the same range as three of their typically developing peers.

These studies provide support for the use of orthography as an effective AAC input system for literate persons with autism. High-functioning persons with autism seem to be able to attend to the visually constant stimuli, encode them, and then respond appropriately. This AAC system would be especially useful for children who are hyperlexic, a specific condition which is found frequently among persons with autism (Ogletree & Oren, 2007). The main characteristic of *hyperlexia* is an above-average reading level paired with a below-average comprehension level for spoken language. Hyperlexic children are often able to learn to speak through extensive repetition and memorization. The condition is closely associated with autism, but there is some debate as to whether it is an autism spectrum disorder or a completely distinct disorder.

Research, however, has not been conducted on the use of orthography as an AAC output system, or as an alternative to verbal speech. That is, empirically controlled research is needed on the use of written material provided by the person with autism to communicate. Such AAC systems might consist of small laptops on which persons with autism can type messages, text messaging apparatuses such as cell phones, and writing.

Picture Schedules

Like orthography, picture schedules are also a visual-constant AAC input system. Picture schedules can be divided into within-task schedules and between-task schedules. In within-task schedules, children learn to follow pictures to complete an activity. For example, Bryan and Gast (2000) taught four children with autism, ages 7 to 8 years, to follow four pictures that sequenced an academic activity (e.g., file-folder games, worksheets). The participants learned to complete the activity using the picture schedule, and after training, the children were able to generalize the skill to a novel activity. Picture schedules can also be used for self-help skills. In Pierce and Schreibman (1994), three low-functioning children with autism, ages 6 to 9 years, were taught a variety of skills such as dressing, setting the table, and doing laundry. Each participant learned three sequences with a picture schedule, completed the sequences even when the therapist was not present, and generalized the skill across setting and task.

Picture schedules can also be used for between-task schedules. These programs help participants learn to transition from one activity to another. For example, MacDuff and colleagues (1993) taught four children, ages 9 to 14 years, to follow a picture activity schedule that included six different after-school activities (e.g., LEGOs, puzzle, TV, handwriting worksheet) and lasted for approximately 60 minutes. The participants were taught to follow their schedules through graduated guidance, which was faded until the teachers were no longer in close proximity to the participants. After training, which ranged from 13 to 27 sessions, the participants maintained the behavior, and generalized the skill to new sequences with the same photographs and to new sequences with different photographs. In a similar study with younger children, the parents of three children with autism, ages 6 to 8 years, learned to help their children follow picture schedules that depicted a variety of home-living tasks. In addition to acquiring the sequences, the children also displayed increases in social initiations and decreases in disruptive behavior, which were maintained for up to 10 months (Krantz, MacDuff, & McClannahan, 1993). These studies seem to indicate that picture schedules are extremely effective visual-constant AAC input systems. However, similar to orthography, picture schedules have not been used as AAC output systems for persons with autism. Although picture schedules may allow other people to communicate with persons with autism, they do not allow persons with autism to communicate with other people. This is an important distinction, because complete communication is bidirectional.

Aided Language Simulation

Aided Language Simulation (ALS) is a visual-constant AAC system that is used for both input and output. Goossens (1989) introduced ALS to teach individuals to both understand and use visual symbols as a means of communication. Through this system, as the communication partner talks to the ALS user, he or she also points to symbols on the user's communication display. For example, the partner might point to the symbol for "ball" while saying, "I see ball." Pairing the visual symbol with the spoken word may increase message saliency and assist in receptive and expressive understanding of vocabulary. In addition to AAC input, AAC output through ALS occurs when the user points to symbols on the communication display. In more advanced stages, the communicative partner responds contingently to the user by scaffolding more advanced communication and language (Goossens et al., 1992). For example, a child may point to a picture of a ball, and in response, the communicative partner would point to picture symbols for "big," "red," and "ball," while saying, "Look, the big, red ball." Although Harris and Reichle (2004) found that three children with moderate cognitive disabilities increased their symbol comprehension and production following ALS implementation, no studies have been published on the effectiveness of ALS with persons with autism.

System for Augmenting Language

The System for Augmenting Language (SAL) is very similar to ALS in that it also emphasizes augmenting both the input of the communication partner and the output of the AAC user. The main difference is that voice-output communication aids (VOCAs) are considered critical to SAL (Romski & Sevcik, 1992). In SAL, each learner's VOCA has a display of visual-graphic symbols. Communication partners are instructed to use the symbols and VOCA to augment their speech input during naturally occurring communication opportunities. For example, at break time, the teacher would push the picture symbols for "Let's play outside" and the VOCA would produce a digitized speech output. Learners are also encouraged to use the device throughout the day (Mirenda, 2001).

Research on the effectiveness of SAL with persons with autism is limited. However, Romski and Sevcik (1996) conducted a 2-year longitudinal study that examined the effectiveness of SAL with 13 students, ages 6 to 20 years, two of which had autism. All of the students were given a VOCA, and communication partners were taught to use the VOCAs, incorporating the components of SAL. At the end of 2 years, all of the participants learned to use SAL, with a total of 20 to 70 symbols mastered. Seven of the participants, including the two with autism, produced messages that consisted of combining two or more symbols. Five years later, all of the participants were still using their VOCAs with an average of 70 symbols (Romski et al., 1999). Although more research with persons with autism is needed, these studies suggest that SAL may be effective for both receptive and expressive communication skills.

Voice-Output Communication Aids (VOCAs)

As described earlier, voice-output communication aids (VOCAs) are electronic devices that produce digitized or synthetic verbal messages when the VOCA user presses a picture, line drawing, or other visual graphic symbol that is on the device board (Mirenda, 2001). In their recent review of VOCAs, Lancioni and colleagues (2007) found that between 1992 and 2006, 16 studies have been published on the use of VOCAs with persons with a range of developmental disabilities, including autism. Out of the 39 students in these studies, all but three succeeded to use VOCAs to varying degrees of success. For example, although some students only learned to use a single message for a single item, other students learned to use a variety of messages to request a range of preferred items (see Datillo & Camarata, 1991; Dyches, 1998; Schepis & Reid, 1995).

Only a few studies have specifically studied the effectiveness of VOCAs with persons with autism. Schepis, Reid, Behrman, and Sutton (1998) used naturalistic teaching strategies to teach four children with autism, ages 3 to 5 years, to use VOCAs during snack and play routines. Over a 1- to 3-month period, all four children demonstrated increases in their communicative interactions. In addition to using their VOCAs to request preferred items, the children also used the AAC system to respond "yes" and "no," to make statements, and to make social comments (e.g., "thank you").

More recently, Sigafoos, Didden, and O'Reilly (2003) taught children with autism or autistic-like characteristics, ages 3 to 13 years, to request objects using a VOCA. All three children were able to request, "I want more" to obtain access to a variety of preferred food, drink, and activity items. The children's requesting behaviors were not affected by the presence or absence of digitized speech output, which was manipulated by the researchers. Furthermore, the digitized speech output did not cause any decreases in the children's verbal speech. In fact, one child began to speak single words toward the end of the study.

Proponents of VOCAs argue that one of their strengths is that the verbal messages can be easily perceived by other people, including those who are unfamiliar with that particular AAC system (Lancioni et al., 2007). Durand (1999) tested this assumption in a study that taught five persons with severe disabilities, ages 3 to 15 years, to use VOCAs through functional communication training. All of the children engaged in severe problem behaviors, such as hand biting, screaming, crying, head banging, and aggressions toward others. With their VOCAs, they were taught to produce alternative communicative behaviors (e.g., "I need help," "I want more") that served the same function as their problem behaviors. After instruction at school, all of the participants were able to independently use their VOCAs in community settings with community members who had never been trained in VOCA use. In another study, however, Dyches, Davis, Lucido, and Young (2002) found contradicting results. Researchers taught an adolescent girl to make requests with a VOCA and with a simple pictographic display and assessed community members' responses to requests made by these two AAC systems. Although the participant was able to generalize both systems to the community settings, community members took slightly longer to acknowledge requests produced by a VOCA as compared to requests made by nonelectronic picture displays. It is unclear if this difference resulted in a qualitatively different communication experience for the user or for the receiver of the communicative act, highlighting the need for more research on the effectiveness of VOCAs when used with untrained community members. Future research should investigate parents' perceived barriers of the effectiveness of VOCAs, including factors such as difficulty with programming, inconsistent reliability, and difficulty using the device in a conversational manner (Bailey et al., 2006).

The Picture Exchange Communication System (PECS)

The Picture Exchange Communication System (PECS) is a visual-constant AAC system that targets communication through the exchange of graphic iconic symbols (Frost & Bondy, 1994). For example, instead of saying, "I want juice," a child who uses PECS may bring a picture of juice to his mom. PECS was developed specifically for children with autism with limited or no functional verbal communication; however, its use has since expanded to include both children and adults with a range of developmental disabilities (Mirenda, 2001). PECS training is divided into six steps that mirror the development of communication and language in typical children (Bondy & Frost, 2001). The training protocol is discussed in detail in the PECS training manuals (Frost & Bondy, 1994, 2002) and is briefly outlined below.

- *Phase I: How to Communicate.* The child learns how to exchange one picture for a desired item with the communication partner.
- *Phase II: Distance and Persistence.* The child learns to travel to the communication book and to the communication partner.
- *Phase III: Discrimination Between Symbols.* The child learns to discriminate between different picture symbols to find the picture symbol of the current preferred item.
- *Phase IV: Using Phrases.* The child learns to combine picture cards to make phrases. For example, the child who wants juice will combine the "I want" picture card with the picture of juice on the sentence strip and exchange the sentence strip with the communication partner.
- *Phase V: Answering a Direct Question.* The child learns to answer questions, such as, "What do you want?"
- *Phase VI: Commenting.* The child learns to comment by combining the "I see" and "I hear" picture cards with other picture symbols. The child also learns to answer other questions, such as "What do you see?"

In addition to relying on a visual-constant modality, PECS training incorporates three other aspects that contribute to its success as a communication intervention for persons with autism. First, PECS is unique in its application of behavioral principles to an AAC intervention that emphasizes functional communication. The developers of PECS view functional communication as "behavior (defined in form by the community) directed to another person who in turn provides related direct or social rewards." (Bondy, 2001, p. 127.) Therefore, there is a link between the communicative act (exchanging a picture of juice) and the child's desire (thirst for juice). By teaching mands (requests) before tacts (comments), the child learns that communication is meaningful because it results in the acquisition of a desired item (Charlop-Christy & Jones, 2006). An emphasis on functional communication that is both meaningful and motivating increases the likelihood that the communicative behavior will occur again (Skinner, 1975).

Second, in addition to emphasizing functional communication, PECS training increases the likelihood that communication will be spontaneous. Unlike other communication interventions that begin training with a verbal prompt (e.g., "Point to what you want"), no verbal prompts are used in PECS training. Instead, a second trainer physically prompts the child from behind. The physical prompter does not socially interact with the child, and only prompts the child to exchange the picture card once he or she indicates a desire for the item (Bondy & Frost, 2001). The physical prompt can be quickly faded through a time delay procedure (e.g. Charlop & Trasowech, 1991). This procedure decreases the likelihood of prompt dependence and ensures that the communicative behavior is child-initiated (Charlop-Christy & Jones, 2006).

Third, PECS recognizes that communication is a social behavior. In typically developing children, communication involves much more than verbal language (Koegel, 2000). In fact, before they learn to speak, typically developing children learn to communicate with their caregivers through other behaviors such as looking, approaching, or pointing (Bondy & Frost, 2001). It is important to recognize the social nature of communication, because social deficits are one of the core features of children with autism (Kanner, 1943). Research indicates that children with autism are either delayed in or lack the social skills (e.g., imitations skills, simple gesturing, social responsiveness, and joint attention) that have been established as critical prerequisites for verbal speech development (Happe, 1994; Koegel, 2000; Schreibmen, 2005). PECS addresses these deficits by ensuring that children with autism learn the basic social elements of communication (e.g., approaching a communication partner and gaining his or her attention) before they learn to discriminate between different pictures (Frost & Bondy, 1994), increasing their likelihood of becoming successful communicators in a social world.

PECS Research

PECS is one of the most widely researched AAC interventions for persons with autism. We will present this literature by dividing it into four main topic areas: *(1)* PECS acquisition, *(2)* PECS generalization and maintenance, *(3)* ancillary benefits of PECS training, and *(4)* comparison studies. The majority of PECS research focuses on PECS acquisition in the training environment. In their review of PECS and VOCA usage with persons with developmental disabilities, Lancioni and colleagues (2007) found that between 1992 and 2006 17 studies have been published on PECS. In these studies, out of a total of 173 participants, only three participants failed to acquire PECS and a fourth participant ended training because of illness. These findings seem promising; however, the authors note that one must be cautious when interpreting PECS success. Although some of the studies only required participants to exchange one picture for a preferred item (e.g., Sigafoos et al., 1996), other studies required participants to learn PECS through Phase V (e.g., Charlop-Christy et al., 2002). A person who has learned to exchange one picture for one preferred item would not seem to have acquired functional communication as defined by Bondy (2001).

A smaller number of studies have taught PECS to persons with autism according to the guidelines in the PECS manual (Frost & Bondy, 1994, 2002). These studies also indicate that, when taught correctly, persons with autism will successfully acquire PECS through Phase III or higher (*see the following for studies that present acquisition data: Charlop-Christy et al., 2002; Ganz & Simpson, 2004; Kravits et al., 2002; Magiati & Howlin, 2003; Tincani et al., 2006*). As characteristic of most skills, duration of PECS training varies for each child. For example, although the three children in Charlop-Christy and colleagues (2002) reached criterion in Phase V after an average of 246 trials, the three children in Ganz and Simpson (2004) reached criterion in Phase IV after an average of 346 trials. In a third study, after 6 months of PECS training in the classroom, the average PECS level for 34 children with autism was between Phases IV and V (Magiati & Howlin, 2003). In conclusion, the research demonstrates that children with autism can easily acquire PECS in the training environment through Phase III or higher.

Fewer PECS studies have included generalization and maintenance measurements. Some of the most rigorous generalization data comes from a study that taught PECS to adults with developmental disabilities (Stoner et al., 2006). In this study, the three adults who learned to use PECS through Phase IV at home also generalized PECS use to fast food restaurants in the community. Studies limited to persons with autism also indicated that participants can generalize PECS use across people (Tincani et al., 2006), across stimuli (Marckel et al., 2006), and across activities (Schwartz et al., 1998). However, more rigorous assessments are needed before we can conclude that persons with autism generalize PECS use outside of the training environment to all naturally occurring settings and situations and with a variety of people. Current research in our lab is assessing children's generalization of PECS use across environments, situations, and people. Initial results indicate that four children with autism who were taught PECS in a workroom generalized spontaneous PECS use to a playroom with a therapist, to their homes with a parent, and to the community with a stranger. One child required minimal training in one of the generalization settings, and the other children did not require any additional training for generalization to occur in all three settings (Greenberg et al., 2010). Furthermore, only one study has included follow-up data on participants' PECS use (Howlin et al., 2007). In this study, classrooms of children with autism were randomly assigned to an immediate treatment group, delayed treatment group, or control group. Treatment consisted of a 2-day PECS workshop for teachers, six half-day school-based training sessions, and 5 months of consultation with a PECS expert. Although both treatment groups showed increases in PECS use immediately after treatment, the children in the immediate treatment group did not maintain these gains 10 months after the consultation had ended. Clearly, more data is needed on PECS maintenance, especially when treatment occurs in 1:1 sessions.

The third area of PECS research presents findings on the ancillary benefits of PECS training. These studies have found that increases in communication with PECS are related to other positive outcomes (Charlop-Christy et al., 2002; Frea et al., 2001; Anderson et al., 2007). After PECS training, the three children in Charlop-Christy and colleagues (2002) showed increases in social behaviors such as eye contact, joint attention, play, requesting, and initiations and decreases in problem behaviors including tantrums, grabbing, out-of-seat behaviors, and disruptions. In another study, a 6-year-old child who learned PECS spent more time playing and less time watching TV (Anderson et al., 2007). Lastly, Frea et al. (2001) demonstrated that once a child learned to communicate effectively with PECS, aggressions toward others decreased. This research demonstrates the importance of functional communication. Once children learn how to use PECS, this form of communication may replace other more maladaptive forms of communication, such as tantrums or aggressions. Furthermore, PECS training reinforces social behaviors such as approaching other people and exchanging pictures with them. These interactions seem to teach PECS users that social interactions can be reinforcing, setting them on the path of becoming social initiators—an important achievement for persons with autism.

The most widely studied ancillary benefit of PECS training concerns concomitant changes in the participants' verbal speech (Anderson et al., 2007; Chalrop-Christy et al., 2002; Carr & Felce, 2007; Ganz & Simpson, 2004; Howlin et al., 2007; Kravits et al., 2002; Liddle, 2001; Magiati & Howlin, 2003; Schwartz et al., 1998; Tincani et al., 2006). Many of these studies report positive results. The three children in Charlop-Christy and colleagues (2002) showed increases in both their imitative and spontaneous speech during free-play and academic sessions. Furthermore, two of the three participants increased their mean-length utterances during and after PECS training. In another single-subject study, PECS training was related to an increase in the number of intelligible words spoken by three children with autism during their PECS training sessions (Ganz & Simpson, 2004). Lastly, although not experimental, Schwartz and colleagues (1998) found that when PECS had been implemented in the classroom for 1 year, 44% of the students showed marked increases in their spoken language.

Although most of the studies indicate that PECS leads to increases in children's verbal speech, some studies have not found such results. In Howlin and colleagues' (2007) randomized group design, PECS training was not related to increases in the frequency of speech or improvements on language test scores for the children in the two treatment groups. Likewise, although Carr and Felce (2007) report that PECS training led to an increase in communicative initiations during classroom observations, this increase was almost entirely accounted for by an increase in the participants' PECS use, not verbal speech. Mixed results indicate the need for more research on the effects of PECS training on learners' verbal speech. Particular attention should be paid to initial differences in the speech profiles between those persons who acquire verbal speech and those who do not. Furthermore, researchers must explicitly describe the sessions in which speech was measured—differences in speech may emerge between PECS training sessions and free-play observations and between sessions in which the PECS book is available or not.

The final area of PECS research compares PECS with other AAC systems such as sign language and VOCAs. Although researchers are now attempting to determine which is the best AAC system for persons with autism, contradictory results indicate that the answer may not be a simple one. Studies comparing PECS and sign language report outcomes such as rate of acquisition, generalization, and the participants' preferred system. Several studies support the use of PECS. For example, Chambers and Rehfeldt (2003) taught four mands to four adults with mental retardation, ages 19 to 40 years, with both sign language and PECS using an alternating-treatments design. Three of the four participants required fewer training sessions to acquire the four mands using PECS than using sign language. The fourth participant did not reach criterion in either modality. Three participants generalized PECS use across settings, and two of the participants generalized sign use across settings. When the items were out of view, all four participants were more likely to request them using PECS than using sign language. Adkins and Axelrod (2002) taught a 7-year-old boy with PDD to request a variety of items with PECS and American Sign Language (ASL). They report that the PECS acquisition rate was faster than the ASL acquisition rate (an average of 7.1 trials for PECS versus an average of 15.7 trials for ASL). These results were consistent even when the same word was taught under both systems. Furthermore, the child was more likely to generalize PECS use outside of training sessions than to generalize ASL.

Results from Tincani (2004) are not so clear-cut. In this study, two children with autism spectrum disorders, ages 5 and 6 years, learned to request items with PECS and sign language in an alternating-treatments design. One participant demonstrated a high percentage of independent mands with sign language after the training was modified to remove modeling prompts. The other participant demonstrated a higher percentage of independent mands with PECS. Both participants were more likely to emit word vocalizations during the sign language sessions. However, once the PECS protocol was modified to include a 4-second delay, the second participant's word vocalization increased to an average of 90% of sessions.

Clearly, these studies do not indicate a clear preference for one AAC system over the other. Some researchers conclude that a student's motor imitation skills should be considered prior to training (Tincani, 2004). This relates to response effort (Richman et al., 2001). If a child has severe fine motor delays, sign language might be less efficient than PECS. It would also be useful to compare the participants' memory skills prior to training. Whereas sign language requires recall memory, the visual symbols in PECS provide constant reminders, and allow the participants to use recognition memory (Mirenda, 2003). Although visual-constant systems might be better adapted to the memory deficits in persons with autism (Charlop-Christy & Jones, 2006), this might not be an issue for persons with high recall memory. Typical of children with autism, there are individual differences that need to be taken into account before determining which AAC system should be used. The treatment of autism has never been "one-size-fits-all."

Other studies have compared the use of PECS and VOCAs. Again, the results are mixed. Although PECS and VOCAs are both visual-constant systems, VOCAs differ in the addition of digitized or synthesized voice output (Lancioni et al., 2007). In their review of PECS and VOCAs, Lancioni and colleagues (2007) describe four studies that compare the use of these two AAC systems (*see Bock et al., 2005; Dyches et al., 2002; Son et al., 2006; Soto et al., 1993*). Two of these studies compared picture boards (instead of PECS) and VOCAs with adults with mental retardation. Whereas the participant in Soto and colleagues (1993) preferred the VOCA, the participant in Dyches and colleagues (2002) preferred the picture board.

Bock and colleagues (2005) taught six nonverbal boys diagnosed with developmental delay, all age 4 years, to request items using PECS and VOCAs in a pull-out room at their schools. Three of the children acquired requesting skills faster with PECS than with their VOCAs. The other three children did not demonstrate differences in acquisition rate between AAC systems. After training, generalization of both systems was assessed in each child's main classroom. During these sessions, both systems were available to the children. Generalization results were mixed; three of the children demonstrated a clear preference for PECS, two of the children demonstrated a clear preference for VOCA, and one child did not show a clear preference for either system.

Only one published study has compared these two AAC systems with children with autism (Son et al., 2006). Three children, ages 3 to 5 years, were taught to request two snack items with both PECS and VOCAs. Acquisition rates did not differ for either system. After training, both systems were available to the children for the preference assessment sessions. One child showed a clear preference for her VOCA, and she chose it in 94% of opportunities. The other two children showed a clear preference for PECS, choosing it in 72% and 98% of opportunities.

As Lancioni and colleagues (2007) note, these studies do not indicate that one AAC system is better than another. Persons with autism are able to acquire both PECS and VOCA when making requests (Son et al., 2006).

Conclusion

Although research on children with autism and AAC systems has made substantial progress since AAC systems were first introduced with this population, the literature has areas of contradiction. It is not yet clear which AAC system is best for the majority of children with autism. However, this does not mean that science cannot inform our decisions. Interventionists should consult the literature to decide which AAC system would be best for each child on an individual basis. This process should involve a thorough consideration of many different factors including the child's strengths and limitations, certain family variables, and other environmental constraints. When evaluating the specific child, important considerations would include the child's communication needs, the child's visual and auditory skill levels, the child's motor abilities, and the child's social skills mastery level. For example, if the child has strong visual discrimination skills and poor fine motor skills, PECS might be a better choice than sign language. If the child can make more complex statements via pictorial representations, then VOCAs might be the best choice.

Interventionists must also recognize that children do not develop in isolation. Children develop in complex environments, which will affect their communication in significant ways. Therefore, environmental variables must also be considered when choosing an AAC system for a specific child (Mirenda, 2003). Several of the most influential environmental variables might stem from the child's parents or primary caregivers. Children's parents are often their primary communicative partners. If an AAC system is going to be successful for the child, then its implementation must also be both supported by and feasible for the parents. In fact, AAC systems are most effective when AAC decisions are family-centered (Bailey et al., 2006). In addition to the child's parents, broader contextual variables should also be considered. Interviews with adult AAC users and their family members identified environmental factors as having the potential to both contribute to and impede AAC effectiveness (Lund & Light, 2007). A significant consideration would be community members' familiarity with different AAC systems. For example, if community members do not know sign language, then PECS or VOCAs might be more effective. Funding might also be of importance. If service providers will not fund more expensive AAC systems, families might not be able to afford VOCAs. Lastly, the educational system's preferences should be factored into the picture. If teachers in a particular school encourage their students to communicate through sign language, they might not support the use of PECS for one child.

In conclusion, AAC decisions for children with autism must be made on an individual basis. Ideally, AAC use will result in functional, spontaneous communication across a variety of settings and with a variety of people (Mirenda, 2003). This goal will only be met if child, family, and environmental characteristics are all taken into consideration. Additionally, researchers should continue to explore the use of AAC systems with children with autism to better inform AAC decisions.

Challenges and Future Directions

The predominant theme throughout this chapter, and in other areas of autism work, is the need for more research. Since AAC systems were first introduced with persons with autism, we have learned a lot about their applications and potential benefits. However, there is still much more to know as most of the literature has been done with non-ASD populations. We end by highlighting three central questions to be addressed by future research.

1. *Which AAC system is best for persons with autism?*

As previously discussed, there is much work to be done in determining the best AAC system for persons with autism. Comparison studies will make important contributions to this field. However, it is essential that these studies follow evidence-based research practices. Most importantly, studies must demonstrate experimental control (Cooper et al., 2007). In comparison studies, experimental control is established when the researchers demonstrate that changes in the participants' communicative behaviors are attributed to the AAC interventions, and not to any other confounding variable. When studying persons with autism, the best experimental method is often single-subject design (Cooper et al., 2007; Simpson, 2003). Single-subject design accounts for the heterogeneity of the population, highlighting variability within the data and between participants (Simpson, 2003). In addition to adhering to empirically validated research practices, researchers must also ensure that they are targeting socially significant behaviors (Cooper et al., 2007). This is especially important when studying AAC systems. Studies that target one request have not demonstrated that the AAC system leads to effective communication. Lastly, more comparison studies should include generalization and maintenance measurements (Schlosser & Lee, 2000). Studies that only compare acquisition rates between two AAC systems will not be able to conclude that one AAC system is more effective than the second AAC system. Truly functional communicative behaviors will be used across environments and maintained over time. Therefore, the most useful comparison studies will also highlight which AAC systems that lead to superior generalization and maintenance over other AAC systems.

2. *What is the relationship between AAC use and the development of verbal speech?*

Although AAC systems should provide persons with autism with a means of communication that is just as effective as verbal speech, many people still view verbal speech as an important milestone for persons with autism. Verbal speech is used by interventionists and researchers to distinguish high-functioning from low-functioning persons with autism (Charlop-Christy, 1987; Schreibman, 2005). Furthermore, many parents are often hesitant to implement AAC systems, fearing that their use will decrease the chances of their children ever speaking (Millar et al., 2006). In their review of the impact of AAC systems on speech production in individuals with autism, Schlosser and Wendt (2008) conclude that AAC systems frequently lead to modest gains in speech production, but that more empirical research is needed to investigate this area. Although more empirical research is needed to confirm that AAC use leads to increases in verbal speech, parents and interventionists should no longer be concerned that AAC use will lead to a decrease in children's verbal speech or prohibit children from ever acquiring verbal speech.

3. *Do AAC systems lead to functional communication?*

Functional communication is achieved when children spontaneously use the skill in naturally occurring settings and situations (Horner & Budd, 1985). Functional communication should be our goal with AAC systems, as it is the only mark of successful communication. If AAC systems are functional, then children will use them to communicate effectively in their everyday lives (Mirenda, 2003). Unfortunately, research to date does not demonstrate that this goal has been met.

Embedded in this definition are two components: *(1)* communication must be spontaneous, and *(2)* communication must generalize. These two aspects are often difficult for persons with autism (Koegel, 2000; Lovaas et al., 1973; Lovaas et al., 1974; Schreibman, 2005). Koegel (2000) notes that although children can easily acquire AAC systems, they may have difficulties with generalization and require prompts in untrained situations. Although several studies have empirically investigated the generalization of AAC systems with persons with autism (e.g., Adkins & Axelrod, 2002; Marckel et al., 2006; Schwartz et al., 1998; Tincani et al., 2006), they have only measured AAC use in a limited number of settings and with a restricted number of people and items; these studies do not give us the complete picture of children's AAC use outside of training and research situations.

Two different lines of research could address these limitations. First, AAC studies should include generalization measurements that attempt to reflect a variety of naturally occurring settings and situations. This implies that generalization probes should be conducted across settings, people, items, and situations. Second, other studies must look beyond these generalization measurements. Although important, generalization probes will not be able to capture all of the situations in which you would expect communication. Furthermore, behavior during research sessions does not always reflect behavior in real-world contexts (Charlop-Christy et al., 2008). Situations are often contrived and the presence of the researcher may influence both the child's and the communication partner's behavior. A generalization probe might indicate that a child frequently uses PECS at home with a parent during 10-minute sessions observed by the researcher, whereas the child might not use PECS as frequently in these real-world contexts during other times when the researcher is not present.

Autism researchers could benefit from looking at research trends outside of our field. Recently, AAC as a discipline has begun to stress the importance of including other outcome measurements. Lund and Light (2006) argue that determining the effectiveness of AAC involves more than looking at how frequently it is being used. If AAC is functional, it will impact the individual's overall communication and functioning. These researchers stress the importance of looking at long-term outcomes across a range of domains, including receptive language, reading comprehension, communicative interaction, functional communication, educational and vocational achievement, self-determination, and quality of life. One way of approaching this issue involves interviewing parents of children who use AAC (Marshall & Goldbart, 2008). One of the major roadblocks to effective AAC use may be difficulty with implementation. AAC use can be expensive for families (especially when buying electronic devices, such as VOCAs), time consuming, and stressful (Lund & Light, 2007). If AAC is not feasible for the parents to implement, then it is unlikely to become functional for the child.

Research on the functionality of AAC systems reminds us of our goal. AAC systems should provide persons with autism with a means of communication—communication that is not prompt-dependent and context dependent, but rather communication that is spontaneous and effective in all situations and settings. This is a lofty goal. However, if achieved, it has the potential of dramatically improving the lives of many persons with autism. It is our hope that these benefits will continue to motivate researchers to study the applications of AAC systems with persons with autism.

SUGGESTED READINGS

Lancioni, G. E., O'Reilly, M. F., Cuvo, A. J., Singh, N. N., Sigafoos, J., & Didden, R. (2007). PECS and VOCAs to enable students with developmental disabilities to make requests: An overview of the literature. *Research in Developmental Disabilities, 28,* 468–488.

Mirenda, P. (2003). Toward functional augmentative and alternative communication for students with autism: Manual signs, graphic symbols, and voice output communication aids. *Language, Speech, and Hearing Services in Schools, 34,* 203–216.

Schlosser, R. W., & Wendt, O. (2008). Effects of augmentative and alternative communication intervention on speech production in children with autism: A systematic review. *American Journal of Speech-Language Pathology, 17,* 212–230.

REFERENCES

Adkins, T., & Axelrod, S. (2002). Topography-versus selection-based responding: Comparison of mand acquisition in each modality. *Behavior Analyst Today, 2,* 259–266.

American Psychiatric Association (2000). *Diagnostic and statistical manual of mental disorders* (Revised 4th ed.). Washington, DC: Author.

American Speech-Language-Hearing Association (1991). Report: Augmentative and alternative communication, *ASHA, 33*(Suppl. 5), 9–12.

Anderson, A., Moore, D. W., & Bourne, T. (2007). Functional communication and other concomitant behavior change following PECS training: A case study. *Behaviour Change, 24*(1), 173–181.

Baer, D. M., Wolf, M. M., & Risley, T. R. (1968). Some current dimensions of applied behavior analysis. *Journal of Applied Behavior Analysis, 1,* 91–97.

Bailey, R. L., Parette, H. P., Stoner, J. B., Angell, M. E., & Carroll, K. (2006). Family members' perceptions of augmentative and alternative communication device use. *Language, Speech, and Hearing Services in Schools, 37,* 50–60.

Barrera, R., Lobatos-Barrera, D., & Sulzer-Araroff, B. (1980). A simultaneous treatment comparison of three expressive language training programs with a mute autistic child. *Journal of Autism and Developmental Disorders, 10*, 21–37.

Barrera, R., & Sulzer-Araroff, B. (1983). An alternating treatment comparison of oral and total communication training programs for echolalic autistic children. *Journal of Applied Behavior Analysis, 16*, 379–394.

Beukelman, D. R., & Mirenda, P. (2005). *Augmentative and alternative communication: Supporting children and adults with complex communication needs* (3rd ed.). Baltimore, MD: Paul H. Brooks Publishing.

Bock, S. J., Stoner, J. B., Beck, A. R., Hanley, L., & Prochnow, J. (2005). Increasing functional communication in non-speaking preschool children: Comparison of PECS and VOCA. *Education and Training in Developmental Disabilities, 40*, 264–278.

Bondy, A. (2001) PECS: Potential benefits and risks. *Behavior Analyst Today, 2*, 127–132.

Bondy, A., & Frost, L. (2001). The Picture Exchange Communication System. *Behavior Modification, 25*, 725–744.

Bonvillian, J. D., & Nelson, K. E. (1976). Sign language acquisition in a mute autistic boy. *Journal of Speech and Hearing Disorders, 41*, 339–347.

Brady, D. O., & Smouse, A. D. (1978). A simultaneous comparison of three methods for language training with an autistic child: An experimental single case analysis. *Journal of Autism and Childhood Schizophrenia, 8*, 271–279.

Bristol, M., Cohen, D., Costello, E., Denckla, M., Eckberg, T., Kallen, R., et al. (1996). State of the science in autism: Report to the National Institutes of Health. *Journal of Autism and Developmental Disorders, 24*, 225–232.

Bryan, L. C., & Gast, D. L. (2000). Teaching on-task and on-schedule behaviors to high-functioning children with autism via picture activity schedules. *Journal of Autism and Developmental Disorders, 30*, 553–567.

Carr, D., & Felce, J. (2007). The effects of PECS teaching to Phase III on the communicative interactions between children with autism and their teachers. *Journal of Autism and Developmental Disorders, 37*, 724–737.

Carr, E., & Dores, P. (1981). Patterns of language acquisition following simultaneous communication with autistic children. *Analysis and Intervention in Developmental Disabilities, 1*, 1–15.

Carr, E., Pridal, C., & Dores, P. (1984). Speech verses sign comprehension in autistic children: Analysis and prediction. *Journal of Experimental Child Psychology, 37*, 587–597.

Chambers, M., & Rehfeldt, R. A. (2003). Assessing the acquisition and generalization of two mand forms with adults with severe developmental disabilities. *Research in Developmental Disabilities, 24*, 265–280.

Charlop, M. H., & Trasowech, J. E. (1991). Increasing autistic children's daily spontaneous speech. *Journal of Applied Behavior Analysis, 24*, 747–761.

Charlop-Christy, M. H., Carpenter, M., Le, L., LeBlanc, L. A., & Kellet, K. (2002). Using the Picture Exchange Communication System (PECS) with children with autism: Assessment of PECS acquisition, speech, social-communicative behaviors, and problem behavior. *Journal of Applied Behavior Analysis, 35*, 213–231.

Charlop-Christy, M. H., & Jones, C. (2006). The Picture Exchange Communication System: A nonverbal communication program for children with autism spectrum disorders. In R. J. McCauley & M. E. Fey (Eds.), *Treatment of language disorders in children* (pp. 105–122). Baltimore, MD: Paul H. Brooks Publishing.

Charlop-Christy, M. H., & Kelso, S. E. (2003). Teaching children with autism conversational speech using a cue card/written script program. *Education and Treatment of Children, 26*, 108–127.

Charlop-Christy, M. H., Le, L., & Freeman, K. A. (2000). A comparison of video modeling with in vivo modeling for teaching children with autism. *Journal of Autism and Developmental Disorders, 30*, 537–552.

Charlop-Christy, M. H., Malmberg, D. B., Rocha, M. L., & Schreibman, L. (2008). Treating autistic spectrum disorder. In R. J. Morris & T. R. Kratochwill (Eds.), *The practice of child therapy*. (4th ed.; pp. 299–335). Mahwah, NJ: Lawrence Erlbaum Associates.

Courchesne, E., Townsend, J., Akshoomoff, N., Saitoh, O., Yeung-Courchesne, R., Lincoln, A. J., et al. (1995). Impairment in shifting attention in autistic and cerebellar patients. *Behavioral Neuroscience, 108*, 848–865.

Cooper, J. O., Heron, T. E., & Heward, W. L. (2007). *Applied behavior analysis* (2nd ed.). Upper Saddle River, NJ: Pearson Prentice Hall.

Datillo, J., & Camarata, S. (1991). Facilitating conversation through self-initiated augmentative communication treatment. *Journal of Applied Behavior Analysis, 24*, 369–478.

Durand, V. M. (1999). Functional communication training using assistive devices: Recruiting natural communities of reinforcement. *Journal of Applied Behavior Analysis, 32*, 247–267.

Dyches, T. T. (1998). Effects of switch training on the communication of children with autism and severe disabilities. *Focus on Autism and Other Developmental Disabilities, 13*, 151–162.

Dyches, T. T., Davis, A., Lucido, B. R., & Young, J. R. (2002). Generalization of skills using pictographic and voice output communication devices. *Augmentative and Alternative Communication, 18*, 124–131.

Fulwiler, R. L., & Fouts, R. S. (1976). Acquisition of American Sign Language by a non-communicating autistic child. *Journal of Autism and Childhood Schizophrenia, 6*, 43–51.

Frea, W. D., Arnold, C. L., & Vittimberga, G. L. (2001). A demonstration of the effects of augmentative communication on the extreme aggressive behavior of a child with autism within an integrated preschool setting. *Journal of Positive Behavior Interventions, 3*, 194–198.

Frost, L. A., & Bondy, A. S. (1994). *PECS: The Picture Exchange Communication System training manual.* Cherry Hill, NJ: Pyramid Educational Consultants.

Frost, L. A., & Bondy, A. S. (2002). *The Picture Exchange Communication System training manual* (2nd ed.). Newark, DE: Pyramid Educational Products.

Ganz, J. B., & Simpson, R. L. (2004). Effects on communicative requesting and speech development of the Picture Exchange Communication System in children with characteristics of autism. *Journal of Autism and Developmental Disorders, 34*, 395–409.

Goossens, C. (1989). Aided communication intervention before assessment: A case study of a child with cerebral palsy. *Augmentative and Alternative Communication, 5*, 14–26.

Goossens, C., Crain, S., & Elder, P. (1992). *Engineering the preschool environment for interactive symbol communication: 18 months to 5 years developmentally.* Birmingham, AL: Southeast Augmentative Communication Conference Publications.

Greenberg, A., Erickson, M. A., & Charlop-Christy, M. H. (2010, May). *Evaluating generalization of the Picture Exchange Communication System in children with autism. Assessing the Picture Exchange Communication System across the lifespan: An evalusation of*

PECS generalization and concomitant increases in vocalizations. Symposium conducted at the Association for Behavior Analysis International annual convention. San Antonio, TX.

Happe, F. (1994). *Autism: An introduction to psychological theory.* London: UCL Press Limited.

Harris, M. D., & Reichle, J. (2004). The impact of aided language simulation on symbol comprehension and production in children with moderate cognitive disabilities. *American Journal of Speech-Language Pathology, 13,* 155–167.

Hermellin, B. (1976). Coding and the sense modalities. In L. Wing (Ed.), *Early childhood autism* (2nd ed.; pp. 135–168). Elmsford, NY: Pergamon.

Horner, R. H., & Budd, C. M. (1985). Acquisition of manual sign use: Collateral reduction of maladaptive behavior, and factors limiting generalization. *Education and Training of the Mentally Retarded, 20,* 39–47.

Howlin, P. (1989). Changing approaches to communication training with autistic children. *British Journal of Disorders of Communication, 24,* 151–168.

Howlin, P. (2006). Augmentative and alternative communication systems for children with autism. In T. Charman & W. Stone (Eds.), *Social and communication development in autism spectrum disorders* (pp. 236–266). New York: Guilford Press.

Howlin, P., Gordon, R. K., Pasco, G., Wade, A., & Charman, T. (2007). The effectiveness of Picture Exchange Communication System (PECS) training for teachers of children with autism: A pragmatic group randomized controlled trial. *Journal of Child Psychology and Psychiatry, 48,* 473–481.

Kanner, L. (1943). Autistic disturbances of affective contact. *Nervous Child, 2,* 217–250.

Koegel, L. K. (2000). Interventions to facilitate communication in autism. *Journal of Autism and Developmental Disorders, 30,* 383–391.

Konstantareas, M., Oxman, J., & Webster, C. (1978). Iconicity: Effects on the acquisition of sign language by autistic and other severely dysfunctional children. In P. Siple (Ed.), *Understanding language through sign language research* (pp. 213–237). New York: Academic Press.

Krantz, P. J., MacDuff, M. T., & McClannahan, L. E. (1993). Programming participation in family activities for children with autism: Parents' use of photographic activity schedules. *Journal of Applied Behavior Analysis, 26,* 137–138.

Krantz, P. J., & McClannahan, L. E. (1993). Teaching children with autism to initiate to peers: Effects of a script-fading procedure. *Journal of Applied Behavior Analysis, 26,* 121–132.

Kravits, T. R., Kamps, D. M., Kemmerer, K., & Potucek, J. (2002). Brief Report: Increasing communication skills for an elementary-aged student with autism using the Picture Exchange Communication System. *Journal of Autism and Developmental Disorders, 32,* 225–230.

La Vigna, G. W. (1977). Communication training in mute autistic adolescents using the written word. *Journal of Autism and Childhood Schizophrenia, 7,* 135–149.

Lancioni, G. E., O'Reilly, M. F., Cuvo, A. J., Singh, N. N., Sigafoos, J., & Didden, R. (2007). PECS and VOCAs to enable students with developmental disabilities to make requests: An overview of the literature. *Research in Developmental Disabilities, 28,* 468–488.

Layton, T. L., & Watson, L. R. (1995). Enhancing communication in non-verbal children with autism. In K. Quill (Ed.), *Teaching children with autism: Strategies to enhance communication and socialization* (pp. 73–104). New York: Delmar.

Layton, T. L. (1988). Language training with autistic children using four different modes of presentation. *Journal of Communication Disorders, 21,* 333–350.

Liddle, K. (2001). Implementing the Picture Exchange Communication System (PECS). *International Journal of Language and Communication Disorders, 36,* 391–395.

Light, J., & Lindsay, P. (1991). Cognitive science and augmentative and alternative communication. *Augmentative and Alternative Communication, 7,* 186–203.

Lincoln, A. J., Courchesne, E., Kilman, B. A., Elmasian, R., & Allen, M. (1988). A study of intellectual abilities in high-functioning people with autism. *Journal of Autism and Developmental Disorders, 18,* 505–524.

Lloyd, L., Fuller, D. R., & Arvidson, H. H. (1997). Introduction and overview. In L. Lloyd, D. R. Fuller, & H. H. Arvidson (Eds.), *Augmentative and alternative communication: A handbook of principles and practices* (pp. 1–7). Boston: Allyn and Bacon.

Lovaas, O. (1977). *The autistic child: Language development through behavior modification.* New York: Wiley.

Lovaas, O. I., Koegel, R., Simmons, J. Q., & Long, J. S. (1973). Some generalization and follow-up measures on autistic children in behavior therapy. *Journal of Applied Behavior Analysis, 6,* 131–166.

Lovaas, O. I., Schreibman, L., & Koegel, R. L. (1974). A behavior modification approach to the treatment of autistic children. *Journal of Autism and Childhood Schizophrenia, 4,* 111–129.

Lund, S. K., & Light, J. (2006). Long-term outcomes for individuals who use augmentative and alternative communication: Part I—What is a "good" outcome? *Augmentative and Alternative Communication, 22,* 284–299.

Lund, S. K., & Light, J. (2007). Long-term outcomes for individuals who use augmentative and alternative communication: Part III—Contributing factors. *Augmentative and Alternative Communication, 23,* 323–335.

MacDuff, G. S., Krantz, P. J., & McClannahan, L. E. (1993). Teaching children with autism to use photographic activity schedules: Maintenance and generalization of complex response chains. *Journal of Applied Behavior Analysis, 26,* 89–97.

Magiati, I., & Howlin, P. (2003). A pilot evaluation study of the Picture Exchange Communication System (PECS) for children with autistic spectrum disorders. *Autism, 7,* 297–320.

Marckel, J. M., Neef, N. A., & Ferreri, S. J. (2006). A preliminary analysis of teaching improvisation with the Picture Exchange Communication System to children with autism. *Journal of Applied Behavior Analysis, 39,* 109–115.

Marshall, J., & Goldbart, J. (2008). "Communication is everything I think." Parenting a child who needs Augmentative and Alternative Communication (AAC). *International Journal of Language and Communication Disorders, 43,* 77–98.

Millar, D. C., Light, J. C., & Schlosser, R. W. (2006). The impact of augmentative and alternative communication intervention on the speech production of individuals with developmental disabilities: A research review. *Journal of Speech, Language, and Hearing Research, 49,* 248–264.

Mirenda, P. (2001). Autism, augmentative communication, and assistive technology: What do we really know? *Focus on Autism and Other Developmental Disabilities, 16,* 141–151.

Mirenda, P. (2003). Toward functional augmentative and alternative communication for students with autism: Manual signs, graphic symbols, and voice output communication aids. *Language, Speech, and Hearing Services in Schools, 34,* 203–216.

Mirenda, P., & Erickson, K. A. (2000). Augmentative communication and literacy. In A. M. Wetherby & B. M. Prizant (Eds.), *Autism spectrum disorders: A transactional approach* (pp. 333–369). Baltimore, MD: Brookes.

Mitchell, P., & Ropar, D. (2004). Visuo-spatial abilities in autism: A review. *Infant and Child Development, 13*, 185–198.

National Research Council (2001). *Educating children with autism.* Washington, DC: National Academy Press.

Ogletree, B. T., & Harn, W. E. (2001). Augmentative and alternative communication for persons with autism: History, issues, and unanswered questions. *Focus on Autism and Other Developmental Disabilities, 16*, 138–140.

Ogletree, B. T., & Oren, T. (2006) *How to use augmentative and alternative communication interventions with individuals with autism spectrum disorders.* Austin, TX: Pro-ed.

Ozonoff, S., Pennington, B. F., & Rogers, S. J. (1991). Executive function deficits in high-functioning autistic individuals: Relationship to theory of mind. *Journal of Child Psychology and Psychiatry, 32*, 1107–1122.

Pierce, K. L., & Schreibman, L. (1994). Teaching daily living skills to children with autism in unsupervised settings through pictorial self-management. *Journal of Applied Behavior Analysis, 27*, 471–481.

Prior, M., & Chen, C. (1976). Short-term and serial memory in autistic, retarded, and normal children. *Journal of Autism and Childhood Schizophrenia, 6*, 121–131.

Quill, K. A. (1997). Instructional considerations for young children with autism: The rationale for visually cued instruction. *Journal of Autism and Developmental Disorders, 27*, 697–714.

Quill, K., & Grant, N. (1996). *Visually cued instruction: Strategies to enhance communication and socialization.* Proceedings of the Autism Society of America National Conference. Milwaukee, WI.

Richman, D. M., Wacker, D. P., & Winborn, L. (2001). Response efficiency during functional communication training: Effects of effort on response allocation. *Journal of Applied Behavior Analysis, 34*, 73–76.

Risley, T., & Wolf, M. (1967). Establishing functional speech in echolaliac children. *Behavior Research and Therapy, 5*, 73–88.

Romski, M. A., & Sevcik, R. A. (1992). Developing augmented language in children with severe mental retardation. In S. F. Warren & J. Reichle (Eds.), *Causes and effects in communication and language intervention* (pp. 113–130). Baltimore, MD: Brookes.

Romski, M. A., & Sevcik, R. A. (1996). *Breaking the speech barrier: Language development through augmented means.* Baltimore, MD: Brookes.

Romski, M. A., Sevcik, R. A., & Adamson, L. (1999). Communication patterns of youth with mental retardation with and without their speech-output communication devices. *American Journal of Mental Retardation, 104*, 249–259.

Rumsey, J. M., & Hamburger, S. D. (1988). Neuropsychological findings in high-functioning men with infantile autism, residual state. *Journal of Clinical and Experimental Neuropsychology, 10* 210–221.

Schlosser, R. W., & Lee, D. L. (2000). Promoting generalization and maintenance in augmentative and alternative communication: A meta-analysis of 20 years of effectiveness research. *Augmentative and Alternative Communication, 16*, 208–226.

Schlosser, R. W., & Wendt, O. (2008). Effects of augmentative and alternative communication intervention on speech production in children with autism: A systematic review. *American Journal of Speech-Language Pathology, 17*, 212–230.

Seal, B. C., & Bonvillian, J. D. (1997). Sign language and motor functioning in students with autistic disorder. *Journal of Autism and Developmental Disorders, 27*, 437–466.

Sherer, M., Pierce, K. L., Paredes, S., Kisacky, K. L., Ingersoll, B., & Schreibman, L. (2001). Enhancing conversational skills in children with autism via video technology: Which is better, "self" or "other" as a model? *Behavior Modification, 25*, 140–159.

Schepis, M. M., & Reid, D. H. (1995). Effects of a voice output communication aid on interactions between support personnel and an individual with multiple disabilities. *Journal of Applied Behavior Analysis, 28*, 73–77.

Schepis, M. M, Reid, D. H., Behrman, M. M., & Sutton, K. A. (1998). Increasing communicative interactions of young children with autism using a voice output communication aid and naturalistic teaching. *Journal of Applied Behavior Analysis, 31*, 561–578.

Schreibman, L. (2005). *The science and fiction of autism.* Cambridge, MA: Harvard University Press.

Schwartz, I. S., Garfinkle, A. N., & Bauer, J. (1998). Communicative outcomes for young children with disabilities. *Topics in Early Childhood Special Education, 18*, 144–159.

Sigafoos, J., Didden, R., & O'Reilly, M. (2003). Effects of speech output on maintenance of requesting and frequency of vocalizations in three children with developmental disabilities. *Augmentative and Alternative Communication, 19*, 37–47.

Sigafoos, J., Laurie, S., & Pennell, D. (1996). Teaching children with Rett syndrome to request preferred objects using aided communication: Two preliminary studies. *Augmentative and Alternative Communication, 12*, 88–96.

Simpson, R. L. (2003). Policy-related research issues and perspectives. *Focus on Autism and other Developmental Disabilities, 18*, 192–196.

Son, S., Sigafoos, J., O'Reilly, M., & Lancioni, G. E. (2006). Comparing two types of augmentative and alternative communication systems for children with autism. *Pediatric Rehabilitation, 9*, 389–395.

Soto, G., Belfiore, P. J., Schlosser, R. W., & Haynes, C. (1993). Teaching specific requests: A comparative analysis on skill acquisition and preference using two augmentative and communication aids. *Education and Training in Mental Retardation, 28*, 169–178.

Stoner, J. B., Beck, A. R., Bock, S. J., Hickey, K., Kosuwan, K., & Thompson, J. R. (2006). The effectiveness of the Picture Exchange Communication System with nonspeaking adults. *Remedial and Special Education, 27*, 154–165.

Sundberg, C. T., & Sundberg, M. L. (1990). Comparing topography-based verbal behavior with stimulus selection-based verbal behavior. *Analysis of Verbal Behavior, 8*, 31–42.

Tincani, M. (2004). Comparing the Picture Exchange Communication System and sign language training for children with autism. *Focus on Autism and Other Developmental Disabilities, 19*, 152–163.

Tincani, M., Crozier, S., & Alazetta, L. (2006). The Picture Exchange Communication System: Effects on manding and speech development for school-aged children with autism. *Education and Training in Developmental Disabilities, 41*, 177–184.

Wechsler, D. (1974). *Wechsler Intelligence Scale for Children–Revised (WISC-R).* New York: Harcourt Assessment.

Wechsler, D. (1981). *Wechsler Adult Intelligence Scale–Revised (WAIS-R).* New York: Harcourt Assessment.

Weitz, C., Dexter, M., & Moore, J. (1997). AAC and children with developmental disabilities. In S. L. Glennen & D. C. DeCoste (Eds.) *Handbook of augmentative and alternative communication* (pp. 395–405). San Diego, CA: Singular Publishing Ltd.

Wilkinson, K. M., & Hennig, S. (2007). The state of research and practice in augmentative and alternative communication for children with developmental/intellectual disabilities. *Mental Retardation and Developmental Disabilities Research Review, 13,* 58–69.

Williams, D. L., Goldstein, G., & Minshew, N. J. (2006). Neuropsychologic functioning in children with autism: Further evidence for disordered complex information-processing. *Child Neuropsychology, 12,* 279–298.

Wraikat, R., Sundberg, C. T., & Michael, J. (1991). Topography-based and selection-based verbal behavior: A further comparison. *Analysis of Verbal Behavior, 9,* 1–18.

Yoder, P., & Layton, T. (1988). Speech following sign language training in autistic children with minimal verbal language. *Journal of Autism and Developmental Disorders, 18,* 217–229.

65 Edward G. Carr†

Positive Behavior Support and Problem Behavior

Since the writing of this chapter, Professor Edward (Ted) Carr passed away following an automobile accident. Dr. Carr was greatly admired by his colleagues and students for his innovation in developing novel and compassionate strategies for improving the quality of life for people with autism. His methods are now practiced worldwide and have been incorporated into the recommendations of the Individuals with Disabilities Education Act, federal legislation that seeks to insure quality education for individuals with disabilities. We are honored to have his work represented in this volume.

Points of Interest

- Problem behavior is the major reason that people with autism spectrum disorders fail to make a good adjustment to society.
- Positive behavior support is effective for reducing problem behaviors and thereby increasing quality of life and adaptation in individuals with autism spectrum disorders.
- Positive behavior support is a transdisciplinary approach that uses educational methods to build life skills and systems and context change methods to redesign an individual's living environment.
- Even the most severe problem behaviors including aggression, self-injury, tantrums, and property destruction can be successfully treated.
- The reconceptualization of autism as a whole-body disorder highlights the necessity for examining the impact of illness and abnormal metabolism on problem behavior. These biological setting events represent new treatment targets that can broaden the scope of intervention.

Problem behavior is the major reason why people with autism spectrum disorders (ASDs) fail to make a good adjustment to society. In this chapter, I will begin by defining problem behavior. Then, I will address the issues of prevalence and clinical significance as well as the nature and relevance of the positive behavior support (PBS) perspective. The five-term contingency, a conceptual scheme for understanding problem behavior, will be presented and related methods for assessing the functions and contexts associated with problem behavior will be discussed. Next, I will highlight the critical linkage between assessment and the systematic, rational development of effective intervention strategies. A tripartite model for conceptualizing interventions—namely, avoid/mitigate/cope—will be described, and the multiple strategies that follow from this conceptualization will be presented. I then discuss the issue of outcome success. Finally, a roadmap for identifying future directions in research and practice will be outlined with respect to knowledge gaps that need to be addressed.

What is Problem Behavior?

Problem behavior includes aggression, property destruction, self-injury, and tantrums as well as noncompliance, pica, stereotypy/self-stimulatory behavior, and a variety of other disruptive behaviors. Although dangerous behaviors such as aggression and self-injury clearly merit close attention from scientists and clinicians, parents report that behavior that is "merely" difficult is often a source of family distress. Thus, elopement, feces smearing, and bizarre vocalizations can—like more dangerous behaviors—generate fear, emotional and physical exhaustion, and public embarrassment on the part of family members (Turnbull & Ruef, 1996). In sum, problem behavior must be defined not only in terms of its topographical characteristics but also in terms of its impact on others.

How Prevalent is Problem Behavior?

Problem behavior can be two or three times more likely to occur in people with developmental disabilities than in the general population (Einfeld & Tonge, 1996). In the absence of intervention, problem behavior generally persists over time and may even become worse (Emerson et al., 2001a).

Epidemiological studies of populations of individuals with an array of developmental disabilities have yielded prevalence rates of problem behavior as low as 2% to as high as 70% (Sigafoos, Arthur, & O'Reilly, 2003). One particularly well-designed total population study reported prevalence rates of

10% to 15% (Emerson et al., 2001b). Variability in prevalence rates across studies reflects differences in sample size, the mix of diagnoses represented in the sample, structural properties of the survey methodology employed, and settings selected for evaluation.

Why is Problem Behavior Important?

Problem behavior is among the leading causes of institutionalization (Bruininks, Hill, & Moreau, 1988). It disrupts family life (Lucyshyn, Dunlap, & Albin, 2002), promotes segregated rather than inclusive education (Janney & Meyer, 1990), and limits employment opportunities (Nisbet & Vincent, 1986). Because problem behavior destroys quality of life, understanding and effectively addressing such behavior requires an approach that is sensitive to broad social, emotional, educational, and ecological contexts. PBS was developed to address these broader concerns.

What is Positive Behavior Support?

PBS is a transdisciplinary approach to understanding and treating problem behavior and other challenges to personal and community adjustment. It uses educational methods to build life skills and systems and context change methods to redesign an individual's living environment (Carr, 2007; Carr & Pratt, 2007). The purpose of all these strategies is to minimize or eliminate problem behavior in ways that promote improved quality of life. Nine elements define the overall approach (Carr et al., 2002).

First, there is a focus on comprehensive lifestyle change and improved quality of life as the ultimate goal of intervention. Lifestyle change results from a broad approach that addresses the multiple dimensions defining quality of life (Hughes et al., 1995): social relationships, personal satisfaction, employment, self-determination, recreation and leisure, community adjustment, and community integration. It is deficiencies in these areas that create the conditions that promote and exacerbate problem behavior (Emerson, McGill, & Mansell, 1994; Koegel & Koegel, 2006; Koegel, Koegel, & Dunlap, 1996). Second, there is a recognition that meaningful support must be provided over protracted time periods. In other words, one must embrace a lifespan perspective to intervention. Third, interventions must have ecological validity—that is, they must be effective in the natural settings of home, school, and community, and they must be implemented by typical support people such as parents, teachers, and job coaches. Fourth, key stakeholders (e.g., parents, teachers, friends) must be involved as collaborators in helping to develop interventions. Fifth, there is an emphasis on social validity of both procedures and outcomes. In other words, typical support people must agree that the intervention strategies selected are practical, desirable, and effective and represent a good fit with their values and needs. Sixth, there is a recognition that the best conceived intervention plans will fail if they are embedded in systems that are disorganized, dysfunctional, or unsympathetic to the broad goals of PBS. Therefore, a signature characteristic of PBS involves systems change and multicomponent intervention. Seventh, there is an emphasis on prevention. This perspective stresses the idea that proactive interventions that build functional skills and redesign environments decrease the likelihood of future episodes of problem behavior. Eighth, there is flexibility with respect to methodological practices. PBS research does not rely exclusively on experimental methodology but, when appropriate, employs correlational analyses, naturalistic observations, and case studies.

The ninth and final feature of PBS is the most distinctive. Specifically, PBS draws information from multiple scientific disciplines and theoretical perspectives (Carr, 2007). A crucial aspect of PBS is its reliance on applied behavior analysis (ABA) and its accompanying operant conceptual framework emphasizing the role of learning principles in building skills and reducing problem behavior. However, no single approach, including ABA, will be able to address all relevant issues. Therefore, PBS has evolved from its ABA roots to embrace other disciplines, including organizational management, community/ecological psychology, cultural psychology, positive psychology, and biomedical science. Thus, altering systems so that they are responsive to human needs requires knowledge of organizational management (Ambrose, 1987). The themes of prevention, social support, and empowerment (all central to PBS practice) are associated with an extensive research literature in community/ecological psychology (Rappaport & Seidman, 2000). Cultural psychology provides essential information about values and customs, family structure, and child-rearing practices relevant to intervention with diverse ethnic groups (Chen, Downing, & Peckham-Hardin, 2002). The emerging field of positive psychology directly addresses quality-of-life issues as well as environmental redesign and, as such, is germane to enhancing PBS efforts (Seligman et al., 2005; Snyder & Lopez, 2005). Finally, biomedical science is a rich source of information about physiological and illness factors that can exacerbate problem behavior and diminish quality of life (Bauman, 2006; Carr & Herbert, 2008; Herbert, 2006).

Not every PBS intervention encompasses all nine of the features just discussed, but PBS, as an integrated field, does. The PBS process is facilitated by having a conceptual framework for understanding problem behavior in a way that leads logically to intervention.

A Five-Term Contingency for Understanding Problem Behavior

Figure 65-1 shows a conceptual framework that can be used to tie together many of the themes relevant to PBS. The framework has five variables. Three of them (systems, setting events,

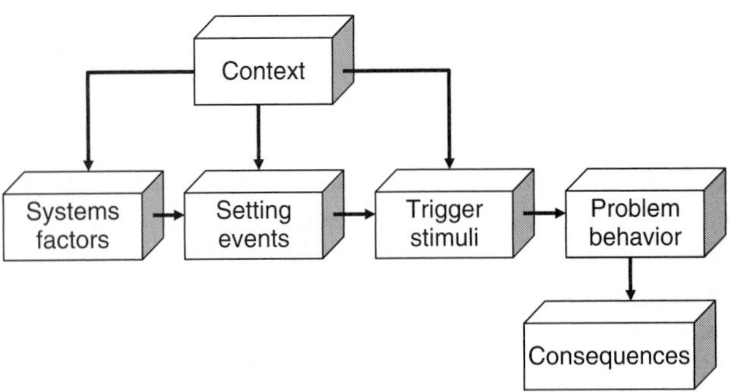

Figure 65–1. A five-term contingency for understanding problem behavior.

trigger stimuli) define the context for problem behavior and are comprised of all variables that precede (are antecedent to) such behavior. One factor, consequences, is comprised of all variables that follow the behavior. The remaining variable is the problem behavior itself, controlled by both antecedents (context) and consequences.

It will be helpful to begin by defining each variable. First, consider context. A trigger (or discriminative) stimulus is a discrete antecedent event that is strongly correlated with reinforcement of behavior. Because it reliably predicts that a specific response (behavior) will be followed by a reinforcer, the presence of the discriminative stimulus is likely to trigger a specific behavior.

A setting event is a variable that influences ongoing discriminative stimulus–response relations. Depending on the nature of the setting event, it can either facilitate or inhibit the likelihood that a given discriminative stimulus will trigger a specific behavior. An important mechanism through which setting events affect behavior is referred to as an "establishing operation" (Michael, 1982). This mechanism works by altering how reinforcing or aversive the consequences of behavior are. That is, the discriminative stimulus is either more or less likely to trigger a given response, depending on whether response consequences have become more reinforcing or more aversive.

Systems refer to broad organizational, ecological, and cultural variables that produce clinically significant settings events (Carr et al., 1998).

Consequences refer to those events that reliably follow a behavior. One major and very important consequence class is referred to as a reinforcer, but it is also variously described as the payoff, motivation, function, purpose, or intent of the behavior.

Finally, there is the behavior itself that, for present purposes, refers to any of the multiple types of problem behavior described and defined earlier, although in intervention, it can also refer to prosocial behavior.

A concrete illustration of the five-term contingency will help clarify its role in understanding problem behavior. Consider a systems variable relevant to organizational management in a school. Specifically, the school has a policy wherein all children who display major problem behavior are put in a special resource classroom. In doing so, an environment is inadvertently created that is noisy, elicits much negative feedback to students from the overstressed teacher, generates high rates of peer teasing and arguments, and promotes student anxiety because of ever-present danger from poorly behaved peers. All of these factors are setting events produced by an ill-conceived policy at the systems level. These setting events, in turn, cause discriminative stimuli related to simple academic assignments (e.g., a teacher request to read a passage from a book and answer questions) to become highly aversive. That is, reading becomes onerous in the context of high noise levels, frequent reprimands, being teased and threatened, and experiencing anxiety. The student responds not by reading but by tearing the book to pieces and screaming at the teacher. In other words, the request to read has become a trigger for aggressive behavior. The teacher responds by allowing the student to escape from having to complete the reading task. Thus, the consequence of aggression is a desired outcome—namely, cessation of the aversive reading task. The student has now learned that aggression in response to an aversive trigger stimulus terminates that stimulus. This series of events, repeated across a variety of academic tasks, compromises learning and will produce a student who displays aggressive behavior throughout the school day.

Types of Consequences (Functions)

Ultimately, people with autism display problem behavior because it serves a function. The research literature suggests two classes of functions: obtaining positive reinforcement and obtaining negative reinforcement. Reinforcement, whether positive or negative, increases the future likelihood of any problem behavior it follows.

Positive reinforcers are consequences that are added (presented) following the display of problem behavior. Attention (e.g., an expression of concern following an act of self-injury) is a common type of positive reinforcer that ensures that the behavior will be repeated in the future (Durand et al., 1989). Another type of positive reinforcer involves the presentation of tangibles (e.g., preferred foods) or access to preferred activities following outbursts of problem behavior, in a vain attempt to mollify the individual (Durand & Crimmins, 1988). Sensory reinforcement (e.g., stroboscopic effects produced by hand-flapping in front of a light source) is a third type of positive reinforcement (Rincover et al., 1979).

Negative reinforcers are consequences that are removed (withdrawn) following the display of problem behavior. These consequences are aversive in nature. Therefore, any problem behavior that is followed by successful avoidance or escape from such consequences is likely to be repeated whenever the individual encounters them in the future. Unfortunately, academic, home, and work tasks are frequently aversive to people with autism, and therefore, their termination following an outburst of problem behavior functions as a negative reinforcer (Carr, Newsom, & Binkoff, 1980). Equally unfortunately, given the nature of autism, social interaction can be very aversive and evoke problem behavior that functions to escape such interaction (Taylor & Carr, 1992).

It is often the case that many different behaviors can serve the same function, and the same behavior can serve multiple functions. Therefore, the most useful analysis of behavior involves an understanding of function and not topography. The "why" of problem behavior (function) is ultimately more important than the "what" of problem behavior (topography).

Types of Antecedents (Contexts)

Function does not exist in a vacuum. It is embedded in and created by specific contexts. Although, as noted, trigger stimuli and setting events can be distinguished on technical grounds, a specific stimulus can function as either, depending on circumstances. For example, a sudden noise can immediately evoke tantrums in a child with auditory hypersensitivity, in which case the noise is functioning as a trigger stimulus. Alternatively, the presence of noise may make an academic task aversive to a child, thereby evoking escape-motivated tantrums, but only when the task is given. In this case, the noise is functioning as a setting event rather than a trigger stimulus (i.e., here, the task, rather than the noise, is the trigger stimulus). Investigators have often focused their attention initially on identifying classes of contextual variables (consisting of both trigger stimuli and setting events) that appear to be closely associated with problem behavior.

Trigger Stimulus/Setting Event Contexts

One plausible way of parsing the research literature on contextual variables is to organize them into one of three categories: social contexts, activity/routine contexts, or biological contexts. Members of each context category have been identified, empirically, as factors that can evoke and/or exacerbate problem behavior. The research literature, although not always uniquely focused on persons with ASDs, nonetheless has great clinical relevance to them. Several examples from each generic category identified in research (e.g., McAtee, Carr, & Schulte, 2004) are briefly noted next and described more fully later.

Social contexts involve factors pertaining to relationships and interpersonal interactions. Thus, problem behavior worsens in the context of poor rapport between people, low levels of attention from others, being denied access to preferred items, and frustration resulting from difficulty in communicating with others.

Multiple aspects of common home and school routines and activities constitute a second category of contexts. Thus, activities that are too difficult, too long, too noisy, or too crowded can set off problem behavior. Activities that involve waiting, unpredictability resulting from changes in routine, and being required to make transitions between settings and activities are also factors related to an increased likelihood of problem behavior.

Biological contexts involving factors related to medication side effects, illness and pain, fatigue, anxiety, and negative mood have all been demonstrated to contribute to problem behavior.

Systemic Contexts

The third aspect of context, systems, represents a topic area that has not, until recently, been the focus of substantive research. Yet, an emerging research base relevant to home (Lucyshyn et al., 2002) and school (Crone & Horner, 2003) highlights the importance of systemic factors in understanding problem behavior.

The core idea behind systemic assessment is that it is necessary to go beyond the person who is displaying problem behavior to fully understand the range of factors influencing such behavior. One set of factors concerns the organizational structure and content of service systems. Another set of factors concerns the structure and characteristics of family systems.

The study of service systems has identified a number of factors reliably associated with problem behavior (Emerson et al., 1994). These include (1) restricting an individual's choices with respect to housing, employment, recreation, and social partners, thereby creating nonpreferred, even aversive, environments; (2) a failure to provide meaningful activities that fully engage the individual; (3) a lack of social support and community networking that isolate the individual, creating barren, unstimulating environments; (4) a lack of resources that results in little opportunity to fully integrate into the broader community (e.g., unavailability of transportation that makes trips to restaurants, movies, sporting events impossible); (5) an insufficient number of competent personnel who know how to create opportunities for enhanced quality of life; and (6) the presence of staff who have conflicting visions of critical service goals; for example, some staff emphasize containment and placidity, whereas others emphasize community integration and personal development.

The study of family systems has likewise identified several factors whose presence severely undermines the ability of parents to effectively manage their child's problem behavior (Singer et al., 2002). Thus, marital discord, parental social isolation, parental depression, parental stress, and poverty or lack of personal resources are all associated with difficulty in behavior management.

A focus on assessing systemic factors at either the service delivery or family level is a hallmark of the PBS approach (Carr et al., 1998) and provides useful information concerning what factors one might focus on in developing broad intervention strategies. Having described the types of contexts and functional consequences that influence problem behavior within a five-term contingency, we can now proceed to answer the question of what assessment strategies are available to identify these factors in real-world settings.

Methods for Assessing Function (Consequences) and Contexts

Three classes of assessment are in common use: indirect observation, direct observation, and experimental (functional analysis). Collectively, these methods are referred to as functional assessment because behavior is a function of both consequences and contexts.

Indirect Observation

Indirect observation is often referred to as informant assessment because it involves gathering information from teachers, parents, and, if possible, the person with ASD (i.e., informants). It can take the form of structured interviews, rating scales, record reviews, and person-centered planning.

The functional assessment interview (FAI) uses a structured format in which informants are asked to respond to questions concerning the nature of the behavior itself, categories of setting events and discriminative stimuli, and putative functions (purposes) of the behavior (O'Neill et al., 1997). The Motivation Assessment Scale (Durand & Crimmins, 1992) and the Contextual Assessment Inventory (McAtee et al., 2004) are rating scales, the former used to identify behavior functions, and the latter, multiple contexts. Record reviews might involve accessing archival information, regarding behavior and its controlling variables, from behavior logs completed by staff (Carr, Ladd, & Schulte, 2008).

Finally, reflecting the PBS emphasis on analyzing broader service and family systems, person-centered planning (Kincaid, 1996) is an interview assessment tool used to identify barriers to and opportunities for choice, engagement, community integration, resources, and family issues, any of which could provide a context for either problem behavior or positive, individual development. Relatedly, structured interviews and rating scales are also available to assess the integrity of living, employment, and recreational environments, all of which impact quality of life and problem behavior (Schalock & Felce, 2004). Family systems factors, which are also critical to quality of life, can be assessed using a variety of instruments (e.g., Abidin, 1997). Thus, assessing marital discord, parental stress, and depression can help identify relationships between the broader family ecology and problem behavior.

Direct Observation

Direct observation does not involve the use of intermediaries. Rather, behavior is observed directly as it is occurring in natural settings. Direct observation most commonly takes the form of A-B-C (antecedent-behavior-consequence) charts, scatter plots, and structured recording of environment–behavior sequences as they unfold in real time.

ABC charts (e.g., Carr et al., 1994) use a format that allows the observer to write down simple narrative descriptions of behaviors (B) as they occur and then to describe the antecedent trigger (discriminative) stimuli (A) as well as the consequences (C) that follow the behavior. A scatter plot (Touchette, MacDonald, & Langer, 1985) involves the use of a grid divided into time-intervals that cover each day of observation (e.g., the entire day may be broken down into half-hour blocks of time). High, low, and zero levels of problem behavior are operationalized and represented by symbols that are entered into the grid, providing a visual pattern of the times of day in which problem behaviors cluster. These times of day are then examined for the presence and type of correlated trigger stimuli and setting events.

Structured recording methods, also referred to as descriptive analysis, provide precise time-based information on A-B-C sequences as they are occurring (e.g., Emerson et al., 1996). Most commonly, the information is presented as frequency counts (e.g., the number of aggressive acts per unit of time) or time samples (e.g., the percentage of 10-second blocks of time, in 1 hour, that contain an aggressive act). Although structured recording is, arguably, the most precise and reliable method of direct observation, it is costly in terms of time and personnel requirements. Also, it is purely correlational in nature, and therefore, one cannot say with certainty that problem behavior is actually controlled by specific antecedents and consequences—only that it is temporally associated with them.

Direct observation at the level of service systems, in contrast to trigger stimuli and/or setting events, is substantially more complex and much less well-developed methodologically. Nonetheless, quality-of-life issues pertaining to systemic factors are an ongoing focus of research. In particular, direct observation methods pertinent to choice, engagement, social activity, and community involvement exist (Felce & Emerson, 2000; Schaloch, 1996). Methods also exist for studying family systems variables related to marital discord, social isolation, depression, and stress. Assessing these factors could yield important insight into the mechanisms responsible for deterioration in problem behavior. For example, research on marital discord demonstrates that it produces inconsistency in child-rearing practices (Downey & Coyne, 1990), a mechanism that could result in poor implementation of intervention strategies that might otherwise decrease the likelihood of problem behavior.

Experimental (Functional Analysis)

Functional analysis involves the experimental manipulation of the antecedents (context) and consequences of problem behavior to identify those variables that have a causal relationship to the behavior. For example, one might manipulate a specific discriminative stimulus (e.g., a task demand) by systematically presenting and withdrawing it. Further, whenever an aggressive behavior (e.g., hitting) occurred, one might allow the child displaying it to escape from the task. If no hitting occurred, then the child would not be allowed to escape. If the child subsequently showed increasing levels of hitting in the presence of the task and little hitting in its absence, then one would have learned two things. First, the function (purpose) of the hitting is to escape from a (likely) aversive task. Second, the task itself is a reliable trigger for hitting. Using variations of this method, it is possible to identify the multiple functions (e.g., attention, escape, tangibles, sensory) and multiple discriminative stimuli that control the behavior (Iwata et al., 1982).

Unlike direct observation, functional analysis can identify causal relationships between environment and behavior. However, it is time-consuming, requires a level of expertise beyond that of many practitioners, raises ethical issues because it involves purposely introducing variables that evoke problem behavior, and is extremely difficult to carry out in complex, natural environments, thereby diminishing its ecological validity (Desrochers, Hile, & Williams-Mosely, 1997).

Best Practices in Assessment

Because each assessment method has limitations as well as strengths, a multi-method approach is the best way to increase the probability of accurately identifying important variables. The three approaches described are commonly used together to ensure that clinically significant information is not missed (Carr et al., 1994). Further, because the variables controlling problem behavior often change over time, best practice dictates ongoing and repeated assessment rather than an initial assessment with no follow-up.

Linking Assessment to Intervention

Several large meta-analyses have found that intervention is about twice as likely to succeed when it is based on a careful functional assessment as when it is not (Carr, Horner et al., 1999; Didden, Duker, & Korzelius, 1997; Scotti et al., 1991). Functional assessment leads directly to an intervention model that focuses on both context and consequences as a general strategy for ameliorating problem behavior.

A Tripartite Model for Conceptualizing Intervention: Avoid/Mitigate/Cope

The key principle of PBS intervention is derived from a knowledge of functional assessment within a five-term contingency. The key principle is that problem contexts produce problem behaviors; therefore, by modifying problem contexts and the behavioral consequences that help create these contexts, we should be able to reduce or eliminate problem behaviors.

There are three generic ways in which problem contexts can be effectively addressed. First, one can avoid the context. Second, one can mitigate the context so that it no longer evokes problem behavior. Third, one can teach skills that allow an individual to cope with the context.

An example will help illustrate the logic of the avoid/mitigate/cope model of intervention. Consider one problematic context noted earlier—namely, having to wait. For example, a child must wait in line at the checkout stand in a grocery store. The child responds to this context with violent tantrums. A parent could address this problematic context by shopping only during "slow" times when lines are very short. This strategy avoids the context by eliminating waiting. When the context cannot be avoided (i.e., the family must shop at a busy time), the parent can introduce highly preferred toys into the routine. This strategy, an example of mitigation, changes the nature of the context by adding new stimuli (toys) that evoke appropriate behavior (playing), thereby replacing inappropriate behavior (tantrums). Finally, when neither avoidance nor mitigation are possible (e.g., busy store and parent did not bring toys), the child can be taught to self-regulate, a coping skill. For example, the child may be instructed to place a checkmark on a piece of paper for every 30 seconds of good behavior and receive a reward (e.g., a special treat) proportional to the number of checkmarks accumulated at the end of the waiting-in-line routine. In this case, a long wait becomes desirable as it presents opportunities for many checkmarks and substantial rewards. Furthermore, self-regulatory behavior replaces tantrums. A discussion of some of the many variations of avoid/mitigate/cope is presented next to illustrate the breadth of the model and its relationship to functional assessment and PBS. Each of these strategies can contribute, incrementally, to various aspects of individual functioning relevant to improving quality of life.

Avoid

An avoid strategy involves eliminating the trigger stimuli and setting events that evoke problem behavior. For example, if noise is a known problem context for a child (O'Reilly, Lacey, & Lancioni, 2000), then a parent may want to avoid unnecessary exposure to this context (e.g., no exposure to loud music, crowded shopping malls, motorcycles). However, complete avoidance is almost never possible in the real world of home, school, and community. Unfortunately, many parents try to approximate complete avoidance by limiting community excursions, by dropping otherwise meaningful home routines, and by shielding their child from certain types of social situations. This tactic impedes the major goal of PBS—namely, developing a good quality of life. In sum, although the judicious and limited use of an avoid strategy may be appropriate in certain circumstances, for the most part, problem contexts will need to be addressed via mitigation or coping.

Mitigate

Mitigation is a generic strategy for reducing problem behavior in which the stimulus properties of the problem context are altered. Specifically, someone other than the individual with ASD introduces new stimuli that evoke nonproblem (appropriate) behavior and/or minimize aspects of the stimulus context that are currently evoking problem behavior. Environmental redesign is a core feature of all mitigation strategies within a PBS model. Several major strategies are discussed next.

Rapport Building

Negative social relationships (poor rapport) can function as a setting event to make common tasks and demands highly aversive, thereby triggering escape-motivated problem behavior (Magito, McLaughlin, & Carr, 2005). In illustration, a female staff member who has a history of negative interactions with a young man with autism asks him to clean his room. The young man responds by trashing his room and the demand is withdrawn. However, when the same demand is presented by a staff member who has excellent rapport with the young man, the result is cheerful compliance. The staff member who has poor rapport with the man is then taught to pair herself with a wide variety of reinforcers (e.g., giving the man his favorite foods, playing his favorite music), to respond positively to his communicative attempts, and to share enjoyable activities with him in a reciprocal, not dominating, manner. The quality of the relationship (a PBS imperative) improves, and problem behavior is virtually eliminated (Magito, McLaughlin, & Carr, 2005). Redesigning the social environment to include many new stimuli that evoke appropriate behavior and that reduce the aversiveness of the interaction brings about the desired change.

Providing and Honoring Choices

Providing choices mitigates the aversiveness of a task situation or activity by allowing the individual to select tasks and activities that are currently more reinforcing or less aversive to him or her. In this manner, the need for escape-motivated problem behavior is undermined and positive engagement with preferred tasks and activities is strengthened. The introduction of choice reconfigures the environment, minimizing stimuli that trigger problem behavior and maximizing stimuli that trigger appropriate behavior (Dunlap et al., 1994).

Social Stories

A social story is a sequence of sentences, sometimes accompanied by pictures, that help an individual to know how to behave in difficult situations (Gray & Garand, 1993). For example, a child finds waiting in line for recess very frustrating and responds by throwing a tantrum to escape from the line and gain access to the playground. In response to this problem, a social story is constructed in which the difficult situation is carefully described (e.g., "At my school, before we go to recess, we wait in line with lots of other children."); specific instructions are given that direct the child on how to behave (e.g., "I have to wait my turn before leaving the building, keep my hands to myself, and not push my classmates out of the way; if I'm having trouble waiting, I can always think of the fun things I'll soon be doing out on the playground."); and the perspectives of other children are clearly stated together with desirable consequences (e.g., "The other children will like that I didn't push them and will want to play with me more once we're outside."). From a functional standpoint, social stories are a series of discriminative stimuli that prompt and trigger appropriate behavior and specify the rules governing when such behavior will be reinforced. Further, social stories greatly enhance the predictability of events, an important consideration given that individuals with autism experience unpredictability as aversive. When a social story is repeatedly rehearsed with a child, evidence suggests that problem behavior may be replaced with socially appropriate behavior (Scattone et al., 2002).

Behavioral Momentum

In this procedure, stimuli that are discriminative for problem behavior (e.g., difficult task demands) are interspersed or embedded among stimuli that are discriminative for socially appropriate behavior (e.g., easy task demands; conversations about pleasant events). Once an individual with autism has been responding appropriately to a series of nonproblematic discriminative stimuli (i.e., a positive behavioral "momentum" has been established), the problematic stimulus is presented (Mace et al., 1988). The result is a reduction in problem behavior. This procedure is likely effective because the presence of many nonproblematic discriminative stimuli evoke appropriate behavior that is positively reinforced by others, and the increase in reinforcement level, in turn, likely mitigates the aversiveness of the problem context (e.g., difficult demands), thereby undermining the motivation for escape-motivated problem behavior.

Curricular Modification

The essence of this strategy is to identify the aversive features of task stimuli (e.g., the academic curriculum) that evoke escape-motivated problem behavior and then to alter those features. For example, one might alter features related to task length and task content. Mitigating the problematic context in this manner can produce a decrease in problem behavior (Dunlap, Kern-Dunlap, & Robbins, 1991).

Noncontingent Reinforcement

If problem behavior functions to access certain reinforcers, then it may be possible to redesign the environment in such a way that the reinforcers are provided noncontingently (i.e., for "free"). In principle, sensory reinforcers, attention, and tangibles could all be provided, as appropriate, after fixed periods of time throughout the day. Thus, if self-injurious behavior is maintained by attention, one could provide attention, intermittently, irrespective of the individual's behavior at any given moment. This "free" attention, in fact, has been shown to reduce self-injurious behavior (Vollmer et al., 1993). Similarly, noncontingent reinforcement (NCR) applied to tangibly motivated problem behavior can reduce that behavior as well (Lalli, Casey, & Kates, 1997). NCR makes problem behavior nonfunctional and unnecessary. Further, the free reinforcers being provided likely also function as discriminative stimuli for appropriate behavior (e.g., when a sought-after tangible object such as a preferred toy is provided, the child will play with the toy; this play behavior replaces the problem behavior).

Altering Setting Events

As noted earlier, affective states involving negative mood, agitation, and irritability can all serve as powerful setting events that increase the likelihood of discriminative stimuli (e.g., academic task demands, home chores) acquiring aversive properties, thereby evoking escape-motivated problem behavior. It would be logical, therefore, to redesign the environment to include countermanding setting events that are associated with positive affect and that have a calming influence. This context-based intervention should decrease the aversiveness of the discriminative stimuli, making escape unnecessary. In fact, research demonstrates that the insertion of countermanding setting events, variously referred to as neutralizing routines (Horner, Day, & Day, 1997) or positive mood induction (Carret al., 2003) and consisting of preferred activities (e.g., pleasant conversation, joking, planning special events), sharply reduces problem behavior and improves affect, a quality-of-life goal consistent with PBS.

Systemic Mitigation

Although there are many narrative accounts concerning the utility of mitigation at the systemic level, there is a dearth of programmatic research demonstrating remediation of problem behavior with this approach. A notable exception to this deficiency is a study of service systems in the United Kingdom (McGill, Emerson, & Mansell, 1994). The investigators implemented broad-based interventions that focused on intensive community integration, structured involvement that included meaningful engagement in housework, occupational and recreational activities, as well as staff development pertaining to effective skills. Environmental redesign produced marked increases in constructive activity and marked decreases in minor and major problem behavior. This investigation can serve as a model for the field as to what can be accomplished from mitigation efforts at the systemic level.

Coping

Coping is a generic strategy for reducing problem behavior in which the individual with ASD acquires a skill that he/she can use to change the stimulus properties of the environment in ways that make problem behavior unnecessary. In mitigation, it is others who initiate constructive stimulus change, whereas in coping, it is the individual with ASD who initiates the change. Coping strategies are often related to the functions of the problem behaviors they are designed to replace. Further, these strategies are consonant with the PBS emphasis on prevention and the paradoxical notion that the best time to deal with problem behavior is when it is not occurring.

Functional Communication Training

This intervention involves teaching an individual specific communicative responses that serve the same function (functional equivalence) as the problem behavior they are intended to replace (Carr & Durand, 1985). In illustration, if functional assessment shows that a child engages in self-injury to attract the attention of an adult, then that child can be taught a communicative phrase (e.g., "Look what I drew, Mom!") that also attracts adult attention. Typically, any attention for self-injury would be withdrawn as well, a process referred to as extinction. Once the communicative phrase is well-established, the child has no need for self-injury anymore and the problem behavior decreases (Carr & Durand, 1985; Wacker et al., 1990). Communication alters the behavior of others, thereby producing a new stimulus environment that supports prosocial behavior.

Self-Management

This strategy involves teaching people three distinct but integrated skills: self-monitoring (i.e., to discriminate their own target behavior—e.g., aggression—and record its presence or absence), self-evaluation (i.e., to make a judgment as to whether their ongoing behavior is prosocial or problematic), and self-reinforcement (e.g., providing themselves with special treats contingent on the presence of prosocial behavior and/or absence of aggression after a period of time has elapsed). This skill can alter the stimulus properties of the environment—that is, because many reinforcers are newly available, these may reduce the aversiveness of the situation in the case of escape-motivated behavior. Further, the prosocial skills themselves may evoke positive reactions from others and this additional attention may, therefore, undermine the need for attention-seeking problem behavior. Several studies have demonstrated that self-management can produce rapid decreases in many problem behaviors, including stereotypy, that are normally quite refractory to intervention (Koegel & Koegel, 1990; Koegelet al., 1992).

Relaxation

As noted previously, anxiety can be a biological setting event. Therefore, it may promote escape-motivated problem behavior in contexts that elicit such anxiety. Progressive muscle relaxation is a skill that can be taught to a range of people with developmental disabilities (Cautela & Groden, 1978). This skill helps the individual to cope with and reduce anxiety and is thus responsive to the functional properties of the problem behavior. Relaxation has been used effectively to reduce even severe problem behavior such as self-injury (Schroeder et al., 1977).

Social Problem-Solving

People with ASDs have deficits in social behavior and problem solving in situations that require sensitivity to the social and emotional cues provided by others. The incomprehensibility of most social situations leads to frustration, failure, and eventual "meltdowns." Therefore, it is useful to teach people with

ASDs how to identify and understand the social and emotional perspectives of others and how to develop and organize strategies for dealing with common social situations. A wealth of pragmatic suggestions and strategies based on clinician experience has been described in detail (Myles & Southwick, 1999).

Multicomponent Intervention: A Best Practice

As we have seen, problem behavior in the natural environment is evoked by many contexts and serves many functions. For this reason, multicomponent intervention and related PBS perspectives have become a best practice in dealing with problem behavior. As noted, each mitigate and cope strategy is proactive, reflecting the PBS emphasis on prevention. However, these strategies are commonly combined when they are used to address problem behavior in the home (Lucyshyn, Albin, & Nixon, 1997), school (Crone & Horner, 2003), workplace (Kemp & Carr, 1995), and community (Vaughn et al., 1997). Further, strategy implementation by natural intervention agents (parents, teachers, job coaches) operating in natural contexts (home, school) highlights the PBS focus on ecological validity. The involvement of key stakeholders (Turnbull & Turnbull, 1996) and a concern with social validity (Carr, Horner et al, 1999)—namely, with the feasibility and acceptability of intervention (both key features of PBS)—are woven into the fabric of multicomponent approaches. Because the variables influencing problem behavior may change over time, the PBS emphasis on lifespan perspective is an important aspect of longitudinal research exploring improvements over a period of years, rather than weeks or even months (e.g., Carr, Levin et al., 1999). The PBS embrace of scientific fields and disciplines beyond applied behavior analysis can be seen in research that focuses on quality-of-life issues related to positive psychology (Dunlap et al., 2003), cultural factors (Wang, McCart, & Turnbull, 2007), organizational management (Sailor et al., 2006), and biomedical influences (Carr & Blakeley-Smith, 2006). In sum, multicomponent intervention is the nexus for the critical features that define PBS and facilitate its effectiveness in addressing problem behavior in complex real-world contexts.

Outcomes: How Well Have We Succeeded?

Several meta-analyses have been conducted examining data across hundreds of studies of problem behavior (Carr, Horner et al., 1999; Didden et al., 1997; Horner et al., 2002; Scotti et al., 1991). Extracting information from the studies most relevant to PBS yields the following conclusions:

1. Even the most severe problem behaviors including aggression, self-injury, tantrums, and property destruction can be successfully treated.
2. There is an 80% or greater reduction from baseline in the level of problem behavior for about two-thirds of the cases, 90% or greater reduction for about one-half of the cases, and a 100% reduction for about one-quarter of the cases (Carr, Horner et al., 1999). It is likely that these figures are underestimates because they only summarize data to 1999 and there have been a large number of successful studies reported since. However, no full-scale meta-analysis exists that captures these more recent data.
3. There are relatively few studies examining and reporting maintenance of intervention effects beyond 1 year. Although durable change has been demonstrated, small sample size mandates cautious interpretation.
4. Improvements in specific aspects of quality of life are well-documented. However, there are relatively few studies examining and reporting multidimensional changes in quality of life related to problem behavior reduction. Although positive change has been noted, small sample size, again, is an issue.

Conclusion

Problem behavior needs to be addressed from a broad perspective that integrates skill building, environmental redesign, systemic influences, and biomedical factors. A conceptual framework that adopts this perspective is most likely to lead to the development of interventions that alter quality of life while at the same time reducing problem behavior. Ultimately, it is an improved quality of life for people with autism and for those who love them.

Challenges and Future Directions

Gaps in the extant literature highlight areas where additional research is needed to further enhance our understanding of problem behavior and increase the number of intervention options available.

- Overwhelmingly, research has focused on externalizing problem behavior. Yet, it is known that internalizing disorders (anxiety, depression) can function as setting events to exacerbate externalizing behavior. Therefore, exploring this linkage through appropriate assessment could help elucidate the potential contribution of cognitive-behavior therapy (Reaven & Hepburn, 2003).
- There is a need to develop algorithms for translating, in a rational and prescriptive manner, complex assessment information from the five-term contingency into intervention development related to the wide array of options stemming from the tripartite model of intervention.
- Long-term maintenance of behavior gains across the lifespan is a function of systems and not procedures (Carr, 2007). An intervention package is effective over time

only if it is applied with integrity over time. Therefore, the factors responsible for sustained intervention efforts must be identified and strengthened.

- The systemic component of the five-term contingency is grossly under-researched. More studies of organizational management and community psychology at the level of service systems (Emerson et al., 1994; Knoster, Villa, Thousand, 2000; Sugai et al., 2000) need to be undertaken to identify the systemic factors responsible for problem behavior and the environmental modifications needed to promote prosocial behavior.
- A sole focus on the individual with ASD does not capture family systems variables that impact problem behavior and intervention sustainability. Relationship discord, personal strengths, parent affective distress, social isolation, and cultural factors must be examined in relation to problem behavior, goal setting, intervention selection, and satisfaction with outcomes. Many of these issues relate to the emerging field of positive psychology (Seligman et al., 2005) that can serve as an additional source of useful concepts and methods.
- The reconceptualization of ASDs as whole-body disorders (Herbert, 2005) highlights the necessity for examining the impact of illness and abnormal metabolism on problem behavior. Problem behaviours may reflect underlying pain and discomfort and may be misinterpreted unless the health of the individual with ASD is considered. These biological setting events represent new treatment targets that can broaden the scope of intervention (Bauman, 2006; Carr & Herbert, 2008).
- The relationship between problem behavior and multiple dimensions of quality of life is likely bidirectional. Research on this relationship, although nascent at present, has the potential for broadening our understanding of the factors that control problem behavior while addressing the central goal of PBS—namely, improving quality of life.
- Research is needed on identifying the factors that lead to the emergence of serious problem behavior. This prevention agenda may be pursued by exploring early developmental processes (Guess & Carr, 1991) and proactive redesign of the environment to eliminate those factors whose cumulative impact over time leads to behavioral deterioration.

SUGGESTED READINGS

Carr, E. G., Dunlap, G., Horner, R. H., Koegel, R. L., Turnbull, A. P., Sailor, W., Anderson, J., Albin, R. W., Koegel, L. K., & Fox, L. (2002). Positive behavior support: Evolution of an applied science. *Journal of Positive Behavior Interventions, 4*, 4–16, 20.

Carr, E. G., Horner, R. H., Turnbull, A. P., Marquis, J. G., Magito McLaughlin, D., McAtee, M. L., et al. (1999). *Positive behavior support for people with developmental disabilities: A research synthesis.* Washington, DC: American Association on Mental Retardation.

Horner, R. H., Carr, E. G., Strain, P. S., Todd, A. W., & Reed, H. K. (2002). Problem behavior interventions for young children with autism. *Journal of Autism and Developmental Disorders, 32*, 423–446.

REFERENCES

Abidin, R. R. (1997). Parenting Stress Index: A measure of the parent-child system. In Zalaquett, C. P. & Wood, R. J. (Eds). *Evaluating Stress: A book of resources* (pp. 277–291). Lanham, MD: Scarecrow Press.

Ambrose, D. (1987). *Managing complex change.* Pittsburgh, PA: Enterprise Group.

Bauman, M.L. (2006). Beyond behavior—Biomedical diagnoses in autism spectrum disorders. *Autism Advocate, 45*(5), 27–29.

Carr, E. G. (2007). The expanding vision of positive behavior support: Research perspectives on happiness, helpfulness, hopefulness. *Journal of Positive Behavior Interventions, 9*, 3–14.

Carr, E. G., & Blakeley-Smith, A. (2006). Classroom intervention for illness-related problem behavior in children with developmental disabilities. *Behavior Modification, 30*, 901–924.

Carr, E. G., Carlson, J. I., Langdon, N. A., Magito McLaughlin, D., & Yarbrough, S. C. (1998). Two perspectives on antecedent control: Molecular and molar. In J. K. Luiselli & M. J. Cameron (Eds.), *Antecedent control: Innovative approaches to behavioral support* (pp. 3–28). Baltimore: Paul H. Brookes.

Carr, E. G., Dunlap, G., Horner, R. H., Koegel, R. L., Turnbull, A. P., Sailor, W., et al. (2002). Positive behavior support: Evolution of an applied science. *Journal of Positive Behavior Interventions, 4*, 4–16, 20.

Carr, E. G., & Durand, V. M. (1985). Reducing behavior problems through functional communication training. *Journal of Applied Behavior Analysis, 18*, 111–126.

Carr, E. G. & Herbert, M. R. (2008). Integrating behavioral and biomedical approaches: A marriage made in heaven. *Autism Advocate, 50 (1)*, 46–52.

Carr, E. G, Horner, R. H., Turnbull, A. P., Marquis, J. G., Magito McLaughlin, D., McAtee, M. L., et al. (1999). *Positive behavior support for people with developmental disabilities: A research synthesis.* Washington, DC: American Association on Mental Retardation.

Carr, E. G., Ladd, M. V., & Schulte, C. (2008). Validation of the Contextual Assessment Inventory (CAI) for problem behavior. *Journal of Positive Behavior Interventions, 10*, 91–104.

Carr, E. G., Levin, L., McConnachie, G., Carlson, J. I., Kemp, D.C., & Smith, C. E. (1994). *Communication-based intervention for problem behavior: A user's guide for producing positive change.* Baltimore: Paul H. Brookes.

Carr, E. G., Levin, L., McConnachie, G., Carlson, J. I., Kemp, D.C., Smith, C. E., & Magito McLaughlin, D. (1999). Comprehensive multisituational intervention for problem behavior in the community: Long-term maintenance and social validation. *Journal of Positive Behavior Interventions, 1*, 5–25.

Carr, E. G., Magito McLaughlin, D., Giacobbe-Grieco, T., & Smith, C. E. (2003). Using mood ratings and mood induction in assessment and intervention for severe problem behavior. *American Journal on Mental Retardation, 108*, 32–55.

Carr, E. G., Newsom, C. D., & Binkoff, J. A. (1980). Escape as a factor in the aggressive behavior of two retarded children. *Journal of Applied Behavior Analysis, 13*, 101–117.

Carr, E. G., & Pratt, C. L. (2007). Positive behavioral supports: Creating meaningful life options for people with ASD. *Autism Advocate, 49 (4)*, 37–43.

Cautela, J. R., & Groden, J. (1978). *Relaxation: A comprehensive manual for adults, children, and children with special needs.* Champaign, IL: Research Press.

Chen, D., Downing, J. E., & Peckham-Hardin, K. D. (2002). Working with families of diverse cultural and linguistic backgrounds. In J. M. Lucyshyn, G. Dunlap, & R. W. Albin (Eds.), *Families and positive behavior support* (pp. 133–154). Baltimore: Paul H. Brookes.

Crone, D. A., & Horner, R. H. (2003). *Building positive behavior support systems in schools.* New York: Guilford.

Desrochers, M. N., Hile, M. G., & Williams-Moseley, T. L. (1997). Survey of functional assessment procedures used with individuals who display mental retardation and severe problem behaviors. *American Journal on Mental Retardation, 101*, 535–546.

Didden, R., Duker, P. C., & Korzilius, H. (1997). Meta-analytic study on treatment effectiveness for problem behaviors with individuals who have mental retardation. *American Journal on Mental Retardation, 101*, 387–399.

Downey, G. & Coyne, J. C. (1990). Children of depressed parents: An integrative review. *Psychological Bulletin, 108*, 50–76.

Dunlap, G., Clarke, C., Carr, E. G., & Horner, R. H. (2003). *RRTC on positive behavior support: Findings from longitudinal case studies.* Paper presented at the annual conference of the Association for Positive Behavior Support, Orlando, FL.

Dunlap, G., dePerczel, M., Clarke, S., Wilson, D., Wright, S., White, R., & Gomez, A. (1994). Choice making and proactive behavioral support for students with emotional and behavioral challenges. *Journal of Applied Behavior Analysis, 27*, 505–518.

Dunlap, G., Kern-Dunlap, L., Clarke, S., & Robbins, F.R. (1991). Functional assessment, curricular revision, and severe behavior problems. *Journal of Applied Behavior Analysis, 24*, 387–397.

Durand, V.M., & Crimmins, D.B. (1988). Identifying the variables maintaining self-injurious behavior. *Journal of Autism and Developmental Disorders, 18*, 99–117.

Durand, V. M., & Crimmins, D. B. (1992). *The Motivation Assessment Scale (MAS) administration guide.* Topeka, KS: Monaco & Associates.

Durand, V.M., Crimmins, D.B., Caulfield, M., & Taylor, J. (1989). Reinforcer assessment I: Using problem behavior to select reinforcers. *Journal of the Association for Persons with Severe Handicaps, 14*, 113–126.

Einfeld, S. L., & Tonge, B. J. (1996). Population prevalence of psychopathology in children and adolescents with intellectual disability: II. Epidemiological findings. *Journal of Intellectual Disability Research, 40*, 99–109.

Emerson, E., Kiernan, C., Alborz, A., Reeves, D., Mason, H., Swarbrick, R., Mason, L., & Hatton, C. (2001a). Predicting the persistence of self-injurious behavior. *Research in Developmental Disabilities, 22*, 67–75.

Emerson, E., Kiernan, C., Alborz, A., Reeves, D., Mason, H., Swarbrick, R., Mason, L., & Hatton, C. (2001b). The prevalence of challenging behaviors: A total population study. *Research in Developmental Disabilities, 22*, 77–93.

Emerson, E., McGill, P., & Mansell, J. (Eds.). (1994). *Severe learning disabilities and challenging behaviours.* London: Chapman & Hall.

Emerson, E., Reeves, D., Thompson, S., Henderson, D., & Robertson, J. (1996). Descriptive analysis of severe challenging behaviour: the application of lag-sequential analysis. *Journal of Intellectual Disability Research, 40*, 260–274.

Felce, D., & Emerson, E. (2000). Observational methods in assessment of quality of life. In T. Thompson, D. Felce, & F. J. Symons (Eds.). *Behavioral observation* (pp. 159–174). Baltimore: Paul H. Brookes.

Gray, C. A., & Garand, J. D. (1993). Social stories: Improving responses of students with autism with accurate social information. *Focus on Autistic Behavior, 8*, 1–10.

Guess, D., & Carr, E. (1991). Emergence and maintenance of stereotypy and self-injury. *American Journal on Mental Retardation, 96*, 299–319.

Herbert, M. R. (2005). Autism: A brain disorder, or a disorder that affects the brain? *Clinical Neuropsychiatry, 2*, 354–379.

Herbert, M. R. (2006). Time to get a grip. *Autism Advocate, 45* (5), 18–25.

Horner, R. H., Carr, E. G., Strain, P. S., Todd, A. W., & Reed, H. K. (2002). Problem behavior interventions for young children with autism. *Journal of Autism and Developmental Disorders, 32*, 423–446.

Horner, R. H., Day, H. M., & Day, J. R. (1997). Using neutralizing routines to reduce problem behaviors. *Journal of Applied Behavior Analysis, 30*, 601–614.

Hughes, C., Hwang, B., Kim, J. H., Eisenman, L. T., & Killian, D. J. (1995). Quality of life in applied research: A review and analysis of empirical measures. *American Journal on Mental Retardation, 99*, 623–641.

Iwata, B. A., Dorsey, M. F., Slifer, K. J., Bauman, K. E., & Richman, G. S. (1982). Toward a functional analysis of self-injury. *Analysis and Intervention in Developmental Disabilities, 2*, 3–20.

Janney, R. E., & Meyer, L. H. (1990). A consultation model to support integrated educational services for students with severe disabilities and challenging behaviors. *Journal of the Association for Persons with Severe Handicaps, 15*, 186–199.

Kemp, D. C., & Carr, E. G. (1995). Reduction of severe problem behavior in community employment using an hypothesis-driven multicomponent intervention approach. *Journal of the Association for Persons with Severe Handicaps, 20*, 229–247.

Kincaid, D. (1996). Person-centered planning. In R. L. Koegel, L. K. Koegel, & G. Dunlap (Eds.), *Positive behavioral support* (pp. 439–466). Baltimore: Paul H. Brookes.

Knoster, T. P., Villa, R. A., & Thousand, J. S. (2000). A framework for thinking about systems change. In R. A. Villa & J. S. Thousand (Eds.), *Restructuring for caring and effective* education (pp. 93–128). Baltimore: Paul H. Brookes.

Koegel, L. K., Koegel, R.L., & Dunlap, G. (1996). *Positive behavioral support.* Baltimore: Paul H. Brookes.

Koegel, L. K., Koegel, R. L., Hurley, C., & Frea, W. D. (1992). Improving social skills and disruptive behavior in children with autism through self-management. *Journal of Applied Behavior Analysis, 25*, 341–353.

Koegel, R. L. & Koegel, L. K. (1990). Extended reductions in stereotypic behavior of students with autism through a self-management treatment package. *Journal of Applied Behavior Analysis, 23*, 119–128.

Koegel, R. L., & Koegel, L. K. (2006). *Pivotal response treatments for autism.* Baltimore: Paul H. Brookes.

Lalli, J. S., Casey, S. D., & Kates, K. (1997). Noncontingent reinforcement as treatment for severe problem behavior: Some procedural variations. *Journal of Applied Behavior Analysis, 30*, 127–137.

Lucyshyn, J. M., Albin, R. W., & Nixon, C. D. (1997). Embedding comprehensive behavioral support in family ecology: An experimental, single-case analysis. *Journal of Consulting and Clinical Psychology, 65,* 241–251.

Lucyshyn, J. M., Dunlap, G., & Albin, R. W. (Eds.). (2002). *Families and positive behavior support.* Baltimore: Paul H. Brookes.

Mace, F. C., Hock, M. L., Lalli, J. S., West, B. J., Belfiore, P., Pinter, E., & Brown, D. K. (1988). Behavioral momentum in the treatment of noncompliance. *Journal of Applied Behavior Analysis, 21,* 123–141.

Magito McLaughlin, D., & Carr, E. G. (2005). Quality of rapport as a setting event for problem behavior: Assessment and intervention. *Journal of Positive Behavior Interventions, 7,* 68–91.

McAtee, M., Carr, E. G., & Schulte, C. (2004). A Contextual Assessment Inventory for problem behavior: Initial development. *Journal of Positive Behavior Interventions, 6,* 148–165.

McGill, P., Emerson, E., & Mansell, J. (1994). Individually designed residential provision for people with seriously challenging behaviours. In E. Emerson, P. McGill, & J. Mansell (Eds.) *Severe learning disabilities and challenging behaviours* (pp. 119–156). London: Chapman & Hall.

Michael, J. (1982). Distinguishing between discriminative and motivational functions of stimuli. *Journal of the Experimental Analysis of Behavior, 37,* 149–155.

Myles, B. S., & Southwick, J. (1999). *Asperger syndrome and difficult moments.* Shawnee Mission, KS: Autism Asperger Publishing Co.

Nisbet, J., & Vincent, L. (1986). The differences in inappropriate behavior and instructional interactions in sheltered and nonsheltered work environments. *Journal of the Association for Persons with Severe Handicaps, 11,* 19–27.

O'Neill, R. E., Horner, R. H., Albin, R. W., Sprague, J. R. Storey, K., & Newton, J. S. (1997). *Functional assessment and program development for problem behavior.* Pacific Grove, CA: Brooks/Cole.

O'Reilly, M. F., Lacey, C., & Lancioni, G. E. (2000). Assessment of the influence of background noise on escape-maintained problem behavior in a child with Williams syndrome. *Journal of Applied Behavior Analysis, 33,* 511–514.

Reaven, J., & Hepburn, S. (2003). Cognitive behavioral treatment of obsessive-compulsive disorder in a child with Asperger Syndrome. *Autism, 7,* 145–164.

Rappaport, J., & Seidman, E. (Eds.). (2000). *Handbook of community psychology.* New York: Kluwer Academic.

Rincover, A., Cook, R., Peoples, A., & Packard, D. (1979). Sensory extinction and sensory reinforcement principles for programming multiple adaptive behavior change. *Journal of Applied Behavior Analysis, 12,* 221–233.

Sailor, W., Zuna, N., Choi, J-H., Thomas, J., & McCart, A. (2006). Anchoring schoolwide positive behavior support in structural school reform. *Research & Practice for Persons with Severe Disabilities, 31,* 18–30.

Scattone, D., Wilczynski, S. M., Edwards, R. P., & Rabian, B. (2002). Decreasing disruptive behaviors of children with autism using social stories. *Journal of Autism and Developmental Disorders, 32,* 535–543.

Schalock, R. L. (Ed.). (1996). *Quality of life. Volume 1. Conceptualization and measurement.* Washington, DC: American Association on Mental Retardation.

Schalock, R. L., & Felce, D. (2004). Quality of life and subjective well-being: Conceptual and measurement issues. In E. Emerson, C. Hatton, T. Thompson, & T. R. Parmenter (Eds.), *The international handbook of applied research in intellectual disabilities* (pp. 423–441). New York: Wiley.

Schroeder, S. R., Peterson, C. R., Solomon, L. J., & Artley, J. J. (1977). EMG feedback and the contingent restraint of self-injurious behavior among the severely retarded: Two case illustrations. *Behavior Therapy, 8,* 738–741.

Scotti, J. R., Evans, I. M., Meyer, L. H., & Walker, P. (1991). A meta-analysis of intervention research with problem behavior: Treatment validity and standards of practice. *American Journal on Mental Retardation, 96,* 233–256.

Seligman, M. E. P., Steen, T. A., Park, N., & Peterson, C. (2005). Positive psychology progress: Empirical validation of interventions. *American Psychologist, 60,* 410–421.

Sigafoos, J., Arthur, M., & O'Reilly, M. (2003). *Challenging behavior and developmental disability.* London: Whurr Publishers.

Singer, G. H. S., Goldberg-Hamblin, S. E., Peckham-Hardin, K. D., Barry, L., & Santarelli, G. E. (2002). Toward a synthesis of family support practices and positive behavior support. In J. M. Lucyshyn, G. Dunlap., & R. W. Albin (Eds.), *Families and positive behavior support* (pp. 155–183). Baltimore: Paul H. Brookes.

Snyder, C. R., & Lopez, S. J. (Eds.). (2005). *Handbook of positive psychology.* New York: Oxford University Press.

Sugai, G., Horner, R. H., Dunlap, G., Hieneman, M., Lewis, T. J., Nelson, C. M., Scott, T., Liaupsin, C., Sailor, W., Turnbull, A. P., Turnbull, H. R., & Wickham, D. (2000). Applying positive behavior support and functional behavior assessment in schools. *Journal of Positive Behavior Interventions, 2,* 131–143.

Taylor, J. C., & Carr, E. G. (1992). Severe problem behavior related to social interaction. II: A systems analysis. *Behavior Modification, 16,* 336–371.

Touchette, P. E., MacDonald, R. F., & Langer, S. N. (1985). A scatter plot for identifying stimulus control of problem behavior. *Journal of Applied Behavior Analysis, 18,* 343–351.

Turnbull, A. P., & Ruef, M. (1996). Family perspectives on problem behavior. *Mental Retardation, 34,* 280–293.

Turnbull, A. P., & Turnbull, H. R. (1996). Group action planning as a strategy for providing comprehensive family support. In L. K. Koegel, R. L. Koegel, & G. Dunlap (Eds.), *Positive behavioral support* (pp. 99–114). Baltimore: Paul H. Brookes.

Vaughn, B. J., Dunlap, G., Fox, L., Clarke, S., & Bucy, M. (1997). Parent-professional partnership in behavioral support: A case study of community-based intervention. *Journal of the Association for Persons with Severe Handicaps, 22,* 185–197.

Vollmer, T. R., Iwata, B. A., Zarcone, J. R., Smith, R. G., & Mazaleski, J. L. (1993). The role of attention in the treatment of attention-maintained self-injurious behavior: Noncontingent reinforcement and differential reinforcement of other behavior. *Journal of Applied Behavior Analysis, 26,* 9–21.

Wacker, D. P., Steege, M. W., Northup, J., Sasso, G., Berg, W., Reimers, T., Cooper, L., Cigrand, K., & Donn, L. (1990). A component analysis of functional communication training across three topographies of severe behavior problems. *Journal of Applied Behavior Analysis, 23,* 417–429.

Wang, M., McCart, A., & Turnbull, A. P. (2007). Implementing positive behavior support with Chinese American families: Enhancing cultural competence. *Journal of Positive Behavior Interventions, 9,* 38–51.

66 Connie Kasari, Jill Locke

Social Skills Interventions for Children With Autism Spectrum Disorders

Points of Interest

- Children with ASDs often experience a variety of social challenges that may hinder their ability to establish meaningful relationships with other children; therefore, increasing social contact and peer interactions for children with autism is an important goal.
- Important active ingredients in successful social skills interventions for children with ASDs include: the context of intervention, methodological approach, facilitation agent, content (target goals), and dose.
- Children with ASDs are responsive to a wide variety of interventions aimed at increasing their social engagement and social skills repertoires. However, there remains a concern regarding the lack of maintenance and generalization of the intervention effect that suggests that acquiring skills may require a longer period of time and additional and continuous social support may be needed.
- Randomized controlled treatment trials need to be conducted on a larger scale in children's natural settings to determine whether a specific intervention type is more efficacious than mere clinical attention or is relevant for the general population of children and adolescents with ASDs.

Given the pressure teachers are under to make academic benchmarks, the social and emotional well-being of children can be overlooked. However, for many children, these social goals are critical to their overall school adjustment. Feeling connected to others can lead to a sense of belongingness that in turn can foster both social-emotional adjustment and academic competence at school (Ladd, Kochenderfer, & Coleman, 1996).

Although all children need to have their social and emotional needs met at school, the needs of some children may be even more challenging. Children with an autism spectrum disorder (ASD) have significant challenges in relating to others, maintaining peer relationships, and making friends. Yet, more and more, parents are requesting full inclusion into general education classrooms for their children with ASDs, in part to promote normalized social interactions, and the possibility of friendships with typically developing children (Kasari et al., 1999). Schools are now beginning to recognize the need to accommodate all children in their classrooms; however, meeting the needs of children with ASDs will take concerted efforts on the part of all involved, including teachers, parents, and peers.

In this chapter we consider what we currently know about the social lives of children with ASDs, including their social interactions with peers and the development of friendships. We identify a number of challenges that children with ASDs face—particularly in school settings with the general population of children—and then examine the effectiveness of current interventions for children with ASDs, with a focus on active ingredients of intervention. Finally, we suggest some avenues for future research in this area.

Characterizing Social Skills and Children With ASD

The term *social skills* is generically used to encompass several domains of social functioning. Matson, Matson, and Rivet (2007) define social skills as interpersonal responses that allow children to adapt to the environment through verbal and nonverbal communication. Children naturally learn and expand their social skills through multiple interactions with others. For children with social deficits, such as children with autism, these natural opportunities are restricted because of a range of impairments in social recognition, communication, and comprehension (American Psychiatric Association, 2000). Broadly, children with ASDs may experience challenges in social reciprocity, initiation of interactions, emotional behavior, eye contact, joint engagement, empathy, and perspective taking. These social deficits affect children's ability to connect with peers and to develop quality relationships with others.

All of these challenges affect how well children with ASDs relate to their peers and others. More than two decades ago, Wing (1988) described three categories of children with ASDs, including those who could be described as "aloof and indifferent," "passive," and "interactive but odd." Children who are aloof and indifferent are the children who tend to ignore others and avoid social contact altogether. An example is the child who becomes engrossed in the slats of the fence surrounding the playground and is oblivious to other children who may try to engage him or her in a game or conversation or the child who may actually leave an area of play when other children enter. The child who is passive tends to accept social contact when it is initiated by others. Such children are sometimes subjected to various roles (e.g., puppy, baby, monster, etc.) in games whether he or she wanted those roles or not. Finally, children classified as "interactive but odd" are motivated to interact with others but typically lack the skill needed to build positive social relationships. They may seek out interactions and then not understand why others avoid them when they do something annoying or unusual.

Given these classifications of children with autism, one might expect that they would be isolated in their classrooms, with limited peer interactions and few friends. At least with young children with autism, this does not seem to be the case. Most higher-functioning children with autism in the primary grades are not isolated in their classroom peer social networks as reported by peer nominations (Chamberlain, Kasari, & Rotheram-Fuller, 2007). Chamberlain et al. (2007) reported that although none of the children with autism in second and third grade classrooms was isolated, these mostly male children were often on the periphery of their classroom social structure. Their connections to others in the class tended to be with a small group of other children, typically female peers. These findings suggest that children with autism are able to establish some social connections with other children in their classroom but may need to be taught specific social skills such as how to hold a conversation, take the perspective of others, and engage in pretend play to be more centrally connected in their class social networks (Scattone, 2007). In addition, many children with autism must learn the subtleties of social interactions, such as developing an awareness of personal space, showing empathy, and reading body language, which may help form stronger connections and higher quality relationships with peers (Scattone, 2007).

Increasing social contact and peer interactions for children with autism is an important goal. However, peer interactions are not the same as developing a selective relationship or friendship with another child. By definition, friendships are "affectionate attachments between two individuals" that are built upon recurring experiences and social interactions (Bukowski, Newcomb, & Hartup, 1996). Friendship has been shown to provide children with a breadth of positive outcomes, including the sense of belongingness and self-worth (Bagwell, Newcomb, & Bukowski, 1998), emotional support, protection from loneliness, isolation, and rejection (Bollmer et al., 2005; Parker & Asher, 1993), and positive school adjustment (Ladd et al., 1996). Thus, it is important to not only promote peer interactions but to also consider friendship development.

Friendships

Friendships are defined by qualities such as companionship, support, closeness, and conflict. Therefore, it is not just whether children have friendships that make a difference in their development and well-being but rather the quality of these friendships that is important (Bukowski, Newcomb, & Hartup, 1996). Friendship quality has been proposed as creating various psychological benefits and costs for children that, in turn, affect their development and adjustment (Ladd et al., 1996).

Multiple reports indicate that more than half of children, adolescents, and adults with autism do not have friends or even acquaintances (Howlin et al., 2004; Orsmond, Krauss, & Seltzer, 2004). These data are derived primarily from parent report, and parents may or may not be privy to their child's innermost feelings about their friends. When researchers have asked children and adolescents themselves, they almost all report having a friend (Bauminger & Kasari, 2000; Chamberlain, Kasari, & Rotheram-Fuller, 2007). When reciprocal nominations are analyzed, however, more than 80% of friends nominated by children with autism are not reciprocated. Thus, a complicated picture emerges in which children may feel they have a friend despite the fact that it is not reciprocated. This may explain why the quality of the friendship is often rated lower than that of typical children (Bauminger & Kasari, 2000; Chamberlain et al., 2007). Thus, non-reciprocated friendships along with poorer reported quality of friendship by children with autism may place children with autism at risk for feelings of isolation and loneliness despite their identification of a friend.

Although truly reciprocal friendships can be difficult to achieve for some children with ASDs, other children are able to succeed. Bauminger and colleagues (2008) are beginning to describe children with reciprocal friendships; for example, in a 2008 study of preadolescent children with high-functioning autism and their reciprocal friends, they found that both groups of children perceived friendship qualities similarly. These data suggest that preadolescents with high-functioning autism have capacities for interpersonal awareness and are similar to typically developing children in their understanding of friendship relationships. Better understanding of how these children came to develop reciprocal friendships will be important in designing interventions for children with ASDs who struggle with establishing friendships.

The foregoing studies typically have examined younger children with ASDs. As children become older, the nature of their peer relationships undergoes significant change as adolescents spend increasingly more time in the company of their same-age friends (Larson & Richards, 1991). During adolescence, friendship gradually deepens in terms of quality features such as closeness, commitment, companionship, intimacy, security, and acceptance of differences among friends (Berndt & Savin-Williams, 1993; Buhrmester, 1990; Marsh et al., 2006; Shulman et al., 1997). As a result, adolescence and young adulthood may be a particularly challenging time for many individuals with autism because of the increasing importance of intimate relationships. Stoddart (1999) has reported that adolescents with Asperger Syndrome experience low self-esteem and have increasing self-awareness of their differences. They also experienced frequent teasing and rejection by their peers, concerns about peers' perceptions, and a lack of ability to make friends (Stoddart, 1999). As a result, adolescence may be an important period for intervention to buffer negative feelings and/or poor psychological outcomes.

An underlying theme that is implicit in several studies regarding friendship quality is the argument that friendship exerts a positive force on development. Nevertheless, there are reasons to expect that the effects of friendship may not always be positive. Certain types of friendships, such as those that are imbalanced, unreciprocated, or marked by conflict, may not provide the sorts of experiences that promote development and well-being (Bukowski, Newcomb, & Hartup, 1996). Conflict and disagreement are common in children's close friendships and may be even more common in friendships where one child has autism. Consequently, several interventions have been developed to enhance social skills and reduce conflict to promote quality friendships in children with autism.

Interventions for Social Skills: Active Ingredients

Unlike most interventions for children with ASDs that are comprehensive and cover all areas of development, social skills interventions tend to be targeted and time limited. With preschool-aged children, particular times during the school day may be targeted for peer interactions, and with older children, a social skills group may be constructed that meets once or twice per week. Whether child-oriented or group-oriented, most interventions search for the active ingredients that will improve children's social skills and ultimately their social connections to others. Aspects of interventions that may be important active ingredients include:

a) the *context* of interventions (e.g., at home or at school during class time or during playground time);
b) *method*—a wide range exists from general applied behavior analysis approaches to more developmental approaches and to specific methods such as video modeling, scripts, social stories, and self-management;
c) the *agent* of intervention, such as sibling-, peer-, or adult-mediated intervention;
d) *content* of interventions, whether focused on, for example, social etiquette, or peer engagement or social knowledge and understanding;
e) *dose*—both intensity and density, such as how often the intervention is delivered and for how long.

It is fair to say that most studies have focused on *method and content*, with content often referring to only a single or limited number of social behaviors that are tested using a single subject design. Agent—who mediates the intervention—becomes important in both the method and context of the intervention. Studies have yet to vary these factors so that it is not possible to determine their importance to social skill development. A number of potential comparisons could be investigated, such as comparing group versus dyad-focused social skills intervention, home- or clinic- versus school-based intervention, and peer-mediated versus adult directed interventions.

Below we discuss the ways in which interventions have addressed these potential active ingredients. We acknowledge however, that we are only at the beginning stages of this work. At this point, we have far too few intervention trials that have varied these different ingredients, so the importance of each ingredient is not well-established. Moreover, many studies examine the combination of a variety of active ingredients, so it is not so easy to separate the importance of each factor.

Context of Intervention

Children's social interactions with others can vary widely by context. For example, children may interact with family members frequently but rarely talk or engage peers at school. Thus, they may appear more socially engaged at home than at school. Agent of intervention (e.g., a family member) may be confounded with context (in this case, home). Overall, very few interventions have been carried out only at home as a way of increasing children's social interactions. An exception is interventions designed to improve the interactions between children with ASDs and their siblings. Far more studies have been carried out in school or community settings. However, even within school settings, the context of intervention can vary from naturalistic interventions on the playground to individualized pull-out sessions with the target child.

Home

Results of the few studies in the home setting have demonstrated that siblings can be effective as trainers and change agents in improving the social interactions of children with autism (Strain & Danko, 1995; Strain et al., 1994). Typically developing siblings have been taught to promote play and play-related speech, to praise play behaviors, and to prompt their siblings with autism to respond to initiations, with skills being generalized and maintained after withdrawing intervention (Bass & Mulick, 2007; Celiberti & Harris, 1993).

In one study, Coe et al. (1991) demonstrated that older elementary children could effectively implement procedures to increase social interactions of younger siblings with autism. Two children with autism received an at-home intervention to increase social behaviors, whereas their typically developing siblings were taught to increase rates of prompts and praise to children with autism for several behaviors. This latter intervention produced increases in targeted behavior for children with autism, as well as increases in the social interactions of children with autism and their older siblings (Coe et al., 1991; McConnell, 2002; Rogers, 2000). Thus, siblings may be valuable intervention agents to foster social skills in children with autism.

Home interventions with siblings may translate to greater social skill with peers in other contexts such as school. However, for the most part, these generalization effects have not been tested. However, one intervention examined an intervention with parents at home and tested the effects of the intervention on their children at school. In this study (Delano & Snell, 2008), the social engagement goals at school for three boys with ASDs were identified and written into individualized social stories that each parent read to their child before and after school. Two of the three boys improved in their prosocial behaviors as a result of the intervention according to observations of children at their school.

School

Efforts to increase social development have led to higher rates of inclusion of children with autism into regular education settings. Despite more exposure to neurotypical peers and more opportunities for social engagement in inclusive settings, research has shown that physical proximity alone does not lead to improved social interactions in children with autism (Myles et al., 1993). Inclusive settings may be a challenging environment for children with autism, particularly during free play or recess times, when children are on the playground and activities may be unstructured and/or unmonitored. Because of the complexity of the playground, some children with autism may feel socially overwhelmed and/or disoriented. As a result, they may spend their free time inside the school buildings (Wainscot et al., 2008) or in the far corners of the playground (e.g., along the edge of the grass, near the fence, etc.) in an attempt to avoid areas of the school that are busy and require good communication skills. Also, the activities that often occur outside the school buildings during break and lunch times typically involve games with multilayered rules such as football, handball, and soccer (Wainscot et al., 2008). These games could pose particular difficulties for children with autism because they are heavily dependent on nonverbal communication and gestures and involve complicated motor coordination. Thus, children with autism can experience difficulties maintaining joint engagement with peers on the playground leading to poor or absent peer relationships. Indeed, more than 90% of children with autism can be discriminated on the playground from children with other disabilities by four behaviors including poor social engagement with peers, lack of respect for personal space, isolation, and inappropriate behavior (Ingram et al., 2007).

Despite the need for interventions on the playground, studies have not directly examined practices that might improve these interactions for children with autism. Most interventions take place inside classrooms. Moreover, in inclusive programs, teachers often are not on the playground; rather, classroom aides or specially hired playground assistants are present to ensure child safety. Aides typically do not directly teach peer play or intervene in children's play, often believing that recess is a "break" from classroom work. Thus, we need further study of children with autism on the playground, both in observational work highlighting individual differences and in effective interventions.

Method (Approach) of Intervention

Because children with autism have varied repertoires of social skills, many different social skills training programs have been designed and implemented. The most commonly applied treatment approach involves applied behavior analysis (ABA) methods. These intervention methods are designed to create multiple learning opportunities and enable high rates of success. The treatment progresses gradually and systematically from relatively simple tasks, such as responding to basic requests made by the instructor to more complex skills that include conversing and interacting with peers. The methods are used by therapists in clinic and home settings as well as by teachers or trained aides in classroom and playground settings.

Although a number of interventions have used very structured and often discrete trials to teach children a particular social skill, such as making eye contact, the trained skill does not always transfer to more naturalistic and unpredictable situations. One issue is that the child's mastery of the skill is tied to the particular teaching context so that the skills do not generalize or transfer to other settings and people. For example, the child may learn to greet his peers in a specialized social group and consistently demonstrate this skill in the confines of the group. However, at school, when faced with a greater diversity of children on the playground and in class, he or she may be unable to generalize greetings. Thus the "mastered skill" fails to be performed.

One response to the lack of generalization from highly structured ABA approaches has been the development of approaches that integrate more traditional methods of ABA into developmental and naturalistic ABA interventions. Pivotal Response Training, Milieu Therapy and Incidental Teaching (Goldstein, 2002) are all examples of approaches that integrate more developmental methods into their ABA teaching strategies. For example, pivotal response training (PRT) focuses on teaching pivotal areas such as motivation, self-management, and self-initiations through multiple cues (Pierce & Schreibman, 1994) and achieves collateral behavior changes not specifically targeted (Koegel & Frea, 1993). Reinforcement is also delivered using natural reinforcers, such as giving the child the ball when he says "ball" rather than a piece of candy. These naturalistic intervention strategies are more likely to facilitate generalization than are strategies that teach skills out of context.

Another common approach for teaching a wide array of skills is video modeling (VM), an instructional process that consists of videotaping behaviors (treatment targets) so children can develop the ability to memorize, imitate, and generalize specific behaviors (Charlop-Christy & Daneshvar, 2003). Using the child in situations in which he or she is successful (video self-modeling [VSM]) as an instructional approach shows particular promise (Bellini & Akullian, 2007). Several studies have shown that VM and VSM may enhance communication skills, academic performance, perspective taking, and social and self-help skills in children with autism (Bellini & Akullian, 2007; Charlop & Milstein, 1989; Charlop-Christy & Daneshvar, 2003; Taylor, Levin, & Jasper, 1999). Many single-subject designs have been conducted on various components of social behavior using ABA, integrative ABA methods, and VM, suggesting that these approaches are effective for teaching social skills. However, generalization continues to be problematic with any approach, highlighting the difficulty in teaching skills that are so subtle and ever-changing depending on context and partner.

Despite the differences among approaches in teaching and delivering social skills interventions, there are also similarities. Almost all studies have focused on the teaching of individual and targeted social skills, such as greeting a peer, entering a group game, and navigating disagreements. The way in which these skills are taught typically involve a number of different strategies, including repetition through discrete trials, role play, and reversal, positive and corrective feedback to improve children's performance, and "homework" assignments to practice learned skills in naturally occurring environments (Matson et al., 2007). Most studies also focus on delivery of the intervention to an individual child with autism that is mediated through others, such as adults (parents, teachers, therapists) or children (peers or siblings).

Thus, in addition to the techniques used to teach social skills, the agent delivering the intervention becomes important to the method and may affect how well the method is delivered. A treatment could be delivered to the child by an expert therapist, a teaching assistant or shadow teacher, a trained peer, or the parent. Although the best approach is to bring everyone into the treatment plan for an individual child, this happens all too rarely.

Agent of Intervention: Adult- vs. Peer-Mediated Social Skills Intervention Approaches

Adult-mediated methodologies have met some success in enhancing interaction with peers (Goldstein & Cisar, 1992), promoting independent play skills (Taylor, Levin, & Jasper, 1999), increasing social initiations (Goldstein & Cisar, 1992), improving perspective taking (Charlop-Christy & Daneshvar, 2003), teaching daily living skills (Pierce & Schreibman, 1994), and promoting generalization across settings (Strain et al., 1994; Koegel et al., 1992; McConnell, 2002; Scattone, 2007). In general, an adult therapist works individually with the target child with autism to increase social skills. The therapist may also train another adult (i.e., teacher, aide, parent) to teach the child social skills.

The most common adult-mediated intervention is to assign a one-on-one aide or shadow teacher to a particular child (Giangreco & Broer, 2006). These aides are only minimally trained but may be systematically supervised by an expert. A cause for concern is that often the least trained person is responsible for a child's intervention in a school setting. In many cases, the teacher may not engage with the child nor see him or herself as responsible for the child's education when an aide is assigned to the child. Aides are often concerned with the amount of responsibility they are given to provide academic and social interventions to the child they are assigned, and the role of expert in which they are often placed (Marks, Schrader, & Levine, 1999).

There is great variability in how aides work; some are assigned to an individual child only, whereas others work with the entire class. Few outcome data exist for this type of intervention some of which suggests that the 1:1 aide may not be effective for facilitating better social interactions for children with ASDs (Giangreco & Broer, 2006; Humphrey & Lewis, 2008). In one study, nearly half of the paraprofessionals believed the child they were assigned to saw them as their primary friend. Children themselves questioned whether the adult who was there to support them marked them in the eyes of their classmates, ultimately interfering with friendship development (Humphrey & Lewis, 2008). Future research studies should more closely examine the efficacy of aide-mediated approaches for promoting social skills and children's close relationships with peers.

A second intervention approach focuses on teaching typically developing peers to engage the child with autism by initiating, prompting, and reinforcing social interactions. Peer-mediated approaches represent the largest and most empirically supported type of social intervention for children with autism (Bass & Mulick, 2007; McConnell, 2002). The use of typically developing peers in social skills interventions as peer tutors or buddies has led to higher rates of eye contact, turn-taking interactions, higher tolerance for waiting (Laushey & Heflin, 2000) and social interaction in young children with autism (Strain & Danko, 1995; Strain et al., 1994). Typically developing peers have assumed a number of roles in peer-mediated intervention studies and have been taught to initiate social interactions and organize play activities (Odom & Strain, 1986), respond to the child with autism (Kamps et al., 2002; Kamps et al., 1992), monitor behavior requests (Morrison et al., 2001), and serve as tutors for schoolwork and recreational activities (Orsmond, Krauss, & Seltzer, 2004). In many paradigms, peers role-play with adults until they have learned the strategies successfully. Subsequently, the peers are cued by the adults to begin to interact with the target children around typical play materials and activities, often on the playground in children's schools, during playdates, or in the community (Bauminger et al., 2008; Harper, Symon, & Frea, 2008; Koegel et al., 2005; Licciardello et al., 2008; Rogers, 2000).

Both the adult-mediated and peer-mediated approaches have demonstrated some success in enhancing or improving children's social skills repertoires; however, many studies employ single-subject designs and have not been subjected to direct comparative research designs in the child's natural environment (Williams White et al., 2007; Bellini et al., 2007). Moreover, we have less evidence of maintenance of learned skills over time, and generalization to new groups of children, or new contexts, thus raising issues of how well the interventions match the needs of children, how teachers motivate children to maintain engagement, and how the environment supports children's social relationships.

Despite the lack of empirical evidence indicating which approach is more effective, one consistent finding is that children with autism are responsive to a wide variety of interventions aimed at increasing their social engagement and social skills repertoires. There remains a question, however, as to whether various approaches lead to maintenance and generalization of the intervention effects. It is likely that children need additional and continuous social support systems (e.g., both child-specific and mediated by others) built into their everyday lives (e.g., in the community, at school, at home, etc.). The answer may lie in targeted school-wide systems change and greater professional development and accountability for teachers if we are to help children with ASDs to acquire, maintain, generalize, and expand their learned social skills.

Group Social Skills Approach

Group social skills programs combine both adult- and peer-mediated approaches. They are commonly implemented outside school settings, such as in clinics with children who often do not attend the same schools or programs. In some intervention programs, these groups are comprised of both typically developing children and children with autism, whereas other studies have utilized groups that consist of only children with autism (Chung et al., 2007; Kroeger, Schultz, & Newsom, 2007; Mackay, Knott, & Dunlop, 2007). Studies of group social skills programs have noted progress in social communication in both reduction of inappropriate talking and increase in appropriate talking (Chung et al., 2007), prosocial behaviors (Kroeger et al., 2007), and social skills and competence (Mackay et al., 2007). Within these settings, curricula are employed that focus on a limited set of social skills, such as entering social groups, starting a conversation, dealing with bullying or rejection, and so forth. Although these groups provide opportunities for peer interaction and practice of these skills, these situations may not generalize to peers outside of the particular environment.

Thus far, there are few large-scale randomized group-based treatment studies and limited application of manualized intervention programs (Lopata et al., 2008; Williams White et al., 2007). Few investigations have utilized group designs to control for confounding factors such as the effects of maturation and time over the course of treatment. In one study, Solomon et al. (2004) utilized a randomized comparative group design to examine the effectiveness of a social enhancement program for 18 children with high-functioning autism. Children participated in small groups for a 20-week intervention with a curriculum that included emotion recognition and understanding, perspective taking, and executive functioning skills. The intervention was effective in increasing emotion recognition and problem solving, and both groups (i.e., intervention and wait-list control) improved in their perspective-taking skills. Although the authors have noted limitations, they have suggested that group social treatments have potentially positive effects for children on the autism spectrum (Lopata et al., 2008; Solomon, Goodlin-Jones, & Anders, 2004). However, until randomized controlled treatment trials are conducted on a larger scale in children's natural settings, it will be difficult to determine whether a specific intervention is more efficacious than mere clinical attention or is relevant for the general population of children and adolescents with autism (Rao et al., 2008).

A major limitation of current studies is the lack of evidence for generalization across contexts, people, and time (Bellini et al., 2007; McConnell, 2002; Rogers, 2000; Williams White et al., 2007). One explanation for the poor generalization and maintenance effects for the various social skills interventions is that a single manualized social skills treatment may not be effective for all children with autism. Because autism is a spectrum disorder, children affected by autism exhibit a variety of symptoms. As a result, one intervention may be particularly effective for one child and ineffective for another child with autism. One issue that has not been dealt with adequately is the content of interventions and the connection of that content for particular children with autism.

Content of Interventions

Most interventions are manualized and cover a number of different skills aimed at initiating and maintaining interactions. Often, a separate topic may be presented at each session, such as greeting peers, initiating conversation, reading emotions, and managing conflicts. These topics may be specific to enhancing peer interactions (Barry et al., 2003), developing friendships (Laugeson et al., 2009), or managing anxiety (Sofronoff, Attwood, & Hinton, 2005; Wood et al., 2009). Given the variability in child repertoires, manualized treatments need to be flexible to meet individual needs to be maximally effective.

Two important factors related to content of social skills interventions are: *(1)* the developmental appropriateness of skills that are taught, and *(2)* flexibility in delivering a manualized, evidence-based intervention. In terms of developmental appropriateness, one concern is the lack of assessment of children in natural settings with peers prior to intervention. Thus, children may attend social skills groups that utilize a manualized intervention, but the topics may not be individually relevant to their particular strengths and weaknesses. Bellini (2006) noted that few treatments connect the focus of the treatment to the individual developmental needs of the child. As an example, a young child may be taught to initiate play with a peer by asking, "Can I play?" but if the child lacks play skills he will not be able to sustain engagement with the peer. In this case, a more appropriate goal may be to teach the child play skills. Indeed, a number of parent and therapist mediated interventions have been developed to teach children joint engagement and play skills with adults (Kasari et al., 2006; Schertz & Odom, 2007), but these types of interventions have rarely been transferred to children and their peers. Play times in classrooms are provided as a break from work times. Play may not be specifically taught, and yet children with autism may be at a loss for how to engage both materials and peers in jointly engaged play routines (Wong, 2007). One question for future research is whether teaching play routines to children with and without autism leads to more peer engagement without teaching discrete skills of social interactions (e.g., asking questions, giving materials, etc).

Although many programs ultimately aim to help children develop friendships, this area of social skills may be particularly important for older children with ASDs and likely needs to be directly targeted. Recent evidence suggests that using a parent-mediated approach is effective in helping adolescents with ASDs to develop friendships (Laugeson et al., 2009). In this approach, groups are held separately for children with ASDs and their parents with sessions focused on how to call friends on the phone and to set up get-togethers. Both parents and children report that the intervention is effective for increasing friendships. Thus, utilizing parent-mediated approaches should be further investigated and potentially included to augment school-based interventions.

A second related issue is the difficulty in meeting the needs of all children with ASDs given the heterogeneity of the disorder and variability in educational opportunities. One way to increase flexibility of treatments for individual children is to use a distillation and matching model for treatment (Chorpita, Daleiden, & Weisz, 2005). *Distillation* refers to finding the common element or technique in a particular set of treatment manuals, such as the use of visual feedback or conflict management techniques. *Matching* refers to the use of the element or technique for a particular child. For example, for children with an anxiety disorder, a common element in most treatment programs is the use of exposure therapy. Thus, using exposure therapy may be a critical element in a social skills program for a child who has high anxiety but may be less effective for a child who does not demonstrate anxiety. Developing a common elements approach to social skills treatments may assist clinicians in individualizing treatment for a particular child, and increasing the flexibility of evidence-based treatments to maximize dissemination.

Exposure therapy is a cognitive behavioral approach to reducing feelings of fear and anxiety in response to certain stimuli or situations. The patient takes part in a program of gradually increasing exposure to the anxiety-inducing factors and, if the approach is successful, eventually becomes habituated to the stimuli.

Future Recommendations

Although socialization deficits associated with ASDs can be severe and may require intervention across the life span, targeted social skills remediation may lead to more favorable prognoses (Scattone, 2007). To date, there are few data suggesting highly efficacious social skills treatments, but there are a number of promising strategies (Williams White et al., 2007).

Given the current state of knowledge, several areas of social skills programs require further research (McConnell, 2002; Rogers, 2000; Williams White et al., 2007). First, there is a need for documentation of the heterogeneity of social deficits for children with ASDs. In their meta-analysis of social skills training, Gresham, Sugai, and Horner (2001) concluded that the traditionally weak treatment effects of many social skills programs may be the result of assessment tools that fail to match identified skill deficits with treatment objectives. As such, the first step of any social skills program should be to identify the specific social skills of the targeted children and, more specifically, the skills that will be the treatment goals of intervention (Bellini, 2006). To determine individualized social skill strengths and weaknesses in children, it is critical that researchers observe children in their natural environments. Using only parent reports may not shed enough light on what the particular issues are for a child on the school playground. Typically, neither parents nor teachers are present on playgrounds. The best informants are likely the child's peers and the playground supervisors (often teaching paraprofessionals). The field needs social skill observational assessments that can be utilized by a variety of professionals and that can be easily implemented. Such information will better inform treatment goals and objectives.

Another essential element of high-quality social skills programming and program accountability requires efficient and effective measurement systems for assessing outcomes in natural environments and within spontaneous interactions (Rogers, 2000). Outcomes should reflect the content of the intervention and have some meaning for the construct under study (Kasari, 2002). Many times, social skills training programs have sought to remediate social skills in a contrived setting such as a clinic where children practice learned skills on adults, not peers. Another issue concerns how change is evaluated and whether the evaluators have access to children in the settings on which they are asked to report. Thus, without the use of meaningful outcome measures, interventions may be found to be inappropriate, insufficient, and/or ineffective (Rao et al., 2008).

Because autism is a spectrum disorder, each child may have vastly different social skills strengths and weaknesses. Some children with autism may need assistance developing social behaviors such as joining a game on the playground, whereas other children may need additional assistance with more subtle social cues like attending to a conversation with a friend. As such, it is imperative that social skills interventions are individualized to the child's developmental needs and target behaviors that can ultimately be used to foster high-quality relationships. One fundamental goal of many social skills training programs is to provide children with autism with the necessary social skills repertoire to be successful in social situations and foster meaningful and long-lasting relationships and friendships with others. Asking children to report on their perceptions of relationship quality has been increasingly utilized in friendship research and provides insightful information that may also address questions relating to children's social awareness. Therefore, it is important to tailor the goals of intervention to each child and provide the necessary skills for children with autism to establish and maintain quality reciprocal relationships, particularly friendships with peers.

Future social skills interventions should also address questions regarding the active ingredients of effective social skills programs (Kasari, 2002). These issues center on dose, content, methods, service delivery, and timing. Most studies of social skills programs have been of low dose (e.g., weekly meetings of short duration), content that is a standard curriculum of specific skills (e.g., greetings, starting conversations), methods that are behavioral in orientation, service delivery that is clinic-driven and typically not in the environment in which social skills need to be executed (e.g., school), and timing that is either late (e.g., when children already show significant distress) or early (e.g., before children are aware of potential peer relationships). The issue of timing raises a number of issues for future studies and requires systematic comparisons to determine when social skills programs may have their greatest impact.

Next, integrating typically developing children into the intervention paradigm has been a key factor in several existing interventions (Bellini et al., 2007; Chung et al., 2007; Laushey & Heflin, 2000; McConnell, 2002; Scattone, 2007) and is an essential component of social skills training for children with autism. Utilizing typical peers has an added benefit in that interventionists have access to social behaviors of age-mates for children with autism so that expectations for the behaviors of children with autism can be realistic. In this way, treatment goals can be established according to the social context and culture of the targeted child with autism.

In many reviews, social skills interventions, treatments, and programs have been criticized for their lack of skills generalization across contexts, people, and time (Bellini et al., 2007; McConnell, 2002; Rogers, 2000; Williams White et al., 2007). Like any intervention program, social skills interventions should document the long-term effects of the intervention for children with autism. Specifically, it is important to evaluate the generalization and maintenance of specific components or social skills learned during the intervention (McConnell, 2002) through follow-up observations, additional evaluations, and/or repeated outcome and/or assessment measures. Furthermore, the use of developmentally generative interventions, where skills and characteristics acquired in treatment lead to ongoing development of increasingly sophisticated social behaviors (McConnell, 2002), may be an effective approach to ensure the use of less intensive social skills training in the future.

Finally, the field needs to develop successful and efficient intervention approaches that are structured, manualized, and packaged for dissemination to a wide variety of community settings (Rogers, 2000). Structured interventions are essential for replication as well as ensuring treatment fidelity (Williams White et al., 2007); however, taking a distillation and matching approach (Chorpita et al., 2005) to treatments increases treatment flexibility, individualization, and potential application by a wide variety of treatment providers.

Conclusion

Much like the nature of ASDs, the existing literature on social skills intervention programs is extremely heterogeneous. Some interventions have shown positive outcomes in children's friendships and knowledge of social skills, but these tend to be poorly maintained and generalized. The future of our understanding depends on well-designed studies that incorporate some of the active elements of treatment. Although we are still at the beginning stages of social skills intervention research, we are hopeful that we can improve the current system so that all children with autism have the opportunities necessary to have rich social experiences.

Challenges and Future Directions

- There is a need to document the heterogeneity of social deficits for children with ASDs as well as to develop and utilize efficient and effective measurement systems for assessing outcomes in natural environments.
- Intervention programs should be individualized to fit the needs of the child, incorporate key active ingredients (i.e., dose, content, methods, service delivery, and timing), and multiple agents of change (i.e., typically developing peers, parents, teachers, and paraprofessionals).
- Finally, we need to document the long-term effects of interventions for children with autism and develop successful and efficient intervention approaches that are structured, manualized, and packaged for dissemination to a wide variety of community settings.

SUGGESTED READINGS

Bellini, S., Peters, J. K., Benner, L., & Hopf, A. (2007). A meta-analysis of school-based social skills interventions for children with autism spectrum disorders. *Remedial and Special Education, 28*, 153–162.

Rao, P. A., Beidel, D. C., & Murray, M. J. (2008). Social skills interventions for children with Asperger's Syndrome or high-functioning autism: A review and recommendations. *Journal of Autism and Developmental Disorders, 38*(2), 353–361.

Williams White, S., Keonig, K., & Scahill, L. (2007). Social skills development in children with autism spectrum disorders: A review of the intervention research. *Journal of Autism and Developmental Disorders, 37*(10), 1858–1868.

ACKNOWLEDGMENT

HRSA Autism Intervention Research - Behavioral Health grant UA3MC11055.

REFERENCES

American Psychiatric Association. (2000). *Diagnostic and statistical manual of mental disorders: Text revision (4th ed., rev.).* Washington, DC: Author.

Bagwell, C. L., Newcomb, A. F., & Bukowski, W. M. (1998). Preadolescent friendship and peer rejection as predictors of adult adjustment. *Child Development, 69*, 140–153.

Barry, T. D., Klinger, L. G., Lee, J. M., Palardy, N., Gilmore, T., & Bodin, S. D. (2003). Examining the effectiveness of an outpatient clinic-based social skills group for high-functioning children with autism. *Journal of Autism and Developmental Disorders, 33*, 685–701.

Bass, J. D., & Mulick, J. A. (2007). Social play skill enhancement of children with autism using peers and siblings as therapists. *Psychology in the Schools. Special Issue: Autism spectrum disorders, 44*, 727–735.

Bauminger, N., & Kasari, C. (2000). Loneliness and friendship in high-functioning children with autism. *Child Development, 71*, 447–456.

Bauminger, N., Solomon, M., Aviezer, A., Heung, K., Gazit, L., Brown, J., et al. (2008). Children with autism and their friends: A multidimensional study of friendship in high-functioning autism spectrum disorder. *Journal of Abnormal Child Psychology, 36*, 135–150.

Bellini, S. (2006). The development of social anxiety in adolescents with autism spectrum disorders. *Focus on Autism and Other Developmental Disabilities, 21*, 138–145.

Bellini, S., & Akullian, J (2007). A meta-analysis of video modeling and video self-modeling for children and adolescents with autism spectrum disorders. *Exceptional Children, 73*, 264–287.

Bellini, S., Peters, J. K., Benner, L., & Hopf, A. (2007). A meta-analysis of school-based social skills interventions for children with autism spectrum disorders. *Remedial and Special Education, 28*, 153–162.

Berndt, T. J., & Savin-Williams, R. C. (1993). Variations in friendships and peer-group relationships in adolescence. In P. T. B. C. (Eds.), *Handbook of clinical research and practice with adolescents* (pp. 203–219). New York: John Wiley.

Bollmer, J. M., Milich, R., Harris, M. J., & Maras, M. A. (2005). A friend in need: The role of friendship quality as a protective factor in peer victimization and bullying. *Journal of Interpersonal Violence, 20*, 701–712.

Buhrmester, D. (1990). Intimacy of friendship, interpersonal competence, and adjustment during preadolescence and adolescence. *Child Development, 61*, 1101–1111.

Bukowski, W. M., Newcomb, A. F., & Hartup, W. W. (1996). *The company they keep: Friendship in childhood and adolescence.* Cambridge: Cambridge University Press.

Celiberti, D. A., & Harris, S. L. (1993). Behavioral intervention for siblings of children with autism: A focus on skills to enhance play. *Behavior Therapy, 24*, 573–599.

Chamberlain, B., Kasari, C., & Rotheram-Fuller, E. (2007). Involvement or isolation? The social networks of children with autism in regular classrooms. *Journal of Autism and Developmental Disorders, 37*, 230–242.

Charlop-Christy, M. H., & Daneshvar, S. (2003). Using video modeling to teach perspective taking to children with autism. *Journal of Positive Behavior Interventions, 5*, 12–21.

Charlop, M. H., & Milstein, J. P. (1989). Teaching autistic children conversational speech using video modeling. . *Journal of Applied Behavior Analysis, 22*, 275–285.

Chorpita, B., Daleiden, E.L., & Weisz, J. R. (2005). Identifying and selecting the common elements of evidence based interventions: A distillation and matching model. *Mental Health Services Research, 7*, 5–16.

Chung, K.-M., Reavis, S., Mosconi, M., Drewry, J., Matthews, T., & Tasse, M. J. (2007). Peer-mediated social skills training program for young children with high-functioning autism. *Research in Developmental Disabilities, 28*, 423–436.

Coe, D. A., Matson, J. L., Craigie, C. J., & Gossen, M. A. (1991). Play skills of autistic children: Assessment and instruction. *Child and Family Behavior Therapy, 13*, 13–40.

Delano, M., & Snell, M. (2008). The effects of social stories on the social engagement of children with autism. *Journal of Positive Behavior Interventions, 8*, 29–42.

Giangreco, M. F., & Broer, S. M. (2007). School-based screening to determine overreliance on paraprofessionals. *Focus on Autism and Other Developmental Disabilities, 22*, 149–158.

Goldstein, H., & Cisar, C. (1992). Promoting interaction during sociodramatic play: Teaching scripts to typical preschoolers and classmates with disabilities. *Journal of Applied Behavior Analysis, 25*, 289–305.

Goldstein, H. (2002). Communication intervention for children with autism: A review of treatment efficacy. *Journal of Autism and Developmental Disorders, 32*, 373–396.

Gresham, F. M., Sugai, G., & Horner, R. H. (2001). Interpreting outcomes of social skills training for students with high-incidence disabilities. *Exceptional Children, 67*, 331–344.

Harper, C. B., Symon, J. B. G., & Frea, W. D. (2008). Recess is time-in: Using peers to improve social skills of children with autism. *Journal of Autism and Developmental Disorders, 38*, 815–826.

Howlin, P., Goode, S., Hutton, J., & Rutter, M. (2004). Adult outcome for children with autism. *Journal of Child Psychology and Psychiatry, and Allied Disciplines, 45*, 212–229.

Humphrey, N., & Lewis, S. (2008). Make me normal: The views and experiences of pupils on the autistic spectrum in mainstream secondary schools. *Autism, 12*, 23–46.

Ingram, D. H., Mayes, S. D., Troxell, L. B., & Calhoun, S. L. (2007). Assessing children with autism, mental retardation, and typical development using the Playground Observation Checklist. *Autism, 11*, 311–319.

Kamps, D., Leonard, B. R., Vernon, S., Dugan, E. P., Delquadri, J. C., Gershon, B. et al. (1992). Teaching social skills to students with autism to increase peer interactions in an integrated first-grade classroom. *Journal of Applied Behavior Analysis, 25,* 281–288.

Kamps, D., Royer, J., Dugan, E., Kravits, T., Gonzalez-Lopez, A., Garcia, J., et al. (2002). Peer training to facilitate social interaction for elementary students with autism and their peers. *Exceptional Children, 68,* 173–187.

Kasari, C. (2002). Assessing change in early intervention programs for children with autism. *Journal of Autism and Developmental Disorders, 32,* 447–461.

Kasari, C., Freeman, S., Bauminger, N., & Alkin, M. (1999). Parental perspectives on inclusion: Effects of autism and Down syndrome. *Journal of Autism and Developmental Disorders, 29,* 297–305.

Kasari, C., Freeman, S., & Paparella, T. (2006). Joint attention and symbolic play in young children with autism: A randomized controlled intervention study. *Journal of Child Psychology and Psychiatry, and Allied Disciplines, 47,* 611–620.

Koegel, L. K., Koegel, R. L., Hurley, C., & Frea, W. D. (1992). Improving social skills and disruptive behavior in children with autism through self-management. *Journal of Applied Behavior Analysis, 25,* 341–353.

Koegel, R. L., & Frea, W. D. (1993). Treatment of social behavior in autism through the modification of pivotal social skills. *Journal of Applied Behavior Analysis, 26,* 369–277.

Koegel, R. L., Werner, G. A., Vismara, L. A., & Koegel, L. K. (2005). The effectiveness of contextually supported play date interactions between children with autism and typically developing peers. *Research and Practice for Persons with Severe Disabilities, 30,* 93–102.

Kroeger, K. A., Schultz, J. R., & Newsom, C. (2007). A comparison of two group-delivered social skills programs for young children with autism. *Journal of Autism and Developmental Disorders, 37,* 808–817.

Ladd, G., Kochenderfer, B. J., & Coleman, C. C. (1996). Friendship quality as a predictor of young children's early school adjustment. *Child Development, 67,* 1103–1118.

Larson, R., & Richards, M. H. (1991). Daily companionship in late childhood and early adolescence: Changing developmental contexts. *Child Development, 62,* 284–300.

Laugeson, E. A., Frankel, F., Mogil, C., & Dillon, A. R. (2009). Parent-assisted social skills training to improve friendships in teens with autism spectrum disorders. *Journal of Autism and Developmental Disorders, 39,* 596–606.

Laushey, K. M., & Heflin, J. (2000). Enhancing social skills of kindergarten children with autism through the training of multiple peers as tutors. *Journal of Autism and Developmental Disorders, 30,* 183–193.

Licciardello, C. C., Harchik, A. E., & Luiselli, J. K. (2008). Social skills intervention for children with autism during interactive play at a public elementary school. *Education and Treatment of Children, 31,* 27–37.

Lopata, C., Thomeer, M. L., Volker, M. A., Nida, R. E., & Lee, G. K. (2008). Effectiveness of a manualized summer social treatment program for high-functioning children with autism spectrum disorders. *Journal of Autism and Developmental Disorders, 38,* 890–904.

Mackay, T., Knott, F., & Dunlop, A. (2007). Developing social interaction and understanding in individuals with autism spectrum disorder: A groupwork intervention. *Journal of Intellectual and Developmental Disability, 32,* 279–290.

Marks, S. U., Schrader, C., & Levine, M. (1999). Paraeducator experiences in inclusive in inclusive settings: Helping, hovering, or holding their own? *Exceptional Children, 65,* 315–328.

Marsh, P., Allen, J. P., Ho, M., Porter, M., & McFarland, F. C. (2006). The changing nature of adolescent friendships: Longitudinal links with early adolescent ego development. *Journal of Early Adolescence, 26,* 414–431.

Matson, J. L., Matson, M. L., & Rivet, T. T. (2007). Social-skills treatments for children with autism spectrum disorders: An overview. *Behavior Modification, 31,* 682–707.

McConnell, S. R. (2002). Interventions to facilitate social interaction for young children with autism: Review of available research and recommendations for educational intervention and future research. *Journal of Autism and Developmental Disorders, 32,* 351–372.

Morrison, L., Kamps, D., Garcia, J., & Parker, D. (2001). Peer mediation and monitoring strategies to improve initiations and social skills for students with autism. *Journal of Positive Behavior Interventions, 3,* 237–250.

Myles, B. S., Simpson, R. L., Ormsbee, C. K., & Erickson, C. (1993). Integrating preschool children with autism with their normally developing peers: Research findings and best practices recommendations. *Focus on Autistic Behavior, 8,* 1–18.

Odom, S. L., & Strain, P. S. (1986). A comparison of peer-initiation and teacher-antecedent interventions for promoting reciprocal social interaction of autistic preschoolers. *Journal of Applied Behavior Analysis, 19,* 59–71.

Orsmond, G. I., Krauss, M. W., & Seltzer, M. M. (2004). Peer relationships and social and recreational activities among adolescents and adults with autism. *Journal of Autism and Developmental Disorders, 34,* 245–256.

Parker, J. G., & Asher, S. R. (1993). Friendship and friendship quality in middle childhood: Links with peer group acceptance and feelings of loneliness and social dissatisfaction. *Developmental Psychology, 29,* 611–621.

Pierce, K. L., & Schreibman, L. (1994). Teaching daily living skills to children with autism in unsupervised settings through pictorial self-management. *Journal of Applied Behavior Analysis, 27,* 471–481.

Rao, P. A., Beidel, D. C., & Murray, M. J. (2008). Social skills interventions for children with Asperger's Syndrome or high-functioning autism: A review and recommendations. *Journal of Autism and Developmental Disorders, 38,* 353–361.

Rogers, S. (2000). Interventions that facilitate socialization in children with autism. *Journal of Autism and Developmental Disorders, 30,* 399–409.

Scattone, D. (2007). Social skills interventions for children with autism. *Psychology in the Schools. Special Issue: Autism spectrum disorders, 44,* 717–726.

Schertz, H. H., & Odom, S. L. (2007). Promoting joint attention in toddlers with autism: A parent-mediated developmental model. *Journal of Autism and Developmental Disorders, 37,* 1562–1575.

Shulman, S., Laursen, B., Kalman, Z., & Karpovsky, S. (1997). Adolescent intimacy revisited. *Journal of Youth and Adolescence, 26,* 597–617.

Sofornoff, K., Atwood, T., & Hinton, S. (2005). A randomized controlled trial of a CBT intervention for anxiety in children with Asperger syndrome. *Journal of Child Psychology and Psychiatry, 46,* 1152–1160.

Solomon, M., Goodlin-Jones, B. L., & Anders, T. F. (2004). A social adjustment enhancement intervention for high functioning autism, Asperger's Syndrome, and pervasive developmental disorder NOS. *Journal of Autism and Developmental Disorders, 34,* 649–668.

Stoddart, K. P. (1999). Adolescents with Asperger Syndrome: Three Case Studies of Individual and Family Therapy. *Autism, 3,* 255–271.

Strain, P. S., & Danko, C. D. (1995). Caregivers' encouragement of positive interaction between preschoolers with autism and their siblings. *Journal of Emotional and Behavioral Disorders, 3,* 2–13.

Strain, P. S., Kohler, F. W., Storey, K., & Danko, C. D. (1994). Teaching preschoolers with autism to self-monitor their social interactions: An analysis of results in home and school settings. *Journal of Emotional and Behavioral Disorders, 2,* 78–89.

Taylor, B. A., Levin, L., & Jasper, S. (1999). Increasing play-related statements in children with autism toward their siblings: Effects of video modeling. *Journal of Developmental and Physical Disabilities, 11,* 253–264.

Wainscot, J. J., Naylor, P., Sutcliffe, P., Tantam, D., & Williams, J. V. (2008). Relationships with peers and use of the school environment of mainstream secondary school pupils with Asperger syndrome (high-functioning autism): A case-control study. *International Journal of Psychology and Psychological Therapy, 8,* 25–38.

Williams White, S., Keonig, K., & Scahill, L. (2007). Social skills development in children with autism spectrum disorders: A review of the intervention research. *Journal of Autism and Developmental Disorders, 37,* 1858–1868.

Wing, L. (1988). The continuum of autistic characteristics. In E. Schopler & G. B. Mesibov (Eds.), *Diagnosis and assessment in autism. Current issues in autism* (pp. 91–110). New York: Plenum Press.

Wong, C. (2007). Play and joint attention of children with autism in the preschool classroom. *Dissertation Abstracts International Section a: Humanities and Social Sciences, 67,* 2534.

Wood, J. J., Drahota, A., Sze, K. M., Har, K., Chiu, A., & Langer, D. (2009). Cognitive behavioral therapy for anxiety in children with autism spectrum disorders: A randomized, controlled trial. *Journal of Child Psychology and Psychiatry, 50,* 224–234.

67 Robin L. Gabriels

Adolescent Transition to Adulthood and Vocational Issues

Points of Interest:

- Entering puberty involves a number of physical, medical, and emotional issues that must be addressed so that the ASD adolescent is able to learn the life skills necessary to transition to adulthood.
- Achieving life skills necessary to enhance independence and quality of life requires targeted interventions for the individual with an ASD in the areas of communication, social behavior, and daily living.
- The few follow-up studies addressing the symptom impairment and abatement in adolescents and adults with an ASD suggest that these individuals can make improvements from childhood to adulthood; however, some experience periods of symptom aggravation and a majority continue to require support services.
- To learn necessary life skills, individuals with an ASD need to be able to attend and focus rather than be distracted by medical or psychiatric issues; therefore, an assessment of the underlying issues or ASD-specific deficits that cause or are driving the behavioral presentation is necessary.
- An understanding of the unique learning characteristics and behaviors of individuals with an ASD can enhance the implementation of interventions to improve their level of functioning in society.

Introduction

Adolescence brings unique challenges to individuals with an autism spectrum disorder (ASD), regardless of his or her level of intellectual ability or the amount and type of early interventions and school-age support services employed. The very fact that the child is now older, larger, and almost physically mature puts him or her at risk for being misunderstood and vulnerable in his or her community. Those unfamiliar with the complexities of autism may have difficulty understanding or ignoring the odd or seemingly rude behaviors of the mature-looking individual with an ASD. Caregivers are also less able to avoid addressing the socially immature behaviors and demands of their adult-sized child with an ASD. Such behaviors may have been tolerated when the individual with an ASD was a young child, but they bring a whole host of problems when the child enters adolescence. Heightened community expectations for increased cognitive, psychological, and social maturity also create challenges for these ASD adolescents. Additionally, entering puberty involves a number of physical, medical, and emotional issues that must be addressed so that the ASD adolescent is able to learn the life skills necessary to transition to adulthood.

Although there are many books related to teaching life skills to individuals with ASDs (*see* Suggested Readings), such teaching can be overwhelming because it is difficult to synthesize this information to address all the unique needs of a given individual with an ASD. Along with this, intervention strategies need to be adjusted to address the developmental strengths and needs of each child as they enter adolescence and continue on to adulthood. This chapter attempts to address this problem by providing a framework for understanding the unique obstacles to helping adolescents with ASDs acquire the life skills needed to enhance their independence and quality of life. The first section of this chapter reviews the current literature regarding the life-course of symptom impairment and abatement that adolescents and adults with ASDs continue to face. Such issues include *communication and social abilities, behavior challenges, daily living skills, and adaptation to community living/vocational environments.* The second section provides a suggested method for approaching life skill instruction with adolescents diagnosed with ASDs by *assessing underlying problems, recognizing the unique ASD learning styles, teaching survival life skills, providing case examples, and addressing issues related to transitioning to residential and vocational settings.*

Life Skills Development for Individuals With Autism Spectrum Disorders

Life Skills

The World Health Organization (WHO, 1999; WHO, 2004) has defined life skills as adaptive and positive behaviors necessary for an individual to deal with the demands of life. Life skills involve problem-solving, decision-making, goal-setting, critical thinking, communication, assertiveness self-awareness, interpersonal skills, and an ability to cope with stress. These are psycho-social and reflective life skills that are particularly difficult for individuals with ASDs because of their qualitative impairments in three core areas: social, communication, and repetitive and stereotyped behaviors and interests (American Psychiatric Association, 2000).

To achieve life skills, the individual with ASD needs to develop specific adaptive living skills (e.g., communication, social behavior, and daily living) necessary to integrate into society. Klin et al. (2007) assert that a "critical indicator of an individual's progress is his or her ability to translate cognitive potential into real-life skills" (i.e., adaptive behaviors) (p. 748). Of concern is the unique and consistent finding that ASD individuals tend to have much lower adaptive functioning abilities compared to their levels of intelligence and that adaptive abilities appear to either level off or decrease as these individuals age (Lockyer & Rutter, 1969; Rumsey et al., 1985; Freeman et al., 1991; Bryson & Smith, 1998; Carter et al., 1998; Bolic & Pousika, 2002; Volkmar, 2003). Having speech by age 5 years and higher childhood intelligence tends to predict a lesser degree of impairment later in life for ASD individuals (e.g., Howlin, 2003; Billstedt et al., 2007; Shattuck et al., 2007). However, these higher functioning individuals can still be handicapped by their inappropriate or odd social behaviors and limited self-care skills (e.g., Ballaban-Gil et al., 1996; Howlin et al., 2004; Gabriels et al., 2007; Klin et al., 2007; Saulnier & Klin, 2007).

A major challenge to life skills intervention and planning for individuals with ASDs is the heterogeneity of symptom impairment across individuals. Individuals with ASDs display variability in the range and severity of the core ASD diagnostic symptoms in the areas of social communication and behavior. For example, some ASD individuals may have limited to no expressive language ability; whereas, others may have a large expressive vocabulary, but have difficulty engaging in reciprocal social conversations. Individuals with ASDs can also differ widely in their social and behavioral presentation from being socially interested but odd in their social interactions with others to engaging exclusively in their restricted interests or odd repetitive behaviors. Individuals with ASDs also display a variety of associated symptom deficits in intelligence and adaptive ability levels, sensory sensitivities, and comorbid medical and psychiatric diagnoses (e.g., Mottron & Burack, 2001; Bolte & Poustka, 2002; Tuchman & Rapin, 2002; Gabriels et al., 2005; Leekam et al., 2006; Leyfer et al., 2006; Klin et al., 2007).

Life Skill Outcomes in Adolescents and Adults With Autism Spectrum Disorders

There have been a limited number of prospective follow-up studies of adolescents and adults with ASDs to assess how children with ASDs function as they enter adolescence and adulthood (Shattuck et al., 2007). The few studies addressing the symptom impairment and abatement in adolescents and adults with ASDs suggest that these individuals can make improvements from childhood to adulthood; however, some experience periods of symptom aggravation. The majority of individuals with ASDs remain significantly impaired and continue to require support services (e.g., Gillberg & Steffenburg 1987; Shattuck et al., 2007; Cederlund et al., 2008; *see also* Seltzer et al., 2004, for a research review). The following section reviews the prospective, retrospective, and cross-sectional studies of adolescents and adults with ASDs. Outcomes in the areas of *communication, social, behavior, and daily living skills* along with *community living and vocational environments will be reviewed.*

Communication

Studies indicate that individuals with ASDs do make improvements in their ability to communicate during adolescence and adulthood; nonetheless, problems remain for ASD individuals with or without speech (*see* Seltzer et al., 2004 for a review). These communication problems involve reciprocal verbal communication and nonverbal communication impairments. For example, in a prospective follow-up study of 105 adolescents and young adults with ASDs and a range of intellectual ability levels, the most common communication problem for this group was a lack of reciprocal verbal communication behaviors such as providing both a response to others and leads for others to follow-up on, in conversations (Billstedt et al., 2007). In everyday life, these conversation difficulties can put the ASD adolescent at risk for social rejection if, for example, the adolescent insists on directing conversations back to their own special interests, without offering comments about what another person wants to talk about. The other common problem in this study's sample was impairment in the use of nonverbal communication skills such as using inappropriate or unvaried facial expression and abnormal voice intonation (Billstedt et al., 2007). A relatively high prevalence of nonverbal communication impairments were also found in a sample of 241 adolescents and adults with ASDs and a range of intellectual ability levels (Shattuck et al., 2007). Nonverbal communication impairments in this ASD population sample included limited use of pointing to express an interest or limited use of head nodding or shaking to communicate as well as restricted use of conventional (e.g., waving) and instrumental gestures (e.g., reaching out for more). These particular nonverbal communication impairments have important implications for predicting the future social interactions of adolescents or adults with ASDs. For example, if an ASD adolescent or adult displays a lack of facial expressions, abnormal voice intonation, and minimal use of gestures, others are likely to misinterpret their intentions, resulting in the ASD individual inadvertently angering or threatening others such as an employer or landlord.

Social

Studies indicate that adolescents and adults with ASDs continue to have significant social problems as reflected by having limited to no friendships or acquaintances and difficulties understanding and engaging in romantic relationships. This difficulty with developing significant social relationships is influenced in part by their social and emotional reciprocity deficits such as their limited ability to share enjoyment or interests with others along with their limited understanding of other's emotional states (*see* Seltzer et al., 2004, for a review). More recent follow-up studies of ASD adolescents and adults with a variety of intellectual abilities similarly indicate persistent problems with social reciprocity in a majority of the individuals studied. These problems were evidenced by limited and inappropriate interactions with same-age peers such as having poor eye contact or unfocused gaze along with a lack of emotional responsiveness, shared enjoyment, understanding of others' emotions (Billstedt et al., 2007; Shattuck et al., 2007).

Studies of higher functioning ASD adolescents have found that higher levels of intelligence are not associated with equally high levels of adaptive social abilities necessary for relationships, college, employment, and independent living (Klin et al., 2007; Saulnier & Klin, 2007). These social impairments of individuals with ASDs may contribute to reports in the literature of the greater likelihood of becoming involved with law enforcement (Curry et al., 1993). For example, a follow-up study that included 70 adolescents and adults with Asperger's Syndrome (AS) found that although the majority of this group was considered law-abiding, 10% had been involved with the law for issues such as fraud, harassment of others, stealing, assault, and sexual abuse (Cederlund, Hagberg et al., 2008). A recent survey of parents of ASD adolescents and adults (ages 13–36 years) compared to parent reports of typical adolescents and adults indicated that along with the younger subset of this sample, older ASD individuals did not necessarily have increased levels of social competence, and that level of social functioning significantly influenced levels of romantic functioning, despite the fact that many of these ASD individuals still had a desire for social and romantic relationships (Stokes, Newton, & Kaur, 2007). In addition to these study findings, the ASD adolescents and adults tended to engage in more inappropriate (e.g., intrusive and threatening) behaviors when in pursuit of romantic relationships with a wider variety of people (e.g., friends, strangers, celebrities) than did the comparison group of typical individuals (Stokes et al., 2007). The fact that problems with social reciprocity have been found to be the most central and persistent problem, regardless of intelligence level, highlights this as a critical area to address when preparing individuals with ASDs for adulthood (Shattuck et al., 2007).

Restricted and Repetitive Behaviors and Interests

Behaviors in this ASD diagnostic domain include stereotyped and repetitive body movements and manipulation of object parts, compulsions and rituals, insistence on things being the same, circumscribed interests, and self-injurious behaviors (Schultz & Berkson, 1995; Lewis & Bodfish, 1998; Bodfish et al., 2000). Studies of these behaviors in adolescents and adults with ASDs indicate mixed results regarding these behavior difficulties (*see* Seltzer et al., 2004, for a review). A recent follow-up study did not find significantly high levels of maladaptive or stereotyped behaviors in their sample of 105 adolescents and adults with ASDs and varying levels of intellectual ability; however, more than half of this sample had problems with engaging in repetitive activities or routines (Billstedt et al., 2007). Another finding was that a majority of this sample (93%) had sensory response problems such as aberrant behavior responses to being touched or when exposed to auditory or visual stimulation (Billstedt et al., 2007). This finding of pervasive sensory response problems in adults with ASDs has been replicated in other studies (e.g., Leekam et al., 2006). Hypotheses have asserted that individuals with ASDs may engage in repetitive behaviors to induce a sensory experience or that repetitive behaviors are a response to a sensory experience (Liss et al., 2006).

A study by Shattuck et al. (2007) of 241 adolescents and adults with ASDs revealed significant improvements in all maladaptive behaviors measured, including improvements in the areas of repetitive activities and restricted interests, with greater likelihood of improvement in individuals age 31 years and older. However, individuals with ASDs and mental retardation (MR) had more maladaptive (e.g., aggression or self-injury) behaviors and less improvement in behaviors over time (Shattuck et al., 2007). An important situation for consideration is that if an ASD individual has communication difficulties and they experience pain related to medical issues or perceive an aversive sensory experience, then this may cause him or her to display an increase in self-injurious or aggressive behaviors. This possibility has implications for the determination of future adult living environments for these ASD individuals. For example, if an ASD individual does not learn more effective means of communicating and his or her behaviors escalate to the point of regularly displaying threatening or dangerous behaviors in response to activities or transitions, then they are not likely to remain in community-based programs (Cox & Schopler, 1993).

Daily Living Skills

As previously mentioned, ASD individuals tend to have higher intelligence levels compared to their levels of adaptive functioning, and they tend to show less of an increase over time in acquiring adaptive skills as compared to typically developing peers (e.g., Lockyer & Rutter, 1969; Rumsey et al., 1985; Freeman et al., 1991; Schatz & Hamdan-Allen, 1995; Bryson & Smith, 1998; Carter et al., 1998; Gillham et al., 2000; Bolic & Pousika, 2002; Gabriels et al., 2007). In autism research, the Vineland Adaptive Behavior Scales (VABS; Sparrow et al., 1984) is often used to measure adaptive skills in the areas of communication, daily living, social, and motor skills. Specific deficits on the VABS have been observed in studies of adolescents and adults with autism with a wide range of intellectual abilities, including limited leisure interests, lack of awareness of the need to dress according to situation, poor motor coordination, problems with receptive and expressive language, difficulties with interpersonal social skills, and dependence on others for daily living activities (Billstedt et al., 2007; Klin et al., 2007; Saulnier & Klin, 2007; Shattuck et al., 2007). Notably, it is important for caregivers and service providers to be aware that adolescents with high-functioning autism or AS will also need formal instruction in life skills, because they may not naturally learn these skills from family members or peers.

Living and Vocational Environments

Over the past 30 years, several studies have examined the types of living and vocational environments that ASD adolescents and adults typically attain. Follow-up studies have revealed that although there is considerable variability in adult role outcomes in areas such as independent living, education, vocations, and relationships, a substantial number of individuals do not live independently, are dependent on their families and service providers for assistance with daily living activities, and have limited social networks. The few individuals who have jobs tend to be poorly paid. (*See* Seltzer et al., 2004, for a review.) There is, however, an estimated 15% to 25% of the ASD population with higher intellectual and language abilities, who have more favorable outcomes in these areas, but more research is needed to investigate the predictors of such outcomes (Seltzer et al., 2004).

Cederlund et al. (2008) conducted one of the first studies to prospectively examine the long-term (i.e., more than 5 years) outcomes of a group of 70 males (ages 16–34 years) diagnosed with AS with higher intellectual and language abilities compared to 70 males (ages 16–36 years) diagnosed with autism, the majority (93%) of whom functioned below the average range of intellectual ability. In the AS group, 27% had what was defined as a "good outcome" by *(1)* being employed or engaged in higher education or vocational training and *(2)* living independently if age 23 years or older or *(3)* having two or more friends if age 22 years or younger. Only 3% of those in the AS group were identified as having "poor outcomes" as defined by having obvious impairments in independent and social functioning but still having communication skills. There were no individuals in the autism group who had "good outcomes," and 56% had "very poor outcomes" as defined by an inability to function independently and having limited communication skills. With regard to living environments, 64% of individuals in the AS group age 23 years and older were living independently, although they were all still dependent on caregivers for support. Only 8% of individuals in the autism group age 23 years and older were living independently, although all were still dependent on caregivers for support. These results support the need to consider providing life skills interventions to ASD individuals regardless of their level of intellectual functioning. In addition, for the ASD individuals who have lower intellectual abilities, it is important to consider the value of specifically targeting interventions to improve communication and independent living skills.

Promoting Optimal Functioning to Learn Life Skills

To learn necessary life skills, ASD individuals need to be able to attend and focus rather than be distracted by medical or psychological issues. For example, sometimes adolescents or adults with ASDs may engage in behaviors involving tantrums, self-injury, aggression toward others, and destruction of property. As a result, life skill teaching environments such as home and community-based school or vocational settings are likely to determine that these individuals are unmanageable. This can then lead to considering more restrictive placements for these individuals where the individual is not expected or allowed to develop life skills to their full capacity.

Behavior problems can affect the ability of an ASD individual to attend to and learn from interventions designed to develop life skills. Addressing an ASD individual's problem behaviors requires an exploration and understanding of the possible underlying *causes* related to such behaviors (e.g., medical or psychiatric co-morbidities). A process of active exploration to determine the underlying causes is warranted, because it is difficult for ASD individuals to spontaneously report or describe their experiences in a way that can be understood by others (Theory of Mind: Baron-Cohen et al., 2000). The iceberg metaphor has been used to provide a visual representation of the "tip-of-the-iceberg" problem behaviors and the underlying medical/psychiatric issues or ASD-specific deficits that may be causing or are driving the behavioral presentation (Cox & Schopler, 1993; Peeters, 1995). This iceberg metaphor serves as a reminder for interventionists to avoid simply attempting to change the visible tip-of-the-iceberg behaviors and instead consider seeking ways to understand and be understood by the individual with an ASD (Morgan, 1996). The following section provides an overview of the myriad of medical or psychiatric issues that are important possible causes or contributors to behavior problems in ASD individuals that should be considered and addressed. (*See* Gabriels & Hill, 2007; Gabriels & Van Bourgondien, 2007; and Goldson & Bauman, 2007, for further discussion about physical, medical, and emotional issues related to individuals with ASDs entering adolescence.)

Medical Health Issues and Autism Spectrum Disorders

Like individuals in the general population, ASD individuals face a wide range of health-care challenges. Deterioration in behaviors or sudden onset of behavioral and emotional disturbances should alert caregivers to the possibility of a physical illness (Wainscott & Corbett, 1996). Compared to the general population, there is a high rate of epilepsy (29%) in individuals with autism who also have lower intellectual functioning, and there is an increased risk of seizures during early childhood and adolescence (Volkmar & Nelson, 1990; Gillberg & Billstedt, 2000; Kielinen et al., 2004). Gastrointestinal (GI) symptoms are prevalent (24%), with chronic diarrhea being the most common (12%) concern in individuals with autism (Molloy & Manning-Courtney, 2001). Along with this, constipation can be a concern because of diet issues or medication side effects. GI symptoms should be taken seriously and investigated because they can cause significant discomfort for the ASD individual, which may result in significant behavior problems (e.g., severe aggression toward self or others) (Goldson & Bauman, 2007).

Abnormal response to sensory input has been documented in numerous studies, and this has implications for the behavioral presentation of ASD individuals (e.g., Baranek et al., 2005). Abnormal sensory responses in ASD individuals can include over- and under-responsiveness to sensory input as well as actively seeking sensory input in all sensory domains (auditory, visual, vestibular, tactile, and oral; Dunn, 1999). It has been hypothesized that along with an individual's perception of sensory information, his or her physical or emotional well-being can affect the intensity of his or her behavioral response (Ayres, 2005; Kerstein, 2008).

Sleep problems resulting from a variety of medical and psychosocial issues are common in ASD individuals and include problems falling asleep and staying asleep, sleeping too much, or experiencing events that interfere with sleep such as seizures (Malow, 2004; Allik et al., 2006). There is an indication that the sleep problems in individuals with ASDs may exacerbate issues such as stereotypic behaviors and communication problems observed during daytime activities (Schreck et al., 2004).

Individuals with ASDs may have more oral conditions (oral injuries, oral sensory defensiveness, and teeth-grinding) compared to children with general developmental delay. These factors can result from a combination of poor daily dental hygiene and inconsistent visits to the dentist, which might increase their risk of developing dental disease (DeMattei et al., 2007). Having dental or other medical problems that may result in general discomfort (e.g., oral sensitivities) or pain (e.g., jaw and headache pain from teeth-grinding), which can result in the ASD individual refusing to eat or engaging in self-injurious behaviors (e.g., head banging). Finally, it is important to help this ASD population access health care on a regular basis to monitor and proactively intervene with medical issues, which, if left untreated, may otherwise result in extreme behavioral exacerbations.

Mental Health Issues

Psychiatric Issues

Deterioration in the behavior functioning from an individual's baseline ASD symptom presentation can signal the onset or worsening of a psychiatric condition. As is the case with medical issues, elevated behavior symptoms can interfere with an individual's capacity to learn life skills and function as independently as possible. Higher rates of affective disorders, particularly depression, have been reported in the ASD population (Chung et al., 1990; Tantam, 1991; Abramson et al., 1992; Ghaziuddin & Greden, 1998; Leyfer et al., 2006). Affective disorders appear to peak in ASD adolescents and young adults and are signaled by behavior deterioration (e.g., increased irritability and aggression) (Gillberg & Billstedt, 2000; Ghaziuddin et al., 2002). Notably, ASD individuals with higher levels of intellectual functioning may be more acutely aware of their social and relationship difficulties, which can contribute to feelings of depression. Higher levels of anxiety disorders have been found in children and adults with ASDs compared to controls (e.g., Lecavalier et al., 2006; Leyfer et al., 2006; Gillott & Standen, 2007). The sources of anxiety for ASD individuals have included situation (e.g., being in a busy mall) and medical (e.g., blood draws) fears (Evans et al., 2005), along with specific phobias (e.g., loud noises) (Leyfer et al., 2006). There is growing evidence that symptoms of repetitive or obsessive behaviors can develop into a separate psychiatric obsessive-compulsive diagnosis in ASD children (Muris et al., 1998; Reaven & Hepburn, 2003) and adults (Szatmari et al., 1989; Tantam, 1991; Ghaziuddin, 2005).

Family Issues

The stress of caring for an ASD individual can impact both the individual and their family members. The unique family system, family life cycle (ASD child entering adolescence), and extended support systems are all important factors that can improve the understanding of an individual's behavior problems and identification of needed family service supports to relieve stress (e.g., respite care, parent training, or support groups) (Head & Abbeduto, 2007). Systems theory asserts that families are interactive systems with each member contributing to, influencing, and being influenced by all aspects of family life and their environment (Minuchin, 1974). Caring for ASD individuals can involve considerable expenditures of time, finances, and effort beyond the typical responsibilities of parenting. Parents of ASD children have reported higher levels of stress, depression, marital discord, and pessimism about their child's future than parents of children with other developmental disabilities. (*See* Head & Abbeduto, 2007, for a literature review.) Specific caregiver concerns that relate to having a child or adolescent with an ASD include the individual's behavior problems (e.g., defiance, disruption, aggression), social and communication deficits, and dependency needs that can restrict family activities (e.g., Fong et al., 1993; Lecavilier, Leone, & Wiltz, 2006).

Parent and sibling factors as well as significant life events are important issues that can affect the behavior presentation of the individual with an ASD. Parents of ASD individuals tend to have elevated levels of psychiatric (Yirmiya & Shaked, 2005) and developmental difficulties (Piven et al., 1997) that can affect how they relate to and engage with the ASD individual. For example, if a caregiver struggles with cycling moods, then this parent may give mixed affective messages that can be extremely frustrating and confusing to the ASD individual, who tends to best understand situations when simple and clear-cut messages are provided. On-going exposure to this kind of environment may result in the ASD individual chronically experiencing high levels of anxiety linked with rage reactions. Sibling relationships (e.g., lack of sibling closeness or positive interactions) can also be a contributing factor to the behavioral expression of the sibling with an ASD, depending on the specific coping patterns (e.g., avoidance of the ASD sibling) adopted by the neurotypical sibling (*see* Orsmond & Seltzer, 2007, for a review.) Finally, exposure to negative life events such as a family move or the death of a family member can be associated with an increase in behavior and mood symptoms (e.g., crying spells, irritability, and sleep and appetite disturbance) expressed by the ASD individual (Ghaziuddin et al., 1995).

Autism Spectrum Disorder Symptom Variability: Hypothetical Case Examples

Individuals with ASDs can present with a wide variability of core ASD social, communication, and behavior symptoms combined with a range of intellectual functioning and associated issues. The following two hypothetical cases provide examples for considering how symptom variability requires an individualized life skill intervention approach. In the first case, AS is the diagnosis; however, it is important to note that current research has not provided evidence that there are clear-cut differences between the impairments and service needs of AS and high-functioning autism. (*See* Kasari & Rotheram-Fuller, 2005, for a review.) These case examples will be discussed again in the life skills intervention section to review possible solutions to address the issues presented here.

Case 1:

Joe is a 13-year-old adolescent male with AS or high-functioning autism with at least average intellectual ability and language skills. Although Joe's *communication* skills include a large vocabulary and ability to engage in conversations about his particular interests, he makes fleeting eye contact and speaks in a monotone voice slightly above the volume level of his peers; his peers are often confused by his facial expression because it rarely changes from looking "serious." When Joe's classmates try to involve him in conversations, they become frustrated by his insistence on guiding conversations back to things of interest to him. *Socially*, Joe has been teased by peers because he sometimes forgets he is in public settings and puts his hands in his pants to touch his genitals. He desperately wants to fit in with a peer group at school and has tried to imitate the behaviors and dress of certain social groups, but he has done so to such an extreme that he has been further rejected. Joe's friendships are limited to a much younger girl in his neighborhood and an e-mail pen pal. Joe likes to figure out how mechanical things work, and sometimes this has resulted in his being accused by others of "breaking" their things. Joe's behavior becomes extremely agitated (e.g., he makes loud remarks or threatens to hurt others) when others try to talk to him about how his behavior impacts them. He also becomes significantly more resistant when he is asked to do something he does not want to do, does not get his way, or if the bell rings to signal time to transition to his next class. In the past, he has been suspended from school because he said he wanted to "blow up the school." At home, Joe has little interest or involvement in *activities of daily living*, including his self-care. He spends a majority of his time on the computer and tinkering with mechanical things around the house. Joe refuses to attempt or assist with simple chores or meal preparation. He prefers to eat variety of unhealthy snacks throughout the day. Joe refuses to shower on a daily basis and he often needs reminding to dress appropriately for weather changes because he prefers to wear shorts or pajama pants all of the time. Because of Joe's interest in tinkering with mechanical things and computers, his parents have considered future *living and vocational* environments that include being in a college living environment with supports to address his self-care and social skills deficits. Within such an environment, they hope Joe might learn skills necessary to work with information technology or mechanical engineering.

Case 2

Sarah is a 15-year-old adolescent female with autism and moderate MR. Sarah *communicates* by using sign language and some simple phrases. However, she uses only a few signs, is not precise in gesturing signs, and her verbalizations tend to be repetitive or echoed. If she is offered a choice, Sarah tends to echo the last thing said to her regardless of her preference. Sarah can also communicate her needs by writing simple sentences, but her primary mode of communication is to grab or throw things. Sarah can read simple words or phrases and understand expectations others have for her if provided with a demonstration or simple written instructions presented with pictures. Sarah enjoys swimming, jumping on the trampoline, and singing in *social* settings. Sarah can take turns with others to play simple board or card games but quickly loses interest. At school and in other community settings, Sarah tends to stand too close to others and will spontaneously touch others or smell their hair. She also tries to take her clothes off or masturbate in public settings. *Behaviorally*, Sarah has a hard time waiting and will begin to bang her head when she is expected to wait too long. She can easily become angry and out -of control when she is simply told "No" or asked to do something. Sarah frequently chews holes in her shirts and hits her face, head, or neck repetitively. These behaviors worsen when she becomes emotionally distressed. Sarah tends to grind her teeth at night and at times during the day. She wakes up several times throughout the night. At home, Sarah's *activities of daily living* are limited to sitting in a rocking chair or swing, watching movies, completing 150-piece puzzles, tearing out magazine pictures and sorting them into piles, or listening to music. Her piles of pictures have cluttered many of the living spaces in her home, but her parents do not move them for fear she will become extremely upset. Sarah's parents also do not engage her in helping with simple chores around the house or cooking, because she needs too much supervision to complete such tasks. Sarah can use the toilet but sometimes needs to be reminded to go to the bathroom and needs help with wiping thoroughly. Sarah needs some assistance with completing the steps involved in bathing and brushing her teeth. She has not been to the dentist in several years because of related emotional distress. Sarah's parents have worried about what they will be facing in terms of finding appropriate *living and vocational environments for Sarah.* They are concerned that Sarah may eventually need to live in a very restricted setting with maximum staff assistance and wonder if she will ever be able to do vocational work.

The next sections review interventions that can be gleaned from the literature regarding the underlying learning styles and needs of individuals with ASDs. Following this, example strategies to address the individual needs and capabilities of these two case examples will be provided.

Teaching Survival Life Skills

What and When to Teach

To determine which survival life skills to teach in preparation for adulthood, it is crucial to identify which behaviors will be needed for the ASD individual to function in a future environment. Following this, it is necessary to systematically teach those behaviors throughout the child's life. During each life stage, systematic teaching of life skills should involve interventions that build on the individual's current behaviors, strengths, and interests while considering questions such as "*How will this skill assist the child in the future?*" Families can be valuable life teachers for ASD individuals by embedding the instruction of life skills into the daily activities of family life. This is an important strategy because ASD individuals have difficulties with skill generalization and function better with predictable routines.

Table 67-1 provides a list of suggested life skills to teach ASD individuals. Skills are summarized under core diagnostic domains. For a more comprehensive guide to life skills for this population, see the Suggested Reading for a list of resources.

School settings should incorporate teaching life skills into the curriculum to prepare ASD individuals for vocational and adult living environments. The individuals with Disabilities Act of 1990 (P.L. 101-476) mandates state and local educational agencies to develop an Individualized Education Plan (IEP) for students with disabilities. The IEP maps out how an individual's unique needs can be met to prepare him or her for further education, employment, and independent living in state and local educational agencies. (*See* Steedman, 2007, for a thorough review of the laws impacting the treatment and long-term care of individuals with ASDs.) Assessment tools such as the *TEACCH Transition Assessment Profile–Second Edition (TTAP)* can assist the IEP intervention planning process by identifying the individual's life skill strengths and weaknesses (Mesibov et al., 2007). The TTAP evaluates the individual's life skills in home and school/work environments in areas such as vocational skills, independent functioning, leisure skills, functional communication skills, and social skills.

How to Teach

Parents may have implemented a variety of best practice behavioral and cognitive-behavioral intervention strategies when the child with an ASD was young but may have discontinued using these strategies when the child enters adolescence, assuming that the child has outgrown such techniques. However, these previously used strategies may still be very important and necessary, because the ASD adolescent is still learning and processing information in the unique ways

Table 67–1.
Suggested life skills to teach

Communication Life Skills	Social Life Skills	Behavior Life Skills
Expressive language skills	*Relationship skills*	*Understanding emotions*
Communication aids, pictures, sign language, or adaptive devices	Friendships (shared enjoyment)	Awareness of levels of internal states
Conversation skills	Sportsmanship	Understanding triggers
Writing skills	Dating	Developing coping skills
Receptive language skills	*Self-care skills*	*Self-regulation skills*
Understanding nonverbal cues, figurative language, and sarcasm	Hygiene	Leisure and sensory-oriented recreation activities
Reading skills	Medical health care	*Safety*
	Diet and meal preparation	Sexuality issues
	Exercise routines	Respecting personal space and property
	Employment	Understanding public versus private behaviors
	Transportation	Dealing with emergencies
	Housing-household chores	
	Managing money	
	Shopping	

particular to this ASD population. This section provides an overview of the unique ASD learning styles and identifies a few key behavioral intervention strategies. This section is not meant to provide an in-depth review or discussion of behavioral intervention theories or methods; rather, this section provides a way to consider extending intervention techniques to match the learning needs of the adolescent with an ASD.

Mesibov (2005) refers to the "culture of autism," which is an extremely useful approach to linking theoretical understandings of this ASD population to intervention approaches. Thinking of autism as a "culture" helps make the tremendous ASD symptom variability comprehensible by focusing on common learning characteristics and patterns of behavior. Such understanding can enhance the implementation of interventions to improve the functioning of ASD individuals in society.

Individuals With an Autism Spectrum Disorder Tend to Think Concretely

Concrete thinking can be evidenced in their difficulties with pragmatic language skills, which involve social, emotional, and cognitive factors that enable an individual to effectively communicate and receive messages (Twachtman-Cullen & Twachtman-Reilly, 2007). Concrete thinking can put an ASD individual at risk for not understanding things such as figurative language (e.g., "Give me a hand"). The ASD individual thus may respond in inappropriate ways or become confused by social situations, social conversations, or school lectures. Intervention techniques such as Social Stories™ (Gray, 2000) are frequently used to teach ASD individuals how to respond and manage their behavior during a variety of social situations. Social Stories™ provide concrete and well-defined social rules and socially appropriate behaviors that the individual can follow to engage more successfully. Social Stories™ have demonstrated some effectiveness in decreasing the negative behaviors in individuals with ASDs (Rust & Smith, 2006; Scattone et al., 2007). Social skills training groups also are an important intervention consideration because they have demonstrated skill improvements in ASD adolescents (e.g., Tse et al., 2007). Teaching ways to deal with bullying can be taught through organizations such as KIDPOWER (www.kidpower.org), an international organization that provides instruction regarding the practical skills needed to address confrontation and victimization (van der Zande, 2007).

Individuals With an Autism Spectrum Disorder Struggle to Understand Others' Intentions, Emotional States, and Behaviors

This struggle has been referred to as "mind-blindness" and described by the Theory of Mind (ToM) (Baron-Cohen, 1995; Baron-Cohen et al., 2000). This impaired mentalizing ability can make it difficult for ASD individuals to infer possibilities based on available information, reflect on how their own behaviors may affect others, and problem-solve ways to change their behaviors to improve their social relationships. For example, an ASD adolescent may become extremely angry if his routine of being picked up by his mother at an appointed time is delayed. This adolescent may be unable to generate more than one possibility to explain why his mother is late; if he could, he may be more forgiving of things he cannot control. Social Stories™ or opportunities to learn by "doing" or role-play can be useful interventions to address this issue. Other techniques derived from behavior learning theory and principles of ABA have evidenced effectiveness with ASD individuals (*see* Matson et al., 1996, for a review of behavioral interventions in autism.) For example, highlighting (e.g., giving social praise) to the ASD individual's appropriate social behaviors whenever they occur serves to both increase the individual's awareness of desired social behaviors and motivate them to display these behaviors more frequently.

Individuals With an Autism Spectrum Disorder Tend to Focus on Details at the Expense of Seeing Things in Context or Getting the "Big Picture"

This difficulty integrating ideas affects the ASD individual's ability to generalize information across situations and has been described by Weak Central Coherence Theory (Frith, 2003). Unfortunately, success in the social world heavily depends on the integration of details such as facial expression, vocal intonation, gestures, body language, and words in context. For example, an ASD individual may not understand the nonverbal or verbal cues of someone else being frustrated with his or her inappropriate remarks; therefore, the ASD individual may continue to escalate his or her inappropriate behavior, misreading the nonverbal cues of another person. One helpful technique to encourage motivation and understanding with ASD individuals is to use the "*First do this, then get that*" behavior teaching strategy. For example, at the first signs the ASD individual is being socially inappropriate, the other person can tell the ASD individual that they will return to talk with them when the ASD individual is engaging in a specific socially desired manner and then immediately remove their attention and engagement. Although ASD individuals may have impaired social interactions, they are still are motivated to engage with others. Being told, "*First do this, than get that*" is a strategy that works well to motivate ASD individuals to do something they may be less interested in doing, such as a chore or a task for another person, because following this, they know they can engage in their preferred activity.

Individuals With Autism Spectrum Disorder Have Difficulty With Organization and Sequencing

This has been as described by the theory of Executive Dysfunction (Ozonoff, 1995; Russell, 1997). Executive functions include cognitive flexibility, an ability to apply social rules flexibly, control impulses, organize, and initiate activities. Individuals with an ASD may have difficulties completing a task unless the steps are clearly outlined for them. They also may have trouble completing activities in a timely manner unless they are provided with specific cues to know when an activity is to be finished. Structured intervention methods such as those developed by Division TEACCH address the poor organization and sequencing skills of ASD individuals (Schopler et al., 1995). For example, the TEACCH approach offers strategies for modifying or structuring the physical environment to enhance comprehension of and cooperation with expectations using such techniques as visual schedules and breaking down multiple-step tasks (e.g., showering) or events (e.g., shopping) into more manageable parts (Krauss et al., 2003). Studies of individuals with ASDs in natural environments have demonstrated that the introduction of external structure (e.g., visual cues like pictures and physical organization) combined with predictable routines can help increase on-task behaviors and completion of work (MacDuff et al., 1993; Hume, 2005). There is also evidence to support alternating activity schedules between preferred (those activities not associated with challenging behaviors) and less preferred activities (activities that evoke challenging behaviors) to decrease the presence of behavior problems (Liptak et al., 2006). *See* previously mentioned "*First do this, then get that*" strategy.

Individuals With an Autism Spectrum Disorder Tend to Be Very Distractible, yet Able to Focus Intensely on Things of Particular Interest to Them (Dawson & Levy, 1989)

They can be abnormally aroused or distracted by sensory input such as sound, touch, smell, taste, or movement (Greenspan & Wieder, 1997; Hirstein et al., 2001; Baranek et al., 2005; Tomchek & Dunn, 2007). An ASD individual's focus on stereotyped or repetitive behaviors can distract him or her from being able to attend to teaching tasks. Preferred or "attractive" sensory stimulus conditions have resulted in a reduction in stereotyped movement behaviors in children with autism (Gal et al., 2002). In addition, it may be easier to motivate and teach new information to ASD individuals if the new skill can be linked to their particular interests or preferred activities (Delmolino & Harris, 2004). Given this information, important intervention strategies for ASD individuals include teaching life skills in learning environments free from aversive sensory input and linking new skills with things that are familiar to or preferred by the ASD individual.

Tables 67-2 and 67-3 provide examples of intervention solutions to some of the issues described in the hypothetical cases presented earlier in this section. Notably, these intervention solutions are not intended to be a comprehensive list of options to consider.

Transitions to Residential and Vocational Training Environments

Ideally, transitions to adulthood should be a gradual planned process that is originally considered when a child is diagnosed, is reconsidered when the child enters puberty, and is then again considered when they reach adulthood. The transition to adulthood has been defined as an "... active process that attends to the medical, psychosocial, and educational-vocational needs of adolescents as they move from child-oriented to adult-oriented lifestyles and systems" (White, 1997, p. 698). Transitions can involve moving from educational to work settings from pediatric to adult health-care providers and from living with the family to living in community settings. Caregivers should make plans and adjustments in their perspectives of eventually having to "let go" during each of these life time periods to minimize having to make (haphazard) decisions in a crisis about issues such as where an ASD individual should live (White, 1997). Such prospective planning can help ensure that life-long social and financial support networks are identified and developed long before the individual reaches adulthood (Aman, 2005). For example, establishing a living will and advanced directives (or mental health plans) can provide guidance to future treatment providers about the child's strengths, needs, and problem behavior warning signs. Organizations such as the *National Alliance on Mental Illness (NAMI)* provides one of the largest network of supports and information for improving the quality of life for individuals with special needs, including supports for helping individuals with an ASD transition to independent living and college (www.nami.org).

Residential Environments

Individuals with ASDs are a diverse group, and although some may be able to live independently, other individuals may require supports to live in a safe and healthy manner. It may be difficult for parents to consider planning alternative living settings during their child's early years, because they may be distracted by the daily life struggles related to managing the ASD child's current needs. However, as early as possible, parents should begin considering future living environments for their child because government and private residential agencies are limited. The *National Association of Residential Providers for Adults with Autism (NARPAA)* is a good resource for finding U.S. agencies that provide residential services (www.NARPAA.org). Parents may consider supervised group homes or other supportive living arrangements. Supportive co-housing arrangements may include setting up an apartment with a hired caregiver or other living arrangements that include a peer roommate who has free or discounted rent in exchange for looking out for the ASD individual. After an ASD individual reaches age 18 years, they may qualify for Supplemental Security Income (SSI) to assist with living expenses, although the individual may still live with their parents (www.ssa.gov). Finally, it is important for parents to consider a special needs trust for their ASD child so that he or she can continue to be cared for after the death of the parents. Notably, some trusts or monies in the child's name may impact the child's continued eligibility for benefits such as SSI.

Table 67–2.
Hypothetical case I solutions for 13-year-old male with Asperger's syndrome

Life Skill Domain	Strengths and Needs	Suggested Interventions	Life Skill Goal
Communication	*Strength:* Interest in computers and how things work	1) After-school clubs involving his interests	Development of prevocational skills and friendships who share interests
	Need: Social conversation skills	2) Social skills groups 3) Individual or group therapy with a speech language pathologist	Increased awareness & understanding of survival social conversation skills
Social	*Strength*: Desire for friendships & ability to imitate others	1) See above social interventions. 2) Involve in a school job	1) See above 2) Provide a defined social engagement role with peers.
	Need: Lacks awareness of private vs. public behaviors, & maintaining appropriate social boundaries	1) Teach what are private vs. public and social boundary behaviors 2) School class addressing sexuality issues	Increased pro-social skills to decrease possible involvement with law enforcement
Behavior	*Strength*: Ability to vocalize frustrations *Needs:* Lacks awareness of levels of internal states, triggers, and coping skills	1) Teach to rate levels of internal states related to triggers on a rating scale. 2) Work with an occupational therapist to identify sensory-related calming/coping strategies.	1) Increased understanding, expression, and ability to cope with frustrations 2) Decrease the possibility of expulsion from community settings.
Activities of daily living	*Strength:* Motivated by computers and tinkering with mechanical things *Needs:* Lacks motivation and possibly an understanding of why or how to engage in variety of self-care and daily living activities	1) Daily written schedule alternating less preferred followed by preferred activity 2) Social story of why it is important to keep the body clean, exercise, and eat healthy food	Increased motivation and understanding to engage in adaptive daily living activities

Table 67–3.
Hypothetical case II solutions for 15-year-old female with autism and mental retardation

Life Skill Domain	Strengths and Needs	Suggested Interventions	Life Skill Goal
Communication	*Strengths:* Understands and uses some sign language and simple phrases. Pictures enhance her understanding *Needs:* Limited ability to consistently communicate in multiple settings	1) Expect and reinforce continued use of sign language and phrase speech 2) Introduce a talking device with pictures and use it with her in multiple settings. Use picture–word schedules. 3) Consult with speech language pathologist	1) Decrease frustrations resulting from a lack of ability to communicate needs or to understand others' expectations. 2) Increase ability to be understood by a variety of individuals in multiple settings.
Social	*Strengths:* Interest in others and in soothing self *Needs:* Lacks understanding of appropriate public vs. private behaviors	1) Teach to use specific location for identified private behaviors. 2) Teach to give handshakes for greetings and to ask to get close to or touch others. 3) Teach variety of leisure skills expanding on sensory and special interests.	Increase pro-social and leisure skills to decrease possible involvement with law enforcement and reduce risk of victimization.

(*Continued*)

Table 67–3. *(Contd.)*

Life Skill Domain	Strengths and Needs	Suggested Interventions	Life Skill Goal
Behavior	*Strengths*: Attempts to occupy self when waiting or soothe self when upset. *Needs:* Difficulty knowing what to do when waiting	1) Use timers (e.g., vibrating watch or hourglass) to signal how long she is to wait. 2) Teach to engage with "waiting" (e.g., sensory-oriented materials made available every time she has to wait.	Increase ability to wait in a pro-social and safe manner.
	Needs: May be experiencing headache and neck pain related to teeth-grinding behaviors	1) See dentist to evaluate condition of teeth. 2) Consult with medical professional about pain management strategies. 3) Consult with occupational therapist to define sensory relieving activities. 4) Provide socially appropriate items to chew such as rubber-type jewelry.	Improve dental health and identify pain management and self-regulation strategies to reduce negative behaviors.
Activities of daily living	*Strengths*: Motivated by swinging, movies, puzzles, and sorting pictures *Needs:* Lacks motivation, and ability to engage in activities of daily living	1) Daily picture schedule alternating less preferred followed by preferred activity 2) Mini picture schedule of the steps to do a skill. 3) Consult with occupational therapist to identify strategies to help engage in daily life activities. 4) Incorporate sorting skills into chore activities.	Increase motivation and ability to engage as independently as possible in a wider variety of daily living activities.

Supportive College Living Programs

There are several programs that provide supportive residential environments where ASD students can receive assistance to develop social and daily living skills while taking courses at a nearby community college. Two examples are The College Internship Program (http://www.collegeinternshipprogram.com) and the College Living Experience (http://www.cleinc.net/home.aspx). Such programs also provide academic assistance to complete college and assistance to prepare the individual for the transition to independent living. Assistance includes helping the ASD individual break down academic and daily living tasks into manageable steps, learn self-regulation stress management skills, develop appropriate friendships, and manage medications, as needed. Other programs provide support to ASD students outside of a residential environment. For example, the AHEADD Model (http://www.aheadd.org) provides continuum of professional staff and peer mentors who serve as liaisons, personal advocates, and coaches to the student with an ASD who is competitively admitted to a college of their choice. Finally, contacting the office for disability services on college campuses can be another resource for services and supports for the ASD individual. *See* Blumberg (2005) for a more in depth discussion of college, career, and residential supports.

Employment Training Programs

Project SEARCH is a high school transition program that provides work training experiences in an effort to increase employment opportunities for individuals with disabilities (http://www.cincinnatichildrens.org/svc/alpha/p/search/). Project SEARCH began at Cincinnati Children's Hospital Medical Center in 1996 and now has more than 106 replication sites across the United States. Although a majority of the SEARCH training programs are within health-care settings, other settings include banks, universities, and manufacturing sites. Project SEARCH provides unpaid year-long vocational preparation internships to high school students (ages 18–21 years) with disabilities. These internships involve hands-on experience in employment settings with highly trained job coaches. The internship focuses on teaching appropriate hygiene, social, and communication skills along with skills related to improving students' ability to take direction, change their behavior, and access public transportation. Admission into the internship program depends on the student's updated immunization record, desire to work, and ability to pass a drug screen and background check. Following the completion of this internship program, there is no commitment by the training site to hire the student, although students typically become employees (Personal Communication Project SEARCH co-founder Erin Riehle, March 13, 2009).

Conclusion

Expanding the possibilities for an optimal quality of life when ASD children grow up necessitates assessment and treatment their medical and psychological health as well as teaching necessary life skills that build on the current behaviors, skills, and interests of the ASD individual. Families can be valuable life teachers for their ASD child by routinely embedding the instruction of life skills into activities of family life, making this teaching a part of routines that are practiced every day. The ASD learning style culture is an important consideration when developing life skills interventions to encourage skill acquisition and generalization across vocational and living environments.

Challenges and Future Directions

- Follow-up studies are needed to evaluate the outcomes of the next generation of adolescents and young adults with ASDs who received intensive early intervention services in the 1990s.
- Studies are needed to assess the actual implementation of life skills preparation in academic environments for ASD individuals along with the impact of these programs on social and vocational outcomes.
- More resources are needed to address the residential and vocational needs of the older adolescent and young adult with an ASD.

SUGGESTED READINGS

Baker, J. (2005). *Preparing for Life: The Complete Guide for Transitioning to Adulthood for Those with Autism and Asperger's Syndrome.* Arlington, TX: Future Horizons.

Gabriels, R., & Hill, D. E. (2007). *Growing Up with Autism: Working with School-Age Children and Adolescents.* New York: Guilford.

Harpur, J., Lawlor, M., & Fitzgerald, M. (2004). *Succeeding in College with Asperger's Syndrome.* London: Jessica Kingsley Publishers.

Hudson, J., & Bixler Coffin, A. (2007). *Out and About: Preparing Children with Autism Spectrum Disorders to Participate in Their Communities.* Shawnee Mission, KS: Autism Asperger Publishing Company.

Palmer, A. (2005). *Realizing the College Dream with Autism or Asperger Syndrome: A Parent's Guide to Student Success.* London: Jessica Kingsley Publishers.

ACKNOWLEDGMENTS

Thanks to Pamela Horne, M.D., Lauren, Kerstein, LCSW, Rebecca Howard, M.A., and John A. Agnew, Ph.D. for their editorial suggestions and support with this chapter.

REFERENCES

Abramson, R. K., Wright, H. H., et al. (1992). Biological liability in families with autism. *Journal of the American Academy of Child and Adolescent Psychiatry, 31*(2), 370–371.

Allik, H., Larsson, J. O., et al. (2006). Sleep patterns of school-age children with Asperger syndrome or high-functioning autism. *Journal of Autism and Developmental Disorders, 36*(5), 585–595.

Aman, M. G. (2005). Treatment planning for patients with autism spectrum disorders. *Journal of Clinical Psychiatry 66*(Suppl 10), 38–45.

American Psychiatric Association, *Diagnostic and Statistical Manual of Mental Disorders, Text Revision (DSM IV - TR).* Vol. IV. 2000, Washington, D.C.: American Psychiatric Association.

Ayres, A. J. (2005). *Sensory Integration and the Child.* Los Angeles, Western Psychological Services.

Ballaban-Gil, K., Rapin, I., et al. (1996). Longitudinal examination of the behavioral, language, and social changes in a population of adolescents and young adults with autistic disorder. *Pediatric Neurology, 15*(3), 217–223.

Baranek, G. T., David, F. J., et al. (2005). Sensory Experiences Questionnaire: Discriminating sensory features in young children with autism, developmental delays, and typical development. *Journal of Child Psychology and Psychiatry, and Allied Disciplines, 47*(6), 591–601.

Baranek, G. T., Parham, L. D., et al. (2005). Sensory and motor features in autism: Assessment and intervention. In Volkmar F., Paul R., Klin A. & Cohen D. J., eds. *Handbook of Autism and Pervasive Developmental Disorders, Third Edition, Volume 2: Assessment, Interventions, and Policy* (pp. 831–861). Hoboken, NJ: John Wiley & Sons.

Baron-Cohen, S. (1995). *Mindblindness: An Essay on Autism and Theory of Mind.* Boston, MIT Press/Bradford Books.

Baron-Cohen, S., Tager-Flusberg, H., et al. (2000). *Understanding Other Minds: Perspectives from Developmental Cognitive Neuroscience.* Oxford: Oxford University Press.

Billstedt, E., Gillberg, I. C., et al. (2007). Autism in adults: Symptom patterns and early childhood predictors. Use of the DISCO in a community sample followed from childhood. *Journal of Child Psychology and Psychiatry, and Allied Disciplines, 48*(11), 1102–1110.

Blumberg, R. (2005). College, career and residential options beyond high school: What parents can do to prepare their son or daughter. In Baker J., ed. *Preparing for Life: The Complete Guide for Transitioning to Adulthood for Those with Autism and Asperger's Syndrome* (pp. 29–45). Arlington, TX, Future Horizons.

Bodfish, J. W., Symons, F. J., et al. (2000). Varieties of repetitive behavior in autism: Comparisons to mental retardation. *Journal of Autism and Developmental Disorders, 30*(3), 237–243.

Bolic, S. & Pousika, R. (2002). The relationship between general cognitive level and adaptive behavior domains in individuals with autism with and without co-morbid mental retardation. *Child Psychiatry and Human Development, 33*, 165–172.

Bolte, S. & Poustka, F. (2002). The relation between general cognitive level and adaptive behavior domains in individuals with autism with and without co-morbid mental retardation. *Child Psychiatry and Human Development, 33*(2), 165–172.

Bryson, S. E. & Smith, I. M. (1998). Epidemiology of autism: Prevalence, associated characteristics and implications for research and service delivery. *Mental Retardation and Developmental Disabilities Research Reviews, 4*, 97–103.

Carter, A. S., Volkmar, F. R., et al. (1998). The Vineland Adaptive Behavior Scales: Supplementary norms for individuals with autism. *Journal of Autism and Developmental Disorders, 28*(4), 287–302.

Cederlund, M., Hagberg, B., et al. (2008). Asperger syndrome and autism: A comparative longitudinal follow-up study more than 5 years after original diagnosis. *Journal of Autism and Developmental Disabilities, 38*(1), 72–85.

Chung, S. Y., Luk, S. L., et al. (1990). A follow-up study of infantile autism in Hong Kong. *Journal of Autism and Developmental Disorders, 20*(2), 221–232.

Cox, R. D. & Schopler, E. (1993). "Aggression and self-injurious behaviors in persons with autism—the TEACCH (Treatment and Education of Autistic and related Communications Handicapped Children) approach." *Acta Paedopsychiatrica, 56*(2), 85–90.

Curry, K., Posluszny, M., et al. (1993). Training Criminal Justice Personnel to Recognize Offenders with Disabilities. Washington, DC, Office of Special Education and Rehabilitative Services.

Dawson, D. & Levy, A. (1989). Arousal, attention and the socioemotional impairments of individuals with autism. In Dawson G., ed. *Autism: Nature, Diagnosis and Treatment,* (pp. 49–74). New York, Guilford Press.

Delmolino, L. & Harris, S. L. (2004). *Incentives for Change: Motivating People with Autism Spectrum Disorders to Learn and Gain Independence.* Bethesda, MD, Woodbine House.

DeMattei, R., Cuvo, A., et al. (2007). Oral assessment of children with an autism spectrum disorder. *Journal of Dental Hygiene, 81*(3), 65.

Dunn, W. (1999). *Sensory Profile.* San Antonio, TX: The Psychological Corporation.

Evans, D. W., Canavera, K., et al. (2005). The fears, phobias and anxieties of children with autism spectrum disorders and down syndrome: Comparisons with developmentally and chronologically age matched children. *Child Psychiatry and Human Development, 36*(1), 3–26.

Fong, L., Wilgosh, L., et al. (1993). The experience of parenting an adolescent with autism. *International Journal of Disability, Development and Education, 40,* 105–113.

Freeman, B. J., Rahbar, B., et al. (1991). The stability of cognitive and behavioral parameters in autism: A twelve-year prospective study. *Journal of the American Academy of Child and Adolescent Psychiatry, 30*(3), 479–482.

Frith, C. (2003). What do imaging studies tell us about the neural basis of autism? *Novartis Foundation Symposium, 251,* 149–166; discussion 166–176, 281–297.

Gabriels, R. & Hill, D. E. (2007). *Growing Up with Autism: Working with School-Age Children and Adolescents.* New York: Guilford.

Gabriels, R. L., Cuccaro, M. L., et al. (2005). Repetitive behaviors in autism: Relationships with associated clinical features. *Research in Developmental Disabilities, 26*(2), 169–181.

Gabriels, R. L., Ivers, B. J., et al. (2007). Stability of adaptive behaviors in middle-school children with autism spectrum disorders. *Research in Autism Spectrum Disorders, 1*(4), 291–303.

Gabriels, R. L. & Van Bourgondien, M. E. (2007). Sexuality and autism: Individual, family and community perspectives and interventions. In Hill D. E., ed. *Growing Up With Autism: Working with School-Age Children and Adolescents.* New York: Guilford Press.

Gal, E., Dyck, M. J., et al. (2002). Sensory differences and stereotyped movements in children with autism. *Behaviour Change, 4,* 207–219.

Ghaziuddin, M. (2005). *Mental health aspects of autism and Asperger syndrome.* London: Jessica Kingsley Publishers.

Ghaziuddin, M., Alessi, N., et al. (1995). Life events and depression in children with pervasive developmental disorders. *Journal of Autism and Developmental Disorders, 25*(5), 495–502.

Ghaziuddin, M., Ghaziuddin, N., et al. (2002). Depression in persons with autism: Implications for research and clinical care. *Journal of Autism and Developmental Disorders, 32*(4), 299–306.

Ghaziuddin, M. & Greden, J. (1998). Depression in children with autism/pervasive developmental disorders: A case-control family history study. *Journal of Autism and Developmental Disorders, 28*(2), 111–115.

Gillberg, C. & Billstedt, E. (2000). Autism and Asperger syndrome: Coexistence with other clinical disorders. *Acta Psychiatrica, Scandinavica, 102*(5), 321–330.

Gillberg, C. & Steffenburg, S. (1987). Outcome and prognostic factors in infantile autism and similar conditions: A population-based study of 46 cases followed through puberty. *Journal of Autism and Developmental Disorders, 17*(2), 273–287.

Gillham, J. E., Carter, A. S., et al. (2000). Toward a developmental operational definition of autism. *Journal of Autism and Developmental Disorders, 30*(4), 269–278.

Gillott, A. & Standen, P. J. (2007). Levels of anxiety and sources of stress in adults with autism. *Journal of Intellectual Disabilities, 11*(4), 359–370.

Goldson, E. & Bauman, M. (2007). Medical health assessment and treatment issues in autism. In Gabriels R. L. & Hill D. E., eds.*Growing Up With Autism: Working with School-Age Children and Adolescents.* New York: Guilford Press.

Gray, C. (2000). *The New Social Story Book Illustrated Edition.* Arlington, TX: Future Horizions.

Greenspan, S. I. & Wieder, S. (1997). Developmental patterns and outcomes in infants and children with disorders in relating and communicating: A chart review of 200 cases of children with autistic spectrum disorder. *Journal of Developmental and Learning Disorders, 1,* 87–141.

Head, L. S. & Abbeduto, L. (2007). Recognizing the role of parents in developmental outcomes: A systems approach to evaluating the child with developmental disabilities. *Mental Retardation and Developmental Disabilities Research Reviews, 13*(4), 293–301.

Hirstein, W., Iversen, P., et al. (2001). Autonomic responses of autistic children to people and objects. *Proceedings. Biological Sciences, 268*(1479), 1883–1888.

Howlin, P. (2003). Outcome in high-functioning adults with autism with and without early language delays: Implications for the differentiation between autism and Asperger syndrome. *Journal of Autism and Developmental Disorders, 33*(1), 3–13.

Howlin, P., Goode, S., et al. (2004). Adult outcome for children with autism. *Journal of Child Psychology and Psychiatry and Allied Disciplines, 45*(2), 212–229.

Hume, K. (2005). Effects of an individual work system on the independent work and play skills in students with autism. *International Meeting for Autism Research (IMFAR).* Boston, May 2005.

Kasari, C. & Rotheram-Fuller, E. (2005). Current trends in psychological research on children with high-functioning autism and Asperger disorder. *Current Opinion in Psychiatry, 18*(5), 497–501.

Kerstein, L. H. (2008). *My Sensory Book: Working Together to Explore Sensory Issues and the Big Feelings They Can Cause.* Shawnee Mission, KS: Autism Asperger Publishing Company.

Kielinen, M., Rantala, H., et al. (2004). Associated medical disorders and disabilities in children with autistic disorder: A population-based study. *Autism, 8*(1), 49–60.

Klin, A., Saulnier, C. A., et al. (2007). Social and communication abilities and disabilities in higher functioning individuals with autism spectrum disorders: The Vineland and the ADOS. *Journal of Autism and Developmental Disorders, 37*(4), 748–759.

Krauss, M. W., Gulley, S., et al. (2003). Access to specialty medical care for children with mental retardation, autism, and other special health care needs. *Mental Retardation, 41*(5), 329–339.

Lecavalier, L., Leone, S., et al. (2006). The impact of behaviour problems on caregiver stress in young people with autism spectrum disorders. *Journal of Intellectual Disability Research, 50*(Pt 3), 172–183.

Leekam, S. R., Nieto, C., et al. (2006). Describing the sensory abnormalities of children and adults with autism. *Journal of Autism and Developmental Disorders, 35*(7), 894–910.

Lewis, M. H. & Bodfish, J. W. (1998). Repetitive behavior disorders in autism. *Mental Retardation and Developmental Disabilities Research Reviews, 4*(2), 80–89.

Leyfer, O. T., Folstein, S. E., et al. (2006). Comorbid psychiatric disorders in children with autism: Interview development and rates of disorders. *Journal of Autism and Developmental Disorders, 36*, 849–861.

Liptak, G. S., Orlando, M., et al. (2006). Satisfaction with primary health care received by families of children with developmental disabilities. *Journal of Pediatric Health Care, 20*(4), 245–252.

Liss, M., Saulnier, C., et al. (2006). Sensory abnormalities in autistic spectrum disorders. *Autism, 10*(2), 152–172.

Lockyer, L. & Rutter, M. (1969). A five- to fifteen-year follow-up study of infantile psychosis. *British Journal of Psychiatry, 115*(525), 865–882.

MacDuff, G. S., Krantz, P. J., et al. (1993). Teaching children with autism to use photographic activity schedules: Maintenance and generalization of complex response chains. *Journal of Applied Behavior Analysis, 26*(1), 89–97.

Malow, B. A. (2004). Sleep disorders, epilepsy, and autism. *Mental Retardation and Developmental Disabilities Research Reviews, 10*(2), 122–125.

Matson, J. L., Benavidez, D. A., et al. (1996). Behavioral treatment of autistic persons: A review of research from 1980 to the present. *Research in Developmental Disabilities, 17*(6), 433–465.

Mesibov, G., Thomas, J. B., et al. (2007). *TTAP: TEACCH Transition Assessment Profile*. Austin, TX: Pro-Ed.

Mesibov, G. B. & Shea, V. (2005). The Cuture of Autism: From Theoretical Understanding to Educational Practice. In Mesibov G. B., Schopler E., & Shea V. *TEACCH Approach to Autism Spectrum Disorders*. New York: Springer.

Minuchin, S. (1974). *Families and Family Therapy*. Cambridge, MA: Harvard University Press.

Molloy, C. A. & Manning-Courtney, P. (2001). *Frequency of gastrointestinal symptoms among children with autism and ASD*. International Meeting for Autism Research, San Diego, California.

Morgan, H. (1996). Appreciating the style of perception and learning as a basis for anticipatng and responding to the challenging behavior of adults with autism. In Morgan H. *Adults with Autism: A Guide to Theory and Practice* (pp. 231–248). New York: Cambridge University Press.

Mottron, L. & Burack, J. A. (2001). *The Development of Autism: Perspectives from Theory and Research*. Mahwah, NJ: Erbaum.

Muris, P., Steerneman, P., et al. (1998). Comorbid anxiety symptoms in children with pervasive developmental disorders. *Journal of Anxiety Disorders, 12*(4), 387–393.

Orsmond, G. I. & Seltzer, M. M. (2007). Siblings of individuals with autism spectrum disorders across the life course. *Mental Retardation and Developmental Disabilities Research Reviews, 13*(4), 313–320.

Ozonoff, S. (1995). Reliability and validity of the Wisconsin Card Sorting Test in studies of autism. *Neuropsychology, 9*, 491–500.

Peeters, T. (1995). *The best treatment of behavior problems in autism is prevention*. European Conference on Autism, University of Athens.

Piven, J., Palmer, P., et al. (1997). Broader autism phenotype, Evidence from a family history study of multiple-incidence autism families. *American Journal of Psychiatry, 154*(2), 185–190.

Reaven, J. & Hepburn, S. (2003). Cognitive-behavioral treatment of obsessive-compulsive disorder in a child with Asperger syndrome: A case report. *Autism, 7*(2), 145–164.

Rumsey, J. M., Rapoport, J. L., et al. (1985). Autistic children as adults: Psychiatric, social, and behavioral outcomes. *Journal of the American Academy of Child Psychiatry, 24*(4), 465–473.

Russell, J. (1997). *Autism as an Executive Disorder*. Oxford: Oxford University Press.

Rust, J. & Smith, A. (2006). How should the effectiveness of Social Stories to modify the behaviour of children on the autistic spectrum be tested? Lessons from the literature. *Autism, 10*(2), 125–138.

Scattone, D., Wilezynski, S. M., Edwards, R. P., & Rabian, B. (2007). Decreasing disruptive behaviors of children with autism using social stories. *Journal of Autism and Developmental Disorders, 32*(6), 535–543.

Saulnier, C. A. & Klin, A. (2007). Brief report, Social and communication abilities and disabilities in higher functioning individuals with autism and Asperger syndrome. *Journal of Autism and Developmental Disorders, 37*(4), 788–793.

Schatz, J. & Hamdan-Allen, G. (1995). Effects of age and IQ on adaptive behavior domains for children with autism. *Journal of Autism and Developmental Disorders, 25*(1), 51–60.

Schopler, E., Mesibov, G. B., et al. (1995). Structured teaching in the TEACCH system. In Schopler E. & Mesibov G. B. *Learning and Cognition in Autism*. New York: Plenum Press, 243–268.

Schreck, K. A., Mulick, J. A., et al. (2004). Sleep problems as possible predictors of intensified symptoms of autism. *Research in Developmental Disabilities, 25*(1), 57–66.

Schultz, T. M. & Berkson, G. (1995). Definition of abnormal focused affections and exploration of their relation to abnormal stereotyped behaviors. *American Journal of Mental Retardation, 99*(4), 376–390.

Seltzer, M. M., Shattuck, P., et al. (2004). Trajectory of development in adolescents and adults with autism. *Mental Retardation and Developmental Disabilities Research Reviews, 10*(4), 234–247.

Shattuck, P. T., Seltzer, M. M., et al. (2007). Change in autism symptoms and maladaptive behaviors in adolescents and adults with an autism spectrum disorder. *Journal of Autism and Developmental Disorders, 37*(9), 1735–1747.

Sparrow, S. S., Balla, D. A., et al. (1984). *Vineland Adaptive Behavior Scales: Interview Edition*. Circle Pines, MN: American Guidance Service.

Steedman, W. (2007). Advocating for services: Legal issues confronting parents and guardians. In Gabriels, R. L. & Hill, D. E., eds. *Growing Up With Autism, Working with School-Age Children and Adolescents*. New York: Guilford Press.

Stokes, M. Newton, N., & Kaur, A. (2007). Stalking and social and romantic functioning among adolescents and adults with autism spectrum disorder. *Journal of Autism and Developmental Disorders, 37*(10), 1969–1986.

Szatmari, P., Bartolucci, G., et al. (1989). A follow-up study of high-functioning autistic children. *Journal of Autism and Developmental Disorders, 19*(2), 213–225.

Tantam, D. (1991). Asperger Syndrome in Adulthood. In Frith, U., ed. *Autism and Asperger Syndrome* (pp. 147–183). Cambridge: Cambridge University Press.

Tomchek, S. D. & Dunn, W. (2007). Sensory processing in children with and without autism: A comparative study using the short sensory profile. *American Journal of Occupational Therapy, 61*(2), 190–200.

Tse, J., Strulovitch, J., et al. (2007). Social skills training for adolescents with Asperger syndrome and high-functioning autism. *Journal of Autism and Developmental Disorders, 37*(10), 1960–1968.

Tuchman, R. & Rapin, I. (2002). Epilepsy in autism. *Lancet Neurology, 1*(6), 352–358.

Twachtman-Cullen, D. & Twachtman-Reilly, J. (2007). Communication and language issues in less-able school-aged children with autism. In Gabriels R. L. & Hill D. E., eds. *Growing Up With Autism, Working with School-Age Children and Adolescents.* New York: Guilford Press.

van der Zande, I. (2007). *The KIDPOWER Book for Caring Adults: Personal Safety, Self-Protection, Confidence and Advocacy for Young People.* Santa Cruz, CA: KIDPOWER Press.

Volkmar, F. (2003). Adaptive skills. *Journal of Autism and Developmental Disorders, 33*(1), 109–110.

Volkmar, F. R. & Nelson, D. S. (1990). Seizure disorders in autism. *Journal of the American Academy of Child and Adolescent Psychiatry, 29*(1), 127–129.

Wainscott, G. & Corbett, J. (1996). Health care of adults with autism. In Morgan H., ed. *Adults with Autism: A Guide to Theory and Practice.* Cambridge: Cambridge University Press.

White, P. H. (1997). Success on the road to adulthood. Issues and hurdles for adolescents with disabilities. *Rheumatic Diseases Clinics of North America, 23*(3), 697–707.

World Health Organization (1999). *Partners in Life Skills Training: Conclusions from a United Nations Inter-Agency Meeting.* Geneva: World Health Organization.

World Health Organization (2004). *Skills for Health: An Important Entry-Point for Health Promoting/Child-Friendly Schools.* Geneva: World Health Organization.

Yirmiya, N. & Shaked M. (2005). Psychiatric disorders in parents of children with autism: A meta-analysis. *Journal of Child Psychology and Psychiatry, 46*(1), 69–83.

68 Family Adaptive Functioning in Autism

Annette Estes, Vanessa Hus, Lauren Elder

Points of Interest

- Families of children with autism spectrum disorders (ASDs) are recognized as being impacted by having a family member with an ASD. Impacts can vary widely and include both negative and positive experiences, ranging from increased resource needs, to higher levels of parenting-related stress, to positive personal growth for family members.
- Families are increasingly appreciated for their crucial role in implementing and supporting early autism intervention. Addressing the needs of children with ASDs thus requires including a focus on the family.
- Family adaptive functioning is proposed as an integrative term for the many specific activities families carry out to support improved outcomes for children with ASDs. These activities include examples such as family-orchestrated child experiences (e.g., summer camps, sports programs), parent–child interaction, and child health and safety functions.
- Early autism intervention can play a role in supporting family adaptive functioning. Evidence suggests intervention that improves child social functioning and decreases problem behavior associated with ASDs may support family adaptive functioning.
- Research is needed to clarify characteristics of intervention programs that lead to improved family adaptive functioning and ways in which family adaptive functioning is related to better outcomes for children with ASDs. Increased attention to measuring clear, well-defined constructs related to the family will support efforts to identify new targets for ASD intervention.

Families of children with ASDs have received increasing attention from autism researchers in recent years. There is a growing appreciation of the potentially daunting hurdles parents may face related to raising a child or children with ASDs. The time of initial diagnosis is often emotionally painful. This process can be complicated by the necessity of initiating early intervention services while concurrently facing the emotional reality of the diagnosis of an ASD. Services are often difficult to access and costly, adding burden to the family. The family context is increasingly understood as a crucial factor to consider in implementing early intervention. Thus, increased attention by research to families of children with ASDs is related in part to an appreciation of the difficulties they face but also to a growing understanding that the success of early intervention may be improved with the support of parents and families.

The Developmental Systems model (DS model; Guralnick, 1998, 2005) provides a framework for understanding the connection between family context, early intervention, and improved outcomes for children with developmental disabilities. This model is centered on developmental principles and places the family—particularly parents—at the center of early intervention programs. The DS model specifies parent–child interaction (e.g., verbal commenting on child play, responsiveness to child initiations, positive physical play), family-orchestrated child experiences (e.g., holiday celebrations, meal time, leisure activities), and child health and safety functions (e.g., medical care, regular sleep patterns, monitoring child whereabouts) as specific functions provided by the family that can improve child outcomes. Within this model, both threats and supports to these central family functions are identified. Family characteristics that may threaten or support family patterns of interaction include personal characteristics of parents (mental health, intellectual ability, and child-rearing attitudes), financial resources, and social supports for the family. Threats also include child characteristics that increase the demands on parents, family resource needs, and distress in the family, as well as decrease confident parenting.

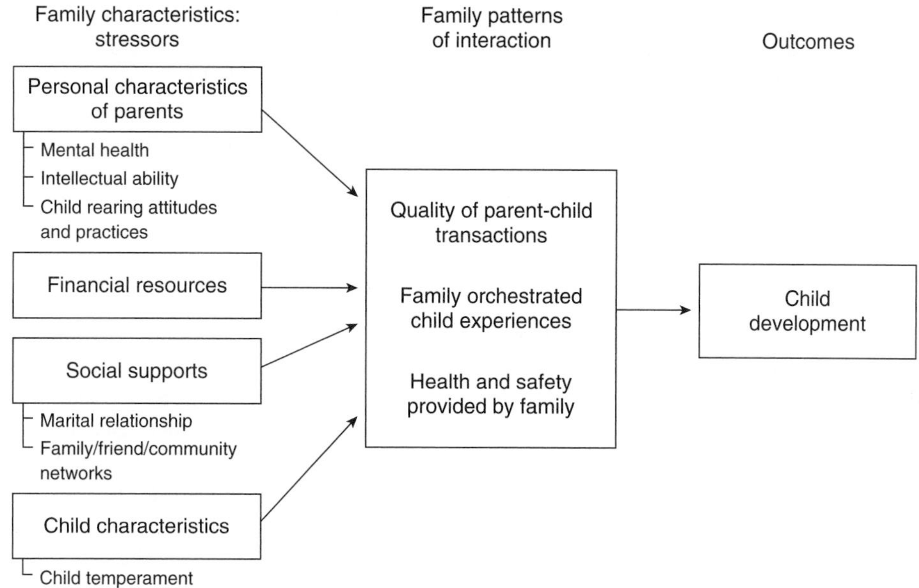

Figure 68–1. Developmental Systems Model. From Guralnick, M. J. (2005). An overview of the developmental systems model for early intervention. In M. J. Guralnick (Ed.), *The developmental systems approach to early intervention* (p. 11). Baltimore: Paul H. Brookes Publishing, Reprinted by permission.

In addition to the functions identified in the DS model, the family system, especially parents, often plays a crucial role in early identification of difficulties for children with ASDs and may be part of an interdisciplinary team approach to implementing early intervention (e.g., Vismara, Colombi, & Rogers, 2009).

There are many complex and heterogeneous constructs that motivate and inform research related to families of children with ASDs. Family adaptive functioning is a concept we propose to use as a framework for the concepts discussed above. Adaptive functioning for an individual is considered the ability of an individual to carry out age-appropriate skills needed to function in daily life, such as dressing, eating, following rules, avoiding accidents, and making friends. The specific activities of families that contribute to improved outcomes for children with ASDs (parent–child interaction, family-orchestrated child experiences, and child health and safety functions in the DS model) can be considered "family adaptive functioning."

Parents are typically the single-most important contributors to family adaptive functioning. Therefore, the first section of this chapter will focus on four constructs related to parental contributors to family adaptive functioning: parenting-related stress, parental psychological distress, parental psychological functioning, and parent coping strategies. Research findings related to these constructs in families with children with ASDs will be discussed, and specific measures of these constructs will be presented. The second section of the chapter will present several key threats and supports to family adaptive functioning: family characteristics, stressful life events, spousal relations, social support, and child characteristics. Measures of each threat and support and relevance to families of children with ASDs will be discussed. The chapter concludes with a discussion of connections between interventions for ASD and family adaptive functioning. Evidence regarding the impact of three types of intervention—early intensive behavioral intervention, parent training, and interventions directly targeting parent stress—on family adaptive functioning is discussed.

Parental Contributors to Family Adaptive Functioning

Parenting-Related Stress

In the extensive literature on parenting, the concept of stress has been used as an umbrella term, integrating a variety of phenomena that may affect parent functioning (Webster-Stratton, 1990). Research on parent stress may include factors that range from extrafamilial (e.g., negative life events), to interparental (e.g., marital distress), to child-related (e.g., difficult child temperament). Stress has also been defined phenomenologically as resulting from the parent's subjective appraisal of the demands placed on them in their role as a parent (Abidin, 1992). The scientific investigation of parent stress is challenging, given the wide variety of concepts the term stress covers. This complexity has resulted in many different constructs being measured, even though they purportedly all relate to parent stress. This has important ramifications for interpreting results of research in this area. For example, Rodrigue, Morgan, and Geffken (1990) found that stress was higher in parents of children with ASDs compared with parents of children with idiopathic developmental delay (DD) and typical development, but only on certain dimensions of parental stress. Perceived parental competence and marital satisfaction were lower in parents of children with ASDs, but self-blame and perceived disruption of finances and activities were equivalent in the ASD and DD groups. In addition, no group differences in family cohesion and mother–child interaction were found between groups. Greenberg and colleagues (2004) found no differences in overall level of optimism, depression, well-being, or health among mothers of adult children with ASDs, Down syndrome, and schizophrenia. Mothers of adults with Down syndrome reported closer relationships with their children compared to mothers of adults with ASDs. The literature strongly supports the notion that parents of children with ASDs experience higher stress (e.g., Dumas et al., 1991; Estes et al., 2009), but it also appears that the way in which stress is defined and measured can offer a more complex picture.

We define *parenting-related stress* as the amount of stress a parent feels related specifically to aspects of parenting their child with ASD. The term parenting-related stress has been used by others (e.g., Abidin, 1992; Hodapp et al., 2003) but with a slightly different meaning. For example, some parenting stress scales include child characteristics, spousal relations, and social support, which we consider as separate constructs. We argue that it is important to attend to these measurement issues so that meaningful comparisons can be made between studies, and models can be objectively tested. In addition, our phenomenological approach emphasizes the parental experience of stress. An underlying assumption of this approach is that stress is subjective and thresholds for experiencing stress vary from person to person. It is important to distinguish between an individual parent's experience of stress (i.e., parenting-related stress) and an investigator's assumptions about the impact of child characteristics on the family. This is because a particular child characteristic may cause great stress for one parent but low stress for another parent. This level of measurement clarity is needed to allow systematic evaluation of the impact of ASD intervention on family adaptive functioning and to increase understanding of moderators of family adaptive functioning. We next review commonly employed rating scales that are used to measure parent-related stress.

One of the most commonly used rating scales to investigate parenting-related stress in families of children with ASDs is the Parenting Stress Index, (PSI; Abidin, 1995) and the PSI-Short Form (PSI-SF, Abidin, 1995). The PSI is based on the theory that the amount of stress a parent experiences is a complex interaction of certain child characteristics, parent characteristics, and situations related to the parenting role. Hence, to assess parent stress levels, the PSI is divided in to two domains; the Child Domain and the Parent Domain. The Parent Domain is relevant to parenting-related stress but also taps into the domains of psychological distress (e.g., Depression) and social support (e.g., Isolation). It comprises seven subscales: Competence, Isolation, Attachment, Health, Role Restriction, Depression, and Spouse. Example items from the Parent Domain are: "I often feel that I cannot handle things very well" and "I feel trapped by my responsibilities as a parent." The entire questionnaire consists of 120 items, rated on a 5-point scale (Strongly Agree to Strongly Disagree). The instrument yields a Total Stress Score, subdomain scores for each of the subscales, and an optional Life Stress score. Using a sample of 534 parents, the PSI demonstrated good reliability on the child domain (0.89), parent domain (0.93), and the Total Stress Score (0.95). Test–retest reliability on a subset of 37 mothers showed adequate reliability on the child domain (0.55) and good reliability on the parent domain (0.70) and Total Stress Score (0.65) after a 1-year interval.

Another frequently used scale is the Questionnaire on Resources and Stress (QRS; Holroyd, 1974). The most frequently used version of the QRS in ASD research appears to be the QRS–Friedrich Short Form (QRS-F; Friedrich, Greenberg, & Crnic, 1983). The QRS-F contains 52 true-false items comprising four subscales: Parent and Family Problems (e.g., "I can go visit with friends whenever I want" and "Other members of the family have to do without things because of ___), Pessimism (e.g., "It bothers me that my son/daughter will always be this way" or "I worry about what will happen to ____ when I can no longer take care of him/her"), Child characteristics (e.g., "I feel tense when I take ____ out in public"), and Physical Incapacitation (e.g., "___can walk without any help"). It has demonstrated good reliability and validity (Honey et al., 2005).

A third questionnaire used in the parent stress literature is the Parenting Daily Hassles Questionnaire (Crnic & Greenberg, 1990). This questionnaire consists of 20 items, each stating a different event that commonly occurs in families with young children (e.g., "Being nagged, whined at, complained to" and "Difficulty getting kids ready for outings and leaving on time"). Each item is rated on a 4-point scale for how often they occur (rarely, sometimes, a lot, or constantly) and on a 5-point scale for intensity (1 being low and 5 being high) of hassle experienced by parents. In a sample of children with three comparison groups: ASD, intellectual disability or language disorder and no clinical concerns, internal consistency between the items on the Frequency and Intensity was 0.86 (Rutgers et al., 2007).

Plant and Sanders (2007) designed two scales that may be useful for investigating the subjective experience of parenting-related stress in families with children with ASDs. The first determines which caregiving tasks parents perceive as most stressful. The second assesses the degree of stress parents associate with each caregiving task. Parents are asked to rate on a 7-point Likert scale (1—not stressful at all, 7—extremely stressful) how stressful they find completing tasks associated with eight caregiving areas: *(1)* direct tasks (e.g., bathing, feeding); *(2)* in-home therapy (e.g., completion of special activities recommended by therapists); *(3)* attending medical appointments, therapy sessions, and educational programs; *(4)* supervision of their child's activities/whereabouts; *(5)* involvement in leisure/play activities; *(6)* education and information about their child's disability; *(7)* advocating for services; and *(8)* managing their child's behavior. The parent's responses in each of the eight areas are added together for a total score, with higher scores indicating greater stress associated with caregiving activities. The authors reported good internal consistency ($r = 0.82$; Plant & Sanders, 2007).

Parental Psychological Distress

Psychological distress is a construct relating to an individual's experience of negative feelings or emotions. There is a wide range of symptoms and emotions investigated in studies of psychological distress, ranging from symptoms of depression and anxiety to pessimism. Research suggests parents of children with ASDs experience increased psychological distress. For example, compared to parents of children without developmental delays, parents of children with ASDs reported higher levels of anxiety (Hamlyn-Wright et al., 2007) and depression (Eisenhower et al., 2005; Hamlyn-Wright et al., 2007). A study by Orsmond and colleagues (2007) has suggested that mothers of adolescents with ASDs have a higher probability of reporting elevated depression and anxiety symptoms compared to normative samples. A variety of studies of parents of children with ASDs have reported increased levels of depression, anxiety, and/or pessimism compared to parents of children with other disabilities, such as Down syndrome, cerebral palsy, intellectual disability, and developmental delay without ASD (Abbeduto et al., 2004; Blacher & McIntyre, 2006; Estes et al., 2009; Hamlyn-Wright et al., 2007). However some, studies do not find elevated levels of psychological distress in parents of children with ASDs compared to parents of typically developing children (Allik et al., 2006; Toth et al., 2007) or children with Fragile X, communicative impairment, developmental delay, or schizophrenia (Abbeduto et al., 2004; Bristol et al., 1993; Herring et al., 2006; Eisenhower et al., 2005; Greenberg et al., 2004; Olsson & Hwang, 2001). Despite the lack of mean group differences, approximately one-third of the mothers of children with ASDs report clinical levels of depressive symptoms—a significantly higher proportion compared to the mothers of children with Fragile X (18.2%) or Down Syndrome (10.3%) (Abbeduto et al., 2004).

Within families affected by ASD, mothers are frequently reported to have higher levels of depressive symptoms (Hastings et al., 2005; Moes et al., 1992, Olsson & Hwang, 2001) and anxiety (Hastings, 2003) compared to fathers. Davis and Carter (2008) have suggested that fewer fathers report depressive symptoms within the clinical range, whereas proportions of mothers and fathers reporting high levels of anxiety were similar. However findings are mixed with regard to depressive versus anxiety symptoms (Hastings, 2003; Hastings et al., 2005; Allik et al., 2006).

Elevated scores on measures of psychological distress may be related to decreased parental quality of life and self-efficacy (e.g., Donenberg & Baker, 1993; Hastings & Brown, 2002; Rodrigue, Morgan, & Geffken, 1992). As such, these findings warrant serious attention from clinicians and researchers. However, it is important to bear in mind that high scores on measures of individual distress may not represent psychopathology (*see* Coyne & Downey, 1991). Furthermore, the relationship between parental psychological distress, parenting-related stress, and child characteristics remains to be delineated. Longitudinal studies investigating these interconnected effects across time will be essential for understanding this complex interaction.

One of the most commonly used measures of psychological distress is the Center for Epidemiologic Studies Depression Scale (CES-D; Radloff, 1977). The CES-D includes 20 items asking the respondent to rate on a scale of 0 (rarely or none of the time) to 3 (most or all of the time) the presence and persistence of depressive symptoms in the last week (e.g., "I had crying spells" and "I was happy.") Internal consistency is reported to range from 0.84 for the general population and 0.90 for the patient sample in the original study (Radloff, 1977) and 0.89 to 0.91 for mothers and fathers of children with ASDs, respectively (Davis & Carter, 2008).

Another frequently used measure is the Hospital Anxiety and Depression Scale (HADS; Zigmond & Snaith, 1983). The HADS consists of 7 items that assess depression (e.g., "I feel as if I am slowed down") and 7 that assess anxiety (e.g., "I get sudden feelings of panic."). Respondents are asked to rate their experience in the last week on a scale of 0 to 3, where higher scores indicate the presence of symptoms and scores greater than 11 suggest the probable presence of a mood disorder. In two samples of parents of children with ASDs, good reliability was reported for both the Anxiety (Cronbach's alpha = 0.86–0.87 for fathers and 0.89–0.90 for mothers) and Depression (0.72–0.74 for fathers, 0.82–0.86 for mothers) scales (Hastings & Brown, 2002; Hastings, 2003).

The Brief Symptom Inventory (BSI; Derogatis, & Melisaratos, 1983) is a 53-item parent self-report measure of psychological distress. Derived from the SCL-90-R (Derogatis, 1983, 1994), the BSI assesses presence of symptoms in nine areas: somatization, obsessive-compulsive, interpersonal sensitivity, depression, anxiety, hostility, phobic anxiety, paranoid ideation, and psychoticism. Respondents are asked to rate items such as "Trouble remembering things" and "Feeling inferior to others" on a scale of 0 ("not at all") to 4 ("extremely"). Scores result in three global indices: the Global Severity Index (level of overall psychological distress), Positive Symptom Distress Index (intensity of symptoms), and Positive Symptom Total (number of symptoms reported). In the original normative sample of 1002 psychiatric outpatients, 719 nonpatient subjects, and 313 psychiatric in-patients, the BSI was found to have good test–retest reliability and internal consistency (0.68–0.91 and 0.71–0.85, respectively, for the 9 dimensions; Derogatis & Melisaratos, 1983). This measure has been used in several studies of parents of children with ASDs (Estes et al., 2009; Toth, et al., 2007; Blackledge & Hayes, 2006).

The Beck Anxiety Inventory (Beck & Steer, 1990) is sometimes used to measure parental anxiety levels. This questionnaire was originally designed as an instrument that would reliably discriminate anxiety from depression and contains 21 items, each representing a different symptom of anxiety (e.g., "Nervous," "Shaky/unsteady," and "Feeling hot"). On a scale from 0 ("not at all") to 3 ("severely bothered"), respondents are asked to rate how much each item has bothered him/her over the past week. Items are summed to produce a total anxiety score. In a sample of parents of toddlers with ASDs, good internal consistency was reported (alpha = 0.86 for mothers and fathers separately; Davis & Carter, 2008).

Parental Psychological Functioning

Parental psychological functioning encompasses facets of individual, psychological well-being or positive emotional functioning in parents. Taken as a whole, investigations suggest that well-being is not simply the opposite of psychological distress, akin to a low score on a Likert scale that ranges from positive to negative emotions. It appears that positive psychological functioning may function relatively independently from psychological distress. For example, parents of children with ASDs may undergo a grieving process related to their child with ASD that entails symptoms of depression and anxiety. However, simultaneously, they may feel personal growth, efficacy, and increased meaning as part of this same process. Greenberg and colleagues (2004) investigated the role of dispositional optimism in mothers of adults with Down syndrome, schizophrenia and autism. They found that maternal optimism was an important mediator of maternal well-being. Smith and colleagues (2008) found that problem-focused coping was associated with increased maternal well-being. Another study found that increased parenting self-efficacy was associated with maternal well-being (Kuhn & Carter, 2006). However, White and Hastings (2004) reported lower social support was associated with anxiety, depression, and parenting-related stress but found no association between social support and a measure of parental well-being. Higgins, Bailey, and Pearce (2005) reported no relationship between coping strategies and measures of self-esteem in parents of children with ASDs.

One measure of well-being that has been used is the Scales of Psychological Well-Being (Ryff, 1989). This measure consists of six subscales (self-acceptance, positive relations with others, autonomy, environmental mastery, purpose in life, and personal growth). Each subscale contains 20 items, divided equally between positive (e.g., "I like most aspects of my personality") and negative items (e.g., "I tend to worry what other people think of me"). Alpha coefficients for the six scales ranged from 0.82 to 0.90 (Schmutte & Ryff, 1997). Several revisions of the measure exist, with subscales ranging from three to six items each. Greenberg and colleagues (2004) used three subscales (personal growth, self-acceptance, and purpose in life) as a measure of positive psychological well-being in a sample of mothers of adults with Down syndrome, ASDs, and schizophrenia and found good internal consistency (0.80–0.88). Smith and colleagues (2008) used a five-item personal growth subscale (e.g., "New experiences are important" and "Life has been continuous learning and growing") in a sample of mothers of toddlers and adolescents with ASDs and reported reliability coefficients of 0.63 and 0.68, respectively (Smith et al., 2008).

Sense of coherence is often measured using the Sense of Coherence Scale (SOC; Antonovsky, 1987). Among several different versions, the SOC-13 has been used in ASD research (Mak et al., 2007; Olsson & Hwang, 2002). The SOC-13 asks respondents to rate 13 statements on a scale of 1 ("very often") to 7 ("very seldom" or "never"). These statements assess cognition (e.g., "Do you ever have very mixed up feelings and ideas?"), emotions (e.g., "How often do you have feelings that you're not sure you can keep under control?"), and hope/meaning (e.g., "How often do you have the feeling that there's little meaning in the things you do in your daily life?"). Internal consistency of the SOC-13 has been reported between 0.78 to 0.87 in samples of parents of children with developmental disabilities and/or ASDs (Mak et al., 2007; Olsson & Hwang, 2002).

Optimism has been measured using a modified version of the Life Orientation Test (LOT; Scheier & Carver, 1992). Greenberg and colleagues used a modified version of the LOT consisting of eight items (e.g., "If something can go wrong for me, it will." and "In uncertain times, I usually expect the best."), rated on a 4-point scale (strongly disagree to strongly agree). In their sample of mothers of children with ASDs, Cronbach's alpha reliability was reported to be 0.87 (Greenberg et al., 2004).

Parental Coping Strategies

Coping is "the process by which individuals respond to threats of stress" (Smith et al., 2008). The style of coping that parents use has been examined in several studies. Many contrast problem-focused coping, which involves trying to solve the problem causing stress, with emotion-focused coping, which involves trying to alleviate the feelings that are a result of the stress. Orsmond et al. (2007) found higher emotion-focused coping in mothers of children with disabilities to be associated with higher anxiety. Stoneman and Payne (2006) reported fathers of children with disabilities who used more problem-focused coping viewed their marriages more positively. Abbeduto and colleagues (2004) found mothers of children with developmental disabilities who used more emotion-focused and less problem-focused coping had higher levels of pessimism and depression. Smith and colleagues (2008) compared coping strategies in mothers of toddlers with ASDs with mothers of adolescents with ASDs. In both groups, greater emotion-focused coping was associated with greater maternal depression and anger. Increased problem-focused coping was associated with decreased depression and increased personal growth. Taken together, these studies indicate that parents of children with disabilities who use more problem-focused coping and less emotion-focused coping may experiences less psychological distress.

The Coping Orientations to Problems Experienced or Multidimensional Coping Inventory (COPE; Carver, Scheier, & Weintraub, 1989) is a 52-item questionnaire used to assess how individuals respond to stressful events. Each item asks the respondent to rate, on a 4-point scale, the frequency with which a particular coping strategy is used during a stressful event. The COPE includes scales measuring emotion-focused coping strategies (e.g., denial, emotionality, disengagement) and problem-focused coping (e.g., active coping, planning, positive reinterpretation, growth). Studies have shown adequate to good internal consistency on the emotion-focused (0.60–0.78) and problem-focused (0.66–0.89) scales with mothers of children with ASDs (Abbeduto et al., 2004; Orsmond et al., 2007; Smith et al., 2008).

The Family Crisis Orientated Personal Evaluation Scales (McCubbin et al., 1991) contains 30 coping behavior items comprising five subscales: reframing (positively reframing events to make them more manageable); passive appraisal (minimization of response to problematic issues); acquiring social support; seeking spiritual support; and mobilizing the family to acquire and accept help from community resources. In a sample of parents of children with ASDs, internal consistency for each of the subscales was reported as follows: reframing (0.82), passive appraisal (0.48), acquiring social support (0.81), seeking spiritual support (0.88), and mobilizing the family (0.59; Honey et al., 2005).

Threats and Supports to Family Adaptive Functioning

Next we turn to several potential threats and supports that may moderate or mediate family adaptive functioning. These include family characteristics, stressful life events, spousal relations, social support, and child characteristics.

Family Characteristics

Particular family characteristics, such as family income and number of children with a disability, may moderate family adaptive functioning in ASD. For example, lower household income predicted higher reported levels of maternal depressive symptoms (Orsmond et al., 2007), whereas higher household income predicted lower parenting-related stress (Mak et al., 2007). Mothers who had one child with ASD and another child with a disability (ASD, ADHD, LD, or other psychiatric condition) reported higher levels of depressive and anxiety symptoms compared to mothers with just one child on the autism spectrum (Orsmond et al., 2007). Parents report less family adaptability and cohesion than U.S. norms (Higgins et al., 2005) and less adaptability than mothers of children with Down syndrome (Rodrigue et al., 1990). Mothers of two children with disabilities reported lower levels of cohesion and adaptability in the family compared to mothers with just one child with ASD (Orsmond et al., 2007). Compared to mothers of children with Down syndrome, mothers of children with ASDs have also reported poorer quality mother–child relationships (Abbeduto et al., 2004). In a study by Greenberg and colleagues (2004), better quality relationships with their child were associated with lower levels of maternal depressive symptoms.

The Family Adaptability and Cohesive Evaluation Scales (FACES-II; Olson et al., 1982) is a 30-item parent-report questionnaire designed to measure the degree of emotional bonding between family members (Cohesion Subscale) and how flexible and able the family system is to change roles and relationships in response to stressors (Adaptability Subscale). The questions assess both positive and negative aspects of family life—for example, “It is easier to discuss problems with people outside the family than with other family members,” and “Family members discuss problems and feel good about the solutions.” Parents are asked to rate each statement on a 5-point scale ranging from 1 (“almost never”) to 5 (“almost always”). In a sample of mothers of adolescent and adult children with ASDs, reliability alphas were 0.72 for both subscales (Orsmond et al., 2007).

The Positive Affect Index (PAI; Bengtson & Schrader, 1982) is a measure of affective closeness used to investigate parents’ perceptions of their relationship with their child. This scale consists of 10 items on a scale of 1 (“not at all”) to 6 (“extremely”). Parents are asked to rate five facets of positive affect: trust, intimacy, understanding, fairness, and mutual respect. Half of the items ask the parent to rate their feelings toward their child in these five areas, whereas the other five items ask the parent to rate the extent to which these five facets are displayed by the child toward the parent. In two samples of mothers with adult children with ASDs, reliability alphas were reported between 0.85 and 0.87 (Greenberg et al., 2004; Lounds et al., 2007).

Stressful Life Events

The occurrence of major life events may impact family adaptive functioning by increasing stress levels in parents of children with ASDs, which in turn may disrupt parenting practices and parent–child interaction. Stressful life events include events that all families may experience, such as the death of a family member, but some such events may be directly related to having a child with autism, such as relocating to access better services. Few studies have systematically explored the influence that life events may have on parents of children with ASDs. Toth and colleagues (2007) reported family changes and stressful events during pregnancy with a younger sibling to the child with autism did not differ significantly between parents of children with autism compared to parents without a child with an ASD. Whether or not life events occur at a higher level in families with a child with ASD, they may be an important consideration when evaluating family adaptive functioning. Furthermore, the impact of stressful life events on parents of children with ASDs may be moderated by social support and coping style (Dunn et al., 2001). The importance of measuring stressful life events in other populations (e.g., Crnic, Greenberg, & Slough, 1986) suggests this is an area that warrants further investigation in families affected by ASDs.

One measure used to assess life events is the Life Experiences Survey (LES; Sarason, Johnson, & Siegel, 1978). The LES is a self-report questionnaire that asks individuals to evaluate the impact of 60 life events on a 7-point scale, ranging from −3 (extremely negative) to +3 (extremely positive). Test–retest reliability correlations were reported to range from 0.19 to 0.53 for the positive change score, 0.56 to 0.88 for the negative change score, and 0.63 to 0.64 for the total score (Sarason et al., 1978). The PSI also contains an optional 19-item Life Stress Scale that asks about the occurrence of potential stressors outside of the parent–child relationship and provides a context for interpreting the PSI scores.

Spousal Relations

There is a well-documented relationship between marital conflict and poorer child outcomes for typically developing children. For example, children exposed to marital conflict may be particularly vulnerable to behavioral and emotional disturbances, social and interpersonal problems, and poorer academic performance (e.g., Grych & Finham, 1990; Jenkins & Smith, 1991; Cummings, Davies, & Simpson, 1994). A small number of studies suggest parents with a child with ASD report lower levels of marital happiness and marital intimacy compared to parents of typically developing children or children with Down syndrome (Fisman et al., 1989; Higgins et al., 2005; Rodrigue et al., 1990). Past research suggested that parents of children with ASDs may be at a higher risk for marital discord (DeMyer, 1979; Donovan, 1988; Rodrigue et al., 1990). In light of studies demonstrating the adverse effects that marital distress can have on children, future research is needed to systematically investigate how the marital relationship is impacted by having a child with ASD.

The Locke-Wallace Marital Adjustment Test (Locke & Wallace, 1959) is a self-report questionnaire of marital adjustment consisting of 15 items, each weighted differently to yield a total possible score of 2 to 158. Total scores have been shown to discriminate between couples referred for intervention (<100) and those who were not at risk for marital difficulties (>100). Of the well-adjusted group tested in the original validation study, 96% achieved scores of 100 or more. Split-half reliability was 0.90.

The Dyadic Adjustment Scale (Spanier, 1976) is a 32-item, self-report measure assessing the quality of the current marriage or relationship with the partner. This scale has been found to have good criterion validity. Marital status (divorced vs. married) significantly correlated with each item ($p < 0.001$) and total scores for married versus divorced significantly differed in a sample of 218 married and 94 divorced individuals. High correlations between the Dyadic Adjustment Scale and the Locke-Wallace Marital Adjustment Test (0.86 for married respondents and 0.88 for divorced; $p \leq 0.001$) also indicated good construct validity. Cronbach's alphas ranged between 0.73 and 0.94 for each subscale and 0.96 for the total scale (Spanier, 1976).

Social Support

Social support may function as a protective factor for parents of children with ASDs. Honey et al. (2005) found that mothers' stress was lower when they rated the helpfulness of informal social support and accessibility of social support as higher. Another study found higher psychological distress in mothers of children with ASDs was associated with lower levels of family social support (Bromley et al., 2004). Parents of children with ASDs rate accessing social support as one of their top coping mechanisms (Luther, Canham, & Cureton, 2005) and report relying on multiple sources of support (Mackintosh, Myers, & Goin-Kochel, 2006). However, mothers of children with ASDs reported emotional support was less available compared with mothers of children intellectual disability and mothers of typically developing children (Weiss, 2002; Rutgers et al., 2007). Data obtained on a web survey from parents indicates that they rely on other parents of children with ASDs more frequently than any other source of support (Mackintosh et al., 2006). Parents reporting higher levels of social support also report lower levels of depression, anxiety, and anger (Benson, 2006; Benson & Karlof, 2008; Gray & Holden, 1994), and mothers with higher self-esteem and higher levels of social support report less depression (Weiss, 2002). Parents who do not seek and receive social support report more relationship problems with their spouse (Dunn et al., 2001). Siklos and Kerns (2006) found that parents of children with ASDs did not differ from parents of children with Down syndrome in the number of family needs. However, parents of children with autism were more likely to report needs relating to professional assistance and ASD intervention, indicating professionals can be an important source of support for parents of children with ASDs.

The Social Support Questionnaire (Sarason et al., 1983) consists of 27 items. For each item, the respondent lists people they can rely on for different aspects of social support (counted to yield N score for item) and rates their satisfaction with these supports on a 6-point scale (S score). Reliability coefficients for N and S scores were 0.97 and 0.94, respectively. This measure has also been used in samples of parents of children with autism (Rodrigue et al., 1990; Rodrigue et al., 1992).

The Family Support Scale (Dunst, Trivette, & Jenkins, 1984) is an 18-item questionnaire asking the parent to rate on a 5-point Likert scale the helpfulness of informal and formal sources of support for raising a young child. This measure can be used to identify the areas in a family's support network that need to be strengthened or accessed to better meet their needs. Based on revised scoring procedures by McConachie and Warings (1997), two scores may be derived from this measure: *(1)* a weighted score for the helpfulness of informal sources (spouse, family, friends, other informal supports) of support available to the family and *(2)* a weighted score for the helpfulness of support from professionals and services available to the family. Dunst et al. (1984) have described good reliability in families of children with disabilities (internal consistency = 0.77, and test–retest reliability = 0.91).

Child Characteristics

Parents face unique challenges related to characteristics of children with ASDs as well as challenges that are common to all parents of children with developmental disabilities. Unlike some other types of developmental disability, ASDs impair social relatedness, which may be particularly emotionally painful for parents. Many children with ASDs also exhibit unusual language and communication patterns, such as stereotyped speech or language delays, and odd and ritualistic behaviors. Researchers have investigated the parents' perceptions of both the negative and positive impact of having a child with ASD on the overall family functioning (Lloyd & Hastings, 2008; Herring et al., 2006; Eisenhower et al., 2005; Hastings et al., 2005; Rodrigue et al., 1990). Problem behaviors, such as irritability, hyperactivity, and self-injury, have consistently emerged as an important child-related source of parental distress for parents of children with ASDs (e.g., Baker et al., 2002; Beck et al., 2004; Hastings, 2002; Hauser-Cram et al., 2001; Hodapp et al., 2003; Konstantareas & Homatidis, 1989). Estes and colleagues (2009) investigated the relationship between behavior problems, adaptive functioning, and maternal distress in preschool-aged children with ASDs and DD without ASDs. Despite the two groups being matched on developmental age, children in the ASD group demonstrated higher levels of problem behavior and lower daily living skills compared with the children in the DD group. Increased levels of child problem behaviors were associated with increased parenting stress and increased psychological distress. However, neither child diagnosis nor daily living skills were significantly associated with parenting stress. Interestingly, parenting stress and child problem behaviors were more strongly correlated in the DD group than in the ASD group, suggesting additional factors may be at play for parents of children with ASDs.

Smith et al. (2008) found that the presence of restricted and repetitive behaviors in adolescents with ASDs, was associated with maternal reports of lower personal growth and less problem-focused coping. Intellectual disability is a child characteristic that does not consistently appear to be associated with parenting stress and psychological function (Baker et al., 2002; Bakeret al., 2003; Johnston et al., 2003). Although a common assumption is that increased intellectual disability is associated with increased parent stress, some research indicates that having a cognitively lower functioning child with developmental disabilities is actually associated with lower parental distress (Gallagher & Bristol, 1989). A related hypothesis is that lower independence (referred to as adaptive functioning) is source of distress for parents. However, results are mixed in terms of the relationship between adaptive function and parental distress, with two studies finding better adaptive skills in children associated with maternal well-being (Fitzgerald, Birkbeck, & Matthews, 2002; Tomanik, Harris, & Hawkins, 2004) and three reporting no association with adaptive skills (Beck et al., 2004; Lecavalier, Leone, & Wiltz, 2006; Estes et al., 2009).

It is beyond the scope of this chapter to review measures of child characteristics. One measure used to assess the child's impact on family functioning is the Family Impact Questionnaire (FIQ; Donenberg & Baker, 1993). This scale measures a parent's perception of the "child's impact on the family compared with the impact other children his/her age have on their families." It comprises 50 items (e.g., "My child's behavior bothers me more," "I enjoy the time I spend with my child more") rated on a scale from 0 ("not at all") to 3 ("very much"). Subscales assess the parent's perception of the child's negative impact (social life, finances, siblings, marriage, and parenting) and positive impact (feelings about parenting) on the family. In a sample of typically developing children and children with various disabilities (including ASD), reliability alphas were reported to be 0.92 for the combined negative impact scales and 0.81 for the positive impact scale (Eisenhower et al., 2005).

The Kansas Inventory of Parental Perceptions Positive Contributions Scale (KIPP-PC; Behr, Murphy, & Summers, 1992) has also been used to assess the parent's belief that the child with disability has a positive impact on the parent (e.g., the child is responsible for the parent learning patience) and positive impact on the family (e.g., the child is responsible for bringing the family closer together). It also has a scale that measures parent belief that their child has positive characteristics (e.g., the child is kind and loving), which may be a measure of child characteristics rather than parent perception on the child's impact on the family. This measure has 50 items, rated on a 4-point scale. In a sample of parents of children with ASDs, the KIPP-PC was shown to have a high level of internal consistency (Cronbach's alpha = 0.95) for both mothers and fathers (Hastings et al., 2005).

Intervention for Autism Spectrum Disorders and Family Adaptive Functioning

Early Intensive Behavioral Intervention

Research has shown that early intensive behavioral intervention (EIBI) leads to improved outcomes for many children with ASDs. A less well-understood, but equally positive set of findings suggests that parents may also benefit from their child's participation in EIBI. It is likely that a complex, transactional relationship exists between parent stress, EIBI, and developmental progress in children with ASDs. Although the mechanisms of change are not well-understood, research does suggest that EIBI can serve to reduce stress in parents. In a study of 65 families with preschool children with ASDs, more intervention hours were associated with a greater improvement in parent stress (Osborne et al., 2007). The children in the study received a variety of interventions, including preschool, speech, EIBI, and parent training for 2 to 40 hours per week. Although improvements in parent stress were reportedly a result of the number of intervention hours received, children with the highest number of intervention hours tended to be receiving EIBI. Thus, additional research is needed to disentangle these results. Schwictenberg and Poehlmann (2007) also found lower depression scores in mothers when their children were receiving more EIBI hours; however, mothers who provided more EIBI hours themselves reported higher levels of personal strain. Salt et al. (2002) compared families of children with ASDs receiving a social-developmental early intervention program with a waitlist control group and found that at follow-up 10 months later, parents of children in the intervention group had lower stress than the control group. However, this difference was not statistically significant, and the number of intervention hours differed between the two groups, making it difficult to reach a conclusion about the effects of the program on parent stress.

EIBI is defined as intervention for children with ASDs that incorporates the behavioral learning principles of ABA, begins prior to age 5 years, and involves 20 to 40 hours per week of intervention.

In one study, parent stress was examined in families with young children (mean age = 28.35 months) with autism and typical development (Baker-Ericzen, Brookman-Frazee, & Stahmer, 2005). In this study, parents participated in an early intervention inclusion program utilizing Pivotal Response Training. Pivotal Response Training is an intervention approach developed and described elsewhere by Koegel and colleagues (e.g., Koegel, Koegel, & Schreibman, 1991; Koegel et al., 1989). Children with autism were enrolled in either a morning or afternoon session for at least 6 months, and each class had four children with autism and eight who were typically developing. Mothers of children with ASDs showed reductions in stress on the Child Domain but not on the Parent Domain on the Parenting Stress Index. Father stress did not change, however. Maternal stress on the Child Domain was predicted by child cognitive functioning and symptoms of autism. There was also a correlation between a child's level of social skills and maternal stress (Parent Domain). This study suggests changes in parent stress may be related specifically to changes in the child's behavior.

Hastings and Johnson (2001) conducted a survey of 141 parents participating in intensive in-home intervention based on Lovaas-style EIBI. The average age of the child was 4.98 years, with an average of 13.47 months of participation in the program. Parent stress was lower in parents who believed in the efficacy of the intervention. In addition, beliefs about treatment efficacy moderated the effects of ASD symptom severity on parents' pessimism. This study highlights the importance of parental beliefs about the effectiveness of their children's intervention services.

Parent stress may also have an impact on the effectiveness of EIBI. Osborne et al. (2007) reported that when children received high levels of intervention, they showed less improvement in educational and adaptive functioning when their parents had high levels of stress. Improvements in IQ were not related to parent stress. Also, a high level of parent stress was not associated with educational outcomes in children who received fewer hours of intervention. The mechanisms behind these reported patterns are not clear. Parenting style, level of treatment involvement, and factors associated with child behavior problems were not investigated but could underlie these findings. It is also important to note that the children with highly stressed parents also demonstrated improvement but not to the same degree as children with less stressed parents.

Parent Training

Several studies have focused on the impact of behavioral parent training programs on reducing parent stress. In one study, 28 mothers of preschool children with ASDs participated in a psycho-educational parent training program or a no-treatment control (Bristol, Gallagher, & Holt, 1993). The treatment consisted of parents and therapists working together to develop an early intervention program using behavior modification and educational techniques for the parents to deliver in the home. Mothers in the treatment group showed decreases in depressive symptoms over time. This was not a randomized trial, as mothers could choose whether or not to participate in the psycho-educational program and the results may be amplified by an uneven distribution of maternal characteristics between the groups. For example, mothers in the treatment group may have been more problem-focused or more efficacious in their problem solving than mothers in the control group.

There has been one randomized trial comparing parent education and behavior management intervention to a parent education and counseling control for parents of children with ASDs (Tonge et al., 2006). Children were 2.5 to 5 years old at the start of the study. All of the children had been diagnosed with ASDs within the previous month. The parent education/behavior management intervention included such topics as general education about ASDs, available services, behavior modification techniques, teaching skills, and stress management for parents. It included rehearsals, modeling, and homework tasks. The control group also received some educational information and discussion; however, the control intervention did not include skills training or homework assignments for the parents. Parents in both groups improved in overall mental health post-intervention and at a 6-month follow-up. The treatment group showed a greater reduction in anxiety, insomnia, somatic symptoms, and family dysfunction at follow-up, suggesting that learning and practicing specific behavior management strategies may be important for reducing parent stress.

The way in which parent training treatment is delivered may be also be an important consideration. In a study using a repeated reversal design with three families with 2-year-old children with ASDs, clinician-directed parent training was compared to parent–clinician partnership parent training (Brookman-Frazee, 2004). Both groups were taught using Pivotal Response Training. In the partnership condition, the clinician asked for parental input and provided choices about target behaviors and how to teach skills. The clinician followed the parent's lead when the parent chose target behaviors or intervention opportunities. In the clinician-directed condition, the clinician chose activities and target behaviors without asking for parent input. Mothers showed decreased stress and increased confidence during parent/clinician partnership periods but not during clinician-directed periods.

Interventions Directly Targeting Parent Stress

Interventions designed to directly target parent stress have been developed and investigated. A review article on interventions for stress in parents of children with intellectual and developmental disabilities suggests that although interventions such as respite care, case management, and parent-led support networks likely reduce stress in parents, cognitive behavioral group interventions have best evidence for reducing stress in mothers (Hastings & Beck, 2004). For example, a support group designed to teach stress management was delivered to mothers of school-aged children with ASDs (Bitsika & Sharpley, 2000). Positive—although not statistically significant—changes were found on measures of anxiety, depression, and stress. A 2-day (14-hour) Acceptance and Commitment Therapy (ACT) workshop was evaluated with a group of 20 parents of children with ASDs and a wait-list control group (Blackledge & Hayes, 2006). ACT "emphasizes acceptance of unpleasant emotions, defusion from difficult thoughts, clarification of the client's personally held values and corresponding goals, and enhancement of the client's effectiveness in moving towards those values and goals" (p. 3). The approach is based on cognitive-behavioral therapy but focuses on mindfulness and acceptance as much as change. Parents in the treatment group showed small but statistically significant improvements in parent stress and depression as measured on the BSI, BDI, and General Health Questionnaire. It remains unclear whether interventions that directly target parent stress will be found to be as effective as interventions targeting child problem behavior, child development, or parenting techniques in families with a child with ASD.

Conclusions

A variety of factors contribute directly and indirectly to family adaptive functioning, but parents are typically the single-most important contributor. Parents of children with ASDs are consistently found to have elevated levels of parenting-related stress and psychological distress, even when compared with parents of children with non-ASD developmental disabilities. It is also the case that positive psychological functioning and effective coping strategies are also often reported in parents of children with ASDs. Potential threats and supports to family adaptive functioning, including socio-economic status, spousal relations, availability of social support, and specific child characteristics, should be considered when designing empirical studies and interventions for children with ASDs. Research on the relationship between family factors (e.g., parenting-related stress) and child-focused interventions (e.g., EIBI, parent training) is still in the early stages. However, it is evident that a child's treatment can have positive impact on parents. Findings suggest that gains in child social functioning and reduction of child problem behavior may reduce parent stress, which, in turn, may improve family adaptive functioning. Factors associated with intervention, such as the number of hours provided, parental beliefs about the efficacy of the intervention, and a collaborative approach to intervention, may also serve to support family adaptive functioning. Further investigation of positive contributors to family adaptive functioning holds promise for increasing the already impressive momentum toward greater understanding and improved outcomes for children with ASDs.

Challenges and Future Directions

- Increased attention to measuring clear, well-defined constructs related to family adaptive functioning is needed. Developing ASD-specific theoretical models of family adaptive functioning and outcomes for children with ASDs and measuring specific components of these models will support innovations in intervention for children with ASDs.
- Research is needed to clarify characteristics of intervention programs that contribute to improved family adaptive functioning. This is particularly challenging because of the transactional nature of the relationship between child behavior, child response to intervention, and family adaptive functioning. However, this line of research is promising and has already suggested intervention targets (such as child problem behavior) and intervention approaches (such as parent–clinician partnership) that may improve family adaptive functioning.
- More work is needed to understand the ways in which family adaptive functioning may positively influence outcomes for children with ASDs and their family members. It will be important to investigate whether these family factors can be targeted directly and whether this will contribute to positive longer-term outcomes for children with ASDs and their families.

SUGGESTED READINGS

Guralnick, M. J. (2005). An overview of the developmental systems model for early intervention. In M. J. Guralnick (Ed.), *The Developmental Systems Approach to Early Intervention* (pp. 3–28). Baltimore: Brookes.

Hastings, R. P., & Beck, A. (2004). Practitioner review: Stress intervention for parents of children with intellectual disabilities. *Journal of Child Psychology and Psychiatry, 45*(8), 1338–1349.

Webster-Stratton, C. (1990). Stress: A potential disruptor of parent perceptions and family interactions. *Journal of Clinical Child Psychology, 19*(4), 302–312.

REFERENCES

Abbeduto, L., Seltzer, M. M., Shattuck, P., Krauss, M. W., Orsmond, G., & Murphy, M. M. (2004). Psychological well-being and coping in mothers of youths with ASD, Down syndrome, or fragile x syndrome. *American Journal of Mental Retardation, 109*(3), 237–254.

Abidin, R. R. (1992). The determinants of parenting behavior. *Journal of Clinical Child and Adolescent Psychology, 21*(4), 407–412.

Abidin, R. R. (1995). *Parenting stress index* (3rd ed.). Odessa, FL: Psychological Assessment Resources.

Allik, H., Larsson, J. O., & Smedje, H. (2006). Health-related quality of life in parents of school-age children with asperger syndrome or high-functioning autism. *Health and Quality of Life Outcomes, 4*(1).

Antonovsky, A. (1987). *Unraveling the mystery of health: How people manage stress and stay well.* London: Jossey-Bass Ltd.

Baker, B. L., Blacher, J., Crnic, K. A., & Edelbrock, C. (2002). Behavior problems and parenting stress in families of three-year-old children with and without developmental delays. *American Journal of Mental Retardation, 107*(6), 433–444.

Baker, B. L., McIntyre, L. L., Blacher, J., Crnic, K., Edelbrock, C., & Low, C. (2003). Pre-school children with and without developmental delay: Behavior problems and parenting stress over time. *Journal of Intellectual Disability Research, 47*(Pt 4-5), 217–230.

Baker-Ericzen, M. J., Brookman-Frazee, L. B., & Stahmer, A. (2005). Stress levels and adaptability in parents of toddlers with and without ASD spectrum disorders. *Research and Practice for Persons with Severe Disabilities, 30*(4), 194–204.

Beck, A., Hastings, R. P., & Daley, D. (2004). Pro-social behaviour and behaviour problems independently predict maternal stress. *Journal of Intellectual and Developmental Disability, 29*(4), 339–349.

Beck, A. T. & Steer, R. A. (1990). *Beck Anxiety Inventory, manual.* San Antonio, TX: Psychological Corporation.

Behr, S. K., Murphy, D. L., & Summers, J. A. (1992). *User's manual: Kansas inventory of parental perceptions (KIPP).* Lawrence, KS: Beach Centre on Family and Disability.

Bengtson, V. L. & Schrader, S. S. (1982). Parent-child relationships. In D. J. Mangon & W. A. Peterson (Eds.), *Research instruments in social gerontology* (Vol. 2, pp. 115–185). Minneapolis: University of Minnesota Press.

Benson, P. R. (2006). The impact of child symptom severity on depressed mood among parents of children with ASD: The mediating role of stress proliferation. *Journal of Autism and Developmental Disorders, 36*, 685–695.

Benson, P. R. & Karlof, K. L. (2008). (e-pub ahead of print). Anger, stress proliferation, and depressed mood among parents of children with ASD: A longitudinal replication. *Journal of Autism and Developmental Disorders.*

Bitsika, V., & Sharpley, C. (2000). Development and testing of the effects of support groups on the well-being of parents of children with autism-II: Specific stress management techniques. *Journal of Applied Health Behaviour, 2*, 8–15.

Blacher, J., & McIntyre, L. L. (2006). Syndrome specificity and behavioral disorders in young adults with intellectual disability: Cultural differences in family impact. *Journal of Intellectual Disability Research, 50*(Pt 3), 184–198.

Blackledge, J. T., & Hayes, S. C. (2006). Using acceptance and commitment training in the support of parents of children diagnosed with ASD. *Child and Family Behavior Therapy, 28*(1), 1–18.

Bristol, M., Gallagher, J., & Holt, K. (1993). Maternal depressive symptoms in ASD: Response to psychoeducational intervention. *Rehabilitation Psychology, 38*(1), 3–10.

Bromley, J., Hare, D. J., Davison, K., & Emerson, E. (2004). Mothers supporting children with autistic spectrum disorders. *Autism, 8*(4), 409–423.

Brookman-Frazee, L. (2004). Using parent/clinician partnerships in parent education programs for children with autism. *Journal of Positive Behavior Interventions, 6*(4), 195–213.

Carver, C. S., Scheier, M. F., & Weintraub, J. K. (1989). Assessing coping strategies: A theoretically based approach. *Journal of Personality and Social Psychology, 56*(2), 267–283.

Coyne, J., & Downey, G. (1991). Social factors and psychopathology: Stress, social support, and coping processes. *Annual Review of Psychology, 42*, 410–425.

Crnic, K. A., & Greenberg, M. T. (1990). Minor parenting stresses with young children. *Child Development, 61*(5), 1628–1637.

Crnic, K. A., Greenberg, M. T., & Slough, N. M. (1986). Early stress and social support influences on mothers' and high-risk infants' functioning in late infancy. *Infant Mental Health Journal, 7*(1), 19–33.

Cummings, E. M., Davies, P. T., & Simpson, K. S. (1994). Marital conflict, gender, and children's appraisals and coming efficacy as mediators of child adjustment. *Journal of Family Psychology, 8*, 141–149.

Davis, N. O., & Carter, A. S. (2008). Parenting stress in mothers and father of toddlers with autism spectrum disorders: Associations with child characteristics. *Journal of Autism and Developmental Disorders, 38*(7), 1278–1291.

DeMeyer, N. (1979). *Parents and children in autism.* Washington, DC: Wiley.

Derogatis, L. R. (1994). *Symptom Checklist-90-R: Administrative scoring and procedures manual.* Minneapolis, MN: NCS Pearson.

Derogatis, L. R., & Melisaratos, N. (1983). The brief symptom inventory: An introductory report. *Psychological Medicine, 13*(3), 595–605.

Donenberg, G., & Baker, B. L. (1993). The impact of young children with externalizing behaviors on their families. *Journal of Abnormal Child Psychology, (21)*, 179–198.

Donovan, A. M. (1988). Family stress and ways of coping with adolescents who have handicaps: Maternal perceptions. *American Journal of Mental Retardation, 92*(6), 502–509.

Dumas, J. E., Wolf, L. C., Fisman, S. N., & Culligan, A. (1991). Parenting stress, child behavior problems, and dysphoria in parents of children with ASD, Down syndrome, behavior disorders, and normal development. *Exceptionality, 2*(2), 97–110.

Dunn, M. E., Burbine, T., Bowers, C. A., & Tantleff-Dunn, S. (2001). Moderators of stress in parents of children with autism. *Community Mental Health Journal, 37*(1), 39–52.

Dunst, C., Jenkins, V., & Trivette, C. (1984). The family support scale: Reliability and validity. *Journal of Individual Family Common Wellness, 1*, 45–52.

Estes, A., Munson, J., Dawson, G. Koehler, E., Zhou, X. H., & Abbott, R. (2009). Parenting stress and psychological functioning among mothers of preschool children with autism and developmental delay. *Autism, 13*(4), 375–387.

Eisenhower, A. S., Baker, B. L., & Blacher, J. (2005). Preschool children with intellectual disability: Syndrome specificity, behavior problems, and maternal well-being. *Journal of Intellectual Disability Research, 49*(Pt 9), 657–671.

Fisman, S., Wolf, L., & Noh, S. (1989). Marital intimacy in parents of exceptional children. *Canadian Journal of Psychiatry, 34*, 519–525.

Fitzgerald, M., Birkbeck, G., & Matthews, P. (2002). Maternal burden in families with children with autistic spectrum disorder. *Irish Journal of Psychology, 33*(1–2), 17.

Friedrich, W. N., Greenberg, M. T., & Crnic, K. (1983). A short form of the questionnaire on resources and stress. *American Journal of Mental Deficiency, 88*, 41–48.

Gallagher, J. J., & Bristol, M. (1989). Families of young handicapped children. In M. C. R. M. C. Wang, & H. J. Walberg (Ed.), *Handbook of special education: Research and practice: Vol. 3* (3rd ed., pp. 295–317). New York: Pergamon.

Gray, D. E., & Holden, W. J. (1994). Psycho-social well-being among the parents of children with autism. *Australian and New Zealand Journal of Developmental Disabilities, 18*(2), 83–93.

Green G., (1996). Early behavioral intervention for autism: What does research tell us? In C. Maurice, G., Green, G., et al. (Eds.); *Behavioral intervention for young children with autism: A manual.* Austin, TX: Pro-Ed.

Greenberg, J. S., Seltzer, M., Krauss, M., Chou, R. J., & Hong, J. (2004). The effect of quality of the relationship between mothers and adult children with schizophrenia, ASD, or Down syndrome on maternal well-being: The mediating role of optimism. *American Journal of Orthopsychiatry, 74*(1), 14–25.

Grych, J. H., & Fincham, F. D. (1990). Marital Conflict and Children's Adjustment: A Cognitive-Contextual Framework. *Psychological Bulletin, 108*(2), 267–290.

Guralnick, M. J. (1998). The effectiveness of early intervention for vulnerable children: A developmental perspective. *American Journal of Mental Retardation, 102*, 319–345.

Guralnick, M. J. (2005). An overview of the developmental systems model for early intervention. In Guralnick M. J. (Ed.), *The developmental systems approach to early intervention* (pp. 3–28). Baltimore: Brookes.

Hamlyn-Wright, S., Draghi-Lorenz, R., & Ellis, J. (2007). Locus of control fails to mediate between stress and anxiety and depression in parents of children with a developmental disorder. *Autism, 11*(6), 489.

Hastings, R. P. (2002). Parental stress and behavior problems of children with developmental disability. *Journal of Intellectual and Developmental Disability, 27*(3), 149–160.

Hastings, R. P. (2003). Child behaviour problems and partner mental health as correlates of stress in mothers and fathers of children with ASD. *Journal of Intellectual Disability Research, 47* (4/5), 231.

Hastings, R. P., & Beck, A. (2004). Practitioner review: Stress intervention for parents of children with intellectual disabilities. *Journal of Child Psychology and Psychiatry, 45*(8), 1338–1349.

Hastings, R. P., & Brown, T. (2002). Behavior problems of children with ASD, parental self-efficacy, and mental health. *American Journal of Mental Retardation, 107*(3), 222–232.

Hastings, R. P., & Johnson, E. (2001). Stress in UK families conducting intensive home-based behavioral intervention for their young child with autism. *Journal of Autism and Developmental Disorders, 31*(3), 327–336.

Hastings, R. P., Kovshoff, H., War, N. J., Espinosa, F. D., Brown, T., & Remington, B. (2005). Systems analysis of stress and positive perceptions in mothers and fathers of pre-school children with autism. *Journal of Autism and Developmental Disorders, 35*(5), 635.

Hauser-Cram, P., Warfield, M. E., Shonkoff, J. P., Krauss, M. W., Sayer, A., & Upshur, C. C. (2001). Children with disabilities: A longitudinal study of child development and parent well-being. *Monographs of the Society for Research in Child Development, 66*(3), serial 266.

Herring, S., Gray, K., Taffe, J., Tonge, B., Sweeney, D., & Einfeld, S. (2006). Behaviour and emotional problems in toddlers with pervasive developmental disorders and developmental delay: Associations with parental mental health and family functioning. *Journal of Intellectual Disability Research, 50*(12), 874–882.

Higgins, D. J., Bailey, S. R., & Pearce, J. C. (2005). Factors associated with functioning style and coping strategies of families with a child with an ASD spectrum disorder. *Autism, 9*(2), 125–137.

Hodapp, R. M., Ricci, L. A., Ly, T. M., & Fidler, D. J. (2003). The effects of the child with Down syndrome on maternal stress. *British Journal of Developmental Psychology, 21*, 137–151.

Holroyd, J. (1974). The questionnaire on resources and stress: An instrument to measure family response to a handicapped family member. *Journal of Community Psychology, 2*, 92–94.

Honey, E., Hastings, R. P., & McConachie, H. (2005). Use of questionnaire on resources and stress (QRS-F) with parents of young children with ASD. *Autism, 9*(3), 246–254.

Jenkins, J. M., & Smith, M. A. (1991). Marital disharmony and children's behaviour problems: Aspects of a poor marriage that affect children adversely. *Journal of Child Psychology and Psychiatry, 32*, 793–810.

Johnston, C., Hessl, D., Blasey, C., Eliez, S., Erba, H., Dyer-Friedman, J., et al. (2003). Factors associated with parenting stress in mothers of children with fragile x syndrome. *Journal of Developmental and Behavioral Pediatrics, 24*(4), 267–275.

Koegel, R. L., Koegel, L. K., & Schreibman, L. (1991). Assessing and training parents in teaching pivotal behaviors. In R. J. Prinz (Ed.), *Advances in behavioral assessment of children and families: A research annual*, Vol. 5 (pp. 65–82). Bristol, PA: Jessica Kingsley.

Koegel, R. L., Schreibman, L., Good, A., Cerniglia, L., Murphy, C., & Koegel, L. K. (1989). *How to teach pivotal behaviors to children with autism: A training manual.* Santa Barbara: University of California.

Konstantareas, M. M., & Homatidis, S. (1989). Assessing child symptom severity and stress in parents of autistic children. *Journal of Child Psychology and Psychiatry, 30*(3), 459–470.

Kuhn, Jennifer C. MA, & Carter, Alice S. PhD. (2006). Maternal self-efficacy and associated parenting cognitions Among mothers of children with ASD. *American Journal of Orthopsychiatry, 76*(4), 564–575.

Lecavalier, L., Leone, S., & Wiltz, J. (2006). The impact of behavior problems on caregiver stress in young people with ASD spectrum disorders. *Journal of Intellectual Disability Research, 50*(Pt 3), 172–183.

Lloyd, T., & Hastings, R. P. (2008). Psychological variables as correlates of adjustment in mothers of children with intellectual disabilities: Cross-sectional and longitudinal relationships. *Journal of Intellectual Disability Research, 52*(1), 37–48.

Locke, H. J. & Wallace, K. M. (1959). Short marital-adjustment and prediction tests: Their reliability and validity. *Marriage and Family Living, 21*, 251–255.

Lounds, J., Seltzer, M. M., Greenberg, J. S., & Shattuk, P. T. (2007). Transition and change in adolescents and young adults with ASD: Longitudinal effects on maternal well-being. *American Journal of Mental Retardation, 112*(6), 401–417.

Luther, E. H., Canham, D. L., & Cureton, V. Y. (2005). Coping and social support for parents of children with autism. *The Journal of School Nursing, 21*(1), 40–47.

Mackintosh, V. H., Myers, B. J., & Goin-Kochel, R. P. (2006). Sources of information and support used by parents of children with autism spectrum disorders. *Journal of Developmental Disabilities, 12*(1), 41–52.

Mak, W. S., Ho, Anna H. Y., & Law, R. W. (2007). Sense of coherence, parenting attitudes and stress among mothers of children with ASD in Hong Kong. *Journal of Applied Research in Intellectual Abilities, (20)*, 157–167.

McConachie H. & Waring M. (1997). *Child psychology portfolio: parental coping and support.* Windsor, UK: NFER-Nelson.

McCubbin, H., Olson, D. & Larsen, A. (1991). F-COPES: Family crisis oriented person evaluation scales. In H. McCubbing & A. Thompson (Eds.), *Family assessment inventories for research and practice* (p. 203). Madison, Wisconsin: University of Wisconsin.

Moes, D., Koegel, R. L., Schreibman, L., & Loos, L. M. (1992). Stress profiles for mothers and fathers of children with autism. *Psychological Reports, 71*(3), 1272–1274.

Olson, D. H., Portner, J., & Bell, R. (1982). Family adaptability and cohesion evaluation scales. In Olson, D. H. et al (Ed.), *Family inventories: Inventories used in a national survey of families across the family life cycle* (pp. 5–24). St. Paul: Family Social Science.

Olsson, M. B., & Hwang, C. P. (2001). Depression in mothers and fathers of children with intellectual disability. *Journal of Intellectual Disability Research, 45*(Pt 6), 535–543.

Olsson, M. B. & Hwang, C. P. (2002). Sense of coherence in parents of children with different developmental disabilities. *Journal of Intellectual Disability Research, 46*(7), 548–559.

Orsmond, G. I., Lin, L., & Seltzer, M. M. (2007). Mother of adolescents and adults with ASD: Parenting multiple children with disabilities. *Intellectual and Developmental Disabilities, 45*(4), 257–270.

Osborne, L. A., McHugh, L., Saunders, J., & Reed, P. (2007). Parenting stress reduces the effectiveness of early teaching interventions for autistic spectrum disorders. *Journal of Autism and Developmental Disorders, 38*(6), 1092–1103.

Plant, K. M., & Sanders, M. R. (2007). Predictors of care-giver stress in families of preschool-aged children with developmental disabilities. *Journal of Intellectual Disability Research, 51*(2), 109–124.

Radloff, L. S. (1977). The CES-D scale: A self-report depression scale for research in the general population. *Applied Psychological Measurement, 1*, 385–401.

Rodrigue, J. R., Morgan, S. B., & Geffken, G. R. (1990). Families of autistic children: Psychological functioning of mothers. *Journal of Clinical Child Psychology, 19*(4), 371–379.

Rodrigue, J. R., Morgan, S. B., & Geffken, G. R. (1992). Psychosocial adaptation of fathers of children with autism, down syndrome, and normal development. *Journal of Autism and Developmental Disorders, 22*(2), 249–263.

Rutgers, A. H., van IJzendoorn, M. H., Bakermans-Kranenburg, M. J., Siwnkels, S. H. N., van Daalen, E., Dietz, C., et al. (2007). Autism, attachment and parenting: A comparison of children with ASD spectrum disorder, mental retardation, language disorder, and non-clinical children. *Journal of Abnormal Child Psychology, 35*, 859–870.

Ryff, C. D. (1989). Happiness is everything, or is it? Explorations on the meaning of psychological well-being. *Journal of Personality and Social Psychology, 57*(6), 1069–1081.

Salt, J., Shemilt, J., Sellars, V., Boyd, S., Coulson, T., & McCool, S. (2002). The Scottish centre for autism preschool treatment programme: II: The results of a controlled treatment outcome study. *Autism, 6*(33), 33–46.

Sarason, I., Johnson, J., & Siegal, J. (1978). Assessing the impact of life changes: Development of the live experiences survey. *Journal of Consulting and Clinical Psychology, 46*, 932–946.

Sarason, I. G., Levine, H. M., Basham, R. B., & Sarason, B. R. (1983). Assessing social support: the social support questionnaire. *Journal of Personality and Social Psychology, 44*, 127–139.

Scheier, M. F., & Carver, C. S. (1992). Effects of optimism on psychological and physical well-being: Theoretical overview and empirical update. *Cognitive Therapy and Research, 16*, 201–228.

Schmutte, P. S., & Ryff, C. D. (1997). Personality and well-being: reexamining methods and meanings. *Journal of Personality and Social Psychology, 3*, 549–559.

Schwichtenberg, A., & Poehlmann, J. (2007). Applied behaviour analysis: does intervention intensity relate to family stressors and maternal well-being? *Journal of Intellectual Disability Research, 51*(8), 598–605.

Siklos, S., & Kerns, K. A. (2006). Assessing need for social support in parents of children with autism and down syndrome. *Journal of Autism and Developmental Disorders, 36*, 921–933.

Smith, L. E., Mailick Seltzer, M., Tager-Flusberg, H., Greenberg, J. S., & Carter, A. S. (2008). A comparative analysis of well-being and coping among mothers of toddlers and mothers of adolescents with ASD. *Journal of Autism and Developmental Disorders, 38*, 876–889.

Spanier, G. B. (1976). Measuring dyadic adjustment: New scales for assessing the quality of marriage and similar dyads. *Journal of Marriage and the Family, 38*(1), 15–25.

Stoneman, Z., & Payne, S. (2006). Marital adjustment in families of young children with disabilities: Associations with daily hassles and problem-focused coping. *American Journal of Mental Retardation, 111*(1), 1–14.

Tomanik, S., Harris, G. E., & Hawkins, J. (2004). The relationship between behaviors exhibited by children with ASD and maternal stress. *Journal of Intellectual and Developmental Disability, 29*, 16–26.

Tonge, B., Brereton, A., Kiomall, M., Mackinnon, A., King, N., & Rinehart, N. (2006). Effects on parental mental health of an education and skills training program for parents of young children with ASD: A randomized controlled trial. *Journal of the American Academy of Child and Adolescent Psychiatry, 45*(4), 561–569.

Toth, K., Dawson, G., Meltzoff, A.N., Greenson, J., & Fein, D. (2007). Early social, imitation, play, and language abilities of young non-autistic siblings of children with autism. *Journal of Autism and Developmental Disorders*, *37*(1), 145–157.

Vismara, L., Columbi, C., & Rogers, S. L. (2009). Can one hour per week of therapy lead to lasting changes in young children with autism? *Autism*, *13*, 93–115.

Webster-Stratton, C. (1990). Stress: A potential disruptor of parent perceptions and family interactions. *Journal of Clinical Child Psychology*, *19*(4), 302–312.

Weiss, M. J. (2002). Hardiness and social support as predictors of stress in mothers of typical children, children with autism, and children with mental retardation. *Autism*, *6*, 115–130.

White, N., & Hastings, R. P. (2004). Social and professional support for parents of adolescents with severe intellectual disabilities. *Journal of Applied Research in Intellectual Disabilities*, *17*(3), 181–190.

Zigmond, A. S., & Snaith, R. P. (1983). The hospital anxiety and depression scale. *Acta Psychiatrica Scandinavia*, *67*, 631–370.

69

Kelly Blankenship, Craig A. Erickson, Kimberly A. Stigler, David J. Posey, Christopher J. McDougle

Psychopharmacological Treatment of Autism

Points of Interest

- Psychostimulants, such as methylphenidate, are less efficacious and cause more adverse events in children with pervasive developmental disorders (PDDs) than in typically developing children with attention deficit hyperactivity disorder.
- The most efficacious class of drugs for the treatment of aggression and irritability in autism and other PDDs is the antipsychotics.
- Based on results from double-blind, placebo-controlled trials, selective serotonin reuptake inhibitors (SSRIs) appear to be more efficacious for improving interfering repetitive behavior and better tolerated in adults compared with children with autism.
- To date, double-blind, placebo-controlled studies have not identified a drug with consistent beneficial effects on the social or communication impairments of autism.

As awareness of autistic disorder (autism) and other pervasive developmental disorders (PDDs) increases, so does research regarding these conditions. The interfering symptoms of these disorders have been recognized for years. More recently, research regarding the treatment of target symptoms associated with PDDs has accelerated. These symptoms include hyperactivity and inattention, irritability and aggression, interfering repetitive behaviors, and social impairment, among others. This chapter focuses on the pharmacologic treatment of these symptom clusters that are commonly disabling in this population. At this time, risperidone and aripiprazole are the only U.S. Food and Drug Administration (FDA) approved pharmacologic agents to treat symptoms associated with autism. There are no other medications that have received FDA approval to treat any of the disabling symptoms of autism or other PDDs. However, in clinical practice, many different drugs are being prescribed to minimize some of the interfering symptoms of PDDs. A priority is placed on discussing randomized, placebo-controlled trials when available, as well as side effects associated with these medications in this diagnostic group. Symptom areas for which controlled trials of medications have not been published, such as mood, anxiety, and sleep difficulties, will not be discussed in this chapter. Also, medications that have been found to be relatively ineffective (e.g., naltrexone and secretin) will not be reviewed in detail.

The "gold standard" design of a drug treatment study includes blinded conditions and placebo control. Random assignment to drug or placebo is critical and a parallel groups approach, rather than crossover approach, can minimize carryover effects. The duration of the trial will be influenced by the time to reach steady state with the particular drug. The choice of the minimum and maximum amount of drug to be administered is also important. The goal is to strike a balance between minimizing potential adverse effects and not missing potential symptom improvement resulting from too low a dose. A particular type or group of symptoms needs to be targeted and a threshold for symptom severity needs to be set. This will allow for the inclusion of a more homogeneous subject sample; age range and diagnostic subtype are also important in this regard. An open-label extension treatment phase is often needed. This allows for a determination of maintenance of response of the drug, as well as an assessment for longer-term adverse events. A blinded discontinuation phase can provide information related to necessary duration of treatment with the drug.

The current optimal approach to measuring symptom change in autism and other PDDs in drug treatment trials includes a variety of parent- and clinician-rated scales. The Aberrant Behavior Checklist (ABC) Irritability and Hyperactivity subscales are parent-rated scales that have been shown to be sensitive to drug treatment effects on symptoms of aggression/self-injury/tantrums and hyperactivity/noncompliance, respectively. The Children's Yale-Brown Obsessive Compulsive Scale for Pervasive Developmental Disorders

(CY-BOCS-PDD) is a clinician-administered scale used to measure change in interfering repetitive behavior. The ADHD Rating Scale is also a clinician-administered scale included because it better reflects inattentiveness and disorganization, which is particularly important in persons with higher-functioning PDDs. Although there are no ideal measures to monitor change in social impairment in autism, the Social Responsiveness Scale is promising, especially given that it only takes parents 20 minutes to complete. The Clinician Global Impression global improvement item score (CGI-I) is based on careful examination of all areas of possible improvement.

Hyperactivity and Inattention

Hyperactivity and inattention are symptoms many individuals with PDDs exhibit. Studies have estimated that as many as 40% to 59% of children diagnosed with PDDs also meet criteria for attention deficit hyperactivity disorder (ADHD) (Gadow, DeVincent, & Pomeroy, 2006; Goldstein & Schwebach, 2004). Interestingly, even with such a high prevalence of diagnosable ADHD within this population, the DSM-IV-TR includes PDD as one of its exclusionary criteria when making an ADHD diagnosis (American Psychiatric Association [APA], 2000).

> Controversy exists as to whether or not ADHD should be an allowable comorbid diagnosis with the PDDs.

Table 69-1 includes published placebo-controlled studies of drugs for motor hyperactivity and inattention in PDDs.

Psychostimulants

For typical children with ADHD, methylphenidate (MPH) and other stimulants are the psychopharmacologic treatments of choice (Greenhill et al., 2002). Response rates to MPH of 70% to 80% have been demonstrated in this population (Greenhill et al., 2001). The data regarding the use of stimulant medication to treat children with PDDs and ADHD symptoms is not as conclusive. Reviews of early studies indicate that children with mental retardation and autism do not respond well to stimulants. There is also a possible increase in stereotypy in this population with stimulant use (Aman, 1982). However, the more recent literature on this topic has come to different conclusions. Quintana et al. (1995) performed a study with 10 DSM-III diagnosed autistic children from the age of 7 to 11 years. The children were given two different MPH doses (10 or 20 mg bid twice a day) in a double-blind crossover study with placebo. Hyperactivity declined a modest but statistically significant degree with MPH. Side effects included irritability, headache, stomachache, lack of appetite, weight loss, and insomnia. Another study was performed with 13 autistic children with ADHD symptoms ages 5.6 to 11.2 years (Handen, Johnson, & Lubetsky, 2000). This was a double-blind, placebo-controlled trial of MPH dosed at 0.3 to 0.6 mg/kg body weight per day. Sixty-two percent of the treated children had a 50% or greater decrease on the Teacher Conners Hyperactivity Index. Improvements in stereotypies and inappropriate speech were also reported. Side effects included depression, irritability, decreased appetite, and drowsiness.

Stigler et al. (2004) performed a retrospective chart review within their clinic on all patients with PDDs treated with a

Table 69–1.
Published placebo-controlled studies of drugs for motor hyperactivity and inattention

Study	Drug	Subjects	Design	Results
Quintana et al., 1995	Methylphenidate	$n = 10$ Age = 7–11	2 weeks Crossover	Methylphenidate > PLA
Handen et al., 2000	Methylphenidate	$n = 13$ Age = 5–11	1 week Crossover	Methylphenidate > PLA 8/13 (62%) responders
RUPP Autism Network, 2005a	Methylphenidate	$n = 72$ Age = 5–14	1 week Crossover	Methylphenidate > PLA
Arnold et al., 2006	Atomoxetine	$n = 16$ Age = 5–15	6 weeks Crossover	Atomoxetine > PLA
Jaselskis et al., 1992	Clonidine	$n = 8$ Age = 5–13	6 weeks Crossover	Clonidine > PLA by teacher and parent, but not clinician 6/8 (75%) responders 2/8 (25%) responders at 1-year follow-up
Fankhauser et al., 1992	Clonidine (transdermal)	$n = 9$ Age = 5–33	4 weeks Crossover	Clonidine > PLA 6/9 (67%) responders

Note: All ages are in years. PLA = placebo. Each study included subjects with autism. RUPP Autism Network, 2005a and Arnold et al., 2006 included subjects with autism and other pervasive developmental disorders.

stimulant. Charts of 195 patients ages 2 to 19 years were reviewed. Sixty-one of the patients had more than one stimulant trial resulting in the analysis of 274 independent stimulant trials. The results indicated that 24.6%, 23.2%, and 11.1% of individuals with a history of one, two, or three stimulant trials, respectively, responded to their first stimulant trial. Patients with autism and PDD not otherwise specified (PDD-NOS) were less likely to respond to stimulants than those with Asperger's Syndrome. However, there was not a link between response and IQ of the patient. Side effects included irritability, dysphoria, weight loss, and agitation. Agitation was seen less often in those with Asperger's Syndrome. The investigators concluded that stimulants were ineffective and not tolerated well in most individuals with PDDs. However, the subtype of PDD may affect the response to stimulants.

The largest randomized, placebo-controlled trial with MPH in children with PDDs to date was funded by the National Institute of Mental Health (NIMH) and performed by the Research Units on Pediatric Psychopharmacology Autism Network (RUPP) (RUPP Autism Network, 2005a). The study included 5 sites throughout the United States. Seventy-two children (ages 5–14 years) with a DSM-IV diagnosis of autism, Asperger's Syndrome, or PDD-NOS and moderate-to-severe hyperactivity entered the study. Before the study began, the children were given test doses of the medication. One day of placebo and 2 days each of ascending low, medium, and high MPH doses were given. Sixty-six children remained in the study following the test dose phase and were able to be randomized to the crossover phase. The children were given placebo and the three doses of MPH, each for 1 week, in a randomized order. The patients that demonstrated a positive response to MPH entered a second phase of the trial. They were given 8 weeks of MPH (open-label) at the determined best dose. Forty-nine percent of the 72 initially enrolled subjects were deemed to be responders. Side effects resulted in 18% (13 of 72) of the subjects discontinuing MPH. Side effects seen more frequently with MPH than with placebo included irritability, decreased appetite, insomnia, and emotional lability. MPH led to lower response rates in autism than in children with Asperger's Syndrome or PDD-NOS. In this study, IQ, age, and weight were not found to be predictive of response. An analysis of the secondary measures of this study led to the conclusion that the medium and high doses were most efficacious, MPH decreased hyperactivity slightly more than inattention symptoms, and worsening of repetitive behavior was not common (Posey et al., 2007a).

The Multimodal Treatment Study of typical Children with ADHD (the MTA study) found that 69% (or 198) of the 289 participants who received MPH were classified as responders. The rate of side effects causing study discontinuation was 1.4% (or 4 of 289 participants) (Greenhill et al., 2001).

The data from the RUPP Autism Network study above combined with those from the MTA study lead to the conclusion that compared with typical developing children, children with PDD are less likely to respond and more likely to have side effects associated with MPH (RUPP Autism Network, 2005a).

Atomoxetine

Atomoxetine is a reuptake inhibitor that is selective for norepinephrine. It is also believed to exert an effect on dopamine in the frontal lobes (Stein, 2004). Atomoxetine is approved by the FDA for the treatment of ADHD. It has been found to be efficacious in treating ADHD symptoms in typically developing children, adolescents, and adults (Pliszka, 2007). There have been several studies performed to determine whether these findings can be extrapolated to individuals with PDDs. Posey et al. (2006) performed an open-label study of 16 children with PDD and ADHD symptoms. The children were given atomoxetine at an average dose of 1.2 mg per kg per day. Twelve of the 16 children (75%) were deemed to be responders. In addition to ADHD symptoms, there was also a more modest improvement in irritability, repetitive speech, social withdrawal, and stereotypy. Two of the 13 children (15%) discontinued the study early because of irritability.

A retrospective study at an outpatient registry identified 20 children with PDD who were placed on atomoxetine for 12 months (Jou, Handen, & Hardan, 2005). Most of these children were also taking at least one other medication. Twelve of the 20 (60%) children were deemed to respond to atomoxetine in the areas of hyperactivity, conduct, learning, and inattention. One patient stopped the medication because of mood swings.

Arnold et al. (2006) performed a double-blind, placebo-controlled, crossover study of atomoxetine in children with PDDs and symptoms of ADHD. Sixteen children were randomized to receive atomoxetine or placebo for 6 weeks. There was a 3-week titration phase, an additional 3 weeks of medication at the titrated dose, a 1-week wash-out period, and then a second treatment phase of atomoxetine or placebo (whichever the patient did not receive in the first phase). Fifty-seven percent of patients were judged to be responders. Three of the 16 stopped the study early—1 because of intolerable side effects and 2 because of efficacy while on placebo. Side effects in this study included appetite suppression and irritability. The authors concluded that similarly to MPH, atomoxetine has a smaller response rate in children with PDDs than in typically developing children. A 10-week, open-label study by Troost et al. (2006) with atomoxetine in 12 children with PDD found a higher rate of intolerable side effects. Five of the 12 children (42%) discontinued because of adverse effects. Sleep problems, fatigue, gastrointestinal symptoms, and irritability were the most common side effects in this study.

Alpha$_2$ Adrenergic Agonists

Clonidine and guanfacine are both central alpha$_2$ agonists that are often prescribed off-label to treat patients with ADHD (Pliszka, 2007). They are thought to work by agonism at the alpha$_2$ adrenergic receptors in the prefrontal cortex of the brain. One of the potential causes of ADHD is dysfunction in this region of the brain (Posey & McDougle, 2007). Studies have been performed to attempt to extrapolate these data to individuals with PDD.

Clonidine and guanfacine are also used to treat high blood pressure.

Clonidine

Two double-blind, placebo-controlled crossover studies have been performed with clonidine in children with PDD. The first involved eight male children with a diagnosis of autism and ADHD symptoms (Jaselskis et al., 1992). These were all children who had not been able to tolerate treatment with neuroleptics, MPH or desipramine. Improvement was found with some of the rating scales used, including the teacher ratings on the ABC and the Parent Conner's scale. Six of the eight children continued treatment after completion of the study. The authors concluded that clonidine was modestly effective for short-term treatment of hyperactivity and mood swings in some autistic children.

A second double-blind, placebo-controlled crossover study was performed with nine autistic males (ages 5–33 years) using transdermal clonidine (Fankhauser et al., 1992). Each individual was either given placebo or a weekly clonidine patch of 0.005 mg per kg per day for 4 weeks. This was followed by a 2-week wash-out period between the two treatment phases. During treatment with clonidine, there was a significant improvement on three (sensory responses, affectual reactions, and social relationships to people) of the five subscales of the Ritvo-Freeman Real Life Rating Scale and on the CGI scale. Sedation and fatigue were seen during the first 2 weeks of treatment.

Guanfacine

There are two published trials with guanfacine in children with PDDs. The first is a retrospective review of 80 children (ages 3–18 years) diagnosed with PDD and treated with guanfacine (Posey et al., 2004). Most children were dosed two to three times daily and were taking one or more other psychotropic medications. The mean dose was 2.6 mg per day. Nineteen of the 80 individuals (24%) were judged to be responders. Three of 6 children had a decrease in tics, 14 of 51 (27%) had an improvement in insomnia, hyperactivity improved in 20 of 75 (27%), and inattention improved in 16 of 76 (21%). Those who responded to treatment were less likely to have been treated with stimulants in the past, less likely to have been tried on multiple other psychotropics, and less aggressive at baseline. Side effects included transient sedation, irritability, constipation, headache, and nocturnal enuresis. No significant change in blood pressure or heart rate was noted. Individuals with PDD-NOS (39.3%) and Asperger's Syndrome (33.3%) were more likely to respond than those with autism (13%).

The second published study was an 8-week, open-label prospective study of guanfacine in 25 children (ages 5–14 years) with PDD and ADHD symptoms who had not responded to or were unable to tolerate MPH (Scahill et al., 2006). Children weighing less than 25 kg started at 0.25 mg at bedtime and were increased to twice the starting dose on day four. Doses were then increased by 0.25 mg every fourth day as tolerated. The maximum dose for this group was 3.5 mg divided three times a day. Children weighing more than 25 kg were given 0.5 mg at bedtime and were increased in 0.5-mg increments. Their maximum dose was 5.0 mg divided in three daily doses. Twelve of the 25 children (48%) were deemed to be responders. In doses ranging from 1 to 3 mg per day there were no serious adverse events and the drug was well-tolerated. Common side effects included sedation, irritability, sleep disturbance, decreased appetite, aggression, agitation, and perceptual disturbance. Three subjects stopped the study early because of irritability.

Irritability and Aggression

Irritability is a common symptom seen in individuals with PDDs (Stigler & McDougle, 2008). Studies have shown that approximately 30% of children and adolescents with PDDs suffer from moderate-to-severe irritability (Lecavalier, 2006). Frequently, the irritability can manifest as aggressive acts toward self or others. When directed toward self (i.e., self-injurious behavior [SIB], such as head banging), serious injury, including retinal detachment or subdural hematoma, can occur (McDougle et al., 2008). The most effective drugs used to treat these symptoms are antipsychotics (both typical and atypical). Clinicians also use mood stabilizers for this purpose. However, their use in this population has not been validated with controlled studies (McDougle et al., 2006). Table 69-2 includes published, placebo-controlled studies of drugs for irritability and aggression in PDDs.

Typical Antipsychotics

Initially, several studies were published using typical antipsychotics to treat children diagnosed as "schizophrenic," "disturbed," and some with "autistic features." Typical antipsychotics studied included chlorpromazine, trifluoperazine, thiothixene, trifluperidol, fluphenazine, and molindone. However, the diagnoses were unclear and the outcome measurements were not standardized, making the generalization of these findings difficult (Posey et al., 2007b).

Haloperidol

The high-potency antipsychotic haloperidol is associated with less cognitive effects and sedation than the lower-potency typical

Table 69–2.
Published placebo-controlled studies of antipsychotics for irritability and aggression

Study	Drug	Subjects	Design	Results
Campbell et al., 1978	Haloperidol	$n = 40$ Age = 2–7 Dx = AUT	10 weeks Parallel groups	Haloperidol > PLA
Cohen et al., 1980	Haloperidol	$n = 10$ Age = 2–7 Dx = AUT	2 weeks Crossover	Haloperidol > PLA
Anderson et al., 1984	Haloperidol	$n = 40$ Age = 2–7 Dx = AUT	4 weeks Crossover	Haloperidol > PLA
Anderson et al., 1989	Haloperidol	$n = 45$ Age = 2–7 Dx = AUT	4 weeks Crossover	Haloperidol > PLA
Naruse et al., 1982	Pimozide Haloperidol	$n = 87$ Age = 3–16 Dx = AUT, PDD	8 weeks Crossover	Pimozide > PLA Haloperidol > PLA Pimozide = Haloperidol
McDougle et al., 1998	Risperidone	$n = 31$ Age = 18–43 Dx = AUT, PDD	12 weeks Parallel groups	Risperidone > PLA 8/14 (57%) Responders
RUPP Autism Network, 2002	Risperidone	$n = 101$ Age = 5–17 Dx = AUT	8 weeks Parallel groups	Risperidone > PLA 34/49 (69%) responders
Shea et al., 2004	Risperidone	$n = 79$ Age = 5–12 Dx = AUT, PDD	8 weeks Parallel groups	Risperidone (64%) > PLA (31%) improvement on ABC-I
Marcus et al., 2009	Aripiprazole	$n = 218$ Age = 6–17 Dx = AUT	8 weeks Parallel groups	Aripiprazole > PLA on ABC-I

Note: All ages are in years. Dx = diagnosis. AUT = autistic disorder. PDD = pervasive developmental disorder not otherwise specified. PLA = placebo. RUPP = Research Units on Pediatric Psychopharmacology. ABC-I = Aberrant Behavior Checklist Irritability subscale.

antipsychotics. It is the most extensively studied of the typical antipsychotics for treating symptoms associated with autism.

The first to perform placebo-controlled studies of haloperidol in autistic children was Magda Campbell. An initial study published in 1978 (Campbell et al., 1978) had the purpose of evaluating the results of behavior therapy and/or haloperidol on behavioral symptoms and language acquisition. Forty autistic children ages 2.6 to 7.2 years were studied using a range of haloperidol dosing of 0.5 to 4.0 mg per day, with a mean dose of 1.65 mg per day. Haloperidol was superior to placebo and the combination of the two treatments was superior to haloperidol alone in acquiring imitative speech. The older children (older than 4.5 years) had a statistically significant response to haloperidol for the symptoms of withdrawal and stereotypy. In this study, side effects were dose-related sedation in 12 of 20 (60%) and dystonic reactions in 2 of 20 (10%).

After this study was performed, several subsequent studies were done to verify and further elucidate the findings. A small placebo-controlled study with nine autistic children was completed with haloperidol by Cohen et al. (1980). This study also found that children receiving haloperidol had significantly reduced rates of stereotypy and increased abilities to orient to the raters of the study. Anderson et al. (1984) subsequently performed a double-blind, placebo-controlled study with haloperidol in 40 children ages 2.3 to 6.9 years with DSM-III diagnosed autism. The haloperidol group (0.5–3.0 mg/day or 0.02–0.22 mg/kg/day) showed a significant decrease in maladaptive behaviors and a trend toward facilitated discriminatory learning. At the above dose range, no adverse effects were noted. Another double-blind, placebo-controlled crossover study with random assignment to treatment sequences with 45 autistic children ages 2.0 to 7.6 years was performed by Anderson et al. (1989). Haloperidol was given over 4 weeks at a dose of 0.25 to 4.0 mg per day. Haloperidol was associated with a statistically significant reduction of symptoms. However, no difference between haloperidol and placebo was found with regards to discrimination learning. No adverse effects were noted.

A secondary analysis performed on the Campbell et al. (1980) and two Anderson et al. (1984, 1989) studies presented above revealed several predictors of response. Higher IQ was predictive of a greater reduction in behavioral symptoms, older children were more likely to respond to haloperidol, and the greater the initial severity of the illness (placebo or treatment group) the more likely there was to be a greater reduction in symptoms. Finally, reduction in symptoms with short-term haloperidol treatment was not related to whether children developed dyskinesias with long-term treatment (Locascio et al., 1991).

A study was performed to determine the long-term efficacy of haloperidol and the effectiveness of discontinuous versus continuous haloperidol administration in 82 autistic children ages 2.3 to 7.9 years (Perry et al., 1989). Sixty children completed the study with doses ranging from 0.5 to 4.0 mg per day. At the start of the study, the children were divided into two groups. Half the children were given continuous haloperidol administration daily. The other half were given haloperidol for 5 days and then placebo for 2 days in a random order for 6 months. After this phase there was a 4-week placebo withdrawal. Drug efficacy did not differ between the continuous and discontinuous haloperidol administration groups. Haloperidol remained effective throughout the placebo withdrawal. Baseline angry and labile affect, uncooperativeness and irritability were symptoms seen in the children that responded best to haloperidol. Twelve of the 60 children (20%) that completed the study had dyskinesias (3 while receiving haloperidol and 9 during drug withdrawal while given placebo).

A longitudinal study was performed to determine the safety of long-term haloperidol use and the risk for haloperidol-related dyskinesias (Campbell et al., 1997). One hundred and eighteen autistic children ages 2.3 to 8.2 years were given 6 months of haloperidol and then 4 weeks of placebo. This schedule was repeated for the children that continued to need haloperidol treatment. The average dose of haloperidol was 1.75 mg per day. Dyskinesias developed in 40 of the 118 children (34%), with 20 of the children developing more than one dyskinetic episode.

Extrapyramidal symptoms (motor side effects) appear to be more common with typical antipsychotics, such as haloperidol, than the newer atypical antipsychotics.

The first episode was tardive dykinesia in 5 of the 40 children and for the other 35 subjects, the first episode was withdrawal dyskinesia. The authors of this study found that female gender may make autistic children more vulnerable to dyskinesias. It was also noted that there may be an increased risk for dyskinesias in those treated longer or with higher total haloperidol doses. The average total Rochester Research Obstetrical Scale score was also found to be significantly higher in those children who developed dyskinesias (Armenteros et al., 1995). Anesthesia use during delivery was also more common in these children. Thus, pre- and perinatal complications may also cause central nervous system dysfunction that may increase susceptibility to dyskinesias.

Pimozide

A double-blind, placebo-controlled study with haloperidol and pimozide (a typical antipsychotic similar to haloperidol) in 87 children with behavioral disturbance (34 of whom were autistic), ages 3 to 16 years, was conducted over 24 weeks (Naruse et al., 1982). Each medication (haloperidol, pimozide, and placebo) was given for 8 weeks with no wash-out period between medications. The dosing ranged between 1 and 9 mg per day for pimozide and between 0.75 and 6.75 mg per day for haloperidol. Response was measured by the Questionnaire on Behavior in Children for parents and guardians and the Rating Scale for Abnormal Behavior in Children for therapists. These were completed prior to the study and then every 4 weeks. The authors concluded that patients with autism respond to both treatments. Pimozide was superior to placebo in the cluster group "abnormal symptoms," especially in sleep disturbance and excretion disorders. This led to the possibility that pimozide could be helpful in social adjustment. There was no significant difference between haloperidol and placebo when measuring "abnormal symptoms." Adverse events seen with both medications included sleepiness.

Atypical Antipsychotics

As described above, there is a significant risk of dyskinesias when treating autistic children with haloperidol. In the United States, atypical antipsychotics have all but replaced the use of typical antipsychotics to treat behavioral disturbances in autism (Posey et al., 2007b). Atypical antipsychotics antagonize the serotonin receptor, in addition to dopamine receptor blockade, and lead to less extrapyramidal symptoms (EPS). They are also thought to be more effective than typical antipsychotics in treating the negative symptoms of schizophrenia, which in some ways resemble the social withdrawal of autism. Thus, there was the consideration that the atypicals could help with this core symptom domain of autism. To date, this hypothesis has not proved to be true (Posey et al., 2008).

Clozapine

There have only been three case reports of clozapine use in this population. All three were described in letters to the editor. One involved a 32-year-old autistic male who had repeat hospitalizations for harming himself as well as others and destroying property. He had been administered multiple treatments with poor responses and severe EPS. He was prescribed clozapine, and the dose was increased to 300 mg per day. Marked improvement was noted after 2 months, with benefits seen in aggressiveness and social interactions continuing beyond 5 years (Gobbi & Pulvirenti, 2001).

Zuddas et al. (1996) described three autistic children who had been treated with clozapine. Two 8-year-old boys and one 12-year-old girl who had been previously treated with neuroleptics with minimal improvement were given increasing doses of clozapine (200–450 mg/day, modified for clinical response). After 3 months of treatment, all three children showed a marked improvement on the Children's Psychiatric Rating Scale.

A 17-year-old Hispanic male with autism and severe mental retardation with increasing aggression toward staff and patients was given clozapine after being administered typical and atypical neuroleptics, mood stabilizers, selective serotonin reuptake inhibitors (SSRIs), and beta blockers with little success (Chen et al., 2001). The clozapine was increased to 275 mg per day over a 15-day period, during which he became more compliant with staff and began to perform some activities of daily living.

Clozapine is not used often clinically for treating those with PDDs, as it has the potential to cause life-threatening agranulocytosis and requires frequent blood draws to monitor the white blood cell count (McDougle et al., 2008). These venipunctures can be very difficult for cognitively impaired individuals to understand and tolerate. There is also the possibility of a lowered seizure threshold when administering clozapine.

Risperidone

Risperidone is an atypical antipsychotic with dopamine and serotonin receptor antagonism. There have been several double-blind, placebo-controlled studies with risperidone in autistic individuals. In the first of these, 31 adults with PDDs received risperidone or placebo for 12 weeks (McDougle et al., 1998). Those that received placebo were then given a 12-week open-label trial of risperidone. Dosages ranged from 1 to 6 mg every day. At the end of the study, 8 of 14 adults (57%) were deemed to be responders to risperidone, whereas none of the adults in the placebo group responded. Of the subjects that initially received placebo and then the 12 weeks of open-label risperidone, 9 of 15 (60%) were found to respond to risperidone. Reductions in repetitive behavior, aggression, anxiety, depression, and irritability were all noted. No change was observed in social behavior or language. Side effects primarily included transient sedation.

A double-blind, placebo-controlled, multisite study of risperidone in autism was conducted with 101 children, ages 5 to 17 years, over 8 weeks by the RUPP Autism Network (RUPP Autism Network, 2002). Dosing ranged from 0.5 to 3.5 mg per day. The children receiving risperidone attained a 56.9% decrease in irritability on the Irritability subscale of the ABC, whereas the placebo-treated group experienced a 14.1% decrease. Of the children who received risperidone, 34 of 49 (69%) had a positive response compared to 6 of 52 (12%) in the placebo group. A positive response was defined as a 25% or greater decrease in irritability as measured by the Irritability subscale of the ABC and a rating of much improved or very much improved on the CGI-I. In the children who responded to risperidone, two-thirds of those who remained in the study maintained the positive response at 6 months. Side effects at 8 weeks included an average weight gain of 2.7 kg (compared to 0.8 kg in the placebo group), increased appetite, fatigue, drowsiness, dizziness, and drooling. It was also noted that there was improvement in the ABC subscales of Stereotypy and Hyperactivity. There was no significant difference between the drug and placebo groups for the subscales of Social Withdrawal and Inappropriate Speech.

Another 8-week double-blind, placebo-controlled trial of risperidone was conducted in Canada with 79 children with PDDs, ages 5 to 12 years (Shea et al., 2004). The dosing of risperidone was 0.01 to 0.06 mg per kg per day with a mean dose of 0.04 mg per kg per day (1.17 mg/day). At the end of 8 weeks, irritability as measured by the ABC Irritability subscale improved by 64% in the risperidone-treated group compared with 31% in the placebo group. Sixty-two percent of the children treated with risperidone showed statistically significant decreases in hyperactivity as measured by the ABC Hyperactivity subscale compared with 39.5% of the placebo group. Adverse effects included somnolence, upper respiratory tract infections, rhinitis, and increased appetite. However, the somnolence eventually resolved in 86% of the cases. There was a statistically significant increase in weight, heart rate (average increase of 8.9 beats per minute), and systolic blood pressure in the children treated with risperidone. There was no significant difference in EPS between groups.

A study to determine the longer-term efficacy of risperidone in 36 autistic children ages 5 to 17 years was performed with a double-blind discontinuation phase (Troost et al., 2005). The children were given an 8-week open-label trial with risperidone. Those children who responded received another 16 weeks of additional treatment. At the end of the 24 weeks, the average daily dose was 1.81 mg per day. After that time, the children were placed in two groups; half received a 3-week taper and then 5 weeks of placebo, and the other half continued to receive risperidone. Relapse occurred in 8 of the 12 subjects (67%) who received placebo and in 3 of the 12 subjects (25%) who continued with risperidone. Adverse effects included weight gain, increased appetite, anxiety, and fatigue.

A second multisite, double-blind discontinuation study to determine the longer-term efficacy and safety of risperidone in autistic children ages 5 to 17 years was performed by the RUPP Autism Network (2005b). Sixty-three children were given 4 months of open-label treatment with risperidone at an average dose of 1.96 mg per day. At the end of 4 months, 38 children who continued to meet response criteria were randomly assigned to continue risperidone at the current dose or receive a gradual placebo substitution. The substitution occurred at a decrease of risperidone by 25% of the original dose per week. The relapse rate for the gradual placebo substitution was 62.5% versus 12.5% for continued risperidone treatment. Side effects associated with risperidone during the 16-week risperidone extension included increased appetite, tiredness, and drowsiness. After 6 months of treatment, the average weight gain was 5.1 kg.

Based in part on the results of these controlled studies performed with risperidone, the FDA approved its use in children diagnosed with autistic disorder ages 5 to 16 years with irritability. This is the first drug to be approved by the FDA for treatment of symptoms associated with autism (McDougle et al., 2008).

Olanzapine

Positive responses to olanzapine in individuals with PDDs have been noted in an open-label study, a case series, and one small placebo-controlled study. The open-label study included 25 children ages 6 to 16 years with PDDs given olanzapine for 3 months at a final average dose of 10.7 mg per day (Kemner et al., 2002). Clinical improvement was noted with the ABC subscales (Irritability, Hyperactivity, and Inappropriate Speech) and TARGET (a checklist of five target symptoms). However, only 3 children were determined to be responders on the CGI-I. EPS occurred in three children but improved with a lower dose. Other side effects included weight gain, increased appetite and loss of strength. The explanation for the low response rate in this study could result from the low average ABC Irritability subscale score (of 11) at study entry. In the two large, placebo-controlled studies of risperidone in children with PDDs, the Irritability subscale scores at study entry were 26 and 20, respectively (McDougle et al., 2008).

Significant weight gain can occur with the atypical antipsychotics, particularly in children and adolescents.

A case series involving seven PDD patients ranging in age from 8 to 52 years that were followed for 52 weeks on olanzapine has been described (Stavrakaki, Antochi, & Emery, 2004). At the end of 6 weeks, four patients had improved (as noted by the CGI-I) and two were much improved (as noted by the CGI-I and the Global Assessment of Functioning scale). At the end of 52 weeks, all the patients had improved to some extent; one was improved, three were much improved, and three were very much improved. The mean dose of olanzapine was 7.1 mg per day. Side effects included sedation and one seizure that was likely not attributable to the medication. Significant weight gain was not experienced. However, all patients received dietary management, behavioral interventions, or both while taking this medication. This could account for the lack of weight gain noted in the study.

Eleven children ages 6 to 14 years with PDDs entered a small double-blind, placebo-controlled study with olanzapine for 8 weeks at an average dose of 10 mg per day (Hollander et al., 2006). The subjects were randomized into parallel treatment groups. Fifty percent in the olanzapine group were noted to be responders judged by the CGI-I compared to 20% in the placebo group. Significant weight gain was noted in the treatment group (7.5 lbs) compared to the placebo group (1.5 lbs).

Quetiapine

The results from studies of quetiapine (an atypical antipsychotic with a mechanism of action similar to clozapine) in the PDD population have been inconsistent. A 16-week open-label study was performed on six children with PDD (mean age: 10.9 years) (Martin, Koenig, Scahill, & Bregman, 1999). Medication dosages ranged between 100 and 350 mg per day (average dose: 225 mg/day). The 16 weeks of treatment were completed by two children who were deemed to be responders on the CGI-I. Three children dropped out early because of lack of efficacy and sedation. One child dropped out early because of a possible seizure. Other adverse effects included behavioral activation, increased appetite, and weight gain.

Another open-label trial was performed using quetiapine administered to nine patients with autism (ages: 10–17 years) for 12 weeks (Findling et al., 2004). Over the initial 6 weeks, the dose of quetiapine was increased to 300 mg per day; dosage could continue to be increased to 750 mg per day. The average dose was 292 mg per day. Six patients were able to finish the trial. Of those, only two patients were deemed to be responders as measured by the CGI-I scale. Side effects included sedation, weight gain, agitation, and aggression.

A retrospective analysis of quetiapine was conducted with a review of 857 charts to find 20 patients with PDD who had been treated for at least 4 weeks with quetiapine and no other antipsychotic or mood-stabilizing drug (Corson et al., 2004). The average dose of quetiapine was 249 mg per day and the average duration of treatment was 60 weeks. The average age of the patients was 12.1 years. Eight of the 20 patients were judged to be responders by the CGI-I scale. Side effects occurred in 10 of the patients and included weight gain, continued sedation, insomnia, and pain. An average weight increase of 5.7 kg was noted. Three of the patients discontinued quetiapine because of weight gain (n = 2) and tardive dyskinesia (n = 1), respectively.

A second retrospective study was performed with 10 PDD patients who were treated with quetiapine for a mean of 22 weeks (Hardan, Jou, & Handen, 2005). The average age was 12 years. The average dose of quetiapine was 477 mg per day. Six of the 10 patients were deemed to be responders by the CGI-I. The Conners Parent Scale was also used to track change. Improvement was seen in the dimensions of conduct, inattention, and hyperactivity. No significant improvement was noted on psychosomatic, learning, or anxiety dimensions. Adverse effects included sedation (n = 3), weight change (average 2.2 lb), mild intention tremor (n = 1), and increased sialorrhea (n = 1). Three children did gain more than 10 pounds with treatment. There were no EPS noted.

Ziprasidone

A case series has been published involving ziprasidone administered to 12 children and adults with PDDs (age range: 8–20 years) who received treatment for at least 6 weeks (McDougle, Kem, & Posey, 2002). The average daily dose was 60 mg with a range of 20 to 120 mg per day. Six of the 12 subjects were responders as judged by the CGI-I. Two of the patients who also had a diagnosis of bipolar disorder were rated as "much worse." The mean weight change for the group was a loss of 5.83 lb. Five of the individuals lost weight, five remained the same weight, and one gained weight (6 lb). The weight loss was believed to be secondary to the discontinuation of prior treatment with other atypical antipsychotics that had resulted in significant weight gain. Transient (in most cases) sedation occurred in eight subjects. Oral dyskinesia was seen in one individual with a history of TD that resolved after ziprasidone was discontinued. No cardiovascular adverse effects were noted.

An open-label retrospective study was conducted in 10 adults with autism who had been switched from another atypical antipsychotic to ziprasidone (Cohen et al., 2004). The average age was 43.8 years, and the average dose was 128 mg per day. The subjects had been treated with ziprasidone for at least 6 months. The reasons for medication change included weight gain, hypercholesterolemia, behaviors, depression, and drowsiness. At the end of 6 months, six subjects were found to have improvement in their behavior, eight lost weight (average 13.1 lb), four of five available cholesterol levels had decreased, and three of five triglyceride levels were reduced. No significant side effects were associated with ziprasidone.

Two case reports have been published describing marked improvement with the use of ziprasidone in autistic children. The first was a 7-year-old male who had not responded to trials of amphetamine, guanfacine, sertraline, and divalproex for symptoms of agitation, impulsivity, irritability, hyperactivity, and intermittent nocturnal awakenings (Goforth & Rao, 2003). The boy responded to 10 mg of ziprasidone nightly. He had less agitation and impulsivity and improvement in his mood. After 8 weeks of treatment, a significant improvement was noted in his language and cognitive performance. He began to use two- to three-word phrases and follow directions. He was rated as "much improved" on the CGI-I. The behavioral and cognitive effects continued to be noted 8 months later. No side effects were reported.

The second case report involved a 15-year-old male with autism, mild mental retardation, and significant ADHD symptoms (Duggal, 2007). He exhibited multiple maladaptive behaviors as well. His symptoms did not respond to MPH alone. Therefore, he was administered risperidone (lack of efficacy) and quetiapine (gained 28 lb over 2 years). Subsequently, he was prescribed ziprasidone at a dose of 20 mg twice a day for the first day, 40 mg twice a day on the second day, and 60 mg twice a day on the third day. After 2 weeks, significant improvement was noted in all of his maladaptive behaviors, including aggressive and disruptive symptoms. His ADHD symptoms (inattention, distraction, hyperactivity, and impulsivity) improved as well. His CGI-I rating was "much improved." MPH was continued at 60 mg per day throughout the titration of ziprasidone. His improvement remained stable over 2 months with no weight gain.

A 6-week open-label study of ziprasidone was performed in 12 adolescents with autism (ages 12.1–18 years; Malone et al., 2007). The average daily dose of ziprasidone was 98 mg (range: 20–160 mg/day). Nine of the 12 individuals (75%) were deemed to be responders based on the CGI-I. There was a significant decrease in total cholesterol (net decrease of 10.2 mg/dl) but not low-density lipoproteins or triglycerides. There was no significant change in weight in this study. The most common side effect was transient sedation. Two patients had dystonic reactions. One was not witnessed by study staff and resolved on its own. The second dystonic reaction occurred after a dose increase, but resolved after 50 mg of diphenhydramine was administered. There was a mean QTc interval (a measurement on the electrocardiogram related to cardiac conduction) increase of 14.7 msec, which was determined to be clinically insignificant.

Aripiprazole

A naturalistic, open-label study of aripiprazole in five males with PDDs (ages 5–18 years) was performed for an average of 12 weeks (range: 8–16 weeks) (Stigler, Posey, & McDougle, 2004). The average dose was 12 mg per day (range: 10–15 mg/day). All five subjects were deemed to be responders as determined by the CGI-I. No EPS or cardiovascular changes were noted. One child gained 1 lb, two children lost weight (likely because of the discontinuation of other atypical antipsychotics), and two of the subjects' weight remained stable. Two of the five subjects demonstrated sedation. One child experienced dizziness.

> Unlike the other atypical antipsychotics, aripiprazole is a partial agonist at the dopamine D_2 and serotonin 5-HT_{1A} receptors.

A retrospective chart review was done with 32 children ages 5 to 19 years with developmental disabilities who had received aripiprazole in an urban setting (Valicenti-McDermott & Demb, 2006). Twenty-four of the children were diagnosed with PDDs and 18 with mental retardation. Target symptoms included aggression, hyperactivity, impulsivity, and SIB. Twenty-eight of the participants had been receiving a different antipsychotic prior to aripiprazole. The average dose was 10.55 mg per day and was administered for 6 to 15 months. Response was noted in 18 of the 32 individuals (56%). However, the drug was reported to be helpful in only 9 of the 24 (37%) children with PDDs. Ten of the 18 (56%) children with mental retardation responded, but only 5 of the 13 (38%) children with both PDDs and mental retardation responded. Side effects were noted in 16 of the 32 (50%) children and caused 7 participants to stop the study. Discontinuation was caused by sleepiness (n = 4), tics (n = 1), increased aggression (n = 2), stiffness (n = 1), myalgias (n = 1), facial dyskinesia (n = 1), and diarrhea (n = 1). Weight gain also occurred with the average body mass index (BMI) increasing from 22.5 to 24.1. The changes in weight were most prominent in those younger than age 12 years, with an average increase in BMI of 21.3 to 23.

A 14-week prospective, open-label trial of aripiprazole (mean dose: 7.8 mg/day) in 25 children and adolescents (mean age: 8.6 years) with Asperger's Syndrome or PDD-NOS was recently reported (Stigler et al., 2009). Twenty-two of 25 subjects (88%), all of whom had significant irritability (aggression, self-injury, tantrums), responded based on the CGI-I. Mild EPS were reported in 9 subjects. Age- and sex-normed BMI increased from a mean value of 20.3 at baseline to 21.1 at endpoint. Prolactin significantly decreased from a mean value of 9.3 at baseline to 2.9 at endpoint. No subject exited the study because of a drug-related adverse event.

Results were recently published from an 8-week, double-blind, placebo-controlled, parallel group, fixed-dose (5, 10, or 15 mg/day) study of aripiprazole in 218 children and adolescents (mean age: 9.7 years) with autism (Marcus et al., 2009). All doses of the drug were significantly better than placebo in reducing mean ABC Irritability subscale scores and improving CGI-I scores at week 8. Discontinuation rates resulting from adverse events were: 7.7% for placebo, 9.4% for 5 mg, 13.6% for 10 mg, and 7.4% for 15 mg. The most common adverse event leading to discontinuation was sedation. At week 8, mean weight change was: +0.3 kg for placebo, +1.3 kg for 5 mg, +1.3 kg for 10 mg, and +1.5 kg for 15 mg. Combined with results from another large placebo-controlled, flexible-dose study of aripiprazole in children and adolescents with autism, this drug was recently granted FDA approval for the treatment of irritability in patients ages 6 to 17 years.

Interfering Repetitive Behaviors

One of the core symptom domains of autism is repetitive and stereotypic behaviors. These can interfere with an individual's ability to function in several different realms. Studies have shown a proven benefit of SSRIs in other disorders such as obsessive-compulsive disorder (OCD) in helping these behaviors (Erickson et al., 2007). A study of 50 adults with autism and 50 age- and sex-matched adults with OCD was performed to compare repetitive thoughts and behaviors between the two diagnostic groups (McDougle et al., 1995). The repetitive thoughts and behaviors of those with OCD differed from what was seen in those with autism. In this study, autistic subjects were much less likely to experience obsessions of contamination, sexual, religious, symmetry, or somatic content. Autistic individuals were more likely to experience compulsions of ordering, hoarding, telling or asking, and touching, tapping, or rubbing when compared with the subjects with OCD. The subjects with OCD were more likely to experience compulsions of cleaning, checking, and counting compared with the autistic subjects.

The repetitive thoughts and behaviors of individuals with autism differ from those with OCD.

There have been multiple studies suggesting significant serotonin abnormalities in those with PDDs. One Dutch study involving 230 patients with PDDs (ages 5–20 years) and their parents revealed an association between the serotonin transporter intron 2 polymorphism and rigid-compulsive behaviors (Mulder et al., 2005). Studies have also found platelet hyperserotonemia in individuals with autism (McBride et al., 1998; Mulder et al., 2004). Another study has suggested that the capacity for autistic children to undergo the normal period of elevated serotonin brain synthesis in childhood is disrupted (Chugani et al., 1999). Although the types of compulsive behaviors may differ between those with OCD and PDD, studies have shown some abnormalities in serotonin function in individuals from both diagnostic groups. As a result, several investigations have assessed the efficacy of SSRIs in the PDD population for improving repetitive and stereotypic behavior. Table 69-3 includes published placebo-controlled studies of SRIs in PDDs.

Clomipramine

Clomipramine is a tricyclic antidepressant with potent serotonin reuptake blocking properties that has been demonstrated to be more effective for OCD than desipramine or placebo. A double-blind study comparing clomipramine, desipramine, and placebo in 30 DSM-III diagnosed autistic individuals ages 6 to 23 years was performed to determine if clomipramine was more effective than the other two for decreasing interfering repetitive and stereotyped behavior (Gordon et al., 1993). Each individual was given a 2-week single-blind, trial of placebo. The individuals with less than a 20% response as measured by the Children's Psychiatric Rating Scale, CGI, Modified NIMH Global OCD and Anxiety scales, Modified NIMH OCD Scale, and Modified Comprehensive Psychopathological Rating Scale OCD subscale were then given a 10-week double-blind, randomized crossover comparison of clomipramine and placebo or clomipramine and desipramine (5 weeks on each agent). The mean dosage of clomipramine was 152 mg per day and that of desipramine was 127 mg per day. At the end of the study, clomipramine was found to be superior to placebo and desipramine in decreasing abnormal behaviors (stereotypies and anger) and obsessive-compulsive behaviors and symptoms (compulsive, ritualized behavior). Hyperactivity improved with both clomipramine and desipramine as compared to placebo. Side effects for clomipramine included prolongation of the corrected QT interval and tachycardia (both improved upon dose reduction). One patient receiving clomipramine suffered a grand mal seizure. Eight of the 12 individuals receiving desipramine suffered from increased irritability, aggression, and temper tantrums.

An open-label study of clomipramine (mean dose: 103.12 mg/day), following a 1-week placebo lead-in, was performed with eight autistic children ages 3.5 to 8.7 years (Sanchez et al., 1996). A 3.5-year-old boy dropped out during the third week because of urinary retention. One child improved moderately and six had worsening behavior as measured by the Clinical Global Consensus Ratings. The authors concluded that clomipramine was not helpful and was associated with serious adverse effects in this young population. Adverse effects included acute urinary retention (n = 1), severe constipation (n = 4), insomnia (n = 4), increased aggression

Table 69–3.
Published placebo-controlled studies of SRIs for interfering repetitive behaviors

Study	Drug	Subjects	Design	Results
Gordon et al., 1993	Clomipramine	$n = 30$ Age = 6–23 Dx = AUT	5 weeks Crossover	Clomipramine > PLA Clomipramine > DMI 19/28 (68%) responders
Remington et al., 2001	Clomipramine Haloperidol	$n = 36$ Age = 10–36 Dx = AUT	7 weeks Crossover	Clomipramine = PLA Clomipramine = Haloperidol
Buchsbaum et al., 2001	Fluoxetine	$n = 6$ Age = 30.5 ± 8.6 Dx = AUT, ASP	8 weeks Crossover	Fluoxetine > PLA 3/6 (50%) responders
Hollander et al., 2005	Fluoxetine	$n = 45$ Age = 5–16 Dx = AUT, ASP	8 weeks Crossover	Fluoxetine > PLA repetitive behavior
McDougle et al., 1996	Fluvoxamine	$n = 30$ Age = 18–53 Dx = AUT	12 weeks Parallel groups	Fluvoxamine > PLA 8/15 (53%) responders
Sugie et al., 2005	Fluvoxamine	$n = 18$ Age = 3–8 Dx = AUT	12 weeks Crossover	Fluvoxamine 5/18 (28%) responders
King et al., 2009	Citalopram	$n = 149$ Age = 5–17 Dx = AUT	12 weeks Parallel groups	Citalopram = PLA

Note: SRIs = serotonin reuptake inhibitors. All ages are in years. AUT = autistic disorder. ASP = Asperger's Syndrome. Dx = diagnosis. PLA = placebo. DMI = desipramine.

and irritability ($n = 4$), drowsiness ($n = 7$), enuresis ($n = 1$), lip-licking ($n = 1$), and diarrhea ($n = 1$).

A 12-week open-label study of clomipramine (mean dose: 139 mg/day) was performed in 35 PDD-diagnosed adults ages 18 to 44 years (Brodkin et al., 1997). Two patients dropped out of the study, one because of agitation and one because of abdominal cramping. Of the 33 patients who finished the study, 18 (55%) were responders as judged by the CGI-I. In the individuals who responded to clomipramine, improvement was noted in repetitive thoughts and behaviors, aggression, and some aspects of social relatedness, such as eye contact and verbal responsiveness. Adverse events seen in 13 of the patients included seizures (2 patients with prior history and 1 with no prior history), constipation ($n = 3$), weight gain ($n = 3$), anorgasmia ($n = 1$), agitation ($n = 1$), and sedation ($n = 2$). No cardiovascular effects or EPS were noted during the study.

A double-blind, placebo-controlled crossover study was conducted to compare clomipramine, haloperidol, and placebo in 36 autistic individuals (ages 10–36 years) who were diagnosed with DSM-IV (Remington et al., 2001). Each individual was randomly placed in one of three sequential treatment groups (clomipramine-placebo-haloperidol, placebo-haloperidol-clomipramine, or haloperidol-clomipramine-placebo). Each medication was given for 7 weeks, with a 1-week wash-out period between medications. The mean daily dose of clomipramine was 128.4 mg and that of haloperidol was 1.3 mg. Haloperidol and clomipramine were statistically comparable for improving irritability and stereotypy in those individuals who completed the trial. However, statistically only 37.5% (12 of 32) of individuals were able to complete the trial of clomipramine, compared with 69.7% (23 of 33) of those given haloperidol. In the clomipramine group, 12 discontinued because of side effects including fatigue ($n = 4$), tremor ($n = 2$), tachycardia ($n = 1$), insomnia ($n = 1$), diaphoresis ($n = 1$), nausea or vomiting ($n = 1$), and decreased appetite ($n = 1$). The other eight discontinued for "behavioral reasons." Seven of the 10 patients discontinued haloperidol because of fatigue ($n = 5$), dystonia ($n = 1$), and depression ($n = 1$). The other three discontinued because of behavior problems.

Fluoxetine

Fluoxetine is an SSRI that has been shown to decrease obsessive-compulsive symptoms in individuals with OCD. There have been several studies performed to determine whether fluoxetine will decrease perseverative, repetitive behaviors in individuals with PDDs. An open-label trial of fluoxetine was performed in 23 autistic individuals (ages 7–28 years) who were diagnosed with DSM-III (Cook et al., 1992). The subjects were started at a dose of 20 mg per day and doses were increased until side effects were seen or it was deemed that no further therapeutic effect would be reached. Ratings were performed after patients had been on medication for an average of 189 days (range: 11–426 days). Fifteen of the subjects had an improvement in the CGI-I. A similar response was seen in the rating on the CGI-I for perseverative and compulsive behaviors.

An open-label study was performed with fluoxetine in 37 autistic children (ages 2–7 years) (Delong, Teague, & Kamran, 1998). Each individual's dosing was between 0.2 and 1.4 mg per kg per day. Twenty-two of the children responded to fluoxetine, with 11 having an "excellent" response that resulted in their being able to be maintained in regular classes. Improvements were noted in behavior, language, cognition, affect, and socialization. Another 11 children improved but not to the same extent.

A pilot study was performed with six PDD patients who had a mean age of 30.5 years to determine the effects of fluoxetine on regional cerebral metabolism in this population (Buchsbaum et al., 2001). Each patient received a 1-week placebo wash-out period. After this they were given fluoxetine for 8 weeks and then placebo for 8 weeks in a randomized crossover design. Doses began at 10 mg per day and increased to 40 mg per day. F^{18}-fluorodeoxyglucose positron emission tomography (PET) with co-registered magnetic resonance imaging was performed at baseline and again after 8 weeks of treatment with fluoxetine. The average Y-BOCS obsessions and Hamilton Anxiety Scale scores showed significant improvement with fluoxetine. The CGI-I was improved in three of the patients and unchanged in the other three. The PET scans revealed increased right frontal lobe metabolic rate after treatment with fluoxetine. The patients whose baseline PET scan showed higher metabolic rates in the medial frontal region and anterior cingulate were more likely to have improvement with fluoxetine.

A double-blind, placebo-controlled crossover study with liquid fluoxetine was performed in 45 individuals with PDD between the ages of 5 and 16 years (Hollander et al., 2005). The trial included two randomized 8-week phases of either fluoxetine or placebo separated by a 4-week wash-out period. The dosage of fluoxetine started at 2.5 mg per day for the first week and then increased if needed. The average dose at the end of the fluoxetine treatment period was 9.9 mg per day. Older children tended to receive higher doses. Fluoxetine was found to be superior to placebo for decreasing repetitive behaviors as measured by the CY-BOCS compulsion scale. Fluoxetine was found to be better than but not statistically superior to placebo on the CGI autism score. The composite measure of global effectiveness (CY-BOCS change and the CGI autism score) was found to be marginally statistically improved by fluoxetine. Adverse reactions were not significantly different between fluoxetine and placebo.

Fluvoxamine

Fluvoxamine has also been studied in subjects with PDDs. A 12-week double-blind, placebo-controlled trial of 30 adults with autism was performed (mean dose: 276.7 mg/day) (McDougle et al., 1996). Eight of the 15 (53%) patients who received fluvoxamine responded as measured by the CGI-I. Improvements were noted in repetitive behaviors, maladaptive behaviors, aggression, and language use. Adverse effects included mild sedation and nausea. No cardiac events or seizures occurred.

As opposed to the preceding results, a 12-week double-blind, placebo-controlled study involving 34 children and adolescents (ages 5–18 years) with PDDs described limited response and poor tolerability with fluvoxamine (McDougle, Kresch, & Posey, 2000). Eighteen of the individuals received fluvoxamine at an initial dose of 25 mg every other day. The dose was increased in 25-mg increments every 3 to 4 days as tolerated. Only 1 child out of 18 responded to fluvoxamine. Side effects were seen in 14 of the children who received fluvoxamine: insomnia (n = 9), hyperactivity (n = 5), agitation (n = 5), aggression (n = 5), increased rituals (n = 2), anxiety (n = 3), anorexia (n = 3), increased appetite (n = 1), irritability (n = 1), decreased concentration (n = 1), and impulsivity (n = 1).

Another study in children and adolescents also showed disappointing results. A 12-week double-blind, placebo-controlled, randomized crossover study with 18 autistic children ages 3 to 8 years was performed with fluvoxamine (Sugie et al., 2005). In addition to testing the response to fluvoxamine, the serotonin transporter gene was also studied to find a correlation between response and serotonin transporter gene promoter region polymorphism (5-HTTLPR). 5-HTTLPR (long [l] or short [s] allele) was measured by the polymerase chain reaction method. Ten of 18 children improved, although "minimally improved" was included as response to treatment. When "much improved" or "very much improved" was used to indicate response, the rate was only 5 of 18 (27.8%) subjects. Superior response to fluvoxamine was noted in those children with the "l" allele.

Sertraline

A 12-week open-label trial with 42 adults (mean age: 26.1 years) with PDDs was conducted with sertraline (mean dose: 122 mg/day) (McDougle et al., 1998). Improvement was noted in 24 of the 42 (57%) patients in aggression and repetitive behaviors. Improvement in social relatedness was not observed. When the percentage was broken down by type of PDD and using the score from the CGI-I, 68% (15 of 22) of the individuals with autism, 0% of the individuals with Asperger's Syndrome (0 of 6), and 64% (9 of 14) of the patients with PDD-NOS improved. Adverse effects included anorexia (n = 1), headache (n = 1), tinnitus (n = 1), alopecia (n = 1), weight gain (n = 3), sedation (n = 1), and anxiety (n = 2). No cardiovascular symptoms, EPS, or seizures occurred.

An open-label case series of nine children (ages 6–12 years) with autism and transition-induced behavior deterioration (panic, anxiety, irritability, or agitation) was conducted with sertraline (Steingard et al., 1997). Eight of the nine (89%) children showed improvement in these symptoms, with sertraline at doses ranging from 25 to 50 mg per day. Response was noted within 3 to 8 weeks of treatment. Two children showed worsening behavior when their medication was raised to 75 mg per day. In three children there was a noted loss of initial response after 3 to 7 months. Adverse effects included stomachache and behavioral activation.

Citalopram and Escitalopram

A retrospective assessment of citalopram (mean dose: 19.7 mg/day) in 14 children and adolescents (ages 4–15 years) with PDDs was performed to determine its efficacy for decreasing aggression, anxiety, stereotypies, and preoccupations (Couturier & Nicolson, 2002). Ten of the 17 subjects (59%) responded as determined by the CGI-I. Adverse events included increased agitation ($n = 2$), insomnia ($n = 1$), and possible tics ($n = 1$).

Another retrospective review of citalopram (mean dose: 16.9 mg/day) in 15 children and adolescents (6–16 years) with PDDs was done to test the effectiveness and tolerability of the drug (Namerow et al., 2003). Eleven of the 15 patients (73%) improved significantly as judged by the CGI-I. Anxiety symptoms improved significantly in 66% and mood symptoms responded in 47% of the individuals.

The NIMH STAART Network recently reported the results of a multisite, double-blind, placebo-controlled trial of citalopram for repetitive behavior in children and adolescents with PDDs (King et al., 2009). A total of 149 subjects (mean age: 9.4±3.1 years) received citalopram (maximum mean dose: 16.5±6.5 mg/day) or placebo for 12 weeks. There was no significant difference in the proportion of responders based on the CGI-I or in the reduction in the Children's Y-BOCS for PDD between groups. Citalopram was significantly more likely to be associated with adverse effects, particularly hyperactivity, increased energy level, impulsivity, and gastrointestinal symptoms.

A 10-week open-label study of escitalopram (mean dose: 11.1 mg/day) was performed in 28 children and adolescents (ages 6–17 years) with PDDs (Owley et al., 2005). There was a forced titration schedule (2.5, 5, 10, 15, and 20 mg) increased weekly unless criteria were met for a decrease in medication dose. All of the ABC subscale scores (Irritability, Social Withdrawal, Stereotypy, Hyperactivity, Inappropriate Speech) and the CGI-I showed improvement. Twenty-five percent of the patients responded to doses less than 10 mg per day. Additionally, 36% of the individuals responded to doses higher than or equal to 10 mg per day. Tolerability and efficacy were not related to weight and correlated only marginally with age. Five children had to discontinue the study because of hyperactivity requiring stimulant use not allowed in this study ($n = 2$), no response ($n = 1$), or disinhibition and aggression ($n = 2$). Side effects seen in other children requiring dose adjustment included irritability ($n = 7$), hyperactivity ($n = 6$), and both hyperactivity and irritability ($n = 5$).

Social Impairment

Core social impairment is one of the distinguishing characteristics of PDDs. Several different theories on the pathobiology of social impairment in PDD have been proposed. One theory includes the brain opioid hypothesis. This idea stems from the similarities seen between the social withdrawal seen in individuals with opioid addiction and the social withdrawal seen in autism (Walters, Barrett, & Feinstein, 1990). A second theory relates to a hypothesized abnormality in the physiology of secretin and its receptors (Köves et al., 2002). This idea was proposed after children receiving secretin injections reportedly displayed improvements in social and behavioral skills (Horvath, 2000). Another theory suggests that autism is associated with hypoglutamateric function. This theory came from observations of the similarities in behavior of autistic individuals and healthy controls who were given an *N*-methyl-D-aspartate (NMDA) antagonist (Carlsson, 1998). Thus medication trials that address these theories have been performed. Table 69-4 presents selected published placebo-controlled trials of drugs for social impairment.

Naltrexone

Several double-blind, placebo-controlled studies of the opioid receptor antagonist naltrexone have been conducted.

Table 69–4.
Published placebo-controlled studies of drugs for social impairment

Study	Drug	Subjects	Design	Results
Belsito et al., 2001	Lamotrigine	$n = 28$ Age = 3–11	12 weeks Parallel groups	Lamotrigine = PLA
King et al., 2001	Amantadine	$n = 39$ Age = 5–19	4 weeks Parallel groups	Amantadine = PLA for primary outcome Amantadine > PLA on clinician-rated hyperactivity and inappropriate speech 9/19 (47%) responders
Posey et al., 2008	D-Cycloserine	$n = 80$ Age = 3–12	8 weeks Parallel groups	D-Cycloserine = PLA

Note: All ages are in years. All studies involved subjects with autistic disorder. PLA = placebo.

Although some of the studies revealed a decrease in hyperactivity and/or irritability, no change in core social impairment was noted (Campbell et al., 1990; Campbell et al., 1993; Willemsen-Swinkels et al., 2005; Feldman, Kolmen, & Gonzaga, 1999).

Secretin

Multiple case reports have described improvement in social skills after intravenous administration of secretin (Horvath et al., 1998). However, a review of 15 double-blind, randomized controlled trials of secretin injection in PDDs revealed that none found secretin to be effective (Sturmey, 2005).

Lamotrigine

Lamotrigine is a drug that modulates glutamate release. Because of its interaction with glutamate, it was hypothesized it could improve social relatedness in individuals with PDDs. A double-blind, placebo-controlled parallel groups study of lamotrigine was performed with 28 children ages 3 to 11 years with autism (Belsito et al., 2001). The children that were given lamotrigine received an increasing dose over 8 weeks to a final dose of 5 mg per kg per day. This dose was continued for an additional 4 weeks. There was a 2-week taper of the drug and then a 4-week drug-free period. Outcome measures after the maintenance phase of lamotrigine included the ABC, the Vineland Adaptive Behavior Scales, the Pre-Linguistic Autism Diagnostic Observation Schedule, and the Childhood Autism Rating Scale. Lamotrigine did not separate from placebo on any of these outcome measures. The most common adverse events included insomnia and hyperactivity. No children discontinued the study because of rashes.

Amantadine

Amantadine hydrochloride has some NMDA noncompetitive antagonist properties. Although it is normally prescribed to treat influenza, herpes zoster, and Parkinson's disease, it has been studied to treat autism. A double-blind, placebo-controlled study of amantadine was performed in 39 autistic children ages 5 to 19 years (King et al., 2001). Children in this study received 2.5 mg every day of either amantadine or placebo for 1 week and then 5 mg twice a day for the next 3 weeks. Results were measured by the ABC and CGI-I. The parent-rated ABC did not show a statistically significant improvement between the two groups. However, the clinician-rated ABC showed statistical significance in the amantadine-treated group for Hyperactivity and Inappropriate Speech. Twice as many patients in the amantadine group versus the placebo group were rated as responders on the CGI-I. Adverse events included insomnia and somnolence.

D-Cycloserine

D-Cycloserine is an antibiotic that is used to treat tuberculosis. It is a partial agonist at the glycine site of the NMDA glutamate receptor. A study with D-cycloserine in schizophrenia showed an improvement in negative symptoms (Goff et al., 1999). Because symptoms of autism have been compared to the negative symptoms of schizophrenia, the idea that D-cycloserine could improve the social impairment of autism was proposed. A pilot study of D-cycloserine was completed in 12 autistic individuals ages 5.1 to 27.6 years (Posey et al., 2004). The patients were given a 2-week placebo lead-in phase and then ascending doses of D-cycloserine of 0.7, 1.4, 2.8 mg per kg per day for 2 weeks each. The ABC and CGI were performed every 2 weeks. Two individuals discontinued the study because of noncompliance ($n = 1$) and increased stereotypic behavior ($n = 1$), respectively. Ten patients completed the study. According to the CGI-I scale, improvement was found to be 0%, 30%, 40%, and 40% for placebo, low, medium, and high doses of D-cycloserine, respectively. The ABC Social Withdrawal subscale also revealed statistically significant improvements. Side effects included increased echolalia and transient motor tics.

More recently, a large-scale 8-week double-blind, placebo-controlled trial of D-cycloserine (1.7 mg/kg/day) was completed in 80 children (67 boys, 13 girls) with autism (ages 3–12 years) (Posey et al., 2008). No significant differences between groups were found on the CGI, ABC Social Withdrawal subscale, or the Social Responsiveness Scale. The drug was well-tolerated. Additional subgroup analyses are being conducted to determine any subject characteristics associated with response.

Memantine

Memantine is FDA-approved for the treatment of Alzheimer's disease.

Memantine is a noncompetitive NMDA receptor antagonist. Open-label add-on treatment with memantine was given to 151 PDD patients ages 2.6 to 26.3 years (Chez et al., 2007). Individuals were started at 5 mg per day. The dose was increased or decreased according to patient response by 2.5 or 5 mg every 4 to 6 weeks. Final dosing ranged from 2.5 to 30 mg per day, with an average dose of 12.67 mg per day. Seventy percent of the patients responded according to the CGI-I scale for language. Seventy-one percent of the patients showed significant improvement in showing interest in others, making efforts in social interaction, and being more cooperative. Twenty-seven patients discontinued the trial, 22 because of an increase in poor behavior and five because of lack of response.

An open-label study of memantine to determine its effectiveness in improving cognitive functioning and behavioral symptoms was initiated in 14 subjects (ages 3 to 12 years) with a diagnosis of PDD (Owley et al., 2006). Memantine was administered at 0.4 mg per kg per day. Twelve subjects completed the study. Significant improvement was seen on memory tests (Children's Significant Scale Dot Learning Subtest) and on three of the ABC subscales: Hyperactivity, Social Withdrawal, and Irritability. There was no significant improvement noted in any subjects on the CGI-I.

A retrospective study of memantine was performed in 18 patients (ages 6 to 19 years) with a diagnosis of PDD (Erickson et al., 2007). Medication doses ranged from 2.5 to 20 mg per day with an average daily dose of 10.1 mg. Sixty-one percent of the patients were rated as responders according to the CGI-I. A significant change from baseline was seen on the CGI-Severity subscale. Side effects were seen in 39% of the patients and included irritability ($n = 4$), rash ($n = 1$), emesis ($n = 1$), increased seizure frequency ($n = 1$), and sedation ($n = 1$). Four of these patients stopped the trial early because of side effects. Two children discontinued the study because of lack of efficacy.

Conclusions

There has been significant progress in the development of pharmacological treatment strategies for target symptoms associated with autism and other PDDs. The large majority of the treatment trials have focused on one target symptom at a time. Utilizing this approach, MPH and alpha$_2$ adrenergic agonists have been shown to be efficacious, to some extent, for inattentive and hyperactive symptoms. The antipsychotics haloperidol, risperidone, and aripiprazole have proven to be even more effective for aggression and irritability. Improvement in interfering stereotypical and repetitive behaviors with SSRIs has been demonstrated to be affected by development, with adults showing more improvement and less adverse events than children. Preliminary work with drugs that affect glutamate function, such as memantine, hold promise for treating aspects of social impairment.

Challenges and Future Directions

The future of pharmacologic treatment development in autism will initially focus on conducting larger-scale, double-blind, placebo-controlled trials of drugs that have shown evidence of effectiveness and safety/tolerability in preliminary pilot studies. For the symptom cluster of hyperactivity and inattention, for example, a randomized controlled trial of atomoxetine is currently underway for children and adolescents with autism and other PDDs. A multisite, controlled study of guanfacine for the same subject population is also likely to begin soon. Preliminary unpublished data suggest that paliperidone, a metabolite of risperidone with purportedly fewer adverse effects than the parent compound, may be effective for treating irritability and aggression in autism. Considering that risperidone is currently one of only two FDA-approved drugs for the treatment of symptoms associated with autism, controlled studies of paliperidone appear to be warranted. Because of the relative lack of efficacy and poor tolerability of SSRIs for children and adolescents with PDDs and interfering repetitive behavior, alternative agents are needed for this symptom cluster. Preliminary data have been published regarding encouraging effects of the glutamatergic drug riluzole in individuals with OCD. Exploratory studies of riluzole should be considered for targeting repetitive behavior in persons with autism and other PDDs. With regard to the more "core" symptom domains of autism (social and communication impairment), controlled studies of particular drugs with effects on glutamate function should be pursued. Based on published pilot data, the NMDA receptor antagonist memantine is one such compound, and a multisite study is currently underway for this purpose. In light of results from systematic studies in adults with anxiety disorders, including simple phobia, social anxiety disorder, and OCD, a combined study of social skills training with intermittent, higher-dose D-cycloserine is also soon to begin. It may be that combining D-cycloserine, a drug with prominent effects on learning and memory, facilitates or enhances the effects of various cognitive therapeutic approaches, including social skills training. In addition, recent publications suggest that the neuropeptide oxytocin, which has been shown to have prominent effects on affiliative behavior in animals, may influence tests of social awareness/judgment in humans. Controlled studies of intranasal oxytocin are currently being pursued as a potential treatment for the impaired social behavior of autism. Beyond this, it will be important for our preclinical colleagues to continue to explore animal models of social impairment, as well as genetic contributions and other molecular approaches in the search for novel biological targets for drug development for the core symptom domains of autism.

Hyperactivity and Inattention
- A double-blind, placebo-controlled trial of atomoxetine
- A double-blind, placebo-controlled trial of guanfacine

Irritability and Aggression
- Pilot study of paliperidone

Interfering Repetitive Behaviors
- Pilot study of riluzole

Social Impairment
- Double-blind, placebo-controlled trial of memantine
- Double-blind, placebo-controlled trial of D-cycloserine + social skills training
- Pilot study of intranasal oxytocin

SUGGESTED READINGS

McDougle, C. J., Posey, D. J., & Stigler, K. A. (2006). Pharmacological treatments. In Moldin, S. O. & Rubenstein J. L. R. (Eds.), Understanding Autism: From Basic Neuroscience to Treatment (pp. 417–442). Boca Raton: CRC Press.

Stigler, K. A., & McDougle, C. J. (2008). Pharmacotherapy of irritability in pervasive developmental disorders. *Child and Adolescent Psychiatric Clinics of North America. 17*, 739–752.

Posey, D. J., Erickson, C. A., & McDougle, C. J. (2008). Developing drugs for core social and communication impairment in autism. *Child and Adolescent Psychiatric Clinics of North America, 17*, 787–801.

ACKNOWLEDGMENTS

Supported in part by the Division of Disability & Rehabilitative Services, Indiana Family and Social Services Administration, (Drs. Blankenship, Erickson, McDougle); National Institute of Health grant K12 UL1 RR025761 Indiana University Clinical and Translational Sciences Institute Career Development Award (Dr. Erickson); Daniel X. and Mary Freedman Fellowship in Academic Psychiatry (Dr. Stigler); National Institute of Mental Health (NIMH) grant K23 MH082119 (Dr. Stigler); NIMH grant R01 MH077600 (Dr. Posey); and NIMH grant R01 MH072964 (Dr. McDougle). Financial Disclosure: Dr. Blankenship (None); Dr. Stigler (Research Grants: Bristol-Myers Squibb Co., Eli Lilly & Co., Janssen Pharmaceutica); Dr. Erickson (Research Grants: Bristol-Myers Squibb Co., F. Hoffman-LaRoche, Ltd., Seaside Therapeutics; Consultant: F. Hoffman-LaRoche, Ltd., Seaside Therapeutics); Dr. Posey (Research Grants: Eli Lilly & Co., Forest Research Institute; Consultant: Bristol-Myers Squibb Co., Eli Lilly & Co., Forest Research Institute; Speaker's Bureau: Janssen Pharmaceutica, Pfizer, Inc.; Common Stock: Shire); Dr. McDougle (Research Grants: Bristol-Myers Squibb Co.; Consultant: Bristol-Myers Squibb Co., Forest Research Institute; Speaker's Bureau: Bristol-Myers Squibb Co.).

REFERENCES

Aman, M. G. (1982). Stimulant Drug Effects in Developmental Disorders and Hyperactivity -Toward a Resolution of Disparate Findings. *Journal of Autism and Developmental Disorders, 12*, 385–396.

American Psychiatric Association (2000). *Diagnostic and Statistical Manual of Mental Disorders*, Fourth Edition, Text Revision. Washington, DC: American Psychiatric Association.

Anderson, L. T., Campbell, M., Gega, D. M., Perry, R., Small, A. M., & Green, W. H. (1984). Haloperidol in the Treatment of Infantile Autism: Effects on Learning and Behavioral Symptoms. *American Journal of Psychiatry, 141*(10), 1195–1202.

Anderson, L. T., Campbell, M., Adams, P., Small, A. M., Perry, R., & Shell, J. (1989). The Effects of Haloperidol on Discrimination Learning and Behavioral Symptoms in Autistic Children. *Journal of Autism and Developmental Disorders, 19*(2), 227–239.

Armenteros, J. L., Adams, P. B., Campbell, M., & Eisenberg, Z. W. (1995). Haloperidol-related Dyskinesias and Pre- and Perinatal Complications in Autistic Children. *Psychopharmacology Bulletin, 31*(2), 363–369.

Arnold, L. E., Aman, M. G., Cook, A. M., Witwer, A. N., Hall, K. L., Thompson, S., et al. (2006). Atomoxetine for Hyperactivity in Autism Spectrum Disorders: Placebo-controlled Crossover Pilot Trial. *Journal of the American Academy of Child and Adolescent Psychiatry, 45*(10), 1196–1205.

Belsito, K. M., Law, P. A., Kirk, K. S., Landa, R. J., & Zimmerman, A. W. (2001). Lamotrigine Therapy for Autistic Disorder: A Randomized, Double-blind, Placebo-controlled Trial. *Journal of Autism and Developmental Disorders, 31*(2), 175–181.

Brodkin, E. S., McDougle, C. J., Naylor, S. T., Cohen, D. J., & Price, L. H. (1997). Clomipramine in Adults With Pervasive Developmental Disorders: A Prospective Open-label Investigation. *Journal of Child and Adolescent Psychopharmacology, 7*(2), 109–121.

Buchsbaum, M. S., Hollander, E., Hazneder, M. M., Tang, C., Spiegel-Cohen, J., Wei, T. C., et al. (2001). Effect of Fluoxetine on Regional Cerebral Metabolism in Autistic Spectrum Disorders: A Pilot Study. *International Journal of Neuropsychopharmacology, 4*(2), 119–125.

Campbell, M., Anderson, L. T., Meier, M., Cohen, I. L., Small, A. M., Samit, C., et al. (1978). A Comparison of Haloperidol and Behavior Therapy and Their Interaction in Autistic Children. *Journal of the American Academy of Child Psychiatry, 17*(4), 640–655.

Campbell, M., Anderson, L. T., Small, A. M., Locascio, J. J., Lynch, N. S., & Choroco, M. C. (1990). Naltrexone in Autistic Children: A Double-blind and Placebo-controlled Study. *Psychopharmacology Bulletin, 26*(1), 130–135.

Campbell, M., Anderson, L. T., Small, A. M., Adams, P., Gonzalez, N. M., & Ernst, M. (1993). Naltrexone in Autistic Children: Behavioral Symptoms and Attentional Learning. *Journal of the American Academy of Child and Adolescent Psychiatry, 32*(6), 1283–1291.

Campbell, M., Armenteros, J. L., Malone, R. P., Adams, P. B., Eisenberg, Z. W., & Overall, J. E. (1997). Neuroleptic-related Dyskinesias in Autistic Children: A Prospective, Longitudinal Study. *Journal of the American Academy of Child and Adolescent Psychiatry, 36*(6), 835–843.

Carlsson, M. L. (1998). Hypothesis: Is Infantile Autism a Hypoglutamatergic Disorder? Relevance of Glutamate–Serotonin Interactions for Pharmacotherapy. *Journal of Neural Transmission, 105*(4–5), 525–535.

Chen, N. C., Bedair, H. S., McKay, B., Bowers, M. B. Jr., & Mazure, C. (2001). Clozapine in the Treatment of Aggression in an Adolescent with Autistic Disorder. *Journal of Clinical Psychiatry, 62*(6), 479–480.

Chez, M. G., Burton, Q., Dowling, T., Chang, M., Khanna, P., & Kramer, C. (2007). Memantine as Adjunctive Therapy in Children Diagnosed with Autistic Spectrum Disorders: An Observation of Initial Clinical Response and Maintenance Tolerability. *Journal of Child Neurology, 22*(5), 574–579.

Chugani, D. C., Muzik, O., Behen, M., Rothermel, R., Janisse, J. J., Lee, J., et al. (1999). Developmental Changes in Brain Serotonin Synthesis Capacity in Autistic and Nonautistic Children. *Annals of Neurology, 45*(3), 287–295.

Cohen, I. L., Campbell, M., & Posner, D. (1980). A Study of Haloperidol in Young Autistic Children: A Within-subjects Design Using Objective Rating Scales. *Psychopharmacology Bulletin, 16*(3), 63–65.

Cohen, S. A., Fitzgerald, B. J., Khan, S. R., & Khan, A. (2004). The Effect of a Switch to Ziprasidone in an Adult Population with Autistic Disorder: Chart Review of Naturalistic, Open-label Treatment. *Journal of Clinical Psychiatry, 65*(1), 110–113.

Cook, E. H. Jr., Rowlett, R., Jaselskis, C., & Leventhal, B. (1992). Fluoxetine Treatment of Children and Adults with Autistic Disorder and Mental Retardation. *Journal of the American Academy of Child and Adolescent Psychiatry, 31*(4), 739–745.

Corson, A. H., Barkenbus, J. E., Posey, D. J., Stigler, K. A., & McDougle, C. J. (2004). A Retrospective Analysis of Quetiapine in the Treatment of Pervasive Developmental Disorders. *Journal of Clinical Psychiatry, 65*(11), 1531–1536.

Couturier, J. L., & Nicolson, R. (2002). A Retrospective Assessment of Citalopram in Children and Adolescents with Pervasive Developmental Disorders. *Journal of Child and Adolescent Psychopharmacology, 12*(3), 243–248.

Delong, G. R., Teague, L. A., & Kamran, M. M. (1998). Effects of Fluoxetine Treatment in Young Children With Idiopathic

Autism. *Developmental Medicine and Child Neurology, 40*, 551–562.

Duggal, H. S. (2007). Ziprasidone for Maladaptive Behavior and Attention-deficit/Hyperactivity Disorder Symptoms in Autistic Disorder. *Journal of Child and Adolescent Psychopharmacology, 17*(2), 261–263.

Erickson, C. A., Posey, D. J., Stigler, K. A., & McDougle, C. J. (2007). Pharmacologic Treatment of Autism and Related Disorders. *Pediatric Annals, 36*(9), 575–585.

Erickson, C. A., Posey, D. J., Stigler, K. A., Mullett, J., Katschke, A. R., & McDougle, C. J. (2007). A Retrospective Study of Memantine in Children and Adolescents with Pervasive Developmental Disorders. *Psychopharmacology, 191*(1), 141–147.

Fankhauser, M. P., Karumanchi, V. C., German, M. L., Yates, A., & Karumanchi, S. D. (1992). A Double-blind, Placebo-controlled Study of the Efficacy of Transdermal Clonidine in Autism. *Journal of Clinical Psychiatry, 53*(3), 77–82.

Feldman, H. M., Kolmen, B. K., & Gonzaga, A. M. (1999). Naltrexone and Communication Skills in Young Children with Autism. *Journal of the American Academy of Child and Adolescent Psychiatry, 38*(5), 587–593.

Findling, R. L., McNamara, N. K., Gracious, B. L., O'Riordan, M. A., Reed, M. D., Demeter, C., et al. (2004). Quetiapine in Nine Youths with Autistic Disorder. *Journal of Child and Adolescent Psychopharmacology, 14*(2), 287–294.

Gadow, K. D., DeVincent, C. J., & Pomeroy, J. (2006). ADHD Symptom Subtypes in Children with Pervasive Developmental Disorder. *Journal of Autism and Developmental Disorders, 36*(2), 271–283.

Gobbi, G., & Pulvirenti, L. (2001). Long-term Treatment with Clozapine in an Adult with Autistic Disorder Accompanied by Aggressive Behavior. *Journal of Psychiatry and Neuroscience, 26*(4), 340–341.

Goff, D. C., Tsai, G., Levitt, J., Amico, E., Manoach, D., Schoenfeld, D. A., et al. (1999). A Placebo-controlled Trial of D-cycloserine Added to Conventional Neuroleptics in Patients with Schizophrenia. *Archives of General Psychiatry, 56*(1), 21–27.

Goforth, H. W., & Rao, M. S. (2003). Improvement in Behavior and Attention in an Autistic Patient Treated with Ziprasidone. *Australian and New Zealand Journal of Psychiatry, 37*(6), 775–776.

Goldstein, S., & Schwebach, A. J. (2004). The Comorbidity of Pervasive Developmental Disorder and Attention Deficit Hyperactivity Disorder: Results of a Retrospective Chart Review. *Journal of Autism and Developmental Disorders, 34*(3), 329–339.

Gordon, C. T., State, R. C., Nelson, J. E., Hamburger, S. D., & Rapoport, J. L. (1993). A Double-blind Comparison of Clomipramine, Desipramine, and Placebo in the Treatment of Autistic Disorder. *Archives of General Psychiatry, 50*(6), 441–447.

Greenhill, L., Beyer, D. H., Finkleson, J., Shaffer, D., Biederman, J., Conners, C. K., et al. (2002). Guidelines and Algorithms for the Use of Methylphenidate in Children with Attention Deficit/Hyperactivity Disorder. *Journal of Attention Disorders, 6*, S89–S100.

Greenhill, L. L., Pliszka, S., Dulcan, M. K., Bernet, W., Arnold, V., Beitchman, J., et al. (2001). Practice Parameter for the Use of Stimulant Medications in the Treatment of Children, Adolescents, and Adults. *Journal of the American Academy of Child and Adolescent Psychiatry, 41*, S26–S49.

Handen, B. L., Johnson, C. R., & Lubetsky, M. (2000). Efficacy of Methylphenidate Among Children with Autism and Symptoms of Attention-deficit Hyperactivity Disorder. *Journal of Autism and Developmental Disorders, 30*(3), 245–255.

Hardan, A. Y., Jou, R. J., & Handen, B. L. (2005). Retrospective Study of Quetiapine in Children and Adolescents With Pervasive Developmental Disorders. *Journal of Autism and Developmental Disorders, 35*(3), 387–391.

Hollander, E., Phillips, A., Chaplin, W., Zagursky, K., Novotny, S., Wasserman, S., et al. (2005). A Placebo Controlled Crossover Trial of Liquid Fluoxetine on Repetitive Behaviors in Childhood Adolescent Autism. *Neuropsychopharmacology, 30*(3), 582–589.

Hollander, E., Wasserman, S., Swanson, E. N., Chaplin, W., Schapiro, M. L., Zagursky, K., et al. (2006). A Double-blind Placebo-controlled Pilot Study of Olanzapine in Childhood/Adolescent Pervasive Developmental Disorder. *Journal of Child and Adolescent Psychopharmacology, 16*(5), 541–548.

Horvath, K. (2000). Secretin Treatment for Autism. *New England Journal of Medicine, 342*(16), 1216.

Horvath, K., Stefanatos, G., Sokolski, K. N., Wachtel, R., Nabors, L., & Tildon, J. T. (1998). Improved Social and Language Skills After Secretin Administration in Patients with Autistic Spectrum Disorders. *Journal of the Association for Academic Minority Physicians, 9*(1), 9–15.

Jaselskis, C. A., Cook, E. H., Fletcher, K. E., & Leventhal, B. L. (1992). Clonidine Treatment of Hyperactive and Impulsive Children With Autistic Disorders. *Journal of Clinical Psychopharmacology, 12*(5), 322–327.

Jou, R. J., Handen, B. L., & Hardan, A. Y. (2005). Retrospective Assessment of Atomoxetine in Children and Adolescents with Pervasive Developmental Disorders. *Journal of Child and Adolescent Psychopharmacology, 15*(2), 325–330.

Kemner, C., Willemsen-Swinkels, S. H., de Jonge, M., Tuynman-Qua, H., & van Engeland, H. (2002). Open-label Study of Olanzapine in Children with Pervasive Developmental Disorder. *Journal of Clinical Psychopharmacology, 22*(5), 455–460.

King, B. H., Wright, D. M., Handen, B. L., Sikich, L., Zimmerman, A. W., McMahon, W., et al. (2001). Double-blind, Placebo-controlled Study of Amantadine Hydrochloride in the Treatment of Children with Autistic Disorder. *Journal of the American Academy of Child and Adolescent Psychiatry, 40*(6), 658–665.

King, B. H., Hollander, E., Sikich, L., McCracken, J. T., Scahill, L., Bregman, J. D., et al. (2009). Lack of Efficacy of Citalopram in Children with Autism Spectrum Disorders and High Levels of Repetitive Behavior: Citalopram Ineffective in Children With Autism. *Archives of General Psychiatry, 66*(6), 583–590.

Köves K., Kausz, M., Reser, D., & Horváth, K. (2002). What May Be the Anatomical Basis That Secretin Can Improve the Mental Functions in Autism? *Regulatory Peptides, 109*(1–3), 167–172.

Lecavalier, L. (2006). Behavioral and Emotional Problems in Young People with Pervasive Developmental Disorders: Relative Prevalence, Effects of Subjects Characteristics and Empirical Classification. *Journal of Autism and Developmental Disorders, 36*(8), 1101–1114.

Locascio, J. L., Malone, R. P., Small, A. M., Kafantaris, V., Ernst, M., Lynch, N. S., et al. (1991). Factors Related to Haloperidol Response and Dyskinesias in Autistic Children. *Psychopharmacology Bulletin, 27*(2), 119–126.

Malone, R. P., Delaney, M. A., Hyman, S. B., & Carter, J. R. (2007). Ziprasidone in Adolescents With Autism: An Open-label Pilot Study. *Journal of Child and Adolescent Psychopharmacology, 17*(6), 779–790.

Marcus, R. N., Owens, R., Kamen, L., Manos, G., McQuade, R. D., Carson, W. H., et al. (2009). A Placebo-controlled, Fixed-dose Study of Aripiprazole in Children and Adolescents With

Irritability Associated With Autistic Disorder. *Journal of the American Academy of Child and Adolescent Psychiatry, 48*(11), 1110–1119.

Martin, A., Koenig, K., Scahill, L., & Bregman, J. (1999). Open-label Quetiapine in the Treatment of Children and Adolescents With Autistic Disorder. *Journal of Child and Adolescent Psychopharmacology, 9*(2), 99–107.

McBride, P. A., Anderson, G. M., Hertzig, M. E., Snow, M. E., Thompson, S. M., Khait, V. D., et al. (1998). Effects of Diagnosis, Race, and Puberty on Platelet Serotonin Levels in Autism and Mental Retardation. *Journal of the American Academy of Child and Adolescent Psychiatry, 37*(7), 767–776.

McDougle, C. J., Kresch, L. E., Goodman, W. K., Naylor, S. T., Volkmar, F. R., Cohen, D. J., et al. (1995). A Case-controlled Study of Repetitive Thoughts and Behavior in Adults With Autistic Disorder and Obsessive-compulsive Disorder. *American Journal of Psychiatry, 152*(5), 772–777.

McDougle, C. J., Naylor, S. T., Cohen, D. J., Volkmar, F. R., Heninger, G. R., & Price, L. H. (1996). A Double-blind, Placebo-controlled Study of Fluvoxamine in Adults with Autistic Disorders. *Archives of General Psychiatry, 53*(11), 1001–1008.

McDougle, C. J., Brodkin, E. S., Naylor, S. T., Carlson, D. C., Cohen, D. J., & Price, L. H. (1998). Sertraline in Adults With Pervasive Developmental Disorders: A Prospective Open-label Investigation. *Journal of Clinical Psychopharmacology, 18*(1), 62–66.

McDougle, C. J., Holmes, J. P., Carlson, D. C., Pelton, G. H., Cohen, D. J., & Price, L. H. (1998). A Double-blind, Placebo-controlled Study of Risperidone in Adults With Autistic Disorder and Other Pervasive Developmental Disorders. *Archives of General Psychiatry, 55*(7), 633–641.

McDougle, C. J., Kresch, L. E., & Posey, D. J. (2000). Repetitive Thoughts and Behavior in Pervasive Developmental Disorders: Treatment With Serotonin Reuptake Inhibitors. *Journal of Autism and Developmental Disorders, 30*(5), 427–435.

McDougle, C. J., Kem, D. L., & Posey, D. J. (2002). Case Series: Use of Ziprasidone for Maladaptive Symptoms in Youths With Autism. *Journal of the American Academy of Child and Adolescent Psychiatry, 41*(8), 921–927.

McDougle, C. J., Stigler, K. A., Erickson, C. A., & Posey, D. J. (2006). Pharmacology of Autism. *Clinical Neuroscience Research, 6*, 179–188.

McDougle, C. J., Stigler, K. A., Erickson, C. A., & Posey, D. J. (2008). Atypical Antipsychotics in Children and Adolescents with Autistic and Other Pervasive Developmental Disorders. *Journal of Clinical Psychiatry, 69* (Suppl 4), 15–20.

Mulder, E. J., Anderson, G. M., Kema, I. P., de Bildt, A., van Lang, N. D., den Boer, J. A., et al. (2004). Platelet Serotonin Levels in Pervasive Developmental Disorders and Mental Retardation: Diagnostic Group Differences, Within-group Distribution, and Behavioral Correlates. *Journal of the American Academy of Child and Adolescent Psychiatry, 43*(4), 491–499.

Mulder, E. J., Anderson, G. M., Kema, I. P., Brugman, A. M., Ketelaars, C. E. J., de Bildt, A., et al. (2005). Serotonin Transporter Intron 2 Polymorphism Associated With Rigid-compulsive Behaviors in Dutch Individuals with Pervasive Developmental Disorders. *American Journal of Medical Genetics. Part B, Neuropsychiatric Genetics, 133B*(1), 93–96.

Namerow, L. B., Thomas, P., Bostic, J. Q., Prince, J., & Monuteaux, M. C. (2003). Use of Citalopram in Pervasive Developmental Disorders. *Journal of Developmental and Behavioral Pediatrics, 24*(2), 104–108.

Naruse, H., Nagahata, M., Nakane, Y., Shirahashi, K., Takesada, M., & Yamazaki, K. (1982). A Multi-center Double-blind Trial of Pimozide (Orap), Haloperidol and Placebo in Children with Behavioral Disorders Using Crossover Design. *Acta Paedopsychiatry, 48*(4), 173–184.

Owley, T., Walton, L., Salt, J., Gutter, S. J. Jr., Winnega, M., Leventhal, B. L., et al. (2005). An Open-label Trial of Escitalopram in Pervasive Developmental Disorders. *Journal of the American Academy of Child and Adolescent Psychiatry, 44*(4), 343–348.

Owley, T., Salt, J., Guter, S., Grieve, A., Walton, L., Ayuyao, N., et al. (2006). A Prospective Open-label Trial of Memantine in the Treatment of Cognitive, Behavioral, and Memory Dysfunction in Pervasive Developmental Disorders. *Journal of Child and Adolescent Psychopharmacology, 16*(5), 517–524.

Perry, R., Campbell, M., Adams, P., Lynch, N., Spencer, E. K., Curren, E. L., et al. (1989). Long-term Efficacy of Haloperidol in Autistic Children: Continuous Versus Discontinuous Drug Administration. *Journal of the American Academy of Child and Adolescent Psychiatry, 28*(1), 87–92.

Pliszka, S. (2007). Practice Parameter for the Assessment and Treatment of Children and Adolescents with Attention-deficit/Hyperactivity Disorder. *Journal of the American Academy of Child and Adolescent Psychiatry, 46*(7), 894–921.

Posey, D. J., Puntney, J. I., Sasher, T. M., Kem, D. L., & McDougle, C. J. (2004). Guanfacine Treatment of Hyperactivity and Inattention in Pervasive Developmental Disorders: A Retrospective Analysis of 80 Cases. *Journal of Child and Adolescent Psychopharmacology, 14*(2), 233–241.

Posey, D. J., Kem, D. L., Swiezy, N. B., Sweeten, T. L., Wiegand, R. E., & McDougle, C. J. (2004). A Pilot Study of D-cycloserine in Subjects With Autistic Disorder. *American Journal of Psychiatry, 161*(11), 2115–2117.

Posey, D. J., Wiegand, R. E., Wilkerson, J., Maynard, M., Stigler, K. A., & McDougle, C. J. (2006). Open-label Atomoxetine for Attention-deficit/Hyperactivity Disorder Symptoms Associated With High-functioning Pervasive Developmental Disorders. *Journal of Child and Adolescent Psychopharmacology, 16*(5), 599–610.

Posey, D. J., & McDougle, C. J. (2007). Guanfacine and Guanfacine Extended Release: Treatment for ADHD and Related Disorders. *CNS Drug Reviews, 13*(4), 465–474.

Posey, D. J., Aman, M. G., McCracken, J. T., Scahill, L., Tierney, E., Arnold, L. E., et al. (2007a). Positive Effects of Methylphenidate on Inattention and Hyperactivity in Pervasive Developmental Disorders: An Analysis of Secondary Measures. *Biological Psychiatry, 61*(4), 538–544.

Posey, D. J., Stigler, K. A., Erickson, C. A., & McDougle, C. J. (2007b). Treatment of Autism with Antipsychotics. In Hollander E. & Anagnostou E. (Eds.). *Clinical Manual for the Treatment of Autism* (pp. 99–120). Washington, DC: American Psychiatric Publishing.

Posey, D. J., Stigler, K. A., Erickson, C. A., & McDougle, C. J. (2008). Antipsychotics in the Treatment of Autism. *Journal of Clinical Investigation, 118*(1), 6–14.

Posey, D. J., Stigler, K. A., Erickson, C. A., Azzouz, F., Mullett, J., Diener, J. T., et al. (2008). A Double-blind Placebo-controlled Study of D-cycloserine in Children With Autistic Disorder. *55th Annual Meeting of the American Academy of Child and Adolescent Psychiatry, Scientific Proceedings*, Abstract P3.53, p. 219.

Quintana, H., Birmaher, B., Stedge, D., Lennon, S., Freed, J., Bridge, J., et al. (1995). Use of Methylphenidate in the Treatment of Children With Autistic Disorder. *Journal of Autism and Developmental Disorders, 25*, 283–294.

Remington, G., Sloman, L., Konstantareas, M., Parker, K., & Gow, R. (2001). Clomipramine Versus Haloperidol in the Treatment of Autistic Disorder: A Double-blind, Placebo-controlled, Crossover Study. *Journal of Clinical Psychopharmacology, 21*(4), 440–444.

Research Units on Pediatric Psychopharmacology (RUPP) Autism Network. (2002). Risperidone in Children With Autism and Serious Behavioral Problems. *New England Journal of Medicine, 347*(5), 314–321.

Research Units on Pediatric Psychopharmacology (RUPP) Autism Network. (2005a). Randomized, Controlled, Crossover Trial of Methylphenidate in Pervasive Developmental Disorders With Hyperactivity. *Archives of General Psychiatry, 62*, 1266–1274.

Research Units on Pediatric Psychopharmacology (RUPP) Autism Network (2005b). Risperidone Treatment of Autistic Disorder: Longer-Term Benefits and Blinded Discontinuation After 6 Months. *American Journal of Psychiatry, 162*(7), 1361–1369.

Sanchez, L. E., Campbell, M., Small, A. M., Cueva, J. E., Armenteros, J. L., & Adams, P. B. (1996). A Pilot Study of Clomipramine in Young Autistic Children. *Journal of the American Academy of Child and Adolescent Psychiatry, 35*(4), 537–544.

Scahill, L., Aman, M. G., McDougle, C. J., McCracken, J. T., Tierney, E., Dziura, J., et al. (2006). A Prospective Open Trial of Guanfacine in Children With Pervasive Developmental Disorders. *Journal of Child and Adolescent Psychopharmacology, 16*(5), 589–598.

Shea, S., Turgay, A., Carroll, A., Schulz, M., Orlik, H., Smith, I., et al. (2004). Risperidone in the Treatment of Disruptive Behavioral Symptoms in Children With Autistic and Other Pervasive Developmental Disorders. *Pediatrics, 114*(5), 634–641.

Stavrakaki, C., Antochi, R., & Emery, P. C. (2004). Olanzapine in the Treatment of Pervasive Developmental Disorders: A Case Series Analysis. *Journal of Psychiatry and Neuroscience, 29*(1), 57–60.

Stein, M. (2004). Atomoxetine (Journal Watch Pediatrics and Adolescent Medicine Web site); http://pediatrics.jwatch.org/cgi/content/full/2004/116/1.

Steingard, R. J., Zimnitzky, B., DeMaso, D. R., Bauman, M. L., & Bucci, J. P. (1997). Sertraline Treatment of Transition-associated Anxiety and Agitation in Children with Autistic Disorder. *Journal of Child and Adolescent Psychopharmacology, 7*(1), 9–15.

Stigler, K. A., Desmond, L. A., Posey, D. J., Wiegand, R. E., & McDougle, C. J. (2004). A Naturalistic Retrospective Analysis of Psychostimulants in Pervasive Developmental Disorders. *Journal of Child and Adolescent Psychopharmacology, 14*(1), 49–56.

Stigler, K. A., Posey, D. J., & McDougle, C. J. (2004). Arpiprazole for Maladaptive Behavior in Pervasive Developmental Disorders. *Journal of Child and Adolescent Psychopharmacology, 14*(3), 455–463.

Stigler, K. A., & McDougle, C. J. (2008). Pharmacotherapy of Irritability in Pervasive Developmental Disorders. *Child and Adolescent Psychiatric Clinics of North America, 17*(4), 739–752.

Stigler, K. A., Diener, J. T., Kohn, A. E., Li, L., Erickson, C. A., Posey, D. J., et al. (2009). Aripiprazole in Pervasive Developmental Disorder Not Otherwise Specified and Asperger's Disorder: A 14-week, Prospective, Open-label study. *Journal of Child and Adolescent Psychopharmacology, 19*(3), 265–274.

Sturmey, P. (2005). Secretin is an Ineffective Treatment for Pervasive Developmental Disabilities: A Review of 15 Double-blind Randomized Controlled Trials. *Research in Developmental Disabilities, 26*(1), 87–97.

Sugie, Y., Sugie, H., Fukuda, T., Ito, M., Sasada, Y., Nakabayashi, M., et al. (2005). Clinical Efficacy of Fluvoxamine and Functional Polymorphism in a Serotonin Transporter Gene on Childhood Autism. *Journal of Autism and Developmental Disorders, 35*(3), 377–385.

Troost, P. W., Lahuis, B. E., Steenhuis, M. P., Ketelaars, C. E., Buitelaar, J. K., van Engeland, H., et al. (2005). Long-term Effects of Risperidone in Children with Autism Spectrum Disorders: A Placebo Discontinuation Study. *Journal of the American Academy of Child and Adolescent Psychiatry, 44*(11), 1137–1144.

Troost, P. W., Steenhuis, M. P., Tuynaman-Qua, H. G., Kalverdijk, L. J., Buitelaar, J. K., Minderaa, R. B., et al. (2006). Atomoxetine for Attention-deficit/Hyperactivity Disorder Symptoms in Children With Pervasive Developmental Disorders: A Pilot Study. *Journal of Child and Adolescent Psychopharmacology, 16*, 611–619.

Valicenti-McDermott, M. R., & Demb, H. (2006). Clinical Effects and Adverse Reactions of Off-label Use of Aripiprazole in Children and Adolescents With Developmental Disabilities. *Journal of Child and Adolescent Psychopharmacology, 16*(5), 549–560.

Walters, A. S., Barrett, R. P., & Feinstein, C. (1990). Social Relatedness and Autism: Current Research, Issues, Directions. *Research in Developmental Disabilities, 11*(3), 303–326.

Willemsen-Swinkels, S., Buitelaar, J. K., Weijen, F. G., & van Engeland, H. (2005). Placebo-controlled Acute Dosage Naltrexone Study in Young Autistic Children. *Psychiatry Research, 58*, 203–215.

Zuddas, A., Ledda, M. G., Fratta, A., Muglia, P., & Cianchetti, C. (1996). Clinical Effects of Clozapine on Autistic Disorder. *American Journal of Psychiatry, 153*(5), 738.

70 Margaret L. Bauman

Autism Spectrum Disorders: Identification and Implications of Associated Medical Conditions

Points of Interest

- Children, adolescents, and adults with ASDs, who experience common medical conditions, may not present with the same signs and symptoms as that exhibited by their neurotypical peers.
- Many nonverbal, sensory disordered persons with ASDs may not be able to express or demonstrate their discomfort or localize pain.
- Many of the medical conditions occurring in individuals with ASDs are treatable.
- Treating medical conditions can improve physical comfort and quality of life and allow the individual to better participate in and benefit from services and interventions.
- Some medical conditions may have genetic implications and may therefore aide in our ability to subtype groups of individuals on the autism spectrum.

Introduction

The autism spectrum disorders (ASDs) are identified by behaviorally defined clinical features characterized by core symptoms of impaired social interaction, delayed and disordered communication/language, and isolated areas of interest. It is now recognized that individuals affected with ASDs are heterogeneous in terms of the cause of their disorder and the degree to which each is affected functionally and neurobiologically. Since its initial description in 1943 (Kanner), a growing body of research has broadened our perspective of the disorder and has created an environment whereby early diagnosis and intervention has become the standard of care, with the realization that in many cases, early identification and intensive therapies can lead to more positive developmental outcomes. With advancements in clinical care has come the observation and appreciation of the fact that many children with ASDs, adolescents and adults have medically relevant health-care issues that may go undetected because of atypical symptom presentation, the inability of the patient to describe or localize discomfort, and often behavioral issues that can make physical examination challenging. However, many of these medical conditions are treatable and, when identified and treated, may improve quality of life for the patient and his/her family and may broaden our understanding of the phenotypic expression of ASDs, leading ultimately to a better defined genotypic subtyping of individuals on the spectrum.

Etiology

Autism is now considered one of the most common disorders of development worldwide. Studies performed by the United States Centers for Disease Control (CDC) in selected communities in 2002 suggest that the current prevalence rates for ASDs are approximately 1 in 150 children (Kuehn, 2007). The increase in the reported prevalence of ASDs has been attributed by some to improved ascertainment, a broadening of the diagnostic definition, and improved public and professional awareness. Others have attributed this upsurge in diagnosis to the contribution of potential, as yet to be identified, environmental factors.

Numerous epidemiologic studies have provided compelling evidence for a genetic basis for autism (Bailey et al., 1995; Bolton et al., 1994). Beginning with the seminal twin study of Folstein and Rutter, published in 1977, the concept of ASDs as a largely genetic disorder has remained in the forefront of autism research. In this study, the authors identified a higher concordance in monozygotic twins than in dizygotic twins. Since that time, numerous linkage studies have been reported, with the most frequently replicated findings being associated with chromosomes 7q, 15q, 22q, and 2q (Schaefer & Mendelsohn, 2008). Additional candidate genes of promise include γ-amino butyric acid (GABA) and serotonin transporter genes, engrailed 2, neuroligin, MECP2, WNT2, PTEN, and MET (Campbell et al., 2006, 2007). Many new loci and genes have been identified, and the reader is referred to the chapters related to genetics in this book for detailed data. Autism is four times more common in males than in females, with a higher ratio in milder forms of the disorder. Further, ASDs are associated with a significant familial recurrence, much higher than that seen in the general population. The reported recurrence risk has been estimated to be approximately 15% in families having one affected child (Landa et al., 2006, 2008; Lauritsen et al., 2005). If the family has two affected children, the recurrence rate for subsequent children increases substantially, up to 25% to 50% (Cook, 2001; Spence, 2004).

Despite modern technology and advanced research, only approximately 6% to 15% of individuals with autism will be found to have an identifiable genetic diagnosis. In addition, a number of syndromes have been associated with ASDs, including Fragile X Syndrome (FXS), tuberous sclerosis, Smith-Lemli-Opitz Syndrome, and Rett Syndrome (MECP2 mutations) (Schaefer et al., 2008; Geschwind, this book). Numerous genes have been investigated as possible candidate genes, but replicated findings are lacking. Current epidemiological studies of ASDs strongly suggest multifactorial inhertitance, including genetic heterogeneity with multiple major gene effects, possible contributing environmental effects, and physiologically linked processes with multiple genes.

One of the many additional potentially important risk factors for ASDs that has gained increased interest is the role of advanced parental age. In a recent study, Durkin et al. (2008) noted that in a study of 1251 children with complete parental age information and who were defined as having ASDs based on DSM-IV criteria, both maternal and paternal age were independently associated with autism. The authors also noted that firstborn offspring of two older parents were three times more likely to develop autism than were later born offspring. A number of potential mechanisms for these effects have been suggested, including age-related chromosomal changes, complications of pregnancy, or possible environmental exposures during pregnancy that could have mutagenic effects. In addition, given the apparent importance of birth order, the authors speculate that these children may be more susceptible to autoimmune responses affecting neurodevelopment or may be affected secondary to maternal exposure to neurotoxic chemicals, passed to the offspring transplacentally or in breast milk, in combination with advanced maternal age. Whatever the mechanisms involved, these observations warrant further investigation in a larger population of children with ASDs.

Clinical Presentation

Although it is now recognized that autism is a clinically and biologically heterogeneous disorder, those affected share a triad of common features that include atypical social interaction, delayed and disordered language, and a markedly restricted repertoire of activities and interests (American Psychiatric Association, 1994). Symptoms can range from relatively subtle and mild to very severe. For example, there may be a qualitative impairment in reciprocal social interaction as opposed to an absolute absence of social interaction. Social behaviors can range from a seemingly total lack of awareness of others to inappropriate eye contact and atypical social responsiveness. Communication skills can span from a total lack of verbal speech and intentional use of gesture to the presence of speech that is associated with atypical intonation, prosody, syntax, and grammar. Although the normal development of single-word receptive and expressive vocabulary may be present, pragmatic language may be significantly impaired. Many affected individuals demonstrate poor eye contact, echolalia, pronoun reversals, stereotypic and repetitive behaviors, sensory processing dysfunction, difficulty dealing with novelty, an obsessive reliance on routine, and some level of cognitive impairment. In very young children, the lack of a pointing response and joint attention and limited pretend play are frequent characteristics as early as age 12 months. Many affected individuals have exceptional islands of rote memory and outstanding isolated talents in the face of otherwise general functional disabilities (Rapin & Katzman, 1998). Although it was initially believed that approximately 75% of those affected with autism functioned in the mentally retarded range, more recent studies have found that fewer than half of affected individuals have significant cognitive impairment (Newschaffer et al., 2007).

Typically, those individuals with nonsyndromic or "essential" autism demonstrate few, if any, dysmorphic features and are generally described as very attractive appearing children. For many years, these children were believed to demonstrate no abnormalities of motor function, or if present, these deficits were believed to be merely associated symptoms. It has now become apparent that gross and fine motor dysfunction is more common than previously appreciated. Numerous clinical studies indicate that children with autism exhibit deficits in skilled motor performance in response to command and with tool use, suggestive of a more generalized dyspraxia (Rogers et al., 1996; Mostofsky et al., 2006). Children with autism often show delays in learning novel complex motor skills such as peddling a tricycle or pumping on a swing with their legs (Gidley Larson & Mostofsky, 2007). Further, in a study of motor impairment in a group of 154 children with ASDs, Ming et al. (2007) noted that hypotonia was the most common motor symptom in this cohort, with motor dyspraxia being more prevalent in younger children than older children. Gross motor delay was reported in 9% and toe-walking in 19%. The etiology of motor dysfunction in ASDs remains uncertain, with abnormalities of the cerebellum, basal ganglia, and/or neural connections across distributed networks being hypothesized (Gidley Larson et al., 2008).

Examination of the autistic child, adolescent, and adult may be complicated by variable levels of cooperation, impaired communication and behavioral issues. Important factors during the physical and neurological assessments should include identification of potential dysmorphic features that might suggest a specific diagnosis or syndrome. Measurements of head circumference throughout childhood has resulted in the observation that a subset of children with ASDs demonstrate a larger than average head circumference, with approximately 20% of these showing a frank macrocephaly of greater than 98% for age and sex. More recent work by Lainhart et al. (2006) highlights the fact that the distribution curve of head size in ASD is similar to that seen in typically developing children but is shifted to the left, suggesting that this unusual head growth may reflect an upregulation of as yet unknown growth factors. The clinical finding of macrocrania is, at this time, without a defined neuropathological correlate.

All patients with autism should have a formal audiogram. Many children with ASDs present with impaired receptive and expressive language and fail to respond to the spoken word, causing some parents to wonder if their child might be deaf. Impaired hearing could alter communication and socialization skills. There is a debate as to the role of electroencephalography (EEG) as part of the routine evaluation of a child with an ASD. Although there are reports of autistic-like symptoms in some children with seizure disorders and an acquired aphasia (Landau Kleffner Syndrome), this disorder is very rare. In general, EEG is probably not indicated as a routine part of the ASD evaluation unless there is a clinical history to suggest a possible seizure disorder. Similarly, cranial imaging studies are not routinely recommended unless abnormalities on neurological examination are observed (Filipek et al., 1999). Additional assessments should include high-resolution karyotype and Fragile X Syndrome studies as an initial step, along with assessments from a speech and language pathologist, an occupational therapist, and a cognitive developmental specialist.

Associated Medical Disorders

Until recently, much of the clinical and basic science research has been focused on the understanding of brain mechanisms that could explain the behavioral, cognitive, social interaction, and communication dysfunction associated with ASDs, with relatively little attention to the possible significance of accompanying medical conditions. Much of this relative neglect may be related to the fact that the physical examination of an individual with autism, particularly children, can be challenging and often limited by poor patient cooperation and difficult office behavior. Further, it now appears that ASD individuals, many of whom are nonverbal or hypo-verbal, may not be able to describe or localize their discomfort. In addition, there is a growing appreciation that persons with ASDs may not present with typical, easily recognized symptoms, making diagnosis in any one circumstance difficult, and therefore overlooked. Research indicates that children with ASDs are more likely than other children with special needs to have difficulty accessing medical care, further compounding the challenge of providing quality routine health care to this population of individuals (Kogan et al., 2008). The fact that a child has autism does not rule out the possibility that he or she may have one or more other illnesses or disorders, similar to those experienced by typically developing children. Identifying and treating these disorders may improve behavior, developmental progress, and quality of life as well as provide leads into potential subsets of individuals with ASD who may have genetic and etiologic implications.

Pain and Discomfort

It is known from the general pediatric literature that typically developing children often show increased rates of problem behaviors in association with physical illness. For example, increased rates of head-banging behavior has been reported in infants who are experiencing middle ear infections (Lissovoy, 1962), and increased frequency of temper tantrums has been observed in toddlers in relationship to upper respiratory infections (Hart et al., 1984). Not surprisingly, physical illness is common in persons with developmental disabilities, and at least one study has suggested that the number of associated medical conditions may be higher for individuals with developmental disabilities than for the general population across the life span (Cooper, 1998). As is the case for typically developing persons, there also appears to be an association between physical illness and problem behaviors in the disabled population. Problem behaviors have been associated with illnesses such as allergies (Taylor et al., 1993), constipation (Lekkas & Lentino, 1978), premenstrual syndrome (Kennedy & Meyer, 1996), and urinary tract and ear infections (Gunsett et al., 1989). Documentation that problem behaviors may be causally linked to physical illness has been provided through studies showing that these behaviors can be significantly reduced as the result of appropriate medical diagnosis and treatment (Ghaziuddin et al., 1993; Peine et al., 1999). It has been suggested that this relationship between physical illness and problem behaviors is not the result of the illness itself but is more likely related to the degree of pain and discomfort experienced by the individual at any given time (Horner et al., 1996; Kennedy & Thompson, 2000).

Determining the causes and source of pain and discomfort can be challenging in nonverbal persons who may not process or localize sensory information accurately. Further, many persons with developmental disabilities, including individuals with ASDs, may not present with the typical signs and symptoms of illness familiar to most primary care physicians and specialists. For example, some ASD persons suffering from gastrointestinal disorders may present with aggression and self-injurious behavior without evidence of vomiting, diarrhea, constipation, or signs of abdominal discomfort (Buie, clinical observation). Thus, a high index of suspicion for some type of medical illness should be raised for any ASD or developmentally disabled patient who presents with an unusual onset or escalation of problem behaviors that have not responded to behavioral and environmental accommodations and that cannot be readily explained. Carr and Owen-DeSchryver (2007) have suggested the use of retrospective and prospective questionnaires, administered by knowledgable informants, to assist in delineating a potential connection between problem behavior and physical illness. In a study of 11 individuals with ASDs, ages 4 to 21 years, the authors noted that retrospective questionnaires alone were often unreliable. The addition of a prospective questionnaire allowed informants to track the association between behaviors and illness-related pain over a period of months and on a daily basis. Informants were supplied with a list of motor and verbal pain indicators derived from the pediatric clinical literature. The resulting data proved reliable in that informants were able to agree among themselves with regard to their observations. Of further concern is the observation that without prevention and prompt intervention, problem behaviors may become more strongly established over time (Horner et al., 2002).

Space does not allow for a detailed description of the multiplicity of possible medical conditions that may affect a person with autism. Therefore, only some of the more common disorders will be briefly highlighted here. These include seizure disorders, sleep disturbances, gastrointestinal disorders, metabolic dysfunction, and hormonal imbalances. However, the primary care and specialty physicians serving persons with ASDs must be constantly alert to a wide range of medical possibilities at any one time.

Seizure Disorders

The prevalence of seizures in adults with autism has been estimated to be between 20% and 35% (Minshew et al., 1997; Tuchman, this book), and in children with ASDs, it has been estimated between 7% and 14% (Rapin, 1996; Tuchman et al., 1991), with peak risk periods occurring in early childhood and adolescence (Volkmar & Nelson, 1990). Although regression of language and cognitive skills in association with seizures has been reported during the teenage years, little is known regarding its etiology or prevalence (Minshew et al., 1997). Seizures may be of any typ,e but partial complex seizures are most frequently reported. The clinical identification of partial complex seizures in autistic individuals can often be complicated by the presence of atypical behavioral patterns and body movements often seen in association with ASDs and frequently attributed to the autism *per se*. Alternatively, not all body movements or mannerisms observed in ASDs are seizure-related and may be manifestations of other medical conditions such as gastroesophageal reflux disease (GERD) (Buie, 2005). Further complicating diagnosis is the fact that there may be a lack of direct correlation between clinical seizures and EEG activity (Minshew et al., 1997). However, any behaviors such as staring, cessation of activity, eye fluttering or aggressive behavior associated with confusion should raise the suspicion of a complex partial seizure and further evaluation pursued. Obtaining a high-quality EEG—especially in toddlers and young children—can be difficult but can be achievable. Prolonged or overnight EEG can often be helpful as well as the use of video tape review of the events recorded in the home or school. A growing number of anticonvulsant medications are now available, and these seizures can usually be brought under control with experienced medical management.

Gastrointestinal Disorders

Although gastrointestinal (GI) dysfunction is believed to be relatively common in autism, the true prevalence of these disorders is unknown (Buie, 2005; Campbell et al., 2009). Similarly, it is not known whether these disorders are more common in persons with ASDs than in typically developing individuals. However, a recent, well-controlled prospective study, using a structured interview, reported a significantly increased prevalence of GI conditions in ASDs as compared to controls (Valicenti-McDermott et al., 2006). Parents often report a number of symptoms in their babies and young children, including diarrhea, constipation, food intolerance, gas, bloating, abdominal pain/discomfort, and a history of reflux (Horvath et al., 1999; Quigley & Hurley, 2000).

Although many children with ASDs present with typical GI track symptoms, others may not and may instead exhibit aggressions and self-injurious behavior, facial grimacing, chest tapping, and the seeking of abdominal pressure (Buie, personal communication). It is well-known that typically developing children can and often do present with behavioral disruptions when not feeling well. There is no reason to believe that children with ASDs should do otherwise. The identification of GERD, gastritis, esophagitis, colitis, inflammatory bowel disease, Crohn's disease and celiac disease have been identified in autistic persons and treatment of these disorders have resulted in improved behavior and better developmental progress (Buie, personal communication), no doubt because the individual is more comfortable and physically well.

Recently, Campbell et al. (2009) have reported that disrupted MET gene signaling may contribute to increased risk for ASDs, including familial GI dysfunction. A functional variant in the promotor of the gene encoding the MET receptor tyrosine kinase has been associated with ASDs, and MET protein expression has been found to be decreased in the temporal lobe cortex in ASD postmortem brain tissue. MET is a pleiotropic receptor that is known to function in both brain development and GI repair. Thus, the identification of medical disorders in ASD individuals (in this case GI disorders) may not only improve quality of life for those affected with ASDs but may lead to improved or more precise definition of genetic and phenotypic subtypes in this complex heterogeneous disorder.

Sleep Disorders

The prevalence of sleep disorders in typically developing children is said to be approximately 30% and appears to be more common in early childhood (Ferber, 1996). In contrast, the prevalence rates among children with autism have been estimated to range from 44% to 83% (Richdale, 1999), and sleep disorders have been reported to be more severe in this population (Malow et al., 2006). It is known that disordered sleep affects daytime health, neurocognitive dysfunction, and behavioral disruptions in a variety of psychiatric and neurologic conditions. In typically developing children, sleep disruption may lead to daytime sleepiness and may manifest itself as hyperactivity, inattention, or aggression (Owens et al., 1998). Insomnia, defined as having trouble initiating and/or maintaining sleep, is the most common feature reported by parents of autistic children. Additional sleep concerns include symptoms of disordered breathing associated with loud snoring, noisy breathing, or occasional pauses or apneas in breathing as well as leg movements and tooth grinding. Occasionally, nocturnal arousals associated with screaming, walking, or confusion have been reported. These sleep disturbances may have multiple causes. Trouble initiating sleep may be related to hyperactivity or medications used to treat hyperactivity. Anxiety, depression, seizure disorders, or abnormalities of circadian rhythm have also been associated with delayed sleep onset.

Although disorders of arousal and behavioral noncompliance may also be factors, one must also consider other medically based disorders. It is known, for example, that GE reflux can contribute to nighttime awakenings in infants as well as older children (Buie, unpublished data). Loud snoring and daytime mouth breathing may suggest enlarged tonsils and/or adenoids as possible factors (Owens et al., 2000). Further, both obstructive and sleep apneas have also been reported in some cases. Given that there is increasing evidence that poor quality and quantity of sleep can have a negative effect on daytime behavior and functioning (Malow et al., 2006), it is important to accurately diagnose and treat reported sleep disruptions in individuals with ASDs.

Metabolic Disorders

Metabolic disorders are considered a rarity among patients with neurodevelopmental disorders, a reported diagnostic yield after initial evaluation varying from 1% to 2.5% (van Karnebeck et al., 2005). Although rare, the effect of correct diagnosis and treatment of a metabolic disorder may have a substantial effect on the patient's developmental outcome. Engbers et al. (2008) performed repeated metabolic studies on a series of 433 subjects with neurodevelopmental disorders whose initial metabolic assessments were said to be normal and identified 12 metabolic diseases (2.8%), some of which were treatable. The prevalence of metabolic disorders in ASDs remains as yet largely unknown with the level of frequency no doubt varying with the specific disorder.

Smith-Lemli-Opitz Syndrome (SLOS) is one of the more common metabolic disorders associated with clinical features of autism (Bukelis et al., 2007). SLOS is an autosomal recessive disorder associated with an inborn error of cholesterol synthesis caused by mutations of the 7-dehydrocholesterol reductase gene (DHCR7) located on chromosome 11q12-13 (Kelley et al., 2001). Cholesterol is essential for neuroactive steroid production, growth of myelin membranes, and normal embryonic and fetal development. It is also believed to modulate oxytocin receptors, ligand activity, and G-protein coupling of the serotonin-1A receptor (Aneia & Tierney, 2008). It has been hypothesized that a deficit in cholesterol may disrupt these biological mechanisms, thereby contributing to clinical features of ASDs as observed in SLOS. The syndrome has an estimated incidence of 1 in 20,000 to 1 in 60,000 births and a carrier frequency of about 1%. Clinical characteristics include developmental delay, facial anomalies (ptosis, upturned nares, small chin, bitemporal narrowing, and microcephaly), and abnormal webbing between the second and third toes. Additional symptoms can include irritability, hyperactivity, self-injury, temper tantrums, and aggression. In mild cases, the physical features may not be readily recognizable. It has been estimated that approximately 50% to 75% of individuals with SLOS may meet criteria for autism. A clinical diagnosis of SLOS can be confirmed by means of biochemical analysis, an elevated level of plasma 7-dehydrocholesterol relative to the cholesterol level establishing the diagnosis. This disorder is not only identifiable but partially treatable with cholesterol supplementation, thus increasing the importance of syndrome recognition.

A number of studies and case reports have suggested that mitochondrial disorders may be a causative factor in a subset of autistic individuals. In 2005, Oliveira et al. published a population-based survey among school-aged children with ASDs and found that 7% of those who underwent a complete metabolic evaluation were diagnosed with a mitochondrial respiratory chain disorder. Further, this group reported that the affected children were clinically indistinguishable from children suffering from ASDs without a mitochondrial dysfunction. More recently, however, Weissman et al. (2008) reported their findings on 25 ASD subjects with biopsy-proven mitochondrial disorder and found that a series of "clinical red flags" could distinguish the affected children from those with idiopathic ASD. These "red flag" characteristics included the involvement of at least one non-neurological organ system, significant gross motor delays, easy fatigability, and repeated regressions after age 3 years. Further, they noted a nearly even distribution between males and females. The authors concluded that with careful clinical and biochemical assessments, children with the co-occurrence of ASDs and mitochondrial dysfunction could be distinguished from those with idiopathic ASDs and that those affected with mitochondrial disorders may represent a significant subset of individuals with autism.

Osteoporosis

Decreased bone mineralization and osteoporosis, once believed to be health issues found in the elderly, is now being recognized with increasing frequency in younger populations, including in childhood. This process is driven to a large extent by nutritional status, calcium, and vitamin D intake (Lehtonen-Veromaa, 2002; Foo et al., 2009; Davies et al, 2005). Thus, conditions associated with poor nutrition during childhood and adolescence, a critical period for bone mass accumulation, may significantly impact on the attainment of healthy peak bone mass. Gastrointestinal disorders appear to be prevalent among children with ASDs and may be more common in this population than among typically developing children (Valicenti-McDermott et al., 2006). Those with ASDs often demonstrate unusual eating patterns, frequently self-initiated, or may be placed on restrictive therapeutic or complementary alternative diets that limit the intake of calcium and vitamin D, the most common being the casein- and/or gluten-free diet. Additional factors may include impaired growth hormone secretion (Ragusa, 1993), low muscle tone (Ming, 2007), limited exercise (Pan, 2008), anticonvulsant medications (Chou et al, 2007; Pack et al., 2008), and the use of psychotropic or stimulant medications to control behaviors that may impact hormonal function, weight gain, and caloric intake (Bostwick et al., 2009; Ziere et al., 2008). Thus, although ASD individuals often have one or more of these well-documented risk factors, there are very few studies that have assessed the impact of any or all of these factors on bone density in ASD. A recent report of decreased cortical bone thickness in ASD children suggests that individuals with autism may be at high risk for the development of osteoporosis (Hediger et al., 2008). Given the potential risk of injury and fractures, as well as general health issues related to under-nutrition in this population, more research is needed.

Obesity

New evidence suggests that children with chronic conditions may be predisposed to being overweight and to obesity. In a recent study, Chen et al. (2009) analyzed reported height, weight, and body mass index (BMI) from 46,707 subjects, ages 10 to 17 years, with the goal of measuring the prevalence of obesity adjusted for demographic and socioeconomic factors. Obesity was defined as 95% or more of the sex-specific BMI for age growth charts. The prevalence of obesity among those without a chronic condition was 12.2%. Among those subjects with chronic conditions, the prevalence of obesity was highest among children with autism (23.4%), followed by those with asthma (19.7%), learning disabilities (19.3%), attention deficit/hyperactivity disorder (18.9%), and hearing/vision conditions (18.4%). The rising rate of obesity in the general population has been attributed to greater nutritional accessibility and more sedentary lifestyles. Although the causes of obesity are recognized to be heterogeneous, environmental and genetic factors have become the focus of intensive research. Numerous national studies have suggested that exposure to television is associated with obesity, lipid disturbances, and poor cardiovascular health during adulthood (Gortmaker et al., 1996; Robinson, 1999). The explanation for this correlation is the concept that television promotes significant lifestyle changes related to an imbalance of caloric intake and expenditure (Coon & Tucker, 2002). Medications that many children, adolescents, and adults with ASDs receive to control seizures, such as valproic acid (Verrotti et al., 2002), or disruptive behavior, such as risperidone (Saddichha et al., 2007), have been associated with excessive weight gain in some cases and may therefore also be contributing factors.

Earlier studies have found similar statistics. For example, a sample of 140 Japanese children with ASDs, ages 7 to 18 years, revealed that 25% were classified as obese (Sugiyama, 1991). In a somewhat later study involving 20,031 children with mental retardation, ages 6 to 17 years, 413 of whom were children with autism, Takeuchi (1994) found the prevalence of obesity to be 22% in boys and 11% in girls. Curtin et al. (2005) more recently reported similar findings in which the overall prevalence for at-risk-for-overweight was 35.7%, and for overweight was 19% among children with ASD. When the data were stratified by age, the prevalence for at-risk-for-overweight and overweight appeared to be highest in the 12- to 17.9-year age group. These observations were echoed in a similar study of 380 boys and 49 girls with autistic disorder. However, the authors noted that at-risk-for-overweight/overweight in autistic children had no relationship to the core features of the disorder and that older age was a predictor of lower height and at-risk-for-overweight among these children (Xiong et al., 2005).

It is well-known that children with autism have different dietary patterns and lifestyles when compared to typically developing children. These factors can affect body growth and nutritional conditions. Although many reports have been directed toward the concern for obesity in ASDs, some studies have reported a tendency toward being underweight among children with autism and Asperger's Syndrome, often associated with delayed physical growth, and generally attributed to low appetite, narrow range of food choices, and digestive disorders (Bolte et al., 2002; Hebebrand et al., 1997; Lesinskiene et al., 2002). Thus, there is significant concern regarding diet, nutrition, physical activity, and therapeutic interventions, which—either separately or in combination—may contribute to serious health-related issues such as diabetes, hypertension, hyperlipidemia, anemia, and osteopenia, to name a few. The role played by potential genetic and environmental factors interacting with dietary and therapeutic approaches will be important topics for future research.

Hearing Impairment

Many children with autism present initially with delays in expressive and receptive language and it is not unusual for a parent to comment that they wondered whether their child might be deaf. Thus, the assessment of auditory abilities in children with ASDs is important in the diagnosis and treatment of this disorder. A small number of studies have investigated the prevalence of hearing impairment within the ASD population. In a study of 199 children with ASDs and adolescents who were audiologically evaluated, mild-to-moderate hearing loss was identified in 7.9% and unilateral hearing loss in 1.6% (Rosenhall et al., 1999). In this same study, profound bilateral hearing loss or deafness was found in 3.5% of all cases. These findings represent a prevalence significantly higher than that observed in the general population and was comparable to that found among individuals with mental retardation. Further, hearing deficits among the ASD subjects occurred at similar rates, regardless of intellectual functioning. Of additional note is the fact that hyperacusis was found in 18.3% of the autism group as compared to 0% in the non-autism comparison group. Similarly, the rate of serous otitis media was found in 23.5% of ASD subjects with a related conductive hearing loss noted in 18.3%, both of which appeared to be increased in persons with autism. Similar concerns have been raised by the more recent study of Tas et al., (2007), raising the suspicion that hearing loss may be more common in children with autism than in typically developing children.

Gynecological Dysfunction in Adolescence

One of the many medical conditions that has not yet been well-studied relates to the potential effects of hormonal imbalance, especially during adolescence, which could be associated with precocious puberty, accelerated or reduced physical growth, and/or behavioral disruptions associated with menstrual pain or discomfort. These factors have been raised in a study published by Carr et al. in 2003, in which both physical discomfort and pain associated with the menstrual cycle were cited as possible causes of problem behaviors in adolescence. The authors, however, also raised the possibility that fluctuations in progesterone and estrogen levels might also be an important variable. This theme has been further expanded in a more recent study in which adolescent girls with autism, Down syndrome, and cerebral palsy were evaluated retrospectively regarding gynecological complaints. Girls with autism were significantly more likely to present with behavioral issues than the other two groups. Management included the use of non-steroidal anti-inflammatory drugs, oral contraceptives, and education (Burke et al., 2009). Further studies are needed in this important area to provide correct diagnoses and appropriate interventions.

Conclusion

Routine medical conditions frequently seen in typically developing individuals, as well as their behavioral implications, have yet to be fully investigated in children, adolescents, and adults with autism (Gilberg, this volume). The frequency and presence of recurrent ear infections, sinusitis, asthma, hypertrophied tonsils and adenoids, urinary tract infections, spastic bladder that be associated with new onset incontinence at any age, attention deficit disorder, disordered sensory processing, allergies, or any other medical condition commonly seen have yet to be carefully considered in autism. These conditions may not always present with the typical signs and symptoms that most physicians have been taught to recognize but should be considered in ASD individuals at any age who present with unexplained and/or changes in behavior. Defining and treating these medical conditions can improve quality of life for the patient as well as his or her family and can be associated with improved developmental gains as the result of better physical health. Further, there is a growing sense that at least in a subset of affected individuals, ASD may involve multiple organ systems. Thus, understanding the biological mechanisms associated with these other organ systems, in addition to expanding our knowledge about the brain in persons with autism, could potentially expand our knowledge and provide insights into the underlying neurobiology of the disorder.

Much progress has been made in the identification and treatment of persons with ASDs, as well as our understanding of the etiologic and biological mechanisms that are or can be associated with the disorder. However, much remains to be unraveled and many questions remain unanswered. With advancing technology and improved medical and diagnostic assessments of those affected with ASDs and their families, it is hoped that diagnoses can be made earlier—potentially at or before birth—and that more effective therapies and interventions will become possible to improve the lives of those affected with autism.

Challenges and Future Directions

- Children, adolescents, and adults with ASDs may not present with the typical signs and symptoms easily recognized by most health-care professionals.
- ASD individuals who present with challenging behaviors such as aggression and self-injury, especially if they are nonverbal, should be evaluated for an underlying medical condition, before assuming that these disruptions are "just behavioral" or "just part of the autism."
- Health-care professionals and caregivers need to learn the signs and symptoms of pain and discomfort in nonverbal or hypo-verbal, sensory-impaired persons with ASDs.
- Some comorbid medical conditions may have genetic and biologic implications that may provide insight into some of the underlying mechanisms related to etiology and phenotypic expression of ASDs and could potentially aide in defining some treatment modalities in the future.

SUGGESTED READINGS:

Buie, T., Campbell, D. B., Fuchs, G. J., et al. (2010). Evaluation, diagnosis and treatment of gastrointestinal disorders in individuals with ASDs: A consensus report. *Pediatrics* (Suppl), *125*, S1–S18.

Coury, D. (2010). Medical treatment of autism spectrum disorders. *Current Opinion in Neurology*, *23*, 131–136.

Oliveira, G., Diogo, L., Grazina, M., et al. (2005). Mitochondrial dysfunction in autism spectrum disorders: A population study. *Developmental Medicine and Child Neurology*, *47*, 185–189.

REFERENCES:

American Psychiatric Association. (1994). *Diagnostic and statistical manual of mental disorders* (4th ed.; DSM-IV). Washington, DC: APA.

Aneia, A., & Tierney, E. (2008). Autism: The role of cholesterol in treatment. *International Review of Psychiatry*, *20*, 165–170.

Bailey, A., Le Couteur, A., Gottesman, I., & Bolton, P. (1995). Autism is a strongly genetic disorder: Evidence from a British twin study. *Psychological Medicine, 25*, 63–77.

Bazar, K. A., Yun, A. J., Lee, P. Y., Daniel, S. M., & Doux, J. D. (2005). Obesity and ADHD may represent different manifestations of a common environmental oversampling syndrome: A model for revealing mechanistic overlap among cognitive, metabolic and inflammatory disorders. *Medical Hypotheses, 66*, 263–269.

Bolte, N., Ozkara, N., & Poustka, F. (2002). Autism spectrum disorders and low body weight: Is there really a systematic association? *International Journal of Eating Disorders, 31*, 349–351.

Bolton, P., MacDonald, H., Pickles, A., Rios, P. et al. (1994). A case-controlled family history study of autism. *Journal of Child Psychology and Psychiatry and Allied Disciplines, 35*, 877–900.

Bostwick, J. R., Guthrie, S. K., & Ellingrod, V. L. (2009). Antipsychotic-induced hyperprolactinemia. *Pharmacotherapy, 29*, 64–73.

Bukelis, I., Porter, F. D., Zimmerman, A. W., & Tierney, E. (2007). Smith-Lemli-Opitz syndrome and autism spectrum disorder. *American Journal of Psychiatry, 164*, 1655–1661.

Burke, L. M., Kalpakjian, C. Z., Smith, Y. R., & Quint, E. H. (2009). Gynecological Issues of adolescents with Down syndrome, autism and cerebral palsy. *Journal of Pediatric and Adolescent Gynecology*, Epub ahead of print. July 28.

Buie, T. M. (2005). Gastrointestinal issues encountered in autism. In: Bauman, M. L. and Kemper, T. L., eds. *The neurobiology of autism* (pp. 103–117). Baltimore: Johns Hopkins University Press.

Campbell, D. B., Sutcliffe, J. S., Ebert, P. J., Militerni, R., Bravaccio, C., & Trillo, S., et al. (2006). A genetic variant that disrupts MET transcription is associated with autism. *Proceedings of the National Academy of Sciences of the United States of America, 103*, 16,834–16,839.

Campbell, D. B., D'Oronzio, R., Garbett, K., Ebert, P. J., Mirnics, K., Levitt, P., et al. (2007). Disruption of cerebral cortex MET signaling in autism spectrum disorder. *Annals of Neurology, 62*, 243–250.

Campbell, D. B., Buie, T. M., Winter, H., Bauman, M. L., Sutcliffe, J. S., Perrin, J. M., et al. (2009). Distinct genetic risk based on association of MET in families with co-occurring autism and gastrointestinal conditions. *Pediatrics, 123*, 1018–1024.

Carr, E. G., & Owen-DeSchryver, J. S. (2007). Physical illness, pain, and problem behavior in minimally verbal people with developmental disabilities. *Journal of Autism and Developmental Disorders, 37*, 413–424.

Carr, E. G., Smith, C. E., Glacin, T. A., Whelan, B. M., & Pancari, J. (2003). Menstrual discomfort as a biological setting event for severe problem behavior: Assessment and intervention. *American Journal of Mental Retardation, 108*, 117–133.

Chen, A. Y., Kim, S. E., Houtrow, A. J., & Newacheck, P. W. (2009). Prevalence of obesity among children with chronic conditions. *Obesity, 10*, 185.

Chou, I. J., Lin, K. L., Wang, H. S., & Wang, C. I. (2007). Evaluation of bone mineral density in children receiving carbamazepine or valproate monotherapy. *Acta Paediatrica Taiwanica, 48*, 317–322.

Cook, E. H. (2001). Genetics of Autism. *Child and Adolescent Psychiatric Clinics of North America, 10*, 333–350.

Coon, K. A., & Tucker, K. L. (2002). Television and children's consumption patterns: A review of the literature. *Minerva Pediatrica, 54*, 430–436.

Cooper, S. (1998). Clinical study of the effects of age on the physical health of adults with mental retardation. *American Journal of Mental Retardation, 102*, 582–589.

Curtin, C., Bandini, L. G., Perrin, E. C., Tyboi, D. J., & Must, A. (2005). Prevalence of overweight in children and adolescents with attention deficit hyperactivity disorder and autism spectrum disorders: A chart review. *BMC Pediatrics, 5*, 48–58.

Davies, J. H., Evans, B. A., & Gregory, J. W. (2005). Bone mass acquisition in healthy children. *Archives of Disease in Childhood, 90*, 373–378.

Durkin, M. S., Maenner, M. J., Newschaffer, C. J., Lee, L. C., Cunniff, C. M., Daniels, J. L., et al. (2008). Advanced parental age and the risk of Autism Spectrum Disorder. *American Journal of Epidemiology, 168*, 1268–1276.

Engbers, H. M., Berger, R., van Hasselt, P., de Koning, T., de Sain-van der Velden, M. G., Kroes, H. Y., et al. (2008). Yield of additional metabolic studies in neurodevelopmental disorders. *Annals of Neurology, 64*, 212–217.

Ferber, R. (1996). Childhood sleep disorders. *Neurologic Clinics, 14*, 493–511.

Filipek, P. A., Accardo, P. J., Baranek, G. T., Cook, E. H., Dawson, G., Gordon, B., et al. (1999). The screening and diagnosis of autistic spectrum disorders, *Journal of Child Psychology and Psychiatry, and Allied Disciplines, 29*, 439–484.

Folstein, S. E., & Rutter, M. (1977). Infantile autism: A genetic study of 21 twin pairs. *Journal of Child Psychology and Psychiatry, 18*, 297–321.

Foo, L. H., Zhang, Q., Zhu, K., Ma, G., Hu, X., Greenfield, H., & Fraser, D. R. (2009). Low vitamin D status has an adverse influence on bone mass, bone turnover, and muscle strength in Chinese adolescent girls. *Journal of Nutrition, 139*, 1002–1007.

Ghaziuddin, M., Elkins, T. E., McNeeley, S. G., & Ghaziuddin, N. (1993). Premenstrual syndrome in women with mental handicap: A pilot study. *British Journal of Developmental Disabilities, 77*, 104–107.

Gidley Larson, J. C., & Mostofsky, S. H. (2006). Motor deficits in autism. In R. Tuchman, I. Rapin, Eds. *Autism: A neurological disorder of early brain development*. London: MacKeith Press.

Gidley Larson, J. C., Bastian, A. J., Donchin, O., Shadmehr, R., & Mostofsky, S. H. (2008). Acquisition of internal models of motor tasks in children with autism. *Brain, 131*, 2894–2903.

Gortmaker, S. L., Must, A., Sobol, A. M., Peterson, K., Colditz, G. A., & Dietz, W. H. (1996). Television viewing as a cause of increasing obesity among children in the United States, 1986–1990. *Archives of Pediatrics and Adolescent Medicine, 150*, 356–362.

Gunsett, R. P., Mulick, J. A., Fernald, W. B., & Martin, J. L. (1989). Brief report: Indications for medical screening prior to behavioral programming for severely and profoundly mentally retarded clients. *Journal of Autism and Developmental Disorders, 19*, 167–172.

Hart, H., Bas, M., & Jenkins., S. (1984). Health and behavior in preschool children. *Child: Care, Health, and Development, 10*, 1–16.

Hebebrand, J., Hennighausen, S., Nau, S., Himmelmann, G. W., Schulz, E., Schafer, H., et al. (1997). Low body weight in male children and adolescents with schizoid personality disorder or Asperger's disorder. *Acta Psychiatrica Scandinavica, 96*, 64–67.

Hediger, M. L., England, L. J., Molloy, C. A., Yu, K. F., Manning-Courtney, P., & Mills, J. L. (2008). Reduced bone cortical thickness in boys with autism or autism spectrum disorder. *Journal of Autism and Developmental Disorders, 38*, 848–856.

Horner, R. H., Vaughn, B. J., Day, H. M., & Ard, W. R., Jr. (1996). The relationship between setting events and problem behavior. In L. K. Koegel, R. L. Koegel and G. Dunlap, Eds. *Positive behavioral support* (pp. 381–402). Baltimore: Brooks.

Horner, R. H., Carr, E. G., Strain, P. S., Todd, A. W., & Reed, H. K. (2002). Problem behavior interventions for young children with autism: A research synthesis. *Journal of Autism and Developmental Disorders, 32*, 423–446.

Horvath, K., Papadimitriou, J. C., Rabsztyn, A., Drachenberg, C., & Tilton, J. T. (1999). Gastrointestinal abnormalities in children with autistic disorder. *Journal of Pediatrics, 135*, 559–563.

Kanner, L. (1943). Autistic disturbances of affective contact. *Nervous Child, 2*, 217–250.

Kelley, R. I., & Hennekam, R. C. H. (2001). Smith-Lemli-Opitz syndrome. In Scriver, C. R., Beaudet, A. L., Valle, D., and Sly, W. S. Eds. *The metabolic and molecular basis of inherited disease* (8th ed., pp. 6183–6201). New York: McGraw-Hill.

Kennedy, C. H., & Meyer, K. A. (1996). Sleep deprivation, allergy symptoms, and negatively reinforced problem behavior. *Journal of Applied Behavioral Analysis, 29*, 133–135.

Kennedy, C. H., & Thompson, T. (2000). Health conditions contributing to problem behavior among people with mental retardation and developmental disabilities. In P. Wehmeyer & J. R. Patton, Eds. *Mental retardation in the 21st century* (pp. 211–231.) Austin, TX: ProEd.

Kogan, M. D., Strickland, B. B., Blumberg, S. J., Singh, G. K., Perrin, J, M., & van Dyck, P. C. (2008). A national profile of health care experiences and family impact of autism spectrum disorder among children in the United States, 2005-2006. *Pediatrics, 122*, 1149–1158.

Kuehn, B. M. (2007). CDC: Autism spectrum disorder common. *Journal of the American Medical Association, 297*, 940.

Lainhart, J. E., Bigler, E. D., Bocian, M., Coon, H., Dinh, E., Dawson, G., et al. (2006). *American Journal of Medical Genetics. Part A, 140*, 2257–2274.

Landa, R. J. & Garrett-Mayer, E. (2006). Development of infants with autism spectrum disorders: A prospective study. *Journal of Child Psychology and Psychiatry and Allied Disciplines, 47*, 629–638.

Landa, R. J. (2008). Diagnosis of autism spectrum disorders in the first 3 years of life. *Nature Clinical Practice Neurology, 4*, 138–147.

Lauritsen, M. B., Pedersen, C. B., & Mortensen, P. B. (2005). Effects of familial risk factors and place of birth on the risk of autism: A nationwide register-based study. *Journal of Child Psychology and Psychiatry and Allied Disciplines, 46*, 963–971.

Lehtonen-Veromaa, M. K., Mottonen, T. T., Nuotio, I. O., Irjala, K. M., Leino, A. E., & Virkari, J. S. (2002). Vitamin D and attainment of peak bone mass among peripubertal Finnish girls: A 3-year prospective study. *American Journal of Clinical Nutrition, 76*, 1446–1453.

Lekkas, C. N., & Lentino, W. (1978). Symptom-producing interposition of the colon: Clinical syndrome in mentally deficient adults. *Journal of the American Medical Association, 240*, 747–750.

Lesinskiene, S., Vilunaite, E., & Paskeviciute, B. (2002). Aspects of the development of autistic children. *Medicina (Kaunas), 38*, 405–411.

Lissovoy, V. (1962). Head banging in early childhood. *Child Development, 33*, 43–56.

Malow, B. A., Marzec, M. L., McGrew, S. G., Wang, L., Henderson, L. M., & Stone, W. I. (2006). Characterizing sleep in children with autism spectrum disorders: A multidimensional approach. *Sleep, 28*, 1559–1567.

Ming, X., Brimacombe, M., & Wagner, G. C. (2007). Prevalence of motor impairment in autism spectrum disorders. *Brain and Development 29*, 565–570.

Minshew, N. J., Sweeney, J. A., & Bauman, M. L. (1997). Neurologic aspects of autism. In D. J. Cohen and F. R. Volkmar, Eds. *Handbook of autism and pervasive developmental disorders* (2nd ed., pp. 344–369), New York: Wiley.

Mostofsky, S., Dubey, P., Jerath, V. K., Jansiewicz, E. M., Goldberg, M. C., & Denkla, M. B. (2006). Developmental dyspraxia is not limited to imitation in children with autism spectrum disorders. *Journal of the International Neuropsychological Society, 6*, 314–326.

Newschaffer, C. J., Croen, L. A., Daniels, J., Giarelli, E., Grether, J. K., Levy, S. E., et al. (2007). *Annual Review of Public Health, 28*, 235–258.

Owens, J., Opipari, L., Nobile, C., & Spirito, A. (1998). Sleep and daytime behavior in children with obstructive apnea and behavioral sleep disorders. *Pediatrics, 102*, 1178–1184.

Owens, L. M., Spirito, A., McGuinn, M., & Nobile, C. (2000). Sleep habits and sleep disturbance in elementary school-aged children. *Journal of Developmental and Behavioral Pediatrics, 21*, 27–36.

Pack, A. M., Morrell, M. I., Randall, A., McMahon, D. I., & Shane, E. (2008). Bone health in young women with epilepsy after one year of antiepileptic drug monotherapy. *Neurology, 70*, 1586–1593.

Pan, C. Y. (2008). Objectively measured physical activity between children with autism spectrum disorders and children without disabilities during inclusive recess settings in Taiwan. *Journal of Autism and Developmental Disorders, 38*, 1292–1301.

Peine, H. A., Rokneddin, D., Adams, K., Blakelock, H., Jenson, W., & Osborne, J. G. (1995). Medical problems, maladaptive behaviors and the developmentally disabled. *Behavioral Interventions, 10*, 149–159.

Quigley, F. M., & Hurley, D. (2000). Autism and the gastrointestinal tract. *American Journal of Gastroenterology, 95*, 2154–2156.

Ragusa, L., Elia, M., & Scifo, R. (1993). Growth hormone deficit in autism. *Journal of Autism and Developmental Disorders, 23*, 421–422.

Rapin, I. & Katzman, R. (1998). Neurobiology of Autism. *Annals of Neurology, 43*, 7–14.

Rapin, I. (1996). Historical data. In I. Rapin, Ed. *Preschool children with inadequate communication: Developmental language disorder, autism, low IQ* (pp. 98–122). London: MacKeith.

Richdale, A. L. (1999). Sleep problems in autism: Prevalence, cause and intervention. *Developmental Medicine and Child Neurology 41*, 60–66.

Robinson, T. N. (1999). Reducing children's television viewing to prevent obesity: A randomized controlled trial. *Journal of the American Medical Association, 282*, 1561–1563.

Rogers, S., Bennetto, L., McEvoy, R., & Pennington, B. (1996). Imitation and pantomime in high-functioning adolescents with autism spectrum disorders. *Child Development, 67*, 2060–2073.

Rosenhall, U., Nordin, V., Sandstrom, M., Ahisen, G., & Gillberg, C. (1999). Autism and hearing loss. *Journal of Autism and Developmental Disorders, 29*, 349–357.

Saddichha, S., Manjunatha, N., Ameen, S., & Akhtar, S. (2007). Effect of olanzapine, risperidone and haloperidol treatment on weight and body mass index in first-episode schizophrenia patients in India: A randomized, double–blind. Controlled, prospective study. *Journal of Clinical Psychiatry, 68*, 1793–1798.

Schaefer, G. B., & Mendelsohn, N. J. (2008). Genetic evaluation for the etiologic diagnosis of Autism Spectrum Disorder. *Genetics in Medicine, 10*, 4–12.

Spence, S. J. (2004). The genetics of autism. *Seminars in Pediatric Neurology, 11*, 196–204.

Sugiyama, T. (1991). A research of obesity in autism. *Japanese Journal on Developmental Disabilities, 13*, 53–58.

Takeuchi, E. (1994). Incidence of obesity among school children with mental retardation in Japan. *American Journal of Mental Retardation, 99*, 283–288.

Tas, A., Yagiz, R., Tas, M., Esme, M., Uzun, C., & Karasalihoglu, A. R. (2007). Evaluation of hearing in children with autism by using TEOAE and ABR. *Autism, 11*, 73–79.

Taylor, D. V., Rush, D., Hetrick, W. P., & Sandman, C. A. (1993). Self-injurious behavior within the menstrual cycle of women with mental retardation. *American Journal of Mental Retardation, 97*, 659–664.

Tuchman, R. F., Rapin, I., and Shinnar, S. (1999). Autistic and dysphasic children. II: Epilepsy. *Pediatrics, 88*, 1219–1225.

Valicenti-McDermott, M., McVicar, K., Rapin, I., Weshill, B. K., Cohen, H., & Shinnar, S. (2006). Frequency of gastrointestinal symptoms in children with autistic spectrum disorders. *Biological Psychiatry, 61*, 492–497.

Verrotti, A., Basciani, F., De Simone, M., Trotta, D., Morgese, G., & Chiarelli, F. (2003). Insulin resistence in epileptic girls who gain weight after therapy with valproic acid. *Journal of Child Neurology, 17*, 265–268.

Volkmar, F. R. & Nelson, D. S. (1990). Seizure disorders in autism. *Journal of the American Academy of Child and Adolescent Psychiatry, 29*, 127–129.

Von Karnebeck, C. D., Jansweijer, M. C., Leenders, A. G., et al. (2005). Diagnostic investigations in individuals with mental retardation: A systematic literature review of their usefulness. *European Journal of Human Genetics, 13*, 6–25.

Weissman, J. R., Kelley, R. I., Bauman, M. L., Cohen, B. H., Murray, K. F., Mitchell, R. L., et al. (2008). Mitochondrial disease in autism spectrum disorder patients: A cohort analysis. *PLoS ONE*, Epub. *3*, e3815.

Xiong, N., Chengye, J., Yong, L., Zhonghu, H., Hongli, B., & Yufeng, Z. (2007). The physical status of children with autism in China. *Research in Developmental Disabilities, 30*, 70–76.

Ziere, G., Dieleman, J. P., van der Cammen, T. J., Hofmann, A., Pols, H. A., & Stricker, B. H. (2008). Selective serotonin reuptake inhibiting antidepressants are associated with an increased risk of non-vertebral fractures. *Journal of Clinical Psychopharmacology, 28*, 411–417.

71 Susan L. Hyman, Susan E. Levy

Dietary, Complementary, and Alternative Therapies

Points of Interest

- Complementary and alternative therapies are used by up to three-fourths of families for their children with ASDs. Up to half of children with ASDs take nutritional supplements and up to one-third use dietary therapies.
- Mind–body therapies like yoga may have an effect on regulating anxiety; music therapy might have a role in encouraging language.
- Biologically based therapies are based on hypotheses related to atypical oxidative stress, gastrointestinal dysbiosis, immunologic dysfunction, and removal of environmental toxins. The potential for side effects of biologic therapies have not been adequately studied.
- Manipulation and body-based therapies like chiropractic are popular, although there are not data to support effectiveness for symptoms of ASDs. The use of massage has been associated with subjective benefits but has not been adequately studied.
- Energy medicine therapies like Qi Gong are being studied for use for symptoms of ASDs.

Although the goal of interventions for autism are to target core and/or concurrent symptoms, conventional medical, psychological, and educational practice have evidence to support their ability to ameliorate only some of the core and concurrent symptoms. The only prescription medications with a package insert with indication for autism treatment are risperidone and apiprazole. Although the effect size for treatment is large, risperidone addresses irritability and not the core symptoms of autism spectrum disorder (ASD) (Scahill et al., 2007). Similarly, conventional educational and behavioral interventions such as early intensive behavioral intervention (Lovaas, 1993) result in improvements by teaching skills but do not address underlying biologic differences. It is not surprising that families of children with ASDs have become increasingly interested in therapies outside conventional treatments to attempt to symptomatically improve, or even cure, their child with ASD.

Complementary and Alternative Medicine Use in Children with Autism Spectrum Disorders

The National Center for Complementary and Alternative Medicine defines complementary and alternative medicine (CAM) as "... a group of diverse medical and health care systems, practices, and products that are not presently considered to be part of conventional medicine." Complementary refers to the use of novel therapies together with conventional medicine. The term *alternative* refers to interventions used in place of conventional practice. Most families of children with ASDs utilize multiple therapeutic approaches simultaneously (Levy & Hyman, 2008). National health information survey statistics (Barnes, 2004) indicate that 20% to 38% of adults and 11% to 21% of children in the United States use CAM therapies. If prayer is included, the overall rate of CAM use in adults increases to 62%. The rates of general CAM use are increasing with availability of information on the internet (V. A. Green et al., 2006) and a culture of increasing participation in medical care decision making (Levy & Hyman, 2008). In 1994, 11% of children were reported to have used CAM (Spigelblatt et al., 1994). By 2003, 45% of children taken for emergency department care had used CAM (Lanski et al., 2003). Little is known, however, of harm that might come from the use of nutritional supplements or other CAM therapies because adverse event reporting is not mandated for products regulated as foods in the case of supplements and not regulated at all for other types of interventions.

Complementary or alternative treatment use is higher among people with chronic illnesses and special health-care needs. Surveys of parents of children with ASDs suggest that reasons for CAM use are similar among families of children with ASDs (Hanson et al., 2007; Wong & Smith, 2006). A survey of CAM use in different chronic disorders reported rates of 9% to 70% (Ernst, 1999). Families of children with ASDs attending a specialized clinic for ASD reported rates of 30% to 70% (Hanson et al., 2007; Levy et al., 2003) The reasons given for pursuing therapies outside of the conventional medical and educational recommendations included fear of side effects (of standard medication treatments), perception of CAM treatments as "natural," hope for cure, belief in theories of disease causation that differ from conventional medicine, and the desire to participate in the choice of therapies (Levy & Hyman, 2008). An internet survey of 552 families of children with ASDs reported an average of seven different treatments, with 27% using a special diet and 43% treating their child with supplements (V. A. Green et al., 2006) CAM use has become so widely used that at one clinic, almost one-third of families had instituted nutritional or other CAM interventions purported to aide symptoms of ASDs before the time of official diagnostic evaluation (Levy et al., 2003).

Reasons Families Pursue *Complementary and Alternative Medicine* Therapies

Although genetic factors are important to the etiology of ASDs, there is increasing evidence that environmental factors may either interact with a genetic predisposition or independently lead to symptoms of ASDs (Bello, 2007). Extrapolation of this line of scientific reasoning leads many proponents of CAM to therapies that purport to remove environmental toxins or modify the effect of environmental agents. Another reason CAM therapies have attained popularity is the slow and tedious progress that may accompany traditional educational approaches and the stepwise approach scientists demand to demonstrate effectiveness of interventions. The symptoms of ASDs change over time with developmental progress and are heterogeneous, so it is often difficult to attribute change to any specific intervention or interventions in clinical practice. It may be difficult to determine which intervention, if any, resulted in perceived improvements. In addition, CAM therapies are perceived as safe by their proponents. This belief is promulgated because many interventions are nonprescription (and thus unregulated by the FDA), are perceived as having an absence of side effects or involve manipulation, or other nonbiologic interventions that many people would see as having no potential for adverse effects. A fourth factor supporting CAM use is the desire by families for more control over treatment choice. Choosing treatment options empowers the family at a time that they may feel that they have little control over the course of their child's diagnosis, treatment, or course. Professionals who counsel families about treatments and the future outcome may be pessimistic regarding resolution of the ASDs, and CAM therapies allow families to hope for a cure for their child. CAM therapies for ASDs purport to treat both core symptoms of autism and medical symptoms such as sleep disruption and gastrointestinal distress that families are concerned about. Finally, CAM therapies may be supported and recommended by celebrities and others in the popular press, sometimes using anecdotal testimony, rather than analysis of scientific evidence, to support safety and efficacy. A culture of distrust has evolved where conventional practitioners may be accused of misleading families by not advocating CAM therapies and being dismissive of observations by families regarding the effectiveness of these therapies. Despite (and perhaps because of) this phenomenon, there is an increasing awareness of CAM practices and an increasing number of clinical trials to examine the safety and efficacy of the interventions.

Integrative Medicine, Pluralism, and Agreeing to Disagree

As therapeutic strategies that were initially popularized as complementary and alternative medicine are examined using scientific techniques, they are making their way into conventional practice as integrative medicine. Integrative medicine is defined as relationship-based care that combines conventional and complementary therapies that have scientific evidence of safety and effectiveness to promote health for the child and family (Kemper, Vohra, Walls, the Task Force on Complementary and Alternative, & the Provisional Section on Complementary, 2008). One alternative treatment that has gained the acceptance of conventional medicine and is often covered by insurance is acupuncture for pain management (Sherman et al., 2006). Some interventions popularized as CAM and integrated into conventional practice have been disproven, such as Gingko Biloba for dementia (Birks & Grimley Evans, 2009) and Vitamins C and E for cardiovascular disease prevention (Sesso et al., 2008). Some CAM therapies may actually have harmful effects. A meta-analysis of antioxidant therapy for prevention of gastrointestinal cancers demonstrated that supplementation was not only not helpful but actually increased mortality (Bjelakovic et al., 2008). There is insufficient scientific data to support many currently used and popular CAM therapies related to ASD treatment. There are no long-term data to know how significant alteration in nutrition might affect health in the future. In 2001, the American Academy of Pediatrics published guidelines to support the respectful discussion of therapies that families wish to investigate while keeping the best interests of the safety of the child as the focus of the medical care provider (American Academy of Pediatrics & Committee on Children With Disabilities, 2001). There are contradictory societal presses: support for the role of families in therapeutic decision making and the desire to advocate for the health of the child; the conflict between tolerance of alternative explanations for conventional theories of pathophysiology and the need for evidence-based practice. A pluralist approach allows for the discussion of therapeutic approaches with the understanding that there may not be agreement among scientists, and clinicians supporting evidence-based practices, and proponents of CAM therapies.

How to Evaluate Therapies

The same standard of evidence-based support should apply for all interventions for children with ASDs. Although CAM therapies are often referred to as "unproven," many of the commonly used treatments for symptoms of ASDs also have modest evidence to support their use (Guyatt et al., 2008). Families and primary care providers need to be educated how to evaluate the information that supports any therapeutic intervention they might elect to pursue. Factors to be considered in examining claims for a therapy include study design, whether the sample size was adequate to support the claims, characterization of the participants, use of valid outcome variables, and standardized implementation of the intervention (Guyatt et al., 2008). The use of placebo-controlled study design is important because caregiver observation may be altered unconsciously by the desire for an effect. Although randomized controlled clinical trials may be the most convincing design in evidence-based practice, useful information for hypothesis generation and clinical care can also be obtained from quasi-randomized design, prospective and retrospective cohort studies, open trials, case series, or systematic reviews.

Complementary and Alternative Medicine Therapies for Autism Spectrum Disorders

Examples of CAM used for ASDs will be discussed for each of the four general areas of CAM categorized by NCCAM. Although extensive, this list is not inclusive of all CAM therapies investigated and implemented for the symptoms of ASDs. The text is organized according to conceptual areas within CAM; however, on a practical level, clinicians and families want to know which therapies are safe and which have data to support their use. Table 70-1 summarizes the CAM therapies discussed in this framework based on the current peer-reviewed literature. Some therapies have insufficient evidence to comment on because lack of data is different than data demonstrating lack of effect.

Mind–Body Therapies

This category of treatments includes combinations of treatments that promote health through the interaction between the mind (psychosocial and physiologic factors) and physical symptoms. Some treatments are less structured and may be individually administered (e.g., relaxation or visual imagery), whereas others may require administration or training in a more procedural fashion. Symptoms such as pain, stress, and anxiety may be more amenable to mind–body therapies (MBTs) using techniques that permit relaxation (Astin, 2004). This hypothesis is in need of confirmation in appropriate clinical trials.

Yoga

Yoga encompasses a system of breathing practices, postures, and physical exercises. Specific controlled trials of yoga in children with autism have not been completed, but there are reports of improvement of symptoms of depression (Kemper, Vohra, Walls, the Task Force on Complementary and Alternative, & the Provisional Section on Complementary, 2008) and improved behavior in a small sample of boys with ADHD who participated in yoga sessions who were also treated with medication (Jensen & Kenny, 2004).

Music Therapy

Music therapy may be administered individually or in a group, with the goal of providing an effective medium for nonverbal social exchange. Core features such as eye contact, joint attention, and social reciprocity (e.g., with turn taking) are features of shared music making (Gold, Wigram, & Elefant, 2006). A recent Cochrane review (Gold, Wigram, & Elefant, 2006) included three small studies (*n* between 4 and 10 subjects) of young boys (age 2–9 years) who received individual music therapy and were compared with a comparison group. The studies described improved gestural and verbal communication skills. It is not clear whether the effects on communicative skills can be generalized to functional use. Kim and colleagues (Kim, Wigram, & Gold, 2008) reported a recent study of the effects of improvisational music therapy on joint attention behaviors in 15 children ages 3 to 5 years. The authors reported improved eye contact duration, turn taking and social approach behaviors in the 10 children who completed the study. This is a promising treatment that is often provided in educational settings, about which more research and data are needed. It is plausible that the imitation, repetition, nonverbal cuing, and use of nonlanguage elements of rhythm and music may render this a plausible therapy (Heaton et al., 2007).

Biologically Based Practices

The CAM therapy most commonly reported by parents are biologically based practices. The Interactive Autism Network (IAN, 2009) reports that more than 50% of the families responding to their online survey reported use of nutritional supplements and almost one-third reported the current use of dietary therapies for treatment of symptoms of autism. Many therapies are used simultaneously. Although little is known regarding effectiveness, less is known regarding the potential for side effects or the effect on conventional medication. Practitioners who advocate biologically based therapies often have claims relative to multiple disorders. They increasingly organize the interventions to fit alternative biologic theories of causation. These theories often extend hypothesis beyond the accepted scientific basis on which they are based.

Table 70–1.
CAM therapies

Treatments	Examples	No Risk and/or Proven to be Effective	Little Risk and/or Possible Benefit	Little Risk and/or No Proven Benefit	Moderate Risk and/or Unclear Benefit and/or No Evidence	High Risk and/or No Benefit an/or Proven Ineffective
Biologically Based Practices						
	Diet: GF/CF*			X		
	Secretin					X
	GI** medication			X		
	Vitamin/Supplements					
	B6/magnesium			X		
	DMG			X		
	Vitamin C		X			
	Carnosine		X			
	Omega 3-fatty acids		X			
	Melatonin	X				
	Methylcobalamin			X		
	Folate			X		
	Immune-Mediated					
	Anti-infectives				X	
	Immunoglobulins				X	
	Chelation					X
	HBOT***					X
Manipulative and Body-Based Practices						
	Massage/QiGong			X		
	Auditory integration			X		
	Vagal nerve stimulation				X	
Mind–Body Practices						
	Meditation, yoga			X		
	Music therapy		X			
	Reiki			X		

* GF/CF = gluten free/casein free.
** GI = gastrointestinal.
*** HBOT= hyperbaric oxygen therapy.

Treatments to Decrease Oxidative Stress

Basic to cellular function is the detoxification of oxygen radicals produced when cells use energy in aerobic metabolism. Oxidative phosphorylation in the mitochondria of cells produces reactive oxygen species that the cell must detoxify. If cellular antioxidant functions do not appropriately regulate production of reactive oxygen species and peroxides, damage can occur to DNA regeneration. This can alter gene function or even lead to cell death. Several CAM therapies are promoted to compensate for suggested abnormalities in metabolic pathways related to the regulation of reactive oxygen species. James et al. (S. Jill James et al., 2004; S. J. James et al., 2006) have reported the observation that children with autism have elevated levels of intermediate compounds in the pathway metabolizing S-adenylhomocysteine (SAH) to adenosine and homocysteine. If adenosine is not removed, then it will inhibit methyltransferase reactions necessary for DNA replication and neurotransmitter production. The SAH is formed from methionine. SAH is transulfurated in another pathway to produce cysteine and glutathione, the primary intracellular antioxidant. The observation of abnormal levels of each of these compounds in children with ASDs compared to controls has led to the hypothesis that there is a primary abnormality in metabolic pathways dealing with oxidative stress in children with ASDs. Several biologic interventions advocated as CAM therapies are intended to address this observation. The progression from biochemical observation to evidence-based treatment requires appropriate clinical trials.

Vitamin B_{12}

Cobalamins are important for nucleic acid metabolism, methyl transfer, blood cell formation, and myelin synthesis and repair. The natural sources of methylcobalamin (Vitamin B_{12}) in the diet include dairy products, meat, and eggs. Folinic acid is typically rapidly reduced to tetrahydrofolate and functions as a folic acid derivative. It is often used as a supplement with cancer chemotherapeutic agents that interfere with the enzymes necessary to metabolize other forms of folate. Subcutaneous administration of Vitamin B_{12} (75 micrograms/kg twice weekly) with 400 micrograms of folinic acid twice daily over 3 months has been reported to significantly increase the cysteine, cysteinylglycine, and glutathione concentrations in 40 children with autism while decreasing the oxidized disulfide form of glutathione (S. J. James et al., 2009). The levels of these transmethylation/transsulfuration metabolites and the glutathione redox status were lower in children with ASDs than control children at baseline and, although increased, remained lower than controls after treatment. Based on the initial observation of this finding (S. Jill James et al., 2004; S. J. James et al., 2006), Vitamin B_{12} administered as an injection, nasal spray, or orally is a popular complementary therapy. James et al. (2004) reported subjective improvement in an open trial. However, the preliminary data on 14 subjects in one small double-blind, placebo-controlled crossover clinical trial did not document behavioral improvement using standard outcome measures (Deprey, 2006). Vitamin B_{12} has no published tolerable upper limit, the amount at which side effects are probable. Folinic acid, on the other hand, is available only by prescription at doses greater than 1 mg because of concerns for abdominal distention, nausea, sleep disturbance, irritability, psychomotor excitation, and increased seizure activity. High doses can also mask a B_{12} deficiency. Dietary sources of *folic acid* which is metabolized to tetrahydrafolate, include leafy green vegetables, fruits, and legumes and peas as well as breads and cereals supplemented with folic acid. The biochemical observation of altered oxidative stress intermediates, and improvement in laboratory values with B_{12} and folinic acid supplementation requires replication and further study to determine if there is an observable therapeutic effect.

Vitamin C

In addition to being an antioxidant, Vitamin C has a role in promoting immune function and the intestinal absorption of iron and potentially affects dopamine binding. It has been evaluated as a treatment for symptoms of ASDs in 18 students in a residential school in a double-blind, placebo-controlled crossover trial. At high doses (8 g/70 kg/day), statistically significant improvements in sensorimotor and stereotyped behaviors were demonstrated (Dolske et al., 1993). This observation has not been replicated to date. Side effects at high doses may include gastrointestinal discomfort, acidification of the urine, or possible negative impact on physiologic antioxidant functions.

Hyperbaric Oxygen Therapy

Increasing ambient air pressure at the same time that oxygen concentration is increased (hyperbaric oxygen therapy [HBOT]) is a conventional treatment for carbon monoxide poisoning, divers who ascend too rapidly (the Bends), and to augment wound healing. It has been examined for the treatment of disorders that are associated with prenatal hypoxic brain injury, such as cerebral palsy. A well-designed trial was unable to identify benefit from HBOT compared to a sham procedure in children with cerebral palsy (Collet et al., 2001). The hypothesis that children with ASDs have areas of hypoxic brain injury stems from single proton emission tomography (SPECT) data demonstrating areas of decreased blood flow in individuals with ASDs (Ohnishi et al., 2000). Although there are children with ASDs and cerebral palsy who experienced hypoxic brain injury, hypoxic brain injury is not a cause of idiopathic autism. A secondary hypothesis suggests that there can be an improvement in oxidative stress by upregulation of enzyme systems related to superoxide dismutase and glutathione peroxidase and increased lipid peroxidation with HBOT treatment (Rossignol et al., 2007). Rossignol and colleagues performed an open trial of HBOT with subjective benefit in 18 participants with ASDs who underwent an average of 40 sessions at either 1.5 or 1.3 atmospheres of pressure and either 100% or 24% oxygen (Rossignol et al., 2007). Blood drawn before the first and after the last session did not identify worsening of oxidative stress in terms of plasma oxidized glutathione levels but did note significantly decreased C reactive protein, which might suggest diminished inflammation. The parents subjectively reported improvement. One child needed alteration of the regimen because of ear pain. The risk for seizures appears to be low. Other potential side effects not observed in this trial include stress with the procedure and the risks inherent in isolating an individual in a chamber. Two double-blind, placebo-controlled trials of HBOT in children with ASDs have been completed with conflicting results. Rossignol et al. (2009) reported improvement in analysis of within-group differences of children with ASDs randomized to HBOT or sham therapy. When the groups were compared, there were no differences on the Aberrant Behavior Checklist (Rossignol et al., 2009). Greenspesheh et al. (2009) found no improvement in a study of children, all of whom had ABA therapy, using similar HBOT procedures. They used valid outcome measures that were corroborated by direct observation data (Greenspesheh et al., 2009). Although ear pain, exacerbation of seizures, and anxiety with the procedure appear to be infrequent, a significant side effect of controversial CAM therapies that is particularly relevant for HBOT is cost. A course of 40 sessions can be $20,000 or more.

Heavy Metal Toxicity

A second but related biologic hypothesis addresses the concern that environmental toxicants from vaccines or other sources lead to the neurologic insult in ASDs. The proposed mechanism includes both disruption of immune function and oxidative stress.

Chelation

Chelating agents bind to heavy metals in the body, such as lead and mercury, and permit elimination of these compounds through the kidney. Chelation is medically indicated in documented occupational and environmental exposures. In pediatric use, this therapy is most commonly indicated for the treatment of elevated lead levels from environmental exposure to lead paint in dust and in older buildings. Although not substantiated by epidemiologic data, there remains a popular belief that children with ASDs could have had neurologic injury from exposure to heavy metals other than lead. This is suggested to be via ethylmercury preservatives and aluminum adjuvants in vaccines and other environmental sources. Proponents of this theory report that individuals with ASDs have an abnormality in the capacity for metal excretion that leads to increased tissue concentrations (Holmes, Blaxill, & Haley, 2003) or have altered metal excretion because of altered gut flora (Adams et al., 2007). Elevated levels of mercury in baby teeth have been reported in children with ASDs. The authors relate this finding to the hypothesis of altered excretion of mercury in children with ASDs (Adams et al., 2007). However, plasma levels are not increased in infants after immunizations preserved with the ethylmercury derivative Thimerosal, suggesting rapid clearance by excretion (Pichichero et al., 2008). Thimerosal has not been used as a preservative in single-use pediatric vaccines since 2001, but environmental sources of elemental mercury include air pollution, and sources of methyl mercury include fish ingestion. Bernard et al. (2001) proposed an etiologic link with mercury exposure and autism. The symptoms of neurologic damage are not convergent with those of autism (Nelson & Bauman, 2003). Heavy metals, if present in an uncomplexed form, may donate electrons to create reactive oxygen species, leading to increased oxidative stress. Urinary excretion of porphyrins was reported to be elevated in children with ASDs compared to siblings with subsequent decrease after chelation therapy (Geier & Geier, 2007). Urinary porphyrins reflect disruption in one potential step in heavy metal excess affecting heme metabolism. Further studies are indicated to explain this observation that includes nutritional and medical characterization of participants. Use of a chelating agent to mobilize mercury as a means of determining the presence of toxicity is not supported by data from studies in unaffected volunteers (Archbold, McGuckin, & Campbell, 2004). Oral agents used for chelation of known heavy metal toxicity include dimercaptosuccinic acid (DMSA) and 2,3-dimercapto-1-propanesulfonic acid (DMPS). Although DMSA has clinical utility in lead poisoning and other heavy-metal toxicity, Na EDTA results in excessive elimination of calcium and has no current clinical indications (Brownet al., 2006). One death of a child with autism has been ascribed to chelation with Na EDTA. The only FDA-approved agent for intravenous chelation of lead is Disodium EDTA Calcium. There are no published randomized clinical trials of chelation for symptoms of ASDs. In rats, it was demonstrated that animals that did not have elevated lead levels had lasting cognitive and affective dysfunction after chelation with succimer, whereas improvement was identified in animals with elevated lead levels (Stangle et al., 2007). A real risk for depletion of iron, calcium, and other metals necessary for routine cellular function exists with chelation treatment. Although proponents often prescribe minerals and other supplements in conjunction with oral, rectal, or topical chelating agents, the efficacy of chelation is unknown and the potential risks great. The unregulated and medically unmonitored use of over-the-counter topical, oral, and rectal chelating agents has never been studied and may be dangerous. Intravenous chelation for symptoms of ASDs is costly and not covered by insurance. The real risk for side effects necessitates medical monitoring if this popular CAM therapy is pursued. There is no evidence in the peer-reviewed literature to support the clinical use of chelation for symptoms of ASDs at this time.

Gastrointestinal

There are several hypotheses regarding the role of intestinal function in the etiology of ASDs or occurrence of symptoms related to discomfort.

Secretin

Secretin is a peptide produced in the pancreas and released into the small intestine to enhance intestinal motility. Secretin receptors have been identified in the brain with potential roles in brain development (Chu, Yung, & Chow, 2006). The popularity of secretin began with a case series of three children with ASDs who were subjectively reported to have improved symptoms after receiving intravenous secretin during endoscopy to evaluate pancreatic function. This report and the resultant publicity led to widespread treatment of children with ASDs with intravenous secretin. Clinical trials ultimately studied more than 600 children with ASDs. None of these trials demonstrated clinical benefit for the core symptoms of ASDs or demonstrated clinical benefit (Williams, Wray, & Wheeler, 2005). Proponents of secretin treatment still maintain that a subgroup of children with GI symptoms may derive benefit from it, although the evidence from well-designed clinical trials overwhelmingly negates claims of clinical effect. The placebo effect may be very potent when there is hope for symptomatic response (Sandler, 2005). Side effects include decreased intestinal motility and the stress and cost of the infusion. Clinical trials data resoundingly refute the use of intravenous, sublingual, or transcutaneous secretin for symptoms of ASDs.

Dietary Intervention

Green et al. (2006) report that almost one-fourth of the respondents to their internet survey were using specialized diets for their children with ASDs. The IAN (2009) reported that almost one-third of their sample reported current use of therapeutic diets for symptoms of ASDs. The most popular therapeutic diet at this time is the gluten-free and casein-free (GFCF) diet. This diet is based on the hypothesis that people with ASDs have a "leaky gut" that permits increased absorption of gluten- and casein-related opiate peptides that function as opioids in the central nervous system and produce symptoms common to autism and opiate exposure (Christison & Ivany, 2006). Increased urinary peptide peaks in the areas expected for caseomorphin and gluteomorphin initially supported this hypothesis. However, recent studies using mass spectroscopy did not identify opioid compounds in the urine to support this hypothesis (Cass et al., 2008). The most recent Cochrane review of the efficacy of the GFCF diet (Millward et al., 2008) reported on two trials with adequate scientific methodology. A single-blind trial compared 10 children with ASDs randomly assigned to a GFCF diet in the community to 10 who were not treated with diet (Knivsberg et al., 2002). General improvements in symptoms related to autism in these subjects suggest the need for further study; however, this study did not examine concurrent therapies or nutrition. Elder et al. (2007) reported a double-blind, placebo-controlled crossover trial in 15 children with ASDs. No behavioral effect could be documented using the Childhood Autism Rating Scale. The nutritional effects of eliminating dairy products may include decreased calcium and Vitamin D intake (Hediger et al., 2007; Johnson et al., 2008).* Risk includes decreased bone density (Herndon et al., 2009). Attention to general nutritional needs is important if a family elects a trial of a restricted diet. Additional studies to examine safety and efficacy are indicated, given the popularity of this intervention and the common use of nutritional supplements in an attempt to compensate for dietary restriction.

Yeast Overgrowth

The hypothesis that yeast overgrowth in the intestine occurs in children with ASDs has resulted in several therapies. Although no excess of candida colonization has been documented by endoscopy in series of children with ASDs (Horvath et al., 1999; Wakefield et al., 2000), there has been one case report of increased urinary organic acids attributed to yeast overgrowth (Shaw, Kassen, & Chaves, 1995). The subjects of the case report had an atypical presentation for idiopathic autism with ataxia and a waxing and waning course. Several approaches are used by proponents of this theory to address yeast production such as decreasing sugar in the diet and treatment with probiotics to alter the intestinal flora. Other approaches are used by proponents of this theory to eliminate yeast already in the intestine, including prescription of the medications nystatin and diflucan. Side effects of this may include altering gut flora to select for resistant strains of yeast and, for diflucan, hepatotoxicity. There are no clinical trials in the literature to support or guide the use of these treatments. There is no biologic basis to support the underlying hypothesis at this time.

Dysbiosis

Alteration of intestinal immune function and gut flora are the basis of the hypothesis that pathologic bacterial species either produce toxins or act in some other way to result in symptoms of ASDs. Finegold et al. (2002) reported different clostridial species in the stool, stomach, and duodena of children with ASDs compared to controls. Bowel inflammation was investigated using two biomarkers: rectal nitrous oxide and fecal calprotectin (Fernell, Fagerberg, & Hellstrom, 2007). Only one (a child who had a history of *C. difficile* infection) of 24 consecutive patients with ASDs studied had elevation of both markers, suggesting that bowel inflammation is infrequent in children with ASDs. A trial of vancomycin was reported to result in subjective improvement in a group of children with ASDs (Sandler et al., 2000). The subjective improvements did not persist. Vancomycin has significant potential side effects when used orally, including pseudomembranous colitis and selection for resistant species of bacteria. In many hospitals, it can only be prescribed after an infectious disease consultation. Off-label use this antibiotic for symptoms of ASDs may contribute to the community selection of bacteria unresponsive to available antibiotics.

Inflammation

Immune and auto-immune phenomena are being investigated by conventional scientists related to both the neurobiology and GI pathology of ASDs. Several complementary therapies in addition to antibiotics and antiyeast agents are purported to affect immune function, including chelation and omega-3 fatty acids. The immune system uses production of reactive oxygen species as part of the mechanism to kill pathogens. Therapies addressing immune-mediated disorders include the approach of replacement of components of the immune system, treatment with interferon to enhance the body's ability to produce an immune response to a known antigen, and the use of anti-infective medications.

IV-IG

Popular interest in infusion of IvIG for symptoms of ASDs followed an initial report of an open trial of pooled human serum immunoglobins to enhance general immune function in children with ASDs, whose authors reported subjective improvement in the participants (Gupta, Aggarwal, & Heads, 1996). Other investigators using more specific clinical trial methodologies have not confirmed the initial positive reports (DelGiudice-Asch et al., 1999; Plioplys, 1998). Autism is not an indication for IvIG administration. Although there is always a small risk in pooled plasma products, mild side effects such as fever and headache are not infrequent. Less common but significant side effects include aseptic meningitis, thrombotic events, and altered renal function. Common immunologic disorders such as atopy, asthma, and food allergy have not been documented to be more common in children with ASDs. Examination of specific alterations in immune function that might affect neurologic development is an active area of current research (Jyonouchi et al., 2005) and is addressing a neurobiologic question related to etiology of altered brain development

Antiviral Agents

Chess (1971) made the observation that children exposed to the rubella virus *in utero* had an increased risk for ASDs. In addition, there are cases of ASDs associated with herpes simplex encephalitis and cytomegalovirus infection. Prenatal bornavirus infection and prenatal maternal influenza infection alter behavior in mice without evidence of a conventional inflammatory response in brain, suggesting that prenatal infection of the mother might result in an immune response that alters fetal brain development (Libbey et al., 2005). In combination with neuropathologic findings of neuroinflammation in isolated brain samples (Vargas et al., 2005), there has been interest by some CAM providers in off-label treatment of children with ASDs with antiviral agents. No clinical trials have been published to judge safety or efficacy of this practice. Side effects of antiviral agents used off label to treat neuroinflammation in children with ASDs include headache, nausea, and abdominal pain. Renal complications can be minimized with adequate hydration. As with antibacterial agents, community use may result in the emergence of viruses with drug resistance. Therefore, in the absence of data to support their use, the public health recommendation would not support off-label use of these agents.

Other Neurobiologic Processes

Because vitamins and herbal products contain ingredients that affect central nervous system function, there is significant interest among families to manage symptoms of ASDs with products that they perceive as safe because they are available over the counter.

Melatonin

As discussed in Chapter 26, sleep disturbances are common among individuals with ASDs. Preliminary studies suggest that children with ASDs may have altered production or release of the hormone melatonin (Tordjman et al., 2005) that is produced by the pineal gland to regulate the sleep–wake cycle. Open-label studies report that treatment with 0.75 to 6 mg of melatonin prior to bedtime improves both sleep-onset and night wakings in children and adolescents with ASDs (Andersen et al., 2008). Observed side effects of melatonin include morning sleepiness and enuresis. No increase in seizures was reported. Melatonin appears to be a safe supplement with a physiologically sound explanation for proposed sleep effect that is currently being evaluated in controlled trials.

Omega-3 Fatty Acids

Omega-3 fatty acids—particularly the long-chain fatty acids eicosapentaenoic acid (EPA) and docosahexaenoic acid (DHA)—have been investigated as treatments for inattention, obsessive compulsive disorder, and other neurologic and psychiatric disorders (Ramakrishnan et al., 2009). Western diets are typically low in this nutrient found in fish and vegetable sources such as flax seeds. Although supplementation has been promoted by CAM providers as a treatment in ASDs to correct dietary deficiency, it is also hypothesized to improve cell membrane fluidity and function, alter neurotransmitter binding, and alter cytokine production to modify inflammatory response. A small double-blind trial in 8 children demonstrated significant improvement in stereotyped behaviors at a dose of 1500 mg/day (Amminger et al., 2007). An open trial in 19 adults with ASDs did not lead to behavioral improvement (Politi et al., 2009). Randomized clinical trials are ongoing to evaluate the effect of treatment. Known side effects are mild and include loose stools, decreased appetite, and aftertaste.

Vitamins and Nutritional Supplements

Vitamins, used as single agents or as combinations, are among the most commonly used complementary therapies for symptoms of ASDs. Green et al. (2006) reported supplement use in 43% of their sample. Various supplements are given to children with ASDs in hopes of enhancing function like Vitamins C and E, minerals such as zinc and selenium, and nutritional supplements such as trimethylglycine (TMG). One of the earliest CAM therapies studied in clinical trials for symptoms for ASDs remains one of the most popular. Vitamin B_6 (pyridoxine) may enhance transulfuration of methionine to cysteine and glutathione; modulate enzyme systems responsible for production of neurotransmitters such as GABA, dopamine, and serotonin; and is involved with immune function because of its role in protein metabolism. Studies to date are inconclusive as to the benefit given the small sample sizes and problems with study design (Nye & Brice, 2005). CAM providers administer this to children with ASDs at high doses with magnesium to decrease hyperactivity and enhance language. Vitamin B_6 is found in a wide variety of foods, including fortified cereals, meat, poultry, fish, and some fruits and vegetables. Potential side effects of excess B_6 include numbness and tingling of the hands as manifestation of a peripheral neuropathy. Magnesium is found in nuts, legumes, whole grains, and green vegetables such as spinach. Excess intake of magnesium may result in decreased appetite, nausea, diarrhea, low blood pressure, cardiac arrhythmias, and changes in mental status. The clinical trials to date do not support recommendation of B_6/magnesium supplementation beyond the RDA.

Clinical trials typically attempt to understand the effect of discrete interventions. Because families of children with ASDs employ seven interventions on average (Green et al., 2006), effectiveness studies will need to examine the interaction of multiple treatment approaches used simultaneously. Adams et al. (Adams & Holloway, 2004) reported subjective improvement in sleep and gastrointestinal function in 20 children with ASDs treated with a multivitamin combination compared to controls. Further research is necessary to examine the safety and efficacy of supplements used concurrently at doses above the Recommended Dietary Allowance. Research in other disorders has cautioned that excess supplementation may be harmful rather than helpful (Bjelakovic et al., 2008). There can be too much of a good thing. For example, it is known that chronic excess intake of Vitamin A can result in fatigue, GI symptoms, and irritability. Excess supplementation with Vitamin E over time is associated with a general increase in mortality and congestive heart failure in adults and is associated with fatigue and GI symptoms. It is difficult to study the effects of nutrient excess as noted previously because the effects occur over long periods of time, the supplements are not regulated so the specific dosage may not be either consistent or known, and multiple agents are often used in conjunction with traditional medications.

Manipulative and Body-Based Therapies

Chiropractic Care

Chiropractic care is the most frequently provided CAM practice in the general population, with children making up 11% of patient visits (Lee, Li, & Kemper, 2000). This care focuses on spinal alignment and body manipulation and its relationship to health (Kemper et al., 2008). The majority of adults who pursue chiropractic care do so for pain or musculoskeletal complaints, with some suggestion of subjective or objective improvement (Kaptchuk & Eisenberg, 1998). A recent review of chiropractic care for non-musculoskeletal conditions (Hawk et al., 2007) summarized results of randomized controlled trials and/or systematic reviews of the efficacy of treatment for medical conditions such as asthma, hypertension, infantile colic, otitis media, and others. Many of the studies suffered from methodologic difficulties and reported some subjective, but few objective, benefits. Similar data about chiropractic treatment of autism are not available. Although very rare, adverse results include delay in appropriate medical care and rare adverse events such as spinal fluid leak (Mathews et al., 2006) or vertebral artery dissection (Chen et al., 2006). Chiropractic care, although not evidence-based or rooted in current scientific understanding of pathophysiology of disease, is covered by most health insurances.

Massage and Therapeutic Touch

Massage is another type of biomechanical treatment that is administered by massage therapists or parents who have been instructed in the techniques. The goals of treatment include addressing sleep difficulties, sensory abnormalities (hyper and hyposensitivity), and improving attention (Escalona et al., 2001). Massage has been demonstrated to be helpful in preterm infants, facilitating growth and earlier discharge (Field, 2002). Hypothesized mechanisms of action include alterations in epinephrine, norepinephrine, serotonin, and cortisol levels (Field et al., 2005) or alteration in vagal tone. Escalona and colleagues (2001) completed a randomized controlled trial of massage versus attention (reading a book to the child) in 20 children with ASDs ages 3 to 6 years. Children randomized to massage therapy had less stereotypic behavior, improved social relatedness, and improved sleep. Further work is needed regarding specific physiologic mechanisms of action and replication of these results using more rigorous study design. No untoward side effects have been reported, and parents reported a feeling of closeness with the children (Cullen, Barlow, & Cushway, 2005). The cost of therapy, time for visits, and direction of resources away from other types of therapies are the potential side effects.

Craniosacral Manipulation

Craniosacral manipulation is another mechanical treatment, which proposes manipulation of bones of the skull to correct the flow of cerebrospinal fluid and promote health. There is no evidence that external manipulation results in alteration of spinal fluid dynamics. Craniosacral manipulation is administered by certain osteopathic physicians, physical therapists, massage therapists, chiropractors, and others. A systematic review of available evidence-based studies revealed few studies, all of which had methodologic difficulties (C. Green et al., 1999) and no support for efficacy for treatment of symptoms of autism beyond the massage component.

Auditory Integration

Auditory integration training is an environmentally administered treatment that was introduced to the United States in the early 1990s, around the time of publication of a book in the popular press describing a "cure" of ASDs using this methodology (Council on Children with Disabilities, 1998). The hypothesis behind this treatment asserts that abnormal sensitivity to certain frequencies of sound are associated with behavior and learning problems (Sinha, et al., 2006) and that training sessions with electronically modified music will improve or cure symptoms. No physiologic mechanism of action has been proposed. A systematic Cochrane review of studies of AIT (Sinha et al., 2004) reported no difference between control and treatment conditions in the larger, more robust studies but suggested improvement in less methodologically sound studies. Potential side effects include exposure to high-output levels of sound and the cost to families in time and money for the therapy.

Vagus Nerve Stimulation

Vagus nerve stimulation is an increasingly accepted treatment for management of intractable epilepsy, despite the fact that the specific mechanism for effectiveness is not known. To administer the treatment, a stimulation system is implanted under general anesthesia. Daniellsson and colleagues (2008) described a case series of 8 children with epilepsy and autism who underwent treatment with vagal stimulation for their intractable epilepsy. They had extensive pre- and post-neuropsychological evaluations. In this open-label pilot study, no child had diminished seizure frequency. Three showed minor improvement in general functioning with no positive cognitive effects. Potential side effects are significant, related to need for general anesthesia and the unknown long-term impact of implantation of the device.

Energy Medicine

Qigong

Qigong is a form of ancient Chinese medical practice used to enhance health with energy realignment of the body with breathing and movement exercises. It has been compared to a moving form of meditation. It is considered a bioenergentic therapy because the technique addresses management of "qi" or specific aspects of energy associated with the body. Silva and colleagues (Silva & Cignolini, 2005; Silva et al., 2007) described several observational case series of children who received medical qigong massage. The authors reported decreased autistic behaviors as well as increased language and sensory function, but methodologic problems include lack of appropriate controls and unblinded analysis of treatment effects.

Reiki

Reiki is a biofield therapy that purportedly affects energy fields that surround and penetrate the human body (Kemper et al., 2008). Reiki grew out of a Japanese tradition where the healer places hands on the subject's body, thus transmitting a healing force (McLean & Kemper, 2006). There are no studies evaluating its effectiveness in treating children with autism.

The Business of Therapy

It has been documented that the annual cost of health care for children with autism is more than seven times greater than children with typical development ($6132 vs. $860) (Liptak, Stuart, & Auinger, 2006). These calculations do not include the significant expense that families of children with autism spend out of pocket on CAM therapies. More than $34 billion dollars are spent annually on CAM therapies in the United States. Cost, however, includes more than the dollar value of the product purchased. It factors in all of the direct costs of the intervention (product, practitioner fees, diagnostic costs, equipment and facility fees), additional nondirect costs (transportation, parents time off from work), indirect costs (parental time off related to the intervention separate from the direct visit, childcare for siblings, lost leisure time), and additional intangible personal costs (discomfort related to the procedures, disappointment if not successful) (Herman, Craig, & Caspi, 2005). Analysis of the cost effectiveness of CAM therapies includes economic, humanistic, and clinical outcomes (Herman, Craig, & Caspi, 2005). Humanistic outcomes are less easily quantifiable than clinical outcome measures and include quality of life, autonomy, safety, comfort, and sense of well-being. Few studies on the cost-effectiveness of CAM have been published. This may be in part because some practitioners are not motivated to examine the cost of therapy. It has also been suggested that demonstration of effectiveness might result in incorporation of these interventions into conventional care and diminish the autonomy of CAM practice (Kelner et al., 2002). The process of CAM itself may have therapeutic benefit in terms of more difficult-to-measure outcomes such as patient empowerment and sense of well-being that are not easily captured in cost–benefit analyses (Herman, Craig, & Caspi, 2005).

The number of uninsured Americans increased from 20% to 23% between 1988 and 1999 and was projected to approach 30% by 2009 (Pagan & Pauly, 2005). These authors reported an increase in CAM use among adults who had decreased access to conventional care because of cost. By extension, CAM use among families of children with ASDs might be increased by difficulty in accessing effective behavioral, and educational therapies. Similarly, emotional or financial investment in CAM therapies may postpone or limit involvement with potentially beneficial therapies.

Research Needs

Families and clinicians need unbiased, well-designed clinical trials that can address both safety and efficacy to inform treatment decisions. This is challenging, given the imperative to treat children during the potential therapeutic window for response, although well-designed studies may take years to be productive of informative results. As with any new pharmacologic or educational intervention, the data from case series and open trials provide information regarding the promise of a therapy that may merit study and may be used to inform sample size determination, choice of valid outcome measures, and study design. Clinical trials are expensive and typically require assessment of each treatment component individually. Commonly used CAM protocols may implement multiple interventions simultaneously. To advance knowledge regarding CAM treatments requires investigation of scientific theories hypothesized as responsible for desired therapeutic effect, commitment of funding for well-designed clinical trials, and education of both families and practitioners about appropriate scientific study design and interpretation of data. A collaborative approach by proponents of CAM and conventional scientists to examine the science and practice of CAM therapy will ultimately benefit the children affected by ASDs and move some therapies from CAM to conventional and others from CAM to history.

Challenges and Future Directions

The challenge to the conventional practitioner is the popular acceptance of many CAM therapies without the evidence that would support their use. This results in mistrust of the medical and scientific establishment by families who find hope in the claims made. It places people with ASDs at potential risk for unanticipated side effects from unregulated therapies. An additional challenge is the defense of conventional therapies that are not supported by the strength of evidence either. To be able to advise patients regarding the safety and efficacy of intervention they might elect, all therapies used for children with ASDs should be examined using the same criteria.

It is plausible that some current therapies considered to be CAM will be demonstrated to have biologic plausibility and will be proven to be effective for specific symptoms of ASDs. It is also plausible that long-term sequelae of CAM intervention not currently thought to have side effects might be identified. Coincident with scientific study of CAM, there needs to be educational efforts for consumers so that family empowerment to participate in the choices for care for their children is done in an informed fashion.

REFERENCES

Adams, J. B., & Holloway, C. (2004). Pilot study of a moderate dose multivitamin/mineral supplement for children with autistic spectrum disorder. *Journal of Alternative and Complementary Medicine, 10*(6), 1033–1039.

Adams, J. B., Romdalvik, J., Ramanujam, V. M., & Legator, M. S. (2007). Mercury, lead, and zinc in baby teeth of children with autism versus controls. *Journal of Toxicology and Environmental Health A, 70*(12), 1046–1051.

American Academy of Pediatrics, & Committee on Children With Disabilities. (2001). Counseling families who choose complementary and alternative medicine for their child with chronic illness or disability. *Pediatrics, 107*(3), 598–601.

Amminger, G. P., Berger, G. E., Schafer, M. R., Klier, C., Friedrich, M. H., & Feucht, M. (2007). Omega-3 fatty acids supplementation in children with autism: A double-blind randomized, placebo-controlled pilot study. *Biologic Psychiatry, 61*(4), 551–553.

Andersen, I. M., Kaczmarska, J., McGrew, S. G., & Malow, B. A. (2008). Melatonin for Insomnia in Children With Autism Spectrum Disorders. *Journal of Child Neurology, 1*, 1.

Archbold, G. P., McGuckin, R. M., & Campbell, N. A. (2004). Dimercaptosuccinic acid loading test for assessing mercury burden in healthy individuals. *Annals of Clinical Biochemistry, 41*(Pt 3), 233–236.

Astin, J. A. (2004). Mind-body therapies for the management of pain. *Clinical Journal of Pain, 20*, 27–32.

Barnes, P. M., Powell-Griner, E., McFann, K., & Nahin, R.L. (2004). *Complementary and alternative medicine use among adults: United States, 2002. Advance Data from vital and health statistics.* Retrieved. from http://www.nccam.nih.gov. Accessed December 6, 2010.

Bello, S. C. (2007). Autism and environmental influences: Review and commentary. *Reviews of Environmental Health, 22*(2), 139–156.

Birks, J., & Grimley Evans, J. (2009). Ginkgo biloba for cognitive impairment and dementia. *Cochrane Database Systematic Reviews* (1), CD003120.

Bjelakovic, G., Nikolova, D., Simonetti, R. G., & Gluud, C. (2008). Antioxidant supplements for preventing gastrointestinal cancers. *Cochrane Database Systematic Reviews* (3), CD004183.

Brown, M. J., Willis, T., Omalu, B., & Leiker, R. (2006). Deaths resulting from hypocalcemia after administration of edetate disodium: 2003–2005. *Pediatrics, 118*(2), e534–536.

Cass, H., Gringras, P., March, J., McKendrick, I., O'Hare, A. E., Owen, L., et al. (2008). Absence of urinary opioid peptides in children with Autism. *Archives of Disease in Childhood, 93*(9), 745–750.

Chen, W. L., Chern, C. H., Wu, Y. L., & Lee, C. H. (2006). Vertebral artery dissection and cerebellar infarction following chiropractic manipulation. *Emergency Medical Journal, 23*(1), e1.

Chess, S. (1971). Autism in children with congenital rubella. *Journal of Autism and Childhood Schizophrenia, 1*(1), 33–47.

Christison, G. W., & Ivany, K. (2006). Elimination diets in autism spectrum disorders: Any wheat amidst the chaff? *Journal of Developmental and Behavioral Pediatrics, 27*(2 Suppl), S162–171.

Chu, J. Y., Yung, W. H., & Chow, B. K. (2006). Secretin: A pleiotrophic hormone. *Annals of the New York Academy of Sciences, 1070*, 27–50.

Collet, J. P., Vanasse, M., Marois, P., Amar, M., Goldberg, J., Lambert, J., et al. (2001). Hyperbaric oxygen for children with cerebral palsy: A randomised multicentre trial. HBO-CP Research Group. *Lancet, 357*(9256), 582–586.

Council on Children with Disabilities. (1998). American Academy of Pediatrics. Committee on Children with Disabilities. Auditory integration training and facilitated communication for autism. *Pediatrics, 102*(2 Pt 1), 431–433.

Cullen, L. A., Barlow, J. H., & Cushway, D. (2005). Positive touch, the implications for parents and their children with autism: An exploratory study. *Complementary Therapeutics in Clinical Practice, 11*(3), 182–189.

Danielsson, S., Viggedal, G., Gillberg, C., & Olsson, I. (2008). Lack of effects of vagus nerve stimulation on drug-resistant epilepsy in eight pediatric patients with autism spectrum disorders: A prospective 2-year follow-up study. *Epilepsy and Behavior, 12*(2), 298–304.

DelGiudice-Asch, G., Simon, L., Schmeidler, J., Cunningham-Rundles, C., & Hollander, E. (1999). Brief report: A pilot open clinical trial of intravenous immunoglobulin in childhood autism. *Journal of Autism and Developmental Disorders, 29*(2), 157–160.

Deprey, L. J. (2006). Double blind placebo controlled cross-over trial of subcutaneous methylcobalamin in autism: Preliminary results (Abstract). *ACAP, 33*, F47.

Dolske, M. C., Spollen, J., McKay, S., Lancashire, E., & Tolbert, L. (1993). A preliminary trial of ascorbic acid as supplemental therapy for autism. *Progress in Neuropsychopharmacology and Biological Psychiatry, 17*, 765–774.

Ernst, E. (1999). Prevalence of complementary/alternative medicine for children: A systematic review. *European Journal of Pediatrics, 158*(1), 7–11.

Escalona, A., Field, T., Singer-Strunck, R., Cullen, C., & Hartshorn, K. (2001). Brief report: Improvements in the behavior of children with autism following massage therapy. *Journal of Autism and Developmental Disorders, 31*(5), 513–516.

Fernell, E., Fagerberg, U. L., & Hellstrom, P. M. (2007). No evidence for a clear link between active intestinal inflammation and autism based on analyses of faecal calprotectin and rectal nitric oxide. *Acta Paediatrica, 96*(7), 1076–1079.

Field, T. (2002). Preterm infant massage therapy studies: An American approach. *Seminars in Neonatology, 7*(6), 487–494.

Field, T., Hernandez-Reif, M., Diego, M., Schanberg, S., & Kuhn, C. (2005). Cortisol decreases and serotonin decreases and dopamine increase following massage therapy. *International Journal of Neuroscience, 115*(10), 1397–1413.

Finegold, S. M., Molitoris, D., Song, Y., Liu, C., Vaisanen, M. L., Bolte, E., et al. (2002). Gastrointestinal microflora studies in late-onset autism. *Clinical Infectious Diseases, 35*(Suppl 1), S6–S16.

Geier, D. A., & Geier, M. R. (2007). A prospective study of thimerosal-containing Rho(D)-immune globulin administration as a risk factor for autistic disorders. *Journal of Maternal-Fetal and Neonatal Medicine, 20*(5), 385–390.

Gold, C., Wigram, T., & Elefant, C. (2006). Music therapy for autistic spectrum disorder. *Cochrane Database Systematic Reviews*(2), CD004381.

Green, C., Martin, C. W., Bassett, K., & Kazanjian, A. (1999). A systematic review of craniosacral therapy: Biological plausibility, assessment reliability and clinical effectiveness. *Complementary Therapeutic Medicine, 7*(4), 201–207.

Green, V. A., Pituch, K. A., Itchon, J., Choi, A., O'Reilly, M., & Sigafoos, J. (2006). Internet survey of treatments used by parents of children with autism. *Research in Developmental Disabilities, 27*(1), 70–84.

Greenspesheh, D., Tarbox, J., Dixon, D. R., Wilke, A. E., Allen, S, Bradsteet J. (2009). Effects of Hyperbaric Oxygen Therapy on Adaptive, Aberrant and Stereotyped Behaviors in Children with Autism; Poster presentation, International Meeting for Autism Research, Chicago May 2009.

Gupta, S., Aggarwal, S., & Heads, C. (1996). Dysregulated immune system in children with autism: Beneficial effects of intravenous immune globulin on autistic characteristics. *Journal of Autism and Developmental Disorders, 26*(4), 439–452.

Guyatt, G. H., Oxman, A. D., Vist, G. E., Kunz, R., Falck-Ytter, Y., Alonso-Coello, P., et al. (2008). GRADE: An emerging consensus on rating quality of evidence and strength of recommendations. *British Medical Journal, 336*(7650), 924–926.

Hanson, E., Kalish, L. A., Bunce, E., Curtis, C., McDaniel, S., Ware, J., et al. (2007). Use of complementary and alternative medicine among children diagnosed with autism spectrum disorder. *Journal of Autism and Developmental Disorders, 37*(4), 628–636.

Hawk, C., Khorsan, R., Lisi, A. J., Ferrance, R. J., & Evans, M. W. (2007). Chiropractic care for nonmusculoskeletal conditions: A systematic review with implications for whole systems research. *Journal of Alternative and Complementary Medicine, 13*(5), 491–512.

Heaton P., Williams K., Cummins O., Happe, F. G. (2007). Beyond perception: Musical representation and on line processing in autism. *Journal of Autism and Developmental Disorders, 37*, 1355–1360.

Hediger, M. L., England, L. J., Molloy, C. A., Yu, K. F., Manning-Courtney, P., & Mills, J. L. (2007). Reduced bone cortical thickness in boys with autism or autism spectrum disorder. *Journal of Autism and Developmental Disorders.*

Herman, P. M., Craig, B. M., & Caspi, O. (2005). Is complementary and alternative medicine (CAM) cost-effective? A systematic review. *BMC Complementary and Alternative Medicine, 5*, 11.

Herndon, A. C., DiGuiseppi, C., Johnson, S. L., Leiferman, J., & Reynolds, A. (2009). Does nutritional intake differ between children with autism spectrum disorders and children with typical development? *Journal of Autism and Developmental Disorders, 39*(2), 212–222.

Holmes, A. S., Blaxill, M. F., & Haley, B. E. (2003). Reduced levels of mercury in first baby haircuts of autistic children. *International Journal of Toxicology, 22*(4), 277–285.

Horvath, K., Papadimitriou, J. C., Rabsztyn, A., Drachenberg, C., & Tildon, J. T. (1999). Gastrointestinal abnormalities in children with autistic disorder. *Journal of Pediatrics, 135*(5), 559–563.

James, S. J., Cutler, P., Melnyk, S., Jernigan, S., Janak, L., Gaylor, D. W., et al. (2004). Metabolic biomarkers of increased oxidative stress and impaired methylation capacity in children with autism. *American Journal of Clinical Nutrition, 80*(6), 1611–1617.

James, S. J., Melnyk, S., Fuchs, G., Reid, T., Jernigan, S., Pavliv, O., et al. (2009). Efficacy of methylcobalamin and folinic acid treatment on glutathione redox status in children with autism. *American Journal of Clinical Nutrition, 89*(1), 425–430.

James, S. J., Melnyk, S., Jernigan, S., Cleves, M. A., Halsted, C. H., Wong, D. H., et al. (2006). Metabolic endophenotype and related genotypes are associated with oxidative stress in children with autism. *American Journal of Medical Genetics. Part B, Neuropsychiatric Genetics, 141*(8), 947–956.

Jensen, P. S., & Kenny, D. T. (2004). The effects of yoga on the attention and behavior of boys with Attention-Deficit/hyperactivity Disorder (ADHD). *Journal of Attention Disorders, 7*(4), 205–216.

Johnson, C. R., Handen, B., Mayer-Costa, M., & Sacco, K. A. (2008). Eating habits and dietary status in young children with autism. *Journal of Developmental and Physical Disability, 20*, 437–448.

Jyonouchi, H., Geng, L., Ruby, A., & Zimmerman-Bier, B. (2005). Dysregulated innate immune responses in young children with autism spectrum disorders: Their relationship to gastrointestinal symptoms and dietary intervention. *Neuropsychobiology, 51*(2), 77–85.

Kaptchuk, T. J., & Eisenberg, D. M. (1998). Chiropractic: Origins, Controversies, and Contributions. *Archives of Internal Medicine, 158*(20), 2215–2224.

Kelner, M. J., Boon, H., Wellman, B., & Welsh, S. (2002). Complementary and alternative groups contemplate the need for effectiveness, safety and cost-effectiveness research. *Complementary Therapies in Medicine, 10*(4), 235–239.

Kemper, K. J., Vohra, S., Walls, R., the Task Force on Complementary, Alternative, M., & the Provisional Section on Complementary,

H. a. I. M. (2008). The use of complementary and alternative medicine in pediatrics. *Pediatrics, 122*(6), 1374–1386.

Kim, J., Wigram, T., & Gold, C. (2008). The effects of improvisational music therapy on joint attention behaviors in autistic children: A randomized controlled study. *Journal of Autism and Developmental Disorders. 38*(9), 1758–1766.

Knivsberg, A. M., Reichelt, K. L., Hoien, T., & Nodland, M. (2002). A randomised, controlled study of dietary intervention in autistic syndromes. *Nutritional Neuroscience, 5*(4), 251–261.

Lanski, S. L., Greenwald, M., Perkins, M., & Simon, H. K. (2003). Herbal therapy use in a pediatric emergency department population: Expect the unexpected. *Pediatrics, 111*, 981–985.

Lee, A. C. C., Li, D. H., & Kemper, K. J. (2000). Chiropractic Care for Children. *Archives of Pediatrics and Adolescent Medicine, 154*(4), 401–407.

Levy, S. E., & Hyman, S. L. (2005). Novel treatments for autistic spectrum disorders. *Mental Retardation and Developmental Disabilities Research and Reviews, 11*(2), 131–142.

Levy, S. E., & Hyman, S. L. (2008). Complementary and alternative medicine treatments for children with autism spectrum disorders. *Child and Adolescent Psychiatry Clinics of North America, 17*(4), 803–820, ix.

Levy, S. E., Mandell, D. S., Merhar, S., Ittenbach, R. F., & Pinto-Martin, J. A. (2003). Use of complementary and alternative medicine among children recently diagnosed with autistic spectrum disorder. *Journal of Developmental and Behavioral Pediatrics, 24*(6), 418–423.

Libbey, J. E., Sweeten, T. L., Mc Mahon, W., & Fujinami, R. S. (2005). Autistic disorder and viral infections. *Journal of Neurovirology, 11*(1), 1–10.

Liptak, G. S., Stuart, T., & Auinger, P. (2006). Health care utilization and expenditures for children with autism: Data from U.S. national samples. *Journal of Autism and Developmental Disorders, 36*(7), 871–879.

Lovaas, O. I. (1993). The development of a treatment-research project for developmentally disabled and autistic children. *Journal of Applied Behavioral Analysis, 26*(4), 617–630.

Mathews, M. K., Frohman, L., Lee, H. J., Sergott, R. C., & Savino, P. J. (2006). Spinal fluid leak after chiropractic manipulation of the cervical spine. *Archives of Ophthalmology, 124*(2), 283.

McLean, T. W., & Kemper, K. J. (2006). Complementary and alternative medicine therapies in pediatric oncology patients. *Journal of the Society for Integrative Oncology, 4*(1), 40–45.

Millward, C., Ferriter, M., Calver, S., & Connell-Jones, G. (2008). Gluten- and casein-free diets for autistic spectrum disorder. *Cochrane Database Systematic Reviews* (2), CD003498.

Nelson, K. B., & Bauman, M. L. (2003). Thimerosal and autism? *Pediatrics, 111*(3), 674–679.

Nye, C., & Brice, A. (2005). Combined vitamin B6-magnesium treatment in autism spectrum disorder. *Cochrane Database Systematic Reviews* (4), CD003497.

Ohnishi, T., Matsuda, H., Hashimoto, T., Kunihiro, T., Nishikawa, M., Uema, T., et al. (2000). Abnormal regional cerebral blood flow in childhood autism. *Brain, 123*(Pt 9), 1838–1844.

Pagan, J. A., & Pauly, M. V. (2005). Access to conventional medical care and the use of complementary and alternative medicine. *Health Affairs (Millwood), 24*(1), 255–262.

Pichichero, M. E., Gentile, A., Giglio, N., Umido, V., Clarkson, T., Cernichiari, E., et al. (2008). Mercury levels in newborns and infants after receipt of thimerosal-containing vaccines. *Pediatrics, 121*(2), e208–214.

Plioplys, A. V. (1998). Intravenous immunoglobulin treatment of children with autism. *Journal of Child Neurology, 13*(2), 79–82.

Politi, O., Cena, H., Comelli, M., Marrone, G., Allegri, C., Emanuele, E., et al. (2009). Behavioral effects of omega-3 fatty acid supplementation of young adults with severe autism: An open label study. *Archives of Medical Research, 39*(7), 682–685.

Ramakrishnan, U., Imhoff-Kunsch, B., & DiGirolamo, A. M. (2009). Role of docosahexaenoic acid in maternal and child mental health. *American Journal of Clinical Nutrition, 89*(3), 958S–962S.

Rossignol, D. A., Rossignol, L. W., James, S. J., Melnyk, S., & Mumper, E. (2007). The effects of hyperbaric oxygen therapy on oxidative stress, inflammation, and symptoms in children with autism: An open-label pilot study. *BMC Pediatrics, 7*(1), 36.

Rossignol, D. A., Rossignol, L. W., Smith, S., Schneider, C., Logerquist, S., Usman, A., Neubrander, J., et al. (2009). Hyperbaric treatment for children with autism: A multicenter, randomized, double-blind, controlled trial. *BMC Pediatrics 9*, doi: 10.1186/1471-2431-9-21.

Sandler, A. (2005). Placebo effects in developmental disabilities: Implications for research and practice. *Mental Retardation and Developmental Disabilities Research Reviews, 11*(2), 164–170.

Sandler, R. H., Finegold, S. M., Bolte, E. R., Buchanan, C. P., Maxwell, A. P., Vaisanen, M. L., et al. (2000). Short-term benefit from oral vancomycin treatment of regressive-onset autism. *Journal of Child Neurology, 15*(7), 429–435.

Scahill, L., Koenig, K., Carroll, D. H., & Pachler, M. (2007). Risperidone approved for the treatment of serious behavioral problems in children with autism. *Journal of Child and Adolescent Psychiatric Nursing, 20*(3), 188–190.

Sesso, H. D., Buring, J. E., Christen, W. G., Kurth, T., Belanger, C., MacFadyen, J., et al. (2008). Vitamins E and C in the prevention of cardiovascular disease in men: The Physicians' Health Study II randomized controlled trial. *Journal of the American Medical Association, 300*(18), 2123–2133.

Shaw, W., Kassen, E., & Chaves, E. (1995). Increased urinary excretion of analogs of Krebs cycle metabolites and arabinose in two brothers with autistic features. *Clinical Chemistry, 41*(8 Pt 1), 1094–1104.

Sherman, K. J., Cherkin, D. C., Deyo, R. A., Erro, J. H., Hrbek, A., Davis, R. B., et al. (2006). The diagnosis and treatment of chronic back pain by acupuncturists, chiropractors, and massage therapists. *Clinical Journal of Pain, 22*(3), 227–234.

Silva, L. M., & Cignolini, A. (2005). A medical qigong methodology for early intervention in autism spectrum disorder: A case series. *American Journal of Chinese Medicine, 33*(2), 315–327.

Silva, L. M., Cignolini, A., Warren, R., Budden, S., & Skowron-Gooch, A. (2007). Improvement in sensory impairment and social interaction in young children with autism following treatment with an original Qigong massage methodology. *American Journal of Chinese Medicine, 35*(3), 393–406.

Sinha, Y., Silove, N., Wheeler, D., & Williams, K. (2004). Auditory integration training and other sound therapies for autism spectrum disorders. *Cochrane Database Systems Review* (1), CD003681.

Sinha, Y., Silove, N., Wheeler, D., & Williams, K. (2006). Auditory integration training and other sound therapies for autism spectrum disorders: A systematic review. *Archives of Disease in Childhood, 91*(12), 1018–1022.

Spigelblatt, L., Laine-Ammara, G., Pless, I. B., & Guyver, A. (1994). The use of alternative medicine by children. *Pediatrics, 94*(6 Pt 1), 811–814.

Stangle, D. E., Smith, D. R., Beaudin, S. A., Strawderman, M. S., Levitsky, D. A., & Strupp, B. J. (2007). Succimer chelation improves learning, attention, and arousal regulation in lead-exposed rats but produces lasting cognitive impairment in the absence of lead exposure. *Environmental Health Perspectives, 115*(2), 201–209.

Tordjman, S., Anderson, G. M., Pichard, N., Charbuy, H., & Touitou, Y. (2005). Nocturnal excretion of 6-sulphatoxymelatonin in children and adolescents with autistic disorder. *Biological Psychiatry, 57*(2), 134–138.

Vargas, D. L., Nascimbene, C., Krishnan, C., Zimmerman, A. W., & Pardo, C. A. (2005). Neuroglial activation and neuroinflammation in the brain of patients with autism. *Annals of Neurology, 57*(1), 67–81.

Wakefield, A. J., Anthony, A., Murch, S. H., Thomson, M., Montgomery, S. M., Davies, S., et al. (2000). Enterocolitis in children with developmental disorders. *American Journal of Gastroenterology, 95*(9), 2285–2295.

Williams, K. W., Wray, J. J., & Wheeler, D. M. (2005). Intravenous secretin for autism spectrum disorder. *Cochrane Database Systematic Reviews* (3), CD003495.

Wong, H. H., & Smith, R. G. (2006). Patterns of complementary and alternative medical therapy use in children diagnosed with autism spectrum disorders. *Journal of Autism of Development Disorders, 36*(7), 901–909.

72 Dilja D. Krueger, Mark F. Bear

The mGluR Theory of Fragile X Syndrome

Points of Interest

- Fragile X Syndrome (FXS) is a single-gene disorder associated with mental retardation and autism that is caused by loss of expression of the fragile X mental retardation protein (FMRP).
- The "mGluR theory of fragile X" postulates that FMRP and group I metabotropic glutamate receptors (mGluRs) act in functional opposition to regulate protein synthesis at the synapse, with mGluRs activating and FMRP repressing translation of FMRP target mRNAs.
- Antagonism of mGluRs is expected to reverse many of the phenotypes resulting from the loss of FMRP and may thus provide a valuable strategy for the treatment of FXS and other autism spectrum disorders (ASDs) linked to excessive synaptic protein synthesis.
- Preclinical studies in animal models of FXS have shown that genetic or pharmacological antagonism of mGluR5 signaling can reverse many of the structural, physiological, and behavioral phenotypes related to FXS.
- Clinical studies are underway to test the efficacy of mGluR5 antagonists in treating patients with FXS.

Synaptic plasticity is an alteration in the strength of synaptic connections between neurons that is believed to be important for long-term information storage in the brain. Several forms of synaptic plasticity exist, including **long-term potentiation (LTP)**, a persistent enhancement of synaptic strength, and **long-term depression (LTD)**, a persistent decrease in synaptic strength. Many different molecular mechanisms are thought to contribute to synaptic plasticity, one of which is the **internalization**, or **endocytosis**, of a class of glutamate receptors known as **AMPA receptors**. The removal of these receptors from the synapse results in a decrease in glutamatergic transmission that may be particularly important for metabotropic glutamate receptor-induced LTD, or **mGluR-LTD**.

Synaptic protein synthesis: also known as **translation**, is the process by which cells generate proteins based on genetic information encoded in the form of messenger RNA, or **mRNA**. Protein synthesis is carried out by large structures called **ribosomes**, which can cluster on mRNAs to form **polyribosomes**. In neurons, the bulk of protein synthesis occurs in the cell body, but certain mRNAs can be translated locally at synapses to generate protein products that are likely to be involved in synapse-specific structural and functional plasticity. These mRNAs are transported into dendrites and stored at synapses in the form of RNA-protein complexes known as **ribonucleoprotein particles** or **RNA granules**. Translation of individual mRNAs can be regulated by proteins that act as **translational activators** or **translational repressors**, and these proteins, in turn, can be regulated by processes such as **phosphorylation** and **dephosphorylation** in response to extracellular signals.

***Fmr1* knockout mice**: Given the difficulty in obtaining information at the molecular and cellular level from human FXS patients, the vast majority of the knowledge summarized in this chapter has been gained from studies conducted in animal models of FXS. The most widely used animal model in fragile X research is an ***Fmr1* knockout mouse**, or ***Fmr1* KO**, that was generated by disrupting exon 5 of the mouse *Fmr1* gene, resulting in loss of expression of the FMRP protein (The Dutch-Belgian Fragile X Consortium et al., 1994).

Introduction

Fragile X Syndrome (FXS) is the most prevalent form of inherited mental retardation, characterized by cognitive and behavioral deficits that include developmental delay, attention deficits and hyperactivity, impulsivity, aggression, sensory hypersensitivity and withdrawal from touch, abnormalities in language and communication, social anxiety, and stereotyped behaviors and interests (Penagarikano et al., 2007; Reiss & Hall, 2007). Approximately 18% to 33% of individuals with FXS are also diagnosed with autism, and the prevalence of FXS in autism is 2% to 4% (Belmonte & Bourgeron, 2006; Zafeiriou et al., 2007), making it one of the most common single-gene disorders associated with autism. Based on this overlap in phenotypes, it has been proposed that there may also be an overlap in the neural mechanisms underlying the two disorders and that understanding how the single-gene alteration in FXS results in autistic-like behaviors may provide valuable insights into potential targets for the research on idiopathic autism (Belmonte & Bourgeron, 2006).

The "mGluR theory of fragile X syndrome" provides a useful example of how basic research into the molecular consequences of such single-gene alterations may produce insights that can be directly translated into therapeutic strategies (Bear et al., 2004). It originated from three basic findings: *(1)* the discovery that activation of a class of neuronal receptors known as metabotropic glutamate receptors, or mGluRs, resulted in the synthesis of new proteins at the synapse (Weiler et al., 1997); *(2)* the subsequent observation that a form of mGluR-induced synaptic plasticity, known as mGluR-dependent long-term depression (LTD), was protein synthesis-dependent (Huber et al., 2000); and *(3)* LTD was exaggerated in a mouse model of FXS (Huber et al., 2002). Together, these findings suggested that FMRP may be a crucial regulator of mGluR-mediated protein synthesis at the synapse and that in the absence of FMRP, mGluR-dependent synaptic maturation and plasticity may be disrupted, resulting in some or all of the phenotypes observed in FXS (Bear et al., 2004). Based on this model, it was proposed that by pharmacologically targeting mGluR function, it might be possible to reverse these phenotypes and develop a treatment strategy for FXS. Since its introduction in 2002, the mGluR theory of fragile X has been extensively investigated, and the results emerging from this research continue to support the notion that mGluRs and their downstream effectors may be promising therapeutic targets for the treatment of FXS.

In this chapter, we first briefly introduce FMRP and metabotropic glutamate receptors. Subsequently, we review the current state of knowledge on the mGluR theory at the level of basic, preclinical, and clinical research. Finally, we discuss the questions that remain to be addressed to ensure that pharmacological interventions based on the mGluR theory have the greatest possible chance of succeeding in clinical trials and providing safe and effective treatments for patients with FXS.

The Fragile X Mental Retardation Protein

Fragile X Syndrome received its name from the observation that individuals with this disorder show a characteristic constriction, or fragile site, at the end of the long arm of chromosome X (Penagarikano et al., 2007). This fragile site was found to result from a CGG trinucleotide repeat expansion located in the first exon of a gene subsequently named *FMR1*, or fragile X mental retardation gene 1 (Verkerk et al., 1991). The triplet repeat expansion causes hypermethylation of the repeat itself and of the surrounding DNA sequence, leading to transcriptional silencing of *FMR1* and hence loss of the *FMR1* gene product FMRP, or fragile X mental retardation protein. Since the initial characterization of this protein 15 years ago (Verheij et al., 1993; Devys et al., 1993), extensive research has focused on identifying its cellular function and the mechanisms by which its disruption results in mental retardation and autism. In this section, we summarize the current understanding of FMRP function and its role in synaptic plasticity and behavior.

Fragile X Mental Retardation Protein Structure and Function

FMRP is expressed widely throughout the body, but it is particularly enriched in the brain and testes. Within the brain, FMRP is expressed almost exclusively in neurons, localizing both to the cell body and to dendrites and synapses (Feng et al., 1997; Christie et al., 2009). Structural analysis of FMRP revealed that it is an mRNA binding protein, containing several characteristic RNA binding motifs, including two KH domains and an RGG box (Siomi et al., 1993; Ashley, Jr. et al., 1993). A comprehensive list of mRNAs targeted by FMRP has yet to be established, but it was estimated that FMRP binds to approximately 4% of all mRNAs present in the brain (Ashley Jr. et al., 1993), and a number of candidates have been identified that will be discussed in more detail in the section on target proteins regulated by FMRP and mGluR signaling.

One important clue regarding the function of FMRP came from the observation that it is associated with polyribosomes, implying a role in the regulation of protein synthesis (Tamanini et al., 1996; Khandjian et al., 1996; Corbin et al., 1997). Based on in vitro assays, FMRP was proposed to function as a repressor of protein synthesis (Laggerbauer et al., 2001; Li et al., 2001), and this is consistent with findings in animal models of FXS showing that basal protein synthesis is increased in the absence of FMRP (Qin et al., 2005; Dolen et al., 2007; Bolduc et al., 2008). Several mechanisms have been proposed by which FMRP may regulate translation (Figure 72-1). In one study, FMRP was found to be associated with stalled, translationally inactive polyribosomes when phosphorylated at residue serine 499, whereas dephosphorylated FMRP was associated with actively translating polyribosomes (Ceman et al., 2003). These findings led to the hypothesis that FMRP-bound mRNAs may be positioned on stalled ribosomes until the arrival of a signal resulting in FMRP dephosphorylation and translational derepression. It has also been proposed that FMRP may be involved in sequestering mRNAs into RNA granules, structures that are thought to represent pools of translationally silent mRNAs that may or may not also contain stalled polyribosomes (Mazroui et al., 2002; Aschrafi et al., 2005). In support of this hypothesis, a decrease in the total number of RNA granules was observed

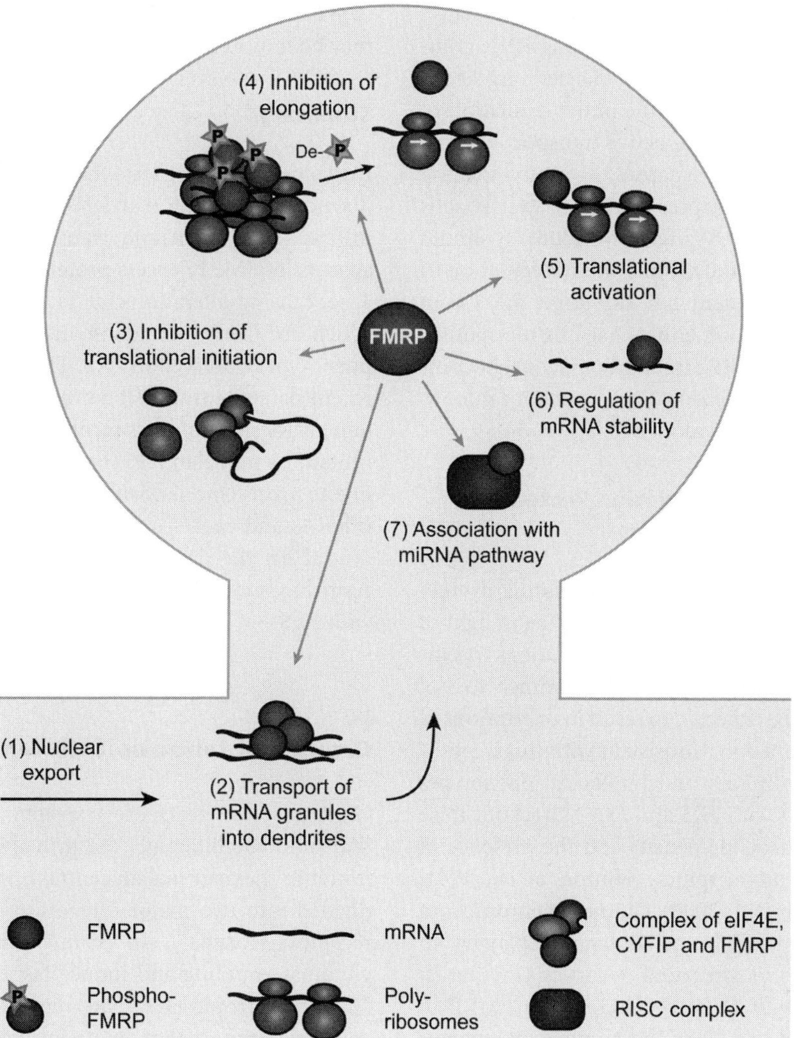

Figure 72–1. Putative roles of FMRP at the synapse. A number of different mechanisms have been proposed by which FMRP may regulate synaptic function and plasticity. These mechanisms include *(1)* Export of target mRNAs from the nucleus, *(2)* Trafficking of mRNA granules into dendrites and synapses, *(3)* Inhibition of translation initiation, *(4)* Inhibition of elongation in response to FMRP phosphorylation, possibly by sequestration of stalled ribosomes into translationally inactive mRNA granules, *(5)* Activation of translation of certain target mRNAs, *(6)* Regulation of stability of target mRNAs, and *(7)* Association with the microRNA pathway. To date, the relative contribution of each of these mechanisms to the regulation of synaptic structure and function remains unknown. It is conceivable that several of these functions occur in parallel at the same synapses or that different mechanisms may play differential roles depending on brain region, Developmental stage, species, or other unknown factors. (See Color Plate Section for a color version of this figure.)

in a mouse model of FXS, consistent with the notion of derepression of mRNAs and increased protein synthesis in the absence of FMRP (Aschrafi et al., 2005). Another more recent model postulates that FMRP may repress translation initiation by recruiting the cytoplasmic FMRP interacting protein 1, or CYFIP1, which in turn was suggested to inhibit the function of the translation initiation factor eIF4E (Napoli et al., 2008). Finally, it has been proposed that FMRP may also regulate protein synthesis by activating, rather than repressing, translation of certain targets (Bechara et al., 2009), by altering the stability of individual mRNAs (Zalfa et al., 2007), and through association with the microRNA pathway (Cheever & Ceman, 2009). Together, these findings imply that FMRP may regulate translation at several levels in parallel or that different mechanisms may be involved under different conditions.

In addition to its role in regulating protein synthesis, FMRP has also been implicated in the transport and localization of mRNAs to dendrites and synapses (Figure 72-1). FMRP contains nuclear import and export signals, and it was proposed to be required for nuclear export of its target mRNAs in ribonucleoprotein particles (Eberhart et al., 1996; Kim et al., 2009). Moreover, FMRP-containing RNA granules were found to be trafficked into neurites in PC12 cells (De Diego Otero et al., 2002) and into dendrites and spines in hippocampal cultures in an activity-dependent manner (Antar et al., 2004; Antar et al., 2005). FMRP was found to interact with kinesins, a class of motor proteins that mediate transport of cargos along microtubules, and this interaction was required for trafficking of FMRP-containing RNA granules to dendrites (Davidovic et al., 2007; Dictenberg et al., 2008). FMRP may thus serve a dual role in the regulation of synaptic mRNAs, first by mediating active transport of RNA granules along microtubules to synapses, and subsequently by repressing translation at synapses until the latter is activated by synaptic stimulation (Wang et al., 2008). It should be noted, however, that one study found no dysregulation of the dendritic localization of putative FMRP target mRNAs in *Fmr1* knockout mice, suggesting either that this mechanism only applies to a subset of FMRP target mRNAs, or that compensatory mechanisms may occur in *Fmr1* knockout mice to replace this function (Steward et al., 1998).

Role of Fragile X Mental Retardation Protein in Synaptic Structure and Plasticity

The identification of a role for FMRP in regulating protein synthesis at the synapse was particularly interesting in light of the increasing evidence linking local protein synthesis to synaptic maturation and plasticity. Given these findings, loss of FMRP expression might be expected to result in disruptions of synaptic structure and function. Consistent with this hypothesis, one of the most prominent morphological phenotypes observed in both patients with FXS and *Fmr1* knockout mice is an increase in dendritic spine density and the presence of abnormal long and tortuous spines (Hinton et al., 1991; Comery et al., 1997; Irwin et al., 2000). Cultured neurons from *Fmr1* knockout mice mimic this phenotype, displaying an increase in the number of structural synapses (Pfeiffer & Huber, 2007). Interestingly, acute replacement of FMRP in these cultures was found to reduce the number of synapses without affecting the function or maturation state of the remaining synapses. Similarly, acute replacement of FMRP in a Drosophila model of fragile X was able to at least partially rescue synaptic structural phenotypes (Gatto & Broadie, 2008). These findings imply that the abnormal increase in spines and synapses observed in the absence of FMRP is not solely an irreversible developmental effect, raising the possibility that acute postnatal manipulations may be able to rescue these deficits and hence provide a viable treatment strategy.

In addition to these effects on synaptic structure, loss of FMRP in animal models has also been shown to affect synaptic plasticity. *Fmr1* knockout mice show exaggerated forms of LTD in hippocampus (Huber et al., 2002) and cerebellum (Koekkoek et al., 2005), consistent with the notion of excess protein synthesis in these mice that underlies the expression of certain forms of LTD (discussed in further detail below). Moreover, several groups have reported a disruption in long-term potentiation (LTP) in the cortex of *Fmr1* knockout mice (Li et al., 2002; Zhao et al., 2005; Desai et al., 2006; Wilson & Cox, 2007), possibly because of an alteration in the threshold for LTP induction (Meredith et al., 2007). Together, these findings suggest that the absence of FMRP causes alterations in synaptic plasticity at synapses throughout the brain, which may be important in the pathogenesis of FXS.

Summary

Evidence to date suggests that the protein disrupted in fragile X syndrome, FMRP, is an RNA-binding protein that regulates mRNA localization and translation at the synapse. In the absence of FMRP, excess protein synthesis occurs at the synapse, causing alterations in synaptic structure and plasticity, which are likely to underlie at least some of the behavioral phenotypes observed in FXS. This hypothesis is supported by recent data showing that administration of low levels of protein synthesis inhibitors reverses memory deficits in a dFmr1 mutant fly model of FXS (Bolduc et al., 2008). Future research on the precise mechanisms by which FMRP regulates synaptic mRNAs and causes excess synaptic protein synthesis will be crucial for the development of therapeutic agents aimed at restoring normal synaptic structure and function in patients with FXS.

Group I Metabotropic Glutamate Receptors

Glutamate receptors are transmembrane receptor proteins that bind to glutamate, the principle excitatory neurotransmitter in the mammalian central nervous system. They can be divided into two major categories: *(1)* ionotropic glutamate receptors (iGluRs), ion channels that open in response to glutamate binding and induce fast excitatory responses, and *(2)* metabotropic glutamate receptors (mGluRs), G-protein coupled receptors that link to intracellular signaling pathways and hence modulate neuronal function. To date there are eight known mGluR subtypes that can be divided into three groups based on sequence homology, pharmacology, and signal transduction mechanisms: group I (mGluR1 and mGluR5), group II (mGluR2 and mGluR3), and group III (mGluR4, mGluR6, mGluR7 and mGluR8). This section will focus on a description of group I mGluRs because of their implication in the pathogenesis of FXS.

Distribution of Group I mGluRs in the Brain

Both mGluR1 and mGluR5 are expressed widely throughout the central nervous system, but they show distinct patterns of enrichment in specific brain regions. mGluR1 expression is most abundant in the cerebellum and the olfactory bulb, as well as in the hippocampus, lateral septum, globus pallidus, thalamus, substantia nigra, and superior colliculus (Martin et al., 1992; Shigemoto et al., 1992). mGluR5 is present at highest levels in cortex, hippocampus, striatum, lateral septum, olfactory bulb, and inferior colliculus (Shigemoto et al., 1993; Romano et al., 1995). In addition to these spatial differences, mGluR1 and mGluR5 show distinct patterns of temporal regulation during postnatal development: mGluR1 expression starts at low levels at birth and increases steadily over the first three postnatal weeks, whereas mGluR5 is highly expressed in the neonatal brain but subsequently decreases in all brain regions except the hippocampus (Catania et al., 1994). Both receptors are found predominantly in dendritic shafts and spines, suggesting a mostly postsynaptic function for group I mGluRs, although some examples of presynaptic expression and function have also been reported.

Function of Group I mGluRs

The discovery of metabotropic glutamate receptors in the late 1980s caused a major shift in the perception of the function of glutamate in the brain (Conn, 2003). Previously, it was believed that glutamate was associated only with fast excitatory neurotransmission, whereas slower modulation of activity in glutamatergic circuits was ascribed to separate neuromodulators such as various monoamines and neuropeptides. The presence of G-protein coupled glutamate receptors at synapses throughout the brain suggested that glutamate itself may also act as a neuromodulator, simultaneously fine-tuning the fast excitatory responses it elicits. This notion became particularly interesting in light of the diversity of mGluR subtypes being identified, implying that these receptors may be involved in a variety of forms of glutamate-induced synaptic modulation. By now, it is known that mGluRs can indeed regulate synaptic plasticity by a plethora of mechanisms throughout the brain (Valenti et al., 2002; Xiao et al., 2006). Here, we will focus on those forms of plasticity that are induced by group I mGluRs and that depend on protein synthesis—that is, those that are potentially most relevant for FXS.

The most thoroughly understood function of group I mGluRs lies in the induction of LTD, a persistent decrease in synaptic strength that occurs in response to prolonged low-frequency stimulation (Figure 72-2). mGluR-dependent LTD is observed in several brain regions, including the hippocampus, cerebellum, striatum, ventral tegmental area, and bed nucleus of the stria terminalis. The molecular mechanisms of this mGluR-induced depression in synaptic strength have been extensively studied in the CA1 subregion of the hippocampus, where LTD can be induced either by specific synaptic stimulation protocols (Oliet et al., 1997; Huber et al., 2000) or by application of the group I mGluR agonist (S)-3,5-dihydroxyphenylglycine (DHPG) (Palmer et al., 1997; Huber et al., 2001). Using these induction protocols, it has been shown that activation of mGluRs causes a rapid internalization of postsynaptic AMPA receptor subunits (Snyder et al., 2001; Xiao et al., 2001), which is believed to underlie, at least in part, the observed decrease in synaptic strength. Both mGluR-LTD and the maintenance of mGluR-induced AMPA receptor internalization are dependent on local protein synthesis at the synapse (Huber et al., 2000; Snyder et al., 2001; Huber et al., 2001), suggesting a mechanism in which mGluR activation leads to the translation of specific proteins required for stabilization of the internalized AMPA receptors. The exact nature of these "LTD proteins" has remained elusive, but one candidate that has recently sparked much interest is the activity-regulated cytoskeletal protein Arc, which is known to be associated with the endocytic machinery (Shepherd et al., 2006; Park et al., 2008; Waung et al., 2008). mGluR-LTD in brain regions other than area CA1 of the hippocampus also appears to be dependent on postsynaptic protein synthesis and AMPA receptor internalization (Karachot et al., 2001; Naie & Manahan-Vaughan, 2005; Yin et al., 2006; Mameli et al., 2007). However, it has been proposed that the nature of the proteins that need to be synthesized and the mechanisms of regulation of local protein synthesis may be specific for each brain region (Bellone et al., 2008). It has also been suggested that the mechanisms of mGluR-LTD are regulated developmentally within the hippocampus and that presynaptic mechanisms that are not protein synthesis-dependent may play a role during certain stages of development (Rammes et al., 2003; Nosyreva & Huber, 2005; Moult et al., 2008).

In addition to mGluR-LTD, several other forms of group I mGluR-induced plasticity have been reported. In area CA1 of the hippocampus, application of subthreshold concentrations of group I mGluR agonists prior to induction of LTP leads to an enhanced magnitude and stability of that LTP, a phenomenon known as LTP priming (Cohen & Abraham, 1996). Conversely, application of the mGluR agonist DHPG to synapses that have already been potentiated by high-frequency stimulation results in loss of that potentiation, a process known as depotentiation (Zho et al., 2002). Like mGluR-LTD, both of these effects are dependent on protein synthesis, and depotentiation also requires AMPA receptor internalization (Raymond et al., 2000; Zho et al., 2002). There have also been reports that certain forms of LTP in hippocampus and cortex may be dependent on mGluR activation (Wilson & Cox, 2007), although the role of protein synthesis in these forms of plasticity is less clear. Finally, DHPG can cause long-lasting alterations of nonsynaptic synchronous neuronal activity in hippocampal slices (Piccinin et al., 2008). The protein synthesis dependence of this effect has not been investigated.

Signaling Pathways Activated by Group I mGluRs.

How does binding of glutamate to group I mGluRs trigger the protein synthesis necessary for mGluR-LTD and other forms of synaptic plasticity (Figure 72-2)? All mGluRs are G-protein coupled receptors, and group I mGluRs are specifically coupled to G proteins containing a $G\alpha_q$ subunit (Hermans & Challiss, 2001; Gerber et al., 2007). Binding of glutamate to the extracellular domain of group I mGluRs results in activation of the $G\alpha_q$ subunit, which in turn results in activation of phospholipase C β (PLCβ), an enzyme that releases the intracellular messengers inositol-1,4,5-trisphosphosphate (IP_3) and diacylglycerol (DAG). IP_3 binds to IP_3 receptors in the endoplasmic reticulum, leading to release of calcium from intracellular stores, whereas DAG (in concert with the released calcium) initiates signaling through the protein kinase C

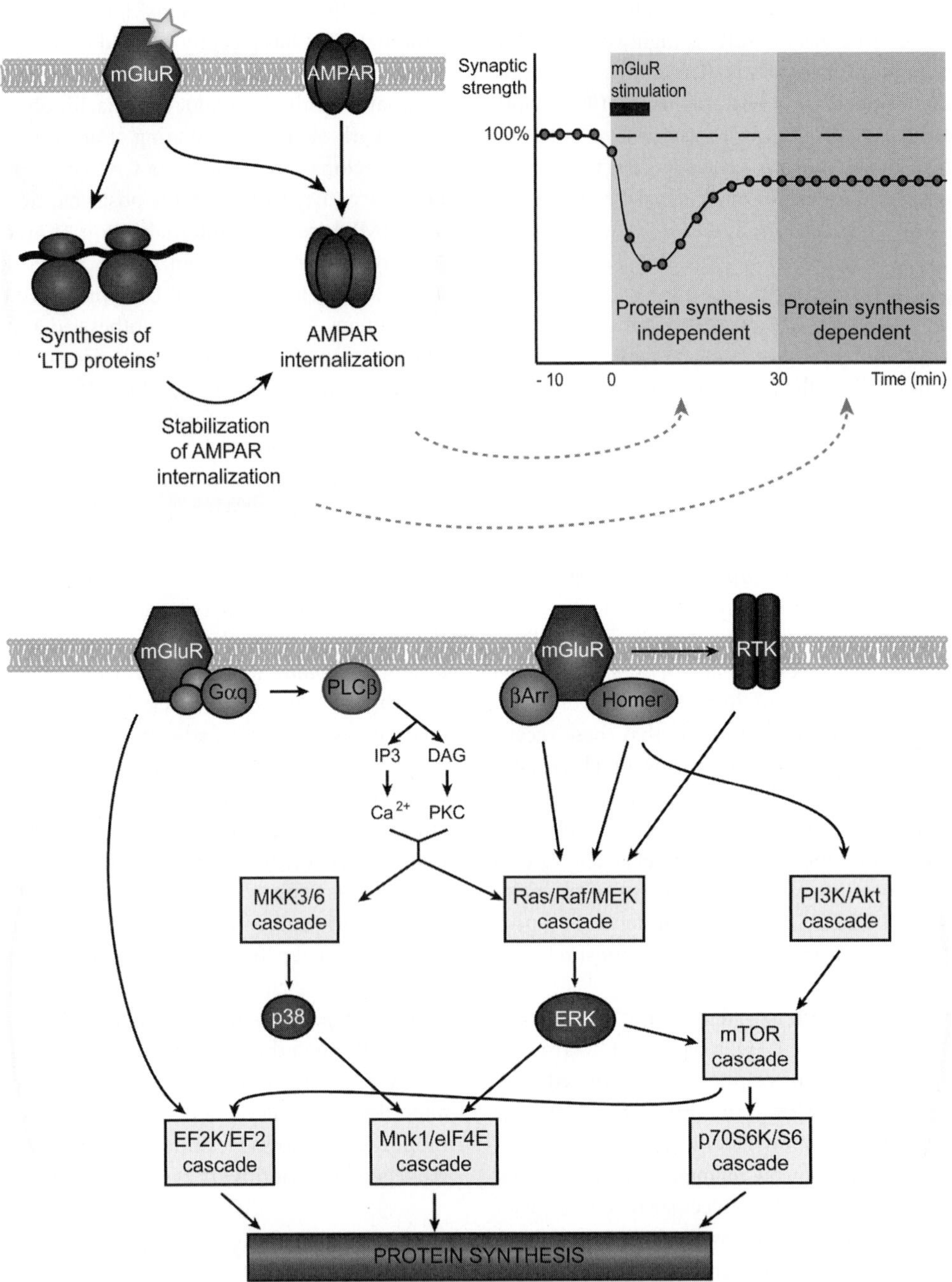

Figure 72–2. Function and signaling of group I mGluRs. *Upper Panel*: Stimulation of group I mGluRs can result in the induction of long-term depression (LTD), a persistent reduction in synaptic strength. Activation of mGluRs causes a rapid internalization of postsynaptic AMPA receptor subunits, which is thought to underlie the initial, protein synthesis-independent, decrease in synaptic strength. Activation of mGluRs also stimulates synaptic protein synthesis, which results in the synthesis of "LTD proteins" that are believed to be required for stabilizing the internalized AMPA receptors. This stabilization of AMPAR internalization is believed to be the basis for the persistent, protein synthesis-dependent, decrease in synaptic strength following induction of LTD. *Lower panel*: Signaling pathways proposed to be activated upon group I mGluR stimulation. To date, the relative contribution of each of these signaling pathways to synaptic protein synthesis remains unknown and is likely to vary depending on factors such as brain region and developmental stage. It should also be noted that research into these signaling pathways is still actively ongoing, and that this schematic may therefore be incomplete. (See Color Plate Section for a color version of this figure.)

(PKC) pathway. The increase in cytosolic calcium levels and the activation of PKC can result in the activation of a number of different downstream signaling pathways (Marinissen & Gutkind, 2001), the details of which appear to somewhat depend on the cell type and preparation under investigation. Both calcium and PKC can initiate a Ras/Raf1/MEK cascade that leads to activation of the extracellular signal-regulated kinase (ERK), and ERK activation has been shown to be required for hippocampal mGluR-LTD and for mGluR-induced activation of global protein synthesis (Gallagher et al., 2004;

Banko et al., 2006; Osterweil et al., 2010). Moreover, the $G\alpha_q$ subunit can activate a MKK3/6 cascade, resulting in activation of p38 MAPK, and this cascade may also be required for mGluR-LTD in area CA1 in adult rats (Moult et al., 2008).

In addition to the canonical G-protein-mediated signal transduction pathway, other signaling cascades have more recently been identified that may also be relevant for group I mGluR-dependent protein synthesis and plasticity. In particular, ERK can be activated by several G-protein- and calcium-independent mechanisms involving interactions with the Homer family of postsynaptic scaffolding proteins, interactions with β-arrestins, or transactivation of receptor tyrosine kinases (Gerber et al., 2007; Wang et al., 2007). Moreover, a transient activation of the PI3K/PDK1/Akt/mTOR pathway was reported to be necessary for mGluR-LTD in area CA1 (Hou & Klann, 2004), and activation of this pathway by group I mGluRs is likely to occur through G-protein-independent mechanisms such as interactions between mGluRs and Homer proteins (Ronesi & Huber, 2008b). Interestingly, activation of the PI3K/Akt/mTOR pathway by mGluRs does not occur under all conditions, and it does not appear to be necessary for mGluR-stimulated global protein synthesis (Osterweil et al., 2010). The functional importance of this pathway thus remains an area of active investigation.

Another important question that remains to be answered concerns the downstream pathways linking mGluR-mediated activation of ERK, p38 MAPK, or Akt to the stimulation of local protein synthesis. Candidates to date include the Mnk1/eIF4E pathway (Banko et al., 2006), the p70S6K/ribosomal protein S6 pathway (Antion et al., 2008), and the EF2K/eEF2 pathway (Park et al., 2008). The relative contribution of each of these pathways remains to be determined and may vary between brain regions and experimental preparations.

Group I mGluRs in Central Nervous System Disorders

In accordance with their key role in regulating synaptic function and plasticity, group I mGluRs have also been implicated in several neurological and psychiatric disorders. Because of their modulation of neuronal excitability, group I mGluRs facilitate epileptiform activity, and administration of pharmacological group I mGluR antagonists has antiepileptogenic and anticonvulsant effects in rodent models of epilepsy (Tang, 2005; Alexander & Godwin, 2006). These antagonists also produce anxiolytic behavioral responses in rodents, as well as decreasing reactivity of the autonomic nervous system to stressful conditions, suggesting a potential use in the treatment of anxiety disorders (Spooren et al., 2000; Pietraszek et al., 2005; Swanson et al., 2005). Similarly, pharmacological or genetic inhibition of mGluR5 results in antidepressant-like effects in rodents (Pilc et al., 2008). Striatal group I mGluRs may play an important role in drug addiction: Reduction of mGluR5 signaling by pharmacological or genetic manipulations abolishes preference for cocaine, morphine, nicotine, and ethanol in rodents, suggesting that group I mGluRs may positively regulate brain reward function (Kenny & Markou, 2004). In one study, a mutation in mGluR5 was linked to a familial case of schizophrenia (Krivoy et al., 2008). Inhibition of group I mGluRs—particularly mGluR1—has been implicated in the treatment of neuropathic pain (Schkeryantz et al., 2007). Finally, aberrant forms of mGluR-dependent striatal plasticity have been described in rodent models of Huntington's disease and Parkinson's disease, suggesting that mGluRs may be a useful target for the treatment of these disorders (Gubellini et al., 2004).

Pharmacological Agents Targeting Group I mGluRs

Because of their potential involvement in several disorders of the CNS, significant efforts are underway to develop pharmacological agents that target group I mGluRs and that may be of widespread therapeutic relevance. The most commonly used antagonist in preclinical research is 2-methyl-6-(phenylethynyl)-pyridine (MPEP), a potent noncompetitive antagonist of mGluR5 that crosses the blood–brain barrier and can be applied in studies both in vitro and in vivo (Lea & Faden, 2006). However, it was subsequently discovered that high doses of MPEP can result in off-target activity at other glutamate receptors, providing a potential caveat to some of the preclinical research on mGluR5 and decreasing its relevance for clinical applications. The more recently developed structural analog 3-((2-methyl-1,3-thiazol-4-yl)ethynyl) pyridine (MTEP) appears to show fewer off-target effects and better CNS penetrability, but it has been less well-characterized in preclinical models to date. Recently, the anxiolytic drug fenobam was shown to be a potent, selective, and noncompetitive antagonist of mGluR5 function (Porter et al., 2005). This important discovery confirmed the role of mGluR5 in anxiety disorders and provided access to a clinically available mGluR5 antagonist. In addition, development of novel modulators of group I mGluR function is underway, and targeting these receptors may soon be a viable treatment strategy for a range of clinical applications.

Summary

Group I mGluRs—particularly mGluR5—play an important role in activity- and protein synthesis-dependent synaptic plasticity throughout the brain, including in areas relevant for the behavioral phenotypes of FXS, such as hippocampus, striatum, cerebellum, and possibly cortex. Dysregulation of group I mGluR function has been linked to several neurological and psychiatric disorders, making these receptors important putative targets for the development of therapeutic interventions. The molecular mechanisms by which group I mGluRs induce protein synthesis and synaptic plasticity are beginning to be elucidated, but further research will be necessary to fully understand these mechanisms and identify potential additional drug targets for mGluR-related disorders.

Basic Research: Fragile X Mental Retardation Protein and mGluR Interactions at the Synapse

The observation that FMRP is a regulator of synaptic protein synthesis, and that mGluR activation induces synaptic protein synthesis that is required for mGluR-dependent plasticity, raised the intriguing possibility that there might be a functional interaction between these two synaptic elements and that the disruption of this interaction in FXS may play a major role in the pathogenesis of the disorder. In this section, we review the evidence that FMRP and mGluR signaling are indeed inter-related at the synapse and summarize what is known about the molecular mechanisms by which this functional interaction occurs.

Regulation of Fragile X Mental Retardation Protein Levels and Localization by mGluR Activation

The initial impetus for studying a role for mGluRs in FXS came from a biochemical screen looking for synaptic mRNAs that change their association with the translational machinery in response to neurotransmitter stimulation. It was shown that chemical stimulation of group I mGluRs in rat cortical synaptoneurosomes (an in vitro preparation that is enriched for synaptic terminals) resulted in an increased association of FMRP mRNA with actively translating ribosomes, as well as an increase in FMRP protein levels (Weiler et al., 1997). Subsequently, this finding was replicated in other experimental preparations, including mouse hippocampal slices (Hou et al., 2006), cultured cortical neurons (Todd et al., 2003a), and in vivo in rat barrel cortex (Todd et al., 2003b). In addition to FMRP synthesis, mGluR activation was also found to regulate the localization of the FMRP mRNA and protein within neurons. In response to stimulation of cultured hippocampal neurons with the group I mGluR agonist DHPG, both FMRP mRNA and protein were shown to translocate from the neuronal cell body into the dendrites, placing them closer to the site of synaptic protein synthesis (Antar et al., 2004). Interestingly, however, there appears to be some debate about the localization of FMRP in dendritic spines, with conflicting reports suggesting that FMRP either moves into spines (Ferrari et al., 2007) or out of spines (Antar et al., 2004) in response to DHPG stimulation. Further research will be required to resolve this issue, but overall it appears clear that the function of FMRP is regulated by mGluR stimulation, although some of the details remain to be investigated.

mGluR-Dependent Plasticity in the Absence of Fragile X Mental Retardation Protein

Following from the observation that FMRP function is regulated by mGluR stimulation, it was hypothesized that this regulation may be a key mechanism in the initiation of mGluR-dependent protein synthesis and plasticity. By this logic, it was proposed that many of the mGluR-induced protein synthesis-dependent plasticity processes described above would be altered in the absence of FMRP. The first evidence in support of this hypothesis was obtained in a study investigating mGluR-LTD in a mouse model of FXS, showing that mGluR-LTD in area CA1 of the hippocampus is exaggerated relative to wild-type controls (Huber et al., 2002). Even more strikingly, mGluR-LTD in the *Fmr1* knockout mice is no longer dependent on protein synthesis, persisting in the presence of the general translation inhibitors anisomycin and cycloheximide, which completely abolish mGluR-LTD in wild-type mice (Nosyreva & Huber, 2006). A similar phenomenon was observed for cerebellar mGluR-LTD in the *Fmr1* knockout mice (Koekkoek et al., 2005). Because one of the mechanisms by which mGluR activation is thought to induce LTD in wild-type animals is by triggering a protein synthesis-dependent internalization of AMPA receptor subunits, it was hypothesized that the excess LTD in the *Fmr1* knockout mice might result from an excess internalization of AMPA receptors. This hypothesis was confirmed using knockdown of FMRP levels by short interfering RNAs in rat hippocampal cultures, resulting in an excess AMPA receptor internalization at prestimulation baseline, which occludes further internalization in response to DHPG stimulation (Nakamoto et al., 2007). Recently, it was shown that another form of mGluR-dependent plasticity, LTP priming, is protein synthesis-independent in *Fmr1* knockout mice (Auerbach & Bear, 2010). The combination of these data led to the theory that under wild-type conditions, FMRP represses the synthesis of certain "plasticity proteins" required for AMPA receptor internalization and other plasticity-related processes until mGluR stimulation relieves this FMRP repression by an unknown mechanism. In the absence of FMRP, it was proposed, these proteins would be synthesized in excess at baseline, eliminating the need for further protein synthesis upon mGluR stimulation and leading to excess protein synthesis-independent plasticity (Figure 72-3). It should be noted that certain forms of synaptic plasticity, such as cortical LTP, appear to be decreased in *Fmr1* knockout mice, arguing against a general exaggeration of all forms of plasticity. It is possible that the coupling mechanisms between group I mGluRs and FMRP may differ between brain regions and synapses or that the decrease in cortical LTP may be a secondary effect of other consequences of FMRP loss.

Overall, the above studies have established a critical role for FMRP in regulating mGluR-dependent synaptic plasticity, presumably through the regulation of mGluR-induced protein synthesis that is required for the subsequent plasticity. Two major questions now arise that will be of fundamental importance in the development of novel therapeutic strategies for FXS: *(1)* At which step does FMRP regulate mGluR-induced protein synthesis, and how is this regulation achieved at the molecular level? and *(2)* What are the "plasticity proteins" and other targets that are synthesized in response to mGluR stimulation and that mediate the mGluR-dependent plasticity? Our current understanding of these questions will be summarized below.

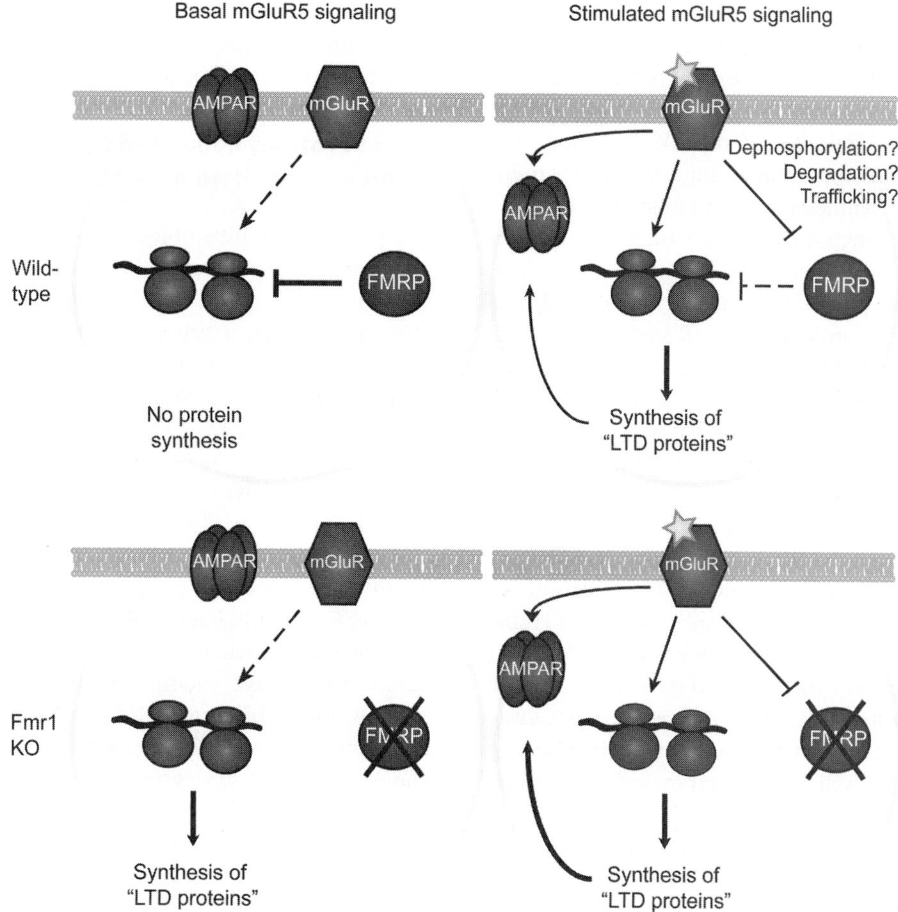

Figure 72–3. Model for the Interaction Between FMRP and Group I mGluRs in Translational Regulation and LTD. *Upper Left Panel*: Under basal conditions in wild-type mice, FMRP acts as a repressor of protein synthesis. As a result, no protein synthesis occurs, despite low levels of basal mGluR signaling. *Upper right panel*: mGluR stimulation in wild-type mice is thought to trigger three events: *(1)* internalization of AMPA receptors, *(2)* upregulation of protein synthesis signaling pathways, and *(3)* relief of FMRP-mediated translational repression by dephosphorylation of FMRP, degradation of FMRP, or translocation of FMRP out of the synapse. This leads to the synthesis of "LTD proteins," which stabilize the internalized AMPA receptors, resulting in protein synthesis-dependent LTD. *Lower left panel*: In *Fmr1* KO mice, FMRP is not present to repress translation, and basal mGluR signaling is therefore sufficient to induce synthesis of LTD proteins. In the absence of AMPA receptor internalization, however, these proteins alone do not result in LTD. *Lower right panel*: Upon mGluR stimulation in *Fmr1* KO mice, AMPA receptors are internalized just as in wild-type mice. However, the LTD proteins are already present in excess, resulting in stabilization of internalized AMPA receptors and hence LTD that is both exaggerated compared to wild-type mice and independent of new protein synthesis. (See Color Plate Section for a color version of this figure.)

Mechanisms of Fragile X Mental Retardation Protein Regulation of mGluR-Induced Protein Synthesis

As discussed above, the details of the molecular function of FMRP remain to be elucidated, and it has consequently proven challenging to determine how FMRP may respond to mGluR activation and participate in the regulation of mGluR-induced protein synthesis. However, a number of recent discoveries have yielded some important clues. Phosphorylation of FMRP was shown to influence the translation state of associated ribosomes (Ceman et al., 2003). Based on this observation, it was proposed that phosphorylated FMRP may act as a translational repressor and that dephosphorylation of FMRP in response to mGluR signaling may be an important switch that leads to the derepression of translation. In accordance with this hypothesis, it was recently shown that stimulation of mGluRs with DHPG in hippocampal cultures results in rapid and temporary (<5 min) dephosphorylation of FMRP by the phosphatase PP2A, and this was proposed to initiate translation (Narayanan et al., 2007). Other potential mechanisms by which FMRP-mediated translational repression may be relieved in response to mGluR activation include the mGluR-induced ubiquitination and degradation of FMRP (Hou et al., 2006) and the translocation of FMRP out of the synapse (Antar et al., 2004). The detailed mechanisms by which dephosphorylation, degradation, or translocation of FMRP are initiated in response to mGluR signaling remain an area of active investigation. Interestingly, it appears that derepression of protein synthesis following mGluR stimulation is a very short-lasting event, because FMRP is rephosphorylated (Narayanan et al., 2007; Narayanan et al., 2008) or newly synthesized (Hou et al., 2006) within 5 minutes of mGluR activation. This implies that it may be important to limit the time window during which protein synthesis can occur following the induction of plasticity, although the extremely brief nature of this time window is somewhat surprising.

Another intriguing phenomenon is that loss of FMRP also appears to cause alterations in the mGluR signaling pathways upstream of FMRP, presumably through complex feedback loops. One study showed that in *Fmr1* knockout mice, mGluR5 receptors are less tightly coupled with synapses and Homer scaffolding proteins, implying an increased lateral motility in the membrane and thus presumably leading to altered signaling properties (Giuffrida et al., 2005). Consistent with this hypothesis, the Homer-dependent activation of mTOR signaling in response to mGluR5 stimulation was absent altogether in *Fmr1* knockout mice (Ronesi & Huber, 2008b). At the same time, basal activation of the PI3K/Akt/mTOR signaling pathway was found to be elevated in *Fmr1* knockout mice (Sharma et al., 2010; Gross et al., 2010). Other groups have reported a slight basal increase in ERK activity (Hou et al., 2006) as well as an aberrant mGluR-induced inactivation of ERK (Kim et al., 2008) in *Fmr1* knockout mice, although these effects are not observed under all conditions (Osterweil et al., 2010).

Target Proteins Regulated by Fragile X Mental Retardation Protein and mGluR Signaling

One of the major areas of focus in fragile X research has been the identification of target mRNAs of FMRP that are dysregulated in the absence of FMRP. Using micro-array studies and other approaches, it was determined that 2% to 4% of all mRNAs in the brain can bind to FMRP via its KH domains and/or its RGG box (Brown et al., 2001; Darnell et al., 2001; Bassell & Warren, 2008). To date, no comprehensive list of all of these targets is available, but we will discuss a number of candidates here based on their potential relevance to mGluR-dependent plasticity (Table 72-1).

Two of the most widely studied FMRP targets are the microtubule-associated protein MAP1B and the elongation factor eEF1A. MAP1B is highly expressed during early postnatal development, where it plays an important role in neurite outgrowth through modulation of microtubule dynamics. MAP1B mRNA binds to FMRP via its RGG domain, and its developmental expression profile is disrupted in *Fmr1* knockout mice, resulting in abnormal microtubule stability

Table 72–1.
List of mRNAs believed to be translationally regulated by both FMRP and group I mGluRs

Protein	Link to FMRP	Link to mGluRs	References
MAP1B	mRNA binds to FMRP Developmental expression time-course is altered in *Fmr1* KO Genetic interaction between dFMR and MAP1B homolog in Drosophila	Synthesized in response to mGluR activation Involved in mGluR-dependent AMPAR endocytosis	Zhang et al., 2001; Lu et al., 2004; Davidkova & Carroll, 2007; Menon et al., 2008
EF1A	mRNA binds to FMRP	Synthesized in response to mGluR activation	Sung et al., 2003; Huang et al., 2005; Antion et al., 2008
Arc	Upregulated in *Fmr1* knockout mice mGluR-stimulated synthesis is abolished in *Fmr1* KO *Fmr1* x Arc double knockout mice have reduced mGluR-LTD	Synthesized in response to mGluR activation Required for mGluR-LTD and AMPAR trafficking	Zalfa et al., 2003; Shepherd et al., 2006; Park et al., 2008; Waung et al., 2008
CaMKII	Upregulated in *Fmr1* KO	Synthesized in response to mGluR activation	Zalfa et al., 2003; Muddashetty et al., 2007
PSD95	mGluR-stimulated synthesis is absent or occluded in *Fmr1* KO Levels downregulated in *Fmr1* KO caused by decreased mRNA stability	Synthesized in response to mGluR activation mGluR stimulation increases mRNA stability	Todd et al., 2003a; Muddashetty et al., 2007; Zalfa et al., 2007
SAPAP3	Upregulated in *Fmr1* KO	Synthesized in response to mGluR activation	Narayanan et al., 2007; Narayanan et al., 2008
APP	Upregulated in *Fmr1* KO	Synthesized in response to mGluR activation	Westmark & Malter, 2007
GluR2/3	Upregulated in *Fmr1* KO	Synthesized in response to mGluR activation	Osterweil et al., unpublished

(Lu et al., 2004; Menon et al., 2008). In Drosophila, loss of dFmr1 leads to synaptic structural defects, and these defects are reversed in double mutants also lacking Futsch, the Drosophila equivalent of MAP1B (Zhang et al., 2001). Recently, it was also shown that MAP1B is synthesized in response to DHPG stimulation in hippocampal cultures, and it is required for DHPG-induced AMPA receptor endocytosis (Davidkova & Carroll, 2007). These findings suggest that alterations in MAP1B regulation may play a role in disrupting axon targeting and synaptogenesis and synaptic plasticity in FXS. eEF1A is a component of the protein synthesis machinery that is responsible for delivering amino acids bound to transfer RNAs to the ribosome. It has been shown that eEF1A mRNA binds to and is repressed by FMRP (Sung et al., 2003) and that eEF1A protein is synthesized in response to DHPG stimulation in hippocampal slices (Huang et al., 2005; Antion et al., 2008). Thus far, the importance of eEF1A synthesis for synaptic plasticity or FXS has not been investigated, but it is conceivable that by expanding the translational machinery, it may contribute to the basal increase in protein synthesis observed in *Fmr1* knockout mice.

Two other candidates that have received much attention are the activity-regulated cytoskeleton-associated protein Arc and the Ca^{2+}/calmodulin-dependent kinase CaMKII α. Arc plays an important role in AMPA receptor trafficking and LTD (Shepherd et al., 2006). *Fmr1* knockout mice reportedly have increased levels of Arc protein, as well as an increased association between Arc mRNA and polyribosomes (Zalfa et al., 2003). Arc is also rapidly upregulated in response to neuronal activity and mGluR-LTD (Waung et al., 2008), and this upregulation (but not a slower, presumably transcriptional event) is abolished in *Fmr1* knockout mice (Park et al., 2008). In *Fmr1* x Arc double knockout mice, mGluR-LTD is reduced (but not abolished). Similar data have been obtained for CaMKIIα, a kinase known to play a crucial role both in synaptic plasticity and in learning and memory. As with Arc, CaMKII α protein levels were found to be increased in *Fmr1* knockout mice, and CaMKII α mRNA showed an increased association with polyribosomes (Zalfa et al., 2003). DHPG stimulation also results in CaMKII α protein synthesis (Muddashetty et al., 2007). Together, these data imply that Arc and CaMKII α may be involved in the altered plasticity observed in *Fmr1* knockout mice.

A somewhat more complicated story has been reported for the regulation of PSD-95, a scaffolding protein that is a major component of the postsynaptic density and that is thought to anchor glutamate receptors and intracellular signaling proteins at the synapse. Like the above candidates, PSD-95 is synthesized in response to DHPG stimulation in cortical cultures and synaptoneurosomes, and this increase is absent or occluded in *Fmr1* knockout mice (Todd et al., 2003a; Muddashetty et al., 2007). However, another study found that in hippocampus of *Fmr1* knockout mice, levels of PSD-95 mRNA are lower than in wild-type mice, and that this results from a decrease in PSD-95 mRNA stability (Zalfa et al., 2007). Moreover, DHPG was shown to increase stability of PSD-95 mRNA in hippocampal cultures from wild-type mice but not from knockout mice. Thus, FMRP may be able to act by several different mechanisms, translationally repressing some mRNAs but increasing the stability of others. Interestingly, another postsynaptic scaffolding protein, SAPAP3, was found to be upregulated both by DHPG stimulation and in the *Fmr1* knockout mouse (Narayanan et al., 2007; Narayanan et al., 2008), indicating that there might be differences in mechanisms of regulation even within categories of similar proteins.

Recently, another target of FMRP was identified in the amyloid precursor protein (APP) that is associated with Alzheimer's disease (Westmark & Malter, 2007). APP levels were increased in synaptoneurosomes and cortical cultures from *Fmr1* knockout mice, and this occluded the further DHPG-induced increase observed in wild-type mice. The physiological function of the APP protein remains somewhat unclear, but it has been implicated in synapse formation and plasticity, and it is conceivable that dysregulation of these events in FXS results in cognitive deficits by mechanisms paralleling those involved in Alzheimer's disease.

Finally, unpublished observations from our laboratory suggest that the AMPA receptor subunit GluR2 may also be an interesting candidate in the search for relevant FMRP targets. Levels of GluR2/3 were found to be increased by DHPG stimulation in hippocampal slices, and this increase was mimicked and occluded in the *Fmr1* knockout mice (Osterweil et al., unpublished). These data are consistent with previous findings showing that the rapid translation of GluR2 is required for mGluR-LTD in the ventral tegmental area (Mameli et al., 2007), suggesting that an excess of mGluR-induced GluR2 synthesis in *Fmr1* knockout mice may contribute to the exaggerated mGluR-LTD phenotype.

Summary

Twelve years after publication of the first study demonstrating a link between FMRP and group I mGluRs, a large body of evidence now supports the model that these two players act in functional opposition to regulate protein synthesis at the synapse, with mGluRs activating and FMRP repressing translation of the majority of target mRNAs. Loss of translational repression by FMRP in FXS appears to result in excess synthesis and dysregulation of target proteins that are required for mGluR-dependent synaptic plasticity, leading to aberrant plasticity that may underlie the behavioral phenotypes observed in FXS. Significant progress has been made in identifying the mechanisms by which mGluR signaling leads to derepression of FMRP-associated protein synthesis and the nature of the relevant target mRNAs. However, it has also become increasingly clear that the interplay between FMRP and mGluRs is far more complex than initially anticipated and that multiple different mechanisms and many essential target proteins may be involved. Further research will be necessary to address both of these crucial questions to fully understand the potential of targeting mGluRs as a pharmacological treatment for FXS and related disorders.

Preclinical Research: Reversal of Fragile X Syndrome Phenotypes by mGluR Antagonism in Animal Models

In light of the growing literature implicating a dysregulation of mGluR signaling in FXS, research efforts have been increasingly aimed at directly testing whether mGluRs might provide a viable therapeutic target for the treatment of FXS. To address this question at the level of preclinical research, a number of groups have used various animal models of FXS to manipulate mGluR signaling and assess whether these manipulations can reverse the deficits observed in these animal models (Table 72-2).

Pharmacological Manipulations in the *Fmr1* Knockout Mouse

One of the first pieces of evidence that mGluRs may indeed provide a promising target for pharmacological interventions in FXS came from a study showing that administration of the mGluR5 antagonist MPEP to *Fmr1* knockout mice reversed the abnormal response of these mice in an open-field test, an experimental measure that is commonly used to assess anxiety-like phenotypes in mouse models (Yan et al., 2005). In addition, *Fmr1* knockout mice show an increase in the probability of audiogenic seizures, a model for the epilepsy frequently observed in fragile X patients, and MPEP administration significantly reduced the probability of these seizures. Consistent with this observation, another group found that *Fmr1* knockout mice showed prolonged epileptiform discharges in area CA3 of hippocampal slices in response to persistently increased synaptic activity and that these prolonged discharges were both protein synthesis-dependent and could be reversed by the application of MPEP (Chuang et al., 2005). These initial studies provided important evidence that mGluR antagonists may at least be able to ameliorate the epilepsy and anxiety phenotypes observed in FXS. More recently, another group was able to reverse a deficit in prepulse inhibition of startle in *Fmr1* knockout mice by acute administration of MPEP (de Vrij et al., 2008). Prepulse inhibition of startle is a functional measure of sensorimotor gating, a process by which sensory information entering the brain is filtered prior to reaching conscious perception.

At the molecular level, *Fmr1* knockout mouse brains were shown to have a decreased number of mRNA granules, which are thought to represent translationally repressed mRNAs,

Table 72–2.
List of studies showing reversal of *Fmr1* knockout phenotypes by antagonism of mGluRs

Study	Animal Model	*Fmr1* Manipulation	mGluR Manipulation	*Fmr1* Knockout Phenotype Studied
Yan et al., 2005	Mouse	*Fmr1* KO	MPEP	Increased exploration in open-field test Increased audiogenic seizures
Chuang et al., 2005	Mouse	*Fmr1* KO	MPEP	Prolonged epileptiform discharges in hippocampal slices
Aschrafi et al., 2005	Mouse	*Fmr1* KO	MPEP	Decrease mRNA granules
McBride et al., 2005	Drosophila	dFmr null	MPEP and others	Deficits in courtship-related behaviors and memory
Tucker et al., 2006	Zebrafish	*Fmr1* knockdown (morpholino)	MPEP	Disruptions in neurite morphology and craniofacial development
Dolen et al., 2007	Mouse	*Fmr1* KO	Cross with mGluR5 heterozygote	Exaggerated ocular dominance plasticity; excessive hippocampal LTD; increased global protein synthesis; increased spine density; increased audiogenic seizures; e3nhanced inhibitory avoidance extinction; increased body weight in young mice
Pan & Broadie, 2007; Pan et al., 2008; Repicky & Broadie, 2009	Drosophila	dFmr null	Cross with dmGluRA knockout	Phenotypes in glutamate receptor trafficking, synaptic plasticity, presynaptic ultrastructure, and coordinated motor behavior
de Vrij et al., 2008	Mouse	*Fmr1* KO	MPEP and fenobam	Deficit in prepulse inhibition: increased dendritic filopodia in hippocampal cultures
Bolduc et al., 2008	Drosophila	dFmr null	MPEP	Deficits in olfactory memory
Chang et al., 2008	Drosophila	dFmr null	MPEP	Increased lethality caused by excitotoxicity
Min et al., 2009	Mouse	*Fmr1* KO	MPEP	Increased GSK3 activation
Osterweil et al., 2010	Mouse	*Fmr1* KO	MPEP	Increased global protein synthesis

and this decrease was reversed by administration of MPEP (Aschrafi et al., 2005). Similarly, the excess protein synthesis observed in hippocampal slices from *Fmr1* knockout mice was corrected by a brief application of MPEP (Osterweil et al., 2010). Hippocampal cultures from *Fmr1* knockout mice showed an abnormal increase in the density of dendritic filopodia, thought to represent aberrant immature synaptic connections, and this increase was reversed by treatment with MPEP or fenobam, another mGluR5 antagonist (de Vrij et al., 2008). Recently, another group reported that glycogen synthase kinase-3, a key signaling enzyme involved in the regulation of many neuronal functions, was hyperactive in *Fmr1* knockout mouse brains and that this hyperactivity could be reversed by acute administration of MPEP (Min et al., 2009).

Genetic Manipulations in the *Fmr1* Knockout Mouse

A complementary strategy to testing whether manipulations of mGluR signaling are able to reverse fragile X-related phenotypes is by genetically decreasing the levels of mGluRs in the *Fmr1* knockout mice. This is particularly important in light of the fact that MPEP has been proposed to have some off-target activity, potentially confounding studies relying solely on this drug. Thus, to take advantage of the specificity of a genetic approach, *Fmr1* knockout mice were crossed with mice heterozygous for the *Grm5* gene—that is, those that had a 50% decrease in mGluR5 levels (Dolen et al., 2007). Using this strategy, seven out of eight fragile X-related phenotypes assessed were reversed in the *Fmr1* x Grm5 crossed mice. In accordance with the data obtained from the above pharmacological approach, genetic reduction of mGluR5 signaling causes a significant decrease in the induction of audiogenic seizures. In addition, this approach reversed the increase in dendritic spines seen in visual cortex of fragile X mice, the increase in protein synthesis in the hippocampus, and the increase in total body weight observed in young fragile X mice. Moreover, the genetic reduction of mGluR5 reduced the excessive hippocampal LTD, as well as an alteration in ocular dominance plasticity, a model for activity-dependent changes in the brain. Finally, the cross rescued an enhanced extinction phenotype in an inhibitory avoidance paradigm, a mouse model for learning and memory. The only phenotype not rescued in this study was macroorchidism, suggesting that other pathways (possibly mGluR1) must be involved in the testicular phenotype.

Manipulation of mGluRs in Other Animal Models of Fragile X Syndrome

Mice are commonly used in the generation of animal models for cognitive disorders because they represent the most highly developed species in which it is currently possible to specifically target and manipulate a gene of interest. However, despite significant progress in the development of techniques for genetic manipulation in mice, it still takes months to years to produce a knockout mouse model for a particular disorder. Moreover, studies are often limited by the spatial requirements for housing large colonies of mice. In contrast, manipulations in invertebrate species such as Drosophila are rapid and require far less space, making them very useful models for initial large-scale screens of mutations or drug effects. This approach was used successfully in the assessment of the effects of targeting mGluRs in a Drosophila model of FXS, in which the Drosophila homolog of the *Fmr1* gene, known alternately as dFmr1 or dfxr1, was disrupted. Male dFmr1 mutant flies showed abnormalities in several behavioral and structural measures of courtship-related learning and memory, and these deficits were reversed by administration of MPEP or other independent mGluR antagonists (McBride et al., 2005). Interestingly, MPEP reversed the deficits in courtship behaviors regardless of whether it was administered during the larval stage, the adult stage, or both, indicating that mGluRs may play a key role both in the development and in the acute function of mGluR-containing synapses. In a subsequent series of studies, another group took a genetic approach in Drosophila using a double knockout of dFmr1 and the only Drosophila mGluR, known as dmGluRA, to assess mechanistic links between these two molecules (Pan & Broadie, 2007; Pan et al., 2008; Repicky & Broadie, 2009). It was shown that dFmr1 and dmGluRA pathways converge to regulate multiple phenotypes, including glutamate receptor trafficking, synaptic plasticity, presynaptic ultrastructure, and coordinated motor behavior, leading the authors to conclude that loss of the receptor at least partially corrects defects caused by impaired translational regulation and vice versa. In other studies, MPEP administration in dFmr1 mutant flies was also able to ameliorate deficits in olfactory memory (Bolduc et al., 2008) and decrease embryonic lethality resulting from excitotoxicity (Chang et al., 2008).

Next to Drosophila, zebrafish embryos are used frequently in developmental studies because they are also easy to manipulate but have the advantage of being a vertebrate species. One group generated *Fmr1* knockdown zebrafish embryos using the morpholino antisense oligonucleotide technology (Tucker et al., 2006). This knockdown of *Fmr1* causes disruptions in neurite morphology in the hindbrain and spinal cord of the embryos, as well as in craniofacial development, including alterations in the cranial cartilage and number of neurons in the trigeminal ganglion. By developing these embryos in medium containing MPEP, the authors were able to restore normal neurite morphology and significantly reduce the number of neurons in the trigeminal ganglion. Together, these data provide evidence that manipulating mGluR signaling can reverse fragile X-related phenotypes across species, indicating that mGluRs may indeed provide a viable target for the treatment of FXS.

Summary

Preclinical studies using diverse animal models and techniques for manipulating group I mGluRs have demonstrated that reductions in signaling through mGluRs—particularly mGluR5—can reverse or ameliorate several phenotypes associated with FXS. These data provide an important proof of concept to indicate that targeting mGluRs may be a valuable strategy for the treatment of FXS. Further research will be necessary to expand the list of phenotypes examined, especially with regard to the many cognitive phenotypes that have thus far received little attention. Moreover, it will be crucial to determine whether there is a specific developmental window of opportunity for targeting mGluRs in FXS and how chronic administration of group I mGluR antagonists would compare to acute treatments in terms of efficacy and potential side effects.

Clinical Research: Targeting mGluRs and Their Downstream Effectors in Fragile X Syndrome Patients

Encouraged by the exciting findings arising from preclinical research, a number of clinical trials have been initiated to test the efficacy of compounds directly or indirectly related to mGluR signaling in treating FXS (Berry-Kravis, 2008; Hagerman et al., 2009). To date, none of these compounds are specifically approved for the treatment of FXS, but promising preliminary results have been obtained, which are summarized below.

mGluR5 Antagonists

The first group I mGluR antagonist to be tested in clinical trials was fenobam, a compound that was originally developed as an anxiolytic with an unknown molecular target and that was subsequently demonstrated to be a selective mGluR5 antagonist (Porter et al., 2005). A phase II clinical trial was recently completed, in which 12 adult patients with FXS received a single dose of fenobam to assess drug safety, pharmacokinetics, and a small number of cognitive and behavioral effects. In this trial, fenobam was found to reduce anxiety and hyperarousal, as well as improving prepulse inhibition of startle and accuracy on a continuous performance task (a measure of sustained attention and impulsivity) in a subset of patients (Berry-Kravis, 2008; Berry-Kravis et al., 2009). Based on these favorable findings, it was concluded that future trials are warranted once the results of this trial have been fully analyzed. Similarly, a recent small open-label trial with acamprosate, a drug with mGluR5 antagonist properties, yielded promising results in 3 young adult patients with FXS (Erickson et al., 2010). In all 3 patients, acamprosate was associated with improved linguistic communication and global clinical benefit as assessed by the CGI-I (clinical global impression-improvement) scale. Other mGluR5 antagonists that have shown promising results in preclinical studies and are currently entering clinical trials include STX107 (Seaside Therapeutics, phase I trial initiated in the United States), AFQ056 (Novartis, phase II trial recently completed in France, Italy, and Switzerland), and RO4917523 (Hoffman-LaRoche, phase II trial initiated in the United States).

Compounds Related to mGluR Signaling

In addition to targeting mGluRs directly, another approach to reducing excessive mGluR-mediated plasticity is to target the signaling pathways downstream of mGluRs. This approach is exemplified by the recent interest in lithium, which is already clinically approved for the treatment of mood disorders. The precise molecular mechanisms of lithium treatment are unclear (Williams et al., 2004), but it is thought to target the phospholipase C pathway, which plays a key role in group I mGluR signaling, as well as glycogen synthase kinase-3, which was found to be hyperactive in *Fmr1* knockout mouse brains in an mGluR5-dependent manner (Min et al., 2009). In a pilot trial on 15 patients with FXS, lithium treatment for 2 months was found to have positive effects on behavioral adaptive skills and one cognitive measure, suggesting that larger-scale clinical trials of this treatment strategy are warranted (Berry-Kravis et al., 2008).

Another study investigated the effects of treatment with the Ampakine CX516, a compound that enhances function of AMPA receptors and may thus counteract the excessive AMPA receptor internalization that underlies the exaggerated mGluR-dependent LTD observed in animal models of FXS (Berry-Kravis et al., 2006). Unfortunately this study did not yield clear positive results on any of the behavioral or cognitive measures tested, although a subset of patients who were also on antipsychotic treatment showed some improvement. This suggests that the dosing may have been inadequate or that targeting AMPA receptors alone may not be an optimal strategy for the treatment of FXS.

General Conclusions and Remaining Questions

Since its inception in 2002, the mGluR theory of FXS has been extensively investigated and validated, based on data ranging from basic in vitro research through in vivo studies in animal models to clinical trials in human patients with FXS. The encouraging nature of these findings, as well as the rapidity with which they have been translated from the bench to preliminary clinical testing, have engendered much excitement in the field, and it is hoped that additional trials may result in effective and clinically approved treatments for FXS in the reasonably near future.

There are a number of important remaining questions that need to be addressed at the preclinical level to direct clinical research toward the most effective intervention strategies. One significant issue is whether the effects of FMRP on synaptic structure and function are largely developmental or whether there is an ongoing acute requirement for FMRP, and hence an opportunity for correction of the synaptic phenotype, throughout adulthood. In the former case, it might be critical to target mGluR signaling as early as possible in post- or even prenatal development. Another major area of active research is the identification of alternative targets for pharmacological intervention that may arise from the mGluR theory. As discussed above, these include signaling pathways downstream of mGluRs, as well as proteins whose mGluR-induced synthesis may be dysregulated as a consequence of the absence of FMRP. In addition, recent studies have suggested that other G_q-coupled receptors (Volk et al., 2007) or indeed any receptors that couple to synaptic translation (Osterweil et al., 2010), may contribute to the excess protein synthesis observed in FXS, and hence may be of interest as therapeutic targets. Finally, it will be of great interest to determine whether the treatment paradigms developed for FXS may also be beneficial to patients with other forms of mental retardation and autism. Several of the single-gene disorders characterized by mental retardation and autism have been linked to protein synthesis pathways at the synapse (Bear et al., 2007; Kelleher & Bear, 2008), and it is conceivable that idiopathic autism in a subset of patients may result from similar disruptions. The mGluR theory may thus have the potential to go far beyond its original scope and provide novel treatment options for a wide range of neurodevelopmental disorders associated with synaptic translation and plasticity.

Challenges and Future Directions

- Identification of developmental versus acute roles of FMRP at synapses: If loss of FMRP function during brain development causes irreversible alterations in synaptic structure and connectivity, then this has significant implications for any therapeutic approaches to FXS, including those based on the mGluR theory.
- Identification of additional drug targets based on the mGluR theory: By increasing our understanding of mGluR signaling pathways and other pathways contributing to synaptic protein synthesis, it may be possible to identify alternative targets for pharmacological intervention that will expand and improve treatment options for FXS.
- Comparison between FXS and other disorders: To determine whether treatment paradigms developed for FXS may also be beneficial to patients with other forms of mental retardation and autism, it will be essential to identify similarities and differences in the molecular and cellular mechanisms underlying these disorders.

SUGGESTED READINGS

Bear, M. F., Huber, K. M., & Warren, S. T. (2004). The mGluR theory of fragile X mental retardation. *Trends in Neurosciences, 27*, 370–377.

Ronesi, J. A. & Huber, K. M. (2008a). Metabotropic glutamate receptors and fragile x mental retardation protein: partners in translational regulation at the synapse. *Science Signaling, 1*, e6.

Bassell, G. J. & Warren, S. T. (2008). Fragile X syndrome: Loss of local mRNA regulation alters synaptic development and function. *Neuron, 60*, 201–214.

ACKNOWLEDGMENTS

The authors are grateful to Dr. Emily Osterweil for helpful comments on the manuscript and to FRAXA, NIH, and HHMI for research support.

REFERENCES

Alexander, G. M. & Godwin, D. W. (2006). Metabotropic glutamate receptors as a strategic target for the treatment of epilepsy. *Epilepsy Research, 71*, 1–22.

Antar, L. N., Dictenberg, J. B., Plociniak, M., Afroz, R., & Bassell, G. J. (2005). Localization of FMRP-associated mRNA granules and requirement of microtubules for activity-dependent trafficking in hippocampal neurons. *Genes, Brain, and Behavior, 4*, 350–359.

Antar, L. N., Afroz, R., Dictenberg, J. B., Carroll, R. C., & Bassell, G. J. (2004). Metabotropic glutamate receptor activation regulates fragile X mental retardation protein and Fmr1 mRNA localization differentially in dendrites and at synapses. *Journal of Neuroscience, 24*, 2648–2655.

Antion, M. D., Hou, L., Wong, H., Hoeffer, C. A., & Klann, E. (2008). mGluR-dependent long-term depression is associated with increased phosphorylation of S6 and synthesis of elongation factor 1A but remains expressed in S6K-deficient mice. *Molecular and Cellular Biology, 28*, 2996–3007.

Aschrafi, A., Cunningham, B. A., Edelman, G. M., & Vanderklish, P. W. (2005). The fragile X mental retardation protein and group I metabotropic glutamate receptors regulate levels of mRNA granules in brain. *Proceedings of the National Academy of Sciences of the United States of America, 102*, 2180–2185.

Ashley, C. T., Jr., Wilkinson, K. D., Reines, D., & Warren, S. T. (1993). FMR1 protein: conserved RNP family domains and selective RNA binding. *Science, 262*, 563–566.

Auerbach, B. D. & Bear, M. F. (2010). Loss of the fragile X mental retardation protein decouples metabotropic glutamate receptor dependent priming of long-term potentiation from protein synthesis. *Journal of Neurophysiology, 104*, 1047–1052.

Banko, J. L., Hou, L., Poulin, F., Sonenberg, N., & Klann, E. (2006). Regulation of eukaryotic initiation factor 4E by converging signaling pathways during metabotropic glutamate receptor-dependent long-term depression. *Journal of Neuroscience, 26*, 2167–2173.

Bassell, G. J. & Warren, S. T. (2008). Fragile X syndrome: Loss of local mRNA regulation alters synaptic development and function. *Neuron, 60*, 201–214.

Bear, M. F., Dolen, G., Osterweil, E., & Nagarajan, N. (2007). Fragile X: Translation in action. *Neuropsychopharmacology, 33*, 84–87.

Bear, M. F., Huber, K. M., & Warren, S. T. (2004). The mGluR theory of fragile X mental retardation. *Trends in Neurosciences, 27*, 370–377.

Bechara, E. G., Didiot, M. C., Melko, M., Davidovic, L., Bensaid, M., Martin, P., et al. (2009). A novel function for fragile X mental retardation protein in translational activation. *PLoS Biology, 7*, e16.

Bellone, C., Luscher, C., & Mameli, M. (2008). Mechanisms of synaptic depression triggered by metabotropic glutamate receptors. *Cellular and Molecular Life Sciences, 65*, 2913–2923.

Belmonte, M. K. & Bourgeron, T. (2006). Fragile X syndrome and autism at the intersection of genetic and neural networks. *Nature Neuroscience, 9*, 1221–1225.

Berry-Kravis, E. (2008). Fragile X research: A status report. *The National Fragile X Foundation Quarterly, 31*, 12–16.

Berry-Kravis, E., Sumis, A., Hervey, C., Nelson, M., Porges, S. W., Weng, N., et al. (2008). Open-label treatment trial of lithium to target the underlying defect in fragile X syndrome. *Journal of Developmental and Behavioral Pediatrics, 29*, 293–302.

Berry-Kravis, E., Krause, S. E., Block, S. S., Guter, S., Wuu, J., Leurgans, S., et al. (2006). Effect of CX516, an AMPA-modulating compound, on cognition and behavior in fragile X syndrome: A controlled trial. *Journal of Child and Adolescent Psychopharmacology, 16*, 525–540.

Berry-Kravis, E. M., Hessl, D., Coffey, S., Hervey, C., Schneider, A., Yuhas, J., et al. (2009). A pilot open-label single-dose trial of fenobam in adults with fragile X syndrome. *Journal of Medical Genetics, 46*, 266–271.

Bolduc, F. V., Bell, K., Cox, H., Broadie, K. S., & Tully, T. (2008). Excess protein synthesis in drosophila fragile X mutants impairs long-term memory. *Nature Neuroscience, 11*, 1143–1145.

Brown, V., Jin, P., Ceman, S., Darnell, J. C., O'Donnell, W. T., Tenenbaum, S. A., et al. (2001). Microarray identification of FMRP-associated brain mRNAs and altered mRNA translational profiles in fragile X syndrome. *Cell, 107*, 477–487.

Catania, M. V., Landwehrmeyer, G. B., Testa, C. M., Standaert, D. G., Penney, J., & Young, A. B. (1994). Metabotropic glutamate receptors are differentially regulated during development. *Neuroscience, 61*, 481–495.

Ceman, S., O'Donnell, W. T., Reed, M., Patton, S., Pohl, J., & Warren, S. T. (2003). Phosphorylation influences the translation state of FMRP-associated polyribosomes. *Human Molecular Genetics, 12*, 3295–3305.

Chang, S., Bray, S. M., Li, Z., Zarnescu, D. C., He, C., Jin, P., et al. (2008). Identification of small molecules rescuing fragile X syndrome phenotypes in Drosophila. *Nature Chemical Biology, 4*, 256–263.

Cheever, A. & Ceman, S. (2009). Translation regulation of mRNAs by the fragile X family of proteins through the microRNA pathway. *RNA Biology, 6*, 175–178.

Christie, S. B., Akins, M. R., Schwob, J. E., & Fallon, J. R. (2009). The FXG: A Presynaptic Fragile X Granule Expressed in a Subset of Developing Brain Circuits. *Journal of Neuroscience, 29*, 1514–1524.

Chuang, S. C., Zhao, W., Bauchwitz, R., Yan, Q., Bianchi, R., & Wong, R. K. S. (2005). Prolonged epileptiform discharges induced by altered group I metabotropic glutamate receptor-mediated synaptic responses in hippocampal slices of a fragile X mouse model. *Journal of Neuroscience, 25*, 8048–8055.

Cohen, A. S. & Abraham, W. C. (1996). Facilitation of long-term potentiation by prior activation of metabotropic glutamate receptors. *Journal of Neurophysiology, 76*, 953–962.

Comery, T. A., Harris, J. B., Willems, P. J., Oostra, B. A., Irwin, S. A., Weiler, I. J., et al. (1997). Abnormal dendritic spines in fragile X knockout mice: Maturation and pruning deficits. *Proceedings of the National Academy of Sciences of the United States of America, 94*, 5401–5404.

Conn, P. J. (2003). Physiological roles and therapeutic potential of metabotropic glutamate receptors. *Annals of the New York Academy of Sciences, 1003*, 12–21.

Corbin, F., Bouillon, M., Fortin, A., Morin, S., Rousseau, F., & Khandjian, E. W. (1997). The fragile X mental retardation protein is associated with poly(A)+ mRNA in actively translating polyribosomes. *Human Molecular Genetics, 6*, 1465–1472.

Darnell, J. C., Jensen, K. B., Jin, P., Brown, V., Warren, S. T., & Darnell, R. B. (2001). Fragile X mental retardation protein targets G quartet mRNAs important for neuronal function. *Cell, 107*, 489–499.

Davidkova, G. & Carroll, R. C. (2007). Characterization of the role of microtubule-associated protein 1B in metabotropic glutamate receptor-mediated endocytosis of AMPA receptors in hippocampus. *Journal of Neuroscience, 27*, 13,273–13,278.

Davidovic, L., Jaglin, X. H., Lepagnol-Bestel, A. M., Tremblay, S., Simonneau, M., Bardoni, B., et al. (2007). The fragile X mental retardation protein is a molecular adaptor between the neurospecific KIF3C kinesin and dendritic RNA granules. *Human Molecular Genetics, 16*, 3047–3058.

De Diego Otero, Y., Severijnen, L. A., van Cappellen, G., Schrier, M., Oostra, B., et al. (2002). Transport of fragile X mental retardation protein via granules in neurites of PC12 cells. *Molecular and Cellular Biology, 22*, 8332–8341.

de Vrij, F. M. S., Levenga, J., van der Linde, H. C., Koekkoek, S. K., De Zeeuw, C. I., Nelson, D. L., et al. (2008). Rescue of behavioral phenotype and neuronal protrusion morphology in Fmr1 KO mice. *Neurobiology of Disease, 31*, 127–132.

Desai, N. S., Casimiro, T. M., Gruber, S. M., & Vanderklish, P. W. (2006). Early postnatal plasticity in neocortex of Fmr1 knockout mice. *Journal of Neurophysiology, 96*, 1734–1745.

Devys, D., Lutz, Y., Rouyer, N., Bellocq, J. P., & Mandel, J. L. (1993). The FMR-1 protein is cytoplasmic, most abundant in neurons and appears normal in carriers of a fragile X premutation. *Nature Genetics, 4*, 335–340.

Dictenberg, J. B., Swanger, S. A., Antar, L. N., Singer, R. H., & Bassell, G. J. (2008). A direct role for FMRP in activity-dependent dendritic mRNA transport links filopodial-spine morphogenesis to fragile X syndrome. *Developmental Cell, 14*, 926–939.

Dolen, G., Osterweil, E., Rao, B. S. S., Smith, G. B., Auerbach, B. D., Chattarji, S., et al. (2007). Correction of fragile X syndrome in mice. *Neuron, 56*, 955–962.

Eberhart, D. E., Malter, H. E., Feng, Y., & Warren, S. T. (1996). The fragile X mental retardation protein is a ribonucleoprotein containing both nuclear localization and nuclear export signals. *Human Molecular Genetics, 5*, 1083–1091.

Erickson, C. A., Mullett, J. E., & McDougle, C. J. (2010). Brief report: acamprosate in fragile X syndrome. *Journal of Autism and Developmental Disorders, 40*, 1412–1416.

Feng, Y., Gutekunst, C. A., Eberhart, D. E., Yi, H., Warren, S. T., & Hersch, S. M. (1997). Fragile X mental retardation protein: nucleocytoplasmic shuttling and association with somatodendritic ribosomes. *Journal of Neuroscience, 17*, 1539–1547.

Ferrari, F., Mercaldo, V., Piccoli, G., Sala, C., Cannata, S., Achsel, T., et al. (2007). The fragile X mental retardation protein-RNP granules show an mGluR-dependent localization in the post-synaptic spines. *Molecular and Cellular Neuroscience, 34*, 343–354.

Gallagher, S. M., Daly, C. A., Bear, M. F., & Huber, K. M. (2004). Extracellular signal-regulated protein kinase activation is required for metabotropic glutamate receptor-dependent long-term depression in hippocampal area CA1. *Journal of Neuroscience, 24*, 4859–4864.

Gatto, C. L. & Broadie, K. (2008). Temporal requirements of the fragile X mental retardation protein in the regulation of synaptic structure. *Development, 135*, 2637–2648.

Gerber, U., Gee, C. E., & Benquet P. (2007). Metabotropic glutamate receptors: intracellular signaling pathways. *Current Opinion in Pharmacology, 7*, 56–61.

Giuffrida, R., Musumeci, S., D'Antoni, S., Bonaccorso, C. M., Giuffrida-Stella, A. M., Oostra, B. A., et al. (2005). A reduced number of metabotropic glutamate subtype 5 receptors are associated with constitutive homer proteins in a mouse model of fragile X syndrome. *Journal of Neuroscience, 25*, 8908–8916.

Gross, C., Nakamoto, M., Yao, X., Chan, C. B., Yim, S. Y., Ye, K., et al. (2010). Excessive phosphoinositide 3-kinase subunit synthesis and activity as a novel therapeutic target in fragile X syndrome. *Journal of Neuroscience, 30*, 10624–10638.

Gubellini, P., Pisani, A., Centonze, D., Bernardi, G., & Calabresi, P. (2004). Metabotropic glutamate receptors and striatal synaptic plasticity: implications for neurological diseases. *Progress in Neurobiology, 74*, 271–300.

Hagerman, R. J., Berry-Kravis, E., Kaufmann, W. E., Ono, M. Y., Tartaglia, N., Lachiewicz, A., et al. (2009). Advances in the Treatment of Fragile X Syndrome. *Pediatrics, 123*, 378–390.

Hermans, E. & Challiss, R. A. (2001). Structural, signalling and regulatory properties of the group I metabotropic glutamate receptors: prototypic family C G-protein-coupled receptors. *Biochemistry Journal, 359*, 465–484.

Hinton, V. J., Brown, W. T., Wisniewski, K., & Rudelli, R. D. (1991). Analysis of neocortex in three males with the fragile X syndrome. *American Journal of Medical Genetics, 41*, 289–294.

Hou, L., Antion, M. D., Hu, D., Spencer, C. M., Paylor, R., & Klann, E. (2006). Dynamic translational and proteasomal regulation of fragile X mental retardation protein controls mGluR-dependent long-term depression. *Neuron, 51*, 441–454.

Hou, L. & Klann, E. (2004). Activation of the phosphoinositide 3-kinase-Akt-mammalian target of rapamycin signaling pathway is required for metabotropic glutamate receptor-dependent long-term depression. *Journal of Neuroscience, 24*, 6352–6361.

Huang, F., Chotiner, J. K., & Steward, O. (2005). The mRNA for elongation factor 1{alpha} is localized in dendrites and translated in response to treatments that induce long-term depression. *Journal of Neuroscience, 25*, 7199–7209.

Huber, K. M., Gallagher, S. M., Warren, S. T., & Bear, M. F. (2002). Altered synaptic plasticity in a mouse model of fragile X mental retardation. *Proceedings of the National Academy of Sciences of the United States of America, 99*, 7746–7750.

Huber, K. M., Kayser, M. S., & Bear, M. F. (2000). Role for rapid dendritic protein synthesis in hippocampal mGluR-dependent long-term depression. *Science, 288*, 1254–1256.

Huber, K. M., Roder, J. C., & Bear, M. F. (2001). Chemical induction of mGluR5- and protein synthesis-dependent long-term depression in hippocampal area CA1. *Journal of Neurophysiology, 86*, 321–325.

Irwin, S. A., Galvez, R., & Greenough, W. T. (2000). Dendritic spine structural anomalies in fragile-X mental retardation syndrome. *Cerebral Cortex, 10*, 1038–1044.

Karachot, L., Shirai, Y., Vigot, R., Yamamori, T., & Ito, M. (2001). Induction of long-term depression in cerebellar Purkinje cells requires a rapidly turned over protein. *Journal of Neurophysiology, 86*, 280–289.

Kelleher, R. J. & Bear, M. F. (2008). The autistic neuron: Troubled translation? *Cell, 135*, 401–406.

Kenny, P. J. & Markou, A. (2004). The ups and downs of addiction: role of metabotropic glutamate receptors. *Trends in Pharmacological Sciences, 25*, 265–272.

Khandjian, E. W., Corbin, F., Woerly, S., & Rousseau, F. (1996). The fragile X mental retardation protein is associated with ribosomes. *Nature Genetics, 12*, 91–93.

Kim, M., Bellini, M., & Ceman, S. (2009). Fragile X mental retardation protein FMRP binds mRNAs in the nucleus. *Molecular and Cellular Biology, 29*, 214–228.

Kim, S. H., Markham, J. A., Weiler, I. J., & Greenough, W. T. (2008). Aberrant early-phase ERK inactivation impedes neuronal function in fragile X syndrome. *Proceedings of the National Academy of Sciences of the United States of America, 105*, 4429–4434.

Koekkoek, S. K. E., Yamaguchi, K., Milojkovic, B. A., Dortland, B. R., Ruigrok, T. J., Maex, R., et al. (2005). Deletion of FMR1 in Purkinje cells enhances parallel fiber LTD, enlarges spines, and attenuates cerebellar eyelid conditioning in fragile X syndrome. *Neuron, 47*, 339–352.

Krivoy, A., Fischel, T., & Weizman, A. (2008). The possible involvement of metabotropic glutamate receptors in schizophrenia. *European Neuropsychopharmacology, 18*, 395–405.

Laggerbauer, B., Ostareck, D., Keidel, E. M., Ostareck-Lederer, A., & Fischer, U. (2001). Evidence that fragile X mental retardation protein is a negative regulator of translation. *Human Molecular Genetics, 10*, 329–338.

Lea, P. M. & Faden, A. I. (2006). Metabotropic glutamate receptor subtype 5 antagonists MPEP and MTEP. *CNS Drug Reviews, 12*, 149–166.

Li, J., Pelletier, M. R., Perez Velazquez, J. L., & Carlen, P. L. (2002). Reduced cortical synaptic plasticity and GluR1 expression associated with fragile X mental retardation protein deficiency. *Molecular and Cellular Neuroscience, 19*, 138–151.

Li, Z., Zhang, Y., Ku, L., Wilkinson, K. D., Warren, S. T., & Feng, Y. (2001). The fragile X mental retardation protein inhibits translation via interacting with mRNA. *Nucleic Acids Research, 29*, 2276–2283.

Lu, R., Wang, H., Liang, Z., Ku, L., O'Donnell, W. T., Li, W, et al. (2004). The fragile X protein controls microtubule-associated protein 1B translation and microtubule stability in brain neuron development. *Proceedings of the National Academy of Sciences of the United States of America, 101*, 15,201–15,206.

Mameli, M., Balland, B., Lujan, R., & Luscher, C. (2007). Rapid synthesis and synaptic insertion of GluR2 for mGluR-LTD in the ventral tegmental area. *Science, 317*, 530–533.

Marinissen, M. J. & Gutkind, J. S. (2001). G-protein-coupled receptors and signaling networks: emerging paradigms. *Trends in Pharmacological Sciences, 22*, 368–376.

Martin, L. J., Blackstone, C. D., Huganir, R. L., & Price, D. L. (1992). Cellular localization of a metabotropic glutamate receptor in rat brain. *Neuron, 9*, 259–270.

Mazroui, R., Huot, M. E., Tremblay, S., Filion, C., Labelle, Y., & Khandjian, E. W. (2002). Trapping of messenger RNA by fragile X mental retardation protein into cytoplasmic granules induces translation repression. *Human Molecular Genetics, 11*, 3007–3017.

McBride, S. M. J., Choi, C. H., Wang, Y., Liebelt, D., Braunstein, E., Ferreiro, D., et al. (2005). Pharmacological rescue of synaptic plasticity, courtship behavior, and mushroom body defects in a drosophila model of fragile X syndrome. *Neuron, 45*, 753–764.

Menon, L., Mader, S. A., & Mihailescu, M. R. (2008). Fragile X mental retardation protein interactions with the microtubule associated protein 1B RNA. *RNA, 14*, 1644–1655.

Meredith, R. M., Holmgren, C. D., Weidum, M., Burnashev, N., & Mansvelder, H. D. (2007). Increased threshold for spike-timing-dependent plasticity is caused by unreliable calcium signaling in mice lacking fragile X gene Fmr1. *Neuron, 54*, 627–638.

Min, W. W., Yuskaitis, C. J., Yan, Q., Sikorski, C., Chen, S., Jope, R. S., et al. (2009). Elevated glycogen synthase kinase-3 activity in Fragile X mice: Key metabolic regulator with evidence for treatment potential. *Neuropharmacology, 56*, 463–472.

Moult, P. R., Correa, S. A. L., Collingridge, G. L., Fitzjohn, S. M., & Bashir, Z. I. (2008). Co-activation of p38 mitogen-activated protein kinase and protein tyrosine phosphatase underlies metabotropic glutamate receptor-dependent long-term depression. *Journal of Physiology, 586*, 2499–2510.

Muddashetty, R. S., Kelic, S., Gross, C., Xu, M., & Bassell, G. J. (2007). Dysregulated metabotropic glutamate receptor-dependent translation of AMPA receptor and postsynaptic density-95 mRNAs at synapses in a mouse model of fragile X syndrome. *Journal of Neuroscience, 27*, 5338–5348.

Naie, K. & Manahan-Vaughan, D. (2005). Investigations of the protein synthesis dependency of mGluR-induced long-term depression in the dentate gyrus of freely moving rats. *Neuropharmacology, 49*, 35–44.

Nakamoto, M., Nalavadi, V., Epstein, M. P., Narayanan, U., Bassell, G. J., & Warren, S. T. (2007). Fragile X mental retardation protein deficiency leads to excessive mGluR5-dependent internalization of AMPA receptors. *Proceedings of the National Academy of Sciences, 104*, 15,537–15,542.

Napoli, I., Mercaldo, V., Boyl, P. P., Eleuteri, B., Zalfa, F., De Rubeis, S., et al. (2008). The fragile X syndrome protein represses activity-dependent translation through CYFIP1, a new 4E-BP. *Cell, 134*, 1042–1054.

Narayanan, U., Nalavadi, V., Nakamoto, M., Pallas, D. C., Ceman, S., Bassell, G. J., et al. (2007). FMRP phosphorylation reveals an immediate-early signaling pathway triggered by group I mGluR and mediated by PP2A. *Journal of Neuroscience, 27*, 14,349–14,357.

Narayanan, U., Nalavadi, V., Nakamoto, M., Thomas, G., Ceman, S., Bassell, G. J., et al. (2008). S6K1 phosphorylates and regulates fragile X mental retardation protein (FMRP) with the neuronal protein synthesis-dependent mammalian target of rapamycin (mTOR) signaling cascade. *Biological Journal of Chemistry, 283*, 18,478–18,482.

Nosyreva, E. D. & Huber, K. M. (2006). Metabotropic receptor-dependent long-term depression persists in the absence of protein synthesis in the mouse model of fragile X syndrome. *Journal of Neurophysiology, 95*, 3291–3295.

Nosyreva, E. D. & Huber, K. M. (2005). Developmental switch in synaptic mechanisms of hippocampal metabotropic glutamate receptor-dependent long-term depression. *Journal of Neuroscience, 25*, 2992–3001.

Oliet, S. H. R., Malenka, R. C., & Nicoll, R. A. (1997). Two distinct forms of long-term depression coexist in CA1 hippocampal pyramidal cells. *Neuron, 18*, 969–982.

Osterweil, E. K., Krueger, D. D., Reinhold, K., & Bear, M. F. (2010). Hypersensitivity to mGluR5 and ERK1/2 leads to excessive protein synthesis in the hippocampus of a mouse model of fragile X syndrome. *Journal of Neuroscience, 30*, 15616–15627.

Palmer, M. J., Irving, A. J., Seabrook, G. R., Jane, D. E., & Collingridge, G. L. (1997). The group I mGlu receptor agonist DHPG induces a novel form of LTD in the CA1 region of the hippocampus. *Neuropharmacology, 36*, 1517–1532.

Pan, L. & Broadie, K. S. (2007). Drosophila fragile X mental retardation protein and metabotropic glutamate receptor A convergently regulate the synaptic ratio of ionotropic glutamate receptor subclasses. *Journal of Neuroscience, 27*, 12,378–12,389.

Pan, L., Woodruff, III E., Liang, P., & Broadie, K. (2008). Mechanistic relationships between Drosophila fragile X mental retardation protein and metabotropic glutamate receptor A signaling. *Molecular and Cellular Neuroscience, 37*, 747–760.

Park, S., Park, J. M., Kim, S., Kim, J. A., Shepherd, J. D., Smith-Hicks, C. L., et al. (2008). Elongation factor 2 and fragile X mental retardation protein control the dynamic translation of Arc/Arg3.1 essential for mGluR-LTD. *Neuron, 59*, 70–83.

Penagarikano, O., Mulle, J. G., & Warren, S. T. (2007). The pathophysiology of fragile X syndrome. *Annual Review of Genomics and Human Genetics, 8*, 109–129.

Pfeiffer, B. E. & Huber, K. M. (2007). Fragile X mental retardation protein induces synapse loss through acute postsynaptic translational regulation. *Journal of Neuroscience, 27*, 3120–3130.

Piccinin, S., Thuault, S. J., Doherty, A. J., Brown, J. T., Randall, A. D., Davies, C. H., et al. (2008). The induction of long-term plasticity of non-synaptic, synchronized activity by the activation of group I mGluRs. *Neuropharmacology, 55*, 459–463.

Pietraszek, M., Sukhanov, I., Maciejak, P., Szyndler, J., Gravius, A., Wislowska, A., et al. (2005). Anxiolytic-like effects of mGlu1 and mGlu5 receptor antagonists in rats. *European Journal of Pharmacology, 514*, 25–34.

Pilc, A., Chaki, S., Nowak, G., & Witkin, J. M. (2008). Mood disorders: Regulation by metabotropic glutamate receptors. *Biochemical Pharmacology, 75*, 997–1006.

Porter, R. H. P., Jaeschke, G., Spooren, W., Ballard, T. M., Buttelmann, B., Kolczewski, S., et al. (2005). Fenobam: A clinically validated nonbenzodiazepine anxiolytic is a potent, selective, and noncompetitive mGlu5 receptor antagonist with inverse agonist activity. *Journal of Pharmacology and Experimental Therapeutics, 315*, 711–721.

Qin, M., Kang, J., Burlin, T. V., Jiang, C., & Smith, C. B. (2005). Postadolescent changes in regional cerebral protein synthesis: an in vivo study in the Fmr1 null mouse. *Journal of Neuroscience, 25*, 5087–5095.

Rammes, G., Palmer, M., Eder, M., Dodt, H. U., Zieglgansberger, W., & Collingridge, G. L. (2003). Activation of mGlu receptors induces LTD without affecting postsynaptic sensitivity of CA1 neurons in rat hippocampal slices. *Journal of Physiology, 546*, 455–460.

Raymond, C. R., Thompson, V. L., Tate, W. P., & Abraham, W. C. (2000). Metabotropic glutamate receptors trigger homosynaptic protein synthesis to prolong long-term potentiation. *Journal of Neuroscience, 20*, 969–976.

Reiss, A. L. & Hall, S. S. (2007). Fragile X syndrome: Assessment and treatment implications. *Child and Adolescent Psychiatric Clinics of North America, 16*, 663–675.

Repicky, S. & Broadie, K. (2009). Metabotropic glutamate receptor-mediated use-dependent down-regulation of synaptic excitability involves the fragile X mental retardation protein. *Journal of Neurophysiology, 101*, 672–687.

Romano, C., Sesma, M. A., McDonald, C. T., O'Malley, K., Van den Pol, A. N., & Olney, J. W. (1995). Distribution of metabotropic glutamate receptor mGluR5 immunoreactivity in rat brain. *Journal of Comparative Neurology, 355*, 455–469.

Ronesi, J. A. & Huber, K. M. (2008a). Metabotropic glutamate receptors and fragile x mental retardation protein: partners in translational regulation at the synapse. *Science Signaling, 1*, e6.

Ronesi, J. A. & Huber, K. M. (2008b). Homer interactions are necessary for metabotropic glutamate receptor-induced long-term depression and translational activation. *Journal of Neuroscience, 28*, 543–547.

Schkeryantz, J. M., Kingston, A. E., & Johnson, M. P. (2007). Prospects for metabotropic glutamate 1 receptor antagonists in the treatment of neuropathic pain. *Journal of Medicinal Chemistry, 50*, 2563–2568.

Sharma, A., Hoeffer, C. A., Takayasu, Y., Miyawaki, T., McBride, S. M., Klann, E., et al. (2010). Dysregulation of mTOR signaling in fragile X syndrome. *Journal of Neuroscience, 30*, 694–702.

Shepherd, J. D., Rumbaugh, G., Wu, J., Chowdhury, S., Plath, N., Kuhl, D., et al. (2006). Arc/Arg3.1 mediates homeostatic synaptic scaling of AMPA receptors. *Neuron, 52*, 475–484.

Shigemoto, R., Nakanishi, S., & Mizuno, N. (1992). Distribution of the mRNA for a metabotropic glutamate receptor (mGluR1) in the central nervous system: an in situ hybridization study in adult and developing rat. *Journal of Comparative Neurology, 322*, 121–135.

Shigemoto, R., Nomura, S., Ohishi, H., Sugihara, H., Nakanishi, S., & Mizuno, N. (1993). Immunohistochemical localization of a metabotropic glutamate receptor, mGluR5, in the rat brain. *Neuroscience Letters, 163*, 53–57.

Siomi, H., Siomi, M. C., Nussbaum, R. L., & Dreyfuss, G. (1993). The protein product of the fragile X gene, FMR1, has characteristics of an RNA-binding protein. *Cell, 74*, 291–298.

Snyder, E. M., Philpot, B. D., Huber, K. M., Dong, X., Fallon, J. R., & Bear, M. F. (2001). Internalization of ionotropic glutamate receptors in response to mGluR activation. *Nature Neuroscience, 4*, 1079–1085.

Spooren, W. P. J. M., Vassout, A., Neijt, H. C., Kuhn, R., Gasparini, F., Roux, S., et al. (2000). Anxiolytic-like effects of the prototypical metabotropic glutamate receptor 5 antagonist 2-methyl-6-(phenylethynyl)pyridine in rodents. *Journal of Pharmacology and Experimental Therapeutics, 295*, 1267–1275.

Steward, O., Bakker, C. E., Willems, P. J., & Oostra, B. A. (1998). No evidence for disruption of normal patterns of mRNA localization in dendrites or dendritic transport of recently synthesized mRNA in FMR1 knockout mice, a model for human fragile-X mental retardation syndrome. *Neuroreport, 9*, 477–481.

Sung, Y. J., Dolzhanskaya, N., Nolin, S. L., Brown, T., Currie, J. R., & Denman, R. B. (2003). The fragile X mental retardation protein FMRP binds elongation factor 1A mRNA and negatively regulates its translation in vivo. *Journal of Biological Chemistry, 278*, 15,669–15,678.

Swanson, C. J., Bures, M., Johnson, M. P., Linden, A. M., Monn, J. A., & Schoepp, D. D. (2005). Metabotropic glutamate receptors as novel targets for anxiety and stress disorders. *Nature Reviews. Drug Discovery, 4*, 131–144.

Tamanini, F., Meijer, N., Verheij, C., Willems, P. J., Galjaard, H., Oostra, B. A., et al. (1996). FMRP is associated to the ribosomes via RNA. *Human Molecular Genetics, 5*, 809–813.

Tang, F. R. (2005). Agonists and antagonists of metabotropic glutamate receptors: anticonvulsants and antiepileptogenic agents? *Current Neuropharmacology, 3*, 299–307.

The Dutch-Belgian Fragile X Consortium, Bakker, C. E., Verheij, C., Willemsen, R., van der Helm, R., Oerlemans, F., Vermey, M., et al. (1994). Fmr1 knockout mice: A model to study fragile X mental retardation. *Cell, 78*, 23–33.

Todd, P. K., Mack, K. J., & Malter, J. S. (2003a). The fragile X mental retardation protein is required for type-I metabotropic glutamate receptor-dependent translation of PSD-95. *Proceedings of the National Academy of Sciences of the United States of America, 100*, 14,374–14,378.

Todd, P. K., Malter, J. S., & Mack, K. J. (2003b). Whisker stimulation-dependent translation of FMRP in the barrel cortex requires activation of type I metabotropic glutamate receptors. *Molecular Brain Research, 110*, 267–278.

Tucker, B., Richards, R. I., & Lardelli, M. (2006). Contribution of mGluR and Fmr1 functional pathways to neurite morphogenesis, craniofacial development and fragile X syndrome. *Human Molecular Genetics, 15*, 3446–3458.

Valenti, O., Conn, P. J., & Marino, M. J. (2002). Distinct physiological roles of the Gq-coupled metabotropic glutamate receptors Co-expressed in the same neuronal populations. *Journal of Cellular Physiology, 191*, 125–137.

Verheij, C., Bakker, C. E., de Graaff, E., Keulemans, J., Willemsen, R., Verkerk, A. J. M. H., et al. (1993). Characterization and localization of the FMR-1 gene product associated with fragile X syndrome. *Nature, 363*, 722–724.

Verkerk, A. J. M. H., Pieretti, M., Sutcliffe, J. S., Fu, Y. H., Kuhl, D. P., Pizzuti, A. et al. (1991). Identification of a gene (FMR-1) containing a CGG repeat coincident with a breakpoint cluster region exhibiting length variation in fragile X syndrome. *Cell, 65*, 905–914.

Volk, L. J., Pfeiffer, B. E., Gibson, J. R., & Huber, K. M. (2007). Multiple Gq-coupled receptors converge on a common protein synthesis-dependent long-term depression that is affected in fragile X syndrome mental retardation. *Journal of Neuroscience, 27*, 11,624–11,634.

Wang, H., Dictenberg, J. B., Ku, L., Li, W., Bassell, G. J., & Feng, Y. (2008). Dynamic association of the fragile X mental retardation protein as a messenger ribonucleoprotein between microtubules and polyribosomes. *Molecular Biology of the Cell, 19*, 105–114.

Wang, J. Q., Fibuch, E. E., & Mao, L. (2007). Regulation of mitogen-activated protein kinases by glutamate receptors. *Journal of Neurochemistry, 100*, 1–11.

Waung, M. W., Pfeiffer, B. E., Nosyreva, E. D., Ronesi, J. A., & Huber, K. M. (2008). Rapid Translation of Arc/Arg3.1 Selectively mediates mGluR-dependent LTD through persistent increases in AMPAR endocytosis rate. *Neuron, 59*, 84–97.

Weiler, I. J., Irwin, S. A., Klintsova, A. Y., Spencer, C. M., Brazelton, A. D., Miyashiro, K., et al. (1997). Fragile X mental retardation protein is translated near synapses in response to neurotransmitter activation. *Proceedings of the National Academy of Sciences of the United States of America, 94*, 5395–5400.

Westmark, C. J. & Malter, J. S. (2007). FMRP mediates mGluR5-dependent translation of amyloid precursor protein. *PLoS Biology, 5*, e52.

Williams, R., Ryves, W. J., Dalton, E. C., Eickholt, B., Shaltiel, G., Agam, G., et al. (2004). A molecular cell biology of lithium. *Biochemical Society Transactions, 32*, 799–802.

Wilson, B. M. & Cox, C. L. (2007). Absence of metabotropic glutamate receptor-mediated plasticity in the neocortex of fragile X mice. *Proceedings of the National Academy of Sciences of the United States of America, 104*, 2454–2459.

Xiao, M. Y., Gustafsson, B., & Niu, Y. P. (2006). Metabotropic glutamate receptors in the trafficking of ionotropic glutamate and GABA(A). Receptors at central synapses. *Current Neuropharmacology, 4*, 77–86.

Xiao, M. Y., Zhou, Q., & Nicoll, R. A. (2001). Metabotropic glutamate receptor activation causes a rapid redistribution of AMPA receptors. *Neuropharmacology, 41*, 664–671.

Yan, Q. J., Rammal, M., Tranfaglia, M., & Bauchwitz, R. P. (2005). Suppression of two major fragile X syndrome mouse model phenotypes by the mGluR5 antagonist MPEP. *Neuropharmacology, 49*, 1053–1066.

Yin, H. H., Davis, M. I., Ronesi, J. A., & Lovinger, D. M. (2006). The role of protein synthesis in striatal long-term depression. *Journal of Neuroscience, 26*, 11,811–11,820.

Zafeiriou, D. I., Ververi, A., & Vargiami, E. (2007). Childhood autism and associated comorbidities. *Brain and Development, 29*, 257–272.

Zalfa, F., Eleuteri, B., Dickson, K. S., Mercaldo, V., De Rubeis, S., di Penta, A., et al. (2007). A new function for the fragile X mental retardation protein in regulation of PSD-95 mRNA stability. *Nature Neuroscience, 10*, 578–587.

Zalfa, F., Giorgi, M., Primerano, B., Moro, A., di Penta, A., Reis, S., et al. (2003). The fragile X syndrome protein FMRP associates with BC1 RNA and regulates the translation of specific mRNAs at synapses. *Cell, 112*, 317–327.

Zhang, Y. Q., Bailey, A. M., Matthies, H. J. G., Renden, R. B., Smith, M. A., Speese, S. D., et al. (2001). Drosophila fragile X-related gene regulates the MAP1B homolog Futsch to control synaptic structure and function. *Cell, 107*, 591–603.

Zhao, M. G., Toyoda, H., Ko, S. W., Ding, H. K., Wu, L. J., & Zhuo, M. (2005). Deficits in trace fear memory and long-term potentiation in a mouse model for fragile X syndrome. *Journal of Neuroscience, 25*, 7385–7392.

Zho, W. M., You, J. L., Huang, C. C., & Hsu, K. S. (2002). The group I metabotropic glutamate receptor agonist (S)-3,5-dihydroxyphenylglycine induces a novel form of depotentiation in the CA1 region of the hippocampus. *Journal of Neuroscience, 22*, 8838–8849.

Commentary

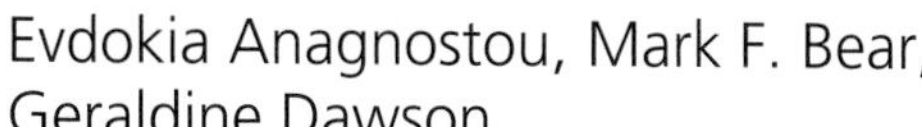

Evdokia Anagnostou, Mark F. Bear, Geraldine Dawson

Future Directions in the Treatment of Autism Spectrum Disorders

The past couple of decades have witnessed a dramatic growth in research on the efficacy of interventions for individuals with autism spectrum disorders (ASD). As described in the chapters in this section, there are now data to support a variety of treatment approaches for individuals with ASD, ranging from pharmacological to behavioral interventions. The state of knowledge pertaining to pharmacological interventions was thoughtfully summarized by the authors in this section. Current data provide support for the use of certain classes of medication for specific target symptoms, such as stimulants and nonstimulants for difficulties in attention/hyperactivity and atypical neuroleptics for irritability and impulsive aggression. Conflicting data were also discussed regarding the efficacy of certain medications, which challenge our current clinical practice and views. The remarkable progress that has been shown in our understanding and treatment of Fragile X was also described, providing an exciting example of the translation of data and insights derived from an animal model to preclinical and clinical research on pharmaceuticals in a relatively brief period of time. Results of studies on behavioral and psychosocial interventions reviewed in the chapters in this section support the efficacy of interventions targeting social skills, sensory motor dysfunction, and the early cognitive and language development of young toddlers with ASD. Thus, some progress in the treatment of ASD has clearly been made. The question before us is: Where do we go from here? In this commentary, we consider current challenges, gaps, and future directions of ASD treatment research, including research on neuropsychopharmacological and behavioral/psychosocial interventions for ASD.

Current Challenges and Gaps in ASD Treatment Research

Neuropharmacological Treatments

The history of neuropsychopharmacology of ASD is characterized by a symptom-focused rather than syndrome-based approach. Symptom domains of ASD that have phenotypic similarity with symptom domains of other neurodevelopmental/neuropsychiatric disorders have been assumed to have similar underlying neurobiology. As such, medications known to have favorable efficacy/safety profiles in other disorders have been "borrowed" and tested in ASD. This approach has had mixed success. The case of risperidone, the first medication to obtain FDA indication for the treatment of a symptom domain associated with ASD, is an example of the success of this approach. Similarly, the positive results of trials testing the efficacy of stimulants and atomoxetine for the treatment of attention-deficit/hyperactivity (ADHD)-like symptoms in autism support such an approach, although the effect sizes for ASD studies are smaller than those observed in ADHD studies. On the other hand, recent data questioning the efficacy of selective serotonin reuptake inhibitors (SSRIs) for the treatment of repetitive behaviors in ASD challenges the notion that phenotypic similarities reflect common neurobiological substrates. As molecular genetics and neuroscience analyses of ASD mature, new approaches are emerging. The exciting development is that for the first time we are in a position to identify novel molecular targets for autism based on the basic science of ASD. Although it is too early to evaluate the ultimate success of such an approach, it is promising that our understanding of the neurobiology of ASD is becoming sophisticated enough that it allows the translation of basic science findings to the development of treatments that target core ASD symptoms and potentially facilitate responses to behavioral interventions. The hope is that by combining autism-specific pharmacological intervention with behavioral interventions, it will be possible to modify the developmental trajectories of individuals with ASD. Still, a series of challenges remains.

Measuring Outcomes

The valid and reliable measurement of outcomes of clinical trials of medications used with individuals with ASD poses significant challenges for the field. Perhaps the biggest challenge is that ASD is a developmental disorder with highly heterogeneous presentation, and as such, it requires measurement of symptom domains across different abilities, developmental and chronological age levels, and symptom severities. Cognitive abilities vary substantially and can influence symptom severity, such as communication ability. Within symptom domains, different behaviors can reflect an underlying core symptom domain. For example, an impairment in social relatedness can be reflected by difficulties in establishing eye contact, peer relationships, and social discourse, and each individual with ASD may have impairments in one or all of these domains. The nature of symptoms, such as an impairment in communication ability, will vary substantially according to developmental level. Even with a relatively small developmental window, such as the elementary school period, children's social abilities can range from just beginning to initiate social contact to engaging in complex social games, for example. In addition to the heterogeneity of symptom expression, another thorny issue is that many of the available outcome measures assess specific skills in a controlled environment, and it is often unclear how to measure performance of the same skills in community settings. There is debate about whether standardized tests, although reliable, correlate with spontaneous use of the skills that they intend to measure.

Another challenge in developing appropriate outcome measures is related to the type of skills we measure. Early intervention researchers have focused on developing measures that target skill acquisition in the areas of cognitive, social, and language abilities, as this is the goal of early intervention. On the other hand, neuropsychopharmacology researchers have focused on developing measures that reflect reduction in maladaptive behavior, since this has been the target of most medications so far. Given that most pharmacological research has targeted school-age children, we lack valid and reliable measures that focus on skills acquisition for this age group that can be used in clinical trials.

Lastly, we lack measures that target the many comorbid psychiatric conditions that are associated with ASD, such as depression and anxiety, which have been validated for use in individuals with autism. The limited availability of outcome measures validated in this population to assess psychiatric comorbidity has also translated into lack of efficacy data on the treatment of psychiatric comorbidities. Similarly, there is a lack of research on effects of such comorbidities on treatment response and side effect generation. Given that the prevalence of anxiety and depression (Ghaziuddin et al., 2002) and ADHD-like symptoms (Gadow et al., 2006) are higher in ASD than the general population, we need to consider the impact of such comorbidities in treatment studies that target core ASD symptoms. In addition, certain comorbid conditions have the potential to produce symptoms that may imitate or contribute to the behavioral symptoms of autism. As such, clarifying the role of such comorbidities in the phenotypic variability of ASD and its effect on treatment response may significantly impact the choice of agents available for the treatment of ASD related symptoms.

Medical Comorbidities

As described in Chapter 74, children with ASD experience a variety of medical issues, including GI disturbance and sleep difficulties. Although the exact link between these medical issues and the pathophysiology of autism remains unclear, there is an urgent need to develop effective treatments for these medical conditions to alleviate suffering, improve behavior, and possibly decrease the amount of psychotherapeutic agents used unnecessarily.

There is emerging evidence to suggest that a wide range of medical conditions or dysfunctions may be conferring risk or even possibly causing an ASD phenotype. Such areas include increased oxidative stress, mitochondrial dysfunction, immune dysregulation, and metabolic disorders. Several rare metabolic syndromes are associated with ASD-like phenotypes (e.g., central folate deficiency, creatine deficiency, Smith-Lemli-Opitz syndrome, PKU), although the incidence of such disorders in children with autism is reported to be low (Zecavati et al., 2009). Research is needed to explore the role of dysfunction in certain systems, such as mitochondrial function or oxidative stress, to determine whether, even in the absence of a diagnosable disorder, such metabolic disorders confer risk for autism, impact treatment response to psychopharmacologic agents, and whether treatment of such conditions improves ASD symptoms (Zecavati et al., 2009).

Alternative and Complementary Treatments

A thorough discussion of alternative treatments is included in Chapter 75. As mentioned by the chapter authors, the data are very limited in regard to both efficacy and safety, but the use of alternative treatments by the ASD community is widespread. The challenges are significant on multiple fronts. With few exceptions, many parents do not have faith in the Western concept of randomized controlled trials. The Western medical community has not invested in testing alternative approaches. Funding to do so has been limited. However, the scientific rationale for many of the alternative treatments needs more rigorous research. Moreover, we know very little about the neurobiological effects of many of the complementary and alternative approaches. An organized effort on all fronts is required to properly test efficacy and safety of alternative approaches and move the field toward integrative, multitradition practice.

Treatments for Adults with ASD

As the first cohorts of children who have received intensive early intervention are crossing into adulthood, it is becoming apparent that we have minimal data on the efficacy of pharmacologic interventions for adults with autism. As such, there are few evidence-based guidelines to help clinicians make informed choices regarding the use of pharmacologic agents in this population. The few available studies are based on very small sample sizes. As mentioned in Chapter 71, the few follow-up studies addressing symptom impairment and abatement in adolescents and adults with an ASD suggest that these individuals improve from childhood to adulthood, but that they still experience periods of symptom aggravation, and a majority continues to require support. The reported rising figures of prevalence of ASD in children will soon reflect increased prevalence of ASD in adults. We are currently not prepared to address their needs given the lack of data for adult oriented interventions, limited understanding of the needs of adults with ASD, and the crucial lack of therapists and physicians with ASD expertise that care for adults.

Heterogeneity of ASD

As described in almost all chapters in the volume, one striking difficulty with developing interventions for ASD is the large individual differences in symptom severity and expression. At this point, we know very little about which characteristics/biomarkers identify distinct subgroups that will respond well to a particular biologic treatment. As such, researchers have found it very difficult to meaningfully stratify the ASD population in intervention studies. Most often, clinical trials try to address this issue by enrolling children who score poorly for the target domain symptom. Other analyses involve examining, and sometimes controlling for, the effect of age and IQ on treatment response. Although such approaches are helpful, they do not fully address the amount of individual variability observed in this population.

We also struggle with how to translate basic science findings that may apply to very small subgroups of children with ASD. The most obvious example is related to rare but causative mutations recently identified. The question arises regarding how the clinical scientist should use the information provided by genetics to develop clinical interventions for a well-known molecular target, when the available sample size for testing this clinical intervention may not allow randomized controlled designs. Suggestions have included grouping mutations that affect similar pathways together, or exploring single subject designs traditionally used by behavioral researchers, but this is a new territory and it will require multidisciplinary input.

Behavioral and Psychosocial Intervention Research

Over the past several decades, we have made tremendous progress in the development of effective behavioral interventions for young children with ASD (Rogers & Vismara, 2008). It is generally agreed that comprehensive, early intensive behavioral interventions can significantly improve the outcomes of preschool aged children with ASD (Reichow & Wolery, 2009). Recently, an early intervention appropriate for toddlers at risk for ASD was shown to be efficacious (Dawson et al., 2009). A randomized controlled trial with children with ASD less than 2 ½ years of age demonstrated that an intensive early intervention that integrates applied behavioral analysis with developmental-relationship approaches, can improve IQ, language, and adaptive behavior, and reduce the severity of diagnosis in young children.

Although progress has been made, significant challenges and gaps in developing behavioral and psychosocial interventions remain. First, similar to neuropharmacological interventions, there is large individual variability in response to behavioral interventions across the life span. For example, although virtually all individuals appear to benefit from early intensive behavioral interventions, some children make extremely rapid progress, while others make slower progress. For those with slow progress, the need for effective alternative or augmented behavioral interventions is great. With the exception of pretreatment IQ, we still have no robust, reliable, and valid clinical or biological indices that predict level of response to behavioral interventions. There is an early literature that provides clues regarding which children with ASD respond well to different types of early behavioral interventions (Sherer & Schreibman, 2005), but there is a great need for more research in this area. Furthermore, the phenomenon of "recovery" or loss of diagnosis, occurring in approximately 10% of children with ASD (Helt et al., 2008), is poorly understood. The biological and/or environmental variables, including treatment variables, that predict recovery from ASD are unknown.

A second challenge is that few studies have yet identified the critical ingredients (mediators) that are responsible for the efficacy of behavioral interventions. For example, although studies have shown that early intensive behavioral intervention is effective for improving outcomes of children with ASD, basic questions pertaining to the optimal dose, age of onset of intervention, and specific treatment modality have not been answered. To date, no study has tested head-to-head whether one approach to early comprehensive behavioral intervention is more effective than another (e.g., ABA using discrete trials teaching versus developmental behavioral approaches).

Third, very few studies have documented the longer-term effects of behavioral intervention. There is a great need for longitudinal studies that examine whether the gains obtained through early intervention are sustained, and if so, what factors account for maintenance of gains. Virtually all randomized controlled trials of comprehensive interventions have been conducted with preschool age children. It is unclear whether children who respond well to these interventions and enter general classroom environments continue to do well during elementary school. It is unknown what specific kinds of ongoing support are needed and what types of residual behavioral challenges these children typically face. The clinical literature suggests that many children who make significant cognitive and language gains as a result of early intensive intervention often experience continued difficulties in the areas of peer relationships, attention, and anxiety. Studies of programs designed to mitigate these difficulties are needed so that early investments in intervention can be of maximum benefit for individuals with ASD.

Fourth, most of the behavioral intervention studies have been conducted by university-based clinical staff, and many of the intervention programs have thus far been developed and evaluated primarily with children with European American backgrounds. To achieve the goal of providing appropriate intervention to all individuals with ASD, it will be important to understand cultural issues pertaining to language barriers, stigma, differences with respect to parenting style, and access to and use of medical and educational services, among others. There is a need to adapt many existing intervention programs to make them more scalable and exportable to the broader community. Mechanisms from training community professionals on a large scale also need to be developed. The use of Web-based and other remote training modalities will need to be tested for their effectiveness.

While progress in the area of early behavioral intervention has been steady, relatively fewer clinical trials designed to test the efficacy of interventions appropriate for school age, adolescent, and adult individuals have been conducted. Reviews of the state of the science regarding social skills interventions (Rao et al., 2008; Reichow & Volkmar, 2009; Williams, et al., 2007) indicate that some promising techniques have been evaluated and manualized. Several studies have shown that social skills during middle and late childhood can be improved through behavioral and psychosocial interventions. It is unclear, however, whether these improvements, which are often taught and assessed in clinic settings, lead to clinically significant improvements in social relationships at home and in the community. Some studies suggest that generalization of learned skills to more complex environments continues to be a challenge. It is unknown, furthermore, whether elementary school–age children who receive social skill interventions are more likely to have satisfying intimate relationships as adolescents and adults. Like other areas of ASD treatment research, research on social skills interventions has been impeded by a lack of valid, reliable measures of social skills that are sensitive to change in treatment studies. In fact, there currently is little consensus on what are the best available measures.

Finally, there is a paucity of research on effective behavioral and psychosocial interventions that can be employed for individuals with ASD during late adolescence and adulthood. A variety of treatment approaches is being used with adults, ranging from social skills groups to job coaching, but the number of published studies that examine the efficacy of such approaches is small. Given the increased prevalence of ASD with many children soon to enter adulthood, it is crucial that more attention be directed toward developing and evaluating behavioral and psychosocial interventions for adults with ASD.

Future Directions in ASD Treatment Research

We have described some of the current challenges and gaps in research on neuropharmacological and behavioral interventions for individuals with ASD. In this section, we highlight some of the future directions in ASD treatment research.

Animal Models to Inform Biological Interventions

Psychiatry has a poor record of translating animal research into new treatments for humans. The traditional approach has been to develop a model in which the animal displays some phenotypes that resemble human symptoms (e.g., depressed mood), and then to validate it by showing that effective treatments in humans can also have beneficial effects in the animal (e.g., fluoxetine). The obvious limitation is that a behavioral phenocopy does not indicate a shared etiology or pathophysiology. Furthermore, showing that a known treatment can be effective in the animal renders the model useful mainly for identifying additional treatments that work by the same mechanism(s) as the known treatments. This approach has not led to new medical breakthroughs in psychiatry. Most existing treatments for neuropsychiatric disorders resulted from a combination of serendipity and astute clinical observation, not animal research. Animal models of ASDs that rely solely on the attempt to phenocopy aspects of the human disease (e.g., impaired social interactions) are not likely to fair any better in furthering discovery of new treatments.

The explosion of knowledge about the human genome and genetic variations that cause or confer risk for disease will change this situation, dramatically (Cowan et al., 2002). Although we are still far from understanding the genetic architecture of ASD, the pace of discovery is quickening. The path from gene discovery to treatment must utilize animals in which the causative mutations can be engineered. It is reasonable to expect that the disruption in brain function by a mutation may manifest differently at the behavioral level in flies, mice, and humans. Yet understanding how neurons function differently in the genetically defined animal model has great potential to reveal core pathophysiological mechanisms and suggest ways that they can be corrected.

Fragile X provides a case in point. Fragile X syndrome (FXS) is manifest in humans in myriad ways—mental retardation, repetitive and autistic behaviors, altered gastrointestinal function, childhood epilepsy. Modeling any one of these behavioral manifestations in wild type mice would not likely reveal the core pathophysiology of Fragile X, or lead to development of a disease-modifying treatment. However, FXS is caused by transcriptional silencing of a single gene, *FMR1*. The homologous gene has been knocked out in both mice and flies, and these Fragile X animal mutants have been studied extensively to understand the functional consequences of the loss of the gene product, FMRP (D'Hulst & Kooy, 2009). Although the story continues to evolve, many of the core deficits in the animal models appear to be caused by excessive downstream consequences of activating metabotropic glutamate receptor 5 (mGluR5). Remarkably, pharmacological or genetic reduction of mGluR5 signaling has been shown to ameliorate or correct a wide array of Fragile X mutant phenotypes in both mice and fruit flies. These findings suggest an evolutionarily conserved relationship between metabotropic glutamate receptors and FMRP. In the absence of FMRP., the consequences of mGluR5 activity are excessive, and this excess can be corrected by reducing mGluR5 activity (Dolen & Bear, 2008). Currently, several human clinical trials are underway using compounds that either reduce glutamate release in the brain or target selectively mGluR5. Preliminary results might be available by the time this book publishes.

Understanding the basic neurobiology in mice of other single gene disorders associated with human autistic behavior and cognitive impairment has also borne fruit. Examples are CNS changes in tuberous sclerosis, which may be ameliorated by inhibitors of the protein kinase mTOR (Ehninger et al., 2009); neurofibromatosis, which may be ameliorated by statins (Acosta et al., 2006); and Rett syndrome, which may be ameliorated by insulinlike growth factor 1 (Tropea et al., 2009); to name a few. Clinical trials based on findings in the animal models are planned or underway.

Single gene mutations that produce behavioral changes on the autism spectrum are rare, and any treatments that derive from these studies may apply to a small fraction of individuals on the autism spectrum. However, there are hints that the mutations responsible for these rare syndromes fall within pathways or networks of proteins with related functions (Kelleher & Bear, 2008). It is entirely possible that a substantial fraction of cases of autism of (currently) unknown etiology may be "Fragile X–like," sharing with FXS excessive glutamate signaling through mGluR5. Others might be "TSC-like" with altered mTOR signaling, and so on. Perhaps the autisms are caused by disruptions of a limited number of functionally related pathways, in which case treatments developed for a rare, genetically defined syndrome may be broadly beneficial. Expansion of ongoing clinical trials for Fragile X, etc, into nonsyndromic autism will be extremely important, as will tests of the "shared pathophysiology" hypothesis in the extant animal models.

We anticipate that the approach of creating a genetically engineered animal model, followed by intensive neurobiological analysis of pathophysiology will be repeated as additional highly penetrant mutations are discovered. One example of this approach is the neuroligin 4 mutant mouse (Jamain et al., 2008). Genetically defined animal models allow neurobiologists to examine how the brain functions differently in autism at a cellular level. This understanding has suggested potential therapeutic targets, and we will soon know how well these insights translate into the clinic. Animal models also allow additional, critical questions to be addressed. These include the degree to which altered brain development and function can be corrected when treatment is initiated in adults, the persistence of benefit if treatments are initiated during early critical periods of development, and the interactions of genes and experience.

Novel Pharmacological Targets

Glutamate System

The glutamate system has become the focus of translational work in recent years. As is described above in detail, the Fragile X model of autism illustrates that manipulation of aspects of this system can lead to a phenotype that includes autistic-like features. In addition to mGluR5 inhibition, there are other possible molecular targets within this system for pharmacologic manipulation. Patients with autism or Asperger's syndrome were found to have raised levels of glutamate in plasma compared to healthy controls in multiple studies (Rolf et al., 1993, Moreno-Fuenmayor et al., 1996, Aldred et al., 2003, Shinohe et al., 2006). Glutamic acid decarboxylase protein, the enzyme responsible for normal conversion of glutamate to GABA in the brain, has been noted to be reduced in the brain of autistic subjects in postmortem studies, suggesting increased levels of glutamate or transporter receptor density in autistic brains (Fatemi et al., 2002). In addition, further postmortem studies have revealed decreased AMPA-type glutamate receptor density in the cerebellum of autistic individuals. In the same study, the mRNA levels of several genes involved in the glutamatergic pathways were significantly increased in autistics, including the excitatory amino acid transporter 1 and the glutamate receptor AMPA 1 (Purcell et al., 2001). Genetic findings are still very preliminary but have so far revealed a mutation in the glutamate receptor gene GRIK2 in 6q21 that is present in 8% of autistic subjects and 4% of controls and seems to be transmitted from mothers to autistic males (Phillipe et al., 1999), a susceptibility mutation in linkage disequilibrium with variants in the metabotropic glutamate receptor 8 gene on chromosome 7 (Serajee et al., 2003), and a single nucleotide polymorphism of the GR1N2A subunit of the NMDA receptor associated with autism (Barnby et al., 2005).

A few medications affecting the NMDA receptor have produced preliminary evidence that encourage further studies in this system. Amantadine, which has NMDA noncompetitive inhibitor activity, was used in a double blind placebo controlled trial in autistic children, was well tolerated, and had modest effects on irritability and hyperactivity (King et al., 2001). Dextromethorphan is an NMDA receptor antagonist. In a series of case studies of children with autism, it was reported to improve problem behaviors such as tantrums and self-injurious behaviors, as well as anxiety, motor planning, socialization, and language (Woodard et al., 2005, Welch et al., 1992, Phillips et al., 1999).

Memantine is a noncompetitive NMDA inhibitor. There have been four open-label studies of this compound reporting on a total of 186 children with autism. Effects of memantine included improvements in irritability, lethargy, hyperactivity, inappropriate speech, stereotypy, memory, and language (Owley et al., 2006, Chez et al., 2007, Niederhofer et al., 2007, Erickson et al., 2007).

The above discussion is encouraging in terms of suggesting that aspects of the glutamate system are possible targets for pharmacological manipulation in individuals with ASD. Well-controlled studies in this area are necessary.

Oxytocin/Vasopressin

Oxytocin (OXT) and the similar peptide vasopressin have been linked to modulation of social cognition and function in both animal models and in humans (see Chapter 34). A number of researchers have hypothesized that OXT may be implicated in autism given that repetitive behaviors and deficits in social interaction are core features of autism, and that this neuropeptide is involved in the regulation of repetitive behaviors and social cognition. Insel et al. (2004) postulated that abnormalities in the neural pathway for OXT could account for many features of autism including the early onset, predominance in males, genetic loading, and neuroanatomical abnormalities. The data for oxytocin involvement in the pathophysiology of autism is still limited although emerging (see Chapter 34). Still, children with autism have lower average levels of blood OXT level in comparison to typically developing children matched for age (Modahl et al., 1998) and may fail to show the normal developmental decrease with age (Green et al., 2001). Differences in OXT peptide processing pathways may result in inactive or less active forms of OXT. Neuropeptide synthesis genes may also be candidates for genetic susceptibility in this disorder. Recent studies suggest a genetic association between the OXT receptor gene and autism (Wu et al., 2005; Ylisaukko-oja et al., 2006; Jacob et al., 2007). Polymorphisms in the AVP receptor have also been linked to autism (Kim et al., 2002; Wassink et al., 2004; and Yirmiya et al., 2006) These findings are consistent with animal studies showing that both OXT and AVP genes are involved in many aspects of social behavior. Hollander et al. (2007) reported that intravenous administration of oxytocin facilitated the retention of social cognition in autism spectrum disorder patients.

Given the above, well-controlled studies manipulating the oxytocin system are warranted. Questions to be still addressed in preparation for large clinical trials are related to the pharmacokinetics/pharmacodynamics of the compound, the mode of administration, and the choice of social cognition outcome measures to be used.

Immune Modulation

Active and ongoing neuroinflammatory process in the cerebral cortex and white matter and cerebellum have been reported in postmortem brain tissue of subjects with ASD. The abnormalities included activation of microglia and astroglia (Vargas et al., 2005). Both microglia and astroglia are integrally involved in cortical organization, neuronal transmission, and synaptic plasticity. Activation of neuroglial cells can produce significant neuronal and synaptic changes that are likely to contribute to CNS dysfunction observed in autism. Increase in CSF proinflammatory factors, including IL-6, interferon-gamma, and MCP-1, have also been reported (Vargas et al., 2005; Pardo et al., 2005; Zimmerman et al., 2006). The changes are consistent with a dysregulated immune response and likely a skewed T helper cell type 1 (TH1/TH2 cytokine profiles), decreased lymphocyte numbers, decreased T cell mitogen response, and the imbalance of serum immunoglobulin levels. Many studies have documented elevated levels of proinflammatory cytokines in patients with ASD, including TNF-alpha/IL-12 (Jyonouchi et al., 2005a, 2005b, 2001); tumor necrosis factor receptor II (Croonenberghs et al., 2002a); IFN-Gamma and IL-1RA (Zimmerman et al., 2005); MCP-1, a macrophage chemoattractant protein (Vargas et al., 2005); and IgG2 and IgG4 (Croonenberghs et al., 2002b). Other studies have found that patients with ASD produce lower levels of IL-10, an important counterregulatory cytokine.

Other evidence possibly linking autism to the immune system comes from immunogenetic studies of the HLA genes, which are important determinants of immune function (Pardo et al., 2005). For example, a particular MHC haplotype (B44-Sc 30-DR4) associated with immune dysfunction has been shown to occur significantly more frequently in individuals with autism or their mothers as compared to unrelated controls (Daniels et al., 1995). Other immune-based genes including HLA-DRB1, complement C4 alleles (Ashwood et al., 2006), and HLA-A2 alleles (Torres et al., 2006) have also been shown to occur with significantly greater frequency in autistic subjects. Finally, evidence is accumulating that autoimmune disorders occur with significantly greater frequency within families of autistic individuals (Sweeten et al., 2003).

There are multiple agents available that may modulate the immune system of children with ASD in favorable way. Of note, this is an area where alternative compounds such as omega 3 fatty acids may be showing as much early promise as Western medications, such as pioglitazone. However, the evidence for any of these is preliminary at best and well-controlled studies are urgently needed.

Back Translation

In this commentary, we have discussed the importance and progress in the translation from basic science to research on treatments. However, "back translation" is also an important strategy for making progress in developing treatments. Findings from clinical trials have the potential to elucidate the pathophysiology of autism. For example, as discussed above, a clinician scientist may consider not only studying the effect of an immune modulating agent on behaviors, but linking such improvements to specific inflammatory biomarkers, thus contributing to our understanding of the nature of possible immunologic abnormalities in this population.

Individual Differences

A significant challenge that needs to be addressed is understanding and predicting individual differences in responses to pharmacological interventions. ASDs are a heterogeneous group of disorders associated with multiple etiologies, clinical presentations, and comorbidities. There is a great need for identification of biomarkers that can predict which individuals will respond to which medications. Genetic and other biomarkers can potentially help predict individual differences in treatment efficacy, pharmokinetics, and side effects profiles.

Future Directions in Early Behavioral Intervention

Intervention with Infants and Toddlers

New advances in very early detection of ASD offer the possibility of intervening before the full syndrome of ASD is present. Thus, for the first time, prevention of ASD is plausible (Dawson, 2008). Genetic and environmental risk factors contribute to an atypical trajectory of brain and behavioral development in ASD that influences the early patterns of interaction between the child and his/her environment, particularly the social environment. Studies of infant siblings of children with ASD have found that many infants who later develop ASD begin to exhibit symptoms during the second half of the first year of life (see Zwaigenbaum, Chapter 5, this volume). Among the earliest symptoms are a lack of attention to other people and a failure to engage in social imitation and communicative babbling. These symptoms influence early interactions between the infant and the social world, thereby limiting the amount and quality of linguistic and social input that may be necessary to promote brain and behavioral development. Thus, early risk factors contribute to *risk processes* resulting in secondary effects of the early symptoms that may contribute to the development of the full ASD syndrome. By intervening early before the full syndrome is present, it might be possible to mitigate the downstream effects of early symptoms on later brain and behavioral development. In this way, prevention of the full syndrome of ASD, at least in some cases, might be possible (Dawson, 2008).

As described by Rogers and Wallace (Chapter 61 in this volume), early interventions that are appropriate for infants at risk for ASD as young as 12 months of age are currently being developed and tested (Dawson et al., 2009). Furthermore, six randomized clinical trials of early interventions for infants and toddlers, funded by Autism Speaks, are currently underway. Although the interventions vary, comparable pretreatment and outcome measures are being used, which will allow for comparing and combining data across the studies. Notably, there are several similarities among the six interventions being tested. They all are parent-delivered, involve individualized approaches that tailor the targeted skills to the developmental level of the child, and address early pivotal skills such as imitation and joint attention that set the stage for later social and communication development. The fact that the interventions are parent-delivered makes these interventions scalable and exportable to the broader parent community.

Combined Behavioral and Pharmacological Interventions

As described above, studies are currently being conducted that examine whether the mechanisms involved in single gene disorders such as FXS (namely, excessive glutamate signaling) may be similar in nonsyndromic ASD. If it is found that there is shared pathophysiology across different genetic subtypes of ASD, it is possible that medications that improve neural signaling would become available for a larger percentage of the ASD population. If such medications become available, it is likely that these will be used in combination with behavioral interventions. Early intensive behavioral interventions facilitate the formation of new connections in the brain that support the development of social behavior and communication. The hope is that medications that improve neural functioning will help individuals with ASD become even more responsive to behavioral interventions. In one of the first randomized clinical trials to examine the efficacy of a combined pharmacological and behavioral approach, Aman and colleagues (2009) found that, in combination, the use of medication and parent training was more effective for reducing serious behavioral problems in children with ASD than medication alone.

In conclusion, emerging data from basic science (neuropathology, genetics/genomics/proteomics, animal models) have made it possible to start identifying neurochemical systems involved in the pathophysiology of autism that can be specifically targeted with neuropsychopharmacological interventions. It is anticipated that, ultimately, pharmacological agents targeting systems involved in the pathophysiology of ASD will be used to facilitate existing behavioral interventions. Research reflecting the reality of providing multimodal interventions will have the largest impact in the care of individuals with autism. Such studies are fairly difficult to do and require significant commitment on the part of funding agencies, researchers, and the autism community. Early data has provided encouragement regarding the feasibility and value of such an approach (Scahill et al., 2009).

REFERENCES

Acosta, M. T., Gioia, G. A., & Silva, A. J. (2006). Neurofibromatosis type 1: New insights into neurocognitive issues. *Current Neurology and Neuroscience Reports*, 6, 136–143.

Aldred, S., Moore, K. M., Fitzgerald, M., & Waring, R. H. (2003). Plasma amino acid levels in children with autism and their families. *Journal of Autism and Developmental Disorders, 33,* 93–97.

Aman, M. G., et al. (2009). Medication and parent training in children with pervasive developmental disorders and serious behaviour problems: Results from a randomized clinical trial. *Journal of the American Academy of Child and Adolescent Psychiatry,* Oct. 23 (Epub ahead of print).

Ashwood, P., & Wakefield, A. J. (2006). Immune activation of peripheral blood and mucosal cd3+ lymphocyte cytokine profiles in children with autism and gastrointestinal symptoms. *Journal of Neuroimmunology, 173,* 126–134.

Barnby, G., Abbott, A., Sykes, N., Morris, A., Weeks, D. E., Mott, R., et al. (2005). Candidate-gene screening and association analysis at the autism-susceptibility locus on chromosome16p: Evidence of association at GRIN2A and ABA. T. *American Journal of Human Genetics, 76,* 950–966.

Chez, M., et al. (2007). Memantine as adjunctive therapy in children diagnosed with ASD. *Journal of Child Neurology, 22,* 574–579.

Cowan, W. M., Kopnisky, K. L., & Hyman, S. E. (2002). The human genome project and its impact on psychiatry. *Annual Review of Neuroscience, 25,* 1–50.

Croonenberghs, J., Bosmans, E., Deboutte, D., Kenis, G., & Maes M (2002a). Activation of the inflammatory response system in autism. *Neuropsychobiology, 45,* 1–6.

Croonenberghs, J., Wauters, A., Devreese, K., Verkerk, R., Scharpe, S., Bosmans, E., et al. (2002b). Increased serum albumin, gamma globulin, immunoglobulin IgG, and IgG2 and IgG4 in autism. *Psychological Medicine, 32*(8), 1457–1463.

D'Hulst, C., & Kooy, R. F. (2009). Fragile X syndrome: From molecular genetics to therapy. *Journal of Medical Genetics, 46,* 577–584.

Daniels, W. W., Warren, R. P., Odell, J. D., Maciulis, A., Burger, R. A., Warren, W. L., et al. (1995). Increased frequency of the extended or ancestral haplotype B44-SC30-DR4 in autism. *Neuropsychobiology, 32*(3), 120–123.

Dawson, G. (2008). Early behavioral intervention, brain plasticity, and autism spectrum disorder. *Development and Psychopathology, 20,* 775–803.

Dawson, G., Rogers, S., Munson, J., Smith, M., Winter, J., Greenson, J., et al. (2009). Randomized, controlled trial of an intervention for toddlers with autism: The Early Start Denver model. *Pediatrics,* Nov. 30 (Epub ahead of print).

Dolen, G., & Bear, M. F. (2008). Role for metabotropic glutamate receptor 5 (mGluR5) in the pathogenesis of fragile X syndrome. *Journal of Physiology, 586,* 1503–1508.

Ehninger, D., de Vries, P. J., & Silva, A. J. (2009). From mTOR to cognition: Molecular and cellular mechanisms of cognitive impairments in tuberous sclerosis. *Journal of Intellectual Disability Research, 53,* 838–851.

Erickson, C. A., et al. (2007). A retrospective study of memantine in children and adolescents with PDD. *Psychopharmacology, 191,* 141–147.

Fatemi, S. H. (2002). The role of reelin in pathology of autism. *Molecular Psychiatry, 7,* 919–920.

Helt, M., Kelley, E., Kinsbourne, M., Pandey, J., Boorstein, H., Herbert, M. et al. (2008) Can children with autism recover? If so, how? *Neuropsychology Review, 18,* 339–366.

Gadow, K. D., DeVincent, C. J., & Pomeroy, J. (2006). ADHD symptom subtypes in children with pervasive developmental disorder. *Journal of Autism and Developmental Disorders, 36*(2), 271–283.

Ghaziuddin, M., Ghaziuddin, N., & Greden, J. (2002). Depression in persons with autism: Implications for research and clinical care. *Journal of Autism and Developmental Disorders, 32*(4), 299–306.

Green, L., Fein, D., Modahl, C., Feinstein, C., Waterhouse, L., & Morris, M. (2001). Oxytocin and autistic disorder: Alterations in peptide forms. *Biological Psychiatry, 50,* 609–613.

Hollander, E., Bartz, J., Chaplin, W., Phillips, A., Sumner, J., Soorya, L., et al. (2007). Oxytocin increases retention of social cognition in autism. *Biological Psychiatry, 61*(4), 498–503.

Insel, T. R., & Fernald, R. D. (2004). How the brain processes social information: Searching for the social brain. *Annual Review of Neuroscience, 27,* 697–722.

Jacob, S., et al. (2007). Association of the oxytocin receptor gene (OXTR) in Caucasian children and adolescents with autism. *Neuroscience Letters, 417,* 6–9.

Jamain, S., Radyushkin, K., Hammerschmidt, K., Granon, S., Boretius, S., Varoqueaux, F., et al. (2008). Reduced social interaction and ultrasonic communication in a mouse model of monogenic heritable autism. *Proceedings of the National Academy of Sciences of the United States of America, 105,* 1710–1715.

Jyonouchi, H., Geng, L., Ruby, A., Reddy, C., & Zimmerman-Bier, B. (2005a). Evaluation of an association between gastrointestinal symptoms and cytokine production against common dietary proteins in children with autism spectrum disorders. *Journal of Pediatrics, 146,* 605–610.

Jyonouchi, H., Geng, L., Ruby, A., & Zimmerman-Bier, B. (2005b). Dysregulated innate immune responses in young children with autism spectrum disorders: Their relationship to gastrointestinal symptoms and dietary intervention. *Neuropsychobiology, 51,* 77–85.

Jyonouchi, H., Sun, S., & Le H (2001). Proinflammatory and regulatory cytokine production associated with innate and adaptive immune responses in children with autism spectrum disorders and developmental regression. *Journal of Neuroimmunology, 120,* 170–179.

Kelleher, R. J., 3rd, & Bear, M. F. (2008). The autistic neuron: Troubled translation? *Cell, 135,* 401–406.

Kim, S. J., et al. (2002).Transmission disequilibrium testing of arginine vasopressin receptor 1A (AVPR1A) polymorphisms in autism. *Molecular Psychiatry, 7*(5), 503–507.

King, B. H., Wright, D. M., Handen, B. L., Sikich, L., Zimmerman, A. W., McMahon, W. M., et al. (2001). Double-blind, placebo-controlled study of amantadine hydrochloride in the treatment of children with autistic disorder. *Journal of the American Academy of Child and Adolescent Psychiatry, 40*(6), 658–665.

Modahl, C., Green, L., Fein, D., Morris, M., Waterhouse, L., Feinstein, C., et al. (1998). Plasma oxytocin levels in autistic children. *Biological Psychiatry, 43,* 270–277.

Moreno-Fuenmayor, H., Borjas, L., Arrieta, A., Valera, V., & Socorro-Candanoza, L. (1996). Plasma excitatory amino acids in autism. *Investigación clínica, 37,* 113–128.

Niederhofer, H. (2007). Glutamate antagonists seem to be slightly effective in psychopharmacologic treatment of autism. *Journal of Clinical Psychopharmacology, 27,* 317.

Owley, T., et al. (2006). A prospective open label trial of memantine in the treatment of cognitive, behavioral and memory dysfunction in PDD. *Journal of Child and Adolescent Psychopharmacology, 16,* 517–524.

Pardo, C. A., Vargas, D. L., & Zimmerman, A. W. (2005). Immunity, neuroglia and neuroinflammation in autism. *International Review of Psychiatry, 17,* 485–495.

Phillipe, A., Martinez, M., Guilloud-Bataille, M., Gillberg, C., Rastam, M., Sponheim, E., et al.(1999). Genome-wide scan for autism susceptibility genes. Paris Autism Research International Sibpair Study. *Human Molecular Genetics, 8*, 805–812.

Purcell, A. E., Jeon, O. H., Zimmerman, A. W., Blue, M. E., & Pevsner, J. (2001). Postmortem brain abnormalities of the glutamate neurotransmitter system in autism. *Neurology, 57*, 1618–1628.

Rao, P. A., Beidel, D. C., & Murray, M. J. (2008). Social skills intervention for children with Asperger syndrome or high-functioning autism: A review and recommendations. *Journal of Autism and Developmental Disorders, 38*, 353–361.

Reichow, B., & Volkmar, F. R. (2009). Social skills interventions for individuals with autism: Evaluation for evidence-based practices within a best evidence synthesis framework. *Journal of Autism and Developmental Disorders, 40*, 149–166.

Reichow, B., & Wolery, M. (2009). Comprehensive synthesis of early behavioral interventions for young children with autism based on the UCLA young autism project model. *Journal of Autism and Developmental Disorders, 39*, 23–41.

Rogers, S. J., & Vismara, L. A. (2008). Evidence-based comprehensive treatments for autism. *Journal of Clinical Child and Adolescent Psychology, 37*, 8–38.

Rolf, L. H., Haarmann, F. Y., Grotemeyer, K. H., & Kehrer, H. (1993). Serotonin and amino acid content in platelets of autistic children. *Acta Psychiatrica Scandinavica, 87*, 312–316.

Scahill, L., Aman, M. G., McDougle, C. J., Arnold, L. E., McCracken, J. T., Handen, B., et al. (2009). Trial design challenges when combining medication and parent training in children with pervasive developmental disorders. *Journal of Autism and Developmental Disorders, 39*, 720–729.

Sherer, M. R., & Schreibman, L. (2005). Individual behavioral profiles and predictors of treatment effectiveness for children with autism. *Journal of Consulting and Clinical Psychology, 73*, 525–538.

Serajee, F. J., Zhong, H., Nabi, R., & Huq, A. H. (2003). The metabotropic glutamate receptor 8 gene at 7q31: Partial duplication and possible association with autism. *Journal of Medical Genetics, 40*, e42.

Shinohe, A., Hashimoto, K., Nakamura, K., Tsujii, M., Iwata, Y., Tsuchiya, K. J., et al., (2006). Increased serum levels of glutamate in adult patients with autism. *Progress in Neuro-psychopharmacology and Biological Psychiatry, 30*(8), 1472–1477.

Sweeten, T. L., Bowyer, S. L., Posey, D. J., Halberstadt, G. M., & McDougle, C. J. (2003). Increased prevalence of familial autoimmunity in probands with pervasive developmental disorders. *Pediatrics, 112*, e420.

Torres, A. R., Sweeten, T. L., Cutler, A., Bedke, B. J., Fillmore, M., Stubbs, E. G., et al. (2006). The association and linkage of the hla-a2 class i allele with autism. *Human Immunology, 67*, 346–351.

Tropea, D., Giacometti, E., Wilson, N. R., Beard, C., McCurry, C., Fu, D. D., et al. (2009). Partial reversal of Rett syndrome-like symptoms in MeCP2 mutant mice. *Proceedings of the National Academy of Sciences of the United States of America, 106*, 2029–2034.

Vargas, D. L., Nascimbene, C., Krishnan, C., Zimmerman, A. W., & Pardo, C. A. (2005). Neuroglial activation and neuroinflammation in the brain of patients with autism. *Annals of Neurology, 57*, 67–81.

Wassink, T. H., et al. (2004). Examination of AVPR1a as an autism susceptibility gene. *Molecular Psychiatry, 9*(10), 968–972.

Welch, L., & Sovner, R. (1992). The treatment of a chronic organic mental disorder with dextromethorphan in a man with severe mental retardation. *British Journal of Psychiatry, 161*, 118–120.

Williams White, S., Keonig, K., & Scahill, L. (2007). Social skills development in children with autism spectrum disorders: A review of the intervention research. *Journal of Autism and Developmental Disorders, 37*, 1858–1868.

Woodard, C., Groden, J., Goodwin, M., & Bodfish, J. A. (2007). Placebo double-blind pilot study of dextromethorphan for problematic behaviors in children with autism. *Autism, 11*(1), 29–41. PubMed PMID: 17175572.

Woodard, C., Groden, J., Goodwin, M., Shanower, C., & Bianco, J. (2005). The treatment of the behavioral sequelae of autism with dextromethorphan: A case report. *Journal of Autism and Developmental Disorders, 35*, 515–518.

Wu, S., et al. (2005). Positive association of the oxytocin receptor gene (OXTR) with autism in the Chinese Han population. *Biological Psychiatry, 58*(1), 74–77.

Yirmiya, N., et al. (2006). Association between the arginine vasopressin 1a receptor (AVPR1a) gene and autism in a family-based study: Mediation by socialization skills. *Molecular Psychiatry, 11*(5), 488–494.

Ylisaukko-oja, T., et al. (2006). Search for autism loci by combined analysis of Autism Genetic Resource Exchange and Finnish families. *Annals of Neurology, 59*(1), 145–155.

Zecavati, N., & Spence, S. J. (2009) Neurometabolic disorders and dysfunction in autism spectrum disorders. *Current Neurology and Neuroscience Reports, 9*(2), 129–136.

Zimmerman, A., Connors, S. L., & Pardo-Villamizar, C. A. (2006). Neuroimmunology and neurotransmitters in autism. In R. Tuchman & I. Rapin (Eds.), *Autism: A neurological disorder of early brain development*, (pp. 141–159). London: MacKeith.

Zimmerman, A. W., Jyonouchi, H., Comi, A. M., Connors, S. L., Milstien, S., Varsou, A., et al. (2005). Cerebrospinal fluid and serum markers of inflammation in autism. *Pediatric Neurology, 33*, 195–201.

Section X

Best Practices in the Diagnosis and Treatment of Autism

73 Best Practices: Early Diagnosis and Psychological Assessment

Zachary Warren, Wendy L. Stone

Points of Interest

- Early diagnosis of ASD provides children and families with more opportunities for accessing specialized intervention services that may promote improved functional outcomes.
- The diagnosis of ASD is often an intense emotional experience for caregivers, and an important aspect of the assessment process involves supporting families and promoting engagement with recommended services.
- In the absence of definitive medical and genetic etiologies, early diagnosis is reliant on understanding a child's behavioral profile in relation to the core symptoms of ASD.
- Additional research is needed to determine the reliability and stability of ASD diagnosis in children under 2 years old.
- Integrative and multidisciplinary approaches hold promise for refining the diagnostic assessment process and enabling service systems to meet the growing needs for appropriate diagnosis at younger ages.

An ever-growing body of scientific literature supports the fact that autism spectrum disorders are not rare. In fact, at an estimated prevalence of 1 in 110, ASD is among the most common of all developmental disabilities (Centers for Disease Control and Prevention [CDC], 2009). At the same time, there is little certainty regarding its etiology, the earliest clinical markers, course, optimal intervention practices, and outcomes for young children with ASD. Complicating this substantially limited scientific knowledge base is the fact that there has been unprecedented popular scientific, political, and media attention paid to ASD in the past decade. Although this attention has in many instances provided substantial benefits on individual, family, and system levels, in the face of scientific uncertainty, this attention has also contributed to a context of confusion and conflict for caregivers and professionals alike in understanding, pursuing, and obtaining appropriate and meaningful diagnostic assessment for ASD at young ages.

> Key Point
>
> - Early diagnosis of ASD can improve functional outcomes for children and families as well as reduce service system demands.

At present, the diagnostic evaluation of young children for ASD represents a public health issue of critical importance. Earlier diagnosis of ASD provides children and families with more opportunities for optimal benefit from intensive and specialized intervention services. Children who enter into autism-specialized intervention services at younger ages may show greater gains in cognitive and adaptive functioning and may be more likely to achieve fully integrated classroom placements at school age than children diagnosed at later ages (Cohen et al., 2006; Dawson & Osterling, 1997; Harris & Handleman, 2000; Remington et al., 2007; Rogers, 1996, 1998; Smith et al., 2000). An early diagnosis may lead to improvements in the quality of life for the child with ASD. When linked with intensive autism-specific intervention, early diagnosis may improve family functioning and ultimately reduce substantial service system demands.

Individuals with ASD were once thought to display comorbid intellectual disabilities and to fail to achieve adaptive independence as adults (Filipek et al., 2000; Howlin et al., 2004). However, recent work suggests that these poor outcomes may not be as prevalent as once thought (Chakrabarti & Fombonne, 2001, 2005). Such changes in the conceptualization of outcomes are complex and are likely to be associated with many factors, including major shifts in diagnostic processes. Thus, we cannot attribute better outcomes solely to the benefits of early diagnosis and intervention. However, all available evidence suggests that early diagnosis and intervention can play a meaningful role in improving outcomes for children with ASD in the short- and long-term. As such, from a public health perspective, early intervention may ultimately reduce the considerable lifetime cost and service system demands associated with providing care and support to individuals with autism and their families (Jacobson & Mulick, 2000; Jarbrink & Knapp, 2001).

Key Points

- Although concerns about ASD are often noticed in the first years of life and professional groups consistently advocate for early screening and intervention, numerous barriers contribute to a significant time gap between first concern and diagnosis.
- There are unique challenges for generating definitive diagnoses of ASD for very young children (i.e., children under 2 years of age).

Despite the public health need and mounting evidence that caregivers of children with ASD are able to identify and report concerns about development to medical professionals by the age of 12 to 18 months (Coonrod & Stone, 2004; DeGiacomo & Fombonne, 1998; Rogers & DilLalla, 1990; Wimpory et al., 2000), currently the average age of diagnosis is around 4 years of age or older in underserved communities and subgroups of children with higher IQs (CDC, 2009; Croen et al., 2002; Mandell et al., 2002; Yeargin-Allsopp et al., 2003). To address the gap between time of first concern and diagnosis and to take advantage of the potential impact of early intervention, several consensus panels involving numerous professional groups—including the American Academy of Neurology (AAN) and American Psychological Society (Filipek et al., 2000), the American Academy of Child and Adolescent Psychiatry (Volkmar et al., 1999), and the American Academy of Pediatrics (AAP) (Johnson & Myers, 2007)—have issued practice parameters endorsing early ASD screening in clinical practice settings. Most notably, recent AAP guidelines endorse formal screening for ASD at 18 and 24 months of age, as well as at any point when caregiver concerns are raised. This mandated screening, in combination with increased caregiver and public awareness of the earliest "red flags" of ASD, are creating a pressing need for diagnostic assessment of very young children (i.e., under 2 years of age). This situation presents a significant challenge to clinical diagnosticians, since the available "gold-standard" diagnostic tools and the judgments of even the most experienced clinicians have been applied in a limited manner to this age group. The field is now facing the critical question of whether and how ASD can be identified and addressed at ages that were not previously thought possible.

It is within the context of unprecedented public awareness, increased mandates and desires for definitive diagnoses of ASD at earlier and earlier ages, and limited empirical evidence surrounding the fundamental early features, course, and treatment of ASD that clinicians and diagnosticians are now operating. This chapter summarizes a wide range of considerations related to the diagnostic assessment process in young children that can optimize our ability to help children with ASD and their families. These issues include not only those related to obtaining an accurate diagnosis in young children, but also those related to the assessment process in general and the provision of optimal clinical care to children and families alike.

Function of Diagnostic Assessment

Key Point

- A meaningful diagnostic assessment of ASD involves understanding a child's unique behavioral profile as well as recommending appropriate interventions based on this profile.

A primary function of a diagnostic assessment for ASD is to understand the child's strengths, challenges, behavioral profile, and their implications for intervention. Ideally, a meaningful diagnosis of a neurobehavioral disorder such as ASD would be tied not only to a specific etiology, but also to specific medical, behavioral, and/or educational interventions, as well as reasonable predictions about the likely individual responses to these interventions (Lord & Richler, 2006). At present, the diagnosis of ASD in young children is not yet sufficiently backed by a body of etiological or intervention research that can reasonably claim to approach this goal. In the vast majority of cases, the field is not yet able to pinpoint specific causes of ASD that can be linked to specific treatments or cures. Likewise, the active ingredients underlying successful ASD treatments have not yet been identified, nor has the field determined whether specific treatments are superior to others, or discovered which treatments are better for whom and when. In the face of this uncertainty, a critical function of the diagnostic assessment process is to link families to individually tailored intervention plans that can be realistically implemented. In this regard, the diagnostic assessment process in young children can often expedite access to services, describe characteristics (e.g., the nature and intensity) of effective treatments, identify key intervention areas, and specify concrete measurable goals for children with ASD and their families.

Key Points

- An important aspect of the diagnostic assessment of ASD involves providing family support and facilitating access to specialized services.
- Parents of young children with ASD often find themselves serving in the role of advocate and resource specialist for their child.
- The diagnostic assessment process can be conceptualized as the initiation of intervention for the child and family.

Apart from providing information about how the child's unique behavioral profile relates to ASD and which services appear appropriate based on such a profile, a meaningful diagnostic assessment should also serve the function of supporting families (Bailey, 2008). The reality of the diagnostic assessment process is that it is often an intense emotional experience that can be quite confusing, frustrating, and frightening for many caregivers. The clinician is not simply focused on establishing a definitive behavioral profile and diagnosis, but is ultimately working toward conveying information about this profile in a manner that promotes optimal understanding, acceptance, and movement toward specific goals. The formal diagnosis of ASD, even when suspected for lengthy intervals of time, contributes to an array of reactions—from relief, to guilt, to loss, to action—in caregivers both in the short- and long-term (Hutton & Caron, 2005). In addition, personal experiences and the increasing variety of accounts of autism in popular media formats often contribute to an array of thoughts and beliefs about the nature of autism (Harrington et al., 2006). The diagnostic assessment process can help address these thoughts and reactions in a manner that helps the family engage proactively in the pursuit of intervention services that available science suggests will benefit the child as well as the family. For example, important components of the diagnostic assessment process include understanding parental beliefs about the causes of their child's ASD and potential attributions of blame and guilt, as well as helping families negotiate the complex landscape of various behavioral, educational, and complementary and alternative treatments. In this regard, the assessment itself may be understood as the initiation of intervention. Specifically, this intervention is provided in the form of helping elucidate and/or reframe the individual strengths and challenges of the child with ASD within larger contexts of what is important to the family to promote optimal developmental trajectories.

Another important aspect of the diagnostic process is the implication a diagnosis holds for obtaining access to desired services. In many instances, a specific ASD diagnosis is required for access to specialized programs, funding, and intervention opportunities (Lord & Richler, 2006). Conversely, the inability to provide a definitive diagnosis because of limitations in our diagnostic methods and understanding at very young ages may prevent families from obtaining certain services. Unfortunately, there is often a gap between the guidelines and laws surrounding interventions, and the availability of community resources and services (Bayley, 2008). As such, families often face significant barriers to accessing interventions. Caregivers are often placed in the extremely difficult role of having to act as expert advocates and resource specialists for their child to secure services that their child needs. Given this situation, the diagnostic assessment represents an entry point for assisting parents in developing effective advocacy and resource procurement skills. Thus, the assessment process not only presents families with overwhelming information about their child's developmental disability, but also conveys the importance of becoming the primary agents for facilitating and implementing service recommendations within complex bureaucracies of existing service systems. Effective diagnostic assessment must balance presentation of information to aid in efficient utilization of available resources in the most time sensitive manner possible (Mash & Hunsley, 2005).

The Assessment Process

Key Points

- Families may have very different experiences, emotions, and expectations that they bring with them to the assessment.
- Incorporating family experiences and input into the assessment from the initial point of entry is critical for establishing a productive working relationship.

Many families seeking a diagnostic evaluation for ASD have already had numerous formal and informal experiences, opinions, and/or evaluations offered by professionals, family, and friends that impact their desire, or lack thereof, for a formal diagnosis of ASD (Goin-Kochel et al., 2006; Mansell & Morris, 2004). Optimally, caregivers have expressed concerns to professionals and individuals within their support networks who have, in turn, been sensitive and supportive in listening to and validating their concerns as well as assisting them in securing a comprehensive diagnostic assessment explicitly for ASD. Even in this ideal circumstance, such support and validation does not eliminate the often intense distress and anxiety that caregivers experience in anticipating an evaluation that might confirm the fears they have about their child. Regrettably, many caregivers do not receive support for their concerns and instead are met with dismissive attitudes by professionals and individuals within family support systems (DeGiacomo & Fombonne, 1998; Goin-Kochel et al., 2006; Liptak et al., 2008). In other circumstances, caregivers may in fact have very limited knowledge or specific concerns about ASD, but have been asked to pursue services by professionals in their care systems. In each of these circumstances, careful attention to the nature and development of the caregivers' concerns—and the reactions of others to these concerns—may promote optimal engagement in the assessment process itself and provide an important springboard to the initiation of treatment.

Whether the caregivers' concerns have been validated, disregarded, or have been minimally present prior to the assessment, it is very important to understand how this mix of experiences and emotions caregivers carry into and through the assessment can impact the primary goal of promoting optimal outcomes for children with ASD. Failure to adequately attend to, discuss, and address such concerns may contribute to potential dismissal, or suboptimal understanding, of the findings and recommendations from the evaluation. This situation may lead to delays in accessing potentially beneficial services, which in turn may impact the child's outcome, disrupt the family system, and increase demands on service systems at later time points. It is therefore extremely important to establish a meaningful working relationship with families from the initial point of contact, and to nurture this relationship throughout the assessment process, the discussion of clinical impressions and recommendations, and the follow-up.

Initial Contact

Key Point

- Conveying appropriate expectations for the assessment process in advance can facilitate the family's comfort and engagement.

The assessment process itself starts with the family's first contact with those affiliated with the clinical assessment system. This contact is not necessarily with the clinician, but more often with nonclinical intake or resource personnel who collect the basic referral information required to determine: *(1)* the appropriateness of a diagnostic evaluation for ASD; and *(2)* the fit between the caregiver's concerns and the resources of the clinical setting. During this process it is critical to balance the need for caregivers to express their concerns and ask questions about the nature of the assessment, with the recognition that they are not usually communicating at this point with the clinicians who will be performing the assessment. This initial contact can be very challenging for intake staff, as caregivers may wish to provide very detailed accounts about their child's history in a manner that may be more specific than necessary at this entry point of the evaluation. Thus, intake staff should make attempts to listen attentively, compassionately, and patiently to caregiver concerns and questions, while also indicating to families which information is actually needed at the time, and what their own limitations are in terms of providing definitive answers to the caregiver's questions.

An important consideration in this initial contact is the emotional state and functioning of the caller. It is a powerful understatement to note that it is quite distressing for caregivers to pursue an evaluation when the question is often explicitly, "Does my child have autism?" Many caregivers are in intense emotional or crisis states when asking this question, and intake personnel should be familiar with strategies for: *(1)* providing reassurance and support to caregivers while gathering the necessary information; and *(2)* offering concrete, pragmatic answers to the most common questions caregivers have about diagnostic evaluations. It can be quite helpful to provide caregivers with specific expectations for the nature of the assessment process, to reduce the uncertainty and distress surrounding this situation (cf., Stone & DiGeronimo, 2006). Specific information may relate to the qualifications of who will perform the assessment, when the assessment will take place, what will happen during the assessment, how long the assessment will last, whether the caregiver(s) can be with the child during the evaluation, whether they should bring along family members and/or support persons, when they will receive the results, and what information they will receive at the end of the evaluation. Family members can also use this information to prepare their children for the evaluation. Specific advance information about the physical nature of the assessment area, including potential difficult situations (e.g., crowded waiting rooms, elevators, parking garages) can avoid unnecessary confusion and facilitate optimal levels of success on the part of the child.

Child and Family Assessment

Key Points

- A good assessment will provide opportunities for the child to demonstrate skills and strengths as well as experience success.
- Families should be active participants in the assessment process.

Optimally, caregivers arrive for comprehensive assessment already having a good understanding of what will happen on that day as well as who will be present during the assessment and why. Even in this circumstance, caregivers are often uncertain as to how they should act and why certain activities are occurring through the course of the assessment day. It is important to make caregivers as comfortable as possible by detailing the main focus of the evaluation, the structure of the day, each assessment tool and its purpose, as well as introducing the members of the assessment team and encouraging caregivers to seek clarification and alert team members to their own or their child's needs whenever they feel necessary.

Many caregivers are concerned about how their child will behave in the assessment environment. For example, they may be worried that their child's behavior will be different than it is in more familiar settings, or that the assessment results may either over- or underestimate the child's true level of skills. Likewise, caregivers may be concerned or embarrassed if the child exhibits challenging behaviors and they may be uncertain about what role they should play in these situations. It is often helpful to let caregivers know that the assessment will be geared toward obtaining optimal performance from the child. Further, it can be beneficial to let caregivers know that all observed behavior will be matched with information from the caregivers themselves about whether these observations are consistent across circumstances that the caretaker observes. Finally, when challenging behaviors manifest themselves, it is helpful to reassure caregivers that the assessment team is comfortable with and adept at addressing these behaviors, and, moreover, that the opportunity to observe such behaviors provides valuable information to the assessment team.

Inviting caregivers to join their children in the assessment room to observe, comment on, and (when appropriate) participate in the assessment process itself can be helpful for many reasons. Their presence often provides the child with a sense of familiarity and comfort, and may also serve a similar function for caregivers themselves. Caregiver participation can offer excellent opportunities to facilitate meaningful discussion about behaviors that both parties have observed. These shared observations provide a framework for discussing behaviors and understanding their significance and impact on family interactions. Some caregivers may be overeager to assist their child in completing activities during the assessment process, but simple reminders about the nature of their participation usually limits any substantial interference in the process (Bailey, 2008). In other circumstances, observations can be quite distressful when caregivers perceive that their child is not passing items or is behaving in a manner that other children might not. In these situations it is important that the clinician provide reassurance to the caregiver and explanations about what they are doing and why, as well as to ensure that the child is given opportunities to experience success and demonstrate positive skills within the context of the assessment. This approach conveys to caregivers that the clinician is not only looking for areas of deficit, but also interested in identifying areas of strength and competence.

Maintaining transparency in the diagnostic assessment process whenever possible can help families understand the assessment from a functional perspective, alleviate any unnecessary uncertainties, and establish a goal-driven alliance between caregivers and clinicians from the outset. When families are included as active participants in the assessment, when their expertise in knowing their children better than anyone else is labeled as critical and important, and when the functions of assessment are clearly explicated, many caregivers will be primed for hearing and accepting information that can be quite difficult to receive. First and foremost, this transparency comes in the form of talking to families about ASD itself. When the referral question relates to the diagnosis of ASD, caregivers should be informed that specific assessment procedures geared toward evaluating the presence or absence of ASD will be conducted. This procedure invites caregivers to start talking about their own concerns and/or preconceptions from the outset, helps alleviate anxiety that could potentially grow over the course of the assessment, and prepares parents for later discussion about ASD diagnosis. Sometimes it is difficult for families themselves to mention the word "autism" as an explicit concern, even when they have sought a referral to an autism-specialized clinic. When this is the case, clinicians should attempt to facilitate the family's discussion of autism at the outset of the assessment process and discuss the term themselves with comfort.

When discussing explicit concerns about autism and the diagnostic process, it can be helpful to provide families with a framework of how and why a diagnosis is established. In the absence of a specific biological or genetic marker for the majority of cases of autism (*See Chapter 40 for details on clinical genetic assessment and Chapter 74 for a description of best practices in medical assessment*), the diagnosis essentially involves creating a behavioral profile of the child's skills and vulnerabilities in the areas of social interaction, communication and language, and repetitive interests and activities. In addition, strengths and challenges in areas not specific to the diagnosis of autism, such as cognitive, motor, and adaptive behavior skills are evaluated to provide a more comprehensive view of the child and help identify areas and target goals for intervention. In circumstances where a specific genetic or biological etiology of ASD is indicated, assessment aims at indexing these same skill areas and the variability related to core ASD symptoms that exist within specific subgroups of children.

Ideally, families should be informed that the assessment will be based on information that they provide as well as behaviors that are observed directly. Explaining that the goal of the assessment is to spend enough time with the child and family to gather an impression of the child's strengths and weaknesses that fits with the family's own experiences can reassure parents about the nature of the process and help create a powerful working alliance. Likewise, describing the often complex names and terms used to refer to specialized clinical tools and procedures can further demystify the assessment process. For example, explaining that the Autism Diagnostic Observation Schedule is a gold standard measure in the assessment of ASD and that it involves talking to and playing with the child so that the clinician can personally experience the child's social and communication skills, can be quite effective in helping families understand a procedure that may otherwise not be transparent. Further, informing families that the behavioral profile of ASD is not characterized merely by the presence or absence of specific behaviors, but also by inconsistencies in displaying developmentally appropriate behaviors across settings, can also be important in facilitating eventual understanding of the diagnostic process. Many families have ideas and stereotypes of individuals with ASD from popular media and personal circumstance that are often focused on the exceptional both in terms of areas of deficit and strength. Finally, conveying information that the ultimate goal of the diagnostic assessment is to provide the family with assistance in ensuring that their child's needs are being met appropriately—regardless of whether a diagnosis is confirmed or disconfirmed—can help those families who may be struggling with the concept of "labeling" and its potential negative effects over time.

Diagnostic Feedback

Key Points

- Disclosure of ASD diagnosis is often an intense emotional experience for families and addressing the varied reactions of caregivers is an important element of successful disclosure.
- Successful feedback must balance the provision of caregiver support with the need to encourage action toward appropriate interventions for the child.

In many circumstances, immediate feedback subsequent to the assessment itself is thought to be ideal. Certainly long delays—and the resulting uncertainty and discomfort associated with waiting—may be extremely difficult to tolerate, and should be minimized whenever possible. However, there may be a number of circumstances under which it might be appropriate to delay feedback. For example, some families may be exhausted from the evaluation day, some may prefer to have other family or supportive individuals with them, and still others may prefer to receive feedback when their child is not with them. It is important to take into account the fact that disclosure of ASD is an event that can have a profound emotional impact for families as well as profound implications for clinical outcomes. Many families may be overwhelmed by disclosure of ASD diagnosis and may benefit from more comprehensive feedback about recommendations and interventions at a later date. Other families may wish to have all the information they can possibly have delivered immediately, so they can move forward with pursuing interventions. It may be hard for families and clinicians alike to know this preference at the outset of the appointment. However, families should be asked explicitly about their preferences, and clinicians should take these preferences into account and be as flexible as possible in offering a follow-up visit to discuss the evaluation results.

Unfortunately, very little empirical work has been conducted regarding effective disclosure of diagnoses of ASD. The existing literature has linked parent satisfaction with ASD diagnosis to factors that are primarily unrelated to the disclosure itself. Specifically, factors such as earlier age at diagnosis, fewer referrals prior to diagnosis, and prior acceptance of concerns by other professionals have been associated with increased satisfaction of disclosure of ASD (Brogan & Knussen, 2003; Mansell & Morris, 2004). A larger body of literature exists regarding the disclosure of diagnostic information about other developmental and physical disabilities (Hasnat & Graves, 1999), but there remain questions as to the applicability of this literature to ASD-specific samples. Notably, a diagnosis of ASD is often delivered later than diagnoses of other physical and developmental disabilities, and there are no specific biological or medical markers of ASD to aid in the diagnosis. With this caveat in place, factors in the disability literature attributed to the successful disclosure of a diagnosis include: interpersonal style, empathetic support and sensitivity, discussion of the whole child, up-to-date knowledge, provision of written material, and opportunities to ask questions (Brogan & Knussen, 2003).

Successful disclosure in many ways should be an end point of an assessment process that has been building from the first point of contact. If families have been prepared for the assessment day itself, the assessment process has been transparent and clearly explained, and families have been involved throughout, then disclosure of a diagnosis can involve revisiting the experiences and observations of the day, reaffirming that the clinician's impression fits with the caregivers' experience of their own child, and placing these impressions within or outside the bounds of a formal ASD diagnosis. Even under ideal circumstances, it is still critical to ask parents about their specific reactions to the diagnosis and their concerns about how and why the diagnosis was made, prior to embarking on a discussion of specific recommendations and resources.

For many parents the emotional reaction of the disclosure necessitates significant pause and/or clinical reassurance. Many parents benefit from the support and validation of their assessment team when clinicians acknowledge the difficulty of considering that their child might have ASD, reinforce the parents' willingness to pursue a diagnostic evaluation, and recognize the impact that disclosure of ASD diagnosis can have on parents. Messages that "normalize" the parents' reactions to this experience, and acknowledge that they have asked perhaps one of the scariest questions possible for the ultimate benefit of their child, should be conveyed. In addition, it is important to convey information to indicate that the diagnosis has not changed their child in any way, but will enable them to access resources that would otherwise have been unavailable. Finally, discussion centering around the numerous areas of child and family strength, in addition to vulnerabilities related to ASD, can assist many families in receiving subsequent information about recommendations and interventions for their children.

Along with providing reassurance and support, effective feedback will also address the specific limitations and vulnerabilities of the child in a manner that promotes involvement with clinically indicated intervention services. Many families will seek reassurance that their child's level of functioning will not necessarily impact or limit them from moving forward. Specifically, many families hold attributions that their child with ASD is "high-functioning," when clinical indicators suggest that there may be significant areas of delay. Although it is important to deliver feedback about strengths and to reassure families experiencing acute distress, ultimately it is important to note the areas of impairment that warrant attention and action in order to help move families toward appropriate resources. Questions regarding level of functioning, including ideas of "recovery" and overcoming challenges, are often driven by projections about the child's future, and the fundamental parental hope for the most positive outcome possible for their child. As such, these questions are ultimately some of the most important for parents, but are very difficult for clinicians to answer for individual children. The ability to predict long-term outcomes for very young children with ASD is quite limited (Chawarska et al., 2007; Lord, Risi, et al., 2006; Stone & Turner, 2007) and this is particularly true for children under 2 years of age. Providing families with quality information about the best group-level predictors and the realistic limitations surrounding diagnostic stability can be quite helpful for families of young children. Currently, these predictors for young children include language capacity, nonverbal abilities, and response to interventions. In addition to child characteristics and intervention factors, it may be that parental and familial factors such as hope, coping strategies, and specific reactions to diagnosis may be strong predictors of outcomes as well, particularly when coupled with clinically informed action. This area is certainly one that warrants significant additional attention, both in terms of research and clinical practice.

Resources and Recommendations

Key Points:

- Accessing appropriate interventions can be challenging for many families and likely requires substantial clinical guidance and follow-up.
- Specific intervention recommendations should be framed within the broader context of best practices for ASD as well as within the community-specific context of what is available.

In addition to seeking answers about long-term implications of ASD diagnosis for their child's development, parents are often looking for more immediate guidance and explicit instruction in garnering help for their child. Unfortunately, even when the results of the diagnostic assessment are quite clear-cut and delivered with certainty, concrete information about how caregivers can best help their child is often lacking. Not only are there limits in terms of the empirical understanding of interventions, but differences in availability of community services and family resources unfortunately impact the quality, intensity, and type of services that many children with ASD will receive. In this context, it falls upon the clinician to deliver realistic information about what the field knows and does not know about effective intervention approaches, which interventions are available through community service systems and which require financial resources, and how parents can augment the impact of interventions via their own expertise and motivation to help their children.

It is beyond the scope of the current chapter to provide an explicit review of specific intervention recommendations for children with ASD; rather, the reader is referred to existing practice parameters (e.g., Myers & Johnson, 2007; National Research Council (NRC), 2001; *See also Chapters 12 and 13 that review interventions for preschool age and infant-toddler age children*). However, several points about conveying such information in the context of the diagnostic assessment process warrant attention. First, it is important to consider that the complex nature of negotiating service systems immediately following ASD diagnosis is overwhelming for most families, even families of substantial means and with copious support. As such, provision of follow-up services aimed explicitly at helping families of young children with ASD secure appropriate intervention appears crucial. When service coordination is lacking in the community, clinicians who schedule follow-up meetings and review intervention programming over time will likely be better able to help families access appropriate services.

It is also extremely important that families be given concrete information about resources, including written materials whenever possible. In addition to supplying timely and understandable evaluation reports, families can often benefit from receiving immediate recommendations or action checklists, in which critical next steps are laid out specifically and concretely. Written materials about ASD and related interventions that are targeted explicitly for parents can be quite helpful for reinforcing action toward clinically indicated services. In the current climate of ASD awareness, many parents have already done copious internet and/or other informal research prior to pursuing a diagnostic evaluation. Although beneficial and empirically supported information is abundant, it is unfortunate that a multitude of information of a much lower quality is widely available as well. Failing to provide families with information or resources for accessing or evaluating this information will leave them in the difficult position of trying to sort out this complex information to make decisions about what may or may not be best for their child. Offering parents a core set of information and encouraging families to seek additional information as needed from other sources can reinforce a model of persistent engagement balanced with clinical support.

In providing feedback about interventions, it must be recognized that in addition to the behavioral and educational interventions recommended in current practice parameters (Myers & Johnson, 2007; NRC, 2001), most parents have questions about complementary and alternative medical (CAM) treatments as well. At present, a majority of children with ASD participate in CAM treatments, with the number of different treatments and their rate of use growing over time (Harrington et al., 2003; Wong & Smith, 2006). Caregivers are often eager to try any potential treatment in search of positive outcomes for their children, and CAM treatments may be more salient, attractive, and alluring than educational and behavioral interventions that actually have more scientific backing (Smith & Wick, 2008). As more children with ASD become involved with CAM treatments, it is important for clinicians to be familiar with these interventions and address them within the context of the assessment. If clinicians hope to assist families more fully in making autonomous, empirically informed decisions about treatments, then they must address questions about CAM treatments in a manner that allows families to feel comfortable reapproaching this issue on an ongoing basis. Materials that provide information in lay terms about the complexity of evaluating treatment effectiveness are sorely needed.

Key Point:

- Addressing the medical complexity of children with ASD is imperative and warrants multidisciplinary collaboration and follow-up.

Finally, young children with ASD are often medically complex and have a variety of needs that go beyond the scope of behaviorally based evaluations for ASD. Diagnostic evaluations should be multidisciplinary in nature, and should include assessment of associated medical conditions (e.g., seizures) and etiologies (e.g., Fragile X Syndrome). Ideally, a pediatrician, neurologist, or psychiatrist should participate in the evaluation to address these medical issues. Although team-based assessments are the ideal, they are not common, and pragmatic challenges related to reimbursement have shifted care systems away from multidisciplinary team models. As such, when evaluations are primarily conducted by a behavioral provider, it is of extreme importance that core medical assessment and consultation be recommended and coordinated as part of that child's ultimate clinical care. In addition, when indicated, referrals should be made to specialists in the areas in which children with autism often have medically related problems (e.g., pediatric sleep specialist, pediatric gastroenterologist, specialist in genetic and metabolic conditions). It is becoming a standard of care to address and discuss issues of genetic vulnerability with families affected by ASD for their own family planning purposes, for the medical care and surveillance of their children, as well as to alleviate parental guilt and/or false attributions about etiology (Johnson & Myers, 2007; Myers & Johnson, 2007). The Autism Treatment Network, a program funded by Autism Speaks, was initiated with the specific goal of developing standards of care for identification, evaluation, and treatment of common medical conditions in children with ASD, such as sleep disorders, seizures, gastrointestinal disorders, and genetic/metabolic disorders. The Autism Treatment Network sites have medical specialists and subspecialists who are experienced in working with children with ASD, and thus represent excellent resources for comprehensive medical care.

Diagnostic Assessment for Children under 2 Years of Age

Key Point:

- Although some children with ASD can be diagnosed under age 2 years, there remain significant questions concerning the reliability and stability of such an early diagnosis using currently available assessment methodologies.

As numerous forces push for accurate ASD diagnoses to be made at younger and younger ages, it is important for those conducting ASD assessments to be aware of the potential limitations that exist regarding our current understanding of the diagnosis in children under 2 years of age. A growing body of work suggests that diagnoses of autism (i.e., autistic disorder) delivered by an expert clinician employing ASD-specific parent report and clinical observation assessment tools at age 24 months are generally reliable and stable up to school age in predicting continued ASD diagnostic classification (Charman et al., 2005; Eaves & Ho, 2004; Lord, Risi, et al., 2006; Stone et al., 1999). However, there appear to be limits to diagnostic stability even at this age. Specifically, there is evidence suggesting that ASD diagnoses fail to achieve optimal stability until 30 months of age (Turner & Stone, 2007) and there is considerable work suggesting that broader ASD classifications (i.e., Pervasive Developmental Disorder – Not Otherwise Specified (PDD-NOS)) are much less stable in young children (Lord et al., 2006; Turner & Stone, 2007). Far less research has been conducted to date examining ASD diagnoses in children under 2 years of age. Consequently, knowledge of the limits of diagnostic classifications is extremely important to understanding optimal assessment practices for ASD in children in this age range.

Accuracy in clinical diagnosis of ASD for children under 2 years of age is, in part, impeded by limitations in our knowledge about specific behavioral manifestations of ASD itself at this time in development. Retrospective studies (see Palomo et al., 2006), prospective studies utilizing at-risk siblings of children with ASD (see Zwaigenbaum et al., 2007 for overview), as well as prospective studies of children failing development screens (Wetherby et al., 2007), have started to identify specific areas of delay that may be characteristic of ASD in the first years of life. This literature suggests that early behavioral markers predictive of a later ASD diagnosis may be present in *some* children as early as the first or second year of life (Bryson et al., 2007; Gamliel et al., 2007; Landa & Garrett-Mayer, 2006; Zwaigenbaum et al., 2005). However, there remain limitations in our certainty resulting from: *(1)* substantial individual variability related to these same markers and subsequent diagnostic outcome, as well as *(2)* mounting evidence for the presence of multiple distinctive developmental trajectories of ASD—characterized by early regressions, decrements, plateaus, slowings, and/or significant improvements—with some children more readily identifiable at specific time points than others (Bryson et al., 2007; Landa et al., 2007). Moreover, there is not yet sufficient evidence that the presence of early social communication vulnerabilities predicts specific ASD-related impairments at all later time points, irrespective of effects of maturation and intervention (Turner & Stone, 2007). Thus, there is sufficient variability in the nature, onset, intensity, and course of these early behavioral markers in young children that the implications for providing a definitive ASD diagnosis or recommending autism-specialized interventions for children under 2 years of age are unclear.

Available tools for detecting symptoms of ASD in children under 2 years old also have serious limitations. Currently, the "gold standard" clinical assessment tools utilized for diagnostic classification are less robust psychometrically for children with a mental age below 24 months, and decline in utility as mental age decreases (Chawarska et al., 2007; Lord, Risi, et al., 2006). Specifically, there are concerns that the Autism Diagnostic Observation Schedule (ADOS) (Lord et al., 2000) and the Autism Diagnostic Interview–Revised (ADI-R) (Rutter et al., 2003)—the leading diagnostic tools with well-established psychometric properties for school-aged children—have questionable diagnostic validity in children under 2 years of age. These tools exhibit tendencies to overclassify nonverbal children and children with mental retardation and to underidentify more verbal children and children without significant repetitive behaviors in their profiles at younger ages (Chawarska et al., 2007; Lord et al., 2006). New algorithms and a toddler module for the ADOS (i.e., ADOS–Toddler Version), may likely improve the utility of this instrument with children below 24 months of age (Gotham et al., 2007), but currently these tools are not widely available, nor is there corresponding empirical work examining the diagnostic validity of these instruments. In addition to instrumentation, there is also a significant discrepancy between the diagnostic classification symptoms as currently described in Diagnostic and Statistical Manual of Mental Disorders (DSM-IV) and markers of ASD in young children (Zwaigenbaum et al., 2007). The DSM-IV symptoms of ASD are most often indicative of ASD symptoms seen in preschool, school-age, and adolescent populations, and their specific extension and application to symptoms of ASD in infancy and toddlerhood is unclear.

Despite these limits, emerging work suggests that ASD can be diagnosed in some children under 2 years old. Specifically, research performed exclusively within the context of high-risk infant sibling samples has, in fact, documented subgroups of children meeting criteria for autistic disorder at 12 to 25 months of age who have retained diagnosis up to a year later (Chawarska et al., 2007; Landa et al., 2007). Again, there appears to be less stability when initial clinical diagnoses are of the broader ASD spectrum, explicitly PDD-NOS (Charwarska et al., 2007; Gamliel et al., 2007). This research offers hope that meaningful, stable ASD diagnosis can be made during the second year of life, at least for certain small groups of children by leading experts in the field of ASD research. However, there remain numerous questions about how such early diagnoses relate to longer-term outcomes and how sensitive early measurements and diagnosis are for larger populations of young children. Specifically, questions remain about whether and how the diagnosis can be made with similar levels of stability, meaning, and impact within broader community settings. This issue is particularly pertinent as current professional guidelines and popular attention push clinicians to screen for and presumably diagnose ASD outside the realm of prospective research studies of high-risk populations and within the context of traditional community pediatric settings.

Key Point:

- The diagnosis of ASD in children under 2 years old should be accompanied by discussion of the limits of our knowledge in terms of diagnostic stability and the need for continued monitoring and follow-up.

In the absence of consensus guidelines of how to interpret DSM-IV criteria for children in this age group, how to utilize early behavioral markers of ASD, as well as how (or whether) to extend available ASD assessment tools to this population, clinicians are left in the challenging position of testing the limits of appropriate classification and diagnosis. At the same time, the existing early intervention and corresponding public health literature make strong arguments that diagnostic classifications, if tied to effective ASD-specific interventions, should be made. Because of the unique challenges of identifying children with ASD under 2 years old, the diagnostic process should be led by a clinician not only experienced with infants and toddlers, but also with symptoms of ASD in infants and toddlers. Ideally, ASD diagnosis in children under 2 years of age should be based on the clinical best judgment of an experienced multidisciplinary team, carefully taking into account a vast array of biopsychosocial information about the child's developmental history and current functioning. The scope of such assessments has been detailed previously (see AAN, 1999; Bishop et al., 2008; Johnson & Myers, 2007; Lord & Richler, 2006) and includes: a medical assessment and physical exam, including evaluation of normal hearing; thorough assessment of developmental level (i.e., evaluation of cognitive, speech/language, communication, and adaptive functioning); direct assessment of spontaneous social communication, play skills, and atypical behaviors matched with extensive clinical interviewing about these same skill domains.

Unfortunately, the current state of our science is that even when such comprehensive methods are undertaken, it may not necessarily be clear that the observed and reported behavioral markers are indicative of the presence or absence of ASD. Even for expert clinicians, it is much more difficult to distinguish ASD from other developmental disorders, including broader spectrum difficulties related to social and communication delays, in children under age 2 years. This fact has been particularly evident within high-risk sibling samples, where subtle and clear differences in social and communication development are clearly present in many children at early ages, but the link between these difficulties and later ASD occurs in a minority of cases (Gamliel et al., 2007; Merin et al., 2007; Presmanes et al., 2007; Stone et al., 2007; Zwaigenbaum et al., 2007). In addition, very young children may present with a range of additional medical and regulatory concerns whose impact on development may be challenging to tease apart in relation to social and communication vulnerabilities. When social-communication impairments are present in very young children, but clinical best estimate diagnostic certainty of ASD is lacking, the constructs of "at risk" and "prevention" may prove useful in acknowledging this developmental uncertainty, while at the same time conveying the needs for immediate intervention services related to core areas of deficit, and for systematic follow-up.

This uncertainty concerning the development of ASD in very young children exists within a context in which parents, clinicians, and service systems want (or need) definitive classifications and answers in order to access specialized services. As such, clinicians are not only confronted with the specific challenge of how to best provide information about how the child's unique behavioral profile relates to the ASD, but also how best to support families in promoting their child's optimal developmental outcome. Clinical best practices dictate that maintaining transparency in the diagnostic assessment process with families is often the ideal. For children under age 2 years, this process includes explicit discussion of the real predictive limits of our science, assessment tools, and diagnostic classification process itself. This presentation of assessment and diagnostic uncertainty can be a particularly challenging process if parents and service systems are expecting clear, authoritative diagnoses on the basis of a one-point-in-time assessment. However, specific value can come from highlighting the limitations of diagnostic assessment within the context of providing reassurance that the assessment process will ultimately result in a richer understanding of the child's behavioral profile of strengths and challenges that can guide specific interventions regardless of whether a definitive diagnosis is issued. Even when primed for and presented with such reassurance during the assessment, it can ultimately be challenging to approach diagnostic ambiguity for families. In assigning concerns of ASD risk, families will likely experience confusion and differing interpretation of whether such assignment warrants specific action or simply increased surveillance and monitoring. As such, it becomes critical for clinicians working in this context to explicitly highlight the warranted interventions to be pursued in the short-term as well as to provide a specific rationale and methods for providing diagnostic clarity as children develop.

Conclusions

All existing evidence powerfully suggests that early diagnoses of ASD and appropriate intervention play a significant role in improving outcomes for children and families. Meaningful diagnostic assessment not only attempts to index ASD-specific concerns in the context of the developmental profile, but also recognizes the critical importance of supporting families to promote engagement in clinically indicated interventions. Ideally, diagnostic assessment also focuses on the complex medical profiles and needs of children with ASD and is multidisciplinary in nature. Currently, limited access to team-based assessments, and limitations of our diagnostic tools themselves for children at very young ages, present potent barriers to early diagnosis and intervention.

Challenges and Future Directions

- The reliance on observable behavioral assessment profiles limits our ability to identify core ASD vulnerabilities at the youngest ages.
- Integrative multidisciplinary tools and procedures may provide an improved assessment methodology for early diagnosis.
- As the limits of ASD diagnosis are pushed younger and younger, it is critical to understand the implications for families and for service systems related to diagnosis and intervention.
- An empirical understanding of the assessment process itself (e.g., how a diagnosis is delivered, family perceptions/attributions) may be powerful in advancing outcomes for individuals with ASD and their families.

The earlier we are able to identify the core vulnerabilities associated with the development of ASD, the closer we will come to understanding the neuroscience, genetics, and etiology of the disorder as well as implementing interventions that promote optimal developmental outcomes for children and their families. Looking ahead, diagnostic assessment may involve the identification of specific genetic and medical etiologies that have direct implications for specific interventions. In absence of such markers at present, provision of exceptional clinical care must balance pressures for definitive diagnoses of ASD at earlier and earlier ages with acknowledgement of the empirical limitations of diagnoses for very young children.

In pushing the limits of ASD diagnosis to include assessments conducted within the first 2 years of life, the viability of the concept of ASD risk may also be important to consider within the realm of community clinical practice. Specifically, regardless of geography and availability of high-quality diagnostic assessment services, the wait for such services is often quite extensive. It is not uncommon for parents of young children to be told that there is a 6-month wait list for services (Zwaigenbaum & Stone, 2006). Waits for evaluations conducted by subspecialists for infants and toddlers would likely prove even longer. As such, the development of assessment tools and pragmatic methods for promoting identification of risk for ASD hold promise. For example, interactive screening tools such as the Screening Tool for Autism in Two-Year-Olds (STAT) (Stone et al., 2000, 2004, 2008) may provide information about risk status as well as immediate intervention goals (Zwaigenbaum & Stone, 2006). The ability to identify risk status and initiate appropriate intervention (or prevention) services has advantages for families faced with long waits for diagnostic evaluations, as well as for clinicians faced with providing definitive diagnoses at a time when it is premature to expect clear-cut meaningful classifications.

Finally, in searching to refine the diagnostic assessment process for young children, researchers must look not only at the earliest social and communicative behavior of ASD in marking atypical development from typical development, but to potential new collaborative methodologies for obtaining diagnoses that incorporate additional sources of information. The inclusion of psychophysiological, functional neuroimaging, and medical and genetic data with early behavioral markers may provide ways for advancing the assessment of ASD in young children. As we wait for such research to add value to our diagnostic process, great care should be taken to utilize our current knowledge to more efficiently identify and serve larger groups of children at risk for ASD as soon as possible. In this regard, benefits will likely come not only from pragmatic revision of assessment, eligibility, and service models for at-risk children, but also from more fully exploring the roles of how diagnostic assessment services can optimally serve families.

SUGGESTED READINGS

Bailey, K. (2008). Supporting families. In K. Chawarska, A. Klin, & F. R. Volkmar (Eds.), *Autism spectrum disorders in infants and toddlers: Diagnosis, assessment, and treatment* (pp. 300–326). New York: Guilford.

Johnson, C. P., & Myers, S. M., (2007). Identification and evaluation of children with autism spectrum disorders. *Pediatrics, 120*, 1183–1215.

Zwaigenbaum, L., & Stone, W. L. (2006). Early screening for autism spectrum disorder in clinical practice settings. In T. Charman & W. Stone (Eds.). *Social and communication development in autism spectrum disorders* (pp. 88–113). New York: Guilford.

REFERENCES

Centers for Disease Control and Prevention (CDC) (2009). Prevalence of Autism Spectrum Disorders-ADDM Network, United States, 2006. *MMWR Weekly Report, 58*, 1–20.

Bailey, K. (2008). Supporting families. In K. Chawarska, A. Klin, & F. R. Volkmar (Eds.), *Autism spectrum disorders in infants and toddlers: Diagnosis, assessment, and treatment* (pp. 300–326). New York: Guilford.

Bishop, S. L., Luyster, R., Richler, J., & Lord, C. (2008). Diagnostic assessment. In K. Chawarska, A. Klin, & F. R. Volkmar (Eds.), *Autism spectrum disorders in infants and toddlers: Diagnosis, assessment, and treatment* (pp. 23–49). New York: Guilford.

Brogan, C. A., & Knussen, C. (2003). The disclosure of a diagnosis of an autistic spectrum disorder: Determinants of satisfaction in a sample of Scottish parents, *Autism, 7*, 31–46.

Bryson, S. E., Zwaigenbaum, L., Brian, J., Roberts, W., Szatmari, P., Rombough, V, et al. (2007). A prospective case series of high-risk infants who developed autism. *Journal of Autism and Developmental Disorders, 37*, 12–24.

Chakrabarti, S., & Fombonne, E., (2001). Pervasive developmental disorders in preschool children. *Journal of the American Medical Association, 285*, 3093–3099.

Chakrabati, S., & Fombonne, E. (2005). Pervasive developmental disorders in preschool children: Confirmation of high prevalence. *American Journal of Psychiatry, 162*, 1133–1141.

Charman, T., Taylor, E., Drew, A., Cockerill, H., Brown, J. A., & Baird, G. (2005). Outcome at 7 years of children diagnosed with autism at age 2: Predictive validity of assessments conducted at 2 and 3 years of age and pattern of symptom change over time. *Journal of Child Psychology and Psychiatry, 46*, 500–513.

Chawarska, K., Klin, A., Paul, R., & Volkmar, F. R. (2007). Autism spectrum disorder in the second year: Stability and change in syndrome expression. *Journal of Child Psychology and Psychiatry, 48*, 128–138.

Cohen, H., Amerine-Dickens, M. S., & Smith, T. (2006). Early intensive behavioral treatment: Replication of the UCLA model in a community setting. *Journal of Developmental and Behavioral Pediatrics, 27*, 145–155.

Coonrod, E. E., & Stone, W. L. (2004). Early concerns of parents of children with autistic and nonautistic disorders. *Infants and Young Children, 17*, 258–268.

Croen, Lisa A., Grether, J. K., & Selvin, S. (2002). Descriptive epidemiology of autism in a California population: Who is at risk? *Journal of Autism and Developmental Disorders, 32*, 217–224.

Dawson, G., & Osterling, J. (1997). Early intervention in autism: Effectiveness and common elements of current approaches. In M. J. Guralnick (Ed.), *The effectiveness of early intervention: Second generation research* (pp. 307–326). Baltimore, MD: Brookes.

DeGiacomo, A., & Fombonne, E. (1998). Parental recognition of developmental abnormalities in autism. *European Child & Adolescent Psychiatry, 7*, 1998.

Eaves, L. C., & Ho, H. H. (2004). The very early identification of autism: Outcome to age 4 ½ to 5. *Journal of Autism and Developmental Disorders, 34*, 367–378.

Filipek, P. A., Accardo, P. J., Baranek, G. T., Ashwal, S., Cook, E. H., Dawson, G., et al., (2000). Practice parameter: Screening and diagnosis of autism: A report of the Quality Standards Subcommittee of the American Academy of Neurology and the Child Neurology Society. *Neurology, 55*, 468–479.

Gamliel, I., Yirmiya, N., & Sigman, M. (2007). The development of young siblings of children with autism from 4 to 54 months. *Journal of Autism and Developmental Disorders, 37*, 171–183.

Goin-Kochel, R. P., Mackintosh, V. H., & Myers, B. J. (2006). How many doctors does it take to make an autism spectrum diagnosis? *Autism, 10*, 439–451.

Gotham, K., Risi, S., Pickles, A., & Lord, C. (2007). The Autism diagnostic observation schedule: Revised algorithms for improved diagnostic validity. *Journal of Autism and Developmental Disorders, 37*, 613–627.

Harris, S. L., & Handleman, J. S. (2000). Age and IQ at intake as predictors of placement for young children with autism: A four-to six-year follow-up. *Journal of Autism and Developmental Disorders, 30*, 137–142.

Harrington, J. W., Rosen, L., Garnecho, A., & Patrick, P. A. (2006). Parental perceptions and use of CAM practices for children with autistic spectrum disorders in private practice. *Journal of Developmental and Behavioral Pediatrics, 27*, 156–161.

Hasnat, M. J., & Graves, P. (1999). Disclosure of developmental disability: A study of parent satisfaction and the determinants of satisfaction. *Journal of Paediatrics and Child Health, 36*, 32–35.

Howlin, P., Goode, S., Hutton, J., & Rutter, M. (2004). Adult outcome for children with autism. *Journal of Child Psychology and Psychiatry, 45*, 212–229.

Hutton, A. M., & Caron, S. L. (2005). Experiences of families of children with autism in rural New England. *Focus on Autism and Other Developmental Disabilities, 20*(3), 180–189.

Jacobson, J. W., & Mulick, J. A. (2000). System and cost research issues in treatments for people with autistic disorders *Journal of Autism and Developmental Disorders, 30*, 585–593.

Järbrink, K., & Knapp, M. (2001). The economic impact of autism in Britain. *Autism, 5*, 7–22.

Johnson, C. P., & Myers, S. M., (2007). Identification and evaluation of children with autism spectrum disorders. *Pediatrics, 120*, 1183–1215.

Landa, R. J., & Garrett-Mayer, E. (2006). Development in infants with autism spectrum disorders: A prospective study. *Journal of Child Psychology and Psychiatry, 47*, 629–638.

Landa, R. J., Holman, K. C., & Garrett-Mayer, E. (2007). Social and communication development in toddlers with early and later diagnosis of autism spectrum disorders. *Archives of General Psychiatry, 64*, 853–864.

Levy, S. E., & Hyman, S. L. (2003). Use of complementary and alternative treatments for children with autistic spectrum disorders is increasing. *Pediatric Annals, 32*, 685–691.

Liptak, G. S., Benzoni, L. B., Mruzek, D. W., Nolan, K. W., Thingvoll, M. A., Wade, C. M., et al. (2008). Disparities in diagnosis and access to health services for children with autism: Data from the National Survey of Children's Health. *Journal of Developmental and Behavioral Pediatrics, 29*, 1–9.

Liptak, G. S., Benzoni, L. B., Mruzek, D. W., Nolan, K. W., Thingvoll, M. A., & Wade, C. M. (2008). Disparities in diagnosis and access to health services for children with autism: Data from the National Survey of Children's Health. *Journal of Developmental and Behavioral Pediatrics, 29*, 152–160.

Lord, C., Rutter, M., DiLavore, P. C., & Risi, S. (1999). *Autism diagnostic observation schedule.* Los Angeles, CA: Western Psychological Services.

Lord, C., & Richler, J. (2006). Early diagnosis of autism spectrum disorders. In T. Charman & W. Stone (Eds). *Social and communication development in autism spectrum disorders* (pp. 35–62). New York: Guilford.

Lord, C. Risi, S., DiLavore, P., Shulman, C., Thurm, A., & Pickles, A. (2006). Autism from 2 to 9 years of age. *Archives of General Psychiatry, 63*, 694–701.

Mandell, D., Listerud, J., Levy, S., & Pinto-Martin, J. (2002). Race differences in the age at diagnosis among Medicaid-eligible children with autism. *Journal of the American Academy of Child and Adolescent Psychiatry, 41*(12), 1447–1453.

Mansell, W., & Morris, K. (2004). A survey of parents' reactions to the diagnosis of an autistic spectrum disorder by a local service. *Autism, 8*, 387–407.

Mash, E. J., & Hunsley, J. (2005). Evidence-based assessment of child and adolescent disorders: Issues and challenges. *Journal of Clinical Child and Adolescent Psychology, 34*, 362–379.

Merin, N., Young, G. S., Ozonoff, S., & Rogers, S. (2006) .Visual Fixation patterns during reciprocal social interaction distinguish a subgroup of 6-month-old infants at risk for autism from comparison infants. *Journal of Autism and Developmental Disorders, 37*, 108–121.

Myers, S. M., & Johnson, C. P. (2007). Management of children with autism spectrum disorders. *Pediatrics, 10*, 1162–1182.

National Research Council (NRC) (2001). *Educating children with autism.* Washington, DC: National Academy Press.

Palomo, R., Belinchón, M., & Ozonoff, S. (2006). Autism and family home movies: A comprehensive review. *Journal of Developmental and Behavioral Pediatrics, 27*, 59–68.

Presmanes, A. G., Wladen, T. A., Stone, W. L., & Yoder, P. J. (2007). Effects of different attentional cues on responding to joint attention in younger siblings of children with autism spectrum disorders. *Journal of Autism and Developmental Disorders, 37*, 133–144.

Remington, B., Hastings, R. P., Kovshoff, H., degli Espinosa, F., Jahr, E., Brown, T., et al. (2007). Early intensive behavioral intervention: Outcomes for children with autism and their parents after two years. *American Journal of Mental Retardation, 112*, 418–438.

Rogers, S. (1996). Brief report: Early intervention in autism. *Journal of Autism and Developmental Disorders, 26*, 243–246.

Rogers, S. J. (1998). Empirically supported comprehensive treatments for young children with autism. *Journal of Clinical Child Psychology, 27*, 168–179.

Rogers, S. J., & DiLalla, D. L. (1990). Age of symptom onset in young children with pervasive developmental disorders. *Journal of the Academy in Child and Adolescent Psychiatry, 29*, 863–872.

Rutter, M., LeCouteur, A., & Lord, C. (2003). *Autism diagnostic interview–revised.* Los Angeles, CA: Western Psychological Services.

Smith, T., Groen, A. D., & Wynne, J. W. (2000). Randomized trial of intensive early intervention for children with pervasive developmental disorder. *American Journal of Mental Retardation, 105*, 269–285.

Smith, T., & Wick, J. (2008). Controversial treatments. In K. Chawarska, A. Klin, & F. R. Volkmar (Eds.), *Autism spectrum disorders in infants and toddlers: Diagnosis, assessment, and treatment* (pp. 243–273). New York: Guilford.

Stone, W. L., Coonrod, E. E., & Ousley, O. Y. (2000). Brief report: Screening Tool for Autism in Two-year-olds (STAT): Development and preliminary data. *Journal of Autism and Developmental Disorders, 30*, 607–612.

Stone, W. L., Coonrod, E. E., Turner, L. M., & Pozdol, S. L. (2004). Psychometric properties of the STAT for early autism screening. *Journal of Autism and Developmental Disorders, 34*, 691–701.

Stone, W. L., & DiGeronimo, T. (2006). *Does my child have autism?: A parent's guide to early detection and intervention in autism spectrum disorders.* San Francisco, CA: Wiley.

Stone, W. L., Lee, E. B., Ashford, L., Brissie, J., Hepburn, S. L., Coonrod, E. E., et al. (1999). Can autism be diagnosed accurately in children under 3 years? *Journal of Child Psychology and Psychiatry, 40*, 219–226.

Stone, W. L., McMahon, C., & Henderson, L. M. (2008). Use of the Screening Tool for Autism in Two-year-olds (STAT) for children under 24 months: An exploratory study. *Autism, 12*, 573–589.

Stone, W. L., McMahon, C. R., Yoder, P. J., & Walden, T. A. (2007). Early social-communicative and cognitive development of younger siblings of children with autism spectrum disorders. *Archives of Pediatric and Adolescent Medicine, 161*, 384–390.

Turner, L. M., & Stone, W. L. (2007). Variability in outcome for children with ASD diagnosis at age 2. *Journal of Child Psychology and Psychiatry, 48*, 793–802.

Volkmar, F., Cook, E. H., Pomeroy, J., Realmuto, G., & Tanguay, P. (1999). Practice parameters for the assessment and treatment of children, adolescents, and adults with autism and other pervasive developmental disorders. *American Academy of Child and Adolescent Psychiatry, 38*, 32–54.

Wetherby, A. M., Watt, N., Morgan, L., & Shumway, S. (2007). Social communication profiles of children with autism spectrum disorders late in the second year of life. *Journal of Autism and Developmental Disorders, 37*, 960–975.

Wimpory, D. C., Hobson, R. P., Williams, J. M. G., & Nash, S. (2000). Are infants with autism socially engaged? A study of recent retrospective parental reports. *Journal of Autism and Developmental Disorders, 30*, 525–536.

Wong, H. H., & Smith, R. G. (2006). Patterns of complementary and alternative medical therapy use in children diagnosed with autism spectrum disorders. *Journal of Autism and Developmental Disorders, 36*, 901–909.

Yeargin-Allsopp, M., Rice, C., Karapurkar, T., Doernberg, N., Boyle, C., & Murphy, C. (2003). Prevalence of autism in a U.S. metropolitan area. *Journal of the American Medical Association, 289*(1), 49–55.

Zwaigenbaum, L., Bryson, S., Rogers, T., Roberts, W., Brian, J., & Szatmari, P. (2005). Behavioral manifestations of autism in the first year of life. *International Journal of Developmental Neuroscience, 23*, 143–152.

Zwaigenbaum, L., & Stone, W. L. (2006). Early screening for autism spectrum disorder in clinical practice settings. In T. Charman & W. Stone (Eds.). *Social and communication development in autism spectrum disorders* (pp. 88–113). New York: Guilford.

Zwaigenbaum, L., Thurm, A., Stone, W. L., Baranek, G., Bryson, S., Iverson, J., et al. (2007). Studying the emergence of autism spectrum disorders in high-risk infants: Methodological and practical issues. *Journal of Autism and Developmental Disorders, 37*, 466–480.

74 Daniel L. Coury

Diagnosis and Assessment of Autism Spectrum Disorders: A Medical Perspective

Points of Interest

- Autism spectrum disorders are associated with several medical syndromes and genetic disorders, and their identification can impact diagnosis, prognosis, and treatment.
- Medical concerns, such as gastrointestinal symptoms and sleep problems, occur commonly and warrant evaluation and management as part of the overall treatment plan.
- Genetic testing consisting of high resolution chromosome analysis and testing for Fragile X syndrome is recommended in all diagnostic evaluations.
- Newer medical treatments have potential to greatly improve core symptoms of ASDs.
- The comprehensive treatment of a person with an ASD can be best provided through the family-centered, coordinated care received in a medical home.

Leo Kanner's original report of what he called "autistic disturbances" in 1943 continues to serve as not only an accurate depiction of the classic form of the disorder now known as autism, but also as a model for reporting the medical and behavioral aspects of psychiatric disorders . His original description of 11 children with similar problems of communication, social relatedness, and repetitive behaviors included careful examination of their progress over an extended period of time. During this ongoing observation, Kanner considered potential underlying medical factors that might have caused the disorder as well as family and social factors. He was most impressed with the parents, who were uniformly highly intelligent but at the same time displayed features similar to their children but in a milder form, and he commented that they were not "warm-hearted." He noted that six of the 11 children had "presented severe feeding difficulty from the beginning of life." He also noted that five of the 11 had relatively large heads. One child had seizures with an abnormal EEG, and the other ten had normal EEGs. One child had a supernumerary nipple, but otherwise there was little in the way of dysmorphic features. As a result of these observations, he concluded that although he could not deny the possible influence of the family unit on the formation of this disorder, he felt that these children came into the world with an innate inability to form typical social relationships. Since that first description, much has been learned regarding the medical or biologic basis for many psychiatric disorders including autism. This chapter will discuss the medical aspects of autism spectrum disorders, and their influence on diagnosis, assessment, and treatment, beginning with a description of the medical evaluation in the context of the autism diagnostic process.

The Medical History

As part of a multidisciplinary diagnostic evaluation for autism, which typically includes a pediatrician, psychologist, speech-language pathologist, and occupational therapist, the medical evaluation is a key component that can inform not only diagnosis but treatment. A thorough developmental and family history should be taken with the goal of identifying risk factors for developmental disorders including autism. The developmental history should include prenatal conditions that affect the developing fetus, perinatal experiences, and conditions or illnesses encountered in infancy and childhood.

Prenatal: A careful history should be obtained of any illness or problems during the pregnancy, such as infections or eclampsia. For example, maternal rubella infection during pregnancy is associated with congenital rubella syndrome, a disorder associated with intellectual disability and potential autistic symptoms (Chess et al., 1978). Other maternal infections, such as flu, have also been shown in rats to increase the risk for behavioral changes similar to those seen in autism (Shi et al., 2003). Toxemia of pregnancy or eclampsia can result in uterine blood flow abnormalities and decreased oxygen supply to the fetus. Preexisting maternal conditions, such as diabetes, can also have effects on the unborn fetus. Maternal seizure disorders requiring treatment with anticonvulsants run the risk of exposing the fetus to potential teratogens such as valproic acid (Rasalam et al., 2005). Exposure to other drugs or alcohol should also be determined. Mothers with preexisting nutritional or metabolic disorders such as hypothyroidism or phenylketonuria (PKU) have increased risks of a child having medical complications. Any unusual maternal dietary habits should also be noted as these may expose the fetus to inadequate or excessive amounts of certain vitamins or minerals.

Perinatal: Premature birth carries many risks of health problems, including respiratory and neurologic sequelae. Recent studies (Kuban et al., 2009; Limperopoulos et al., 2008) have indicated an increased risk of displaying symptoms associated with autism among graduates of neonatal intensive care units. Intrapartum fetal distress, birth asphyxia, intraventricular hemorrhage, sepsis, and meningitis are a few of the disorders affecting developmental outcome in this age group. Early feeding problems may be associated with later diagnosis of an ASD, perhaps reflecting early motor problems often associated with ASDs.

Postnatal: Medical difficulties during the first year of life can have significant effects on the developing central nervous system. Evidence of adequate growth and nutrition should be obtained through past growth charts or identified dates with heights and weights. Head growth trajectory should be noted, as it has been shown that atypical head growth characterized by accelerated growth beginning at about 4 months of age has been associated with ASDs (Webb et al., 2007). Deceleration of head growth after a period of normal growth has been associated with Rett syndrome (Huppke et al., 2003). Hospitalizations and surgeries should be documented. Reports of early developmental milestones are useful in considering first signs of a problem. Descriptions of social behavior during infancy, such as vocalizations, smiling, and interacting are important, as are difficulties noted with feeding or cuddling. Reports of any potential head trauma resulting in loss of consciousness should be noted.

Developmental History: The child's attainment of typical developmental milestones is an important part of the diagnostic process (*see Chapters 5 and 73 in this volume for detailed information about developmental signs often observed during the first and second year of life*). Delays in language can be caused by several conditions other than autism, such as hearing loss, specific language delay, or as part of a global developmental delay. The child's progress in social, communication, and motor domains should be queried as well as observed during the assessment. A history of developmental regression, or loss of skills, is of concern when reported by parents. This can suggest either a specific condition such as childhood disintegrative disorder, or a progressive metabolic or neurodegenerative disorder.

Family History: A family history focused on developmental and behavioral disorders should be elicited. A family history of autism spectrum disorders is of value, as the risk is increased significantly in subsequent children if a sibling has an ASD (Muhle et al., 2004). ASDs have also been found to be associated with a family history of autoimmune disorders (Ashwood & Van de Water, 2004). Other disorders associated with ASDs include Fragile X syndrome, Rett syndrome, and tuberous sclerosis. A family history of several males affected by mental retardation may suggest Fragile X syndrome; a history of several members with epilepsy, brain tumors or other tumors can be indicative of tuberous sclerosis complex. Early infant mortality in siblings or first-degree relatives can be seen in some metabolic disorders. Apart from the emphasis on disorders associated with autism, the history should inquire about usual family medical history concerns such as autoimmune, cardiac, gastrointestinal, pulmonary, endocrine and renal disorders, and cancer.

Review of Systems

In addition to assessing the primary concern leading to evaluation of a child or adolescent for ASDs, the medical assessment also should address any coexisting functional complaints. Concerns seen most frequently in children with ASDs include gastrointestinal (GI) and related nutritional status, sleep issues, innate immunity or risk for infectious diseases, and general behaviors such as stereotypies or hyperactivity. Psychiatric comorbidities such as ADHD, anxiety, and depression are very common, especially in older children and adolescents. Although the behavioral concerns usually are related to ASD diagnostic criteria, the other symptoms are more likely to be seen by many physicians as problematic but not related to the diagnostic visit. Medical problems such as GI distress, sleep disturbances, and so on, have been found to be significant problem areas for the child and family (Limoges et al., 2005; Nikolov et al., 2009; Tuchman & Rapin, 2002). Moreover, many of these problems have successful treatments and can, therefore, have a significant and immediate impact on quality of life and behavioral functioning. Best medical practice dictates that these should be reviewed and assessed accordingly as part of a thorough evaluation.

Gastrointestinal Concerns

Gastrointestinal symptoms including abdominal pain, diarrhea, gaseousness, and constipation are frequently reported by parents of children with ASDs. Numerous studies have examined these complaints through a wide range of surveys and with varying attempts at comparison or control groups. Reports of the incidence of gastrointestinal symptoms range from 17% (Taylor et al., 2002), to 85% (Horvath & Perman, 2002). A recent study of a well-characterized sample from the Research Units on Pediatric Psychopharmacology

(RUPP) reported a 22.7% incidence rate (Nikolov et al., 2009). Most frequent among the symptoms are diarrhea and constipation, often reported as alternating episodes in the same child. Abdominal pain may be clearly communicated by the child, or may be interpreted by the family to be present based on the child's behaviors. For example, a child experiencing pain may be more irritable, aggressive, or self-injurious. Parents may note certain behaviors occurring within a short time period of eating or elimination, and identify these as indicative of discomfort or of food intolerance or allergy. Their child's limited diet or food preferences may be interpreted as the child's response to food intolerances in an effort to reduce discomfort. Conversely, parents often describe implementing a variety of dietary changes in response to their child's gastrointestinal symptoms. In addition to diet manipulations that any parent might make in response to their child's complaints or symptoms, there are many nontraditional approaches parents may elect to use directed at treating these gastrointestinal symptoms, such as a gluten-free, casein-free diet, digestive enzyme supplementation, or probiotics.

Sleep Concerns

Sleep problems in individuals with autism spectrum disorders are frequently seen. They include delayed sleep onset, night waking, early awakening, obstructive sleep apnea, sleep epilepsy, and reduced need for sleep. A large population-based, case-controlled study of young ASD children (ages 2 to 5 years) found that 56% of children had at least one frequent sleep problem, with night waking and sleep onset problems the most prominent, a rate similar to children with other developmental disorders, but higher than typically developing children (Hansen et al., 2008). Although there are many reported sleep problems, difficulties with obtaining proper polysomnographic studies in this population have resulted in fewer studies using objective measures to define the sleep disorder. Studies using these methods frequently do find sleep abnormalities confirming what is commonly reported by parents (Richdale, 1999; Malow, 2004).

The Physical Examination

Although the diagnosis of an ASD continues to be a behavioral diagnosis at this time, there are medical conditions that may predispose to its development or that may occur as comorbidities. The medical evaluation is important in helping to ascertain etiology of the patient's ASD, and in the establishment of a comprehensive treatment plan that addresses all medical conditions along with the nonmedical treatment of the patient's ASD.

General: The child's affect, gait, and interactions with parents and staff should be observed as the child and parent are brought back to the examining room. Reports by the parents of a change or worsening in gait or mobility should be correlated with these observations. Any special concerns, such as extreme responses to loud noises or marked fearfulness, should be noted. The child's responses to office staff, to others in the waiting room, and to requests to come to the exam room can give initial clues as to ability to hear and understand requests and questions, and verbal language in responses, as well as willingness to comply and ability to transition from waiting room to exam room. The child's responses to recording of height, weight, and vital signs should be similarly observed. Throughout these early minutes in the assessment visit, attention should be paid to the child's ability to make and maintain eye contact, to communicate appropriately for age, and any obvious patterns of behavior or stereotypies.

Head and Neck: Head circumference should be recorded, as a large percentage of children with ASDs have macrocephaly. Recent findings suggest a correlation of macrocephaly in patients with autism and mutations in the phosphatase and tensin (PTEN) gene (Varga et al., 2009). If macrocephaly is identified, the head circumference of both parents should also be obtained, as the most common cause of macrocephaly is familial and nonpathologic. Attention should be paid to the presence of any dysmorphic features—eyes, ears, nose, oral cavity—that would suggest a specific medical syndrome. Limited ability to abduct the eyes or presence of facial asymmetry may suggest Moebius syndrome, which may accompany autism in 25 to 40% of cases (Gillberg & Steffenburg, 1989; Johansson et al., 2001). A flattened appearance to the nose and face may indicate midfacial hypoplasia, which can be seen in several syndromes. The prominence of the philtrum and upper lip may be clues to fetal alcohol exposure.

Skin: There should be an examination for café au lait spots (hyperpigmented) or ash leaf marks (hypopigmented), as may be seen in neurofibromatosis and tuberous sclerosis, respectively. A Wood's lamp may be useful in this process. *Wood's light*, or ultraviolet light, is used to highlight pigmentary changes in the skin. It can help differentiate hypomelanotic macules from similar appearing lesions caused by topical fungal infections. Inspection for shagreen patches on the trunk, or adenoma sebaceum on the face should be made, as these are seen in tuberous sclerosis. Palpation of the skin for fibromas should be done as part of screening for neurofibromatosis.

Abdominal: Examination should be done for enlargement of the liver or spleen, as this may be seen in certain metabolic disorders. Attention should be paid to palpating for stool to support a history of constipation.

Genito-Urinary: The presence of hyperpigmented macules on the penis may suggest PTEN mutation. Macro-orchidism may indicate Fragile X syndrome.

Neurologic: The neurologic examination should document status of reflexes, muscle tone, and strength. Any abnormalities of muscle size or lateralizing findings should be noted. Examination of the cranial nerves may be done as part of the head and neck exam, and may be difficult to fully ascertain if the patient is uncooperative.

Extremities: Documentation should be made of range of motion and any dysmorphic features—syndactyly, arachnodactyly, contractures, etc.—which might suggest a specific syndrome.

Cardiac and pulmonary exams should be completed as the child allows. Although there are no specific findings associated with autism in these portions of the physical, their inclusion is part of a thorough medical exam.

An important point to note is that many children with ASDs are difficult to examine in comparison to typically developing children. If the child is tired and uncooperative, some components of the examination may be deferred to a second visit. Although oppositional behavior may limit the documentation of physical findings, the type of resistance the child displays during the medical exam process often contributes to the diagnostic process in terms of documenting behavioral criteria for an ASD. A patient and gentle approach is usually best, and much appreciated by both patient and parents, and can set a positive tone for other parts of the diagnostic process and ongoing care. A child's sensitivity to touch, sound, and lights can influence the willingness of the child to be cooperative with the exam.

Associated Medical Conditions

There are several medical conditions for which their association with ASDs is clearly higher than that of the general population. Although the developmental-behavioral phenotype for these medical conditions may include symptoms meeting the diagnostic criteria for autism, such cases are often referred to as "secondary" autism; that is, their medical condition is believed to play a role in the causation of their autism. This etiology has been estimated to occur in up to 10% of cases (Barton & Volkmar, 1998; Battaglia & Carey, 2006). Improved understanding of these associated disorders can shed light on the underlying pathophysiology seen in the more common idiopathic ASDs.

Fragile X Syndrome

Fragile X syndrome is caused by a trinucleotide repeat on the X chromosome (Oberle & Rousseau, 1991; Verkerk et al., 1991). The gene defect occurs at the 5' end of the gene for FMR-1 protein. This repeat segment results in hypermethylation of the gene and subsequently failure to produce the FMR-1 protein. The syndrome is characterized by mental retardation, short stature, large ears and long face with prominent jaw, and macro-orchidism. Language development is particularly affected, and can be affected in female carriers (Bennetto et al., 2001). This is related to the number of trinucleotide repeats and the proportion of inactivated affected X chromosomes; the spectrum of the phenotype is related to the total amount of FMR-1 protein production.

Fragile X syndrome occurs in approximately 1 in 4,000 males in the general population (Sherman, 2002). Studies of Fragile X in autism populations suggest an incidence of up to 5%. Conversely, estimates of the rate of ASDs in Fragile X syndrome has been reported to be as high as 15 to 33% (Rogers et al., 2001). Although Fragile X is not a major cause of autism, autism or autistic symptomatology is a common complication of Fragile X. The autistic phenotype seen with Fragile X syndrome males tends to feature significant gaze aversion, hyperactivity, and increased sensory sensitivity. In affected females there is a tendency toward severe social anxiety. Both have a common pattern of "cluttered" speech, with episodes of rapidly speaking and verbal perseverations.

Beyond the behavioral and neurocognitive phenotype, individuals with Fragile X syndrome have an increased rate of other medical conditions. Joint laxity is seen in the majority, and hypotonia is common in the early years. As a result, complications such as scoliosis and hernias may occur. Seizures are reported in approximately 20% of cases, and there is an increasing identification of cardiac problems as they mature into adulthood. Most commonly this presents as mitral valve prolapse, and is seen in up to half of cases (Hagerman, 2002). Identification of medical complications of the disorder is important to the provision of comprehensive care to the patient.

Tuberous Sclerosis

Tuberous sclerosis complex (TSC) is an autosomal dominant disorder with primary manifestations in the nervous system. The textbook presentation is one of angiofibromas on the face, epilepsy, and mental retardation. The disorder is named for the cortical tubers that develop, which are assumed to be the principal cause for the patient's epilepsy. Epilepsy is the most common component, occurring in up to 90% of individuals with TSC. The TSC gene function is related to regulation of cell growth and proliferation, along with abnormal organogenesis. Loss of function of the gene, as happens in tuberous sclerosis complex, leads to uncontrolled cellular growth and the development of hamartomas throughout the body. The most easily identified dermatologic manifestations include angiofibroma of the face, hypomelanotic macules (often referred to as *ash leaf spots*), and a shagreen patch. Angiofibroma of the face, seen in 75% of cases, typically develop from about age 4 or 5 years onward, and are frequently mistaken for acne. The shagreen patch is less frequent, occurring in less than one-fourth of patients, and gives the skin an orange-peel texture. It is usually seen on the trunk or back, and may appear in children as young as age 2 years. Hypomelanotic macules are present on the trunk in nearly 90% of patients and can be identified in the first year of life, thus encouraging a thorough inspection of the skin in the diagnostic assessment of a young child for autism. A Wood's lamp, or ultraviolet lamp, is often useful in highlighting these lesions in infants and toddlers. Presence of hypomelanotic macules is not diagnostic of TSC, but is one of the findings that, when assembled, may point to this diagnosis.

It has been thought that the cortical tubers are the primary cause of epilepsy and mental retardation in cases of TSC. However, newer research suggests that cognitive and neurobehavioral aspects have a much more complex etiology than this.

If diagnosed, TSC has significant implications for ongoing medical management and monitoring. The pathognomonic hamartomatous lesions can occur in numerous organs and tissues. Brain manifestations such as cortical tubers, subependymal nodules, and giant cell astrocytomas can cause significant neurological symptoms. Although these are rarely malignant, their presence and growth can impinge on other brain structures and result in hydrocephalus or other complications. Rhabdomyomas of the heart and retinal phakomas occur in more than half of subjects, and angiomyolipomas frequently occur in the kidney.

15q 11q13 Duplication Syndrome

The region of chromosome 15 q11q13 has received significant attention since the mid-1990s. Various deletions, insertions, inversions, and duplications have been identified (Battaglia, 2005). Deletions are associated with Angelman's syndrome and Prader-Willi syndrome (Christian et al., 1999). The duplication referred to as inv dup (15) presents a consistent pattern of intellectual disability and hypotonia. A strong association has been found between isodicentric chromosome 15 and autistic features (Rineer et al., 1998; Borgatti et al., 2001). These children present with extreme gaze avoidance and social withdrawal, with a range of self-stimulatory behaviors directed at objects in their vicinity such as spinning objects, shiny objects, and water. Expressive language is poor and stereotypies are very common. Cognitive function is usually overall delayed, and significant hypotonia is present from birth and contributes to late acquisition of motor milestones. Although these children have some mild dysmorphic features, they do not have a characteristic appearance. Epilepsy appears to be a common complication (Battaglia et al., 1997).

Differential Diagnosis and Laboratory Workup

Laboratory studies and ancillary testing and consultation should be conducted to confirm or rule out conditions and diagnoses suggested by the history and physical examination. Some studies are recommended in all cases because of the significance of the result in formulating a diagnosis and treatment (e.g., obtaining an electrocardiogram (ECG) in any person over age 50 years with chest pain). Other studies are conducted only when the presentation—presenting concern, detailed history, and physical examination—suggests potential diagnoses that may rule out the presenting concern (e.g., not an ASD but a communication disorder) or that may need to be addressed as part of the overall treatment plan. Recommendations for laboratory evaluations in ASD assessments are changing rapidly as new information is acquired and new technologies become available.

Audiology: The presentation of a child who does not speak or seem to listen, as seen in suspected ASD, requires evaluation of hearing in all cases. This is currently recommended as part of the evaluation of any child with developmental delay.

Lead Screening: The known effects of lead exposure on development, the increased risk of exposure associated with younger children who examine much of their environment through the mouthing of objects, and the potential to provide treatment that can improve function all support the screening for lead with a blood lead level.

Genetic Screening: The yield for genetic testing continues to increase as newer techniques are introduced and genetic correlates of medical conditions are identified. Current recommendations are for high resolution chromosome studies and for DNA analysis for Fragile X syndrome in all children with developmental delay. Newer techniques such as microarray technologies are developing rapidly. These methods are capable of locating copy number variants (CNVs) of smaller and smaller size, and of screening for larger and larger numbers of these CNVs on a single array—well over 5 million and quickly rising. However, many of the CNVs identified through this process are of no known significance. Performing this testing at this time often leads to uncomfortable discussions with the family about finding an abnormality and not knowing what it means. Until more is known, this procedure is not considered routine or mandatory, but this field is rapidly advancing and recommendations could change in the near future.

Metabolic Screening: Mandatory screening for numerous inborn errors of metabolism is done in most developed countries. In the United States, all states screen for 27 different disorders and vary in their requirements to screen up to a total of 51 disorders. Although children with some metabolic disorders such as PKU can display symptoms of an ASD, the majority of metabolic conditions present earlier in life with significant medical symptoms such as failure to thrive, seizures, and recurrent infections. There is no recommendation for routine metabolic screening in an ASD evaluation. Testing should be done only if clinically indicated, such as abnormal state of consciousness, repeated episodes of vomiting, dysmorphic features, and family history of a metabolic disorder. Questionable screening at birth, as in an immigrant child, is another indication.

Electroencephalography (EEG): Children and adolescents with ASDs do have an increased incidence of epilepsy, and studies have shown a rate of EEG abnormalities higher than the general population. However, these abnormalities are largely nonspecific and do not impact on care. Similarly, at this time there is no evidence to support treating EEG abnormalities in the absence of clinical seizure activity. There is no recommendation for routine EEG testing in ASD evaluations. Testing should be done in any child with a history of suspicious spells or episodes. It is also recommended in cases with a history of regression, particularly language, because of the possibility of identifying Landau Kleffner syndrome, a treatable disorder.

Neuroimaging Studies: Similar to EEG findings, computed tomography (CT) and magnetic resonance imaging (MRI) studies have shown an increased incidence of intracranial abnormalities compared to more typically developing children. Again, these abnormalities have failed to accumulate into recognizable ASD phenotypes and rarely require any specific intervention. The presence of macrocephaly alone, with normal neurologic findings and no indication of intracranial process are not adequate to justify neuroimaging. There is no recommendation for routine neuroimaging in ASD evaluations but this field also is rapidly progressing and this may change in the near future.

Other Studies: The laboratory evaluation of a number of other minerals, hormones, and micronutrients, urinary peptides, food allergy testing, and hair analysis and heavy metal exposure are not recommended. Immunologic testing for celiac antibodies or signs of inflammation, stool analysis for yeast, and other neurochemical testing for glutathione disorders are also not recommended. The scientific evidence for conducting these studies fails to support them at this time.

Psychological and Speech-Language Testing: These evaluations are recommended as a required component of a diagnostic workup for ASDs. Psychologists routinely administer the standardized behavioral diagnostic tests, such as the Autism Diagnostic Observation Schedule (Lord et al., 2000). In addition, psychological testing is needed to establish levels of intellectual disability and pinpoint specific patterns of cognitive strengths and weaknesses, such as specific problems in auditory processing, memory, attention, and social comprehension. Speech-language evaluations are important for understanding the causes and nature of language delay, such as problems in the areas of oral motor functioning, phonemic discrimination, verbal memory, receptive versus expressive language, gestural development, and pragmatic language. These assessments are necessary for confirming the diagnosis and for establishing the treatment plan. More detailed neuropsychological testing should be done if standard testing fails to provide adequate detail regarding the child's cognitive abilities and if concerns about educational progress and strategies are present.

Medical Treatments

Treatment of Gastrointestinal Symptoms

It is possible that gastrointestinal symptoms can contribute to behavioral disturbance and can exacerbate the child's ASD symptoms (e.g., self-injurious behavior that may increase in response to pain). Thus, treatment of the gastrointestinal problem can have positive effects on reducing ASD-related symptoms and improve the child's ability to engage in and profit from behavioral and educational interventions. Some have theorized that core ASD symptoms can be directly related to GI-related problems (Reichelt, Ekrein, & Scott, 1990). The theory postulates that ASD symptoms are a manifestation of food intolerance, with gluten and/or casein sensitivity the most commonly identified culprit. This theory suggests that peptides from gluten and casein have a significant role in the origins of autism and that some of the physiology and psychology of autism might be explained by excessive opioid activity linked to these peptides. Frequently there is no traditional laboratory or research evidence of celiac disease or casein sensitivity to support the use of a gluten-free, casein-free diet in these children, with some having no gastrointestinal symptoms, but the diet is safe and effective for use in patients with celiac disease. Proponents also point out that some cases of celiac disease also fail to have traditional laboratory-supporting evidence. As a result, the diet can be followed as a therapeutic trial. It is important to help parents understand that it can be difficult to determine whether the diet is actually helping their child, especially if it is initiated along with other interventions. Thus, it is helpful to identify a person, such as the child's teacher or therapist, who is unaware of when the trial was initiated who can provide objective feedback regarding whether the child's behavior has improved.

Reichelt, Ekrein, and Scott (1990) identified 15 children with autism and abnormal urinary protein patterns. These were hypothesized to reflect gluten or casein protein absorption abnormalities, with more protein absorption and subsequent increased urinary excretion. A gluten-free and casein-free diet was implemented for these children for several years in an open-label fashion. The authors reported improvement in the children's behavior over time as rated by both parents and teachers. Similar findings were reported by several small studies (Knivsberg et al., 1995; Knivsberg et al., 2002; Knivsberg et al., 2003). Ratings from families participating in the Autism Research Institute collection of data regarding use of diets report improvement of symptoms in 66%, no change in 31%, and worsening in 3% (Autism Research Institute, 2009).

Many studies of the gluten-free casein-free diet that have reported improvement in areas other than the gastrointestinal tract suffer from methodologic problems including inconsistent diagnostic criteria, small numbers of children treated, lack of an appropriate comparison group, and failure to control for other therapies the child might be receiving for their autistic disorder (Reichelt et al., 1990; Knivsberg et al., 1995; Lucarelli et al., 1995; Whiteley et al., 1999; Knivsberg et al., 2002). As a result, it is difficult to clearly discern the true efficacy or lack thereof for this treatment, as noted in a recent review (Christison & Ivany, 2006). A recent Cochrane review was unable to compare the studies identified in their literature review because of a lack of common outcome measures, making a meta-analysis impossible. The reviewers were only able to identify two small, randomized, controlled trials, totaling less than three dozen subjects. Their review concluded that evidence for efficacy of this treatment is poor and that larger, randomized, controlled trials were needed (Millward et al., 2008). When there has been evidence of celiac disease, dietary changes have reduced gastrointestinal symptoms, but not the core behavioral symptoms of the child's autistic disorder (Barcia et al., 2008).

The gluten-free, casein-free diet most often includes a regimen of vitamin and other nutritional supplements as a comprehensive approach to treating autism. To consider it as solely a treatment for gastrointestinal symptoms as described here does not give credit to the overall intent of the therapy. It is discussed in further detail in Chapter 71.

The presence of gastrointestinal symptoms in children with autism spectrum disorders may someday have diagnostic or prognostic benefit and should be evaluated. Recent genetic studies into potential causes for autism spectrum disorders has indicated a role for the autism spectrum disorder met receptor tyrosine kinase (MET) promoter variant rs1858830 in individuals with co-occurring autism spectrum disorder and gastrointestinal conditions (Campbell et al., 2009). The authors examined 918 individuals from 214 families to determine the association of MET alleles with autism spectrum disorder and the presence of gastrointestinal symptoms. They found an association in 118 families with at least one child with both an ASD and gastrointestinal conditions, but no association in the 96 families lacking this association. More recently, it has been seen that the MET gene is also associated with the social and communication domains of ASDs in these cases (Campbell et al., 2009). Further research in this area may someday characterize a clinical phenotype, which may then lead to a more specific treatment regimen. Studies such as this help emphasize the significance of family histories in better defining clinical phenotypes of ASDs, and as an important part of the medical assessment.

At the present time, the existence of a distinct gastrointestinal condition occurring in ASDs has not been clearly documented. There is heated controversy regarding what has been called autistic enterocolitis and how it should be managed if it indeed exists. What has been clearer is that families report many gastrointestinal symptoms but frustration with the evaluation and treatment these symptoms receive by the managing physician. In developing best practices for the management of gastrointestinal symptoms in children and adolescents with ASDs, at this time the recommendation is to follow existing best practice parameters for the symptom in question. Heeding parental concerns and addressing them in the same manner one would for a typically developing child will likely serve the child and family well in the majority of cases (Buie et al., 2010). The Autism Treatment Network (ATN) was founded in 2005 with a goal of expanding knowledge and expertise in the treatment of medical conditions associated with autism spectrum disorders. This network now consists of over a dozen autism centers across the United States and Canada, each following a multidisciplinary philosophy of evaluation and treatment for patients on the autism spectrum. Part of the work of these medical centers is focused on establishing and testing clinical guidelines for the assessment and treatment of various medical comorbidities seen in children and adolescents with autism. Guidelines for assessment and treatment of GI and other medical problems are being developed by these clinicians, along with testing of these recommendations in clinical practice (Coury et al., 2009).

Treatment of Sleep Problems

Johnson and Malow (2008) have noted that most sleep problems are multifactorial, and have strongly recommended that behavioral interventions be instituted prior to any trials of pharmacotherapy. Reed and colleagues (2009) have examined the use of behavioral interventions to promote sleep in 20 children ages 3 to 10 years with autism. Direct parental instruction was given covering effective daytime and nighttime habits, initiating a bedtime routine, and optimizing parental interactions at bedtime and during night wakings. Actigraphy documented an improvement in sleep latency, and insomnia symptoms showed improvement on several subscales of a standardized questionnaire. An important point of this study was its addition to available evidence that sleep problems can often be managed through nonpharmacologic methods, even in children with significant developmental disorders.

Melatonin, a sleep-promoting chemical secreted by the pineal gland in response to levels of darkness, is viewed by many as a natural and safe treatment for sleep latency problems, where delayed or reduced melatonin release may be present. Melatonin use in treating insomnia in children with developmental problems has been described in several studies with improvement reported in the majority of patients (Anderson et al., 2008; Johnson & Malow, 2009). It has also been shown effective in adults with autism and chronic sleep problems, most frequently sleep latency concerns (Galli-Carminati et al., 2009). However, delayed or reduced melatonin release is rarely confirmed or documented in clinical practice, so melatonin use is largely empiric. Ideally, it should be initiated following a formal sleep evaluation with polysomnography and carefully monitored. Difficulties obtaining such studies in children with ASDs tend to limit this practice.

Failure to improve sleep symptoms with melatonin often leads clinicians to use other medications to promote sleep onset and maintenance. In the general pediatric population and in children and adolescents with ASDs, the medications that are FDA-approved and indicated for treatment of sleep disorders are typically not used as first-line treatments. Physicians report the practice of prescribing medications such as antihistamines (diphenhydramine, brompheniramine), alpha agonists (clonidine, guanfacine), benzodiazepines (clonazepam, lorazepam), and trazodone for their sedating side effects to treat the sleep issues rather than for the medications' primary indications. In some circumstances, clinicians report prescribing other medications such as risperidone with a goal of treating other symptoms associated with autism, such as irritability or repetitive behaviors, as well as the sleep problem.

A major concern in this area is the use of pharmacotherapeutic agents, some of which have significant potential adverse effects, without a clear definition of the underlying etiology of the child's sleep problem. Moreover, there are very few systematic studies of the use of these treatments specifically for sleep problems. For example, there is one open-label study of the use of clonidine for sleep disturbance (Ming et al., 2008). Work by the Autism Treatment Network to improve evaluation and understanding of the pathophysiology underlying sleep problems in children and adolescents with autism spectrum disorders, and the Network's capacity to conduct multisite research will hopefully lead to better and more specific treatments. Early work done by Network investigators (Reed et al., 2009) has demonstrated the benefit of educating parents by providing direct instruction in sleep hygiene, as opposed to simply providing written information regarding bedtime routines. Additional research into the underlying causes of sleep problems could help avoid unnecessary medication as well as identifying what medications might be appropriate and in which situations.

Psychopharmacology for Associated and Core Symptoms of ASDs

Many of the core symptoms of ASDs bear resemblance to other known disorders—stereotypies are reminiscent of obsessive-compulsive behaviors, gaze aversion appears to manifest anxiety symptoms, unfocused overactive behavior looks much like the hyperactivity seen in attention deficit hyperactivity disorder (ADHD). Furthermore, it is recognized that individuals with ASDs suffer from comorbid psychiatric conditions, such as ADHD, obsessive-compulsive disorder, anxiety, and depression. When behavioral and other therapies are not sufficient in treating these manifestations, or when these behaviors severely limit the effectiveness of behavioral and other therapies, pharmacologic treatments are often considered. These tend to be used empirically, based on the patient's major symptom presentation. The stimulant medications typically used to treat attention difficulties and hyperactivity in individuals with ADHD can be effective in treating these same symptoms in ASDs, although they tend to have a lower efficacy rate and a higher rate of adverse effects (Aman et al., 2008; Posey et al., 2007). The same is true for anxiolytic medications for anxiety symptoms (Kolevson, 2006). The antipsychotic class of medications has been used for decades, and is known for reducing overactive behavior and aggression. The newer atypical antipsychotics have had significant study and are often effective for symptoms such as self-injurious behavior, aggression toward others, and repetitive behaviors. Their well-known calming effect has also been shown efficacious in treating the irritability seen in many children with ASDs (McCracken et al., 2002; Filipek et al., 2006).

Future Medical Treatments

The tremendous heterogeneity in symptom presentation among individuals with ASDs suggests multiple causes and multiple neurobiologic pathways. Although behavioral and educational treatments have been shown to be most effective for promoting development and decreasing symptoms of autism, improved understanding of etiology and biological mechanisms and the resulting medical treatments have great potential to accelerate improvement for ASDs. Research in this area offers promise that eventually medications will be available that can: *(1)* treat core ASD symptoms, *(2)* treat more specific neurotransmitter pathways, and *(3)* alter the expression of specific target genes found to be involved.

Treatment of Core ASD symptoms

Various medications currently used in mainstream medical practice are focused on symptomatic treatment of specific ASD-associated target symptoms such as repetitive behaviors. There is continued progress in pharmacologic compounds with more specific neurotransmitter targets, better-defined therapeutic effects and fewer adverse effects. There will be new and improved stimulants, antipsychotics and anxiolytics. One novel approach being investigated is aimed at treatment of core symptoms, such as those in the social domain (Andari et al., 2010). Oxytocin, a naturally occurring neuropeptide, is known to promote social behavior and its deficiency in mouse models results in abnormal social behaviors similar to those seen in autism. A medication that is able to ameliorate the core social domain would have a tremendous impact on the efficacy of behavioral treatments. Reduction of social deficits could allow greater focus on language therapy and management of repetitive and perseverative behaviors. An enhancement in the social domain would likely improve the important factor of innate motivation and desire to please others, key elements of success in promoting positive behavior and learning.

Fragile X Syndrome

The GABAergic and glutamatergic neurotransmitter systems have been implicated in autism (Fatemi, Folsom, et al., 2009; Fatemi, Reutiman, et al., 2009). Gamma-amino butyric acid (GABA) receptors play a role in inhibitory neurotransmission, and influence the developmental and functional plasticity of the brain. Recent work in animal models has shown that blocking GABA-B receptors can inhibit glutamate signaling and subsequently reduce metabotropic glutamate receptor (mGluR) mediated protein synthesis, which is increased because of lack of Fragile X mental retardation -1 (FMR-1) protein-suppressing production (Bear et al., 2004). Multiple aspects of Fragile X syndrome appear to be related to this excess activation. Treatment with GABA-B receptor agonists in drosophila fly models of Fragile X have shown significant improvement in courtship behavior and impaired memory (McBride et al., 2005). Treatment given to drosophila during development resulted in correction of neuroanatomical defects seen in the untreated group. Studies in adult drosophila demonstrated improvement in social behavior and memory also, but no correction of neuroanatomic structures. Clinical trials in humans are underway.

Tuberous Sclerosis Complex (TSC)

Research in the genetics of TSC has led to better understanding of how the normal protein complex TSC1 functions to inhibit the mammalian target of rapamycin (mTOR) cascade, which is known to govern cell growth (O'Callaghan et al., 2004). When the TSC genes fail to function as is seen in TSC, the result is continuous oversignaling, resulting in cell overgrowth and the characteristic tumors. This increased signaling appears to also be involved in the modification of synapses that occurs during learning, and leads to memory impairments (Goorden et al., 2007). Studies in mouse models have shown that rapamycin have shown clear improvement in cognitive abilities even in adult mice (Ehninger et al., 2008).

Other Disorders

The recent advances in our understanding of the neurochemical and molecular basis of ASDs and related conditions, and the subsequent development of novel treatments for the specific disorders mentioned above, represent a massive shift in the medical treatment paradigm. Similar discoveries have been made in mouse models for phosphatise tensin homolog (PTEN) mutants and Rett syndrome (methyl CpG binding protein 2 (MECP2) mutation) (Kwon et al., 2003; Shabazian et al., 2002). Even more exciting is the experimental work in these animal models demonstrating significant improvement in adult animals, and the potential for reversing many cognitive and social symptoms (Zhou et al., 2009; Guy et al., 2007). Most research geared toward acquiring better understanding of the etiology of a disorder is done with the hope of identifying a way to eventually prevent the disorder. The findings in these adult animal models hold hope for effective treatments for humans with ASDs and a variety of neurodevelopmental disorders. Given the evidence supporting these multiple—and not always overlapping—etiologies, it is likely that personalized treatments incorporating several modalities will be developed for each person with an ASD.

The Need for Comprehensive Care: The Medical Home

Diagnosis and assessment of the child, adolescent, or adult with an ASD requires multidisciplinary evaluation. Most commonly involved are psychologists, psychiatrists, neurologists, and developmental pediatricians, as well as speech and language pathologists and occupational therapists. Various medical specialists may also be consulted for specific aspects, such as pediatric sleep specialists, gastroenterologists, and medical geneticists. The treatment plan is built around appropriate behavioral therapy and educational programming, with medical treatments as necessary for associated symptoms or conditions.

Health care expenses for families with a child with an ASD are higher than those for typically developing children (Mandell et al., 2006). Costs can be as much as ten times that of other families. Much of this is because of costly inpatient psychiatric care. When this inpatient care is excluded, the remaining ambulatory care costs suggest that children with ASDs are not receiving additional primary-care services that would be indicative of appropriately coordinated services, as suggested by the medical home model. Families with a child with an ASD experience significant difficulties accessing the care their child needs (Ruble et al., 2005). Many factors that lead to lack of access, such as race and education, could be mollified by systems and policies that provide a structure within which available services can be coordinated by personnel acquainted with ASDs and the network of agencies and programs needed. A medical home, discussed in more detail below, would meet this need. Kogan et al. (2008) reviewed data from the *2005–2006 National Survey of Children with Special Health Care Needs* and identified over 2,000 children with ASDs. They found that this population is more likely to have a variety of unmet needs, including specific health-care needs, difficulty receiving referrals, and delayed or foregone care. They concluded that receiving primary care through a medical home model could reduce financial impacts and the burden on employment and time spent coordinating care. Homer et al. (2008) have reviewed the literature on the effectiveness of the medical home and found it does indeed support improved health-related outcomes for children with special health-care needs.

The medical home is a primary-care practice—a pediatrician or family physician and support staff—that provides family-centered, comprehensive, community-based, coordinated care. The medical home communicates with specialty providers, service providers, and community agencies to coordinate the patient's care. The medical home also coordinates coverage for services with the patient's health insurance provider, and provides ongoing monitoring and management of the patient's care with input from involved specialists and ancillary service providers. Patients receiving care through a medical home have reduced unnecessary duplication of services and fewer unmet medical needs.

Materials are available from a variety of sources on how primary-care providers can incorporate medical home services in their practices (American Academy of Pediatrics: www.medicalhomeinfo.org; Waisman Center: www.waisman.wisc.edu/nmhai/). These resources include guidelines for initiating discussion and promoting interaction and collaboration with service providers for ASD children and their families. The medical care for children and adolescents with ASDs will only increase with the advances in medical treatment under development. Promotion of the medical home philosophy on a broader scale is needed.

Conclusions

The diagnosis of an autism spectrum disorder is based purely on behavioral observations. Rapid advances in our understanding of the etiology of various "autisms" are increasingly calling for new laboratory tests to help identify medical conditions that may have a causative role. These advances will lead to a larger role for the medical component in the diagnosis and assessment of autism disorders. In addition, the potential for more and better medical treatments for core autism symptoms, as well as for associated conditions, will broaden the medical portion of autism management. The need for coordination of medical treatments with behavioral and other intervention approaches needed by the ASD population can be met through the further development of the medical home comprehensive care model, which promotes patient-centered, community-based, comprehensive care.

Challenges and Future Directions

- Further understanding of the relationship between medical symptoms such as gastrointestinal complaints and autism spectrum disorders can lead to healthier lives and better outcomes.
- Genetic testing techniques such as microarrays are rapidly evolving, and as their costs decrease and their usefulness increases they will become one of the most important parts of the medical evaluation.
- As the scope of medical treatments for autism increases, there will be challenges in keeping primary-care physicians up-to-date and competent in using these treatments. The medical home model provides a good framework for coordinating the care that persons with ASDs require.

SUGGESTED READING

Nikolov, R. N., Bearss, K. E., Lettinga, J., Erickson, C., Rodowski, M., Aman, M. G., et al. (2009). Gastrointestinal symptoms in a sample of children with pervasive developmental disorders. *Journal of Autism and Developmental Disorders, 39*, 405–413.

Johnson, K. P., & Malow, B. A. (2008). Assessment and pharmacologic treatment of sleep disturbance in autism. *Child and Adolescent Psychiatric Clinics of North America, 17*(4), 773–785.

Campbell, D. B., Buie, T. M., Winter, H., Bauman, M., Sutcliffe, J. S., Perrin, J. M., et al. (2009). Distinct genetic risk based on association of MET in families with co-occurring autism and gastrointestinal conditions. *Pediatrics, 123*(3), 1018–1024.

REFERENCES

Aman, M. G., Farmer, C. A., Hollway, J., & Arnold, L. E. (2008). Treatment of inattention, overactivity, and impulsiveness in autism spectrum disorders. *Child and Adolescent Psychiatric Clinics of North America, 17*(4), 713–738, vii.

American Academy of Pediatrics (2010). Autism information. Available at http://www.medicalhomeinfo.org/health/autism.html Accessed December 13, 2010.

Andari, E., Duhamel, J. R., Zalla, T., Herbrecht, E., Leboyer, M., & Sirigu, A. (2010). Promoting social behavior with oxytocin in high-functioning autism spectrum disorders. *Proceedings of the National Academy of Sciences of the United States of America March, 2; 107*(9), 4389–4394.

Andersen, I. M., Kaczmarska, J., McGrew, S. G., & Marlow, B. A. (2008). Melatonin for insomnia in children with autism spectrum disorders. *Journal of Child Neurology, 23*(5), 482–485.

Ashwood, P., & Van de Water, J. (2004). Is autism an autoimmune disease? *Autoimmunity Reviews, 3*, 557–562.

Autism Research Institute (2009). *Parent ratings of behavioral effects of biomedical interventions.* Available at http://autism.com/fam_ratingsbehaviorbiomedical.asp. Accessed December 13, 2010.

Barcia, G., Posar, A., Santucci, M., & Parmeggiani, A. (2008). Autism and coeliac disease. *Journal of Autism and Developmental Disorders, 38*(2), 407–408.

Barton, M., & Volkmar, F. (1998). How commonly are known medical conditions associated with autism? *Journal of Autism and Developmental Disorders, 28*, 273–278.

Battaglia, A., Gurrieri, F., Bertini, E., Bellacosa, A., Pomponi, M. G., Paravatou-Petsotas, M., et al. (1997). The inv dup(15) syndrome: A clinically recognizable syndrome with altered behaviour, mental retardation and epilepsy. *Neurology, 48*, 1081–1086.

Battaglia, A. (2005). The inv dup(15) or idic(15) syndrome: A clinically recognisable neurogenetic disorder. *Brain and Development, 27*(5), 365–369.

Battaglia, A., & Carey, J. C. (2006). Etiologic yield of autistic spectrum disorders: A prospective study. *American Journal of Medical Genetics. Part C, Seminars in Medical Genetics, 142C*, 3–7.

Bear, M. F., Huber, K. M., & Warren, S. T. (2004). The mGluR theory of fragile X mental retardation. *Trends in Neurosciences, 27*, 370–377.

Bennetto, L., Pennington, B., Taylor, A., & Hagerman, R. J. (2001). Profile of cognitive functioning in women with the fragile X mutation. *Neuropsychology, 15*(2), 290–299.

Borgatti, R., Piccinelli, P., Passoni, D., Dalpra, L., Miozzo, M., Micheli, R., et al. (2001). Relationship between clinical and genetic features in "inverted duplicated chromosome 15" patients. *Pediatric Neurology, 24*, 111–116.

Buie, T., Fuchs, G. J., III, Furuta, G. T., Kooros, K., Levy, J., Lewis, J. D. et al. (2010) Recommendations for evaluation and treatment of common gastrointestinal problems in children with ASDs. *Pediatrics, 125*(Suppl 1), S19–29.

Campbell, D. B., Buie, T. M., Winter, H., Bauman, M., Sutcliffe, J. S., Perrin, J. M., et al. (2009). Distinct genetic risk based on association of MET in families with co-occurring autism and gastrointestinal conditions. *Pediatrics, 123*(3), 1018–1024.

Campbell, D. B., Warren, D., Sutcliffe, J. S., Lee, E. B., & Levitt, P. (2010). Association of MET with social and communication phenotypes in individuals with autism spectrum disorder. *American Journal of Medical Genetics. Part B, Neuropsychiatric Genetics, 153B*(2), 438–446.

Chess, S., Fernandez, P., & Korn, S. (1978). Behavioral consequences of congenital rubella. *Journal of Pediatrics, 93*(4), 699–703.

Christian, S. L., Fantes, J. A., Mewborn, S. K., Huang, B., & Ledbetter, D. (1999). Large genomic duplicons map to sites of instability in the Prader-Willi/Angelman syndrome chromosome region (15q11–q13). *Human and Molecular Genetics, 8*, 1025–1037.

Christison, G. W., & Ivany, K. (2006). Elimination diets in autism spectrum disorders: Any wheat amidst the chaff? *Journal of Developmental and Behavioral Pediatrics, 27*(Suppl 2), S162–171.

Coury, D., Jones, N., Klatka, K., Winklosky, B., & Perrin, J. (2009). Healthcare for children with autism: The Autism Treatment Network. *Current Opinion in Pediatrics, 21*, 828–832.

Ehninger, D., Han, S., Shilyansky, C., Zhou, Y., Li, W., Kwiatkowski, D. J., et al. (2008). Reversal of learning deficits in a Tsc2+/- mouse model of tuberous sclerosis. *Nature Medicine, 14*, 843–848.

Fatemi, S. H., Folsom, T. D., Reutiman, T. J., & Thuras, P. D. (2009). Expression of GABA(B) receptors is altered in brains of subjects with autism. *Cerebellum, 8*(1), 64–69.

Fatemi, S. H., Reutiman, T. J., Folsom, T. D., & Thuras, P. D. (2009). GABA(A) receptor downregulation in brains of subjects with autism. *Journal of Autism and Developmental Disorders, 39*(2), 223–230.

Filipek, P. A., Steinberg-Epstein, R., & Book, T. M. (2006). Intervention for autistic spectrum disorders. *NeuroRx, 3*(2), 207–216.

Galli-Carminati, G., Deriaz, N., & Bertschy, G. (2009). Melatonin in treatment of chronic sleep disorders in adults with autism: A retrospective study. *Swiss Medical Weekly, 139*(19–20), 293–296.

Gillberg, C., & Steffenburg, S. (1989). Autistic behavior in Moebius syndrome. *Acta Paediatrica Scandinavica, 78*, 314–316.

Goorden, S. M., van Woerden, G. M., van der Weerd, L., Cheadle, J. P., & Elgersma, Y. (2007). Cognitive deficits in Tsc1+/- mice in the absence of cerebral lesions and seizures. *Annals of Neurology, 62*, 648–655.

Guy, J., Gan, J., Selfridge, J., Cobb, S., & Bird, A. (2007). Reversal of neurological defects in a mouse model of Rett syndrome. *Science, 315*, 1143–1147.

Hagerman, R. J. (2002). Physical and behavioral phenotype. In R. J. Hagerman & P. J. Hagerman (Eds.), *Fragile X syndrome: Diagnosis, treatment and research* (3rd ed.) (pp. 3–109). Baltimore, MD: The Johns Hopkins University Press.

Hansen, R. L., Ozonoff, S., Krakowiak, P., Angkustsiri, K., Jones, C., Deprey L. J., et al. (2008). Regression in autism: Prevalence and associated factors in the CHARGE Study. *Ambulatory Pediatrics, 8*(1), 25–31.

Homer, C. J., Klatka, K., Romm, D., Kuhlthau, K., Bloom, S., Newacheck, P., et al. (2008). A review of the evidence for the medical home for children with special health care needs. *Pediatrics, 122*(4), e922–937.

Horvath, K., & Perman, J.A. (2002). Autism and gastrointestinal symptoms. *Current Gastroenterology Reports, 4*(3), 251–258.

Huppke, P., Held, M., Laccone, F., & Hanefeld, F. (2003). The spectrum of phenotypes in females with Rett syndrome. *Brain Development, 25*(5), 346–351.

Johansson, M., Wentz, E., Fernell, E., Strömland, K., Miller, M., & Gillberg, C. (2001). Autistic spectrum disorders in Möbius sequence: A comprehensive study of 25 individuals. *Developmental Medicine and Child Neurology, 43*(5), 338–345.

Johnson, K. P., & Malow, B. A. (2008). Sleep in children with autism spectrum disorders. *Current Treatment Options in Neurology, 10*(5), 350–359.

Johnson, K. P., & Malow, B. A. (2009). Assessment and pharmacologic treatment of sleep disturbance in autism. *Child and Adolescent Psychiatric Clinics of North America, 17*(4), 773–785.

Kanner, L. (1943). Autistic disturbances of affective contact. *The Nervous Child, 2*, 217–250.

Knivsberg, A. M., Reichelt, K. L., Nodland, N., & Hoien, T. (1995). Autistic syndrome and diet: A follow-up study. *Scandinavian Journal of Education and Research, 39*, 223–236.

Knivsberg, A. M., Reichelt, K. L., Hoien, T., & Nodland, M. (2002). A randomized, controlled study of dietary intervention in autistic syndromes. *Nutritional Neuroscience, 5*(4), 251–261.

Knivsberg, A. M., Reichelt, K. L., Hoien, T., & Nodland, M. (2003). Effect of dietary intervention on autistic behavior. *Focus on Autism Other Developmental Disabilities, 18*(4), 247–256.

Kogan, M. D., Strickland, B. B., Blumberg, S. J., Singh, G. K., Perrin, J. M., & van Dyck, P. C. (2008). A national profile of the health care experiences and family impact of autism spectrum disorder among children in the United States, 2005–2006. *Pediatrics, 122*(6), e1149–1158.

Kolevzon, A., Mathewson, K. A., & Hollander, E. (2006). Selective serotonin reuptake inhibitors in autism: A review of efficacy and tolerability *Journal of Clinical Psychiatry, 67*(3), 407–414.

Kuban, K. C., O'Shea, T. M., Allred, E. N., Tager-Flusberg, H., Goldstein, D. J., & Leviton, A. (2009). Positive screening on the Modified Checklist for Autism in Toddlers (M-CHAT) in extremely low gestational age newborns. *Journal of Pediatrics, 154*(4), 535–540.

Kwon, C. H., Zhu, X., Zhang, J., & Baker, S. J. (2003). mTor is required for hypertrophy of Pten-deficient neuronal soma in vivo. *Proceedings of the National Academy of Sciences of the United States of America, 100*, 12923–12928.

Limoges, E., Mottron, L., Bolduc, C., Berthiaume, C., & Godbout, R. (2005). Atypical sleep architecture and the autism phenotype. *Brain, 128*, 1049–1061.

Limperopoulos, C., Bassan, H., Sullivan, N. R., Soul, J. S., Robertson, R. L. Jr., Moore, M., et al. (2008). Positive screening for autism in ex-preterm infants: Prevalence and risk factors. *Pediatrics, 121*(4), 758–765.

Lord, C., Risi, S., Lambrecht, L., Cook E. H., Jr., Leventhal, B. L., DiLavore, P. C., et al. (2000). The autism diagnostic observation schedule-generic: A standard measure of social and communication deficits associated with the spectrum of autism. *Journal of Autism and Developmental Disorders, 30*(3), 205–223.

Lucarelli, S., Frediani, T., Zingoni, A., Ferruzzi, F., Giardini, O., Quintieri, F., et al. (1995). Food allergy and infantile autism. *Panminerva Medica, 37*(3), 137–141.

Malow, B. A. (2004). Sleep disorders, epilepsy, and autism. *Mental Retardation and Developmental Disabilities Research Reviews, 10*(2), 122–125.

Mandell, D. S., Cao, J., Ittenbach, R., & Pinto-Martin, J. (2006). Medicaid expenditures for children with autistic spectrum disorders: 1994 to 1999. *Journal of Autism and Developmental Disorders, 36*(4), 475–485.

McBride, S. M., Choi, C. H., Wang, Y., Liebelt, D., Braunstein, E., Ferreiro, D., et al. (2005). Pharmacological rescue of synaptic plasticity, courtship behavior, and mushroom body defects in a drosophila model of fragile X syndrome. *Neuron, 45*, 753–764.

McCracken, J. T., McGough, J., Shah, B., Cronin, P., Hong, D., Aman, M. G., et al. (2002). Research Units on Pediatric Psychopharmacology Autism Network. Risperidone in children with autism and serious behavioral problems. *New England Journal of Medicine, 347*(5), 314–321.

Millward, C., Ferriter, M., Calver, S., & Connell-Jones, G. (2008). Gluten- and casein-free diets for autistic spectrum disorder. *Cochrane Database of Systematic Reviews, 16*(2). DOI: 10.1002/14651858.CD003498.pub3.

Ming, X., Gordon, E., Kang, N., & Wagner, G. C. (2008). Use of clonidine in children with autism spectrum disorders. *Brain and Development, 30*(7), 454–460.

Muhle, R., Trentacoste, S. V., & Rapin, I. (2004). The genetics of autism. *Pediatrics, 113*(5), e472–486.

Nikolov, R. N., Bearss, K. E., Lettinga, J., Erickison, C., Rodowski, M., Aman, M. G., et al. (2009). Gastrointestinal symptoms in a sample of children with pervasive developmental disorders. *Journal of Autism and Developmental Disorders, 39*, 405–413.

Oberle, I., & Rousseau, R. (1991). Instability of a 550 base pair DNA segment and abnormal methylation in fragile X syndrome. *Science, 252*, 1097–1102.

O'Callaghan, F. J., Harris, T., Joinson, C., Bolton, P., Noakes, M., Presdee, D., et al. (2004). The relation of infantile spasms, tubers, and intelligence in tuberous sclerosis complex. *Archives of Diseases of Childhood, 89*, 530–533.

Posey, D. J., Aman, M. G., McCracken, J. T., Scahill, L., Tierney, E., Arnold, L. E., et al. (2007). Positive effects of methylphenidate on inattention and hyperactivity in pervasive developmental disorders: An analysis of secondary measures. *Biological Psychiatry, 61*(4), 538–544.

Rasalam, A., Hailey, H., Williams, J. H. G., Moore, S. J., Turnpenny, P. D., Lloyd, D. J., et al. (2005). Characteristics of fetal anticonvulsant syndrome associated autistic disorder. *Developmental Medicine and Child Neurology, 47*(8), 551–555.

Reed, H. E., McGrew, S. G., Artibee, K., Surdkya, K., Goldman, S. E., Frank, K., et al. (2009). Parent-based sleep education workshops in autism. *Journal of Child Neurology, 24*(8), 936–945.

Reichelt, K. L., Ekrein, J., & Scott, H. (1990). Gluten milk proteins and autism: Dietary intervention effects on behavior and peptide secretion. *Journal of Applied Nutrition, 42*, 1–11.

Richdale, A. L. (1999). Sleep problems in autism: Prevalence, cause, and intervention. *Developmental Medicine and Child Neurology, 41*(1), 60–66.

Rineer, S., Finucane, B., & Simon, E. W. (1998). Autistic symptoms among children and young adults with isodicentric chromosome 15. *American Journal of Medical Genetics, 81*, 428–433.

Rogers, S., Wehner, E., & Hagerman, R. J. (2001). The behavioral phenotype in fragile X: Symptoms of autism in very young children with fragile X syndrome, idiopathic autism, and other developmental disorders. *Journal of Developmental and Behavior Pediatrics, 22*, 409–417.

Ruble, L., Heflinger, C., Renfrew, J., & Saunders, R. (2005). Access and service use by children with autism spectrum disorders in Medicaid managed care. *Journal of Autism and Developmental Disorders, 35*(1), 3–13.

Shahbazian, M., Young, J., Yuva-Paylor, L., Spencer, C., Antalffy, B., Noebels, J., et al. (2002). Mice with truncated MeCP2 recapitulate many Rett syndrome features and display hyperacetylation of histone H3. *Neuron, 35*, 243–254.

Sherman, S. (2002). Epidemiology. In R. J. Hagerman, & P. J. Hagerman (Eds.), *Fragile X syndrome: Diagnosis, treatment and research* (3rd ed.) (pp. 363–427). Baltimore, MD: The Johns Hopkins University Press.

Shi, L., Fatemi, S. H., Sidwell, R. W., & Patterson, P. H. (2003). Maternal influenza infection causes marked behavioral and pharmacological changes in the offspring. *Journal of Neuroscience, 23(1)*, 297–302.

Taylor, B., Miller, E., Lingam, R., Andrews, N., Simmons, A., & Stowe, J. (2002). Measles, mumps, and rubella vaccination and bowel problems or developmental regression in children with autism: Population study. *British Medical Journal, 324*(7334), 393–396.

Tuchman, R., & Rapin, I. (2002). Epilepsy in autism. *Lancet Neurology, 1*, 352–358.

Varga, E. A., Pastore, M., Prior, T., Herman, G. E., & McBride, K. L. (2009). The prevalence of PTEN mutations in a clinical pediatric cohort with autism spectrum disorders, developmental delay, and macrocephaly. *Genetics in Medicine, 11*(2), 111–117.

Verkerk, A. J., Pieretti, M., Sutcliffe, J. S., Ying-Hui, F., Kuhl, D., Pizzuti, A., et al. (1991). Identification of a gene (FMR-1) containing a CGG repeat coincident with a breakpoint cluster region exhibiting length variant in fragile X syndrome. *Cell, 65*, 905–914.

The Waisman Center (2008). Available at http://www.waisman.wisc.edu/nmhai/. Accessed December 13,2010.

Webb, S. J., Nalty, T., Munson, J., Brock, C., Abbott, R., & Dawson, G. (2007). Rate of head circumference growth as a function of autism diagnosis and history of autistic regression. *Journal of Child Neurology, 22*(10), 1182–1190.

Whiteley, P., Rodgers, J., & Savery, D. (1999). A gluten-free diet as an intervention for autism and associated spectrum disorder: preliminary findings. *Autism, 3*, 45–65.

Zhou, J., Blundell, J., Ogawa, S., Kwon, C. H., Zhang, W., Sinton, C., et al. (2009). Pharmacological inhibition of mTORC1 suppresses anatomical, cellular, and behavioral abnormalities in neural-specific Pten knock-out mice. *Journal of Neuroscience, 29*, 1773–1783.

75 Kara Hume, Samuel L. Odom

Best Practice, Policy, and Future Directions: Behavioral and Psychosocial Interventions

Points of Interest

- Though individuals with ASDs have been receiving behavioral and psychosocial interventions for over 50 years, it has been difficult to clearly identify what practices are effective across age levels and skill domains.
- The National Professional Development Center on ASD, a federal initiative, has recently identified 24 evidence-based practices (EBP) for individuals with ASDs across domains and age levels.
- The National Standards Project, an initiative of the National Autism Center, identified 11 established practices for individuals with ASDs across domains and age levels and also conducted an evaluation of comprehensive treatment models serving individuals with ASDs.
- Once best practices are identified, implementation of the practices should be a systematic process that includes clear assessments of fidelity, as well as plans for sustainability.

Intervention for individuals with ASDs has a long and varied history—beginning primarily with psychodynamic therapy in the mid-1900s (Ruttenberg, 1971). Once deemed ineffective in treating ASDs, as the understanding of autism's cause began to shift, behavioral intervention emerged as an effective treatment in the early 1960s (Lovaas, 1971). Behavioral intervention refers to treatment derived from the field of applied behavior analysis, which includes a systematic application of behavioral principles and procedures. This type of intervention was first implemented under highly structured conditions (e.g., discrete trial training) and has more recently been applied in naturalistic settings and across skill domains. Psychosocial interventions, which are defined more broadly as any nonpharmacological treatment aimed at improving the functioning of individuals with ASDs, then followed (Seida et al., 2009). Psychosocial interventions include treatments in the fields of developmental and clinical psychology, cognitive-social learning theory, and sensory integrative therapy (Mesibov et al., 2005; Schreibman & Ingersoll, 2005).

Despite the long history, the efficacy of and evidence base for a number of behavioral and psychosocial interventions for individuals with ASDs, remains inexact. Selecting and implementing evidence-based practices for individuals with ASDs pose a number of challenges for practitioners across disciplines, as well as families selecting interventions for their child. Though mandated through educational policy (e.g., No Child Left Behind), professional standards (e.g., National Association of School Psychologists), and ethics conduct codes (e.g., Association for Behavior Analysis), the identification and usage of scientifically proven practices in the field of ASD can be difficult. Factors contributing to this difficulty include the wide variety of interventions available, the difficulty in discerning "true" evidence from potentially biased information touted by intervention developers, and the sheer volume of information available to practitioners and families via mass media. In addition, universally agreed upon standards by which to identify a practice as evidence-based have not yet been developed and often little guidance is provided to practitioners and families in finding and selecting evidence-based practices. Finally, once EBPs are identified, support for implementation is limited and policies related to adoption and usage are scant. The purpose of this chapter is to identify behavioral and psychosocial interventions and comprehensive treatment models that have evidence of efficacy for learners with ASDs, describe the implications of implementation science for promoting the use of efficacious practices and models in programs, and highlight current challenges to the service provision based on EBPs.

Efforts to Identify Efficacious Practices

To address these challenges, national professional organizations, researchers, and practitioners have begun to identify practices from the research literature that are evidence-based. In 2000, the National Academy of Sciences convened a committee to review research on educational practices for children with ASDs and their families, which subsequently generated general recommendations for practice (National Research Council, 2001). Some states, such as New York (www.health.state.ny.us/community/infants_children/early_intervention/autism/index.htm), have followed systematic processes for identifying intervention and educational practices for children with ASDs.

Scholarly reviews of the literature, reviews of reviews, and program evaluations have been conducted as well. For example, Iovannone, Dunlap, Huber, and Kincaid (2003) reviewed four studies (including the National Academy of Sciences report) and identified six core components of effective programs for individuals with ASDs. The identified components (e.g., individualized supports and services) were broad-based, however, and did not include recommendations for specific practices or treatment models. A number of additional reviews focus only on specific domains (e.g., problem behavior: Horner et al., 2002), research designs (e.g., single subject: Odom et al., 2003), and/or specific interventions (e.g., video modeling: Bellini & Akullian, 2007). Most recently, a systematic review of 30 research reviews related to behavioral and psychosocial interventions revealed a number of positive outcomes for many interventions (including behavioral and communication interventions) (Seida et al., 2009). However, the authors noted the difficulty in comparing and summarizing intervention effects across different outcomes with the use of different measures, and indicated that "uncertainty remains about best practices for the treatment of autism." (Seida et al., 2009, p. 103)

Classifying Interventions: A Note

When examining the evidence across behavioral and psychosocial interventions, an important distinction in intervention practices should be made. Two types of practices appear in the literature: focused intervention practices and comprehensive treatment models (Wolery & Garfinkle, 2002).

A *focused intervention* is a procedure designed to be utilized for a relatively brief period with the aim of producing specific behavioral and developmental changes related to targeted behaviors or skills (Odom, Collet-Klinenberg, et al., 2010). Focused interventions are utilized for a fairly brief period (e.g., several months) with the clear objective of changing targeted behaviors or skills (e.g., verbal language, attention to task). Ideally, focused interventions are based on explicit practitioner behavior that can be described and measured, such as prompting, reinforcement, discrete trial teaching, or use of visual schedules.

A *Comprehensive Treatment Model* (CTM) is a set of practices of relatively intense and lengthy duration designed to have a broad impact on a core deficit by using multiple components to target skills across multiple domains.

Comprehensive treatment models (CTMs) consist of a set of practices designed to achieve a broader learning or developmental impact on the core deficits of ASD, as described in previous chapters (National Research Council, 2001). They occur over an extended period of time (e.g., a year or years), are intense in their application (e.g., 25 hours per week), and usually have multiple components targeting skills across multiple domains. CTMs have been in existence for over 30 years and new models continue to be created. Examples of historic CTMs are the UCLA Young Autism Project (now the Lovaas Institute), Treatment and Education of Autistic and Communication Handicapped Children (TEACCH), the Denver Model, and the Princeton Child Development Institute (PCDI). When reviewing interventions, the National Professional Development Center on Autism Spectrum Disorders (NPDC) focused solely on focused interventions, while the National Standards Project (NSP) reviewed both focused interventions and CTMs.

Focused Intervention Practices

Two national centers have recently conducted independent and complementary reviews of focused intervention practices for individuals with ASDs. These national centers were charged with reviewing the intervention research literature, identifying standards for determining research quality evaluating research designs, categorizing evidence-based practices, and disseminating that information to practitioners and families. In 2007, the Office of Special Education Programs in the U.S. Department of Education funded the NPDC to promote the use of EBPs in programs for infants, children, and youth with ASDs and their families. An initial activity of this center has been to identify EBPs. In addition, the NSP, an initiative of the National Autism Center, has recently completed an exhaustive review of the strength of evidence for psychosocial and behavioral interventions for individuals with ASDs (NSP, 2009). These two efforts are the most current, comprehensive, evaluative reviews of the literature on focused intervention practices for learners with ASDs.

Criteria for Evidence

Several professional organizations have established criteria for determining whether an intervention is efficacious or evidence-based (Chambless & Hollon, 1998; Kratochwill & Stoiber, 2002; Odom et al., 2004). The criteria converge around several common indicators for the level of evidence provided by experimental/quasi-experimental group designs or single-case designs. The NPDC's criteria was drawn from the work of Nathan and Gorman (2007), Rogers and Vismara (2008), Odom and colleagues (2004), Horner and colleagues (2005), and Gersten and colleagues (2005).

In order for the NPDC to accept evidence about a practice from a particular study, the study had to: *(1)* have been conducted with participants diagnosed with ASDs who were between birth and 22 years of age, *(2)* have outcomes for those participants as dependent measures, *(3)* clearly demonstrate that the use of the practice was followed by gains in the targeted teaching skills, and *(4)* have adequate experimental control so that one could rule out most threats to internal validity (Gersten et al., 2005; Horner et al., 2005). When a research study met these criteria, it could qualify as evidence for a specific practice. For a specific practice to meet NPDC criteria for an EBP, the practice had to have evidence from: *(a)* at least two experimental or quasi-experimental group design studies carried out by independent investigators, *(b)* at least five single-case design studies from at least three independent investigators, or *(c)* a combination of at least one experimental/ quasi-experimental study and three single-case design studies from independent investigators.

The NSP developed a model for evaluating the research literature based on the work of health and psychology fields (Agency for Health Research and Quality, 2002; American Psychological Association Presidential Task Force on Evidence-based Practices, 2003). Similar to the NPDC, studies included in the NSP's review had to: *(1)* have been conducted with participants diagnosed with ASDs who were between birth and 22 years of age and *(2)* have outcomes for those participants as dependent measures. A Scientific Merit Rating Scale was developed and eligible studies were scored from 0 to 5 across five dimensions: *(1)* experimental rigor of the research design, *(2)* quality of the dependent variable, *(3)* evidence of treatment fidelity, *(4)* demonstration of participant ascertainment, and *(5)* generalization data collection. For example, when rating the design of the study, NSP reviewers scored items related to the number of participants, the number of groups, whether data were lost, and the overall study design. These scores were weighted and combined with a treatment effects rating (from beneficial to adverse) to produce a total strength of evidence classification system. Interventions were then assigned a classification of established, emerging, unestablished, or ineffective/harmful based on their scores.

Search Practices

Both the NPDC and the NSP conducted extensive and broad-based literature searches to locate peer-reviewed articles describing behavioral and psychosocial interventions and outcomes for individuals with ASDs. Detailed descriptions of the search processes can be found in work by Odom, Collet-Klinenberg, et al. (2010) and in the NSP's findings and conclusions (2009).

Identified Practices

NPDC

From their review of the literature, investigators with the NPDC have identified 24 EBPs, listed in Table 75-1. The practices are briefly defined in the table and further information about a number of the practices can be found in previous chapters (e.g., Chapter 59). Two sets of practices are grouped within a larger descriptor. The first subgroup is *Behavioral Teaching Strategies*, which are fundamental intervention techniques (e.g., prompting, reinforcement) based on the principles of applied behavior analysis. These strategies appear as parts of other focused interventions (e.g., prompting and reinforcement is a part of *Discrete Trial Training*), but they also have sufficient evidence to be listed independently. Second, NPDC grouped a set of strategies used primarily to reduce or eliminate interfering behaviors (e.g., tantrums, disruptive behavior, aggression, self-injury, repetitive behavior) under a general classification of *Positive Behavior Support* (PBS). The general PBS approach consists of individual focused interventions, organized around the results of functional behavioral assessment and ordered in level of intensity (Horner et al., 2002). In this grouping, NPDC included *Differential Reinforcement of Other Behavior* (DRO/A/I) as a special application of the use of reinforcement to the reduction of interfering behavior. The additional practices are listed alphabetically.

In Table 75-2, each EBP is listed in a domain by age-level matrix. This matrix allows one to see what EBPs have evidence of efficacy for teaching skills in specific educational domains, and across what age level the intervention is deemed evidence-based. For example, for naturalistic intervention, the table indicates that this practice has demonstrated efficacy across the three age groupings for teaching communication and social skills.

NSP

The NSP has identified 11 behavioral and psychosocial interventions as established and they are listed in alphabetical order in Table 75-3. An established intervention is defined by the NSP as one that "has sufficient available evidence to confidently determine that it produces favorable outcomes for individuals with ASD." (NSP, 2009, p. 10.) These interventions have several published, peer-reviewed studies that received a Scientific Merit Rating Scale score of 3, 4, or 5 (described above) and produced beneficial treatment effects for specific targets. The NSP has also grouped interventions into packages, such as the Antecedent Package (e.g., priming, teacher presence, choice), Behavioral Package (e.g., differential reinforcement, discrete trial training, token economy), and a Peer Training Package (e.g., Integrated Play Groups, circle of friends). In Tables 75-4 and 75-5, the established practices are presented across domains and age levels. These are presented as separate tables, as the domain by age level by practice data are not yet available.

Similarities and Differences in Findings between NPDC and NSP

Table 75-6 outlines the similarities between the findings of the two projects. Nineteen of the 24 interventions (79%) recognized as evidence-based by the NPDC are also considered

Table 75–1.
NPDC Identified evidence-based practices with descriptors

Evidence-Based Practice	Descriptor
Behavioral Strategies	
Prompting	Behaviorally based antecedent teaching strategy.
Reinforcement	Behaviorally based consequence teaching strategy.
Task analysis and chaining	Behaviorally based antecedent teaching strategy that breaks down steps and links them for prompting.
Time delay	Behaviorally based antecedent teaching strategy that promotes errorless learning.
Computer-aided instruction	The use of computers for varied instruction.
Discrete trial training (DTT)	One-to-one instructional strategy that teaches skills in a planned, controlled, and systematic manner.
Naturalistic interventions	A variety of strategies that closely resemble typical interactions and occur in natural settings, routines, and activities.
Parent-implemented interventions	Strategies that recognize and utilize parents as the most effective teachers of their children.
Peer-mediated instruction/intervention (PMII)	Strategies designed to increase social engagement by teaching peers to initiate and maintain interactions.
Picture Exchange Communication System (PECS)™	A system for communicating that uses the physical handing over of pictures or symbols to initiate communicative functions.
Pivotal Response Training (PRT)	An approach that teaches the learner to seek out and respond to naturally occurring learning opportunities.
Positive Behavioral Support Strategies	
Functional Behavior Assessment (FBA)	A systematic approach for determining the underlying function or purpose of behavior.
Stimulus control/Environmental modification	The modification or manipulation of environmental aspects known to impact a learner's behavior.
Response interruption/redirection	The physical prevention or blocking of interfering behavior with redirection to more appropriate behavior.
Functional Communication Training (FCT)	A systematic practice of replacing inappropriate or ineffective behavior with more appropriate or effective behaviors that serve the same function.
Extinction	Behaviorally based strategy that withdraws or terminates the reinforcer of an interfering behavior to reduce or eliminate the behavior.
Differential Reinforcement (DRA/I/O/L)	Behaviorally based strategies that focus reinforcement on alternative, incompatible, other, or lower rates of the interfering behavior in order to replace it with more appropriate behavior.
Self-management	A method in which learners are taught to monitor, record data, report on, and reinforce their own behavior.
Social narratives	Written narratives that describe specific social situations in some detail and are aimed at helping individuals to adjust to the situation or adapt their behavior.
Social skills training groups	Small group instruction with a shared goal or outcome of learned social skills in which participants can learn, practice, and receive feedback.
Structured work systems	Visually and physically structured sequences that provide opportunities for learners to practice previously taught skills, concepts, or activities.
Video modeling	Utilizes assistive technology as the core component of instruction and allows for prerehearsal of the target behavior or skill via observation.
Visual Supports	Tools that enable a learner to independently track events and activities.
VOCA/Speech Generating Devices (SGD)	Electronic, portable devices used to teach learners communication skills and as a means of communication.

From Odom, S., Collet-Klinenberg, L., Rogers, S., & Hatton, D. (2010). Evidence-based practices in interventions for children and youth with autism spectrum disorders. *Preventing School Failure, 54,* 275–282. Reproduced with permission.

Table 75–2.
NPDC EBP, X Learner outcome & age level matrix key

	Academics & Cognition			Behavior			Communication			Play			Social			Transition		
Evidence-Based Practices	EC	EL	MH	EC	EL	MH	EC	EL	MH	EC	EL	MH	EC	EL	MH	EC	EL	MH
Computer assisted anstruction	■	■	■															
Differential reinforcement				■	■	■	■	■	■				■	■	■			
Discrete trial training	■	■		■	■		■	■		■	■		■	■				
Extinction				■	■	■												
Functional Behavioral Assessment				■	■	■	■	■	■									
Functional Communication Training				■	■		■	■										
Naturalistic interventions							■	■	■				■	■	■			
Parent-implemented interventions				■	■		■	■		■	■		■	■				
Peer mediated instruction/intervention							■	■	■				■	■	■			
Picture Exchange Communication System				■	■	■	■	■	■				■	■	■			
Pivotal Response Training	■	■	■	■	■	■	■	■	■	■	■	■	■	■	■			
Prompting	■	■	■	■	■	■	■	■	■									
Reinforcement	■	■	■	■	■	■	■	■	■									
Response interruption & redirection	■	■	■	■	■	■												
Self-management	■	■	■	■	■	■	■	■	■	■	■	■	■	■	■	■	■	■
Social narratives	■	■	■	■	■	■	■	■	■	■	■	■	■	■	■			
Social skills groups							■	■	■				■	■	■			
Speech generating devices (VOCA)							■	■	■									
Stimulus control	■	■	■	■	■	■												
Structured work systems	■	■	■							■	■	■				■	■	■
Task analysis	■	■	■	■	■	■	■	■	■				■	■	■			
Time delay		■						■			■			■				
Video modeling	■	■	■				■	■	■	■	■	■	■	■	■			
Visual supports	■	■	■	■	■	■	■	■	■	■	■	■	■	■	■	■	■	■

EC = Early Childhood, ages 0 to 5 years.
EL = Elementary, ages 6 to 11 years.
MH = Middle/High, ages 12 to 22 years.
Notes: Shading indicates that there is an evidence base for a specific practice.
Colett-Klingenberg, L. & National Professional Development Center on ASD. (2009). *Matrix of evidence-based practice, outcomes, and age of participants with ASD.* Unpublished figure from presentation. Madison, WI: National Professional Development Center on ASD.

Table 75–3.
NSP-identified established practices with NSP descriptors

Established Practice	Descriptor
Antecedent package	Modification of situational events that precede challenging behavior.
Behavioral package	Interventions to reduce challenging behavior and teach functional alternatives.
Comprehensive behavioral treatment for young children	Comprehensive treatment programs that use a combination of behavioral analytic approaches.
Joint attention intervention	Interventions focused on teaching referencing/regulating others' behavior.
Modeling	Interventions using peers or adults to model appropriate target skill.
Naturalistic teaching strategies	Child-directed interactions occurring in natural settings.
Peer training package	Teaching children without disabilities how to elicit target behavior in children with ASDs.
Naturalistic interventions	A variety of strategies that closely resemble typical interactions and occur in natural settings, routines and activities.
Pivotal Response Treatment (PRT)	Teaching pivotal behaviors in natural environment producing naturalized behavioral improvements.
Schedules	Task list that communicates a series of activities.
Self-management	Teaching individuals to regulate their own behaviors.
Story-based intervention package	Written descriptions of a situation that assist in eliciting target behavior.

Table 75–5.
NSP-established practices, X age level matrix key

Established Practices	E C	E L	M H
Antecedent package			
Behavioral package			
Comprehensive behavioral treatment for young children			
Joint attention intervention			
Modeling			
Naturalistic teaching strategies			
Peer training package			
Pivotal response treatment (PRT)			
Schedules			
Self-management			
Story-based intervention package			

Notes: Shading indicates that there is an evidence base for a specific practice.

established practices by the NSP. Four of the NPDC's evidence-based practices (computer-aided instruction, Picture Exchange Communication System, social skills training groups, speech generating devices) are deemed "emerging" by the NSP report, while one of the NPDC's practices is not identified as "established" or "emerging" practices by the NSP (parent-implemented interventions). In addition, the NSP identified one focused intervention practice that was not identified by the NPDC (joint attention intervention and comprehensive behavioral treatment for young children, as the NPDC did not review comprehensive treatment models).

Table 75–4.
NSP-established practices, X learner outcome matrix key

	Academics & Cognition	Behavior	Communication	Play	Interpersonal	Self-Regulation
Established practices						
Antecedent package						
Behavioral package						
Comprehensive behavioral treatment for young children						
Joint attention intervention						
Modeling						
Naturalistic teaching strategies						
Peer training package						
Pivotal response treatment (PRT)						
Schedules						
Self-management						
Story-based intervention package						

Notes: Shading indicates that there is an evidence base for a specific practice.

Table 75–6.
Similarities between NPDC and NSP

	NSP Established Practices										
	Antecedent Package	Behavioral Package	CBTYC[3]	Joint Attention[3]	Modeling	Naturalistic	Peer Training	PRT	Schedules	Self-Management	Story-Based
Prompting	X										
Reinforcement	X										
Task analysis		X									
Time delay	X										
Computer-aided instruction[1]											
DTT		X									
Naturalistic interventions						X					
Parent-implemented[2]											
PMI							X				
PECS[1]											
PRT								X			
FBA		X									
FCT		X									
Stimulus control	X										
Response interruption		X									
Extinction		X									
Differential reinforcement		X									
Self-management										X	
Social narratives											X
Social skills training groups[1]											
Structured work systems									X		
Video modeling					X						
Visual supports									X		
SGD[1]											

X = Practice is recognized by both NPDC and NSP.
1 = Recognized by NSP as an emerging practice.
2 = Not recognized by NSP as established or emerging.
3 = Not recognized by NPDC as an EBP.

Comprehensive Treatment Models

As described previously, there remains a scarcity of evaluation or comparative evaluation information about CTMs. In their review of the literature, members of the National Academy of Sciences Committee on Educating Children with Autism (National Research Council, 2001) identified a set of widely acknowledged comprehensive treatment models and common features that exist across models, but they did not examine efficacy of the models. In a recent critical review of CTMs for young children with ASDs and their families, Rogers and Vismara (2008) evaluated the current research on comprehensive treatments for young children with ASDs, finding limited evidence of efficacy for all but the Lovaas model, with some limited support for Pivotal Response Treatment (PRT) (Koegel et al., 1999). Focusing only on a single model, Reichow and Wolery (2009) documented substantial support for the UCLA Young Autism Project Model (the Lovaas model), especially when the researchers were trained by model developers, hours of therapy were high, and the duration of the intervention was long. A second independent review by Howlin, Magiati, and Charman (2009) drew similar conclusions, but also found that documentation of the fidelity of implementation of the CTMs in the studies was often limited.

The previous summaries of the empirical evidence suggested that one may draw practical recommendations by examining features of CTMs that appear to be efficacious (National Research Council, 2001; Rogers & Vismara, 2008). Working with Autism Guidelines Project funded by the State of California Department of Development Services and with assistance from the National Standards Project, Odom, Boyd, Hall, and Hume (2010) conducted a multidimensional evaluation to examine features of CTMs. The purpose of the evaluation was to supply information to service providers so that they could make decisions about adopting a CTM, family members could make decisions about selecting a CTM for the individual with the ASD within their family, or a researcher could determine questions for future research. This process is summarized in the subsequent sections.

Criteria for Evidence

Odom, Boyd and colleagues (2010) defined CTMs by six criteria, which represent the inclusion/exclusion criteria. First, a description of the model and its components had to be published in a refereed journal article, book chapter, or book. Second, at least a single procedural guide, manual, curriculum, or description should exist to define the model. Third, the model must have a clear theoretical or conceptual framework. This framework must be published in one of the formats noted previously. Fourth, the model must address multiple developmental or behavioral domains that, at a minimum, represent the core features of autism spectrum disorder (i.e., social competence, communication, repetitive behaviors). Fifth, the model must be intensive. Intensity is defined by the number of hours the model is implemented per week (e.g., National Academy of Sciences Committee recommended 25 hours or more), longevity (e.g., model implementation extends across a period equal to or greater than a typical school year, which is usually 9 to 10 months), and/or engagement (i.e., a planned set of activities or procedures actively engage the child/person with autism in learning experiences consistent with the model). Finally, the sixth criterion was that the CTM must have been implemented in at least one site in the United States.

When a CTM was identified as having met the inclusion criteria, evaluators assembled a portfolio of evidence needed for evaluating the model, including published journal articles and/or chapters, web pages, books, curricula, and/or procedural manuals. Models were scored on a 0 to 5 rating scale on each of six domains: *(1)* operationalization, *(2)* implementation measures, *(3)* replication, *(4)* type of empirical evidence, *(5)* quality of the research methodology, and *(6)* complementary evidence from studies of focused interventions.

Search Practices

CTMs were located through several sources. First, a systematic and thorough review of the literature was conducted. A search in PsychINFO and EBSCO was initiated using the keywords *autism, comprehensive, treatment, program description,* and *intervention*. CTMs also tend to be described in book chapters and literature reviews, so the NSP surveyed well-known books that include chapter identifications of such models (e.g., Handleman & Harris, 2006, 2008), books that have reviewed the evidence from the field (e.g., National Research Council, 2001), and highly visible handbooks (e.g., Volkmar et al., 2005). Evaluators presented the information from this project in public forums and at conference presentations. Audience members were asked to review the list of CTMs identified, and to recommend models that were missed.

Identified Models

Evaluators identified a total of 30 CTMs using the inclusion criteria previously described. The ratings for each model are presented in Table 75-7. For more detailed descriptions of the models, please refer to Odom, Boyd, et al. (2010). As noted, the ratings range from 0 to 5, with 5 being the highest. Rather than generating a single summary score, this review established a profile across dimensions of the evaluation. This profile depicts the CTMs that have the stronger and weaker evidence for each dimension. Models that have ratings of 4 or 5 across dimensions of the evaluation have stronger evidence of what NSP calls "model development." That is, they are procedurally well-documented, they have been replicated, and there is some evidence of efficacy, even if limited. These models include: Denver, Learning Experiences: an Alternative Program for preschoolers and parents (LEAP), Lovaas Institute, May Institute, and Princeton Child Development Institute (PCDI). There are other models

Table 75–7.
NSP's ratings of CTMs

Program	Operationalization	Fidelity	Replication	Outcome data	Quality	Additional studies
Alpine	5	3	5	3	N/A	2
Autism Partnerships	5	3	5	0	N/A	1
CARD	5	4	4	3	N/A	2
Children's Toddler	2	3	1	5	3	2
Developmentally Appropriate Treatment for Autism (DATA)	3	1	5	3	N/A	2
Denver	5	4	5	5	2	0
DIR	5	3	5	4	2	0
Douglass	5	3	0	5	3	5
Eden	3	2	0	0	N/A	0
Hanen	2	0	1	3	N/A	2
Higashi	2	0	2	3	N/A	0
Institute for Child. Development	3	2	0	3	N/A	0
Lancaster	2	0	0	0	N/A	0
LEAP	4	5	5	4	2	5
Lovaas Institute	5	4	5	5	3	5
May Institute	5	4	5	4	2	5
Miller	3	1	5	4	0	1
PCDI	5	4	5	4	2	5
PRT	4	3	5	4	2	5
Pyramid	2	3	4	3	N/A	5
Responsive Teaching	3	3	0	5	3	0
Relationship Development Intervention (RDI)	5	3	0	4	2	0
SCERTS	5	0	0	0	N/A	4
Son Rise	3	0	0	2	N/A	0
Strategies for Teaching Based on Autism Research (STAR)	5	3	5	4	2	0
Summit	3	4	0	0	N/A	0
TEACCH	3	3	5	5	2	2
Therapeutic Pathways	5	4	3	4	3	0
Valley	3	3	5	0	N/A	0
Walden	4	3	4	3	N/A	2

Odom, S. L., Boyd, B. A., Hall, L. J., & Hume, K. (2010). Evaluation of comprehensive treatment models for individuals with Autism Spectrum Disorders. *Journal of Autism and Developmental Disorders. 40,* 425–436. Reproduced with permission.

Note: Errata information from Odom, Boyd, et al. (2010) has been incorporated in this table.

that have ratings of 4 or 5 on less than four domains, but there remain features of the model that could be strengthened. These include: Autism Partnerships, Center for Autism and Related Disorders, Inc (CARD), Children's Toddler Program, Developmental, Individual-Difference, Relationship-Based Model (DIR), Douglass, Responsive Teaching, Social Communication and Emotional Regulation, and implementing Transactional Supports (SCERTS), and Treatment and Education of Autistic and related Communication handicapped CHildren (TEACCH). Also, there are some models that received very low evaluation ratings across the board. These included Hanen, Higashi, Eden, Summit, Lancaster, and Son Rise. Again, potential consumers may use this as a general guide when determining the degree of model development and level of efficacy evidence that exists for individual CTMs.

As a group, CTMs were strongest in the operationalization of their models. Given the strength of the operationalization dimension, it was surprising that measurement of implementation was relatively weak in comparison. When CTMs are designed as models that may be adopted by service providers, the availability of implementation instruments would be a critical feature because they would allow: *(a)* the developer to observe and document the use of their model, and *(b)* the adopter to evaluate their own implementation. This is a much-needed direction for future developers of CTMs.

As a group, CTM projects reported frequent replications by individuals outside of the central project. Nearly half the CTM developers (14 out of 30) reported that two or more independent sites had replicated their model. Some sites reported replication by dozens of programs (e.g., TEACCH, Lovaas, DIR, LEAP). Across CTMs, the published evidence of efficacy was not strong. Over half (16 out of 30) of the CTMs had no publication of efficacy in peer-reviewed journals, although often they did report efficacy data in book chapters or from their program reports. Some models (Lovaas Institute, Responsive Teaching, Children's Toddler School, TEACCH) had at least two publications of efficacy in peer-reviewed journals, and among these the Lovaas Institute has the most extensive record of publications, which as noted earlier, had been found also by other authors (Howlin et al., 2009; Reichow & Wolery, 2009; Rogers & Vismara, 2008).

Promoting the Use of Evidence-Based Practices and Comprehensive Treatment Models: Implementation Science

The science of intervention has led to the identification of focused intervention practices and comprehensive treatment models having evidence that they produce positive developmental and learning outcomes for learners with ASDs and their families. A summary of these findings appears in previous sections. A common and naive assumption from some scientists is that if effective practices are identified, then service providers will employ them in their work with learners with ASDs. This logic fails in two ways. First, the professional development literature indicates that having a practitioner read about a practice or model of treatment or even learn about it in a workshop does not usually lead to use in classrooms, homes, or community (Joyce & Showers, 2002). Second, even if service providers use a practice or comprehensive treatment model, the key features of the practice or model have to be delivered in the way that they were delivered in the research documenting that documented their efficacy (Durlak & DuPre, 2008). Both of these issues, adoption of a practice to be used in a program and fidelity of implementation, are central constructs of an emerging field in human services called *implementation science*. In this section, we will describe implementation science, as it is employed in a range of disciplines for promoting wide-scale implementation.

Implementation Science

"Implementation research is the scientific study of methods to promote the systematic uptake of research findings and other EBP into routine practice, and, hence, to improve the quality and effectiveness of health services and care." (Eccles & Mittman, 2006, p. 1.) The definition of implementation and its measurement are factors associated with use in classrooms. Purveyors (i.e., EBP or CTM developers) have typically taken two approaches to assessing implementation at the program level. First, they may assess the amount of an intervention a learner with an ASD receives. O'Donnell (2008) referred to this as a structural approach to implementation. The metric may be number of lessons completed, number of trials delivered, or number of minutes in intervention. For example, the National Academy of Sciences' Committee on Educating Children with Autism proposed that children with autism receive at least 25 hours of an intensive intervention program each week (National Research Council, 2001).

Second, purveyors assess implementation by observing and rating the quality of implementation, which O'Donnell (2008) noted as a process approach to implementation measurement. For example, in their research on the relative treatment effects for preschool-age children with ASDs for two CTMs (i.e., TEACCH and LEAP), Hume and colleagues (2009) developed implementation measures describing the key features of each program model, and conducted 194 observations using the measures across 34 classrooms. Internal consistency reliability analyses and descriptive discriminant analyses were conducted and the measures were found to be reliable (total alphas ranged across measure from .93 to .94) and to clearly discriminate the models from one another and from a "business as usual" classroom not using either CTM.

Unfortunately, assessment of implementation occurs rarely in the ASD literature. In their review of the intervention literature from 1970 to the early 1990s, Wolery and Garfinkle (2002) found that only 13% of the studies reported procedural fidelity information. When reviewing only single-case design studies (SCDs) involving young children with ASD and published from 1990 to 2003, Odom and colleagues (2003) found that 32% of the studies had fidelity measures. For CTMs, Odom, Boyd and colleagues (2010) found that 22 of the 30 models have some form of implementation assessment, but only nine could provide evidence of inter-rater agreement, and only one had documented the internal consistency form of reliability for their measures.

In addition to the importance of having fidelity of implementation measures for documenting the actual implementation of EBPs, such measures may prove to be useful tools for providing feedback to teachers (e.g., through coaching or consultation) on their use of specific EBPs or their implementation of the CTM. In addition, they may be used to assist service providers in self-monitoring their own use of practices. The NPDC has developed implementation checklists for each of the practices it has identified as having an evidence base (Odom, Colett-Klingenberg et al., 2010), and the checklists are currently placed in modules that will appear on the website of the Ohio Center for Autism and Low Incidence Disabilities (http://www.ocali.org/aim/).

From Implementation to Scaling up and Sustainability

To move science into practice on a broader-than-single-classroom scale, implementation scientists have elaborated on the ecological systems models of Bronfenbrenner (1979) and others to determine the factors in distal (from the learner and classroom) levels of an organization that may affect the "uptake" of EBPs and be sustainable across time (Durlak & DuPre, 2008). Fixsen, Naoom, Blase, Friedman, and Wallace (2005) proposed a multilevel model of implementation that has core implementation features (e.g., training, coaching) at the center, but is seated within a second system level of organizational components (e.g., site selection, administration), and a third even more distal level of influence factors (e.g., economic, political). They propose that implementation at a school district or system level is a six-phase process, beginning with exploration and adoption and ending with sustainability. For working with early childhood special education programs, Kahn and colleagues (2009) have articulated a model for achieving long-term systems change to support high-quality early-intervention practices for all children with disabilities, which involves establishing a multilevel plan that includes state infrastructure, professional development systems, local infrastructure, and local context (e.g., classroom or program).

To promote service providers' use of EBPs with learners having ASDs, the NPDC has developed a multisystem approach to promoting service providers' use of EBPs for children with ASDs. Basing their conceptual framework on the work by Fixsen and colleagues (2005), Kahn and colleagues (2009) and others, the process begins with states applying to work with the NPDC and completing a detailed plan of their involvement and the infrastructure support they would provide. Over a 2-year period, project staff work with state planning teams to share research information about the assessment of quality in programs, EBPs, the process for linking learner goals and specific EBPs, and the process for documenting learner progress. NPDC staff and technical assistance support team collaborate in the first year to provide the coaching and consultation to classroom staff for promoting use of EPBs. The NPDC team systematically withdraws it support from the state's planning and technical assistance teams during the second year of their involvement. The efficacy of this type of support for producing changes at the state, classroom, and child levels is now being evaluated.

Future Trends and Directions

An active research literature on focused intervention practices and comprehensive treatment models now fuels the potential for increasing the quality of services provided to learners with ASDs and the prospect for more positive outcomes. This literature, and the glaring absences that exist in parts of the literature, provide insights into possible future directions in intervention research and service provision. In this concluding section, we will examine the types of models that are currently being developed or will need to be developed in the future, the changing demographics of the populations of the United States and its implications for ASDs, and the necessary economic and professional infrastructure needed for providing high-quality services.

EBPs and CTM Development

Identification of EBPs from the research literature is like shooting at a moving target. There are many journals that publish intervention research on ASDs, so even when a thorough review is conducted, its currency is limited and ongoing updates are necessary. For example, the newest literature in the reviews conducted by the NSP and the NPDC will be 3 years old by the time this chapter reaches publication. Documented practices will not necessarily go out of date, but literature will begin to support new practices. For example, when Odom and colleagues (2003) conducted their review, the social stories intervention was identified as an emerging practice but there had not yet been a sufficient number of studies demonstrating its efficacy, but when the NPDC conducted their review in 2007, a sufficient number of studies had been published to support it as an EBP (Odom, Colett-Klingenberg, et al., 2010). For the field, ongoing surveillance of the literature will be necessary to benefit from the most current science.

As illustrated in Table 75-2, which showed the ages of children for which there was efficacy evidence for focused intervention practices, most evidence was grouped around the preschool and elementary age ranges. Similarly, for CTMs identified by Odom, Boyd, and colleagues (2010), the majority focused on preschool-age and elementary-age children. Focused intervention research and model development in the future will clearly need to be designed for participants younger than or older than the preschool and elementary age range. Already there is much activity at the infant/toddler level. Drawing from the summary by Odom, Boyd, and colleagues (2010) of CTMs, Boyd, Odom, Humphreys, and Sam (2010) identified five CTMs that have been developed specifically for infants and toddlers. In the future, major contributions to the infant/toddler intervention area will be publication of efficacy studies from projects within the Toddler Treatment Network, which has been funded by Autism Speaks (www.autismspeaks.org/science/research/initiatives/toddler_treatment_network.php). Along with a concerted focus on early screening and identification (Boyd et al., 2010), the possibility of efficacious services being available for infants and toddlers with autism is bright, although the caveat will come with funding, which will be described subsequently.

A glaring weakness in the field is evidence-based focused intervention practices and CTMs for middle-school and high-school students with ASDs (Odom, Colett-Klingenberg, et al., 2010). Practices identified for younger children can be effective with older learners with ASDs, but they must be adapted for developmental differences, a broad range of expectations, and a variety of contexts. Models that support students with ASDs attending inclusive middle- and high-school classes and school-to-work models that prepare students for the future in the community are largely underresearched. The National Institutes of Health Interagency Autism Coordinating Committee (2008) has identified as a priority the development and evaluation of practices and models for adolescents with ASDs, so this may well be a direction for research and development in the future.

Population Demographics and Provision of Services

The population demographics of the United States is changing, with our citizenry becoming more racially, ethnically, and linguistically diverse. Although it appears that ASDs are not associated with racial, cultural, and socioeconomic status (Fombonne, 2003), that does not mean that racial and cultural issues do not have an effect on the development and skills acquisition for children of color with ASDs. In their demographic analysis of a surveillance study for ASDs, Mandell and colleagues (2009) significant disparities in the frequency of diagnoses of ASDs, with African-American and Latino children significantly underdiagnosed. In reviews of interventions for participants with ASDs and other developmental disabilities, often information about the ethnic or racial characteristics of participants is not provided at all. In reviews by Odom and colleagues (2003) and Karasu and Odom (2009), the authors found few studies reported racial or ethnic information. Although it is likely that the central features of EBPs and CTMs will be effective for learners from diverse ethnic, racial, and linguistic backgrounds, ways in which interventions are delivered, information is shared, and families are involved may be different for children and families from some racially, ethnically, and linguistically different groups. The challenge for the field will be to build procedural systems that will allow implementation of key features of intervention in different cultural contexts.

Necessary Infrastructure with States to Support Use of Evidence-Based Practices

As noted previously, a large-scale movement to support the use of EBPs requires an infrastructure that will support professional development and implementation within states. The National Academy of Science Committee report (National Research Council, 2001) described previously noted that building such an infrastructure was a feature to promoting the quality of services for learners with ASDs. Such an infrastructure would ideally provide training to service providers, but importantly, also establish a system of ongoing coaching and consultation at the local level (Hall, 2009). It may also incorporate the rapidly advancing use of technology (e.g., web-based training modules, telemedicine), communities of practice, and peer coaching (Odom, 2009). Some states have invested in such an infrastructure (e.g., Indiana, Pennsylvania), while others are in the process of building such supports (e.g., states now working with the NPDC). However, without such support from this distal-system level, substantial change at the local district and classroom level is likely to be limited.

Conclusion

In recent years, considerable effort has been placed on identifying practices having scientific evidence of efficacy in producing positive outcomes for learners with ASDs. Reviews of the literature have found focused intervention practices and comprehensive treatment model programs that are evidence-based. Yet, a challenge for the field will be to support the use of efficacious practices in programs for learners with ASDs. Models for scaling up the use of practices have emerged from the field of implementation science and may well provide a basis for supporting the use of evidence-based practices in services for learners with ASDs. Yet, there are continued challenges for the field. These include the following:

- Ongoing surveillance of the literature to identify new practices that supported are by future research (especially for infant/toddler and middle-school/high-school programs) and further substantiation of EBPs and CTMs already identified;
- Development of EBPs and CTMs for adolescents and young adults with ASDs will be important;
- Creation of focused intervention and CTM procedures appropriate for and effective with learners with ASDs and their families who are racially, ethnically, and/or linguistically different from the majority culture in the United States;

- Establishment of infrastructure within states to promote the high-quality services and use of evidence-based practices at the local level.

SUGGESTED READINGS

National Autism Center's National Standards Project (2009). Findings and conclusions. Available at http://www.nationalautismcenter.org/ (accessed October 21, 2009).

Odom, S. L., Boyd, B. A., Hall, L. J., & Hume, K. (2010). Evaluation of comprehensive treatment models for individuals with Autism Spectrum Disorders. *Journal of Autism and Developmental Disorders. 40*, 425–436.

Odom, S., Collet-Klinenberg, L., Rogers, S., & Hatton, D. (2010). Evidence-based practices in interventions for children and youth with autism spectrum disorders. *Preventing School Failure, 54*, 275–282.

ACKNOWLEDGMENTS

The production of this chapter was supported by Project No. H32G070004 from the Office of Special Education Programs and Project No. R324B070219 from the Institute of Education Sciences, both within the U.S. Department of Education. Also, the authors express their appreciation to Dr. Susan Wilczynski and the National Standards Project for their assistance.

REFERENCES

Agency for Health Research and Quality (2002). Systems to rate the strength of scientific evidence. In S. West, V. King, T. Carey, K. Lohr, & N. McKoy (Eds.), *Evidence Report/Technology Assessment No. 47*. Research Triangle Park, NC : Prepared by the Research Triangle Institute.

American Psychological Association Presidential Task Force on Evidence-Based Practices (2003). *Report of the Task Force on Evidence-Based Interventions in School Psychology*. Available at http://www.madison.k12.in.us/MCSWeb/CSSU/EBI%20Manual.pdf (accessed on July 9, 2009).

Bellini, S., & Akullian, J. (2007). A meta-analysis of video modeling and video self-modeling interventions for children and adolescents with autism spectrum disorders. *Exceptional Children, 73*, 264–287.

Boyd, B. A., Odom, S. L., Humphreys, B. P., & Sam, A. M. (2010). Infants and toddlers with autism spectrum disorder: Early identification and early intervention. *Journal of Early Intervention, 32*, 75–98.

Bronfenbrenner, U. (1979). *The ecology of human development*. Cambridge, MA: Harvard University Press.

Chambless, D. L., & Hollon, S. D. (1998). Defining empirically supported therapies. *Journal of Consulting and Clinical Psychology, 66*, 7–18.

Colett-Klingenberg, L. & National Professional Development Center on ASD. (2009). *Matrix of evidence-based practice, outcomes, and age of participants with ASD*. Unpublished figure from presentation. Madison, WI: National Professional Development Center on ASD.

Durlak, J. A., & DuPre, E. P. (2008). Implementation matters: A review of research on the influence of implementation on program outcomes and the factors affecting implementation. *American Journal of Community Psychology, 41*, 327–350.

Eccles, M. P., & Mittman, B. S. (2006). Welcome to *Implementation Science. Implementation Science, 1*, 1–3.

Fixsen, D. L., Naoom, S. F., Blase, K. A., Friedman, R. M., & Wallace, F. (2005). *Implementation research: A synthesis of the literature*. Tampa, FL: University of South Florida, Louis de la Parte Florida Mental Health Institute, The National Implementation Network (FMHI Publication 231).

Fombonne, E. (2003). Epidemiological surveys of autism and other pervasive developmental disorders: An update. *Journal of Autism and Developmental Disorders, 33*, 365–382.

Gersten, R., Fuchs, L. S., Compton, D., Coyne, M., Greenwood, C., & Innocenti, M. S. (2005). Quality indicators for group experimental and quasi-experimental research in special education. *Exceptional Children, 71*, 149–164.

Hall, L. J. (2009). *Autism spectrum disorders: From theory to practice*. Columbus, OH: Merrill Publishing Co.

Handleman, J. S., & Harris, S. L. (Eds.) (2008). *Preschool education programs for children with autism*. Austin, TX: PRO-ED.

Handleman, J. S., & Harris, S. L. (Eds.) (2006). *School-age education programs for children with autism*. Austin, TX: PRO-ED.

Horner, R. H., Carr, E. G., Halle, J., McGee, G., Odom, S., & Wolery, M. (2005). The use of single-subject research to identify evidence-based practice in special education. *Exceptional Children, 71*, 165–179.

Horner, R. H., Carr, E. G., Stain, P. S., Todd, A. W., & Reed, H. K. (2002). Problem behavior interventions for young children with autism: A research synthesis. *Journal of Autism and Developmental Disorders, 32*, 423–446.

Howlin, P., Magiati, I., & Charman, T. (2009). Systematic review of early intensive behavioral interventions for children with autism. *American Journal of Intellectual and Developmental Disabilities, 114*, 23–41.

Hume, K, Boyd, B., Coman, D., Gutierrez, A., Shaw, E., Sperry, L., et al. (2009, May). *Discriminant analysis and reliability evaluation of fidelity measures for comprehensive treatment models serving young children with ASD*. International Meeting for Autism Research. Chicago, IL.

Interagency Autism Coordinating Committee (2008). *The Interagency Autism Coordinating Committee strategic plan for ASD research*. Washington, DC: National Institute of Mental Health. (retrieved from http://iacc.hhs.gov/strategic-plan/2008/rfi-on-draft-strategic-plan-asd-research-august.shtml on July 13, 2009).

Iovannone, R., Dunlap, G., Huber, H., & Kincaid, D. (2003). Effective educational practices for students with autism spectrum disorders. *Focus on Autism and Other Developmental Disabilities, 18*, 150–166.

Joyce, B., & Showers, B. (2002). *Student achievement through staff development* (3rd ed.). Alexandra, VA: Association for Supervision and Curriculum Development.

Kahn, L., Hurth, J., Kasperzak, C. M., Diefendorf, M. J., Goode, S. E., & Ringwalt, S. S. (2009). The National Early Childhood Technical Assistance Center model for long-term systems change. *Topics in Early Childhood Special Education, 29*, 24–40.

Karasu, N., & Odom, S. L. (2009). *Evidence-based interventions to promote sound and communication skills: A meta-analysis of single subject design studies*. Manuscript submitted for publication.

Kratochwill, T. R., & Stoiber, K. C. (2002). Evidence-based interventions in school psychology: Conceptual foundations of the Procedural and Coding Manual of Division 16 and the Society for the Study of School Psychology. *School Psychology Quarterly, 17*, 341–389.

Lovaas, I. (1971). Considerations in the development of a behavioral treatment program for psychotic children. In D. Churchill, G. Alpern, & M. DeMyer (Eds.), *Infantile autism: Proceedings of the Indiana University Colloquium* (pp. 124–144). Springfield, IL: Charles C. Thomas.

Mandell, D. S., Wiggins, L. D., Carpenter, L. A., Daniels, J., DiGuisepppi, C., Durkin, M. S., et al., (2009). Racial/ethnic disparites in the identification of children with autism spectrum disorders. *American Journal of Public Health, 99*, 493–498.

Mesibov, G., Shea, V., & Schopler, E. (2005). *The TEACCH approach to autism spectrum disorders*. New York: Plenum Press.

Nathan, P. E., & Gorman, J. M. (2007). *A guide to treatments that work* (3rd ed.). New York: Oxford University Press.

National Autism Center's National Standards Project (2009). Findings and conclusions. Available at http://www.nationalautismcenter.org/(accessed October 21, 2009).

National Research Council (2001). *Educating children with autism*. Washington, DC: National Academy Press.

Odom, S. L. (2009). The tie that binds: Evidence-based practice, implementation science, and child outcomes. *Topics in Early Childhood Special Education, 29*, 53–61.

Odom, S. L., Boyd, B. A., Hall, L. J., & Hume, K. (2010). Evaluation of comprehensive treatment models for individuals with Autism Spectrum Disorders. *Journal of Autism and Developmental Disorders, 40*, 425–436.

Odom, S. L., Brantlinger, E., Gersten, R., Horner, R. D., Thompson, B., Harris, K. (2004). *Quality indicators for research in special education and guidelines for evidence-based practices: Executive summary*. Arlington, VA: Council for Exceptional Children Division for Research.

Odom, S. L., Brown, W. H., Frey, T., Karasu, N., Smith-Carter, L., & Strain, P. S. (2003). Evidence-based practices for young children with autism: Evidence from single subject design research. *Focus on Autism, 18*, 176–181.

Odom, S., Collet-Klinenberg, L., Rogers, S., & Hatton, D. (2010). Evidence-based practices in interventions for children and youth with autism spectrum disorders. *Preventing School Failure, 54*, 275 –282.

Odom, S. L., Hanson, M. J., Lieber, J., Diamond, K., Palmer, S., Butera, G., et al. (in press). Prevention, early childhood intervention, and implementation science. In B. Doll, W. Pfohl, & J. Yoon (Eds.), *Handbook of youth prevention science*. New York: Routledge.

O'Donnell, C. L. (2008). Defining, conceptualizing, and measuring fidelity of implementation and its relationship to outcomes in K-12 curriculum intervention research. *Review of Educational Research, 78*, 33–84.

Reichow, B., & Wolery, M. (2009). Comprehensive synthesis of early intensive behavioral interventions for young children with autism based on the UCLA young autism project model. *Journal of Autism and Developmental Disorders, 39*, 23–41.

Rogers, S., & Vismara, L. (2008). Evidence-based comprehensive treatments for early autism. *Journal of Clinical Child and Adolescent Psychology, 37*, 8–38.

Ruttenberg, B. A. (1971). A psychoanalytic understanding of infantile autism and its treatment. In D. Churchill, G. Alpern, & M. DeMyer (Eds.), *Infantile autism: Proceedings of the Indiana University Colloquium* (pp. 145–184). Springfield, IL: Charles C. Thomas.

Seida, J., Ospona, M., Karkhaneh, M., Hartling, L., Smith, V., & Clark, B. (2009). Systematic reviews of psychosocial interventions for autism: An umbrella review. *Developmental Medicine and Child Neurology, 51*, 95–104.

Schreibman, L., & Ingersoll, B. (2005). Behavioral interventions to promote learning in individuals with autism. In F. Volkmer, R. Paul, A. Klin, & D. Cohen (Eds.), *Handbook of autism and pervasive developmental disorders* (pp. 882–896). Hoboken, NJ: John Wiley & Sons.

Volkmar, F., Paul, R., Klin, A., & Cohen, D. (Eds.) (2005). *Handbook of autism and pervasive developmental disorders* (3rd ed.). Hoboken, NJ: John H. Wiley and Sons, Inc.

Wolery, M., & Garfinkle, A. N. (2002). Measures in intervention research with young children who have autism. *Journal of Autism and Developmental Disorders, 32*, 463–478.

76 James T. McCracken

Pharmacotherapy for Autism Spectrum Disorders

Points of Interest

- Studies of dopamine, serotonin, glutamate, and acetylcholine in ASDs suggest drug targets.
- Effective treatments have been demonstrated for two targets of severe irritability and hyperactive-impulsive behaviors.
- Clinical monitoring tools have emerged from the methods of clinical trials.
- Core ASD domains are largely untouched by current drug treatments.

Introduction

Children, adolescents, and adults with the full range of the ASDs are frequently referred for possible pharmacologic treatment for an array of associated difficult-to-manage behaviors, and to support adaptation and progress from other forms of interventions. Indeed, recent surveys of individuals with ASDs have documented an increasing acceptance of psychotropic medications as an often-reached-for component of treatment, with as many as 3/4 of individuals with ASDs reportly receiving a psychotropic medication within the past year (Esbensen et al., 2009). Furthermore, the use of multiple psychotropic medications, and other complementary and alternative treatments, is commonplace. These survey data observe that the frequency of use of psychotropic medications in the context of ASDs may be continuing to increase substantially (Esbensen et al., 2009; Martin et al., 1999). Such widespread use of pharmacotherapy for individuals with ASDs demands a careful appreciation of the evidence base for these treatments. In this chapter, we review the available evidence for each of the major drug classes, as well as information regarding their safety and optimal use. In addition, we discuss current recommendations based on the best evidence available for the largest and most commonly presented targets for treatment in individuals with ASDs. Lastly we describe future directions for drug development in ASDs based on emerging models of etio-pathophysiology of ASDs and related conditions.

Neurobiology of ASDs and Co-Occurring Maladaptive Behaviors: Relevant Studies

Although the fundamental pathophysiology remains unknown for "idiopathic" ASDs, a variety of investigations have attempted to uncover changes in relevant neurochemical systems that also represent sites of action of many commonly prescribed psychotropics. Many of these ASD-related neurobiologic differences may be more germane to understanding specific dimensions of behavior or associated behaviors rather than core features of ASDs; nevertheless they form the basis for some arguments for consideration of particular drug classes. The bulk of these studies of the neurobiology of autism has been directed toward investigating changes in the serotonin (5-hydroxytryptamine; 5-HT), dopamine (DA), cholinergic, and glutamatergic systems.

Research demonstrating changes in the functioning of the serotonin system in individuals with ASDs has a long history dating back to the observation of elevated levels of whole blood 5HT in the periphery of children with autism (Schain & Freedman, 1961). This finding, observed in approximately 30 to 50% of individuals with ASDs, has been frequently replicated (Anderson et al., 1987), although the confounding of this relationship with degrees of intellectual disability complicates its interpretation. A variety of other research approaches have probed changes in the 5HT system in individuals with ASDs; observations of blunted prolactin release following acute administration of the 5HT indirect agonist fenfluramine have been noted in ASD versus controls (Hoshino et al., 1984; McBride et al., 1989); decreased 5HT2A receptor subtype binding in leukocytes has been reported in hyperserotonemic individuals with ASDs (Cook et al., 1993), and acute dietary tryptophan depletion was found to exacerbate autistic symptoms in a controlled study of three adults with ASDs (McDougle, Naylor, Cohen, Aghajanian, et al., 1996). More refined dimensional analyses of the core domain of repetitive behavior in ASDs provided support for a relationship with gene variants in SLC6A4 (serotonin transporter protein) (Brune et al., 2006), which is intriguing given that SLC6A4 is the principal site of action of serotonin reuptake inhibiting (SRI) antidepressants, which are standard treatments for Obsessive-Compulsive Disorder (OCD). However, these data have often been critiqued as too indirect to glean conclusions regarding central nervous system (CNS) 5HT functioning. Yet bolstering the validity of these reports, studies utilizing positron emission tomography (PET) scanning have uncovered more direct evidence for altered serotonin synthesis patterns in children with ASDs (Chugani et al., 1999). The interpretation of these data is complex too; individuals with autism showed changes in the lateralization of 5HT synthesis and differences in the developmental trajectories of increases in early childhood followed by subsequent decreases in synthesis capacity comparable to adult levels, in some analyses correlating with language skill acquisition. Given the widespread regulatory influence of 5HT on a broad range of systems and behaviors including mood, activity, sleep, and repetitive behavior, such data cited above have been used as an argument for consideration of the use of many psychotropics thought to interact with 5HT function. Overall, 5HT function may differ in ASDs compared to typically developing children, but such changes in 5HT may be related more to dimensions of ASDs, rather than serving as a marker for ASD diagnostic status.

The dopamine (DA) system has also been the subject of some investigation in individuals with ASDs. The elevation of mean levels of cerebrospinal fluid (CSF) homovanillic acid (HVA) (Gillberg et al., 1983) suggested a possible relationship between increased DA function and hyperkinetic movements in ASDs including stereotypic behaviors, however most studies contrasting subject groups of autism versus controls have not found differences (Anderson & Hoshino, 1997). Again, negative studies have focused on small case-control comparisons; DA function may hold more importance in its possible association with motor activity and other specific domains of the ASD phenotype.

More direct information has been obtained from postmortem analyses of brain tissue from individuals with ASDs. *The cholinergic system*, a widespread and key component of learning and memory functions, has been investigated in studies assaying receptor expression in various areas of the cerebral cortex. Cholinergic muscarinic receptor-1 (M1 subtype) binding was found to be reduced by up to 30% in samples from subjects with ASDs. Nicotinic receptor binding was even more prominently reduced (65 to 73%) in the frontal and parietal cortical regions (Perry et al., 2001), in the cerebellum (Lee et al., 2002), but not in the basal forebrain (Perry et al., 2001). Such data on cholinergic changes are in need of replication, but have been interpreted to suggest cholinergic agonists as a possible suggested treatment path.

Overlapping problems in social communication and autistic features are common to females with Rett Syndrome, where evidence for abnormalities in glutamatergic transmission is known, so glutamatergic changes have been suggested to be possibly relevant to other individuals on the autism spectrum. Such data from studies of Rett Syndrome include the findings of increased CSF glutamate, and alterations in metabotropic glutamate receptors (mGluRs), depending on age (Armstrong, 2005). The role of glutamate also arises in the detailed molecular pathway analyses of Fragile X Syndrome (FXS), where the reduction in expression of the Fragile X Mental Retardation Protein (FMRP) releases inhibitory control on protein synthesis, and where mGluR5 antagonist agents have been shown to reverse effects and "rescue" the organism from preclinical FXS phenotypes in vivo (Dolen & Bear, 2008).

The possible role of alterations in neuropeptide hormone systems such as oxytocin and vasopressin in ASDs has been raised by extensive literature uncovering the influences of these hormones on social behaviors in both animals and humans. Oxytocin receptor knockout mice show disruptions of their usual social behavior, and acute administration of oxytocin to normal control adults has been shown to modulate behaviors such as trust, affect toward others, and social perception in experimental paradigms. Although other molecular signaling pathways such as ERK and PI3K are under consideration for their possible role in aspects of the physiology of ASDs (Levitt & Campbell, 2009), the above form the crux of observations of neurochemical systems that have formed the indirect arguments for the use of a number of common psychotropic agents as described below.

Prior to considering the common uses of psychotropic agents for individuals with ASDs, it is crucial to emphasize that currently drug therapy takes on an adjunctive role, mainly targeting associated maladaptive and specific impairing ASD symptoms. With few exceptions (noted below), little change has been noted in broader core symptoms of ASDs (e.g., social ability) from psychotropic drug treatment. However, the negative impact of common maladaptive behaviors and symptoms such as aggression, hyperactivity, self-injury, and disordered mood can be marked, interfering with educational and other therapeutic efforts, necessitating more restrictive schooling or living environments, and posing real threats to the safety of some individuals with ASDs and their family members. Therefore, drug therapy can play an important role, but needs to be considered in the context of a multimodal therapeutic approach, complementing educational, behavioral, and social habilitative efforts.

Review of Drug Classes for the Treatment of ASDs

Antidepressants

The antidepressants continue to be the most widely prescribed category of psychotropic agents for individuals with ASDs for more than the past decade. Among the antidepressants, the selective serotonin reuptake inhibiting agents (SSRIs) are the most frequently utilized. Although a relatively large number of reports are found in the literature for this class, including fluxoamine (Luvox), fluxoetine (Prozac), citalopram (Celexa), escitalopram (Lexapro), sertraline (Zoloft), and paroxetine (Paxil), overall the number of rigorous controlled studies (those obtaining ratings of change from individuals "blinded" to treatment and comparisons to placebo groups) is small. One of the initial studies of the SSRIs, which generated much enthusiasm for these agents, examined the effects of fluvoxamine in 30 adults with autism. In a randomized placebo-controlled, double-blind design, substantial global clinical improvement was seen in 53% of adults randomized to fluvoxamine vs. 0% assigned to placebo group over 12 weeks of observation, with average fluvoxamine doses between 200 to 300 milligrams (mg) per day. Improvements included reduced repetitive behaviors by 36% from baseline, decreased aggression, improved language use, overall reduced maladaptive behavior ratings, and with good tolerability (McDougle, Naylor, Cohen, Volkmar, et al., 1996). These results generated the clinical hypothesis that many of the repetitive behaviors seen in individuals with ASDs could be considered analogs of OCD symptoms. However, an attempt to replicate these findings in a controlled trial with fluvoxamine in a group of children and adolescents with autism was unsuccessful; moreover, adverse events were pronounced and raised significant concerns about poor tolerability and safety of the agent in the majority of children who received the active drug. At present, these contradictory findings are unexplained but may relate to prominent developmental effects on treatment response in ASDs possibly specific to the 5HT system, given the alterations in developmental trajectories of 5HT synthesis cited above.

Fluoxetine has also been examined in a number of open-label reports and two controlled trials. Utilizing a low dose (less than 10 mg/day) designed to avoid adverse effects in children and adolescents with ASD, fluoxetine was demonstrated to be associated with an improvement in measures of repetitive behavior versus placebo and clinical global impression of severity (Hollander et al., 2005). However, closer inspection of the magnitude of change observed showed the extent of the improvement to be modest on the primary outcome of repetitive behaviors, and global improvement was not observed, leaving the clinical significance of the results uncertain. Also, even in this low dose range, 19% of subjects required a dose reduction because of side effects, mainly activation. A naturalistic study from clinic experience of open-label treatment with fluoxetine in 129 young children with autism suggested benefit in over 66% (DeLong et al., 2002), but the study is limited by the absence of controls and little descriptive information. In another open-label study of fluoxetine using doses of 10 to 80 mg/day, 65% of subjects were defined as responders using a global measure of severity (Cook et al., 1992). Similarly, additional pilot studies and clinical observations with fluoxetine have suggested possible benefits in symptoms such as irritability, depressed mood, and repetitive behaviors (Fatemi et al., 1998), however such reports lack the comparison to a placebo or inactive control, leaving them vulnerable to the likely effects of expectancy bias. Side effects of activation have been commonly noted in studies of fluoxetine, including hyperactivity, agitation, insomnia, and aggression. Lastly, a recent large, industry-sponsored, multisite, double-blind, placebo-controlled trial of fluoxetine for the treatment of ASDs associated with high levels of repetitive behavior was reported to show no benefit of fluoxetine over placebo. (personal communication from L. Scahill, 2009).

Citalopram has been suggested to be beneficial on several outcome domains in association with ASDs. However, in one of the largest controlled treatment trials in children and adolescents with ASDs for any agent, citalopram was found to have no benefit versus placebo in a total sample of 149 children (mean age of 9 years old) given average daily doses of 10 to 20 mg/day, on measures of repetitive behavior and global improvement (King et al., 2009). Secondary analyses suggest that caregiver strain may serve as a moderator of placebo response in the sample. Plasma citalopram levels were comparable to concentrations observed in efficacious adult antidepressant studies. The trial included sensitive and systematic examination of adverse events and results revealed increased rates of gastrointestinal symptoms and insomnia in citalopram-treated subjects versus those assigned to placebo. Moreover, nearly 1/3 of children randomized to citalopram displayed signs and symptoms of "activation," including increased activity, irritability, and dysregulated behavior, frequently leading to dose reductions and in some instances discontinuation of treatment. Analyses of secondary measures revealed little, if any, evidence for beneficial effects of citalopram across a wide range of symptom domains. One report has examined the benefits of escitalopram in a 10-week study for children and adolescents (mean age of 10 years) with ASDs and moderate levels of irritability (tantrums, aggression, mood lability), examining benefits on irritability as a target. In this report, 61% of subjects were noted to be good responders to doses of 20 mg or less per day. Adverse events were common, including extensive irritability and hyperactivity, and many subjects required dose reductions because of the emergence of side effects. Nearly 20% of the sample dropped out because of adverse effects or worsening behaviors; overall however, completing subjects showed solid improvement, with a 50% reduction in ratings of irritability from baseline for the entire sample (Owley et al., 2005). A follow-up report on an expanded sample of 58 subjects with ASDs noted similar improvements; analyses suggest gene variants in the 5HT transporter gene (SLA6A4) may relate to initial improvement but there is no clear-cut association with ultimate response (Owley et al., 2009).

Sertraline has been reported in open-label studies to possibly have benefit for ASD-associated behaviors of aggression, repetitive behavior, anxiety, and irritability. Open-label treatment (average dose of 122 mg/day) observations in 42 adults with ASDs with varying profiles of maladaptive behaviors over 12 weeks reported improvement in 57% of subjects (McDougle, Brodkin, et al., 1998) though changes in symptoms assessed such as repetitive behaviors were modest (20 to 30% decrease from baseline); interestingly the smaller number of subjects with Asperger's Syndrome showed little improvement. A smaller case series described the experience of sertraline treatment in nine children with ASDs and anxiety/agitation, with the majority described as improved (Steingard et al., 1997). Overall, these uncontrolled reports have suggested good tolerability for sertraline in individuals with ASDs, though agitation, insomnia, and gastrointestinal (GI) symptoms are common. However, no controlled trials are available.

Tricyclic Antidepressants

Three tricyclic antidepressants—clomipramine, nortriptyline, and despiramine—have been studied in autism spectrum disorders. Observations of effects of clomipramine and despiramine were obtained in two small, well-controlled crossover comparisons of 12 children and adolescents with ASDs (Gordon et al., 1993). Clomipramine was superior to placebo and to desipramine with respect to ratings on the Children's Psychiatric Rating Scale (CPRS) autism subscale; capturing withdrawal, odd relating, and limited communication, and measures of repetitive behaviors were also noted to improve. Desipramine was equivalent to clomipramine on a measure of hyperactivity with a large reductions from 25 to 50% versus placebo ratings, but clomipramine was noted to produce a greater side-effect burden. Nevertheless, a remarkable 80% of subjects chose to continue clomipramine post-study. Improvements in hyperactivity were also noted in an open-label study of nortiptyline in 16 children with autism. However, the adverse event data from the above studies, as well as subsequent open-label reports, have documented the challenges to tolerability because of the tricyclic anticholinergic and antiadrenergic properties, which are associated with problems of urinary retention, irritability, cardiovascular effects, and fatigue in some individuals. Clomipramine may also lower the seizure threshold at doses above 3 mg/kg/day. Such adverse events coupled with concerns of cardiac effects of the tricyclics have undercut interest in further investigations of these agents, and the use of these drugs remains very limited.

Mirtazapine has been reported to have possible benefits for children and adults with ASDs from open-label clinical experience. Mean daily doses of 7.5 to 45 mg/day were noted to yield positive responses in 35% of 26 individuals receiving at least 4 weeks of treatment, based on improvement in a range of symptoms such as aggression, self-injury, hyperactivity, anxiety, and insomnia (Posey et al., 2001). Venlafaxine, a mixed reuptake inhibitor, was also noted in two case series of patients to yield apparent improvement in symptoms like those of attention deficit hyperactivity disorder (ADHD) (Carminati et al., 2006; Hollander et al., 2000), but the use of venlafaxine for ADHD symptom management is limited in typically developing children as well because of lack of evidence.

Taken together, rigorous studies of the effects of antidepressants in children and adolescents with ASDs do not confirm benefits suggested by wide community use, or by smaller scale, open-label treatment reports, regardless of the targeted symptoms or endpoints. Side effects are common including GI, weight gain, sleep, agitation, and activation, which can range from mild to severe, and must be considered against the limited benefits in the literature. Some adult data appear to suggest better efficacy in adults than in children, but data are sparse. Unfortunately, methodologic limitations in the measurement of mood and anxiety symptoms in ASDs have impeded more thorough study of these agents for these symptom targets. However, the common observations of dysphoric mood, anxiety symptoms, and in some instances diagnoses of depression and anxiety in individuals with ASDs continue to appear to prompt their consideration; the field awaits a large-scale controlled trial which specifically targets anxiety and mood in individuals with ASDs. Careful and slower titration of low doses of these agents is advised if they are to be prescribed at all. The use of side-effect rating scales may indicate early warning signs of activation and other potentially severe adverse effects. The risk of significant side effects of these agents added to the current limited evidence of benefit should lead to more restricted use of these medications.

Antipsychotics

As a drug class, the antipsychotics have emerged as the second most commonly prescribed class of agents in community surveys, with substantial increases in recent use despite cautions relating to adverse effects of long-term exposure. The apparent broad short-term benefits of the antipsychotics, particularly members of the second-generation antipsychotic drugs (SGAs), have led to several large-scale controlled trials and resulting approval from the FDA for two members of this class for the specific target of severe irritability and aggression associated with autistic disorder. Table 76-1 lists available rigorous controlled trials for these agents in ASDs.

The SGAs represent a diverse group of compounds (McGough, 2005). Most of these agents share prominent effects on both the 5HT and DA systems. In addition however, the majority of this class displays high affinity for a wide range of other neurotransmitter receptor targets, including histaminic, adrenergic, cholinergic, and other receptors (Nasrallah, 2008). These broad neuropharmacologic profiles are likely associated with the wide range and varying mix of commonly associated side effects of these agents.

Table 76–1.
Randomized, controlled trials of antipsychotics in autism disorders

Agent	Sample	Design	Average Dose	Outcomes
Risperidone, (McDougle 1998)	n = 31, autism 55%; PDD 45% 28 years.	12-week placebo vs. risperidone parallel groups.	2.9 mg	57% response to risperidone, 0% to placebo, 9/15 responders continued drug.
Risperidone (McCracken [RUPP], 2002)	n = 101, autism and severe irritability, 9 years (5 to 16).	8-week placebo vs. risperidone parallel groups.	1.8 mg	75% response to risperidone, 12% response to placebo.
Risperidone (Shea 2004)	n = 79, autistic d/o 68%, PDD, NOS, 7.5 years.	8-week placebo vs. risperidone.	1.2 mg	87% response to risperidone vs. 40% placebo.
Risperidone (Aman, 2009)	n = 124, ASD, (4 to 13).	16-week med-only vs. med + behavior therapy.	2.0 to 2.25 mg	Significant decreases in ABC-Irritability: No difference CGI-Improvement ratings.
Risperidone (Troost, 2005)	n = 24, ASD.	9-week open-label, 8-week double-blind placebo discontinued.	1.7 mg	No group effects on symptoms; risperidone group better on vigilance tasks.
Olanzapine (Hollander, 2006)	n = 11.	8-week placebo vs. olanzapine.	10 mg	Responders: 50% olanzapine vs. 20% placebo.
Aripiprazole (Owen, 2009)	n = 98, 9 years (6 to 17).	8-week placebo vs. aripiprazole.		Responders: 52% aripiprazole vs. 14% placebo.
Aripiprazole (Marcus, 2009)	n = 218, autistic disorder and irritability 9 years (6 to 17).	8-week placebo vs. aripiprazole fixed dose.	5 mg, 10 mg, 15 mg	Responders (CGI-I much or very much improved): Placebo: 35% ; 5mg: 56% (significant vs placebo); 10mg: 49% (non-significant); 15mg: 53% (non-significant).

Risperidone is the most widely investigated member of the SGAs in ASDs. Following a number of case reports and open-label trials suggesting possible beneficial effects of risperidone, risperidone has been studied in four large-scale controlled trials in ASDs. The National Institute of Mental Health (NIMH) Research Units in Pediatric Psychopharmacology (RUPP) Autism Network (2002) reported on the first major controlled trial of risperidone in children with autism. Risperidone demonstrated significant benefits versus placebo during a double-blind 8-week acute treatment phase involving 101 children and adolescents with autistic disorder with moderate to severe levels of irritability, aggression, and self-injurious behavior. Blind ratings of global improvement showed 75% of those treated with risperidone to show a clinically significant response versus 15% in the placebo group, with a mean daily dose of 1.8 mg/day. In a 4-month open-label extension phase, benefits observed in the acute phase were maintained in over 85% of subjects, with no requirement of increasing risperidone daily doses. A unique feature of this study was the final phase of a placebo-controlled discontinuation study of a subsample of 32 individuals completing 6 months of risperidone treatment. Placebo substitution was associated with a significant return of symptoms of irritability and aggression in 62.5% of subjects versus 12.5% of individuals maintained on their prior dose of risperidone for an additional 2 months, supporting durability of treatment for up to 6 months of treatment; this also suggests that some individuals can successfully interrupt treatment without relapse after short-term treatment. Subsequent studies have confirmed these observations using similar designs. Two additional large-scale studies have provided similar evidence of benefit for the target symptoms of agitation, aggression, and severe irritability (Aman et al., 2009; Shea et al., 2004). A study of 79 children from 5 to 12 years of age with any ASD diagnosis reported over 80% showing clinical improvement with a mean daily dose of 1.2 mg/day (Shea et al., 2004). Further studies involving risperidone administration have provided additional support for therapeutic effects on endpoints of aggression, irritability, and agitation. A large NIMH-supported controlled trial compared the benefits of risperidone monotherapy to risperidone plus weekly parent behavioral management treatment (Aman et al., 2009). Overall, risperidone led to marked decreases in ratings of irritability from baseline, and the addition of behavior management training was associated with further decreases in ratings of irritability, reduced ratings of noncompliant behavior, and a modest decrease in average daily dose of risperidone from 2.25 to 2.0 mg/day (Aman et al., 2009). Relative to community dosing practices, the robust effects of low doses in the above studies represent an important statement to clinicians to question the clinical need for daily doses of greater than 2 to 3 mg per day in most children and adolescents treated with risperidone. The research model of this study, which evaluated the effects of combined treatments, both pharmacologic and behavioral, represents the possible beginning of a needed, new generation of research. Many questions remain about whether the benefits of accepted but lengthy and time-intensive behavioral, social, and educational interventions can be accelerated or enhanced by combined drug therapies; these are crucial questions for the field of ASD intervention research.

Interestingly, examination of secondary endpoints from the placebo-controlled trials suggest that other ASD symptom domains show significant improvements as well, as also reflected in a smaller controlled trial in adults with ASDs showing broad improvements (McDougle, Holmes, et al., 1998). Hyperactivity ratings and measures of repetitive behaviors have been found to display significantly greater improvements versus placebo, at times achieving reductions of 35 to 50% from baseline ratings, depending on the endpoints; however no trial has prospectively specifically tested the effects of any of the SGAs on the core ASD domain of repetitive behaviors.

Risperidone exposure is linked to a number of common side effects—increased appetite and weight gain (nearly 3 kg in 8 weeks), drowsiness and sedation, drooling, tremor, and dizziness. Longer-term metabolic effects of concern include the development of metabolic syndrome and diabetes, and unknown effects of prolonged hyperprolactinemia. Although data are sorely limited, smaller-scale investigations do not observe negative effects on cognitive functioning (Aman et al., 2005). Clinical recommendations based on the literature support initiating treatment at low doses (0.5 mg/day) and if needed by continued symptomatology, gradually titrating in no greater than 0.5 mg increments over 4 to 8 weeks, up to a recommended maximum dose range of 3 to 4 mg per day, with most individuals responding to doses as low as 1 to 2 mg per day.

Aripiprazole has been studied in two large-scale placebo-controlled trials as a treatment for aggression, severe tantrums, and self-injurious behavior associated with autistic disorder. Overall, those subjects assigned to aripiprazole treatment showed decreases in ratings of irritability between 43 and 50% with approximately 50% subjects treated with aripiprazole rated as "much" or "very much" improved versus 35% for those in the placebo group during the 8-week acute trial. Fixed-dose assignments of 5, 10, and 15 mg per day in one trial did not strongly point to a recommended or superior daily dose; open label and case series reports suggest improvements as well, with doses varying considerably between 2.5 to 15 mg per day over periods of treatment up to 15 months of exposure, and with improvements most evident observed in aggression, severe tantrums, and agitation. Limited published information is available for longer-term treatment with aripiprazole. Side effects include fatigue, gastrointestinal symptoms, somnolence, weight gain, and extrapyramidal symptoms (EPS) such as akathisia. Weight gain of nearly 1.5 to 2.0 kg over an 8-week exposure have been noted in studies of aripiprazole, and not were strongly correlated to overall daily dose. Based on the above data, aripriprazole has also received FDA approval for the treatment of severe irritability associated with autism in children and adolescents. Effective doses appear to vary widely, and careful titration over the wide ranges tested in clinical trials is often needed. Clinicians should be aware of the possibility of clinical confusion between akathisia versus worsening clinical symptoms. Other mild symptoms of EPS such as drooling, slowed gait, increased motor tone, agitation, or cogwheeling should trigger consideration of dose reduction or addition of treatments for EPS.

Other than risperidone and aripiprazole, few controlled trial and systematic studies are available for other SGAs. Olanzapine was contrasted using random assignment to open-label treatment with olanzapine or haloperidol in one report involving 11 children and adolescents with ASDs. Overall, global response was found to be superior with those treated with olanzapine versus those receiving haloperidol. Improvements were noted across several outcomes including global ratings, agitation, hyperactivity, and language usage. However, weight gain was significantly greater in subjects treated with olanzapine even during the 6-week study period. Two open-label studies of olanzapine, both describing 12-week response to moderate mean doses of 7.5 to 10 mg/day found varying rates of improvement. Benefits were suggested to be observed in hyperactivity, irritability, anxiety, and mood symptoms, although the number of responders ranged from 12 to 86% (Potenza et al., 1999). One small double-blind placebo-controlled study of 11 children with ASDs suggested superior global response rates for those assigned to olanzapine (50%) versus those receiving placebo (20%), although symptom severity ratings did not differ between groups (Hollander et al., 2006). Quetiapine has been noted in open-label reports to be associated with limited benefit and tolerability. No controlled trial studies have been reported with quetiapine. A range of side effects has been noted including increased appetite, weight gain, sedation, possible sedation, drooling, and possible reduction in seizure threshold. Ziprasidone has been described in two open-label reports to have possible benefit on symptoms of aggression, agitation, and irritability; limited safety and tolerability observations are available. Target doses for ziprasidone are not well-defined; wide doses ranges from 20 to 160 mg per day are associated with improvement in 50 to 75% of individuals in the reports. Improvement has been most notably observed in relationship to maladaptive behavior, disruptive behavior, aggression, and hyperactivity. In contrast to most of the members of the SGAs, ziprasidone has shown little evidence for associated weight gain, even in individuals followed for up to 6 months of exposure. Extrapyramidal symptoms have been noted to occur in association with ziprasidone. Although no symptoms suggesting common adverse effects on cardiac function have been described in individuals with ASDs, one open-label report documented an increase of 15 milliseconds in the Q-T wave interval, corrected for heart rate (QTC).

The oldest second-generation antipsychotic clozapine, has been subjected to little investigation for use in individuals with ASDs, mainly because of concerns about the risk of agranulocytosis requiring frequent blood monitoring and longer-term tolerability challenges. Case reports have noted possible improvement in aggression, hyperactivity, and stereotypic behavior with doses of 200 to 450 mg/day (Zuddas et al., 1996), with sedation, weight gain, enuresis, and drooling appearing frequently in these uncontrolled reports.

Typical Antipsychotics

Although less commonly utilized in clinical practice, haloperidol has a history of controlled study for the treatment of children with autism, with work dating back several decades. In double-blind placebo-controlled trials with low doses of haloperidol (less than 2 mg/day) in children from 2 to 8 years of age with a mixture of diagnoses (including what would fall into ASDs today), improvements were noted across a range of domains including reduced social withdrawal, stereotypy, and hyperactivity. Longer-term observations of continued haloperidol treatment suggested that benefits were maintained over time, however systematic studies examining outcomes in children where haloperidol was periodically withdrawn at 6-month intervals suggested that the frequency of dyskinesias observed was surprisingly high. Up to 1/3 of all subjects enrolled in these studies demonstrated withdrawal dyskinesias, which were more common in those subjects receiving higher daily doses of haloperidol. Although the reports documented the eventual resolution of dyskinesias in all cases, the high frequency of this adverse event has raised serious concerns about long-term exposure to potent dopamine antagonists such as haloperidol (Anderson et al., 1984; Campbell et al., 1978; Campbell et al., 1997; Perry et al., 1989). Low-potency typical antipsychotics, such as chlorpromazine, in individual doses from 12.5 to 50 mg are sometimes utilized for the short-term management of severe aggressive rage outbursts, but sedation, anticholinergic effects, EPS, dyskinesia risk, and potential cardiovascular effects such as orthostatic hypotension lower the benefit/risk ratio of this group of drugs as a maintenance treatment.

Overall, research on the clinical effects of the antipsychotics in children with ASDs possesses areas of substantial depth, though many agents have not yet been carefully studied. The methodology for investigating the clinical utility of these drugs for their common targets of agitation, aggression, irritability, and self-injury is sound and now widely accepted, and many of the measures used in the clinical trials of the FDA-approved agents have utility in the clinical monitoring of these agents (Aberrant Behavior Checklist, Community Version; Abnormal Involuntary Movement Scale; Parent Side Effect Rating Scale; Parent Target Symptom Ratings). Clinicians faced with individuals with ASDs with moderate to severe aggressive behaviors, rage outbursts, agitation, and self-injury have two approved choices for treatment with a supporting evidence base. Along with tools for systematic monitoring of drug effects on behaviors comes recommendations for safety monitoring for these agents, including baseline and periodic fasting glucose, lipids, weight, and cardiovascular parameters (Correll, 2008).

Stimulants

The category of psychostimulants has been noted in community surveys to be frequently prescribed in as many as 15% of individuals with ASDs, usually for treatment of associated behaviors of hyperactive, inattentive, impulsive behaviors common to individuals with ASDs. Indeed, it has been less well-appreciated until recently that the disruptive behaviors may represent the most common impairing associated constellation of symptoms in individuals with ASDs, arguably conceived of as one aspect of an "expanded phenotype." (McCracken, in press) However, despite the frequent overlap of disruptive behaviors with ASDs, little information has been available until recently as to whether standard treatments for ADHD (in typically developing individuals) possess efficacy and safety in individuals with ASDs.

Small-scale studies, most with brief treatment periods and few with placebo controls, suggested modest benefit on ADHD symptoms but raised concerns about tolerability because of common side effects of social withdrawal, mood lability, motor tics, and even cases of apparent psychotic symptoms associated with stimulant exposure.

The largest controlled study of psychostimulants in children and adolescents with ASDs was conducted by the NIMH RUPP Autism Network, which enrolled 72 subjects (mean age of 9 years) with a range of ASD diagnoses (74% with DSM-IV autistic disorder). Subjects were entered into a double-blind placebo-controlled 4-week crossover trial, following a brief open-label period to establish tolerability. Average daily doses of methylphenidate were conservative (0.125, 0.25, 0.5 mg per kg tid; afternoon doses were halved). Overall results suggested solid benefit in 49% of the subjects enrolled in the trial as defined by substantial reductions in hyperactivity of greater than 25 to 30% from teacher and/or parent ratings, and study clinician ratings of clinical global improvement. However, nearly one of five subjects was unable to complete the brief trial because of intolerance of methylphenidate, with prominent adverse events of mood lability, social withdrawal, and decreased appetite frequently observed. Interestingly, secondary analyses of structured observational data obtained from a substudy of younger subjects in the trial suggested methylphenidate at best dose was associated with increases in some measures of joint attention behaviors and self-regulation (Jahromi et al., 2009). The observation represents one of the few suggestions of improvements in a core deficit of ASD associated with medication exposure, but requires replication.

Atomoxetine

Several small-sized open-label reports and one proof-of-concept controlled study suggest the possible benefit of atomoxetine on ADHD symptoms in individuals with ASDs, most prominently on hyperactive and impulsive symptoms. Open-label treatment with atomoxetine for an average of 20 weeks was associated with reductions from baseline in overall parent ratings of ADHD symptoms, with average reductions in the range of 25%; 60% of subjects were described as "much improved" or "very much improved" by clinician ratings, though no comparison treatments exist to balance expectancy bias (Jou et al., 2005). Two other open-label pilot studies also provided some evidence for possible benefit for atomoxetine. One report of 12 children with ASDs suggested improvements of parent ratings of ADHD symptoms, however 42% of these subjects discontinued because of adverse events, and some measures did not evidence statistically significant decreases in ADHD symptoms (Troost et al., 2006). An additional 8-week open-label study of 16 children with ASDs recorded more substantial decreases in ADHD symptom ratings; a drop of nearly 50% in parent and teacher ratings of inattentive and hyperactive behaviors from baseline during the 8-week trial were present, with mean doses reached of 1.2 mg per kg per day (Posey et al., 2006). However, no change in repeated testing with a computerized performance task of sustained attention was observed (Posey et al., 2006). One small study reported on results of a double-blind placebo comparison trial of atomoxetine of children with ASDs (Arnold et al., 2006). Although those subjects assigned to atomoxetine achieved nearly double the responder rate vs. placebo (56% vs. 25%) the improvement in symptoms appeared to be limited to decreases observed in hyperactive-impulsive symptoms. Taken together these data suggest possible modest benefit of atomoxetine for the treatment of ADHD-like behaviors in ASDs, but with questions about tolerability and disappointing impact on problems of inattention and concentration, clearly important because of the cognitive deficits common to individuals with ASDs (Ventola & Tsatsanis, in press). Dosing also remains uncertain, as most of the extant reports in samples with ASDs use relatively lower average daily doses than those found most efficacious in typically developing children with ADHD.

Alpha-2 Adrenergic Agonists/ Antihypertensives

Clonidine and guanfacine have been explored in small studies in mixed groups of subjects of autism spectrum disorders. Both exert effects through CNS cortical and subcortical alpha-2 receptors, which in a variety of experimental models have been noted to have beneficial effects on measures of cognitive performance. Two small but well-controlled studies have reported on clonidine's possible benefit on disruptive behavior symptoms on individuals with autism spectrum disorders. Using the clonidine transdermal patch in a crossover design, Clinical Global Impression (CGI) improvement ratings suggested superior benefit for the clonidine treatment phase in subjects including children and adults, despite no significant difference in disruptive behavior symptoms as rated by parents (King et al., 2001), leaving estimation of overall benefit uncertain. Another study of clonidine also used a double-blind placebo-controlled crossover design with eight subjects with ASDs (Jaselskis et al., 1992). Although ADHD symptoms were rated by parents to be significantly lower during the clonidine phase, teacher ratings documented more modest improvements with estimated effect sizes in the moderate range (mean daily doses of 0.15 to 0.2 mg/day).

Guanfacine has been described as possibly beneficial in individuals with ASDs with prospective and open-label studies. A review of treatment experience of 80 subjects, primarily children, suggested improvement in global severity ratings by treating clinicians. A multisite 8-week course of guanfacine with average daily doses in the range of 1.5 to 2.5 mg per day in 25 children with ASDs and high levels of hyperactive-impulsive behavior suggested large improvements by both parent and teacher ratings of hyperactive-impulsive behavior (Scahill et al., 2006). Fifty-eight percent of subjects were rated "much improved" or "very much improved" by study clinicians. Overall, guanfacine has been well-tolerated, but adverse events are common and include sedation and fatigue, mood lability, headache, hypotension, bradycardia, and sleep changes. Too little data exists to rigorously assess the utility of the alpha agonists in ASDs at this time, and the level of indication is rated at best as "possibly indicated."

Mood Stabilizers and Anticonvulsants

The frequent co-occurrence of seizure disorders in 10 to 20% of individuals with ASDs often provides a clear indication for the use of antiepileptic drugs (AEDs). Additional associations of mood lability, mood swings, nonspecific EEG abnormalities, and rage outbursts have fueled interest in examining the benefits of mood stabilizers and AEDs in ASD. Unfortunately, little evidence from rigorous experimental studies is available, however an open-label report of the effects of divalproex sodium suggested benefits in five of 14 individuals across a wide age span (Hollander et al., 2001). A controlled trial of lamotrigine in 28 children with ASDs, found no significant benefits versus placebo-assigned subjects in an 8-week study, although the subjects entered the trial with only mild to moderate ratings of disruptive and maladaptive behaviors, perhaps limiting the potential of observing an effect of lamotrigine versus placebo. An additional report described treatment experience in a mixed sample of 50 children, in whom 13 children with autism were noted; global improvements were noted in several areas in terms of benefits for attention and maladaptive behaviors.

A chart review of treatment experience in 15 children with ASDs noted the possible benefit of topiramate in eight of 15 (53%) based on treating clinician ratings (Hardan et al., 2004). Benefits were found in symptom ratings of inattention and hyperactivity, where decreases from 30 to 38% were noted compared to pretreatment ratings. Another case series of topiramate use in doses in 2.5 mg per kg per day was noted to be beneficial in two of 5 children with autism and maladaptive behaviors (Mazzone & Ruta, 2006).

Levetiracetam has been described anecdotally as a treatment for maladaptive behaviors in 10 children with ASDs. Benefits were described as widespread, particularly for problems of aggression, hyperactivity, irritability, and impulsive behavior. However, a 10-week double-blind placebo-controlled study of levetiracetam in 20 children and adolescents with autism found no drug versus placebo differences that achieved significance, and adverse events were common at a mean daily dose of 862.5 mg per day (Rugino & Samsock, 2002; Wasserman et al., 2006). Overall, the benefits of several diverse AEDs have not conclusively emerged from systematic studies, despite the promise suggested by anectodal reports and the association of seizures and abnormal EEG activity in many individuals with ASDs. Taken together, the disappointing results for AEDs in placebo-controlled trials provide another sobering example of the possible overestimation of drug effects in the absence of stringently controlled research designs.

Naltrexone

Naltrexone has been investigated in a number of reports, most commonly as a potential treatment targeting self-injurious behavior. Outcome measures of self-injurious behavior, language use, and social behavior have not documented significant effects of naltrexone especially versus placebo, but interestingly, ratings of hyperactivity have been noted to be reduced compared to baseline measures or placebo controls in most reports. Side effects have been confined to mild sedation. Naltrexone and related compounds may deserve additional examination as alternatives to stimulants and atomoxetine for the treatment of ADHD-like behaviors associated with ASDs.

Amantadine

Amantadine is a compound with multiple neurochemical effects from inhibition of the dopamine transporter and from N-methyl-D-aspartic acid (NMDA) receptor antagonist properties. Prior case series suggested benefits for treatment of individuals with ASDs. A well-controlled double-blind placebo-controlled study of amantadine hydrochloride in children and adolescents with ASDs, found few differences for amantadine versus placebo during the 4-week study period. However, blind investigator ratings of hyperactivity symptoms revealed significant improvement versus placebo in the amantadine-treated subjects (King et al., 2001). Benefits for younger children and higher-dose treatment are suggested by these results, given the maturation of the glutamate system and the low rate of adverse events described in the study.

Memantine

Memantine shares with amantadine antagonist effects at NMDA receptors; given the evidence of glutamatergic excess in Rett Syndrome and Fragile X Syndrome, some anecdotal experience with memantine in ASD has been described in two open-label studies. One report of experience in 14 children and adolescents with ASDs found no prominent benefits on cognition but behavioral improvements were noted on scales on hyperactive behavior and social behavior (Owley et al., 2005). In a chart review of clinical experience with 18 subjects with ASDs, 61% were described by treating clinicians as responders based on global improvement with possible decreases noted in ratings of hyperactivity (Erickson et al., 2007) . However, increases in activity and behavioral worsening have also been noted in conjunction with memantine exposure even at low doses, leaving considerable uncertainty about whether safety and efficacy can be established for memantine in children with ASDs.

Cholinesterase Inhibitors

Because of reports cited above of postmortem tissue analysis suggesting reduced nicotinic receptors and reductions of other components of the cholinergic system, preliminary studies of acetylcholinesterase inhibitors have been completed. Retrospective reports of donepezil have suggested improvements in disruptive behaviors in one clinical report. Galantamine, another acetylcholinesterase inhibitor with more prominent effects on nicotinic receptors was tested in a randomized placebo-controlled crossover study of 20 children with ASDs. Modest benefits favoring galantamine were observed on outcomes of mood lability, aggression, hyperactivity, and inappropriate speech. An open-label study of 12 weeks of galantamine in 13 children with ASDs was noted to show improvement as measured by ratings of irritability and social withdrawal symptom scales, however these improvements were small; 23% could not complete the 12 weeks because of adverse effects, and disruptive behavior symptoms were not noted to decrease from baseline. Rivastigmine is another acetylcholinesterase inhibitor. Open-label clinical treatment experience for rivastigmine over 12 weeks was described in one report for 32 children with ASDs. Comparisons to baseline ratings suggested improvement in overall ratings of autism symptoms and on ratings of hyperactive and impulsive behavior. Although these similar agents have been associated with modest behavioral gains in children with ASDs, the extent of the symptom changes appear to fall short from providing pronounced global improvements; the utility of increasing tonic cholinergic tone in ASD remains to be determined.

Targeted Treatment Using Psychotropics in ASDs: Potential Guidelines

How to incorporate the observations reviewed above into individual patient recommendations is a definite challenge for clinicians who seek to reduce pronounced maladaptive behaviors not manageable by behavioral interventions alone. In the following section, we attempt to synthesize the available evidence, as it may be applied to specific and commonly identified targets for treatment in individuals with ASDs. Each suggested pathway, with few exceptions, would at the present time be considered off-label treatment based on varying levels of evidence as summarized above. However, as demonstrated by two FDA approvals of agents for children and adolescents with autistic disorder and severe irritability, data are accumulating. A few general clinical recommendations are warranted. First and foremost, the use of psychotropic medication should always be considered as only one component of a multimodal plan incorporating psychosocial treatments, educational and rehabilitative interventions, and environmental manipulations. Efforts should always be made to reduce medication exposure to the least amount possible and for the shortest duration. Overall, the goals of treatment need to be clearly specified in advance, with suitable monitors of treatment impact on the designated targets acquired both pretreatment and at key intervals during the course of ongoing drug therapy. Goals for treatment should be behaviorally based and should be specified in advance, preferably utilizing observations obtained from multiple sources. Depending on the class of medication and the specific agent prescribed, pretreatment monitoring, including physical examination as well as possible lab studies, may be indicated. Overall, consideration of the possible benefits of any drug therapy should be weighed against the identified risks of such treatment, and particularly for longer-term exposure. As noted below, with the exception of treatments targeting repetitive behaviors, the benefits of pharmacological treatment appear to be limited to associated features, leaving most core features of the ASD, such as social and language impairments, untouched. It is of note that few moderators of drug therapy have been identified despite many efforts to reveal them. Neither IQ, sex, ASD subtype, nor pubertal status has been found to influence treatment response. However, one exception to the above is the identification in studies of risperidone of the moderating effect of 5' nucleotidase, a marker of zinc status (Farmer et al., in press). However, additional efforts to identify moderators have been limited by the relatively small number of treatment samples available; in that regard it may be of interest that some studies of adults with ASDs note apparently greater improvement than that observed in parallel studies of children and adolescents. Such age differences are unexplained; treatment samples in adult studies may differ from child studies with the inclusion of higher-functioning individuals; other unknown influences on treatment outcome may be active.

Presented in graphical form are two suggested clinical pathways for treatment selection: one for ASD associated with frequent, moderate to severe aggression, mood lability, and agitation (Figure 76-1), and one for ASD accompanied by high levels of ADHD symptoms (Figure 76-2). Treatment selection for these two sets of target behaviors can be argued to be solidly informed by research evidence, as synthesized in the pathways shown. What about other common targets of repetitive behaviors, anxiety, and insomnia? Unfortunately, data available fall short of clear and usual standards for even "probable indications." The failure of SSRIs to reduce repetitive behaviors in multiple trials raises questions about their application; the clinician is encouraged to assess carefully for other indicators which may be drug-responsive such as rage outbursts or hyperactivity. Anxiety is often invoked as an explanation for maladaptive behaviors in ASD, but is challenging to assess in the population; possible treatments may include antidepressants, AEDs, and even low-dose SGAs (*see Chapter 69, this volume*). Interventions for insomnia to be considered might include behavioral therapy, melatonin, atypical antidepressants, and alpha agonists (*see Chapter 69, this volume*).

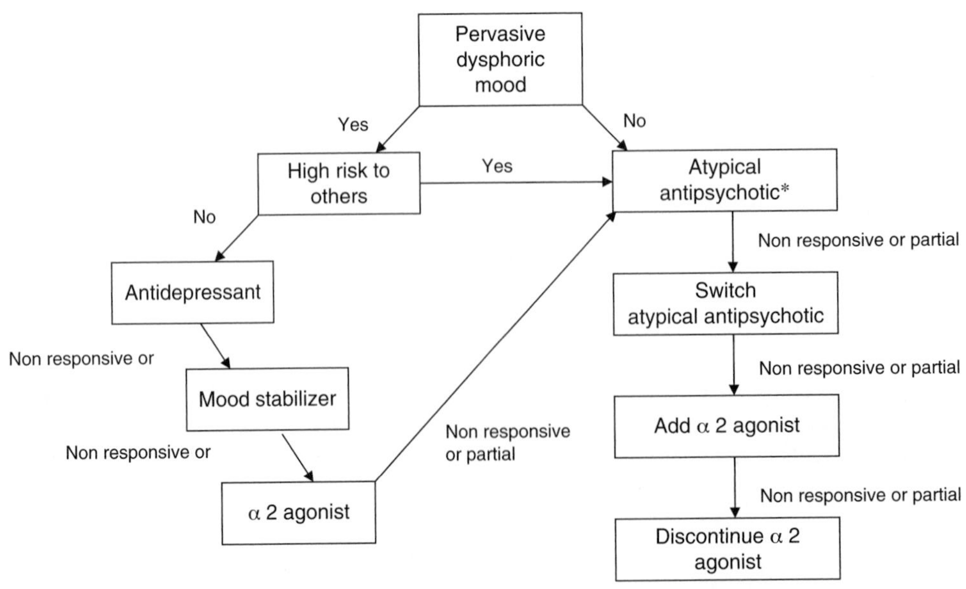

Figure 76–1. Targeted pharmacotherapy for ASD rage outbursts, severe irritability, aggression. * Risperidone, aripiprazole FDA-approved.

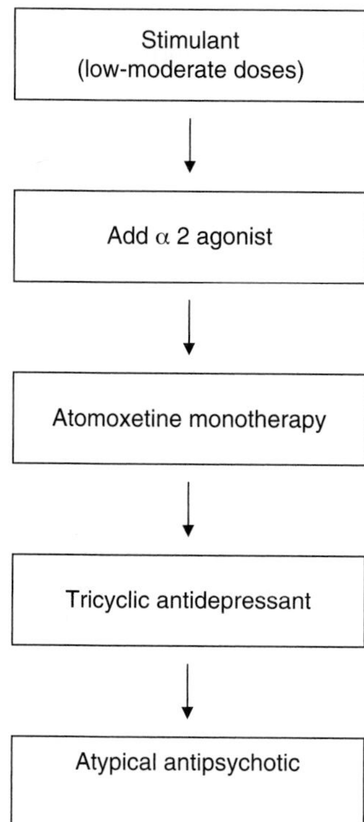

Figure 76–2. Targeted pharmacotherapy for ASDs, hyperactive-impulsive, inattentive.

Conclusion

As can been gleaned from the review above, there is much work to do in developing and testing new possible pharmacotherapies for both associated and core features of ASDs. Significant progress has been made delineating reliable and relatively sensitive measures for most of the common associated maladaptive behaviors, and efforts are underway to improve on measures of core domains of the ASDs, which would be suitable for use in a clinical trial context. Given the hoped-for progress in identifying the molecular pathophysiology of autism, there is reason for continued optimism in the search for treatments that may have even more significant impact on functioning, overall outcome, and in reducing the morbidity of these disorders.

A major unmet need is to identify drugs that may have significant benefit in ameliorating the wide range of cognitive impairments seen in individuals with ASDs. Although ASDs are notable for their wide variability in cognitive functioning, even individuals in the "high-functioning" range are frequently noted to demonstrate impairments in a variety of basic cognitive skills, including judgment and planning, working memory, cognitive flexibility, organization, and social cognition. Besides cognition, the major gap in identified treatments to date has been the lack of obvious benefit of available drug therapies on social and communicative functioning of individuals with ASDs. Despite a robust preclinical science effort, to date no treatments explored in individuals with ASDs have been found to reliably improve global measure of social functioning. However, two recent examples suggest continued optimism. Acute administration of intranasal oxytocin in small but well-controlled experimental studies has identified improvements in measures of social perception and cognition, in normal volunteers and in a small number of adults with ASDs. Given the possible role of neuropeptides in regulating aspects of social functioning, such findings have generated strong interest, but clinical applicability of such a treatment approach is far from certain. In addition, the improvements in measures in social communication, in particular joint attention-initiating behaviors and emotion regulation ratings, observed in the small controlled trial of methylphenidate versus placebo in children with ASDs also suggests that these core deficits within the ASD may be both tractable and malleable targets for treatment.

Lastly, the greatest optimism is based upon the promise of an ultimate revealing of the underlying molecular pathophysiology in ASD, which is expected to be quite varied across large numbers of individuals with these conditions, likely reflecting the impact of multiple pathways, multiple genetic risk variants, as well as multiple possible environmental influences. However, once individual molecular pathways can be identified, targeted treatments become possible. Although such efforts to extrapolate from gene pathways to clinical treatment have not always proven to be foolproof in principle (witness Fragile X and neurofibromatous 1 treatment failures despite preclinical models), a molecular-based intervention science for ASD is just beginning.

Challenges and Future Directions

- Inadequate knowledge of important molecular pathways disrupted in ASDs.
- Need for identified drug treatments for core domains.
- Need for improved outcome measures and biomarkers of treatment response.

SUGGESTED READING

Aman, M., et al. (2009). Medication and parent training in children with pervasive developmental disorders and serious behavior problems: Results from a randomized clinical trial. *Journal of the American Academy of Child and Adolescent Psychiatry*, October, 2009 epub.

Correll, C. U. (2008). Assessing and maximizing the safety and tolerability of antipsychotics used in the treatment of children and adolescents. *Journal of Clinical Psychiatry*, *69*(Suppl 4), 26–36.

Scahill, L. (2008). How do I decide whether or not to use medication for my child with autism? Should I try behavior therapy first? *Journal of Autism and Developmental Disorders*, *38*(6), 1197–1198.

ACKNOWLEDGMENTS

Preparation of the manuscript was supported in part by grants to JTM from NICHD HD055784, UA3MC11055, and NIMH P50 MH077248.

REFERENCES

Aman, M. G., Arnold, L. E., McDougle, C. J., Vitiello, B., Scahill, L., Davies, M., et al. (2005). Acute and long-term safety and tolerability of risperidone in children with autism. *Journal of Child and Adolescent Psychopharmacology, 15*(6), 869–884.

Aman, M. G., Hollway, J. A., Leone, S., Masty, J., Lindsay, R., Nash, P., et al. (2009). Effects of risperidone on cognitive-motor performance and motor movements in chronically medicated children. *Research in Developmental Disabilities, 30*(2), 386–396.

Anderson, G. M., Freedman, D. X., Cohen, D. J., Volkmar, F. R., Hoder, E. L., McPhedran, P., et al. (1987). Whole blood serotonin in autistic and normal subjects. *Journal of Child Psychological Psychiatry, 28*(6), 885–900.

Anderson, G. M., & Hoshino, Y. (1997) Neurochemical studies of autism. In D. J. Cohen, F. R. Volkmar (Eds.), *Handbook of autism and pervasive developmental disorders* (2nd ed., pp. 325–343). New York: John Wiley.

Anderson, L. T., Campbell, M., Grega, D. M., Perry, R., Small, A. M., & Green, W. H. (1984). Haloperidol in the treatment of infantile autism: Effects on learning and behavioral symptoms. *American Journal of Psychiatry, 141*(10), 1195–1202.

Armstrong, D. D. (2005). Neuropathology of Rett syndrome. *Journal of Child Neurology, 20*(9), 747–753.

Arnold, L. E., Aman, M. G., Cook, A. M., Witwer, A. N., Hall, K. L., Thompson, S., et al. (2006). Atomoxetine for hyperactivity in autism spectrum disorders: Placebo-controlled crossover pilot trial. *Journal of the American Academy of Child and Adolescent Psychiatry, 45*(10), 1196–1205.

Arnold, L. D., Farmer, C., Chmura, K. H., Davies, M., Witwer, A., Chuang, S., et al. (in press). Moderators, mediators, and other predictors of risperidone response in children with autistic disorder and irritability. *Journal of Child and Adolescent Psychopharmacology.*

Brune, C. W., Kim, S. J., Salt, J., Leventhal, B. L., Lord, C., & Cook, E. H., Jr. (2006). 5-HTTLPR Genotype-specific phenotype in children and adolescents with autism. *American Journal of Psychiatry, 163*(12), 2148–2156.

Campbell, M., Anderson, L. T., Meier, M., Cohen, I. L., Small, A. M., Samit, C., et al. (1978). A comparison of haloperidol and behavior therapy and their interaction in autistic children. *Journal of the American Academy of Child Psychiatry, 17*(4), 640–655.

Campbell, M., Armenteros, J. L., Malone, R. P., Adams, P. B., Eisenberg, Z. W., & Overall, J. E. (1997). Neuroleptic-related dyskinesias in autistic children: A prospective, longitudinal study. *Journal of the American Academy of Child and Adolescent Psychiatry, 36*(6), 835–843.

Carminati, G. G., Deriaz, N., & Bertschy, G. (2006). Low-dose venlafaxine in three adolescents and young adults with autistic disorder improves self-injurious behavior and attention deficit/hyperactivity disorders (ADHD)-like symptoms. *Progress in Neuropsychopharmacology and Biological Psychiatry, 30*(2), 312–315.

Chugani, D. C., Muzik, O., Behen, M., Rothermel, R., Janisse, J. J., Lee, J., et al. (1999). Developmental changes in brain serotonin synthesis capacity in autistic and nonautistic children. *Annals of Neurology, 45*(3), 287–295.

Cook, E. H., Jr., Arora, R. C., Anderson, G. M., Berry-Kravis, E. M., Yan, S. Y., Yeoh, H. C., et al. (1993). Platelet serotonin studies in hyperserotonemic relatives of children with autistic disorder. *Life Sciences, 52*(25), 2005–2015.

Cook, E. H., Jr., Rowlett, R., Jaselskis, C., & Leventhal, B. L. (1992). Fluoxetine treatment of children and adults with autistic disorder and mental retardation. *Journal of the American Academy of Child and Adolescent Psychiatry, 31*(4), 739–745.

Correll, C. U. (2008). Monitoring and management of antipsychotic-related metabolic and endocrine adverse events in pediatric patients. *International Review of Psychiatry, 20*(2), 195–201.

DeLong, G. R., Ritch, C. R., & Burch, S. (2002). Fluoxetine response in children with autistic spectrum disorders: Correlation with familial major affective disorder and intellectual achievement. *Developmental Medicine and Child Neurology, 44*(10), 652–659.

Dolen, G., & Bear, M. F. (2008). Role for metabotropic glutamate receptor 5 (mGluR5) in the pathogenesis of fragile X syndrome. *Journal of Physiology, 586*, 1503–1508.

Erickson, C. A., Posey, D. J., Stigler, K. A., Mullett, J., Katschke, A. R., & McDougle, C. J. (2007). A retrospective study of memantine in children and adolescents with pervasive developmental disorders. *Psychopharmacology (Berl), 191*(1), 141–147.

Esbensen, A. J., Greenberg, J. S., Seltzer, M. M., & Aman, M. G. (2009). A longitudinal investigation of psychotropic and non-psychotropic medication use among adolescents and adults with autism spectrum disorders. *Journal of Autism and Developmental Disorders, 39*(9), 1339–1349.

Fatemi, S. H., Realmuto, G. M., Khan, L., & Thuras, P. (1998). Fluoxetine in treatment of adolescent patients with autism: A longitudinal open trial. *Journal of Autism and Developmental Disorders, 28*(4), 303–307.

Gillberg, C., Svennerholm, L., & Hamilton-Hellberg, C. (1983). Childhood psychosis and monoamine metabolites in spinal fluid. *Journal of Autism and Developmental Disorders, 13*(4), 383–396.

Gordon, C. T., State, R. C., Nelson, J. E., Hamburger, S. D., & Rapoport, J. L. (1993). A double-blind comparison of clomipramine, desipramine, and placebo in the treatment of autistic disorder. *Archives of General Psychiatry, 50*(6), 441–447.

Hardan, A. Y., Jou, R. J., & Handen, B. L. (2004). A retrospective assessment of topiramate in children and adolescents with pervasive developmental disorders. *Journal of Child and Adolescent Psychopharmacology, 14*(3), 426–432.

Hollander, E., Dolgoff-Kaspar, R., Cartwright, C., Rawitt, R., & Novotny, S. (2001). An open trial of divalproex sodium in autism spectrum disorders. *Journal of Clinical Psychiatry, 62*(7), 530–534.

Hollander, E., Kaplan, A., Cartwright, C., & Reichman, D. (2000). Venlafaxine in children, adolescents, and young adults with autism spectrum disorders: An open retrospective clinical report. *Journal of Child Neurology, 15*(2), 132–135.

Hollander, E., Phillips, A., Chaplin, W., Zagursky, K., Novotny, S., Wasserman, S., et al. (2005). A placebo controlled crossover trial of liquid fluoxetine on repetitive behaviors in childhood and adolescent autism. *Neuropsychopharmacology, 30*(3), 582–589.

Hollander, E., Wasserman, S., Swanson, E. N., Chaplin, W., Schapiro, M. L., Zagursky, K., et al. (2006). A double-blind placebo-controlled pilot study of olanzapine in childhood/adolescent pervasive developmental disorder. *Journal of Child and Adolescent Psychopharmacology, 16*(5), 541–548.

Hoshino, Y., Yamamoto, T., Kaneko, M., Tachibana, R., Watanabe, M., Ono, Y., et al. (1984). Blood serotonin and free tryptophan concentration in autistic children. *Neuropsychobiology, 11*(1), 22–27.

Jahromi, L. B., Kasari, C. L., McCracken, J. T., Lee, L. S., Aman, M. G., McDougle, C. J., et al. (2009). Positive effects of methylphenidate on social communication and self-regulation in children with pervasive developmental disorders and hyperactivity. *Journal of Autism and Developmental Disorders, 39*(3), 395–404.

Jaselskis, C. A., Cook, E. H., Jr., Fletcher, K. E., & Leventhal, B. L. (1992). Clonidine treatment of hyperactive and impulsive children with autistic disorder. *Journal of Clinical Psychopharmacology, 12*(5), 322–327.

Jou, R. J., Handen, B. L., & Hardan, A. Y. (2005). Retrospective assessment of atomoxetine in children and adolescents with pervasive developmental disorders. *Journal of Child and Adolescent Psychopharmacology, 15*(2), 325–330.

King, B. H., Hollander, E., Sikich, L., McCracken, J. T., Scahill, L., Bregman, J. D., et al. (2009). Lack of efficacy of citalopram in children with autism spectrum disorders and high levels of repetitive behavior: Citalopram ineffective in children with autism. *Archives of General Psychiatry, 66*(6), 583–590.

King, B. H., Wright, D. M., Handen, B. L., Sikich, L., Zimmerman, A. W., McMahon, W., et al. (2001). Double-blind, placebo-controlled study of amantadine hydrochloride in the treatment of children with autistic disorder. *Journal of the American Academy of Child and Adolescent Psychiatry, 40*(6), 658–665.

Lee, M., Martin-Ruiz, C., Graham, A., Court, J., Jaros, E., Perry, R., et al. (2002). Nicotinic receptor abnormalities in the cerebellar cortex in autism. *Brain, 125*(Pt 7), 1483–1495.

Levitt, P., & Campbell, D. B. (2009). The genetic and neurobiologic compass points toward common signaling dysfunctions in autism spectrum disorders. *Journal of Clinical Investigation, 119*(4), 747–754.

Martin, A., Scahill, L., Klin, A., & Volkmar, F. R. (1999). Higher-functioning pervasive developmental disorders: Rates and patterns of psychotropic drug use. *Journal of the American Academy of Child and Adolescent Psychiatry, 38*(7), 923–931.

Mazzone, L., & Ruta, L. (2006). Topiramate in children with autistic spectrum disorders. *Brain and Development, 28*(10), 668.

McBride, P. A., Anderson, G. M., Hertzig, M. E., Sweeney, J. A., Kream, J., Cohen, D. J., et al. (1989). Serotonergic responsivity in male young adults with autistic disorder. Results of a pilot study. *Archives of General Psychiatry, 46*(3), 213–221.

McCracken, J. T., McGough, J., Shah, B., Cronin, P., Hong, D., Aman, M. G., et al. (2002). Risperidone in children with autism and serious behavioral problems. *New England Journal of Medicine, 347*(5), 314–321.

McCracken, J. T. (2011). Disruptive behaviors in children with autism spectrum disorders. In E. Hollander, A. Kolevzon, & J. T. Coyle (Eds.), *Textbook of autism spectrum disorders* (pp. 159–167). New York: American Psychiatric Publishing.

McDougle, C. J., Brodkin, E. S., Naylor, S. T., Carlson, D. C., Cohen, D. J., & Price, L. H. (1998). Sertraline in adults with pervasive developmental disorders: A prospective open-label investigation. *Journal of Clinical Psychopharmacology, 18*(1), 62–66.

McDougle, C. J., Holmes, J. P., Carlson, D. C., Pelton, G. H., Cohen, D. J., & Price, L. H. (1998). A double-blind, placebo-controlled study of risperidone in adults with autistic disorder and other pervasive developmental disorders. *Archives of General Psychiatry, 55*(7), 633–641.

McDougle, C. J., Naylor, S. T., Cohen, D. J., Aghajanian, G. K., Heninger, G. R., & Price, L. H. (1996). Effects of tryptophan depletion in drug-free adults with autistic disorder. *Archives of General Psychiatry, 53*(11), 993–1000.

McDougle, C. J., Naylor, S. T., Cohen, D. J., Volkmar, F. R., Heninger, G. R., & Price, L. H. (1996). A double-blind, placebo-controlled study of fluvoxamine in adults with autistic disorder. *Archives of General Psychiatry, 53*(11), 1001–1008.

McGough, J. J. (2005). Attention-deficit/hyperactivity disorder pharmacogenomics. *Biological Psychiatry, 57*(11), 1367–1373.

Nasrallah, H. A. (2008). Atypical antipsychotic-induced metabolic side effects: Insights from receptor-binding profiles. *Molecular Psychiatry, 13*(1), 27–35.

Owley, T., Brune, C. W., Salt, J., Walton, L., Guter, S., Ayuyao, N., et al. (2009). A pharmacogenetic study of escitalopram in autism spectrum disorders. *Autism Research, 3*(1), 1–7.

Owley, T., Walton, L., Salt, J., Guter, S. J., Jr., Winnega, M., Leventhal, B. L., et al. (2005). An open-label trial of escitalopram in pervasive developmental disorders. *Journal of the American Academy of Child and Adolescent Psychiatry, 44*(4), 343–348.

Perry, E. K., Lee, M. L., Martin-Ruiz, C. M., Court, J. A., Volsen, S. G., Merrit, J., et al. (2001). Cholinergic activity in autism: Abnormalities in the cerebral cortex and basal forebrain. *American Journal of Psychiatry, 158*(7), 1058–1066.

Perry, R., Campbell, M., Adams, P., Lynch, N., Spencer, E. K., Curren, E. L., et al. (1989). Long-term efficacy of haloperidol in autistic children: Continuous versus discontinuous drug administration. *Journal of the American Academy of Child and Adolescent Psychiatry, 28*(1), 87–92.

Posey, D. J., Guenin, K. D., Kohn, A. E., Swiezy, N. B., & McDougle, C. J. (2001). A naturalistic open-label study of mirtazapine in autistic and other pervasive developmental disorders. *Journal of Child and Adolescent Psychopharmacology, 11*(3), 267–277.

Posey, D. J., Wiegand, R. E., Wilkerson, J., Maynard, M., Stigler, K. A., & McDougle, C. J. (2006). Open-label atomoxetine for attention-deficit hyperactivity disorder symptoms associated with high-functioning pervasive developmental disorders. *Journal of Child and Adolescent Psychopharmacology, 16*(5), 599–610.

Potenza, M. N., Holmes, J. P., Kanes, S. J., & McDougle, C. J. (1999). Olanzapine treatment of children, adolescents, and adults with pervasive developmental disorders: An open-label pilot study. *Journal of Clinical Psychopharmacology, 19*(1), 37–44.

Rugino, T. A., & Samsock, T. C. (2002). Levetiracetam in autistic children: An open-label study. *Journal of Developmental and Behavioral Pediatrics, 23*(4), 225–230.

Scahill, L., Aman, M. G., McDougle, C. J., McCracken, J. T., Tierney, E., Dziura, J., et al. (2006). A prospective open trial of guanfacine in children with pervasive developmental disorders. *Journal of Child and Adolescent Psychopharmacology, 16*(5), 589–598.

Schain, R. J., & Freedman, D. X. (1961). Studies on 5-hydroxyindole metabolism in autistic and other mentally retarded children. *Journal of Pediatrics, 58*, 315–320.

Shea, S., Turgay, A., Carroll, A., Schulz, M., Orlik, H., Smith, I., et al. (2004). Risperidone in the treatment of disruptive behavioral symptoms in children with autistic and other pervasive developmental disorders. *Pediatrics, 114*(5), e634–641.

Steingard, R. J., Zimnitzky, B., DeMaso, D. R., Bauman, M. L., & Bucci, J. P. (1997). Sertraline treatment of transition-associated anxiety and agitation in children with autistic disorder. *Journal of Child and Adolescent Psychopharmacology, 7*(1), 9–15.

Troost, P. W., Steenhuis, M. P., Tuynman-Qua, H. G., Kalverdijk, L. J., Buitelaar, J. K., Minderaa, R. B., et al. (2006). Atomoxetine for attention-deficit/hyperactivity disorder symptoms in children with pervasive developmental disorders: A pilot study. *Journal of Child and Adolescent Psychopharmacology, 16*(5), 611–619.

Ventola, P., & Tsatsanis, K. D. (2011). Neuropscyhological characteristics. In E. Hollander, A. Kolevzon, & J. T. Coyle (Eds.), *Textbook of autism spectrum disorders* (pp. 196–204). New York: American Psychiatric Publishing.

Wasserman, S., Iyengar, R., Chaplin, W. F., Watner, D., Waldoks, S. E., Anagnostou, E., et al. (2006). Levetiracetam versus placebo in childhood and adolescent autism: A double-blind placebo-controlled study. *International Clinical Psychopharmacology, 21*(6), 363–367.

Zuddas, A., Ledda, M. G., Fratta, A., Muglia, P., & Cianchetti, C. (1996). Clinical effects of clozapine on autistic disorder. *American Journal of Psychiatry, 153*(5), 738.

77 Best Practices: Pediatrics

Mary Catherine Aranda, Sarah J. Spence

Points of Interest

- Current recommendations call for developmental surveillance at every well-child check and the use of autism-specific screening tools at 18 months and 24 months of age, as well as when there is any developmental concern.
- Many resources regarding early detection and management of autism spectrum disorders have been developed in recent years including easy-access internet websites such as www.cdc.gov/autism, www.firstsigns.org, www.aap.org, and www.autismspeaks.org.
- The primary-care evaluation of a child with an ASD should include a comprehensive history including birth, developmental, medical, and detailed family histories, and a complete physical exam including observations of the child's interactions, communication, and behaviors.
- The primary-care physician (PCP) should consider the following medical issues when caring for a child with an ASD: seizures, sleep disturbance, gastrointestinal dysfunction, feeding and nutritional issues, immune problems, tics and Tourette Syndrome, and genetic abnormalities. Children with ASDs are also at increased risk for intellectual disabilities, a history of regression, sensory-motor abnormalities, behavioral problems, and other psychiatric disorders.
- Research suggests that intensive early intervention can substantially improve outcomes in children with ASDs.
- Although behavioral and educational therapies are the mainstay of treatments, there is a vast array of therapeutic options currently in practice. Unfortunately, there is very little evidence regarding what therapeutic technique is best for a given child.

Introduction

With the rise in the prevalence of ASDs in the last 20 years to approximately 1 in a 110 children (CDC, 2007; Fombonne, 2009), primary-care pediatricians must rise to meet the challenge of recognizing, screening, evaluating, and managing children with ASDs in their practice. Media concern, parental awareness, and an expanding research agenda have pushed this group of diagnoses to the forefront of child development. Most primary-care providers are aware that autism involves the core deficits of an autism spectrum disorder, which include qualitative impairments in social interaction and communication, and restricted, repetitive, and stereotyped patterns of behavior, interests, and activities (Association, 2000). Because it has been shown that children with ASDs can make significant developmental gains with intense early intervention, parents and pediatric providers must recognize children at risk for ASDs as early as possible, be knowledgeable about intervention, and be able to make proper referrals for further workup and management if necessary.

This chapter is dedicated to the description of what would be considered "best practices" for pediatricians and PCPs. Unfortunately, the state of research into most medical issues in ASD is not well enough developed to have established truly evidence-based practice parameters. Here we summarize much of what has been presented in detail in previous chapters in this volume and synthesize the elements into a guide for caring for a patient on the autism spectrum. We describe the importance of developmental surveillance, the usage and timing of specific ASD screening tools, and the gold standards for diagnosis and thorough assessments. A synopsis of the latest research and best practices for evaluation and management of common medical conditions, psychiatric and cognitive comorbidities, and their workups will also be presented all in the context of providing a medical home for children with ASDs. Finally, we provide brief descriptions of the available interventions so the PCP can be familiar with the family's options and help them navigate the system.

Developmental Surveillance and Screening

For over 10 years, professional groups have published consensus guidelines, practice parameters, and clinical reports to help PCPs recognize, evaluate, and manage children with suspected ASDs. Although each group has a slightly different focus, there is a clear consensus regarding the role of the PCPs in surveillance and screening. The PCP has a unique role as the point of first contact for most children. The practice of developmental surveillance at every well-child visit and the further use of general and autism-specific screening tools at specific time points is clearly important, but is not in widespread use (Myers & Johnson, 2007). Unfortunately, it is still common to see delays in screening and diagnosis that result in slower referrals to intervention and may adversely affect developmental outcome. Some of these practice recommendations and tools designed to help the PCPs recognize early signs of ASDs are reviewed below.

The first publication regarding guidelines for screening and diagnostic referral came from a meeting of leaders in the research and clinical community sponsored by the Cure Autism Now (CAN) foundation (Geschwind et al., 1998). Shortly thereafter, practice parameters were released by the American Academy of Child and Adolescent Psychiatry (Volkmar et al., 1999), the Child Neurology Society and the American Academy of Neurology (Filipek et al., 2000; Filipek et al., 1999) and the American Academy of Pediatrics (AAP) (AAP, 2001). Most recently the AAP has put out detailed clinical reports regarding identification and evaluation (Johnson & Myers, 2007) and management of children with ASDs (Johnson & Myers, 2007). Each of these publications reviews the current evidence and makes recommendations that can be used in the primary-care setting.

There have been mixed results regarding the accuracy of clinical judgment alone in estimating the developmental progress of a child (Sices et al., 2003; Smith, 1978). In one study, 80% of the children who were eventually diagnosed with ASDs were not initially flagged for concern by their physicians (Robins, 2008). Thus, as the rate of identification of children with ASDs increases, so has the evidence for the importance of screening. Evidence has shown that general screening tools may not be sensitive enough to pick up all ASDs hence the need for ASD-specific screening at specific intervals (Pinto-Martin et al., 2008).

Current recommendations from the AAP call for developmental surveillance to be done at every well-child visit and suggest the use of validated developmental screening tests at specific visits: 9 months, 18 months, and either 24 or 30 months of age (AAP, 2006). Crucial elements of surveillance include careful attention to parental concerns, knowing relevant risk factors, following developmental milestones, and close observation of the child. Risk factors for ASDs include family history of ASD, certain genetic syndromes, or any loss of skills. The AAP report recommends ASD-specific screening testing at the 18-month and 24-month visits, the latter of which is required to identify the child who experienced developmental regression between 18 and 24 months of age (Johnson & Myers, 2007).

There are a number of standardized screening tests available for use in the primary-care setting (*see Chapter 5*). Some are general developmental screening tests, including: the Ages and Stages Questionnaire (ASQ), the BRIGANCE Screens, the Child Development Inventories (CDI), and the Parents' Evaluation of Developmental Status (PEDS). Others are ASD-specific, including: the Modified Checklist for Autism in Toddlers (M-CHAT), the Pervasive Developmental Disorders Screening Test 11 (PDDST-11), and the Social Communication Questionnaire (SCQ).

Increasing Awareness and Knowledge of ASDs

In response to poor consistency in screening for ASDs, several organizations have worked diligently to increase and enhance knowledge for professionals and for parents. These organizations provide valuable tools for use in the primary-care practice.

The Centers for Disease Control and Prevention (CDC) (www.cdc.gov/autism) has been closely tracking the prevalence of ASDs since 1996. A public awareness campaign called "Learn the Signs. Act Early" (www.cdc.gov/actearly) launched in 2004 has reached tens of millions of health-care providers, parents, child-care providers, and community supports. First Signs, an organization begun by a parent of a child with autism, is dedicated to guiding parents and practitioners through developmental monitoring, red flags for ASDs, screening, diagnosis and treatment. In 2007, First Signs and Autism Speaks teamed up to make a very useful ASD video glossary, which has video clips of typically developing children as well as children on the autism spectrum (www.firstsigns.org).

The AAP has released several publications and developed a resource toolkit to educate practitioners in recognizing the early signs of ASDs. They also help practitioners educate parents on both typical and atypical child development by giving them examples of when to be concerned (red flags). The "Autism A.L.A.R.M." flyer informs primary-care physicians that ***A**utism is prevalent, **L**isten to parents, **A**ct early, **R**efer, and **M**onitor*, and includes the AAP surveillance and screening algorithm for ASDs[1]. With this algorithm, pediatric primary-care providers implement a risk assessment point system to guide proper follow-up and evaluation of children who may have characteristics of an ASD. An AAP introductory booklet, "Understanding Autism Spectrum Disorders," is also available for parents and primary-care providers. The AAP Autism toolkit (2007)[2] is another valuable resource for physicians containing the surveillance and screening algorithm, ASD-specific screening tests, ASD evaluation checklists, physician information sheets, and parent handouts on autism-specific topics such as vaccines, therapies, and complementary therapies.

Autism Speaks (www.autismspeaks.org) is a private foundation dedicated to raising awareness and funding a global biomedical research agenda on the genetics, causes, early detection, diagnosis, and treatment of autism spectrum disorders. Their website is another resource for PCPs with general information about ASDs, reviews of various treatments and therapies, and research updates. They created the "100-Day Kit" for parents, a booklet published in both English and Spanish, which helps families organize and set priorities immediately after an autism diagnosis.

All of these tools are valuable to the PCP for their own use and to share with families.

Diagnosis and Assessment

Following the screening guidelines and employing these tools will allow the PCP to identify children suspected to have an ASD, but what then? Diagnostic criteria delineated in the Diagnostic and Statistical Manual of Mental Disorders from the American Psychiatric Association (DSM-IV or DSM IV-tr) (American Psychiatric Association, 1994 & 2000) can be used to confirm the suspicion or at least to narrow the diagnostic possibilities. In cases where the diagnosis is clear, the child can be immediately referred for early intervention services specific to autism. In other cases, practitioners may feel a referral for further ASD diagnostic testing is necessary but should be simultaneously recommending early intervention services. But PCPs need to understand that because of the heterogeneity of the disorder a diagnosis alone is insufficient. A thorough assessment of each child that can evaluate potential genetic causes, identify comorbid medical conditions, and delineate an individual's strengths and challenges is often the most important piece for families, and is essential for treatment planning.

The "gold standard" ASD assessments are usually performed at clinical centers that employ a multidisciplinary team of experts in the field. Teams are often comprised of some combination of child psychologists, child psychiatrists, child neurologists, pediatric developmentalists, speech-language pathologists, and occupational therapists. Ideally, in addition to specific ASD diagnostic testing, the assessment should include thorough evaluation of behavior, cognition, speech and language, and sensorimotor function. A medical assessment should also be performed and appropriate referrals to specialists such as in neurology, genetics or gastroenterology can be made. Unfortunately the access to these centers is often limited.

Primary-Care Evaluation for Children with ASDs

The primary-care evaluation of a child with an ASD is based on routine primary-care practice guidelines with special attention to specific issues characteristic of ASDs (*see Table 77-1*). Ideally, office visits should take into account the child's core deficits (e.g., poor social communication skills and resistance to change/need for routine) and PCPs should be aware that exams will often be limited by behavioral difficulties and visits may take longer (Myers & Johnson, 2007).

A comprehensive history includes a developmental history and three-generation pedigree. A complete medical history should include the typical review of systems but with special focus on problems that appear to be increased in children with ASDs: neurological issues (i.e., seizures), sleep difficulties, and GI problems. Birth history is also important because babies with prematurity, low birth weight, and perinatal difficulties appear to be at increased risk (Limperopoulos et al., 2008). Developmental history needs to query more than the simple language and motor milestones and should focus on social communication skills (e.g., back and forth sharing of sounds, eye contact, responding to name, imitating others, pointing) as well as any maladaptive behaviors (e.g., rocking, hand or finger mannerisms, spinning). Any sensory difficulties (e.g., sensitivity to loud noises, certain textures, certain tastes) should be elicited from the parent. A history of any loss of any

TABLE 77–1.
Keys to history and physical exam in a child with an ASD

- Thorough history
  - Query medical and behavioral issues past and present
  - Query developmental history
  - Query family history to include a three-generation pedigree
- Complete physical exam
  - Observe child in exam room
  - Measure growth parameters, especially head circumference
  - Conduct dysmorphology evaluation
  - Evaluate skin with Wood's lamp
  - Conduct neurological exam
- Studies for all children with developmental delays
  - Conduct audiologic evaluation
  - Screen for lead
- Studies to consider in ASD
  - Genetic testing
  - Metabolic testing
  - EEG
  - MRI

skills or regression should be documented. Given the strong genetic component of autism, the child's family history should be queried for any ASD diagnosis, genetic disorder, neurological disorders (seizures), psychiatric history (obsessive-compulsive disorder, anxiety or mood disorders), language delay or disability, and other learning difficulties.

Beyond its importance for routine health care, a physical exam is an opportunity for direct observation of a child's behavior allowing a preliminary assessment of eye contact, joint attention, and the child's main form of communication and expressive language skills. Any repetitive or stereotyped behaviors in the exam room should also be recorded. Noting the presence or absence of certain physical findings is essential. Although macrocephaly is not specific to autism, providers should be aware that this is overrepresented in this disorder with 20% showing head circumferences above the 98% (Fombonne et al., 1999). Examining the child for any dysmorphic features (face, limbs, stature, genitalia) can also yield clues to various genetic syndromes and diagnoses associated with ASDs. Because there is a higher incidence of autism in children with tuberous sclerosis, a careful evaluation of a child's skin for neurocutaneous lesions such as hypopigmented macules or ash-leaf spots (using a *Wood's lamp* or ultraviolet light source) is important. A neurological exam focusing on reflexes, abnormal movements, strength, tone, and coordination will assist the physician in ruling out neurological and muscle disorders that may be contributing to the core deficits of an ASD.

There are certain studies and labs that should be done in every child with developmental delay including an ASD. A formal audiologic hearing evaluation is recommended for all children with developmental delays (ASHA, 2004) to rule out hearing problems that could contribute to communication deficits. Lead screening is also recommended for all child showing signs of developmental delay, even if the child does not have pica or an oral fixation (CDC, 1997). Although not implicated in causing autism, lead poisoning can lead to learning disabilities, cognitive deficits, and behavioral problems. Many children on the autism spectrum, especially children with intellectual disabilities, remain in the oral-motor phase of development, placing them at a higher risk for lead poisoning (Cohen et al., 1976; Shannon & Graef, 1996).

Recommendations regarding additional medical testing are inconsistent (Johnson & Myers, 2007) and often based on clinical practice experience and expertise. PCPs need to recognize that further workup may have two different functions: diagnostic testing warranted by current health-related issues and testing for possible etiologies. This latter issue is often the most important to parents.

Tests to consider include EEG, MRI, and genetic testing. Some neurologists will use EEG for routine screening although the practice standards only call for it if there is a clinical suspicion of seizures or developmental regression. Brain MRIs are currently only recommended in the case of an abnormal neurological exam (Filipek et al., 2000). Many of the existing practice guidelines call for basic genetic testing in ASDs including high-resolution chromosome analysis and DNA for Fragile X. Many will also do fluorescence in situ hybridization (FISH) for the 15q region looking for duplication. The newer microarray technology is more sensitive in identifying abnormalities in individuals with ASDs (Shen et al., 2010) and is likely to replace karyotypes in the very near future. The presence of moderate to severe intellectual disability and syndromic features greatly increases the yield of genetic testing. Discovery of a genetic abnormality is especially important because of genetic counseling implications.

Although any additional testing may not be done in a primary-care setting, it is important for practitioners to be aware of the possible comorbidities in this disorder and to have a low threshold for making subspecialty referrals appropriate for each child. All too often, issues are ignored because they are simply attributed to "the autism."

Establishment of a Medical Home

Despite the fact that a child may receive the diagnosis of an ASD outside of his primary care, a child's medical home will usually continue to remain with his PCP. For this reason, patients and families will be greatly benefited by a provider who is knowledgeable about ASDs. Navigating the world of autism can be extremely difficult for parents and children. They deserve to have a primary-care physician who will recognize and manage common medical problems seen with ASDs, facilitate early intervention and school issues, help sort through various therapies and treatments, and ultimately aid in planning for various transitions such as entering school, beginning adolescence, and venturing into adulthood.

It is especially important to remember that these children need the same standard of care as children with typical development. They need to be treated for the same childhood illnesses, receive appropriate anticipatory guidance, and have their immunizations kept up-to-date.

Medical Issues to Consider

Seizures

One of the most frequent medical comorbidities is epilepsy. It is commonly stated that 1/3 of individuals with ASDs will have seizures, although reported rates are variable, probably resulting from sample ascertainment differences. Large population-based samples show rates ranging from 5 to 26% (Fombonne, 1999). Risk factors for epilepsy include moderate to severe intellectual disability, comorbid neurological and neurogenetic conditions (e.g., cerebral palsy, Tuberous Sclerosis Complex, 15q duplication syndrome), and female gender (Spence & Schneider, 2009). Age of seizure onset is bimodal (early childhood vs. adolescence or early adulthood) (Volkmar & Nelson, 1990), and there is variability in the type and severity of seizures.

The diagnosis of epilepsy is made more challenging because the behavior exhibited during a seizure can be confused with typical ASD behaviors. For instance, absence (petit mal) and complex partial seizures are characterized by periods of unresponsiveness. However, failing to answer to your name is one of the hallmarks of ASD behavior. Complex partial seizures can also demonstrate behavioral automatisms that could be confused with autistic stereotypical behaviors.

Any suspicion of seizures should prompt a neurology referral for further workup including EEG. Although a prolonged or overnight EEG (including natural sleep) is more sensitive to abnormalities than a routine office study, these are often more difficult to obtain in children with behavioral difficulties. Seizure treatment in ASD has the same goals as for all pediatric epilepsy: the best efficacy with the lowest side-effect profile; but with special consideration of behavioral side effects of anticonvulsants, both negative (behavioral dysregulation) and positive (mood stabilization).

Finally, there is growing awareness and interest in the occurrence of background EEG abnormalities—especially epileptiform discharges—in ASDs, even in the absence of clinical seizures. Some studies have shown epileptiform discharges in up to 60% of individuals (Chez et al., 2006; Kim et al., 2006). What to do about these abnormalities is not yet known but there are practitioners prescribing anticonvulsant medication based on the idea that discharges could negatively affect cognition or behavior. Although there are some small studies from other childhood epilepsy syndromes that suggest that these treatments could be beneficial (Spence & Schneider, 2009), more empiric data are needed to determine if these will eventually be considered among best practices in ASD.

Sleep Issues

Parents report significant sleep disorders as one of the most common comorbidities in ASDs. Sleep problems include insomnia, delayed sleep onset, sleep fragmentation, and early-morning awakening (Johnson & Malow, 2008) and appear to occur more frequently in children with ASDs than typical children (DeVincent et al., 2007; Polimeni et al., 2005). Although problems may be even more common in ASD children with comorbid intellectual disability, they are also prevalent for those with normal intelligence (Malow et al., 2006). PCPs must consider the multitude of causes for sleep difficulty including comorbid medical issues (seizures, gastrointestinal disturbance) or psychiatric issues (anxiety), medications (stimulants, asthma treatments) and/or behavioral/environmental issues. Finding the cause(s) and offering appropriate treatment may significantly improve daytime functioning (Johnson & Malow, 2008).

Gastrointestinal Dysfunction

Results from studies investigating the relationship between gastrointestinal (GI) symptoms and ASDs have been conflicting, leading to much discussion and debate. Initial reports of significant GI symptoms in children with ASDs (e.g., frequent constipation, loose stools or diarrhea, reflux, abdominal pain and bloating) suffered from selection bias and lack of control populations, calling into question whether this is an issue unique to autism. But a more recent study demonstrated significantly higher symptom rates in the ASD children compared to those with typical development and other developmental disabilities (70% versus 28% and 42%, respectively) (Valicenti-McDermott et al., 2006), supporting the idea that GI dysfunction is an associated condition of ASDs.

There have also been reports of abnormalities on endoscopy. In a now infamous study[3] published in the *Lancet* in 1998, a group of GI specialists performed endoscopy in a small number of patients with ASDs and reported ileal lymphoid hyperplasia in these children (Wakefield et al., 1998b). Another group found esophagitis, gastritis, and duodenitis (Horvath et al., 1999). Further studies from the Wakefield group have postulated an immune-mediated pathology (Furlano et al., 2001; Torrente et al., 2002). However, interpretation of the findings is limited by lack of proper controls and biased recruitment of children with known GI symptoms, which may not be representative of the general population of children with ASDs. There is further disagreement regarding whether these histological changes are specific to ASDs or even pathological (MacDonald & Domizio, 2007).

At this time, there are no specific recommendations regarding GI workup or treatment in children with an ASD diagnosis. However, the Autism Speaks' Autism Treatment Network, a group of clinicians from 15 hospitals serving children with autism, is currently developing guidelines for GI assessment in autism. For ASD patients with GI symptoms, a closer evaluation of the GI system is certainly warranted. Dependent on the severity of the condition, a GI referral may be necessary. Anecdotal evidence suggests that GI discomfort can contribute to aberrant behavior and that behavioral improvement can be seen with proper medical treatment.

Feeding and Nutritional Issues

Food selectivity is frequently described in children with ASDs. Sensory as well as behavioral issues and rigid mealtime routines have been implicated. However, data on nutrient intake of these children is both limited and conflicting. One study demonstrated no differences in nutrient intake between children with and without ASDs (Lockner et al., 2008). Another showed inadequate vitamin intake in children with ASDs (Cornish, 1998). Anecdotally the authors have seen patients where strict food preferences have actually contributed to malnutrition and required intervention via tube feeding.

Many children with ASDs will be placed on modified diets and/or given supplements (Hanson et al., 2007; Levy & Hyman, 2003). Concern for food allergies may drive special diet choices but there has been limited research proving any overlap of non-IgE-mediated food allergies and autism (Jyonouchi, Geng, Ruby, Reddy, et al., 2005; Jyonouchi, Geng, Ruby, & Zimmerman-Bier, 2005). Families may confuse what they see as adverse behavioral reactions to a given food with a true allergy. This is not to say that children with ASDs never have food allergies, but these may not be related to the autism diagnosis (Murch, 2005). The pediatrician should be aware of the child's diet and should help supervise any exclusion diet or vitamin supplementation to ensure there are no significant nutritional deficiencies or significant side effects from high doses of vitamins. If close monitoring of diet and supplements is beyond the scope of practice for the practitioner, a referral to a nutritionist might be beneficial.

Immune Problems

Involvement of the immune system in autism is currently a very active research area (*see Chapter 24*), but most of the work has been done in the basic science arena investigating etiology. From a clinical perspective the data are limited. Counter to anecdotal reports, there is no evidence for increased rates of infection in the early lives of children with autism (Rosen et al., 2007). Some studies have suggested higher rates of autoimmune disorders in family members of children with autism (Sweeten et al., 2003). Immunological profiling of children with ASDs has yielded inconsistent evidence of immune dysregulation (Ashwood & Van de Water, 2004) and the clinical significance of this remains unknown. Because auto-immunity has been implicated (Wills et al., 2007), some practitioners are advocating immune-mediated treatments (steroids or intravenous immunoglobulins). Although this may eventually prove to be an important treatment mechanism in ASDs, at this time there is scant evidence to support efficacy.

Tics and Tourette Syndrome

Studies have shown significantly higher rates of tics and Tourette Syndrome in individuals with ASDs than would be expected by chance co-occurrence alone. In samples of ASD patients tics have been reported in up to 22% and Tourette Syndrome in 8 to 20% (Baron-Cohen et al., 1999; Burd et al., 1987; Canitano & Vivanti, 2007).

One difficulty for practitioners is to differentiate tics (especially complex tics) from the motor and vocal stereotypies seen in ASDs. Tics tend to be brief and occur abruptly out of the context of typical or normal behavior. Stereotypies such as hand flapping, spinning, and hopping are repetitive or ritualistic movements that are typically more rhythmic and continuous than tics. Tics tend to have a waxing and waning course and can change in type and frequency while stereotypies will often remain constant for many years. Although children with autism will likely have stereotypies, it is important for pediatricians to be aware of the increased risk of tics and Tourette syndrome in ASDs because of the treatment implications. Children on the autism spectrum with comorbid tic disorders may have worsening tics when started on stimulant medications. Neuroleptic medications, often used in patients with a primary tic disorder, may be beneficial to the child on the spectrum with comorbid tics but will likely be less effective for the stereotypies.

Genetic Abnormalities

Although the etiology of autism remains largely unknown, it is clear that there is a strong genetic component, and recurrence risk within families is estimated at approximately 10%. Certain genetic syndromes or neurogenetic disorders are also known to be overrepresented in individuals with ASDs. Neurological or genetic disorders may account for up to 10 to 20% of autism cases (Barton & Volkmar, 1998; Kielinen et al., 2004; Oliveira et al., 2007) and chromosomal abnormalities are present in 3 to 9% using standard cytogenetic testing (karyotyping) (Fombonne et al., 1997; Wassink et al., 2001). Newer genetic testing methodologies using microarrays are now able to detect copy number variations (CNVs), which demonstrate microdeletion and duplications in the genome, postulated to be etiologically related to ASDs in a subset of patients (Sebat et al., 2007; Szatmari et al., 2007).

The most frequent associations are with Fragile X Syndrome, Tuberous Sclerosis Complex, and 15q duplication syndrome, each of which is thought to be present in 1 to 3% of individuals with autism. Rett Syndrome also shares phenotypic features with autism (at least at the early stages) and should especially be considered in girls with regression. A microdeletion and/or duplication syndrome involving a region on chromosome 16 (16p11) has also been reported (Kumar et al., 2008; Weiss et al., 2008). Autism has also been seen in patients with other neurogenetic syndromes, including: Neurofibromatosis, Hypomelanosis of Ito, Moebius Syndrome, Prader-Willi and Angelman, Joubert, Down Syndrome, Williams Syndrome, Sotos Syndrome; muscular dystrophy, Cowden Syndrome, Cohen Syndrome, Velocardiofacial Syndrome, ARX mutations, and Timothy syndrome (Spence, 2004). Obviously each of these syndromes must be considered in the context of its typical clinical presentation beyond autism symptoms.

There are also reports of an autism phenotype in some patients with metabolic disorders such as untreated Phenylketonuria (PKU) (Baieli et al., 2003), disorders of purine metabolism, biotinidase deficiency, disorders of cerebrospinal fluid (CSF) neurotransmitters including deficiency of folic acid (Moretti et al., 2008), and Smith-Lemli-Opitz syndrome (SLOS) (Tierney et al., 2001), and others (Manzi et al., 2008). Although these are rare conditions, detection is crucial because they may represent treatable entities.

There has also been interest in the overlap between mitochondrial disorders and ASDs, which is highlighted in a case report questioning the role of vaccines in the autistic regression of a child later found to have an underlying mitochondrial disorder (Poling et al., 2006). Published literature would suggest that these cases are rare, but clues to possible mitochondrial dysfunction include significant hypotonia, seizures, and severe delays (Filiano et al., 2002; Oliveira et al., 2005).

Other Associated Conditions

Intellectual Disabilities

Historically the literature has stated that approximately 70% of individuals with autism have comorbid intellectual disability

(Fombonne, 1999; Rapin, 1997). However, there have been more recent studies that have shown lower rates (Fombonne, 2009) and this may result from the inclusion of children on the milder end of the autism spectrum, availability of intervention, and improved testing of cognitive abilities in nonverbal children.

Cognitive abilities can be difficult to measure because of behavioral difficulties that interfere with testing and the fact that tests often rely heavily on language, a core deficit in this disorder. Therefore, low scores may not be completely reflective of true deficits. In tests that attempt to separate out nonverbal and verbal abilities, there is often a significant discrepancy between verbal and nonverbal scores. Although the trend has been either similar scores on these domains or higher scores on the nonverbal domains (Munson et al., 2008), higher verbal scores have been found in some studies of children with high-functioning autism or Asperger Disorder (Miller & Ozonoff, 2000).

Knowing the cognitive level of an individual with an ASD impacts several factors, including diagnostic clarity, treatment, and prognosis. Clinicians often have a difficult time differentiating autism core features in a child with severe intellectual disability. Because children with very low IQs will often be nonverbal and have limited social awareness, one might confuse this with autism. Therefore, clinicians must evaluate a child's social abilities in relation to their developmental age before diagnosing an ASD.

Individuals with ASDs and intellectual disability also have an increased risk of comorbid disorders such as epilepsy (Spence & Schneider, 2009), psychiatric disorders (attention-deficit/hyperactive disorder, mood disorders, catatonia) (McCarthy, 2007) and genetic syndromes (especially in dysmorphic individuals) (Battaglia & Carey, 2006; Miles & Hillman, 2000; Shevell et al., 2001). Furthermore, correct assessments of cognitive abilities are crucial for educational planning. Overall intelligence and particularly nonverbal cognitive ability tends be one of the strongest predictors of outcomes in general (Helt et al., 2008), in studies investigating pretreatment variables in predicting the success of behavioral treatments (Howlin et al., 2009), and in studies extending to adulthood (Howlin et al., 2004).

There are children on the autism spectrum with extraordinary splinter skills in areas such as math or art who may be considered savants, but these situations are rare and poorly understood.

Regression

Approximately 1/5 to 1/3 of children with ASDs will experience some type of regression of previously acquired skills. This typically occurs between 15 and 24 months of age (Turner et al., 2006; Werner & Dawson, 2005). Severe regression occurring after a 2-year period of typical development is diagnostic of Childhood Disintegrative Disorder, a rare pervasive developmental disorder (Association, 1994; Mouridsen, 2003).

Regression can be in the form of loss of verbal skills, loss of social skills (eye contact, play behaviors) or loss of gestural communication (waving bye-bye, pointing) (Lord et al., 2004; Meilleur & Fombonne, 2009; Stefanatos et al., 2002) and can occur in children with typical development or even more often, in the setting of already delayed milestones (Meilleur & Fombonne, 2009). Some studies have suggested a poorer cognitive outcome for children with ASDs and regression, with these children having more intellectual disability (Hoshino et al., 1987; Kobayashi & Murata, 1998).

The astute clinician should not automatically attribute signs of regression to psychosocial stressors (such as a family move or a new sibling), but rather further investigate the nature and severity of the regression. Epileptic disorders such as infantile spasms or Landau-Kleffner Syndrome or rare metabolic disorders need to be considered in the differential diagnosis.

Sensory-Motor Abnormalities

Although not part of the core features of autism, sensory and motor dysfunction is common in children with ASDs. Odd behaviors appear to indicate either decreased or increased interest or sensitivity to the sensory world (Rogers et al., 2003). These occur in all senses, including visual (close visual inspection, peering out of the corners of the eyes), auditory (intolerance to noises, holding hands over the ears), somatosensory (repetitive feeling of surfaces, intolerance to certain sensations) or olfactory systems (needing to sniff objects).

More interest is also being paid to subtle motor deficits in these children. There have been reports of motor delays (Mayes & Calhoun, 2003), hypotonia (Ming et al., 2007), gait and balance issues (Kielinen et al., 2004; Minshew et al., 2004), clumsiness (Ghaziuddin & Butler, 1998), and dyspraxia (Dziuk et al., 2007; Mandelbaum et al., 2006) in individuals with ASDs (*see Chapter 22*).

Behavior Problems

Many children with ASDs have challenging behaviors such as significant tantrums, aggression toward others, and self-injury, which often interfere with educational programs, community involvement, and family life. These may be more prevalent in individuals with comorbid intellectual disability (Bodfish et al., 2000; Schroeder et al., 2001).

A role for the PCP is to evaluate the child for medical reasons that may be contributing to these behaviors (Bosch et al., 1997), as a number of medical problems may negatively influence behavior. A careful history and examination is essential for their identification, especially because individuals with autism may not be able to communicate specific symptoms. The following medical issues should be considered: infections (otitis media, pharyngitis, dental abscess, UTI, URI); GI problems (constipation, reflux); sleep disturbances; undetected injuries (even fractures); hormonal fluctuations during puberty. Those medical issues that are amenable to treatment should be treated accordingly. In addition to common medical issues, medications or supplements that the child may be taking may produce behavioral side effects. Finally, possible environmental or situational causes of the behaviors should be explored with the family. As with typically developing children, transitions, family events, certain places, and new siblings can be possible reasons for exacerbation of problem behaviors.

PCPs can also help families with behavioral intervention by requesting a functional behavioral analysis to be accomplished by a child psychologist or qualified professional in the school system. This analysis should not only assist in discovering the antecedents and triggers for the behaviors, but should also facilitate a behavioral plan to decrease and/or manage behaviors. In severe cases, physicians should consider referral to a specialist for medication management (a developmental-behavioral pediatrician, child psychiatrist, or child neurologist).

Other Psychiatric Disorders

It is important for the PCP to be aware that children with autism can and do present with comorbid psychiatric disorders. Although current DSM criteria preclude a diagnosis of Attention Deficit Hyperactivity Disorder (ADHD) in the setting of ASD, it is clear that many children on the spectrum have significant difficulty with attention and hyperactivity. Similarly, mood disorders and anxiety can be common. Given the complexities of teasing out behaviors that result from the autism vs. these other disorders, most PCPs will want to consider referral to a child psychiatrist for further evaluation and treatment. (*See Chapters 15–18, 20, 22, 69, and 76 for more detail.*)

Interventions

As soon as a child is suspected of having an ASD, early intervention services should be initiated as research suggests that intensive early intervention substantially improves outcomes (Sallows & Graupner, 2005). A panel convened by the National Research Council defined intensive early intervention as at least 25 hours per week of instruction with year-round services (Lord & McGee, 2001). Although a PCP may not be responsible for setting up therapy, understanding the options and educating families on their rights is important. A brief overview is presented below.

Navigating the Educational System

Federal regulations ensure that all children with disabilities be offered funded educational programming either through an Individualized Family Service Plan (IFSP) or an Individualized Education Plan (IEP). A state-funded IFSP will document and guide the early-intervention process for the family with a child under 3 years old with a suspected or diagnosed ASD. When the child turns 3 years old, the local school system takes over the child's educational services. IEPs outline the education services to include needed therapies (behavioral, speech, occupational, physical) for learning purposes as well as specific short-term and long-term goals for the child with an ASD. However, these programs are not mandated to offer the 25 hours per week of instruction or year-round services, so the child's pediatrician should be aware of other community services and therapies to supplement the child's early-intervention experience. Local programs vary tremendously and many families will choose to go beyond the funded programs to obtain more intensive or different services.

Available Behavioral Interventions

Behavioral and educational therapies are the mainstay of treatments. Unfortunately, the literature regarding the efficacy of various therapies lags behind the growing number of children needing services. Although there are certainly differences between treatment programs in technique and even underlying theory (e.g., strict behaviorist vs. more developmental or naturalistic), there is some agreement on some common elements including the need for: immediate access, intensive therapy, low student–teacher ratios, parent training, exposure to typically developing peers, frequent evaluation, structure and predictability, and opportunities for generalization (Myers & Johnson, 2007). (*For more detail on these therapies, see Chapter 58–66, and 75 in this volume.*)

Applied Behavior Analysis (ABA) techniques have been the best-studied and have demonstrated efficacy for creating significant developmental and cognitive gains (Lovaas, 1987; McEachin et al., 1993; Sallows & Graupner, 2005). ABA therapy strives to increase and enhance social communication as well as teach cognitive skills and decrease problem behaviors through a variety of behavioral analytic methods to include, but not limited to: repetition, positive reinforcement, shaping, prompting, and fading.

The Treatment and Education of Autistic and Related Communication-Handicapped Children (TEACCH) program is a special education model tailored to the individual's needs, similar to ABA. The focus of TEACCH is a structured physical, social, and communicating environment, especially helpful for the visual learner (www.teacch.com). Another team-based educational model is Social Communication, Emotional Regulation and Implementing Transactional Supports (SCERTS). This model uses a variety of behavioral interventions including ABA, visual supports, and augmentative communication (www.scerts.com).

The Developmental, Individual-difference, Relationship-based (DIR) model contains "Floor-time" therapy. The Floor-time model involves the parent engaging the child at his or her current developmental level and allowing the child to lead the interaction (www.floortime.org). The Relationship Development Intervention (RDI) method is another parent-based therapy (Gutstein et al., 2007) with a goal of having the child make social improvements in everyday functioning and relationships through a variety of social activities (www.rdiconnect.com). These interventions, although popular, have not yet been empirically validated to be efficacious.

Responsive teaching (RT) (Mahoney & Perales, 2005) and Pivotal Response Training (PRT) (Koegel et al., 2001) are intervention models that encourage parents to be the primary interventionists and are applied in the child's natural environment, such as home and school.

Other approaches to augment behavioral therapies are also frequently employed. Speech and language therapy works on verbal and nonverbal skills as well as teaching other modalities of communication such as sign language or use of augmentative communication devices or systems. For children with fine motor delays, delayed self-help skills, or significant sensory issues, occupational therapy may be beneficial. Therapists often use sensory integration therapy for children with ASDs and sensory issues, although efficacy data are lacking. Another commonly used technique (especially for higher-functioning children) is social skills training, which may help with joint attention, social communication, and understanding of nonverbal cues.

The bulk of published evidence supports the efficacy of early intervention based on applied behavior analysis. Unfortunately, there is very little evidence regarding what therapeutic technique is best for a given child. This leaves many families struggling with which model to choose or being forced to go with what is available in their community.

Psychopharmacological Treatment

Although pediatricians may not be prescribing medications, they should be aware of those agents in most common usage for individuals with ASDs. Treatments are currently targeted on specific symptoms and medication choices are based on usage in other childhood psychiatric disorders. But as reviewed in this volume (*see Chapter 69 and 76*) there is limited empiric evidence for efficacy specifically in autism. At the same time, psychoactive medication usage is very common and increasing over time in this population with reported rates over 50% (Aman et al., 2003; Mandell et al., 2008; Oswald & Sonenklar, 2007).

Stimulants and alpha-adrenergic blockers target hyperactivity and attentional problems. Antidepressants (especially serotonergic) are commonly used for mood, anxiety, and the obsessive-compulsive type behaviors (restricted interests, repetitive behaviors). Various mood stabilizers (including anticonvulsants) are used for mood lability and outbursts. Antipsychotic or neuroleptic agents are most often employed for aggression and irritability. In fact, risperidone is currently the only agent with specific FDA approval for use in ASDs. Melatonin and a variety of sedative agents have been used for sleep problems.

Complementary and Alternative Medicine (CAM)

It is imperative for the pediatrician to appreciate the high rate of CAM use in individuals with ASDs. Studies estimate that up to 75 to 95% of ASD families may be using some form of CAM (Harrington et al., 2006; Levy & Hyman, 2003; Wong & Smith, 2006). So in order to provide optimal care, physicians need to be asking families about CAM use. One role for the PCP is to encourage families to carefully evaluate the scientific evidence (or lack thereof) for these treatments and to point out those with "red flags" that would make us question their validity, such as claims of immediate benefit, cure, and total lack of side effects (Myers & Johnson, 2007). Parents also need to know that so-called "natural" treatments may produce adverse effects and affect other medications that the child is taking. Although a full review of the available CAM therapies is beyond the scope of this chapter (*see Chapter 71 for a complete review*), awareness of the most common treatments is important.

The gluten-free casein-free diet is one of the most commonly used special diets. Anecdotally parents report not only improved GI symptoms, but also improved behavior and communication skills. Unfortunately, this diet has not yet been rigorously tested for efficacy and small studies show conflicting results (Elder et al., 2006; Knivsberg et al., 1995; Knivsberg et al., 2002). Parents need to know that this diet is still unproven in children with ASDs.

Supplements are another common CAM therapy. There are a multitude of products marketed for children with autism, including vitamins, minerals, fatty acids and amino acids, and even enzyme preparations. Some are recommended in homeopathic doses, others in supratherapeutic amounts. Again, there are very few studies to support their use, but the PCP must be aware of what patients are taking and educate families on possible side effects such as those seen with high doses of certain vitamins (e.g., A, D, E, B-3, B-6, and C) (Rosenbloom, 2007).

Practitioners and families may find the National Center for Complementary and Alternative Medicine (NCCAM, www.nccam.nih.gov) to be a helpful resource for investigating various alternative therapies for ASDs.

Conclusions

Given the prevalence of autism, PCPs will inevitably be taking care of patients on the autism spectrum. Best practices would dictate that the child with an ASD is cared for in the context of a medical home where the practitioner is knowledgeable about everything from screening and diagnosis, to workup and management, to interventions and family support. This is obviously a lofty goal for many primary-care providers in the current practice setting but we hope the information provided in this chapter can get them closer to a realization of this goal.

Unfortunately, the state of the scientific literature is not at the point where truly evidence-based practice parameters can be devised for most of the problems encountered by individuals with ASDs in the primary-care setting, but we should be heartened by the fact that there are groups working on this issue. As mentioned above, the Autism Treatment Network[4] is a collection of autism centers around the country and in Canada that is dedicated to collecting the data necessary to create practice parameters for medical workup and treatment of children with ASDs. As data are collected, practice standards and, later, true evidence-based practice parameters will be created and shared with the primary-care community. Until that time, PCPs are left with the enormous challenge of keeping up-to-date with a fast-moving and complex field.

Challenges and Future Directions

- Creation of a medical home in the primary-care setting for all individuals with autism that would greatly improve care practices for children and their families.
- Improved access to autism diagnosis and evaluation centers and subspecialty referrals for all families to reduce burden on primary-care providers.
- Improved data on prevalence of various medical and other comorbidities in ASDs that would allow for better education for families on the risks of these entities.
- Establishment of practice standards and eventually evidence-based practice parameters for management of medical issues in ASDs.

NOTES

1 Website: http://www.medicalhomeinfo.org/health/Autism%20downloads/AutismAlarm.pdf

2 More information at http://www.aap.org/publiced/autismtoolkit.cfm

3 The real controversy came with the comment that these children had experienced a behavioral regression after their MMR vaccine, implying that the vaccination may have been causally related to autism (Kawashima et al., 2000; Wakefield et al., 1998a), a controversy that played out in the media. However, in 2004 allegations of scientific misconduct were brought to the Lancet editors (Horton, 2004) and a partial retraction was printed by 10 of 13 authors (S. H. Murch et al., 2004). Many further studies have failed to demonstrate a causal relationship between MMR and ASD (Chen, Landau, Sham, & Fombonne, 2004; Dales, Hammer, & Smith, 2001; DeStefano, Bhasin, Thompson, Yeargin-Allsopp, & Boyle, 2004; Hornig et al., 2008; Richler et al., 2006; Taylor et al., 1999). Unfortunately, because of the media frenzy, there are still concerns about the possible link between the MMR and autism in the lay community.

4. Website: http://www.autismspeaks.org/science/programs/atn/. Funded by Autism Speaks and a grant from the Health Resources and Services Administration (HRSA).

SUGGESTED READING

Johnson, C. P., & Myers, S. M. (2007). Identification and evaluation of children with autism spectrum disorders. *Pediatrics, 120*(5), 1183–1215.

Myers, S. M., & Johnson, C. P. (2007). Management of children with autism spectrum disorders. *Pediatrics, 120*(5), 1162–1182.

ACKNOWLEDGMENTS

The authors wish to thank Susan Swedo, Audrey Thurm, and Geoff Smith for helpful comments on this manuscript.

Disclaimer: This work was written as part of our official duties as Government employees. The article is freely available for publication without a copyright notice, and there are no restrictions on its use, now or subsequently. The views expressed in this chapter are the private views of the authors and are not to be construed as official or reflecting the views of the NIMH, NIH, HHS, Department of the Army, Department of Defense, or the United States Government.

REFERENCES

AAP (2001). The pediatrician's role in the diagnosis and management of autistic spectrum disorder in children. *Pediatrics, 107*, 1221–1226.

AAP (2006). Identifying infants and young children with developmental disorders in the medical home: An algorithm for developmental surveillance and screening. *Pediatrics, 118*(1), 405–420.

Aman, M. G., Lam, K. S., & Collier-Crespin, A. (2003). Prevalence and patterns of use of psychoactive medicines among individuals with autism in the Autism Society of Ohio. *Journal of Autism and Developmental Disorders, 33*(5), 527–534.

American Psychiatric Association. (1994). *Diagnostic and Statistical Manual of Mental Disorders* (4th ed.; DSM-IV). Washington, DC.

American Psychiatric Association. (2000). *Diagnostic and Statistical Manual of Mental Disorders* (4th ed., text rev.; DSM-IV-TR). Washington, DC.

ASHA (1991). *Guidelines for the audiologic assessment of children from birth through 36 months of age.* American Speech-Language-Hearing Association. (www.asha.org/policy)

Ashwood, P., & Van de Water, J. (2004). A review of autism and the immune response. *Clinical and Developmental Immunology, 11*(2), 165–174.

Baieli, S., Pavone, L., Meli, C., Fiumara, A., & Coleman, M. (2003). Autism and phenylketonuria. *Journal of Autism and Developmental Disorders, 33*(2), 201–204.

Baron-Cohen, S., Scahill, V. L., Izaguirre, J., Hornsey, H., & Robertson, M. M. (1999). The prevalence of Gilles de la Tourette syndrome in children and adolescents with autism: A large scale study. *Psychological Medicine, 29*(5), 1151–1159.

Barton, M., & Volkmar, F. (1998). How commonly are known medical conditions associated with autism? *Journal of Autism and Developmental Disorders, 28*(4), 273–278.

Battaglia, A., & Carey, J. C. (2006). Etiologic yield of autistic spectrum disorders: A prospective study. *American Journal of Medical Genetics. Part C, Seminars in Medical Genetics, 142C*(1), 3–7.

Bodfish, J. W., Symons, F. J., Parker, D. E., & Lewis, M. H. (2000). Varieties of repetitive behavior in autism: Comparisons to mental retardation. *Journal of Autism and Developmental Disorders, 30*(3), 237–243.

Bosch, J., Van Dyke, C., Smith, S. M., & Poulton, S. (1997). Role of medical conditions in the exacerbation of self-injurious behavior: An exploratory study. *Mental Retardation, 35*(2), 124–130.

Burd, L., Fisher, W. W., Kerbeshian, J., & Arnold, M. E. (1987). Is development of Tourette disorder a marker for improvement in patients with autism and other pervasive developmental disorders? *Journal of the American Acadamy of Child and Adolescent Psychiatry, 26*(2), 162–165.

Canitano, R., & Vivanti, G. (2007). Tics and Tourette syndrome in autism spectrum disorders. *Autism, 11*(1), 19–28.

CDC (1997). *Screening young children for lead poisoning: Guidance for state and local public health officials.* Atlanta, Centers for Disease Control and Prevention.

CDC (2009). *Prevalence of autism spectrum disorders—Autism and developmental disabilities monitoring network,* United States, 2006. *Morbidity and Mortality Weekly Report Surveillance Summary, 58*(10), 1–20.

Chen, W., Landau, S., Sham, P., & Fombonne, E. (2004). No evidence for links between autism, MMR and measles virus. *Psychological Medicine, 34*(3), 543–553.

Chez, M. G., Chang, M., Krasne, V., Coughlan, C., Kominsky, M., & Schwartz, A. (2006). Frequency of epileptiform EEG abnormalities in a sequential screening of autistic patients with no known clinical epilepsy from 1996 to 2005. *Epilepsy and Behavior, 8*(1), 267–271.

Cohen, D. J., Johnson, W. T., & Caparulo, B. K. (1976). Pica and elevated blood lead level in autistic and atypical children. *American Journal of Diseases of Children, 130*(1), 47–48.

Cornish, E. (1998). A balanced approach towards healthy eating in autism. *Journal of Human Nutrition and Dietetics, 11,* 501–509.

Dales, L., Hammer, S. J., & Smith, N. J. (2001). Time trends in autism and in MMR immunization coverage in California. *Journal of the American Medical Association, 285*(9), 1183–1185.

DeStefano, F., Bhasin, T. K., Thompson, W. W., Yeargin-Allsopp, M., & Boyle, C. (2004). Age at first measles-mumps-rubella vaccination in children with autism and school-matched control subjects: A population-based study in metropolitan Atlanta. *Pediatrics, 113*(2), 259–266.

DeVincent, C. J., Gadow, K. D., Delosh, D., & Geller, L. (2007). Sleep disturbance and its relation to DSM-IV psychiatric symptoms in preschool-age children with pervasive developmental disorder and community controls. *Journal of Child Neurology, 22*(2), 161–169.

Dziuk, M. A., Gidley Larson, J. C., Apostu, A., Mahone, E. M., Denckla, M. B., & Mostofsky, S. H. (2007). Dyspraxia in autism: Association with motor, social, and communicative deficits. *Developmental Medicine and Child Neurology, 49*(10), 734–739.

Elder, J. H., Shankar, M., Shuster, J., Theriaque, D., Burns, S., & Sherrill, L. (2006). The gluten-free, casein-free diet in autism: Results of a preliminary double blind clinical trial. *Journal of Autism and Developmental Disorders, 36*(3), 413–420.

Filiano, J. J., Goldenthal, M. J., Rhodes, C. H., & Marin-Garcia, J. (2002). Mitochondrial dysfunction in patients with hypotonia, epilepsy, autism, and developmental delay: HEADD syndrome. *Journal of Child Neurology, 17*(6), 435–439.

Filipek, P. A., Accardo, P. J., Ashwal, S., Baranek, G. T., Cook, E. H., Jr., Dawson, G., et al. (2000). Practice parameter: Screening and diagnosis of autism: Report of the Quality Standards Subcommittee of the American Academy of Neurology and the Child Neurology Society. *Neurology, 55*(4), 468–479.

Filipek, P. A., Accardo, P. J., Baranek, G. T., Cook, E. H., Jr., Dawson, G., Gordon, B., et al. (1999). The screening and diagnosis of autistic spectrum disorders. *Journal of Autism and Developmental Disorders, 29*(6), 439–484.

Fombonne, E. (1999). The epidemiology of autism: A review. *Psychological Medicine, 29*(4), 769–786.

Fombonne, E. (2009). Epidemiology of pervasive developmental disorders. *Pediatric Research, 65*(6), 591–598.

Fombonne, E., Du Mazaubrun, C., Cans, C., & Grandjean, H. (1997). Autism and associated medical disorders in a French epidemiological survey. *Journal of the American Academy of Child and Adolescent Psychiatry, 36*(11), 1561–1569.

Fombonne, E., Roge, B., Claverie, J., Courty, S., & Fremolle, J. (1999). Microcephaly and macrocephaly in autism. *Journal of Autism and Developmental Disorders, 29*(2), 113–119.

Furlano, R. I., Anthony, A., Day, R., Brown, A., McGarvey, L., Thomson, M. A., et al. (2001). Colonic CD8 and gamma delta T-cell infiltration with epithelial damage in children with autism. *Journal of Pediatrics, 138*(3), 366–372.

Geschwind, D. H., Cummings, J. L., Hollander, E., DiMauro, S., Cook, E. H., Lombard, J., et al. (1998). Autism screening and diagnostic evaluation: CAN consensus statement. *CNS Spectrums, 3*(3), 40–49.

Ghaziuddin, M., & Butler, E. (1998). Clumsiness in autism and Asperger syndrome: A further report. *Journal of Intellectual Disabilities Research, 42*(Pt 1), 43–48.

Gutstein, S. E., Burgess, A. F., & Montfort, K. (2007). Evaluation of the relationship development intervention program. *Autism, 11*(5), 397–411.

Hanson, E., Kalish, L. A., Bunce, E., Curtis, C., McDaniel, S., Ware, J., et al. (2007). Use of complementary and alternative medicine among children diagnosed with autism spectrum disorder. *Journal of Autism and Developmental Disorders, 37*(4), 628–636.

Harrington, J. W., Rosen, L., Garnecho, A., & Patrick, P. A. (2006). Parental perceptions and use of complementary and alternative medicine practices for children with autistic spectrum disorders in private practice. *Journal of Developmental and Behavioral Pediatrics, 27*(2 Suppl), S156–161.

Helt, M., Kelley, E., Kinsbourne, M., Pandey, J., Boorstein, H., Herbert, M., et al. (2008). Can children with autism recover? If so, how? *Neuropsychology Reviews, 18*(4), 339–366.

Hornig, M., Briese, T., Buie, T., Bauman, M. L., Lauwers, G., Siemetzki, U., et al. (2008). Lack of association between measles virus vaccine and autism with enteropathy: A case-control study. *PLoS ONE, 3*(9), e3140.

Horton, R. (2004). A statement by the editors of The Lancet. *Lancet, 363*(9411), 820–821.

Horvath, K., Papadimitriou, J. C., Rabsztyn, A., Drachenberg, C., & Tildon, J. T. (1999). Gastrointestinal abnormalities in children with autistic disorder. *Journal of Pediatrics, 135*(5), 559–563.

Hoshino, Y., Kaneko, M., Yashima, Y., Kumashiro, H., Volkmar, F. R., & Cohen, D. J. (1987). Clinical features of autistic children with setback course in their infancy. *Japanese Journal of Psychiatry and Neurology, 41*(2), 237–245.

Howlin, P., Goode, S., Hutton, J., & Rutter, M. (2004). Adult outcome for children with autism. *Journal of Child Psychology and Psychiatry and Allied Disciplines, 45*(2), 212–229.

Howlin, P., Magiati, I., & Charman, T. (2009). Systematic review of early intensive behavioral interventions for children with autism. *American Journal on Intellectual and Developmental Disabilities, 114*(1), 23–41.

Johnson, C. P., & Myers, S. M. (2007). Identification and evaluation of children with autism spectrum disorders. *Pediatrics, 120*(5), 1183–1215.

Johnson, K. P., & Malow, B. A. (2008). Assessment and pharmacologic treatment of sleep disturbance in autism. *Child and Adolescent Psychiatric Clinics of North America, 17*(4), 773–785, viii.

Jyonouchi, H., Geng, L., Ruby, A., Reddy, C., & Zimmerman-Bier, B. (2005). Evaluation of an association between gastrointestinal symptoms and cytokine production against common dietary proteins in children with autism spectrum disorders. *Journal of Pediatrics, 146*(5), 605–610.

Jyonouchi, H., Geng, L., Ruby, A., & Zimmerman-Bier, B. (2005). Dysregulated innate immune responses in young children with autism spectrum disorders: Their relationship to gastrointestinal symptoms and dietary intervention. *Neuropsychobiology, 51*(2), 77–85.

Kawashima, H., Mori, T., Kashiwagi, Y., Takekuma, K., Hoshika, A., & Wakefield, A. (2000). Detection and sequencing of measles virus from peripheral mononuclear cells from patients with inflammatory bowel disease and autism. *Digestive Diseases and Sciences, 45*(4), 723–729.

Kielinen, M., Rantala, H., Timonen, E., Linna, S. L., & Moilanen, I. (2004). Associated medical disorders and disabilities in children with autistic disorder: A population-based study. *Autism, 8*(1), 49–60.

Kim, H. L., Donnelly, J. H., Tournay, A. E., Book, T. M., & Filipek, P. (2006). Absence of seizures despite high prevalence of epileptiform EEG abnormalities in children with autism monitored in a tertiary care center. *Epilepsia, 47*(2), 394–398.

Knivsberg, A. M., Reichelt, K., Nodland, N., & Hoein, T. (1995). Autistic syndrome and diet: A follow-up study. *Scandinavian Journal of Educational Research, 39*, 223–236.

Knivsberg, A. M., Reichelt, K. L., Hoien, T., & Nodland, M. (2002). A randomised, controlled study of dietary intervention in autistic syndromes. *Nutritional Neuroscience, 5*(4), 251–261.

Kobayashi, R., & Murata, T. (1998). Setback phenomenon in autism and long-term prognosis. *Acta Psychiatrica Scandinavica, 98*(4), 296–303.

Koegel, R. L., Koegel, L. K., & McNerney, E. K. (2001). Pivotal areas in intervention for autism. *Journal of Clinical Child Psychology, 30*(1), 19–32.

Kumar, R. A., KaraMohamed, S., Sudi, J., Conrad, D. F., Brune, C., Badner, J. A., et al. (2008). Recurrent 16p11.2 microdeletions in autism. *Human Molecular Genetics, 17*(4), 628–638.

Levy, S. E., & Hyman, S. L. (2003). Use of complementary and alternative treatments for children with autistic spectrum disorders is increasing. *Pediatric Annals, 32*(10), 685–691.

Limperopoulos, C., Bassan, H., Sullivan, N. R., Soul, J. S., Robertson, R. L., Jr., Moore, M., et al. (2008). Positive screening for autism in ex-preterm infants: Prevalence and risk factors. *Pediatrics, 121*(4), 758–765.

Lockner, D. W., Crowe, T. K., & Skipper, B. J. (2008). Dietary intake and parents' perception of mealtime behaviors in preschool-age children with autism spectrum disorder and in typically developing children. *Journal of the American Dietetic Association, 108*(8), 1360–1363.

Lord, C., & McGee, J. P. (2001). *Educating children with autism.* Washington, DC: National Academy Press.

Lord, C., Shulman, C., & DiLavore, P. (2004). Regression and word loss in autistic spectrum disorders. *Journal of Child Psychology and Psychiatry, 45*(5), 936–955.

Lovaas, O. I. (1987). Behavioral treatment and normal educational and intellectual functioning in young autistic children. *Journal of Consulting and Clinical Psychology, 55*(1), 3–9.

MacDonald, T. T., & Domizio, P. (2007). Autistic enterocolitis: Is it a histopathological entity? *Histopathology, 50*, 371–379.

Mahoney, G., & Perales, F. (2005). Relationship-focused early intervention with children with pervasive developmental disorders and other disabilities: A comparative study. *Journal of Developmental and Behavioral Pediatrics, 26*(2), 77–85.

Malow, B. A., Marzec, M. L., McGrew, S. G., Wang, L., Henderson, L. M., & Stone, W. L. (2006). Characterizing sleep in children with autism spectrum disorders: A multidimensional approach. *Sleep, 29*(12), 1563–1571.

Mandelbaum, D. E., Stevens, M., Rosenberg, E., Wiznitzer, M., Steinschneider, M., Filipek, P., et al. (2006). Sensorimotor performance in school-age children with autism, developmental language disorder, or low IQ. *Developmental Medicine and Child Neurology, 48*(1), 33–39.

Mandell, D. S., Morales, K. H., Marcus, S. C., Stahmer, A. C., Doshi, J., & Polsky, D. E. (2008). Psychotropic medication use among Medicaid-enrolled children with autism spectrum disorders. *Pediatrics, 121*(3), e441–448.

Manzi, B., Loizzo, A. L., Giana, G., & Curatolo, P. (2008). Autism and metabolic diseases. *Journal of Child Neurology, 23*(3), 307–314.

Mayes, S. D., & Calhoun, S. L. (2003). Ability profiles in children with autism: Influence of age and IQ. *Autism, 7*(1), 65–80.

McCarthy, J. (2007). Children with autism spectrum disorders and intellectual disability. *Current Opinion of Psychiatry, 20*(5), 472–476.

McEachin, J. J., Smith, T., & Lovaas, O. I. (1993). Long-term outcome for children with autism who received early intensive behavioral treatment. *American Journal of Mental Retardation, 97*(4), 359–372, discussion 373–391.

Meilleur, A. A., & Fombonne, E. (2009). Regression of language and non-language skills in pervasive developmental disorders. *Journal of Intellectual Disability Research, 53*(2), 115–124.

Miles, J. H., & Hillman, R. E. (2000). Value of a clinical morphology examination in autism. *American Journal of Medical Genetics, 91*(4), 245–253.

Miller, J. N., & Ozonoff, S. (2000). The external validity of Asperger disorder: Lack of evidence from the domain of neuropsychology. *Journal of Abnormal Psychology, 109*(2), 227–238.

Ming, X., Brimacombe, M., & Wagner, G. C. (2007). Prevalence of motor impairment in autism spectrum disorders. *Brain and Development, 29*(9), 565–570.

Minshew, N. J., Sung, K., Jones, B. L., & Furman, J. M. (2004). Underdevelopment of the postural control system in autism. *Neurology, 63*(11), 2056–2061.

Moretti, P., Peters, S. U., Del Gaudio, D., Sahoo, T., Hyland, K., Bottiglieri, T., et al. (2008). Brief report: Autistic symptoms, developmental regression, mental retardation, epilepsy, and dyskinesias in CNS folate deficiency. *Journal of Autism and Developmental Disorders, 38*(6), 1170–1177.

Mouridsen, S. E. (2003). Childhood disintegrative disorder. *Brain and Development, 25*(4), 225–228.

Munson, J., Dawson, G., Sterling, L., Beauchaine, T., Zhou, A., Elizabeth, K., et al. (2008). Evidence for latent classes of IQ in young children with autism spectrum disorder. *American Journal of Mental Retardation, 113*(6), 439–452.

Murch, S. (2005). Diet, immunity, and autistic spectrum disorders. *Journal of Pediatrics, 146*(5), 582–584.

Murch, S. H., Anthony, A., Casson, D. H., Malik, M., Berelowitz, M., Dhillon, A. P., et al. (2004). Retraction of an interpretation. *Lancet, 363*(9411), 750.

Myers, S. M., & Johnson, C. P. (2007). Management of children with autism spectrum disorders. *Pediatrics, 120*(5), 1162–1182.

Oliveira, G., Ataide, A., Marques, C., Miguel, T. S., Coutinho, A. M., Mota-Vieira, L., et al. (2007). Epidemiology of autism spectrum disorder in Portugal: Prevalence, clinical characterization, and medical conditions. *Developmental Medicine and Child Neurology, 49*(10), 726–733.

Oliveira, G., Diogo, L., Grazina, M., Garcia, P., Ataide, A., Marques, C., et al. (2005). Mitochondrial dysfunction in autism spectrum disorders: A population-based study. *Developmental Medicine and Child Neurology, 47*(3), 185–189.

Oswald, D. P., & Sonenklar, N. A. (2007). Medication use among children with autism spectrum disorders. *Journal of Child and Adolescent Psychopharmacology, 17*(3), 348–355.

Pinto-Martin, J. A., Young, L. M., Mandell, D. S., Poghosyan, L., Giarelli, E., & Levy, S. E. (2008). Screening strategies for autism spectrum disorders in pediatric primary care. *Journal of Developmental and Behavioral Pediatrics, 29*(5), 345–350.

Polimeni, M. A., Richdale, A. L., & Francis, A. J. (2005). A survey of sleep problems in autism, Asperger's disorder and typically developing children. *Journal of Intellectual Disability Research, 49*(Pt 4), 260–268.

Poling, J. S., Frye, R. E., Shoffner, J., & Zimmerman, A. W. (2006). Developmental regression and mitochondrial dysfunction in a child with autism. *Journal of Child Neurology, 21*(2), 170–172.

Rapin, I. (1997). Autism. *New England Journal of Medicine, 337*(2), 97–104.

Richler, J., Luyster, R., Risi, S., Hsu, W. L., Dawson, G., Bernier, R., et al. (2006). Is there a 'regressive phenotype' of autism spectrum disorder associated with the Measles-Mumps-Rubella vaccine? A CPEA Study. *Journal of Autism and Developmental Disorders, 36*(3), 299–316.

Robins, D. L. (2008). Screening for autism spectrum disorders in primary care settings. *Autism, 12*(5), 537–556.

Rogers, S. J., Hepburn, S., & Wehner, E. (2003). Parent reports of sensory symptoms in toddlers with autism and those with other developmental disorders. *Journal of Autism and Developmental Disorders, 33*(6), 631–642.

Rosen, N. J., Yoshida, C. K., & Croen, L. A. (2007). Infection in the first 2 years of life and autism spectrum disorders. *Pediatrics, 119*(1), e61–69.

Rosenbloom, M. (2007). *Toxicity, vitamin [electronic version].* emedicine.com.

Sallows, G. O., & Graupner, T. D. (2005). Intensive behavioral treatment for children with autism: Four-year outcome and predictors. *American Journal of Mental Retardation, 110*(6), 417–438.

Schroeder, S. R., Oster-Granite, M. L., Berkson, G., Bodfish, J. W., Breese, G. R., Cataldo, M. F., et al. (2001). Self-injurious behavior: Gene-brain-behavior relationships. *Mental Retardation and Developmental Disabilities Research Reviews, 7*(1), 3–12.

Sebat, J., Lakshmi, B., Malhotra, D., Troge, J., Lese-Martin, C., Walsh, T., et al. (2007). Strong association of de novo copy number mutations with autism. *Science, 316*(5823), 445–449.

Shannon, M., & Graef, J. W. (1996). Lead intoxication in children with pervasive developmental disorders. *Journal of Toxicology and Clinical Toxicology, 34*(2), 177–181.

Shen, Y., Dies, K. A., Holm, I. A., Bridgemohan, C., Sobeih, M. M., Caronna, E. B., et al. with Autism Consortium Clinical Genetics/DNA Diagnostics Collaboration. (2010). Clinical genetic testing for patients with autism spectrum disorders. *Pediatrics, 125*(4), e727–35.

Shevell, M. I., Majnemer, A., Rosenbaum, P., & Abrahamowicz, M. (2001). Etiologic yield of autistic spectrum disorders: A prospective study. *Journal of Child Neurology, 16*(7), 509–512.

Sices, L., Feudtner, C., McLaughlin, J., Drotar, D., & Williams, M. (2003). How do primary care physicians identify young children with developmental delays? A national survey. *Journal of Developmental and Behavioral Pediatrics, 24*(6), 409–417.

Smith, R. D. (1978). The use of developmental screening tests by primary-care pediatricians. *Journal of Pediatrics, 93*(3), 524–527.

Spence, S. J. (2004). The genetics of autism. *Seminars in Pediatric Neurology, 11*(3), 196–204.

Spence, S. J., & Schneider, M. T. (2009). The role of epilepsy and epileptiform EEGs in autism spectrum disorders. *Pediatric Research, 65*(6), 599–606.

Stefanatos, G. A., Kinsbourne, M., & Wasserstein, J. (2002). Acquired epileptiform aphasia: A dimensional view of Landau-Kleffner syndrome and the relation to regressive autistic spectrum disorders. *Child Neuropsychology, 8*(3), 195–228.

Sweeten, T. L., Bowyer, S. L., Posey, D. J., Halberstadt, G. M., & McDougle, C. J. (2003). Increased prevalence of familial autoimmunity in probands with pervasive developmental disorders. *Pediatrics, 112*(5), e420.

Szatmari, P., Paterson, A. D., Zwaigenbaum, L., Roberts, W., Brian, J., Liu, X. Q., et al. (2007). Mapping autism risk loci using genetic linkage and chromosomal rearrangements. *Nature Genetics, 39*(3), 319–328.

Taylor, B., Miller, E., Farrington, C. P., Petropoulos, M. C., Favot-Mayaud, I., Li, J., et al. (1999). Autism and Measles, Mumps, and Rubella vaccine: No epidemiological evidence for a causal association. *Lancet, 353*(9169), 2026–2029.

Tierney, E., Nwokoro, N. A., Porter, F. D., Freund, L. S., Ghuman, J. K., & Kelley, R. I. (2001). Behavior phenotype in the RSH/Smith-Lemli-Opitz syndrome. *American Journal of Medical Genetics, 98*(2), 191–200.

Torrente, F., Ashwood, P., Day, R., Machado, N., Furlano, R. I., Anthony, A., et al. (2002). Small intestinal enteropathy with epithelial IgG and complement deposition in children with regressive autism. *Molecular Psychiatry, 7*(4), 375–382, 334.

Turner, L. M., Stone, W. L., Pozdol, S. L., & Coonrod, E. E. (2006). Follow-up of children with autism spectrum disorders from age 2 to age 9. *Autism, 10*(3), 243–265.

Valicenti-McDermott, M., McVicar, K., Rapin, I., Wershil, B. K., Cohen, H., & Shinnar, S. (2006). Frequency of gastrointestinal symptoms in children with autistic spectrum disorders and association with family history of autoimmune disease. *Journal of Developmental and Behavioral Pediatrics, 27*(2 Suppl), S128–136.

Volkmar, F., Cook, E. H., Jr., Pomeroy, J., Realmuto, G., & Tanguay, P. (1999). Practice parameters for the assessment and treatment of children, adolescents, and adults with autism and other pervasive developmental disorders. American Academy of Child and Adolescent Psychiatry Working Group on Quality Issues. *Journal of the American Academy of Child and Adolescent Psychiatry, 38*(12 Suppl), 32S–54S.

Volkmar, F. R., & Nelson, D. S. (1990). Seizure disorders in autism. *Journal of the American Academy of Child and Adolescent Psychiatry, 29*(1), 127–129.

Wakefield, A. J., Murch, S. H., Anthony, A., Linnell, J., Casson, D. M., Malik, M., et al. (1998a). Ileal-lymphoid-nodular hyperplasia, non-specific colitis, and pervasive developmental disorder in children. *Lancet, 351*(9103), 637–641.

Wakefield, A. J., Murch, S. H., Anthony, A., Linnell, J., Casson, D. M., Malik, M., et al. (1998b). Ileal-lymphoid-nodular hyperplasia, non-specific colitis, and pervasive developmental disorder in children [see comments]. *Lancet, 351*(9103), 637–641.

Wassink, T. H., Piven, J., & Patil, S. R. (2001). Chromosomal abnormalities in a clinic sample of individuals with autistic disorder. *Psychiatric Genetics, 11*(2), 57–63.

Weiss, L. A., Shen, Y., Korn, J. M., Arking, D. E., Miller, D. T., Fossdal, R., et al. (2008). Association between microdeletion and microduplication at 16p11.2 and autism. *New England Journal of Medicine, 358*(7), 667–675.

Werner, E., & Dawson, G. (2005). Validation of the phenomenon of autistic regression using home videotapes. *Archives of General Psychiatry, 62*(8), 889–895.

Wills, S., Cabanlit, M., Bennett, J., Ashwood, P., Amaral, D., & Van de Water, J. (2007). Autoantibodies in autism spectrum disorders (ASD). *Annals of the New York Academy of Sciences, 1107*, 79–91.

Wong, H. H., & Smith, R. G. (2006). Patterns of complementary and alternative medical therapy use in children diagnosed with autism spectrum disorders. *Journal of Autism and Developmental Disorders, 36*(7), 901–909.

Commentary

Holly K. Tabor

Bioethical Considerations in Autism Research and Translation: Present and Future

What Does Bioethics Have to Do with Autism?

Bioethics is a field of study focused on ethical controversies in science and medicine. Bioethics is often classified into clinical ethics, or ethical decision-making in a clinical setting, and research ethics, or ethical decision-making in the context of biomedical research. Both areas involve consideration of the four principles of bioethics, as described by Tom Beauchamp and James Childress in their book *Principles of Biomedical Ethics*: (1) autonomy, or respect for individual decision-making; (2) beneficence, or doing good and providing benefit; (3) nonmaleficence, or avoiding harm; and (4) justice, or treating individuals and groups equitably and fairly (Beauchamp & Childress, 2008).

Bioethics is more colloquially understood to be figuring out what is the "right thing" or "moral thing" to do in medicine and biomedical research. In this context, bioethicists are sometimes perceived to be the "ethics police" who look for wrongdoing and try to correct it, thereby slowing down the progress of science. This view of bioethics is distorted in several ways. First, most bioethicists act in advisory and commentary roles, and do not have enforcement authorities. Second, the role of bioethics is to work together with researchers, clinicians, institutions, and other stakeholders to think critically about emerging challenges in biomedicine, and to help develop tools and strategies to meet them and innovate when necessary. Bioethics as a discipline can help frame ethical challenges related to new technological advances in both research and therapeutic contexts. Bioethics can also help frame the debate when there exist conflicting societal values surrounding controversial issues in biomedicine.

One important context for bioethics is the area of research ethics, or advocating for the four principles of bioethics in the conduct of research. This means using the lens of bioethics to protect the individual rights of research participants (autonomy); balance benefit, or doing good (beneficence), with avoiding doing harm (nonmaleficence); and advocate for treating individuals and groups fairly, particularly groups whose perspectives are not always voiced or represented (justice).

In this commentary, I argue that autism, as a diagnosis and a field of study, has several features that may make it more susceptible to research ethics challenges than many other areas of study. Autism research is primarily conducted in children, adolescents, and adults who have challenges with communication and comprehension. There are many existing challenges to conducting research in children, and particularly research on new approaches with possible risks. As autism research proliferates, more individuals with autism and their typical siblings are being enrolled in studies, and therefore some of these challenges will be magnified. Additionally, the increasing prevalence of autism and the absence of firm etiological explanations of its causes, effective treatments, or preventions lead researchers and families to place extraordinarily high expectations on research as providing immediate and future benefit.

It is beyond the scope of this article to examine all of the bioethical challenges in autism, or even in autism research. Some of these challenges have been discussed elsewhere (Chen, Miller, & Rosenstein, 2003; McMahon, Batym, & Botkin, 2006). Bioethical challenges in autism would likely be framed and prioritized somewhat differently by different stakeholders and are likely to change over time. In this chapter will highlight several key and emerging challenges in research and in the shifting boundaries between research and clinical translation, which are likely to influence the practice of clinicians and researchers, as well as the experiences of families, in the near future. The first area examined is the challenge of obtaining meaningful assent for children with autism. While I examine this issue in a research context for children under the age of 18 years, many of the same issues will be applicable for adults with autism because of the communication difficulties associated with the disorder, and will also be relevant for informed consent in a clinical context.

The second area examined is the research ethics involved with the enrollment of typically developing siblings of children with autism in research. The third area examined is the risk of therapeutic misconception in autism research. The fourth area examined is the potential for challenges associated with accelerated translation of research findings into clinical practice, using the example of array comparative genomic hybridization (array CGH) testing for autism.

Rethinking Meaningful Assent for Children with Autism

A fundamental principle of bioethics is the respect for autonomy, or the right of an individual to make decisions for oneself about medical care and about participation in research. One of the key tools for respecting autonomy in research is the process of informed consent. In research involving children, it is required that parents participate in informed consent and be told all of the possible benefits and risks to the child of participating in the research, ranging from possible physical harms to psychological harms. In addition, federal regulations from the Office for Human Research Protections (OHRP) require that researchers make every attempt to obtain assent from children. Assent is defined as "a child's affirmative agreement to participate in research" (US Code of Federal Regulations TITLE 45—Public Welfare, Department of Health and Human Services Part 46, Protection of Human Subjects, 46.402).

The concept of autonomy is challenging in autism because of the features of the condition. Children and adults with autism often have significant communication challenges both in terms of what they can communicate and what they can understand. Yet, a fundamental principle of autonomy is the right to know what is involved in a research protocol or clinical procedure, and being able to decide whether to participate.

Given the communication and comprehension challenges in autism, how should we assess what children with autism can understand or decide? Federal regulations suggest that IRBs and researchers should take into consideration the decision-making capacity of the target research population of children, including factors such as age, maturity, and psychological state. According to the regulations, the assessment of capacity for decision-making can be made for all the children to be enrolled in a particular study, or for each individual child. The guidelines recognize that not all children can be involved in the assent process. They state that the IRB may determine that assent is not a necessary condition for proceeding with research if "the capability of some or all of the children is so limited that they cannot be reasonably consulted" (US Code of Federal Regulations TITLE 45—Public Welfare, Department of Health and Human Services Part 46, Protection of Human Subjects, 46.408(a)).

Can children with autism, perhaps even severely affected children, be reasonably consulted about research participation? How can or should we assess their capacity for assent? There are no published accounts of assessment protocols, and anecdotal accounts of current practices seem to vary. When data already exist about the anticipated cognitive abilities of the children to be recruited (e.g., mental age levels), sometimes a rule, such as a mental age cutoff, can be used to determine which children can or cannot assent. However, it is likely that mental age measures, which are derived from IQ tests, will not be available for many children, and may not always accurately reflect the ability to understand simple explanations of procedures.

Alternatively, a verbal approach is sometimes used, where a consent form is explained in its most basic outline verbally to a child with autism. Pictures and photographs that explain the study can also be used. However, given the communication and attention challenges of some autistic children, this may not be the most effective method of delivering information. Still another approach that may be applied is to not require assent from children with autism, due to their limited capabilities. This solution, however, seems imperfect and not in keeping with the ethical principle of respect for autonomy behind the requirement for pediatric assent.

While some children with autism may not be able to understand the details of the goals of the research or the consent form, respecting the autonomy of children with autism requires that at least an effort be made to explain what the child will be required to do, and the possible risks and benefits of those procedures. The same commitment to autonomy requires that some effort be made to use data about best practices for communicating with children across the autism spectrum in order to develop, validate, and disseminate tools and protocols for assent that are more likely to be successful with this research population.

Increasing numbers of children with autism are being recruited to participate in research studies, often through a person or institution with whom they also have a clinical relationship. It is possible that the current and future scope of autism research will involve more children with communicative and intellectual disabilities than any other kind of disease research to date. True respect for autonomy in autism research requires new and creative approaches to assent for children and adolescents with autism.

There are some data from other studies suggesting that investment in this kind work might be successful. First, we need to develop autism-specific tools for measuring decisional capacity. Several papers have described such tools for clinical research in individuals with impairments such as schizophrenia (Jeste et al., 2007; Dunn et al., 2007; Andre-Barron, Strydom, & Hassiotis, A, 2008). There are also data indicating that the capacity to consent to research may vary across patients with different neuropsychiatric disorders, suggesting that some disease- and impairment-specific tools may need to be developed, as well as tools that may address different impairments on the autism spectrum (Palmer et al., 2005).

Second, there is also a need to develop tools for communicating with children and adolescents with autism about what is involved in research as part of the assent process. A recent study demonstrated that use of multimedia consent tools improved the capacity to consent among adult patients with schizophrenia (Jeste et al., 2009). This suggests that the development of autism-specific multimedia consent tools might also improve assent among pediatric autism research participants.

Autism researchers, policymakers, and families have the opportunity to help biomedical research more broadly by developing and incorporating new tools for respecting autonomy of people with disabilities and challenges like those seen in autism. The fact that communication and understanding are challenging for many children and adults with autism, and may be impossible for some, should not be seen as implying that meaningful assent in children, or consent in adults, is not possible or not worthwhile for all individuals with autism. New assessment tools will need to incorporate evolving strategies from research and from educational strategies about communicating with children with autism, ranging from graphics and pictures to the use of adaptive technologies. Such an effort would require commitment and funding from government and from advocacy organizations. It would also require creative and dedicated researchers who are willing to take the time and energy to implement and disseminate the tools developed, and families who are willing to participate in research to validate and test the tools.

What About the Siblings? Research Ethics Involving Siblings of Children with Autism

Another significant ethical challenge in autism relates to the involvement of typically developing siblings in many autism research projects. Many autism studies specifically recruit siblings for research. These range from family-based genetic studies to studies of infant siblings that are designed to assess early signs and developmental trajectories of young siblings who are at increased risk for autism due to genetic liability (Rogers, 2009). Siblings may be asked to participate in research in a variety of ways, ranging from providing a DNA sample, to more complex psychological, developmental, and medical assessments. The time commitment for involvement may range from a single visit to visits spanning much of their childhood.

Dr. Douglas Diekema has written an excellent article about the specific federal requirements regarding the level of risk allowed in research in children. In this article, he describes how federal regulations require that research in children "can only be justified if the level of risk entailed in the research is very low, or if there is the potential for direct benefit to the child by participating in the research project" (Diekema, 2006, p. S7). Research that does not fit these criteria can be approved for patients who have a specific condition or disorder "if the research is likely to yield generalizable knowledge about the subject's disorder or condition… *and* the risk of research represents no more than a minor increase over minimal risk" for that group of patients (Diekema, 2006, S7).

Given this framework, it is unclear how to evaluate the risk to siblings of children with autism who are recruited to participate in studies. Unaffected siblings of children with autism are not in the same category of receiving direct benefit or benefiting *themselves* from generalizable knowledge coming from the study, although their siblings and family members may receive such benefits. It can be argued that siblings may receive some indirect benefits, including access to early screening for ASD-related phenotypes. They also may, in the present or in the future, experience positive feelings from participating in research on a disease that affects their sibling or their whole family. However, these benefits are likely smaller, less direct, and possibly more variable, than those for children with autism who are enrolled in research.

Another important ethical question is whether siblings of children with autism are exposed to risks, and possibly unique risks, when they are recruited to participate in research studies. On the one hand, giving a blood sample or having one's parents fill out a questionnaire reasonably might be described as posing minimal risk. On the other hand, having one's DNA sequence shared in a publically available database, or having one's behavioral assessment disclosed to others might be characterized as a greater than minimal risk.

Studies on siblings suggest that there may be other more complicated risks that are specific to unaffected family members of children with autism who participate in research (Dawson et al., 2002; Dawson et al, 2007; Toth, Dawson, Meltzoff, Greenson, & Fein, 2008). A Pubmed search using the terms "autism" and "siblings" revealed three articles examining nonautism phenotypes in siblings, including complex immune dysfunction (Sarasella et al., 2009), dysfunctions in the prefrontal cortex (Kawakubo et al., 2009), and emotional problems (Petalas, Hastings, Nash, Lloyd, & Downey, 2009). In each of these articles, results were described as evidence of autism endophenotypes, or genetic components of traits related to autism. An additional article examined the phenotypic features of siblings of individuals with autism with the rare CNV on chromosome 16p11.2, which were described as ranging from "apparently healthy" to "meeting criteria for ASD" (Fernandez et al., 2009). This kind of article represents a new kind of "genotype-driven" research, where previously undiagnosed family members who share genetic variants are examined more closely to see if they have any features that might be related to autism.

This sampling of recent articles represents a trend in autism research toward examining the phenotypic traits of unaffected siblings as a primary outcome in a way that may not be described in the original informed consent documents and process. There may be a risk to siblings of being identified as having traits both related and unrelated to autism when they and their parents were not aware that this activity was part of the scope of research. These risks may be psychosocial, for example, being categorized by the researchers as having "emotional problems" or impaired cognition. They may experience stigma by having the research be interpreted broadly by society to mean that siblings of children with autism have emotional problems or brain dysfunctions, or perhaps undiagnosed autism. Alternatively, they may experience risks related to confidentiality. Siblings may not wish information about whether they carry a rare CNV to be published and possibly linked to them through the publication of detailed information about their family.

These concerns may not be unique to autism research, but they are becoming increasingly prevalent in autism studies. There are certainly compelling scientific reasons to study the siblings of children with autism. I would argue, however, that researchers, funding agencies, and IRBs need to carefully weigh the risks and benefits of this kind of research, not just to children and families with autism, but also to healthy siblings. Researchers need to tailor consent forms and perhaps pursue reconsent as the research objectives change to specifically address the unique risks to "healthy" siblings. It also seems critical to reconsent healthy siblings when they reach 18 and allow them the possibility to withdraw from the research. This may be particularly important for genetic research using samples in biobanks or repositories collected from children (Burke & Diekema, 2006), as a recent study suggests that 46% of participants would want to be recontacted as adults for consent for continued research use of samples collected when they were children (Goldenberg, Hull, Botkin, & Wilfond, 2009). As genetic research evolves, it may be more likely that siblings of children with autism are recruited for additional research specifically because of their genotypic information (McGuire & McGuire, 2009). This kind of genotype-driven recruitment may increase potential burden, both practical and psychological, on siblings, in a way that was not anticipated at the time of initial study recruitment and enrollment.

There is also evidence that siblings of children who participate themselves in genetic research may experience risks of psychosocial harms from participating in some kinds of research. In one study, siblings of children with ataxia telangiectasia (A-T) who were enrolled in genetic linkage studies before the age of 18 were interviewed retrospectively about their feelings about the research. The siblings described fear of the procedure involved in the blood draw, apprehension around reporting of carrier results, and confusion about the possibility of having A-T. The visit with the researcher represented "a highly charged event in the lives of these individuals" that increased anxiety, but also offered an opportunity to relay concerns or discuss information (Fanos, 1999, 276). While A-T is a very different disease in presentation and inheritance patterns than autism, this study suggests that siblings of children with autism who are asked to enroll in research may also feel anxiety and confusion, and that the psychosocial impact of their participation may be long-lasting.

There are also emerging data about how parents and children decide to participate in research that may impact assent in autism research. A recent study by Varma, Jenkins, and Wendler surveyed 117 parent-child pairs where the child was enrolled in clinical research or receiving clinical care for asthma or cancer. Among the respondents, 90.5% of pediatric patients believed they should be involved in making research enrollment decisions. Only 61.5% of the parents believed that children should be involved in making research enrollment decisions. The authors suggest that these findings highlight how parents and children can disagree about research participation, and suggest that researchers need to be aware of and address these possible disagreements when they enroll and obtain assent (Varma, Jenkins, & Wendler, 2008).

More research is needed about the experience of siblings in autism research, both at the time of the research and after they have reached adulthood, to characterize the possible risks involved. Researchers, bioethicists, and IRBs may need to develop tools to minimize these kinds of harms to siblings if they exist. In the meantime, researchers and funding agencies should consider the possible risks to unaffected siblings enrolled in research. Increasingly, academic medical centers are establishing research ethics consult services to support researchers in addressing ethical challenges such as these as they arise in the course of research planning and implementation (Cho et al., 2008; Pilcher, 2006).

How Can This Research Study Help My Child? Risk of Therapeutic Misconception in Autism Research

A third significant ethical challenge in autism research is the potential for therapeutic misconception, fundamental confusion among researchers and/or research participants between the goals of research, or generalizable knowledge, and the goals of clinical care, or improving the health of an individual person (Cho & Magnus, 2007; Applebaum, Roth, & Lidz, 1982). Essentially, research participants believe that the goal of research is to provide clinical care that will benefit them personally, rather than to produce generalizable knowledge that may help them and others. While therapeutic misconception is a challenge in many diseases and areas of research, I argue that families with autism may be more likely to have therapeutic misconception about research than families with other diseases.

The potential for therapeutic misconception in autism needs to be framed in the current context of the treatment and diagnosis of autism. A great deal of autism research is conducted at academic medical centers with "autism centers" or autism researchers who are considered experts in their field. Very often, these researchers are also clinicians and wear both "hats," with a range of overlapping clinical and research responsibilities and relationships. Frequently, parents bring their children to these centers to obtain access to expertise, advice, and treatment from experts that will help their child.

This occurs against a backdrop of a medical system that provides very little in the way of treatment for families with autism. Parents are often desperate to find medical guidance that they cannot find through their regular pediatrician or through any services that they get from government and school agencies. They may also find it challenging to get the services that they believe their child may need, like applied behavior analysis (ABA) interventions, because their medical insurance will not pay for it and their school district will not provide it.

Parents may be invited to have their children participate in research studies about autism, as patients at autism academic medical centers. These studies may be peripheral to their care. However, they may actually provide certain services or evaluations for free as part of the research, or on a faster timeline than might be available by remaining on a clinic waitlist. These kinds of services may range from diagnostic reports that can be shared with schools in order to access services, to access to experimental pharmaceutical therapies that might not be available elsewhere, to the provision of free behavioral interventions. In some situations, families may actually first come to the autism academic medical centers not as patients but as willing research participants, specifically in order to get access to these kinds of services and expertise which they cannot get access to elsewhere or as quickly.

This may not seem to be a serious problem. In fact, giving back information and expertise to research participants is an important aspect of respect for research participants and upholding the value of reciprocity. It also may be ethically incumbent on researchers to return research results that may have clinical utility outside the research context.

The challenge lies in the potential for therapeutic misconception: families may misunderstand the procedures, risks, and benefits of research, and may choose to participate based on this misunderstanding, believing that research fulfills the same goals as medical care. In autism, families may be more likely agree to participate in research specifically because they believe it will provide a direct clinical benefit to their child. When the standard recommendation for intervention is not available to them, they may be more likely to seek research studies as a means to obtain clinical interventions for their child. This may increase the likelihood of confusion about the goals of the research and the role of the clinician researcher.

Therapeutic misconception may influence how parents perceive the balance of risks and benefits in a particular research study. For example, if they will receive a diagnostic report from an autism "expert" at an academic medical center for free in exchange for their participation, they may be more willing to allow their child with autism, or their unaffected children, to participate in research protocols that they might not otherwise have considered beneficial, or that they might even consider potentially harmful. There are some data supporting this hypothesis specifically in autism. One recent study by Vitiello and colleagues assessed the understanding of parents whose children were enrolled in a randomized placebo controlled trial for risperidone. While parents showed accurate understandings of the main research components of the study, approximately one fourth seemed unaware that treatment was randomly assigned and not personalized, suggesting that parents believe that even in a research context, one of the goals is to optimize the treatment of their child, rather than to produce generalizable knowledge (Vitiello et al., 2003).

We need more empirical research about whether parents of children with autism who enroll in research experience therapeutic misconception, how, and what to do about it. One recent study used a qualitative interview guide to measure therapeutic misconception in research by focusing on research participants' understandings of the purpose of research in juxtaposition to their motivation for participating (Kim et al., 2009). This approach may be particularly useful in the context of autism. In the meantime, researchers and IRBs need to be very cautious about the significant potential for therapeutic misconception in autism research, specifically when individuals act both as researchers and as clinicians. This may require more careful consideration of recruitment strategies, informed consent processes, and clear delineation of clinical and research roles and decisions by providers.

Research Payoffs? Accelerated Translation of Research Results into Clinical Practice

The goal of autism research is to develop generalizable knowledge that can be then applied to screening, treatment, or prevention protocols and benefit the lives of individuals with autism. The pace of research often seems very slow, and it can take many years, even decades, for findings to be translated into the clinical setting. This is frustrating to researchers and clinicians, but is especially frustrating to families.

In the last few years, there have been efforts across biomedical research to more rapidly translate research findings into effective clinical therapies. Autism has been no exception to this trend. Rapid translation has the potential for great benefits. However, the rush to accelerate translation also has potential risks and harms that merit caution.

One recent example of accelerated translation is the adoption of array CGH testing for copy number variants as part of the evaluation for autism. In array CGH, the DNA from a patient sample and a normal reference sample are each labeled with different fluorescent dyes. The two samples are then hybridized to a glass slide containing several thousand probes that include most of the coding and noncoding regions of the genome. The ratio of the fluorescence intensity of the patient sample to that of the reference samples is measured and calculated for each probe to measure the number of copies present in that part of the genome. This method allows for smaller sizes of DNA sequences and structural variants to be detected than using older techniques, and therefore is much higher resolution and able to detect many more duplications and deletions.

Despite over two decades of genetic research in autism, very few genetic factors have been identified that are significantly associated with autism. This has been a great source of frustration to researchers, clinicians, and families. In 2007, using array CGH, CNVs were identified as structural variants in the genome that existed commonly among individuals, but varied in their location, size, and the genes involved. Researchers quickly developed projects to examine the possible role of CNVs in autism, by applying array CGH and analyzing genotyping results from existing studies.

Articles were published in 2007 and 2008 by several groups using different samples and techniques. Cook and Scherer described these CNV findings in their review in *Nature* in October 2008. Generally, the studies found that CNVs were rare, but that there were more CNVs in autism cases than in controls. They found that up to 40% of family-specific CNVs were found to be inherited from a parent without autism spectrum disorder. They also found that in several cases, unrelated individuals carried de novo or inherited CNVs at the same locus (Cook & Scherer, 2008).

One of the affected loci identified was a microdeletion or microduplication at chromosome 16p11.2. A CNV at this location was replicated across 3 studies. In these studies, a CNV was found in 1% of autism cases. Individuals with the CNV at 16p11.2 also had facial dysmorphology. The CNV at 16p11.2 was also found in non-ASD cases with developmental delay or mental retardation and in some controls (Cook & Scherer, 2008). The deletion was also found in individuals with language or psychiatric disorders, although at lower frequency (0.1%), as well as in the general population (0.01%) (Weiss et al., 2008). An additional recent study found a deletion in 16p11.2 in seven individuals with intellectual disability (Mefford et al., 2009). Other studies have found that the deletion is not specific to autism but is also enriched in patients with mental retardation, developmental delay, or schizophrenia without autistic features (Mefford et al., 2009; Itsara et al., 2009; Biljsma et al., 2009). These papers suggest substantial phenotypic heterogeneity and diversity among individuals with CNVs at 16p11.2.

One of the key steps in the translational pathway for genomics is careful consideration of each potential clinical application of scientific findings. In translating genetic research findings into the clinical setting, stakeholders, including researchers, clinicians, companies, families, and policymakers, must decide whether or not there is sufficient evidence to justify the broad application of a genetic test. From an ethics perspective, this requires weighing the possible risks and benefits to families from using the test. Translation requires consideration of who should get the test and when, who should give the test, and perhaps most importantly, how positive and negative results should be interpreted.

The story of the translation of testing of CNVs for autism in the last two years is a story of a kind of "accelerated translation" that is becoming more common in genetics and genomics, but that may also be becoming more prevalent in autism. Specifically, new genomic technologies, like array CGH, are being translated into broad clinical practice on a much more accelerated timeline than research results, or genetic results, have been in the past. Translation seems to be accelerated in situations like autism when there is a large possible target population for the test. Less than a year after the published findings on CNVs and autism, several companies came out with specific array CGH testing for autism. For example, Baylor College of Medicine advertised their "Genetic Testing for Autism" in the abstract book for the 2008 meeting of the American Society of Human Genetics, with the statement that "Through [*sic*] genetic evaluation of patients with Autism Spectrum Disorders (ASD) is critical for appropriate medical management and family counseling" (Baylor College of Medicine).

The advertisement referred to the 2008 Practice Guidelines from the American College of Medical Genetics (ACMG) on "Clinical genetics evaluation in identifying the etiology of autism spectrum disorders." The guidelines state that, "Defining the etiology of an ASD can be of great benefit to the parent and family. Information gained from an identified etiology can help with family counseling, medical management, preventive health strategies, and empowerment of the family" (Schaefer, Mendelsohn, & the ACMG Professional Practice and Guidelines Committee, 2008). The guidelines state that, "A genetic consultation should be offered to all persons and families with ASDs. Evaluations should be considered for any individual along the full autism spectrum" (304).

This is a dramatic recommendation. While autism has long been thought to have a substantial genetic component, genetic evaluation had been previously limited to ruling out known syndromes with autistic-like features, such as Fragile X, and was not considered part of standard practice (Abdul-Rahman & Hudgins, 2006). In this Practice Guideline, the ACMG suggests that array CGH testing will provide significant benefits to enough families that it is worthwhile to recommend it as part of standard practice.

It is unclear, however, whether the promise of these benefits is supported by the existing research evidence (Tabor & Cho, 2007). Given the very small proportion of autism that may be explained by CNVs, it is important to examine the claims of the ACMG Practice Guidelines and advertisements for testing services like the one from Baylor. The guidelines suggest that family counseling around CNVs is important, yet, given the phenotypic heterogeneity of autism, as well as the incomplete penetrance and heterogeneity of cases with specific CNVs, it is unclear what kind of counseling can really be given to families about how specific CNVs will manifest in phenotypic traits or what the recurrence risks are for future siblings. It is also unclear, at least until there is further research, how knowledge of the presence of a CNV in a child would affect medical management or preventive health strategies, such as targeting of early interventions. Finally, the ACMG guidelines suggest that this kind of genetic testing can provide "empowerment of the family" (Schaefer, Mendelsohn, & the ACMG Professional Practice and Guidelines Committee, 2008, 164). However, it is unclear what kind of empowerment they refer to, and toward what end. Furthermore, if the information linking CNVs to autism is determined in the future to be incorrect or incomplete, it is unclear what potential harms might occur.

It is possible that future research will provide enough evidence to support integration of CNV testing into evaluation of all cases of autism. However, I would argue that the ACMG Practice Guidelines and their adoption may be premature in their optimism and enthusiasm. In an effort to translate the possible benefits of testing as quickly as possible, there may in fact be some unanticipated harms created. Genetic testing is very expensive, and may not be covered by insurance in all situations or even available for some families. By recommending testing for all families, clinicians, researchers, and organizations might be placing a significant financial burden on some of those families. Given the limited state of research data, it is not clear how families should be counseled about either positive or negative results. There is a chance that parents might interpret positive results to mean that they should not have more children, when the pattern of inheritance and penetrance of CNVs for autism is very ambiguous. If they receive negative results, families may decide that they do not have a genetic predisposition to autism, which may also be inaccurate.

What can the example of CNV testing for autism tell us about translation of autism research more generally? Certainly every effort should continue to be made to rapidly translate research findings to achieve the maximum benefit for patients and families. Yet, even as these efforts proceed, it is important to be cautious about the potential risks of accelerated translation, and not assume that rapid widespread translation of tests, services, and information is always an unmitigated good. It is critical for stakeholders, ranging from researchers, to clinicians, institutions, and professional organizations, to carefully consider the possible harms created by accelerated or premature translation. These harms, if anticipated, can be planned for and minimized, and procedures can be developed to monitor the translation process, its successes and challenges or failures, and modify practices and guidelines as needed.

Conclusion

In conclusion, there are specific features of autism and autism research that may make it more susceptible to certain research ethics challenges. The current expansion of autism research presents an opportunity for the field to take initiative and leadership in meeting these challenges and developing standard tools and practices to improve the respect for autonomy of children with autism and their typically developing siblings who participate in research. It also presents an opportunity for the community of stakeholders to evaluate the promises of research, and make sure that safeguards are in place to minimize therapeutic misconception, while still enhancing access to care and research participation. Finally, as autism research identifies potential leads in understanding etiology, all stakeholders must temper their exuberance and eagerness to facilitate rapid translation by developing processes to ensure a thoughtful and deliberative process that will provide maximum benefit while minimizing potential harms of this translation.

ACKNOWLEDGMENTS

Dr. Tabor would like to acknowledge funding from NHGRI Grant #5ROOHG004316-03 and the Institute for Translational Health Sciences Grant number 1 UL1 RR 025014-01. She would also like to thank Drs. Heather Mefford, Douglas Diekema, and David Magnus for their input and Ms. Kaiti Carpenter, Ms. Anjali Truitt and Ms. Julia Crouch for their editorial assistance.

REFERENCES

Abdul-Rahman, O. A., & Hudgins, L. (2006). The diagnostic utility of a genetics evaluation in children with pervasive developmental disorders. *Genetics in Medicine*, *8*, 50–54.

Andre-Barron, D., Strydom, A., & Hassiotis, A. (2008). What to tell and how to tell: A qualitative study of information sharing in research for adults with intellectual disability. *Medical Ethics*, *34*, 501–506.

Applebaum, P., Roth, L., & Lidz, C. (1982). The therapeutic misconception: Informed consent in psychiatric research. *International Journal of Law and Psychiatry*, *5*, 319–329.

College of Medicine. Advertisement. American Society of Human Genetics Program Book, October 2008.

Beauchamp, T. L., & Childress, J. L. (2008). *Principles of biomedical ethics*. New York: Oxford University Press.

Bijlsma, E. K., Gijsbers, A. C., Schuurs-Hoeijmakers, J. H., van Haeringen, A., Fransen van de Putte, D. E., et al. (2009). Extending the phenotype of recurrent rearrangements of 16p11.2: Deletions in mentally retarded patients without autism and in normal individuals. *European Journal of Medical Genetics*, *52*, 77–87.

Burke, W., & Diekema, D. S. (2006). Ethical issues arising from the participation of children in genetic research. *Journal of Pediatrics*, *149*(1 Suppl), S34–38.

Chen, D. T., Miller, F. G., & Rosenstein, D. L. (2003). Ethical aspects of research into the etiology of autism. *Mental Retardation and Developmental Disabilities Research Reviews*, *9*, 48–53.

Cho, M. K., & Magnus, D. (2007, September 27). Therapeutic misconception and stem cell research. *Nature Reports Stem Cells*. Published online: doi:10.1038/stemcells.2007.88.

Cho, M. K., Tobin, S. L., Greely, H. T., McCormick, J., Boyce, A., & Magnus, D. (2008). Research ethics consultation: The Stanford experience. *IRB*, *30*, 1–6.

Cook, E. H., Jr., & Scherer, S. W. (2008). Copy-number variations associated with neuropsychiatric conditions. *Nature*, *455*, 919–923.

Dawson, G., Webb, S., Schellenberg, G. D., Dager, S., Friedman, S., Aylward, E., et al. (2002). Defining the broader phenotype of autism: Genetic, brain and behavioral perspectives. *Development and Psychopathology*, *14*, 581–611.

Dawson, G., Estes, A., Munson, J., Schellenberg, G., Bernier, R., & Abbott, R. (2007). Quantitative assessment of autism symptom-related traits in probands and parents: Broader phenotype autism scale. *Journal of Autism and Developmental Disorders, 37*, 523–536.

Diekema, D. S. (2006). Conducting ethical research in pediatrics: A brief historical overview and review of pediatric regulations. *Journal of Pediatrics, 149*(1 Suppl), S3–11.

Dunn, L. B., Palmer, B. W. Applebaum, P. S., Saks, E. R., Aarons, G. A., & Jeste, D. V. (2007). Prevalence and correlates of adequate performance on a measure of abilities related to decisional capacity: Differences among three standards for the MacCAT-CR in patients with schizophrenia. *Schizophrenia Research, 89*, 1–3.

Fanos, J. H. (1999). The missing link in linkage analysis: The well sibling revisited. *Genetic Testing, 3*, 273–278.

Fernandez, B. A., Roberts, W., Chung, B., Weksberg, R., Meyn, S., Szatmari, P., et al. (2009, September 15). Phenotypic spectrum associated with de novo and inherited deletions and duplications at 16p11.2 in individuals ascertained for diagnosis of autism spectrum disorder. *Journal of Medical Genetics* [Epub ahead of print].

Goldenberg, A. J., Hull, S. C., Botkin, J. R., & Wilfond, B. S. (2009). Pediatric biobanks: Approaching informed consent for continuing research after children grow up. *Journal of Pediatrics, 155*, 578–583.

Itsara, A., Cooper, G. M., Baker, C., Giriraian, S., Li, J., Absher, D., et al. (2009). *American Journal of Human Genetics, 84*, 148–161.

Jeste, D. V., Palmer, B. W., Applebaum, P. S., Golshan, S., Glorioso, D., Dunn, L. B., et al. (2007). A new brief instrument for assessing decisional capacity for clinical research. *Archives of General Psychiatry, 64*, 966–974.

Jeste, D. V., Palmer, B. W., Golshan, S., Eyler, L. T., Dunn, L. B., Meeks, T., et al. (2009). Multimedia consent for research in people with schizophrenia and normal subjects: A randomized controlled trial. *Schizophrenia Bulletin, 35*, 719–729.

Kawakubo, Y., Kuwabara, H., Wantanabe, K., Minowa, M., Someya, T., Minowa, I., et al. (2009). Impaired prefrontal hemodynamic maturation in autism and unaffected siblings. *PLoS One, 3*, e6881.

Kim, S. Y., Schrock, L., Wilson, R., Frank, S. A., Holloway, R. G., Kieburtz, K., et al. (2009). An approach to evaluating the therapeutic misconception. *IRB, 31*, 7–14.

McGuire, S. E., & McGuire, A. L. (2008). Don't throw the baby out with the bathwater: Enabling a bottom-up approach to genome-wide association studies. *Genome Research, 18*, 1683–1685.

McMahon, W. M., Baty, B. J., & Botkin, J. (2006). Genetic counseling and ethical issues for autism. *American Journal of Medical Genetics C Seminar Medical Genetics, 142C*, 52–57.

Mefford, H. C., Cooper, G. M., Zerr, T., Smith, J. D., Baker, C., Shafer, N., et al. (2009). A method for rapid, targeted CNV genotyping identifies rare variants associated with neurocognitive disease. *Genome Research, 19*, 1579–1585.

Palmer, B. W., Dunn, L. B., Applebaum, P. S., Mudaliar, S., Thal, L., Henry, R., et al. (2006). Assessment of capacity to consent to research among older persons with schizophrenia, Alzheimer disease, or diabetes mellitus: Comparison of a 3-item questionnaire with a comprehensive standardized capacity instrument. *Archives of General Psychiatry, 62*, 726–733.

Petalas, M. A., Hastings, R. P., Nash, S., Lloyd, T., & Dowey, A. (2009). Emotional and behavioural adjustment in siblings of children with intellectual disability with and without autism. *Autism, 13*, 471–483.

Pilcher, H. (2006). Bioethics: Dial "E" for ethics. *Nature, 440*, 1104–1105.

Rogers, S. G. (2009). What are infant siblings teaching us about autism in infancy? *Autism Research, 2*, 125–137.

Saresella, M., Marventano, I., Guerinin, F. R., Mancuso, R., Ceresa, L., Zanzottera, M., et al. (2009, August 21). An autistic endophenotype results in complex immune dysfunction in healthy sibling of autistic children. *Biological Psychiatry* [Epub ahead of print].

Schaefer, G. B., Mendelsohn, N. J., & the ACMG Professional Practice and Guidelines Committee. (2008). Clinical genetics evaluation in identifying the etiology of autism spectrum disorders. *Genetics in Medicine, 10*, 301–305.

Tabor, H. K., & Cho, M. K. (2007). Ethical implications of array comparative genomic hybridization in complex phenotypes: Points to consider in research. *Genetics in Medicine, 9*, 626–631.

Toth, K., Dawson, G., Meltzoff, A. N., Greenson, J., & Fein D. (2007). Early social, imitation, play and language abilities of young non-autistic siblings of children with autism. *Journal of Autism and Developmental Disorders, 37*, 145–157.

US Code of Federal Regulations TITLE 45—Public Welfare, Department of Health and Human Services Part 46, Protection of Human Subjects. Revised June 23, 2005; Effective June 23, 2005.

Varma, S., Jenkings, T., & Wendler, D. (2008). How do children and parents make decisions about pediatric clinical research? *Journal of Pediatric Hematology and Oncology, 30*, 823–828.

Vitiello, B., Aman, M. G., Scahill, L., McCracken, J. T., McDougie, C. G., Tierney, E., et al. (2003). Research knowledge among parents of children participating in a randomized clinical trial. *Journal of the American Academy of Child and Adolescent Psychiatry, 44*, 145–149.

Weiss, L. A., Shen, Y., Korn, J. M., Arking, D. E., Miller, D. T., Fossdal, R., et al., Autism Consortium. (2008). Association between microdeletion and microduplication at 16p11.2 and autism. *New England Journal of Medicine, 358*, 667–675.

Wendler, D., & Grady, C. (2008). What should research participants understand to understand they are participants in research? *Bioethics, 22*(4), 203–208.

Section XI

Public Policy

78 The Economic Costs of Autism: A Review

Djesika Amendah, Scott D. Grosse, Georgina Peacock, David S. Mandell

Points of Interest

- This chapter takes a lifespan approach and construes costs broadly to incorporate those of individuals with ASDs and their families. We consider cost in four domains: medical, nonmedical, productivity, and caregiver time.
- Estimates of incremental mean medical expenditures range from $2,100 to $11,200 per person per year.
- Annual estimates of nonmedical costs include $40,000 to $60,000 for intensive behavioral interventions for children prior to school age, $13,000 for special education services from ages 6 to 21 years, and $60,000 to $128,000 for residential services, although the proportion of persons using this last service is unknown.
- Estimates of the loss of productivity among adults with ASDs are less robust, and rely on convenience samples. Among adults with high-functioning autism, at least half are employed, but little is known about their skills level and earnings. The real productivity losses of adults with ASDs are unknown.
- The only recent U.S. population-based estimate suggests an annual loss of parental productivity of $6,000 per child, or $7,400 from the societal perspective.
- Most cost data on children and adults with ASDs is decades old. A full, contemporary understanding of the economic costs of autism and the cost-effectiveness of interventions is missing.

In the United States, the estimated prevalence of autism spectrum disorders in 2006 ranged from 4.2 to 12.1 per 1000, with an average prevalence of 9.0 per 1,000 (95% confidence interval 8.6–9.3) (ADDM 2009). This high prevalence provides a sense of urgency regarding the cost of care for persons with ASDs. There is much debate as to how public and private systems will bear the costs associated with the intensive interventions recommended for children with ASDs and the long-term supports needed by many adults with ASDs. Accurate assessment of the cost of care for individuals with ASDs allows for appropriate system planning and provides a baseline against which to measure the effectiveness of interventions designed to improve outcomes and community integration.

Most U.S.-based studies of ASD-related costs estimate medical expenditures, which represent only a small percentage of total costs, between 3% and 5% of the total (Ganz, 2007; Järbrink et al., 2003; Järbrink, 2007). Few studies have evaluated nonmedical costs, including productivity costs incurred by persons with ASDs or their parents. Most estimates of nonmedical costs have relied on data from European countries, which are not necessarily representative of the United States. Published estimates of total lifetime costs for a child with an ASD, including an often-cited estimate of $3.2 million (Ganz, 2007) rely on speculative assumptions. In this chapter, we critically assess these assumptions in the light of available data. We review both the peer-reviewed literature and additional sources for information on the costs of care for individuals with ASDs, with a focus on the United States. We take a lifespan approach, and construe costs broadly to incorporate those of individuals with ASDs and their families. We also make recommendations regarding the next steps in assessing costs of care for individuals with these complex lifelong disorders.

Methods

We conducted a literature search though the following databases: PubMed, EconLit, ERIC, and Google™. We used the keyword *autism*, paired with the following keywords: *cost, service utilization,* and *employment.* We also examined references of articles identified using these searches to identify additional documents addressing autism costs. Although we did not limit the search by language or date of publication, we did not identify relevant publications in languages other than English.

We identified seven studies that estimate per capita medical costs or expenditures for individuals with ASDs in the United States (Table 78-1). For nonmedical expenditures, we included studies regardless of country of origin, owing to a scarcity of U.S.-based studies. We included studies that compared health care or educational service utilization between persons with and without ASDs (Tables 78-2–78-3). We also included studies with data on behavioral therapies, residential care, supported employment, and employment of individuals with ASDs or their caregivers, few of which reported expenditures or costs (Tables 78-4–78-9). Finally, we included studies on total annual and lifetime costs (Tables 78-10–78-11). Documents included in this review represent 40 studies.

In this review, we focused on the incremental cost of ASDs, defined as the difference between average (mean) costs incurred by persons with ASDs and the mean costs incurred by persons of the same age without ASDs. In other words, all cost estimates in this chapter are expressed as the net cost per person with ASD. When we refer to the "total" cost of ASD we refer to the sum of all types of cost, expressed on a per capita basis. The aggregate cost of ASD in a population can be calculated as the per capita cost multiplied by the number of people with an ASD.

We consider four cost components: medical, nonmedical, productivity, and caregiver time costs. Medical costs refer to the value of medical care provided by physicians, physician extenders (physician assistants, nurse practitioners), nurses, pharmacists, allied health professionals, and staff working under their supervision, as well as prescription medications and laboratory tests. We exclude studies of complementary or alternative medicines. Nonmedical expenditures include educational and early-intervention services, behavioral, occupational, and speech and language therapies, residential care and other items such as home modifications, travel to medical appointments, or supported employment.[1] Note that many therapies can be offered through either the educational or health-care systems. The distinction between medical and nonmedical costs largely reflects how services are typically paid for in the United States.

Studies of medical costs typically report expenditures, the amounts for which providers are reimbursed for a service. In the United States, reimbursements are negotiated between the payer, which usually is an insurance company, and the provider, and they vary in the extent to which they take into account all of the costs associated with providing a service or good. Few studies (e.g., Croen et al., 2006) have analyzed medical costs from the provider perspective, which is the value of resources (e.g., labor, supplies, facility costs) used to produce a service.

Productivity costs represent the lost value of gross earnings of an affected individual resulting from unemployment or underemployment. These might be caused by the inability of persons with ASDs to acquire skills needed for a higher-paying job or to work full-time and in a typical environment when they have those skills. The productivity losses include also the value of fringe benefits and taxes. Caregiver time costs typically refer to the income lost by parents and other familial caregivers because of competing caregiving demands.

In this review, all monetary estimates were converted to 2003 U.S. dollars,[2] adjusting for differences in currencies and inflation. Estimates in other currencies were first converted to U.S. dollars using Purchasing Power Parity values for the year in which the study reported monetary estimates. These values are calculated as the relative prices of a bundle of goods and services purchased in different countries in a given year[3] and are more stable than foreign exchange rates. U.S. dollar estimates for medical expenditures from different years were adjusted to 2003 values using the Medical Care Consumer Price Index. The Employment Cost Index of total compensation for state and local government workers[4] was used to adjust other nonmedical costs. All expenditure figures in the text were rounded to the nearest $100.

Results

Medical Expenditures

Five recent U.S. studies used either insurance claims or administrative data to calculate either medical expenditures or costs for persons with ASDs age 21 years or less. Two of these studies used the International Classification of Diseases, Clinical Modification (ICD-9-CM) codes 299.0 and 299.8 to characterize ASDs (Croen et al., 2006; Shimabukuro et al., 2008). Three others used all 299 three-digit codes, which encompass small numbers of children with disintegrative disorders and psychoses (Flanders et al., 2006, 2007; Leslie & Martin, 2007; Mandell et al., 2006). These latter three studies calculated mean expenditures for children with ASDs but only Mandell et al. reported expenditures for children without ASDs. The latter is required to calculate the incremental expenditures for children with ASDs relative to typically developing children.

Shimabukuro et al. (2008) used the MarketScan® Commercial Claims and Encounters database on Americans with private employer-sponsored insurance for the year 2003. They calculated incremental mean and median expenditures associated with ASDs in individuals 1 to 21 years of age of $4,700 and $2,600, respectively. The composition of expenditures in those data varied by age, with prescription medications comprising a larger proportion for adolescents and young adults (Oswald & Sonenklar, 2007). Croen et al. (2006) analyzed administrative data from one California health-management organization from July 2003 to June 2004. They calculated incremental mean and median expenditures per person with an ASD to the organization of $1,800 and $700, respectively. Mandell et al. (2006) used Medicaid claims to compute ASD expenditures in a metropolitan county in Pennsylvania for the years 1994 through 1999. The incremental mean expenditure was $10,500 per person with an ASD.

Other studies used information from household surveys to calculate medical expenditures. Liptak et al. (2006) examined parent-reported expenditures and health-care utilization from the Medical Expenditure Panel Survey for the years 1997 to 2000. The authors calculated the incremental mean and median expenditures per child with an ASD to be $2,100 and $1,400, respectively. In 1985 to 1986, Birenbaum et al. (1990) conducted the only U.S. national survey of individuals with ASDs or intellectual disabilities under the age of 25 years. Their sample relied on the national census of children receiving

Table 78–1.
Summary of studies on annual total medical expenditures for children with ASDs in the United States

Authors, Year, Data Source	Sample Composition		Included Expenditures	Annual Expenditures in 2003 (U.S. $ per Child)
	ASD	Comparison group		
Shimabukuro et al. (2008). MarketScan claim data, multistates, ICD-9 code 299.0 and 299.8.	Age 1 to 21 years in 2003; ASD size = 3,481.	Similar children without ASD, size = 1,199,380.	Sum (inpatient, outpatient, and pharmacy).	ASD: Mean $5,930, Median $2,870; Comparison: Mean $1,230, Median $320; Incremental: Mean $4,700, Median $2,550.
Croen et al. (2006). Private insurance capitated claim data in California, ICD-9 code 299.0 and 299.8.	Age 2 to 18 years between July 2003 and June 2004; ASD size = 3,053.	Similar children without ASD, size = 30,529.	Sum (hospital laboratory, radiology, outpatient home health utilization).	ASD: Mean $2,715, Median $1,058; Comparison: Mean $896, Median $335; Incremental: Mean $1,819, Median $723.
Mandell et al. (2006). Public insurance Medicaid claim data in metro county in Pennsylvania, ICD-9 code 299.	Age 0 to 21 years; 1994 to 1999 ASD size = 334.	Similar children without ASD and without Intellectual Disability, frequency = 183,488.	Sum (ambulatory care, emergency care, hospitalization, psychiatric hospitalization and psychiatric outpatient care).	ASD: Mean $11,832; Comparison: Mean $1,306; Incremental: Mean $10,525.
Liptak et al. (2006) Medical Expenditure Panel Survey (MEPS) parental reports.	MEPS 1997 to 2000, age ≤19 years with ASD size = 31; weighted size = 340,158.	Similar children without ASD, depression, and without mental retardation. size = 14,413, weighted = 152,293,614.	Sum (inpatient, outpatient, emergency room, physician, nonphysician, home health care, pharmacy, other).	ASD: Mean $2,423, Median $1,463; Comparison: Mean $340, Median $86; Incremental: Mean $2,083, Median $1,377.
Birenbaum et al. (1990). Nationally representative survey based on school and special education districts and 1980 censuses.	Survey period June 1985 to June 1986. Sample under age 18 years, size = 235; age 18 to 24 years, size = 58.	National Medical Care Utilization and Expenditures Survey [NMCUES] 1980. Age 0 to 16 years and 17 to 44 years. Excludes individuals with disabilities.	Annual health-care expenditures.	Under 18 years of age. ASD:Mean $2,435, Median< $1,218; Comparison: Mean $974; Incremental: Mean $1,461.
Flanders et al. (2006). 20% of 2.08 million on Medicaid California, PDD:ICD-9 299 and 330.8.	Age 3 to 17 years at the time of diagnosis. Period: from January 1, 1996 to June 30, 2002 (365 days after diagnosis); Size = 731 children with Pervasive Development Disorders (PDDs).	Similar children without Pervasive Development Disorders; size=731 with asthma and 731 with diabetes.	Sum (inpatient, outpatient, prescription); Special costs = sum (emergency department, home visit, outpatient, laboratory, speech therapy, radiology, surgery).	In the first 12 months after diagnosis; PDD: Mean $6,235, Median $1,177.
Leslie et al. (2006). MarketScan, Privately insured in U.S, ICD-9 code 299	Year: 2003 Age ≤ 17 years, ASD size = 2,411.	Persons with other mental health disorders.	Sum (inpatient, outpatient, and prescription).	ASD: Mean $6,073, Median $3,416.

ICD-9: International classification of diseases 9th edition.

special education, including those in private schools. The estimated prevalence of ASD at the time was 5 per 10,000 children. The comparison group consisted of individuals in the 1987 Medical Care Utilization and Expenditures Survey. They estimated incremental mean costs of $1,500 for children under the age 18 years and $1,700 for persons ages 19 to 24 years.

Summary. The incremental mean medical expenditures estimated in the five recent U.S. studies range from $2,100 to $11,200 per person per year. Differences in health-care expenditures across studies can result from a variety of factors. These include differences in who makes diagnoses or how they are reported, for example, medical vs. educational records, and administrative records vs. parental survey. Differences can also be associated with the type of insurance plan and methodological differences. Population-based surveys are likely to report lower average expenditures of ASD per person than health insurance administrative data for at least two reasons. First, children with medical diagnoses are likely to incur higher medical expenditures than children who were identified outside the medical system and did not have an ASD diagnosis confirmed by a physician. Second, surveys rely on parental reports, which are subject to inaccurate recall of expenditures. Järbrink et al. (2003) found that when parents were asked to recall expenditures, they underestimated them by 34% compared to diaries kept by parents in which costs were recorded as they occurred.

The type of insurance plan affects estimates of expenditures or costs. Children enrolled in a staff model managed-care organization incurred lower average costs (Croen et al., 2006) than privately-insured children enrolled in fee-for-service plans (Shimabukuro et al., 2008). In general, public insurance programs reimburse at a lower rate than private insurance programs (Reinhardt, 2006). Moreover, covered services can differ between various payers. A few state Medicaid programs, including Pennsylvania, reimburse for behavioral therapy delivered in schools, and this might account for the particularly high expenditures reported by Mandell et al. (2006).

Another methodological issue relates to the composition of the comparison group involved in the calculation of incremental costs. For instance, Shimabukuro et al. (2008) and Croen et al. (2006) consider all children without ASDs as the comparison group while Liptak et al. (2006) and Mandell et al. (2006) used children without ASDs and without intellectual disabilities as the comparison group. Excluding other costly conditions from the comparison group could increase the incremental costs of ASDs.

Utilization of Health-Care Services

Not all studies have collected data on medical costs associated with ASDs; some surveys of parents only collected information about service utilization (Ganz, 2006; Gurney et al., 2006). Estimates of ratios of health-service utilization between persons with and without ASDs can also be used to approximate relative medical costs. Two recent U.S. studies found that children with ASDs had about twice as many nonemergency outpatient clinic visits on average, and to a lesser extent, a greater number of emergency department (ED) visits as their typically developing counterparts (Croen et al., 2006; Gurney et al., 2006). A third study estimated that children with ASDs had almost 13 times as many nonemergency outpatient visits as typically developing children and twice as many ED visits

Table 78–2.
Summary of studies on utilization of health-care services by children with ASDs in the United States

Authors, Year, Data Source	Sample Composition		Inclusion	Comparison
	ASD	Comparison Group		
Gurney et al. (2006). National Survey for Children's Health (NSCH).	483 children with autism; age range: 3 to 17 years; period: January 2003 to July 2004.	Similar children without ASD, frequency = 84,789 others.		Parents of children with autism reported more conditions: depression, anxiety, behavioral, and ADHD. Also more allergies.
Ruble et al. (2005). Medicaid managed care from Tennessee.	1,474 children with ASD. Age range: 0 to 17 years; period: July 1994 to June 2000.	None.	Family, individual, and group therapy, residential and inpatient services, medication management, day treatment, case management.	Number of children receiving service with ASD diagnosis increased by 171% but number of service days increased only by 74%. Mean number of service days decreased by 40%.
Leslie & Martin (2007). MarketScan, Privately insured in U.S, ICD-9 code 299.	Year: 2002 to 2004 Age ≤ 17 years, ASD size = 2,411.	Persons with other mental health disorders.	Inpatient, outpatient, and prescription care.	20% increase between 2000 and 2004.

(Liptak et al., (2006). The reason for the discrepancy in numbers of nonemergency outpatient visits is unclear and parallels the variation in reported medical expenditures or costs.

Data on trends in health-care utilization by children with ASDs are also inconsistent across studies. For example, the mean number of service days per child with an ASD enrolled in Medicaid in Tennessee decreased by 40% between 1994 and 2000 (Ruble et al., 2005). In contrast, a time-trend analysis of MarketScan data reported an increase of 20% in average health-care utilization among privately insured individuals with ASDs between 2000 and 2004, based on expenditures adjusted for inflation (Leslie & Martin, 2007). This finding suggests variability in the policy and practice of different payers regarding health-care delivery to children with ASDs.

Nonmedical Expenditures

As described earlier in this chapter, nonmedical expenditures include educational services, behavioral, occupational, and speech and language therapies, residential care, etc. Educational costs associated with ASDs depend on how services are delivered. Residential schools, which are much more costly, appear to be commonly used in Sweden (Järbrink, 2007) but not in the United States. In the United States, more children with ASDs receive behavioral therapy services in schools than in medical settings (Ruble et al., 2005; Yeargin-Allsopp et al., 2003). The Special Education Expenditures Project, commissioned by the U.S. Department of Education for the 1999-to-2000 school year, calculated mean expenditures for pupils receiving publicly funded special education services for different disabilities. They found the mean incremental expenditures for ASDs as a qualifying condition were $12,900 per student receiving services for an ASD, the second-highest cost for any condition (Chambers et al., 2004, 2003). Children with multiple disabilities educated outside the public school system and reimbursed by special education services incurred a mean incremental expenditure of $20,000 (Chambers et al., 2003). Many children with ASDs receive special education services under a different qualifying condition, such as a specific learning disability or emotional disturbance, which is associated with lower costs. On the other hand, some children with ASDs receive services through the multiple disabilities qualification, which is associated with higher costs (Chambers et al., 2003).

In Sweden, the mean incremental cost of educating children with ASDs was reported to be $25,100. This estimate was based on a survey in four municipalities involving 33 families with children with ASDs and using unit costs reported by the school authorities (Järbrink, 2007). The strength of this Swedish study lies in the fact that it is a population survey. However, most of the higher cost estimate was associated with the use of separate schools for seven of the 33 children with ASDs, which is not characteristic of U.S. children with ASDs.

Behavioral interventions are generally recommended for children with ASDs and are more effective if started early, ideally before age 3 years (Butter et al., 2003). Early intensive behavioral intervention based on applied behavior analysis is one commonly used form of behavioral intervention. In this approach, the standard of care is for children with ASDs to receive about 35 to 40 hours per week of one-on-one teaching for 2 to 4 years. As originally conceptualized (Lovaas, 1987),

Table 78–3.
Summary of studies on nonmedical expenditures for children with ASD: Education

Authors, Year, Country	Sample Composition		Inclusion	Annual Expenditures in 2003 (U.S. $ per Child)
	ASD	Comparison Group		
Chambers et al. (2003, 2004). United States	Survey of U.S. approximately 5000 special education providers, 1000 schools, and 300 local education authorities; year: 1999 to 2000; children with disabilities.	Children without any disabilities.	School-related expenses for children by disability category, regular and special education classes, resources, specialists, related services, other special education services.	Mean ASDs: $18,790; Mean Comparison: $6,556; Mean Incremental: $12,854. Mean, Speech and language Disorders: $11,513; Mean comparison $6,888; Mean Incremental: $4,625. Education outside public school system, Mean ASDs: $26,876; Mean Comparison: $6,888; Mean Incremental: $19,989.
Järbrink (2007). Sweden	Population-based survey in four municipalities; 33 children in 2005. Average age: 11.6 years, range 4 to 18 years.	Other children without ASD.	All school-related expenditures. Unit cost obtained from schools. No more detail provided.	Mean $25,099.

this intervention costs on average $40,000 per year per child but can exceed $60,000 depending on family participation, economy of scale, and other factors (Butter et al., 2003; Chasson et al., 2007; Jacobson et al., 1998; Sallows & Graupner, 2005). We could find no cost estimates associated with other common behavioral intervention methods in the peer-reviewed literature, such as Treatment and Education of Autistic and related Communication-handicapped Children (TEACCH), floor time (Thomas et al., 2007a, b), or other applied behavioral analysis methods.

The costs of residential care for adults with ASDs are difficult to estimate, partly because of the lack of information on residential arrangements for representative samples. Residential options for persons with ASDs range from independent living with supports to institutional care for those with severe disabilities. Between these two extremes exists a range of options, such as group homes, supported living, semi-independent living services, and living with a family member or in a foster-care setting. In order to estimate average residential costs for persons with ASDs, the first requirement is to estimate the distribution of adults with ASDs in these different settings. Krauss et al. (2005) found that 67 of 133 (50%) U.S. adults with ASDs (mean age of 32 years), 96.5% of whom had autistic disorder, lived in a staffed residential setting and an additional 11% were in semi-independent living. An additional 51 (38%) lived with family members, and one lived in foster care. Similarly, Eaves and Ho (2008) found that 23 of 47 (47%) young adults (mean age of 24 years) with ASDs in Canada lived in residential facilities. In a Swedish survey of young adults with ASDs, most with Asperger's Syndrome, two of 19 (11%) individuals lived in a group home (Järbrink et al., 2007).

An older study from North Carolina (Wall, 1990) reported the costs of residential care for persons with ASDs living in 11 group homes affiliated with TEACCH, one home for children, two for adolescents and eight for adults. These homes served 52 clients at any given time. The cost per person with an ASD was $56,600 and $34,000 for federally or state-funded homes, respectively.[5] A recent analysis (Lakin et al., 2008) reported average Medicaid expenditure for U.S. adults with intellectual disabilities, including persons with ASDs, of $128,300 for those living in residential facilities and $61,800 for those receiving home- and community-based services, mostly residing in group homes. Residential costs for adults with high-functioning autism (HFA) are presumably much lower as they may require less supervision. The Swedish study cited above reported mean expenditures of only $2,200 per person per year for all HFA adults, most of whom did not require residential care (Järbrink et al., 2007).

Children with ASDs and their families often require services such as respite care, home modification, or socialization services. Two studies calculated that mean annual expenditures for these types of nonmedical services ranged from $5,500 in a pilot study of 17 children in the United Kingdom (Järbrink et al., 2003) to $15,400 in Sweden (Järbrink, 2007).

Adults with ASDs may benefit from supported employment services "such as assessment and diagnosis, counseling, job search assistance, assistive technology, and on-the-job training" as they may increase job retention (Hagner & Cooney, 2005; Lawer et al., 2008) and decrease loss of productivity. In Sweden, Järbrink et al. (2007) evaluated the cost of community support and employment service for adults with ASDs, mostly Asperger's Syndrome,[6] at $9,800 per year. The annual mean cost of supported employment in a 2-year U.K. program was $20,400 per person (Mawhood & Howlin, 1999). The largest supported employment program in the United States is operated by the Rehabilitative Services Administration. In 2005, approximately 2,000 adults with ASDs received vocational rehabilitation services through it, less than 1% of the total served, at an average cost of $3,300 per person (Lawer et al., 2008).

Table 78–4.
Summary of studies on nonmedical expenditures for children with ASD: Behavioral therapy

Authors, Year, Country	Sample: Children with ASD	Annual Expenditures in 2003 (U.S. $ per Child)
Jacobson et al. (1998). United States	Children receiving Early Intensive Behavioral Intervention in Pennsylvania in 1996.	Mean $33,000.
Butter et al. (2003). United States	Children receiving Lovaas therapy.	Mean exceeds $60,000.
Chasson et al. (2007). United States	Cost of Applied Behavioral Analysis based on Sallows and Graupner (2005).	Mean: $40,000 to $60,000.
Sallows & Graupner (2005). United States	Lovaas therapy, 24 children, Age 2 to 3½ years at start.	Mean Exceeds $50,000.
Järbrink (2007). Sweden	Population-based survey in four municipalities; 33 children in 2005. Average age: 11.6 years, range 4 to 18 years.	Mean $25,099.

Loss of Productivity among Individuals with ASDs

Persons with ASDs often incur loss of productivity resulting from unemployment or underemployment; the latter occurs if they either work less than full-time or earn less than the average wage because they lack appropriate work or social skills. Lawer et al. (2008) found that 42% of U.S. adults with ASDs who received vocational rehabilitative services were competitively employed and 2.1% were in a sheltered employment. One of the few empirical estimates of average productivity

Table 78–5.
Summary of studies on residential care use and costs

Authors, Year, Country	Sample: Persons with ASD	Residential Options	Annual Expenditures in 2003 (U.S. $ per Person)
Birenbaum et al. (1990). United States	Nationally representative survey based on school and special education districts and 1980 censuses. Survey period June 1985 to June 1986. Sample under age 18 years, size = 235; age 18 to 24 years, size = 58.	5% of children and 19% of young adults in group home.	N/A
Krauss (2005). United States	135 adults, mostly with autistic disorder; average age 31.9 years.	53% in group home; 11% in semi-independent care.	N/A
Eaves & Ho (2007). Canada	47 adults with ASD; mean age 24 years.	47% in residential care.	N/A
Howlin (2000). International	Review of studies on HFA Mean age across studies ranges 18 to 38 years.	16% to 50% living semi/ independent.	N/A
Järbrink et al. (2007). Sweden	19 adults mostly with high-functioning ASD, Mean age 29.6; two waves of collection: 2000 to 2001 and 2002 to 2003.	Two in residential care (10%).	Mean: $2,199.
Wall (1990). North Carolina, United States	11 group homes for 52 persons with ASD.		State funded: $56,688; Federally funded: $33,959.
Lakin et al. (2008). United States	1,421 persons with intellectual disabilities receiving Medicaid from four states.		Medicaid-funded residential facility: $128,275; Medicaid-funded home and community based services: $61,770.

N/A: Not Available.

Table 78–6.
Summary of studies on other nonmedical expenditures specific to person with ASD

Authors, Year, Country	Sample: Children with ASD	Inclusion	Annual Expenditures in 2003 (U.S. $ per Child)
Birenbaum et al. (1990). United States	Nationally representative survey based on school and special education districts and 1980 censuses. Survey period June 1985 to June 1986. Sample under age 18 years, size = 235; age 18 to 24 years, size = 58.	Child care, special programs, after school, day care, weekend program, summer school, overnight respite, travel to medical appointments, home and car modification, damage replacements.	Mean $362.
Järbrink (2007). Sweden	Population-based survey in four municipalities; 33 children in 2005. Average age: 11.6 years, range 4 to 18 years.	Home placement, respite care, camp, domestic support worker, day outings, personal assistant, befriending service.	Mean $15,390.
Järbrink & Knapp (2003). United Kingdom	17 children, convenience sample for pilot study.	Damages, extra help, transport, special activities, extra cost for siblings, court cases, other.	ASD mean range: $5,505 to $8,366; median range: $4,678 to $6,106.

costs comes from Sweden and included 19 adults with HFA (average age of 29.6 years) who could work and were enrolled in a project that offered support for employment. Järbrink et al. (2007) found that about 50% of the sample had a paid job and the average loss of potential income was $16,400 per person per year, accounting for almost half of the annual cost of ASD in that study. A published review of six studies of adults with HFA by Howlin (2000) found that the percentage of individuals in paid employment ranged from 5% to 55%, depending on the survey sample, the geographic location,

Table 78–7.
Summary of studies on supported employment

Authors, Year, Country	Sample Composition		Inclusion	Annual Expenditures in 2003 (U.S. $ per Child)
	ASD	Comparison Group		
Järbrink et al. (2007). Sweden	Adults mostly with ASD, mean age 29.6 years, data collection in 2000 and 2003.		Community support, employment service.	Mean $9,768.
Mawhood & Howlin (1999). United Kingdom	30 adults with ASD, average age 31.1 years, collection in 1994 to 1996.	20 adults without ASD, average age 28 years.	Supported employment.	Mean: $20,445.
Rogers et al. (1995). United States		19 adults with severe psychiatric disabilities, average age 36 years, range 18 to 55 years; collection in 1990.	Supported employment.	Mean: $7,731.
Cones (2008). United States		Adults with intellectual and developmental disabilities.	Supported employment.	Mean: $4,334.

the type of support available to persons with ASDs, and how employment was defined. A survey of 117 adults (no age information provided) with HFA who were clients of a U.K. job placement service found that 54% to 100% of clients were in paid employment (Howlin et al., 2005), but that was not a representative survey of the population of adults with HFA. Two Canadian studies based on convenience samples reported that the majority of adults with ASDs who were interviewed were employed for pay, but with variable earnings. Eaves and Ho (2007) studied 47 young adults in Canada (mean age of 24 years) with ASDs and found that 4% were independent and held a job, 49% were "generally in work" and 47% held a low-paying, part-time, or a volunteer work position (personal communication from Linda Eaves, October 17, 2007).[7] Among a sample of nine young adults in Canada with Asperger's syndrome (average age of 20.3 years) who were not students, three had never held a paid job, three had part-time employment, and the other three held full-time jobs (Jennes-Coussens et al., 2006). An international review of the labor market participation of low-functioning individuals with ASDs indicated that 2% to 18% of adults were employed (Synergies Economic Consulting, 2007).

Generally, these studies suggest that at least 50% of adults with HFA are employed; however adults with a lower level of functioning are less likely to be employed. These results are based on convenience samples of adults. None of the studies cited in this section reported whether persons with ASDs worked in a capacity commensurate to their skills, except that one study noted that average earnings among those who had paid jobs were lower (Jennes-Coussens et al., 2006). Thus, their substantial losses of productivity are not well-measured. Also, it should be acknowledged that the availability of government benefits can deter people with disabilities from being employed for pay, although the Ticket to Work and Work Incentive Improvement Act of 1999 (Public Law 106–170) attempts to reduce the disincentives to employment among individuals receiving Social Security disability benefits.

Loss of Productivity of Caregivers

Parenting children with ASDs requires extra time that could otherwise be spent in paid work or other activities. Parents in one U.K. survey[8] were reported to spend an average of 40 extra hours per week caring for their young child with an ASD (Järbrink et al., 2003); this is a very high estimate relative to those from other studies. A representative, national U.S. survey found that 27% of families of a child with an ASD (ages 3 to 17 years) reported spending 10 or more hours per week providing care or coordinating care for their child (Kogan et al., 2008). Family caregivers in Sweden during 2002 to 2003 reported spending about 2 hours per week caring for an adult child with an ASD (Järbrink et al., 2007).

Other researchers have estimated the loss of hours of paid work and earnings (Grosse, 2010). The majority (57%) of a sample of 2,088 U.S. families of children or youth ages 3 to 17 years with ASDs in the 2005–2006 National Survey of Children with Special Health Care Needs reported that a family member reduced or stopped employment because of their child's condition (Kogan et al., 2008). An analysis of data from the 2003–2004 National Survey of Children's Health found that 39% of 82 families of preschool-age children with ASDs reported that child-care considerations had led a family member to quit work, change jobs, or alter type of work in the last 12 months, compared with 9% of 14,079 families with typically developing children (Montes & Halterman, 2008b).

Estimates of the loss in earnings require the collection of detailed information for representative samples of families of children with and without ASDs. Using the 2005 National Household Education Survey of After School Programs and Activities, Montes and Halterman (2006) found that mothers

Table 78–8.
Summary of studies on loss of productivity of persons with ASD

Authors, Year, Country	Sample: Adults with ASD	Percentage of Individuals with ASD in Work	Mean Annual Productivity Loss
Järbrink et al. (2007). Sweden	Survey: 19 adults with functioning ASD in Sweden, Mean age 29.6; two waves of collection: 2000 to 2001 and 2002 to 2003.	50%.	$16,413.
Howlin (2000). Canada, Denmark, U.K., U.S.	Review of studies on high-functioning autism (HFA); mean age across studies ranges from 18 to 38 years.	5% to 100%.	
Howlin et al. (2005). United Kingdom	117 adults; No age provided .	54% to 100%.	
Eaves & Ho (2008). Canada	47 adults; mean age 24 years, range 19 to 31 years.	4% independent. 49% "generally in work." 47% low-pay, part-time, or volunteer.	
Jennes-Coussens et al. (2006). Canada	12 adults with HFA, mean age 20.3 years among the nonstudents.	33% full-time. 33% part-time.	
Synergie Consulting review (2007). Australia	Review of international studies. Low-functioning adults with ASD.	2% to 18%.	

of children with ASDs in grades kindergarten through eight were less likely to be employed than other mothers, (53% vs. 67%). Like mothers, fathers of children with ASDs were less likely to be employed (82% vs. 93%), and more likely to be working part-time. Montes and Halterman (2008a) calculated the mean loss of parental income in this sample to be $6,000 per year for each child with an ASD. To be equivalent to the total loss of productivity from a societal perspective, one should multiply this estimate by 1.31 to adjust for employer-paid fringe benefits and payroll taxes (Grosse et al., 2009), or approximately $7,900 per year in 2003 dollars.

In Sweden, Järbrink (2007) evaluated parental time loss for paid work to be $5,400 per child. For young adults with ASDs in Sweden, parental loss of earnings was much lower, averaging about $103 per person (Järbrink et al., 2007). In the United Kingdom, Järbrink et al. (2003) estimated the loss of income for caregivers of young children with an ASD to be $19,300 per year. The median parental income loss amounted to $16,700 per year.

Generally, these studies suggest that parents of children with ASDs spend more time caring for their children than parents of typically developing children, but the time required for care seems to decrease as children with ASDs age. In the United States, this extra parenting time translates into a loss of earned income of $6,000 according to Montes and Halterman (2008a), which is equivalent to 17% of median income of a married U.S. worker in 2003 (Bureau of Labor Statistics, 2004)[9].

Mean Annual Total Cost

Mean annual total costs provide a useful summary as the distribution of cost may vary depending on local policies and the age of the persons with ASDs and whether they have an intellectual disability or not. In the United Kingdom, Knapp et al. (2009) calculated that the mean annual expenditures per child with an ASD without intellectual disability age 4 to 17 years was $33,100, and education and respite care account for 89% of it. For children with intellectual disability, the cost rose from $36,900 for those ages 4 through 11 years to $63,200 for those ages 12 to 17 years. Together, education and respite care account for 58% and 89% of those expenditures, respectively. In an earlier study in the U.K., the mean and median annual costs per child were respectively $57,600 and $54,200 in a small pilot survey of 17 children with ASDs (Järbrink et al., 2003). Medical costs accounted for 3%, nonmedical costs accounted for 63% (53% for education and behavioral therapy), and parental loss of income represented 34%. In Sweden, the annual per capita costs of ASD in a sample of 33 children were $54,500 (Järbrink, 2007). Medical-care costs represented 5% of the total, nonmedical care accounted for 80%, of which education alone accounted for 51% of total costs, and caregiver costs were 15% of total costs.

Annual expenditures for adults are generally higher than those of children. In the United Kingdom, Järbrink and Knapp (2001) found that annual expenditures per adult with an ASD and intellectual disability is $116,500 and the cost per adult without intellectual disability was about 58% of that at $67,900. In Sweden, the mean annual cost for 19 young adults with ASDs ages 19 to 39 years was calculated to be $35,600 per person (Järbrink et al., 2007). Medical-care costs constituted 16% of total costs, nonmedical care accounted for 30%, productivity losses accounted for 49%, and parental earnings losses were 5% of the total costs. In Australia, the mean total incremental costs for individuals of all ages with ASDs were

Table 78–9.
Summary of studies on parental loss of productivity

Authors, Year, Country	Sample Composition	Percentage of Parents Who Work		Incremental Time Spent on Care	Annual Productivity Loss
		ASD	Comparison		
Järbrink et al. (2003). United Kingdom	17 children, convenience sample for pilot study.			40 hours per week.	Mean: $19,297. Median: $16,707.
Järbrink et al. (2007). Sweden	Survey: 19 adults with functioning ASD in Sweden, Mean age 29.6; two waves of collection: 2000 to 2001 and 2002 to 2003.	N/A	N/A	48 hours per month.	Mean: $103.
Järbrink et al. (2007). Sweden	Population-based survey in four municipalities; 33 children in 2005. Average age: 11.6 years, range 4 to 18 years.	N/A	N/A		Mean: $5,430.
Montes & Halterman (2006). United States	National Household Education Survey, after school (2005) kindergarten to eighth grade, 131 children with ASD and 11,573 otherwise similar children.	Mothers: 53%, Fathers: 82%.	Mothers: 67%, Fathers: 93%.		Mean: $6,046.
Birenbaum et al. (1990). United States	See Table 78-1.	Mothers: 35%.	Mothers: 53%.		

N/A: Not Available.

estimated based on a compilation of literature and modeling to be $38,000 per person. Medical costs represented 3%, nonmedical costs 25%, productivity losses represented 49%, and caregiver costs accounted for 23% of the total costs (Synergies Economic Consulting, 2007).

Lifetime Costs

Three published studies estimated the lifetime cost of ASDs using modeling techniques to address gaps in information. First, Ganz (2007, 2006) estimated a lifetime cost of $3.2 million for a typical child with an ASD, calculated using a 3% per year discount rate to discount costs incurred in the future to present values, as is standard practice in U.S. health economics analyses. He assumed that a child would be diagnosed at age 3 years and receive behavioral therapy for 4 years, special education and child care through age 22 years, and adult care from age 23 years to the end of life. Ganz assumed that 10% to 35% of adults with ASDs engage in supported employment in which they receive specific work-related help and coaching and earn 20% of average national income[10] but that no adult with an ASD works independently. Ganz assumed that 10% to 20% of fathers and 55% to 60% of mothers of children with ASDs were out of the workforce. Further, 50% of adults with ASDs were assumed to live in a specialized institution. On the basis of these assumptions, Ganz projected lifetime medical expenditures of approximately $100,000 (3%), nonmedical expenditures of $1,185,100 (37%), loss of productivity of $971,100 (30%) and parental loss of productivity of $904,600 (28%).

Several of these cost components appear overstated. First, Ganz assumed that a "typical" child would receive intensive behavioral therapy at a cost of $40,000 per year for 4 years. However, few children with ASDs currently have access to these intensive therapies (Thomas, et al., 2007b). Second, Ganz made pessimistic assumptions about the employment of both individuals with ASDs and their parents. The author assumed that no adult with an ASD works independently, whereas as many as one-half of HFA adults are employed (Eaves & Ho, 2007; Howlin, 2000; Howlin et al., 2005; Järbrink et al., 2007; Jennes-Coussens et al., 2006). Ganz (2007) assumed an average parental loss of annual earnings of $43,000 per year, which is seven times higher than a subsequent empirical estimate of $6,000 per year (Montes & Halterman, 2008a). It should be noted that the median yearly earnings of a married U.S. worker in 2003 was just over $36,000 (Bureau of Labor Statistics, 2004).[11]

Earlier, Järbrink and Knapp (2001) evaluated lifetime costs in the United Kingdom. They assumed that 25% of persons with an ASD have HFA and 75% have an intellectual disability in addition to an ASD. During their lifetime, persons with HFA were projected to cost $1.3 million and those with lower-functioning autism about $4.7 million, without discounting costs in future years. "Living support" or residential care represented about 40% of the cost for persons with HFA and 73% of the total costs for low-functioning individuals. A maximum of 35% of adults with HFA were assumed to live independently and it was assumed that all others would need living support. Also, it was assumed that 60% of persons with ASDs and intellectual disability would be in residential care by 20 years

Table 78–10.
Summary of studies on annual total cost of ASD

Authors, Year, Country	Sample: Persons with ASD	Total per Person with ASD	Distribution			
			Medical	Nonmedical	Productivity Loss	Parental Productivity Loss
Järbrink et al. (2007), Sweden.	Population sample of 33 children.	Mean: $54,546.	5%	80%	0%	15%
Järbrink et al. (2007), Sweden.	Pilot study of 17 children.	Mean: $57,572; Median: $54,246.	3%	63%	0%	34%
Järbrink et al. (2003), United Kingdom.	Literature review.	Mean: $35,603.	16%	30%	49%	5%
Synergie Consulting review(2007), Australia.	Literature review.	Mean: $38,045.	3%	25%	49%	23%
Knapp et al. (2009), United Kingdom.	Literature review;					
	children age 4 to 11 years with ID;	Mean: $36,947;	33%	59%	0%	8%
	children age 12 to 17 years with ID;	Mean: $63,245;	6%	89%	0%	5%
	children age 4 to 17 years without ID;	Mean: $33,078;	10%	89%	0%	1%
	adults with ID;	Mean: $116,481;	7%	59%	2%	32%
	adults without ID.	Mean: $67,861, respectively.	34%	15%	45%	7%

ASD: Autism Spectrum Disorders; ID: Intellectual disability.

of age and the others by 55 years of age. It was assumed that the majority of adults with ASDs could not live independently during their adulthood, an assumption based on a sample of adults who received autism-specific services.

Third, Knapp et al. (2009) calculated lifetime cost estimates for the United Kingdom for individuals with ASDs with and without intellectual disability, assuming a 45:55 split. Using a 3.5% discount rate, as is now standard practice in U.K. health economic analyses, the lifetime cost was estimated to be $1,221,366 for those without intellectual disability and $1,893,400 for those with intellectual disability. Neither estimate included any loss of parental earnings resulting from informal caregiving. Knapp and colleagues assumed that 79% of adults with an ASD without intellectual disability live in private households, compared with 35% of adults with an ASD and intellectual disability. These estimates appear more in line with prior findings than the assumptions in the previous U.K. cost study by Järbrink and Knapp (2001).

Overall, the Ganz estimate of lifetime costs assumed optimal patterns of care for children with ASDs but the worst possible outcomes in terms of lost productivity. Access to early intensive therapy and appropriate education should improve long-term outcomes and reduce both productivity costs and residential costs (Jacobson et al., 1998; Motiwala et al., 2006). All of the studies cited appear likely to overstate service utilization and expenditures among adults, especially for residential care, because they did not account for adults who had an ASD diagnosis as children but did not continue to receive ASD-related services as adults.

Conclusion

In the United States, there are a number of fairly precise estimates of mean incremental medical expenditures for children with ASDs, although there is substantial variation among these different estimates. Recent estimates of annual medical expenditures per individual range from $2,100 to $11,200 and represent 3% to 5% of the estimated total annual cost for a child with an ASD. For nonmedical costs, the mean annual incremental cost of educating a child with an ASD as a qualifying condition for special education is about $13,000. Intensive behavioral interventions cost between $40,000 and $60,000 per child per year. Recent U.S. estimates of other nonmedical costs such as home transformation or respite services are not readily available.

There is a dearth of empirical data on costs for adults with ASDs, particularly residential-care costs, loss of productivity, and cost to parents or other caregivers, which most likely represent the bulk of ASD-related lifetime costs. The only one of these with a recent U.S. population-based estimate suggests an annual loss of parental productivity of $6,000 per child, or $7,400 from the societal perspective. This calculation needs to be replicated with other surveys. Estimates of residential costs per person with an ASD or learning disabilities range from $60,000 to $128,000 per year, but estimates of the proportion of persons who need these services do not exist. Our review indicates that estimates of the loss of productivity of adults with ASDs mostly rely on convenience samples. Among adults

Table 78–11.
Summary of studies on lifetime cost of ASD

Authors, Year, Country	Sample: Persons with ASD	Total Mean per Person	Distribution			
			Medical	Nonmedical	Productivity Loss	Parental Productivity Loss
Ganz (2007, 2006), United States.	Societal perspective: literature review, all children received appropriate care but with worst possible outcomes. Discount cost.	$3,200,000.	3%	37%	31%	29%
Järbrink & Knapp (2001), Sweden.	Societal perspective: literature review, no discounting.	Low-functioning: $4,700,000; HFA: $1,300,000.	Low-functioning: 3.4%; HFA: 9%.	Low-functioning: 95.3%; HFA: 71.7%.	Low-functioning: 0%; HFA: 17.5%.	Low-functioning: 1.3%; HFA: 1.8%.
Knapp et al. (2009), United Kingdom.	Societal perspective: literature review, discounted cost.	With intellectual disability: $1,893,373; without intellectual disability: $1,221,366.	Not available from published paper.	Not available from published paper.	Not available from published paper.	Not available from published paper.

HFA: high-functioning autism

with HFA, at least half are employed but we do not know much about their skills level and their earnings. The real productivity losses of adults with ASDs are unknown. Thus, we lack reliable estimates of total yearly or lifetime costs of ASDs in the United States.

Cost components are affected by the time period of the data, the services considered, sample size and representativeness, and the organization and financing of care, as well as how ASDs are diagnosed and ascertained. Most studies cited in this chapter were not based on population samples, and self-selection may bias the results. The only U.S. national survey to collect cost data on children and adults with ASDs (Birenbaum et al., 1990) was conducted more than two decades ago. New, population-based surveys are needed. The 2005–2006 National Survey of Children with Special Health Care Needs collected qualitative information on impacts of ASDs for a representative sample of more than 2,000 families with a child or youth with an ASD but did not collect cost data (Kogan et al., 2008) and did not address costs for adults with ASDs.

ASD describes a continuum in which some persons require a high level of lifelong support but others function independently or with little support. Consequently, it is necessary to collect cost and service utilization data for representative samples of individuals with ASDs. Such data could be used as a reliable baseline to measure the cost-effectiveness of interventions and to guide policymakers in allocating resources for the care of persons with ASDs.

Challenges and Future Directions

- We do not have a reliable estimate of the overall lifetime costs associated with ASDs for an individual child or for a nation. Some cost estimates include implausible assessments of productivity losses.
- We lack standardized cost estimates for both ASDs and other developmental conditions or disabilities that would allow for comparability in estimates of the economic impacts of these disorders.
- The biggest gap in data is the lack of information from representative samples of parents of children with ASDs on out-of-pocket expenditures and use of therapies, particularly alternative therapies.
- We lack data on large, representative samples of adults with ASDs to document costs associated with productivity losses and personal care/housing.
- The greatest need for economic data on ASDs is to quantify the economic impact of early-intervention programs. However, this requires cost estimates that are sensitive to differences in functioning, which can be affected by such

intervention programs. We do not have such data at the present time.

ACKNOWLEDGMENTS

We acknowledge helpful comments received from Coleen Boyle, Cynthia Cassell, Clark Denny, Christine Prue, Paul Shattuck, and Marshalyn Yeargin-Allsopp.

The findings and conclusions in this report are those of the authors and do not necessarily represent the official position of the Centers for Disease Control and Prevention.

NOTES

1 Children in the United States with ASDs are entitled to services mandated under the special education law "Individual with Disabilities Education Act (IDEA)" from birth until the age 21 years.

2 We chose 2003 because it is the modal year of data in the U.S.-based papers reviewed.

3 Purchasing Power Parity are conversion rates from the Organisation for Economic Cooperation and Development that equalize the purchasing power of different currencies. http://www.oecd.org/department/0,3355,en_2649_34357_1_1_1_1_1,00.html accessed on 4/7/2008.

4 See www.bls.gov accessed on 9/20/2007.

5 The author did not provide the years covered by his study and attempts to contact him were unsuccessful. We therefore assume that those costs are effective in 1990, the year in which the paper was published.

6 The study is described in more detail below in the productivity section.

7 Linda Eaves reported that persons with ASDs in British Columbia were eligible for public support of C$800 per month and that public support could reduce their incentives for labor market participation.

8 Data collection dates not clear, but study offer prices of 1999 to 2000.

9 Median usual weekly earnings of full-time wage and salary workers by selected characteristics, 2003 annual averages. The weekly earning of a married worker with spouse present equals $697, or $36,244 per year.

10 Unpublished appendix obtained from Michael Ganz, personal communication, December 5, 2007.

11 See Notes 9

REFERENCES

Autism and Developmental Disabilities Monitoring Network Surveillance Year 2006 Principal Investigators, Centers for Disease Control and Prevention (CDC). (2009). Prevalence of autism spectrum disorders–Autism and Developmental Disabilities Monitoring Network, United States, 2006. *Morbidity and Mortality Weekly Report Surveillance Summaries, 58*(SS10), 1–20.

Birenbaum, A., Guyot, D., & Cohen, H. J. (1990). Health care financing for severe developmental disabilities. *Monographs of the American Association on Mental Retardation, 14*, 1–150.

Bureau of Labor Statistics (2007) *Consumer Price Index-All urban consumers. Series ID:CUSR0000SAM.* Retrieved September 18, 2007 from www.bls.gov.

Bureau of Labor Statistics (2006). *New ECI news release table structure, by new table numbers. Table 11. Employment Cost Index for wages and salaries, for state and local government workers, by occupational group and industry.* Retrieved September 20, 2007, from http://www.bls.gov/ncs/ect/naicscrswlk.htm.

Bureau of Labor Statistics (2004). *Highlights of women's earnings in 2003.* Retrieved September 20, 2007, from http://www.bls.gov/cps/cpswom2003.pdf.

Butter, E., Wynn, J., & Mulick, J. A. (2003). Early intervention critical to autism treatment. *Pediatric Annals, 32*, 677.

Chambers, J. G., Parrish, T. B., & Harr, J. J. (2004). *What are we spending on special education services in the United States, 1999-2000?* Washington, DC: American Institutes for Research for United States Department of Education Office of Special Education Programs.

Chambers, J. G., Shkolnik, J., & Pérez, M. (2003). *Total expenditures for students with disabilities, 1999–2000: Spending variation by disability*: Washington, DC: American Institutes for Research for United States Department of Education, Office of Special Education Programs.

Chasson, G. S., Harris, G. E., & Neely, W. J. (2007). Cost comparison of early intensive behavioral intervention and special education for children with autism. *Journal of Child and Family Studies, 16*, 401–413.

Cone, A. A. (2008). *Fact sheet: Supported employment.* Retrieved August 27, 2008, from http://www.aaidd.org/Policies/faq_supported_employ.shtml.

Croen, L. A., Najjar, D. V., Ray, T., Lotspeich, L., & Bernal, P. (2006). A comparison of health care utilization and costs of children with and without autism spectrum disorders in a large group-model health plan. *Pediatrics, 118*, e1203–1211.

Eaves, L. C., & Ho, H. H. (2008). Young adult outcome of autism spectrum disorders. *Journal of Autism and Developmental Disorders, 38*, 739–747.

Flanders, S. C., Engelhart, L., Pandina, G. J., & McCracken, J. T. (2007). Direct health care costs for children with pervasive developmental disorders: 1996–2002. *Administration and Policy in Mental Health and Mental Health Services Research, 34*, 213–220.

Flanders, S. C., Engelhart, L., Whitworth, J., Hussein, M. A., Vanderpoel, D. R., & Sandman, T. (2006). The economic burden of pervasive developmental disorders in a privately insured population. *Managed Care Interface, 19*, 39–45.

Fombonne, E. (2003). Epidemiological surveys of autism and other pervasive developmental disorders: An update. *Journal of Autism and Developmental Disorders, 33*, 365–382.

Ganz, M. L. (2006). The costs of autism. In S. Moldin & J. Rubenstein (Eds.), *Understanding autism: From neuroscience to treatment* (pp. 476–502). Boca Raton, FL: Taylor and Francis Group.

Ganz, M. L. (2007). The lifetime distribution of the incremental societal costs of autism. *Archives of Pediatrics and Adolescent Medicine, 161*, 343–349.

Grosse, S. D. (2010). In R. Urbano (Ed.), Sociodemographic characteristics of families of children with Down syndrome and the economic impacts on families of child disability. *International Review of Research in Mental Retardation, 39*, 257–294.

Grosse, S. D., Krueger, K. V., & Mvundura, M. (2009). Economic productivity by age and sex: 2007 estimates for the United States. *Medical Care, 47*, S94–S103.

Gurney, J. G., McPheeters, M. L., & Davis, M. M. (2006). Parental report of health conditions and health care use among children with and without autism: National survey of children's health. *Archives of Pediatrics and Adolescent Medicine, 160*, 825–830.

Hagner, D., & Cooney, B. F. (2005). "I do that for everybody": Supervising employees with autism. *Focus on Autism and Other Developmental Disabilities, 20*, 91–97.

Howlin, P. (2000). Outcome in adult life for more able individuals with autism or Asperger syndrome. *Autism, 4*, 63–83.

Howlin, P., Alcock, J., & Burkin, C. (2005). An 8 year follow-up of a specialist supported employment service for high-ability adults with autism or Asperger syndrome, *Autism, 9*, 533–549.

Hume, K., Bellini, S., & Pratt, C. (2005). The usage and perceived outcomes of early intervention and early childhood programs for young children with autism spectrum disorder. *Topics in Early Childhood Special Education, 25*, 195–207.

Jacobson, J. W., Mulick, J. A., & Green, G. (1998). Cost-benefit estimates for early intensive behavioral intervention for young children with autism: General model and single state case. *Behavioral Interventions, 13*, 201–226.

Järbrink, K. (2007). The economic consequences of autistic spectrum disorder among children in a Swedish municipality. *Autism, 11*, 453–463.

Järbrink, K., Fombonne, E., & Knapp, M. (2003). Measuring the parental, service and cost impacts of children with autistic spectrum disorder: A pilot study. *Journal of Autism and Developmental Disorders, 33*, 395–402.

Järbrink, K., & Knapp, M. (2001). The economic impact of autism in Britain. *Autism, 5*, 7–22.

Järbrink, K., McCrone, P., Fombonne, E., Zandén, H., & Knapp, M. (2007). Cost-impact of young adults with high-functioning autistic spectrum disorder. *Research in Developmental Disabilities, 28*, 94–104.

Jennes-Coussens, M., Magill-Evans, J., & Koning, C. (2006). The quality of life of young men with Asperger syndrome. *Autism, 10*, 403–414.

Knapp, M., Romeo, R., & Beecham, J. (2009). Economic cost of autism in the UK. *Autism. 13*, 317–336.

Kogan, M. D., Strickland, B. B., Blumberg, S. J., Singh, G.K., Perrin, J. M., & van Dyck, P. C. (2008). A national profile of the health care experiences and family impact of autism spectrum disorder among children in the United States, 2005–2006. *Pediatrics, 122*, e1149–1158.

Krauss, M. W., Seltzer, M. M., & Jacobson, H. T. (2005). Adults with autism living at home or in non-family settings: Positive and negative aspects of residential status. *Journal of Intellectual Disability Research, 49*, 111–124.

Lakin, K. C., Doljanac, R., Byun, S. Y., Stancliffe, R. J., Taub, S., & Chiri, G. (2008). Factors associated with expenditures for Medicaid home and community based services (HCBS) and intermediate care facilities for persons with mental retardation (ICF/MR) services for persons with intellectual and developmental disabilities. *Intellectual and Developmental Disability, 46*, 200–214.

Lawer, L., Brusilovskiy, E., Salzer, M. S., & Mandell, D. S. (2008). Use of vocational rehabilitative services among adults with autism. *Journal of Autism and Developmental Disorders, 39*, 487–494.

Leslie, D. L., & Martin, A. (2007). Health care expenditures associated with autism spectrum disorders. *Archives of Pediatrics and Adolescent Medicine, 161*, 350–355.

Liptak, G., Stuart, T., & Auinger, P. (2006). Health care utilization and expenditures for children with autism: Data from U.S. national samples. *Journal of Autism and Developmental Disorders, 36*, 871–879.

Lovaas, O. I. (1987). Behavioral treatment and normal educational and intellectual functioning in young autistic children. *Journal of Consulting and Clinical Psychology, 55*, 3–9.

Mandell, D. S., Cao, J., Ittenbach, R., & Pinto-Martin, J. (2006). Medicaid expenditures for children with autistic spectrum disorders: 1994 to 1999 [Electronic Version]. *Journal of Autism and Developmental Disorders, 36*, 265–275.

Mandell, D. S., Novak, M. M., & Zubritsky, C. D. (2005). Factors associated with age of diagnosis among children with autism spectrum disorders. *Pediatrics, 116*, 1480–1486.

Mawhood, L., & Howlin, P. (1999). The outcome of a supported employment scheme for high-functioning adults with autism or Asperger syndrome. *Autism, 3*, 229–254.

Montes, G., & Halterman, J. (2006). Characteristics of school-age children with autism. *Journal of Developmental and Behavioral Pediatrics, 27*, 379–385.

Montes, G., & Halterman, J. S. (2008a). Association of childhood autism spectrum disorders and loss of family income. *Pediatrics, 121*, e821–826.

Montes, G., & Halterman, J. S. (2008b). Child care problems and employment among families with preschool-aged children with autism in the United States. *Pediatrics, 122*, e202–208.

Motiwala, S. S., Gupta, S., Lilly, M. B., Ungar, W. J., & Coyte, P. C. (2006). The cost effectiveness of expanding behavioural intervention to all autistic children in Ontario. *Healthcare Policy, 1*, 135–151.

OECD (2008). *Purchasing Power Parities (PPPs) for OECD countries since 1980.* Retrieved April 7, 2008 from OECD: http://www.oecd.org/department/0,3355,en_2649_34357_1_1_1_1_1,00.html.

Oswald, D. P. & Sonenklar, N. A. (2007). Medication use among children with autism spectrum disorders. *Journal of Child and Adolescent Psychopharmacology, 17*, 348–355.

Reinhardt, U. E. (2006). The pricing of U.S. hospital services: Chaos behind a veil of secrecy. *Health Affairs, 25*, 57–69.

Rogers, E. S., Sciarappa, K., MacDonald-Wilson, K., & Danley, K. (1995). A benefit-cost analysis of a supported employment model for persons with psychiatric disabilities. *Evaluation and Program Planning, 18*, 105–115.

Ruble, L., Heflinger, C., Renfrew, J., & Saunders, R. (2005). Access and service use by children with autism spectrum disorders in Medicaid Managed Care. *Journal of Autism and Developmental Disorders, 35*, 3–13.

Sallows, G. O., & Graupner, T. D. (2005). Intensive behavioral treatment for children with autism: Four-year outcome and predictors. *American Journal of Mental Retardation, 110*, 417–438.

Shimabukuro, T. T., Grosse, S. D., & Rice, C. (2008). Medical expenditures for children with an autism spectrum disorder in a privately insured population. *Journal of Autism and Developmental Disorders, 38*, 546–552.

Synergies Economic Consulting (2007). *Economic costs of autism spectrum disorders.* Retrieved September 10, 2007, from www.synergies.com.au.

Thomas, K. C., Ellis, A. R., McLaurin, C., Daniels, J., & Morrissey, J. P. (2007a). Access to care for autism-related services. *Journal of Autism and Developmental Disorders, 37*, 1902–1912.

Thomas, K. C., Morrissey, J. P., & McLaurin, C. (2007b). Use of autism-related services by families and children. *Journal of Autism and Developmental Disorders, 37*, 818–829.

Wall, A. J. (1990). Group homes in North Carolina for children and adults with autism. *Journal of Autism and Developmental Disorders, 20*, 353–366.

Yeargin-Allsopp, M., Rice, C., Karapurkar, T., Doernberg, N., Boyle, C., & Murphy, C. (2003). Prevalence of autism in a U.S. metropolitan area. *Journal of the American Medical Association, 289*, 49–55.

79 Future Directions: Setting Priorities to Guide the Federal Research Effort

Thomas R. Insel, Susan A. Daniels

Points of Interest

- The Interagency Autism Coordinating Committee, a federal advisory committee composed of federal and public members, issued the first federal strategic plan for autism research in 2009 and an updated strategic plan in 2010.
- The strategic plan and its first update were developed through an extensive process involving input from federal agencies, scientific experts, advocacy and research organizations, people with ASD and their families, and the public.
- The 2010 IACC Strategic Plan for ASD Research is organized according to seven key consumer-based questions that are critically important to people with ASD and their families. The plan spans a broad range of topics in ASD biomedical and services-related research.
- The National Institutes of Health (NIH), the primary federal agency that conducts biomedical research on autism, has had a steadily rising autism research budget from 1997 to 2009.
- The NIH is currently conducting autism research through its extramural and intramural programs, and is providing critical research resources to the scientific community to foster autism research.
- With the framework provided by the IACC strategic plan and judicious use of funds such as those provided by the American Recovery and Reinvestment Act (ARRA) of 2009 to support a diverse portfolio of science, the federal autism research effort is poised to address critical needs of people with ASD and their families.

Several federal agencies have been involved in research or services for individuals affected by ASD for the past three decades. The Children's Health Act of 2000 (P.L. 106-310) established the IACC to integrate the commitment of most of the involved agencies under the leadership of the Department of Health and Human Services (DHHS). As research and service budgets for ASD grew during the years following the enactment of the Children's Health Act, the IACC provided a forum not only for coordination of federal research efforts, but also for research planning, public input, and documentation of the increasing need for services. The national Autism Summit Conference, held in November 2003, focused on the federal government's role in biomedical autism research, and provided a public forum to disseminate, evaluate, and integrate the latest practice- and science-based autism information among federal, academic, and community participants. The conference, attended by the Secretary of Health and Human Services, the Secretary of Education, and several members of Congress, described the importance of increasing awareness about autism and launched a research matrix to guide the field toward specific short- and long-term goals for ASD research (Autism Summit Conference Summary, 2003). Progress on these goals was described in the report, "Evaluating Progress on the IACC Autism Research Matrix," published by the IACC in 2006. Among key findings from the report were that the science of autism had recently begun to converge on the concept of ASD as a group of brain disorders, that several prominent gaps remained in research to understand the causes and molecular bases of autism, that more randomized clinical trials of individual comprehensive intervention approaches were needed, and that more emphasis on research was needed to enhance services and supports for individuals with ASD and their families.

The Combating Autism Act (CAA) of 2006 (P.L. 109-416) reauthorized Title 1 of the Children's Health Act and expanded coordination of federal activities in autism. The CAA mandated the reestablishment of the IACC to coordinate all efforts concerning autism spectrum disorders across the DHHS and required a more specific composition of the committee. Up to two-thirds of the committee was required to be composed of representatives of federal agencies, and at least one-third was to be composed of public members, including at least one individual with a diagnosis of an autism spectrum disorder, at least one parent or legal guardian of an individual with an autism spectrum disorder, and at least one member who is a representative of a leading research, advocacy, or service organization for individuals with autism spectrum disorder. This partnership between federal agencies and members of the public provides a meaningful way to include public input in government priority setting. Currently, IACC membership includes two individuals with ASD, several parents of children with ASD, and individuals who are leaders of national autism advocacy groups (Autistic Self Advocacy Network, Autism Society, Autism Speaks, and Coalition for SafeMinds), representatives of private national research organizations (Autism Science Foundation, Simons Foundation, the U.C. Davis M.I.N.D. Institute), as well as officials from the following federal agencies that deal with autism research or services: Centers for Disease Control and Prevention (CDC), the Department of Education, the Centers for Medicare and Medicaid Services (CMS), the HHS Office on Disability, Substance Abuse and Mental Health Services Administration (SAMHSA), the Administration for Children and Families (ACF), the Health Resources and Service Administration (HRSA), five Institutes of the National Institutes of Health and the NIH director. The federal partners cover different parts of the ASD landscape. For instance, scientists at the CDC focus on epidemiology and public awareness, different institutes of the NIH cover the biology of and interventions for ASD, and CMS provides support to states for ASD services. Similarly, the public members represent a variety of viewpoints and perspectives. The IACC serves as a forum for representatives of each agency and public members to inform each other, as well as the general public, about the challenges and opportunities for ASD research and services as seen from different corners of the community. The IACC also regularly invites speakers to discuss current findings in scientific and services research to present at its meetings, holds public workshops, and collects public input through events such as town hall meetings and formal Requests for Information (RFI). As the new IACC was established in accordance with the Federal Advisory Committee Act, all meetings are open to the public and all decisions are advisory to the federal government.

The responsibilities of the IACC under the CAA include development of a research strategic plan for autism spectrum disorders, annually updating the strategic plan to reflect advances in science and newly identified research opportunities and needs, monitoring of federal activities related to autism, preparation of a summary of biomedical and services research advances in autism spectrum for Congress, and making recommendations to the Secretary of HHS and the Director of NIH regarding the strategic plan for autism research and federal activities related to autism.

A Research Strategic Plan for ASD

Building on the experience of developing the matrix for autism research in 2003, the new IACC developed the first federal strategic plan for ASD research, which documents recent progress in autism research, identifies current research gaps and opportunities, and recommends a series of research objectives spanning biomedical science and services that can be supported through the activities of federal agencies, private foundations, or public–private partnerships.

The original 2009 plan was developed through an extensive process engaging a variety of federal agencies, scientific experts, and public stakeholders. In December 2007, the IACC issued a public RFI to solicit high-priority research questions within the areas of autism: risk factors, biology, diagnosis, and treatment (IACC Request for Information, 2007). The IACC used the input received to inform a series of scientific workshops that involved over 60 scientists, clinicians, and autism advocates, where a series of research objectives for the strategic plan were developed. A town hall meeting and other RFIs were used to gather additional public input as the draft plan continued to take shape (IACC Town Hall Meeting, 2008; IACC Request for Information, 2008). The language of the draft plan was meticulously reviewed and revised by the IACC in a series of public meetings that took place between November 2008 and January 2009 (IACC Meetings and Events, 2009). This first IACC strategic plan was finalized in January 2009 and submitted to the Congress, the Secretary of Health and Human Services and the Director of NIH, as required by the CAA (*IACC Strategic Plan for ASD Research*, 2009; IACC News Release, 2009).

In January 2010, the IACC completed an update of the strategic plan (*IACC Strategic Plan for ASD Research*, 2010; IACC News Update, 2010). This revised plan more fully addresses the needs of the people with ASD across the spectrum, from young children to adults, and places new emphasis on both nonverbal and cognitively impaired people with ASD. The committee also decided to create a new seventh chapter in the plan on surveillance and infrastructure in order to focus attention on the need for expanded and enhanced research infrastructure—from bio-repositories to better surveillance—to bolster ASD research. Input for the 2010 plan was gained through a variety of means, including a formal RFI soliciting public input on additional topics that could be addressed in the 2010 update of the plan, a town hall meeting on services for people with ASD, and a 2-day scientific workshop involving ASD researchers, clinicians, advocates, people with ASD and family members of people with ASD (IACC, Request for Information, 2009; IACC Services Town Hall Meeting, 2009; IACC Scientific Workshop, 2009).

An important part of the strategic planning effort leading to the first IACC strategic plan and the 2010 update of the plan was the consideration of the historical and current funding landscape for ASD research. The largest funder of ASD research worldwide is the U.S. National Institutes of Health.

Figure 79-1 illustrates the levels of NIH funding for autism research over the past two decades, showing a steady increase in funding starting in 1996. The American Recovery and Reinvestment Act, signed into law by President Obama on Feb. 17, 2009, provided funds to many federal agencies to stimulate the economy. NIH used a portion of the ARRA funds it received to support new initiatives to advance research on ASD. As shown in Figure 79-1, the NIH official funding commitment for ASD-related research reached an all-time high of approximately $196 million in 2009, encompassing $64 million in ARRA funds and $132 million in non-ARRA research funds (NIH RePORT website, 2010).

The IACC and NIMH Office of Autism Research Coordination (OARC), the office that provides logistical and policy support to the IACC, undertook the first ever comprehensive analysis of the research portfolios of government and private funders of ASD research in 2009, looking back into 2008 funding data. Table 79-1 shows the research funders who provided information for the portfolio analysis, their ASD research budgets, numbers of projects and average funding per project. In 2008, these funders supported over $222 million in ASD research. The analysis of the autism research portfolio showed that approximately 65% of the overall funding was provided by government agencies, while private funders contributed approximately 35% (see Figure 79-2). When examining how these funds were distributed in relation to the 2009 IACC Strategic Plan for ASD Research, the greatest proportion of funding was found to have been allocated to research on risk factors for ASD (37%), followed by treatments and interventions (24%), the underlying biology of autism (18%) and diagnosis (13%) (see Figure 79-3). Services research and research on lifespan issues lagged behind at 1% and 5%, respectively, indicating a need for increased research efforts in these areas.

The mission of the IACC Strategic Plan is to "focus, coordinate, and accelerate high-quality research and scientific discovery in partnership with stakeholders to answer the urgent questions and needs of people on the autism spectrum and their families." In keeping with this mission, the research objectives recommended by the IACC in their 2010 update of

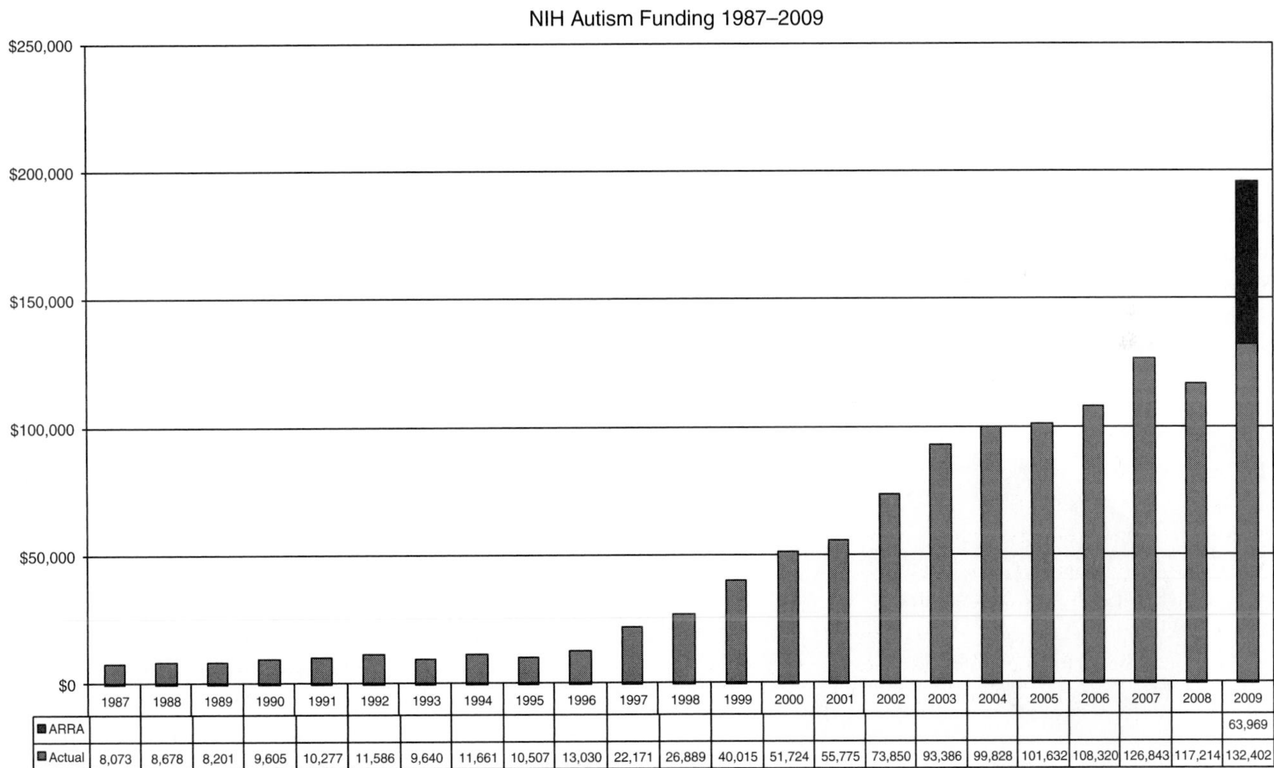

	1987	1988	1989	1990	1991	1992	1993	1994	1995	1996	1997	1998	1999	2000	2001	2002	2003	2004	2005	2006	2007	2008	2009
ARRA																							63,969
Actual	8,073	8,678	8,201	9,605	10,277	11,586	9,640	11,661	10,507	13,030	22,171	26,889	40,015	51,724	55,775	73,850	93,386	99,828	101,632	108,320	126,843	117,214	132,402

Figure 79–1. Autism funding at the NIH has greatly increased over a 22-year span. Over the past decade, general NIH funding for ASD research more than tripled from approximately $40 million in 1999 to over $132 million in 2009. With an addition of almost $64 million from the American Recovery and Reinvestment Act (ARRA) in 2009, NIH funding for autism research reached its highest level yet at $196 million. Please note that funding levels prior to 2008 were calculated using the former NIH coding system. Since 2008, the NIH has used the automated Research Condition and Disease Categorization (RCDC) system to standardize how NIH-funded projects are categorized as autism research. The change from the old NIH coding system to the new RCDC system results in what appears to be a decrease in funding in 2008 from 2007, but this dip actually only represents a change in how specific projects were counted toward the autism funding total and not an actual decrease in funding of projects. Source: NIH RePORT website.

Table 79–1.
2008 Autism spectrum disorder research funding by funding agency/organization

Funding Agency/Organization	Number of Projects Funded	Average Funding Per Project	Total Funding
National Institutes of Health	340	$346,970	$117,969,770
Simons Foundation	77	$558,256	$42,985,684
Autism Speaks	200	$154,141	$30,828,116
Centers for Disease Control and Prevention	27	$682,855	$15,022,812
Health Resources and Services Administration	3	$2,030,264	$6,090,792
Department of Education	7	$491,292	$3,439,047
Autism Consortium	22	$100,683	$2,215,017
Department of Defense	8	$147,223	$1,177,781
Center for Autism and Related Disorders	26	$31,369	$815,581
Organization for Autism Research	16	$45,625	$730,000
Autism Research Institute	13	$40,085	$521,099
Southwest Autism Research & Resource Center	5	$79,000	$395,000
Centers for Medicare and Medicaid Services	1	$24,643	$24,643
Grand Total	**745**	**$300,291**	**$222,215,342**

Notes: This table lists the total funding provided by the agencies and organizations included in the IACC/OARC 2008 portfolio analysis, as well as number of projects funded, and the average funding per project. Together the agencies and organizations funded over $222 million in research in 2008. The NIH project number shown reflects unique NIH projects. NIH projects cofunded by more than one NIH institute were combined and counted only as a single project. This approach differs from that used by the NIH RePORTER system, where each cofund is counted as a separate project.

Please note that research projects included are those identified by the agencies and organizations as funded in the most recent 12 months for which data were available. The NIH project number shown reflects unique NIH projects. Projects funded by more than one NIH institute ("cofunds") were combined and only counted as a single project. This approach differs from that used in the NIH RePORT Expenditures and Results (RePORTER) system, where each cofund is counted as a separate project.
Source: IACC Portfolio Analysis, 2008.

the ASD strategic plan are organized around seven general questions that are commonly asked by individuals and families when facing the challenges of ASD (see Table 79-2).

The plan includes not only research opportunities, but short- and long-term objectives with metrics for evaluating progress, and proposed budgetary requirements. The proposed budgetary requirements are professional judgment estimates for how much each project or program associated with a specific objective would potentially cost. The budgets are provided as advisory figures to guide agencies and organizations that may be involved in implementing various objectives from the plan. Importantly, the IACC does not have its own budget for research. It can accelerate, focus, and coordinate research efforts, but funding to accomplish the research must be provided by the government agencies and private organizations represented on the Committee, as well as by other members of the community who wish to support these efforts.

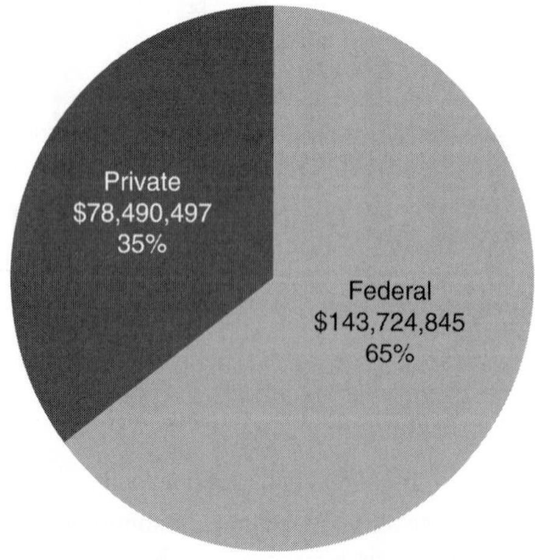

Figure 79–2. Contributions of Federal and Private ASD Research Funders to ASD Research in 2008. Of the $222 million spent on ASD research in 2008, 65% came from federal sources, while 35% of funding came from private organizations. Source: IACC Portfolio Analysis, 2008.

Although most scientists recognize that many important scientific discoveries have been made through serendipity resulting from investigator-initiated projects, targeted research initiatives are another approach used by government agencies to fund science—particularly in cases where there are clear research gaps that need to be filled to move the science forward. The IACC Strategic Plan for ASD Research lays out a series of targeted research objectives that correspond to consumer-focused questions and that reflect the urgency of ASD as a public health issue. The plan's logically organized research objectives chart a course toward needed breakthroughs in autism research, while also providing a framework for accountability. The completion of the initial 2009 plan just before the passage of the American Recovery and Reinvestment Act of 2009 was fortuitous, as some of the new funds appropriated to

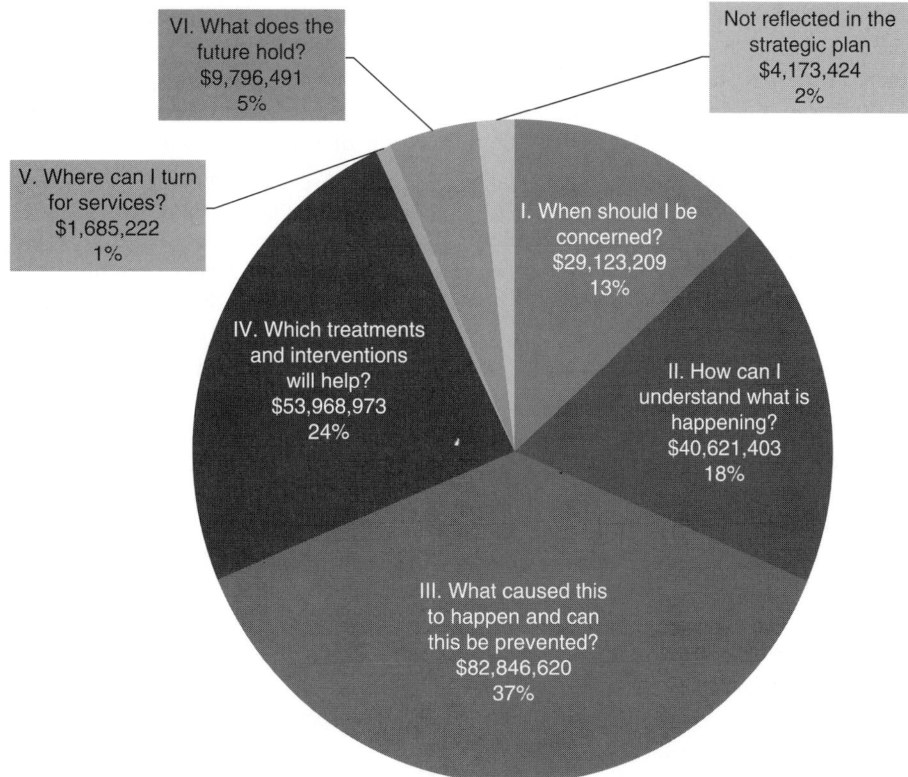

Figure 79–3. 2008 Autism Spectrum Disorder (ASD) Research Funding Categorized According to the 2009 IACC Strategic Plan for ASD Research. In 2008, the largest proportion of research funding (37%) from 13 U.S. funding agencies and organizations was devoted to risk factors for ASDs, reflected in the IACC strategic plan question, "What caused this to happen and can this be prevented?" Twenty-four percent of the research addressed interventions and treatments, 18% related to the underlying biology of ASDs and 13% related to diagnosis. Research on services and lifespan issues garnered the smallest proportion of funding. Source: IACC Portfolio Analysis, 2008.

Table 79–2.
The structure of the 2010 IACC strategic plan for ASD research

Question/Strategic Plan Chapter	Scientific Categories
1. When should I be concerned?	Diagnosis
2. How can I understand what is happening?	Biology of ASDs
3. What caused this to happen and can this be prevented?	Genetic and environmental risk factors
4. Which treatments and interventions will help?	Treatments and interventions
5. Where can I turn for services?	Comparative effectiveness and implementation research, access to services
6. What does the future hold, particularly for adults?	Services and supports that improve quality of life across the lifespan
7. What other infrastructure and surveillance needs must be met?	Infrastructure to support research, the research workforce and to conduct ASD surveillance

Notes: The 2010 IACC Strategic Plan for ASD Research is divided into seven chapters, each of which is named for a critical consumer-based question regarding autism research, indicated in the left-hand column. The plan's recommended research objectives correspond to these questions and fall into the scientific categories indicated in the right-hand column. Source: 2010 IACC Strategic Plan for Autism Spectrum Disorder Research.

NIH were able to be committed to implementing the plan in 2009 and 2010. Indeed, a series of autism-focused initiatives were successful in soliciting a large new pool of autism research projects, amounting to over $64 million in new research in 2009 to jumpstart implementation of the IACC Strategic Plan, with an additional infusion of over $20 million anticipated in 2010. New projects include studies to develop new screening tools, identify biomarkers, conduct deep sequencing and epigenomic studies to identify genetic and environmental risk factors, conduct clinical studies to test behavioral therapies, assess various service modalities such as telehealth, and characterize the impacts of autism in the second half of life. The new ARRA funds, as well as increases in non-ARRA spending on autism, resulted in more than a 50% increase in the NIH budget for autism in 2009 relative to 2007. While the ARRA funds are only a 2-year addition that will not continue in future years, it is expected that general/base (non-ARRA) NIH autism funding levels will keep pace with, and hopefully exceed, the trends of overall NIH funding levels over time. Future NIH funding for autism will, as always, be dependent on Congressional appropriations.

Intramural ASD Research

Roughly 90% of NIH research funds are awarded to institutions around the nation outside of NIH where scientists engage in what is called "extramural" research. The remaining 10% are invested in the "intramural" research program, where laboratory research is conducted by NIH scientists at the agency's main campus in Bethesda, Maryland. The NIH intramural program exists for high-risk research, for a rapid response to emerging public health problems (i.e., SARS, AIDS), and for the development of unique tools and resources to serve scientific investigators across the nation.

In the summer of 2006, the National Institute of Mental Health (NIMH) launched an intramural effort specifically focused on ASD. Early goals of this program included identifying subtypes of ASDs with a focus on regression (using cerebrospinal fluid [CSF] proteomics, magnetic resonance imaging [MRI], sleep electroencephalography [EEG], and testing of novel interventions [e.g., minocycline, riluzole, donepezil]). By January 2010, over 500 children had been screened and over 100 had been enrolled in one of the protocols. Studies in the intramural program can recruit patients from across the nation and provide extensive clinical and research testing without charge. Current protocols include a study of children who reportedly have recovered from ASD.

Services for ASD

Complex service systems present a challenge to people with ASD and their families. The emerging field of health-services research, sometimes called implementation science, is helping to meet this challenge. *Health-services research* plays a critical role in evaluating the effectiveness of interventions in community settings, identifying best practices for broad dissemination of research findings into clinical practice, and informing policy on ASD services and supports. Research in areas such as comparative effectiveness studies of evidence-based practices can inform health-care quality, health-care reimbursement, and educational policies. Participation by families and people affected by ASD is critical to the success of this research if it is to optimize the quality and accessibility of needed services for the autism community.

The 2009 IACC Strategic Plan for ASD Research identified the need for research related to autism services, and the 2010 edition of the plan added several new objectives to better address services needs across the full lifespan and including people of varying levels and types of disability. Because states differ in the services offered, the IACC called for an initial "state of the states" report, currently underway at the Centers for Medicare and Medicaid Services, to describe the variation in policies and resources across the states. This variation also provides an opportunity for naturalistic experiments to determine which policies and which resources are providing the most value in communities. NIH currently supports a portfolio of research on services for people with ASD, which was expanded using a portion of the funds received through ARRA, but there is a need to continue to increase this effort to ensure that the best science on autism informs the services offered to diverse populations.

The National Database for Autism Research

In addition to the IACC research strategic plan, the National Database for Autism Research (NDAR) will be a critical tool in fostering communication throughout the global ASD research community (National Database for Autism Research, 2010). NDAR is a secure biomedical informatics platform created by the NIH for scientific collaboration and data sharing for investigators who collect genotypic, phenotypic, imaging, pedigree, and other relevant ASD research data. Beyond providing investigators with significant technical capabilities for their data, NDAR has developed strategies to assure protection of research subjects, ensure data quality, and harmonize compatibility across other publicly and privately funded ASD research data sources.

NDAR uses a secure system of computer-generated codes called *Global Unique Identifiers* (GUIDs) to allow the association of a single research participant's genetic, imaging, clinical assessment, and other information even if the data were collected at different locations or through different studies. The use of GUIDs keeps direct personal identifiers from ever being transmitted or stored in the NIH NDAR records and thus minimizes risks to study participants. As many subjects have been enrolled in multiple studies (often from different funding sources), the GUID ensures that each individual can be tracked across multiple research projects. NDAR is scheduled to begin to provide data available for broad research access in 2010. NDAR agreements with 54 NIH-supported studies should ultimately yield data from 45,000 human subjects, and by federating with other federal and private databases, NDAR anticipates acquiring data from another 25,000 people with ASD. This wealth of data will serve to stimulate ASD research and research collaborations not only in the United States, but also around the world.

Research Gaps and Opportunities

What is missing in the current federal approach to ASD? As noted above, ASD research is supported by many groups, both federal and private. The increase in private funding for ASD research and the success of advocacy groups in educating families about ASD research and services attests to the importance of a combined public–private effort to: *(a)* provide synergy for areas of need, *(b)* reduce redundancy in funding, and *(c)* to identify gaps that may be served better by either private or public funding. For instance, the need for biobanks for ASD research can be fulfilled by a combined outreach effort from advocacy groups using federal funds to supply the needed infrastructure for storing and distributing tissue. In the future, the coordination that has developed via the IACC for federal partnerships needs to be extended to ensure close working relationships with private funding organizations.

In contrast to many other childhood-onset disorders, such as Type 1 diabetes or asthma, there is relatively little investment in autism research within either the biotechnology or the pharmaceutical sectors. This may reflect the state of the science—there are no molecular targets yet for drug development—or it may reflect a historical bias toward behavioral and rehabilitative approaches to ASDs. Increasing private interest in Fragile X syndrome and Rett syndrome suggests that the emergence of molecular targets for autism will instigate growing interest in ASD from biotechnology and pharmaceutical companies in the near future. This is particularly important given the absence of medications for the core symptoms of ASD. Although NIH research traditionally identifies potential new targets for medications, the private sector has usually taken the lead in product development efforts.

Finally, much of the surge in NIH funding of ASD research was made possible with ARRA money which arrived just after the release of the IACC strategic plan. ARRA funds are, however, limited to 2009 and 2010. Although there has been an increase in NIH funding of ASD research using non-ARRA funds, this increase will not substitute for the loss of ARRA in 2011. This means that a decrease in total funding for ASD research is expected at NIH just as new scientific opportunities and needs arise from updates of the strategic plan. Following the ARRA surge in funding, the IACC may need to set priorities for its objectives in order to advise funding agencies about the optimal use of funds.

Conclusions

Most discussions of the federal role in ASD research focus on funding. Although money is necessary for scientific breakthroughs, it is never sufficient. Some of the most important medical advances of the past century, such as the polio vaccine, have used little federal money (Oshinsky, 2005) and others were serendipitous or resulted from small clinical studies, such as the discovery of the bacterial cause of peptic ulcers (Marshall & Warren, 1983, 1984). Base funding for ASD research at NIH has more than tripled in the past decade. If the the additional funds provided by ARRA are also taken into account, the overall increase in NIH funding for ASD was nearly fivefold between 1999 and 2009.

Enhanced funding has the potential to increase the number of scientists working on ASD and attract scientists from other fields into ASD research, but it cannot ensure breakthroughs. We have learned from other areas of biomedical science that basic science, often seemingly unrelated to a clinical problem, can reveal the critical opportunity. Translational science that builds on basic insights and uses new tools, such as induced pluripotent stem cells (Takahashi et al., 2007; Yu et al., 2007) can be the bridge between the laboratory and the clinic. And paradoxically, clinical research, which seems the most urgent and most likely to yield immediate benefit, may be the most frustrating in the search for breakthroughs. Nevertheless, clinical research will be the only way to discover biomarkers, to demonstrate the efficacy of a new treatment, or to understand which intervention will be best for any specific individual with an ASD. The federal ASD research enterprise, in partnership with private funders and with guidance from the IACC, aims to support a diverse portfolio of science, from basic to clinical, with a coordinated, strategic approach that ensures that the available funds are used for optimal public good.

Challenges and Future Directions

- Supporting a diverse portfolio of basic to clinical research to enable advances in: diagnosis, understanding the underlying biology of ASD, identifying risk factors and biomarkers, developing effective treatments and interventions, services research, and research on lifespan issues.
- Building new partnerships between federal agencies and private organizations to enable both research and the development of needed research infrastructure (i.e., database networks and biobanks).
- Identifying molecular targets for potential drug therapies, which would bring biotechnology and pharmaceutical companies in as partners.
- Judiciously using federal funds and partnering with private organizations to build on the discoveries made through ARRA-funded grants, whose funding was a special 2-year opportunity enabled by the American Recovery and Reinvestment Act of 2009.

SUGGESTED READING

IACC (2010). The IACC Website: www.iacc.hhs.gov.

IACC (2010). *2010 IACC Strategic Plan for Autism Spectrum Disorder Research*. Retrieved from http://iacc.hhs.gov/strategic-plan/.

REFERENCES

Interagency Autism Coordinating Committee (2003). *Autism summit conference summary.* Retrieved from the Department of Health and Human Services Interagency Autism Coordinating Committee website at http://iacc.hhs.gov/reports/2003/autism-summit-conference-nov.shtml.

Interagency Autism Coordinating Committee (2009). *2008 IACC autism spectrum disorder research portfolio analysis report.* Retrieved from the Department of Health and Human Services Interagency Autism Coordinating Committee website at http://iacc.hhs.gov/portfolio-analysis/2008/index.shtml.

Interagency Autism Coordinating Committee (2009). *2009 IACC Strategic plan for autism spectrum disorder research.* Retrieved from the Department of Health and Human Services Interagency Autism Coordinating Committee website at http://iacc.hhs.gov/reports/2009/iacc-strategic-plan-for-autism-spectrum-disorder-research-jan26.shtml.

Interagency Autism Coordinating Committee (2010). *2010 IACC strategic plan for autism spectrum disorder research.* Retrieved from the Department of Health and Human Services Interagency Autism Coordinating Committee website at http://iacc.hhs.gov/strategic-plan/2010/.

Interagency Autism Coordinating Committee (2006). *Evaluating progress on the IACC autism research matrix.* Retrieved from the Department of Health and Human Services Interagency Autism Coordinating Committee website at http://iacc.hhs.gov/reports/2006/evaluating-progress-autism-matrix-nov17.shtml.

Interagency Autism Coordinating Committee (September 30-October 1, 2009). *IACC scientific workshop agenda, materials, transcript and videocast on IACC meeting and events webpage.* Retrieved from the Department of Health and Human Services Interagency Autism Coordinating Committee website at http://iacc.hhs.gov/events/.

Interagency Autism Coordinating Committee (July 24, 2009). *IACC services town hall meeting agenda, analysis, transcript and videocast on IACC meeting and events webpage.* Retrieved from the Department of Health and Human Services Interagency Autism Coordinating Committee website at http://iacc.hhs.gov/events/.

Interagency Autism Coordinating Committee (2008, May 3). *IACC town hall meeting agenda and summary on IACC meeting and events webpage.* Retrieved from the Department of Health and Human Services Interagency Autism Coordinating Committee website at http://iacc.hhs.gov/events/.

Interagency Autism Coordinating Committee (2009). *Meetings and events website.* Retrieved from the Department of Health and Human Services Interagency Autism Coordinating Committee website at http://iacc.hhs.gov/events/.

Interagency Autism Coordinating Committee (2009). *News release: Advisory panel releases first federal strategic plan for autism research.* Retrieved from http://iacc.hhs.gov/strategic-plan/advisory-panel-releases-first-federal-strategic-plan-for-autism-research.shtml.

Interagency Autism Coordinating Committee (2010). *News update: New 2010 IACC strategic plan emphasizes research infrastructure, non-verbal people with ASD and the full spectrum from young children to adults.* Retrieved from http://iacc.hhs.gov/strategic-plan/advisory-panel-releases-first-federal-strategic-plan-for-autism-research.shtml.

Interagency Autism Coordinating Committee (2007). *Request for information soliciting public input on ASD research priorities.* Retrieved from the Department of Health and Human Services Interagency Autism Coordinating Committee website at http://iacc.hhs.gov/public-comment/archive.shtml and http://iacc.hhs.gov/strategic-plan/2007/rfi-on-asd-research-priorities-dec19.shtml.

Interagency Autism Coordinating Committee (2008). *Request for information soliciting public input on the IACC strategic plan for ASD research.* Retrieved from the Department of Health and Human Services Interagency Autism Coordinating Committee website at http://iacc.hhs.gov/public-comment/archive.shtml and http://grants.nih.gov/grants/guide/notice-files/NOT-MH-08-021.html.

Interagency Autism Coordinating Committee (2009). *Request for information soliciting public input on the IACC strategic plan for ASD research.* Retrieved from the Department of Health and Human Services Interagency Autism Coordinating Committee website at http://iacc.hhs.gov/public-comment/2009/.

Marshall, B. J., & Warren, J. R. (1983). Unidentified curved bacillus on gastric epithelium in active chronic gastritis. *Lancet, 1*(8336), 1273–1275. PMID 6134060.

Marshall, B. J., & Warren, J. R. (1984). Unidentified curved bacilli in the stomach patients with gastritis and peptic ulceration. *Lancet, 1*(8390), 1311–1315. PMID 6145023.

National Database for Autism Research (NDAR) Website. (2010). National Institutes of Health. Retrieved from http://ndar.nih.gov/ndarpublicweb/.

National Institutes of Health Report (2010). Retrieved from http://report.nih.gov/.

Oshinsky, D. M. (2005). *Polio: An American story.* New York: Oxford University Press.

Public Law 106-310, The Children's Health Act of 2000. (October 17, 2000). Retrieved from Government Printing Office at http://frwebgate.access.gpo.gov/cgi-bin/getdoc.cgi?dbname=106_cong_public_laws&docid=f:publ310.106.pdf.

Public Law 109-416, the Combating Autism Act of 2006. (December 19, 2006). Retrieved from Government Printing Office at http://frwebgate.access.gpo.gov/cgi-bin/getdoc.cgi?dbname=109_cong_public_laws&docid=f:publ416.109.pdf.

Research, Condition, and Disease Categories (RCDC). (2009). *Autism.* Retrieved from the National Institutes of Health Research Portfolio Online Reporting Tool website at http://report.nih.gov/rcdc/categories/.

Takahashi, K., Tanabe, K., Ohnuki, M., Narita, M., Ichisaka, T., Tomoda, K., et al. (2007). Induction of pluripotent stem cells from adult human fibroblasts by defined factors. *Cell, 131* (5), 861–872. doi:10.1016/j.cell.2007.11.019. PMID 18035408.

Yu, J., Vodyanik, M. A., Smuga-Otto, K., Antosiewicz-Bourget, J., Frane, J. L., Tian, S., et al. (2007). Induced pluripotent stem cell lines derived from human somatic cells. *Science, 318* (5858), 1917–1920. doi:10.1126/science.1151526. PMID 18029452.

80 Craig Snyder, Peter Bell

To Petition the Government for a Redress of Grievances

Two anecdotes, separated in time by a little more than a decade, illustrate just how far the autism community has come in advocating for the attention and assistance of the federal government.

October 1997—Just 2 years after it was founded, and with a total budget hovering around a million dollars, the autism advocacy organization, Cure Autism Now (CAN) had just hired a Washington lobbyist to try to get the government of the United States to do something, do anything, about the clearly growing number of children being diagnosed with autism.

CAN's cofounders—Jonathan Shestack and Portia Iversen—were seasoned Hollywood figures, whose world came crashing down in 1994 when their 2-year-old son, Dov, was diagnosed with autism. They had been shocked to find that very little was known about the causes of autism. To make things worse, the only effective treatment available, Applied Behavior Analysis (ABA), wasn't even covered by health insurance.

No group in America, not even 13-year-old girls swooning over the latest boy band, was more gaga over mixing with celebrities than the powerful lawmakers of Washington. Elected officials have a sort of fame themselves, but no glamour. And these people who actually run the world are drawn, as if by gravity, to the orbit of the stars residing on the Left Coast (a.k.a. Hollywood).

So a young lobbyist—1 month into private practice following a stint as chief of staff for a prominent U.S. senator—managed to get an audience with the new chairman of the Senate Health, Education, Labor and Pensions (HELP) Committee, Senator Bill Frist (R–TN). One year prior, Senator Frist had become the first medical doctor elected to the Senate in a century. The meeting took place in an uncommon venue. Not in the chairman's Capitol office, but rather he was invited to a VIP tour of the set of the NBC television series *ER*. He was a fan of the popular show, and the opportunity to hold our meeting in the fictitious doctor's lounge on the *ER* set, hosted by "Dr. Green" (played by actor Anthony Edwards), was irresistible.

Senator Frist didn't know much about autism. Being a doctor in an unrelated field (heart surgery in his case), in those days, barely gave one a leg up in background on the subject over any layman. The essential reference point on autism at that time was still Dustin Hoffman's character in the 1988 movie *Rain Man*.

But Senator Frist was a good listener and quick study. It was clear—much to the surprise of a liberal Democrat like Shestack (who expected nothing could really get done for autism while Republicans controlled Congress)—that this man, who went to Africa during Congressional recesses to operate by flashlight on the sickest of kids in the remotest of villages, wanted to walk the talk of his professed Christian Conservatism in his new role as America's most powerful legislator on health policy.

"Okay," he said, "I got it. There's a new epidemic of autism. No one knows why. The NIH is spending very little on research. The CDC isn't even trying to figure out accurate prevalence numbers. The federal government has a role, a responsibility."

"But what do you want specifically?" he asked.

"A law about autism," we told him. "A piece of legislation detailing and authorizing funds for a federal effort to combat autism."

"Impossible," he replied. "Congress doesn't, won't, just can't pass 'single-disease' bills. My Lord, if Congress started doing this, it would be all we ever did. And we shouldn't do it. Politicians shouldn't start telling scientists what to do based on which group of sufferers screams the loudest, hires the best lobbyists and—irony noted—gets the best celebrity meat to promote their cause."

"Still, this autism thing sounds bad," he added. "Work with my staff. We'll figure something out."

October 2008—It's the Thursday before the Tuesday of Election Day, the final weekend before America will choose its 44th president.

Barack Obama probably has the race won but his campaign is taking no chances. His disciplined, methodical staff will leave no votes on the table that may still be persuadable.

Polls show six states still too close to call. Theoretically, their electoral votes constitute enough uncertainty to determine the outcome by some models. One of these states is Nevada, where a prominent autism advocate is pressing the Obama team for more detail on the candidate's platform about autism than had hitherto been published. So Obama's staff releases to this parent activist a previously undisclosed draft bill.

In his capacity as a sitting senator, Obama (D–IL) has written a bill to expand and intensify the federal fight against autism. Most notably, the proposed legislation includes a provision to mandate that all health insurance policies in the nation must provide coverage for autism services, including the current, expensive, gold standard of care, Applied Behavior Analysis.

The internet lights up with the news. Short of a cure, the greatest single relief possible for the families grappling with autism is an insurance mandate. Providing coverage for evidence-based, medically necessary therapies would end the nearly universal discrimination against people with autism and help those suffering from the disorder to lead lives of the highest possible quality.

Within hours, supporters of Senator John McCain (R–AZ) within the autism community have the Obama bill in front of GOP vice presidential candidate, Alaska Governor Sarah Palin (R–AK), whose sister has a child with autism, and the McCain campaign is pondering a response.

At the highest levels of American politics, within the inner circles of both major party candidates for president of the United States, among the final tactical decisions being discussed during this historic race, are about autism—not about cancer, AIDS, Alzheimer's, not even solely about Iraq or the economy—but about autism.

The next day, which happens to be Halloween, the Obama campaign offers a final pre-election treat to America's kids with autism, and all of those who love them—the Obama platform statement on autism, published on www.ObamaForAmerica.com, is amended to promise that, as president, Obama will "mandate insurance coverage of autism treatment...."

So we've come quite a distance in just a decade, along the path of securing a public policy commitment to fight autism—from a bizarre meeting with a senator, caring, but largely naive about autism, to substantial attention from the new President of the United States.

How did it happen?

The most powerful source of the progress is nothing to celebrate. It is the autism epidemic itself. It is the fact that parents find themselves in every corner and at every level of American society—from West Nowhere to the West Wing of the White House—raising kids with autism, in such numbers and with such social and economic impact, that the problem can simply no longer be ignored.

Prevalence produces awareness. But that alone is no guarantee of the kind of consciousness that ignites action. And on this score there is much for the autism community to be proud.

The United States Constitution guarantees to every American the right to petition the government for the redress of grievances, and many do so with passion and conviction. On most days, the Capitol complex in Washington, D.C. seems under siege with people wearing this or that hat, ribbon, or sash, lobbying for this or that cause. It's inspiring and infuriating at the same time.

But for more than a decade now, ever since that meeting on a Hollywood sound stage with Senator Frist, no group of ordinary Americans has more consistently and capably petitioned their government than the families affected by autism—whether their "kid" is 2 or 42 years old.

Of course, parents of this recent generation (children born in the 1990s and after)—with all of their fervor and refusal to accept defeat—have stood on the shoulders of the even more isolated and ignored generations of parents who raised their children with autism when it was considered rare and the result of bad parenting. These earlier advocates helped establish special education in our schools and saved many children from our society's shameful waste pail.

And, against that truly heroic backdrop, the present generation of parents—more numerous and more connected (by technology)—have worked, rallied, and sang. They have written, faxed, and emailed. They have testified with poignancy, argued with rigor, and dug deep to contribute to friends. They have been marvelous and utterly unflappable.

And with no disrespect to many other worthy and effective lobbying groups, heaven help the politician who gets in the way of a mom trying to help her child with autism.

In one instance, symbolizing countless others, Elizabeth Emken, a CAN volunteer from Northern California and mother to then 6-year-old Alex with autism (later vice president for government relations at Autism Speaks (AS) and a self-taught lobbyist, in the way Abe Lincoln was a self-taught country lawyer), went to meet with Senator Arlen Specter (R–PA). Specter then chaired the Appropriations Subcommittee, which funds all federal health agencies and, as such, is constantly lobbied by representatives of every disease that afflicts the human race.

Senator Specter has been a tireless and singularly effective champion for expanded funding for biomedical research, being largely responsible, along with Senator Tom Harkin (D–IA), for more than doubling the budget of the NIH from $12 billion to $30 billion per year.

He is, however, equally legendary on the Hill for his brilliance and for his temper, and Ms. Emken first met him on a bad day.

It turned out the inopportune moment for this meeting was just following an interview of the senator by ABC News in which he was ambushed and harshly criticized for supposedly dividing up medical research dollars based on which diseases had the biggest celebrity spokespeople. When Ms. Emken tried to present her case, with actor/autism advocate Anthony Edwards at her side, the senator cut her off in mid-sentence and, red-faced, excoriated her for being before him with a request on autism funding levels.

Mama lion had no thought of herself, only of her cub. She got very close to the senator's face and said with as much grace as tenacity, "Are you telling me that the mother of a sick child has no right to ask for help from the people elected to serve our nation, no right to come here and educate you about the needs of these suffering families and, about the proper role of your office in overseeing what the bureaucrats are doing with my dollars?"

The senator, who was in truth already on Elizabeth's side, has been even more so ever since. Through the work of so many parents, in so many meetings, is how autism became a national public health priority, at least in Congress.

And the emergence of autism as such marks a good moment both to look back on accomplishments in autism advocacy to date and also to look forward to the continuing agenda.

Why Lobby?

Why has it been necessary for parents to march and mobilize and for lobbyists to be engaged and deployed on autism? Surely the federal government agencies charged with the public health of the nation—principally the CDC and the NIH—should have detected the coming tsunami, understood its social and economic costs, and set about to do their jobs. Well, maybe not.

At a minimum, it is the CDC's job to know about trends in morbidity, to count Americans who suffer from various maladies and track patterns as they take shape. A host of federal programs—from Medicaid to various programs relating to housing and vocational training—are responsible for assisting disabled Americans to live their lives with the highest quality possible, given their limitations. And, of course, it is the job of the NIH to find the causes and ultimately the treatments and cures for disease, so the other agencies will have fewer to count and rescue.

Before the late 1990s, when the autism community began to aggressively lobby for more research in Washington, virtually none of this was happening. The CDC had no plan to undertake epidemiological work on autism prevalence or patterns, the human service agencies had no focused efforts on autism and the NIH was spending, at best, about $5 million to $10 million per year on autism research. Although using very meager funds, scientists had made significant progress in developing reliable diagnostic instruments, defining the symptoms and characteristics of the disorders, documenting its association with certain biological features and a genetic etiology, and developing what remains to this day the most effective intervention for autism (Applied Behavioral Analysis), their efforts before the 1990s were greatly hampered by a lack of adequate funding and awareness of autism as a major public health problem. Because of the lobbying efforts that began in the mid-1990s that led to enhanced funding, as well as the advent of a wide range of new technologies that allowed scientists for the first time to study brain function and explore the genome in detail, a new era of autism research has emerged that rests on the foundation built by earlier science. This research holds the promise to discover the causes, more effective treatments, and hopefully, a cure for autism.

Before the late 1990s, there simply was no federal recognition of the urgency of the growing autism epidemic and no plan to respond with appropriate resources. Almost everything that has been done recently to combat autism results from parents lobbying Congress and Congress therefore compelling the executive agencies to do what needs to be done—with those agencies, inexplicably continuing to this very day, fighting a rear-guard action against the mandate of Congress to take autism more seriously.

In this story lies a perfect case study of the failure of bureaucratic institutions to remain true to their missions. The federal public health apparatus has failed the autism community and the nation at large with every effort they have made to avoid or minimize work on autism, displaying a greater concern for maintaining their fiefdoms as independent centers of power than for doing the very things they are in business to do.

On autism, we should all be thankful for the American right to lobby. The ability of the autism community to persuade Congress to pass pieces of legislation dealing with autism, and to appropriate funds to carry out autism activities has been the locomotive of autism progress.

Foundational Accomplishments

Thus far, autism advocates have convinced the federal government to pass two landmark bills that have benefited their loved ones with autism—the Children's Health Act of 2000 and the Combating Autism Act of 2006. The community has also won the attention and action of the Pentagon by obtaining critical funds for autism research through the Congressionally Directed Medical Research Programs (CDMRP).

These acts of legislation and appropriations constitute a federal declaration of war on autism, the disorder and not those living with autism. They embody national recognition of the urgency of the autism epidemic and they begin the process of deploying a scale of resources appropriate to the problem.

The Children's Health Act of 2000

Senator Frist's brilliant (in the "through-the-looking-glass" world of Washington) solution to the problem of how to legislate on autism, when Congress can't and shouldn't legislate about a "single disease" (his view and the "rule" until then), was to put together a bill about many single diseases.

The Children's Health Act of 2000 (CHA) had more than 20 titles, each in essence a wholly distinct piece of legislation about a separate disease. In addition to autism, which was given the honor of being Title I, the law cobbled together previously separate proposals on things ranging from infant hearing screening to asthma to head injuries.

The autism advocates, frankly, didn't care. Frankenstein might not be handsome, but he did come to life. Likewise, what they wanted—a law to kick-start federal efforts on biomedical research and epidemiology on autism—would get signed into law by the president.

The main features of the CHA title on autism included:

- Direction to the NIH to expand, intensify, and coordinate the activities of the NIH with respect to research on autism.
- Establishment of Autism Centers of Excellence to conduct basic and clinical research into autism and required communication and cooperation among centers.
- Requirement of NIH to provide for a program under which samples of tissues and genetic materials that are of use in research on autism are donated, collected, preserved, and made available for such research.
- Mandating a means through which the public can obtain information on the existing and planned programs and activities of NIH with respect to autism.
- Direction to the CDC to establish three regional centers of excellence in autism and pervasive developmental disabilities epidemiology for the purpose of collecting and analyzing information on the number, incidence, correlates, and causes of autism.
- Creation of a clearinghouse within the CDC for the collection and storage of data generated from the monitoring programs established by the act.
- Establishment of an Autism Coordinating Committee to coordinate all efforts within the Department of Health and Human Services concerning autism.

The path to the enactment of the CHA was the proverbial "long and winding road." There are no straight lines between a policy objective and a public law, but the course of the CHA was extraordinarily complicated because it involved so many distinct interests.

At first, the effort faced the usual obstacles that cause so many bills to languish. Most importantly, there is the conventional wisdom (and the cold reality on which that wisdom is based) that the vast majority of legislation introduced in each Congress simply dies. Added to that was the sense that the CHA was especially ambitious.

If there was any one area in which the Clinton White House and the Republican Congress had never seen eye-to-eye—and therefore in which little policy making actually got done—it was health care.

Therefore, the early phase of autism community lobbying for the CHA had to follow the motto of "slow and steady." Relationships had to be built and cosponsors were added one office visit at a time.

Although Senator Frist had come up with the concept of the CHA—putting together a number of previously free-standing legislative proposals loosely related to one another around the concept of children's health—autism advocates thought it best for there to be a separate, free-standing autism bill for which they could seek cosponsors, in order to show a significant and always growing number of supporters in both the House and Senate.

The free-standing bill—which then became Title I of the CHA—was called the "Advancement in Pediatric Autism Research Act." It was first introduced in the Senate, by Senator Slade Gorton (R–WA), and next in the House, by Congressman Jim Greenwood (R–PA).

Interesting events accompanied both introductions.

What happened on the Senate side—the run-up to Senator Gorton's introduction of the country's first piece of legislation about autism—was both dramatic in real life and later dramatized (overly dramatized, actually) in an episode of the NBC television series *The West Wing*.

The choice to ask Senator Gorton to take the lead on autism issues in the Senate was made for sound but prosaic reasons. He was known as smart and hard-working and as a tough conservative. Sponsorship by someone on the right, we thought, would send a strong message that concern for autism was not simply another bleeding-heart federal-spending exuberance.

He was a member of the committee of jurisdiction, the HELP Committee. He was friends with the majority leader, Senator Trent Lott (R–MS) (and the leader would ultimately decide, as anyone in that position does for any bill, whether it would ever be brought to a vote on the floor of the Senate). Additionally, some members of CAN's lobbying team had experienced past friendly dealings with Senator Gorton's chief of staff, Tony Williams. This increased the probability of getting a fair hearing in trying to persuade the senator to become their champion.

The initial meeting with Mr. Williams produced the unexpected turn-of-events, which ultimately would lead to a portrayal on national television.

Mr. Williams listened, with less than his usual patience, to the presentation of the policy concepts behind the proposed autism legislation. He then asked the legislative assistant who handled health matters for Senator Gorton to leave the room. After the door closed, he asked "How did you find out?"

It seems that a grandchild of the senator's had recently been diagnosed with autism—a fact that had not yet been publicly reported and which the senator and his family were not at that moment ready to reveal.

The honest truth—still doubted by many more than a decade later—is that the advocates had no idea.

Call it luck, karma, or just coincidence, but the autism advocates had stumbled into asking a powerful member of the Senate to sponsor the first ever piece of legislation about autism just as he was coming to grips with life as the Senate's only grandfather of a child with autism.

They never learned all of the personal details—and never asked—but it was soon clear that the senator's wife and daughter would accept nothing less than that he enthusiastically support the proposed legislation. And he did just that.

On the House side, the drama to give birth to the first autism bill was much more commonplace, and yet more potentially harmful to the project.

Congressman Jim Greenwood was a highly regarded "moderate" Republican, a member of the Health Subcommittee of the House Commerce Committee, and someone with a long record of work on children's health issues. Prior to serving in Congress, he was a social worker who had close contact with children and adults on the autism spectrum. He was a natural target for the autism advocates as the leading House player on the bill.

However, Congressman Chris Smith (R–NJ) wanted in on the action. Representative Smith's district includes Brick Township in New Jersey, where in the late 1990s, alarms had gone off, heard around the nation, about an unusually high rate of autism–a so-called "cluster." Naturally, wanting to serve his constituents, Congressman Smith saw himself as leading any House efforts on autism. Indeed, he eventually created—along with Congressman Mike Doyle (D–PA)—a Congressional Autism Caucus known as Coalition for Autism Research and Education (C.A.R.E.), which members of Congress could join as an expression of their concern about autism as a public health issue.

Going to Greenwood was never meant to disrespect Smith. Nonetheless, a turf struggle emerged.

As in many such instances, the path of political compromise often does coincide with doing the right thing.

The initial version of Representative Greenwood's bill had only included provisions relating to biomedical research at the NIH. Representative Smith's separate bill, however, required action by the CDC—meaningful epidemiology on autism.

In committee, it was agreed to combine the two bills and to speak of the new product, as was correct, as having been jointly authored by Congressmen Greenwood and Smith.

This combined Greenwood/Smith bill became the one introduced by Senator Gorton in the Senate. And that, in turn, became Title I of the Children's Health Act, once Senator Frist had agreed to go forward in that fashion.

There is a curious thing in the life cycle of a legislative initiative in Washington. Often, the chances for enactment of a bill go from being impossible to inevitable with nothing apparent in between.

And so it was with the CHA.

Many of the disparate interests whose causes stood to benefit from passage of the bill formed a coalition to get it done. There was strength in numbers. As a result of this multi-pronged lobbying effort, many members of Congress became cosponsors—perhaps not agreeing with or even being fully aware of all of the provisions of the bill—but committed to the enactment of some particular piece within it.

Even though the CHA was now "real," with a perceived high chance of passage, another curious legislative phenomenon kicked in—people throwing unrelated baggage onto the moving train, some of which contained bombs that could have derailed the whole vehicle.

In the end game of the passage of the CHA, the fall of 2000 was of course an election year, and the CHA became, at times, a hostage, and a potential murder victim, of both the Right and the Left.

The strongly pro-life Chairman of the House Commerce Committee, Representative Tom Bliley (R–VA), insisted that the bill include a provision promoting adoption (but also involving very controversial requirements for counseling women seeking abortions regarding adoption). The liberal lion (and Dean of the House of Representatives) Representative John Dingell (D–MI) insisted that that bill include his favorite provisions aimed at stopping Americans from smoking and various forms of gun control.

With fights over abortion and guns—there were certainly moments when it seemed all too much weight for our program to improve and expand research on autism to bear.

But the momentum of the moving train proved quite strong. In the end, everyone compromised—Bliley and the pro-choice groups reached an accommodation on language (through spectacular negotiating by Jim Greenwood) and Congressman Dingell relented under a crushing pressure of public support for passing the CHA.

President Clinton signed the CHA into law during the transition after the election of President Bush. It was widely heralded as the only significant health-care legislation which the combination of the Clinton administration and the Republican Congress had been able to achieve.

In his signing message, President Clinton gave credit for the bill to his wife—who was then just about to become a candidate for Senate from New York.

In truth, Mrs. Clinton, as first lady, had limited involvement in the process. But the autism community welcomed her desire to become a champion of the cause—something she went on to embrace with enthusiasm and skill as a senator and a candidate for president in more recent years.

The Combating Autism Act of 2006

The CHA was a breakthrough, to be sure. Without question, additional funds were spent on autism research—both biomedical and epidemiological—than would have been absent the law and the continued advocacy throughout its 5-year term to appropriate the authorized amounts. The work of the Autism Centers of Excellence (ACE Centers), created by the act, helped build the cadre of scientists willing to work on autism and, in turn, basic medical knowledge about the disorder which those scientists generated. CHA funds also got the CDC into the autism surveillance business in a measurable way and led to the first standard data point for autism—that one in 150 children in America have an autism diagnosis.

By the end of the 5-year authorization of the CHA, autism awareness, both popular and political, had grown enough that the advocates were confident about seeking to reauthorize and expand the federal autism legislative commitment through the vehicle of a true "single-disease" bill.

By this time, a new powerhouse of an organization, Autism Speaks, had been created and brought great resources to the table, both material and perceptual, than the prior organizations. CAN and Autism Speaks entered into a formal partnership, which would become a prelude to their ultimate merger, and the whole proved greater than the apparent sum of the parts.

At the beginning of the effort, it was still very much an uphill battle. The arguments we had heard from Senator Frist, back in 1997, about why Congress couldn't and shouldn't pass such bills were still the position of all the Congressional leaders and committee chairmen who would be relevant for this process. Still, life is easier when you have no choice, and we faced the apparent "catch 22" that although single-disease bills were still a taboo, we were also told there was no appetite for another multidisease Frankenstein like the CHA.

The lobbying effort took two years and, just like its predecessor, had many twists and turns. The bill died far more times than it passed.

Perhaps the two most notable obstacles that had to be overcome were Senator Tom Coburn (R–OK) and Congressman Joe Barton (R–TX).

Bills like this—which are wrongly perceived as special-interest favors—are almost never brought to the Senate floor for a full-fledged process of debate, potential amendment, and a vote on final passage. They are passed by *Unanimous Consent* (UC). That means that any single senator can kill a piece of legislation by withholding his or her consent.

In the fall of 2006, with a Congressional election upon us and Republicans justifiably nervous about substantial losses, owing to the rapidly declining popularity of President Bush and the war in Iraq, the business of the Senate had stalled, even more than usual.

The Combating Autism Act (CAA) had prime sponsorship by Senator Rick Santorum (R–PA), the third-highest ranking member of the Majority Republican Caucus, who was in deep trouble in his own re-election effort. Generally, someone in a position like that gets whatever he wants from other members of his party.

The CAA also had the support of HELP Committee Chairman, Senator Mike Enzi (R–WY), whose staff had labored diligently and brilliantly to produce a single-disease bill for which it was worth breaking "the rule." It also had the support of the majority leader—the position to which autism's old friend Senator Frist had risen.

On the Democratic side, Senate Minority Leader Harry Reid (D–NV), committee ranking member, Senator Edward Kennedy (D–MA), and original Democratic bill sponsor Senator Chris Dodd (D–CT) all wanted to get the bill passed—defying the conventional approach of wanting to deny the vulnerable Santorum anything good on which to campaign back in Pennsylvania.

With such a constellation of supporters, what could go wrong?

Tom Coburn.

Senator Coburn—a hard conservative and budget hawk, believed the rule against single-disease bills should remain unbroken. He also believed that the new spending authorized in the bill—slightly over $1 billion during the 5-year term— was too much money. He was impervious to all arguments about the growing prevalence and public costs of autism. He was just against any new government spending, on pretty much anything.

Senator Coburn was approached by Majority Leader Frist and cajoled by Committee Chairman Enzi, to no avail. Finally, just before the Senate would recess for the 2006 elections, Senator Coburn was begged by Senator Santorum, and he traded something—we still don't know precisely what. Senators Santorum, Enzi, and Frist agreed to reduce the authorized spending levels in the bill by $100 million, bringing the total under $1 billion and Coburn agreed to release his hold.

The details of the dollar cut were executed between staff, on the floor of the Senate and with autism advocates on the telephone. There was no rational basis for the cuts. It was pure sausage-making.

But the bill passed the Senate unanimously.

When transmitted to the other side of the Capitol, it was dead on arrival. The Chairman of the House Commerce Committee, Representative Joe Barton, shared the same beliefs about single-disease bills as did Senator Coburn, and he had the gavel of the committee, which would have to act on the bill before it could ever get to the floor of the House.

The autism community was frankly merciless and relentless in its efforts to persuade Mr. Barton.

Protestors staged acts of civil disobedience in his district offices and used the then-new technology of YouTube to show the world images of their being arrested for trying to visit with their congressman on the subject of their sick kids.

A group of Texas moms protested the arrival of the Speaker of the House, Congressman Denny Hastert (R–IL), at a fundraiser on behalf of Barton's re-election campaign.

The constant deluge of phone calls to the Barton offices overwhelmed the switchboards and reduced receptionists to tears.

And last, but certainly not least, radio and television personality Don Imus practically burned Barton in effigy on his national airwaves every day for more than a month.

In the end, there was an accommodation. Congressman Barton was able to maintain the principle, as he saw it, that Congress should not authorize appropriations for the NIH to conduct research on a specific disease. Instead, the bill as passed by the Senate was modified in the House to authorize appropriations for the purposes of the act—including biomedical research by the NIH—with the appropriations authorized to be spent under the control of the secretary of Health and Human Services, rather than the director of the NIH.

Another "perfect 10" Washington gymnastics routine. Just as Senator Frist had been willing to pass a bill about a bunch of different diseases because he was unwilling to pass a bill about any single disease, Barton was willing to pass a bill that gave the Department of Health and Human Services (of which the NIH is an organic and subordinate part) authorization to spend money on autism because that money was not specifically identified to be spent by the NIH.

More sausage, but another historic victory.

The CAA is arguably the most comprehensive single-disease bill ever adopted into law. Its main features include:

- Elevation of ownership of the federal response to autism from the NIH director to the HHS secretary.
- Authorization of nearly $1 billion over 5 years to combat autism through research, screening, early detection, and early intervention—at least a 50% increase.
- Expansion and intensification of biomedical research on autism, including an essential focus on possible environmental causes.
- Broadening of training opportunities to increase the number of sites able to diagnose—under such program, trainees receive a balance of academic, clinical, and community opportunities.
- Promotion of research into best practices and to determine evidence-based interventions.
- Requirement of the CDC to support collection, analysis, and reporting of state data and award grants for regional centers of excellence.
- Direction to the Interagency Autism Coordinating Committee (IACC) to provide information and recommendations on programs, and to develop and annually update a strategic plan for autism research, including proposed budgetary requirements.
- Requirement of the IACC to have increased and mandatory public representation—at least 1/3 of the committee—including an individual with an autism spectrum disorder (ASD), a parent of an individual with an ASD, and a representative of leading research, advocacy, and service organizations for individuals with ASDs.

Department of Defense Funding

In the early 1990s, advocates for increased federal spending on breast cancer research came up with a brilliant—even if theoretically questionable—strategy. There is only so much money in the NIH and it is hand-to-hand combat among the disease groups for control of that money.

Despite the pretense that the NIH allocates funds based only on scientific promise, the process is intensely political—actually involving many kinds of politics, among which any alleged meddling by elected officials may well be the least intrusive and offensive.

The kinds of politics that determine disease funding include: which universities have more clout and better relationships, which individual scientists establish themselves as thought leaders in their fields, and which bureaucrats within the NIH are better at building their individual power bases.

Given all the limits—both in terms of aggregate dollars and in terms of the number and sharpness of knives slicing up the NIH pie—breast cancer advocates looked to the Department of Defense (which, of course, has historically spent significant sums on battlefield-related medical research and the actual provision of healthcare) as fertile ground for an end-run around the NIH.

These advocates got an astounding $150 million appropriated to be spent by the Pentagon on research for breast cancer. That sum has been reappropriated—and grown—every year now for the better part of almost two decades.

Thus was born the Congressionally Directed Medical Research Programs (CDMRP) in the Pentagon's budget—a mini-NIH for the diseases whose supporters can get Congress to pony up.

On the very general argument that the America that was once defended with a force of volunteers no longer primarily sends to war unattached 18-year-old men, but rather has an obligation to the needs of the families of servicemen and service-women who are, in effect, part of our current fighting forces, nearly any health-care research can be justified as potentially effecting the morale and readiness of the troops.

Led by the National Alliance for Autism Research (NAAR) (another major pre-Autism Speaks research and advocacy group, since also merged into AS) that was what the autism community repeated in order to finally be admitted to this club in fiscal year 2007.

Current best estimates are that there are approximately 8,000 minor children of active-duty military personnel afflicted with autism. The pressures on kids with autism participating in military life, with frequent moves from base to base, even country to country, are enormous. So the Pentagon budget now includes support for autism research.

One of the unique aspects of the CDMRP for autism research is that consumer advocates (consumers) are active participants in virtually all aspects of the program execution. The consumers represent the voice and vision of individuals affected by autism and they work collaboratively with leading scientists and clinicians in setting program priorities, reviewing proposals, and contributing their unique perspectives and a sense of urgency to program processes.

To date, about $30 million has been appropriated to the Department of Defense (DOD) Autism Research Program. The program mission is to "promote innovative research that advances the understanding of autism spectrum disorders and leads to improved treatment outcomes." Importantly, the research funded by this group is perceived by the autism community as being more innovative, cutting edge, and more likely to produce significant findings than research funded by the NIH. Autism advocates now have, by virtue of the demonstrated success of this program, nothing less than the Department of Defense at their backs to urge similar innovation in autism research at the NIH.

All That Remains

The platform promise by Presidential candidate Barack Obama to secure a federal guarantee of autism insurance coverage was, without doubt, a huge symbolic victory for the community. As already noted, ending the discrimination against those with autism by the health insurance industry— getting coverage for ABA and other medically necessary, evidence-based treatments for autism—will be the single most important improvement in the quality of life of those facing autism, short of dramatic medical breakthroughs. As of this writing, and following three years of battles, 23 state laws have been enacted along these lines. Collectively, these states represent almost half of the US population. However, this is less than meets the eye, as the reach of each state's regulatory authority over health insurance is generally about 15% to 30% of its own population.

Certainly, despite the great and continuing success of the autism community's state-based lobbying on this issue, the answer to the problem still must be found at the federal level.

In the context of the heated legislative process - the mother of all legislative battles - which led to the national health care reform bill passed in June 2010, the autism community secured language (through the championship of Senator Robert Menendez (R–NJ) and Congressman Mike Doyle) which includes a requirement for the coverage of "behavioral health treatments" in the "essential benefits" package which the law mandates for all those who will purchase their insurance through the newly created health insurance "state-based exchanges".

This is a far cry from a universal federal mandate - principally because the law does not cover the benefits which must be provided by companies which self-insure (and are regulated under the pre-existing ERISA federal statute). This omission occurred as the political popularity of the President's proposals plummeted between the time the House of Representatives passed its version of health reform and the time of the final passage of the bill which became law, through the Senate.

It is not that the appetite of Congress and the President for autism coverage shrank but politics being the art of the possible, the ultimate provision of coverage for autism treatments in the final bill simply shrunk with the downsizing of the overall scope of the legislation.

It therefore remains a principal objective of the autism community going forward to achieve in federal law a universal guarantee of autism insurance coverage. Clearly, those political winds have turned forcefully against any further expansion of federal intervention in the health insurance arena. But autism insurance discrimination remains wrong and the community will continue to seek redress for this grievance.

Beyond insurance, the time is already upon us - and work has already been in progress, as of this writing, for over a year, on the reauthorization of the CAA, with key provisions due to expire in September 2011.

Senator Christopher Dodd, retiring from the Senate as of January 2011, and long time autism champions in the House, Mike Doyle and Chris Smith, have once again signed on to initiate the legislative process for reauthorization.

The principle new facets being sought by the community in the second coming of the CAA include:

- Further reform and rationalization of the administration of federal autism research efforts. Although most lobbying in Washington can really be reduced to every group wanting more money, the autism community has come to understand that without a more thoughtful approach to how research dollars are spent, greater spending by itself might well produce almost nothing tangible for those living with autism.
- Expand (to a scale equal to the challenge) and coordinate federal service delivery efforts with respect to the lifelong needs of those with autism. From housing, to transportation and vocational training, people on the autism spectrum have needs that change throughout their lifespan that our society has an obligation to address. Providing appropriate services can also reduce overall social costs by maximizing not only the quality of life of adults with autism, but their ability to be productive members of their communities.

In addition to insurance and the CAA, the ambitious, but warranted, agenda of the autism community for continued expansion in the federal response to autism also includes the enactment of a tax-preferred savings vehicle for the long-term financial needs of those with autism. At present, the federal tax code provides preferential treatment to the most able and advantaged of America's children—those who will go on to 4-year colleges. Yet the code offers nothing to help with the long-term financial needs of America's disabled children, including those with autism. Again, this is an area where the equities and efficiencies of the policy position urged by the autism community are both clear.

Conclusion

By the relevant standards of comparison, the autism community's advocacy efforts in Washington have been fantastically successful over the last decade. The community now is perceived to have a degree of political clout that leads to the ability to get things done.

Still, as the autism epidemic has progressed, with no cure yet in sight, the work is just beginning.

As all sides in the titanic debate over health reform—perhaps the only thing on which they do—is that the greatest long-term threat to the economic health of the United States is unfunded liabilities for medical (and related social) needs in the middle of this century. Certainly, the aging of our population is one of the main factors in this looming crisis. But so is autism. With at least one in 110 Americans born today predicted to be diagnosed with autism (1 in 70 boys), there is a surging cadre of people with a lifetime of expensive necessities.

Public policy to respond to these threats—and all the other problems we face as a nation—tends to be made in ways that aren't pretty. But, so far, autism advocacy has achieved great things in notably honorable ways. And it needs to keep doing so.

81 Temple Grandin

Top Priorities for Autism/Asperger's Research: Perspectives from a Person with Autism

Points of Interest

- A top research priority is sensory oversensitivity.
- Research participants with autism or Asperger's Syndrome must be assigned to studies based on their specific sensory problems.
- The different type of sensory problems are visual, auditory, tactile, taste, and vestibular problems.
- Individuals on the autism/Asperger's spectrum need to be taught job skills such as being on time, doing things that other people want, and good manners.
- Factors that help individuals to be successful are using obsessions to motivate learning job skills and having mentors who provide instruction in career-relevant skills.
- The three kinds of specialized minds are: *(1)* Photo-realistic visual thinkers, *(2)* Pattern thinkers (music and math minds), and *(3)* Verbal specialists (facts minds).

I was born in 1947 before many doctors knew what autism was. Fortunately, when I was 2 ½ year old, I was taken to Boston Children's Hospital to see Dr. Bronson Cruthers, a well-known child neurologist. I had all the symptoms of autism—no speech, rocking, a lack of tolerance for being hugged, and no social relatedness. Instead of recommending institutionalization, she referred me to a small speech therapy school that had two dedicated teachers who ran it out of their modest home. Within a year, I was talking. At 3 years of age, my mother hired a nanny who played constant turn-taking games with me and my sister. My early educational program was as good as many programs used today. In this chapter, I offer my perspective, as a person affected by autism, on what I view as the three highest priorities for future autism research: sensory oversensitivity, employment, and cognitive styles.

Top Research Priority 1: Sensory Oversensitivity

Since the mid-1980s, I have been giving talks on my experiences with autism throughout the U.S. and other countries. From a research perspective, I believe a top priority is doing research on sensory oversensitivity problems. Sensitivity to noise, fluorescent lights, scratchy clothes, or strong smells is a serious problem for many individuals with autism and Asperger's Syndrome (Grandin, 1995/2006; Williams, 1994, 1996; Barron & Barron, 1992; Joliffe et al., 1992). Sensory problems are very variable from a minor nuisance to completely debilitating. For some individuals, a noisy restaurant, a sporting event, or a busy office cannot be tolerated. Socializing and employment are extremely difficult for an individual if they are not able to tolerate the environments in which these activities occur.

I have been talking about sensory oversensitivity problems for over 20 years. Why have many researchers overlooked sensory problems? They have done hundreds of research studies on theory of mind and only a handful of studies on sensory issues. The time has now come to change the ratio of the studies. There need to be hundreds of studies on sensory issues and only a handful of studies on theory of mind. Problems with sensory oversensitivity can completely wreck the lives of some individuals on the autism spectrum.

Why are Sensory Issues Neglected?

I think a major reason why sensory issues are neglected is that people who have a normal sensory system are not able to imagine an alternate reality, where a loud noise hurts like a dentist's drill or scratchy clothes cause a burning sensation. Normal people have a huge deficit in sensory theory of mind. They are not able to empathize with an overwhelming intense sensory experience. First-person accounts published during the last 25 years have described the sensory issues. In my book *Thinking in Pictures*, I reviewed every first-person account I could find that was published before 1995 (Grandin, 1995/2006). There were a bunch of them. Sensory issues are not a new issue. Today on the internet, people on the spectrum describe their battles with sensory oversensitivity.

Oversensitivity vs. Scrambling

Sensory problems are very variable and can range from mild problems with overly sensitive touch to sensory scrambling. Recent studies show that the sensory systems in autism are very abnormal (Kern et al., 2007; Van der Smagt et al., 2007; Leekam et al., 2007 ; Boddart et al., 2004 ; Wiggens et al., 2009). Parents have reported many sensory symptoms (Rogers et al., 2003). In my own case, I have difficultly screening out background noise, and the school bell ringing was like a dentist's drill hitting a nerve. Another individual reported that when other kids spoke, his hearing would either fade out or their voices sounded like bullets (White & White, 1987). Many individuals report that they can see the flicker of fluorescent lights. They say it is like being at a disco and it makes paying attention in a class really difficult. One of my students was a severe dyslexic and fluorescent lights made many classrooms and office environments intolerable for her. She would get so spaced out that she could not think. Another friend of mine who has autism told me that certain rough fabric created a burning sensation on her skin. When I was little, I could not tolerate the feeling of being hugged. I wanted to feel the good feeling of being hugged but the stimulus was too overwhelming. It was like a tidal wave engulfing me (Grandin & Scariano, 1986).

Donna Williams, in her many books, describes becoming overcome with sensory overload and conversations would turn into "blah blah" meaningless noise (Williams, 1994, 1996). When she gets overstimulated she may see colored blobs instead of the objects in the room around her. Sinclair (1992) describes problems with his senses getting mixed up. Other people have described that their hearing fades in and out like a bad mobile telephone connection. Many nonverbal individuals can say only the vowel sounds. I have heard this myself and many parents have reported it. I think the reason why they say vowel sounds results from not being able to hear the consonants.

When I was little, one of my first words was "ba" for ball. My speech teacher helped me to hear consonant sounds by slowing down and enunciating hard consonants. She would say, "c...c... u... p...p," so I could hear the consonants stretched out, and she said each word more slowly. When grown-ups talked quickly to each other I could only hear the vowels. When I was little, I thought grown-ups had a special language that they used with each other. People who remain nonverbal often rely on touch and smell because seeing and hearing is so scrambled and does not provide accurate information. This is why they often smell and constantly touch things. Tito, a nonverbal adult with autism, told me (via typing) that he saw colors and disjointed shapes. Both Tito (Iverson, 2006; Muckhopadhyay, 2004, 2008) and my dyslexic student are auditory learners. Their visual system often gives them scrambled information so they rely on hearing because there is less distortion. Ceasaron and Garber (1991) and Williams (1994, 1996) all describe a sensory system that is monochannel. Seeing and hearing at the same time is difficult. Sensory information coming to one sense may get mixed up with another sense and one of the sense systems partially shuts down.

Research Difficulties

The extreme variability of autism/Asperger's sensory issues makes research studies difficult. If you examined 20 children labeled with autism, maybe only five or six would have severe visual processing problems like Donna Williams. In my own case, vision is normal. To do meaningful research on sensory issues requires assignment of subjects to experiments by their *specific* sensory problems instead of broad labels such as autism or Asperger's Syndrome. When the general labels are used, a person with major visual processing problems is put into the same study with people like me who have mainly touch and sound sensitivity problems.

The variability of autism spectrum disorders has also made many brain studies difficult. Amaral et al. (2008) reviewed neuroanatomical studies and many studies have had conflicting results. For both sensory and brain studies, autism spectrum subgroups should be identified and assigned to separate studies. Mixing apples and oranges together in the same study introduces so much variability that getting consistent results becomes more difficult.

Occupational therapists have worked for years doing sensory therapies that use deep pressure, swinging, or balancing activities to help individuals with autism to function better. The pioneer in this field was Jean Ayres (1979). People who work directly with individuals with autism know that these therapies are effective but many professionals reject them because hard scientific data are lacking on their effectiveness. This probably results from the great variability in sensory problems. A particular sensory therapy may really help improve the functioning of one individual and have little effect on another. Below is an outline of my three recommendations for sensory research.

1. Participants with autism and Asperger's Syndrome must be assigned to all studies based on their *specific* sensory problem(s). This will reduce variability of the data and make a study more likely to show significant results. Assignment to studies with labels such as autism or Asperger's Syndrome will introduce excessive variability into the data.
2. Studies need to be done with brain scans and other brain function technologies to determine how the brain is malfunctioning compared to a normal child or adult.

A few good studies have already been done. More studies like these need to be funded.

3. Studies need to be done to test therapies for treating sensory problems. Subjects must be assigned to the study by the sensory modality that is abnormal. Individuals should be grouped in categories such as *visual processing problems* or *auditory processing problems*.

How to Identify Sensory Problems

Identifying sensory problems as a tool for assigning subjects to a study can be done with a simple questionnaire and observation of the subjects. Even if these assessment tools are crude, they will be more precise than assigning subjects strictly by autism or Asperger's Syndrome labels. My suggestions below are based on over 20 years of experience talking to individuals on the spectrum and reading first-person accounts.

Signs of Visual Processing Problems

1. Finger flicking near the eyes (nonverbal).
2. Tilts head when reading, looks out the corner of his eye.
3. Avoids fluorescent lights. If the child or adult is verbal, they will tell you that fluorescent lights flicker and bother them (Williams, 1994, 1996). Most likely to be a problem with fluorescents that operate at 50 to 60 cycles. Higher frequencies may have less effect. In the individual who is nonverbal, he will perform more poorly in rooms with fluorescent lights and may have more tantrums. Tantrums may occur more often in rooms or stores with fluorescents.
4. Fears escalators. Individuals with visual processing problems often get scared because they have difficulty figuring out how to get on and off the moving stairway.
5. Acts blind. –The individual may act like a blind person when she goes up or down a strange stairway they are *not* familiar with.
6. Print "wiggles." Verbal individual may report that black print on a white page wiggles or vibrates.
7. Poor night perception. If the individual drives, they often hate driving at night.
8. Dislikes rapid movement. Avoids automatic sliding doors and other things that move rapidly.
9. Dislikes high contrast of light and dark. Bright contrasting colors are avoided. Dislikes multicolored floor tiles and anything that forms a lattice or grid pattern.

From my many conversations with individuals on the autism spectrum, 50- to 60-cycle fluorescent lights are the number one visual sensitivity problem. Another common symptom is the print moving on the page.

Signs of Auditory Processing Problems

1. Auditory threshold for hearing sounds or tones is normal or close to normal but sometimes the individual appears deaf.
2. Cannot hear when there is a lot of background noise (Geder-Salejarvi et al., 2005).
3. Difficulty hearing hard consonants. Hears vowels more easily. Mixes up words that have vowel sound that are similar (e.g., cat, bat, and sat).
4. Verbal individuals have abnormal test results on tests of central auditory processing. The results of my auditory tests are covered in *Thinking in Pictures* (Grandin, 1995/2006). I was shocked at how abnormal they were.
5. Child or adult covers his ears when loud sounds occur. More sensitive auditory threshold (Tharpe et al., 2006).
6. Tantrums are frequent in noisy places such as a train station, sporting events, or very loud movies.
7. Verbal individuals will tell you that their ears hurt from certain sounds such as smoke alarms, firecrackers, balloons popping, or fire alarms (Grandin, 1995/2006).
8. Verbal individuals will tell you that sometimes their hearing will shut off or change volume, especially when they are in overstimulating environments (White and White, 1987). Their hearing may sometimes seem like a bad mobile phone connection.
9. Difficulty localizing the source of a sound (Teder-Salejarvi et al., 2005).

Signs of Touch Sensitivity and Abnormal Tactile Sensitivity

1. The child pulls away when hugged by a familiar adult.
2. Constantly takes off all his/her clothes or only certain articles of clothing. Wool and other scratchy materials cause the most problems.
3. A verbal individual will tell you certain fabrics cannot be tolerated against her skin. I could not tolerate wool clothes. More sensitive individuals may not be able to tolerate cotton socks that have a coarse texture.
4. The child or adult may seek deep-pressure stimulation and get under heavy pillows, carpets or roll herself up in blankets. The individual may wedge herself in a tight spot such as between the mattress and the box spring. Deep pressure is calming (Edelson et al., 1999; Grandin & Scariano, 1986).
5. The individual may lash out or tantrum when suddenly touched by another person.

Signs of Olfactory Sensitivity and Abnormal Smell

1. Smells of certain substances are avoided.
2. Attracted to certain strong smells.
3. Certain smells can trigger a tantrum.

Signs of Taste Sensitivity

1. Restricted diet; eats only certain foods.
2. May avoid foods with certain textures (Barron & Barron, 1992).

Signs of Balance, Vestibular and Motor Problems

1. Clumsy and/or poor gross motor skills.
2. Difficulty balancing. Tandem walking is difficult (like walking on a tightrope).
3. Does not get dizzy easily after doing activities that would normally cause dizziness.
4. Very sloppy handwriting.

Sensory problems are very variable. I think there is a tendency for the nonverbal individuals on the autism/Asperger's spectrum to have more severe sensory problems. However, I have met many very intelligent high-functioning individuals who have severe debilitating problems with sensory oversensitivity. People like me who think in pictures may have more sensory oversensitivity problems than the type of individual with Asperger's Syndrome who is a more verbal, nonvisual thinker. These verbal individuals know lots of facts about their favorite subjects and are poor at visual skills such as drawing. People like me who are good at visual skills such as drawing often have more sensory problems and higher levels of fear and anxiety.

Research on Sensory Therapies

Problems with visual and auditory oversensitivity need to be researched first because they cause the most problems and can make functioning in a normal work or social environment so painful that the individual withdraws. If a visual therapy such as Irlen colored lenses is studied, only subjects who have visual problems should be included. I should be left out of this study because my answers are all "No" on the visual processing problem symptoms. My dyslexic student really benefited from Irlen lenses and answered "Yes" to all nine of the vision questions. Irlen lenses are pale colored lenses. The person tries on many different colored lenses until he/she finds a color where the print no longer jiggles on the page he/she read. Each person has to pick out the color that works best for them. I have talked to many other people on the autism spectrum who said that they would answer "Yes" on all the questions. If a study is done on auditory problems, I should definitely be included. In my own case, my answers are "Yes" on all the auditory questions except question 8, which asks about hearing shutting off or the volume changing. This occurs in individuals that have more severe problems than I do. To conclude this section, individuals *must* be assigned to studies based on the sensory modality that has a problem. To be involved in a study, the subject should have a "Yes" answer on at least half of the questions. Sensory problems are highly variable. One individual may have severe visual processing problems and another does not.

Practical Tips for Sensory Problems that People Can Do Themselves

These tips have come mostly from my own experiences, as well as those of other individuals on the autism/Asperger's spectrum. The books by Biel and Peska (2004) and Kranowitz (1998) provide additional information.

Visual Processing Problems

1. Wear a hat with a brim when in rooms with florescent lights.
2. Use a lamp with an old-fashioned incandescent light bulb to block out florescent lights at your desk.
3. In a room with florescent lights, sit next to a window.
4. Get Irlen lenses or experiment with different pale-colored sunglasses (Lightson et al., 1999; Evans & Joseph, 2002).
5. Print reading materials on tan, light blue, gray, light green, or other pastel paper to reduce contrast or use transparent-colored overlays.
6. Get a laptop computer to reduce screen flicker. TV monitors and flat panels lit with florescent lights flicker like a strobe. All new computer screen technologies should be compared to a laptop when a person with visual processing problems buys a new computer screen.

Sound Sensitivity

1. Wear earplugs in noisy places. Take them off for at least half the day to prevent hearing from getting more sensitive.
2. Record sounds that hurt the ears on a recording device. The individual with the sound sensitivity problem should play them back at a reduced volume.
3. Loud sounds and noise will be more easily tolerated when the person is rested and not tired.
4. Loud sounds are better tolerated when the individual on the spectrum initiates them.

Touch Sensitivity

1. Deep pressure can help desensitize an individual to touch sensitivity. Most individuals with autism spectrum disorders (ASDs) can be desensitized and learn to tolerate being hugged.
2. Sensitivity to scratchy clothing is more difficult to desensitize. I cannot tolerate anything scratchy against my skin. Washing all new clothing that touches the skin several times before wearing it will make it more comfortable. Remove all tags and wear underwear inside out to get the seams away from the skin.
3. Sensitivity to medical examinations can sometimes be desensitized by applying deep pressure to the area that has to be examined.

Medication Research on Cognition

Some people on the spectrum really need medication. Medication saved me and stopped horrible anxiety and panic attacks (Grandin, 1995/2006). When medication is used, doctors must be careful to choose medications that do not interfere with the ability of a person to use his brain. I have speculated that visual thinkers like me can often benefit from taking Prozac or Zoloft to stop panic attacks and anxiety. These medications are good because they do not affect the person's ability to work and design things. To avoid agitation and insomnia, people on the autism/Asperger's Syndrome spectrum often need much lower doses of antidepressants.

Some medications could wreck a person's career. I tried Buspar for anxiety and it made me so "spacey" that I would not think clearly. After 1 week, I stopped taking it. Several other people had memory problems when they took Paxil. There is a need for doing research on the effects of medication on cognitive functions. The right medications can work wonders, but the wrong medications could have the person walking around in a fog.

Behavior Problems and Sensory Oversensitivity

When a child or adult has a behavior problem, the question that should be asked is—is the problem caused by sensory problems or is it simply bad behavior? When I was growing up in the 1950s, autism was never used as an excuse for rude behavior or having no table manners. In the 1950s, all kids were taught to have manners and say "please" and "thank you". My strict 1950s upbringing was an important key to my success. My mother recognized my problems with sensory issues and that certain noises terrified me. She knew I could learn to behave myself at a formal Sunday dinner at Granny's because her apartment was quiet. At the circus, I had a big tantrum because of the noise. My mother was observant enough to determine when I misbehaved because of a sensory issue and when I misbehaved because of bad behavior. Sensory issues were never punished. Bad behavior had consequences and the consequence for such behavior was no TV for 1 night. This emphasizes the importance of structure in the upbringing of a normal child, which may even be more important in an autistic child.

Top Research Priority 2: Prepare for Successful Employment

One of my greatest concerns is many individuals with a diagnosis of Asperger's Syndrome may be held back by the label. I was shocked when some social service agency said that only 20% of the people with Asperger's Syndrome can get good stable employment. I do not believe that the prevalence of Asperger's Syndrome has increased. In the past, people with Asperger's Syndrome were called "geeks" and "nerds." Most of the older people with Asperger's Syndrome who were born before 1970 are in the workforce in good jobs they have kept for many years. I can remember kids I went to school with who may be labeled as having Asperger's Syndrome today. One has a good job as a psychologist with a PhD and the other has kept good retail jobs with full health benefits. He is a valued member of the store's staff because he can talk to customers about every product in the store.

In the meat industry, I have worked with many successful individuals who are all undiagnosed Asperger's Syndrome. One of them is the head engineer at a large meat plant. He has kept his job even though his bosses have changed many times. He keeps the plant running and his social life is with the other persons with Asperger's Syndrome and "nerds" who work in the plant maintenance department.

Young Individuals with Asperger's Syndrome are Getting Fired from Jobs

I have talked to numerous young people with Asperger's Syndrome who have been fired from countless jobs that the older individuals with Asperger's Syndrome have managed to keep. I think that today's less structured methods of upbringing children are to blame. They are getting fired for doing stupid things that I learned not to do when I was 9 years old. All the table manners and polite social skills that I learned when I was little really helped me. Below are the skills I learned as a child that have helped me keep jobs.

1. *Being on time.* By the time I was 8 years old, I learned to be on time. When I entered first grade at age 6 years, mother taught me to use an alarm clock and to lay out my clothes the night before so I could get dressed quickly in the morning. Many individuals have Asperger's Syndrome lost good jobs they were good at because they were always late to work. Nobody had taught them to be on time when they were little.
2. *Learn to do things others want.* A major key for successful employment is learning to do tasks that will please other people. In the year 2010, I am hearing too many individuals with Asperger's Syndrome saying things like, "I have authority issues with the boss." They never learned that sometimes they have to obey other people. In the 1950s I was taught that sometimes you have to do things the grown-ups want, such as demonstrating good table manners. My mother motivated me by making sure I got real recognition when I did a really good job. I was thrilled when I was allowed to sing a solo at an adult concert. I knew this was a special privilege and the audience loved it. When I painted a really nice watercolor of the beach, mother framed it in a real frame with glass. I responded to this recognition, and later on it translated into doing work that other people appreciated and wanted. In high school, I painted signs for many different people. I learned that when I made a sign for a hair salon, I had to paint a design the client would like. John Robison, the Asperger's Syndrome author of *Look Me in the Eye*, has had good employment all his life. He started out in high school and college where he became an expert at fixing tape recorders

and record players. Other people appreciated his skill with electronics (Robison, 2007).

3. *Teach job skills young.* I am seeing too many individuals with Asperger's Syndrome graduating from college with no job skills. When I was 13 years old, my mother got me a seamstress job for two afternoons a week. I worked for a dressmaker out of her home. This was the first time I earned money at a job and I bought some crazy shirts with it. During high school I worked summers at my aunt's ranch. Even though I talked nonstop about things that bored people, everyone loved the horse bridles I made. In college, I had two summer intern jobs at a research lab and at a school for children with autism. These work experiences were extremely beneficial.

In Silicon Valley, there are young people with Asperger's Syndrome who get good jobs in computers or the tech industry. These kids are successful because their parents taught them career-relevant programming skills starting at 10 to 12 years of age. They were apprenticed into the industry.

1. *Use mentors.* When I was in high school I was an unmotivated student who seldom studied. I saw no point in studying until I had a goal of becoming a scientist. Many successful individuals with Asperger's Syndrome, both diagnosed and undiagnosed, became successful because they had either a parent or a teacher instruct them in career-relevant skills such as electronics, programming, scientific research, journalism, or auto mechanics. I have talked to many successful people with Asperger's Syndrome who have skilled jobs. In most cases, a mentor gave them formal instruction in computer programming, photography, or some other vocation. Young people will fool around with computers but they need a mentor to get them turned on to learning programming. Formal instruction is needed to get a teenager with Asperger's Syndrome focused about learning a career.
2. *Teach turn taking.* When I was a child, all the games and activities that were fun required participation and taking turns with another child. We played lots of board games and table hockey. Another big problem I observe today is that many young people with Asperger's Syndrome do not know how to take turns. This can cause many problems at work. Turn taking must be taught to all children on the spectrum. Board games and card games are good methods. Turn-taking skills learned in childhood will translate into being able to get along well with other people in the workplace.
3. *Avoid multitasking.* Many of the entry-level jobs such as waiter in a busy restaurant or working in a big grocery store require too much multitasking. Myself and many other people on the autism/Asperger's spectrum cannot multitask. All the good job experiences I had in high school and college did not require multitasking. My work on livestock equipment design has no multitasking.
4. *Sell your work, not yourself.* People thought I was weird, but they were impressed when they saw a portfolio of my drawings and photos of completed projects. People respect abilities (Grandin & Duffy, 2004). I used attractive brochures and portfolios to sell my design services.
5. *Develop areas of strength.* Many educators put too much emphasis on deficits and not enough emphasis on development of areas of strength. My ability in art and drawing was *always encouraged.* I think it is really unfortunate that many U.S. schools have stopped classes in art, wood shop, electronics, auto mechanics, and other hands-on jobs. A child that is bored taking elementary math should be allowed to take advanced math, but he may need special education in reading (Grandin & Duffy, 2004).
6. *Expose children and teenagers to interesting things.* I became interested in cattle when I went to my aunt's ranch. A high-school experimental psychology class that featured lots of fascinating optical illusions stimulated my initial interest in becoming a scientist. These experiences stimulated my interest in both psychology and cattle behavior. Kids are not going to get interested in things that they are not exposed to. Children and teenagers on the spectrum need to be exposed to many interesting things.
7. *Use obsessions to motivate learning and job skills.* Obsessions are great motivators. A creative teacher can channel them into career-relevant skills. If a child likes trains, read a book about trains and do math with trains. My obsessions with my squeeze machine were used to motivate scientific study. My science teacher told me that if I wanted to figure out why pressure was relaxing, I had to learn how to read scientific journal articles. He taught me to read real scientific papers when I was a teenager and I learned that scientists did not use the *Encyclopedia Britannica.* Today, I am really worried about kids who get so addicted to video games that it is difficult to get them interested in other things. Playing video games should be limited to 1 hour per day. However, career-relevant skills such as programming a game can be done for much longer periods. Take a video game obsession and broaden it. One parent encouraged development of artistic ability by having her son draw pictures of video-game characters.
8. *Do not make rude comments or discuss controversial subjects at work.* Many brilliant individuals with Asperger's Syndrome have been fired from jobs because they made rude comments about the appearance of coworkers and customers. When I was about 8 years old, I learned that calling somebody "Fatso" was not appropriate. People are losing good jobs because they made rude comments to customers. My old-fashioned 1950s upbringing stopped me from losing a job because of stupid rude comments.

I also was taught to avoid controversial subjects such as religion and politics at work. These subjects should only be discussed with intimate friends. I follow the advice that was on an old stagecoach sign:"No discussion of politics or religion while riding in the coach."

Worried About a Handicapped Mentality

I am very concerned that some teenagers and adults with Asperger's Syndrome and high-functioning autism are getting into a "handicapped mentality." Asperger's Syndrome is sometimes used as an excuse to not be successful. Recently I talked to a college student with Asperger's Syndrome who asked for so many accommodations from the disability office that it had become ridiculous. People on spectrum do need some accommodations such as a quiet place for sleep and study and a little more time to take tests. The problems with florescent lights also need to be addressed. Asking for a room free from 50- to 60-cycle florescent lights may be required for some individuals for taking tests. One girl told me that it drove her crazy when another student was typing text messages on her phone in class. She wanted the disability office to do something about it. I told her to sit in another part of the classroom. The law says that *reasonable* accommodations should be made. Her requests were no longer reasonable.

I am seeing too many smart young people with Asperger's Syndrome on Social Security disability pay who would be perfectly capable of working. John Robison, author of *Look me in the Eye*, has made the same observation during many of his speaking tours. We are both concerned about young people with an Asperger's Syndrome label using it as an excuse to not succeed. Both John and I were called "retards" when we were little. This very negative label motivated me in my early 20s to prove to other people that I was not stupid. John now has a very successful car dealership and he has had good employment his whole life.

Top Research Priority 3: Research on Different Kinds of Minds

Another area that needs to be researched is the different specialized ways that different people on the autism spectrum think. Through reading other personal accounts and talking to many individuals on the spectrum, I have observed that there are three basic kinds of specialist cognitive types (Grandin, 2009). They all share the common trait of having a skill in one area and a huge deficit in another area.

1. *Photo-realistic visual thinkers:* This is my type and it is described in detail in *Thinking in Pictures* (Grandin, 1996/2006). When I wrote this book in 1995, I thought all people on the spectrum were visual thinkers. I have discovered that this is not true. All my thoughts are in photo-realistic pictures. I can search the database in my head like searching the internet with an internet search engine set for finding photos. My weak area is algebra and foreign language. Algebra made no sense because there was no way to convert it to pictures.

At conferences I have talked to several individuals who could not do algebra but could do geometry and trigonometry. I never got a chance to try geometry because I failed algebra. Another interesting thing I have found about visual thinkers is that they seldom have severe visual processing problems. I think this would interfere with putting clear pictures into memory.

2. *Pattern thinker with a (music and math mind):* This is a more abstract form of visual thinking. Instead of seeing photo-realistic pictures in their imaginations, they see patterns and relationships between numbers. The first-person accounts of Jerry Newport and Daniel Tammett are good examples of pattern thinking (Newport & Newport, 2007; Tammett, 2006).

Interestingly, some of these individuals also had difficulty with algebra, but they can do many higher forms of math. I have talked to many pattern thinkers. Some have severe visual processing problems. They have told me that they see or hear sound patterns. A woman with autism named Michelle Dawson has teamed up with researcher Laurent Mottron from the University of Montreal. A groundbreaking paper published in 2007 clearly shows that people with autism have intelligence skills that may be different than normal people (Dawson et al., 2007). When a normal child takes the WISC IQ test and the Raven's Progressive Matrices, they get similar scores on both tests. When children with autism took both tests, the Raven's scores were an average of 30 percentile points higher than the WISC scores. The Raven's is a test that measures pattern thinking. It tests the ability to see sameness and differences in a series of complex patterns. The WISC measures pattern thinking in the block design text, but many of the other subtexts require good language skills.

3. *Verbal specialist with a (facts mind):* There are the individuals who know all the verbal facts about their favorite subject. They are definitely not visual thinkers and often their math skills are only average. Many children and adults with this cognitive pattern love history. Some of these people make great journalists or legal researchers. They also may run fantastic fun websites about their favorite star or book.

Match Skills to Job Title

There needs to be more research on matching the individual's cognitive type to the right jobs. Visual thinkers can be really good at art, graphic design, photography, animal behavior, architecture, cartooning, industrial design, and other jobs that utilize visual skills. The pattern thinkers excel at engineering computer programming, math, statistics and other technical jobs. The verbal thinkers make excellent journalists, and researchers who are good at finding information in vast archives of data. Any job that requires meticulous record keeping would also be a good occupation.

Is Mild Asperger's Syndrome Really a Disability?

Simon-Baron Cohen has asked this question many times (Baron-Cohen, 2000). None of our technology or computers would exist if Asperger's Syndrome and autism traits were eliminated. The really social people did not invent the first stone spear. They spent all their spare time talking to each other and socializing. In fact, many famous scientists such as Einstein or Tesla (who invented the power plant) would probably be diagnosed with autism today. Mozart, Carl Sagan, Thomas Jefferson, and many others probably had Asperger's Syndrome (Ledgin, 2002; Fitzgerald & O'Brien, 2007). Brain research is showing that maybe there is a wide range of brain types ranging from hyper-social to a brain better suited for solving scientific or technical problems, which requires more attention to detail.

How I Conceptualize the Neurobiology of Autism

The research of Manual Casanova at the University of Knoxville really got me thinking (Cassanova et al., 2007). His research showed that three famous neuroscientists and people with autism both have had more *mini-columns* per square inch of brain gray matter (Casanova et al., 2006). Mini-columns are analogous to the brain's microprocessor units. Maybe additional mini columns helps people with autism and scientists process detailed information. The work of Dr. Nancy Minshew and her colleagues at the University of Pittsburgh indicates that the normal mind may drop out the details (Minshew et al., 2007; Minshew et al., 2002). Another study showed that people with autism use the visual parts of the brain more for processing verbal language (Kana et al., 2006). Eric Courchesne has suggested that local circuits in the brain may be enhanced and long-distance circuits may be poor. The work of Bruce Miller and his colleagues also provides great insight into how the brain works. In the normal person, language and abstract reasoning may cover up visual, math, and music skills. Patients with frontal temporal lobe dementia, a form of presenile dementia, sometimes have art and music talents emerge when the frontal cortex areas are destroyed (Miller et al., 2000; Miller et al., 1998). The paintings done by several of these patients resemble autistic savant art.

From reading all of these research studies, I hypothesize that there is a continuum of brain types. At one end, the highly social emotional brain would have super-efficient, long-distance connections between different brain regions to process rapidly changing social cues. The disadvantage of this brain is that details would get left out. At the other end of the spectrum would be a brain that has poor long-distance connections, but local connections with extra wiring. This would provide the ability to pay attention to details, but the processing speed would be much slower. It is likely that in an earlier era, people with Asperger's Syndrome and high-functioning autism would have been highly valued as scribes, artisans, stone masons, and other highly specialized trades. I had an interesting conversation with a mother from India. She said, "In our culture we recognize that kids labeled with Asperger's Syndrome are smart and sometimes naughty, and we prepare them for engineering and computer jobs starting at an early age." Getting a good job is important. The happy people on the spectrum have interesting work they can do with other people similar to them. One computer programmer with Asperger's syndrome said to me, "I am with my own people."

Conclusions

Autism/Asperger's Syndrome research needs to branch out into new areas. These areas include sensory oversensitivity problems, employment, and cognitive types. As described above, sensory problems can be extremely debilitating and make normal socializing impossible because the person is not able to tolerate a noisy restaurant or sports stadium. Florescent lights that operate at 50 to 60 cycles, cause serious problems for some individuals because they can see the flicker. For some individuals, fluorescents really interfere with learning or work. Sensory problems need to be researched to find ways to treat them. Research projects will be more likely to have significant results if subjects are assigned to studies based on the type of sensory symptoms instead of just broad labels such as autism. Sensory problems are extremely variable. Some individuals have noise sensitivity and others may have visual problems.

A second top priority research area is how to promote successful employment for people with Asperger's Syndrome and high-functioning autism. Intervention programs that help develop vocational skills and assess the types of job a specific individual is likely to succeed in are needed. In addition, techniques that offer mentoring and role-modeling, such as job coaches, should be studied.

A third topic area that needs studied is cognitive subgroups. People on the autism spectrum have areas of strength and areas of deficits. The cognitive types are: *(1)* photo-realistic visual thinkers, *(2)* pattern thinkers (music and math minds), and *(3)* verbal specialists (facts minds). Steps must be taken to improve employment of individuals on the spectrum. My highly structured upbringing in the 1950s really helped me. I was taught manners, turn taking, and other social skills that really helped me in the workplace. It is also essential to develop the individual's area of strength into employment and a career.

REFERENCES

Amaral, D. G., Schumann, C. M., & Nordahl, C. W. (2008). Neuroanatomy of autism. *Trends in Neurosciences, 31*, 137–145.

Ayres, J. A. (1979). *Sensory integration and the child.* Los Angeles, CA: Western Psychological Services.

Baron-Cohen, S. (2000). Is Asperger's Syndrome and high functioning autism necessarily a disability? *Developmental Psychopathology, 12*, 480–500.

Barron, J., & Barron, S. (1992). *There's a boy in here*. New York, NY: Simon and Schuster.

Biel, L., & Peske, N. (2004). *Raising a sensory smart child, the definitive handbook for helping a child with sensory integration issues*. New York, NY: Penguin Books.

Boddaert, N., Chabane, N., Belin, P., Bourgeois, M., Royer, V., Barthelemy, C., et al., (2004). Perception of complex sounds in autism: Abnormal auditory cortical processing in children. *American Journal of Psychiatry, 161*, 2117–2120.

Casanova, M. E., Kooten, I. A. J. van, Switala, A. E., Engeland, H. van, Heinsen, H., Steinbusch, H. W. M., et al. (2006). Minicolumnar abnormalities in autism. *Acta Neuropathologica 112*,187–303.

Casanova, M. E., Switala, A. E., Tripp, J., & Fitzgerald, M. (2007). Comparative minicolumnar morphopetry of three distinguished scientists. *Autism, 11*(6), 557–569.

Ceasaroni, L., & Garber, M. (1991). Exploring the experience of autism through firsthand accounts. *Journal of Autism and Developmental Disorders, 21*, 303–312.

Dawson, M., Soulieres, I., Gernsbacher, M. A., & Mottron, L. (2007). The level and nature of autistic intelligence. *Psychological Science, 18*, 657–662.

Edelson, S. M., Edelson, M. G., Kerr, D. C., & Grandin, T. (1999). Behavioral and physiological effects of deep pressure on children with autism: A pilot study evaluating the efficacy of Grandin's Hug Machine. *American Journal of Occupational Therapy, 53*, 145–152.

Evans, B. J., & Joseph, F. (2002). The effect of coloured filters on the rate of reading in an adult student population. *Ophthalmic Physiological Optometry, 22*, 535–545.

Fitzgerald., M., & O'Brien, B. (2007). *Genius genes*. Shawnee Mission, KS: Autism Asperger Publishing Co.

Grandin, T., & Scariano, M. (1986). *Emmergence: Labelled autistic*. Novato, CA: Academic Therapy Publications.

Grandin, T. (1996/2006). *Thinking in pictures* (Expanded Edition). New York, NY: Vintage (Random House).

Grandin, T. (2009). How does visual thinking work in the mind of a person with autism? A personal account, *Philosophical Transactions of the Royal Society, 364*, 1437–1442.

Grandin, T., & Duffy, K. (2004). *Developing talents*. Shawnee Mission, KS: Autism Asperger Publishing.

Iverson, P. (2006). *Strange son*. New York, NY: Riverhead Books (Division of Penguin).

Joliffe, T., Lakesdown, R., & Robinson, C. (1992). Autism: A personal account. *Communication, 26*(3), 12–19.

Kana, R. K., Keller, T. A., Cherkassky, V. L., Minshew, N. J., & Just, M. A. (2006). Sentence comprehension in autism: Thinking in pictures with decreased functional connectivity. *Brain, 129*(9), 2484–2493.

Kern, J. K., Trivedi, M. H., Grannemann, B. D., Garver, C. R., Johnson, D. G., Andrews, A. A., et al. (2007). Sensory correlations in autism. *Autism, 11*, 123–134.

Kranowitz, C. S. (1998). *The out of synch child*. New York, NY: Penguin Books, Skylight Press.

Ledgin, N. (2002). *Aspergers and self esteem*. Arlington, TX: Future Horizons.

Lightstone, A., Lightstone, T., & Wilkins, A. (1999). Both coloured overlays and coloured lenses can improve reading fluency, but their optimal chromaticities differ. *Opthalmic Physiological Optometry, 19*, 274–285.

Leekam, S. R., Nieto, C., Libby, S. J., Wing, L., & Gould, J. (2007). Describing the sensory abnormalities of children and adults with autism. *Journal of Autism and Developmental Disorders, 37*, 894–910.

Miller, B. L., Boone, K., Cummings, J. L., Read, S. L., & Mishkin, F., (2000). Functional correlates of musical and visual ability in fronto-temporal dementia. *British Journal of Psychiatry, 176*, 458–463.

Miller, B. L., Cummings, J., Michkin, J., Boone, K., Prince, F., Ponton, M., et al. (1998). Emergence of art talent in frontotemporal dementia. *Neurology, 51*, 978–981.

Minshew, N. J., Meyer, J., & Goldestein, C. (2002). Abstract reasoning in autism: A dissociation between formation and concept identification. *Neuropsychology, 16*, 327–334.

Minshew, N. J., & Williams, D. L. (2007). The new neurology of autism. *Archives of Neurology, 64*, 945–950.

Muckhopadhyay, T.R. (2004). *The mind tree*. New York, NY: Arcade Publishing.

Muckopadhyay, T. R. (2008). *How can i talk if my lips don't move?* New York, NY: Arcade Publishing.

Newport, J., & Newport, M. (2007). *Mozart and the whale*. New York, NY: Touchstone Books.

Robison, J. E. (2007). *Look me in the eye*. New York, NY: Crown Publishers.

Rogers, S. J., Hepburn, S., & Welner, E. (2003). Parent reports of sensory symptoms in toddlers with autism and those with other developmental disorders. *Journal of Autism and Development Disorders, 33*, 631–642.

Sinclair, J. (1992). Bridging the gaps on inside view of autism. In E. Schopler & G. B. Mesibov (Eds.), *High-functioning individuals with autism* (pp. 294–302). New York, NY: Plenum Press.

Tammet, D. (2006). *Born on a blue day*. New York, NY: Free Press.

Teder-Salejarvi, W. A., Pierce, K. L., Courchesne, E., & Hillyard, S. A. (2005). Auditory spatial localization and attention deficits in autistic and adults. *Cognitive Brain Research, 23*, 221–234.

Tharpe, N. M., Bess, F. H., Sladen, D. P., Schissel, H., Couch, S., & Schery, T. (2006). Auditory characteristics of children with autism. *Ear and Hearing, 27*, 430–441.

Van der Smagt, M. J., van Engeland, H., & Kemmer, C. (2007). Brief report: Can you see what is not there? Low level auditory-visual integration in autism spectrum disorder. *Journal of Autism and Developmental Disorders, 37*, 2014–2019.

Wiggens, L. D., Robins, D. L., Bakeman, R., & Adamson, L. B. (2009). Brief Report: Sensory abnormalities as a distinguishing symptom of autism spectrum disorders in young children, *Journal of Autism and Developmental Disorders, 39*, 1087–1091.

White, D. B., & White, M. S. (1987). Autism from the inside. *Medical Hypotheses, 24*, 223–229.

Williams, D. (1994). *Somebody somewhere*. New York, NY: Time Books.

Williams, D. (1996). *Autism—An inside-out approach*. London, England: Jessica Kingsley.

INDEX

Note: Page references followed by "*f*" and "*t*" denote figures and tables, respectively.

F

G

J

U

V